Pathophysiology
Concepts of Human Disease

Matthew Sorenson, PhD, APN, ANP-C
Director, School of Nursing
Associate Professor, Nursing
DePaul University College of Science and Health
Chicago, Illinois

Laurie Quinn, PhD, RN, FAAN, FAHA, CDE
Clinical Professor, College of Nursing
Biobehavioral Health Science
University of Illinois at Chicago
Chicago, Illinois

Diane Klein, PhD, RN
Associate Professor, Nursing
Marcella Niehoff School of Nursing
Loyola University
Chicago, Illinois

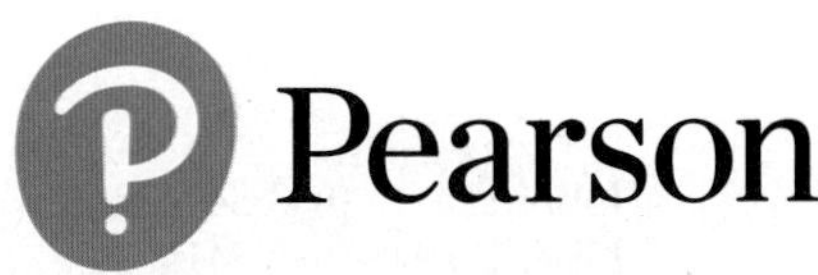

330 Hudson Street, NY NY 10013

Vice President, Health Science and TED: Julie Levin Alexander
Director of Portfolio Management: Katrin Beacom
Executive Portfolio Manager: Pamela Fuller
Development Editor: Laura S. Horowitz, York Content Development
Portfolio Management Assistant: Erin Sullivan
Vice President, Content Production and Digital Studio: Paul DeLuca
Managing Producer, Health Science: Melissa Bashe
Content Producer: Bianca Sepulveda
Project Monitor: Sue Hannahs
Operations Specialist: Maura Zaldivar-Garcia
Creative Director: Blair Brown
Creative Digital Lead: Mary Siener
Managing Producer, Digital Studio, Health Science: Amy Peltier
Digital Studio Producer, REVEL and e-text 2.0: Ellen Viganola
Digital Content Team Lead: Brian Prybella
Digital Content Project Lead: William Johnson
Vice President, Field Marketing: David Gesell
Executive Product Marketing Manager: Christopher Barry
Sr. Field Marketing Manager: Brittany Hammond
Full-Service Project Management and Composition: SPi Global
Project Manager: Thomas Russell
Inventory Manager: Vatche Demirdjian
Interior Design: Studio Montage
Cover Design: Studio Montage
Printer/Binder: LSC Communications, Inc.
Cover Printer: Phoenix Color/Hagerstown

Library of Congress Cataloging-in-Publication Data

Names: Sorenson, Matthew, author. | Quinn, Laurie, author. | Klein, Diane, 1947-2017, author.
Title: Pathophysiology : concepts of human disease / Matthew Sorenson, Laurie Quinn, Diane Klein.
Description: Hoboken, New Jersey : Pearson Education, 2017. | Includes bibliographical references and index.
Identifiers: LCCN 2017055102| ISBN 9780133414783 | ISBN 0133414787
Subjects: | MESH: Disease | Pathologic Processes–physiopathology | Nurses' Instruction
Classification: LCC RB127 | NLM QZ 140 | DDC 616/.047--dc23
LC record available at https://lccn.loc.gov/2017055102

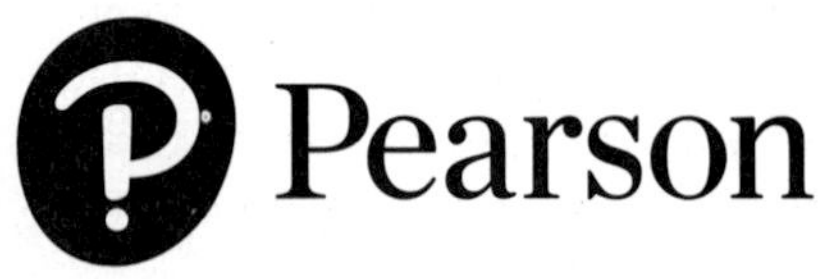

ISBN 10: 0-13-341478-7
ISBN 13: 978-0-13-341478-3
1 18

About the Authors

Matthew Sorenson, PhD, APN, ANP-C

The pre-nursing career of Matthew Sorenson includes experience as a recovery room orderly, paramedic, and child care worker and an initial collegiate major in history. His nursing career began with a BSN degree from Northern Illinois University (with a minor in history). After graduation, he worked primarily in physical rehabilitation, focusing on neurologic conditions and injury, an area in which he remains active. He holds an MS in Applied Family and Child Studies (Focus on Abuse and Neglect) and an MS in Nursing (Community Health Focus).

His doctorate is from Loyola University Chicago, where he studied stress-related changes in immunologic function in those with multiple sclerosis. Postdoctoral education includes a three-year fellowship with the neurology service at Edward Hines Jr. VA Hospital (focus on multiple sclerosis) and a year-long fellowship in Disability Ethics through the Rehabilitation Institute of Chicago. He is an Adult Nurse Practitioner. His time as a nurse practitioner is spent primarily with street outreach programs targeting the homeless and working poor. His research focuses on immunologic correlates of fatigue, particularly in those with multiple sclerosis. He is currently funded to investigate viral epigenetics in multiple sclerosis. He teaches physical assessment, pharmacology, medical-surgical nursing, and pathophysiology. Academically, Dr. Sorenson teaches at DePaul University with an additional appointment in the School of Medicine (Physical Medicine and Rehabilitation) at Northwestern University. He served as a program director for several years and was recently named Director of the School of Nursing.

To my grandmother, Gertrude, for her inspiration. To my parents, Robert and Joyce, for their encouragement and support. Janet, your love and support was and always will be the cornerstone of my life.

Laurie Quinn, PhD, RN, FAAN, FAHA, CDE

Laurie Quinn is a Clinical Professor in the Department of Biobehavioral Health Science in the College of Nursing at the University of Illinois at Chicago (UIC). Dr. Quinn earned her PhD from UIC in Nursing Science and has been on the UIC College of Nursing faculty for 20 years. Her primary research focus is the study of metabolic alterations associated with diabetes mellitus, especially their role in the development of cardiovascular disease. Her research has focused on examining the effect of aerobic exercise on the metabolic derangements of both type 1 and type 2 diabetes. She is currently part of an interdisciplinary team from University of Chicago, Illinois Institute of Technology, and UIC that is developing an artificial pancreas.

Dr. Quinn is a Certified Diabetes Educator and worked as a Clinical Nurse Specialist at Rush University Medical Center. She has received several awards for teaching excellence and has lectured in graduate and undergraduate physiology, pathophysiology, and pharmacology classes. She has published and presented extensively in research and clinical practice venues on diabetes-related topics.

Dr. Quinn is an active member of the American Diabetes Association and American Heart Association. She has been a healthcare coordinator at an American Diabetes Association summer camp for children with diabetes for several years. In this role, she has cared for numerous children with type 1 diabetes and helped to educate clinical staff and students from various healthcare specialties on the treatment of type 1 diabetes.

To my parents Lauretta and Thomas Quinn and sister Margaret Quinn for all of their support throughout the years.

Diane Klein, PhD, RN

Diane Klein earned a BSN degree from Loyola University Chicago and then worked as a nurse in the trauma unit and later in a medical unit at Cook County Hospital. During her clinical practice, she became interested in research, which led her to earn a PhD in physiology from the University of Illinois at the Medical Center Campus in Chicago. Her dissertation research focused on intracellular signaling systems in cancer cell growth. Her research interests as a faculty member at Loyola University Chicago included the role of cyclic nucleotides in altered lung metabolism during septic shock, myocardial metabolism and function during septic shock, effects of chronic ethanol intake on metabolic alterations during sepsis, and the use of nebulized morphine in the treatment of dyspnea.

Dr. Klein was an Associate Professor in the School of Nursing at Loyola University Chicago, where she taught undergraduate and graduate pathophysiology courses for over 30 years. She believed that nursing students require a strong foundation in pathophysiology because it is the basis for their understanding of pharmacology and the rationale for clinical assessments and interventions. In addition to pathophysiology courses, Dr. Klein taught undergraduate adult health clinical courses, undergraduate and graduate pharmacology, advanced physiology for clinical practice, and stress in health and illness.

In addition to teaching pathophysiology courses, Dr. Klein presented topics related to pathophysiology at local and national meetings of both nursing and basic science organizations. Selected topics presented included resources for teaching genetics and genomics, problems of mechanically ventilated patients, biotrauma, the immune system and sepsis, fluid and electrolyte imbalances associated with trauma, effects of endotoxin and cyclic nucleotides on lung glucose oxidation, pathophysiology update for practicing nurses, and oxidative stress in critical illness and therapeutic strategies.

Diane Klein passed away in July of 2017, just as this book, on which she had worked for almost 10 years, was going to press. This book would not have existed if not for Diane's interest and hard work. Matthew Sorenson, Laurie Quinn, and the staff at Pearson are grateful for Diane's contributions and commitment to this project.

Thank You

Our appreciation first and foremost goes to Pamela Fuller for believing in this project. Without the editorial skill and patience of Laura Horowitz, this project would not have seen final fruition. We would be remiss if we did not acknowledge the valuable work of the contributors who provided time, energy, and depth to this work. The feedback of the reviewers was also crucial in shaping this book. Finally, thanks go to the students in our classrooms whose energy, questions, and drive for knowledge provided the genesis of this project.

Matthew Sorenson
Laurie Quinn
Diane Klein

Contributors

Michael P. Adams, PhD
Adjunct Professor of Biological Sciences
Pasco-Hernando State College
Hillsborough Community College
Formerly Dean of Health Professions
Pasco-Hernando State College
New Port Richey, Florida

Omar AL-Rawajfah, PhD, RN
Dean, Faculty of Nursing
AL AL-Bayt University
Mafraq, Jordan

Kyle T. Bergan, DNP, MS, RN, EMT-B, CEN
Clinical Adjunct Faculty
DePaul University
Chicago, Illinois
Staff Nurse, Emergency Department
West Suburban Medical Center
Oak Park, Illinois

Jean K. Berry, PhD, APN
Clinical Associate Professor Emerita
University of Illinois
College of Nursing,
Department of Biobehavioral Health Science
Chicago Illinois

Linda Blevins, DNP, MFA, ELS, RN
Board-Certified Editor in the Life Sciences
President, Charis Communications LLC
Springboro, Ohio

Adam M. Boise, MS, APRN
Concord Surgical Associates
Concord Hospital
Concord, New Hampshire

Neftali Cabezudo, PhD, RN-BC
VA Program Co-Director & Faculty, VANAP USF
Nursing Education & Professional Development
VA Northern California Health Care System
Mather, California

Marcy Caplin, PhD, RN, CNE
RN/BSN & Graduate Nurse Educator Programs
Kent State University
Kent, Ohio

Margaret-Ann Carno, PhD, MBA, MJ, RN, CPNP,D, ABSM, FAAN
Professor of Clinical Nursing and Pediatrics
School of Nursing
University of Rochester
Rochester, New York

Patricia Caudle, DNSc, CNM, FNP-BC
Associate Professor
Frontier Nursing University
Hyden, Kentucky

Will Chapleau, EMT-P, RN, TNS
Director of Performance Improvement
American College of Surgeons
Chicago, Illinois

Claire DeCristofaro, MD
Clinical Assistant Professor, DNP Program
The Medical University of South Carolina
Charleston, South Carolina

Suzanne DeYoung, MSN, DNP
Assistant Professor
Greenville Technical College
Greenville, South Carolina

Carolyn J. Driscoll, PhD RN FNP-C
Nurse Practitioner
Hepatology Section
Division of Gastroenterology, Hepatology, and Nutrition
Virginia Commonwealth University Health System
Richmond, Virginia

Hon-Vu Q. Duong, MD
Clinical Instructor of Ophthalmology
Westfield Eye Center
Las Vegas, Nevada
Senior Lecturer of Neurosciences, Anatomy & Physiology
Nevada State College
Henderson, Nevada

Julie Eggert, PhD, GNP-BC, AGN-BC, AOCN, FAAN
Professor and Coordinator, Healthcare Genetics Doctoral Program
Mary Cox Professor
Clemson University
Clemson, South Carolina

Jennifer S. Eisenstein, DNP, APRN, FNP-C
Nurse Practitioner
The Eisenstein Clinic
Arlington Heights, Illinois

Mary Alice Estes, RN, MSN, CNE
Instructor - Associate Degree Nursing
Alvin Community College
Alvin, Texas

Sarah Schwarz Farabi, PhD, RN
Postdoctoral Fellow
University of Colorado, School of Medicine
Denver, Colorado

Katherina Fontanilla, DNP, RN
Nursing Instructor
College of Southern Nevada
Henderson, Nevada

Sarah Gabua, DNP, RN, CNE
Nursing Instructor
Aspen University
Denver, Colorado

Lisa Gaston, MSc, ACNP
Manager, Clinical Nurse Consultant
Celgene
Melrose Park, Illinois

Matthew W. Gifford, OD
Red Eye Eyewear
Chicago, Illinois

Eileen D. Hacker, PhD
Associate Professor Emerita of Biobehavioral Health Science
University of Illinois at Chicago
Chicago, Illinois

Rebecca Hernandez, MSN, APRN, FNP-BC
Clinical Assistant Professor
School of Nursing
The University of Texas – Rio Grande Valley
Edinburg, Texas

Jeanne B. Hewitt, PhD, RN
Associate Professor, College of Nursing
Director, Community Outreach and Engagement Core
Children's Environmental Health Sciences Core Center
University of Wisconsin
Milwaukee, Wisconsin

Karen Hill, RN, BS, MN, PhD
Associate Professor
Southeastern Louisiana University
Hammond, Louisiana

Barbara J. Holtzclaw, PhD, RN, FAAN
Professor
Associate Dean for Research
Earl and Fran Ziegler College of Nursing
University of Oklahoma Health Sciences
Oklahoma City, Oklahoma

Art Hsieh, MA, NRP
Emergency Care Program
Santa Rosa Junior College
Santa Rosa, California

Immaculata Igbo, PhD, MSc
Professor
Pathophysiology & Pharmacology
Prairie View A&M University – College of Nursing
Houston, Texas

Linda Janusek, PhD, RN, FAAN
Professor
Niehoff Endowed Chair for Research
Department of Health Promotion
Loyola University Chicago
Maywood, Illinois

Rita W. Kaspar, PhD, RN, CNP
Columbus, Ohio

Linda J. Keilman, DNP, GNP-BC, FAANP
Associate Professor
Gerontological Nurse Practitioner
Michigan State University
College of Nursing
East Lansing, Michigan

Amy Mitchell Kennedy, MSN, RN
Nursing Content Manager
Newport News, Virginia

Vicki Keough, PhD, APRN-BC, ACNP, FAAN
Dean and Professor
Marcella Niehoff School of Nursing
Loyola University Chicago
Maywood, Illinois

Joanne Kouba, PhD, RDN
Associate Professor
Marcella Niehoff School of Nursing
Loyola University Chicago
Maywood, Illinois

Susan Krawczyk, CRNA, DNP
NorthShore University Health System
School of Nurse Anesthesia
Park Ridge, Illinois

Bhuma Krishnamachari, PhD
Assistant Dean of Research
New York Institute of Technology College of Osteopathic Medicine
Glen Head, New York

Christina M. Lattner, MSN Ed, ECRN, AGNP-C, ANP-BC, RN-BC
Assistant Clinical Professor
School of Nursing, College of Science and Health
DePaul University
Chicago, Illinois

Kathy Lauer, PhD, RN
Assistant Professor
College of Nursing
Rush University
Chicago, Illinois

MariJo Letizia, PhD, APN/ANP-BC, FAANP
Professor
School of Nursing
Loyola University Chicago
Maywood, Illinois

Pamela F. Levin, PhD, APHN-BC
Professor
College of Nursing
Rush University
Chicago, Illinois

Laura Logan, MSN, RN, CCRN
Clinical Instructor
DeWitt School of Nursing
Stephen F. Austin State University
Nacogdoches, Texas

Shari J. Lynn, MSN, RN
Faculty
Department of Acute and Chronic Care
Johns Hopkins School of Nursing
Baltimore, Maryland

Dawna Martich, MSN, RN
Nursing Education Consultant
Pittsburgh, Pennsylvania

Herbert L. Mathews, PhD
Department of Microbiology and Immunology
Loyola University Chicago
Maywood, Illinois

Patricia McCarthy, PhD
Professor
Associate Chair & Program Director
Department of Communication Disorders & Sciences
Rush University
Chicago, Illinois

Daniel R. Mead, MSN, RN
Student Nurse Practitioner- Internal Medicine/Geriatrics
University of Cincinnati
Charge Nurse-Telemetry
Norwegian American Hospital
Adjunct Faculty
DePaul University
Chicago, Illinois

Elizabeth Moxley, PhD, RN
Assistant Professor
School of Nursing
DePaul University
Chicago, Illinois

Cathy Marie Murks, RN, APN-NP
Nurse Practitioner
The University of Chicago Medicine
Chicago, Illinois

Martha Olson, DNP, MSN
Professor
Iowa Lakes Community College
Emmetsburg, Iowa

Cynthia Parkman, PhD, RN
Faculty
School of Health and Human Services -- Nursing
National University
San Diego, California

Matthew Pastore, MS, LGC
Genetic Counselor Lead
Clinical Assistant Professor of Pediatrics
Nationwide Children's Hospital
Columbus, Ohio

Lynn Perkins, PhD, MSN, RN
Nursing Faculty
Minneapolis Community and Technical College
Minneapolis, Minnesota

Tammy Poma, ANP-BC, CNN-NP
Nephrology Nurse Practitioner
University of Chicago
Chicago, Illinois

Peter T. Pons, MD
PHTLS Associate Medical Director
Brighton, Colorado

Jori Reigle, MS, RN
Lecturer/Adjunct Clinical Instructor
School of Nursing
University of Michigan
Flint, Michigan

Judith L. Reishtein, PhD, MS, RN
Course Facilitator
College of New Rochelle
The State University of New Jersey
New Rochelle, New Jersey

Bernadette T. Roche, APN, CRNA, EdD
Adjunct Associate Professor
School of Nursing
DePaul University
Chicago, Illinois

Laura Robbins-Frank, MSN, RNC, APN
Instructor
Marcella Niehoff School of Nursing
Loyola University Chicago
Chicago, Illinois

Kathryn Wirtz Rugen, PhD, FNP-BC, FAANP
National Nurse Practitioner Consultant,
Centers of Excellence in Primary Care Education
Veterans Health Administration
Clinical Associate Professor
University of Illinois at Chicago
Chicago, Illinois

Karen L. Saban, PhD, RN, APRN, CNRN, FAHA
Associate Professor
Associate Dean for Research
Loyola University Chicago
Maywood, Illinois

Deborah Saber, PhD, RN, CCRN-K
Assistant Professor
School of Nursing
The University of Maine
Orono, Maine

Jessica Simmons, MSN, APN, FNP-C, CWON, DNC
Nurse Practitioner - Internal Medicine
Mercy Health
Rockford, Illinois

Marsha Snyder, PHD, PMHNP/CNS, BC, CADC
Clinical Associate Professor
University of Illinois
Chicago, Illinois

Angela Starkweather, PhD, RN, ACNP-BC, CNRN, FAAN
Director, Center for Advancement in Managing Pain
Professor
University of Connecticut
Storrs, Connecticut

Marcia Stout, DNP, APN, FNP-C, CWON, CHSE
Adjunct Assistant Professor
College of Health Professions
Rosalind Franklin University of Medicine and Science
North Chicago, Illinois

Amy K. Winston, AuD
Clinical Audiologist
Assistant Professor
Department of Communication Disorders and Sciences
Rush University Medical Center
Chicago, Illinois

Reviewers

Jean K. Berry, PhD, APN
Clinical Associate Professor Emerita
College of Nursing, Department of Biobehavioral Health Science
University of Illinois
Chicago, Illinois

Sophia Beydoun, MSN, RN
Nursing Faculty
Henry Ford College
Dearborn, Michigan

Theresa Capriotti, DO, MSN, CRNP
Clinical Associate Professor
Villanova University
Villanova, Pennsylvania

Hilary Carlson, RN, CPNP
Adjunct Clinical Instructor
School of Nursing
Columbia University
New York, New York

Margaret-Ann Carno, PhD, MBA, MJ, D, CPNP, ABSM, FAAN
Professor of Clinical Nursing and Pediatrics
School of Nursing
University of Rochester
Rochester, New York

Lori Ciafardoni, MSN/ED, RN
Assistant Professor
State University of New York
Delhi, New York

Anne Clayton, MS
Instructor
College of Nursing
Michigan State University
East Lansing, Michigan

Barbara E. Connell, RN, MSN
Program Director
Southwestern Community College
Sylva, North Carolina

Ann Crawford, PhD, RN, CNS, CEN, CPEN
Professor, College of Nursing
University of Mary Hardin-Baylor
Belton, Texas

Diane Daddario, DNP, ANP-C, ACNS-BC, RN-BC, CMSRN
Nursing Faculty
Pennsylvania State University
University Park, Pennsylvania

Jean E. DeMartinis, PhD, FNP-BC
Associate Professor, College of Nursing
University of Massachusetts
Amherst, Massachusetts

Fernande E. Deno, MSN, RN, CNE
Nursing Instructor
Anoka-Ramsey Community College
Coon Rapids, Minnesota

David J. Derrico, RN, MSN, CNE
Clinical Assistant Professor
College of Nursing
University of Florida
Gainesville, Florida

Kirsty Digger, DNS, RN, CEN
Associate Professor
School of Nursing
State University of New York
Delhi, New York

Julie B. Doyle, EdD, RN
Faculty
Geisinger Lewistown Hospital School of Nursing
Lewistown, Pennsylvania

Tonya Eddy, PhD, RN
Assistant Professor
University of Central Missouri
Warrensburg, Missouri

Abimbola Farinde, PharmD, PhD
Professor
Columbia Southern University
Orange Beach, Alabama

Rebecca A. Fountain, PhD, RN
Assistant Professor
University of Texas
Tyler, Texas

Karla Hanson, MS, RN
Instructor
College of Nursing
South Dakota State University
Sioux Falls, South Dakota

Pamela G. Harrison, EdD, RN, CNE
Professor
Indiana Wesleyan University
Marion, Indiana

Patty Hawley, MSED
Instructor
Ferris State University
Big Rapids, Michigan

Deborah Henry, PhD(c), RN
Director of Nursing
Blue Ridge Community College
Flat Rock, North Carolina

Barbara J. Holtzclaw, PhD, RN, FAAN
Professor / Associate Dean for Research
University of Oklahoma Health Sciences Center
Earl and Fran Ziegler College of Nursing
Oklahoma City, Oklahoma

Arthur Hsieh, MA, NRP
Paramedic Program Director
Santa Rosa Junior College
Windsor, California

Immaculata Ngozi Igbo, PhD, MSc, BSc
Professor
College of Nursing
Prairie View A&M University
Houston, Texas

Linda J. Keilman, DNP, GNP-BC, FAANP
Associate Professor, College of Nursing
Michigan State University
East Lansing, Michigan

Christine Kleckner, MA, MAN, RN
Nursing Instructor
Minneapolis Community and Technical College
Minneapolis, Minnesota

Barbara Lane, MSN, RN-BC
Program Coordinator
School of Nursing
Lincoln University
Fort Leonard Wood, Missouri

Claire M. Leonard, PhD
Professor, Biology
Pre-Professional Advisor College Science & Health
William Paterson University
Wayne, New Jersey

Laura Logan, MSN, RN, CCRN
Clinical Instructor, DeWitt School of Nursing
Stephen F. Austin State University
Nacogdoches, Texas

Terrence Miller, PhD, BS
Biology Instructor
Central Carolina Community College
Sanford, North Carolina

Jeremy Morse, PhD, ARNP, ANP-C
Director of Institutional Support & Donor Relations
Palm Beach Atlantic University
West Palm Beach, Florida

Janet Pinkelman, MSN, RNC-MNN
Professor of Nursing
Owens Community College
Toledo, Ohio

Colleen M. Quinn, EdD, MSN, RN
Professor
Broward College
Pembroke Pines, Florida

Christine Recktenwald, MSN, RN
Assistant Teaching Professor
University of Missouri
St. Louis, Missouri

Jori Anne Reigle, BA, MS, RN
Lecturer/Adjunct Clinical Instructor
School of Nursing
University of Michigan
Flint, Michigan

Tara Rich, RN, MSN
Department Head
ADN/PN Program Director
James Sprunt Community College
Kenansville, North Carolina

Carol Rizer, CRNA, DNP
Assistant Professor
The University of Texas
Tyler, Texas

Janet Czermak Russell, DNP, APN-BC
Associate Professor of Nursing
Essex County College
Newark, New Jersey

Leighsa Sharoff, EdD, RN, PMHNP/CNS, AHN-BC
Associate Professor
Simulation Coordinator
Hunter College, City University of New York
New York, New York

Monica L. Tenhunen, DNP, RN, GNP-BC, ANP-C
Assistant Professor
Department of Nursing
Texas A&M University
Commerce, Texas

Kimberly Valich, MSN, RN
Assistant Professor
Medical Surgical III Course Coordinator
Department of Nursing
University of Saint Francis
Crown Point, Indiana

Preface

Why We Wrote This Text

One of the challenges of teaching pathophysiology is helping students understand the underlying concepts behind the details. This book started with conversations on how best to facilitate student understanding. We chose to create this book as a way of fostering student learning and clinical application.

The goals of *Pathophysiology: Concepts of Human Disease* are not only to provide students with the latest information about pathophysiology that is relevant to clinical practice, but also to empower students with competencies that will endure throughout their nursing career. The approach we have taken to pathophysiology reflects the shift in focus of healthcare from mainly understanding diseases in their later stages to understanding risk factors and interventions that can maintain good health and slow progression of disease in humans. For example, obesity, lack of regular physical activity, and tobacco use are risk factors for many common diseases such as diabetes mellitus, hypertension, atherosclerosis, cancer, and asthma. Therefore, we address risk behaviors that underlie leading causes of morbidity and mortality. The focus of this book will enhance students' understanding of disease processes and their ability to explain and motivate patients in their care to make therapeutic lifestyle changes.

Because of the rapid expansion of knowledge related to pathophysiology and the content saturation experienced by students in pathophysiology courses as well as other nursing courses, the concept-based approach for organization of content is used *Pathophysiology: Concepts of Human Disease*. This will help students to understand the elements common to many disease states. An explanation of the major physiologic concept addressed in each chapter and a list of related concepts are provided in the Chapter Overview of each chapter. The concepts we have used include the following:

Acid–Base Balance
Addiction
Cellular Regulation
Cognition
Comfort and Pain
Elimination
Energy Balance
Environment
Fluid and Electrolyte Balance
Hemostasis
Immunity
Infection
Inflammation and Oxidative Stress
Intracranial Regulation
Metabolism
Mobility
Mood and Affect
Nutrition and Digestion
Oxygenation
Perfusion
Reproduction
Sensory Perception
Sexuality
Stress and Coping
Thermoregulation
Tissue Integrity
Trauma

The most extensive coverage for each concept addressed is given to conditions, risk factors, and behaviors underlying the leading causes of morbidity and mortality. This ensures that the most prevalent disorders are given the most coverage. Identification of the conditions emphasized in the book is based on the Centers for Disease Control and Prevention's National Center for Health Statistics (http://www.cdc.gov/nchs/index.htm) and the national healthcare agenda as described in *Healthy People 2020*, published by the National Institutes of Health (NIH). According to the NIH, "The leading health indicators reflect the major health concerns in the U.S. at the beginning of the 21st century. The leading health indicators were selected based on their importance as public health issues." Chapter content related to *Healthy People 2020* focus areas is highlighted in special boxes. Summary tables are used to cover less common conditions.

The Cover

Starting with the cover, we emphasize the major focus of this text: human beings. Pathophysiology does not occur in a vacuum. Diseases, disorders, and syndromes occur in people—in individuals—and happen to neonates and infants, to children and adolescents, to men and women, to older adults. We call them "patients," but they are people first: parents, workers, students, lovers, siblings. The people shown on the cover appear as patients in case studies in the text.

Connor Whelan

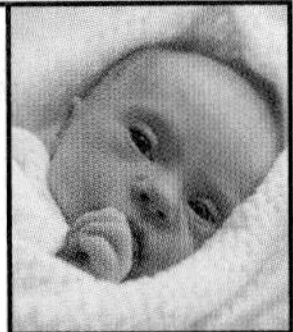

Connor Whelan is the infant son of parents who are delighted to welcome him to the world. Connor has Down syndrome and a congenital heart defect. You will meet Connor in Chapter 25, "Cardiac Structural Disorders."

Angela Wang

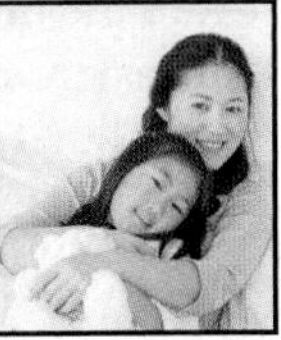

Jennifer Yang hears from her daughter's school that Angela should be tested for cognitive difficulties. The tests reveal possible toxins. You will meet Jennifer and Angela in Chapter 3, "Environmental Influences on Disease and Injury."

Matthew Horn

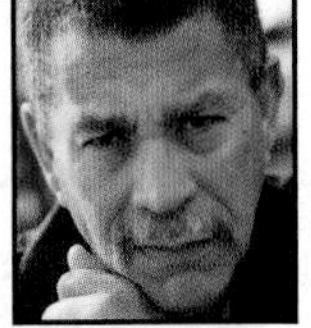

Matthew Horn visits his healthcare provider for an annual checkup and complains that his right hand shakes when he's just sitting around or watching TV. The shaking seems to disappear when he's actively using his hand. That, along with other symptoms, leads to a suspicion of Parkinson disease. You will meet Matthew in Chapter 34, "Disorders Affecting Motor Function."

Irene Rollins

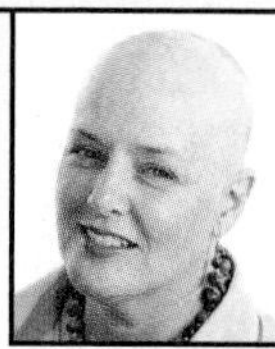

Irene Rollins, age 67, has ovarian cancer and is near the end of her life. You will meet Irene in Chapter 53, "Pathophysiology at the End of Life."

The background image on the cover depicts a strain of the influenza virus. Influenza is a contagious respiratory illness that can be mild, moderate, or deadly. Every year in the United States, millions of people are infected with an influenza virus, hundreds of thousands are hospitalized, and tens of thousands die.

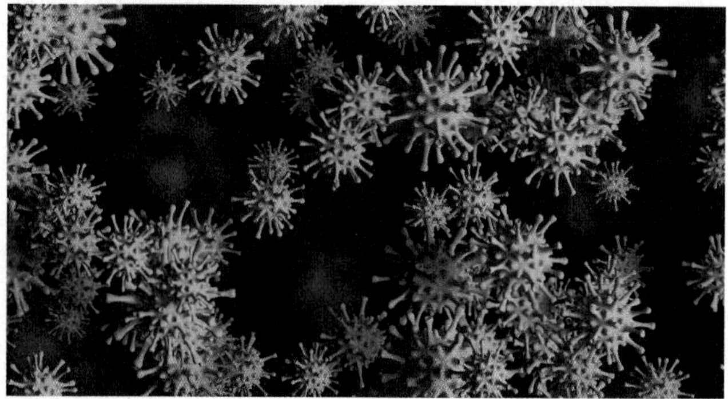

The individuals featured on our cover highlight another important aspect of *Pathophysiology: Concepts of Human Disease*: We cover the lifespan from birth to death. Information specific to infants and children, pregnant women, and older adults is highlighted with icons to draw attention to these specific populations.

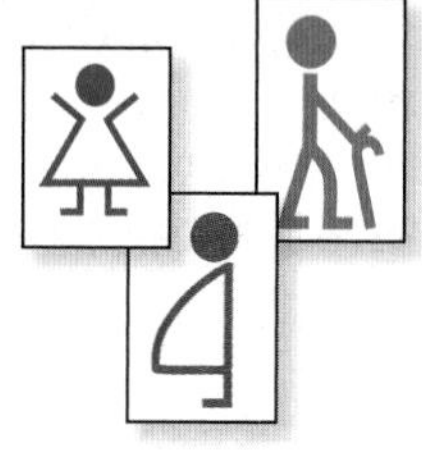

Unit Structure

Pathophysiology: Concepts of Human Disease comprises 53 chapters divided into 15 units. The first four units provide in-depth coverage of pathophysiologic mechanisms; the rest of the units cover disorders, diseases, syndromes, and injuries grouped by concept. On each unit opener there is a visual that summarizes the content of the unit. These are great tools for students to review the unit.

Unit I: Foundations of Pathophysiology

Unit I introduces students to the foundational concepts and key components of the study of pathophysiology, including everything from terminology to genetics and the influence of the environment and stress on the human condition.

- **Chapter 1: Introduction to the Basics of Pathophysiology** introduces the readers to the basics of pathophysiology, including essential terminology, an overview of health and illness, the leading indicators of morbidity and mortality, and the importance of evidence-based practice. It also provides an overview of the structure of the chapters and features. With the Human Genome Project ushering in an era of genomics and proteomics, healthcare providers require increased understanding of the molecular biologic aspects of disease. This includes not only genetics, (e.g., inherited single-gene disorders), but also genomics, which involves the interactions among many genes in the human genome and the influence of environment and lifestyle on gene expression.
- **Chapter 2: Genetics, Genomics, and Epigenomics** addresses new knowledge and technologies related to genomics being used in molecular diagnostic and predisposition testing, as well as ways to increase customization of preventive strategies and treatment regimens for people with different phenotypes of many acute and chronic conditions.
- **Chapter 3: Environmental Health Influences on Disease and Injury** covers environmental influences on disease and injury. This topic is essential to pathophysiology but is rarely included in textbooks. The impact of the environment on the development of disease in humans is enormous. This chapter covers everything from environmental hazard classifications to the impact of the environment on assessing patients to the pathophysiologic mechanisms underlying alterations caused by environmental hazards.
- **Chapter 4: Stress and Adaptation** is another topic that is underrepresented in other pathophysiology texts. The effects of stress on physical and mental health are a key component of human disease, and we cover it in detail.

Unit II: Risks Underlying the Leading Causes of Morbidity and Mortality

Unit II stresses one of the major themes of *Pathophysiology: Concepts of Human Disease*: health promotion and disease prevention. Each of the major risk categories underlying the leading causes of morbidity and mortality are covered in this unit. Again, most other pathophysiology texts devote little or no coverage to these important topics.

- **Chapter 5: Health Risks of Obesity and Physical Inactivity**
- **Chapter 6: Risks Related to Substance Use Disorders**
- **Chapter 7: Risks Related to Sleep Alterations**

Unit III: Fluid, Electrolyte, and Acid–Base Imbalances

Unit III covers the critical content of fluid and electrolyte balance and acid–base balance, both of which are key factors in maintaining health.

- **Chapter 8: Fluid and Electrolyte Imbalances**
- **Chapter 9: Acid–Base Imbalances**

Units IV: Cell Injury, Inflammation, and Alterations of Cell Growth and Regulation

Unit IV completes the foundational content by covering cell injury and aging, inflammation, and neoplasia.

- **Chapter 10: Mechanisms of Cell Injury and Aging**
- **Chapter 11: Inflammation**
- **Chapter 12: Neoplasia**

Units V through XIV

In Units V through XIV **(Chapters 13 – 49)**, we cover the most prevalent disorders within each concept. We have endeavored to cover the essential "need to know" content and to keep "nice to know" material to a minimum in an effort to combat the content saturation students face. Each unit covers one or more concepts:

- **Unit V: Infection and Disorders of Immunity**
- **Unit VI: Disorders of Oxygenation**
- **Unit VII: Disorders of Perfusion**
- **Unit VIII: Disorders of Mood and Cognition**
- **Unit IX: Disorders of Sensory Perception and Thermoregulation**
- **Unit X: Disorders of Mobility**
- **Unit XI: Disorders of Endocrine Regulation**
- **Unit XII: Altered Tissue Integrity**
- **Unit XIII: Disorders of Digestion, Metabolism, and Elimination**
- **Unit XIV: Disorders of Sexuality and Reproduction**

Unit XV: Trauma and Multisystem Conditions

The last unit is unique to *Pathophysiology: Concepts of Human Disease*. Trauma is a major cause of morbidity and mortality, but it is not covered in most other pathophysiology texts. And our last chapter covers a phenomenon that every patient and every nurse will experience. It is an important topic that is often overlooked, but we have covered it in detail.

- **Chapter 50: Mechanisms of Traumatic Injury**
- **Chapter 51: The Pathophysiology of Primary and Secondary Traumatic Injury**
- **Chapter 52: Biologic, Chemical, and Radiologic Agents of Disease**
- **Chapter 53: Pathophysiology at the End of Life**

Unique Content

Pathophysiology: Concepts of Human Disease endeavors to cover all topics related to human disease and injury, including many that are rarely covered in pathophysiology textbooks. Our unique chapters include:

- **Chapter 3: Environmental Health Influences on Disease and Injury**
- **Chapter 6: Risks Related to Substance Use Disorders**
- **Chapter 7: Risks Related to Sleep Alterations**
- **Chapter 29: Emotional Regulation and Mood**
- **Chapter 30: Neurocognitive and Neurodevelopmental Disorders**
- **Chapter 50: Mechanisms of Traumatic Injury**
- **Chapter 51: The Pathophysiology of Primary and Secondary Traumatic Injury**
- **Chapter 52: Biologic, Chemical, and Radiologic Agents of Disease**
- **Chapter 53: Pathophysiology at the End of Life.**

In-Chapter Assessments

While developing this first edition of *Pathophysiology: Concepts of Human Disease,* the authors – who are experienced classroom teachers – wanted to build in many opportunities for students to assess their understanding of the material as they are reading the content. Therefore, every chapter includes the following sets of questions:

- **Check Your Progress:** Found at the end of each numbered section, these questions are designed to assess students' understanding of the content.
- **Case Studies:** Each part of each case study ends with questions that cover the content in the section as well as the content of the case study.
- **Review Questions:** These are NCLEX-style questions found at the end of each chapter. They are written at the Understand, Apply, Analyze, and Evaluate levels of Bloom's taxonomy.

Answers to the Check Your Progress and Case Study questions are in the instructor resources for the print book and are pop-ups in the student eText. Answers for the Review Questions are in Appendix A in the print book and are given, along with rationales, as the student answers the questions in the eText.

Chapter Guide

The chapters in **Pathophysiology: Concepts of Human Disease** have been developed in a consistent structure to facilitate learning. Readers will see the same basic format used throughout the book.

Each chapter starts with **Chapter Outline and Learning Outcomes,** a list of the numbered sections in the chapter along with the learning outcome for each.

Chapter 5

Health Risks of Obesity and Physical Inactivity

Jean Barry

Chapter Outline and Learning Outcomes

5.1 Chapter Overview and Case Studies
Outline the global prevalence of, medical conditions associated with, and concepts related to obesity and physical inactivity.

5.2 Etiology and Pathophysiology of Obesity
Describe the etiology of obesity and outline the pathophysiologic consequences, including chronic diseases and metabolic syndrome.

5.3 Health Risks of Obesity
Outline the health risks and functional outcomes associated with obesity.

5.4 Health Risks of Physical Inactivity
Discuss the role of physical inactivity/activity in the development and progression of chronic diseases and recommendations for physical activity.

Key Terms and Abbreviations come next. Each Key Term is included in the glossary at the end of the print book and is hyperlinked to its definition in the eText. The Abbreviations list contains the abbreviations specific to the topic that are used throughout the chapter.

KEY TERMS

Adipocytes, 12
Anorexigenic, 5
Body mass index (BMI), 11
C-reactive protein, 10
Epigenetics, 8
Exercise, 16
Hepatomegaly, 13
Hyperinsulinemia, 8
Insulin resistance, 8
Metabolic equivalent of task (MET), 17
Metabolic syndrome, 10
Monogenic, 7
Nonalcoholic fatty liver disease (NAFLD), 13
Nonalcoholic steatohepatitis, 13
Obesity, 3
Orexigenic, 5
Physical fitness, 16
Polygenic, 7
Polymorphisms, 7
Reactive oxygen species (ROS), 8
Satiety, 6
Steatohepatitis, 13
Steatosis, 13
Visceral adiposity, 8

ABBREVIATIONS

α-MSH—α-melanocyte stimulating hormone
AGE—advanced glycosylation end product
AGRP—agouti-related peptide
ARC—arcuate nucleus
BMI—body mass index
CART—cocaine and amphetamine-regulated transcript peptide
CCK—cholecystokinin
GLP-1—glucagon-like peptide-1
HDL—high-density lipoprotein
IL-6—interleukin 6
LDL—low-density lipoprotein
MC4R—melanocortin 4 receptor
NAFLD—nonalcoholic fatty liver disease
NPY—neuropeptide Y
POMC—pro-opiomelanocortin
ROS—reactive oxygen species
PYY—peptide YY
T2D—type 2 diabetes mellitus
TNFα—tumor necrosis factor alpha

5.1 Chapter Overview and Case Studies 3

5.1 Chapter Overview and Case Studies

One of the major challenges of the 21st century is the prevention and treatment of obesity. The World Health Organization (WHO) defines **obesity** as abnormal or excessive fat accumulation that may impair health.[1,2] More than 33% of U.S. adults and 17% of U.S. children are obese.[3] Obesity is a factor in the development of a number of medical conditions, including diabetes, cardiovascular disease (coronary artery disease, myocardial infarction, angina pectoris, heart failure, stroke, hypertension, and atrial fibrillation), metabolic syndrome, cancer, arthritis and disability, gallbladder disease, acute pancreatitis, nonalcoholic fatty liver disease, pulmonary complications, and depression.[4] One of the goals of *Healthy People 2020* is to promote good health through nutrition and maintenance of a healthy body weight.

There has been a dramatic increase in the prevalence of obesity in the United States over the last two decades. Prevalence estimates of obesity in 2014 by state ranged from 20 to 35%[5] (**Figure 5.1**). The total excess cost related to the current prevalence of overweight and obesity among adolescents is estimated to be $254 billion.[6] This number includes $208 billion in lost productivity secondary to premature morbidity and mortality and $46 billion in direct medical costs.[6] If current trends in the development of overweight and obesity continue, the total healthcare costs related to obesity could reach $861–$957 billion by 2030; this would account for 16–18% of U.S. health expenditures.[6]

The first section in each chapter is **Chapter Overview and Case Studies**. Here the authors introduce the topic, explain the concepts related to each topic, and present the case studies that will be threaded throughout the chapter.

Check Your Progress: Section 5.1

1. How does the World Health Organization define the term *obesity*?
2. What are some of the major health problems associated with obesity?
3. What are the current trends in physical activity among U.S. adults and adolescents?

The main sections are double-numbered with a matching learning outcome. At the end of each section, there is a **Check Your Progress** box that features two or three open-ended questions about the content just presented.

Carrilyn Proust: Introduction

Carrilyn Proust, age 43, presents to her primary care provider's office complaining of a chronic, nonproductive cough and shortness of breath with even minor physical activities, such as climbing stairs. Ms. Proust was recently diagnosed with a viral upper respiratory tract infection, which was treated symptomatically. She suspects that her shortness of breath is secondary to her viral respiratory infection. She states that her primary concern is her chronic cough, which is preventing her from sleeping at night. She has been taking an over-the-counter cough suppressant, but she reports that this treatment is not effectively reducing her cough. She is afebrile and denies any recent history fever or chills. She reports that she has been "coughing so hard that sometimes blood comes up." Ms. Proust has a 20 pack-year history of cigarette smoking. She began smoking at age 21 and quit smoking at age 41. She denies allergies to any medications or foods. Her vital signs are within normal limits.

Carrilyn Proust: Application

Ms. Proust's primary care provider orders a chest x-ray, which reveals a mass in the lower lobe of Ms. Proust's right lung. For further evaluation, the primary care provider schedules Ms. Proust for a pulmonary computed tomography (CT) scan. In addition, a sputum sample is collected for analysis. Ms. Proust's sputum sample contains a moderate amount of blood. Ms. Proust's CT reveals an abnormal mass approximately 1 centimeter in diameter in the lower lobe of her right lung. Cytology of her sputum sample reveals suspected malignant cells. Ms. Proust is referred to an oncologist for further evaluation and treatment.

3. On the basis of her gender, what type of lung cancer does Ms. Proust most likely have?
4. What finding in Ms. Proust's history and physical examination suggests that Ms. Proust does not have small cell carcinoma?

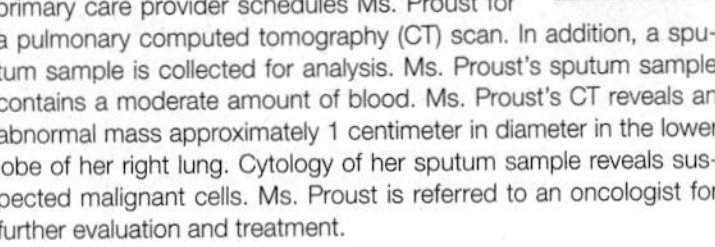

Carrilyn Proust: Outcome

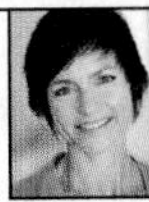

Ms. Proust's oncologist diagnoses her with stage 0 NSCLC—specifically, adenocarcinoma. Clinical staging reveals that the that malignancy appears to be confined to the 1-cm mass in her right lower lung field. No lymph node involvement or metastasis is identified. Ms. Proust undergoes uncomplicated surgical excision of the tumor. Postoperative pathologic staging reveals no apparent lymph node involvement or cancer metastasis. However, because of Mrs. Proust's smoking history and subsequent increased risk for cancer recurrence, radiation and chemotherapy are added to her treatment plan to help reduce her risk for cancer recurrence.

5. Discuss the rationale for pathologic staging in Ms. Proust's treatment.
6. Although Ms. Proust has a small tumor with no lymph node involvement or metastasis, explain the rationale for adding chemotherapy and radiation therapy to her surgical treatment.

Each **Case Study** appears multiple times in the chapter with an **Introduction**, one or more **Applications**, and an **Outcome** section. The patients featured in the case studies reflect the diversity of the population of the United States across all age groups.

Etiology and Pathogenesis

The primary cause of lung cancer is cigarette smoking, th result of the carcinogenic character of multiple chemica in cigarette smoke. The chemicals bind and mutate DN (see the feature on Genetics and Genomics for Clinic Practice).[12] There is a linear relationship between the inter sity of smokin other cancers,

Clinical Manifestations

Most patients with lung cancer do not seek medical car until they after they become symptomatic. The most com mon symptom is a persistent cough with or without spu tum production. Cough is not a specific symptom for lun cancers, and initially it is typically attributed to cigarett commo streake

Linking Pathophysiology to Diagnosis and Treatment

Diagnostic tests for lung cancer include chest x-ray, computed tomography (CT), sputum cytology, and directly sampling cells from the tumor or pleural fluid. An abnormal chest x-ray often triggers the diagnostic workup for lung cancer.

- CT scan of the thorax is done to identify tumors larger than 1 cm in diameter and to better visualize tumors

Each disorder that is covered has been chosen for its prevalence, i.e., the authors focused on the disorders that healthcare providers will see most often in clinical practice. For every disorder, the content is broken into three sections: **Etiology and Pathogenesis**, **Clinical Manifestations**, and **Linking Pathophysiology to Diagnosis and Treatment**.

Obesity in childhood and adoles public health problem associated long-term complications. Obese likely to have risk factors for cardiovasc diabetes, such as hyper resistance. Additionally at risk for musculosk

Obesity during pregnancy is a increased maternal and fetal risks. N cations include pregnancy-induce gestational diabetes, respiratory compli thromboembolism, preterm delivery, cesa etic complication ate include conge

In older adults, overweight and o ated with higher levels of functi when compared with normal-w Although obesity in older adults is asso adverse outcomes described in this chapt evidence that the risk of adverse outcomes

Lifespan Considerations are highlighted with icons for children, pregnant women, and older adults.

Chapters end with a **Chapter Summary** that gives a bulleted list of highlights for each numbered section/learning outcome.

26 Chapter 19 Neoplastic, Infectious, and Pulmonary Vascular Respiratory Disorders

CHAPTER SUMMARY

19.1 Chapter Overview and Case Studies

Describe the primary considerations and concepts related to pulmonary vascular, neoplastic, and infectious respiratory disorders.

- Pulmonary disorders include alterations caused by neoplastic growths, infectious diseases, abscesses, and vascular disorders.
- Neoplastic growths may be malignant or benign.
- Malignant growths are composed of cancerous cells that are capable of metastasizing (spreading) from the site of origin to other body sites or invading local body sites and causing tissue destruction.
- Benign growths contain cells that are nonmalignant (noncancerous). Infectious diseases that serve as sources of pulmonary disorders include a variety of alterations that may affect either the upper respiratory tract, the lower respiratory tract, or both.
- Pulmonary vascular disorders include alterations of blood flow within the lungs or to or from the pulmonary circuit.

19.2 Malignant Lung Cancer

Differentiate the causes, classification, underlying pathogenesis, and clinical manifestations of malignant lung cancers and approaches to diagnosis and treatment of these conditions across the lifespan.

- Cigarette smoking is the primary risk factor for lung cancer. There is a 15- to 20-year delay between starting smoking and development of lung cancer.
- Other smoke exposures (cigars, pipes, passive exposure) and exposures to environmental and occupational carcinogens (radon or asbestos) also increase the risk for lung cancer.
- Genetic susceptibility, benign chronic lung disorders, and diet contribute to lung cancer risk.
- Histologically, carcinomas are classified as adenocarcinoma, squamous cell carcinomas, and large cell carcinomas (all three of which are considered non–small cell carcinomas) and small cell car
- Adenocarcinoma and squam classified as differentiated (ret features, but cell division is u entiated (retaining enough fe but cell division is faster and t
- Adenocarcinomas are glandu the lung periphery. They grow tasize early because of invasi lymphatics.
- Squamous cell carcinomas usually originate in medial bronchial mucosa at bronchial bifurcations and metastasize to adjacent lymph nodes and lung tissue.
- Large cell carcinomas often present as big, bulky solitary tumors in the lung periphery.
- Small cell carcinomas are aggressive, highly malignant, and fast-growing tumors that metastasize early and widely.
- Symptoms initiating a diagnostic workup include obstructive pneumonia, dyspnea with a pleural effusion, hemoptysis, pain, hoarseness, or a paraneoplastic disorder.
- Initial lung cancer symptoms are often nonspecific with a persistent cough that is attributed to another cause.
- Diagnostic tools include sputum cytologic analysis, CT scan of the thorax, bronchoscopy, fine needle aspiration, thoracentesis, and mediastinoscopy.

19.3 Benign Lung Lesions

Differentiate the causes, classification, underlying pathogenesis, and clinical manifestations of benign lung lesions and approaches to diagnosis and treatment of these conditions across the lifespan.

- Pulmonary granulomas are formed to control an inhaled antigen that cannot be digested or in response to an autoimmune inflammatory process.
- Macrophages engulf the antigen, and helper T cells surround the macrophages, preventing a chronic inflammatory response.
- As macrophages die, the exposed antigen stimulates a further granulomatous inflammatory response.
- Tuberculosis is caused by the rod-shaped aerobic *M. tuberculosis* bacillus, which is protected by a waxy capsule. Transmission is primarily through inhalation of infected droplets by a susceptible person.
- *M. tuberculosis* can remain latent and in a state of dormancy for years; individuals with latent TB are not infectious.
- Active TB is symptomatic and communicable to other individuals.
- Reactivation of latent TB (secondary TB) occurs when

Review Questions are NCLEX-style to give the students practice with the format.

20 Chapter 5 Health Risks of Obesity and Physical Inactivity

6. You are placed in charge of an intervention for the students of a local elementary school. You know that a key factor for change in children's association with food is to address:
   a. the parents because they are all making incorrect food choices.
   b. the food insecurity that these children experience because it affects their food choices.
   c. the city parks and rec department because there are not enough state-of-the-art activities at the local YMCA.
   d. None of the above, since you are just one person.
7. Mr. Xi is scheduled to undergo a Roux-en-Y gastric bypass. He wants to know what he should expect from the procedure. You explain that:
   a. he will not be restricted in his diet post procedure.
   b. he will be monitored for increased hepatic glucose production.
   c. he will have improved insulin sensitivity and thus improved beta-cell function.
   d. he will need to use more diabetic medication because of the surgery.
8. A new nurse is teaching a class at the local YMCA. The students are older adults from the community. The nurse's topic is the importance of weight management as the individuals age. Understanding of this material is noted by a student who says:
   a. "Weight gain will not affect my ability to care for myself."
   b. "Weight loss will not help if I have joint pain."
   c. "Weight gain will affect my ability to do simple tasks, such as turning in bed, by myself."
   d. "Weight loss can increase my change of diabetes and its complications."

Answers to Review Questions can be found in Appendix A. Answers to Check Your Progress and Case Study questions will be found online for the print book and will be pop-ups in the eText.

ANSWERS

Answers to Review Questions can be found in Appendix A. Answers to Case Study and Check Your Progress questions are available on the faculty resources site. Please consult with your instructor.

Recommended Websites and **References** round out the offerings.

RECOMMENDED WEBSITES

Centers for Disease Control and Prevention: Childhood Overweight and Obesity
https://www.cdc.gov/obesity/childhood/index.html

Physical Activity Guidelines for Americans
https://health.gov/paguidelines/guidelines

REFERENCES

1. Maggi, S., Busetto, L., Noale, M., Limongi, F., & Crepaldi, G. (2015). Obesity: Definition and epidemiology. In A. Lenzi, S. Migliaccio, & L. M. Donini (Eds.), *Multidisciplinary approach to obesity: From assessment to treatment* (pp. 31–39). New York, NY: Springer.
2. World Health Organization. (2014). *Overweight and obesity*. Available at http://www.who.int/mediacentre/factsheets/fs311/en
3. Ogden, C. L., Carroll, M. D., Kit, B. K., & Flegal, K. M. (2014). Prevalence of childhood and adult obesity in the United States, 2011–2012. *JAMA, 311*(8), 806–814.
4. Pi-Sunyer, X. (2009). The medical risks of obesity. *Postgraduate Medicine, 121*(6), 21–33.
5. Centers for Disease Control and Prevention. (2016). *Overweight and obesity*. Available at http://www.cdc.gov/obesity/data/prevalence-maps.html
6. Go, A. S., Roger, V. L., Benjamin, E. J., et al. (2013). Heart disease and stroke statistics—2013 update: A report from the American Heart Association. *Circulation, 127*, e6–e245.
7. Centers for Disease Control and Prevention. (2014). *Facts about physical activity*. Available at http://www.cdc.gov/physicalactivity/data/facts.html
8. U.S. Department of Health and Human Services. (2017). *Physical activity*. Available at http://www.healthypeople.gov/2020/topics-objectives/topic/physical-activity
9. Gurevich-Panigrahi, T., Panigrahi, S., Wiechec, E., & Los, M. (2009). Obesity: Pathophysiology and clinical management. *Current Medicinal Chemistry, 16*(4), 506–521.
10. Yu, J. H., & Kim, M. S. (2012). Molecular mechanisms of appetite regulation. *Diabetes and Metabolism Journal, 36*(6), 391–398.
11. Sam, A. H., Troke, R. C., Tan, T. M., & Bewick, G. A. (2012). The role of the gut/brain axis in modulating food intake. *Neuropharmacology, 63*(1), 46–56.
12. Molina, P. E. (2013). *Endocrine physiology* (4th ed.). New York, NY: McGraw-Hill Medical.
13. Kanaya, A., & Vaisse, C. (2011). Obesity. In D. G. Gardner & D. M. Shoback (Eds.), *Greenspan's basic and clinical endocrinology* (pp. 699–709). New York, NY: McGraw Hill.
14. Skolnik, N. S, & Ryan, D. H. (2014). Pathophysiology, epidemiology, and assessment of obesity in adults. *Journal of Family Practice, 63*(7), S3–S10.
15. Filippatos, T. D., Elisaf, M. S. (2013). Effects of glucagon-like peptide-1 receptor agonists on renal function. *World Journal of Diabetes, 4*(5), 190–201.

19.6 Pulmonary Vascular Disorders 31

GLOSSARY

Acute bronchitis A very common, self-limited lower respiratory tract inflammation; often referred to as a "chest cold."

Adenocarcinoma A common form of lung cancer that starts in the lining of the glands.

Antigenicity The ability to stimulate the formation of antibodies.

Bacillus Calmette-Guérin (BCG) Tuberculosis vaccine that is one of the most widely used vaccines throughout the world.

Benign In reference to a tumor, one that does not spread to, invade, and destroy surrounding tissue.

Blastomycosis A fungal infection caused by *Blastomyces dermatitidis*, an uncommon fungus that is found in Ohio, the Great Lakes region, and the Mississippi River valley; it is common in dogs in endemic areas but also occurs in horses, cows, and bats, and infections in animals can serve as an indicator of human disease.

Bronchiolitis A condition characterized by inflammation of the bronchioles.

Coccidiodomycosis A fungal infection caused by *Coccidioides immitis*, which is endemic in the soil in the southwestern United States but can also be found throughout the world; it grows best in bird feces; also known as *San Joaquin Valley fever*.

Hospital-acquired pneumonia (HAP) A classification of pneumonia in which the infection was not incubating at the time of hospital admission and develops 48 hours or more after hospital admission.

Influenza A highly contagious viral infection that sweeps through a geographic region as an epidemic that lasts 6–8 weeks during the winter months.

Pertussis A highly contagious respiratory infections usually caused by *Bordetella pertussis* that has been controlled in children through pertussis vaccination; also known as whooping cough.

Pneumonia An inflammation of the lung parenchyma that is typically characterized by lung consolidation with alveoli filled with exudate.

Pulmonary arterial hypertension (PAH) A primary disorder of increased blood pressure in the pulmonary arteries; characterized by an increased pulmonary arterial resistance in the absence of left ventricular failure or chronic thromboembolism.

Pulmonary embolism (PE) Occurs when a substance or object (e.g., blood clot, fat globule, air bubble, bone fragment, or foreign matter) is pumped from the right heart into progressively smaller pulmonary arteries until it wedges in a vessel that is too small for

At the end of the book, students will find a complete **Glossary**.

Chapter Features

To enhance the content offered within the usual structure, we have feature boxes throughout:

Healthy People 2020 features highlight the role of the Healthy People initiative and the topics and objectives for healthcare that in contains.

Healthy People 2020

Nutrition and Weight Status

The overall goal of the Nutrition and Weight Status objectives for *Healthy People 2020* is to promote health and reduce the risk of chronic disease through healthful diets and the achievement and maintenance of healthy body weights. In addition, these objectives emphasize that efforts to modify diet and weight should address individual behaviors along with the policies and environments that support these behaviors. Those objectives are broadly divided into the following categories: HealthCare and Worksite Settings, Weight Status, Food Insecurity, Food and Nutrient Consumption, and Iron Deficiency.[1] The primary objectives are as follows:

- Increase the number of states with nutrition standards for foods and beverages provided to preschool-aged children in child care.
- Increase the proportion of schools that offer nutritious foods and beverages outside of school meals.
- Increase the number of states that have state-level policies that incentivize food retail outlets to provide foods that are encouraged by the Dietary Guidelines for Americans.
- Increase the proportion of Americans who have access to a food retail outlet that sells a variety of foods that are encouraged by the Dietary Guidelines for Americans.

Healthcare and Worksite Settings

- Increase the proportion of primary care physicians who regularly measure the body mass index of their patients.
- Increase the proportion of physician office visits that include counseling or education related to nutrition or weight.
- Increase the proportion of worksites that offer nutrition or weight management classes or counseling.

Weight Status

- Increase the proportion of adults who are at a healthy weight.
- Reduce the proportion of adults who are obese.
- Reduce the proportion of children and adolescents who are considered obese.
- Prevent inappropriate weight gain in youth and adults.

Food Insecurity

Food insecurity is the inability to access sufficient safe, nutritious food that is needed to maintain a healthy and active life.[2]

- Eliminate very low food security among children.
- Reduce household food insecurity and in doing so reduce hunger.

Food and Nutrient Consumption

- Increase the contribution of fruits to the diets of the population aged 2 years and older.
- Increase the variety and contribution of vegetables to the diets of the population aged 2 years and older.
- Increase the contribution of whole grains to the diets of the population aged 2 years and older.
- Reduce consumption of calories from solid fats and added sugars in the population aged 2 years and older.
- Reduce consumption of saturated fat in the population aged 2 years and older.
- Reduce consumption of sodium in the population aged 2 years and older.
- Increase consumption of calcium in the population aged 2 years and older.

Iron Deficiency

- Reduce iron deficiency among young children and females of childbearing age.
- Reduce iron deficiency among pregnant females.

References

1. U.S. Department of Health and Human Services. (2017). *Nutrition and weight status*. Available at http://www.healthypeople.gov/2020/topics-objectives/topic/nutrition-and-weight-status
2. World Health Organization. (2014). *Trade, foreign policy, diplomacy and health*. Available at http://www.who.int/trade/glossary/story028/en

Impact of Current Research on Clinical Practice

Treatment of Fatigue with a Central Nervous System Stimulant

Description: Fatigue and depression are common near the end of life and have a negative effect on the person's quality of life. In a double-blind investigation in which neither clinicians nor patients knew whether the patient received the investigational medication or placebo, 30 hospice patients in either inpatient or outpatient settings were randomized to receive treatment with either methylphenidate (Metadate, Ritalin), a mild central nervous system stimulant that increases the levels of norepinephrine and dopamine in the brain, or a placebo. The placebo was a tablet that looked identical to methyphenidate but contained starch instead of the medication. The research study nurse conducted the physical assessments and administered the symptom assessment scales. While all patients reported fatigue, no differences in severity scores were observed between the treatment and placebo groups at the beginning of the study.

Clinical Practice: A statistically significant decrease in the severity of fatigue was observed by day 14 in the group treated with methylphenidate. No improvement in fatigue was experienced by patients in the placebo group. Patients treated with methylphenidate who had clinically significant depression at the beginning of the study experienced improvement in depression based on three depression self-report scales; less improvement was noted in the placebo group. These results support the use of the central nervous system stimulant methylphenidate to improve the quality of life of patients experiencing fatigue or depression associated with terminal illness.

Research Study: Kerr, C., Drake, J., Milch, R., et al. (2012). Effects of methylphenidate on fatigue and depression: A randomized, double-blind, placebo-controlled trial. *Journal of Pain and Symptom Management, 43*(1), 68–77.

Impact of Current Research on Clinical Practice features show students how research is used clinically to highlight the importance of evidence-based practice.

Impact of Nutrition in Clinical Practice features highlight the importance of nutrition in health promotion, disease prevention, and nursing management of patients.

Impact of Nutrition in Clinical Practice

Nutrition at the End of Life

Joanne Kouba

At the end of life, the goal is for the patient to eat for pleasure and satisfaction. Dietary restrictions are eliminated, and patients are encouraged to eat and drink whatever foods and fluids appeal to them. Patients and family members must receive information about anorexia and cachexia as an expected consequence of end-stage disease. They should be informed that better care or increased effort to feed the patient will not reverse cachexia because the process of muscle protein degradation is not due just to decreased caloric intake and therefore does not respond to interventions such as supplemental nutrition or high-calorie foods. Enteral feedings via gastrostomy or nasogastric tubes are limited to patients who state that they are hungry but do not have the mechanical ability to eat.

Artificial hydration and nutrition at the end of life is a subject of considerable controversy. The benefits must be weighed against the burdens of such treatment, including the associated risks of fluid overload, peripheral and pulmonary edema, electrolyte imbalances, infection, and aspiration into the lungs. A decrease in food and fluid intake is part of the normal process of dying; as death approaches, parenteral and enteral feeding does not improve symptoms or prolong life.

Genetics and Genomics for Clinical Practice

DNA Mutation in Lung Cancer

A variety of oncogenes (e.g., *MYC*, *KRAS*, *EGFR*, *c-MET*, and *cKIT*), deleted or mutated tumor suppressor genes such as *p53*, fusion genes such as *EML4-ALK*,[12] and activated signal transduction molecules have been associated with lung cancer. The pattern for specific genetic alterations varies with the type or subtype of lung cancer. For example, *KRAS* is most common genetic mutation in adenocarcinomas in women who smoke, while epidermal growth factor receptor gene (*EGFR*) occurs more commonly in adenocarcinomas in women who do not smoke and Asians; *p53* mutations occur most commonly in squamous cell carcinomas but also are present in small cell carcinomas.[12] The *EML4-ALK* fusion gene in non–small cell lung cancer does not exist with *EGFR* or *KRAS* mutations, and its presence identifies a subset of individuals with non–small cell lung cancer that will respond to ALK-targeted agents but not *EGFR* tyrosine kinase inhibitors.[12] The importance of this genetic research is that it will allow targeting of the specific sensitivities of a tumor with oncology medications that will interfere with tumor growth.[12,13]

CLINICAL POINT: Cigarette smoking has been directly linked to DNA mutations by a specific metabolite of benzo(a)pyrene in cigarette smoke that damages three specific loci on the *p53* tumor suppressor gene. The *p53* tumor suppressor gene mutations are present in approximately 60% of all lung cancers. Cigarette smoke contains over 200 carcinogens that act as initiators (polycyclic aromatic hydrocarbons), promoters (phenol derivatives), and contaminants such as radioactive elements, arsenic, nickel, molds, and additives. ■

Genetics and Genomics for Clinical Practice features demonstrate the foundational importance of genetics and genomics in the study of pathophysiology.

Visuals

All of the artwork in **Pathophysiology: Concepts of Human Disease** has been specifically created for this text. It is attractive, realistic, and accurate. Visual learners in particular will be delighted to see the detailed illustrations.

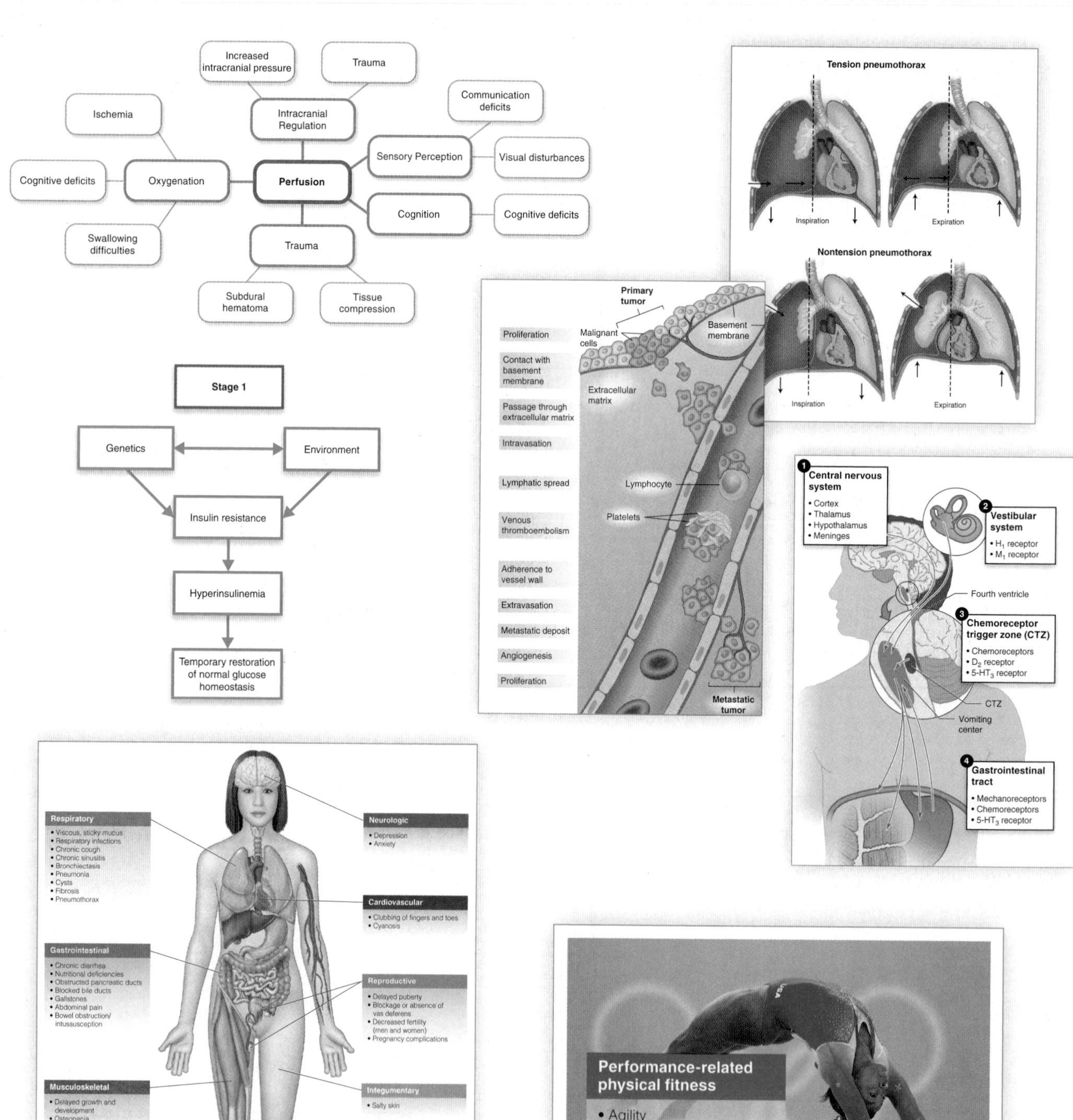

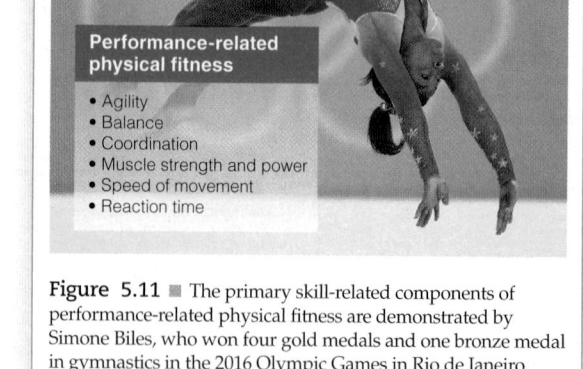

Figure 5.11 ■ The primary skill-related components of performance-related physical fitness are demonstrated by Simone Biles, who won four gold medals and one bronze medal in gymnastics in the 2016 Olympic Games in Rio de Janeiro.

MyLab Nursing

MyLab Nursing is an online learning and practice environment that works with the text to help students master key concepts, prepare for the NCLEX-RN exam, and develop clinical reasoning skills. Through a new mobile experience, students can study *Pathophysiology: Concepts of Human Disease* anytime, anywhere. New adaptive technology with remediation personalizes learning, moving students beyond memorization to true understanding and application of the content. MyLab Nursing contains the following features:

Dynamic Study Modules

New adaptive learning modules with remediation that personalize the learning experience by allowing students to increase both their confidence and their performance while being assessed in real time.

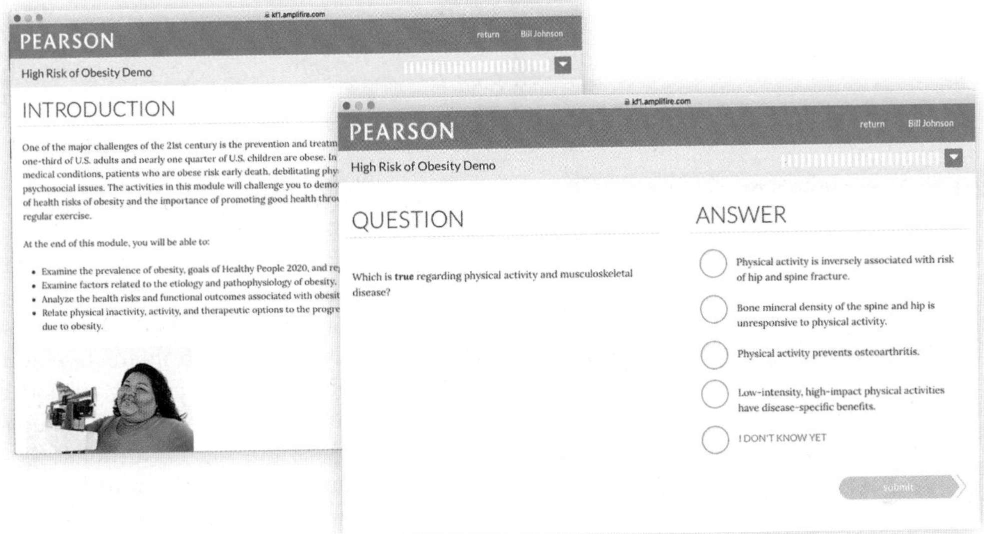

NCLEX-Style Questions

Practice tests with more than 1000 NCLEX-style questions of various types build student confidence and prepare them for success on the NCLEX-RN exam. Questions are organized by Chapter.

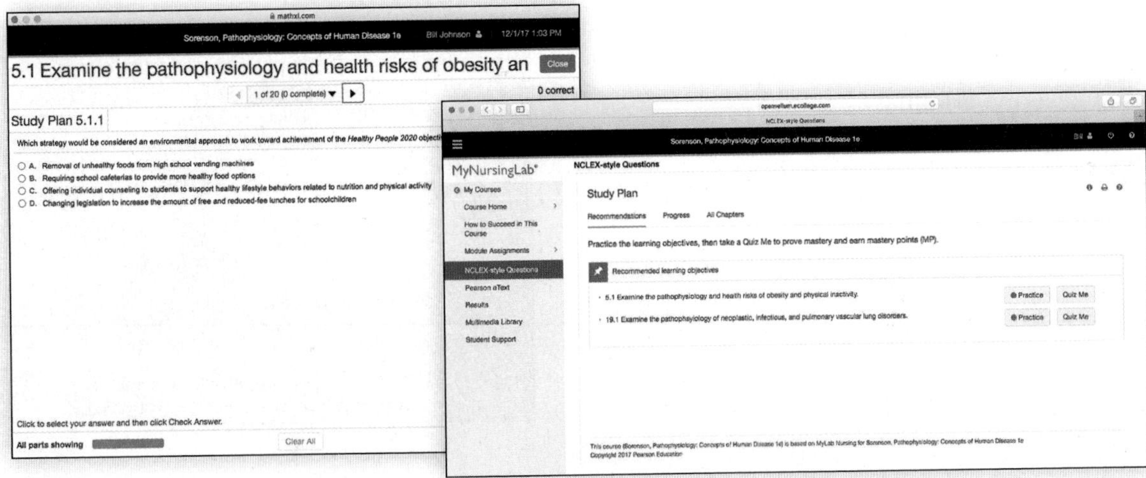

Decision Making Cases

Clinical case studies that provide opportunities for students to practice analyzing information and making important decisions at key moments in patient care scenarios. These 15 unfolding case studies are designed to help prepare students for clinical practice.

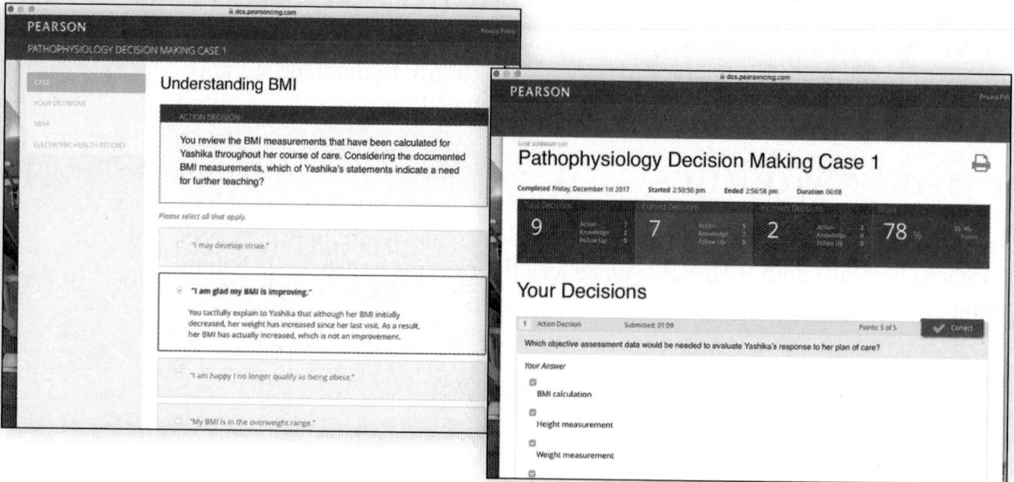

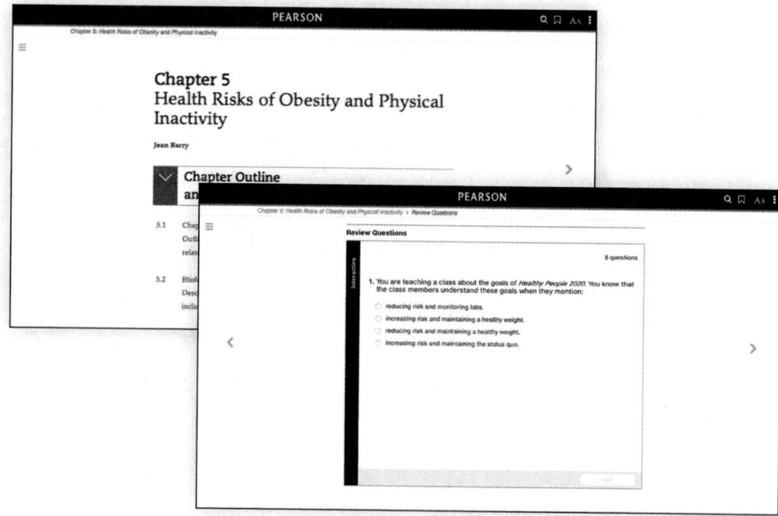

Pearson eText

Enhances student learning both in and outside the classroom. Students can take notes, highlight, and bookmark important content, or engage with interactive and rich media to achieve greater conceptual understanding of the text content. Interactive features include audio clips, pop-up definitions, figures, questions and answers, the nursing process, hotspots, and video animations. Some examples of video animations include:

- **Congenital Heart Defect Animations** illustrate the many congenital heart defects that may occur in new-borns and provide students the opportunity to see, hear, and understand how congenital heart defects impair the correct functioning of the heart and how they may be corrected.

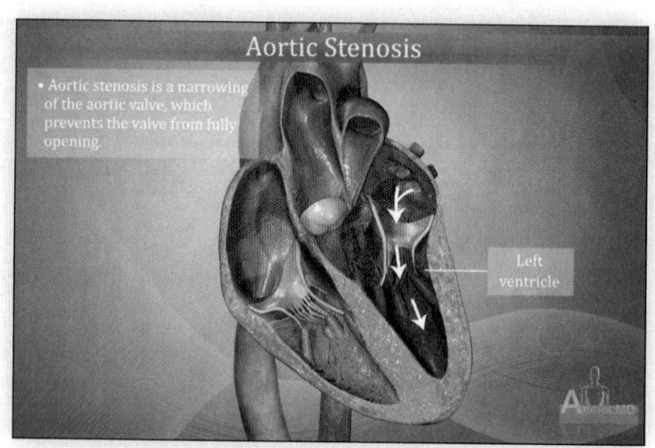

Instructor Resources

Instructor Resource Manual
Lecture Note Power Points
Test bank

Contents

Unit III: Fluid, Electrolyte, and Acid–Base Imbalances 168

Unit IV: Cell Injury, Inflammation, and Alterations of Cell Growth and Regulation 236

Unit V: Infection and Disorders of Immunity 324

Pathophysiology

Concepts of Human Disease

Unit I
Foundations of Pathophysiology

Pathophysiology is the study of functional alterations at the molecular, cellular, tissue, and organ system levels that are involved in disease states, and also involves the study of the impact of alterations in one organ system on the function of others. Understanding these alterations is the basis for understanding the mechanisms that are responsible for clinical manifestations of disease, both those noted by the healthcare provider on physical assessment or through diagnostics, such as x-rays, and those that the patient reports to the provider.

Underneath all physiologic mechanisms, there are basic principles at play. Through understanding these basic principles, or concepts, a healthcare professional can apply that knowledge across different situations and disease states. For example, Down syndrome is a genetic disorder caused by trisomy of chromosome 21. It can result in miscarriage or in a live-born child with a combination of congenital birth defects, characteristic facial features, and variable degrees of mental impairment. The degree of impairment may be influenced by environmental variables, such as the mother's prenatal health and prenatal nutrition.[1,2] Impairment may also be affected after birth by the family's ability to afford and access early intervention services, appropriate nutrition, and healthcare for the child. In other words, the quality of services and care available in the family's social environment will affect the child's long-term health and ability to interact with other people and function in his environment.

Stress and adaptation also play a role. The ability of the child's parents to respond to the stresses of having a child with Down syndrome will affect their own physical and mental health and that of all their children. The first and possibly the most important stressor for the family of a child with Down syndrome is the time of diagnosis, which can initiate a period of intense feelings of grief and loss.[3] The degree of the child's impairment in turn affects the family environment and stress levels. In children with disabilities such as Down syndrome, co-occurring seizures, anxiety, irritability, and greater extent of disability in the affected child all have been linked to increased financial and employment strain on parents and caregivers.[4] To close the circle, cultural variables, another aspect of social environment, also play a role. A family's understanding of why their child has Down syndrome may be culturally influenced. Further, if a family receives poor treatment from healthcare providers who lack cultural competency, the family may be reluctant to continue return for further treatment.[5]

The chapters in this unit address key factors that inform pathophysiology and, in turn, inform the care of patients. Underlying pathophysiology of an illness can be influenced by any combination of individual and family behaviors and lifestyles (including cultural beliefs and preferences), physical and mental wellness states, genetic and epigenetic factors, environmental factors at both the individual and population levels, and the neurologic and physiologic mechanisms that regulate how—and how well—the individual reacts and adapts to stress.

References

1. Coppedé, F. (2016). Risk factors for Down syndrome. *Archives of Toxicology, 90*(12), 2917–2929.
2. Hildebrand, E., Kallen, B., Josefsson, A., Gottvall, T., & Blomberg, M. (2014). Maternal obesity and risk of Down syndrome in the offspring. *Prenatal Diagnosis, 34*(4), 310–315.
3. Nelson Goff, B. S., Springer, N., Cline Foote, L., Frantz, C., Peak, M., Tracy C., Veh, T., Bentley, G. E., & Cross, K. A. (2013). Receiving the initial Down syndrome diagnosis: A comparison of prenatal and postnatal parent group experiences. *Intellectual and Developmental Disabilities, 51*(6), 446–457.
4. Ouyang, L., Grosse, S. D., Riley, C., Bolen, J., Bishop E., Raspa, M., & Bailey, D. B., Jr. (2014). A comparison of family financial and employment impacts of fragile X syndrome, autism spectrum disorders, and intellectual disability. *Research in Developmental Disabilities, 35*(7), 1518–1527.
5. Spector, R. (2017). *Cultural diversity in health and illness* (9th ed.). New York, NY: Pearson.

Social Environment Factors

- Financial resources
- Access to health and mental health services
- Community resources

Individual and Family Behaviors

- Substance use
- Abuse and neglect
- Parenting styles
- Communication styles
- Activity levels

Physical Environment Factors

- Prenatal health of the mother
- Prenatal nutrition
- Newborn and early childhood nutrition and feeding practices
- Safe environment

Genetic and Epigenetic Factors

- Family history of physical or mental illness
- Susceptibility for genetic disorders

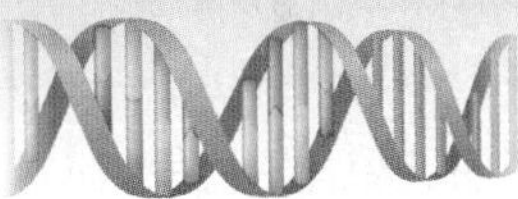

Stress and Adaptation

- Number and nature of stressors
- Response and adaptation
- Coping mechanisms and resources

Physical and Mental Wellness

- Healthy behaviors
- Presence of chronic physical or mental illness in the home
- Trauma history

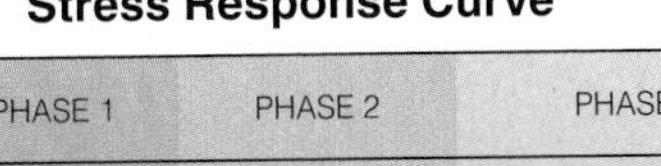

Stress Response Curve

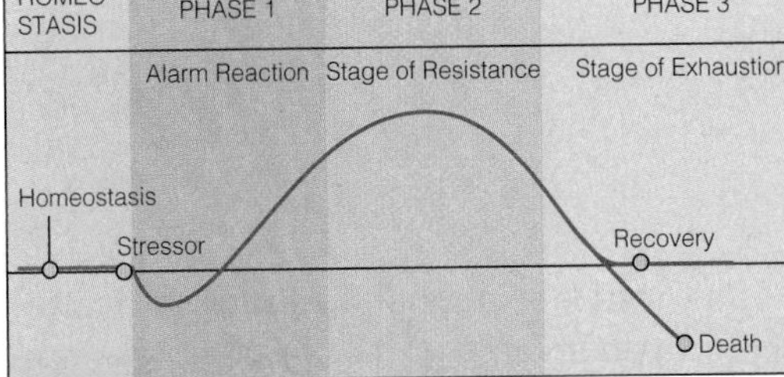

Chapter 1

Introduction to the Basics of Pathophysiology

Matthew Sorenson, Laurie Quinn, and Diane Klein

Chapter Outline and Learning Outcomes

1.1 The Language of Pathophysiology
Define the conceptual basis for and the language used in the study of pathophysiology.

1.2 Overview of Health and Illness
Describe characteristics of risk factors associated with health and illness.

1.3 The Structure of *Pathophysiology: Concepts of Human Disease*
Outline the structure of this book/eText, including the pathogenesis and etiology of disease; the clinical manifestations of disorders; how pathophysiology is linked to diagnosis and treatment; and the impact of genetics, nutrition, and lifespan on health and illness.

1.4 Leading Indicators of Morbidity and Mortality
Describe the study of epidemiology, and outline the leading indicators of morbidity and mortality in the United States.

1.5 The Importance of Evidence-based Practice
Explain the importance of evidence-based practice.

KEY TERMS

Clinical manifestations, 10
Disease, 8
Disorder, 8
Epidemiology, 14
Epigenomics, 11
Etiology, 10
Evidence-based practice (EBP), 17
Exacerbation, 11
Genetics, 11
Genomics, 11
Health, 8
Iatrogenic, 10
Idiopathic, 10
Illness, 8
Incidence, 14
Injury, 8
Ischemia, 7
Hypertension, 8
Modifiable risk factor, 9
Morbidity, 15
Mortality, 15
Nonmodifiable risk factor, 9
Pathogenesis, 10
Pathology, 5
Pathophysiology, 5
Prevalence, 14
Public health, 14
Remission, 11
Risk factor, 9
Sign, 10
Symptom, 10
Syndrome, 9

ABBREVIATIONS

CDC—Centers for Disease Control and Prevention
DALY—disability-adjusted life-year
EBP—evidence-based practice
IOM—Institute of Medicine
NIH—National Institutes of Health
WHO—World Health Organization

1.1 The Language of Pathophysiology

Essential Terminology

Pathophysiology is the study of functional alterations at the molecular, cellular, tissue, and organ system levels that are involved in disease states. Because many organ systems are interrelated, pathophysiology also involves the study of how alterations in one organ system can affect the function of others. Understanding these alterations is the basis for understanding the mechanisms responsible for clinical manifestations of disease noted on physical assessment or reported by the patient. In other words, pathophysiology is important in order to understand *why* alterations happen rather than just *what* happens.

Understanding pathophysiology requires knowledge of the principles of normal anatomy and physiology. These principles are briefly reviewed at the beginning of each relevant chapter. By understanding the normal physiology of the renal system, for example, it is possible to reason out at least some of the expected alterations in the individual as a result of impaired renal function, such as acute or chronic renal failure. The focus in this book is the concepts underlying the physiologic and pathophysiologic changes seen in association with disease.

Pathology is a medical discipline that focuses on structural alterations in tissues and organs and is closely related to pathophysiology. This discipline involves the analysis of specimens, such as tissue, blood, urine, and sputum removed from patients for the purpose of aiding in the diagnosis of certain diseases and assessing their progression. Other scientific disciplines contribute to the process of understanding the pathogenic process of disease. Histology is a subdivision of pathology that studies the microscopic anatomy of cells and tissues either in the form of samples from a patient or grown outside the body in tissue culture. Specialized stains are used in histologic studies to identify various cell types, the organization of the cells, and intracellular contents as viewed with the aid of light or electron microscopy. These interrelated disciplines of pathophysiology, pathology, and histology are all important in understanding disease processes.

The Conceptual Basis of Pathophysiology

Underneath all physiologic mechanisms, there are basic principles at play. Through understanding these basic principles, or concepts, a healthcare professional can apply that knowledge across different situations and disease states.

For a listing of concepts featured in this book, see **Table 1.1** ■. Each primary concept has related subconcepts that reflect related biophysiologic processes. Examples of disease states that reflect the pathogenic concept are also provided.

Pharmacologic therapies and nursing interventions are based on the conceptual mechanisms that underlie a pathogenic process. For example, in the treatment of

Table 1.1 Biophysiologic Concepts

Biophysiologic Concepts	Subconcept	Examples of Diseases/Conditions Related to the Concept
Acid–base balance	Excretion	Metabolic acidosis/alkalosis Respiratory acidosis/alkalosis
Addiction	Dependence Loss of control Tolerance Withdrawal	Alcohol abuse or dependence Behavioral addiction (e.g., gambling, gaming, shopping) Opiate abuse or dependence
Cellular regulation	Cell differentiation Cell growth	Cellular aging Cellular injury Neoplasia Tissue and wound healing
Cognition	Behavior Judgment Memory	Dementia Delirium Depression and anxiety Thought disorders
Comfort	Acute pain Chronic pain	Headache Neuropathy
Elimination	Bowel and bladder function Hydration Nutrition	Acute kidney injury Bowel obstruction Ulcerative colitis Urinary incontinence
Energy balance	Environment Metabolism Nutrition Thermoregulation	Cachexia Fatigue Obesity Wasting syndrome
Environment	Culture Hydration Nutrition Society	Air pollution Lead poisoning Mercury poisoning Food-borne infections Lifestyle risk factors

(Continued)

Table 1.1 Biophysiologic Concepts *Continued*

Biophysiologic Concepts	Subconcept	Examples of Diseases/Conditions Related to the Concept
Fluid and electrolyte balance	Excretion Hydration Nutrition	Diabetes insipidus Hyponatremia/hypernatremia Hypokalemia/hyperkalemia Hypocalcemia/hypercalcemia
Hemostasis	Bleeding Coagulation	Pulmonary emboli Disseminated intravascular coagulation Thrombocytopenia
Immunity	Hypersensitivity Infection Inflammation	Autoimmune disorders HIV infection and AIDS Pneumonia Septic shock
Infection	Energy balance Hydration Infection control Nutrition Tissue integrity	Bacterial abscess Common cold Colitis Healthcare-associated infections Lower/upper respiratory infections Sepsis
Inflammation and oxidative stress	Coagulation Infection Tissue integrity	Asthma Inflammatory bowel disease Rheumatoid arthritis
Intracranial regulation	Cerebral autoregulation Fluid and electrolyte balance Trauma Ventilation	Cerebrovascular accident Hydrocephalus Seizure disorders Traumatic brain injury
Metabolism	Energy balance Hormonal regulation	Diabetes mellitus Metabolic syndrome Hypothyroidism Obesity
Mobility	Ambulation Balance	Spinal cord injury Stroke
Mood and affect	Coping Culture Emotion Social support Stress	Anxiety Depression Postpartum depression
Nutrition and digestion	Diet Malabsorption Fluid balance	Iron deficiency anemia Atherosclerosis Obesity Ulcers GI bleeding
Oxygenation	Hypoxia Ischemia Respiration Ventilation	Asthma Anemia Carbon monoxide poisoning Heart failure Acute respiratory distress syndrome Shock
Perfusion	Ischemia Vasoconstriction	Heart failure Atherosclerosis Thromboembolic disorders
Sensory perception	Hearing Smell Taste Touch Vision	Hearing loss Glaucoma Retinopathy Vision loss
Sexuality	Culture Gender Hormonal balance Sexual orientation	Erectile dysfunction Impotence Pelvic floor dysfunction
Reproduction	Sexuality	Infertility Female genitourinary issues Male genitourinary issues Sexually transmitted infections
Stress and coping	Appraisal Coping Stressor	Homeostasis/allostasis Allostatic load Acute stress disorder Posttraumatic stress disorder

Biophysiologic Concepts	Subconcept	Examples of Diseases/Conditions Related to the Concept
Tissue integrity	Thermoregulation Sensation Wounds	Pressure injury
Thermoregulation	Fever Hypothermia Hyperthermia	Fever Hypothermia Malignant hyperthermia Burns
Trauma	Consciousness Mobility Perfusion Sensation Oxygenation	Blunt trauma Penetrating trauma Burns

hypertension, one of the options is using a medication that decreases the strength with which the heart contracts. Calcium channel blockers stop the movement of calcium into cardiac tissue and thereby lessen the contractile force of the heart, lowering blood pressure.

Understanding the conceptual basis of pathogenesis then aids in understanding pharmacologic actions and nursing interventions. Turning a patient to help prevent pressure injuries is based on principles of blood flow and tissue ischemia. Developing that understanding provides the rationale for turning a patient on a schedule and highlights the importance of performing that basic nursing action. Two brief examples are provided to further demonstrate the importance of these biophysical concepts.

Example 1: Myocardial Ischemia and Infarction. Tissue integrity is a major concept explored in this text. A decrease in blood flow to tissue means that there is a decrease in the amount of oxygen and glucose to tissue. The decrease in oxygen can then result in death, or infarction, of the tissue. Decreases in glucose deprive cells of a major energy source and can disrupt cellular regulation. This decrease in oxygen and glucose is called **ischemia**. A related term is *hypoxia*, which refers to a lack of oxygen to tissue. This can occur from disruptions of the respiratory system.

The oxygen levels in the blood may stimulate constriction of blood vessels, decreasing the flow of blood. Such narrowing of blood vessels is seen in conditions of atherosclerosis, a condition in which the presence of lipids plays a major role. The immune system also plays a role in how quickly lipids accumulate and thus reduce the diameter of blood vessels.

Other illness states such as diabetes, an alteration in hormonal release with effects on metabolism, can influence the relative thickness or viscosity of blood, further slowing circulation. Therefore, pathophysiology is best viewed as a series of interrelated concepts that help to explain how a disease state affects health. In this situation, inflammation, oxygenation, perfusion, and metabolism are all involved in the pathogenesis of myocardial infarction in a patient with diabetes. See **Figure 1.1** ■ for a diagram of the relationships between these concepts.

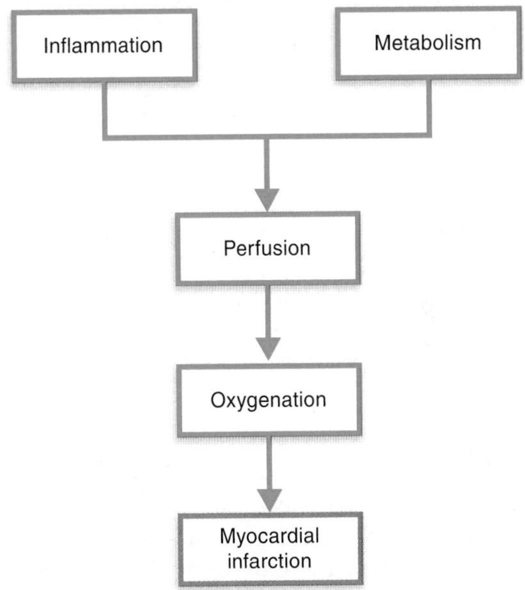

Figure 1.1 ■ Concepts related to the pathogenesis of myocardial infarction in an individual with diabetes.

Example 2: Asthma. Oxygenation is the main concept associated with asthma. Asthma is a condition of reactive airway constriction. In other words, parts of the respiratory tract are sensitive to the presence of allergens. In the presence of an environmental allergen, such as cat hair, parts of the respiratory tract constrict, restricting the flow of air into the lung. The reduction in air flow leads to decreases in the concentration of oxygen in the bloodstream. The allergen stimulates the immune system, which releases inflammatory mediators. The resulting inflammation contributes to the reduction of airflow. Obesity, an alteration of metabolism, is a state of chronic inflammation that can worsen asthma. Obesity also can make it harder for an individual to breathe properly, owing to pressure on the lungs and the person's relative lack of fitness. There are nervous pathways that influence the constriction and dilation of the respiratory system. In this example, oxygenation reflects the concentration of oxygen but is under the influence of other concepts such as inflammation and immunity, along with other concepts such as metabolism (obesity) that can influence the degree of inflammation. See **Figure 1.2** ■ for a diagram of the relationships between these concepts.

Case Studies

Case studies are used throughout this book/eText to help the reader apply the chapter content to clinical situations.

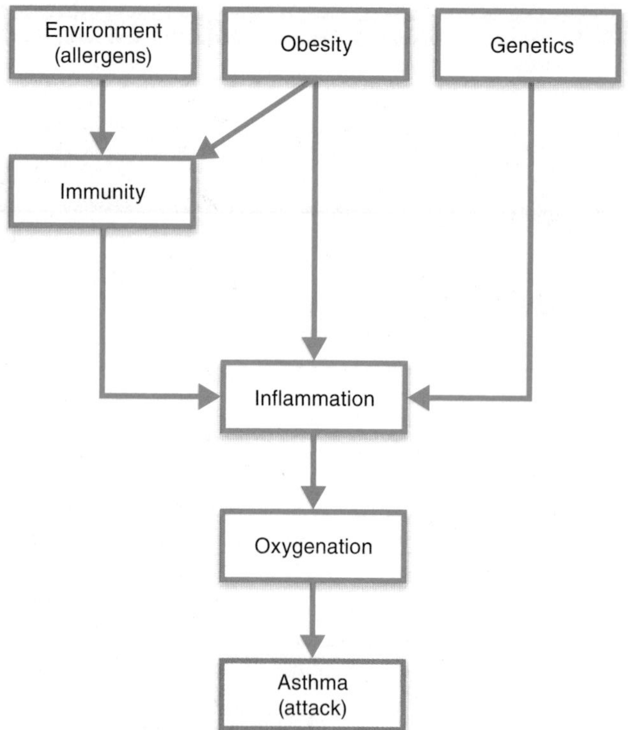

Figure 1.2 ■ Concepts related to an asthma attack.

Each case study focuses on one patient, who is followed throughout the chapter. Most chapters have two or three case studies. The following case study will be addressed throughout this chapter to introduce the reader to the format of the case studies used in the book.

Frank Smith: Introduction

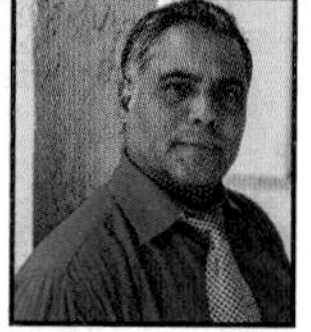

Frank Smith, age 55, presents at the clinic with a chief complaint of headache with blurred vision over the past 3 hours. He describes his headache as bitemporal and throbbing. Lying down makes it worse. Mr. Smith's medical history includes hypertension, for which he was prescribed two medications. He states that he ran out of his medication 4 days ago and has not been able to afford the prescription. His blood pressure is 190/110, and he has a pulse of 68 with a strong character.

1. What characteristics of Mr. Smith's chief complaint support the idea that alterations in one system can affect the function of others?
2. What major biophysiologic concepts should the nurse focus on during the assessment of Mr. Smith?

Knowledge of pathophysiology is important for healthcare providers, including nurses, physicians, pharmacists, dieticians, and physical and occupational therapists. It provides a foundation for other courses, such as pharmacology and nutrition, as well as for clinical practice. Pathophysiology is the basis for understanding the current health status of patients and for early detection and appropriate intervention in response to changes in the clinical course. Pathophysiology is also used in teaching patients about their conditions and about health promotion, risk reduction, and prevention of complications. One of the purposes of this chapter is to introduce the concepts of health and illness along with terminology used in describing disease progression along with the leading causes of morbidity and mortality. An additional concern that will emerge in later chapters is the concept of injury. **Injury** is damage caused to the body by an external force.

Check Your Progress: Section 1.1

1. How does the conceptual basis of pathophysiology help in the process of assessment and diagnosis?
2. What is the difference between pathophysiology and pathology?
3. How do nurses apply pathophysiology in daily practice?

1.2 Overview of Health and Illness

Characteristics of Health and Illness

Generally, the use of the word **health** refers to an absence of disease or functional changes that can result in disease. Health and illness are then terms best viewed as points along a continuum (**Figure 1.3** ■). Throughout life, the individual can be situated at different points along the continuum, moving back and forth between wellness and illness.

The terms *illness*, *disease*, and *condition* are often used almost interchangeably. Even in healthcare and nursing settings, the terms may be used as synonyms. However, there are some distinct differences to consider. The term **disease** can refer to a situation that is impairing functional ability in some way. For example, **hypertension** (a sustained elevation in blood pressure) is a disease with clear diagnostic criteria that can lead to a number of symptoms and complications.

The word **illness** is often used as a synonym for disease, but in healthcare, it is used to describe the individual experience that a person has with a disease. How each person responds to disease is different, and the subjective interpretation of the disease is influenced by the person's prior beliefs, knowledge, cultural factors, and overall state of health (**Figure 1.4** ■). For example, a healthy individual who catches a cold may feel miserable for a few days, but the disease will run its course, life will go back to normal, and the individual would not describe herself as "ill." On the other hand, if an individual with asthma catches a cold, it can exacerbate the asthma, may change the medication regimen, and could even require hospitalization. So, a patient with asthma who has a cold may feel quite ill.

If hypertension and the common cold are diseases that can result in illness, a different term is needed for the functional changes that can occur as a result the disease. In healthcare, the term **disorder** is used to describe a disruption of physiologic or psychologic function. As an example,

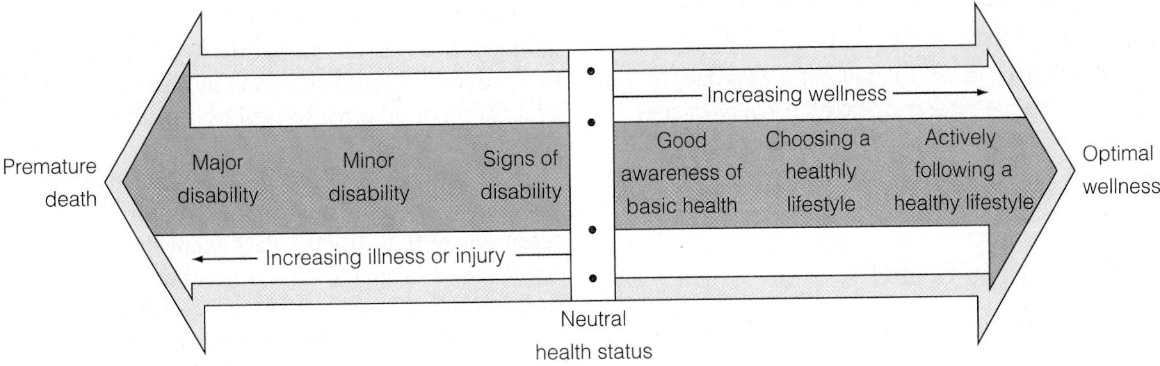

Figure 1.3 ■ An illness–wellness continuum.

several genetic variations can lead to disruptions of classes of immune cells. These disruptions can result in what is referred to as an immunoproliferative disorder. In other words, the continuing production or growth of certain cell types can lead to a loss of other cells or the release of immature cells. Leukemia is an example of such a disorder or disruption of normal cellular regulation.

The term **syndrome** usually refers to a group of signs and symptoms that emerge from a disease state. An example is acute coronary syndrome, which manifests as angina accompanied by changes in the electrophysiology of the heart resulting from a decrease in blood flow to the heart. This decrease in blood flow reduces the amount of oxygen that the heart receives, resulting in ischemia. With acute coronary syndrome, there are several potential causes, and different electrocardiogram abnormalities can be found.[1] Thus, a syndrome can have varying etiologic factors and some variation in diagnostic findings. The commonalities are in the cluster of signs and symptoms along with a shared underlying pathogenic mechanism.

Risk Factors

A **risk factor** is anything that puts a person at a greater risk for developing a particular disease. Risk factors emerge from a number of sources. One is the genetic blueprint provided to each of us at birth, and another is lifestyle factors. Lifestyle factors reflect decisions about diet, exercise, smoking and other variables that influence health. Another phrase that may be heard in healthcare courses is *social determinants of health*. Social determinants of health are factors related to where one lives, educational level, income, availability of fresh food, public transportation, and a number of other considerations that can affect health. These factors are often bound within society and are not as readily influenced as lifestyle risk factors.

Risk factors are traditionally classified as modifiable or nonmodifiable. A **modifiable risk factor** is one that the individual can change, such as diet or smoking. A **nonmodifiable risk factor** is one that cannot be altered, such as age, race, and genetic characteristics. The relationship between risk factors and disease is discussed in Section 1.3.

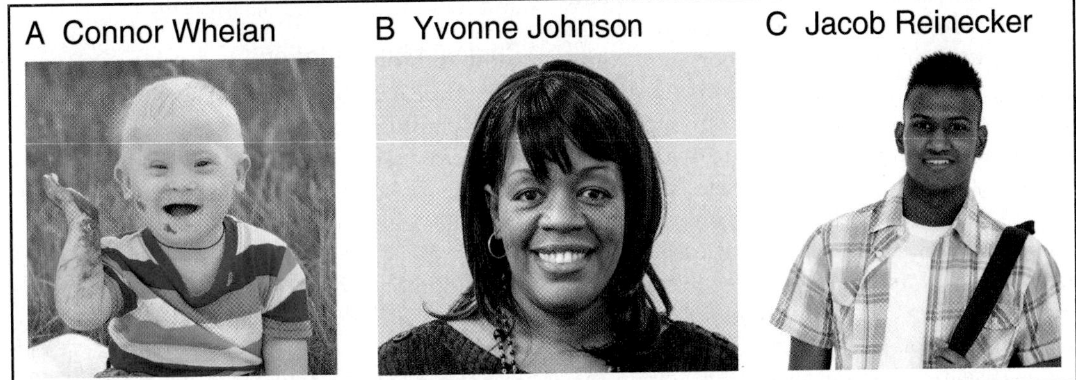

Figure 1.4 ■ **A.** Connor Whelan is an infant. He has Down syndrome and a congenital heart defect that will need to be corrected when he is 12 months old. **B.** Yvonne Johnson is a 35-year-old woman experiencing joint swelling, pain, and fatigue. The pain and fatigue are beginning to affect her ability to work. Her family physician has not been able to identify a cause. **C.** Jacob Reinecker is a 22-year-old college student who came to the emergency department after experiencing a sudden, stabbing pain in his chest with resulting shortness of breath. As you read the rest of this chapter, think about these questions: (1) Are these patients healthy or ill? (2) Are their conditions acute or chronic? (3) What risks factors does each patient have that might shed some light on the patient's conditions?

Check Your Progress: Section 1.2

1. Should obesity be considered a condition or a disease?
2. What is the difference between a disorder and a syndrome?
3. Is family history a modifiable or nonmodifiable risk factor?

1.3 The Structure of *Pathophysiology: Concepts of Human Disease*

Presentation of Disorders and Conditions

Throughout this book/eText, the presentation of a condition or disorder will follow a certain structure. First, information will be presented about the *Etiology and Pathogenesis* of a condition. Then, a section will present information on the *Clinical Manifestations* of that condition or disorder. A third section will provide information *Linking Pathophysiology to Diagnosis and Treatment*.

Etiology and Pathogenesis

The **etiology** of a disease or injury is its cause. For some conditions, only one etiologic factor or agent is involved. For example, the etiology of the common cold is a rhinovirus. The etiology of other conditions is multifactorial, that is, several factors contribute to causation. For example, the etiology of hypertension involves various combinations of factors such as genetic predisposition, dietary intake of sodium and lipids, stress, atherosclerosis, and lifestyle choices such as cigarette smoking. The etiology of most clinical conditions is multifactorial.

Etiologic agents may be exogenous, that is, arising from the external environment, such as chemical, physical, and infectious agents. Examples of chemical etiologic agents are alcohol, lead, mercury, air pollutants, carbon monoxide, pesticides, and adverse effects of medications. Examples of physical etiologic agents are extremes in environmental temperatures, radiation, trauma, and electricity. Examples of infectious etiologic agents are bacteria, viruses, fungi, and helminths. Not all individuals who have been exposed to exogenous etiologic agents will develop a disease because that depends on intensity and duration of exposure along with other factors such as the individual's preexisting health status and the person's genetics and genomics.

Endogenous disease etiologies arise from within the body. Examples are abnormal immune reactions, gene mutations, coagulation defects, stress, and metabolic abnormalities. An abnormal substance present in the body is not necessarily the etiologic agent. For example, in sickle cell disease there is an abnormal type of hemoglobin (hemoglobin S) present. The etiology of sickle cell disease is inheritance of a mutated gene that codes for production of hemoglobin S. This abnormal type of hemoglobin is the result of the mutated gene.

When the cause of a disease cannot be determined, its etiology is said to be **idiopathic**. The etiology of conditions that are caused unintentionally by a treatment, a diagnostic procedure, or an error caused by a healthcare provider are called **iatrogenic**.

The pathogenesis of a disease refers to origin of, or the underlying mechanisms responsible for, the clinical manifestations of that disease. **Pathogenesis** is the origin of the sequence of events to structural and/or functional alterations in cells, tissues, or organs resulting in disease. The following example will help in distinguishing etiology from pathogenesis.

Example 3: Diarrhea Associated with *Clostridium difficile*. In cases of diarrhea associated with *Clostridium difficile* (abbreviated as *C. difficile* and often called *C. diff*), the etiology of the diarrhea is infection with *C. difficile*, which is a gram-positive, spore-forming bacterium. The pathogenesis of *C. difficile* diarrhea involves the interaction of multiple environmental and host factors.[2] The pathogenesis begins with exposure of the individual to an environmental source of the bacterial spores and their entry into the gastrointestinal tract, where host defense factors and the intestinal microbiota (microorganisms that are normally present) determine whether the spores become activated and the ability of the bacteria to replicate and injure the intestinal wall. The use of antibiotics that alter the host's microbiome, preventing the normal intestinal flora from keeping the *C. difficile* organisms under control, is the most common cause. Pathogenic factors that influence whether diarrhea develops and its severity and whether the bacterial toxins enter the systemic circulation are multifactorial. They include bacterial virulence factors, the host's innate and adaptive immune responses, secretion of inflammatory cytokines, recruitment of phagocytic cells, increased permeability of the intestinal epithelial layer, intestinal epithelial cell death, and loss of water and electrolytes.

Clinical Manifestations

The **clinical manifestations** of a disease include the signs and symptoms associated with it as well as alterations in diagnostic tests, such as imaging studies and biochemical analyses of body fluids. Clinical manifestations can change over the course of a disease in both the types of manifestations present and their characteristics. A **sign** is an objective indication of disease that is observable by the person conducting a physical assessment. Examples of signs include abnormal heart or lung sounds, rash, fever, a change in the respiratory or heart rate, sluggish or absent pupil reaction to light, and changes in skin color.

A **symptom** is a subjective sensation indicative of disease that is perceived by the affected individual but not observable by the person examining the individual. Examples of symptoms include pain, nausea, dyspnea, and numbness. Patients are questioned about their symptoms during the health history. A variety of tools are available to assist patients in rating the severity and other characteristics of certain symptoms.

Common presenting signs or symptoms that cause an individual to seek attention by a healthcare provider include pain, persistent cough, fever, rash, fatigue, difficulty breathing, mood alterations, gastrointestinal changes such as constipation or diarrhea, bleeding, dizziness, impaired sleep, and visual or hearing deficits. Some diseases, especially in the early stages, are asymptomatic, that is, the patient experiences no symptoms. Examples of asymptomatic conditions are hypertension, diabetes, and coronary artery disease. Some clinical manifestations are the direct result of the disease; others are the result of the body's attempt to compensate for the disease. For example, tachycardia (increased heart rate) can be due to an alteration in the site of generation or conduction of electrical impulses in the heart, or it can be due to the body's attempt to compensate for anemia or a decreased circulating blood volume. A decrease in urine output can be due to renal failure or to renal retention of water as compensation for a fluid deficit.

CLINICAL POINT: To determine whether an intervention is required, it is important to differentiate body responses that are harmful, maladaptive responses from those that are adaptive and currently compensatory responses. ■

A syndrome consists of the signs and symptoms that are present in combination and are characteristic of a particular disease. Examples of clinical syndromes are acquired immunodeficiency syndrome, acute respiratory distress syndrome, Down syndrome, fetal alcohol syndrome, metabolic syndrome, and nephrotic syndrome.

Acute and Chronic. The temporal course of a disease or injury is often referred to as *acute* or *chronic*. An acute injury or disease is one that appears quickly; a chronic condition has an enduring quality with lasting implications. An important point is that neither of these terms relates to severity or degree of injury or disease. For example, when an individual sprains an ankle, an acute injury, the injury is sudden but might not have significant lasting implications. In contrast, with a chronic disease, there are several states that may be enduring and lasting (such as a mild case of osteoarthritis) but without significant impairment of functional ability. That said, in general in discussing acute or chronic conditions in healthcare, the focus is usually on conditions that require intervention or care, that is, conditions of a more severe nature.

Exacerbations and Remissions. The clinical course of some chronic diseases is characterized by alternating periods of exacerbations and remissions that have variable durations. During an **exacerbation**, there is an increase in the severity of a disease. The exacerbation can be detected by a worsening of the patient's symptoms and/or signs, including laboratory and other diagnostic tests. During a **remission**, there is a decrease in the severity of a disease. In a partial remission, some clinical manifestations of the disease are present; however, they have decreased in severity. In a total remission, there is complete disappearance of detectable manifestations of the disease. For some chronic diseases, such as leukemia and rheumatoid arthritis, there are specific criteria that define a remission. If a complete remission lasts the number of years specified for a particular disease, such as cancer, the patient is considered cured. Examples of chronic diseases characterized by alternating periods of exacerbations and remissions are cancer, infection with the human immunodeficiency virus, and autoimmune disorders such as inflammatory bowel disease, multiple sclerosis, and rheumatoid arthritis.

Linking Pathophysiology to Diagnosis and Treatment

Throughout this book/eText, information will be provided that ties the pathophysiologic concepts to clinical diagnosis and treatment. All treatment strategies have a basis in the physiologic and pathophysiologic mechanisms. As an example, the renin-angiotensin-aldosterone system is one of the major regulatory systems in the body. This system regulates sodium and fluid balance, in turn controlling blood pressure. Many of the pharmacologic therapies for hypertension target particular aspects of this regulatory system, serving to decrease blood pressure. When the text provides information about the etiology of disease, the relative incidence and prevalence of a condition are often discussed. To provide an understanding of those concepts and their relation to health, a brief overview of epidemiology is presented in Section 1.4.

Genetics and Genomics

Through **genetics**, the role of specific genes is studied. This study involves examining how genetic variations are passed through familial inheritance. A related term, **genomics**, refers to the study of the function of groups of genes in terms of mediating physiologic function. Throughout this book/eText, information will be provided as to how an inherited genetic trait, such as sickle cell trait, influences the likelihood that an individual will develop sickle cell disease. Information will also be provided on current research demonstrating how genomic pathways are being found that can predispose an individual to illness or health. Techniques have been developed that allow for the study of all genetic variations or modifications that have influenced a particular cell. This area of study is referred to as **epigenomics**, in that the focus is on the broader picture in terms of studying a complete set of modifications to cellular DNA. Throughout this book/eText, features called *Genetics and Genomics for Clinical Practice* will provide an example of current research and how the studies of heritability (genetics), function (genomics), and overall variation (epigenomics) have relevance for the pathophysiologic mechanism under discussion. See the Genetics and Genomics for Clinical Practice feature.

Nutrition

Nutrition is an area often identified as a modifiable risk factor. The consumption of a diet that is high in carbohydrates and fat can place an individual at increased risk for the development of diabetes, while increased consumption of sodium can have adverse implications for cardiovascular health. Throughout this text, Impact of Nutrition in Clinical Practice features are provided to aid in understanding how dietary choices and influences can impact the development of disease.

Genetics and Genomics for Clinical Practice

Human Genome Project

Rita Kaspar

The pursuit of the mystery of trait inheritance began when Gregor Mendel presented series of experiments on plant hybridization in 1865. It took a significant leap forward in 1952 when Rosalind Franklin made the distinct helical pattern of DNA visual in photographs and in 1953 when James Watson and Francis Crick modeled the double helix. In the following decades, the process of DNA-driven protein synthesis was deciphered, rapid DNA sequencing and amplification techniques were established, and several disease-causing genes were identified. These advances set the stage for the Human Genome Project (HGP), which officially began in 1990 and was completed in 2003, an unprecedented international effort to map out and understand all genes of our species, *Homo sapiens*.[1,2]

Using blood samples from a diverse pool of anonymous volunteers, the HGP aimed to identify the order of the some 3 billion DNA base pairs in all 23 pairs of chromosomes. Human DNA was fragmented and cloned into bacteria, which were then grown in large quantities for sequencing. As the human genome was being mapped and a torrent of data was being obtained, the genomes of five model organisms were also being sequenced. The knowledge of human genetics and genomics reveals biological variations among individuals and populations but also introduces the challenges of interpreting gene–gene and gene–environment interactions associated with health and pathology.[3] On a broader scale, the Ethical, Legal and Social Implications Research Program, an integral part of the HGP, fosters inquiries that help to shape the foundations of healthcare beliefs, practices, and policies in the genomic era. Healthcare has embarked on a one-way journey to personalized medicine since the beginning of the HGP, and we are eager to welcome a new generation of custom-made lifestyle and pharmacologic interventions that work for every individual.

References

1. Nature (London). (2001). What a long, strange trip it's been. . . . *Nature, 409*, 756–757, doi:10.1038/35057286
2. National Human Genome Research Institute and the Smithsonian National Museum of Natural History. (n.d.). *Timeline of the human genome.* Available at https://unlockinglifescode.org/timeline
3. Collins, F. S., McKusick, V. A., & Jegalian, K. (2012). *Implications of the genome project for medical science*. Available at https://www.genome.gov/25019925/online-education-kit-implications-of-the-genome-project-for-medical-science

Impact of Nutrition in Clinical Practice

2015–2020 Dietary Guidelines for Americans: User-friendly and Evidence-based

Joanne Kouba

The Institute of Medicine (IOM) has established recommendations for 14 vitamins, 15 minerals, and 7 subgroups of macronutrients. Fortunately, this complex information is translated into a roadmap for eating healthfully in the *Dietary Guidelines for Americans 2015–2020* (DGA). The eighth edition of this iconic resource by the U.S. Department of Agriculture and the U.S. Department of Health and Human Services includes five guidelines, to encourage healthy food choices for individuals 2 years of age and older with a focus on nutrient adequacy and diet-related, chronic disease prevention:[1]

1. **Follow a healthy eating pattern across the lifespan.** A key theme is the concept of *eating pattern*, which acknowledges that meals, snacks, and beverages all contribute to energy and nutrient intakes. Optimal eating patterns should be fostered early in life and continued through the aging years. The DGA outlines three eating pattern options—Healthy U.S.-Style, Healthy Mediterranean-Style, and Healthy Vegetarian—with resources such as MyPlate, MyWins campaign, and ChooseMyPlate.gov to help consumers translate the science into food choices.[1,2]
2. **Focus on variety, nutrient density, and amount.** Beyond the need to manage calorie intake for energy balance, Americans should maximize food value by choosing foods that are nutrient-dense. The following recommendations will help Americans increase their intake of shortfall nutrients, specifically potassium, fiber, calcium, and vitamin D, while reducing risk of cardiovascular diseases, hypertension, and diabetes. Adults are advised to consume at least 4.5 cups of fruits and vegetables daily for a variety of vitamins, minerals, phytochemicals, and fiber. The more highly pigmented the fruits and vegetables are, the better. Beets, spinach, squash, and berries are all good picks.

   Most adults do not consume the recommended amounts of vegetables and fruit.[2] Because mixed dishes are common, one strategy to improve this is to incorporate more vegetables into mixed dishes such as tacos, sandwiches, soup, casseroles, and pastas.[2]

   At least half of our daily intake of grains should be whole grains. The words "whole wheat" as the first ingredient indicates a whole grain product. Other good choices are common foods as oatmeal and popcorn. Less familiar grains such as quinoa or whole-grain couscous could also be included. Whole grains are nutrient-dense, promote satiety, moderate calorie intake, and lower the risk of chronic disease. Most Americans should consume two to three servings of low-fat dairy foods such as milk, yogurt, or low-fat cheese daily. Emphasis is placed on protein choices that are lower in fat (such as dried peas or beans) and opting for fish rather than red meat or poultry.

   Consumers should consult the nutrition facts label on packaged foods for serving size guidance.
3. **Limit calories from added sugars and saturated fats, and reduce sodium intake.** The triple threat of an obesogenic diet is characterized by these items. Solid fats, which are primarily saturated, and added sugars are collectively termed SoFAS and are targeted as "empty calories" that provide minimal nutrient value and promote weight gain. Solid fats include butter, animal fat, and shortenings. Saturated fat should be limited to less than 30% of energy intake, and trans fats should be minimized to lower the risk of heart disease. Added sugars appear on food labels as high-fructose corn syrup, anhydrous dextrose, sucrose, maltodextrins, and more. Cakes, cookies, chips, sweetened beverages, and ice

cream are examples of foods that are high in SoFAS. Sodium should be limited to 2,300 mg/day for individuals younger than 51 years of age and less than 1,500 mg/day for those 51 years of age or older, African Americans, and individuals with hypertension, diabetes, or chronic kidney disease. This means limiting processed foods and using the Nutrition Facts Label to make food decisions.

4. **Shift to healthier food and beverage choices.** Americans are encouraged to find items from and within all food groups that appeal to their personal and cultural preferences with the understanding that small changes may have a big impact if repeated many times over a year.
5. **Support healthy eating patterns for all.** This item encourages the development of food policies, systems, and environments that make healthy eating patterns effortless and the norm where we learn, play, work and shop. Creative partnerships with community partners, health care providers, policymakers, food service managers, and manufacturers can foster these initiatives. Examples include revisions of the Nutrition Facts Panel that increase consumer awareness about SoFAS and of the National School Lunch meal standards to include only whole grains and nutrient-dense vegetables.

The U.S. Department of Agriculture website provides additional detailed information on the *Dietary Guidelines for Americans 2015–2020*, including information for particular groups such as pregnant women and older adults. This can be accessed at http://www.cnpp.usda.gov/publications/dietaryguidelines/2010/policydoc/policydoc.pdf.

References

1. U.S. Department of Health and Human Services & U.S. Department of Agriculture. (2015). *2015–2020 Dietary Guidelines for Americans* (8th ed.). Available at http://health.gov/dietaryguidelines/2015/guidelines
2. Schap, T. E., Kucsynski, K. J., Ciampo, M. A., & Chang, S. A. (2016). Food choices: Small shifts, large gains. *Journal of the Academy of Nutrition and Dietetics, 116*(11), 1747–1749.

Lifespan Considerations

Throughout the lifespan, there are variations in physiologic function that influence health and illness. Often, nursing textbooks and other content focus on the adult condition. In actual practice, however, nurses are responsible for caring for newborns, infants, children, adolescents, adults, and older adults. In short, nurses are responsible for providing care across the lifespan. It is important to give consideration to all lifespan situations, including issues specific to infants and children, changes associated with pregnancy, and issues tied to the older adult population.

In the pediatric population, genetic variables can significantly influence fetal development, leading to a number of alterations in physiologic functions. In addition, several disease states have increased incidence and prevalence in pediatric populations. Examples include tetralogy of Fallot (a series of cardiac defects) and sickle cell disease.

Separately, pregnancy induces a host of physiologic changes with impact on pathogenesis of illness and disease. These changes put the mother at risk for developing several disease states such as gestational diabetes and preeclampsia.

With aging, there are separate considerations requiring awareness. It is therefore important to pay attention to age-related changes in physiology. Also, certain conditions are associated with long-term consequences, leading to increased incidence and prevalence in the older adult population. In each chapter of this book, examples of considerations that must be given in relation to pediatric, pregnancy and geriatric conditions are provided. Following are examples of these considerations utilizing concepts presented in this text.

Genetic variables shape the development of the heart, causing several cardiac defects in children. These defects significantly influence perfusion and oxygenation, leading to alterations in cognitive function and developmental delay.[3] ■

Early in pregnancy, hormonal increases result in lower glucose levels and increased appetite. As pregnancy progresses, there are gradual increases in after-meal glucose levels. This is concurrent with decreasing sensitivity to the effects of insulin, placing the mother at risk for developing gestational diabetes. The mother's social environment may also influence food availability and choices, making an evaluation of nutritional options during pregnancy an important nursing consideration.[4] ■

Certain conditions are more likely to occur in older adults. Dietary patterns in combination with genetic factors contribute to the incidence of atherosclerosis, a narrowing of arterial diameter as a result of lipid accumulation. This influences the flow of blood and thus oxygen to the brain. Hypertension and heart failure also affect the flow of blood to the brain, altering perfusion and oxygenation. The development of several small areas of ischemia in the brain as a result can led to a disruption of memory and cognition. These changes reinforce the need for a detailed physical examination on the part of the nurse working with older adults. ■

Frank Smith: Application

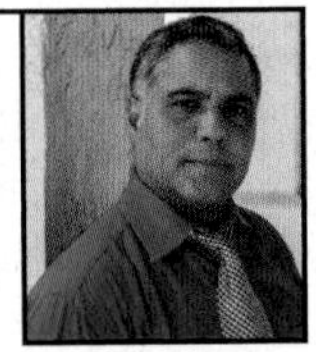

Mr. Smith has a prior history of hypertension for which he does not currently have the necessary prescriptions. A nursing assessment needs to include dietary considerations along with questions about the availability of his healthcare provider and financial status. His racial/ethnicity status should also be determined to evaluate for the presence of possible genetic risks.

3. In addition to asking Mr. Smith about the types of food he consumes, why would it be informative to ask him about who prepares his food?
4. If Mr. Smith has a genetic risk for hypertension, in what other ways may this information be used to inform the management of his disease?

Check Your Progress: Section 1.3

1. What is the difference between the etiology and pathogenesis of a disease?
2. When a patient presents with shortness of breath, is this a sign or a symptom?
3. Why is it important to consider the development stage of the individual during assessment of a patient's presenting signs and symptoms?

1.4 Leading Indicators of Morbidity and Mortality

The Study of Epidemiology

Epidemiology is broadly defined as the study of how disease is distributed in populations and identification of the factors influencing the distribution.[5] Through epidemiology, information is obtained that identifies the frequency of disease in a particular population. The frequency of disease is classified in two ways: incidence and prevalence. **Incidence** is the number of new cases of a disease or condition within a defined period and for a defined population, such as the number of individuals who experienced a spinal cord injury within the past 12 months in the United States. Other defined populations could include adults, children, and athletes. Incidence provides a sense of frequency of occurrence in a particular group or population. **Prevalence** is the number of individuals of a defined population who already have a disease or condition, such as the number of adults in the United States with a spinal cord injury. Throughout this text, information will be provided regarding the incidence and prevalence of many of the conditions covered.

In the study of epidemiology, a number of statistical techniques are used that aid healthcare providers in understanding how rapidly a condition may be developing in a population. One of these is a technique referred to as *relative risk*, which is the probability of developing a certain disease in the presence of select risk factors. As an example, a relative risk ratio could be calculated to identify the probability that smokers will develop lung cancer. This can then help to identify a relationship between certain risk factors and the probability of a disease developing.

The results of epidemiologic studies are used to plan and evaluate strategies to prevent health-related problems and to guide to treatment of people with these health problems. The science of epidemiology is data-driven, incorporating systematic and unbiased approaches to the collection, analysis, and interpretation of data.[6] The objectives of epidemiology are to identify the cause of the disease and the risk factors, to determine the extent of the disease in the community, to study the natural history and the prognosis of the disease, to evaluate both existing and newly developed preventive and therapeutic measures and modes of health care delivery, and to provide the basis for developing public policy related to a variety of measures.[5]

Example 4: Type 2 Diabetes in Youth. Type 1 diabetes (T1D) is caused by autoimmune-mediated destruction of the pancreatic beta cell; type 2 diabetes (T2D) is characterized by insulin resistance and a relative decrease in insulin secretion from the pancreatic beta cell.[7] Historically, diabetes that developed during childhood or adolescence was usually diagnosed as T1D, and diabetes that developed in adulthood was usually diagnosed as T2D. In the mid-1990s, it became apparent that the number of young people with T2D was increasing; however, the data supporting this increase were based on anecdotal evidence, clinical reports, registries, and small cross-sectional studies. An understanding of the incidence and prevalence of T1D and T2D in youth has important clinical, social, and economic implications that extend into adulthood; therefore, an assessment of the scope of diabetes among youths was needed.

In 2000, the Centers for Disease Control and Prevention (CDC) and the National Institutes of Health (NIH) implemented an observational multicenter study, the SEARCH for Diabetes in Youth, to determine the status of diabetes among youths with diabetes in the United States. One of the primary goals of SEARCH study was to estimate the number of new and existing childhood diabetes cases by type, age, sex, and racial or ethnic group. Another important goal was to characterize key risk factors for diabetes complications according to race/ethnicity and diabetes type.[8]

Epidemiologic data published in 2009 estimated that there were 191,986 people age 20 years or younger with diabetes in the United States.[9] There were 166,984 with T1D, 20,262 with T2D, and 4,740 with other types of diabetes. The prevalence of diabetes increased with age and was slightly higher in females. Diabetes was most prevalent in non-Hispanic Whites and least prevalent in Asian/Pacific Islanders. The highest prevalence of T2D was observed among Native Americans and Black youths. Other findings noted that the prevalence of multiple cardiovascular disease risk factors was high among youths with diabetes, especially those younger than 10 years of age.[10] The SEARCH investigators compared complication rates between youths with type 1 and 2 diabetes and noted that microalbuminuria (excretion of 30–300 mg of albumin over 24 hours) and hypertension were significantly more common in those with T2D than in those with T1D. Microalbuminuria, suggesting the presence of early kidney disease, was found in more than 25% of patients with T2D, compared with 6% of subjects with T1D. Hypercholesterolemia and hypertriglyceridemia were more frequent in subjects with T2D. Rates of peripheral and autonomic neuropathy were similar in both groups; however, only retinopathy was less common in subjects with T2D.[8] These data support the early development of diabetic complications among youths with diabetes and early interventions to decrease risk.

Public Health

Public health is the science of protecting and improving the health of families and communities through promotion of healthy lifestyles, research for disease and injury prevention, and detection and control of infectious diseases.[11]

The goal of public health initiatives is to improve the life of each individual; however, the central site of activity for the majority of public health interventions is within communities. There are public health issues that are localized in the community, and their reach is contained within the local area. However, there are many public health problems that extend beyond the individual or local community. Infectious diseases can extend beyond local boundaries. Natural disasters can cause a multitude of public health problems and can spread locally, nationally and globally. Such problems may require the involvement of organizations at the national and international levels, and it is crucial that public health agencies communicate with each other to address such issues.

The ability to track the burden of disease is necessary to understand and meet challenges to improving health.[12] A core epidemiologic function is public health surveillance, which is defined as a continuing and systematic collection, analysis, and interpretation of health data that guide decisions about health and assist in determining plans of action.[6] Morbidity and mortality reports are useful sources of public surveillance data. **Mortality** is defined as the number of deaths in a given population; **morbidity** is defined as a departure from physiologic or psychologic well-being and encompasses disease, injury, and disability.[6] Major sources of morbidity and mortality data include public and private health care providers, clinicians, laboratories, and hospitals that are responsible for reporting to health departments.[6] For example, the CDC's National Notifiable Diseases Surveillance System (NDSS) is a public health disease surveillance system that facilitates the collection, management, analysis, interpretation, and dissemination of health-related data for diseases that have been designated as necessary for national notification.[13] Among the major functions of the NDSS is to publish summaries of data findings throughout local, national, and territorial jurisdictions weekly and annually in the journal *Morbidity and Mortality Weekly Report (MMWR)*.[13] From the MMWR, the leading causes of death in the United States are outlined in **Table 1.2** ■.

Table 1.2 Leading Causes of Death in the United States in 2015

Cause	Number of Deaths
Heart disease	614,348
Cancer (all forms)	591,699
Chronic lower respiratory diseases	147,101
Accidents (unintentional injuries)	136,053
Stroke (cerebrovascular diseases)	133,103
Alzheimer disease	93,541
Diabetes	76,488
Influenza and pneumonia	55,227
Nephritis, nephrotic syndrome, and nephrosis	48,146
Intentional self-harm (suicide)	42,773

SOURCE: National Center for Health Statistics. (2016). *Health, United States, 2015: With special feature on racial and ethnic health disparities*. Hyattsville, MD: National Center for Health Statistics.

The World Health Organization (WHO) Global Burden of Disease (GBD) study was designed to provide an ongoing and comprehensive method of assessing the global burden of disease, injuries and risk factors. In particular, the GBD describes the leading causes of morbidity and mortality in specific populations. In the GBD study, morbidity was reported in disability-adjusted life-years (DALYs). The DALYs for a disease or health condition are defined as the years of potential life lost due to premature mortality and the years of productive life lost due to disability for people living with the health condition or its sequelae. One DALY is considered to be one lost year of "healthy" life. Mortality rate is a measure of the frequency of the occurrence of death in a defined population within a specified time interval.[12]

Chronic Disease

The CDC defines chronic diseases as prolonged noncommunicable illnesses that are seldom cured or spontaneously resolved.[14] Currently 50% of U.S. adults live with at least one chronic illness.[15] The most prominent chronic illnesses in the U.S. are heart disease, cancer, chronic lower respiratory diseases, stroke, Alzheimer disease, diabetes, and nephritis/nephrotic syndrome/nephrosis. Approximately 7 of 10 deaths among people living in the United States result from one of these chronic diseases. Heart disease, cancer, and stroke account for more than 50% of all deaths each year. Diabetes is the leading cause of kidney failure, nontraumatic lower extremity amputations, and blindness among U.S. adults.[16] Arthritis remains the most common cause of disability and limits activity for 19 million U.S. adults. Over the past few decades, obesity has emerged as a major contributor to chronic illness. Approximately 33% of U.S. adults and 20% of youths are obese. Obesity is independently and indirectly associated with morbidity and mortality.

The four most important modifiable health risk behaviors are physical inactivity, poor nutrition, tobacco use, and excessive alcohol consumption.[17] Unfortunately, more than one third of all U.S. adults fail to meet minimum recommendations for aerobic physical activity, and only 33% of U.S. high school students participate in daily physical education classes. Tobacco use remains a major risk factor for disease and disability. An estimated 20% of adults and high school students in the United States are smokers. Nutritional intake can contribute to poor health outcomes. For example, only 24% of U.S. adults and 20% of U.S. high school students eat five or more servings of fruits and vegetables per day, and over 60% of U.S. youths eat more than the recommended daily amounts of saturated fat. Approximately 16% of U.S. adults participate in binge drinking, and a reported 45% of U.S. high school students report having consumed at least one drink of alcohol in the previous month.[15]

Many factors contribute to the development of chronic diseases and associated morbidity and mortality. Age, gender, and racial/ethnic differences are among the primary factors contributing to the complexity of chronic diseases.

Age

The number of U.S. children and adolescents with a chronic disease has increased over the past several decades, from 1.8% in the 1960s to more than 7% in 2004.[15] The most common chronic disorders in U.S. youths are asthma, diabetes, obesity, hypertension, dental disease, mental illness, attention-deficit/hyperactivity disorder, sickle cell anemia, cystic fibrosis, genetic diseases, and birth defects.[15]

The most common diseases in older adults are cardiovascular and cerebrovascular disorders, malignancy, neurogenerative disorders, pulmonary disorders, endocrine and metabolic disorders, and chronic renal diseases with renal failure.[16] People are living longer, often entering older age with chronic diseases that developed in youth or middle age. As mortality rates decline and the population ages, the presence of multimorbidity, defined as the coexistence of two or more chronic conditions, is very common among older adults.[18] The complex relationship between chronic disease and aging has become a focus of intense research. The influence of previous life exposures (e.g., diseases, injuries, environmental influences) on the development of chronic diseases in older age is a prevailing theme in several investigations. Some examples include exploring the relationship between obesity in midlife and cognitive abilities in late life[19] and the relationship between T2D and risk of Alzheimer disease.[20] There are other ongoing investigations into identifying biological markers of aging, such as leukocyte telomere length.[21] Such biomarkers could be used to develop and guide treatments for older adults.

Gender

There are significant gender disparities in morbidity and mortality. In most countries, life expectancy is lower in men than in women.[22] This gender disparity persists irrespective of race, ethnicity, or place of residence. In general, men have higher morbidity and mortality from disease such as coronary heart disease, hypertension, diabetes, and cancer. Additionally, coronary heart disease, hypertension, and diabetes develop at earlier ages in men than in women. This longer duration of disease likely contributes to the increased morbidity and mortality in men.[22]

4 Chronic conditions or diseases can influence maternal and fetal outcomes during pregnancy. Obesity increases the risk for a number of chronic diseases, such as gestational diabetes, hypertension, and preeclampsia (high blood pressure and proteinuria).[23,24] Smoking during pregnancy is associated with increased risk for a variety of adverse outcomes, such as placental abruption (partial or total separation of the uterus from the fetus), preterm rupture of membranes, low infant birth weight, and preterm delivery. Women who had type 1 or type 2 diabetes before becoming pregnant can have a variety of adverse fetal and maternal outcomes, such as increased risk for preeclampsia, hypertension during pregnancy, cesarean delivery, miscarriage, birth defects, preterm delivery, macrosomia (very large baby), hypoglycemia, fetal death, and infant death. Hypertension before pregnancy is associated with an increased risk for maternal (e.g., preeclampsia, placental abruption, and gestational diabetes) and fetal (e.g., preterm delivery, small for gestational age) outcomes.[23] ■

Ethnicity

Health disparities influence the development and trajectory of chronic disease. Certain racial and ethnic variables can place individuals at a significant increased risk for developing major chronic disease. Tied into health disparities are socioeconomic determinants of health, in that individuals in lower socioeconomic groups are more likely to develop chronic disease.[17] These health disparities are present regardless of age. The percentage of children with a chronic disease has increased dramatically over the past several decades with racial and ethnic minority youths having higher likelihood for disorders such as asthma, diabetes, cancer, and mental illness.[15]

Healthy People 2020

Introduction

Healthy People is a health promotion program developed by U.S. Department of Health and Human Services that provides 10-year national objectives for improving the health of people in the United States. During the past several decades, the *Healthy People* program has identified goals and monitored progress toward achieving these goals.[24] *Healthy People 2020* contains 42 topic areas with approximately 600 objectives. More specifically, there are 26 Leading Health Indicators organized under 12 topics:

1. Access to Health Services
2. Clinical Preventive Services
3. Environmental Quality
4. Injury and Violence
5. Maternal, Infant, and Child Health
6. Mental Health
7. Nutrition, Physical Activity, and Obesity
8. Oral Health
9. Reproductive and Sexual Health
10. Social Determinants
11. Substance Abuse
12. Tobacco

A summary of *Healthy People 2020* objectives and health indicators will be presented throughout the chapters whenever applicable to guide the reader in assessing high-priority areas of preventive health and/or treatment.

Reference

1. HealthyPeople. (2017). *Leading health indicators.* Available at https://www.healthypeople.gov/2020/Leading-Health-Indicators

Check Your Progress: Section 1.4

1. What information about disease in society do incidence and prevalence provide?
2. How could findings from the SEARCH study be used to guide public health measures?
3. Of the top 10 causes of mortality, how many are due to a chronic condition?

1.5 The Importance of Evidence-based Practice

The most common definition of **evidence-based practice (EBP)** is from Dr. David Sackett, who stated that EBP is "the conscientious, explicit and judicious use of current best evidence in making decisions about the care of the individual patient. It means integrating individual clinical expertise with the best available external clinical evidence from systematic research."[25] The underlying principle is that practice decisions should be based on research studies that have been evaluated by using a set of consistent criteria. The expression emerged from the arena of evidence-based medicine in recognition of the need for other healthcare professions, such as nursing, to utilize profession specific research to guide practice.[26] Often, findings are compiled into sets of practice guidelines. These guidelines provide a base for identifying healthcare procedures and techniques that are supported by direct clinical evidence.

Beyond evidence-based guidelines lies a process of integration of guidelines and recommendations into clinical practice. This process relies on melding clinical expertise with existing research evidence in providing care that also respects the values and preferences of the patient. Without acknowledging patient preferences and experience, the healthcare provider could implement interventions supported by the literature but find a patient who is not adhering to the recommendations because of different goals or values. Therefore, all evidence-based practice requires careful patient interviewing and assessment to identify values and expectations before selection a treatment intervention. The treatment intervention should then be selected on the basis of available clinical research and findings.

Frank Smith: Outcome

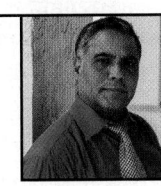

There is a set of evidence-based guidelines to guide the treatment of Mr. Smith's hypertension. For a male patient 55 years of age without any prior medical history except the hypertension, the newest practice guidelines recommend as the treatment goal a systolic blood pressure of less than 150 mmHg and a diastolic blood pressure of less than 90 mmHg.[26] The pharmacologic treatment choices depend on the patient's age, race, and gender. Other important factors are the initial numeric reading of the blood pressure and the presence of comorbid conditions.[27] On the basis of these variables, a pharmacologic therapy would be initiated. Nursing interventions would then include medication education, monitoring of blood pressure, and education about lifestyle modifications and the pathogenic process of hypertension.

Health and illness are points on a continuum. The presence of other diseases influences the treatment choices for the management of hypertension. Also, although the individual may have hypertension, it is imperative to evaluate for the presence of other conditions. The individual may be relatively healthy with the exception of the one disease state, and effective treatment can limit or reduce the development of adverse consequences that could emerge from the disease process. The nurse should assess for the presence of other health risks and provide the necessary education to help reduce the possibility that Mr. Smith will develop long-term complications from hypertension, such as vision loss and kidney disease.

5. What additional information should be used to select the pharmacologic treatment intervention for Mr. Smith's hypertension?
6. Given that Mr. Smith's initial problem arose because he wasn't able to afford his medication, in what additional ways can the nurse support his ability to adhere to the prescribed treatment?

Check Your Progress: Section 1.5

1. What is the underlying principle of evidence-based practice?
2. How can evidence-based practice guidelines be applied to clinical practice?
3. What additional information is important to consider before selecting an evidence-based treatment intervention?

CHAPTER SUMMARY

1.1 The Language of Pathophysiology

Define the conceptual basis for and the language used in the study of pathophysiology.

- Pathophysiology is the study of functional alterations at the molecular, cellular, tissue, and organ system levels that are involved in disease states.
- Pathology is a medical discipline that focuses on structural alterations in tissues and organs and is closely related to pathophysiology. This discipline involves the analysis of specimens, such as tissue, blood, urine, and sputum removed from patients for the purpose of aiding in the diagnosis of certain diseases and assessing their progression.
- Underneath all physiologic mechanisms, there are basic principles at play. Through understanding these basic principles, or concepts, a healthcare professional can apply that knowledge across different situations and disease states.
- Pharmacologic therapies and nursing interventions are based on the conceptual mechanisms that underlie a pathogenic process.

- As an example, in the treatment of hypertension, one of the options is using a medication that decreases the strength with which the heart contracts. Calcium channel blockers stop the movement of calcium into cardiac tissue and thereby lessen the contractile force of the heart, lowering blood pressure.
- Understanding the conceptual basis of pathogenesis then aids in understanding pharmacologic actions and nursing interventions.

1.2 Overview of Health and Illness

Describe characteristics of and risk factors associated with health and illness.

- Health refers to an absence of disease or functional changes that can result in disease.
- Health and illness are best viewed as points along a continuum.
- Disease refers to the impairment of functional ability in some fashion.
- Illness is the individual experience a person has with a disease.
- A syndrome is a group of signs and symptoms that emerge from a disease state.
- Risk factors are things that place a person at greater risk for developing disease. They may be modifiable or nonmodifiable.

1.3 The Structure of *Pathophysiology: Concepts of Human Disease*

Outline the structure of this book/eText including the pathogenesis and etiology of disease; the clinical manifestations of disorders; how pathophysiology is linked to diagnosis and treatment; and the impact of genetics, nutrition, and lifespan on health and illness.

- Etiology refers to the cause of a disease or injury.
- Etiologic agents may arise from the external environment, such as chemical, physical, and infectious agents.
- Endogenous disease etiologies arise from within the body. Examples are abnormal immune reactions, gene mutations, coagulation defects, stress, and metabolic abnormalities.
- The pathogenesis of a disease refers to the underlying mechanisms that are responsible for the clinical manifestations of that disease. Pathogenesis is the sequence of events in response to the etiologic agents(s) involving structural and/or functional alterations in cells, tissues, or organs that result in disease.
- The clinical manifestations of a disease include the signs and symptoms associated with it as well as alterations in diagnostic tests, such as imaging studies and biochemical analyses of body fluids.
- Clinical manifestations can change over the course of a disease in both the types of manifestations present and their characteristics.
- A sign is an objective indication of disease that is observable by the person conducting a physical assessment.
- A symptom is a subjective sensation indicative of disease that is perceived by the affected individual but not observable by the person examining the individual.
- Some clinical manifestations are the direct result of the disease; others are the result of the body's attempt to compensate for the disease.
- An acute injury or disease is one that appears quickly; a chronic condition has an enduring quality with lasting implications.
- During an exacerbation, there is an increase in the severity of a disease.
- During a remission, there is a decrease in the severity of a disease.
- Through genetics, the role of specific genes is studied.
- Genomics refers to the study of the function of groups of genes in terms of mediating physiologic function.
- In the pediatric population, genetic variables can significantly influence fetal development, leading to a number of alterations in physiologic functions. In turn, several disease states see increased incidence and prevalence in pediatric populations.
- Pregnancy induces a host of physiologic changes that may affect the pathogenesis of illness and disease. These changes place the mother at risk for the development of several disease states, such as gestational diabetes and preeclampsia.

1.4 Leading Indicators of Morbidity and Mortality

Describe the study of epidemiology, and outline the leading indicators of morbidity and mortality in the United States.

- Epidemiology is broadly defined as the study of how disease is distributed in populations and identification of the factors influencing the distribution.
- Public health is the science of protecting and improving the health of families and communities through promotion of healthy lifestyles, research for disease and injury prevention, and detection and control of infectious diseases.
- The goal of public health initiatives is to improve the life of each individual; however, the central site of activity for most public health interventions is in communities.
- Morbidity and mortality reports are useful sources of public surveillance data. Mortality is defined as the number of deaths in a given population; morbidity is defined as a departure from physiologic or psychologic well-being and encompasses disease, injury, and disability.

- Many factors contribute the development of chronic diseases and associated morbidity and mortality. Age, gender, and racial/ethnic differences are among the primary factors contributing to the complexity of chronic diseases.
- *Healthy People* is a health promotion program developed by U.S. Department of Health & Human Services that provides 10-year national objectives for improving the health of people in the United States. During the past several decades, the *Healthy People* program has identified goals and monitored progress toward achieving these goals.

1.5 The Importance of Evidence-based Practice

Explain the importance of evidence-based practice.

- The most common definition of evidence-based practice is "the conscientious, explicit and judicious use of current best evidence in making decisions about the care of the individual patient. It means integrating individual clinical expertise with the best available external clinical evidence from systematic research."
- Evidence-based practice decisions should be based on research studies evaluated using a set of consistent criteria.
- Beyond evidence-based guidelines lies a process of integration of guidelines and recommendations into clinical practice. This process relies on melding clinical expertise with existent research evidence in providing care that also respects the values and preferences of the patient.

REVIEW QUESTIONS

1. Understanding that intracranial regulation is an important concept in patients with traumatic brain injury, the nurse knows that a priority subconcept includes which of the following?
   a. Fluid and electrolytes
   b. Hormone balance
   c. Appraisal
   d. Social support
2. The nurse shows understanding of the difference between modifiable and nonmodifiable risk factors when she develops a specific intervention focused on which of the following?
   a. The higher rate of women affected by rheumatoid arthritis
   b. An increased incidence of sickle cell disease in African Americans
   c. The prevalence of Gaucher disease in people with Ashkenazi Jewish ancestry
   d. A smoking cessation program geared toward young adults
3. The nurse is considering the etiology of a client with spinal cord injury who developed a bed sore (pressure injury). What information provided explains the etiology?
   a. The area of skin breakdown became red and started to drain a clear exudate.
   b. After the breakdown occurred, the skin became infected with *Staphylococcus aureus*.
   c. The client's nutritional status is poor, and shearing forces were applied during transfer to and from the bed.
   d. A transparent dressing was applied to help reduce skin breakdown.
4. A client with breast cancer is being seen during her treatment and reports to the nurse that she has experienced extreme fatigue over the past few days. Which of the following information represents a clinical sign that may be considered as the etiology of the client's fatigue?
   a. She complains of dry, itchy skin across her torso and back.
   b. Her hemoglobin count is 7.5 g/dL.
   c. Her memory is not as good as it used to be, and she almost forgot her appointment.
   d. She describes being nauseated every time she attempts to eat.
5. A nurse is assessing a clinical population composed of Native Americans to determine the risk of developing diabetes in clients with high cholesterol. Which of the following types of data would tell the nurse the information that he needs to know?
   a. Prevalence
   b. Incidence
   c. Relative risk
   d. DALYs
6. An older adult male with heart failure is being seen by his nurse in the outpatient clinic. Which of the following information would indicate that the client's cardiovascular system is adapting to the condition of his heart?
   a. His blood pressure is 120/80 mmHg.
   b. The nails of his fingers are clubbed.
   c. He has a bluish tinge to his lips.
   d. His pulse oximeter reads 85%.

7. The nurse is providing free health screenings in his community. He demonstrates knowledge about the most important modifiable health risk behaviors when he addresses which factor with his clients?
   a. Obtaining a screening mammogram
   b. Getting the influenza vaccination
   c. Reducing periods of physical inactivity
   d. Brushing teeth twice per day and flossing
8. The nurse is discussing evidence-based treatment options for a client with diabetes. Which of the following questions reflects that the nurse understands how to apply evidence-based decisions?
   a. "Do you have a plan for how you will follow the prescribed treatment?"
   b. "How will you afford all the medications that you will be taking?"
   c. "Of the treatment goals we've discussed, which one do you value the most?"
   d. "Are you going to involve your spouse in your daily treatment routine?"

ANSWERS

Answers to Review Questions can be found in Appendix A. Answers to Case Study and Check Your Progress questions are available on the faculty resources site. Please consult with your instructor.

RECOMMENDED WEBSITES

Centers for Disease Control and Prevention
https://www.cdc.gov

Genetics Home Reference: Your Guide to Understanding Genetic Conditions
https://ghr.nlm.nih.gov

Global Burden of Disease
http://www.who.int/topics/global_burden_of_disease/en

HealthyPeople
https://www.healthypeople.gov

Morbidity and Mortality Weekly Report (MMWR)
https://www.cdc.gov/mmwr/index.html

World Health Organization
http://www.who.int/en

REFERENCES

1. Meier, P., Lansky, A. J., & Baumbach, A. (2014). Almanac 2013: Acute coronary syndrome. *Acta Cardiologica, 69*(1), 100–108.
2. Peniche, A. G., Savidge, T. C., & Dann, S. M. (2013). Recent insights into Clostridium difficile pathogenesis. *Current Opinion in Infectious Disease, 26*(5), 447–453.
3. Marino, B. S., Lipkin, P. H., Newburger, J. W., Peacock, G., Gerdes, M., Gaynor, J. W., Mussatto, K. A., Uzark, K., Goldberg, C. S., Johnson, W. H., Jr., Li, J., Smith, S. E., Bellinger, D. C., Mahle, W. T., American Heart Association Congenital Heart Defects Committee, Council on Cardiovascular Disease in the Young, Council on Cardiovascular Nursing, & Stroke Council. (2012). Neurodevelopmental outcomes in children with congenital heart disease: Evaluation and management. *Circulation, 126*(9), 1143–1172.
4. Colicchia, L. C., Parviainen, K., & Chang, J. C. (2016). Social contributors to glycemic control in gestational diabetes mellitus. *Obstetrics & Gynecology, 128*(6), 1333–1339.
5. Gordis, L. (2014). *Epidemiology* (5th ed.). Philadelphia, PA: Elsevier.
6. Centers for Disease Control and Prevention. (2011). *Principles of epidemiology in public health practice: An introduction to applied epidemiology and biostatistics* (3rd ed.). Available at https://www.cdc.gov/ophss/csels/dsepd/ss1978
7. American Diabetes Association. (2013). Diagnosis and classification of diabetes mellitus. *Diabetes Care, 36*(Suppl. 1), S67–S74.
8. Mayer-Davis, E. J., Bell, R. A., Dabelea, D., et al. (2009). The many faces of diabetes in American youth: Type 1 and type 2 diabetes in five race and ethnic populations: The SEARCH for Diabetes in Youth Study. *Diabetes Care 32*, S99–S101.
9. Pettitt, D. J., Talton, J., Dabelea, D., et al. (2014). Prevalence of diabetes in U.S. youth in 2009: The SEARCH for Diabetes in Youth Study. *Diabetes Care 37*, 402–408.
10. Rodriguez, B. L., Fujimoto, W. Y., Mayer-Davis, E. J., et al. (2006). Prevalence of cardiovascular disease risk factors in U.S. children and adolescents with diabetes: The SEARCH for Diabetes in Youth Study. *Diabetes Care, 29*, 1891–1896.
11. CDC Foundation. (2016). *What is public health?* Available at http://www.cdcfoundation.org/content/what-public-health
12. Murray, C. J., & Lopez, A. D. (2013). Measuring the global burden of disease. *New England Journal of Medicine, 369*, 448–457.
13. Centers for Disease Control and Prevention. (2013). *National Notifiable Diseases Surveillance System 2013*. Available at http://wwwn.cdc.gov/nndss/default.aspx
14. Centers for Disease Control and Prevention. (2009). *Chronic diseases: The power to prevent, the call to control*. Available at http://purl.access.gpo.gov
15. Price, J. H., Khubchandani, J., McKinney, M., & Braun, R. (2013). Racial/ethnic disparities in chronic diseases of youths and access to health care in the United States. *BioMed Research International, 2013*, 787616.
16. Akushevich, I., Kravchenko, J., Ukraintseva, S., Arbeev, K., & Yashin, A. I. (2012). Age patterns of incidence of geriatric disease in the U.S. elderly population: Medicare-based analysis. *Journal of the American Geriatrics Society, 60*, 323–327.
17. National Center for Health Statistics. (2016). *Health, United States, 2015: With special feature on racial and ethnic health disparities*. Hyattsville, MD: National Center for Health Statistics.
18. Salive, M. E. (2013). Multimorbidity in older adults. *Epidemiologic Reviews, 35*, 75–83.

19. Dahl, A. K., & Hassing, L. B. (2013). Obesity and cognitive aging. *Epidemiologic Reviews, 35*(1), 22–32.
20. Vagelatos, N. T., & Eslick, G. D. (2013). Type 2 diabetes as a risk factor for Alzheimer's disease: The confounders, interactions, and neuropathology associated with this relationship. *Epidemiologic Reviews, 35*(1), 152–160.
21. Sanders, J. L., & Newman, A. B. (2013). Telomere length in epidemiology: A biomarker of aging, age-related disease, both, or neither? *Epidemiologic Reviews, 35*(1), 112–131.
22. Pinkhasov, R. M., Shteynshlyuger, A., Hakimian, P., Lindsay, G. K., Samadi, D. B., & Shabsigh, R. (2010). Are men shortchanged on health? Perspective on life expectancy, morbidity, and mortality in men and women in the United States. *International Journal of Clinical Practice, 64*, 465–474.
23. Centers for Disease Control and Prevention. (2011). *Preventing and managing chronic disease to improve the health of women and infants*. Available at http://www.cdc.gov/reproductivehealth/womensrh/ChronicDiseaseandReproductiveHealth.htm
24. U.S. Department of Health and Human Services. (2012). *About Healthy People*. Available at http://www.healthypeople.gov/2020/about/history.aspx.
25. Sackett, D., Rosenburg, W. M .C., Gray, A. M., Haynes, R. B., & Richardson, W. S. (1996). Evidence based medicine: What it is and what it isn't. *BMJ, 312*, 71. Available at http://www.bmj.com/content/312/7023/71
26. Dale, A. E. (2006). Determining guiding principles for evidence-based practice. *Nursing Standard, 20*(25), 41–46.
27. James, P. A., Oparil, S., & Carter, B. L., et al. (2014). 2014 evidence-based guideline for the management of high blood pressure in adults: Report from the panel members appointed to the Eighth Joint National Committee (JNC 8). *JAMA, 311*(5), 507–520.

Chapter 2

Genetics, Genomics, and Epigenomics

Bhuma Krishnamachari and Matthew Pastore

Chapter Outline and Learning Outcomes

2.1 Chapter Overview and Case Studies

Describe the impact of genetics, genomics, and epigenomics on personalized healthcare, and explain the concepts related to them.

2.2 Molecular Basis of Gene Expression

Identify components of the genetic code and the organization of genes on chromosomes.

2.3 The Human Genome, Genomics, and Epigenomics

Understand the differences between the human genome and epigenome and the mechanisms by which epigenetic modifications occur and affect gene expression.

2.4 Gene Replication, Transcription, and Translation

Explain the function and sequence of events involved in gene replication during mitosis and meiosis, transcription, and translation.

2.5 Mutations

Compare single-nucleotide polymorphisms and the various types of gene mutations, including point mutations, insertions, deletions, and translocations, in regard to their characteristics and possible clinical consequences.

2.6 Categories of Genetic Disorders

Compare the characteristics and patterns of inheritance of genetic disorders caused by abnormalities of chromosome number or structure to those caused by autosomal, X-linked, and mitochondrial disorders.

2.7 Phenotypic Variations in Human Disease

Differentiate the mechanisms responsible for phenotypic variations in human disease.

2.8 Genes and Neoplasia/Malignancies

Understand the role of genetic and epigenomic factors in cancer.

2.9 Genetic- and Genomic-based Diagnostic Tests

Apply the following tests to the appropriate clinical situation: karyotyping, fluorescence in situ hybridization, single-gene testing, and genome-wide association studies.

2.10 Linking Pathophysiology to Treatment: Genetic- and Genomics-based Therapies

Apply the following genetic-based therapies to appropriate clinical situations: gene replacement therapy, pharmacogenomics, antisense nucleotides, and transcription factor modulation.

2.11 Advances in Human Genomics

Analyze the impact of advances in genomics and epigenomics on personalized healthcare.

KEY TERMS

Allele, 26
Aneuploidy, 34
Antisense oligonucleotide, 41
Barr body, 26
Central dogma, 28
Chromosome, 25
Chromosome nondisjunction, 34
Codon, 31
Cytogenetics, 39
Deoxyribonucleic acid (DNA), 25
Diploid cells, 28
DNA replication, 28
Double helix, 25
Down syndrome, 34
Epigenetics, 23
Epigenome, 27
Epigenomics, 23
Exons, 30
Fluorescence in situ hybridization (FISH), 39
Gene, 23

Key Terms continue on next page.

Genetic imprinting, 33
Genetics, 23
Genome-wide association studies (GWAS), 41
Genomics, 23
Genotype, 35
Gonadal cells, 28
Haploid cells, 29
Heterozygous, 35
Homozygous, 35
Introns, 31
Karyotyping, 39
Marfan syndrome, 36
Meiosis, 28
Messenger RNA (mRNA), 29
Missense mutation, 33
Mitochondrial DNA (mtDNA), 37
Mitosis, 28
Mosaicism, 34
Mutation, 33
Neurofibromatosis, 35
Nonsense mutation, 33
Nucleotide, 25
Oogenesis, 29
Pedigree, 35
Penetrance, 35
Pharmacogenomics, 40
Phenotype, 35
Point mutation, 33
Preimplantation genetic diagnosis, 39
Proto-oncogene, 38
Punnett square, 35
Ribonucleic acid (RNA), 28
Ribosomal RNA (rRNA), 29
Silent mutation, 33
Single-nucleotide polymorphism (SNP), 34
Somatic cells, 28
Spermatogenesis, 29
Splicing, 30
Transcription, 29
Transcription factors, 30
Transcription factor modulators, 41
Transfer RNA (tRNA), 29
Translation, 31
Triploidy, 34
Tumor suppressor gene, 38
Variable expressivity, 35

ABBREVIATIONS

DNA—deoxyribonucleic acid
FISH—fluorescence in situ hybridization
GWAS—genome-wide association studies
mRNA—messenger RNA
mtDNA—mitochondrial DNA
RNA—ribonucleic acid
rRNA—ribosomal RNA
SNP—single-nucleotide polymorphism
tRNA—transfer RNA

2.1 Chapter Overview and Case Studies

Our bodies function through a complex interaction between genes and environment. A **gene** is segment of DNA that codes for the production of a certain protein. To understand this interaction, we will first review basics of genetics. **Genetics** is the study of individual genes and their impact on inheritance and on single-gene and chromosomal disorders. **Genomics** is the study of the structure, function, and analysis of the human genome together. **Epigenetics** is the external modification of DNA that affect gene expression, and **epigenomics** is the study of the chemical compounds that instruct the genome where and when genes are expressed within a cell. Additionally, a description of genetic- and genomic-based diagnostic tests and treatment strategies will be described in this chapter.

With the completion of the Human Genome Project and discovery of numerous genes related to common diseases and gene-related diagnostic and treatment technologies, genetics and genomics have enhanced pediatric and adult healthcare in fields including geriatrics, oncology, endocrinology, cardiology, neurology, mental health, immunology, and critical care. This increases the importance of having at least a basic understanding of genetic and genomic concepts and their use in clinical practice. In fact, members of a variety of federal agencies that developed *Healthy People 2020* added a goal related to genomics (see the Healthy People box).

The goal of this chapter is to provide a basic understanding of genetic and genomic concepts to guide nursing practice. Additional attention is paid to resources that can allow for updating of knowledge as the fields of genetics and genomics advance.

Concepts Related to Genetics and Genomics

Genetics are a primary influence on health, including genetic mutations that cause diseases such as ovarian cancer, sickle cell disease, autoimmune disorders, and depression. **Figure 2.1** ■ is a map of concepts related to genetics and genomics.

Case Studies

To assist in the application of content in this chapter to clinical practice, three case studies are introduced here, and the pathophysiology involved and clinical significance of the information will be addressed throughout the chapter.

Healthy People 2020

Genomics

Goal: "Improve health and prevent harm through valid and useful genomic tools in clinical and public health practices."[1]

Overview: This is a new goal that was not in the *Healthy People 2010* healthcare agenda for the nation. It was added on the basis of research evidence that substantiates the benefits of taking a family health history and the use of genetic and genomic tests to identify risk factors, diagnose disease, and guide the use of screening tests and treatment options. "Genomics plays a role in 9 out of 10 of the leading causes of death including heart disease, cancer, stroke, diabetes, and Alzheimer's disease."[1] Genomics also plays a role in a variety of neuromuscular, immune, vision, and hearing disorders. Evidence-based guidelines are needed to improve the use of the increasing number of genomic tests that are available to healthcare professionals and direct to the consumer.

Objectives: The two objectives of *Healthy People 2020* related to genomics target cancer and are to "increase the proportion of women with a family history of breast and/or ovarian cancer who receive genetic counseling" and "increase the proportion of persons with newly diagnosed colorectal cancer who receive genetic testing to identify familial colorectal cancer syndromes."[2] One purpose of these objectives is to increase the early diagnosis and treatment of asymptomatic individuals who have breast, ovarian, or colorectal cancer, thereby improving survival. Another purpose is to identify individuals at risk who need more frequent screening, such as mammography or colonoscopy, or who need administration of medications that are available in some cases to decrease risk of development of certain types of cancer.

References

1. Healthy People 2020. (2017). *Topics and objectives: Genomics*. Available at http://www.healthypeople.gov/2020/topicsobjectives2020/overview.aspx?topicid=15
2. Healthy People 2020. (2017). *Topics and objectives: Genomics objectives*. Available at https://www.healthypeople.gov/2020/topics-objectives/topic/genomics/objectives

Michelle Kane: Introduction

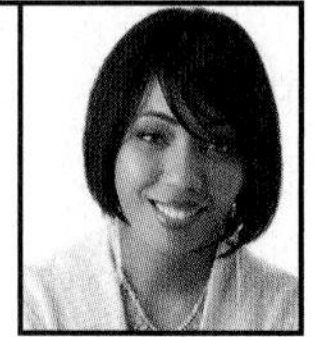

Michelle Kane is a 37-year-old woman who comes to her internist's office for a routine physical examination. During the history and physical, she mentions that her mother died of breast cancer at the age of 45 and that her mother's sister died of ovarian cancer at the age of 60. Ms. Kane's only sister is alive at age 50 but had breast cancer at age 30. Additionally, Ms. Kane mentions that both her father and her paternal grandfather have had heart attacks in their 60s. There is also a paternal grandmother who had breast cancer at age 80. Ms. Kane is worried about her own risk of breast cancer and heart disease and whether there is some way to assess her hereditary risk.

Ms. Kane wonders whether genetic testing would provide any useful information. She thinks that she already had genetic testing to assess these risks previously during pregnancy when testing was performed to look for problems in her baby. Finally, Ms. Kane mentions that she heard on the news that a new heart disease gene was discovered and wonders whether she should have testing for it.

1. How do the new *Healthy People 2020* goals related to genomics affect Ms. Kane?
2. What possible genetic risk factors can you identify in Ms. Kane?

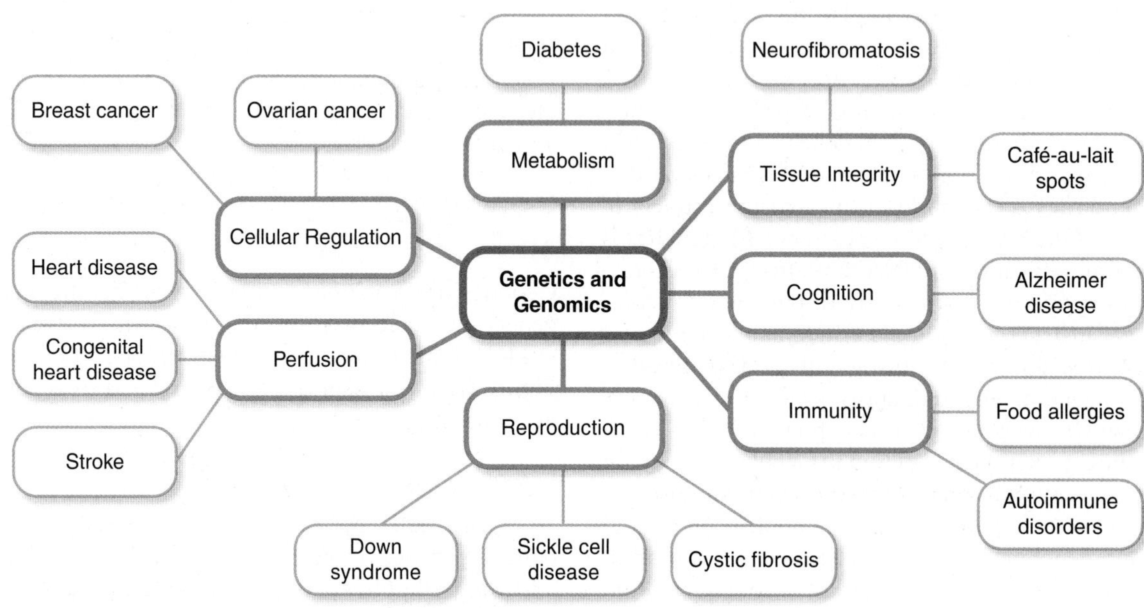

Figure 2.1 ■ Concepts related to alterations of genetics.

John Barrows: Introduction

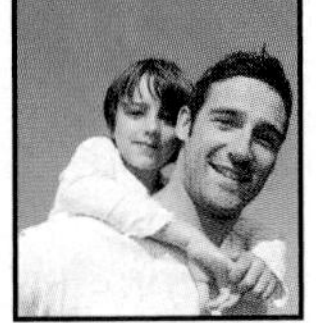

John Barrows is a 45–year-old male who brings his 10-year-old son Devin to a genetics clinic after Devin's pediatrician points out several clinical features suggestive of neurofibromatosis 1 (NF1), specifically eight café-au-lait macules and a plexiform neurofibroma. Devin's diagnosis of NF1 is confirmed after a clinical exam by the medical geneticist. The geneticist points out that Mr. Barrows may also have NF1. Mr. Barrows states that while he does have similar skin markings, he could not have a diagnosis of NF1 because he does not have all of the other clinical features seen in his son.

1. What is the field of study that will help Mr. Barrows understand the relationship between NF1 in himself and in his son?
2. On the basis of the clinical manifestations of NF1 in Mr. Barrows and his son, what might his family history reveal?

Bianca Vasquez: Introduction

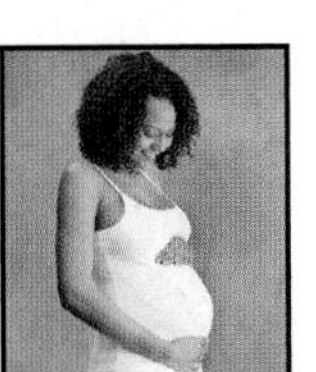

Bianca Vasquez is a 25-year-old female who has food allergies. She recently learned that she is pregnant and is concerned that her newborn will inherit her allergies. She saw a brief report on the news about reducing her baby's genetic risk through an epigenetic approach. She was advised by her genetic counselor that recent studies suggest that increased intake of polyunsaturated fatty acids from fish oil during pregnancy may modify inflammatory and immune mechanisms and reduce sensitivities to common food allergens. Ms. Vasquez was also told that individual responses to fish oil supplements may differ, owing to the uniqueness of each person's genome.

1. What is epigenetics?
2. What advice might the genetic counselor give Ms. Vasquez about news reports of genetic breakthroughs?

Check Your Progress: Section 2.1

1. What is epigenomics?
2. How has the Human Genome Project affected the health of children and adults?
3. What was the purpose of adding a genomic goal to *Healthy People 2020*?

2.2 Molecular Basis of Gene Expression

The building block of human's genetic material is **deoxyribonucleic acid (DNA)**. In the DNA are 22,000 genes that provide instructions for how our bodies should work. Each gene is made up of a sequence of **nucleotides**, which are made up of three components: a phosphate, a deoxyribose, and one of four nitrogenous bases—adenine, guanine, cytosine, and thymine (**Figure 2.2** ■).

Structurally, DNA consists of two separate strands of consecutive nucleotides joined by chemical bonds. The two strands bind together as a **double helix** by hydrogen bonds between nucleotides[1] (**Figure 2.3** ■). Adenine and guanine are called purine bases. Cytosine and thymine are called pyrimidine bases. These terms refer to the nitrogen ring structure found in each type of base. A purine base can pair only with a pyrimidine base and vice versa; specifically, thymine (T) always pairs with adenine (A), and guanine (G) always pairs with cytosine (C).

The double helix is combined with proteins called histones and is compacted to form structures called **chromosomes** (see **Figure 2.4** ■). Each chromosome contains many genes. Thus, each chromosome is a bookshelf

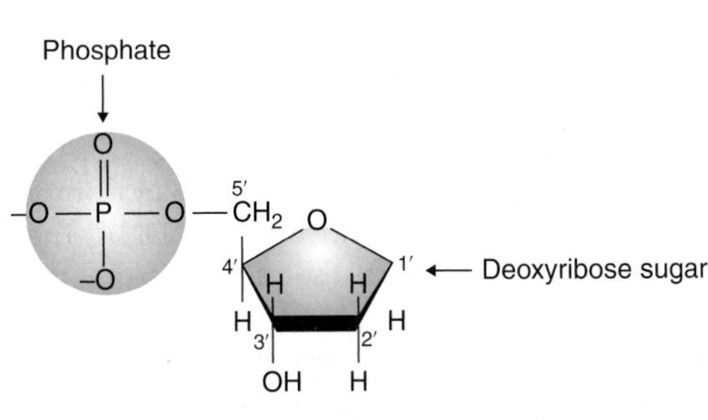

Purine nucleotides

Nitrogen base Adenine (A)

Guanine (G)

Pyrimidine nucleotides

Cytosine (C)

Thymine (T)

Figure 2.2 ■ Components of DNA.

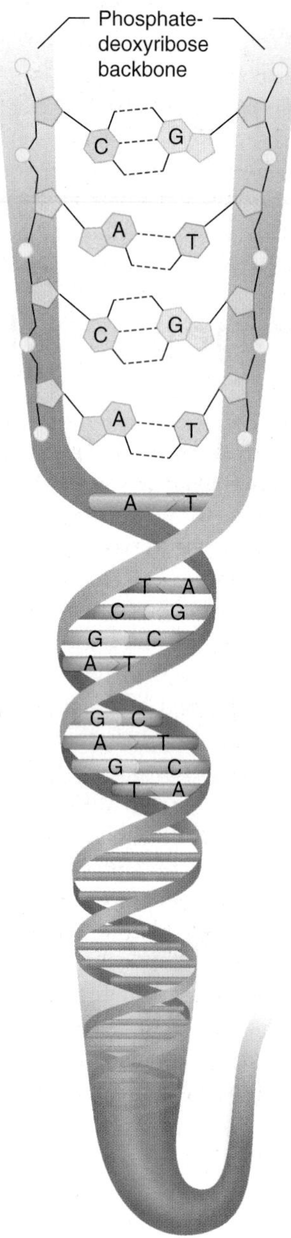

Figure 2.3 ■ DNA base pairing.

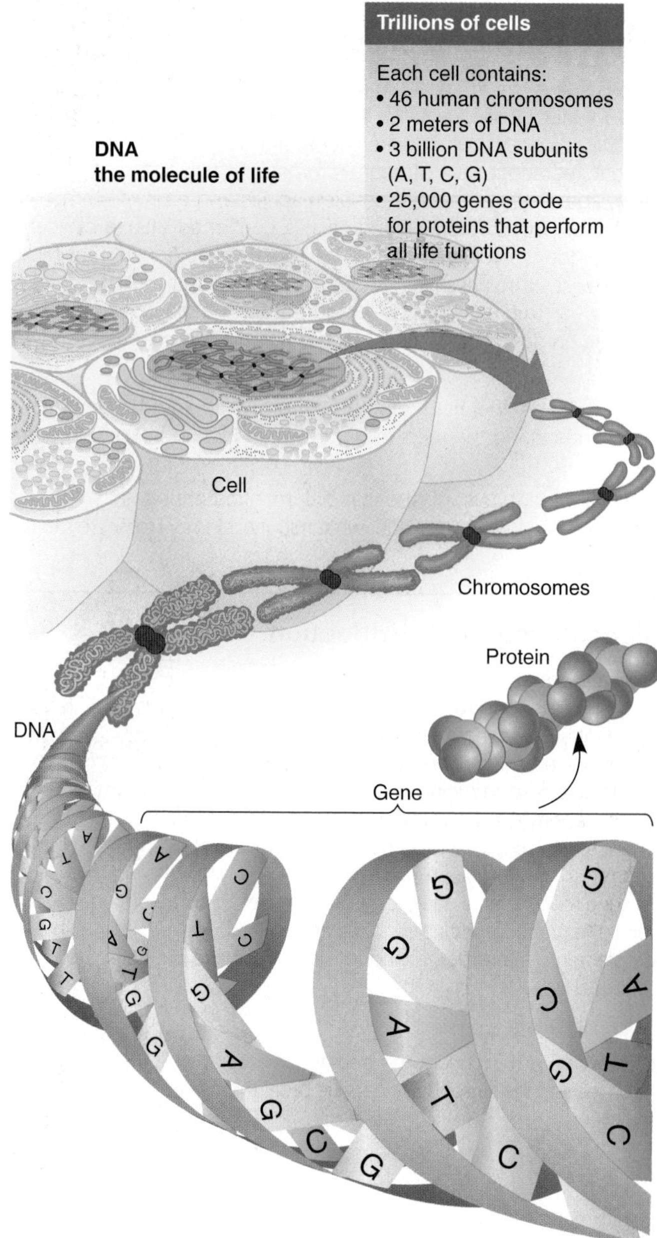

Figure 2.4 ■ Structure of a chromosome.

containing instruction manuals (genes), the DNA being the letters used to write the instructions.[1]

Humans have a total of 46 chromosomes in most cells of the body, which are grouped in 23 pairs. For each pair of chromosomes, an individual inherits one from each parent. The 23rd pair are the sex chromosomes and are designated either X or Y. Individuals with two X chromosomes are female, and those with an X chromosome and a Y chromosome are male. Chromosomes are located inside the nucleus of the cell. Red blood cells do not contain chromosomes because they lose their nucleus before leaving the bone marrow.[1]

Egg and sperm cells contain only 23 chromosomes, consisting of one chromosome of each pair. At conception, they join to make a complete set of 46 chromosomes. Because there are two copies of each chromosome, each person has two copies of each gene. Alternative forms of an individual gene are called **alleles** (**Figure 2.5** ■). Mitochondria have their own circular DNA that is always maternally inherited.[1] Because several important metabolic genes exist in mitochondrial DNA, there are many hereditary disorders that result from mitochondrial mutations.[2]

With males having just one X chromosome compared to females having two, there must be a mechanism for gene dosage compensation for genes on the X chromosome. X inactivation allows for one of the two X chromosomes in each cell of the female to be turned off, allowing for equal expression of genes in males and females. The inactivated X chromosome in each cell is called the **Barr body**.[1,3]

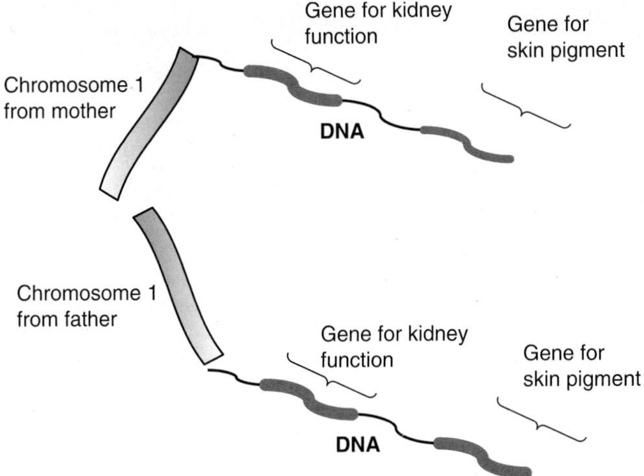

Figure 2.5 ■ For each chromosome type in the body, there are two copies. One is from the mother, and one is from the father. Therefore, for each gene in the body, there are two copies. Each copy of the same gene type is called an allele.

> **Check Your Progress: Section 2.2**
> 1. What are the four nitrogen bases?
> 2. Describe the function of the Barr body.
> 3. What is an allele?

2.3 The Human Genome, Genomics, and Epigenomics

The Genome and Genomics

The genome is an organism's complete set of DNA. With the exception of mature red blood cells, which do not have nuclei, every human cell possesses the entire genome. Genome sizes vary greatly from one organism to another, and the genomic DNA sequence is 99.9% identical among all humans. The size of the human genome is 3.2 billion base pairs including all 22,000 genes. However, the known genes make up only 2% of the genome. To date, the functions of approximately half of the identified genes remain unknown. The remaining 98% of the genome does not encode proteins but is responsible for maintaining chromosome structure and directing gene expression.

Genomics is a rapidly emerging field of science that examines mechanisms of health and disease by studying the entire genome versus individual genes. The Human Genome Project officially began in 1990 and ended in 2003 and successfully sequenced the human genome, identified and mapped the genes within it,[4] and sequenced model organisms used in research. This has allowed scientists to comparatively study the structure, function, interaction and evolution of genes and genomes.

Epigenetics and the Epigenome

Unlike mutations, epigenetic mechanisms can affect gene function without changing the underlying DNA sequence. The term *epigenetics* (*epi-* means "above") means "the study of changes in gene function that are mitotically- and/or meiotically-heritable and that do not entail a change in DNA sequence."[5] Similarly, the term *epigenome* means "above the genome." The **epigenome** is the collection of the chemical compounds (not part of genomic DNA) that instruct the genome where and when genes are expressed within a cell. These modifications can be passed on during cell division or inherited. For example, studies using animal models have shown that maternal dietary supplementation of folic acid, vitamin B_{12}, choline, and betaine altered the offspring's coat color phenotype through DNA methylation changes in the epigenome.[6,7] The plasticity of the epigenome allows reprogramming to occur throughout an individual's lifetime with alterations of lifestyle (e.g., nutrition, air pollution, the aging process). In particular, the epigenome is the most vulnerable to deregulation during gestation, neonatal and puberty development, and old age.[8]

Epigenetic modifications play an essential role in many biological processes, including cell differentiation and response to external factors in the environment, such as chemicals in food and medications. Biochemical processes such as DNA or histone methylation, chromatin remodeling, and RNA interference are epigenetic mechanisms of modifying gene function[9] (see **Figure 2.6** ■). In DNA methylation, a methyl group (CH_3) is attached to a promoter region in a gene, which can result in silencing of a gene. This can be beneficial if the gene that is silenced is harmful, such as an oncogene. Certain chemicals in foods cause epigenetic modification by methylation of DNA or histones. In chromatin remodeling, structural change in chromatin affects DNA transcription (the formation of RNA from DNA) or chromosome segregation during cell division. RNA interference is a process whereby small interfering strands of RNA bind to a complementary mRNA sequencing to prevent translation. RNA interference allows expression of only the genes that are needed for functioning of a particular cell type. The most researched epigenetic phenomena are X chromosome inactivation in females[10,11] and genomic imprinting[12,13] (genes that are expressed only on the basis of which parent the gene is inherited from).

CLINICAL POINT: Failure of RNA interference can result in a cell type producing an unexpected protein. For example, certain lung cancers synthesize and secrete antidiuretic hormone, which is normally synthesized in the brain. Research is ongoing to determine whether interfering RNA strands could silence genes that promote cancer cell division. ■

The discoveries of epigenetics and the epigenome have raised key questions that are being actively investigated.[9] These questions include the following:

- Which genes result in enhanced disease susceptibility when epigenetically deregulated by environmental factors?

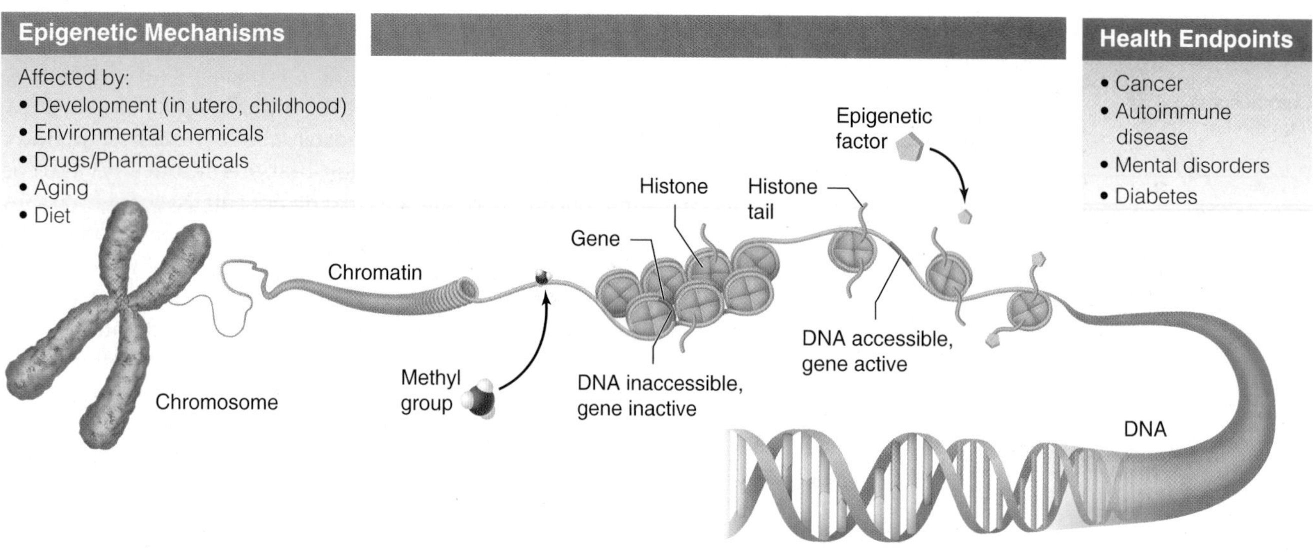

Figure 2.6 ■ Epigenetic mechanisms of modifying gene expression. The epigenome can mark DNA in two ways, both of which play a role in turning genes off or on. The first occurs when certain chemical tags called methyl groups attach to the backbone of a DNA molecule. The second occurs when a variety of chemical tags attach to the tails of histones, which are spool-like proteins that package DNA neatly into chromosomes. This action affects how tightly DNA is wound around the histones.

- What environmental factors at what dose deleteriously alter the epigenome?
- What role does the epigenome have in reproduction, development, and disease etiology?
- What nutrients at what dose reduce the harmful effects of chemical and physical environmental factors on the epigenome?
- Can epigenetic biomarkers be identified that will allow for early-stage disease detection and treatment?
- Can technologies be developed that will allow for a quick and accurate genome-wide assessment of the epigenome?

Check Your Progress: Section 2.3

1. Describe how DNA methylation can be beneficial in fighting disease.
2. What is the biochemical process of chromatin remodeling?
3. Explain the biochemical process of RNA interference.

2.4 Gene Replication, Transcription, and Translation

DNA is the set of instructions for how the body should work. At conception, we start out as one cell, created by the joining of a sperm and an egg. This cell and the DNA within it must be replicated over and over again to make all of the cells in the body. From the DNA, **ribonucleic acid (RNA)** is formed. It is similar in structure to DNA except that the sugar component (ribose) of the nucleotides contains an extra oxygen molecule and uracil is used a base instead of thymine. RNA is then used to synthesize proteins that are used to create the body's tissues and organs. This process of DNA to RNA to protein is called the **central dogma**. Each portion of the central dogma involves a series of chemical reactions that will be explained in the following sections.

Cell Division and DNA Replication

Each cell of the body must have all 46 chromosomes and the genes they carry, with the exception of some specialized cells. The process of cell division used to create identical copies of a cell is called **mitosis** (**Figure 2.7** ■). Since **gonadal cells**, that is egg and sperm cells, must have only half of this genetic information (one of each chromosome pair), or 23 chromosomes total, cell division occurs differently by a process called **meiosis**.[1]

The basic process of cell division, whether it is mitosis or meiosis, is the same. Before a cell divides, DNA replication must occur. During **DNA replication**, the double-stranded DNA is unwound, and then replication occurs along both DNA strands, resulting in two double-stranded DNA molecules. After all of the chromosomes have been replicated, the cell undergoes mitosis and divides into two cells with identical DNA. Mitosis occurs in all **somatic cells** (everything that's not an egg or sperm).[1]

In **meiosis**, egg and sperm cells are created for reproduction. Meiosis initially begins with a cell that has 46 total chromosomes, two of each chromosome type (**Figure 2.8** ■). This is called a **diploid cell**. Replication of DNA occurs just as it does in mitosis. However, the goal here is to place *one* of every chromosome pair into a cell. This occurs by following DNA

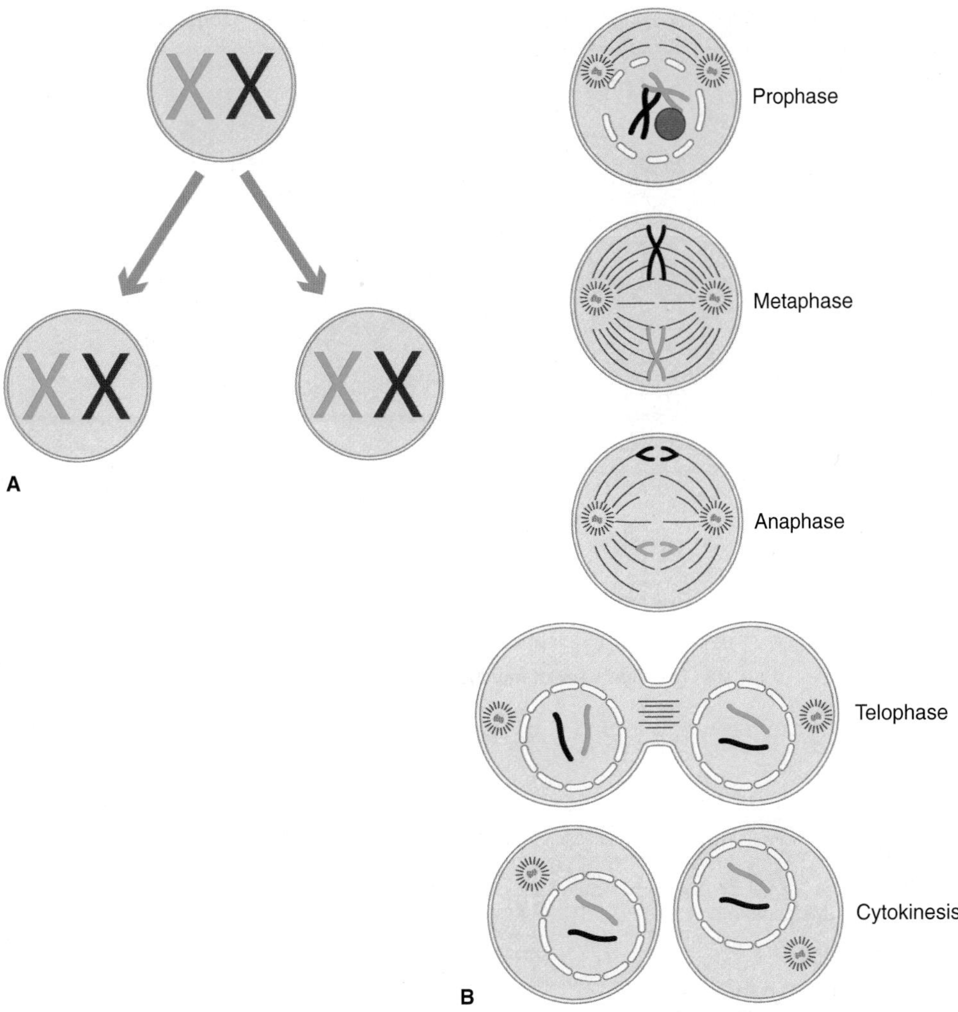

Figure 2.7 ■ The purpose of mitosis is to take diploid cells and make two identical clones. **A** shows a simplified version and **B** shows a detailed version. This process is used to make all the somatic cells of the body. Thus, all the cells have identical genetic content. Different tissue types and organs are created by turning on different genes in different areas of the body.

replication with two sets of cell divisions, and the end product is four daughter cells, each with a total of 23 chromosomes, one of each chromosome pair. These are called **haploid cells**. Meiosis ensures a unique combination of, and variation in, physical and behavioral traits in each new generation.

The process of meiosis differs slightly between sperm and eggs. In **spermatogenesis**, the creation of sperm, a diploid cell undergoes meiosis I (the first cell division in meiosis) and then meiosis II (the second cell division) shortly afterwards to make four haploid sperm. **Oogenesis** is the process of making eggs. Diploid cells in the female ovaries remain in prophase I, the first step of meiosis I until puberty. At this time, one ovum is released per menstrual cycle and completes meiosis I, resulting in one functional secondary oocyte and a nonfunctional polar body. This polar body does not undergo further cell divisions. If the secondary oocyte is not fertilized, it will be expelled from the body during menstruation. If fertilized, the secondary oocyte will undergo meiosis II; one of the two daughter cells will become the egg cell, and the other will become a second, nonfunctional polar body. In nondisjunction, improper separation of chromosomes results in the egg or sperm having an incorrect number of chromosomes, which can ultimately result in an imbalance in a fetus (see **Figure 2.9** ■).

Transcription

The process of "reading" a gene is called **transcription**, in which an RNA strand is formed from a template strand of DNA. There are three different types of RNA, each with a unique function. **Messenger RNA (mRNA)** is used as a template for protein synthesis. **Transfer RNA (tRNA)** carries appropriate amino acids to the template mRNA strand during protein formation. **Ribosomal RNA (rRNA)** helps to make the ribosomes, the machinery for protein formation to occur. The proteins are then utilized for regular body function.[1] The process of protein formation is discussed later in this chapter.

Despite cells in the body having identical genetic material, different genes are used or "turned on" depending on

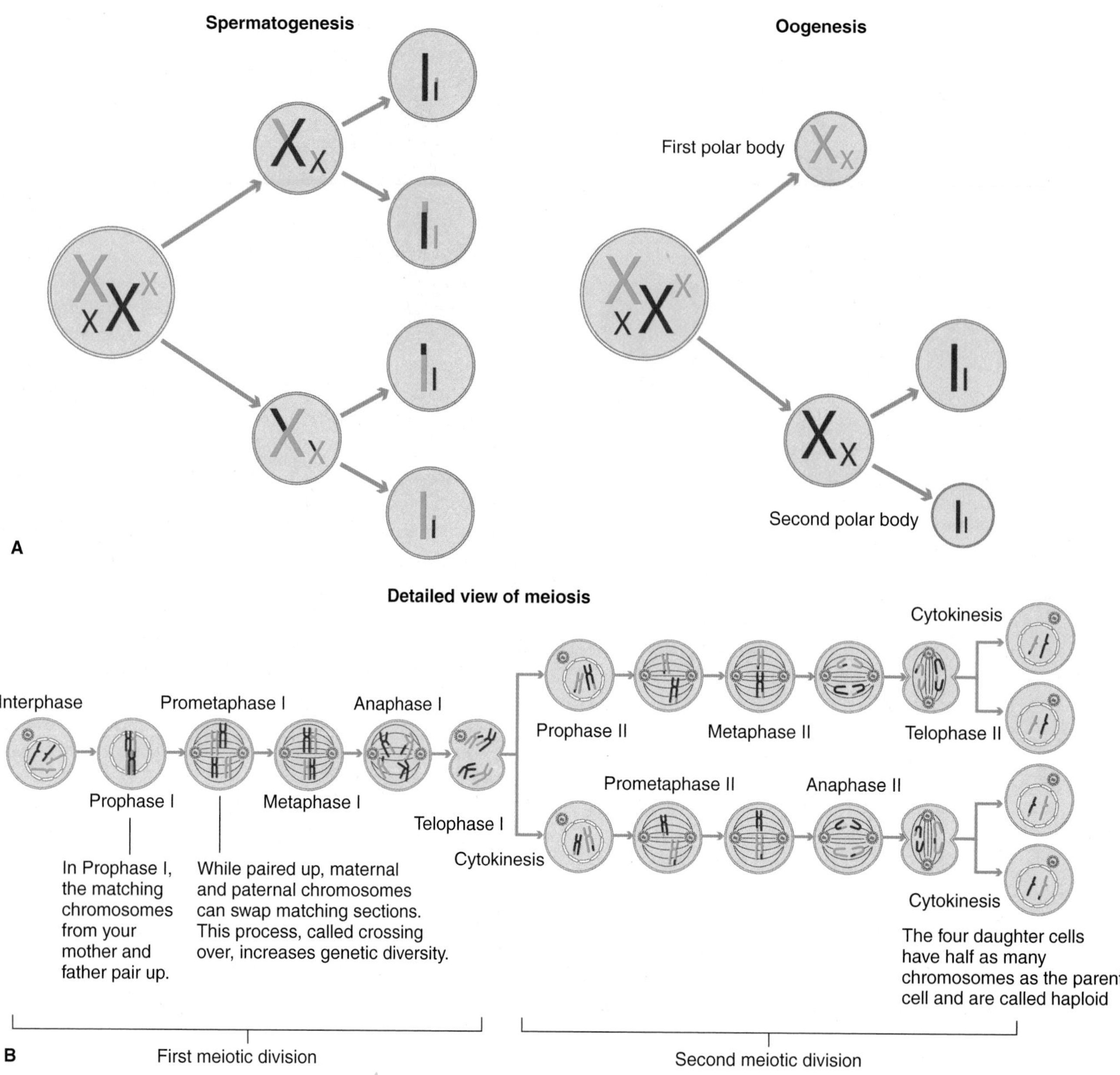

Figure 2.8 ■ Meiosis is used to make sperm and egg cells. **A** shows a simplified version and **B** shows a detailed version. During meiosis, a cell's chromosomes are copied once, but the cell divides twice. For simplicity, we have illustrated cells with only three pairs of chromosomes. The purpose of meiosis is to make haploid germ cells from diploid cells. In males, four haploid germ cells will be made by one meiotic division. In females, only one of the two cells created at the first cell division will go on to further cell divisions. The other is lost as a polar body. That cell will complete only the second cell division if fertilization occurs, and one of the two newly created cells will be expelled as a polar body.

tissue type. For instance, the kidneys will use only genes that are important for kidney function. The genes that are necessary for heart function exist in the kidney cells, but they are suppressed (not turned on). For transcription to begin, a series of **transcription factors**, or regulatory proteins, must bind to the promoter region at the beginning of the gene. While human disease can occur as a result of mutations, or changes, in the DNA, disease can also occur as a consequence of faulty transcription. For example, inflammatory disorders are the result of a change in transcription of several genes.[14,15] (Refer to Chapter 6 for more information about inflammation.)

The RNA transcribed from DNA is used for making a protein. The process of making RNA is very similar to the process of DNA replication except that only one strand of RNA is made per double-stranded DNA. See **Figure 2.10** ■, which depicts the sense and antisense strands of DNA and their role in DNA transcription. Messenger RNA (mRNA) carries a message instructing how the gene product is made. The mRNA is initiated at a universal start sequence and is terminated at a set stop sequence (see **Figure 2.11** ■).[1]

The initial mRNA transcript needs to go through a process called **splicing** (**Figure 2.12** ■) to become a mature message. Each gene has exons and introns. The **exons** are

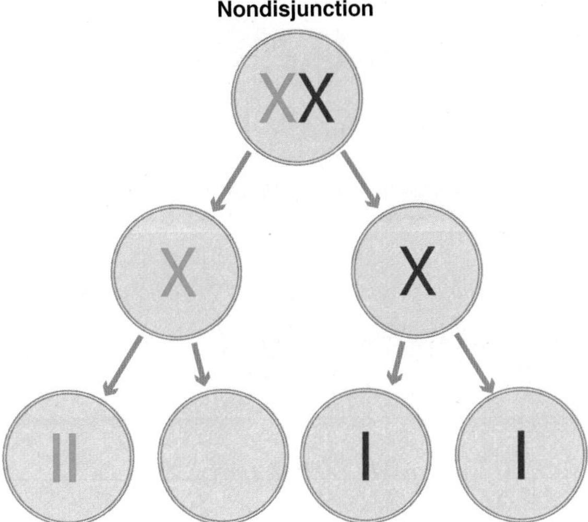

Figure 2.9 ■ If nondisjunction (the improper separation of chromosomes) occurs during meiosis, the eggs or sperm may have an incorrect number of chromosomes. If the germ cell with an improper number of chromosomes is fertilized, the resulting fetus will have the wrong number of chromosomes. This can lead to miscarriage or a live-born child with health problems.

the "useful" coding parts of the gene. Interspersed between the exons are noncoding **introns**. The purpose of these noncoding introns is not known, but they may hold regulatory sequences for proper gene function. To create a protein, the noncoding parts of mRNA (the introns) are removed, or spliced, and the coding exons are joined together. Splicing involves a series of chemical reactions to remove the introns and attach all of the exons. The same gene may have different splicing patterns in different cells of the body or even in the same cell so that multiple variations of a protein can be made from the same gene. Incorrect splicing and thus an aberrant protein product can result in disease.[1,16]

Translation

Messenger RNA leaves the nucleus of the cell and travels to the ribosomes, where translation occurs (**Figure 2.13** ■). **Translation** is the process of protein synthesis with mRNA directing assembly of a string of amino acids to create a protein product. Every three nucleotides in mRNA code are grouped together as a **codon**. Each codon corresponds to an amino acid. There are 64 possible codons in the human body but only 20 corresponding amino acids, allowing for more than one codon to correspond to an amino acid. One specific codon serves as the start codon to initiate protein formation, while three different codons serve as stop codons to signal the end of a protein. tRNA transports individual amino acids to the ribosome, and amino acids are sequentially added to create the initial protein chain.[17]

Modifications occur via protein folding, in which the amino acid chain gets its three-dimensional structure, which a key determinant of how well the protein will function. Any disruption in conformation, even a single amino acid change, can potentially cause disease. In sickle cell disease, one amino acid change causes the hemoglobin molecule to fold improperly. This alters the shape of the red blood cells when oxygen levels decrease, which prevents the red cells from passing through capillaries, resulting in tissue ischemia.[1,17]

Check Your Progress: Section 2.4

1. What is the difference between mitosis and meiosis.
2. Describe the difference between haploid and diploid cells.
3. Compare the roles of messenger RNA, transfer RNA, and ribosomal RNA.

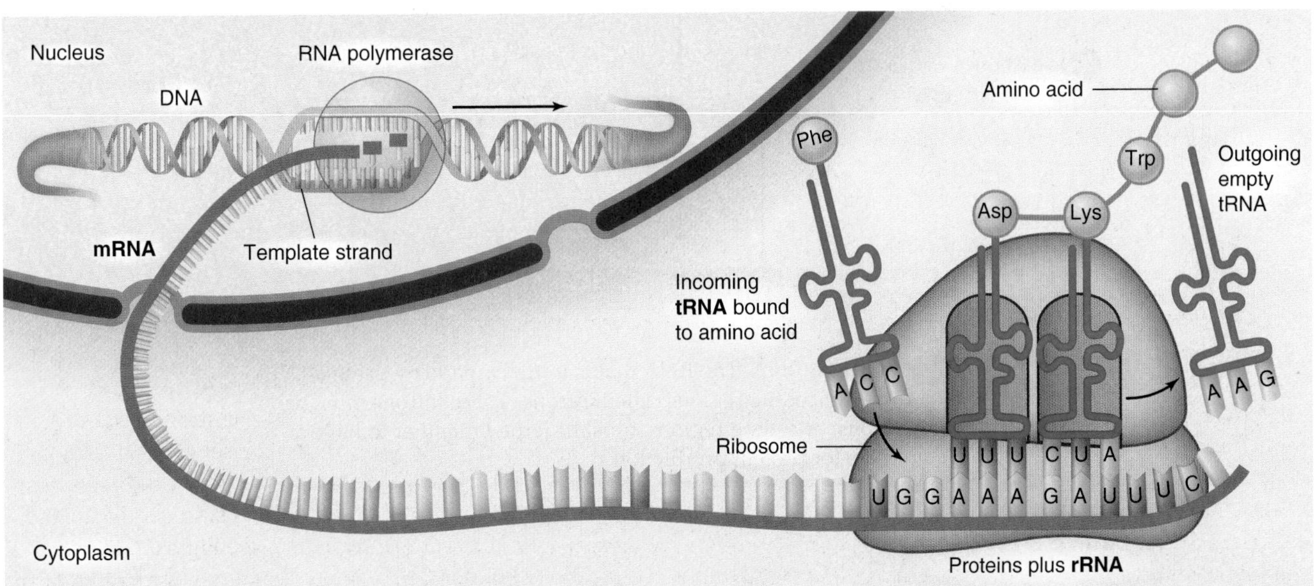

Figure 2.10 ■ Transcription of messenger RNA (mRNA).

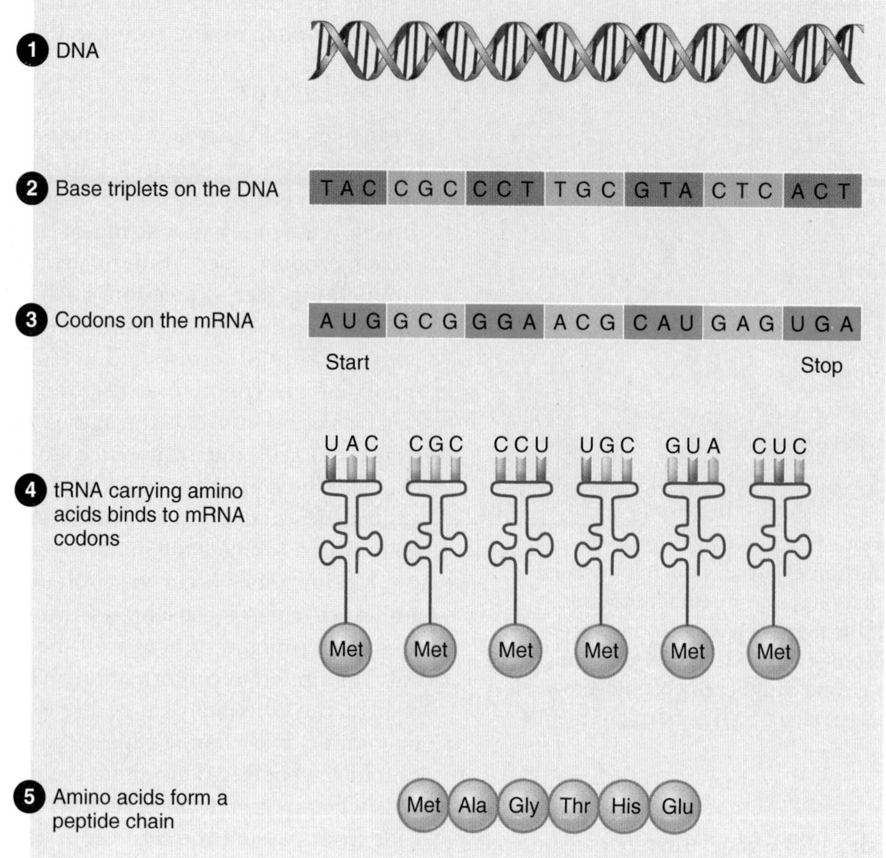

Figure 2.11 ■ Relationship of a DNA base sequence to peptide structure.

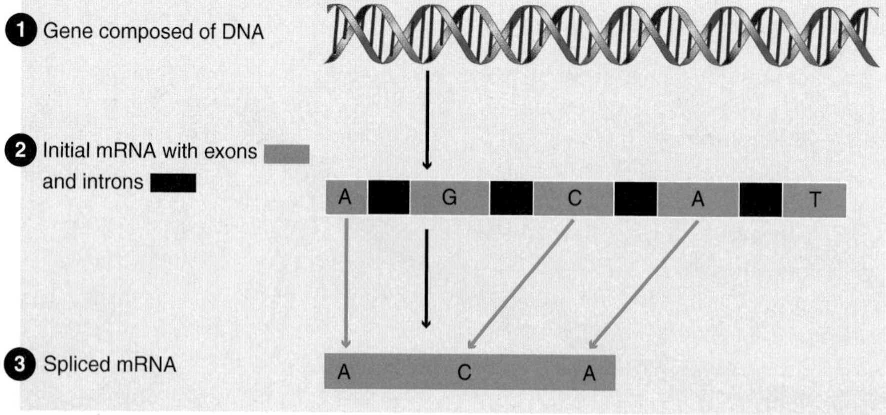

Figure 2.12 ■ Splicing of mRNA. The RNA that is initially made by using a DNA template has numerous noncoding regions called introns. These introns must be spliced out, and the exons, or coding regions, must be joined together to have a functional RNA template for protein production.

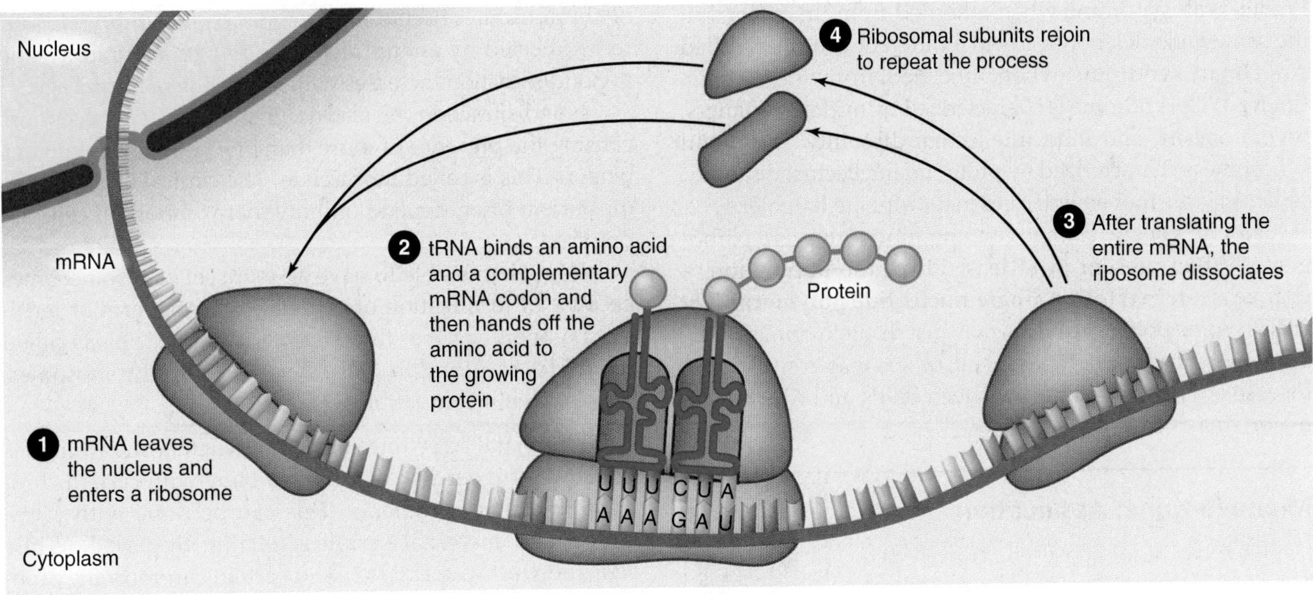

Figure 2.13 ■ Translation of mRNA.

2.5 Mutations

A **mutation** is a grammatical error in a gene, which can be of varying types and severity (**Figure 2.14** ■). Ultimately, any amino acid change, disruption of a start or stop codon, or incorrect splicing can be potentially harmful. Although most mutations are corrected by repair mechanisms, an uncorrected mutation can be transmitted on through generations.[1]

A **point mutation** is a change in one nucleotide. This can have varying levels of severity. If the amino acid is not changed by a point mutation, it is a **silent mutation**. However, a **missense mutation** causes a change in the amino acid sequence. The clinical significance depends on whether the new protein product is ultimately functional. Many amino acid changes can be benign, but as was mentioned above with sickle cell disease, one amino acid change can also result in dramatic changes that have serious clinical consequences. In some cases, a point mutation changes a codon into a premature stop codon. This is called a **nonsense mutation**, which results in little or no protein produced and almost always results in serious clinical consequences.[1]

Insertion and deletion of nucleotides affect the gene's entire triplet codon reading frame. That is, inserting or deleting nucleotides will cause the wrong amino acids to be used at every point after the mutation. This type of mutation, depending on the location in the gene, almost always has significant clinical effects.[1] Mutations can also occur at the chromosome level, including multigene deletions, duplications, and translocations (rearrangements) (see Figure 2.14), which often results is a clinically severe presentation.[1]

In **genetic imprinting**, some genes have differential expression based on the parent from whom the genes are inherited. Disrupting epigenetic mechanisms such as methylation can lead to human disease. For example, a deletion of a portion of chromosome 15 leads to a disorder called

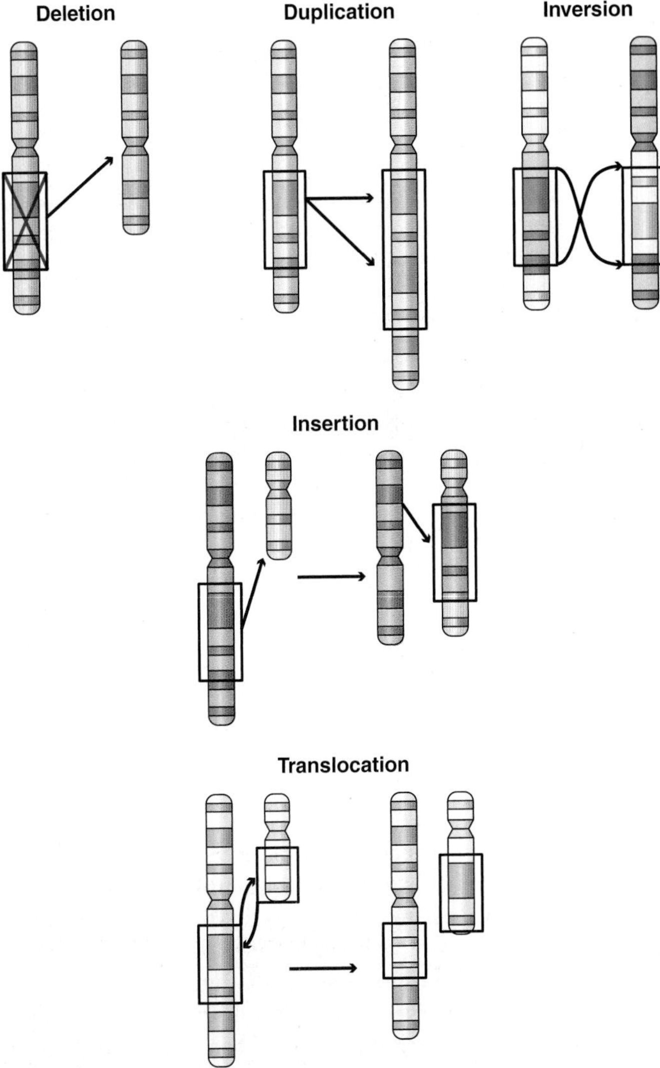

Figure 2.14 ■ Types of mutations.

Prader-Willi syndrome when inherited from the father, but the same gene deletion leads to a different condition called Angelman syndrome when inherited from the mother. Prader-Willi syndrome is characterized by muscle weakness, severe obesity, and mild intellectual disability. Angelman syndrome is characterized by profound intellectual disability, seizures, jerky movements, and inappropriate laughter.[1]

Not all genetic changes among individuals are pathogenic. When present in at least 1% of the population, a change is referred to as a **single-nucleotide polymorphism (SNP)**. Some polymorphisms may just result in human variation with no clinical impact at all; others may contribute to disease.[1,18] The association between SNPs and disease is a major area of current study.[1,19]

Michelle Kane: Application

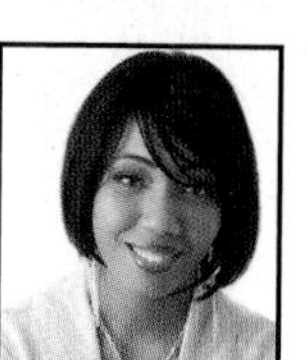

Ms. Kane has heard about the discovery of a new heart disease gene. Genetics researchers may find an association between a SNP and a disease, but they might not immediately know its specific role, if any, in the disease. Therefore, announcements made in the news about "new genes" rarely have an immediate impact on clinical care. It may take a long time for new genetic knowledge to be translated into clinical practice. Therefore, it is important for healthcare providers to be aware not only of new gene discoveries but also of their clinical application.

3. How should a healthcare provider describe an SNP to Ms. Kane?
4. Because Ms. Kane has a family history of heart disease, she wants to know whether she should have testing for the new heart disease gene that was just discovered. What should her healthcare provider advise her?

Check Your Progress: Section 2.5

1. Compare the four types of mutations.
2. What are the consequences of genetic imprinting?
3. Describe the results of insertion or deletion of nucleotides.

2.6 Categories of Genetic Disorders

Genetic disorders can be caused by chromosomal or single-gene disorders or be of multifactorial origin. These modes of inheritance are described in the following sections.

Chromosomal Disorders

The most basic type of genetic disorder results from an abnormality of chromosome number or structure. Sometimes chromosomes don't separate out properly during cell division, resulting in the wrong number of chromosomes going into a cell. This is called **chromosome nondisjunction**. Nondisjunction in an egg or sperm can cause an embryo to have an extra (trisomy) or missing chromosome (monosomy), which most often can result in an early miscarriage but in some cases can result in a live-born baby.[1,20] When the wrong number of chromosomes occurs in a pregnancy, the embryo is said to be affected by **aneuploidy**. The risk of aneuploidy due to nondisjunction increases with increasing maternal age.[1,21]

Nondisjunction can also occur shortly after conception, causing the presence of more than one genetic cell line in a person. This is called **mosaicism**. The clinical effects of the mosaicism often depend on how many abnormal cells are present.[1]

It is also possible to have an extra set of chromosomes because of fertilization of one egg by two sperm or fertilization of an egg that then divides into two. This is called **triploidy**, resulting in an embryo with 69 chromosomes. This is often incompatible with life.[22]

4 Prenatal screening can assess whether the woman is at a higher risk of having a baby with certain chromosomal problems. This can be done with ultrasound and maternal serum screening by blood. While screening tests can assess risk of certain chromosome problems, diagnosis can occur only with the use of invasive procedures, such as chorionic villus sampling or amniocentesis. Both procedures obtain cells from the growing fetus to assess fetal chromosome number and structure. ■

Women age 35 years and older who are pregnant are routinely offered prenatal diagnostic testing.[20,23] Both procedures carry a small risk of miscarriage. Thus, pregnant women must be appropriately counseled about what could be found, and informed consent must be obtained before either procedure is done. **Down syndrome** (trisomy 21) can result in miscarriage but can also result in a live-born child. Down syndrome is associated with a combination of birth defects, characteristic facial features, and variable degrees of intellectual disability[1,23] (see **Figure 2.15** ■). Trisomies 13 and 18 are rarer but much more severe, resulting in severe intellectual disability and numerous congenital abnormalities; more than 90% of children born with trisomy 13 or trisomy 18 die within the first year of life.[1,20,23]

Sex chromosome aneuploidies are often compatible with life. Males with Klinefelter syndrome have two X chromosomes and a Y chromosome. Clinical symptoms can be subtle, though most individuals with Klinefelter syndrome will ultimately present with infertility.[1,24] Females with Turner syndrome have only one X chromosome; they often present with short stature and infertility.[1,20]

Structural anomalies, both sporadic and inherited, can also occur, including translocations (when segments of one or more chromosomes break and reattach to another chromosome), ring chromosomes, inversions, and chromosome deletions. Several distinct chromosome deletion syndromes have been described in the medical literature.[1]

Mendelian Pattern of Inheritance: Single-gene Disorders

Numerous genetic disorders are caused by single-gene mutations and inherited in different patterns. Four main inheritance patterns will be discussed in this chapter: autosomal dominant, autosomal recessive, X-linked recessive, and mitochondrial.

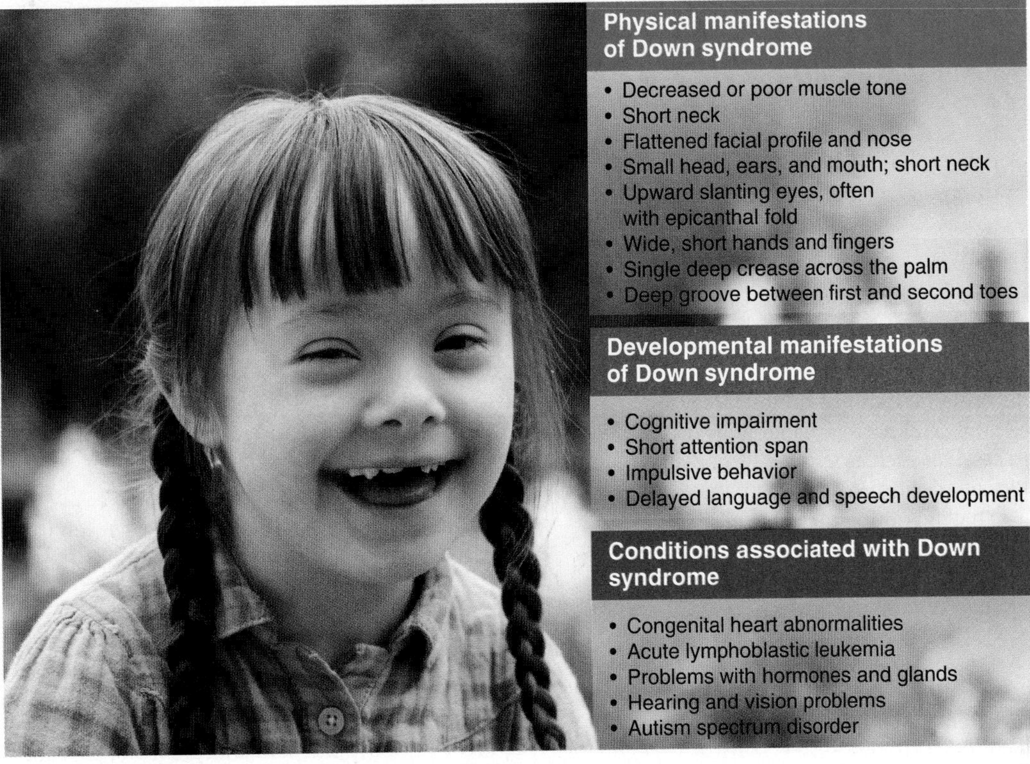

Physical manifestations of Down syndrome
• Decreased or poor muscle tone
• Short neck
• Flattened facial profile and nose
• Small head, ears, and mouth; short neck
• Upward slanting eyes, often with epicanthal fold
• Wide, short hands and fingers
• Single deep crease across the palm
• Deep groove between first and second toes
Developmental manifestations of Down syndrome
• Cognitive impairment
• Short attention span
• Impulsive behavior
• Delayed language and speech development
Conditions associated with Down syndrome
• Congenital heart abnormalities
• Acute lymphoblastic leukemia
• Problems with hormones and glands
• Hearing and vision problems
• Autism spectrum disorder

Figure 2.15 ■ Clinical manifestations of Down syndrome.

When an individual has identical alleles for a given gene, they are **homozygous**. Two different versions of the gene are **heterozygous**. **Genotype** is the actual genetic code in a person, whereas **phenotype** is the clinical expression related to the genotype.[1]

The process of identifying mutations and their association with human disease is not always straightforward, since the relationship between genotype and phenotype is often inconsistent. The clinical phenotype in individuals with mutations in the same gene can be different. This is called **variable expressivity**. Reduced **penetrance** means that not everyone who inherits a mutation will have clinical symptoms. Diseases that have variable expressivity or reduced penetrance can be difficult to recognize in a family because the pattern of disease may be inconsistent. A genetic disorder can also be due to a new mutation, which means that a mutation occurred in an individual for the first time. Even with no family history of the condition, the affected individual will be at increased risk to pass the mutation down to subsequent generations. **Neurofibromatosis**, an autosomal dominant condition that causes numerous cutaneous lesions (see **Figure 2.16** ■), such as those described for the 10-year-old son of Mr. Barrows in the case study, has a 50% new mutation rate, meaning that half the individuals diagnosed will have no prior family history.

CLINICAL POINT: In clinical practice, it is often useful to draw a genetic **pedigree** through several generations so that the pattern of genetic disease can be visualized. In these pedigrees, circles represent women, and squares represent men. Individuals of the same generation are on one row, and their offspring are drawn in a row below, connected by a vertical line to their parents. Individuals who have had children together are linked by a horizontal line. Examples of pedigrees are described in the following section. ■

Autosomal Recessive Inheritance

The word *autosomal* means that the gene of interest is on one of the non-sex chromosomes. Thus, males or females can be affected. Recessive inheritance indicates that both copies of a gene must not be working to express the trait. A person who inherits only one copy of a mutated gene will be a carrier but will not express the trait. When both parents are carriers of a gene mutation, there is a 25% chance in each pregnancy that the child will inherit two mutated genes and thus have the disease. A **Punnett square** is used to determine the probability of the genotype that children will inherit on the basis of the genotype of the parents. **Figure 2.17** ■ shows a Punnett square for recessive inheritance represented by a mutated gene (a) where both parents are carriers (Aa). Examples of recessive diseases include cystic fibrosis (which is covered in Chapter 18) and sickle cell disease (which is

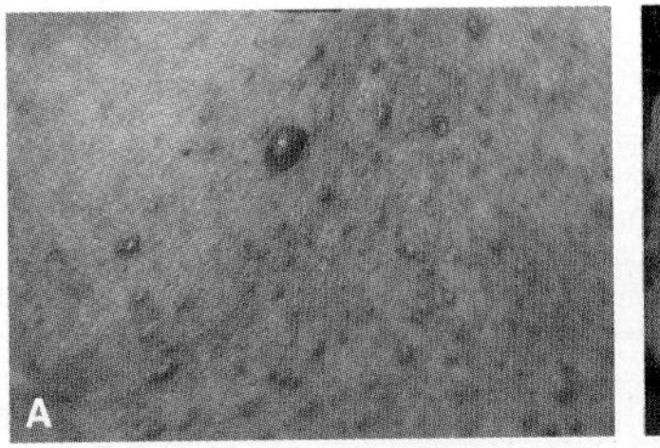

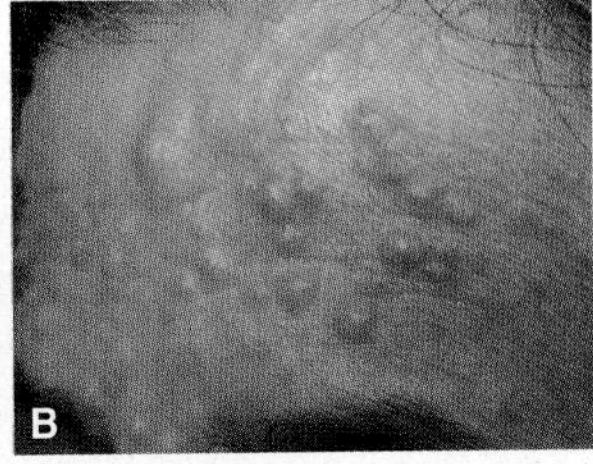

Figure 2.16 ■ Cutaneous lesions of neurofibromatosis. **A.** Café-au-lait spots. **B.** Neurofibromas.

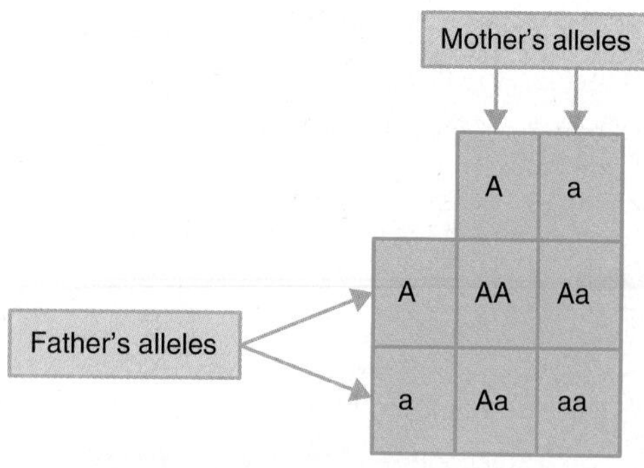

Figure 2.17 ■ Punnett square. In this example, both the mother and the father are heterozygous (Aa) for a mutated gene (a) that is recessive, such as the one responsible for sickle cell disease. When both parents are carriers of a gene mutation, each child they have will have a 25% chance of inheriting the two mutated genes (aa) and therefore manifesting a recessive disease.

covered in Chapter 21). Carrier frequencies for recessive diseases vary among different ethnic groups.

CLINICAL POINT: It is standard of care to offer appropriate carrier screening based on ethnic background to couples who are considering pregnancy and also to construct a genogram in many clinical settings. ■

Figure 2.18 ■ shows a classic pedigree for an autosomal recessive disease. Note that often in an autosomal recessive condition, there is not a family history of the condition. The disease occurs only when two carriers have a child together and both carriers pass on the mutation to that child.

Autosomal Dominant Inheritance

In autosomal dominant inheritance, males or females can be affected. Dominant inheritance indicates that only one copy of a mutated gene is required to cause disease. When a parent has an autosomal dominant gene mutation, there is a 50% chance in each pregnancy that the child will inherit the mutation and manifest disease. Examples of autosomal dominant diseases include Huntington disease, hereditary nonpolyposis colon cancer syndrome, and **Marfan syndrome**, a connective tissue disorder that causes pathogenic skeletal, ocular, and cardiac features. **Figure 2.19** ■ shows a classic pedigree for an autosomal dominant disease. Note that if an individual has a new mutation, there will be no prior family history of the disease in the pedigree.

X-linked Inheritance

X-linked (or sex-linked) diseases refer to mutations that occur on the X chromosome. Females have two copies of the X chromosome. Remember that for many of the genes on the X chromosome, only one copy of the gene needs to be expressed. Therefore, for females, one of the two X chromosomes in every cell is turned off. With males having only one copy of the X chromosome, a male with a mutation in an X-linked gene will manifest the disease. A female can pass an X-linked mutation to a son or daughter, but only the son will manifest the severe form of the disease. A father cannot pass on the X-linked condition to his sons because a male inherits his X chromosome from his mother and the Y chromosome from his father. Therefore, in an X-linked condition, it is likely that only males will be affected, and the condition can be traced through the maternal lineage.[1]

However, more recently, it has been identified that female carriers of an X-linked condition may manifest

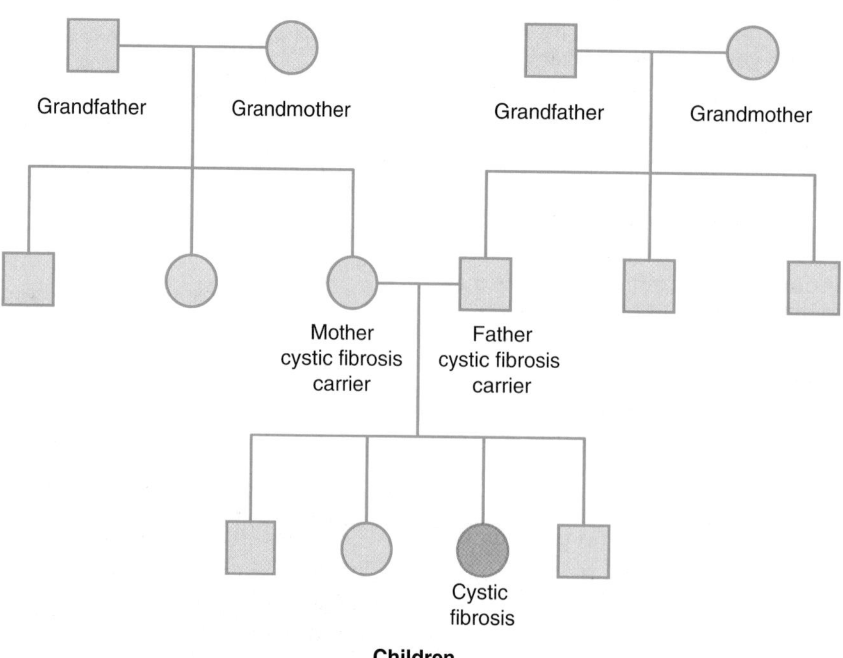

Figure 2.18 ■ Example of a genetic pedigree of the autosomal recessive disease cystic fibrosis.

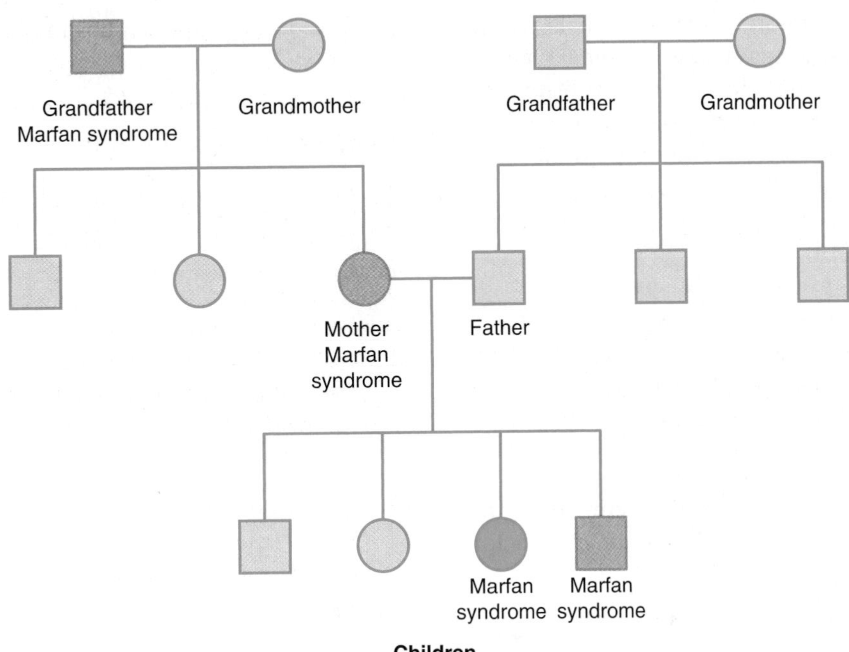

Figure 2.19 ■ Example of a genetic pedigree of the autosomal dominant disease Marfan syndrome.

some clinical symptoms but to a milder extent than is seen in males. Affected males with fragile X syndrome have intellectual disability and characteristic facial features and behaviors. In female carriers, premature ovarian failure or even learning problems can occur. **Figure 2.20** ■ shows a pedigree of fragile X syndrome.[1]

Mitochondrial Inheritance

Mitochondrial DNA (mtDNA) is the DNA located in mitochondria, cellular organelles that convert chemical energy from food into adenosine triphosphate (ATP). Mitochondrial DNA is inherited exclusively from the mother as the fertilized oocyte contains enzymes that degrade mitochondrial

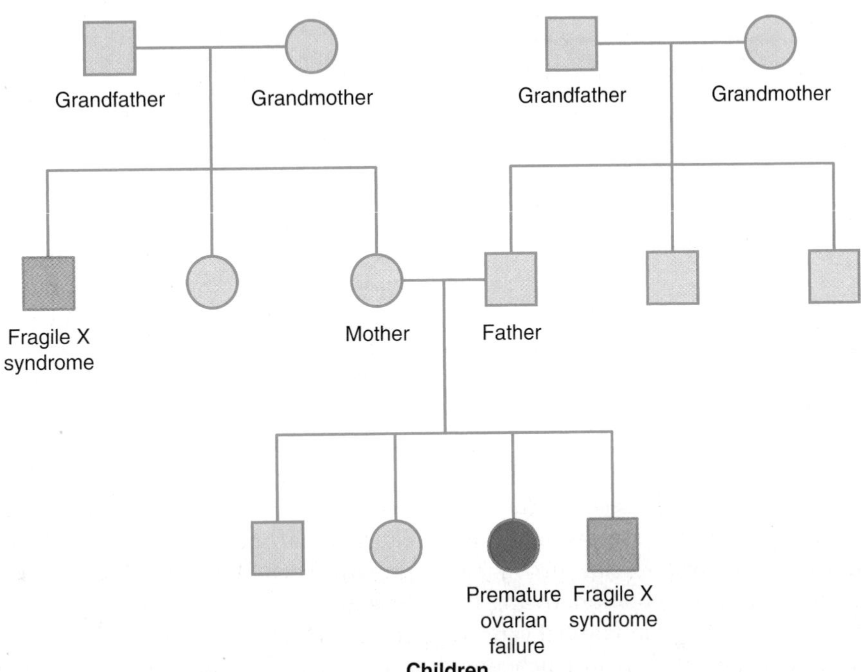

Figure 2.20 ■ Pedigree of fragile X syndrome.

DNA in the sperm.[1] Therefore, an affected male will not pass on the condition, whereas an affected female can pass it on up to 100% of the time. Many proteins responsible for mitochondrial function are encoded by nuclear genes as well. Therefore, some mitochondrial disorders are inherited in an autosomal pattern.[1,25]

Multifactorial Genetic Disease

Most human diseases are a result of an interaction between both genes and environment. Multiple cases of a disease in one family do not implicate a purely genetic cause, since families usually share both genes and environment. Hypertension, inflammatory bowel disease and diabetes are prime examples, with clear hereditary components but numerous important environmental factors as well. For multifactorial diseases, clinical genetic testing alone may be less useful than modification of environmental factors, like diet.[26]

Michelle Kane: Application

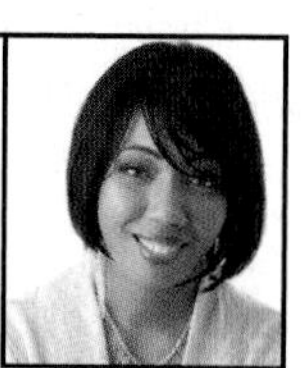

Ms. Kane has a valid concern about her family history of heart disease. Heart disease certainly has hereditary components, though the majority are not known and those that are known might be tested only through a genome-wide association study (discussed later in this chapter), which currently has limited clinical utility. Heart disease is often multifactorial, and a single gene test alone would not be an accurate predictor of disease. Ms. Kane would be best served by using exercise and a healthy diet as her means to avoid heart disease and making sure her healthcare providers are aware of her family history so that they can order appropriate screening.

5. What effect might the environment have on Ms. Kane's risk for heart disease?
6. What advice should the healthcare provider give Ms. Kane to address her concerns about heart disease?

Check Your Progress: Section 2.6

1. What is the difference between genotype and phenotype?
2. How does variable expressivity make it difficult to recognize mutations in a family?
3. What is the significance of recessive inheritance to offspring when one or both parents carry the mutation?

2.7 Phenotypic Variations in Human Disease

Manifesting multifactorial disease depends on multiple genes, environmental influences, and lifestyle choices. Therefore, significant variation in disease presentation exists. However, single-gene disorders can also have quite a bit of variation in clinical presentation, owing to factors such as reduced penetrance, as in familial cancer syndromes, and variable expressivity,[1] as in Duchenne and Becker muscular dystrophies. However, for several genetic syndromes, variations in phenotype remain unexplained.[1,27,28]

John Barrows: Outcome

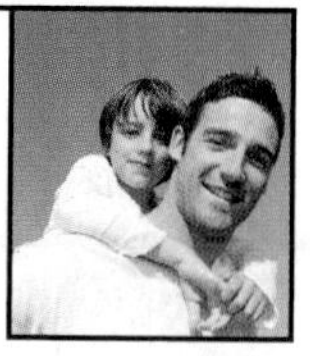

Mr. Barrows questions the possibility that he may be affected with NF1, since his clinical features are not identical to his son's. However, NF1 is known to have variable expressivity. Therefore, a diagnosis of NF1 cannot be ruled out for Mr. Barrows until he has had a medical genetics evaluation. He may have NF1 but have a milder clinical presentation than his son's.

3. How does variable expressivity explain Mr. Barrows's confusion about not having the same clinical features as his son for NF1?
4. What is the relationship between genotype and phenotype in Mr. Barrows and his son?

Check Your Progress: Section 2.7

1. How do single-gene disorders exhibit clinical variation?
2. What factors are involved in multifactorial disease presentation?

2.8 Genes and Neoplasia/Malignancies

The genetic basis of cancer warrants its own discussion, since cancer is always caused by a disruption of normal gene function, though this occurs in a number of ways. More information about the role of genetics and genomics in cancer can be found in Chapter 12 and in chapters throughout the book that cover specific types of cancers. Cancer most often occurs as a result of mutations in genes responsible for controlling cell growth. These genes generally fall into one of two categories: **proto-oncogenes** and **tumor suppressor genes**. Proto-oncogenes regulate cell proliferation. These genes may code for transcription factors, growth factors, or other growth-promoting agents. These genes become cancer-promoting (oncogene) when they acquire a gain of function, that is, when they are expressed more than they should be. Conversely, tumor suppressors are responsible for curbing cell growth. Loss of function of these genes promotes tumorogenesis.[29] Most hereditary cancer conditions are due to germ line mutations in tumor suppressor genes, especially those involved in DNA repair. Mutations in these genes predispose the person to cancer because of the inability to repair later-occurring mutations in other genes.[30]

Generally, cancer occurs after a series of mutations cause a particular group of cells to have unregulated growth. There are several mechanisms by which a regulatory gene can be disrupted. One mechanism is through a chromosome translocation (see Figure 2.14), in which the breakage and joining of two different chromosomes creates a fusion gene that promotes aberrant cell growth. The creation of genetic sequences that can target and bind the fusion gene is one basis of combating cancer with targeted medications.[1]

When a hereditary cancer is suspected, clinical genetic testing may be indicated. For example, while most cases of breast cancer are not due to a hereditary susceptibility, up to 5% of cases are due to autosomal dominant inheritance of a mutation in either the *BRCA1* or *BRCA2* gene. Having a *BRCA1* or *BRCA2* mutation confers a very high lifetime risk of both breast cancer and ovarian cancer. Even males with a *BRCA1* or *BRCA2* gene mutation have an increased risk of breast cancer. Early identification of a gene mutation may allow for enhanced screening and some prophylactic options for early detection and/or decreasing the risk of cancer.[1]

Michelle Kane: Application

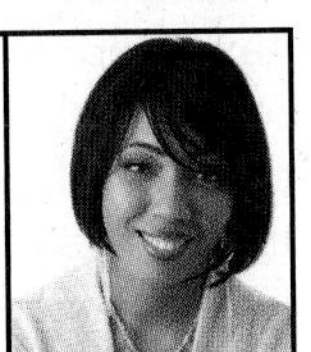

Ms. Kane has a valid concern about her risk for breast cancer. Cancer in multiple generations of a family with early ages of onset should trigger a concern for a hereditary cancer syndrome, such as hereditary breast and ovarian cancer caused by a mutation in either *BRCA1* or *BRCA2*. The later-onset breast cancer in Ms. Kane's paternal grandmother is less concerning in terms of a hereditary cause. A later-onset cancer is likely due to a series of acquired mutations in proto-oncogenes and tumor suppressor genes that ultimately led to carcinogenesis.

7. If Ms. Kane's mother has the *BRCA1* or *BRCA 2* gene, what is Ms. Kane's chance of having the breast cancer gene?
8. How would having the breast cancer gene change Ms. Kane's medical care?

Check Your Progress: Section 2.8

1. What is the role of mutations in proto-oncogenes and tumor suppressor genes in promoting cancer?
2. How does chromosome translocation cause cancer?
3. What is the cause of most hereditary cancers?

2.9 Genetic- and Genomic-based Diagnostic Tests

There is no single genetic test that will detect every type of genetic disorder or risk factor. Therefore, it is important to apply the appropriate genetic test for the situation and to ensure that results are properly interpreted and explained to patients. Genetic testing can occur at a wide range of ages, even at the earliest stage of development. **Preimplantation genetic diagnosis** involves the screening of embryos that are produced through in vitro fertilization for the presence of genetic or chromosome abnormalities. The embryos that do not carry the genetic error can be implanted in the mother's uterus. Genetic testing can raise ethical issues. For example, it is not appropriate to offer genetic testing in childhood for an adult-onset hereditary cancer syndrome, especially if there are no preventive measures that can be taken during childhood. Different categories of genetic testing are reviewed here.

Cytogenetics

Cytogenetics is a laboratory field involving the characterization of chromosome structure and number. **Karyotyping** is a test used to examine the visual appearance of chromosome structure and number (see **Figure 2.21** ■). This type of genetic testing can identify aneuploidy and triploidy as well as translocations and other gross chromosomal structural abnormalities. However, it cannot detect single-gene mutations.

Fluorescence in situ hybridization (FISH) has been utilized both for rapid detection of chromosome number and for targeting specific DNA sequences. This test can detect small deletions or structural abnormalities that are not seen in standard karyotyping. In this process, a probe that has the target DNA sequence will attach to the chromosome if the sequence is present. A fluorescent tag on the probe signals when the DNA sequence has been identified. If a FISH test shows three signals for a chromosome 21 probe, then this indicates trisomy 21 (Down syndrome). Similarly, failure of the probe to attach indicates a chromosome deletion.[1]

Single-gene Testing

Single-gene sequencing is designed to detect nucleotide changes anywhere in the gene. A limitation of sequencing is it will not detect deletions or rearrangements. Other technologies, such as Southern blotting, are used to detect deletions and rearrangements. The many techniques used to detect different types of single-gene mutations are not explored here, as that is beyond the scope of this textbook. However, new technologies to detect different types of single-gene mutations are constantly evolving, including simultaneous multigene panel testing by using next-generation sequencing.

Michelle Kane: Outcome

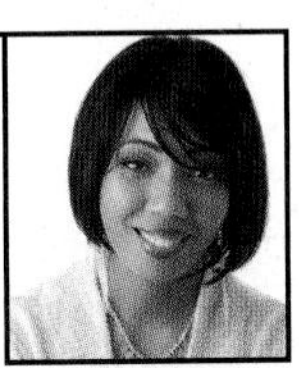

Ms. Kane was not certain which genetic tests had already been performed on her. The genetic testing that was done when she was pregnant would not have included the *BRCA* genes. That test was most likely a prenatal diagnostic test to look for chromosome abnormalities in her fetus. Pretest informed consent is critical to obtain so that patients are aware of what a test can identify and its limitations.

9. What is an ethical issue that might arise from testing a child for an adult-onset genetic disorder such as *BRCA*-related breast cancer?
10. If Ms. Kane had prenatal karyotyping, what type of abnormalities might be detected in the fetus?

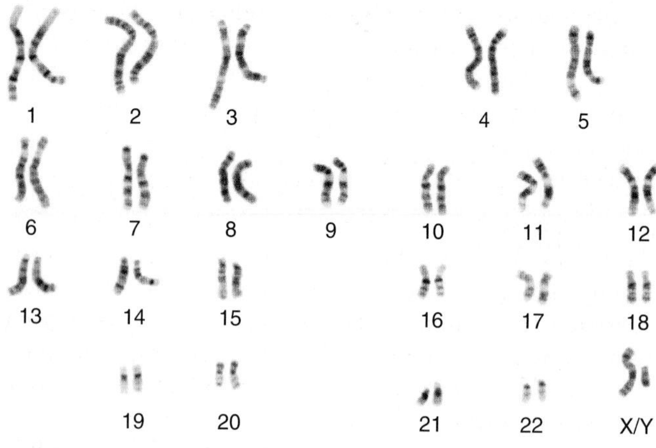

Figure 2.21 ■ Normal karyotype of a human male.

Gene Expression Testing

Gene expression tests evaluate how expression levels affect cell function and influence progression of disease by measuring the mRNA produced. For example, patterns of expression that are not amenable to chemotherapy can allow some cancer patients to be spared from having ineffective chemotherapy and suffering from its severe adverse effects.[31]

Genetic Detection of Infections

Genetic technologies have many applications beyond looking for hereditary disease. Many infectious microorganisms, particularly viruses, can be identified in the human body by their genetic sequence. Like humans, infectious agents such as bacteria and viruses employ DNA and RNA to encode their functions. Specific chemical or radioactively labeled genetic probes can be created to identify their genetic sequence.

There are a number of clinical and investigative applications based on the polymerase chain reaction (PCR). These techniques are used to detect a sequence of interest, even in very small amounts.[1,32] PCR is used to monitor the viral load and its response to medications in individuals infected with the human immunodeficiency virus. Many medications made to combat infectious agents are created by targeting its genetic sequence. In response, infectious agents often acquire drug resistance by altering a single nucleotide of their gene sequence and thus escape recognition by a particular medication. Molecular techniques are also useful in identifying these single-nucleotide changes to identify the potential for drug resistance.[1,32]

Check Your Progress: Section 2.9

1. What is the rationale for preimplantation genetic testing?
2. What type of information can be gained from karyotyping?
3. What are the indications for fluorescence in situ hybridization (FISH)?

2.10 Linking Pathophysiology to Treatment: Genetic- and Genomic-based Therapies

Gene Replacement Therapy

A major focus on gene replacement therapy began in the 1990s. The idea behind this therapy was to express or silence genes that are implicated in disease processes. DNA or RNA is engineered to be delivered (often via virus) into an individual so that target cells take up the gene and then express its protein product. Over the years, researchers have modified viral vectors to preserve only minimal components of the viral genome, allowing space to package the therapeutic recombinant DNA or RNA and deliver it to the target cells of interest.[33] While this therapy seems promising, challenges include the potential for harm from the virus itself and having the healthy gene integrate itself before getting cleared by the body.[34]

Pharmacogenomics and Personalized Medicine

Variability in drug efficacy and safety among individuals is a major challenge in clinical practice, drug development, and drug regulation. The discipline that blends pharmacology with genomic capabilities is called **pharmacogenomics**. A recent focus has been on identifying genetic variants in drug metabolic pathways to predict medication response, allowing for customized prescribing based on genotype.

The U.S. Food and Drug Administration maintains a list of approved drugs for which pharmacogenomic information is available, allowing for personalized treatment plans as a standard practice. Screening known biomarkers allows for prediction of treatment tolerance, risk for toxicity, and dose response before starting chemotherapy and facilitates making appropriate dose adjustments or choice of drug.[35] Additionally, non–cancer drugs such as warfarin, valproic acid, and acetaminophen all have readily accessible pharmacogenomics information in their prescribing information.

Bianca Vasquez: Outcome

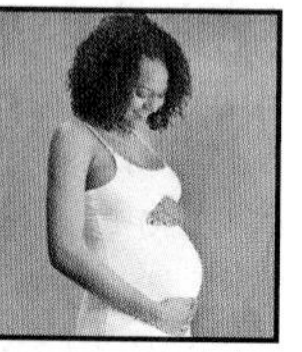

Mrs. Vasquez, who wants to minimize the chance that her baby will inherit her allergies, was informed that research is ongoing to further understand the underlying mechanisms of fish oil use and why results of taking fish oil supplements vary from person to person.

3. How can the study of pharmacogenetics help Mrs. Vasquez reduce her baby's risk of inheriting her allergies.
4. What resource is available to provide pharmacogenetic information?

Antisense Oligonucleotides

Cancer treatments have been developed in which an **antisense oligonucleotide** (sequence of complementary nucleotides) is used to directly bind the DNA or RNA to block the aberrant gene product. Gleevec (Imatinib) is the most publicized example of this approach in the treatment of chronic myelogenous leukemia, which is caused by the *BCR-ABL* fusion gene,[36] and it has now has been investigated for its therapeutic use in other cancers.[37]

Transcription Factor Modulation

Transcription factor modulators selectively increase or decrease transcription levels of certain genes. The corticosteroid prednisone can have beneficial anti-inflammatory effects but also detrimental weight gain and bone loss. Not being cell specific, transcription modulation must be used carefully, considering the potential side effects,[38] but these may be limited in the future by cell-specific targeting.[39]

Check Your Progress: Section 2.10

1. What is the pharmacogenomics?
2. Describe the action of antisense oligonucleotides in the treatment of cancer.
3. What are the limitations of transcription factor modulators?

2.11 Advances in Human Genomics

Genomic technologies have become dramatically cheaper and faster. Readouts of 250 billion bases of DNA, compared to only 25,000 in 1990, can now be generated within 1 week, allowing more efficient gene and disease pathway discovery. Since the completion of the Human Genome Project, more than 1800 disease-associated genes have been identified, and some 2000 diagnostic genetic tests are now available. With data and technologies generated from the Human Genome Project, a worldwide collaborative study of different ancestries to develop a haplotype map of the human genome, called the International HapMap Project, was undertaken.

International HapMap Project

A haplotype is a set of alleles on the same chromosome that are tightly linked and usually transmitted together during meiosis. The Human Genome Project revealed that humans are genetically 99.9% identical, and the International HapMap Project focuses on analyzing the 0.1% of the genomic elements that make us different from one another.[40] Data from the International HapMap Project revealed 3.1 million common SNPs in the human genome across geographically diverse populations.[41] These projects have profound implications for understanding human biology and for detection of risk factors and diagnosis of both rare and common disorders.

Genome-wide Association Studies

Genome-wide association studies (GWAS) are genomic tests used in both research and clinical practice that were originally designed to identify relationships between common genome variation and particular traits of interest. GWAS seek to identify SNPs that are associated with specific traits. Recent technologic innovations, specifically hybridization technology using DNA microarrays, have allowed hundreds of thousands of SNPs to be analyzed simultaneously in a GWAS.[42]

A microarray is a glass chip with targeted DNA probes that is used to examine genetic changes or gene expression levels of thousands of genes at once instead of having to test each individually. This can be clinically useful when there are several possible genes associated with a given disease. Because of the thousands of genes that can be studied at once using GWAS, it is referred to as high-throughput technology. In GWAS, DNA samples from a large number of healthy (control) and diseased (case) individuals are obtained and then color labeled. Equal amounts of genomic DNA from the control and case samples are then hybridized to the same microarray chip. Identical portions of the two genomes are be visualized as yellow (versus red or green) on a DNA probe, making it easy to identify where the two genomes are similar and different, with sophisticated statistical procedures and software utilized to identify significant differences. When the study is carefully designed and implemented, results of GWAS can identify common genomic variants that contribute to complex traits and disorders.

Descriptions of the increasing clinical applications of GWAS relevant to both rare and common disorders can be found at the Genome Advance of the Month section at the National Human Genome Research Institute's website, with more being reported every month. The June 2011 article titled "Transforming Clinical Care with Whole Genome Sequencing" described situations in which GWAS saved the lives of individuals when other diagnostic tests had not detected their disorder. In one case, a 4-year-old boy was severely underweight at 20 pounds with life-threatening colon ulcerations and fistulas that caused fecal material to collect under his skin. He was thought to have an inflammatory bowel disease resembling Crohn disease, but the usual treatment did not provide long-term improvement. Despite numerous evaluations, surgical procedures, antibiotics, blood transfusions, and an episode of life-threatening sepsis, standard diagnostic tests did not identify the cause. Finally, a GWAS identified a rare X-linked inhibitor of apoptosis deficiency that caused increased apoptosis (programmed cell death) in the child's intestinal cells leading to the ulcerations as well as accelerated death of his immune cells. He was treated with hematopoietic stem cell transplantation, and 42 days after transplantation, he was able to eat and drink normally with no recurrence of intestinal symptoms.[43]

In another report, the use of GWAS allowed discovery of a new disease in which affected individuals have calcifications in the arteries of their lower extremities and hands that obstruct blood flow. GWAS identified a mutation that caused increased levels of the enzyme alkaline phosphatase that resulted in calcium phosphate deposits in their arteries, and the affected individuals were able to be treated successfully.[44]

Check Your Progress: Section 2.11

1. What are the health implications of genome-wide association studies (GWAS)?
2. What is a haplotype?
3. What are the implications of the International HapMap Project?

CHAPTER SUMMARY

2.1 Chapter Overview and Case Studies

Describe the impact of genetics, genomics, and epigenomics on personalized healthcare, and explain the concepts related to them.

- Genetics is the study of individual genes, their impact on inheritance, and single-gene and chromosomal disorders.
- Genomics is the study of all genes in the structure, function, and analysis of the human genome together.

2.2 Molecular Basis of Gene Expression

Identify components of the genetic code and the organization of genes on chromosomes.

- The genetic code in DNA is made up of four nucleotides (adenine, guanine, cytosine, thymine), which are used to create the sequence for each gene. The genome is the complete set of DNA for an individual.
- Two DNA strands are bound together to create a double helix, which wraps around histones and is compacted to form chromosomes.
- Each chromosome contains a large amount of DNA and thousands of genes.
- Humans have a total of 46 chromosomes in most cells in their body. Egg and sperm cells contain one chromosome of each pair for a total of 23 chromosomes each. When egg and sperm combine, the resulting cell has a total of 46 chromosomes.

2.3 The Human Genome, Genomics, and Epigenomics

Understand the differences between the human genome and epigenome and the mechanisms by which epigenetic modifications occur and affect gene expression.

- The Human Genome Project identified and mapped the location of all genes in the human genome.
- The epigenome consists of factors that regulate gene expression without changing the genetic code.

2.4 Gene Replication, Transcription, and Translation

Explain the function and sequence of events involved in gene replication during mitosis and meiosis, transcription, and translation.

- The process of cell division that is used to create identical copies of a cell is called mitosis.
- The cell division process that is used to place genetic material in the gonadal cells is called meiosis.
- There are three types of RNA: Messenger RNA (mRNA) carries information from DNA in the nucleus to the ribosome. Transfer RNA (tRNA) transfers amino acids to mRNA on the ribosome. Ribosomal RNA (rRNA) is in charge of synthesizing ribosomes.
- Transcription involves creating mRNA from a template strand of DNA.
- Translation uses RNA as a template to create a series of amino acids, which are then used to create a protein product.

2.5 Mutations

Compare single-nucleotide polymorphisms and the various types of gene mutations, including point mutations, insertions, deletions, and translocations, in regard to their characteristics and possible clinical consequences.

- A mutation is a coding error in a gene. A point mutation is a change in one nucleotide of a gene sequence. If the amino acid is not changed by a point mutation, then the change is a silent mutation. If the amino acid is changed, then this is a missense mutation. If the amino acid change results in a stop codon, then this is a nonsense mutation.
- Insertion and deletion of nucleotides in a gene will almost always have serious consequences.

2.6 Categories of Genetic Disorders

Compare the characteristics and patterns of inheritance of genetic disorders caused by abnormalities of chromosome number or structure to those caused by autosomal, X-linked, and mitochondrial disorders.

- Genotype is the genetic code. Phenotype is the expression of the genetic code but is also affected by environmental factors that affect gene expression.
- Most human disease is a result of an interaction between both genes and environment.
- The most basic type of genetic disorder results from an abnormality in chromosome number or structure.
- Many genetic disorders are the result of a mutation in a single gene.
- There are four main inheritance patterns: autosomal dominant, autosomal recessive, X-linked recessive, and mitochondrial.
- A Punnett square is used to predict the percentage of children who are likely to inherit a particular genotype based on the genotype of their parents.
- A genetic pedigree is drawn through several generations so that the pattern of genetic disease can be visualized.

2.7 Phenotypic Variations in Human Disease

Differentiate the mechanisms responsible for phenotypic variations in human disease.

- Multifactorial diseases depend on multiple genes as well as environmental influences. Therefore, there are bound to be variations in how individuals present with disease.
- Single-gene disorders can also have quite a bit of variation in clinical presentation, owing to reduced penetrance and variable expressivity.
- The reasons for variations in phenotype in many diseases remain unexplained.

2.8 Genes and Neoplasia/ Malignancies

Understand the role of genetic and epigenomic factors in cancer.

- All cancers are caused by disruption of normal gene function that results in excessive cell division.
- Some viruses cause cancer by activating a proto-oncogene.
- Most cancers that have a hereditary basis are the result of germ line mutation in tumor suppressor genes or genes involved in repair of DNA.
- Clinical genetic testing for some hereditary cancer syndromes is available.

2.9 Genetic- and Genomic-based Diagnostic Tests

Apply the following tests to the appropriate clinical situation: karyotyping, fluorescence in situ hybridization, single-gene testing, and genome-wide association studies.

- Cytogenetics uses tests such as karyotyping and fluorescence in situ hybridization (FISH) to detect alterations in chromosome number and structure.
- Single-gene tests detect alterations in nucleotide sequence. Gene expression tests detect the level of products produced.
- Genetic technologies, such as PCR, are used to detect and quantify certain microorganisms in the body.

2.10 Linking Pathophysiology to Treatment: Genetic- and Genomic-based Therapies

Apply the following genetic-based therapies to appropriate clinical situations: gene replacement therapy, pharmacogenomics, antisense nucleotides, and transcription factor modulation.

- Genetic-based therapies include gene replacement therapy, in which a normal gene is carried into cells by viral vector; treatment with antisense oligonucleotides, which bind to DNA or RNA to prevent protein production; and transcription factor modulation, which is used to activate or suppress protein production.
- Pharmacogenomics studies how genetic variants affect an individual's drug metabolic pathways in order to predict medication responses with the goals of providing the most effective treatment and minimizing adverse drug effects.

2.11 Advances in Human Genomics

Analyze the impact of advances in genomics and epigenomics on personalized healthcare.

- Genome-wide association studies (GWAS) are used to identify the relationships between the most common type of genome variation and particular traits of interest.

REVIEW QUESTIONS

1. The nurse is caring for a client with neurofibromatosis. Which statement by the client indicates that further teaching is needed?
   a. "I can't pass this disorder on to my children."
   b. "The disease may show up differently in my children."
   c. "Café-au-lait spots are harmless signs of the disease."
   d. "The disease can cause neurofibromas."

2. A pregnant woman underwent genetic testing and was told that her fetus has aneuploidy. On the basis of this information, the nurse explains that:
   a. the pregnancy will end in a miscarriage.
   b. a mutation of a single cell is present.
   c. the cells have an abnormal number of chromosomes.
   d. there will be no clinically significant consequences.
3. Genetic testing indicates that a pregnant woman is the carrier of an autosomal dominant gene mutation but her partner does not carry the gene. Which of the following would the nurse explain to the woman and her partner?
   a. There is a 25% chance that the child will have the disease.
   b. There is a 50% chance that the child will have the disease.
   c. There is a 100% chance that the child will manifest the disease.
   d. There is no chance that the child will manifest the disease.
4. Genetic testing indicates that one partner has an X-linked disease. The nurse explains that:
   a. a son will manifest the disease.
   b. a daughter will have a more severe form of the disease.
   c. a son will inherit the disease from his father.
   d. a daughter can receive the disease only from her mother.
5. The genetic counselor is explaining preimplantation genetic diagnosis to a couple. Which of the following does the counselor tell the couple?
   a. It involves genetic testing of both partners before conception.
   b. It involves screening embryos that are produced through in vitro fertilization.
   c. It involves the screening of eggs before in vitro fertilization.
   d. It involves intrauterine genetic testing of the fetus.
6. Genetic testing reveals that both parents are carriers of an autosomal recessive gene mutation. Which of the following statement made by a parent indicates understanding of the nurse's teaching?
   a. "There's a 25% chance that our baby will manifest the recessive disorder."
   b. "There's a 50% chance that our baby will manifest the recessive disorder."
   c. "There's a 100% chance that our baby will manifest the recessive disorder."
   d. "There's no chance that our baby will manifest the recessive disorder."
7. The nurse is teaching two parents who are both carriers for an autosomal recessive disorder. The nurse explains that which of the following will be used to determine the chance that each child will manifest the disorder?
   a. Pedigree
   b. Punnett square
   c. Karyotype
   d. FISH
8. Which of the following statements would be made by the nurse to a patient with an X-linked disorder?
   a. "Females mainly utilize one of their two X chromosomes."
   b. "Males do not use their X chromosome."
   c. "The X chromosome carries most of the same genes as the Y chromosome."
   d. "Females inactivate both of their X chromosomes."

ANSWERS

Answers to Review Questions can be found in Appendix A. Answers to Case Study and Check Your Progress questions are available on the faculty resources site. Please consult with your instructor.

RECOMMENDED WEBSITES

Centers for Disease Control and Prevention: Public Health Genomics
https://www.cdc.gov/genomics/resources/index.htm

Cincinnati Children's Hospital Medical Center: Genetics Education Program for Nurses
https://www.cincinnatichildrens.org/education/clinical/nursing/genetics

Genetic Testing Registry
https://www.ncbi.nlm.nih.gov/sites/gtr

Genetics 101 for Health Care Professionals
https://www.genome.gov/27527637

International Society of Nurses in Genetics
http://www.isong.org/index.php

Medscape Genomic Medicine Resource Center
http://www.medscape.com/resource/genomic-medicine

National Human Genome Research Institute of NIH (NHGRI)
https://www.genome.gov

Oncology Nursing Society: Genetics Clinical Resource Area
https://www.ons.org/tags/genetics-and-genomics-0

REFERENCES

1. Nussbaum, R., McInnes, R., and Willard, H. (2016). *Thompson and Thompson genetics in medicine* (8th ed.). New York, NY: Elsevier.
2. Skorecki, K., & Mandel, H. (2015). Mitochondrial DNA and heritable traits and diseases. In A. Fauci, E. Braunwald, D. Kasper, et al. (Eds.), *Harrison's principles of internal medicine* (19th ed.). New York, NY: McGraw-Hill.
3. Balaton, B. P., & Brown, C. J. (2016). Escape artists of the X chromosome. *Trends in Genetics, 32*(6), 348–359.
4. Collins, F., Morgan, M., & Patrinos, A. (2003). The Human Genome Project: Lessons from large-scale biology. *Science, 300*(5617), 286–290.
5. Wu, C. T., & Morris, J. R. (2001). Genes, genetics, and epigenetics: A correspondence. *Science, 293*(5532), 1103–1105.
6. Wolff, G. L., Kodell, R. L., Moore, S. R., & Cooney, C. A. (1998). Maternal epigenetics and methyl supplements affect agouti gene expression in Avy/a mice. *FASEB Journal, 12*, 949–957.
7. Waterland, R. A., & Jirtle, R. L. (2003). Transposable elements: Targets for early nutritional effects on epigenetic gene regulation. *Molecular and Cellular Biology, 23*, 5293–5300.
8. Dolinoy, D. C., & Jirtle, R. L. (2008). Environmental epigenomics in human health and disease. *Environmental and Molecular Mutagenesis, 49*(1), 4–8.
9. Jirtle, R., & Skinner, M. (2007). Environmental epigenomics and disease susceptibility. *Nature Reviews Genetics, 8*(4), 253–262.
10. Thorvaldsen, J. L., Verona, R. I., & Bartolomei, M. S. (2006). X-tra! X-tra! News from the mouse X chromosome. *Developmental Biology, 298*, 344–353.
11. Huynh, K. D., & Lee, J. T. (2005). X-chromosome inactivation: A hypothesis linking ontogeny and phylogeny. *Nature Reviews Genetics, 6*, 410–418.
12. Lewis, A., & Reik, W. (2006). How imprinting centres work. *Cytogenetic and Genome Research, 113*, 81–89.
13. Reik, W., & Walter, J. (2001). Genomic imprinting: Parental influence on the genome. *Nature Reviews Genetics, 2*, 21–32.
14. Bahrami S., & Drabløs F. (2016). Gene regulation in the immediate-early response process. *Advances in Biological Regulation, 62*, 37–49.
15. Deutschman, C. (2005). Transcription. *Critical Care Medicine, 33*(12), S400–S403.
16. van den Hoogenhof, M. M., Pinto, Y. M., & Creemers, E. E. (2016). RNA splicing: Regulation and dysregulation in the heart. *Circulation Research, 118*(3), 454–468.
17. Rodnina, M. V. (2016). The ribosome in action: Tuning of translational efficiency and protein folding. *Protein Science, 25*(8), 1390–1406.
18. Ott, J., Kamatani, Y., & Lathrop, M. (2011). Family-based designs for genome-wide association studies. *Nature Reviews Genetics, 12*(7), 465–474.
19. Jiang, Z., Wang, H., Michal, J. J., Zhou, X., Liu, B., Woods, L., & Fuchs R. A. (2016). Genome wide sampling sequencing for SNP genotyping: Methods, challenges and future development. *International Journal of Biological Sciences, 12*(1), 100–108.
20. Metcalfe, A., Hippman, C., Pastuck, M., & Johnson, J. A. (2014). Beyond trisomy 21: Additional chromosomal anomalies detected through routine aneuploidy screening. *Journal of Clinical Medicine, 3*(2), 388–415.
21. Chard, R. L., & Norton, M. E. (2016). Genetic counseling for patients considering screening and diagnosis for chromosomal abnormalities. *Clinics in Laboratory Medicine, 36*(2), 227–236.
22. Witters, G., Van Robays, J., Willekes, C., Coumans, A., Peeters, H., Gyselaers, W., & Fryns, J. P. (2011). Trisomy 13, 18, 21, triploidy and Turner syndrome: The 5T's. Look at the hands. *Facts Views & Vision in ObGyn, 3*(1), 15–21.
23. Evans, M. I., Andriole, S., & Evans, S. M. (2015). Genetics: Update on prenatal screening and diagnosis. *Obstetrics & Gynecology Clinics of North America, 242*(2), 193–208.
24. Bird, R. J., & Hurren, B. J. (2016). Anatomical and clinical aspects of Klinefelter's syndrome. *Clinical Anatomy, 29*(5), 606–619.
25. Mishra, P., & Chan, D. C. (2014). Mitochondrial dynamics and inheritance during cell division, development and disease. *Nature Reviews Molecular Cell Biology, 15*(10), 634–646.
26. Legaki, E., & Gazouli, M. (2016). Influence of environmental factors in the development of inflammatory bowel diseases. *World Journal of Gastrointestinal Pharmacology and Therapeutics, 7*(1), 112–125.
27. Campos, F. G. (2014). Surgical treatment of familial adenomatous polyposis: Dilemmas and current recommendations. *World Journal of Gastroenterology, 20*(44), 16620–16629.
28. Mah, J. K., Korngut, L., Dykeman, J., Day, L., Pringsheim, T., & Jette, N. (2014). A systematic review and meta-analysis on the epidemiology of Duchenne and Becker muscular dystrophy. *Neuromuscular Disorders, 24*(6), 482–491.
29. Abreu Velez, A. M., & Howard, M. S. (2015). Tumor-suppressor genes, cell cycle regulatory checkpoints, and the skin. *North American Journal of Medical Sciences, 7*(5), 176–188.
30. Prakash, R., Zhang, Y., Feng, W., & Jasin, M. (2015). Homologous recombination and human health: the roles of BRCA1, BRCA2, and associated proteins. *Cold Spring Harbor Perspectives in Biology, 7*(4), a016600.
31. Schmidt, K. T., Chau, C. H., Price, D. K., & Figg, W. D. (2016). Precision oncology medicine: The clinical relevance of patient specific biomarkers used to optimize cancer treatment. *Journal of Clinical Pharmacology, 56*(12), 1484–1499.
32. Agut, H., Bonnafous, P., & Gautheret-Dejean, A. (2015). Laboratory and clinical aspects of human herpesvirus 6 infections. *Clinical Microbiology Reviews, 28*(2), 313–335.
33. Ferrari, F., Xiao, X., McCarty, D., & Samulski, R. (1997). New developments in the generation of Ad-free, high-titer rAAV gene therapy vectors. *Nature Medicine, 3*(11), 1295–1297.
34. Quasim, W., Gaspar, H., & Thrasher, A. (2007). Update on clinical gene therapy in childhood. *Archive of Disease in Childhood, 92*, 1028–1031.
35. U.S. Department of Health and Human Services. (2017). *Table of pharmacogenomic biomarkers in drug labeling*. Available at https://www.fda.gov/drugs/scienceresearch/researchareas/pharmacogenetics/ucm083378.htm
36. Fausel, C. (2007). Targeted chronic myeloid leukemia therapy: Seeking a cure. *American Journal of Health-System Pharmacy, 64*(Suppl. 15), S9–S15.

37. Oosteron, A., Judson, I., Verweij, J., et al. (2001). Safety and efficacy of imatinib (STI571) in metastatic gastrointestinal stromal tumors: A phase I study. *Lancet, 358*, 421–1423.
38. Janeway, C., Travers, P., Walport, M., et al. (2001). *Immunobiology* (5th ed.). New York, NY: Elsevier.
39. Morishita, R., Gibbons, G., Horiuchi, M., et al. (1995). A gene therapy strategy using a transcription factor decoy of the E2F binding site inhibits smooth muscle proliferation in vivo. *Proceedings of the National Academy of Sciences, 92*, 5855–5859.
40. International HapMap Consortium. (2003). The International HapMap Project. *Nature (London), 426*(6968), 789–796.
41. Frazer, K., Ballinger, D., Cox, D., et al. (2007). A second generation human haplotype map of over 3.1 million SNPs. *Nature (London), 449*(7164), 851–861.
42. Hinds D. A., et al. (2005). Whole-genome patterns of common DNA variation in three human populations. *Science, 307*, 1072–1079.
43. Worthey, E., Mayer, A., Syverson, G., et al. (2011). Making a definitive diagnosis: Successful clinical application of whole exome sequencing in a child with intractable inflammatory bowel disease. *Genetics in Medicine, 13*(3), 255–262. doi:10.1097/GIM.0b013e3182088158
44. St. Hilarie, C., Ziegler, S., Markello, T., et al. (2011). NT5E mutations and arterial calcifications. *New England Journal of Medicine, 364*, 432–442.

Chapter 3

Environmental Health Influences on Disease and Injury

Jeanne Beauchamp Hewitt, Pamela F. Levin, and Omar Al-Rawajfah

Chapter Outline and Learning Outcomes

3.1 Chapter Overview and Case Studies

Describe the relationship between social environment, physical environment, built environment, genetic endowment, and health outcomes, and discuss concepts related to environmental health.

3.2 Environmental Hazard Classification

Classify environmental hazards according to their nature, transport media, routes of exposure, and outcomes.

3.3 Key Concepts of Environmental Health from Related Sciences

Discuss how key concepts from environmental health related sciences are applied in the assessment, intervention, and evaluation process to control or prevent environmental health problems.

3.4 Environmental Epidemiology

Explain how environmental epidemiology is used to understand and protect the health of individuals, communities, and populations regarding environmental hazards.

3.5 Pathophysiologic Mechanisms

Explain the basic pathophysiologic mechanisms underlying alterations caused by environmental hazards.

3.6 Hazards and Health Effects of Environmental Agents

Analyze the relationship between various hazardous agents and the health effects they produce.

KEY TERMS

Built environment, 48
Dose-response relationship, 63
Engineering controls, 62
Environmental hazard, 51
Environmental health, 48
First-pass effect, 63
Industrial hygiene, 62
Mode of transmission, 61
Physical environment, 48
Precautionary principle, 71
Protective factors, 53
Risk assessment, 71
Risk factors, 53
Route of exposure, 52
Sentinel health event, 54
Social environment, 48
Surveillance, 53
Susceptibility, 59
Toxicant, 49
Transport media, 52
Vulnerability, 59
Xenobiotics, 61

ABBREVIATIONS

NHANES—National Health and Nutrition Examination Survey
PCBs—polychlorinated biphenyls
PPE—personal protective equipment
ppm—parts per million

3.1 Chapter Overview and Case Studies

This chapter presents a framework and key concepts for understanding environmental health. Health practitioners use this knowledge base to recognize, control, and prevent diseases, injuries, and other problems related to environmental factors. Three case studies illustrate how healthcare professionals can apply the knowledge base generated from epidemiology, microbiology, toxicology, industrial hygiene, and environmental health. To aid in recognizing environmental and occupational health hazards, the chapter also reviews prevalent biological, chemical, physical, and psychosocial agents and their health effects.

Definition of Environmental Health

The National Environmental Health Association defines **environmental health** as "the science and practice of preventing human injury and illness and promoting well-being by identifying and evaluating environmental sources and hazardous agents and limiting exposures to hazardous physical, chemical, and biological agents in air, water, soil, food, and other environmental media or settings that may adversely affect human health."[1] This definition includes as parts of the environment not only the outdoors, but also the insides of homes, workplaces, schools, and other enclosed community settings. As defined, environment affects the health of both individuals and populations. **Figure 3.1** ■ illustrates the dynamic effects of the environment on the health of individuals, communities, and populations.

Individual Level

According to the classic Evans and Stoddart ecological model (see Figure 3.1), the social and physical environments are key determinants of an individual's health.[2] The **social environment** includes both social and psychosocial factors in the environment such as gender, education, employment status, social networks, and interpersonal interactions. The **physical environment** includes the places where people live, work, and play. The physical environment can interact with the individual's genetic endowment, called gene–environment interaction,[3] as well as with other factors. In addition to gene–environment interactions, there is increasing interest in understanding the role of environmental chemicals in inducing nongenomic imprinting (e.g., DNA methylation, which alters transcription) that changes phenotypic expression from parent to offspring and subsequent generations in the absence of further exposure.[4,5] This is called epigenetic transgenerational inheritance.[5]

Community Level

At the local community level, the social environment includes neighborhood and community factors such as social networks and resources (social capital) as well as the level of shared commitment toward and respect for the values and rights of others (social cohesion). Also included in the social environment are the general level of wealth or impoverishment of the community, the level of psychosocial stress, and the availability and accessibility of goods (e.g., sufficient food) and services, including health and education. The physical environment at the community level includes air and water quality; nutritional quality and safety, which in turn depend on the quality of soil, air, and water; and the built environment. The **built environment** is human-made (rather than natural) conditions of housing and other buildings; transportation of goods and people, including transportation systems (e.g., public transportation, streets and highways); physical safety hazards (e.g., traffic patterns, violence); and accessibility to recreational venues such as parks, sidewalks, and paths. Together, the social and physical environments of local communities affect the health of populations.

Population Level

At the population level, the sum of the effects of environmental factors can be dramatic. For example, within the framework of pathophysiology, environmental factors contribute significantly to 83% of the 102 major diseases, injuries, and fatalities tracked by the World Health Organization.[6] Nearly three fourths of the global burden of disease and death is attributed to 22 conditions; the leading causes include acute respiratory illnesses, diarrhea, perinatal

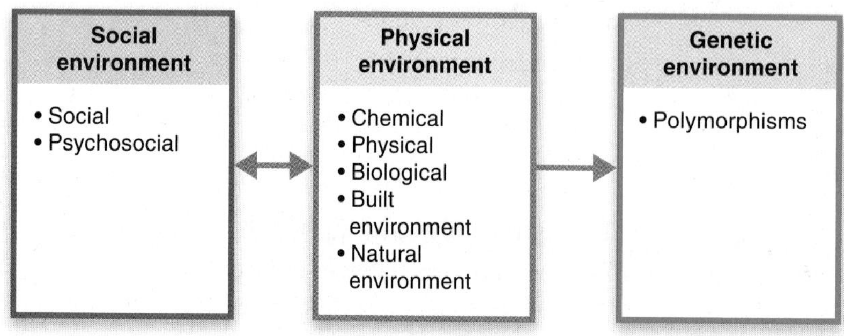

Figure 3.1 ■ Ecological model for environmental health.

SOURCE: Based on Evans, R. G., & Stoddart, C. J. (1990). Producing health, consuming health care. *Social Science and Medicine, 31*, 1347–1363.

conditions, vaccine-preventable infections in children, cancer, depression, ischemic heart disease, and cerebral vascular disease.[7] Excluding personal behaviors such as cigarette smoking, the environment causes approximately 8–10% of all ischemic heart disease through air pollution and occupational exposures. Environmental determinants such as housing conditions and air pollution, which include environmental tobacco smoke (secondhand smoke), cause 40–60% of acute respiratory illnesses. Environmental hazards contribute substantially to the global burden of disease and injury.[8,9]

Nationally, environmental health is a prominent component of the Healthy People initiative. One of the four overarching goals for *Healthy People 2020* is "creating social and physical environments that promote good health for all."[10] Fifty percent of the 42 topic areas specifically target environmental health or incorporate environmental health objectives aimed at reducing associated risk of disease, injury, or death.

Concepts Related to Environmental Health

The environment is related to many other concepts, as is depicted in **Figure 3.2** ■. Air quality has a major impact on pulmonary function and thus on oxygenation. Inhalation of chemicals such as carbon monoxide, air pollutants, and cigarette smoke contribute to a variety of lung diseases, including asthma, emphysema, and lung cancers. Inhalation of pathogenic bacteria, viruses, or fungi in the environment can result in pulmonary infections.

Certain environmental **toxicants** (toxic substances) contribute to development of atherosclerosis and its complications, including hypertension, ischemic heart disease, and

Healthy People 2020

Environmental Health

Goal: "Promote health for all through a healthy environment."[1]

Overview: "Humans interact with the environment constantly. These interactions affect quality of life, years of healthy life lived, and health disparities. Environmental health consists of preventing or controlling disease, injury, and disability related to the interactions between people and their environment."[1] According to a World Health Organization news release on March 15, 2016, approximately 12.6 million people died in 2012 as a result of living or working in an unhealthy environment, which accounts for nearly one in four deaths worldwide.[2]

Objectives: There are 24 Healthy People objectives that target the following six environmental health issues.

1. ***Outdoor Air Quality:*** Air pollution contributes to premature death from cancer and from cardiovascular and respiratory diseases. Improvement in air quality is still needed. In 2015, approximately 121 million people lived in U.S. counties that did not meet the national standards for air quality.[3] Healthy People objectives to improve air quality include increased use of alternative modes of transportation such as walking, bicycling, and mass transit to decrease emissions from motor vehicles.
2. ***Surface and Ground Water Quality:*** Surface water and ground water include water used for drinking and recreation, such as aquifers, lakes, and oceans. Environmental hazards, including infectious organisms and toxic chemicals in water, can cause acute or chronic illness. Examples of Healthy People objectives related to water quality are to increase the number of people served by drinking water that meets the standards set by the Safe Drinking Water Act[4] and to increase the number of days when beaches are open and safe.
3. ***Toxic Substances and Hazardous Wastes:*** Objectives in this area include reductions in lead blood levels in children, illness-related pesticide exposures, and pollutants released into the air.
4. ***Healthy Homes and Communities:*** To improve the quality of home and community environments, Healthy People objectives include reduction of indoor mouse and cockroach allergens, increasing the percentage of new homes built with radon-reducing features in areas with high radon risk, and increasing the percentage of schools that have policies and practices that promote a healthy school environment.
5. ***Infrastructure and Surveillance:*** Healthy People objectives related to infrastructure and surveillance include increasing the number of U.S. states, districts, and territories that monitor for diseases that can be caused by lead, pesticides, mercury, arsenic, cadmium, and carbon monoxide poisonings.
6. ***Global Environmental Health:*** Safe water is a global issue not only for individuals who travel to other countries, but also because of the impact of water quality on domestic and foreign food sources and the fact that some lakes, oceans, and rivers are shared by different countries. The one Healthy People objective related to this issue is reduction of the global burden of diseases caused by poor water quality, sanitation, and insufficient hygiene.

Current levels and specific targets related to all the environmental health objectives are located at the *Healthy People 2020* website.[5]

References

1. Healthy People 2020. (2017). Environmental health overview. Available at https://www.healthypeople.gov/2020/topics-objectives/topic/environmental-health
2. World Health Organization. (2016). An estimated 12.6 million deaths each year are attributable to unhealthy environments. Available at http://www.who.int/mediacentre/news/releases/2016/deaths-attributable-to-unhealthy-environments/en
3. U.S. Environmental Protection Agency. (2017). Air quality: National summary. Available at https://www.epa.gov/air-trends/air-quality-national-summary
4. U.S. Environmental Protection Agency. Safe drinking water act (SDWA). (2016). Retrieved from at https://www.epa.gov/sdwa
5. Healthy People 2020. (2017). Environmental health objectives. Available at https://www.healthypeople.gov/2020/topics-objectives/topic/environmental-health/objectives

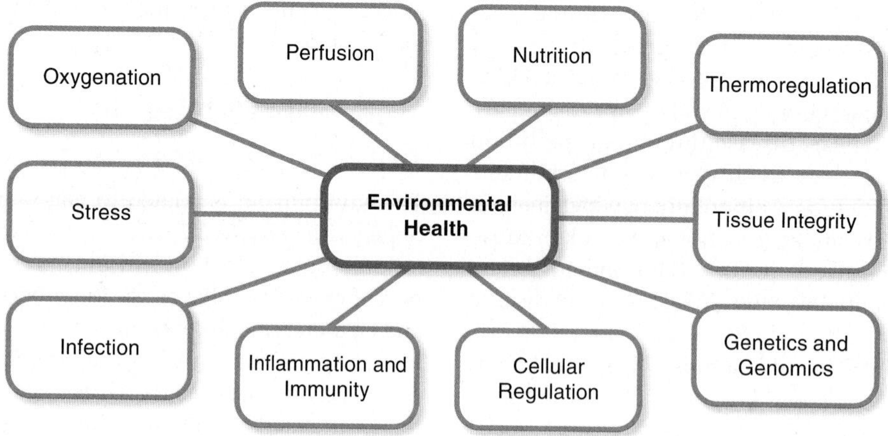

Figure 3.2 ■ Concepts related to environmental health. The environment is a source of substances, such as oxygen, water, and nutrients that are essential for life. However, biological, physical, chemical, and psychosocial hazards in the environment are contributing factors to most diseases and injuries. The types of interactions among these concepts are described briefly in the chapter overview and in more detail in this and other chapters.

peripheral vascular disease, which impair perfusion. Soil and water quality affect the nutritional value and safety of food and water. Changes in environmental temperature activate compensatory warming or cooling mechanisms to keep body temperature within a narrow normal range. Extremes of age and certain diseases limit these compensatory mechanisms. Excessive environmental heat or cold can result in dysfunctional thermoregulation, resulting in hyperthermia or hypothermia, respectively, both of which can be lethal.

Integrity of the skin and mucous membranes is essential for protection against pathogenic microorganisms in the environment. Environmental agents, such as plant toxins and abrasive chemicals, can alter the integrity of the skin or mucous membranes, increasing the risk for infections. Elements of the built environment and social interactions resulting in violence are sources of traumatic injuries.

Environmental carcinogens and physical hazards, such as radiation, can cause genetic mutations, which involve an alteration in gene structure. Numerous chemicals derived from food, medications, or environmental toxicants are capable of causing epigenomic alterations that alter the activation and/or suppression of genes. Either a mutation or an epigenomic alteration can affect genes that regulate cell growth (oncogenes and tumor suppressor genes), leading to cancer. The environment is a source of numerous chemical agents, such as air pollutants, heavy metals, and carcinogens, as well as physical agents, such as radiation and electricity, that can adversely affect the regulation of cell functions including metabolism and proliferation. Environmental agents that come into contact with the skin or mucous membranes or are inhaled or ingested and cause irritation or infection of the skin or internal tissues trigger the inflammatory response to limit the spread of injury and the immune response to eradicate infections. The immune response can react in a maladaptive manner to environmental agents such as allergens, resulting in hypersensitivity reactions. Exposure to nonpathogenic microorganisms in the environment is necessary for normal development of the immune system and the protective normal flora in the body. The environment is also a source of numerous species of pathogenic microorganisms that can cause infections.

It is not just the physical attributes of the environment that affect health. An individual's perception of the physical or social environment as being unpleasant or threatening can elicit the stress response, with potential adverse effects on health.

Case Studies

Environmental health is influential at global, local, and individual levels, as reflected in the definition of environmental health. Furthermore, statistics show that environmental conditions contribute significantly to disease, injury, and death.[6,8,9] The following case studies, which continue throughout this chapter, illustrate the effects of the environment on human health.

Angela Yang: Introduction

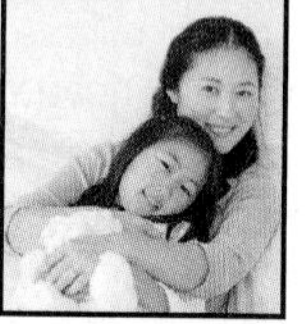

Jennifer Yang received a note from the school nurse recommending that her 5-year-old daughter, Angela, be tested for possible medical reasons underlying some cognitive difficulties. Angela's blood test revealed a lead level of 3.7 μg/dL, which is below the 5.0 μg/dL blood lead level of concern.[11]

1. Discuss a possible reason that may have prompted Angela's healthcare provider to test Angela's blood for lead.
2. Besides lead poisoning, what environmental health influences may affect Angela at the community level?

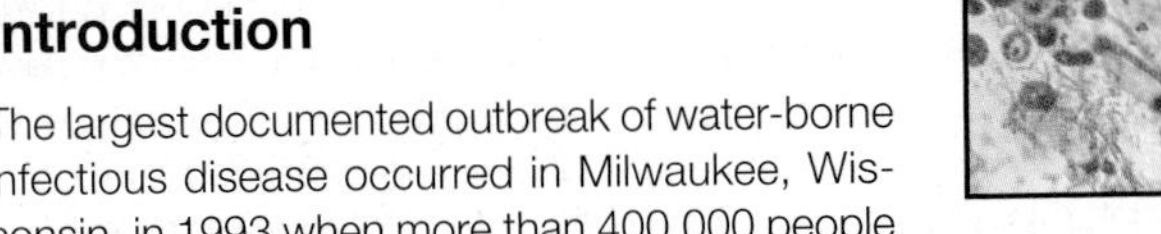

Milwaukee, Wisconsin: Introduction

The largest documented outbreak of water-borne infectious disease occurred in Milwaukee, Wisconsin, in 1993 when more than 400,000 people became ill with cryptosporidiosis.[12] Animal waste runoff from farms and nearby slaughterhouses was the suspected cause of the outbreak. (Note: The case study image shows *Cryptosporidium spp.* oocysts, which are acid-fast, stained red, and yeast cells, which are not acid-fast, stained green.)

1. Using the hazard classification schema in **Table 3.1** ■, identify how animal waste runoff could have produced widespread illness in Milwaukee, Wisconsin.
2. What physical factors, other than *Cryptosporidium* in the water supply, might have affected the Milwaukee community?

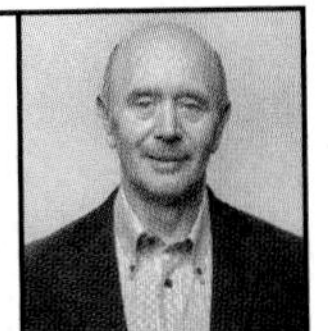

Richard Mara: Introduction

Richard Mara, age 65, retired from his job in the printing industry and relocated to a warm climate. During his first visit to the clinic near his new home, the healthcare provider noticed that Mr. Mara asked her to repeat several questions during his health history. Suspecting hearing loss, the healthcare provider focused on questions related to lifetime exposures to noise, smoking, alcohol use, occupational exposures to neurotoxins (e.g., solvent and heavy metal exposures), hobbies and home maintenance (e.g., leaded glass-making and other arts and crafts, woodwork and furniture refinishing, painting), and history of using ototoxic medications (e.g., aminoglycosides, erythromycin, high-dose vancomycin, nonsteroidal anti-inflammatory drugs, cisplatin, furosemide, and high-dose salicylates such as aspirin). During the environmental health history, Mr. Mara described several environmental exposures to noise, including weekly mowing, occasional snowmobiling, a military history involving rifle firing (approximately 10 rounds per week for 24 months), and a minimal exposure to neurotoxic chemicals used by himself or other household members in hobbies, recreation, or home maintenance. Mr. Mara had used nonsteroidal anti-inflammatory drugs occasionally for headaches and musculoskeletal soreness or pain, mostly related to overexertion at work; however, he denied use of any of the other ototoxic medications listed by his healthcare provider. The provider also noted that Mr. Mara was a lifelong nonsmoker.

1. Which factors in Mr. Mara's history affected the quality of air in his environment?
2. Identify factors in Mr. Mara's occupational history that have had an impact on his health.

Check Your Progress: Section 3.1

1. According to the Evans and Stoddart ecological model, what environments are key determinants of an individual's health?
2. Identify the six environmental health issues targeted by 24 of the *Healthy People 2020* objectives.
3. What social environmental factors at the community level affect population health?

Table 3.1 Hazard Classification

Classification Schema	Types
Nature of the hazard	Biological Chemical Physical Psychosocial
Transport media	Air Water Soil Food
Routes of exposure	Inhalation Ingestion Dermal absorption Transplacental
Settings	Home Workplace School Community
Outcomes	Mutagen Teratogen Carcinogen Organ- or system-level agent that can produce an adverse outcome, such as • Cardiotoxicant • Immunotoxicant • Hepatotoxicant • Nephrotoxicant • Neurotoxicant • Reproductive toxicant • Pulmonary toxicant • Vasculotoxicant

3.2 Environmental Hazard Classification

Methods of classifying **environmental hazards** can be (1) by nature of the hazard, (2) by transport media, (3) by routes of exposure, (4) by setting, and (5) by outcomes (see Table 3.1).[13] As new agents are constantly emerging, understanding the standard classification approaches allows timely development of interventions.

Nature of the Hazard

The traditional approach to classifying environmental hazards is by nature, which includes biological, chemical, physical, and psychosocial categories. More recently, the built environment has been added.[14] Biological hazards are primarily exposures to microorganisms and parasites. These include bacteria (e.g., tuberculosis, anthrax), viruses (e.g., rabies, hepatitis), protozoa (e.g., malaria, toxoplasmosis), fungi (e.g., *Aspergillus*, *Candida*), and helminths (e.g., tapeworms or roundworms), as well as the more recently recognized prions. Biological hazards also include allergens (e.g., pollens) and toxins produced by fish, microorganisms, plants, and algae, such as dinoflagellates ("red tide").[13,15] See Chapter 13 for more detail.

Chemical hazards consist of both inorganic and organic (i.e., carbon-based) agents. Inorganic health hazards include corrosive agents, such as ozone and ammonia; halogens, such as chlorine and iodine; and heavy metals, such as lead, mercury, and cadmium. Hazardous organic substances include alcohols (e.g., ethanol, methanol), glycols (e.g., ethylene glycol), aldehydes (e.g., formaldehyde, glutaraldehyde), halogenated hydrocarbons (e.g., carbon tetrachloride, trichloroethylene, dichlorodiphenyltrichloroethane [DDT]), and other organic solvents (e.g., benzene, octane).[13]

Transfer of energy in the environment poses a physical hazard. Sources of energy include electricity, kinetic (mechanical) forces, light, radiation, sound waves, and thermal energy. For example, kinetic energy that results in injury is released during a fall, an automobile crash, or repetitive muscular movements. High- and low-intensity sound waves and extremes of temperature are hazardous forms of energy. Radiation hazards are categorized as ionizing or nonionizing. Ionizing radiation has sufficient energy to eject electrons that are tightly bound to atoms and includes radiation from nuclear testing, radon, and x-rays.[16] Ionizing radiation is capable of causing mutations. Nonionizing radiation has sufficient energy to cause atoms to vibrate but not enough energy to eject electrons. Nonionizing radiation is emitted from electromagnetic fields and visible and ultraviolet light, among other sources. Psychosocial hazards are stressors resulting from human interaction with the social environment that produce uncertainty, anxiety, or lack of control, often referred to as stress. Stress may result from crowded living conditions; threatened or actual loss of income, housing, transportation, food, or other necessities; interpersonal conflict and violence; noise; or high-demand/low-control jobs. Stress also may be the result of experiencing a natural disaster or living near a hazardous waste site.[17–19]

Transport Media and Routes of Exposure

Transport media and routes of exposure are interrelated. **Transport media** are the means through which environmental hazards are transported to people; these include air, soil, water, and food. The actual **route of exposure**—how the contaminant contacts of enters the human body—can be through inhalation, ingestion, dermal absorption, or transplacentally.[13,20] The primary route of exposure to chemicals in the environment (e.g., at home, at school, during recreational activities) is ingestion; the main route in occupational settings is inhalation. Food and water serve as the primary media for unintentional ingestion of chemical contaminants. Other factors increase the risk of inadvertent exposures. Smoking cigarettes or using other tobacco products such as snuff, applying makeup, chewing gum, eating and drinking, and any other hand-to-mouth behavior in contaminated areas pose additional hazards through inadvertent ingestion. Absorption of chemicals through the skin and mucous membranes also is an important route of exposure.

Angela Yang: Application

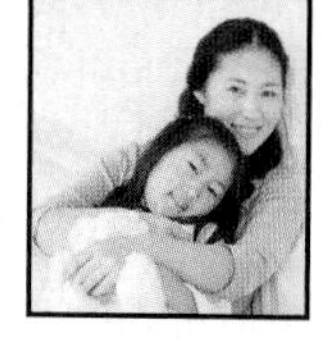

Although there is no safe level of lead, the Yangs' family physician ruled out lead as a cause of Angela's cognitive problems. But this blood lead level prompted the physician to conduct a thorough review of Angela's health history. Findings included that the family eats fish frequently and the mother ate fish regularly when she was pregnant with Angela. Mercury is a neurotoxicant that is found to some degree in most fish and seafood in the form of methylmercury. On the basis of Angela's health history, the physician ordered tests of her blood mercury level. Angela's blood mercury level was 2.3 μg/dL. She may have been exposed to methylmercury first prenatally through transplacental transfer, then during lactation, and later during childhood by ingesting contaminated fish. Fish become contaminated with methylmercury when mercury enters oceans, lakes, and rivers from natural (e.g., volcanoes, forest fires) and industrial (primarily coal-burning) sources. **Figure 3.3** ■ diagrams several possible routes of exposure.

3. Describe the routes of exposure in Angela's history that may have resulted in elevated mercury levels.
4. Which transport media may be involved in Angela's elevated mercury levels?

Settings

Hazards exist across all settings, whether in the home, the workplace, the school, or the larger community. In the home, exposures can be through inhalation of such hazardous substances as tobacco smoke or animal dander or through ingestion (e.g., pesticides on food, eating lead-based paint chips) and dermal absorption (e.g., household cleaning products).

4 The fetus is exposed transplacentally when environmental agents that are present in the woman's body, such as lead, carbon monoxide, or mercury, cross the placenta. Fetal alcohol syndrome is caused by transplacental exposure to ethanol.[20] ■

Exposures in schools are often the result of biological (e.g., mold, viruses, *Escherichia coli* strains), chemical (e.g., asbestos, volatile organic compounds in adhesives), physical (e.g., noise, playground or shop equipment), or psychosocial (e.g., stress, bullying) hazards.[17,20] In the surrounding community, environmental hazards contaminate the air (e.g., ozone, nitrogen dioxide), water (e.g., mercury, *Cryptosporidium* spp.), soil (e.g., lead-based paint, pesticides, *Clostridium* spp.), and food (e.g., *Salmonella*, antibiotic and hormone supplements fed to animals).[15,20,21] Workplace exposures to environmental hazards are currently the best documented. Possible exposures vary with the type of workplace. For example, probable exposures in healthcare facilities include antineoplastic drugs used in cancer chemotherapy and ethylene oxide (chemical); lifting and noise (physical); shift work and stress (psychosocial); and HIV, hepatitis B and C, *Mycobacterium tuberculosis*, and methicillin-resistant *Staphylococcus aureus* (biological).

Outcomes

Another method of classification uses the type of outcome associated with a chemical, physical, or biological agent. Sometimes the effect is named on the basis of the system that is affected, such as neurotoxicant, cardiotoxicant, and pulmonary toxicant (see Table 3.1). Other names reflect the effect of the agent, such as mutagen, an agent that alters genetic information; teratogen, a cause of birth defects; carcinogen, a cause of cancer; and pulmonary fibrotic agent. A single agent may cause more than one disease or illness; for example ionizing radiation is a mutagen, a teratogen, and a carcinogen. For this reason, this classification method is more useful for policy-making than for clinical or public health practice.[13,21]

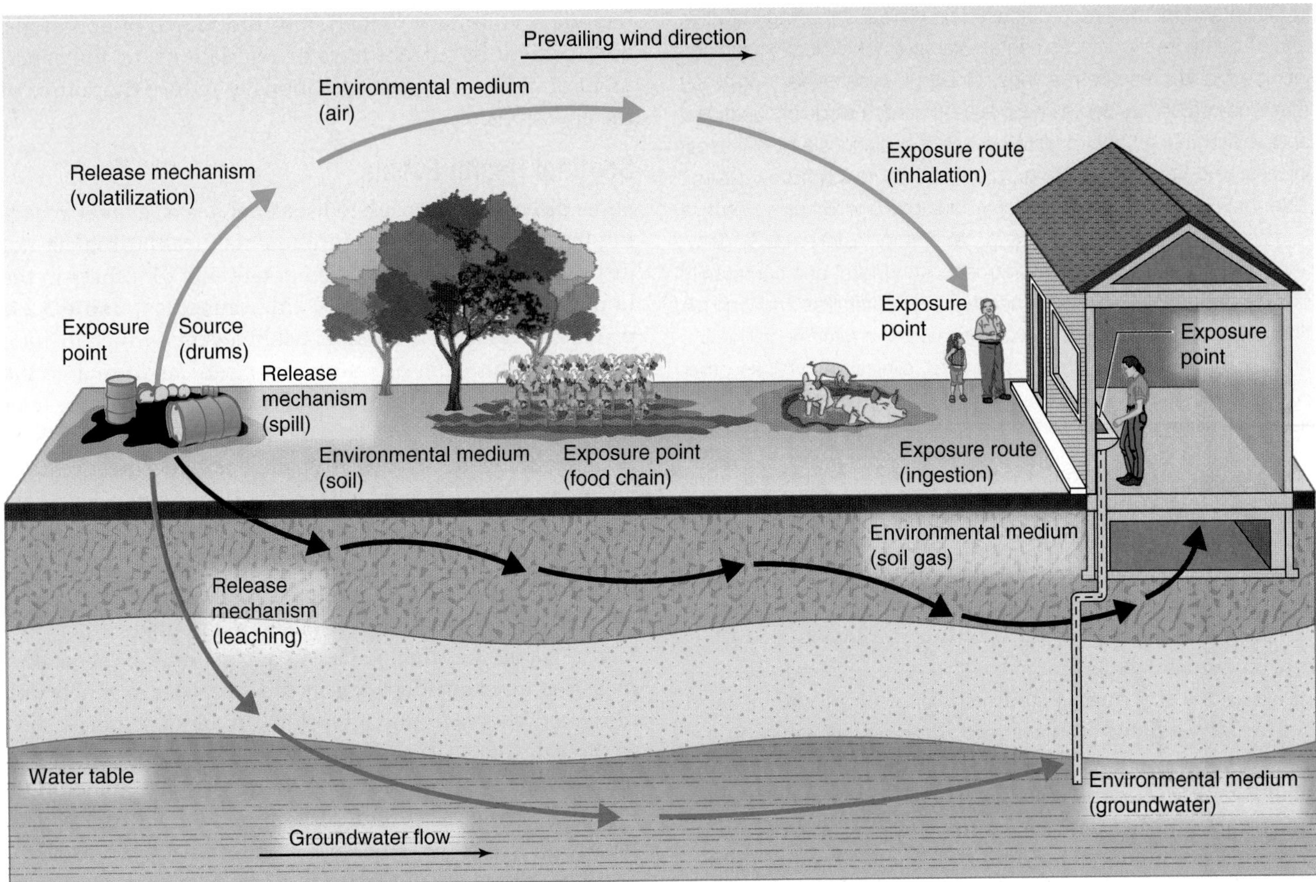

Figure 3.3 ■ Exposure pathways.

SOURCE: Based on Agency for Toxic Substances and Disease Registry. (2005). Exposure evaluation: Evaluating exposure pathways. In: *Public health assessment guidance manual.* Atlanta, GA: Centers for Disease Control and Prevention. Available at https://www.atsdr.cdc.gov/hac/phamanual/ch6.html/

Check Your Progress: Section 3.2

1. Describe the four routes of exposure for environmental hazards.
2. Describe the environmental hazards faced by children in the school setting.
3. Identify the difference between ionizing and nonionizing radiation hazards.

3.3 Key Concepts of Environmental Health from Related Sciences

As environmental health is inherently interdisciplinary, related terminology and key concepts are drawn from basic and applied sciences, especially epidemiology, microbiology, toxicology, and industrial hygiene.

Epidemiology

Epidemiology is the study of the distribution of the health status and outcomes in defined populations, associated factors of influence, and interventions to prevent or control health problems on the basis of epidemiologic findings (see Chapter 1).[22] Factors that determine health include **risk factors**, which increase the chances of disease or injury such as vulnerability and susceptibility, as well as **protective factors** that decrease the same chances. Epidemiology provides scientific evidence about the toxicity (or benefits) of chemicals and the risks and benefits of physical and biological agents, natural and built environment features, and psychosocial exposures.[23] Many of the methods that are used in epidemiologic studies also are used to monitor the health of populations.

Surveillance

Surveillance, as practiced, for example, by the Centers for Disease Control and Prevention, is an important public health function in which health data on populations are systematically collected, analyzed, and interpreted on an ongoing basis and used to design and implement interventions to prevent and control health problems.[24,25] Surveillance includes monitoring (screening) individuals for exposure to hazards and disease and injury outcomes.[26] It uses various data sources, including clinical and occupational records, disease registries, birth and death records, and environmental monitoring.[26,27]

CLINICAL POINT: Health professionals perform an important role in epidemiology and surveillance activities through the assessment and recording of the health of individuals. They typically record such data in health and medical records based on clinical screening activities and in-depth health assessments. Examples of clinical screenings include blood pressure readings, blood glucose levels, and body mass index (BMI). In-depth health assessments include occupational and environmental health histories and the diagnosis of diseases, injuries, and health states (e.g., pregnancy) through history taking, diagnostic procedures, pathology findings, and other subjective (e.g., symptoms) and objective (e.g., laboratory tests) data. Similarly, assessments of the home environment, workplace, and community provide important data on the health status of families and populations. Nurses in public health, occupational and environmental health, home health, and ambulatory care (e.g., clinics), as well as other health professionals in various settings, perform these broader-based assessments. ■

Health professionals and others collect, record, and transmit clinical and other relevant data to the public health system for use in birth and death records, registries of birth defects and cancer, and other population-based record-keeping systems.[27] Additionally, the public health system and businesses (e.g., water utilities, employers, hospitals and emergency departments) collect data such as indicators of air and water quality and records of employment- and community-related injuries and illnesses. These data are used for epidemiologic studies, including public health surveillance. For example, Seattle researchers correlated routine air monitoring data for ozone, nitrogen dioxide, sulfur dioxide, carbon monoxide, and particulate matter required under the Clean Air Act with hospitalizations for asthma in children and adults.[28] The researchers followed this descriptive surveillance-based study with an additional epidemiologic study conducted in seven cities, which showed that children with asthma experienced a significantly increased risk of symptoms and use of rescue inhalants two days after carbon monoxide or nitrogen dioxide levels increased in their local communities.[29] An essential component of surveillance is the implementation of interventions, followed by evaluation to determine whether the interventions are effective. These examples of the effect of air pollution on worsening asthma symptoms require interventions that include a voluntary reduction in the source of emissions, enforcement of current laws or regulations, or the enactment of more stringent regulations to reduce the source of the emissions.

Sentinel Health Events

Some diseases are considered **sentinel health events**, meaning that they herald an environmental health problem not just for an individual, but also potentially for others in the home, work, and community environments.[27] **Table 3.2** ■ provides examples of sentinel health events, which include mesothelioma from asbestos, clear cell carcinoma of the vagina from diethylstilbestrol, and angiosarcoma of the liver from vinyl chloride exposures.[13,27] Other environmental sentinel health events involve atypical health occurrences and are more likely to be recognized through population-based surveillance conducted by public health agencies.[27] An example is bladder cancer that develops in people without risk factors of smoking or occupational exposure to bladder carcinogens (e.g., aniline dyes used in tanning leather)[13] or having a younger-than-expected age at onset. Other examples of sentinel health events include a cluster in genetically unrelated people living or working in the same place, such as three or more cases of lung cancer in nonsmokers or primary liver cancer in people without evidence of hepatitis B or C or cirrhosis. Certain rare cancers would be atypical, particularly if multiple cases are observed, such as rhabdomyosarcoma, myelogenous leukemia, acute leukemia in children, or acute granulocytic leukemia in adults.[27] Additionally, public health experts should consider and investigate new diseases or asthma in low-risk children who, for example, have no allergies and live in households without exposure to environmental tobacco smoke.

CLINICAL POINT: Alert nurses and other primary healthcare providers are in the best position to recognize acute poisonings from lead and other metals, pesticides, and nitrates, which may cause methemoglobinemia; neuropathies from toxic exposures; precocious onset of puberty or breast development due to endocrine disruptors; and cancers with clear environmental links. ■

Table 3.2 Environmental/Occupational Sentinel Health Events

Hazard	Examples of Industries and Occupations with Potential Exposures	Sentinel Condition
Biological Hazards		
Mycobacterium tuberculosis	Healthcare personnel, including laboratory workers	Pulmonary tuberculosis
Silica and *Mycobacterium tuberculosis*	Quarry workers, sandblasters, miners, metal foundry workers, ceramic workers	Silico-tuberculosis
Yersinia pestis	Shepherds, farmers, ranchers, hunters, field geologists	Plague
Francisella tularensis, Pasteurella tularensis	Hunters, ranchers, fur handlers, sheep industry workers, veterinarians, laboratory workers, soldiers, cooks	Tularemia
Bacillus anthracis	Shepherds, farmers, veterinarians, butchers, handlers of imported hides or fibers, weavers	Anthrax
Brucella abortus suis	Shepherds, farmers, veterinarians, laboratory workers, slaughterhouse workers, field officers	Brucellosis

Hazard	Examples of Industries and Occupations with Potential Exposures	Sentinel Condition
Mycobacterium marinum	Aquarium workers/cleaners/breeders, longshoremen	Fish-fancier finger
Herpes simplex virus	Healthcare workers	Herpetic whitlow
Clostridium tetani	Farmers, ranchers	Tetanus
Human immunodeficiency virus	Healthcare workers	Human immunodeficiency virus (HIV)
Rubella virus	Healthcare workers	Rubella
Hepatitis A virus	Daycare center personnel, staff in orphanages or other group homes, healthcare workers	Hepatitis A
Hepatitis B virus	Healthcare workers, daycare center personnel, staff in orphanages or other group homes	Hepatitis B
Hepatitis C virus	Healthcare workers, daycare center personnel, staff in orphanages or other group homes	Hepatitis C
Rabies virus	Veterinarians, animal and game wardens, laboratory workers, farmers, ranchers, trappers	Rabies
Chlamydia psittaci	Psittacine bird breeders, pet shop staff, poultry producers/workers, veterinarians, zoo staff	Ornithosis
Rickettsia rickettsii	Laboratory workers, virologists, microbiologists, physicians	Rocky Mountain spotted fever
Leptospira	Farmers, laborers	Leptospirosis
Histoplasma capsulatum	Bridge maintenance workers	Histoplasmosis
Sporothrix schenckii	Nursery workers, foresters, florist, equipment operators	Sporotrichosis
Flour	Bakers	Asthma
Red cedar (plicatic acid) and other wood dusts	Woodworkers, furniture makers	Asthma
Bacillus-derived exoenzymes	Detergent formulators	Asthma
Unknown	Crab, prawn, snow crab processing workers	Asthma
Psyllium dust (plant-based fiber source used medicinally)	Hospital and long-term care nurses, laxative manufacturing and packing workers	Asthma
Aspergillus clavatus	Maltworkers	Maltworker lung
Pasteurized compost	Mushroom farmers/workers	Mushroom worker's lung
Erwinia herbicola (Enterobacter agglomerans)	Grain handlers	Grain handler lung
Redwood sawdust *Thuja plicata*	Red cedar mill workers, woodworkers, sawmill and joinery workers	Sequoiosis
Cinnamon dust, cinnamaldehyde	Cinnamon processing workers	Unspecified allergic alveolitis
Aspergillus fumigatus	Distillery, vegetable compost plant worker	Unspecified allergic alveolitis
Unknown	Sawmill worker	Unspecified allergic alveolitis
Alternaria, wood dust	Paper manufacture/wood room	Unspecified allergic alveolitis
Unknown	Snow crab processing worker	Unspecified allergic alveolitis
Chemical Hazards		
Chlorophenols	Carpenter, cabinet maker, sawmill worker, lumberjack, electrician, fitter	Malignant neoplasm of nasopharynx
Vinyl chloride monomer	Workers in the vinyl chloride polymerization industry	Hemangiosarcoma of liver
Asbestos	Workers involved in the manufacture or use of asbestos or asbestos products such as carpenters, other construction workers	Mesothelioma of the peritoneum and/or pleura
Hardwood dusts	Woodworkers, cabinet and furniture makers	Malignant neoplasm of the nasal cavities
Unknown	Boot and shoe industry	Malignant neoplasm of the nasal cavities
Chromates	Chromium producers, processors, users	Malignant neoplasm of the nasal cavities
Nickel	Nickel smelting and refining	Malignant neoplasm of the nasal cavities
Chlorophenols	Sawmill worker, carpenter	Malignant neoplasm of the nasal cavities
Asbestos	Asbestos industries and utilizers	Malignant neoplasm of larynx
Asbestos	Workers in the mining, manufacture, or use of asbestos	Malignant neoplasm of larynx
Coke oven emissions	Topside coke oven workers	Malignant neoplasm of larynx
Chromates	Chromium producers, processors, and users	Malignant neoplasm of larynx

(Continued)

Table 3.2 Environmental/Occupational Sentinel Health Events *Continued*

Hazard	Examples of Industries and Occupations with Potential Exposures	Sentinel Condition
Chemical Hazards *Continued*		
Nickel	Nickel smelters, processors, and users	Malignant neoplasm of larynx
Arsenic, arsenic trioxide	Smelters	Malignant neoplasm of larynx
Mustard gas	Mustard gas formulators	Malignant neoplasm of larynx
Bis(chloromethyl)ether, chloromethyl methyl ether	Ion exchange resin makers, chemists	Malignant neoplasm of larynx
Pesticides, herbicides, fungicides, insecticides	Plant protection workers/agronomists	Malignant neoplasm of larynx
Unknown	Welders	Malignant neoplasm of larynx
Inorganic arsenic, sulfur dioxide, copper, lead, sulfuric acid, arsenic trioxide	Copper smelter and roaster workers	Malignant neoplasm of larynx
Asbestos, hexavalent chromium	Welders, gas cutters	Malignant neoplasm of larynx
Polyaromatic hydrocarbons	Foundry floor molders and casters	Malignant neoplasm of larynx
Unknown	Dichromate production floor molders and casters	Malignant neoplasm of larynx
Chromium dust	Chromate production workers	Malignant neoplasm of larynx
Lead chromate, zinc chromate	Chromate pigment production workers	Malignant neoplasm of larynx
Zinc chromate dust	Pigment production workers	Malignant neoplasm of larynx
Unknown	Steel industry furnace and foundry workers	Malignant neoplasm of larynx
Unknown	Rubber reclamation operations workers	Malignant neoplasm of larynx
Mineral/cutting oils	Automatic lathe operators, metalworkers	Malignant neoplasm of scrotum
Soots/tar/tar distillates	Coke oven workers, petroleum refiners, tar distillers	Malignant neoplasm of scrotum
Mineral oil, pitch, tar	Tool setters, fitters, cotton spinners, chimney sweeps, machine operators	Malignant neoplasm of scrotum
Benzidine, alpha- and beta-naphthylamine, magenta, auramine, 4-aminobiphenyl, 4-nitrophenyl	Rubber and dye workers	Malignant neoplasm of bladder
Coke oven emissions	Coke oven workers	Malignant neoplasm of kidney, other, and unspecified urinary organs
Unknown	Rubber industry workers	Lymphoid leukemia, acute
Benzene	Workers exposed to benzene	Myeloid leukemia, acute
Benzene	Workers exposed to benzene	Erythroleukemia
Copper sulfate	Whitewashing and leather industry workers	Hemolytic anemia, nonautoimmune
Arsine	Electrolytic processing workers, arsenical ore mining workers	Hemolytic anemia, nonautoimmune
Timellitic anhydride	Plastics industry workers	Hemolytic anemia, nonautoimmune
Naphthalene	Dye, celluloid, resin industries workers	Hemolytic anemia, nonautoimmune
Trinitrotoluene	Workers employed in the manufacture of explosives	Aplastic anemia
Benzene	Workers exposed to benzene	Aplastic anemia
Benzene	Workers exposed to benzene	Agranulocytosis or neutropenia
Phosphorus	Explosives and pesticide industries workers	Agranulocytosis or neutropenia
Inorganic arsenic	Workers in pesticide, pigment, and pharmaceuticals industries	Agranulocytosis or neutropenia
Aromatic amino and nitro compounds (e.g., aniline, trinitrotoluene, nitroglycerine)	Workers in explosives and dye industries	Methemoglobinemia
Aniline, o-toluidine, nitrobenzene	Workers in the rubber industry	Methemoglobinemia
Lead	Battery, smelter, and foundry workers	Toxic encephalitis
Inorganic and organic mercury (e.g., methylmercury)	Electrolytic chlorine production workers, battery makers, fungicide formulators	Toxic encephalitis
Manganese	Manganese processing workers, battery makers, welders	Parkinson disease, secondary
Carbon monoxide	Workers in internal combustion engine industries	Parkinson disease, secondary
Toluene	Workers in the chemical industry using toluene	Cerebellar ataxia
Organic mercury (e.g., methylmercury)	Electrolytic chlorine production workers, battery makers, fungicide formulators	Cerebellar ataxia

Hazard	Examples of Industries and Occupations with Potential Exposures	Sentinel Condition
Methyl methacrylate monomer	Dental technicians	Mononeuritis of upper limb and mononeuritis multiplex
Arsenic, arsenic compounds	Pesticide industry workers, pigment industry workers, pharmaceutical formulators	Inflammatory and toxic neuropathy
Hexane	Furniture refinishers	Inflammatory and toxic neuropathy
Methyl n-butyl ketone	Plastic-coated-fabric workers	Inflammatory and toxic neuropathy
Trinitrotoluene	Explosives industry workers	Inflammatory and toxic neuropathy
Carbon disulfide	Rayon manufacturing workers	Inflammatory and toxic neuropathy
Tri-o-cresyl phosphate	Plastics, hydraulics, coke industries workers	Inflammatory and toxic neuropathy
Inorganic lead	Battery, smelter, and foundry workers	Inflammatory and toxic neuropathy
Inorganic mercury	Dentists, chloralkali workers	Inflammatory and toxic neuropathy
Organic mercury	Chloralkali plant workers, fungicide makers, battery makers	Inflammatory and toxic neuropathy
Acrylamide	Workers in plastics and paper manufacturing industries	Inflammatory and toxic neuropathy
Ethylene oxide	Ethylene oxide sterilizer operator in manufacturing or health care	Inflammatory and toxic neuropathy
Trinitrotoluene	Explosives industry workers	Cataract
Naphthalene	Moth repellent formulators, fumigators	Cataract
Dinitrophenol, dinitro-o-cresol	Workers in explosives, dye, herbicide, and pesticide industries	Cataract
Ethylene oxide	Ethylene oxide sterilizer operator, microbiology supervisors, inspectors	Cataract
Vinyl chloride	Vinyl chloride polymerization industry workers	Raynaud phenomenon, secondary
Platinum	Jewelry, alloy, and catalyst makers	Asthma
Isocyanates	Polyurethane, adhesive, paint workers	Asthma
Chromium, cobalt	Alloy, catalyst, refinery workers	Asthma
Aluminum soldering flux	Solderers	Asthma
Phthalic anhydride	Plastic, dye, insecticide makers	Asthma
Formaldehyde	Foam workers, latex makers, biologists	Asthma
Gum arabic	Printing industry workers	Asthma
Nickel sulfate	Nickel plater	Asthma
Trimellitic anhydride	Workers in plastics industry, manufacture of organic chemicals	Asthma
Coal dust	Coal miners	Coal worker pneumoconiosis
Asbestos	Workers involved in the manufacture or use of asbestos or asbestos products such as carpenters, other construction workers	Asbestosis
Silica	Quarry workers, silica processors, sandblasters, miners, metal foundry workers, ceramic workers	Silicosis
Talc	Talc processing, soapstone mining/milling, polishing, cosmetics industry	Talcosis
Beryllium	Beryllium alloy workers, ceramic and cathode ray tube makers, nuclear reactor workers	Chronic beryllium disease of the lung
Cotton, flax, hemp, and cotton-synthetic dusts	Cotton industry workers	Byssinosis
Ammonia	Workers in refrigeration, fertilizer, oil refining industries	Acute bronchiolitis, pneumonitis, and pulmonary edema due to fumes and vapors
Chlorine	Workers in alkali and bleach industries	Acute bronchiolitis, pneumonitis, and pulmonary edema due to fumes and vapors
Nitrogen oxides	Silo fillers, arc welders, nitric acid industry workers	Acute bronchiolitis, pneumonitis, and pulmonary edema due to fumes and vapors
Sulfur dioxide	Workers in paper and refrigeration industries, oil refining	Acute bronchiolitis, pneumonitis, and pulmonary edema due to fumes and vapors
Cadmium	Cadmium smelters, processors	Acute bronchiolitis, pneumonitis, and pulmonary edema due to fumes and vapors
Trimellitic anhydride	Plastics industry workers	Acute bronchiolitis, pneumonitis, and pulmonary edema due to fumes and vapors

(Continued)

Table 3.2 Environmental/Occupational Sentinel Health Events *Continued*

Hazard	Examples of Industries and Occupations with Potential Exposures	Sentinel Condition
Chemical Hazards *Continued*		
Vanadium pentoxide	Boilermakers	Acute bronchiolitis, pneumonitis, and pulmonary edema due to fumes and vapors
Trimellitic anhydride	Workers in organic chemicals manufacturing	Acute bronchiolitis, pneumonitis, and pulmonary edema due to fumes and vapors
Carbon tetrachloride, chloroform, tetrachloroethane, trichloroethylene, tetrachloroethylene	Workers who use solvents, including drycleaners and those in the plastics industry	Toxic hepatitis
Phosphorus, trinitrotoluene	Workers in explosives and dye industries	Toxic hepatitis
Chloronaphthalenes	Fire and waterproofing additive formulators	Toxic hepatitis
Methylenedianiline	Plastics formulators	Toxic hepatitis
Ethylene dibromide	Fumigators, gasoline and fire extinguisher formulators	Toxic hepatitis
Cresol	Disinfectant, fumigant, synthetic resin formulators	Toxic hepatitis
Inorganic lead	Battery makers, plumbers, solderers	Acute or chronic renal failure
Arsine	Workers in electrolytic processes, arsenical ore smelting	Acute or chronic renal failure
Inorganic mercury	Battery makers, plumbers, solderers	Acute or chronic renal failure
Carbon tetrachloride	Fluorocarbon formulators, fire extinguisher makers	Acute or chronic renal failure
Ethylene glycol	Antifreeze manufacturing workers	Acute or chronic renal failure
Inorganic lead	Chromate pigment production workers	Acute or chronic renal failure
Kepone	Kepone formulators	Infertility, male
Dibromochloropropane	Dibromochloropropane (DBCP) producers, formulators, and applicators	Infertility, male
Irritants (e.g., cutting oils, phenol, solvents, acids, alkalis, detergents); allergens (e.g., nickel, chromates, formaldehyde, dyes, rubber products)	Workers in leather tanning, poultry dressing plants, fish packing, adhesives and sealant industries, boat building and repair	Contact and allergic dermatitis
Cryolite (Na_2AlF_6)	Cryolite workers (grinding room)	Skeletal fluorosis
Cryolite (Na_2AlF_6)	Cryolite refining workers	Skeletal fluorosis
Physical Hazards		
Radium	Radium chemists, processors, radium dial painters	Malignant neoplasm of the nasal cavities, bone
Radon decay products	Uranium and fluorspar miners, iron ore (underground) miners	Malignant neoplasm of the trachea, bronchus, and lung
Ionizing radiation	Radiologists, radium chemists, and radium dial painters	Acute lymphoid or myeloid leukemia, aplastic anemia, cataract
Microwaves	Microwave and radar technicians	Cataract
Infrared radiation	Blacksmiths, glass blowers, bakers	Cataract
Cumulative trauma	Meatpackers, deboners	Carpal tunnel syndrome
Cumulative trauma	Poultry processing workers, meatpackers, deboners	Mononeuritis of upper limb and mononeuritis multiplex
Whole body or segmental vibration	Lumberjacks, sawyers, grinders, chippers, rock drillers, stone cutters, jackhammer operators, riveters	Raynaud phenomenon, secondary

CLINICAL POINT: Exposures that pose a risk to one person (e.g., elevated blood lead level in a construction worker) should trigger either greater vigilance in looking for other cases or active investigation to determine whether the person's coworkers and household members are similarly affected (exposure or health outcome). An important part of surveillance is to implement intervention(s) to identify (i.e., screen) and treat people early in the disease process and to prevent exposures, and thus disease and injury, in the population. Interventions to prevent exposures are discussed later in this chapter. ■

Angela Yang: Application

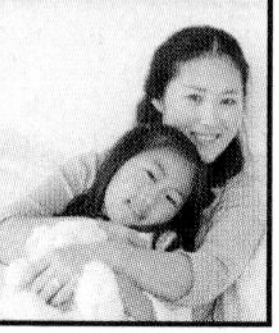

Because of Angela's health history, the Yangs' family physician requested that the other child in the household be screened for mercury levels (as well as lead).

5. Describe the role of surveillance in screening the children in the Yang household.
6. How do the lead and mercury levels of the Yang family act as a sentinel health event?

Vulnerability

The U.S. Environmental Protection Agency's Cumulative Risk Framework suggests that an individual or a population is more **vulnerable** to adverse health risks from environmental exposures on the basis of several factors, including differential exposure, the interrelated factors of preparedness and ability to recover, and susceptibility.[30] As **Figure 3.4** ■ details, response to exposures varies by life state (e.g., pregnant, young, old), preexisting conditions, nutritional status, and cultural practices. Previous exposures to physical and chemical hazards or cumulative exposures over a lifetime result in heightened risk of injury and disease. These include exposures to noise and ultraviolet radiation as well as exposures to carcinogens, use of immunosuppressant drugs, or conditions (e.g., end-stage renal disease, HIV/AIDS). In addition, differences in exposures increase vulnerability. Multiple exposures to different toxicants are one example; the risk of lung cancer for people who have been exposed to radon is as much as 25 times greater in those who smoke cigarettes.[31] In developing countries, the World Health Organization reports gender differences in mortality from unsafe water and indoor smoke, presumably because women in these countries have the primary responsibility for collecting and using water and for cooking.[32]

As Figure 3.4 indicates, differences in preparedness and ability to recover are interrelated vulnerability factors, concerned with the ability to withstand and recover from an exposure. Locally and globally, socially and economically disadvantaged populations are disproportionately exposed to hazards, resulting in higher disease burden from environmental exposures. Individuals with lower educational levels often work in lower-wage jobs with higher exposure risks and lower insurance coverage. Aggregate living conditions for older or developmentally delayed populations are meant to enhance well-being. However, this type of setting increases the risk for exposures to biological hazards in populations whose immune systems are often less able to cope with the exposure.

CLINICAL POINT: Some cultural practices involve the use of herbal and other remedies to treat symptoms of diseases, which result in environmental exposures. The most frequently cited example of cultural remedies is the use in Mexican cultures of lead (*azarcón*) or mercury (*greta*) powders to treat an abdominal disorder (*empacho*).[33] ■

A key vulnerability factor is **susceptibility**, which denotes characteristics that increase the risk of individuals for environmental disease or injury.[30] Such characteristics include age, gender, race/ethnicity, stage of development, and genetic predisposition. While exposures occur across the age spectrum, the two extremes (fetuses and young children and aged people) are at greatest risk because of normal differences in their physiologic functioning. In fetuses and children, such differences are related to immaturity, whereas in older adults, they are associated with the normal aging process.

During pregnancy, the developing fetus is susceptible to environmental toxicants via the transplacental route. This is a critical period of susceptibility. Known teratogens include pharmaceuticals and other drugs that affect fetal development. Their effects depend on transport of the toxicant to the fetal circulation, the relative inability of the fetus to biotransform the toxicant, and the timing of exposure. Examples include the effect of maternal ingestion of thalidomide on fetal limb development and diethylstilbestrol taken by the mother before the 18th week of gestation on the fetal reproductive system.[13,20] The mother's ingestion of ethanol affects cell migration, leading to changes in fetal brain development. Other toxicants that cross the placenta and affect fetal development include lead, methylmercury, and components of cigarette smoke (e.g., polycyclic aromatic hydrocarbons, lead, cadmium, carbon monoxide). ■

As organ growth and development continue through childhood, children who are exposed to toxicants are susceptible to physiologic alterations. Exposure of children to environmental tobacco smoke slows the growth of lung function. Children have a higher metabolic rate than adults, coupled with higher levels of absorption of toxicants through the integumentary, pulmonary, and gastrointestinal systems. Children consume more oxygen and produce more carbon dioxide per kilogram of body weight than adults, which leads to greater sensitivity to air pollution. Because the child's surface-to-body mass ratio is 2–3 times greater than an adult's, a child absorbs more toxicants kilogram per kilogram than an adult does.[20] Lead is stored in the bone (biological sanctuary). Because children absorb far more lead than adults (50% versus 10%), lead stored in the bone during childhood and beyond serves as a reservoir for low-dose, chronic exposure even when the primary source of exposure has been removed.

Hand-to-mouth exploratory behaviors in toddlerhood increase the likelihood of ingestion of toxicants such as lead paint dust or arsenic from treated wood in playground equipment. Being shorter than adults, their breathing zone is closer to the floor, where chemicals that are heavier than air and dust particles (e.g., lead) concentrate. Children also are exposed to workplace toxicants on the clothes of adults. The classic case is childhood mesothelioma—cancer of the pleura, peritoneum, or both—resulting from children being exposed to asbestos through their parents, who wear and launder contaminated work clothes at home. ■

At the other end of the age spectrum, the normal aging process increases older adults' susceptibility to the health effects of environmental hazards. Age-related physiologic changes occur in the cardiac, hepatic, immune, integumentary, pulmonary, and renal systems.[34] For example, diminished cardiac output and diminished blood flow to the liver and kidneys result in reduced ability to detoxify and eliminate toxicants. Decline in cell-mediated immunity increases older adults' risks for viruses and cancer. Chemicals are more easily absorbed through the skin because of changes to the stratum corneum. Increased adipose tissue

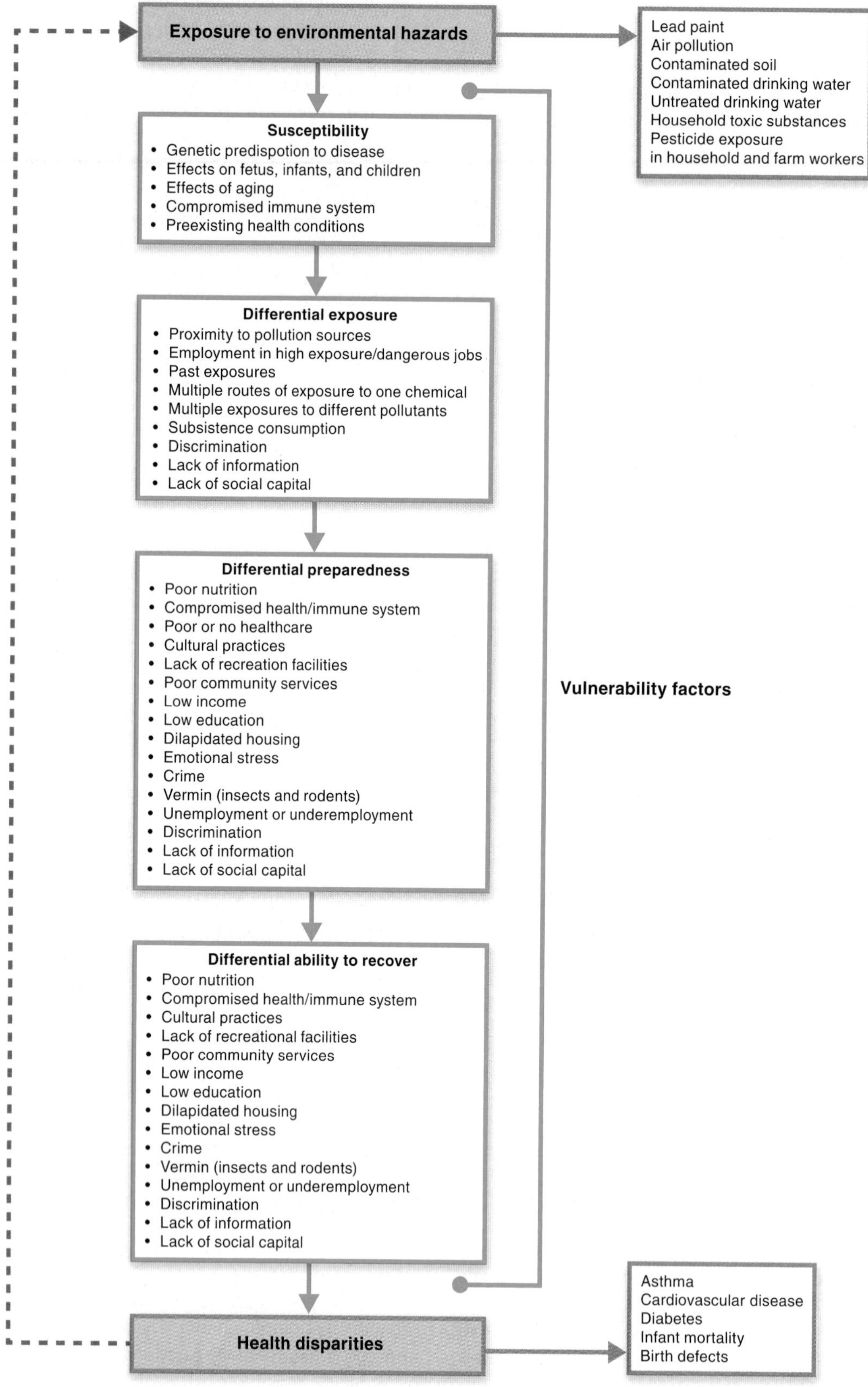

Figure 3.4 ■ Cumulative risk framework.

SOURCE: Based on National Environmental Justice Advisory Council to the U.S. Environmental Protection Agency. (2004). *Ensuring risk reduction in communities with multiple stressors: Environmental justice and cumulative risks/impacts*. Available at https://www.epa.gov/sites/production/files/2015-04/documents/ensuringriskreducationnejac.pdf mass in conjunction with decreased lean body mass alter the distribution of toxicants and pharmaceuticals in the body. Although diminished functions in older adults are usually attributed to normal aging only, environmental exposures may also contribute to the decline in function. For example, hearing loss can result from exposures to noise and to some chemicals, including solvents and lead.[13,35] ■

Microbiology

Microorganisms are present in vast numbers in moist, organic environments and even in arid environments. While many of these microorganisms are nonpathogenic (do not cause diseases), some are pathogenic. The presence of pathogenic microorganisms alone, however, is not enough to cause disease. For infection to occur, a series of events must occur[15]:

1. An appropriate **mode of transmission** or transferral of the microorganism in sufficient numbers from source to host
2. Presence of pathogenic organisms of sufficient virulence (able to cause infection)
3. A susceptible host whose resistance to the pathogenic microorganism(s) is not sufficient to mount an immune response to clear the body of the microorganism without causing disease.

The mode of transmission is important to consider in environmental health. Infections are transmitted from environments to people through pathogens in airborne droplets or nuclei, in water or food, and through contact with contaminated inanimate surfaces or animals (see Chapter 13).[15] Other sources of infectious diseases in human populations include waste generated by humans (e.g., sewage), animals (in agriculture and the wild), and hospitals and clinics, as well as by individuals in the community (e.g., used syringes).

From an environmental perspective, animal waste and raw or inadequately treated sewage are primary sources of contamination of water used for irrigation of crops, recreation, and drinking and are potential sources of exposure to disease-causing organisms.[36] Individual and community wells can become contaminated by human or animal waste when septic systems or sewer pipes are located too close to wells or when agricultural runoff contaminates the well water directly. Because well water typically is not treated, the water may become contaminated and cause illness if consumed. In contrast, surface water (i.e., water from lakes, rivers, and streams) in developed countries is treated for human consumption and then distributed to households and businesses through large underground pipes. Either inadequate treatment of surface water or contamination in the water distribution system can result in water-borne infectious disease. In developing countries, shallow wells, which are highly susceptible to contamination, and the lack of water treatment of surface water are the norm and result in a very high rate of gastrointestinal illnesses such as diarrhea.[37,38] However, water-borne diseases have occurred even when the treatment of drinking water was considered adequate.[39]

Milwaukee, Wisconsin: Application

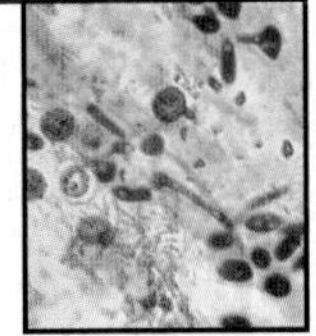

In the cases of water-borne infectious disease in Milwaukee, Wisconsin, subsequent DNA evidence revealed that *Cryptosporidium hominis*, which is known to be harbored in the human intestine, was the culprit of the outbreak.[36] Food-borne infections can result from contamination with pathogens at any point in the growing, processing, distribution, storage, preparation, cooking, and serving of food.[40] Water- and food-borne infections often share the same pathogens. For example, approximately 90% of cases of cryptosporidiosis result from water-borne infection. The remainder of cases are attributed to contamination of food, direct person-to-person transmission, and zoonotic (animal-to-human) transmission.[40,41]

3. Which age groups in Milwaukee, Wisconsin, may be particularly susceptible to cryptosporidiosis?
4. What role might health professionals play in the surveillance activities that could detect water-borne disease in the Milwaukee community?

Medical waste, which includes laboratory animal waste, pathology waste, blood and blood products, selected isolation waste, and sharps, is another potential source of environmentally caused infectious disease.[42] Medical waste generated in healthcare facilities is an occupational hazard primarily for janitorial and laundry staff members, nurses, emergency medical personnel, and refuse workers, not the general public. Nevertheless, sharps used in home healthcare, by people with chronic medical problems (e.g., diabetes, hepatitis C, draining wounds), or by users of intravenous drugs pose risks to refuse workers and the general public. Effective treatment of medical waste includes chemical decontamination, heat (autoclaving and incineration), irradiation, and sanitary landfill. Improper management of medical waste, including incomplete combustion and beach wash-ups, can contaminate the general environment and pose health risks to the community. Public health policies that promote appropriate collection and disposal of sharps contribute to the reduction of risk among workers and the public.[43]

Toxicology

Toxicology is the study of the harmful effects of **xenobiotics**, or exogenous chemical agents.[13] Toxicology includes research to understand the mechanisms by which chemicals produce adverse effects. In humans, exposure to chemicals provides the opportunity for biological absorption and potential adverse health effects.[13,18] In the United States, an expansive exposure surveillance program was initiated in 1999 to examine many different types of exposures to toxic chemicals in the U.S. population.[11,44] This surveillance program, the National Health and Nutrition Examination Survey (NHANES), is designed so that findings are generalizable to the U.S. population.

Angela Yang: Application

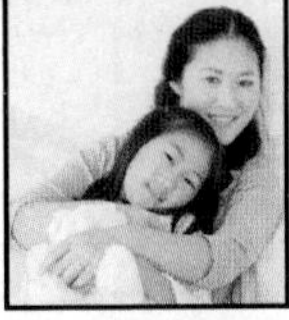

Angela has cognitive deficits that are possibly attributable to methylmercury exposure. Methylmercury would be considered the hazard, and Angela's cognitive difficulties are one manifestation of neurotoxicity induced by an environmental exposure.[45,46]

Much of what is known about the human health effects of methylmercury comes from a large epidemiologic study of 1022 children in the Faroe Islands (located in the Norwegian Sea), whom researchers have followed since birth in 1987–1988.[45,46] The researchers used maternal hair and blood taken at the time of birth and cord blood to measure prenatal exposure of the children to mercury. They examined the children at age 7 years and again at age 14 years for neurobehavioral performance on standardized tests. These studies found an association between prenatal mercury exposures and deficits in motor and verbal skills and attention at ages 7 and 14 years.

Angela's blood lead level was 3.7 μg/dL. According to NHANES data from 2009–2012[11] (**Table 3.3** ■), this lead level was above the 95th percentile for children her age and well above the geometric mean. Although the blood lead level did not reach poisonous levels (i.e., 5 μg/dL), ample evidence shows that lead levels below 5 μg/dL also adversely affect cognition—estimated to be a mean decrement of 7.4 IQ points for a shift from 1 μg/dL to 10 μg/dL.[47] Therefore, the physician's conclusion that lead did not contribute to Angela's cognitive problems may not be accurate.

According to the same NHANES data[11] (see Table 3.3), Angela's blood mercury level of 2.3 μg/dL exceeded the 95th percentile for children ages 1–5 years and was well above the geometric mean. Mercury levels below those currently considered safe have been shown to adversely affect language, attention, and memory and, to a lesser degree, visual, spatial, and motor functions.[45,46] Cord blood (prenatal exposure) is the biomarker most closely correlated with these cognitive deficits. Thus, both lead and mercury may have contributed to Angela's cognitive difficulties.

7. How does the concept of biological sanctuary possibly correlate with Angela's future health even if the sources of lead are removed?
8. What role do the NHANES data play in the care of Angela?

Fish and seafood are the primary source of methylmercury exposure.[48] Nevertheless, methylmercury is not a normal constituent of fish and seafood. It gets there through a chain of events. Natural occurrences such as volcanic eruptions and forest fires release elemental mercury into the atmosphere. Since the Industrial Revolution, human activities have increasingly emitted mercury into the environment. While coal-burning power plants are the major source of human-made environmental contamination, the incineration of mercury-containing wastes from other industries (including the healthcare sector) and the general public also contribute. Particles and mercury vapor released into the air get deposited into oceans, lakes, and rivers and sink into the sediment layer, where anaerobic microorganisms form methylmercury out of carbon atoms and mercury (see **Figure 3.5** ■). Methylmercury bioconcentrates from the lowest to the highest plants and animals on the food chain. In other words, it bioconcentrates from bacteria and plankton to small fish, which eat the plankton, to bigger fish and fowl, which feed on smaller fish, all the way to humans. Larger fish and fish that are higher on the food chain bioconcentrate the methylmercury deposits found in the muscle tissue of their prey. In turn, sea mammals, fowl, and humans who eat fish, especially fish or seafood that is high on the food chain, also bioconcentrate methylmercury. Neither the preparation nor the cooking method can decrease the amount of methylmercury in fish and seafood because mercury binds tightly to protein that forms the muscle tissue, which is consumed. (In contrast, polychlorinated biphenyls [PCBs] and other highly fat-soluble molecules are concentrated in the skin and fat tissues of fish and largely can be removed before cooking and eating.)

The example of methylmercury illustrates the concept of bioconcentration: that humans at the top of the food chain have the highest levels of the toxicant from food sources. Another concept, bioaccumulation, occurs when the rate of biological uptake exceeds the rate of excretion. Bioaccumulation is more likely with fat-soluble (i.e., lipophilic) toxicants or when toxicants are stored, such as with lead sequestered in bone. Several principles of toxicology apply broadly to understanding the effect of chemicals on human health. The principles of toxicology and pharmacology are identical and can be used to illustrate some concepts (see **Box 3.1**).

Industrial Hygiene

Industrial hygiene is the science related to anticipating, recognizing, controlling, and evaluating hazards that arise in or from the workplace that may affect the health and well-being of workers and members of the community.[35] Principles of industrial hygiene include the concept of a hierarchy of controls that ranks engineering controls as first and foremost and administrative controls/education and personal protective equipment (PPEs) as important but not to be used instead of engineering controls. **Engineering controls** consist of a set of methods to control exposures by modifying the source of contaminants or reducing the quantity of contaminants released into the environment. The primary intervention strategy should be to eliminate or reduce the hazard when possible or to apply other engineering controls; examples are listed in **Box 3.2**.[35] These principles apply broadly to environmental health.[18]

Table 3.3 Select Data[1] on Blood Lead (μg/dL) and Total Blood Mercury (μg/L) Levels in Children from the National Health and Nutrition Examination Survey (2009–2012)

		2009–2010		2011–2012	
Toxicant	Age Group (Years)	Geometric Mean	95th Percentile	Geometric Mean	95th Percentile
Lead	1–5	1.17	3.37	.970	2.91
	6–11	.838	2.01	.681	1.89
Mercury	1–5	*	1.30	.262	.990
	6–11	*	1.88	.330	1.40

[1]NHANES data available at http://www.cdc.gov/biomonitoring/pdf/FourthReport_UpdatedTables_Feb2015.pdf

*Not calculated; proportion of results less than the limit of detection was too high to provide valid results.

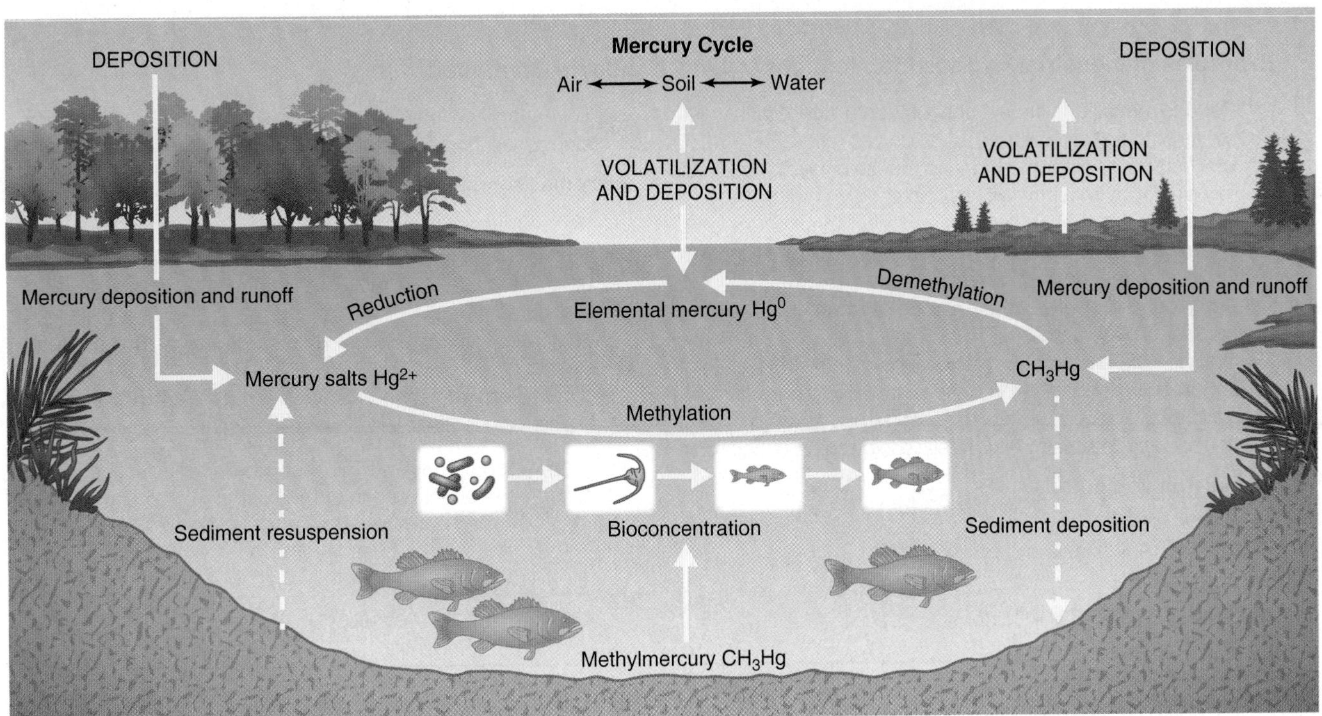

Figure 3.5 ■ The mercury cycle. Various sources emit elemental mercury into the air, which settles into bodies of water where methylmercury, the most toxic form of mercury, is formed by bacteria in the water. In this cycle, mercury is changed from its elemental form into its ionic form as well as the organic methylmercury form. Small fish eat phytoplankton, which have accumulated methylmercury; larger fish eat smaller fish. When larger fish eat smaller fish, the methylmercury bioconcentrates in the fish that are higher on the food chain. Humans, who are highest on the food chain, eat fish and are inadvertently exposed to methylmercury in the muscle tissue of the fish.

Box 3.1
General Principles of Toxicology

- A general axiom in toxicology is that "the dose makes the poison."[13] For toxicants, the risk of toxicity generally increases as the dose increases (i.e., a **dose–response relationship**). There may be some "low" dose (i.e., threshold) that does not produce observed adverse effects. An exception to "the dose makes the poison" applies when chemical and physical agents alter genetic material.
- Lipophilic (i.e., hydrophobic or fat-soluble) chemicals have longer half-lives ($T_{1/2}$) than less lipophilic or hydrophilic (i.e., water-soluble) chemical compounds do. Small nonionic molecules and lipophilic chemicals readily cross membranes, including the blood–brain barrier and the placenta. Chemicals will bioaccumulate when the rate of excretion is less than the rate of uptake. Because of their longer half-lives, lipophilic chemicals have greater potential than more water-soluble chemicals to bioaccumulate. Bioaccumulation increases the internal dose and therefore the risk of adverse effects.
- Toxicants that are indirect-acting agents must be biotransformed to one or more metabolites, which are chemically active (i.e., toxic). Toxicants (as well as pharmaceuticals) that are ingested are transported from the stomach through the hepatic portal vein to the liver, where biotransformation occurs (called the **first-pass effect**).[13] Many environmental chemicals require bioactivation. Some pharmaceuticals such as cyclophosphamide, which is used primarily to treat cancer, also require bioactivation. Conversely, because of the first-pass effect, ingestion of direct-acting toxicants reduces their toxicity.

Box 3.2
Examples of Industrial Hygiene Interventions to Limit Exposure

Engineering Controls

- Eliminate or reduce the use of hazardous substances.
- Replace hazardous substances with less harmful or toxic materials.
- Change operating processes (e.g., adding ozonation to the water treatment process that uses filtration and chlorination).
- Employ general ventilation (e.g., open windows) inside homes and other buildings, as well as local exhaust ventilation (hoods), particularly in workplaces.
- Contain hazards in enclosures to minimize the escape of vapors, gases, dusts, particles, or microbiological agents into the general breathing environment.

(Continued)

Box 3.2
Examples of Industrial Hygiene Interventions to Limit Exposure *Continued*

- Reduce emissions to air and effluents (industrial waste streams) to soil and water.
- Use barriers or other measures to reduce or eliminate injuries resulting from uncontrolled physical energy.
- Use mechanical lifting devices and align the work or other environment to the person and task to minimize ergonomic stresses to the musculoskeletal system.
- Apply good housekeeping in indoor environments; clean up outdoor environments.
- Optimize the design and maintenance of infrastructure (e.g., sewer and water distribution systems, transportation systems) to minimize infiltration of biological, chemical, and radiation hazards and uncontrolled energy (e.g., kinetic energy in vehicle collisions).

Administrative Controls

- Policymaking
- Enforcement of laws and policies
- Education and training of workers, including public health employees, as well as the general public.

Personal Protective Equipment

PPE are devices that serve as barriers to hazards. Examples include the following:

- Sunglasses to reduce the risk of cataracts from ultraviolet light exposure
- Seat belts to reduce the severity of injuries in motor vehicle crashes
- Gloves, respirators, and chemical-resistant gowns to reduce exposure to biological and chemical agents.

Although important, use of PPE depends on individual behavior, which limits the effectiveness of PPE compared to engineering controls, which do not depend on voluntary compliance.

Angela Yang: Outcome

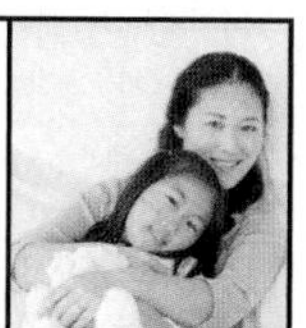

The neurologic effects of lead and mercury exposure are permanent.[45–47] Therefore, Angela's schools will need to assist her to maximize her learning potential, taking into account her cognitive challenges. Primary population-level control measures would focus on reducing the use of coal-burning power plants to generate electricity (a major source of mercury emissions), the use of efficient scrubbers (i.e., engineering controls) to capture mercury before it is released into the air, switching from coal to solar or wind power, and reduction in the use of mercury or the substitution of a less harmful chemical in various products. Examples of such products include electrical switches, medical equipment such as thermometers, and mercury in medicines (e.g., thimerosal [ethylmercury] as an antiseptic in vaccines). People can influence the marketplace by selecting products without mercury and by reducing their consumption of methylmercury in fish and seafood, substituting less contaminated fish species for more contaminated species. Generally, small fish with small mouths from less polluted source waters are less contaminated.[49]

9. What is the rationale behind the public health nurse's recommendation that the Yang family consume smaller fish with smaller mouths?
10. How does the concept of bioaccumulation relate to Angela's lead levels?

Milwaukee, Wisconsin: Outcome

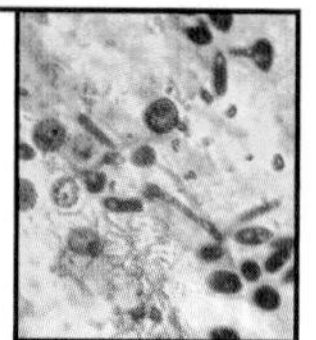

After the 1993 cryptosporidiosis outbreak, the City of Milwaukee implemented additional engineering controls. The city extended the intake pipe into Lake Michigan to minimize potential contamination of the source water with wastewater. The city also changed the water treatment processes to include the use of ozone, which, unlike chlorine, kills protozoan oocytes, including *Cryptosporidium* spp. These engineering controls have drastically diminished the risk of large-scale water-borne gastrointestinal disease outbreaks in Milwaukee.[36]

5. What is the purpose of the engineering controls put in place by the City of Milwaukee?
6. What administrative controls by the City of Milwaukee would be helpful in reducing the risk of water-borne disease outbreaks?

Richard Mara: Application

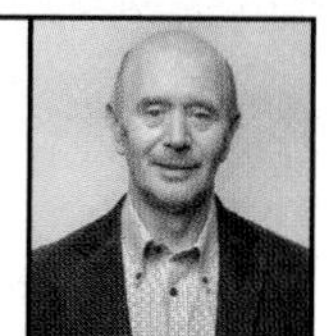

Mr. Mara's occupational history revealed that he worked as a printer in a small printing business for 40 years. During that time, continuous noise from the printing press required workers to talk loudly to hear one another. His work also involved the direct use of inks, which contain heavy metals used as pigments and also contain various solvents, including toluene. The place of employment did not use engineering controls, such as enclosure of the printers and insulation to reduce noise and vibration. General ventilation consisted of opening windows when the weather permitted, but no local ventilation (hood) was available. There were no occupational health services either on site or through contractual arrangements with an occupational medicine clinic. The employer did not provide hearing protection, such as earmuffs or earplugs. The employer did provide gloves (of unknown material) and rubber aprons, which Mr. Mara used regularly to reduce staining of his hands and clothes.

3. According to the principles of industrial hygiene, which intervention to limit exposure to environmental hazards would have the highest priority?
4. While PPE serve as barriers to hazards, what administrative controls are needed to ensure that PPE is effective?

Check Your Progress: Section 3.3

1. What role do healthcare workers play in epidemiology and surveillance?
2. Explain why children are more susceptible to toxicants than adults are.
3. How does the first-pass effect affect the toxicity of ingested chemicals.

3.4 Environmental Epidemiology

Environmental epidemiology is broad and complex because of the many exposures and range of outcomes discussed previously. Exposures may lead to outcomes that are acute (e.g., carbon monoxide poisoning) or chronic (e.g., lead and mercury poisonings, cancer, asthma, chronic pulmonary diseases). Directly linking causative environmental agents to a specific health effect can be challenging because of the web of causation (discussed in Chapter 1). In addition, except for injuries, there is no single comprehensive database on the prevalence, incidence, and mortality attributed to environmental agents, nor does one definitive source show what proportion of environmental diseases (e.g., infectious diseases, cancer, developmental problems, asthma) is attributable to certain environmental agents (e.g., microorganisms, chemicals, radiation). This section provides some background on the epidemiology of injuries (physical agents), infectious diseases (biological agents), and some chronic health problems caused in whole or in part by physical agents and chemical exposures.

Injury Epidemiology

Injuries result from the release of physical energy sufficient to cause tissue damage or death. The source of the energy can vary greatly, such as exposure to excessive heat (i.e., thermal burns), radiation (i.e., radiation burns), and physical force including trauma linked to violence (e.g., bullets as projectiles) or ergonomic injuries from falls or repeated trauma to the musculoskeletal system. (e.g., back strain). Features of the built environment can affect the risk of injury. For example, the presence or absence of sidewalks and bicycle paths affects the risk of injury to pedestrians and bicyclists.

The usually short time between exposure to a physical force such as kinetic, thermal, or radiant energy and injury more clearly links injuries to the causative exposure. Consequently, it is more feasible to conduct surveillance and formal epidemiologic studies of injuries than of other outcomes associated with biological and chemical agents. As a result, more is known about the incidence, mortality, and risk factors associated with acute injuries among workers and the general population than about other environmentally related health outcomes.

Epidemiologists distinguish injuries on the basis of whether they are intentional (suicide, homicide, and intentional nonfatal injuries) or unintentional (all other types). In 2014 in the United States, unintentional injuries ranked as the fourth leading cause of death overall and the leading cause for persons ages 1–44 years.[50] Common unintentional nonfatal injuries in 2014 included those due to falls, being struck by or against objects, overexertion, motor vehicle occupancy, being cut or pierced, poisoning, bites or stings, and assault (other than sexual), but the leading causes differed by age group.[51] Motor vehicle crashes were the fourth leading cause of nonfatal injuries overall, accounting for more than 2.4 million injuries.[52] In 2014, suicide was the second leading cause of death for people ages 10–34 years and the fourth leading cause for those ages 35–54 years.[50] In 2014, homicide was the third leading cause of death for people ages 1–4 years and 15–34 years, the fourth leading cause for children ages 5–9, and the fifth leading cause for children ages 10–14 and adults ages 35–44 years. In that same year, more than 2.1 million violence-related nonfatal injuries also occurred.[52]

Infectious Disease Epidemiology

The Centers for Disease Control and Prevention tracks more than 50 reportable diseases, including HIV/AIDS, cryptosporidiosis, Lyme disease, pertussis, salmonellosis, and tuberculosis.[53] Acute infectious diseases such as influenza and many gastrointestinal illnesses may be characterized by predictable patterns (e.g., seasonal) or may result from less predictable outbreaks (e.g., spikes related to food- or waterborne contamination).[54] With easier and more affordable travel and the globalization of the economy, large numbers of people and vast quantities of food and other products move around the world and can result in an outbreak, a rapid spread of emerging or reemerging infectious disease. Examples include severe acute respiratory syndrome, avian influenza, and salmonella infection from eggs.[54,55]

Surveillance Using Environmental Epidemiology Principles

One of the main epidemiologic methods to determine environmental exposures and health outcomes is through surveillance. The NHANES surveillance program takes comprehensive health histories, conducts thorough physical examinations, and performs various anthropometric measurements and health tests including hearing and cognition. In addition, an important component of NHANES is the extensive biomonitoring program that it has conducted since 1999 through blood and urine samples.[44] The biomonitoring program detects the uptake of more than 200 environmental toxicants such as lead, mercury, cadmium, PCBs, dioxins, and phthalates (plasticizers) in the U.S. population. Epidemiologists use statistical methods to examine the relationships between toxicants and other environmental agents and health outcomes using NHANES or other data.

Findings from environmental epidemiologic studies have been used to determine which outcomes best serve as sentinel health events. Table 3.2 presents a summary of environmental/occupational sentinel health events cross-classified by type of hazard. Of the environmental sentinel health events outlined in Table 3.2, only precocious onset of puberty/breast development and clear cell carcinoma of the vagina are not represented. Precocious development would indicate endocrine disruption; clear cell carcinoma of the vagina in young women is clearly linked to the hormone diethylstilbestrol[56] and to endocrine disruption.[57]

A cost analysis of four environmental health problems—lead poisoning, asthma, cancer, and neurobehavioral disorders—illustrates their magnitude among U.S. children.[58] In this analysis, environmental exposure was considered to be the source of 100% of lead poisonings; 30% of cases of asthma; 5% of cancers; and 10% of cases of autism, cerebral palsy, and mental retardation (intelligence quotient [IQ] below 85). The annual costs of lead poisoning in 5-year-olds were projected to be $43.4 billion US dollars in 2000 ($60.2 billion in 2016). Annual projected costs for asthma were $2.0 billion

Impact of Current Research on Clinical Practice

Detecting Lead in Drinking Water

Description: The contamination of drinking water with lead in Flint, Michigan, is an example of environmental epidemiology that combined regularly collected surveillance data with additional hazard evaluation. On April 25, 2014, the drinking water source for Flint, Michigan's approximately 99,000 residents was switched from Lake Huron (through the Detroit Water Authority) to the Flint River (through the Flint Water System). Despite residents' complaints of very poor water quality, the Flint Water System used no corrosion control. As a result, lead was leached out from the pipes into the drinking water. Other research showed that the drinking water was contaminated with lead. Between January 3, 2015, and October 5, 2015, a water advisory was issued encouraging residents to use bottled water. The prevalence of childhood lead poisoning ($\geq 5\ \mu g/dL$) was examined on the basis of 9422 samples. Venous or capillary blood samples were collected before the switch, during the early changeover to Flint River water, after the water advisory (bottled water use) while Flint River water continued to be used, and after the switch back to Lake Huron as the water source. The prevalence of lead poisoning in children during these time periods was 3.1%, 5.0%, 3.9%, and 1.4%, respectively.

Clinical Practice: The blood lead levels show an elevated prevalence of lead poisoning among young children when Flint River water was used for drinking, cooking, and other activities; it decreased once the use of bottled water or filtered drinking water had been strongly encouraged. The widespread reporting of childhood lead poisoning due to drinking water in Flint, Michigan, served as a sentinel health event for the rest of the nation.

Research Study:
Kennedy, C., Yard, E., Dignam, T., et al. (2016). Blood lead levels among children aged < 6 years: Flint, Michigan, 2013–2016. *MMWR, 65*. doi: http://dx.doi.org/10.15585/mmwr.mm6525e1.

($2.8 billion); for cancer, $332 million ($460 million); and for mental retardation, autism, and other neurobehavioral outcomes, $9.2 billion ($12.8 billion). In a separate analysis, Trasande et al.[59] estimated that mercury emissions affect between 300,000 and 600,000 infants each year through lowered IQ. Over a lifetime, such decreased IQ was estimated to result in lost economic productivity of $8.7 billion ($12 billion) for affected children born each year. ■

Animal laboratory studies provide invaluable experimental evidence about exposure–disease associations that have been identified in epidemiologic studies of human populations. When epidemiologic and laboratory data are essentially consistent, the laboratory findings lend support to the results from epidemiologic studies. Furthermore, laboratory studies are critical, as they aid in our understanding of pathophysiologic mechanisms.

Check Your Progress: Section 3.4

1. Why is it easier to connect injuries to causative exposure than it is to connect infectious diseases to causative exposure?
2. What is the difference between intentional and unintentional injuries?
3. Describe the impact of globalization and easier travel on the spread of disease.

3.5 Pathophysiologic Mechanisms

Exposure to one or more environmental agents may trigger multiple mechanisms that can interfere with normal cell growth and function. Such interference may involve genomic mutations, oxidative stress, inflammation and tissue repair, endocrine/hormonal disruption, and oxygen deprivation.[13] These mechanisms may operate alone, simultaneously, or sequentially, and they ultimately result in local or systemic pathology, such as the health problems noted in Table 3.2 and those discussed later in this chapter. For example, metabolic processes and environmental agents such as xenobiotics and ionizing radiation produce oxidative stress. Oxidative stress includes the production of oxygen-based free radicals, which can cause DNA damage that, if unrepaired, ultimately result in health problems such as cancer or developmental disorders. Oxidative stress may also trigger the production of reactive nitric oxide species in asthma and chronic obstructive pulmonary diseases.[60] Endocrine disruptors and other hormonally active agents in the environment mimic or block endogenous cell signals. Signal transduction, as it is called, has been linked in experimental animals with structural and functional abnormalities in the reproductive tract and abnormal development.[57] Disruption of signal transduction also has been shown experimentally to enhance fibrosis in chronic pulmonary disease and in bronchitis and asthma.[61] Both lead and mercury are well-known neurotoxicants.[13,20,45,47] It is less widely recognized but accurate that lead and mercury function as endocrine disruptors.[62,63] Hearing loss due to noise has been shown to be induced by decreased blood flow and free radical formation in the cochlea.[64] Carbon monoxide results from incomplete combustion of fossil fuel.[65] Carbon monoxide interferes with the normal uptake of oxygen by binding to hemoglobin with a much higher affinity than oxygen, thereby displacing oxygen in tissue and cells.[66] In the United States each year, an estimated 15,000 emergency department visits and 500 deaths due to asphyxia are attributed to carbon monoxide poisoning.[65]

Epigenetic mechanisms due to environmental exposures have received increasing attention. Epigenetics has been defined as "molecular factors/processes around the DNA that regulate genome activity independent of DNA sequence."[67] These processes are stable during cell division.

Known epigenetic processes consist of DNA methylation, histone modification, functional noncoding RNA, and chromatin structure. Research has shown that endocrine-disrupting agents and other environmental toxicants as well as some pharmaceuticals, nutrition (e.g., caloric restriction), and stress can promote disease susceptibility through epigenetic mechanisms.[67–69] Epigenetic transgenerational inheritance due to environmental exposures results in altered epigenetic information of the germ line that is passed on to subsequent generations without continued environmental exposures.[67] Thus, exposure of a pregnant woman to such an agent can result in epigenetic-induced changes that may be passed on to successive generations (i.e., great-grandchildren and beyond) whether or not they are exposed to the culpable agent.[68] Diethylstilbestrol's effect on genital tract abnormalities of offspring is one example. Multigenerational epidemiologic studies are needed to systematically examine epigenetic effects in human populations.

Thus, as the above examples illustrate, a variety of mechanisms in different cells and tissues are involved in the development of pathophysiologic responses that may ultimately result in disease. The chapters in Unit II, Risks Underlying the Leading Causes of Morbidity and Mortality, review some of these pathophysiology mechanisms. In addition, social and psychosocial stressors are linked to many disease states, including asthma, hypertension, cardiovascular disease, immunosuppression, preterm birth, depression, and violence to self and others, but the pathophysiologic mechanisms for many of these diseases are not yet well understood. For additional background, the reader is referred to Chapter 4 on psychosocial factors related to stress and disease.

Check Your Progress: Section 3.5

1. What role did epigenetic transgenerational inheritance play in the effects of diethylstilbestrol in offspring of women who took this drug during pregnancy?
2. Explain how lead and mercury function as endocrine disruptors.
3. What is the relationship between oxidative stress and cancer?

3.6 Hazards and Health Effects of Environmental Agents

The range of environmental hazards and associated health effects is daunting. Data in **Table 3.4** illustrate the links among environmental agents, specific exposures to hazards, associated health effects, and at-risk environments/occupations, all strongly based on epidemiologic evidence. Many more exposure–disease associations remain to be discovered by alert clinicians using the procedures described here.

Table 3.4 Examples of Environmental Agents, Sources of Exposure or Energy, Routes of Entry, Primary Systems Affected, and Primary Health Effects

Agent	Sources of Exposure	Routes of Entry	Primary Systems Affected	Primary Health Effects
Microbiological Agents				
Staphylococcus aureus	In healthcare settings: intravenous catheters, urinary catheter; endogenous in immunocompromised patients	Primary: intravenous route; secondary: infection (spread from other infections, such as wound infections)	Bloodstream (bacteremia, causing spread to all body organs)	Multiple organ dysfunction syndrome, fever
Streptococcus	Endogenous sources: gastrointestinal (GI) and genitourinary tracts; exogenous sources: contaminated medical devices	Primary: intravenous route; secondary: infection (spread from other infections, such as wound infections and respiratory infections)	Bloodstream (bacteremia, causing spread to all body organs)	Multiple organ dysfunction syndrome, infective endocarditis, fever
Hepatitis A	Food and water contaminated by hepatitis A virus; person-to-person transmission	Ingestion, infected blood, sexual contact	Liver	Jaundice, hepatitis, GI symptoms, fever
Hepatitis B and C	Infected blood and other body fluids; mother to newborn at time of delivery	Direct blood-to-blood contact, unprotected sex, unsterile needles, from an infected woman to her newborn during vaginal birth	Liver	Jaundice, acute and chronic hepatitis, liver cirrhosis, liver failure, fever
HIV	Infected blood and other body fluids; mother to newborn at time of delivery	Direct blood-to-blood contact, unprotected sex, unsterile needles, from an infected woman to her newborn during vaginal birth or through breastfeeding	Immune system	Opportunistic infections, AIDS wasting, anemia, multiple organ failure

(Continued)

Table 3.4 Examples of Environmental Agents, Sources of Exposure or Energy, Routes of Entry, Primary Systems Affected, and Primary Health Effects *Continued*

Agent	Sources of Exposure	Routes of Entry	Primary Systems Affected	Primary Health Effects
Microbiological Agents *Continued*				
Fungemia: *Candida* spp.	In healthcare settings: immunocompromised patients (e.g., low-birth-weight babies, HIV and oncology patients), central venous catheter	Endogenous, intravenous therapy	Bloodstream (bacteremia, causing spread to all body organs	Multiple organ failure; disseminated candidiasis lesions including papules, pustules, nodules, and folliculitis; *Candida*; endophthalmitis; fever
Cryptosporidium parvum and *Cryptosporidium hominis*	Water, food contaminated by animal and/or human waste	Ingestion	Gastrointestinal	Diarrheal illness; may also cause non-GI symptoms including arthritis, cholangitis, pancreatitis, hepatitis, and pulmonary cryptosporidiosis
E. coli O157:H7	Primarily food (especially inadequately cooked ground beef) or water contaminated by animal and/or human waste	Ingestion	Gastrointestinal, renal	Diarrheal illness, frequently with bloody stool; hemolytic uremic syndrome
Influenza viruses	Infected person in community, workplace	Inhalation	Pulmonary	Influenza
Mycobacterium tuberculosis	Infected person in community or workplace; consumption of unpasteurized milk or milk products (e.g., cheese, yogurt) from *M. tuberculosis*–infected cattle	Inhalation, ingestion	Pulmonary	Pulmonary tuberculosis infection or disease, disseminated tuberculosis (nonpulmonary tissues)
Salmonella	Food, water contaminated with *S. typhi*, which is shed from the intestinal tract of infected humans	Ingestion	Gastrointestinal, renal	Diarrheal illness, bacteremia, involving systemic infection with *Salmonella typhimurium* or other *Salmonella* spp. and Reiter syndrome, a form of chronic arthritis, are potential complications.
Chemical Agents				
Antineoplastic drugs	Medication	Ingestion, parenteral	Hematologic, reproductive, neurologic, gastrointestinal	Leukemias and other cancers, adverse developmental and reproductive outcomes in workers; cognitive impairment and nausea, vomiting, diarrhea in patient populations
Methylmercury	Fish and seafood	Ingestion	Neurologic, reproductive	Cognitive impairment, adverse developmental and reproductive outcomes
Carbon monoxide	Incomplete combustion of fossil fuels in home, workplace	Inhalation	Blood	Acute symptoms include headache, drowsiness, light-headedness, slurred speech, irritability, impaired gait, stupor, rapid loss of consciousness, coma, seizures, and death.
Atrazine (synthetic herbicide)	Atrazine is a herbicide sprayed on farm crops, nursery crops such as fir trees, and roadways, that may contaminate well water	Inhalation, ingestion of atrazine-contaminated water or atrazine by-products	Endocrine, reproductive	Teratogen and reproductive toxin; liver, kidney, and heart damage has been observed in animal models.
Trichloroethylene	Dry cleaning processing, paints, adhesives, varnishes	Inhalation, dermal absorption	Nervous, skin, cardiovascular	Acute CNS depression, peripheral and cranial neuropathy, dermatitis, arrhythmias
Lead	Paint, storage batteries, pottery glazes and glassware that contain lead; cultural practices in which lead is a component or ingredient	Ingestion of dust, inhalation of dust or fumes	Hematologic, renal, gastrointestinal, neuromuscular, CNS, reproductive	Anemia, nephropathy, abdominal pain, palsy (wrist drop), encephalopathy

Agent	Sources of Exposure	Routes of Entry	Primary Systems Affected	Primary Health Effects
Physical Agents				
Ionizing radiation	Radon, x-ray, dirty bomb	Inhalation, ingestion, dermal absorption	Pulmonary, hematologic, integumentary, gastrointestinal, reproductive	Cancer (lung, stomach, leukemia), bone marrow suppression, alopecia, sterility (male, female)
Noise	Sound waves and vibration	Auditory, whole-body absorption	Neurologic, cardiovascular, immune	Hearing loss, tinnitus, psychologic stress, sleep disturbances, hypertension, myocardial infarction, increase in adrenergic hormones
Nonionizing radiation	Ultraviolet A, ultraviolet B, electromagnetic fields	Absorption	Integumentary, neurologic, hematologic, immune	Erythemia, sunburn, nonmelanoma skin cancer, cutaneous malignant melanoma, cataracts, leukemia (possibly), immunosuppression
Physical force	Kinetic	Absorption	All, depending on type of injury	
Repetitive motion	Kinetic/biomechanical	Absorption	Musculoskeletal, peripheral nervous	Carpal tunnel syndrome, bursitis, tenosynovitis, ganglion cyst, tendinitis
Temperature extremes	Thermal	Absorption	Integumentary, central nervous system	Heat rash, exhaustion, stroke, frostbite, hypothermia, trench foot
Vibration	Mechanical	Absorption	Vascular, musculoskeletal, neurologic	Raynaud phenomenon, tenosynovitis, hearing loss
Psychosocial Agents				
Stress	Conflict in family, work, social relationships; interaction with natural and built environment; workload demands	Intrapersonal, interpersonal	Neurologic, immune, cardiovascular, pulmonary, gastrointestinal	Mental health (anxiety, depression, substance abuse); immune dysfunction; hypertension; changes in heart rate/rhythm; cardiovascular disease; asthma; gastritis; ulcers
Violence	Conflict in family, work, social relationships; social, political, economic conflict; war	Intrapersonal, interpersonal, collective (social, political, economic)	Nonphysical: same as for stress Physical: depends on the severity and location of injury	Nonphysical: same as for stress Physical: same as for stress; varies by severity and location of injury

SOURCES: Adapted from Mullan, R. J., & Murthy, L. I. (1983). Occupational sentinel health events: An up-dated list for physician recognition and public health surveillance. *American Journal of Industrial Medicine, 19*, 775–799; cross-validated against Rutstein, D. D., Mullan, R. J., Frazier, T. M., et al. (1983). Sentinel health events (occupational): A basis for physician recognition and public health surveillance. *American Journal of Public Health, 73*(9), 1054–1062. Murthy, L. I. (1997). Two NIOSH resources for implementing workplace safety and health surveillance. *Annals of the New York Academy of Sciences, 837*, 319–352.

Detecting Exposures to Environmental Hazards

The patient's health history is the most critical means to determine exposures to environmental agents.[70] To be effective, the health history must include details about exposures to biological, chemical, physical, and psychosocial agents at work, in the home, and in the community for both present and past exposures. In addition, the health history should elicit information regarding the degree to which engineering, work practices, and PPE are and were used to control hazards.

CLINICAL POINT: The healthcare provider must ask not only about the person's current occupation, but also about the tasks and procedures involved in the job, which often reveal practices that increase the risk of exposure to hazards. Sometimes, it is informative to ask patients to demonstrate how they do the task and the environment in which the task is performed (e.g., crowded, noisy, dusty). In addition, the history of past exposures should include temporary work (e.g., employment or volunteer work) as well as summer and after-school jobs in childhood or adolescence. While temporary, these jobs can entail many hazards. Examples include thermal and electrical burns; falls on wet or greasy floors; cuts and other injuries; possibly sleep deprivation if there are competing demands from school, home, and work; chemical exposures; and stress from working in fast-paced jobs as at fast-food restaurants. Inquiring about hobbies and recreation, including these activities done by others in the home, is necessary to determine possible exposures such as exposure to solvents during refinishing furniture and pesticides during gardening. ■

Depending on the health history, biomonitoring of actual exposures (biological uptake) may be done. Most biomonitoring is done on worker populations. For biomonitoring of workers, venous blood, urine samples, or other specimens (depending on the chemical or metabolites measured) should be taken at the end of a work shift.[71] As an example, toluene is a commonly used solvent in industry and is also recreationally used in "glue sniffing." In one study, workers who had been exposed to an average air concentration of 34 parts per million (ppm) (compared with the Occupational Safety and Health Administration's Permissible Exposure Limit [air] of 200 ppm) during an 8-hour shift had a mean blood toluene level of 45.7 μg/dL.[72] In the same study, the general population had a mean blood toluene level of 0.1 μg/dL, which meets the criterion level for unexposed populations.[73]

Except for lead levels, biomonitoring of children is seldom done. However, studies have shown that children are exposed to pesticides at home and school that raise concerns about the short- and long-term health consequences of pesticides and other toxicants.[74,75] ■

There are a myriad of biomonitoring tests, and the reader is referred to the CDC's National Biomonitoring Program (https://www.cdc.gov/biomonitoring/about.html) for information on specific tests. Healthcare providers should use knowledge of a patient's current and past exposures to hazards to guide the physical examination.

Detecting Diseases, Injuries, and Other Health Problems

The physical examination, whether head-to-toe or focused, provides initial evidence of possible health problems.

CLINICAL POINT: Deviations from normal detected in the physical examination may result from environmental exposures (alone or interacting with other exposures), genetic predisposition, or both. When information obtained from the health history and results of the physical examination converge, the data lend credence to an environmental etiology. An absence of corroboration may warrant more detailed examination or testing and appropriate referrals. Diagnostic testing may consist of laboratory tests, diagnostic imaging, electrophysiologic tests, or other tests as indicated by the particular system(s) involved. ■

The following case study examines a clinical situation with respect to essential environmental health principles. The discussion that follows reviews how the inclusion of environmental health principles in the history and physical examination affects the plan for the patient.

Richard Mara: Application

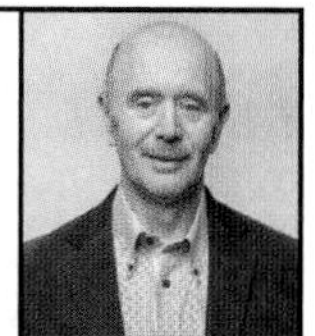

Richard Mara's healthcare provider was able to detect a possible health problem—noise-induced hearing loss—via the health history by considering possible environmental hazard exposures. Nevertheless, background knowledge of possible environmental health hazards was necessary for the provider to incorporate relevant health history questions. For example, the provider was aware that each year, 30 million workers are exposed to noise sufficient to cause hearing loss.[76,77] Noise also is a common environmental exposure. Other exposures, however, also contribute to hearing loss. The provider knew that exposures to solvents, heavy metals, and possibly cigarette smoking at work, at home, or during recreational activities can induce sensorineural hearing loss, particularly in combination with noise.[77–80]

Mr. Mara's healthcare provider took a thorough health history that included data about occupational and environmental sources of exposure to noise and toxicants known to contribute to hearing loss. The provider also performed hearing screening tests (whisper-and-watch, Rinne, and Weber tests) as a part of the physical examination.

5. In addition to hearing loss, the healthcare provider should assess Mr. Mara for what other health effects due to long-term exposure to noise?
6. Why does the healthcare provider not rely solely on Mr. Mara's subjective report of reduced hearing from the health history to diagnose hearing loss?

The case study of Richard Mara provides an example of the interaction of a physical hazard (noise) and one or more chemical hazards (solvents and heavy metals) that can increase the risk of hearing loss more than either hazard alone. The case study also illustrates that a hazard such as noise can have two or more different health effects. Using the hazard classification by nature, which was discussed earlier, the following sections present common biological, chemical, physical, and psychosocial environmental agents and the corresponding known health effects (see also Table 3.4).

Biological Hazards

The extent of environmentally acquired infections in the United States is difficult to track. In occupational settings, many biological agents are associated with sentinel health events (see Table 3.2).[15] Because food- and water-borne infections are prevalent environmental health problems afflicting the U.S. population, the following discussions focus on these infections and the role of endotoxins in chronic respiratory diseases.

According to surveillance and hospitalization data and taking into account the estimated underreporting of food-borne illnesses, the U.S. population experiences more than 38 million cases of food- and water-borne illnesses each year.[41] Almost 60% of these illnesses are attributed to noroviruses (formerly called Norwalk-like viruses).[41,81] Noroviruses are predominantly water-borne (60%).[41] Bacterial, parasitic, and viral organisms vary in the proportion that are food-borne, from 10% for *Cryptosporidium* spp. and *Giardia lamblia* to 100% for *Bacillus cereus*, food-borne botulism, *Clostridium perfringens*, staphylococcal food poisonings, streptococcal food-borne illnesses, and *Trichinella spiralis*. In 2014, the FoodNet Surveillance System reported that the case fatality rate was highest for *Listeria monocytogenes* (15%), followed by *Yersinia* spp. (1.0%) and *Vibrio* spp. (1.0%).[82]

Substantial progress in tracking food- and water-borne illnesses has been made, but challenges remain. Most (72%) food-borne outbreaks do not have a recognized etiology,[81] and the FoodNet surveillance system identified only 19,507 laboratory-confirmed cases in 2014.[82]

Biological agents are not limited to organisms that cause infectious disease. One of the best examples is endotoxins, which consist of lipopolysaccharide elements from the outer membrane of gram-negative bacteria. Recent research has demonstrated the importance of endotoxins in triggering asthma or asthma-type symptoms in children independent of other asthma triggers.[83,84] Endotoxins are also present in workplaces.[85] They serve as an excellent illustration of a ubiquitous biological agent that affects indoor air quality and poses health risks to children and adults alike.

Chemical Hazards

More than 80,000 synthetic chemical compounds have been developed in the United States over the past 50 years.[86] Annually, 15,000 of these chemicals are produced in excess of 10,000 pounds per year, while an additional

2800 chemicals are produced in excess of 1 million pounds. Fewer than half (43%) of the high-volume chemicals have undergone toxicity testing, and only a small proportion (7%) has been tested for developmental toxicity.[20,87]

Risk assessment characterizes the potential adverse health effects on humans as a consequence of exposures to hazardous substances or situations.[13] Risk assessment uses information about the structure and function of chemicals, in vitro assays of genotoxicity, in vivo studies using suitable animal models, and epidemiologic studies of human health effects. An alternative approach to risk assessment is called the **precautionary principle**, which asserts that interventions must be undertaken when an environmental threat to human health is feasible, even if scientific evidence is not conclusive.[88]

Much of what is known about human health effects of chemicals is based on studies of occupational groups at higher doses than are typically found in the general population. For example, epidemiologic studies have shown that the risk of mesothelioma (cancer of the pleural and peritoneal linings of the thoracic and abdominal cavities, respectively) is significantly elevated in workers who have been exposed to asbestos, such as shipbuilders[89] and insulation workers.[90] Relatively few studies have been reported on mesothelioma, lung cancer, or asbestosis (a chronic fibrotic lung disease) in non–occupationally exposed people, such as residents of Libby, Montana, who were exposed to asbestos-contaminated vermiculite from 1920 to 1990. However, Miller more recently reported on 32 cases of mesothelioma in household members of shipbuilders, insulators, and other asbestos-exposed workers.[91] The household members' diagnoses of mesothelioma were attributed to asbestos that was taken home on work clothes and shoes. Radiologic evidence of asbestosis also has been reported in wives, sons, and daughters of asbestos-exposed shipyard workers.[92]

Physical Hazards

Physical hazards are both natural and human-made, depending on the source of energy. Exposure to ionizing radiation, for example, occurs naturally with radon and artificially through x-ray devices. Temperature extremes, which occur for various reasons, are another type of physical hazard. Locally, temperature extremes in weather increase as the global climate changes. At the micro level, many manufacturing processes generate extreme temperatures in the workplace, such as heat during steel fabrication or cold as part of food refrigeration. The outcomes of exposure to physical hazards range from immediate health effects (e.g., sunburn, heat stroke, frostbite, tinnitus) to effects that emerge after prolonged exposure, such as cataracts (ultraviolet light), carpal tunnel syndrome (biomechanical), sensorineural hearing loss (noise), and lung cancer (radon). An emerging issue related to physical hazards is the built environment, which serves as a health hazard when land use and transportation avenues do not support health.

Physical inactivity and obesity are more common in children in geographical areas where there are fewer recreational facilities.[93] ■

Richard Mara: Outcome

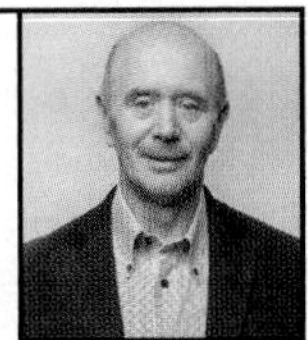

The findings of Mr. Mara's examination indicated bilateral sensorineural hearing loss. His healthcare provider discussed with Mr. Mara cost–benefit considerations for referral. Hearing aids are effective only for conductive hearing loss, and sensorineural hearing loss is usually permanent and cumulative over a lifetime. It is preventable, however, so the decision was to emphasize avoidance of further noise and chemical exposures, because continued exposure to noise and neurotoxicants would contribute to even greater hearing loss. The healthcare provider used concepts from toxicology (see Box 3.2) as the basis for counseling Mr. Mara on how to minimize exposures that would likely increase his hearing loss.

Knowing that noise is associated not only with hearing loss, but also with other health problems, including hypertension (see Table 3.4 and refer to Chapter 31), the healthcare provider paid particular attention to these systems during the physical examination. For Mr. Mara, blood pressure, sleep patterns, stress level, and cardiovascular indicators were within normal limits. So, the plan was to monitor his health at 6-month intervals as he gets established in his new environment.

In reflecting on Mr. Mara's former workplace, the healthcare provider realized that the lack of occupational health services at work contributed not only to Mr. Mara's hearing loss and potentially other adverse outcomes (see Tables 3.1 and 3.4), but also to health problems among many other workers. Had a good occupational health service been operating, engineering controls could have prevented the high levels of sustained noise, exposures to chemicals through inhalation and dermal exposure, and subsequent health problems. The work site management could have conducted regular surveillance programs, consisting of a hearing conservation program that follows the Occupational Health and Safety Administration regulations, measurements of contaminants in the air, and biological monitoring to ensure that the engineering controls and work practices were effective as part of an occupational health/industrial hygiene program.

7. Using administrative controls from the concepts of toxicology in Box 3.2, how might the healthcare provider counsel Mr. Mara to minimize exposures that would likely increase his hearing loss?
8. What engineering controls could have been put in place to prevent or reduce Mr. Mara's hearing loss?

Psychosocial Hazards

Exposure to psychosocial hazards can occur in any setting: home (e.g., abuse, stress), school (e.g., bullying, harassment), work (e.g., harassment, stress from rotating shifts, job demands), and the community at large, such as with road rage, natural disasters, terrorist events, or war. These exposures can have deleterious effects in multiple systems. Immediate psychologic effects may include anxiety disorders, depression, or posttraumatic stress disorder. Physiologic ramifications may include increases in heart rate, blood pressure, and respiration as well as increased production of stress hormones (e.g., epinephrine, cortisol) and decreased digestive motility (refer to Chapter 4 for specifics). Health outcomes also may include injuries resulting from violence, which can range from minor bruises to multisystem trauma and death. Psychologic responses (e.g., depression) may result from exposures to neurotoxicants such as lead, mercury, or solvents[13] and therefore warrant a careful exposure history to determine appropriate intervention.

The most common psychosocial agent is stress, and daily exposure to stress occurs in well-resourced countries as well as in under-resourced ones. As with chemical agents, exposure to stress may be acute or chronic, and health outcomes may vary with type or duration of exposure. For example, in most natural disasters, stress responses are transient. Longer-term responses, such as depression and posttraumatic stress disorder, are more likely to emerge in people who live near contaminated sites when there is a continued perceived danger, little sense of control, continued media coverage, and personal involvement in or a relationship with someone directly affected by the contamination.[18]

Check Your Progress: Section 3.6

1. A health history to detect exposure to environmental hazards should elicit what key information?
2. What is the purpose of biomonitoring?
3. Describe the relationship between the health history and the physical examination in detecting environmental injuries.

CHAPTER SUMMARY

3.1 Chapter Overview and Case Studies

Describe the relationship between social environment, physical environment, built environment, genetic endowment, and health outcomes, and discuss concepts related to environmental health.

- Environmental health is determined by the social (social and psychologic hazards) and physical environments (physical, chemical, and biological hazards, and the natural and built environments) that interact with each other and with the individual's genetic endowment.
- Multiple mechanisms are involved in the pathogenesis of environmentally related diseases and injuries.
- Exposure to environmental hazards is common and occurs in the context of where people live, work, play, and go to school.
- Case studies were used to apply the chapter concepts to prevent and intervene early in the pathogenesis of environmental diseases, injuries, and other health problems.
- The main physiologic concepts related to environmental health are oxygenation, perfusion, nutrition, thermoregulation, tissue integrity, genetics and genomics, cellular regulation, inflammation, immunity, infection, and stress.

3.2 Environmental Hazard Classification

Classify environmental hazards according to their nature, transport media, routes of exposure, and outcomes.

- Hazards are classified by using several approaches based on the type of hazard and exposure; these approaches include nature, transport media, route, setting, and outcomes.
- Classification of environmental hazards according to their nature includes biological, chemical, physical, and psychosocial hazards.
- Air, water, soil, and food are types of transport media for hazards.
- Routes of exposure to hazards are inhalation, ingestion, dermal absorption, and transplacental.
- Settings in which hazard exposures occur are the home, workplace, school, and community.
- Hazards are also classified according to their outcomes, such as mutagen, teratogen, or carcinogen, or by the organ system that is adversely affected (e.g. cardiotoxicant, neurotoxicant).

3.3 Key Concepts of Environmental Health from Related Sciences

Discuss how key concepts from environmental health–related sciences are applied in the assessment, intervention, and evaluation process to control or prevent environmental health problems.

- Although environmental hazards are ubiquitous, some segments of the population are at more risk of exposure and resulting environmental diseases, injuries, and health problems than are others.
- Some segments of the population are particularly vulnerable to environmental hazards. Examples include fetuses; children; older adults; and people with differential exposure, preparedness, and ability to recover.
- Surveillance, epidemiology, microbiology, toxicology, and industrial hygiene form the basis for assessment, intervention, and evaluation of progress made to assess, control, and prevent environmental health problems.
- Exposures to biological, chemical, physical, and psychosocial hazards underlie preventable diseases, injuries, and other health problems.
- Sentinel health events herald an environmental health problem not just for the individual but also potentially for others in the home, work, and community environments.

- Control of hazards, and therefore, environmental health problems, depends on the recognition and application of various environmental health interventions.
- Environmental health interventions include surveillance, hazard evaluations, epidemiology, engineering controls, education, and policymaking.

3.4 Environmental Epidemiology

Explain how environmental epidemiology is used to understand and protect the health of individuals, communities, and populations regarding environmental hazards.

- Environmental diseases, injuries, and health problems are prevalent, costly, and often fatal.
- Surveillance for environmental hazards and formal epidemiologic studies benefit from the availability of biomonitoring data and the linkage of these data with health outcomes using databases (e.g., NHANES) and other epidemiologic studies.

3.5 Pathophysiologic Mechanisms

Explain the basic pathophysiologic mechanisms underlying alterations caused by environmental hazards.

- Multiple pathophysiologic mechanisms including genomic mutation, epigenetic effects, oxidative stress, inflammation and tissue repair, endocrine/hormonal disruption, and oxygen deprivation are involved in environmental diseases, injuries, and health problems.
- Pathophysiologic mechanisms involved in different environmental diseases function alone, sequentially, or simultaneously.

3.6 Hazards and Health Effects of Environmental Agents

Analyze the relationship between various hazardous agents and the health effects they produce.

- This chapter provided examples of the many environmental hazards and resulting adverse health outcomes, including sentinel health events.
- Environmental and occupational sentinel health events represent a wide range of health outcomes and biological, chemical, and physical hazards are identified as causative environmental agents.
- Environmental health histories are critical in detecting exposures to environmental hazards and potential environmental diseases, injuries, and other health problems.
- Environmental health histories and physical examinations are used to recognize sentinel health events and to recognize new environmental health problems.
- Awareness of biological, chemical, physical, and psychosocial hazards is key to early recognition, control, and prevention of environmental health problems.

REVIEW QUESTIONS

1. The public health nurse is assessing the environmental health of a community. Which of the following would the nurse assess?
   a. Financial resources
   b. Physical environment
   c. Public school system
   d. Recreational resources

2. The nurse is teaching a class on environmental safety for new parents. The nurse teaches that the primary route of exposure of chemicals in the home is which of the following?
   a. Inhalation
   b. Ingestion
   c. Dermal absorption
   d. Intraplacental

3. Young children are more susceptible than adults to environmental disease or injury for which of the following reasons?
   a. Many chemicals cross the placenta.
   b. Blood flow to the liver is diminished.
   c. Surface-to-body mass is reduced.
   d. Metabolism is higher.

4. When elevated lead levels are detected in one child in a family, the nurse explains that the other children also need to be tested. Which of the following statements by the mother indicates that the mother understands the nurse's instruction?
   a. "My other children are at risk because they are exposed to the same hazards in the home."
   b. "My other children are not at risk because they attend different schools."
   c. "There's no need to test the other children because we have removed the lead paint."
   d. "There is no need to test my other children because they are not showing any signs of elevated lead levels."

5. Which of the following actions by the public health nurse is an example of epidemiology?
   a. Providing care to a child with an elevated mercury level
   b. Teaching parents about the effects of high mercury levels in children
   c. Evaluating the effectiveness of measures to clean the drinking water for a town
   d. Campaigning for safe drinking water laws

6. The occupational health nurse in a large industrial plant is answering questions after a presentation to management on the routes of exposure to the chemicals that are used in the plant. Which of the following statements indicates that the nurse needs to clarify concepts?
   a. "Food in the cafeteria does not need to be protected from airborne contamination."
   b. "We need to make sure that all workers on the plant floor are wearing respirators."
   c. "Workers handling chemicals need to wear protective gloves."
   d. "Workers need to wear eye protection when working with gases or vapors."

7. Having noticed that there are many children in the community with asthma, the public health nurse starts to collect data on families in the community. Which of the following functions is the nurse engaged in?
   a. Surveillance
   b. Assessment of environmental hazards
   c. Prevention
   d. Hazard control

8. Which of the following is an epidemiologic function of the public health nurse?
   a. Identifying health hazards for asthma in a home
   b. Teaching a program on living with asthma
   c. Evaluating risk factors for asthma in a community
   d. Determining the effectiveness of asthma treatment in an adult

ANSWERS

Answers to Review Questions can be found in Appendix A. Answers to Case Study and Check Your Progress questions are available on the faculty resources site. Please consult with your instructor.

RECOMMENDED WEBSITES

Agency for Toxic Substances and Disease Registry
https://www.atsdr.cdc.gov

American Nurses Association
http://nursingworld.org

Centers for Disease Control and Prevention
https://www.cdc.gov

Environmental Health Perspectives
https://ehp.niehs.nih.gov

Health Care Without Harm
https://noharm.org

National Center for Environmental Health
https://www.cdc.gov/nceh/default.htm

National Toxicology Program
https://ntp.niehs.nih.gov

Occupational Safety and Health Administration
https://www.osha.gov

Pocket Guide to Chemical Hazards
https://www.cdc.gov/niosh/npg

The Luminary Project: Nurses Lighting the Way to Environmental Health
http://www.theluminaryproject.org

U.S. Environmental Protection Agency
https://www.epa.gov

REFERENCES

1. National Environmental Health Association. (2016). *Definitions of environmental health.* Retrieved from http://www.neha.org/about-neha/definitions-environmental-health
2. Evans, R. G., & Stoddart, G. L. (1990). Predicting health, consuming health care. *Social Science & Medicine, 31*, 1347–1363.
3. Simonds, N. I, Ghazarian, A. A., Pimentel, C. B., et al. (2016). Review of the gene-environment interaction literature in cancer: What do we know? *Genetic Epidemiology, 40*(5), 356–365. doi: 10.1002/gepi.21967
4. Skinner, M. K. (2008). What is an epigenetic transgenerational phenotype? F3 or F2. *Reproductive Toxicology, 25*, 2–6.
5. Pembry, M. E. (2010). Male-line transgenerational responses in humans. *Human Fertility, 13*, 268–271.
6. Pruss-Ustün, A., & Corvalan, C. (2006). *Preventing disease through healthy environments: Towards an estimate of the environmental burden of disease.* Geneva, Switzerland: World Health Organization. Available at http://www.who.int/quantifying_ehimpacts/publications/preventingdisease.pdf
7. Smith, R. R., Corvalan, C. F., & Kjellstrom, T. (1999). How much global ill health is attributable to environmental factors? *Epidemiology, 10*, 573–584.
8. GBD 2013 Mortality and Causes of Death Collaboration. (2015). Global, regional, and national age-sex specific all-cause and cause-specific mortality for 240 causes of death, 1990–2013: A systematic analysis for the global burden of disease study 2013. *Lancet*, 385(9963), 117–171.
9. Global Burden of Disease Pediatrics Collaboration. (2016). Global and national burden of diseases and injuries among children and adolescents between 1990 and 2013: Findings from the Global Burden of Disease 2013 Study. *JAMA Pediatrics, 2170*(3), 267–287. doi: 10.1001/jamapediatrics.2015.4276

10. U.S. Department of Health and Human Services. (2016). *Healthy People 2020*. Available at https://www.healthypeople.gov
11. Centers for Disease Control and Prevention. (2015). *Fourth national report on human exposure to environmental chemicals: Updated tables*. Available at http://www.cdc.gov/biomonitoring/pdf/FourthReport_UpdatedTables_Feb2015.pdf
12. MacKenzie, W. R., Hoxie, N. J., Proctor, M. E., et al. (1994). A massive outbreak in Milwaukee of Cryptosporidium infection transmitted through the public water supply. *New England Journal of Medicine, 331*, 151–167.
13. Klaassen, C. D. (Ed.). (2013). *Casarett and Doull's toxicology: The basic science of poison* (8th ed.). New York, NY: McGraw Hill.
14. Srinivasan, S., O'Fallon, L. R., & Dearry, A. (2003). Creating healthy communities, healthy homes, healthy people: Initiating a research agenda on the built environment and public health. *American Journal of Public Health, 93*, 1446–1450.
15. Nester, E., Anderson, D., Roberts, C. E., Jr., & Nester, M. (2009). *Microbiology: A human perspective* (6th ed.). Boston, MA: McGraw-Hill Higher Education.
16. U.S. Environmental Protection Agency (n.d.). *Ionizing and non-ionizing radiation*. Available at https://www.epa.gov/radiation/radiation-basics.
17. Pope, A. M., Snyder, M. A., & Mood, L. H. (Eds.). (1995). *Nursing, health, & the environment*. Washington, DC: National Academy Press.
18. Frumkin, H. (2016). *Environmental health: From global to local* (3rd ed.). San Francisco, CA: John Wiley & Sons.
19. Tucker, P. (2001). Scientific research continues on the psychological responses to toxic contamination. *Hazardous Substances & Public Health, 10*, 1–3.
20. Etzel, R. A., & Balk, S. J. (Eds.). (2012.) *Pediatric environmental health* (3rd ed.). Elk Grove Village, IL: American Academy of Pediatrics.
21. Rom W. N., & Markowitz S. B. (Eds.). (2007). *Environmental and occupational medicine* (4th ed.). Philadelphia, PA: Lippincott, Williams, & Wilkins.
22. Gordis, L. (2014). *Epidemiology* (5th ed.). Philadelphia, PA: Saunders.
23. Thomas, D. C. (2009). *Statistical methods in environmental epidemiology*. New York, NY: Oxford University Press.
24. Rutstein, D. D., Mullan, R. J., Frazier, T. M., et al. (1983). Sentinel health events (occupational): A basis for physician recognition and public health surveillance. *American Journal of Public Health, 73*, 1054–1062.
25. Mullan R. J., & Murthy L. I. (1991). Occupational sentinel health events: An up-dated list for physician recognition and public health surveillance. *American Journal of Industrial Medicine, 19*, 775–799.
26. Halperin, W., & Baker, E. L. (Eds.). (1992). *Public health surveillance*. New York, NY: Van Nostrand Reinhold.
27. Shy, C., Greenberg, R., & Winn, D. (1994). Sentinel health events of environmental contamination: A consensus statement. *Environmental Health Perspectives, 102*, 316–317.
28. Sheppard, L., Levy, D., Norris, G., Larson, T. V., & Koenig, J. Q. (1999). Effects of ambient air pollution on nonelderly asthma hospital admissions in Seattle, Washington, 1987–1994. *Epidemiology, 10*(1), 23–30.
29. Schildcrout, J. S., Sheppard, L., Lumley, T., et al. (2006). Ambient air pollution and asthma exacerbations in children: An eight-city analysis. *American Journal of Epidemiology, 64*, 505–517.
30. National Environmental Justice Advisory Council to the U.S. Environmental Protection Agency. (2004). *Ensuring risk reduction in communities with multiple stressors: Environmental justices and cumulative risks/impacts*. Available at http://www.epa.gov/compliance/ej/resources/publications/nejac/nejac-cum-risk-rpt-122104.pdf
31. Darby, S., Hill, D., Auvinen, A., et al. (2005). Radon in homes and risk of lung cancer: Collaborative analysis of individual data from 13 European case-control studies. *BMJ 330*, 1–6. doi: 10.1136/bmj.38308.477650.63
32. World Health Organization. (2002). *The world health report 2002: Reducing risks, promoting healthy life*. Geneva, Switzerland: WHO. Available at http://www.who.int/whr/2002/en/whr02_en.pdf?ua=1
33. Baer, R. D., Garcia de Alba, J., Leal, R. M., et al. (1998). Mexican use of lead in the treatment of empacho: Community, clinic, and longitudinal patterns. *Social Science & Medicine, 47*, 1263–1264.
34. Abrass, I. B. (1990). The biology and physiology of aging. *Western Journal of Medicine, 153*, 641–645.
35. Levy, B. S., Wegman, D. H., Baron, S. L., & Sokas, R. K. (2011). *Occupational and environmental health: Recognizing and preventing disease and injury* (6th ed.). New York, NY: Oxford University Press.
36. Hewitt, J. B. (2007). Cryptosporidiosis. In F. R. Lashley & J. D. Durham (Eds.), *Emerging infectious diseases: Trends and issues* (2nd ed., pp. 95–110). New York, NY: Springer.
37. Egorov, A., Frost, F., Muller, T., et al. (2004). Serological evidence of Cryptosporidium infections in a Russian city and evaluation of risk factors for infections. *Annals of Epidemiology, 14*, 129–136.
38. Rowland, M. G. (1986). The Gambia and Bangladesh: The seasons and diarrhoea. *Dialogue on Diarrhoea, 26*, 3.
39. Goldstein, S. T., Juranek, D. D., Ravenholt, O., et al. (1996). Cryptosporidiosis: An outbreak associated with drinking water despite state-of-the-art water treatment. *Annals of Internal Medicine, 124*, 459–468.
40. Centers for Disease Control and Prevention. (2004). Diagnosis and management of foodborne illnesses: A primer for physicians and other health care professionals. *MMWR, 53*(RR-4), 1–40.
41. Mead, P. S., Slutsker, L., Dietz, V., et al. (1999). Food-related illness and death in the United States. *Emerging Infectious Diseases, 5*, 607–625.
42. Lichtveld, M. Y., Rodenbeck, S. E., & Lybarger, J. A. (1992). The findings of the Agency for Toxic Substances and Disease Registry Medical Waste Tracking Act Report. *Environmental Health Perspectives, 98*, 243–250.
43. Turnberg ,W. L., & Jones, T. S. (2002). Community syringe and disposal policies in 16 states. *Journal of the American Pharmacists Association*, 42, S99–S104.
44. Centers for Disease Control and Prevention. (2009). *Fourth national report on human exposures to environmental chemicals*. Available at http://www.cdc.gov/exposurereport/pdf/FourthReport.pdf
45. Grandjean, P., Weihe, P., White, R. F., et al. (1997). Cognitive deficit in 7-year-old children with prenatal exposure to methylmercury. *Neurotoxicology and Teratology, 19*, 417–428.
46. Debes, F., Budtz-Jorgensen, E., Weihe, P., et al. (2006). Impact of prenatal methylmercury exposure on neurobehavioral function at age 14 years. *Neurotoxicology and Teratology, 28*, 536–547.
47. Canfield, R. L., Henderson, C. R., Jr., Cory-Slechta, D. A., et al. (2003). Intellectual impairment in children with blood lead concentrations below 10 μg per deciliter. *New England Journal of Medicine, 348*(16), 1517–1526.
48. Mahaffey, K. R., Clickner, R. P., & Bodurowl, C. C. (2004). Blood organic mercury and dietary mercury intake: National Health and Nutrition Examination Survey, 1999 and 2000. *Environmental Health Perspectives, 112*, 562–570.
49. Thigpen, K. G., & Petering, D. H. (2004). Beyond the bench: Fish tales to ensure health. *Environmental Health Perspectives*, 112(13), A738–A739.
50. Centers for Disease Control and Prevention. (2016). *10 leading causes of death and injury, 2014*. Available at http://www.cdc.gov/injury/wisqars/LeadingCauses.html
51. Centers for Disease Control and Prevention. (2016). *10 leading causes of non-fatal injuries, 2014*. Available at http://www.cdc.gov/injury/wisqars/LeadingCauses.html
52. Centers for Disease Control and Prevention. (2015). *Non-fatal injury reports, 2001–2014*. Available at http://webappa.cdc.gov/sasweb/ncipc/nfirates2001.html
53. Centers for Disease Control and Prevention. (2016). *Nationally notifiable conditions: Annual list of infectious conditions*. Available at https://wwwn.cdc.gov/nndss/conditions/notifiable/2016
54. Centers for Disease Control and Prevention. (2010). *Multistate outbreak of human* Salmonella *enteritidis infections associated with shell eggs (final update)*. Available at http://www.cdc.gov/salmonella/enteritidis

55. Lashley, F. R., & Durham, J. D. (Eds.). (2007). *Emerging infectious disease: Trends and issues* (2nd ed.). New York, NY: Springer.
56. Herbst, A. L., Ulfelder, H., & Poskanzer, D. C. (1971). Adenocarcinoma of the vagina: Association of maternal stilbestrol therapy with tumor appearance in young women. *New England Journal of Medicine, 284*, 878–881.
57. Institute of Medicine. (1999). *Hormonally active agents in the environment.* Washington, DC: National Academy Press.
58. Landrigan, P. J., Schechter, C. B., Lipton, J. M., et al. (2002). Environmental pollutants and disease in American children: Estimates of morbidity, mortality, and costs for lead poisoning, asthma, cancer, and developmental disabilities. *Environmental Health Perspectives, 110*(7), 721–728.
59. Trasande, L., Schechter, C., Haynes, K. A, et al. (2006). Applying cost analyses to drive policy that protects children: Mercury as a case study. *Annals of the New York Academy of Sciences, 1076*, 911–23.
60. Ricciardolo, F. L., Nijkamp, F. P., & Folkerts, G. (2006). Nitric oxide synthase (NOS) as therapeutic target for asthma and chronic obstructive pulmonary disease. *Current Drug Targets, 7*, 721–735.
61. Ingram, J. L., & Bonner, J. C. (2006). EGF and PDGF receptor tyrosine kinase as therapeutic targets for chronic lung diseases. *Current Molecular Medicine, 6*, 409–421.
62. Klaper, R., Rees, C. B., Drevnick, P., et al. (2006). Gene expression changes related to endocrine function and decline in reproduction in fathead minnow (*Pimephales promelas*) after dietary methylmercury exposures. *Environmental Health Perspectives, 114*, 1337–1343.
63. Schantz, S. L., & Widholm, J. J. (2001). Cognitive effects of endocrine-disrupting chemicals in animals. *Environmental Health Perspectives, 109*, 1197–2006.
64. Le Prell, C. G., Yamashita, D., Minami, S., Yamasoba, T., & Miller, J. M. (2007). Mechanisms of noise-induced hearing loss indicate multiple methods of prevention, *Hearing Research, 226*, 22–43.
65. King, M., & Bailey, C. (2007). Carbon monoxide-related deaths: United States 1999–2004. *MMWR, 56*, 1309–1312.
66. Beckett, W. S. (2007). Chemical asphyxiants. In W. N. Rom & S. Markowitz (Eds.), *Environmental and occupational medicine* (4th ed., pp. 561–569). Philadelphia, PA: Lippincott Williams & Wilkins.
67. Skinner, M. K. (2014). Endocrine disruptor induction of epigenetic transgenerational inheritance of disease. *Molecular and Cell Endocrinology, 398*(1–2), 4–12. doi: 10.1016/j.mce.2014.07.019
68. Nilsson, E. E., & Skinner, M. K. (2015). Environmentally induced epigenetic transgenerational inheritance of reproductive diseases. *Biology of Reproduction, 93*(6), 145, 1–8, doi: 10.1095/biolreprod.115.134817
69. Yao, Y., Robinson, A. M., Zucchi, F. C., Robbins, J. C., Babenko, O., Kovalchuk, O., Kovalchuk, I., Olson, D. M., & Metz, G. A. (2014). Ancestral exposure to stress epigenetically programs preterm birth risk and adverse maternal and newborn outcomes. *BMC Medicine, 12*, 121. doi: 10.1186/s12916-014-0121-6
70. Agency for Toxic Substances and Disease Registry (ATSDR). (2015). *Case studies in environmental medicine: Taking an exposure history.* Available at https://www.atsdr.cdc.gov/csem/csem.asp?csem=33&po=0
71. National Institute of Occupational Safety and Health. (2016). *Pocket guide to chemical hazards* Available at http://www.cdc.gov/niosh/npg
72. Brugnone, F., Gobbi, M., Ayyad, K., et al. (1995). Blood toluene as a biological index of environmental toluene exposure in the "normal" population and in occupationally exposed workers immediately after exposure and 16 hours later. *International Archives of Occupational and Environmental Health, 66*, 421–425.
73. Agency for Toxic Substances and Disease Registry. (2015). *Toxicological profile for toluene.* Available at http://www.atsdr.cdc.gov/ToxProfiles/TP.asp?id=161&tid=29
74. Alarcon, W. A., Calvert, G. M., Blondell, J. M., et al. (2005). Acute illnesses associated with pesticide exposure at schools. *JAMA, 294*, 455–465.
75. Lu, C., Knutson, D. E., Fisker-Andersen, J., et al. (2001). Biological monitoring survey of organophosphorous pesticide exposure among preschool children in the Seattle metropolitan area. *Environmental Health Perspectives, 109*, 299–303.
76. Occupational Safety & Health Administration. (n.d.). Safety and health topics: Occupational noise exposure. Available at https://www.osha.gov/SLTC/noisehearingconservation/index.html
77. Chang, S. J., Chen, C. J., Lien, C. H., et al. (2006). Hearing loss in workers exposed to toluene and noise. *Environmental Health Perspectives, 114*, 1283–1286.
78. Helzner, E. P, Cauley J. A, Pratt S. R, et al. (2005). Race and sex differences in age-related hearing loss: The Health, Aging and Body Composition Study. *Journal of the American Geriatrics Society, 53*, 2119–2127.
79. Mizoue, T., Miyamoto, T., & Shimizu, T. (2003). Combined effect of smoking and occupational exposure to noise on hearing loss in steel factory workers. *Occupational and Environmental Medicine, 60*, 56–59.
80. Morata, T. C, Fiorini A. C, Fischer F. M, et al. (1997). Toluene-induced hearing loss among rotogravure printing workers. *Scandinavian Journal of Work, Environment & Health, 23*, 289–298.
81. Widdowson, M. A., Sulka, A., Bulens, S. N., et al. (2005). Norovirus and foodborne disease, United States, 1991–2000. *Emerging Infectious Diseases, 11*(1), 95–102.
82. Centers for Disease Control and Prevention. (2014). *Foodborne Diseases Active Surveillance Network (FoodNet): FoodNet surveillance report for 2014 (final report).* Atlanta, GA: U.S. Department of Health and Human Services. Available at http://www.cdc.gov/foodnet/pdfs/2014-foodnet-surveillance-report.pdf
83. Dales, R., Miller, D., Ruest, K., et al. (2006). Airborne endotoxin is associated with respiratory illness in the first 2 years of life. *Environmental Health Perspectives, 114*, 610–614.
84. Thorne, P. S., Kulhánková, K., Yin, M., et al. (2005). Endotoxin exposure is a risk factor for asthma: The national survey of endotoxin in U.S. housing. *American Journal of Respiratory and Critical Care Medicine, 172*, 1371–1377.
85. Lee, J. A., Johnson, J. C., Reynolds S. J., Thorne, P. S., & O'Shaughnessy, P. T. (2006). Indoor and outdoor air quality assessment of four wastewater treatment plants. *Journal of Occupational and Environmental Hygiene, 3*, 36–43.
86. U.S. Environmental Protection Agency. (1996). *Environmental threats to children's health.* Washington, DC: U.S. Environmental Protection Agency.
87. Goldman, L. R., & Koduru, S. (2000). Chemicals in the environment and developmental toxicity to children: A public health and policy perspective. *Environmental Health Perspectives, 108*(Suppl. 3), 443–448.
88. Grandjean, P. (2004). Implications of the precautionary principle for primary prevention and research. *Annual Review of Public Health, 25*, 199–223.
89. Bang, K. L. M., Pinheiro, G. A., Wood, J. M., et al. (2006). Malignant mesothelioma mortality in the United States, 1999–2001. *International Journal of Occupational and Environmental Health, 12*, 9–19.
90. Ulvestad, B., Kjaerheim, K., Martinsen, J. I., et al. (2004). Cancer incidence among members of the Norwegian trade union of insulation workers. *Journal of Occupational and Environmental Medicine, 46*, 84–89.
91. Miller, A. (1990). Mesothelioma in household members of asbestos-exposed workers: 32 United States cases since 1990. *American Journal of Industrial Medicine, 47*, 458–462.
92. Kilburn, K. H., Warshaw, R., & Thorton, J. C. (1985). Asbestosis, pulmonary symptoms and functional impairment in shipyard workers. *Chest, 88*, 254–259.
93. Sallis, J. F., Floyd, M. F., Rodriquez, D. A., & Saelens, B. E. (2012). The role of built environments in physical activity, obesity, and CVD. *Circulation, 125*(5), 729–737.

Chapter 4

Stress and Adaptation

Matthew Sorenson, Linda Janusek, and Herbert L. Mathews

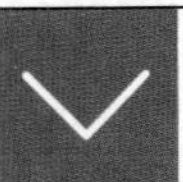

Chapter Outline and Learning Outcomes

4.1 Chapter Overvew and Case Studies

Define stress, coping, and adaptation, and list concepts related to stress.

4.2 Conceptualizations of Stress

Summarize the major conceptual approaches to the study of stress.

4.3 The Body in Balance

Compare and contrast homeostasis and allostasis.

4.4 The Body Responding to Stress

Compare and contrast the various models of stress response.

4.5 The Effects of Stress on Health

Explain the pathogenesis and clinical manifestations of stress.

4.6 Stress and Mental Health

Explain the mechanisms whereby stress contributes to the development or exacerbation of psychiatric disorders such as depression, anxiety, and post-traumatic stress disorder.

4.7 Stress and Physical Health

Explain the mechanisms whereby stress contributes to the development or exacerbation of physiologic disorders such as multiple sclerosis, inflammatory bowel disease, and coronary artery disease.

KEY TERMS

Adaptation, 78
Allostasis, 82
Allostatic load, 82
Catecholamines, 83
Coping, 78
Cortisol, 81
General adaptation syndrome (GAS), 82
Homeostasis, 79
Psychoneuroimmunology, 91
Stress, 78
Stressor, 82

ABBREVIATIONS

ACTH—adrenocorticotropic Hormone
ASD—acute stress disorder
CRF—corticotropin-releasing factor
GAS—general adaptation syndrome
HPA—hypothalamic–pituitary–adrenal
HSV—herpes simplex virus
IL—interleukin
LC/NE—locus coeruleus–norepinephrine
MS—multiple sclerosis
NK—natural killer
PTSD—posttraumatic stress disorder
SNS—sympathetic nervous system

4.1 Chapter Overview and Case Studies

The origins of stress as a concept can be found in the work of early philosophers and physicians who speculated about the influence of emotion on physical health. **Stress** is the psychologic and physiologic response of an organism to an event that is often perceived as a threat or challenge. Most conceptualizations of stress propose that this negative perception produces a state of physiologic arousal that ultimately has adverse health consequences for the individual. **Coping** is the dynamic process through which individuals apply psychologic and behavioral measures to handle internal and external stress demands. **Adaptation** comprises the physiologic and psychologic processes used in response to stress. This chapter provides a general overview of stress and the consequences of stress. Additionally, this chapter covers conceptual definitions and models of stress, including the theoretical concept of allostasis.

Concepts Related to Stress

The term *stress* is best seen as describing a complex relationship among an individual's physiologic and psychologic processes and environment. Ultimately, stress results from situations in which the individual encounters environmental events that require a degree of adaptation. The individual's ability to adapt depends on the resources that are available and the coping strategies that can be implemented at the time. If the demands posed by an event exceed the individual's coping ability and resources, stress occurs. This stress can then elicit responses, either physiologic or psychologic (e.g., smoking, substance use), that can place the individual at risk for disease (**Figure 4.1** ■).

Case Studies

The consequences of stress are followed through the chapter through presentation of select case studies. The case of Alexander Cho examines the impact of stress in the context of a psychologic condition. The case of Ella Fraser focuses on the relationship between stress and the worsening of asthma, a physiologic condition.

Alexander Cho: Introduction

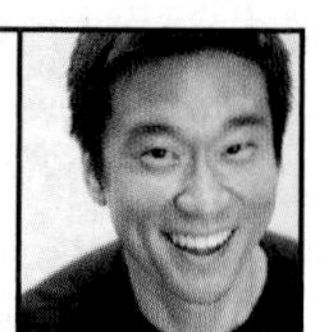

Alexander Cho, age 40, reports decreased sleep, nightmares, and difficulty concentrating. The symptoms have been occurring over the past 4 months, ever since he witnessed an accident in which his best friend was killed at a commuter train crossing. He reports feeling detached from his daily life and says that his symptoms have been interfering with his ability to work. He avoids taking routes to work that come near train stations, and he reports heightened anxiety to the point of chest pain, sweating, and intense feelings of anxiety when he hears a train whistle or has to travel over train tracks. He denies any other significant medical history.

1. If Mr. Cho's symptoms were to continue without relief, what could result?
2. What physiologic symptoms is Mr. Cho manifesting secondary to his stress response?

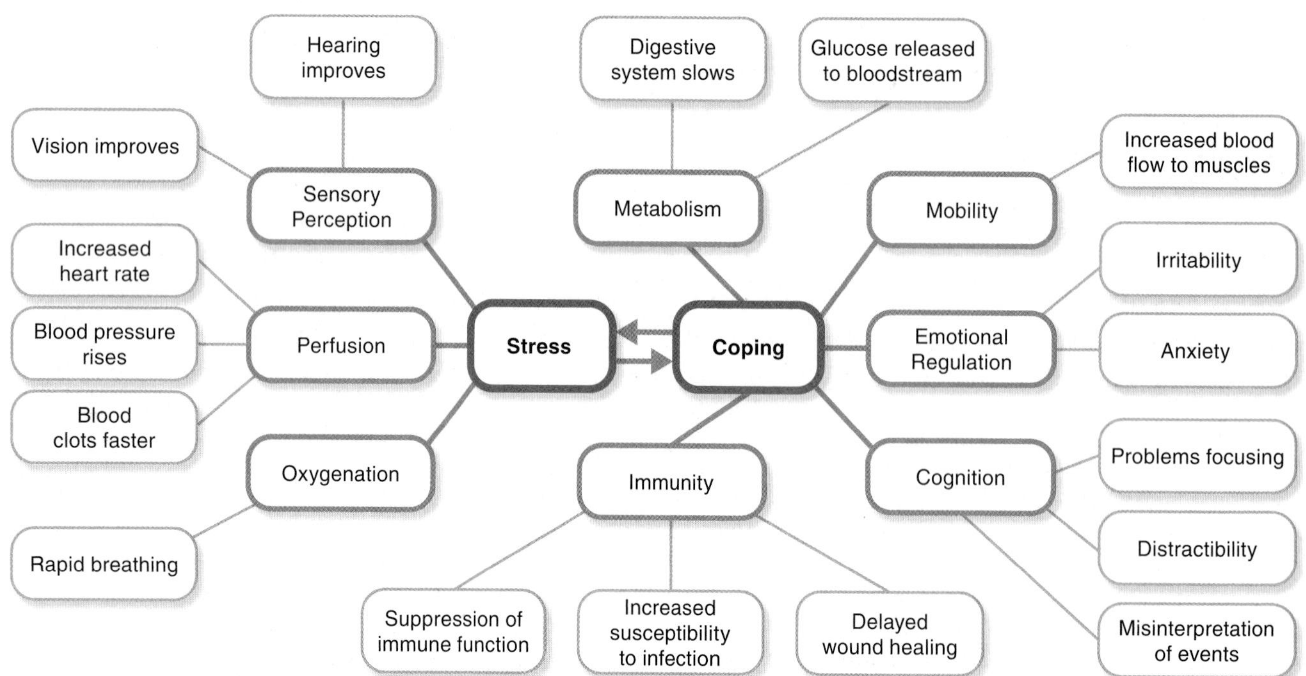

Figure 4.1 ■ Concepts related to stress and coping.

Ella Fraser: Introduction

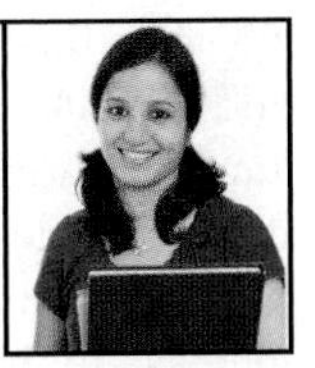

Ella Fraser is a 21-year-old student with a history of intermittent asthma. She recently moved across the country to start graduate school. Since beginning the semester, she reports an increase in nighttime coughing to approximately three nights per week, and she is often awakened by coughing. She is feeling fatigued with chest tightness during the day and feels short of breath two to three times per week.

1. What is the stress trigger for Ms. Fraser's intermittent asthma?
2. What is complicating Ms. Fraser's coughing at night that affects her functioning during the day?

Check Your Progress: Section 4.1

1. What term describes the physiologic or psychologic response to an event that is often perceived as a threat or challenge?
2. What is coping?
3. What is the relationship between adaptation and stress?

4.2 Conceptualizations of Stress

An underlying assumption of all approaches to stress is that over time, human beings have developed means of responding to external threats through a process of sympathetic arousal that provides the energy for either engaging in combat with a threatening situation or taking flight from a stimulus (known as the fight-or-flight response). Such response patterns are no longer adaptive in most situations in a culture that presents demands of a more subtle and intricate psychologic nature. For example, if a staff nurse were reprimanded by a manager for neglecting to document a patient's care, the nurse might experience a state of physiologic arousal that cannot be relieved by exercise, running away, or fighting in the midst of that situation. The evolutionary pattern of human development has reinforced physiologic response patterns that provide the body with certain mechanisms that may no longer be useful in many situations.

Conceptual models of stress tend to focus on a particular aspect of this larger process of stress. The larger process, which has been referred to as the stressful experience, would need to take into account coping patterns, lifestyle, genetic influences, health, nutritional state, and other factors in attempting to provide a complete picture of stress. Using smaller conceptual models can provide a more detailed view of aspects of stress. These models focus on characteristics of the events or conditions that produce stress and can be viewed as describing the environment from which the stress arises—social (stimulus), psychologic (transactional), and physiologic (response)—with differing explanations of the nature of stress and resources within each environment.[1] Regardless of the nomenclature used, the focus is on characteristics of the events or conditions that produce a degree of stress (stress as environmental stimulus), the individual's response to events (stress as physiologic response), or the mental and psychologic appraisal processes involved in the emergence of a state of stress (stress as transaction between individual and environment). Fundamental to these approaches is the idea of a state of balance, of **homeostasis** or allostasis. Clinically, understanding the conceptual approaches to stress can help understand how life events influence health. An additional consideration is that internal events (e.g., infection, organ failure) can also be viewed as stressful stimuli to which the individual must respond. In such cases, nursing actions and interventions are trying to help the individual return to a state of homeostasis. Acute stress results in numerous physiologic effects, mediated mainly by sympathetic response (**Figure 4.2** ■). Of particular interest to health are effects on the immune system.

Stressors can have significant effects on a host's immune response to microbial pathogens; the extent of the effects depends on the type, duration, and intensity of the stressor. These effects result from activation of various central nervous system (CNS) pathways, including the hypothalamic–pituitary–adrenal (HPA) axis, the sympathetic nervous system (SNS), and the endogenous opioid pathway. Activation of these pathways increases the levels of neuroendocrine hormones, which subsequently lead to suppressed innate and adaptive immune responses. Chronic stress produces profound immune suppression due to increased production of glucocorticoids and catecholamines.[2] These modulate lymphocyte trafficking and immune function through leukocyte receptors.

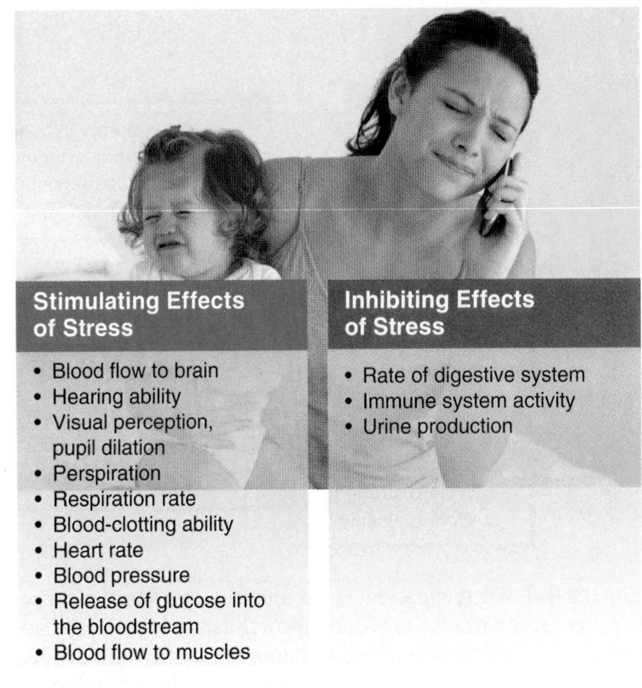
Stimulating Effects of Stress
• Blood flow to brain
• Hearing ability
• Visual perception, pupil dilation
• Perspiration
• Respiration rate
• Blood-clotting ability
• Heart rate
• Blood pressure
• Release of glucose into the bloodstream
• Blood flow to muscles
Inhibiting Effects of Stress
• Rate of digestive system
• Immune system activity
• Urine production

Figure 4.2 ■ Bodily effects of stress.

Although the word *stress* generally has negative connotations, stress is a familiar aspect of life, being a stimulant in some situations but a burden in others. For human beings, an acute stress response can have health-promoting effects. The duration of a stressor is thought to be important in considering its impact on an individual. For example, differences exist in the ways in which acute (short-term) and chronic (long-term) stressors affect the immune system. Chronic stress significantly suppresses delayed-type hypersensitivity responses (e.g., response to a skin test) and decreases leukocyte mobilization to the skin. Acute stress enhances the delayed-type hypersensitivity response and increases leukocyte mobilization.[3] Although stress is typically thought to be immunosuppressive, acute stress can result in immune enhancement that can promote protection from infections but alternatively could contribute to the exacerbation of immunopathology (**Figure 4.3** ■). In response to immunologic challenge, acutely stressed individuals show significantly greater leukocyte infiltration and enhanced production of chemokines (chemoattractant proteins for leukocytes) and cytokines such as interleukin 1 (IL-1), IL-6, tumor necrosis factor, and interferon gamma (pro-inflammatory and Th1) (see **Figure 4.4** ■).

As a further example, acute stress enhances maturation and trafficking of dendritic cells to sites of antigenic challenge. Dendritic cells are efficient antigen-presenting cells that promote activation and recruitment of T lymphocytes during the initial antigen challenge, inducing a long-term increase in immunologic memory. This means that on second exposure to an antigen, the individual will have a more pronounced immune response, resulting in enhanced protection and more rapid healing. On the other hand, stress can worsen certain disease states (e.g., autoimmune or inflammatory disease) by inducing increased responses on the part of the immune system.

The ability of acute stress to enhance immune response is considered an evolutionary advantage. In an encounter with a physical stressor, the individual could experience wounding and infection, and the stress response could promote a beneficial antigen-specific immune response. During such an immune response, factors such as leukocyte trafficking, antigen presentation, helper T-cell function, leukocyte proliferation, cytokine and chemokine function, and effector cell function would be receptive to stress hormone-mediated immune enhancement. Thus, acute stress has adaptive immune-enhancing effects that

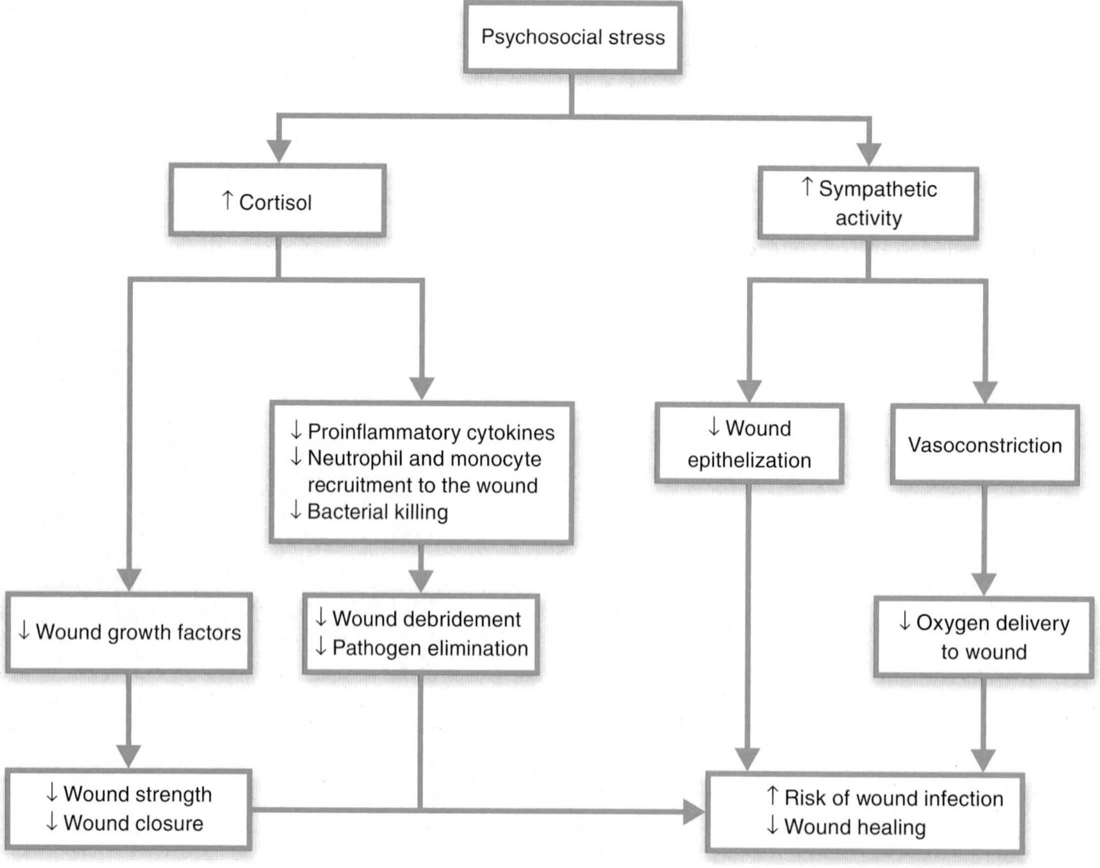

Figure 4.3 ■ Psychosocial stress affects wound healing through the release of cortisol and by activation of the SNS. Cortisol suppresses the release of wound growth factors that decrease wound strength and impair wound closure. Cortisol also reduces the production of pro-inflammatory cytokines needed in the early phase of wound healing. Cortisol also decreases the recruitment of neutrophils and monocytes to the wound and impairs bacterial killing by these phagocytic cells, thus impairing pathogen elimination. Sympathetic activity decreases wound epithelialization and reduces oxygen delivery to the wound. As a result, not only is there a decrease in wound healing, but also psychosocial stress can increase the risk for wound infection.

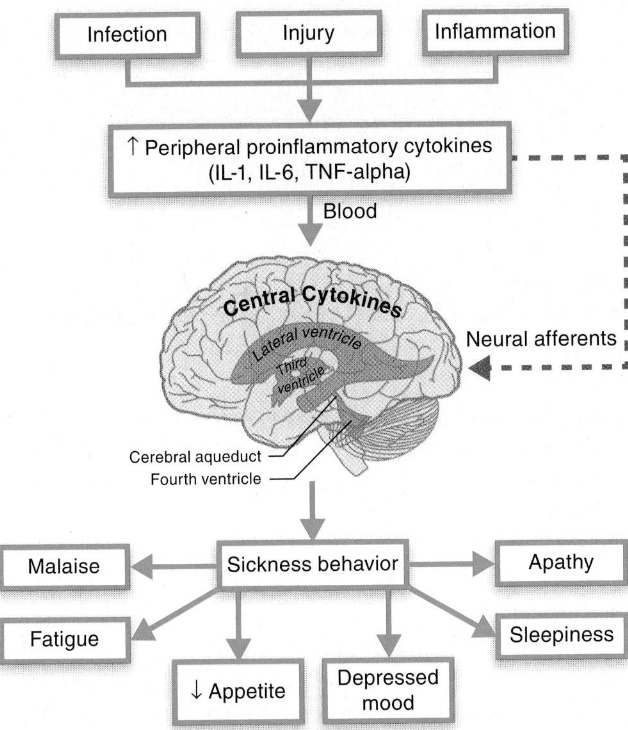

Figure 4.4 ■ Immune-to-brain signaling occurs in response to infection, injury, and inflammation that occur in peripheral organs and tissues. These pathologic processes result in macrophage activation and the release of pro-inflammatory cytokines (IL-1, IL-6, and tumor necrosis factor alpha [TNF-alpha]). Although too large to directly stimulate key brain areas that mediate behavioral changes, these cytokines are able to trigger elevations in central (brain) cytokines, which in turn activate key brain areas that mediate sickness behavior. Peripherally produced pro-inflammatory cytokines can initiate this through the blood that circulates around the circumventricular organs, which lie outside of the blood–brain barrier or by being transported from the blood across the blood–brain barrier via a specialized transporter system. Also, peripherally produced cytokines can activate neural afferents that are present in the local area of tissue infection, inflammation or injury. Activation of these neural afferents signal areas of the brain that mediate sickness behavior.

are beneficial. The effects of stress (acute or chronic) on immune function are especially important to understand because stress is a ubiquitous fact of life and stress hormones are important components of an individual's physiologic response to the environment.

Alexander Cho: Application

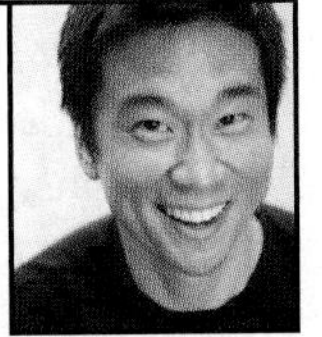

A significant life event occurred to Mr. Cho that involved a previous sense of closeness or friendship with the victim of a train accident. Mr. Cho now perceives stimuli associated with the train as threatening and has attempted to cope by avoiding train crossings and routes over railroad tracks. The coping strategies have been ineffective, and Mr. Cho is still experiencing a significant degree of stress, which is producing effects on his memory and generating a state of physiologic arousal. Eventually, if the condition is not be treated, Mr. Cho's overall health and functioning will deteriorate.

3. As Mr. Cho's chronic sense of physiologic arousal continues, what factors are being activated?
4. As Mr. Cho's immune response continues as a chronic condition, what substances will indicate immunopathology?

Ella Fraser: Application

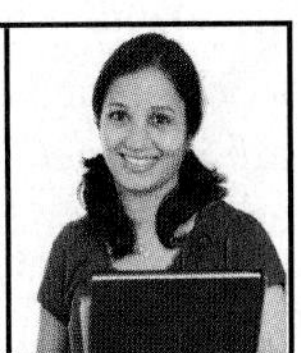

Relocation and starting a new program of study can engender a significant degree of stress. This stress can influence immunologic and respiratory function to a degree that can lead to a worsening of asthma symptomatology. Ms. Fraser's increased difficulty in breathing at night with an increase in nighttime coughing indicates an exacerbation of asthma.

3. Is Ms. Fraser showing pulmonary signs of inflammation? If so, why?
4. How can Ms. Fraser's symptomatology be explained?

Check Your Progress: Section 4.2

1. What is the sympathetic arousal mechanism that is activated by a stressful situation?
2. How does the stress response affect the immune system?
3. How does stress affect the autoimmune response?

4.3 The Body in Balance

Homeostasis

Emotional states can trigger a defensive response by stimulating arousal of the SNS. This sympathetic response could be seen as causing the body to deviate from a normal resting or set point. Other physiologic mechanisms are then brought into play in an attempt to return to the body to the set point—to a state of balance. The term *homeostasis* was first used by Walter Cannon to describe this process.[2] Maintenance of homeostasis involves several mechanisms that provide protection by helping to return the body to a more normative state after the appearance of a demand.

Homeostasis indicates the presence of an internal state of balance. This state of balance is maintained through a process of feedback that functions similar to that of a thermostat. **Cortisol** is a hormone that is released during the stress response. The presence of cortisol in the bloodstream then serves as a negative regulator to prevent further release of cortisol. The concept of homeostasis is built around this idea of negative feedback. The presence of a physiologic mediator can serve to shut off its own release or the release of another mediator.

Allostasis

Homeostasis implies a degree of internal stability. The presentation of a stress-evoking stimulus requires a response to return the body to a state of consistency or balance. This concept has been viewed as limited in that it addresses only feedback mechanisms that attempt to return the body to a particular uniform threshold. However, in dealing with the context of daily life, a person is in a continual state of flux, with some physiologic mechanisms in play and others at rest, so the body must respond appropriately to a multitude of environmental demands. This state of flux is referred to as **allostasis**. Allostasis is not necessarily a dramatic departure from homeostasis; allostasis still employs mechanisms that are involved in the response to internal or external stimuli and mechanisms that are involved in the eventual suppression of that response. The physiologic mechanisms under investigation remain the same: primarily the SNS and the HPA axis.[4]

The concept of allostasis can be extended beyond physiologic parameters to behavioral ones. Certain behavioral activities or emotions are experienced along a normative spectrum. At either end of the spectrum, there are psychopathologic states. Lifestyle choices involving substance use, dietary influences, and exercise can also influence one's psychologic state as well as having ramifications for the physiologic state. Some of these choices may even be adaptive in dealing with subjective feelings of stress in the short term (such as exercising for an hour each day) but could result in adverse health consequences with protracted use (such as overtraining to the point of becoming ill or injured).[4]

The mechanisms involved in responding to stress can experience a state of exhaustion, fail to cease function after removal of the stressing event, or falter in providing a response to the initial event. When these situations occur, the individual is experiencing a state of allostatic load.[4] **Allostatic load** includes more than the effects of stress responses. The physiologic mechanisms involved in the stress response interact with genetic determinants for disease, nutritional influences, and the existing state of the organism. Stress responses are viewed as occurring not within a physiologic vacuum but rather in the context of the individual's life and stress history. There are four methods by which allostasis can contribute to allostatic load:

1. The individual experiences multiple stressors that may be novel or to which the individual cannot attach appropriate meaning. The experience of uncertain or novel events puts the individual in the position of experiencing repeated stressful events, each of which evokes a stress response.
2. Adaptation fails, and the individual is no longer capable of adapting or adjusting to environmental events.
3. The stress response is inappropriately prolonged, and the normative suppressing mechanisms fail.
4. The individual's physiologic response is inadequate to meet the imposed demands. This leads to a process of secondary activation of other mediator mechanisms in an attempt to respond to the demand.[4]

Allostatic load may be viewed as the sum total of the wear and tear that an individual has experienced. The outcome of this load is organ damage.

Check Your Progress: Section 4.3

1. Define homeostasis and allostasis.
2. Name three maladaptive responses to stress.
3. One form of allostatic load occurs when adaptation fail. Explain this type of allostatic load.

4.4 The Body Responding to Stress

Models of stress as response focus on the biologic or physiologic response to a state of stress. The events that evoke such stress are often considered, but the main emphasis is on the response.

The General Adaptation Syndrome

One model of stress that focuses on the physiologic response is the **general adaptation syndrome (GAS)** model, developed by Hans Selye. In the GAS model, the term *stress* describes a theoretical construct to depict an individual's response to a clearly defined event or stimulus, called a **stressor**.[5] The theoretical construct was depicted as one in which the use of the term *stress* was considered analogous to the use of the term in physics, in which stress is a deforming force, with strain the resultant change. Stress is thus an event or demand that produces a degree of strain.[5] This could be considered a stimulus approach, in that the term *stress* refers to events that occur outside the body. However, the work of Selye and the GAS model are clearly focused on the individual's response. The GAS itself in many ways reflects a failure by an individual to respond appropriately to the stressor.[6] Response conceptualizations of stress focus on the physiologic or psychologic changes that may occur; little attention is paid to the stimulus that causes the changes or to determining its characteristics. The focus is on what happens within the individual.

The GAS is best viewed as an adaptive response to stress that consists of three distinct stages: a pattern of alarm followed by a stage of resistance as the individual attempts to compensate for changes induced by the stage of alarm (see **Figure 4.5** ■). A stage of exhaustion can follow if the individual cannot successfully adapt to the physiologic changes that occur during the stage of resistance.[6] The GAS been defined as "the sum of all non-specific systemic reactions of the body which ensue upon long-continued exposure to systemic stress."[5]

- ***Stage of alarm:*** Alarm is a pattern of physiologic activation originally conceptualized as occurring in response to the injection of noxious agents or physical stressors. Physical stressors include issues that reflect overall health and can place the individual at increased risk. Malnutrition, dehydration, sleep deprivation, and environmental extremes of heat and cold all reflect physical conditions that put stress on the individual. During this period, there is a rapid production of

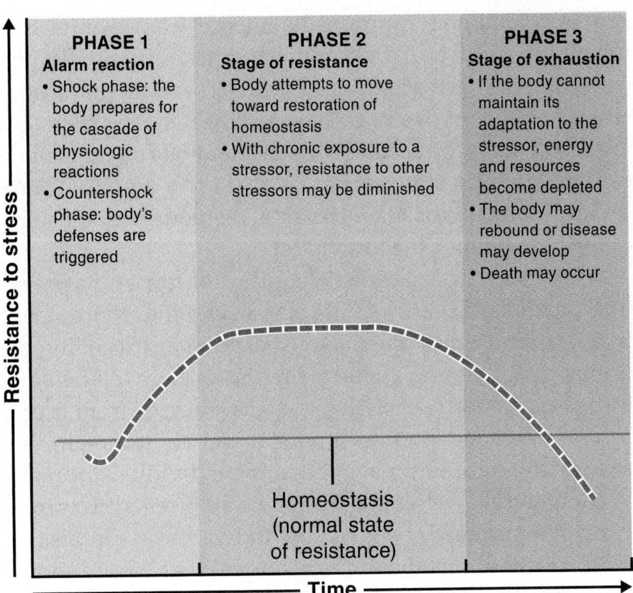

Figure 4.5 ■ General adaptation syndrome.

catecholamine. This catecholamine surge is believed to have an effect on heart rate and blood pressure as well as a variety of effects on the increased mobilization of energy. The sympathetic system is responsible for the release of **catecholamines** (norepinephrine, epinephrine), which activate the fight-or-flight response. Marked increases are seen in central and peripheral levels of norepinephrine in the presence of stress-inducing stimuli. In response to this surge, there is also a rapid release of cortisol, prolactin, and growth hormone. Changes in the release of catecholamines are believed to manifest in increases in both heart rate and mean arterial blood pressure, which are commonly found in response to stress-producing stimuli. These changes are even found to occur in anticipation of a stressor, as when an individual becomes anxious before a test.[6]

- *Stage of resistance:* An individual cannot tolerate the physiologic changes that occur during the stage of alarm for long. The pattern of response that is seen in the stage of alarm is eventually countered by the release of cortisol and other mediators in the stage of resistance. This stage could be viewed as a period of homeostasis. However, because the individual remains under stress, this period of homeostasis or brief adaptation does not last, and exhaustion occurs. Selye referred to an adaptive capacity, the internal resources that an individual has in meeting the demand placed by a stressor. This adaptive capacity is ultimately exceeded.
- *Stage of exhaustion:* In the stage of exhaustion, the individual has lost the capacity to sustain a defense against stress. The organs are no longer able to release balancing mediators, and organ damage begins to occur. Ultimately, what Selye referred to as diseases of adaptation occur in response to sustained stress.

The presence of social supports and a sense of controllability can have moderating effects on stress, which can be viewed as coping. Selye referred to these interacting constructs as "conditioning factors" and theorized that such factors are learned or developed through life as one experiences and adapts to stress.[5] The initial event may still be viewed as threatening, but there may be effective adaptation when the person feels supported and confident that the situation can be managed.

Stress as a Stimulus

Stimulus conceptualizations of stress highlight the situation. Stress is seen as an environmental threat or danger that requires response, such as a physical threat or the death of a loved one. Certain societal or cultural values are attached to events that give these events value. Events that are seen as posing a threat or that require a significant degree of life change are seen as stressors. The focus in stimulus approaches is on determining the characteristics of events that serve as stressors. With life events, the operative premise is that transition or change, requires psychologic and physiologic responses that, if they endure, can lead to the development of illness. The presence of life events is not necessarily positive or negative in nature. It is the sum total of the nature of these experiences that influences health. Negative events may require a greater degree of change than do events that are viewed as positive.

The individual perceives the stress-evoking event to have certain elements that represent a threat to some aspect of the person. The event may manifest as a need for change or adaptation on the part of the individual,[7] a disruption of the individual's worldview,[8] or a threat or danger, or it may represent an unmet psychologic need. Ultimately, how the event is interpreted leads to a physiologic response. The sympathetic fight-or-flight response is viewed as a protective response of the body to an emotional state. If an individual fails to resolve feelings of anxiety emerging from conflict, physiologic consequences can result.

Stress as a Transaction

The conceptualization of stress as a transaction emphasizes individual perception (or appraisal) of the given event as the most significant factor in the process. The response depends on how the event or situation interacts with the individual's existing coping resources and the perceived meaning of the event. Before the physiologic response occurs, there must be a perception of the event as stressful. Perception of meaning on the part of the individual has two bases:

1. Elements that are present in the environment or stimulus, such as an individual receiving a diagnosis of cancer
2. Elements within the individual, such as the individual's ability to cope with the news.

Perceived threat emerges from the interaction between the two.[9] However, the appraisal of an event as a threat, while necessary, is not sufficient to produce stress. Primary appraisal is an evaluation of the salience of the event to well-being.[9] After the value judgment of threat has been made (primary appraisal), another judgment is made of the resources that are available to the individual in coping with the effects of the initial value judgment (secondary appraisal) (see **Figure 4.6** ■).

The process can also be described as depending on whether the individual appraises the situation as being benign, neutral, or stressful, stressful events being appraised as loss, threat, or challenge.[9] As in the work of Selye, there can be positive aspects to stress through the interpretation of a stimulus as a challenge. Both challenge and threat appraisals are seen as initiating the coping process. Challenge appraisals emerge from events that inherently evoke positive emotional states, such as a desired job promotion or a wedding. Threat appraisals result from situations that evoke negative emotional states, such as a job layoff or a serious illness. Such situations could include examinations or other situations that carry an implication of harm. The important element is the perceived meaning of the situation for the individual.[9]

The classic transactional definition of stress is "a particular relationship between the person and the environment that is appraised by the person as taxing or exceeding his or her resources and endangering his or her well-being."[9] In this definition, psychologic stress emerges from a process of interaction between person and environment that eventually presents an event that the individual appraises as endangering well-being in some way. Stress results from a relative mismatch between the individual's appraisal of the demand or threat and the resources that the individual perceives as available. In the transactional view, the experience of stress comes from the cognitive appraisal of a stimulus as taxing or exceeding one's available resources with a resultant perceived threat to psychologic or physical well-being.[9]

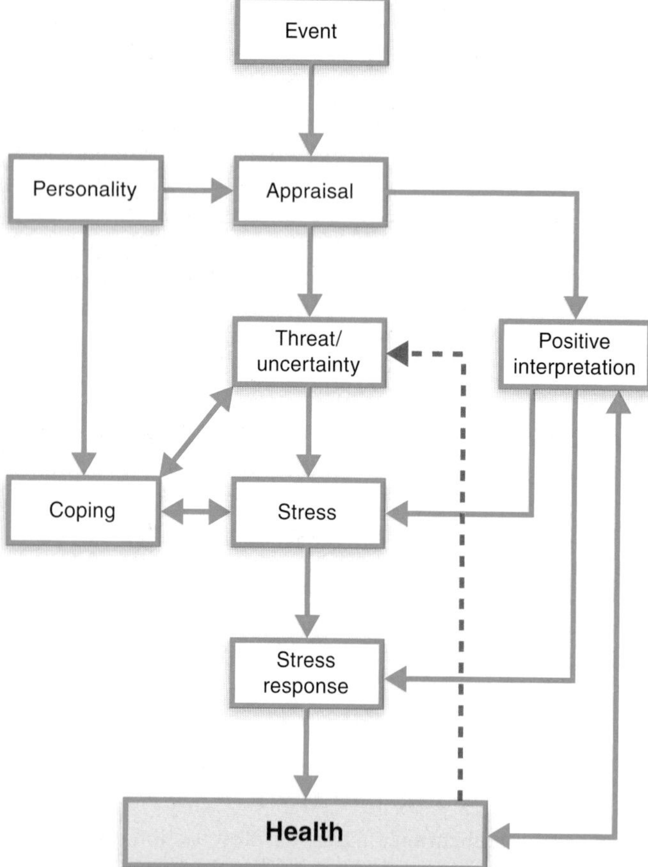

Figure 4.6 ■ Components of the transactional nature of stress. In transactional models of stress, dispositional aspects influence the individual's response to an internal or external event. Such dispositional aspects include personality and physical health. An event that is perceived as life threatening is processed immediately in a manner akin to stimulus–response processing. Events that are not perceived as life threatening result in a degree of cognitive dissonance or discomfort and undergo a degree of cognitive interpretation before the development of stress. The initial stress response depends on the coping resources available to the individual; in turn, the presence of coping resources influences health outcome. However, stress of sufficient intensity can immediately influence health outcome without the mediation of coping.

Alexander Cho: Application

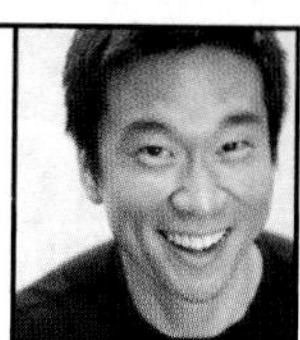

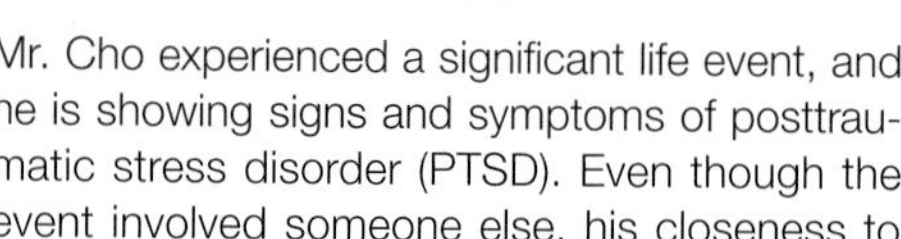

Mr. Cho experienced a significant life event, and he is showing signs and symptoms of posttraumatic stress disorder (PTSD). Even though the event involved someone else, his closeness to the victim makes him feel that he is at risk for harm when he is near a train. The diagnostic criteria for PTSD involve three main categories: (1) a reexperiencing of the traumatic event, (2) feelings of detachment or emotional numbness, and (3) increased arousal. Mr. Cho is interpreting the event as a threat and will attempt to avoid situations that remind him of the event. If he is unable to do so, he will experience an increase in symptoms. The case displays the factors discussed in the conceptual models: a significant life event, an interpretation of an event as a threat, and a pattern of sympathetic activation in response to stimuli that Mr. Cho associates with the traumatic event. The presence of sympathetic symptoms reflects the stage of alarm. Mr. Cho's attempts to cope with these symptoms reflects the stage of resistance. The presence of reoccurring symptoms that intrude on his rest and impair his work performance reflects aspects of the stage of exhaustion.

5. What changes in vital signs may Mr. Cho manifest in the stage of alarm?
6. Describe the factors that may have a mediating effect on Mr. Cho's response to stress.

Check Your Progress: Section 4.4

1. Explain the stage of exhaustion in the general adaptation syndrome.
2. In the transactional view of stress, what are the two individual appraisals that will guide the physiologic stress response?
3. How is the fight-or-flight response triggered in the stage of alarm?

4.5 The Effects of Stress on Health

A hallmark of stress is the presence of a degree of emotional arousal concordant with physiologic arousal. The individual's response is measured in terms of physiologic response (heart rate, blood pressure) or psychologic response (anxiety, tension).

The Etiology and Pathogenesis of Stress

The physiologic response to stress involves two primary mechanisms: the HPA axis and the sympathetic adrenal medullary system, also known as the locus coeruleus–norepinephrine (LC/NE) system. The HPA axis and LC/NE systems are not necessarily exclusive of one another. These systems interact and are capable of initiating each other, and each is inhibited by the endogenous opioid system and the presence of gamma-aminobutyric acid. Each of these mechanisms is capable of producing differing degrees of response depending on intensity of the stressor and/or perceived situational control. Activation of these two systems leads to the pattern of sympathetic activation that is seen in response to stress.[10,11]

The HPA axis affects the secretion of hormones from the pituitary and adrenal glands and is involved in the release of cortisol. The interpretation of an event as stressful stimulates the release of corticotropin-releasing factor (CRF) from the hypothalamus. CRF elicits the release of adrenocorticotropic hormone (ACTH) from the anterior pituitary. ACTH stimulates the release of cortisol from the adrenal cortex. The presence of cortisol in the bloodstream serves to restrict the release of further CRF from the hypothalamus, providing a negative feedback loop. Cortisol affects energy metabolism through effects on protein utilization and blood glucose.[12]

The LC/NE system is a group of neurons located in the pons. They have connections to the limbic system, the hypothalamus, the thalamus, and parts of the spinal cord. These neurons regulate the release of norepinephrine and control alertness, arousal, and vigilance. The LC/NE system is believed to play a role in the coordination of the CNS during the response to stress.[10,11]

The adaptive stress response involves the HPA, dopaminergic, and noradrenergic systems along with the amygdala, hippocampus, prefrontal cortex, and hypothalamus (**Figure 4.7** ■). Each of these areas mediates the stress response in some way. Beyond the CNS, the major glands involved in the response to stress are the pituitary and adrenals. Cells within the hypothalamus secrete CRF, which

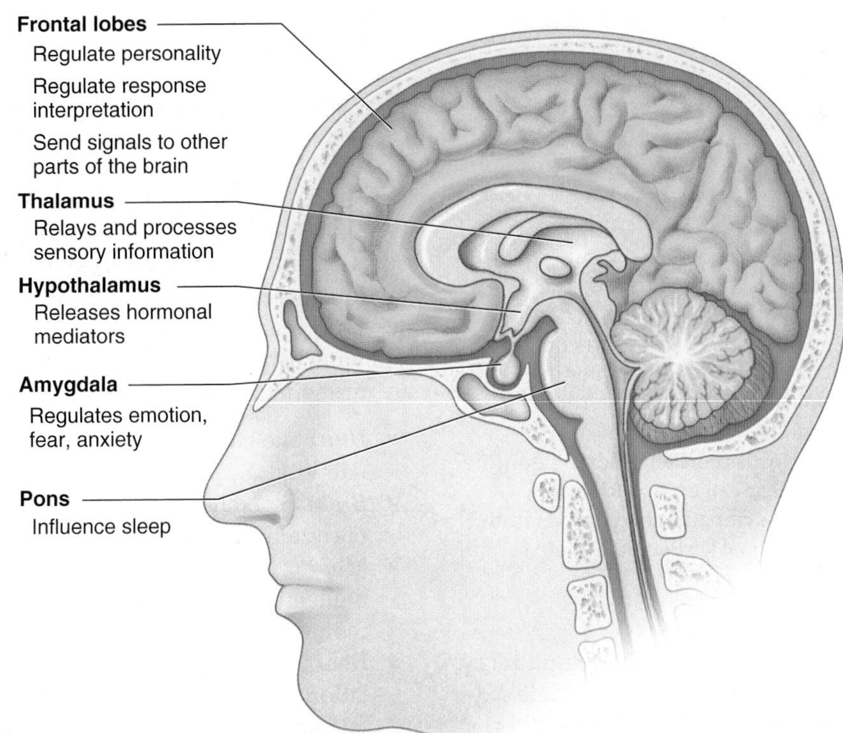

Figure 4.7 ■ Several parts of the brain are involved in the interpretation of stress and responses on the part of the individual. The frontal lobes are involved in personality regulation and response interpretation, sending signals to other parts of the brain such as the thalamus and hypothalamus. The amygdala plays a role in the regulation of emotion and regulates fear and anxiety. The hypothalamus releases hormonal mediators that have end effects on other organs, such as the adrenals. The pons is part of the brainstem and influences sleep, as does the reticular activating system.

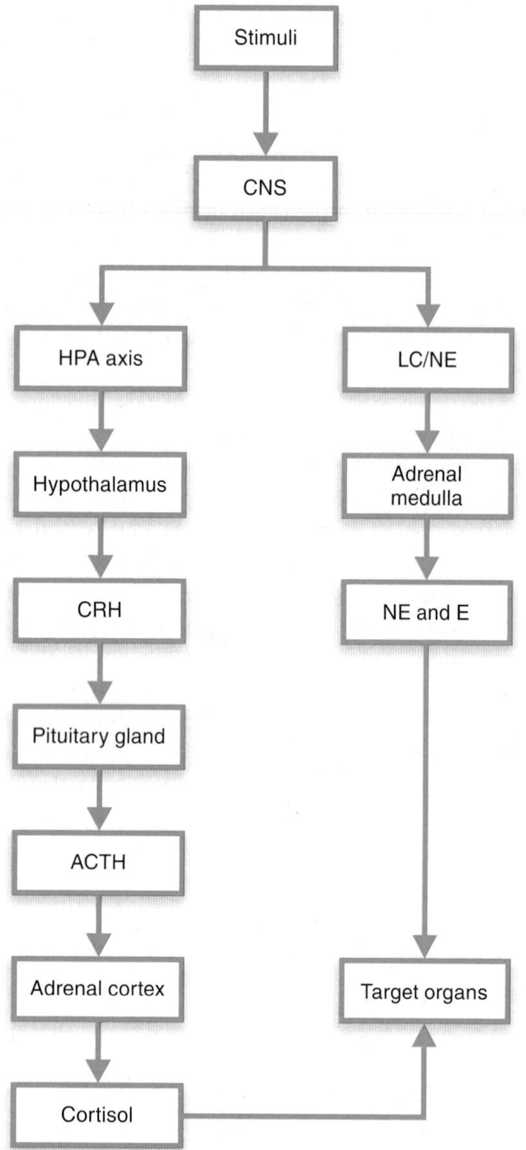

Figure 4.8 ■ The stress response involves several pathways, which begin with a signaling stimulus. The hypothalamic–pituitary–adrenal (HPA) axis involves the hypothalamus, which regulates the release of corticotropin-releasing hormone (CRH), which in turn stimulates the release of adrenocorticotropic hormone (ACTH) from the pituitary. ACTH in turn stimulates the release of cortisol from the adrenal glands. The locus coeruleus–norepinephrine (LC/NE) system evokes the release of epinephrine and norepinephrine, which leads to sympathetic responses from target organs (heart, gastrointestinal system, lungs, etc.).

stimulates the release of ACTH from the anterior pituitary gland.[12] Other cells within the hypothalamus secrete oxytocin and vasopressin and innervate directly the posterior pituitary (**Figure 4.8** ■).

The pituitary gland is located at the base of the brain immediately below the hypothalamus and has two parts: the anterior and the posterior. The adrenal glands are located on top of each kidney and have two parts: the medulla, which is involved in the release of catecholamine, and the cortex, which is involved in the expression of steroids. In response to stimulation, the adrenal gland releases epinephrine and norepinephrine, which are the major players in the sympathetic response to stress. These catecholamines stimulate the amygdala, which mediates the emotional response to an event. The hippocampus is also activated; this activation is believed to hold cues to which characteristics of an event are seen as a threat or not.[11] Activity in the frontal cortex is reduced, narrowing focus to the threatening event.

Acute psychologic stress conditions have been demonstrated to increase the circulating levels of epinephrine, norepinephrine, cortisol, ACTH, and beta-endorphin. Cortisol elevations are typically found to occur later than the elevation of catecholamines and to have a more lasting pattern of elevation.

The CNS provides the link between environmental events and physiologic responses. The brain not only provides a means for the interpretation of stimuli, but also is subject to the effects of stress hormones. Stress can contribute to the development of neurochemical changes within the CNS that lead to the development of psychologic or physiologic disorders. Stress has been associated with the development or exacerbation of psychiatric disorders, especially depressive disorders. Posttraumatic stress disorder is conceptualized as resulting from exposure to an event that is viewed as threatening to the safety of the individual or of those valued by the individual. The event either overwhelms the individual's coping defense or is of such an unremitting, recurring nature that the individual cannot escape the stress.

Clinical Manifestations of Stress Throughout the Body

The response to stress affects every body system and is associated with a number of health-related conditions. Stress can also lead to lifestyle choices such as smoking, substance use and abuse, nutritional changes, and risk taking that can influence management of an existing disease condition. The following list shows where the effects of stress on the body are most often seen (see also **Figure 4.9** ■):

- *Hair:* The effects can result in psychogenic patterns of hair loss.
- *Brain:* Blood flow to the brain increases, and the release of certain hormones increases.
- *Mouth:* Oral symptoms include bruxism (grinding of the teeth), disorders of the temporomandibular joint, mouth sores, and gum disease.
- *Heart:* The heart beats faster, and sympathetic stimulation causes an increase in contractile strength. This results in an increase in blood flow to the body.
- *Lungs:* Most people breathe faster with constriction of the upper airways.
- *Muscles:* The skeletal muscles tense and can be become rigid.
- *Digestive tract:* Blood flow is shunted to high-priority areas of the body, such as the lungs, heart, and brain.

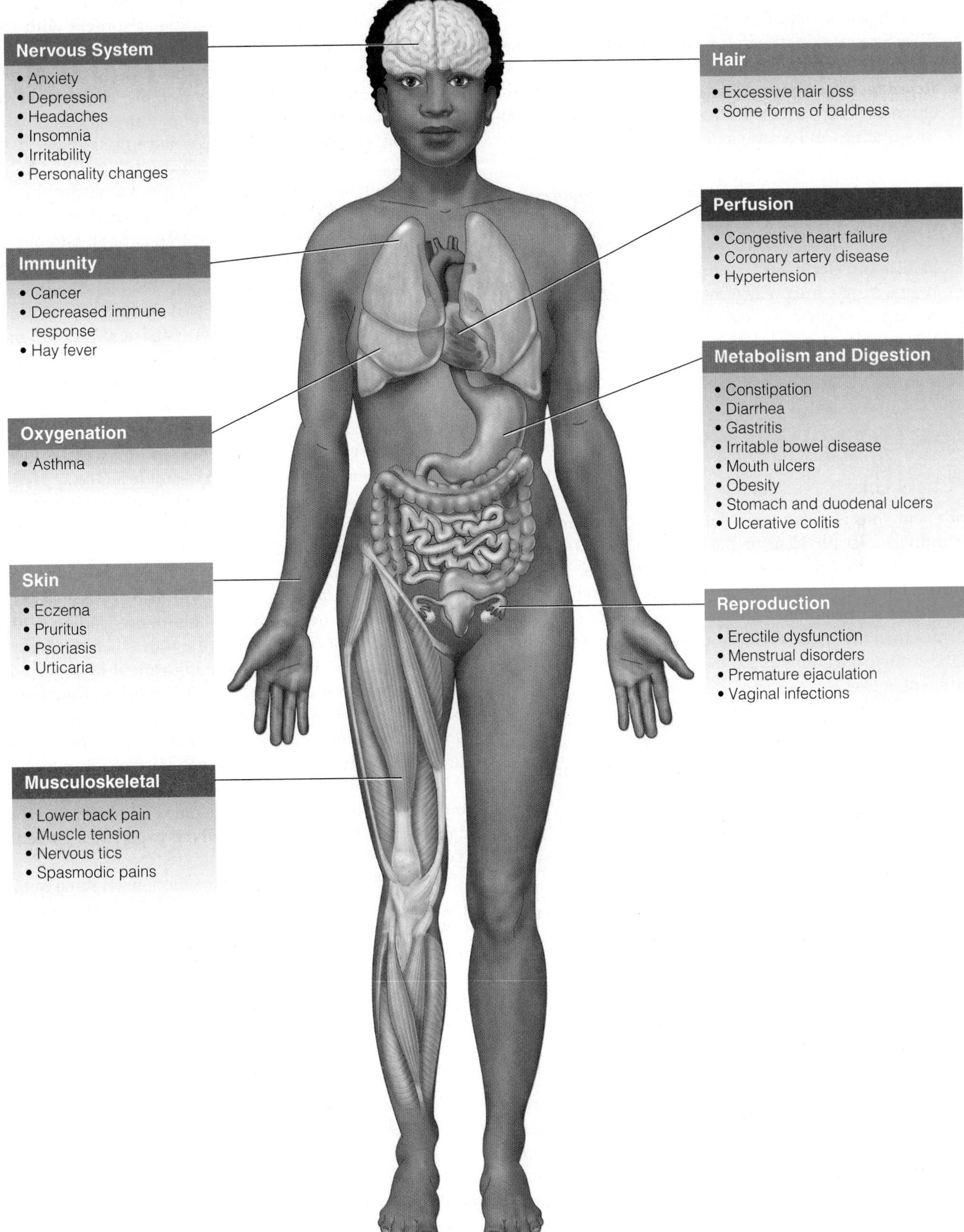

Figure 4.9 ■ Disorders and conditions that can be caused or aggravated by stress.

This decreases blood flow to the digestive system and slow digestion; nausea may result.

- *Skin:* Several skin diseases, such as eczema and psoriasis, can be exacerbated.
- *Reproductive organs:* Hormone levels can be influenced by long periods of stress, resulting in menstrual irregularities and a drop in testosterone.

Check Your Progress: Section 4.5

1. What hormones are released from the anterior pituitary and the adrenal cortex in response to stress?
2. What is the stress response of the digestive tract?
3. Name the two glands that release hormones in response to HPA axis activation.

4.6 Stress and Mental Health

An event that is perceived as extremely threatening to an individual's physical or psychologic well-being can produce feelings of intense fear, helplessness, or even horror. These emotional responses can overwhelm the individual's physiologic and psychologic defenses. An event is then traumatic by virtue of the perceived meaning of the event to the individual and the affective response that the event evokes.

Depression and Anxiety

The negative affective states that are most commonly considered to be responses to stress are depression and/or anxiety. The explanatory theory for the role of anxiety is that a traumatic event is an external stressor that produces a state of anxiety with which the individual is unable to cope. Threat is posed to the individual's psychologic, integrity and is of such a nature that it is overwhelming. States of anxiety are also associated with certain signs and symptoms that are reflective of sympathetic activation.

There is a pattern of research that demonstrates the effects of stress on depressive states.[13] The relationship between stress and depression has often been unclear and reciprocal in nature. An existing state of depression may influencing event perceptions, and depression may manifest as a result of failed coping. As an individual attempts to cope and the attempts fail, feelings of helplessness and worthlessness may emerge.[13]

It is difficult to determine when an individual experiences a pathologic level or degree of stress. While there are certain consequences from normative levels of stress, clinicians and researchers are often concerned about the point at which the threshold is crossed when the response continues for an extended period of time or at a level of intensity beyond that normally expected.

The fifth edition of the *Diagnostic and Statistical Manual of Mental Disorders* (DSM-5) lists two disorders with the term *stress* in the diagnostic label: posttraumatic stress disorder (PTSD) and acute stress disorder (ASD). The difference occurs in the onset of symptoms. In ASD, symptoms are expected to occur within 1 month of the traumatic event, and symptoms are not expected to last longer than 4 weeks. In PTSD, symptoms are expected to take longer than 1 month to develop.[14]

ASD and PTSD are psychiatric disorders characterized by the continual reexperience of a traumatic situation. The recollection of the event is accompanied by symptoms of increased arousal and by attempts to avoid stimuli that may be associated with the original event. Three distinct criteria define ASD and PTSD: (1) persistent reexperiencing of the traumatic event through flashbacks or dreams, (2) persistent attempts to avoid stimuli perceived to be associated with the traumatic event in combination with a general lack of interest in activities along with a lack of affect, and (3) persistent symptoms of increased arousal. These disorders are considered to result from the appraisal of an event as extremely traumatic in conjunction with an initial response that consisted of feeling "intense fear, helplessness, or horror."[14]

Distinct from ASD or PTSD are adjustment disorders. These conditions develop after exposure to a clearly defined stressor of a less intense nature than those leading to the development of ASD or PTSD. As with other psychiatric conditions, the individual with adjustment disorder will display significant disruption in the ability to function in society, along with a feeling of distress. Disruptions in daily functioning are expected to occur within 3 months of exposure to an event, and symptoms are not typically expected to occur for longer than 6 months. Adjustment disorders could be characterized as the outcome of maladaptive coping responses by an individual who is experiencing a sense of distress.[14]

An encounter with significant emotional trauma can be seen as an exemplar of a particular kind of learning, one in which a variety of chemicals are released in the body that eventually lead to structural changes in the brain. The impact of the trauma, an event that involves a conditioned emotional memory, ensures the frequent release of high-intensity emotional signals that may eventually result in neuronal changes and ultimately an enduring psychiatric condition.

Memory

The individual's emotional responses can have effects on memory. Memory begins with the registration of information from the environment. This process may be automatic and occur at a perceptual level without conscious awareness. Information from the senses is organized by comparison with perceptual maps and then forwarded to higher cortical levels, where a meaning or semantic interpretation is given to the registered event. After this initial period of encoding, in which a memory trace is formed, a process of consolidation occurs in which the permanence of the memory trace is set.

The process of associating a stimulus with a memory begins with the hippocampus, which along with an aspect of the thalamus, is associated with explicit memory. The hippocampus at the time of retrieval aids in bringing together elements of the memory trace from several neocortical areas. The hippocampal component of memory cannot distinguish between cues that pose a genuine threat and cues that may be similar but nonthreatening. This then allows for unconscious misinterpretation of a message or environmental stimulus.[15]

Individuals with pathologic stress responses often reexperience the original trauma. The reexperiencing of initial trauma triggers the initial acute stress response with activation of the SNS. This acute stress state leads to increased release of norepinephrine within the hippocampus and other brain areas, which in turn affects the encoding and retrieval of memory.[15]

The HPA axis also plays a role in affecting the memory of individuals with PTSD. The experiencing of intrusive thoughts and memories in a manner beyond the person's control may result in increased cortisol levels. A period of exposure to levels of cortisol often associated with psychologic and physical stress has been shown to produce reversible alterations of declarative memory, which governs the conscious recall of long-term memories. Involved in the anticipation of a stimulus is the prefrontal cortex. The release of dopamine from the prefrontal cortex is enhanced in the presence of stressors of great intensity or long duration. This release of dopamine has been thought to contribute to the development of PTSD through effects on neurons in the prefrontal cortex, leading a state of hypervigilance. The prefrontal cortex also is involved in the development of coping strategies. A functional defect in this area could then impair the ability to develop and use effective coping strategies in the face of stress.[15,16]

Exposure to stressful environments early in life can have long-term implications for neurologic and cognitive development. The release of hormonal mediators as part of the stress response leads to changes in brain structure. Areas associated with fear and avoidance can be enlarged, leading to higher levels of anxiety with impaired decision making.[17] ■

Heightened stress levels during pregnancy are associated with lower fetal birth weight and preterm birth. Higher levels of stress are tied to postpregnancy maternal levels of anxiety and depression.[18] ■

Selective attention, hypervigilance, and an orientation toward certain stimuli are influenced by the noradrenergic brain systems that are involved in the production and release of catecholamine. Stressors that are seen as uncontrollable may lead to a sensitization of catecholamine receptors that manifests as hypervigilance, increased autonomic nervous system hyperreactivity, and increased startle response.[19,20] These effects on memory are by no means restricted to PTSD and other psychiatric conditions. Stress can affect daily functioning by influencing spatial memories, causing an individual to forget the location of common items such as keys or forgetting to perform certain tasks. Depending on its nature and timing, stress can enhance or inhibit retention of information.[21]

Alexander Cho: Outcome

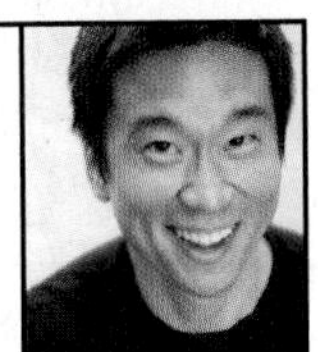

Mr. Cho experiences sleep disturbance and difficulty concentrating. He is displaying symptoms of PTSD after witnessing the traumatic death of a friend. The coping strategies Mr. Cho may have had previously were insufficient to deal with the significant stress that resulted. Nurses are well positioned to help identify maladaptive coping patterns and assist in the search for better strategies. While treating PTSD requires the aid of trained therapists, strategies that are often used include support groups and relaxation training.

The use of meditation or guided imagery can helpful to enhance coping ability through changing aspects of interpretation and psychologic responses. Starting a program of regular exercise can also be helpful in providing an outlet for energy, improving overall cardiovascular fitness, and mediating physiologic responses. Writing, talking with others, and blogging are ways of sharing concerns and obtaining support from others. Social support can helpful in dealing with stress, and the cathartic experience of sharing feelings and concerns is often helpful.

7. How can meditation or guided imagery help to mediate stress responses?
8. What role does cardiovascular fitness play in helping the patient with a stress disorder?

Check Your Progress: Section 4.6

1. What are the differences between ASD, PTSD, and adjustment disorders?
2. How do the hippocampus and thalamus work together when false threats are interpreted as real threats?
3. How does dopamine contribute to PTSD?

4.7 Stress and Physical Health

Respiratory Disease

Through activation of sympathetic pathways, stress results in increased respiratory and heart rates. This results in an increase in the rate of oxygen consumption. There is evidence that psychologic stress can worsen asthma through the induction of respiratory constriction.[22] Such stress-induced inflammation could be associated with increased stress responsivity on the part of certain asthma patients.[23]

Ella Fraser: Outcome

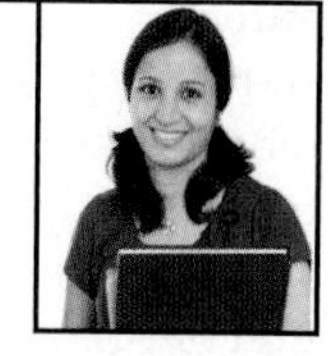

Ms. Fraser recently moved across the country and started graduate school. She is facing multiple sources of stress that can lead to suppression of immune function, leaving her more prone to the development of respiratory infections that may contribute to the worsening of asthma. Increased levels of stress may alone be associated with increased bronchoconstriction leading to emergence of more symptoms. Her relocation may also have exposed her to a different set of antigens in the surrounding environment, leading to increased inflammation.

Treatment of intermittent asthma generally relies on the use of albuterol, a smooth muscle bronchodilator to alleviate constriction. When symptoms increase, a steroidal therapy may be given for a few days in either oral or inhaled form until symptoms decrease. In case of true worsening of asthma, a combination inhaler may be provided to the patient to help maintain airway opening. It is important to consider techniques designed to facilitate stress reduction and coping. By using these methods to help cope with the stress that Ms. Fraser is experiencing, additional pharmacologic treatments can be avoided, or their use can be minimized.

5. How might sources of stress affect Ms. Fraser's asthma?
6. What strategies other than medication could Ms. Fraser use to decrease her stress levels?

Neurologic Disease

In recent years, an increasing body of knowledge has made it clear that the brain and the endocrine and immune systems are intimately linked by a complex feedback network. Working in conjunction, these systems produce a number of cytokines, hormones, and neuropeptides in common and share receptors for many of these molecules. It is hypothesized that many of the observed alterations in immune function that occur in response to stress may be related to alterations at the cytokine level. Cytokines are soluble proteins released by immune cells that have pro-inflammatory and anti-inflammatory properties. Disruptions of immune function, particularly in cytokine function, could contribute to the development of neurologic disease.

The uncertainty that surrounds a chronic disease such as multiple sclerosis (MS) can pose a threat to the individual and may induce stress. Individuals with MS often report a belief that psychologic stress precipitates exacerbations of the disease. Much of the early literature on MS reflects this belief. MS may develop from inappropriate stress responses that could exacerbate a dysregulation of cytokine production. The cytokines that are associated with inflammatory processes and with pronounced T-cell–mediated immune responses are referred to as Th1 cytokines. Cytokines associated with antibody production and the suppression of inflammatory responses are referred to as Th2 cytokines. Production of Th1 cytokines through feedback mechanisms influences the production of Th2 cytokines and vice versa. In individuals with MS, the interplay or equilibrium among cytokines is believed to be disrupted. Individuals with MS have demonstrated a cytokine profile characterized by elevated levels of select pro-inflammatory cytokines, such as IL-12, interferon gamma, IL-6, and tumor necrosis factor alpha, in conjunction with decreased production of anti-inflammatory (particularly IL-10) cytokines.[24] These pro-inflammatory mediators are believed to contribute to the destruction of myelin and the death of oligodendrocytes. The release of the pro-inflammatory cytokines is associated with the presence of stress. Psychologic stress has been shown to be associated with an increase in the production of pro-inflammatory cytokines.

The production of these inflammatory mediators is believed to be involved in the development of other disease states, particularly cardiovascular and gastrointestinal diseases. The release of these immune mediators known as cytokines, particularly those with inflammatory properties such as tumor necrosis factor alpha, IL-1, and IL-6, stimulate the HPA axis. This stimulation is then normally countered by the release of cortisol. In individuals with MS, there may be a deficiency in the normal suppressive aspects of the immune system, leading to a continuation of inflammatory responses that damage myelin.

Gastrointestinal Disease

The experience of life events is associated with the development or worsening of inflammatory bowel disease, peptic ulcer disease, and gastroesophageal reflex disease. Both acute and chronic stress conditions have been found to contribute to the development of these disorders. Acute onset can represent exposure to a traumatic event. Chronic onset could reflect years of anxiety or inappropriate lifestyle choices such as poor nutrition or caffeine or other drug consumption that could reflect attempts to deal with stress.

Stress has been shown to slow gastric emptying and to increase motility of the colon. The development of a pattern of increased sympathetic responsiveness to stress may play a role in the development of inflammatory bowel disease. A state of hypervigilance and increased catecholamine production can contribute to the development of inflammatory bowel disease by increasing motor activity of the colon. In turn, a blunted HPA response may be present in individuals with inflammatory bowel disease, contributing to disease by the individual's inability to limit the sympathetic response to stress. The presence of inflammatory mediators may occur in an unrestricted fashion, contributing to gastrointestinal disease. Stress-related changes in neuroanatomic structures of the CNS may play a role by contributing to a pattern of ongoing epinephrine and norepinephrine release. This ongoing pattern of sympathetic response may also contribute to hypersecretion of gastric acid. Over time, the circulation of the gastrointestinal tract can be disrupted, contributing to localized ischemia and further damage.[25]

Cardiovascular Disease

Cognitive stress states have been reported to have effects on the cardiovascular system. A degree of stress could promote the development of either good health or disease. Such changes depend on the individual's current health status and vulnerability. The development of illness relies to a great degree on the individual's health status, both physiologic and psychologic. For the individual who is already at risk the changes induced by stress may worsen an existing disease condition. Individuals with coronary artery disease have been demonstrated to experience episodes of myocardial ischemia in response to mental stress occurring during the performance of routine daily activities. Positive emotional states are associated with lower levels of aortic calcification and with a lowered risk of ischemic events. These findings suggest a different mechanism of action for positive emotions than for negative ones.[26]

Psychosocial stress has been found to be a major contributing factor to acute myocardial infarction.[27] The presence of increased levels of hostility and anxiety are associated with the incidence of coronary artery disease, and individuals whose personality is characterized by increased negative affect are more likely to experience increased cardiovascular mortality and morbidity.[28] The presence of this personality type may be seen as a form of chronic stress. This state of chronic stress then stimulates the sympathetic and HPA systems, ultimately producing a state of chronic inflammation. This chronic inflammation contributes to the development of atherosclerosis, placing the organism at an increased risk for cardiovascular disease.[29]

CLINICAL POINT: The presence of stress, either physical (such as postoperative or posttraumatic) or psychologic, can lead to elevations in blood glucose level. Such elevations do not mean that the patient had developed diabetes; they indicate transient elevations due to the release of cortisol influencing the production and release of glucose. ■

Stress and the Immune System

The interplay between stress and immune function is well established and acknowledged, and several fields of research are investigating stress in relation to particular body systems or disease states. Terms such as *psychoendocrinology* and *psychoneuroimmunology* can be found throughout the scientific literature. **Psychoneuroimmunology** is the study of how emotional states influence immunologic and neurologic function. One focus in the field is investigating the influence of stress on immunologic responses and how these responses contribute to disease. It is not surprising that stress has been found to have several effects on immunologic function and infection.

Aging of the immune system is referred to as *immunosenescence*. The age-related changes lead to a less effective immune response that places older adults at an increased risk for infection and poor wound healing. In addition, stress can further reduce the functional ability of the immune system and lead to increased levels of anxiety and depression.[30] ■

Effects of Stress on the Immune Response to Microorganisms

One of the best-characterized immune functions that is affected by exposure to chronic stress is natural killer (NK) cell activity. In addition to anti-tumor effects, NK cells constitute the body's first line of defense against virus infections. These cells are a component of the innate immune system and play a key role in controlling and lysing virus-infected cells during the early phase of a viral infection. Greater NK cell numbers and/or greater cytolytic activity increases one's natural resistance to viruses. Protection against viral infections is also mediated by two arms of the adaptive immune system. One of these is the cell-mediated immune response, which against viral infections is primarily mediated by cytotoxic T lymphocytes (CD8+). The other arm of the adaptive immune system is the humoral immune response by B lymphocytes (CD19+), which produce antibodies. Chronic stress results in lowered innate and adaptive immune responses in humans and is associated with increased incidence, duration, and severity of infection and decreased survival (e.g., the annual morbidity and mortality associated with influenza infections).

Another good example of the effect of stress on the immune system is the reactivation of latent viral infections. The immunosuppressive effect of chronic stress promotes reactivation of latent viruses such as herpes simplex virus (HSV)-1 and HSV-2. Stressors as diverse as an academic examination and marital distress have been linked to apparent latent virus reactivation, as judged by higher levels of circulating antibody specific for HSV-1, HSV-2, cytomegalovirus, and Epstein-Barr virus.[31,32] Each of these viruses is latent in that the virus exists within the host in a quiescent state as a result of continued and specific cell-mediated immunity directed against virus-infected somatic cells. However, if cell-mediated immunity is reduced (e.g., by stress), these viruses reactivate and replicate, leading to viral shedding and stimulation of the humoral immune response. Shed virus is antigenic and stimulates B lymphocytes to respond to the virus with the production of antibody, resulting in a subsequent increase in antibody levels specific for that virus. Hence, an increase in specific antibody within the circulation is an indication of viral shedding, resulting from the effect of stress on the cell-mediated immune function that normally controls viral replication and shedding.[33]

It has been clearly established that suppression of the immune response increases mycotic and bacterial infections. However, there is no clear-cut empirical evidence that psychologic stress increases the incidence and severity of bacterial and mycotic human infections, although the association of emotional stress with infectious mycologic disease is suspected. Fungal infections are well known to be associated with the stressful conditions of surgical trauma, cancer, organ transplants, long-term antibiotic use, corticosteroid therapy, diabetes mellitus, critical illness, and pregnancy. Stress hormones such as cortisol and catecholamines are known to enhance pathogenesis of experimental fungal disease. For example, *Candida albicans* and related fungi are endogenous opportunists; infections with these fungi are typically associated with debilitating and/or predisposing conditions. *Candida* infections have become the first symptom of active AIDS to appear in HIV-positive individuals. One factor shared by AIDS patients and other susceptible individuals is hormonal imbalance resulting from HPA and SNS activation. Candidiasis also appears frequently in people undergoing surgery, a unique form of stress that involves emotional stressors (anxiety), chemical stressors (anesthesia), physical stressors (surgery), and often the stress of pain. Similarly, emotional stress has been positively correlated with increased incidence of carrying *Candida*, and psychosocial factors, particularly stress, have been implicated in vulvovaginitis caused by *Candida albicans*.[34] Interestingly, somatic factors did not influence the occurrence or relapse with this infectious agent, and antimycotic treatment influenced only the symptoms of the illness, not its cause. Women with recurrent vulvovaginal candidiasis have been shown to have a blunted rise in morning cortisol levels and lower mean levels of salivary cortisol after awakening as well as locally compromised immune function. These observations suggest a role for stress in the incidence and susceptibility of these women to this fungal infection.

Invasion of the body by disease causing microorganisms is not necessarily sufficient to actually cause the disease. Disease occurs only when the infectious agent is pathogenic and the immune system is compromised or unable to recognize the invading microorganism. Psychologic stress can alter the immune response, but it is unclear whether such an alteration is sufficient to influence the body's ability to fight infectious disease. To address this issue, a series of human viral challenge studies were conducted in which psychologic parameters were assessed and volunteers were then exposed to one of five viruses that cause the common cold.[35] The participants were monitored for infection and illness. The results showed that the greater the psychologic stress, the greater the probability for clinical manifestations of a viral infection. Two types of psychologically stressful life events were strongly associated with greater illness susceptibility: enduring (1 month or longer) interpersonal problems with family or friends and enduring problems related to work (underemployment or unemployment). Moreover, across all types of events, the longer the stressful life event lasted, the greater was the risk for developing a clinical illness. In these studies, higher levels of epinephrine and norepinephrine were related to a greater risk of developing a cold. However, neither catecholamines nor immune effector mechanisms were associated with the duration or clinical manifestations of viral infection. In a separate study, influenza virus challenge of volunteers showed that those with higher psychologic stress had greater symptomatology, greater accumulation of nasal mucus, and higher amounts the pro-inflammatory cytokine IL-6. The IL-6 response was temporally related to illness expression, indicating that IL-6 acted as a major mediator through which stress was associated with symptoms of illness.[36] The effect of stress in this highly controlled human challenge model did not appear to be due to stress-elicited suppression of immune function. Instead, chronic stress appeared to interfere with the immune system's ability to respond to hormonal signals that turn off the release of pro-inflammatory cytokines. Individuals under stress may overrespond (e.g., produce too much IL-6), which triggers and prolongs the symptoms of upper respiratory infections. In other words, stress did not reduce the immune response to viral challenge; rather, it amplified the IL-6 response. It may be that adults facing a severe chronic stressor have a diminished capacity to suppress IL-6 production because of stressor-induced glucocorticoid resistance. It is important to note that such data are derived from a controlled but artificial challenge paradigm and that the results are based on correlations. However, the relationship of stress to immune outcome is a complex one in that further investigation has demonstrated positive emotional style to be associated with a lower risk of developing an upper respiratory infection. Individuals with a positive emotional style had fewer symptoms and signs of respiratory viral infection and with fewer upper respiratory tract symptoms. Understanding the contribution of positive emotions to immunity and protection from disease has become an active area of psychoneuroimmunology research.

Since stress influences the immune system in healthy populations, it is plausible that stress and other psychosocial factors may play a role in the immune abnormalities associated with HIV infections.[37] HIV-infected individuals display physiologic changes that are consistent with chronic elevations of resting levels of cortisol, as evidenced by muted cortisol responsivity (due to downregulated receptors), and a flattened cortisol circadian rhythm. (Note that cortisol is secreted in a circadian pattern, with high levels in the morning that decrease to low levels at bedtime.) Elevated cortisol levels predict accelerated immune decline and development of AIDS in individuals who are HIV-positive. Furthermore, HIV-positive men show signs of SNS activation and a diminished capacity to suppress HIV plasma viral load as well as a poorer CD4+ T-cell recovery when treated with highly active antiretroviral therapy. SNS activation results in downregulation of lymphocyte and NK cell function, and chronic SNS activation with release of norepinephrine alters lymphocyte trafficking, cytokine production, and cytotoxicity and facilitates HIV replication. HIV-positive individuals assigned to cognitive behavior stress management (CBSM) demonstrate less activation of HPA axis–mediated stress responses, better immunologic control of the virus, and increased immune system reconstitution with decreased HIV viral RNA in peripheral blood. These biological changes were associated with reductions in depression and increases in relaxation and social support during the stress management intervention. CBSM reduces anxiety, depression, and social isolation by lowering physical tension, increasing a sense of control and self-efficacy, and building interpersonal skills necessary to maintain adequate, effective social relationships.[38] These psychologic effects are hypothesized to improve regulation of peripheral catecholamines and cortisol via changes in the SNS and HPA axis, respectively, and in turn lead to better immune control of the HIV virus.[39]

The Influence of Stress on Vaccination Outcomes

Psychologic stress can modulate the humoral immune response to vaccination.[40] Prospective longitudinal studies demonstrate that people who report higher levels of stress exhibit lower levels of protective antibodies against microbial pathogens including influenza, hepatitis B, and pneumonia.[41–43] From a clinical perspective, these findings suggest that stress may diminish the efficacy of vaccination procedures and thereby increase vulnerability to pathogens that give rise to infectious disease. The most robust evidence is derived from studies of older adults who experienced chronic stress as caregivers for family members suffering from dementia.[44] These caretakers exhibit blunted antibody responses to influenza and to bacterial pneumonia vaccines when compared to matched control individuals. The deficits in antibody response persisted years after the family member had died, suggesting that chronic severe stressors may have long-term adverse consequences on the immune system. Despite evidence that the presence of stress is associated with poorer antibody response, little is known about the mechanisms responsible for this phenomenon. Models of stress and immunity suggest that dysregulated hormone secretion or maladaptive health practices could operate as mediational pathways. Of these hormones, cortisol was shown to be most consistently associated with poorer antibody responses. Individuals who secreted the most cortisol, either over the period of a day or in response to a stressor, exhibited the poorest antibody responses to vaccination.[40] In contrast to the chronic stress of caregiving, an acute laboratory stress prior to influenza vaccination was shown to increase subsequent antibody titers in vaccinated women. Interestingly, distress on the days after the vaccination contributed to a reduced antibody response to vaccination. Hence, the timing of vaccination with regard to a stressor may have a significant effect on the outcome of vaccination. These observations demonstrate that the nature of stress, whether acute or chronic, influences the immune response and in this case the response to vaccination.

Check Your Progress: Section 4.7

1. What is the effect of stress on vaccination outcomes?
2. What is the relationship between personality and heart disease?
3. Describe how stress affects inflammatory bowel disease.

CHAPTER SUMMARY

4.1 Chapter Overview and Case Studies

Define stress, coping, and adaptation, and list concepts related to stress.

- Stress is a term used to denote the psychologic and physiologic response of an organism to an environmental event that is often perceived as negative.
- Coping is the dynamic process through which individuals apply psychologic and behavioral measures to handle internal and external demands.
- Adaptation incorporates both physiologic and psychologic processes used in response to stress.
- Concepts related to stress include, but are not limited to, oxygenation, perfusion, sensory perception, metabolism, mobility, emotional regulation, cognition, and immunity.

4.2 Conceptualizations of Stress

Summarize the major conceptual approaches to the study of stress.

- The response to external threats involves sympathetic arousal that provides the energy for fight-or-flight responses.
- The response to stress involves coping, lifestyle choices, genetic influences, and overall health.
- Conceptual models of stress describe select mechanisms of the larger process of responding to stress.
- Stress can be describe as resulting from an event (stimulus) or from a pattern of interaction between the perception of the individual and characteristics of the environment (transaction).
- Concepts of stress as a response tend to examine physiologic patterns of response.
- Stress responses can have differing effects on the immune system. Acute stress activates the immune system; chronic stress suppresses immune responses.

4.3 The Body in Balance

Compare and contrast homeostasis and allostasis.

- The response to stress can affect a state of physiologic balance, or homeostasis.
- The theoretical concept of allostasis views the body as being in a dynamic state of flux and views physiologic responses along a continuum.
- Allostatic load is the sum total of the wear and tear experienced by an individual.

4.4 The Body Responding to Stress

Compare and contrast the various models of stress response.

- The general adaptation syndrome (GAS) represents the response of the organism to long-term stress.
- The GAS has three stages: alarm, resistance, and exhaustion. Alarm represents the immediate response to stress. Resistance is a period of adaptation. Exhaustion is the depletion of stress mediators, resulting in organ damage.
- Life event approaches to stress view events as inducing change. If enough change is demanded, whether positive or negative, stress results.
- The transaction approach to stress conceptualizes stress as occurring when the organism rates a situation as exceeding available resources and posing a risk for harm.

4.5 The Effects of Stress on Health

Explain the pathogenesis and clinical manifestations of stress.

- A cardinal sign of stress is emotional arousal concordant with physiologic arousal.
- The physiologic response to stress involves two primary mechanisms: the hypothalamic–pituitary–adrenal (HPA) axis and the sympathetic adrenal medullary system, also known as the locus coeruleus–norepinephrine (LC/NE) system.
- The HPA axis affects the secretion of hormones from the pituitary and adrenal glands and is involved in the release of cortisol.
- Cortisol has effects on energy metabolism through effects on protein utilization and blood glucose.
- The LC/NE system is a group of neurons located in the pons that mediate the sympathetic response.
- Acute stress condition increases circulating levels of epinephrine, norepinephrine, cortisol, ACTH, and beta-endorphin.
- The response to stress affects every body system and is associated with a number of health-related conditions.

4.6 Stress and Mental Health

Explain the mechanisms whereby stress contributes to the development or exacerbation of psychiatric disorders such as depression, anxiety, and posttraumatic stress disorder.

- The CNS is the mediating link between environmental events and response.
- Stress can lead to the development of psychiatric states known as acute stress disorder (ASD) and post-traumatic stress disorder (PTSD). These disorders are characterized by a continued state of hyperarousal and reexperiencing of the trauma.
- The release of cortisol and catecholamine can induce lasting changes in parts of the brain involved in the stress response. These changes can affect memory and may induce increased responsiveness to future stress.

4.7 Stress and Physical Health

Explain the mechanisms whereby stress contributes to the development or exacerbation of physiologic disorders such as multiple sclerosis, inflammatory bowel disease, and coronary artery disease.

- Through activation of sympathetic pathways, stress results in increased respiratory rate and heart rate. Physiologic responses also lead to increased inflammation. Through these mechanisms, stress can worsen respiratory disease.
- Illness-related uncertainty is often a source of stress. Through influence on immune activation, stress can play a role in disease exacerbations in individuals with multiple sclerosis.
- The experience of life events is associated with the development or worsening of inflammatory bowel disease, peptic ulcer disease, and gastroesophageal reflex disease. Stress slows gastric emptying and increases motility of the colon. Increased sympathetic responsiveness to stress may play a role in the development of inflammatory bowel disease.
- Increased sympathetic activation in response to stress leads to activation of the cardiovascular system. Heart rate and blood pressure increase in relation to stress, and stress has been found to be a major contributing factor to acute myocardial infarction
- Stress suppresses the activity of natural killer cells. This leads to increased susceptibility to viral infections. Antibacterial defenses of the body are also reduced in response to chronic stress, leading a state of immunosuppression. Yet acute stress situations activate elements of the immune system, boosting defenses for a short period.
- Individuals who are under a significant degree of stress have decreased responses to vaccinations, producing lower levels of antibodies.

REVIEW QUESTIONS

1. Which of the following responses indicates that the client understands what the nurse has taught about stress?
   a. "Stress is always harmful."
   b. "Stress can be an environmental or psychologic threat."
   c. "Happy life events are not stressful."
   d. "Stress is the same across cultures."
2. The nurse is caring for a client with herpes simplex virus. The nurse understands that chronic stress can cause which of the following conditions?
   a. Increased cell-mediated immunity
   b. Inactivation of the humoral immune response
   c. Reduction in the levels of circulating antibody for HSV
   d. Reactivation of the latent virus
3. The nurse is caring for a client with a high level of cortisol. Which of the following manifestations should the nurse expect to find?
   a. Increased blood glucose level
   b. Hypotension
   c. Bradycardia
   d. Vasodilation
4. The nurse is caring for a client with an infection. The nurse anticipates which of the following effects of chronic stress on this client?
   a. A suppressed innate immune response
   b. A heightened immune response
   c. No effect on the immune system
   d. An intensified adaptive immune response
5. Which of the following health effects is likely to be seen in a client experiencing chronic stress?
   a. Enhanced delayed-type hypersensitivity
   b. Suppressed delayed-type hypersensitivity
   c. Increased leukocyte mobilization
   d. Enhanced antigen-specific immune response
6. A client in the stage of alarm would most likely exhibit which of the following?
   a. Exhaustion
   b. Organ damage
   c. Increased mean arterial blood pressure
   d. Bradycardia
7. An assessment of a client with posttraumatic stress disorder is likely to reveal symptoms that:
   a. occur within 1 month of the event.
   b. last less than 4 weeks.
   c. take longer than 1 month to develop.
   d. are resolved within a year of the event.
8. A client with posttraumatic stress disorder is most likely to experience which of the following?
   a. Persistent attempts to face the traumatic stimuli
   b. Persistent repression of the traumatic event so that it will not show up in dreams
   c. Persistent symptoms of dampened arousal
   d. Persistent lack of interest in activities

ANSWERS

Answers to Review Questions can be found in Appendix A. Answers to Case Study and Check Your Progress questions are available on the faculty resources site. Please consult with your instructor.

RECOMMENDED WEBSITES

American Psychological Association
www.apa.org/topics/stress/index.aspx

Franklin Institute
https://www.fi.edu/brain/stress.htm

National Institute for Occupational Safety and Health
https://www.cdc.gov/niosh/topics/stress

REFERENCES

1. Semmer, N. K., McGrath, J. E., & Beeher, T. A. (2005). Conceptual issues in research on stress and health. In C. L. Cooper (Ed.), *Handbook of stress medicine and health* (pp. 1–43). Boca Raton, FL: CRC Press.
2. Rohleder, N. (2012). Acute and chronic stress induced changes in sensitivity of peripheral inflammatory pathways to the signals of multiple stress systems—2011 Curt Richter Award winner. *Psychoneuroendocrinology, 37*(3), 307–316.
3. Dhabhar, F. S., Saul, A. N., Daugherty, C., Holmes, T. H., Bouley, D. M., & Oberyszyn, T. M. (2010). Short-term stress enhances cellular immunity and increases early resistance to squamous cell carcinoma. *Brain, Behavior, and Immunity, 24*(1), 127–137.
4. McEwen, B. S. (2004). *The end of stress as we know it*. Washington, DC: Joseph Henry Press.
5. Selye, H. (1978). *The stress of life* (rev. ed.). New York, NY: McGraw-Hill.
6. McCarty, R., & Pacak, K. (2007). Alarm phase and general adaptation syndrome. In G. Fink (Ed.), *Encyclopedia of stress* (2nd ed., pp. 119–123). San Diego, CA: Academic Press.
7. Horowitz, M. J. (1998). *Cognitive psychodynamics: From conflict to character*. New York, NY: John Wiley & Sons.
8. Janoff-Bulman, R. (1995). Victims of violence. In S. George, J. Everly, & J. M. Lating (Eds.), *Psychotraumatology: Key papers and core concepts in post-traumatic stress* (pp. 73–86). New York, NY: Plenum.
9. Lazarus, R. S., & Folkman, S. (1984). *Stress, appraisal, and coping*. New York, NY: Springer.
10. Kolcz, J. (2012). Neuroendocrine regulation of stress response in clinical models. In T. Sumiyoshi (Ed.), *Neuroendocrinology and behavior*. Rijeka, Croatia: InTech. doi:10.5772/48533
11. Tort, L., & Teles, M. (2011). The endocrine response to stress: A comparative view. In F. Akin (Ed.), *Basic and clinical endocrinology up-to-date* (pp. 263–286). Rijeka, Croatia: InTech. doi:10.5772/21446
12. Tsigos, C., & Chrousos, G. P. (2002). Hypothalamic-pituitary-adrenal axis, neuroendocrine factors and stress. *Journal of Psychosomatic Research, 53*(4), 865–871.
13. Sickmann, H., Li, Y., Mørk, A., Sanchez, C., & Gulinello, M. (2014). Does stress elicit depression? Evidence from clinical and preclinical studies. *Current Topics in Behavioral Neurosciences, 18*, 123–159.
14. American Psychiatric Association. (2013). Trauma- and stressor-related disorders. In *Diagnostic and statistical manual of mental disorders* (5th ed., pp. 265–290). Arlington, VA: American Psychiatric Association.
15. Lindau, M., Almkvist, O., & Mohammed, A. H. (2010). Learning and memory, effects of stress on. In G. Fink (Ed.), *Stress consequences: Mental, neuropsychological and socioeconomic* (pp. 365–371). San Diego, CA: Academic Press.
16. Etkin, A., Egner, T., & Kalisch, R. (2011). Emotional processing in anterior cingulate and medial prefrontal cortex. *Trends in Cognitive Sciences, 15*(2), 85–93.
17. Shonkoff, J. P., Garner, A. S., et al. (2012). The lifelong effects of early childhood adversity and toxic stress. *Pediatrics, 129*(1), e232–e246.
18. Dunkel Schetter, C., & Tanner, L. (2012). Anxiety, depression and stress in pregnancy: Implications for mothers, children, research, and practice. *Current Opinion in Psychiatry, 25*(2), 141–148.
19. Harvey, B. H., Brand, L., Jeeva, Z., & Stein, D. J. (2006). Cortical/hippocampal monoamines, HPA-axis changes and aversive behavior following stress and restress in an animal model of post-traumatic stress disorder. *Physiology & Behavior, 87*(5), 881–890.
20. Harvey, B. H., Naciti, C., Brand, L., & Stein, D. J. (2004). Serotonin and stress: Protective or malevolent actions in the biobehavioral response to repeated trauma? *Annals of the New York Academy of Sciences, 1032*(1), 267–272.
21. Schwabe, L., Wolf, O. T., & Oitzl, M. S. (2010). Memory formation under stress: Quantity and quality. *Neuroscience & Biobehavioral Reviews, 34*(4), 584–591.
22. Ritz, T. (2012). Airway responsiveness to psychological processes in asthma and health. *Frontiers in Physiology, 5*(3), 343.
23. Rosenkranz, M. A., Busse, W. W., Sheridan, J. F., Crisafl, G. M., & Davidson, R. J. (2012). Are there neurophenotypes for asthma? Functional brain imaging of the interaction between emotion and inflammation in asthma. *PloS One, 7*(8), e40921.
24. Amedei, A., Prisco, D., & D'Elios, M. (2012). Multiple sclerosis: The role of cytokines in pathogenesis and in therapies. *International Journal of Molecular Sciences, 13*(10), 13438–13460.
25. Konturek, P. C., Brzozowski, T., & Konturek, S. J. (2011). Stress and the gut: Pathophysiology, clinical consequences, diagnostic approach and treatment options. *Journal of Physiology and Pharmacology, 62*(6), 591–599.
26. Matthews, K. A., Owens, J. F., Edmundowicz, D., Lee, L., & Kuller, L. H. (2006). Positive and negative attributes and risk for coronary and aortic calcification in healthy women. *Psychosomatic Medicine, 68*(3), 355–361.
27. Jiang, W., Samad, Z., Boyle, S., et al. (2013). Prevalence and clinical characteristics of mental stress–induced myocardial ischemia in patients with coronary heart disease. *Journal of the American College of Cardiology, 61*(7), 714–722.
28. Kupper, N., Pedersen, S. S., Hofer, S., Saner, H., Oldridge, N., & Denollet, J. (2013). Cross-cultural analysis of type D (distressed) personality in 6222 patients with ischemic heart disease: A study from the International HeartQoL Project. *International Journal of Cardiology, 166*(2), 327–333.
29. Libby, P. (2012). Inflammation in atherosclerosis. *Arteriosclerosis, Thrombosis, and Vascular Biology, 32*(9), 2045–2051.
30. Heffner, K. L. (2011). Neuroendocrine effects of stress on immunity in the elderly: Implications for inflammatory disease. *Immunology and Allergy Clinics of North America, 31*(1), 95–108.
31. Glaser, R., & Kiecolt-Glaser, J. K. (1997). Chronic stress modulates the virus-specific immune response to latent herpes simplex virus type 1. *Annals of Behavioral Medicine, 19*(2), 78–82.
32. Pariante, C. M., Carpiniello, B., Orru, M. G., et al. (1997). Chronic caregiving stress alters peripheral blood immune parameters: The role of age and severity of stress. *Psychotherapy and Psychosomatics, 66*(4), 199–207.
33. Gouin, J. P., Hantsoo, L., & Kiecolt-Glaser, J. K. (2008). Immune dysregulation and chronic stress among older adults: A review. *Neuroimmunomodulation, 15*(4), 251–259.
34. Meyer, H., Goettlicher, S., & Mendling, W. (2006). Stress as a cause of chronic recurrent vulvovaginal candidosis and the effectiveness of the conventional antimycotic therapy. *Mycoses, 49*(3), 202–209.
35. Pedersen, A., Zachariae, R., & Bovbjerg, D. H. (2010). Influence of psychological stress on upper respiratory infection: A meta-analysis of prospective studies. *Psychosomatic Medicine, 72*(8), 823–832.
36. Cohen, S., Alper, C. M., Doyle, W. J., Treanor, J. J., & Turner, R. B. (2006). Positive emotional style predicts resistance to illness after experimental exposure to rhinovirus or influenza a virus. *Psychosomatic Medicine, 68*(6), 809–815.
37. Cole, S. W. (2008). Psychosocial influences on HIV-1 disease progression: Neural, endocrine, and virologic mechanisms. *Psychosomatic Medicine, 70*(5), 562–568.
38. Antoni, M. H., Carrico, A. W., Duran, R. E., et al. (2006). Randomized clinical trial of cognitive behavioral stress management on human immunodeficiency virus viral load in gay men treated with highly active antiretroviral therapy. *Psychosomatic Medicine, 68*(1), 143–151.

39. Jones, D., Owens, M., Kumar, M., Cook, R., & Weiss, S. M. (2013). The effect of relaxation interventions on cortisol levels in HIV-sero-positive women. *Journal of the International Association of Providers of AIDS Care, 13*(4), 318–323.
40. Pedersen, A. F., Zachariae, R., & Bovbjerg, D. H. (2009). Psychological stress and antibody response to influenza vaccination: a meta-analysis. *Brain, Behavior, and Immunity, 23*(4), 427–433.
41. Cohen, S., Janicki-Deverts, D., Doyle, W. J., et al. (2012). Chronic stress, glucocorticoid receptor resistance, inflammation, and disease risk. *Proceedings of the National Academy of Sciences of the United States of America, 109*(16), 5995–5999.
42. Effros, R. B. (2011). Telomere/telomerase dynamics within the human immune system: Effect of chronic infection and stress. *Experimental Gerontology, 46*(2–3), 135–140.
43. Fagundes, C. P., Glaser, R., & Kiecolt-Glaser, J. K. (2013). Stressful early life experiences and immune dysregulation across the lifespan. *Brain, Behavior, and Immunity, 27*(1), 8–12.
44. Bauer, M. E., Vedhara, K., Perks, P., Wilcock, G. K., Lightman, S. L., & Shanks, N. (2000). Chronic stress in caregivers of dementia patients is associated with reduced lymphocyte sensitivity to glucocorticoids. *Journal of Neuroimmunology, 103*(1), 84–92.

Unit II
Risks Underlying the Leading Causes of Morbidity and Mortality

The primary risk factors for the leading causes of morbidity and mortality include obesity and physical inactivity; using tobacco, alcohol, and other legal and illegal substances; and alterations in sleep. A number of factors and processes contribute to shorten the life expectancy of individuals with alterations in these areas, but three systems or pathways discussed frequently in the literature are the sympathetic nervous system (SNS), inflammation, and metabolism.

- As outlined in Chapter 4, chronic stress—either physiological or psychological—stimulates the SNS and the HPA axis, leading to chronic inflammation and insulin resistance, which in turn contribute to atherosclerosis and diabetes. Further, long-term stress responses such as anxiety and negative affect increase the risk for cardiovascular events and mortality.[1,2]
- BMI above normal is strongly associated with diabetes, coronary disease, stroke, and respiratory disease mortality, decreasing longevity of the individual.[3,4] In addition, obesity increases risk for psychological stress due to functional consequences to physical activity[5] and emotional consequences of stigma.[6]
- Chronic alcohol and drug use lead to self-neglect and impair physiological and psychological health in many ways. For example, chronic use of alcohol and drugs impacts SNS responses, increasing risk for arrhythmia, stroke, and other cardiovascular alterations; and it is associated with a broad range of personal and socioeconomic issues.
- Both obesity and alcohol use are independent risk factors for obstructive sleep apnea (OSA). Impaired breathing and ventilation of OSA increase SNS activity, leading to transient but recurring cardiovascular changes. Left untreated, these may result in organ damage and eventual death.

Obesity, alcohol and drug use, and sleep dysfunction alone are sufficient to tax physiological systems and affect morbidity and mortality rates. But any combination of these will overwhelm systems, increase mortality, and shorten lifespan. For example, an overweight patient with diabetes and a history of cardiac illness (e.g., stroke and myocardial infarction) faces a reduced life expectancy between 12 and 15 years. Add alcohol abuse to the mix, and an individual might face a reduction in life expectancy of as much as 23 years.[3,4]

The chapters in this unit will explore in detail the relationship between obesity and physical inactivity; nicotine, alcohol, and drug use; and sleep impairment on individual mortality and morbidity. Knowledge of the pathophysiological and neurobiological processes involved in these energy imbalances will help nurses better assess and care for their clients, as well as help them develop client education for individual clients and activities aimed at helping individuals and communities prevent the complications that arise from obesity, substance use, and alterations in sleep.

References

1. Matthews, K. A., Owens, J. F., Edmundowicz, D., Lee, L., & Kuller, L. H. (2006). Positive and negative attributes and risk for coronary and aortic calcification in healthy women. *Psychosomatic Medicine, 68*(3), 355–61.
2. Jiang. W., Samad, Z., Boyle, S., et al. (2013). Prevalence and clinical characteristics of mental stress–induced myocardial ischemia in patients with coronary heart disease. *Journal of the American College of Cardiology, 61*(7), 714–722.
3. The Emerging Risk Factors Collaboration. (2015). Association of cardiometabolic multimorbidity with mortality. *JAMA, 314*(1), 52–60.
4. The Global BMI Mortality Collaboration. (2016). Body-mass index and all-cause mortality: individual-participant-data meta-analysis of 239 prospective studies in four continents. *The Lancet, 388,* 776–786. Retrieved from http://www.thelancet.com/pdfs/journals/lancet/PIIS0140-6736(16)30175-1.pdf
5. Lim, S. S., Norman, R. J., Davies, M. J., & Moran, L. J. (2013). The effect of obesity on polycystic ovary syndrome: a systematic review and meta-analysis. *Obesity Reviews, 14*(2), 95–109.
6. Luppino, F. S., de Wit, L. M., Bouvy, P. F., et al. (2010). Overweight, obesity, and depression: a systematic review and meta-analysis of longitudinal studies. *Archives of General Psychiatry, 67*(3), 220–229.

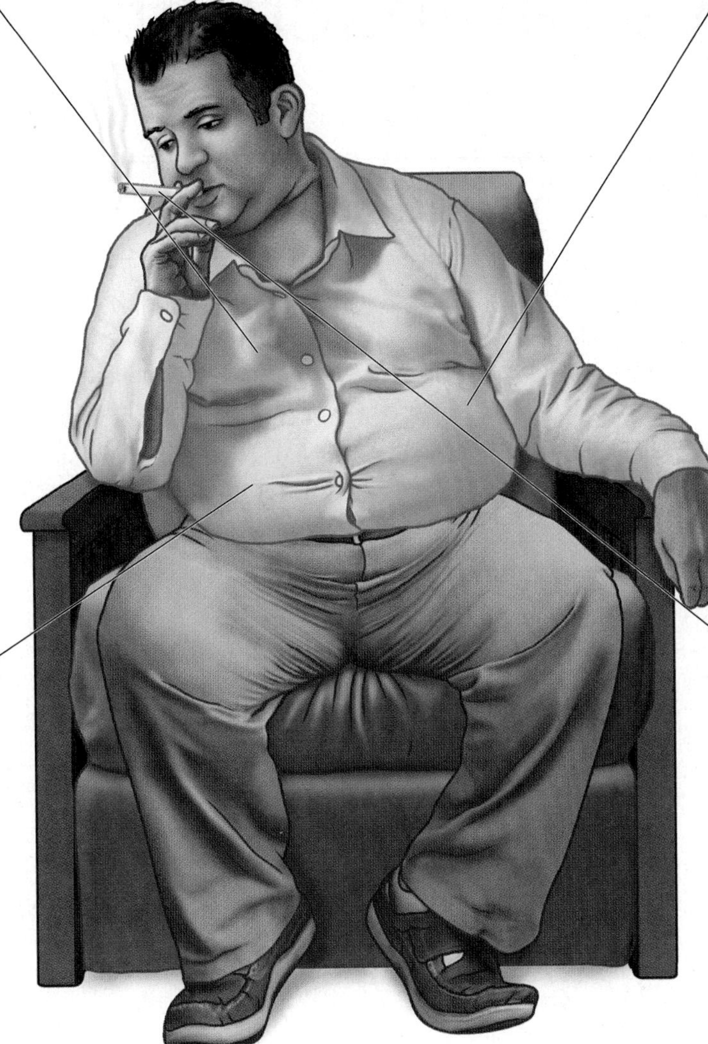
EFFECTS OF CHRONIC INFLAMMATION

SNS Responses
• Erectile dysfunction
• Increased blood pressure
• Increased heart rate
• Increased sweating
• Release of epinephrine and norepinephrine
• Release of glucose
• Respiratory distress

Chronic Inflammatory Responses
• Atherosclerosis
• Autoimmune disorders
• Endothelial dysfunction
• Hyperinsulinemia
• Hyperleptinemia
• Hypertension
• Impaired blood glucose regulation
• Insulin resistance
• Oxidative stress
• Systemic inflammatory response syndrome

RISK FACTORS

Obesity and Physical Inactivity
• Cancer
• Coronary disease
• Diabetes
• Metabolic disease
• Musculoskeletal stress
• Psychological stress
• Respiratory disease
• Stroke
• Premature death

Substance Abuse
• Cancer
• Cardiovascular disease
• Chronic obstructive pulmonary disease
• Cognitive dysfunction
• Dysrhythmia
• Gastrointestinal disorders
• Liver disease
• Mental illness
• Physical injury
• Respiratory disease
• Stroke
• Premature death

Sleep Dysfunction
• Attention deficit
• Cardiovascular disease
• Chronic pain
• Cognitive decline
• Emotional lability
• Falling/injury
• Hypertension
• Inflammation
• Insulin resistance
• Mental illness
• Respiratory disease
• Stroke
• Substance abuse
• Premature death

Chapter 5

Health Risks of Obesity and Physical Inactivity

Jean K. Berry

Chapter Outline and Learning Outcomes

5.1 Chapter Overview and Case Studies

Outline the global prevalence of, medical conditions associated with, and concepts related to obesity and physical inactivity.

5.2 Etiology and Pathophysiology of Obesity

Describe the etiology of obesity and outline the pathophysiologic consequences, including chronic diseases and metabolic syndrome.

5.3 Health Risks of Obesity

Outline the health risks and functional outcomes associated with obesity.

5.4 Health Risks of Physical Inactivity

Discuss the role of physical inactivity/activity in the development and progression of chronic diseases and recommendations for physical activity.

KEY TERMS

Adipocytes, 110
Anorexigenic, 103
Body mass index (BMI), 109
C-reactive protein, 108
Epigenetics, 106
Exercise, 114
Hepatomegaly, 111
Hyperinsulinemia, 106
Insulin resistance, 106
Metabolic equivalent of task (MET), 115
Metabolic syndrome, 108
Monogenic, 105
Nonalcoholic fatty liver disease (NAFLD), 111
Nonalcoholic steatohepatitis, 111
Obesity, 101
Orexigenic, 103
Physical fitness, 114
Polygenic, 105
Polymorphisms, 105
Reactive oxygen species (ROS), 106
Satiety, 104
Steatohepatitis, 111
Steatosis, 111
Visceral adiposity, 106

ABBREVIATIONS

α-MSH—α-melanocyte stimulating hormone
AGE—advanced glycosylation end product
AGRP—agouti-related peptide
ARC—arcuate nucleus
BMI—body mass index
CART—cocaine and amphetamine-regulated transcript peptide
CCK—cholecystokinin
GLP-1—glucagon-like peptide-1
HDL—high-density lipoprotein
IL-6—interleukin 6
LDL—low-density lipoprotein
MC4R—melanocortin 4 receptor
NAFLD—nonalcoholic fatty liver disease
NPY—neuropeptide Y
POMC—pro-opiomelanocortin
ROS—reactive oxygen species
PYY—peptide YY
T2D—type 2 diabetes mellitus
TNFα—tumor necrosis factor alpha

5.1 Chapter Overview and Case Studies

One of the major challenges of the 21st century is the prevention and treatment of obesity. The World Health Organization (WHO) defines **obesity** as abnormal or excessive fat accumulation that may impair health.[1,2] More than 33% of U.S. adults and 17% of U.S. children are obese.[3] Obesity is a factor in the development of a number of medical conditions, including diabetes, cardiovascular disease (coronary artery disease, myocardial infarction, angina pectoris, heart failure, stroke, hypertension, and atrial fibrillation), metabolic syndrome, cancer, arthritis and disability, gallbladder disease, acute pancreatitis, nonalcoholic fatty liver disease, pulmonary complications, and depression.[4] One of the goals of *Healthy People 2020* is to promote good health through nutrition and maintenance of a healthy body weight.

There has been a dramatic increase in the prevalence of obesity in the United States over the last two decades. Prevalence estimates of obesity in 2014 by state ranged from 20 to 35%[5] (**Figure 5.1** ■). The total excess cost related to the current prevalence of overweight and obesity among adolescents is estimated to be $254 billion.[6] This number includes $208 billion in lost productivity secondary to premature morbidity and mortality and $46 billion in direct medical costs.[6] If current trends in the development of overweight and obesity continue, the total healthcare costs related to obesity could reach $861–$957 billion by 2030; this would account for 16–18% of U.S. health expenditures.[6]

Healthy People 2020

Nutrition and Weight Status

The overall goal of the Nutrition and Weight Status objectives for *Healthy People 2020* is to promote health and reduce the risk of chronic disease through healthful diets and the achievement and maintenance of healthy body weights. In addition, these objectives emphasize that efforts to modify diet and weight should address individual behaviors along with the policies and environments that support these behaviors. Those objectives are broadly divided into the following categories: HealthCare and Worksite Settings, Weight Status, Food Insecurity, Food and Nutrient Consumption, and Iron Deficiency.[1] The primary objectives are as follows:

- Increase the number of states with nutrition standards for foods and beverages provided to preschool-aged children in child care.
- Increase the proportion of schools that offer nutritious foods and beverages outside of school meals.
- Increase the number of states that have state-level policies that incentivize food retail outlets to provide foods that are encouraged by the Dietary Guidelines for Americans.
- Increase the proportion of Americans who have access to a food retail outlet that sells a variety of foods that are encouraged by the Dietary Guidelines for Americans.

Healthcare and Worksite Settings

- Increase the proportion of primary care physicians who regularly measure the body mass index of their patients.
- Increase the proportion of physician office visits that include counseling or education related to nutrition or weight.
- Increase the proportion of worksites that offer nutrition or weight management classes or counseling.

Weight Status

- Increase the proportion of adults who are at a healthy weight.
- Reduce the proportion of adults who are obese.
- Reduce the proportion of children and adolescents who are considered obese.
- Prevent inappropriate weight gain in youth and adults.

Food Insecurity

Food insecurity is the inability to access sufficient safe, nutritious food that is needed to maintain a healthy and active life.[2]

- Eliminate very low food security among children.
- Reduce household food insecurity and in doing so reduce hunger.

Food and Nutrient Consumption

- Increase the contribution of fruits to the diets of the population aged 2 years and older.
- Increase the variety and contribution of vegetables to the diets of the population aged 2 years and older.
- Increase the contribution of whole grains to the diets of the population aged 2 years and older.
- Reduce consumption of calories from solid fats and added sugars in the population aged 2 years and older.
- Reduce consumption of saturated fat in the population aged 2 years and older.
- Reduce consumption of sodium in the population aged 2 years and older.
- Increase consumption of calcium in the population aged 2 years and older.

Iron Deficiency

- Reduce iron deficiency among young children and females of childbearing age.
- Reduce iron deficiency among pregnant females.

References

1. U.S. Department of Health and Human Services. (2017). *Nutrition and weight status*. Available at http://www.healthypeople.gov/2020/topics-objectives/topic/nutrition-and-weight-status
2. World Health Organization. (2014). *Trade, foreign policy, diplomacy and health*. Available at http://www.who.int/trade/glossary/story028/en

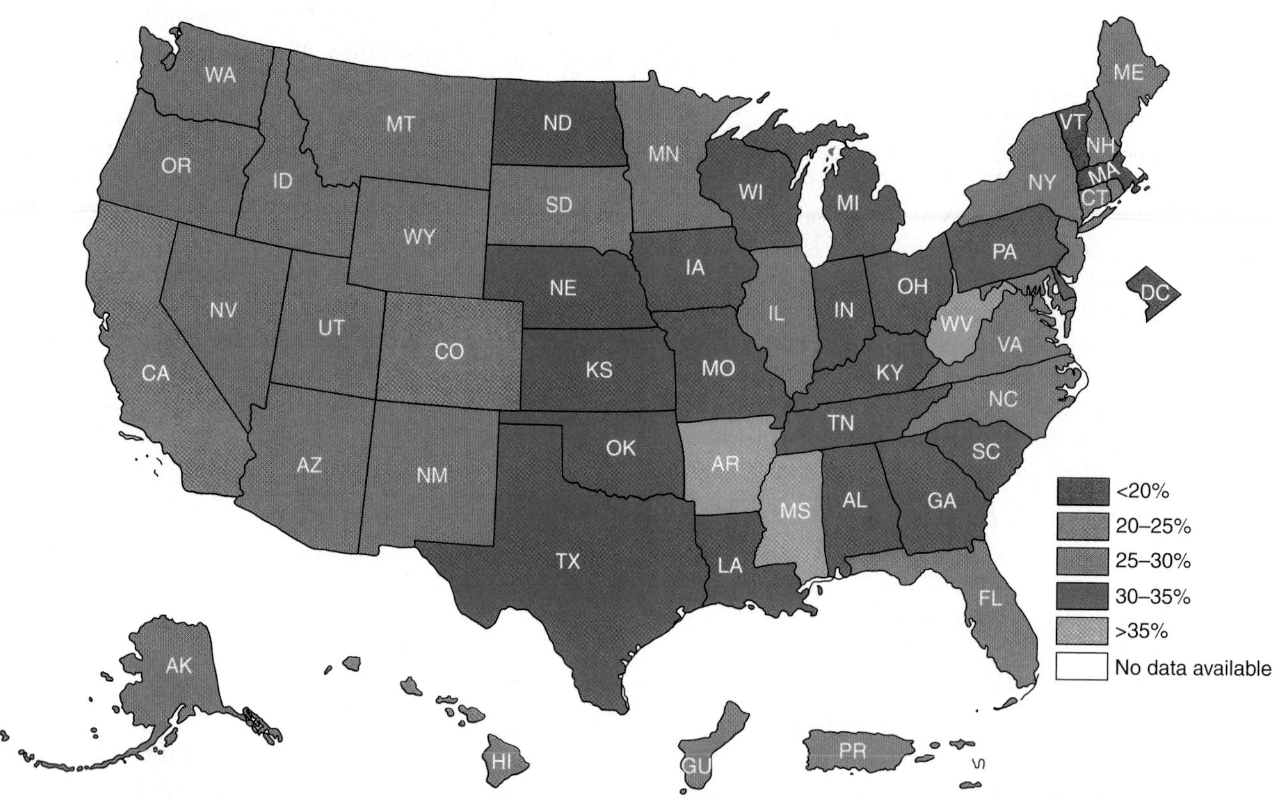

Figure 5.1 ■ Prevalence rates of obesity in the United States, 2014.

SOURCE: CDC: Obesity prevalence maps. Retrieved from http://www.cdc.gov/obesity/data/prevalence-maps.html.

Obesity arises from multiple genetic, behavioral, metabolic, environmental, and socioeconomic factors. These factors are also associated with the development of a physically inactive and sedentary lifestyle. Physical inactivity contributes to the development of chronic disorders both independently and through its association with obesity. Only 48% of all adults in the United States meet the recommended minimum of 150 minutes of moderate-intensity exercise or 75 minutes of vigorous-intensity exercise per week.[7,8] Fewer than 3 in 10 high school students get the recommended 60 minutes of physical activity every day.[7,8] This chapter explores the risks related to obesity and physical inactivity.

Concepts Related to Obesity and Physical Inactivity

The major concept governing this chapter is energy balance (**Figure 5.2** ■). The process of energy balance is regulated by food intake, energy expenditure, and energy storage. Decreased physical activity, metabolic rate, and thermogenesis (heat production) reduce energy expenditure and increase energy storage in the form of adipose tissue.[9] Additionally, the amount of adipose tissue is regulated by neural and hormonal signals to the brain.[9] Adipose tissue hormones, gastrointestinal hormones, and classical endocrine hormones sense this information and signal the hypothalamus, which integrates the information, subsequently influencing food intake and energy expenditure. Dysregulation of these signals results in increased adiposity and obesity, which, in turn, affect concepts such as cellular regulation, inflammation, mood and affect, oxygenation, perfusion, sleep, and tissue integrity.

Case Studies

The following cases will be addressed throughout the chapter to assist in application of chapter content to clinical situations that involve individuals with obesity.

Thomas Johnson: Introduction

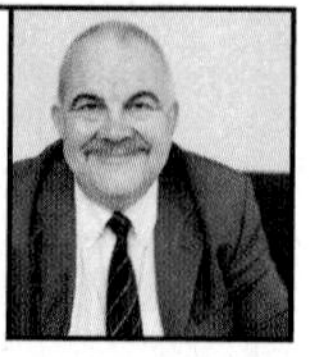

Thomas Johnson is a 45-year-old male who states that he has always been in "good health." He has just started a new job as a salesperson for a large computer company after having been unemployed for several months. The nurse practitioner in his new company's employee health office referred Thomas to his primary healthcare provider for a workup of hypertension, obesity, and possible diabetes, noting that he had not seen a healthcare provider in approximately 5 years.

1. According to the Healthcare and Worksite settings objectives, what is a key factor for the nurse practitioner to observe in looking at Mr. Johnson's height and weight?
2. What effect could further disease processes have on Mr. Johnson's life?

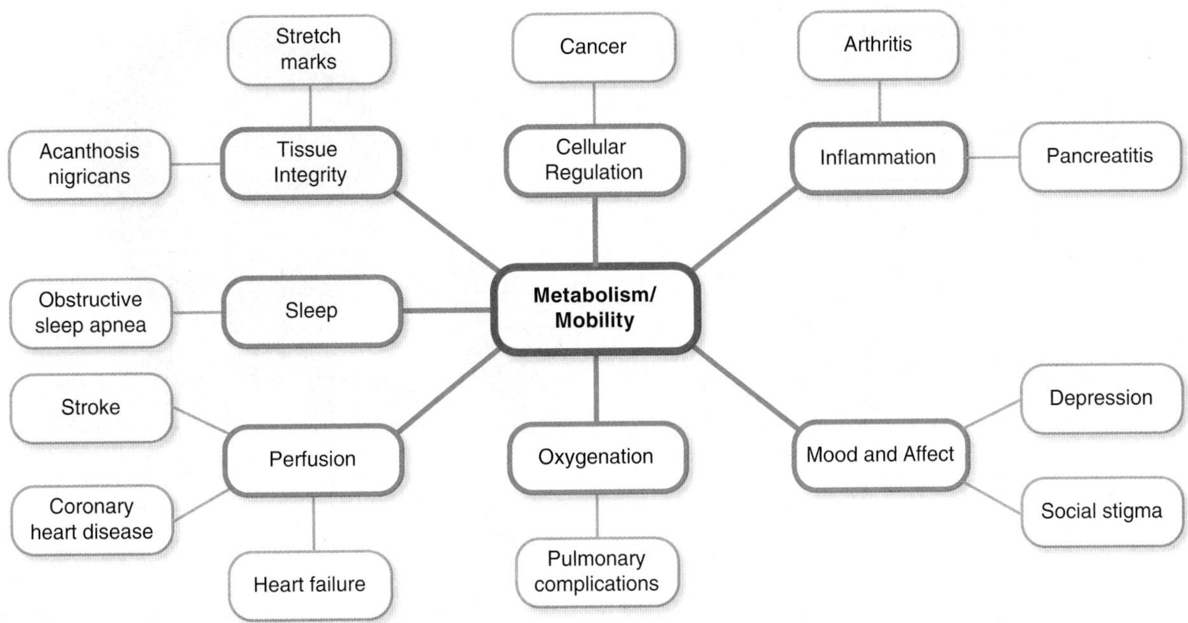

Figure 5.2 ■ Concepts related to obesity and physical inactivity.

Yashika Devon: Introduction

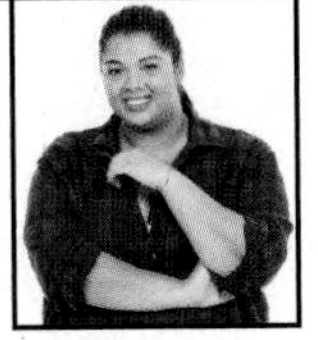

Yashika Devon is a 16-year-old female who has gained approximately 40 pounds over the previous year. There is no apparent medical reason for her weight gain (e.g., hypothyroidism); her vital signs and all diagnostic and laboratory tests are normal. She avoids participating in physical activity and sports programs at her high school for a variety of reasons, including self-consciousness about her physical appearance. Her diet consists largely of high-fat foods, and she routinely snacks all evening on cookies, pretzels, and chips.

1. Yashika has already been deemed obese. What would be the first objective assessments necessary to create a baseline plan of care for her?
2. Yashika is known to consume high-fat and high-calorie foods. What is the recommended caloric intake for her age and lifestyle (sedentary)?

Check Your Progress: Section 5.1

1. How does the World Health Organization define the term *obesity*?
2. What are some of the major health problems associated with obesity?
3. What are the current trends in physical activity among U.S. adults and adolescents?

5.2 Etiology and Pathophysiology of Obesity

Energy homeostasis is regulated primarily by the brain, gastrointestinal tract, other organ systems, and adipose tissue with the purpose of controlling food intake, satiety, and energy expenditure. These processes involve a variety of chemical mediators in both central and peripheral neurochemical pathways (**Figure 5.3** ■).

Regulation of Food Uptake

The hypothalamus is the regulating center of appetite and energy homeostasis. It receives input from all peripheral organs along with neural pathways from the brainstem. Appetite is stimulated and depressed within the arcuate nucleus (ARC) of the hypothalamus. Appetite is stimulated by the activation of **orexigenic** (appetite stimulating) neurons expressing neuropeptide Y (NPY) and agouti-related protein (AGRP). And it is depressed by **anorexigenic** (appetite depressing) neurons, which express α-melanocyte stimulating hormone (α-MSH) derived from pro-opiomelanocortin (POMC), and cocaine and amphetamine-regulated transcript peptide (CART). Neural afferents and hormonal signals from the periphery signal to higher brain center signals (e.g., those relaying reward) to regulate the hedonic or pleasurable aspects of food ingestion. Signals regarding smell, sight, memory of food, and the social context under which it was eaten are also integrated. Additionally, hormones can modulate hypothalamic gene expression and modulate energy intake. These hormones and their roles in energy intake are described in **Figure 5.4** ■ and in the following sections.

Selected Adipose Tissue Hormones Involved with Food Intake and Obesity

Leptin is an adipocyte-derived secretory product that provides signals to the brain about the amount of adipose tissue energy reserves. Leptin is synthesized in white adipocytes and released into the systemic circulation; it is then transported across the blood–brain barrier and binds to specific

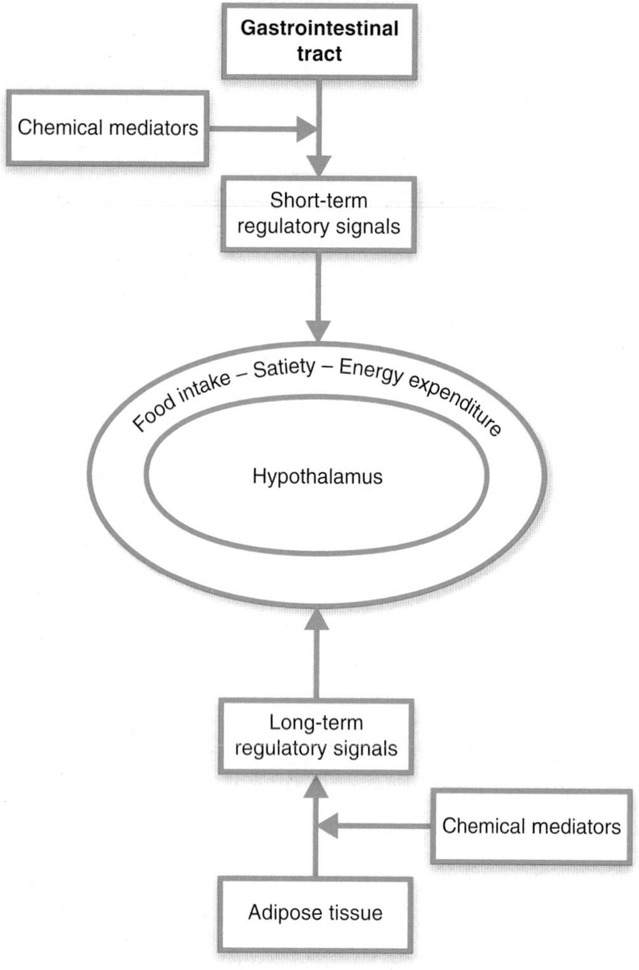

Figure 5.3 ■ Energy homeostasis is regulated primarily by the brain, gastrointestinal tract, other organ systems, and adipose tissue with the purpose of controlling food intake, satiety, and energy expenditure. These processes involve a variety of chemical mediators in both central and peripheral and central neurochemical pathways.

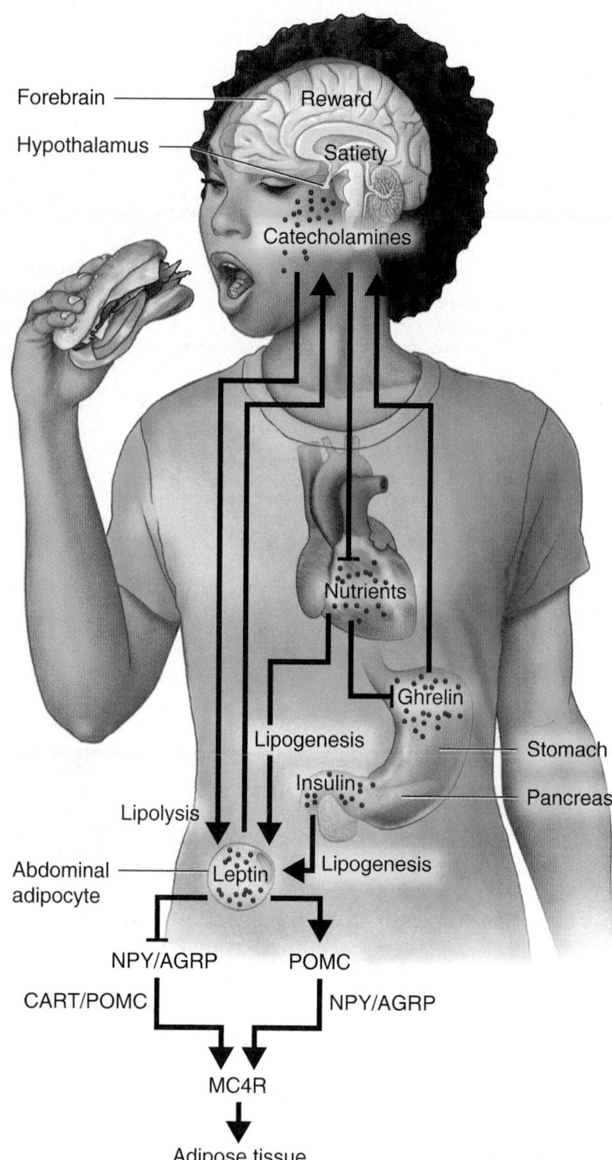

Figure 5.4 ■ Selected hormones and their role in energy intake.

leptin receptors on the hypothalamus, inhibiting appetite.[10–12] More specifically, leptin acts on leptin receptors in the ARC of the hypothalamus to regulate the production and release of peptides involved in food intake.[11,12] Outside of the hypothalamus, leptin interacts with the mesolimbic dopamine system, which is involved in motivation and reward of feeding.

The binding of leptin to its receptors activates gene transcription resulting in *reduced* expression of NPY and AGRP, peptides that increase food intake. Leptin also *enhances* the expression of POMC, the source of α-MSH, and CART, peptides that decrease food intake.[10] The two groups of neurons (NPY/AGRP and POMC/CART) have projections that extend to the paraventricular nucleus of the hypothalamus that contains a dense neuronal population expressing the melanocortin 4 receptor (MC4R). The binding of leptin to its receptors on POMC neurons results the release of α-MSH, a cleavage product from the larger POMC peptide. The binding of MC4R in the paraventricular nucleus by α-MSH results in reduced food intake. Additionally, AGRP competes α-MSH for binding to MC4R. When AGRP binds to MC4R, food intake increases. Since leptin activates POMC neurons and inhibits AGRP neurons, it acts in an integrated manner to increase activation of MCR4 by α-MSH and decrease activation of MCR4 by AGRP. The result is an overall decrease in food intake.[13] This process is termed the leptin–melanocortin pathway of energy balance (**Figure 5.5** ■).

Selected Gastrointestinal Hormones Involved with Food Intake and Obesity

A number of gastrointestinal hormones are involved in normal food intake. These hormones exert their effects on a variety of systems, especially those related to hunger, **satiety** (the feeling of being full after eating), and energy balance. The gastrointestinal hormones that exert the most significant effects on obesity include the following.

- *Cholecystokinin (CCK)* is a peptide produced by I-type cells in the duodenum and small intestine in response

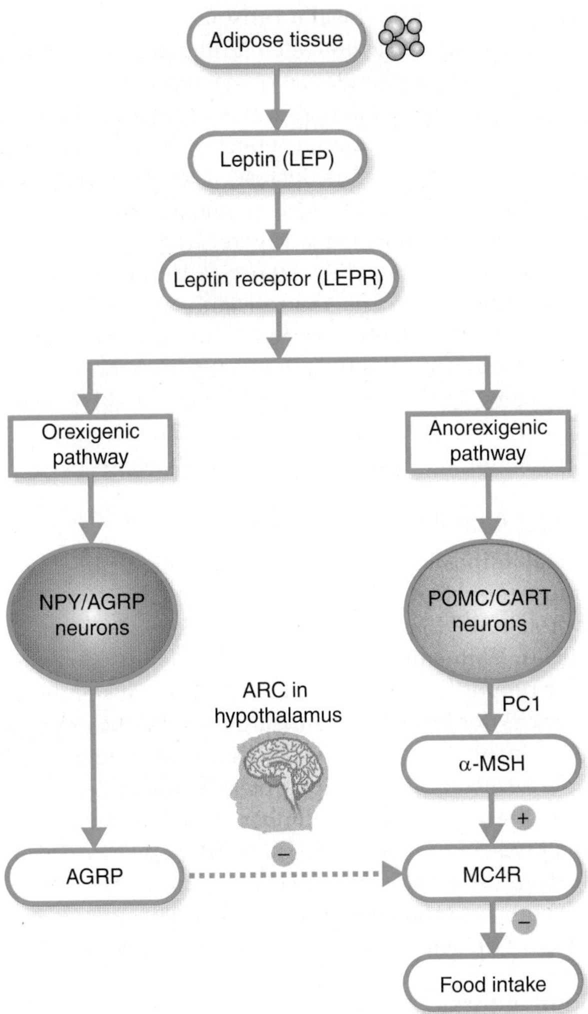

Figure 5.5 ■ The leptin–melanocortin pathway of energy balance.

to fat and protein, stimulating gut motility, contraction of the gallbladder, pancreatic enzyme secretion, gastric emptying, and acid secretion. Additionally, CCK binds to CCK receptors located on the vagus nerve, transferring satiety signals to the hypothalamus.[10,12]

- ***Glucagon-like peptide-1 (GLP-1)*** is a peptide produced in the L-cells of the ileum and colon, exerting anorexigenic effects through the GLP-1 receptors, which are distributed in the brain, gastrointestinal tract, and pancreas. Additionally, GLP-1 amplifies glucose-dependent insulin secretion from the pancreatic β-cells.
- ***Peptide YY (PYY)*** is a peptide secreted by the L cells of the distal small bowel and colon in response to food ingestion and the presence of fat in the intestinal lumen, reducing appetite and food intake. The major form of circulating PYY (PYY3-36) binds to hypothalamic receptors and reduces food intake.
- ***Ghrelin*** is a peptide produced in the stomach that stimulates appetite. Ghrelin levels increase before meals and decrease after a meal. Ghrelin production is stimulated by fasting and suppressed by intake of food, acting in part by modulating the orexigenic hypothalamic neurons PPY and AGRP neurons in the hypothalamus.
- ***Adiponectin*** has several effects, including decreased fatty acids and muscle triglycerides, decreased hepatic triglycerides, increased hepatic insulin action, increased glucose stimulated insulin secretion, decreased visceral adipose tissue, and decreased inflammation.[14]

CLINICAL POINT: For many years, it was noted that plasma insulin levels following oral ingestion of glucose were higher than after receiving an intravenous injection of glucose. This was termed the *incretin effect*. This effect was attributed to the release of gastrointestinal hormones, including GLP-1. A compound found in the saliva of the Gila monster, a large lizard native to the southwestern United States, was used to develop the first GLP-1 agonist. This pharmaceutical preparation, exenatide (Byetta®), was the first in a class of medications called *incretins* and was approved by the U.S. Food and Drug Administration in 2005. This is an injectable medication available by prescription for people with type 2 diabetes mellitus (T2D). When food is eaten, GLP-1 is released into the blood by the intestine in response to food intake. GLP-1 slows food absorption, increases satiety, and improves insulin responsiveness.[15] ■

Factors in the Etiology and Pathophysiology of Obesity

The current epidemic of obesity has spurred intense research into unraveling the factors underlying the complex etiology and pathophysiology of obesity.

Genetics

The genetic contribution to obesity has been explored extensively over the past few decades. Research has helped to elucidate genes associated with **monogenic** (single-gene) or the more common **polygenic** (multiple-genes) causes of obesity. Single gene mutations are often associated with severe obesity syndromes resulting from alterations in central or peripheral appetite control mechanisms. The interaction of several **polymorphisms** (the presence of two or more alternative forms of genes)[1] and epigenetic modifications are associated with the more common form of obesity.[16]

The discovery of leptin in 1994[17] and the identification of the leptin–melanocortin pathway initiated extensive research into the genetics of obesity. Genetic disorders associated with disruption of the leptin–melanocortin pathway are rare, affecting only 1–5% of obese people[18]; however, they have provided valuable information on body weight regulation. The first genetic defect that was identified was congenital leptin deficiency.[19] People with this defect can be successfully treated with subcutaneous injections of recombinant leptin. Homozygous mutations in the gene encoding for leptin are associated with severe obesity, hyperphagia (an abnormal increase in appetite), and impaired satiety.[18] Mutations in the leptin receptor are also associated with severe obesity and hyperphagia,[20] and mutations in leptin and the leptin receptor are associated with delayed puberty and hypogonadic hypogonadism.[18] In addition, a number of rare genetic syndromes include severe obesity as a prominent characteristic. For example, Prader-Willi syndrome, which is associated with a genetic alteration in chromosome 15, is characterized by diminished fetal activity, obesity, muscular hypotonia, mental retardation, short stature, hypogonadic hypogonadism, and small hands and feet.[13]

There is a significant proportion of genetic heritability in common obesity (40–70%).[13] Classic twin and adoptee studies have provided evidence of the role of genetics in the heritability of obesity. When the contributions of genetic factors and family environment to obesity were explored in a sample of adult Danish adoptees divided into four weight classes (thin, median weight, overweight, and obese), a strong relationship was found between the weight class of the adoptees and the body mass index (BMI) of their biologic parents but not their adoptive parents.[21] A study of identical and fraternal twins who were either reared apart or reared together concluded that genetic influences on BMI have substantial influence, whereas the childhood environment has little or no influence.[22]

A number of genes have been linked to obesity through genome-wide association scans, and the possible roles of such genes are an area of investigation. There is intense interest in the role of epigenetics in obesity. **Epigenetics** is the study of the molecular control of gene expression that is not caused by changes in DNA sequence. Epigenetic factors can be can be passed on through mitosis and meiosis. Environmental exposures in critical developmental periods of intrauterine and extrauterine life can affect the epigenetic effects and produce obesity.[23]

Inflammation

Obesity is known to be associated with chronic inflammation.[24] The relationship between obesity and inflammation has been widely researched; however, the exact mechanisms mediating the link between inflammation and obesity have not been delineated. The initial step in the development of adiposity-related obesity likely begins with increased nutrient intake and decreased physical activity. The adipocyte becomes lipid-laden and hypertrophied in response to increased caloric load and decreased energy expenditure. The resulting cellular stress causes adipocytes, endothelial cells, and immune cells in adipose tissue to produce proinflammatory cytokines, endothelial adhesion molecules, pro-atherogenic mediators, and chemotactic mediators (e.g., interleukin 6 [IL-6], tumor necrosis factor alpha [TNFα], IL-1β, monocyte chemoattractant protein-1, and plasminogen activator inhibitor-1).[25] Chemoattractant and endothelial adhesion molecules bind chemokine and integrin receptors on monocytes and recruit them into adipose tissue.[25] Monocytes differentiate into macrophages within the adipose tissue, where they secrete and produce proinflammatory mediators and contribute to systemic and local inflammation.[25]

Insulin Resistance

Insulin resistance is defined as the inability of insulin to achieve its expected biological response. Obesity causes insulin resistance in cells such as those found in adipose tissue, liver, and muscle and is a strong risk factor for the development of T2D. Insulin resistance in the obese individual is a result of several altered functions of insulin target cells and the accumulation of macrophages that secrete proinflammatory mediators. In this cellular environment, there is a less-than-expected effect of insulin on insulin receptors in tissues. Thus, increased levels of insulin are required to keep glucose levels within a normal range. As this process becomes more severe, hyperglycemia may develop, with ensuing T2D. **Hyperinsulinemia** (increased insulin secretion) and insulin resistance are related to obesity and are also classic characteristics of impairments in glucose tolerance. Weight gain increases insulin resistance and impairs glucose transport into insulin-sensitive cells. As BMI increases, so does the secretion of endogenous insulin in an attempt to maintain normal blood glucose levels.

Visceral Adiposity

Visceral adiposity, or central fat distribution, also contributes to the development of higher levels of small, low-density lipoprotein (LDL) particles rather than large, buoyant LDL particles. With equal cholesterol values, individuals with higher proportions of small, dense LDL are at significantly higher risk for heart disease than those with lower proportions of small LDL. Each LDL particle of either type contains one single molecule of apolipoprotein B protein. This protein is used for estimating the number of LDL particles and is also a predictor of risk for coronary artery disease. In addition, increased body weight increases cardiac work and may contribute to cardiomyopathy and heart failure even in the absence of diabetes, hypertension, or atherosclerosis.

Oxidative Stress

Reactive oxygen species (ROS) are highly reactive, unstable molecules that interact with and damage other molecules (including proteins, lipid, carbohydrates, and DNA). They also impair receptors on cell membranes and alter intracellular signaling pathways. The body's antioxidant defenses include vitamins, such as vitamins E and C, and plant flavonoids present in bright-colored fruits and vegetables, such as strawberries, blueberries, tomatoes, and broccoli. Also part of the antioxidant defense system are enzymes, such as superoxide dismutase and glutathione peroxidase, that inactivate ROS, convert very toxic to less toxic reactive oxygen molecules, or repair the damage done by the ROS. Oxidative stress is present when there is an increased production of ROS relative to the body's antioxidant defenses. Refer to the section on oxidative stress in Chapter 10 for additional information on the production and types of ROS and antioxidant defenses. The causes of oxidative stress associated with overweight and obesity include hyperglycemia, increased production of ROS, decreased levels of antioxidant defenses, chronic inflammation, increased lipid levels, and hyperleptinemia

Hyperglycemia, caused by insulin resistance associated with obesity, activates several pathways that produce ROS. Advanced glycosylation end products (AGEs) are formed from proteins, lipids, and nucleic acid in the presence of hyperglycemia.[26] These AGEs activate receptors and intracellular signal pathways, including those in adipose cells, which produce ROS. There is also increased production of ROS by skeletal muscle of obese individuals. Increased oxygen consumption results from the mechanical load of bearing excessive weight during exercise. The increased oxygen consumption and electron transport activity in mitochondria results in some of the additional oxygen being converted to ROS.

Leptin levels increase with increasing adiposity, and leptin can stimulate the production of ROS, including hydrogen peroxide and the hydroxyl radical, by vascular endothelial cells. Decreased levels of antioxidants in obesity add to the oxidative stress. Antioxidant levels are decreased as a result of poor nutritional habits consisting of a decreased intake of foods rich in antioxidants plus the depletion of antioxidants as they are consumed in the body's attempt to inactivate the increased amount of ROS present.

Obesity is associated with increased plasma and tissue levels of triglycerides and free fatty acids due to increased dietary fat intake. The excessive lipid levels increase mitochondrial electron transport, resulting in increased production of ROS, and stimulate white blood cells to increase their production of ROS. Lipids are targets of ROS; the more lipids are present, the more substrate is available for lipid peroxidation, which involves a chain reaction of increasingly more lipid free-radical formation. As explained previously, obesity (especially visceral obesity) is a pro-inflammatory state with increased production of adipocytokines. There is a link between inflammation and oxidative stress. Pro-inflammatory cytokines, such as TNFα and IL-6 produced in fat-laden adipose tissue, stimulate inflammatory cells (macrophages and neutrophils) to produce ROS, including hydrogen peroxide, hydroxyl radical, and hypochlorous acid. An example of how oxidative stress can begin in childhood and lead to progressive damage throughout life is shown in (**Figure 5.6** ■).

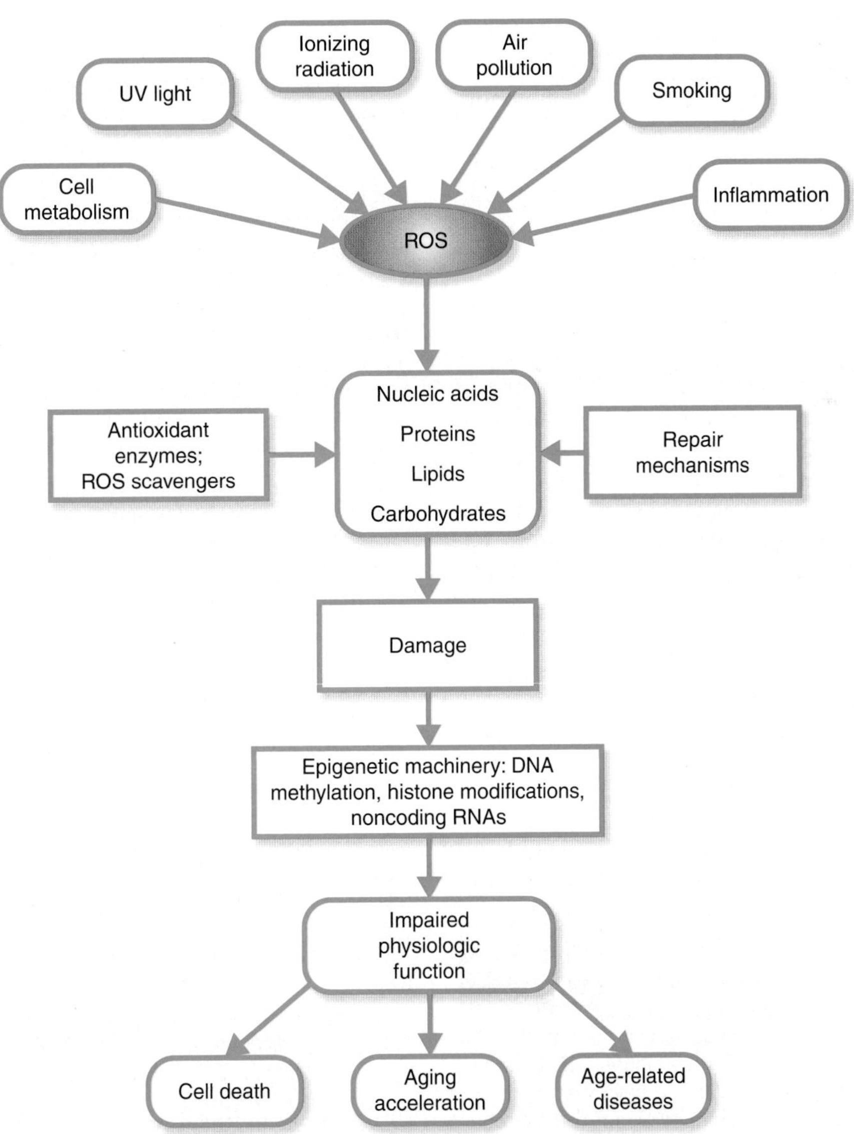

Figure 5.6 ■ Oxidative stress can begin in childhood and lead to progressive damage throughout life. ROS = reactive oxygen species; UV = ultraviolet.

Metabolic Syndrome

Metabolic syndrome is a condition characterized by insulin resistance, increased visceral fat, increased release of free fatty acids (which impair insulin clearance by the liver), and alterations in peripheral metabolism.[27] The National Cholesterol Education Program Adult Treatment Panel III has provided five criteria defining metabolic syndrome.[28] An individual who has three of the five criteria has metabolic syndrome.

1. Increased waist circumference: men > 40 inches; women > 35 inches
2. Elevated triglyceride levels: ≥ 150 mg per dL
3. Elevated blood pressure: ≥ 130/85 mmHg
4. Elevated fasting glucose level: ≥ 100 mg per dL
5. Reduced high-density lipoprotein (HDL) cholesterol levels: men < 40 mg/dL; women < 50 mg/dL

The increased visceral adiposity results in increased levels of IL-6, TNFα, and **C-reactive protein** (a serum marker of systemic inflammation) and reduced levels of adiponectin and interleukin 10, setting up a milieu that leads to insulin resistance and endothelial dysfunction, which lead to metabolic syndrome, diabetes, and atherosclerosis. The constellation of abnormalities in metabolic syndrome includes central adiposity, hypertension, insulin resistance, hyperinsulinemia, glucose intolerance, dyslipidemias (hypertriglyceridemia, decreased HDL cholesterol and small LDL diameter), and increased plasminogen activator inhibitor-1.[27]

What do obesity, metabolic syndrome, insulin resistance, T2D, and cardiovascular disease have in common that can explain why several of these conditions frequently develop in the same individuals? The answer is that the pathophysiologic mechanisms of inflammation and oxidative stress are involved in all those conditions. Adipose tissue is no longer viewed as just a storage depot for fat. Adipose tissue has endocrine functions, and excess fat has a role in these interrelated disease states. With this background information about the pathophysiology of obesity, the next two sections discuss the adverse health consequences of obesity: problems related to metabolic changes due to excess fat cells and problems related to increased fat mass.

Thomas Johnson: Application

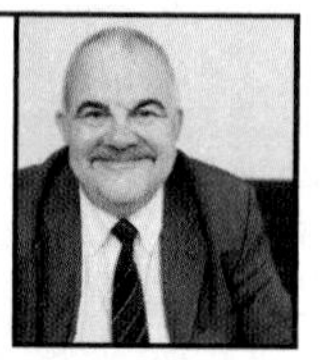

Thomas Johnson reports no significant health problems to his healthcare provider, but on further questioning, he notes that he had a severe episode of gout in his left foot approximately 3 years ago. He also reports that he has gained 55 pounds over the previous 3 years. His current weight is his highest adult weight. He eats a high-fat, high-cholesterol diet and says that he drinks two to three beers per day. He has smoked a pack of cigarettes per day for 20 years. He describes his work as very stressful. He travels frequently and has limited physical activity. He reports that his mother died at 56 years of age from diabetes. His father is 75 years old and has a history of a stroke and chronic heart failure. Mr. Johnson has four sisters (ages 33, 48, 52, and 56) who have diabetes. One sister is on dialysis. One sister is morbidly obese and has had gastric bypass surgery.

On physical examination, Mr. Johnson's vital signs are as follows: pulse 99, respirations 24, temperature 98.6°F, blood pressure 150/92 (right arm, sitting), 160/96 (left arm, sitting).

His weight and height are as follows: weight 237 pounds, height 68 inches, BMI 36 kg/m^2, waist circumference 45 inches.

His laboratory values are as follows:

Test	Result	Normal Range
C-reactive protein	3.5 mg/L	< 0.8 mg/L
Fasting blood glucose	105 mg/dL	< 100 mg/dL
Total cholesterol	275 mg/dL	100–199 mg/dL
Fasting triglycerides	180 mg/dL	< 150 mg/dL
High-density lipoprotein	35 mg/dL	40–50 mg/dL (men)
		50–59 mg/dL (women)
Low-density lipoprotein	210 mg/dL	< 100 mg/dL

Mr. Johnson is at high risk for diabetes and cardiovascular disease. He has an elevated blood glucose consistent with prediabetes, an elevated blood pressure consistent with hypertension, dyslipidemia (elevated total cholesterol, elevated LDL cholesterol, elevated fasting triglycerides, and low HDL), evidence of systemic inflammation (elevated C-reactive protein); is obese; has an increased waist circumference; and meets the criteria for metabolic syndrome. He has a family history of diabetes. His diet is poor. He smokes and has a stressful lifestyle with little physical activity.

Mr. Johnson meets with the healthcare team, which develops a plan of care that is directed toward weight loss, increasing physical activity, nutrition modification, and dealing with stress. He is taught how to take his blood pressure and begins an antihypertensive medication. He has a schedule of follow-up appointments with his physician, his nurse practitioner, and a nutritionist.

3. Mr. Johnson's BMI is 36. This places him in the obese category. What will the nurse practitioner first talk about with Mr. Johnson concerning his weight?
4. Mr. Johnson verbalizes that he does not have a daily routine, since he was unemployed for several months. What recommendation would the nurse practitioner give him?

Yashika Devon: Application

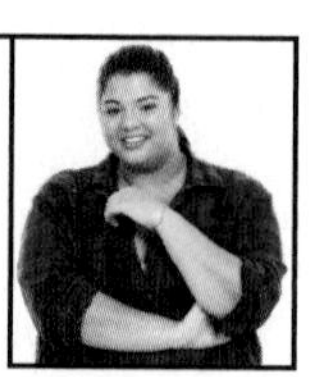

Yashika Devon's mother is concerned about Yashika's health and schedules an appointment with the pediatrician. As was noted previously, Yashika has had a recent 40-pound weight gain, has poor nutritional habits, and does little exercise. She reports that she is self-conscious about her weight and about exercising. Additionally, her mother and 25-year-old sister are both obese and have T2D.

On physical examination, Yashika's vital signs are as follows: pulse 76, respirations 20, temperature 98.6°F, blood pressure 110/70 (right arm, sitting), 110/72 (left arm, sitting).

Her height and weight are as follows: weight 200 pounds, height 64 inches, BMI 34.3 (98th percentile for girls age 16 years 0 months.) The healthcare provider notes a velvety pigmented rash at the nape of Yashika's neck.

Her laboratory results are as follows:

Test	Result	Normal Range
Fasting blood glucose	90 mg/dL	< 100 mg/dL
Total cholesterol	180 mg/dL	100–199 mg/dL
Fasting triglycerides	125 mg/dL	< 150 mg/dL
High-density lipoprotein	55 mg/dL	40–50 mg/dL (men)
		50–59 mg/dL (women)
Low-density lipoprotein	90 mg/dL	< 100 mg/dL

At this time, Yashika's biochemical laboratory values are within the normal range. The presence of the velvety hyperpigmented rash (acanthosis nigricans) is consistent with hyperinsulinemia and insulin resistance. Yashika is at risk for diabetes and cardiovascular disease.

Yashika meets with her family nurse practitioner, and together they structure a plan to work on increasing physical activity. They set realistic goals for increasing physical activity through increased participation in school and community physical activity programs. Additionally, Yashika is referred to the nutritionist for dietary education.

3. Yashika avoids participation in activities at school. What would you counsel her about this aspect of her health?
4. What kind of statement from Yashika indicates understanding of the education and counseling that was given to her?

Check Your Progress: Section 5.2

1. What adipose tissue hormones and gastrointestinal hormones are involved in the regulation of food uptake?
2. What are some of the genetic components of obesity?
3. What foods contain high levels of the antioxidants vitamin E and vitamin C?

5.3 Health Risks of Obesity

Obesity is known to increase the risk for many diseases, reduce quality of life and functional capacity, and shorten the lifespan. Health risks of obesity include not only the pathologic risks for morbidity and mortality that are increased with obesity, but also the functional and psychosocial risks that occur with increasing body weight. In 2008, the Obesity Society defined obesity as a disease.[29] Obesity is associated with the development of a range of disorders, especially T2D, but also many other systemic and orthopedic disorders, which are covered more thoroughly in other chapters. This descriptive terminology has widespread ramifications for the public's understanding of obesity and social stigma as well as treatment, reimbursement, education, and consumer protection programs. This designation as a disease is based on the recognition that obesity is a complex condition with multiple causes, many of which are beyond the individual's control. In addition, obesity causes suffering, ill health, societal stigma, discrimination, and early mortality.

Obesity is conceptually defined as an excess of body fat and is clinically defined by the **body mass index (BMI).** BMI (calculated as the weight in kilograms divided by the square of height in meters) is classified as follows[30]:

Normal: 18.5–24.9
Overweight: 25.0–29.9
Obese: ≥ 30.0

A BMI above 40 kg/m^2 is considered extreme or morbid obesity. Patients who have greater than 30.0 BMI are further subdivided into three obesity classes:[30]

Obese class I: 30–34.99 kg/m^2
Obese class II: 35–39.9 kg/m^2
Obese class III: ≥ 40 kg/m^2

CLINICAL POINT: For children and adolescents (aged 2–19 years), the BMI value is plotted on the CDC growth charts to determine the BMI-for-age percentile. In this classification, overweight is defined as a BMI at or above the 85th percentile and lower than the 95th percentile. Obesity is defined as a BMI at or above the 95th percentile for children of the same age and sex.[31] A child's weight status is determined on an age- and sex-specific percentile for BMI rather than by the BMI categories used for adults. Classifications of overweight and obesity for children and adolescents are determined in this way because children's body composition varies by age and gender. A calculator for determining BMI status for children and adolescents can be found at https://www.cdc.gov/obesity/childhood/defining.html ■

Obesity in childhood and adolescence is a major public health problem associated with short- and long-term complications. Obese youths are more likely to have risk factors for cardiovascular disease and diabetes, such as hypertension, dyslipidemia, and insulin resistance. Additionally, obese children and adolescents are at risk for musculoskeletal problems, sleep apnea, and social and psychologic problems. The approach to the prevention, treatment, and management of obesity is multifactorial. Children and adolescents' physical activity and dietary behaviors are influenced by many factors; these include (but are not limited to) families, communities, schools, healthcare providers, faith-based institutions, government agencies, and the media.[32] As for adults, lifestyle interventions including dietary and physical activity modifications and behavioral strategies make up the framework for effective prevention and treatment of obesity. Of greatest importance, however, is parental and familial involvement with family behavioral therapy; this has been cited as the most widely supported treatment for children.[33] ■

Obesity during pregnancy is associated with increased maternal and fetal risks. Maternal complications include pregnancy-induced hypertension, gestational diabetes, respiratory complications, venous thromboembolism, preterm delivery, cesarean deliveries, and surgical and anesthetic complications.[34] Examples of risks to the fetus and neonate include congenital abnormalities, neonatal hypoglycemia, premature delivery, miscarriage, and stillbirth.[34] Obesity-associated maternal hyperglycemia due to diabetes can cause increased fetal insulin secretion, resulting in increased nutrient storage and macrosomia (large body size). Large fetal size can necessitate a cesarean delivery or trigger premature labor. Other complications are associated with inflammation and oxidative stress induced by obesity and diabetes.[35] Oxidative stress can cause vascular endothelial injury, placental inflammation, and altered gene expression. Furthermore, the effects of maternal obesity extend beyond the perinatal period. Children of obese women have an increased rate of hospitalization during the first 5 years of life, particularly for infections and nervous system, metabolic, and respiratory conditions.[36] Because of the risks to both mother and fetus associated with obesity during pregnancy, it is important for overweight and obese women to have weight counseling before conception so that they can achieve weight loss before becoming pregnant. ■

In older adults, overweight and obesity are associated with higher levels of functional limitations when compared with normal-weight adults.[37] Although obesity in older adults is associated with the adverse outcomes described in this chapter, there is some evidence that the risk of adverse outcomes lessens with age and mild obesity.[38] In fact, increases in adiposity appear to have a protective effect on frail older adults and those with chronic diseases.[38] ■

Health Risks Due to Excess Fat

Conceptually, the general definition of obesity utilizing BMI cut points does not specify where the excess fat is stored, as it can be either excess total body fat or a specific area of excess fat deposition, such as the abdomen. In addition, the **adipocytes** may be enlarged in morphology to produce this excess fat. Regardless, the clinical system of classification by BMI is useful for describing and identifying people at risk, as well as for formulating and developing interventions targeting those risks. However, ethnic and racial differences have been noted in the accuracy of the original BMI formulas, and several specific equations have been tested for particular groups of people.[39] In addition, it is known that central obesity includes metabolically active adipocytes and is more highly related to obesity-related diseases than is obesity, that occurs primarily in the hips, legs, or arms.

Type 2 Diabetes Mellitus

The risk of T2D increases dramatically with increased weight and with a more central distribution of body fat, reflecting visceral adiposity. Several early classic studies examined the relationship between obesity and T2D; the results have been replicated in more recent studies. The classic Nurses' Health Study examined a large sample of women and demonstrated that the risk of T2D was lowest in women with a BMI less than 22. A steady increase in the relative risk of developing T2D with increasing BMI was noted; at a BMI of 31 or more, women had an age-adjusted relative risk of 40 or greater.[40] In men participating in the Health Professionals Follow-up Study, a similar relationship was noted, the lowest risk of developing diabetes being associated with a BMI of less than 23 and the greatest risk with a BMI of 35 or more.[41] Diabetes mellitus is discussed in more detail in Chapter 37.

Weight gain over the lifespan also increases the risk of diabetes. Weight gained after age 18 years contributes to an increased risk for diabetes, while weight loss is associated with a reduction in relative risk. Interestingly, weight gain seems to precede the onset of diabetes. The National Health and Nutrition Examination Survey (NHANES)[42] clearly demonstrated an increasing incidence of diabetes associated with increasing levels of obesity. The incidence of T2D ranged from 8% for normal-weight individuals to 43% for individuals with a BMI of 40 or more.[42]

Dyslipidemias

Dyslipidemias such as high levels of low-density lipoproteins are obesity-related and known to be linked with deposition of atheromatous plaques, which can contribute to the development of several types of cardiovascular and heart disease. Dyslipidemias are covered in Chapters 23 and 24.

Hypertension

Hypertension occurs frequently in overweight and obese individuals.[43] In a large meta-analysis of comorbidities related to overweight and obesity, the pooled relative risk for hypertension in men with overweight or obesity was found to be 1.28 and 1.84, respectively. In women, the risk for overweight or obese individuals was 1.65 and 2.42, respectively.[43] In addition, hypertension is closely associated with T2D, impaired glucose tolerance, hypertriglyceridemia, and hypercholesterolemia. Hypertension is covered in Chapter 23.

Heart Disease

Heart disease is the most common cause of death in the United States.[44] Major factors associated with heart disease include increased levels of BMI and dyslipidemias. It is known that a low level of HDL cholesterol places an individual at greater risk for coronary artery disease than does an elevated triglyceride level.[28] An interesting and seemingly contradictory finding is the obesity paradox, which is evidence that overweight and obese patients who survive an initial medical occurrence, such as a cardiovascular event (e.g., myocardial infarction) sometimes have improved outcomes. This paradox is based on the premise that a known risk factor is transformed into a protective factor after an initial occurrence.[45] Although there has been no explanation of this phenomenon, it has been documented that most of the obese patients in studies examining this paradox were younger than the normal-weight cohort patients. Advancing age is a predictor of higher cardiovascular risk, and this may be a partial explanation for the obesity paradox.[46] The obese patients in these studies were younger than the patients in the normal-weight cohort group, and they did not have significant age-related comorbidities, Thus, the younger obese patients had higher survival rates than the older normal-weight cohort patients, but the advantage was most probably conferred by younger age rather than by obesity. A recent study of diabetic patients found no support for the obesity paradox, with no association between BMI and mortality comparing obese diabetic patients to a normal-weight cohort of diabetic patients.[47] Research on this phenomenon is ongoing.

Metabolic Syndrome

Metabolic syndrome is a major factor in the development of cardiovascular disease. While the cut points for evaluating levels of specific lipids on which to base treatment are being challenged and the definition of metabolic syndrome varies slightly between national organizations, metabolic syndrome is now recognized as a pathologic entity that seems to confer greater morbidity and mortality risks than the individual factors alone would contribute.[28]

Nonalcoholic Fatty Liver Disease

Nonalcoholic fatty liver disease (NAFLD) and **nonalcoholic steatohepatitis** are terms that describe a group of liver abnormalities associated with obesity. These abnormalities include **hepatomegaly** (enlarged liver) and elevated liver enzymes and, in the case of nonalcoholic steatohepatitis, include abnormal changes in the histology of the liver, including fibrosis and cirrhosis. Collectively, these abnormal changes can lead to **steatosis** (fatty changes), **steatohepatitis** (inflammation and fatty changes in the liver), and fatal cirrhosis (**Figure 5.7** ■). The prevalence of NAFLD is not well defined in the Americas but is estimated at 20–30% worldwide.[48] More information on liver disease can be found in Chapter 44.

Gallbladder Disease

Gallbladder disease is the most common hepatobiliary pathology associated with overweight and obesity. The relationship between gallbladder disease and obesity appears to lie in the increased cholesterol turnover related to total body fat. Cholesterol production is linearly related to body fat, and the increased cholesterol is excreted in the bile. Higher levels of cholesterol concentrations in relation to bile acids and phospholipids in the bile increase the chance of precipitation of cholesterol gallstones in the gallbladder. Obesity increases the relative risk for gallbladder disease, as noted in a meta-analysis.[43] Across categories of BMI, the relative risk estimates were 1.09 for overweight and 1.43 for obesity.[40] More information on gallbladder disease can be found in Chapter 43.

Endocrine Changes

Endocrine changes that occur with obesity include irregular menses and frequent anovular cycles in women, along with a decreased rate of fertility in both men and women.[49] There have also been reports of increased rates of toxemia, hypertension, and cesarean sections in pregnant obese women. In addition, hirsutism in women is commonly seen with obesity, indicating altered reproductive and endocrine status.[49]

Polycystic ovary syndrome is another common condition associated with obesity. It appears to be involved with aberration in gonadotropin secretion and is related in an unclear manner to abnormalities of blood glucose control associated with obesity.[50]

Cancer

Cancers of specific types have demonstrated a relationship with obesity. Cancers of the colon, rectum, and prostate are more common in obese males. Cancers of the reproductive system and gallbladder are more common in obese women.[43] In women, this relationship may be explained partially by increased production of estrogen from adipose tissue stromal cells. More information about cancers can be found in Chapter 12.

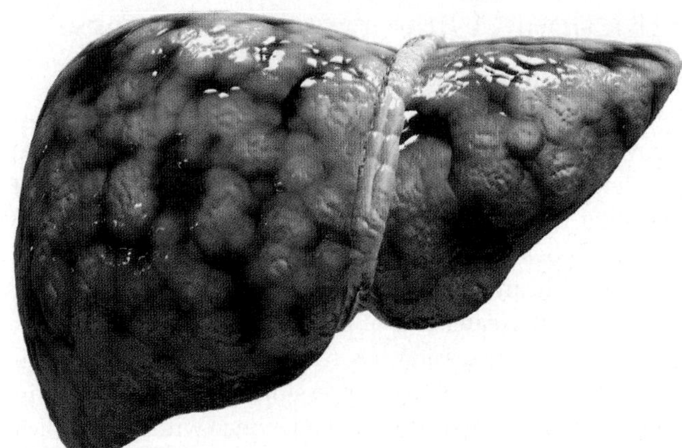

Figure 5.7 ■ Fatty changes in the liver.

Obstructive Sleep Apnea

Obstructive sleep apnea is more prevalent in overweight or obese individuals than in those with normal body weight; however, the relationship between obesity and obstructive sleep apnea is highly complex.[51] Increased neck circumference and fat deposits in the pharyngeal area may lead to a smaller lumen and a greater propensity for collapse, increasing blood pressure and decreasing in oxygen levels during sleep. Truncal obesity can cause increased abdominal pressure on the diaphragm, which may lead to reduced lung compliance and decreased residual lung volume. In addition, there are likely interactions related to the presence of increased visceral obesity influencing obstructive sleep apnea.[51] More information about sleep apnea can be found in Chapter 7.

Musculoskeletal and Skin Disorders

Diseases of bones, joints, muscles, connective tissue, and skin associated with excess weight include osteoarthritis with cartilage changes, particularly in the knees and ankles. In non-weight-bearing joints, there are also changes in cartilage and bone metabolism that are independent of weight bearing. The global burden of hip and knee changes have been studied and ranked as the 11th highest contributor to global disability.[52] The relative risk of joint replacement related to being overweight or obese was increased 2.76 and 4.20, respectively, for men and 1.80 and 1.96, respectively, for women.[43] Skin changes such as stretch marks (striae) as well as deepening pigmentation (acanthosis nigricans) in the folds of the neck, knuckles, and extensor surfaces occur in many overweight individuals (see **Figures 5.8** ■ and **5.9** ■).

Acanthosis nigricans is associated with insulin resistance and is most common in obese children with T2D. ■

Functional Outcomes Due to Obesity

Psychosocial Impairment

Psychosocial function may be impaired in obese individuals. While this difficulty is often not considered a medical problem, it may impair the individual as much as some of the other obesity-associated problems or even more. The stigma of obesity is damaging, affecting education, employment, healthcare, and other aspects of life. Obese women seem to be at greater risk of psychologic dysfunction than obese men.[53] Depression has shown a reciprocal relationship with obesity. While depression is more common in overweight and obese women than in men with similar BMI categories, the overall relative risk for depression in obesity is increased, with an odds ratio of 1.55.[53]

Weight bias exists across the lifespan, with stereotyping in all decades of life. A recent study evaluated the perceptions that 5- to 21-year-old individuals have toward members of their own age group. Viewing pictures of 20-, 40-, and 60-year-old faces on slender, large, and very large bodies, participants evaluated the pictures on six dimensions used in obesity stereotyping research. In all decades of life, heavier women were rated more negatively than thinner women on all dimensions examined. While older women were rated more negatively than younger women on attractiveness, they were rated more positively on every other dimension.[54] For adults with severe obesity, stigma is associated with the need for oversized chairs, scales, beds, wheelchairs, and other pieces of equipment that are designed for normal-weight individuals.

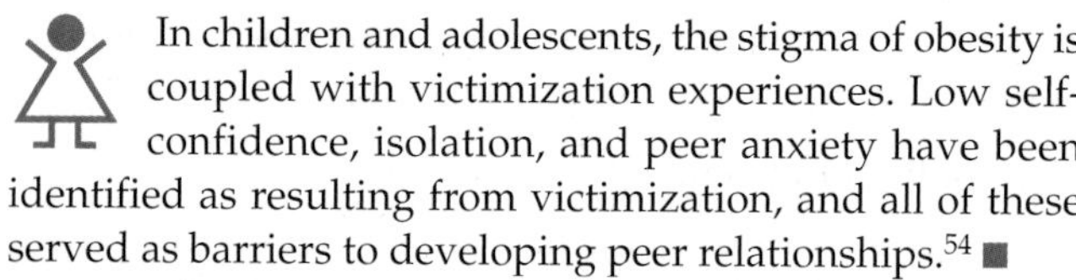

In children and adolescents, the stigma of obesity is coupled with victimization experiences. Low self-confidence, isolation, and peer anxiety have been identified as resulting from victimization, and all of these served as barriers to developing peer relationships.[54] ■

Functional Limitations

Functional limitations occur with the more extreme stages of obesity. As BMI increases, the ability to perform necessary activities of daily living becomes compromised. Difficulties with bending down to put on shoes or to care for feet are common in early stages of obesity. Eventually, working outside the home, shopping, bathing, and walking independently become difficult if not impossible. Late-stage obesity is characterized by additional disabilities, including confinement to bed and the inability to turn over without assistance.

Lifespan Considerations

Lifespan decreases occur with excess body fat, as this condition introduces a mortality rate increase, with an estimate of between 280,000 and 325,000 deaths attributable to obesity annually in the United States.[55] More than 80% of these deaths occurred in people with a BMI greater than 30. The American Cancer Society's Prevention Study I noted increased rates of death from all causes and from cardiovascular disease in both men and women with a greater BMI up to the age of 75 years. These findings were supported in a subsequent study by the American Cancer Society, with a consistently higher relative risk of death in all individuals with elevated BMI values. The years of life lost data taken from the Framingham Study indicate that nonsmoking

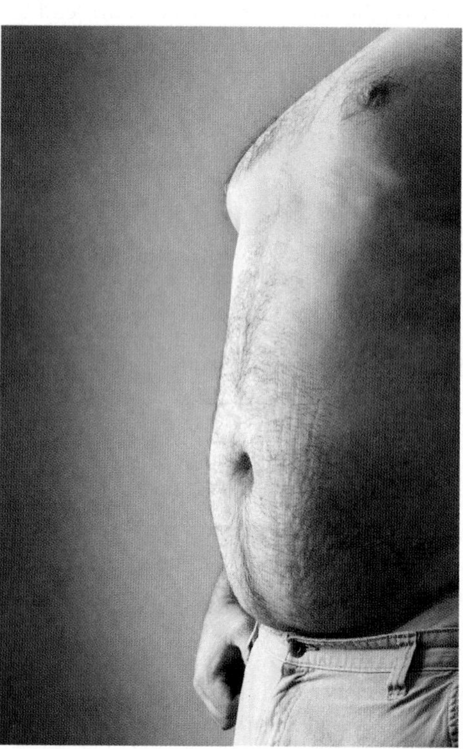

Figure 5.8 ■ Obese individual with stretch marks (striae).

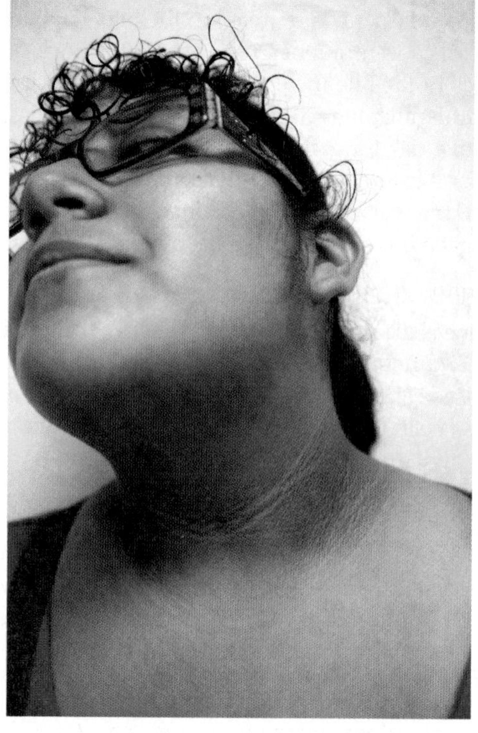

Figure 5.9 ■ Overweight individual with acanthosis nigricans.

women with BMI greater than 25 at age 40 lost 3.3 years and male nonsmoking men lost 3.1 years compared with normal-weight peers.[56]

Linking Pathophysiology to Treatment: Interventions to Achieve Weight Loss

Weight loss addresses a number of risk factors, as changes that lower blood pressure and triglycerides correspond to a 5–10% weight loss. HDL cholesterol increases with weight loss of this magnitude, and there is evidence that T2D rates decrease significantly with weight reduction. While the exact mechanisms of pathology are not clearly defined, weight loss appears to be the best treatment for this increasingly prevalent disease.

Interventions that can reduce fat mass and the associated inflammation and oxidative stress in obese individuals, as well as improve insulin sensitivity, are lifestyle changes, medications, antioxidant supplements, and surgery.

Lifestyle Changes

Lifestyle changes include caloric restriction with limitation of fat intake and increased ingestion of foods that are rich in antioxidants, such as fruits and vegetables (**Figure 5.10** ■). For additional information on specific types of antioxidants found in various foods, refer to the section on oxidative stress in Chapter 10. In addition to food sources of antioxidants, numerous antioxidant supplements are available for purchase by prescription and over the counter. Clinical trials are needed to determine the efficacy of treating overweight and obese individuals with these supplements.

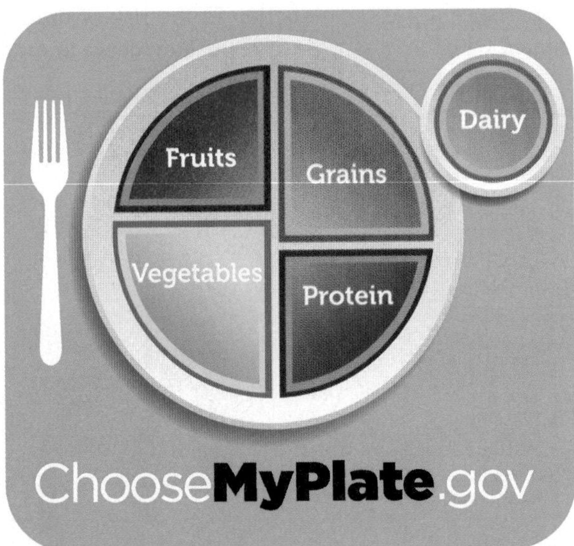

Figure 5.10 ■ ChooseMyPlate is a program developed by the U.S. Department of Agriculture to help individuals adopt and maintain a healthy eating style. For more information, visit the program's website at https://www.choosemyplate.gov/MyPlate.

Medications

In addition to the widely used lipid-altering medications, such as the statins, new medications are under investigation for improving the metabolic profile and decreasing inflammation and oxidative stress associated with overweight and obesity.

Surgery

Surgical procedures, such as gastric banding, achieve weight loss by decreasing stomach size, thereby decreasing the amount of food that the individual can comfortably ingest. These procedures carry risks associated with surgery, including adverse reactions to anesthetic agents, infections, and bleeding. However, a surgical intervention is the only effective means for some obese individuals to lose weight and achieve the metabolic benefits of the reduction in fat mass and associated reduction in inflammation and oxidative stress.

Thomas Johnson: Outcome

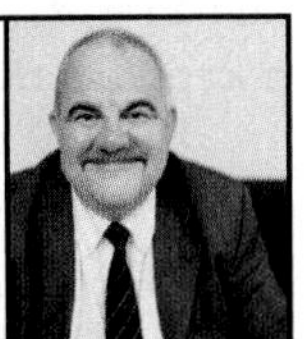

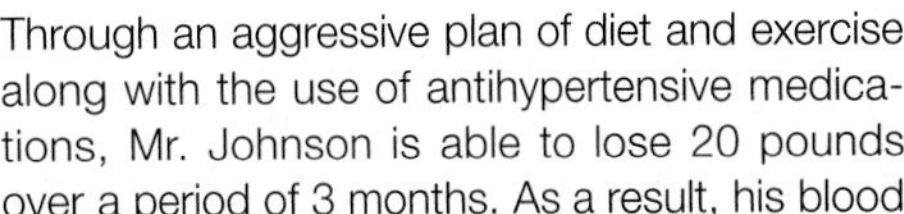

Through an aggressive plan of diet and exercise along with the use of antihypertensive medications, Mr. Johnson is able to lose 20 pounds over a period of 3 months. As a result, his blood pressure, glucose, lipids, and inflammatory markers improve. His healthcare provider encourages him to continue his weight loss and exercise and suggests that he consider joining a weight loss or exercise group to help him stay with his plan.

5. Mr. Johnson is educated and counseled on his weight. By the end of his visit, he should understand what factors can cause obesity. What statement from Mr. Johnson would indicated understanding of these factors?
6. What other effects could Mr. Johnson's obesity have had on his health?

Yashika Devon: Outcome

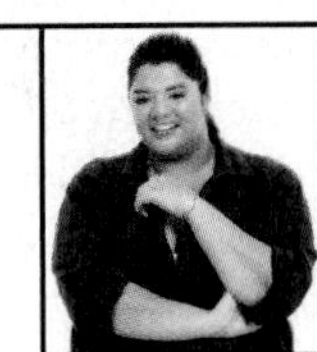

Through an aggressive plan of diet and exercise, Yashika is able to lose 30 pounds over a period of 3 months. As a result, her blood pressure, glucose, lipids, and inflammatory markers improve. In addition, the velvety rash at the nape of her neck has cleared, suggesting a reduction in her insulin resistance. Yashika discusses her happiness with this weight loss but also worries about her ability to maintain the rigorous schedule. Her nurse practitioner refers her to a support group for teenagers working on weight loss.

5. Yashika asks why weight gain affects her mood. How do you respond?
6. Yashika has listened to you and wants to know what kind of activity she can do in her room and how much and how often she needs to do it to keep seeing results. What education do you give her?

Check Your Progress: Section 5.3

1. Describe the relationship between obesity and social stigma.
2. How does social stigma influence personal, social, and economic plans for obesity treatment?
3. What are the benefits of weight loss in obesity?

5.4 Health Risks of Physical Inactivity

Historically, high levels of physical activity have been associated with improved health outcomes. The first comprehensive and influential reports on the role of physical activity in health and disease, *Physical Activity and Health: A Report of the Surgeon General*, was published in 1996.[57] This report provided historical background and discussed the evolution of physical activity recommendations, addressing the physiologic responses and long-term adaptations to exercise, the effects of physical activity on health and disease, patterns and trends in physical activity, and the role of physical activity in health promotion activities. The report concluded that people of all ages could benefit from regular physical activity. Unfortunately, the number of people participating in physical activity programs since the publication of this report has not increased substantially.

The U.S. Department of Disease Prevention and Health Promotion published the first edition of the *Physical Activity Guidelines for Americans* in 2008; the second edition of these guidelines are in development. They were developed and synthesized from review of scientific evidence on the health benefits of physical activity.[58] These guidelines reflect the consensus of several experts on physical activity recommendations and provide the emphasis for health promotion initiatives to address the growing problem of physical activity and sedentary lifestyles. The *Physical Activity Guidelines for Americans* can be accessed at http://www.health.gov/paguidelines.

Before discussing the relationship between physical inactivity and various health conditions, it is important to review the conceptual definitions of physical activity, physical fitness, and exercise. The terms *physical activity* and *exercise* are often used interchangeably; however, there are commonalities and differences between the two concepts. Both physical activity and exercise involve bodily movement produced by contraction of skeletal muscle that increases energy expenditure above basal levels. This energy expenditure is measured in kilocalories ranging on a continuum from low to high. Physical activity and exercise are characterized according to mode, intensity, and purpose (e.g., occupational, leisure-time, household). **Exercise** is a subcategory of physical activity that is planned, structured, and repetitive and with a goal of improvement or maintenance of one or more components of physical fitness as the objective.[59]

The term **physical fitness** has been defined in a number of ways. The most accepted definition is "the ability to carry out daily tasks with vigor and alertness, without undue fatigue and with ample energy to enjoy leisure-time pursuits and meet unforeseen emergencies."[59] Physical fitness can be divided into two major components: health-related and performance-related physical fitness. The goal of health-related physical fitness is to improve some aspect(s) of health; the goal of performance-related physical fitness is to improve some aspect of athletic performance. The primary components of health-related physical fitness include cardiorespiratory endurance, skeletal muscle endurance, skeletal muscle strength, body composition, and flexibility. The primary components of performance-related physical fitness include agility, balance, coordination, muscle strength and power, speed of movement, and reaction time (**Figure 5.11** ■). There are interrelationships between health-related physical fitness and performance-related physical fitness. For example, physical balance may be a component of performance-related fitness in athletes; however, physical balance may also be a component of health-related fitness in patients with a neurologic disorder. The individual importance of any component depends on the health- or performance-related goal.

Physical Activity and Health-Related Physical Fitness

Higher levels of physical activity are associated with lower mortality rates for adults of all ages; those who are moderately active on a regular basis have lower mortality rates than those who are less active. Physical activity has a number of important physiologic effects, particularly on the cardiorespiratory, metabolic, endocrine, and musculoskeletal systems and on mental health. In addition, physical activity is used to prevent and treat of a number of chronic diseases, such as cancer.

All-Cause Mortality

There is a large body of scientific evidence regarding the relationship between physical activity and all-cause mortality rates. Studies examining these relationships are usually large longitudinal cohort studies. In such studies, groups of individuals may be followed over long periods of time to examine trends and effects associated with variables such as physical activity. Available data consistently show an inverse relationship between physical activity and all-cause mortality; during follow-up observation, the most active individuals experience a greater reduction in the risk of mortality compared with the least active.[58] There is evidence to suggest

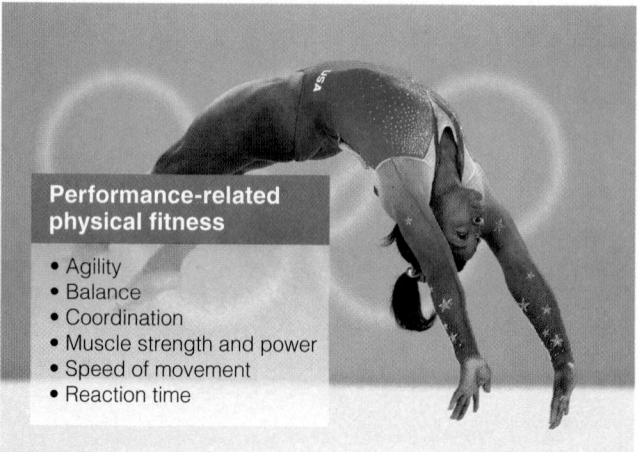

Figure 5.11 ■ The primary skill-related components of performance-related physical fitness are demonstrated by Simone Biles, who won four gold medals and one bronze medal in gymnastics in the 2016 Olympic Games in Rio de Janeiro.

that it is the overall volume of energy expended, not the type of activity, that is most important to the lower risk of mortality. In addition, there appears to be a dose effect that confers such benefits on all-cause mortality; the greatest benefits were achieved with a greater volume of energy expended.

Cardiorespiratory Disease

Routine moderate- to vigorous-intensity aerobic exercise can result in improvements in cardiorespiratory fitness (VO_2 max), exemplified by an increase in the ability of the cardiorespiratory system to transport oxygen to skeletal muscles and the ability of skeletal muscles to utilize the oxygen. There is convincing evidence to suggest that there is a beneficial relationship between aerobic exercise and cardiovascular health outcomes, including morbidity and mortality from coronary artery disease, stroke, hypertension, atherogenic dyslipidemia, and vascular function.[60] In addition, aerobic exercise is considered a standard of therapy for improving functional performance in patients with peripheral arterial disease.[60]

The most favorable cardiorespiratory outcomes are noted when the volume of physical activity exceeds 800 MET-minutes per week. A **metabolic equivalent of task (MET)** is defined as the ratio of metabolic rate (rate of energy consumption) during a specific physical activity to a reference rate of metabolic rate at rest. For example, 800 MET-minutes per week is equivalent to approximately 12 miles per week of walking or jogging; however, this amount can be achieved through a combination of exercise bouts with different intensities, durations, and frequencies.[60] Energy expenditure at a given exercise intensity is highly dependent on baseline fitness level, sex, type of activity, and other factors, such as the presence of chronic illness. An individualized exercise prescription can be developed on the basis of such factors. The risk of injury and cardiovascular events increases with higher volumes of exercise, so the exercise prescription should be approached gradually on starting a program, especially in initially sedentary individuals.

Metabolic Disease

Exercise is associated with increased insulin sensitivity and enhanced glucose transport into muscle cells. Physical activity and exercise play an essential role in preventing T2D. The role of exercise in the prevention of T2D has been studied extensively over the past two decades. Data from clinical trials have established that increasing moderate physical activity up to 150 minutes per week reduces the risk of developing T2D in patients with impaired glucose tolerance. The reduction in risk is greater with weight loss, which emphasizes the relationship between obesity and impairments in glucose tolerance.

Cancer

High levels of physical activity are associated with reduced risk of developing several cancers. A recent meta-analysis concluded that physical activity may prevent breast cancer in postmenopausal women.[61] Additional evidence suggests that leisure-time physical activity is associated with a reduction is colon cancer.[62] Whether there is a relationship between physical activity and cancer recurrence is unknown.

Musculoskeletal Disease

Physical activity is beneficial for musculoskeletal health. For example, physical activity is inversely associated with risk of hip and spine fracture.[58] Bone mineral density in the spine or the hip is responsive to exercise training. For example, the bone mineral density in the spine or the hip can be increased or the rate of decline can be modified by exercise training. In addition, physical activity can increase skeletal muscle mass, strength, power, and neuromuscular activation. There is no evidence to support the idea that physical activity or exercise can prevent osteoarthritis; however, patients participating in moderate-intensity, low-impact physical activity have noted disease-specific benefits such as decreased pain, increased physical function, and improved quality of life.[58]

Mental Health

Physical activity appears to protect against symptoms of depression and the cognitive decline associated with aging, including the onset of dementia.[58] Higher levels of physical activity also may enhance feelings of well-being. In addition, physical activity may reduce the symptoms of anxiety, poor quantity and quality of sleep, feelings of distress, and fatigue.[58]

Linking Pathophysiology to Treatment

Interventions to Increase Physical Activity to Prevent Diabetes

The Diabetes Prevention Program (DPP) was a major multicenter clinical research trial designed to discover whether modest weight loss through dietary changes and increased physical activity or treatment with an oral diabetes medication (metformin) could prevent or delay the onset of T2D. All of the study participants had prediabetes at the beginning of the study. Participants in the lifestyle intervention group, who received intensive individual counseling and behavioral support on effective diet, exercise, and behavior modification, reduced their risk of developing T2D by 58%, while participants in the medication group reduced their risk for developing T2D by 31%. The integration of increased physical activity through programs like the DPP has major implications for preventing disease.[63] This program has become a model for the prevention of T2D.

Pharmacologic Interventions to Promote Weight Loss in Obesity

While it is widely accepted that lifestyle modifications as described above are the best way to approach weight loss, pharmacologic and surgical interventions are available to assist in the treatment of obesity. Pharmacologic interventions are described in **Table 5.1** ■.

A variety of surgeries are used in the treatment of weight loss; the most common are laparoscopic adjustable gastric banding, Roux-en-Y gastric bypass, and laparoscopic or open sleeve gastrectomy.[3] In the laparoscopic adjustable

Table 5.1 Pharmacologic Treatments That Assist in Weight Loss

Medication	Description
Drugs Acting on the Gastrointestinal System	
Orlistat	Orlistat inhibits pancreatic and gastric lipase, decreasing the hydrolysis of ingested triglycerides; leads to reduced fat absorption.[64]
Drugs Acting on the Central Nervous System (CNS)	
Lorcaserin	Lorcaserin is a selective serotonin 2c receptor (5-HT_{2C}) that produces hypophagia through action on hypothalamic neurons, resulting in decreased food consumption and satiety.[64,65]
Phentermine plus topiramate	This is a fixed combination of phentermine, a nonselective monoamine-releasing agent acting as an appetite suppressant, and topiramate, an anticonvulsant used for prevention of migraine headaches. Together they produce an anorexic effect.[64]
Bupropion plus naltrexone	This is a fixed combination of bupropion, a selective dopamine and norepinephrine-reuptake inhibitor used for smoking cessation and depression, and naltrexone, an opioid agonist used for treatment of opioid addiction.[64,65]
Drugs Acting on the Gastrointestinal System and the CNS	
Liraglutide	Liraglutide is a glucagon-like peptide receptor agonist that was originally approved for treatment of T2D that increases glucose-dependent insulin secretion, decreases excessive and inappropriate glucagon secretion, slows gastric emptying, and increases satiety. In higher doses, liraglutide is associated with weight loss.[65]

gastric banding procedure, an adjustable silicone band is placed around the upper stomach. A pouch is created above the band, while there is a narrowing of the upper stomach diameter below.[3] In the Roux-en-Y gastric bypass, a small pouch is created from the stomach and remains attached to the esophagus at one end and a section of the small intestine at the other. This bypasses the remaining part of the stomach and the initial loop of the small intestine.[3] In the laparoscopic or open sleeve gastrectomy procedure, the stomach is divided vertically, and its size is reduced by 75%. The pyloric valve remains in place so that digestion and stomach function remain unchanged.[3]

There appear to be a wide range of physiologic changes following bariatric surgery that result in the prevention or remission of diabetes or improvements in glycemic control. The physiologic and molecular mechanisms underlying these changes are not clearly understood. These mechanisms appear to be both acute and chronic and related to the type of surgery.[66] A variety of postsurgical effects, such as caloric restriction, rapid emptying of nutrients, and enhanced nutrient/bile delivery to the mid/distal jejunum and ileum, lead to reduced hepatic glucose production, increased tissue glucose uptake, improved insulin sensitivity, and enhanced pancreatic β-cell function.[66] These metabolic improvements are mediated additional factors, such as weight loss, altered gut microbiome (collection of all the microorganisms located in the gut), gut hormones, bile acids, and neural signaling.[66] Unraveling the physiologic and molecular change following bariatric surgery will help in understanding the mechanisms underlying obesity and developing treatments.

Check Your Progress: Section 5.4

1. Why are programs like the Diabetes Prevention Program so successful in preventing T2D?
2. Summarize the effect that the different bariatric surgeries have on the body and why they are effective with weight loss.
3. What kind of pharmacologic treatments are effective for weight loss and why?

CHAPTER SUMMARY

5.1 Chapter Overview and Case Studies

Outline the global prevalence of, medical conditions associated with, and concepts related to obesity and physical inactivity.

- Obesity is a complex condition with multiple causes, resulting in suffering, ill health, early mortality, societal stigma, and discrimination.
- Obesity is conceptually defined as an excess of body fat. In adults, body fat is clinically defined by specific BMI categories designated as normal, overweight, or obese.
- More than 33% of U.S. adults and 17% of U.S. children are obese.
- Obesity is a factor in the development of a number of medical conditions, including diabetes, cardiovascular disease (coronary artery disease, myocardial infarction, angina pectoris, heart failure, stroke, hypertension, and atrial fibrillation), metabolic syndrome, cancer, arthritis, gallbladder disease, acute pancreatitis, NAFLD, pulmonary complications, and depression.

5.2 Etiology and Pathophysiology of Obesity

Describe the etiology of obesity and outline the pathophysiologic consequences, including chronic diseases and metabolic syndrome.

- Obesity arises from multiple genetic, behavioral, metabolic, environmental, and socioeconomic factors.
- Adipose tissue hormones and gastrointestinal hormones involved with food intake and obesity are associated with obesity.
- The multiple abnormalities lead to inflammation, insulin resistance, visceral adiposity, and oxidative stress, which are major contributors to chronic diseases and metabolic syndrome.

5.3 Health Risks of Obesity

Outline the health risks and functional outcomes associated with obesity. The health risks include the following:

- T2D
- Dyslipidemias
- Hypertension
- Heart disease
- Metabolic syndrome
- NAFLD
- Gallbladder disease
- Endocrine changes
- Cancer
- Obstructive sleep apnea
- Musculoskeletal and skin disorders.

The functional outcomes due to obesity include the following:

- Psychosocial impairment, including depression and effects on education, employment, and healthcare
- Functional limitations, such as difficulty performing ADLs
- Increased mortality rates and higher risk of death in all individuals with elevated BMI values.

5.4 Health Risks of Physical Inactivity

Discuss the role of physical inactivity/activity in the development and progression of chronic diseases and recommendations for physical activity.

- Higher levels of physical activity are associated with lower mortality rates for adults of all ages.
- Physical activity has a number of important physiologic effects related to cardiorespiratory, metabolic, endocrine, cancer, musculoskeletal, and mental health.

REVIEW QUESTIONS

1. You are teaching a class about the goals of *Healthy People 2020*. You know that the class members understand these goals when they mention:
   a. reducing risk and maintaining a healthy weight.
   b. increasing risk and maintaining a healthy weight.
   c. reducing risk and monitoring labs.
   d. increasing risk and maintaining the status quo.
2. The nurse identifies the criteria that classify a female client with metabolic syndrome. Which of the following criteria does the nurse list?
   a. Waist circumference of 32 inches
   b. Triglycerides of 150
   c. HDL of 68
   d. Fasting glucose level of 109 mg/dL
3. You are asked why obesity occurs with respect to hormones. You know that obesity occurs as a result of defects in:
   a. GLP-3.
   b. PZZ.
   c. peptide cholecystokinin.
   d. amylase.
4. A teacher is asked to educate parents about healthy weights of children and adults. She is able to do both, using a BMI chart. How is childhood obesity categorized differently from adult obesity?
   a. Childhood obesity is plotted by age.
   b. Childhood obesity is plotted by age and race.
   c. Childhood obesity is plotted by age, height, and weight.
   d. Childhood obesity is plotted by age, height, and race.
5. A 45-year-old female has been referred to you for treatment of obesity. What is the first treatment you initiate?
   a. You recommend OTC diet pills to be taken daily.
   b. You recommend a diet change from 2500 calories to 1000 calories.
   c. You recommend joining an elite gym of competitive weight lifters.
   d. You recommend 30 minutes of brisk walking 5 times a week.

6. You are placed in charge of an intervention for the students of a local elementary school. You know that a key factor for change in children's association with food is to address:
   a. the parents because they are all making incorrect food choices.
   b. the food insecurity that these children experience because it affects their food choices.
   c. the city parks and rec department because there are not enough state-of-the-art activities at the local YMCA.
   d. None of the above, since you are just one person.
7. Mr. Xi is scheduled to undergo a Roux-en-Y gastric bypass. He wants to know what he should expect from the procedure. You explain that:
   a. he will not be restricted in his diet post procedure.
   b. he will be monitored for increased hepatic glucose production.
   c. he will have improved insulin sensitivity and thus improved beta-cell function.
   d. he will need to use more diabetic medication because of the surgery.
8. A new nurse is teaching a class at the local YMCA. The students are older adults from the community. The nurse's topic is the importance of weight management as the individuals age. Understanding of this material is noted by a student who says:
   a. "Weight gain will not affect my ability to care for myself."
   b. "Weight loss will not help if I have joint pain."
   c. "Weight gain will affect my ability to do simple tasks, such as turning in bed, by myself."
   d. "Weight loss can increase my change of diabetes and its complications."

ANSWERS

Answers to Review Questions can be found in Appendix A. Answers to Case Study and Check Your Progress questions are available on the faculty resources site. Please consult with your instructor.

RECOMMENDED WEBSITES

Centers for Disease Control and Prevention: Childhood Overweight and Obesity
https://www.cdc.gov/obesity/childhood/index.html

Physical Activity Guidelines for Americans
https://health.gov/paguidelines/guidelines

REFERENCES

1. Maggi, S., Busetto, L., Noale, M., Limongi, F., & Crepaldi, G. (2015). Obesity: Definition and epidemiology. In A. Lenzi, S. Migliaccio, & L. M. Donini (Eds.), *Multidisciplinary approach to obesity: From assessment to treatment* (pp. 31–39). New York, NY: Springer.
2. World Health Organization. (2014). *Overweight and obesity*. Available at http://www.who.int/mediacentre/factsheets/fs311/en
3. Ogden, C. L., Carroll, M. D., Kit, B. K., & Flegal, K. M. (2014). Prevalence of childhood and adult obesity in the United States, 2011–2012. *JAMA, 311*(8), 806–814.
4. Pi-Sunyer, X. (2009). The medical risks of obesity. *Postgraduate Medicine, 121*(6), 21–33.
5. Centers for Disease Control and Prevention. (2016). *Overweight and obesity*. Available at http://www.cdc.gov/obesity/data/prevalence-maps.html
6. Go, A. S., Roger, V. L., Benjamin, E. J., et al. (2013). Heart disease and stroke statistics—2013 update: A report from the American Heart Association. *Circulation, 127*, e6–e245.
7. Centers for Disease Control and Prevention. (2014). *Facts about physical activity*. Available at http://www.cdc.gov/physicalactivity/data/facts.html
8. U.S. Department of Health and Human Services. (2017). *Physical activity*. Available at http://www.healthypeople.gov/2020/topics-objectives/topic/physical-activity
9. Gurevich-Panigrahi, T., Panigrahi, S., Wiechec, E., & Los, M. (2009). Obesity: Pathophysiology and clinical management. *Current Medicinal Chemistry, 16*(4), 506–521.
10. Yu, J. H., & Kim, M. S. (2012). Molecular mechanisms of appetite regulation. *Diabetes and Metabolism Journal, 36*(6), 391–398.
11. Sam, A. H., Troke, R. C., Tan, T. M., & Bewick, G. A. (2012). The role of the gut/brain axis in modulating food intake. *Neuropharmacology, 63*(1), 46–56.
12. Molina, P. E. (2013). *Endocrine physiology* (4th ed.). New York, NY: McGraw-Hill Medical.
13. Kanaya, A., & Vaisse, C. (2011). Obesity. In D. G. Gardner & D. M. Shoback (Eds.), *Greenspan's basic and clinical endocrinology* (pp. 699–709). New York, NY: McGraw Hill.
14. Skolnik, N. S, & Ryan, D. H. (2014). Pathophysiology, epidemiology, and assessment of obesity in adults. *Journal of Family Practice, 63*(7), S3–S10.
15. Filippatos, T. D., Elisaf, M. S. (2013). Effects of glucagon-like peptide-1 receptor agonists on renal function. *World Journal of Diabetes, 4*(5), 190–201.

16. Rojas, J., Aguirre, M., Velasco, M., & Bermudez, V. (2013). Obesity genetics: A monopoly game of genes. *Amercian Journal of Therapeutics, 20*(4), 399–413.
17. Zhang, Y., Proenca, R., Maffei, M., Barone, M., Leopold, L., & Friedman, J. M. (1994). Positional cloning of the mouse obese gene and its human homologue. *Nature, 372*(6505), 425–432.
18. Farooqi, I. S. (2014). EJE Prize 2012: Obesity: From genes to behaviour. *European Journal of Endocrinology, 171*(5), R191–R195.
19. Montague, C. T., Farooqi, I. S., Whitehead, J. P., et al. (1997). Congenital leptin deficiency is associated with severe early-onset obesity in humans. *Nature, 387*(6636), 903–908.
20. Hager, J., Dina, C., Francke, S., et al. (1998). A genome-wide scan for human obesity genes reveals a major susceptibility locus on chromosome 10. *Nature Genetics, 20*(3), 304–308.
21. Stunkard, A. J., Sørensen, T. I. A., Hanis, C., et al. (1986). An adoption study of human obesity. *New England Journal of Medicine, 314*(4), 193–198.
22. Stunkard, A. J., Harris, J. R., Pedersen, N. L., & McClearn, G. E. (1990). The body-mass index of twins who have been reared apart. *New England Journal of Medicine, 322*(21), 1483–1487.
23. Herrera, B. M., Keildson, S., & Lindgren, C. M. (2011). Genetics and epigenetics of obesity. *Maturitas, 69*(1), 41–49.
24. Marseglia, L., Manti, S., D'Angelo, G., et al. (2014). Oxidative stress in obesity: A critical component in human diseases. *International Journal of Molecular Sciences, 16*(1), 378–400.
25. Blüher, M. (2016). Adipose tissue inflammation: A cause or consequence of obesity-related insulin resistance? *Clinical Science, 130*(18), 1603–1614.
26. Gaens, K. H., Stehouwer, C. D., & Schalkwijk, C. G. (2013). Advanced glycation endproducts and its receptor for advanced glycation endproducts in obesity. *Current Opinion in Lipidology, 24*(1), 4–11.
27. Bluher, M., & Mantzoros, C. S. (2015). From leptin to other adipokines in health and disease: Facts and expectations at the beginning of the 21st century. *Metabolism, 64*(1), 131–145.
28. Alberti, K. G., Eckel, R. H., Grundy, S. M., et al. (2009). Harmonizing the metabolic syndrome: A joint interim statement of the International Diabetes Federation Task Force on Epidemiology and Prevention; National Heart, Lung, and Blood Institute; American Heart Association; World Heart Federation; International Atherosclerosis Society; and International Association for the Study of Obesity. *Circulation, 120*(16), 1640–1645.
29. Allison, D. B., Downey, M., Atkinson, R. L., et al. (2008). Obesity as a disease: A white paper on evidence and arguments commissioned by the Council of the Obesity Society. *Obesity (Silver Spring), 16*(6), 1161–1177.
30. Jensen, M. D., Ryan, D. H., Apovian, C. M., et al. (2014). AHA/ACC/TOS guideline for the management of overweight and obesity in adults: A report of the American College of Cardiology/American Heart Association Task Force on Practice Guidelines and the Obesity Society. *Circulation, 129*(25, Suppl. 2), S102–S138.
31. Centers for Disease Control and Prevention. (2014). *Overweight and obesity: Basics about childhood obesity*. Available at http://www.cdc.gov/obesity/childhood/basics.html
32. Centers for Disease Control and Prevention. (2015). *Childhood obesity facts*. Available at http://www.cdc.gov/healthyyouth/obesity/facts.htm
33. Altman, M., & Wilfley, D. E. (2015). Evidence update on the treatment of overweight and obesity in children and adolescents. *Journal of Clinical Child and Adolescent Psychology, 44*, 521–537.
34. Harper, A. (2014). Reducing morbidity and mortality among pregnant obese. *Best Practice & Research Clinical Obstetrics & Gynaecology, 29*(3), 427–437.
35. Jarvie, E., Hauguel-de-Mouzon, S., Nelson S. M., Sattar, N., Catalano, P. M., & Freeman, D. J. (2010). Lipotoxicity in obese pregnancy and its potential role in adverse pregnancy outcome and obesity in the offspring. *Clinical Science, 119*(3), 123–129.
36. Cameron, C. M., Shibl, R., McClure, R. J., Ng, S. K., & Hills, A. P. (2014). Maternal pregravid body mass index and child hospital admissions in the first 5 years of life: Results from an Australian birth cohort. *International Journal of Obesity, 38*(10), 1268–1274.
37. Vasquez, E., Batsis, J. A., Germain, C. M., & Shaw, B. A. (2014). Impact of obesity and physical activity on functional outcomes in the elderly: Data from NHANES 2005.2010. *Journal of Aging and Health, 26*(6), 1032–1046.
38. Woo, J. (2015). Obesity in older persons. *Current Opinion in Clinical Nutrition and Metabolic Care, 18*(1), 5–10.
39. Goh, L. G., Dhaliwal, S. S., Welborn, T. A., Lee, A. H., & Della, P. R. (2014). Ethnicity and the association between anthropometric indices of obesity and cardiovascular risk in women: A cross-sectional study. *BMJ Open, 4*(5), e004702.
40. Colditz, G. A., Willett, W. C., Rotnitzky, A., & Manson, J. E. (1995). Weight gain as a risk factor for clinical diabetes mellitus in women. *Annals of Internal Medicine, 122*(7), 481–486.
41. Chan, J. M., Rimm, E. B., Colditz, G. A., Stampfer, M. J., & Willett, W. C. (1994). Obesity, fat distribution, and weight gain as risk factors for clinical diabetes in men. *Diabetes Care, 17*(9), 961–969.
42. Nguyen, N. T., Nguyen, X. M., Lane, J., & Wang, P. (2011). Relationship between obesity and diabetes in a US adult population: Findings from the National Health and Nutrition Examination Survey, 1999–2006. *Obesity Surgery, 21*(3), 351–355.
43. Guh, D. P., Zhang, W., Bansback, N., Amarsi, Z., Birmingham, C. L., & Anis, A. H. (2009). The incidence of co-morbidities related to obesity and overweight: A systematic review and meta-analysis. *BMC Public Health, 9*, 88.
44. Centers for Disease Control and Prevention. (2014). *Heart disease facts*. Available at http://www.cdc.gov/heartdisease/facts.htm
45. Katsnelson, M., & Rundek, T. (2011). Obesity paradox and stroke: Noticing the (fat) man behind the curtain. *Stroke, 42*(12), 3331–3332.
46. Ghoorah, K., Campbell, P., Kent, A., Maznyczka, A., & Kunadian, V. (2014). Obesity and cardiovascular outcomes: A review. *European Heart Journal: Acute Cardiovascular Care, 5*(1), 77–85.
47. Tobias, D. K., Pan, A., Jackson, C. L., et al. (2014). Body-mass index and mortality among adults with incident type 2 diabetes. *New England Journal of Medicine, 370*(3), 233–244.
48. Lopez-Velazquez, J. A., Silva-Vidal, K. V., Ponciano-Rodriguez, G., et al. (2014). The prevalence of nonalcoholic fatty liver disease in the Americas. *Annals of Hepatology, 13*(2), 166–178.
49. Unuane, D., Tournaye, H., Velkeniers, B., & Poppe, K. (DATE). Endocrine disorders & female infertility. *Best Practice & Research Clinical Endocrinology & Metabolism, 25*(6), 861–873.
50. Lim, S. S., Norman, R. J., Davies, M. J., & Moran, L. J. (2013). The effect of obesity on polycystic ovary syndrome: A systematic review and meta-analysis. *Obesity Reviews, 14*(2), 95–109.
51. Romero-Corral, A., Caples, S. M., Lopez-Jimenez, F., & Somers, V. K. (2010). Interactions between obesity and obstructive sleep apnea: Implications for treatment. *Chest, 137*(3), 711–719.
52. Cross, M., Smith, E., Hoy, D., et al. (2014). The global burden of hip and knee osteoarthritis: Estimates from the Global Burden Of Disease 2010 study. *Annals of the Rheumatic Diseases, 73*(7), 1323–1330.
53. Luppino, F. S., de Wit, L. M., Bouvy, P. F., et al. (2010). Overweight, obesity, and depression: A systematic review and meta-analysis of longitudinal studies. *Archives of General Psychiatry, 67*(3), 220–229.
54. Puhl, R. M., & Heuer, C. A. (2012). Obesity stigma: Important considerations for public health. *Health, 24*, 252.
55. Lim, S. S., Norman, R. J., Davies, M. J., & Moran, L. J. (2013). The effect of obesity on polycystic ovary syndrome: A systematic review and meta-analysis. *Obesity Reviews, 14*(2), 95–109.
56. Peeters, A., Barendregt, J. J., Willekens, F., Mackenbach, J. P., Al Mamun, A., & Bonneux, L. (2003). Obesity in adulthood and its consequences for life expectancy: A life-table analysis. *Annals of Internal Medicine, 138*(1), 24–32.
57. Centers for Disease Control and Prevention. (1996). *Physical activity and health: A report of the Surgeon General*. Available at https://www.cdc.gov/nccdphp/sgr/

58. Physical Activity Guidelines Advisory Committee. (2008). *Physical activity guidelines advisory committee report*. Washington, DC: U.S. Department of Health and Human Services.
59. Caspersen, C. J., Powell, K. E., & Christenson, G. M. (1985). Physical activity, exercise, and physical fitness: Definitions and distinctions for health-related research. *Public Health Reports, 100*(2), 126–131.
60. U.S. Department of Health and Human Services. (2008). *Physical activity guidelines for Americans.* Available at http://www.health.gov/paguidelines/guidelines/default.aspx
61. Goncalves, A. K., Dantas Florencio, G. L., Maisonnette de Atayde Silva, M. J., Cobucci, R. N., Giraldo, P. C., & Cote, N. M. (2014). Effects of physical activity on breast cancer prevention: A systematic review. *Journal of Physical Activity and Health, 11*(2), 445–454.
62. Anzuini, F., Battistella, A., & Izzotti, A. (2011). Physical activity and cancer prevention: A review of current evidence and biological mechanisms. *Journal of Preventive Medicine and Hygiene, 52*(4), 174–180.
63. Ruggiero, L., Castillo, A., Quinn, L., & Hochwert, M. (2012). Translation of the diabetes prevention program's lifestyle intervention: Role of community health workers. *Current Diabetes Report, 12*(2), 127–137.
64. Dietz, W. H., Baur, L. A., Hall, K., et al. (2015). Management of obesity: Improvement of health-care training and systems for prevention and care. *Lancet, 385*, 2521–2533.
65. Bragg, R., & Crannage, E. (2016). Review of pharmacotherapy options for the management of obesity. *Journal of the American Association of Nurse Practtitoners, 28*(2), 107–115.
66. Batterham, R. L., & Cummings, D. E. (2016). Mechanisms of diabetes improvement following bariatric/metabolic surgery. *Diabetes Care, 39*(6), 893–901.

Chapter 6

Risks Related to Substance Use Disorders

Marsha Snyder and Laurie Quinn

Chapter Outline and Learning Outcomes

6.1 Chapter Overview and Case Studies

Identify common substances of abuse and related pathophysiology concepts.

6.2 Anatomy and Neurobiology of the Brain

Describe the neurobiology of the brain and how it relates to substance use disorders.

6.3 Alcohol Use Disorder

Differentiate the causes, classification, underlying pathogenesis, and clinical manifestations of and the general treatment strategies for alcohol use disorder.

6.4 Tobacco Use Disorder

Differentiate the causes, classification, underlying pathogenesis, and clinical manifestations of and the general treatment strategies for tobacco use disorder.

6.5 Cannabis Use Disorder

Differentiate the causes, classification, underlying pathogenesis, and clinical manifestations of and the general treatment strategies for cannabis use disorder.

6.6 Stimulant Use Disorders

Differentiate the causes, classification, underlying pathogenesis, and clinical manifestations of and the general treatment strategies for stimulant use disorder.

6.7 Hallucinogen Use Disorder

Differentiate the causes, classification, underlying pathogenesis, and clinical manifestations of and the general treatment strategies for hallucinogenic use disorder.

6.8 Opioid Use Disorder

Differentiate the causes, classification, underlying pathogenesis, and clinical manifestations of and the general treatment strategies for opioid use disorder.

KEY TERMS

Agonist, 134
Alcohol intoxication, 128
Alcohol overdose, 128
Alcohol withdrawal syndrome, 128
Alcohol use disorder, 126
Benzodiazepines, 125
Binge drinking, 128
Blood alcohol concentration (BAC), 127
Cannabis, 134
Cannabis use disorder, 134
Cirrhosis, 129
Depressant, 127
Dopamine, 122
Glutamate, 127
Hallucinogen persisting perception disorder (HPPD), 138
Hallucination, 138
Hallucinogens, 138
Marijuana, 134
Mesolimbic pathway, 131
Methamphetamine, 136
Naloxone, 139
Neurotransmitter, 124
N-methyl-D-aspartate (NMDA) receptor, 127
Norepinephrine, 136
Opioid use disorder, 139
Physical dependence, 124
Psychoactive drugs, 122
Psychologic dependence, 124
Reward pathway, 124
Secondhand smoke (SHS), 133
Serotonin, 125
Smokeless tobacco, 133
Tetrahydrocannabinol (THC), 134
Tobacco use disorder, 131
Tolerance, 124
Vaping, 131
Wernicke-Korsakoff syndrome, 129

ABBREVIATIONS

BAC—blood alcohol content
GABA—gamma-aminobutyric acid
HPPD—hallucinogen persisting perception disorder
NMDA—N-methyl-D-aspartate
SHS—secondhand smoke
THC—tetrahydrocannabinol
VTA—ventral tegmental area

6.1 Chapter Overview and Case Studies

The most common substance use disorders are alcohol use disorder, tobacco use disorder, cannabis use disorder, stimulant use disorder, hallucinogen use disorder, and opioid use disorder. Alcohol, tobacco, and cannabis are among the most commonly used psychoactive substances in the Western world. Increasing concern about the use of these substances is the co-occurrence of the use of these substances with other substance use, mental health problems, and associated medical problems. Studies report that as many as 80% of people who abuse alcohol smoke regularly; rather than dying from alcohol-related diseases, the majority of these people die from smoking-related diseases. In addition, **psychoactive drugs** (i.e., drugs that can affect emotions, mind, and behavior) impose a substantial health burden on society. Drug-related deaths have more than doubled since the early 1980s, one in four deaths being attributed to alcohol, tobacco, and illicit drug use. Substance abuse is related to more deaths, illness, and disability than is any other preventable disease.[1]

Concepts Related to Substance Use Disorders

Substance use disorder involves the recurrent use of alcohol, tobacco and nicotine, prescription drugs, or illegal drugs such that the user experiences clinical and functional impairment.[2] Examples of such impairment include health problems and disability as well as the inability to manage overall responsibilities of daily life. The term *addiction* refers to the most chronic stage of substance use disorder, which is characterized by loss of self-control, as demonstrated by compulsive drug taking despite the desire to discontinue use of the drug.[2] The terms *substance use disorder* and *addiction* are often used interchangeably.

When neurobiology is used as the overall model, the major concepts associated with addiction include binge and intoxication, withdrawal and negative affect, and preoccupation and anticipation.[2] *Binge* and *intoxication* are associated with increased release of **dopamine** and activation of the brain's reward system. *Withdrawal* is associated with activation of the brain regions associated with emotions, resulting in increased sensitivity to stress and negative emotions. *Preoccupation* is associated with decreased function of the prefrontal cortex. During preoccupation, the individual attempts to balance the desire for the drug, the will to abstain, the possibility of relapse, and the continued cycle of addition.[2] Intoxication and binging, withdrawal, and preoccupation are recurring stages, associated with neuroadaptations and changes in neurocircuitry, and are influenced by genetic, environmental, and social factors.[2]

Individuals with substance use disorders will have alterations in other concepts as well, some of which depend on the particular substance being abused. Some related concepts are shown in **Figure 6.1** ■.

Case Studies

The pathophysiology and clinical significance of the symptoms experienced by the individuals in the cases will be addressed throughout the chapter to assist in applying chapter content to clinical situations involving individuals with substance use disorders.

Juliet Hernandez: Introduction

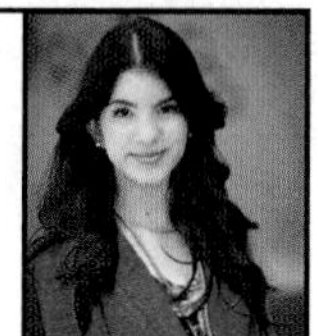

Ms. Hernandez is a 25-year-old struggling artist. She is seen at her primary care provider's office. Ms. Hernandez states that she has not had a physical examination in several years. She is seeking medical help for a sinus problem and sores around her mouth.

1. Ms. Hernandez self-identifies as a struggling artist. What is a possible barrier to obtaining routine preventive healthcare services?
2. Ms. Hernandez's chief complaint is sinus problems and sores around her mouth. These symptoms may result from what type of substance exposure?

James Wilson: Introduction

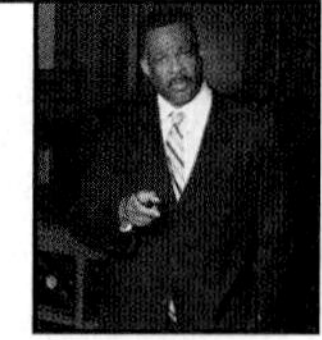

James Wilson, 65 years old, lives alone; his wife Joan died recently. He was brought to the hospital by his son, who reports finding Mr. Wilson on the kitchen floor with a large bruise on his left temple. Mr. Wilson appears to have injured his wrist in the fall.

1. What part of the social history raises your suspicion that Mr. Wilson may be under unusual stress?
2. Because Mr. Wilson suffered a fall, you suspect a syncopal episode. What important questions in the social history may give you information that could help to explain a loss of consciousness?

Check Your Progress: Section 6.1

1. What are the most commonly used psychoactive substances in the Western world?
2. Activation of the dopamine and reward system in the brain is associated with which aspects of substance use disorder?
3. Decreased activity of the prefrontal cortex is associated with which aspect of substance use disorder?

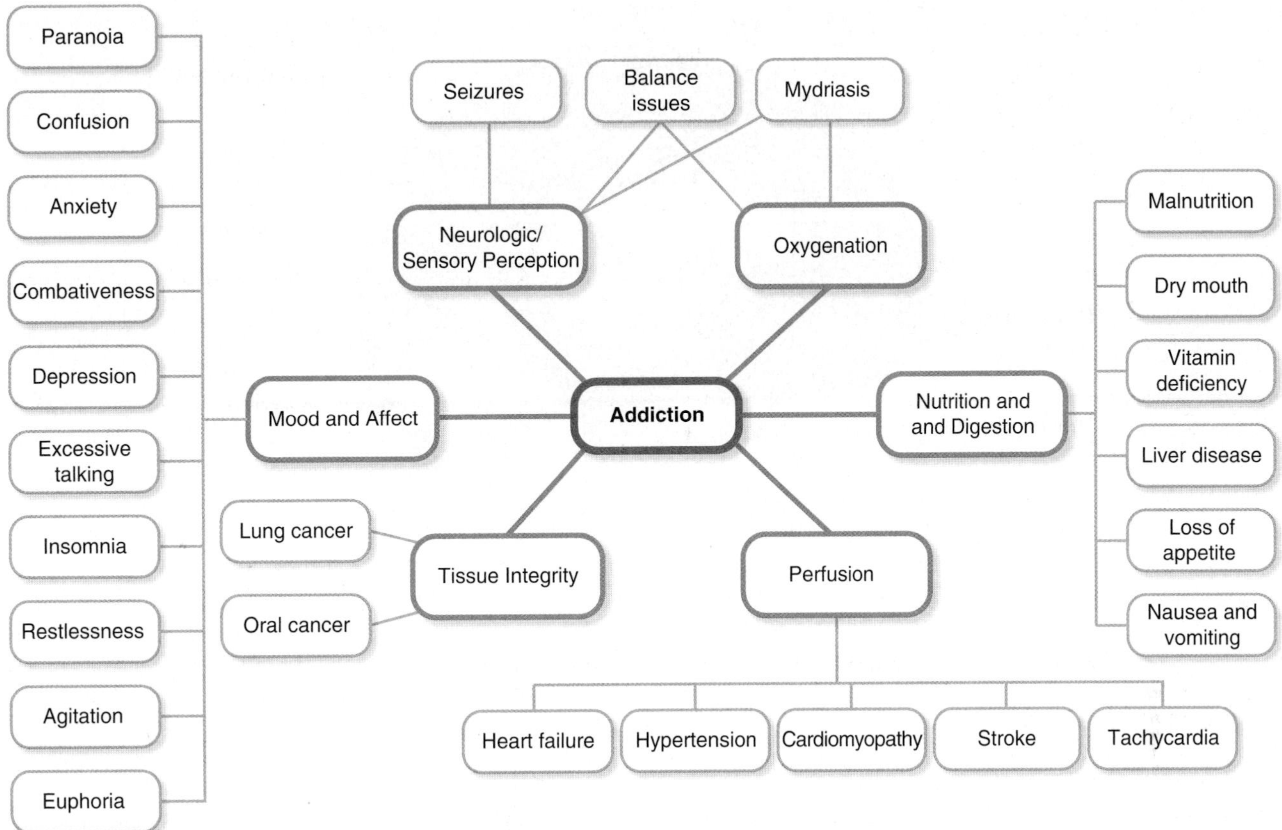

Figure 6.1 ■ Concepts related to substance abuse.

6.2 Anatomy and Neurobiology of the Brain

An understanding of the pathophysiology of substance use disorders is based on an understanding of anatomic structure and neurobiology of the brain. Major concepts in anatomy and neurobiology are reviewed briefly in the following paragraphs.

Anatomy and Physiology of the Brain

The major regions the brain include the brainstem, cerebellum, limbic system, diencephalon, and cerebral cortex. The brainstem controls basic functions critical to life, such as heart rate and breathing. The cerebellum is located above the brainstem and has important functions in motor control. The limbic system is located on top of the brainstem and within the cortex. The limbic system contains the brain's reward center and links brain structures that control and regulate feelings of pleasure (e.g., the amygdala and hippocampus). The hippocampus, a large limbic structure, has the role of sending memories out to the appropriate part of the cerebral hemisphere for long-term storage and retrieving them when necessary. The roles of storage and retrieval and storage of memory are of great importance in substance use disorders. Sensory (visual, auditory, tactile) information arrives at the lateral aspect of the amygdala within the limbic system and is processed and conveyed to the central nucleus, which projects to several parts of the brain involved in responses to fear (see **Figure 6.2** ■). The amygdala generates emotions from perceptions that may be generated through interaction with the hypothalamus and prefrontal cortex. It is also responsible for determining what memories are stored and the location for storage.

The diencephalon, located beneath the cerebral hemispheres, contains the thalamus and the hypothalamus. The primary role of the hypothalamus is regulation of basic drives such as hunger, thirst, pain response, pleasure, sexual satisfaction, anger, and aggressive behavior. The hypothalamus is also involved with the autonomic nervous system in regulation of pulse, blood pressure, breathing, and arousal in response to emotional circumstances. The thalamus is involved in sensory perception and regulation of motor functions (i.e., movement), connecting areas of the cerebral cortex that are involved in sensory perception and movement with other parts of the brain and spinal cord that also have roles in sensation and movement. The cerebral cortex covers most of the brain structures and is divided into right and left hemispheres. The cerebral cortex is also divided into sensory, motor, and association areas, which control specific functions; for example, the sensory areas receive and process information from the senses. The cerebral cortex is composed of the frontal, parietal, occipital, and temporal lobes. Each of these lobes has specific functions; for

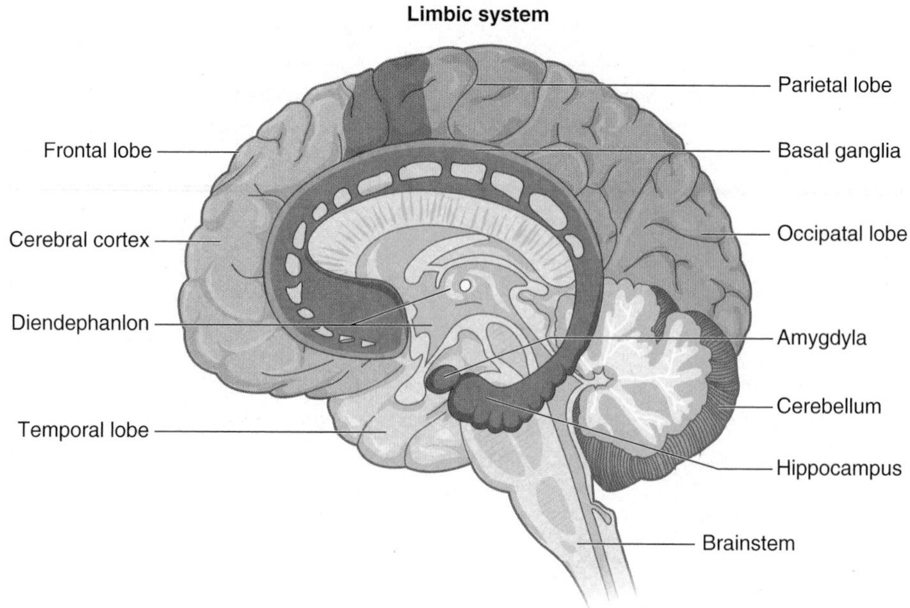

Figure 6.2 ■ Structures of the brain related to substance abuse.

example, the frontal cortex is involved in thinking, planning, problem solving, and decision making.

Excitable cells communicate with each other through a synapse, which is a specialized structure that allows communication from one cell to another; these synapses can be electrical or chemical. In an electrical synapse, the cells communicate through a gap junction that allows communication between cells through direct passage of ionic currents from one cell to another. In chemical synapses, the presynaptic neuron releases a **neurotransmitter**, or chemical substance that binds to a specific receptor on the cell membrane of the postsynaptic cell. This stimulates or inhibits an electrical response in that cell. A number of neurotransmitters in the neurobiology of substance disorders reinforce the effects of drugs; some examples are dopamine, opioid peptides, gamma-aminobutyric acid (GABA), glutamate, serotonin, and acetylcholine.

Neurobiology Related to Substance Use

A group of neurons that are located in the midbrain called the ventral tegmental area (VTA) connect to a variety of places within the limbic system; the important connection is to the nucleus accumbens in the basal ganglia (**Figure 6.3** ■). The basal ganglia are a large, complex set of structures within the limbic system that function in generating movements, some cognitive functions, and emotional and motivational activities. When a drug activates the VTA neurons, these neurons release the neurotransmitter dopamine into the nucleus accumbens, and the person feels pleasure. The nucleus accumbens, a primitive brain structure in the basal ganglia, and the VTA, part of the midbrain, are closely associated with the **reward pathway** along with dopamine, forming what is considered the final common pathway for drugs such as cocaine, morphine, and alcohol. In the median forebrain, nerves connected to the septum, amygdala, and nucleus accumbens communicate with the hypothalamus and the VTA. The median forebrain acts as a power source for brain reward, releasing dopamine into brain networks.[3]

Increased levels of dopamine are associated with the feelings of well-being, exhilaration, and pleasure; consequently, the formation of positive memories and reinforcement for continued substance use occurs, leading to **psychologic dependence**. If the drug is unavailable, a state of uneasiness or dissatisfaction occurs, and the person may experience emotional or motivational withdrawal symptoms. In some cases, the reinforcement results in **physical dependence** on the substance to function in everyday life. **Tolerance** occurs as the body attempts to maintain homeostasis. But if the body is held in a depressive state, as is seen in regular alcohol use, the brain compensates by reducing the inhibitory neurotransmitter GABA from being released or by reducing the number of receptor sites for this neurotransmitter. This does not occur immediately; but after repeated use, the drug does not produce the same central nervous system (CNS) effect as it did before. More of the drug is needed to achieve the desired effect, but the homeostatic mechanisms respond by further decreasing the release of GABA or decreasing the number of receptor sites. If the drug is abruptly stopped, symptoms of withdrawal occur as the levels of the substance fall below the usual dosage.[3] Symptoms of withdrawal, which vary among substances,

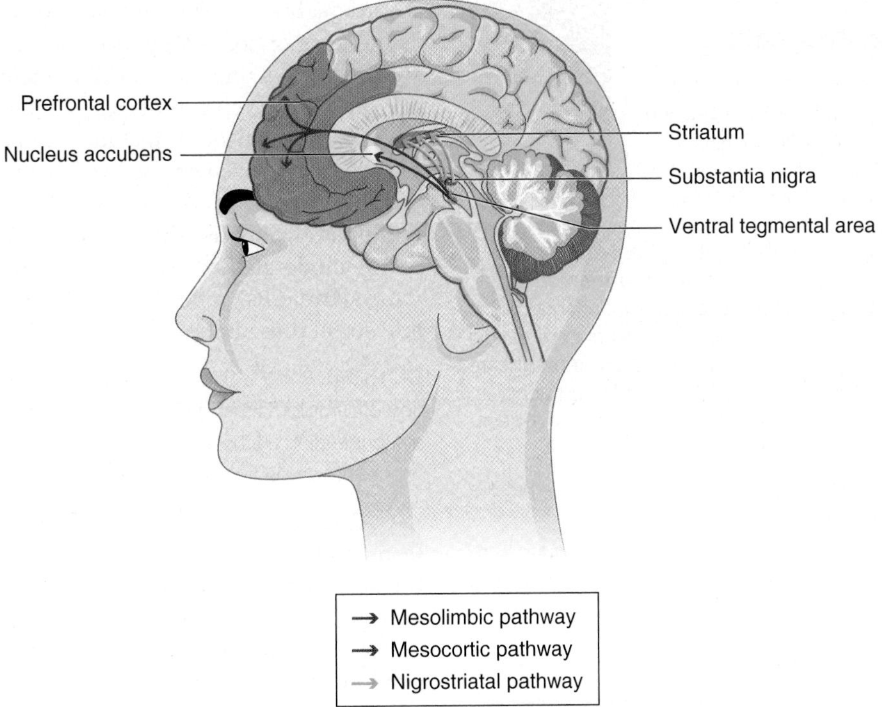

Figure 6.3 ■ Dopamine reward pathways.

are the defining characteristic of physical dependence on a substance.

While increased dopamine is the primary reward pathway, other neurotransmitters such as **serotonin** may modulate motivational factors that are associated with drug acquisition and also may help to regulate release of dopamine at the VTA of the brain. GABA, another neurotransmitter, is involved in modulation of dopamine through inhibitory effects on dopamine release onto dopaminergic neurons. Drugs such as alcohol, barbiturates, and **benzodiazepines** interact at the GABA receptor sites, inhibiting the release of GABA onto the dopaminergic receptors. This allows dopamine to flood the receptor sites; the end result is the euphoric sense of well-being and relaxation that people who use drugs seek. Mental illnesses and substance abuse tend to co-occur, since people will self-medicate to relieve mental distress or illness. Drug use increases the risk for mental illness, especially in individuals with a genetic predisposition or other vulnerabilities.[3,4]

Genetics and Genomics for Clinical Practice

Vulnerability to Dependency

Rita Kaspar

The biological differences that may make one person more vulnerable to dependency and another person less vulnerable may be associated with genetic differences. However, substance use disorders are complex diseases, making identification of the genes associated with the particular substance dependence very challenging. As is the case with other diseases, vulnerability to substance use and dependence is a complex trait. Many inherited and environmental factors determine the likelihood that someone will become dependent on a substance. Substance dependence often runs in families. Research suggests that variation in a key serotonin receptor gene can be linked to greater dopamine release in the anterior region of the brain, suggesting an association with the rewarding effects of dopamine and the crucial role it plays in continued drug use. The following genetic markers have been identified:

1. The A1 allele of the dopamine receptor gene *DRD2* occurs more often in people who are dependent on alcohol or cocaine.
2. Nonsmokers are more likely than smokers to carry a protective allele of the *CYP2A6* gene, which causes them to feel nauseated and dizzy when they smoke tobacco products, and findings identified a cluster of three nicotinic receptor subunit genes ($\alpha3$ $\alpha5$ $\beta4$) linked to smoking quantity, nicotine dependence, and the risk of two smoking-related diseases: lung cancer and peripheral arterial disease.
3. Alcoholism is rare in people with two copies of the *ALDH*2* gene variation.[5]

Juliet Hernandez: Application

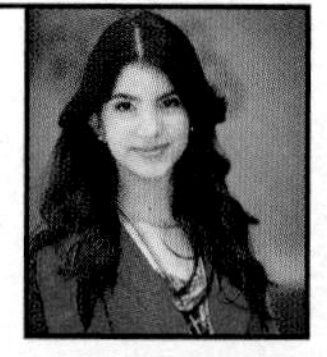

An evaluation of Ms. Hernandez begins with a thorough history and physical examination. She reports that she is currently unemployed and struggling as an artist, and she is living with her grandmother. She indicates needing financial help. She reports that both of her parents were addicted to drugs, and she experienced physical, sexual, and emotional abuse at their hands throughout her childhood. Her father died of liver disease at the age of 37. Ms. Hernandez reports smoking a pack of cigarettes daily but denies substance use except for drinking a few glasses of wine and smoking a few joints of marijuana with friends on weekends. The healthcare provider notes that Ms. Hernandez appears irritable and nervous. Her eyes are glassy, and she is unable to sit still during the assessment interview.

3. On the basis of the history given by Ms. Hernandez, what are her risk factors for substance use disorder?
4. What findings during physical examination cause you to suspect that Ms. Hernandez's substance use may be more than she described in her history?

Check Your Progress: Section 6.2

1. What is the function of the frontal cortex?
2. The ventral tegmental area (VTA) and nucleus accumbens are part of which neural circuit in the brain?
3. Which is the primary neurotransmitter involved in activating the reward circuit in the brain?

6.3 Alcohol Use Disorder

Excessive alcohol use is a leading cause of preventable death. This dangerous behavior accounted for approximately 88,000 deaths per year from 2006 to 2010.[6] Heavy alcohol use has been associated with increased risk for breast cancer, liver disease, heart disease, gastrointestinal disorders, brain abnormalities, and cognitive dysfunction. The effects of consuming a large amount of alcohol in a short period of time may result in violence, alcohol poisoning, and motor vehicle crashes.[7] Risk factors for developing an alcohol use disorder include interaction among genetic, psychologic, and environmental factors. The *Diagnostic and Statistical Manual of Mental Disorders*, Fifth Edition (DSM-5) identifies **alcohol use disorder** as mild (two or three symptoms), moderate (four or five symptoms), or severe (six or more symptoms), reflecting subclassifications of behavioral and social presentations.[8]

CLINICAL POINT: Because this is a progressive disorder, presentation of symptoms and general appearance will vary among individuals, depending on the amount they ingest and the period of time over which that amount is consumed. ■

Alcoholic beverages are made through a process of fermentation and distillation. Fermentation is the basis for all alcoholic beverages. The process of fermentation occurs with the action of yeast on sugar in the presence of water. Yeast combines with carbon, hydrogen, and oxygen from sugar into ethyl alcohol and carbon dioxide; thus, $C_6H_{12}O_6$ (glucose) is transformed into C_2H_5OH (ethyl alcohol + CO_2 [carbon dioxide]). Common alcohol products include beer, table wine, fortified wine (wine to which a distilled liquor has been added), distilled liquor, liqueurs, cordials or aperitifs, malt liquor, and alcopop (flavored alcohol products).[9] The amount of alcohol varies among these products (**Figure 6.4** ■).

Some of the alcohol that is ingested is absorbed in the stomach, but the majority is absorbed within the small intestine. The rate of absorption depends on both the concentration of alcohol in the beverage and whether it is taken with a meal. Upon ingestion, alcohol consumed with a meal remains in the stomach for digestive action, where protein in the food retains the alcohol along with the food. When alcohol is taken with water, the water decreases the concentration and slows the absorption of alcohol. However, carbonated liquids will speed up absorption because carbon

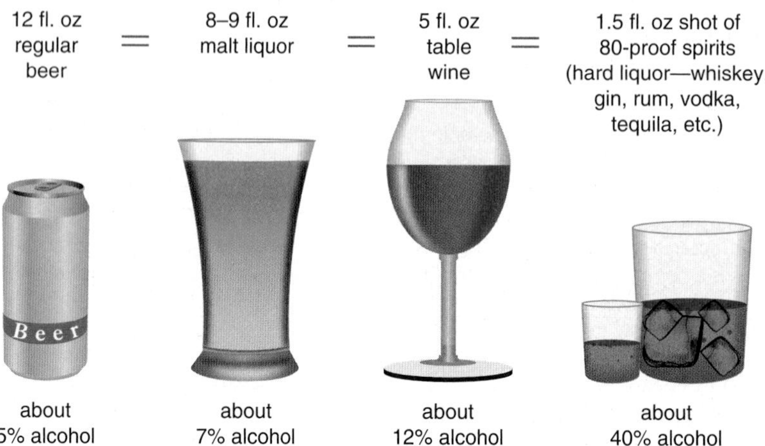

Figure 6.4 ■ One standard drink = 1/2 ounce of ethyl alcohol.

dioxide acts to move everything within the stomach rapidly into the small intestine. Thus, sparkling wines and champagne have a faster onset than wine.[3]

Unlike food, alcohol requires no digestion and is absorbed unchanged into the bloodstream. However, energy that is formed when alcohol is absorbed cannot be converted to lipids or protein and stored for later use. For this reason, when alcohol is in the system, other calories are not burned, and the rate at which fat is burned for energy decreases. Once alcohol has been absorbed, it remains in the bloodstream with other body fluids until it is metabolized in the liver. The metabolic process in the liver occurs when the enzyme alcohol dehydrogenase converts alcohol to acetaldehyde. In turn, acetaldehyde is rapidly converted to acetic acid by aldehyde dehydrogenase. Alcohol is removed from the body at a constant rate at about 0.25–0.03 ounces per hour, depending on the activity of the enzyme alcohol dehydrogenase. This metabolic rate is stable regardless of the blood alcohol concentration, exercise, or caffeine intake.

About 2% of the alcohol is excreted unchanged in breath, and a small amount is excreted through the skin and urine.[3] Heavy alcohol ingestion results in changes in the level of microsomal enzymes and higher blood levels of acetaldehyde that are normally at low levels to manage the usual intake. If an individual is taking other medications, these drugs are metabolized more slowly because alcohol is given first preference for metabolism. Once alcohol has been fully removed from the body, enzyme levels remain high, increasing medication metabolism.[3] Chapter 44 covers the effects of alcohol on the liver.

In the legal system, the **blood alcohol concentration (BAC)** is used to determine when an individual is under the influence of alcohol. The BAC measures the percentage of alcohol in the blood. In all 50 U.S. states, a BAC of 0.08 is considered too drunk to drive. **Table 6.1** ■ outlines various BACs and the effect of alcohol on the body at each level.

Etiology and Pathogenesis

Neurotransmitters can be excitatory or inhibitory, increasing or decreasing the brain's electrical activity, respectively. Alcohol enhances the effects of the inhibitory neurotransmitter GABA in the brain. At the same time, alcohol decreases the effects of the excitatory neurotransmitter **glutamate**. Alcohol also increases the concentration of dopamine in the brain's reward center. Ligand-gated ion channels also mediate the effects of alcohol. Of these channels, type A GABA receptors ($GABA_A$) appear to play a central role in mediating the effects of alcohol in the CNS. Since GABA is the primary inhibitory neurotransmitter, activation of $GABA_A$ receptors by GABA tends to decrease neuronal excitability. Additionally, the **N-methyl-D-aspartate (NMDA) receptor** is a glutamate-gated ion channel associated with excitatory neurotransmission in the brain.

Consumption of even small amounts of alcohol elicits a pleasant response because of alcohol's effect on the brain reward centers in the basal forebrain and in particular the nucleus accumbens and the amygdala. Alcohol is a sedative and a **depressant**, and when the drug is removed, the body recovers from CNS depression by rebounding with overstimulation, irritability, and nervousness. Alcohol use even in small amounts interrupts REM (rapid eye movement) sleep, making it difficult for the drinker to recover both physically and psychologically. As the amount of alcohol in the blood decreases, altered electrolytes and decreased blood glucose can lead to hand tremors and seizures in chronic heavy drinkers.

One major concern during pregnancy is fetal alcohol spectrum disorders, a group of conditions that can occur in an individual whose mother drank alcohol during pregnancy. Presentation of the disorder can include a mix of physical, behavior, and learning problems. Other risks to the fetus include cerebral palsy, premature birth, miscarriage, and stillbirth. The exact amount of alcohol that is safe to drink during or while considering pregnancy is unknown. Therefore, abstinence from all alcohol products, including beer and wine, is encouraged during pregnancy to promote healthy fetal development. While many pregnancies are unplanned and women typically do not know

Table 6.1 Effects of Blood Alcohol Concentration

BAC	Effects of BAC on the Drinker
0.02–0.03	Slight euphoria and loss of shyness Mildly relaxed; possibly ligh-theaded No loss of coordination
0.04–0.06	Feeling of well-being and euphoria Lowered inhibitions Relaxed with a sensation of warmth Minor impairment of reasoning and memory
0.07–0.09	Euphoria increases; judgment and self-control decrease Some impairment of balance, speech, vision, reaction time, hearing Caution, reason, and memory impaired Illegal to drive in all states
0.10–1.25	Continued euphoria Significant impairment of judgment and motor coordination Slurred speech; impaired balance, vision, reaction time, hearing
0.13–0.15	Euphoria decreases; dysphoria begins Gross impairment of motor skills and physical coordination Blurred vision; major loss of balance Judgment and perception severely impaired
0.16–0.19	Dysphoria increases Nausea may occur "Sloppy" drunk behavior
0.20–0.24	Dazed, confused, disoriented May need help to stand or walk Nausea and vomiting Blackouts may occur
0.25–0.29	All mental, physical, and sensory functions severely impaired Risk of asphyxiation from choking on vomit
0.30–0.34	Stupor Little comprehension of surroundings
0.35–0.39	Coma is possible
0.40 and up	Onset of coma Possible death due to respiratory arrest

that they are pregnant for the first 4–6 weeks, women are encouraged to stop drinking as soon as they are aware that they are pregnant, since the sooner they stop drinking, the lower are the health risks for the fetus.[10] ■

The developmental stage of adolescence is a time of experimentation and rapid physical and emotional changes. Adolescents and young adults ages 12–20 years drink 11% of all alcohol consumed in United States.[11] In adolescence, regular alcohol use or binge drinking tends to occur along with smoking, substance use, and risky sexual behavior, and the combination frequently causes biopsychosocial problems. ■

The National Institute on Alcohol Abuse and Alcoholism defines **binge drinking** as a pattern of drinking that brings BAC levels to 0.08 g/dL.[12] Probably the most critical area that is affected by early alcohol use is the disruption in normal growth and development and changes that occur in brain development. The adolescent brain is still developing, and alcohol use can increase the risk for mental health and neurocognitive problems that can persist into adulthood. Individuals who begin drinking at an early age are more likely as adults to engage in heavy alcohol use and develop dependence on the substance, which can further develop into more mental health and social problems.[13,14] Young people who drink alcohol are more likely to present with social and academic problems associated with arrests for driving while intoxicated, physically hurting or killing another person while drunk, and risky behaviors such as unprotected sexual activity and abuse of other drugs. Increased morbidity and mortality in this age group is associated with car crashes, falls, burns, drowning, and other unintentional injuries as well as alcohol poisoning and higher risk for suicide.[15]

Clinical Manifestations

The clinical manifestations of alcohol use vary with the amount of alcohol consumed and the frequency of consumption. Clinical manifestations depend on the BAC, as outlined in Table 6.1. In healthcare, alcohol use is categorized as **alcohol intoxication** (i.e., the BAC is sufficient to produce physical abnormalities consistent with behavioral changes) or **alcohol overdose** (i.e., the BAC is sufficient to produce impairments that increase the risk of harm, including death). Chronic abusers of alcohol will have clinical manifestations that tend to occur 24–72 hours after cessation of drinking, which is termed **alcohol withdrawal syndrome**.[3] The etiology and clinical manifestations and a brief description of diagnosis and treatment of alcohol abuse can be found in **Table 6.2** ■.

Table 6.2 Etiology and Clinical Manifestations of Alcohol Abuse

Etiology	Clinical Manifestations	Linking Pathophysiology to Diagnosis and Treatment
Alcohol Intoxication		
Alcohol intoxication is the consequence of alcohol entering the bloodstream faster than it can be metabolized by the liver, which breaks down the alcohol into nonintoxicating by-products.	Euphoria and relaxation Behavior changes; risky behavior Lowered inhibitions Cognitive impairment Ataxia (motor incoordination) Nausea, vomiting Blackouts Tachycardia Elevated blood pressure	Many of the effects of alcohol intoxication are the result of $GABA_A$ receptor activation and enhancement of serotonin and nicotinic acetylcholine receptors. Diagnosis is based on clinical symptoms (the history may be unreliable) along with a serum ethanol level and basic electrolytes. The general treatment includes rest, hydration, preventing access to alcohol, and protecting the person from injury.
Alcohol Overdose		
In an overdose situation, a dangerously high concentration of alcohol in the blood occurs. Situations in which there is naive use, such as in teenage binge drinking, can result in dangerous toxicity.	Unconsciousness Coma Respiratory depression Death	This is a medical emergency and is different from alcohol intoxication. It is important to discriminate when alcohol becomes a toxin to which the body cannot adapt. General diagnostic tests include serum alcohol and glucose, CBC, arterial blood gases, comprehensive metabolic panel, electrolytes, and urinalysis. Treatment includes supportive care, including close monitoring, strategies to prevent aspiration (e.g., elevating the head of the bed), oxygen therapy, intravenous fluids, vitamins, and glucose.
Alcohol Withdrawal Syndrome		
Severe life-threatening symptoms occur 24–72 hours after the last drink or reduction of use. Excessive drinking excites the nervous system. When a person drinks daily, over time the body becomes dependent on alcohol. When this happens, the CNS can no longer adapt easily to the lack or lowered amount of alcohol.	***Mild:*** Insomnia, irritability, anxiety, headache, nausea, anorexia, mild hypertension, mild tachycardia, tremors (mild) flushing, slight sweating, no confusion, oriented ***Moderate:*** Visibly tremulous, restless, and very anxious. Insomnia, nightmares, nausea and vomiting, variable confusion, transient hallucinations, elevated blood pressure, pulse 100–120, obvious sweating ***Severe:*** Uncontrollable shaking, agitation, intense fear, total wakefulness, dry heaves, vomiting, marked sweating, elevated blood pressure, pulse 120–140, confusion and disorientation, hallucinations and illusions, seizures, death	General diagnostic tests include serum glucose, CBC, arterial blood gases, comprehensive metabolic panel, electrolytes, and urinalysis. Symptoms of withdrawal are often treated with sedatives (benzodiazepines) to gradually assist the body in readapting to functioning without alcohol. Individuals withdrawing from alcohol are not always dehydrated, and overhydration with parenteral fluid can be harmful. Hypoglycemia is a danger during detoxification. Inclusion of carbohydrates in oral fluid (e.g., orange juice) is helpful. Fever should be monitored and its presence indicates a need for additional medication in the detoxification medication schedule. Assess for infection. Drug interaction may occur with the detoxification medication and other prescribed drugs.

Every organ in the body is affected by the toxic effects of alcohol or by its primary metabolite, acetaldehyde. Many heavy drinkers have chronic malnutrition. Fatty acids are the usual fuel for the liver, but when alcohol is present, alcohol is used as fuel instead, leading to fatty acid storage in the liver. This process can usually be reversed; but over time, with sustained heavy drinking and prolonged high levels of alcohol intake, destruction and inflammation can occur, with alcoholic hepatitis as the end result. Cirrhosis, another liver disease, can occur with prolonged alcohol use. In **cirrhosis**, liver cells are replaced by fibrous tissue, changing the composition of the liver such that the results are inadequate blood flow and impaired liver function. (See Chapter 44 for more information on alcoholic hepatitis and cirrhosis.)

Cancer is associated with heavy alcohol use not only in the liver but also in the mouth, tongue, pharynx, larynx, esophagus, stomach, lung, pancreas, colon, and rectum. Possible sources for tumor growth include direct tissue irritation from alcohol contact, nutritional deficiencies, suppression of the immune system, and induction of activating enzymes. Many drinkers also smoke cigarettes. The interaction of alcohol and cigarette smoke is associated with increased incidence of cancers in the oral cavity, pharynx, and larynx. Both cigarette smoking and heavy alcohol use are common suppressors of the immune system, increasing the risk for infectious diseases such as tuberculosis, pneumonia, hepatitis B, and HIV infection. Alcohol causes the bronchi to become irritated, inflamed, and susceptible to infection. Heavy drinkers have decreased ability to fight infections, owing to suppression of the immune system (decreased WBCs and macrophages). Alcohol has a numbing effect, and overly sedated drinkers find it difficult to expectorate. As a direct toxin to lung tissue, alcohol destroys alveoli, contributing to decreased lung air capacity and loss of elasticity. Chronic obstructive pulmonary disease (COPD) is common in this population and contributes to respiratory infections.[3] Long-term heavy drinking can cause alcoholic cardiomyopathy, hypertension, and stroke. Binge drinking and heavy drinking can lead to stroke through exacerbation of hypertension, arrhythmias, and cardiomyopathy.[3]

Hormonal changes associated with chronic alcohol use include decreased testosterone and increased estrogen in males. Decreased plasma testosterone results in decreased fertility and atrophic (shrunken) testes. Increased estrogen results in feminization features (loss of facial hair, possible breast enlargement); this often occurs in heavy chronic alcohol users.

Probably the largest area of concern is the effect of alcohol on the brain that is seen in heavy drinkers. Brain imaging through CT scans and MRI demonstrate tissue loss that is probably the direct result of alcohol toxicity rather than malnutrition. Excessive drinking does not kill brain cells directly but inhibits normal communication between brain cells by damaging dendrites at sites where they connect to another cell body through electrochemical stimulation; thus, communication among brain cells is interrupted. Organic brain syndrome, often seen in heavy drinkers, reflects a global decline in intellect, impaired problem solving ability, difficulty with fine motor skills, difficulty with swallowing, and abnormal electroencephalograms.

Two types of organic brain syndrome are commonly seen in **Wernicke-Korsakoff syndrome**. In Wernicke disease, symptoms of confusion, ataxia, and abnormal eye movements are associated with vitamin B_1 deficiency. These symptoms can be reversed through vitamins and improved diet. Most individuals with Wernicke disease also exhibit symptoms of Korsakoff psychosis, which includes difficulty remembering recent events or decreased ability to learn new information. This syndrome makes alcohol recovery difficult, given that the drinker cannot remember not to drink.

Vitamin deficiency, especially of thiamine (vitamin B_1), leads to peripheral neuropathy (tingling and numbness in the hands and feet) and to impaired production of the enzymes needed for maintaining myelination of the axon part of the nerve cell. This loss of covering causes destruction to nerve cells that culminates in tingling and numbness as well as muscle weakness. This nerve damage results in loss of balance and coordination, as seen in the characteristic wide-based gait that is used to maintain balance.[3]

James Wilson: Application

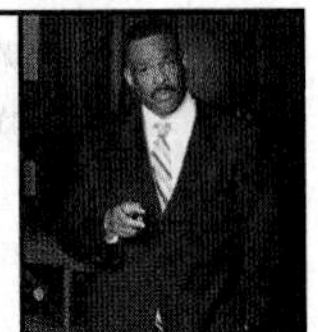

On examination, Mr. Wilson's vital signs are pulse 100, respirations 30, temperature 101°F, blood pressure 150/90, with labored breathing and shortness of breath. He has yellowish sclera, agitation, and confusion, and he had an episode of hematemesis while in the emergency department. Mr. Wilson is a thin man with weight 110 pounds and height 62 inches. Physical examination reveals hepatomegaly, pitting edema in both extremities, and an enlarged abdomen. Mr. Wilson's son reports, "After my mother died, Dad took it hard and seemed to drink more than his usual each night to cope with his grief." The son further elaborates that his father had a 15-year history of regular alcohol drinking (about a quart of beer daily) along with a pack or more of cigarettes a day.

3. What may have been the source of Mr. Wilson's hematemesis in the emergency department?
4. How has smoking cigarettes added to Mr. Wilson's medical issues?

Linking Pathophysiology to Diagnosis and Treatment

Either directly or indirectly, alcohol affects every organ in the body. For this reason, excessive alcohol use is a major health concern that continues to challenge healthcare providers and members of our society. The serious medical complications are numerous. The Centers for Disease Control and Prevention (CDC) reports that among adults ages 20–65 years, 1 in 10 deaths are due to excessive alcohol use.[16] Too often, a problem with alcohol is not addressed until physical symptoms develop. While alcohol use disorder is a chronic and progressive illness, the early symptoms are generally behavioral and not physical, and the behavior symptoms are easier to ignore. The majority of medical problems typically appear in the late, chronic stage of the illness.

CLINICAL POINT: Diagnosing the problem early before physical conditions occur enables early intervention and recovery from the disease. ■

Table 6.3 Common Laboratory Tests to Ascertain Level of Alcohol Use

Lab Test	Definition	Normal Values
Gamma-glutamyl transferase (GGT)	A liver enzyme that is increased by heavy alcohol intake and also by many other conditions that affect the liver. Most commonly used as a traditional biomarker. Primarily reflects liver damage that is often related to alcohol consumption. Performs best in adult ages 30–60 years. Low levels of GGT may indicate a magnesium deficiency.	Generally between 4300 and 10,800 cells/mm^3
Mean corpuscular volume (MCV)	Measures the size of red blood cells. May increase over time in heavy drinkers but may also be affected by many other conditions.	Normal range: 86–98 μm^3
Aminotransferases	Enzymes that are found primarily in the liver. Drinking too much alcohol, certain drugs, liver disease, and bile duct disease can cause high levels in the blood. Hepatitis is another problem that can raise these levels. Low levels of SGPT and SGOT may indicate deficiency of vitamin B6.	SGOT (AST): 5 to 40 units per liter of serum SGPT (ALT): 7–56 units per liter of serum
Bilirubin	A by-product of the routine destruction of red blood cells occurring in the liver, normally released as bile in the feces. Elevation of the bilirubin can suggest liver dysfunction. Other conditions with increased destruction of red blood cells can cause elevated bilirubin levels despite normal liver function.	0.1–1.0 mg/dL
Albumin level	A common protein found in the blood with a variety of functions. It is produced only in the liver, and lower than normal levels can be suggestive of chronic liver disease or liver cirrhosis. Many conditions other than liver disease also may cause low albumin levels.	3.5–5 g/dL
Coagulation panel or prothrombin time (PT or INR)	A measure of the blood's ability for normal clotting and prevention of bleeding and bruising; clotting factors are normally produced in the liver	9.5–13.8 seconds
Blood alcohol concentration (ethanol test)	Ethanol testing is used to determine the extent of a person's recent drinking but does not diagnose alcohol use disorder. A blood sample is more accurate than a level of alcohol found in the breath. See Table 6.1.	50–75 mg

A summary of common laboratory tests to ascertain the level of alcohol use can be found in **Table 6.3** ■.

In general, the treatments for alcohol use disorders include behavioral treatments (e.g., cognitive–behavioral therapy, motivational enhancement therapy, marital and family counseling); medications (e.g., naltrexone, acamprosate, disulfiram); and mutual support groups (e.g., Alcoholics Anonymous [AA]).[17] The major aim of such treatments is for the patient to stop drinking. Naltrexone can be used to stop the craving for alcohol; acamprosate can help people maintain alcohol abstinence; and disulfiram causes unpleasant effects (e.g., flushing of the face, headache, nausea, vomiting) when even small amounts of alcohol are consumed. Programs such as AA provide peer support for people whose goal is abstinence from alcohol.

Alcohol may have different effects on older people than on younger people. Adults over the age of 65 years are more likely to be affected by at least one chronic illness, many of which can make them more vulnerable to the negative effects of alcohol consumption. Older adults have a decrease in body water, increased sensitivity and decreased tolerance to alcohol, and decreased metabolism of alcohol in the gastrointestinal tract; as a result, a small amount of alcohol leaves them quickly feeling euphoric and overly relaxed. This may lead to impaired judgment, placing the individual at risk for automobile accidents, falls, and fractures. In addition, alcohol can cause brain changes that can be mistaken as signs of Alzheimer disease, as the older drinker may present with memory difficulties or become easily confused. Older adults and family may not recognize a change in drinking behavior, and the older adult may deny alcohol use when questioned by healthcare providers. Concerns may arise only after serious health or social problems emerge. Drinking in advanced age can facilitate the development of some cancers and liver damage, affect the immune system, and compromise existing conditions such as osteoporosis, diabetes, hypertension, ulcers, and altered cardiac status.

There is high comorbidity of alcohol use disorder with depression and anxiety, and rates for both increase in adults ages 50 years and older, increasing the risk for alcohol problems and misuse of prescription medication. Women in particular seem to be more affected by negative mood states, increasing their risk for depression and their vulnerability for alcohol use disorders.[18,19] Barriers to treatment for older adults vary depending on each person's situation and perspective on the healthcare system. Lack of available transportation can present barriers to attending hospital or clinic appointments or to regular AA attendance. Diminished social networks offer fewer friends for support or possibly for rides. Many older adults complain that they feel discounted or not listened to because many clinics do not focus services on the unique needs of older adults, such as hearing loss or ambulation limitations. In addition, many older people have limited time to attend regularly scheduled appointments, since they may be involved in the care of another family member or are caring for grandchildren. ■

James Wilson: Outcome

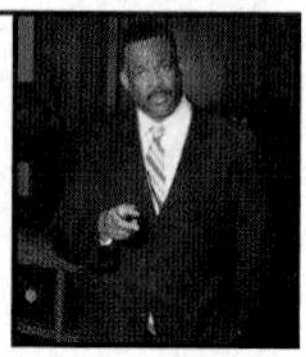

Mr. Wilson was admitted to the hospital after the blood tests and x-ray of his hand were completed in the emergency department. The results of his laboratory tests included elevated liver enzymes and slightly elevated creatinine and BUN. In addition, he was noted to be mildly anemic, with an increased MCV and decreased magnesium. Mr. Wilson was diagnosed with alcoholic liver disease and mild renal insufficiency. He was treated conservatively with fluids and electrolytes, including magnesium, and was started on thiamine. The physician decided to forgo a liver biopsy at this time. After consultation with the healthcare team, Mr. Wilson was discharged to home with instructions to begin attending AA meetings. The hospital social worker gave Mr. Wilson literature about local meetings and explored with him whether he had transportation to the meeting. At a 6-month follow-up visit, Mr. Wilson reports that he has stopped drinking, attends AA meetings regularly, and has moved into his son's home, where he enjoys helping to care for his grandchildren. His biochemical profile, including liver enzymes, has improved, and there is no immediate need for a liver biopsy.

5. What data will you use to track how serious Mr. Wilson's medical status is in relation to his drinking and smoking?
6. What factors contributed to Mr. Wilson's substance abuse?

Check Your Progress: Section 6.3

1. In all 50 states, at what BAC level is someone legally considered too drunk to drive?
2. How does alcohol ingestion affect sleep?
3. A pregnant woman has heard from her friends that drinking alcohol in moderation is permissible during pregnancy. What patient education is important?
4. What medications are used for treatment of alcohol use disorder?

6.4 Tobacco Use Disorder

Historically tobacco as an herb was considered to be useful for treating a number of disorders. As early as 1529 A.D., tobacco was reported to be helpful in the treatment of headaches, the common cold, and sores on the head.[3] **Tobacco use disorder** is characterized by the harmful consequences of persistent tobacco use, a pattern of compulsive tobacco use, and (sometimes) physiologic dependence on tobacco (i.e., tolerance and/or withdrawal). Current evidence supports that smokers compared to nonsmokers suffer from poorer general health beginning at an early age and extending throughout adult life. While a decline in cigarette smoking among adults from 42% in 1965 to 18% was reported in 2012, more than 42 million Americans continue to smoke tobacco. Trends in the United States suggest that particularly for youth and young adults, the use of multiple tobacco products has increased, and **vaping** (use of e-cigarettes) by middle and high school students has increased by 50%.[20]

Tobacco is a leafy plant, and dried tobacco leaves can be shredded and smoked in cigarettes, cigars, and pipes; ground into snuff and sniffed through the nose; made into chewing tobacco; or moistened, ground, or shredded into dip and placed in the mouth between the lip and gum.[21] Tobacco is an addictive substance because it contains the chemical nicotine. Addiction to nicotine makes it very difficult to quit smoking and the use of other tobacco products.[21] Current research demonstrates that nicotine may not be the only ingredient in tobacco that influences the addictive potential of tobacco. Since 2000, the content of the cigarettes has been different from that of the cigarettes of the previous decades. In 1950, the required content for 1000 cigarettes was 2.5 pounds (1.2 kg) of leaf tobacco; today, only about 1.34 pounds (0.8 kg) are required to produce the same number of cigarettes. Today, there are approximately 600 ingredients in cigarettes that when burned create more than 7000 chemicals. A list of common substances found in tobacco products can be found in **Table 6.4** ■.

Adolescent brains maybe more vulnerable to the effects of the chemical changes caused by tobacco use and more susceptible to the addictive potential. ■

The peak plasma concentration of nicotine depends on the method of delivery. For example, smoking (inhalation) is associated with the fastest and highest peak plasma concentrations; while delivery from other systems, such as smokeless tobacco, is much slower. When nicotine is inhaled through smoking, it is rapidly absorbed into the pulmonary venous circulation and circulated via the arterial circulation to the brain. Nicotine diffuses into brain tissue, where it binds to nicotinic cholinergic receptors (nAChRs) located in the **mesolimbic pathway**, which is the dopaminergic, or reward, system of the brain.[22] The absorption of nicotine through the mucous membranes is modulated by pH. Since nicotine is a weak base, absorption is enhanced by increasing the pH. Chewing tobacco and snuff are formulated with alkalizing chemicals to increase the absorption of nicotine.[22] Nicotine is rapidly metabolized in the liver by the cytochrome P450 system, specifically CYP2A6 and to a lesser extent the CYP2B6 and CYP2E1 enzymes, and then to cotinine. Nicotine has a half-life of 1–2 hours. The clearance of the CYP2A6 enzyme appears to be influenced by a variety of factors, including genetic, racial, and hormonal factors. For example, genetically slow metabolism of nicotine may be associated with decreased dependence. Cotinine is excreted in the urine, has a half-life of

Table 6.4 Selected Chemicals Found in Tobacco Smoke

Chemicals Found in Tobacco Smoke	Other Uses for These Chemicals
Acetone	Found in nail polish remover
Acetic acid	An ingredient in hair dye
Ammonia	A common household cleaner
Arsenic	Used in rat poison
Benzene	Found in rubber cement
Butane	Used in lighter fluid
Cadmium	Active component in battery acid
Carbon monoxide	Released in car exhaust fumes
Formaldehyde	Embalming fluid
Hexamine	Found in charcoal lighter fluid
Lead	Used in batteries
Naphthalene	An ingredient in moth balls
Methanol	A main component in rocket fuel
Nicotine	Used as insecticide
Tar	Material for paving roads
Toluene	Used to manufacture paint

approximately 19 hours, and is widely used a biomarker of nicotine exposure.[22]

Etiology and Pathogenesis

Most smokers consistently smoke cigarettes at a rate that provides about 1–2 micrograms of nicotine per kilogram of body weight with each drag on the cigarette. This seems to be the dose that is required to stimulate the cerebral cortex. In tasks that require rapid information processing or alert attention, nicotine increases performance through activation of areas of the brain associated with visual attention, arousal, and motor activation.[23] Repeated exposure to nicotine over time results in the development of tolerance, the condition in which higher doses of a drug are required to produce the same initial effect. The rapid metabolism of nicotine requires frequent dosing to maintain a steady level of nicotine. During the period spent in sleep, the smoker is nicotine free and some tolerance is lost, prompting smokers to report that the first cigarette in the morning is the best or strongest smoke of the day. As the day progresses, tolerance is reestablished, and later cigarettes have less effect, so the person requires more frequent dosing to achieve that first cigarette effect and to alleviate anxiety associated with the lowering nicotine level in the brain.[3]

The effect of nicotine extends to areas outside of the CNS as it mimics acetylcholine occupying the cholinergic receptor, thus preventing incoming impulses and blocking further transmission of information into the synapses. Nicotine acts as both a stimulant and a sedative. Once exposed to nicotine, the smoker experiences the stimulant effect caused partly by nicotine's stimulation of release of epinephrine from the adrenal glands as well as other sympathetic nervous system (SNS) sites. This sudden increase of epinephrine causes a corresponding increase in serum glucose, blood pressure, heart rate, and respiration. As a result of this release of epinephrine, there is increased coronary blood flow, vasoconstriction in the skin, and increased heart rate and blood pressure. This increase in heart rate increases the need for oxygen but does not increase the oxygen supply, placing increased stress on the cardiovascular system.[3]

CLINICAL POINT: Smoking is linked to a number of chronic conditions, including respiratory infections, COPD, and malignant diseases such as lung cancer.[3] The immune system is also compromised by tobacco. Smokers are at increased risk for infections such as pneumonia, respiratory infections, bloodborne viruses, and sexually transmitted diseases, especially individuals who may already have compromised immune systems.[24] ■

4 Smoking tobacco has serious effects on reproductive health. Smoking can make it difficult for a woman to get pregnant and increases the risk for miscarriage for those who continue to smoke during pregnancy. Serious complications that may be related to maternal tobacco smoking during pregnancy include premature birth, certain birth defects such as cleft lip or cleft palate, low birth weight, and infant death. Women who smoke can experience other medical problems during pregnancy such as separation of the placenta from the uterus too early, which causes dangerous bleeding and health risks to both mother and baby. ■

Clinical Manifestations

Initially, the signs and symptoms of tobacco use may be attributed not directly to use of tobacco but to another problem, such as a mental disorder or respiratory problem. A general assessment of a patient may reveal signs consistent with tobacco use such as clothing that smells of smoke, a bottle for chew or dip spit, cigarette packs, stained teeth or fingernails, wrinkles, or a hoarse voice (**Figure 6.5** ■).[25] Some immediate effects of nicotine use are tachycardia, hypertension, and increased respiration.[25] Signs and symptoms of tobacco withdrawal are not life threatening. In general, they are characterized by four or more of the following: irritability/frustration/anger, anxiety, difficulty concentrating, increased appetite, restlessness, depressed mood, and insomnia.

Among adolescents and adults who smoke tobacco, there is high psychiatric comorbidity, including abuse of other substances. It is estimated that individuals with psychiatric disorders buy approximately 44% of all cigarettes sold in the United States. The rate of depression in young adults is highest among smokers and lowest in individuals who quit or never started smoking. In adults, there is an increased incidence of anxiety disorders among tobacco users, but this may be associated with withdrawal symptoms. The largest comorbidity exists among people with serious mental illness (i.e., schizophrenia, bipolar disorder), in whom rates of smoking are as high as 90%.[26]

In its early stages, use of tobacco rarely causes interruption in employment, meeting home obligations, or

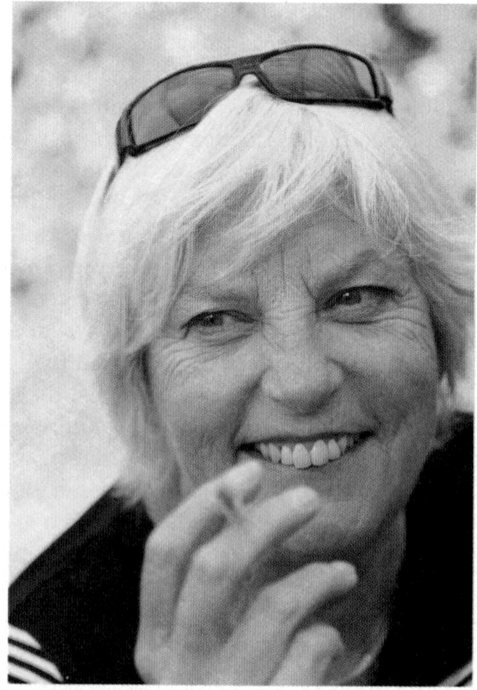

Figure 6.5 ■ Smoking speeds up the aging process of the skin. Nicotine causes narrowing of the blood vessels in the outermost layer of the skin, which impairs oxygenation of the skin, leading to wrinkles. Smokers often have stained teeth and fingers.

social problems. Medical complications develop gradually, first with an acute cough and later with chronic respiratory problems. Tobacco use disorder is diagnosed only when tobacco use becomes persistent and causes significant occupational and social issues (e.g., arguments about smoking, smoking in restricted areas, frequent sick calls) or when the use is physically hazardous (e.g., smoking in bed, smoking around flammable chemicals) or results in legal difficulties.

Smoking is linked to a number of chronic conditions, including respiratory infections, COPD, and malignant diseases such as lung cancer.[3] The immune system is also compromised by tobacco. Smokers are at increased risk for infections such as pneumonia, respiratory infections, bloodborne viruses, and sexually transmitted diseases, especially tobacco users who may already have compromised immune systems.[24]

In youths who smoke, those who have behavioral problems are at increased risk for mental disorders such as conduct disorders and attention-deficit/hyperactivity disorder. Increased depression and anxiety increase the risk for suicide, especially in adolescent users.[26,27] ■

Linking Pathophysiology to Diagnosis and Treatment

Although the medical consequences are typically not evident until age 40, smokers begin to show effects that continue to multiply over time. Reversing medical harm needs to occur early and can be facilitated by smoking cessation aids and nicotine replacement medication that does not appear to cause harm. The most common diseases connected to smoking are cardiovascular disorders, COPD, and cancers. Smoking during pregnancy increases the risk of low birth weight and miscarriage. Individuals who suffer from mental illness are at a higher risk of developing a tobacco use disorder.

CLINICAL POINT: It is well known that half of all smokers will die from tobacco-related disease if they do not quit. ■

Smokeless tobacco, a type of tobacco that is not burned to provide its effect, such as various forms of chewing tobacco and snuff. has advantages over smoking, as it is unlikely to cause lung cancer. However, it is not without risks, given that the smokeless tobacco products are absorbed from the mouth or nose along with other compounds in the tobacco. While not burned during use, these products contain potent carcinogens, including nitrosamines. The greatest concern in nonsmoked tobacco products is increased risk for cancer of the mouth, tongue, cheek, gums, pharynx, and esophagus. Other risks associated with smokeless tobacco include stomach and pancreatic cancer, leukopenia (from white sores in the mouth that can become cancer), bone loss around the roots of the teeth, tooth loss, stained and discolored teeth, and bad breath. E-cigarettes are a recent development in the smokeless tobacco movement and have not been fully studied.

CLINICAL POINT: Exposure to **secondhand smoke (SHS)**, that is, smoke from tobacco that is being smoked by someone else, is suggested to be the cause of more deaths due to cardiovascular disease than to lung cancer in nonsmoking adults as well as serious health conditions in children, including sudden infant death syndrome, respiratory infections, and more severe asthma.[23,28] ■

While lung cancer is the most prominent culprit in morbidity related to tobacco use in the United States, cardiovascular disease claims more lives of smokers 35 years of age and older every year.

Treatments for smoking cessation include individual and group behavioral therapy, over-the-counter products (nicotine gum); prescription nicotine replacement products (nicotine patch, inhaler, nasal spray); and prescription nonnicotine products (bupropion).

The 2012 Surgeon General's Report indicates that about 90% of all smokers first tried cigarettes as teens; reflecting that, about three of every four teen smokers continue smoking into adulthood.[29] ■

Impact of Current Research on Clinical Practice

Identifying Disease Risk and Possible Outcome

Description: The study of a novel intervention, REFRESH, which is aimed at reducing children's exposure to SHS in their homes, included 59 smoking mothers with at least one child younger than 6 years. The randomized feasibility study included four home visits over a 1-month period, which involved two 24-hour measurements of home air quality and a motivational interview to encourage changes in smoking behavior within the home to reduce child SHS exposure. The enhanced group received their air quality data as part of their motivational interview at visit two; the control group received that information at visit four.

Clinical Practice: On being interviewed, the mothers reported that they were able to understand the data they were shown and were shocked by the values measured in their homes despite having been aware of the effects of SHS exposure. They appreciated the intervention taking place in their homes, as it allowed them to have personalized data. In response to the information and encouragement through motivational interviewing, many of the mothers changed their smoking behaviors in their home and in particular were motivated to protect their own children as a result of the knowledge they had gained. This approach can be used in home visits to encourage behavior change in homes where smoking occurs and small children reside.

Research Study:

Wilson, I., Semple, S., Mills, L. M., et al. (2013). REFRESH—Reducing families' exposure to secondhand smoke in the home: A feasibility study. *Tobacco Control, 22*(5), e8.

Check Your Progress: Section 6.4

1. What effects does nicotine have on brain function?
2. What are the effects of cigarette smoking on pregnancy?
3. What is the relationship between cigarette smoking and serious mental illness?

6.5 Cannabis Use Disorder

Cannabis, a flowering plant in the genus *Cannabaceae*, is the source of the most-used drug after alcohol and tobacco in the United States. In 2014, about 22.2 million people ages 12 years and up reported having used marijuana during the past month.[30] In that same year, 2.6 million people in the same age range reported having used marijuana for the first time within the past 12 months.[30]

Marijuana is a greenish-gray mixture of the dried, shredded leaves and flowers of cannabis, the hemp plant. It may consist of *Cannabis sativa*, *Cannabis indica*, or a hybrid of the two. The main psychoactive chemical in marijuana is delta-9-tetrahydro-cannabinol, commonly called **tetrahydrocannabinol (THC)**.[31] Marijuana can be smoked via hand-rolled cigarettes, pipes, water pipes, or cigars. Additionally, marijuana can be mixed into foods such as brownies, cookies, or candies. Concentrated resins and oils containing high doses of THC and/or another active ingredient, cannabidiol, are increasingly popular for both medical and recreational use.[31]

Classic studies on the pharmacologic properties of marijuana were done during the 1980s and 1990s.[32,33] THC, the active ingredient in marijuana, is one of a group of chemicals called cannabinoids. The metabolic and absorption properties of THC depend on the delivery method. Approximately 50% of the THC in a marijuana cigarette is inhaled through smoke, is absorbed in the lungs, and rapidly enters the bloodstream, reaching the brain within minutes.[34] The bioavailability of THC following oral ingestion is reduced in comparison to smoking the same dose. In addition, oral ingestion of THC has a delayed response and longer duration. THC and other cannabinoids are lipid soluble and accumulate in fatty tissues; they reach peak concentrations within 4–5 days.[34] The tissue elimination half-life of THC is approximately 7 days. Total elimination of a single dose takes approximately 30 days.[33]

Etiology and Pathogenesis

There are cannabinoid receptors, CB1 and CB2, located throughout the body. These receptors are activated by endogenous cannabinoids and are located in the CNS (basal ganglia, hippocampus, cerebellum, and cortex) and peripheral sites (immune cells and spleen).[35] The mechanism of action of marijuana results from the binding of cannabis to CB1 and CB2 receptors. This binding results in psychoactive and systemic effects in the peripheral tissues.[35] THC, in particular, has been shown to release dopamine from the nucleus accumbens and prefrontal cortex that may increase the rewarding properties of the drug.[35] Since THC affects the frontal cortex areas of the brain, judgment can become impaired, and the individual may engage in risk-taking behaviors such as driving while high on marijuana or risky sexual behaviors. A recent study that followed people from ages 13 to 38 years found that those who were heavy marijuana users in their teens had up to an 8-point drop in IQ even if they quit in adulthood, highlighting the effect of marijuana on hippocampus function.[36]

Clinical Manifestations

Marijuana's immediate effects include distorted perception, difficulty with thinking and problem solving, and loss of motor coordination. Psychoactive symptoms may include anxiety, paranoia, poor eye contact, agitation, both grandiose and paranoid delusions, and psychosis. Physiologic effects of marijuana intoxication include conjunctival injection, tachycardia, diaphoresis, and dry mouth. Heavy marijuana use in youth has been linked to increased risk for developing mental illness and poorer cognitive functioning. Some symptoms of **cannabis use disorder** include disruptions in functioning due to cannabis use, the development of tolerance, cravings for cannabis, and the development of withdrawal symptoms, such as the inability to sleep, restlessness, nervousness, anger, or depression within a week of ceasing heavy use.[36] Long-term use of the drug can contribute to respiratory infection, impaired memory, and exposure to cancer-causing compounds.[35]

CLINICAL POINT: Synthetic cannabinoids refer to a growing number of synthetic psychoactive chemicals that are sprayed on dried, shredded plant material for smoking or are sold as liquids to be vaporized and inhaled in e-cigarettes and other devices. These chemicals are called synthetic cannabinoids because they are related to chemicals found in the marijuana plant. Synthetic cannabinoids represent a group of new psychoactive substances that are erroneously called synthetic marijuana and are purported to be safe.[37] These are synthetic compounds with cannabinoid-like actions but not necessarily a cannabinoid chemical structure. They may be pure **agonists** with high affinity at the CB1 receptor, differing from THC, which is a partial agonist at both the CB1 and CB2 receptors.[38] These synthetic cannabinoids can produce intense, prolonged adverse effects characterized by signs and symptoms such as tachycardia, agitation, sedation, and psychosis that sometimes require hospitalization.[38,39] However, there is a role for regulated and FDA-approved synthetic cannabinoids in the treatment of various disorders. For example, the U.S. Food and Drug Administration (FDA) has approved dronabinol and nabilone for oral administration in the treatment of anorexia associated with weight loss in patients with AIDS and for nausea and vomiting associated with cancer chemotherapy in patients who have not responded to traditional antiemetic treatments.[38] ■

Linking Pathophysiology to Diagnosis and Treatment

There are specific diagnostic criteria in DSM-5 for cannabis intoxication, cannabis withdrawal, and cannabis use disorders.[8] A general overview of these criteria is provided below. The diagnostic criteria for *cannabis intoxication* specifies that the patient experiences at least two of the following signs or symptoms within a 2-hour period of using cannabis that cannot be attributed to any other drug or medical condition:

conjunctival injection, increased appetite, dry mouth, and tachycardia.[8] *Cannabis withdrawal* is diagnosed by the following criteria: cessation of frequent and prolonged cannabis usage that has been daily over the period of several months along with the exhibition of three or more of the following signs and symptoms over the course of approximately 1 week: irritability, anger, or depression; nervousness or anxiety; sleep difficulty (e.g., insomnia); decreased appetite or weight loss; restlessness; depressed mood; and at least one physical symptom causing discomfort (e.g., sweating, fever, chills, headache).[8] These psychologic and/or physical symptoms must cause significant impairment to important areas of life functioning (e.g., social and occupational).

Cannabis use disorder is the significant impairment or distress in multiple areas of functionality and also development of tolerance and withdrawal to the drug over a 12-month period. DSM-5 provides a comprehensive list of areas of life functioning that may be impaired by cannabis use, such as persistent use of cannabis negatively affecting the individual's ability to fulfill roles at work, school, or home; or persistent use of cannabis in physically hazardous conditions. The diagnosis of cannabis use disorder may be classified as mild, moderate, or severe. The treatment for cannabis use disorder involves approaches such as cognitive–behavioral therapy (CBT). CBT is a form of psychotherapy that allows people to identify strategies to correct problematic behaviors such as drug use.[40]

Medical use of cannabis is now legal in 29 states and the District of Columbia, and recreational use is legal in 8 states and the District of Columbia. Medically, cannibis is used to increase appetite and decrease nausea, to lessen the severity of seizures, and to reduce pain and inflammation. Research is ongoing in areas such as treating brain cancer, autoimmune diseases, HIV/AIDS, and multiple sclerosis (see Impact of Research on Clinical Practice).[41–43]

Check Your Progress: Section 6.5

1. What psychoactive substance is found in cannabis?
2. Does cannabis use in adolescence have a permanent effect on the individual?
3. What are some of the potential medical uses of cannabis as a therapeutic agent?

6.6 Stimulant Use Disorders

While stimulants encompass a large range of substances, the most commonly abused stimulants are amphetamines, synthetic cathinones, methamphetamine, and cocaine.[30] In 2014, the Substance Abuse and Mental Health Services Administration reported that an estimated 913,000 people age 12 years and older had a stimulant use disorder due to cocaine use; 569,000 people in the United States age 12 years and older reported using methamphetamines in the past month; and an estimated 476,000 people had a stimulant use disorder as a result of using other stimulants besides methamphetamines.[30]

Stimulants can be synthetic (such as amphetamines) or plant-derived (such as cocaine). They may be inhaled through the nose or taken orally or intravenously.[30] Amphetamines were originally developed as nasal decongestants and were eventually used as weight loss drugs. Amphetamine sulfates and related drugs (e.g., ephedra) have a long history of abuse in the United States. Cathinones are amphetamine analogs; the newer synthetic cathinones (known as bath salts) have become sources of abuse along with methamphetamines.[44] Cocaine, derived from the leaves of the *Erythroxylum coca* plant, is a major source of addiction in the United States.[45]

The understanding of synthetic cathinones remains limited, but they are thought to have characteristics similar to

Impact of Current Research on Clinical Practice

Medical Uses of Cannabis

Description: As early as 1975, researchers were able to show that there were positive medicinal uses for oral THC, particularly antiemetic properties. The FDA approved the cannabinoid medication dronabinol in 1985 for use in helping patients with cancer who were on chemotherapy to gain weight and in 1992 for appetite stimulation in patients with AIDS.[41] A recent National Institutes of Health report on medical marijuana indicates that most marijuana that is sold as medicine has the same quality and carries the same health risks as street-grade marijuana.[42] Scientist are also interested in the marijuana chemical cannabidiol (CBD), an oil form of the drug that may be less desirable for recreational use, since it is not intoxicating. Plants are bred to produce this oil in the hope of using it to treat conditions such as childhood epilepsy. Other work being conducted includes animal studies that have shown that marijuana extracts can destroy certain cancer cells and reduce the size of others. Some evidence supports the use of purified extracts from whole-plant marijuana that can help in the treatment of some of the most serious types of brain tumors. Other areas of research include using extracts to treat autoimmune diseases, HIV/AIDS, and multiple sclerosis.[43]

Clinical Impact: It is important to know the laws of the state in which you will practice healthcare. When you know what is and is not legal in your state, you are better prepared to help your patients.

Research Studies:

National Institute on Drug Abuse. (2016). *Monitoring the future.* Available at https://www.drugabuse.gov/related-topics/trends-statistics/monitoring-future

National Institute on Drug Abuse. (2014). *Drugs, brains, and behavior: The science of addiction.* Available at https://www.drugabuse.gov/publications/drugs-brains-behavior-science-addiction/preface

National Institute on Drug Abuse. (2015). *Drug facts: Is marijuana medicine?* Available at https://www.drugabuse.gov/publications/drugfacts/marijuana-medicine

those of amphetamines.[46] Since amphetamines are lipophilic, they are able to cross the blood–brain barrier and produce a rapid onset of effects when they are injected or inhaled. Oral ingestion of amphetamines leads to peak concentrations within 2 hours, while cathinone peaks following oral ingestion within 1 hour.[46] The half-lives of amphetamines and cathinones differ by specific drug; they range from 3 to 24 hours but can extend to 30 hours. Amphetamines are metabolized by the liver and eliminated through the kidney.[46]

Methamphetamine is readily absorbed after administration via oral, pulmonary, nasal, intramuscular, intravenous, rectal, and vaginal routes.[43] Methamphetamine is lipophilic, so it readily crosses the blood–brain barrier. The onset of action occurs within seconds after smoking or injecting; the effects may be observed within 5 minutes after intranasal use or within 20 minutes following oral ingestion.[46] Peak plasma concentrations are achieved approximately 30 minutes after intravenous or intramuscular administration and up to 2–3 hours after ingestion. Although methamphetamine has a plasma half-life of 12–34 hours, the duration of its effect commonly persists beyond 24 hours.[46] Elimination of methamphetamine occurs through several hepatic and renal pathways, including cytochrome CYP2D6. Of interest is that polymorphisms of CYP2D6 have been implicated in cases of unanticipated toxicity.[46] Additionally, the degradation of methamphetamine can result in active metabolites that can accumulate with repeated, frequent, or binge use.[46]

Illegal cocaine exists in two forms: base (also known as crack or freebase) and salt.[47] While each of these forms of cocaine exerts the same pharmacologic actions on reaching the brain or target organ, they differ in important properties that are associated with the route of administration. For example, cocaine base can be smoked because it has a relatively low melting point (98°C) and is relatively insoluble in water. This makes it difficult to dissolve for injection administration. Cocaine salt, in contrast, cannot be smoked because it melts at 195°C.[47] Cocaine salt can be injected or inhaled through the nose. In contrast to cocaine base, cocaine salt is highly water soluble and can be used for injection purposes and facilitating absorption across mucous membranes.[47]

Cocaine is readily absorbed through the mucous membranes of the nose and mouth and from the genitourinary, gastrointestinal, and respiratory tracts. The onset of action for cocaine depends on the route of administration. Intravenous or inhaled administration of cocaine results in an onset of action within seconds; intranasal or gastrointestinal administration result in slower onsets of 20–30 minutes and up to 90 minutes, respectively.[48] The effects of intravenous or inhaled cocaine administration usually lasts 15–30 minutes; the effects of intranasal and gastrointestinal administration last approximately 1 hour and 3 hours, respectively.[48] Cocaine is metabolized primarily in the liver. The primary metabolite is benzoylecgonine, which is the metabolite found in highest concentration in urine and is detectable in the urine for up to 8 days after cocaine consumption. It is this metabolite that is measured in urine drug tests for cocaine.[48]

Etiology and Pathogenesis

Amphetamines and Cathinones. The primary pharmacologic use of amphetamines is for its CNS effects. Amphetamines have been approved by the FDA for the treatment of narcolepsy and attention-deficit/hyperactivity disorder.[49] Though appropriate for use in treating these conditions, they have become a source of abuse for nonprescribed users. The primary activity of amphetamines is to increase the synaptic activity of neurotransmitters (dopamine and **norepinephrine**). Synthetic cathinones are synthetic drugs that are chemically related to cathinone, a stimulant found in the khat plant. The khat plant is native to East Africa and the Arabian peninsula, and its leaves are chewed for their mild stimulant effects. The synthetic variants of cathinone can be much stronger than the khat plant and can be very dangerous.[50]

Methamphetamine. Methamphetamine (meth) is closely related to amphetamines. **Methamphetamine** is a psychostimulant that causes an increase in the synapse of monoamines, including dopamine, norepinephrine, and serotonin, whose primary effects are mediated through the dopamine reward system. Long-term use of methamphetamine is associated with significant health problems. Chronic methamphetamine users may be unable to function in social and occupational settings. The course of methamphetamine abuse can be lengthy and prolonged with periodic episodes of intense use followed by periods of sobriety and then relapse.

Cocaine. Cocaine exerts its effects by blocking reuptake of the neurotransmitters dopamine and norepinephrine in the central and peripheral nervous system, thus enhancing the activity of these neurotransmitters. Chronic use may result in pronounced pulmonary, cardiovascular, and CNS changes along with overdose and death. While the initial effects may include euphoria, enhanced self-esteem, and increased libido, more chronic effects may include paranoia, confusion, and decreased libido. Conditions associated with visits to the emergency department include chest pain, palpitations, psychiatric conditions, seizures, delirium, suicidal ideation, and overdose.[30]

Clinical Manifestations

Neuropsychiatric signs and symptoms can exist in both amphetamine and cathinone use; however, they are more common and pronounced in cathinone intoxication. This is especially true of the violent and self-harming behaviors. **Table 6.5** ■ presents the signs and symptoms of stimulant use disorder by concepts and body system for each type of stimulant.

Linking Pathophysiology to Diagnosis and Treatment

The cardiovascular symptoms of acute cocaine intoxication must be emphasized. The cardiovascular consequences of cocaine use are extensive and can be deadly. Cocaine-induced SNS effects include increased sensitivity to norepinephrine; inhibition of catecholamine reuptake; and increased heart rate, blood pressure, myocardial

Table 6.5 Signs and Symptoms of Stimulant Use Disorders

Systems/Concepts Affected by Stimulant Intoxication	Amphetamine and Cathinone Intoxication	Methamphetamine Intoxication	Cocaine Intoxication
Cardiovascular symptoms/Perfusion	Tachycardia Palpitations Hypertension Dysrhythmias	Tachycardia Hypertension Arrhythmias Chest pain Hypotension Acute and chronic cardiomyopathy	Chest pain Tachycardia Hypertension Myocardial ischemia Myocardial infarction Heart failure Hemorrhagic or ischemic stroke Dysrhythmias Thrombus formation
Renal symptoms/Elimination	Acute kidney injury	Acute renal failure	Kidney failure
Fluid and Electrolyte Balance	Hypokalemia Hyponatremia Hypermagnesemia	Dehydration Metabolic acidosis	
Neurologic symptoms/Intracranial Regulation	Tremors Seizures Myoclonus Intracerebral hemorrhage	Seizures Focal neurologic defects Choreiform movements	Seizures
Mood, affect, cognition, and trauma/ Emotional Regulation	Combativeness Hallucinations Confusion Violent behavior Self-inflicted injury	Alertness Agitation Euphoria Disorganized thinking Increased energy Increased sexual urges Disrupted sleep patterns Excessive talking Mood changes Psychosis	Anxiety Euphoria Panic attack Irritability Paranoia Restlessness Altered sexual function Increased energy Excited and exuberant speech
Musculoskeletal and skin disorders/Mobility and Tissue Integrity	Cellulitis Abscess formation Necrotizing fasciitis (from injection)	Tightened jaw muscles Grinding teeth Tooth decay Thermal burns (from drug preparation)	Muscle pain Damage to nose and sinus tissues
Nutrition and gastrointestinal symptoms/ Nutrition and Digestion, Metabolism, and Elimination		Dry mouth Loss of appetite Nausea and vomiting Diarrhea	Perforated gastric ulcers Ischemic colitis Intestinal infarction
Thermoregulation and Sensory Perception	Hyperthermia Diaphoresis Mydriasis	Hyperthermia Diaphoresis	Mydriasis

contractility, and myocardial oxygen demand.[51] Cocaine-induced effects on cardiomyocytes include mitochondrial damage and cell death, disruption in excitation coupling, and blockade of sodium and potassium channels. Cocaine-induced effects on vasculature include vasoconstriction and a prothrombotic state, increased platelet aggregation, endothelial dysfunction, thrombosis, and decreased myocardial oxygen supply.[51] The long-term cardiovascular consequences include atherosclerosis, cardiomyopathy and heart failure, aortic dissection, and endocarditis.[51]

Juliet Hernandez: Outcome

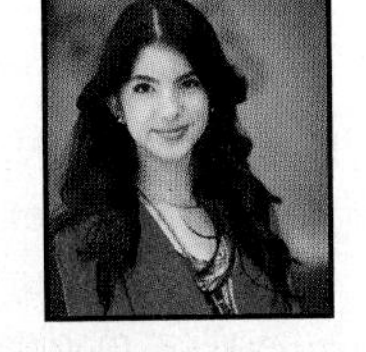

Her grandmother finds Ms. Hernandez in a confused, euphoric state and calls emergency medical services. The paramedics note that Ms. Hernandez has dilated pupils and is bleeding from her nose. She is hypertensive, and her pulse is irregular and rapid. An electrocardiogram shows a cardiac dysrhythmia with possible evidence of myocardial ischemia. The paramedics begin oxygen therapy, and an intravenous line is secured. Suspecting a drug overdose from an unknown substance, the paramedics administer naloxone, an opioid antagonist, and transport Ms. Hernandez to the emergency department. There, she begins to seize, and benzodiazepines are administered. She is diagnosed with acute cocaine toxicity and is hospitalized for 3 days. A cardiac workup is negative for a myocardial infarction. Ms. Hernandez is discharged to an inpatient rehabilitation facility. Despite inpatient and outpatient therapy, she has multiple relapses and is brought to the emergency department after a cardiac arrest. She is successfully resuscitated. Afterward, she begins her rehabilitation in earnest and is successful in abstaining from cocaine.

5. What complications of cocaine abuse did Ms. Hernandez exhibit when she was brought to the emergency department?
6. What pathologic effects of cocaine on cardiovascular physiology led to Ms. Hernandez's cardiac arrest?

There are a number of general treatments for stimulant use disorders, such as medications, individual and group counseling, inpatient and residential treatment, intensive outpatient treatment, peer supports and 12-step programs.[52] Replacement or substitute medications have been used in treating other substance use disorders. The substitute drug must have effects similar to those of the abused drug but with a lower potential for abuse, allowing the patient to take advantage of behavioral and social treatments. Opioids have been used as a substitution for heroin. However, no such medications have been approved for cocaine use disorder. A recent Cochrane review investigated whether treatment with psychostimulants with less addictive potential (e.g., amphetamine sulfate) could be an effective therapy for treatment of cocaine use disorders.[52] The authors concluded that efficacy of psychostimulants for cocaine dependence was not entirely clear; however, there was evidence that the use of psychostimulants deserved further investigation.[53]

Check Your Progress: Section 6.6

1. What are two medical conditions that are treated with amphetamines?
2. List the cardiovascular complications of cocaine abuse.
3. Which type of illegal cocaine is inhaled and which type is smoked?

Table 6.6 Hallucinogen Signs and Symptoms

Systems/Concepts Affected by Hallucinogen Intoxication	Signs and Symptoms
Cardiovascular system/Perfusion	Tachycardia Palpitations Hypertension/hypotension
Neurologic system/Intracranial Regulation	Tremors Hyperreflexia
Mood, affect, cognition, and trauma/Emotional Regulation	Paranoia Suicidal ideation Anxiety Depression Euphoria Intensification of feelings Acute cognitive impairments Megalomania Depersonalization Acute neurophysiologic impairment
Musculoskeletal/Mobility	Motor incoordination
Nutrition and gastrointestinal symptoms/Nutrition and Digestion, Metabolism, and Elimination	Nausea and vomiting
Thermoregulation and Sensory Perception	Diaphoresis Mydriasis

6.7 Hallucinogen Use Disorder

In 2014, an estimated 1.2 million people in the United States (0.4% of the population) reported having used hallucinogens in the past month. In that same year, 246,000 people in the United States had a hallucinogen use disorder.[30] **Hallucinogens**, which are substances that can alter sensory perception, mood, and thought patterns, have been used throughout history, especially in religious activities.[54] Psilocybin (mushrooms), mescaline, and peyote are hallucinogens that occur naturally; lysergic acid diethylamide (LSD) is an older hallucinogen that is synthetically produced. There are newer hallucinogenic such as phencyclidine (PCP) and 3,4-methylenedioxy methamphetamine (MDMA) that are increasingly being used.[54] However, LSD remains the prototypical and most widely studied hallucinogen.

In general, hallucinogens are consumed orally and are rapidly absorbed from the gastrointestinal tract.[54] For example, LSD has an onset of action, peak effect, and duration of action of 30–90 minutes, 3–5 hours, and 6–12 hours, respectively; PCP has an onset of action, peak effect, and duration of action of 30–60 minutes, 1–4 hours, and 4–6 hours, respectively.[54] Hallucinogens have different properties based on the specific drug and the method of administration.

Etiology and Pathogenesis

The neurobiology of hallucinogens is highly complex and incompletely understood; however, it appears to involve the interaction of serotonin, dopamine, and glutamate neurotransmitters.[54] A **hallucination** occurs when a person exhibits sensory perceptions without any external stimuli to precipitate them. Individuals using hallucinogens may experience trips and flashbacks. The term *trip* refers to the symptoms that occur during an acute period of intoxication, while the term *flashback* refers to symptoms that occur after the acute effects have dissipated. Flashbacks can occur months and even years after the acute intoxication.[54]

Clinical Manifestations

In addition to hallucinations, patients may report a heightened perception of sensory input, a distorted sense of time, euphoria, feelings of expansiveness, and enhanced spiritual experiences. These sensations are often referred to as psychedelic experiences. Common signs and symptoms associated with hallucinogens are listed in **Table 6.6** ■.[55] Note that these symptoms are primarily related to enhanced SNS, neuropsychiatric, and gastrointestinal symptoms.

Linking Pathophysiology to Diagnosis and Treatment

Although flashbacks can occur for weeks to months after ingestion of the drugs, they usually become less frequent over time. These occasional flashbacks can be differentiated from **hallucinogen persisting perception disorder (HPPD)**, in which the hallucinations occur unpredictably, interfere with daily activities, and cause anxiety and depression. There are no approved medications to treat hallucinogen use disorders. As in all substance use disorders, behavioral therapy and counseling may be effective.

Check Your Progress: Section 6.7

1. How long after an acute hallucinogen intoxication can flashbacks occur?
2. What medications are used to treat hallucinogen use disorder and hallucinogen persisting perception disorder?
3. Physical signs and symptoms of hallucinogen use are related to which division of the autonomic nervous system?

6.8 Opioid Use Disorder

Opioids are a class of drugs with a chemical structure similar to alkaloids that are found in opium poppies.[30] Opioids have analgesic effects and are used for pain relief; however, they have tremendous potential for abuse. Opioid use disorder can be associated with misuse of prescription opioid medications, use of opioid medications prescribed for other individuals, or use of illegally obtained heroin.[56] **Opioid use disorder** is a chronic, relapsing illness of a pattern of opioid use that is associated with negative health consequences. In 2014, an estimated 1.9 million people in the United States had an opioid use disorder related to prescription pain relievers; an additional 586,000 people had an opioid use disorder that was related to heroin use.[30]

Opioids are natural and synthetic substances that interact at one of three receptor main opioid receptor systems (mu, kappa, and delta).[56] There are a number of naturally occurring (e.g., morphine and codeine), semisynthetic (e.g., hydromorphone, oxycodone, hydrocodone, and heroin), and synthetic forms of opioids (e.g., meperidine, methadone, tramadol, and fentanyl).[56]

There are differences in pharmacokinetics between specific opioid preparations; however, a few generalizations can be made. There is tremendous variability in the serum half-life of opioid preparations.[57] For example, morphine, hydrocodone, and methadone have half-lives of 1.9 ± 0.5 hours, 4.24 ± 0.99 hours, and 27 ± 12 hours, respectively. Most opioids are metabolized by the liver to active metabolites and are eliminated through renal mechanisms.[57] The route of administration (i.e., intravenous, intranasal, inhaled, or oral) influences the bioavailability of the drug and desired effects. For example, low-purity heroin can produce euphoria when given intravenously. The majority of heroin overdoses occur with intravenous administration.

Etiology and Pathogenesis

The actions of opioids are mediated through the interaction of transmembrane proteins (mu, kappa, and delta) that are located in the central and peripheral nervous system. Opioids have potent analgesic and CNS depressive effects and can produce euphoria.[56] Opioids are highly addictive with rapid progression to physiologic dependence followed by the development of tolerance and subsequent withdrawal in the absence of such drugs.[58] Over the past few decades, illicit drugs such as heroin and prescription drugs such as oxycodone have caused substantial morbidity and mortality among the U.S. population. In 2014, 4.3 million people in the United States had engaged in nonmedical use of prescription painkillers in the past month, 1.9 million people in the United States met criteria for prescription use disorder based on their use of prescription painkillers in the past year, 212,000 people age 12 years or older had used heroin for the first time within the past 12 months, and approximately 435,000 people were regular users of heroin.[59] These addictions are associated with increased mortality, particularly mortality associated with overdose and trauma.

Clinical Manifestations

An overdose of opioids is a life-threatening emergency. General clinical manifestations of opioid toxicity include the following:

- Decreased or unchanged heart rate
- Decreased or unchanged blood pressure
- Decreased respiratory rate
- Decreased or unchanged temperature
- Decreased bowel sounds
- Sedation or coma
- Seizures
- Miosis.

Chronic clinical manifestations of intravenous opioid abuse include track marks, which are calluses that follow the track of a vein that has been frequently injected.[56] Chronic clinical manifestations of intranasal opioid use include a perforated nasal septum. Chronic opioid use may be associated with signs and symptoms of other chronic diseases, such as HIV and hepatitis C; this is especially true of opioids that are injected intravenously.[56]

CLINICAL POINT: **Naloxone** (Narcan) is an opioid antagonist medication that rapidly reverses the effects of an opioid overdose. Naloxone has been prescribed for use in community settings as part of overdose education and prevention programs and can be administered by families, caregivers, and emergency personnel.[60] Most U.S. states have passed legislation authorizing healthcare providers to provide naloxone through standing orders to such individuals and protection from penalties related to practicing medicine without a license.[60] The medication can be administered intravenously, intramuscularly, or subcutaneously, and an intranasal spray has been approved.[60] ■

Linking Pathophysiology to Diagnosis and Treatment

The use of opioid prescription medications has produced a dilemma among clinicians. While these medications have the potential for abuse, they also have tremendous abilities to reduce pain and increase physical functioning among people who are afflicted with chronic pain. Clinicians have long tried to balance the potential for substance use disorders with relieving pain.

The CDC has established guidelines for clinicians regarding use of opioid medications. The CDC's recommendations stress that nonopioid therapy is preferred for treatment of chronic pain. Opioids should be prescribed only when the benefits for reducing pain and increasing function outweigh the risks; they should be prescribed at the lowest effective dosage with careful reassessment when an increase in dosage is considered; and concurrent use of opioids and benzodiazepines should be avoided whenever possible. Additionally, clinicians should evaluate benefits and harms of chronic opioid therapy with patients every 3 months or more often and should review prescription drug monitoring program data for high-risk combinations or dosages.[61] For individuals with opioid disorders, clinicians should offer evidence-based treatment such as medication-assisted treatment with buprenorphine or methadone.[61]

CLINICAL POINT: Starting in 1999 and continuing until today, a drug epidemic in the United States has killed more than half a million individuals.[62] In 2015, 52,404 people died of drug overdoses, and 33,000 of those were due to opioids.[63] From 1999 to 2013, the number of prescriptions written for opioids quadrupled. The CDC has guidelines for prescribing opioids for chronic pain to help improve practices in primary care settings.[63] ■

Check Your Progress: Section 6.8

1. What are the physical findings in chronic opioid abuse?
2. What are the key points in using opioids to manage pain?
3. What types of opioids are commonly used in opioid use disorder?

CHAPTER SUMMARY

6.1 Chapter Overview and Case Studies

Identify common substances of abuse and related pathophysiology concepts.

- The most common substance use disorders are alcohol use disorder, tobacco use disorder, cannabis use disorder, stimulant use disorder, hallucinogen use disorder, and opioid use disorder.
- Abuse of tobacco, alcohol, and other substances is associated with crime, lost productivity, and increased healthcare utilization.
- Risk factors for substance abuse include the dynamic interaction of genes, the environment, and peer pressure.

6.2 Anatomy and Neurobiology of the Brain

Describe the neurobiology of the brain and how it relates to substance use disorders.

- Alcohol, tobacco, cannabis, stimulants, and hallucinogens are the most commonly used psychoactive substances.
- Death from tobacco-related disease is more common than death resulting from use of any other substance.
- Dependence on psychoactive substances is generally related to the dopamine reward pathway.
- The nucleus accumbens and ventral tegmental area along with neurotransmitters form the common pathway for psychoactive substances.
- The major behaviors associated with addiction include binging and intoxication, withdrawal and negative effect, and preoccupation and anticipation.

6.3 Alcohol Use Disorder

Differentiate the causes, classification, underlying pathogenesis, and clinical manifestations of and the general treatment strategies for alcohol use disorder.

- Alcohol products are readily absorbed in the stomach and intestine but are metabolized in the liver.
- Alcohol increases the inhibitory neurotransmitter GABA and inhibits communication among neurons.
- Long-term heavy drinking can result in tissue damage to multiple organ systems.
- Acute withdrawal symptoms can be life threatening.
- Alcohol use poses risks to the unborn infant.
- Treatments for alcohol use disorders include behavioral treatments (e.g., cognitive–behavioral therapy), medications (e.g., naltrexone, acamprosate, disulfiram), and mutual support groups (e.g., Alcoholics Anonymous).

6.4 Tobacco Use Disorder

Differentiate the causes, classification, underlying pathogenesis, and clinical manifestations of and the general treatment strategies for tobacco use disorder.

- The reinforcing properties of nicotine are enhanced by the other chemicals found in smoked tobacco; they also cause destruction of lung tissue.
- Use of tobacco products is linked to chronic respiratory disorders, cancers, and a compromised immune system.
- Smokeless tobacco products and secondhand smoke are associated with health risks similar to those experienced by the tobacco smoker.
- Treatments for smoking cessation include individual and group behavioral therapy, over-the-counter products (nicotine gum); prescription nicotine replacement products (nicotine patch, inhaler, nasal spray); and prescription nonnicotine products (bupropion).

6.5 Cannabis Use Disorder

Differentiate the causes, classification, underlying pathogenesis, and clinical manifestations of and the general treatment strategies for cannabis use disorder.

- Marijuana (cannabis) is the most-used drug in the United States after alcohol and tobacco.
- THC, the principal active ingredient in marijuana, is one of a group of chemicals called cannabinoids.
- The mechanism of action of marijuana results from the binding of cannabis to cannabinoid receptors, CB1 and CB2.
- Marijuana's immediate effects include distorted perception, difficulty with thinking and problem solving, and loss of motor coordination.
- Psychoactive symptoms of cannabis use may include anxiety, paranoia, poor eye contact, agitation, grandiose and paranoid delusions, and psychosis.
- The treatment for cannabis use disorder involves behavioral approaches such as cognitive–behavioral therapy.

6.6 Stimulant Use Disorders

Differentiate the causes, classification, underlying pathogenesis, and clinical manifestations of and the general treatment strategies for stimulant use disorder.

- The most commonly abused stimulants are amphetamines and synthetic cathinones, methamphetamine, and cocaine.
- In general, stimulants can be taken orally, inhaled, or administered intravenously. They cross the blood–brain barrier and produce a rapid onset of effects.
- The primary activity of amphetamines is to increase the synaptic activity of neurotransmitters (i.e., dopamine and norepinephrine).
- Methamphetamine causes an increase in the synapse of monoamines, including dopamine, norepinephrine, and serotonin.
- Cocaine exerts its effects by blocking reuptake of the neurotransmitters dopamine and norepinephrine in the central and peripheral nervous system, thus enhancing the activity of these neurotransmitters.
- A variety of symptoms are associated with stimulant use disorders; the most common are the cardiovascular and neuropsychiatric symptoms.
- Cocaine use, in particular, is associated with acute (e.g., myocardial ischemia, myocardial infarction, and stroke) and long-term (e.g., atherosclerosis) cardiovascular disease.
- There are a number of general treatments for stimulant use disorders, such as medications, individual and group counseling, inpatient and residential treatment, intensive outpatient treatment, peer supports and 12-step programs.

6.7 Hallucinogen Use Disorder

Differentiate the causes, classification, underlying pathogenesis, and clinical manifestations of and the general treatment strategies for hallucinogenic use disorder.

- There are a number of naturally occurring hallucinogens (e.g., psilocybin and mescaline). However, lysergic acid diethylamide (LSD), an older synthetic hallucinogen, remains the prototypical and most widely studied hallucinogen.
- The neurobiology of hallucinogens is highly complex and incompletely understood; it appears to involve the interaction of serotonin, dopamine, and glutamate.
- Patients with hallucinogen use disorders may report a heightened perception of sensory input, a distorted sense of time, euphoria, feelings of expansiveness, and enhanced spiritual experiences.
- Patients may report flashbacks for months or years after use of hallucinogens.
- Occasional flashbacks can be differentiated from hallucinogen persisting perception disorder, in which the hallucinations occur unpredictably and interfere with daily activities and mood.
- There are no approved medications to treat hallucinogen use disorders. As in all substance use disorders, behavioral therapy and counseling may be effective.

6.8 Opioid Use Disorder

Differentiate the causes, classification, underlying pathogenesis, and clinical manifestations of and the general treatment strategies for opioid use disorder.

- There are a number of naturally occurring (e.g., morphine and codeine), semisynthetic (e.g., hydromorphone, oxycodone, hydrocodone, and heroin), and synthetic forms of opioids (e.g., meperidine, methadone, tramadol, and fentanyl).
- Opioids have potent analgesic and CNS depressive effects and can produce euphoria.
- Opioids are highly addictive with rapid progression to physiologic dependence followed by the development of tolerance and subsequent withdrawal in the absence of such drugs.
- Acute opioid addiction is a medical emergency; chronic opioid addiction (particularly intravenous drug administration) often is associated with other chronic illness, such as HIV and hepatitis C.
- Clinicians are obligated to balance the risks and benefits of opioid treatment for patients with chronic pain. This involves periodic structured monitoring and evaluation of the patient with respect to the efficacy of dosing, side effects, and tolerance.
- For patients with an opioid disorders, clinicians should offer evidence-based treatment such as medication-assisted treatment with buprenorphine or methadone.

REVIEW QUESTIONS

1. Vitamin B_1 (thiamine) is given to clients with chronic alcohol use disorder (chronic alcoholism). What conditions will benefit from administering this treatment?
   a. Wernicke disease
   b. Korsakoff psychosis
   c. Peripheral neuropathy
   d. All of the above

2. The amygdala is responsible for:
   a. regulation of basic drives such as hunger and thirst.
   b. the fear response and generating emotions.
   c. motor control.
   d. control of basic functions that are critical to life, such as respiration and heart rate.

3. An individual has used alcohol regularly for several months. Care of this individual recognizes the need to monitor for withdrawal symptoms if alcohol intake is suddenly discontinued because the client has developed:
   a. physical dependence.
   b. tolerance.
   c. liver cirrhosis.
   d. alcohol overdose.
4. All of the following are true about alcohol metabolism and action EXCEPT:
   a. sparkling wines and champagne have a faster onset of alcohol action.
   b. most ingested alcohol is absorbed in the small intestine.
   c. alcohol decreases the effect of the inhibitory brain neurotransmitter GABA.
   d. alcohol dehydrogenase enzyme converts alcohol to acetaldehyde in the liver.
5. All of the following are true about the use of tobacco products EXCEPT:
   a. use of smokeless tobacco does not cause cancer.
   b. cigarette smoking raises the risk of various cancers.
   c. inhaled cigarette smoke contains thousands of chemicals in addition to nicotine.
   d. smoking cessation medications include nicotine replacement products.
6. The brain actions of cannabis are due to:
   a. binding of the active chemical in cannabis to cannabinoid receptors (CB1 and CB2).
   b. release of dopamine in the nucleus accumbens that activates the reward circuit.
   c. THC action in the prefrontal cortex.
   d. all of the above.
7. Which of the following is true about methamphetamine use?
   a. Methamphetamine acts as a depressant in the central nervous system.
   b. Chronic methamphetamine use has few or no adverse health consequences.
   c. Monoamines such as dopamine, serotonin, and norepinephrine are increased in the brain with methamphetamine use.
   d. Methamphetamine action in the brain has no effect on the reward system.
8. Which of the following is true about opioid use disorder?
   a. Most overdoses occur as a result of intravenous administration of drug.
   b. A hallmark of overdose is an increased respiratory rate.
   c. It is rare that prescription opioid analgesic drugs are diverted for illicit use.
   d. Because of the risk of opioid use disorder, opioids should never be used as analgesics in medical therapeutics.

ANSWERS

Answers to Review Questions can be found in Appendix A. Answers to Case Study and Check Your Progress questions are available on the faculty resources site. Please consult with your instructor.

RECOMMENDED WEBSITES

National Council on Alcoholism and Drug Dependence Inc.
https://ncadd.org

National Institute on Drug Abuse
http://www.drugabuse.gov

Substance Abuse and Mental Health Services Administration: Prevention
http://www.samhsa.gov/ebp-web-guide/substance-abuse-prevention

REFERENCES

1. National Institute on Drug Abuse. (2012). *Medical consequences of drug abuse*. Available at https://www.drugabuse.gov/related-topics/medical-consequences-drug-abuse/mortality
2. Volkow, N. D., Koob, G. F., McLellan, & A. T. (2016). Neurobiologic advances from the brain disease model of addiction. *New England Journal of Medicine, 374*(4), 363–371.
3. Hart, C. L., & Ksir, C. (2013). *Drugs, society, & human behavior* (15th ed.). New York: McGraw-Hill.
4. National Institute on Drug Abuse. (n.d.). *Addiction science: From molecules to managed care*. Available at https://www.scribd.com/presentation/83408958/Addiction-Science-From-Molecules-to-Managed-Care
5. Mroziewicz, M., & Tyndale, R. F. (2010). Pharmacogenetics: A tool for identifying genetic factors in drug dependence and response to treatment. *Addiction Science & Clinical Practice, 5*(2), 17–29.

6. Stahre, M., Roeber, J., Kanny, D., Brewer, R. D., & Zhang, X. (2014). Contribution of excessive alcohol consumption to deaths and years of potential life lost in the United States. *Preventing Chronic Disease, 26*(11), 130293.
7. Centers for Disease Control and Prevention. (2014). *Alcohol deaths*. Available at http://www.cdc.gov/features/alcohol-deaths/index.html
8. American Psychiatric Association. (2013). *Diagnostic and statistical manual of mental disorders* (5th ed.). Washington DC: American Psychiatric Association.
9. National Institute on Drug Abuse. (2016). *Commonly abused drug charts*. Available at https://www.drugabuse.gov/drugs-abuse/commonly-abused-drugs-charts
10. Centers for Disease Control and Prevention. (2016). *Fetal alcohol spectrum disorders (FASDs): Alcohol use in pregnancy*. Available at https://www.cdc.gov/ncbddd/fasd/alcohol-use.html
11. Centers for Disease Control and Prevention (CDC). (2016). *Fact sheets: Underage drinking*. Available at http://www.cdc.gov/alcohol/fact-sheets/underage-drinking.htm
12. National Institute on Alcohol Abuse and Alcoholism. (2015). *Alcohol & your health: Overview of alcohol consumption*. Available at https://www.niaaa.nih.gov/alcohol-health/overview-alcohol-consumption/moderate-binge-drinking
13. Marshall, E. J. (2014). Adolescent alcohol use: Risks and consequences. *Alcohol and Alcoholism, 49*(2), 160–164.
14. Skala, K., & Walter, H. (2013). Adolescence and alcohol: A review of the literature. *Neuropsychiatrie, 27*(4), 202–211.
15. Centers for Disease Control and Prevention (CDC). (2014). *Underage drinking*. Available at http://www.cdc.gov/alcohol/fact-sheet/underage-drinking.html
16. Centers for Disease Control and Prevention (CDC). (2014). *Fact sheets: Alcohol use and your health*. Available at http://www.cdc.gov/alcohol/fact-sheets/alcohol-use.htm
17. National Institute on Alcohol Abuse and Alcoholism. (2016). *Alcohol facts and statistics*. Available at https://www.niaaa.nih.gov/alcohol-health/overview-alcohol-consumption/alcohol-facts-and-statistics
18. Satre, D. D., Sterling, S. A., Mackin, R. S., & Weisner, C. (2011). Patterns of alcohol and drug use among depressed older adults seeking outpatient psychiatric services. *American Journal of Geriatric Psychiatry*, 19(8), 695–703.
19. National Institute on Aging. (2016). Alcohol use in older people. *Health and Aging*. Available at https://www.nia.nih.gov/health/publication/alcohol-use-older-people
20. Centers for Disease Control and Prevention. (2016). *Youth and tobacco use*. Available at http://www.cdc.gov/tobacco/data_statistics/fact_sheets/youth_data/tobacco_use/
21. U.S. Department of Health & Human Services. (2017). *Tobacco and nicotine*. Available at http://betobaccofree.hhs.gov/about-tobacco/tobacco-and-nicotine/index.html
22. Benowitz, N. L. (2008). Clinical pharmacology of nicotine: Implications for understanding, preventing, and treating tobacco addiction. *Clinical Pharmacology and Therapeutics, 83*(4), 531–541.
23. Myers, C. S., Taylor, R. C., Salmeron, B. J., Waters, A. J., & Heishman, S. J. (2013). Nicotine enhances alerting, but not executive, attention in smokers and nonsmokers. *Nicotine & Tobacco Research, 15*(1), 277–281.
24. American Lung Association. (2015). *Marijuana and lung health*. Available at http://www.lung.org/stop-smoking/smoking-facts/marijuana-and-lung-health.html
25. Camenga, D. R., & Klein, J. D. (2016). Tobacco use disorders. *Child and Adolescent Psychiatric Clinics of North America, 25*(3), 445–460.
26. National Institute on Alcohol Abuse. (2013). *Tobacco use and comorbidity*. Available at https://www.drugabuse.gov/publications/research-reports/tobacco/tobacco-use-comorbidity
27. National Institute on Drug Abuse. (2016). *What is marijuana?* Available at https://www.drugabuse.gov/publications/research-reports/marijuana/what-marijuana
28. Wilson, I., Semple, S., Mills, L. M., et al. (2013). REFRESH—Reducing families' exposure to secondhand smoke in the home: A feasibility study. *Tobacco Control*, 22(5), e8.
29. U.S. Surgeon General. (2012). *Preventing tobacco use among youth and young adults*. Available at https://www.surgeongeneral.gov/library/reports/preventing-youth-tobacco-use/
30. Substance Abuse and Mental Health Services Administration. (2015). *Substance use disorders*. Available at http://www.samhsa.gov/disorders/substance-use
31. MedlinePlus. (2017). *Marijuana*. Available at https://medlineplus.gov/marijuana.html
32. Agurell, S., Halldin, M., Lindgren, J. E., et al. (1986). Pharmacokinetics and metabolism of delta 1-tetrahydrocannabinol and other cannabinoids with emphasis on man. *Pharmacological Reviews, 38*(1), 21–43.
33. Maykut, M. O. (1985). Health consequences of acute and chronic marihuana use. *Progress in Neuro-Psychopharmacology & Biological Psychiatry*, 9(3), 209–238.
34. Ashton, C. H. (2001). Pharmacology and effects of cannabis: A brief review. *British Journal of Psychiatry, 178*, 101–106.
35. Simpson, A. K., & Magid, V. (2016). Cannabis use disorder in adolescence. *Child and Adolescent Psychiatric Clinics of North America, 25*(3), 431–443.
36. Meier, M. H., Caspi, A., Ambler, A., et al. (2012). Persistent cannabis users show neuropsychological decline from childhood to midlife. *Proceedings of the National Academy of Sciences of the United States of America, 109*(40), E2657–2664.
37. National Institute on Drug Abuse. (2015). *Synthetic cannabinoids*. Available at https://www.drugabuse.gov/publications/drugfacts/synthetic-cannabinoids
38. Gorelick, D. A., Saxon, A., & Hermann, R. (2016). Cannabis use and disorder: Epidemiology, comorbidity, health consequences, and medico-legal status. *UpToDate*. Available at https://www-uptodate-com.proxy.cc.uic.edu/contents/cannabis-use-and-disorder-epidemiology-comorbidity-health-consequences-and-medico-legal-status
39. Wang, G. (2016). Synthetic cannabinoids: Acute intoxication. *UpToDate*. Available at http://www.uptodate.com/contents/synthetic-cannabinoids-acute-intoxication
40. National Institute on Drug Abuse. (2016). *Available treatments for marijuana use disorders*. Available at https://www.drugabuse.gov/publications/research-reports/marijuana/available-treatments-marijuana-use-disorders
41. National Institute on Drug Abuse. (2015). *Montoring the future 2015 survey results*. Available at https://www.drugabuse.gov/related-topics/trends-statistics/infographics/monitoring-future-2015-survey-results
42. National Institute on Drug Abuse. (2014). *Drugs, brains, and behavior: The science of addiction*. Available at https://www.drugabuse.gov/publications/drugs-brains-behavior-science-addiction/preface
43. Hart, C. L., Ksir, C., & Ray, O. S. (2009). *Drugs, society, and human behavior* (13th ed.). New York, NY: McGraw-Hill.
44. Paulus, M. (2016). Methamphetamine use disorder: Epidemiology, clinical manifestations, course, assessment, and diagnosis. *UpToDate*. Available at http://www.uptodate.com/contents/methamphetamine-use-disorder-epidemiology-clinical-manifestations-course-assessment-and-diagnosis
45. Gorelick, D. A. (2015). Cocaine use disorder in adults: Epidemiology, pharmacology, clinical manifestations, medical consequences and diagnosis. *UpToDate*. Available at http://www.uptodate.com/contents/cocaine-use-disorder-in-adults-epidemiology-pharmacology-clinical-manifestations-medical-consequences-and-diagnosis
46. Arnold, T. C., & Ryan, M. L. (2014). Acute amphetamine and synthetic cathinone ("bath salt") intoxication. *UpToDate*. Available at http://www.uptodate.com/contents/acute-amphetamine-and-synthetic-cathinone-bath-salt-intoxication
47. Hatsukami, D. K., & Fischman, M. W. (1996). Crack cocaine and cocaine hydrochloride: Are the differences myth or reality? *Jama, 276*(19), 1580–1588.

48. Kampman, M. D. (2016). Pharmacotherapy for stimulant use disorders in adults. *UpToDate.* Available at http://www.uptodate.com/contents/pharmacotherapy-for-stimulant-use-disorders-in-adults
49. Park, T. M., & Haning, W. F., 3rd. (2016). Stimulant use disorders. *Child and Adolescent Psychiatric Clinics of North America, 25*(3), 461–471.
50. National Institute of Drug Abuse. (2016). *DrugFacts: Synthetic cathinones ("bath salts").* Available at https://www.drugabuse.gov/publications/drugfacts/synthetic-cathinones-bath-salts
51. Stankowski, R. V., Kloner, R. A., & Rezkalla, S. H. (2015). Cardiovascular consequences of cocaine use. *Trends in Cardiovascular Medicine, 25*(6), 517–526.
52. Substance Abuse and Mental Health Services Administration. (2016). *Treatments for substance use disorders.* Avaliable at https://www.samhsa.gov/treatment/substance-use-disorders
53. Castells, X., Cunill, R., Perez-Mana, C., Vidal, X., & Capella, D. (2016). Psychostimulant drugs for cocaine dependence. *Cochrane Database of Systematic Reviews, 9,* CD007380.
54. Delgado, J. (2016). Intoxication from LSD and other common hallucinogens. *UpToDate.* Available at http://www.uptodate.com/contents/intoxication-from-lsd-and-other-common-hallucinogens
55. Hardaway, R., Schweitzer, J., & Suzuki, J. (2016). Hallucinogen use disorders. *Child and Adolescent Psychiatric Clinics of North America, 25*(3), 489–496.
56. Strain, E. (2015). Opioid use disorder: Epidemiology, pharmacology, clinical manifestations, course, screening, assessment, and diagnosis. *UpToDate.* Available at http://www.uptodate.com/contents/opioid-use-disorder-epidemiology-pharmacology-clinical-manifestations-course-screening-assessment-and-diagnosis
57. Stolbach, A., & Hoffman, R. S. (2016). Acute opioid intoxication in adults. *UpToDate.* Available at http://www.uptodate.com/contents/acute-opioid-intoxication-in-adults
58. Sharma, V., Biyani, G., & Bhatia, P. K. (2015). Opioids induced serotonin toxicity? Think again. *Indian Jorunal of Anaesthesia, 59*(7), 463.
59. Substance Abuse and Mental Health Services Administration. (2015). *Behavioral health trends in the United States: Results from the 2014 National Survey on Drug Use and Health.* HHS Publication No. SMA 15-4927, NSDUH Series H-50. Available at https://www.samhsa.gov/data/sites/default/files/NSDUH-FRR1-2014/NSDUH-FRR1-2014.pdf
60. Coffin, P. (2016). Prevention of lethal opioid overdose in the community. *UpToDate.* Available at http://www.uptodate.com/contents/prevention-of-lethal-opioid-overdose-in-the-community
61. Dowell, D., Haegerich, T. M., & Chou R. (2016). CDC guideline for prescribing opioids for chronic pain—United States, 2016. *Jama, 315*(15), 1624–1645.
62. Lopez, G., & Frostenson, S. (2017). How the opioid epidemic became America's worst drug crisis ever, in 15 maps and charts. Retrieved from http://www.vox.com/science-and-health/2017/3/23/14987892/opioid-heroin-epidemic-charts.
63. Centers for Disease Control and Prevention (CCD). (2017). Opioid overdose. Retrieved from https://www.cdc.gov/drugoverdose/

Chapter 7
Risks Related to Sleep Alterations

Judith L. Reishtein

Chapter Outline and Learning Outcomes

7.1 Chapter Overview and Case Studies

Describe sleep and concepts related to sleep.

7.2 Normal Sleep

Discuss the characteristics of normal sleep and the regulation of body rhythms and sleep.

7.3 Measurement of Sleep

Explain what measures are used to assess sleep and its outcomes.

7.4 Sleep Deprivation

List physiologic, psychologic, and sociologic consequences of insufficient and disturbed sleep.

7.5 Insomnia

Describe factors leading to insomnia and how it is diagnosed and treated.

7.6 Sleep-Disordered Breathing

Differentiate the causes, classification, underlying pathogenesis, and clinical manifestations of sleep-disordered breathing and approaches to diagnosis and treatment of these conditions across the lifespan.

7.7 Narcolepsy

Differentiate the causes, classification, underlying pathogenesis, and clinical manifestations of narcolepsy and approaches to diagnosis and treatment of this condition across the lifespan.

7.8 Restless Legs Syndrome

Differentiate the causes, classification, underlying pathogenesis, and clinical manifestations of restless legs syndrome and approaches to diagnosis and treatment of this condition across the lifespan.

7.9 Parasomnias

Identify and define selected parasomnias, and describe the causes, pathogenesis, and clinical manifestations of these conditions and approaches to their diagnosis and treatment across the lifespan.

KEY TERMS

Apnea–hypopnea index (AHI), 155
Bruxism, 162
Cataplexy, 160
Central sleep apnea (CSA), 159
Circadian rhythm, 147
Continuous positive airway pressure (CPAP), 158
Electrocardiogram (ECG), 151
Electroencephalogram (EEG), 147
Electromyelogram (EMG), 151
Electro-oculogram (EOG), 151
Enuresis, 162
Homeostatic mechanism, 147
Hypnagogic hallucination, 160
Hypnogram, 151
Hypnopompic hallucination, 160
Hypocretin, 148
Hypopnea, 156
Insomnia, 153
Jet lag, 153
Melatonin, 147
N1, 148
N2, 148
N3, 148
Narcolepsy, 160
Night terrors, 162
Non-rapid eye movement sleep (NREM sleep), 148
Obstructive sleep apnea (OSA), 155
Parasomnia, 162
Polysomnography (PSG), 150
Rapid eye movement sleep (REM sleep), 148
Restless legs syndrome (RLS), 161
Shift work disorder, 152
Sleep, 147
Sleep-disordered breathing, 155
Sleep latency, 148
Sleep onset rapid eye movement period (SOREMP)s, 160
Sleep paralysis, 160
Sleep phase delay, 153
Somnambulism, 162
Suprachiasmatic nucleus (SCN), 147
Zeitgeber, 152

ABBREVIATIONS

AHI—apnea–hypopnea index
CPAP—continuous positive airway pressure
CSA—central sleep apnea
ECG—electrocardiogram
EEG—electroencephalograph
EMG—electromyelogram
EOG—electro-oculogram
MSLT—multiple sleep latency test
NREM—non-rapid eye movement
OSA—obstructive sleep apnea
PSG—polysomnography
REM—rapid eye movement
RLS—restless leg syndrome
SCN—suprachiasmatic nucleus
SOREMP—sleep onset rapid eye movement period
SWS—slow wave sleep

7.1 Chapter Overview and Case Studies

Sleep is an essential part of life. What happens during sleep affects the body and brain in ways that have only recently been understood and appreciated. In fact, if a person chronically experiences insufficient sleep, the brain will try to make up for that lack by going to sleep for a few microseconds at a time. These episodes are so short that the individual does not notice them, but they disrupt concentration, prolong reaction times, and can lead to accidents and critical injury.

Insufficient sleep is very common in the developed world. It is most often related to sociologic causes such as shift work, jet lag, staying up to watch TV, using electronic devices, and socializing. However, insufficient sleep can also be secondary to sleep disrupted by a sleep disorder, such as sleep apnea, narcolepsy, restless legs syndrome, or, more commonly, nightmares or sleepwalking.

This chapter will discuss what happens during normal sleep and how sleep is assessed. Following a presentation on sleep deprivation and insomnia, several relatively common sleep disorders will be discussed: sleep-disordered breathing (including sleep apnea), narcolepsy, and restless legs syndrome. For each disorder, the underlying pathophysiologic mechanisms will be explained; clinical manifestations, including signs, symptoms, and physical and diagnostic findings will be linked to the pathophysiology; and treatment modalities will be reviewed in light of the pathophysiology.

Concepts Related to Sleep

Our understanding of sleep has evolved over the past several decades. Sleep is now viewed as an actively regulated process; it is not simply the result of diminished waking.[1] Sleep is a complex behavior that alternates with periods of wakefulness in a cyclic pattern that is associated with a rhythm over a 24-hour day. The cortical activation necessary for maintenance of wakefulness is supported by an extensive network of subcortical pathways and structures; the initiation and maintenance of sleep requires suppression of activity in ascending arousal systems.[2] There are two specific types of sleep: rapid eye movement (REM) sleep and non-rapid eye movement (NREM) sleep. The two types of sleep are associated with differing effects on cardiorespiratory and thermoregulatory functioning under the influence of the autonomic nervous system, while transitions between REM and NREM states are initiated by neurons within the brainstem.[2] Additionally, sleep and wake states have distinct hormonal patterns that influence metabolism.

Sleep is necessary for good health and well-being; alterations in sleep can result in adverse health outcomes. A conceptual model of sleep health developed by Buysse suggests that there are relationships among dimensions of sleep (satisfaction, alertness, timing, efficiency, and duration); genetic, epigenetic, molecular, and cellular processes; system-level processes (inflammation, sympathetic nervous system activation, hormonal responses, and neural circuitry); and health, disease, and function[3] (**Figure 7.1** ■). In this model, sleep dimensions influence genetic, epigenetic, molecular, and cellular processes, which in turn influence system-level

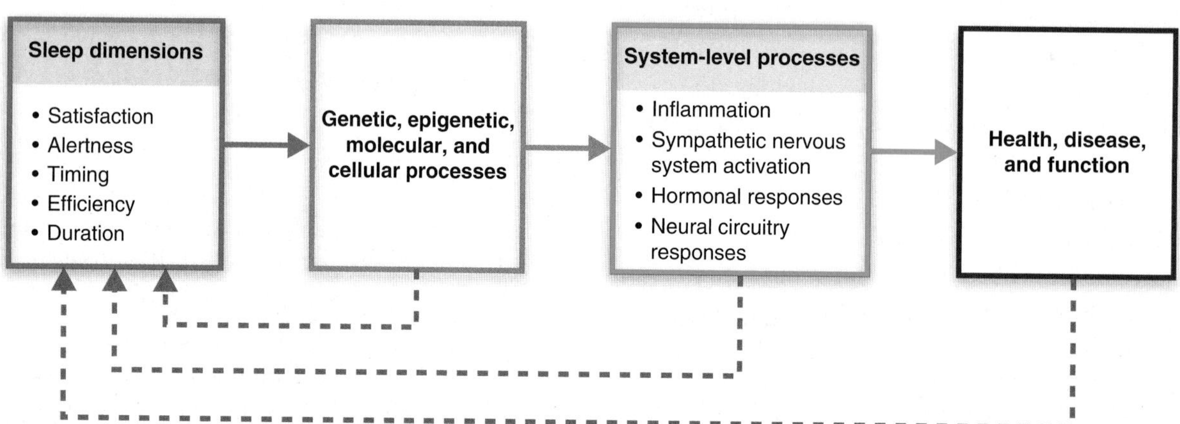

Figure 7.1 ■ Conceptual model of sleep health.

processes that affect health disease and function. Most important, there are reciprocal relationships among these processes such that just as sleep influences health, disease, and function, health disease and function influence sleep.

Case Studies

The following cases will be addressed throughout the chapter to assist in application of chapter content to clinical situations that involve individuals with disorders of sleep.

Kelly Chambliss: Introduction

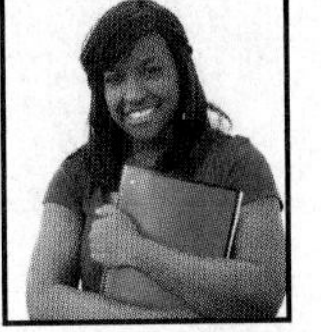

Kelly Chambliss is a third-year nursing student who sleeps about 5 hours a night. Her worries about clinical performance and tests often make it difficult for her to fall asleep. This has caused her to fall asleep in class, and she often finds her mind drifting when she wants to pay attention in her clinical setting.

1. What psychologic factor is affecting Ms. Chambliss ability to fall asleep?
2. Why is Ms. Chambliss falling asleep in class?

Stuart Jackson: Introduction

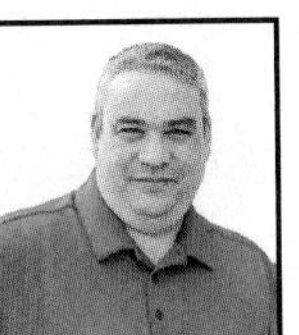

Stuart Jackson is an overweight middle-aged man who snores every night. His wife has noticed that he snores, snorts in his sleep, and occasionally wakes up gasping for breath. Because of his snoring, Mr. Jackson now sleeps in a separate bedroom. Mr. Jackson wakes up feeling tired and has fallen asleep several times at work.

1. What physical factor is contributing to Mr. Jackson's snoring?
2. Why does Mr. Jackson wake up feeling tired every day?
3. What other potential mental function impairments may occur as a result of Mr. Jackson's sleep problems?

Ann Rebo: Introduction

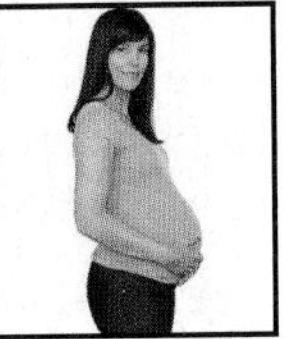

Ann Rebo, who is 7 months pregnant, is bothered by tingling and prickling in her legs whenever she lies down, especially at night. These sensations affect her ability to fall asleep, and they wake her up during the night. The only way to relieve these leg sensations is to get up and walk around.

1. Ms. Rebo has symptoms that suggest a condition called restless legs syndrome (RLS). What factor in her health history may be contributing to the development of this condition?
2. In educating Ms. Rebo about her complaint, would you tell her that her symptoms are a normal part of pregnancy and she shouldn't worry about them? Why or why not?
3. Ms. Rebo says that she thought her leg symptoms were simple leg cramps, and she is not clear on what RLS is. What patient education should be provided?

Check Your Progress: Section 7.1

1. Which part of the brain controls transitioning between NREM sleep and REM sleep?
2. What are some examples of sleep disorders?
3. To initiate sleep, what change must occur to the ascending neurologic arousal systems?

7.2 Normal Sleep

Sleep has been defined as a reversible state of detachment from the environment in which the individual neither senses nor responds to the surroundings. Its easy reversibility differentiates sleep from coma.

Sleep is regulated by two interacting processes: the homeostatic mechanism and the circadian rhythm (**Figure 7.2** ■). The **homeostatic mechanism** consists of physiologic processes that detect changes from a set baseline. During wake time, adenosine builds up in the brain, inhibiting acetylcholine and glutamine, two excitatory neurotransmitters. Caffeine helps alertness by blocking adenosine receptors in the brain. As the time since waking increases, so does the homeostatic need for sleep.

Circadian rhythm, the approximately 24-hour cycle of body processes, is regulated by the body's "master clock," the **suprachiasmatic nucleus (SCN)**, which is located in the anterior hypothalamus. The SCN controls secretion of **melatonin** (a sleep-inducing hormone produced by the pineal gland), triggering its release just before a person's normal bedtime. Melatonin release drops over the course of the sleep period. Exposure to light causes melatonin release to lessen (**Figure 7.3** ■).

Current guidelines divide normal sleep into four stages, based on the **electroencephalogram (EEG)**, a recording of the electrical activity of the brain.[4] The period between going to bed and the first stage of sleep is referred to as

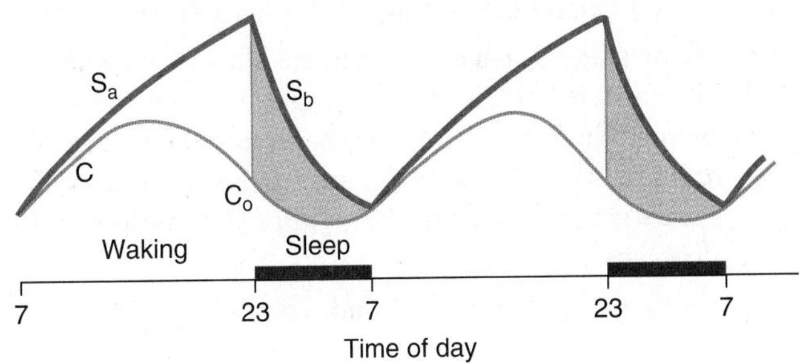

Figure 7.2 ■ This model, developed by Borbély and Ackerman in 1980, depicts how the circadian rhythm (process C) and homeostatic mechanism (process S) interact to regulate timing of sleep. As one spends time awake, the need for sleep builds up, creating sleep pressure (S_a). During sleep, this sleep pressure dissipates as the brain fulfills its need for sleep (S_b). The circadian process (C), by contrast, is the approximately 24-hour daily rest and activity rhythm of the body. When the circadian time for sleep onset (C_o) matches a high level of sleep pressure, the individual falls asleep. (If sleep does not occur at this time, the need and drive for sleep will continue to build until it is impossible to ignore. If the setting is inappropriate for sleep, the brain will go to sleep, though for only a few seconds. These micro sleeps are momentarily restorative to the brain but not noticeable by the individual.) During sleep, both the homeostatic and circadian drives for sleep decrease, and when they reach a minimum, the person awakens.

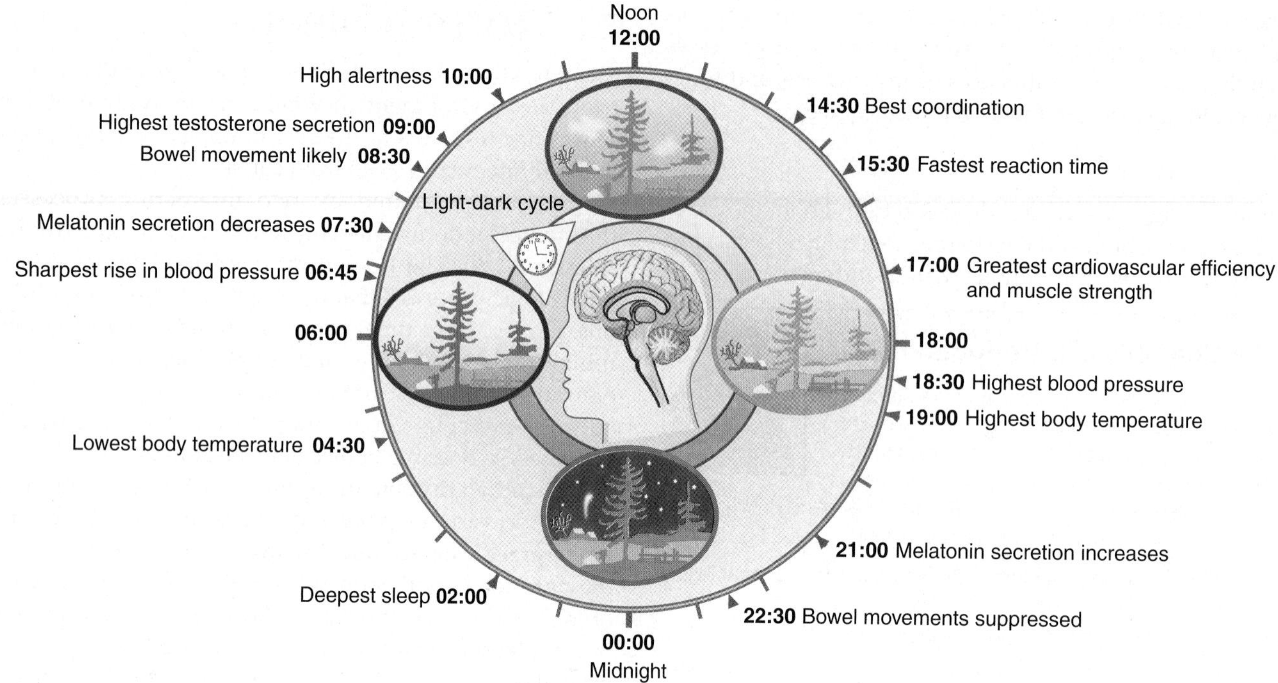

Figure 7.3 ■ Human biological clock.

sleep latency. The four sleep stages are as follows (see also **Figure 7.4** ■):

1. **N1** or stage 1, is sometimes called light sleep. The individual drifts from the awake state into sleep, and slow rolling movements of the eye may be observed. The EEG shows low-amplitude mixed-frequency waves usually in the range of 4–7 hertz (theta waves).
2. **N2** or stage 2, is considered the start of true sleep. The individual becomes disengaged from the environment, the respiratory and heart rates become more regular, the body temperature drops, and the EEG shows stage-specific features called K complexes and sleep spindles.
3. **N3** or stage 3, is also called deep sleep. Breathing becomes even slower. It is often referred to as delta sleep or slow wave sleep (SWS) because of the slow brain waves that are seen on the EEG.[1] Despite relaxation of muscles and a drop in blood pressure, the blood supply to the muscles increases during this stage. Restorative processes during this stage of sleep include renewal of energy, repair of tissues, and storage of short-term memories as long-term memories. Certain hormones, such as growth hormone, are released at this time. N1 through N3 are responsible for about 75% of sleep time in a normal healthy young adult and are collectively called **non-rapid eye movement sleep (NREM sleep)**.
4. In **rapid eye movement sleep (REM sleep)**, the eyes move back and forth rapidly. The brain is very active during this stage. An EEG performed during REM sleep is indistinguishable from an EEG performed on an awake individual, though eye movements and muscle tone differ in awake and asleep individuals.

   During REM sleep, voluntary muscles relax and do not respond to nervous stimuli. REM sleep is also required for learning and formation of long-term memories. Dreaming occurs primarily during this stage.

During the night, the brain cycles through the stages of sleep. The first cycle lasts about an hour and a half to 2 hours, with the first REM period beginning about 90 minutes after sleep onset. Subsequent cycles are shorter. N3 sleep occurs primarily in the first half of the night, while more REM sleep takes place in the second half of the night. The number of minutes spent in each stage of sleep changes across the lifespan (see **Figure 7.5** ■).

Infants spend 50–80% of their sleep time in REM sleep. As children grow, their sleep begins to transition to the pattern shown in adults, with relatively more N1 and N2 sleep and about 25% REM sleep. ■

Older adults have shorter sleep cycles and spend a smaller proportion of their sleep time in N3 and REM sleep. They also take longer to fall asleep, tend to wake up during their sleep more frequently and to stay awake longer when they do, and typically nap more than younger adults do. ■

Several hormones contribute to the regulation of sleep and wakefulness. Gamma-aminobutyric acid (GABA), a neurotransmitter that is widely distributed throughout the brain, enhances SWS, while norepinephrine helps to regulate REM sleep. Dopamine interacts with acetylcholine to increase wakefulness. The hormone **hypocretin** (also called orexin), which is produced in the hypothalamus, stimulates waking activity as well as regulating energy use, appetite, emotional behavior, and reward-seeking behaviors.

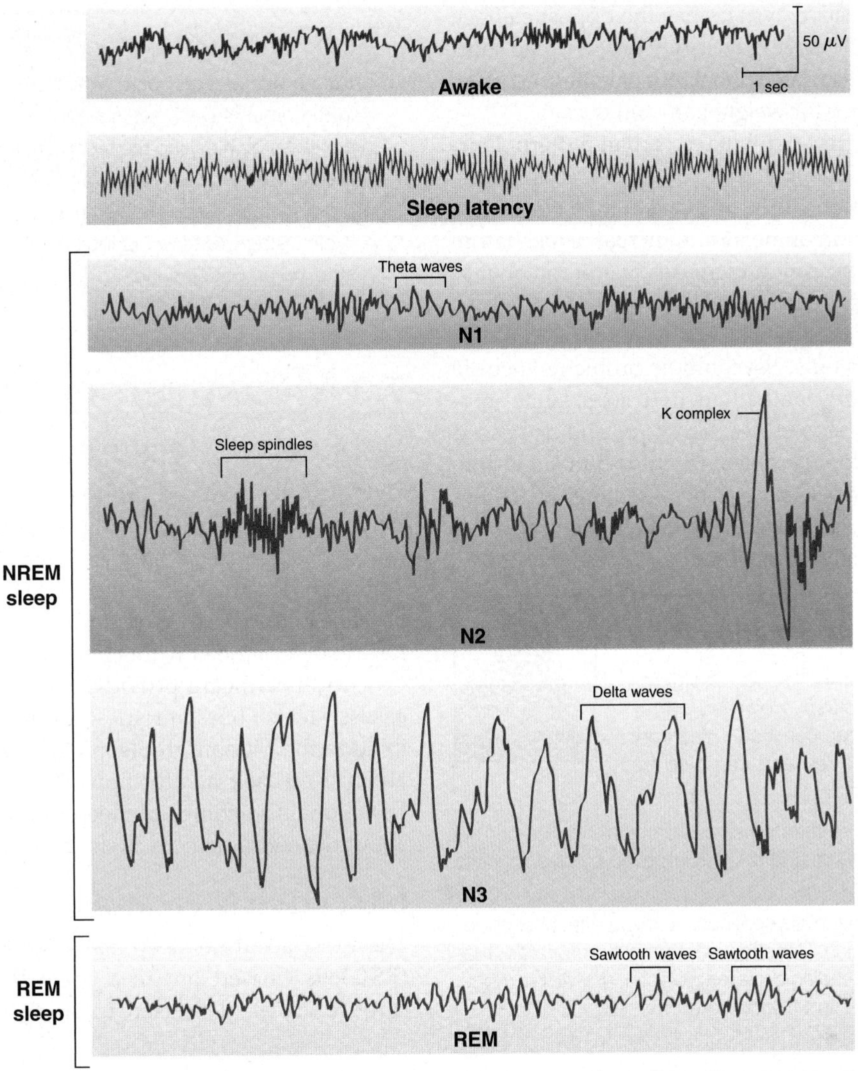

Figure 7.4 ■ Stages of sleep.

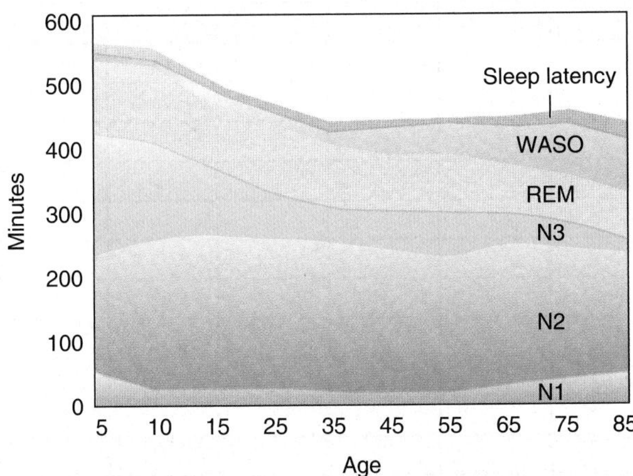

Figure 7.5 ■ Relative changes in distribution of sleep stages over the lifespan. WASO = wake after sleep onset.

During sleep, neurologic responses to changes in respiration decrease. The blunted response to changes in blood O_2 and CO_2 levels causes mild hypoventilation.

CLINICAL POINT: Hypoventilation can lead to hypercapnia (increased blood level of CO_2) and hypoxemia (decreased blood level of oxygen) in people who have COPD or heart failure and in those with sleep-disordered breathing. On awakening, it may take up to an hour for their blood oxygen and CO_2 to be restored to their usual baseline levels. ■

Many maintenance processes take place during sleep. Memories are stabilized, and recent memories are sorted and stored, important emotional context being saved and emotional content deemed unimportant being deleted. For this to happen, the individual needs at least 6 hours of sleep that includes both deep sleep (N3) and REM sleep. Physical coordination and performance of new skills also improve as the brain moves control of these actions to areas other than those used in learning the skills. Sleep also enables an individual to discern patterns and make inferences from information previously learned.[5]

Sleep is also intimately connected with metabolism. People who have short sleep duration experience both decreased leptin levels and increased ghrelin levels. Leptin, a hormone produced in adipose tissue, decreases the appetite and increases the amount of energy used; ghrelin, a hormone produced by the digestive system, has the opposite effect, increasing appetite and saving energy. Thus, chronic short sleep, because of the associated imbalance of leptin and ghrelin levels, is a risk factor for weight gain and obesity.

Other hormones also exhibit a circadian pattern. During sleep, secretion of prolactin and growth hormone increases, and secretion of thyroid-stimulating hormone decreases. The secretion of melatonin increases just before sleep, while cortisol secretion increases just before awakening in the morning (see Figure 7.3).

Lack of sleep, or sleep deprivation, leads to psychologic and physiologic problems. Psychologic problems include memory loss, irritability, inattention, delusions, labile emotions, slurred speech, slowed reaction time, and decreased coordination. Physiologic problems include blurred vision, dysfunctional hormone secretion, increased energy expenditure, weight gain, impaired blood cell function, and impaired immune system function.

Kelly Chambliss: Application

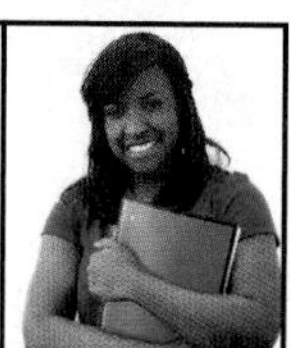

Kelly Chambliss believes that school problems are interfering with her sleep. However, it may be the opposite: Poor sleep can lead to memory problems and falling grades and can also be responsible for weight gain.

3. Ms. Chambliss is suffering memory problems. What normal process that occurs during sleep is impaired by sleeping less than 6 hours per night?
4. If Ms. Chambliss insomnia continues, it might affect her endocrine system function. Describe the normal hormonal fluctuations during the circadian cycle for prolactin, growth hormone, melatonin, cortisol, and thyroid hormone.

Check Your Progress: Section 7.2

1. During our waking hours, which neurotransmitter builds up in the brain and causes sleepiness? (Hint: Caffeine causes alertness by blocking the receptors for this chemical.)
2. Melatonin is a sleep-inducing hormone. Which part of the brain synthesizes this substance?
3. Which stage of sleep is indistinguishable from the awake state on an EEG tracing?

7.3 Measurement of Sleep

Subjective Measures

Sleep can be assessed both subjectively and objectively. Anyone who is experiencing a sleep problem should be asked to keep a sleep diary for several weeks (**Figure 7.6** ■). Although sleep diaries are known to be inexact, they provide baseline information on routine bedtimes and wake time and help to determine how much (or little) a person is sleeping.

Any healthcare provider can use written surveys to assess sleep characteristics. Examples of such surveys include the Pittsburgh Sleep Quality Index,[6,7] which asks about sleep itself, and the Epworth Sleepiness Scale[8] and the Functional Outcomes of Sleep Questionnaire,[9] which ask about the consequences of sleep.

Objective Measures

The most accurate sleep assessment, a **polysomnogram (PSG)**, is carried out in a specialized sleep laboratory (**Figure 7.7** ■). It is used to study normal sleep and to

Sleep Diary	Name:						
	Week of:						
Morning Questions	Mon.	Tues.	Wed.	Thurs.	Fri.	Sat.	Sun.
What time did you go to bed last night?							
What time did you fall asleep?							
How many times did you wake up last night?							
How long were you awake during the night?							
Was your sleep good, fair, or poor?							
Did you wake up before your alarm?							
How many times did you hit the snooze button?							
How do you feel this morning?							
Evening Questions	Mon.	Tues.	Wed.	Thurs.	Fri.	Sat.	Sun.
Did you drink any caffeine today?							
How much?							
Did you exercise today?							
How many minutes?							
How many times did you nap today?							
Did you drink any alcohol today?							
How much?							

Figure 7.6 ■ Example of a sleep diary.

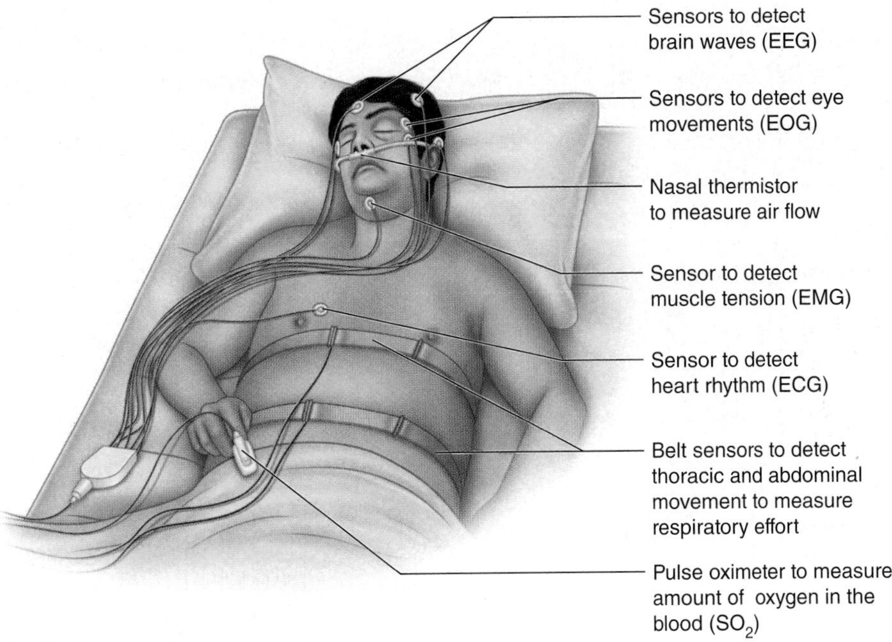

Figure 7.7 ■ Polysomnography setup.

diagnose sleep–wake disorders. The PSG consists of a battery of instruments, each of which measures a different sleep parameter:

- An EEG detects brain waves, necessary for identifying sleep stages.
- An **electromyelogram (EMG)** records muscle tension and relaxation.
- An **electro-oculogram (EOG)**, recording of eye movement, identifies REM sleep.
- An **electrocardiogram (ECG)** measures cardiac activity.
- A nasal thermistor measures nasal air flow to determine respirations.
- Thoracic and abdominal movement detectors measure respiratory effort.
- A pulse oximeter measures oxygen saturation (SO_2).
- Leg sensors detect body position and limb movements.

Home (ambulatory) sleep studies, which measure two to four of the parameters, are often used to screen for sleep disorders or in research.[10] They have been approved by the Centers for Medicare and Medicaid Services since 2008 for use in the adult population.

The findings of a PSG can be represented by a sleep histogram, or **hypnogram**, a diagram that depicts the stages of sleep (**Figure 7.8** ■ and **Figure 7.9** ■).

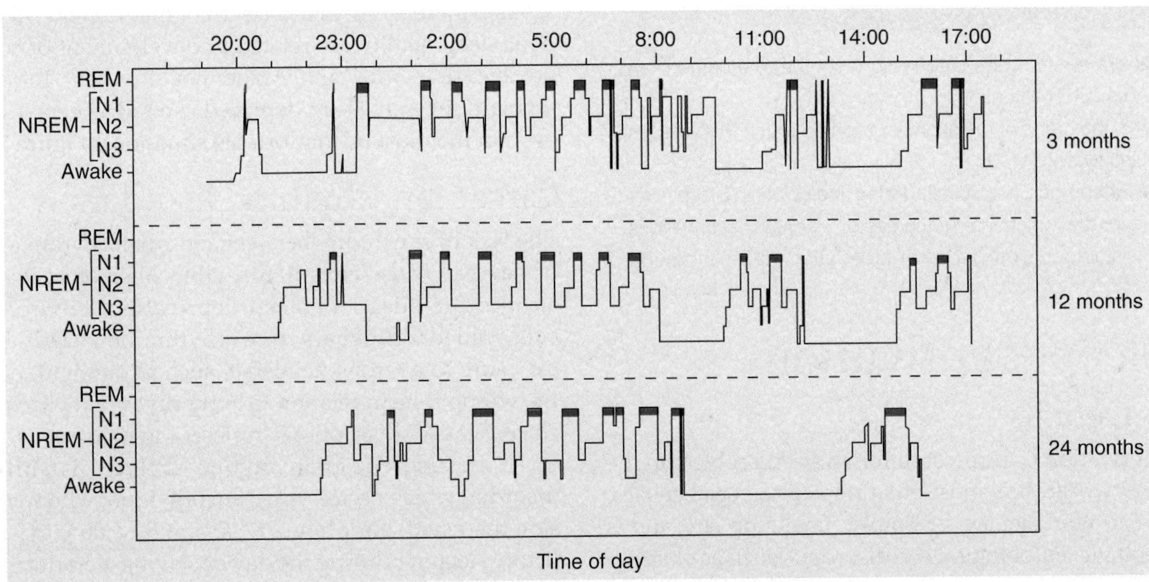

Figure 7.8 ■ Sample hypnograms of an infant at ages 3, 12, and 24 months.

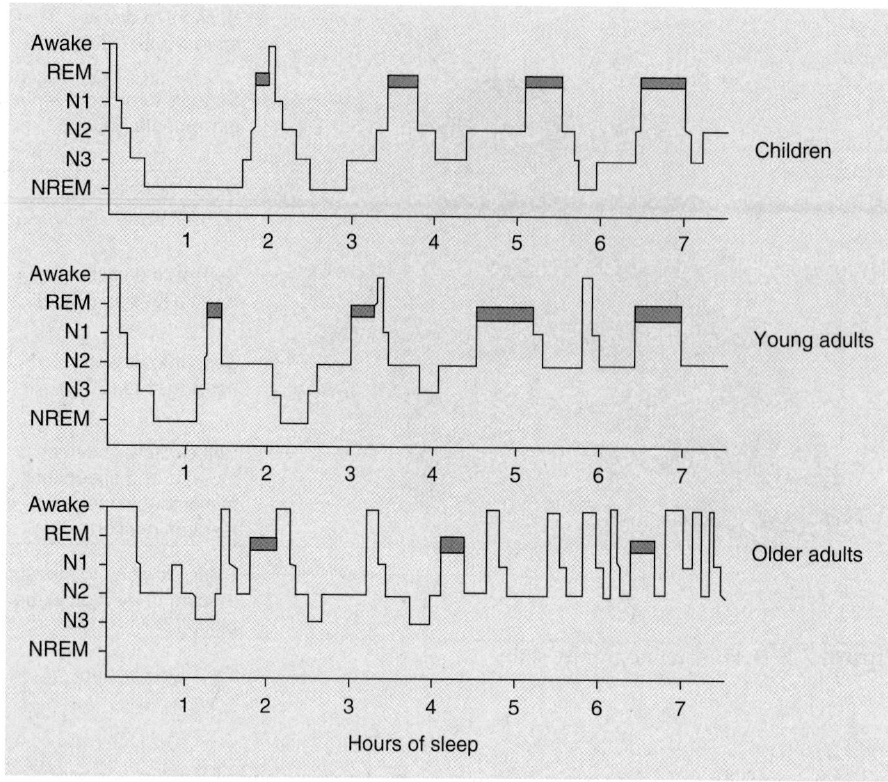

Figure 7.9 ■ Sample hypnograms of children, young adults, and older adults.

Other objective ways of studying sleep include pulse oximetry and actigraphy. An ambulatory pulse oximeter, which measures both the SO_2 and the pulse, can be used to screen for sleep apnea, although it cannot be used for diagnosis. An actigraph, or motion sensor, detects periods of activity and rest. Its data can be used as estimates of sleep characteristics, such as consecutive hours of sleep, number and length of awakenings during sleep period and total sleep time.

Check Your Progress: Section 7.3

1. What are some of the diagnostic tests that are carried out during a PSG evaluation?
2. What is the name of the chart or graph on which PSG results are displayed?
3. If the Pittsburgh Sleep Quality Index, the Epworth Sleepiness Scale, or the Functional Outcomes of Sleep Questionnaire is administered to a patient, what information will be obtained?

7.4 Sleep Deprivation

Sleep Deficits

Sleep deprivation is the most common sleep problem in the developed world. It is most often related to social causes, such as shift work, jet lag, or simply staying up late, and is not pathologic. Pathologic sleep disorders, such as obstructive sleep apnea and narcolepsy, also lead to insufficient sleep, causing sleep deprivation. Although not a pathologic condition itself, any kind of sleep deprivation is a risk factor for several diseases. Short sleep duration and sleep disruption from any cause are associated with changes in inflammatory markers, increased insulin resistance, hypertension and other cardiovascular problems, stroke, and increased all-cause mortality (**Figure 7.10** ■).[11]

Neurobehavioral consequences of sleep deprivation include emotional lability, prolonged reaction time, inability to pay close attention to a task for a prolonged period, and deficits in functions (such as making decisions). There is also increasing evidence that insufficient sleep and poor sleep quality are related to development of cognitive decline, dementia, and Alzheimer disease.[12] Individuals who are severely sleep deprived can fall asleep anywhere, even in the most uncomfortable situations (**Figure 7.11** ■).

Circadian Rhythm Disorders

The lack of synchrony between circadian rhythm and time of day can cause circadian rhythm mismatch, leading to sleep difficulties and sleep deprivation. Environmental cues, called **zeitgebers**, reset rhythm on a daily basis. If exposure to a strong zeitgeber, such as sunlight, occurs at the wrong time in relation to body rhythm, the lack of synchrony causes disruptions in sleep and alertness.

One such circadian rhythm problem is **shift work disorder**, which occurs when an individual who works outside the usual work hours (7:00 a.m. to 6:00 p.m.) has difficulty sleeping during the day or staying alert during work hours. Shift workers are often exposed to sunlight on their way to or from work, which resets their circadian rhythm.

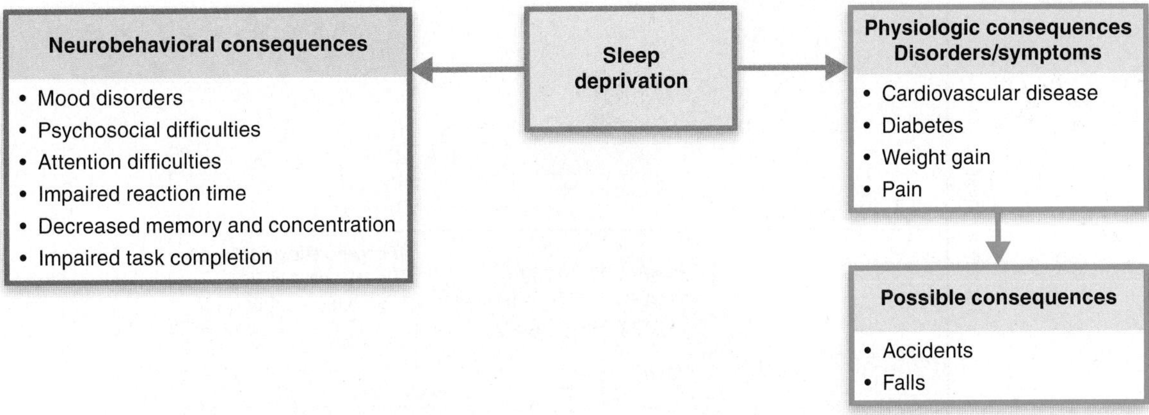

Figure 7.10 ■ Consequences of sleep deprivation include neurobehavioral and physiologic issues that can result in increased consumption of healthcare resources.

The resulting sleep deprivation predisposes the individual to accidents and errors at work and at home.

Adolescents often experience a shift in circadian rhythm called **sleep phase delay**. They go to sleep later, and consequently, they wake up later when permitted. This phase delay is secondary to two factors that occur during puberty: (1) Melatonin secretion starts later in the day, and (2) the need to sleep (homeostatic sleep drive) builds up more slowly. Nonetheless, adolescents' sleep requirement remains 8.5–9.5 hours per night, and they can easily accumulate significant sleep debt, which affects physical and mental health, accident rates, and academic performance. The American Academy of Pediatrics recommends that middle schools and high schools start after 8:30 a.m.[13] ■

Rapid travel across several time zones leads to sleep alterations and **jet lag** because the person's internal circadian rhythm is not synchronous with the outside world. Generally, the body can adapt to a change of 1 hour without difficulty.

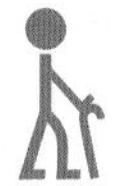

Jet lag becomes more difficult to adjust to as a person ages. ■

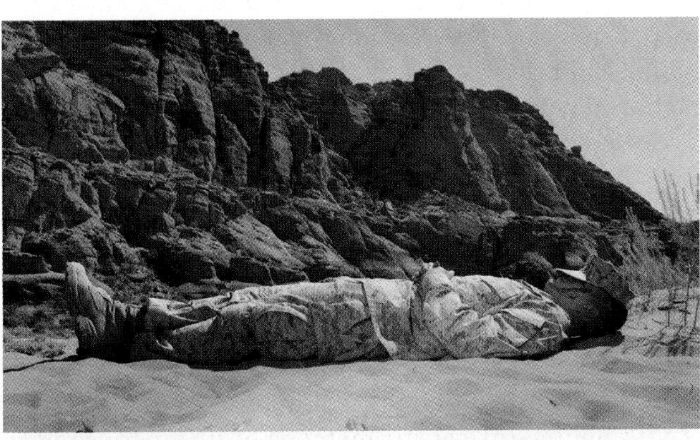

Figure 7.11 ■ Individuals who are severely sleep deprived can fall asleep anywhere, as demonstrated by this U.S. soldier in Afghanistan.

Although there is no perfect treatment for jet lag, several actions can help. Because exposure to sunlight is the strongest zeitgeber, it is advisable to spend time outside during daylight at the destination. Taking melatonin or a melatonin agonist, such as ramelteon (Rozerem), about 5–30 minutes before going to bed at the destination can help, as can using a short-acting hypnotic, such as zolpidem (Ambien) or zaleplon (Sonata). Stimulants such as caffeine, modafinil (Provigil), or armodafinil (Nuvigil) may help during the day.

Check Your Progress: Section 7.4

1. What shift in the circadian rhythm is seen in adolescents?
2. What strong zeitgeber may reset the circadian rhythm of individuals with shift work disorder?
3. Traveling across several time zones rapidly can cause what circadian rhythm disorder?

7.5 Insomnia

Insomnia, having difficulty initiating or maintaining sleep, is a highly prevalent condition, affecting about 30–50% of the adult population.

Etiology and Pathogenesis

Almost everyone experiences insomnia at some time. Three types of factors are implicated in the development of insomnia: predisposing factors, precipitating factors, and perpetuating factors (**Figure 7.12** ■).[14] Predisposing factors relate to the individual's tendency to have difficulty sleeping, such as hyperarousal or frequently worrying. Precipitating factors, such as loss of a job, a death in the family, or other stressful event, trigger a period of poor sleep. Most episodes of insomnia are acute and last only 3–4 weeks. However, in individuals who have perpetuating factors, such as inadequate coping skills or poor sleep habits, which contribute to prolongation of the episode, the insomnia may last over a month, becoming chronic.

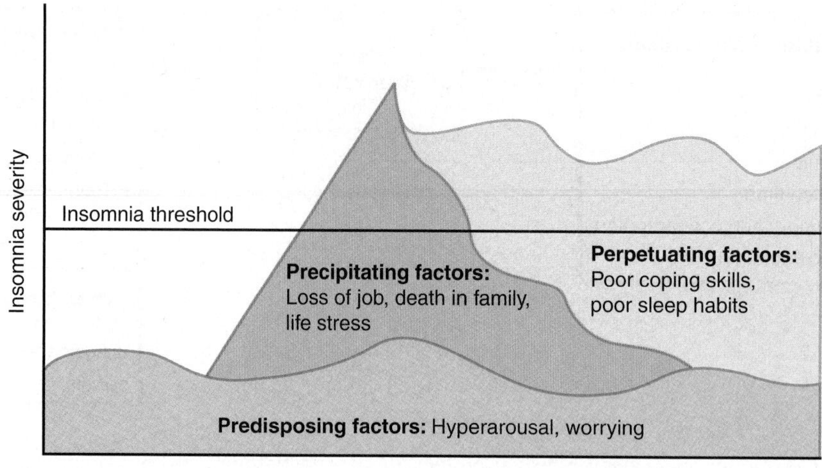

Figure 7.12 ■ Individual predisposing factors exist in the person's daily life but usually cause no problems. When a precipitating factor occurs, such as an unusual stress, the person will experience insomnia that will continue at varying levels for a few weeks and then disappear. However, if the individual experiences any perpetuating factors, such as anxiety related to poor sleep, after about 4 weeks the insomnia may become chronic, and it may last for years.

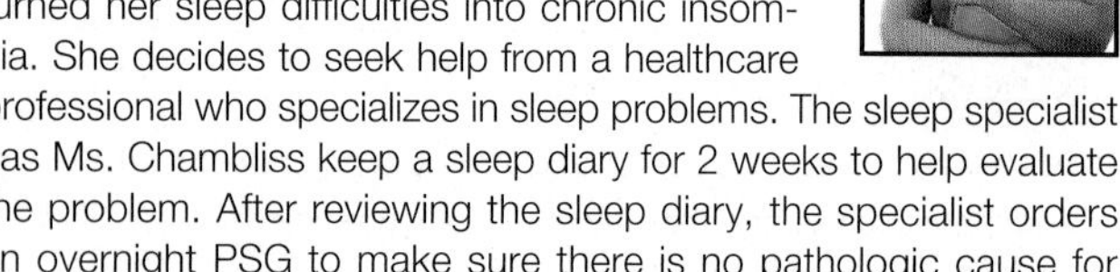

Kelly Chambliss: Application

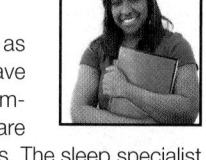

The ongoing stresses of school are acting as perpetuating factors for Ms. Chambliss and have turned her sleep difficulties into chronic insomnia. She decides to seek help from a healthcare professional who specializes in sleep problems. The sleep specialist has Ms. Chambliss keep a sleep diary for 2 weeks to help evaluate the problem. After reviewing the sleep diary, the specialist orders an overnight PSG to make sure there is no pathologic cause for Ms. Chambliss sleeplessness.

5. Ms. Chambliss's PSG report indicates increased sleep latency. What does this term imply?
6. Ms. Chambliss asks you whether she will be able to stop falling asleep or suffering loss of attention during the day. What do you tell her?
7. Ms. Chambliss tells you that she is not sure she will be able to maintain her sleep hygiene, since she is so busy with school. She doesn't believe that insomnia will hurt her over time. What patient education do you provide?

Clinical Manifestations

Insomnia can have significant effects on an individual. It is a risk factor for several mental disorders, particularly major depression, anxiety disorders, and substance abuse. Chronic insomnia is also associated with decreased cognitive ability and impaired performance of monotonous tasks, particularly driving.[15] Physiologic effects include decreased immune function. Insomnia-related fatigue and irritability can lead to decreased exercise and social isolation. Insomnia has been implicated as a risk factor for type 2 diabetes, chronic pain, hypertension, and cardiovascular disease. The cost of insomnia in the United States is over $1 billion a year, consisting of the direct costs of healthcare visits and medications and the indirect costs of accidents, decreased work productivity, and absenteeism from work.[10]

Linking Pathophysiology to Diagnosis and Treatment

Diagnosis of insomnia is based on patient report. When someone complains of insomnia, it is necessary to perform a complete assessment to ascertain whether or not the insomnia is the presenting symptom of another sleep or medical disorder. PSG is not performed to evaluate insomnia, but it may be used to rule out other sleep disorders as the cause of the poor sleep. Additionally, examination of a 2-week sleep diary (see Figure 7.6) is necessary. Use of a subjective tool to measure sleep quality, such as the Pittsburgh Sleep Quality Index[6] or the Insomnia Severity Index[16,17] will aid in the diagnosis. Actigraphy can be used as an objective measure and to validate the information on the sleep diary.

Acute insomnia may be treated with a short course of a hypnotic, such as a benzodiazepine receptor agonist (e.g., zolpidem, zopiclone, zaleplon, eszopiclone). Newer drugs, including melatonin receptor agonists (e.g., ramelteon) or a histamine receptor antagonist (e.g., doxepin), can also be used. Benzodiazepines are not recommended because they inhibit REM sleep and increase the risk of falls during the night and next-day drowsiness.

Mindfulness meditation, t'ai chi, and cognitive–behavioral therapy have all been used to treat chronic insomnia.[18] A 3- to 6-week course of cognitive–behavioral therapy is the most successful treatment. If the individual has a pronounced shift in circadian rhythm, phototherapy will be used to reset the internal clock in the suprachiasmatic nucleus.

Insomnia in older adults is frequently related to chronic disease and medication use. For this reason, nonpharmacologic methods of treating insomnia, particularly cognitive–behavioral therapy, are preferred. Although t'ai chi is also effective in improving sleep quality, fatigue, and depressive symptoms, it is not as effective in older adults as cognitive–behavioral therapy.[18] ■

Kelly Chambliss: Outcome

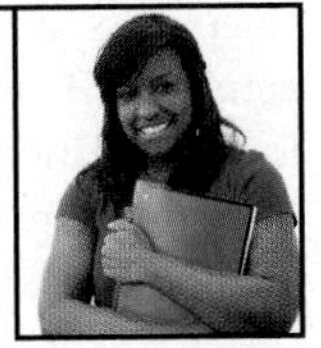

Ms. Chambliss's sleep diary, actigraphy, and PSG show prolonged sleep latency and prolonged wake times during the middle of the night. Ms. Chambliss starts cognitive–behavioral therapy, which begins with developing better sleep hygiene. Within 2 months, she begins sleeping better, her grades are starting to improve, and she is able to continue the sleep improvement program on her own.

8. Over time, Ms. Chambliss's symptoms have improved with treatment methods such as improved sleep hygiene and cognitive–behavioral therapy. Will she have to remain under active clinical care, or can she maintain these methods on her own?
9. If Ms. Chambliss had not sought treatment for her insomnia, would she be at risk of any physical complications of chronic sleep deprivation?
10. Ms. Chambliss had a predisposing factor to developing insomnia: frequent worrying. Her perpetuating factors that created a chronic condition included the stress of school. She has asked whether there is a possibility of having episodes of insomnia in the future. What is your reply?

Check Your Progress: Section 7.5

1. What is the term for something that can trigger the development of insomnia?
2. An impairment in the performance of monotonous tasks such as driving, with the resultant increase in automobile accidents, occurs in what common sleep disorder?
3. With which complementary/alternative therapies has insomnia been successfully treated?

7.6 Sleep-Disordered Breathing

Sleep-disordered breathing occurs when respiratory airflow is disrupted either as a result of airway constriction or collapse (obstructive sleep apnea) or because of impaired neurologic control of respiration (central sleep apnea). Sleep-disordered breathing is the most common primary sleep disorder in the United States. It can range from simple, uncomplicated snoring to life-threatening obstructive sleep apnea.

Obstructive Sleep Apnea

Obstructive sleep apnea (OSA) is a condition in which breathing repeatedly stops and starts during sleep. This may happen up to 60 (or more!) times an hour secondary to airway constriction or collapse. It is estimated that about 26% of adults between the ages of 30 and 70 years in the United States have OSA as defined as a decrease or cessation of airflow five or more times an hour during sleep.[19]

It is estimated that approximately 50% of the elderly experience some form of sleep-disordered breathing.[11] Because sleep-disordered breathing is a risk factor for falls, cognitive impairments, and increased mortality, every older adult patient should be asked about symptoms. ■

Risk factors for OSA include being male, overweight, and middle-aged or older and having an anatomic abnormality of the upper airway, such as a fat tongue or a thick neck. Although men are 3–4 times as likely as women to experience OSA, being postmenopausal increases a woman's risk of this condition. Being edentulous (lacking teeth) increases the risk, and the **apnea–hypopnea index (AHI)**, the number of times airflow stops or decreases per hour of sleep, increases if dentures are removed for sleep.

Etiology and Pathogenesis

Excess body weight leads to enlargement of fat pads, which narrow the pharyngeal airway. Fat deposition in the chest or abdominal wall increases the work of breathing and leads to hypoventilation and increased secretion of leptin, which influences breathing. Abnormal craniofacial anatomy (such as decreased anterior–posterior space at the base of the cranium; lowered location of the hyoid; long soft palate; enlarged tongue, tonsils, or adenoids; small lower jaw; or lower jaw behind the plane of the upper jaw) can decrease airway size, thereby increasing the risk of OSA (**Figure 7.13** ■). Other risk factors include use of alcohol or sedative or hypnotic drugs.

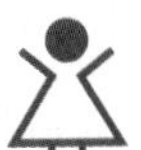

In children, OSA is usually secondary to enlarged tonsils or facial or upper airway malformation. ■

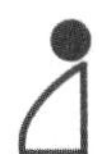

The increased risk for OSA in pregnant women is thought to be related to their increased weight and to swelling of the nasal mucosa. ■

In individuals with Alzheimer disease, a decrease in the activity of cholinergic neurons, which help to regulate respiratory drive and upper airway motor activity, may also increase the OSA risk. ■

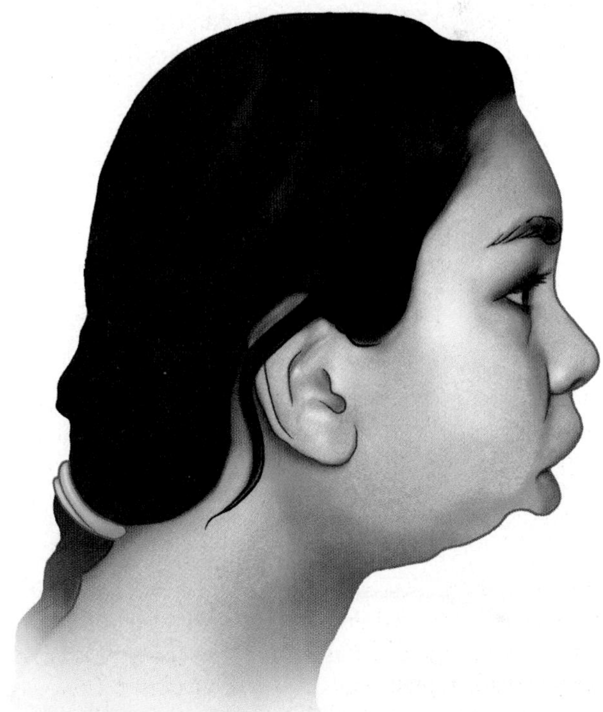

Figure 7.13 ■ A young woman with retrognathia (lower jaw behind the plane of the upper jaw).

During wake periods, normal muscle tone in the pharyngeal dilator muscles holds the upper airway open. However, when muscle tone is lost during sleep (especially during REM sleep), the airway can collapse, leading to blockage (**Figure 7.14** ■). In people who have OSA, decreased muscle tone may be secondary to a decrease in nervous stimulation of these muscles or to an anatomic abnormality in the airway. In people who sleep on their backs, the tongue may relax and fall backwards, leading to airway narrowing or blockage. If the airway is partially blocked, the individual may snore without any change in the blood oxygen level (SO_2) or may experience a transient drop in the SO_2 (**hypopnea**). If the problem is more severe, the airway may be totally blocked, and air flow ceases, leading to a drop in SO_2 that lasts for several seconds. To be classified as an apnea for an adult, the cessation of airflow must last at least 10 seconds.

CLINICAL POINT: It is important to note that during an obstructive apnea event, ventilatory efforts continue, and both abdominal and thoracic movements can be observed. These movements of the abdomen and thorax are termed paradoxical because they are opposite to each other; as the chest rises, the abdomen sinks, and vice versa. ■

The rise in blood CO_2 (hypercapnia) and drop in blood O_2 (desaturation) cause the individual to momentarily arouse, and airway muscle tone returns. The individual then takes a breath and falls back to sleep, and the cycle begins again. Although the individual may gasp for air or snort during the associated arousal, these arousals are too short for the individual to remember on wakening in the morning. However, they may be noticed by the sleep partner, who often reports having witnessed breathing pauses, gasping, or snorting. The brief awakenings interrupt the sleep cycle, and many people who have OSA experience almost no deep sleep or REM sleep, leading to complaints of sleep that is not restful, morning headaches or dry throat, daytime sleepiness, and even falling asleep at work or during social activities. This drowsiness can lead to accidents; there is an increased incidence of automobile accidents in people who have untreated OSA.[20] Nocturia and erectile dysfunction also occur more often in people who have OSA.

In children, OSA does not always present with signs of sleepiness. Rather, children with OSA, like other children who have insufficient sleep, are usually hyperactive and inattentive and exhibit behavior problems. ■

The frequent desaturation–awakening–reoxygenation events have distinct pathophysiologic consequences. Because sympathetic nervous system activity increases, the heart rate rises briefly, leading to an increase in venous return, which in turn causes a transient rapid rise in blood pressure. This process repeats itself several hundred times a night and is thought to lead over the course of years to permanent thickening of arteriolar walls, narrowed arteriolar lumens, increased peripheral resistance, and hypertension that is resistant to treatment.

The reoxygenation that follows hypoxia leads to a surge in production of free radicals, particularly reactive oxygen species, which combine with nitric oxide, causing a decrease in circulating nitric oxide. The combination of increased reactive oxygen species and decreased nitric oxide causes oxidative stress, which leads to increased levels of inflammatory mediators (cytokines, adipokines, and adhesion molecules) and decreased circulating antioxidants. The resulting inflammation and endothelial dysfunction constitute another cause of treatment-resistant hypertension and atherosclerosis.[21] This intermittent hypoxemia causes greater physiologic stress on the body than an equivalent uninterrupted period of hypoxemia. Over and above its effect on blood pressure, untreated OSA is an independent risk factor for coronary heart disease, myocardial infarctions, and strokes.

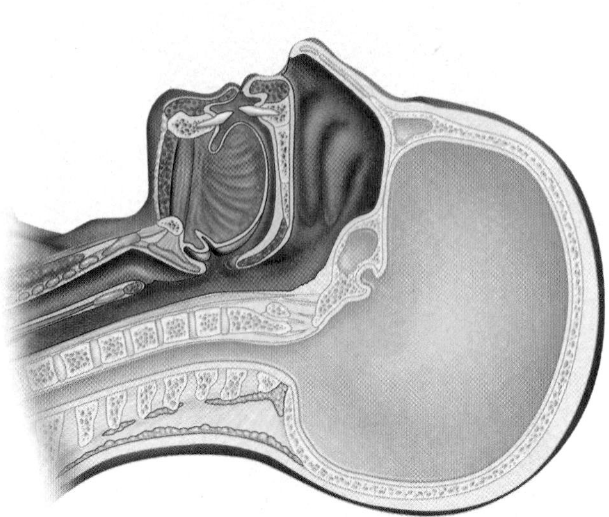

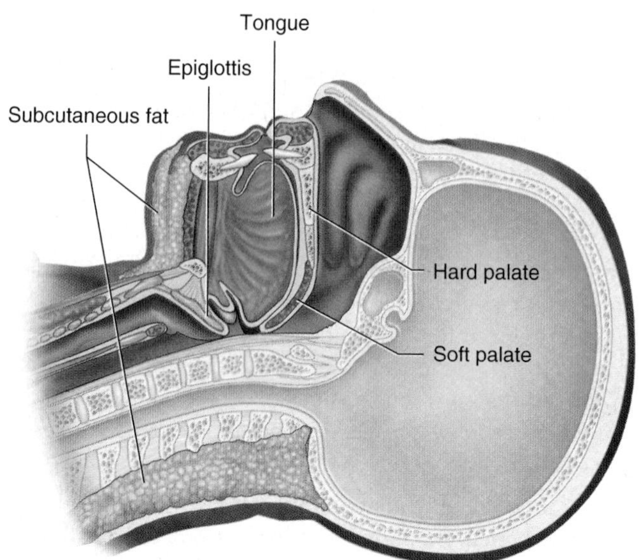

Figure 7.14 ■ Illustration of the anatomy of a normal subject (**A**) and a patient with sleep apnea (**B**). The upper airway is smaller and the soft palate is longer in the patient with sleep apnea, clearly blocking the airway. The amount of subcutaneous fat (shown in yellow at the back of the neck and under the chin) is greater in the apneic patient than in the normal subject.

Clinical Manifestations

Because of its effect in decreasing SWS and REM, in addition to the effects of decreased oxygenation of the brain during sleep, sleep apnea has multiple effects on cognitive and neurobehavioral functions. The individual with untreated OSA will have poor short-term memory, decreased ability to convert short-term to long-term memory, decreased ability to maintain attention when performing tasks over time, increased reaction time, difficulty planning or carrying out plans, and problems processing information. These consequences may also be responsible for the higher rates of delirium in postoperative patients who have untreated OSA. The major social effect of OSA is social isolation. Erectile dysfunction is also more common in men who have OSA than in men with normal sleep.[8]

Because of apnea-induced hypoxia, untreated OSA can lead to poor fetal growth, small placenta, and babies that are small for gestational age at birth. Therefore, women with OSA risk factors or pregnancy-associated problems such as hypertension, preeclampsia, and gestational diabetes, or slow intrauterine growth should be screened for the condition. ■

Stuart Jackson: Application

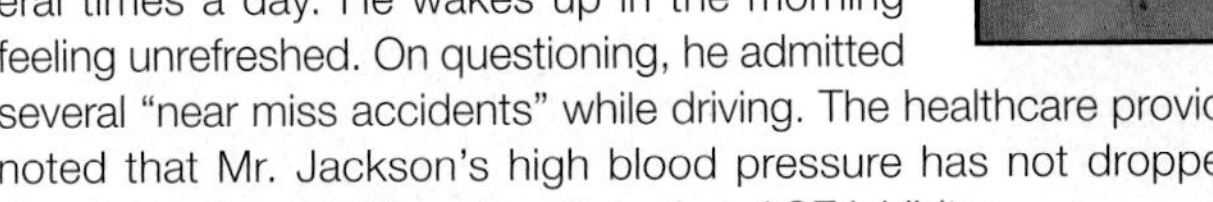

Mr. Jackson told his healthcare provider that he has difficulty concentrating and falls asleep several times a day. He wakes up in the morning feeling unrefreshed. On questioning, he admitted several "near miss accidents" while driving. The healthcare provider noted that Mr. Jackson's high blood pressure has not dropped, despite treatment with a diuretic and an ACE inhibitor.

4. If Mr. Jackson were not middle-aged but were 65 years old or older, why would you ask about snoring as part of the health history?
5. You receive the PSG report on Mr. Jackson when he comes to the sleep clinic for his follow-up visit. He asks what types of results on the PSG confirmed his diagnosis of OSA. What would be expected on the PSG report for someone with OSA?
6. What possible postoperative anesthesia complication is increased for someone like Mr. Jackson who has untreated OSA?

Linking Pathophysiology to Diagnosis and Treatment

People are sometimes screened for sleep apnea by using overnight pulse oximetry at home. If the pulse oximetry shows multiple desaturations lasting more than a few seconds or if the assessment and health history indicate the probability of sleep apnea, the person should undergo full overnight PSG in a sleep laboratory or use a portable PSG at home. PSG is required for definitive diagnosis and for differentiation among OSA, central sleep apnea, and other sleep disorders. The major diagnostic criterion is the AHI. In OSA, respiratory efforts in the form of chest and abdominal movements are seen throughout the periods that show no airflow; in central sleep apnea, there is complete absence of respiratory efforts during airflow absence. The PSG will often show a pattern of Cheyne-Stokes breathing. **Table 7.1** ■ compares the PSG findings for OSA, central sleep apnea, and other sleep disorders.

Lifestyle changes are often recommended for people with mild sleep apnea. Since most people who have OSA are overweight, weight loss is usually recommended. Although this helps to alleviate the problem, people with OSA tend not to be able to lose enough weight to resolve the problem. Bariatric surgery has improved OSA in morbidly obese patients (those with a body mass index [the weight in kilograms divided by the square of the height in meters] $\geq$ 40), but the improvement is not usually sufficient to preclude the need for further OSA therapy. Other lifestyle changes that may help people with OSA include smoking cessation and developing better sleep habits (such as not eating a heavy meal before bedtime

Table 7.1 Comparison of PSG Findings in Sleep Disorders

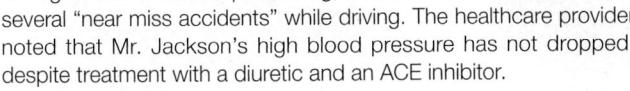

Condition and Sleep Architecture	PSG Findings
Obstructive sleep apnea Decreased SWS and REM sleep; frequent arousals following O_2 desaturations	**EEG:** Frequent periods of N1 and microarousals **Oximetry:** Periods of desaturation lasting at least 10 seconds for hypopneas; for an apneic event, there does not have to be a desaturation **Airflow:** Decreased during periods of desaturation (hypopnea); measured or absent (apnea) **EOG:** Normal **Muscle tension:** Normal **Chest and abdominal wall movement:** Continue through desaturation periods; paradoxic movements often noted (chest and abdomen expand and contract oppositely) **Visual (video camera feed):** Paradoxical respiratory movements during desaturation (chest and abdomen expand and contract oppositely) **AHI:** The total number of obstructive apneas and hypopneas divided by the total sleep time provides the apnea–hypopnea index (AHI) *Severity (for adults):* • AHI 5 to < 15/hour: mild OSA • AHI 15 to < 30/hour: moderate OSA • AHI ≥ 30/hour: severe OSA
Central sleep apnea Decreased SWS and REM sleep	**EEG:** Frequent periods of N1 and microarousals **Oximetry:** can have periods of desaturation **Airflow:** absent for at least 10 seconds without any effort for each event **EOG:** Normal **Muscle tension:** Normal **Chest and abdominal movement:** Absent during event **Visual:** No abdominal or chest movement seen during desaturation periods

(*Continued*)

Table 7.1 Comparison of PSG Findings in Sleep Disorders *Continued*

Condition and Sleep Architecture	PSG Findings
Narcolepsy REM periods at onset of sleep during a Multiple Sleep Latency Test	**EEG:** Short sleep latency; frequent awakenings **Oximetry:** Normal **Airflow:** Normal **EOG:** Normal **Muscle tension:** Normal **Chest and abdominal movement:** Normal **Visual:** Normal
REM behavior disorder Normal	**EEG:** Normal during all sleep stages **Oximetry:** Normal **Airflow:** Normal **EOG:** Normal **Muscle tension:** No atonia during REM sleep **Chest and abdominal movement:** Normal **Visual:** Movement seen during REM sleep: sleepwalking, sleep eating, acting out of dreams

NOTE: EEG = electroencephalogram; EOG = electro-oculogram

SOURCES: Data from Ahmed, I., & Thorpy, M. (2010). Clinical features, diagnosis and treatment of narcolepsy. *Clinics in Chest Medicine, 31*(2), 371–381; Bloom, H. G., Ahmed, I., Alessi, C. A., et al. (2009). Evidence-based recommendations for the assessment and management of sleep disorders in older persons. *Journal of the American Geriatrics Society, 57*(5), 761–789; Gooneratne, N. S., & Vitiello, M. V. (2014). Sleep in older adults: Normative changes, sleep disorders, and treatment options. *Clinics in Geriatric Medicine, 30*(3), 591–627; Roth, T., Dauvilliers, Y., Mignot, E., et al. (2013). Disrupted nighttime sleep in narcolepsy. *Journal of Clinical Sleep Medicine, 9*(9), 955–965; Berry, R. B., Brooks, R., Gamaldo, C. E., Harding, S. M., Lloyd, R. M., Marcus, C. L., & Vaughn, B. V. (2016). *The AASM manual for the scoring of sleep and associated events: Rules, terminology and technical specifications* (Version 2.3). Darien, IL: American Academy of Sleep Medicine; Silber, M. H. (2013). Sleep-related movement disorders. *CONTINUUM: Lifelong Learning in Neurology, 19*(1 Sleep Disorders), 170–184.

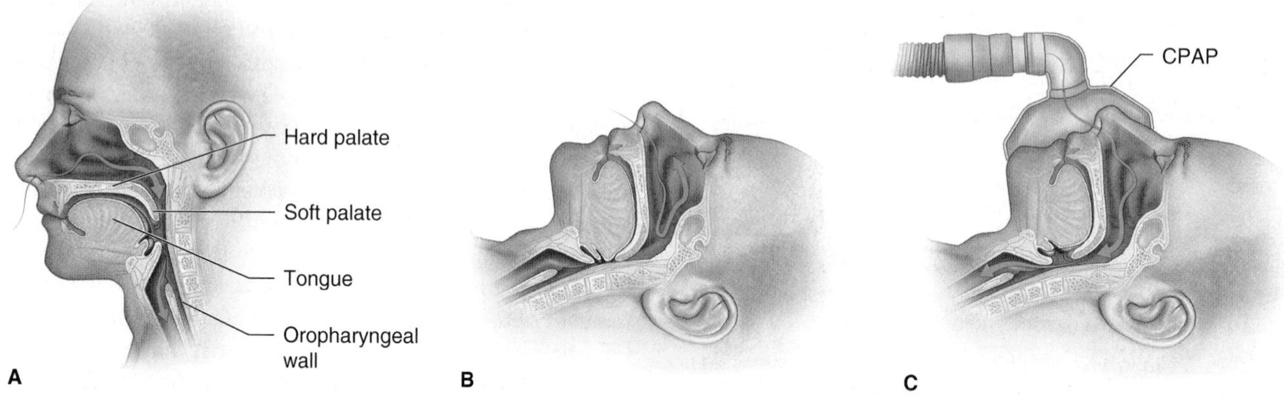

Figure 7.15 ■ How nasal CPAP therapy works in OSA. **A.** In the awake individual, muscle tone maintains an open airway against negative pressure during inspiration. **B.** When the individual is asleep, the tongue, soft palate, and oropharyngeal walls collapse, closing off the airway. **C.** Positive pressure, supplied by CPAP, acts as a splint to keep the airway open regardless of the sleeper's position.

and a decrease or elimination of alcohol use in the evening). For the few patients who have apneas only when they sleep on their backs, measures to prevent back sleeping (such as putting hard pillows behind them in bed or sewing a tennis ball in the neck of their pajamas) may prevent the apneas.

The most effective treatment for OSA is nasal **continuous positive airway pressure (CPAP)** (**Figure 7.15** ■ and **Figure 7.16** ■). The CPAP machine provides a flow of air at a preset pressure, which acts as a splint to hold the airway open. The proper pressure for an individual is determined during a PSG in which the pressure is adjusted upward (titrated) until the apnea–hypopnea rate is decreased by 90%. Most CPAP machines have a built-in heater/humidifier unit to prevent dry nose and throat problems associated with constant high air flow through the airway.

Oral appliances are another option for treating OSA, particularly in people with simple snoring or mild to moderate OSA and in people who either refuse CPAP treatment or have been unsuccessful in using it. These appliances expand

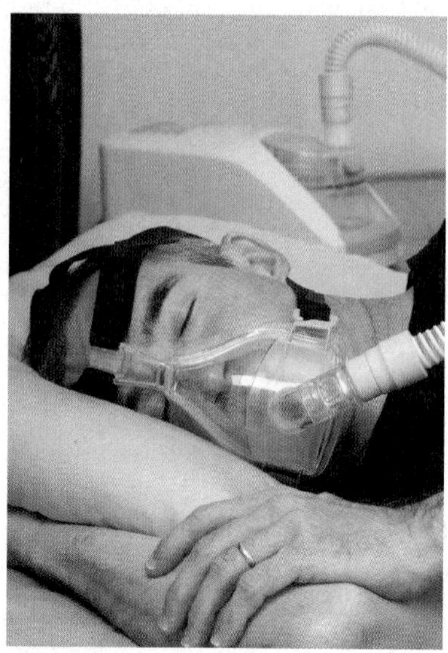

Figure 7.16 ■ CPAP in use.

the upper airway by moving the lower jaw or tongue forward and possibly by increasing airway muscle tone.

A fourth option for treating OSA is surgery to correct the anatomy of the individual's upper airway. The oldest treatment for OSA is surgical creation of a permanent tracheotomy, which bypasses the collapsible upper airway. Nasal reconstruction can be performed if the blockage is within the nose or nasopharynx. Uvulopalatopharyngoplasty (surgery to remove the uvula and parts of the soft palate and soft tissues of the pharynx), laser-assisted uvulopalatoplasty, and procedures to decrease the size or position of the base of the tongue have all been used to increase the size of the airway. Adverse effects associated with these procedures are serious, however, and the procedures themselves may not be effective in curing the OSA. See the Research feature for more information on the treatment of OSA and its relationship with hypertension.

In children, OSA is often secondary to enlarged tonsils and/or adenoids, and removal of the tonsils or adenoids may cure the condition. However, the child should undergo repeat PSG 3–6 months after surgery to verify that there are no residual apneas. ■

Stuart Jackson: Outcome

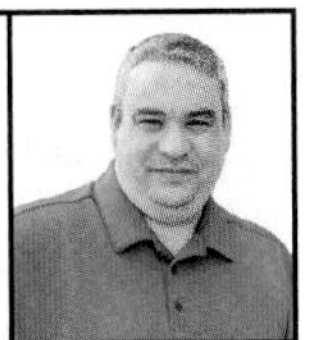

Although Mr. Jackson does not like the idea of using CPAP every night for the rest of his life, the idea of surgery is even less appealing. He decides to try the CPAP machine and uses it about 4–5 hours a night most nights of the week. After a month, he reports that he is feeling more energetic, that he can stay awake at work and at home in the evening, and that his wife has started sleeping as his bed partner again.

7. Mr. Jackson is feeling upset that he has the diagnosis of OSA. He wonders whether this condition is common. What do you tell him?
8. Mr. Jackson is happy with the results of his CPAP treatment but asks whether there are any other interventions that can help him with his OSA. He does not want medication, surgery, or other appliances. What do you tell him?
9. Mr. Jackson would like to know why his blood pressure is finally responding to his hypertension medication. He wonders why his blood pressure remained elevated before he began his CPAP therapy. What patient education should you provide in response to his query?
10. Mr. Jackson would like to know what other options he would have for treatment of his OSA if for some reason the CPAP didn't work or he couldn't continue using CPAP. Patient education would include what information?

Central Sleep Apnea

Central sleep apnea (CSA) is a cessation in breathing secondary to a decrease in respiratory center output. It is generally caused by a neurologic or cardiac problem, such as stroke, renal failure, or congestive heart failure or by sleeping at high altitude. In central sleep apnea, no respiratory effort is made, unlike OSA, in which chest and abdominal muscles continue to make respiratory efforts despite a blocked airway. As with OSA, being male and being older are risk factors for CSA. Risk factors specific for CSA include systolic heart failure, atrial fibrillation, and hypocapnia.

The apneic episode in CSA starts with a rise in dissolved blood CO_2 (pCO_2), which triggers a brief period of hyperventilation. This, in turn, causes the pCO_2 to drop below the level required by chemoreceptors in the medulla to stimulate an inhalation, and apnea results. This apnea causes the pCO_2 to rise until another hyperventilatory response occurs.

It should be noted that people who experience CSA often have some degree of OSA as well. Treatment of either type of sleep apnea may result in unmasking the other one. Therefore, in screening for sleep-disordered breathing, both OSA and CSA should be kept in mind. After treatment for OSA has begun, the clinician should remain alert for complaints of CSA, such as worsening heart failure or reports by the sleep partner of breathing pauses and gasps.

CLINICAL POINT: OSA and CSA can exist simultaneously; this condition is called mixed apnea. Often, when one condition is treated, the other one is unmasked. ■

Impact of Current Research on Clinical Practice

Treatment for OSA and Its Relationship to Hypertension

Description: Obesity is a risk factor for both hypertension and OSA, and OSA is an independent risk factor for hypertension. Prior epidemiologic studies and research on animal models have shown a relationship between weight loss and improvements in both OSA and hypertension, as well as between positive pressure treatment for OSA and hypertension improvement. Two studies looked at the relationship between treatment for moderate to severe OSA and blood pressure. Chirinos et al. found that either CPAP or weight loss caused significant reduction in systolic pressure after 2 months and after 6 months, but larger reductions occurred in patients who combined weight loss and CPAP treatment. The biggest reduction in systolic BP occurred in those who used CPAP at least 4 hours a night on 70% of the nights. Prasad et al. found that people who were treated with CPAP had experienced significant decreases in both mean systolic and diastolic pressure at 6 and at 12 months.

Clinical Practice: Prasad et al. looked at retrospective data on people with OSA to demonstrate this relationship. In a prospective interventional study, Chirinos et al. found that treating OSA leads to small lowering of blood pressure. Therefore, it is prudent for people who have difficult-to-control hypertension and risk factors for OSA, such as overweight or advancing age, to perform a complete evaluation for OSA (including PSG) and to be treated for the condition if it is found.

Research Studies:

Chirinos, J. A., Gurubhagavatula, I., Teff, K., et al. (2014). CPAP, weight loss, or both for obstructive sleep apnea. *New England Journal of Medicine, 370*(24), 2265–2275.

Prasad, B., Carley, D. W., Krishnan, J. A., Weaver, T. E., & Weaver, F. M. (2012). Effects of positive airway pressure treatment on clinical measures of hypertension and type 2 diabetes. *Journal of Clinical Sleep Medicine, 8*(5), 481–487.

The first step in treatment of CSA is optimal treatment of the underlying cause. Use of medications, such as ACE inhibitors, beta blockers, and diuretics, and cardiac resynchronization where appropriate, can also improve CSA. CPAP has improved the condition of many people with CSA, although other forms of positive pressure work better for some patients. These include biPAP (higher inspiratory pressure with lower expiratory pressure) and noninvasive positive pressure ventilation (CPAP with a backup respiratory rate that delivers a breath in the absence of inspiratory effort).

Check Your Progress: Section 7.6

1. What are the three types of sleep apnea?
2. During an apneic episode from OSA, what blood gas abnormalities cause the individual to awaken?
3. Which therapy is the most effective treatment for OSA and has been shown to have a beneficial effect on the blood pressure?

7.7 Narcolepsy

Narcolepsy, one of the most serious sleep disorders, is characterized by excessive daytime sleepiness and sudden inappropriate bouts of sleep.[22] Other signs of narcolepsy are **cataplexy** (a sudden brief loss of voluntary muscle tone), hypnagogic hallucinations, and sleep paralysis. People with narcolepsy sleep poorly at night and may complain of insomnia. Because unexpected sleep episodes and cataplexy are unpredictable, the narcoleptic person may have difficulty remaining employed or meeting family responsibilities. Anxiety or depression is not uncommon.

Etiology and Pathogenesis

Narcolepsy occurs in about 0.04% of the population, approximately equally in males and females. Narcolepsy has a hereditary component; it is found about 30 times more often in first-degree relatives of a narcoleptic person than in relatives of unaffected people. Two human leukocyte antigens are associated with narcolepsy with cataplexy. These genes are thought to interact with environmental and developmental factors such as infection or head trauma to cause the condition.[8]

Clinical Manifestations

Excessive daytime sleepiness and fatigue are the first symptoms of narcolepsy, usually appearing in adolescence. They cause frequent bouts of sleep, which last a few seconds to several minutes and occur at any time or place, including while eating, talking, or driving. The short naps are refreshing and partially compensate for poor nighttime sleep. The individual can then maintain wakefulness for several hours. Because of disturbed sleep, the individual will also complain of insomnia or fatigue.[23]

Cataplexy generally appears within 5 years of the initial symptoms. It is usually triggered by laughter or other strong emotion, such as anger, surprise, or sexual arousal, and affects part or all of the body. It can range from a feeling of weakness to complete muscular collapse. Cataplexy seems like an absence seizure, but the person remains conscious of the surroundings.

The short sleep latency that is seen in narcolepsy is secondary to nighttime sleep loss. People with narcolepsy often go directly from wakefulness to REM sleep; these periods are called **SOREMPs** (sleep onset rapid eye movement periods). Patients with narcolepsy experience a **hypnagogic hallucination** (a vivid dreamlike experience at the wake-to-sleep transition) or a **hypnopompic hallucination** at the sleep-to-wake transition because there is no sense of transition between waking and sleep.

Sleep paralysis, a transient inability to move, occurs during transitions to or from sleep. It can be frightening until the individual realizes that it ends quickly. Sleep paralysis and SOREMPs can also occur in a healthy person who is sleep deprived but will disappear with sufficient sleep in these individuals.

Although narcolepsy can occur in young children, it is both rare and difficult to diagnose. Children may be unable to describe symptoms. Excessive daytime sleepiness may be difficult to diagnose because napping is expected. In school-age children, behavior problems, inattention, poor school performance, or lack of energy may mask excessive sleepiness. The child may describe strange hallucinations. ■

There are three types of narcolepsy:

1. **Narcolepsy with cataplexy:** In narcolepsy with cataplexy, the PSG demonstrates fragmented sleep. A daytime PSG, the Multiple Sleep Latency Test (MSLT), will show episodes of sleep beginning soon after the individual lies down in a dark room and SOREMPs. Because this type of narcolepsy is usually caused by the loss of neurons that produce hypocretin (orexin) in the hypothalamus, a spinal tap will show an abnormally low level of hypocretin-1 (< 110 pg/mL).
2. **Narcolepsy without cataplexy:** In narcolepsy without cataplexy, the individual also has excessive daytime sleepiness, but the hypocretin levels are usually above 110 pg/mL.
3. **Secondary narcolepsy:** For a diagnosis of secondary narcolepsy, the individual must exhibit excessive daytime sleepiness as well as a medical condition that accounts for it. The person must also demonstrate the same findings on PSG and MSLT as in the other types of narcolepsy, or the hypocretin level in the cerebrospinal fluid must be less than 110 pg/mL.

Other neurotransmitters may play a role, including GABA, norepinephrine, and dopamine. They all regulate aspects of sleep and alertness and thus may influence the symptoms of narcolepsy.

The major negative effects of narcolepsy involve safety. Affected people should not drive or engage in other activities in which sudden sleep or loss of motor control could lead to accident or serious injury.

Linking Pathophysiology to Diagnosis and Treatment

The best diagnostic test for narcolepsy is all-night PSG (recording a minimum 6 hours of sleep) followed by a daytime MSLT. The PSG of someone who has narcolepsy will show no signs of another sleep disorder that could explain the symptoms. It will also show short sleep latency, SOREMPs, increased overall N1 (stage 1 sleep), and frequent arousals.[24]

During the MSLT, the individual is put into a quiet dark room for 20 minutes several times during the day and is told to sleep. A person with narcolepsy will fall asleep in 8 minutes or less, and the PSGs of at least two of the naps will show a SOREMP.

Treatment is focused on symptom management. Patient education is crucial. The patient should take two to four scheduled naps daily lasting 15–30 minutes each, be encouraged to maintain regular sleep habits, and avoid sleep deprivation. Safety should be stressed, and the patient should be warned about the dangers of driving or other hazardous activities.

Medication is necessary to manage symptoms. Stimulants such as, modafinil (Provigil), armodafinil (Nuvigil), amphetamines, and methylphenidate (Ritalin) are used to manage daytime sleepiness. Sodium oxybate (Xyrem) is a central nervous system depressant but has been shown, when taken at night, to decrease the number of cataplexy attacks during the day and to decrease excessive daytime sleepiness. Sodium oxybate is the pharmacologic form of GABA, which is normally produced in small amounts in the brain. Sodium oxybate is thought to work at the level of the noradrenergic, dopaminergic, and thalamocortical neurons. This activity leads to an increase in deep (N3) sleep, consolidated periods of REM, fewer arousals from sleep, and decreased SOREMPs. Better sleep at night leads to less daytime sleepiness. Sodium oxybate is also effective against cataplexy but must be used with care because of its respiratory depression and abuse potential.

Check Your Progress: Section 7.7

1. Which neurotransmitter is found to be decreased in the cerebrospinal fluid in individuals suffering from narcolepsy with cataplexy?
2. Patients with narcolepsy may experience a vivid dreamlike experience during the wake-to-sleep or sleep-to-wake transition. What are these experiences called?
3. What diagnostic tests are used in the evaluation of an individual for a possible diagnosis of narcolepsy?

7.8 Restless Legs Syndrome

Strange sensations in the legs and an accompanying need to move the legs when the person is resting or lying still is termed **restless legs syndrome (RLS)**. The sensations have been described as pain, itching, tingling, or pins and needles and in other imaginative ways. RLS can affect only one leg or the chest, arms, or face. These sensations can be relieved temporarily by purposeful movement, such as walking. The need to move leads to sleep disruption, feeling unrested in the morning, excessive daytime sleepiness, fatigue, and decreased ability to concentrate. The leg movements can even disrupt the bed partner's sleep.

RLS affects about 10–11% of people.[25] Risk factors include diabetes, pregnancy, anemia, overweight, use of caffeine, smoking, having a sedentary lifestyle, and use of some medications.

RLS is classified as either primary or secondary. Primary (idiopathic) RLS is thought to have a hereditary component because more than half of patients diagnosed with RLS have a family history. But primary RLS may occur in people who have no risk factors. Secondary RLS tends to occur in people with a condition that predisposes them to iron-deficiency anemia, such as pregnancy, end-stage renal disease, or use of certain antidepressants, dopamine antagonists, and antihistamines.

RLS is three times as common in pregnant women as in nonpregnant women. Even women who have normal levels of folate, hemoglobin, serum iron, and ferritin before pregnancy or who are taking prenatal vitamin supplements may develop RLS as a result of increased needs. ■

Ann Rebo: Application

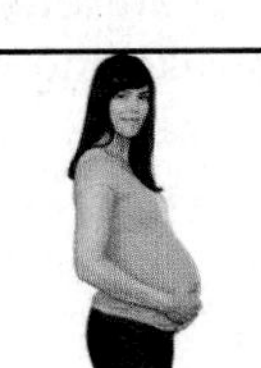

Poor sleep during the last trimester of pregnancy is well documented. Ms. Rebo may find it comfortable to sleep in only one position. This could lead to muscle stiffness and cramping or pain, which may wake her up. The pains can be relieved by changing position or dorsiflexing the foot. Ms. Rebo's description of her leg sensations does not sound like muscle cramps, so her healthcare provider orders blood tests for iron and ferritin levels.

4. What health conditions or other health history are important to consider in the assessment of an individual who may have RLS?
5. It is said that RLS is a diagnosis of exclusion. What does this mean?
6. You are drawing blood to check Ms. Rebo for anemia. She asks why this test is necessary. What information do you give her?

Etiology and Pathogenesis

RLS is both a sleep disorder and a motor disorder. It is related to a low level of iron in the brain, which affects dopamine metabolism. This can occur even when the serum iron level is normal. (Although anemia does not occur until the serum transferrin level drops to 10–12 ng/mL, RLS can develop when the serum transferrin level is 50 ng/mL.) Because iron is a cofactor in the production of dopamine, a deficit of iron in the substantia nigra leads to a decrease in the dopamine transporter. Additionally, the number of transferrin receptors is decreased in RLS (opposite to what is found in anemia), and there is an insufficient amount of the iron regulatory protein 1 (IRP1).

Clinical Manifestations

The major manifestations of RLS—the strange sensations and need to move the legs—are often accompanied by twitching or jerking of the legs or, in some cases, the arms or trunk during sleep or occasionally during wake time. Additionally, the condition cannot be explainable by an alternative cause, such as positional discomfort or leg cramps.

CLINICAL POINT: For a diagnosis of RLS, four symptoms must be present. They can be remembered by using the mnemonic **URGE**:

Urge to move legs, usually accompanied by unpleasant sensations

Rest provokes symptoms.

Getting active (moving) relieves symptoms.

Evening and night worsen symptoms. ■

Linking Pathophysiology to Diagnosis and Treatment

RLS is a diagnosis of exclusion because many other diseases can cause similar symptoms, and diagnosis is based on meeting symptomatology criteria. A PSG is used only to eliminate another sleep disorder

About 2–4% of children have RLS.[26] Children ages 2 to 12 years must meet the four criteria for adult RLS diagnosis and must describe the leg sensations in their own words. ■

Sometimes the Suggested Immobility Test is performed. During waking hours, the person is seated in chair in a quiet darkened room with legs outstretched. Several EEG sensors are placed on the scalp to monitor alertness, and EMG sensors are attached to the legs. The person is then told to stay awake and not to move the legs. Subjective rating of leg sensations and objective measurements of leg movements and muscle tension confirm the diagnosis.

Because stimulants such as caffeine, nicotine, and theophylline can exacerbate RLS, patients should decrease the use of these substances, especially late in the day. If the person is taking a dopamine antagonist (e.g., some antihistamines, antiemetics, calcium channel blockers, or others), the medication should either be discontinued or changed to one without antidopaminergic properties.

Low iron and serum ferritin levels should be corrected. Even people with RLS who have normal ferritin levels may benefit from iron supplementation.

The mainstay of RLS therapy in adults is dopamine supplementation in the form of a dopamine agonist, such as pramipexole (Mirapex), ropinirole (Requip), or rotigotine (Neupro). Other medications that can be used as needed include low-dose opioids, the anticonvulsant gabapentin enacarbil (Horizant), and benzodiazepines.

Pharmacologic treatment tends to become less effective with time. Dopaminergic medications exhibit augmentation (symptoms occur earlier in the evening or the afternoon, spread to other extremities, or get worse) and rebound (symptoms get worse in early morning). These medication side effects have led many people with RLS to seek alternative treatments for the condition, particularly the herb valerian (*Valeriana officinalis*). Because randomized clinical trials of valerian have not clearly demonstrated its effectiveness, more research is needed before its use can be either recommended or discouraged.

Anne Rebo: Outcome

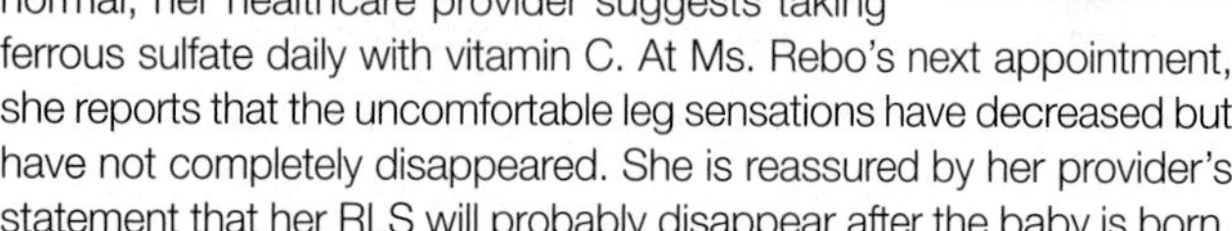

Ms. Rebo is diagnosed with RLS. Because of her pregnancy, she is unwilling to take any medication. Despite her serum iron and ferritin levels being normal, her healthcare provider suggests taking ferrous sulfate daily with vitamin C. At Ms. Rebo's next appointment, she reports that the uncomfortable leg sensations have decreased but have not completely disappeared. She is reassured by her provider's statement that her RLS will probably disappear after the baby is born.

7. Ms. Rebo asks why she has developed RLS and worries about a genetic contribution to this disorder. Patient education includes what information?
8. What lifestyle changes can Ms. Rebo implement to help reduce the symptoms of her RLS?
9. Why is Ms. Rebo's iron supplementation given with vitamin C?
10. Ms. Rebo has heard that "natural" herbal remedies might be helpful for her RLS. What response is appropriate?

Check Your Progress: Section 7.8

1. An individual with RLS may be able to relieve the uncomfortable sensations in the extremities by which simple action?
2. What type of RLS may have a hereditary component?
3. In evaluating an individual with symptoms of RLS, what diagnostic test can help to confirm the diagnosis?

7.9 Parasomnias

Any transient abnormal event that occurs during sleep may be called a **parasomnia**. Parasomnias can occur during the transition from waking to sleep, during NREM and REM sleep. Safety is one of the key issues with parasomnias, as people may injure themselves or someone else during the event. Parasomnias include **bruxism** (grinding one's teeth during sleep), **somnambulism** (sleep walking), nightmares, **enuresis** (bedwetting), sleep paralysis, REM sleep behavior disorder, **night terrors** (also called sleep terrors), and other phenomena.

During a night terror, the person seems to wake from NREM sleep terrified, sits up with open eyes, cries out, may speak incoherently, and is unresponsive to outside stimuli. There is often the feeling of a malevolent presence, called by different names in different cultures, such as succubus, alien, or old lady. The individual remains asleep and does not remember the night terror the following morning.

Night terrors occur in about 1–6% of children, usually between the ages of 4 and 12 years.[27] Because the child returns to sleep and does not remember the event on awakening, these are more upsetting to the parents than to the child. ■

For information on these and other relatively common sleep problems, see **Table 7.2** ■.

Check Your Progress: Section 7.9

1. A night terror may appear very frightening to an observer. What does the child who has the night terror experience on awakening the next morning?
2. What is the priority consideration in management of sleepwalking (somnambulism)?
3. An enuretic alarm is a nondrug intervention that uses a moisture detection pad with an alarm that sounds if the pad becomes wet. What childhood sleep problem can be managed with this device?

Table 7.2 Selected Sleep Problems

Etiology and Pathogenesis	Clinical Manifestations	Linking Pathophysiology to Diagnosis and Treatment
REM sleep behavior disorder (RBD): Lack of somatic muscle atonia during REM, leading to acting out dream content		
Common causes of chronic RBD: neurologic disorder; depression or destruction of neurons in the pons and locus coeruleus areas responsible for REM atonia; reduced activity or destruction of serotonergic and noradrenergic areas of brainstem responsible for inhibiting activity during REM. May be related to development of neurologic disease (Parkinson, ALS, Alzheimer, demyelinating disease), stroke, or traumatic brain injury; toxicity from psychotropic medications or excessive caffeine. Occurs in about 0.5% of the population, more men than women; there may be a familial tendency.	Seemingly purposeful, often vigorous or violent movements during REM sleep, which can lead to injury of self or others. May be reported by the individual or the sleep partner.	Clonazepam (reduces some REM muscle activity) and melatonin (suppresses REM motor activity) may be helpful. Patient safety measures: lock windows and bedroom door, remove firearms and sharp objects from room. If actions are violent, the individual should not sleep with a bed partner.
Sleepwalking (somnambulism)		
More common in childhood; occurs in 1–17% of children, peaks at 11–12 years; more boys than girls; about 4% of adults; may be related to family history, fever, sleep deprivation, physical activity, emotional stress, or use of medications such as sedatives, hypnotics, stimulants, and antihistamines. Functional dissociation of locomotion centers in CNS from waking centers.	Individual appears to awaken, may sit on edge of bed, walk, and/or talk. The eyes are open, but the facial expression is blank. Generally no memory of the activity the next day.	Diagnosis by report of witnesses. No treatment; care should be taken for the safety of known sleepwalkers, including locking doors and windows and blocking stairways. Tricyclic antidepressants and benzodiazepines may be helpful if the activity is dangerous. Anticipatory wakening of children may be helpful. Comorbid sleep disorders can exacerbate or provoke sleepwalking, so evaluate for other sleep disorders and treat them.
Sleep inertia (sleep drunkenness): Drowsiness and poor performance immediately after waking; classified as an arousal disorder		
More prominent when sleep is preceded by a period of sleep deprivation. It is affected by the stage of sleep immediately before waking (greatest on waking from N2) and by where it occurs in relation to individual's circadian rhythm. May be related to differential restoration of blood flow to areas of brain on awakening. Blood flow to the brainstem and thalamus is reactivated first; blood flow to areas responsible for alertness and performance increases more slowly, leading to slower reactivation of functions.	Decreased cognitive ability and vigilance after awakening from sleep or nap; lasts 30–120 minutes depending on the duration of wakefulness before the sleep episode.	Use of caffeine improves recovery; chewing gum containing 100 mg caffeine improves immediate performance and response time but does not completely restore it to normal waking level.
Night terrors (sleep terrors): Form of dissociated sleep in which there are abrupt awakenings from sleep with signs of panic and anxiety		
Occurs in about 3% of prepubertal children, subsides in adolescence, rare in adults.	Individual sits up during sleep, screaming, sweating, tachycardic, tachypneic, does not respond to verbal stimuli, is difficult to fully arouse; amnesia of event when the person awakens.	Occurs spontaneously or related to significant trauma or psychopathology. Generally occurs during partial arousals from N3 sleep. May be triggered by another sleep disorder or by a loud noise or other stimuli. No treatment; the individual gradually calms down and returns to sleep.
Nightmare (dream anxiety attack): Intense dream that arouses bad feelings		
Lifetime prevalence estimated at 100%, More common in children, although many adults report at least one per month; frequently occur in people with PTSD. Seem to involve troubling feeling or experience that has not been adequately integrated into normal mental functioning, resulting in unpleasant emotion. May occur in stressful situations in normally functioning individuals.	Nightmare disorder: repetitive episodes of awakenings from sleep with recall of intensely disturbing dream involving fear, anxiety, anger, sadness. The individual is fully alert on awakening from the nightmare, recalls the dream clearly, falls back asleep slowly. Typically occurs in second half of sleep.	No treatment necessary for occasional nightmares. Because persistent nightmares are associated with mental health problems (e.g., PTSD, anxiety disorder), psychotherapy and psychotropic drugs may be necessary.
Enuresis (bedwetting): Nocturnal bedwetting during sleep		
Frequent in childhood, occurs in 0.5% of adults. Cause unknown, may be manifestation of nocturnal seizures Not associated with any specific pathology; may be related to genetic, behavioral, psychologic or physiologic factors (e.g., bladder size, decreased vasopressin release, delayed development)	Urination without awaking during sleep (although sensations of having voided or a wet bed may lead to awakening).	Conditioning with liquid detecting pad and bell may help. Tricyclic antidepressants may be used for short term only. Vasopressin analog (Desmopressin) taken intranasally helps in some cases.

SOURCES: Data from Newman, R. A., Kamimori, G. H., Wesensten, N. J., Picchioni, D., & Balkin, T. J. (2013). Caffeine gum minimizes sleep inertia. *Perceptual & Motor Skills, 116*(1), 280–293. Howell, M. J. (2012). Parasomnias: An updated review. *Neurotherapeutics, 9*(4), 753–775. Redeker, N. S., & McEnany, G. P. (2011). *Sleep disorders and sleep promotion in nursing practice*. New York, NY: Springer. Sateia, M. (Ed). (2014). *International classification of sleep disorders* (3rd ed.). Darien IL: American Academy of Sleep Medicine.

CHAPTER SUMMARY

7.1 Chapter Overview and Case Studies

Describe sleep and concepts related to sleep.

- Sleep is a vital part of life. If a person does not get enough sleep, the brain will sleep for short periods that the individual does not detect.
- The most common cause of insufficient sleep in the developed world is sociologic, but pathologic sleep disorders are also important.

7.2 Normal Sleep

Discuss the characteristics of normal sleep and the regulation of body rhythms and sleep.

- Normal sleep cycles through several phases, divided into NREM sleep (stages N1, N2, N3) and REM sleep.
- The first sleep cycle of the night lasts about 90 minutes; subsequent cycles are shorter. The relative amount of each stage of sleep varies according to age. Infants' sleep has a high proportion of REM, while older adults have lower proportions of both N3 (SWS) and REM sleep.
- Sleep is regulated by the interaction of the body's circadian rhythm and the homeostatic drive for sleep.
- The circadian rhythm is regulated by the internal clock, which is reset by zeitgebers, time cues. The strongest zeitgeber is sunlight, but eating and other activities also contribute.
- The homeostatic drive is dependent on the length of time the individual has been awake, as adenosine builds up in the brain over the course of the time awake.

7.3 Measurement of Sleep

Explain what measures are used to assess sleep and its outcomes.

- Objective aspects of sleep can be measured by using actigraphy and PSG, which is the most comprehensive measure.
- Sleep and consequences of sleep can be examined subjectively by using a sleep diary or survey tool

7.4 Sleep Deprivation

List physiologic, psychologic, and sociologic consequences of insufficient and disturbed sleep.

- Insufficient sleep can lead to poor memory, increased reaction time, poor executive function, poor immune system function, weight gain, blurred vision, and disrupted hormone secretion.

7.5 Insomnia

Describe factors leading to insomnia and how it is diagnosed and treated.

- Acute insomnia is the result of a precipitating factor, usually an acute stressor such as illness or a death in the family.
- Chronic insomnia is related to a perpetuating factor, such as unemployment or poor coping skills.
- Diagnosis is through history, including a sleep diary and, if necessary, a PSG to rule out pathologic sleep disorder.
- Insomnia is best treated with cognitive–behavioral therapy.

7.6 Sleep-Disordered Breathing

Differentiate the causes, classification, underlying pathogenesis, and clinical manifestations of sleep-disordered breathing and approaches to diagnosis and treatment of these conditions across the lifespan.

- Sleep-disordered breathing can range in severity from simple snoring through mild hypopneas to OSA and CSA, in which respiration actually ceases for short periods of time throughout the sleep period.
- In OSA, the airway is blocked, usually by collapse secondary to poor muscle tone or excess fat in the pharyngeal walls.
- In CSA, neurologic stimulation of the respiratory muscles is disrupted secondary to a cardiac or neurologic problem.
- In both types of apnea, the SO_2 level falls during the night, and the resulting intermittent hypoxemia leads to hypertension resistant to treatment, atherosclerosis, heart disease, and stroke.
- The most effective treatment for obstructive sleep apnea is positive pressure ventilation, Other treatments include interventions to open the airway through dental treatment to advance the jaw or tongue, surgery to decrease tissue surrounding and partially blocking the airway, and weight loss for obese patients.
- CSA is managed by first treating the underlying cause. Positive pressure ventilation may be used cautiously with the addition of a backup respiratory rate.

7.7 Narcoplepsy

Differentiate the causes, classification, underlying pathogenesis, and clinical manifestations of narcolepsy and approaches to diagnosis and treatment of this condition across the lifespan.

- Narcolepsy, an arousal disorder, seems to be caused by an autoimmune process in a person with a hereditary disposition to the condition. It is caused by a lack of hypocretin.

- Narcolepsy manifests itself as excessive daytime sleepiness accompanied by unpredictable bouts of sleep as well as hypnagogic and hypnopompic hallucinations, sleep paralysis, and sometimes cataplexy.
- Interventions include lifestyle adjustments such as a regular sleep schedule, including naps, and protection of patient safety. Medications are used to increase alertness (e.g., amphetamines, modafinil), consolidate sleep (e.g., sodium oxybate, SSRIs), and inhibit cataplexy (e.g., sodium oxybate).

7.8 Restless Legs Syndrome

Differentiate the causes, classification, underlying pathogenesis, and clinical manifestations of restless legs syndrome and approaches to diagnosis and treatment of this condition across the lifespan.

- RLS is caused by a defect in dopamine metabolism, generally brought on by a deficit in brain iron, transferrin, and/or ferritin).
- RLS is manifested as unusual leg sensations, accompanied by a need to move the legs, when resting or lying down, usually in the evening. The sensation is described by words such as pain or itching or even more imaginatively.
- Treatment consists of increasing iron stores and administration of dopamine agonist.

7.9 Parasomnias

Identify and define selected parasomnias, and describe the causes, pathogenesis, and clinical manifestations of these conditions and approaches to their diagnosis and treatment across the lifespan.

- Relatively common parasomnias include REM behavior disorder (muscles do not relax during REM, leading to acting out dreams), somnambulism (complex behavior occurring during N3 SWS), sleep inertia (difficulty reestablishing waking alertness following sleep), night terrors (abrupt awakenings from sleep accompanied by inescapable fear or terror), nightmares (dreams that cause fear or distress), and enuresis (bedwetting).

REVIEW QUESTIONS

1. Diagnostic testing for RLS includes laboratory tests for anemia and iron levels. The reason for this diagnostic test in RLS evaluation is that low iron levels:
   a. cause muscle cramping.
   b. cause muscle weakness.
   c. reduce dopamine activity in the brain.
   d. indicate a poor diet.
2. An EEG may be used to determine the stage of sleep. Which of the following is correct?
   a. Healthy young adults spend most of their sleep time in NREM sleep.
   b. Restorative sleep is REM sleep.
   c. Infants spend most of their sleep time in NREM sleep.
   d. A person with obstructive sleep apnea typically has snoring episodes during NREM sleep.
3. You are discussing an upcoming plane flight with your 70-year-old client, who will be visiting family. The travel plans include flying from the east coast of the United States (Florida) to the west coast (California). Your patient is concerned about the possibility of jet lag because he had a bad case of jet lag 15 years ago when he took a similar trip. Which of the following is an appropriate response?
   a. "Jet lag occurs only with north to south travel, so you do not need to worry."
   b. "There is not much you can do about jet lag. You'll just have to suffer through it."
   c. "You are lucky. As one gets older, jet lag becomes less severe, and your symptoms won't be as bad as they were when you were younger."
   d. "Spending time in the sunlight at your destination will help, and there are also medications that may be helpful."
4. Your client with OSA has returned to the clinic after being on CPAP therapy for the past month. Before he began CPAP, his hypertension was not responding to antihypertensive medication, and he was very overweight. You:
   a. ask whether his sleep partner reports less snoring and encourage continued use of the CPAP.
   b. expect that regular use of the CPAP will result in an improvement of his hypertension.
   c. check his weight as part of the physical evaluation and encourage weight loss to achieve a normal weight.
   d. All of the above
5. Your 75-year-old client has suffered a fall. Luckily, she did not fracture any bones or have a serious injury from the fall. Which of the following is correct?
   a. You explain that prevention of future falls is a priority.
   b. Evaluation should include a consideration of heart failure or other cardiac problem.
   c. A disturbed sleep pattern is a potential nursing diagnosis.
   d. All of the above

6. A 22-year-old man is being seen in the clinic because he has been falling asleep two or three times a day for the past few years. Yesterday, he also experienced profound muscle weakness. You expect that:
   a. a spinal tap will be performed to check his hypocretin levels.
   b. there is no family history of similar symptoms.
   c. his sudden sleep attacks are due to boredom with his life activities.
   d. no other diagnostic tests are needed to confirm his diagnosis.
7. Your 35-year-old patient complains that when her alarm clock awakens her in the morning on work days, she feels very sleepy for at least an hour and she has difficulty concentrating and getting ready for work. Drinking coffee helps her alertness somewhat. You suspect a diagnosis of:
   a. narcolepsy.
   b. restless legs syndrome (RLS).
   c. REM sleep behavior disorder (RBD).
   d. sleep inertia (sleep drunkenness).
8. A 40-year-old man is brought to the health center by his wife. The man suffered a traumatic brain injury 6 months ago, and since then he has had multiple episodes of violent movements during sleep, which worry his wife, who is his bed partner. Which of the following is correct?
   a. His wife should be encouraged to continue sleeping as his bed partner so that she can restrain him when he has these episodes.
   b. You feel confident that these episodes are occurring during NREM sleep stage.
   c. You suspect REM sleep behavior disorder (RBD).
   d. His symptoms are unrelated to his history of TBI.

ANSWERS

Answers to Review Questions can be found in Appendix A. Answers to Case Study and Check Your Progress questions are available on the faculty resources site. Please consult with your instructor.

RECOMMENDED WEBSITES

American Academy of Sleep Medicine (AASM)
http://www.aasmnet.org

American Sleep Apnea Association
http://www.sleepapnea.org

National Institutes of Health NINDS: information on narcolepsy, restless legs syndrome, sleep apnea
https://www.ninds.nih.gov/disorders/disorder_index.htm

National Sleep Foundation
https://sleepfoundation.org

NHLBI: information on CPAP, narcolepsy, Pickwickian syndrome (obesity-hypoventilation syndrome), restless legs syndrome, and sleep apnea
https://www.nhlbi.nih.gov/health/health-topics/by-alpha

Sleep education.com
http://www.sleepeducation.org

Stanford University Center for Narcolepsy
http://med.stanford.edu/narcolepsy.html

REFERENCES

1. Hobson, J. A. (2005). Sleep is of the brain, by the brain and for the brain. *Nature, 437*(7063), 1254–1256.
2. Carley, D. W., & Farabi, S. S. (2016). Physiology of sleep. *Diabetes Spectrum, 29*(1), 5–9.
3. Buysse, D. J. (2014). Sleep health: Can we define it? Does it matter? *Sleep, 37*(1), 9–17.
4. Berry, R. B., Brooks, R., Gamaldo C. E., Harding S. M., Lloyd R. M., Marcus C. L., & Vaughn B. V. (2016). *The AASM manual for the scoring of sleep and associated events: Rules, terminology and technical specifications* (Version 2.3). Darien IL:American Academy of Sleep Medicine.
5. Stickgold, R. (2012). To sleep: Perchance to learn. *Nature Neuroscience, 15*(10), 1322–1323.
6. Buysse, D. J., Reynolds, C. F., Monk, T. H., Berman, S. R., & Kupfer, D. J. (1989). The Pittsburgh Sleep Quality Index: A new instrument for psychiatric practice and research. *Psychiatric Research, 28*, 193–213.
7. Smyth, C. (2012). *The Pittsburgh sleep quality index (PSQI)*. New York, NY: Hartford Institute for Geriatric Nursing.
8. Johns, M. W. (1991). A new method for measuring daytime sleepiness: The Epworth Sleepiness Scale. *Sleep, 14*, 540–545.
9. Weaver, T. E., Laizner, A. M., Evans, L. K., et al. (1997). An instrument to measure functional status outcomes for disorders of excessive sleepiness. *Sleep, 20*(10), 835–843.
10. Collop, N. (2012). Home sleep testing: Appropriate screening is the key. *Sleep, 35*(11), 1445–1446.

11. Buysse, D. J., Grunstein, R., Horne, J., & Lavie, P. Can an improvement in sleep positively impact on health? *Sleep Medicine Reviews, 14*(6), 405–410.
12. Spira, A. P., Chen-Edinboro, L. P., Wu, M. N., & Yaffe, K. (2014). Impact of sleep on the risk of cognitive decline and dementia. *Current Opinion in Psychiatry, 27*(6), 478–483.
13. Adolescent Sleep Working Group, Committee on Adolescence, & Council on School Health. (2014). School start times for adolescents. *Pediatrics, 134*, 642–649.
14. Gooneratne, N. .S, & Vitiello, M. V. (2014). Sleep in older adults: Normative changes, sleep disorders, and treatment options. *Clinics in Geriatric Medicine, 30*(3), 591–627.
15. Perrier, J, Bertran, F., Sullivan, M., Coque, C., Bulla, J., Denise, P., & Bocca, M.-L. (2014). Impaired driving performance associated with effect of time duration in patients with primary insomnia. *Sleep, 37*(9), 1565–1573.
16. Bastien, C. H., Vallières, A., & Morin, C. M. (2001). Validation of the Insomnia Severity Index as an outcome measure for insomnia research. *Sleep Medicine, 2*, 297–307.
17. Morin, C. M., Belleville, G., Bélanger, L., & Ivers, H. (2011). The Insomnia Severity Index: Psychometric indicators to detect insomnia cases and evaluate treatment response. *Sleep, 34*(5), 601–608.
18. Irwin, M. R., Olmstead, R., Carrillo, C., et al. (2014). Cognitive behavioral therapy vs. tai chi for late life insomnia and inflammatory risk: A randomized controlled comparative efficacy trial. *Sleep, 37*(9), 1543–1552.
19. American Academy of Sleep Medicine. (2014). Rising prevalence of sleep apnea in U.S. threatens public health. *National Healthy Sleep Awareness Project*. Available at http://www.aasmnet.org/articles.aspx?id=5043
20. Strohl K. P., Brown D. B., Collop, N., et al. (2013). An official American Thoracic Society clinical practice guideline: Sleep apnea, sleepiness, and driving risk in noncommercial drivers. *American Journal of Respiratory & Critical Care Medicine, 187*(11), 1259–1266.
21. Reishtein J. L. (2011). Obstructive sleep apnea: A risk factor for cardiovascular disease. *Journal of Cardiovascular Nursing, 20*(2), 106–116.
22. Sateia, M. (Ed). (2014). *International classification of sleep disorders* (3rd ed.). Darien, IL: American Academy of Sleep Medicine.
23. Ahmed, I., & Thorpy, M. (2010). Clinical features, diagnosis and treatment of narcolepsy. *Clinics in Chest Medicine, 31*(2), 371–381.
24. Roth, T., Dauvilliers, Y., Mignot, E., et al. (2013). Disrupted nighttime sleep in narcolepsy. *Journal of Clinical Sleep Medicine, 9*(9), 955–965.
25. Silber, M. H. (2013). Sleep-related movement disorders. *CONTINUUM: Lifelong Learning in Neurology, 19*(1 Sleep Disorders), 170–184.
26. Picchietti, D. L., Bruni, O., de Weerd, A., Dumer, J. S., Kotagel, S., Owens, J. A., & Simakajomboon, N. S. (2013). Pediatric restless legs syndrome diagnostic criteria: An update by the International Restless Legs Syndrome Study Group. *Sleep Medicine, 14*(12), 1253–1259.
27. Spratt, E .G. (2016). Sleep terrors. *Medscape*. Available at http://emedicine.medscape.com/article/914360-overview#a5

Unit III

Fluid, Electrolyte, and Acid–Base Imbalances

Chapter 8
Fluid and Electrolyte Imbalances

Chapter 9
Acid–Base Imbalances

The mechanisms that regulate fluid, electrolyte, and acid–base balances in the body are essential to homeostasis. Even slight changes to fluid, electrolyte, or acid–base balance can result in symptoms that impair function and threaten safety.

Fluid and electrolyte balance has a reciprocal relationship with acid–base balance in that certain specific combinations of imbalance in fluids and electrolytes can result in acid–base imbalance, and acid–base imbalance can, in turn, affect fluid and electrolyte balance. For example, one pathway to metabolic alkalosis is through excessive vomiting. The resulting loss of gastric fluid creates deficits in water, chloride, and potassium. These volume deficits stimulate the production of aldosterone, which causes sodium and water to be resorbed into the blood, further perpetuating the metabolic alkalosis.

Fluid, electrolyte, and acid–base balance are often impaired by illness or injury. For example, respiratory compensation is limited by lung disease, by hypoxemia that develops with decreased ventilation occurring as compensation for metabolic alkalosis, and by the fatigue of respiratory muscles associated with prolonged rapid and deep breathing in compensation for metabolic acidosis. In addition, the lungs cannot compensate for an acid–base imbalance if they are the cause of the imbalance.

In hospital settings, healthcare providers must be especially vigilant. Postoperative vomiting or nasogastric suctioning can combine with hyperventilation due to pain or anxiety to result in both metabolic and respiratory acidosis, owing to the combination of volume deficit, loss of gastric acid, and increased elimination of CO_2. Other acute conditions that can result in acid–base imbalances can be found in Table 9.2.

Sudden alterations in level of consciousness (LOC) or central nervous system activity may signal disruption of fluid and electrolyte or acid–base imbalance. For example:

- Dehydration: confusion, lethargy, light-headedness, headache, difficulty paying attention
- Hypocalcemia: irritability, anxiety, seizures
- Respiratory acidosis: drowsiness, dizziness, disorientation
- Metabolic alkalosis: decreased level of consciousness, dizziness, irritability.

The clinical implications of any meaningful change in these homeostatic mechanisms are many. Risk for injury related to changes in LOC or neuromuscular alterations is present in even mild states of imbalance.[1] Infants, young children, older adults, and patients with chronic illnesses such as diabetes or respiratory disease are at particular risk for increased morbidity and mortality if imbalances are not corrected quickly. In critically ill patients, risk for imbalance may be related to the underlying illness, current therapies, or a combination of the two.[2] Early assessment of arterial blood gases is an essential component of a thorough evaluation of the patient.

References

1. Corbett, J. V., & Banks, A. D. (2013). *Laboratory tests and diagnostic procedures with nursing diagnoses* (8th ed.). Upper Saddle River, NJ: Pearson.
2. Kowk, M. H., Norris, S. H. L., Williams, T. A., Harahsheh, Y., Chapman, A. R., Dobb, G. J., & Magder, S. (2016). A comparison of prognostic significance of strong ion gap (SIG) with other acid–base markers in the critically ill: A cohort study. *Journal of Intensive Care, 4*, 43.

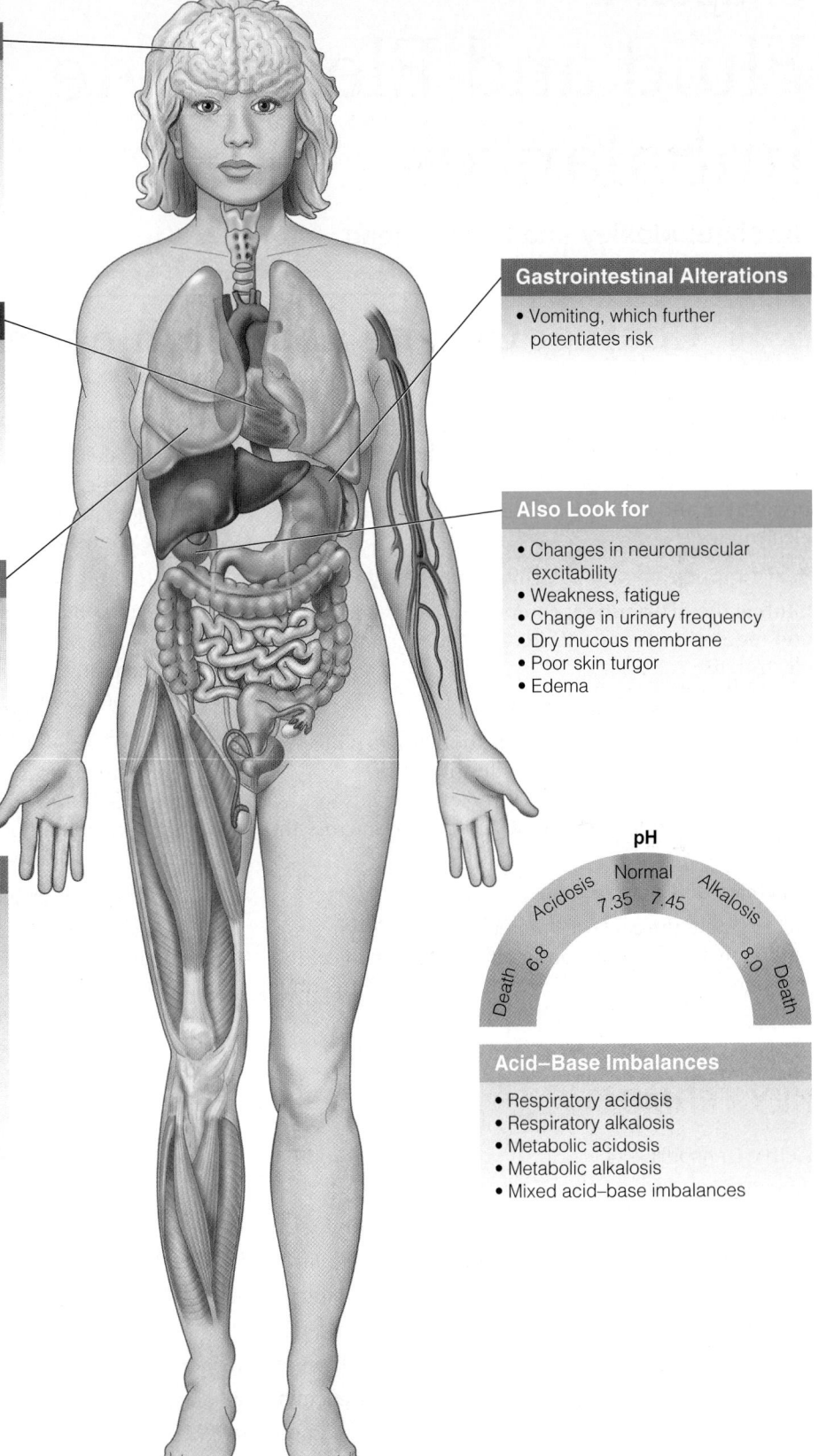

Neurologic Alterations

- Altered mental status
- Irritability, restlessness
- Dizziness
- Confusion, disorientation
- Drowsiness, lethargy
- May progress to coma if untreated

Cardiovascular Alterations

- Changes in cardiac contractility
- Increase or decrease in circulating blood volume
- Hypertension or hypotension
- Arrhythmias
- Myocardial ischemia

Respiratory Alterations

- Changes in ABGs
- Change in rate and/or depth of breathing (i.e., signs of compensation)
- Increased work of breathing
- Hypercapnia or hypocapnia

Fluid and Electrolyte Imbalances

- Fluid volume excess
- Fluid volume deficit
- Hypernatremia
- Hyponatremia
- Hyperchloremia
- Hypochloremia
- Hyperkalemia
- Hypokalemia
- Hypercalcemia
- Hypocalcemia
- Hyperphosphatemia
- Hypophosphatemia
- Hypermagnesemia
- Hypomagnesemia

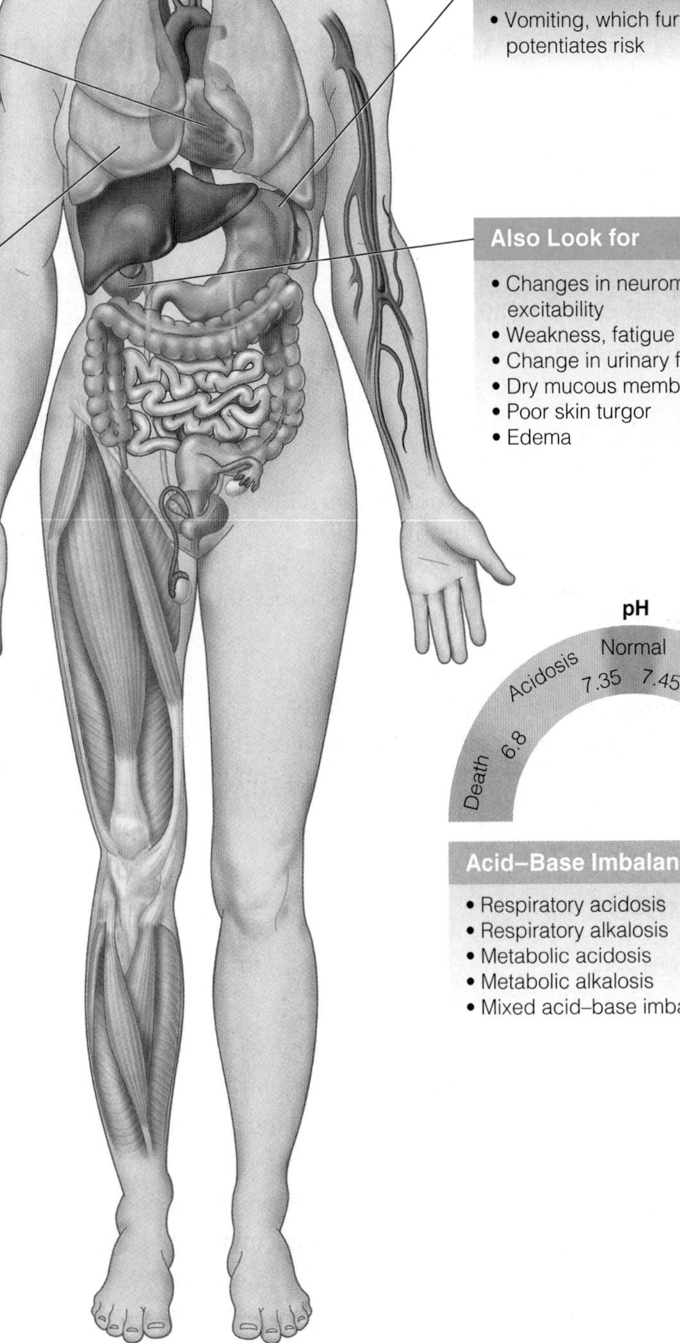

Gastrointestinal Alterations

- Vomiting, which further potentiates risk

Also Look for

- Changes in neuromuscular excitability
- Weakness, fatigue
- Change in urinary frequency
- Dry mucous membrane
- Poor skin turgor
- Edema

Acid–Base Imbalances

- Respiratory acidosis
- Respiratory alkalosis
- Metabolic acidosis
- Metabolic alkalosis
- Mixed acid–base imbalances

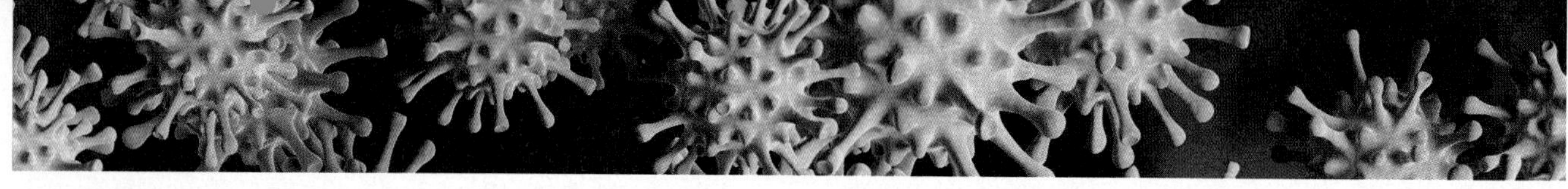

Chapter 8
Fluid and Electrolyte Imbalances

Elizabeth Moxley and Daniel Mead

Chapter Outline and Learning Outcomes

8.1 Chapter Overview and Case Studies

Describe the normal fluid and electrolyte balance, the results of inappropriate fluid and electrolyte imbalance, and concepts related to fluids and electrolytes.

8.2 Composition and Distribution of Body Fluids

Outline the distribution, composition, movement, and regulation of body fluids and the regulation of electrolytes.

8.3 Water and Sodium Imbalances

Differentiate the causes, classification, underlying pathogenesis, and clinical manifestations of water and sodium imbalances and approaches to diagnosis and treatment of these conditions across the lifespan.

8.4 Chloride Imbalances

Differentiate the causes, classification, underlying pathogenesis, and clinical manifestations of chloride imbalances and approaches to diagnosis and treatment of these conditions across the lifespan.

8.5 Potassium Imbalances

Differentiate the causes, classification, underlying pathogenesis, and clinical manifestations of potassium imbalances and approaches to diagnosis and treatment of these conditions across the lifespan.

8.6 Calcium Imbalances

Differentiate the causes, classification, underlying pathogenesis, and clinical manifestations of calcium imbalances and approaches to diagnosis and treatment of these conditions across the lifespan.

8.7 Phosphorus Imbalances

Differentiate the causes, classification, underlying pathogenesis, and clinical manifestations of phosphorus imbalances and approaches to diagnosis and treatment of these conditions across the lifespan.

8.8 Magnesium Imbalances

Differentiate the causes, classification, underlying pathogenesis, and clinical manifestations of magnesium imbalances and approaches to diagnosis and treatment of these conditions across the lifespan.

KEY TERMS

Active transport, 174
Aldosterone, 181
Anion, 177
Atrial natriuretic peptide (ANP), 182
Brain natriuretic peptide (BNP), 182
Calcium, 188
Cation, 177
Chloride, 185
Chvostek sign, 190
Colloid osmotic pressure, 174
Diffusion, 173
Edema, 174
Electrolyte, 171
Extracellular fluid (ECF), 173
Hydrostatic pressure, 174
Hypercalcemia, 189
Hyperchloremia, 185
Hyperkalemia, 186
Hypermagnesemia, 192
Hypernatremia, 179
Hyperphosphatemia, 190
Hypertonic, 179
Hypocalcemia, 189
Hypochloremia, 185
Hypokalemia, 188
Hypomagnesemia, 192
Hyponatremia, 178
Hypophosphatemia, 191
Hypotonic, 179
Intracellular fluid (ICF), 172

Key Terms continue on next page.

ABBREVIATIONS

ADH—antidiuretic hormone
ANP—atrial natriuretic peptide
BNP—brain natriuretic peptide
ECF—extracellular fluid
ICF—intracellular fluid
PTH—parathyroid hormone
RAAS—renin–angiotensin–aldosterone system
TBW—total body water

8.1 Chapter Overview and Case Studies

A dynamic process of homeostasis is maintained through consistent fluid and electrolyte adjustments according to the needs of the cellular environment. (An **electrolyte** is any substance that dissociates into ions in water.) These requirements involve the renal system, hormones, and neural function of the body. Fluid fluctuations affect cellular function, blood volume, and hemodynamics. The composition of electrolytes affects cellular changes and the electrical potential of cells, and results in fluid shifts. Alterations in pH disrupt the function of enzyme systems and may result in cellular injury. Fluid and electrolyte imbalances may result in life-threatening complications.[1] A thorough understanding of fluid and electrolyte function and alterations, as well as the ability of the body to compensate, is essential for choosing and applying appropriate treatment options for these pathophysiologic conditions.

Concepts Related to Fluid and Electrolytes

The amount of fluid in the body affects the overall workload of the heart, and alterations in fluid levels often manifest in significant changes in vital signs. An excess of fluid causes an increase in blood pressure as the heart works harder to compensate for the increased amount of fluid in the circulation. Fluid can then begin to leak out of the circulation, resulting in edema. In addition, fluid can accumulate in the lungs, affecting oxygenation. When there is a deficit of fluid, the heart has to beat faster to circulate the reduced volume of blood, resulting in an elevated heart rate even in the face of a decreased blood pressure, leading to changes in perfusion. The concentration of electrolytes, in turn, influences the generation and propagation of electrical signals throughout the body, certain electrolytes having pronounced effects on cardiovascular function. The presence of electrolyte concentrations is evaluated through blood chemistry testing; certain values identify low or high concentrations. Normal electrolyte values are outlined in **Table 8.1** ■ and selected concepts related to alterations of fluids and electrolytes are shown in **Figure 8.1** ■.

Table 8.1 Normal Electrolyte Values

Serum Component	Values
Electrolytes	
Sodium (Na^+)	135–145 mEq/L
Chloride (Cl^-)	95–105 mEq/L
Bicarbonate (HCO_3^-, total carbon dioxide)	22–30 mEq/L
Calcium (Ca^{2+}) (total)	4.5–5.5 mEq/L (9–11 mg/dL)
Potassium (K^+)	3.5–5.3 mEq/L
Phosphorus (PO_4^{3-})	1.7–2.6 (mEq/L (2.5–4.5 mg/dL)
Magnesium (Mg^{2+})	1.5–2.5 mEq/L (1.8–3.0 mg/dL)
Serum osmolality	
	280–300 mOsm/kg

SOURCES: Data from Kee, J. (2013). *Pearson handbook of laboratory and diagnostic tests with nursing implications* (7th ed.). Hoboken, NJ: Pearson. Longo, D. L., Fauci, A. S., Kasper, D. L., Hauser, S. L., Jameson, J. L., & Loscalzo, J. (2012). *Harrison's principles of internal medicine* (18th ed., Vols. 1–2). New York, NY: McGraw-Hill. Martini, F. H., & Ober, W. C. (2015). *Visual anatomy and physiology*. Hoboken, NJ: Pearson.

Case Studies

The following case studies are integrated throughout the chapter to assist in application of chapter content to clinical situations that involve individuals with alterations in fluids and electrolytes.

Heather Manuel: Introduction

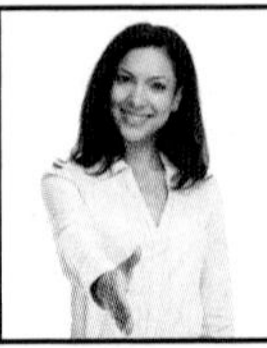

Heather Manuel, age 44, has a long medical history, including type 1 diabetes mellitus since age 6, hypertension, peripheral neuropathy in her feet, and chronic renal failure for 4 years requiring hemodialysis 3 times a week for the past 2 years. She has an arteriovenous (AV) fistula that is currently nonfunctional. She has had three surgical procedures for AV fistulas, and after a short time, the AV fistulas become nonfunctional.

1. Considering Ms. Manuel's medical history, what would you anticipate her plasma potassium level to be?
2. What risk factors exist within the medical history of Ms. Manuel that could contribute to the development of renal failure?

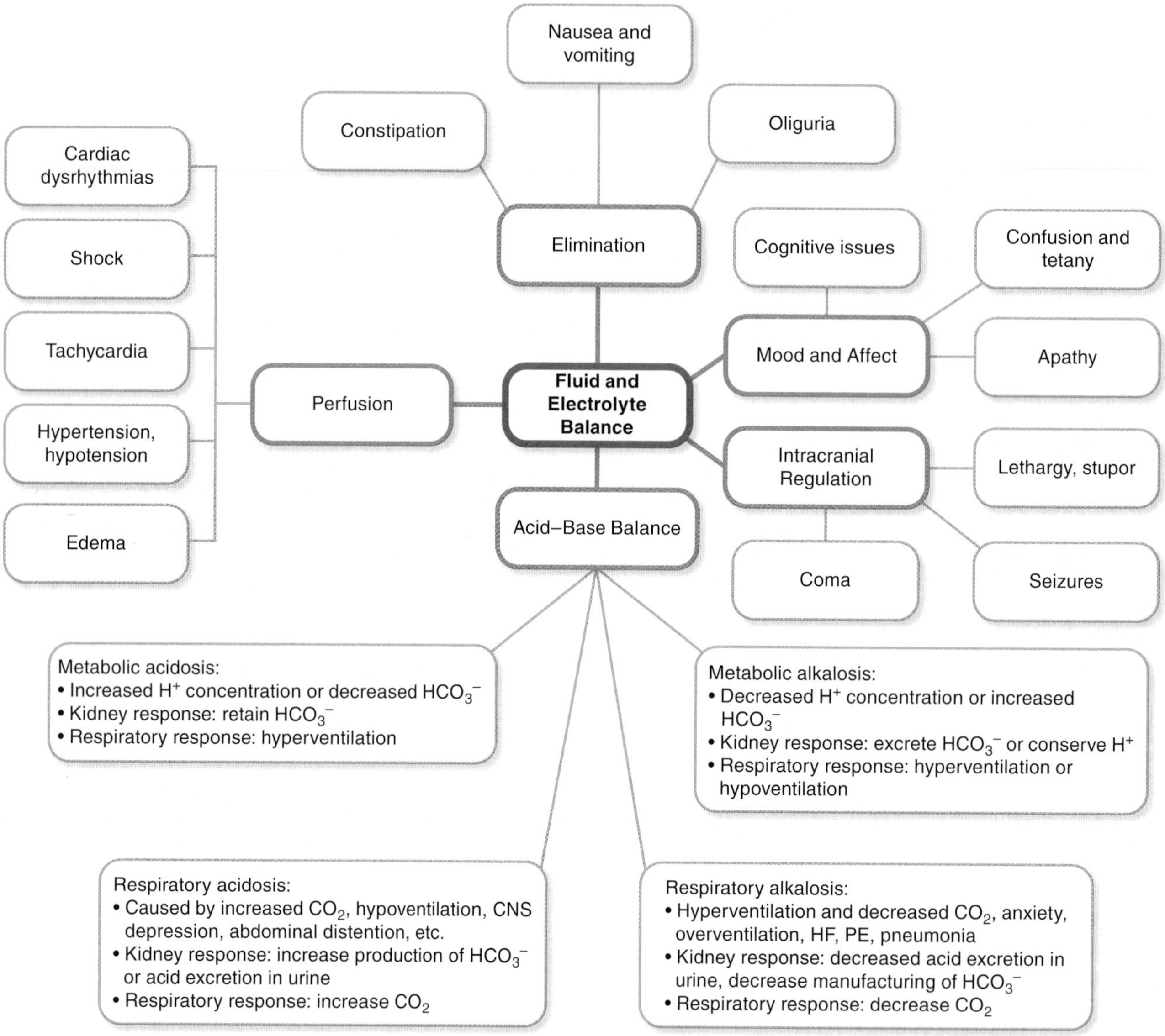

Fluid and Electrolyte Balance

Elimination
- Nausea and vomiting
- Constipation
- Oliguria

Perfusion
- Cardiac dysrhythmias
- Shock
- Tachycardia
- Hypertension, hypotension
- Edema

Mood and Affect
- Cognitive issues
- Confusion and tetany
- Apathy

Intracranial Regulation
- Lethargy, stupor
- Coma
- Seizures

Acid–Base Balance

Metabolic acidosis:
- Increased H^+ concentration or decreased HCO_3^-
- Kidney response: retain HCO_3^-
- Respiratory response: hyperventilation

Metabolic alkalosis:
- Decreased H^+ concentration or increased HCO_3^-
- Kidney response: excrete HCO_3^- or conserve H^+
- Respiratory response: hyperventilation or hypoventilation

Respiratory acidosis:
- Caused by increased CO_2, hypoventilation, CNS depression, abdominal distention, etc.
- Kidney response: increase production of HCO_3^- or acid excretion in urine
- Respiratory response: increase CO_2

Respiratory alkalosis:
- Hyperventilation and decreased CO_2, anxiety, overventilation, HF, PE, pneumonia
- Kidney response: decreased acid excretion in urine, decrease manufacturing of HCO_3^-
- Respiratory response: decrease CO_2

Figure 8.1 ■ Concepts related to alterations in fluids and electrolytes.

Grace Vincent: Introduction

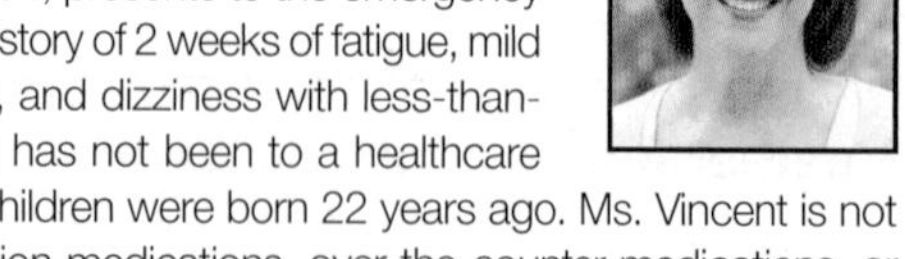

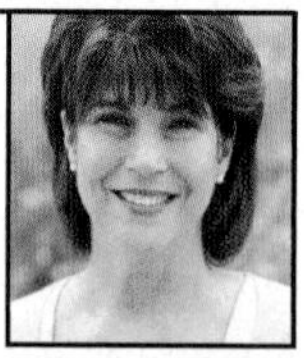

Grace Vincent, age 54, presents to the emergency department with a history of 2 weeks of fatigue, mild shortness of breath, and dizziness with less-than-normal activity. She has not been to a healthcare provider since her children were born 22 years ago. Ms. Vincent is not taking any prescription medications, over-the-counter medications, or herbal supplements. Her family history is unknown, as she was adopted.

1. Considering Ms. Vincent's age and lack of health screening for 22 years, what could be causing her symptoms?
2. Considering Ms. Vincent health history, what could be contributing to the symptom of dizziness and mild shortness of breath?

Check Your Progress: Section 8.1

1. Name two electrolytes found in plasma.
2. What are the signs of hypovolemia?
3. What are the signs of hypervolemia?
4. What is the impact of fluid excess on blood pressure?

8.2 Composition and Distribution of Body Fluids

The fluid in the body constitutes total body water (TBW), which varies according to the individual's age and amount of body fat. Fat contains less water than muscle, so lean individuals have more body water by proportion than individuals with greater fat content. Similarly, younger individuals have a greater percentage of TBW compared with those who are older. TBW is typically equivalent to 60%, or 42 liters of fluid for a 70-kilogram adult male. At birth, infants are composed of 70% TBW, decreasing to 61% at 12 months (approximately the same as the adult). The volume and concentration of body fluid are maintained in three functional compartments, which are traditionally divided across two categories: intracellular fluid and extracellular fluid (**Figure 8.2** ■).

Distribution and Composition of Body Fluids

Intracellular Fluid Component

By far the largest portion of fluid spacing in the body can be categorized as **intracellular fluid (ICF)**. The normal distribution of ICF involves approximately 63–70% of the total volume of body fluid. ICF is maintained within the cellular membrane, that is, in the cellular cytoplasm. ICF is dense and contains water, proteins, and electrolytes.[2]

Extracellular Fluid Component

The **extracellular fluid (ECF)** component includes the remaining 30–37% of the fluid volume in the body. The ECF can be divided into three subcategories: intravascular, interstitial, and transcellular volumes. **Sodium**, a naturally occurring metallic element, is the primary cation in ECF and has several physiologic functions, including effects on nerve impulse conduction.[3]

Intravascular. The intravascular component of the ECF is composed of the constituents of the whole blood. Intravascular fluid consists mainly of blood plasma and the ECF fluid, lymph, and transcellular fluid. This intravascular component has high concentrations of potassium, magnesium, phosphate, and proteins.

Interstitial. The interstitial fluid is another component of the ECF and represents the fluid in tissues and surrounding the cells. Interstitial fluid is a transport mechanism for nutrients, waste products, and gas exchange from the intracellular component to the filtration systems (i.e., the kidneys, liver, and lymphatic system).

Transcellular. The smallest component of the ECF is the transcellular component. This reflects fluid found in defined spaces, such as the cerebral spinal fluid, synovial fluid in joints, and fluid in body cavities. Transcellular fluid is rich in sodium, chloride, and bicarbonate.

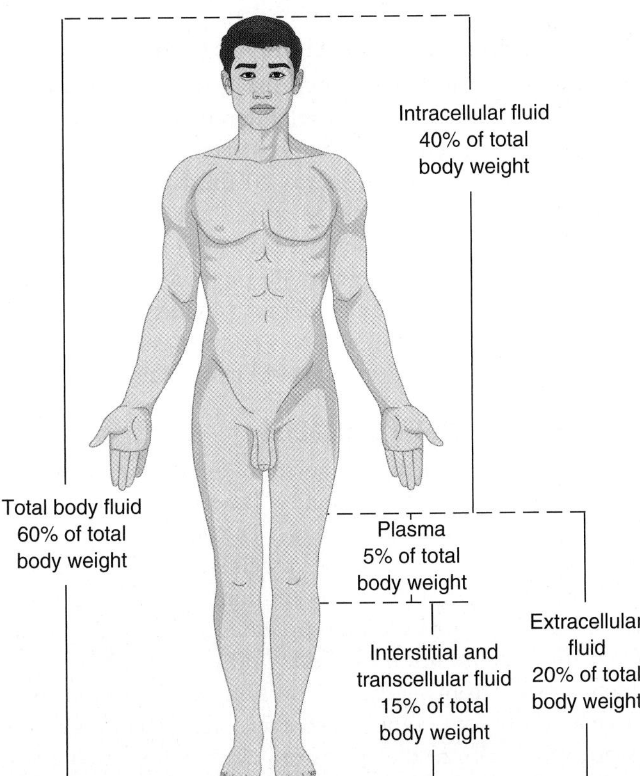

Figure 8.2 ■ Distribution of fluid compartments in the body.

Movement of Body Fluid

To maintain homeostasis, solutes are transported through semipermeable membranes. The movement of water between the ICF and ECF occurs through three mechanisms: osmosis, diffusion, and active transport (**Figure 8.3** ■). In **osmosis**, water molecules move from the less concentrated area to the more concentrated area in an attempt to equalize the concentration of solutions on two sides of a membrane (see Figure 8.3a). The movement of water between the ICF and ECF compartments is primarily a function of osmotic forces. The combined solute concentration in water is osmolarity, the number of solute particles per liter of solution. This concentration in body fluids is similar to **osmolality**, or the amount of solute per kilogram of solution. The amount of fluid leaving the capillary network is maintained close to equilibrium with the fluid that is resorbed. The tendency toward equilibrium across bodily compartments is achieved primarily from the movement of water rather than solute. This movement maintains a balance between the hydrostatic pressure of the blood and the capillary colloid osmotic pressure. Water is transported through water channels called aquaporins to maintain the composition of water in a state of equilibrium. Sodium is mainly responsible for the osmotic balance of the ECF, while potassium affects the osmotic balance in the ICF.[4]

The concentration of solutes in body fluids is traditionally expressed as osmolality. Osmolality is determined by the total solute concentration within a fluid compartment and is measured as parts of solute per kilogram of water. Sodium is the greatest determinant of osmolality; glucose and urea also contribute. Plasma osmolality (measured in milliosmoles per kilogram, or mOsm/kg) can therefore be estimated according to the formula 2[serum Na] + [Glucose]/18 + [BUN]/2.8. Normal serum osmolality is 275–295 mOsm/kg; hyperosmolar is greater than 295 mOsm/kg, and hypo-osmolar is less than 275 mOsm/kg.[5]

In **diffusion**, molecules move through a semipermeable membrane from an area of higher concentration to an area of lower concentration (see Figure 8.3b). Substances that are too large to cross the cellular membrane by diffusion, such as proteins, are transported out of the cell by **active transport**, a system that requires energy in the form of ATP to assist electrons to flow uphill (see Figure 8.3c).

Solutes that diffuse freely have less of an effect on the osmotic balance; those that are restricted to one primary compartment, such as sodium or potassium, have more osmotic activity. Sodium is mainly responsible

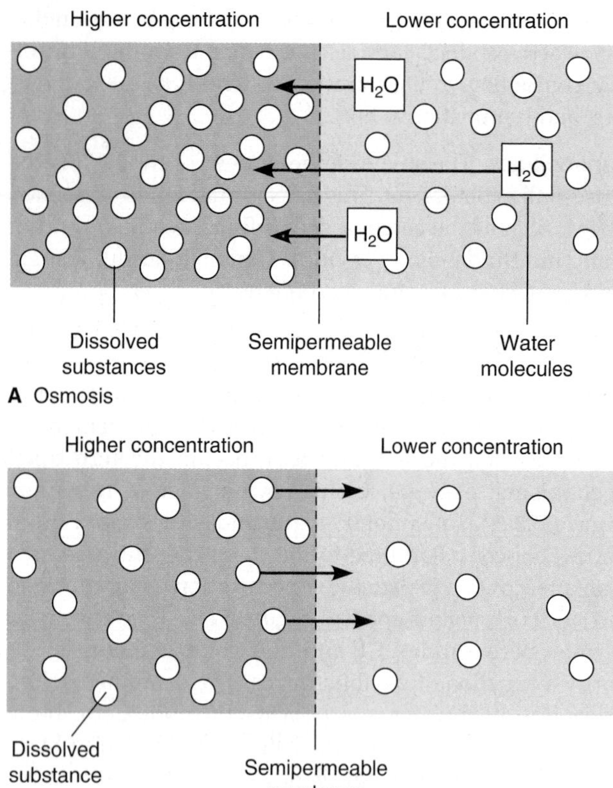

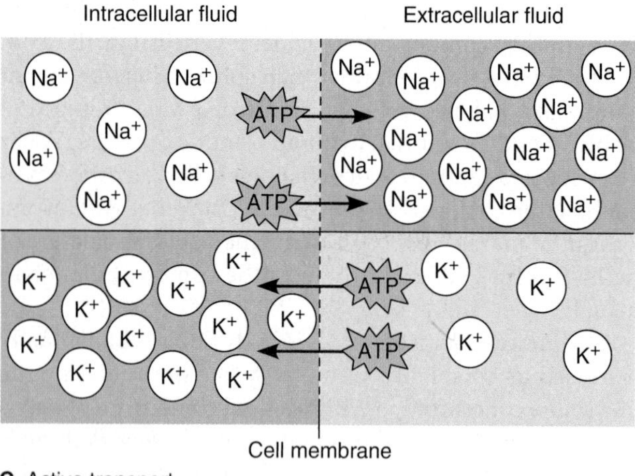

Figure 8.3 ■ Movement of fluids in the body is accomplished by **A.** osmosis, **B.** diffusion, or **C.** active transport.

for the osmotic balance of the ECF, whereas potassium affects the osmotic balance in the ICF. Diffusion involves the even distribution of molecules. Substances that are too large to cross the cellular membrane by diffusion, such as proteins, are transported out of the cell by active transport. Active transport moves solutes against the electrochemical gradient according to cellular requirements. The movement of water or blood passing through a membrane by a force, such as pressure, is filtration.[6] As a result of the flow of blood from the arterial to the venous end of the capillary, various forces determine whether the movement of fluid involves filtration or resorption. These forces include osmotic or hydrostatic pressures between the capillary and interstitial space.[3]

Hydrostatic pressure (the pressure of fluids or their properties when in equilibrium) is greater than **colloid osmotic pressure** (also known as *oncotic pressure*), which is the concentration of proteins, particularly albumin, that gives rise to water-pulling forces of a particular compartment at the arterial end of the capillary, resulting in the movement of fluid to the interstitial space. At the venous portion of the capillary, fluid moves into the capillary, owing to a higher colloid osmotic pressure than hydrostatic pressure. The net effect is filtration at the arterial end of the capillary and resorption at the venous end. Interstitial hydrostatic pressure promotes the movement of approximately 10% of the interstitial fluid along with a small amount of protein into the lymphatic system, eventually returning the fluid to the circulation. The integrity of the capillary membrane is an important factor in the filtration of fluid. Plasma proteins may potentially move into the interstitial space because of changes in membrane permeability.[3]

Edema

Edema is the accumulation of interstitial fluid volume. Typically, edema results from an increase in capillary hydrostatic pressure or capillary membrane permeability, a decreased colloid osmotic pressure, lymphatic obstruction, an excess of sodium and body water, or a combination of more than one mechanism.

Increased Capillary Hydrostatic Pressure

An increase in the capillary hydrostatic pressure occurs as a result of sodium and water retention that may be caused by venous obstruction. Venous obstruction contributes to localized edema from an increased fluid pressure in the capillaries, resulting in leakage of fluid into the interstitial space. Venous obstruction may result from the presence of clots. Increased capillary hydrostatic pressure usually results from an increased systemic venous pressure due to heart failure. Renal failure that involves an increased blood volume also contributes to an increased hydrostatic pressure.

Increased Capillary Permeability

Damage to the integrity of the endothelium may increase capillary membrane permeability. Trauma and burns may contribute to endothelial damage. The effects from hyperemia (an excess of blood in the vessels supplying an organ) and inflammation initiated by immune system responses cause localized, and in certain situations generalized, edema from the accumulation of fluids and proteins. Localized edema results from allergens or swelling in an affected area; edema may become generalized if an anaphylactic response is precipitated from the effects of inflammatory mediators such as histamine.

Decreased Colloid Osmotic Pressure

Edema may also occur from decreases in colloid osmotic pressure that contributes to the accumulation of fluid in the tissues from the effects of filtration. Plasma proteins maintain fluid resorption and therefore an adequate inward force preventing fluid accumulation in the tissues. Plasma protein depletion, primarily albumin, results in a decrease in central blood volume, contributing to the movement of fluid into the interstitial space and edema. Hepatic or renal disease involving damage to glomeruli or protein loss from malnutrition due to gastrointestinal (GI) losses contributes to low levels of protein in the bloodstream, resulting in challenges in osmotic pressure.[3]

Obstruction in the Lymphatic System

Lymphatic obstruction results in the accumulation of fluid and plasma proteins in the interstitial space. Often, the edema is localized, and lymphedema results. The surgical removal of lymph nodes and vessels often contributes to lymphatic obstruction. Other causes of lymphatic obstruction are trauma, radiation, metastasis, and inflammation.

Excess Body Water and Sodium

Excess body water and sodium result from the decreased cardiac output from heart failure or an inadequate excretion of sodium in renal failure. Compensatory mechanisms contribute to the retention of sodium and water as a result of the decreased cardiac output from heart failure. The retention of sodium causes an increased circulating plasma volume, contributing to an increased capillary pressure. Because of the heart's diminished ability to increase force of contraction in response to the increased volume, edema occurs from the shift of fluid into the interstitial space. Hypovolemia (a decreased volume of circulating blood in the body) occurs as a result of inadequate sodium excretion by the kidneys.[7]

Classification of Edema

Edema is often defined according to how it is manifested in the body, and the distribution of edema contributes to the etiology. Edema within an area of tissue from an injury, infection, or obstruction is more commonly localized. Generalized edema is often uniformly distributed and may accumulate in gravity-dependent positions. Edema from heart failure may increase in the extremities in response to positioning, whereas edema may be pronounced throughout the body if the etiology is hypoproteinemia. Dependent edema, or edema found in the dependent portions of the body, is typically found in disease processes that result in fluid volume excess. Edema is rarely found in situations of fluid volume deficiency.

Fluid spacing is a term used to classify the distribution of water in the body. *First spacing* refers to the normal distribution of fluid in the ICF and ECF. *Second spacing* is the excess accumulation of fluid in the interstitial spaces, referred to as edema. **Third spacing** involves the accumulation of fluid in areas (typically the intestinal space) that normally have no fluid or a minimal amount of fluid. Fluid lost from the intravascular space into the nonfunctional spaces can occur through several mechanisms, such as the loss of colloid osmotic pressure. This loss of the colloid osmotic pressure stems from deficits caused by either decreased intake or malproduction of proteins such as albumin. The loss of the concentration of protein in the intravascular fluid results in the loss of the water-pulling forces of colloid osmotic pressure. Examples of third spacing include ascites and edema that is associated with burns.

Clinical Manifestations

Edema is essentially the accumulation of interstitial fluid in a bodily space. This produces swelling that may be palpable and that compresses surrounding tissue and circulatory structures.[8] Clinical manifestations depend on the bodily space in which edema occurs. In the respiratory system, particularly the lungs, pulmonary edema results in shortness of breath due to a lack of adequate oxygenation of blood. In the extremities, edema is more readily notable and palpable. This palpable quality is then graded on a scale of 1–4, the higher score indicating more serious and enduring edema (**Figure 8.4** ■).

Linking Pathogenesis to Diagnosis and Treatment

Because the accumulation of fluid prevents the exchange of gases and leads to tissue compression, treatment is focused on removal of the fluid. Typically, diuretic therapy is used to aid in excretion of fluid from the body. Depending on the location of the edema, select intravenous solutions may be used in aid in pulling fluid from the tissue so that it can be excreted.

Regulating Body Fluids

Water intake is regulated by the thirst mechanism. Hypothalamic receptors are triggered in response to an increased serum osmolality or decreased circulating volume, such as decreased blood pressure, to facilitate water movement into or out of the capillaries between the plasma and the interstitial fluid. Vasopressin (antidiuretic hormone, or ADH) is released from the posterior pituitary and kidney excretion of water. The water intake decreases serum osmolality, thereby inhibiting ADH secretion, so the kidneys produce dilute urine (**Figure 8.5** ■).

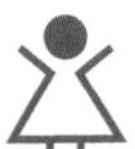

Newborns and infants have a high percentage of body weight composed of water, especially ECF, which can be lost from the body easily (**Figure 8.6** ■). The most common causes of dehydration in infants and children are severe diarrhea and vomiting. Signs of dehydration in infants and children include dry mouth and tongue, a lack of tears when crying, no wet diapers for 3 hours, sunken eyes and cheeks, sunken fontanels, listlessness, and irritability.[9] ■

Older adults have smaller fluid reserves, their ability to conserve water is reduced, and their sense of thirst is less acute. Often, they do not feel thirsty until they are already dehydrated. Chronic diseases, mobility issues, and certain medications also affect older adults' water intake. Older adults should increase their fluid intake during hot weather and when they are ill.[9] ■

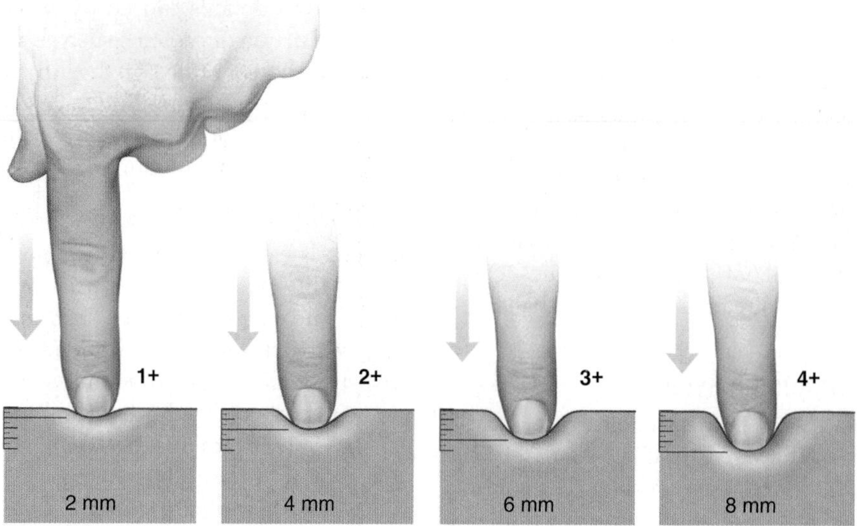

Figure 8.4 ■ Grading pitted edema.

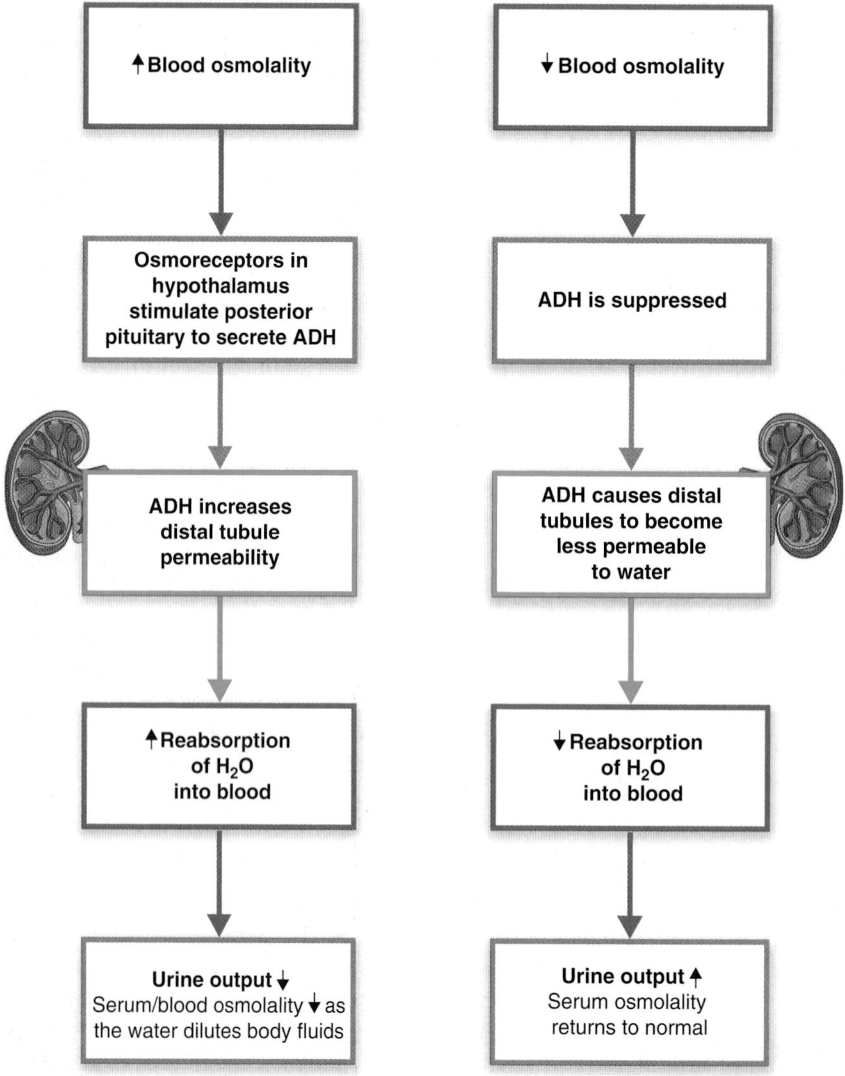

Figure 8.5 ■ Antidiuretic hormone regulates water excretion from the kidneys.

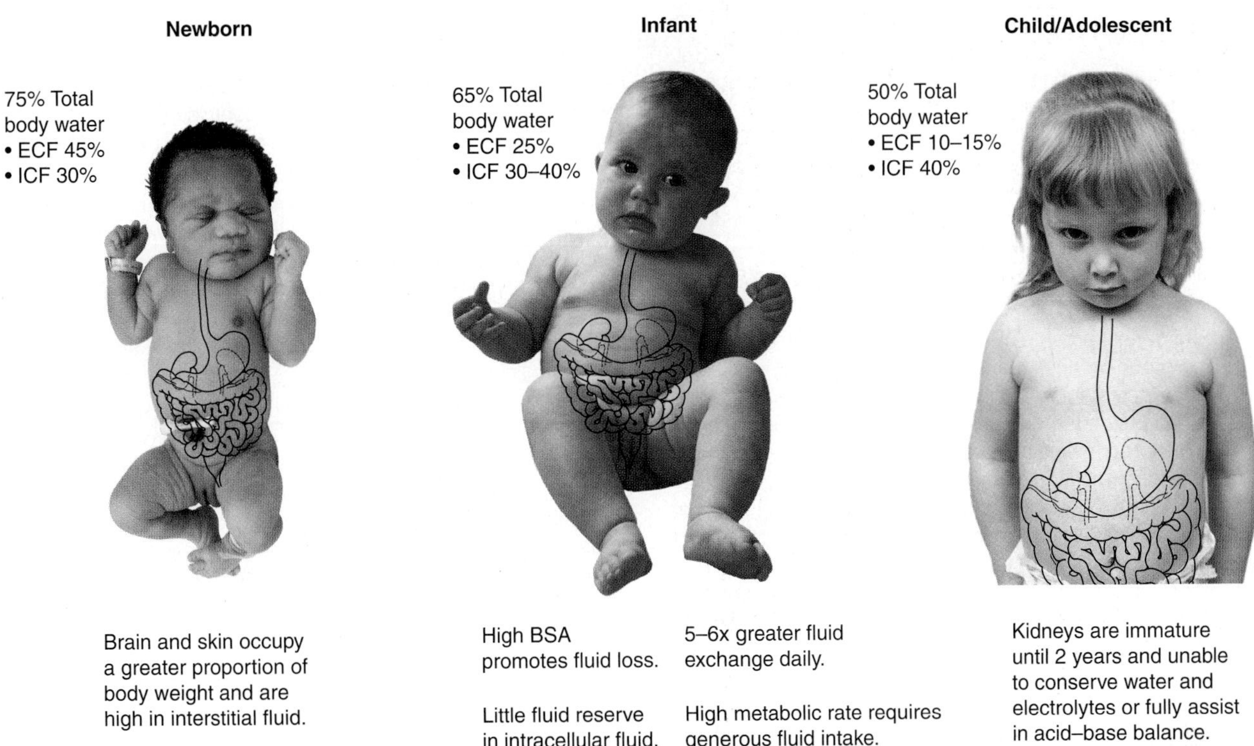
Newborn
Infant
Child/Adolescent
75% Total
body water
• ECF 45%
• ICF 30%
65% Total
body water
• ECF 25%
• ICF 30–40%
50% Total
body water
• ECF 10–15%
• ICF 40%
Brain and skin occupy a greater proportion of body weight and are high in interstitial fluid.
High BSA promotes fluid loss.
5–6x greater fluid exchange daily.
Little fluid reserve in intracellular fluid.
High metabolic rate requires generous fluid intake.
Kidneys are immature until 2 years and unable to conserve water and electrolytes or fully assist in acid–base balance.

Figure 8.6 ■ Newborns, infants, and children have a high percentage of body weight composed of water, especially ECF.

Regulating Electrolytes

In water, electrolytes dissociate into ions. **Cations** (positively charged electrolytes) include sodium (Na^+), potassium (K^+), calcium (Ca^{2+}), and magnesium (Mg^{2+}). **Anions** (negatively charged electrolytes) include bicarbonate (HCO_3^-), chloride (Cl^-), and phosphate (PO_4^{3-}).

Sodium concentration is regulated by renal and hormonal mechanisms and by natriuretic peptides that arise from cardiac tissue. Several factors identified include atrial natriuretic peptide (ANP), brain natriuretic peptide (BNP) and C-type natriuretic peptide (CNP). However, the main regulatory mechanism of renal sodium excretion is the renin–angiotensin–aldosterone system, which is explained in the next section. Water is regulated by ADH and the osmotic gradient that results from the concentration of sodium. Sports drinks and energy drinks, which are marketed as a means for restoring electrolyte balance, can actually disrupt electrolyte concentrations if consumed when the individual is not experiencing a concentration deficit[3,10] (see Impact of Nutrition in Clinical Practice).

Check Your Progress: Section 8.2

1. What is the definition of edema?
2. Name the two major fluid compartments of the body.
3. How does the kidney regulate fluid balance?

Impact of Nutrition in Clinical Practice

Thirsty for the Facts on Popular Drinks?

Joanne Kouba

The names of sports drinks and energy drinks tempt consumers to "buy me." But their ingredient lists say, "Buyer beware." Sports drinks are marketed to suggest that they will enhance athletic performance and maintain hydration by replacing nutrients lost during exercise.[1] These drinks generally contain carbohydrates, minerals, electrolytes, flavoring, and vitamins. Ads for energy drinks, which are not the same as sports drinks, suggest that they will boost energy, reduce fatigue, heighten mental function, and increase concentration.[1] Along with the nutrients found in sports drinks, energy drinks include nonnutritive additives such as caffeine, guarana, ginseng, ginkgo, and taurine.[1,2]

Water is essential to maintain hydration and many metabolic functions. Daily fluid needs are variable and depend on factors such as sweat loss from physical activity. The American Academy of Pediatrics (AAP) recommends water, moderate juice intake, and low-fat milk as regular fluid sources for hydration in young people during normal daily activities.[1] Water should be the first beverage

(Continued)

Impact of Nutrition in Clinical Practice *Continued*

choice for children during school and for most physical activity. Concerns that dehydration can lead to fatigue, impaired performance, cognitive lapses, electrolyte imbalances, and heat illness should be considered for anyone who performs strenuous physical activity. Hydration management is important for these individuals especially in conditions of high temperatures and humidity. In these situations, sports drinks may be indicated. However, sports drinks are not indicated during periods of sedentary activity. The AAP does not recommend energy drinks at all for children or adolescents.[1]

Carbohydrates provide the primary source of energy for most age groups. Other than milk and some juice, additional carbohydrate-containing beverages are generally not needed except when prolonged vigorous activity depletes muscle glycogen. This situation makes blood glucose an important fuel source to maintain performance and prevent fatigue. A sports drink with carbohydrate would be appropriate in these situations. However, if carbohydrate-containing sports and/or energy drink intake is not necessary, then excess calorie and sugar intake occurs, contributing to risk of obesity and dental caries. Intake of sports drinks is not recommended during meals, with snacks, or as a substitute for milk or water.

Protein is added to some sports drinks to aid with "muscle recovery" after a strenuous workout or event. For most individuals, a well-balanced, varied diet should provide adequate protein. Low-fat milk is a common food with protein and good for a "recovery" meal or snack. If nothing else is available, a sports drink that contains protein could be used. Drinks that contain individual amino acids are another matter. Glutamine, arginine, taurine, and other amino acids are heavily marketed as ergogenic additives to boost immune function, vasodilatation, lipolysis, and the action of caffeine.[1] However, their benefits are not supported by scientific literature, and they are discouraged for children and adolescents.[1]

Caffeine, which is routinely added to energy drinks, is thought to increase endurance and strength and reduce fatigue in adults. Other effects include increased heart rate, blood pressure, motor activity, attentiveness, diuresis, and temperature; sleep disturbances, dysrhythmias, and increased anxiety in individuals with anxiety disorders.[1] These effects have not been well evaluated in children. Concerns about caffeine in children include its effect on neurologic and cardiovascular tissues and dependence. Recent case reports suggest that atrial fibrillation occurs in healthy adolescents as a result of using highly caffeinated drinks.[3] A 16-year-old boy died in April 2017 after drinking a café latte, a large Diet Mountain Dew, and an energy drink in a 2-hour period, causing an arrhythmia. He had no underlying heart disease.[4] Seizures have also been reported in healthy youths and adults after ingestion of multiple energy drinks in a short time period.[5,6] Caffeine toxicity is not a rare phenomenon in our society, especially since caffeine-containing beverages are readily available, poorly regulated, and heavily marketed. The American Association of Poison Control Centers received 5156 calls about energy drinks in 2014, 40% were about children younger than age 6.[7] Some energy drinks contain 500 milligrams of caffeine per container.[1] This is about 14 times the amount in a can of cola. For these reasons, the AAP discourages any caffeine intake in all children.

Some products contain dangerous combinations of alcohol, high doses of caffeine, and other stimulants. While these are clearly not appropriate for children and adolescents, they are popular with young adults.[8] Their use has been associated with episodes of loss of consciousness and aggression, resulting in sales bans by certain states and colleges, and they are riskier to drink than alcohol alone.[8]

Evocative names and vibrant packaging suggest excitement and life in the fast lane for consumers of these products. However, scrutiny of label ingredients has led experts to raise concerns about excessive calorie intake, dental caries, reliance on caffeine, unrealistic expectations, substitution of these drinks for nutrient-dense foods, stimulant toxicity, and even cardiac and neurologic events. Water, low-fat milk, and moderate juice intake should provide enough fluids for most individuals at any age. Sports drinks can be used selectively for those who are engaged in vigorous, sustained physical activity. Energy drinks are not recommended for youths. Healthcare professionals should be aware of the wide range of ingredients in popular beverages and their health effects.

References

1. Committee on Nutrition and the Council on Sports Medicine and Fitness. (2011). Clinical report—Sports drinks and energy drinks for children and adolescents: Are they appropriate? *Pediatrics, 127*(6), 1182–1189.
2. Iyadurai, S. J., & Chung, S. S. (2007). New-onset seizures in adults: Possible association with consumption of popular energy drinks. *Epilepsy & Behavior, 10*(3), 605–508.
3. DiRocco, J. R., During, A., Morelli, P. J., et al. (2011). Atrial fibrillation in healthy adolescents after highly caffeinated beverage consumption: Two case reports. *Journal of Medical Case Reports, 5*, 18. Available at http://www.jmedicalcasereporrts.com/content/5/1/18
4. Lynch, J., & Goldschmidt, D. Teen dies from too much caffeine, coroner says. *CNN.* Retrieved from http://www.cnn.com/2017/05/15/health/teen-death-caffeine/index.html
5. Babu, K. M., Zuckerman, M. D., Cherkes, J. K., et al. (2011). First-onset seizure after use of 5-hour ENERGY. *Pediatric Emergency Care, 27*, 539–540.
6. Trabulo, D., Marques, S., & Pedroso, E. (2011). Caffeinated energy drink intoxication. *Emergency Medicine Journal, 29*(8), 712–714.
7. American Heart Association. (2014). Poison control data show energy drinks and young kids don't mix. Retrieved from http://news.heart.org/tag/american-association-of-poison-control-centers-national-poison-data-system/
8. Marczinski, C. A. (2015). Can energy drinks increase the desire for more alcohol? *Advances in Nutrition, 6*, 96–101. Retrieved from http://advances.nutrition.org/content/6/1/96.full 1292.

8.3 Water and Sodium Imbalances

Water and sodium imbalances can be categorized on the basis of etiology. A volume imbalance, also referred to as an isotonic imbalance, involves equal alterations in the sodium and water concentrations, whereas osmolar imbalances involve an alteration in the concentration between water and sodium or other solutes in the ECF. Isotonic fluid imbalances may involve hypervolemia or hypovolemia; however, the sodium level remains normal in either imbalance.[1,4,11]

Sodium is the main cation in the ECF. Normal ECF sodium concentrations are maintained between 135 and 145 mEq/L. Sodium is a primary determinant of ECF osmolality, and concentrations below 135 mEq/L constitute **hyponatremia**, whereas concentrations greater than 145 mEq/L constitute **hypernatremia**. Sodium is essential

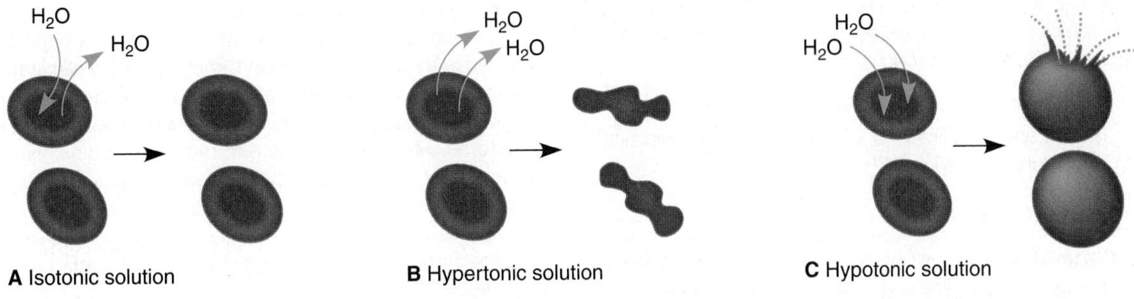

Figure 8.7 ■ Depiction of cell transformations in isotonic, hypertonic, and hypotonic solutions.

for transmission of nerve and muscle impulses, and it combines with the bicarbonate radical as part of acid and base regulation.[1]

Water balance may be classified as isotonic, hypertonic, or hypotonic (**Figure 8.7** ■):

- **Isotonic** solutions have the same osmolality as body fluids. Normal saline (0.9% sodium chloride) is an isotonic solution.
- **Hypertonic** solutions have a higher osmolality than body fluids. An example of a hypertonic solution is 3% sodium chloride.
- **Hypotonic** solutions have a lower osmolality than body fluids. An example of a hypotonic solution is 0.45% sodium chloride.

Plasma contains 9% sodium. An equivalent osmolality between the plasma and sodium is isotonic, as the concentrations of concentration of plasma and sodium are equivalent. A higher or lower sodium or fluid concentration results in alterations.

Clinical manifestations of fluid volume excess and fluid volume deficit are compared in **Table 8.2** ■.

Isotonic Fluid Volume Excess

Isotonic fluid volume excess typically results from ECF volume excess, or hypervolemia. Fluid and electrolyte concentration increases at a rate equivalent to that of the ECF. The same osmolality is maintained in a state of hypervolemia rather than euvolemia.

Etiology and Pathogenesis

Isotonic fluid volume excess or volume overload typically occurs simultaneously with or after an increase in extracellular sodium levels. An excess volume generally refers to an increased ECF volume, which in most cases is related to a decreased excretion of water and sodium, as in acute kidney injury or chronic kidney disease (both of which are covered in Chapter 46). Renal sodium retention leads to an increased bodily sodium content with a subsequent increase in excess volume in varying degrees. This may occur in individuals with Cushing syndrome, heart failure, renal failure, liver cirrhosis, or during drug therapy. However, the underlying etiology may be derived from a significant increase in enteral or parenteral sodium ingestion.[1,7]

Excess fluid may result from an excessive administration of intravenous fluids or hypersecretion of adrenocorticoid hormones, such as aldosterone. Aldosterone acts directly on the kidneys to increase the retention of both sodium and water; thus, hypersecretion can lead to an isotonic fluid volume excess. Disease states such as heart failure, liver failure, or malnutrition may also contribute to isotonic fluid volume excess. On a biochemical level, fluid will move out of the ECF into the cells, causing them to swell. In extreme circumstances, this swelling can lead to cell lysis. Common etiologies include heart failure, liver failure, cirrhosis, excessive sodium intake, and select drug therapy such as vasopressin or angiotensin-converting enzyme inhibitors.

Table 8.2 Clinical Manifestations of Fluid Volume Excess and Fluid Volume Deficit

Clinical Manifestation	Fluid Volume Excess	Fluid Volume Deficit
Blood pressure	Increased	Decreased systolic Postural hypotension
Heart rate	Increased	Increased
Pulse amplitude	Increased	Decreased
Respirations	Moist crackles Wheezing	Normal
Jugular vein	Distended	Flat
Edema	Dependent	Rare
Skin turgor	Taut	Loose, poor
Urine output	Low or normal	Low, concentrated
Urine specific gravity	Low	High
Weight	Gain	Loss

Grace Vincent: Application

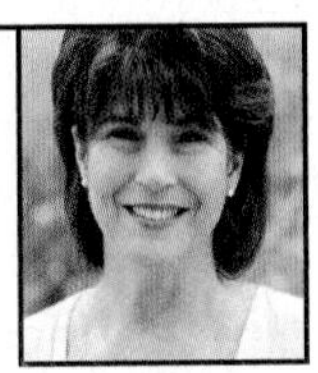

Ms. Vincent's vital signs are pulse 104 and irregular, respirations 28, temperature 99.1°F, blood pressure 162/94, SpO_2 90%. Body measurements are height 5′5″, weight 235 pounds, and BMI 39.1. Ms. Vincent states that her weight 2 weeks ago was 215 pounds. On assessment, she is awake, alert, and oriented × 4. She is in mild to moderate respiratory distress and started on 2 L/min oxygen via nasal cannula to supplement her poor SpO_2 saturation. Cardiovascular assessment demonstrates an irregular pulse bilaterally, and the point of maximal impulse is displaced laterally. Ms. Vincent is placed on a cardiac monitor that shows atrial fibrillation. After initial interventions, she continues to complain of dyspnea on exertion, though she does feel better with the supplemental oxygen.

There are bilateral crackles on auscultation in the lower lung lobes. The lower extremities both have 2+ edema with weak pulses. The lower extremities are cool to the touch.

3. What is the likely cause of Ms. Vincent's pedal edema?
4. What factors are most likely contributing to the development of hypertension in Ms. Vincent?

Clinical Manifestations

The clinical manifestations of isotonic fluid volume excess are weight gain, a decreased serum hematocrit, and decreased plasma protein from the dilutional effect of excess plasma (see Table 8.2). Assessment findings may reveal distended neck veins, increased blood pressure, and increased capillary hydrostatic pressure, contributing to the presence of edema.

Linking Pathophysiology to Diagnosis and Treatment

Isotonic fluids have a solute content much like that of the human body (i.e., equivalent osmolality). In isotonic fluid volume excess, the water and solutes in the human body are increasing at equivalent rates, resulting in the same osmolality in hypervolemic form rather than euvolemia.[4]

As solutes and fluid are increasing, serum levels will show a decreased hematocrit, and a decrease in blood urea nitrogen (BUN) levels indicates the presence of artificial dilution. In the face of declining serum laboratory values, the overall body weight will increase as a result of additional fluid volume. If a urinalysis is performed, a very low specific gravity will be found, owing to excessive fluid excretion. Vital signs and hemodynamic measures will reflect a high cardiac output; these will include hypertension, high central venous pressure, and/or high pulmonary capillary wedge pressure. X-rays may show findings such as pulmonary vascular congestion, pleural effusion, pericardial effusion, and ascites.

Treatment is aimed at restricting fluid intake and correcting the underlying etiology. Returning the osmolality to normal will aid in creating an euvolemic state. Loop diuretics such as furosemide may be indicated to promote the excretion of sodium and fluid. Optimal nursing care of the patient with isotonic fluid excess includes monitoring fluid intake and output, weighing the patient daily, assessing respirations to listen for crackles in fluid volume overload, assessing the skin for peripheral edema, monitoring responses to medication therapy with diuretics, promoting rest, and utilizing semi-Fowler positioning for orthopnea in symptomatic patients.[12–14]

Grace Vincent: Outcome

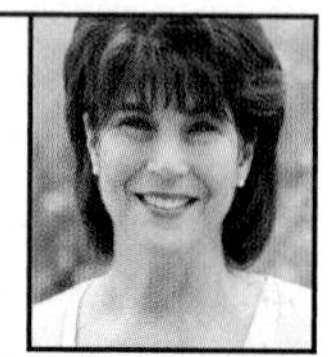

Ms. Vincent is diagnosed with heart failure. One of the major indicators is her rapid weight gain over a relatively short period of time. A rule of thumb used with heart failure patients is that they should call their provider if they experience either a 3-pound weight gain in 1 day or a 5-pound weight gain in 1 week. The physical findings of crackles in the lungs, displaced point of maximal impulse, and peripheral edema support the diagnosis of heart failure.

Ms. Vincent was ultimately started on furosemide for fluid retention and warfarin for atrial fibrillation, given compression stockings, and provided with dietary education targeted toward eliminating excessive sodium intake. She was also further educated on the signs and symptoms of heart failure and to be aware of worsening signs and symptoms. Ms. Vincent was referred to a cardiologist for further management of blood pressure, heart failure, and atrial fibrillation. Prognosis will depend on a multitude of factors such as whether Ms. Vincent adheres to therapy, whether her atrial fibrillation can be converted back to normal sinus rhythm, and control of high blood pressure.

5. Explain the pathophysiology of the crackles and dyspnea experienced by Ms. Vincent in relation to heart failure.
6. Discuss the rationale for the use of furosemide and warfarin for the management of heart failure, atrial fibrillation, and hypertension.

Isotonic Fluid Volume Deficit

Etiology and Pathogenesis

Isotonic fluid volume deficits occur when water and electrolytes are lost or depleted in a symmetric fashion. Typical causes of isotonic fluid volume deficit include, but are not limited to, hemorrhage, vomiting, diarrhea, fever, excess sweating, burns, diabetes insipidus, and uncontrolled diabetes mellitus. Isotonic fluid volume deficit is associated with dehydration and/or hypovolemia. The water and the solute content of the body's fluid are depleted at equivalent rates. On a biochemical level, the fluid moves out of the cells into the dehydrated (higher serum osmolality) ECF, and the cells ultimately shrink as a result of osmosis.[4]

Clinical Manifestations

Isotonic fluid volume deficit results in hypovolemia with a normal serum sodium level. Clinical symptoms include a decrease in urine output, weight loss, and an increased hematocrit. Clinical manifestations include tachycardia, decreased skin turgor and blood pressure, and, potentially, hypovolemic shock.

A priority of treatment is addressing the cause of the fluid deficit and replacing lost volume. Daily weighing and strict intake and output management are pivotal to monitoring the fluid volume status of an at-risk patient. Neurologic assessments can show a decreased level of consciousness with a decreased fluid volume status. Regular respiratory assessments are warranted to auscultate for pulmonary edema. Rales may indicate that the patient is in fluid volume overload after being rehydrated. Monitoring for skin and tongue turgor is also important; poor turgor and dry mucous membranes indicate that the patient is still in isotonic fluid volume deficit.

Linking Pathophysiology to Diagnosis and Treatment

Maintaining the balance of fluid and electrolytes is crucial to the care of patients across the continuum, and healthcare providers must be cognizant of key electrolytes, their function in the body, normal values, signs and symptoms of imbalances, treatment modalities, and monitoring and assessment parameters.[6] In isotonic fluid deficit, the water and the solute content of the body's fluid are depleted at equivalent rates. Overall, isotonic fluid volume deficit is associated with dehydration and/or hypovolemia. On a pathophysiologic level, the fluid moves out of the cells into the dehydrated (higher serum osmolality) ECF, and the cells ultimately shrink as a result of osmosis of the fluid.[3,15]

Laboratory values from the patient's serum and urine will be of great importance in determining the etiology and treatment of an isotonic fluid volume deficit. Like many fluid imbalances, addressing the underlying cause is the most efficient mode of treatment. In patients with isotonic fluid volume deficit, blood serum values will show increased hematocrit, increased blood urea nitrogen:creatinine ratio, and increased serum osmolality. Urinalysis may show increased urine osmolality and increased specific gravity depending on the underlying etiology. Nursing staff will note an overall decrease in urine production.

Typically, in mild cases of isotonic fluid volume deficit, the patient will be managed with increased oral fluid. A clinical example is viral gastritis, in which the patient can have profound diarrhea, and supplemental fluid will likely be the treatment. In young, healthy patients, the fluid volume deficit can be managed on an outpatient basis with treatment of symptoms and increased oral fluid intake (**Figure 8.8** ■). Patients with moderate to severe isotonic fluid volume deficit or patients who cannot take oral fluid rehydration may need to be given intravenous rehydration to correct the deficit. In most cases, an isotonic fluid such as 0.9% saline is given intravenously until the patient's blood pressure and heart rate have been stabilized. Then the isotonic fluid can be continued, or the patient can be switched to a hypotonic fluid such as 0.45% saline to replenish the fluid status.[11]

CLINICAL POINT: Patients who are treated with intravenous hydration need to be monitored to ensure that overreplacement of water leading to fluid volume excess does not occur. ■

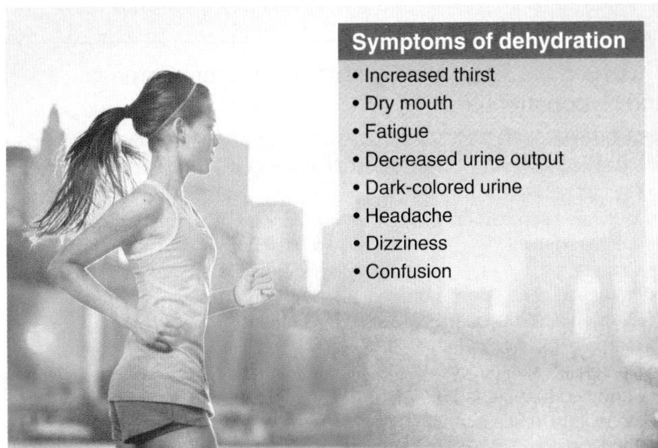

Figure 8.8 ■ When exercising outdoors, especially on a hot, sunny day, it is important to stay adequately hydrated.

Typical nursing management of an isotonic fluid deficit is much like that for other fluid pathologies. Assessment of the patient's vital signs is important to ensure that hypovolemia has been corrected and the patient is hemodynamically stable. If the patient has a severe deficit, ICU admission and monitoring fluid volume status with a central venous catheter may be needed.[3,15]

With pediatric patients, careful monitoring of hemodynamic status should occur with isotonic fluid volume deficit. Children have a much greater risk of physiologic compromise, owing to their relative percentage of TBW. The percentage of fluid volume that makes up the body typically decreases with age. Therefore, isotonic fluid deficit will need to be corrected with both volume and electrolytes along with the hemodynamic monitoring. The amount of replacement and the thoroughness of monitoring will depend on the severity of the isotonic fluid volume deficit. ■

Careful monitoring should be included in managing older adults with isotonic fluid volume deficit. These patients typically have a smaller percentage of TBW than younger patients. At any age, physical assessment should include assessment of the vital signs for hypovolemia, skin assessment for poor skin turgor, and generalized weakness and confusion, which suggest impaired cardiac output. Symptoms can be more profound in older adults and children. ■

Sodium Imbalances

Sodium, a primary determinant of ECF osmolality, is regulated through various mechanisms. Hormonal regulation involves **aldosterone** (a mineralocorticoid synthesized and secreted by the adrenal cortex), which is secreted in response to hemodynamic changes. A decreased blood pressure will stimulate the secretion of renin and subsequent activation of the **renin–angiotensin–aldosterone system (RAAS)**, resulting in sodium retention, increased fluid volume and subsequent blood pressure increase.

The RAAS responds to low blood pressure and low serum sodium (**Figure 8.9** ■).[16] Low serum sodium is important because water follows sodium. The RAAS helps to increase blood pressure by using the mechanisms to change one chemical into another to produce a reaction. The first step happens when the kidneys detect a drop in blood pressure (hypotension) or a decrease in sodium. When the kidneys detect hypotension or low sodium, the juxtaglomerular cells release renin into the bloodstream.[16] Renin meets up with angiotensinogen, which is produced by the liver. When renin and angiotensinogen meet, they react and form angiotensin I.[17] Angiotensin I then passes through the lungs and hooks up with the angiotensin-converting enzyme and becomes angiotensin II.[17] Angiotensin II is a potent arterial vasoconstrictor. Because the vessels (*vaso-*) become narrower (*constrict*), this increases blood pressure. Angiotensin II continues to the adrenal glands, and aldosterone is formed. Aldosterone increases the retention of sodium, which increases blood volume. It is also important

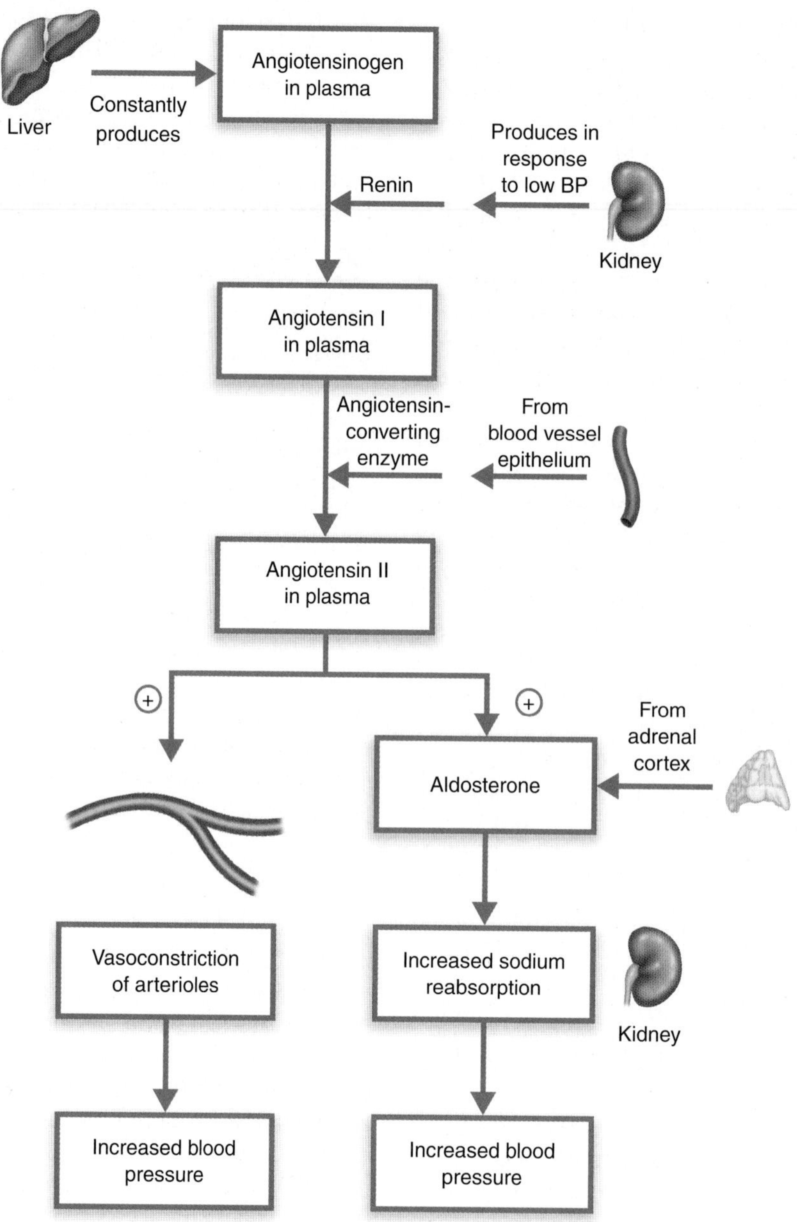

Figure 8.9 ■ The renin–angiotensin–aldosterone pathway.

to remember that while aldosterone is saving sodium, it is removing potassium from the body through urination.

The natriuretic peptides, **atrial natriuretic peptide (ANP)** produced by atrial cells and **brain natriuretic peptide (BNP)** originating from ventricular cells are then released in response to the elevated atrial pressure resulting from the increased circulating volume, due to sodium retention. These substances also stimulate the release of urodilatin from the kidney that antagonizes the RAAS, thereby lowering ANP and BNP levels.

The signs and symptoms of sodium imbalances are listed in **Table 8.3** ■.

Table 8.3 Signs and Symptoms of Hypernatremia and Hyponatremia

Hypernatremia	Hyponatremia
• Plasma sodium > 145 mEq/L • Increased serum osmolality • Increased thirst • Oliguria • Increased urine specific gravity • Dry skin and mucous membranes • Decreased skin turgor • Furrowed tongue and dry mouth • Headache, restlessness • Tachycardia • Hypotension • Vascular collapse • Seizures, coma	• Plasma sodium < 135 mEq/L • Decreased serum osmolality • Muscle cramps, weakness • Headache • Anxiety • Lethargy, stupor • Anorexia • Nausea and vomiting • Hypotension • Shock • Coma

Hypernatremia

Hypernatremia involves an increased sodium concentration, greater than 145 mEq/L.

Etiology and Pathogenesis

The most common cause of hypernatremia is an increased output or decreased intake of water. An increased sodium consumption may also cause this imbalance; thirst impairments or water deprivation, inappropriate treatment, diarrhea, burns, and heat stroke are all possible etiologies. Hypernatremia may be due to secondary effects that occur as a manifestation of disease processes, such as diabetes insipidus. Isotonic fluid volume deficits may occur early, along with hypernatremia from a lack of ADH or insufficient renal responses to ADH later in the disease process. Other causes of hypernatremia are fever and infection that contribute to an increased respiratory rate and dehydration.[12]

Clinical Manifestations

Hyperosmolality often results from hypernatremia; water moves to the ECF, resulting in ICF dehydration. Clinical presentation includes thirst, fever, dry membranes, hypotension, tachycardia, low jugular venous pressure, and restlessness. Pulmonary edema occurs when water shifts from the ICF to the interstitial space. Central nervous system (CNS) symptoms may include muscle twitching, hyperreflexia, confusion, coma, convulsions, and cerebral hemorrhage. The effects on the CNS are considered the most serious.[18]

Linking Pathophysiology to Diagnosis and Treatment

In evaluating the serum levels in a patient, hypernatremia will reflect an increased serum sodium and increased serum osmolality. The urinalysis will show an increase in urine specific gravity. A stool culture would be beneficial to collect for a patient with watery diarrhea to identify a potential underlying infectious cause that can be treated. Serum ADH can be found in central diabetes insipidus; however, it can be decreased or normal in nephrogenic diabetes insipidus.

Medical management of hypernatremia is aimed at decreasing the serum sodium content. Typically, this is done with hypotonic fluids such as 0.3% saline and dextrose 5% in water or with isotonic fluids such as 0.9% saline. If the etiology is diabetes insipidus, treatment with desmopressin acetate, a synthetic form of ADH, is warranted. Proper intake and output management with appropriate documentation is needed along with daily body weight measurement to assess the fluid volume status in the patient with hypernatremia. The nurse should monitor for signs and symptoms of thirst or fever. Administration of appropriate fluids and increasing intake should be done if the patient lacks intake or has increased water excretion, as in diabetes insipidus. Patients with hypernatremia should be placed on seizure precautions.[14]

Hyponatremia

Hyponatremia is a common cause of a hypotonic fluid imbalance that may occur from sodium concentrations below 135 mEq/L.

Etiology and Pathogenesis

Hyponatremia is a typical electrolyte abnormality in hospitalized individuals and is due to serum sodium deficits due to the loss of body fluids through various etiologies or extracellular volume that dilutes the sodium level. Fluid loss commonly results from vomiting and diarrhea or other GI depletion, or an effect from medications (diuretics). Inadequate excretion results from renal dysfunction, adrenal insufficiency (i.e., Addison disease), syndrome of inappropriate antidiuretic hormone secretion, or diabetic ketoacidosis. Hypotonic fluid administration postoperatively as well as oral water intoxication as is the case with psychogenic polydipsia are also potential etiologies.[14]

Fluid shifts from the ICF to the ECF in a variety of situations, including hyperglycemia and electrolyte imbalances. The underlying mechanism is the fluid shifting from an area of high concentration of fluid to an area of low concentration of fluid. In hyperglycemia, the fluid is moving to the ECF to dilute the high amounts of sugar in the blood. Ultimately, this fluid shift will dilute the sodium in the intravascular space.

Clinical Manifestations

Hyponatremia contributes to symptoms of hypovolemia. As a result of abnormal sodium concentrations, intracellular sodium deficits occur, resulting in neurologic sequelae. Clinically, characteristic neurologic effects include lethargy, headache, confusion, seizures, and coma. The loss of sodium that results in hypovolemia contributes to symptoms of hypotension, tachycardia, and a deceased urine output, similar to symptoms of dehydration (see Table 8.3).

Linking Pathophysiology to Diagnosis and Treatment

The diagnostic procedures in cases of low sodium levels are aimed at identifying both the hyponatremia and the underlying cause in a secondary disease process. Serum laboratory values can show decreased serum sodium, chloride, and bicarbonate levels and increased hematocrit. Urinalysis can show low urine specific gravity. Increased potassium, BUN, and creatinine levels can also be found in renal insufficiency. An elevated BNP level occurs with heart failure. A decreased serum cortisol level can reflect adrenal insufficiency.

Correcting the underlying etiology of the hyponatremia is as important as returning the sodium concentration to within the normal range. Establishing stable hemodynamic status is a priority if the individual is hemodynamically unstable.

Mild hyponatremia can be managed with oral sodium replacement through increasing dietary sodium chloride intake or pharmacologic therapy with sodium bicarbonate. Many healthcare providers elect to utilize a water restriction of 1–2 L/day with or without corresponding fluid volume excess. Moderate hyponatremia will likely need to be managed with intravenous fluids such as lactated Ringer's or isotonic saline.

For severe hyponatremia, the healthcare provider may elect to utilize hypertonic fluids (2–3% sodium chloride), which will rapidly replenish the serum sodium. However, this course of treatment raises many safety concerns, owing to the risk of causing hypernatremia. To prevent overcorrection, constant monitoring is required while using hypertonic fluids.

As with other fluid volume and electrolyte issues, nursing management of intake and output along with daily body weight measurement is imperative to assess the patient's fluid volume status. Serum sodium will need to be monitored periodically to evaluate the degree of correction in the serum sodium. Dietary sodium and fluid intake management and education are important, especially when the patient is at particularly high risk of hyponatremia. Seizure precautions should be initiated for patients with either hyponatremia or hypernatremia (**Figure 8.10** ■).

Timely diagnosis and proper treatment are important for children with hyponatremia. The symptoms vary little at different ages; however, the loss of serum sodium concentration will have amplified effects on younger patients. ■

Hyponatremia is highly prevalent in older adults. Even minor chronic clinical hyponatremia can result in a higher incidence of falls and cognitive impairment. Hyponatremia has a rather high incidence, owing to a multitude of underlying conditions, and clinically significant cases are usually multifactorial. For example, thiazide

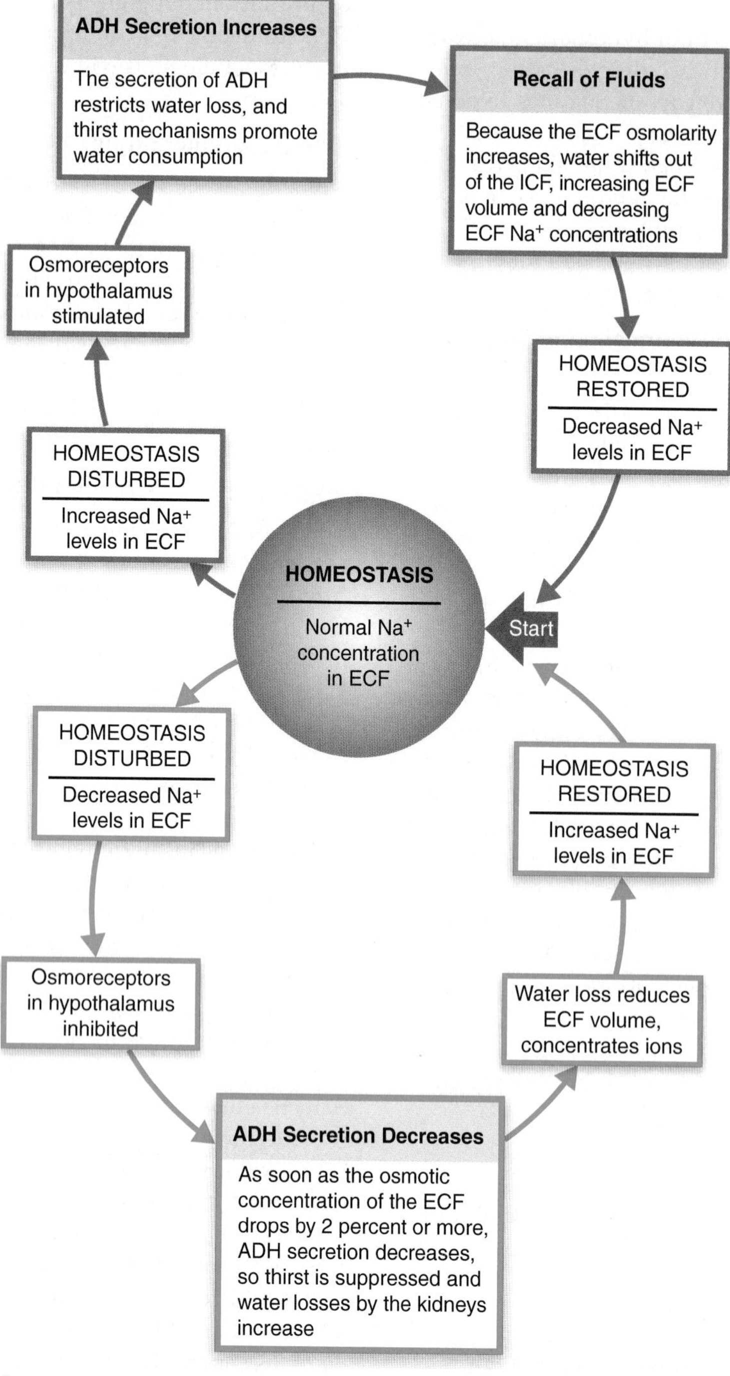

Figure 8.10 ■ Physiologic mechanisms maintaining serum sodium balance.

type and loop diuretics have a tendency to cause hyponatremia. These are both common medications used to treat disease processes such as hypertension, heart failure, and some genitourinary pathologies. The increasing use of these medications will cause a higher incidence of clinical complications such as hyponatremia. ■

Check Your Progress: Section 8.3

1. Give an example of a patient at risk for developing hypernatremia.
2. How does ADH help the kidney to regulate fluid balance?
3. An increase in plasma osmolality can influence fluid movement from ICF into ECF. Explain the link between the underlying physiology and why this would occur.

8.4 Chloride Imbalances

Chloride, a naturally occurring anion, is the primary ECF anion, with normal concentrations ranging from 96 to 106 mEq/L. Sodium and water balances are intimately related, and the concentration of chloride is generally proportional to that of sodium. Chloride is involved in the maintenance of ECF osmolality and acid–base regulation, and it is inversely related to the concentration of bicarbonate (HCO_3^-). Chloride is found in the stomach, as a component of hydrochloric acid, and is essential for carbon dioxide transport in red blood cells. High levels of chloride are found in the cerebrospinal fluid, bile, and pancreatic juices. Signs and symptoms of chloride imbalances are listed in **Table 8.4** ■.

Hyperchloremia

Etiology and Pathogenesis

Hyperchloremia is an abnormally high plasma concentration of chloride ions. Potential etiologies of hyperchloremia include metabolic acidosis (which is the most common etiology), water loss, dehydration, head injury that causes endocrine abnormalities, hypernatremia, severe diarrhea, respiratory alkalosis, and hyperparathyroidism. Chloride imbalances are usually transient, along with the acute etiology. For example, if the underlying etiology is dehydration with more fluid loss than electrolyte loss, the sodium chloride in the serum will be in proportionally higher concentration, owing to the dehydration.

Table 8.4 Signs and Symptoms of Chloride Imbalances

Hyperchloremia	Hypochloremia
• Chloride > 107 mEq/L • Often asymptomatic • Dehydration • Polydipsia • Rapid, labored breathing • Muscular weakness	• Chloride < 97 mEq/L • Generally has features similar to those of metabolic alkalosis • Confusion • Sweating • Tetany • Slow, shallow respirations • Muscular weakness • Seizures

Clinical Manifestations

Clinical manifestations of hyperchloremia resemble those of hypernatremia, presenting like dehydration. Typically, symptoms will be tied to the underlying fluid volume association of hyperchloremia. Fluid volume deficit can have symptoms relating to dehydration: headache, thirst, poor skin turgor, decreased urine output, dry skin, and dry mucous membranes.

Linking Pathophysiology to Diagnosis and Treatment

Serum chemistry panel values will show high levels of chloride and may show high sodium levels as well. Arterial blood gases reveal metabolic acidosis or respiratory alkalosis. Elevated parathyroid hormone (PTH) can be found in hyperparathyroidism. The BUN:creatinine ratio will be elevated in water loss and dehydration. The medical care of the patient with hyperchloremia is focused on utilizing intravenous hypotonic fluids, lactated Ringer, sodium bicarbonate (in acid–base imbalances), and diuretic therapy with concurrent hypernatremia. Many providers opt to restrict both sodium and chloride in the diet to help correct the hyperchloremia and possible concurrent hypernatremia. Patient care should be centered on restricting chloride and sodium when appropriate, administering ordered intravenous fluids, and providing patient education on the etiology of hyperchloremia and how to prevent further episodes.

Hypochloremia

Etiology and Pathogenesis

Hypochloremia (an abnormally low concentration of chloride ions in the blood) is usually caused by a loss of GI secretions as a result of vomiting and/or diarrhea or nasogastric suctioning. Other etiologies of hypochloremia may include an elevated bicarbonate level, as in alkalosis, burns, or, on rare occasions, decreased consumption of dietary sources of chloride. Although hypochloremia can occur as a lone process, that is rare.

Chloride usually decreases in response to volume depletions (with and without sodium depletion). Usually, the kidney will attempt to retain more sodium and bicarbonate ions to restore chloride balance. Ultimately, this process will lead to metabolic alkalosis as a result of the relative increase in serum pH. The administration of diuretics can result in hypochloremia through effects on fluid volume, as can the administration of certain hormones particularly steroidal therapies due to their influence on fluid balance and movement.

Clinical Manifestations

The clinical manifestations of hypochloremia resemble those of hyponatremia in some respects. Acute fluid volume excess associated with dilutional hypochloremia can lead to cerebral edema with altered mental status, confusion, and convulsions. Other symptoms may include headache, weakness, nausea, tetany, weight gain, and, in some cases, increased urine output.

Linking Pathophysiology to Diagnosis and Treatment

Serum chemistry will show low chloride levels, and many patients with hypochloremia have low sodium levels as well. An elevated BUN:creatinine ratio will possibly occur with GI losses and burns. Arterial blood gases can reveal metabolic alkalosis. Other laboratory studies can be completed if the underlying etiology is unclear.

Depending on the etiology, the treatment plan can consist of isotonic saline or hypertonic saline as well as replacement with oral sodium chloride. Changing the patient from a loop diuretic therapy to another class of drugs may be beneficial in preventing further hypochloremia. Recall that loop diuretics act on the ascending portion of the loop of Henle, which prevents sodium, potassium, and chloride resorption, therefore contributing to hypochloremia.

CLINICAL POINT: Ammonium chloride can be given to a patient with metabolic acidosis. However, this medication should be avoided for patients with hepatic or renal impairment. ■

If intravenous fluid therapy is initiated, monitoring of fluid intake and output along with daily weight measurement is important to assess fluid volume status. Serum electrolyte levels should be monitored periodically to ensure adequate replacement. The nurse should educate the patient about chloride-rich foods such as tomato juice, bananas, dates, eggs, cheese, milk, salty broth, canned vegetables, and processed meals. Further education such be given to the patient if pharmacologic therapy is being altered away from the use of loop diuretics.

Check Your Progress: Section 8.4

1. Sodium is considered the primary ECF cation. What is the primary ECF anion?
2. List three causes of hypochloremia.
3. List three functions of chloride.
4. How does the use of loop diuretics contribute to the onset of hypochloremia?

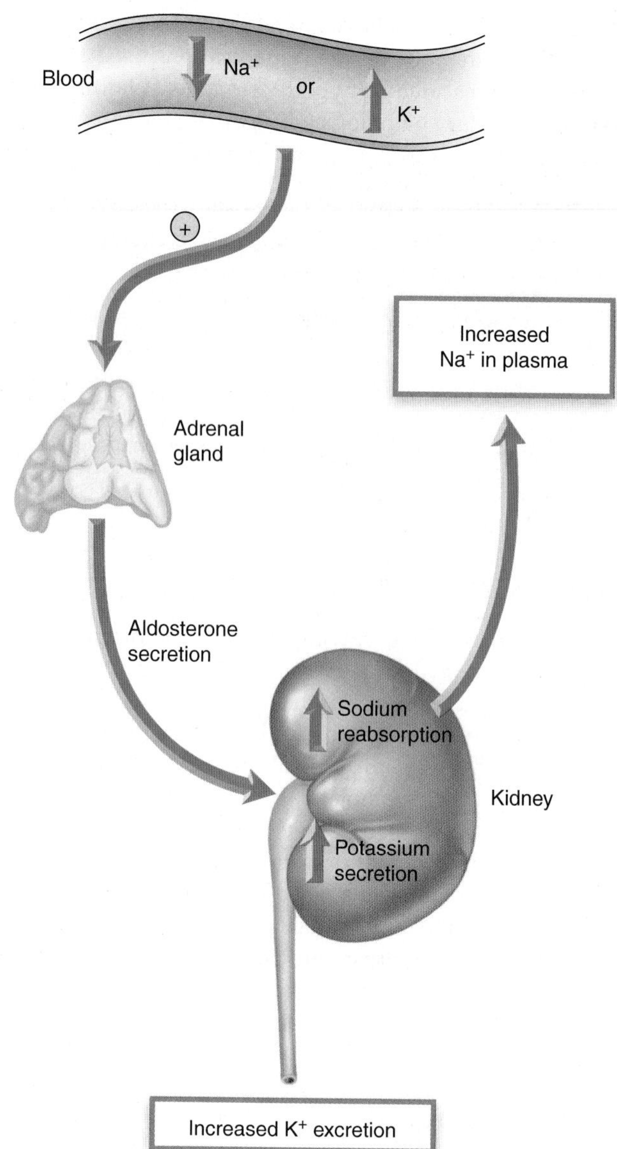

Figure 8.11 ■ Renal regulation of sodium and potassium balance.

8.5 Potassium Imbalances

Potassium is the predominant ICF ion with a normal level between 3.5 and 5.0 mEq/L. Potassium regulates ICF osmolality and is involved in maintaining the resting membrane potential. It is also an essential component in the Na^+/K^+ pump, is exchanged for H^+ as part of the buffering mechanism to maintain blood pH, and facilitates glycogen storage in liver and skeletal muscle cells (**Figure 8.11** ■). Potassium contributes to osmotic pressure in the ICF, and any imbalance requires prompt medical attention as it can quickly result in lethal clinical manifestations.[7,19] Signs and symptoms of potassium imbalances are listed in **Table 8.5** ■.

Hyperkalemia

Hyperkalemia is an abnormally high plasma concentration of potassium ions. ECF potassium concentrations

Table 8.5 Signs and Symptoms of Potassium Imbalances

Hyperkalemia	Hypokalemia
• ECG changes: peaked T waves, prolonged PR interval, absent P wave with widened QRS complex • Bradycardia • Heart blocks • Cardiac arrest • Anxiety • Tingling • Numbness • Muscle weakness • Renal failure • Nausea • Vomiting • Diarrhea • Abdominal pain	• ECG changes: flattened T waves, presence of U waves, ST segment depression, prolonged QT interval • Weak/thready pulses • Ventricular fibrillation • Cardiac arrest • Orthostatic hypotension • Lethargy • Fatigue • Confusion • Paresthesias • Decreased deep tendon reflexes • Nausea • Vomiting • Abdominal distention • Ileus • Renal failure • Weakness • Respiratory arrest • Bladder dysfunction

above 5.5 mEq/L constitute hyperkalemia. Hyperkalemia can stress the cardiovascular system, leading to lethal arrhythmias and a multitude of other pathologic consequences.[7,19]

Etiology and Pathogenesis

Common causes of hyperkalemia include oversupplementation, renal failure resulting in decreased excretion, tissue trauma and breakdown, hypoxia, acidosis, and insulin deficiency. Each of these situations results in the movement of potassium from ICF to the ECF, resulting in a change in cellular membrane permeability.

Endocrine abnormalities such as hypoaldosteronism, as in the case of Addison disease, or the effects from medications such as potassium-sparing diuretics (spironolactone) are also contributing factors. A gradual change occurs in the body's ability to adjust to increased potassium levels. In hypoaldosteronism, the adrenal cortex fails to secrete adequate amounts of aldosterone, which ultimately causes decreased renal excretion of potassium, leading to excessive accumulations of potassium in the serum. Other manifestations of hypoaldosteronism can be hyponatremia due to insufficient retention from the kidneys and ultimately hypotension from poor fluid retention.[7,19]

Disorders that contribute to a change in membrane permeability include burns, massive crush injuries, and trauma. In a state of hypoxia, the elevated H^+ replaces ICF potassium, resulting in hyperkalemia.

Heather Manuel: Application

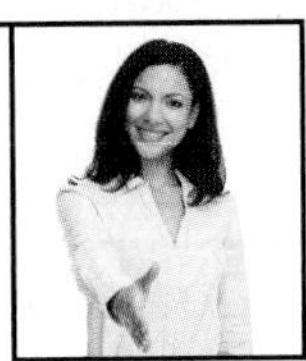

Ms. Manuel presented this morning at the emergency department, confused and lethargic. She has symptoms of nausea, vomiting, weakness, tingling in the fingers, and muscle twitching. Vital signs and signs are pulse 103, respirations 24, temperature 99.0°F, blood pressure 180/110, SpO_2 94%. The ECG reveals sinus tachycardia and tall, peaked T waves. Her deep tendon reflexes are hyperactive.

3. What is the significance of the ECG changes experienced by Ms. Manuel?
4. Nausea and vomiting are risk factors for what electrolyte imbalance?

Clinical Manifestations

Symptoms of hyperkalemia vary; muscle weakness, paralysis, and dysrhythmias are common manifestations. CNS effects such as neuromuscular irritability may occur and may progress to the extreme state of paralysis. The symptom severity is proportional to the degree of hyperkalemia and rate of potassium increase in the ECF. Various additional clinical situations may also further exacerbate hyperkalemia.[20]

Serum levels of potassium will be greater than 5 mEq/L. In heart failure and/or renal failure, elevated BNP, BUN, and creatinine levels are likely to coincide with the elevated potassium level. Hypoaldosteronism will likely have a decreased serum cortisol level accompanying the elevated serum potassium level. An electrocardiogram can show tachycardia, bradycardia, tall or peaked T waves, ST segment depression, widened QRS, and, in severe cases, cardiac arrest.[20]

Linking Pathophysiology to Diagnosis and Treatment

Typically, patients with hyperkalemia are given sodium polystyrene sulfonate to help reduce the serum potassium by enhancing GI loss through increased stool excretion. Hemodialysis may be necessary in patients with severe hyperkalemia to avoid lethal cardiac arrhythmias. It may be necessary to switch diuretics if the patient is taking a potassium-sparing diuretic such as spironolactone.[20]

Intravenous calcium gluconate can be given to counteract the lethal cardiac effects of hyperkalemia and should be used promptly with impending or current arrhythmias. Intravenous sodium bicarbonate can be used with corresponding metabolic acidosis. Hypertonic dextrose solution such as a D50% intravenous push followed by regular insulin can temporarily reduce the serum potassium level. This mechanism uses the extra blood sugar and insulin available to force the excess potassium available into the intracellular matrix. Ultimately, the sodium–potassium pump will restore the intracellular balance and force the potassium out of the cell back into the ECF; however, this treatment will give the clinician extra time to treat the patient with other methods and avoid potential arrhythmias. Loop diuretics such as furosemide (Lasix) can be administered to help inhibit resorption of sodium, potassium, and chloride, which in turn facilitates the excretion of these electrolytes and excess fluid in disease processes such as heart failure and renal failure.[20]

Intake and output management for patients with heart, hepatic, or renal failure is imperative to assess the functioning of these filtration systems. Observation for signs of muscle weakness can indicate worsening hyperkalemia or development of other electrolyte abnormalities. Dietary potassium should be limited in patients who are currently receiving therapy for hyperkalemia and patients who are at risk for hyperkalemia. Dietary education should be aimed at limiting or avoid foods that are high in potassium such as avocados, bananas, green leafy vegetables, yams, yogurt, white beans, squash, apricots, and mushrooms. Patients who are receiving dialysis must be encouraged to adhere to their dialysis schedule and not miss treatments.

Heather Manuel: Outcome

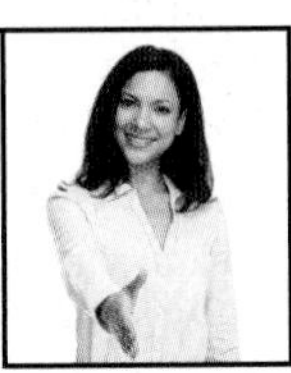

The recurrent malfunction of Ms. Manuel's AV fistula site most likely has led to a situation of inadequate hemodialysis. Her symptoms and examination indicate hyperkalemia, hypocalcemia, metabolic acidosis, and uremia, which will be confirmed with serum studies showing high potassium, BUN, and creatinine levels and a low calcium level. Arterial blood gases demonstrate metabolic acidosis from the lack of filtration of waste products from the renal insufficiency. A temporary hemodialysis catheter is placed in the jugular vein to provide emergent hemodialysis. Ms. Manuel is referred to a surgical specialist for revision of the fistula.

5. Why are the serum levels of BUN and creatinine increased in patients with chronic renal disease?
6. Low calcium levels and hyperkalemia are electrolyte imbalances associated with what disorder?

Hypokalemia

Hypokalemia (abnormally low concentration of potassium ions in the blood) can be just as lethal as hyperkalemia because of the potential cardiac arrhythmias. Hypokalemia occurs when the serum K^+ concentration is less than 3.5 mEq/L.

Etiology and Pathogenesis

A potential cause of hypokalemia is a decreased potassium intake; other etiologies include GI loss through suctioning, incomplete potassium replacement, and excessive use of laxatives. Other causes of hypokalemia include fluid overload, effects from medications such as loop diuretics causing excessive renal excretion, and hyperaldosteronism (Cushing disease). The regulation of pH or clinical situations that result in the shift of potassium into the ICF, such as respiratory alkalosis or the administration of insulin, may contribute to hypokalemia. In the context of hyperaldosteronism, excessive aldosterone is secreted by the adrenal cortex, ultimately leading to excessive renal excretion of potassium and other issues such as hypertension and excessive sodium retention.

Clinical Manifestations

In hypokalemia, serum potassium will be low, typically under 3.5 mEq/L. In Cushing disease, elevated blood sugar and elevated serum cortisol may be present if assessed. In GI losses, the serum results may reflect dehydration. In heart or renal failure, elevated BNP, BUN, and creatinine levels may accompany hypokalemia. Electrocardiographic findings can include flattened T wave, U wave development, and cardiac arrest in severe cases (< 2 mEq/L).

Linking Pathophysiology to Diagnosis and Treatment

Treatment of hypokalemia is typically aimed at correcting the underlying pathophysiology and administering acute or chronic supplementation for selected patients. Oral potassium supplements can be prescribed for patients with slight hypokalemia or poor dietary intake, and intravenous potassium supplements may be prescribed for patients with significant hypokalemia and those who cannot take oral supplementation. Corresponding hypotension should be corrected promptly. If the patient is taking a loop or thiazide type diuretic and cannot take oral potassium supplements, switching to a potassium-sparing diuretic such as spironolactone may be considered.[20]

Monitoring for cardiac arrhythmias should occur before adequate supplementation; on initial supplementation, patients will likely be admitted to the ICU or a telemetry setting for monitoring of cardiovascular function, primarily through continuous electrocardiography. The intravenous access site should be monitored for burning and pain; potassium is irritating to the tissues around the intravenous access point and can cause infiltration and discomfort. Patients receiving digoxin should be monitored for signs and symptoms of digoxin toxicity, since hypokalemia can potentiate the effects of digoxin. Dietary education should be focused on increasing intake of foods that are high in potassium such as fruit juices, bananas, melons, citrus fruits, vegetables, lean meats, milk, and whole grains. Ensure that patients who are receiving diuretic therapy with thiazide type or loop diuretics have adequate supplementation to counteract potassium loss. Ensure that the patient has an adequately functioning genitourinary system. If the patient has minimal urinary output, potassium supplementation can lead to hyperkalemia.[20]

Children are at great risk of hypokalemia when they experience excessive vomiting and diarrhea. The usual cause is loss of potassium along with fluid volume. Careful potassium replacement is needed to avoid overreplacement and hyperkalemia. ■

Like hyponatremia, hypokalemia can occur from diuretic use in adults. Older adults are at greater risk of hypokalemia as a result of alterations in nutrition and renal function. Typically, older adult patients are treated with acute and/or chronic potassium supplementation to counteract iatrogenic or physiologic hypokalemia. Potassium replacement should be monitored carefully because of the relative risk of overreplacement in older adults with renal disease. Patients with renal disease can have decreased clearance of potassium, leading to hyperkalemia. Renal disease is the most common cause of hyperkalemia in older adults. ■

Check Your Progress: Section 8.5

1. Why is hypoaldosteronism a risk factor for hyperkalemia?
2. Hypokalemia affects membrane excitability, particularly cardiac excitation. How does hypokalemia affect cardiac rhythm?
3. Older patients are most likely to be at risk for decreased or increased potassium levels. Explain why.

8.6 Calcium Imbalances

Calcium is a cation that exists in the body in an active form as ionized calcium and as a protein-bound molecule (40%). While serum calcium concentrations are rigidly controlled between 9.0 and 10.5 mg/dL, the majority of calcium is found in the bone and a fraction in the blood (40–50% bound to albumin). The form of calcium that had the most significant physiologic effect is the ionized, or free, calcium.[21]

Calcium is found primarily in bones and teeth, and it is essential for coagulation, muscular contraction of certain types of muscle, and cellular electrophysiology and membrane potential, and it acts as a second messenger in hormonal and neurotransmitter pathways. The normal calcium level in the blood ranges between 8.5 and 10.5 mg/dL. The level of serum calcium affects the function of other electrolytes, such as phosphate and sodium, and its cellular function varies depending on these levels. Signs and symptoms of calcium imbalances are listed in **Table 8.6** ■.

Hypercalcemia

Etiology and Pathogenesis

Hypercalcemia is an abnormally high plasma concentration of calcium ions. Common causes of hypercalcemia include malignancy, hyperparathyroidism that increases PTH levels, immobilization (leading to excessive bone loss), thiazide diuretics, thyrotoxicosis, and excessive ingestion of calcium and/or vitamin D. In the context of hyperparathyroidism, excessive amounts of parathyroid hormone are produced, which causes increased calcium release from bones and also enhances kidney resorption of calcium, thus increasing serum calcium levels by multiple mechanisms. Free or ionized calcium levels increase in acidotic states, whereas alkalosis contributes to increased protein binding, thereby lowering ionized calcium levels.[22,23]

Clinical Manifestations

Calcium imbalances in the body can lead to a variety of pathologic consequences. Cardiac, musculoskeletal, and neuromuscular effects are most commonly associated with increased morbidity and mortality. Hypercalcemia may decrease the action of sodium in skeletal muscles, resulting in decreased excitability of muscles and nerves. This occurs through blockage of sodium channels by calcium leading to effects on muscle and nerve depolarization. Clinical symptoms include fatigue, weakness, lethargy, and possibly nausea. Hypercalcemia is also associated with decreased phosphate levels due to hyperparathyroidism.[22,23]

Linking Pathophysiology to Diagnosis and Treatment

Elevated serum calcium levels will be found on serum studies. An elevated parathyroid hormone level can be found in hyperparathyroidism or renal failure. Vitamin D levels can be elevated in oversupplementation or misdiagnosis of vitamin D deficiency. TSH, T3, and T4 should be evaluated to determine whether hyperthyroidism is a factor in the patient's hypercalcemia. Electrocardiographic findings can include a shortened QT interval, a shortened ST segment, or various tachyarrhythmias.[24]

Table 8.6 Signs and Symptoms of Calcium Imbalances

Hypercalcemia	Hypocalcemia
• Serum calcium level > 5.5 mEq/L)	• Serum calcium level < 4.5 mEq/L)
• Increased thirst	• Numbness and tingling
• Increased urine output	• Muscle cramping
• Anorexia	• Hyperactive reflexes
• Nausea and vomiting	• Tetany
• Constipation	• Laryngeal spasms
• Muscle weakness	• Positive Chvostek sign
• Increased BP	• Positive Trousseau sign
• AV block	• Decreased BP
• Lethargy	• Ventricular dysrhythmias
• Coma	• Bone pain, fractures

In patients with either hyperparathyroidism and/or hypercalcemic crisis (a serum calcium level greater than 17 mg/dL) treatment with intramuscular calcitonin is warranted. Calcitonin will reduce serum calcium by increasing the deposition of calcium and phosphorus into bones as well as enhancing urinary excretion of calcium. This is particularly useful in heart failure and renal failure to avoid calcification of soft tissues. In most patients, the use of intravenous fluids both assists in diluting serum calcium and enhancing renal excretion. Loop diuretics such as furosemide (Lasix) are also helpful in facilitating renal excretion of calcium. Administration of intravenous phosphorus can help to cause a reciprocal reduction in serum calcium. However, this must be done with extreme caution because of the possibility of causing hypocalcemia and/or calcification of susceptible tissues. Oral bisphosphonates can be used to inhibit osteoclast activity and prevent further bone breakdown in the etiologies of hyperparathyroidism and certain cancers. Corticosteroids can also be of use to decrease bone turnover in the same pathologies. Consider reevaluation of vitamin D deficiency and selected therapy if the patient is receiving vitamin D supplementation.[24]

Hypocalcemia

Etiology and Pathogenesis

Hypocalcemia (abnormally low concentration of chloride ions in the blood) is particularly common in patients with renal failure as a result of several mechanisms discussed earlier in the chapter. **Figure 8.12** ■ shows a depiction of the human body's normal physiologic mechanisms to balance

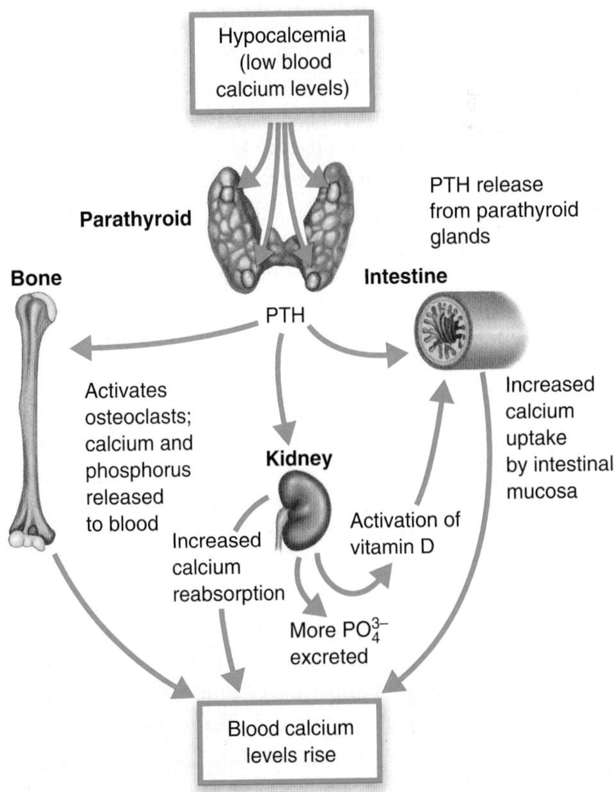

Figure 8.12 ■ Normal physiologic mechanisms of the body that restore homeostasis to the balance of serum calcium.

serum calcium. If any one of these mechanisms breaks down, hypocalcemia can ensue. Other causes include parathyroid gland removal, hypoparathyroidism, hypomagnesemia, hyperphosphatemia, hypoalbuminemia, vitamin D deficiency, pancreatitis, alkalosis, and side effects of medications such as loop diuretics. Interventions such as blood transfusion may cause hypocalcemia.

Clinical Manifestations

Marked CNS and neuromuscular excitability are major implications of hypocalcemia. Tingling, spasms, tetany, and possibly convulsions in extreme hypocalcemia may occur. Two clinical signs of neuromuscular excitability are the Chvostek sign and Trousseau sign. Tapping on the facial nerve below the temple can elicit a twitch or spasm of the nose or lip on the ipsilateral side of tapping; this action is known as the **Chvostek sign**. The **Trousseau sign** can be elicited by occluding the arterial blood flow of the arm for 5 minutes, eventually causing a contraction of the arm and hand. This is typically done with a blood pressure cuff.

Other clinical manifestations of hypocalcemia are ECG changes (such as prolonged QT interval leading to ventricular arrhythmias and cardiac arrest), tetany (manifesting as laryngospasm), intestinal cramping, hyperactive bowel sounds, and osteoporosis with or without pathologic fractures.[24]

Linking Pathophysiology to Diagnosis and Treatment

In the serum, total and ionized calcium levels will be decreased. In hypoparathyroidism or parathyroid gland removal, low to undetectable levels can be found on laboratory studies. Corresponding hypomagnesemia and hyperphosphatemia can occur as well. Amylase and lipase levels can be elevated with a pancreatitis etiology.

In severe hypocalcemia, utilization of intravenous calcium salts such as calcium gluconate and calcium chloride to replace serum calcium is required. Vitamin D supplementation should occur in vitamin D deficiency. Vitamin D enhances calcium absorption from the GI tract. Dietary management is required for a host of reasons, including increasing intake of calcium-containing foods and decreasing intake of phosphorus-containing food. Avoiding the use of isotonic saline is optimal, since isotonic saline can enhance renal secretion of calcium. Treatment of hypoparathyroidism starts with vitamin D and calcium supplementations. Phosphate-binding agents such as sevelamer may be required to reduce serum phosphorus in patients with chronic renal failure.[24]

Patients need dietary education to increase calcium-containing foods such as dairy products, green leafy vegetables, canned salmon, sardines, and fresh oysters. The nurse should encourage patients to adhere to vitamin D supplementation, which helps to enhance absorption of calcium through the GI tract. Decreasing intake of phosphorus-containing food may be required to sustain adequate levels of serum calcium. Education should be given about avoiding excessive alcohol and caffeine intake. Excessive intake of either substance can inhibit calcium absorption. Excessive smoking can increase urinary calcium excretion, further worsening hypocalcemia. Teach the patient to avoid excessive use of phosphorus-containing laxatives, which can decrease calcium absorption and/or decrease the serum calcium level. It is important to note that rapid infusion of calcium salts can cause cardiac arrest or bradycardia and can potentiate the effects of digoxin, leading to digoxin toxicity. Calcium salts should be diluted for administration. Seizure precautions should be initiated in severe cases of hypocalcemia. Weight-bearing exercises can be considered to decrease bone calcium loss.

Hypocalcemia has similar pathophysiologic mechanisms and symptomatology in children and adults; however, the signs and symptoms are more profound in children. Neuromuscular excitability and laryngeal spasm are far more serious in children and can happen much more easily. Weakness and confusion may occur very shortly after the calcium builds up to the threshold of hypercalcemia in the younger patient. ■

Hypocalcemia is common in older adults with renal disease. Renal disease can lead to decreased clearance of phosphate in the serum, which directly opposes serum calcium concentrations. Decreased PTH production can lead to decreased levels of serum calcium as well, through excess bone resorption of calcium. Hypercalcemia is rarer; however, when it occurs, it can signify a significant disease process such as bone metastasis. ■

Check Your Progress: Section 8.6

1. List three risk factors for hypercalcemia.
2. A positive Trousseau sign is an assessment for what electrolyte disorder?
3. Hypocalcemia in an older adult with chronic renal failure is a risk factor for what disorder?

8.7 Phosphorus Imbalances

Phosphorus is a naturally occurring element in the human body that plays a role in bone formation. The normal range for phosphorus is between 2.5 and 4.5 mg/dL. Phosphate acts as a buffer in acid–base regulation; is a component in bone and ATP formation and thereby provides energy for muscle contraction; is involved in glucose, fat, and protein metabolism in DNA, RNA, and phospholipids; and, as part of PTH regulation, maintains control of calcium and phosphate concentrations and vitamin D regulation. In addition, phosphorus is involved in red blood cell, white blood cell, and platelet function.[25–27] Signs and symptoms of phosphorus imbalances are listed in **Table 8.7** ■.

Hyperphosphatemia

Etiology and Pathogenesis

Hyperphosphatemia is an abnormally high concentration of phosphate ions in the blood. The most common etiology of hyperphosphatemia in both primary and acute care is chronic renal failure. Other causes of hyperphosphatemia

Table 8.7 Signs and Symptoms of Phosphorus Imbalances

Hyperphosphatemia	Hypophosphatemia
• Serum phosphate level > 4.5 mg/dL (> 2.6 mEq/dL) • Paresthesias • Muscle weakness • Nausea and vomiting • Dysphagia • Tetany • Decreased blood pressure • Cardiac dysrhythmias	• Serum phosphate level < 2.5 mg/dL (< 1.7 mEq/L) • Intention tremor, paresthesias • Confusion, stupor • Bone pain • Joint stiffness • Bleed disorders (platelet dysfunction) • Impaired white blood cell function • Seizures

include respiratory acidosis, metabolic acidosis, hypocalcemia (coincides hyperphosphatemia in chronic renal failure), vitamin D excess, and chemotherapy (hyperphosphatemia from tumor lysis). Calcium has an inverse relationship with phosphorus. In hyperphosphatemia, hypocalcemia can be a common associated finding. In renal failure, decreased renal function causes an elevated serum phosphorus, which in turn causes a reciprocal drop in serum calcium. Osteopenia and/or osteoporosis and pathologic fractures ensue.[25–27]

Clinical Manifestations

The symptoms of hyperphosphatemia typically correlate with those of hypocalcemia. Tingling, spasms, tetany, and possibly convulsions in extreme hyperphosphatemia may occur, mainly as a result of the development of hypocalcemia from the etiology of hyperphosphatemia. Both the Chvostek sign and Trousseau sign can be elicited. Decreased blood pressure and cardiac arrhythmias can occur in extreme cases.

Linking Pathophysiology to Diagnosis and Treatment

A key indicator is an elevated phosphorus level in blood chemistry studies. Patients with chronic renal failure will have corresponding elevated BUN and creatinine levels as well as elevated PTH and decreased calcium levels. Arterial blood gases can show metabolic acidosis or respiratory acidosis.

Most healthcare providers suggest restriction of dietary phosphate, with the goal of decreasing serum phosphate levels over time. Vitamin D preparations such as calcitriol (intramuscular and intravenous) can be given to increase the calcium absorbed through the GI tract, which in turn causes a reciprocal drop in serum phosphorus. Other treatment modalities include phosphate-binding agents such as sevelamer, and aluminum hydroxide or loop diuretic therapy can enhance renal excretion of phosphorus. In selected patients, isotonic saline can be of benefit to increase volume; this can help renal excretion purely as a result of the increased volume to be excreted. In profound hyperphosphatemia, hemodialysis may be indicated if not already in use.

Hypophosphatemia

Etiology and Pathogenesis

Typical causes of **hypophosphatemia** (an abnormally low concentration of phosphate ions in the blood) include malnutrition, alcohol withdrawal, heat stroke, respiratory alkalosis, hepatic encephalopathy, major burns, hyperparathyroidism, chronic diarrhea, and vitamin D deficiency. In hyperparathyroidism, excessive parathyroid hormone is produced and released, causing an enhancement of calcium release from the bones, thus causing a reciprocal drop in serum phosphate.[25–27]

Clinical Manifestations

Clinical manifestations of hypophosphatemia correlate with those of hypercalcemia. Extreme symptoms include red blood cell and platelet dysfunction, neuromuscular dysfunction, altered mental status, convulsions, excessive bone resorption, and possible respiratory failure.

Linking Pathophysiology to Diagnosis and Treatment

Decreased serum phosphorus will be found on serum chemistry. In malnutrition, the patient can be cachectic and have low serum albumin and prealbumin levels. Arterial blood gases can show respiratory alkalosis. Elevation in liver enzymes and serum ammonia can occur in hepatic encephalopathy. Elevated PTH hormone levels can be found in hyperparathyroidism.

Mild to moderate hypophosphatemia can usually be corrected with oral phosphorus, along with an increase in phosphorus-containing food. Severe cases of hypophosphatemia (serum level less than 1 mg/dL and no GI function) are dangerous and need prompt correction with IV phosphorus. Like treating hyponatremia with hypertonic saline, administration with intravenous phosphorus needs to be managed with caution. Rapid infusion of intravenous phosphorus can cause overreplacement, which can result in a dangerous reciprocal drop in serum calcium. Assessment of a patient with hypocalcemia can show tetany and calcification of sensitive tissues (blood vessels, heart, lung, kidneys, and eyes). Dietary education should include increasing consumption of food such as pumpkin seeds, squash seeds, cheeses, salmon, shellfish, Brazil nuts, pork, beef, low-fat dairy, tofu, beans, and lentils.

Check Your Progress: Section 8.7

1. Explain how vitamin D supplementation can affect the plasma phosphate level.
2. Hypophosphatemia can be linked to nutritional imbalance and consumption of what?
3. What electrolyte is concurrently affected by hyperphosphatemia?

8.8 Magnesium Imbalances

Magnesium is a major intracellular cation and is principally regulated by PTH. A normal magnesium level is between 1.3 and 2.1 mg/dL. Magnesium is a cofactor in enzymatic reactions, and it has a role in ATP generation, DNA replication, and mRNA production and translation. Magnesium also prevents potassium from exiting from the cardiac cells and is a smooth muscle relaxant. An important function of magnesium in the body includes neuromuscular integrity.[22,23,28] Signs and symptoms of magnesium imbalances are listed in **Table 8.8**.

Table 8.8 Signs and Symptoms of Magnesium Imbalances

Hypermagnesemia	Hypomagnesemia
• Serum magnesium level > 3.0 mg/dL (> 2.5 mEq/L) • Confusion and lethargy • Hypotension • Cardiac dysrhythmias • Coma • Cardiac arrest	• Serum magnesium level < 1.8 mg/dL (< 1.5 mEq/L) • Personality changes • Nystagmus • Positive Chvostek and Trousseau signs • Hypertension • Tachycardia • Cardiac dysrhythmias

Hypermagnesemia

Etiology and Pathogenesis

Hypermagnesemia (an abnormally high concentration of magnesium ions in the blood) is relatively rare, but when observed clinically, it often results from renal failure and is more pronounced if magnesium-containing antacids are consumed. The use of laxatives may contribute to hypermagnesemia, as can increased dietary intake, diabetic ketoacidosis, lithium toxicity, burns, trauma, and shock. A common iatrogenic cause of hypermagnesemia is an overreplacement with supplements or overuse of magnesium-containing laxatives, which can be exacerbated in patients with renal failure.[22,23,28]

Clinical Manifestations

Serum levels of magnesium will be elevated. Patients with renal failure may also have increased BUN and creatinine levels along with other electrolyte disturbances. The true danger with hypermagnesemia relates to the cardiovascular system. An electrocardiogram can reveal several disturbing findings: bradyarrhythmias, tall T wave, widened QRS, prolonged QT interval, atrioventricular blocks, and finally cardiac arrest.

Linking Pathophysiology to Diagnosis and Treatment

The first step in treatment of hypermagnesemia is stopping all medications that contain magnesium and finding alternative medications in order to prevent further elevation of serum magnesium levels. In severe cases, mechanical ventilation or other ventilator support may be needed if the patient is in respiratory depression. Intravenous calcium gluconate can be administered to reverse neuromuscular symptoms. Emergency hemodialysis may be warranted for patients with severe symptoms. Loop diuretics with either sodium chloride or lactated Ringer will help to promote excretion of magnesium in patients with adequate renal function.

Hypotension, shallow respirations, decreased deep tendon reflexes, and decreased level of consciousness can be signs of hypermagnesemia. Nutritional education should aim at decreasing magnesium intake by avoiding foods such as beans, nuts, whole grains, and green leafy vegetables, especially in renal insufficiency because of the increased risk they pose. Patients who use or overuse magnesium-containing laxatives should be counseled on their appropriate use. Alternative treatment may be needed to avoid further instances of hypermagnesemia.

Hypomagnesemia

Etiology and Pathogenesis

Hypomagnesemia is an abnormally low concentration of magnesium ions in the blood. Causes of hypomagnesemia include hypocalcemia, hypokalemia, decreased albumin level, decreased dietary intake, decreased absorption in the small intestine, GI losses, acute pancreatitis, starvation, diuretic therapy, and diabetic ketoacidosis. The most common cause is excessive alcohol intake. Hypomagnesemia in patients who abuse alcohol is typically due to malabsorption.[22,23,28]

Clinical Manifestations

The level of serum magnesium will be decreased in hypomagnesemia. Similar to the clinical concerns that result from hypermagnesemia, the cardiovascular sequelae are most worrisome and may affect mortality. An electrocardiogram will reveal premature ventricular contractions, ventricular tachycardia, ventricular fibrillation, and torsades de pointes. Other manifestations include changes in mental status and personality along with nystagmus and hypertension.[22,23,28]

Linking Pathophysiology to Diagnosis and Treatment

Diet management alone can usually correct mild hypomagnesemia by increasing foods with a magnesium content. Moderate cases of hypomagnesemia can be managed with dietary magnesium and/or oral magnesium oxide or magnesium gluconate. Severe hypomagnesemia is usually managed initially with intravenous magnesium sulfate and usually oral magnesium oxide if the underlying cause cannot be fully corrected. Intravenous replacement of magnesium is usually required in parenteral nutrition.

Magnesium replacement can cause diarrhea (some magnesium salts are the basis for endoscopy preps and laxatives), so assessment of fluid volume status is imperative for ensuring that the patient is hemodynamically stable. Ensure slow administration of intravenous magnesium to avoid cardiac arrhythmias or conduction abnormalities such as heart blockade or asystole. Calcium gluconate can be given to treat hypermagnesemia stemming from overreplacement and/or rapid replacement. Dietary management includes foods that are high in magnesium such as green leafy vegetables, nuts, seeds, legumes, whole grains, seafood, peanut butter, and cocoa. Monitoring patients for excessive alcohol use is important, since patients who drink a lot of alcohol can be at high risk for hypomagnesemia. Serum magnesium should be periodically monitored to ensure adequate replacement. Seizure precautions should be implemented in severe cases of hypomagnesemia.

CLINICAL POINT: Magnesium has sedating effects on the various systems of the body. Hypermagnesemia produces respiratory depression, decreased deep tendon reflexes, decreased level of consciousness, bradyarrhythmias, and hypotension. Hypomagnesemia causes the opposite symptoms: increased deep tendon reflexes, hypertension, and tachyarrhythmias. ■

Hypomagnesemia may coincide with chronic alcoholism in older adults. It would be wise to complete a screening for alcohol abuse on patients who are suspected of hypomagnesemia secondary to chronic alcoholism. It is also important to note that hypermagnesemia is common in renal failure and magnesium-containing laxative abuse. Many older adults frequently use over-the-counter laxatives, many of which contain magnesium. ■

Check Your Progress: Section 8.8

1. List three risk factors for hypermagnesemia.
2. How would you generally classify the impact of hypomagnesemia on body functions?
3. How does the degree of alcohol use affect the magnesium plasma level?

CHAPTER SUMMARY

8.1 Chapter Overview and Case Studies

Describe the normal fluid and electrolyte balance, the results of inappropriate fluid and electrolyte imbalance, and concepts related to fluids and electrolytes.

- An electrolyte is any substance that dissociates into ions in water.
- The regulation of electrolytes is heavily dependent on renal function.
- Disruptions of fluid regulation influence electrolytes concentrations as well as cellular function.
- Cardiac output is heavily dependent on the amount of fluid in the body.
- Excessive amounts of fluid increase preload, or the amount of fluid the heart must contend with.
- A fluid deficit will require increases in heart rate to circulate the reduced volume effectively.

8.2 Composition and Distribution of Body Fluids

Outline the distribution, composition, movement, and regulation of body fluids and the regulation of electrolytes.

- Total body water can vary according to age and body mass index.
- Infants have a higher percentage of body water than adults.
- Fluid is contained in three compartments representing intracellular and extracellular fluids.
- Intracellular fluid represents the largest fluid space in the body.
- Extracellular fluid comprises three subdivisions: intravascular, interstitial, and transcellular.
- Intravascular fluid is composed of whole blood.
- Interstitial fluid represents fluid in tissue.
- Transcellular is fluid in spaces such as joints and cavities.
- Fluid moves through the body in accordance with the principles of osmosis, diffusion, and active transport.
- Osmolality refers to the concentration of solutes in fluid.

8.3 Water and Sodium Imbalances

Differentiate the causes, classification, underlying pathogenesis, and clinical manifestations of water and sodium imbalances and approaches to diagnosis and treatment of these conditions across the lifespan.

- Fluid imbalances related to volume are isotonic imbalances.
- An isotonic imbalance involves equal alterations in the sodium and water concentrations.
- Sodium is the main cation in the ECF.
- Normal ECF sodium concentrations are maintained between 135 and 145 mEq/L.
- Higher than normal levels of sodium are referred to as hypernatremia.
- Lower than normal levels of sodium are referred to as hyponatremia.
- Isotonic fluid volume excess typically occurs simultaneously with or after an increase in extracellular sodium levels.
- Renal sodium retention leads to an increased bodily sodium content with a subsequent increase in excess fluid volume in varying degrees.
- The clinical manifestations of isotonic fluid volume excess are weight gain, a decreased serum hematocrit, and decreased plasma protein from the dilutional effect of excess plasma. Assessment findings may reveal distended neck veins, increased blood pressure, and increased capillary hydrostatic pressure, contributing to the presence of edema.
- Treatment is aimed at restricting fluid intake and correcting the underlying etiology.

8.4 Chloride Imbalances

Differentiate the causes, classification, underlying pathogenesis, and clinical manifestations of chloride imbalances and approaches to diagnosis and treatment of these conditions across the lifespan.

- Chloride, a naturally occurring anion, is the primary ECF anion.
- Chloride is involved in the maintenance of ECF osmolality and acid–base regulation.

- Higher or lower than normal levels of chloride influence respiratory function and muscular strength.
- Hyperchloremia is an abnormally high plasma concentration of chloride ions.
- Clinical manifestations of hyperchloremia resemble those of hypernatremia.
- Hypochloremia (an abnormally low concentration of chloride ions in the blood) is usually caused by a loss of GI secretions from vomiting and/or diarrhea or nasogastric suctioning.

8.5 Potassium Imbalances

Differentiate the causes, classification, underlying pathogenesis, and clinical manifestations of potassium imbalances and approaches to diagnosis and treatment of these conditions across the lifespan.

- Potassium is the predominant ICF ion with a normal level between 3.5 and 5.0 mEq/L.
- Potassium regulates ICF osmolality and is involved in maintaining the resting membrane potential.
- Lower or higher than normal levels of potassium can have significant effects on cardiovascular function.
- Hyperkalemia is an abnormally high plasma concentration of potassium ions.
- Common causes of hyperkalemia include oversupplementation, renal failure resulting in decreased excretion, tissue trauma and breakdown, hypoxia, acidosis, and insulin deficiency.
- Hyperkalemia is typically treated with sodium polystyrene sulfonate to help reduce the serum potassium by enhancing gastrointestinal loss through increased stool excretion.
- Hypokalemia (abnormally low concentration of potassium ions in the blood) can be just as lethal as hyperkalemia to a patient, owing to the potential for cardiac arrhythmias.
- A potential cause of hypokalemia is a decreased potassium intake. Other etiologies include gastrointestinal loss through suctioning, incomplete potassium replacement, and excessive use of laxatives.
- The management of hypokalemia is typically aimed at correcting the underlying pathophysiology and administering acute or chronic supplementation in some patients.

8.6 Calcium Imbalances

Differentiate the causes, classification, underlying pathogenesis, and clinical manifestations of calcium imbalances and approaches to diagnosis and treatment of these conditions across the lifespan.

- Calcium is a cation that exists in the body in an active form as ionized calcium.
- Serum calcium concentrations are rigidly controlled between 9.0 and 10.5 mg/dL.
- Calcium is found primarily in the bones and teeth. It is essential for coagulation, muscular contraction of types of muscle, and cellular electrophysiology and membrane potential, and it acts as a second messenger in hormonal and neurotransmitter pathways.
- The normal calcium level in the blood ranges between 8.5 and 10.5 mg/dL. The level of serum calcium affects the function of other electrolytes.
- Hypercalcemia is an abnormally high plasma concentration of calcium ions.
- Calcium imbalances in the body can lead to a variety of pathologic consequences. Cardiac, musculoskeletal, and neuromuscular effects are most commonly associated with increased morbidity and mortality.
- Hypocalcemia (abnormally low concentration of chloride ions in the blood) is particularly common in renal failure.
- Marked central nervous system and neuromuscular excitability are major implications of hypocalcemia.

8.7 Phosphorus Imbalances

Differentiate the causes, classification, underlying pathogenesis, and clinical manifestations of phosphorus imbalances and approaches to diagnosis and treatment of these conditions across the lifespan.

- The normal range for phosphorus is between 2.5 and 4.5 mg/dL.
- Phosphate acts as a buffer in acid–base regulation, and it is a component in bone and ATP formation.
- Hyperphosphatemia is an abnormally high concentration of phosphate ions in the blood.
- The most common etiology of hyperphosphatemia in both primary and acute care is chronic renal failure.
- The symptoms of hyperphosphatemia typically correlate with those of hypocalcemia. Tingling, spasms, tetany, and possibly convulsions in extreme hypocalcemia may occur, mainly resulting from the development of hypocalcemia from the etiology of hyperphosphatemia.
- Typical causes of hypophosphatemia (an abnormally low concentration of phosphate ions in the blood) include malnutrition, alcohol withdrawal, heat stroke, respiratory alkalosis, hepatic encephalopathy, major burns, hyperparathyroidism, chronic diarrhea, and vitamin D deficiency.

8.8 Magnesium Imbalances

Differentiate the causes, classification, underlying pathogenesis, and clinical manifestations of magnesium imbalances and approaches to diagnosis and treatment of these conditions across the lifespan.

- Magnesium is a major intracellular cation.
- A normal magnesium level is between 1.3 and 2.1 mg/dL.

- Magnesium is a cofactor in enzymatic reactions, and it has a role in ATP generation, DNA replication, and mRNA production and translation.
- Magnesium prevents potassium from exiting from the cardiac cells and is a smooth muscle relaxant. Hypermagnesemia (an abnormally high concentration of magnesium ions in the blood) is relatively rare, but when observed clinically, it often results from renal failure and is more pronounced if magnesium-containing antacids are consumed.
- The true danger in hypermagnesemia relates to the cardiovascular system. An electrocardiogram can reveal several disturbing findings: bradyarrhythmias, tall T wave, widened QRS, prolonged QT interval, atrioventricular blocks, and finally cardiac arrest.
- Hypomagnesemia is an abnormally low concentration of magnesium ions in the blood.
- Causes of hypomagnesemia include hypocalcemia, hypokalemia, decreased albumin level, decreased dietary intake, decreased absorption in small intestine, GI losses, acute pancreatitis, starvation, diuretic therapy, and diabetic ketoacidosis.
- Similar to the clinical concerns that result from hypermagnesemia, the cardiovascular sequelae are most worrisome and may affect mortality.

REVIEW QUESTIONS

1. An elderly client is brought to the ER with a history of vomiting for 2 days. The client appeared confused and weak. The client is most likely experiencing:
   a. hypernatremia and fluid volume excess.
   b. hyponatremia and fluid volume excess.
   c. hyponatremia and fluid volume excess.
   d. hyponatremia and fluid volume deficit.
2. A nurse is reviewing a client's lab result values. The nurse should associate a serum sodium level of 158 mEq/L with which imbalance and clinical manifestation?
   a. Hyponatremia and hypotension
   b. Hypernatremia and increased thirst
   c. Hyperkalemia and weight gain
   d. Hypokalemia and peaked T wave
3. A client has a serum phosphate concentration of 1.8 mg/dL. Which assessment findings will the nurse expect to observe?
   a. Hypocalcemia
   b. Hyperactive bowel sounds
   c. Muscle weakness and numbness
   d. Peripheral edema
4. A nurse is caring for an older adult who is experiencing a fluid imbalance. Which age-related change should the nurse associate with fluid imbalance?
   a. Efficient temperature regulation
   b. Higher percentage of total body water than younger adults
   c. Decreased thirst perception
   d. Improved renal excretory function
5. A client is receiving intravenous infusion of magnesium sulfate for the prevention of seizures. What assessment finding would indicate to the nurse that the rate of infusion is too fast?
   a. Sunken eyeballs
   b. Hypomagnesemia
   c. Diminished deep tendon reflexes
   d. Dry mucosa and skin
6. Which of the following clients is at greatest risk for developing hypernatremia?
   a. A client with hypoaldosteronism
   b. A client with dehydration
   c. A client with vomiting
   d. A client with diuretic use
7. A 65-year-old male is diagnosed with electrolyte imbalance following diarrhea for 3 weeks. His personal history indicates that he is an alcoholic. Which signs and symptoms should the nurse expect?
   a. Positive Chvostek and hypercalcemia
   b. Oliguria with hyponatremia
   c. Muscle cramping and hypomagnesemia
   d. Tingling with hypophosphatemia
8. The family of a client with hypercalcemia expresses concern that the client is "not acting like himself." The nurse should do further assessment of:
   a. anxiety.
   b. carpal spasms.
   c. seizure activity.
   d. personality alteration.

ANSWERS

Answers to Review Questions can be found in Appendix A. Answers to Case Study and Check Your Progress questions are available on the faculty resources site. Please consult with your instructor.

RECOMMENDED WEBSITES

MedLinePlus: Fluid and Electrolyte Balance
https://medlineplus.gov/fluidandelectrolytebalance.html#cat51

Merck Manual: Electrolyte Disorders
http://www.merckmanuals.com/professional/endocrine-and-metabolic-disorders/electrolyte-disorders

New England Journal of Medicine: Disorders of Fluids and Electrolytes
http://www.nejm.org/page/fluids-and-electrolytes

Nurses Labs: Fluid and Electrolytes
https://nurseslabs.com/fluid-and-electrolytes

REFERENCES

1. Harring, T. R., Deal, N. S., & Kuo, D. C. (2014). Disorders of sodium and water balance. *Emergency Medicine Clinics of North America, 32*(2), 379–401. doi:10.1016/j.emc.2014.01.001
2. Martini, F. H., & Ober, W. C. (2015). *Visual anatomy & physiology* (2nd ed.). Boston, MA: Pearson.
3. Garrett, B. M. (2017). *Fluids and electrolytes: Essentials for nursing and healthcare practice*. Boca Raton, FL: CRC Press.
4. Danziger, J., & Zeidel, M. L. (2015). Osmotic homeostasis. *Clinical Journal of the American Society of Nephrology, 10*(5), 852–862. doi:10.2215/cjn.10741013
5. Kee, J. L. (2017). *Pearson handbook of laboratory and diagnostic tests with nursing* (8th ed.). Hoboken, NJ: Pearson.
6. Walker, M. D. (2016). Fluid and electrolyte imbalances: Interpretation and assessment. *Journal of Infusion Nursing, 39*(6), 382–386. doi:10.1097/NAN.0000000000000193
7. Pohl, H. R., Wheeler, J. S., & Murray, H. E. (2013). Sodium and potassium in health and disease. *Metal Ions in Life Sciences, 13*, 29–47. doi:10.1007/978-94-007-7500-8_2
8. Stearns, R. H. (2016). Clinical manifestations and diagnosis of edema in adults. *UpToDate.* Available at http://www.uptodate.com/contents/clinical-manifestations-and-diagnosis-of-edema-in-adults
9. Mayo Clinic. (2016). *Dehydration.* Available at http://www.mayoclinic.org/diseases-conditions/dehydration/symptoms-causes/dxc-20261072
10. Martini, F., Ober, C. E., Welch, K., & Hutchings, R. T. (2018). *Visual anatomy & physiology* (3rd ed.). New York, NY: Pearson.
11. Harrison, T. R., & Longo, D. L. (2013). *Harrison's manual of medicine* (18th ed.). New York, NY: McGraw-Hill Medical.
12. Agrawal, V., Agarwal, M., Joshi, S. R., & Ghosh, A. K. (2008). Hyponatremia and hypernatremia: Disorders of water balance. *Journal of the Association of Physicians of India, 56*, 956–964.
13. Lindner, G., & Funk, G. C. (2013). Hypernatremia in critically ill patients. *Journal of Critical Care, 28*(2), 216.e11-20. doi:10.1016/j.jcrc.2012.05.001
14. Morley, J. E. (2015). Dehydration, hypernatremia, and hyponatremia. *Clinics in Geriatric Medicine, 31*(3), 389–399. doi: 10.1016/j.cger.2015.04.007
15. Aditianingsih, D., & George, Y. W. (2014). Guiding principles of fluid and volume therapy: Best practice & research. *Clinical Anaesthesiology, 28*(3), 249–260. doi:10.1016/j.bpa.2014.07.002
16. Rahimi, Z., Moradi, M., & Nasri, H. (2014). A systematic review of the role of renin angiotensin aldosterone system genes in diabetes mellitus, diabetic retinopathy and diabetic neuropathy. *Journal of Research in Medical Sciences, 19*(11), 1–15.
17. Underwood, P. C., & Adler, G. K. (2013). The renin angiotensin aldosterone system and insulin resistance in humans. *Current Hypertension Reports, 15*(1), 59–70. doi:10.1007/s11906-012-0323-2
18. van der Jagt, M. (2016). Fluid management of the neurological patient: A concise review. *Critical Care (London, England), 20*(1), 126. doi:10.1186/s13054-016-1309-2
19. Suarez-Rivera, M., & Bonilla-Felix, M. (2014). Fluid and electrolyte disorders in the newborn: Sodium and potassium. *Current Pediatric Reviews, 10*(2), 115–122.
20. Ashurst, J., Sergent, S. R., & Sergent, B. R. (2016). Evidence-based management of potassium disorders in the emergency department. *Emergency Medicine Practice, 18*(11), 1–24.
21. Zofkova, I. (2016). Hypercalcemia: Pathophysiological aspects. *Physiological Research, 65*(1), 1–10.
22. Felsenfeld, A. J., Levine, B. S., & Rodriguez, M. (2015). Pathophysiology of calcium, phosphorus, and magnesium dysregulation in chronic kidney disease. *Seminars in Dialysis, 28*(6), 564–577. doi:10.1111/sdi.12411
23. Hoorn, E. J., & Zietse, R. (2013). Disorders of calcium and magnesium balance: A physiology-based approach. *Pediatric Nephrology, 28*(8), 1195–206. doi:10.1007/s00467-012-2350-2
24. Chang, W. T., Radin, B., & McCurdy, M. T. (2014). Calcium, magnesium, and phosphate abnormalities in the emergency department. *Emergency Medicine Clinics of North America, 32*(2), 349–366. doi:10.1016/j.emc.2013.12.006
25. Geddes, R. F., Finch, N. C., Syme, H. M., & Elliott, J. (2013). The role of phosphorus in the pathophysiology of chronic kidney disease. *Journal of Veterinary Emergency and Critical Care, 23*(2), 122–133. doi:10.1111/vec.12032
26. Huang, C. L., & Moe, O. W. (2013). Clinical assessment of phosphorus status, balance and renal handling in normal individuals and in patients with chronic kidney disease. *Current Opinion in Nephrology and Hypertension, 22*(4), 452–458. doi:10.1097/MNH.0b013e328362483a
27. Nadkarni, G. N., & Uribarri, J. (2014). Phosphorus and the kidney: What is known and what is needed. *Advances in Nutrition, 5*(1), 98–103. doi:10.3945/an.113.004655
28. Gonzalez, W., Altieri, P. I., Alvarado, S., et al. (2013). Magnesium: The forgotten electrolyte. *Boletin de la Asociacion Medica de Puerto Rico, 105*(3), 17–20.

Chapter 9
Acid–Base Imbalances

Diane Klein

Chapter Outline and Learning Outcomes

9.1 Chapter Overview and Case Studies

Describe the importance of maintaining acid–base balance and concepts related to acid–base balance.

9.2 Characteristics of Acids and Bases and Their Daily Production in the Body

Differentiate the characteristics of acids and bases and their sources in the body.

9.3 Measures of Hydrogen Ion Concentration

Explain pH and its relation to the hydrogen ion concentration.

9.4 Regulation of Acid–Base Balance

Compare the roles and limitations of chemical buffers, the kidneys, and the lungs in the maintenance of acid–base balance in the extracellular fluid, and explain the regulation of intracellular pH.

9.5 Types and Effects of Acid–Base Imbalances

Describe the four types of simple acid–base imbalances, and explain the basis for the clinical manifestations of acidosis and alkalosis.

9.6 Laboratory Tests Used in Assessment of Acid–Base Status

Interpret arterial and venous blood gas results, the anion gap, and base excess values.

9.7 Respiratory Acidosis

Differentiate the causes, underlying pathogenesis, and clinical manifestations of respiratory acidosis and approaches to diagnosis and treatment of this condition across the lifespan.

9.8 Respiratory Alkalosis

Differentiate the causes, underlying pathogenesis, and clinical manifestations of respiratory alkalosis and approaches to diagnosis and treatment of this condition across the lifespan.

9.9 Metabolic Acidosis

Differentiate the causes, underlying pathogenesis, and clinical manifestations of metabolic acidosis and approaches to diagnosis and treatment of this condition across the lifespan.

9.10 Metabolic Alkalosis

Differentiate the causes, underlying pathogenesis, and clinical manifestations of metabolic alkalosis and approaches to diagnosis and treatment of this condition across the lifespan.

9.11 Mixed Acid–Base Imbalances

Describe common clinical conditions that result in mixed acid–base imbalances.

9.12 Stepwise Analysis of Acid–Base Imbalances

Utilize a stepwise approach in the analysis of simple acid–base imbalances, and differentiate simple from mixed acid–base imbalances using equations for expected compensation.

KEY TERMS

Key Terms continue on next page.

ABBREVIATIONS

ABGs—arterial blood gases
BE—base excess
H^+—hydrogen ion
HCO_3^-—bicarbonate ion
$PaCO_2$—partial pressure of carbon dioxide in arterial blood
PCO_2—partial pressure of carbon dioxide
pH—negative log of the hydrogen ion concentration
pHi—intracellular pH
pKa—the dissociation constant of the weak acid
$PvCO_2$—partial pressure of carbon dioxide in venous blood
TCO_2—total CO_2

9.1 Chapter Overview and Case Studies

Maintenance of acid–base balance in order to regulate the hydrogen ion (H^+) concentration in body fluids is essential for normal cell and organ function and therefore for survival. Hydrogen ions are present in body fluids in much smaller amounts than other electrolytes such as calcium, sodium, and potassium; however, hydrogen ions are highly reactive, and their concentration must be precisely regulated within a narrow normal range. When there is an alteration in the H^+ concentration, proteins either gain or lose hydrogen ions; this alters the charge distribution on the protein, resulting in a change in its three-dimensional structure and ability to function. For example, enzymes, which are proteins that catalyze metabolic reactions, function optimally only within a narrow range of H^+ concentrations. Above or below this normal range, there will be impaired ability of enzymes to regulate cellular reactions, including those involved in metabolism and energy production. A disruption in acid–base balance also interferes with the function of proteins that are components of receptors, ion channels, and ion pumps. Because acid–base imbalances often result in alterations in compartmental distribution of potassium and calcium, the functions regulated by those electrolytes, such as nerve conduction and muscle contraction are also disrupted.

There are several mechanisms that, within limits, regulate the concentration of acids and bases in body fluids. These mechanisms are essential, since there are potential variations in the daily load of acids and bases due to differences in their dietary intake, metabolic production, and elimination. Many disease states, certain medications, and some therapeutic interventions can disrupt acid–base balance. Examples include kidney, liver, lung, and gastrointestinal disorders; diabetes mellitus; heart failure; shock; administration of intravenous fluids; and gastric suctioning.

This chapter addresses the normal regulation of acid–base balance in intracellular and extracellular fluids, the use of laboratory test results in the assessment of acid–base status, and the causes, clinical manifestations, and general principles of treatment of acidosis and alkalosis. More details about specific effects of the many disease states that can cause acid–base imbalances are addressed in subsequent chapters.

Concepts Related to Acid–Base Balance

The concept of acid–base balance is related to several other concepts, as shown in **Figure 9.1** ■. These relationships are briefly described here and explained in more detail later in this chapter. Because the H^+ concentration affects the structure and function of proteins, including enzymes, cell membrane receptors, and ion channels, it has a major impact on the regulation of a variety of cell functions. Alterations in the concentration of H^+ alter the compartmental distribution of some other electrolytes, including potassium and calcium, resulting in altered neuromuscular excitability. Changes in acid–base balance alter the level of electrolytes that affect neuromuscular excitability and therefore muscle contraction and mobility. Cognition is affected by changes in H^+ concentration because that alters the diameter of cerebral blood vessels and the volume of blood reaching the brain and because changes in H^+ concentration alter intracellular pH and the function of neurons. Acids are produced as by-products of metabolic reactions. Changes in the H^+ concentration can alter the activity of enzymes involved in metabolic reactions that produce ATP.[1]

The lungs regulate the elimination of carbon dioxide, which is a source of carbonic acid, and the kidneys regulate the elimination of both H^+ and the base bicarbonate. Lung or kidney disorders can cause acid–base imbalances. On the other hand, acid–base imbalances can change the rate and depth of breathing by way of their effect on central and peripheral chemoreceptors. Changes in acid–base balance also affect the amount of both H^+ and bicarbonate ions that are eliminated by the kidneys.

Adequate tissue perfusion that delivers oxygen and nutrients to cells is required to maintain aerobic metabolism and prevent accumulation of lactic acid and a subsequent acid–base imbalance. Because changes in H^+ concentration alter the compartmental distribution of potassium and calcium, which affects contraction of smooth muscle in blood vessels, they can cause vasoconstriction or

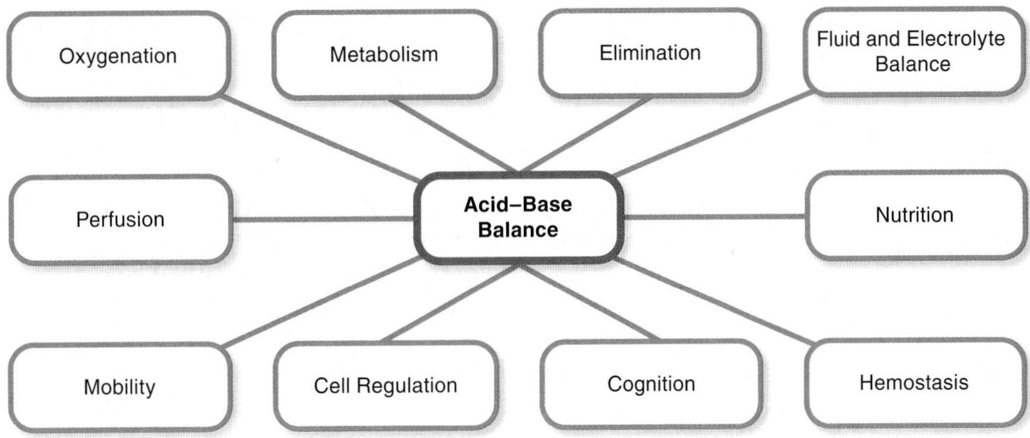

Figure 9.1 ■ Concepts related to acid–base imbalances.

vasodilation, thereby affecting tissue perfusion.[2] The H^+ concentration affects oxygenation because it alters the ability of hemoglobin to bind and transport oxygen and its ability to release oxygen to cells. Decreased oxygenation results in an acid–base imbalance because it leads to anaerobic metabolism and accumulation of lactic acid. Severe **acidosis** (a condition of below-normal blood pH due to an excess of acid relative to base) impairs activation of coagulation factors and contributes to blood loss in states such as trauma.

Foods and drinks are sources of acids and bases that can change the body's acid–base balance if they are not buffered or adequately eliminated. For example, foods that are high in acid include citrus fruits, which contain ascorbic and citric acids, and carbonated beverages, which contain carbonic and phosphoric acids. Examples of foods that are high in base, such as phosphate, include broccoli and raisins.

Case Studies

The following cases are addressed throughout the chapter to assist in the application of chapter content to clinical situations.

Jordon Washington: Introduction

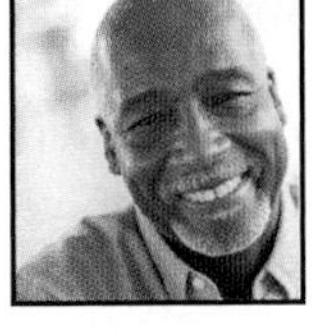

Jordon Washington, age 64, has emphysema, a chronic obstructive lung disease that is caused by a long history of cigarette smoking. He is currently hospitalized because he developed pneumonia and increased difficulty breathing. His arterial blood gas values are pH 7.24. $PaCO_2$ 68 mmHg, PaO_2 55 mmHg, BE +10 mEq/L.

1. What acute and chronic conditions contributed to Mr. Washington's acid–base imbalance?
2. How are the lab values used to determine the type of acid–base imbalance that is present?

Vivian Lee: Introduction

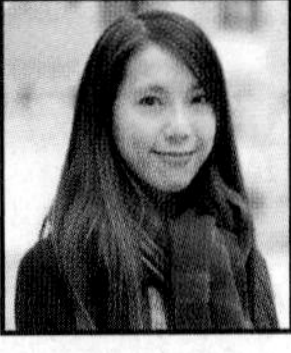

Vivian Lee is a 19-year-old college student who has maintained a straight A average in all her courses so far, and she and her parents are very proud of this. However, she has been struggling to keep an A grade in her biology course and has been feeling very stressed during the current semester. She experiences a panic attack at the beginning of the final exam in her biology course. Her respiratory rate is very rapid at 42 breaths per minute, and she becomes dizzy. She is taken to the emergency department, and her initial lab test results are pH 7.56, $PaCO_2$ 26 mmHg, PaO_2 104 mmHg, HCO_3^- 24 mEq/L.

1. What type of acid–base imbalance does Ms. Lee have, and what caused her dizziness?
2. What short- and long-term treatment strategies are appropriate for managing Ms. Lee's condition?

Sabrina Russell: Introduction

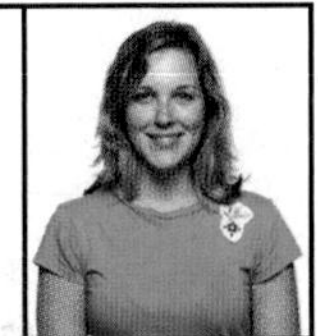

Sabrina Russell, age 28, has type 1 diabetes mellitus and requires daily injections of insulin. She has stopped taking her insulin because she has been gaining weight and is concerned about fitting into her bridesmaid dress for a friend's wedding that will take place in 3 weeks. Ms. Russell has also been inducing vomiting after eating in order to lose weight. As a result of these actions, she develops a decreased level of consciousness and an acetone odor to her breath. She is admitted to a hospital with the following initial venous blood values: pH 7.4, $PaCO_2$ 35 mmHg, HCO_3^- 22 mEq/L. Her plasma glucose is 612 mg/dL, serum chloride 86 mEq/L, serum potassium 3.1 mEq/L, and serum sodium 148 mEq/L.

1. On the basis of Ms. Russell's history and lab values ,could she have an acid–base imbalance even though her pH is within the normal range?
2. If so, what is causing Ms. Russell's acid–base imbalance?

Check Your Progress: Section 9.1

1. Why is it physiologically important to maintain pH within a narrow range?
2. Name two major body systems that are involved in maintaining acid–base balance.

9.2 Characteristics of Acids and Bases and Their Daily Production in the Body

An **acid** is a substance that dissociates into an H^+ and a conjugate base (B^-), which is an anion, as shown by the equation

HB	↔	$H^+ + B^-$
Acid	Hydrogen ion	Conjugate base

An H^+ is a proton, that is, the nucleus of a hydrogen atom that has lost its only electron. Hydrogen ions are highly reactive and seek to combine with negative charges on other substances in order to replace their missing electron. Strong acids dissociate to a greater extent than weak acids and release large amounts of H^+. Hydrochloric acid (HCl) and sulfuric acid (H_2SO_4) are examples of strong acids. Weak acids, by contrast, bind more tightly to their H^+ and only partially dissociate, releasing smaller amounts of H^+. Examples of weak acids are carbonic acid (H_2CO_3) and lactic acid ($CH_3CHOHCOOH$).

Both volatile and nonvolatile acids are produced in the body. A **volatile acid** can dissociate, forming a gas that is eliminated by the lungs. The volatile acid produced in the body is **carbonic acid** (H_2CO_3). It is a volatile acid because the carbon dioxide (CO_2) released from H_2CO_3 is a gas that is eliminated by the lungs. CO_2 is formed during aerobic metabolism of lipids, carbohydrates, and proteins. Approximately 15,000–20,000 mmol of CO_2 are produced in the body each day.[3] Even though CO_2 itself is not an acid, it is a source of acid in the body because some of the CO_2 in body fluids combines with water to form carbonic acid, as shown by the following reversible reaction:

$$CO_2 + H_2O \leftrightarrow H_2CO_3 \leftrightarrow H^+ + HCO_3^-.$$

H_2CO_3 can dissociate into H^+ (acid) and the base bicarbonate (HCO_3^-). Accumulation of carbon dioxide increases carbonic acid levels, making body fluids more acidic even though carbonic acid can dissociate into an H^+ and a base because the addition of H^+ causes a relatively greater percent increase in H^+, which are normally in much lower concentration than the base bicarbonate HCO_3^-. **Nonvolatile acids** (also called *fixed acids*) are not gases and therefore cannot be eliminated by the lungs. Nonvolatile acids are normally eliminated mainly by the kidneys in the urine and to a lesser degree by the gastrointestinal intestinal tract. Approximately 50–100 mEq of nonvolatile acids are produced each day, including lactic acid, ketoacids, sulfuric acid, and phosphoric acid.[4] Because of the much lower daily production of nonvolatile acids compared to volatile acids, it takes longer to reach a comparable degree of acidity (decrease in pH) in kidney failure than in respiratory failure.

A **base** is an H^+ acceptor. The presence of a base in a solution containing H^+ will lower the concentration of H^+ because the base binds to the H^+ ions, neutralizing them. The stronger the base, the greater is its affinity for binding H^+. An example of a strong base is sodium hydroxide (NaOH), which dissociates to release hydroxyl ions (OH^-). An example of a weak base is **bicarbonate (HCO_3^-)**, which can combine with free H^+ to form carbonic acid, which is a weak acid. The term *alkali*, in its strictest sense, refers to a base containing one of the alkaline metals, such as sodium or potassium, and a very basic ion such as the hydroxyl ion forming a base such as NaOH or KOH. In general usage, however, the term *alkali* is used synonymously with the term *base*. Therefore, when the blood is more basic than normal, the condition is called **alkalosis**.

Check Your Progress: Section 9.2

1. Give examples of a volatile acid and a nonvolatile acid.
2. What is a base?

9.3 Measures of Hydrogen Ion Concentration

The H^+ concentration of most body fluids is very low. For example, the H^+ concentration of arterial blood is approximately 0.0000004 mEq/L. To eliminate the need for cumbersome numbers, the H^+ concentration can be expressed in scientific notation, for example, as 4×10^{-7} mol/L for arterial blood. To further simplify the expression of H^+ concentration, the concept of pH was introduced. The **pH** of a solution is the negative logarithm or power (the "p" in "pH") to which the number 10 must be raised to equal the concentration of H^+ (the "H" in "pH") in milliequivalents per liter (mEq/L) as follows: H^+ concentration $= 1 \times 10^{-pH}$ or $pH = -\log[H^+]$. The pH scale extends from 0 to 14, with a midpoint of 7.00 representing chemical neutrality. It is important to remember that because pH is the negative logarithm of the hydrogen ion concentration, it is inversely related to the hydrogen ion concentration. That is, as pH values decrease, the H^+ concentration and acidity increase, and as pH values increase, the H^+ concentration and acidity decrease.

The measurement of H^+ concentration in terms of pH is in common use. However, the expression of H^+ concentration in terms of its actual concentration is receiving increasing support from clinicians because it more explicitly reflects the magnitude of change in hydrogen ion concentration. Because the concentration of H^+ in body fluids is much lower than the concentration of other electrolytes, such as sodium, which has a normal range of 135–145 mEq/L, or potassium, with a normal range of 3.5–5.0 mEq/L, H^+ concentration is expressed in terms of nanoequivalents per liter (nEq/L) rather than milliequivalents per liter. One nEq is approximately equal to one millionth of a milliequivalent. The relationship between pH and actual H^+ concentration and the pH of various body fluids is shown in **Table 9.1** ■. There is a narrow range of H^+ concentration that is compatible with life. Extreme arterial blood pH values of 7.8 (16 nEq/L of H^+) and 6.8 (160 nEq/L of H^+) represent a difference of only 0.4–0.6 pH unit above

Table 9.1 Relationship between pH and Hydrogen Ion Concentration

pH	H^+ Concentration (nEq/L)	Body Fluid Example* (pH)
1	100,000,000	Gastric fluid (1–3)
2	10,000,000	
3	1,000,000	
4	100,000	
5	10,000	
6	1,000	Urine usually (4.0–8.0)
6.8	160	
6.9	126	
7.0	100	Pure water
7.1	80	
7.2	64	
7.3	50	Venous blood (7.3–7.4); cerebrospinal fluid (7.33)
7.4	40	Arterial blood (7.35–7.45)
7.5	32	
7.6	26	
7.7	20	
7.8	16	
8	10	Pancreatic fluid (7.6–8.2)
9	1	

* Numbers in parentheses indicate the pH range for that body fluid.

or below a normal pH of 7.4. An arterial pH of 6.8 or below or 7.8 or above is not compatible with life for any extended period. There is a much smaller range of change in $[H^+]$ that is compatible with life compared to the normal range of other electrolytes.

Check Your Progress: Section 9.3

1. A change in pH by 1 actually means what change in H^+ concentration?
2. Is small intestinal pH lower or higher than gastric pH?

9.4 Regulation of Acid–Base Balance

Several compensatory mechanisms function to maintain the pH of body fluids within a narrow normal range despite moment-to-moment fluctuations in H^+ concentration resulting from the daily ingestion, metabolic production, and utilization of acids and bases. These compensatory mechanisms can also restore the pH to normal or near normal in disease states, at least for a while; however, they do not reverse the underlying cause of the imbalance. The compensatory mechanisms consist of the following:

- Intracellular and extracellular chemical buffers that neutralize excess acids and bases
- The respiratory system, which regulates the amount of carbonic acid by eliminating it in the form of carbon dioxide in exhaled air
- The renal system, which regulates the excretion of bicarbonate and H^+ from nonvolatile acids.

Good tissue perfusion is also important for local acid–base balance, since adequate blood flow will carry away metabolically produced carbon dioxide and nonvolatile acids and thus prevent their local accumulation.

Chemical buffer systems consist of a weak acid and a weak base and react almost immediately to a change in H^+ concentration in body fluids.[5] Chemical buffers in most body fluids consist of the bicarbonate buffer system, the phosphate buffer system, and intracellular and extracellular proteins. Extracellular chemical buffering reaches maximum efficacy within about an hour after the onset of an acid–base imbalance. The reaction that occurs when the bicarbonate buffer system reacts with a strong acid or base and converts it to a weaker acid or base, resulting in a lesser change in pH, is demonstrated by what happens when hydrochloric acid is added to a solution ($NaHCO_3 + HCl \leftrightarrow H_2CO_3 + NaCl$), resulting in production of the weaker acid H_2CO_3 and sodium chloride. By contrast, when a strong base such as sodium hydroxide is added, it is converted to a weak base as shown in the following reaction:

$$H_2CO_3 + NaOH \leftrightarrow NaHCO_3 + H_2O$$

The pH of a buffer system can be calculated by using the Henderson–Hasselbalch equation:

$$pH = pKa + \log_{10}\frac{[A^-]}{[HA]}$$

[HA] is the concentration of the undissociated weak acid in the buffer system. The acid can dissociate into H^+ and a conjugate base, which is an anion with its concentration depicted as $[A^-]$. For the bicarbonate–carbonic acid buffer system, the Henderson–Hasselbalch equation is

$$pH = pKa + \log_{10}\left(\frac{[HCO_3^-]}{[H_2CO_3]}\right)$$

OR

$$pH = 6.1 + \log_{10} (24\ mEq/L/1.2\ mEq/L)$$

OR

$$pH = 6.1 + 1.3 = 7.4$$

Normally, the ratio of the base bicarbonate (HCO_3) to carbonic acid (H_2CO_3) is 20:1 (**Figure 9.2** ■). As long as that ratio is maintained, the pH stays within the normal range. For example, if the concentration of both bicarbonate and carbonic acid doubled, the ratio would still be 20:1.

The **pKa** is the dissociation constant of the weak acid. It is the pH at which half the acid in a solution is dissociated and half is undissociated; that is, half is in the form of a weak acid (HA), and half is in the form of the conjugate base (A^-). For an ideal buffer system, the pKa of the buffer system is approximately equal to the pH of the solution in which it is present. Although the pKa of the bicarbonate

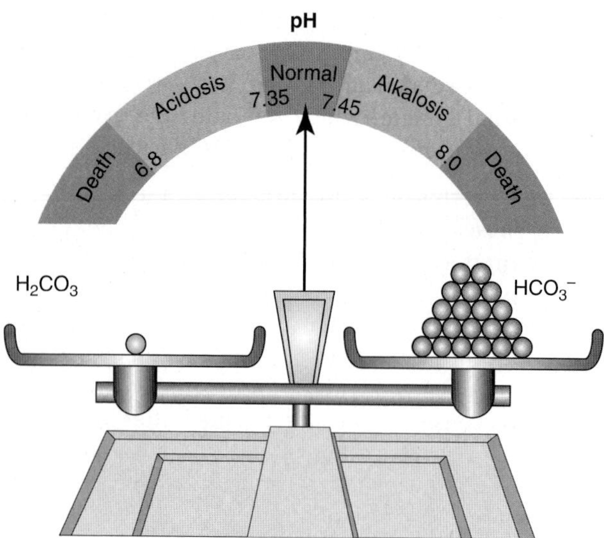

Figure 9.2 ■ The pH scale and relationship between bicarbonate and carbonic acid. As long as the ratio of the base bicarbonate (HCO_3^-) to carbonic acid (H_2CO_3) is 20:1, the pH of arterial blood will be in the normal range of 7.35–7.45.

buffer system is 6.1 and the pH of blood is approximately 7.4, the bicarbonate buffer system is still an important extracellular fluid buffer because the lungs can regulate the level of carbonic acid and the kidneys can regulate the level of bicarbonate in this buffer system.

CLINICAL POINT: The pKa is relevant not only to physiologic buffer systems but also to pharmacology. Most medications are in the form of a weak acid or a weak base and have a pKa value. The pKa is a characteristic of the medication that determines its degree of dissociation and therefore ionization in body fluids with different pH values. The undissociated and nonionized form of the medication is lipid soluble and able to cross the lipid bilayer in cell membranes and therefore enter intracellular fluid and cross the blood–brain barrier. The dissociated and ionized form of the medication is water soluble but not lipid soluble and therefore is unable to cross cell membranes. The pH of urine affects the elimination of medications because those that are ionized at the pH of the urine will not be able to be resorbed across the lipid bilayer of cell membranes of renal tubular cells and so will be eliminated in the urine. On the other hand, medications that are nonionized at the pH of urine will move across the renal tubular cells and be resorbed back into the blood and possibly accumulate to toxic levels. Therefore, changes in the pH of body fluids, such as blood and urine, affect the distribution of medications to various body compartments and their elimination in the urine. ■

The phosphate buffer system also consists of a weak base, which is disodium hydrogen phosphate (Na_2HPO_4), and a weak acid, which is dihydrogen sodium phosphate (NaH_2PO_4). The phosphate buffer system functions similarly to the bicarbonate buffer system in that it converts strong acids and bases to weak acids and bases thereby minimizing the degree of change in pH. The concentration of the phosphate buffer system in extracellular fluid is much lower than that of the bicarbonate buffer system and therefore is less effective in buffering the extracellular fluid. However, the phosphate buffer system has an important role in intracellular buffering and in buffering H^+ that is excreted in the urine.

Plasma proteins and intracellular proteins, including hemoglobin in red blood cells and albumin, can buffer H^+, which binds to negative charges on proteins. The carboxyl group (COOH) on proteins can release a H^+, and the amino group (NH_2) can accept a H^+. Intracellular buffering also consists of ionic pumps on cell membranes that regulate H^+ and HCO_3^- movement across cell membranes. This will be described in more detail in the section on regulation of intracellular pH.

Bone tissue can also buffer H^+. H^+ ions move into bones to be buffered by bone hydroxyapatite and carbonates, such as sodium bicarbonate, calcium bicarbonate, and calcium carbonate, resulting in the release of calcium and phosphate from bone.[5] The prolonged high level of H^+ in chronic acidosis activates osteoclasts, which cause bone resorption.[6] The loss of these electrolytes from bone and the activation of osteoclasts result in bone demineralization and increased risk of fractures in states of chronic metabolic acidosis, as in chronic kidney failure.

Respiratory Regulation of Acid–Base Balance

The respiratory system plays a major role in acid–base balance because it regulates the elimination of CO_2, which is continuously produced as a waste product of cell metabolism in tissues throughout the body. Normal lungs have a large surface area over which CO_2 diffuses from the blood in the pulmonary capillaries into the alveoli, from which it is then eliminated in exhaled air. Normally, the respiratory system maintains a partial pressure of CO_2 in the arterial blood ($PaCO_2$) of 35–45 mmHg. If CO_2 accumulates, the hydrogen ion concentration of body fluids increases because approximately 3% of CO_2 in body fluids combines with water to form carbonic acid (H_2CO_3), which then dissociates and releases a H^+ and a HCO_3^- as shown in the following equation:

$$CO_2 + H_2O \leftrightarrow H_2CO_3 \leftrightarrow H^+ + HCO_3^-$$

As is seen in the equation, when there is an alteration in the concentration of carbon dioxide and thus carbonic acid, there is a change not only in the concentration of H^+ but also in the concentration of HCO_3^-. Usually, this source of HCO_3^- is ignored because it represents only a small percentage change in the total HCO_3^- concentration. On the other hand, because the H^+ concentration in body fluids is normally very low, much lower than that of bicarbonate, the change in H^+ concentration derived from CO_2 reacting with water represents a much larger percentage change. Therefore, the predominant result of an alteration in CO_2 level is an alteration in H^+ concentration.

Not only does respiration affect the levels of CO_2 and H^+, but CO_2 and H^+ also regulate respiration because of their effect on the respiratory center in the brainstem. There is a feedback mechanism that operates between the respiratory center and the lungs. When there is an excess of H^+, it is detected by the respiratory center, and a neural reflex is triggered that causes an increase in the rate and force of contraction of the muscles of respiration. The result is an increase in the rate and depth of breathing with increased elimination of CO_2 and thus a decrease in carbonic acid, which brings the pH back up toward normal. However, in extreme acidosis, that is, when pH is below 7.00, this compensatory reflex mechanism begins to fail, and the hyperventilation ceases. In states of H^+ deficit or base excess, the opposite reaction occurs. That is, ventilation becomes depressed, and CO_2 accumulates, resulting in an increase in carbonic acid, which brings the pH back down toward normal. This compensatory hypoventilation is not very marked because the hypoxemia and hypercapnia that develop as a result of the hypoventilation will eventually stimulate respiration.[7] The lungs compensate for metabolic acid–base imbalances; maximal compensation takes 24–48 hours.[8]

If the lungs are the cause of acidosis or alkalosis, as in respiratory acidosis or respiratory alkalosis, they cannot compensate to help restore acid–base balance. If the acidosis or alkalosis is of nonrespiratory origin, that is, it has a metabolic cause, respiratory compensation for metabolic acidosis or alkalosis begins within minutes when the chemoreceptors detect a change in hydrogen ion concentration. The slight delay is due to the time it takes to transport blood with an altered pH to the respiratory center in the brainstem and to then initiate the reflex response. It takes up to several hours for respiratory compensation to reach maximal effectiveness.[5] The respiratory system can be quite effective in compensating for an acid–base imbalance and returning the pH to near normal. However, respiratory compensation is usually not complete; that is, the pH is not returned all the way back to normal because as the pH approaches normal, the stimulus that is driving the respiratory center diminishes, and the compensatory effort stops. The respiratory response to an acid–base imbalance is effective for only a few days. Fortunately, most forms of metabolic acidosis are acute and stand to benefit the most from short-term respiratory compensation. In individuals with lung disease or a neuromuscular disease that interferes with the ability of the lungs or the muscles of respiration to respond to reflex neural control, there will be a decreased capacity for respiratory compensation of a metabolic acid–base imbalance. The expected changes in $PaCO_2$ for metabolic acidosis and metabolic alkalosis are shown in **Table 9.2** ■.

There are limitations in the capacity of the lungs to compensate for metabolic acid–base imbalances. Hypoventilation can occur as a compensatory response to metabolic alkalosis. As the lungs retain more carbon dioxide, more carbonic acid is formed from the combination of carbon dioxide and water. However, this response is limited by the subsequent hypoxemia that results from hypoventilation. In other words, respiratory compensation for metabolic alkalosis does not get to the point at which life-threatening hypoxemia develops. Extreme respiratory buffering for metabolic acidosis, as with Kussmaul respirations (very deep respirations), cannot continue indefinitely because it leads to respiratory muscle fatigue. The presence of acute or chronic respiratory disorders, such as pneumonia or chronic obstructive pulmonary disease, limits the ability of the lungs to compensate for metabolic acid–base imbalances.

Renal Regulation of Acid–Base Balance

The renal system is essential for the maintenance of acid–base balance because it is the only regulator of the levels of bicarbonate and nonvolatile acids. Normally, the pH of urine is acidic because most of the products of cell metabolism are excreted in the urine are acids. However, when there is a state of base excess, the kidneys can excrete urine that is alkaline. The pH of urine can range from 4.00 to 8.00 and usually averages around 6.00.

The kidneys contribute to acid–base balance by three mechanisms that take place along the tubules of the nephron:

- The conservation of HCO_3^- by the resorption of bicarbonate from the renal tubule lumen back into the blood
- Secretion of H^+ into the urine and synthesis of new bicarbonate
- Excretion of H^+ buffered by ammonia.[1,4,7]

Table 9.2 Primary Imbalance and Expected Compensation for Acid–Base Disorders

Primary Disorder	pH	Alteration Responsible for the Change in pH	Compensatory Change	Expected Compensation
Respiratory acidosis	↓	↑$PaCO_2$	↑HCO_3^-	
Acute				$\Delta\ HCO_3^- = 0.10\ \Delta\ PaCO_2$
Chronic				$\Delta\ HCO_3^- = 0.35\ \Delta\ PaCO_2$
Respiratory alkalosis	↑	↑$PaCO_2$	↓HCO_3^-	
Acute				$\Delta\ HCO_3^- = 0.20\ \Delta\ PaCO_2$
Chronic				$\Delta\ HCO_3^- = 0.50\ \Delta\ PaCO_2$
Metabolic acidosis	↓	↓HCO_3^-	↓$PaCO_2$	$\Delta\ PaCO_2 = 1.2\ \Delta\ HCO_3^-$
Metabolic alkalosis	↑	↑HCO_3^-	↑$PaCO_2$	$\Delta\ PaCO_2 = 0.9\ \Delta\ HCO_3^-$

The symbol Δ in the equations means "change in."

SOURCES: Hasan, A. (2013). *Handbook of blood gas/acid-base interpretation* (2nd ed., p. 257). New York, NY: Springer; Marini, J., & Wheeler, A. (2010). *Critical care medicine: The essentials* (4th ed., p. 234). Philadelphia, PA: Lippincott Williams & Wilkins; Marino, P. (2014). *Marino's The ICU book* (4th ed.). Philadelphia, PA: Lippincott Williams & Wilkins.

These renal mechanisms take longer to respond to an acid–base imbalance than do either the chemical buffers or the respiratory system. The renal system takes 8–12 hours to begin to have an effect and might not reach maximum effectiveness for 4–6 days. Despite its slow response time, the renal system is the most effective in compensating for an acid–base imbalance because it can excrete and thus eliminate H^+ or bicarbonate ions when necessary. The kidneys are capable of returning the pH all the way back to normal. The expected changes in bicarbonate level when the kidneys compensate for respiratory acidosis and respiratory alkalosis are shown in Table 9.2. However, the kidneys will not be able to compensate if their function is impaired as a result of disease or if they are the cause of the acid–base imbalance.

Renal Conservation of Bicarbonate

One mechanism by which the kidneys regulate acid–base balance is the conservation of HCO_3^- by a process of resorption of filtered HCO_3^- back into the blood coupled with the excretion of H^+ into the urine. HCO_3^- must be recycled this way, or else it will be lost from the body, resulting in a base HCO_3^- deficit. Because HCO_3^- ions are charged, they do not readily cross cell membranes, and since there is no HCO_3^- ion pump in the renal tubules to assist in their transport out of the urine in the renal tubule lumen, HCO_3^- ions must be resorbed indirectly in the form of carbon dioxide (CO_2) in the sequence of events, which is illustrated in **Figure 9.3** ■. Water formed in the process of resorption of HCO_3^- is either excreted in the urine or resorbed, depending on the fluid needs of the body at the time. Note that the H^+ are secreted into the tubule lumen and subsequently excreted in the urine by a process that is coupled to the resorption of sodium (Na^+) from the lumen into the tubule cell by the action of a sodium–hydrogen exchanger.

CLINICAL POINT: This explains why in states of volume deficit, which stimulate aldosterone secretion causing sodium and water resorption, increased amounts of H^+ are lost in the urine, resulting in metabolic alkalosis. ■

The net effect of all the reactions shown in Figure 9.3 is that for each H^+ secreted into the urine, a HCO_3^- ion is resorbed and returned to the blood, thereby maintaining the plasma HCO_3^- concentration. Normally, most of the bicarbonate that is filtered into the urine is resorbed. However, when there is a HCO_3^- excess, the HCO_3^- ions enter the urine in the renal tubular lumen, where there are not enough H^+ to combine with them and go through the reactions necessary for HCO_3^- resorption. Therefore, the excess HCO_3^- ions combine instead with Na^+ or other cations and are excreted in the urine.

Secretion of H^+ into the Urine and Synthesis of New Bicarbonate

In addition to the resorption of HCO_3^-, the kidneys can synthesize new HCO_3^- and add it to the blood during the process of secretion of H^+ into the renal tubules by an ATP-dependent pump in cells of the collecting ducts (**Figure 9.4** ■). This new bicarbonate is needed to replace what was used up in the buffering of the daily load of H^+. There is a limit to the amount of free H^+ that can be eliminated in the urine

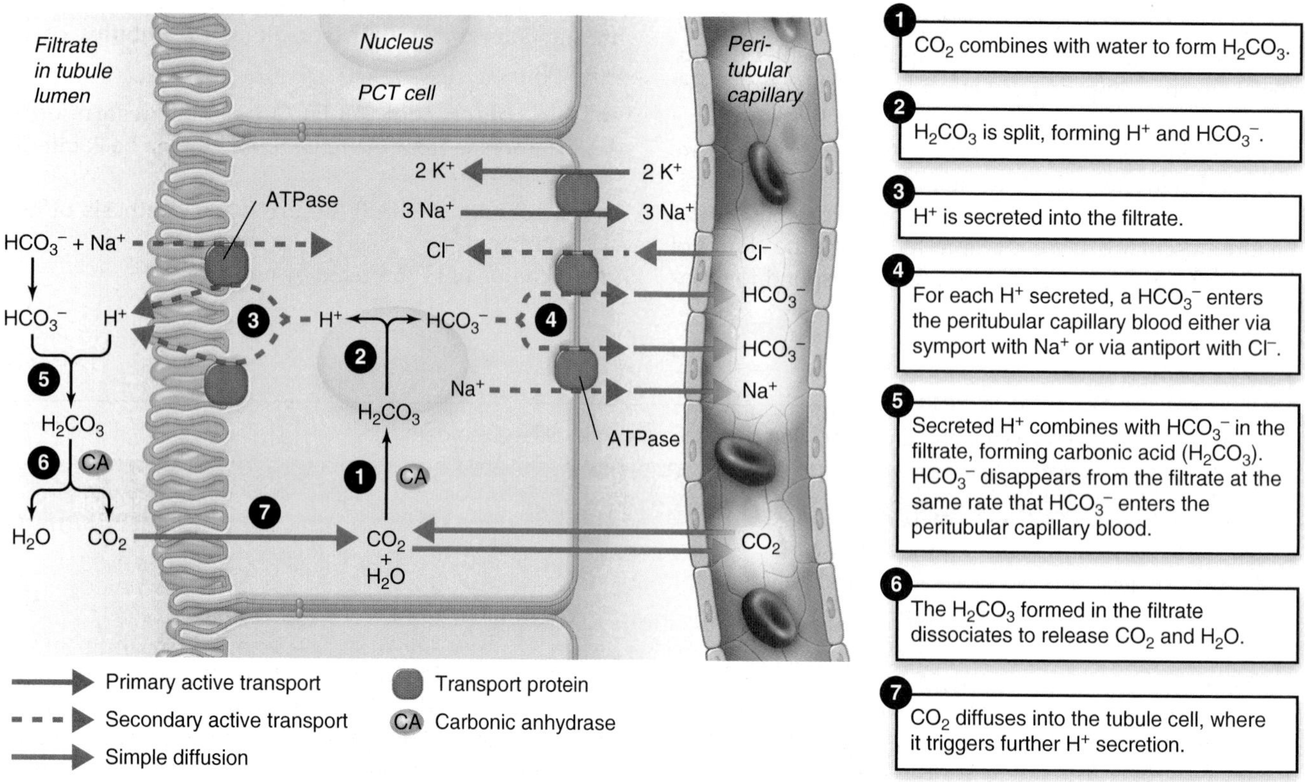
Filtrate in tubule lumen
Nucleus
PCT cell
Peri-tubular capillary
2 K+
3 Na+
ATPase
HCO3− + Na+
Cl−
HCO3−
H+
HCO3−
Na+
H2CO3
CA
H2O
CO2
CO2 + H2O
ATPase
1 CO2 combines with water to form H2CO3.
2 H2CO3 is split, forming H+ and HCO3−.
3 H+ is secreted into the filtrate.
4 For each H+ secreted, a HCO3− enters the peritubular capillary blood either via symport with Na+ or via antiport with Cl−.
5 Secreted H+ combines with HCO3− in the filtrate, forming carbonic acid (H2CO3). HCO3− disappears from the filtrate at the same rate that HCO3− enters the peritubular capillary blood.
6 The H2CO3 formed in the filtrate dissociates to release CO2 and H2O.
7 CO2 diffuses into the tubule cell, where it triggers further H+ secretion.
Primary active transport
Secondary active transport
Simple diffusion
Transport protein
CA Carbonic anhydrase

Figure 9.3 ■ Conservation of bicarbonate ions.

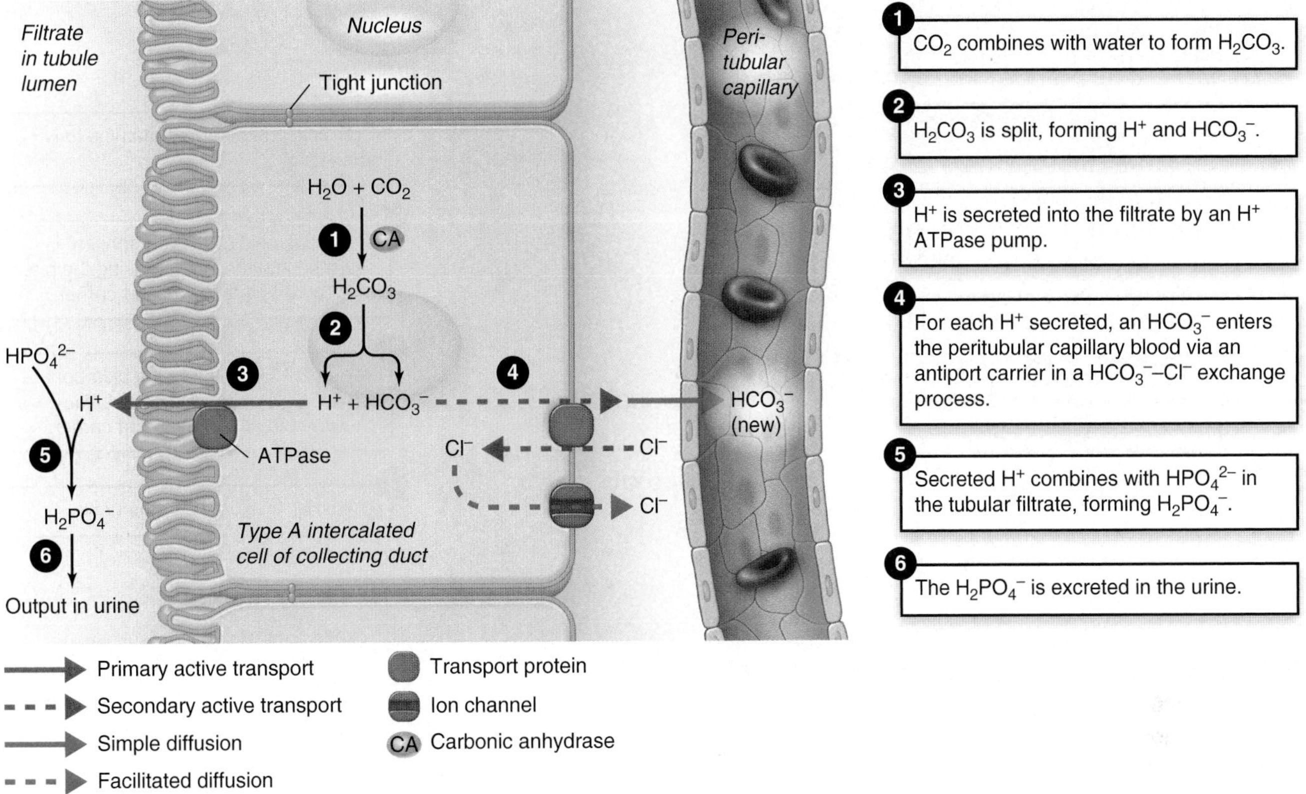

Figure 9.4 ■ Secretion of H^+ in the urine and synthesis of new HCO_3^-.

because a large amount in the urine will cause the urine pH to fall below 4.0, resulting in damage to structures of the renal tract as a direct result of the high acidity. By combining with H^+, renal buffers allow the kidneys to excrete excess H^+ while preventing the urine pH from falling low enough to cause renal cell injury. Because of its relatively high concentration and effectiveness as a buffer at the usual acid pH of urine, the phosphate buffer system has an important role in renal buffering. Some hydrogen ions that are secreted into the renal tubule lumen combine with monohydrogen phosphate (HPO_4^{-2}) to form dihydrogen phosphate ($H_2PO_4^-$), as shown in Figure 9.4. The negative charge on $H_2PO_4^-$ makes it lipid insoluble and unable to diffuse across the renal tubule cell membrane and back into the blood. Therefore, the $H_2PO_4^-$ ions become trapped in the renal tubule and are excreted in the urine. However, the phosphate buffer system is not very effective when extreme acid loads cause the pH of urine to fall below 4.5.

Excretion of H^+ Buffered by Ammonia

Ammonia (NH_3), which is produced from the metabolism of the amino acid glutamine, is another important renal buffer. Ammonia is a base that can combine with H^+ to form an ammonium ion (NH_4^+). NH_4^+ combines with chloride in the urine, forming ammonium chloride (NH_4Cl). For each H^+ excreted in the urine in the form of NH4$^+$, an HCO3$^-$ ion is resorbed back into to the blood (**Figure 9.5** ■). The effectiveness of this buffer system is related to the solubility characteristics of NH_3 and NH_4^+. NH_3 is not ionized and is therefore lipid soluble and able to easily cross cell membranes. As the NH_3 produced in the renal tubule cells accumulates, a concentration gradient develops, causing NH_3 to diffuse out of the tubule cells into the tubule lumen fluid, where it can combine with H^+ ions to form NH_4^+. Because NH_4^+ is ionized, it is not lipid soluble and cannot diffuse out of the tubule lumen and is subsequently excreted in the urine. The pH of the urine affects the diffusion rate of NH_3 into the tubule lumen. As the pH of urine becomes more acidic as a result of the increased amount of H^+ ions, NH_3 combines with those H^+ to a greater extent to form more NH_4^+. This keeps the concentration of NH_3 in the urine low, which promotes the diffusion of more NH_3 out of the tubule cells, so more is available to buffer H^+. If a chronic increase in acid load develops, the excretion of H^+ as NH_4^+ can increase. It takes several days for this mechanism to have its maximum effect. The delay is related to the time it takes the renal tubule cells to synthesize large amounts of the enzyme needed for ammonia production. The ammonia-buffering mechanism is especially important when the urine is very acidic because the other buffers in the renal tubule fluid become ineffective below pH 4.5.

Maintenance of pH within the normal range is critical for fetal development and survival. Chemical buffers that maintain acid–base balance in the fetus are similar to those in the adult. In the adult, both the lungs and the kidneys are important physiologic buffer systems. However, in the fetus, the lungs are nonfunctional, and the kidneys are not fully developed. In the fetus, the placenta takes the place of the lungs in delivery of oxygen and removal of

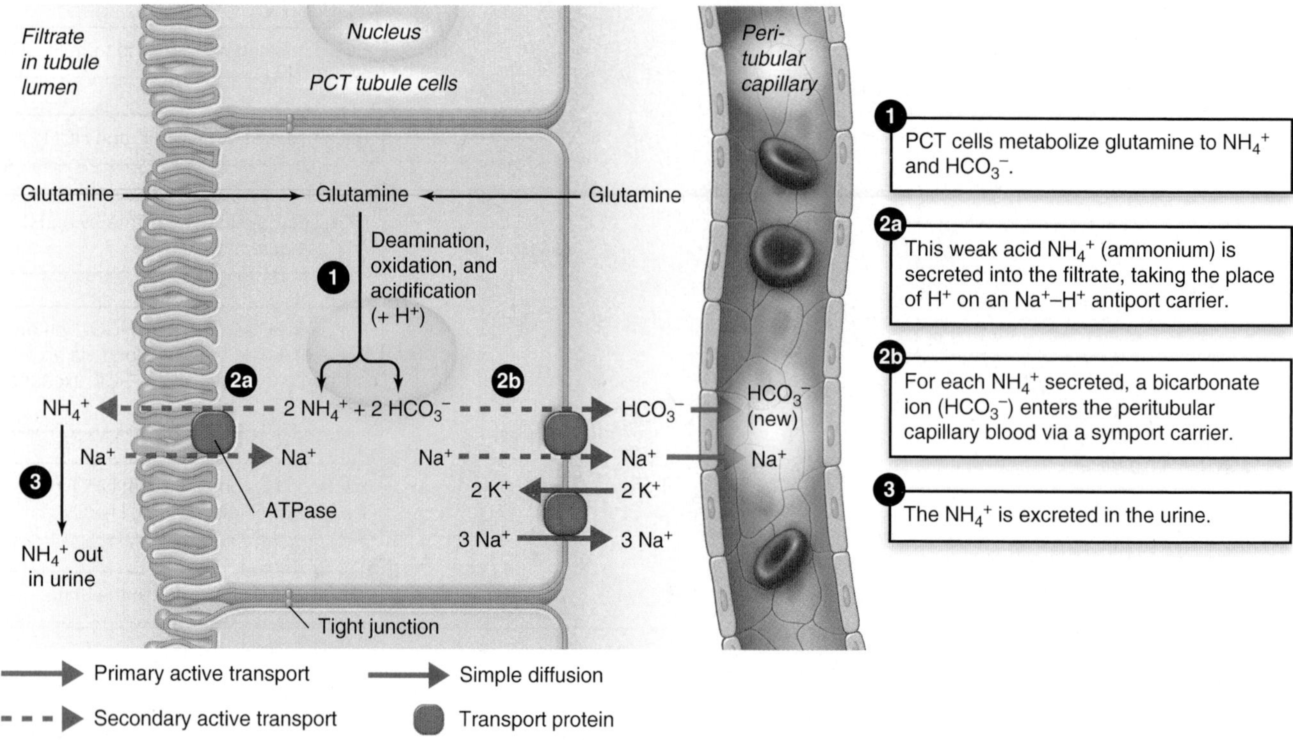
Filtrate
in tubule
lumen
Nucleus
PCT tubule cells
Peri-
tubular
capillary
Glutamine
Glutamine
Glutamine
1
Deamination,
oxidation, and
acidification
(+ H+)
2a
2b
NH4+
2 NH4+ + 2 HCO3−
HCO3−
HCO3−
(new)
Na+
Na+
Na+
Na+
Na+
3
ATPase
2 K+
2 K+
3 Na+
3 Na+
NH4+ out
in urine
Tight junction
Primary active transport
Simple diffusion
Secondary active transport
Transport protein
1 PCT cells metabolize glutamine to NH4+ and HCO3−.
2a This weak acid NH4+ (ammonium) is secreted into the filtrate, taking the place of H+ on an Na+–H+ antiport carrier.
2b For each NH4+ secreted, a bicarbonate ion (HCO3−) enters the peritubular capillary blood via a symport carrier.
3 The NH4+ is excreted in the urine.

Figure 9.5 ■ Excretion of H^+ buffered by ammonia.

CO_2 and shares the role of the kidneys in eliminating H^+ from nonvolatile acids.[2] CO_2 crosses cell layers of the placenta rapidly; however, nonvolatile acids cross much more slowly. The fetus is less able to compensate for acid–base imbalances compared to adults. ■

Compensation versus Correction of Acid–Base Imbalances

Compensation for and correction of an acid–base imbalance are not the same. **Compensation** is present when various chemical buffers and renal or respiratory function return the pH closer to or actually back within the normal range; however, the underlying disease process responsible for the acid–base imbalance is still present. **Correction** of an acid–base imbalance occurs when the condition responsible for the acid–base imbalance is controlled or no longer present and the pH is within the normal range. For example, if metabolic acidosis is caused by accumulation of lactic acid as a result of hypoxia, the condition would be compensated by increased CO_2 elimination by the lungs and corrected when oxygen levels and lactic acid production return to normal. Another example is respiratory acidosis caused by pneumonia with compensation resulting from the kidneys adding more of the base HCO_3^- to the blood and correction of the acid–base imbalance resulting from eradication of the infection that caused the pneumonia by the administration of an antibiotic.

Regulation of Intracellular pH

The intracellular pH (pHi) has a major impact on cell functions, including enzymes, ion channels, and neuronal activity.[9] Intracellular fluid must be protected against changes in the H^+ concentration that occur in the cell and changes that occur in the extracellular fluid, which affect the pHi. The pHi varies with different cell types and ranges from 7.08 to 7.31,[10] which is lower than the extracellular fluid pH because of production of CO_2 and nonvolatile acids in cells as by-products of metabolic reactions. Because it is not feasible to measure pHi in clinical settings, the pH of extracellular fluids, such as blood, urine, and cerebrospinal fluid, is measured as an assessment of acid–base status.

There are several mechanisms that function to regulate pHi. Buffering in intracellular fluid is accomplished mainly by the phosphate buffer system, intracellular proteins, and hemoglobin in red blood cells. CO_2 is very lipid soluble and readily crosses cell membranes. However, the cell membrane has low permeability to most electrolytes, including H^+ and $HCO3^-$, and special transport mechanisms are required to move them across cell membranes. There are transporters in cell membranes that regulate the exchange of electrolytes across the membrane. An **antiport** is a transport molecule that moves two different electrolytes in opposite directions across a cell membrane and a **symport** is a transport molecule that moves two different electrolytes in the same direction across a cell membrane. Various antiports and symports present in cell membranes involved in the regulation of pHi are shown in **Figure 9.6** ■. Some of these transporters require energy in the form of ATP. That results in increased utilization of ATP in certain acid–base imbalances and impaired buffering capacity in the presence of hypoxia because of decreased oxygen availability to synthesize ATP. Some of the ion exchange transporters do not require ATP. For example, energy for ion exchange for the Na^+–H^+ exchanger is derived from the electrochemical gradient that favors the diffusion of

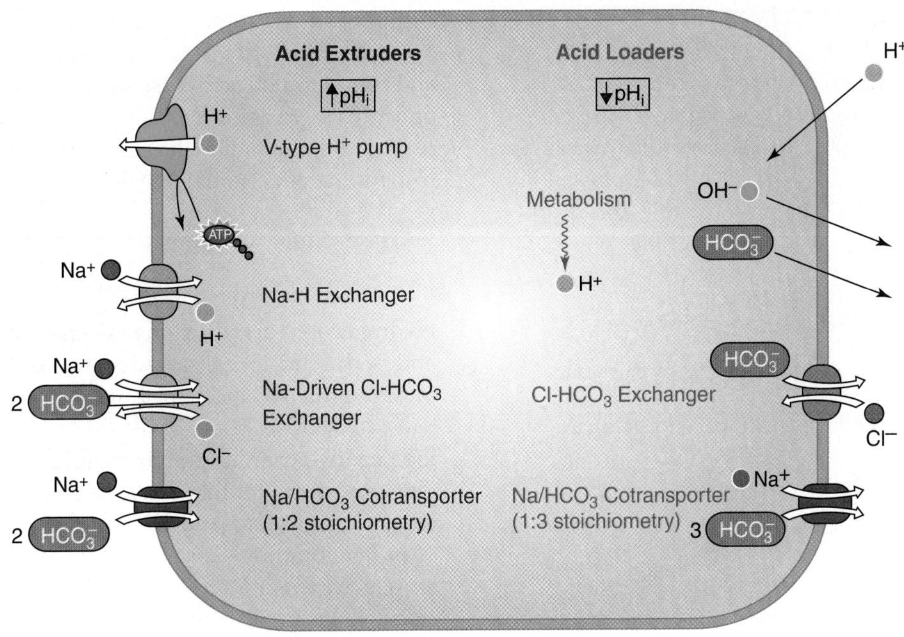

Figure 9.6 ■ Regulation of intracellular pH (pHi).

sodium into cells and that causes hydrogen ions to move out of the cells.[10,11] The Na^+–H^+ exchanger is an antiport that is regulated by pHi, and when it reaches normal, the Na^+–H^+ exchanger turns off. Normally, H^+ from fixed acids produced as a by-product of metabolism are removed from cells by antiports such as the Na^+–H^+ exchanger, and the extruded H^+ are carried away by the normally rapid blood flow, which maintains a diffusion gradient to remove more H^+. However, when there is decreased perfusion, H^+ ions accumulate both inside and outside cells.

HCO_3^- does not readily diffuse across cell membranes, and a transporter is required to move it across cell membranes. However, HCO_3^- takes much longer to enter cells than does carbon dioxide.

CLINICAL POINT: The slow transport of HCO_3^- across cell membranes has significant implications related to the use of buffers to treat acidosis. Bicarbonate, administered as sodium bicarbonate, reacts with H^+ from fixed acids such as lactic acid or ketoacids in the extracellular fluid, producing carbon dioxide as a by-product. The carbon dioxide readily enters cells and reacts with intracellular water, forming carbonic acid. Therefore, even though administration of sodium bicarbonate in states of metabolic acidosis with elevated levels of fixed acids, such as lactic acid, results in a change in blood pH back up toward normal, the pHi becomes more acidic. That is why administration of sodium bicarbonate for treatment of metabolic acidosis is used much less frequently than it was in the past. ■

Membrane transporters that regulate pHi can be affected by certain medications. For example, nonsteroidal anti-inflammatory drugs (NSAIDs), especially the older first-generation ones such as aspirin and ibuprofen, have strong effects on cell membrane transporters.[12] NSAIDs inhibit the Na^+–H^+ exchanger and thereby decrease pHi. NSAIDs also inhibit the chloride–bicarbonate (Cl^-–HCO_3^-) antiport in gastric epithelial cells, resulting in decreased bicarbonate secretion into the layer of mucus that normally protects the stomach lining from digestion by hydrochloric acid secreted by gastric cells (**Figure 9.7** ■). The first-generation NSAIDs and to a lesser extent the second-generation ones can cause erosive gastritis and ulcers by these mechanisms.

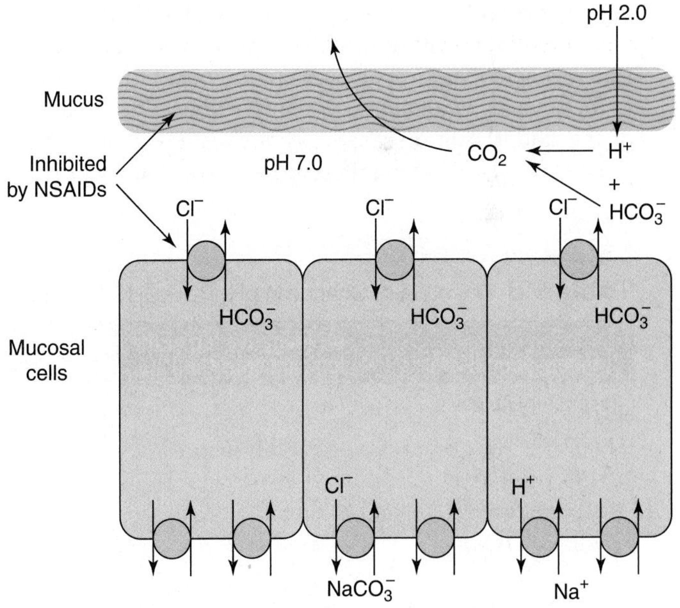

Figure 9.7 ■ Effect of nonsteroidal anti-inflammatory drugs (NSAIDs) on bicarbonate secretion by gastric cells. NSAIDs, especially those of the first generation such as aspirin and ibuprofen, have strong effects on hydrogen ion pumps. NSAIDs inhibit the Na^+–H^+exchanger (antiport) and thereby decrease intracellular pH. They also inhibit the chloride–bicarbonate (Cl^-–HCO_3^-) antiport in gastric epithelial cells, resulting in decreased bicarbonate secretion into the layer of mucus that normally protects the stomach lining from digestion by gastric acid. The first generation, and to a lesser extent the second generation, NSAIDs can cause erosive gastritis and ulcers by these mechanisms.

Check Your Progress: Section 9.4

1. How does kidney disease contribute to acid–base imbalance?
2. Salicylate (aspirin) overdose has been associated with respiratory alkalosis. Explain the mechanism that contributes to this.

9.5 Types and Effects of Acid–Base Imbalances

There are four types of simple acid–base imbalances:

- Respiratory acidosis
- Respiratory alkalosis
- Metabolic acidosis
- Metabolic alkalosis.

A **simple acid–base imbalance** is the presence of one type of acid–base imbalance. Respiratory acid–base imbalances are due to alterations in CO_2 elimination by the lungs. Metabolic acid–base imbalances are due to alterations in the level of nonvolatile acids or the base HCO_3. In respiratory and metabolic acidosis, the pH is decreased, and the H^+ concentration is increased. In respiratory and metabolic alkalosis, the pH is increased, and the H^+ concentration is decreased. The causes of these acid–base imbalances are covered in later sections in this chapter. The alterations in physiologic functions and resulting clinical manifestations that occur in states of acid–base imbalances are the result of the effects of the acidosis or alkalosis on cell functions plus the effects of the underlying disease process causing the acid–base imbalance as well as manifestations of respiratory or renal compensation. Refer to **Table 9.3** ■ for the direction of change in blood gas parameters in states of uncompensated and compensated acid–base imbalances. Many of the effects of acidosis are similar whether the acidosis is caused by a respiratory or a metabolic acid–base imbalance. This is also true for the effects of alkalosis.

Effects of Acidosis and Alkalosis on Neuromuscular Function

Hydrogen ions and calcium ions are both positively charged, and both bind to varying degrees to negative charges on plasma proteins, such as albumin, and to intracellular proteins. In acidosis, some of the excess hydrogen ions bind to the negative charges on intracellular and extracellular proteins. As a result of this, fewer calcium ions can bind to proteins. Calcium ions and H^+ compete for a limited number of protein binding sites. The result is that in acidosis, there is an increased amount of free, ionized (non–protein-bound) calcium. It is free calcium that is active and able to participate in a variety of physiologic functions. The excess free calcium caused by acidosis blocks sodium channels in nerve and muscle cells, impairing sodium entry, which normally occurs during the action potential, as shown in **Figure 9.8** ■. The result is decreased neuromuscular excitability. The decreased neuromuscular activity causes muscle weakness and weak reflexes. Decreased contractility of the diaphragm can contribute to the development or worsening of respiratory failure. Decreased sodium entry into vascular smooth muscle leads to vasodilation with subsequent increased cerebral blood flow, which can increase intracranial pressure and result in coma in more serious cases. Vasodilation in the cerebral circulation also causes headache due to stretching of the cerebral arteries, confusion, and behavioral alterations.

Table 9.3 Direction of Change in pH, PCO_2, HCO_3^-, and BE in Acid–Base Imbalances

Compensation State	pH (negative log of the hydrogen ion concentration)	Serum HCO_3^- (bicarbonate ion)	PCO_2 (partial pressure of carbon dioxide)	BE (base excess)
Respiratory Acidosis				
Uncompensated	Decreased	Normal	Increased	Normal
Partially compensated	Less decreased	Increased	Increased	Increased
Fully compensated	Normal	Increased more	Increased	Increased more
Respiratory Alkalosis				
Uncompensated	Increased	Normal	Decreased	Normal
Partially compensated	Less increased	Decreased	Decreased	Decreased
Fully compensated	Normal	Decreased more	Decreased	Decreased more
Metabolic Acidosis				
Uncompensated	Decreased	Decreased	Normal	Decreased
Partially compensated	Less decreased	Decreased	Decreased	Decreased
Fully compensated	Near normal	Decreased	Decreased More	Decreased
Metabolic Alkalosis				
Uncompensated	Increased	Increased	Normal	Increased
Partially compensated	Less increased	Increased	Increased	Increased
Fully compensated	Near normal	Increased	Increased more	Increased

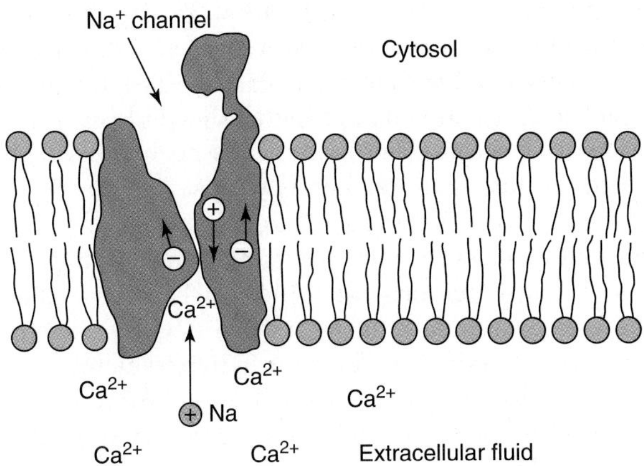

Figure 9.8 ■ Alterations in neuromuscular activity caused by changes in free, ionized calcium levels. The lipid bilayer in nerve or muscle cell membranes with a sodium channel are shown on the left. Normally, during an action potential, the sodium channel would open, allowing sodium to rush into the cell, causing depolarization. Free, ionized calcium can occupy space in the extracellular portion of the sodium channel, thereby interfering with sodium entry. The more free calcium is available, the greater the degree of obstruction of the sodium channels. Acidosis results in increased levels of free calcium, which impairs sodium entry into nerve and muscle cells and decreases neuromuscular excitability. Alkalosis results in decreased levels of free calcium, which results in more sodium entry into nerve and muscle cells, increasing neuromuscular excitability.

In alkalosis, there are fewer H^+ competing with calcium ions for protein binding sites. Therefore, more calcium is bound to protein and therefore inactive. With less calcium blocking sodium channels, there is increased neuromuscular activity. The clinical manifestations of this include positive Chvostek and Trousseau signs (**Figure 9.9** ■), hyperactive reflexes, paresthesias, convulsions, laryngospasm, and tetany.

Effects of Acidosis and Alkalosis on the Central Nervous System

Generally, there is a lower intracellular pH for a given extracellular pH in acute respiratory acidosis than in metabolic acidosis because of higher cell permeability to carbon dioxide than to hydrogen ions. Therefore, for any particular blood pH in acidosis, clinical manifestations, especially those affecting the central nervous system (CNS), may be worse in respiratory acidosis than in metabolic acidosis before compensation. In addition to the intracellular acidosis, CNS manifestations of acidosis, such as confusion, headache, seizures, and coma, are also the result of vasodilation-induced increased cerebral blood flow, which can increase intracranial pressure and result in manifestations such as papilledema (swelling of the optic disc).[1,5]

As with acidosis, there are more profound changes in intracellular pH during alkalosis in respiratory alkalosis than in metabolic alkalosis because of the high permeability of cell membranes to carbon dioxide. Increased intracellular pH as well as vasoconstriction and decreased cerebral blood

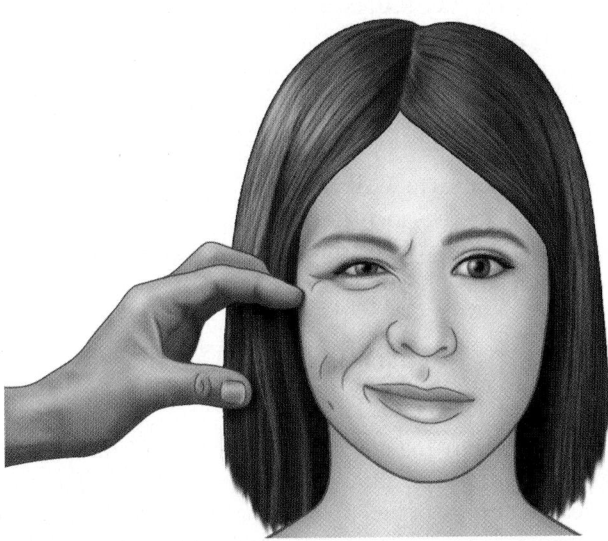

A Chvostek sign

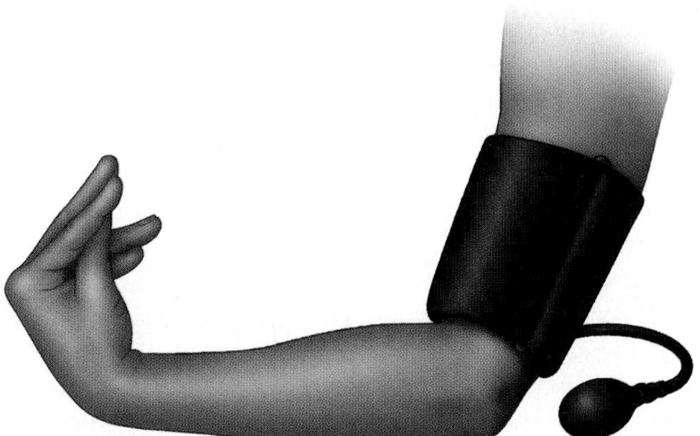

B Trousseau sign

Figure 9.9 ■ Both Chvostek sign, **A**, and Trousseau sign, when positive, **B**, indicate increased neuromuscular excitability when the level of free, ionized calcium is decreased, as occurs in alkalosis. Chvostek sign can be elicited by tapping the face in front of the ear just below the temple where the facial nerve is located; when there is increased neuromuscular excitability, the facial nerve causes contraction of the lips, nose, and face on the side that was tapped. Trousseau's sign is elicited by increasing pressure on nerves in the arm by inflating a blood pressure cuff just above the systolic pressure for a few minutes. If increased neuromuscular excitability is present, the pressure will result in a carpal spasm of the hand.

flow and decreased unloading of oxygen from hemoglobin in severe alkalosis all contribute to impaired CNS function. Respiratory alkalosis can result in a decrease in cerebral blood flow by 35–40% of baseline when the $PaCO_2$ decreases by about 20 mmHg. CNS manifestations of alkalosis include dizziness, anxiety, seizures, confusion, and coma.

Vivian Lee: Application

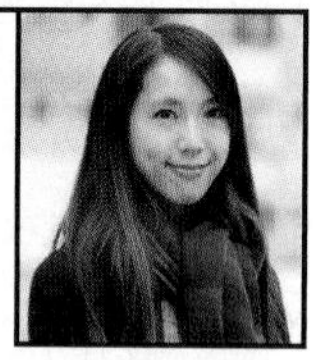

The dizziness caused by the panic attack that Ms. Lee experienced during a final exam was the result of constriction of cerebral blood vessels and decreased unloading of oxygen to neurons in the central nervous system, causing them to become hypoxic.

3. What are the symptoms of respiratory alkalosis?
4. Explain the meaning of "decreased unloading of oxygen to neurons" as it contributes to the symptoms of alkalosis.

Effects of Acidosis and Alkalosis on Perfusion

Acidosis has adverse effects on both the heart and the vasculature that contribute to decreased perfusion.[13–15] Acidosis has a negative inotropic effect on the heart; that is, it decreases cardiac contractility. H^+ ions interfere with excitation–contraction coupling and decrease the sensitivity of troponin C on actin (the thin filament of muscle fibers) for calcium. Increased sympathetic tone can initially help to compensate somewhat for the negative inotropic effect of acidosis but will not be effective in a denervated heart, such as a transplanted heart, or in the presence of beta-blocker medications or when the pH is less than 7.20. The stimulation of the sympathetic–adrenal system is counteracted by the decreased responsiveness of adrenergic receptors to catecholamines in acidosis. Impaired sodium entry into vascular smooth muscle causes vasodilation, resulting in a decreased effective circulating blood volume; hypotension; and warm, flushed skin.

In alkalosis, there is increased neuromuscular activity in vascular smooth muscle leading to vasoconstriction, which decreases cerebral blood flow. However, this effect is transient, lasting only a few hours. The effect of alkalosis on cardiac contractility is biphasic, with an increase in contractility up to a pH of 7.7 and decreased cardiac contractility with pH levels greater than 7.7.[16] Hypokalemia associated with alkalosis can cause atrial and ventricular tachydysrhythmias. Alkalosis has variable effects on systemic vascular resistance (SVR); vasodilation and decreased SVR occur with pH values up to 7.65, and vasoconstriction and increased SVR occur with pH values greater than 7.65. The increased vascular reactivity can cause coronary artery vasospasm, resulting in myocardial ischemia and angina. Chest pain of noncardiac origin occurring in alkalosis is often the result of spasms of esophageal muscles.

Effects of Acidosis and Alkalosis on Electrolyte Levels

Hydrogen ions can move into and out of cells in exchange with other electrolytes in response to changes in the extracellular H^+ concentration. H^+ and potassium ion exchange across cell membranes occurs as part of compensation for certain types of acid–base imbalances (**Figure 9.10** ■). In states of metabolic acidosis that are caused by an excess of inorganic acids, such as hydrochloric acid (occurring, for example, with severe diarrhea) or with an excess of sulfuric acid as occurs in kidney failure, some of the excess H^+ enter cells in exchange for the movement of potassium ions out of the cell. This ion exchange is necessary to maintain the normal negative electrical charge in cells; however, it results in hyperkalemia. When metabolic acidosis is caused by accumulation of organics acids, such as lactic acid as occurs with hypoxia, or ketoacids, such as beta-hydroxybutyric acid as occurs in diabetic ketoacidosis, hyperkalemia is not caused by the acidosis. That is because both the H^+ and the anion that forms when the organic acid dissociates can enter cells, for example, H^+ and lactate from lactic acid. When both a positive and a negative charge enter the cell, the intracellular charge is not changed, and potassium efflux is not required. In metabolic alkalosis, H^+ ions move out of cells into the extracellular fluid in exchange for the movement of potassium into cells, resulting in hypokalemia. In respiratory acid–base imbalances, which involve changes in CO_2 levels, there is usually only a slight change in serum potassium levels. In acidosis, there is an increase in serum phosphate because glycolysis is depressed during acidosis, and there is decreased utilization of phosphate in metabolic reactions. As was explained in the discussion of the effects of acidosis and alkalosis on neuromuscular function, the free, ionized calcium level is increased in acidosis and decreased in alkalosis.

Effects of Acidosis and Alkalosis on Metabolism

Activity of the enzyme phosphofructokinase is depressed as a result of acidosis, which impairs glycolysis and ATP production. Decreased availability of ATP as an energy source contributes to weakness and fatigue during acidosis. By contrast, there is increased activity of phosphofructokinase in alkalosis, which stimulates glycolysis, resulting in increased use of phosphate.

Effects of Acidosis and Alkalosis on Oxygenation

The hemoglobin–oxygen dissociation curve shifts to the right in acidosis, as shown in **Figure 9.11** ■, because of decreased affinity of hemoglobin for oxygen and increased unloading of oxygen to cells, which can be beneficial in acidosis.[5] In alkalosis, the hemoglobin–oxygen curve shifts to the left, as shown in Figure 9.11, because of increased affinity of hemoglobin for oxygen, resulting in decreased unloading of oxygen to cells.[5] This decrease in cellular oxygenation contributes to the adverse effects of alkalosis. The effects of acidosis and alkalosis are summarized in **Table 9.4** ■.

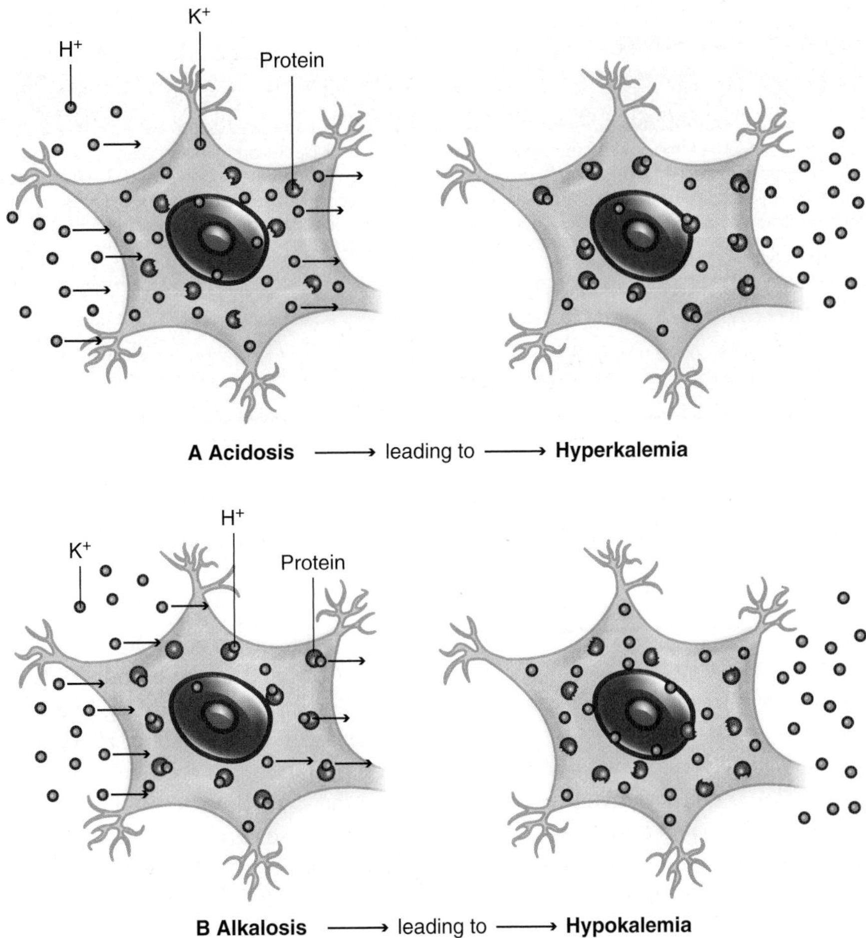

Figure 9.10 ■ The relationship between acid–base imbalances and potassium imbalances. Potassium diffuses out of cells in states of respiratory acidosis and metabolic acidosis associated with accumulation of inorganic acids. In metabolic acidosis caused by accumulation of organic acids, both the H^+ and the anion from the dissociated acid can diffuse into cells; therefore, K^+ exit from the cell is not needed to maintain the electrical charge in the cell.

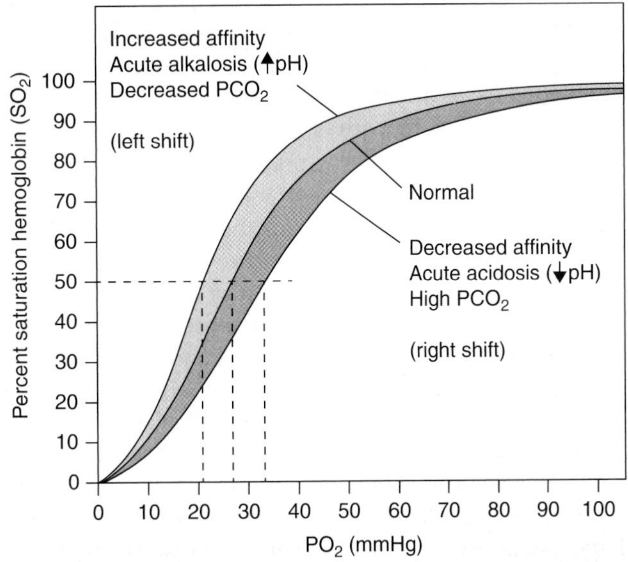

Figure 9.11 ■ Effects of acidosis and alkalosis on the oxyhemoglobin dissociation curve. The graph shows the relationship between changes in PO_2 (partial pressure of oxygen) and SO_2 (saturation of hemoglobin with oxygen). The line in the middle represents the normal hemoglobin saturation with oxygen at various PO_2 levels. In acidosis, the curve shifts to the right of normal, so at any given PO_2 value, the SO_2 is less than normal because of decreased affinity of hemoglobin for oxygen and easier unloading of oxygen to tissues. In alkalosis, the hemoglobin–oxygen curve shifts to the left because of increased affinity of hemoglobin for oxygen, resulting in decreased unloading of oxygen to cells.

Table 9.4 Effects of Acidosis and Alkalosis

Physiologic Function	Effects of Acidosis	Effects of Alkalosis
Electrolyte balance	• Increased amount of free, ionized (non–protein-bound) calcium due to increased H^+ binding to proteins • Hyperkalemia due to movement of potassium out of cells in exchange for entry of H^+ into cells	• Decreased amount of free, ionized (non–protein-bound) calcium due to decreased H^+ binding to proteins. • Hypokalemia due to movement of potassium into cells in exchange for movement of H^+ out of cells
Neuromuscular activity	• Decreased neuromuscular excitability due to increased level of free calcium blocking sodium channels	• Increased neuromuscular excitability due to decreased level of free calcium blocking sodium channels
Metabolism	• Impaired glycolysis resulting in decreased ATP production	• Increased glycolysis and utilization of phosphate
Oxygenation	• Decreased affinity between hemoglobin and oxygen resulting in increased unloading of oxygen to cells	• Increased affinity between hemoglobin and oxygen resulting in decreased unloading of oxygen to cells
Perfusion	• Decreased cardiac contractility • Vasodilation resulting in hypotension	• Increased cardiac contractility up to arterial pH of 7.70 and decreased contractility with pH above 7.70 • Vasoconstriction with pH above 7.65
CNS (neural regulation)	• Increased intracranial pressure due to vasodilation resulting in increased cerebral blood volume	• Impaired cerebral oxygenation due to decreased cerebral blood flow caused by vasoconstriction and decreased unloading of oxygen from hemoglobin

Check Your Progress: Section 9.5

1. Explain how metabolic alkalosis might manifest clinically by numbness and tingling.
2. The blood work of a patient with metabolic acidosis indicates a rise in potassium level above normal (5.8 mEq/L). As the nurse, how would you explain the change in electrolyte to a student nurse shadowing you?

9.6 Laboratory Tests Used in Assessment of Acid–Base Status

Laboratory tests used in the assessment of acid–base status include arterial blood gases, venous blood gases, the base excess, and the anion gap. These laboratory tests, along with assessment of the patient's risk factors for a particular type of acid–base imbalance and their clinical manifestations, are used in the detection of acid–base imbalances and identification of the underlying cause of the imbalance.

Arterial Blood Gases

Arterial blood gases (ABGs) are the measure of the pH, $PaCO_2$, PaO_2, and bicarbonate in the arterial blood. The parameters included in the ABGs provide information about gases that are dissolved in the blood ($PaCO_2$ and PaO_2) as well as other substances, including pH and bicarbonate. The normal range for the pH of arterial blood is 7.35–7.45. Remember that the lower the pH, the higher is the H^+ concentration. An arterial pH below 7.35 indicates acidosis, and a pH above 7.45 indicates alkalosis. In clinical settings, the terms *acidosis* and *acidemia* and the terms *alkalosis* and *alkalemia* are often used interchangeably; however, they do not have the exact same meanings. *Acidosis* refers to the pathophysiologic process resulting in an excess amount of H^+ in the body. *Acidemia* refers to a state of excess H^+ and base deficit (low pH) in the blood. *Alkalosis* refers to the pathophysiologic process resulting in a deficit of H^+ in the body. *Alkalemia* refers to a state of H^+ deficit and base excess (elevated pH) in the blood. Acidosis and alkalosis can be present at the same time because an individual can have two or more processes present at the same time that are driving the pH in opposite directions. For example, a person could have respiratory alkalosis due to anxiety and metabolic acidosis due to lactic acidosis. Respiratory alkalosis will decrease the level of carbon dioxide (and thus carbonic acid) and raise the pH, while the lactic acidosis will increase the H^+ concentration and lower the pH. The resultant pH of the blood can be either high or low, depending on which process is more severe, or the pH could be within the normal range if the two opposing acid–base imbalances are pulling the pH in opposite directions to a similar degree. That is why you cannot assume that a patient's acid–base status is normal just because the pH is within the normal range.

The partial pressure of carbon dioxide in the arterial blood ($PaCO_2$) is the pressure exerted by carbon dioxide dissolved in the plasma in arterial blood. The normal range for the $PaCO_2$ in arterial blood is 35–45 mmHg. Carbonic acid levels change in the same direction as the $PaCO_2$ because 3% of carbon dioxide dissolved in plasma combines with water to form carbonic acid. When the pH is below normal and the $PaCO_2$ is increased, it indicates respiratory acidosis. When the pH is above normal and the $PaCO_2$ is decreased, it indicates respiratory alkalosis. The $PaCO_2$ can also be increased or decreased if the lungs are compensating for a metabolic acid–base imbalance. Whether a change in $PaCO_2$ is due to the primary respiratory acid–base imbalance or a result of respiratory compensation for a metabolic imbalance can be determined by looking at both the pH and the $PaCO_2$ level. For example, if the pH is low as a result of metabolic acidosis, the lungs compensate by decreasing the $PaCO_2$. In that case, a low $PaCO_2$ level, which also means a low carbonic acid level, could not be the cause of the low pH; it must therefore be a compensatory change.

Bicarbonate HCO_3^- is a base with the normal range of 22–26 mEq/L in arterial blood. Its level is primarily regulated by the kidneys, as was explained in the discussion of compensation. When the pH is below normal and the HCO_3^- is decreased, it indicates metabolic acidosis. When the pH is above normal and the HCO_3^- is increased, metabolic alkalosis is indicated. The HCO_3^- can also be increased or decreased, if the kidneys are compensating for a respiratory acid–base imbalance. Whether a change in HCO_3^- is due to a primary metabolic acid–base imbalance or a result of renal compensation for a respiratory imbalance can be determined by looking at both the pH and the HCO_3^- level. For example, if the pH is low as a result of respiratory acidosis, the kidneys compensate by increasing the serum HCO_3^- level. In that case, the increased HCO_3^- level could not be the cause of the low pH because HCO_3^- is a base; therefore, the increased HCO_3^- must be a compensatory change.

Some clinical laboratories report the **total CO_2 (TCO_2)** rather than the bicarbonate level. The TCO_2 is slightly higher than the bicarbonate level because it is a measure of carbon dioxide in the form of HCO_3^- ions, H_2CO_3, and CO_2 attached to proteins such as hemoglobin, as well as the CO_2 dissolved in plasma (**Figure 9.12** ■). Approximately 90% of the total CO_2 consists of CO_2 in the form of HCO_3^- ions. To determine the TCO_2, acid is added to a blood sample, which causes CO_2 gas to be liberated from these sources and measured. The normal value for the TCO_2 is 23–29 mmol/L.

The partial pressure of oxygen in arterial blood (PaO_2) represents the pressure of oxygen molecules dissolved in the plasma in arterial blood. Although the PaO_2 does not provide the direct information about acid–base status that the $PaCO_2$ and bicarbonate levels do, it is included in the ABG report because it provides information about the ability of the lungs to oxygenate the blood. The PaO_2 can help to point to the cause if acidosis is present; for example, lactic acidosis is likely present as a result of anaerobic metabolism if the PaO_2 is very low. The normal range for the PaO_2 in older children and adults, other than older adults, is 80–100 mmHg. The normal range for the PaO_2 is lower in newborns, at 60–70 mmHg.

Because of the physiologic alterations that occur with aging, older adults, even those without lung disease, usually have a PaO_2 value lower than that in younger adults. The equation for calculating the expected PaO_2 value in older adults is $PaO_2 = 100-(\text{age} \times 0.3)$. Therefore, for example, an 80-year-old adult would be expected have a PaO_2 of 76 mmHg. ■

Approximately 3% of carbon dioxide in body fluids combines with water to form carbonic acid (H_2CO_3). Laboratories usually do not measure or report the H_2CO_3 because it can be easily calculated by multiplying $PCO_2 \times 0.03$. The normal range for H_2CO_3 is 1.05–1.35 mEq/L.

Venous Blood Gases

Venous blood gases are a measure of the pH, $PaCO_2$, PaO_2, and bicarbonate in the venous blood. Arterial blood has long been used as the gold standard in the assessment of acid–base balance. However, venous blood is increasingly being used to assess acid–base status for the following reasons: Several research studies have shown that venous blood can substitute for arterial blood in some circumstances with

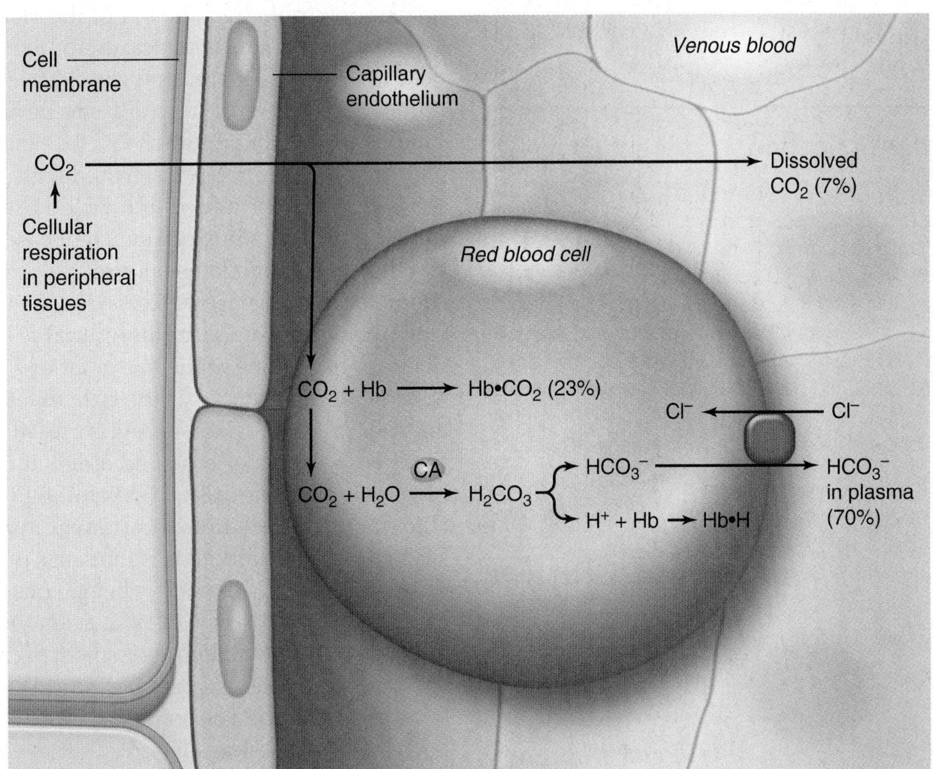

Figure 9.12 ■ Forms of carbon dioxide in the blood.

lower risk of complications, and in states of cardiovascular collapse, venous blood provides better information than arterial blood about acid–base status at the cellular level. There are several advantages to the use of venous blood for determination of pH and bicarbonate. A venipuncture causes less pain than an arterial puncture, which needs to be done if the patient does not have an indwelling arterial line, because more force is needed to puncture an artery.[17] There is also a lower risk of bleeding, aneurysm or hematoma formation, and thrombosis and blood vessel spasm resulting in tissue ischemia with a venipuncture compared to an arterial puncture.[18] To use venous blood as a substitute for arterial blood in the assessment of acid–base status, venous blood must accurately reflect changes that are occurring simultaneously in the arterial blood of the individual. Several research studies have shown a high degree of correlation between arterial and venous pH, bicarbonate, and base excess in patients with a variety of acute and chronic respiratory and metabolic disorders who were in emergency departments or critical care units.[17–21] Normal values of venous blood gases are shown in **Table 9.5** ■.

Arterial and venous blood gases do not always provide the same information. Venous blood gas values are a better indicator of what is occurring at the cellular level; arterial blood gas values reflect primarily what the lungs have added to or removed from the blood.[22] In conditions of circulatory collapse, there can be marked differences and poor correlation between arterial and venous blood gas values. For that reason, venous blood gases are sometimes measured in addition to arterial blood gases during cardiopulmonary resuscitation. Because of medications administered into the arterial system and mechanical ventilation, arterial blood gases may not show the severity of acid–base imbalances during cardiac arrest as well as do venous blood gases, which reflect cell activity.[5,7,23]

Sabrina Russell: Application

Ms. Russell's venous blood was sampled to assess her acid–base status. Her blood was sampled in an emergency department, and she did not have an arterial line in place. Therefore, if arterial blood gases were to be analyzed, an arterial puncture would have to be performed, which would be more painful and associated with the risk of more complications than would be the case for a venous puncture. Research has shown that venous blood pH and HCO_3^- are comparable to those variables measured in arterial blood in patients with diabetic ketoacidosis, which was Ms. Russell's diagnosis.

3. Why was venous blood used rather than arterial blood to assess Ms. Russell's acid–base status?
4. How does the pulmonary system compensate for metabolic acidosis?
5. Diabetic ketoacidosis is an example of what kind of acid–base disorder?

Base Excess

The **base excess (BE)** is a measure of all bases in the blood, including bicarbonate, phosphate, and proteins such as albumin and hemoglobin. Although it is called the base excess, this laboratory test detects either a base excess or a base deficit. Since the bicarbonate level is measured in the base excess, the base excess and bicarbonate level usually change in the same direction. Some clinical laboratories report the bicarbonate level; others report the base excess. Either can be used in the assessment of acid–base status.

The presence of a base excess or a base deficit is determined by the amount of acid or base that needs to be added to 1 liter of blood to titrate the blood pH to 7.40. Actually only a few milliliters of blood are removed from the patient and tested, and the amount of acid or base that has to be added to one liter of blood is calculated. In this test, the blood sample is exposed to a PCO_2 of 40 mmHg so that any respiratory condition that may have been present in the patient does not affect the pH of the blood sample. Therefore, the base excess is a measure of the metabolic component of acid–base status and is not affected by respiratory buffering. If nonvolatile acid has to be added to the blood sample to bring the pH down to 7.40, it indicates an excess of base, and the amount is designated with a positive number. If base needs to be added to the blood sample to bring the pH up to 7.40, it indicates a deficit of base and is designated by a negative number. The normal value for the base excess should be zero, that is, no excess or deficit of base. However, since the normal range for the arterial pH is 7.35–7.45 and it does not have to be at the midpoint of 7.40, as used in this test, the normal range for the base excess is between −2.0 and +2.0 mEq/L. A base excess is present in states in which there is an excess of base and a deficit of H^+ as occurs in metabolic alkalosis caused by vomiting with loss of hydrochloric acid. A base deficit is present in metabolic acidosis when a loss of bicarbonate is the cause of the metabolic acidosis or when bicarbonate is being consumed in buffering H^+ from fixed acids such as lactic acid or ketoacids. The base excess test is often used in assessment of critically ill patients with metabolic acidosis because the pH might not reflect the severity of the acidosis because the pH is brought partially back to normal as a result of respiratory compensation.[24]

When the kidneys add the base bicarbonate to the blood as compensation for respiratory acidosis, there will

Table 9.5 Normal Ranges for Arterial and Venous Blood Acid–Base Parameters

Acid–Base Parameter	Arterial Blood	Peripheral Venous Blood
pH	Adult and child: 7.35–7.45 Newborn: 7.32–7.49 2 months to 2 years: 7.34–7.46	7.32–7.38
PCO_2	Adult and child: 35–45 mmHg Under 2 years: 26–41 mmHg	40–50 mmHg
TCO_2	Adult and child: 23–29 mmol/L	23–30 mmol/L
HCO_3^-	Adult and child: 22–26 mEq/L Newborn: 22–30 mEq/L	21–22 mEq/L
PO_2	Adult and child: 80–100 mmHg Newborn: 60–70 mmHg	40–50 mmHg
BE	−2.0 to +2.0 mEq/L	−2.0 to +2.0 mEq/L

Impact of Current Research on Clinical Practice

Use of Venous Blood in the Assessment of Acid–Base Status

Description: Byrne and colleagues conducted a systematic review of the literature for research studies published up to December 2012 that compared peripheral venous blood gas with arterial blood gas analysis in individuals over the age of 16. A meta-analysis of the 18 studies found was conducted. A meta-analysis is a statistical method for combining the results of many research studies to identify trends in and increase the power of the results. There were a total of 1,768 patients in the studies with a variety of conditions in various clinical settings. The meta-analysis found that pH obtained from peripheral venous blood compared well with that of arterial blood, the arterial blood pH typically being 0.03 pH unit higher than that of venous blood. There was too much variation between arterial and venous blood PCO_2 for them to be considered comparable. As was expected, there was a significant difference between the PO_2 values in arterial and venous blood, the PO_2 of arterial blood typically being about 40 mmHg higher than that of venous blood.

Clinical Practice: The results of this study support the use of peripheral venous blood samples in many clinical situations to assess pH in individuals over the age of 16, thereby eliminating exposure to the pain and risk of complications associated with an arterial puncture. Because of the large difference in PO_2 between arterial and venous blood even in healthy individuals, venous blood cannot be used as a substitute for arterial blood to determine PO_2. However, arterial blood sampling to assess PaO_2 is not always necessary because pulse oximetry allows for noninvasive assessment of oxygenation by measurement of hemoglobin saturation with oxygen. The study did not include pediatric patients or those with circulatory collapse, and the results cannot be generalized to those populations.

Research Study:

Byrne, A., Bennet, M., Chatterji, R., et al. (2014). Peripheral venous and arterial blood gas analysis in adults: Are they comparable? A systematic review and meta-analysis. *Respirology, 19*, 168–175.

be a base excess; when the kidneys are compensating for respiratory alkalosis by eliminating more bicarbonate in the urine, there will be a base deficit. If a metabolic acid–base imbalance can cause a base excess or a base deficit and renal compensation for a respiratory imbalance can also cause a base excess or base deficit, how can you know whether an alteration in the base excess is due to a primary metabolic acid–base imbalance or to renal compensation for a respiratory imbalance? The answer is that you need to look at the pH and the $PaCO_2$ as well as the base excess. For example, if the pH is below normal, the $PaCO_2$ is normal or below normal depending on whether respiratory compensation is present, and there is a base deficit (negative BE value), these conditions indicate the presence of metabolic acidosis. On the other hand, if the pH is above normal, the $PaCO_2$ is below normal, and there is a base deficit (negative BE value), these conditions indicate respiratory alkalosis with renal compensation (kidneys excreting more bicarbonate to compensate for the deficit of carbonic acid).

Anion Gap

The **anion gap** is used in the assessment of acid–base imbalances when the type of imbalance is not clear from the patient's history and blood gases and to assist in differentiating the cause of metabolic acidosis due to accumulation of fixed acids from metabolic acidosis due to bicarbonate deficit.[25–27] It is also helpful in determining whether a mixed acid–base imbalance is present. The pH is not always decreased when there is acidosis if another imbalance causing alkalosis is also present. So the anion gap can detect acidosis even if the pH is within the normal range.

The anion gap is based on the principle of electroneutrality of extracellular fluid. That is, the sum of the concentration of cations in the extracellular fluid equals the sum of the concentration of the anions. Because sodium (Na^+) is the most abundant cation in extracellular fluid and chloride (Cl^-) and bicarbonate (HCO_3^-) are the most abundant anions, they are used to simplify calculation of the anion gap and are referred to as the measured cations and anions.

$$\text{Anion gap} = Na^+ - (Cl^- + HCO_3^-).$$

The sum of the anions $Cl^- + HCO_3^-$ is less than the Na^+ concentration. As can be seen in the bar graph in **Figure 9.13**, this difference (i.e., the anion gap) consists of the unmeasured anions, and the sum of the concentration of all the cations is equal to the sum of the concentration of all the anions. The normal range for the anion gap is often considered to be 8–16 mEq/L, with 12 as the midpoint.

CLINICAL POINT: If you look only at the anion gap and do not take into consideration the patient's albumin level, you can miss the presence of acidosis. Albumin, which is an anion, makes up part of the anion gap. So if a patient has a low albumin level (hypoalbuminemia), a common finding in critically ill patients, the anion gap will be lower than normal. Each decrease in serum albumin by 1 g/dL (from the normal of 4.5 g/dL) decreases the anion gap by 2.5 mEq/L.[25,26] If the patient with hypoalbuminemia then becomes hypoxic and lactic acidosis develops, for example, the accumulation of lactate anions increases the anion gap back to normal. The normal anion gap in this case could cause the clinician to misdiagnose the cause of the patient's problems. To correct the anion gap for low albumin levels, the adjusted anion gap is calculated by using the following equation: Adjusted anion gap = observed anion gap + 2.5 × (normal albumin in g/dL − observed albumin in grams per deciliter). If the albumin is given in grams per liter, multiply by 0.25 instead of 2.5. The value for the adjusted anion gap should be normal if the anion gap is altered only as a result of a low albumin level.

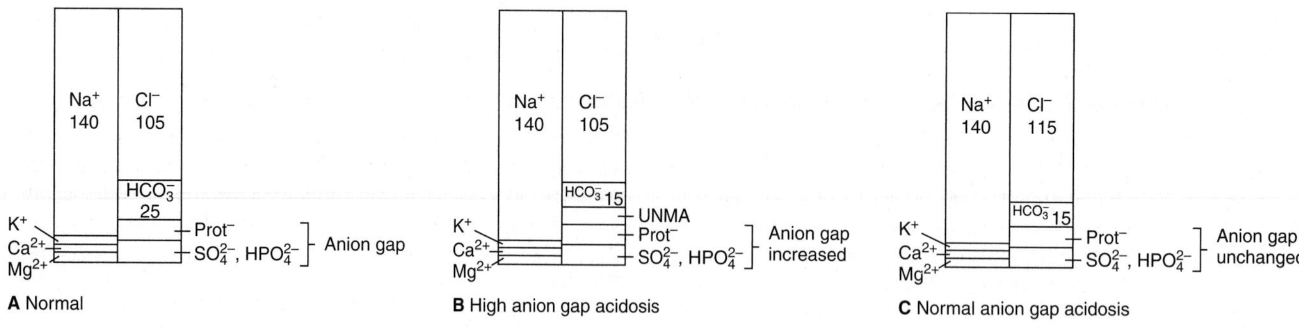

Figure 9.13 ■ Normal and elevated anion gap metabolic acidosis.

Lactic acidosis, ketoacidosis, and renal failure are the most common causes of a high anion gap metabolic acidosis. These conditions are all associated with an increased production or accumulation of nonvolatile acids. The anion gap becomes elevated when these nonvolatile acids dissociate, releasing an H^+ and an anion (see Figure 9.13). For example, when lactic acid dissociates, the lactate anion (lactate$^-$) and an H^+ are released. Anions released in various conditions are listed in **Table 9.6** ■.

Metabolic acidosis can occur with a normal anion gap, as shown in Figure 9.13. In this situation, the chloride level is increased (hyperchloremia), and the base HCO_3^- level is below normal. There is a reciprocal relationship between the two anions chloride and HCO_3^-; that is, if one goes up, there will be increased excretion of the other to maintain electrical neutrality in the extracellular fluid. If the chloride level increases, for example from administration of chloride in intravenous solutions, the kidneys will eventually decrease the HCO_3^- level, resulting in a hyperchloremic metabolic acidosis, which is a type of normal anion gap metabolic acidosis.

Table 9.6 Anions Produced from Nonvolatile (Fixed) Acids

Condition	Acids That Accumulate	Anions Produced When the Acid Dissociates
Lactic acidosis	Lactic acid	Lactate$^-$
Diabetic ketoacidosis	Acetoacetic acid and beta-hydroxybutyric acid	Acetoacetate$^-$ and beta-hydroxybutyrate$^-$
Kidney failure	Sulfuric acid, phosphoric acid, and uric acid	Sulfate$^-$, phosphate$^-$, and urate$^-$
Salicylate poisoning (e.g., aspirin overdose)	Salicylic acid and lactic acid	Salicylate$^-$ and lactate$^-$
Ethylene glycol poisoning	Glycolic acid, glycoxylic acid, and oxalic acid	Glycolate$^-$, glycoxylate$^-$, and oxalate$^-$
Methanol poisoning	Formic acid	Formate$^-$

Check Your Progress: Section 9.6

1. Base excess implies what change in acid–base balance?
2. What anion is excreted in exchange for bicarbonate (HCO_3^-)?

9.7 Respiratory Acidosis

Respiratory acidosis is a state of elevated CO_2 (hypercapnia) and H_2CO_3 and decreased blood pH. Hypercapnia results in increased H_2CO_3 levels because 3% of carbon dioxide dissolved in body fluids combines with water to form H_2CO_3. The increase in H_2CO_3 decreases the pH of the arterial blood below 7.35 and the venous blood below 7.32 and decreases the ratio of bicarbonate to carbonic acid below 20:1.

Etiology and Pathogenesis

Respiratory acidosis is caused by conditions that impair alveolar ventilation or diffusion of carbon dioxide from the blood into the alveoli in the lungs and conditions in which there is increased production of carbon dioxide without an increase in ventilation to eliminate the excess carbon dioxide (**Table 9.7** ■). Conditions that cause respiratory acidosis are either acute conditions, such as pneumonia, acute asthma exacerbation, and acute respiratory distress syndrome, or chronic conditions, such as emphysema and chronic bronchitis. The differentiation between acute and chronic respiratory acidosis is based on whether or not the kidneys have had time to compensate for the acidosis, as evidenced by the expected increase in serum bicarbonate levels. Acute respiratory acidosis is present before renal compensation. Chronic respiratory acidosis is present after renal compensation is complete (usually beyond 48 hours after the initiation of hypercapnia). Individuals who have compensated respiratory acidosis due to a chronic condition can develop an acute condition that exacerbates the respiratory acidosis. A brief description of some of the conditions that cause respiratory acidosis is provided here. More detail about these conditions is provided in Chapters 17 through 20.

Decreased Central Drive to Breathe. Breathing is regulated by a complex interaction of neural centers in the brainstem that receive input from higher brain centers and peripheral chemoreceptors and send neural signals out to the muscles of respiration. A variety of factors can interfere with the regulation of breathing, resulting in hypoventilation, hypercapnia, and respiratory acidosis. Examples of medications acting on the CNS that can impair the central drive to breathe are general anesthetics, barbiturates, and opioid analgesics such as morphine and codeine. These medications are not likely to cause respiratory depression

Table 9.7 Causes of Respiratory Acidosis

Cause	Examples
Decreased central drive to breathe	• Drug-induced respiratory depression (e.g., opioids, barbiturates, alcohol) • Increased intracranial pressure • Central sleep apnea • Prolonged apnea associated with prematurity
Lung parenchymal disorders	• Restrictive lung disorders (e.g., atelectasis, pulmonary fibrosis, pleural effusion) • Obstructive lung disorders (e.g., emphysema, asthma, cystic fibrosis, chronic bronchitis) • Lung cancer • Pulmonary edema • Pneumonia • Infant respiratory distress syndrome • Acute lung injury and acute respiratory distress syndrome
Upper airway obstruction	• Aspiration of a foreign object into the trachea • Laryngospasm
Disorders affecting the chest wall or muscles of respiration	• Chest trauma • Phrenic nerve injury • Myasthenia gravis (autoimmune destruction of acetylcholine receptors on skeletal muscles) • Guillain-Barré syndrome (inflammatory condition of nerves that innervate skeletal muscles) • Kyphoscoliosis (combination of kyphosis, which is a flexion curvature of the vertebral column resulting in a humpback shape, and scoliosis, which is a lateral curvature of the vertebral column) • Severe hypokalemia • Severe hypophosphatemia

when used properly in the therapeutic dose range. However, the respiratory depressant effect is dose dependent; that is, the higher the amount of the medication in the body, the more likely that respiratory depression will occur. Respiratory depressant effects are additive, which means that if a person is taking more than one substance that can depress the respiratory center, such as alcohol and a barbiturate, a lower amount of each drug in combination could cause respiratory depression compared to the amount needed if that drug were used alone. Additional conditions associated with a decreased central drive to breathe are increased intracranial pressure compressing the brainstem resulting from a brain tumor or head trauma, periods of cessation of breathing due to prolonged sleep apnea or apnea occurring in premature newborns, and cardiopulmonary arrest.

Lung Tissue and Neuromuscular Disorders. Disorders that restrict lung expansion, such as atelectasis and pulmonary fibrosis, and disorders that obstruct airflow, such as asthma or cystic fibrosis, are common causes of respiratory acidosis. Neurologic or muscular disorders that affect the nerves or muscles involved in breathing cause impaired ventilation even if the lung tissue itself is normal. The skeletal muscles that are normally involved in breathing are the diaphragm, the intercostal muscles between the ribs, and, to a lesser extent, the abdominal muscles. Any disease process that impairs innervation or contractility of these muscles, such as phrenic nerve injury or myasthenia gravis, can cause hypoventilation severe enough to result in respiratory acidosis. Obesity and abdominal distention due to fluid accumulation in the abdominal cavity limit the ability of the diaphragm to contract and move downward during inspiration, resulting in restriction of lung expansion.

Electrolyte Imbalances. Severe hypokalemia causes respiratory acidosis because low potassium in the extracellular fluid causes some potassium to move out of cells, leaving the charge inside the cell more negative and farther from its threshold potential. Therefore, muscles involved in breathing such as the diaphragm will have decreased contractility, leading to hypoventilation. With severe hypophosphatemia there is decreased availability of phosphate, which is needed for synthesis of adenosine triphosphate which is the energy source for muscle contraction. Therefore, a severe phosphate deficiency also leads to decreased contractility of muscles of respiration leading to respiratory acidosis.

Increased CO_2 Production without Increased CO_2 Elimination. High fevers, seizures, sepsis, and thyrotoxicosis are examples of conditions associated with increased body temperature, which increases the metabolic rate and production of CO_2 as a by-product. Overfeeding with carbohydrates generates a large amount of CO_2. If increased ventilation (an increased rate and/or depth of breathing) does not occur along with the increased production of CO_2, then excessive amounts of H_2CO_3 will be formed, resulting in respiratory acidosis.

Permissive Hypercapnia. Permissive hypercapnia is an increase in $PaCO_2$ that is allowed to develop in patients who are being treated with mechanical ventilation with low tidal volumes.[28] Mechanical ventilation with a low tidal volume of 6 mL/kg body weight, for example, is a lung protective ventilation strategy because it does not cause the degree of alveolar overdistention, alveolar rupture, and lung inflammation associated with ventilation with higher tidal volumes.[29] This low tidal volume ventilation can result in various degrees of hypercapnia and subsequent respiratory acidosis. Causes of permissive hypercapnia are summarized in **Table 9.8** ■.

Jordon Washington: Application

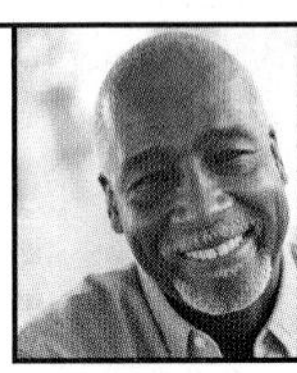

Mr. Washington's arterial pH of 7.24 indicates acidosis, and his elevated $PaCO_2$ of 68 mmHg indicates that it is of respiratory origin. His BE of +10 mEq/L is due to an increased amount of base HCO_3^-, most likely a reflection of renal compensation for his chronic lung disease that was present before he developed pneumonia. The fact that he developed an acute respiratory disease (pneumonia) that impairs gas exchange in the lungs even further caused his pH to fall to a very low level (7.24) and his $PaCO_2$ to become very high at 68 mmHg. Because of this and the presence of hypoxemia (PaO_2 55 mmHg), Mr. Washington has been hospitalized to treat the pneumonia and the respiratory acidosis. Because the pneumonia is of acute onset, his kidneys have not had time to add additional HCO_3^- to the blood to compensate for the additional CO_2 retention due to pneumonia.

3. What is COPD, and what are its signs and symptoms?
4. Explain how pneumonia infection affects alveolar gas exchange, thus contributing to hypoxemia.

Table 9.8 Causes of Permissive Hypercapnia

Causes	Examples
Limitation of diaphragm movement	• Obesity with decreased alveolar ventilation • Ascites (fluid accumulation in the abdominal cavity)
Increased CO_2 production without an increase in ventilation	• High fevers • Seizures • Sepsis • Thyrotoxicosis • Overfeeding with carbohydrates (produces large amount of CO_2)

Clinical Manifestations

The manifestations of respiratory acidosis include changes in blood gases, signs of compensation, and other manifestations of acidosis that are mainly the result of decreased neuromuscular excitability, as was explained in the previous section. Most conditions that cause CO_2 retention and respiratory acidosis also cause hypoxemia; therefore, manifestations of decreased blood oxygen and tissue hypoxia will likely also be present. There will also be manifestations of the underlying condition responsible for the respiratory acidosis, such as chest trauma or pneumonia. In uncompensated respiratory acidosis, the arterial blood pH is below 7.35, the $PaCO_2$ is increased above 45 mmHg, and the HCO_3^- and BE are within the normal range. As the kidneys compensate for respiratory acidosis by retaining more bicarbonate, the serum HCO_3^- level and BE increase, and the pH moves back up toward normal. The degree to which the serum HCO_3^- level is expected to increase as compensation for various changes in $PaCO_2$ in acute and chronic respiratory acidosis is shown in Table 9.2. As a sign of compensation, the urine becomes more acidic, owing to increased excretion of hydrogen ions and increased resorption of bicarbonate back into the blood.

Linking Pathophysiology to Diagnosis and Treatment

The diagnosis of respiratory acidosis is based on the patient's history of the presence of a condition that causes respiratory acidosis (see Table 9.7), manifestations of acidosis, and assessment of blood gases. Arterial blood will most likely be sampled instead of venous blood when respiratory acidosis is suspected in order to obtain information about the ability of the lungs to oxygenate the blood in addition to the pH and CO_2 level in the blood.

The best intervention to reverse respiratory acidosis is to improve ventilation in order to increase elimination of carbon dioxide, thereby decreasing the level of carbonic acid. Ventilation may need to be improved, for example by suctioning mucus out of the airway, removing edema fluid from the lungs by the use of diuretics to increase renal excretion of water, reversal of bronchospasm by the use of bronchodilator drugs, or intubating the patient's trachea and placing the patient on mechanical ventilation. Oxygen administration to reverse hypoxemia accompanying hypercapnia will not increase elimination of carbon dioxide. Administration of buffers, such as sodium bicarbonate, to increase the blood pH is generally contraindicated for treatment of patients with respiratory acidosis who are breathing on their own because as the buffer increases, the pH of the blood chemoreceptor stimulation of breathing diminishes, so less CO_2 is eliminated. Some physicians recommend the administration of sodium bicarbonate in cases of respiratory acidosis to attenuate adverse hemodynamic effects of acidosis for patients with severe acidosis ($pH < 7.1$) who are mechanically ventilated or for patients with coexisting renal failure who will not have renal compensation for their acidosis.[30]

Jordon Washington: Outcome

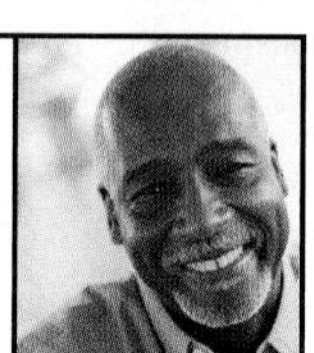

Mr. Washington's pneumonia is diagnosed with a chest x-ray and a sputum sample. The sputum sample is sent to the microbiology lab for a culture and sensitivity test to identify the causative microorganism and its sensitivity to antimicrobial medications. Mr. Washington responds well to treatment with oxygen therapy to reverse his hypoxemia and the appropriate antibiotic to treat his streptococcal pneumonia. After 4 days, he is discharged from the hospital with an appointment for a follow-up clinic visit in 2 weeks.

5. Considering Mr. Washington's history of COPD, what precaution will the nurse adhere to in administering oxygen as ordered?
6. What other medications have the potential to be used in managing Mr. Washington's pulmonary diseases?

Check Your Progress: Section 9.7

1. List three risk factors for respiratory acidosis.
2. Why is hypokalemia a risk factor for respiratory acidosis?

9.8 Respiratory Alkalosis

Respiratory alkalosis is a state of decreased CO_2 (hypocapnia) and carbonic acid and increased pH caused by hyperventilation. **Hyperventilation** is increased alveolar ventilation in excess of carbon dioxide production as a result of an increased rate and/or depth of breathing. Hypocapnia can be detected as below-normal levels of carbon dioxide in both arterial blood ($PaCO_2$) and venous blood ($PvCO_2$). The carbon dioxide deficit results in a deficit of carbonic acid, which elevates the pH of the arterial blood above 7.45 and increases the ratio of bicarbonate to carbonic acid above 20:1. On the other hand, the hypocapnia that occurs when the lungs compensate for metabolic acidosis functions to normalize the pH and does not result in respiratory alkalosis or an above-normal pH. The distinction between acute and chronic respiratory alkalosis is based on whether or not enough time has passed for renal compensation to occur. Acute respiratory alkalosis is the presence of hypocapnia before renal compensation. Chronic respiratory alkalosis is the presence of hypocapnia after renal compensation is complete (usually beyond 48 hours after the initiation of hypocapnia).

Etiology and Pathogenesis

Conditions that cause respiratory alkalosis stimulate the respiratory center in the brain either directly or indirectly, resulting in hyperventilation (**Table 9.9** ■). In conditions in which there is decreased oxygen delivery to the peripheral chemoreceptors in the aortic arch and the carotid arteries, such as in hypoxemia, in which the PaO_2 falls below 60 or 70 mmHg, or in severe hypotension, hypovolemia, or anemia, there is reflex activation of the respiratory center due to neural input from the peripheral chemoreceptors. This results in a reflex increase in ventilation as the body attempts to normalize the oxygen content in the blood; however, this also leads to excessive elimination of carbon dioxide, resulting in respiratory alkalosis. Hypoxemia is not the only cause of respiratory alkalosis in some lung diseases such as pulmonary fibrosis, pulmonary edema, and pulmonary embolism. Mechanoreceptors located in the chest wall, the airways, and interstitial tissue in the lung transmit neural signals into the respiratory center in the brain that cause reflex hyperventilation and respiratory alkalosis. For example, irritant receptors in the epithelial cell lining of the airways are stimulated by inhaled irritants and by airway inflammation. Pulmonary emboli and pulmonary edema cause a reflex hyperventilation resulting from pressure-induced activation of juxtacapillary receptors located between the pulmonary capillary and alveolar walls.

Respiratory alkalosis is also caused by stimulation of the respiratory center in the brainstem by emotions, accumulation of certain endogenous substances produced in the body, some medications, and brain lesions. A common cause of respiratory alkalosis is hyperventilation resulting from psychologic factors such as extreme emotional states of anxiety, fear, or anger. This occurs because areas of the cerebral cortex and limbic system, which are involved in emotions, have neural connections to the respiratory center in the brainstem. In some cases of extreme emotional upset, a person can hyperventilate to the point of unconsciousness, after which the respiratory pattern usually returns to normal. Increased levels of certain endogenous substances, such as ammonia and progesterone, stimulate the respiratory center. Respiratory alkalosis secondary to hyperventilation occurs in patients with liver failure; the factors that are thought to be involved are elevated levels of ammonia and progesterone resulting from the inability of the severely diseased liver to clear these substances from the blood. Both ammonia and progesterone stimulate the respiratory center in the brain.

Progesterone levels increase during pregnancy, the highest levels occurring during the third trimester. The progesterone-induced hyperventilation decreases the $PaCO_2$, with levels of 28–31 mmHg considered normal near the end of pregnancy. This decrease in $PaCO_2$ facilitates the transfer of CO_2 from the fetus to the mother's blood. Therefore, a $PaCO_2$ of 44, for example, indicates hypercapnia in a pregnant woman even though a $PaCO_2$ of 44 is within the normal range for a nonpregnant adult.[31] Does this mean that all women have an elevated pH in the third trimester of pregnancy? No, because the kidneys compensate for the chronic respiratory alkalosis by excreting more bicarbonate in the urine, which normalizes the pH. ■

A commonly used category of medication that stimulates the respiratory center when ingested in high amounts is salicylates, such as aspirin and methyl salicylate. In the brain, high amounts of salicylates uncouple oxidative phosphorylation, resulting in increased glucose utilization and carbon dioxide production, which stimulates the central chemoreceptors, resulting in respiratory alkalosis.[32] Brain tumors, ischemia, infections such as meningitis, or intracranial bleeding can cause hyperventilation due to irritation, increased temperature, or increased lactic acid production near the central chemoreceptors in the respiratory center.

Hypermetabolic states, as occur with fevers and hyperthyroidism, can cause hyperventilation, resulting in respiratory alkalosis. These conditions are associated with increased body temperature, increased metabolic rate, and increased production of carbon dioxide, all of which stimulate ventilation. The increased ventilation in states of increased body temperature serves as a way to lose heat in exhaled air. Several mechanisms are involved in respiratory alkalosis that develops in sepsis, which is a serious systemic infection. These mechanisms include hypoxemia and hypotension, which cause a reflex increase in alveolar ventilation, due to decreased delivery of oxygen to peripheral chemoreceptors, and fever, which activates the respiratory center in the brain.

Mechanical ventilation, which is used to treat severe hypoxemia, can cause respiratory alkalosis if the respiratory rate is set higher than that needed for normal elimination of carbon dioxide. Carbon dioxide is more soluble and more easily crosses the alveolar capillary membrane, so ventilator settings such as a high respiratory rate that might be needed to oxygenate the blood can cause excessive elimination of carbon dioxide, resulting in respiratory alkalosis.

Table 9.9 Causes of Respiratory Alkalosis

Causes	Examples
Stimulation of peripheral chemoreceptors	• Hypoxemia • Anemia • High altitude without acclimation
Stimulation of respiratory center in the brain (central chemoreceptors)	• Psychologic factors (e.g., anxiety, pain, fear, stress) • Fever • Brain lesions (e.g., head injury, tumors, stroke, infections) • Drugs (e.g., salicylates, nicotine) • Elevated level of endogenous substances (e.g., progesterone, ammonia)
Stimulation of pulmonary irritant, stretch, or juxtacapillary receptors	• Pulmonary embolism • Pulmonary edema • Pulmonary hypertension • Pulmonary fibrosis • Airway inflammation
Mechanical ventilation	• Inappropriate ventilator setting • Therapeutic induction of hypocapnia for treatment of increased intracranial pressure

Vivian Lee: Application

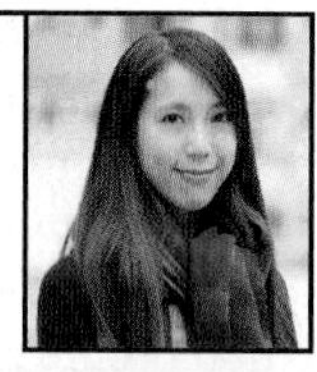

Ms. Lee is currently in an emergency department and has a pH of 7.56, indicating alkalosis. Her decreased $PaCO_2$ of 26 mmHg indicates that the alkalosis has a respiratory cause. The fact that Ms. Lee has a very rapid respiratory rate of 42 is another indicator of respiratory alkalosis. Her HCO_3^-, and BE values are normal because not enough time has elapsed for significant renal compensation to occur. Therefore, she has uncompensated respiratory alkalosis. After a few days, when her kidneys have had time to compensate, the HCO_3^- should increase above 28 mEq/L, and the pH should decrease and be at the high end of the normal range. However, Ms. Lee is receiving treatment in an emergency department for her panic attack, and the respiratory alkalosis will be corrected, making renal compensation unnecessary.

5. How does renal compensation for respiratory alkalosis result in a decrease in the HCO_3^- level?
6. Why was Ms. Lee diagnosed with uncompensated respiratory alkalosis?

Clinical Manifestations

The manifestations of respiratory alkalosis include changes in blood gases, signs of compensation, and other manifestations that are mainly the result of increased neuromuscular excitability. In uncompensated respiratory alkalosis, the arterial blood pH is above 7.45, the venous blood pH is above 7.38, the $PaCO_2$ is decreased below 35 mmHg, and the serum bicarbonate is within the normal range. As the kidneys compensate for respiratory alkalosis by excreting more bicarbonate, the serum bicarbonate level decreases, and the pH goes back down toward normal. The degree to which the serum bicarbonate level is expected to decrease as compensation for acute and chronic respiratory alkalosis is shown in Table 9.2. Clinical manifestations caused by the alkalosis were described in the section titled "Clinical Manifestations of Alkalosis." Remember that many of the clinical manifestations of respiratory alkalosis, including dizziness, paresthesias, tetany, and hyperactive reflexes, are the result of increased entry of sodium into nerve and muscle because of decreased levels of free, ionized calcium, which causes increased neuromuscular excitability. Acute onset of hypocapnia causes contraction of smooth muscle in cerebral arteries, resulting in dizziness and confusion due to decreased cerebral blood flow. The increased work associated with an increased rate and/or depth of breathing during respiratory alkalosis can be sensed by patients as an increased effort to breathe, causing dyspnea, which patients often express as shortness of breath or difficulty breathing. The clinical manifestations due to the alkalosis are more severe in acute respiratory alkalosis because in chronic respiratory alkalosis, renal compensation has returned the pH closer to normal. Manifestations of the underlying condition responsible for the respiratory alkalosis, such as pneumonia or salicylate overdose, will also be present.

CLINICAL POINT: It is important to recognize the presence of respiratory alkalosis not only in order to quickly intervene to normalize the pH but also because respiratory alkalosis could be occurring as a result of hypoxemia caused by a potentially life-threatening condition such as a pulmonary embolus or sepsis. ■

Linking Pathophysiology to Diagnosis and Treatment

The diagnosis of respiratory alkalosis is based on the patient's history of the presence of a condition that causes respiratory alkalosis (see Table 9.9), manifestations of alkalosis, and assessment of blood gases.

The preferred treatment for respiratory alkalosis is identification and treatment of the underlying cause. For example, if respiratory alkalosis is caused by hyperventilation as a reflex response to hypoxemia, therapy with supplemental oxygen as well as treatment of the cause of the hypoxemia is indicated. If hypoxemia is caused by a severe asthma attack, it is treated with a bronchodilator and supplemental oxygen. Hypoxemia caused by pneumonia is treated with an antimicrobial medication and supplemental oxygen. Respiratory alkalosis caused by excessive ventilation of a patient on mechanical ventilation can be reversed by decreasing the rate and/or tidal volume settings on the ventilator. For individuals who are prone to hyperventilate in response to anxiety or other strong emotions, providing a soothing environment, reassurance, and coaching the person to breathe more slowly are helpful in stopping the hyperventilation. Prevention of respiratory alkalosis in these patients can be achieved by teaching them to recognize the manifestations of hyperventilation and to breathe more slowly and regularly at its onset. These individuals also need assistance to recognize and cope with the situations that trigger them to hyperventilate. For extremely anxious and symptomatic patients, antianxiety medication may be necessary along with psychotherapy.

Rapid normalization of the carbon dioxide level can be accomplished by having the patient breathe into a closed system such as a mask with a carbon dioxide reservoir or a paper bag or even cupped hands held closed around the mouth and nose. This will cause the patient to rebreathe exhaled air containing more carbon dioxide than is in atmospheric air. Treatments that increase carbon dioxide in the inhaled air can quickly relieve symptoms of respiratory alkalosis, such as dizziness; however, they do not correct the underlying condition that is causing the hyperventilation. Rebreathing exhaled air is not the treatment of choice for patients with lung disease and hypoxemia because that could lower their blood oxygen levels more than it is already lowered as a result of the lung disease.

Calcium chloride or calcium gluconate can be used if tetany develops as a result of low levels of ionized calcium causing a severe increase in neuromuscular excitability. If respiratory alkalosis is severe enough to cause tetany secondary to increased neuromuscular activity, calcium can be administered in the form of calcium chloride (faster acting) or calcium gluconate (slower acting because the gluconate has to be metabolized to release the calcium). Remember that in alkalosis, more calcium is bound to protein, and there is less free, ionized calcium blocking sodium channels, resulting in increased neuromuscular activity.

Vivian Lee: Outcome

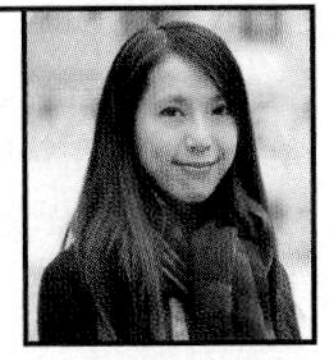

Ms. Lee's respiratory alkalosis, which was caused by a panic attack ,was treated with a face mask that forced her to rebreathe some of the CO_2 that she was exhaling at an excessive rate. The nurse encouraged Ms. Lee to breathe more slowly. A psychiatry consult was ordered to determine the circumstances related to her episode of extreme anxiety. After normalization of her blood gases, Ms. Lee was counseled to meet with her college academic advisor to discuss strategies related to time management and exam preparation in order to avoid the recurrence of a panic attack. She was then discharged to home.

7. Explain the link between Ms. Lee's hyperventilation and her dizziness.
8. How else can Ms. Lee manage her anxiety issue?

Check Your Progress: Section 9.8

1. Severe alkalosis is associated with tetany. This symptom can be explained to be as a result of decreased level of what?
2. How can use of antacids contribute to metabolic alkalosis?

9.9 Metabolic Acidosis

Metabolic acidosis is a state of H^+ excess, bicarbonate deficit, and decreased blood pH and a decreased ratio of bicarbonate to carbonic acid below 20:1 caused by accumulation of nonvolatile (fixed) acids or excessive loss of the base bicarbonate.

Etiology and Pathogenesis

There are two major categories of metabolic acidosis: elevated anion gap metabolic acidosis, which is caused by conditions that increase production or decrease elimination of fixed (nonvolatile) acids, and normal anion gap metabolic acidosis, which is caused by conditions that increase base bicarbonate losses from the body or conditions that decrease production or renal resorption of bicarbonate.

Causes of Elevated Anion Gap Metabolic Acidosis. The most common causes of elevated anion gap metabolic acidosis are lactic acidosis, diabetic and alcoholic ketoacidosis, renal failure, and certain poisons.

Lactic acidosis is a type of elevated anion gap metabolic acidosis. Type A lactic acidosis is caused by conditions that cause hypoxia, thereby decreasing oxygen availability to cells and resulting in anaerobic metabolism and accumulation of lactic acid. Type A lactic acidosis is due to conditions that cause an imbalance between oxygen demands and oxygen supply. Conditions such as seizures can cause hypoxia if the increased oxygen demand is not met by an increased oxygen supply. The causes of type B lactic acidosis are conditions other than hypoxia that result in increased levels of lactic acid. Causes of type B lactic acidosis include renal failure, salicylate poisoning, alcohol poisoning, and ingestion of certain medications.

Ketoacidosis is caused by abnormal lipid metabolism resulting in increased production of ketoacids such as acetoacetic acid and beta-hydroxybutyric acid. Ketoacidosis occurs in starvation as a result of increased metabolism of lipids mobilized from adipose tissue. Diabetic ketoacidosis is the result of a serious insulin deficiency or decreased cell responsiveness to insulin causing deranged metabolism of carbohydrates and lipids. Diabetic ketoacidosis is explained in more detail in Chapter 37. Alcoholic ketoacidosis results from excessive ingestion of beverages containing ethanol, such as beer, wine, vodka, and whiskey. Cases of accidental or intentional ethanol toxicity have also occurred from ingestion of solutions such as mouthwash that contain ethanol. Most of the ethanol ingested undergoes hepatic metabolism by the enzyme alcohol dehydrogenase to produce acetaldehyde. Acetaldehyde is then oxidized to acetyl coenzyme A, which enters the Krebs cycle (also known as the citric acid cycle or the tricarboxylic acid cycle) to produce fatty acids and ketones, the basis for alcoholic ketoacidosis.

Elevated anion gap metabolic acidosis present in acute and chronic renal failure is the result of decreased glomerular filtration rate impairing the excretion of the daily load of nonvolatile acids. Another factor contributing to acidosis in renal failure is decreased renal production of ammonia and thereby decreased ability to excrete H^+ buffered in the urine. Examples of substances ingested in poisonings that can cause increased anion gap metabolic acidosis are salicylates and ethylene glycol. Salicylates, such as aspirin, are one of the most extensively used medications worldwide. They are used therapeutically, by prescription or over the counter, for their antipyretic, anti-inflammatory, analgesic, and antiplatelet effects. They are a common cause of accidental and intentional poisonings.

Salicylates cross the placenta and are secreted into breast milk and can therefore result in fetal, neonatal, or infant poisoning if ingested in excess by a pregnant or lactating woman. ■

The highest mortality rate from salicylate overdose is among older adults who take a salicylate routinely for treatment of a medical condition, such as arthritis, and then take additional amounts or another product containing a salicylate to treat an acute problem, such as a cold or the flu. ■

An early effect of salicylate overdose is stimulation of the respiratory center in the brainstem, resulting in respiratory alkalosis. Many of the other clinical manifestations of salicylate overdose are due to their ability to inhibit cell enzymes, thereby impairing oxidative metabolism and ATP production; this results in accumulation of fixed acids such as lactic acid and ketoacids, thereby producing metabolic acidosis.

Ethylene glycol is an odorless, colorless, water-soluble alcohol that is a component in antifreeze and de-icing agents. It has a sweet taste and a CNS depressant effect similar to that caused by ethanol and is therefore a palatable substitute for ethanol. It is sometimes used by alcohol-dependent individuals because it is less expensive than ethanol or by those who are trying to hide their ingestion of ethanol. It has also been ingested intentionally in suicide attempts and accidentally by children. Metabolism of ethylene glycol, as with the other alcohols, occurs mainly in the liver by action of the enzyme alcohol dehydrogenase. Ethylene glycol is metabolized to glycoaldehyde, which is then further metabolized to glycolic acid, glycoxylic acid, and oxalic acid (**Figure 9.14** ■). It is these metabolites of ethylene glycol that are responsible for its toxicity by causing an increased anion gap metabolic acidosis. Methanol is another type of alcohol that is not intended for human consumption; however, when it is consumed, it is metabolized to formic acid, causing an increased anion gap metabolic acidosis.

A common cause of acidosis in the fetus is decreased perfusion of the placenta caused by maternal conditions such as hemorrhage, sepsis, or severe hypertension or compression of the umbilical cord.[33] The decreased placental blood flow causes hypoxia in the fetus, leading to anaerobic metabolism and accumulation of lactic acid, which results in elevated anion gap metabolic acidosis. Decreased perfusion of the placenta also results in accumulation of CO_2 in the fetus and increased production of carbonic acid, resulting in respiratory acidosis. ■

A way to help remember many causes of high anion gap metabolic acidosis is to remember the word **MULEPAK** because the letters in this word are the first letter of causes of high anion gap metabolic acidosis:

- Methanol
- Uremia (caused by renal failure)
- Lactic acidosis
- Ethylene glycol
- Paraldehyde (and other drugs)
- Aspirin (and other salicylates)
- Ketoacidosis.

Sabrina Russell: Application

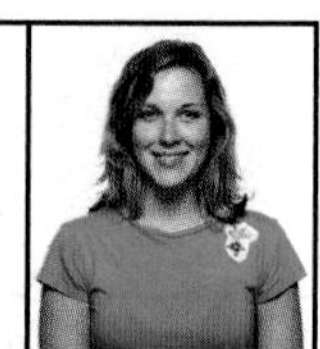

On the basis of Ms. Russell's history and clinical manifestations, she is diagnosed with diabetic ketoacidosis, a condition that causes acidosis; however, her pH is within the normal range. This is a situation in which calculating the anion gap can help to determine what is going on. Remember that the anion gap = $Na^+ - (Cl^- + HCO_3^-)$. On the basis of Ms. Russell's lab values, her anion gap = 148 − (86 + 22) = 40 mEq/L. That value indicates an elevated anion gap metabolic acidosis. Ms. Russell's pH is in the normal range, which did not indicate the acidosis present because she has also been vomiting, resulting in loss of gastric acid

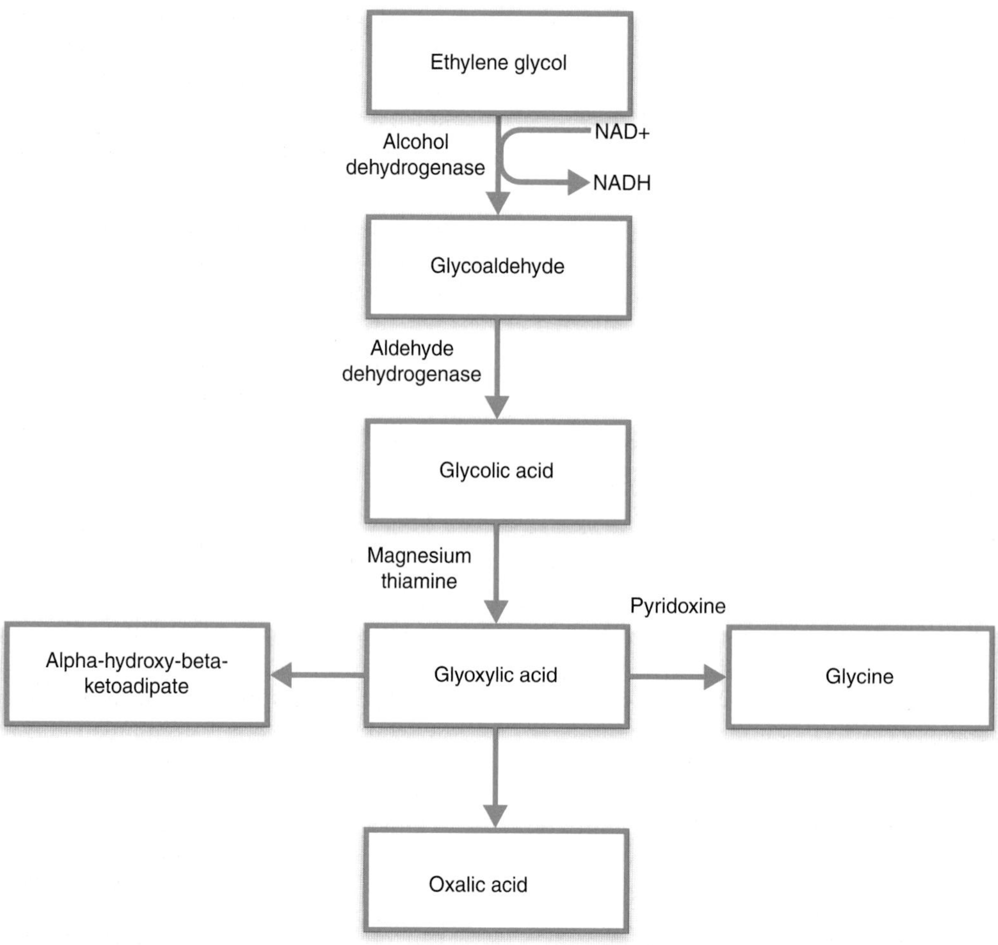

Figure 9.14 ■ Acid products of metabolism of ethylene glycol and methanol.

and metabolic alkalosis, which drove the pH up. The mechanisms involved in Ms. Russell's alkalosis are explained in the section on metabolic alkalosis.

6. Is it correct to say that Ms. Russell had a mixed metabolic acidosis and alkalosis? Justify your answer.
7. Ms. Russell had an anion gap of +40 mEq/L. What does an anion gap of −40 mEq/L imply?

Causes of Normal Anion Gap Metabolic Acidosis. Normal anion gap metabolic acidosis is caused by conditions associated with loss of HCO_3^--rich intestinal fluid or impaired HCO_3^- resorption in the kidneys. Intestinal fluid is rich in bicarbonate, and watery diarrhea or intestinal drainage results in HCO_3^- loss, which, when severe enough, causes metabolic acidosis. Increased renal loss of bicarbonate occurs with use of acetazolamide (Diamox), which is a medication that inhibits the enzyme carbonic anhydrase, thereby impairing renal resorption of bicarbonate. The function of carbonic anhydrase in renal regulation of HCO_3^- is explained in Figure 9.3. In **hyperchloremic metabolic acidosis**, increased chloride levels, for example secondary to administration of intravenous fluids containing chloride, can cause metabolic acidosis if the chloride accumulates because the increase in chloride results in increased renal excretion of HCO_3^-.

The basis for this is the reciprocal relationship between the anions chloride and HCO_3^-; that is, when chloride increases, bicarbonate decreases, owing to increased renal excretion to maintain electrical neutrality in the extracellular fluid (**Figure 9.15** ■). Different types of renal tubular acidosis cause metabolic acidosis. In type 1 (distal) renal tubular acidosis, there is a defect in the H^+ pump in the distal convoluted tubule in the nephrons, resulting in impaired ability to secrete H^+ ions into the urine. In type 2 (proximal) renal tubular acidosis, there is impaired resorption of bicarbonate in the proximal convoluted tubule. The causes of metabolic acidosis are summarized in **Table 9.10** ■.

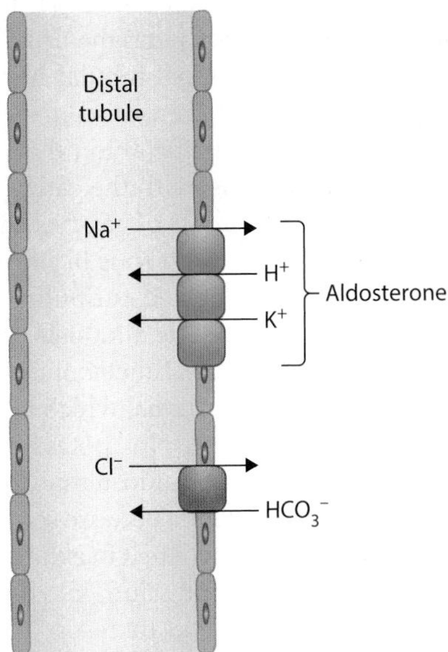

Figure 9.15 ■ Chloride and bicarbonate exchange in the renal tubules and effect of aldosterone on excretion of H^+. In the distal tubule and collecting duct, bicarbonate secretion into the urine is coupled to chloride resorption. Aldosterone causes sodium resorption in exchange for $H^+$and K^+secretion into the renal tubular lumen.

Clinical Manifestations

The manifestations of metabolic acidosis include changes in venous and arterial blood gases, signs of compensation, and other manifestations that are mainly the result of decreased neuromuscular excitability. In uncompensated metabolic acidosis, the arterial blood pH is below 7.35, the peripheral venous pH is below 7.32, the $PaCO_2$ is normal, and the serum bicarbonate is less than 22 mEq/L. Signs of compensation include increased rate and depth of breathing as the lungs eliminate more than the normal amount of carbon dioxide. Kussmaul respirations, which are very deep and rapid respirations, are present in more severe cases of metabolic acidosis. As the lungs compensate for metabolic acidosis by increased elimination of CO_2, the serum carbonic acid level decreases, and the pH moves back up toward normal. The degree to which the $PaCO_2$ level is expected to decrease as compensation for metabolic acidosis is shown in Table 9.2. Clinical manifestations caused by the acidosis were described earlier in the chapter. Many of the clinical manifestations of metabolic acidosis are due to decreased neuromuscular excitability. Manifestations of the underlying condition responsible for the metabolic acidosis, such as hyperkalemia, hypoxemia, or kidney failure, will also be present.

Linking Pathophysiology to Diagnosis and Treatment

The diagnosis of metabolic acidosis is based on the patient's history of the presence of a condition that causes metabolic acidosis (see Table 9.10), manifestations of acidosis, and assessment of blood gases.

If impaired perfusion of the fetus and subsequent hypoxia causing metabolic acidosis are suspected at the time of birth, umbilical cord blood is sampled to assess acid–base status immediately after delivery of the fetus in order to make decisions about care of the newborn.[2,34] ■

Metabolic acidosis is best treated by interventions that control the underlying cause of the acidosis. Some buffers that are used to increase plasma pH for treatment of metabolic acidosis generate various amounts of CO_2. That fact

Table 9.10 Causes of Metabolic Acidosis

Sign	Examples
Elevated anion gap	Lactic acidosis Ketoacidosis (diabetic, alcoholic) Renal failure Salicylate toxicity Ethylene glycol ingestion
Normal anion gap	Hyperchloremia Renal tubular acidosis Diarrhea Acetazolamide administration

needs to be taken into consideration in choosing a buffer to treat different causes of metabolic acidosis. Sodium bicarbonate is a buffer that was used in the past and is still used to a lesser degree to treat metabolic acidosis. Injection of sodium bicarbonate increases the pH of extracellular fluids, since it is a base. However, it does not readily enter cells and therefore does not increase the pHi and can even decrease it. The resultant intracellular acidosis impairs cell functions. If sodium bicarbonate is used to treat high anion gap metabolic acidosis, CO_2 is produced and easily enters cells, where it combines with water to form carbonic acid (H_2CO_3) in the following reaction:

$$\text{Lactate} + H^+ + NaHCO_3 \rightarrow \text{Na lactate} + H_2O + CO_2$$

Carbicarb is a buffer mixture of sodium bicarbonate and sodium carbonate (Na_2CO_3). Tham is a buffer that crosses cell membranes and therefore buffers intracellular fluid as well as extracellular fluid. Controversy still exists about the best buffer, timing of administration, and dosing to use in treatment of different causes of metabolic acidosis.

Check Your Progress: Section 9.9

1. Another definition of metabolic acidosis is deficiency of what?
2. Compensatory mechanisms help to modify acid–base changes but do not correct the cause. Explain.

9.10 Metabolic Alkalosis

Metabolic alkalosis is a state of H^+ deficit, bicarbonate excess, increased blood pH, and increased ratio of bicarbonate to carbonic acid above 20:1 caused by excessive loss of nonvolatile (fixed) acids or excessive accumulation of the base HCO_3^-.

Etiology and Pathogenesis

Metabolic alkalosis is caused by three types of conditions:

- Excessive loss of hydrogen ions
- Excessive intake of base
- Excessive renal retention of bicarbonate.

Metabolic alkalosis involves factors that initiate the alkalosis in the generation phase and factors that sustain the alkalosis in the maintenance phase. The generation and maintenance phases of metabolic alkalosis often overlap in time. The factor(s) that generate metabolic alkalosis may be the same as or different from the factor(s) that maintain metabolic alkalosis. Metabolic alkalosis is generated by an increased amount of bicarbonate in the extracellular fluid resulting from excessive loss of hydrogen ions from the extracellular fluid, increased intake of base, excessive renal retention of bicarbonate, or loss of extracellular fluid volume without comparable loss of bicarbonate (**contraction alkalosis**). Because of the tremendous capacity of the kidneys to excrete bicarbonate in the presence of excess bicarbonate levels, a condition that impairs the kidneys' ability to excrete bicarbonate must be present to maintain the alkalosis. Factors that impair renal excretion of bicarbonate, thereby maintaining metabolic alkalosis, are circulating fluid volume deficit, potassium or chloride deficiency, and high aldosterone levels. The two most common causes of metabolic alkalosis—loss of gastric fluid and use of diuretics—will be explained to illustrate the interaction of factors that generate and factors that maintain metabolic alkalosis.

Parietal cells in the gastric wall secrete hydrochloric acid, which functions in the digestion of food. Since gastric fluid contains a high amount of H^+ and Cl^- ions, an obvious mechanism contributing to development of metabolic alkalosis as a result of loss of gastric fluid due to vomiting or nasogastric suctioning is the loss of H^+ from the body. However, additional factors are involved in this. Normally, when hydrochloric acid secreted by the stomach reaches the intestines, it stimulates pancreatic secretion of bicarbonate into the intestinal lumen to neutralize the H^+. When hydrochloric acid is lost by vomiting or nasogastric suctioning and therefore does not reach the intestines, bicarbonate is not secreted into the intestines and is retained and enters the circulation (**Figure 9.16** ■). Now there is an addition of bicarbonate to the extracellular fluid as well as a loss of H^+ that is generating metabolic alkalosis.

The maintenance of metabolic alkalosis associated with loss of gastric fluid is due to the deficit of water, chloride, and potassium that occurs with loss of gastric fluid. Volume deficits stimulate aldosterone secretion from the adrenal gland. Aldosterone causes sodium (Na^+) and water resorption from urine in the renal tubular lumen back into the blood (see Figure 9.15). Aldosterone activates the Na^+–H^+ antiport (see Figure 9.5), which increases renal tubular Na^+ resorption in exchange for secretion of H^+ ions into the urine. When Na^+ is resorbed from urine in the renal tubular lumen, it must be accompanied by resorption of an anion in order to maintain electrical neutrality. Cl^- is the anion that is normally resorbed in the largest amount with the cation Na^+. However, the Cl^- deficit due to the loss of gastric fluid results in the next most abundant anion, which is bicarbonate, being resorbed with Na^+. Chloride deficit contributing to alkalosis is called **hypochloremic metabolic alkalosis**. Another factor contributing to maintenance of metabolic alkalosis due to loss of gastric fluid is hypokalemia, which is the result of loss of potassium in gastric fluid plus potassium secretion into urine caused by the elevated aldosterone level. Alkalosis also contributes to hypokalemia because some H^+ moves out of cells, to replace the H^+ ion deficit in extracellular fluid, in exchange for movement of potassium into cells. The kidneys respond to potassium deficits by resorbing potassium in exchange for increased secretion of H^+ into the urine by way of the H^+–K^+ exchanger (see Figure 9.5). This results in acidic urine despite the presence of metabolic alkalosis.

CLINICAL POINT: Even if vomiting stops or nasogastric suctioning is discontinued, thereby terminating the loss of gastric water and H^+, Cl^-, and K^+ ions, metabolic alkalosis will not resolve unless the water and electrolyte deficits are corrected. The reason is that those deficits are responsible for maintenance of the metabolic alkalosis because they impair the ability of the kidneys to eliminate bicarbonate and retain H^+ ions. ■

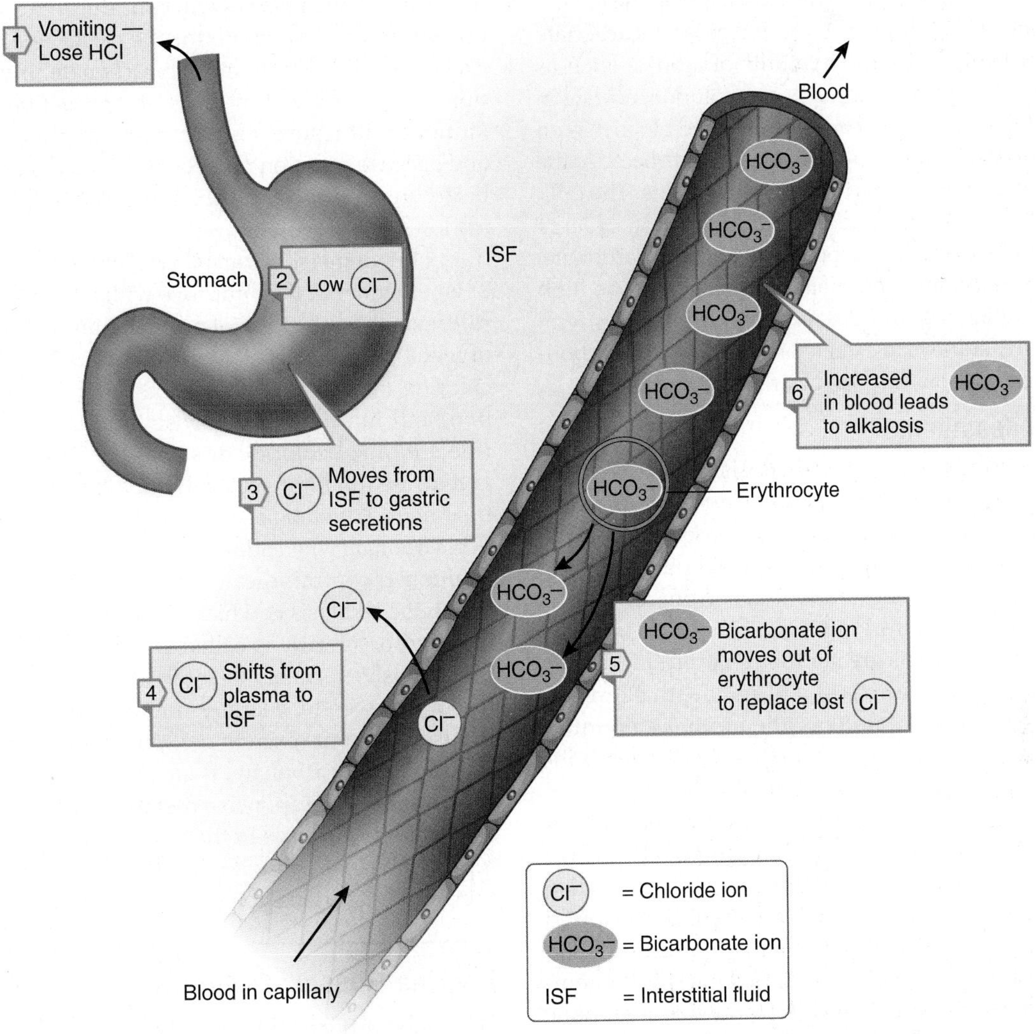

Figure 9.16 ■ Mechanisms involved in production of metabolic alkalosis due to loss of gastric fluid.

Sabrina Russell: Application

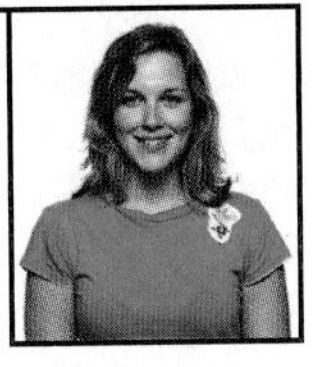

With the explanation of factors that generate and maintain metabolic alkalosis, you should now understand why Ms. Russell developed metabolic alkalosis as a result of self-induced vomiting in her attempt to lose weight.

8. How did the self-induced vomiting induce metabolic alkalosis in Ms. Russell?
9. Gastric acid loss decreases bicarbonate secretion by the pancreas. What impact will that have on acid–base balance?

Diuretic administration is another common cause of metabolic alkalosis. Two categories of diuretics—loop diuretics and thiazide diuretics—result in metabolic alkalosis due to factors that generate alkalosis and factors that maintain the alkalosis. These diuretics cause increased renal excretion of water and several electrolytes, including K^+, H^+, and Na^+ ions. Diuretic-induced loss of the cation Na^+ in the urine is accompanied by an approximately equal loss of the anion Cl^- in the urine. Hypovolemia caused by these diuretics stimulates aldosterone secretion. Aldosterone then has the same effects that function in maintenance of metabolic alkalosis, as described previously in the section on gastric fluid loss, including volume contraction alkalosis, increased renal bicarbonate resorption, and increased secretion of H^+ into the urine.

Other causes of metabolic alkalosis include excessive or too rapid correction of acidosis and ingestion or administration of large amounts of bicarbonate or other bases. For example, in chronic respiratory acidosis, the kidneys compensate by retaining an increased amount of bicarbonate. In this situation, when the $PaCO_2$, and thus carbonic acid, is quickly lowered, for example by placing the patient on mechanical ventilation, the elevated bicarbonate has less acid to buffer, resulting in metabolic alkalosis. This condition is called posthypercapnic metabolic alkalosis. Because it takes the kidneys several days to decrease the amount of bicarbonate that had been retained, it is important to avoid excessively rapid normalization of the $PaCO_2$ in individuals with chronic respiratory acidosis. Increased intake of large amounts of the base bicarbonate in the form of baking soda or bicarbonate-containing antacids causes metabolic alkalosis if the kidneys cannot excrete the increased bicarbonate load. Administration of large amounts of anions, such as lactate$^-$ in lactated Ringer's intravenous solution, acetate in hyperalimentation solutions, or citrate in stored blood, has an effect similar to the administration of bicarbonate because the liver metabolizes these anions forming bicarbonate. The milk alkali syndrome, which is caused by the ingestion of large amounts of milk and antacids containing calcium carbonate, results in hypercalcemia and metabolic alkalosis. The high calcium content in milk and certain antacids interferes with the ability of the kidneys to excrete bicarbonate, and carbonate in the antacid is converted to bicarbonate in the liver.

Clinical Manifestations

The manifestations of metabolic alkalosis include changes in blood gases, signs of compensation, and other manifestations that are mainly the result of increased neuromuscular excitability. In uncompensated metabolic alkalosis, the arterial blood pH is above 7.45, the peripheral venous blood pH is above 7.38, the $PaCO_2$ level is normal, and the serum bicarbonate level is greater than 26 mEq/L. Signs of compensation include decreased rate and depth of breathing as the lungs retain more than the normal amount of carbon dioxide. As the lungs compensate for metabolic alkalosis by decreased elimination of CO_2, the serum carbonic acid level increases, and the pH decreases back toward normal. The degree to which the $PaCO_2$ level is expected to increase as compensation for metabolic alkalosis is shown in Table 9.2. Clinical manifestations caused by the alkalosis were described earlier in the section titled "Types and Effects of Acid–Base Imbalances." Remember that many of the clinical manifestations of metabolic alkalosis are due to increased neuromuscular excitability. Manifestations of the underlying condition responsible for the metabolic alkalosis, such volume depletion or hypokalemia, will also be present. Manifestations of fluid and electrolyte deficits are described in Chapter 8.

Linking Pathophysiology to Diagnosis and Treatment

The diagnosis of metabolic alkalosis is based on the patient's history of the presence of a condition that causes metabolic alkalosis (**Table 9.11** ■), manifestations of alkalosis, and assessment of blood gases.

As with all acid–base imbalances, it is important to identify and treat the underlying cause of metabolic alkalosis. For example, an electrolyte imbalance such as hypochloremia or hypokalemia needs to be corrected; if it is left uncorrected, the kidneys will continue to resorb chloride or potassium to compensate for the electrolyte deficit and, in exchange, will excrete more bicarbonate. If volume depletion is not corrected in cases of contraction alkalosis, the kidneys will resorb sodium and water as compensation, and because an anion must be resorbed along with sodium, bicarbonate will be resorbed, especially if chloride levels are low.

States of metabolic alkalosis are categorized on the basis of whether or not they improve with administration of chloride, usually in the form of normal saline (0.9% NaCl). States of metabolic alkalosis that are associated with depletion of chloride, such as loss of gastric fluid or diuretic administration, and improve in response to administration of chloride are called chloride or saline responsive. The carbonic anhydrase inhibitor acetazolamide (Diamox) is used in the treatment of metabolic alkalosis to increase renal excretion of bicarbonate when added volume from infusion of a saline solution is contraindicated. On the other hand, a state of metabolic alkalosis in which alkalosis persists despite treatment with chloride is called chloride (saline) resistant or unresponsive form of metabolic alkalosis. An adrenal gland tumor that secretes a large amount of aldosterone, resulting in sustained renal excretion of potassium and resorption of sodium and bicarbonate, is an example of a condition that causes saline unresponsive metabolic alkalosis. Resolution of metabolic alkalosis in that condition requires potassium replacement, possibly an aldosterone antagonist medication, and/or surgical removal of the tumor.

Table 9.11 Causes of Metabolic Alkalosis

Signs	Examples
Chloride (saline) responsive	Loss of gastric fluid Diuretic administration Volume deficit Posthypercapnia
Chloride (saline) resistant	Aldosterone-producing tumors Hypokalemia

Sabrina Russell: Outcome

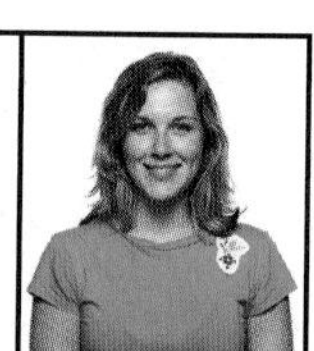

Ms. Russell had a mixed acid–base imbalance (the presence of two or more acid–base imbalances at the same time). Because she stopped taking her insulin injections, she has developed diabetic ketoacidosis, which is a form of elevated anion gap metabolic acidosis. She has also developed metabolic alkalosis caused by self-induced vomiting, which she did in an attempt to lose weight. These two imbalances pulled the pH in opposite directions, resulting in a pH within the normal range. She is treated with intravenous insulin to achieve rapid normalization of her blood glucose and fatty acid metabolism. Ms. Russell's diabetic ketoacidosis is successfully treated. Her nurse meets with Ms. Russell before her discharge to discuss the importance of adhering to the diabetes treatment regimen, including the injections of insulin and exercise options to improve weight control and her overall health. The nurse also explains the dangers associated with self-induced vomiting. The hospital dietitian meets with Ms. Russell to discuss nutritious meal preparation that will help to control her weight.

10. What are the dangers of regular self-induced vomiting?
11. What dietary modifications will support a healthy body weight and better control of Ms. Russell's blood glucose level?

Check Your Progress: Section 9.10

1. List three risk factors for metabolic alkalosis.
2. In hypokalemia, the renal response leads to increased renal acid excretion. Explain this statement.

9.11 Mixed Acid–Base Imbalances

A **mixed acid–base imbalance** consists of two or more types of acid–base imbalances in an individual at the same time. A number of pathophysiologic processes driving the pH in the same direction or in different directions can be present at the same time. For example, the presence of two conditions causing acidosis or two conditions causing alkalosis or the presence of one condition causing acidosis and another causing alkalosis is common. Can acidemia and alkalemia be present in an individual at the same time? No, since acidemia and alkalemia refer to the pH of the blood. The pH of arterial or venous blood cannot be both alkalemic and acidemic at the same time. If there are two or more processes occurring at the same time in an individual that cause acid–base imbalance, the pH will reflect the sum of the effects of all the acid–base imbalances. The pH may be low, high, or even within the normal range, depending on the overall effects of the various imbalances. Examples of conditions in which there is a mixed acid–base imbalance are presented in **Table 9.12** ■.

You might be wondering how to know whether a mixed acid–base imbalance is present, since you realize that it is important to identify and treat all the disorders causing acid–base imbalances. The detection of mixed acid–base imbalances is aided by knowing the clinical conditions present in an individual and their effects on acid–base status plus calculation of the anion gap and use of equations for expected compensation. There are limits to the degree of change that can occur in $PaCO_2$ as compensation for metabolic acidosis or alkalosis. There are also limits to the degree of change in bicarbonate that can occur as compensation for respiratory acidosis or alkalosis. The expected compensatory changes are shown in Table 9.2. If a change in bicarbonate or $PaCO_2$ exceeds the normal limits of compensation, it usually indicates the presence of a mixed acid–base imbalance.

Check Your Progress: Section 9.11

1. Considering the different case studies presented in this chapter, which of the patients presented with a mixed acid–base imbalance?
2. A patient with type 1 diabetes and COPD is likely to present with what type of mixed acid–base imbalance?

Table 9.12 Examples of Causes of Mixed Acid–Base Imbalances

Conditions	Mixed Acid–Base Imbalances Present	Pathophysiologic Mechanisms Involved
Cardiopulmonary arrest	1. Respiratory acidosis 2. Metabolic acidosis 3. Hypercapnic metabolic acidosis	1. CO_2 accumulation from respiratory failure 2. Lactic acidosis due to poor tissue perfusion causing anaerobic metabolism 3. Decreased elimination of CO_2 resulting from circulatory collapse and impaired delivery of CO_2 to the lungs
Postoperative vomiting or nasogastric suctioning plus hyperventilation due to pain or anxiety	1. Metabolic alkalosis 2. Respiratory alkalosis	1. Volume deficit and loss of gastric acid 2. Increased elimination of CO_2
Renal failure plus vomiting	1. Metabolic acidosis 2. Metabolic alkalosis	1. Impaired renal excretion of fixed acids 2. Volume deficit and loss of gastric acid
Liver failure	1. Respiratory alkalosis 2. Metabolic acidosis	1. Stimulation of the respiratory center by elevated ammonia level 2. Impaired hepatic clearance of lactate
Diabetic ketoacidosis plus vomiting	1. Metabolic acidosis 2. Metabolic alkalosis	1. Insulin deficiency causing abnormal metabolism with increased production of ketoacids (e.g., beta-hydroxybutyric acid) 2. Loss of gastric acid due to vomiting
Diabetic ketoacidosis plus lactic acidosis	1. High anion gap metabolic acidosis 2. High anion gap metabolic acidosis	1. Insulin deficiency causing abnormal metabolism with increased production of ketoacids (e.g., beta-hydroxybutyric acid) 2. Poor tissue perfusion from volume depletion resulting in lactic acidosis from anaerobic metabolism
Chronic obstructive pulmonary disease plus excessive use of a diuretic drug	1. Respiratory acidosis 2. Metabolic alkalosis	1. Decreased elimination of CO_2 2. Increased urinary loss of water, sodium, and chloride stimulates aldosterone secretion, resulting in increased HCO_3 resorption
Septic shock plus acute respiratory distress syndrome	1. Metabolic acidosis 2. Respiratory acidosis	1. Lactic acidosis due to poor tissue perfusion causing anaerobic metabolism 2. Inflammation causing pulmonary edema and decreased elimination of CO_2
Salicylate (e.g., aspirin) overdose	1. Respiratory alkalosis 2. Metabolic acidosis	1. Salicylate stimulation of the respiratory center resulting in increased elimination of CO_2 2. Salicylate impairment of aerobic metabolism resulting in anaerobic metabolism and accumulation of lactic acid

9.12 Stepwise Analysis of Acid–Base Imbalances

An acid–base imbalance should be suspected on the basis of the patient's clinical manifestations, history, and lab data, including ABGs or venous blood gases. The first step is to check the blood pH to determine whether acidemia (pH < 7.35 in arterial blood, pH < 7.32 in venous blood) or alkalemia (pH > 7.45 in arterial blood, pH > 7.38 in venous blood) is present. If the pH is within the normal range, it could be due to normal acid–base status, complete compensation for an acid–base imbalance, or the presence of a mixed imbalance with pathophysiologic processes pulling the pH in opposite directions. The next step is to determine whether the imbalance is of respiratory or metabolic origin on the basis of changes in PCO_2 and bicarbonate (HCO_3) as shown in **Figure 9.17**. The word **ROME** can help to determine whether the acid–base imbalance is of respiratory or metabolic origin. The letters *RO* stand for "respiratory opposite"; that is, in respiratory acid–base imbalances, the pH and the CO_2, which is the primary cause of the imbalance, are changed in opposite directions. For example, in respiratory acidosis, the pH is decreased and the CO_2 is increased. The letters *ME* stand for "metabolic equal," which means that in metabolic imbalances, the pH and the bicarbonate change in the same direction. For example, in metabolic acidosis, both the pH and the bicarbonate decrease.

Respiratory acid–base imbalances
Opposite (The pH and PCO_2, which is the cause of the imbalance, move in opposite directions. Respiratory acidosis: ↓ pH because of ↑ PCO_2. Respiratory alkalosis: ↑ pH because of ↓ pCO_2
Metabolic acid–base imbalances
Equal (The pH and HCO_3^-, which is the cause of the imbalance, move in the same direction. Metabolic acidosis: ↓ pH because of ↓ HCO_3^-. Metabolic alkalosis: ↑ pH because of ↑ HCO_3^-.

The equations for expected compensation (Table 9.2) are used to determine whether a mixed acid–base imbalance is present. For an example of analysis of a mixed acid–base imbalance, consider a patient with metabolic acidosis with an HCO_3^- level of 16 mEq/L (the HCO_3^- level is low because it is a base and is used up in buffering acids) and a $PaCO_2$ level of 21 mmHg. The expected change (decrease in this case) in $PaCO_2$ as a result of respiratory compensation is calculated by using the following formula from Table 9.2:

$$\text{Expected } \Delta\, PaCO_2 \text{ for metabolic acidosis} = 1.2\, \Delta\, HCO_3$$

$$\Delta\, PaCO_2 = 1.2 \times (24 - 16)$$

$$\Delta\, PaCO_2 = 10 \text{ mmHg}$$

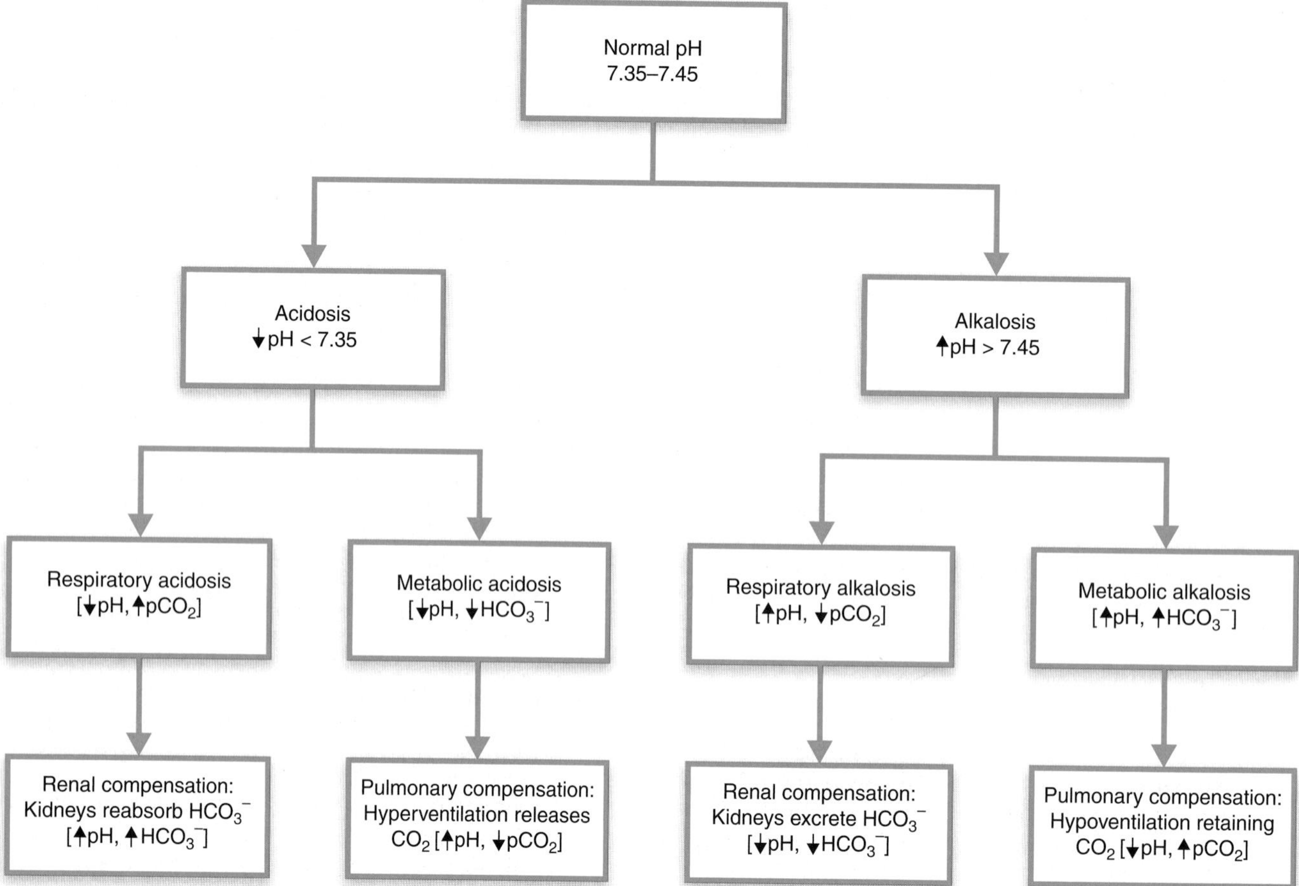

Figure 9.17 Assessment of acid–base imbalances.

The expected $PaCO_2$ in this case is then $40 - 10 = 30$ mmHg. However, the patient's actual $PaCO_2$ was 21 mmHg, indicating that the carbon dioxide is lower than expected because of compensation alone and that a respiratory alkalosis is also likely present. Using the equations for expected compensation helps clinicians to determine whether appropriate compensation is occurring and whether more than one acid–base imbalance is present that will require its cause to be identified and treated.

Check Your Progress: Section 9.12

1. What does "ME" in the mnemonic ROME mean in analyzing ABG data?
2. By applying ROME, indicate how you would analyze these ABG data: pH 7.55, pCO_2 32, and HCO_3^- 22.

CHAPTER SUMMARY

9.1 Chapter Overview and Case Studies

Describe the importance of maintaining acid–base balance and concepts related to acid–base balance.

- Hydrogen ions (H^+) are highly reactive and bind to negative charges on proteins, which alters protein structure and function. Changes in the H^+ concentration alter the compartmental distribution of some other electrolytes, thereby affecting physiologic functions regulated by those electrolytes, including nerve conduction, muscle contraction, and secretion of cell products.
- Regulation of H^+ concentration in both the extracellular and intracellular fluid compartments is critical for survival.
- Detection and treatment of acid–base imbalances are important not only because of the adverse effects of the acidosis or alkalosis but also because of the harm caused by the underlying condition causing the acid–base imbalance.

9.2 Characteristics of Acids and Bases and Their Daily Production in the Body

Differentiate the characteristics of acids and bases and their sources in the body.

- An acid is a substance that donates H^+ ions to a solution. When an acid dissociates, it releases a H^+ ion and its conjugate base, which is an anion. For example, when lactic acid dissociates, it releases a H^+ ion and the lactate$^-$ anion into a solution.
- A base is a H^+ ion acceptor. When most bases bind to a H^+ ion, they become a cation.
- Volatile acids are gases that can be eliminated in exhaled air from the lungs. Carbonic acid is the volatile acid produced in the body, and when it dissociates, it forms CO_2 and water with the CO_2 eliminated by the lungs.
- Nonvolatile (fixed) acids are eliminated from the body mainly by the kidneys.
- Both volatile and nonvolatile acids are produced daily during metabolic reactions, and acids and bases are ingested from dietary sources.
- Any excess acids or bases must be eliminated from the body or buffered in order to maintain acid–base balance.

9.3 Measures of Hydrogen Ion Concentration

Explain pH and its relation to the hydrogen ion concentration.

- pH is the negative logarithm of the H^+ ion concentration and is inversely related to the hydrogen ion concentration. The lower the pH number, the higher the H^+ concentration. The higher the pH number, the lower the H^+ concentration.
- Because the H^+ concentration in body fluids is much lower than that of other electrolytes, its concentration is expressed in nanoequivalents per liter (nEq/L) rather than milliequivalents per liter (mEq/L) or as the pH.
- Expression of the actual concentration of H^+ in nEq/L provides a more accurate indication of the acidity or alkalinity of body fluids. However, pH is still commonly used in clinical practice.
- Acidosis is present when the pH of arterial blood is less than 7.35; alkalosis is present when the pH of arterial blood is above 7.45.
- An arterial pH of 6.8 or below or 7.8 or above is not compatible with life for any extended period.

9.4 Regulation of Acid–Base Balance

Compare the roles and limitations of chemical buffers, the kidneys, and the lungs in the maintenance of acid–base balance in the extracellular fluid, and explain the regulation of intracellular pH.

- Compensation for an acid–base imbalance occurs when the degree of change in pH is minimized by the action of chemical and/or physiologic buffer systems.
- Correction of an acid–base imbalance occurs when the underlying cause of the imbalance is no longer present.

- The body's compensatory mechanisms, which include chemical buffer systems, the lungs, and the kidneys, limit the degree of change in pH caused by daily fluctuations in H^+ concentration and by disorders that cause acid–base imbalances.
- Chemical buffer systems in body fluids minimize the change in H^+ concentration that occur when an acid or a base is added by neutralizing the acid or base or by converting a strong acid or base to a weaker acid or base that dissociates to a lesser degree.
- Chemical buffers act almost immediately to changes in pH; however, these buffers have limited availability.
- The most important chemical buffer system in extracellular fluids is the bicarbonate–carbonic acid system. If the ratio of bicarbonate to carbonic acid is maintained at 20:1, the pH will be within the normal range.
- The lungs regulate the level of the volatile acid carbonic acid, which dissociates into water and CO_2, and the CO_2 is eliminated in exhaled air.
- As compensation for metabolic acidosis, the rate and/or depth of breathing increases, thereby eliminating more CO_2 and lowering carbonic acid levels, thereby increasing pH back toward normal. The opposite occurs with decreased ventilation, which compensates for metabolic alkalosis.
- The lungs begin to react within minutes of the onset of a change in pH but take 12–36 hours for maximum compensation.
- Respiratory compensation is limited by the presence of lung disease, hypoxemia that develops with decreased ventilation occurring as compensation for metabolic alkalosis, and the fatigue of respiratory muscles associated with prolonged rapid and deep breathing occurring as compensation for metabolic acidosis. Also, the lungs cannot compensate for an acid–base imbalance if they are the cause of the imbalance.
- The kidneys regulate bicarbonate levels and H^+ from nonvolatile acids by controlling the amount of H^+ secreted into urine in the renal tubules and the amount of HCO_3^- resorbed from the urine back into the blood as well as the addition of newly synthesized bicarbonate to the blood.
- H^+ are excreted in the urine buffer by phosphate or ammonia so that the pH of urine does not fall low enough to injure the renal tubular epithelial cells.
- The kidneys are very effective in compensating for acid–base imbalances; however, it takes 4–6 days to reach their maximal buffering capacity.
- The kidneys cannot compensate for an acid–base imbalance if they are contributing to it, and renal compensation will be less effective in the presence of kidney disease.
- Regulation of intracellular pH is critical for normal cell metabolism and other cell functions and is achieved by the phosphate buffer system, intracellular proteins, and a variety of transporters that facilitate exchange of H^+ and bicarbonate across cell membranes.
- The cell membrane is very permeable to CO_2, which easily diffuses into cells, where it combines with water to form carbonic acid.

9.5 Types and Effects of Acid–Base Imbalances

Describe the four types of simple acid–base imbalances, and explain the basis for the clinical manifestations of acidosis and alkalosis.

- A simple acid–base imbalance occurs when only one of the four types of imbalances is present, that is, respiratory acidosis, respiratory alkalosis, metabolic acidosis, or metabolic alkalosis.
- The effects of acidosis are similar in respiratory and metabolic acidosis, and the effects of alkalosis are similar in respiratory and metabolic alkalosis.
- Neuromuscular activity is altered in acid–base imbalances because H^+ and calcium ions compete for binding sites on proteins. In acidosis, more hydrogen ions bind to proteins with fewer sites available for calcium binding, which increases the level of free, ionized calcium. The increased free calcium blocks sodium channels in nerve and muscle, decreasing neuromuscular activity and resulting in manifestations such as muscle weakness and vasodilation. The opposite occurs in alkalosis, in which there is increased neuromuscular activity resulting in manifestations such as hyperactive reflexes, positive Chvostek and Trousseau signs, laryngospasm, and tetany.
- CNS alterations in acidosis and alkalosis are due to the change in pH in the CNS as well as changes in cerebral blood flow. Decreased neuromuscular activity in acidosis results in vasodilation of cerebral blood vessels and increased cerebral blood flow, which can increase intracranial pressure. Increased neuromuscular activity in alkalosis causes vasoconstriction, which reduces cerebral blood and oxygen delivery to the brain.
- In metabolic acidosis caused by an excess of inorganic acids, such as sulfuric acid, and in respiratory acidosis, some of the excess H^+ enter cells in exchange for the movement of potassium out of cells in order to maintain the normal intracellular electrical charge. This explains the hyperkalemia associated with acidosis.
- In metabolic acidosis caused by accumulation of organic acids, such as lactic acid, both the H^+ and anion (in this case lactate$^-$) move into the cell, so the exit of K^+ is unnecessary.
- In respiratory and metabolic alkalosis, some H^+ move out of cells to replace the extracellular deficit of H^+ in exchange for potassium movement into cells, resulting in hypokalemia.
- Changes in unloading of oxygen from hemoglobin affect cellular oxygenation in acid–base imbalances.

The hemoglobin–oxygen dissociation curve shifts to the right in acidosis, which means that there is decreased affinity of hemoglobin for oxygen and increased unloading of oxygen to cells. In alkalosis, the hemoglobin–oxygen curve shifts to the left, which means that there is increased affinity of hemoglobin for oxygen, resulting in decreased unloading of oxygen to cells.

- In severe acidosis, there is vasodilation and decreased cardiac contractility due to decreased neuromuscular excitability, resulting in hypotension, decreased tissue perfusion, and decreased oxygenation.
- Severe alkalosis causes decreased cellular availability of oxygen because of vasoconstriction, which decreases tissue perfusion, and decreased unloading of oxygen from hemoglobin.

9.6 Laboratory Tests Used in Assessment of Acid–Base Status

Interpret arterial and venous blood gas results, the anion gap, and base excess values.

- In addition to assessment of the clinical manifestations of acidosis and alkalosis, laboratory tests are used in the diagnosis of acid–base imbalances, including arterial or venous blood gases, the base excess (BE), and the anion gap.
- The information from arterial blood gases (ABGs) that is most useful for assessment of acid–base status includes the pH (normal = 7.35–7.45), $PaCO_2$ level (normal = 35–45 mmHg), and HCO_3^- level (normal = 22–26 mEq/L).
- Venous blood samples can be obtained with fewer complications than may occur in arterial blood sampling. Venous blood can be used as a substitute for arterial blood to measure pH and HCO_3^- to assess a variety of respiratory and metabolic acid–base imbalances.
- The normal ranges for the pH of venous blood (7.3–7.41) and the HCO_3^- level in venous blood (21–22 mEq/L) are slightly lower than those found in arterial blood.
- In states of cardiovascular collapse such as during cardiopulmonary resuscitation, venous blood gas values are much lower than those in arterial blood and cannot substitute for arterial blood gases. However, venous blood gases can also be measured to provide a better assessment of acid–base status at the cellular level.
- A blood pH below normal indicates acidosis; a blood pH above normal indicates alkalosis.
- The $PaCO_2$ level is above normal during respiratory acidosis and during respiratory compensation for metabolic alkalosis. The $PaCO_2$ level is below normal during respiratory alkalosis and during respiratory compensation for metabolic acidosis.
- The HCO_3^- level is below normal during metabolic acidosis and during renal compensation for respiratory alkalosis. The HCO_3^- level is above normal during metabolic alkalosis and during renal compensation for respiratory acidosis
- The total CO_2 (TCO_2) is a measure of all forms of CO_2 in the blood, including bicarbonate (HCO_3^-), carbonic acid (H_2CO_3), CO_2 attached to hemoglobin, and CO_2 dissolved in plasma (PCO_2).
- The base excess (BE) test detects either an excess of base, designated by a positive number, or a deficit of base, designated by a negative number. The base excess or base deficit is a measure of all bases in the blood. When the BE is a positive number greater than 2.0 mEq/L, it indicates an elevated amount of base and can be due to metabolic alkalosis or renal compensation for respiratory acidosis. When the BE is more negative than –2.0 mEq/L, it indicates a below-normal amount of base and can be due to metabolic acidosis or renal compensation for respiratory alkalosis.
- The anion gap is used to detect the presence of an increased amount of anions produced when nonvolatile acids dissociate, as occurs in metabolic acidosis .
- The anion gap is calculated by subtracting the sum of the anions chloride and bicarbonate from the concentration of the cation sodium. The difference is the anion gap and consists of anions formed when fixed acids dissociate, such as albumin$^-$, sulfate$^-$, phosphate$^-$, lactate$^-$, acetoacetate$^-$, and beta hydroxybutyrate$^-$.
- An elevated anion gap metabolic acidosis is caused by the presence of an elevated amount of fixed acids. The three most common causes of elevated anion gap metabolic acidosis are lactic acidosis, ketoacidosis, and kidney failure.
- The most common cause of normal anion gap metabolic acidosis is hyperchloremia, which causes a fall in the concentration of the base bicarbonate.

9.7 Respiratory Acidosis

Differentiate the causes, underlying pathogenesis, and clinical manifestations of respiratory acidosis and approaches to diagnosis and treatment of this condition across the lifespan.

- Respiratory acidosis is caused by impaired elimination of CO_2 by the lungs and is characterized by blood pH below 7.35, elevated $PaCO_2$, normal serum bicarbonate level, and a decreased ratio of bicarbonate to carbonic acid below 20:1.
- Renal compensation for respiratory acidosis takes several days and consists of increased resorption of bicarbonate from urine in the renal tubules and increased renal excretion of H^+, resulting in a bicarbonate level greater than 28 mEq/L in arterial blood.
- Effects of respiratory acidosis are primarily related to increased levels of free calcium, which blocks sodium channels, resulting in decreased neuromuscular excitability.
- Respiratory acidosis is best treated by interventions that improve alveolar ventilation and return elimination of CO_2 to normal.

9.8 Respiratory Alkalosis

Differentiate the causes, underlying pathogenesis, and clinical manifestations of respiratory alkalosis and approaches to diagnosis and treatment of this condition across the lifespan.

- Respiratory alkalosis is caused by any condition resulting in hyperventilation, which results in excess elimination of CO_2 and is characterized by an increased blood pH, a decreased pCO_2 level, a normal HCO_3^- level, and an increased ratio of bicarbonate to carbonic acid above 20:1.
- Expected renal compensation for respiratory alkalosis is decreased resorption of bicarbonate from renal tubular fluid and decreased renal excretion of H^+, resulting in a serum bicarbonate level less than 21 mEq/L.
- Effects of respiratory alkalosis are primarily related to decreased levels of free calcium, resulting in increased neuromuscular excitability and impaired cell oxygenation due to decreased unloading of oxygen from hemoglobin.
- Respiratory alkalosis is best treated by interventions that restore ventilation to normal.
- Rebreathing exhaled CO_2 can normalize the $PaCO_2$; however, additional interventions are needed to reverse the underlying cause of the hyperventilation.

9.9 Metabolic Acidosis

Differentiate the causes, underlying pathogenesis, and clinical manifestations of metabolic acidosis and approaches to diagnosis and treatment of this condition across the lifespan.

- Metabolic acidosis is characterized by a decreased arterial and venous blood pH, a decreased blood HCO_3^- level, a normal $PaCO_2$ level, and a decreased ratio of bicarbonate to carbonic acid below 20:1.
- Causes of metabolic acidosis are categorized according to their effect on the anion gap. Elevated anion gap metabolic acidosis is caused by conditions, such as lactic acidosis, ketoacidosis, and renal failure, that result in accumulation of nonvolatile acids. Normal anion gap metabolic acidosis is caused by conditions, such as hyperchloremia, diarrhea, and renal tubular acidosis, that result in excessive loss of HCO_3^-.
- Expected respiratory compensation for metabolic acidosis is an increased rate and/or depth of breathing resulting in a decreased $PaCO_2$ level, which decreases the level of carbonic acid and returns the pH back up toward normal.
- Effects of metabolic acidosis are primarily related to increased levels of free calcium resulting in decreased neuromuscular excitability.
- Treatment of metabolic acidosis is directed at reversing the underlying cause. Use of the buffer sodium bicarbonate is reserved for treatment of life-threatening normal anion gap metabolic acidosis.

9.10 Metabolic Alkalosis

Differentiate the causes, underlying pathogenesis, and clinical manifestations of metabolic alkalosis and approaches to diagnosis and treatment of this condition across the lifespan.

- Metabolic alkalosis is characterized by an increased blood pH, an increased HCO_3^- level, a normal $PaCO_2$ level, and an increased ratio of bicarbonate to carbonic acid above 20:1.
- Generation of metabolic alkalosis is due to excessive loss of H^+ ions or intake of base.
- Because the kidneys are normally able to excrete large amounts of bicarbonate, for metabolic alkalosis to be maintained, a condition must be present that impairs renal excretion of bicarbonate, such as hypokalemia, hypochloremia, or volume deficit.
- Causes of metabolic alkalosis are categorized according to whether or not they respond to administration of chloride. Causes of chloride-responsive metabolic alkalosis are loss of gastric fluid, volume depletion, diuretics, and too rapid correction of chronic hypercapnia. Causes of chloride-resistant metabolic acidosis include hypokalemia and aldosterone-producing tumors.
- Expected respiratory compensation for metabolic alkalosis is decreased rate and/or depth of breathing resulting in an increased $PaCO_2$, which increases the level of carbonic acid and returns the pH back down toward normal.
- Effects of metabolic alkalosis are primarily related to decreased levels of free calcium resulting in increased neuromuscular excitability and impaired cell oxygenation due to decreased unloading of oxygen from hemoglobin.
- Treatment of metabolic alkalosis is directed at reversing the underlying cause and correcting any fluid, potassium, or chloride deficits that drive continued HCO_3^- loss in the urine.

9.11 Mixed Acid–Base Imbalances

Describe common clinical conditions that result in mixed acid–base imbalances.

- In a mixed acid–base imbalance, two or more types of acid–base imbalances are present at the same time in an individual.
- The imbalances that are present in states of mixed acid–base imbalances can be two conditions that cause acidosis, such as respiratory and metabolic acidosis, or two conditions that cause alkalosis, such as respiratory and metabolic alkalosis.
- The imbalances that are present in states of mixed acid–base imbalances can be one condition that causes acidosis and one that causes alkalosis, such as metabolic acidosis and respiratory alkalosis or metabolic alkalosis and respiratory acidosis.

- In a mixed acid–base imbalance with one condition causing acidosis and another causing alkalosis, the pH may be low, high, or even within the normal range depending on the degree to which the conditions alter the pH.

9.12 Stepwise Analysis of Acid–Base Imbalances

Utilize a stepwise approach in the analysis of simple acid–base imbalances and differentiate simple from mixed acid–base imbalances using equations for expected compensation.

- The type of acid–base imbalance that is present is determined by the patient's history of a condition that can cause acidosis or alkalosis, clinical manifestations, and laboratory test results that include arterial or venous blood gas data.
- The pH is assessed to determine whether it is normal, decreased (indicating acidosis), or increased (indicating alkalosis).
- Whether the cause of the imbalance is of respiratory or metabolic origin is determined next by assessment of the $PaCO_2$ and HCO_3^- levels.
- The mnemonic ROME, which stands for **R**espiratory **O**pposite **M**etabolic **E**qual, can be used to remember the direction of change of values in respiratory and metabolic acid–base imbalances.
- In respiratory acid–base imbalances the pH and the $PaCO_2$, which is the primary cause of the imbalance, move in opposite directions. In metabolic acid–base imbalances, the pH and the HCO_3^-, which is the primary cause of the imbalance, move in the same direction.
- The presence of mixed acid–base imbalances is diagnosed by the same information used for simple acid–base imbalances plus use of equations for expected compensation for acid–base imbalances.
- If the amount of change in $PaCO_2$ or HCO_3^- is above or below the value for expected compensation, it indicates the presence of an additional acid–base imbalance responsible for contributing to the change in CO_2 or HCO_3^-.

REVIEW QUESTIONS

1. A female patient is admitted with a diagnosis of COPD. What arterial blood gas (ABG) result should the nurse expect?
   a. pH 7.45, $PaCO_2$ 38, HCO_3 31
   b. pH 7.31, $PaCO_2$ 36, HCO_3 16
   c. pH 7.33, $PaCO_2$ 49, HCO_3 23
   d. pH 7.47, $PaCO_2$ 35, HCO_3 18

2. A client presents in the hospital with pneumonia. His ABG results are pH 7.48, $PaCO_2$ 31 mmHg, HCO_3 28 mEq/L, PaO_2 88 mmHg. How would the nurse interpret this result?
   a. Mixed respiratory and metabolic alkalosis
   b. Mixed respiratory and metabolic acidosis
   c. Metabolic acidosis
   d. Respiratory alkalosis

3. A 70-year-old female presents to her primary care provider and reports dizziness, confusion, and tingling in the extremities. Blood tests reveal pH 7.47, PCO_2 32, and HCO_3 16. Which of the following is the most likely diagnosis?
   a. Metabolic alkalosis with respiratory compensation
   b. Metabolic acidosis with respiratory compensation
   c. Respiratory alkalosis with renal compensation
   d. Respiratory acidosis with renal compensation

4. A 49-year-old male with a long history of smoking complains of excessive tiredness, shortness of breath, and overall ill feelings. Lab results reveal decreased pH 7.31, $PaCO_2$ 47 mmHg, and HCO_3 24. These findings help to confirm the diagnosis of:
   a. metabolic alkalosis.
   b. metabolic acidosis.
   c. respiratory alkalosis.
   d. respiratory acidosis.

5. A patient is admitted, and the blood lab results indicate metabolic acidosis and hyperkalemia. Which of the following diseases would be associated with these changes?
   a. Respiratory failure
   b. Renal failure
   c. Liver failure
   d. Hypertension

6. The nurse is teaching a student nurse about body buffer systems involved in acid–base balance. Which of the following buffer pairs is considered the major plasma buffering system?
   a. Sodium–potassium
   b. Potassium–hydrogen ion
   c. Carbonic acid–bicarbonate
   d. Hemoglobin–protein

7. A 36-year-old woman has presented to the emergency department following a panic attack. Her blood pressure, respiratory rate, and heart rate are all highly

elevated, while her temperature and oxygen saturation are within normal ranges. How will her body try to deal with the resulting change in pH?
a. Increased respiratory rate
b. Decreased respiratory rate
c. Increased excretion of H^+ by the kidneys
d. Decreased resorption of HCO_3 by the kidneys

8. Regulation of acid–base balance achieved through the removal or retention of volatile acids is accomplished by which of the following systems?
a. Renal
b. Hepatobiliary
c. Integumentary (skin)
d. Pulmonary

ANSWERS

Answers to Review Questions can be found in Appendix A. Answers to Case Study and Check Your Progress questions are available on the faculty resources site. Please consult with your instructor.

RECOMMENDED WEBSITES

6 easy steps to acid-base interpretation at: http://www.youtube.com/watch?v=6stANI3zNA0&feature=related

Alan Grogono of Tulane University Department of Anesthesiology: Acid-Base Tutorial http://www.acid-base.com/index.php

Eric Strong at Stanford University: Elevated Anion Gap Metabolic Acidosis (ABG Interpretation: Lesson 8) https://www.youtube.com/watch?v=CmQOtP3pFus

Eric Strong at Stanford University: Normal Acid-Base Regulation (ABG Interpretation: Lesson 2) https://www.youtube.com/watch?v=LFiU5hKDBpU

Merck Manual: Acid-Base Balance https://www.merckmanuals.com/professional/endocrine-and-metabolic-disorders/acid-base-regulation-and-disorders/acid-base-regulation

University of Connecticut: Acid Base Online Tutorial http://fitsweb.uchc.edu/student/selectives/TimurGraham/Welcome.html

REFERENCES

1. Halperin, M., Kamel, K., & Goldstein, M. (2010). *Fluid, electrolyte, and acid-base physiology: A problem-based approach* (4th ed.). Philadelphia, PA: Elsevier.
2. Cunningham, F., Leveno, K., Bloom, S., et al. (2014). The newborn. In F. G. Cunningham, K. J. Lenovo, S. L. Bloom, C. Y. Spong, J. S. Dashe, B. L. Hoffman, B. M. Casey, & J. S. Sheffield (Eds.), *Williams obstetrics* (24th ed., pp. 624–636). New York, NY: McGraw-Hill.
3. Parrillo, J., & Delinger, R. (2014). Acid-base, electrolyte, and metabolic abnormalities. In J. Parrillo & R. Dellinger (Eds.), *Critical care medicine: Principles of diagnosis and management in the adult* (4th ed., pp. 993–1028). Philadelphia, PA: Elsevier.
4. Rennke, H., & Denker, B. (2014). *Renal pathophysiology: The essentials* (4th ed.). Philadelphia, PA: Lippincott Williams and Wilkins.
5. Hasan, A. (2013). *Handbook of blood gas/acid-base interpretation* (2nd ed.). New York, NY: Springer.
6. Arnett, T. (2010). Acidosis, hypoxia, and bone. *Archives of Biochemistry and Biophysics, 503*, 103–109.
7. Hall, J. (2016). Acid-base regulation. In J. Hall (Ed.), *Guyton and Hall textbook of medical physiology* (13th ed., pp. 409–426). Philadelphia, PA: Elsevier
8. Marini, J., & Wheeler, A. (2010). Acid-base disorders. In J. Marini & A. Wheeler (Eds.), *Critical care medicine: The essentials* (4th ed., pp. 227–244). Philadelphia, PA: Lippincott Williams & Wilkins.
9. Ruffin, V., Salameh, A., Boron, W., & Parker, M. (2014). Intracellular pH regulation by acid-base transporters in mammalian neurons. *Frontiers in Physiology, 5*, 1–11.
10. Salameh, A., Ruffin, V., & Boron, W. (2014). Effects of metabolic acidosis on intracellular pH responses in multiple cell types. *American Journal of Physiology: Regulatory, Integrative, and Comparative Physiology, 307*, R1413–R1427.
11. Giebisch, G., & Windhager, E. (2009). Transport of acids and bases. In W. Born & E. Boulpaep (Eds.), *Medical physiology: A cellular and molecular approach* (pp. 851–865). Philadelphia, PA: Elsevier.
12. Tonnessen, T. I. (2000). Intracellular pH and electrolyte regulation. In A. Grenvik, S. Ayers, P. Holbrook, & W. Shoemaker (Eds.), *Textbook of critical care* (4th ed., pp. 507–522). Philadelphia, PA: W.B. Saunders.
13. Kellum, J. (2011). Acid-base disorders. In J.-L. Vincent, E. Abraham, F. Moore, P. Kochanek, & M. Fink (Eds.), *Textbook of critical care* (6th ed., pp. 43–52). Philadelphia, PA: Elsevier.
14. Kraut, J., & Madias, N. (2012). Treatment of acute metabolic acidosis: A pathophysiologic approach. *Nature Reviews Nephrology, 8*, 589–601.
15. Palmer, B. (2013). Respiratory acid-base disorders. In D. Mount, M. Sayegh, & A. Singh (Eds.), *Core concepts in the disorders of fluid, electrolytes and acid-base balance* (pp. 297–306). New York, NY: Springer.
16. Barnett, V., and Schmidt, G. (2005). Acid-base disorders. In J. Hall, G. Schmidt, & L. Wood (Eds.), *Principles of critical care* (3rd ed., pp. 1169–1181). New York, NY: McGraw-Hill.
17. Kelly, A.-M., Klim, S., & Rees, S. (2014). Agreement between mathematically arterialized venous versus arterial blood gas values in patients undergoing non-invasive ventilation: A cohort study. *Emergency Medicine Journal, 31*, e46–e49.
18. Heidari, K., Hatamabadi, H., Ansarian, N., et al. (2013). Correlation between capillary and arterial blood gas parameters in an ED. *American Journal of Emergency Medicine, 31*, 326–329.

19. Herrington, W. G., Nye, H. J., Hammersley, M. S., & Watkinson, P. J. (2014). Are arterial and venous samples clinically equivalent for the estimation of pH, serum bicarbonate and potassium concentration in critically ill patients? *Diabetic Medicine, 29*, 32–35.
20. Kelly, A.-M. (2010). Review article: Can venous blood gas analysis replace arterial in emergency medical care. *Emergency Med Australasia, 22*, 493–498.
21. Menchine, M., Probst, M., Agy, C., et al. (2011). Diagnostic accuracy of venous blood gas electrolytes for identifying diabetic ketoacidosis in the emergency department. *Academic Emergency Medicine, 18*, 1105–1108.
22. Strehlow, M. C. (2010). Early identification of shock in critically ill patients. *Emergency Medicine Clinics of North America, 28*(1), 57–66.
23. Androgue, H., Rashad, N., Gorin, A., et al. (1989). Assessing acid-base status in circulatory failure. *New England Journal of Medicine, 320*, 1312–1316.
24. Dries, D. (2014). Traumatic shock and tissue hypoperfusion: Nonsurgical management. In J. Parrillo & R. Dellinger (Eds.), *Critical care medicine: Principles of diagnosis and management in the adult* (4th ed., pp. 409–431). Philadelphia, PA: Elsevier.
25. Kraut, J., & Madias, N. (2007). Serum anion gap: Its uses and limitations in clinical medicine. *Clinical Journal of the American Society of Nephrology, 2*, 162–174.
26. Marino, P. (2014). *Marino's The ICU book* (4th ed.). Philadelphia, PA: Lippincott Williams & Wilkins.
27. Vichot, A., & Rastegar, A. (2014). Use of anion gap in the evaluation of a patient with metabolic acidosis. *American Journal of Kidney Diseases, 64*(4), 653–657.
28. Ijland, M., Heunks, L., & Van der Hoven, J. (2010). Bench to bedside review: Hypercapnic acidosis in lung injury—from permissive to therapeutic. *Critical Care, 14*, 237–246.
29. Acute Respiratory Distress Syndrome Network. (2000). Ventilation with lower tidal volumes as compared with traditional tidal volumes for acute lung injury and the acute respiratory distress syndrome. *New England Journal of Medicine 342*, 1301–1308.
30. Hassett, P., Contress, M., & Laffey, J. (2008). Hypercapnia: Permissive, therapeutic, or not at all? In J. L. Vincent (Ed.), *Intensive care medicine: Annual update* (pp. 269–281). New York, NY: Springer.
31. Monga, M., & Mastrobattista, J. (2014). Maternal cardiovascular, respiratory, and renal adaptation to pregnancy. In K. Creasy, R. Resnik, J. Iams, C. Lockwood, T. Moore, & M. Greene, (Eds.), *Creasy & Resnik's maternal-fetal medicine principles and practice* (7th ed., pp. 93–99). Philadelphia, PA: Elsevier.
32. Weiner, S. (2014). Toxicologic acid-base disorders. *Emergency Medicine Clinics of North America, 32*, 149–116.
33. Creasy, K., Resnik, R., Iams, J., Lockwood, C., Moore, T., & Greene, M. (Eds.). (2014). *Creasy & Resnik's maternal-fetal medicine principles and practice* (7th ed.). Philadelphia, PA: Elsevier.
34. Cantu, J., Szychowski, J., Li, X., et al. (2014). Predicting fetal academia using umbilical venous cord gas parameters. *Obstetrics & Gynecology, 124*(5), 926–932.

Unit IV

Cell Injury, Inflammation, and Alterations of Cell Growth and Regulation

Manifestations of illness and injury are categorized as either signs or symptoms. Signs are objective in that they can be observed or elicited on examination or can be determined by laboratory or diagnostic tests. Clinical signs of illness or injury include the wheezing a healthcare provider may hear when auscultating the lungs of a client with asthma or the visible swelling and warmth that indicate a sprained ankle. Symptoms, which are manifestations that only the client can perceive and describe, include pain and anxiety, although these may result in observable signs if severe enough. For example, pain is a symptom, but the client in pain may guard the affected area, and the client with anxiety may have elevated blood pressure.

All clinical manifestations of illness and injury have one thing in common: They signal the occurrence of a pathophysiologic process at the cellular level. The process may be reversible in that the affected area returns to normal when the stimulus is removed and the injury to cells is mild. For example, a sprained ankle returns to full functioning after sufficient rest, which allows inflammatory mediators to clear the injurious stimuli and replace injured cells. Nonreversible cell injury indicates that pathologic cell changes are permanent. In some cases, they may lead to cell death. An example of nonreversible cell injury is the tissue necrosis associated with ischemia in the client with diabetes who develops gangrene in a toe or foot.

Two physiologic processes that play roles in helping the body achieve homeostasis after the onset of illness or injury are free radical production and inflammation. Unfortunately, they can also lead to further illness or injury at the cellular level. When there is an imbalance between free radical production and reactive metabolites, the reactive oxygen species (ROS) and their elimination by the protective mechanisms of antioxidants, oxidative stress occurs. Oxidative stress can cause damage to surrounding cellular components, leading to an inflammatory response. If the inflammation does not resolve and becomes chronic, the mast cells and leukocytes recruited for damage control require an elevated oxygen uptake. This uptake leads to a "respiratory burst" with accumulation of ROS at the damaged site. Inflammatory cells are also attracted to the damaged site and initiate processes that further recruit inflammatory cells, which then produce chemical mediators that also play a role in ROS. This sustained and cyclic inflammatory/oxidative environment cascade causes more damage to the neighboring healthy cells. Over time, this leads to carcinogenesis. Cancer-associated inflammatory processes then continue the inflammatory cycle as microphages that attempt to respond to and destroy the cancer cells are also being used by the tumor to support its continued survival.[1]

Knowledge of these physiologic processes has direct implications for nursing. The nurse who identifies early that a client is not achieving full and timely return to functioning after an illness or injury may be instrumental in disrupting a more severe pathology, such as ischemia or hypoxia, preventing it from becoming chronic or from exacerbating a comorbid illness.

Knowledge of cellular mechanisms is also essential in identifying risk for illness or injury. Nurses have long understood that caregiver role strain has implications for health and mental health outcomes for both the client and the informal caregiver. Research is finally catching up with clinical practice by illuminating physiologic pathways that are affected by the strains of caregiving. In a study of women caregivers caring for veterans who were recovering from a traumatic brain injury, caregivers reported higher levels of anger and blame had higher levels of tumor necrosis factor alpha, a proinflammatory cytokine.[2] The strains of long-term caregiving may well increase the caregiver's risk for inflammatory disorders. Nurses who are able to assist caregivers access support groups, respite care, and financial and other resources may help caregivers to lower their risk for involvement of inflammatory processes related to the burdens of caregiving.

References

1. Hanahan, D., & Weinberg, R. A. (2011). Hallmarks of cancer: The next generation. *Cell, 144*(5): 646–674. doi:10.1016/j.cell.2011.02.013
2. Saban, K. L., Mathews, H. L., Collins, E. G., et al. (2016). The man I once knew: Grief and inflammation in female partners of veterans with traumatic brain injury. *Biological Research for Nursing, 18*(1), 50–59.

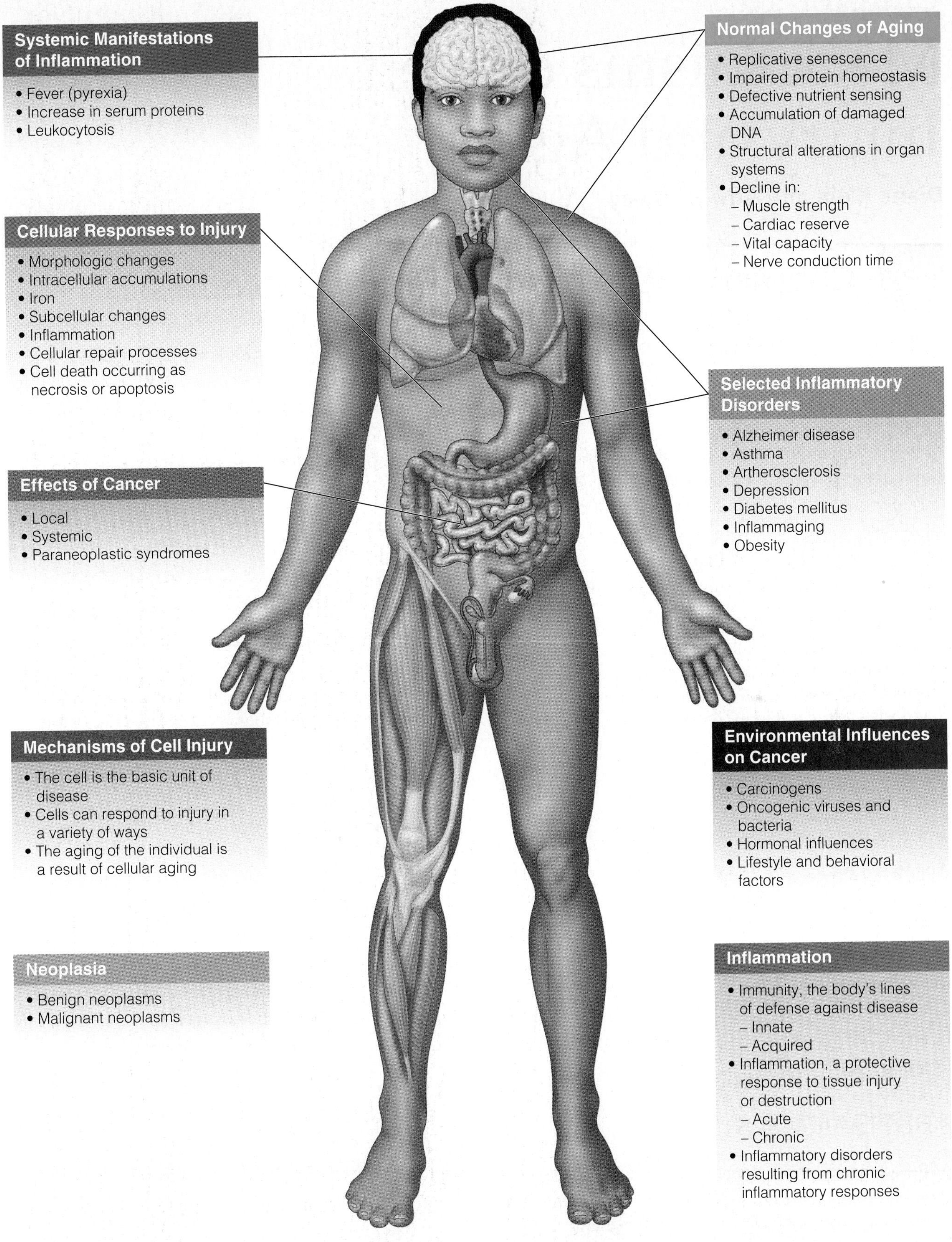

Systemic Manifestations of Inflammation

- Fever (pyrexia)
- Increase in serum proteins
- Leukocytosis

Cellular Responses to Injury

- Morphologic changes
- Intracellular accumulations
- Iron
- Subcellular changes
- Inflammation
- Cellular repair processes
- Cell death occurring as necrosis or apoptosis

Effects of Cancer

- Local
- Systemic
- Paraneoplastic syndromes

Mechanisms of Cell Injury

- The cell is the basic unit of disease
- Cells can respond to injury in a variety of ways
- The aging of the individual is a result of cellular aging

Neoplasia

- Benign neoplasms
- Malignant neoplasms

Normal Changes of Aging

- Replicative senescence
- Impaired protein homeostasis
- Defective nutrient sensing
- Accumulation of damaged DNA
- Structural alterations in organ systems
- Decline in:
  - Muscle strength
  - Cardiac reserve
  - Vital capacity
  - Nerve conduction time

Selected Inflammatory Disorders

- Alzheimer disease
- Asthma
- Artherosclerosis
- Depression
- Diabetes mellitus
- Inflammaging
- Obesity

Environmental Influences on Cancer

- Carcinogens
- Oncogenic viruses and bacteria
- Hormonal influences
- Lifestyle and behavioral factors

Inflammation

- Immunity, the body's lines of defense against disease
  - Innate
  - Acquired
- Inflammation, a protective response to tissue injury or destruction
  - Acute
  - Chronic
- Inflammatory disorders resulting from chronic inflammatory responses

Chapter 10

Mechanisms of Cell Injury and Aging

Diane Klein and Amy Kennedy

Chapter Outline and Learning Outcomes

10.1 Chapter Overview and Case Studies

Differentiate reversible from nonreversible cell injury, cellular adaptation, and concepts related to cell injury and aging.

10.2 The Cell as the Basic Unit of Disease

Summarize cell structures and functions, and describe the consequences of injury to the cell membrane and organelles.

10.3 Common Causes of Cell Injury

Explain the common causes of cellular injury.

10.4 Environmental Factors That Cause Cell Injury

Differentiate the causes, classification, underlying pathogenesis, and clinical manifestations of cell injury caused by environmental factors and approaches to diagnosis and treatment of these injuries across the lifespan.

10.5 Impact of Injury on Cell Types Present in Many Organs

Describe the impact of injury on endothelial and epithelial cells in various organs.

10.6 Cellular Responses to Injury

Summarize the cellular responses to injury and the cellular repair process.

10.7 Cell Death

Compare and contrast the causes and effects of cell death due to necrosis and cell death due to apoptosis.

10.8 Aging of the Individual as a Result of Cellular Aging

Describe the normal lifespan, the molecular basis of aging, and the changes that occur with aging in the human body.

KEY TERMS

Antioxidants, 248
Apoptosis, 264
Atrophy, 258
Autophagy, 259
Carbon monoxide (CO), 250
Cellular adaptation, 239
Channelopathies, 241
Dysoxia, 247
Dysplasia, 259
Eukaryotic cell, 240
Gangrene, 263
Hyaline, 261
Hyperplasia, 259
Hypertrophy, 259
Hypoxemia, 245
Hypoxia, 245
Ionizing radiation, 255
Lead, 253
Lipofuscin, 261
Melanin, 261
Metaplasia, 259
Necrosis, 262
Nonionizing radiation, 254
Oxidative stress, 247
Reactive oxygen species (ROS), 248
Replicative senescence, 265

ABBREVIATIONS

ATP—adenosine triphosphate
CO—carbon monoxide
ECM—extracellular matrix
ER—endoplasmic reticulum
IGF-1—insulin-like growth factor 1
IIS—IFG-I signaling
ROS—reactive oxygen species
SER—smooth ER

10.1 Chapter Overview and Case Studies

Cells are the smallest structural and functional unit of an organism. The most pressing need for any free living cell is to establish a structural and functional barrier between its internal milieu and a hostile environment. Cells encounter many stressors as a result of changes in their internal and external environments. Changes made in the cell in response to these stressors that favor cell survival are termed **cellular adaptation**. The goal of this adaptation is to maintain homeostasis. To avoid injury, cells adapt to stressors, in general by conserving resources, decreasing or ceasing differentiated functions and focusing exclusively on their own survival.

Maladaptive cellular changes lead to cell injury, the cellular basis of disease. There are two basic types of cell injury: reversible and nonreversible (**Figure 10.1** ■). Reversible cell injury denotes pathologic changes that can revert back to normal. This reversal occurs when the stimulus is removed and the injury is mild or of short duration. It is important to note that cell injury is reversible up to a certain point. Nonreversible cell injury indicates that pathologic cell changes are permanent and may lead to cell death.

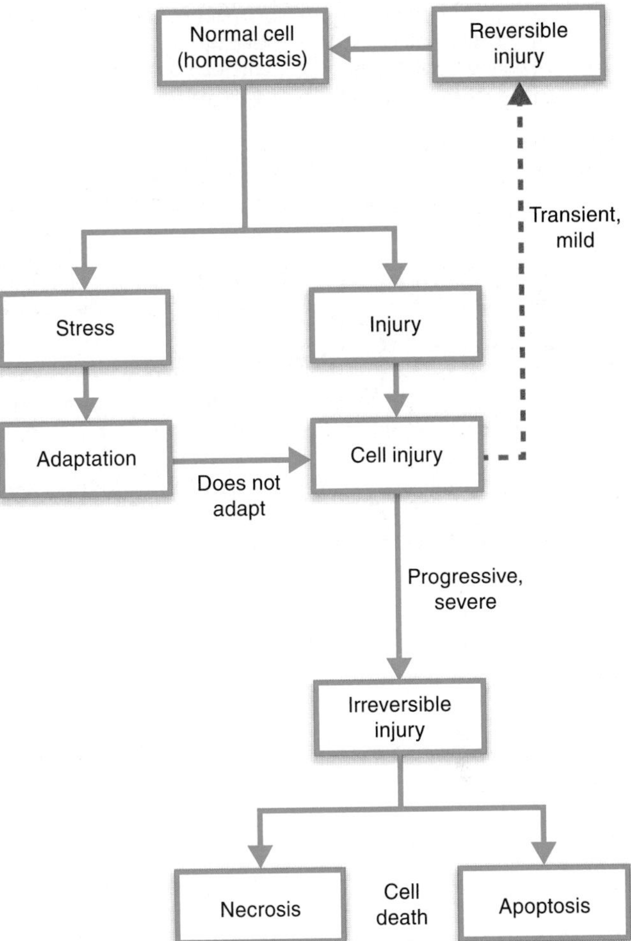

Figure 10.1 ■ Reversible and nonreversible cell injury.

Concepts Related to Cell Injury and Aging

Cell injury, along with aging, affects the entire body. The primary concepts involved in cell injury and aging include cellular regulation along with inflammation and oxidative stress. Cell injury and aging can affect any organ system and therefore impair processes associated with any physiologic concept, such as oxygenation, perfusion, immunity, metabolism, neural or endocrine regulation, and elimination (**Figure 10.2** ■). For example, cell injury that occurs when myocardial cells are deprived of oxygen results in reversible injury when the blood supply is compromised for 10 to 15 minutes. The heart muscle will be injured; however, it can recover to normal function. When blood supply is compromised for a longer period of time, the myocardial cells die, leading to nonreversible injury and necrosis resulting in decreased cardiac contractility. In this example of cell injury, acid–base balance, comfort, fluid and electrolyte balance, and perfusion are all concepts affected as a result of myocardial cell injury.

Case Studies

The following cases will be addressed throughout the chapter to assist in application of chapter content to clinical situations that involve mechanisms of cell injury and aging.

Samuel Murphy: Introduction

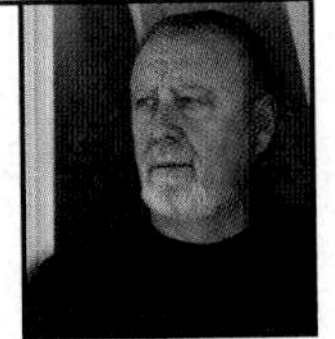

Samuel Murphy is a 65-year-old male whose wife recently died from cancer. Mr. Murphy worked as a manual laborer in the construction industry for over 40 years before retiring this past winter. Mr. Murphy, a smoker since adolescence, was diagnosed with chronic obstructive pulmonary disease at the age of 48. Concurrent diagnoses include hypertension and hyperlipidemia, which are controlled with medication and diet. Mr. Murphy has two adult children and five grandchildren who visit him often.

1. What factors in Mr. Murphy's history place him at risk for cellular injury?
2. Describe the general pathophysiologic process by which smoking leads to cell injury.

Sophia Velazquez: Introduction

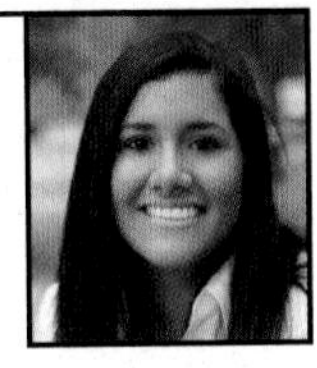

Sophia Velazquez, age 17, was home alone overnight while her parents were attending an out-of-town wedding. When they returned on Sunday afternoon, they found Sophia unresponsive in her bed. Mr. Velazquez called 9-1-1 for an ambulance while Mrs. Velazquez tried to awaken Sophia.

When the paramedics arrive, they are directed to Sophia's bedroom. The paramedics note that both parents are feeling unwell with complaints of nausea, weakness, and headache. Suspecting carbon monoxide poisoning, the paramedics immediately open the windows and remove Sophia and her parents from the home. As soon as they get outdoors and start breathing fresh air, Sophia's parents start to feel better. In the ambulance, Sophia's hemoglobin saturation with oxygen in arterial blood (SaO_2) measured with a standard pulse oximeter is 94%. Her respirations are rapid and shallow. Her heart rate is 110 beats/minute, and her blood pressure is 72/54. A paramedic intubates Sophia and administers 100% oxygen.

1. Is Sophia most likely experiencing reversible or nonreversible cell injury?
2. What are the consequences to Sophia of nonreversible cell injury?

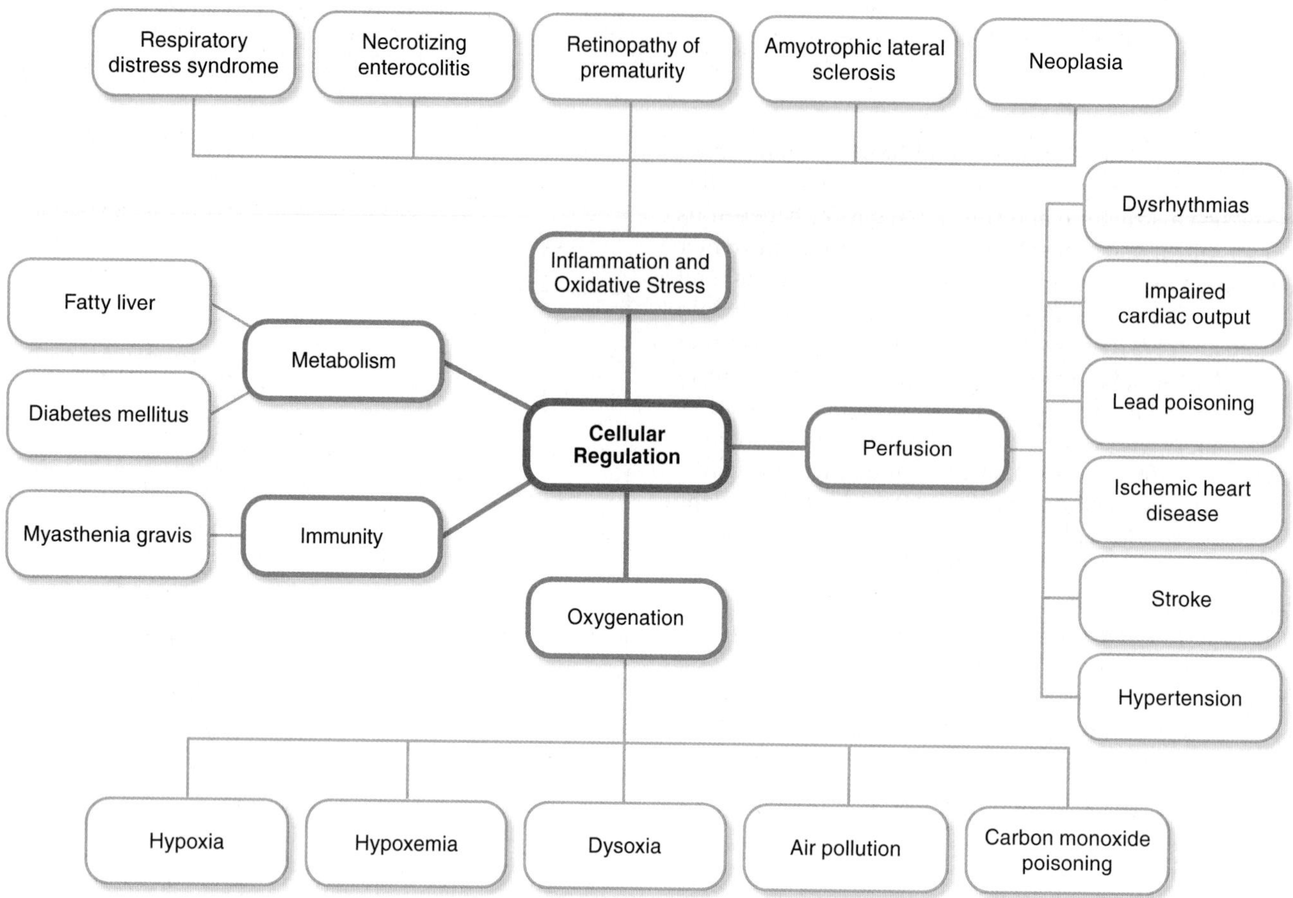

Figure 10.2 ■ Concepts related to cell injury and aging.

> **Check Your Progress: Section 10.1**
>
> 1. Define cellular adaptation.
> 2. What is the difference between reversible and nonreversible cell injury?
> 3. Describe the effect of cell injury and aging on the body.

10.2 The Cell as the Basic Unit of Disease

All **eukaryotic cells** (those with a true nucleus) have common structures that perform specific, unique functions. The primary components include the nucleus, cytoplasm, and the cell membrane, also known as the plasma membrane (**Figure 10.3** ■). The nucleus, the largest organelle in the cell, is referred to as the control center. It is a rounded, elongated structure containing the genome along with the enzymes that are necessary for deoxyribonucleic acid (DNA) and ribonucleic acid (RNA) transcription. The cell membrane is a dynamic and fluid structure that consists of an organized arrangement of lipids, carbohydrates, and proteins. The cytoplasm, which lies inside the cell membrane, contains membrane-enclosed organelles along with the cytoplasmic matrix, or inclusions, in the aqueous gel. This matrix contains a variety of solutes, including inorganic ions (Na^+, K^+, Ca^+) and organic molecules (carbohydrates, lipids, proteins, and RNA).

Cells can be injured in a variety of ways leading to immediate and often severe consequences. Injury to the cell membrane places both the outer plasma membrane and internal organelles at risk, as such injury results in abnormal ion fluxes and dysfunction of the organelles.

Cell Membranes

The cell membrane, or plasma membrane, is one of the most important parts of the cell (**Figure 10.4** ■). The primary function of the cell membrane is to act as a semipermeable structure that separates the intracellular and extracellular environments. Injury to the cell membrane places both the membrane and internal organelles at risk, as such injury results in abnormal ion and water fluxes and dysfunction of the organelles. Other functions include providing receptors for hormones, neurotransmitters, and other biologically active substances; participating in the electrical events that occur in both nerve and muscle cells; and aiding in the regulation of cell growth and proliferation. There are two main factors that alter membrane potentials and excitability: the difference in the concentration of ions between the inside and outside of the membrane and the permeability of the membrane to these ions. Cell membrane permeability is a quality that permits the passage of solutes and solvents into and out

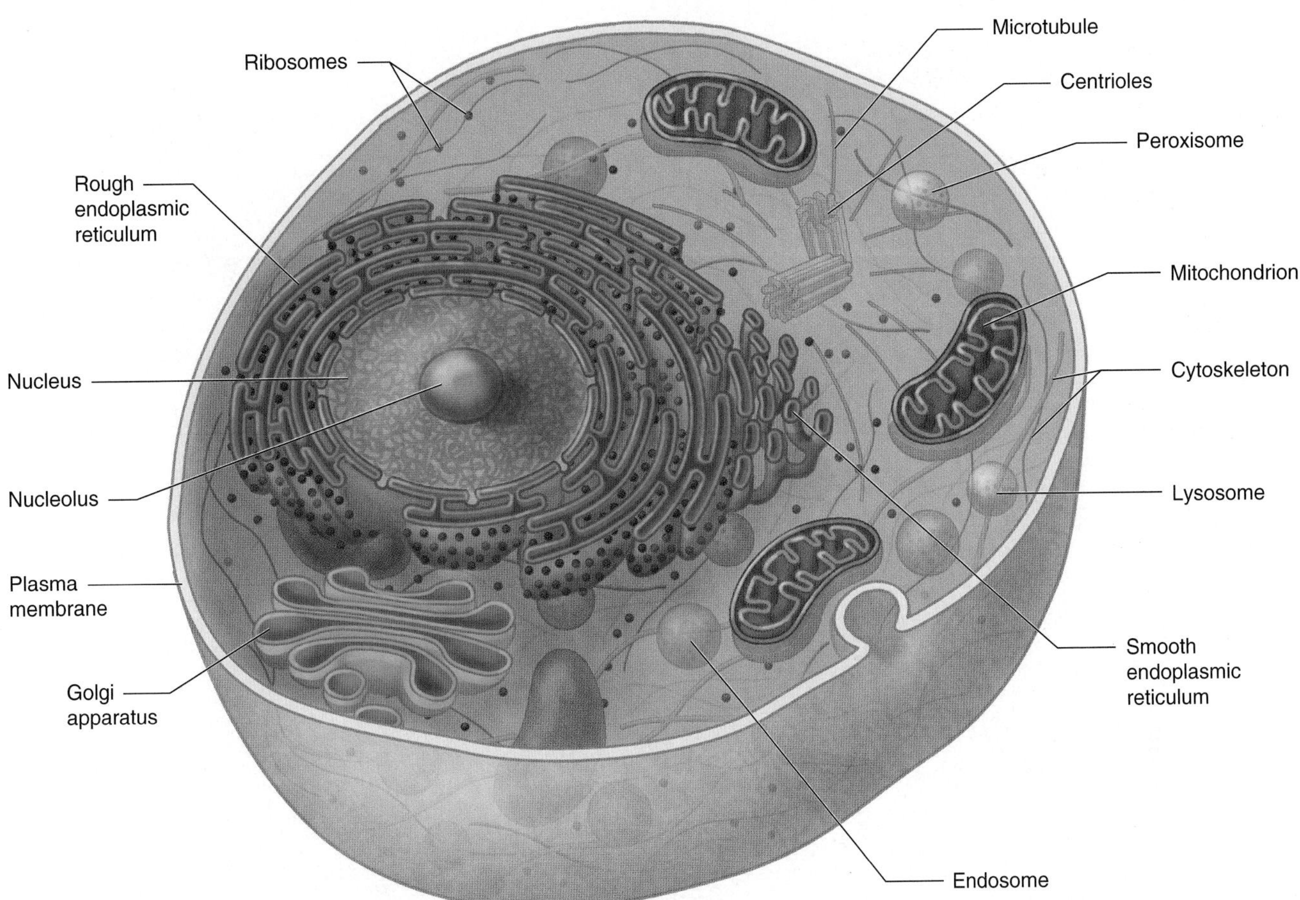

Figure 10.3 ■ All eukaryotic cells (those with a true nucleus) have common structures that perform specific, unique functions. The primary components include the nucleus, cytoplasm, and the cell membrane, or plasma membrane.

of the cell. The metabolic rate affects cell membrane permeability. For example, reduced ATP (adenosine triphosphate) causes acute cell swelling due to the failure of the energy-dependent sodium–potassium pump. Specifically, intracellular potassium levels decrease, and sodium and water accumulate in the cell.

There are many integral transmembrane proteins that form ion channels located on cell membranes or the surface of intracellular organelles. These channel proteins have complex structures and are selective with respect to the type of ion, such as sodium, potassium, calcium, and magnesium, that they allow to move through the channel. Ion channels function in a variety of cell activities, such as release of neurotransmitters that regulate nerve conduction and muscle contraction, regulation of water movement and cell volume, and secretion of cell products, including hormones, growth factors, and inflammatory mediators. **Channelopathies** are disorders caused by dysfunction of a channel protein or one or more of its subunits. Since ion channels are present in a variety of cell types, the various channelopathies can affect many different cell functions. A channelopathy is either a genetic disease caused by inheritance of a mutated gene that codes for production of a channel protein or one of its subunits or an acquired disease caused, for example, by an autoimmune attack against an ion channel protein. Channelopathies can cause an increase in function or a decrease in function and may affect various organ systems. More detailed information about several of these conditions can be found in later chapters.

Since ion channel function is critical for nerve conduction and muscle contraction, it is not surprising that channelopathies are responsible for a number of neuromuscular disorders, including some forms of epilepsy, migraine headaches, and movement disorders ranging from muscle paralysis to muscle hyperexcitability.[1] Pain channelopathies result from a mutation in ion channels in nociceptors (pain receptors) and result in either excessive pain or insensitivity to pain even in response to tissue injury. Cardiac channelopathies are responsible for many types of inherited dysrhythmias that cause altered heart rate and/or rhythm impairing cardiac output and tissue perfusion.

Recently discovered cardiac channelopathies include those that cause up to 30% of cases of sudden infant death syndrome (SIDS), which is unexpected death of an apparently healthy infant.[2] ■

Endocrine channelopathies result in alterations in hormone secretion, such as familial hyperaldosteronism and familial hyperinsulinemic hypoglycemia. Renal channelopathies affect water or ion secretion or resorption along the

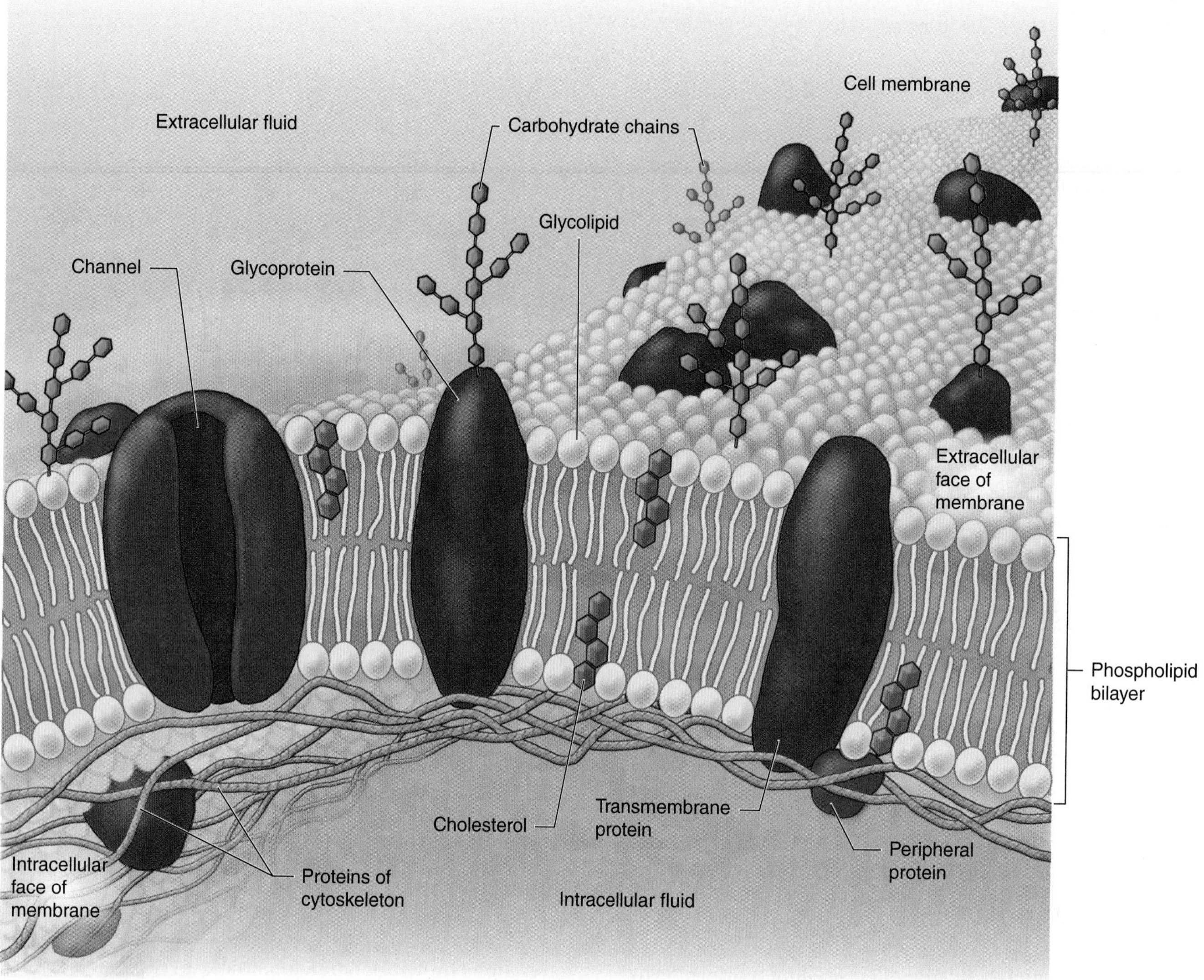

Figure 10.4 ■ The primary function of the cell membrane is to act as a semipermeable structure that separates the intracellular and extracellular environments.

nephron. An example of a renal channelopathy is nephrogenic diabetes insipidus, in which there is decreased responsiveness to antidiuretic hormone, resulting in loss of large amounts of water in the urine and dehydration.[3] Respiratory channelopathies are involved in asthma and cystic fibrosis.[4] Asthma is a common disorder in children and adults that involves airway inflammation and bronchoconstriction. The channelopathy in asthma affects calcium transport in airway smooth muscle cells. In cystic fibrosis, the primary defect is in an abnormal chloride channel, resulting in increased sodium and water resorption that causes respiratory tract secretions to thicken and occlude the airways. An example of an acquired channelopathy caused by autoimmunity is myasthenia gravis, in which the immune system destroys ion channels that normally respond to the neurotransmitter acetylcholine and cause skeletal muscle contraction. In myasthenia gravis, there is progressive weakness of skeletal muscles including the diaphragm that can result in respiratory failure.

Cell Organelles

The cell organelles are contained in the cytoplasm. The organelles, along with their functions and results of dysfunction, are described in **Table 10.1** ■.

Cell Metabolism

Cell metabolism, which is also called energy metabolisms, is defined as a set of chemical processes that help an organism respond to its surroundings. Cell metabolism is mainly involved in the production and utilization of energy that is used for activities such as cell growth and cell or tissue repair. The cells produce energy by metabolism of carbohydrates, amino acids, and lipids.

There are two types of energy metabolism. *Catabolism* consists of breaking down stored nutrients and body tissues to produce energy; *anabolism* is a constructive process by which complex molecules are formed from simpler ones. These biological responses are essential for an organism to

Table 10.1 Function and Dysfunction of Cell Organelles

Organelles	Function of Organelles	Results of Dysfunction
Ribosomes	Synthesize proteins and other materials needed for cell function.	Results in ribosomopathies, in which genetic abnormalities cause impaired biogenesis and function resulting in specific clinical phenotypes.
Endoplasmic reticulum (ER)	Functions as a tubular communication system for the transportation of various substances from one part of the cell to another and provides the machinery for a major share of the cell's metabolic functions.	Interferes with the synthesis of pancreatic digestive enzymes and liver plasma proteins along with glycogen storage and the metabolism of lipid-soluble drugs, leading to a variety of clinical manifestations.
Golgi complex	Modifies the substances synthesized in the ER and packages them into secretory granules or vesicles along with receiving proteins and other substances from the cell surface by a retrograde transport mechanism.	Defects in the microtubules result in a rare and severe group of genetic disorders that result in a lack of growth hormone, leading to skeletal system abnormalities.
Mitochondria	Supplies the energy in the form of ATP needed by the cell.	Leads to decrease in the energy production within the cell that is needed to sustain life and support growth, causing cell injury or cell death. If the damage is repeated throughout the body, whole systems can fail.
Lysosomes	Function as part of the cell's digestive system.	Molecules that are supposed to be broken down accumulate as a result of a deficiency in on the lysosomal enzymes, causing Tay-Sachs disease.
Peroxisomes	Function as part of the cell's digestive system.	Fatty acids accumulate, stripping these cells of their fatty sheaths, which are vital to nerve transmission.

synthesize complex molecules and convert nutrient molecules into other usable forms for future use.

Abnormalities with cell metabolism can have catastrophic effects. Without this process, the cell lacks energy to carry out biological reactions, which can lead to cell death. The percentage of cells that have to die before there is organ dysfunction varies with the organ.

Cell-to-Cell Connections and Interactions

Direct interactions between cells are critical for the development and function of multicellular organisms. Cells communicate with each other and with the internal and external environments through a number of different mechanisms. Interactions between cells can be stable, such as those that occur through cell junctions. These junctions are involved in the communication and organization of cells within a particular tissue by way of both electrical and chemical signaling systems that control not only electrical potentials, but also the overall function of the cell and gene activity that is required for cell division and cell replication (**Figure 10.5** ■).

Other cell-to-cell interactions are transient or temporary. This type of interaction occurs between cells of the immune system and with the interactions that are involved with the inflammatory process (refer to Chapter 11). The loss of communication between cells can result in uncontrolled cells growth and the development of cancer (refer to Chapter 12). These types of intercellular interactions are distinguished from other types, including those that occur between cells and the extracellular matrix.

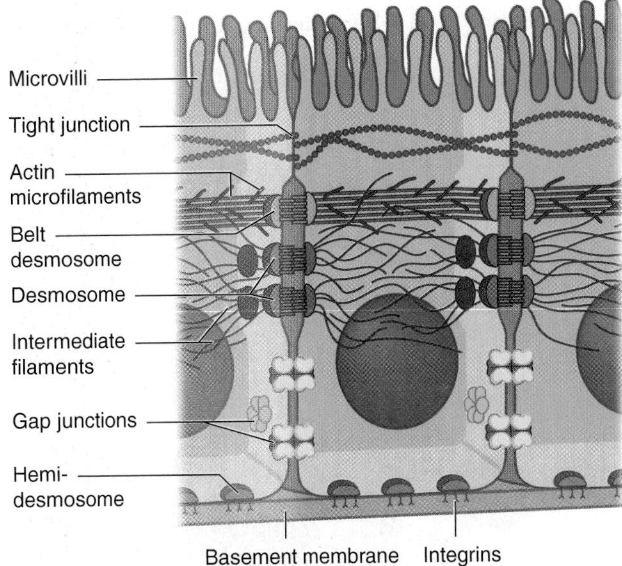

Figure 10.5 ■ Cell-to-cell interactions.

Extracellular Matrix

The extracellular matrix (ECM) is nonliving material that is secreted by cells (**Figure 10.6** ■). It is composed of secreted proteins and polysaccarides. The ECM can be either semi-fluid or rigidly solid and hard, and it fills space between the cells in tissue. The ECM provides structural support to cells and tissues along with playing a substantial role in regulating the behavior of cells in multicellular organisms. Also the ECM is a substrate that guides cell migration during the process of embryonic development and wound healing.

Abnormal ECM dynamics can be catastrophic. Dysfunction of the ECM leads to deregulated cell proliferation and invasion, failure of cell death, and loss of cell differentiation. This results in not only congenital defects but also pathologic processes, including tissue fibrosis and cancer. It is essential to understanding ECM remodeling and regulation to develop new interventions for disease processes.

Cell Signaling Systems

Cell signaling systems consist of receptors that reside either in the cell membrane or within the cells (**Figure 10.7** ■). Receptors residing in the cell membrane are referred to as surface receptors; receptors within the cell are referred

Epithelium
Integrins
Basement membrane
Fibroblast
Integrins
Endothelial cells
Capillary
Adhesive glycoproteins
Integrins
Fibroblast
Interstitial matrix
Proteoglycan
Type IV collagen
Laminin
Cross-linked collagen triple helices
Proteoglycan

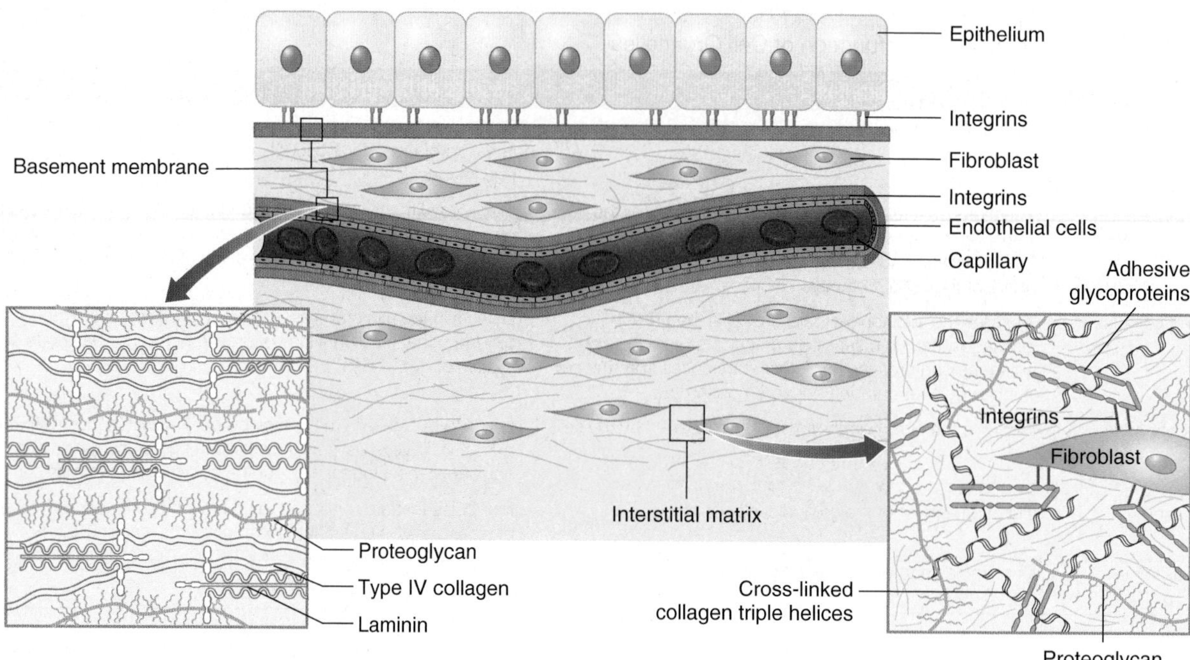

Figure 10.6 ■ The extracellular matrix is nonliving material secreted by the cells.

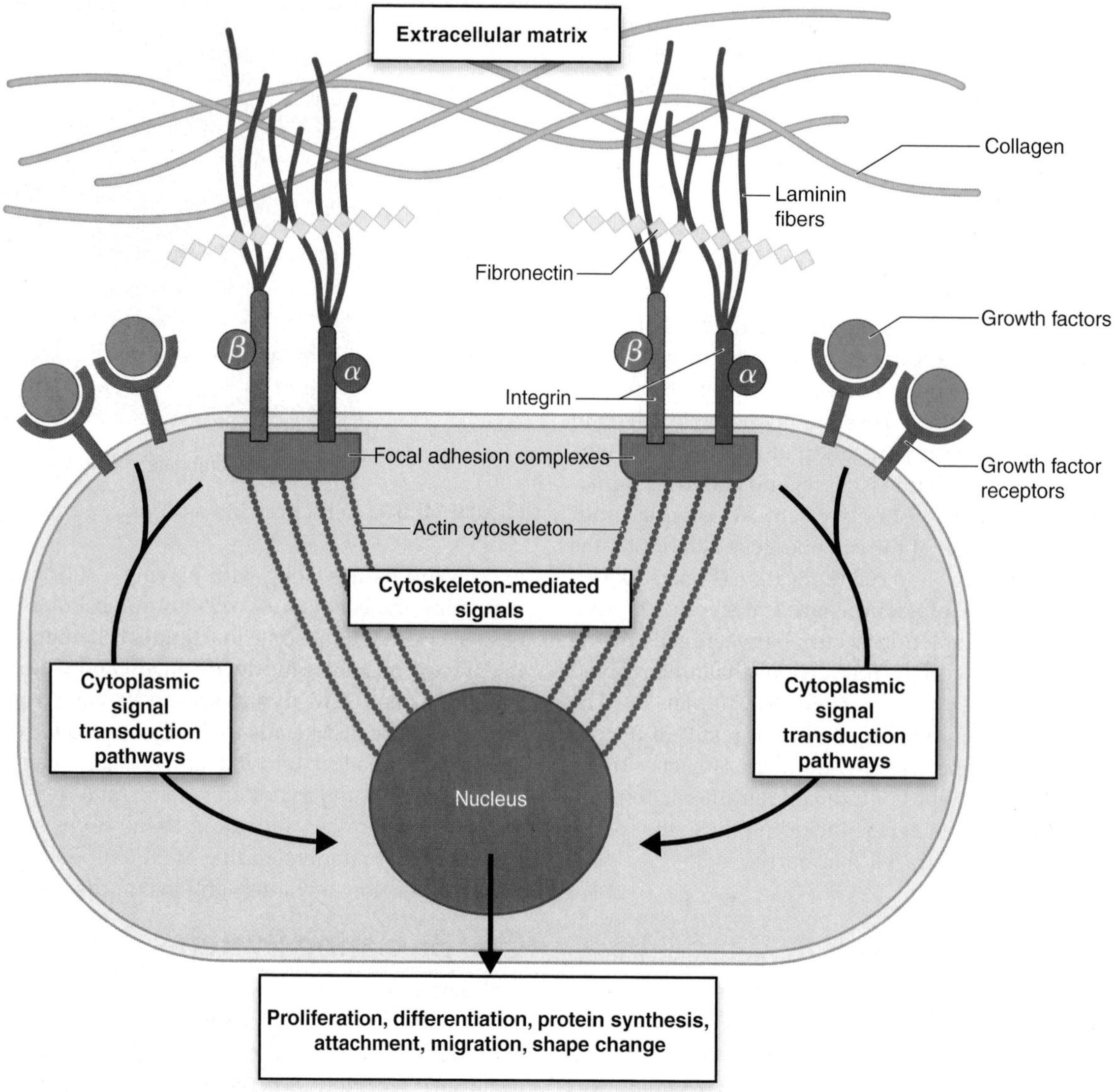

Extracellular matrix
Collagen
Laminin fibers
Fibronectin
Growth factors
β
α
β
α
Integrin
Focal adhesion complexes
Growth factor receptors
Actin cytoskeleton
Cytoskeleton-mediated signals
Cytoplasmic signal transduction pathways
Cytoplasmic signal transduction pathways
Nucleus
Proliferation, differentiation, protein synthesis, attachment, migration, shape change

Figure 10.7 ■ Cell signaling pathways.

to as intracellular receptors. These receptors are activated by a variety of extracellular signals, or first messengers, including neurotransmitters, protein hormones, growth factors, steroids, inflammatory mediators, and other chemical messengers. This pathway may also include additional intercellular mechanisms known as second messengers. Transducers and effectors of these signaling systems are responsible for physiologic responses.

The type of cell signaling abnormality is responsible for different disease processes within the body. Cell signals can be lost, be hyperactive, not reach or be ignored by the target, or experience a combination of these.

CLINICAL POINT: Hyperactive signals due to increased levels of excitatory neurotransmitters occur with strokes, which are also called brain attacks. The immediate response is death of the nearby brain cells; however, the most catastrophic event comes when the dying cells release large amounts of the signaling molecule glutamate, which is toxic to the cells when produced in excess, leading to widespread brain damage. ■

When cell signals do not reach their target, the affected nerve cells can no longer transmit signals from one area to another. This is the etiology of multiple sclerosis, a disease in which the protective wrappings around nerve cells in the brain and spinal cord are destroyed, leading to many problems. Signals that are ignored have the same impact as those that do not reach their target. A specific example of this is type 2 diabetes mellitus. With this disease process, the insulin signals are being sent; however, the target cells are ignoring (or are resistant) to these signals, causing hyperglycemia to occur.

Many mechanisms maintain appropriate cell growth, including cell division in response to external signals, enzymes that repair damaged DNA, and cells making connections with neighboring cells. When cell communication breaks down, this causes uncontrolled cell growth, often leading to cancer. Cancer begins when a cell gains the ability to grow and divide, even in the absence of a signal. Ordinarily, this unregulated growth triggers a signal for self-destruction. However, with cancer, the cell loses its ability to respond to death signals, divides out of control, and forms a tumor. In turn, cell communication events cause blood vessels to grow into the tumor, which enables it to grow larger and communicate with, and spread to, other parts of the body.

Check Your Progress: Section 10.2

1. What are the common structures found in eukaryotic cells?
2. Describe the primary function of a cell membrane.
3. What is the correlation between channelopathy and cystic fibrosis?

10.3 Common Causes of Cell Injury

Cell injury, which can be reversible (allowing the cell to recover) or irreversible (causing cell death) can occur in a variety of different ways. Common causes of cell injury that will be explored here are hypoxia, dysoxia, and oxidative stress. Other causes of cell injury include factors such as the environment; genetics, genomics, and epigenomics; infectious agents; immune reactions; nutritional imbalances; and trauma. Some of these causes of cell injury are covered in the next section, with additional topics explored in other chapters in this text.

Hypoxia

When the body does not have enough oxygen, the result is hypoxia or hypoxemia. **Hypoxia** is defined as low oxygen in the tissues; **hypoxemia** is defined as low oxygen in the blood. These terms can be used interchangeably in certain circumstances. Hypoxic events deprive the cell of oxygen and interrupt oxidative metabolism and the generation of ATP (**Figure 10.8** ■). Hypoxia can result from insufficient oxygen in the air, respiratory disease, decreased perfusion due to vasoconstriction or other caused of vascular obstruction, anemia, edema, or the inability of the cell to use the oxygen that is available. A short time margin exists between reversible and nonreversible cell damage. The actual time necessary to produce irreversible cell damage depends on the degree of oxygen deprivation and the specific metabolic needs of the cell.

Types of Hypoxia

There are four basic types of hypoxia:

1. ***Hypoxemic hypoxia.*** The most common type of hypoxia is hypoxemic hypoxia. Hypoxemic hypoxia occurs when the PaO_2 is below normal (less than 80 mmHg) because either the alveolar PO_2 is reduced (for environmental reasons such as altitude) or the blood cannot fully equilibrate with the alveolar air (owing to lung disease with diffusion impairment such as emphysema or fibrosis).
2. ***Ischemic hypoxia.*** In ischemic, or stagnant, hypoxia, the tissue is not receiving enough oxygen because of decreased perfusion caused by a cardiac or vascular disorder.
3. ***Anemic hypoxia.*** In anemic hypoxia, the lungs can be in perfect working condition; however, the oxygen-carrying capacity of the blood is reduced. This type of hypoxia often occurs with anemia and can also occur as a result of carbon monoxide poisoning. The carbon monoxide binds with the hemoglobin, preventing oxygen from binding, which reduces the oxygen-carrying capacity of the blood. In this type of anemia, the tissues do not get sufficient oxygen to maintain their metabolic needs because of decreased oxygen transport in the blood.
4. ***Histoxic hypoxia.*** The term *histoxic* means that the cells have been poisoned. In histoxic hypoxia, there is no problem getting the oxygen to the tissue, but the tissue is unable to use the oxygen. This type of hypoxia is often caused by exposure to cyanide, which prevents mitochondrial enzymes from using oxygen to create energy.

Cellular Effects of Hypoxia

Hypoxia causes a power failure in the cell. This causes widespread effects on the cell's structural components

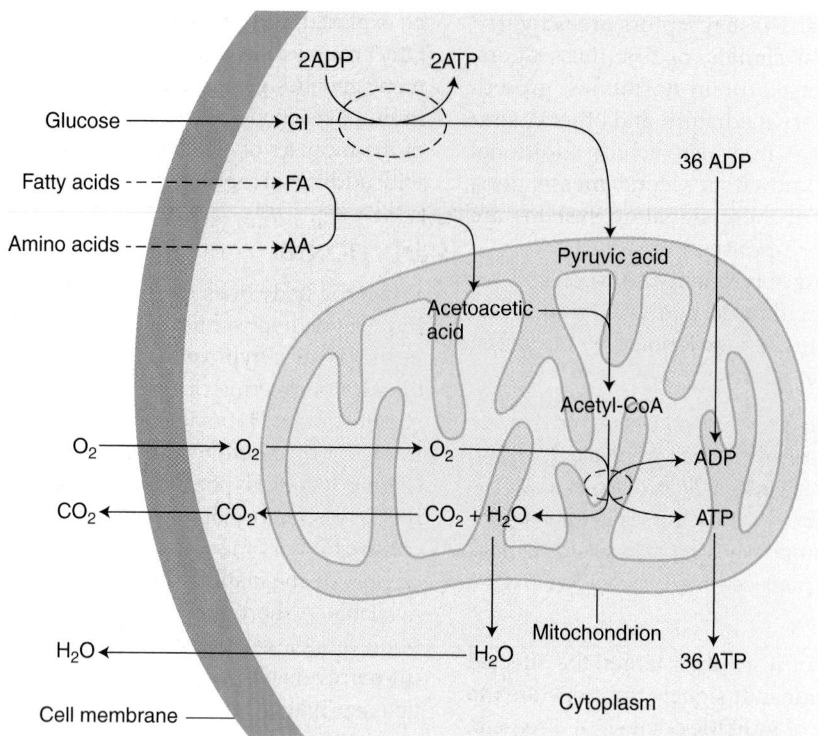

Figure 10.8 ■ Formation of adenosine triphosphate (ATP) in the cell, showing that most of the ATP is formed in the mitochondria. ADP = adenosine diphosphate; CoA = coenzyme A.

and functions (see Figure 10.8). As the oxygen tension in the cell falls, oxidative metabolism decreases, causing the cell to revert to anaerobic metabolism. When this occurs, the cell will attempt to use its limited glycogen stores to maintain vital functions. However, as the cellular pH falls, lactic acid accumulates in the cell. This acidic environment can have adverse effects on both intercellular structures and biochemical reactions, including alterations in the cell membrane, causing chromatin clumping and cell volume changes.

Hypoxia leads to reduced ATP, which can cause acute cell swelling caused by the failure of the energy-dependent sodium/potassium–adenosine triphosphatase membrane pump. This extrudes sodium from, and returns potassium to, the cell. With impaired functioning of this pump, intracellular potassium levels decrease, and sodium and water accumulate in the cell. This movement of water and ions into the cells is associated with dilation of the endoplasmic reticulum, increased membrane permeability, and decreased mitochondrial function.

Cellular changes caused by hypoxia are reversible, to a point, if oxygenation is restored. If the oxygen supply is not restored, there is a continued loss of enzymes, proteins, and ribonucleic acid through the hyperpermeable cell membrane. Injury to the lysosomal membranes results in the leakage of destructive lysosomal enzymes in the cytoplasm, causing enzymatic digestion of cell components. Leakage of the intracellular enzymes through the permeable cell membrane into the extracellular fluid provides an important clinical indicator of cell injury and death, which are measured by laboratory blood tests.

Variations in Organ Susceptibility to Hypoxia

Tissues vary considerably in their sensitivity to hypoxia. Mechanisms that allow tolerance to hypoxia and prevent tissue damage are poorly understood. Neurologic cells tolerate hypoxia for only a few minutes, while the bladder smooth muscle may survive for several days with decreased oxygen. This has important implications in the management of oxygen transport and monitoring of tissue hypoxia in critically ill patients.

Hypoxia can cause failure of the energy-dependent membrane channels, leading to a subsequent loss of membrane integrity, changes in cellular calcium homeostasis, and changes in cellular enzyme activity. An enzyme's sensitivity to hypoxia is a function of the oxygen concentration at which it has half maximum activity (KmO_2).[5]

Cellular tolerance to hypoxia may involve a reduction in the metabolic rate, increased extraction of oxygen from the blood and surrounding tissues, and adaptations of enzymes to allow metabolism at low partial pressures of oxygen. Anaerobic energy production is important to the survival of some tissues despite this insufficiency. Skeletal muscle increases glucose update by 600% during hypoxia, and bladder smooth muscle has the capacity to generate up to 60% of total energy requirement by anaerobic glycolysis alone. In cardiac cells, anaerobic glucose use protects the integrity of the cell membrane by maintaining energy-dependent potassium channels.[6]

Specific differences with regard to susceptibility to hypoxia vary significantly. Survival times of various tissues during hypoxia are as follows:

- Brain: less than 3 minutes
- Kidney and liver: 15–20 minutes
- Skeletal muscle: 60–90 minutes
- Vascular smooth muscle: 24 to 72 hours
- Hair and nails: Several days

Maintenance of blood flow to the most hypoxia-sensitive organs should be a primary therapeutic goal.[7]

Samuel Murphy: Application

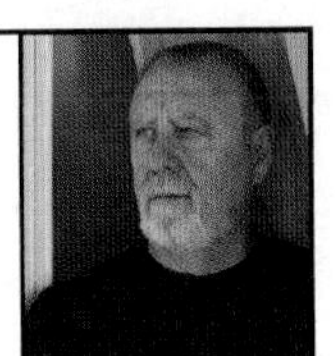

Mr. Murphy presents at the emergency department (ED) because his symptoms of flu have continued to worsen. Mr. Murphy tells the nurse that while he usually has a productive cough, the sputum is normally clear or white. In the past several days, the sputum was a yellowish-green color. He complains of fatigue that has been interfering with this ability to complete activities of daily living, stating, "I just can't seem to catch my breath when I am doing anything other than sitting in my living room." Vital signs and pertinent assessment data on admission to the ED include the following: pulse 86, respiratory rate 32, temperature 102°F, blood pressure 176/90, pulse oximetry 88% on room air. Rhonchi were noted on auscultation of the lung fields throughout, and +2 edema was noted in bilateral lower extremities. Mr. Murphy states that he takes a water pill for swelling but it doesn't appear to be working as it normally does.

The healthcare provider orders oxygen by nasal cannula to be administered at 2 L/min and a chest x-ray. Laboratory orders include a complete blood count, a culture and sensitivity (C&S) of Mr. Murphy's sputum, and an arterial blood gas analysis. Mr. Murphy is admitted to the hospital to treat the exacerbation of chronic obstructive pulmonary disease (COPD) and to rule out a diagnosis of pneumonia.

3. On the basis of Mr. Murphy's history, which type of hypoxia does he most likely have?
4. What are potential causes of Mr. Murphy's hypoxia?
5. Because of Mr. Murphy's dysoxia, what changes may be needed in his plan of care regarding activities of daily living?

Dysoxia: Imbalance Between Oxygen Supply and Demand

Dysoxia is an imbalance between oxygen supply and oxygen demand. It occurs when there is either a decreased supply of or an increased demand for oxygen. Conditions that cause dysoxia are explored further below.

Decreased Oxygen Supply

Conditions that cause a decreased oxygen supply include respiratory, cardiac, and vascular disorders. Respiratory disorders that block the exchange of oxygen at the alveolar capillary membrane include pneumonia, pulmonary edema, asthma, and drowning. A decreased supply of oxygen can also occur when the body cannot transport an adequate amount of oxygen to the target tissues because of a cardiac disorder such as heart failure, a vascular disorder such as atherosclerosis, or a hematologic disorder such as anemia.

Increased Oxygen Demand

An increased metabolic rate increases the demand for oxygen. The level of oxygenation declines when the systems of the body cannot meet this demand. An increased metabolic rate is normal in pregnancy, wound healing, and exercise because the body is using energy or building tissue. Most individuals are able to meet the increased demand for oxygen and do not display symptoms of dysoxia.

Dysoxia also occurs when a patient is unable to increase oxygen supply to match the increase in oxygen demand. Pathologic conditions, including shivering and fever that can occur with viral or bacterial sepsis, physical agitation, and seizure activity, can cause dysoxia to occur. An oxygen supply that may be adequate at rest will not be adequate if the need for oxygen increases.

CLINICAL POINT: An increase in the need for oxygen can occur during routine hospital care activities such as turning, bathing, or linen changes. The most vulnerable patients are those whose supply system is unable to meet oxygen demands even in the resting state. Therefore, it is important for the nurse to assess oxygenation variables and pace activities that affect the susceptible patient's oxygenation. ■

Samuel Murphy: Outcome

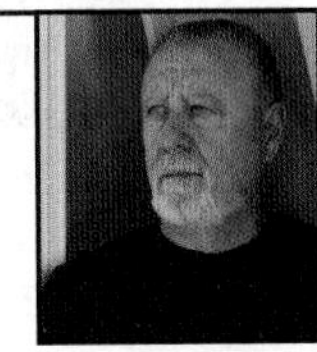

Mr. Murphy's pulse oximetry reading continues to remain below 90% despite the 2 L/min of oxygen that was administered via nasal cannula. Arterial blood gas results indicate respiratory acidosis, and the chest x-ray indicates a diagnosis of pneumonia. Although the sputum C&S is pending, a broad-spectrum antibiotic is prescribed via the intravenous route, and the first dose is administered after the C&S has been obtained. Mr. Murphy's respiratory status continues to worsen, and he is mechanically ventilated and transferred to the intensive care unit. Despite these interventions, Mr. Murphy experiences cardiac arrest and dies during the night shift.

6. What factors in Mr. Murphy's history may have caused dysoxia?

Oxidative Stress

Oxidative stress is an imbalance between the production of reactive oxygen species (ROS), such as free radicals, and the ability of the body to counteract, or detoxify, their harmful effects through neutralization by antioxidants (**Figure 10.9** ■). Free radicals are highly reactive chemical species with an unpaired electron in the outer orbit of the molecule. This unpaired electron causes the free radicals to be unstable and to react nonspecifically with molecules in the vicinity, causing chain reactions that cause the generation of new free radicals. In the cells and tissues, these free radicals react with proteins, lipids, and carbohydrates, not only causing damage to the cell membrane, but also inactivating enzymes and damaging the nucleic acids that make up DNA. This condition occurs when the generation of ROS exceeds the ability of the body to neutralize or eliminate the ROS or repair the damage they have caused.

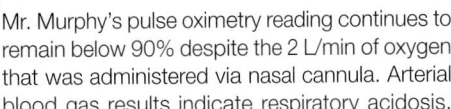

Oxidative stress is of utmost importance in providing care to the neonate. Healthy, mature neonates can tolerate the drastic change is oxygen concentration that occurs with the transition from fetal circulation

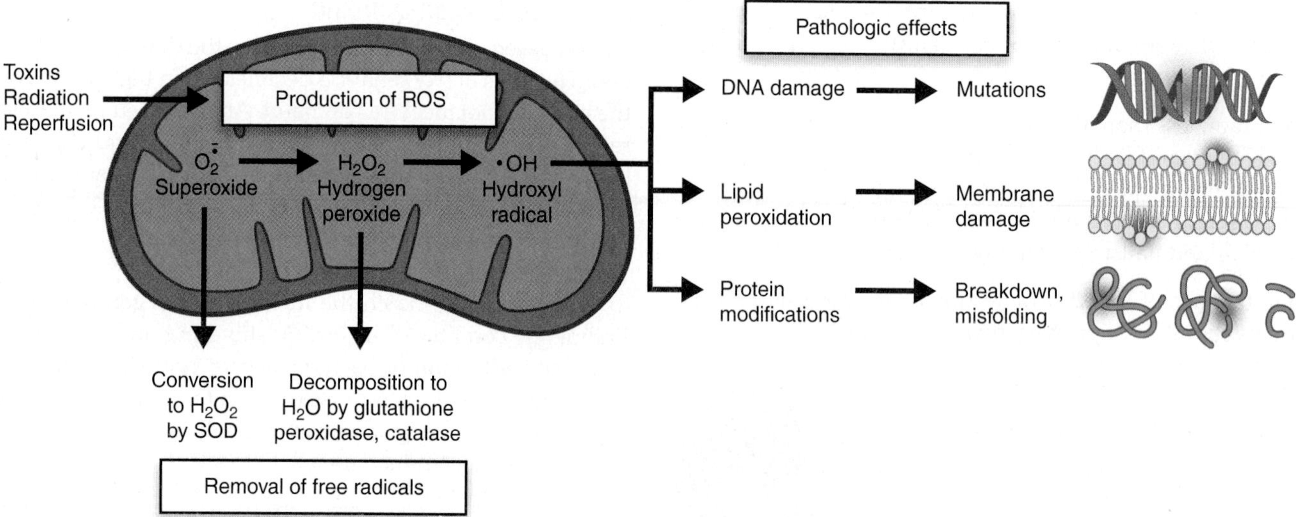

Figure 10.9 ■ The generation, removal, and role of reactive oxygen species (ROS) in cell injury. The production of ROS is increased by many injurious stimuli. These free radicals are removed by spontaneous decay and by specialized enzymatic systems. Excessive production or inadequate removal leads to accumulation of free radicals in cells, which may damage lipids (by peroxidation), proteins, and deoxyribonucleic acid (DNA), resulting in cell injury. SOD = superoxide dismutase.

to newborn circulation. An oxidant–antioxidant imbalance in neonates is implicated in the pathogenesis of the major complications associated with prematurity, including respiratory distress syndrome (RDS), necrotizing enterocolitis, chronic lung disease, retinopathy of prematurity, and intravascular hemorrhage. These disorders are accompanied by inflammatory processes with free radial generation and oxidative stress.

In newborns with RDS, respiratory failure due to deficient alveolar development and the production of surfactant are complicated by diminished antioxidant stores and enzymatic antioxidant inducibility. The premature neonate's lungs are particularly susceptible to oxidant stress because there are many sources of ROS production and a general lack of antioxidant defenses. The full-term neonate is armed with sufficient defenses, but the preterm neonate is not. Therefore, it is critical to ensure that the neonate's lungs are resistant to high oxygen tensions, which are required in the treatment of RDS. ■

Effects of ROS

Reaction oxygen species (ROS) are oxygen-containing molecules that include free radicals such as superoxide (O_2^-) and hydroxyl (OH^-) radicals and nonradicals such as hydrogen peroxide (H_2O_2). Oxidative stress can lead to oxidation of cell components, activation of signal transduction pathways, and changes in both gene and protein expression. DNA modification and damage can also occur as a result of oxidative stress. Current research suggests that mitochondrial DNA is also a target of oxidation causing mitochondrial dysfunction.[8]

Although ROS and oxidative stress are associated with cell and tissue damage, recent evidence suggests that ROS do not always act in a damaging manner. Current research indicates that ROS are important signaling molecules that are used in healthy cells to regulate and maintain normal activities and functions including vascular tone, endothelial growth factor, and insulin signaling, and as a preconditioning function to protect cells from injury when there are high levels of ROS.[9] It is important to note that ROS can also serve both intracellular and intercellular messengers.

Situations in Which ROS Are Produced

It was originally thought that ROS are produced endogenously only by normal metabolic processes and cell activity, including the metabolic burst that accompanies phagocytosis. However, ROS are formed by several different mechanisms including the interaction of ionizing radiation with biological molecules and as an unavoidable byproduct of cellular respiration. Other situations can also produce ROS, including the administration of high levels of supplemental oxygen and during reperfusion after an ischemic event and during inflammatory response.

The damage caused by oxidative stress has been implicated in many disease processes. Pathogenic mutations in the gene for superoxide dismutase are associated with amyotrophic lateral sclerosis (ALS). Oxidative stress is also thought to play a role in the development of cancer. The reestablishment of blood flow after loss of perfusion that occurs with heart attack and stroke is also associated with oxidative injury to vital organs. Oxidative stress also contributes to endothelial dysfunction that contributes to the development, progression, and prognosis of cardiovascular disease. Age-related functional declines have also been linked to the damage caused by oxidative stress.

Antioxidant Defense Mechanisms

Antioxidants are natural and synthetic molecules that either inhibit the reactions responsible for production of ROS or neutralize ROS. Antioxidants include both enzymatic and nonenzymatic compounds. Enzymes that are known to function as antioxidants include superoxide dismutase, catalase, glutathione peroxidase, and thioreductase. Nonenzymatic antioxidants include vitamins such as A (carotenes), E (tocopherols), and C (ascorbate). Other nonenzymatic antioxidants are glutathione and flavonoids along with

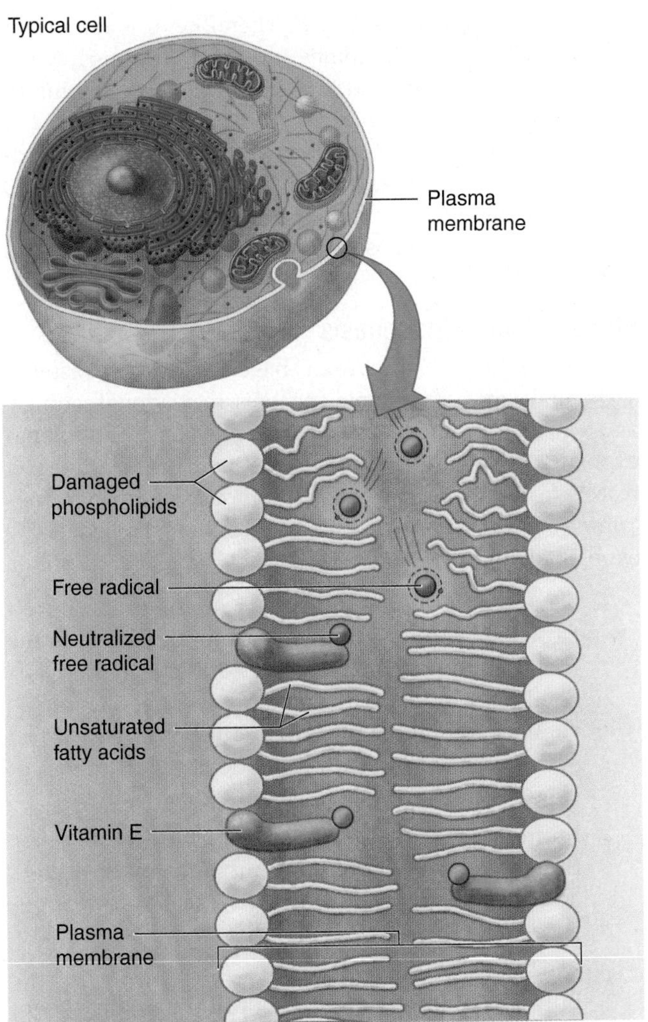

Figure 10.10 ■ Mechanisms of action of vitamin E, one of the most important lipid-soluble antioxidants.

micronutrients such as selenium and zinc. Vitamin C is the most important water-soluble antioxidant in the extracellular fluid. It helps to neutralize ROS in the aqueous phase before it can attack the lipids. Vitamin E is the most important lipid-soluble antioxidant, as it can protect the membrane fatty acids from lipid peroxidation (**Figure 10.10** ■).[10]

Because oxidants play a role in many diseases, many medications have an antioxidant action that may contribute to their pharmacologic activity. Some examples include calcium channel antagonists, beta-adrenoreceptor antagonists, antiarrhythmic drugs, and statins. All of these drugs are used in the treatment of cardiovascular diseases.

Check Your Progress: Section 10.3

1. Which vitamins play an antioxidant role?
2. Explain the pathologic process by which carbon monoxide poisoning leads to anemic hypoxia.
3. Describe the role of oxidative stress in the development of respiratory distress syndrome in premature babies.

10.4 Environmental Factors That Cause Cell Injury

There are certain environmental factors that contribute to cell injury. This section discusses air pollution, carbon monoxide poisoning, lead poisoning, and radiation. In Chapter 3, selected biological, chemical, and physical hazards are discussed. Additional biologic, chemical, and radiologic agents of disease are covered in Chapter 52. Chapter 33 covers temperature extremes.

Air Pollution

The six most common pollutants in the air across the United States are carbon monoxide, lead, nitrogen dioxide, ozone, particulate matter, and sulfur dioxide.[11] The Environmental Protection Agency (EPA), as required by the Clean Air Act, sets national air quality standards for these pollutants. Despite improvements in air quality resulting from these regulations, significant amounts of pollutants continue to be released into the air, and many areas in the United States have air pollution levels that exceed national standards at various times of the year.[12] These air pollutants are derived mainly from the combustion of fossil fuels by motor vehicles and various industrial processes. Fossil fuels, such as oil, coal, and natural gas, are organic matter derived from decomposition of formerly living sources. Because air pollutants are inhaled directly into the lungs, their main adverse effect is respiratory impairment. These substances irritate cells in the airways causing inflammation, oxidative stress, bronchoconstriction, and increased mucus secretion that causes various degrees of airway obstruction and clinical manifestations including coughing, wheezing, and dyspnea (shortness of breath). Individuals with conditions that decrease oxygenation, such as respiratory and cardiac disorders, are most susceptible; however, high levels of air pollution can be hazardous to everyone. Some components of air pollution have also been implicated in causing lung cancer. Individuals with coronary artery disease have increased risk of chest pain and myocardial infarction (heart attack) from air pollution because the respiratory impairment can decrease the amount of oxygen reaching the blood and delivered to the heart. Higher exposure to air pollution occurs in individuals who live near areas with heavy motor vehicle traffic, such as expressways, people who work in high-traffic areas such as road maintenance crews, and those who engage in physical activity outdoors, which is associated with deeper and faster breathing, resulting in increased inhalation of any pollutants present in the air.

Chronic exposure to sublethal amounts of carbon monoxide in outdoor air can have adverse effects, especially for individuals with cardiovascular or respiratory disease. The mechanism of carbon monoxide's adverse effects is the same as that described previously for acute carbon monoxide poisoning: the ability of carbon monoxide to bind to hemoglobin and myoglobin, thereby decreasing oxygen delivery to tissues. Lead gets into the air from the soil and industrial facilities such as utility and lead battery plants. The harmful effects of inhaled lead are similar to those explained earlier for lead that has been ingested. Nitrogen dioxide (NO_2) and sulfur dioxide (SO_2) are very reactive gases present in polluted air that cause airway irritation, inflammation, and bronchoconstriction. Nitrogen dioxide participates in reactions that produce ground-level ozone and sulfur dioxide can be converted to sulfuric acid. Ozone (O_3) is a gas produced by a reaction in the presence of heat and sunlight between nitrogen oxides and volatile organic compounds emitted from gasoline vapor, chemical solvents, air conditioners, power plants, and some factories. Ozone is the main component of what is commonly referred to as smog. The ozone layer that occurs naturally in the atmosphere 10–30 miles above the earth is protective because it decreases the amount of harmful ultraviolet radiation from the sun that reaches the earth's surface. So you may be wondering why ozone is considered a hazardous air pollutant. A statement about ozone by the EPA is "good up high bad nearby."[13] Ground-level ozone is harmful because it causes adverse effects on the respiratory and cardiovascular systems similar to those described previously for other air pollutants. Particle pollution, also called particulate matter, consists of particles of solids and liquid in the air. They are classified either as fine particles that have a diameter less than 2.5 μm in diameter ($PM_{2.5}$) or as coarse particles that have a diameter between 2.5 and 10 μm (PM_{10}). The coarse particles are derived from wind-blown soil, dust, pollen, and spores, and because of their large size, they penetrate only into the trachea and bronchi when inhaled. Fine particles are derived mainly from fuel combustion, and because of their small size, they can penetrate into smaller airways and into alveoli, where they can cross the alveolar capillary membrane and enter the circulation. In addition to inflammation and oxidative stress in the airways, fine particles have been implicated in causing lung cancer.

CLINICAL POINT: The air quality index is a report of daily air quality in over 300 cities in the United States based on the level of common air pollutants. Information about the air quality index should be given to individuals with asthma and other respiratory disorders or cardiovascular disorders to help them plan the safest time to be outdoors and to adjust their outdoor activity level to minimize worsening of symptoms caused by air pollution. Because air quality can change daily, the EPA updates and posts information at its AirNow website. ■

A map at the EPA's AirNow website shows air quality throughout the United States represented by colors as shown in **Figure 10.11** ■. There is a link for healthcare providers at the website that contains brief fact sheets that can be printed and distributed to patients with information about air pollution and how to use the air quality index to decrease their risk of exposure. Also, anyone can sign up at the website for the EnviroFlash system that sends daily emails with notification of the current and forecasted air quality in your area.

Carbon Monoxide Poisoning

Carbon monoxide (CO) is a tasteless, odorless, colorless gas, so its presence cannot be directly detected by the person or people affected by it. Therefore, it is important to have CO detectors in homes and other buildings. Acute poisoning due to elevated levels of CO causes cell injury due to hypoxia, inflammation, and oxidative stress. CO causes more than half of all deaths from poisoning worldwide.[14] In the United States each year, an estimated 20,000 emergency department visits and 400 unintentional deaths not related to CO exposure in fires are attributed to CO poisoning.[15]

Etiology and Pathogenesis

Toxic and lethal exposures to CO have occurred as a result of accidental exposure in homes, schools, recreational settings, and workplaces and in fires and as a result of intentional exposure in suicide attempts. Exogenous CO production results from incomplete combustion of fossil (carbon containing) fuel.[15] Common sources of potentially lethal CO exposure include the following:

1. Car exhaust fumes from a car motor running in a closed space and exhaust fumes from boats with the motor running. Children and adults have died as a result of swimming behind a boat that had its motor running to operate the air conditioning or electrical system. The CO in these situations caused a loss of consciousness, and then the individuals drowned.
2. Improperly ventilated appliances, including furnaces, fireplaces, gas, kerosene, or propane space heaters and gasoline-powered generators used to run appliances during power outages that are placed too close to a home.
3. Burning buildings in which burning cotton, wood, paper, or synthetic substances produce CO.

The adverse effects of CO include its ability to decrease oxygen availability to cells by the following three mechanisms:

1. CO binds to hemoglobin, forming carboxyhemoglobin, which prevents the normal amount of oxygen from binding to hemoglobin. CO has an affinity for hemoglobin that is 200 times greater than the affinity between oxygen and hemoglobin.
2. CO binds to the most labile sites on the hemoglobin molecule, leaving only the stronger binding sites available for oxygen, resulting in a decreased unloading of oxygen to cells.
3. CO binds to myoglobin in skeletal and cardiac muscle, forming carboxymyoglobin. Myoglobin is a pigment similar to hemoglobin that functions to transport oxygen in cardiac and skeletal muscle cells. CO binding to myoglobin results in decreased oxygen transport in muscle.

Additional mechanisms of CO toxicity include its ability to bind to cytochrome oxidase, which is a mitochondrial enzyme that normally transfers electrons from oxygen to hydrogen to form ATP during aerobic metabolism.[16] If oxygen can't bind to cytochrome oxidase, electron transfer is inhibited, and ATP production is decreased. The binding

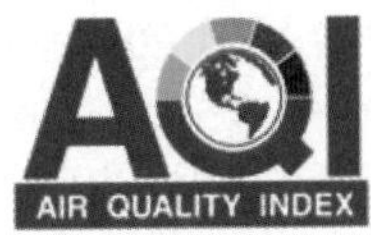

Air Quality Index Levels of Health Concern	Numerical Value	Meaning
Good	0 to 50	Air quality is considered satisfactory, and air pollution poses little or no risk.
Moderate	51 to 100	Air quality is acceptable; however, for some pollutants there may be a moderate health concern for a very small number of people who are unusually sensitive to air pollution.
Unhealthy for Sensitive Groups	101 to 150	Members of sensitive groups may experience health effects. The general public is not likely to be affected.
Unhealthy	151 to 200	Everyone may begin to experience health effects; members of sensitive groups may experience more serious health effects.
Very Unhealthy	201 to 300	Health alert: everyone may experience more serious health effects.
Hazardous	301 to 500	Health warnings of emergency conditions. The entire population is more likely to be affected.

Figure 10.11 ■ The air quality index.

of CO to cytochrome oxidase can last for days after exposure and explains why clinical symptoms can persist even after carboxyhemoglobin levels have decreased, especially in tissues with high oxygen and ATP demands such as the heart and brain. Cell injury resulting from hypoxia and decreased ATP leads to inflammation and oxidative stress, which cause further cell injury.

CO inhaled by a pregnant woman crosses the placenta and enters the fetal circulation. Because fetal hemoglobin has an affinity for CO higher than that of adult hemoglobin and because of the high metabolic rate and oxygen demands during the fetal period, CO exposure is especially hazardous to the fetus. Depending on the period of gestation when the fetus is exposed and the severity of the exposure, CO toxicity can cause anatomic malformations, intrauterine fetal death, cerebral palsy, seizures, and/or other neurologic alterations.[14] ■

Clinical Manifestations

Low levels of CO are normally present in the body because CO is a by-product of some metabolic reactions and results in carboxyhemoglobin levels in the range of 1–2% in nonsmokers. CO inhaled from cigarette smoking results in elevated carboxyhemoglobin levels of up to 10% depending on the number of cigarettes smoked each day. Carbon monoxide inhaled from tobacco products such as cigarettes contributes over time to vascular endothelial cell damage and atherosclerosis and to lung injury.

Acute, mild CO poisoning may initially resemble the flu with nausea, vomiting, and weakness. The throbbing headache caused by CO is the result of vasodilation of cerebral blood vessels. Nitric oxide is a vasodilator released by platelets and neutrophils that are activated as a result of inflammation caused by CO poisoning.[17] The increased cerebral blood flow resulting from vasodilation can contribute to cerebral edema and increased intracranial pressure, which causes neurologic alterations. Other manifestations of more severe CO poisoning, such as dyspnea, confusion, cardiac dysrhythmias, and coma, are a reflection of hypoxia caused by the decreased amount of oxygen transported in the blood. The binding of carbon monoxide to the heme pigment in hemoglobin can give a pink color to the skin and mucus membranes; a cherry red color is seen only in severe cases, usually just before death. **Table 10.2** ■ shows the relationship between clinical manifestations and the carboxyhemoglobin level.

Table 10.2 Clinical Manifestations Associated with Various Carboxyhemoglobin Levels

% Carboxyhemoglobin	Clinical Manifestations
1–2	No symptoms: normal level produced from catabolism of hemoglobin
3–10	Levels found in tobacco smokers that can exacerbate respiratory and cardiac disorders
10–30	Headache, exertional dyspnea, dizziness, nausea, fatigue
30–50	Confusion, nausea, vomiting, syncope, tachypnea
50–60	Severe headache, tachycardia, hypotension, syncope, coma and/or seizures
60–80	Coma, cardiac and/or respiratory failure, death imminent
> 80	Death within minutes unless immediate intervention occurs

SOURCES: Data from Betterman, K., & Patel S. (2014). Neurologic complications of carbon monoxide intoxication. *Handbook of Clinical Neurology, 120*(3), 971–979; Bleecker, M. (2015). Carbon monoxide intoxication. *Handbook of Clinical Neurology, 131*(3), 191–203; Fenton, J. (2002). Toxic gases. In *Toxicology: A case-oriented approach* (pp. 257–282). Boca Raton, FL: CRC Press.

CLINICAL POINT: There is not always a good correlation between the carboxyhemoglobin level and the clinical manifestations; that is, the clinical manifestations can be more severe than expected from the carboxyhemoglobin level at the time. The reason for this disparity is that the carboxyhemoglobin level may have been much higher before the time when the patient is being observed and may have already caused a significant degree of hypoxia and organ damage. By the time the patient reaches the hospital, the patient will likely have been treated with supplemental oxygen, which will lower the carboxyhemoglobin levels. Also, the carboxyhemoglobin level does not indicate the duration of exposure to carbon monoxide or the degree of binding of carbon monoxide to cytochrome oxidase or myoglobin. The clinical signs and symptoms provide a better indication of the severity of poisoning than the carboxyhemoglobin level at any one time point. ■

Sophia Velazquez: Application

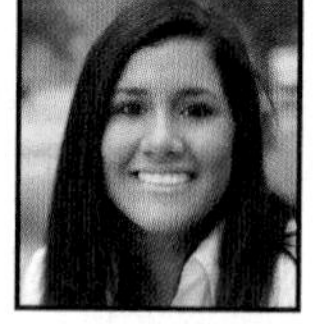

Sophia is still comatose and hypotensive on arrival in the emergency department. She remains intubated and is mechanically ventilated. Vasopressors are administered to improve her blood pressure. The following assessment data are obtained.

Arterial blood gases: pH = 7.28, $PaCO_2$ = 48 mmHg, PaO_2 = 52 mmHg, HCO_3^- = 15 mEq/L

SaO_2 measured with a multiwavelength pulse oximeter: 61%

Carboxyhemoglobin level: 48%

Cardiac evaluation: Elevated levels of creatine kinase and troponin I (markers of cardiac injury); electrocardiogram showed ST elevation (indicative of cardiac hypoxia); echocardiogram showed severely impaired cardiac output

Computed tomography (CT) scan of the brain shows cerebral edema.

Chest x-ray reveals pulmonary edema.

3. What clinical manifestations would be expected with a carboxyhemoglobin level of 48%?
4. What may account for the discrepancy between Sophia's carboxyhemoglobin level and her clinical manifestations?

Linking Pathophysiology to Diagnosis and Treatment

Diagnosis of CO poisoning is made by ascertaining the circumstances in which the individual was found, measurement of carboxyhemoglobin levels in the blood, and assessment for the clinical signs and symptoms of CO poisoning and of oxygenation.

CLINICAL POINT: It is important to understand that in assessing oxygenation parameters in a patient with CO poisoning, the saturation of hemoglobin with oxygen in arterial blood (SaO_2) measured by standard pulse oximeters will give a falsely elevated level. Standard pulse oximeters use only two wavelengths of light, which are designed to measure the ratio between hemoglobin saturated with oxygen (oxyhemoglobin) and desaturated hemoglobin (deoxyhemoglobin). These dual-wavelength pulse oximeters do not detect the presence of carboxyhemoglobin and will overestimate the oxygen saturation. To obtain an accurate oxygen saturation reading, a multiwavelength pulse oximeter that measures oxyhemoglobin, deoxyhemoglobin, and carboxyhemoglobin should be used.[16] ■

The affected individual needs to be removed immediately from the source of CO. Oxygen should be administered as soon as possible because CO exerts its toxic effects by binding to sites on hemoglobin, myoglobin, and cytochrome oxidase that are normally occupied by oxygen. The rationale is to increase the availability of oxygen molecules to compete with CO for binding sites and facilitate the elimination of CO from the body. When a person is breathing room air, which has an oxygen concentration of approximately 21%, the half-life ($T_{1/2}$) of CO is 4–6 hours;[14] that is, it takes 4–6 hours for the CO level to decrease by half (50%) of what it was originally. When a person is breathing 100% oxygen with a face mask, the half-life of CO is decreased to 40 to 90 minutes.[14] In life-threatening cases of CO poisoning, it can be necessary to decrease the half-life and increase the clearance of carbon monoxide at an even faster rate by the use of hyperbaric oxygen, usually at 3 atmospheres, which can decrease the half-life of CO to approximately 20 minutes.[14] In a hyperbaric oxygen chamber, 100% oxygen is breathed at a greater than atmospheric pressure in a closed chamber. The beneficial effects of hyperbaric oxygen are due to the increased pressure, which forces more oxygen to dissolve in the plasma, helping to sustain cell metabolism until the CO is released from hemoglobin and other binding sites and eliminated from the body. Recovery from CO poisoning can lag behind normalization of carboxyhemoglobin levels, so oxygen therapy is continued until the patient's signs and symptoms improve. Full recovery can occur within a few days. On the other hand, some patients who survive serious carbon monoxide poisoning develop delayed neurologic sequelae with problems such as memory deficits, hearing impairment, seizures, gait abnormalities, and behavioral changes often secondary to demyelination of certain neurons in the brain.

Fetal elimination of CO lags behind that of the mother because the fetal lungs are nonfunctional and do not participate in elimination of CO. Therefore, to normalize fetal carboxyhemoglobin levels, the pregnant woman should receive oxygen therapy for 5 times longer than that needed to normalize her own carboxyhemoglobin level.[14] ■

Sophia Velazquez: Outcome

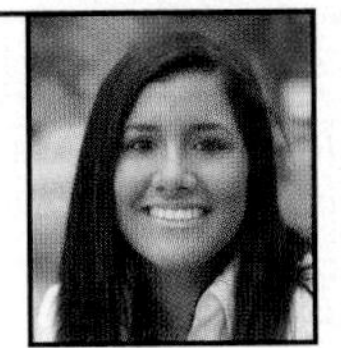

In addition to treatment with supplemental oxygen, Sophia is treated with hyperbaric oxygen therapy. Over the next 24 hours, her oxygenation parameters and carboxyhemoglobin levels normalize, and she regains consciousness. She is eventually discharged to home in the care of her parents. She has an appointment for follow-up in the neurology clinic in 2 weeks to assess for delayed neurologic sequelae.

Assessment in the family's home for the cause of the carbon monoxide poisoning reveals a blocked combustion opening in the furnace and rust in the ventilation system. The home has a battery-operated carbon monoxide detector, but it is not functioning and the parents admit to not changing the batteries for several years. The Velazquezes were given the recommendations to have their furnace checked by a licensed technician at the beginning of each season and to install several electric-powered carbon monoxide detectors with battery backups.

5. What is the role of hyperbaric oxygen in the treatment of Sophia's carbon monoxide?
6. What neurologic deficits might Sophia experience as a result of her carbon monoxide poisoning?

Lead Poisoning

Lead is a heavy metal that occurs naturally as part of the earth's crust and can be toxic to most organs. Despite government regulations, such as banning lead-based house paints and phasing out leaded gasoline, there are still several environmental sources of lead. According to the Centers for Disease Control and Prevention (CDC), "Today at least 4 million households have children living in them that are being exposed to high levels of lead. There are approximately half a million U.S. children ages 1 to 5 with blood lead levels above 5 μg/dL, the reference level at which the CDC recommends public health action be initiated."[18]

Etiology and Pathogenesis

Lead can be absorbed into the blood from the gastrointestinal tract after ingestion of a substance containing lead, from the respiratory tract after inhalation of lead dust, and from the skin after dermal contact.[19] Lead contamination occurs in the air and soil from certain factory emissions, and exposure to lead-containing waste and water has occurred from pipes that contain lead or the lead used in soldering copper pipes together. Refer to Chapter 3 for a description of the lead contamination of the water in Flint, Michigan. Lead dust is released during renovations or demolition of old homes that were originally painted with lead-based paint. Lead can enter food products when they are grown in lead-contaminated soil and when food is served from dishes, cups, or other pottery made with lead-containing (non-food-grade) paints or glazes or from lead crystal. Some imported foods, such as spices or candy containing lead that is not properly tested, can make their way into the market. Also, certain herbal remedies used by some cultures have been found to contain lead. Occupational exposure to lead includes the manufacturing of batteries and ammunition, car repairs, soldering, and welding.

Young children exhibit hand-to-mouth behavior, and a common source of lead toxicity occurs when children pick up and eat paint chips containing lead that have fallen from walls in older homes or put imported lead-containing toys, which have occasionally reached store shelves in the United States, into their mouths. Lead tastes sweet, so once it starts, children will continue with the behavior. Also lead-containing dust can be brought into the home by a parent who has occupational exposure to lead that contaminates their clothing. ■

Lead is very toxic and can adversely affect many organ systems. One of the mechanisms underlying lead's toxicity and responsible for many of the associated clinical manifestations is lead's interference with calcium and the many functions regulated by calcium. Both calcium (Ca^{+2}) and lead (Pb^{+2}) are cations with two positive charges. Lead can occupy sites, such as on enzymes and in nerve terminals, where calcium normally binds, thereby preventing calcium from activating enzymes or neurotransmitter release from neurons. Intracellular lead impairs cell signaling systems that are normally regulated by calcium. Antioxidant enzymes, such as superoxide dismutase and glutathione peroxidase, are inhibited by lead, resulting in oxidative stress.[20] The reactive oxygen molecules that are produced in states of oxidative stress can damage all cell components, including proteins, lipids, carbohydrates, and DNA. Lead also activates apoptosis (genetically programmed cell death), resulting in progressive cell loss in various organs.[21] Anemia caused by lead results from its ability to inhibit the enzyme involved in synthesis of the heme component of hemoglobin, impair iron absorption from the intestines, and produce oxidative stress that damages erythrocyte membranes resulting in premature lysis. The resulting decrease in the amount of oxygen transported in the blood causes hypoxia in many organs.

Clinical Manifestations

Lead crosses the blood–brain barrier, and many of the clinical manifestations of lead toxicity are due to its ability to cause hypoxia and oxidative stress and impair neurotransmitter function in the nervous system. Neurologic manifestations of lead poisoning include seizures, movement disorders, delirium, vomiting, coma, and issues with cognition and attention span that result in learning disabilities. Lead is excreted by the kidneys, where it damages nephrons and can cause renal kidney injury. Refer to **Figure 10.12** ■ for effects of lead correlated with blood lead levels.

As with other toxic chemicals, the embryo, fetus, and young child are more susceptible to the harmful effects of lead than are older children and adults. Lead is transferred across the placenta from maternal to fetal circulation. Because lead accumulates in bone and is slowly released from bone into the circulation over many years, a pregnant woman who was exposed to lead as a child can be a source of lead to her fetus. Lead impairs enzyme function involved in formation of the myelin sheath on neurons, thereby altering nerve conduction. Most myelination of nerves occurs in the first few months of life; therefore, early lead exposure can impair development of the nervous system.[22] ■

10 µg/dL	30 µg/dL	50 µg/dL	70 µg/dL	90 µg/dL	110 µg/dL	130 µg/dL	150 µg/dL
Developmental toxicity	Decreased calcium homeostasis Decreased then increased vitamin D metabolism Increased risk of HTN in adulthood	Decreased hemoglobin synthesis Colic	Anemia	Nephropathy Encephalopathy	Encephalopathy	Encephalopathy	Death

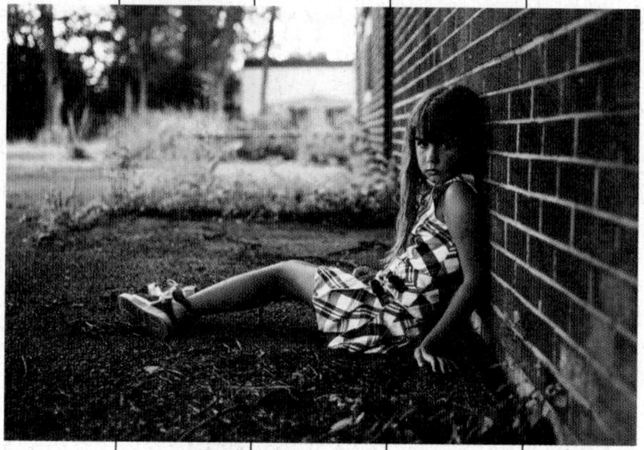

Figure 10.12 ■ Effects associated with various blood levels of lead in children.

Linking Pathophysiology to Diagnosis and Treatment

Lead poisoning is most often diagnosed by screening procedures done in high-risk populations, risk being determined by the likelihood of lead exposure in the home or associated with an occupation.[20] Poisoning is confirmed with a blood lead level (see Figure 10.12); however, the blood level does not reflect the total body lead content. Blood lead levels are measured in whole blood rather than in plasma or serum because most of the lead in blood is in the erythrocytes.[23] Because of impaired synthesis of heme caused by lead, levels of free erythrocyte protoporphyrin, a precursor of heme, increase as a result of chronic lead toxicity.[19] If the free erythrocyte protoporphyrin level is normal in the presence of an elevated blood lead level, the lead toxicity is most likely acute. Imaging studies can be used to differentiate acute and chronic lead exposures. Abdominal x-rays can detect radiopaque substances such as lead recently ingested with paint chips. Bone x-rays can detect dense bands referred to as lead lines that occur with chronic poisoning.

When acute or chronic lead poisoning is suspected, the individual should be removed immediately from the source of lead, and the source should be removed from the individual's environment. Education about how to prevent lead exposure should be provided. A dietary assessment should be performed, and recommendations should be made to ensure adequate intake of calcium and iron because lead interferes with the actions of these substances. For acute ingestion of lead resulting in blood lead levels above 44 µg/dL, a chelating medication is recommended, which will bind to lead in the gastrointestinal tract and decrease its absorption.[19,20] This will decrease progression of symptoms and can be lifesaving. However, chelating medications are not effective in removing lead that has accumulated in bone and other organs. Blood lead levels can increase several days to weeks after therapy with a chelating medication as a result of lead diffusing out of bone.

Radiation

Radiation is a physical environmental hazard and comprises a wide spectrum of wave-propagated energy, including ionizing gamma rays to radiofrequency waves. Radiation is a form of energy emitted from a source and then absorbed by the body. It is a common environmental agent encountered locally and globally. Radiation hazards are categorized as nonionizing or ionizing (**Figure 10.13** ■). **Nonionizing radiation** has enough energy to cause atoms to vibrate but not enough to eject electrons. Sources of nonionizing radiation include ultraviolet (UV) radiation and electromagnetic fields.[24] The most common source of UV radiation is sunlight; however, the proliferation of lasers and tanning salons are emerging additional sources of this hazard. While sunlight contains UV-A, UV-B, and UV-C radiation, UV-A and UV-B are most concerning, because naturally occurring UV-C does not reach the earth's surface. UV-A penetrates deeper into the skin layer and is responsible for long-term skin damage. The well-documented health effects of UV-B exposure are skin cancers and cataracts. The effects of ultraviolet radiation from the sun in causing skin cancer are described in Chapter 41. UV-C is a potential hazard for workers who are exposed to this higher-energy form of ultraviolet radiation that is used primarily in industrial processes and as a germicide. Electromagnetic radiation is emitted from sources such as microwave ovens, electric power lines, electric machinery, and cell phones. The World Health Organization's International Agency for Research on Cancer concluded that electromagnetic radiation is possibly carcinogenic to humans, as the epidemiologic data

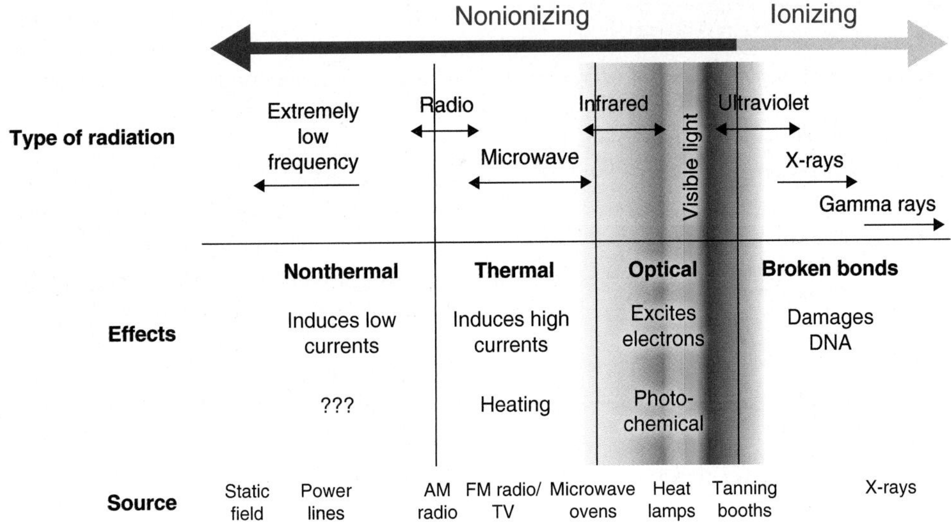

Figure 10.13 ■ Types of ionizing and nonionizing radiation.

consistently report an association between electromagnetic radiation and the risk of childhood leukemia.[24]

Ionizing radiation has enough energy to eject electrons that are tightly bound to atoms. This produces two types of electrically charged ions; the electrons released are negatively charged, and the molecules from which the electrons are removed are positively charged. Sources of ionizing radiation exposure include x-ray devices, atomic or dirty bombs, nuclear testing, radon, and work-related exposures to radium and thorium.[25] Radon, produced from the natural radioactive decay of radium, is found in soil, rocks, and water from wells. Radon concentration varies geographically; the New England, Appalachian, and Rocky Mountain states of the United States have the highest national concentrations. Radon is harmless when present in the diluted outdoor air but poses a health risk in confined spaces such as well-insulated homes, where the gas can accumulate to hazardous levels. Exposure occurs via inhalation of radon gas and ingestion of contaminated water. Radon is the second leading cause of lung cancer deaths and a significant risk factor for stomach cancer.[26] Ionizing radiation has the potential to cause damage to all cells in the body; however, more rapidly dividing cells, such as blood cell precursors in the bone marrow and epithelial cells lining the gastrointestinal tract, are most susceptible to the damaging effects of radiation. That explains the early onset of anemia and gastrointestinal alterations caused by radiation exposure.

4 The embryo, fetus, and young child are especially susceptible to the harmful effects of radiation because of the rapid rate of cell division occurring in these developmental stages. Therefore, avoiding radiation exposure as much as possible is especially important during pregnancy and early childhood. ■

Some cell damage caused by ionizing radiation can be reversed by cellular repair mechanisms; however, not all damage is reversible. Ionizing radiation that damages the genome is capable of causing mutations. These mutations can impair the ability to regulate cell proliferation and may result in cancer. Cell injury caused by ionizing radiation also results in inflammation and oxidative stress, owing to production of reactive oxygen molecules, that can activate apoptosis (genetically programmed cell death) resulting in loss of functional cells and progressive organ dysfunction. **Table 10.3** ■ lists the adverse effects of acute exposure to various high levels of ionizing radiation. For information regarding radiation used as a weapon of mass destruction refer to Chapter 52.

Table 10.3 Health Effects of Acute Exposure to High Levels of Ionizing Radiation

Exposure (rem)*	Health Effect	Time to Onset (without treatment)
5–10	Changes in blood chemistry (e.g., anemia)	Hours
50	Nausea	
55	Fatigue	
70	Vomiting	
75	Hair loss	2–3 weeks
90	Diarrhea	
100	Hemorrhage	
400	Possible death	Within 2 months
1000	Destruction of intestinal lining, internal bleeding, death	1–2 weeks
2000	Damage to central nervous system,	
	loss of consciousness,	Minutes
	and death	Hours to days

* A rem is a measure of the dose of radiation in terms of the amount deposited in the body. For the purpose of comparison, most individuals receive 0.3 rem annually from exposure to natural sources of radiation in the environment.

SOURCE: Data from Environmental Protection Agency. (n.d.). *Radiation protection*. Available at http://www.epa.gov/radiation/understand/health_effects.html.

Check Your Progress: Section 10.4

1. Describe the protective and harmful effects of ozone on health.
2. Why is use of a pulse oximeter not accurate in measuring oxygen saturation in the patient with carbon monoxide poisoning?
3. What neurologic manifestations may be seen in a child with lead poisoning?

10.5 Impact of Injury on Cell Types Present in Many Organs

Epithelia are formed of cells that line the cavities in the body and also cover flat surfaces. Of the four major tissue types, the epithelial cells are by far the most prolific, as many types of epithelial tissue retain the ability to differentiate and undergo rapid proliferation for replacing injured cells. Nothing can enter or leave the body without passing through or between the cells that form the epithelial boundary.

Endothelial cells line the blood vessels and act as a gatekeeper to the tissue compartment. These cells selectively facilitate an enhanced vascular and tissue response to injury and inflammation (**Figure 10.14**). Endothelial cells present a barrier to excess injurious cells and agents, thus protecting the vasculature and tissue.

Injury to Endothelial Cells

Endothelial dysfunction is a systemic pathologic state that can be defined as an imbalance between vasodilating and constricting substances that are produced by or acting on the endothelium. Endothelial cell injury can be triggered by a number of different mechanisms. These mechanisms include bacterial or viral infection; oxidative stress through abnormal regulation of ROS, hypoxia, turbulent blood flow and shear stress; environmental irritants such as tobacco products; and hyperlipidemia. These factors all lead to the generation of an inflammatory process and the endothelial cell activation.

The endothelial response to injury can be divided into two levels of response: first, an initial rapid response and then a slower, phenotypic response. The initial rapid response involves changes in levels of nitric oxide, prostaglandins, ET-1, von Willebrand factor, and tissue plasminogen activator. The slower response, however, depends on fundamental changes in the characteristics of the cell surface along with alterations in the underlying basement membrane and the smooth muscle cells that surround the endothelium. These changes are caused by molecules that are potent growth factors involved in the deposition of ECM

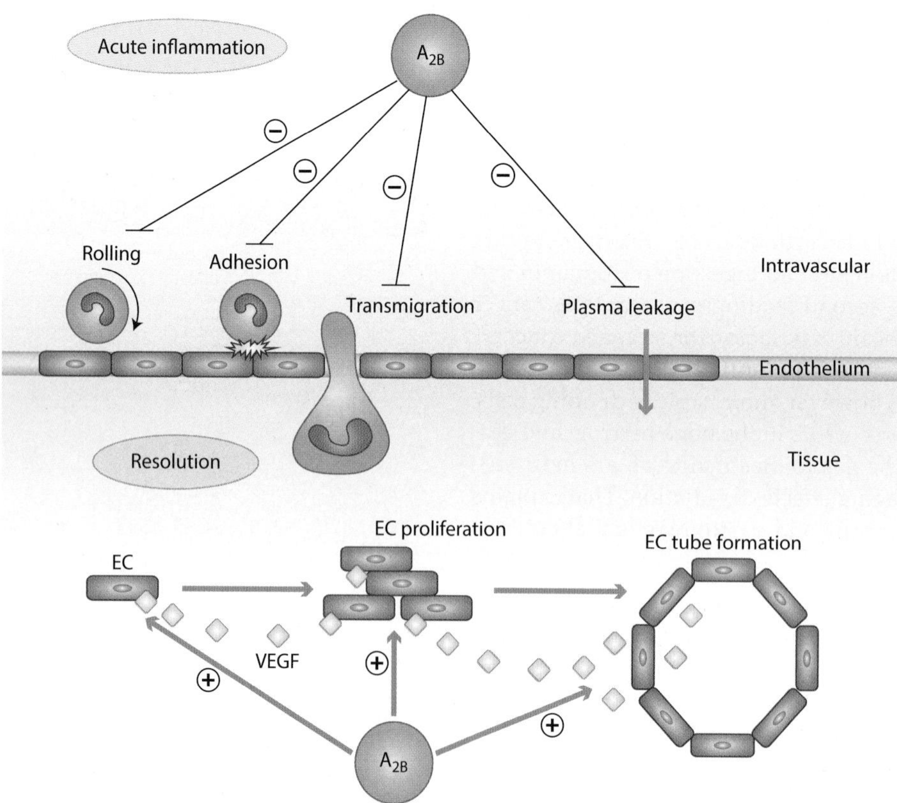

Figure 10.14 ■ Regulatory effects of the vascular endothelium in normal and pathologic states.

and the activation and proliferation of the vascular smooth muscle cells, pericytes, and other mesenchymal cell types associated with the blood vessel. This ultimately results in vessel remodeling, including profound changes in cellular architecture.[27]

Impairment of endothelial function causes certain clinical manifestations, including edema, hypertension, abnormal vasoconstriction or vasodilation, and hypercoagulability. Impaired endothelial function is thought to be the initial step in atherogenesis, which leads to ischemic heart disease and thrombolytic strokes. Impaired endothelial function is also associated with hypertension, diabetes mellitus, and heart failure. It is important to note that research is inconclusive as to whether the endothelial dysfunction is a cause or a consequence of these disorders. Understanding specific endothelial function is likely the key to modifying risk factors associated with cardiovascular disease and their sequelae.

Injury to Epithelial Cells

The location of many epithelial tissues, which are in contact with the external environment, exposes them to a variety of insults. These insults range from mechanical damage from cuts and scrapes to active penetration from mosquitoes, parasites, and hypodermics to bacterial and fungal attacks to poisoning by toxic chemicals. When an epithelial cell is injured (e.g., from insect bites, scrapes, or cuts), blood may leak out, and microorganisms may be allowed to enter. Such injury results in the release of factors that activate fibroblasts, which results in the production of collagen and fibronectin to plug the compromised epithelium (**Figure 10.15** ■). Certain epithelia, such as those in the gastrointestinal and respiratory tracts, are continually recycled, new cells being created by mitotic activity while old cells are sloughed off. Many additional epithelial cells (not just those on the skin and intestine) have the ability to respond to the stimulus of an injury with mitotic activity and cell migration to regenerate the tissue following damage. This confers on most epithelia an automatic ability to deal effectively with injury by replacing lost tissue with new growth from undamaged edges.

When the epithelial cells' ability to divide is stimulated inappropriately, it can result in the formation of a tumor. Cells in epithelial tumors often retain their basic epithelial characteristics, remaining attached to one another and differentiating to form layered structures. As long as the neoplastic cells respect the basement membrane, the tumor will remain localized. However, once cells break through this boundary, they can enter the circulation and metastasize.

Check Your Progress: Section 10.5

1. What diseases are associated with impaired endothelial function?
2. What is the role of the basement membrane in controlling epithelial tumors?
3. What are the two levels of response to injury by endothelial cells?

10.6 Cellular Responses to Injury

The cell undergoes adaptive changes when confronted with stressors that endanger normal structure and function. These adaptive changes permit survival and maintenance

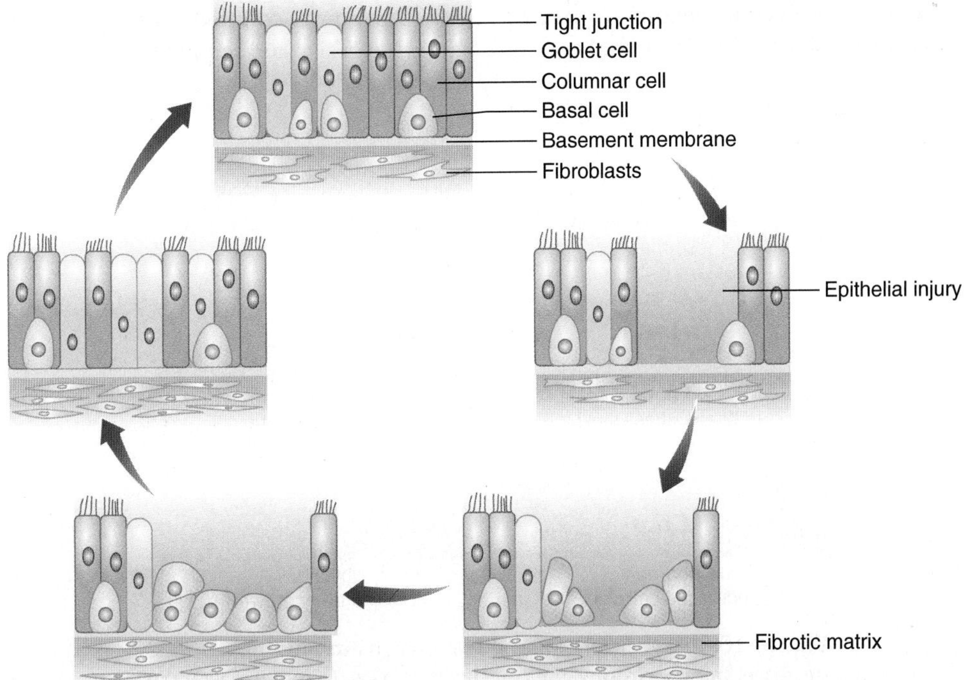

Figure 10.15 ■ Epithelial injury and repair in airway disease.

of cell function. It is only when the stress is overwhelming or adaptation is ineffective that cell injury and death occur.

Morphologic Changes

Morphologic cell changes occur in response to reversible injury. These responses include plasma membrane alterations, mitochondrial changes, dilation of the endoplasmic reticulum (ER), and nuclear alterations. These morphologic changes allow the cell to adapt to the insult and recover structure and function.

Two specific morphologic changes that occur with reversible cell injury are cell swelling and fat accumulation. Cell swelling occurs whenever the cells are incapable of maintaining ionic and fluid homeostasis. It is the result of energy-dependent ion pumps in the plasma membrane. Fat accumulation occurs in hypoxic, along with various forms of toxic and metabolic cell, injury. It is manifested by the appearance of lipid vacuoles in the cytoplasm and is often seen in hepatocytes and myocardial cells.

Cells are able to adapt to increased work demands or threats to survival. Normal cellular adaptation occurs in response to an appropriate stimulus and then ceases when the adaptation is no longer required. These adaptive changes often include alteration in cell size, number, and type. These adaptive changes may occur in isolation or in combination. These changes are implemented without compromising the normal function unless the cell becomes overwhelmed. The specific cell changes include changes in size (atrophy and hypertrophy), changes in number (hyperplasia), and changes in form (metaplasia, dysplasia, and autophagy), all of which are depicted in **Figure 10.16** ■.

Atrophy

Atrophy is a decrease in cell size. Atrophy occurs when there is a decrease in work demands (physiologic atrophy) or as a result of adverse environmental conditions (pathologic atrophy). Most cells are able to revert to a smaller size, with a lower and more efficient level of function that is compatible with survival. Atrophied cells decrease their use of oxygen by decreasing the number and size of organelles and other cell structures, including mitochondria, myofilaments, and ER structures. When a sufficient number of cells have atrophied, the entire tissue or organ atrophies.

Cell size, particularly in muscle tissue, is related to workload. As the workload of the cell decreases, oxygen consumption and protein synthesis also decrease. Proper muscle mass is maintained by sufficient levels of insulin and insulin-like growth factor 1 (IGF-1). When these substances are low or catabolic signals are present, muscle atrophy occurs. Mechanisms responsible for this atrophy include reduced synthetic processes, increased proteolysis by the ubiquitin–proteasome system, and apoptosis or genetically programmed cell death. In the ubiquitin–proteasome system, the intracellular proteins that are destined for destruction are covalently bonded to a small protein referred to as ubiquitin. When this occurs, the intracellular proteins are degraded by small cytoplasmic organelles referred to as proteasomes.

The general causes of atrophy are grouped into five categories: disuse, denervation, loss of endocrine stimulation, inadequate nutrition, and decreased perfusion. Disuse atrophy occurs where there is a reduction of skeletal muscle activity. For example, when a cast is used in the treatment of a fractured bone, the extremity is encased, causing disuse atrophy. Because atrophy is adaptive and reversible, muscle size is restored after the cast has been removed and use of the muscle resumes.

Another form of atrophy is denervation atrophy. This occurs in the muscles of paralyzed limbs. Atrophy may also result from a lack of endocrine stimulation. This occurs in women experiencing menopause due to the loss of estrogen stimulation resulting in atrophy of reproductive organs. Atrophy can also occur as a result of malnutrition. When malnutrition is coupled with decreased perfusion, cells decrease in size and require less energy in order to survive.

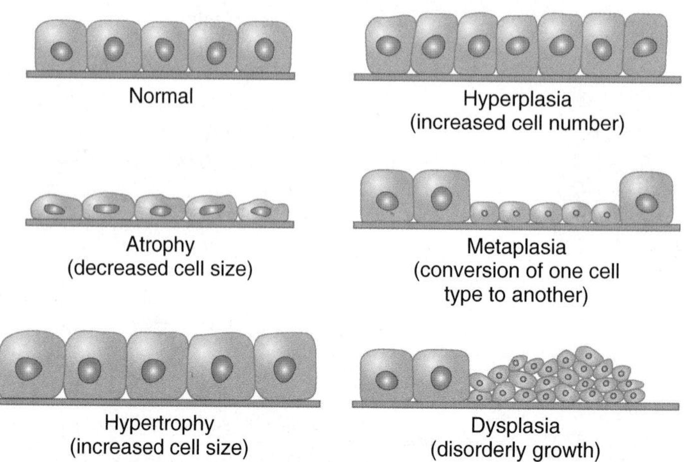

Figure 10.16 ■ Morphologic alterations. In atrophy, the cell sizes decrease. In hypertrophy, the cell size increases. In hyperplasia, the number of cells increases. In metaplasia, one type of cell converts to another. In dysplasia, the cell growth is disorderly.

Hypertrophy

An increase in cell size that is coupled with an increase in the amount of functioning tissue mass is referred to as **hypertrophy**. This occurs from an increased workload and often manifests in the cardiac and skeletal muscle tissue. This tissue cannot adapt to an increase in workload through mitotic cell division and formation of more cells. When hypertrophy occurs, it involves an increase in cell size and the functional components of the cell that allows equilibrium between demand and functional capacity. For example, when muscle cells atrophy, additional actin and myosin filaments, cell enzymes, and ATP are synthesized.

Hypertrophy can occur as a result of normal physiologic processes and as a result of pathologic conditions. When muscle mass increases with exercise, this is an example of physiologic hypertrophy. Pathologic hypertrophy is the result of disease conditions and can be either adaptive or compensatory. For example, the thickening of the urinary bladder from long-continued obstruction of urinary outflow occurs as a result of a pathologic condition. Another example of pathologic hypertrophy, myocardial hypertrophy, occurs from conditions such as valvular heart disease or hypertension. Hypertrophy can also occur for compensatory reasons, such as the loss of an organ, either because it was surgically removed or because it was rendered inactive as a result to disease. An example of this type of hypertrophy occurs when an individual has only one functioning kidney. The remaining kidney hypertrophies as a compensatory mechanism.

Hyperplasia

When there is an increase in the number of cells in an organ or tissue this is referred to as **hyperplasia**. Hyperplasia occurs in tissues with cells that are capable of mitotic division, including the epidermis, intestinal epithelium, and glandular tissue. Other cells, such as neurons, rarely divide and have little capacity for hyperplasia. Hyperplasia, like the other adaptive cell responses, is a controlled process that occurs in response to a stimulus. When the stimulus is removed, the hyperplasia ceases to occur.

Hyperplasia can occur as a result of physiologic and nonphysiologic processes. There are two types of physiologic hyperplasia: hormonal and compensatory. Hormonal hyperplasia occurs during pregnancy, causing breast and uterine enlargement due to estrogen stimulation. Hyperplasia also occurs when an individual has a partial hepatectomy, or removal of the liver. The regeneration that occurs is an example of compensatory hyperplasia. Hyperplasia also occurs during wound healing via proliferating fibroblasts and blood vessels, which contribute to the wound healing process.

While hypertrophy and hyperplasia are two distinct processes, they often occur together and may be triggered by the same mechanisms.

A woman's uterus experiences both hypertrophy and hyperplasia during pregnancy. Both are the result of estrogen stimulation. ■

Metaplasia

Metaplasia is a reversible change in which one adult cell type, such as epithelial or mesenchymal, is replaced by another type of adult cell. This change is thought to involve the reprogramming of undifferentiated stem cells that are present in the tissue that is experiencing metaplastic changes. Metaplasia often occurs in response to chronic irritation and inflammation. It allows for substitution of cells that are better able to survive under circumstances that would cause more fragile cells to become weakened.

Metaplasia never oversteps the boundaries of the primary tissue type. This means that while one type of epithelial cell may be converted to another type of epithelial cell, it will not be converted to a connective tissue cell. An example of this process is the adaptive substitution of stratified squamous epithelial cells for the ciliated columnar cells in the trachea and large airways for an individual who smokes cigarettes. The squamous epithelium is better able to survive in this situation; however, the individual loses the protective function that the ciliated epithelium provides for the respiratory tract. Any individual who has continued exposure to influences that cause metaplasia to occur is at an increased risk for cancerous transformation of the metaplastic epithelium.

Dysplasia

Dysplasia is characterized by deranged cell growth of specific tissue. It results in cells that vary in size, shape, and organization. A minor degree of dysplasia occurs with chronic irritation or inflammation. For example, dysplasia is often encountered in areas of metaplastic squamous epithelium of the respiratory tract and uterine cervix. Although this dysplasia is abnormal, it is adaptive in that it is potentially reversible. Once the irritating cause has been removed, the dysplasia dissipates.

Dysplasia is often a precursor to cancer, especially of the respiratory tract and uterine cervix. Dysplastic changes in these areas have been found adjacent to the foci of cancerous transformation. Cervical cancer is routinely screened through the use of the Papanicolaou (Pap) smear. This test develops a series of incremental epithelial changes ranging from severe dysplasia to invasive cancer. Dysplasia is an adaptive process; therefore, its presence does not necessarily lead to cancer. Dysplastic cells can revert to their former structure and function once the stimulus causing it has been removed.

Autophagy

Autophagy is a normal physiologic process in the body that deals with the destruction of cells within the body. This process maintains homeostasis, or normal functioning. Autophagy occurs through protein degradation and the turnover of the destroyed cell organelles. These processes allow for new cell formation to occur.

The autophagy process is enhanced and increased during times of stress to meet the needs of the body. Cellular stress is caused in any circumstance that causes a deprivation of nutrients and/or growth factors available. Therefore, autophagy provides an alternative source of intracellular building blocks and substrates. This provides the cell with energy and the ability to survive during times of stress.[28]

Autophagy is also associated with pathophysiologic conditions in which this cellular process plays either a cytoprotective or a cytopathic role. This role is assumed in response to a stress. These stressors include metabolic, inflammatory, neurodegenerative, and therapeutic stress. Research indicates that modulating the activity of autophagy, through targeting specific regulatory molecules in the autophagy machinery, may affect disease processes. Therefore, autophagy may represent a new pharmacologic target for the development of drugs, along with other therapeutic interventions, for various human disorders, including cancer. The induction or suppression of this process may exert therapeutic effects by programming cell survival or cell death.[29]

Intracellular Accumulations

Intracellular accumulations represent the buildup of substances that cells cannot immediately use or eliminate. These substances accumulate in the cytoplasm, lysosomes, or nucleus. In some instances, the accumulation may be an abnormal substance that the cell has produced. In other cases, the cell may be storing exogenous material, or products, of pathologic processes that are occurring elsewhere in the body. These substances may accumulate transiently or permanently and may be harmless or toxic. The most common intracellular accumulations include water, lipids, calcium, glycogen, hyaline, and pigments, illustrated in **Figure 10.17** ■.

Water

The accumulation of water, termed *hydropic degeneration*, occurs in response to reversible cell injury. This accumulation of water, which causes cellular swelling, is the first manifestation of almost all forms of cell injury. Hydropic degeneration is caused by ischemia and chemical aging.

There is a specific process leading to hydropic change due to ischemia. First, there is a lack of blood supply, which leads to decreased oxygen tension within the cell. This causes ATP depletion and failure of the sodium–potassium pump. The failure of the sodium–potassium pump leads to increased intracellular sodium and water along with increased extracellular potassium. This combination allows the cell to swell.

Ischemia also causes an activation of the anaerobic pathway due to an accumulation of phosphates and lactates, which are collectively referred to as catabolites. This accumulation causes an increased osmotic load. The increased osmotic load is responsible for the cell swelling.

Exposure to chemical agents can also precipitate hydropic change. This chemical exposure can be either direct or indirect. Directly acting chemicals cause increased cell membrane injury. Examples of chemicals causing direct hydropic change include cyanide, mercury, antineoplastic drugs, and antibiotics. Indirectly acting chemicals, such as carbon tetrachloride, release highly toxic and reactive free radicals. This leads to lipid peroxidation and cell membrane damage. This damage increases the influx of sodium and water into the cell, resulting in cell swelling.[30]

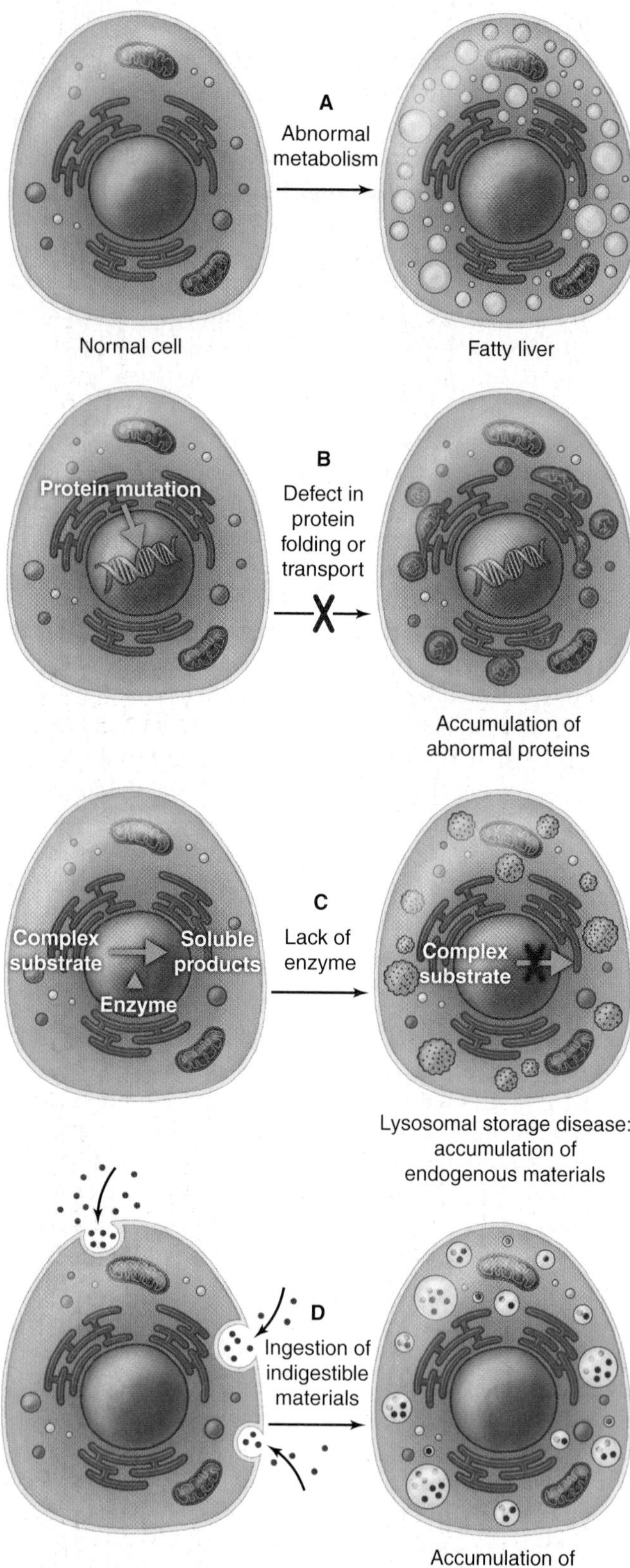

Figure 10.17 ■ Mechanisms of intracellular accumulations.

Lipid

Fatty change, or the accumulation of lipids, is the abnormal accumulation of triglycerides in the parenchymal cells. This often occurs in the liver, the major organ for fat metabolism. Accumulation of lipids can also occur in the cardiac muscle and the kidneys. The causes of lipid accumulation include toxins (e.g., alcohol), protein malnutrition, diabetes mellitus, anoxia, starvation, and obesity.

Several mechanisms are involved with each of the causes associated with lipid accumulation. When alcohol is the cause, the metabolites act as hepatotoxins that alter the actions of the mitochondria and microsomes. The leads to increased synthesis and a decreased breakdown of lipids. With protein malnutrition, the synthesis of apoproteins is reduced.

When diabetes mellitus or starvation occurs, there is an increased mobilization of free fatty acids from the peripheral tissues of the liver. With anoxia, the oxidation of fatty acid is inhibited. When obesity is the cause, there is an increased intake of dietary fat, leading to the increased transport of free fatty acids to the periphery.[31]

Calcium

Pathologic calcification is the abnormal deposition of calcium salts. These depositions also include small amounts of magnesium, iron, and other minerals mixed with the calcium. There are two basic types of pathologic calcifications: dystrophic and metastatic.

Dystrophic calcification is the deposition of calcium salts in dead or dying tissues that lack any calcium metabolism abnormalities. The common sites for dystrophic calcification include atheromas, damaged heart valves, tuberculous lymph nodes, papillary carcinoma of the thyroid or ovaries, and meningiomas. Dystrophic calcification can also occur in dead parasites and in fetuses. Metastatic calcification occurs in normal tissues in the presence of hypercalcemia. There are three primary causes for metastatic calcification: increased secretion of the parathyroid gland, destruction of bone tissue, and renal failure.

Increased secretion of the parathyroid gland is caused primarily by adenoma, hyperplasia, or carcinoma. Another cause is ectopic secretion of parathyroid hormone in response to protein. For example, this occurs as a result of squamous cell carcinoma of the lung; with breast, ovarian, or renal cell carcinoma; and with adult T-cell leukemia or lymphoma. Destruction of bone tissue is another cause of metastatic calcification. This occurs as a result of a primary tumor of the bone marrow, such as leukemia and multiple myeloma; skeletal metastasis; the increased bone turnover that occurs with Paget disease; or prolonged immobilization. Renal failure is also a cause for metastatic calcification. Specifically, renal failure causes phosphate retention, which causes secondary hyperparathyroidism.[32]

Glycogen

Excessive intracellular accumulation of glycogen occurs as a result of diabetes mellitus and glycogen storage diseases, which are termed glycogenoses. Diabetes mellitus is the most common and important disorder of glucose metabolism. Glycogen is found in epithelial cells of the distal portions of the proximal tubules and the Henle loops, referred to as Armani cells. Glycogenoses, on the other hand, are a group of diseases characterized by excessive accumulation of glycogen. This accumulation can be normal, or it can be abnormal as a result of an inherited deficiency of any of the enzymes that are responsible for glycogen synthesis or degradation. Clinical effects of glycogenoses include enlarged liver or kidney, bleeding tendencies, painful cramps in the skeletal muscles during exercise, and cardiomegaly.[33]

Hyaline

The term **hyaline** refers to an alteration within the cells or in the extracellular space resulting in protein-containing cell debris that has a pink to red appearance when stained with hematoxylin and eosin. Hyaline changes give a homogeneous, glassy, or pink to red appearance to the cells. It is often used as a descriptive histologic term rather than to define a specific marker for cell injury. This color change is produced by a variety of alterations; however, it does not represent a specific pattern of accumulation. The intracellular accumulations of protein, including resorption droplets and tumoral hyaline globules, are examples of intracellular hyaline deposits. Extracellular hyaline is difficult to analyze; however, it often occurs as a result of a decrease in vascularity and an increase in the thickness of collagen fibers, such as those in old scars. Two examples are hyaline arteriosclerosis that occurs in the small arteries and capillaries of the kidney as a result of diabetes mellitus and hyalinization of damaged glomeruli.[34]

Pigments

Pigments are substances occurring in living matter that absorb visible light. There are three classifications: endogenous pigments, artifact pigments, and exogenous pigments. The two specific endogenous pigments that accumulate in the intracellular space are lipofuscin and melanin.

Lipofuscin is a granular yellow-brown pigment composed of lipid-containing residues of lysosomal digestion. It is considered an aging pigment found in the liver, kidney, cardiac muscle, retina, adrenals, nerve cells, and ganglion cells. **Melanin** is a nonhemoglobin brown-black pigment synthesized in melanocytes. This pigment protects the nuclei of basal epidermal cells from ultraviolet light. It is formed when the enzyme tyrosinase catalyzes the oxidation of tyrosinase to dihydroxylphenylalanine.[35]

Iron

Hemosiderin is an endogenous blood-derived golden yellow to brown granular, or crystalline, pigment. Hemochromatosis is an excess accumulation of hemosiderin in the cells caused by iron excess. This excess of iron can be either local or systemic. The systemic excess is caused by excessive intake of iron, frequent blood transfusions, or hemolytic anemia.

When there is a systemic excess of iron, it is stored in the mononuclear phagocytic cells of the bone marrow, spleen, liver, and lymph nodes. Iron is also taken up by macrophages that are scattered in different organs, including the skin, pancreas, and kidneys. When iron accumulates, it is stored in parenchymal cells of the heart, liver, and pancreas, causing damage to these cells. The damage to the myocardium can lead to heart failure, damage to the liver leads to fibrosis, and damage to the pancreas leads to diabetes mellitus.[36]

Subcellular Changes

Certain agents and stresses cause distinct alterations that involve the subcellular organelles. The organelles that are affected include the smooth ER (SER), the mitochondria, and the cytoskeleton. While some of these alterations can occur in acute lethal injury, others occur either in chronic forms of cell injury or as adaptive responses.

Hypertrophy of the SER is a subcellular change caused by cell injury. The SER is involved in the metabolism of various chemicals. The cells that are exposed to these chemicals show hypertrophy of the SER as an adaptive response. Alterations in the number, size, shape, and function of the mitochondria can also occur. Cell hypertrophy causes an increased number of mitochondrial cells; atrophy causes a decreased number of these same cells. The cytoskeleton may also change as a result of cell injury. Certain drugs and toxins interfere with the assembly and function of the cytoskeletal filaments, resulting in an abnormal accumulation. These abnormalities often manifest as unusual appearance and function of the cells, aberrant movements of the intracellular organelles, defective cell locomotion, or intracellular accumulations of fibrillary material.

Inflammation

When cellular contents leak out through the damaged plasma membrane, inflammation occurs. This inflammation is the result of the free radicals that are produced by leukocytes that enter the tissues. Inflammation also occurs with necrosis. Cellular necrosis is often the result of adjacent; caseous necrosis, which is often enclosed within a distinct inflammatory border that occurs with granulomas. For more information on inflammation refer to Chapter 11.

Cellular Repair Processes

During the repair process, a cell must clear out damaged proteins and produce new functional molecules. The cell contains lysosomes, which are organelles that contain enzymes that break down biological molecules. These small subunits are reused to produce new molecules via cellular recycling. The cells are constantly manufacturing new proteins. These proteins are needed to replace damaged ones and to perform new functions the cell may be called on to perform. This process takes place through gene expression. It involves using information from a gene to manufacture proteins. These complicated biochemical processes occur continually in most cells. Many cells are able to survive long periods of time because they can repair moderate damage and produce new molecules. These processes require adequate nutrition and energy.

Check Your Progress: Section 10.6

1. What role does atrophy play in cellular adaptation?
2. Identify the five categories of general causes of atrophy.
3. What is the difference between hypertrophy and hyperplasia?

10.7 Cell Death

The mechanisms of cell injury are capable of producing two outcomes: sublethal and reversible cell damage or irreversible injury with cell destruction and death. Cell destruction and removal usually involve necrosis or apoptosis, as shown in **Figure 10.18** ■. Death of the entire organism, known as somatic death, is covered in Chapter 53.

Necrosis

Necrosis is cell death in an organ or tissue that is still part of a living organism. It involves unregulated enzymatic digestion of cell components, loss of cell membrane integrity (causing an uncontrolled release of the products into the extracellular space), and the initiation of the inflammatory response. Necrosis often interferes with cell replacement and tissue regeneration.

Characteristics of Necrosis

Necrotic cell death causes marked changes in the appearance of the cytoplasmic contents and the nucleus. However, these changes are often not visible under the microscope for hours after cell death occurs. Infarction, or tissue death, occurs when an artery supplying an organ or part of the body becomes occluded and no other source of blood supply exists. The shape of the infarction is conical and corresponds to the distribution of the artery and its branches. The artery may be occluded by an embolus, a thrombus, disease of the arterial wall, or pressure from outside the vessel.

Types of Necrosis

The dissolution of the necrotic cell or tissue can follow several paths: coagulative necrosis, liquefactive necrosis, caseous necrosis, fat necrosis, or gangrenous necrosis. During the process of coagulative necrosis, the cell can be transformed to a gray, firm mass. Coagulative necrosis is a characteristic of hypoxic injury and is seen in infarcted areas. Acidosis often develops with coagulative necrosis, causing denaturation of the enzymatic and structural proteins of the cell. During liquefactive necrosis, the cell undergoes liquefaction. This type of necrosis occurs when some of the cells die but their catalytic enzymes are not destroyed. An example of this type of necrosis is the softening of the center of an abscess with discharge of its contents. Caseous necrosis is a distinctive form of coagulation necrosis. With this type of necrosis, the dead cells persist indefinitely as soft, cheese-like debris. Caseous necrosis is most commonly found in the center of tuberculosis granulomas and is thought to be the result of immune mechanisms.

Fat necrosis, or death of adipose tissue, is a form of liquefactive necrosis. This type of necrosis is often caused by trauma and is affected by lipolytic enzymes. Fat necrosis is characterized by the formation of small, dull, chalky, gray or white foci. These manifestations represent small quantities of calcium soaps formed in the affected tissue when fat is hydrolyzed into glycerol and fatty acids. Fat necrosis most commonly occurs in the breasts and subcutaneous areas. It may also occur in the abdominal cavity after an episode of pancreatitis as a result of the release of enzymes from the pancreas.

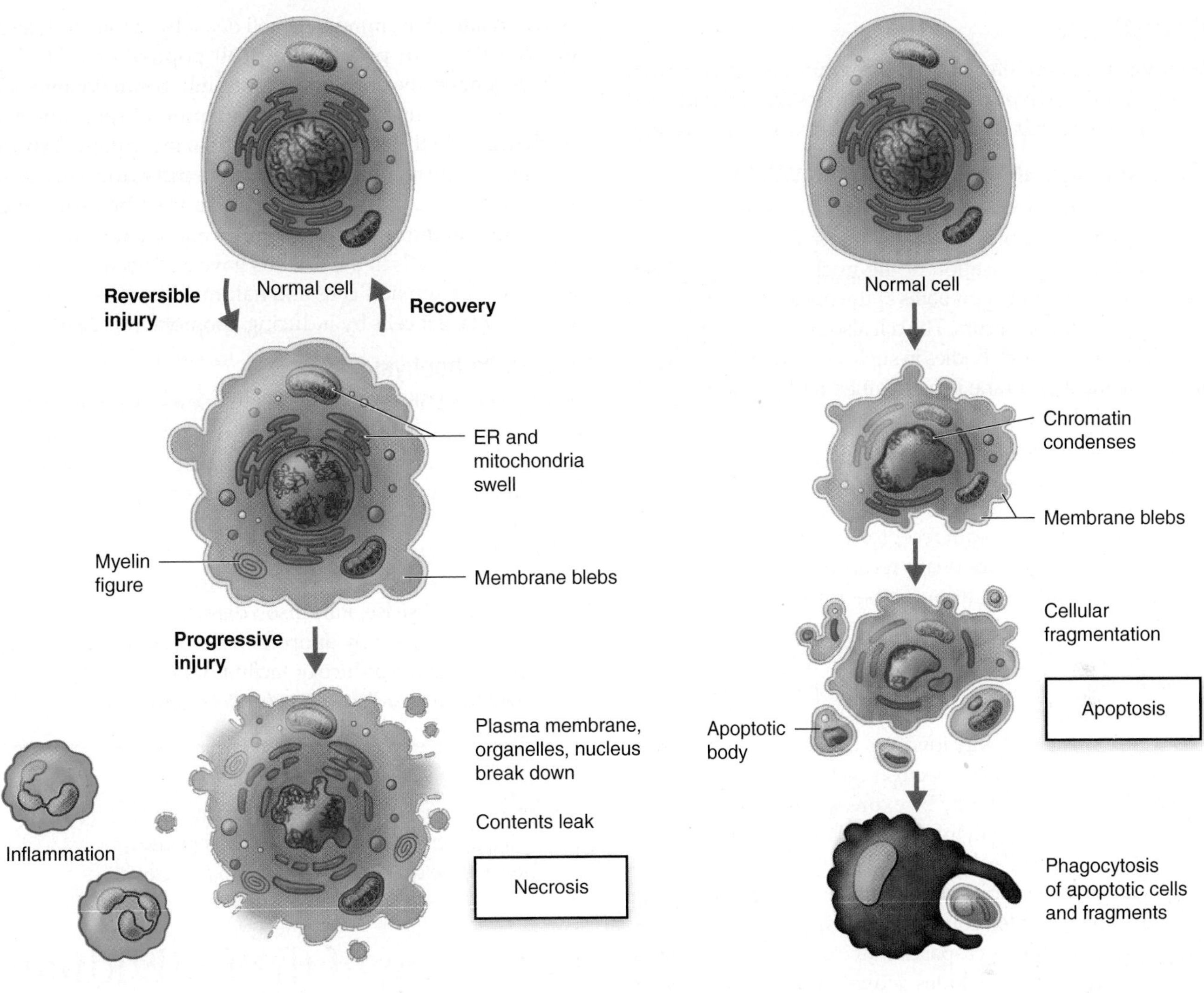

Figure 10.18 ■ Schematic illustration of the morphologic changes in cell injury culminating in **A** necrosis or **B** apoptosis. ER = endoplasmic reticulum.

The term **gangrene** is used to describe a mass of necrotic tissue. Gangrenous necrosis is a form of coagulation necrosis. There are two types of gangrene: dry and wet. With dry gangrene, the tissue becomes dry, appears wrinkled, and shrinks. The color changes to dark brown or black. The spread of dry gangrene is slow. The irritation caused by the dead tissue produces a line of inflammatory reaction between the dead gangrenous tissue and the healthy tissue. This is often referred to as the line of demarcation. Dry gangrene often results from interference with the arterial blood supply to tissue without interference with venous return. It is confined almost exclusively to the extremities.

With wet gangrene (also known as moist gangrene), the area is cold, swollen, and pulseless. The skin is moist and black and appears to be under tension. Blebs often form on the surface, liquefaction occurs, and a foul odor is noted if the gangrene is caused by bacterial action. Wet gangrene has no line of demarcation between normal and diseased tissue; therefore, the spread of tissue damage is rapid. Systemic symptoms are often severe, and death may occur unless the condition can be arrested.

Wet gangrene results primarily from interference with venous return. Bacterial invasion plays a role in the development of this type of gangrene and is often responsible for many of its prominent symptoms. Wet gangrene can affect the extremities and internal organs. Bacterial invasion is often the reason when dry gangrene is converted to wet gangrene.

Gas gangrene is a specific type of gangrene that results from infection of devitalized tissues by one of several *Clostridium* bacteria, most commonly *Clostridium perfringens*. Gas gangrene is often the result of trauma and compound fractures. The bacteria produce toxins that dissolve cell membranes. This causes death of muscle cells, massive spreading edema, hemolysis of red blood cells, hemolytic anemia, hemoglobinuria, and renal failure. Characteristic of gas gangrene are the bubbles of hydrogen sulfite gas that form in the muscle.

Gas gangrene is serious and potentially fatal. Antibiotics are prescribed to treat the infection, and surgical intervention may be required to remove the infected tissue. In the most serious cases, amputation may be required to prevent the spread of infection.

Apoptosis

Apoptosis is often referred to as programmed cell death. It is a highly selective process that eliminates injured and aged cells. In other words, apoptosis controls tissue regeneration.

Characteristics and Pathways of Activation

Cells undergoing apoptosis have characteristic morphologic features along with biochemical changes. During apoptosis, shrinking and condensation of the nucleus and cytoplasm occur. The chromatin aggregates at the nuclear envelope and DNA fragmentation occurs. The cell also becomes fragmented into multiple apoptotic bodies in such a way that the integrity of the plasma membrane is maintained and inflammation is not initiated. The changes in the plasma membrane induces phagocytosis of the apoptotic bodies by macrophage, along with other cells, which completes the degradation process.

There are two basic pathways for apoptosis: extrinsic pathways (which are death receptor dependent) and intrinsic pathways (which are death receptor independent) (see Figure 10.18). The execution phase for both pathways is carried out by proteolytic enzymes referred to as caspases. These enzymes are present in the cell as procaspases. They are activated by cleavage of an inhibitory portion of their polypeptide chain.

The extrinsic pathway involves the activation of certain receptors, including tumor necrosis factor (TNF) and the Fas ligand. The Fas ligand may be expressed on the surface of certain cells, including cytotoxic T cells, or may appear in a soluble form. When Fas ligand binds to its receptor, proteins congregate at the cytoplasmic end to form a death-initiating complex. This complex converts procaspase-8 to caspase-8, activating a cascade of caspases that execute the process of apoptosis. The result includes activation of endonucleases that cause fragmentation of DNA and cell death.

In addition to TNF and Fas ligand, other signaling molecules have the ability to activate the extrinsic pathway. These signaling molecules include TNF-related apoptosis-inducing ligand, the cytokine interleukin 1, and lipopolysaccharide. Lipopolysaccharide is the endotoxin found in the outer cell membrane of gram-negative bacteria.

The intrinsic pathway of apoptosis, also referred to as the mitochondrion-induced pathway, is activated by certain conditions, including DNA damage, ROS, hypoxia, decreased ATP levels, cellular senescence, and activation of the p53 protein by DNA damage. This pathway involves the opening of the mitochondrial permeability pores with the release of cytochrome c from the mitochondria into the cytoplasm.

Cytoplasmic cytochrome c activates caspases, including caspase-3. This step occurs in both the extrinsic and intrinsic pathways. Activation, or increased levels, of proapoptotic proteins, including *Bid* and *Bax*, after caspase-8 activation in the extrinsic pathway can lead to the mitochondrial release of cytochrome c. This bridges the two pathways to apoptosis.

Normal Physiologic Role

Apoptosis is responsible for several normal physiologic processes, including the programmed destruction of cells during embryonic development, hormone-dependent involution of tissues, death of immune cells, cell death by cytotoxic T cells, and cell death in proliferating cell populations. During embryogenesis, the development of a number of organs such as the heart occurs as a result of apoptosis. Apoptotic cell death occurs in the hormone-dependent involution of endometrial cells during the menstrual cycle and in the regression of breast tissue after weaning an infant from breastfeeding. The control of immune cells numbers and the destruction of autoreactive T cells in the thymus have also been credited to apoptosis. Cytotoxic T cells and natural kill cells are thought to destroy target cells by inducing apoptotic cell death.

Role in Pathophysiology

Apoptosis continues to be an active area of investigation in order to better understand and treat a variety of disease processes. For example, interference with apoptosis is a contributing factor to carcinogenesis and the development of autoimmune disorders. Apoptosis is also involved in the cell death associated with viral infections, including hepatitis B and C. Several neurodegenerative disorders, including Alzheimer disease, Parkinson disease, and ALS, are also thought to be caused by apoptosis. The therapeutic actions of certain drugs can induce or facilitate apoptosis. Apoptosis continues to be an active area of investigation.

Check Your Progress: Section 10.7

1. What is the difference between necrosis and apoptosis?
2. Compare and contrast wet and dry gangrene.
3. Describe the characteristics of caseous necrosis.

10.8 Aging of the Individual as a Result of Cellular Aging

Like adaptation and injury, aging is a process that involves the cells and tissue of the body. A number of theories have been proposed to explain the cause of aging. These theories are not mutually exclusive, as aging is likely complex with multiple causes. The main theories about the aging process can be categorized as evolutionary, molecular, cellular, or systems-level explanations.

Normal Lifespan

The normal lifespan of a cell depends on the type of cell it is along with the function, location, and overarching purpose of the cell. There are approximately 200 types of cells in the human body. The average lifespan varies from a few hours to several months. Degenerative conditions, illness, and other conditions can affect the lifespan of a cell. In most cases, it is helpful to think about cell life, death, and regeneration along a spectrum.

The cells that have the shortest lifespan typically exist for just a few hours, sometimes days. Many bacteria fall into this category, especially those that require a host to survive. Most human blood cells have a lifespan of a few weeks. Neutrophils, however, generally live for only a few hours. Taste receptor cells often live about 10 days, and the cells that line the gut live about 5 days. Many cells often live somewhere between a few weeks and a few months, such as human skin cells, which constantly regenerate. When these cells die, they are replaced by new cells within a month.

Cells within organs work constantly; therefore, these cells typically have a lifespan of weeks to months. Liver cells, for example, usually live from 8 to 16 months, and most red blood cells live approximately 4 months. Immune cells, such as T cells, often last for a few days; however, if these cells are fighting infection, they could live several months at a time.

There are many different types of muscle cells. Most have an average lifespan of approximately 25 years. Examples of muscle cells include cardiac cells, skeletal cells, and smooth muscle cells. Most muscle cells contain protein filaments that aid in contraction and relaxation and are responsible for movement. While muscle cells do eventually die, they often grow with a person for a significant portion of the individual's life.

Some cells have a lifespan that is equal to the lifespan of the person. This does not mean that the cells will never die or regenerate. Nerve cells, or neurons, are an example of this type of cell. Nerve cells specialize in conducting electrical impulses; however, these cells do not self-replicate. This is also true for certain brain cells, especially those in the cortex and the brain stem. Some of these cells are with a person at birth. Many of these cells do not die until the individual dies.[37]

Molecular Basis of Aging

The evolutionary theories about the aging process focus on genetic variation and reproductive success. After the reproductive years have passed, however, it is not clear that continued longevity contributes to the fitness of the species. Therefore, anti-aging genes would not necessarily be selected, preserved, and prevalent in the gene pool.

The molecular theories of cellular aging focus on the mutations, or changes, in gene expression. Because of the appearance, properties, and function of the cells depend on gene expression, this aspect is likely involved in the aging process. Recent attention is being given to the so-called aging gene that has been identified in model systems.

Replicative Senescence

Replicative senescence refers to the limitation in the number of times that cells can divide. This process is a basic feature for most somatic cells with the exception of tumor cells and some stem cells. With this process, the cell divisions counting mechanism is posited to exist as a consequence of a telomere-shortening hypothesis.

A number of cellular theories of senescence are under investigation. Some of these theories focus on telomere shortening, free radical injury, and apoptosis. Evidence from the 1960s indicates that many cells in culture exhibit a limit in replicative capacity. This is referred to as the Hayflick limit of about 50 population doublings. This limit seems to be related to the length of the telomeres, which are DNA sequences at the ends of the chromosomes. Each time a cell divides, the telomeres shorten until a critical minimal length is attained. Once this occurs, senescence ensues, and further replication of the cell does not occur. Some cells have telomerase that prevent senescence and contribute to the cellular immortality seen in cancer. Therefore, telomere shortening appears to be related to other theories of the cellular causes of aging. For example, free radicals and oxidative damage can kill cells and hasten telomere shortening. Calorie restriction, which increases longevity, is thought to be related to reduced mitochondrial free radical generation caused by reduced methionine or other dietary amino acid intake.

Defective Protein Homeostasis

Aging, along with some aging-related disease processes, causes impaired protein homeostasis, or proteostasis. An array of quality control mechanisms preserve the stability and the functionality of their proteomes. Proteostasis involves mechanisms for the stabilization of correctly folded proteins. These mechanisms include the heat-shock family of proteins along with mechanisms for the degradation of proteins by proteasome or the lysosome. There are also regulators of age-related proteotoxicity. These regulators act through an alternative pathway that is distinct from molecular chaperones and proteases. All of these systems function in a coordinated fashion to restore the structure of misfolded polypeptides or to remove and degrade them completely. This prevents the accumulation of damaged components and ensures the continuous renewal of intracellular proteins.

Many studies have demonstrated that proteostasis is altered with aging. In addition, the chronic expression of unfolded, misfolded, or aggregated proteins contributes to the development of several age-related pathologies, including Alzheimer disease, Parkinson disease, and cataracts.[38]

Defective Nutrient Sensing

IGF-1 and insulin signaling are referred to as the insulin and IGF-I signaling (IIS) pathway. The IIS pathway is the most conserved aging-controlling pathway in evolution. Genetic polymorphisms or mutations that reduce the function of the IIS have been linked to longevity.

Levels of both growth hormone and IGF-1 decline during normal gaining. Therefore, a decreased IIS level is a common characteristic of physiologic and accelerated aging. Organisms with a constitutively decreased IIS can survive longer, owing to lower rates of both cell growth and metabolism. These lower rates of growth and metabolism are also associated with lower rates of cellular damage.

Physiologically and pathologically aged organisms decrease IIS in an attempt to extend their lifespan. This defensive response against aging could eventually become deleterious; therefore, aggravating the aging process. Therefore, extremely low levels of IIS signaling are incompatible with life.[38]

Accumulation of Damaged DNA

DNA plays a central role in life; therefore, it is implicated in aging. One hypothesis is that DNA damage and/or mutation accumulation causes aging. Because DNA damage is seen as a broader theoretical framework than mutations and DNA damage can lead to mutations, the current focus is on DNA damage. Therefore, the theory is referred to as the DNA damage theory of aging.

DNA mutations and alterations and chromosomal abnormalities increase with age. Evidence suggests that DNA damage accumulates with age in some types of stems cells and may contribute to loss of function with age. Correlations have also been found between DNA repair mechanisms and the rate of aging. Even a slight increase in the DNA repair rate over a long period of time and hundreds of cell divisions will have major consequences and could contribute to determining the rate of aging.

An emerging hypothesis is that only specific types of DNA changes are crucial in aging. This explains why mutations in some DNA repair genes affect aging while others do not. Emerging evidence also suggests that DNA damage that contributes to mutations and/or chromosomal abnormalities increases the risk of cancer. However, the DNA damage that interferes with transcription appears to contribute to aging as a result of the effects on cellular aging and cell signaling.[39]

Functional and Structural Changes That Occur with Aging and Effects on Organ Systems

Aging is a complex but natural process in which physiologic and structural alterations occur in almost all organ systems. Beginning in the fourth decade of life, even in the absence of disease, there is a progressive decline in muscle strength, cardiac reserve, vital capacity, nerve conduction time, and glomerular filtration rate. Although the biological basis of aging is poorly understood, there is a general consensus that the clarification should be sought at the cellular level. Many cell functions decline with age. A reduction is noted in oxidative phosphorylation by the mitochondria and synthesis of nucleic acids and transcription factors along with cell receptors and cell proteins.

The system-level theories center on the decline of integrative organ systems, specifically immunologic and neuroendocrine systems. These systems are necessary for overall control of other body systems. The immune system may decline with age or be less effective in protecting the body, due to infection or cancer. In addition, mutations and manipulations of certain genes cause significant changes in longevity. The mechanisms that regulate aging are thought to be complex and multifactorial; therefore, any interventions to prolong aging are apt to also be both complex and multifactorial. ■

Check Your Progress: Section 10.8

1. How do evolutionary theories explain aging?
2. What factors affect the lifespan of a cell?
3. Describe the possible role of telomere shortening in senescence.

CHAPTER SUMMARY

10.1 Chapter Overview and Case Studies

Differentiate reversible from nonreversible cell injury, cellular adaptation, and concepts related to cell injury and aging.

- Reversible cell injury involves pathologic changes that can be reversed.
- In nonreversible cell injury, pathologic cell changes are permanent and may lead to cell death.
- The goal of cellular adaptation is to maintain homeostasis.
- The primary concepts that are affected by cell injury and aging include cellular regulation along with inflammation and oxidative stress.

10.2 The Cell as the Basic Unit of Disease

Summarize cell structures and functions, and describe the consequences of injury to the cell membrane and organelles.

- The primary components of a cell include the nucleus, cytoplasm, and plasma membrane.
- Cells can be injured in a variety of ways that may lead to immediate and often severe consequences.
- The primary function of the plasma membrane is to act as a semipermeable structure that separates the intracellular and extracellular environments.
- The cell organelles are contained in the cytoplasm. These organelles are analogous to the organs of the body. Each organelle has a specific function. Organelle dysfunction can result in a variety of disease processes.
- Cell signaling systems consist of receptors that reside either in the cell membrane or within the cells.
- Different types of cell signaling abnormality are responsible for different disease processes within the body. Cell signals can be lost, be hyperactive, not reach or be ignored by the target, or a combination.
- Cell metabolism is mainly involved in the extraction of energy that is used for activities such as cell growth or cell and tissue repair. Abnormalities that occur with cell metabolism could cause the cell to lack the energy needed to carry out biological reactions, which can lead to cell death.
- Direct interactions between cells are critical to the development and function of multicellular organisms. The loss of communication between cells can result in uncontrolled cells growth and the development of cancer.
- The extracellular matrix (ECM) provides structural support to cells and tissues and plays a substantial role in regulating the behavior of cells in multicellular

organisms. Dysfunction of the ECM leads to deregulated cell proliferation and invasion, failure of cell death, and loss of cell differentiation.

10.3 Common Causes of Cell Injury

Explain the common causes of cellular injury.

- Hypoxic events deprive the cell of oxygen and interrupt oxidative metabolism and the generation of ATP.
- There are four basic types of hypoxia: hypoxic hypoxia, ischemic (stagnant) hypoxia, anemic hypoxia, and histotoxic hypoxia.
- Hypoxia causes a power failure in the cell. This causes widespread effects on the cell's structural and functional components.
- In dysoxia, tissues cannot make full use of the oxygen that is available to the cells. It occurs when there is a decreased supply of or demand for oxygen.
- Oxidative stress is an imbalance between the production of free radicals and the ability of the body to counteract, or detoxify, their harmful effects through neutralization by antioxidants.

10.4 Environmental Factors That Cause Cell Injury

Differentiate the causes, classification, underlying pathogenesis, and clinical manifestations of cell injury caused by environmental factors and approaches to diagnosis and treatment of these injuries across the lifespan.

- The six most common pollutants in the air across the United States are carbon monoxide, lead, nitrogen dioxide, ozone, particulate matter, and sulfur dioxide. Because air pollutants are inhaled directly into the lungs, their main adverse effect is respiratory impairment. These substances irritate cells in the airways, causing inflammation, oxidative stress, bronchoconstriction, and increased mucus secretion, which cause various degrees of airway obstruction.
- Carbon monoxide is a tasteless, odorless, colorless gas, so its presence cannot be directly detected by the person or people affected by it. Acute poisoning due to elevated levels of CO causes cell injury due to hypoxia, inflammation, and oxidative stress. CO causes more than half of all deaths from poisoning worldwide. The affected individual needs to be removed immediately from the source of CO. Oxygen should be administered as soon as possible because CO exerts its toxic effects by binding to sites on hemoglobin, myoglobin, and cytochrome oxidase that are normally occupied by oxygen.
- Lead is a heavy metal that can be absorbed into the blood from the gastrointestinal tract after ingestion of a substance containing lead, from the respiratory tract after inhalation of lead dust, and from the skin after dermal contact. Lead is very toxic and can adversely affect many organ systems. It crosses the blood–brain barrier, and many of the clinical manifestations of lead toxicity are due to its ability to cause hypoxia and oxidative stress and to impair neurotransmitter function in the nervous system.
- Radiation is a physical environmental hazard and comprises a wide spectrum of wave-propagated energy, including ionizing gamma rays to radiofrequency waves. Nonionizing radiation has enough energy to cause atoms to vibrate but not enough to eject electrons. Ionizing radiation has enough energy to eject electrons that are tightly bound to atoms.

10.5 Impact of Injury on Cell Types Present in Many Organs

Describe the impact of injury on endothelial and epithelial cells in various organs.

- The endothelial response to injury can be divided into two levels of responses: an initial rapid response and a slower, phenotypic response.
- When an epithelial cell is injured (e.g., from insect bites, scrapes, or cuts), blood may leak out and microorganisms may be allowed to enter. This injury results in the release of factors that activate fibroblasts. This results in the production of collagen and fibronectin to plug the compromised epithelium.

10.6 Cellular Responses to Injury

Summarize the cellular responses to injury and the cellular repair process.

- Morphologic cell changes occur in response to reversible injury. These changes allow the cell to adapt to the insult and recover structure and function. The specific cell changes include changes in size (atrophy and hypertrophy), changes in number (hyperplasia), and changes in form (metaplasia, dysplasia, and autophagy).
- Intracellular accumulations represent the buildup of substances that cells cannot immediately use or eliminate. The most common intracellular accumulations include water, lipids, calcium, glycogen, hyaline, and pigments.
- Hemochromatosis is an excess accumulation of hemosiderin in the cells caused by iron excess. When iron accumulates, it is stored in parenchymal cells of the heart, liver, and pancreas, causing damage to these cells.
- Certain agents and stresses cause distinct alterations that involve the smooth ER, the mitochondria, and the cytoskeleton. Some of these alterations can occur in acute lethal injury; others occur in either chronic forms of cell injury or as adaptive responses.
- When cellular contents leak out through the damaged plasma membrane, inflammation occurs. This inflammation is the result of the free radicals that are

produced by leukocytes that enter the tissues. Inflammation also occurs with necrosis.

- During the repair process, a cell must clear out damaged proteins and produce new functional molecules. These complicated biochemical processes occur continually in most cells. Many cells are able to survive for long periods of time because they can repair moderate damage and produce new molecules.

10.7 Cell Death

Compare and contrast the causes and effects of cell death due to necrosis and cell death due to apoptosis.

- Necrosis refers to cell death in an organ or tissue that is still part of a living organism. It involves unregulated enzymatic digestion of cell components, loss of cell membrane integrity (causing an uncontrolled release of the products into the extracellular space), and the initiation of the inflammatory response.
- Apoptosis is often referred to as programmed cell death. It is a highly selective process that eliminates injured and aged cells.

10.8 Aging of the Individual as a Result of Cellular Aging

Describe the normal lifespan, the molecular basis of aging, and the changes that occur with aging in the human body.

- The normal lifespan of a cell depends on the type of cell it is along with the function, location, and overarching purpose of the cell. Some cells exist for just a few hours; others live for weeks, months, or years; cells such as neurons may live as long as the individual.
- The evolutionary theories about the aging process focus on genetic variation and reproductive success. The molecular theories of cellular aging focus on the mutations, or changes, in gene expression. A number of cellular theories of senescence are also under investigation.
- Aging is a complex but natural process in which there are physiologic and structural alterations in almost all organ systems. Many cell functions decline with age. A reduction is noted in oxidative phosphorylation by the mitochondria and synthesis of nucleic acids and transcription factors along with cell receptors and cell proteins.

REVIEW QUESTIONS

1. The nurse is teaching a community class on home safety. Which of the following does the nurse teach about carbon monoxide poisoning?
   a. Carbon monoxide has a distinct onion-like smell.
   b. Carbon monoxide has no taste or smell.
   c. Carbon monoxide produces a yellow haze.
   d. Carbon monoxide causes burning of the eyes.
2. A client is admitted to the hospital with a carboxyhemoglobin level of 15% after inhaling carbon monoxide. Which of the following manifestations is the nurse most likely to assess?
   a. Headache, exertional dyspnea, dizziness
   b. Confusion, nausea, vomiting
   c. Severe headache, tachycardia, seizures
   d. Coma, cardiac and/or respiratory arrest
3. Which of the following is the nurse likely to assess in a child with lead poisoning?
   a. Short attention span
   b. Wheezing in all lung fields
   c. Hearing loss
   d. Cardiac arrhythmias
4. Which of the following treatments does the nurse anticipate in a child with acute lead poisoning?
   a. Blood transfusion
   b. Large volume intravenous fluids
   c. Hemodialysis
   d. Chelation therapy
5. The nurse is teaching a community class on disease prevention. The nurse recommends avoiding which of the following types of radiation from the sun to reduce the risk of cataracts?
   a. UV-A
   b. UV-B
   c. UV-C
   d. Electromagnetic
6. Which of the following laboratory values would be elevated in the client with hemochromatosis?
   a. Mercury
   b. Lead
   c. Iron
   d. Calcium
7. A client with dry gangrene of a lower extremity will exhibit which of the following manifestations?
   a. Coldness, swelling, and pulselessness
   b. No line of demarcation
   c. Wrinkled and shrunken tissue
   d. Blebs
8. A worker in an industrial plant exposed to 50 rem of ionizing radiation will most likely exhibit:
   a. nausea.
   b. fatigue.
   c. vomiting.
   d. hair loss.

ANSWERS

Answers to Review Questions can be found in Appendix A. Answers to Case Study and Check Your Progress questions are available on the faculty resources site. Please consult with your instructor.

RECOMMENDED WEBSITES

Atlas of Pathology: Cell Injury and Adaptation
http://www.pathologyatlas.ro/cell-injury-adaptation.php

Environmental Protection Agency (EPA)
https://www.airnow.gov/

Medline Plus: Antioxidants
https://medlineplus.gov/antioxidants.html

REFERENCES

1. Spillane, J., Kullmann, D., & Hanna, M. (2016). Genetic neurological channelopathies: Molecular genetics and phenotypes. *Journal of Neurology, Neurosurgery, and Psychiatry, 87*, 37–48.
2. Cannizzaro, L. (2015). Developmental and genetic diseases. In D. Stayer, E. Rubin, J. Saffitz, & A. Schiler (Eds.), *Rubin's pathology: Clinicopathologic foundations of medicine* (7th ed., pp. 243–298). Philadelphia, PA: Wolters Kluwer Health.
3. Loudon, K., & Fry, A. (2014). The renal channelopathies. *Annals of Clinical Biochemistry, 51*(4), 441–458.
4. 4. Kim, J.-B. (2014). Channelopathies. *Korean Journal of Pediatrics, 57*(1), 1–18.
5. Hirota, K. (2015). Involvement of hypoxia-inducible factors in the dysregulation of oxygen homeostasis in sepsis. *Cardiovascular & Hematological Disorders Drug Targets, 15*(1), 29–40. doi:10.2174/1871529X15666150108115553.
6. McKeown, S. R. (2014). Defining normoxia, physoxia and hypoxia in tumours: Implications for treatment response. *British Journal of Radiology, 87*(1035), 20130676. doi:10.1259/bjr.20130676.
7. McNamee, E. N., Johnson, D. K., Homann, D., & Clambey, E. T. (2013). Hypoxia and hypoxia-inducible factors as regulators of T cell development, differentiation, and function. *Immunologic Research, 55*(0):58–70. doi:10.1007/s12026-012-8
8. Mikhed, Y., Daiber, A., & Steven, S. (2015). Mitochondrial oxidative stress, mitochondrial DNA damage and their role in age-related vascular dysfunction. *International Journal of Molecular Sciences*, 16(7): 15918–15953.
9. Ray, P.D., Huang, B-W., & Tsuji, Y. (2012). Reactive oxygen species (ROS) homeostasis and redox regulation in cellular signaling. *Cellular Signaling*, 24(5): 981–990.
10. Mandal, A. (2013). What are antioxidants? *Medical News: Life Sciences & Medicine*. Available at http://www.news-medical.net/health/What-are-Antioxidants.aspx
11. Environmental Protection Agency. (2017). *What are the six common air pollutants?* Available at http://www.epa.gov/airquality/urbanair
12. Environmental Protection Agency. (2017). *Air pollution: Current and future challenges*. Available at https://www.epa.gov/clean-air-act-overview/air-pollution-current-and-future-challenges#common
13. Environmental Protection Agency. (2014). Good up high bad nearby: What is ozone? *AirNow*. Available at https://cfpub.epa.gov/airnow/index.cfm?action=gooduphigh.index
14. Friedman, P., Guo, X., Stiller, R., & Laifer, S. (2015). Carbon monoxide exposure during pregnancy. *Obstetrical & Gynecological Survey, 70*(11), 705–712.
15. Centers for Disease Control and Prevention. (2015). *Carbon monoxide poisoning*. Available at https://www.cdc.gov/co/faqs.htm
16. Maloney, G. (2016). Carbon monoxide. In J. Tintinalli, S. Stapczynski, O. Ma, et al. (Eds.), *Tintinalli's emergency medicine* (8th ed., pp. 1437–1440). New York, NY: McGraw-Hill Education.
17. Guzman, J. (2012). Carbon monoxide poisoning. *Critical Care Clinics, 28*, 537–548.
18. Centers for Disease Control and Prevention. (2017). *Lead*. Available at http://www.cdc.gov/nceh/lead
19. Dapul, H., & Laraque, D. (2014). Lead poisoning in children. *Advances in Pediatrics, 61*, 313–333.
20. Markowitz, M. (2016). Lead poisoning. In R. Kliegman, B. Stanton, J. Geme, & N. Schor (Eds.), *Nelson textbook of pediatrics* (pp. 3431–3435). New York, NY: Elsevier.
21. Lidsky, T., & Schneider, J. (2003). Lead neurotoxicity in children: Basic mechanisms and clinical correlates. *Brain, 126*, 5–19.
22. Allen, K. (2015). Is prenatal lead exposure a concern in infancy? What is the evidence? *Advances in Neonatal Care, 15*(6): 416–420.
23. Fleming, M. (2015). Disorders of iron and copper metabolism, the sideroblastic anemias, and lead toxicity. In S. Orkin, D. Fisher, D. Ginsburg, et al. (Eds.), *Nathan and Oski's hematology and oncology of infancy and childhood* (pp. 344–381). New York, NY: Elsevier.
24. World Health Organization. International Agency for Research on Cancer. (2011). *IARC classifies radiofrequency electromagnetic fields as possibly carcinogenic to humans*. Available at http://www.iarc.fr/en/media-centre/pr/2011/pdfs/pr208_E.pdf.
25. Environmental Protection Agency. (2017). Radionuclide basics: Radium. *Radiation Protection*. Available at https://www.epa.gov/radiation/radionuclide-basics-radium.
26. American Cancer Society. (2015). *Radon and cancer*. Available at https://www.cancer.org/cancer/cancer-causes/radiation-exposure/radon.html.
27. Elisa, T., Antonio, P., Giuseppe, P., et al. (2015). Endothelin receptors expressed by immune cells are involved in modulation of inflammation and in fibrosis: Relevance to the pathogenesis of systemic sclerosis. *Journal of Immunology Research, 2015*, 147616. doi:10.1155/2015/147616
28. Mandal, A. (2016). What are antioxidants? *Medical News: Life Sciences & Medicine*. Available at http://www.news-medical.net/health/What-are-Antioxidants.aspx
29. Cheng, Y., Ren, X., Hait, W. N., & Yang, J. M. (2013). Therapeutic targeting of autophagy in disease: Biology and pharmacology. *Pharmacological Reviews, 65*(4), 1162–1197. doi:10.1124/pr.112.007120
30. howMed. (n.d.). *Hydropic change*. Available at http://howmed.net/pathology/hydropic-chage
31. howMed. (n.d.) *Fatty change*. Available at http://howmed.net/pathology/fatty-change

32. howMed. (n.d.). *Calcification*. Available at http://howmed.net/pathology/calcification
33. howMed. (n.d.). *Intracellular accumulations*. Available at http://howmed.net/pathology/intracellular-accumulations
34. Meriden, Z., Shi, C., Edil, B. H., et al. (2011). Hyaline globules in neuroendocrine and solid-pseudopapillary neoplasms of the pancreas: A clue to the diagnosis. *American Journal of Surgical Pathology, 35*(7), 981–988. doi:10.1097/PAS.0b013e31821a9a14
35. howMed. (n.d.). *Intracellular accumulations of melanin*. Available at http://howmed.net/pathology/intracellular-accumulation-of-melanin
36. howMed. (n.d.). *Hemosiderosis*. Available at http://howmed.net/pathology/hemosiderosis/ N.D.
37. Reece, T. (n.d.). Physiology of self renewal: When physiology shapes anatomy, lifespan of body parts. *Medical Science Navigator*. Available at http://www.medicalsciencenavigator.com/physiology-of-self-renewal
38. López-Otín, C., Blasco, M. A., Partridge, L., Serrano, M., & Kroemer, G. (2013). The hallmarks of aging. *Cell, 153*(6), 1194–1217. doi:10.1016/j.cell.2013.05.039
39. de Magalhaes, J. P. (2014). Damage-based theories of aging. *senescense.info*. Available at http://www.senescence.info/causes_of_aging.html

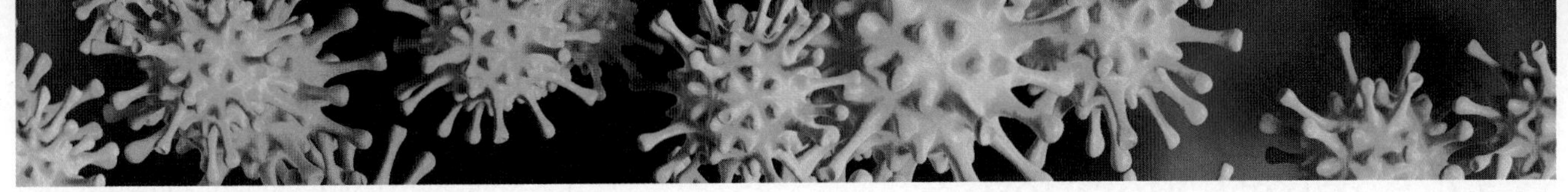

Chapter 11 Inflammation

Karen Saban

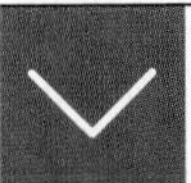

Chapter Outline and Learning Outcomes

11.1 Chapter Overview and Case Studies

Recognize the complex role that inflammation plays in defending the body from injury and promoting healing.

11.2 Functions of the Inflammatory Response in Health and Disease

Describe the inflammatory response as a key component of the body's defense system.

11.3 Acute Inflammatory Response

Discriminate the characteristics of the acute inflammatory response.

11.4 Regulation and Termination of Acute Inflammation

Explain the regulation and resolution of the acute inflammatory process.

11.5 Morphologic Types and Outcomes of Acute Inflammation

Discuss the primary morphologic types of acute inflammation and the four possible outcomes of acute inflammation.

11.6 Chronic Inflammation

Identify the conditions under which chronic inflammation may arise, and explain the process of chronic inflammation and its possible outcomes.

11.7 Systemic Manifestations of Inflammation

Describe the causes and processes associated with systemic inflammation.

11.8 Impaired and Excessive Inflammation

Discuss the potential causes and consequences of impaired and excessive inflammation.

11.9 Overview of Disorders Associated with Chronic Inflammation

Recognize key disorders in which inflammation is an important contributing factor.

11.10 Linking Pathophysiology to the Diagnosis and Treatment of Inflammation

Identify primary treatments for inflammation.

KEY TERMS

Acquired (adaptive) immunity, 274
Acute-phase response, 284
C-reactive protein (CRP), 274
Cardinal signs of inflammation, 276
Chemokines, 279
Chemotaxis, 277
Complement proteins, 279
Cytokines, 279
Eicosanoids, 279
Fibrinous inflammation, 282
Inflammasome, 279
Inflammation, 272
Innate immunity, 274
Kinins, 280
Leukocyte, 277
Pattern recognition receptors, 281
Purulent (suppurative) inflammation, 282
Scarring, 282
Serous inflammation, 282
Shift to the left, 274
Systemic inflammatory response syndrome (SIRS), 284
Suppuration, 282
Ulceration, 282
Vasodilation, 277

ABBREVIATIONS

CRP—C-reactive protein
HPA—hypothalamic–pituitary–adrenal
hsCRP—high-sensitivity C-reactive protein
NK—natural killer
SIRS—systemic inflammatory response syndrome

11.1 Chapter Overview and Case Studies

Survival depends on the ability of the human body to recognize and remove infectious organisms, toxins, and damaged tissues and to eliminate them without significant harm to the surrounding normal cells. **Inflammation** (from the Latin word for "to set on fire") is defined as a protective tissue response to tissue injury or destruction of tissues. Words ending in "itis," such as "appendicitis, "cellulitis," and "osteomyelitis," denote an inflammatory disease process. Inflammation is not synonymous with infection. Infection is the invasion of body tissue by a disease-causing organism. Inflammation is the body's immunovascular response to the disease-causing organism. However, inflammation may also be a response to tissue injury that is not related to a disease-causing organism. For example, inflammation may occur in association with a sprain or bone fracture.

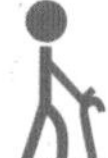

Inflammation is the common denominator of many chronic age-related diseases such as arthritis, gout, Alzheimer disease, and diabetes. ■

The goals of inflammation are to eliminate the initial cause of injury, remove dead cells, and begin the process of tissue repair. In most circumstances, beneficial effects are accomplished by the inflammatory process, as is seen with healing of a wound and recovery from the common cold. However, sometimes the components of inflammation may result in harm to healthy tissue or inflammation can become chronic (see the Impact of Current Research on Clinical Practice).

This chapter addresses the functions of the inflammatory response; provides a review of the acute inflammatory response; discusses regulation, termination, and outcomes of the acute inflammatory response; and identifies morphologic types of acute inflammation. In addition, chronic inflammation and systemic inflammation are addressed. The process of impaired and excessive inflammation is examined. Finally, an overview of disorders associated with inflammation is provided.

Concepts Related to Inflammation

A patient with an alteration in inflammation will have alterations in related concepts (**Figure 11.1** ■). When bacteria or a virus enters the body and causes an infection, it triggers the inflammatory response. The normal process of inflammation neutralizes the antigen and initiates healing. Widespread infection prompts a widespread inflammatory response, the manifestations of which include generalized pain and fever. A localized infection results in a limited inflammatory response that causes redness and tenderness at the affected site. An acute inflammatory response usually resolves when the invading pathogen has been eradicated. When acute inflammation persists, chronic inflammation may develop. With chronic inflammation, the inflammatory response may be disproportionate to the initial insult and can lead to more damage than would be expected from the initial cause. Examples of chronic inflammatory disorders include Crohn disease and ulcerative colitis. Related concepts include infection and elimination.

Many of the blood cells and components of the inflammatory response are mediated by the immune system, which also protects the body from harm. In autoimmune diseases, inflammation and immune responses are mistakenly initiated against normal healthy tissue. The symptoms of an autoimmune disease depend on the tissue that

Impact of Current Research on Clinical Practice

The Chronic Stress of Caregiving

Description: Cuijpers demonstrated that about half of people who provide informal care to loved ones develop depressive symptoms associated with the chronic stress of caregiving.[1] Studies by Vitaliano and colleagues demonstrate that in addition to the psychologic impact of caregiving, informal caregivers experience altered immune function[2] and increased levels of stress-related hormones.[3] Saban and colleagues showed altered hypothalamic–pituitary–adrenal function in female caregivers of stroke survivors[4]; and in a study of women caregivers caring for veterans who were recovering from a traumatic brain injury, caregivers who reported higher levels of anger and blame had higher levels of tumor necrosis factor alpha (TNF-α), a pro-inflammatory cytokine.[5]

Clinical Practice: Because higher levels of TNF-α have been shown to be associated with inflammatory-related diseases such as cardiovascular disease,[6] TNF-α may be an important biomarker for identifying caregivers who are at risk for developing chronic inflammatory-related disease.

Research Studies:

1. Cuijpers, P. (2005). Depressive disorders in caregivers of dementia patients: A systematic review. *Aging & Mental Health, 9*(4), 325–330.
2. Vitaliano, P. P., Scanlan, J. M., Krenz, C., Schwartz, R. S., & Marcovina, S. M. (1996). Psychological distress, caregiving, and metabolic variables. *Journals of Gerontology Series B: Psychological Sciences & Social Sciences, 51*(5), 290–299.
3. Vitaliano, P. P., Zhang, J., & Scanlan, J. M. (2003). Is caregiving hazardous to one's physical health? A meta-analysis. *Psychological Bulletin, 129*(6), 946–972.
4. Saban, K. L., Mathews, H. L., Bryant, F. B., O'Brien, T. E., & Janusek, L. W. (2012). Depressive symptoms and diurnal salivary cortisol patterns among female caregivers of stroke survivors. *Biological Research for Nursing, 14*(4), 396–404.
5. Saban, K. L., Mathews, H. L., Collins, E. G., Hogan, N. S., Tell, D., Bryant, F. B., Pape, T. L., Griffin, J. M., & Janusek, L. W. (2015). The man I once knew: Grief and inflammation in female partners of veterans with traumatic brain injury. *Biological Research for Nursing, 18*(1), 50–59.
6. Zhang, H,. Park, Y., Wu, J., et al. (2009). Role of TNF-alpha in vascular dysfunction. *Clinical Science, 116*(3), 219–230.

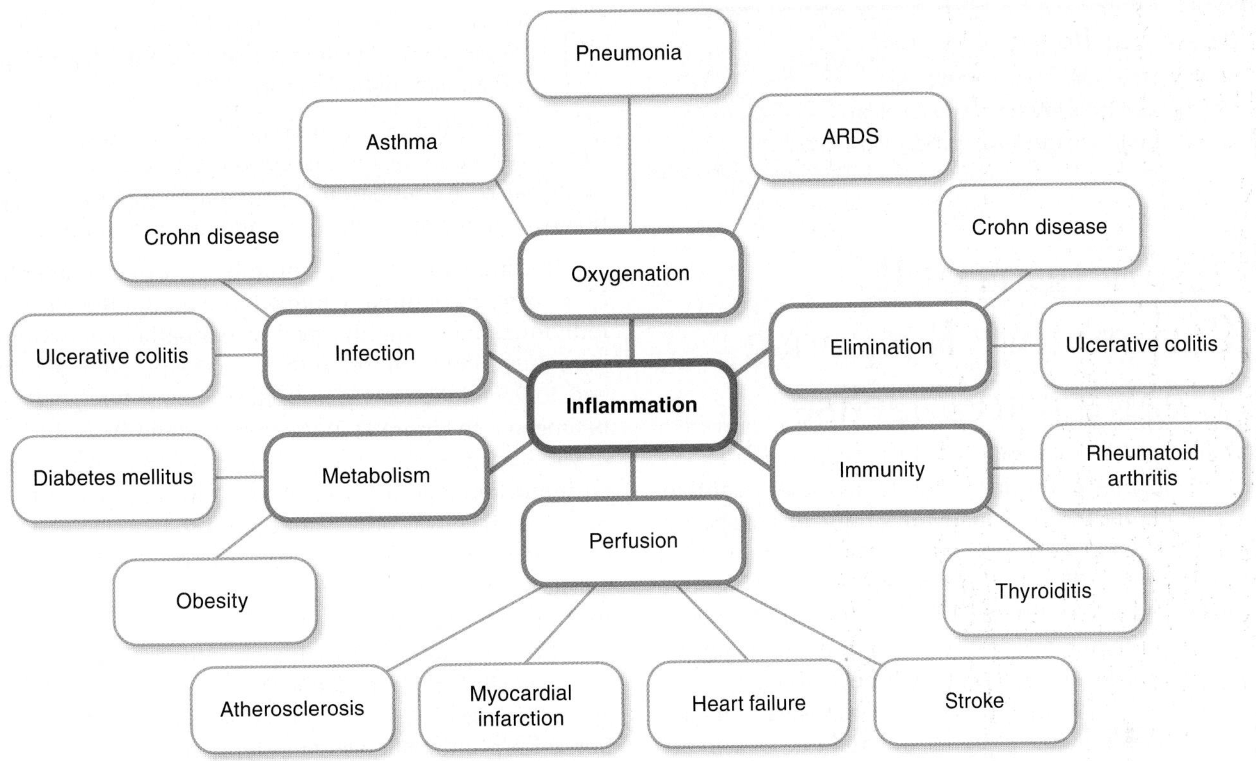

Figure 11.1 ■ Concepts related to inflammation.

is affected. Patients with rheumatoid arthritis experience joint pain, stiffness, and loss of function. If the thyroid is attacked, tiredness and weight gain result. Related concepts include comfort, mobility, and metabolism.

In asthma, the inflammatory response causes constriction of smooth muscle in the airways and increased mucus production, resulting in decreased oxygenation. The narrowed airway requires the client to exert more effort to move air into and out of the lungs. Common triggers of this response include pollen, particles from dust mites, and animal dander. Related concepts include oxygenation.

Case Studies

The pathophysiologic process of inflammation is demonstrated in two case studies woven throughout this chapter to assist with application of knowledge to clinical practice.

Timothy White: Introduction

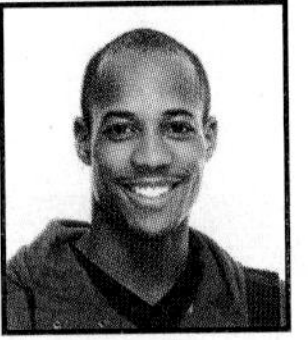

Timothy White is a 28-year-old reportedly healthy male who teaches high school chemistry. He presents to the emergency department (ED) with sharp pain in his lower right abdomen. He states that he has had a loss of appetite for the past 2 days and has vomited four times over the past 12 hours. He denies diarrhea or traveling outside of the United States. His vital signs are pulse 96, respirations 24, temperature 101.1°F, blood pressure 108/78. Mr. White is alert and oriented but appears to be anxious. He rates his abdominal pain as an 8 on a scale of 0–10, with 0 being minimal pain and 10 being very severe pain. On examination, he exhibits rebound tenderness on deep pressure to the lower abdomen.

1. Which cardinal signs of inflammation does Mr. White demonstrate?
2. Does Mr. White's condition appear to be acute inflammation or chronic inflammation? Explain.

Lucia Morales: Introduction

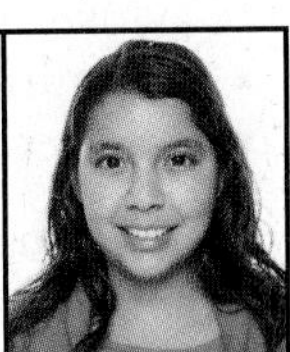

Lucia Morales is a 13-year-old female with a history of asthma since she was a young child. She presents to her pediatrician complaining of episodes of coughing and wheezing during increased physical activity over the past week. She recently joined the seventh grade cross-country team at her junior high school. Her mother gives a history of four severe asthma attacks over the course of Lucia's life in which she required admission to the emergency department for nebulizer treatments and intravenous corticosteroids. Over the past year, Lucia's asthma has been well controlled with beclomethasone inhaler taken twice a day with no need to use her rescue bronchodilator inhaler (albuterol). However, since joining the cross-country team 2 weeks ago, Lucia reports using her rescue inhaler two to three times a day for chest tightness and coughing that occurs when she is running or doing intense physical activity. She requires three puffs of the rescue inhaler for relief of her symptoms. Currently, she denies shortness of breath, chest tightness, or wheezing. Her vital signs are all within normal limits. On auscultation, mild wheezes are heard bilaterally on expiration. No rhonchi or rales are heard.

1. Compare and contrast Lucia's case to Timothy White's case.
2. What are the characteristics of chronic inflammation?

Check Your Progress: Section 11.1

1. What are the goals of inflammation?
2. List four concepts related to inflammation.
3. Compare and contrast inflammation and infection.

11.2 Functions of the Inflammatory Response in Health and Disease

Inflammation is a complex, tightly regulated process that encompasses both innate and acquired, or adaptive, immunity (**Table 11.1** ■). **Innate immunity**, or nonspecific immunity, is the defense system with which an individual is born. It provides the first line of defense in the immune response, protecting the host during the time between exposure to the antigen and generation of the adaptive immune response. Innate immunity is not learned, and it is not permanently changed as a result of exposure to microorganisms. Components of the innate immune system are depicted in **Figure 11.2** ■ and include the following:

- Physical barriers such as skin, mucous membranes, and mucus
- Enzymes in epithelial and phagocytic cells
- Inflammation-related proteins in the blood such as **C-reactive protein (CRP)**, which is a marker for inflammation in the body
- Toll-like receptors that help to sense pathogens and signal a response
- Cells that release inflammatory mediators, such as cytokines
- Antimicrobial peptides
- Phagocytes.

The signs of inflammation under the control of the innate immune system include redness, swelling, heat, and pain.

The child's immune system response to insult differs significantly from that of the adult. In pediatric patients, macrophages are more responsive to pro-inflammatory molecules, increasing the production of additional inflammatory mediators. In addition, infants are less able than adults to produce anti-inflammatory mediators. ■

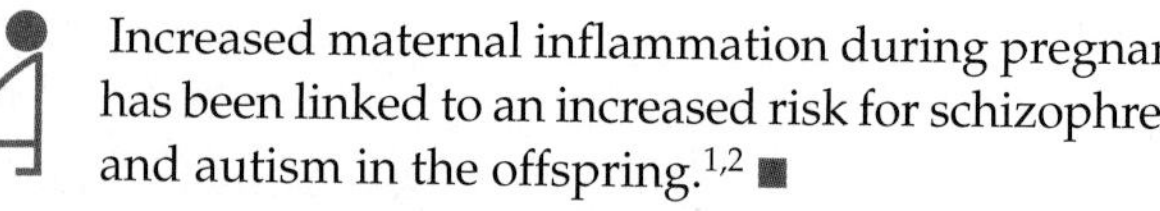

Increased maternal inflammation during pregnancy has been linked to an increased risk for schizophrenia and autism in the offspring.[1,2] ■

The aging of the immune system is likely a major determinant for susceptibility to diseases. It may also be foundational in sustaining chronic conditions due to the associated pro-inflammatory profile. ■

In contrast to innate immunity, **acquired** or **adaptive immunity**, is continually refined throughout the life of the individual and is highly specific to a pathogen. Acquired immunity allows an individual, once exposed to a pathogen, to have long-lasting protection against that particular pathogen (see Figure 11.2). Acquired immunity is the basis of vaccination. Lymphocytes (both B cells and T cells) play an important role in carrying out the acquired immune response. B cells produce antibodies that attach to a specific antigen allowing immune cells to destroy the antigen. T cells directly attack the antigen as well as help to control the immune response.

Inflammation can be divided into two basic categories: acute and chronic (**Table 11.2** ■). Acute inflammation is characterized by a brisk onset of relatively short duration with prominent systemic signs, such as fever, chills, and malaise. Examples of acute inflammatory processes include infections, tissue injury (trauma, physical, or chemical), response to foreign bodies, and immune reactions (such as hypersensitivity). Typically, systemic responses of acute inflammation (fever, leukocytosis, and plasma protein synthesis) and local responses (swelling, redness, heat, pain) are prominent. Usually in adults, there are more than 11,000/μL white blood cells with an increased level of immature neutrophils in the circulation (also known as a **shift to the left**). Acute inflammation can sometimes precede chronic inflammation. However, in many cases chronic inflammation is not a sequel to acute inflammation but rather an independent response.

In pediatric patients, structural differences in the airway increase the risk for obstruction, especially in the event of airway inflammation. In comparison to adults, children have a larger tongue relative to the oral cavity, decreased airway muscle tone, a shorter epiglottis, a more anteriorly positioned larynx, a shorter and narrower trachea, and prominent adenoid and lymphoid tissue. These differences are especially evident when the child is supine; because of the child's proportionately larger head and

Table 11.1 Characteristics of Innate and Acquired Immunity

Characteristics	Innate Immunity	Acquired Immunity
Line of defense	First line of defense	Second line of defense
Timing of defense	Immediate response	Delay between exposure to antigen and response. Can take days to weeks. Once acquired immunity is developed to a specific antigen has developed, response is immediate.
Specificity	Broad	Specific response to specific antigen
Memory	No memory involved	Memory involved
Cells involved	Mast cells, granulocytes (neutrophils, eosinophils, basophils), monocytes, macrophages, natural killer cells, platelets, endothelial cells	T and B lymphocytes, macrophages, dendritic cells

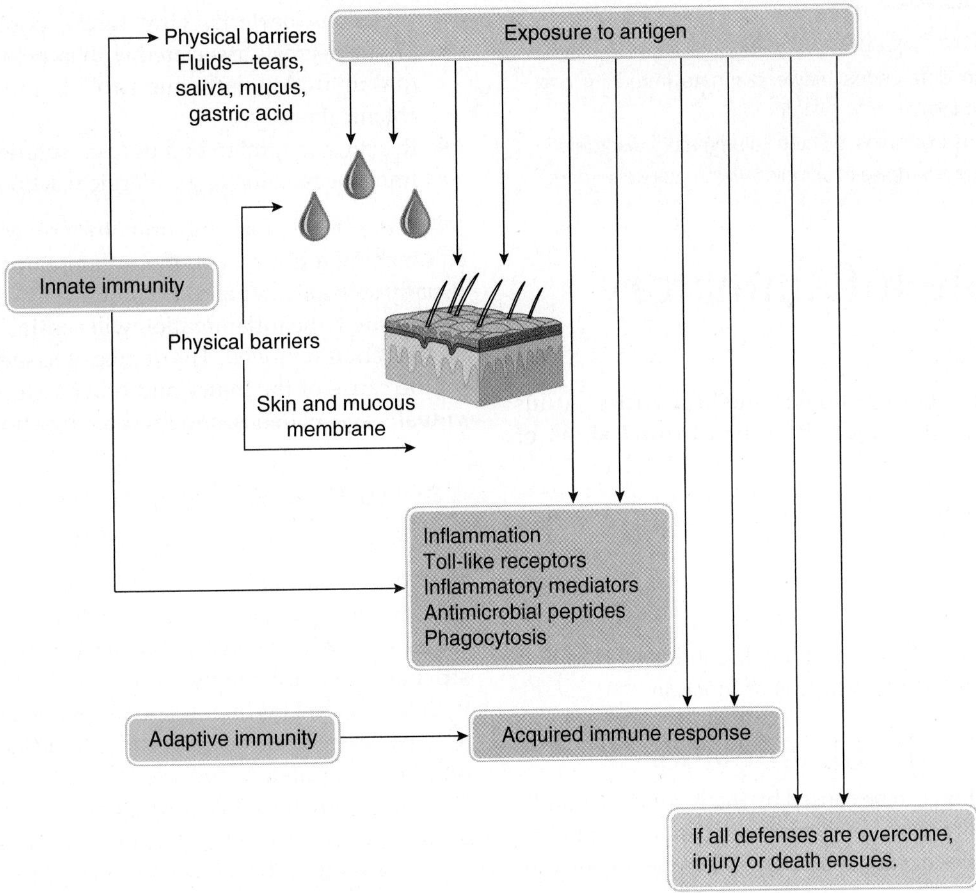

Figure 11.2 ■ Inflammation is a complex, tightly regulated process that encompasses both innate and acquired, or adaptive, immunity.

occiput compared to those of adults, hyperflexion of the neck further narrows the airway. ■

Chronic inflammation is defined as persisting at least 2 weeks and is characterized by high levels of lymphocytes, macrophages, and monocytes. The signs and symptoms associated with chronic inflammation are typically less severe than those of acute inflammation. Common chronic inflammatory diseases include diabetes mellitus, atherosclerosis, and chronic obstructive pulmonary disease. In addition, inappropriate inflammation may occur when there is no foreign substance to fight off and leads to autoimmunity. Examples of autoimmune disorders include multiple sclerosis, systemic lupus erythematosus, and Hashimoto thyroiditis.

Overall, the functions of the acute inflammatory response are to protect the organism and to repair damaged tissue. Specifically, these functions include the following:

1. Interaction with the acquired immune system to bring about a more specific response to contain and destroy the pathogen through the influx of macrophages and lymphocytes
2. Prevention of further damage of tissue by diluting the toxins produced by the pathogen
3. Prevention of the spread of infection or tissue injury by walling off the area
4. Preparation of the area for healing.

Table 11.2 Characteristics of Acute and Chronic Inflammation

Feature	Acute Inflammation	Chronic Inflammation
Onset and duration	Fast onset (minutes to hours) and relatively short duration	Slow onset: over days to weeks and lasting at least 2 weeks
Cellular infiltrate	↑Neutrophils	↑Monocytes ↑Macrophages ↑Lymphocytes
Degree of tissue injury	Usually mild and self-limiting	Persistent and progressive
Predominant process	Vascular and exudative	New connective tissue formation
Local and systemic signs	Prominent	Less severe

Check Your Progress: Section 11.2

1. What are the differences between innate immunity and acquired immunity?
2. What are some examples of acute inflammatory disorders?
3. What are some examples of chronic inflammatory disorders?

11.3 Acute Inflammatory Response

Over 2000 years ago, the Roman medical writer, Aulus Cornelius Celsus described the four **cardinal signs of inflammation**:

- Redness (rubor)
- Heat (calor)
- Swelling (tumor)
- Pain (dolor).

A fifth consequence of inflammation, identified by Rudolph Virchow in the 19th century, is loss of function.

Causes of Acute Inflammation

Acute inflammation can be caused by many different conditions. Any type of tissue injury may elicit an inflammatory response. Examples of causes of acute inflammation include the following:

- Infections (bacterial, viral, fungal, parasitic)
- Tissue necrosis associated with ischemia (e.g., myocardial infarction, ischemic stroke), trauma, physical or chemical injury
- Reaction to foreign bodies (e.g., splinter, prosthesis)
- Immune reaction (e.g., allergic reaction).

If the cause of the inflammatory process is brief (such as touching a hot stove), the inflammatory response will usually subside after about 48 hours. However, if the cause is persistent, the inflammation will continue until the causative agent is removed. The degree of tissue injury depends on the cause of the injury and other factors such the individual's age, genetics, and immune function.

Vascular Events in the Acute Inflammatory Response

Most of the essential components of the inflammatory process are found in the circulatory system. Immediately after the tissue insult, the precapillary arterioles temporarily constrict as a defense against potential blood loss associated with the injury. This brief vasoconstriction phase is followed by a prolonged period of vasodilation that lasts throughout the inflammatory process. As a result of tissue injury, chemical mediators (histamine, complement, kinins, prostaglandins, etc.) as well as leukocytosis-inducing factor are released (**Figure 11.3** ■). The release of chemical mediators initiates the following:

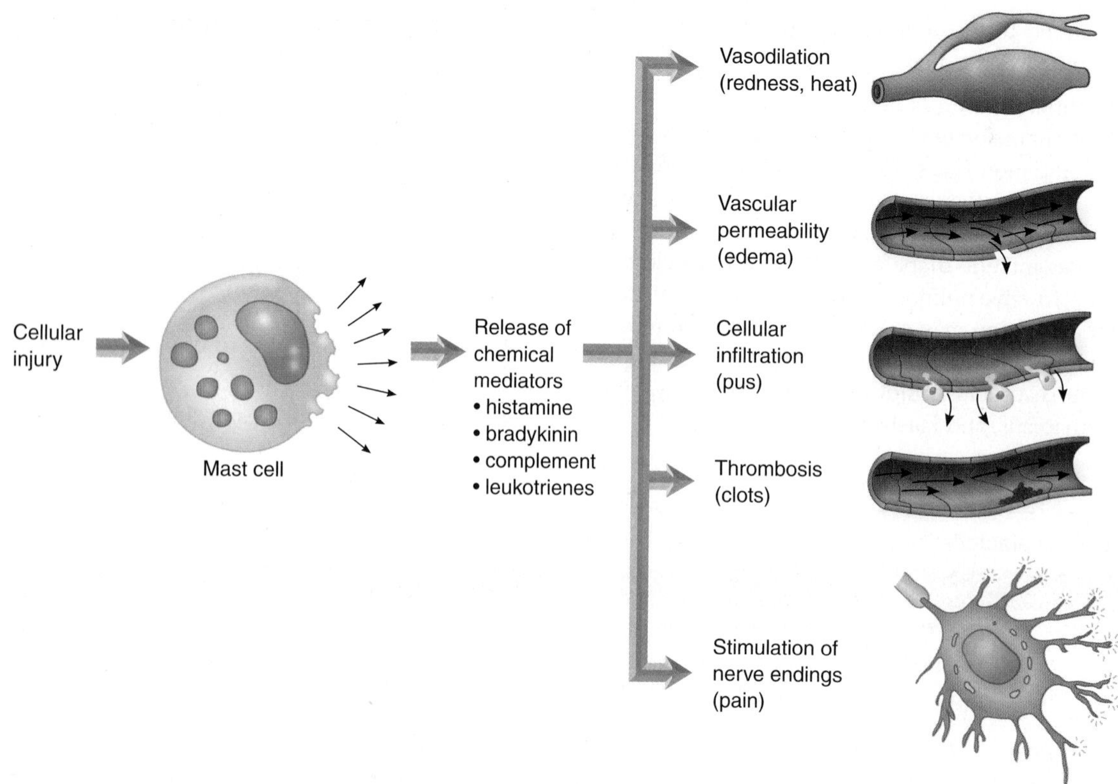

Figure 11.3 ■ Vascular events in the acute inflammatory process.

1. **Vasodilation**, or enlargement of the vessel wall lumen, which slows blood velocity, increases blood flow with oxygen and nutrients to the injured tissue. Increased tissue perfusion causes redness and warmth at the site.
2. Increased capillary permeability allows formation of an early transudate (which is protein poor) to an exudate (which is protein rich) in the extracellular tissue as well as enabling clotting proteins to prevent injury to surrounding healthy tissue. Accumulation of fluid as a result of increased permeability results in edema or swelling.
3. Neutrophils, monocytes, and lymphocytes migrate through the enlarged junctions between the endothelial lining and the surrounding tissue. **Chemotaxis** (movement of an organism in response to a chemical stimulant) causes **leukocytes** (white blood cells) to move.
4. In addition to chemical mediators, leukocytosis-inducing factors increase the number of white blood cells in the bloodstream. Chemical mediators and adhesion factors allow white blood cells to migrate through vessel walls in a multistep process. The leukocytes first roll on the vessel wall, detaching and binding again. Eventually, the leukocytes adhere to the vessel wall lining up along the inside of the vessel wall. This process, called *margination*, is imperative to the inflammatory process. Subsequently, the leukocytes transmigrate (also called *diapedesis*) across the vessel wall toward the source of injury (see **Figure 11.4** ■).

CLINICAL POINT: The circulating leukocyte count can decrease in conditions of severe inflammation, such as in acute respiratory distress syndrome, because of the large number of leukocytes that are attached to the vascular wall or have migrated into tissues. ■

CLINICAL POINT: Individuals with a rare genetic disorder called leukocyte adhesion deficiency syndrome are unable to mount an adequate inflammatory response because their leukocytes are unable to adhere to vessel walls.[3] Consequences of this syndrome include recurrent infections, leukocytosis, and delayed wound healing. ■

Once at the injured site, the leukocyte cells destroy the pathogen through phagocytosis. See **Figure 11.5** ■. Phagocytosis is completed in a three-step process:

1. Recognition of the pathogen to be destroyed by the leukocyte
2. Engulfment of the pathogen by the leukocyte
3. Killing or degrading of the pathogen. Phagocytosis stimulates that production of hydrogen peroxide within the lysosomes of the phagocyte, which causes the pH to decrease, enhancing the action of the enzymes.

As phagocytosis proceeds from the initial binding of a target to actin-dependent internalization and ultimately to degradation of the target in the phagolysosome, myeloid cells acquire information about the target through a variety of mechanisms. At the cell surface, receptors sample the chemical constituents of the particle, and membrane dynamics facilitate an assessment of its physical properties. Additional information is gathered as the phagosome pinches off from the plasma membrane and as it matures through interactions with other intracellular compartments. Finally, the degradation of the target exposes ligands that were not previously accessible and releases ligands into the cytosol for detection by intracellular receptors. The information gathered by all of these processes is integrated to shape the ensuing immune response.

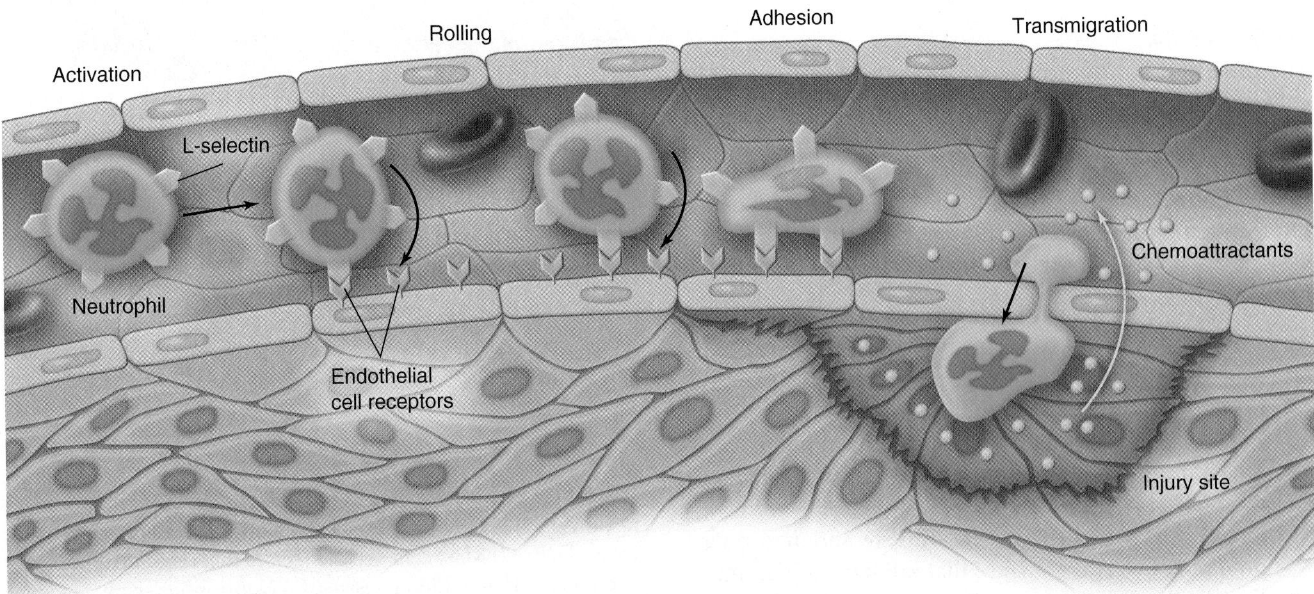

Figure 11.4 ■ The process of margination.

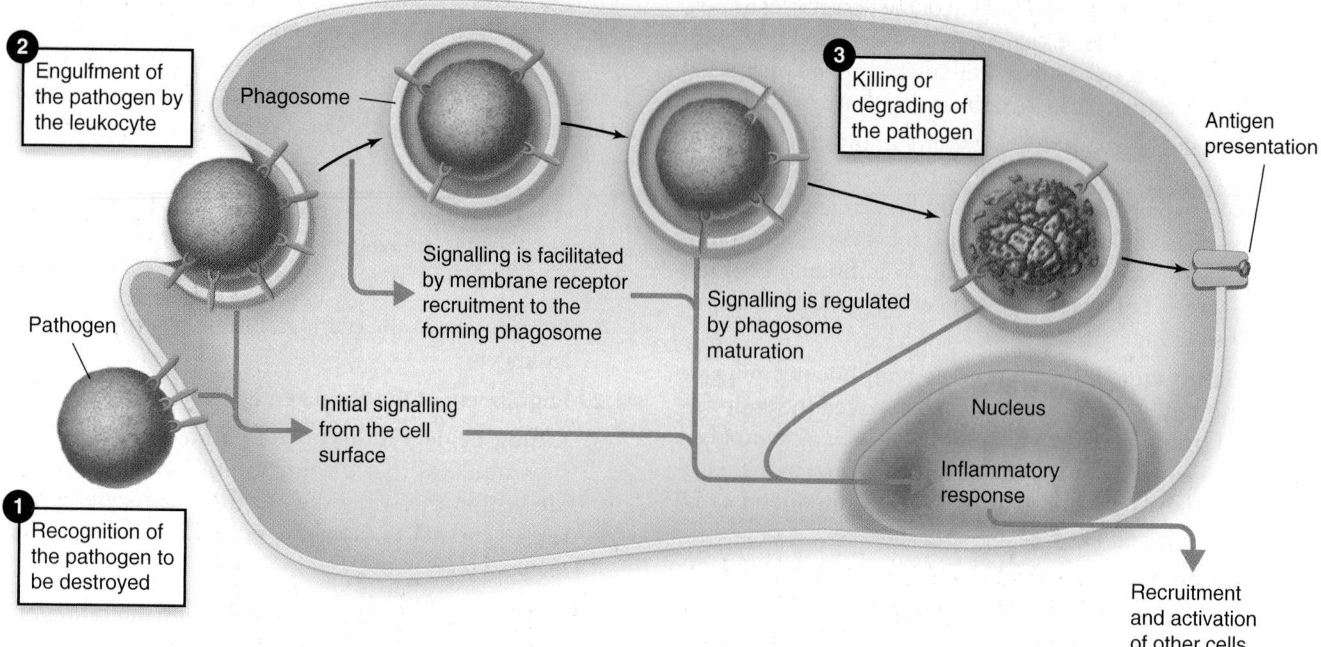

Figure 11.5 ■ The process of phagocytosis.

Cell Types and Cellular Events Involved in the Acute Inflammatory Response

The acute inflammatory response involves many different cell types (**Figure 11.6** ■). However, the leukocytes are the primary components of inflammatory response. There are three major types of leukocytes: lymphocytes, granulocytes and monocytes. Lymphocytes consist of T cells, B cells, and natural killer cells (NK cells). Granulocytes (also called myeloid leuokocytes) include neutrophils, esoinphils, and basinophils/mast cells. Monocytes include monocytes, macrophages and dendritic cells.

Lymphocytes

The three types of lymphocytes—T cells, B cells, and NK cells—originate from the common lymphoid cell in the bone marrow and make up about 20% of the white blood cell count. T cells mature in the thymus, and B cells mature in the bone marrow. Both T cells and B cells are responsible for acquired immunity. NK cells, part of the innate immune system, are released into the circulation after forming in the bone marrow.

- *T cells:* There are two distinct types of T cells that can be differentiated by the presence of CD4 and CD8 surface proteins. T cells that have CD4 on their surfaces are T-helper cells and are responsible for producing cytokines that mediate the immune response. T cells that have CD8 on their surfaces are cytotoxic T cells. Cytotoxic T cells recognize specific antigens and in response produce powerful enzymes that kill the antigen cell.
- *B cells:* B cells are responsible for providing humoral immunity and produce large amounts of antibodies in response to specific antigens.
- *Natural killer cells:* Natural killer cells, part of the innate immune system, are large granular lymphocytes that are activated by the cytokines released by T cells. They are able to kill tumor cells and cells infected with viruses without prior exposure to the antigen. Natural killer cells contain perforin and granzyme, which activate cell apoptosis via cell membrane receptors.

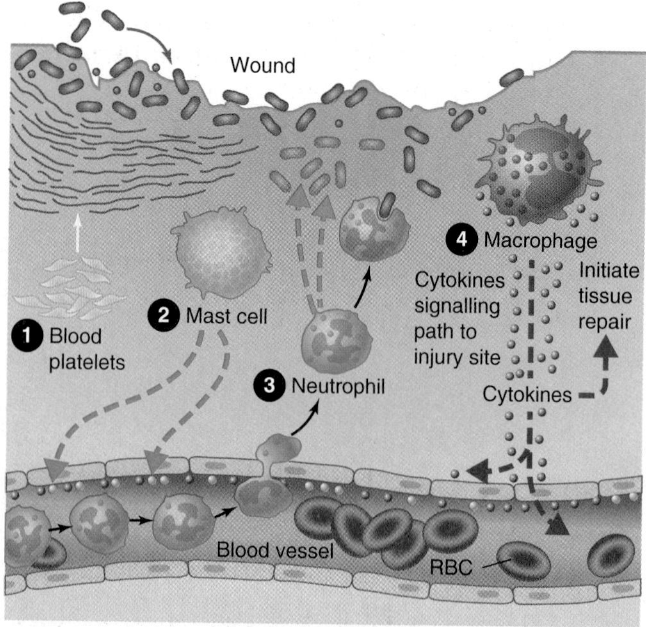

Figure 11.6 ■ Types of cells involved in the inflammatory response. (1) Platelets release blood-clotting proteins at the wound site. (2) Mast cells secrete factors that mediate dilation and constriction of blood vessels. (3) Neutrophils secrete factors that kill or degrade pathogens. Neutrophils and macrophages secrete factors that remove pathogens by phagocytosis. (4) Macrophages secrete cytokines that attract immune system cells.

Granulocytes

Granulocytes are characterized by the presence of granules in their cytoplasm and are sometimes referred to as polymorphonuclear leukocytes. The three types of granulocytes are neutrophils, eosinophils, and basophils or mast cells.

- *Neutrophils:* Neutrophils are the most common type of white blood cell, comprising 60–70% of circulating leukocytes, and generally live for about 5 days in the circulation. Neutrophils are typically the first responders to an infection or injury and are found in abundant amounts at the site. They are the major component of pus related to acute inflammation. They actively phagocytose bacteria and generate oxygen (hydrogen peroxide) and nitric oxide that expedite the destruction of pathogens.[4] During severe acute infection, immature neutrophils, called band cells, are released into the circulation.
- *Eosinophils:* Eosinophils account for about 4% of all leukocytes. Their primary roles include defending against parasitic infections and responding to allergic reactions. Their granules contain a protein that is a potent toxin against parasites.
- *Basophils and mast cells:* Basophils make up only about 1% of leukocytes. Their primary function is to release histamine and other vasoactive amines in response to infection, injury, or allergic reaction. They are also involved in wound healing and chronic inflammation. Basophils and mast cells are similarly structured except that basophils circulate in blood vessels and mast cells are found in connective tissue, particularly near blood vessels.

Monocytes

Monocytes do not have granules in their cytoplasm and include monocytes, macrophages, and dendritic cells.

- *Monocytes and macrophages:* Monocytes and macrophages develop from bone marrow stem cells. Monocytes are immature macrophages or dendritic cells (they differentiate into either class) and make up about 6% of circulating leukocytes. They are irregularly shaped; are found primarily in the blood; and target bacteria, viruses, and debris and destroy them by phagocytosis. Macrophages are large and irregularly shaped and contain a large bean-shaped nucleus. When monocytes enter tissue from the circulation, they are called macrophages. In contrast to neutrophils, which also phagocytose pathogens, monocytes live for months. The cell surface of macrophages are covered with receptor proteins, which allows them to locate antigens that have been coated by antibodies.
- *Dendritic cells:* Dendritic cells are antigen-presenting cells found in tissue that has contact with the external environmnent, such as the skin and linings of the nose, bronchi, and gastroinestinal tract. Their primary function is to process antigen material and present it on the cell surface to the T cells, helping to shape the adaptive immune response.

Chemical Mediators of Inflammation

Mediators of inflammation, which are secreted by cells or produced from plasma proteins, are chemicals that regulate the inflammatory response.

Cell-Derived Mediators

Cell-derived mediators are maintained in intracellular granules and can be quickly released or produced in response to tissue injury. Primary cell types that produce mediators during acute inflammation are macrophages, dendritic cells, and mast cells. For example, histamine is quickly released from mast cells in response to tissue damage. However, neutrophils, endothelial cells, and platelets can also produce mediators. In general, mediators that are produced in response to specific stimuli are short-lived and can stimulate the release of other mediators, thereby amplifying the inflammatory response. The major types of mediators related to acute inflammation are vasoactive amines (e.g., histamine), lipid mediators (e.g., prostaglandins and leukotrienes), cytokines and chemokines, and lysosomal components (e.g., oxygen free radicals, nitric oxide).

- *Vasoactive amines*: The two major vasoactive amines are histamine and serotonin. Both of them are among the first mediators to be released in response to inflammation and affect blood vessels. Histamine, which is found in mast cells, basophils, and platelets, is quickly released in response to injury and allergic reactions. Release of histamine results in vasodilation, increased vascular permeability, and endothelial activation. Serotonin, which is stored in platelets and neuroendocrine cells in the gastrointestinal tract, is a vasoconstrictor.
- *Lipid mediators:* Lipid mediators include prostaglandins, leukotrienes, and lipoxins, which are derived from arachidonic acid. They are also known as **eicosanoids**. Prostaglandins are primarily responsible for vasodilation; leukotrienes promote increased vascular permeability, chemotaxis, and leukocyte adhesion. Lipoxins decrease inflammation by suppressing the recruitment of neutrophils.
- *Cytokines, inflammasomes, and chemokines:* **Cytokines** are small proteins that are either pro-inflammatory or anti-inflammatory by nature. There are many different cytokines but the most well studied cytokines in relationship to acute inflammation are listed in **Table 11.3** ■. **Inflammasomes** are complex proteins that promote the production of pro-inflammatory cytokines such as interleukin 1β (IL-1β), IL-18, and IL-33. **Chemokines** are a group of small signaling proteins that act as chemoattractants to recruit leukocytes to areas of damaged tissue. They also control migration of cells during normal processes of tissue maintenance. They are classified into four main groups: CXC, CC, CXC3C, and XC.

Plasma Protein Systems

There are three primary plasma protein systems that are involved in the inflammatory response: complement system, coagulation system, and kinin system. These systems

Table 11.3 Common Cytokines Related to Acute Inflammation

Cytokine	Main Source	Primary Action
TNF-α	Macrophages, mast cells, T lymphocytes	Regulates immune cells, induces fever, cachexia
IL-1	Macrophages, endothelial cells, epithelial cells	Group of 11 cytokines with both pro-inflammatory and anti-inflammatory properties
IL-6	Macrophages	Has both pro-inflammatory and anti-inflammatory effects; plays a role in mediating fever
IL-17	T lymphocytes	Mediates pro-inflammatory response; associated with allergic reactions

are sometimes referred to as cascades because each component of the system is activated sequentially.

1. ***Complement system:*** The complement system consists of over 20 distinct plasma proteins, known as **complement proteins**, that normally circulate in the blood in an inactive form but are activated in response to inflammation. The complement system can be activated by either the innate or the acquired immune response. As a result of activation, a cascade of events is triggered via three different pathways through which complement is activated on cell surfaces: classical, lectin, and alternative (**Figure 11.7** ■). The classical pathway is usually produced by IgG or IgM antigen–antibody complexes. The lectin pathway can be triggered by first exposure to the antigen and consists of lectin binding to bacterial cell walls. The alternative pathway is activated as part of the innate immune system and can also be triggered on first exposure to the antigen. These three pathways amplify the inflammatory process to increase vascular permeability, enhance phagocytosis, and promote vasodilation.
2. ***Coagulation system:*** There is a bidirectional relationship between inflammation and coagulation. Inflammatory mediators, such as cytokines, can activate coagulation. For example, the release of IL-6, a cytokine, stimulates production of platelets.[5] In addition, mediators involved in the clotting or coagulation system can stimulate and perpetuate the inflammatory process. Plasma proteins are activated by factor XII, also known as Hageman factor, which promotes the formation of bradykinin and kallikrein. Furthermore, protease-activated receptors provide an important link between inflammation and coagulation and may contribute to endotoxic shock and sepsis.[6]
3. ***Kallikrein–kinin system:*** The kallikrein–kinin system (also known as the kinin system) is a cascade of metabolic events that interacts with the clotting system and plays an important role in the inflammatory process. The kinin system is initiated by the Hageman factor (factor XII). Bradykinin and kallidin are two of the many kinins produced by this system. **Kinins** are potent vasodilators, regulators of the inflammatory process, and are also involved in pain sensation and cell growth.[7]

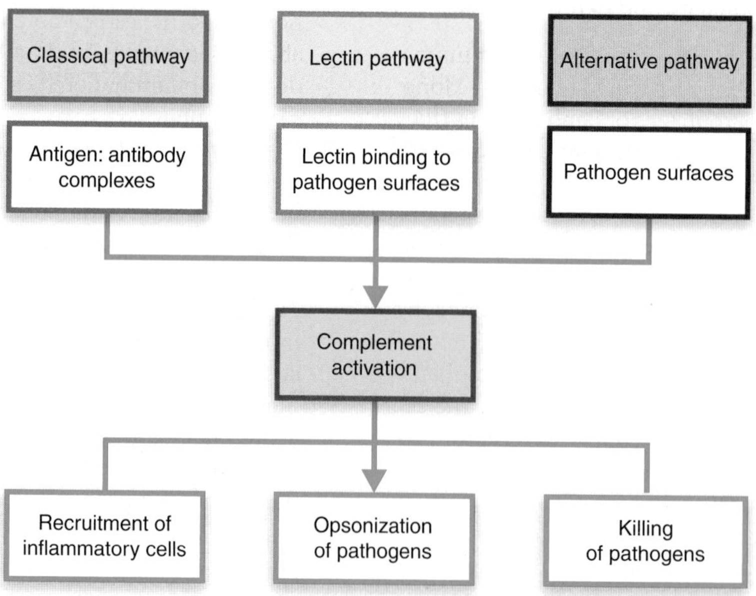

Figure 11.7 ■ The complement system can be activated by either the innate or the acquired immune response. As a result of activation, a cascade of events is triggered by either the classical, lectin, or alternative pathway.

Timothy White: Application

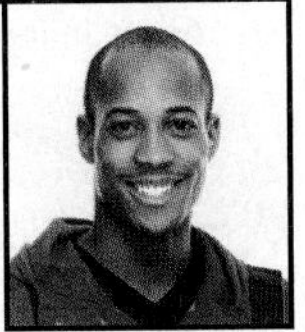

Mr. White is in the ED. He is now rating his pain a 7 out of 10. An intravenous catheter is placed, and he is given medication for pain. After blood has been drawn for a complete blood count (CBC) and urine has been collected for a urinalysis, he is transported to radiology for a CT scan of his abdomen. The CBC with differential is unremarkable except for moderate leukocytosis (14,000/mm^3) with a shift to the left (20% band cells). The urinalysis results are normal. An abdominal CT scan demonstrates acute suppurative appendicitis with a markedly enhanced and thickened inflamed appendix.

3. Explain why the leukocytes are high in the CBC differential.
4. What signs might signal worsening of the infection?

Check Your Progress: Section 11.3

1. What are examples of lymphocytes?
2. What are some examples of myeloid leukocytes?
3. What are the three types of plasma protein systems?

11.4 Regulation and Termination of Acute Inflammation

The inflammatory process is induced by factors that are exogenous (e.g., pathogens) and factors that are endogenous (chemicals released from the injured cells) to the individual. These inducing agents interact with **pattern recognition receptors** (e.g., toll-like receptors) on specialized cells such as macrophages, dendritic cells, and mast cells that help to identify pathogen-associated molecular patterns, leading to the production and release of cytokines and other chemicals that mediate the response of the cells causing inflammation.[8] If the inflammatory response is not regulated (i.e., by the production and release of cytokines) and terminated appropriately, tissue damage leading to impaired organ failure and even death may ensue. The regulation and termination of inflammation involve several well-integrated processes that help to return the system to homeostasis. A primary method by which inflammation is regulated is via anti-inflammatory pathways.[8] An example of an important anti-inflammatory pathway is the hypothalamic–pituitary–adrenal (HPA) axis, which controls the release of glucocorticoids and anti-inflammatory cytokines (e.g., IL-10, TGF-β) (**Figure 11.8** ■). In general, glucocorticoids attenuate inflammation.

In addition to the HPA axis, the sympathetic nervous system (SNS) (also known as the adrenergic system) and the parasympathetic nervous system (PNS) (also known as the cholinergic system) play critical roles in regulating the inflammatory response. Lymph node–related organs, such as the spleen, thymus, bone marrow, and lymph nodes, are innervated primarily by the SNS. The SNS releases neurotransmitters, such as norepinephrine, to downregulate the production of pro-inflammatory cytokines (e.g., IL-6, TNF-α) and upregulate the production of anti-inflammatory cytokines

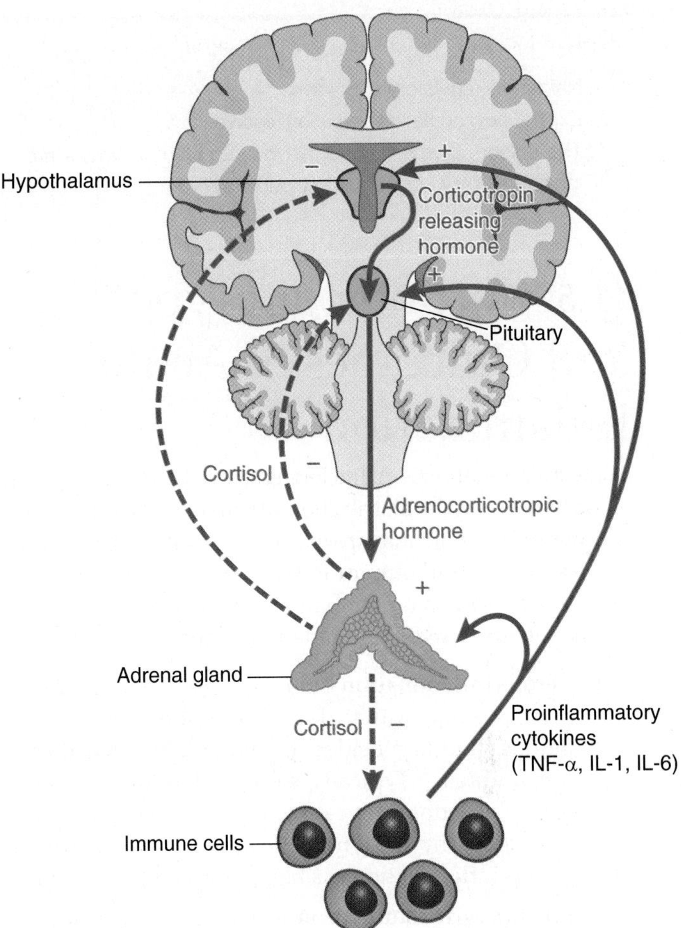

Figure 11.8 ■ The hypothalamic–pituitary–adrenal axis.

(e.g., IL-10).[9,10] In addition, the SNS promotes recruitment of leukocytes and increases blood and lymph flow.

The inflammatory reflex is a neurologic mechanism that regulates the immune response to tissue damage. This reflex consists of the vagus nerve transmitting information about peripheral inflammation to the brain (sensory arc) and then relaying an action potential through the descending pathway (motor arc) to inhibit pro-inflammatory cytokine production in the spleen. The cholinergic anti-inflammatory pathway (in the PNS) is the descending or motor pathway of this reflex. In addition to inhibiting cytokine release, the cholinergic anti-inflammatory pathway decreases neutrophil activation.[11]

Timothy White: Application

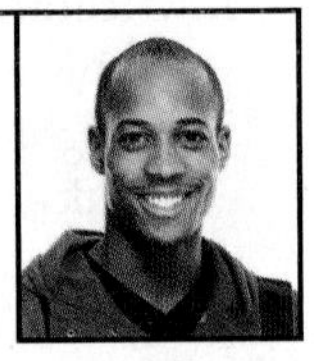

Mr. White is taken to the operating room for an appendectomy. The next day, he is resting comfortably in his hospital room. He complains of moderate incisional pain when he moves. The incision is dry with no redness or swelling. He denies nausea and vomiting and is on a clear liquid diet. His CBC with differential is normal, his breath sounds are clear, and he has been able to take a short walk.

5. What are indications that Mr. White's inflammatory response to the infection is resolving?
6. What places Mr. White at risk of developing chronic inflammation?

Check Your Progress: Section 11.4

1. Name two regulatory pathways.
2. Explain how acute inflammation resolves.
3. The spleen, thymus, bone marrow, and lymph nodes are innervated by which regulatory pathway?

11.5 Morphologic Types and Outcomes of Acute Inflammation

Acute inflammation is characterized by vasodilation of small blood vessels and redistribution of leukocytes and fluid to extravascular tissue in response to tissue injury. Patterns of morphology of inflammation are typically classified into four groups: serous inflammation, fibrinous inflammation, purulent (supportive) inflammation or abscess, and ulcers.

1. **Serous inflammation** is fluid accumulation as a result of tissue injury that does not contain many cells. Serous fluid is considered exudative because it contains proteins. Typically, serous inflammation is not severe and does not cause significant destruction. It is resorbed by the lymphatic system. An example of serous inflammation is a blister formed from a burn.
2. **Fibrinous inflammation** is the result of increased vascular permeability that allows fluid with large proteins (e.g., fibrinogen) to leak out of the vessels into the surrounding tissue. Fibrinous inflammation develops when the vascular leak is large and is considered to be more severe than serous inflammation. An example of fibrinous inflammation is fibrinous pericarditis.
3. The main characteristic of **purulent (suppurative) inflammation** is the formation of pus, which contains many neutrophils, cellular debris, and edema fluid. The formation of pus, or **suppuration**, may occur if the pathogen is difficult to eliminate or severe. Pyogenic bacteria, such as *Staphylococcus*, commonly causes pus formation. Appendicitis and suppurative tonsillitis are examples of acute supportive inflammation.
4. **Ulceration** results from very severe inflammation and is a local defect caused by necrosis of cells and sloughing of necrotic tissue. A common example of an ulceration is gastric ulceration. If the acute ulcer is replaced with connective tissue or scarring, it becomes a chronic ulcer. It is important to note that not all ulcers are caused by inflammation; some may result from a malignancy.

The outcome of acute inflammation depends on many different factors (see **Figure 11.9** ■). These factors include the following:

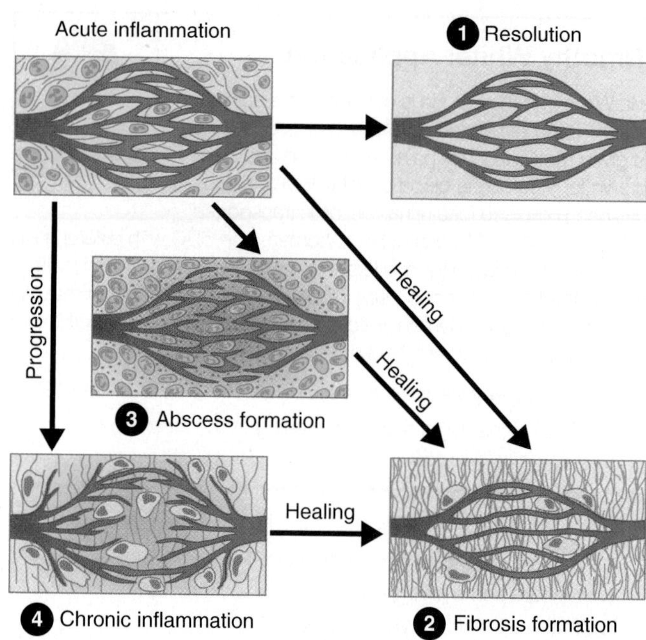

Figure 11.9 ■ The possible outcomes of acute inflammation are (1) resolution, (2) fibrosis, (3) abscess formation, and (4) chronic inflammation.

1. ***Resolution*** of the inflammatory process and healing of the injured tissue. No permanent destruction of normal tissue. Examples include complete wound healing and recovery from the common cold.
2. ***Fibrosis formation*** or scarring may develop if there is significant tissue damage. **Scarring** occurs when epithelial cells are replaced by fibroblasts. Depending on the location of the scarring, it may permanently impair physical functioning. For example, a myocardial infarction results in necrotic tissue that is replaced by fibroblasts. This scar tissue in the heart cannot function as it once did.
3. ***Abscess formation*** may occur. An abscess, usually caused by bacteria, is a cavity that contains pus. Redness and edema often extend around the abscess in the surrounding tissues.
4. ***Chronic inflammation*** may develop following acute inflammation if the cause is not eradicated.

Timothy White: Application

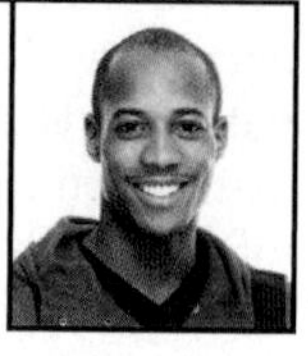

Mr. White is getting ready to be discharged from the hospital. His nurse is providing him with discharge instructions, which include a list of signs and symptoms he should monitor and when to notify his physicians. The nurse instructs Mr. White to call his physician if he experiences fever or chills or notices any drainage or increased redness around his incision.

Several days after Mr. White is discharged, he develops a fever of 101°F and abdominal pain. He calls his physician, who advises him to go directly to the ED. On examination, Mr. White's vital signs are as follows: pulse 108, temperature 101.4°F, blood pressure 98/60. He has purulent drainage at his wound site. His CBC with differential reveals a WBC of moderate leukocytosis (18,000/mm^3) with a shift to the left (30% band cells). He is diagnosed with a wound infection and is placed on antibiotics.

7. What are the four possible outcomes of acute inflammation?
8. What signs of systemic inflammation is Mr. White demonstrating?

Check Your Progress: Section 11.5

1. What are the four primary classifications of morphology associated with inflammation?
2. Which type of morphology is associated with pus formation?
3. What type of morphology is associated with necrosis?
4. What is an abscess?
5. Which type of outcome is associated with scar formation?

11.6 Chronic Inflammation

Chronic inflammation is defined as inflammation that lasts more than 2 weeks. It may follow acute inflammation or may develop as an independent disease process. In general, chronic inflammation is more insidious than acute inflammation and has a prolonged duration.

Causes

The following are potential causes of chronic inflammation:

- ***Unresolved or repeated acute infections*** may develop into chronic inflammation. Unresolved infections from particular viruses, bacteria, fungi, or parasites that are difficult to eliminate may lead to chronic inflammation. Some infectious organisms may elicit a delayed hypersensitivity reaction that may develop into a granulomatous reaction.
- ***Autoimmune diseases*** are caused by an excessive and inappropriate response of the immune system and may result in chronic inflammation. Examples include rheumatoid arthritis and multiple sclerosis. Inappropriate immune responses may also result from an unregulated response to a microbe (e.g., inflammatory bowel disease). In addition, an inappropriate immune response to common environmental exposures may also lead to chronic allergic inflammation (e.g., asthma).[12]
- ***Prolonged exposure to irritants*** that may be either exogenous or endogenous. Silicosis is an example of a chronic inflammatory disease affecting the respiratory system that results from long-term inhalation of silica.

Risks for developing chronic inflammation include poor blood supply, malnutrition, abnormal neutrophil function, and prolonged use of anti-inflammatory medications such as corticosteroids.

Morphologic Types

A characteristic of chronic inflammation is infiltration of macrophages and lymphocytes instead of the influx of neutrophils commonly associated with acute inflammation. In addition, chronic inflammation is associated with tissue destruction and replacement of damaged tissue with fibrous tissue via angiogenesis (blood vessel formation).

Cells Involved

Several cell types are involved in the leukocyte infiltration, tissue damage, and fibrosis associated with chronic inflammation:

- ***Macrophages*** are the primary cells involved in chronic inflammation. They are derived from monocytes in the circulating blood, are active in phagocytosis, and secrete a wide variety of biologically active chemicals, including cytokines and growth factors. In addition to destroying and eliminating microbes and debris, they initiate the process of tissue repair and contribute to scar formation.
- ***Lymphocytes*** are often present in chronic inflammation. In particular, lymphocytes contribute to autoimmune and other hypersensitivity disorders. They secrete cytokines and promote inflammation.
- ***Eosinophils*** play an important role in hypersensitivity reactions and parasitic infections. They contain granules that are highly toxic to parasites but also destructive to surrounding tissues.
- ***Mast cells*** are involved in both chronic and acute inflammation. They are primarily involved in hypersensitivity reactions such as allergic reactions and response to venom. They secrete several cytokines that promote and propagate inflammation associated with chronic inflammation.
- ***Neutrophils***, although they are primarily involved in the acute inflammatory response, also play a role chronic inflammation. An example of this is the chronic bacterial infection osteomyelitis, which can persist for several months.

Granulomatous Inflammation

Granulomatous inflammation is a distinct type of chronic inflammation that is characterized by the formation of granulation tissue. It usually results as a protective response to some type of injury or tissue damage such as chronic infection or a foreign body. Examples of disease that involve granulomatous inflammation are tuberculosis, histoplasmosis, syphilis, sarcoidosis, and schistosomiasis. Foreign bodies such as asbestos fibers may also cause granulomatous inflammation. Granulomatous inflammation involves three cell types:

- ***Epithelioid cells***, consisting of macrophages that are similar to epithelial cells.
- ***Multinucleated (Langhans) giant cells***, which result from the combination of macrophage and epithelioid cells
- ***Lymphocytes***, which form a ring around the granuloma.

Outcomes of Chronic Inflammation

Chronic inflammation that continues for months or years can lead to significant health problems. For example, inflammatory bowel disease can eventually lead to colon cancer. The chronic inflammation associated with asthma and recurring asthma exacerbations can lead to denudation of the airway epithelium and enhanced airway hyperreactivity.

Lucia Morales: Outcome

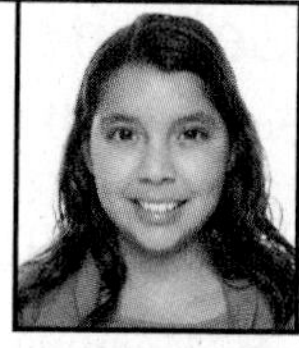

On further questioning, Lucia reports that she has been running with her team in a forest preserve. The physician thinks that Lucia should further investigate an environmental allergic reaction as the basis for Lucia's asthma exacerbation, so he refers her to an allergist.

3. What types of cells do you think are involved in Lucia's inflammatory response?
4. What are some possible causes of Lucia's asthma exacerbation?

Check Your Progress: Section 11.6

1. What are potential causes of chronic inflammation?
2. What is the primary or most common cell involved in the leukocyte infiltration, tissue damage, and fibrosis associated with chronic inflammation?
3. What factors put a person at risk for developing chronic inflammation?

11.7 Systemic Manifestations of Inflammation

Inflammation is a localized process; however, the chemical mediators (e.g., cytokines) in inflammation can cause systemic effects. This reaction is known as the **acute-phase response**. Effects include fever, increase in serum proteins, and leukocytosis.

- ***Fever*** or pyrexia is defined as an elevation in body temperature and occurs as a result of specific cytokines (e.g., IL-1) being released from neutrophils and macrophages. These cytokines are known as endogenous pyrogenes because they are produced from within the body, in comparison to exogenous pyrogenes which are produced by pathogens. Pyrogenes stimulate the synthesis and release of prostaglandins, which affect the hypothalamus to induce fever.[13]

CLINICAL POINT: Medications such as aspirin and other nonsteroidal anti-inflammatory drugs reduce fever by inhibiting prostaglandin synthesis. ■

In many cases, fever is beneficial, since some pathogens are highly sensitive to even slight rises in temperature.[14] It is also believed that fever may induce heat shock proteins, which promote lymphocytic response to pathogens.[15] More details about fever are covered in Chapter 33.

- ***An increase in serum proteins*** occurs during the acute-phase response. These proteins are synthesized predominantly in the liver through stimulation by cytokines (e.g., IL-1, IL-6, TNF-α) and may increase many times over in response to tissue injury. The most common serum proteins are CRP, fibrinogen, and serum amyloid. CRP acts by binding to microbial cell walls and facilitates phagocytosis.

CLINICAL POINT: Measurement of CRP in the blood is often used clinically to determine the degree to which an individual may be experiencing inflammation. For example, if an individual is experiencing shoulder pain, a CRP measurement may help to determine whether the shoulder pain is related to inflammation. In addition, high-sensitivity CRP (hs-CRP) is a valuable marker for risk of myocardial infarction in patients with atherosclerosis.[16] The erythrocyte sedimentation rate (ESR) also provides a nonspecific measure of inflammation. ■

Fibrinogen, which binds to red blood cells, causing them to aggregate more readily, plays an important role in the ESR level. The ESR level is often used to monitor response to antibiotic treatment in osteomyelitis.[17]

- ***Leukocytosis*** is defined as an increase in white blood cells. The normal white blood count ranges from 4000 to 10,000 cells/μL. In acute inflammation, especially when it is caused by a bacterial infection, the white blood cell (WBC) count may range from 15,000 to 20,000 cells/μL. The WBC differential is important in determining causes of infection. In general, increased neutrophils suggest acute inflammation, while increased monocytes indicate chronic inflammation. Increased levels of eosinophils most likely reflect an allergic reaction. See **Table 11.4** ■ for more details related to the WBC differential. In addition, often, during an infection, immature to mature neutrophils, such as band cells, may be present in greater numbers as a result of the body trying to quickly respond to the infection. This greater proportion of immature neutrophils compared to mature neutrophils is known as a shift to the left.

Systemic Inflammatory Response Syndrome

Systemic inflammatory response syndrome (SIRS) is a severe systemic response to inflammation. When SIRS is due to an infection, it is considered to be sepsis. Other causes of SIRS include pulmonary embolism, anaphylaxis, and adrenal insufficiency. SIRS can frequently lead to a number of complications, including shock and multiple organ failure. In 1992, the American College of Chest Physicians/Society of Critical Care Medicine Consensus Conference outlined the criteria for the diagnosis of SIRS.[18] In adults, two of the following criteria must be met: (1) body temperature less than 36°C or greater than 38°C; (2) heart rate greater than 90 beats per minute; (3) respiratory rate greater than 20 breaths per minute or arterial partial pressure of carbon dioxide less than 32 mmHg; and (4) WBC count less than 4000 cells/mm^3 or greater than 12,000 cells/mm^3 or the presence of greater than 10% immature neutrophils. However, this definition has been criticized for lack of sensitivity, face validity, and construct validity[19,20] and is currently being considered for revision.

Table 11.4 Possible Causes of High and Low WBC Differential Results

Type of WBC and Normal Range	Examples of Causes of a High Count	Examples of Causes of a Low Count
Neutrophils Normal range in adults: 2.0–7.0 × 10^9/L (40–80%)	Known as neutrophilia • Acute bacterial infections and some infections caused by viruses and fungi • Chronic inflammation (e.g., inflammatory bowel disease, rheumatoid arthritis) • Tissue death caused by trauma, major surgery, myocardial infarction, burns • Physiologic (stress, rigorous exercise) • Smoking • Pregnancy: last trimester or during labor • Chronic leukemia (e.g., myelogenous leukemia)	Known as neutropenia • Myelodysplastic syndrome • Severe infection (e.g., SIRS, septic shock) • Drug reaction (e.g., phenytoin) • Autoimmune disorders • Chemotherapy • Aplastic anemia
Lymphocytes Normal range in adults: 1.0–3.0 × 10^9/L (20–40%)	Known as lymphocytosis • Acute viral infections (e.g. chicken pox) • Certain bacterial infections (e.g., pertussis, tuberculosis) • Lymphoma	Known as lymphopenia or lymphocytopenia • Autoimmune disorders (e.g., lupus, rheumatoid arthritis) • Infections (e.g., HIV, hepatitis, influenza) • Bone marrow damage (e.g., chemotherapy, radiation therapy) • Immune deficiency
Monocytes Normal range in adults: 0.2–1.0 × 10^9/L (2–10%)	Known as monocytosis • Chronic infections (e.g., tuberculosis, fungal infection) • Infection within the heart (bacterial endocarditis) • Collagen vascular diseases (e.g., lupus, scleroderma, rheumatoid arthritis, vasculitis) • Inflammatory bowel disease • Myelogenous leukemia • Chronic myelomonocytic leukemia • Juvenile myelomonocytic leukemia	Known as monocytopenia Usually, one low count is not medically significant. Repeated low counts can indicate: • Bone marrow damage or failure • Hairy-cell leukemia
Eosinophils Normal range in adults: 0.02–0.5 × 10^9/L (1–6%)	Known as eosinophilia • Asthma, allergies such as hay fever • Drug reactions • Inflammation of the skin (e.g., eczema, dermatitis) • Parasitic infections • Inflammatory disorders (e.g., celiac disease, inflammatory bowel disease) • Certain malignancies/cancers	Known as eosinopenia This is often difficult to determine because numbers are normally low in the blood. One or an occasional low number is usually not medically significant.
Basophils Normal range in adults: 0.02–0.1 × 10^9/L (<1–2%)	Known as basophilia • Rare allergic reactions (e.g., hives, food allergy) • Inflammation (rheumatoid arthritis, ulcerative colitis) • Some leukemias	Known as basopenia As with eosinophils, numbers are normally low in the blood, so an occasionally low number is usually not medically significant.

SOURCES: Curry, C. V. (2015). Differential blood count. *Medscape*. Retrieved from http://emedicine.medscape.com/article/2085133-overview; American Association for Clinical Chemistry. (2015). *Lab tests online: WBC differential*. Retrieved from https://labtestsonline.org/understanding/analytes/differential/tab/test; Mayo Clinic. (2015). Test ID: CBC. Retrieved from http://www.mayomedicallaboratories.com/test-catalog/Clinical+and+Interpretive/9109.

Timothy White: Outcome

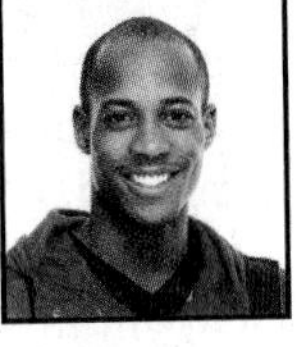

Mr. White completes his course of antibiotics for his wound infection, and comes to his physician's office 2 weeks after discharge for a postoperative follow-up examination. He is afebrile, and his incision is healing well. He reports minimal pain. His CBC with differential is unremarkable.

10. What type of acute inflammation did Mr. White experience?
11. What could have occurred if Mr. White had not sought medical attention when he first experienced abdominal pain?

Check Your Progress: Section 11.7

1. What are the primary signs of systemic inflammation?
2. List three potential causes of SIRS.
3. What are the criteria for diagnosing SIRS?

11.8 Impaired and Excessive Inflammation

Usually inflammation is a normal response to an injury or pathogen. However, when it occurs in a dysregulated or inappropriate manner, excessive tissue damage and disease occur.

Impaired or excessive inflammation is characterized by overexpression of leukocyte adhesion molecules, production of excessive pro-inflammatory cytokines, and damage to tissues. Overproduction of TNF-α, IL-6, and IL-1β is associated with many inflammatory-related diseases such as acute respiratory distress syndrome, rheumatoid arthritis, and inflammatory bowel disease.[21–25] (These disorders are covered in Chapters 20, 36, and 42, respectively.) An autoimmune disease develops when the body mounts an inflammatory response to normal tissue. It is thought that many autoimmune disorders are genetically based.[26] Autoimmune disease may be organ specific, as in the case of autoimmune thyroiditis, in which the body perceives the thyroid gland and thyroid-related hormones to be foreign.[27] Alternatively, an autoimmune disease may be tissue specific. An example of a tissue-specific autoimmune disease is alopecia areata, an autoimmune disorders that attacks the hair follicle and causes hair loss, which is covered in Chapter 41.[28]

There are several theories regarding the pathophysiology of autoimmune diseases. Some researchers have suggested impaired clearance of apoptotic cells as the underlying mechanism in autoimmune disorders and other chronic inflammatory diseases.[29] Removal of dead cells by phagocytosis is a necessary process to maintain tissue homeostasis. Normally, this process does not trigger the immune response or inflammation. However, genetic anomalies or a persistent disease state may result in inappropriate apoptotic clearance of these cells. If dead cells are not efficiently cleared, they may leak intracellular antigens and DNA, which can provoke an autoimmune response, as occurs in systemic lupus erythematosus.[30]

Check Your Progress: Section 11.8

1. What do organ-specific and tissue-specific autoimmune disorders have in common?
2. Review trustworthy Internet sites, and find examples of organ-specific autoimmune disorders.
3. What can happen if dead cells are not sufficiently cleared?

11.9 Overview of Disorders Associated with Chronic Inflammation

Chronic inflammation is an important contributing factor in several disorders, such as Alzheimer disease, asthma, atherosclerosis, depression, diabetes mellitus, and obesity. A brief overview of selected examples will be provided. The reader is referred to other chapters for more detailed information about these disorders. **Table 11.5** ■ lists selected conditions involving inflammation and their related concepts.

Table 11.5 Conditions Involving Inflammation and Their Related Concepts

Concept	Conditions Involving Inflammation
Cellular regulation	Cancer
Cognition and mood	Alzheimer disease, dementia, depression
Elimination	Inflammatory bowel disease (Crohn disease, ulcerative colitis)
Immunity	Infections, hypersensitivity reactions, autoimmune disorders
Metabolism	Diabetes mellitus, obesity
Mobility	Rheumatoid arthritis, physical inactivity
Oxygenation	Asthma, pneumonia, emphysema, acute respiratory distress syndrome
Perfusion	Atherosclerosis, myocardial infarction, heart failure, vasculitis, septic shock, stroke
Thermoregulation	Fever, frostbite
Tissue integrity	Trauma, burns, wound healing

Alzheimer Disease

Alzheimer disease (AD), a type of dementia, is a progressive neurodegenerative disorder characterized by progressive memory loss and functional impairment that eventually leads to death. The hallmarks of AD are the accumulation of beta-amyloid peptide plaques and neurofibrillary tangles in the brain. Evidence demonstrates that activation of the immune system accompanies the development and progression of AD.[31,32] It is theorized that the neuroinflammation observed in AD is primarily driven by immune-related cells, such as microglia, in the brain.[33] Some researchers posit that a bacterial infection may trigger an inflammatory cascade associated with the development of AD.[34] Research is being done to develop approaches to detecting immune alterations before the onset of AD in order to identify individuals who are at high risk and to develop tailored early interventions to deter progression of the disease.[35] Alzheimer disease is covered in more depth in Chapter 30.

Asthma

Asthma is a disease of the airways that involves chronic airway inflammation, dysfunction of the airways, and tissue remodeling.[36] Asthma is believed to be caused by both genetic predisposition to the disease and environmental factors, including exposure to allergens and infection. Studies have shown that a genetic predisposition to respond to an allergen with a local mucosal immunoglobulin type E (IgE) is a significant risk factor for developing asthma. Chronic inflammation associated with asthma is directed by complex interactions between the innate and acquired immune systems. Asthma is covered in depth in Chapter 18.

Poorly controlled or severe asthma has been associated with adverse maternal and fetal outcomes. Adverse maternal outcomes include preeclampsia, pregnancy-induced hypertension, and uterine hemorrhage; adverse outcomes for infants include preterm labor, premature birth, congenital anomalies, fetal growth restriction, low birth weight, and neonatal hypoglycemia, seizures, and tachypnea.[37] ■

Atherosclerosis

For many years, atherosclerosis was believed to be to the result of endothelial injury that led to platelet aggregation and eventually an atherosclerotic plaque. Only recently has atherosclerosis been recognized as a chronic inflammatory disease.[38] Although the process is still not fully understood, atherosclerosis is believed to be due to a chronic inflammatory response (involving both innate and acquired immunity systems) of leukocytes (mostly monocytes and macrophages) to low-density lipoproteins particles in the walls of the arteries that begins in childhood. Mast cells have also been recently identified as playing an important role the development of atherosclerosis by releasing vasoactive histamine and other products. On the basis of new knowledge about atherosclerosis as a chronic inflammatory disease, research has identified several inflammatory biomarkers that can assist in predicting the risk of cardiovascular disease, such as hsCRP. Atherosclerosis is covered in depth in Chapter 23.

Depression

Extensive evidence demonstrates that depression is associated with chronic inflammation.[39,40] A recent meta-analysis found higher levels of IL-6 in individuals with major depressive disorder than in those without depression.[41] Furthermore, studies demonstrate that psychosocial stressors may stimulate the production of pro-inflammatory cytokines, such as IL-6 and TNF-α.[42,43] It is hypothesized that higher levels of pro-inflammatory cytokines associated with chronic psychosocial stress may promote the development of depression.[44] Furthermore, pro-inflammatory cytokines are decreased with antidepressant therapy.[45] Depression is covered in depth in Chapter 29.

Diabetes Mellitus

Type 2 diabetes mellitus (T2D) is a metabolic disorder characterized by insulin resistance and pancreatic β-cell dysfunction resulting in hyperglycemia. Chronic inflammation and alterations in the immune system play important roles in T2D.[46] Studies have demonstrated elevated levels of CRP, cytokines, chemokines, fibrinogen, and haptoglobin in individuals with T2D.[47–50] In particular, IL-6 and CRP are strongly associated with T2D.[51] Multiple mechanisms contribute to inflammation in T2D. One process is that excess levels of glucose and free fatty acids from overnutrition stress the pancreatic islets as well as insulin-sensitive tissues in adipose tissue and the liver. This leads to production and secretion of cytokines and chemokines, contributing to tissue inflammation.[51] Another potential mechanism is that hypoxia and cell death of adipose tissue as a result of adipose tissue growth exceeding vascular supply, may induce systemic inflammation, leading to diabetes.[52] Other potential mechanisms of T2D include a defect in anti-inflammatory system that regulates IL-1RA, chemokines secreted by adipose tissue, and activation of NF-κB and JUN N-terminal kinase (JNK) pathways.[51] Type 2 diabetes is covered in depth in Chapter 37.

Inflammaging

Inflammaging is chronic, low-grade inflammation associated with aging.[53] One cause of inflammaging may be damaged cells that accumulate with age. This debris can mimic bacterial products and activate the immune system, resulting in chronic inflammation. Another potential cause of inflammaging is the gut's inability, with age, to adequately respond to harmful substances produced by gut microbiota. Genes are believed to play a significant role in determining the extent to which inflammaging occurs. Current research is exploring interventions to ameliorate the effects of inflammaging.

Obesity

There is a plethora of evidence that adipose tissue, previously believed to be an inert tissue, is a metabolically dynamic organ that secretes hormones, cytokines, chemokines, growth factors, and complement proteins.[54,55] Adipose tissue is also implicated in the development and progression of many chronic inflammatory disorders such as diabetes,[56,57] depression,[58] asthma,[59] and atherosclerosis.[60–62] Obesity is covered in depth in Chapter 5.

Check Your Progress: Section 11.9

1. Provide examples of disorders associated with chronic inflammation.
2. Identify commonalities among these disorders.
3. Choose a condition and research the relationship between the immune response and the condition.

11.10 Linking Pathophysiology to the Diagnosis and Treatment of Inflammation

Treatment of inflammation depends on the underlying cause of the inflammation and is aimed at decreasing redness, swelling, pain, heat, and loss of function. A common treatment for inflammation related to injury for many years was the RICE protocol, which consists of Rest, Ice, Compression, and Elevation (RICE). Typically, ice is applied for 20 minutes every 2–3 hours, and the injured area is compressed and elevated above the heart as appropriate. However, recent research has brought into question the effectiveness of applying ice to an injured area. In a review of studies examining the effectiveness of using the RICE protocol for ankle sprains, researchers found that randomized controlled trials found insufficient evidence for the effectiveness of the RICE protocol for ankle sprains.[63] Furthermore, findings from this review suggest that mobilization of the ankle rather than rest may promote healing.

Medications used to treat inflammation include aspirin, acetaminophen, nonsteroidal anti-inflammatory drugs (NSAIDs), cyclooxygenase (COX) inhibitors, and prednisone (**Table 11.6** ■). It is important to note that these medications do not treat the cause of the inflammation; instead, they treat the symptoms associated with inflammation: redness, heat, swelling, pain, and loss of function.

Nutritional factors can either promote inflammation or have anti-inflammatory effects, as described in the Impact of Nutrition in Clinical Practice box.

Check Your Progress: Section 11.10

1. Explain treatments to reduce inflammation.
2. Describe common pharmacologic treatments for inflammation.
3. Name five foods that are identified as phytochemicals, which confer anti-inflammatory actions in the human body.

Table 11.6 Common Medications Used to Treat Inflammation

	Aspirin	Acetaminophen	NSAIDs	Cyclooxygenase Inhibitors	Prednisone	Medications That Target Specific Mediators
Actions	Anti-inflammatory Analgesic Antipyretic	Analgesic Antipyretic	Anti-inflammatory Analgesic Antipyretic	Anti-inflammatory Analgesic Antipyretic	Anti-inflammatory Suppresses immune system	Used for more serious types of inflammation such as rheumatoid arthritis (e.g., adalimumab)
Precautions	Alters blood clotting and increases risk for bleeding Should not be given to children	May damage kidney and/or liver in high doses	Delays blood clotting	May increase risk for heart disease Should not be used in people allergic to sulfonamides	Increased risk of infection Increased blood pressure and edema Osteoporosis and skeletal wasting with long-term use	Increase risk of developing lymphoma Should not be used if infection is present such as tuberculosis

Impact of Nutrition in Clinical Practice

Nutritional Perspectives on Inflammation

Joanne Kouba

Plant-based foods contain bioactive compounds, referred to as phytochemicals, which have anti-inflammatory actions in the human body. These compounds reduce free radical production and oxidative stress, modulate sympathetic activity, control pro-inflammatory cytokine production, and regulate signaling pathways protecting cells against chronic inflammation.[1] Observational and randomized controlled feeding trials in both humans and animal models have demonstrated that phytochemical antioxidants reduce the aging process and the risk of several conditions associated with inflammation, including some cancers, cardiovascular disease, diabetes, multiple sclerosis, Crohn disease, possibly depression and Alzheimer disease.[1-3]

Key to minimizing chronic inflammation is a dietary pattern that promotes a healthy body weight while containing generous amounts of foods with natural antioxidants from fruits and vegetables, whole grains, and omega-3 fatty acids balanced with modest amounts of refined starches, sugar, saturated and trans fats, which are considered pro-inflammatory.[1,4] The following table provides examples of major phytochemical categories and food examples. The primary anti-inflammatory mechanism of fruits and vegetables is the provision of antioxidants, which dampen the activation of the NF-κB, which is a nuclear factor that activates genes that code for production of inflammatory mediators. Omega-3 fatty acids from foods such as fish, walnuts, and flax reduce synthesis of pro-inflammatory compounds derived from the omega-6 fatty acid, arachidonic acid. Whole grains contribute more phytochemical antioxidants.

Both type and quantity of dietary fat can influence inflammation. Specific fatty acids that are considered pro-inflammatory, such as arachidonic acid, are found in refined corn, soy, sunflower, and safflower oils and in saturated and trans fats.[1,3-5] These fats increase pro-inflammatory cytokines IL-1, TNF-α, and IL-6.[3] Obesity is associated with metabolic derangements collectively known as metabolic syndrome, characterized by insulin resistance, hyperlipidemia, and hypertension. Excess energy intake associated with obesity results in hypertrophic and dysfunctional adipocytes, which repress mitochondrial function, resulting in disruption of insulin signaling, and increase macrophage activity, resulting in inflammation.[5]

The Mediterranean diet is one that combines the concepts described and encourages a dietary pattern rich in fruits and vegetables, whole grains, nuts, olive oil, and fish while discouraging intake of pro-inflammatory dietary factors. Increasing evidence suggests that the Mediterranean diet increases anti-inflammatory cytokines, increases anti-inflammatory biomarkers, improves endothelial function, and regulates genetic polymorphisms associated with atherosclerosis, resulting in reduced chronic inflammation and protection from chronic disease.[2,6] This approach to lifestyle behaviors that protect against inflammation focuses on a plant-based diet with variety and moderation.

Selected Phytochemical Categories with Compound and Food Examples

Category of Phytochemical	Compound Examples	Food Examples
Carotenoids	α-, β-, γ-carotenes; lycopene; lutein	Carrots, pumpkin, tomato, grapefruit, mango, papaya
Flavonoids	Anthocyanin, quercitin	Apples, citrus fruits, cranberry
Glucosinolates	Allium compounds	Garlic, onions, leeks, scallions
Indoles	Sulforaphane	Broccoli, cauliflower, brussels sprouts, cabbage
Isoflavones	Saidzein, genestein	Soy, legumes
Polyphenols	Kaempferol, resveratrol	Tomato, tea, red wine
Terpenes	Limonene, carnosol	Citrus fruit peel, rosemary

SOURCE: American Institute for Cancer Research. (n.d.). *Phytochemicals: Cancer fighters in the foods we eat.* Available at http://www.aicr.org/reduce-your-cancer-risk/diet/elements_phytochemicals.html

References

1. Prasad S., Bokyung S., & Aggarwal, B. B. (2012). Age-associated chronic disease require age-old medicine: Role of chronic inflammation. *Preventive Medicine, 54,* S29–S37.
2. Gotsis, E., Anagnostis P., Mariolis A., et al. (2014). Health benefits of the Mediterranean diet: An update of research over the last 5 years. *Angiology, 66*(4), 304–318.
3. Galland, L. (2010). Diet and inflammation. *Nutrition in Clinical Practice, 25*(6), 634–640.
4. Kiecolt-Glaser, J. K. (2010). Stress, food, and inflammation: Psychoneuroimmunology and nutrition at the cutting edge. *Psychosomatic Medicine, 72*(4), 365–369.
5. Chalkiakaki A., & Guarente L. (2012). High-fat diet triggers inflammation-induced cleave of SIRT1 adipose tissue to promote metabolic dysfunction. *Cell Metabolism, 16,* 180–188.
6. Schwingshackl, L., & Hoffmann, G. (2014). Mediterranean dietary pattern, inflammation and endothelial function: A systematic review and meta-analysis of intervention trials. *Nutrition Metabolism & Cardiovascular Diseases, 24*(9), 929–939.

CHAPTER SUMMARY

11.1 Chapter Overview and Case Studies

Recognize the complex role that inflammation plays in defending the body from injury and promoting healing.

- Innate immunity, or nonspecific immunity, is the defense system that an individual is born with.
- Components of the innate immunity system include physical barriers, enzymes in epithelial and phagocytic cells, inflammatory related proteins in blood, toll-like receptors that help sense pathogens, inflammatory mediators such as cytokines, antimicrobial peptides, and phagocytes.
- Acquired or adaptive immunity is continually refined throughout life and is specific to a pathogen.
- Lymphocytes, which include B and T cells, play an important role in acquired immunity.
- The acute and chronic inflammatory responses differ in speed of onset, duration, cellular infiltrates, degree of injury, and predominance of systemic inflammatory involvement.

11.2 Functions of the Inflammatory Response in Health and Disease

Describe the inflammatory response as a key component of the body's defense system.

- The functions of the inflammatory response are to contain and destroy the pathogen, prevent further damage to tissue, and initiate the healing process.

11.3 Acute Inflammatory Response

Discriminate the characteristics of the acute inflammatory response.

- The cardinal signs associated with acute inflammation are redness, heat, swelling, pain, and loss of function.
- Acute inflammation can be caused by many different conditions. Examples include infections, tissue necrosis associated with ischemia, and reaction to a foreign body.
- Most essential acute inflammatory components are found in the circulatory system.
- Following tissue injury, chemical mediators and leukocytosis-inducing factors are released, resulting in vasodilation, increased capillary permeability, and chemotaxis.
- In addition, white blood cells migrate through the vessel walls in a multistep process involving transmigration and margination.
- Once at the injury site, leukocytes destroy pathogens through phagocytosis.
- Phagocytosis is a three-step process: (1) recognition of the pathogen, (2) engulfment of the pathogen by leukocytes, and (3) killing or degrading of the pathogen.
- Many cell types are involved in the acute inflammatory response, including lymphocytes (T cells, B cells, and NK cells) and granulocytes (neutrophils, eosinophils, basophils and mast cells) and leukocytes (monocytes, macrophages, and dendritic cells).
- Primary types of cell-derived mediators include vasoactive amines (e.g., histamine), lipid mediators (e.g., prostaglandins and leukotrienes), cytokines and chemokines, and lysosomal components (e.g., oxygen free radicals, nitric oxide).
- Plasma protein systems are also involved in mediating the inflammatory response. The three primary systems are the complement system, the clotting system, and the kallikrein–kinin system.

11.4 Regulation and Termination of Acute Inflammation

Explain the regulation and resolution of the acute inflammatory process.

- Regulation and termination of inflammation involve several well-integrated processes that help the system return to homeostasis.
- Anti-inflammatory pathways play a primary role in regulation of inflammation. An example is the HPA axis, which controls release of glucocorticoids and anti-inflammatory cytokines.
- The SNS and PNS play important roles in regulating inflammation.

11.5 Morphologic Types and Outcomes of Acute Inflammation

Discuss the primary morphologic types of acute inflammation and the four possible outcomes of acute inflammation.

- Patterns of morphology are classified into four groups: serous inflammation, fibrinous inflammation, purulent inflammation or abscess, and ulcers.
- Four possible outcomes of acute inflammation are resolution, fibrosis formation, abscess formation, and chronic inflammation.

11.6 Chronic Inflammation

Identify the conditions under which chronic inflammation may arise, and explain the process of chronic inflammation and its possible outcomes.

- Causes of chronic inflammation include unresolved or repeated acute infections, autoimmune diseases, and prolonged exposure to irritants.
- A characteristic of chronic inflammation is infiltration of macrophages and lymphocytes.
- In addition to macrophages and lymphocytes, eosinophils, mast cells, and neutrophils may also be involved in chronic inflammation.
- Granulomatous inflammation is a distinct type of chronic inflammation characterized by the formation of granulation tissues. An example is tuberculosis.
- Granulomatous inflammation involves epithelioid cells, multinucleated (Langhans) giant cells and lymphocytes.

11.7 Systemic Manifestations of Inflammation

Describe the causes and processes associated with systemic inflammation.

- The systemic response is known as the acute-phase response.
- The acute-phase response include fever, an increase in serum proteins, and leukocytosis.
- Systemic inflammatory response syndrome (SIRS) is a severe systemic response to inflammation and can lead to shock and multiple organ failure.

11.8 Impaired and Excessive Inflammation

Discuss the potential causes and consequences of impaired and excessive inflammation.

- Impaired or excessive inflammation can lead to tissue damage and disease.
- Autoimmune disease develops when the body mounts an inflammatory response to normal tissue.
- It is theorized that autoimmune disorders are genetically based.

11.9 Overview of Disorders Associated with Inflammation

Recognize key disorders in which inflammation is an important contributing factor.

- Examples of disorders associated with chronic inflammation include Alzheimer disease, asthma, atherosclerosis, depression, diabetes mellitus, and obesity.

11.10 Linking Pathophysiology to Diagnosis and Treatment of Inflammation

Identify primary treatments of inflammation.

- Medications used to treat inflammation include aspirin, acetaminophen, nonsteroidal anti-inflammatory drugs, cyclooxygenase inhibitors, and prednisone.

REVIEW QUESTIONS

1. A client presents to an urgent care setting after cutting her hand while chopping vegetables in her kitchen. The cut does not require stitches. When thinking about the healing process, you understand which of the following statements to be true?
   a. The wound is expected to heal through localized, chronic inflammatory response.
   b. The wound is expected to heal through an autoimmune response.
   c. The wound is expected to heal through a localized, acute inflammatory response.
   d. The wound is expected to heal after a widespread inflammatory response.
2. A client is receiving a unit of packed red blood cells. The client's vital signs before the transfusion started were pulse 100, respirations 20, temperature 98°F, blood pressure 90/50. After 15 minutes of receiving the transfusion, the client appears to be having an acute inflammatory response to the blood product. Which of the following sets of vital signs indicate this type of response?
   a. Pulse 98, respirations 18, temperature 98.2°F, blood pressure 90/52
   b. Pulse 102, respirations 20, temperature 98.9°F, blood pressure 94/54

c. Pulse 103, respirations 21, temperature 98.2°F, blood pressure 94/56
d. Pulse 100, respirations 18, temperature 101.6°F, blood pressure 94/90

3. Sepsis develops after the complement system's initial response has been amplified. During activation of the coagulation system, inflammatory mediators can activate coagulation. With this in mind, which of the following goals should be included in the care plan of a client with sepsis?
   a. The client and family will define the complement system, coagulation system, and kallikrein–kinin system.
   b. Tell the client to inform you of any pain in the calf area.
   c. Inform the client and family about the risks of developing a deep vein thrombosis.
   d. The client will not develop signs or symptoms of a deep vein thrombosis during hospitalization.

4. A client presents after suffering a scalding burn from canning tomatoes at home. When assessing the client's burn, you note pink and red areas of skin and some blisters. You document the presence of
   a. a serosanguinous blister.
   b. ulceration.
   c. serous inflammation.
   d. purulent inflammation.

5. A client with chronic inflammation asks you to differentiate between the different types of cells that are involved in the inflammation process. Which of the following would you include?
   a. Macrophages are the primary cells involved in chronic inflammation. They destroy and eliminate microbes and debris along with beginning tissue repair. In comparison, mast cells are involved in acute and chronic inflammation.
   b. Lymphocytes are not often involved in chronic inflammation. They secrete cytokines and promote inflammation. In comparison, mast cells are involved in acute and chronic inflammation.
   c. Mast cells are involved in acute and chronic inflammation. They are involved in hypersensitivity reactions, while neutrophils are involved only in chronic inflammation such as chronic bacterial infections and osteomyelitis.
   d. Neutrophils are the primary cells involved in chronic inflammation, while eosinophils are the primary cells involved in acute inflammation.

6. A client receiving chemotherapy asks you to review her lab work. You anticipate which of the following findings?
   a. Neutrophils of greater than 7.0×10^9/L (40–80%)
   b. Neutrophils of less than 7.0×10^9/L (40–80%)
   c. No change in the neutrophils or 7.0×10^9/L (40–80%)
   d. No change in the neutrophils or $0.2–1.0 \times 10^9$/L (2–10%)

7. A client with a sprained ankle has received a prescription for ibuprofen. He tells you that he has had problems with his liver in the past and wonders whether it is okay to take the medication. What is your best response?
   a. "Ibuprofen is better than Tylenol for your ankle sprain."
   b. "Acetaminophen is the medication that is hard on your liver."
   c. "Ibuprofen can delay blood clotting. Let's talk to the physician."
   d. "The pharmacist is the best person to talk to about that."

8. Which of the following statements is true about the relationship between nutrition and inflammation?
   a. There is no relationship between nutrition and inflammation. This myth has been debunked.
   b. Plant-based foods contain bioactive compounds, which reduce the risk of several conditions associated with inflammation.
   c. Only the type of dietary fat can influence inflammation.
   d. Excess energy reduces macrophage activity, resulting in increased inflammation.

ANSWERS

Answers to Review Questions can be found in Appendix A. Answers to Case Study and Check Your Progress questions are available on the faculty resources site. Please consult with your instructor.

RECOMMENDED WEBSITES

American Academy of Allergy, Asthma & Immunology
http://www.aaaai.org/home.aspx

American Association for Clinical Chemistry
https://www.aacc.org

Center for Disease Control and Prevention
https://www.cdc.gov

Center for Human Immunology, Autoimmunity, and Inflammation
https://chi.nhlbi.nih.gov/web

Inflammation Research Association
http://inflammationresearch.org

Psychoneuroimmunology Research Society
https://www.pnirs.org

REFERENCES

1. Cassels, C. (2014). Inflammation in pregnancy strongly linked to schizophrenia. Available at http://www.medscape.com/viewarticle/831135
2. National Institutes of Health. (2013). Prenatal inflammation linked to autism risk. *News Releases*. Available at http://www.nih.gov/news-events/news-releases/prenatal-inflammation-linked-autism-risk
3. van de Vijver, E., van den Berg, T. K., & Kuijpers, T. W. (2013). Leukocyte adhesion deficiencies. *Hematology/Oncology Clinics of North America, 27*(1), 101–116, viii.
4. Reddy, R. C., & Standiford, T. J. (2010). Effects of sepsis on neutrophil chemotaxis. *Current Opinion in Hematology, 17*(1), 18–24.
5. Kaser, A., Brandacher, G., Steurer, W., et al. (2001). Interleukin-6 stimulates thrombopoiesis through thrombopoietin: Role in inflammatory thrombocytosis. *Blood, 98*(9), 2720–2725.
6. van der Poll, T., de Boer, J. D., & Levi, M. (2011). The effect of inflammation on coagulation and vice versa. *Current Opinion in Infectious Diseases, 24*(3), 273–278.
7. Hillmeister, P., & Persson, P. B. (2013). The kallikrein-kinin system. *Acta Physiologica, 206*(4), 215–219.
8. Medzhitov, R. (2010). Inflammation 2010: New adventures of an old flame. *Cell, 140*(6), 771–776.
9. Burnstock, G. (2013). Cotransmission in the autonomic nervous system. *Handbook of Clinical Neurology, 117*, 23–35.
10. de Montmollin, E., Aboab, J., Mansart, A., & Annane, D. (2009). Bench-to-bedside review: Beta-adrenergic modulation in sepsis. *Critical Care (London, England), 13*(5), 230.
11. Huston, J. M., & Tracey, K. J. (2010). The pulse of inflammation: Heart rate variability, the cholinergic anti-inflammatory pathway and implications for therapy. *Journal of Internal Medicine, 269*(1), 45–53.
12. Barnes, P. J. (2011). Pathophysiology of allergic inflammation. *Immunological Reviews, 242*(1), 31–50.
13. Moltz, H. (1993). Fever: Causes and consequences. *Neuroscience & Biobehavioral Reviews, 17*(3), 237–269.
14. Launey, Y., Nesseler, N., Malledant, Y., & Seguin, P. (2011). Clinical review: Fever in septic ICU patients—friend or foe? *Critical Care (London, England), 15*(3), 222.
15. Repasky, E., & Issels, R. (2002). Physiological consequences of hyperthermia: Heat, heat shock proteins and the immune response. *International Journal of Hyperthermia, 18*(6), 486–489.
16. Kim, H., Yang, D. H., Park, Y., et al. (2006). Incremental prognostic value of C-reactive protein and N-terminal proB-type natriuretic peptide in acute coronary syndrome. *Circulation Journal, 70*(11), 1379–1384.
17. Michail, M., Jude, E., Liaskos, C., et al. (2013). The performance of serum inflammatory markers for the diagnosis and follow-up of patients with osteomyelitis. *International Journal of Lower Extremity Wounds, 12*(2), 94–99.
18. Bone, R. C., Balk, R. A., Cerra, F. B., et al. (1002). Definitions for sepsis and organ failure and guidelines for the use of innovative therapies in sepsis. The ACCP/SCCM Consensus Conference Committee. American College of Chest Physicians/Society of Critical Care Medicine. *Chest, 101*(6), 1644–1655.
19. Balk, R. A. (2014). Systemic inflammatory response syndrome (SIRS): Where did it come from and is it still relevant today? *Virulence, 5*(1), 20–26.
20. Kaukonen, K. M., Bailey, M., Pilcher, D., Cooper, D. J., & Bellomo, R. (2015). Systemic inflammatory response syndrome criteria in defining severe sepsis. *New England Journal of Medicine, 372*(17), 1629–1638.
21. Li, T., Luo, N., Du, L., Liu, J., Gong, L., & Zhou, J. (2012). Early and marked up-regulation of TNF-alpha in acute respiratory distress syndrome after cardiopulmonary bypass. Frontiers in *Medicine, 6*(3), 296–301.
22. Semerano, L., Thiolat, A., Minichiello, E., Clavel, G., Bessis, N., & Boissier, M. C. (2014). Targeting IL-6 for the treatment of rheumatoid arthritis: Phase II investigational drugs. *Expert Opinion on Investigational Drugs, 23*(7), 979–999.
23. Tanaka, T., Narazaki, M., & Kishimoto, T. (2014). IL-6 in inflammation, immunity, and disease. *Cold Spring Harbor Perspectives in Biology, 6*(10), a016295.
24. Lissner, D., & Siegmund, B. (2011). The multifaceted role of the inflammasome in inflammatory bowel diseases. *Scientific World Journal, 11*, 1536–1547.
25. Masters, S. L. (2013). Specific inflammasomes in complex diseases. *Clinical Immunology, 147*(3), 223–228.
26. Cotsapas, C., & Hafler, D. A. (2013). Immune-mediated disease genetics: The shared basis of pathogenesis. *Trends in Immunology, 34*(1), 22–26.
27. Pyzik, A., Grywalska, E., Matyjaszek-Matuszek, B., & Rolinski, J. (2015). Immune disorders in Hashimoto's thyroiditis: What do we know so far? *Journal of Immunology Research, 2015*, 979167.
28. Gilhar, A., & Kalish, R. S. (2006). Alopecia areata: A tissue specific autoimmune disease of the hair follicle. *Autoimmunity Reviews, 5*(1), 64–69.
29. Szondy, Z., Garabuczi, É., Joós, G., Tsay, G. J., & Sarang, Z. (2014). Impaired clearance of apoptotic cells in chronic inflammatory diseases: Therapeutic implications. *Frontiers in Immunology, 5*, 354.
30. Munoz, L. E., Lauber, K., Schiller, M., Manfredi, A. A., & Herrmann, M. (2010). The role of defective clearance of apoptotic cells in systemic autoimmunity. *Nature Reviews Rheumatology, 6*(5), 280–289.
31. Krstic, D., Madhusudan, A., Doehner, J., et al. (2012). Systemic immune challenges trigger and drive Alzheimer-like neuropathology in mice. *Journal of Neuroinflammation, 9*, 151.
32. Zhang, B., Gaiteri, C., Bodea, L. G., et al. (2013). Integrated systems approach identifies genetic nodes and networks in late-onset Alzheimer's disease. *Cell, 153*(3), 707–720.
33. Prinz, M., Priller J., Sisodia S. S., & Ransohoff R. M. (2011). Heterogeneity of CNS myeloid cells and their roles in neurodegeneration. *Nature Neuroscience, 14*(10), 1227–1235.
34. Bibi, F., Yasir, M., Sohrab, S. S., et al. (2014). Link between chronic bacterial inflammation and Alzheimer disease. *CNS & Neurological Disorders—Drug Targets, 13*(7), 1140–1147.
35. Heppner, F. L., Ransohoff, R. M., & Becher, B. (2015). Immune attack: The role of inflammation in Alzheimer disease. *Nature Reviews Neuroscience, 16*(6), 358–372.
36. Murdoch, J. R., & Lloyd, C. M. (2010). Chronic inflammation and asthma. *Mutation Research, 690*(1–2), 24–39.
37. Little, M. (2014). Asthma in pregnancy. *Medscape*. Available at http://emedicine.medscape.com/article/796274-overview
38. Libby, P. (2012). Inflammation in atherosclerosis. [Review]. *Arteriosclerosis, Thrombosis & Vascular Biology, 32*(9), 2045–2051.
39. Horowitz, M. A., & Zunszain, P. A. (2015). Neuroimmune and neuroendocrine abnormalities in depression: Two sides of the same coin. *Annals of the New York Academy of Sciences, 1351*, 68–79.
40. Zalli, A., Jovanova, O., Hoogendijk, W. J., Tiemeier, H., & Carvalho, L. A. (2016). Low-grade inflammation predicts persistence of depressive symptoms. *Psychopharmacology, 233*(9), 1669–1678.
41. Haapakoski, R., Mathieu, J., Ebmeier, K. P., Alenius, H., & Kivimaki, M. (2015). Cumulative meta-analysis of interleukins 6 and 1beta, tumour necrosis factor alpha and C-reactive protein in patients with major depressive disorder. *Brain, Behavior, and Immunity, 49*, 206–215.
42. Coe, C. L., & Laudenslager, M. L. (2007). Psychosocial influences on immunity, including effects on immune maturation and senescence. *Brain, Behavior, and Immunity, 21*(8), 1000–1008.
43. Maes, M., Song, C., Lin, A., et al. (1998). The effects of psychological stress on humans: Increased production of pro-inflammatory cytokines and a Th1-like response in stress-induced anxiety. *Cytokine, 10*(4), 313–318.

44. Berk, M., Williams, L. J., Jacka, F. N., et al. (2013). So depression is an inflammatory disease, but where does the inflammation come from? *BMC Medicine, 11*, 200.
45. Maes, M., Song, C., Lin, A. H., et al. (1999). Negative immunoregulatory effects of antidepressants: Inhibition of interferon-gamma and stimulation of interleukin-10 secretion. *Neuropsychopharmacology, 20*(4), 370–379.
46. Hameed, I., Masoodi, S. R., Mir, S. A., Nabi, M., Ghazanfar, K., & Ganai, B. A. (2015). Type 2 diabetes mellitus: From a metabolic disorder to an inflammatory condition. *World Journal of Diabetes, 6*(4), 598–612.
47. Wang, X., Bao, W., Liu, J., et al. (2013). Inflammatory markers and risk of type 2 diabetes: A systematic review and meta-analysis. *Diabetes Care, 36*(1), 166–175.
48. Spranger, J., Kroke, A., Mohlig, M., et al. (2003). Inflammatory cytokines and the risk to develop type 2 diabetes: Results of the prospective population-based European Prospective Investigation into Cancer and Nutrition (EPIC)-Potsdam Study. *Diabetes, 52*(3), 812–817.
49. Pickup, J. C., Mattock, M. B., Chusney, G. D., & Burt, D. (1997). NIDDM as a disease of the innate immune system: Association of acute-phase reactants and interleukin-6 with metabolic syndrome X. *Diabetologia, 40*(11), 1286–1292.
50. Hu, F. B., Meigs, J. B., Li, T. Y., Rifai, N., & Manson, J. E. (2004). Inflammatory markers and risk of developing type 2 diabetes in women. *Diabetes, 53*(3), 693–700.
51. Donath, M. Y., & Shoelson, S. E. (2011). Type 2 diabetes as an inflammatory disease. *Nature Reviews Immunology, 11*(2), 98-107.
52. Hosogai, N., Fukuhara, A., Oshima, K., et al. (2007). Adipose tissue hypoxia in obesity and its impact on adipocytokine dysregulation. *Diabetes, 56*(4), 901–911.
53. Franceschi, C., & Campisi, J. (2014). Chronic inflammation (inflammaging) and its potential contribution to age-associated diseases. *Journals of Gerontology Series A: Biological Sciences and Medical Sciences, 69*(Suppl. 1), S4–S9.
54. Calabro, P., & Yeh, E. T. (2007). Obesity, inflammation, and vascular disease: The role of the adipose tissue as an endocrine organ. *Subcellular Biochemistry, 42*, 63–91.
55. Galic, S., Oakhill, J. S., Steinberg, G. R. (2010). Adipose tissue as an endocrine organ. *Molecular and Cellular Endocrinology, 316*(2), 129–139.
56. Aguilar-Valles, A., Inoue, W., Rummel, C., & Luheshi, G. N. (2015). Obesity, adipokines and neuroinflammation. *Neuropharmacology, 96*(Pt. A), 124–134.
57. Kotas, M. E., & Medzhitov, R. (2015). Homeostasis, inflammation, and disease susceptibility. *Cell, 160*(5), 816–827.
58. de Wit, L., Luppino, F., van Straten, A., Penninx, B., Zitman, F., & Cuijpers, P. (2010). Depression and obesity: A meta-analysis of community-based studies. *Psychiatry Research, 178*(2), 230–235.
59. Leiria, L. O., Martins, M. A., & Saad, M. J. (2015). Obesity and asthma: Beyond T(H)2 inflammation. *Metabolism, 64*(2), 172–181.
60. Lovren, F., Teoh, H., & Verma, S. Obesity and atherosclerosis: Mechanistic insights. *Canadian Journal of Cardiology, 31*(2), 177–183.
61. Lubrano, V., & Balzan, S. (2015). Consolidated and emerging inflammatory markers in coronary artery disease. *World Journal of Experimental Medicine, 5*(1), 21–32.
62. Luna-Luna, M., Medina-Urrutia, A., Vargas-Alarcon, G., Coss-Rovirosa, F., Vargas-Barron, J., & Perez-Mendez, O. (2015). Adipose tissue in metabolic syndrome: Onset and progression of atherosclerosis. *Archives of MedicalResearch, 46*(5), 392–407.
63. van den Bekerom, M. P., Struijs, P. A., Blankevoort, L., Welling, L., van Dijk, CN., & Kerkhoffs, G. M. (2012). What is the evidence for rest, ice, compression, and elevation therapy in the treatment of ankle sprains in adults? *Journal of Athletic Training, 47*(4), 435–443.

Chapter 12

Neoplasia

Julie Eggert and Matthew Sorenson

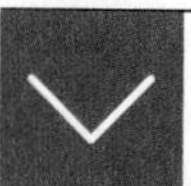

Chapter Outline and Learning Outcomes

12.1 Chapter Overview and Case Studies

Define neoplasia and cancer, and discuss concepts related to the development of malignant tumors.

12.2 Cell Cycle and Cellular Differentiation

Compare and contrast cell cycles for normal and malignant cells.

12.3 Molecular Basis of Cancer

Identify how genetic factors interact to affect the molecular changes associated with a malignancy.

12.4 Carcinogenesis

Explain the multistep process of carcinogenesis, incorporating angiogenesis, mechanisms of altered cellular differentiation, and cancer growth rates.

12.5 Cancer Invasion and Metastasis

Analyze how the mechanisms of cancer invasion and metastasis affect the patterns of spread of cancer cells.

12.6 Epidemiology of Cancer

Determine the epidemiology of cancer and how factors such as age, gender, race/ethnicity, and the effect of geographic location affect the incidence of different cancers.

12.7 Clinical Manifestations of Cancer

Identify clinical manifestations commonly associated with different forms of cancer.

12.8 Linking Pathophysiology to Diagnosis and Treatment

Explain the link between the pathophysiology of cancer and the different treatment modalities across the lifespan.

KEY TERMS

Angiogenesis, 296
Aneuploidy, 301
Apoptosis, 296
Benign, 295
Biopsy, 313
Cancer, 295
Cell cycle, 297
Cell cycle checkpoints, 297
Carcinogenesis, 303
Chromosome translocation, 300
Cluster of differentiation, 317
Differentiation, 298
Fibronectin, 306
Gene amplification, 301
Gene product, 299
Germ line mutations, 296
Growth factors, 302
Initiation, 305
Loss of heterozygosity, 302
Malignant, 295
Metastasize, 296
microRNAs (miRNA), 302
Mutation, 296
Mutator genes, 300
Neoplasia, 295
Neoplasm, 295
Oncogene, 300
Paraneoplastic syndromes, 312
Primary tumor, 306
Progression, 305
Promotion, 305
Proto-oncogene, 300
Somatic mutations, 296
Targeted therapy, 317
Tumor, 295
Tumor markers, 313
Tumor necrosis factor (TNF), 312
Tumor suppressor genes, 300

ABBREVIATIONS

EGFR—epidermal growth factor receptor
GFR—growth factor receptor
HLA—human leukocyte antigen
HPV—human papillomavirus
miRNA—microRNA
ObGF—osteoblast growth factor
OcAF—osteoclast activating factor
TNF—tumor necrosis factor
TNM—tumor–node–metastasis
VEGF—vascular endothelial growth factor

12.1 Chapter Overview and Case Studies

Neoplasia is a term that refers to the process of abnormal growth of cells. The abnormal growth of cells is called a **tumor** or a **neoplasm**. A growing mass of cells can cause compression damage to blood vessels and neighboring tissue but might not invade neighboring tissues or spread to other sites in the body. A **benign** tumor is one that might not be harmless but is localized and does not invade other tissues or spread to other parts of the body. The invasion of surrounding tissue or spread to other parts of the body is what characterizes a tumor as **malignant**. When a tumor develops malignancy, it is often referred to as *cancerous*.

The term **cancer** encompasses more than 200 diseases that occur at different ages with different rates of growth, differentiation, detection evasiveness, and capacities to spread to adjacent tissue and/or metastasize to distant sites, treatment responses, and prognosis. However, at the cellular and molecular levels, researchers and clinicians are beginning to view cancer as a condition caused by genetic alterations and defective cell functions that are actually very similar among differing forms.[1,2] These alterations can be associated with nature (innate characteristics such as genetics), for example, inherited cancer syndromes such as hereditary breast and ovarian cancer syndrome or immune deficiencies. Alternatively, the genetic alterations associated with cancer can be caused by nurture (life experiences, including exposure to environmental factors), which includes factors such as obesity, poor diet, and smoking.

A malignant growth is the result of changes in the structure of deoxyribonucleic acid (DNA) and/or gene transcription or translation. The resultant defective protein or proteins that are produced lead to transformation of normal cell components into forms that cause uncontrolled cell proliferation, spread to adjacent tissues, and/or metastasis to distant sites in the body. This chapter focuses on explaining the changes cells undergo when they become malignant. Knowledge of this process will provide a foundation for understanding the growth of cancers, their detection, and their treatment.

Benign and Malignant Neoplasms

There are a number of terms that are unique to the understanding of neoplasia and cancer. The differentiation between benign and malignant is an important concept to explore in detail, as there are characteristics that differentiate benign and malignant neoplasms (**Table 12.1** ■). The characteristics of the cells from the tumor are assessed in a pathology laboratory to determine whether the histologic changes are due to a benign or a malignant (cancerous) growth.[3]

Benign neoplasms are growths that are not cancer, typically develop slowly, and are encased by a connective tissue capsule. These abnormal growths do not spread into adjacent tissue or invade other organs. A benign tumor ends with the suffix *-oma*, as in adenoma.[3] While a benign tumor is usually nonthreatening to the host, it can cause life-threatening problems if it impinges on the function of important structures in the body such as the lungs, spinal cord, or brain. Examples of benign tumors are acoustic neuroma (tumor of the acoustic nerve) and pneumocytoma (tumor of the pneumocytes, which are the epithelial cells lining the alveoli of the lung).

A cancerous neoplasm is also called a malignancy. Description of malignant tissue will also begin with the cell type or tissue of origin but will include a different suffix. Malignant tissue originating from epithelial tissue is designated by the suffix *-carcinoma*. Malignant tissue from mesenchymal tissue is indicated by the suffix *-sarcoma*. Hematopoietic or lymphoid tissue neoplasms are called leukemias or lymphomas.[4] An example of a malignant tumor is a ductal adenocarcinoma of the breast.

Malignant cells have an abnormal appearance with large nuclei and abnormal amounts of DNA, limited cytoplasm, and an immature appearance when viewed under a microscope.[4] This abnormal collection of cells grows rapidly,

Table 12.1 Comparison of Benign and Malignant Neoplasms

Benign	Malignant
Not a cancer	Cancerous
Rarely life-threatening	May be life-threatening
Encapsulated	Typically unencapsulated
Grow locally	Ability to spread to surrounding tissue or invade other organs
Well differentiated, maintains specialization	Poorly differentiated or wide range of cellular changes, loss of specialization
Normal mitosis	Mitotic count varies, abnormal mitosis
Minimal nuclear variation in size and shape	Variation in nuclear variation is minimal to marked, often variable
Organized	Disorganized
Diploidy	Range of ploidy statuses
Cells typically grow slowly (slow doubling time)	Typically includes fast-growing cells (rapid doubling)

does not usually have a capsule, aggressively invades the surrounding tissue, and will **metastasize** (spread) to other organs. Even though a metastatic cancer may be located in another organ site, the cells still have histologic similarity to the tissue of origin, at least initially. For example, a breast cancer that has spread to the bone will still have characteristics of a breast cell and not those of a bone cell. In addition, cancers of a specific tissue type seem to prefer to metastasize to the same organ sites. For example, breast cancers will spread to the lungs, liver, and bones. A lung cancer is more likely to spread to the adrenal glands.[4]

Over time, malignant tissue loses the characteristics of a normal cell. Multiple changes on and in the cellular membrane promote the ability of the cancer cell to easily invade locally and spread distantly. Messages from the cellular membrane to the nucleus promote alternative signaling pathways and result in loss of control for cell division and proliferation, resulting in the immortalization of the cell. Immune surveillance is fooled by other cell changes that allow the malignant cell to masquerade as a normal cell and escape destruction by the immune response.[4]

Concepts Related to Cancer

All cancer is genetic, resulting from damaged DNA or RNA, whether the damage occurs in germ line (egg or sperm) or somatic cells (non–germ line). The term **mutation** is used to denote the process causing permanent alteration in a DNA sequence. **Germ line mutations** occur in eggs or sperm and are therefore inherited. **Somatic mutations** affect DNA after conception and are generally not inherited.

Some cancer-causing mutations are known as *drivers* and others as *passengers*. The drivers are mutations in genes that are known to be associated with cancer or genes that are known to serve a tumor-suppressing role. Drivers provide excellent targets for cancer treatment. Passenger mutations are considered to have no impact on changes occurring in the cancer cell and only accompany the drivers.[5]

The gene products of the altered DNA sequences yield a different outcome depending on the signaling pathways affected. These include changes in cell division and proliferation, programmed cell death (**apoptosis**), vascularization of the tumor (**angiogenesis**), and an alternative form of energy production (aerobic glycolysis). Taken together, alterations affect cell circuitry both separately and collectively, creating an altered environment capable of supporting a malignant tumor.[2]

Maintenance of the immune system is important to prevent cancer. If immune function is depleted as a result of foreign attackers or illness or is limited, owing to an inherited disease, the lack of an orchestrated immune response can leave an individual open to the development of a malignancy. The normal immune system performs a process of constant surveillance of the human body, looking for damaged cells being formed on a daily and a moment-to-moment basis with attack mechanisms ready to identify and destroy such cells.[3,6] These defense mechanisms are part of the innate immune system, and they engage inflammatory mechanisms in defense of the individual. Unfortunately, the longer an inflammation persists, the higher is the risk of developing a cancer. Because chronic inflammation lasts over a longer period of time, cells that are normally recruited in the process of immunologic control and repair (such as mast cells and leukocytes) require an elevation in oxygen uptake. This uptake leads to a respiratory burst with accumulation of reactive oxygen species at the site of damage. In turn, other inflammatory cells are attracted to the site and produce metabolites of arachidonic acid, cytokines, and chemokines that further propagate inflammatory response and elicit chemical mediators that also play a role in oxidative stress. This sustained inflammatory and oxidative environment becomes cyclic, causing more damage to the neighboring healthy cells and, over time, leading to neoplasia.[2] Selected concepts related to neoplasia are outlined in **Figure 12.1** ■.

Case Studies

To assist in the application of content in this chapter to clinical practice, two case studies are introduced here, and the pathophysiology involved and clinical significance of the information are addressed throughout the chapter.

Laura Beckman: Introduction

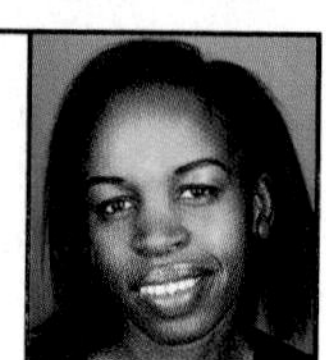

Laura Beckman, age 32, recently noticed a lump in her left breast. No one on her mother's side of the family has had a diagnosis of breast cancer, so Ms. Beckman believes that the lump is related to her menstrual period. After her next period, she still feels the lump and thinks it has grown. Ms. Beckman makes an appointment to see her healthcare provider, believing that the lump is the result of an infection in a milk duct, as she had after the delivery of her first child approximately 18 months ago. She hopes the provider will prescribe an antibiotic to solve the problem. When talking with the nurse, Ms. Beckman states that the lump is not painful and feels larger, but it does not seem to increase or decrease in size with her menses.

1. How should the nurse respond when Ms. Beckman asks about the difference between a benign tumor and a malignant tumor?
2. What should the nurse say if Ms. Beckman asks how she can reduce her risk of cancer?

Edgar Graham: Introduction

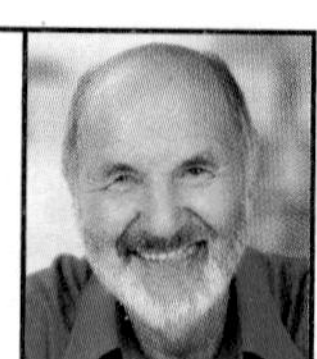

Edgar Graham is 66 years old and has inflammatory bowel disease and hemorrhoids, both of which were diagnosed 12 years ago. Several months ago, he noticed blood in the toilet after a bowel movement but was not concerned, thinking that it was due to the hemorrhoids. Today, Mr. Graham noted more blood in the toilet bowl and realized that it was not in association with a bowel movement, and he has not noticed any of the pain typically associated with his hemorrhoids. Because of continued gastrointestinal bleeding, he makes an appointment with his healthcare provider to be assessed for colon cancer.

1. What role may Mr. Graham's inflammatory bowel disease play in the development of cancer?
2. How should the nurse respond when Mr. Graham expresses fear that he has cancer?

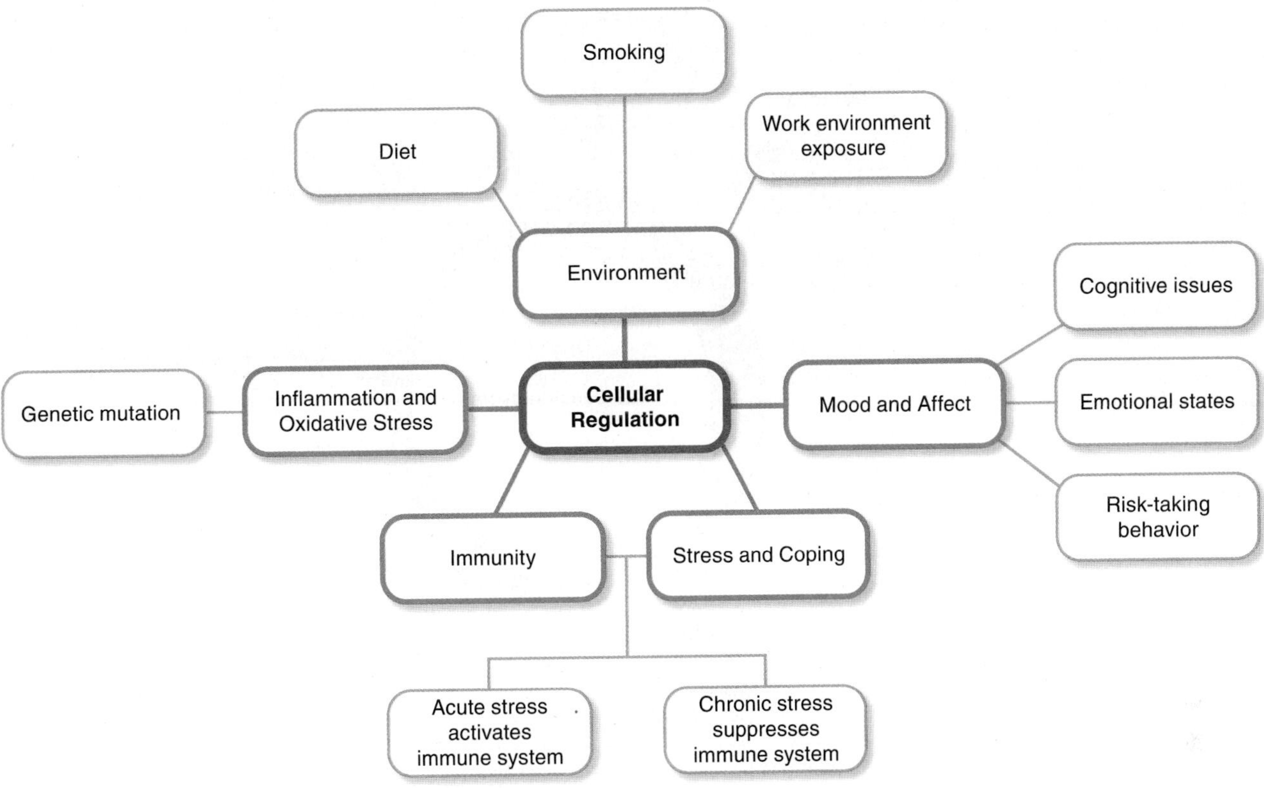

Figure 12.1 ■ Concepts related to cancer affect the types of cancer, their risks, and interventions that can both increase and decrease the risks.

Check Your Progress: Section 12.1

1. Explain how a benign tumor can become life-threatening.
2. What is the difference between a germ line mutation and a somatic mutation?
3. Compare driver mutations with passenger mutations.

12.2 Cell Cycle and Cellular Differentiation

It is through the cell cycle that DNA damage truly becomes cancerous. The **cell cycle** is the period of time from one cell division to the next. It is regulated by several checkpoints, which are necessary because the conditions for cell division are often not ideal and can result in errors in DNA replication or in alterations of chromosomes. Once the cell receives the signals that activate cell division, the cell begins to go through the various stages of the cell cycle, ending in replication of cell contents, including the genome, and division into two identical daughter cells.[7] The length of the cell cycle differs among cell types in the body. Cancer cells do not necessarily have shorter cell cycles; however, they move through the cell cycle many more times than normal cells without performing normal functions of that tissue. Also in cancer cells, error-prone DNA repair allows accumulation of genetic errors that affect normal cell cycle control mechanisms. This allows the cell cycle to function without the normal cell proliferations controls.[2,7]

The Normal Cell Cycle and Its Checkpoints

In the normal cell cycle, a well-controlled sequence of events occurs during the phases of gap 1 (G1), DNA synthesis (S), gap 2 (G2), mitosis (M), and gap zero (G0) (**Figure 12.2** ■). **Cell cycle checkpoints** function to ensure that the process of DNA replication occurs in the correct sequence, that errors are corrected, and that one event is completed before the next is started.[2,7] The cell cycle checkpoints involve specific genes that code for the following three types of proteins:

- Enzymes called cyclin-dependent kinases act like a gas pedal, enhancing passage through phases of the cell cycle by phosphorylating proteins that drive the cell cycle forward.
- Cyclins, such as cyclin A and cyclin B, bind to and activate the cyclin-dependent kinases.
- A variety of proteins that inhibit the cyclin-dependent kinases, such as p17, p21, and p53, function as brakes to stop the cell cycle.

The two main cell cycle checkpoints are at the transition from the gap 1 to the DNA synthesis phase and at the transition from gap 2 to the mitosis phase (see Figure 12.2).[7]

The first phase of the cell cycle is gap 1 (G1), during which the cell grows and DNA is prepared to be copied. During the checkpoint at the end of the G1 phase, the cell takes an inventory of the materials needed to replicate DNA, such as enzymes and nucleotides, and searches for any needed repair of defects before DNA replication. Entry into

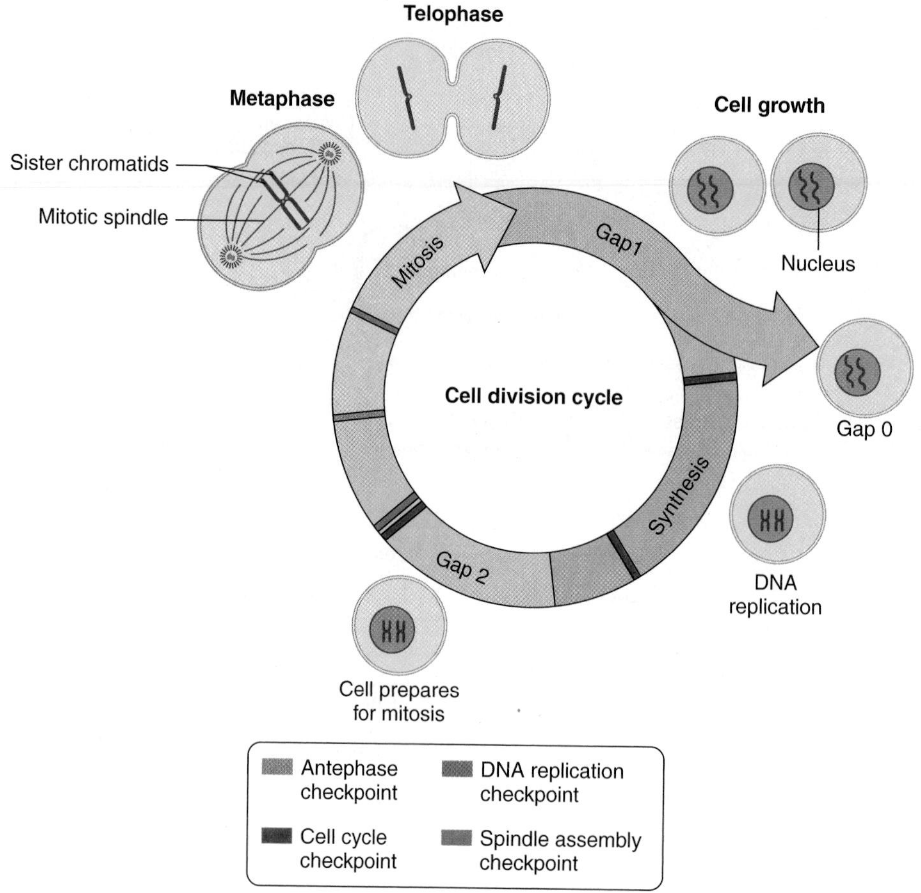

Figure 12.2 ■ The normal cell cycle and each of its growth phases, demonstrating the checkpoints where DNA is monitored for correctness and the G0 phase where the cell rests from replication yet continues to perform its metabolic functions.

the DNA synthesis (S) phase is carefully restricted by this checkpoint to prevent replication of DNA damage, which is important in maintaining the integrity of the human genome. At this checkpoint, there is a tumor suppressor protein, called the retinoblastoma protein, that functions as a brake, stopping cell cycle progression. Any changes in this protein must be removed for the cell cycle to progress. The retinoblastoma protein is so named because if both of the alleles of the retinoblastoma gene are mutated, it results in retinoblastoma, a tumor of the retina in the eye.[2,7]

When cell sensors determine that the cell is ready to progress through the cycle, there is activation of certain cyclin-dependent kinases, which remove the retinoblastoma brake by phosphorylating it. When the brake is removed, genes are expressed that code for products needed for DNA synthesis in the next phase. If the cell is not ready to progress, the *TP53* gene is activated and codes for production of the p53 tumor suppressor protein, which has been called the guardian of the cell cycle because of the ways in which it maintains the integrity of the genome. For example, p53 activates the gene that produces p21 (an inhibitor of several cyclin-dependent kinases) and can activate apoptosis if damage is too severe to be repaired.[8]

The second phase of the cell cycle is the synthesis (S) phase, in which the synthesis of DNA occurs, creating an exact copy of all chromosomes in the cell that will later be divided between two daughter cells. At the S checkpoint, the cell takes another inventory to determine whether each segment of DNA has been copied properly and whether the correct number of chromosomes is present. If an error is detected, p53 tumor suppressor levels increase, stopping progression of the cell cycle and activating DNA repair enzymes. If the damage is too severe to be repaired, p53 activates apoptotic pathways that program for cell death.[2,8,9]

After the DNA has been copied, the cell progresses to the gap 2 (G2) phase and prepares for mitosis by producing the mitotic spindle and proteins necessary for cell division. During the phase of mitosis (M), the two copies of chromosomes separate, and the cell divides into two daughter cells, leaving each new cell with a full set of 46 chromosomes (cytokinesis). After completing the previous four phases, the daughter cells enter gap 0 (G0), which is a temporary or permanent rest from cell division, and perform normal cellular functions.[9]

Any chromosomal abnormalities at the end of the cell cycle could be due to defects in checkpoint surveillance. For example, mutations of the cyclin-dependent kinase inhibitors in somatic cells are present in a large percentage of cancers. Mutations of cyclin-dependent kinase inhibitors in germ cells are associated with inherited forms of cancer

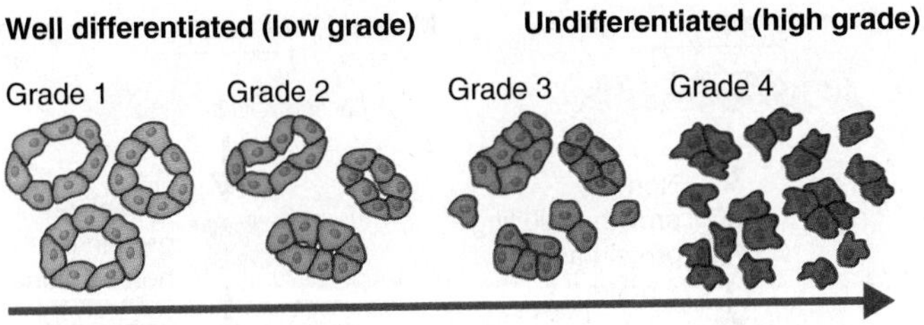

Figure 12.3 ■ The different grades of cellular differentiation as the cell moves from maturity and differentiation back into an immature cell that is dedifferentiated. Grading of differentiation is important during the diagnosis discussions before cancer treatment.

risk. Acquiring genomic damage permits evolving populations of precancerous cells to gain functional capabilities associated with malignant transformation. These include (1) self-sufficiency in growth signals, (2) insensitivity to antigrowth signals, (3) evasion of apoptosis, (4) sustained angiogenesis (growth of new blood vessels), (5) tissue invasion and metastasis, and (6) limitless replicative potential.[10]

Cell Differentiation and Cancer

The maturation of a normal cell to one with distinct morphology and specialized functions is known as **differentiation**. The most immature cell is labeled as a blast cell or dedifferentiated cell. Cancer cells lose their specialized or differentiated appearance and become so undifferentiated as to appear similar to blast cells.

CLINICAL POINT: The term *blast crisis* describes a state of rapid proliferation of immature blast cells in the bone marrow and/or blood that occurs in the late stage of certain leukemias such as chronic myelogenous leukemia. ■

Grading of the level of differentiation of cancer cells compared to cells from the tissue of origin is done with microscopic examination. The levels are identified as grades 1 through 4; the lower number refers to well-differentiated cells with specialized function and the higher number refers to poorly differentiated cells with very little specialized function (**Figure 12.3** ■). GX is used to indicate tissue that cannot be assessed.[11]

Check Your Progress: Section 12.2

1. What is the importance of cell cycle checkpoints?
2. What is the role of the checkpoint at the end of the G1 phase?
3. Describe cell differentiation in cancer cells.

12.3 Molecular Basis of Cancer

Although the transformation of normal cells into a cancer is initiated at the genetic level, there are many factors, such as environmental variables, oxidative stress, hormonal influences, lifestyle factors, and chronic inflammation, that occur outside the cell and can alter the **gene products** (proteins) and therefore change the activity and function of the cell or tissue. Interactions of genes with the above variables can initiate and promote the change from normal cellular mechanisms to those found in malignant cells.[6] This revised "spelling" of the genetic code is led by mutations in DNA that cause altered RNA messaging, modified amino acids in the protein products of DNA, and ultimately changed proteins, creating misdirection for a variety of functions of the cell.[2,4] All cancer is caused by multiple mutations in many different genes that control growth of cells and their ability to survive, repair DNA, motility, and angiogenesis.

Genetic Mutations

The most common type of mutation is a point mutation, which occurs when a single nucleotide base of DNA is substituted for another base. One example could be replacement of an adenine (A) with a guanine (G). Silent, missense, and nonsense mutations are types of point mutations in DNA sequences that encode proteins:

- ***Silent point mutations*** are a base substitution in the third position of a codon. This causes a mutation that usually results in the generation of an amino acid that is the same as the one generated by the original codon spelling. Thus, the gene product is unaltered.
- ***Missense point mutations*** occur when an amino acid in the sequence of the protein has been replaced. This may or may not result in a deleterious (disease-causing) gene product, depending on the amino acid that has been substituted. If the structure and properties of the normal and substituted amino acids are similar, no deleterious gene products will result. If the structure and properties of the two amino acids are very different, a deleterious or nonfunctional gene product may result.
- ***Nonsense point mutations*** are deleterious mutations. Some codons are used as "stop" and "start" messages to initiate gene product expression. When a base substitution results in the generation of a stop codon, meaning that the gene product will be truncated (spliced off) and probably nonfunctional, a nonsense point mutation occurs.

Deletions and insertions are other types of mutations that are frequently associated with cancers:

- ***Deletion mutations*** occur when at least one base pair is lost from a sequence of DNA. One way to think of reading a codon sequence is to think of a "reading frame," a window through which you always see three—and only three—bases. If brackets represent the reading frame, then a sequence might be read as UUA [AAU] GAU. Deletion of one or two bases changes the reading frame of the sequence; the frame grows to allow a view of three bases, but they might not be the same three that were in the frame before the deletion. In the above example, if AA were removed, the reading frame would shift, and the sequence would become [UGA]. The result would be an altered amino acid called a frameshift mutation. The gene product of such a mutation is usually nonfunctional.

- *Insertion mutations* of additional base pairs also may lead to a frameshift mutation, depending on whether multiples of three base pairs are inserted. It is possible for an insertion to restore the reading frame of a gene with a deletion mutation (or vice versa). The gene product would contain a garbled amino acid order between the insertion and deletion, but it would otherwise be correct.

A graphic depiction of genetic mutations is shown in **Figure 12.4**.

Tumor Suppressor Genes

Tumor suppressor genes are normally responsible for inhibiting cell replication or braking cell growth (**Figure 12.5**). If there is one functioning copy of the gene, the protein is produced, and normal braking occurs. The inactivation or loss of the second allele (gene) causes loss of function (loss of braking), and the cell begins to replicate without interruption, allowing it to become immortalized. Deletions in a sequence of DNA, therefore, are a hallmark of defective tumor suppressor (TS) genes.[2]

The *TP53* gene is considered the guardian of the genome. When changed with deletions and mutations, the *TP53* gene (located on chromosome 17) is associated with a wide range and number of cancers, including lung, breast, esophageal, liver, bladder, and ovarian carcinomas; brain tumors; sarcomas; lymphomas; and leukemias. The germ line mutations of *TP53*, transmitted in an autosomal dominant fashion, are a hallmark of Li-Fraumeni syndrome. This syndrome is caused by inheritance of the mutated *TP53* gene, and individuals with this condition have an increased risk of developing a variety of cancers at a younger age than the general population. Somatic mutations of the *TP53* gene are found in the tumors of every type of cancer with an incidence ranging from 30% to 60%.[2,8]

There are other tumor suppressor genes that encode for proteins in the cytoplasm. The normal *NF1* (neurofibromatosis gene) is a tumor suppressor that encodes a protein similar to the proteins that modify *RAS* function. With the loss of the *NF1* tumor suppressor function, the *RAS* gene may become activated and prolong the signal, allowing continued cell proliferation. Loss of other tumor suppressor genes may also cause cellular disorganization that leads to abnormal cell proliferation; an example is colon cancer associated with the *APC* gene.[12] Other tumor suppressor genes that code for proteins with unclear cellular function include the breast–ovarian cancer genes *BRCA1* and *BRCA2*. These genes are associated with inherited breast, ovarian, pancreatic, prostate, and melanoma cancers.

Normal amino acid	The fat cat sat for the rat
Missense mutation	The far cat sat for the rat
Insertion mutation	The fea tca tsa tfo rth era t
Deletion mutation	The ftc ats atf ort her at

Figure 12.4 Various types of genetic mutations.

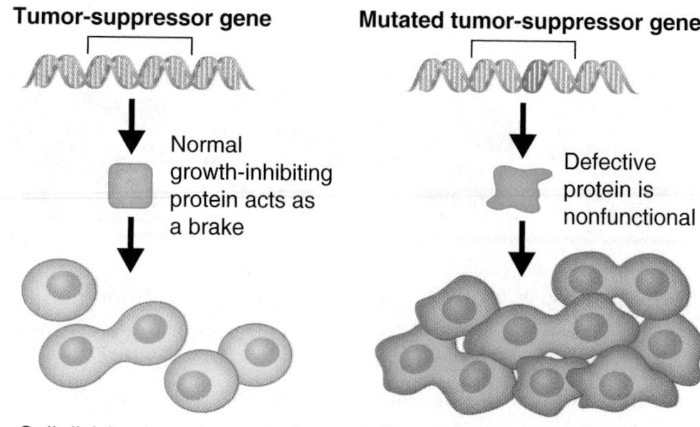

Figure 12.5 Tumor suppressor genes act like a brake on cell function. The second figure example shows a mutation in the tumor suppressor gene that allows the continued function of the gene and production of its protein product.

Oncogenes

Proto-oncogenes are normal genes that are responsible for regulation of proliferation of cells, such as in tissue healing after injury. Because the proto-oncogene stimulates tissue growth, such as in wound healing, it is known as the "gas pedal" of proliferation. Once healing is complete, the "gas pedal" is turned off. The mutated form of the gene is called an **oncogene**, and it can allow continuous and ongoing cell growth. While the tumor suppressor genes require "two hits," or loss of heterozygosity affecting both alleles of the gene, the oncogene mutation is a dominant mutation and needs the loss of only one allele for cancer to be enabled.[12]

A **chromosome translocation** occurs when a piece of one chromosome breaks off and fuses to another chromosome. Chromosomal translocations primarily affect oncogenes. Translocations cause oncogene overexpression such as that found in chronic myelogenous leukemia. Reciprocal translocations involve exchange of genetic material between two chromosomes or within the same chromosome. One example of a cancer caused by a translocation is Burkitt lymphoma, in which 80% of cases have a translocation of the long arms of chromosomes 8 and 14. This translocation causes activation of another oncogene, *MYC*, which also results in continuous cell cycling and apoptosis.

CLINICAL POINT: Translocations are the hallmarks of leukemias and lymphomas.[13] An acquired translocation associated with activation of oncogenes is common with a majority of chronic myelogenous leukemia cases. This particular translocation of DNA in white blood cells found in the bone marrow is called the Philadelphia chromosome (Ph+). The translocation involves the breaking off of the long arm tip of chromosome 9 with fusion to the long arm tip of chromosome 22. The fusion creates a gene (*BCR-abl*) that deregulates proliferation and allows uncontrolled cell growth, or immortality of abnormal white blood cells (**Figure 12.6**).

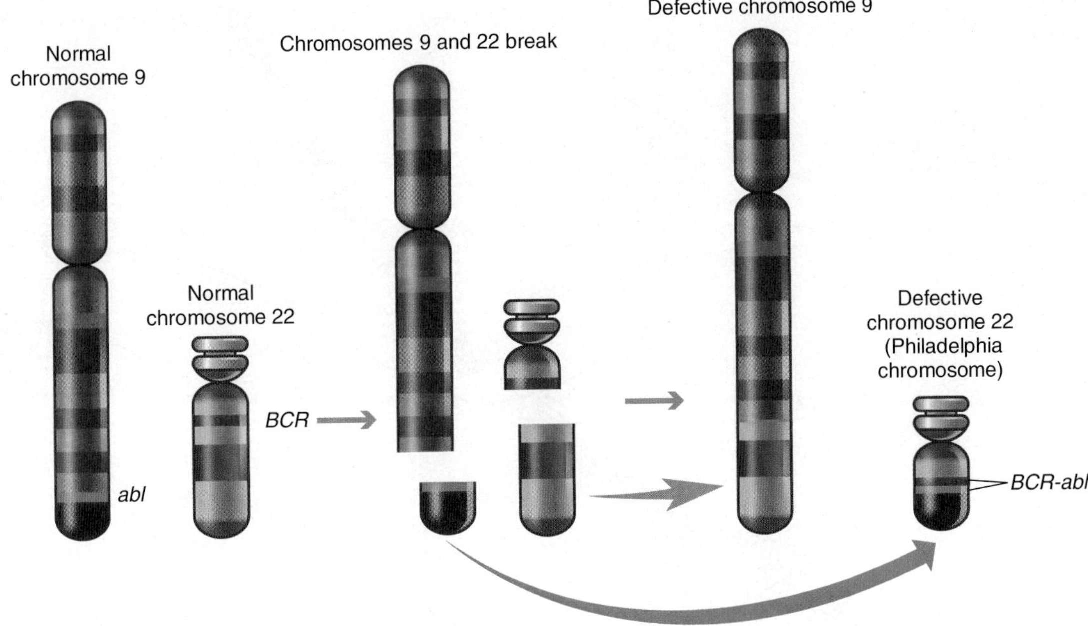

Figure 12.6 The pieces of chromosome 9 and 22 translocate to form the Philadelphia chromosome, which is used to diagnose chronic myelogenous leukemia.

Mutator Genes

There are more than 20,000 events each day that damage DNA. While **mutator genes** (DNA repair genes) can be oncogenes or tumor suppressor genes, they are not part of cell regulatory pathways. Instead, mutator genes prevent genetic instability through their repair role. Mutator genes encode error correction systems that check DNA for damage or mismatched base pairs. Mutations in these genes lead to inefficient replication or repair of DNA.[3,14]

Additional Genetic Alterations in Cancer Cells

In addition to mutations, the genetic alterations associated with cancer include chromosomal abnormalities, amplification, and defects in mismatch repair.

Chromosomal Abnormalities

Cancer cells typically have a bizarre, unstable chromosomal structure that comprises many gains, losses, or rearrangements of chromosomes. Only a few of these abnormalities appear to be causally linked to cancer. The specific genes responsible for chromosomal instability have not yet been identified, though many have been identified as drivers.[3,14]

Recurrent structural chromosomal rearrangements are a common feature of most cancers. How these rearrangements develop may be attributed to genetic weak points or chromosomal fragile sites. Chromosomal fragile sites are regions on chromosomes that are particularly sensitive to forming nonrandom gaps or breaks when DNA synthesis is interrupted.[15]

Chromosomal deletions are associated most often with solid tumors. The most common deletion is in specific gene sequences, which result in the loss of a chromosomal band or the loss of heterozygosity of a specific allele.[16] Deletions, as was noted previously, are the hallmark alteration occurring in tumor suppressor genes. The same chromosome deletions can be seen in tumors of different cellular origin.[2,16]

Aneuploidy is an abnormal chromosome number and can involve a gain or a loss of chromosome(s). As changes in the DNA accumulate, tumor formation progresses with gross changes in chromosome number, consistent with malignant transformation. For example, in most colorectal cancers, aneuploidy is found and associated with genetic instability.[2,17]

Gene amplification, an increase in the number of gene copies, results in elevations of the protein (gene product) without modification of the gene itself. Amplification of certain genes may be related to the development of cancer. As tumor cells progress, they lose cell cycle control and tumor suppressor gene activity. This allows uncontrolled cell proliferation and development of other qualities of the malignant cell.[2,16]

CLINICAL POINT: These amplified gene sequences can result in increased numbers of cell membrane receptors, such as HER2/neu, which are used as markers of breast cancer subtype and progression and to guide personalized cancer treatment. ■

Normal synthesis of DNA relies on a backup signal to differentiate between a parental strand and a daughter strand of DNA that contains a replication error. In normal DNA synthesis, specific repair proteins recognize and bind to the mismatch. The result is a process that essentially unwinds DNA in the direction of the mismatch, degrades the damaged DNA strand, and seals the nick that degradation causes in the strand. Sometimes, however, the wrong nucleotide incorporates into the strand during DNA strand synthesis, and DNA's normal editing system fails to correct the error. Defects in genes that encode the mismatch repair proteins most often have been associated with hereditary

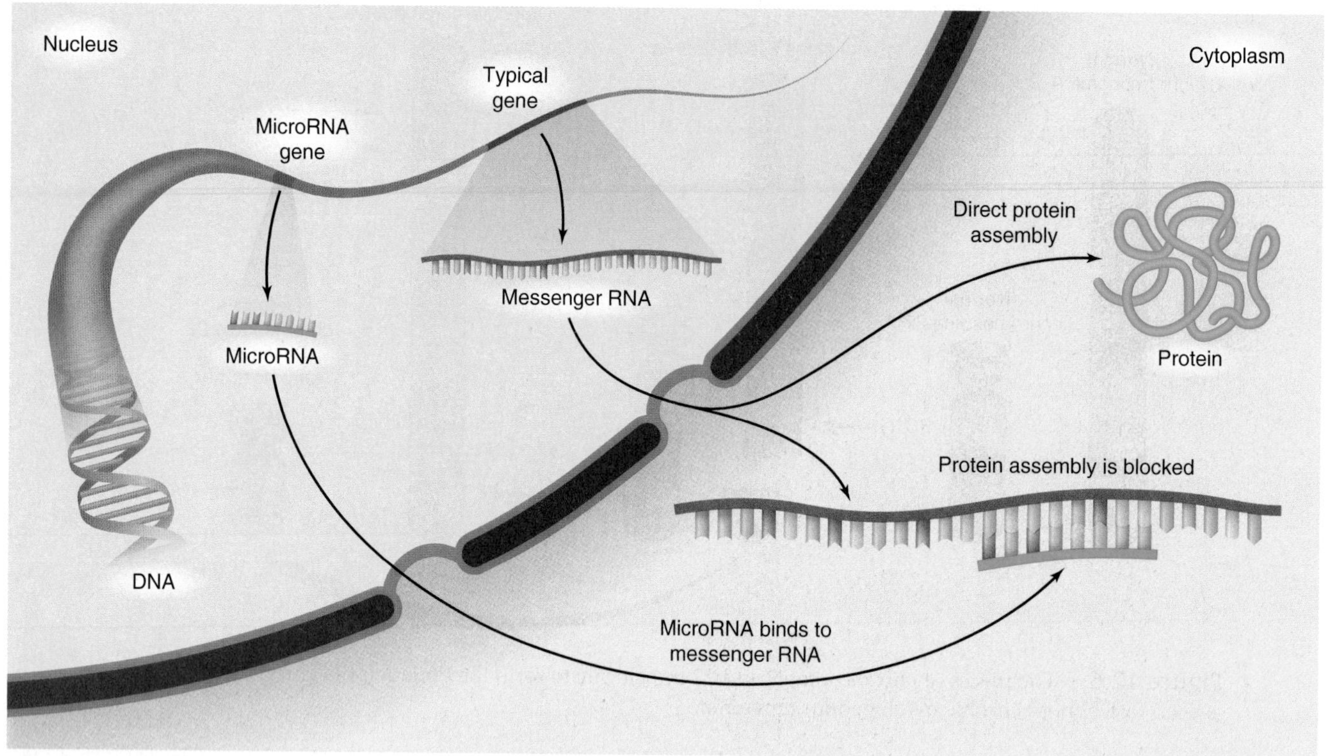

Figure 12.7 ■ The small piece of microRNA controls the translation of messenger RNA into an altered protein product.

nonpolyposis colorectal cancer. Most patients with hereditary nonpolyposis colorectal cancer show widespread alterations in the DNA base sequences, or microsatellite sequences (expanding sequences of tandem repeats of 2–6 DNA base pairs), distributed throughout the genome. For example, CGC would expand to CGCCGCCGC. These sequences may be associated with defects in mismatch repair and may be highly unstable and prone to single-nucleotide deletion or insertion.[2,18]

Very small pieces of noncoding RNA, about 20–23 nucleotides in length and named **microRNAs** (miRNA, or miR [pronounced "mere"]), control gene expression in many cellular processes (**Figure 12.7** ■). By downregulating and/or degrading messenger RNA (mRNA), the miR is involved in gene silencing, especially of genes involved in apoptosis and cell proliferation.[19] Either mechanism causes interference in the ability to produce protein that is important to signaling pathways for metabolism, apoptosis, cell differentiation, and development. MicroRNAs have also have been linked to tumor formation. Research indicates that miRNAs act primarily as tumor suppressors.[19]

Growth Factors

Most **growth factors** are proteins that act outside the cell as chemical signals to regulate cellular behavior. Cell growth, differentiation, and survival and the architecture and morphology are all controlled by growth factors. In signaling pathways, growth factors activate the signal across the cell membrane, into the cytoplasm, and perhaps into the nucleus. Growth factors must interact with specific receptors to accomplish signaling (**Figure 12.8** ■).

Membrane-Associated G proteins

Guanine nucleotide-binding proteins (G proteins) act as signal transducers—on–off switches—for cell surface growth factor receptors (GFRs). G proteins disrupt part of the signal cascade that flows into the cell cytoplasm. As part of the 50-member *RAS* proto-oncogene superfamily, when mutated, these oncogenes are known to cause malignant transformation. Normal *RAS* gene proteins transmit signals from GFRs to proteins to activate signaling pathways. Mutant *RAS* gene proteins activate signaling pathways even when unprompted by GFRs. Found in virtually all types of human cancer, the mutant *RAS* gene occurs in approximately two thirds of all malignant tumors. There are three isoforms (mRNAs with the same gene locus but with different protein coding DNA sequences), each associated with different types of cancer. These include *NRAS*, *KRAS*, and *HRAS*.[20] The incidence of these oncogenes in tumors vary widely by tissue type.

Loss of Heterozygosity

The first inherited mutation of a tumor suppressor gene is commonly a small change confined to the actual gene with recessive status. This creates heterozygosity with one normal (wild type) and one mutated gene, yielding normal protein expression. When the second mutation on the other allele involves the loss of all or part of a chromosome, there is an allelic loss of any marker close to the tumor suppressor gene, or **loss of heterozygosity**. Thus, if a patient with cancer is heterozygous for a specific genetic marker located close to the tumor suppressor gene, the tumor tissue loses this heterozygosity with the second mutation.[16] Most tumor specimens with loss of heterozygosity contain a mixture of

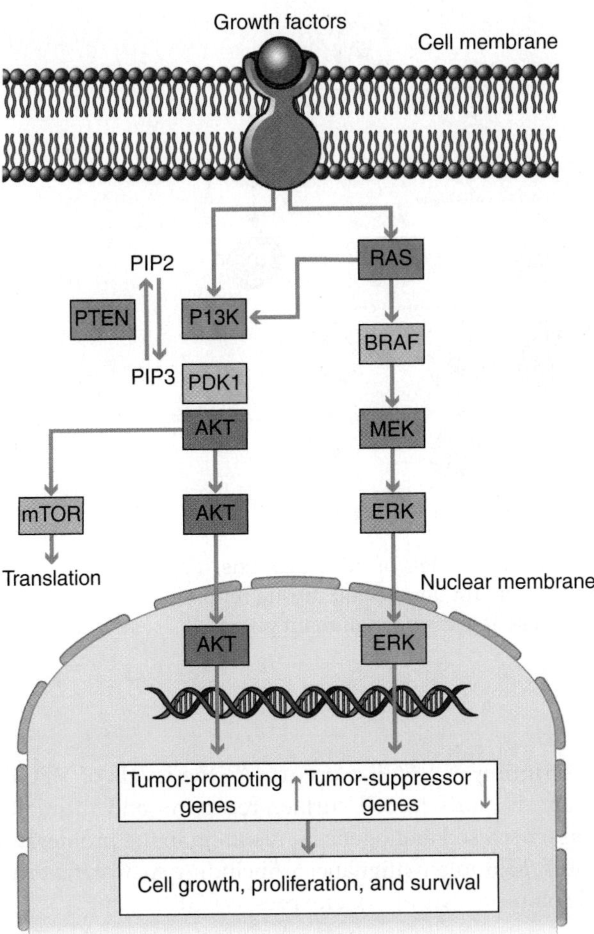

Figure 12.8 ■ Growth factors bind to receptors on the cell membrane and stimulate a signal that follows a circuitry of signaling pathways to initiate important cell functions such as duplication, angiogenesis, and apoptosis.

tumor and nontumor tissue, indicating a decreased relative intensity of tumor rather than a total loss of the band from one allele.[16]

Edgar Graham: Application

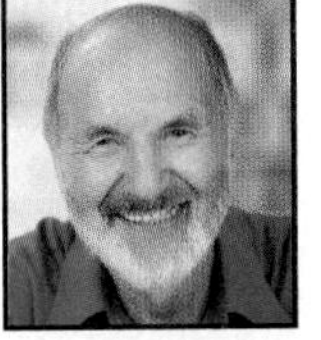

Mr. Graham is being evaluated for the presence of a hereditary nonpolyposis colorectal cancer. The healthcare provider performs a genogram as part of the screening assessment, and Mr. Graham reports that two cousins and an uncle have been diagnosed with this condition. This cancer is associated with a high incidence in the family tree and is associated with a genetic mismatch repair. This leads to the development of multiple mutations resulting in tumor formation. A screening history is crucial to determine whether the individual is at risk for development of this disease. The evaluative criteria include consideration of the number of family members diagnosed with this cancer.

3. What is the relationship between mismatch repair proteins and hereditary nonpolyposis colorectal cancer, such as Mr. Graham's diagnosis?
4. What factors outside the cell may affect Mr. Graham's gene proteins inside his cells, leading to cancer?

Check Your Progress: Section 12.3

1. Describe silent point mutations.
2. Why are proto-oncogenes known as the "gas pedal" of cell proliferation?
3. What is the role of mutator genes in promoting genetic stability?

12.4 Carcinogenesis

The term **carcinogenesis** refers to the process whereby normal cells develop into cancer cells. The process occurs in several stages and involves structural and functional changes in cells.

Mechanisms of Altered Cell Differentiation

The evolution of a cancer is based on two models: stochastic and cancer stem cell (**Figure 12.9** ■). The stochastic model describes cancer cells with much heterogeneity such that each cancer cell has the ability to proliferate and form a variety of new tumors from the same tissue of origin. The cancer stem cell model suggests that most cells have a limited ability to proliferate, while a few cells, the stem cells, are responsible for forming sites for growth of new tumors, especially after long lengths of time since remission.[2]

Cancer stem cells are a small subpopulation of cancer cells. Depending on the tissue type of origin, they can vary in number from 1 in 10,000 to 1 in 100. Cancer stem cells, like normal stem cells, have the ability to self-renew, differentiate, express telomerase, activate antiapoptosis, migrate, and metastasize.[2] Of special note, they remain in the G0 phase. Since cancer stem cells are not rapidly dividing, they are insensitive to chemotherapy and radiation. Thus, a patient who has been in remission from a cancer for decades may suddenly have an exacerbation, with return of signs and symptoms of the cancer. This is caused when the stem cell moves out of G0 phase and begins to move through the cell cycle toward continued division.[2,21] As cancer cells proliferate, more are detectable as they cause systemic effects for the patient.

Angiogenesis

As tumor cells are established and begin to proliferate, the mutations and cellular disorganization cause restrictions in oxygen supply, leading to areas of hypoxia. For the clump of cells to survive, glucose uptake and glycolysis are needed to generate energy. As in any other cell, lactate is produced and results in decreased adenosine triphosphate (ATP) production and ultimately contributes to the fatigue experienced by patients with a malignancy.[22] This lack of oxygen also curtails the proliferation of the malignant cells.[2,23] For tumors to grow to a larger size, they need to develop a microcirculatory system.[2,24] Vascular endothelial growth factor (VEGF) causes the growth of new vessels, forming a microcirculatory system to and within a tumor. This process is called angiogenesis (**Figure 12.10** ■). With tumor cell induced hypoxia,

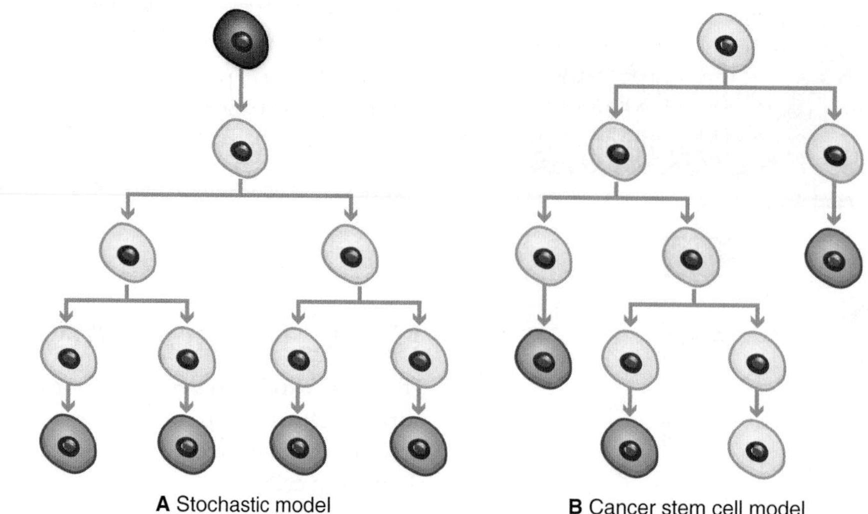

A Stochastic model
B Cancer stem cell model

Figure 12.9 ■ Comparison of the **A** stochastic and **B** stem cell models of carcinogenesis, depicting how cancer cells (shown in green) may be able to remain undetected during remission or grow into a heterogeneous group of cells with more or less aggressive malignant potential.

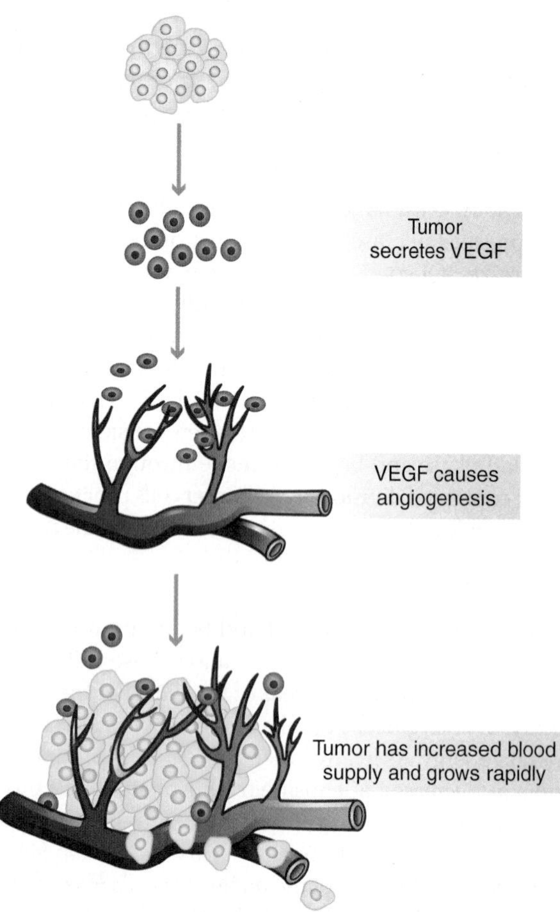

Tumor secretes VEGF
VEGF causes angiogenesis
Tumor has increased blood supply and grows rapidly

Figure 12.10 ■ Angiogenesis occurs when VEGF stimulates growth of blood vessels from the vascular system to provide nutrients to the tumors.

transcription of VEGF-α occurs. As the levels of VEGF-α elevate, it binds to cell surface receptors and ultimately causes increased angiogenesis, resulting in the proliferation of cells. Multiple malignancies, including metastatic breast and colorectal cancers, overexpress VEGF.[22]

Cancer Growth Rates

Like normal cells, cancer cells duplicate and grow according to their time in and movement through the cell cycle. Depending on the tissue of origin, cell growth may be rapid (e.g., hair, mucous membrane, hematopoietic cells) or slow (e.g., endometrial and neurologic tissues). The rates can also be affected by variables such as the pH of the cell; the amount of oxygen, glucose, and other nutrients available; or the existing space in which to grow. Once the growth factor binds to a receptor on or across the cell membrane, a signaling pathway is activated and communicates with other molecules in the cytoplasm until the message signal finally reaches the nucleus to direct cell growth, differentiation, and survival. Any alteration to the gene may cause different protein expression and, ultimately a different outcome in cell proliferation and survival.

The primary cause of altered growth and proliferation of a cancer cell is the change in proliferative signals. If there is increased tyrosine kinase activity, reactions occur to stimulate mitotic cell division, allowing rapid and continued growth of the malignancy.[23] Growth factor receptors that are known to be oncogenic when overexpressed include epidermal growth factor receptor (EGFR), human epidermal growth factor receptor 2 (HER2/neu), and transforming growth factor beta (TGF-β). Overexpression of EGFR is associated with some lung cancers and breast, ovarian, and colorectal cancers. Almost all (80–100%) head and neck cancers overexpress EGFR; it is also associated with decreased survival rates. More aggressive breast and ovarian cancers are linked to elevated expression of HER2/neu. Tumor relapse and poor survival rates are associated with expression of both EGFR and TGF-β.[23]

Multistep Process of Carcinogenesis

The three-step theory of carcinogenesis is widely used to explain how cancer develops from a normal cell in a multistep process (**Figure 12.11** ■). In this theory, **initiation** is the first step and is set off when a cancer-causing agent damages the DNA. As a result, the DNA attempts to repair; if it is successful, there is no initiating step. If repair does not occur, the damage becomes permanent, a mutation, but it requires a promoter to transform into a malignant cell.

During **promotion**, the second step of carcinogenesis, carcinogens (promoters) are introduced to the cell. Promoters may cause genetic alteration or inhibit apoptosis of the cell. They can also cause reversible or irreversible DNA damage. If the damage is reversible, there are factors that inhibit the promoters. Cancer-reversing or cancer-suppressing agents such as vitamins, flavonoids, and indoles can modify cancer risk.[24] Immune function, age, or hormonal factors of the host may inhibit the promoters. Time or dosage limits of exposure to the promoter may not be enough to cause the transforming alteration to the cell. Characteristics of promoters include (1) having the ability to induce tumors in initiated cells, (2) causing tumors only when applied *after* the initiating factor, (3) having a threshold level with both dose and time interval between dosing, or (4) being both an initiator and a promoter (e.g., cigarette smoke, alcohol, asbestos). There is clonal expansion with tumor growth.[24]

If there is irreversible damage to the DNA, the outcome is **progression** with accumulation of mutations and continued cellular transformation with increasing potential for local invasion and/or metastasis.[24] Specific symptoms associated with progression are based on the cancer type and site of invasion or metastasis.

Adults and children can develop cancers in the same parts of the body, but the time of onset and types of symptoms may vary. Childhood cancers tend to originate in mesenchymal (connective, bone, cartilage, circulatory, and lymphatic systems) tissue or neural tissue and are not recognizable at a premalignant stage. They have short latency periods, grow rapidly, and are aggressively invasive. ■

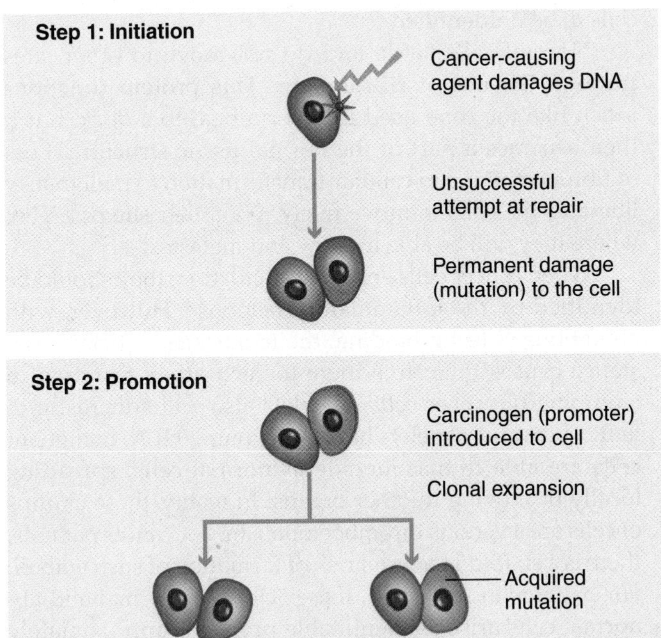

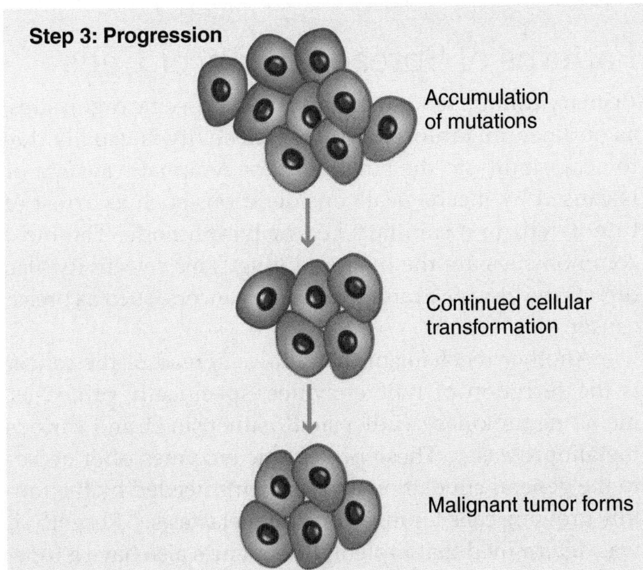

Figure 12.11 ■ The three-step theory of carcinogenesis.

Check Your Progress: Section 12.4

1. What is the difference between the stochastic and cancer stem cell models of cancer?
2. How do cancer stem cells produce an exacerbation after years of a remission?
3. Why do cancers grow more rapidly and aggressively in children than in adults?

12.5 Cancer Invasion and Metastasis

Once the cellular DNA has accumulated driver mutations, the normal cell begins transforming and gaining traits that enable it to grow, spread locally, invade the lymphatic system, and metastasize to other areas of the body (**Figure 12.12** ■). Mechanisms of cancer invasion are described below. The patterns of spread of cancer cells may depend on the type of cancer and the host's immune status.

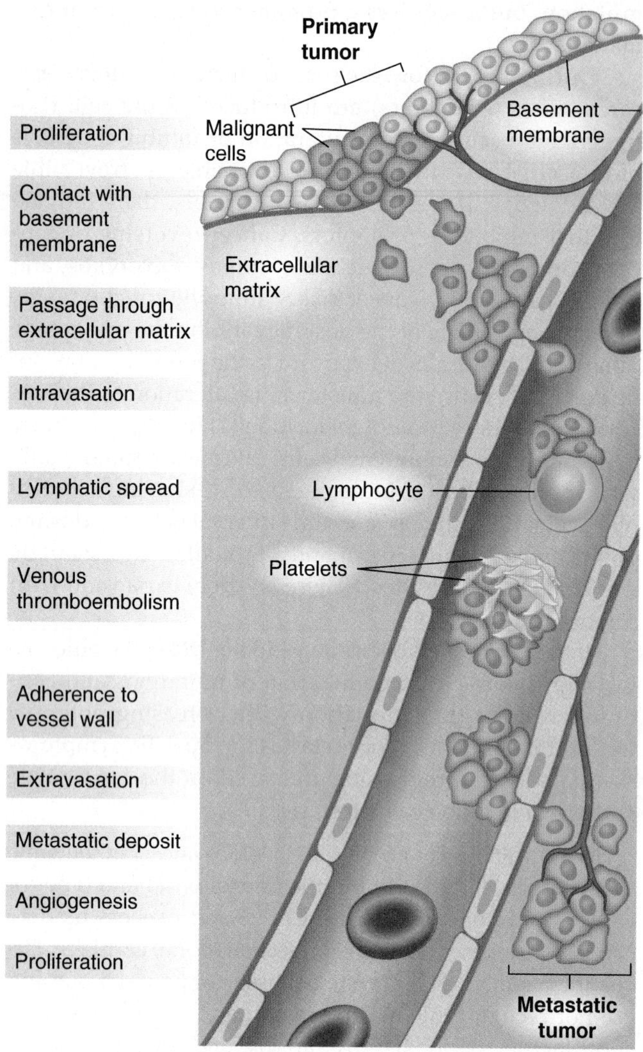

Figure 12.12 ■ Cancer invasion and metastasis. Transformed cells initially remained confined to their site or origination (in situ). As the cells lose their fibronectin and cellular matrix (including the cytoskeleton infrastructure), they gain the ability to intravasate into the circulatory systems of the blood and lymphatics. Cells then become trapped in confined spaces and begin the process of angiogenesis and cell growth in a secondary site.

Mechanisms of Cancer Invasion and Metastasis

After transformation, a malignant cell begins to exhibit a number of changes in cellular functions. Altered cytoskeletal control causes the cell to lose internal and external functions. Internally, the loss of cytoskeleton structure prevents normal function of the microtubules, which are responsible for chromosome separation before division of the cell.[25] The modification of external cytoskeleton causes the cell to lose rigidity, making it more amenable to continued proliferation.[25] Once normal cells have finished replication, they come into contact with adjacent cell membranes, and their growth should be inhibited. Malignant cells lose this trait, and even though they are in contact with the cell next to them, they continue to grow and proliferate. As was noted above, the repetitive movement through the cell cycle allows the malignancy to have continued replication; thus, they appear to grow faster than a normal cell even though their time through a cell cycle is the same.

The proteins, glycoproteins, and glycolipids on the surface of the cellular membrane have enhanced mobility, perhaps owing in part to loss of cytoskeletal control. Normally, the human leukocyte antigen (HLA) is responsible for participating in recognition and targeting nonself-antigens for destruction. In cancer, it may have an inhibitory effect on natural killer cells, dendritic cells, and T cells, inducing these cells to be tolerant of foreign tissue, much like that seen with tolerance of the fetus during pregnancy. Finally, the HLA can be lost from the cell surface, allowing cancer cells to be unidentified.[2,26]

Normal cells settle and do not move to other sites through the use of **fibronectin**. This protein functions much like the rope used to moor a boat to a dock, but it then becomes a part of the normal tissue structure. Loss of fibronectin due to cellular transformation to malignancy liberates the cells to move freely to another site or organ, where they will be able to grow and metastasize.[27]

When cancer cells enter the circulation, they should be identified by the inflammatory response. However, with alterations in lectin binding, the leukocytes' "sticky" substance causes them to adhere to each other, resulting in clumping of cancer cells. Platelets also will adhere. Since leukocytes and platelets have functioning HLA, malignant cells are able to masquerade as normal cells, spreading locally or moving to other organs. In reality, these clumps of cells are a venous thromboembolism. For cancer patients, there is a sixfold increased risk of formation of such emboli. For patients in remission, these "clots" of normal and abnormal cells arise as identifiable problems approximately 6 months before a diagnosed exacerbation of the malignant disease.[28]

Patterns of Spread of Cancer Cells

Primary tumors tend to metastasize to specific organ sites, as outlined in **Table 12.2** ■. The selectivity is usually due to accessibility to the circulatory or lymphatic system or is caused by mechanical considerations such as arrest of tumor cells in a capillary bed or lymph node. The most common sites are the liver and lung. This selectivity also directs the biopsy strategy for some cancers, such as breast cancer.

Another mechanism that allows spread of the cancer is the secretion of lytic enzymes, specifically proteases, including urokinase, cathepsin B, cathepsin D, and various metalloproteases. These proteolytic enzymes offer access to the general circulation and nutrients needed by the rapidly growing cells for invasion and metastasis.[29] Recently, it was determined that proteolytic enzymes also have a function in the development of cancer.[2,30] The metalloproteases exert their effects by degrading structural components of

Table 12.2 Common Sites of Spread for Metastatic Tumors

Primary Tumor Site	Most Common Metastatic Sites
Breast	Axillary regional lymph nodes, contralateral breast via lymphatics, lung, pleura, liver, bone, brain
Colon	Regional lymph nodes, liver, lung, direct spread to urinary bladder or stomach, peritoneum
Kidney	Lung, liver, bone, adrenal gland
Ovary	Peritoneum, regional lymph nodes, lung, liver
Pancreas	Liver, stomach by direct spread, colon, lung peritoneum
Prostate	Bone, regional lymph nodes, adrenal gland
Stomach	Liver, lung, peritoneum
Testis	Regional lymph nodes, lung, liver
Thyroid	Bone, liver, lung
Urinary bladder	Direct spread to rectum, colon, prostate, ureter, vagina, bone, regional lymph nodes, lung, peritoneum, liver, brain
Uterus	Regional lymph nodes, lung, liver, ovary, vagina, bone

SOURCES: Based on Criscitiello, C., Andre, F., Thompson, A., et al. (2014). Biopsy confirmation of metastatic sites in breast cancer patients: Clinical impact and future perspectives. *Breast Cancer Research, 16*, 205, doi:10.1186/bcr3630; Riihimaki, M., Hemminki, A., Fallah, M., Thomsen, H., Sundquist, K., Sundquist, J., & Hemminki, K. (2014). Metastatic sites in lung cancer. *Lung Cancer, 86*, 78–84; Weidle, U. H., Maisel, D., Klostermann, S., Weiss, E. H., & Schmitt, M. (2011). Differential splicing generates new transmembrane receptor and extracellular matrix-related targets for antibody-based therapy of cancer. *Cancer Genomics & Proteomics, 8*, 211–226.

the extracellular matrix while regulating growth factors, cell adhesion molecules and other proteinases, allowing transformation into a malignant cell.[30] Another group of proteases, the ADAMS family, cause shedding of the extracellular domains of growth factors, cytokines, and adhesion proteins, so they cannot bind along the outside of the plasma membrane of the cell (**Figure 12.13** ■). This prevents remodeling of the cell. Because protein receptors are not bound to the membrane for initiation of the signaling process, this leads to lack of intracellular signaling, allowing malignant transformation of a cell through angiogenesis and enhanced cellular proliferation.[29,30]

Once malignant cells are able to leave their site of origin and metastasize to different organ or tissue sites, some of their pattern of spread depends on the ectopic hormones produced by the cancer. See also, the discussion of paraneoplastic syndromes later in the chapter. For example, prostate and breast cancers secrete osteoblast growth factors (ObGFs), and breast cancer will also secrete osteoclast activating factors (OcAFs). Increased ObGFs cause increased pressure within the bone, owing to more bone being laid down, resulting in a pathogenic fracture. Increased OcAFs cause more breaking down of the bone network, owing to loss of bony matrix, resulting in a fragile structure and ultimately pathogenic fracture. Hence, pathogenic fractures in patients with cancer occur but are caused by two different mechanisms.

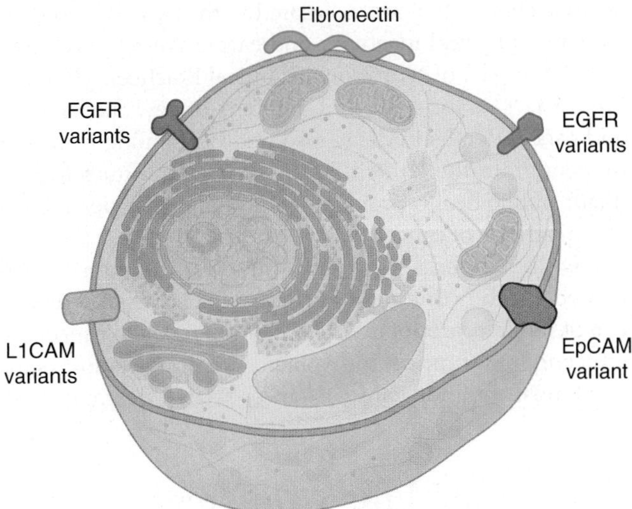

Figure 12.13 ■ ADAMS proteases cause changes to the matrix of the cell by inhibiting cell adhesion to the membrane and shedding the extracellular domains of growth factors and fibronectin so the cell cannot adhere, causing diminished ability for growth factor–induced signaling, allowing transformation of the malignant cell.

Laura Beckman: Application

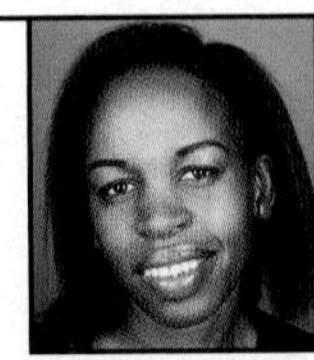

The nurse encourages Ms. Beckman to come to the office to talk with the physician and have a clinical breast examination. Ms. Beckman agrees to make the appointment. She also decides to search the Internet for information about "breast lumps" and learns some frightening information about cancer and metastasis. Her left arm hurts, and she is certain that a malignancy has spread to her bones and she will soon have a broken arm. By the time of her appointment with the physician, she is crying and certain that she will need to have both breasts removed and will die before her 18-month-old daughter is 3 years old.

3. What is a possible reason that Ms. Beckman's breast lump has increased in size?
4. Explain the pathophysiology that led Ms. Beckman to believe that she will soon have a broken arm.

Check Your Progress: Section 12.5

1. Why are cancer patients at an increased risk for developing thromboemboli?
2. Primary tumors of the kidney commonly metastasize to which organs?
3. What is the role of human leukocyte antigen (HLA) in cancer proliferation?

12.6 Epidemiology of Cancer

Globally, cancer is the leading cause of death in economically developed countries and the second leading cause of death in developing countries.[31] These statistics are attributed to growth of the aging population in addition to lifestyle choices that are associated with cancer. Of note are smoking, physical inactivity, and eating Westernized diets (see the Impact of Nutrition in Clinical Practice).[31] Refer to **Figure 12.14** ■ for estimated numbers of new cancer cases and cancer deaths in developed and developing countries by gender. In the United States, cancer continues to be a major public health problem, with one in four deaths due to a diagnosis of cancer.[31-33]

For both men and women, the most common cancer-related death is due to lung cancer, often associated with use of tobacco products. The second is prostate cancer for men and breast cancer for women. Colorectal cancer is the third most common cause of cancer-related death for both genders.[34]

Gender and Ethnic Differences in Cancers

For all races, breast cancer is the most common type of cancer in women, and prostate cancer is the most common type in men. Black men have the highest overall cancer incidence and death rates; Asian and Pacific Islander men have the lowest rates. Cancer incidence and mortality rates for all cancers except kidney cancer are higher for black men than for white men. Major factors that contribute to racial disparities affecting health vary by cancer site and include frequency of the risk factor and availability of excellent healthcare.[35] For men of all races except those of Hispanic origin, cancer of the lung remains the most commonly diagnosed malignancy (64.7%), though the incidence has dropped, probably as a result of intensive antismoking and lung cancer prevention campaigns. Nevertheless, the cancer with the highest death rate for males and females continues to be lung cancer.[36] Refer to **Figure 12.15** ■ for the estimated incidence of the ten leading cancer types in males and females in the United States in 2012.

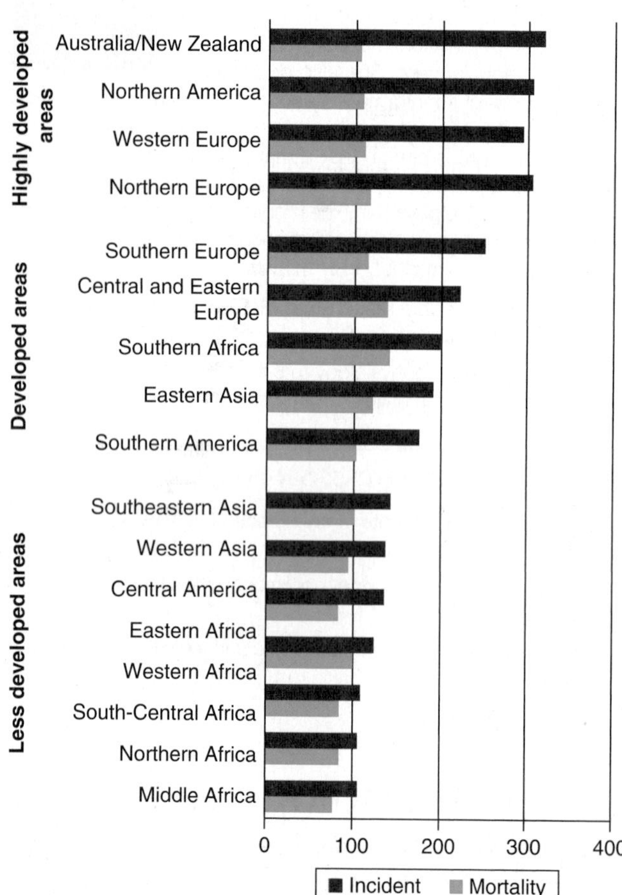

Figure 12.14 ■ Cancer cases and deaths in developed and developing countries.

For women of reproductive age, cancer is the second most common cause of death. The incidence of cancer during pregnancy is approximately 0.07–0.1%. The four cancers that occur most commonly during pregnancy are cervical cancer, breast cancer, melanoma, and lymphoma (mostly Hodgkin lymphoma).[37–39] ■

Cancer across the Lifespan

For children between 1 and 14 years of age, cancer is the second most common cause of death, but it is still relatively rare for children in this age range. Leukemias are the most commonly diagnosed malignancy during childhood, at 30%. Brain tumors and other nervous system tumors are second, at 20%.[38] ■

In children, teenagers, and adults younger than 39 years of age, leukemia is the most common cancer-related cause of death. Young women are the exception from the ages of 20 to 39 years, when the most common cause is breast cancer.

In men 40–59 years of age, the most common cause of death is lung cancer.[35] In the United States, cancer is the second leading cause of death, behind heart disease, in individuals older than 85 years of age. For those younger than 85 years of age, cancer is now the leading cause of death. ■

Effect of Geographic Location on Incidence of Different Cancers

A variety of factors affect the geographic variation of cancer occurrence globally, including the prevalence of risk factors, availability and use of screening, treatment availability, and age. Many of the leading cancers in the world are due to infection (15% of all cancers). In women, these include cervical cancer caused by the human papillomavirus (HPV), approximately 70% being associated with types 16 and 18. Vaccines are available for adolescent females, but screening continues to be important, since HPV types 6 and 11 are not affected by the vaccine.[33] Liver cancer is commonly associated with hepatitis B virus (HBV). Globally, 60% of cases of this cancer are associated with developing countries. The highest rates are found in parts of Asia and sub-Saharan Africa, where approximately 8% of the population is chronically infected with HBV.[13] HBV infections continue to rise in many parts of the world including the United States and Central Europe.

Impact of Nutrition in Clinical Practice

Cancer Prevention: Parsley, Sage, Rosemary, and Thyme

Joanne Kouba

Research studies on the role of nutrition in cancer prevention often evaluate a specific nutrient with regard to cancer risk, such as fat intake and the risk for breast cancer. However, research trends have shifted to assessment of broader patterns of food intake. Recent reviews have reported that diets with at least five daily helpings of a variety of fruits and vegetables low in starch were "probable" to prevent cancers of the mouth, pharynx and larynx, esophagus, stomach, and lung. There was "limited" evidence that these natural foods would prevent cancers of the nasopharynx, lung, colorectum, ovary, endometrium, pancreas, or liver.[1] Evidence does suggest an association between high dietary intake of fiber and prevention of colorectal cancer.[2] To be sure, this adds layers of complexity. The first is measurement issues. Many people are not aware of what spices and herbs are in mixed dishes, their form, source, and so on. Another issue is that a single ingredient may contain several bioactive compounds; for instance, ginger contains curcumin, zingiberone, ingeral, and paradol. Put another way, a single bioactive compound can be found in multiple ingredients; curcumin, for example, is present in turmeric, ginger, and mustard.[3]

Despite these concerns, research indicates that bioactive ingredients in spices and herbs are involved in reducing cancer risk through antimicrobial, antioxidant, and anticarcinogenic effects. Potential mechanisms for the antibacterial action of herbs and spices may be disruption of the bacterial phospholipid cell membrane, resulting in permeability, loss of cellular compounds, and damage to genetic material. Studies report antimicrobial effects of herbs and spices on gram-negative and gram-positive bacteria. However, this effect varies, depending on the form of herbs and spices used (e.g., fresh, dried, ground) or the combinations of herbs and spices. Several strains of *Helicobacter pylori* bacteria increase the risk of stomach, liver, gallbladder and intestinal cancers. Interestingly, oil extracted from cinnamon bark contains potent bactericidal inhibitors of *H. pylori*.[2]

An imbalance of the oxidant–antioxidant environment in the human body is hypothesized to impair cell immunity, damage DNA, and cause mutations that contribute to development of cancer. Many herbs and spices have antioxidant properties and are therefore the focus of research. Potent antioxidant activity has been reported in both dried (cloves, oregano, ginger, cinnamon, allspice, cumin, ginger) and fresh (sage, peppermint, thyme) herbs and spices. Physiologic alterations due to inflammation can increase the risk for cervical, liver, esophageal, and colorectal cancers, particularly in the presence of other genetic or immunologic factors. Reduction of inflammatory response may reduce the risk for cancer. Herbs and spices are the subject of research related to this potentially protective mechanism against cancer, especially considering adverse effects of anti-inflammatory medications.

The nuclear transcription factor NF-kappa promotes expression of genes involved in cancer cell survival, angiogenesis, and cancer proliferation. Curcumin inhibits activation of NF-kappa. Other laboratory and animal studies suggest that turmeric, coriander, fennel, cumin, saffron, and quercitin are involved in similar pathways that may limit tumor division and metastasis.[3]

For thousands of years, herbs and spices have been used to enhance taste. Results from laboratory and animal studies of the role of herbs and spices in cancer prevention or treatment are interesting and promising, and this role is the subject of current research. However, the research is clouded by issues of valid measurement, lack of standardized preparations, questionable molecular targets, variable dosing, and undocumented toxicities. Healthcare providers can anticipate the development of evidence-based recommendations when this information is obtained; in the meantime, we should all enjoy a bounty of fruits and vegetables flavored with a variety of herbs and spices.

References

1. God, J., Tate, P. L., Larcom, L. L. (2011). Red raspberries have antioxidant effects that play a minor role in the killing of stomach and colon cancer cells. *Nutrition Research, 30*(11), 777–782.
2. American Cancer Society. (2017). Can colorectal cancer be prevented? Retrieved from https://www.cancer.org/cancer/colon-rectal-cancer/causes-risks-prevention/prevention.html
3. Blackadar, C. B. (2016). Historical review of the causes of cancer. *World Journal of Clinical Oncology 7*(1), 54–86.

Globally, stomach cancer is the most common infection-associated cancer. This incidence is more common in developing countries (25%) than in countries classified as developed (8%) economically.[33] Stomach cancer caused by *Helicobacter pylori* infection is twice as common in men as in women. The significant decrease in the global incidence of stomach cancer is believed to be due to the availability of refrigeration for fresh fruits and vegetables and the introduction of more sensitive screening in countries such as Japan.[33]

Globally, research shows that as individuals age, they are more at risk for being diagnosed with cancer, likely because of a longer duration of exposure to carcinogenic agents. Newly diagnosed cancer cases (78%) occur more frequently in economically developed countries than in developing countries (58%). Because of environmental carcinogen exposure, certain regions may have an increased incidence of certain cancers. Leukemia is associated with occupations in radiology, some cancers in farmers are associated with exposure to pesticides, and some cancers in funeral directors are associated with exposure to formaldehyde. People who spend a lot of time in the sun without protective barriers, such as farmers, ski instructors, and welders, are at higher risk for skin cancers.[40]

Because of the burden of cancer in the United States, cancer reduction continues to be one of the goals of the *Healthy People 2020* agenda.

Check Your Progress: Section 12.6

1. What factors contribute to the high incidence of cancers in Western countries?
2. What are the three focus areas of *Healthy People 2020* in relation to prevention and early detection of cancer?
3. How does ethnicity affect cancer incidence and mortality?

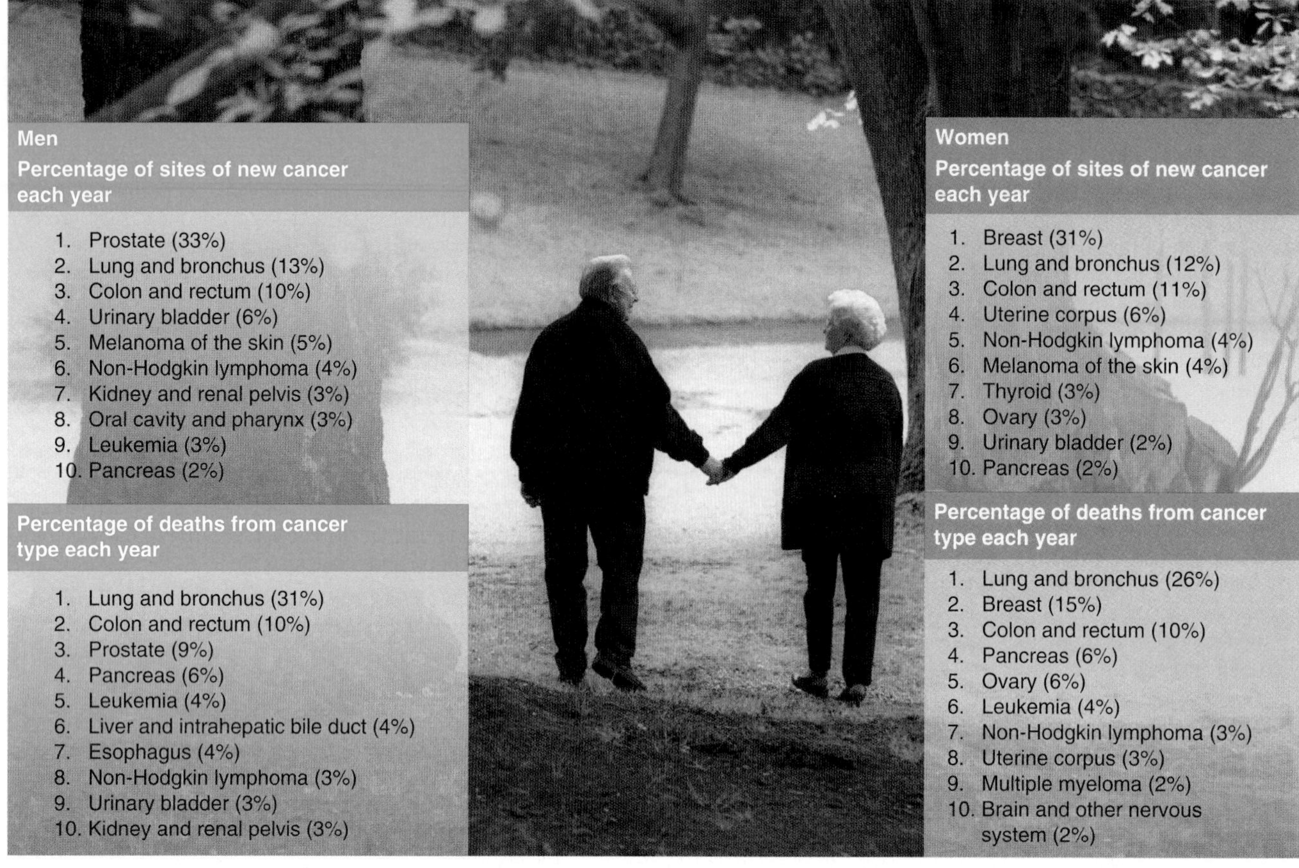
Men
Percentage of sites of new cancer each year
1. Prostate (33%)
2. Lung and bronchus (13%)
3. Colon and rectum (10%)
4. Urinary bladder (6%)
5. Melanoma of the skin (5%)
6. Non-Hodgkin lymphoma (4%)
7. Kidney and renal pelvis (3%)
8. Oral cavity and pharynx (3%)
9. Leukemia (3%)
10. Pancreas (2%)
Percentage of deaths from cancer type each year
1. Lung and bronchus (31%)
2. Colon and rectum (10%)
3. Prostate (9%)
4. Pancreas (6%)
5. Leukemia (4%)
6. Liver and intrahepatic bile duct (4%)
7. Esophagus (4%)
8. Non-Hodgkin lymphoma (3%)
9. Urinary bladder (3%)
10. Kidney and renal pelvis (3%)
Women
Percentage of sites of new cancer each year
1. Breast (31%)
2. Lung and bronchus (12%)
3. Colon and rectum (11%)
4. Uterine corpus (6%)
5. Non-Hodgkin lymphoma (4%)
6. Melanoma of the skin (4%)
7. Thyroid (3%)
8. Ovary (3%)
9. Urinary bladder (2%)
10. Pancreas (2%)
Percentage of deaths from cancer type each year
1. Lung and bronchus (26%)
2. Breast (15%)
3. Colon and rectum (10%)
4. Pancreas (6%)
5. Ovary (6%)
6. Leukemia (4%)
7. Non-Hodgkin lymphoma (3%)
8. Uterine corpus (3%)
9. Multiple myeloma (2%)
10. Brain and other nervous system (2%)

Figure 12.15 ■ A comparison of the ten leadings cancers in men and women in the United States. Note that non-melanoma skin cancers are not included.

SOURCE: Data from American Cancer Society. (2016). *Cancer facts & figures 2016*. Available at http://www.cancer.org/acs/groups/content/@research/documents/document/acspc-047079.pdf.

Healthy People 2020

Cancer Reduction

Goal: "Reduce the number of new cancer cases, as well as the illness, disability, and death caused by cancer."[1]

Why Is Cancer Important?

Despite advances in understanding of the pathophysiology of cancer, which have led to new treatments that have resulted in decreases in incidence and mortality from cancer, cancer is still the second leading cause of death in the United States.[2] As the Healthy People website states, "Many cancers are preventable by reducing risk factors such as use of tobacco products, physical inactivity and poor nutrition, obesity, and ultraviolet light exposure."[1] Also many cases of cervical cancer can be prevented by vaccination against human papillomavirus, and many cases of liver cancer can be prevented by vaccination against hepatitis B virus. Cancer risk reduction involves education of the public and access to screening tests and to programs such as smoking cessation and weight reduction programs.

Objectives: The *Healthy People 2020* objectives focus on the prevention and early detection of cancer, which increase the likelihood of long-term survival. The three focus areas are as follows:

- Reduction in cancer death rates for lung, breast, cervical, colorectal, prostate, and oropharyngeal cancers and melanoma, the most aggressive of the skin cancers
- Increasing the percentage of individuals who are counseled for and receive screening for breast, cervical, colorectal, and prostate cancer based on the most current evidence-based guidelines available for screening for these cancers
- Increasing the percentage of individuals who decrease their exposure to ultraviolet radiation from sunlight and artificial ultraviolet light used in tanning salons.

Based on current statistics, such as 50.6 lung cancer deaths occurring per 100,000 individuals each year, a reasonable objective for improvement over the decade is determined. For example, a Healthy People objective is to achieve a 10% reduction in lung cancer deaths to 45.5 deaths per 100,000 individuals each year. At the Healthy People website, there are links to information for guidance in achieving each objective. These include a link to the U.S. Preventive Services Task Force (https://www.uspreventiveservicestaskforce.org) with information about risk assessment and screening tests recommended for various types of cancer.

References

1. Healthy People. (2017). *Topics and objectives: Cancer*. Available at https://www.healthypeople.gov/2020/topicsobjectives2020/overview.aspx?topicid=5
2. Kochanek, K. D., Murphy, S. L., Xu, J., & Tejada-Vera, B. (2016). Deaths: Final data for 2014. Available at https://www.cdc.gov/nchs/data/nvsr/nvsr65/nvsr65_04.pdf

12.7 Clinical Manifestations of Cancer

The effects and symptoms associated with cancer will depend on the location and size of the tumor. Most cancers will be painless in the initial stage of the malignant process. However, as the tumor enlarges, presses on nerves, and impinges on space, other effects will emerge. Symptoms associated with the cancer will depend on factors such as the role of the tissue in primary body function (e.g., gastrointestinal) or space available for tumor growth, inflammation related to the cancer, or angiogenesis. Common signs of cancer are weight loss and cachexia due to the metabolic demands of the malignancy.[2]

The disease of cancer is similar in children and adults. The malignancies are due to accumulation of genetic alterations and have the capability of moving from the primary site of origin to a metastatic region. A diagnosis of metastatic disease carries a poor prognosis for both adults and children. For both patient populations, multimodality treatments with or without adjuvant therapy can be beneficial, depending on the tumor type and stage of diagnosis. Once a tumor has been "cured," or pushed into remission, there are still late effects that may become issues for child or adult survivors.

Common Clinical Manifestations of Cancer

The American Cancer Society developed the acronym **CAUTION** to assist the public in remembering common signs and symptoms of cancer.[40] Each letter in the word refers to the first initial of the following phrases:

Change in bowel or bladder habits
A sore that does not heal
Unusual bleeding or discharge
Thickening or lump in the breast or any part of the body
Indigestion or difficulty swallowing
Obvious change in a mole
Nagging cough or hoarseness.

While these do not address each type of cancer, they do target lung, breast, colon, prostate, and skin cancers. Many people do not know that the most common type of cancer is skin cancer.[40]

Another misconception is that a cancer will be painful and therefore obvious to the patient and healthcare providers. In reality, an early-stage cancer does not cause pain unless it is pressing against a nerve or blood supply, causing hypoxia in the area. Many times, early-stage cancers are painless, allowing the false belief that seeing a doctor is not necessary. This leads to diagnosis of a cancer at a later time when it could have been diagnosed early. An example of a cancer that causes pain only during certain times of the day is osteosarcoma, which is a rare cancer that may be associated with pain at the site of the cancer at night. This is because the muscles and tendons that provide support during the day are relaxed at night, allowing pressure from the tumor to inflict discomfort at the site of origin.

Common signs and symptoms associated with childhood cancers can be remembered by using the first letters in the words **CHILDHOOD CANCER** to assist in remembering the clinical manifestations[41]:

Continued, unexplained weight loss
Headaches, frequently with early morning vomiting
Increased swelling or persistent pain in the bones, joints, back, or legs
Lump or mass, especially in the abdomen, neck, chest, pelvis, or armpits
Development of excessive bruising, bleeding, or rash
Hard time sleeping due to persistent pain at night
Obvious paleness
Occur suddenly and persist
Diseases that are uncommon.

Constant infections
A whitish color behind the pupil
Nausea that persist or vomiting without nausea
Constant tiredness
Eye or vision changes
Recurring or persistent fevers of unknown origin. ■

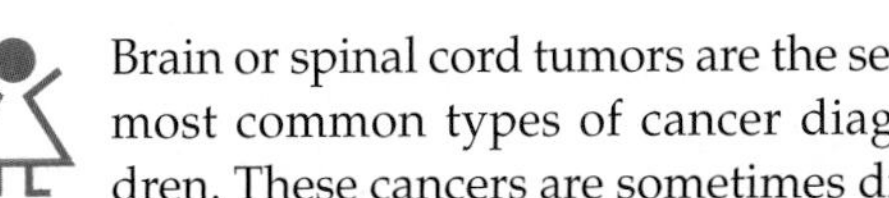

Brain or spinal cord tumors are the second and third most common types of cancer diagnosed in children. These cancers are sometimes difficult to diagnose because symptoms are not the same for every child and are frequently associated with other childhood disorders. Common brain tumor symptoms include morning headache or headache that goes away after vomiting; frequent nausea and vomiting without temperature elevation or stomach discomfort; loss of balance and trouble walking; unusual changes in personality or behavior; and vision, hearing, and speech problems. Symptoms for spinal cord tumors include back pain or pain that spreads from the back toward the arm or legs, trouble urinating, change in bowel habits, weakness in the legs, and trouble walking.[42] All of these symptoms are due to increasing intracranial pressure or spinal cord compression. Depending on the symptoms, a biopsy may be attempted to remove a sample of tissue, using a needle, which may be guided by imaging diagnostics such as computerized tomography (CT) or magnetic resonance imaging (MRI). ■

Pregnant woman often ignore many symptoms of a potential cancer, attributing them to physiologic changes associated with pregnancy. Multiple factors have the potential to affect the pregnancy and natural history of the tumor. The diagnosis and cancer staging workup and treatment of cancer in pregnant women will affect the woman, the unborn fetus (or multiple fetuses), and perhaps the woman's future fertility and/or early menopause.[39] ■

Laura Beckman: Application

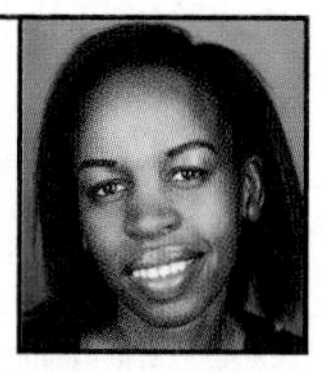

Ms. Beckman's history reveals information consistent with the signs and symptoms summarized by the acronym used with cancer. The development of a lump is a significant sign, and it is important to note that although the lump is present, it is not tender and does not fluctuate in relation to her menstrual cycle. On physical examination, no discharge is noted, and the site does not elicit tenderness on palpation. No lumps are noted in the axillary region. It is important to provide information to Ms. Beckman about other physiologic changes that can occur and to provide additional information about the diagnostic procedures that will be recommended. An ultrasound will generally precede a mammogram, with the possibility of other diagnostic evaluations.

5. How should the nurse respond when Ms. Beckman says that her breast lump cannot be cancerous because it is not painful?
6. When Ms. Beckman asks what signs and symptoms of cancer she should report, how should the nurse reply?

Edgar Graham: Application

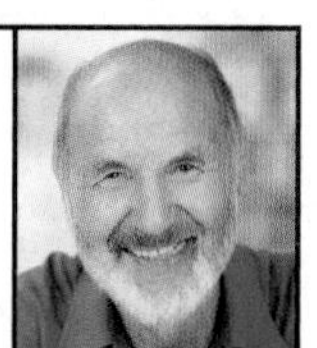

The presence of rectal bleeding not associated with hemorrhoids is one of the warning signs provided in the above acronym. The presence of unusual bleeding requires careful follow-up and evaluation, particularly in situations in which a number of family members already had a hereditary cancer. For an individual at high risk, such as Mr. Graham, education should be provided about the diagnostic testing that will be recommended.

5. Besides bleeding, what other CAUTION signs and symptoms should Mr. Graham report that are likely directly related to his risk for colon cancer?
6. Because of the risk of metastasis from the colon, what other CAUTION signs and symptoms should Mr. Graham report?

Local Effects

Local effects of cancer are linked to the tissue source of the tumor; the increase in size of the tumor and pressure it exerts on surrounding cells, blood vessels, and nerves; and the location of the tumor. For example, tumors of the lung may grow and block the bronchus, causing shortness of breath. A brain tumor may cause personality changes, blindness, headache, or tremors, depending on the location of the tumor in the brain. Leukemia will cause symptoms based on the type of blood cell involved; impaired leukocyte functions will lead to increased infection, platelet alterations result in bruising and bleeding, and if the red blood cell number is increased, there can be an increased possibility of blood clots. Other cancers, such as multiple myeloma, might cause hypercalcemia, and liver cancers can cause jaundice.[2]

Systemic Effects

Systemic effects associated with cancer are primarily due to cytokines secreted by the tumor. Two common cytokines are tumor necrosis factor and interleukin 6, which cause fever, cachexia, and fatigue. **Tumor necrosis factor (TNF)** is secreted by several different cell types, particularly those associated with the immune system. As these phagocytic cells burst into a feeding frenzy, as when activated by cancer cells, they begin to secrete more and more TNF. Consider a person who has been diagnosed with a terminal cancer. The macrophages are both functioning as part of the inflammatory response, trying to search out and destroy the invading tumor cells, and also being activated and used by the cancer cells to secrete factors needed for cancer cell survival, such as those needed to support angiogenesis. As the tumor grows in size and number of metastases, the macrophages continue to divide but also are secreting TNF, which is a cytokine associated with cachexia and muscle wasting in individuals with cancer and other chronic illnesses. Interleukin 6 is secreted during inflammation. As the inflammatory and immune responses combat the malignancy, this interleukin causes fatigue associated with many cancers both in the early stages before diagnosis and especially when the patient's condition becomes terminal.[2]

Paraneoplastic Syndromes

Infrequently, a malignancy will produce hormones, peptides, or cytokines or will cross-react with normal tissues to cause symptoms distant from the tumor or its metastasis. These are thought to be produced ectopically (out of place, i.e., by cells that do not normally produce the substance) or due to antibodies produced by the immune system and directed against the tumors that cross-react with and damage other tissues.[43] On the basis of clusters of symptoms, these conditions are labeled **paraneoplastic syndromes**, and at times, they are the first indication that an individual has an undiagnosed cancer. The four primary types of syndromes are endocrine, hematologic, dermatologic, and neurologic. Cancers that are most commonly associated with paraneoplastic syndromes are small cell lung cancer, breast cancer, gynecologic tumors, and hematologic malignancies. Treatment of paraneoplastic syndromes with symptomatology are directed toward the malignancy but also to correct immunosuppression, electrolyte imbalance, and hormonal instability.[43]

Endocrine paraneoplastic syndromes are commonly seen with malignancies such as small cell lung cancer, pancreatic cancers, and breast cancer. Cushing syndrome may be due to ectopic production of adrenocorticotropic hormone (ACTH) or ACTH-like molecules and is most likely to be linked with small cell cancer of the lung. The symptoms of Cushing syndrome are due to cortisol excess leading to hyperglycemia, hypokalemia, hypertension, central obesity, and moon facies. The central obesity common to Cushing syndrome is not found with paraneoplastic Cushing syndrome.[44]

Syndrome of inappropriate antidiuretic hormone (SIADH) secretion is an endocrine paraneoplastic syndrome most commonly associated with small cell cancer of the lung and is seen in 1–2% of all patients with cancer. While this seems to be a rare syndrome, it affects up to 45% of patients with a diagnosis of small cell cancer of the lung. Because antidiuretic hormone leads to water resorption in the kidneys, the syndrome causes increased water in all fluid compartments and a normal or elevated blood volume and hyponatremia without edema. Mild symptoms include headache, weakness, and memory difficulties progressing to altered mental status, seizures, coma, respiratory collapse, and death.[44]

Hypercalcemia associated with malignancy occurs in up to 10% of terminal cancer patients and carries a 30-day mortality rate of almost 50%. The cause is a parathyroid hormone (PTH)–related protein secreted by tumor cells most commonly linked with squamous cell tumors. When this protein binds to the PTH receptors in the bone and kidney, phosphate and calcium regulation is affected. Metastasis to the bone of some cancers increases osteolytic activity, causing hypercalcemia. These cancers include breast cancer, multiple myeloma, and lymphomas. Very rarely, vitamin D may be secreted by lymphomas, or there may be ectopic production of PTH.[44]

Paraneoplastic hematologic syndromes cause anemia of chronic disease, leukocytosis, thrombocytosis, eosinophilia, basophilia and disseminated intravascular coagulation. Problems with the red blood cells are seen with renal cancers and hepatomas. Monoclonal gammopathies are also seen with plasma cell cancers such as multiple myeloma, but many are labeled as MGUS (monoclonal gammopathies of unknown significance).

The neurologic paraneoplastic syndromes include types of peripheral neuropathies and cerebellar and other central neurologic paraneoplastic syndromes.[43,44] These syndromes are rare in cancer, affecting only 1% of all patients with cancer.[43] Patients with small cell cancer of the lung, lymphomas or multiple myelomas are at highest risk to develop these syndromes. The most common peripheral neuropathy is a distal sensorimotor polyneuropathy causing mild motor weakness, sensory loss, and absent distal reflexes. The symptoms are the same as those associated with chronic illness. Other paraneoplastic syndromes include the Hodgkin-associated Guillain-Barré syndrome and small cell cancer of the lung–associated Eaton-Lambert syndromes.[43,44]

Progressive bilateral leg and arm ataxia with dysarthria may be associated with subacute cerebellar degeneration. Dementia, nystagmus, and an extensor plantar sign such as a Babinski sign can also result from this neurologic paraneoplastic syndrome.

Dermatologic paraneoplastic syndromes cause a variety of cutaneous symptoms. Itching, which is the most common, is especially associated with leukemia and lymphomas. Flushing is due to vasoactive substances from the tumors. Ichthyosis is a desquamation of the extensor surface of the extremities and is found with lymphomas and with cancers of the lung, breast, ovary, and cervix.[44]

Check Your Progress: Section 12.7

1. What common symptoms are associated with a brain tumor in children?
2. What is the underlying cause of hypercalcemia in some patients with malignancies?
3. What is the mechanism that produces local cancer effects?

12.8 Linking Pathophysiology to Diagnosis and Treatment

Cancer screening, diagnosis, and follow-up in response to treatment involve assessment of clinical manifestations of cancer, measurement of tumor markers in body fluids, examination of biopsy samples in a pathology laboratory, and radiographic tests.

Tumor Markers

Tumor markers are molecules in the blood, urine, or other body fluids that indicate a change in the status of tumor growth. Because some, such as carcinoembryonic antigen (CEA), are also found with normal tissue or inflammation, they are used as a baseline for comparison after diagnosis and treatment of a cancer. Sometimes they are specific to a cancer, such as HER2 and breast cancer, and are used to determine treatment, or they can indicate progression of disease (such as CEA). CA-125 is commonly used to track for detection and follow-up after ovarian cancer treatment.

Biopsies and Histologic Findings

A **biopsy** is extraction of a tissue sample to more closely evaluate the presence or status of a disease. The initial surgical biopsy provides the tissue sample for pathologic analysis of a tumor or lesion (abnormal growth). There are several types of biopsies, including fine needle aspiration (use of a needle to aspirate disaggregated cells from a solid lesion), core needle biopsy (removal of a tissue sample in the lumen of a needle), incisional biopsy (surgical removal of a small sample of suspicious tissue), and excisional biopsy (removal of the entire tissue sample). Some surgical biopsy procedures use ultrasound or radiologic diagnostics to guide the collection of abnormal tissue. Careful examination of the tissue by a pathologist provides the histology grade of the tumor, which is needed for planning treatment.[45]

One type of biopsy includes identification of the sentinel lymph node to screen for metastasis. A radiographic dye or radioactive isotope is injected around the tumor site. The surgeons wait for the sentinel lymph node or nodes that drain the tumor site to take up the dye or radioactive isotope. (The lymph node is labeled the *sentinel node* because it is the first to be reached with lymphatic drainage from the tumor.) The node or nodes that take up the dye are biopsied. If there are no metastatic cells, there is no reason to schedule the more extensive axillary dissection, which carries a risk of infection and future lymphedema.[46]

Laura Beckman: Application

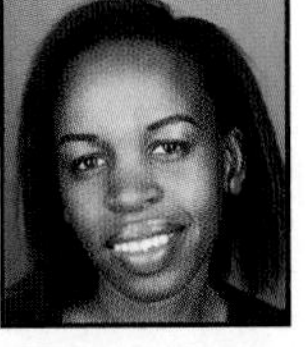

Ultrasound reveals a solid mass in Ms. Beckman's breast. To provide diagnostic certainty, a needle biopsy is scheduled to remove a small piece of tissue for analysis. Considering the high degree of concern Ms. Beckman is already displaying about the possibility of cancer, it is important to allow her the time to share her concerns and provide information about each test along the way, particularly because it will generally take 7–14 days to receive a result from the pathology laboratory.

7. What is the role of a biopsy in the diagnosis of Ms. Beckman's tumor?
8. How should the nurse respond when Ms. Beckman asks whether the needle biopsy is a surgical procedure?

Radiographic Tests

Positron emission tomography (PET) is used to identify increased metabolism. In oncology, this test will identify distant metastatic lesions to determine how many there are and where they are located, information that will be used for future treatment and/or follow-up planning.

X-ray computerized tomography (CT) uses a computer to construct a series of cross-sectional scans obtained by examining body organs with x-ray. Contrast can be added to distinguish between benign and malignant tumors and between high- and low-grade tumors (based on angiogenesis present in high-grade tumors). The CT can also be combined with the PET to increase the sensitivity and specificity of cancer detection.[47]

Edgar Graham: Application

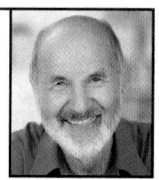

Mr. Graham requests that genetic testing be performed to help identify whether he has developed colorectal cancer. Such testing usually produces more reliable findings in individuals younger than 35 years of age, and given Mr. Graham's family history, it may not provide any additional information. A virtual colonoscopy may be ordered, in which air is injected into the colon and a CT scan is performed.

7. What is the purpose of a CT scan in the diagnosis of cancer in Mr. Graham?
8. On the basis of Mr. Graham's family history of colon cancer, would he be more likely to have a germ line mutation or a somatic mutation?

Staging and Grading of Cancers

As was noted above, cancer is a group of diseases that share specific characteristics associated with malignancy. To clearly communicate information about cancer to professionals, the American Joint Committee on Cancer developed a mechanism to report evidence-based anatomic staging using a classification system. The original tissue type differentiates a cancer from other types; the anatomic extent of disease and the histologic type of tissue are also included.[48] Recent progress in the molecular biology of cancer and genetics has created a need for specific markers, such as mitotic count or certain oncogenes, to be included in the staging of cancers internationally. Currently, however, the basis of cancer staging often continues to be the anatomic extent of the disease.

Malignant tumors are divided into solid tumors and hematologic tumors. Solid tumors are categorized as carcinomas or sarcomas. Prefixes identify the source (e.g., *osteo-* from bone). Hematologic malignancies originate from cells of the blood components.

There are multiple cancer staging systems, including the Jewett staging of bladder cancer, Duke's staging of colorectal cancer, and the International Federation of Gynecology and Obstetrics (FIGO) staging for gynecologic cancers. Factors that are common to each of these systems is the primary tumor location, tumor size, number of tumors, presence or absence of lymph node involvement, cell type and tumor grade, and presence or absence of metastasis.[48] In the 1980s, the tumor–node–metastasis (TNM) staging system was selected to be used globally. In the TNM staging system, "T" stands for the primary tumor, "N" denotes the absence or presence and the extent of regional lymph node involvement, and "M" represents the presence or absence of distant metastasis (**Table 12.3** ■).[48] Numbers (0–3) are used with the TNM letters to communicate the size or extent of the tumor in addition to the amount of metastasis that is present. The letter X is used to designate that a category has not been or cannot be evaluated. The *AJCC Cancer Staging Manual, 2016* provides a guide to the TNM classification for each specific tumor and histologic types.[49]

Table 12.3 TNM Characters Used in Staging System

Stage	Description
Primary Tumor (T)	
TX	Primary tumor cannot be evaluated
T0	No evidence of primary tumor
Tis	Carcinoma in situ (early cancer that has not spread to neighboring tissue)
T1, T2, T3, T4	Size and/or extent of the primary tumor
Regional Lymph Nodes (N)	
NX	Regional lymph nodes cannot be evaluated
N0	No regional lymph node involvement
N1, N2, N3	Involvement of regional lymph nodes (number and/or extent of spread)
NOTE: The suffix SN indicates that the lymph node is a sentinel node only, not a node from a complete axillary or regional dissection. The sentinel node may be either positive (+) or negative (−) for disease. See the example below.	
Distant Metastasis (M)	
M0	No distant metastasis
M1	Distant metastasis present
NOTE: The designation of M1 to indicate distant metastasis may be further specified with one or more of the following subscripts to specify sites of metastasis.	
Pulmonary	PUL
Osseous	OSS
Hepatic	HEP
Brain	BRA
Lymph nodes	LYM
Bone marrow	MAR
Pleura	PLE
Peritoneum	PER
Adrenal	ADR
Skin	SKI
Other	OTH
Example: T3 N1SN + M1PUL	

SOURCE: Reprinted with permission from *AJCC Cancer Staging Manual, Eighth Edition* (2016) published by Springer Science and Business Media LLC, www.springerlink.com.

Five classifications are used for each tumor site:

- *Clinical staging* is completed during the initial workup of the disease.
- *Pathologic staging* is completed from information identified by the pathologist.
- *Posttherapy* information is based on information after treatments (such as neoadjuvant or primary chemotherapy and radiation treatment) but before surgery.
- *Retreatment staging* is based on information obtained after exacerbation or progression of disease after treatment and a period of remission.
- *Autopsy staging* is completed by the medical examiner on the death of the patient when there was no known cancer but it was discovered postmortem.

Most treatments for cancer are designed to destroy or remove the malignant tumor or cells. The foundational knowledge of how cancer cells replicate, how they move through the cell cycle, and the growth rates for different tissue types is important to understand so that the nurse is aware of what patients are experiencing and can educate them about what to expect in regard to symptoms and needs at home as well as to monitor for adverse effects associated with treatment. Many oncology nurses work in a special care unit, and their patients require high-level and intensive care and other work in clinic or home care settings. Frequently, there are emergencies that occur in the ambulatory oncology setting.

CLINICAL POINT: Understanding the link between the pathophysiology of cancer and treatment assists healthcare providers in anticipating the physical and educational needs of patients and their families. ■

Cancers in childhood respond well to standard modalities of treatment, especially chemotherapy, with an encouraging outcome of greater than 5-year survival rates for over 80% of childhood cancers. Most young patients are cured. Leukemia, brain cancer, germ cell and trophoblastic tumors, gonad neoplasms, and renal tumors have the largest numbers of survivors.[50] ■

Cancer during pregnancy is uncommon, though as women delay childbearing to older ages, more women are being diagnosed during gestation. Breast cancer, melanoma, and cervical cancer are the most commonly diagnosed cancers during pregnancy, followed by the hematologic malignancies. The diagnostic workup is typically the same as that for nonpregnant women, based on age- and stage-matched counterparts. Once a cancer has been diagnosed, the patient should be referred to an institution that has experience working with cancer patients who are also pregnant. A multidisciplinary team approach is suggested, including an obstetrician and a neonatologist on the oncology team.

The three types of treatment for breast cancer are chemotherapy, surgery, and irradiation. The regimen should be chosen on the basis of the staging of the tumor. The results of one study identified that decisions about termination of the pregnancy, cancer treatment, or no treatment, depended on the gestational trimester, with pregnancy termination occurring in the first and second trimester.[51] ■

Surgery

Recognized as the oldest and most researched therapy for treating cancer, surgery is still the most successful method of diagnosing, treating, and curing malignancies. Surgical treatment for cancers is useful for intervention at the initial (primary) site, regional locations, or distant metastasis. When used for rehabilitation and/or palliative care (symptom control), surgery can be combined with nonsurgical interventions to improve cancer treatment, survival, quality of life and long term outcomes. Compared to earlier surgical procedures, the current protocols are more limited in the amount of tissue removed, conservative, and multimodal (use of more than one treatment strategy) due to advances in the knowledge of the biology of cancer, techniques in pathology, new genetic knowledge, and innovative clinical trial research.[45]

Chemotherapy

The use of chemotherapy, also called antineoplastic therapy, as a pharmacologic treatment for cancer is based on the principle that it will target rapidly proliferating cancer cells. Cancers proliferate rapidly because they progress continuously through the phases of the cell cycle without pausing to carry out their normal metabolic functions in the G0 phase or to repair DNA damage at checkpoints during the G1 and G2 phases of the cell cycle. This gives the impression that the cells grow more rapidly than the surrounding tissue, when in reality, the cancer and the tissue of origin have the same cell cycling time. The growth difference between normal and malignant tissue occurs because the cancer does not rest from replication but is continually moving through the cell cycle again and again. Normal tissue rests from cell division to perform specialized functions, causing the appearance of prolonging the cycling time in comparison to cancer cells originating in the same tissue. The cancer tissue has a more rapid growth rate because more cells are undergoing cell division at any one time in comparison to the normal tissue from which the cancer originated.[52]

Most chemotherapy agents target the cell cycle or specific phases in the cycle (**Table 12.4** ■). This targeting of the growth and cell division of the cancer cell causes it to be destroyed or go through apoptosis. Unfortunately, the cells of the normal tissue also have a cell cycle, and chemotherapy treatments affect normal cells with rapid growth rates, such as the hematopoietic cells, mucous membranes throughout the alimentary tract, and hair follicles. Each repetitive protocol will decrease the number of cancer cells but also destroy the normal rapidly proliferating cells, causing toxic side effects such as anemia (low red blood cells), thrombocytopenia (low platelet levels) or increased risk of infection due to neutropenia (decrease in number of phagocytic neutrophils).[52] Frequently, patients lose their hair (alopecia) as a result of the systemic effects of chemotherapy.

Chemotherapy is the treatment of choice for hematopoietic malignancies and solid tumors that have spread or metastasized beyond the borders of the tissue of origin. Typically, chemotherapy is a systemic treatment used to target proliferating cells that have spread to others areas of the body. There are several classifications of chemotherapeutic

Table 12.4 Classifications of Antineoplastic Agents and Mechanism of Action

Antineoplastic Agents	Mechanism of Action
Antimetabolite	Inhibit protein synthesis, substitute incorrect metabolites during DNA synthesis Inhibit DNA synthesis Cell-cycle specific, S phase
Alkylating agents	Cross-link DNA strands Cell-cycle nonspecific
Antitumor antibiotics	Interfere with RNA and DNA synthesis Cell-cycle nonspecific
Nitrosoureas (subtype of alkylating agent)	Interfere with DNA replication and repair Cell-cycle nonspecific Cross the blood–brain barrier
Plant alkaloids	Mitotic spindle poison Most cell-cycle specific, M phase
Topoisomerase I inhibitors	Prevent realignment of DNA strands Maintain single strand breaks

SOURCES: Data from National Cancer Institute. (2015). *Chemotherapy*. Available at https://www.cancer.gov/about-cancer/treatment/types/chemotherapy; Muehlbauer, P., et al. (2014). Principles of antineoplastic therapy. In M. Polovich, J. M. Whitford, & C. LeFebvre (Eds.), *Chemotherapy and biotherapy guidelines and recommendations for practice* (4th ed., pp. 25–47). Pittsburgh, PA: ONS Publishing Division; NIH NCI: (2016). *A to Z list of cancer drugs*. Available at https://www.cancer.gov/about-cancer/treatment/drugs.

medications, each of which works a little differently from the others, such as binding the DNA, cross-linking DNA, or destroying mitotic spindles.[52]

Pregnant women should not be given chemotherapy during the first trimester, as it is associated with congenital malformations in up to 20% of delivered infants. If there is a need for initiation of chemotherapy during the first trimester, termination should be considered. Second and third trimester administration of chemotherapy agents is safer and not associated with the long-term fetal effects noted during first trimester administration. If chemotherapy is the treatment of choice, the fact that the pregnancy could affect the pharmacokinetics of the agents needs to be considered. For the pregnant women newly diagnosed with breast cancer, the hormone marker status of the breast tumors (HER2-positive or triple negative hormone status) could affect the targeted therapy or timing of chemotherapy. If the infant is born prematurely, either naturally or by induced labor, there are some risks, such as immaturity of the lungs.[53] Typically, to avoid hematologic complications at the time of delivery due to excessive bleeding, chemotherapy should not be given after week 35 of pregnancy or within 3 weeks of a planned delivery.[53] ■

Radiation

Radiation therapy is used to treat localized cancers. High-energy radioactive substances are used to shrink malignant tumors and kill cancer cells. The most commonly used energy particles are electromagnetic, and they release energy in waves of varying lengths and frequency. Radio waves have the least amount of energy, followed by microwave, infrared, visible light, ultraviolet light, x-rays and finally gamma rays. Gamma waves have the greatest amount of electromagnetic energy, with the shortest waves and highest frequency. Those with the highest energy cause differing degrees of ionization (ability to remove an atom from a molecule, causing life-threatening biologic damage to surrounding tissue) and can penetrate to deep levels in the body.[54] Electrons can minimally penetrate the body; beta particles can penetrate more deeply; and photons (gamma particles) are able to penetrate to different and deepest depths.

Radiation treatment uses controlled ionized particles and targets the cancerous area as narrowly as possible to minimize injury to surrounding tissue. Ionizing radiation can be delivered from inside or outside the body. External beam treatments target the cancer and pass through the body (breast or brain). Internal radiation uses a source of radiation that is either ingested into the body and circulated to the target organ (e.g., thyroid) or placed close to the cancer target (e.g., prostate gland), where it emits the ionizing energy.[54]

Adverse effects of radiation therapy depend on the size of the dose and the part of the body that is treated.

CLINICAL POINT: Careful monitoring is needed to assess for adverse effects, which can include loss of appetite, hyperpigmentation of the skin with wet or dry desquamation, tooth decay, bone marrow depression, or damage to internal organs or structures such as the lungs (during breast cancer treatment) or cerebral arteries (during treatment for brain tumor). Some effects, such as hyperpigmentation, can last for a year and have recall (return of reddening and skin irritation in previously treated areas of the body) when the skin is unprotected and in the sun for prolonged periods of time. Of note, if gamma rays are used for treatment, both the entrance and exit sites of the body will need to be assessed.[55] ■

Radiation therapy should be avoided during the first trimester of pregnancy because of potential harm to the fetus. During the second and third trimesters, radiation can be used if the uterus is carefully shielded. Endocrine therapy should be avoided during the pregnancy because of potential harm to the fetus.[53] ■

Biologic Therapies

Biologic therapies, or biotherapies, enhance the ability of the body to use its natural defenses to fight cancer. Succinctly, the immune system is utilized through stimulating treatments to stop the growth of the cancer by increasing the immune system cells so that they can destroy the cancer cells or keep the cancer from spreading to other sites. The current theory is that these biologic treatments augment the immune cells through three mechanisms:

- This augmentation can increase the cell numbers so the specialized leukocytes can use their own destructive weaponry, such as immunoglobulin or complement, to destroy the malignancy.
- Another mechanism stimulates the immune cell itself to phagocytize or cause lyses of the cancer cells.
- A third mechanism is injection of a cytokine that can activate an immune cell to target and/or orchestrate a reaction against the malignant tumor.

Because biologic therapies use normal secretions or cells of the body, the theory was that there would be minimal adverse effects. In reality, some have been life threatening and/or have diminished the patient's quality of life.[56]

Targeted Therapies

Targeted therapy for cancer has moved the focus of treatment from an "empiric guess to a predictive choice."[57] These agents, also termed *personalized medicine*, target the hallmarks of cancer growth with less toxicity than conventional chemotherapy. Currently, there are FDA-approved medications that target tumor angiogenesis, growth signals and signaling pathways, and cell cycle apoptosis. Primarily, these therapies inhibit or block the targeted receptor or pathway, thus preventing cell growth and promoting death of the immortalized malignant cell.[57]

Gene Therapy

The desire to correct the altered genes causing the cancer has been a goal since it became obvious that genes were the drivers behind the development and progression of cancer. The experimental procedure of gene therapy focuses on the use of genes to treat or prevent disease. Most commonly a normal gene is inserted, using a variety of placement techniques, to replace an abnormal gene. Other possibilities include repairing an abnormal gene or altering the amount by which a gene can be turned "on" or "off." Currently, research directions include killing cancer cells by replacing or knocking out the gene; incorporating genes that will boost the immune system, which will in turn destroy the cancer; utilization of viruses that occur naturally (such as retroviruses that cause the common cold) to selectively infect cancer cells and then cause them to be destroyed; and injection of viruses that will replicate

Impact of Current Research on Clinical Practice

HPV Vaccinations

Description: Because of the global incidence of cervical human papillomavirus (HPV) infections and the diagnosis of cancer in the female genitalia, HPV was historically identified as an infectious contagion responsible for the transformation of normal cervical cells into a malignancy. Research studies identified that types 6, 11, 16, and 18 caused cancers of the vulva, vagina, penis, anus, colon, oropharynx, oral cavity, and tonsils in both males and females. In 2006, the U.S. Food and Drug Administration (FDA) approved the quadrivalent HPV vaccine for use in females to prevent cancers induced by those four types of the HPV.[1] Five years later, the Centers for Disease Control and Prevention recommended the use of the quadrivalent HPV vaccine for males 16–26 years of age.[2]

Clinical Practice: Even with the new vaccines, cervical cancer continues to be a common but preventable cancer for women living in low- and middle-income countries. Because providing sustainable programs for this population is difficult, the incidence, prevalence, and mortality rates continue to be aggravated, with sad outcomes for many families.[3] The HPV-related cancers, including oropharyngeal and anal cancers, continue to be on the rise in males and females.[3] The newly approved Gardasil-9 vaccine has expanded the coverage to the nine most common HPV types causing cancer, with the likely ability to prevent 90% of cervical cancers and 78% of anal cancers. Continued discussions about HPV vaccination are vital in order to focus on its primary purpose: cancer prevention.[4] Many cancer-focused organizations stress the importance of the need to increase the proportion of adolescent boys and girls receiving the HPV vaccine. Data from studying HPV and other vaccines strongly support the ability to increase HPV vaccination rates through improved education, reduced cost, better provider reimbursement, more structured vaccination programs, increased involvement of oncologists in advocating for these issues, and additional research, which could lead to complete eradication of HPV-related cancers in men and women.[4]

A study by Wilson and colleagues found that awareness is already high (near saturation) in target populations, so there is no need to focus on this area of education. There are other factors, such as strong and consistent follow-up physician recommendations, that are more likely to affect follow-through with vaccination. Finally, their results strongly recommend the need for discussions of risk assessment that are tailored to the young adult population.[5]

Healthcare providers in a university health center implemented a quality improvement program to increase HPV vaccination rates. The initiatives included interventions to prevent missed opportunities for vaccination, offering strong recommendations for vaccination, use of patient reminders, use of campus reminders, and marketing on the campus. After 16 weeks, the electronic health record and feedback surveys were used for evaluation. Results identified a 13-fold increase in administered vaccines during the intervention period. Provider recommendations were identified as having the most impact on the decision to vaccinate.[6]

Research Studies:

1. Giuliano, A. R., Palefsky, J. M., Goldsteon, S., et al. (2011). Efficacy of quadrivalent HPV vaccine against HPV infection and diseases in males. *New England Journal of Medicine, 364*(5), 401–411.
2. Centers for Disease Control and Prevention. (2011). Recommendations on the use of quadrivalent HPV vaccine in males—Advisory Committee on Immunization Practices. *Morbidity and Mortality Weekly Report, 60*(50), 1705–1708.
3. American Cancer Society. (2016). *Cancer facts & figures*. Available at http://www.cancer.org/acs/groups/content/@research/documents/document/acspc-047079.pdf
4. Bailey, H., Chuang, L., DuPont, N., et al. (2016). American Society of Clinical Oncology statement: Human papillomavirus vaccination for cancer prevention. *Journal of Clinical Oncology, 34*, 1–17.
5. Wilson, A., Hashib, M., Bodson, J., et al. (2016). Factors related to HPV vaccine uptake and 3-dose completion among women in a low vaccination region of the USA: An observational study. *BMC Women's Health, 16*, 41.
6. Daly, K., Halon, P., Aronowitz, T., & Ross, G. (2016). A university health initiative to increase human papillomavirus vaccination rates. *Journal of the Nurse Practitioner, 12*(6), e281–e286.

selectively in the cancer cells and then destroy the cancer cells or perhaps not even allow replication and just induce cell death. Gene therapy is currently available only through clinical trials.[58,59]

Stem Cell Transplantation

Stem cell transplantation uses multiple types of cancer treatment to promote a better outcome. Initially, patients receive chemotherapy and a growth factor to cause hematopoietic stem cells to be released from the bone marrow into the peripheral circulation. These could be identified with a **cluster of differentiation** cell marker (a cell surface marker used to identify leukocytes in the laboratory) and then collected and frozen for future use. Next, patients receive high doses of chemotherapy and total body radiation designed to destroy the cancer throughout the body and the brain. Radiation therapy is used primarily to target the brain, since most chemotherapy agents do not cross the blood–brain barrier. The chemotherapy and radiation therapy are so toxic that the hematopoietic cells are obliterated, and the hematopoietic stem cells are needed to rescue the patient from tissue or organ toxicities or death. Once the treatment is complete and the patient's stem cells (autologous hematopoietic stem cell transplantation [HSCT]) have been collected, they are reinfused.[60] Sometimes, bone marrow from another individual is used for the transplant (allogeneic transplantation) after careful crossmatching.[61] Multiple early complications are common after HSCT. These include nausea, vomiting, diarrhea mucositis, myelosuppression, and liver and renal toxicity.[60] Both acute and chronic graft-versus-host disease (GVHD) can occur in allogeneic transplantation patients. In the first few weeks after transplantation, acute GVHD can occur. Chronic GVHD occurs later and includes pulmonary complications such as cryptogenic organizing pneumonia. Long-term issues of fertility and sexuality should be discussed early in the transplant decision-making process.[60,61]

Common malignant indications for stem cell transplantation include leukemia, lymphoma, multiple myeloma, and high-risk solid tumors such as neuroblastoma, germ cell tumors, and Ewing sarcoma. Patients with high-risk solid tumors that require high doses of chemotherapy to achieve a potential cure may receive autologous transplantations in some cases.[60]

Laura Beckman: Outcome

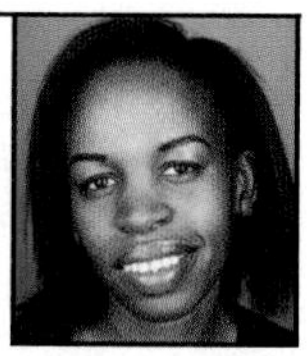

Ms. Beckman had a fine needle biopsy that determined the lump was a fibrocystic lump, referred to as a fibroadenoma. These tumors are benign formations that are not considered cancerous and generally appear after age 30. At this time, Ms. Beckman is given the option of removing the lump or leaving it in place. Removal would occur through cryoablation (freezing) or the use of radiofrequency ablation (sound waves to break up the lump). Regardless of her choice, Ms. Beckman will require close monitoring and follow-up.

9. How should the nurse respond if Ms. Beckman asks whether she can assume that all future breast lumps will be fibroadenomas?
10. What should the nurse tell Ms. Beckman when she asks whether cryoablation is a cure for fibroadenomas?

Edgar Graham: Outcome

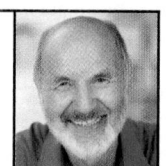

The presence of a significant family history of colorectal cancer in combination with an inflammatory bowel disorder implies a significant risk for the development of hereditary nonpolyposis colorectal cancer. There is a clear genetic risk along with the presence of an inflammatory state that also contributes to the development of cancer. The genetic testing confirms the presence of colorectal cancer. Unfortunately, removal of the colon is the only method that has been shown to prevent further growth of the tumor. Mr. Graham is scheduled for removal of the colon with subsequent ileostomy. Before surgery, a significant amount of teaching and counseling will be necessary to prepare Mr. Graham for the dietary changes he will need to make and for how to maintain the stoma site.

9. What role will oncology nurses play in Mr. Graham's treatment and recovery?
10. What potential genetic defect might have contributed to Mr. Graham's hereditary nonpolyposis colorectal cancer?

Check Your Progress: Section 12.8

1. What is the role of a sentinel node in the diagnosis of cancer?
2. What factors are included in the TNM staging system?
3. Using current theory, what are the three mechanisms used by biologic treatments to enhance the immune system to fight cancer?

CHAPTER SUMMARY

12.1 Chapter Overview and Case Studies

Define neoplasia and cancer, and discuss concepts related to the development of malignant tumors.

- Cellular regulation is controlled by somatic and germ line DNA.
- The gene products of the altered DNA sequences yield a different outcome for the multiple signaling pathways they affect.
- The longer an inflammation persists, the higher is the risk of developing a cancer.
- If an individual's immune system is depleted owing to foreign attackers or illness or is limited as a result of an inherited disease, the lack of an orchestrated immune response can leave an individual open to development of a malignancy.
- Research shows that stress and poor coping mechanisms can lead to a lack of exercise, weight gain, and

poor nutritional practices and lifestyle strategies, including increased alcohol intake.

- Nutrition, alcohol intake, and exercise each have the potential to prevent or potentiate the risk of cancer.

12.2 Cell Cycle and Cellular Differentation

Compare and contrast cell cycles for normal and malignant cells.

- Division of the cell is regulated by the cell cycle.
- The phases of the normal cell cycle are gap 1 (G1), DNA synthesis (S), gap 2 (G2), mitosis (M), and gap 0 (G0), also called the resting phase.
- Each phase of the cell cycle has a specific function related to DNA replication and cell division.
- Checkpoints function during the cell cycle to check DNA replication for accuracy before committing to replication and division.
- Malignant cells dedifferentiate with altered similarity to the tissue of origin and a lack of specialized functions.

12.3 Molecular Basis of Cancer

Identify how genetic factors interact to affect the molecular changes associated with a malignancy.

- Most cancers are sporadic; caused by accumulation of driver mutations.
- A small percentage of cancers are the result of inherited mutations in the germ line.
- Oncogenes are gain of function mutations, and tumor suppressor genes are loss of function mutations; both lead to cancer.
- The *TP53* gene is the best-known tumor suppressor gene and is associated with a wide variety of cancers.
- Multiple genetic alterations are commonly found in cancer cells and include mutations, chromosomal translocations; deletions; aneuploidy; gene amplification; and defects in mismatch repair, including MSI.
- The miRNA can silence a gene by downregulating or degrading the messenger RNA.
- There are a variety of growth factors that regulate cell behavior such as cell growth, angiogenesis, differentiation, and survival.
- The G protein is associated with the *RAS* superfamily of genes, which are known to cause malignant transformation when mutated.
- Loss of heterozygosity occurs when one allele is a mutation and the other is a wild type.

12.4 Carcinogenesis

Explain the multistep process of carcinogenesis, incorporating angiogenesis, mechanisms of altered cellular differentiation, and cancer growth rates.

- There are two models that describe the evolution of cancer: stochastic and cancer stem cell.
- Cancer stem cells may remain in the G0 phase for extended periods of time, causing patients to remain free of symptoms of their malignancy after treatment but to experience return of symptoms at some unanticipated point in the future.
- The stochastic model states that multiple hits are required for a cell to mutate and transform into a malignancy.
- Angiogenesis is an important factor in malignant transformation using vascular endothelial growth factor.
- Normal and malignant cells from the same tissue of origin have identical growth rates, traveling through the cell cycle at the same rate. However, the malignant cells do not go into the resting (G0) phase, and this causes them to appear to proliferate faster than the normal cell.
- Accumulations of mutations create altered proteins (gene expression) that change the proliferative signals, allowing malignant cells to avoid death and continue proliferating.
- Carcinogenesis is a multistep process of initiation, promotion, and progression.

12.5 Cancer Invasion and Metastasis

Analyze how the mechanisms of cancer invasion and metastasis affect the patterns of spread of cancer cells.

- In cancer, human leukocyte antigen may be immunotolerant or lost.
- Multiple proteins, such as fibronectin and lectin, affect the adhesion to the cell membrane and "stickiness" of cells.
- Tissue selectivity of malignant cells guides diagnosis and treatment.
- The metalloproteases cause separation of structural components of the extracellular matrix, growth factor binding proteins, growth factor precursors, tyrosine kinases, cell adhesion molecules, and other proteinases, so signals to the intracellular organelles are lost or incomplete, allowing transformation into a malignant cell.

12.6 Epidemiology of Cancer

Determine the epidemiology of cancer and how factors such as age, gender, race/ethnicity, and the effect of geographic location affect the incidence of different cancers.

- Cancer is the leading cause of death in economically developed countries. One in four deaths in the United States is due to cancer.
- Men have a higher probability of being diagnosed with cancer by the age of 60 than women do.
- Cancer is the number one cause of death in people younger than 85 years of age and the second most

common cause of death for individuals older than 85 years of age.

- The second most common cause of death in children is cancer. Cancers in children have a better cure rate than those in adults. Leukemias are the most common childhood cancers.
- Overall, mortality and incidence rates for most cancers are higher in African Americans except for cancers of the breast, lung, and kidney.
- Many of the leading cancers in the world are linked to infections, 15% of all cancers being due to contagion.
- Geographic location is an important factor for cancers such as mesothelioma, leukemia, and skin cancers.
- The incidence of cancer during pregnancy is approximately 0.1%.

12.7 Clinical Manifestations of Cancer

Identify clinical manifestations commonly associated with different forms of cancer

- Local effects of cancer are linked to the tissue source of the tumor, the increase in size of the tumor, and the location.
- Systemic effects are due to the cytokines secreted by the tumor and tissue changes the tumor has caused, such as obstruction of the superior vena cava by a rapidly growing lung cancer.
- Paraneoplastic syndromes are caused by hormones, peptides, or cross-reaction with normal tissues to cause symptoms distant from the tumor or its metastasis.
- Follow-up guidelines for monitoring late effects for survivors of childhood cancers are associated with age at diagnosis, type of malignancy, treatment that included a combination of chemotherapy plus radiation, and an earlier treatment era. Survivors with 15 years of disease-free survival rarely experience a relapse.
- The acronym CAUTION is used as an aid in remembering the common clinical manifestations of cancer and to promote the early detection of cancer.
- Childhood and adult cancers differ in type of tissue where the cancer originated, onset of symptoms, and outcome.
- Common clinical manifestations of cancer include change in bowel or bladder habits, a sore that does not heal, unusual bleeding or discharge, thickening or lump in the breast or any part of the body, indigestion or difficulty swallowing, an obvious change in a mole, and/or a nagging cough or hoarseness.

12.8 Linking Pathophysiology to Diagnosis and Treatment

Explain the link between the pathophysiology of cancer and the different treatment modalities across the lifespan.

- Early detection of cancer does not include pain at the site of concern.
- Tumor markers are molecules from the blood, urine, or other body fluids that indicate a change in the status of tumor growth.
- A variety of biopsy approaches are used to gain a tissue sample to be evaluated for signs of malignant transformation.
- PET, CT, and MRI scans are used to identify tumors in the body.
- The staging system uses the TNM approach with numbers 1 through 3 and X to designate size or extent of the tumor or lymph node invasion in addition to the presence of metastasis.
- Most treatments for a cancer target the rapidly proliferating cells.
- Surgery may be used for cure, control, or palliative interventions to treat the symptoms of cancer.
- Chemotherapy targets rapidly proliferating cells and may be used for cure or palliation of disease.
- The side effects of chemotherapy can be anticipated, as it targets rapidly proliferating cells of the GI tract, bone marrow, and hair.
- Chemotherapy should not be given to a pregnant patient in the first trimester, after week 35 of pregnancy, or within 3 weeks of a planned delivery to avoid hematologic complications at the time of delivery.
- Radiation is used to treat localized cancers or treat symptoms that occur because of terminal illness.
- Biologic therapies enhance the ability of the body to use its natural defense to fight cancer.
- Targeted therapies are personalized medicine, using medications that target tumor angiogenesis, growth signals and signaling pathways, and cell cycle apoptosis.
- Stem cell transplantation uses multiple types of cancer treatment to promote a better outcome.

REVIEW QUESTIONS

1. The nurse is caring for a client with colon cancer. Which of the following would the nurse expect to see on the client's pathology report?
   a. No encapsulation
   b. No lymph node involvement
   c. Large cell size with normal cytoplasm
   d. Enlarged nuclei with large amounts of DNA

2. The nurse explains to a client with colon cancer that a staging of T1N2MX indicates:
   a. no metastatic lesions.
   b. that the metastatic status could not be evaluated.
   c. that one lymph node is involved.
   d. no evidence of primary tumor.
3. A woman who had a hysterectomy for the treatment of ovarian cancer is being seen for her annual follow-up examination. Which laboratory value would be assessed at this visit?
   a. CEA
   b. HER2 receptor status
   c. CA-125
   d. AFP
4. Which paraneoplastic syndrome finding should be anticipated in a client diagnosed with a lymphoma?
   a. Hypercalcemia
   b. Itching
   c. Thrombocytopenia
   d. Peripheral neuropathy
5. Which of the following statements made by a client in the process of diagnostic testing for osteosarcoma indicates to the nurse that the client needs more instruction?
   a. "A sarcoma is benign."
   b. "Cancer may spread to other organs."
   c. "Cancer cells are fast-growing."
   d. "Benign tumors stay local."
6. Which of the following manifestations would the nurse expect to assess in a child with a brain tumor?
   a. A nighttime headache
   b. A headache that persists after vomiting
   c. Vomiting associated with a fever
   d. Frequent nausea and vomiting
7. The nurse is teaching a client with positive *BRCA1* and *BRCA2* genes that these genes are associated with which of the following cancers?
   a. Breast, ovarian, and lung
   b. Prostate, testicular, and melanoma
   c. Ovarian, pancreatic, and melanoma
   d. Melanoma, breast, and lung
8. A client is receiving radiation therapy for breast cancer treatment. Which of the following adverse effects requires immediate treatment?
   a. Loss of appetite
   b. Hyperpigmentation of the skin
   c. Bone marrow depression
   d. Skin desquamation

ANSWERS

Answers to Review Questions can be found in Appendix A. Answers to Case Study and Check Your Progress questions are available on the faculty resources site. Please consult with your instructor.

RECOMMENDED WEBSITES

American Cancer Society
https://www.cancer.org

Cancer SurvivorLink
http://www.cancersurvivorlink.org

Children's Oncology Group
www.survivorshipguidelines.org

Genes-Environment Interaction
https://www.niehs.nih.gov/health/topics/science/gene-env/index.cfm

National Children's Cancer Society
https://www.thenccs.org

NCI Cancer Mortality Maps
https://ratecalc.cancer.gov

Pediatric Oncology Resource Center
http://www.ped-onc.org

REFERENCES

1. National Cancer Institute. (2015). *Dictionary of cancer terms*. Available at http://www.cancer.gov/publications/dictionaries/cancer-terms?cdrid=45164
2. Hanahan, D., & Weinberg, R. A. (2011). Hallmarks of cancer: The next generation. *Cell, 144*(5), 646–674. doi:10.1016/j.cell.2011.02.013
3. National Cancer Institute. (2013). *What is metastatic cancer?* Available at http://www.cancer.gov/about-cancer/understanding/what-is-cancer/metastatic-fact-sheet#q3
4. Longo, D. L. (2012). Cancer cell biology and angiogenesis. In D. L. Longo, A. S. Fauci, D. L. Kasper, et al. (Eds.), *Harrison's principles of internal medicine* (18th ed., pp. 672–688). New York, NY: McGraw-Hill.
5. Mired, S. K., Goranskaya, D., & Alexeyenko, A. (2014). Distinguishing between driver and passenger mutations in individual cancer genomes by network enrichment analysis. *BMC Bioinformatics, 15*, 308–329. doi:10.1186/1471-2105-15-308

6. National Cancer Institute. (2015). *What is cancer?* Available at http://www.cancer.gov/about-cancer/understanding/what-is-cancer#differences-cancer-cells-normal-cells
7. Bertoli, C., Skotheim, J. M., & de Bruin, R. (2013). Control of cell cycle transcription during G1 and S phases. *Nature Reviews Molecular Cell Biology, 14*(8), 518–528. doi:10.1038/nrm3629
8. Muller, A. J., & Vousden, K. H. (2013). p53 mutations in cancer. *Nature Cell Biology, 15*(1), 1–8.
9. Williams, G. H., & Stoeber, K. (2012). The cell cycle and cancer. *Journal of Pathology, 2*, 352–364. doi:10.1002/path.3022
10. Hanahan D., & Weinberg, R. A. (2000). The hallmarks of cancer. *Cell, 100*, 57–70.
11. National Cancer Institute. (n.d.). *SEER training modules*. Available at http://training.seer.cancer.gov/coding/guidelines/rule_g.html
12. National Cancer Institute. (2104). *Cancer types: Breast cancer treatment and pregnancy*. Available at http://www.cancer.gov/types/breast/hp/pregnancy-breast-treatment-pdq#link/_104_toc.
13. Ranjan, A., Penninga, E., Jelsig, A. M., Hasselbalch, H. C., & Bjerrum, O. W. (2013). Inheritance of the chronic myeloproliferative neoplasms: A systematic review. *Clinical Genetics, 83*(2), 99–107.
14. Loeb, L. A. (2011). Human cancers express mutator phenotypes: Origin, consequences and targeting. *Nature Reviews Cancer, 11*, 450–457.
15. Jiang, Y., Lucas, I., Le Beau, & M. M. (2015). Common chromosomal fragile sites and cancer. In J. D. Rowley, M. M. Le Beau, & T. H. Rabbitts (Eds.), *Chromosomal translocations and genome rearrangements in cancer* (pp. 73–94). New York, NY: Springer.
16. Burrell, R. A., McGranahan, N., Bartek, B., & Swanton, C. (2013). The causes and consequences of genetic heterogeneity in cancer evolution. *Nature, 501*(19), 338–345.
17. Gordon, D. J., Resio, B., & Pellman, D. (2012). Causes and consequences of aneuploidy in cancer. *Nature Reviews Genetics, 13*, 189–203.
18. National Cancer Institute. (2016). *Genetics of colorectal cancer (PDQ®)—Health professional version*. Available at http://www.cancer.gov/types/colorectal/hp/colorectal-genetics-pdq#link/_6_toc
19. Farazi, T. A., Hoell, J. I., Morozov, P., & Tuschl, T. (2013). MicroRNAs in human cancer. *Advances in Experimental Medical Biology, 774*, 1–20.
20. Prior, I., Lewis, P., & Matto, C. (2012). A comprehensive survey of *RAS* mutations in cancer. *Cancer Research, 72*(10), 2457–2467.
21. Kreso, A., & Dick, J. (2014). Evolution of the cancer stem cell model. *Cancer Stem Cell, 14*(3), 175–191. doi:10.1016/j.stem.2014.02.006
22. Goel, H. & Mercurio, A. (2013). VEGF targets the tumor cell. *Nature Reviews Cancer, 13*, 871–882 (2013) doi:10.1038/nrc3627
23. Kolch, W., Halasz, M., Granovskaya, M., & Kholodenko, B. (2015). The dynamic control of signal transduction networks in cancer cells. *Nature Reviews Cancer, 15*, 515–527. doi:10.1038/nrc3983
24. CancerQuest. (2016). Cancer initiation, promotion and progression. Available at https://www.cancerquest.org/cancer-biology/cancer-development#initiation.
25. Fife, C. M., McCarroll, J. A., & Kavallaris, (2014). M. Movers and shakers: Cell cytoskeleton in cancer metastasis. *British Journal of Pharmacology, 171*(24), 5507–5523.
26. Schreiber, R. D, Old, L. J, & Smyth, M. J. (2011). Cancer immunoediting: Integrating immunity's roles in cancer suppression and promotion. *Nature, 331*, 1565. doi:10.1126/science.1203486
27. Singh, P., Carraher, C., & Schwarzbauer, J. E. (2010). Assembly of fibronectin extracellular matrix. *Annual Review of Cell and Developmental Biology, 26*, 397–419. doi:10.1146/annurev-cellbio-100109-104020
28. Horsted, F., West, J., & Grainge, M. J. (2012). Risk of venous thromboembolism in patients with cancer: A systematic review and meta-analysis. *PLOS Medicine, 9*, e1001275.
29. Duffy, M. G., Mullooly, M., O'Donovan, N., Sumainizah, S., Crown, J., Pierce, A., & McGowan, P. M. (2011). The ADAMS family of proteases: New biomarkers and therapeutic targets for cancer. *Clinical Proteomics, 8*, 1–13.
30. Hadler-Olsen, E., Winberg, J.-O., & Uhlin-Hansen, L. (2013). Matrix metalloproteinases in cancer: Their value as diagnostic and prognostic markers and therapeutic targets. *Tumor Biology, 34*(4), 2041–2051 doi:10.1007/s13277-013-0842-8
31. Jemal, A., Center, M., Ferlay, J., Ward, E., & Forman, D. (2011). Global cancer statistics. *CA: A Cancer Journal for Clinicians, 61*(2), 69–90.
32. God, J., Tate, P. L., & Larcom, L. L. (2011). Red raspberries have antioxidant effects that play a minor role in the killing of stomach and colon cancer cells. *Nutrition Research, 30*(11), 777–782.
33. Blackadar, C. B. (2016). Historical review of the causes of cancer. *World Journal of Clinical Oncology 7*(1), 54–86.
34. Seigel, R., Naishadham, D., & Jemal, A. (2012). Cancer statistics, 2012. *CA: A Cancer Journal for Clinicians, 62*, 10–29.
35. Siegel, R., Miller, K., & Jemal, A. (2015). Cancer statistics. *CA: A Cancer Journal for Clinicians, 65*(1), 5–29.
36. Desantis, C., Ma, J., Bryan, L., & Jemal, A. (2014). Breast cancer statistics, 2013. *CA: A Cancer Journal for Clinicians, 64*(1): 52–62.
37. Nambiar, M. J., & Rema, T. (2016). Cancer in pregnancy. In A. Gandhi, N. Malhotra, J. Malhotra, N. Gupta, & N. M. Bora (Eds.), *Principles of critical care in obstetrics* (pp. 289–293). New Delhi, India: Springer India.
38. Silva, C., & Chung, F. S. (2012). Pregnancy and cancer. *Reproductive Health and Cancer in Adolescents and Young Adults, 732*, 89–102. doi:10.1007/978-94-007-2492-1_7
39. Cardonick, E., Dougherty, R., Grana, G., Gilmandyar, D., Ghaffar, S., & Usmani, A. (2010). Breast cancer during pregnancy: Maternal and fetal outcomes. *Cancer Journal, 16*(1), 76–82.
40. American Cancer Society. (2016). *Cancer facts & figures*. Available at http://www.cancer.org/acs/groups/content/@research/documents/document/acspc-047079.pdf
41. Ped-Onc Resource Center. (2015). *Signs of childhood cancer*. Available at http://www.ped-onc.org/diseases/SOCC.html
42. National Cancer Institute. (2014). *Cancer in children and adolescents*. Available at http://www.cancer.gov/cancertopics/factsheet/Sites-Types/childhood.
43. Pelosof, L. C., & Gerber, D. E. (2010). Paraneoplastic syndromes: An approach to diagnosis and treatment. *Mayo Clinic Proceedings, 85*(9), 838–854. doi:10.4065/mcp.2010.0099
44. Chabner, B. A., & Thompson, E. C. (2008). Overview of cancer: Paraneoplastic syndromes. In *The Merck Manual for Health Professionals*. Kenilworth, NJ: Merck Sharp & Dohme. Available at http://www.merckmanuals.com/professional/hematology_and_oncology/overview_of_cancer/paraneoplastic_syndromes.html
45. National Cancer Institute. (2015). *Types of treatment: Surgery*. Available at http://www.cancer.gov/about-cancer/treatment/types/surgery
46. National Cancer Institute. (2011). *Diagnosis and staging: Sentinel lymph node biopsy*. Available at http://www.cancer.gov/about-cancer/diagnosis-staging/staging/sentinel-node-biopsy-fact-sheet
47. National Cancer Institute. (2015). *Diagnosis: Imaging*. Available at http://www.cancer.gov/about-cancer/diagnosis-staging/diagnosis
48. National Cancer Institute. (2015). *Diagnosis and staging*. Available at http://www.cancer.gov/about-cancer/diagnosis-staging/staging
49. American Joint Committee on Cancer. (2016). *AJCC cancer staging manual* (8th ed.). New York, NY: Springer International.
50. Phillips, S. M., Padgett, L., Leisenring, W. M., et al. (2015). Survivors of childhood cancer in the United States: Prevalence and burden of morbidity. *Cancer Epidemiology Biomarkers & Prevention, 24*, 653–663. doi:10.1158/1055-9965.EPI-14-1418
51. National Comprehensive Cancer Network. (2016). *Guidelines: Breast cancer during pregnancy*, version 2.2016. Available at

https://www.nccn.org/professionals/physician_gls/pdf/breast.pdf

52. National Cancer Institute. (2015). *Chemotherapy*. Available at http://www.cancer.gov/about-cancer/treatment/types/chemotherapy
53. Peccatori, F., Azim, H., Hoekstra, H., Pavidis, N., Kesic, V., & Pentheroudakis, G. (The Esmo Guidelines Working Group). (2013). Cancer, pregnancy and fertility: ESMO clinical practice guidelines for diagnosis, treatment and follow-up. *Annals of Oncology, 24*(Suppl. 6), 160–170. doi:10.1093/annonc/mdt199
54. Baskar, R., Lee, K. A., Yeo, R., & Yeoh, K.-W. (2012). Cancer and radiation therapy: Current advances and future directions. *International Journal of Medical Sciences, 9*(3), 193–199.
55. Haubner, F., Ohmann, E., Pohl, F., Strutz, J., & Gassner, H. (2012). Wound healing after radiation therapy: Review of the literature. *Radiation Oncology, 7*, 162.
56. Al-Lazikani, B., Banerji, U., & Workman, P. (2012). Combinatorial drug therapy for cancer in the post-genomic era. *Nature Biotechnology, 30*(7), 1–13.
57. Vanneman, M., & Dranoff, G. (2012). Combining immunotherapy and targeted therapies in cancer treatment. *Nature Reviews Cancer, 12*, 232–251.
58. U.S. National Library of Medicine. (2016). Gene therapy. Available at https://ghr.nlm.nih.gov/search?query=gene+therapy
59. Amer, M. (2014). Gene therapy for cancer: Present status and future perspective. *Molecular and Cellular Therapies, 2*, 27
60. Perumbeti, A. (2016). Hematopoietic stem cell transplantation. *Medscape*. Retrieved from http://emedicine.medscape.com/article/208954-overview
61. Bensinger, W. (2012). Allogeneic transplantation: Peripheral blood versus bone marrow. *Current Opinions in Oncology, 24*(2), 191–196.

Unit V

Infection and Disorders of Immunity

The immune system by and large protects individuals from the myriad of pathogenic microorganisms that are encountered as a part of daily living. Because the immune system has developed specifically for this protective role, any dysregulation of the immune system can lead to increased susceptibility to particular types of infectious agents.

Protection from pathogens depends greatly on the integrity of the skin and mucosal surfaces to prevent entry of microorganisms, the effectiveness of the inflammatory response to prevent the spread of infection throughout the body, and the effectiveness of the body's immune response to eradicate pathogenic microorganisms. Exposure to infectious organisms or infectious materials triggers a cascade of inflammatory and immune events that are designed to help protect the body from harm, including an increase in the production of specialized white blood cells and chemical mediators that fight infection.

One example is that of primary immunodeficiencies (PIs), a heterogeneous group of genetic disorders that affect all components of immune system function. Overall, the most common manifestations of PI are recurrent, severe, and/or persistent or unresponsive bacterial and viral infections involving both common and opportunistic pathogens or infections with unexpected or severe complications.[1] These infections occur most often in the sinuses, middle ear, bronchi, lungs, and gastrointestinal tract. Individuals with PI are susceptible to a variety of autoimmune or inflammatory diseases and malignancies.

In another example, recent studies suggest that atopic individuals (those with type 1, or immediate, hypersensitivity, also known as allergies) may experience dysfunction of the skin barrier leading to hypersensitization to antigens, resulting in an array of allergic responses up to and including the airway hyperreactivity that is common in patients with asthma.[2] This theory supports the idea of the atopic march, a progressive development of type 1 hypersensitivity response that begins with atopic dermatitis (AD) in infancy and progresses through childhood to the development of allergic rhinitis and later asthma. More recent findings suggest that the progressive development of additional allergic disease may not always occur in this sequence and is seen not only in childhood.[2,3] Individuals with asthma are at increased risk for developing respiratory infection and increased risk for experiencing more acute symptoms if they develop an infection.[4] Infection exacerbates symptoms by continuing or increasing bronchoconstriction of the airway.

Viruses, toxins, and other insults can all cause disruption in cellular regulation. In turn, disruptions in cellular regulation increase the individual's susceptibility to infection and resulting illness or functional impairment. For example, with leukemia and multiple myeloma, the proliferation of malignant cells disrupts the production of erythrocytes, neutrophils, and thrombocytes.

Nurses provide care to patients with infection and disorders of immunity and cellular regulation during acute exacerbations, assist in preventing the development of chronic illness or dysfunction through timely assessment and interventions, and provide health education related to prevention. For example, patients with an autoimmune disorder or a disorder such as leukemia require teaching about infection prevention. Patients with type 1 hypersensitivity need education related to avoiding known triggers. As with any chronic illness, patients with these disorders benefit from medication education to prevent exacerbations and reduce side effects. Patients with acute and chronic conditions also benefit from discussions about alternating periods of activity with periods of rest to reduce fatigue and activity intolerance, both of which affect quality of life. Knowledge of the pathophysiologic processes involved in each specific disorder will help the nurse tailor patient teaching more specifically to each patient's needs.

References

1. Younger, E. M., Epland, K., Zampelli, A., Hintermeyer, M. K. (2015). Primary immunodeficiency diseases: A primer for PCPs. *Nurse Practitioner, 40*(2), 1–7.
2. Bantz, S. K., Zhu, Z., & Zheng, T. (2014). The atopic march: Progression from atopic dermatitis to allergic rhinitis and asthma. *Journal of Clinical Cellular Immunology, 5*(2), 202. Available at https://www.ncbi.nlm.nih.gov/pmc/articles/PMC4240310/pdf/nihms629575.pdf
3. Dharmage, S. C., Lowe, A. J., Matheson, M. C., Burgess, J. A., Allen, K. J., & Abramson, M. J. (2014). Atopic dermatitis and the atopic march revisited. *Allergy: European Journal of Allergy and Clinical Immunology, 69*(1), 17–27.
4. American Academy of Allergy, Asthma, and Immunology. (2014). When the sneeze becomes a wheeze. Available at https://www.aaaai.org/global/latest-research-summaries/New-Research-from-JACI-In-Practice/infections-asthma

Autoimmune Disease

- Loss of self-tolerance
- Hereditary and environmental causes
- Systemic lupus erythematosus

Events Involved in Infection

- Pathogens live in reservoirs
- Pathogens leave reservoirs via portal of exit
- Transmission occurs through direct, indirect, or vector methods
- Pathogen enters host through portal of entry

Hypersensitivity Disorders

- Type I, immediate
- Type II, antibody-mediated
- Type III, immune complex-mediated
- Type IV, cell-mediated

Immunity

Immune system
- Innate
- Adaptive (acquired)

Immunodeficiencies
- Primary (inherited)
- Secondary (induced)

Host protection
- Passive immunity
- Active immunity
  - Natural
  - Vaccination

AIDS

- Secondary immunodeficiency
- Caused by infection with HIV

Associated conditions
- Cytomegalovirus diseases
- Tuberculosis
- Kaposi sarcoma
- AIDS-related lymphoma

White Blood Cell Disorders

- Acute myelogenous leukemia
- Acute lymphocytic leukemia
- Chronic myelogenous leukemia
- Chronic lymphocytic leukemia
- Non-Hodgkin lymphoma
- Hodgkin lymphoma
- Multiple myeloma

Agents of Infectious Disease

- Bacteria
- Viruses
- Parasites
- Prions
- Fungi
- Protozoa
- Helminths

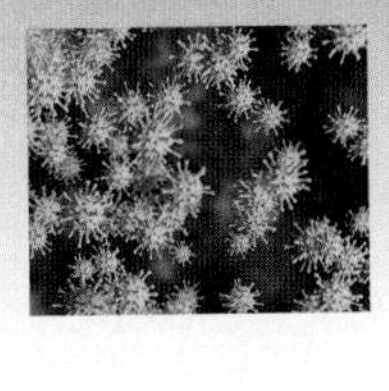

Chapter 13
Mechanisms of Infection and Host Protection

Linda Janusek, Herbert L. Mathews, and Linda Blevins

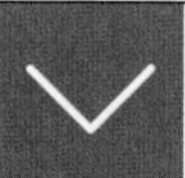

Chapter Outline and Learning Outcomes

13.1 Chapter Overview and Case Studies

Identify factors that increase the global threat of infectious disease and explain concepts related to infection, such as immunity, inflammation, tissue integrity, environment, thermoregulation, perfusion, and oxygenation.

13.2 The Host–Microbe Relationship

Explain the mutual beneficial relationship between the human host and commensal microorganisms.

13.3 From Pathogen to Infectious Disease

Describe the series of events that allow a microbial pathogen to exit an environmental reservoir and to produce infectious disease in humans, and list examples of microbial virulence factors.

13.4 Microbial Agents of Infectious Disease

Contrast the characteristic features of bacteria, viruses, fungi, prions, protozoa, and helminths, and explain the steps of viral invasion and replication within a human host cell.

13.5 The Innate and Adaptive Immune Response to Infectious Microorganisms

Compare and contrast the components of the innate immune system versus the components of the adaptive immune system.

13.6 Resistance to Infectious Disease

Explain the protective immune mechanisms that defend against viral pathogens.

13.7 Resistance to Different Microbial Pathogens as Mediated by Different Host Protective Mechanisms

Describe the means by which microorganisms are opsonized by the immune system and identify the effective form of adaptive immunity that protects against intracellular pathogenic microorganisms such as *Mycobacterium tuberculosis*.

13.8 Immune Deficient/Susceptible Host

Explain the differential etiology of primary and secondary immune deficiencies.

13.9 Protection from Infectious Disease by Vaccination

Explain the difference between passive and active immunity and describe how vaccination provides immunity to infectious agents.

KEY TERMS

Active immunity, 355
Adaptive (acquired) immune system, 350
Alarmone, 337
Antigenic drift, 344
Antigenic shift, 345
Bacteria, 336
Biofilm, 335
Colonization, 333
Commensal microorganism, 330
Cytokine, 336
Dendritic cells, 352
Emerging infectious disease, 327
Endotoxemia, 336
Endotoxin, 336
Epidemic, 344
Eukaryote, 337
Exotoxin, 336
Fomite, 340
Fungi, 348
Gram-negative bacteria, 337
Gram-positive bacteria, 337
Healthcare-associated infections (HAIs), 330
Helminths, 349
Herd immunity, 356
Host, 329

Key Terms continue on next page.

Immunodeficiency, 354
Incubation period, 345
Infectious disease, 333
Innate (natural) immune system, 350
Latent viral state, 346
Major histocompatibility complex (MHC) proteins, 352
Mutualism, 330
Mycobacteria, 338
Natural immunity, 355
Neurotoxin, 336
Obligate intracellular parasite, 342
Opportunistic pathogens, 339
Opsonization, 350
Pandemic, 344
Passive immunity, 355
Pathogen, 330
Pathogen-associated molecular pattern, 350
Pattern-recognition receptors, 350
Portal of entry, 331
Portal of exit, 331
Primary immunodeficiency, 354
Prion, 348
Prodrome, 345
Prokaryote, 337
Protozoa, 349
Pyogenic cocci, 340
Reservoir, 331
Secondary immunodeficiency, 354
Spirillia, 340
Spirochete, 339
Spore, 337
Superantigens, 336
Transmission, 331
Tropism, 344
Vaccination (immunization), 355
Vector, 331
Vehicle, 333
Virulence, 333
Virulence factors, 333
Virus, 342
Zoonosis, 333

ABBREVIATIONS

AIDS—acquired immune deficiency syndrome
HAI—healthcare-associated infection
HIV—human immunodeficiency virus
HPV—human papillomavirus
MHC—major histocompatibility complex
MRSA—methicillin-resistant *Staphylococcus aureus*
SARS—severe acute respiratory distress syndrome
TB—tuberculosis
VAP—ventilator-associated pneumonia
VRSA—vancomycin-resistant *Staphylococcus aureus*

13.1 Chapter Overview and Case Studies

Humans have always been afflicted with infectious disease, as is dramatically shown by the "black death," a plague that swept through Europe in the mid 14th century and killed an estimated 25 million people. Since that time, vast improvements in sanitation and public health measures have remarkably reduced the incidence and spread of infectious disease. This, coupled with the advent of vaccines and antibiotics for the prevention and treatment of infection, led to widespread belief that the scourge of infectious disease had been conquered. This optimism was shattered at the end of the 20th century with the emergence and reemergence of several major infectious threats as well as the development of antibiotic-resistant strains of microorganisms It is now clear that infectious disease remains a perpetual challenge.[1]

An **emerging infectious disease** is one that is newly identified in a population or a disease that has significantly increased in incidence or geographic range. The emergence in the 1980s of the human immunodeficiency virus (HIV),which is the cause of acquired immune deficiency syndrome (AIDS), the spread of severe acquired respiratory syndrome (SARS) across Asia and into Toronto in the 1990s, the global threat of avian flu, the 2007 and 2015 outbreaks of Zika virus, and the 2014 outbreak of Ebola have dramatically reemphasized the dangers that infectious disease pose to human health and well-being.

Resistance to antibiotic drugs has greatly contributed to the reemergence of infectious diseases that were once thought to have been nearly eliminated, as seen by the reemergence of pulmonary tuberculosis in the 1980s.[1] Population crowding and global travel facilitate the spread of infectious disease across continents and put humans at greater risk.[2] Infectious threats are further compounded by the menace of bioterrorism, as evidenced by the intentional and surreptitious mailing of anthrax spores within the U.S. postal system in 2001 that killed five people.[3]

The website of the Centers for Disease Control and Prevention (CDC) contains a section titled Emergency Preparedness and Response, which includes information on microorganisms that have been and can be used in acts of bioterrorism.[4] There, you can search a list of microorganisms for information on their mode of transmission and incubation period, control of spread of the infection, treatment after exposure and after infection, photographs of the organism and clinical manifestations of the infection, diagnostic testing, and where to report the infection.

The threat of infectious disease looms even larger because microorganisms have become resistant to many antimicrobial medications by genetic alteration of their structure and/or metabolism so they are now resistant to the antimicrobial mechanisms of these drugs (i.e., the microbes have developed multidrug resistance).[1] Overuse of antimicrobials has contributed significantly to this resistance by selectively pressuring microorganisms to mutate in order to evade the lethal consequences of these drugs. For instance, *Staphylococcus aureus* bacteria have evolved resistance to methicillin (methicillin-resistant *Staphylococcus aureus*, or MRSA) and vancomycin (vancomycin-resistant *Staphylococcus aureus*, or VRSA) and are difficult to treat. Penicillins such as methicillin exert their effects by binding to penicillin-binding proteins, which are enzymes used by the bacteria to construct the peptidoglycans in their cell walls. MRSA strains have acquired a gene (MecA) that encodes for an alternative penicillin-binding protein, which is not bound by penicillins. Hence, these strains are resistant to these antibiotics as well as to all beta-lactam antibiotics, including other types of penicillin, cephalosporin, and carbapenem antibiotics. Infections caused by these "superbugs" (so called because they are exceedingly resistant to antibiotics) are not limited to the hospital environment but are now becoming more prevalent in the community (i.e., community-acquired MRSA), such as in the homeless and prison populations.[5] Community-acquired MRSA also occurs in football and wrestling teams, in nursing home residents, and even in skinned knees of children.

The study of infectious disease agents has become increasingly interesting because a number of microorganisms have now been recognized to play important roles in the pathogenesis of human diseases, other than those that are typically thought to be infectious diseases. For example, *Helicobacter pylori* bacteria can cause peptic ulcer disease and certain forms of stomach cancer, hepatitis B and C viral infections increase the risk of liver cancer, and the human papillomavirus (HPV) causes the majority of cervical cancers in women.[6] Often, the immune response elicited by microorganisms plays an important role in disease. This is best illustrated in cardiovascular disease, in which chronic infection and/or inflammation leads to release of inflammatory mediators that promote the development of atherosclerotic plaques.[7] However, even though the immune system can play a role in disease development, it is the immune system that by and large protects the mammalian host from the myriad pathogenic microorganisms that are encountered as a part of daily living. The immune system has specifically developed for such a protective role; therefore, any dysregulation of that system can lead to increased susceptibility to particular types of infectious agents.

This chapter provides an introduction to bacteria, viruses, fungi, and parasites with an emphasis on the interaction of these microorganisms with the human host, that is, the host–microbe relationship. General microbiological concepts such as microbial structure, growth, and replication are placed in a clinically relevant context. The importance of pathogenic or virulence factors and the role of these factors in the pathophysiology of infectious disease is developed. The response of the host to the infectious agent and the means by which the human host is protected from infectious disease are described.

Concepts Related to Infection

Infection is related to numerous concepts, including inflammation, immunity, cellular regulation, tissue integrity, thermoregulation, nutrition, stress, perfusion, and oxygenation. Protection from pathogens depends greatly on the integrity of the skin and mucosal surfaces to prevent entry of microorganisms, the effectiveness of the inflammatory response to prevent the spread of infection throughout the body, and the effectiveness of the body's immune response to eradicate pathogenic microorganisms. Exposure to infectious organisms or materials triggers a cascade of inflammatory and immune events that are designed to help protect the body from harm, including an increase in the production of specialized white blood cells and chemical mediators that fight infection. Adequate nutrition in regard to protein, vitamin, and mineral intake is needed both to maintain tissue integrity and to support the function of inflammatory and immune cells. Fever, which is a thermoregulatory response, is commonly associated with infection and increases the body's metabolic rate. Both the immune response and the thermoregulatory response to infection lead to an increase in oxygen consumption. Adequate oxygenation is required for the function of inflammatory and immune cells and for the production of reactive oxygen molecules used by phagocytic cells to destroy microorganisms. Perfusion is required to deliver oxygen, nutrients, and inflammatory and immune cells to sites of infection. Stress affects the ability to fight infection because glucocorticoids that are released during the stress response have anti-inflammatory and immunosuppressant effects. **Figure 13.1** ■ illustrates concepts related to infection.

Case Studies

The pathophysiology involved and the clinical significance of the information in the following cases will be addressed throughout the chapter to assist in application of chapter content to clinical situations.

J.D. Clarkson: Introduction

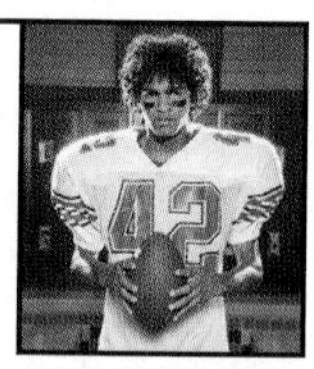

J.D. Clarkson is a 17-year-old male who plays tight end on his high school football team. After a Friday night football game, J.D. complains to the team trainer that his knee hurts and he thinks that he may have been bitten by a spider. On examination, the trainer observes several red bumps that resemble pimples located in the vicinity of a previous knee abrasion. J.D. admitted that he borrowed his teammate's unlaundered knee pads last week during practice, even though sharing team equipment is against the school's athletic policy. The trainer washes the affected area with soap, applies an antibacterial ointment, and covers the area with a large gauze pad. On Saturday night, J.D. awakens at 3 a.m. with severe pain in his knee and a high fever. His parents bring him to the emergency department. He presents with a swollen knee that is red and warm to touch. The red bumps are now dramatically increased in size and appear as large pus-filled boils. J.D. is given an intramuscular injection of penicillin and sent home on oral penicillin. He returns 48 hours later with an abscessed wound. The physician notes cellulitis (inflammation of the skin and subcutaneous tissue) with an area of erythema (redness) and induration (hardness) over J.D.'s knee. The

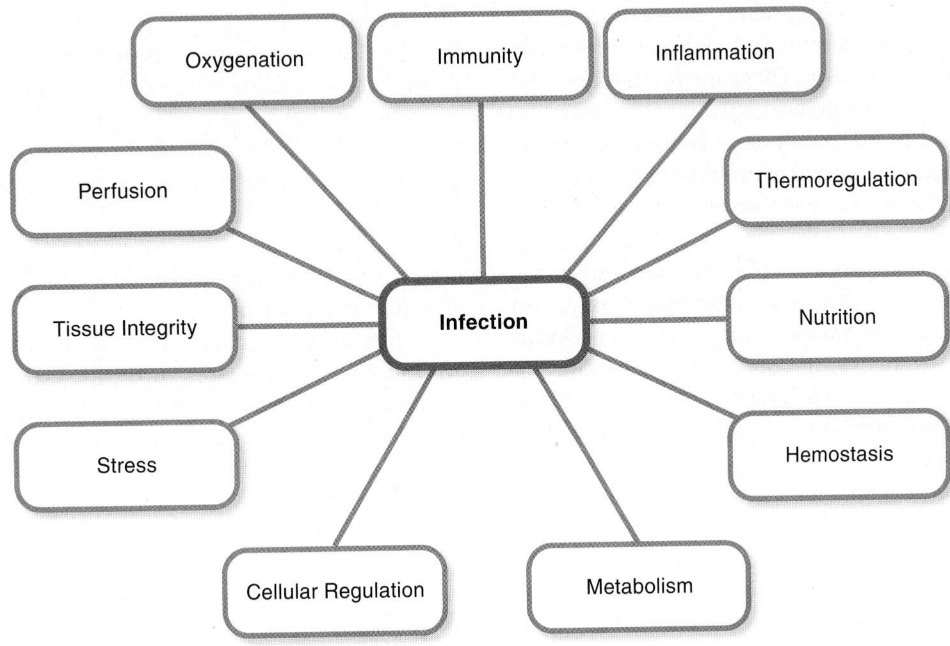

Figure 13.1 ■ Concepts that are related to infection include oxygenation, immunity, inflammation, thermoregulation, nutrition, hemostasis, metabolism, cellular regulation, stress, tissue integrity, and perfusion.

affected area is incised and drained, and a specimen is sent for Gram staining and culture and antibiotic sensitivity testing. Results reveal gram-positive cocci arranged in yellowish clusters, consistent with *Staphylococcus aureus*. Two days later, the antibiotic susceptibility tests confirm that the organism is resistant to penicillin and oxacillin and therefore represents a MRSA. J.D. is admitted to the hospital for treatment.

1. Describe the process of development of resistant strains of microorganisms.
2. Explain how penicillin works to fight infection.

Bernard Reinberg: Introduction

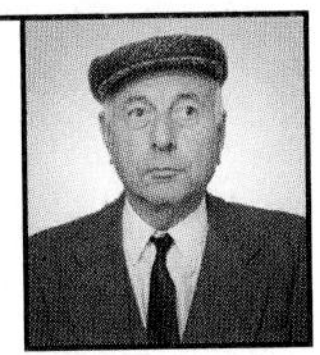

Bernard Reinberg, age 75, is transported by ambulance from his assisted living facility to the emergency department in acute respiratory distress. At admission, he is agitated and dyspneic and appears undernourished. He complains of "a knifelike pain whenever he takes a deep breath," and on coughing, he produces a yellowish sputum. Before this acute situation, he had a 10-day history of fever, malaise, myalgia, and nonproductive cough. Other significant medical history reveals that Mr. Reinberg smoked 10 cigarettes a day for 40 years. He also has type 2 diabetes mellitus and coronary artery disease. When asked whether he had the "flu shot" (i.e., influenza vaccine), Mr. Reinberg stated, "I had the flu shot five years ago, but I still keep getting the flu every year." Vital signs at hospital admission are as follows: temperature 39°C, heart rate 145 beats/minute, respiratory rate 18 breaths/minute, and blood pressure 98/54 mmHg. His oxygen saturation while breathing room air is 82% (normal is 95–100%). Laboratory evaluations reveal an elevated white blood cell count of 14,000 cells/μL^3 (30% bands and 18% polymorphonuclear cells). Auscultation of his chest reveals reduced breath sounds in the left lung. His chest x-ray shows infiltrates in the middle and lower lobes of his left lung. Serologic testing shows evidence of influenza A. Blood and sputum samples for microbial culture are ordered, and Mr. Reinberg is placed on oxygen therapy and broad-spectrum antibiotics. His final diagnosis is influenza complicated by a secondary bacterial pneumonia caused by *Streptococcus pneumoniae*.

1. What are the mechanisms that protect a person from pathogens?
2. Why does Mr. Reinberg's undernourished condition place him at risk for infection?

Check Your Progress: Section 13.1

1. What is an emerging infectious disease?
2. What factors have led to the reemergence of diseases that were thought to have been nearly eliminated?
3. Give an example of a microorganism that can cause a disease other than infection.

13.2 The Host–Microbe Relationship

Humans have an intimate and dynamic relationship with microbes (microorganisms). Microorganisms are diverse and abundant inhabitants of our environment, and they often coexist upon and within us. Humans serve as **hosts** for microorganisms because we provide the appropriate environmental conditions (temperature, pH, etc.) and a steady supply of nutrients that support microbial growth.

The vast majority of microorganisms that populate the human host do not cause harm or disease but reside within the host as persistent colonists. These microorganisms are referred to as **commensal microorganisms**. They make up the commensal flora or normal flora or, as they have more recently been termed, the normal microbiota of the host. For instance, microorganisms such as *Staphylococcus epidermidis* commonly reside on the epithelial surface of the skin. Other commensals populate the mucosa of the mouth and reside on the mucosal surfaces of the respiratory, urogenital, and intestinal tracts. The composition of the normal flora is influenced by a person's genetics, age, sex, diet, and hygiene.

The mucosal surfaces are technically outside the body. Many of these microorganisms can cause disease if they enter the sterile organs or tissues of the body. For example, commensal microorganisms that populate the gastrointestinal tract, such as the *Enterococci* and *Bacteroides*, are normally contained within the intestinal lumen by the intestinal barrier, which consists of tight junctions between epithelial cells and surface coatings such as mucins. However, certain pathophysiologic conditions, such as intestinal ischemia that can occur in burn, shock, and trauma victims, can disrupt the intestinal barrier and allow bacteria to breach the barriers of the intestines and enter the circulation. Outside of the intestinal confines, enteric bacteria can harm the host; indeed, the dissemination of these bacteria can play a role in sepsis and septic shock. Commensal microorganisms not only derive benefit from the host but also confer benefit to the host. By occupying attachment sites within tissues such as the intestines and vagina, commensal bacteria prevent colonization by pathogenic bacteria and can also provide essential vitamins, such as K and B_{12}, and may play an important role in the development of the immune system. This mutually beneficial relationship is termed **mutualism**.

The term *microbiome* refers to all the genes of the commensal microorganisms on and in the human body. The Human Microbiome Project focuses on the study of microbial genes and gene products in the human body and their relationship to maintenance of health and variations in the microbiome that are associated with production of diseases such as inflammatory bowel disease, type 1 diabetes mellitus, obesity, atherosclerosis, cancer, asthma, and allergies. Expanding knowledge of the microbiome in health and disease will likely lead to new forms of treatment for a variety of diseases by nurturing commensal microorganisms and eliminating pathogenic ones.

Microorganisms that harm the host or produce disease are known as **pathogens**. Infectious disease is the third leading cause of death in the United States, but worldwide, infectious disease is the leading cause of death. Infectious disease afflicts individuals both in the community and in the acute care or hospital setting. For example, the large majority of infectious diseases such as pneumonia, tuberculosis, and hepatitis are transmitted within the community. Infections that are acquired within a hospital or other healthcare setting are called **healthcare-associated infections (HAIs)**. See the feature on *Healthy People 2020* for information about the national agenda to decrease HAIs, and see the Impact of Research on Clinical Practice feature for information on causes and prevention of healthcare-associated pneumonia.

To control infectious disease, epidemiologists investigate the causes, geographic, ecologic, and ethnic distribution, and method of spread of infections. Control of infectious disease requires worldwide surveillance of infectious outbreaks and coordination of healthcare professionals in order to treat and control the spread of infectious disease. Implementation of infection control measures is necessary for the prevention of infection. Good hand hygiene, including proper hand washing and use of gloves, is a simple but effective way to control the spread of infection, and there are evidence-based guidelines for

Healthy People 2020

Healthcare-Associated Infections

Goal: "Prevent, reduce, and ultimately eliminate healthcare-associated infections (HAIs)."[1]

Overview: HAIs are infections that develop as a result of being treated in a healthcare facility such as a hospital, outpatient clinic or surgical center, rehabilitation center, or nursing home. Common types of HAIs are urinary tract infections associated with bladder catheterization, surgical wound infections, pneumonia associated with being intubated and mechanically ventilated, and bloodstream infections associated with a central line, such as one placed in the subclavian vein or superior vena cava to facilitate frequent blood sampling or for administration of medications. HAIs can be transmitted from one patient to another by means such as the contaminated hands or gloves of healthcare providers; contaminated equipment such as portable x-ray machines, needles, and catheters; and failure to use aseptic technique in caring for surgical wounds or endotracheal tubes. In the United States, HAIs are one of the leading causes of preventable deaths.[1] In hospitals, HAIs increase the length of hospital stays and exponentially increase the cost of medical care. Implementation of existing preventive guidelines is estimated to decrease the incidence of certain HAIs by up to 70%, leading to a significant reduction in medical costs.[1]

Objectives: There are two objectives related to healthcare-associated infections. The first is to reduce central line–associated bloodstream infections. The second is to reduce invasive healthcare-associated MRSA infections.[2] Specific targets related to these objectives and strategies to achieve the targets are outlined on the *Healthy People 2020* website.[2]

References

1. *Healthy People 2020.* (2017). *Healthcare-associated infections: Overview.* Available at https://www.healthypeople.gov/2020/topics-objectives/topic/healthcare-associated-infections
2. *Healthy People 2020.* (2017). *Healthcare-associated infections: Objectives.* Available at https://www.healthypeople.gov/2020/topics-objectives/topic/healthcare-associated-infections/objectives

Impact of Current Research on Clinical Practice

Taking the Bite Out of Ventilator-Associated Pneumonia

Description: Healthcare-associated pneumonia is one of the most common healthcare-associated infections in the critically ill individual. Individuals in the intensive care unit (ICU) who are intubated and mechanically ventilated are at greatest risk for development of a type of healthcare-associated pneumonia called ventilator-associated pneumonia (VAP). Normally, the lower respiratory tract is sterile. However, bacterial colonization of the lower respiratory tract can occur more readily in a mechanically ventilated individual because placement of an endotracheal tube allows direct entry of bacteria into the lower respiratory tract. Pathways by which microorganisms enter the respiratory tract include aspiration of oropharyngeal or gastric contents, inhalation of contaminated air, and hematogenous seeding,[1] which is the spread of infection from one site to another site by way of circulating blood. Bacterial colonization of the airway, which is a causative factor for VAP, may be linked to microaspiration of oropharyngeal secretions or gastric contents.[1]

Also, mechanically ventilated ICU individuals are critically ill and have a reduced cough reflex and an impairment of the mucociliary clearance mechanism that normally keeps microorganisms from entering and colonizing the lower respiratory tract. Clearance of the oral cavity is also compromised because these individuals are often given medications that reduce salivary flow and produce xerostomia (dry mouth). Within days after admission, the oral flora of ICU individuals changes from the normal gram-positive flora to primarily gram-negative organisms. The bacteria that are mainly responsible for VAP are *Acinetobacter baumanii*, *P. aeruginosa*, *K. pneumoniae*, *E. coli*, and *S. aureus*.[2] These bacteria are often resistant to standard antibiotics and complicate treatment.

Clinical Practice: In a study published in 2011, Berry et al. concluded that implementation of a standardized oral hygiene protocol using a toothbrush for mechanical cleaning of the teeth may significantly reduce the colonization of dental plaque with respiratory pathogens.[3] As an extension of these findings, the researchers hypothesized that using a toothbrush to perform oral hygiene care for mechanically ventilated patients may reduce the incidence of VAP.[3] However, in 2014, on the basis of a review of 16 randomized controlled studies and 9 meta-analyses, Klompas et al. concluded that the use of chlorhexidine for routine oral care may be more effective in lowering VAP rates among patients who had undergone cardiac surgery.[4] More research is needed to evaluate the efficacy of chlorhexidine in preventing VAP among mechanically ventilated patients.

Research Studies:

1. Luna, C. M., Bledel, I., & Raimondi, A.(2014). The role of surveillance cultures in guiding ventilator-associated pneumonia therapy. *Current Opinion in Infectious Diseases, 27*(2), 184–193.
2. Tedja, R., & Gordon, S. (2013). *Hospital-acquired, health care–associated, and ventilator-associated pneumonia*. Available at http://www.clevelandclinicmeded.com/medicalpubs/diseasemanagement/infectious-disease/health-care-associated-pneumonia
3. Berry, A. M., Davidson, P. M., Masters, J., Rolls, K., & Ollerton, R. (2011). Effects of three approaches to standardized oral hygiene to reduce bacterial colonization and ventilator associated pneumonia in mechanically ventilated patients: A randomised control trial. *International Journal of Nursing Studies, 48*(6), 681–688.
4. Klompas, M., Branson, R., Eichenwald, E. C., et al. (2014). Strategies to prevent ventilator-associated pneumonia in acute care hospitals: 2014 update. *Infection Control and Hospital Epidemiology, 35*(8), 915–936.

healthcare workers' hand hygiene practices.[8] Unfortunately, lack of compliance with hand hygiene guidelines remains problematic.[9]

Check Your Progress: Section 13.2

1. Describe the relationship between a commensal microorganism and the host.
2. How are healthcare-associated infections transmitted?
3. Describe the role of brushing teeth in the prevention of ventilator-associated pneumonia (VAP).

13.3 From Pathogen to Infectious Disease

The production of infectious disease in humans involves a series of events and interactions between the potential pathogenic microorganism and the susceptible host. These events involve movement of the microorganism from its source or reservoir, transmission to the host, adhesion to host cells or tissues, colonization and propagation of the microorganism, damage to the host cells and tissues, and evasion of host defense mechanisms. The pathogenicity, or ability of the microorganism to produce disease, depends on completing some or all of these steps.

Events Involved in Infection

Microbial pathogens live, grow, and multiply in a variety of environments called **reservoirs** that can serve as a source of infection to humans. Soil, water, food, and inanimate surfaces in the environment can harbor pathogenic microorganisms. A number of microorganisms multiply in animals or insects, which in turn serve as vectors of infection to humans. **Vectors** are living intermediaries that convey an infectious agent from its reservoir to a susceptible host. Humans also serve as microbial reservoirs, and human-to-human transmission is a major mode of infection. Potential pathogens can exit these reservoirs via pathways referred to as **portals of exit**, such as coughing or sneezing through the mouth or nose, and enter the host and initiate the process of infection.

Transmission of infection is the passage of a pathogen from an infected host to a previously noninfected host via direct or indirect contact. Microbial pathogens are transmitted to the host in a variety of ways. The means by which a pathogen enters the host is called the **portal of entry**. Portals of entry include direct entry, ingestion, inhalation, and parenteral (injected) entry. Direct entry of a pathogen may occur when an individual incurs a wound that is contaminated with soil containing the spores of *Clostridium tetani* (which causes tetanus) or when an individual is subjected to a needlestick contaminated with a pathogen, such as HIV. Respiratory pathogens are commonly transmitted from droplets of fluid that are released into the environment by an infected person during activities such talking, coughing, spitting, sneezing, or even singing. The infectious agents in these droplets enter the body of another person through the eyes, nose, or mouth. The distance that the droplets can travel is usually less than 1 meter. However, if the droplets are light enough, they can become airborne and remain suspended for long periods of time and travel distances greater than 1 meter. Whether an infection occurs by airborne transmission depends on the resistance of the pathogen to environmental conditions that influence the duration that the pathogen remains airborne, such as sunlight and drying as well as atmospheric conditions including humidity and air circulation. **Table 13.1** ■ provides a summary of common respiratory infections.

Table 13.1 Common Respiratory-Associated Infections

Disease	Organism	Commentary
Bacterial		
Typical pneumonia	*Streptococcus pneumoniae* • Gram-positive cocci • Antiphagocytic capsule	Most common cause of community-acquired pneumonia in adults.
Typical pneumonia	*Staphylococcus aureus* • Gram-positive cocci • Forms clusters resembling grapes	Some strains may be methicillin resistant (MRSA).
Typical pneumonia	*Bacillus anthracis* • Gram-positive bacilli • Antiphagocytic capsule • Produces exotoxins • Forms spores	Infection occurs through contact with infected animal products or spore-contaminated dust. Spores are highly resistant to chemical and physical destruction. Spores can be weaponized and present potential bioterrorism threat.
Typical pneumonia	*Klebsiella pneumoniae* • Bacilli • Antiphagocytic capsule • Part of GI microbial flora	Primarily infects individuals compromised by alcoholism, diabetes, or chronic obstructive pulmonary disease.
Typical pneumonia	*Haemophilus influenzae* • Gram-negative coccobacilli • Part of respiratory microbial flora	Type b has capsule and produces most serious, invasive disease. Primarily produces pneumonia in older adults and immuno-compromised.
Typical pneumonia	*Escherichia coli* • Gram-negative • Part of microbial flora of colon	Neonates are at greater risk when *E. coli* escapes the colon and enters sterile body sites and overwhelms their immature immune system.
Pneumonic plague	*Yersinia pestis* • Gram-negative • Antiphagocytic capsule	Animal reservoir; transmitted by fleas. Primarily southwestern United States. Potential biological weapon.
Whooping cough	*Bordetella pertussis* • Gram-negative • Antiphagocytic capsule	Causes paroxysms of coughing followed by "whoop" as the individual inspires rapidly. Pertussis vaccine given in childhood
Chronic pneumonia Tuberculosis	*Mycobacterium tuberculosis* • Acid-fast • Resistant to drying	Leading cause of worldwide death by infection. Survives and grows in host macrophages, where it remains viable but quiescent for decades; immunosuppression can reactivate it.
Atypical pneumonia	*Legionella pneumophila* • Gram-negative • Antiphagocytic capsule • Flagella	Inhabitant of water and soil. Colonizes humidifiers, air conditioners, water distribution systems. Resists chlorine disinfection.
Atypical pneumonia	*Mycoplasma pneumoniae* • Contains membrane-associated adhesion molecules that bind to bronchial epithelial cells and inhibits ciliary action	Most common cause of atypical pneumonia in adults. Called "walking pneumonia" due to minimal signs and symptoms.
Pharyngitis and Tonsillitis	*Streptococcus pyogenes* • Gram-positive cocci	Most common cause of sore throats. Release of exotoxin can also cause scarlet fever.
Diphtheria	*Corynebacterium diphtheriae* • Gram-positive • Produces exotoxin that inhibits protein synthesis and mediates its effects	Initially produces local throat infection with productive thick, grayish exudates; can obstruct airway. Vaccine part of childhood recommended vaccine schedule.
Viral		
Common cold	Rhinovirus • RNA virus • 100 serotypes makes vaccine development unrealistic	Virus requires lower temperature and hence replicates in nasal passages.
Common cold	Influenza virus • RNA virus • Type A and B cause disease	Surface displays two membrane protein spikes (HA-hemagglutinin; NA-neuraminidase). These membrane proteins vary from one flu season to the next. (See Figure 13.8.)
Pharyngitis and Tonsillitis	Adenovirus • DNA virus	Throat infections may progress to viral pneumonia.

Enteric (gastrointestinal) pathogens enter the host by ingestion of contaminated food or liquids. Certain foods are more suitable for microbial growth, and under appropriate environmental conditions, this growth is nourished. Common cases of food poisoning occur in this manner when pathogens such as *Salmonella* or *E. coli* are transmitted from eating undercooked eggs or meats or contaminated fruits or vegetables. Other bacteria, such as *Clostridium botulinum*, grow best in anaerobic acidic foods. Infectious diseases can be transmitted by vectors. Some pathogens are transmitted and enter the host by vectors such as the bite of an insect. For instance, West Nile disease and some forms of meningitis are transmitted by mosquitoes, and Lyme disease is transmitted by the bite of the deer tick. Animals may also transmit infectious disease to humans. **Zoonosis** refers to any disease that can be passed from animals to humans. For example, cats can spread toxoplasmosis, which can be very dangerous to pregnant woman. Animal bites can transmit diseases such as plague and rabies.

Other pathogens, such as HIV, *Herpes*, and *Chlamydia* can enter the host's urogenital tract during sexual activity. **Table 13.2** ■ lists common sexually transmitted infections. Inanimate objects can also serve as vehicles of transmission. **Vehicles** are nonliving intermediaries that convey the infectious agent from its reservoir to a susceptible host. This occurs when a sick individual touches an object and leaves behind fluid or cells containing the pathogen. This pathogen is passed along to a healthy person who touches the object. Proper hand hygiene and gloving are important practices that stop the chain of transmission.[8]

Colonization refers to the establishment of microorganisms within the body. Once a pathogen enters a host, occupies an ecologic niche, and proliferates, it is said to have colonized the host. Colonization depends on characteristics of both the host and the pathogen. The human body has many favorable niches that are warm and moist and have nutritional sources that favor microbial growth.

On the other hand, the human host has a variety of host defense mechanisms to counter microbial colonization and invasion. The pathogen must evade or overcome these host defense mechanisms. For example, an enteric pathogen must be able to survive passage through the acidic environment of the stomach before colonizing the intestines. If successful, the microorganism will be capable of adhering to host cells at the portal of entry, proliferating, and potentially causing an infection.[10]

J.D. Clarkson: Application

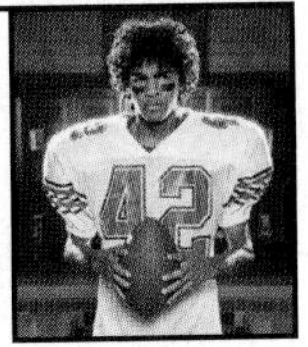

J.D. wore his teammate's MRSA-contaminated knee pads over his knee abrasion. This provided a warm, moist environment that facilitated the colonization of MRSA, allowing the pathogen to increase in sufficient number and cause infection.

3. Explain how the contaminated knee pad acted as a vehicle for infection.
4. What role did colonization play in J.D.'s infection?

Infection and Virulence

Infection occurs when the microorganisms multiply in a body part or tissue. **Infectious disease** occurs when the pathogen multiplies in sufficient quantities to cause tissue damage and impairment of function of the host. **Virulence** is the degree to which a microorganism is capable of causing infectious disease. Virulence varies across types and strains of microorganisms. For example, both *Shigella* and *Vibrio* can cause gastrointestinal infections, but *Shigella* is more virulent than the bacteria that cause cholera. It is estimated that it takes fewer than 200 *Shigella* bacilli to produce disease, compared to 100 million *Vibrio cholerae* bacilli. Microorganisms are equipped with a variety of mechanisms that assist them to infect the host and potentially cause infectious disease. Factors that enhance the pathogenicity of a microorganism are called **virulence factors**. In general,

Table 13.2 Common Sexually Transmitted Infections

Disease	Organism	Commentary
Bacterial		
Gonorrhea	*Neisseria gonorrhoeae* • Gram-negative cocci	Pili facilitate attachment to host; pyrogenic
Syphilis	*Treponema pallidum* • Spirochete	Flagella propel in corkscrew manner; facilitates host invasion
Viral		
Acquired immune deficiency syndrome AIDS	Human immunodeficiency virus (HIV-1 and HIV-2) • RNA virus/	Uses the enzyme reverse transcriptase to covert RNA to DNA for replication
Genital herpes	Herpes simplex (HSV-2) • DNA virus	Enters a latent viral state in the host and can be reactivated to produce recurring disease
Genital (venereal) warts	Human papillomavirus (HPV) • DNA virus	Increases risk of cervical cancer; HPV vaccine approved
Fungal		
Vaginal yeast infection	*Candida albicans*	Produces thick white discharge; debilitated and immunosuppressed individuals at greater risk for recurrent infections; also infection occurs when antibacterial antibiotics allow yeast to overgrow

virulence factors include factors that facilitate a microorganism's ability to adhere to host cells and invade host tissues as well as the means by which a microorganism evades the host's immune defense mechanisms. **Table 13.3** provides examples of the main virulence factors.[10]

Adhesion is a pivotal early step in the infectious process. Without adhesion, potential pathogens can be swept from the body, such as by the upward sweeping action of ciliated cells that line the respiratory tract or by the flushing motion of fluids, such as urine, that flow from the body. Some pathogens, such as *S. pneumoniae*, which causes infection of the lungs or pneumonia, are surrounded by a slime layer that help them to stick to the respiratory mucosa. Similarly, the influenza virus uses a protein (hemagglutinin) on its outer surface to adhere or stick to the mucosa of the respiratory tract. Other microorganisms have pili or fimbrae that project from their surface and facilitate adherence. *Escherichia coli* and *N. gonorrhoeae* are examples of

Table 13.3 Examples of Characterized Virulence Factors

Organism	Virulence/Pathogenic Factor	Pathogenic Mechanism
Toxins		
Bacillus anthracis	Anthrax toxin	Induces cytokines that mediated cell death
Bordetella pertussis	Pertussis toxin	Reduces phagocytosis Destroys blood cells (i.e., hemolysis and leukolysis)
Clostridium botulinum	Botulism toxin	Flaccid paralysis
Clostridium tetani	Tetanus toxin	Spastic paralysis
Corynebacterium diphtheriae	Diphtheria toxin	Blocks protein synthesis, resulting in cell death
Escherichia coli	Heat-labile toxin	Diarrhea
Pseudomonas aeruginosa	Exotoxin A	Inhibits protein synthesis, resulting in cell death
Salmonella species	Enterotoxin	Diarrhea
Staphylococcus aureus	Heat-stable enterotoxins Toxic shock toxin Exfoliatin	Diarrhea Cytokine release that leads to fever and inflammation Causes separation of the layers within the epidermis and is the causative agent of scalded skin syndrome in newborns
Shigella dysenteriae	Shiga toxin	Diarrhea Hemolytic colitis Hemolytic uremia
Streptococcus pyogenes	Erythrogenic/pyrogenic toxin Streptolysin S Streptolysin O	Erythema Lyses leukocytes, platelets, and RBCs Lyses leukocytes, platelets, and RBCs
Vibrio cholera	Cholera toxin	Diarrhea
Neisseria gonorrhoeae *Neisseria meningitidis*	Lipid A	Inflammation
Adhesins (facilitate binding to host cells and invasion)		
Escherichia coli	Pili (uropathogenic *E. coli*) Fimbriae	Binds to mannose-containing receptors on host cells and facilitates invasion Allows binding to galactose-containing glycolipids and glycoproteins present on epithelial cells and facilitates invasion
Streptococcus pyogenes	M proteins Lipoteichoic acids	Binds extracellular matrix
Adenovirus	Penton base and a fiber. The fiber contains the viral attachment proteins.	Binds class I major histocompatibility complex (MHC)
Salmonella enterica	Fimbriae	Binds to M cells within the intestines.
Human immunodeficiency virus (HIV)	Gp120	Binds CD4 and coreceptors: CXCR4 CCR5
Rhinovirus	Capsid	Binds to ICAM-1
Influenza A	Hemagglutinin	Binds to sialic acid
Poliovirus	Capsid	Binds to glycoprotein known as CD155
Neisseria gonorrhoeae	Fimbriae, pilin	Binds to GD_1 ganglioside
Treponema pallidum	P1, P2, P3	Binds fibronectin
Mycoplasma pneumoniae	Protein P1	Binds to sialic acid
Vibrio cholerae	Type 4 pili	Binds fucose and mannose

Organism	Virulence/Pathogenic Factor	Pathogenic Mechanism
Capsule		
Neisseria meningitidis *Escherichia coli* *Klebsiella pneumoniae* Group B streptococci	Distinct complex polysaccharide capsular material	Antiphagocytic
Haemophilus influenzae	Polyribosyl ribitol phosphate	Antiphagocytic
Streptococcus pyogenes	Hyaluronic acid	Antiphagocytic
Streptococcus pneumoniae	Complex polysaccharide	Antiphagocytic
Tissue/Cellular Destruction		
Clostridium perfringens	Phospholipase C, collagenase protease, hyaluronidase	Degradative enzymes that break down tissue structure
Staphylococcus aureus	Hyaluronidase, fibrinolysin lipases	
Streptococcus sp.	Streptolysins S and O, hyaluronidase, DNases, streptokinases	Enzymes that facilitate the development of infection and spread into the tissue.
Polioviruses, herpes simplex virus, togaviruses, poxviruses	Damage of cells by replicating virus	Inhibition of cellular protein synthesis, leading to cell destruction.
Herpes simplex virus, varicella-zoster virus, paramyxoviruses, HIV	Damage of cells by replicating virus	Cellular fusion, which allows the virus to easily move from cell to cell, evading the immune system.
Enveloped viruses	Damage as a consequence of immunologic recognition of viral protein	Alteration of cell membrane structure
Adenovirus	Fibers	Toxic for mammalian cells
Evade/Resist Immune System		
Streptococcus pyogenes	M protein	Inhibit phagocytosis
Staphylococcus aureus	Protein A	Inhibit opsonization
Legionella spp., *Mycobacterium tuberculosis*, *Chlamydia* spp.	Surface structures	Inhibition of phagolysosome fusion
Salmonella typhimurium, *Mycobacterium leprae*, *Leishmania* spp.	Surface structures	Resistance to lysosomal enzymes
Herpes simplex virus, varicella-zoster virus, paramyxoviruses, HIV	Damage of cells by replicating virus	Cell-to-cell infection via syncytia formation, which is a multinucleate mass of cytoplasm produced by the merging of cells Latent infection
HIV, influenza virus	Due to mutation frequency	Antigenic variation
Adenovirus Epstein-Barr virus	Encoded protein	Blocks production of interferon, an antiviral cytokine
Measles		Impairment of dendritic cell function, reducing antigen presentation
Herpes simplex virus Human immunodeficiency virus Measles virus	Encoded protein	Impairment of lymphocyte function
Adenovirus 12 Cytomegalovirus Herpes simplex virus	Encoded protein	Reduces class I MHC expression on host cell membranes

pathogens that have pili and subsequently can more readily adhere to the mucosa of the urogenital tract and cause either bladder or genital tract infections. Certain bacteria are encased in a capsule, which not only facilitates adhering to host cells but also protects them from being phagocytosed and subsequently killed by polymorphonuclear leukocytes or macrophages.[10]

Because *S. aureus* has a unique affinity for endothelium (lining blood vessels and cardiac valves), it also may lead to the development of vasculitis and endocarditis. Once established in the host, *S. aureus* produces a variety of tissue-degrading enzymes such as hyaluronidase that facilitate its invasiveness into host tissues. Other damaging toxins produced by *S. aureus* include hemolysins and leukocidins, which dissolve red and white blood cells, respectively. Other toxins produced by *S. aureus* mediate tissue damage and include alpha toxin, superantigens, and exfoliative toxins. See Table 13.3.

Often, bacteria can form biofilms. A **biofilm** consists of a community of bacteria that colonize together within a sticky web of extracellular material. Biofilms develop on surfaces within the host and serve to protect the microorganisms from host elimination and antibiotic treatment.[11] For example, *Streptococcus mutans* form biofilms within dental plaque that can develop around the tooth surface; these bacteria are implicated in tooth decay. Biofilms exist in wounds, and evidence suggests that their presence interferes with wound healing.[11] Biofilms can also form on inert medical devices such as surgical appliances, artificial valves, or other prostheses that are implanted within the body and hence can serve as a breeding ground for infectious disease.

Once microorganisms have successfully found a niche and adhered to the host, they will propagate and form a colony. In the case of bacteria, as they grow in number, they often release byproducts of metabolism, such as acids or gases, that damage host tissues. The microbes and the substances they produce can elicit an inflammatory response characterized by host cell release of chemical mediators called pro-inflammatory cytokines and chemokines. In excess, inflammatory mediators can also damage the host.

Once they have formed a colony, microorganisms can invade and spread throughout the host's tissues. This is facilitated by the release of enzymes such as collagenase and hyaluronidase that destroy connective tissue. Other bacteria produce substances that promote their uptake into host cells. For instance, the invasion protein of certain enteric pathogens (*Shigella*, *Salmonella*, and *Yersinia*) promotes their binding to M cells of the colon. M cells, in turn, invaginate and take in these bacteria.

The components of the bacterial cell wall can also increase its virulence or ability to cause damage to the host. An excellent example of this is **endotoxin**, which is a lipopolysaccharide molecule located within the cell wall of gram-negative bacteria.[12] Endotoxin produces a wide range of host responses that play a role in the inflammatory process, as well as the pathogenesis of sepsis and septic shock that can occur with widespread gram-negative bacteremia). **Endotoxemia**, which is characterized by excessive levels of endotoxin in the blood, is associated with consumption of a high-fat diet.[12] Other bacteria can produce exotoxins, which consist of proteins secreted by either gram-positive or gram-negative bacteria. **Exotoxins** are polypeptide proteins that are primarily produced by gram-positive bacteria; some forms of gram-negative bacteria may produce exotoxins as well.[13] Enteric (gastrointestinal) pathogens such as cholera and Shiga toxins produce exotoxins that alter intestinal cell water balance and cause profound watery diarrhea. **Neurotoxins** are natural or artificial substances that destroy all or part of a neuron. Botulinum and tetanus toxin are examples of natural neurotoxins. Botulinum inhibits the release of acetylcholine at the neuromuscular synapse, which inhibits nerve impulses from activating muscles, hence producing a flaccid paralysis. The tetanus toxin inhibits glycine release, which inactivates inhibitory neurons to muscle, producing a rigid paralysis.

Some bacteria have molecules on their surface called superantigens. **Superantigens**, which are specialized toxins, activate T lymphocytes and lead to massive production of cytokines that damage host tissues.[10] Superantigens produced by *S. aureus* are responsible for toxic shock syndrome, which was linked in the early 1980s to tampon use by menstruating women[10] *S. aureus* is able to multiply in the hyperabsorbent tampons and release toxins into the blood that stimulate massive cytokine release, which in turn, produces an abrupt onset of fever, hypotension, and multiple organ dysfunction syndrome. A warning about this risk now accompanies tampon products.[14]

Cytokines are chemical messenger molecules such as interleukins and interferon that are produced by immune cells, as well as other cells. Cytokines mediate communication among immune system cells and between immune system cells and the rest of the body.

J.D. Clarkson: Outcome

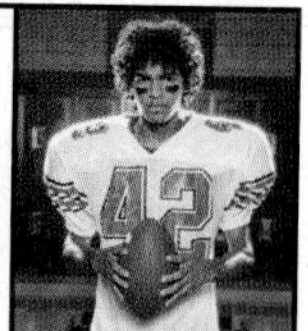

J.D. contracted a MRSA skin infection by using his teammate's soiled knee pads. Culture and sensitivity of wound drainage reveal the causative organism to be *S. aureus*, which has a number of virulence factors that enhance its pathogenicity. J.D.'s wound infection progressed to form an abscess, which walled off the infection and protected the bacteria from host defense mechanisms.

J.D.'s course of treatment includes incision and drainage of his abscess as well as a full course of treatment with the antibiotic clindamycin. Because his clindamycin is administered intravenously, his course of care requires a peripherally inserted central venous catheter (PICC) as well as numerous clinic visits for administration of the medication. J.D.'s infection resolves without further complications; however, his scenario illustrates the ease with which the MRSA epidemic is propagated in the community. At present, public health guidelines are in place to reduce the spread of community-acquired MRSA among athletes and within schools.[15]

5. Describe the role of pathogen adhesion early in J.D.'s infectious process.
6. Explain how *S. aureus* damages host tissues.

Check Your Progress: Section 13.3

1. Describe the role of superantigens in the development of toxic shock syndrome.
2. What role do cytokines play in the infectious process?
3. How does biofilm promote infection?

13.4 Microbial Agents of Infectious Disease

Organisms that cause infections in humans include bacteria, viruses, fungi, prions, protozoa, and helminths. Examples of these organisms and the mechanisms whereby they cause infections are described in the following sections.

Bacteria

Bacteria are small unicellular organisms that are important causes of infectious disease in humans. They are informally categorized on the basis of their response to Gram staining, their shape, and their distinctive physiologic characteristics. This method of grouping bacteria is based not on genetic analysis but rather on visual characteristics seen on microscopic examination of tissues and fluids derived from infected individuals. As illustrated in **Figure 13.2** ■, bacteria exist in a variety of shapes. Spherical bacteria are called cocci (singular: coccus), and some cocci exist in pairs (*S. pneumoniae*) or clusters (*Staphylococcus*). Others appear as rods, such as *E. coli*. Spirochetes are spiral or coiled

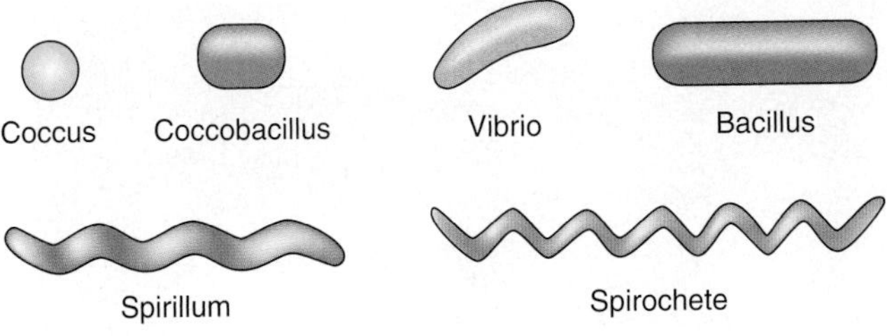

Figure 13.2 ■ The general shapes of bacteria.

organisms such as *Treponema pallidum*, which causes syphilis. Certain bacteria can form filamentous branches (e.g., *Nocardia* and *Actinomyces*).[16]

Bacteria are **prokaryotes**, which do not have distinct membrane-bound cell organelles and do not have nuclei or mitochondria (see **Figure 13.3** ■). In contrast, mammalian cells (as well as fungi, protozoa, helminths, and plants) have distinct cell organelles and are classified as **eukaryotes** (Greek for "true nucleus"). Since bacteria do not have a nuclear membrane, their chromosome, consisting of DNA, lies freely within the cytoplasm. Bacterial DNA is double-stranded and circular. The non–nuclear-bound DNA is believed to simplify protein synthesis by coupling transcription of mRNA directly to its translation into proteins. Bacteria also have structures called plasmids, which are small circular extrachromosomal DNA. Plasmids are thought to give bacteria a selective advantage because they encode resistance to many antibiotics. Resistance genes can be passed from one bacterial species to another. Bacteria reproduce by simple binary fission, producing two equivalent daughter cells. Bacterial growth is characterized by an initial lag (no growth) period, when the bacteria are adapting to their environment; the log phase, when bacteria are increasing in number exponentially; and a stationary phase, when there is no change in living bacterial cell numbers. The lack of nutrients and the buildup of toxic by-products triggers the production of **alarmones**, which halts bacterial metabolic processes and can lead to death of the bacteria or spore formation.[17]

Certain bacteria are capable of converting into dehydrated structures called **spores**. Spores represent a dormant or nonvegetative state of the bacteria. They are formed when bacteria are nutrient deprived and/or in harsh environmental conditions, such as extremes of temperature or osmolarity. Spores are highly resilient structures that can survive for centuries, and they are resistant to infection control measures such as disinfectants. Spores can germinate back to the vegetative state, or original bacteria cell, when water and nutrients become available. Examples of spore-forming bacteria include *B. anthracis* (the etiologic agent of anthrax) and *C. tetani* (the etiologic agent of tetanus).[17]

Bacteria have distinctive features (**Figure 13.4** ■). For instance, *Streptococci, Staphylococci, Micrococcus*, and *Neisseria* are cocci (Figure 13.4A), and *Bacillus, E. coli, Salmonella*, and *Vibrio* are bacilli (Figure 13.4B). A distinctive feature of bacteria is that they are surrounded by a cell wall. The presence of a cell wall is important to bacterial survival because it allows them to grow in an often hostile environment (high osmotic pressure, extreme temperatures or dryness, and limited energy sources). Bacteria are grouped as either gram-positive or gram-negative on the basis of a laboratory technique called Gram staining. When stained with crystal violet, **gram-positive bacteria** retain the stain after acid washing and appear purple (purple-positive) (see Figure 13.4A); **gram-negative bacteria** do not retain the crystal violet stain after an acid wash and can be counterstained, typically with safranin, allowing for the appearance of red-colored bacteria microscopically (see Figure 13.4B). Gram staining takes about 10 minutes to complete and is a quick and easy way to group bacteria and assist in making decisions related to antibiotic drug choice.[13] As examples, *S. pneumoniae* is a gram-positive coccus, *C. perfringens* is a

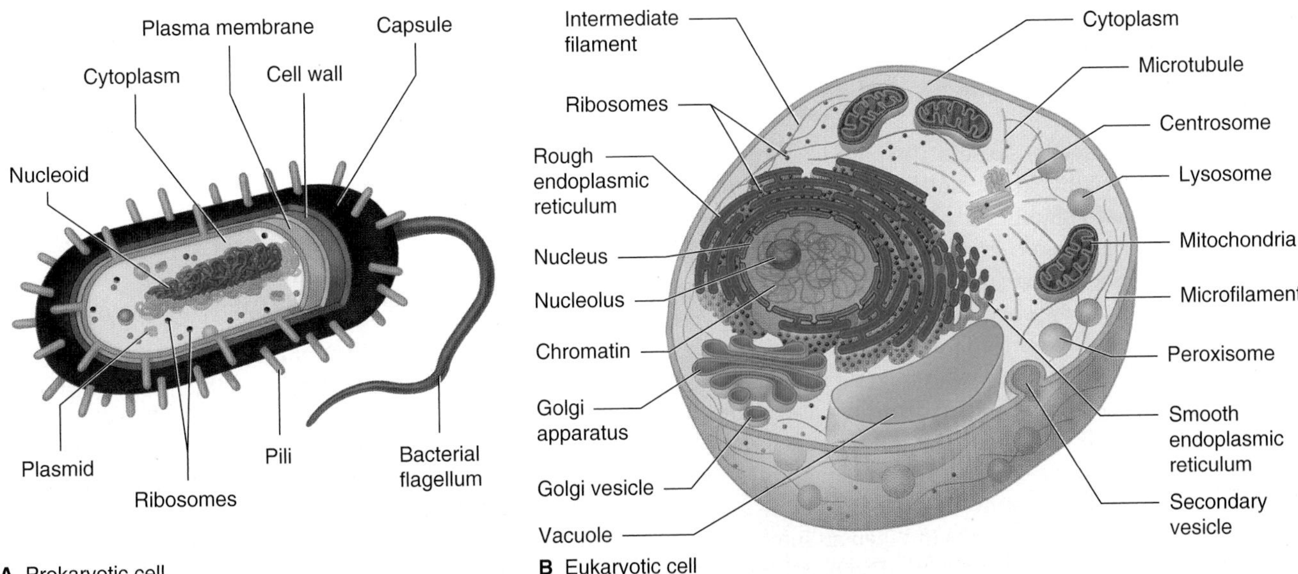

Figure 13.3 ■ **A**. Bacteria are classified as prokaryotes, which lack a distinct nucleus, mitochondria, and distinct membrane-bound cellular organelles. **B**. Mammalian cells, fungi, protozoa, and helminths are eukaryotes.

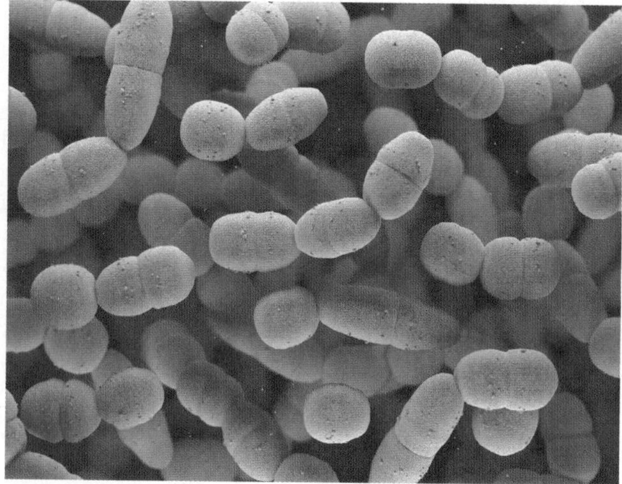

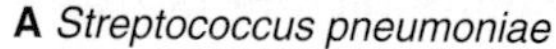

A *Streptococcus pneumoniae*

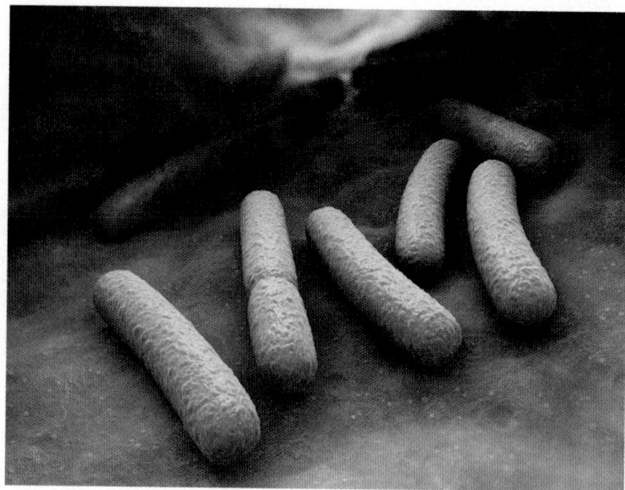

B *Escherichia coli*

Figure 13.4 ■ Scanning and transmission electron micrographs of bacteria. **A**. Cocci. *S. pneumoniae*, demonstrating pairs and short chains, is gram-positive. **B**. Bacilli. *E. coli*, showing single cells, is gram-negative.

gram-positive bacillus, *E. coli* is a gram-negative bacillus, and *N. meningitidis* is a gram-negative coccus.

The cell wall of gram-positive organisms is mainly composed of a large polysaccharide-protein polymer called peptidoglycan. The interlocking molecular chains provided by peptidoglycan forms a meshlike exoskeleton protective layer, yet it is porous enough to allow for diffusion of nutrients. It also contains teichoic acids that enhance virulence and lipoteichoic acids that can exert weak endotoxin-like effects in the host. In contrast, the cell wall of gram-negative organisms has a thin peptidoglycan layer but contains an outer layer of lipopolysaccharide or endotoxin.[17] Endotoxin is a key mediator of sepsis and endotoxin shock that can occur with gram-negative infections.

Mycobacteria are acid-fast bacteria, meaning that they cannot be decolorized easily with acid solutions. They are slow growing and have a waxy cell wall that is rich in complex lipids, making these organisms resistant to phagocytosis as well as to detergents and common antibiotics. *Mycobacterium tuberculosis* causes pulmonary tuberculosis (TB), a leading cause of infection and infection-related deaths worldwide.

TB is a global infectious disease; one third of the world's population is infected.[18] In the United States, the incidence of TB had decreased significantly by the early 1980s, but a resurgence in cases was observed in 1985. This was due in part to the emergence of the human immune deficiency virus (HIV). The immune deficiency associated with HIV infection places the individual at risk for TB as a result of reductions in the number of $CD4^+$ lymphocytes. Immigration to the United States from countries where TB is endemic has also increased the prevalence of TB in this country. TB remains problematic in prisons, homeless shelters, and nursing homes. The tubercle bacilli are spread from person to person by droplet nuclei released into the environment when an infected person coughs, sneezes, speaks, or sings. The bacilli multiply in the alveoli of the lungs and may migrate to other parts of the body such as the kidney, brain, or bone. Alveolar macrophages phagocytize the bacilli and on activation can eliminate small foci of the bacilli. Larger groups of the bacilli become incorporated into an encasement called a granuloma. Pulmonary granulomas can be large, necrotic, and/or caseous, and when encapsulated with fibrin, the bacilli contained within are protected from macrophage killing. These bacilli can remain dormant for the rest of the individual's life or can be reactivated years later in old age or under other circumstances that result in immunosuppression. Currently, a prolonged multidrug regimen is used to treat TB. Persistent problems of drug-resistant strains of the tubercle bacilli make TB a continuing healthcare challenge.[19]

Escherichia coli are enteric gram-negative rods that inhabit the intestinal tract and are members of the family *Enterobacteriaceae*. Levels of *E. coli* are monitored as an indicator of fecal contamination of drinking water systems, swimming areas, and public food sources. *E. coli* is also an important cause of urinary tract infections. Urinary tract infections are more common in women than men because the urethra is shorter in women and bacteria are more capable of ascending the urinary tract. Infectious pathogens that cause urinary tract infections are listed in (**Table 13.4** ■).

Certain strains of *E. coli*, such as the O157:H7 strain, cause serious gastrointestinal tract disease that can be life-threatening in the very young and in older adults because of their inefficient immune systems. ■

A variety of microbial pathogens are implicated in gastrointestinal infections, some of which are transmitted through contaminated food. For example, *E. coli* O157:H7 is often transmitted after ingestion of contaminated and undercooked ground beef.[20] The family Enterobacteriaceae includes several other genera that cause primary infections of the human gastrointestinal tract and foodborne illness. The most prominent are *Salmonella* and *Shigella*. Like *E. coli*, these enteric bacteria are gram-negative facultative anaerobic rods.

Table 13.4 Common Bacterial Causes of Urinary Tract Infections

Organism	Commentary
Escherichia coli • Gram-negative rod • Fimbriae mediate adherence	Most common cause of urinary tract infections, including cystitis and pyelonephritis. Women at greater risk Transmission most commonly from intestinal flora
Pseudomonas aeruginosa • Gram-negative rod • Pili mediate adherence • Grows in aqueous environment	Primarily a result of healthcare-associated infection in hospitalized individuals, acquired through urinary catheters
Staphylococcus saprophyticus • Gram-positive cocci • Part of vaginal microbial flora	Frequent cause of cystitis in women Transmission commonly from vaginal flora Also common hospital-acquired infection due to urinary catheters
Other enterobacteria • *Klebsiella*, *Enterobacteriaceae*, *Proteus*, and *Serratia* • Part of gut microbial flora	Primarily opportunistic organisms that are important causes of hospital-acquired infection Commonly colonize hospitalized individuals who have indwelling catheters, have had invasive procedures, and are on antibiotics that lead to overgrowth of gut microbial flora. Also, critical illness leads to disruption of the gut barrier and systemic release of these pathogens, which then invade sterile body sites.

According to genetic studies, there is a single species of *Salmonella* (*Salmonella enterica*). However, there are a very large number of antigenic types of *Salmonella*, only a few of which are commonly associated with human disease. These types are referred to as *Salmonella enteritidis*, *Salmonella choleraesuis*, and *Salmonella typhi*. Salmonellosis is transmitted by contaminated food (such as poultry and eggs). It does not have a human reservoir and usually presents as a gastroenteritis (nausea, vomiting, and nonbloody stools). The disease is usually self-limiting and lasts 2–5 days. The microorganisms invade the epithelium and do not produce systemic infection. In uncomplicated cases of salmonellosis, which are the vast majority, antibiotic therapy is not useful. *S. cholerae-suis* (seen much less commonly) causes septicemia after invasion. In this case, antibiotic therapy is required.

The severest form of salmonella infections, enteric fever ("typhoid"), which is caused by *S. typhi*, is rarely seen in the United States today, although it caused widespread epidemics in the past and is still a significant pathogen in the developing world. The microorganism is transmitted from a human reservoir, in the water supply (if sanitary conditions are poor), or in contaminated food. It initially invades the intestinal epithelium; during this acute phase, gastrointestinal symptoms are apparent. The microorganism penetrates (usually within the first week) and passes into the bloodstream and is disseminated by macrophages. This septicemia is usually temporary, and the organism finally lodges in the gallbladder. Organisms are shed into the intestine for some weeks. At this time, the gastroenteritis (including diarrhea) is the major symptom. Antibiotic therapy is essential.

Shigella flexneri, *Shigella boydii*, *Shigella sonnei*, and *Shigella dysenteriae* all cause bacillary dysentery or shigellosis (bloody feces associated with intestinal pain). Humans are the only reservoir. The organisms invade the epithelial lining of the gut but do not penetrate it. Usually within 2–3 days, dysentery results from bacteria damaging the epithelial layers lining the gut, often with the release of mucus and blood (found in the feces) and attraction of leukocytes (also found in the feces as "pus"). Watery diarrhea is frequently observed with Shiga toxin, a pathogenic factor that causes cellular toxicity by inhibition of protein synthesis.[21] Dehydration is of primary concern, and replacement of lost fluids and salts may be the only treatment that is needed. Individuals with severe dysentery are usually treated with antibiotics. However, some *Shigella* bacteria have become drug-resistant.[22]

Shigellosis is primarily a disease of young children, occurring by fecal–oral contact. Outbreaks have been reported in daycare centers.[23] Adults can catch this disease from children, and infected adult food handlers who contaminate food can also transmit it. The source in each case is unwashed hands. ■

Pseudomonas are gram-negative encapsulated rods and are widely distributed in nature in water, soil, plants, and animals. *P. aeruginosa* is an important opportunistic pathogen that is a leading cause of healthcare-acquired infections. **Opportunistic pathogens** are microorganisms that use the opportunity to infect a host that has weakened defense mechanisms, such as individuals with AIDS, transplant recipients, and individuals with an autoimmune disease on immunosuppressive therapy. *Pseudomonas* frequently contaminates watery environments, such as hot tubs, wet intravenous tubing, or other water-containing receptacles. *P. aeruginosa* is a frequent cause of healthcare-associated pneumonia, urinary tract infections, wounds, and burns. Debilitated, older, and other immunosuppressed individuals with indwelling lines that offer an easy portal of entry are at greatest risk.[24]

Some bacteria have flagella that facilitate their mobility. For example, **spirochetes** are thin, flexible spiral-shaped bacteria that have endoflagella, which are made up of axial filaments. These filaments can rotate and allow the cell to bend and rotate during movement (i.e., snakelike movement). Clinically important spirochetes include *Treponema pallidum*, which causes the sexually transmitted infection syphilis, and *Borrelia burgdorferi*, which causes Lyme disease. Lyme disease is transmitted by the bite of a tick, commonly found in animal reservoirs such as rodents and deer. Early Lyme disease is manifested by flulike symptoms. This condition is commonly associated with the development of a red lesion with a clear center, resembling a bull's-eye. However, half or more of the individuals who have Lyme disease will not develop a bull's-eye lesion.[25] If untreated, the organism can spread by way of the lymph or blood to secondary sites (musculoskeletal, skin, brain, etc.) and produce systemic disease, including arthritis, cardiac, and neurologic symptoms.[25]

Spirillia are spiral-shaped bacteria that also have flagella. *Helicobacter pylori* are spirillia and are capable of colonizing the acidic environment of the stomach; unless treated, the colonization will persist for life. *H. pylori* causes most cases of peptic and duodenal ulcers; if untreated, the associated chronic inflammation increases the risk for gastric cancer. Also belonging to the spirillia is *Campylobacter jejuni*, which causes diarrhea. *C. jejuni*, the leading cause of bacterial food-borne infection in developed countries, is most often transmitted by consumption of contaminated chicken meat.[26]

Pyogenic cocci are spherical bacteria that can cause suppurative (pus-producing) infections. These include gram-positive cocci, such as *S. aureus*, *Streptococcus pyogenes*, and *S. pneumoniae*, and gram-negative cocci, such as *N. gonorrhoeae* and *N. meningitidis*. These bacteria are clinically important causes of bacterial infections in humans. Staphylococci produce a wide range of infections, ranging from localized skin and wound infections to systemic disease such as pneumonia and endocarditis. Staphylococci are gram-positive, spherical bacteria that form clusters similar to a bunch of grapes that are hardy and resist heat and drying. As a result, they can persist for long periods of time as **fomites**, which are inanimate objects or substances by which an infectious organism can be transmitted from one individual to another, such as on doorknobs and surfaces in individual care areas, individual gowns, and bed linens. *Staphylococcus aureus* is a leading cause of infections in humans. *Staphylococcus epidermidis* (typically considered a part of the normal flora (microbiota) of human skin, nasal mucosa, and the gastrointestinal tract) is less pathogenic but can be associated with human infections as well.[27] Research suggests that *S. epidermidis* may have a role in the development of certain forms of rosacea.[28]

Staphylococcus aureus is visually recognized in culture by its characteristic gold pigmentation. It is notorious for the wide range of infections it can produce in humans. It is pyogenic and can produce suppurative skin infections, and it is often the cause of wound infections. Other skin infections due to *S. aureus* include impetigo, furuncles, and carbuncles. Impetigo is characterized by pus-containing vesicles that rupture and then form a yellowish crust. Furuncles, also called boils, are infections that usually originate in a gland or hair follicle in the skin. Carbuncles are infections in the subcutaneous area of the skin that form connecting pockets of infection. *S. aureus* toxins mediate food poisoning, toxic shock syndrome, and scalded skin syndrome, which is seen most often in infants. *S. aureus* also produces systemic infections such as pneumonia, septic arthritis, osteomyelitis, and acute endocarditis. It is noteworthy that *S. aureus* is a cause of HAIs and is often transmitted from the hands of healthcare workers who have been colonized from their own reservoir or from contact with an infected individual. *S. aureus* can also be transmitted from insertion of devices such as vascular catheters, resulting in bacteremias.[27]

A number of virulence factors enhance the pathogenicity of *S. aureus*. These include a capsule and surface proteins that resist phagocytosis. The surface proteins facilitate adherence by binding to extracellular matrix molecules (i.e., fibronectin, collagen) of the host. For example, a breach in the normal barrier of the mucosa or skin, such as through wounding or irritation, exposes host proteins such as fibronectin and allow *S. aureus* to bind. These binding proteins also allow *S. aureus* to colonize the plastic surfaces of medical devices such as catheters. *S. aureus* produces enzymes, such as coagulase, that convert the clotting factor fibrinogen to fibrin, forming a fibrin mesh around a collection of bacteria and tissue debris, resulting in formation of an abscess. Abscesses wall off the infection and also protect the bacteria from host defense mechanisms. Because *S. aureus* has a unique affinity for endothelium, which is the lining of blood vessels and cardiac valves, it can produce vasculitis and endocarditis. Once established in the host, *S. aureus* produces a variety of tissue-degrading enzymes, such as hyaluronidase, which breaks down hyaluronic acid and facilitates its invasiveness into host tissues.[13]

Staphylococcus aureus produces damaging toxins, such as hemolysins and leukocidins, which dissolve red and white blood cells, respectively. Other toxins produced by *S. aureus* mediate tissue damage and include alpha toxin, superantigens, and exfoliative toxins.

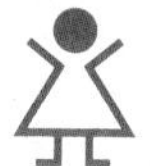

Exfoliative toxins produce skin erythema and separation, as manifested in staphylococcal scalded skin syndrome, which can occur in infants.[27] ■

Staphylococcus aureus produces enterotoxin B, which causes 20% of cases of acute food poisoning. Foods are typically contaminated during food preparation. Under the appropriate conditions, *S. aureus* can multiply within a few hours and release sufficient toxin to result in food poisoning. Commonly implicated foods include custards, potato salad, tuna salad, processed (salted) meats, and ice cream. Contaminated foods are normal in appearance, odor, and taste. Heating kills the bacteria but does not inactivate the toxin.[27]

Food-related illnesses are a major health burden in the United States, as outbreaks can sicken large segments of the population, and death may occur in those who are most susceptible, such as older adults. ■

Most of these illnesses are preventable, and each outbreak is analyzed to determine its cause and to institute preventive measures. The CDC collects data on foodborne disease outbreaks through the Foodborne Disease Outbreak Surveillance System.[29] In addition to *S. aureus*, a number of other microorganisms are associated with infections or intoxications via the gastrointestinal tract, as seen in **Table 13.5** ■. Each of these pathogenic microorganisms produces infections or intoxications as a consequence of virulence factors associated with the individual microorganism.

Table 13.5 Common Microorganisms That Cause Gastrointestinal and Infections or Intoxications

Disease/Symptoms	Organism	Commentary
Bacterial		
Food poisoning	*Staphylococcus aureus*	Typically due to contamination of mayonnaise or dairy products
Food poisoning Flaccid paralysis	*Clostridium botulinum* • Gram-positive • Obligate anaerobe • Spore forming	Spores found in soil. Produces exotoxin that blocks acetylcholine release at neuromuscular junction leading to paralysis
Cholera Diarrhea	*Vibrio cholera* • Gram-negative rod • Cholera toxin initiates fluid movement into the intestine, with eventual loss of this fluid from the body as diarrhea.	Transmitted by contaminated food and water Profuse watery diarrhea (rice–water stools) Causes massive loss of fluid and electrolytes from the body High mortality if untreated
Inflammatory gastroenteritis Diarrhea	*Escherichia coli* • Enterotoxigenic	Common cause of "traveler's diarrhea" Transmitted by contaminated food and water
Inflammatory gastroenteritis Diarrhea	*Escherichia coli* • Enteropathogenic • Destroys intestinal microvilli	Important cause of infant diarrhea in developing countries
Inflammatory gastroenteritis Diarrhea Vomiting	*Escherichia coli* • Enteroaggregative	Dehydration (primarily of infants) Aggregative pattern of adhesion due to fimbriae
Pseudomembranous colitis	*Clostridium difficile* • Gram-positive rod • Spore forming • Produces toxins A and B • Minor part of gut microbial flora	Overgrows in colon of an individual on antibiotics, which disrupt balance of gut flora Characterized by explosive diarrhea with pseudomembrane formation in the colon
Invasive gastroenteritis Fever Cramping	*Shigella* spp. • Gram-negative rod • Low infectious dose • Shiga toxin produced	Characterized by bloody diarrhea and painful abdominal cramping Very young children and older adults at risk
Invasive gastroenteritis Fever	*Salmonella enterica* • Gram-negative rod • Adheres to and invades enterocytes of intestine, leading to a profound inflammatory response.	"Food poisoning" Transmitted from human to human by oral–fecal route or by contaminated food products (uncooked poultry, raw eggs) Pets (turtles) can transmit. Young children and older adults at risk
Invasive gastroenteritis Diarrhea	*Escherichia coli* • Enteroinvasive	Ingestion of contaminated food and water Plasmid-mediated invasion of epithelial cells
Invasive gastroenteritis Bloody diarrhea	*Escherichia coli* • Enterohemorrhagic • Exotoxin produced • Serotype O157:H7 most common	Profuse bloody diarrhea and acute renal failure (hemolytic uremic syndrome) Mainly transmitted in undercooked ground beef
Bloody diarrhea	*Campylobacter jejuni* • Gram-negative spiral rod	Transmission by oral–fecal route and via contaminated meat (poultry) or water. Causes ulcerative, inflammatory lesions
Gastric and duodenal ulcers	*Helicobacter pylori* • Gram-negative rod • Curved or spiral • Flagella motile	Colonizes mucosal cells of the stomach. Secreted urease produces ammonium ions, which neutralize acid pH Transmitted from person to person
Viral		
Invasive gastroenteritis Diarrhea	Rotavirus • RNA virus (reovirus) • Nonenveloped	Severe gastroenteritis primarily in infants and children Infects epithelial cells of small intestine primarily the jejunum Microvilli disrupted and malabsorption syndrome (lack of nutrient absorption) occurs Incubation 48 hrs or less
Invasive gastroenteritis Vomiting	Norwalk agent • RNA virus (nonenveloped)	Replicated in GI tract; shed in feces; transmission by oral–fecal route after ingestion of contaminated food or water Cause of gastroenteritis in schools, camps, prison, cruise ships, etc. Symptoms short-lived (24–48 hours)
Hepatitis	Hepatitis A, B, C, D, E	Caused by immunopathology of hepatocytes by immune response to virus
Parasitic		
Inflammatory gastroenteritis Diarrhea	*Giardia lamblia*	Most common parasitic intestinal disease in U.S. Generally clinically mild
Inflammatory gastroenteritis Diarrhea	*Cryptosporidium parvum* • Intracellular parasite that lives in the villi of the lower small intestine	Transmission in drinking water contaminated by feces of domestic animals and farm runoff Usually mild but more severe in immunocompromised individuals

Streptococci are gram-positive cocci arranged in chains that cause significant infectious disease in humans. They are able to survive on dry surfaces and are pathogenic because they exhibit antiphagocytic capsules and secrete exotoxins. *Streptococci* can reside on the skin and nasopharynx and can be transmitted from infected individuals and also from healthy human carriers. *S. pyogenes* can cause acute pharyngitis (strep throat), which is the most common streptococcal infection. Postinfection sequelae can occur, including acute rheumatic fever and glomerulonephritis. *S. pyogenes* can also cause purulent skin infections such as impetigo. *Streptococcus pneumoniae* is the most common cause of pneumonia and otitis media and can also cause meningitis. Some forms of *S. pneumoniae* are encapsulated, which makes them very resistant to phagocytosis.[13] Moreover, there are 90 different capsular types of pneumococci.[30] The streptococci and other respiratory pathogens are summarized in Table 13.1, and their virulence factors are outlined in Table 13.3.

Individuals over 65 years of age at risk for streptococcal pneumonia should be vaccinated with a vaccine that targets 23 of the capsular types, which represent 85 -90% of those that cause invasive disease.[30,31] ■

For children, a pneumococcal vaccine is available that targets 13 of the capsular subtypes.[30] This vaccine is recommended for administration in a series of four doses for children beginning at the age of 2 months, with the final dose administered between 12 and 15 months of age. For children who do not receive the pneumococcal vaccine before age 15 months, the vaccine is still recommended. However, for these children, a primary care provider will determine the number and frequency of vaccine doses.[30] ■

Other clinically significant streptococcal pathogens include *Streptococcus agalactiae*, which resides in the vaginal tract of female carriers and the urethral mucus membranes of male carriers.

Women colonized with *Streptococcus agalactiae* can transmit this microbe to newborns during passage through the birth canal. *S. agalactiae* can cause septicemia and meningitis in the newborn, with a high mortality rate. ■

Neisseria are gram-negative pyogenic (pus-producing) cocci that on microscopic observation look like a pair of kidney beans. They have hairlike appendages called pili that facilitate their attachment to host epithelial and mucosal cells. *Neisseria gonorrhoeae* causes the sexually transmitted infection gonorrhea. *N. meningitidis* is one of the most frequent causes of meningitis. It is transmitted through inhalation of respiratory droplets. Its pili permit adherence to the nasopharyngeal mucosa, and its outer capsule resists phagocytosis. Outbreaks occur more often in winter and early spring and in facilities such as schools and dormitories where crowding and close contact are common. Onset is rapid with great intensity.[32]

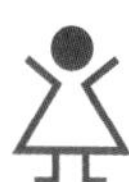

Meningococcal vaccine is routinely recommended for all children between 11 and 12 years of age, with a booster dose administered at age 16. This vaccine also is recommended for certain high-risk children ages 2 through 10 years.[33] ■

Some bacteria are **obligate intracellular parasites**, which they can grow only inside host cells. These include bacteria such as the gram-negative *Rickettsia*. *Rickettsia* are transmitted by bites from arthropods such as ticks, fleas, and lice and produce diseases including typhus fever, Rocky Mountain spotted fever, and Q fever. *Rickettsia* infect the endothelial cells that line capillaries, leading to focal thrombi in the skin and numerous other organs. If untreated, myocardial failure or renal failure can occur.[34] *Chlamydia* are also obligate intracellular parasites.[35] They are unable to produce ATP in adequate amounts and in that sense are energy parasites. *Chlamydia trachomatis* causes the most common sexually transmitted infection in the United States, which affects both men and women. Women may develop infection of the cervix and pelvic inflammatory disease. Repeated infection can lead to sterility. *C. trachomatis* can also cause an eye infection known as trachoma, which is prevalent in developing countries.

Bernard Reinberg: Application

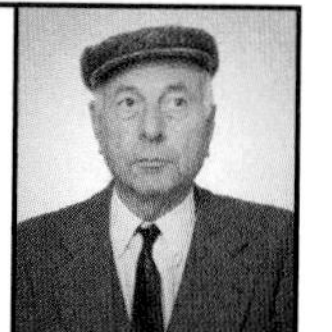

Bernard Reinberg had not received the pneumococcal vaccine, He developed streptococcal pneumonia subsequent to his influenza, which made his lungs more susceptible to a secondary bacterial infection. He also has a history of smoking, which weakens his immune response as well as his ability to clear potential pathogens from his respiratory tract.

3. Why are older adults with influenza, such as Mr. Reinberg, at risk for secondary bacterial infection?
4. Laboratory testing revealed that Mr. Reinberg had a gram-positive coccus. What is the significance of this finding?

Viruses

Viruses are major causes of infectious disease in humans. They are nonliving obligate intracellular parasites that can replicate only in living cells, as they lack the capacity to produce energy and to make proteins.

Structural Features of Viruses

As a group, viruses are much smaller than bacteria. Yet within the group of medically important viruses, viral size extends from the small parvovirus (18 nm) to the large poxviruses (300 nm). A comparison of viral size relative to bacteria is shown in **Figure 13.5** ■. Viruses exist in a range of structures from very simple spheres to complex geometric shapes that display precise symmetry. For example, the rabies virus is a rhabdovirus whose form takes on a helical shape. The outer surfaces of other viruses form an icosahedron, which is composed of 12 pentamer units fitted together into a precise geometric arrangement. The geometric exterior of the herpes virus is even more complex and resembles a soccer ball (icosahedral symmetry). The names of viruses are based on their characteristic shape, the tissue they preferentially infect, or the geographic area where the virus first surfaced as a cause of disease. For example, the togavirus is so named because it is covered by a toga-like

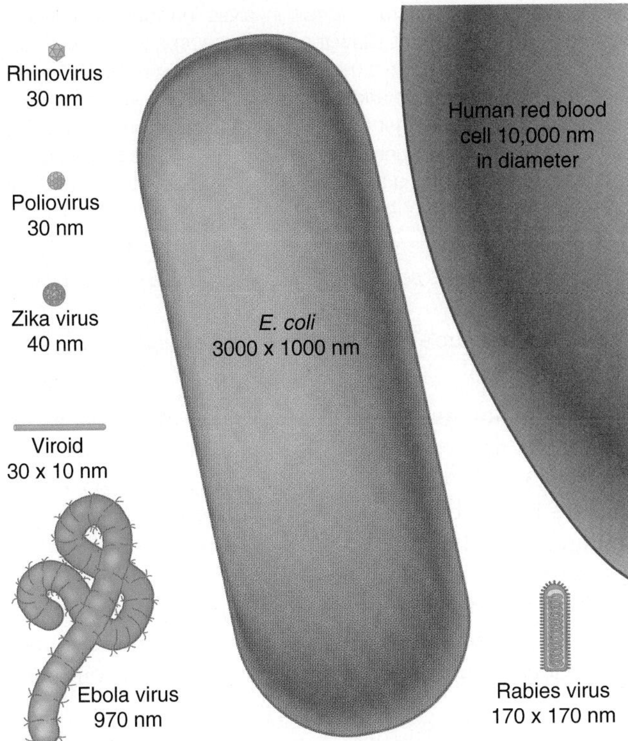

Figure 13.5 ■ A comparison of the relative sizes of bacteria and viruses.

mantle or envelope, while the hepatitis and rhinovirus are so named because they infect the liver and the nasal passages, respectively. Viruses named after geographic areas of infectious outbreak include the West Nile virus (the West Nile district of Northern Uganda), the Sendai virus (Sendai, Japan), the Norwalk virus (Norwalk, Ohio), the Coxsackie virus (Coxsackie, New York), and the Zika virus (the Zika forest in Uganda).[36]

The genome (nucleic acid) of a virus consists of either DNA or RNA. Viral DNA or RNA can be either single stranded or double stranded and either circular or linear. The general structure of a virus is illustrated in **Figure 13.6** ■. The genome of a virus is surrounded by a protein coat called a capsid. The capsid packages, protects, and facilitates the delivery of the viral genome. The genome plus the capsid is called the nucleocapsid. Host defense mechanisms, such as antibodies, are often directed against capsid surface proteins. The nucleocapsid of some viruses is covered with an outer envelope (i.e., enveloped viruses), while others are nonenveloped. Viral envelopes are derived from mammalian cell membranes when they are released from the host cell. Viral envelopes consist of lipids, proteins, and glycoproteins. Enveloped and nonenveloped viruses differ not only in their structural characteristics but also in their infectivity. Compared to nonenveloped viruses, enveloped viruses are environmentally labile. Their membrane can be preserved only if they are in an aqueous environment. Consequently, they spread in large droplets and secretions or via blood transfusions. Examples are the influenza virus and the HIV virus. In contrast, nonenveloped viruses are hardier and can survive adverse environments. Nonenveloped viruses can withstand the harsh conditions of the gastrointestinal tract and are resistant to common disinfectants. They also survive inadequate sewage treatment. Enteric viruses that cause gastrointestinal infections are nonenveloped.[36]

Viral Invasion and Replication in the Human Host

Viruses replicate within the host cell and use the host as a source of substrate, energy, and other components necessary to manufacture viral proteins and to replicate the viral genome. The process of viral replication consists of eight steps, divided into an early phase and a late phase. The early phase includes (1) viral recognition of the host target cell, (2) attachment to the host cell, (3) penetration of the host cell membrane, and (4) release and uncoating of the viral genome into the host cell's cytoplasm. The late phase consists of (5) viral genome transcription (replication), (6) synthesis of viral structural components, (7) assembly of new viral particles, and (8) release of new viruses from the host cell. When its genome is uncoated, a virus loses its infectivity; hence, the period of time from viral uncoating to release of new viruses is referred to as the eclipse period. The latent period refers to the time during which extracellular viruses cannot be detected. The latent period includes the eclipse period and ends with the release of newly formed virus.

The first two steps in viral replication include recognition and attachment to the host target cell. The glycoproteins

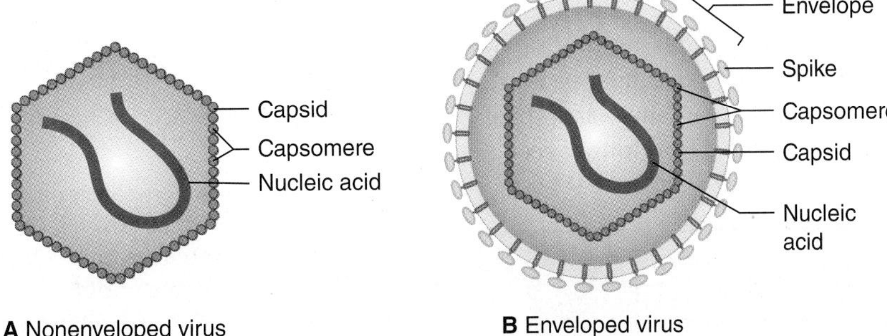

Figure 13.6 ■ General structure of a virus. **A**. Viruses can be nonenveloped (icosahedral nucleocapsid) or enveloped, **B**. where the nucleocapsid is encased within a membrane that may be studded with surface proteins.

(gp) on the outer surface of the virus serve as viral attachment proteins. Viral attachment proteins facilitate viral binding to host tissues. For example, the HIV virus is an enveloped virus whose outer envelope is studded with gp120, which mediates HIV's attachment to host target cells. Some viruses display canyon-like clefts or "keyholes" on their surface that are used to bind to a receptor on the host target cells. When binding to host cells, viruses exhibit the property of **tropism**—the preference of virus to bind to specific targets or host cells. For instance, the virus that causes rabies has a tropism for nervous tissue, as it will selectively bind to the acetylcholine receptor of neurons, whereas the HIV virus selectively binds to cells with the CD4 receptor, such a T lymphocytes. Some viruses bind to receptors that are located on cells common to many host tissues. This property characterizes the influenza virus, which binds to sialic acid receptors of epithelial cells that are widely distributed throughout the body. The susceptible host target cell defines the tissue tropism and, in turn, the manifestations of the disease caused by the virus.[36]

Once the virus has attached to the host cell, it will penetrate and enter the cell. Depending on the virus, this can occur by endocytosis, by fusion of the viral cell membrane with that of the host, or by direct penetration into the host cell. Once internalized, the viral genome is delivered to the site of replication, and the viral capsid or envelope is removed (uncoating). The genome of most DNA viruses is delivered to the host cell nucleus, whereas RNA viruses replicate in the cytoplasm. Uncoating may be initiated by attachment to the host cell receptor or by the acidic environment of the endosome or lysosome proteases. The viral genome will then direct the synthesis of new viral RNA or DNA and viral capsid proteins, and these will be assembled into the newly formed viruses or viral progeny. Some viruses form an empty capsid, and then the genome is inserted during assembly; others form their capsids around the genome. Following assembly, the progeny viruses are released from the host cell. Enveloped viruses are released by budding from the host cell membrane, which is used to form the viral envelope; nonenveloped viruses are released passively on lysis and death of the host cell.[13] The general sequence of viral replication is illustrated in **Figure 13.7** ■.

Viral replication, especially RNA viral replication, occurs at a fast rate, and this rapid replication leads to an increased rate of errors, which cause genetic mutations. As a result, viruses readily change their structure, producing new strains of virus that are able to evade host immune defense mechanisms. Viral mutations can alter viral structure in such a way that the viral type is no longer recognized by a previously immunized host's immune system.

Bernard Reinberg: Application

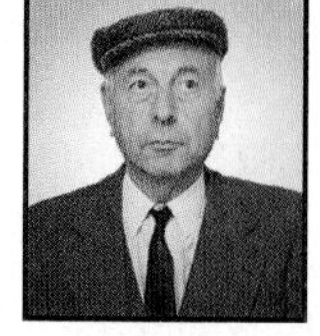

Mr. Reinberg did not get the current seasonal influenza vaccination. His most recent vaccination from 5 years ago was not effective, owing to changes in viral structure that occur in the genes that regulate expression of two major influenza viral surface antigens, hemagglutinin A and neuraminidase, involved in viral attachment to host cells. Such mutations allow the virus to escape detection by the host's immune system. Because the influenza virus is an RNA virus, it replicates at a rapid rate and is prone to errors that lead to genetic mutations. Commonly, genes regulating the structure of antigens on the surface of the influenza virus mutate from season to season, so these surface proteins are altered in such a way that previously formed antibodies are not effective against past strains of influenza virus.

5. How do viruses such as the influenza viruses use the host to replicate?
6. Describe the role of hemagglutinin A and neuraminidase in viral attachment.

The major genetic mutations that alter the influenza virus are termed *antigenic drift* and *antigenic shift* (**Figure 13.8** ■). **Antigenic drift** is characterized by minor changes in the structure of viral hemagglutin A and neuraminidase and this may result in an influenza epidemic.[13] An **epidemic** is a widespread outbreak of an infectious disease in which many people are infected simultaneously. A **pandemic** occurs when an epidemic becomes very widespread and affects a whole region, a continent,

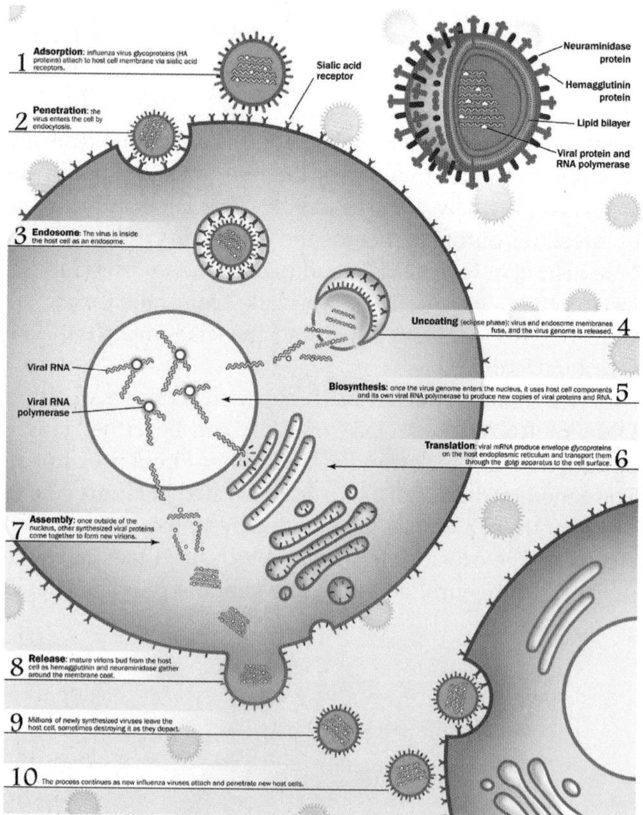

Figure 13.7 ■ The general steps of viral replication: (1) recognition of host target cell, (2) attachment to host cell receptor, (3) penetration of host cell membrane, (4) uncoating of viral genome, (5) transcription of the viral genome, (6) synthesis of viral structural proteins, (7) replication of the viral genome, (8) viral assembly, (9) viral release from the host cell. (10) Enveloped viruses bud from the host cell membrane and form the viral envelope; nonenveloped viruses are released on lysis of the host cell.

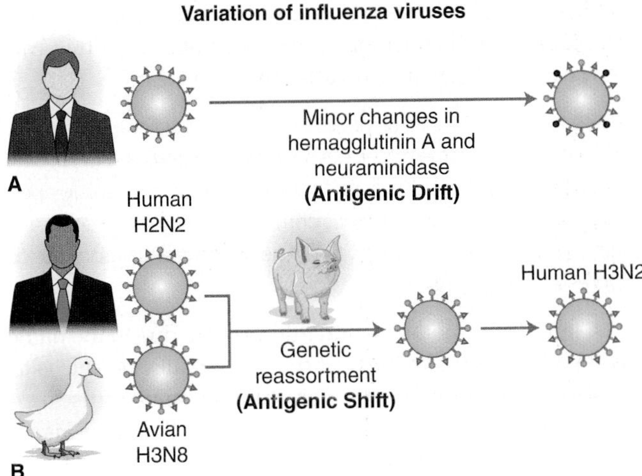

Figure 13.8 ■ **A**. Antigenic drift. **B**. Antigenic shift.

or the world, such as the 1918 H1N1 influenza pandemic, which killed an estimated 40 million people in less than a year.[37] In contrast, an **antigenic shift** occurs when there is a major genetic change that enables the influenza virus to jump from one species to another.[37] For example, this can occur when an avian (bird) influenza strain undergoes a genetic change that allows it to directly infect humans, that is from bird to human. This can also occur when an avian virus passes to an intermediate host, such as a pig that is simultaneously infected with a human influenza virus. The intermediate host allows mixing of viral genes (reassortment) from the two viral species producing a new strain of virus that can then infect humans and evade any previously established host defense. The major changes in viral antigens that occur with antigenic shift may result in a pandemic.

CLINICAL POINT: Since the influenza virus undergoes frequent antigenic drift, a new flu vaccine must be developed yearly. Based on the predicted yearly strains for influenza A, B, and C, which are the three forms of influenza virus that cause disease in humans,[38] a new vaccine is made to provide protection against the predicted strain of influenza viruses. It is important that individuals who are at risk for influenza obtain the influenza vaccine every year. ■

Individuals who are at risk for influenza include older adults, the immunocompromised, and those with chronic respiratory and/or cardiac conditions. These individuals are not only at risk for influenza but also more prone to the complications of influenza virus infection, which include the development of primary viral or secondary bacterial pneumonia. The influenza virus impairs the cilia that line the bronchioles and keep bacteria from adhering and colonizing the lung. As a result, influenza infection increases the risk of secondary bacterial pneumonias, especially in older adults and debilitated individuals. Healthcare workers are also highly encouraged to receive the yearly influenza vaccine because of their increased risk of contracting and spreading this communicable disease among their patients.

Bernard Reinberg: Outcome

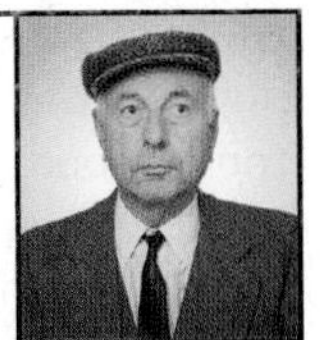

Mr. Reinberg has many risk factors that predispose him to secondary bacterial pneumonia. As an older adult, he is subject to an age-related decline in immune response. He has a history of smoking, and cigarette smoking damages cilia and impairs alveolar macrophages, allowing the virus to reach the lower lobes of the lung and colonize. Furthermore, he has diabetes, and comorbidities such as diabetes are known to decrease the immune response. Also, residing in an assisted living facility increases the number of contacts with other people who may transmit respiratory pathogens.

Treatment of individuals who contract influenza may include administration of a neuraminidase inhibitor, such as oseltamivir (Tamiflu), zanamivir (Relenza), or peramivir (Rapivab). However, for maximum effectiveness, these antiviral agents must be administered within 48 hours of symptom onset. Because Mr. Reinberg's onset of symptoms occurred approximately 10 days before his hospital admission, administration of a neuraminidase inhibitor was not included in his care. Treatment of his influenza was symptomatic and included administration of intravenous fluids, aerosolized bronchodilators, and antipyretic medications to control his fever. Treatment of his secondary bacterial pneumonia caused by *S. pneumoniae* required a course of antibiotics. In total, his recovery necessitated a 12-day hospitalization, after which he was transferred back to the assisted living facility.

7. How does Mr. Reinberg's history of smoking contribute to his risk of developing a secondary bacterial infection?
8. Why should Mr. Reinberg receive an annual influenza vaccine?

Depending on viral and host factors, infection with a virus may not be immediately accompanied by clinical signs and symptoms of infection. This asymptomatic period occurs during the time of viral replication or amplification of viral number. This can also include the time during which the virus spreads to a secondary site of infection. Spread of a viral infection to a secondary site occurs by way of the blood or lymphatic system. For instance, the varicella virus enters the host through the respiratory mucosa and initially causes pulmonary symptoms (primary infection). This virus then migrates to the skin by way of lymph nodes and produces a secondary infection marked by vesicular lesions of the skin (chickenpox). The brain can be a secondary site of viral infection, as some viruses gain access to the brain from the bloodstream, cerebral spinal fluid or infected macrophages that migrate into the central nervous system. Not all viruses extend to a secondary site; some may remain localized at the site of primary infection.

The asymptomatic period of viral infection is also called the **incubation period**. Depending on the virus, the time period of incubation varies widely. For example, the incubation period for influenza is 1–2 days, whereas the incubation period for hepatitis B is 50–150 days. Particularly striking is the incubation time for HIV, which ranges from 1 to 10 years. Many viral infections are first manifested by a **prodrome**, which consists of nonspecific symptoms such as lethargy, headache, and fever. The prodrome symptoms are due to the release of immune products, such as interferon and interleukins. The prodrome is followed by the more specific symptoms associated with the infecting virus (e.g., enteric viruses produce gastrointestinal distress, whereas respiratory viruses produce cough and symptoms of pulmonary congestion). Some viruses are never eliminated from the body but reside in a **latent viral state**. This means that the virus is harbored in the body in an inactive state but can be reactivated under certain conditions and cause active disease. This is well illustrated by the herpes simplex virus, which causes herpes labialis ("cold sores"). When the herpetic lesion is cleared by the immune system, the herpes virus retreats to the trigeminal nerve ganglia and remains quiescent. Conditions such as sunlight, stress, or fever can reactivate the herpes virus, causing it to move from the nerve to the lip epithelium and produce an active case of herpes labialis. As a consequence, individuals infected with *Herpes labialis* suffer repeated outbreaks of infection.[39]

Varicella zoster, the virus that causes chickenpox, can also cause a disease called shingles. Shingles is most common in individuals over 60 years of age. After an active case of chickenpox, varicella zoster assumes a latent state and remains present but inactive in the nerve ganglia along the spinal cord. For a number of reasons, the latent virus can become reactivated and will travel along the nerve fibers back to the skin to cause shingles. Shingles begins as a burning or itching sensation on one side of the face or body, followed in 3–5 days by a vesicular rash that is very painful and lasts several weeks. Some individuals are left with chronic pain in the form of postherpetic neuralgia that can last for weeks or even years after the rash clears.

CLINICAL POINT: Antiviral medications are most effective if started early in the course of the disease. A vaccine (Zostavax) is now recommended for individuals 60 years or older who have had chickenpox and whose immune system is not compromised by other diseases, such as HIV infection or cancer, or by medications such as immunosuppressive drugs.[40] ■

Clinical symptoms of viral infection are due to the damage the virus causes to the host cells and tissues as well as to the host's immune response. For example, some viruses are lytic, meaning that they kill the target cells that they infect. Viruses such as HIV can cause fusion of the host's cells into multinucleated giant cells called syncytia. Syncytia permit the virus to spread from cell to cell without being detected by the host's immune system. Certain viruses are oncogenic; that is, they increase the risk for cancer. An example of an oncogenic virus is HPV, which causes genital warts. HPV is capable of inactivating cell growth regulatory proteins and can cause cervical cancer. A vaccine is now available to prevent HPV infections and lower the risk of developing cervical cancer.[41] (See the Impact of Research on Clinical Practice feature.)

Impact of Current Research on Clinical Practice

Vaccination Against Human Papillomaviruses and Prevention of Cervical Cancer

Description: Human papillomaviruses (HPVs) are a group of more than 100 viruses. They are called papillomaviruses because some of them cause warts, or papillomas, which are benign tumors. The HPVs that cause the common warts that grow on hands and feet are different from those that cause growths in the throat or genital area. Of the more than 100 types of HPV, over 40 types can be passed from one person to another through sexual contact.[1]

In the United States, approximately 79 million Americans currently have HPV, and an estimated 14 million new genital HPV infections occur each year.[2] Most HPV infections occur without any symptoms and are eliminated without any treatment over the course of a few years. However, HPV infection sometimes persists for many years, and such persistent infections may lead to cervical abnormalities that can lead to cervical cancer. Cervical cancer strikes nearly half a million women each year worldwide, claiming more than a quarter of a million lives, and is the second most common cancer in women. Studies suggest that HPVs play a role in cancers of the anus, vulva, vagina, and penis and some cancers of the oropharynx, the base of the tongue, and the tonsils. Moreover, HPV is the most common sexually transmitted infection in the United States.

Most people never even know that they have had HPV because the virus usually does not cause any symptoms. For most people, the body's immune system will clear the virus, and the infected person will not develop related health problems. Although most HPV infections clear and do not lead to cancer, virtually all cases of cervical cancer are clearly associated with and likely caused by HPV infection. As a consequence, investigations were undertaken to determine whether a vaccine could be developed to boost the body's immune response to these virus types in order to prevent the cancer-causing infection. Genetic engineering was used to create the vaccine, which is made up of noninfectious virus-like particles that trigger an antibody response that is capable of protecting the body against infection by HPV types 16 and 18, which cause approximately 70% of cervical cancers, and against HPV types 6 and 11, which cause approximately 90% of genital warts.

Clinical Practice: The U.S. Food and Drug Administration approved the HPV vaccine in June 2006 for females ages 9–26 years. This was the first vaccine licensed specifically to prevent cervical cancer, and research suggests that it is a highly effective preventive measure. In clinical trials, the HPV vaccine demonstrated nearly 100% protection against precancerous variations of HPV as well as for HPV4, which causes genital warts. Since 2006, HPV infections among teenage girls in the United States have decreased by 56%.[1]

A three-dose HPV vaccine series is recommended for all children at 11 or 12 years of age. Teenage males and females who have not previously received the vaccine are encouraged to receive it. The vaccine is recommended for women who are younger than 27 years old and for men who are younger than 21 years old, including any male who has sex with men. The HPV vaccine also is recommended for young males who are immunocompromised (including those who have HIV or AIDS) through age 26 years if previous vaccination has not been completed.[1]

Research Studies:

Centers for Disease Control and Prevention. (2016). *Human papillomavirus (HPV): Questions and answers*. Available at https://www.cdc.gov/hpv/parents/questions-answers.html

Centers for Disease Control and Prevention. (2016). *Human papillomavirus (HPV)*. Available at https://www.cdc.gov/std/hpv/STDFact-HPV.htm

Current Issues in Emerging Infectious Disease: Ebola Virus Disease, Enterovirus D68, and Zika Virus

In recent years, viruses have gained heightened significance from the standpoint of emerging infectious disease. In particular, the Ebola virus, enterovirus D68, and Zika virus have raised serious health concerns.

Ebola Virus Disease. In West Africa, 2014 marked history's largest outbreak of Ebola, followed by the emergence of the world's first Ebola epidemic.[42] As of December 2014, Ebola virus disease had been linked to four deaths in the United States.[43] Internationally, however, the death toll was much higher. By December 2014, a total of 20,206 confirmed, suspected , and probable cases of Ebola virus disease and 7905 deaths were reported in eight countries: Sierra Leone, Liberia, Guinea, Mali, Senegal, Nigeria, Spain, and the United States.[44]

Formerly known as Ebola hemorrhagic fever,[45] Ebola virus disease may be caused by several viral pathogens in the *Filoviridae* family of viruses, known as filoviruses.[46] The most recent outbreak of Ebola virus disease has been linked to *Zaire ebolavirus*. However, this organism is only one of several pathogens that are considered to be Ebola viruses; in total, the ebolavirus family includes five species of viruses.[46]

The Ebola virus, which is one of the most lethal viruses in history, attacks and cripples immune cells, triggering an outpouring of chemicals. This flood of chemical release, which is called a cytokine storm, causes the death of other immune cells.[46] A closer look at the mechanism of action of the Ebola virus involves consideration of RNA, glycoprotein, and replication.[47]

The Ebola virus is an enveloped package that contains RNA. Glycoprotein, which protrudes from the viral cell membrane, binds to receptors on the cellular surface. In turn, receptor binding by glycoprotein triggers macropinocytosis, which causes the virus to be engulfed by the cell membrane. After entering the cell, the RNA of the Ebola virus is uncoated, allowing the virus to take control of the human cell's proteins and to replicate. After new viral particles are produced, they travel to the cell membrane and undergo a budding process, during which they can be transported to other cells and continue the process of infection.[47]

Ebola virus can spread via direct contact with infected body fluids, including saliva, urine, feces, sweat, semen, breast milk, and vomit. Portals of entry include skin and mucous membranes.[48] Transmission of Ebola virus may also occur by way of contact with contaminated materials, objects, and surfaces. Early manifestations of Ebola virus disease include fever, chills, fatigue, and other flulike symptoms. Late manifestations include profuse bleeding from body orifices and organ failure. Treatment is supportive, as there is no known cure.[48]

Enterovirus D68. In recent years, enterovirus D68 (EV-D68) has been identified as an emerging infectious disease. EV-D68 was originally identified in 1962 via analysis of a throat culture obtained from a child who was diagnosed with pneumonia.[49] Since its identification, this virus has been linked to a very limited number of infections. Between 1970 and 2005, only 26 cases of EV-D68 were reported.[50] However, by 2012, outbreaks in Japan, the Netherlands, the Philippines, and the United Kingdom prompted concerns about an epidemic.[51] In 2014, the United States experienced a nationwide outbreak of EV-D68. Between August and December 2014, a total of 1152 individuals in 49 states and the District of Columbia were reportedly infected with this virus.[52]

Children are especially susceptible to EV-D68. Primary disease sequelae include respiratory-related manifestations that may range from mild coldlike symptoms to severe respiratory distress.[11] In rare cases, EV-D68 has been linked to severe neurologic impairment, including flaccid paralysis.[49] ■

The precise mechanism of action of EV-D68 has not yet been determined. However, researchers believe the ability of this virus to invade lymphocytes provides a mechanism for its spread to secondary target organs.[49] Although routes of transmission for EV-D68 are not fully understood,[49] transmission is believed to occur via exposure to contaminated respiratory secretions, including sputum, saliva, and nasal mucus. Therefore, potential modes of transmission may include sneezing, coughing, or contacting a surface that is contaminated with the virus.[53] Treatment is supportive, as no definitive cure has been identified.[49]

Zika Virus Infection. The Zika virus is an emerging pathogen. It is an RNA arbovirus first isolated from a monkey in the Zika forest in Uganda in 1947 and then in the *Aedes* mosquito a year later. Zika virus infection in humans was identified in the early 1950s in Africa and Asia, and for many years, there were only sporadic cases, limited to a few countries. Then outbreaks of Zika virus infections started occurring in other areas, including Micronesia in 2007, French Polynesia in 2013, Brazil in 2015, and Florida in 2016. The Zika virus has now spread to many other areas in South and Central America, the Caribbean, Mexico, and the United States. In February 2016, the World Health Organization declared the Zika virus pandemic a public health emergency of international concern.

Zika virus infection is transmitted primarily by the bite of infected *Aedes* mosquitoes. However, Zika virus has been found in the semen of infected men and in vaginal secretions of infected women, and several cases of sexual transmission have been confirmed.[54] The transmission of Zika virus by blood transfusions from infected donors, including those who were asymptomatic, was initially found during the outbreak in French Polynesia.[55] The U.S. Food and Drug Administration has recommended that all donations of whole blood and blood components be tested to prevent transmission of Zika virus through transfusions. Perinatal transmission of Zika virus from an infected pregnant woman to her fetus is of major concern because the virus has teratogenic effects.[54]

Individuals infected with Zika virus can either be asymptomatic or have mild symptoms including fever, muscle aches, rash, headache, conjunctivitis, and arthralgia that can last up to a week. Although manifestations of Zika virus infection are often mild and self-limiting, two serious neurologic conditions have been linked to Zika virus infection: Guillain-Barré syndrome in adults and microcephaly in fetuses and newborns. Guillain-Barré syndrome is a type of peripheral neuropathy caused by inflammation and demyelination of nerve fibers leading to impaired nerve conduction, which results in weakness and paralysis. It can affect the muscles involved in breathing and may lead to respiratory failure. Guillain-Barré syndrome is known to be triggered by other infections that stimulate production of antibodies that cross-react with myelin, resulting in its immune-mediated destruction. Increases in the incidence of the previously rare Guillain-Barré syndrome have been linked to several outbreaks of Zika virus infection.

The dramatic increase in the incidence of microcephaly, an abnormally small head size due to impaired brain development, has been linked to Zika virus infection during pregnancy. The virus has been isolated from placental and brain tissue during autopsy of affected fetuses. Laboratory studies have confirmed that the Zika virus can infect and kill neural precursor cells grown in culture; this appears to be the basis for its neurotropic properties. The Zika virus can be isolated from amniotic fluid of infected pregnant women and from their blood, and microcephaly can be detected by an ultrasound.

The basis for diagnosis of Zika virus infection includes the person's clinical manifestations and history of travel to or residence in an area with active Zika virus infection. However, since the clinical manifestations of Zika virus infection resemble those of several other viral infections, such as West Nile virus, and because locations with a Zika virus epidemic may also have outbreaks of other viral infections, confirmation of the diagnosis is based on detection of Zika virus RNA in the blood or urine.

Because the virus is largely transmitted by mosquitoes, prevention of Zika virus infection involves environmental control of mosquitoes by use of insecticides and removal of stagnant water, where mosquitoes lay eggs.

Insect repellents can be used to prevent mosquito bites; however, they should be approved by the Environmental Protection Agency for safety and efficacy. Wearing long pants and tops with long sleeves and using screens in windows also help to reduce mosquito bites. Several Zika virus vaccines are under development; they are in various stages of clinical trials. The vaccine developed by scientists at the National Institute of Allergy and Infectious Diseases is a DNA vaccine that contains genes that code for Zika virus proteins. When injected into humans, the genes are transcribed into viral proteins, and an immune response is activated, which will destroy the virus if it enters the body.[56] Another vaccine that is under investigation contains live, attenuated (weakened) Zika virus. However, several years of study of the safety, effect on the immune response, and ability to prevent infection will be needed before a Zika virus vaccine is commercially available.

Because of the potential serious harm to the fetus caused by Zika virus, pregnant women should avoid travel to regions with Zika virus transmission. Women living in regions with active Zika virus infections are advised to consider avoiding pregnancy until the epidemic is controlled or a vaccine becomes available. ■

No antiviral medications are currently available to treat Zika virus infection; however, research to develop a safe and effective medication is under way. One of the medications under development is a caspase inhibitor. Zika virus increases activity of the caspase enzyme in neural cells, resulting in cell death.[57] Treatment of symptomatic individuals with Zika virus infection involves supportive care such as maintenance of fluid and electrolyte balance and nutritional support.

Prions

The word *prion* is short for "proteinaceous infectious particles." **Prions** are nonliving particles that are transmitted to mammals and cause neurodegenerative disease. Prions are notoriously known to cause bovine spongiform encephalopthy, also known as "mad cow disease." An outbreak of bovine spongiform encephalopthy in the United Kingdom occurred in 1985. This outbreak and the link to human neurodegenerative disease triggered public alarm about the safety of ingesting beef from cattle with bovine spongiform encephalopthy. This led to a widespread ban on importation of beef from countries where bovine spongiform encephalopthy has been identified. To minimize risk and limit spread, the United States now implements severe restrictions on the importation of live animals such as cattle, sheep, and goats.[58] Ingestion of prion-contaminated beef can cause a human disease called new variant Creutzfeldt–Jakob disease, a central nervous system degenerative disease. Prions are able to infect host cells and convert normal host cell protein into dangerous proteins simply by inducing these normal proteins to change their conformation or shape (without changing their amino acid sequence). In turn, these abnormal host proteins infect additional nerve cells and lead to widespread disease. The immune system does not recognize these altered proteins as foreign; hence, there is no immune response. As prions multiply they aggregate into amyloid rods (fibrils). Neurons take them up, and they accumulate in cell vacuoles. This causes the cells to appear spongy and impairs neural function. Creutzfeldt–Jakob disease has a long latent period; it requires years or decades before symptoms, such as dementia, are manifested.[58]

Fungi

Fungi are microorganisms that have rigid chitin- or cellulose-based cell walls that reproduce primarily by sporulation. Fungi include the molds, yeasts, and higher fungi (e.g., *Histoplasma*, *Cryptococcus*, and *Candida*). All fungi are gram-positive and eukaryotic, and they have sterols but not peptidoglycan in their cell membrane. Most fungi are multicellular, although some, such as yeasts, are unicellular. Fungi can cause infections that are superficial and localized to the skin, the hair, or the nails and cause such diseases as athlete's foot or ringworm, which is also known as tinea. Lung infections caused by fungi can be more serious. For example, histoplasmosis is a mild to severe lung infection caused by *Histoplasma capsulatum* transmitted by bat or bird droppings. Pneumocystitis is an infection of the lung caused by *P. jiroveci* (formerly called *P. carinii*) that can cause a fatal pneumonia in individuals with AIDS. Cryptococcosis is a systemic infection caused by the yeast *Cryptococcus neoformans*. The most common manifestation is a subacute or chronic form of meningitis resulting from the inhalation of the microorganism. Yeasts of the *Candida* genus are opportunistic pathogens that may cause diseases such as vaginal yeast infections and thrush (a throat infection that is often found in infants) among people who are immunocompromised or undergoing antibiotic therapy. Antibiotics reduce the bacterial population that is normally present in the vagina and throat, allowing the yeast to grow unchecked. Another opportunistic fungus is *Aspergillus fumigatus*, which can infect the lungs, inner ear, and sinuses of immunosuppressed individuals and can disseminate throughout the body.[59]

Protozoa and Helminths

Protozoa are unicellular, eukaryotic microorganisms that include the familiar amoeba and paramecium. Protozoa do not have cell walls and are typically acquired through contaminated food or water or from the bite of an infected arthropod such as a mosquito. Two common protozoa, *Giardia lamblia* and *Cryptosporidium parvum*, can cause diarrheal disease.[43] Malaria is a tropical illness that is caused by several species of the protozoan *Plasmodium*. Malaria is an important global public health problem; in 2015, there were 95 countries and territories with ongoing malaria infections with approximately 3.2 billion individuals at risk.[60]

4 *Toxoplasma gondii* is an intracellular protozoon that is responsible for toxoplasmosis, which is an infection that poses a serious threat in immunosuppressed individuals and pregnant women (who are characteristically immunocompromised due to hormonal changes during pregnancy). The microorganism infects cats and small rodents and can be transferred to humans from those animals. In immunocompromised individuals, infection results in generalized involvement of brain, liver, lung and other organs, and often death. Another reason why exposure to *T. gondii* during pregnancy is dangerous is because it crosses the placenta and can be transmitted from the blood of an infected pregnant woman to her fetus, resulting in congenital toxoplasmosis. Adverse effects associated with congenital toxoplasmosis can include hearing loss, impaired vision, seizures, and altered cardiac and renal function. To decrease the risk of exposure to *T. gondii* from cats during pregnancy, pregnant women should limit their exposure to cats, especially to those who have been outdoors or eat raw meat, and should avoid emptying cats' litter boxes. ■

Helminths are simple, invertebrate animals, some of which are infectious parasites. They are multicellular, and their physiology is similar in many ways to that of humans. This makes helminth infections difficult to treat because drugs that kill helminths are frequently very toxic to human cells. Many helminths have complex, multistage reproductive cycles that require a vertebrate host and an invertebrate host. An example is the genus *Schistosoma*, which is a flatworm. One species of *Schistosoma* causes swimmer's itch; another species causes the much more serious disease schistosomiasis, which is endemic in Africa and Latin America. Schistosome eggs hatch in freshwater, and the resulting larvae infect snails. When the snails shed these larvae, the larvae attach to and penetrate human skin. They feed, grow, and mate in the human bloodstream. Damage to human tissue is caused by the accumulation of schistosome eggs, which have sharp spines; they produce disease symptoms such as diarrhea and abdominal pain. Liver and spleen involvement is common.[61] Another disease due to a helminth is trichinosis, caused by the roundworm *Trichinella spiralis*. This infectious agent is typically ingested in improperly cooked pork from infected pigs. Early disease symptoms include vomiting, diarrhea, and fever; later symptoms include intense muscle pain because the larvae grow and mature in muscle tissue. Fatal cases often show congestive heart failure and respiratory paralysis. The medically important protozoa and helminths are termed parasites. Parasitic infections are increasing throughout the world, in part because of increased host susceptibility due to the impact of HIV on the immune system of infected individuals. Additional factors, including climate change as a consequence of global warming and increased international travel, also increased the spread of parasitic infections.[62] Starvation and the breakdown in sanitation that accompanies war have resulted in the reemergence of other parasitic infections.[63]

Check Your Progress: Section 13.4

1. What is the recommended schedule for pneumococcal vaccination in children?
2. How are bacteria categorized?
3. What is the key difference between cells of bacteria and those of mammals?

13.5 The Innate and Adaptive Immune Response to Infectious Microoorganisms

Most infectious agents do not penetrate the body surface; they are prevented from doing so by a variety of biochemical and physical barriers (**Figure 13.9** ■). However, if infectious agents do penetrate the body, there is a dynamic interplay between the immune system, which attempts to limit the infectious agent, and the infectious agent, which attempts to invade and replicate within the host. There are two major compartments of the immune response that protect from invasive microorganisms: the innate and adaptive immune

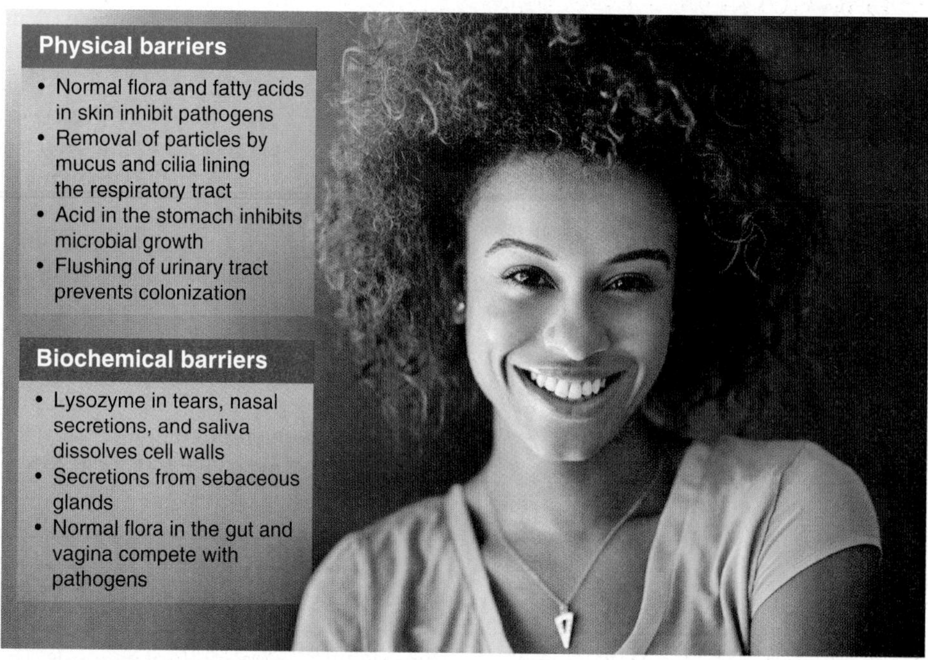

Physical barriers
• Normal flora and fatty acids in skin inhibit pathogens
• Removal of particles by mucus and cilia lining the respiratory tract
• Acid in the stomach inhibits microbial growth
• Flushing of urinary tract prevents colonization
Biochemical barriers
• Lysozyme in tears, nasal secretions, and saliva dissolves cell walls
• Secretions from sebaceous glands
• Normal flora in the gut and vagina compete with pathogens

Figure 13.9 ■ Biochemical and physical barriers to penetration by infectious microorganisms.

systems. The **innate (natural) immune system** comprises antigen-nonspecific defense mechanisms that quickly respond after exposure to an infectious agent. This is the immunity that one is born with and is the body's initial response to prevent infection. Unlike adaptive immunity, innate immunity does not recognize every possible antigen. Instead, it is designed to recognize a few highly conserved structures that are present in many different microorganisms. The structures that are recognized are known as **pathogen-associated molecular patterns**; they include lipopolysaccharide of gram-negative bacteria, peptidoglycan of both gram-negative and gram-positive bacteria, lipoteichoic acids from the gram-positive bacteria, bacterial DNA, double-stranded RNA from viruses, and glucans from fungi. Many host defense cells (e.g., phagocytes and dendritic cells) have **pattern-recognition receptors** (many of which are known as toll-like receptors) for these common pathogen-associated molecular patterns, which mediate an immediate response against the invading microorganism.[63] Components of the innate immune system are summarized in **Table 13.6** ■.

The **adaptive (acquired) immune system** comprises antigen-specific defense mechanisms. On initial exposure to an antigen, the adaptive immune system requires several days to become host protective. Unlike the innate immune system, the adaptive immune system is capable of targeting specific pathogens. Antibodies produced by the adaptive immune system are designed to react with and eliminate a particular antigen.[63] This is the immunity that one develops throughout life, and it usually improves on repeated exposure to a given antigen or infectious agent, such as by vaccination or actual infection. Components of the adaptive immune system are antigen-specific B lymphocytes that produce antibodies as well as antigen-specific T lymphocytes that can produce cytokines or can be cytotoxic for cellular targets that display the specific antigen (**Figure 13.10** ■). Different types of infectious agents stimulate distinct patterns of immune response that typically are host protective and result in adaptive and specific immunity to the infectious agent. The principal protective immune response against extracellular bacteria (those invading extracellular spaces) and bacteria in the circulation is specific antibody that opsonizes bacteria for phagocytosis by macrophages and polymorphonuclear leukocytes. During the process of **opsonization**, a pathogen is marked by complement proteins for phagocytic ingestion and destruction.[64,65] Specific

Table 13.6 Components of the Innate Immune System

Component	Examples
Anatomic, mechanical, and chemical barriers	Skin, flow of air or fluids, salivary lysozyme, fatty acids of the skin, antimicrobial peptides
Phagocytic cells	Polymorphonuclear leukocytes, monocytes, and macrophages
Cells that release inflammatory mediators	Basophils, mast cells, and eosinophils
Lymphocytes	Natural killer cells
Molecules of innate immunity	Complement proteins, acute-phase proteins

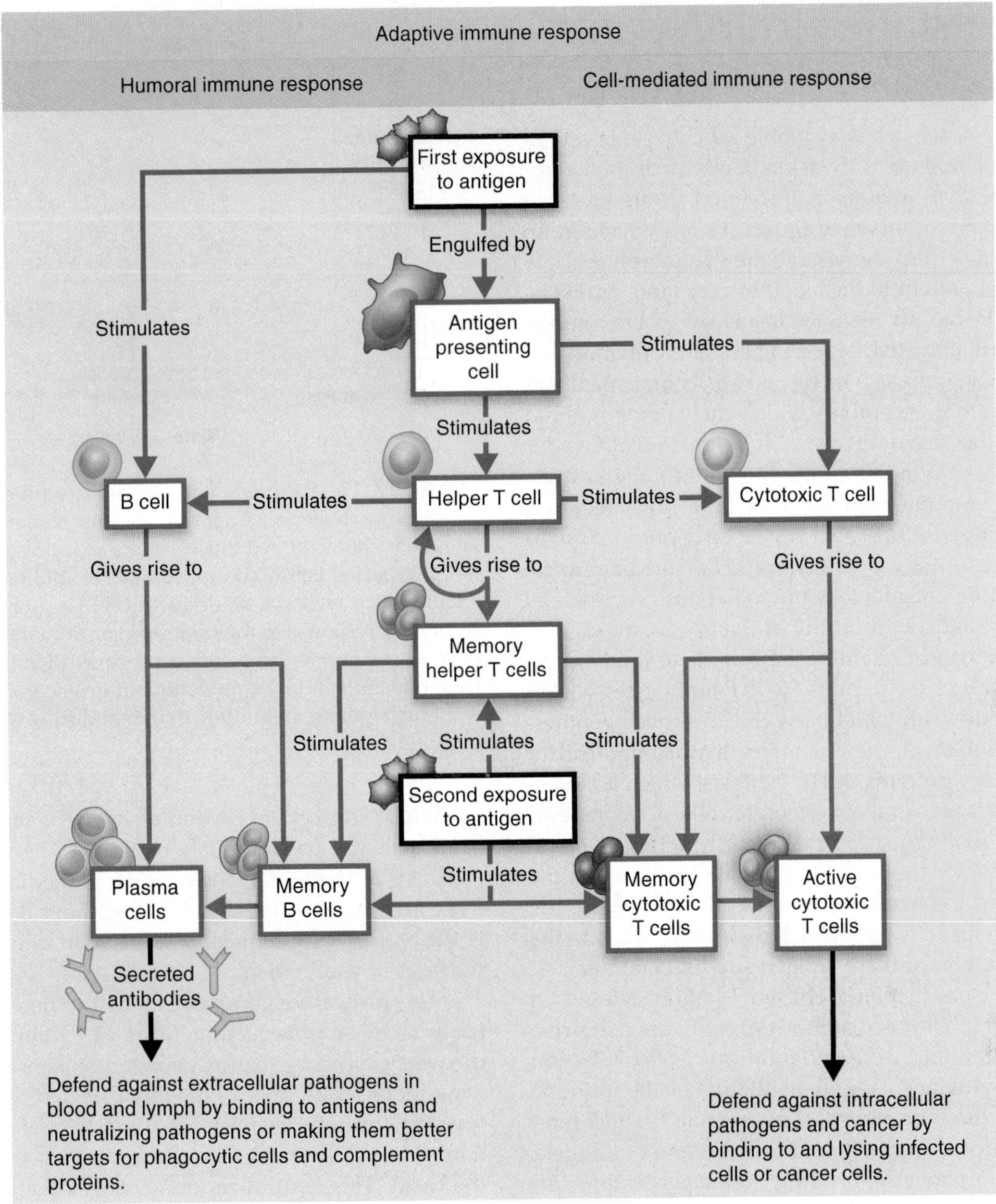

Figure 13.10 ■ Adaptive immune response to an infectious microorganism.

antibody and complement opsonize both gram-positive and gram-negative bacteria and can lyse gram-negative bacteria. Complement comprises over 20 different serum proteins, some of which can bind to antibodies or to membrane components of cells.[49] When bound, these complement proteins are cleaved enzymatically, yielding fragments that can lyse or opsonize bound cells as well as induce directed chemotaxis of other cell populations. Intracellular bacteria survive and replicate within host cells, including phagocytes, because these microorganisms have developed mechanisms for resisting intracellular degradation. Immunity against these bacteria is principally cell-mediated and consists of T-helper lymphocytes that activate macrophages by the production of cytokines. In contrast to bacteria, viruses are obligatory intracellular infectious agents. Adaptive immunity against viruses consists of specific cytotoxic T lymphocytes that lyse virally infected cells and may contribute to tissue injury even when the infectious virus is not cytopathic by itself. Adaptive immunity against viruses also consists of specific antibodies and T-helper lymphocytes that provide cytokines for the growth and differentiation of effector T and B lymphocytes.

Check Your Progress: Section 13.5

1. Describe the difference between the innate immune system and the adaptive immune system.
2. What are the five components of the innate immune system?
3. What are the components of the adaptive immune system?

13.6 Resistance to Infectious Disease

Immediate host defense is available quickly (in less than an hour) after microbial invasion. Cells such as macrophages are resident in almost all tissues and are found in particularly large numbers at mucosal sites, which are in contact with the external environment. Polymorphonuclear leukocytes are present in the blood in very large numbers, and they can be rapidly recruited to any site where complement has been activated. Macrophages and polymorphonuclear leukocytes possess receptors (e.g., complement and pattern-recognition receptors), which enable them to bind and phagocytize microorganisms. If the microbial invader evades these components of the innate immune system, the adaptive immune response to the infectious agents is induced (see Figure 13.10). During the early phase of adaptive host defense, antigen-presenting cells called **dendritic cells**[66] engulf or phagocytose microbial antigen, such as viral antigen, and degrade the antigen into small peptides. These antigen-presenting cells traffic to local lymph nodes and present the peptides to T lymphocytes within the lymph node via interaction with cell surface peptide-presenting proteins known as **major histocompatibility complex (MHC) proteins**. MHC proteins, which are present on the surfaces of most vertebrate cells, allow natural killer cells to distinguish normal cells from target cells.[63] This process allows the rare (1 in a million) antigen-specific T lymphocytes to encounter the presented peptide. The antigen (peptide) activation of T lymphocytes leads to the clonal proliferation of these antigen-specific lymphocytes, resulting in the production of effector T lymphocytes, such as T-helper lymphocytes that produce cytokines that drive the proliferation and differentiation of cytotoxic T lymphocytes.[67] Cytokines (soluble mediators of the immune response) produced by other antigen-specific T-helper lymphocytes induce the growth and proliferation of antigen-activated B lymphocytes, resulting in the generation of a primary and then a secondary antibody response to the infectious agent.[66] Specific antibody plays an important role in clearing many primary infections. The presence of IgM (characteristic of the primary response) begins to be detectable in the circulation 3–4 days after antigen entry and peaks between 2 and 3 weeks. The IgG response (characteristic of the secondary response) is delayed 5–7 days and persists much longer. See **Figure 13.11** ■. Host protection from the infectious agent is a result of this adaptive immunity. Subsequent encounters with the same infectious agent will also be vigorously mounted. This secondary or adaptive immune response, which is mediated by long-lived memory T lymphocytes and memory B lymphocytes, is the basis for subsequent protective immunity, which is the basis of vaccination.

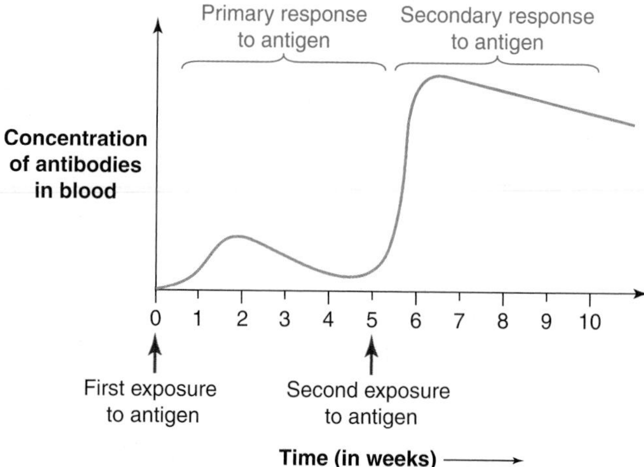

Figure 13.11 ■ Primary and secondary antibody response to antigenic challenge. Adaptive immune response to antigen is characterized during the primary response by a long lag period before the appearance of antibody in the circulation as well as a predominant IgM response. The secondary response to the same antigen is characterized by a shorter lag period before appearance of antibody in the circulation and by a predominant IgG response that is of a much greater magnitude than that during the primary immune response.

The protective components of the host response to bacteria are summarized in **Table 13.7** ■. In addition, for diseases caused by exotoxigenic organisms (microorganisms that secrete toxins, such as *C. tetani*, which causes tetanus), the immune response functions not only to eliminate the invading microorganism but also to neutralize the toxin. This neutralization occurs as the result of specific antibody blocking the interaction of the toxin with its mammalian cell surface target. In the case of tetanus toxin, the antibody blocks the toxin from binding to neurons. Without antibody, the toxin causes sustained muscle contraction, tetany. The immune protective mechanisms listed in Table 13.7 are also protective when the host is infected with a virus. Other protective mechanisms that are employed in the host defense against viruses are listed in **Table 13.8** ■.

Table 13.7 Direct Mechanisms by Which the Immune Response Combats Bacterial and Viral Infectious Agents

Immune System Component	Target	Effector Mechanism
Neutrophils and macrophages	Intact microorganism	Phagocytosis and intracellular destruction
Antibody	Surface antigen of a microorganism	Blocks adsorption of the microorganism to host tissue
Antibody + complement	Surface antigen of a microorganism	Enhanced phagocytosis by neutrophils and macrophages
Antibody + complement	Host cell surface antigen	Lysis of infected cell
Activated macrophages	Engulfed microorganism	Enhanced intracellular destruction

Table 13.8 Direct Mechanisms by Which the Immune Response Combats Viral but Not Bacterial Infectious Agents

Immune System Component	Target	Effector Mechanism
Cytotoxic T lymphocytes	Cell surface presented viral peptides	Cytolysis
Natural killer cells	Virally infected host cells	Cytolysis
Interferons	Nonvirally infected host cells	Cellular antiviral state

Check Your Progress: Section 13.6

1. Describe the immediate host defense reaction after a microbial invasion.
2. Compare the responses of IgM and IgG in response to a microbial invasion.
3. What role do dendritic cells play in the early phase of adaptive host defense?

13.7 Resistance to Different Microbial Pathogens as Mediated by Different Host Protective Mechanisms

The immune system must cope with a spectrum of pathogenic microorganisms, which have distinct lifestyles. Different arms of the immune system are needed for protection from these differing microorganisms. In addition, many pathogenic microorganisms have evolved specific countermeasures, which limit or inhibit the effectiveness of the immune response. The general types of microbial pathogens are classified as either extracellular or intracellular microorganisms.

Resistance to Extracellular Microorganisms

Bacteria

Bacteria are probably the simplest type of microorganisms for the immune system to combat. In many cases, phagocytes are able to clear such infectious agents. Specific antibody is highly effective, both by directing complement-mediated lysis of gram-negative bacteria and by opsonization of gram-negative and gram-positive bacteria. A good example of a gram-negative bacterium is *N. meningitidis*, which causes meningitis. A good example of a gram-positive bacterium is *S. aureus*, which causes skin infections. Some bacteria, such as *S. pneumoniae*, which causes pneumonia, have evolved antiphagocytic capsules, which prevent recognition by innate immune mechanisms. Effective removal requires both antibody and complement to promote efficient opsonization and clearance by phagocytes. IgA plays an important role in the removal of microorganisms that infected mucosal surfaces (respiratory tract, gut, genitourinary tract). Secretory IgA can protect from *N. gonorrhoeae*, which causes gonorrhea.

Fungi

Phagocytic cells primarily handle these microorganisms, particularly cytokine-activated phagocytes. An excellent example of a fungus that is handled by the immune system in this way is *C. albicans*, which is a fungus that causes yeast infections.

Parasites

Large, multicellular parasites present a special problem to the immune system and indeed are rather poorly eliminated. The mechanisms that are deployed include antibody-directed complement-mediated destruction and antibody-dependent cellular cytotoxicity (antibodies specific for the parasite are bound to receptors on the effector cells) mediated by eosinophils derived from the peripheral blood. Innate immunity is generally ineffective. The parasites employ many evasion strategies, including complement inhibitors, release of large quantities of soluble antigen, and acquisition of host proteins.

Resistance to Intracellular Microorganisms

Bacteria and Protozoa

Many microorganisms have evolved resistance to the constitutive killing mechanisms used by phagocytes. These pathogens actively replicate inside mammalian cells, either in the phagosome or in the cytoplasm. An excellent example is *M. tuberculosis*, which causes tuberculosis. These types of microorganisms cannot be eliminated by the innate immune system. T-cell activation is required, and a T-helper lymphocyte response, which results in the production of cytokines that activate phagocytes (in this case, alveolar macrophages), is necessary for clearance of the microorganism.[68] Antibody is generally ineffective in eliminating such infections. What is effective is the development of a delayed type hypersensitivity reaction to proteins derived from mycobacteria. See **Figure 13.12** ■. This reaction demonstrates the importance of cytokine producing T-helper lymphocytes that are responsive to the mycobacteria, and such a reaction correlates with exposure to the antigen and probable protective immunity. Resistance to the protozoan *T. gondii* is mediated in the same manner, and active destruction of the protozoan occurs in activated macrophages.

Viruses

Viruses are a very diverse group of obligate intracellular pathogens. Almost every form of immunity comes into play against some type of virus. Enveloped viruses can

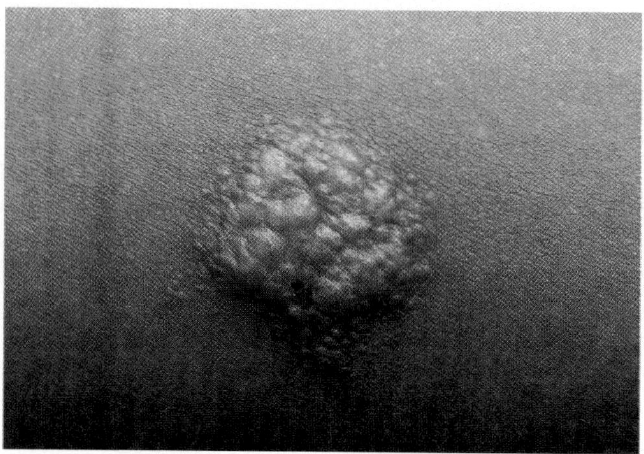

Figure 13.12 ■ A positive delayed type hypersensitivity response to a protein extracted from mycobacteria 48 hours after intradermal injection of the antigen. The injection site becomes indurated in a person with a positive reaction.

be damaged by complement. Phagocytes can take up and destroy antibody- and complement-coated viruses. Other key players in antiviral immunity are interferons, which produce an antiviral state in neighboring host cells; natural killer cells, which directly lyse infected cells; antibody, which functions to eliminate virus in the circulation; cytotoxic T lymphocytes, which destroy infected cells through cytotoxic mechanisms; and T-helper lymphocytes, which produce cytokines that orchestrate the immune response to the virus. Influenza virus is an excellent example of a virus that commonly infects humans.

Check Your Progress: Section 13.7

1. What role do capsules play in resistance?
2. What is the mechanism that the immune system uses against fungi?
3. What are the mechanisms used by parasites to avoid elimination?

13.8 Immune Deficient/ Susceptible Host

The importance of the immune system in protection from infectious agents is most dramatically illustrated in individuals with immune deficiencies. **Immunodeficiency** is a consequence of a defect in one or more components of the immune system. Immunodeficiencies are classified as either **primary** (inherited) or **secondary** (induced as a consequence of disease, disease treatment, or malnutrition).

Primary immunodeficiency diseases present as recurrent or overwhelming infections in very young children and are identified by the individual defective immunologic component: antibody, T lymphocyte, combined T and B lymphocyte, or phagocytic. The defect in each condition leads to preferential susceptibility to certain types of microorganisms. Typically, antibody (B-lymphocyte) deficiency results in susceptibility to bacterial infection. T-lymphocyte deficiency results in susceptibility to viral and fungal infections. ■

Secondary immunodeficiencies are acquired and are a result of infectious disease, systemic disease (e.g. cancer, diabetes mellitus), drug or radiotherapeutic treatment for disease (e.g., treatment of cancer and autoimmune disease), and injury (e.g., burns, trauma, splenectomy). A well-known example of a secondary immunodeficiency is infection with HIV, which leads to the acquired immune deficiency syndrome resulting from a deficiency of $CD4^+$ lymphocytes. Another prevalent example of secondary immunodeficiency is the use of immunosuppressive drugs and/or radiation therapy for treatment of cancer and certain autoimmune diseases. Such treatment results in a generalized immune suppression that is not confined to a single component of the immune system. Another example worth noting is individuals who have been splenectomized. These individuals are very susceptible to bacteria that require opsonizing antibodies for effective elimination. These individuals have a lifelong risk of sudden onset sepsis and should be vaccinated against such bacteria (e.g., *S. pneumoniae*, *N. meningitidis*, and *H. influenzae* type b).

Other groups that are at higher risk for infectious disease include the very young and older adults. Infants, especially premature infants, are at high risk for a variety of infections owing to the immaturity of their immune systems. Older adults are at risk because of their age-related decline in immune function and the frequent presence of other comorbidities (e.g., diabetes) that also suppress immune defenses. ■

Intravenous drug users place themselves at greater risk for infection because of shared and often unsanitary drug paraphernalia, direct microbial entry at intravenous sites, and often a general state of debilitation that impairs their immune defense mechanisms. As a group, critically ill individuals in intensive care units are at risk for infections, which often are resistant to standard antibiotic therapy. These individuals readily become colonized with resistant microorganisms and are at risk for infection due to the presence of indwelling lines and devices that breech host defense barriers and allow direct colonization of the individual by these pathogenic microorganisms.

Check Your Progress: Section 13.8

1. What is the difference between primary immunodeficiency and secondary immunodeficiency?
2. Why are individuals at the extreme ends of the lifespan more susceptible to infection?
3. Why are IV drug users at high risk for infection?

13.9 Protection from Infectious Disease by Vaccination

Immunity to the development of infectious disease can be either passive or active. **Passive immunity** is the provision of temporary protection from an infectious agent by the administration of exogenous antibody to a recipient. Passive immunity also occurs when anti-toxin (antibody specific for the toxin) is provided therapeutically to a recipient. The purpose of this form of passive immunity is to prevent disease after known exposure, such as a needlestick, or to ameliorate symptoms of an ongoing disease.

Passive immunity occurs when maternal preformed antibody is transferred across the placenta to the developing fetus. Only antibody that is of the size and structure capable of crossing the placental barrier (i.e., IgG) can be transferred. Also, only antibody to infectious agents to which the mother has previously been exposed will be transferred. Maternal antibody provides temporary, albeit limited, immune defense during the early newborn period. ■

In contrast, **active immunity** to infectious agents is immunity that develops as a result of activation of the host's own immune system. Active immunity can occur by either natural or artificial means. **Natural immunity** occurs when an individual experiences an infectious disease naturally and immune memory cells are formed. These memory cells are capable of more readily responding to this specific infectious agent on reexposure to the same agent. Depending on the infectious agent as well as host factors, natural immunity may last a lifetime. Active immunity is induced artificially with vaccination. **Vaccination (immunization)** is the administration of a dead or attenuated (weakened) infectious agent or its components to an individual with the purpose of inducing an immune response and forming memory cells that are sensitive to this infectious agent, hence protecting the individual on future exposure.[69]

The development of vaccines and the process of vaccination represent a major milestone in the prevention of infectious disease. For example, vaccination against smallpox led to the eradication of this disease in 1980, and vaccination is no longer required. However, because of the danger of bioterrorism, smallpox remains an infectious threat, and certain at-risk groups (e.g., military personnel, certain healthcare workers) can be vaccinated against smallpox. Increasing rates of immunization against other diseases is a priority of *Healthy People 2020*. Research using genomics to develop more effective vaccines is a high priority in infectious disease control, as discussed in the Genetics and Genomics feature.

Healthy People 2020

Immunization and Infectious Diseases

Goal: "Increase immunization rates and reduce preventable infectious diseases."[1]

Overview: Infectious diseases continue to be a significant cause of illness, disability, and death among people in the United States. National immunization recommendations target 17 vaccine-preventable illnesses that affect individuals of all ages.[1] Individuals might not receive immunizations because they lack access to healthcare, fear adverse effects of an immunization, or lack insurance coverage and cannot pay for vaccines and do not know about the availability of vaccines at no cost. The Vaccines for Children program provides vaccines without cost for eligible children.[2]

Immunizations have a major role in reduction of morbidity and mortality caused by certain infectious diseases. In the United States, an estimated 42,000 adults and 300 children die each year from vaccine-preventable diseases.[1] An increased risk for outbreaks of vaccine-preventable illnesses exists in small groups of unvaccinated and undervaccinated populations.[1] An example of an outbreak of vaccine-preventable disease occurred in Minnesota in 2011. As reported in the CDC's *Morbidity and Mortality Weekly Report (MMWR)*, measles was confirmed in an infant, and subsequent investigation identified 13 additional cases of measles, including children and adults, several of whom required hospitalization.[3] The outbreak originated from a 30-month-old child who was born in the United States and developed measles after returning from a trip to Kenya. Locations where the infection was transmitted to others included household contacts, a child care center, an emergency department, and a living facility for homeless individuals.[3] The affected individuals who were not vaccinated for measles included five infants who were too young to be vaccinated and several others who were not vaccinated because of concerns related to the safety of the vaccine.[3]

Objectives: There are 33 *Healthy People 2020* objectives related to improving vaccinations for children, adolescents, and adults to achieve the goal of reducing vaccine-preventable diseases.[4] Examples of the objectives are to increase the percentage of children and adults who are vaccinated annually against seasonal influenza, to increase the number of adults who are vaccinated against pneumococcal infection, and to achieve effective vaccination coverage for universally recommended vaccines among young children.

References

1. *Healthy People 2020*. (2017). *Immunization and infectious diseases: Overview*. Retrieved from https://www.healthypeople.gov/2020/topics-objectives/topic/immunization-and-infectious-diseases
2. Centers for Disease Control and Prevention. (2016). *Vaccines for children program (VFC)*. Retrieved from https://www.cdc.gov/vaccines/programs/vfc/index.html
3. Centers for Disease Control and Prevention. (2011). Notes from the Field: Measles Outbreak—Hennepin County, Minnesota, February–March 2011. *Morbidity and Mortality Weekly Report (MMWR), 60*(13), 421. Retrieved from http://www.cdc.gov/mmwr/preview/mmwrhtml/mm6013a6.htm
4. *Healthy People 2020* (2017). *Immunization and infectious diseases: Objectives*. Retrieved from https://www.healthypeople.gov/2020/topics-objectives/topic/immunization-and-infectious-diseases/objectives

Genetics and Genomics for Clinical Practice

Vaccine Development Using Genomics

Ever since 1796, when Edward Jenner began to use live cowpox virus to vaccinate people against smallpox, vaccination has been an important means by which to limit infectious disease. Inactivated, live attenuated, and subunit vaccines have been used as effective medical interventions to prevent and limit the spread of pathogenic microorganisms. The effectiveness of these developed vaccines has been impressive. However, preparation by conventional approaches has not resulted in effective vaccines for all significant pathogenic microorganisms. These limitations are being overcome in dramatic fashion by first obtaining the complete genome of the infectious agent, identifying candidate genes, expressing those genes, and then using the expressed proteins to screen for effective vaccine candidates. This approach is known as reverse vaccinology, and it reduces the time and cost required for the identification of novel antigens that could be used as targets for vaccines.[1] Reverse vaccinology has been used to identify new candidate antigens for preclinical and clinical studies for numerous pathogens, including serogroup B *N. meningitidis*, *S. pyogenes*, *S. agalactiae*, *S. pneumoniae*, and pathogenic *E. coli*.[2] More recently, reverse vaccinology has been used to develop vaccines against parasites including *Plasmodium falciparum* and *Schistosoma*. This has been more difficult because parasites have larger genomes than bacteria or viruses do.[3]

Reverse vaccinology is a promising technique that will likely be exploited to design vaccines for viral and bacterial pathogens for which vaccines do not currently exist, including recently identified pathogens (e.g., hepatitis C virus), emerging pathogens (e.g., H1N1 flu and coronavirus), and variant forms of antibiotic-resistant pathogens (e.g., *S. aureus* and *M. tuberculosis*).[4]

References

1. Menakha, M., & Manoharan, C. (2011). Application of reverse vaccinology in designing a common vaccine for bacterial endocarditis. *International Journal of Pharmaceutical Sciences Review and Research, 11*(1), 95–101.
2. Seib, K. L., Zhao, X., & Rappuoli, R. (2012). Developing vaccines in the era of genomics: A decade of reverse vaccinology. *Clinical Microbiology and Infection, 18*(Suppl. 5), 109–16.
3. Lew-Tabor, A., & Valle, M. (2016). A review of reverse vaccinology approaches for the development of vaccines against ticks and tick borne diseases. *Ticks and Tick-borne Diseases, 7*, 573–585.
4. Rappuoli, R., Pizza, M., Del Giudice, G., & De Gregorio, E. (2014). Vaccines, new opportunities for a new society. *Proceedings of the National Academy of Sciences, 111*(34), 12288–12293.

CLINICAL POINT: A vaccine attempts to mimic the host's natural immune response to the actual infectious agent. Therefore, vaccine development requires knowledge of not only the characteristics of the pathogen but also the type of human immune response it elicits. ■

Often, vaccines must be administered again as a booster to restimulate the host's immune response and replenish the store of memory cells. For example, the tetanus toxoid is given as a booster every 10 years. Despite having a measles vaccine since 1962, an outbreak of measles in college dormitories and preschools led to the revaccination of at-risk individuals. More than 10 years after the introduction of the varicella vaccine in 1995, cases of breakthrough varicella (chickenpox) have emerged in children, including children who had received the vaccine. It is important to realize that vaccination is not 100% effective, and many individuals remain undervaccinated, and some do not receive vaccination at all. Nevertheless, vaccination provides **herd immunity** when a significant portion of a population is immunized, thus reducing the number of susceptible hosts enough to slow or halt the spread of an infectious agent.

Table 13.9 ■ lists the main types of vaccines. Some vaccines consist of inactivated or killed pathogens that are administered to the recipient. For example, a virus is

Table 13.9 The Main Types of Vaccines

Type of Vaccine	Definition	Examples
Inactivated (killed)	Pathogen is treated with a chemical so it no longer can reproduce.	Salk polio, hepatitis A, influenza, rabies
Attenuated (weakened)	Pathogen is grown under conditions that make it less virulent.	Sabin oral polio vaccine, measles, mumps, rubella, nasal influenza vaccine, varicella, and smallpox, *Mycobacterium bovis* bacille Calmette-Guérin
Subunit	Contains purified antigens rather than whole organisms.	Pertussis, hepatitis B
Toxoids	Toxins are treated with chemicals to remove toxic components yet retain antigenicity.	Tetanus toxoid, botulinum toxoid, diphtheria
Conjugate	Antigen is linked to a protein carrier (conjugate) to increase the vaccine's effectiveness.	*Haemophilus influenza B, Streptococcus pneumoniae, Neisseria meningitidis, Salmonella typhi*
Recombinant	Genes from a pathogen are inserted into a vector, usually a virus, that has very low virulence, and either the vector or the peptide produced by the vector is administered in a vaccine.	Hepatitis B surface antigen produced from a gene transfected into yeast cells and purified for injection as a subunit vaccine
DNA	The DNA of the pathogen is administered to the host. The host cells produce the pathogen's antigens; in turn, an immune response to these antigens is elicited.	Experimental; trials ongoing for HIV and influenza vaccines. Introduce pathogen DNA by bombarding the skin with DNA-coated gold particles; also possible to introduce DNA in nose drops.

grown in tissue culture and treated with a chemical, such as formaldehyde, so that it cannot reproduce. Attenuated vaccines are produced when the pathogen is grown under conditions that make it less virulent; an example is the measles, mumps, and rubella vaccine. The vaccine for the hepatitis B virus is a synthetic recombinant vaccine. A recombinant vaccine is made by first isolating the gene that encodes for an antigen of the targeted pathogen. This gene is then transfected into a recombinant system, such as yeast, that has been genetically engineered to make large quantities of the targeted antigen. The produced recombinant antigen is then purified and used for vaccine production. There are many other types of vaccines, and scientists are actively investigating newer and more efficient ways of vaccine development for existing and emerging infections.

Check Your Progress: Section 13.9

1. What is herd immunity?
2. What is the difference between inactive vaccines and attenuated vaccines?
3. Why do some vaccines require a booster vaccine?

CHAPTER SUMMARY

13.1 Chapter Overview and Case Studies

Identify factors that increase the global threat of infectious disease and explain concepts related to infection such as immunity, inflammation, tissue integrity, environmental health, thermoregulation, nutrition, perfusion, and oxygenation.

- In the United States, infectious disease is the third leading cause of death, and worldwide infectious disease is the leading cause of death.
- Infectious disease remains a major cause of human disease because (a) new microorganisms continue to emerge, (b) prior infectious threats that were once thought to have been eliminated reemerge as infectious threats, (c) microorganisms are able to develop resistance to antimicrobial therapy, (d) population crowding and global travel increase the worldwide spread of infectious disease, and (e) infectious agents might be used as agents of bioterrorism.
- Concepts related to infection include immunity, cellular regulation, oxygenation, nutrition, inflammation, thermoregulation, tissue integrity, perfusion, hemostasis, and environmental health.

13.2 The Host–Microbe Relationship

Explain the mutual beneficial relationship between the human host and commensal microorganisms.

- The commensal flora consists of the microorganisms that are normal inhabitants of human hosts (on the skin and mucosal surfaces).
- The microbiome is all the genes of the commensal microorganisms in and on the body and functions in maintenance of health. Alterations in the normal microbiome contribute to a variety of diseases.
- Healthcare-associated infections are infections that are contracted in a hospital setting or other healthcare setting.
- The portal of entry is the means by which an infectious pathogen enters the human host, such as direct entry, ingestion, inhalation, and parenteral.
- Colonization is the establishment of microorganisms within an ecologic niche within the body.

13.3 From Pathogen to Infectious Disease

Describe the series of events that allow a microbial pathogen to exit an environmental reservoir and to produce infectious disease in humans, and list examples of microbial virulence factors.

- Infection occurs when the microorganisms multiply in a body part or tissue. Infectious disease occurs when the pathogen multiplies in sufficient quantities to cause tissue damage and impairment of function of the host.
- Virulence is defined as the degree to which a microorganism is capable of causing infectious disease. Virulence factors include substances produced by microorganisms that facilitate adhesion to host cells, invasion of host tissues, toxins that lead to destruction of host cells and tissues, and ways by which the microorganism evades the host's immune defense mechanisms.
- An endotoxin is a large lipopolysaccharide molecule located on the outer surface of the cell wall of gram-negative bacteria. Exotoxins consist of toxic substances secreted by either gram-positive or gram-negative bacteria.

13.4 Microbial Agents of Infectious Disease

Contrast the characteristic features of bacteria, viruses, fungi, prions, protozoa, and helminths, and explain the steps of viral invasion and replication within a human host cell.

- Bacteria are small unicellular organisms surrounded by a cell wall. They belong to the grouping called prokaryotes. Prokaryotes do not have distinct membrane-bound cell organelles and do not have nuclei or mitochondria. Eukaryotes (mammalian cells, fungi, protozoa, helminths, and plants) have distinct cell organelles.

- Certain bacteria can convert into dormant dehydrated structures known as spores when in harsh environmental conditions. Spores are highly resistant structures and can survive many years.
- Because of the different components within their cell walls bacteria can be grouped as either gram-positive or gram-negative when stained by a laboratory technique called Gram staining. Gram-positive bacteria retain the crystal violet stain after an acid wash and appear purple; gram-negative bacteria do not retain the stain and appear red after a counterstain with saffron.
- Mycobacteria, such as the *M. tuberculosis*, represent a separate category of bacteria called acid-fast bacteria, which cannot be decolorized easily with acid solutions.
- Opportunistic pathogens are microorganism that uses the opportunity to infect a host who has weakened defense mechanisms (e.g., immunocompromised individuals such as those with AIDS or transplant recipients on immunosuppressive therapy).
- *Staphylococcus* bacteria are a major causes of infection in humans, including skin and wound infections, pneumonia, endocarditis, and food poisoning. *Staphylococcus aureus* frequently contaminates the hospital environment and causes hospital-acquired or healthcare-associated infections.
- Certain bacteria have mutated so that they are no longer susceptible to antibiotics and are difficult to treat. An example is MRSA, which causes significant hospital-acquired as well as community-acquired infections.
- *Streptococcus* bacteria cause infections such as acute pharyngitis (strep throat) and can also cause infections such as skin infections and pneumonia.
- Some bacteria are obligate intracellular parasites; they can grow only inside host cells. Examples include the *Rickettsia*, which are transmitted by arthropods, and the *Chlamydia*, which cause the most common sexually transmitted disease in the United States.
- Viruses are obligate intracellular parasites that can replicate only in living cells, as they lack the capacity to produce energy and to make protein. The genome of a virus is composed of either RNA or DNA.
- Enveloped viruses have an external membrane that covers their nucleocapsids and are environmentally labile; nonenveloped viruses are hardier and can survive conditions such as the harsh environment of the gastrointestinal tract. Enteric viruses that cause gastrointestinal infections are nonenveloped.
- Viral replication includes the following steps: recognition and attachment to the host target cell, penetration of the host cell membrane, release (uncoating) of the viral genome, replication of the viral genome, synthesis of viral structural proteins, viral assembly, and viral release form the host cell.
- Viral tropism is the preference of the virus to bind to specific targets or host cells (i.e., selective binding or attachment).
- Antigenic drift involves minor changes in a viral antigen that can lead to an epidemic; antigenic shift involves major changes in viral genetics that allow the antigen to jump from one species to another. Antigen shifts can lead to pandemics or global epidemics. The clinical course of viral infections can include an asymptomatic period called the incubation period. The prodrome consists of early nonspecific symptoms of viral infection such as lethargy, headache, and fever.
- Certain viruses, such as the herpes virus, can enter a latent viral state after producing an acute infection. During a latent state, a virus remains within the host in an inactive state but can be reactivated and produce an acute infection under certain conditions, such as stressful life events.
- Prions are nonliving particles that are transmitted to mammals and cause neurodegenerative disease. Prions have been implicated as the cause of bovine spongiform encephalopathy (mad cow disease).
- Fungi, protozoa, and helminths are eukaryotic microbial infections agents that can be pathogenic in humans.

13.5 The Innate and Adaptive Immune Response to Infectious Microorganisms

Compare and contrast the components of the innate immune system versus the components of the adaptive immune system.

- The innate and adaptive immune systems function together to eliminate infectious microbial agents.
- The innate immune system comprises anatomical barriers, phagocytic cells, cells that release inflammatory mediators, natural killer cells, and complement.
- The adaptive immune system comprises antigen-specific B lymphocytes that produce antibodies and antigen-specific T lymphocytes that can produce cytokines or can be cytotoxic for cellular targets displaying specific antigen.

13.6 Resistance to Infectious Disease

Explain the protective immune mechanisms that defend against viral pathogens.

- Immune resistance to extracellular bacteria is mediated primarily by antibody, complement, and phagocytic cells.
- Immunity to intracellular bacteria and fungi is mediated primarily by cytokine-activated phagocytes.

- Immune resistance to viruses is mediated by antibody, complement, phagocytic cells, interferons, natural killer cells, antibody, cytotoxic T lymphocytes, and T-helper lymphocytes, which produce cytokines that orchestrate the immune response to the virus.

13.7 Resistance to Different Microbial Pathogens as Mediated by Different Host Protective Mechanisms

Describe the means by which microorganisms are opsonized by the immune system and identify the effective form of adaptive immunity that protects against intracellular pathogenic microorganisms such as *M. tuberculosis*.

- Passive immunity is the provision of temporary protection from an infectious agent through the administration of exogenous antibody to a recipient; active immunity is protection that results from activation of the person's own immune system.

13.8 Immune Deficient/ Susceptible Host

Explain the differential etiology of primary and secondary immune deficiencies.

- Immunodeficiency is a consequence of a defect in one or more components of the immune system. Immunodeficiencies are classified as either primary (inherited) or secondary (induced as a consequence of disease, disease treatment, or malnutrition).
- Secondary immunodeficiencies are acquired and are a result of infectious disease, systemic disease, drug or radiotherapeutic treatment for disease, and injury. An example of a secondary immunodeficiency is infection with HIV, which leads to the acquired immune deficiency syndrome (AIDS).
- Populations that are at increased risk for infection include critically ill individuals in intensive care units, especially patients whose care requires insertion of invasive lines and devices. Intravenous drug users are at greater risk for infection owing to shared and often unsanitary drug paraphernalia, direct microbial entry at intravenous sites, and physical debilitation that impairs their immune defense mechanisms.

13.9 Protection from Infectious Disease by Vaccination

Explain the difference between passive and active immunity and describe how vaccination provides immunity to infectious agents.

- Active immunity to infectious agents results from activation of the host's own immune system. Active immunity can occur by either natural or artificial means (i.e., vaccination).
- Passive immunity, which is temporary, results from administration of exogenous antibody to a recipient
- Natural immunity occurs when an individual experiences an infectious disease naturally and immune memory cells are formed.
- Vaccination is the administration of a dead or attenuated (weakened) infectious agent or its components to an individual with the purpose of inducing an immune response and forming memory cells to this infectious agent, hence protecting the individual on future exposure.

REVIEW QUESTIONS

1. A patient has developed methicillin-resistant *Staphylococcus aureus*. Which of the following is the most likely cause?
   a. Poor hand hygiene by the healthcare team
   b. Overuse of antibiotics
   c. Inadequate nutrition
   d. A compromised immune system

2. An urgent care clinic has treated many patients over the past week for symptoms of influenza. The nurse reports to the nursing director that the clinic may be experiencing which of the following?
   a. A pandemic
   b. Antigenic shift
   c. Antigenic drift
   d. An epidemic

3. The nurse is teaching a patient ways to avoid contracting respiratory infections. Which statement indicates that the patient understands the mode of transmission?
   a. "I can get a respiratory infection by eating contaminated food."
   b. "I can get a respiratory infection when someone sneezes."
   c. "I can get a respiratory infection from sweat on equipment at the gym."
   d. "I can get a respiratory infection through an open wound."

4. Which of the following patients, who have had chickenpox, should receive Zostavax, a vaccine against shingles?
   a. A 60-year-old man in good health
   b. A 60-year-old man with HIV
   c. A 60-year-old man taking immunosuppressive drugs
   d. A 60-year-old man with non-Hodgkin lymphoma

5. The school nurse is teaching parents about the HPV vaccine. Which statement by a participant indicates that she understands the education?
   a. "A three-dose vaccine is needed starting at 9 months of age."
   b. "My 11-year-old son should receive the HPV vaccination."
   c. "All women over age 30 should receive the HPV vaccine."
   d. "Immunocompromised young men should not receive the HPV vaccine."

6. Which of the following is an appropriate schedule for the meningococcal vaccine?
   a. A single dose administered at age 16
   b. A single dose administered at 6 months of age
   c. One dose at age 11 and a booster at age 16
   d. One dose at age 6 months and a booster at age 16

7. What recommendation should the nurse give to a pregnant woman who wants to travel to a country with Zika virus?
   a. It is safe to travel to a region with Zika virus after the first trimester.
   b. Avoid travel to a region with Zika while pregnant.
   c. Travel to a Zika region is safe while pregnant if a mosquito repellent is used.
   d. Wait until after the second trimester to travel to a Zika region.

8. Which of the following should the nurse tell a patient with herpes simplex virus?
   a. An episode of herpes simplex offers lifetime immunity.
   b. Herpes simplex virus can be reactivated under stressful conditions.
   c. There are no symptoms during the prodromal phase.
   d. Sunlight can help to inactivate the virus.

ANSWERS

Answers to Review Questions can be found in Appendix A. Answers to Case Study and Check Your Progress questions are available on the faculty resources site. Please consult with your instructor.

RECOMMENDED WEBSITES

Antibiotic / Antimicrobial Resistance
https://www.cdc.gov/drugresistance

Antimicrobial Resistance: Fact sheet
http://www.who.int/mediacentre/factsheets/fs194/en

Bioterrorism Agents/Diseases
https://emergency.cdc.gov/agent/agentlist.asp

Doctor Fungus: On-line Reference to All Things Mycological
http://mycosesstudygroup.org/

Global Health Protection and Security
httpz://www.cdc.gov/globalhealth/healthprotection/index.html

Immune System 101
https://www.aids.gov/hiv-aids-basics/just-diagnosed-with-hiv-aids/hiv-in-your-body/immune-system-101

Mycology Online
http://www.mycology.adelaide.edu.au

National Institute of Allergy and Infectious Diseases
https://www.niaid.nih.gov

Overview of the Immune System
https://www.niaid.nih.gov/research/immune-system-overview

Virusworld
http://www.virology.wisc.edu/virusworld/viruslist.php

Vaccines & Immunizations
https://www.cdc.gov/vaccines/index.html

Whatever Happened to Polio?
http://amhistory.si.edu/polio

REFERENCES

1. Fauci, A. S., & Morens, D. M. (2012). The perpetual challenge of infectious diseases. *New England Journal of Medicine, 366*, 454–461.
2. Khan, K., McNabb, S. J., Memish, Z. A., et al. (2012). Infectious disease surveillance and modelling across geographic frontiers and scientific specialties. *Lancet Infectious Diseases, 12*(3), 222–230.
3. Centers for Disease Control and Prevention. (2015). *Anthrax*. Available at http://www.cdc.gov/anthrax
4. Centers for Disease Control and Prevention. (2016). *Bioterrorism agents/diseases*. Available at https://emergency.cdc.gov/agent/agentlist.asp
5. Uhlemann, A. C., Otto, M., Lowy, F. D., & DeLeo, F. R. (2014). Evolution of community-and healthcare-associated methicillin-resistant Staphylococcus aureus. *Infection, Genetics and Evolution, 21*, 563–574.
6. American Cancer Society. (2016). *Infections that can lead to cancer*. Available at http://www.cancer.org/acs/groups/cid/documents/webcontent/002782-pdf.pdf
7. Libby, P. (2012). Inflammation in atherosclerosis. *Arteriosclerosis, Thrombosis, and Vascular Biology, 32*, 2045–2051.

8. Centers for Disease Control and Prevention. (2016). *Hand hygiene in healthcare settings: Guidelines*. Available at http://www.cdc.gov/handhygiene/Guidelines.html
9. Longtin, Y., Farquet, N., Gayet-Ageron, A., Sax, H., & Pittet, D. (2012). Caregivers' perceptions of patients as reminders to improve hand hygiene. *Archives of Internal Medicine, 172*(19), 1516–1517.
10. Murray, P. R., Rosenthal, K. S., & Pfaller, M. A. (2013). Mechanisms of bacterial pathogenesis. In *Medical microbiology* (7th ed., pp. 138–146). Philadelphia, PA: Mosby/Elsevier.
11. Metcalf, D. G., & Bowler, P. G. (2013). Biofilm delays wound healing: A review of the evidence. *Burn Trauma, 1*(1), 5–12.
12. Pendyala, S., Walker, J. M., & Holt, P. R. (2012). A high-fat diet is associated with endotoxemia that originates from the gut. *Gastroenterology, 142*(5), 1100–1101.
13. Parija, S. C. (2012). *Textbook of microbiology & immunology* (2nd ed.). Puducherry, India: Reed Elsevier India.
14. Vostral, S. L.(2011). Rely and toxic shock syndrome: A technological health crisis. *Yale Journal of Biology and Medicine, 84*, 447–459.
15. Occupational Safety and Health Administration. (2016). *Healthcare wide hazards: Infection*. Available at https://www.osha.gov/SLTC/etools/hospital/hazards/infection/infection.html
16. Murray, P. R., Rosenthal, K. S., & Pfaller, M. A. (2013). Bacterial classification, structure, and replication. In *Medical microbiology* (7th ed., pp. 109–121). Philadelphia, PA: Mosby/Elsevier.
17. Murray, P. R., Rosenthal, K. S., & Pfaller, M. A. (2013). Bacterial metabolism and genetics. In *Medical microbiology* (7th ed., pp. 122–137). Philadelphia, PA: Mosby/Elsevier.
18. Centers for Disease Control and Prevention. (2015). *Tuberculosis (TB): Data and statistics*. Available at http://www.cdc.gov/tb/statistics/default.htm
19. Centers for Disease Control and Prevention. (2016). *Tuberculosis (TB)*. Available at http://www.cdc.gov/tb/webcourses/CoreCurr/TB_Course/Menu/frameset_internet.htm.
20. Centers for Disease Control and Prevention. (2015). E. coli *(*Escherichia coli*): General information*. Available at http://www.cdc.gov/ecoli/general/index.html.
21. Murray, P. R., Rosenthal, K. S., & Pfaller, M. A. (2013). Enterobacteriaceae. In *Medical microbiology* (7th ed., pp. 258–272). Philadelphia, PA, Mosby/Elsevier.
22. Mayo Clinic. (2015). *Shigella infection: Treatments and drugs*. Available at http://www.mayoclinic.org/diseases-conditions/shigella/basics/treatment/con-20028418
23. Sjölund Karlsson, M., Bowen, A., Reporter, R., Folster, J. P., et al. Outbreak of infections caused by *Shigella sonnei* with reduced susceptibility to azithromycin in the United States. *Antimicrobial Agents and Chemotherapy, 57*, 1559–1560.
24. Centers for Disease Control and Prevention. (2014). Pseudomonas aeruginosa *in healthcare settings*. Available at http://www.cdc.gov/hai/organisms/pseudomonas.html
25. Donta, S. T. (2012). Issues in the diagnosis and treatment of Lyme disease. *Open Neurology Journal, 6*, 140–145.
26. Humphrey, S., Chaloner, G., Kemmett, K., et al. (2014). *Campylobacter jejuni* is not merely a commensal in commercial broiler chickens and affects bird welfare. *mBio, 5*(4), e01364–14.
27 Murray, P. R., Rosenthal, K. S., & Pfaller, M. A. (2013). Staphylococcus and related gram-positive cocci. In *Medical microbiology* (7th ed., pp. 174–187). Philadelphia, PA: Mosby/Elsevier.
28. Whitfeld, M., Gunasingam, N., Leow, L. J., Shirato, K., & Preda, V. (2011). *Staphylococcus epidermidis*: A possible role in the pustules of rosacea. *Journal of the American Academy of Dermatology, 64*(1), 49–52.
29. Centers for Disease Control and Prevention. (2015). *Foodborne outbreak tracking and reporting: Surveillance for foodborne disease outbreaks*. Available at http://www.cdc.gov/foodsafety/fdoss/surveillance/index.html
30. Centers for Disease Control and Prevention. (2016). *Pneumococcal vaccine*. Available at https://www.cdc.gov/vaccines/vpd-vac/pneumo/
31. Blasi, F., Mantero, M., Santus, P., & Tarsia, P. (2012). Understanding the burden of pneumococcal disease in adults. *Clinical Microbiology and Infection, 18*(Suppl. 5), 7–14.
32. Murray, P. R., Rosenthal, K. S., & Pfaller, M. A. (2013). Neisseria and related genera. In *Medical microbiology* (7th ed., pp. 248–257). Philadelphia, PA: Mosby/Elsevier, Philadelphia, PA, 2013:248–257.
33. Centers for Disease Control and Prevention. (2015). *Meningococcal vaccination*. Available at http://www.cdc.gov/vaccines/vpd-vac/mening/default.htm
34. Murray, P. R., Rosenthal, K. S., & Pfaller, M. A. (2013). Rickettsia and Orientia. In *Medical microbiology* (7th ed., pp. 368–374). Philadelphia, PA: Mosby/Elsevier, Philadelphia, PA, 2013:368-374.
35. Moore, E. R., & Ouellette, S. P. (2014). Reconceptualizing the chlamydial inclusion as a pathogen-specified parasitic organelle: An expanded role for Inc proteins. *Frontiers in Cellular and Infection Microbiology, 4*, 157. doi: 10.3389/fcimb.2014.00157
36. Murray, P. R., Rosenthal, K. S., & Pfaller, M. A. (2013). Viral classification, structure, and replication. In *Medical microbiology* (7th ed., pp. 393–409). Philadelphia, PA: Mosby/Elsevier.
37. Murray, P. R., Rosenthal, K. S., & Pfaller, M. A. (2013). Orthomyxoviruses. In *Medical microbiology* (7th ed., pp. 524–533). Philadelphia, PA: Mosby/Elsevier.
38. Centers for Disease Control and Prevention. (2014). *Types of influenza viruses*. Available at http://www.cdc.gov/flu/about/viruses/types.htm
39. Murray, P. R., Rosenthal, K. S., & Pfaller, M. A.. (2013). Mechanisms of viral pathogenesis. In *Medical microbiology* (7th ed., pp. 410–420). Philadelphia, PA: Mosby/Elsevier.
40. Centers for Disease Control and Prevention. (2015). *Shingles (herpes zoster) vaccination*. Available at http://www.cdc.gov/vaccines/vpd-vac/shingles/default.htm
41. Centers for Disease Control and Prevention. (2016). *Genital HPV infection: Fact sheet*. Available at http://www.cdc.gov/std/hpv/stdfact-hpv.htm
42. Centers for Disease Control and Prevention. (2015). *Ebola (Ebola virus disease)*. Available at http://www.cdc.gov/vhf/ebola/outbreaks/index.html
43. Centers for Disease Control and Prevention. (2016). *2014 Ebola outbreak in West Africa: Case counts*. Available at http://www.cdc.gov/vhf/ebola/outbreaks/2014-west-africa/case-counts.html
44. World Health Organization. (2016). *Ebola situation reports*. Available at http://www.who.int/csr/disease/ebola/situation-reports/en
45. World Health Organization. (2016). *Ebola virus disease*. Available at http://www.who.int/mediacentre/factsheets/fs103/en/
46. Hayden, C. E. (2014). (2014). The Ebola questions. *Nature, 514*, 554–557.
47. Mulherkara, N., Raabenb, M., de la Torrec, J. C., Whelanb, S. P., & Chandrana, K. (2011). The Ebola virus glycoprotein mediates entry via a non-classical dynamin-dependent macropinocytic pathway. *Virology, 2*(25), 72–83.
48. MedlinePlus. (2014). *Ebola virus disease*. Available at http://www.nlm.nih.gov/medlineplus/ency/article/001339.htm.
49. Foster, C. B. (2015). Enterovirus D68: A clinically important respiratory enterovirus. *Cleveland Clinic Journal of Medicine, 82*(1), 26–31.
50. Khetsuriani, N., LaMonte-Fowlkes, A., Oberst, S., & Pallansch, M. A. (2006). Enterovirus surveillance—United States, 1970–2005. *MMWR Surveillance Summaries, 55*(8), 1–20.
51. Renois, F., Bouin, A., & Andreoletti, L. (2013). Enterovirus 68 in pediatric patients hospitalized for acute airway diseases. *Journal of Clinical Microbiology, 51*(2), 640–643.
52. Centers for Disease Control and Prevention. (2016). *Enterovirus D68 for health care professionals*. Available at https://www.cdc.gov/non-polio-enterovirus/hcp/ev-d68-hcp.html
53. Centers for Disease Control and Prevention. (2016). *Enterovirus D68*. Available at https://www.cdc.gov/non-polio-enterovirus/about/ev-d68.html

54. Centers for Disease Control and Prevention. (2016). *Zika virus: Transmission & risks*. Available at https://www.cdc.gov/zika/transmission/index.html
55. Musso, D., Nhan, T., Robin, E., et al. (2014). Potential for Zika virus transmission through blood transfusion demonstrated during an outbreak in French Polynesia, November 2013 to February 2014. *Eurosurveillance, 19*(14), article 2. doi:10.2807/1560-7917.ES2014.19.14.20761
56. National Institutes of Health. (2016). *News release: NIH begins testing investigational Zika vaccine in humans*. Available at https://www.nih.gov/news-events/news-releases/nih-begins-testing-investigational-zika-vaccine-humans
57. Xu, M., Lee, E., Wen, Z., et al. (2016). Identification of small-molecule inhibitors of Zika virus infection and induced neural cell death via a drug repurposing screen. *Nature Medicine, 22*(10),1101–1107. doi:10.1038/nm.4184
58. Centers for Disease Control and Prevention. (2015). *Variant Creutzfeldt-Jakob disease (vCJD)*. Available at http://www.cdc.gov/prions/vcjd/index.html
59. Murray, P. R., Rosenthal, K. S., & Pfaller, M. A. (2013). Pathogenesis of fungal disease. In *Medical microbiology* (7th ed., pp. 611–618). Philadelphia, PA: Mosby/Elsevier.
60. World Health Organization. (2016). *Malaria*. Available at http://www.who.int/mediacentre/factsheets/fs094/en.
61. World Health Organization. (2016). *Schistosomiasis*. Available at http://www.who.int/mediacentre/factsheets/fs115/en
62. Weaver, H. J. (2014). Climate change and human parasitic disease. In C. D. Butler (Ed.), *Climate change and global health* (pp. 95–104). Wallingford, UK: CABI.
63. Russell, P., Hertz, P., & McMillan, B. (2014). Defenses against disease. In *Biology: The dynamic science* (3rd ed., pp. 1002–1023). Belmont, CA: Brooks/Cole.
64. Murray, P. R., Rosenthal, K. S., & Pfaller, M. A. (2013). Innate host responses. In: *Medical Microbiology* (7th ed., pp. 47–60). Philadelphia, PA: Mosby/Elsevier.
65. Denyer, S. P., Hodges, N. A., Gorman, S. P., & Gilmore, B. F., eds. (2011). *Hugo & Russell's pharmaceutical microbiology* (8th ed.). Chichester, UK: Wiley-Blackwell.
66. Murray, P. R., Rosenthal, K. S., & Pfaller, M. A. (2013). Elements of host protective responses. In *Medical microbiology* (7th ed., pp. 47–60). Philadelphia, PA: Mosby/Elsevier.
67. Murray, P. R., Rosenthal, K. S., & Pfaller, M. A. (2013). Antigen-specific immune responses. In *Medical microbiology* (7th ed., pp. 61–79). Philadelphia, PA: Mosby/Elsevier.
68. Murray, P. R., Rosenthal, K. S., & Pfaller, M. A. (2013). Mycobacterium. In *Medical microbiology* (7th ed., pp. 235–247). Philadelphia, PA: Mosby/Elsevier.
69. Centers for Disease Control and Prevention. (2012). *Vaccines: The basics*. Available at http://www.cdc.gov/vaccines/vpd-vac/vpd-vac-basics.htm

Chapter 14

Hypersensitivity and Autoimmune Disorders

Diane Klein and Amy Kennedy

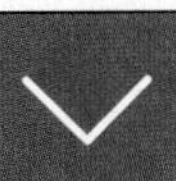

Chapter Outline and Learning Outcomes

14.1 Chapter Overview and Case Studies

Describe the normal immune response, the results of inappropriate immune response, and concepts related to the immune response.

14.2 Hypersensitivity Disorders

Differentiate the causes, classification, underlying pathogenesis, and clinical manifestations of hypersensitivity disorders and the diagnosis and treatment of these conditions across the lifespan.

14.3 Autoimmune Disease

Differentiate the causes, classification, underlying pathogenesis, and clinical manifestations of autoimmune disease and the diagnosis and treatment of these conditions across the lifespan.

KEY TERMS

Allergen, 367
Allergic reactions, 367
Anaphylaxis, 368
Antigen, 365
Atopic, 369
Central tolerance, 374
Hypersensitivity reaction, 367
Immune response, 365
Immunity, 364
Immunologically ignorant, 375
Peripheral tolerance, 374
Primary immune response, 365
Rhinoconjunctivitis, 369
Secondary immune response, 365
Self-tolerance, 374
Systemic lupus erythematosus (SLE), 375

ABBREVIATIONS

CTL—cytotoxic T lymphocyte
DTH—delayed-type hypersensitivity
IC—immune complexes
MHC—major histocompatibility complex
SLE—systemic lupus erythematosus
Th1—type 1 T-helper cells
Th2—type 2 T-helper cells

14.1 Chapter Overview and Case Studies

The cells of the immune system are present in large quantities in the central and peripheral lymphoid organs. These tissues and organs are widely distributed in the body. They provide different and often overlapping functions (**Figure 14.1** ■).

The central lymphoid organs, which consist of the bone marrow and the thymus, provide an environment for the production and maturation of immune cells. The lymphoid organs are composed of a type of supporting connective tissue referred to as *reticular tissue*. Reticular tissue provides a framework for the lymphoid organs and allows leukocytes and other cells to circulate and encounter antigens. The peripheral lymphoid organs recognize and process antigens. In addition, these organs promote the cellular interactions necessary for the development of adaptive immune responses. The peripheral lymph node organs include the lymph nodes, spleen, tonsils, appendix, and Peyer patches in the intestine along with the mucosa-associated lymphoid tissue in the respiratory, gastrointestinal, and reproductive systems.

The lymphoid organs are connected by networks of lymph channels, blood vessels, and capillaries that allow the immune cells to continuously circulate through the various tissues and organs throughout the body. This circulation allows the cells to seek out and destroy foreign material, thus allowing immunity and immune responses to occur. Examples of foreign material include infectious agents such as bacteria and viruses, toxins such as urushiol (the toxin found in poison ivy), and substances such as pollen, dust, or transplanted tissue. Foreign material is, essentially, anything from outside the body.

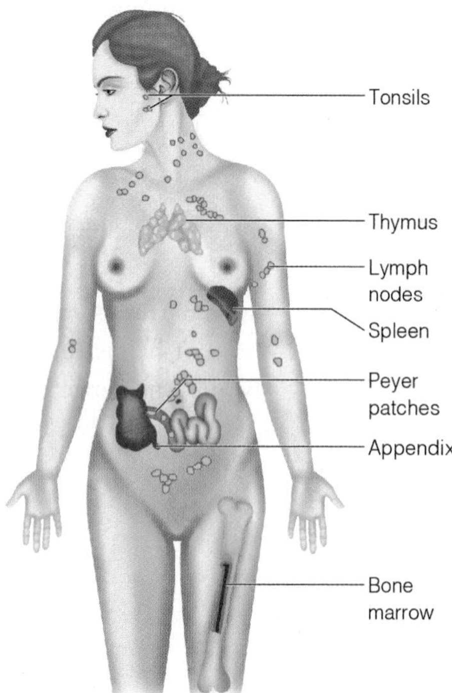

Figure 14.1 ■ The lymphoid system, showing the central organs of the thymus and bone marrow and the peripheral organs, including the spleen, tonsils, lymph nodes, and Peyer patches.

The term **immunity** means protection from infectious disease. The coordinated and collective response of the immune system's cells and molecules in the body is referred to as an **immune response**. The immune response is how the body recognizes and defends against bacteria and viruses as well as other foreign and harmful substances.

Specifically, the immune system protects the body by recognizing and responding to foreign materials, which are collectively called **antigens**. Antigens are molecules, often composed of lipids or proteins, located on the surface of cells. These molecules bind to receptors in the body and generate a response from the immune system. The immune system, when working properly, recognizes and destroys substances that contain antigens.

As described in Chapter 13, two basic immune responses occur in response to antigens: humoral immunity and cellular immunity. While both responses stimulate division, humoral immunity primarily occurs in body fluids and cellular immunity occurs in body cells. During the **primary immune response**, there is a latent period before the antibody is detected in the blood. The latent period involves antigen processing by the APCs and recognition by the T-helper cells. After recognition, the T-helper cells become activated and produce cytokines (**Figure 14.2** ■). These cytokines stimulate and direct the immune response. The activation process takes 7–14 day. Once antibodies are generated and become detectable, their level continues to rise for several weeks. Individuals often recover from infectious disease during the primary immune response because the antibody concentration is reaching its peak.

IgG crosses the placenta during the last few weeks of pregnancy and is stored in fetal tissue. As a result of this transfer, a neonate born to an HIV-positive mother tests positive for antibodies. It is important to note, however, that the child is not necessarily infected with the virus.[1] ■

Newborns are protected against antigens during the first month of life, owing to the passive transfer of maternal antibodies through the placenta. Protection is prolonged if the infant is breastfed, as IgA is transferred through breast milk.[1] ■

The **secondary immune response**, also called *memory immune response*, occurs on subsequent exposure to the antigen. During the secondary immune response, the rise in antibody occurs faster and reaches higher levels, owing to available memory cells. This occurs because the memory cells recognize the antigen and mount a more efficient response, producing a specific antibody. This memory response is used in the administration of booster immunizations, such as tetanus. For the individual who has been previously immunized, the booster shot provides an almost

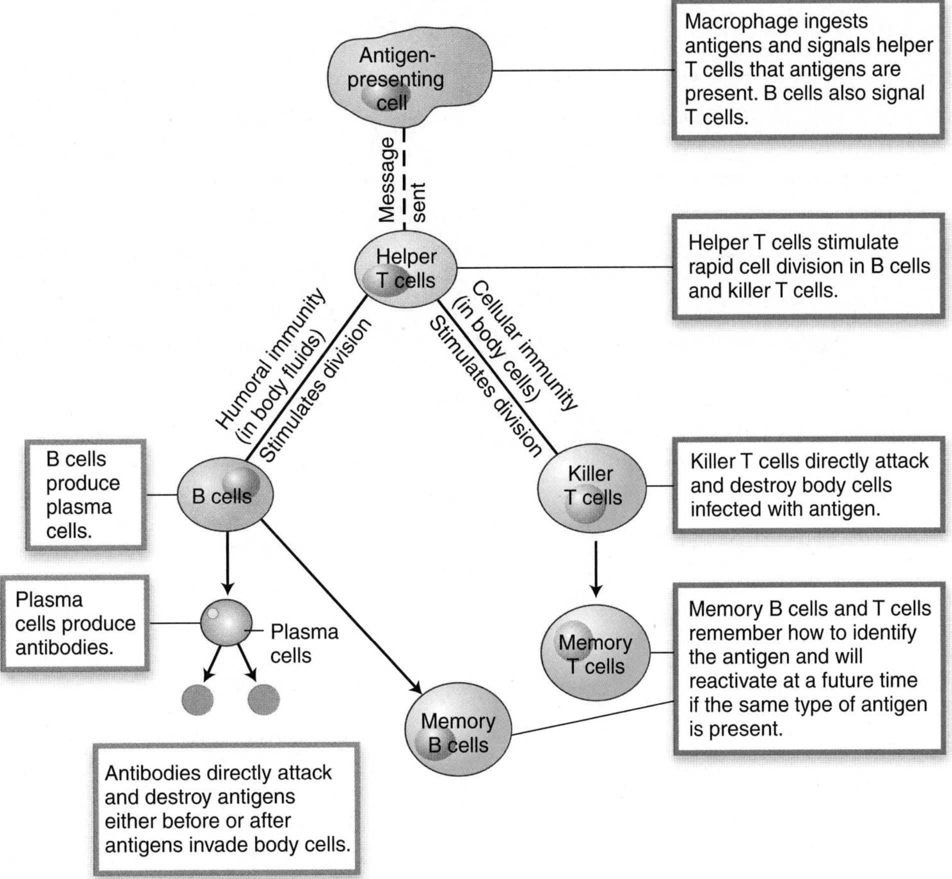

Figure 14.2 ■ The primary immune response encompasses a cascade of events that involve humoral immunity and cellular immunity.

immediate rise in the antibody to a level that is sufficient to prevent the development of the disease.

The immune system is a multifaceted defense network. It has evolved to perform the following functions:

- Protect against invading microorganisms
- Prevent cancer cell proliferation
- Mediate the healing of damaged tissue.

Under normal circumstances, the body's immune response deters disease. There are certain situations in which there is inadequate, inappropriate, or misdirected activation of the immune system. This can lead to debilitating and even life-threatening illnesses, which include immunodeficiency states, allergic or hypersensitivity reactions, transplantation rejection, and autoimmune disorders. This chapter focuses on the pathophysiology of hypersensitivity reactions along with autoimmune disorders.

Aging is responsible for changes in immune responsiveness that affect both cell-mediated and humoral immune responses. Older adults are more susceptible to infection and have a higher incidence for cancer. See Chapter 10 for more information.[2] ■

Concepts Related to Immune Response

The immune system protects the body; therefore, it affects, and is affected by, other systems in the body. This means that the concept of immune response is related to several other important concepts. The concepts that are most often related to immune response include comfort, inflammation and oxidative stress, and tissue integrity (**Figure 14.3** ■).

Owing to the rapid and often dramatic nature of the immune response, the body experiences a variety of both localized and systemic discomforts. Because the skin is the body's primary barrier to foreign bodies and antigens, skin discomfort is common in the immune response and stems from a variety of sources, including allergic reactions, inflammation, and wound healing.

Inflammation and oxidative stress reactions occur in reaction to an insult, injury, or antigen in the circulatory system. These reactions cause fluid and cells to move out of the bloodstream to the affected tissue to eliminate the infectious agent. Inflammation and oxidative stress often resolve when the threat has been eliminated. However, abscess, scar formation, and persistent inflammation can lead to chronic inflammation.

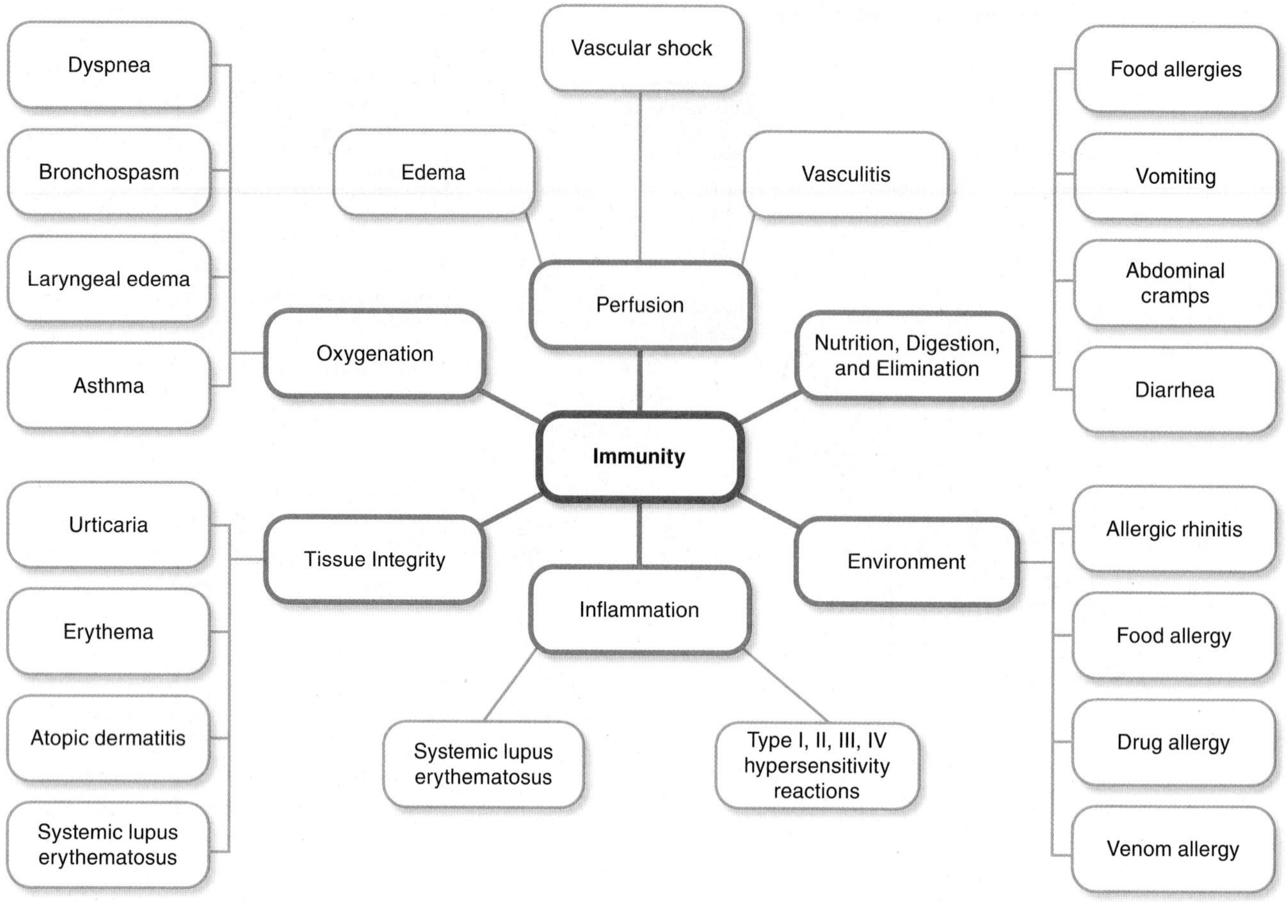

Immunity

- Oxygenation
  - Dyspnea
  - Bronchospasm
  - Laryngeal edema
  - Asthma
- Perfusion
  - Edema
  - Vascular shock
  - Vasculitis
- Nutrition, Digestion, and Elimination
  - Food allergies
  - Vomiting
  - Abdominal cramps
  - Diarrhea
- Tissue Integrity
  - Urticaria
  - Erythema
  - Atopic dermatitis
  - Systemic lupus erythematosus
- Inflammation
  - Systemic lupus erythematosus
  - Type I, II, III, IV hypersensitivity reactions
- Environment
  - Allergic rhinitis
  - Food allergy
  - Drug allergy
  - Venom allergy

Figure 14.3 ■ Concepts related to the immune response.

Tissue integrity has a two-way relationship with the immune response. When tissue integrity is impaired, the immune response is triggered. For example, burns, traumatic injury, and certain cancer therapies impair tissue integrity. This allows infectious agents a portal of entry into the body.

The reverse is also true in that certain immune responses can lead to impaired tissue integrity. An allergic reaction can cause clinical manifestations such as contact dermatitis. The tissue integrity issues are treated concurrently with the underlying issue. Patient education about proper skin care is essential.

Case Studies

The following cases are addressed throughout the chapter to assist in application of chapter content to clinical situations that involve individuals with disorders of immune response.

Nicolas Lopez: Introduction

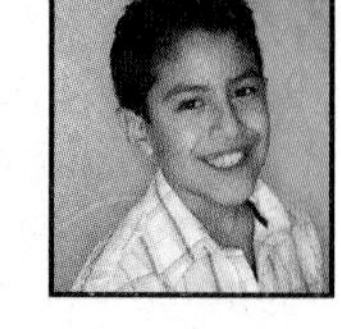

Nicolas Lopez is a 10-year-old boy who was diagnosed with a severe peanut allergy as a preschooler. He presents at the pediatric urgent care clinic at 6:30 on a Sunday evening with his father. Mr. Lopez states that Nicolas was at a birthday party and when Mr. Lopez came to pick him up, Nicolas reported difficulty swallowing. On further inspection, Mr. Lopez noted a wheal-like rash on Nicolas's arms and neck. Mr. Lopez does not have access to the boy's prescribed epinephrine autoinjector, and Nicolas's mother won't be picking the child up until after school on Monday. Mr. Lopez states, "I tried to call her to pick up his medication, but she didn't answer the phone. My only choice was to come here."

1. What medical condition does Mr. Lopez suspect that prompted him to bring his son to the pediatric urgent care clinic on a Sunday evening?
2. Could prior patient and family education have helped to avoid the visit to the pediatric urgent care clinic?

Yvonne Johnson: Introduction

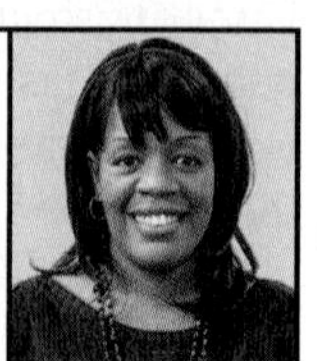

Yvonne Johnson, age 35, is a single mother to her 15-year-old son Randall. She receives child support from Randall's father, who is active in his son's life. Ms. Johnson completed a bachelor's degree in marketing 5 years ago. However, she has been unable to find a job in this field that does not require relocation. She is currently an administrative assistant for a law firm, but she is not satisfied with this job. She cannot quit until she finds another job with health benefits. Ms. Johnson's parents and siblings live in the area and are supportive.

Over the past 4 years, Ms. Johnson has experienced unexplained mild to moderate generalized symptoms of joint swelling, pain, and fatigue. Several trips to her family healthcare provider have not revealed a cause for the problem. Ms. Johnson leads a sedentary lifestyle and is overweight. However, her mother says there is no reason that a healthy woman would be experiencing these symptoms. Ms. Johnson's mother makes an appointment for Ms. Johnson to see her primary care physician but is unable to get an appointment that is not several weeks away.

1. Ms. Johnson perceives herself to be healthy yet has intermittent symptoms of an unusual nature that prompt her mother's concern. What barriers to regular healthcare are highlighted in this case study?
2. What questions might be important for Ms. Johnson to ask her mother before the visit with the primary care physician?

Check Your Progress: Section 14.1

1. Why is skin discomfort often one of the symptoms in disorders involving the immune system?
2. The immune system is there to protect us against foreign antigens and injury, but how might such an immune response impair the body's protective mechanisms?
3. What are some potential complications of an immune response that may require clinical attention and treatment?

14.2 Hypersensitivity Disorders

Hypersensitivity disorders result from inappropriate activation of the immune system. While activation of the immune system leads to the production of antibodies and T-cell responses as a protective mechanism again microorganisms, individuals who experience hypersensitivity disorders experience tissue damage and injury. The disorders caused by this inappropriate immune response are referred to as **hypersensitivity reactions**.

There are four basic types of hypersensitivity reactions:

- Type I reactions are IgE-mediated disorders.
- Type II reactions are antibody-mediated disorders.
- Type III reactions are complement-mediated immune disorders.
- Type IV reactions are T-cell–mediated disorders.

These reactions differ in terms of the type of immune response causing the injury along with the nature of the location of the antigen that is the target of the reaction. For example, a latex allergy can result from either an IgE-mediated or a T-cell–mediated hypersensitivity reaction.

Type I: Immediate Hypersensitivity Disorders

Type I reactions often occur within minutes of an antigen challenge. These reactions are referred to as **allergic reactions**. In the context of an allergic response, the antigens are often referred to as **allergens**. Allergens that are associated with this type of response include the protein in pollen, house dust mites, animal dander, foods, and chemicals like the antibiotic penicillin.

Exposure to the allergen can occur in many ways, including inhalation, ingestion, injection, or skin contact. The specific portal of entry often determines whether the individual will experience a local, or atopic, reaction or a systemic reaction. Local reactions are often annoying, such as those seen with seasonal allergies. Local reactions can also be debilitating, such as those seem with asthma. A type I reaction can be life threatening, as there is the potential for anaphylactic shock to occur.

Three types of cells are central to a type I hypersensitivity reaction. These cells include the T-helper cells, mast cells, and basophils. There are two subsets of T-helper cells. These cells develop from the same precursor CD4+ T lymphocyte. The type 1 T-helper (Th1) cells differentiate in response to microbes. This stimulates the differentiation of B cells into IgM- and IgG-producing plasma cells. The Th2 cell differentiation occurs in response to allergens and helminths (intestinal parasites), causing the secretion of cytokines (i.e., IL-4, IL-5, IL-13). This stimulates the differentiation of B cells into IgE-producing plasma cells. The IgE cells act as growth factors for mast cells along with the recruitment and activation of eosinophils.

Mast cells (tissue cells) and basophils (blood cells) are derived from hematopoietic precursor cells located in the bone marrow. The mast cells and basophils have granules that contain mediators. These mediators are released to initiate the early events in type I hypersensitivity reactions. Mast cells are normally distributed throughout connective tissue. Large numbers of mast cells are found in areas beneath the skin and mucous membranes of the respiratory, gastrointestinal, and genitourinary tracts and adjacent to blood and lymph vessels. Because of their location, mast cells are exposed to environmental antigens and parasites. Mast cells located in different parts of the body, or even in a single site, can have significant differences in mediator content and sensitivity to agents that produce mast cell degranulation.

Type I hypersensitivity reactions begin with the sensitization (or priming stage) of the mast cell or basophil. When this occurs, allergen-specific IgE antibodies attach to receptors on the surface of these cells. With subsequent exposure, the sensitizing allergen binds to the cell-associated IgE, triggering a series of events that lead to degranulation of the sensitized mast cells or basophils. This ultimately causes the release of their preformed mediators (**Figure 14.4** ■). Mast cells are also the source of lipid-derived membrane products, including prostaglandins and leukotrienes, along with cytokines, which participate in the continued response to the allergen.

Many type I hypersensitivity reactions have two well-defined phases. The first phase, often referred to as the *primary response* or the *initial-phase response*, is characterized by vasodilation, vascular leakage, and smooth muscle contraction. The second, or late-phase, response causes more intense infiltration of tissues with eosinophils and other acute and chronic inflammatory cells. This causes tissue destruction in the form of epithelial cell damage.

The first phase usually occurs within 5–30 minutes of exposure to antigen and subsides within 60 minutes of

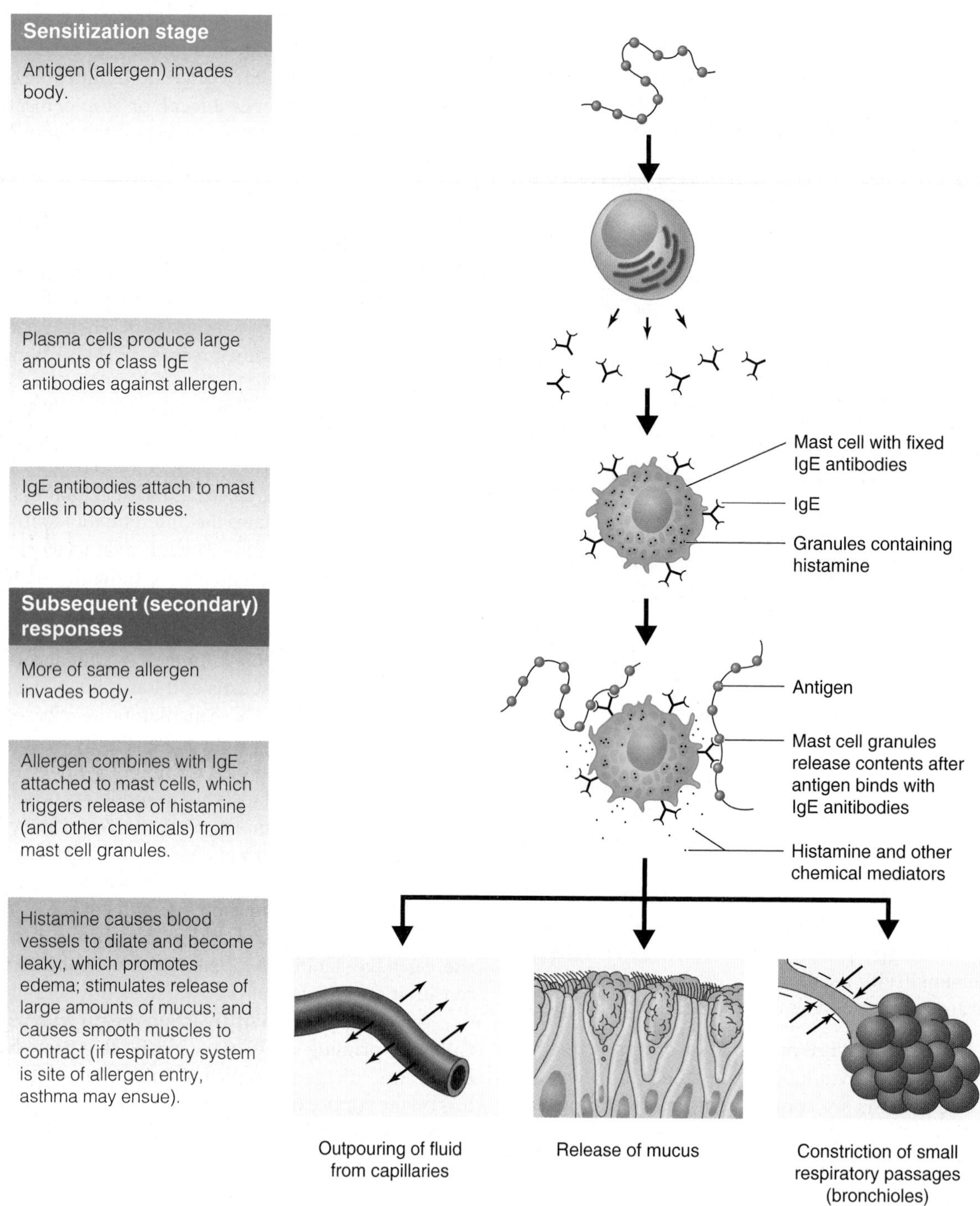
Sensitization stage
Antigen (allergen) invades body.
Plasma cells produce large amounts of class IgE antibodies against allergen.
IgE antibodies attach to mast cells in body tissues.
Mast cell with fixed IgE antibodies
IgE
Granules containing histamine
Subsequent (secondary) responses
More of same allergen invades body.
Allergen combines with IgE attached to mast cells, which triggers release of histamine (and other chemicals) from mast cell granules.
Antigen
Mast cell granules release contents after antigen binds with IgE anitibodies
Histamine and other chemical mediators
Histamine causes blood vessels to dilate and become leaky, which promotes edema; stimulates release of large amounts of mucus; and causes smooth muscles to contract (if respiratory system is site of allergen entry, asthma may ensue).
Outpouring of fluid from capillaries
Release of mucus
Constriction of small respiratory passages (bronchioles)

Figure 14.4 ■ Type I (IgE-mediated) hypersensitivity reaction.

exposure. It is mediated by mast cell degranulation along with the release of mediators, including histamine, acetylcholine, adenosine, chemotactic mediators, and enzymes (such as chymase and trypsin). The mediators cause the generation of kinins. Histamine, a potent vasodilator, increases the permeability of the capillaries and venules, leading to smooth muscle contraction and bronchial constriction. Acetylcholine produces bronchial smooth muscle contraction and dilation of small blood vessels. The kinins, a group of potent inflammatory peptides, require activation through the modification of enzymes. Once the kinins have been activated, vasodilation and smooth muscle contraction occur.

The secondary phase occurs approximately 2–8 hours after the first phase and may last for several days. It results from the action of lipid mediators and cytokines that are involved in the inflammatory response. The lipid mediators are derived from mast cell membrane phospholipids, which are broken down to form arachidonic acid. Arachidonic acid is the parent compound that synthesizes leukotrienes and prostaglandins. The leukotrienes and prostaglandins produce responses that are similar in nature to those of histamine and acetylcholine; however, their effects are delayed and prolonged by comparison. Mast cells also produce cytokines and chemotactic factors, prompting the influx of eosinophils and leukocytes to the site of allergen contact, which further contributes to the inflammatory response.

Not all IgE-mediated responses produce discomfort and disease. Late-phase type I hypersensitivity reactions play a protective role in the control of parasitic infections. IgE antibodies directly damage the larvae of these parasites by recruiting inflammatory cells and causing antibody-dependent cell-mediated cytotoxicity. This particular type I hypersensitivity reaction is particularly important in developing countries, where much of the population is infected with intestinal parasites.

Anaphylactic Reactions

Anaphylaxis is a systemic life-threatening type I hypersensitivity reaction.[3] It results from the presence of an antigen introduced by injection, insect sting, or absorption through the epithelial surface of the skin or gastrointestinal mucosa. Clinical manifestations include widespread edema, vascular shock due to vasodilation, and difficulty breathing. The level of severity depends on the level of sensitization. Even a small amount of antigen, such as the presence of peanut residue on equipment that has been used for preparing foods containing peanuts, can be sufficient to cause an anaphylactic reaction.

Within minutes of exposure, the individual experiences itching, urticaria (hives), and skin erythema. This is followed by bronchospasm and respiratory distress. Vomiting, abdominal cramps, diarrhea, and laryngeal edema and obstruction follow. Anaphylaxis is a medical emergency that requires immediate intervention to prevent shock and even death.

CLINICAL POINT: The initial management of anaphylaxis focuses on establishing a stable airway and intravenous access along with the administration of epinephrine. Individuals with a history of anaphylaxis should be provided with preloaded epinephrine syringes. Education should include appropriate technique for administering the epinephrine along with seeking immediate professional care. Prevention of exposure to potential triggers that cause anaphylaxis is essential. Finally, all individuals with the potential for anaphylaxis should be taught to wear or carry a medical alert bracelet, necklace, or other identification to inform emergency personnel of the possibility of anaphylaxis. ■

When a child has a history of anaphylaxis, it is essential to train all family members, along with other caregivers, in the procedure for administering injectable epinephrine, using either an Epi-Pen or an Adrenaclick.[1] ■

Atopic Reactions

Atopic, or local, reactions often occur when an antigen is confined to a particular site of exposure. The term **atopic** refers to a genetically determined hypersensitivity to common environmental allergens mediated by an IgE–mast cell reaction. Individuals with atopic reactions are often allergic to more than one (and often many) environmental allergens. The most common atopic disorders are urticaria, allergic rhinitis (hay fever), atopic dermatitis, food allergies, and some forms of asthma.

CLINICAL POINT: Susceptibility to immediate hypersensitivity disorders tends to be genetically determined, and a positive family history of allergy is found in about 50% of atopic individuals. Therefore, it is essential to include this topic in the health history of all individuals to determine susceptibility. ■

Allergic Rhinitis

Allergic rhinitis is characterized by symptoms of sneezing, itching, and **rhinoconjunctivitis** (watery discharge from the nose and eyes). Typical allergens include pollens from ragweed, grasses, trees, and weeds; fungal spores; house dust mites; animal dander; and feathers. This condition not only produces nasal symptoms but frequently is associated with other chronic airway disorders, such as sinusitis and bronchial asthma. Severe attacks may be accompanied by systemic malaise, fatigue, and muscle soreness from sneezing. Fever is absent. Sinus obstruction may cause headache.

There are two types of allergic rhinitis: perennial and seasonal allergic. Diagnosis is based on the chronology of symptoms. Individuals with perennial allergic rhinitis experience symptoms throughout the year, while those with seasonal allergic rhinitis (i.e., hay fever) are plagued with intense symptoms in conjunction with periods of high allergen (e.g., pollens, fungal spores) exposure. Symptoms that become worse at night suggest a household allergen, and symptoms that disappear on weekends suggest occupational exposure.

Allergic rhinitis is diagnosed by history and physical examination, microscopic identification of an increased number of eosinophils on a nasal smear, and skin testing to identify the offending allergens (**Figure 14.5** ■). When possible, avoidance of the offending allergen is recommended. Treatment is symptomatic and includes the use of oral antihistamines along with oral or topical decongestants. Tolerance and rebound congestion may occur when topical decongestants are used for longer than 1 week. Intranasal corticosteroids often are effective when used appropriately. Intranasal cromolyn, a drug that stabilizes mast cells and prevents their degranulation, may be useful, especially when administered before expected contact with an offending allergen. A program of specific immunotherapy ("allergy shots") may be used when symptoms are

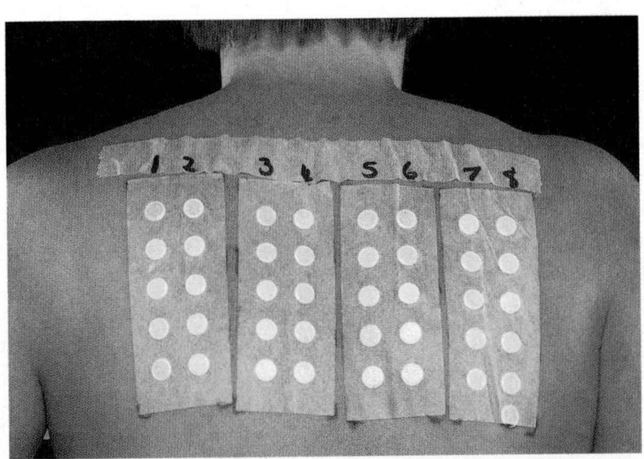

Figure 14.5 ■ A patch test for allergies.

particularly bothersome. Desensitization involves frequent (usually weekly) injections of the offending antigens. The antigens, which are given in increasing doses, stimulate production of high levels of IgG, which acts as a blocking antibody by combining with the antigen before it can combine with the cell-bound IgE antibodies.[4]

Food Allergy

Any food can cause an allergic reaction. The foods that are most commonly associated with a type I hypersensitivity reaction in children are milk, eggs, peanuts, soy, tree nuts (e.g., walnuts, almonds, pecans, cashews, hazelnuts), fish, and shellfish. In adults, foods commonly attributed to allergy are peanuts, shellfish, and fish. The allergenicity of a food may be changed by heating or cooking. For example, an individual may have an allergic reaction after drinking milk but not have symptoms after eating cooked foods that contain milk.

The primary target of food allergy may be the skin, the gastrointestinal tract, or the respiratory system. Reactions can be either acute or chronic. Acute reactions include hives and anaphylaxis. Chronic reactions often include asthma, atopic dermatitis, and gastrointestinal disorders. Anaphylaxis occurs as a multiple-organ response associated with IgE-mediated hypersensitivity. The foods most responsible for anaphylaxis are peanuts, tree nuts, and shellfish.

Food allergies tend to develop during childhood. The allergic response is thought to occur after contact between a specific food allergen and sensitizing IgE in the intestinal mucosa. This causes both the local and systemic release of histamine along with other mediators of the allergic response. The allergens are often food proteins and partially digested food products. Carbohydrates, lipids, or food additives such as preservatives, colorings, or flavorings also are potential allergens. Closely related food groups can contain common cross-reacting allergens. For example, some people are allergic to all legumes (beans, peas, and peanuts).[5] ■

CLINICAL POINT: It is important to know that individuals with an allergy history may have cross-reactivities to other substances. In the case of penicillin allergy, cross-reactivity to other related classes of antibiotics is possible, so extreme precautions must be taken before administering parenteral antibiotics. This is also true of other allergies, such as latex allergy and some foodstuffs (banana, avocado, kiwi, and chestnut together with papaya, fig, potato, and tomato); 30–80% of people with latex allergy experience symptoms when they eat one or more of these foods. ■

Food allergies are diagnosed by a careful food history and provocative diet testing. Provocative testing involves eliminating a suspected allergen from the diet for a time. If the symptoms disappear and then reoccur when the food is reintroduced, an allergy is diagnosed. Only one food should be tested at a time.

Treatment focuses on avoidance of any food responsible for the allergy. However, avoidance may be difficult for people who are exquisitely sensitive to a particular food protein, as foods may be contaminated by the protein during processing or handling of the food. For example, contamination may occur when chocolate candies without peanuts are processed with the same equipment that is used for making candies with peanuts. Even using the same spatula to serve cookies with and without peanuts can cause enough contamination to produce a severe reaction.

Nicolas Lopez: Application

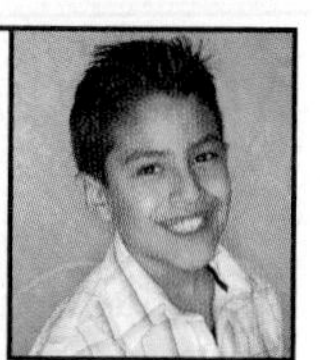

As the nurse working at the pediatric urgent care clinic, you conduct an initial assessment and patient interview with Nicolas and Mr. Lopez. Nicolas reports that he did not knowingly eat anything with peanuts. However, he did have a piece of birthday cake, and that is when he began to "feel funny." Mr. Lopez states, "I don't usually take him to birthday parties for his friends, so I didn't know that I need to say anything about his allergy. His mother usually takes care of that when accepting the invitation."

You observe red welts on Nicholas's face, neck, trunk, and arms. The skin appears irritated because Nicolas has been scratching the welts. His lips appear slightly swollen. Vital signs indicate a slightly decreased blood pressure and rapid heart rate for his age. You note wheezing on auscultation of his lungs. The healthcare provider prescribes a corticosteroid injection and an albuterol inhaler, which you administer as prescribed.

3. What pathophysiologic processes are causing Nicolas to have decreased blood pressure and increased heart rate?
4. How will the mechanism of action of the prescribed medications help to relieve Nicolas's symptoms?

Type II: Antibody-Mediated Disorders

Type II hypersensitivity reactions are often referred to as *antibody-mediated reactions*. These reactions are mediated by IgG or IgM antibodies directed against target antigens on cell surfaces or in connective tissues. The antigens may be endogenous (present on the membranes of body cells) or exogenous (absorbed on the membrane surface) (**Figure 14.6** ■). Three different types of antibody-mediated mechanisms are involved in type II reactions:

- Complement- and antibody receptor–mediated phagocytosis
- Complement- and antibody receptor–mediated inflammation
- Antibody-mediated cellular dysfunction.

Examples of each type are outlined in **Box 14.1**.

Type III: Immune Complex–Mediated Disorders

Type III, or immune complex, allergic disorders are mediated by the formation of insoluble antigen–antibody complexes, complement fixation, and localized inflammation (**Figure 14.7** ■). Immune complexes that are formed in the circulation produce damage when in contact with the vessel lining or are deposited in tissues, including the renal glomerulus, skin venules, lung, and joint synovium. Once deposited, the immune complexes elicit an inflammatory response

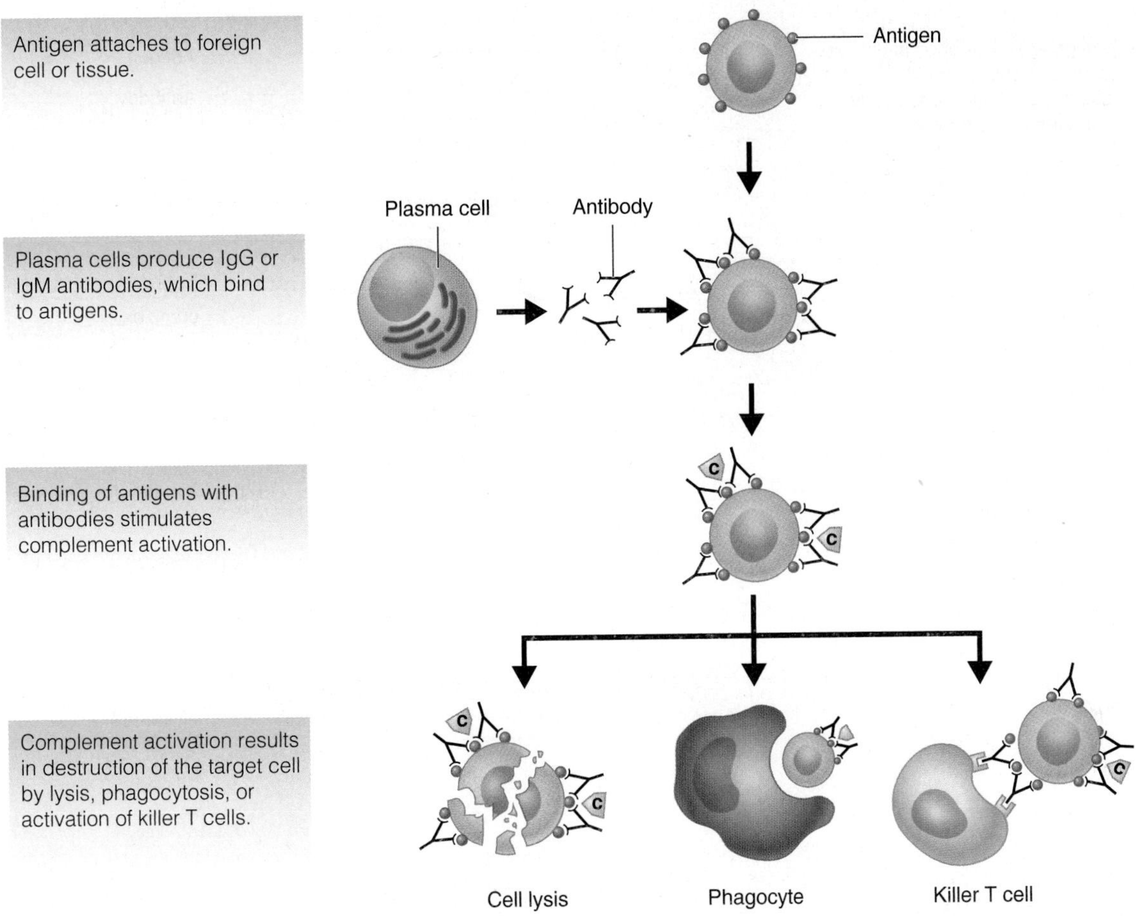

Figure 14.6 ■ Type II (cytotoxic) hypersensitivity reaction.

by activating complement. This leads to chemotactic recruitment of neutrophils and other inflammatory cells. The activation of these inflammatory cells by immune complexes and complement, accompanied by the release of potent inflammatory mediators, is directly responsible for the injury.

Immune complex–mediated reactions are responsible for the vasculitis seen in certain autoimmune diseases such as systemic lupus erythematosus (SLE) or the kidney damage seen with acute glomerulonephritis. Type III immune complex disorders can be generalized, or systemic, if the

Box 14-1

Type II Antibody-Mediated Disorders

Complement- and Antibody Receptor–Mediated Phagocytosis

- This occurs with mismatched blood transfusion reactions, with hemolytic disease of the newborn due to ABO or Rh incompatibility, or with certain drug reactions.
- With drug reactions, the binding of the drug (or its metabolites) to the surface of red or white blood cells causes an antibody response that lyses the drug-coated cells.

Complement- and Antibody Receptor–Mediated Inflammation

- Inflammation occurs when antibodies are deposited in the extracellular tissues, such as basement membranes and matrix.
- The activated leukocytes release injurious substances, such as enzymes and reactive oxygen intermediates, causing inflammation and tissue damage.
- This type of inflammation is responsible for the tissue injury seen in glomerulonephritis and vascular rejection in organ transplantation.

Antibody-Mediated Cellular Dysfunction

- Antibody binding causes a change in cell function.
- In Graves disease, an autoantibody is directed against thyroid-stimulating hormone (TSH) receptors on thyroid cells, which stimulates thyroxine production, leading to hyperthyroidism.
- In myasthenia gravis, autoantibodies to acetylcholine receptors on the neuromuscular end-plates either block the action of acetylcholine or mediate internalization or destruction of receptors, causing decreased neuromuscular function.

Antigens invade body and bind to antibodies in circulation. Antigen–antibody complexes are formed.
Antigen
Antibody
Antigen–antibody complex
Antigen–antibody complexes are deposited in the basement membrane of vessel walls and other body tissues, activating complement.
C
Basement membrane
Complement activation leads to release of inflammatory chemical mediators. Infiltration of polymorphonuclear leukocytes (PMNs) is followed by release of lysozymes. Tissue damage may be extensive.
Polymorphonuclear leukocyte
Lysosome
Chemical mediators
Release of lysosomal granules

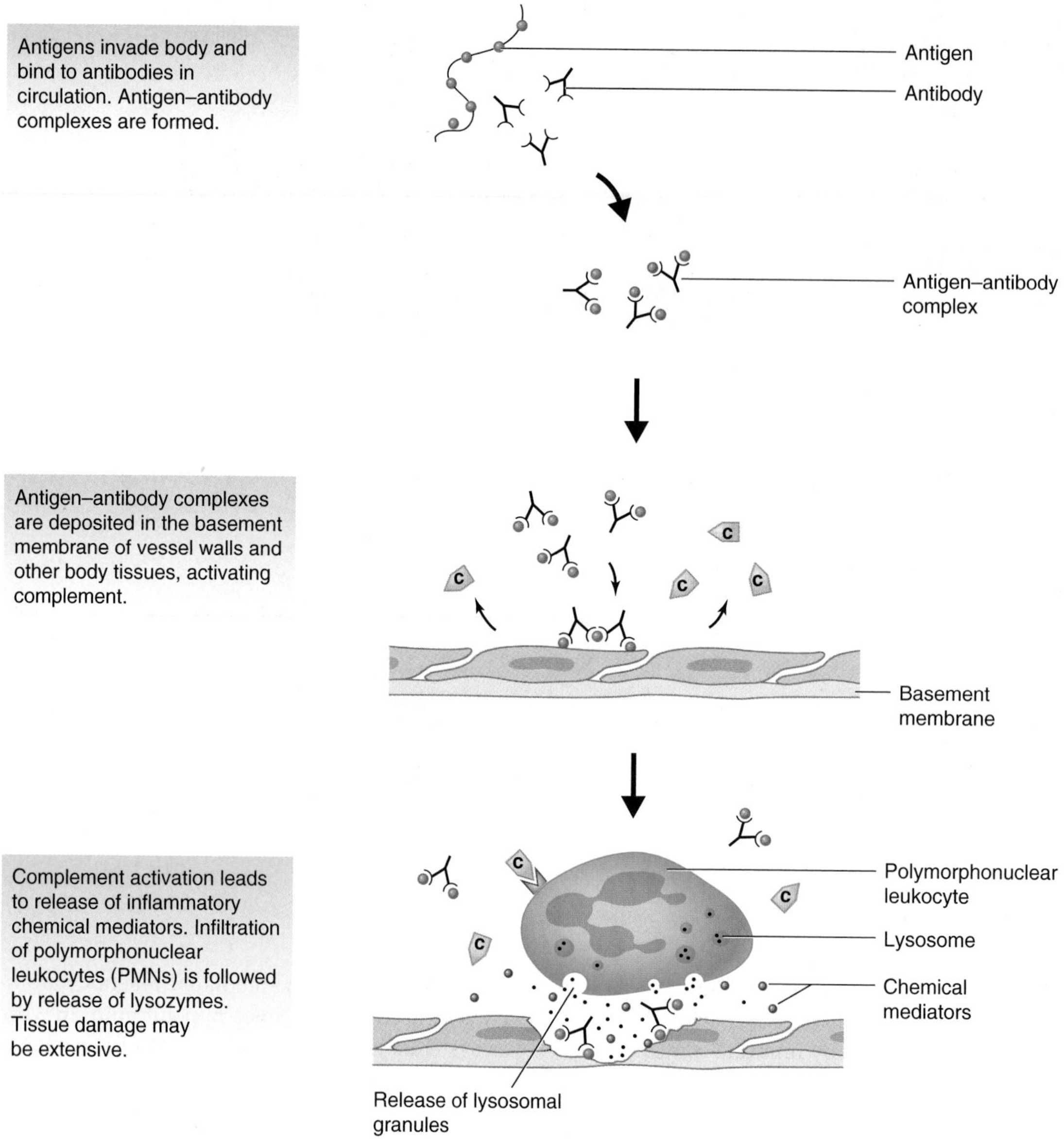

Figure 14.7 ■ Type III (immune complex–mediated) hypersensitivity reaction.

immune complexes are formed in the circulation and deposited in many organs. One example is serum sickness, which is described in **Box 14.2**. These disorders can also be localized to one organ. The organs that are often affected include the kidney, joints, and small blood vessels of the skin. Another example is Arthus reaction, also described in Box 14.2.

Box 14.2

Type III Immune Complex-Mediated Disorders

Serum sickness: Serum sickness is a disorder that occurs when the immune system reacts to medicines that contain foreign proteins used to treat immune conditions:

- Deposited complexes activate complement, increase vascular permeability, and recruit phagocytic cells, promoting focal tissue damage and edema.
- It is caused by antibiotics (e.g., penicillin), other drugs, various foods, and insect venom.
- Damage is often temporary, with symptoms resolving in a few days.

Arthus reaction: Arthus reaction is a disorder that involves previous sensitization or experience with an antigen and the formation of immune complexes after intradermal injection of the antigen, such as a vaccination:

- Arthus reaction involves localized tissue necrosis (usually the skin) caused by immune complexes.
- Injected antigen diffuses into local blood vessels, where it comes into contact with IgG, causing localized vasculitis.
- Arthus reaction is often caused by drug reaction.

CLINICAL POINT: Treatment for serum sickness is directed to remove the sensitizing antigen and provide relief from symptoms. Pharmacologic treatment often includes aspirin for joint pain and antihistamines for pruritus. For severe reactions, epinephrine or systemic corticosteroids may be prescribed. ■

Type IV: Cell-Mediated Hypersensitivity Disorders

Type IV hypersensitivity reactions involve cell-mediated immune responses. This type of reaction is the principal mechanism of response to a variety of microorganisms, including intracellular pathogens such as *Mycobacterium tuberculosis* and viruses, as well as extracellular agents such as fungi, protozoa, and parasites. It can cause cell death and tissue injury in response to chemical antigens (contact dermatitis) or self-antigens (autoimmunity).

Type IV hypersensitivity reactions are mediated by specifically sensitized T lymphocytes. There are two specific types of type IV reactions. These reactions include direct cell-mediated cytotoxicity and delayed-type hypersensitivity (**Figure 14.8** ■).

In direct cell-mediated cytotoxicity, CD8+ cytotoxic T lymphocytes (CTLs) directly kill target cells that express peptides derived from cystosolic antigens that are presented in association with class I major histocompatibility complex (MHC) molecules. For example, in viral infections, CTL responses can lead to tissue injury by killing infected target cells even if the virus itself has no cytotoxic effects. Some viruses directly injure infected cells and are said to be cytopathic; other, noncytopathic viruses do not. Because CTLs cannot distinguish between cytopathic and noncytopathic viruses, they kill virtually all infected cells, regardless of whether the infection is harmful. In certain forms of hepatitis, for example, the destruction of liver cells is due to the host CTL response and not the virus.

Delayed-type hypersensitivity (DTH) reactions occur in response to soluble protein antigens.[6] These reactions primarily involve antigen-presenting cells such as macrophages and CD4+ T-helper cells of the Th1 type. During the reaction, Th1 cells are activated and secrete an array of cytokines. These cytokines recruit and activate monocytes, lymphocytes, fibroblasts, and other inflammatory cells. These T-cell–mediated responses require the synthesis

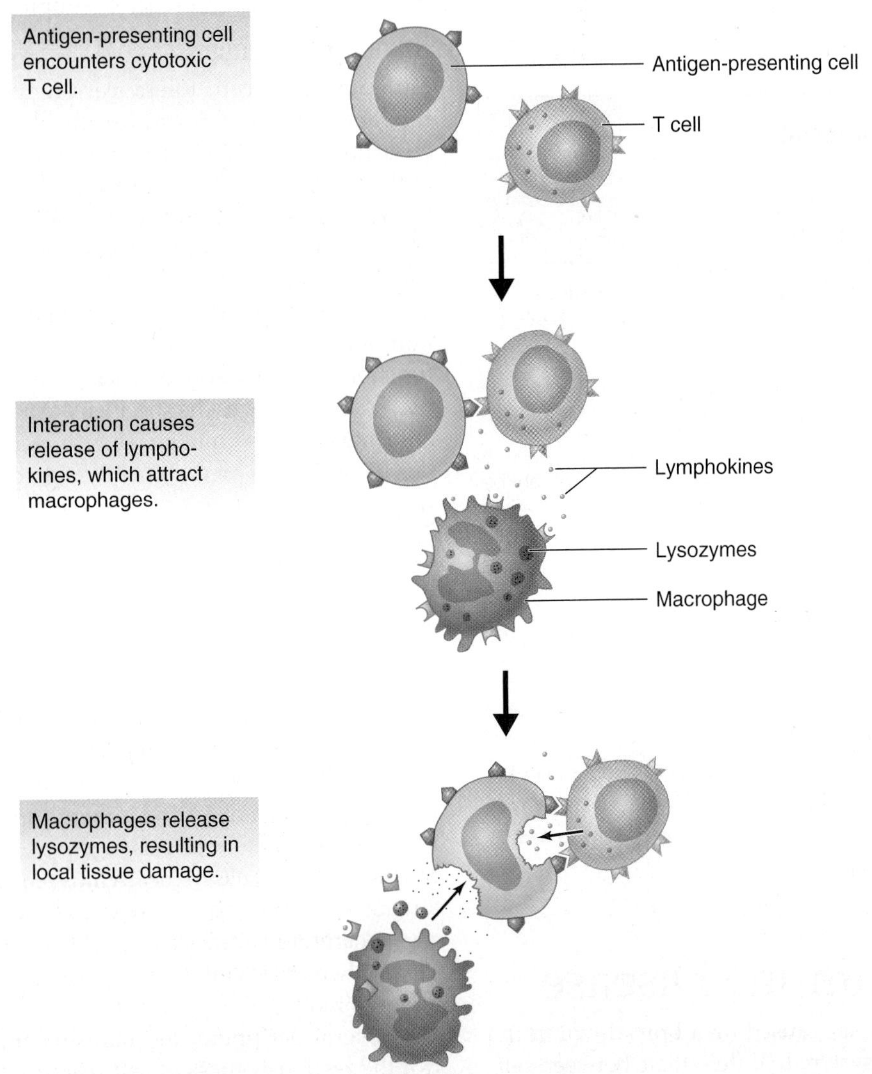
Antigen-presenting cell encounters cytotoxic T cell.
Antigen-presenting cell
T cell
Interaction causes release of lymphokines, which attract macrophages.
Lymphokines
Lysozymes
Macrophage
Macrophages release lysozymes, resulting in local tissue damage.

Figure 14.8 ■ Type IV (delayed) hypersensitivity reaction.

of effector molecules and often take 24–72 hours to develop; therefore, they are called delayed-type hypersensitivity disorders. The best-known DTH response is the reaction to the tuberculin test, in which inactivated tuberculin or purified protein derivative is injected under the skin.

The immune response is often diminished in older adults, owing to changes in the immune system that occur with age. This diminished responsiveness is called anergy, and it an result in a negative TB skin test, even when the patient has active disease. ■

In addition to its beneficial protective role, DTH can be the cause of disease. Examples include allergic contact dermatitis, hypersensitivity pneumonitis (a rare disorder that affects the lungs, also known as bird fancier's lung), and latex allergy. DTH may also play a role in transplant rejection and autoimmune disorders.

Diagnosis of contact dermatitis is made by observing the distribution of lesions on the skin surface. This will allow the practitioner to associate any pattern with exposure to possible allergens. If a specific allergen is suspected, a patch test may be prescribed to confirm the suspicion. Treatment is often limited to removal of the irritant and application of topical preparations to relieve symptomatic skin lesions and prevent secondary bacterial infections. Severe reactions, however, may require systemic corticosteroid therapy.

Nicolas Lopez: Outcome

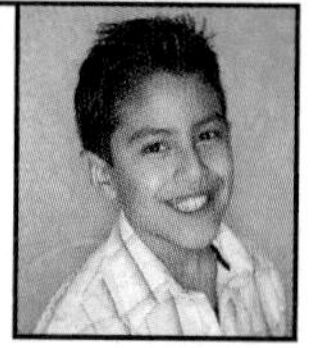

Within 10 minutes of administration of the prescribed medications, Nicolas's lungs are clear to auscultation, his swallowing improves, and the urticaria appears to be resolving. The provider instructs Mr. Lopez to follow up with Nicholas's allergist for further evaluation and writes a prescription for medication that should be kept with Nicolas at all times in case of future incidents.

5. What are examples of the types of medications that Nicolas is prescribed to keep available at all times in case of future incidents of severe food allergy reaction?
6. In addition to prescribed medication, what measures might be taken to safeguard Nicolas's health?

Check Your Progress: Section 14.2

1. What are some examples of antigens that are allergens and have the potential to cause a type I hypersensitivity reaction?
2. What are the more common types of foods that can cause food allergies in children and adults?
3. You have just administered an allergy shot to your patient who has seasonal allergic rhinitis. Your patient asks why she needs to receive these shots every week for the next year. What is your response?

14.3 Autoimmune Disease

Autoimmune diseases are caused by a breakdown in the ability of the immune system to differentiate between self- and nonself-antigens.[7] These diseases can affect any cell or tissue in the body. Autoimmune disorders include Hashimoto thyroiditis, which is tissue specific, and SLE, which can affect multiple organs and systems.

Immune Tolerance

For the immune system to function properly, it must be able to differentiate foreign antigens from self-antigens. This ability is referred to as **self-tolerance**. Several chemical messengers (i.e., interleukins) and costimulatory signals are essential to the activation of immune responses and the preservation of self-tolerance. It results from both central and peripheral mechanisms that delete self-reactive immune cells that cause autoimmunity or render their response ineffective in destroying self-cells and self-tissue.

Central tolerance refers to the elimination of self-reactive T cells and B cells in the central lymphoid organs (i.e., the thymus for T cells and the bone marrow for B cells). **Peripheral tolerance** occurs from the deletion or inactivation of autoreactive T cells or B cells that escaped elimination in the central lymphoid organs. Peripheral tolerance involves mechanisms such as receptor editing, absence of necessary costimulatory signals, production of immunologic ignorance by separating self-reactive immune cells from target tissues, and the presence of suppressor immune cells.

Humoral Tolerance

Humoral, or B-cell, tolerance refers to the loss of self-tolerance that occurs as a result of the development of autoantibodies. Humoral tolerance is characteristic of many autoimmune disorders. For example, hyperthyroidism in Graves disease is due to autoantibodies to the TSH receptor.

Several mechanisms are available to filter autoreactive B cells out of the B-cell population. These mechanisms include clonal deletion of immature B cells in the bone marrow; deletion of autoreactive B cells in the spleen or lymph nodes; functional inactivation, or anergy; and receptor editing, a process that changes the specificity of a B-cell receptor when autoantigen is encountered. There is increasing evidence that B-cell tolerance is predominantly due to help from T cells.

Cellular Tolerance

The central mechanisms of cellular, or T-cell, tolerance involve the deletion of self-reactive T cells in the thymus. T cells develop from bone marrow–derived progenitor cells that migrate to the thymus, where they encounter self-peptides bound to MHC molecules. T cells that display the host's MHC antigens and T-cell receptors for a nonself-antigen mature in the thymus. This process is often referred to as *positive selection*. T cells that have a high affinity for host cells are sorted out and undergo apoptosis (cell death). This process is referred to as *negative selection*. The deletion of self-reactive T cells in the thymus requires the presence of autoantigens. Many autoantigens are not present in the thymus. Therefore, self-reactive T cells may escape the thymus, so peripheral mechanisms that participate in T-cell tolerance are required.

Several peripheral mechanisms are available to control the responsiveness of self-reactive T cells. Sometimes the host antigens are not available in the appropriate immunologic form or are separated from the T cells. This is the case with the blood–brain barrier. When this occurs, the corresponding T cells remain **immunologically ignorant** of the presence of the antigens.

In other cases, the autoreactive T cell encounters its corresponding antigen in the absence of the costimulatory signals that are necessary for its activation. The peripheral activation of T cells requires two signals: recognition of the peptide antigen in association with the MHC molecules on the APCs and a set of secondary costimulatory signals. Because costimulatory signals are not strongly expressed on most normal tissues, the encounter of the autoreactive T cells and their specific target antigens frequently results in anergy.

Another mechanism of cellular tolerance involves the apoptotic death of autoreactive T cells. It is mediated by an apoptotic cell surface receptor (called Fas) that is present on the T cell and a soluble membrane messenger molecule (Fas ligand) that binds to the apoptotic receptor and activates the death program. The expression of the apoptotic Fas receptor is markedly increased in activated T cells; therefore, coexpression of the Fas messenger molecule by the same cohort of activated autoreactive T cells may serve to induce their death.

Suppressor T cells, some of which have the ability to downregulate the function of autoreactive T cells, are also thought to play a role in peripheral T-cell tolerance. These cells are believed to be a distinct subset of CD4+ and CD8+ T cells. However, the mechanism by which these T cells exert their suppressor function is not clear. Hypotheses include that they may secrete cytokines that suppress the activity of self-reactive immune cells, or they may delete the self-reactive T-cell clones.

Autoimmune Disease Mechanisms

Autoimmunity is caused by a loss of self-tolerance. The exact mechanism by which this occurs, however, is largely unknown. It is believed that genetics, environmental factors, and even gender play a role in the activation of self-reactive lymphocytes. Autoimmune diseases are complex; therefore, it is unlikely that any one factor is to blame for the development of these diseases.[7]

Factors

Two primary factors are believed to cause autoimmune diseases: heredity and environment.[7] Genetic factors increase the incidence and severity of autoimmune diseases. The molecular basis for this association is unknown. Because autoimmunity does not develop in all individuals who have a genetic predisposition, it is believed that other factors precipitate the altered immune state. This is often referred to as a *trigger event*. A trigger event may be a virus, a microorganism, a chemical substance, or a self-antigen from a body tissue that has been hidden from the immune system during the development of an autoimmune disease.

Environmental factors, such as an infectious agent, are often involved in the pathogenesis of an autoimmune disorder. However, their precise role in initiating the autoreactive response is largely unknown. Proposed mechanisms involved in the loss of self-tolerance include the breakdown of T-cell anergy, the release of sequestered antigens, molecular mimicry, and superantigens.

Diagnosis and Treatment

The criteria for determining an autoimmune disorder is determination that immunologic findings are not caused by another condition, along with the lack of other identified causes for the disorder. The specific diagnosis of autoimmune disease is currently based on clinical findings and serologic testing. In the future, these disorders are likely to be diagnosed by directly identifying the genes that are responsible for the condition.

The basis for serologic assays is the demonstration of antibodies that are directed against tissue antigens or cellular components. The detection of these autoantibodies in the laboratory is accomplished by one of three methods: indirect fluorescent antibody assays, enzyme-linked immunosorbent assays, or particle agglutination of some kind. The rationale for each of these methods is similar in that the individual's serum is diluted and allowed to react with an antigen-coated surface. For most serologic assays, the individual's serum is serially diluted until it no longer produces a reaction. This is referred to as a *positive titer*.

Treatment of autoimmune disease is based on the tissue or organ that is affected, the effector mechanism involved, and the magnitude and chronicity of effector processes. In ideal circumstances, treatment focuses on the specific mechanism underlying the autoimmune disorder. Immunosuppressive drugs and corticosteroids may be used to arrest or reverse the downhill course that often occurs with autoimmune disorders. Plasmapheresis may be used to purge autoreactive cells from the immune repertoire for patients who experience severe cases of autoimmunity. Research into the development of vaccines that target critical pathways in the emergence of autoimmune responses is ongoing.

Systemic Lupus Erythematosus

Systemic lupus erythematosus (SLE), often referred to simply as *lupus*, is a chronic autoimmune disease that causes generalized inflammation. In addition to affecting the skin and joints, SLE affects other organs in the body such as the kidneys, the pleura, the pericardium, and the brain. Most individuals diagnosed with SLE experience fatigue, rashes, arthritis, and fever. SLE flares vary in severity from mild to serious. Most individuals experience periods of exacerbation followed by periods of remission.

Etiology and Pathogenesis

The etiology of SLE is clearly multifocal but is not fully known.[8] Lupus is more common in women than in men and manifests most often between the ages of 15 and 44 years. It affects African Americans and people of Asian descent more than individuals of other races and ethnicities. Drug-induced SLE is caused by the body's overreaction in response to certain medications, such as isoniazid, hydralazine, and procainamide. Drug-induced SLE often manifests after an individual takes these and other drugs for at least 3–6 months.[9]

Although the exact etiology of SLE remains unclear, many of the clinical manifestations of SLE are mediated both directly and indirectly by antibody formation and the creation of immune complexes (IC). The pathogenic potential of IC varies, depending on several variables. The first variable is the characteristics of the antibody, including specificity, affinity, charge, and the ability to activate complement or other mediators of inflammation. The second variable is the nature of the antigen, including its size and charge. Next, the ability of the IC to be solubilized by the complement and bond to the complement receptor on the red blood cells. It is important to note that both systems may be defective in SLE. Finally, the rate at which the IC are cleared by immunoglobulin receptors on monocytes or macrophages in the liver and spleen from circulation is often genetically impaired in SLE.[9]

Clinical Manifestations

There are several different categories of clinical manifestations that are often seen in individuals diagnosed with SLE. Constitutional symptoms are those that most individuals diagnosed with SLE will experience at some point after diagnosis. These constitutional symptoms include fatigue, fever, myalgia, and weight change. A hallmark symptom for most individuals diagnosed with SLE includes acute cutaneous lupus erythema, commonly referred to as a *butterfly rash* (**Figure 14.9** ■). This rash presents as erythema in a malar distribution over the cheeks and nose. The rash spares the nasolabial folds and often occurs after sun exposure. Other clinical manifestations of SLE are presented by system in **Figure 14.10** ■.[10]

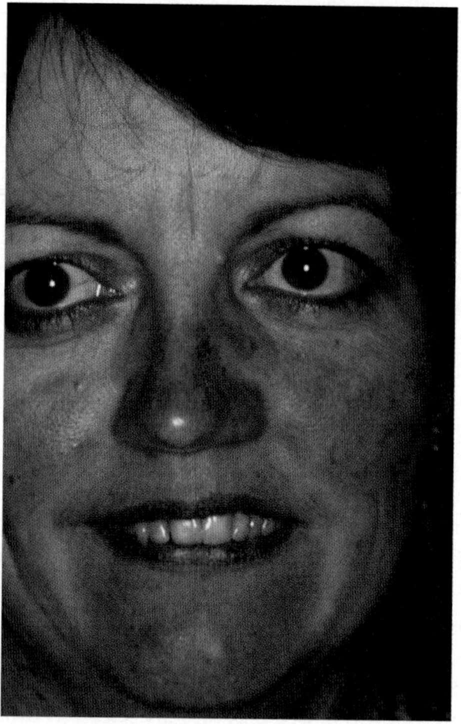

Figure 14.9 ■ The butterfly rash of systemic lupus erythematosus.

Yvonne Johnson: Application

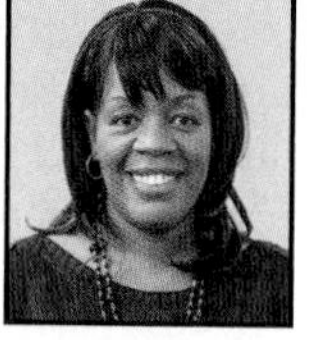

Ms. Johnson checks in for her appointment with the family practice healthcare provider, and the nurse begins the health history and physical examination. Ms. Johnson shares that she has had pain in her hands for several months. When the nurse asks more about the pain, Ms. Johnson states, "I would rate my pain as a 6 out of 10 on most days. When I get out of bed in the morning, I feel like my hips are on fire." She elaborates by saying, "My finger and hip joints often feel hot when I touch them. Look at this redness and swelling!" Ms. Johnson's finger joints are edematous with noted erythema. The nurse notes that Ms. Johnson's maternal aunt has a history of rheumatoid arthritis.

The nurse asks about other symptoms, and Ms. Johnson mentions that she has been experiencing swelling not only in her hands but also in her feet for approximately 4 years. She also states that she does not feel rested when she wakes up and often needs a nap when she gets home in the evening after work. She states, "I feel tired all the time!" On assessment of vital signs, the nurse notes that Ms. Johnson's blood pressure is slightly elevated (134/92 mmHg) and her body mass index (BMI) is 28, indicating that she is overweight. A dietary assessment indicates that Ms. Johnson is ingesting too much sodium. She also has reddened areas on her cheeks, although they are barely noticeable because of her dark complexion. When asked about her skin, Ms. Johnson says, "Some days are worse than others, but I usually have red cheeks." The nurse documents a butterfly rash in the medical record.

The healthcare provider suggests that Ms. Johnson begin taking ibuprofen, 800 mg every 8 hours for pain and inflammation management. The nurse provides education on ways to lower her sodium intake and decrease overall calorie consumption for weight management. The healthcare provider believes that Ms. Johnson's elevated blood pressure is attributed to a combination of her race, diet, and overweight status. Ms. Johnson is given a referral to a rheumatologist to further explore the generalized inflammation noted during the health history and physical assessment and to assess for a possible autoimmune disorder.

3. How will the mechanism of action of the ibuprofen alleviate Ms. Johnson's symptoms?
4. Ms. Johnson is referred to a rheumatologist for further evaluation. What types of conditions are managed by a rheumatologist?

Linking Pathophysiology to Diagnosis and Treatment

The diagnosis of SLE is based on clinical judgment after alternative diagnoses have been excluded. In the absence of SLE diagnostic criteria, clinicians use the SLE classification criteria to identify the salient clinical manifestations when making the diagnosis. Diagnosis with serologic data is important in suggesting the possibility of SLE. Certain antibodies (such as the anti–double-stranded DNA and anti-Smith) are highly correlated with SLE.[11]

Treatment for SLE focuses on ensuring long-term survival, achieving the lowest possible disease activity, preventing organ damage, minimizing drug toxicity, improving quality of life, and educating patients about their role in disease management. Treatment for patients diagnosed with SLE is individualized on the basis of preference, clinical manifestations, disease activity and severity, and any comorbidities. Individuals who have been diagnosed with SLE must be monitored at

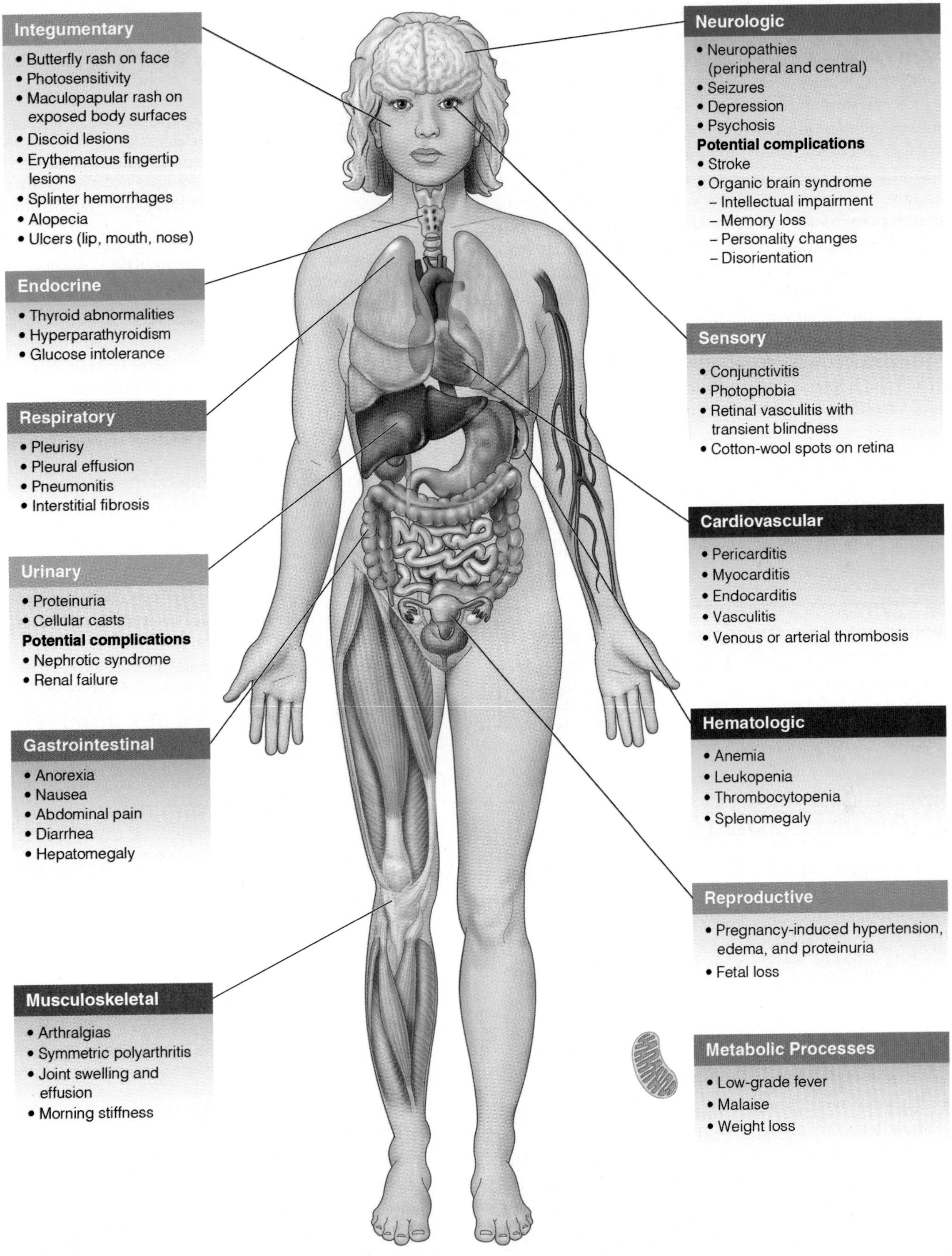

Integumentary
• Butterfly rash on face
• Photosensitivity
• Maculopapular rash on exposed body surfaces
• Discoid lesions
• Erythematous fingertip lesions
• Splinter hemorrhages
• Alopecia
• Ulcers (lip, mouth, nose)
Endocrine
• Thyroid abnormalities
• Hyperparathyroidism
• Glucose intolerance
Respiratory
• Pleurisy
• Pleural effusion
• Pneumonitis
• Interstitial fibrosis
Urinary
• Proteinuria
• Cellular casts
Potential complications
• Nephrotic syndrome
• Renal failure
Gastrointestinal
• Anorexia
• Nausea
• Abdominal pain
• Diarrhea
• Hepatomegaly
Musculoskeletal
• Arthralgias
• Symmetric polyarthritis
• Joint swelling and effusion
• Morning stiffness
Neurologic
• Neuropathies (peripheral and central)
• Seizures
• Depression
• Psychosis
Potential complications
• Stroke
• Organic brain syndrome
– Intellectual impairment
– Memory loss
– Personality changes
– Disorientation
Sensory
• Conjunctivitis
• Photophobia
• Retinal vasculitis with transient blindness
• Cotton-wool spots on retina
Cardiovascular
• Pericarditis
• Myocarditis
• Endocarditis
• Vasculitis
• Venous or arterial thrombosis
Hematologic
• Anemia
• Leukopenia
• Thrombocytopenia
• Splenomegaly
Reproductive
• Pregnancy-induced hypertension, edema, and proteinuria
• Fetal loss
Metabolic Processes
• Low-grade fever
• Malaise
• Weight loss

Figure 14.10 ■ Multisystem effects of systemic lupus erythematosus.

regular intervals by a rheumatologist to optimize nonpharmacologic and pharmacologic therapies. It is not uncommon for the individual to require a multidisciplinary approach to care, owing to multiorgan system involvement.[12]

Several nonpharmacologic measures, along with other medical interventions, are important in the comprehensive management of SLE. Individuals who have been diagnosed with SLE are taught the importance of protection from sunlight, maintaining adequate nutritional intake, getting enough exercise, stopping smoking, and receiving appropriate immunizations. It is essential that appropriate care be administered in the treatment of any comorbidities that may exacerbate symptoms associated with SLE and that the patient avoid any medications (such as sulfa antibiotics) known to exacerbate the symptoms of SLE.[12]

The choice of pharmacologic therapy is highly individualized and depends on the predominant symptoms, organ involvement, response to previous therapies, and disease activity and severity. In general, all individuals diagnosed with SLE are treated with hydroxychloroquine to provide relief of constitutional manifestation and symptoms associated with the musculoskeletal and mucocutaneous systems. Additional pharmacologic therapy is determined by the severity of the disease process and the combination of clinical manifestations.[12]

Yvonne Johnson: Outcome

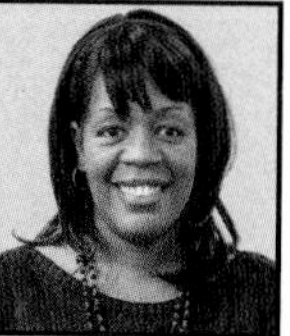

Ms. Johnson sees a rheumatologist to determine whether she might have an autoimmune disorder. Blood is drawn for lab work, and Ms. Johnson tests positive for anti-DNA antibody, anti-Smith antibody, and antinuclear antibody. An initial diagnosis of connective tissue disease is made. The rheumatologist states, "This is often the initial diagnosis for individuals who have symptom of an autoimmune disorder. I believe that, over time, you will be diagnosed with systemic lupus erythematosus (SLE)."

Because Ms. Johnson's blood pressure remains elevated, the rheumatologist prescribes hydrochlorothiazide for management and advises Ms. Johnson to continue the prescribed ibuprofen. She is also prescribed a 14-day taper of prednisone and hydroxychloroquine. Ms. Johnson makes an appointment to return for a follow-up visit in 4 weeks.

Because these medications suppress the immune system, the nurse educates Ms. Johnson about the risks of being immunocompromised. These risks include the potential for infection, gastrointestinal upset, and systemic rash.

Ms. Johnson begins feeling better almost immediately after beginning this regimen. Within a few days, the pain and swelling are almost completely gone. She continues to be monitored by the rheumatologist and will require follow-up care for the foreseeable future.

5. Why does the rheumatologist tell Ms. Johnson that she eventually will probably have a diagnosis of systemic lupus erythematosus?
6. What patient education about self-care for immunocompromised does the nurse give Ms. Johnson?

Check Your Progress: Section 14.3

1. What is a trigger event in the development of an autoimmune disorder?
2. Why do we normally not develop autoantibodies to our own tissues and cells?
3. What are some examples of autoimmune disorders?

CHAPTER SUMMARY

14.1 Chapter Overview and Case Studies

Describe the normal immune response, the results of inappropriate immune response, and concepts related to the immune response.

- The central lymphoid organs consist of the bone marrow and the thymus, which provide an environment for the production and maturation of immune cells.
- The peripheral lymphoid organs concentrate and produce antigens along with promoting cellular interactions necessary for the development of adaptive immune responses. These organs include the lymph nodes, spleen, tonsils, appendix, Peyer patches in the intestine, and the mucosa-associated lymphoid tissue in the respiratory, gastrointestinal, and reproductive systems.
- The immune system protects the body by recognizing and responding to antigens.
- Two basic immune responses occur in response to antigens: humoral immunity and cellular immunity.
- The concepts that are most often related to immune response include comfort, inflammation and oxidative stress, and tissue integrity.

14.2 Hypersensitivity Disorders

Differentiate the causes, classification, underlying pathogenesis, and clinical manifestations of hypersensitivity disorders and the diagnosis and treatment of these conditions across the lifespan.

- The disorders caused by this inappropriate immune response are referred to as hypersensitivity reactions.
- Type I reactions are IgE-mediated disorders. Examples include anaphylaxis, allergic rhinitis, and food allergies.
- There are three other types of hypersensitivity reactions. Type II reactions are antibody-mediated disorders. Type III reactions are complement-mediated immune disorders. Type IV reactions are T-cell–mediated disorders. The reactions differ in terms of the type of immune response causing the injury along with the nature of the location of the antigen that is the target of the reaction.

14.3 Autoimmune Disease

Differentiate the causes, classification, underlying pathogenesis, and clinical manifestations of autoimmune disease and the diagnosis and treatment of these conditions across the lifespan.

- Autoimmune disease is caused by a breakdown in the ability of the immune system to differentiate between self- and nonself-antigens.
- For the immune system to function properly, it must be able to differentiate foreign antigens from self-antigens. This ability is referred to as self-tolerance. Central tolerance refers to the elimination of self-reactive T cells and B cells in the central lymphoid organs. Peripheral tolerance occurs from the deletion, or inactivation of, autoreactive T cells or B cells that escaped elimination in the central lymphoid organs.
- Humoral, or B-cell, tolerance refers to the loss of self-tolerance occurring as a result of the development of autoantibodies. The central mechanisms of cellular, or T cell, tolerance involve the deletion of self-reactive T cells in the thymus.
- Autoimmunity is caused by a loss of self-tolerance. The exact mechanism by which this occurs is largely unknown. It is believed that genetics, environmental factors, and even gender play a role in the activation of self-reactive lymphocytes.
- Systemic lupus erythematosus (SLE or lupus) is a chronic autoimmune disease that causes generalized inflammation. In addition to affecting the skin and joints, SLE affects other organs in the body such as the kidneys, the pleura, the pericardium, and the brain.

REVIEW QUESTIONS

1. Your instructor is stung by a bee while searching for a cell phone signal in her front yard. She experiences a severe allergic reaction, with difficulty breathing as a result of airway edema, and has to go to the hospital. The nurse providing care realizes that this type I hypersensitivity reaction is the result of the action of which immunoglobulin?
   a. IgE
   b. IgA
   c. IgM
   d. IgG
2. A 41-year-old man has been seen several times by his primary care provider for rhinoconjunctivitis and other complaints consistent with a diagnosis of allergic rhinitis. After taking a 2-week vacation, the man realizes that his symptoms have disappeared. This suggests:
   a. food allergy.
   b. occupational exposure.
   c. autoimmune disease.
   d. infection.
3. A pathophysiology student recalls that the mast cell, a major activator of inflammation, initiates the inflammatory response through the process of:
   a. chemotaxis.
   b. endocytosis.
   c. pinocytosis.
   d. degranulation.
4. A hiker is seen in the clinic on Tuesday after having gone hiking on Saturday. He has a poison ivy rash on his extremities, face, and buttocks. This condition is an example of which type of hypersensitivity reaction?
   a. IgE-mediated hypersensitivity reaction (type I hypersensitivity reaction)
   b. Immune complex–mediated hypersensitivity reaction (type III hypersensitivity reaction)
   c. Cell-mediated delayed hypersensitivity reaction (type IV hypersensitivity reaction)
   d. Innate immunity
5. An older adult patient has just been admitted to a nursing home with symptoms suggestive of tuberculosis (TB). Her tuberculin skin test is negative (nonreactive), although the chest x-ray is positive for TB infection and a sputum sample confirms the diagnosis on laboratory testing. The patient's family asks the nurse why her TB skin test is negative. They are concerned that the diagnosis is an error. Which of the following explanations provided by the nurse will help to explain the need for isolation and treatment despite the negative (nonreactive) TB test?
   a. "We treat all our new nursing home patients for TB."
   b. "In older adults, diminished immune function can result in a negative TB skin tests, even when the patient has active disease."
   c. "The TB skin test is not reliable and should not be trusted."
   d. "It is a complete mystery why her TB skin test is negative."
6. A patient with known anaphylaxis to penicillin receives an injection of a cephalosporin antibiotic. Within minutes, his blood pressure drops, and he experiences difficulty breathing. On examination, he has perioral edema and wheezing on pulmonary auscultation. Which of the following is true?
   a. The patient is experiencing anaphylaxis to the cephalosporin antibiotic due to cross-reactivity.
   b. Someone must have injected him with penicillin by mistake.
   c. This type of reaction is minor and will resolve by itself without any clinical intervention.
   d. The patient is experiencing a purely psychologic reaction due to his fear of injections.

7. A blood transfusion reaction due to mismatched donor and recipient blood, and hemolytic disease of the newborn are both examples of which type of hypersensitivity reaction?
   a. Type I hypersensitivity reaction
   b. Type II hypersensitivity reaction
   c. Type III hypersensitivity reaction
   d. Type IV hypersensitivity reaction
8. A young boy was brought to a new clinic yesterday for healthcare, and his parents did not have his vaccination record. They had a vague recollection that he was recently given a vaccination but could not remember exactly which vaccine was given or exactly when it was administered. Despite this lack of information, the child received a tetanus–diphtheria booster vaccination on his upper arm at the clinic. This morning, he wakes up with pain, swelling, induration (hardening of the skin), and edema at the vaccination site. He has no other symptoms. Which of the following is true?
   a. This is a serum sickness reaction.
   b. This is an Arthus reaction.
   c. This is an infection at the vaccination site.
   d. The reaction is due to poor skin care at the vaccination site.

ANSWERS

Answers to Review Questions can be found in Appendix A. Answers to Case Study and Check Your Progress questions are available on the faculty resources site. Please consult with your instructor.

RECOMMENDED WEBSITES

American Academy of Allergy Asthma & Immunology
https://www.aaaai.org

Lupus Foundation of America
http://www.lupus.org

Merck Manuals: Overview of the Immune System
http://www.merckmanuals.com/home/immune-disorders/biology-of-the-immune-system/overview-of-the-immune-system

REFERENCES

1. Ball, J. W., Bindler, R. C., Cowen, K., & Shaw, M. (2017). *Principles of pediatric nursing: Caring for children* (7th ed.). Hoboken, NJ: Pearson Education.
2. National Institute on Aging. (2015). *Immune system: Can your immune system still defend you as you age?* Available at https://www.nia.nih.gov/health/publication/biology-aging/immune-system-can-your-immune-system-still-defend-you-you-age
3. Mustafa, S. S. (2016). Anaphylaxis. *Medscape*. Available at http://emedicine.medscape.com/article/135065-overview
4. University of Texas, Department of Otorhinolaryngology–Head & Neck Surgery. (2017). *Understanding the mechanism of allergen immunotherapy*. Available at https://med.uth.edu/orl/newsletter/understanding-mechanism-allergen-immunotherapy
5. American Academy of Pediatrics. (2015). *Food allergies in children*. Available at https://www.healthychildren.org/English/healthy-living/nutrition/Pages/Food-Allergies-in-Children.aspx
6. Abramson, S. L. (2015). Delayed hypersensitivity reactions. *Medscape*. Available at http://emedicine.medscape.com/article/136118-overview
7. Vojdani, A. (2014). A potential link between environmental triggers and autoimmunity. *Autoimmune Diseases, 2014*, Article IJ 437231. Available at https://www.hindawi.com/journals/ad/2014/437231
8. Schuer, P. H., & Hahn, B. H. (2016). Epidemiology and pathogenesis of systemic lupus erythematosus. *UpToDate*. Available at https://www.uptodate.com/contents/epidemiology-and-pathogenesis-of-systemic-lupus-erythematosus
9. U.S. National Library of Medicine. (2015). Drug-induced lupus erythematosus. *Medline Plus*. Available at https://medlineplus.gov/ency/article/000446.htm
10. Gladman, D. D. (2015). Overview of the clinical manifestations of systemic lupus erythematosus in adults. *UpToDate*. Available at https://www.uptodate.com/contents/overview-of-the-clinical-manifestations-of-systemic-lupus-erythematosus-in-adults?source=search_result&search=clinical%20manifestations%20of%20SLE&selectedTitle=1~150
11. Wallace, D. J. (2015). Diagnosis and differential diagnosis of systemic lupus erythematosus in adults. *UpToDate*. Available at https://www.uptodate.com/contents/diagnosis-and-differential-diagnosis-of-systemic-lupus-erythematosus-in-adults?source=see_link
12. Wallace, D. J. (2015). Overview of the management and prognosis of systemic lupus erythematosus in adults. *UpToDate*. Available at https://www.uptodate.com/contents/overview-of-the-management-and-prognosis-of-systemic-lupus-erythematosus-in-adults?source=search_result&search=diagnosis%20and%20treatment%20of%20SLE&selectedTitle=1~150

Chapter 15
Immunodeficiency Disorders

Kathy Laurer and Linda Blevins

Chapter Outline and Learning Outcomes

15.1 Chapter Overview and Case Studies

Describe the types of immunodeficiency disorders and concepts related to immunodeficiency.

15.2 HIV and AIDS

Differentiate the causes, classification, underlying pathogenesis, and clinical manifestations of acquired immunodeficiency syndrome and approaches to diagnosis and treatment of the condition across the lifespan.

15.3 Common Conditions Associated with HIV/AIDS

Differentiate the causes, classification, underlying pathogenesis, and clinical manifestations of common conditions associated with HIV and AIDS and approaches to diagnosis and treatment of these conditions across the lifespan.

15.4 Primary Immunodeficiencies

Differentiate the causes, classification, underlying pathogenesis, and clinical manifestations of primary immunodeficiencies and approaches to diagnosis and treatment of these conditions across the lifespan.

KEY TERMS

Acquired immunodeficiency syndrome (AIDS), 389
AIDS-related lymphoma, 392
Antiretroviral therapy (ART), 390
CD4 receptor, 386
Chemokine receptors, 387
Cytomegalovirus (CMV), 391
Dendritic cells, 387
Distal symmetric polyneuropathy (DSP), 392
Granuloma, 391
Heterozygous, 387
Highly active antiretroviral therapy (HAART), 390
HIV-associated lipodystrophy syndrome (HALS), 392
Human immunodeficiency virus (HIV), 383
Integrase, 387
Kaposi sarcoma (KS), 392
Lentiviruses, 385
Long terminal repeat (LTR), 387
Opportunistic infection (OI), 391
Primary immunodeficiency (PI), 393
Provirus, 387
Retrovirus, 385
Reverse transcriptase, 387
Seroconversion, 389
Transmitted drug resistance (TDR), 390
Tropism, 385
Tuberculosis (TB), 391
Viral set point, 387
Window period, 389

ABBREVIATIONS

AIDS—acquired immunodeficiency syndrome
ART—antiretroviral therapy
CMV—cytomegalovirus
CVID—common variable immunodeficiency
DSP—distal symmetric polyneuropathy
EBV—Epstein-Barr virus
GI—gastrointestinal
HAART—highly active antiretroviral therapy
HALS—HIV-associated lipodystrophy syndrome
HIV—human immunodeficiency virus
INSTI—integrase strand transfer inhibitor
IVIG—intravenous immunoglobulin
KS—Kaposi sarcoma
LTR—long terminal repeat
mRNA—messenger RNA
NK—natural killer

Abbreviations continue on the next page.

NNRTI—nonnucleoside reverse transcriptase inhibitor
NRTI—nucleoside reverse transcriptase inhibitor
OI—opportunistic infection
PI—primary immunodeficiencies
RTV—resistance to ritonavir
SCID—severe combined T-cell and B-cell immunodeficiency
SIV—simian immunodeficiency virus
TB—tuberculosis
TDR—transmitted drug resistance

15.1 Chapter Overview and Case Studies

Immunodeficiency disorders include a heterogeneous group of abnormalities of B-lymphocyte (humoral or antibody-mediated), T-lymphocyte (cell-mediated), phagocytic, and complement-related immune function, thus affecting both innate and adaptive immunity, maintenance of self-tolerance, and cancer cell surveillance. These disorders may be secondary or primary.

Secondary or acquired immunodeficiency disorders are more common than primary disorders. Secondary immunodeficiency disorders may result from a wide variety of internal and external factors, including aging, stress, nutritional deficiencies, selected malignancies, infection, and immunosuppressive treatment modalities. Worldwide, nutritional deficiencies are the most common cause of secondary immunodeficiency. However, the most common life-threatening cause of secondary immunodeficiency, especially in developing nations, is acquired immunodeficiency syndrome (AIDS). As of 2013, approximately 35 million individuals worldwide were infected with human immunodeficiency virus (HIV), the majority of them in sub-Saharan Africa.[1] Despite advances in diagnosis and treatment, AIDS remains a fatal disease in much of the world.

Primary immunodeficiencies (PIs) comprise more than 250 diseases,[2] most of which have been proven to be or are suspected of being the result of genetic mutations; the majority of these are inherited. In general, these disorders generally appear to be rare, although they are more frequent in selected populations. The most commonly reported disorders include selective IgA deficiency, X-linked agammaglobulinemia, hypogammaglobulinemia, common variable immunodeficiency, specific antibody deficiency, and transient hypogammaglobulinemia of infancy.[3] A fourth disorder, severe combined immunodeficiency (also known as "bubble boy" disease), is the most serious primary immunodeficiency (PID) and is considered a pediatric emergency; unless it is treated by stem cell transplantation, death within the first or second year of life often occurs.

Concepts Related to Immunodeficiency

Immunodeficiency can adversely affect every body system and all facets of life. In most cases, the severity of adverse effects is directly relate to the nature and degree of immunodeficiency. For example, candidiasis (thrush), an opportunistic oral fungal infection related to HIV, can lead to dysphagia (difficulty swallowing) and loss of appetite,[4] which can negatively affect the individual's nutrition status and lead to metabolic alteration. Medications used in treating immunodeficiency disorders have side effects that may include nausea, vomiting, and diarrhea, all of which can contribute to impaired elimination. Opportunistic respiratory infections associated with HIV such as *Pneumocystis jiroveci* pneumonia, histoplasmosis, and coccidioidodomycosis can produce a variety of effects, including impaired gas exchange leading to decreased oxygenation and impaired perfusion of tissues and organs.[4] **Figure 15.1** ■ illustrates concepts related to immunodeficiency.

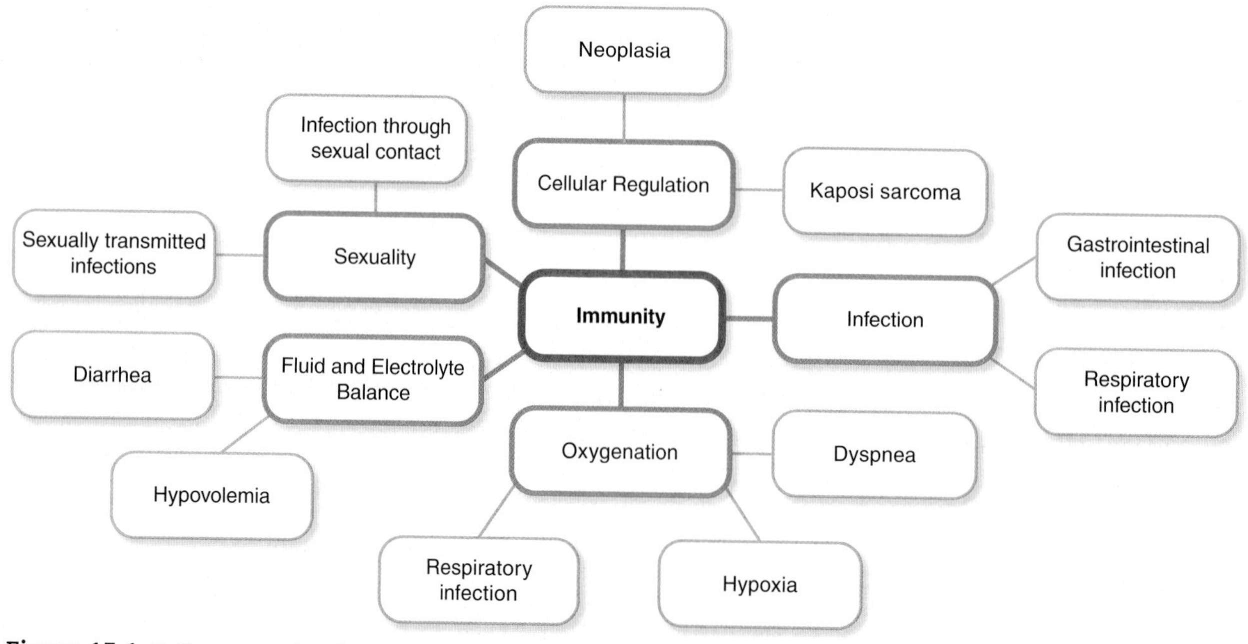

Figure 15.1 ■ Concepts related to immunodeficiency disorders.

There is a diverse range of immunodeficiencies. These can result in select deficits in immunologic defense and may range to complex genetic disorders with corresponding effects on cardiovascular status and function. There are also links between immunodeficiencies and the development of autoimmune diseases. Ultimately, the primary concern is a lack of immunologic defense, resulting in an increased risk of infection. Depending on the site of infection, several potential consequences may emerge. Respiratory infections can lead to consolidation with lung tissue, preventing effective gas exchange. This in turn leads to issues with oxygenation and resultant hypoxia. Gastrointestinal infections can result in issues related to the absorption of nutrients, influencing nutritional status and function. Diarrhea and related fluid loss from gastrointestinal (GI) infections can affect fluid and electrolyte status. Pronounced immunodeficiencies can result in the development of opportunistic infections and several forms of neoplasia.

Case Studies

The following cases will be addressed throughout the chapter to assist in application of chapter content to clinical situations that involve individuals with immunodeficiency disorders.

DeShawn Ruffin: Introduction

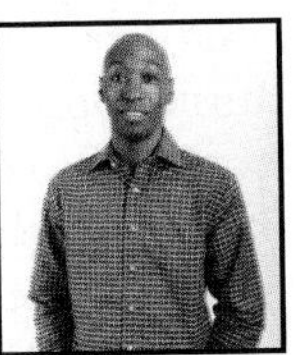

DeShawn Ruffin, age 39, first tested seropositive for HIV at age 35. Mr. Ruffin visited his primary care physician at the time because he was experiencing recurrent ear and throat infections along with swollen cervical lymph nodes. Initially, he was prescribed antibiotics for his recurrent infections. However, over the course of a year, the primary care physician recognized Mr. Ruffin's pattern of increasingly severe symptoms. The physician recommended an enzyme immunoassay screening; when the results came back, Mr. Ruffin learned that he had tested positive for HIV antibodies. At that time, his $CD4^+$ T-lymphocyte count was 570 cells/mm^3. Over the past month, Mr. Ruffin has experienced worsening shortness of breath as well as a cough. Two days ago, Mr. Ruffin developed hemoptysis (coughing up blood). At that time, he scheduled an appointment with his primary care provider.

1. Why are Mr. Ruffin's recurrent ear and throat infections of concern?
2. Explain whether HIV is a primary or secondary immunodeficiency disorder.

Stassi Laramore: Introduction

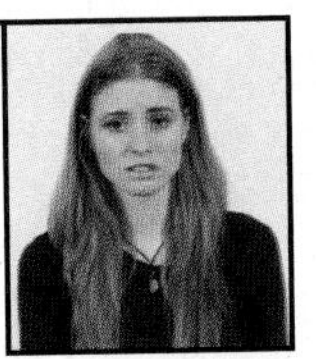

Stassi Laramore is 21 years old. One year ago, during a routine screening for sexually transmitted infections, Ms. Laramore tested positive for HIV. She was prescribed antiretroviral therapy, but she has been intermittently noncompliant because of a lack of financial resources and low tolerance for the medications' side effects. Her $CD4^+$ T-lymphocyte count has been relatively stable at 760 cells/mm^3. Since her initial diagnosis, Ms. Laramore has been in a monogamous relationship. She and her partner use condoms for prevention of HIV transmission as well as for birth control. However, Ms. Laramore has scheduled an appointment with her primary care provider because her menstrual period is 4 weeks overdue and she is concerned that she might be pregnant.

1. What are some of the side effects caused by medications to treat immunodeficiency disorders that Ms. Laramore may experience?
2. How can a therapeutic relationship between Ms. Laramore and the nurse help to improve Ms. Laramore's compliance with treatment?

Check Your Progress: Section 15.1

1. What are immunodeficiency disorders?
2. Describe secondary or acquired immunodeficiency disorders.
3. Explain primary immunodeficiency disorders.

15.2 HIV and AIDS

Since its identification in 1981, the acquired immunodeficiency syndrome (AIDS) has been responsible for over 39 million deaths worldwide.[1] Although current treatment strategies have dramatically reduced morbidity and mortality rates in industrialized nations, AIDS remains a leading cause of death in developing nations.

The causative agent of AIDS is the **human immunodeficiency virus (HIV)**, a retrovirus that infects key cells in the immune system and induces defects in cellular and humoral immunity. Two strains of HIV have been recognized: HIV-1 and HIV-2. HIV-1 is responsible for most HIV infections worldwide and is the causative agent of AIDS. HIV-2 is genetically similar to HIV-1 but is less pathogenic.[5] HIV likely evolved from a related virus, the simian immunodeficiency virus (SIV), which is believed to have crossed into the human population from chimpanzees in the second half of the 20th century.[6]

HIV infection encompasses a continuum of clinical and immunologic manifestations that range from asymptomatic infection to AIDS, a life-threatening condition characterized by profound immunologic dysfunction, opportunistic infections, and malignancies. Disease progression is highly variable. Some individuals progress to AIDS within a few years of infection; others remain relatively asymptomatic after 20 or more years of infection. Variability in disease progression has been shown to correlate with individual differences in efficiency of immune responses as well as genetic differences in the infecting viral subtype.[5]

Although antiretroviral drugs have dramatically prolonged the survival of HIV-infected people, current treatments are inadequate to completely eradicate the virus from an infected host, resulting in lifelong infection. Therefore, nurses for generations to come will be challenged to manage HIV infection and its associated morbidities.

Epidemiology of and Risk Behaviors for HIV and AIDS

Worldwide, of the estimated 35 million individuals who are HIV-positive, an estimated 19 million are not aware they have the virus.[1] HIV/AIDS is the world's leading cause of death among adults aged 15–59.[7] Sub-Saharan Africa is the worldwide epicenter of the HIV and AIDS epidemic, accounting for nearly 80% of all deaths related to AIDS or HIV-associated illnesses.[7]

In North America, an estimated 1.3 million people were living with HIV infection at the end of 2014, and 20,000 AIDS-related deaths were reported in that year.[8] Approximately 39,000 new infections were recorded in the United States in 2015.[9] The introduction of antiretroviral therapy medications in the mid-1990s has led to an increase in life expectancy among individuals who are HIV-positive as well as a significant decrease in AIDS-related deaths.[10] Still, HIV and AIDS pose serious health threats.

In the United States, African Americans account for a disproportionate number of new HIV cases. In 2014, African Americans, who make up only 12% of the American population, accounted for 44% of new HIV infections[9] (**Figure 15.2** ■).

HIV is transmitted through exchange of body fluids. It has been isolated from most bodily fluids, including blood, semen, cervicovaginal secretions, cerebrospinal fluid, saliva, tears, and breast milk.[11] However, HIV is not known to be transmitted by way of tears or saliva.[12] There are five requirements for HIV transmission from an infected host to an uninfected individual:

1. There must be an infected host.
2. There must be infectious viral particles in a body fluid.
3. There must be a bolus of infectious particles.
4. Infectious particles must encounter target cells in an uninfected individual.
5. Infected cells must escape clearance from the immune system.

The primary mode of transmission worldwide is through sexual contact. The most efficient sexual transmission modes are penile–anal intercourse and penile–vaginal intercourse. The presence of genital ulcers increases the risk of infection by providing a portal of viral entry as well as serving as a site for the congregation of target immune cells.[12] Viral transmission from infected females to their partners is less efficient than transmission from males, most likely owing to the lower concentration of infectious virus particles in cervicovaginal secretions than in seminal fluid.[13] The efficiency of sexual transmission is enhanced when plasma HIV titers are high; thus, antiretroviral therapy may reduce the risk of transmission to uninfected partners.[14]

Nonsexual transmission can occur via exchange of blood through transfusion of contaminated blood products, injection drug use, or occupational needlestick injuries. Since the introduction of nucleic acid testing of all donated blood products in the 1990s, the risk of transfusion-related infection has been reduced to 1 in 1–1.5 million units transfused.[15] The risk of needlestick transmission has been shown to be approximately 0.3%[14]; needlestick transmission is most likely to occur if the wound is deep, if there is visible blood on the instrument, and if the source person has a high viral titer. Postexposure prophylaxis should be instituted as quickly as possible if the source person is known to be HIV-positive.

Vertical, or mother to infant, transmission accounts for more than 300,000 new infections annually, mostly in developing countries. HIV can be transmitted to the infant prepartally via transplacental passage, intrapartally via exposure of the infant to maternal blood and vaginal secretions, and postpartally via ingestion of breast milk. Research conducted in 1994 suggested that antiretroviral therapy during pregnancy reduced the risk of vertical transmission from 25% to 8%.[14] Adherence to current recommendations—including administering antiretroviral medications to HIV-positive mothers during pregnancy, during delivery, and while breastfeeding—can reduce the risk of vertical transmission by 90%.[14]

Stassi Laramore: Application

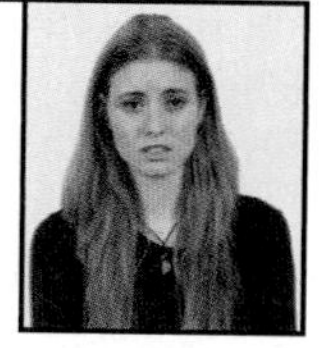

Ms. Laramore's pregnancy test is positive. Because of her stable CD4$^+$ T-lymphocyte count and barriers to following her prescribed medication regimen, Ms. Laramore hopes that she will not need to take antiretroviral medications during a pregnancy. She reports that she experiences severe nausea and diarrhea in response to the medications; her symptoms are sometimes so severe that she is unable to work. Along with the medication side effects,

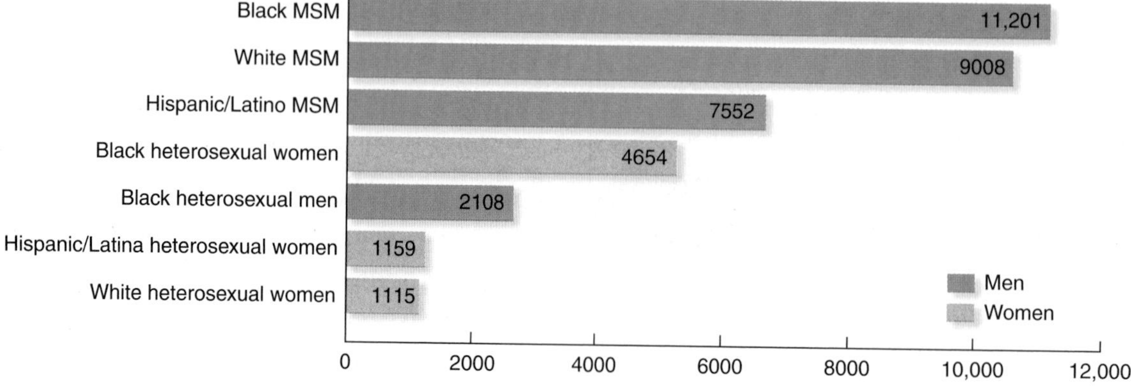

Figure 15.2 ■ Estimated new HIV diagnoses in the United States for the most-affected populations, 2014. MSM = men who have sex with men.

SOURCE: Based on CDC. (2016). *HIV in the United States: At a glance*. Retrieved from http://www.cdc.gov/hiv/statistics/overview/ataglance.html>

Ms. Laramore tells the nurse that she simply cannot afford to pay for the medications, especially if she is going to be challenged by the added expenses of raising a child.

3. Explain the process of vertical transmission of HIV from mother to infant that may occur with Ms. Laramore.
4. Through what possible routes might Ms. Laramore have contracted HIV?

Etiology and Pathogenesis of HIV Infection

HIV is a **retrovirus**, meaning that its genetic material is composed of RNA. HIV belongs to a family of retroviruses known as **lentiviruses**. Lentiviruses infect cells of the immune system and cause immunodeficiency. Because they escape immune clearance, lentiviruses cause persistent infections that are characterized by long incubation periods and delayed symptom onset.

HIV Structure

HIV is spherical and consists of an outer phospholipid envelope that contains two glycoproteins: gp41, which spans the envelope, and gp120, which is attached to gp41 and lies outside the envelope. The inner surface is lined with the p17 matrix protein, which stabilizes the virus. The center of the virus is a cone-shaped core that is composed of the p24 capsid protein. The core contains two strands of RNA and reverse transcriptase enzymes necessary for viral replication (**Figure 15.3** ■).

HIV Genes

The HIV genome contains approximately 10,000 nucleotides contained within nine genes. Three genes encode for structural and enzymatic proteins: *env*, *pol*, and *gag*. The *env* gene encodes for gp160, a large polyprotein precursor that is cleaved into gp41 and gp120. The *pol* gene encodes for three enzymes that mediate viral replication: reverse transcriptase, integrase, and protease. The *gag* gene encodes for a polyprotein that is cleaved into the matrix (p17) and capsid (p24) proteins. In addition to encoding for structural and enzymatic proteins, the HIV genome encodes several regulatory proteins, two of which are essential for viral replication: tat and rev.[16]

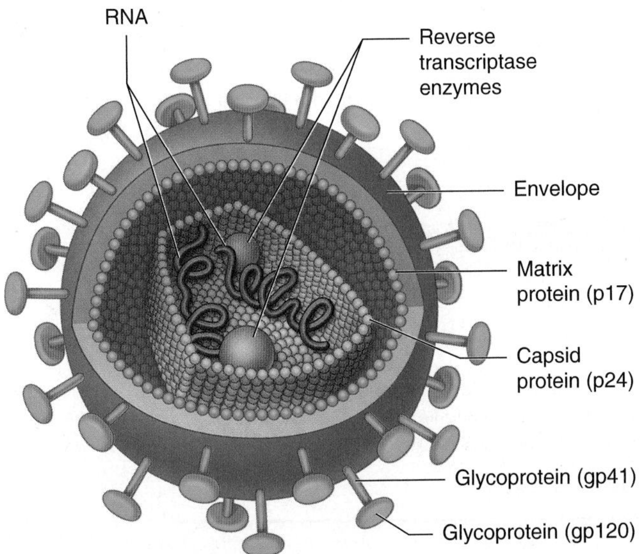

Figure 15.3 ■ Structure of HIV.

HIV-1 Subtypes

HIV-1 can be categorized into four phylogenetic groups: the M (major) group, the O (outlier) group, the N (non-M/non-O) group, and the P group. These groups likely represent four different introductions of SIV into the human population. Group M accounts for most HIV infections worldwide. Groups O, N, and P have been identified only in African countries. Within Group M, there are 11 subtypes, or clades, based on genetic similarities: A, B, C, D, E, F, G, H, I, J, and K. In North America and Europe, clade B predominates; in sub-Saharan Africa, clade C predominates. Individuals who are coinfected with two clades can develop recombinant viral subtypes called circulating recombinant forms. The genetic diversity of HIV has been a major limitation to developing a prophylactic vaccine that will be effective worldwide.[17]

HIV Tropism

HIV differs in its **tropism**, or ability to infect target cells. The major target cells of HIV are CD4-expressing T-helper lymphocytes and macrophages. While all HIV isolates are capable of infecting $CD4^+$ T lymphocytes, some additionally infect macrophages and are known as macrophage tropic strains (M tropic). Other viral isolates are capable of infecting only T lymphocytes and are known as T-cell tropic strains (T tropic). Although multiple viral isolates can be transmitted in a single exposure to infected body fluids, M tropic strains nearly always establish the initial infection.[18]

Classification of HIV Disease

The Centers for Disease Control and Prevention (CDC) system of classifying the severity of HIV infection is based on age-specific $CD4^+$ T-lymphocyte count or $CD4^+$ T-lymphocyte percentage of total lymphocytes (**Table 15.1** ■). Stages of HIV infection range from 0 to 3. Staging of HIV infection is based on the individual's $CD4^+$ T-lymphocyte count, which takes precedence over the CD4

Table 15.1 HIV Infection Stage Based on Age-specific $CD4^+$ T-lymphocyte Count or $CD4^+$ T-lymphocyte Percentage of Total Lymphocytes

	Age at Time of $CD4^+$ T-lymphocyte Test					
	< 1 Year		1–5 Years		≥ 6 Years	
Stage	Cells/μL	%	Cells/μL	%	Cells/μL	%
1	≥ 1500	≥ 34	≥1000	≥ 30	≥ 500	≥ 26
2	750–1499	26–33	500–999	22–29	200–499	14–25
3	< 750	< 26	< 500	< 22	< 200	< 14

SOURCE: Centers for Disease Control and Prevention. (2014). Revised surveillance case definition for HIV infection—United States, 2014 recommendations and reports. *Morbidity and Mortality Weekly Report (MMWR), 63*(RR03), 1–10. Available at http://www.cdc.gov/mmwr/preview/mmwrhtml/rr6303a1.htm?s_cid=rr6303a1_e

T-lymphocyte percentage. The CD4 T-lymphocyte percentage is considered only when the CD4$^+$ T-lymphocyte count is unavailable.[19]

In the CDC classifications of severity of HIV infection, criteria for stage 0 comprise sequential test results that are suggestive of early HIV infection; specifically, these criteria apply to situations in which an indeterminate or negative result is obtained within 180 days of a positive result. Criteria for stage 0 supersede and are considered independent of criteria used for stages 1, 2, and 3. Additional considerations related to CDC criteria for staging of HIV infection include the following:

- If the criteria for stage 0 are met, then the stage is 0 regardless of criteria for other stages (e.g., CD4$^+$ T-lymphocyte test results and presence of opportunistic illnesses).
- If the criteria for stage 0 are not met and a stage 3–defining opportunistic illness has been diagnosed, then the stage is 3 regardless of the CD4$^+$ T-lymphocyte count.
- If the criteria for stage 0 are not met and the criteria for other stages are unavailable, then the stage is classified as unknown.[19]

HIV Lifecycle

The HIV lifecycle is depicted in **Figure 15.4** ■.

HIV Receptors

HIV infects cells that express the **CD4 receptor** on their surface. The CD4 molecule is the receptor for the major histocompatibility complex class II molecule on antigen-presenting cells.[20] The interaction between CD4 and major

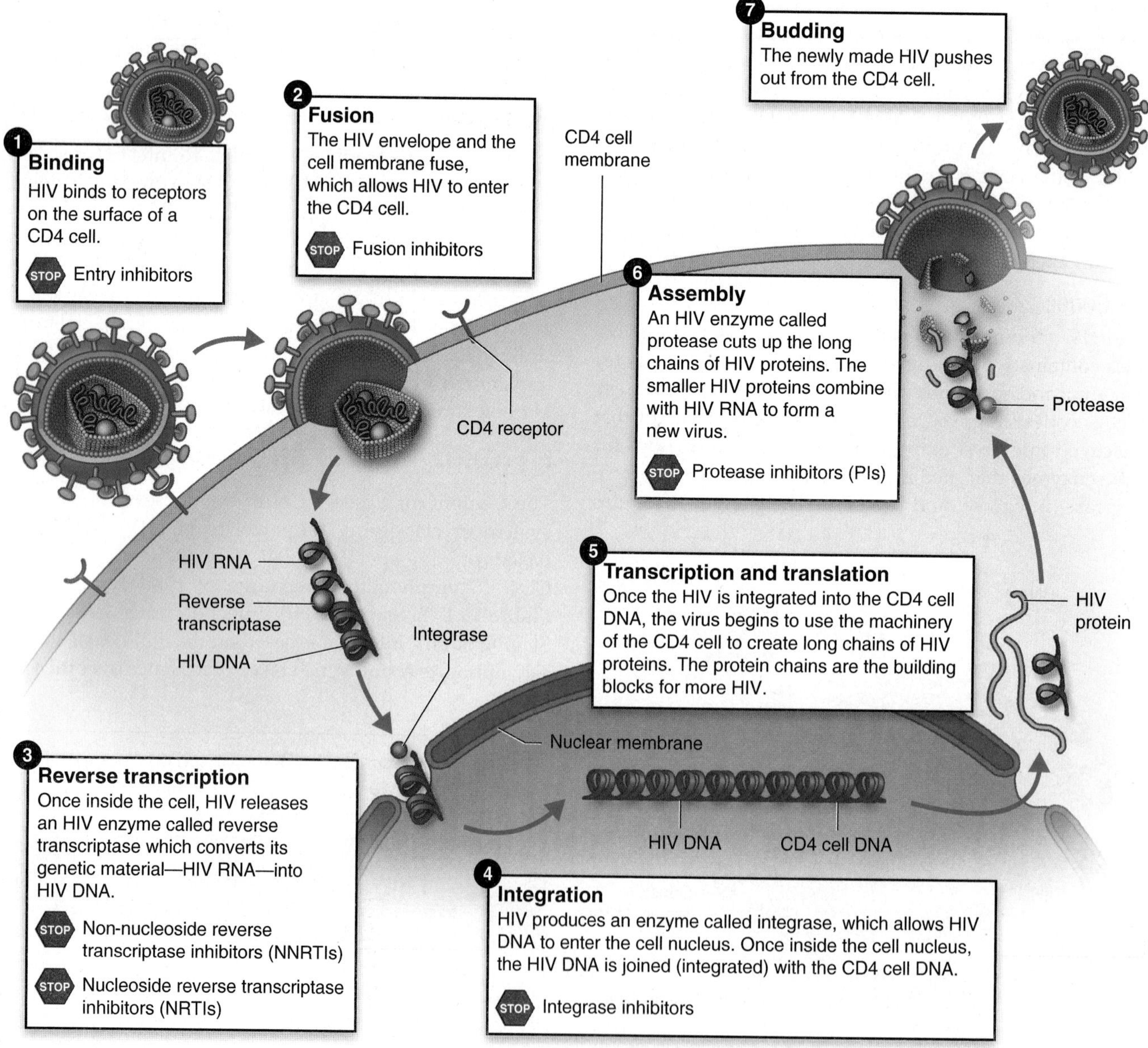

Figure 15.4 ■ The HIV lifecycle.

histocompatibility complex (MHC) class II molecules is necessary for T cells to recognize antigens. $CD4^+$ cells that are susceptible to HIV infection include the helper subset of T lymphocytes, monocytes/macrophages, dendritic, and brain microglial cells.[18]

HIV uses **chemokine receptors** as coreceptors to gain entry into target cells. Chemokine receptors are G-protein–coupled receptors whose activation mediates leukocyte extravasation and migration. Two chemokine receptors have been identified as coreceptors for HIV infection: CXCR4, which mediates infection by T tropic viral isolates, and CCR5, which mediates infection by M tropic viral isolates.[21] Approximately 20% of Caucasians fail to express the CCR5 receptor, owing to a 32-base-pair deletion in the encoding gene, and are thus resistant to infection with M tropic isolates.[18] Individuals who are **heterozygous** for this mutation (i.e., they have received one mutated copy and one normal copy from their parents) are susceptible to infection with M tropic isolates but show slower disease progression.[16,18]

Attachment, Fusion, and Entry

The gp120 envelope protein is responsible for viral attachment to target cells. Viral attachment involves two binding events. The first event is binding of gp120 to the CD4 molecule (**Figure 15.4**, event 1). This induces conformational changes in gp120 that permit the second event, binding to the chemokine coreceptor. It is believed that binding of the chemokine receptor triggers conformational changes that expose a gp41 region called the fusion peptide, which is then inserted into the host cell membrane. The gp41 protein then folds back on itself and pulls the viral envelope and host cell membranes together, resulting in fusion of the two membranes (**Figure 15.4**, event 2). Following fusion, the virus sheds its core protein coat and releases the core contents into the target cell cytoplasm.[16–18]

Reverse Transcription and Integration

Reverse transcriptase is a viral polymerase that generates two copies of DNA using the viral RNA as a template. DNA strand synthesis does not proceed from one end of the viral RNA template to the other. Instead, the DNA strand is partially transcribed at one end of the RNA template and then jumps to the other end of the template. It then continues its transcription in the opposite direction until a complete strand has been transcribed (**Figure 15.4**, event 3). Because the HIV-1 genome is approximately 10,000 nucleotides long, each replication cycle may produce up to 10 mutations per viral genome. As a result, there is great potential for genetic diversity among viral strains.[22]

The DNA copies are flanked at each end by structures called **long terminal repeats (LTRs)** that contain binding sites for viral proteins that regulate replication. The viral DNA and the enzyme **integrase** migrate to the cell nucleus through nuclear pores (**Figure 15.4**, event 4). Integrase covalently links the LTRs into the host DNA in a random fashion; the integrated viral DNA is known as the **provirus**. Viral genes are now part of the host's chromosomes and will replicate each time the infected cell replicates.[23]

Transcription, Translation, Assembly, and Budding

Proviral transcription occurs in activated cells (**Figure 15.4**, event 5). Quiescent cells are latently infected and do not transcribe provirus. Activation of an infected cell stimulates host cell RNA polymerase II to transcribe proviral genes into messenger RNAs (mRNAs). The early mRNA transcripts that are synthesized are too short to support replication of complete virus particles, but they do contain sequences that encode for the regulatory proteins tat and rev. Thus, tat and rev are the first viral proteins that are synthesized. Tat binds to the early short mRNA transcripts and promotes their elongation; rev mediates the transport of mRNAs from the nucleus to the cytoplasm.[23]

Once in the cytoplasm, the mRNAs are translated into polyprotein precursors at the ribosome. These polyproteins are gag, pol, and env, and they will serve as the structural and regulatory proteins that make up new viral particles. Some of the full-length RNA strands do not undergo translation and will be packaged into the core of new viral particles. The polyproteins accumulate at the host cell membrane and assemble into nascent viral particles (**Figure 15.4**, event 6). The particles bud from the host cell and acquire their lipid envelopes from the cell membrane (**Figure 15.4**, event 7). Once extruded into the environment, the viral protease cleaves the polyproteins into their functional forms, thus creating mature and infectious virions.[23]

Viral Replication Dynamics

HIV generally enters the body through mucosal surfaces, where it is trapped by **dendritic cells**. Dendritic cells are antigen-presenting cells located in the mucosal lining of tissues. Following viral trapping, dendritic cells travel to regional lymph nodes and infect resident $CD4^+$ T lymphocytes.[24] After the initial infection, there is a rapid rise in plasma viral load to levels that often exceed 1 million RNA copies/mL of blood.[25] Since the host has not yet mounted an effective HIV-specific immune response, the virus can rapidly disseminate to anatomic and cellular tissue reservoirs, including the brain, spleen, and peripheral lymph nodes.[26] During this period, there is a precipitous decline in $CD4^+$ T-lymphocyte numbers. After a few weeks, the host develops HIV-specific humoral and cell-mediated immune responses that induce reduction in plasma viremia and partial restoration of $CD4^+$ T-lymphocyte counts.[6] However, HIV-specific immune responses cannot be directed against provirus in quiescent memory cells, which constitute a major reservoir of latent virus. Thus, the virus can elude immune clearance, resulting in persistent infection (**Figure 15.5** ■).[26]

In untreated individuals, the viral load tends to stabilize approximately 6 months after infection. This stable viral load is known as the **viral set point**, and higher levels have been shown to correlate with rapid $CD4^+$ T-lymphocyte depletion and subsequent disease progression.[27] Research is inconclusive with regard to the long-term effects of early antiretroviral treatment on the viral set point. Some studies suggest that initiation of antiretroviral therapy during early HIV infection reduces the viral set point and thus may delay disease

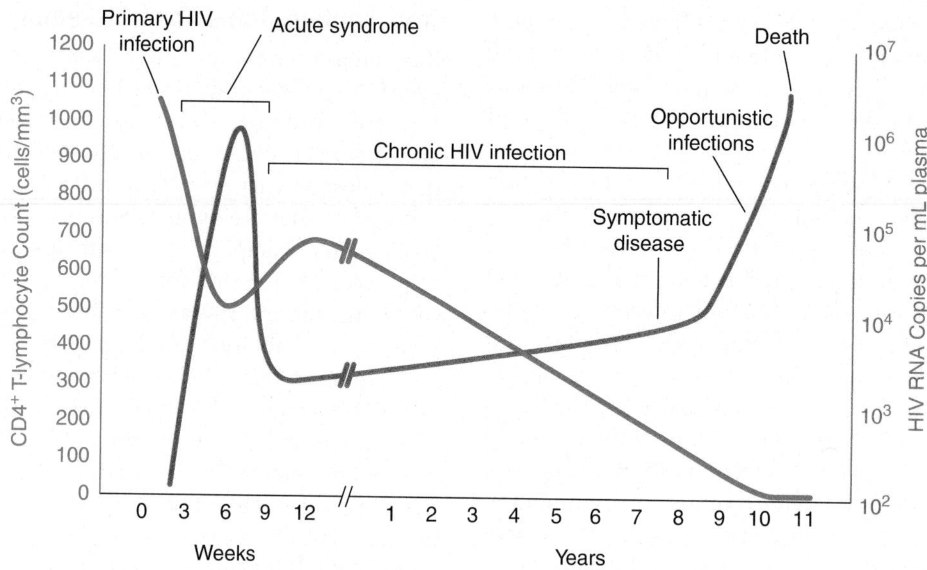

Figure 15.5 ■ Clinical time course of untreated HIV infection.

progression. However, other research studies have concluded that early treatment of HIV infection with antiretroviral therapy does not have long-term effects on the viral set point.[28]

Mechanisms of CD4$^+$ T-lymphocyte Depletion

The mechanisms underlying HIV-induced depletion of CD4$^+$ T lymphocytes have not been completely characterized. In vitro studies suggest that the mechanism of CD4$^+$ T-lymphocyte destruction during viral integration depends on the activation of DNA-dependent protein kinase, which is a primary factor involved in the DNA damage response.[29]

From a broad perspective, research suggests that the death of infected CD4$^+$ T lymphocytes is caused by one of three primary mechanisms:

- Pyroptosis,[30] which is a type of programmed cell death that is associated with inflammatory processes triggered by the presence of microorganisms
- Activation of an integrase-initiated DNA damage response in cells that have integrated the virus[31]
- Induction of apoptosis (programmed cell death) in cells that are productively infected and, as such, produce progeny virions.[32]

Emergence of Viral Resistance

HIV is characterized by rapid genetic evolution that diminishes the effectiveness of both host immune responses and antiretroviral medications. Several factors contribute to genetic mutations in the virus. A major factor is the absence of a proofreading mechanism in reverse transcriptase that can detect and correct misincorporated nucleotides. It is estimated that each progeny virus particle differs from the parent virus by at least one nucleotide. Because HIV contains only ~10,000 nucleotides and as many as 10 billion virus particles are produced daily in an untreated individual, the potential for the rapid emergence of viral heterogeneity is enormous.

Another factor is genetic recombination. Coinfecting viral strains can combine in vivo and produce heterogeneous viral species within a single individual. Inadequate adherence to HIV medication regimens is a major factor in the emergence of viral mutants. Current standards suggest that adherence to antiretroviral medication regimens must be maintained at a level of 90–95% to prevent plasma drug concentrations from dropping to suboptimal levels and subsequent breakthrough replication of drug-resistant mutants.[33]

Clinical Manifestations of HIV Infection

HIV infection may be primary, chronic, or advanced, AIDS being the most advanced form of HIV infection. The following sections provide an overview of the manifestations associated with each of these categories of HIV infection.

Primary HIV Infection

Primary HIV infection is a nonspecific, acute syndrome that occurs 2–4 weeks after viral infection and lasts for 1–2 weeks. It is estimated that 40–90% of HIV-infected individuals exhibit signs and symptoms of primary infection. The most common signs and symptoms are fever, fatigue, headache, lymphadenopathy, arthralgias, and a maculopapular rash that affects the face and trunk (**Figure 15.6** ■).[34,35]

Because an effective immune response has not yet been mounted, viral titers are typically very high, ranging from 10^5 to 10^6copies/mL.[18,35] During this period of high viremia, high concentrations of HIV are present in plasma and genital secretions; as a result, infected individuals are highly contagious.[34] Also during this viremic period, a transient decrease in CD4$^+$ T-lymphocyte count occurs.[18]

Within a few weeks, there is a marked clonal expansion of HIV-specific cytotoxic T lymphocytes, which corresponds with a dramatic decline in viral load and a rebound in CD4$^+$ T-lymphocyte counts, although they do not rise to preinfection levels.[18]

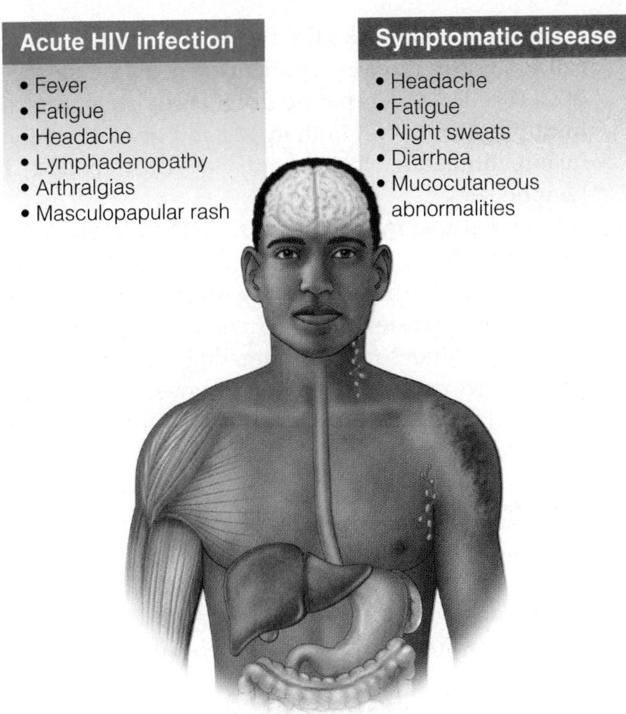

Figure 15.6 ■ Clinical manifestations of HIV infection in the primary and symptomatic phases of infection.

Seroconversion occurs when neutralizing antibodies appear, generally within a few weeks to a few months after infection. The period between infection and the appearance of neutralizing antibodies is called the **window period**. During this time, HIV testing will detect only HIV antibodies; therefore, individuals with early acute HIV infection may test falsely negative for the infection. To document seroconversion when acute HIV infection is suspected, the individual should undergo repeat serologic testing over the next 3–6 months.[35]

Chronic HIV Infection

After the acute infection subsides, most individuals show no clinical manifestations of HIV infection for several years, even in the absence of treatment. However, during this prolonged asymptomatic period, HIV actively replicates, and there is an intense reduction in the half-life of circulating $CD4^+$ T lymphocytes. The average duration of this asymptomatic period is 10 years, although there is considerable variability.[18]

Several host factors can influence the duration of the asymptomatic period. Older age is associated with accelerated progression to AIDS, while heterozygotes for the CCR5 32-base-pair deletion show delayed progression. Behavioral factors, such as smoking, poor nutrition, depression, and unprotected anal intercourse have been shown to correlate with more rapid progression to AIDS. Genetic variations in $CD8^+$ T lymphocytes, which are involved in the immune response to HIV, also are believed to affect the rate of progression from acute HIV infection to AIDS.[18]

Symptomatic Disease

HIV-related conditions develop as $CD4^+$ T-lymphocyte counts decline. Early conditions are generally non–life-threatening and include headache and fatigue. Over time, the conditions become more severe and include fever, night sweats, diarrhea, and mucocutaneous abnormalities.[18] The most advanced stage of HIV infection is AIDS. **Acquired immunodeficiency syndrome (AIDS)** is characterized by severe immunodeficiency (i.e., $CD4^+$ T-lymphocyte count < 200 cells/mm^3), opportunistic infections, and/or malignancies.[18,34] **Table 15.2** ■ lists laboratory tests that are commonly used to diagnose and treat and HIV and AIDS. Although AIDS was once a uniformly fatal disease, highly active antiretroviral therapy, which was introduced in late 1995, has dramatically improved survival rates.

Compared to adults and adolescents, infants and young children who are HIV-positive differ with regard to the diagnosis, clinical manifestations, and treatment of HIV infection. Adolescents, children, and infants for whom HIV infection is suspected or confirmed should be referred to primary care providers who are skilled in managing the care of pediatric patients who are HIV-positive.[34] ■

Table 15.2 Common Laboratory Tests for HIV/AIDS

Test and Purpose	Comments	Normal Range
HIV ELISA: To detect the presence of anti-HIV antibodies	Sensitivity and specificity rates > 98%; if reactive, results are confirmed with Western blot	Nonreactive
Western blot: To confirm seropositive HIV ELISA results	Positive Western blot shows presence of antibodies directed against either gp120/160 and gp41 or gp120/160 and p24.	Nonreactive
HIV RNA: To quantitate viral load in plasma	Used to diagnose primary HIV infection and to monitor response to antiretroviral therapy	Undetectable
Lymphocyte subset analyses: To stage disease and monitor disease progression	Characterized by high biological variability	800–1050 cells/mm^3
Phenotypic resistance analyses: To determine viral susceptibility to antiretroviral agents	Reverse transcriptase and protease genes from patient viral isolates are inserted into a laboratory viral clone, and replication at various drug concentrations is measured.	Not applicable
Genotypic resistance assay: To determine viral susceptibility to antiretroviral agents	Reverse transcriptase and protease genes from patient viral isolates are sequenced and compared with known resistance mutations.	Not applicable

Older adults are among the populations for whom diagnosis of HIV infection tends to be delayed. Many HIV-positive older adults develop AIDS-defining illnesses within 1 year of an initial diagnosis of HIV infection. To promote prompt recognition and treatment of HIV infection, essential measures to promote early identification and treatment of HIV infection include adherence to recommended screening protocols and education.[36] ■

Linking Pathophysiology to the Treatment of HIV Infection

Antiretroviral therapy (ART) is the cornerstone for the treatment of HIV infection. Typically, treatment of HIV combines a minimum of three medications that diminish viral replication. Use of a combination of antiretroviral drugs, which is sometimes referred to as **highly active antiretroviral therapy (HAART)**, helps to decrease viral resistance to the medications. The following sections summarize the pharmacologic effects of current classifications of ART medications and provide an overview of approaches to pharmacotherapy.

Pharmacologic Agents

In most cases, treatment of individuals who are infected with HIV involves a combination of three ART medications from at least two different pharmacologic classes. To date, there are six classes of antiretroviral medications that can be combined in HAART regimens.[37] Collectively, these drugs target three different stages in the HIV lifecycle.

- ***Nucleoside reverse transcriptase inhibitors (NRTIs)*** were the first class of antiretroviral medications approved for use in the United States. After undergoing intracellular phosphorylation, NRTIs are structural analog of the cellular nucleotides that compose the DNA strands copied from viral RNA. They compete with cellular nucleotides for reverse transcriptase–mediated incorporation into growing DNA chains. By blocking reverse transcriptase, NRTIs inhibit HIV replication.[37]
- ***Nonnucleoside reverse transcriptase inhibitors (NNRTIs)*** bind to reverse transcriptase and later cause a conformational change in the enzyme that inhibits its activity. As a result, HIV replication is inhibited.[37]
- ***Protease inhibitors*** act at a late stage in the viral lifecycle. They bind to the active site of HIV protease and block the proteolytic cleavage of viral polyproteins that occurs immediately after budding. The resulting viral particles are immature and incapable of infecting new cells. Protease inhibitors are among the most potent inhibitors of HIV replication.[18]
- ***Entry inhibitors*** (also known as fusion inhibitors) include chemokine coreceptor (CCR5) antagonists. These medications inhibit HIV's ability to enter the cell through binding to or blocking proteins involved in the process. Because binding to CCR5 is necessary for HIV's entry into the target cell, CCR5 antagonists can block HIV from invading the target cell by binding to a receptor present on the surface of CD4 cells.[37,38] A separate drug, enfuvirtide, acts at multiple sites within both gp120 and gp41 to inhibit fusion, ultimately blocking entry of HIV into $CD4^+$ T lymphocytes.[17]
- ***Integrase strand transfer inhibitors (INSTIs)*** block the enzyme integrase, which is necessary for HIV to accomplish viral replication. Following reverse transcription, viral strand transfer of HIV occurs. A major effect of INSTI medications involves targeting the strand transfer reaction and, by blocking integrase, preventing the insertion of HIV's DNA into the DNA of $CD4^+$ T lymphocytes.[18]

Approaches to Pharmacotherapy

Current treatment guidelines recommend offering HAART to all individuals who are infected with HIV.[36] For patients with early-stage HIV infection, primary treatment goals include suppression of plasma HIV RNA to undetectable levels.

To guide the choice of medications, treatment of individuals who have early-stage HIV infection should be preceded by genotypic antiviral resistance testing.[39] Exposure to HAART medications may yield HIV mutations and subsequent development of drug-resistant strains of HIV, rendering previously effective HIV medications ineffective.[40,41] Transmission of drug-resistant forms of HIV, or **transmitted drug resistance (TDR)**, has emerged as a significant public health threat. TDR may be more prevalent among individuals with acute HIV infection than among those with chronic HIV infection.[41]

For cases in which genotypic antiviral drug resistance testing is unavailable, HAART still may be initiated. Resistance to ritonavir (RTV)-boosted protease inhibitors typically develops slowly, and NRTIs are not prone to clinically significant TDR. As such, a combination of RTV-boosted PIs and NRTIs is recommended for individuals who do not undergo genotypic antiviral drug resistance testing.[35]

Interruption of antiretroviral therapy typically is not recommended, as cessation of treatment may result in viral rebound, leading to even more pronounced immunosuppression and worsening of the individual's overall health status.[39] Despite these risks, certain circumstances may necessitate interruption of the HAART regimen, such as cases of severe medication toxicity. Illnesses that interfere with oral intake of food or GI absorption (such as gastroenteritis or pancreatitis) also may result in temporary cessation of HAART, as certain antiretroviral medications must be taken with food.[39]

Although HAART is indicated for all individuals with HIV,[36] early treatment is associated with both positive and negative effects. The potential benefits for early therapy include preservation of immune function, prolongation of clinical latency, and a possible reduced risk of transmission. Potential risks of early therapy include drug toxicities, possible development of drug-resistant mutants that will limit treatment options in symptomatic disease, and the risk of transmitting drug-resistant mutants to uninfected individuals, thus limiting their treatment options.[35]

4 Because HIV antibody is transferred from mother to fetus by way of the placenta, positive serum tests for HIV antibodies are anticipated in all infants who are born to HIV-positive mothers, whether or not the infant is actually infected. For infants who are younger than 18 months, a conclusive diagnosis of HIV infection usually includes HIV nucleic acid testing.[34] ■

DeShawn Ruffin: Application

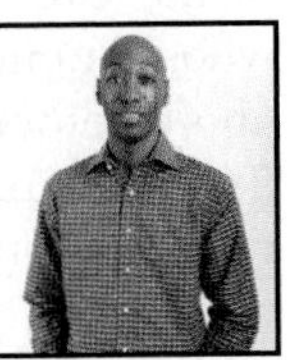

Mr. Ruffin's HIV is being managed on a combination drug regimen that includes two NRTIs and one PI. His viral load is currently 50,000 copies/mL; 3 months ago, his viral load was undetectable. His CD4$^+$ T-lymphocyte count is 526 cells/mm^3, down from 680 cells/mm^3 3 months ago. Although he has been following his HAART regimen, he has experienced multiple complications, including several opportunistic infections. In light of his medical history, Mr. Ruffin is especially concerned about his shortness of breath and hemoptysis.

3. What is the mechanism of action of the NRTI drugs that Mr. Ruffin is taking for his HIV?
4. What is the rationale for the use of combined drug therapy in the treatment of HIV?

Stassi Laramore: Outcome

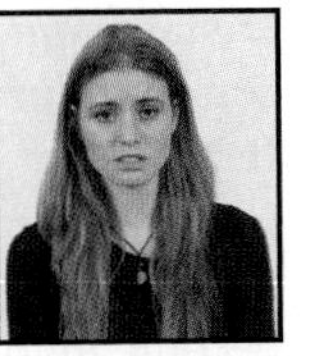

Ms. Laramore's primary care provider counsels her about the risks of vertical transmission of HIV and explains the benefits of following a HAART regimen during pregnancy, including a potential 90% reduction in the risk of vertical transmission. The primary care provider also explains to Ms. Laramore that her infant likely will require prophylactic treatment for prevention of HIV. After considering the benefits of HAART, Ms. Laramore verbally consents to adhere to the medication regimen. The primary care provider refers Ms. Laramore to a social services agency to develop a plan for financial assistance with paying for the medications.

5. How is a diagnosis of HIV infection made in infants born to HIV-positive mothers?
6. Explain why strict adherence to the HAART regimen is so important for Ms. Laramore.

Check Your Progress: Section 15.2

1. What are the five requirements for HIV transmission?
2. Describe the signs and symptoms of primary HIV infection.
3. Why is the HIV-infected person highly contagious in the 2- to 4-week period following viral infection?

15.3 Common Conditions Associated with HIV/AIDS

Conditions that are commonly associated with HIV infection and AIDS include opportunistic infections, certain malignancies, and neuropathic disorders. Selected examples of each condition are described in the following sections.

Opportunistic Infections

An **opportunistic infection (OI)** is an infection that occurs with increased frequency or greater severity as a result of the host's weakened or compromised immune response. In a healthy individual whose immune response is intact, the causative organisms of OIs—which include bacteria, viruses, fungi, and protozoa—usually do not cause illness. Among individuals who are infected with HIV, commonly occurring OIs include cytomegalovirus diseases and tuberculosis.

Cytomegalovirus Diseases

Cytomegalovirus (CMV) is a double-stranded DNA virus that is carried by 60% of the U.S. population. It can be found in blood, saliva, semen, cervical secretions, and urine. Normally, the immune system inhibits CMV replication. However, in individuals with severe immunosuppression (typically when the CD4$^+$ T-lymphocyte count drops below 50 cells/mm^3), active viral replication can occur with dissemination to target tissues such as the retina, gut, lungs, and the central nervous system. CMV retinitis is the most common CMV infection, accounting for 80–90% of all CMV infections among AIDS patients.

Valganciclovir, a guanine nucleoside analog, is the treatment of choice for CMV infections. It terminates viral DNA elongation; thus, its mechanism of action is similar to that of NRTIs. The optimal duration of maintenance therapy with valganciclovir has not yet been established.[42]

Tuberculosis

Tuberculosis (TB) is an acid-fast bacillus that is transmitted through aerosolized droplets. Upon inhalation, the bacilli are transported to the pulmonary alveoli, where they are ingested and walled off in granulomas by alveolar macrophages. A **granuloma** is a mass of fused macrophages that sequester persistent infectious agents and prevent their activation and dissemination. While HIV infection does not confer increased risk for acquiring TB infection, it does increase the risk of activation of latent disease and subsequent dissemination. Among individuals who are infected with HIV, TB is the leading cause of death[43]; therefore, all HIV-infected individuals should undergo annual tuberculin testing.

The sputum of individuals with active TB infection will contain dead *M. tuberculosis*. In individuals whose immune systems are compromised, including those with HIV, sputum testing for TB may yield a false negative result, owing to the weakened immune system's inability to destroy the bacteria.

First-line drugs of choice for TB include isoniazid and a rifamycin in combination with pyrazinamide and ethambutol. Second-line drugs used in the treatment of TB include fluoroquinolones and aminoglycosides.[44] However, emerging strains of this pathogen include multidrug-resistant TB, which is resistant to first-line medications, including isoniazid and rifamycin. Extensively drug-resistant TB demonstrates resistance to both first- and second-line drugs of choice.[42] Treatment of extensively drug-resistant TB includes administration of bedaquiline fumarate, though this medication is not universally recommended, owing to serious adverse effects.[45]

DeShawn Ruffin: Outcome

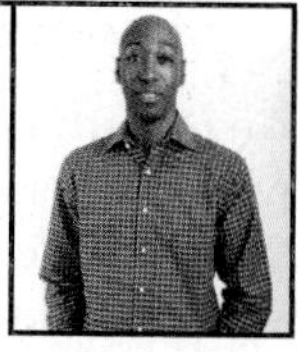

Mr. Ruffin's physician orders a sputum culture and sensitivity, as well as a chest x-ray. Although the sputum smear is negative for *M. tuberculosis*, the blood sample and chest x-ray are both positive for the disease. Sensitivity testing suggests that the form of *M. tuberculosis* that is causing Mr. Ruffin's infection is not a multi-drug-resistant strain. He is treated with a combination of isoniazid, rifamycin, pyrazinamide, and ethambutol for 2 months, immediately followed by a 4-month course of isoniazid and rifamycin. He recovers successfully, but several of his family members who tested positive for latent TB require treatment as well.

5. Why might Mr. Ruffin's sputum be negative for *M. tuberculosis* despite his chest x-ray and blood cultures being positive for the disease?
6. Explain why Mr. Ruffin is at increased risk for opportunistic infections.

Malignancies

Malignancies associated with HIV infection and AIDS include Kaposi sarcoma and certain forms of lymphoma.

Kaposi Sarcoma

Kaposi sarcoma (KS) is the most common AIDS-associated malignancy (**Figure 15.7** ■). The etiologic agent, human herpesvirus 8, has been isolated in all forms of KS. The cell of origin is unknown, although mesenchymal cells, smooth muscle cells, and fibroblasts may be the sites of tumor initiation. While tumors generally manifest in the skin, they can also develop in the oral cavity, gut, lymph nodes, brain, and visceral organs. Histologically, all forms of KS are characterized by interwoven bands of spindle cells and vascular structures contained within a network of collagen and reticular fibers. Dermatologic lesions can present as localized or disseminated plaques and/or nodules that are brown, red, or purple. The clinical course of disease is highly variable, and HAART-induced immunoreconstitution has been associated with regression of lesions. Therapies may include involve intralesional injections of vinblastine or, for widespread disease, radiation therapy and systemic treatment with cytotoxic agents.[46]

AIDS-Related Lymphoma

AIDS-related lymphoma is a heterogeneous collection of B-cell malignancies that occur in extranodal sites, including the central nervous system, GI tract, and liver. AIDS-related lymphoma may also manifest as primary effusions in the pleural, pericardial, and peritoneal cavities. CNS lymphomas typically manifest when the $CD4^+$ T-lymphocyte count is less than 50 cells/mm^3. Systemic lymphomas can occur in individuals with higher counts.

The etiologic agent of AIDS-related lymphoma is Epstein-Barr virus (EBV), also known as human herpesvirus 4, which is carried by approximately 90–95% of adults in the United States.[47] Immunocompetent individuals, whose immune systems can control EBV replication, show no symptoms of infection. However, the T-cell dysfunctions that are characteristic of HIV infection lead to uncontrolled EBV replication and dysregulated B-cell proliferative responses. The expanded pool of B cells can become infected with EBV and undergo genetic transformations that culminate in malignancy.[48] Treatment involves chemotherapy in combination with HAART.

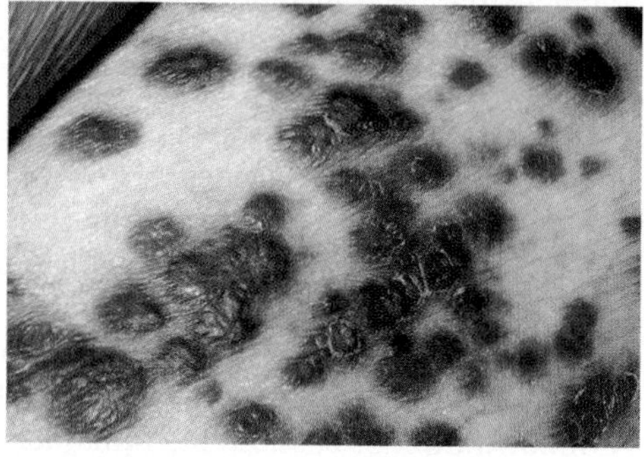

Figure 15.7 ■ Kaposi sarcoma lesions on an individual with AIDS.

Other Conditions

HIV is associated with numerous neurologic and metabolic alterations, including distal symmetric polyneuropathy, and HIV-associated lipodystrophy syndrome.

Distal Symmetric Polyneuropathy

Distal symmetric polyneuropathy (DSP) is one of the most common forms of HIV-associated peripheral neuropathy. It has been shown to affect up to 50% of HIV-infected persons.[49] It is a sensory axonal neuropathy that involves the toes and soles of the feet; the fingers and hands may become involved over time. The most common manifestations of DSP involve absent or diminished ankle jerks and diminished vibration and pinprick sensations in the distal lower extremities.[49] Patients also may present with aching, stabbing, burning, or tingling sensations in the affected regions. Although DSP typically affects only the lower extremities at first, disease progression may lead to the involvement of the upper extremities as well.[49]

Distal symmetric polyneuropathy can be a direct sequela of HIV infection, or it can result from treatment with neurotoxic drugs. The pathogenesis likely involves the elaboration of pro-inflammatory and neurotoxic factors, such as tumor necrosis factor alpha, by activated immune cells in peripheral nerves. Nerve biopsy generally reveals axonal degeneration of myelinated and unmyelinated fibers.

Neuropathic pain is poorly responsive to opioids or nonsteroidal anti-inflammatory drugs. Adjuvant agents have been shown to provide partial relief and are the treatment of choice. They include antidepressants, anticonvulsants, and corticosteroids.[49]

HIV-Related Lipodystrophy Syndrome

HIV-associated lipodystrophy syndrome (HALS) refers to a collection of morphologic and metabolic abnormalities that include insulin resistance, glucose intolerance, dyslipidemia, and fat redistribution (i.e., truncal obesity and peripheral wasting). The prevalence of HALS has been difficult to estimate, owing to the lack of a consensus definition, although approximately 50% of HIV-infected people exhibit at least one of these abnormalities.

The etiology of HALS is not fully understood. Dyslipidemia and fat redistribution had been described in the pre-HAART era, but the incidence of metabolic conditions dramatically increased with the introduction of the protease inhibitors. Because HALS likely represents several metabolic disturbances that can occur independently, several pathogenetic mechanisms have been postulated. Etiologic factors that are recognized as being central to the development of HALS include HAART-induced adipocyte inflammation, oxidative stress, macrophage infiltration, mitochondrial toxicity, and impaired adipocyte function.[50]

Check Your Progress: Section 15.3

1. What role do T lymphocytes play in the development of AIDS-related lymphoma?
2. What is the mechanism for the development of CMV disease in patients with immunosuppression?
3. How does distal symmetric polyneuropathy develop in people with HIV?

15.4 Primary Immunodeficiencies

Primary immunodeficiencies (PIs) represent a heterogeneous group of genetic disorders affecting all components of immune system function, including phagocytic and complement activity as well as B-lymphocyte, T-lymphocyte, and natural killer (NK) cell function (**Figure 15.8** ■). Antibody deficiencies predominate. The characteristic result of PI is an increased susceptibility to infection.

Because of their hereditary nature, the majority of PIs present at birth or during early childhood; however, some forms of PI are not diagnosed for many years unless they are life-threatening. Currently, more than 250 primary immunodeficiency disorders have been documented.[2] In spite of the large number of PIs that have been identified in the clinical literature, these disorders appear to be rare within the general population, affecting approximately 500,000 individuals in the United States.[51]

CLINICAL POINT: The Jeffrey Modell Foundation and the American Red Cross have identified 10 warning signs of PI in an attempt to assist individuals, families, and healthcare providers with early detection.[52] If an individual has two or more of the following, a diagnosis of PI should be considered:

1. Four or more new ear infections within 1 year
2. Two or more serious sinus infections within 1 year
3. Two or more months on antibiotics with little effect
4. Two or more pneumonias within 1 year
5. Failure of an infant to gain weight or grow normally
6. Recurrent deep skin or organ abscesses
7. Persistent thrush or fungal infection on skin
8. Need for intravenous antibiotics to clear infection
9. Two or more deep-seated infections including septicemia
10. A family history of PI. ■

Overall, the most common manifestations of PI are recurrent, severe, and/or persistent/unresponsive bacterial and viral infections involving both common and opportunistic pathogens or infections with unexpected or severe complications.[3] These infections most often occur in the sinuses, middle ear, bronchi, lungs, and GI tract. In addition, because of the role of the immune system in the maintenance of tolerance to self-antigens and surveillance

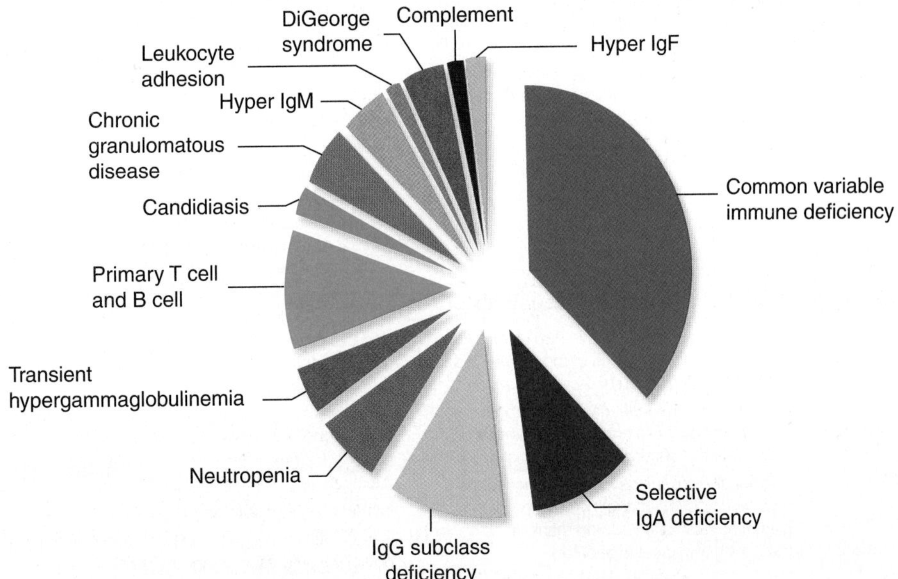

Figure 15.8 ■ Relative distribution of the primary immunodeficiencies.

for cancerous cells, individuals with PI are also susceptible to a variety of autoimmune or inflammatory diseases and malignancies.

In children with PI, alterations in growth and development may represent the first manifestation of acute complications. Infants and young children should be assessed every 3 months; wellness visits may be alternated with immunologist appointments. For school-age children and adolescents, assessment is recommended every 6 months.[3] ■

Table 15.3 ■ summarizes five selected primary immunodeficiencies: two common B-cell immunodeficiencies, selective IgA deficiency and IgG subclass deficiency; one T-cell immunodeficiency, DiGeorge syndrome/anomaly; and two combined B-cell and T-cell immunodeficiencies, common variable immunodeficiency (CVID) and severe combined T-cell and B-cell immunodeficiency (SCID). More detailed and comprehensive information about primary immunodeficiencies can be found in the Recommended Readings and Recommended Websites sections at the end of this chapter.

Check Your Progress: Section 15.4

1. What are the most common manifestations of primary immunodeficiencies?
2. Identify the warning signs of primary immunodeficiency as identified by the Jeffrey Modell Foundation and the American Red Cross.
3. What are the early manifestations of severe combined immunodeficiency (also known as "bubble boy" disease)?

Table 15.3 Selected Primary Immunodeficiency Disorders

Definition/Etiology	Pathophysiologic Mechanism	Clinical Manifestations	Treatment
Primary B-cell Deficiency: Selective IgA Deficiency			
Most common antibody deficiency, with incidence of 1 in 400–3000 Defined as a serum IgA concentration of less than 7 mg/dL with normal IgM and IgG levels in individuals older than 4 years of age The mode of inheritance varies and may be autosomal recessive, autosomal dominant, or multifactorial Occurs in both males and females and shows a familial pattern	Selective IgA deficiency results from a failure of B cells carrying IgA to mature and differentiate into plasma cells capable of secreting IgA Pathophysiologic mechanism is essentially unknown, but a number of possibilities have been proposed, including intrinsic B-cell defects, maternal anti-IgA antibodies, impaired antibody switching, T-cell suppression of IgA, and/or insufficient T-helper cell function	Often asymptomatic and undiagnosed Up to $\frac{1}{3}$ of affected individuals demonstrate recurrent upper respiratory infections (e.g., sinusitis, otitis media), bronchial asthma, and GI infections (mucosal surfaces unprotected by IgA) Increased prevalence with chronic lung disease Associated autoimmune diseases (e.g., rheumatoid arthritis, lupus erythematosus, idiopathic thrombocytopenia purpura, Crohn disease, ulcerative colitis) Strong association with allergy (e.g., bronchial asthma and food allergies)	Prophylactic and/or episodic antibiotics Cautious use (some individuals may have anti-IgA antibodies) immunoglobulin therapy (IVIG)
Primary B-cell Deficiency: IgG Subclass Deficiency			
Incidence and prevalence not well established Defined as an abnormally low level of one or more of three of four IgG subclasses (IgG2, IgG3, IgG4); diagnostic level defined as 2 or more standard deviations below the age-adjusted mean in individuals with normal or near normal levels of IgG and IgM 15–20% may also have IgA deficiency	The underlying pathophysiologic mechanism(s) underlying deficiencies poorly understood; genetic deletions, transcriptional, posttranscriptional, and/or translational defects may be involved Each type of subclass deficiency leaves a person vulnerable to specific types of infections	Majority of cases are asymptomatic and often undiagnosed Most common manifestations include recurrent upper respiratory infections (e.g., sinusitis, otitis media, mastoiditis), bronchial asthma, bronchiectasis, and pneumonia caused by encapsulated organisms; IgG2 and IgG4 deficiencies most often associated with recurrent pulmonary infections May manifest as environmental allergies Associated with other primary and secondary immunodeficiencies, such as ataxia-telangiectasia, Wiskott-Aldrich syndrome, HIV/AIDS, and after bone marrow transplantation	Prophylactic and/or episodic antibiotics Cautious use of IVIG for individuals more seriously ill and/or not responsive to antimicrobial therapy
Primary T-cell Deficiency: DiGeorge Syndrome/Anomaly with or Without 22q11.2 Deletion			
Variable T-cell deficiency caused by defective embryologic development of the third and fourth pharyngeal pouches; leads to hypoplasia or aplasia of the thymus and parathyroid glands; incidence of 1 in 4000 with deletion Cases based on environmental exposures (e.g., fetal alcohol syndrome) have also been identified Occurs in both males and females but rarely familial Most individuals demonstrate mild to moderate T-cell deficit; severe T-cell deficit in ~0.3%	Chromosomal deletion within 22q11, producing absence of hypoplasia of the thymus gland, resulting in interruption of T-cell maturation. Cell-mediated immune responses are absent or diminished. B-cell numbers are normal or increased, but antibody production is subnormal. Additionally, organs developing at the same embryonic period as the thymus and parathyroid glands are also affected and manifest as abnormal palate and cardiac anomaly	Wide variation in organ involvement exists related to the amount of genetic material lost Prolonged viral infections and secondary bacterial infections are common; the presence of abnormal palate anatomy (occurring in about $\frac{1}{3}$) increases the risk of upper respiratory infections (e.g., sinusitis, otitis media) Increased risk of autoimmune disease. Cardiac defects (e.g., truncus arteriosus, tetralogy of Fallot) present in about 75–90%. Hypocalcemic tetany is present in ~50–60% and most often manifests within 24–48 hours after birth	Stem cell transplantation Transplantation of mature thymic epithelial tissue

Definition/Etiology	Pathophysiologic Mechanism	Clinical Manifestations	Treatment
Primary T-cell Deficiency: Primary T-cell and B-cell Immunodeficiency			
Mixed group of disorders primarily involving B-cell dysfunction with incidence of ~1/25,000–1/100,000 in primarily Caucasian individuals of European ancestry Defined as the presence of markedly decreased serum Ig levels with significant depression of IgM and IgA Polygenic causation suspected Can occur at any age, but average age at onset is 25–30 years of age	Blocked B-cell maturation and differentiation; B-cell count usually normal, but cells fail to mature into antibody-secreting plasma cells May involve an intrinsic B-cell defect, increased numbers of CD8 suppressor T-cell activity, decreased CD4 helper T-cells function, decreased ratio of CD4/CD8 T-cells, and/or inadequate/dysfunctional B-cell/T-cell interaction	Hypogammaglobulinemia Recurrent bacterial pneumonia; also recurrent upper respiratory infections (e.g., sinusitis, otitis media), bronchial asthma, and bronchiectasis ~50% manifest GI malabsorption, chronic diarrhea, and/or weight loss Hypertrophy of lymphoid tissues is a frequent feature Unique feature, in terms of development of noncaseating granulomas in liver, spleen, lymph nodes, lung, and skin	IVIG Prophylactic and/or episodic antibiotics Cautious use of corticosteroid therapy for autoimmune or granulomatous complications
Severe Combined Immunodeficiency (SCID): "Bubble Boy" Disease			
The most severe form of primary immunodeficiency A mixed group of rare, and potentially fatal, genetic disorders; overall incidence of 1/50,000–100,000 live births Phenotype varies with underlying pathophysiologic mechanism Defined as profound deficiencies of T- and B-cell and sometimes natural killer cell function Diverse genetic origins, either inherited or de novo mutations	There are two major forms of SCID: 1. **X-linked SCID (SCID-X1)** accounts for ~44–60% of cases SCID. Absence of mature T and NK lymphocytes; B cells increased (but poorly functional) Mutation of IL-2 receptor gene that encodes for a common gamma-chain receptor shared by several cytokine receptors, resulting in faulty intracellular signal transduction 2. **Autosomal recessive SCID** can be caused by a number of genetic abnormalities: Deficiency of gene responsible for adenosine deaminase, resulting in accumulation of metabolites that directly or indirectly lead to apoptosis of thymocytes and circulating lymphocytes Deficiency of the major signal transducer for common gamma-chain receptor shared by several cytokine receptors, leading to absence of mature T and NK lymphocytes; B-cell numbers normal or increased but not fully functional Deficiency of Artemis gene product (Athabascan SCID); mapped to chromosome 10; absence results in inability to repair DNA.	In first few months of life, recurrent, severe, and/or persistent episodes of diarrhea, pneumonia, otitis media, sepsis, and skin infections caused by a variety of common and opportunistic bacteria and viruses; usually disseminated and often fatal; accompanied by failure to thrive At risk for graft-versus-host disease from maternal T lymphocytes crossing placenta or from nonirradiated blood products or allogenic bone marrow Severe lymphopenia; immunoglobulin levels diminished to absent Small, often undetectable, thymus; thymus-dependent parts of spleen depleted of lymphocytes, while lymph nodes, tonsils, and adenoids are absent or extremely underdeveloped	Death occurs before first or at the latest second birthday if the patient does not undergo allogenic bone marrow or stem cell transplantation Gene therapy for SCID due to gamma-chain deficiency or adenosine deaminase deficiency IVIG therapy Prophylactic and/or episodic antibiotics

SOURCES: Data from Ballow, M. (2002). Primary immunodeficiency disorders: Antibody deficiency. *Journal of Allergy and Clinical Immunology, 109*, 581–591. Bayry, J., Hermine, O., Webster, D. A., Levy, Y., & Kaveri, S. V. (2005). Common variable immunodeficiency: The immune system in chaos. *Trends in Molecular Medicine, 11*, 370–376. Bonilla, F. A., Bernstein, I. L., Khan, D. A., et al. (2005). Practice parameter for the diagnosis and management of primary immunodeficiency. *Annals of Allergy, Asthma, & Immunology, 94*, S1–S63. Buckley, R. H. (2002). Primary cellular immunodeficiencies. *Journal of Allergy and Clinical Immunology*, 109, 747–757. Chapel, H., Geha, R., & Rosen, F. (2003). Primary immunodeficiency diseases: An update. *Clinical and Experimental Immunology, 132*, 9–15. Cooper, M. A., Pommering, T. L., & Koranyi, K. (2003). Primary immunodeficiencies. *American Family Physician, 68*, 2001–2008, 2011. Cunningham-Rundles, C. (2006). Selective IgA deficiency. In E. R. Stiehm, H. D. Ochs, & J. A. Winkelstein (Eds.), *Immunologic disorders in infants and children* (5th ed., pp. 427–446). Philadelphia, PA: Elsevier Saunders. Fischer, A. (2000). Severe combined immunodeficiencies (SCID). *Clinical and Experimental Immunology, 122*, 143–149. Fischer, A., & Notarangelo, L. D. (2006). Combined immunodeficiencies. In E. R. Stiehm, H. D. Ochs, & J. A. Winkelstein (Eds.), *Immunologic disorders in infants and children* (5th ed., pp. 289–355). Philadelphia, PA: Elsevier Saunders. Gennery, A. R., & Cant, A. J. (2001). Diagnosis of severe combined immunodeficiency. *Journal of Clinical Pathology, 54*, 191–195. Hammerstrom, L., Vorechovsky, I., & Webster, D. (2000). Selective IgA deficiency (SIgAD) and common variable immunodeficiency (CVID). *Clinical and Experimental Immunology, 120*, 225–231. Notarangelo, L., Casanova, J. L., Fischer, A., et al. (2004). Primary immunodeficiency diseases: An update. *Journal of Allergy and Clinical Immunology, 114*, 677–687. Ochs, H. D., Stiehm, E. R., & Winkelstein, J. A. (2006). Antibody deficiencies. In E. R. Stiehm, H. D. Ochs, & J. A. Winkelstein (Eds.), *Immunologic disorders in infants and children* (5th ed., pp. 356–426). Philadelphia, PA: Elsevier Saunders. O'Shea, J. J., Husa, M., Li, D., et al. (2004). Jak3 and the pathogenesis of severe combined immunodeficiency. *Molecular Immunology, 41*, 727–737. Riminton, D. S., & Limaye, S. (2004). Primary immunodeficiency diseases in adulthood. *Internal Medicine Journal, 34*, 348–354. Sneller, M. C. (2001). Common variable immunodeficiency. *Southern Society for Clinical Investigation, 321*, 42–48. Stiehm, E. R., Ochs, H. D., & Winkelstein, J. A. (2006). Immunodeficiency disorders: General considerations. In E.R. Stiehm, H. D. Ochs, & J. A. Winkelstein (Eds.), *Immunologic disorders in infants and children* (5th ed., pp. 289–355). Philadelphia, PA: Elsevier Saunders.

CHAPTER SUMMARY

15.1 Chapter Overview and Case Studies

Describe the types of immunodeficiency disorders and concepts related to immunodeficiency.

- Immunodeficiency disorders may be primary or secondary and include a heterogeneous group of abnormalities of B-lymphocyte (humoral or antibody-mediated), T-lymphocyte (cell-mediated), phagocytic, and complement-related immune function.
- Immunodeficiency disorders affect both innate and adaptive immunity, maintenance of self-tolerance, and cancer cell surveillance.
- The most common life-threatening cause of secondary immunodeficiency, especially in developing nations, is acquired immunodeficiency syndrome (AIDS).
- Secondary or acquired immunodeficiency disorders are more common than primary disorders. Secondary immunodeficiency disorders may arise as a result of a wide variety of internal and external factors.
- Primary immunodeficiencies (PIs) comprise more than 250 diseases, most of which are proven to be or suspected of being the result of genetic mutations; the majority of these are inherited.

- Immunodeficiency can adversely affect all facets of life and every body system. The concepts related to immunodeficiency include immunity, infection, perfusion, oxygenation, mobility, metabolism, tissue integrity, cognition, and cellular regulation.

15.2 Acquired Immunodeficiency Syndrome

Differentiate the causes, classification, underlying pathogenesis, and clinical manifestations of acquired immunodeficiency syndrome and approaches to diagnosis and treatment of the condition across the lifespan.

- HIV is transmitted through exchange of body fluids.
- The primary modes of transmission are sexual contact, injection drug use, and mother-to-child (vertical) transmission.
- HIV is a retrovirus whose genetic material is contained in RNA.
- HIV is characterized by genetic heterogeneity, thus limiting vaccine development.
- There are two tropic strains of HIV: macrophage tropic (M tropic), which preferentially infect macrophages and establish the initial infection, and T-cell tropic (T tropic), which infect T lymphocytes.
- The major targets for HIV infection are $CD4^+$ T lymphocytes, monocytes/macrophages, and dendritic cells.
- HIV uses the chemokine receptors CCR5 and CXCR4 as coreceptors to gain entry into target cells.
- The HIV enzyme reverse transcriptase generates two copies of DNA using the viral RNA as a template.
- The viral DNA is incorporated into the host cell's chromosomes; thus, viral genes replicate each time the infected cell replicates.
- Approximately 6 months after infection, the plasma viral load stabilizes at a level known as the viral set point. The viral set point is prognostically significant and correlates with rate of $CD4^+$ T-lymphocyte depletion and disease progression.
- HIV-induced mechanisms of $CD4^+$ T-lymphocyte depletion include direct cytopathic effects, syncytia formation, reduced thymic production of new cells, and activation of apoptotic pathways.
- Inadequate adherence to HIV medications (< 90–95% adherence) is a major factor in the emergence of viral mutants.
- The goal of HAART is to achieve suppression of HIV replication to undetectable levels.
- Initiation of HAART is recommended for all individuals who are infected with HIV.
- Resistance testing can be used to select optimal HAART regimens in treatment-experienced individuals.

15.3 Common Conditions Associated with HIV/AIDS

Differentiate the causes, classification, underlying pathogenesis, and clinical manifestations of common conditions associated with HIV and AIDS and approaches to diagnosis and treatment of these conditions across the lifespan.

- Cytomegalovirus (CMV) retinitis is the most common CMV infection in HIV/AIDS. CMV infections are treated with valganciclovir therapy; the optimal duration of treatment has not yet been established.
- HIV infection increases the risk of activation of latent tuberculosis (TB) and dissemination. All HIV-infected individuals should undergo annual tuberculin testing.
- Kaposi sarcoma (KS), the most common AIDS-associated malignancy, is caused by infection with human herpesvirus 8.
- AIDS-related lymphoma is a group of B-cell malignancies that involves extranodal sites, such as the central nervous system, GI tract, and liver. It is caused by infection with the Epstein-Barr virus.
- Distal symmetric polyneuropathy (DSP) is a sensory axonal neuropathy that affects up to 50% of HIV-infected individuals. It can be the direct result of HIV infection or a complication of antiretroviral therapy.
- HIV-related lipodystrophy is a collection of morphologic and metabolic abnormalities. It includes insulin resistance, glucose intolerance, and fat redistribution.

15.4 Primary Immunodeficiencies

Differentiate the causes, classification, underlying pathogenesis, and clinical manifestations of primary immunodeficiencies and approaches to diagnosis and treatment of these conditions across the lifespan.

- Over 250 primary immunodeficiencies (PIs) have been identified, but the overall incidence and prevalence are low.
- Primary immunodeficiencies are primarily hereditary and are often diagnosed in infancy and childhood. However, better diagnosis and treatment have led to a significant increase in the number of adults living with PI.
- The most commonly identified primary immunodeficiencies are selective IgA deficiency and IgG subclass deficiency (both B-cell deficiencies) as well as common variable immunodeficiency (CVID) (both T-cell and B-cell deficiency).
- The most common manifestations of PIs are recurrent, severe, and/or persistent/unresponsive bacterial and viral infections involving both common and opportunistic pathogens or infections with unexpected or severe complications.

- Individuals with PI are at increased risk for a variety of autoimmune or inflammatory diseases and malignancies.
- See Table 15.3 for specifics on selected primary immunodeficiency disorders.

REVIEW QUESTIONS

1. A client with a positive ELISA is scheduled for a Western blot analysis. The nurse explains which of the following to the client?
   a. ELISA measures antibody, while Western blot measures antigen.
   b. The specificity of the reacting antibodies in an ELISA is not known.
   c. Clumping of viral antigens can result in a falsely positive ELISA.
   d. ELISA is less sensitive than the Western blot.
2. The nurse is assessing a client with primary HIV infection. Which of the following is the nurse most likely to observe?
   a. Lymphadenopathy
   b. Night sweats
   c. Diarrhea
   d. Fever
3. The $CD4^+$ T-lymphocyte count for a client with AIDS is 150 cells/mm^3. The nurse understands that this client:
   a. is in remission.
   b. is asymptomatic.
   c. has opportunistic infections.
   d. is no longer contagious.
4. Which of the following statements made by a client on HAART therapy indicates understanding of the regimen?
   a. "I can stop these pills once my symptoms are gone."
   b. "It is important to take drug holidays to prevent resistance."
   c. "I need to take these medications exactly as prescribed."
   d. "These medications will cure me of HIV."
5. The nurse is assessing an infant with DiGeorge syndrome with 22q11.2 deletion. Which of the following is the nurse most likely to observe?
   a. Narrow nasal bridge
   b. Upward slant (mongoloid) of eyes
   c. Underdeveloped mandible
   d. Cleft palate
6. The nurse is caring for a client with HIV and CMV. Which of the following signs is the nurse most likely to assess?
   a. Retinitis
   b. Respiratory infections
   c. Skin lesions
   d. Lymphadenopathy
7. The nurse caring for a client diagnosed with AIDS is most likely to assess which of the following conditions?
   a. $CD4^+$ T-lymphocyte count $>$ 200 cells/mm^3
   b. Opportunistic infection
   c. Distal symmetric polyneuropathy
   d. HIV-associated lipodystrophy syndrome
8. Which of the following would the nurse expect when caring for an infant with SCID?
   a. A normal thymus gland
   b. A life-threatening infection
   c. Overdeveloped tonsils
   d. Lymphadenopathy

ANSWERS

Answers to Review Questions can be found in Appendix A. Answers to Case Study and Check Your Progress questions are available on the faculty resources site. Please consult with your instructor.

RECOMMENDED WEBSITES

AIDSinfo
    https://aidsinfo.nih.gov

The Complete HIV/AIDS Resource
    http://www.thebody.com

HIV InSite
    http://hivinsite.ucsf.edu

Immune Deficiency Foundation
    http://primaryimmune.org

Eunice Kennedy Shriver National Institute of Child Health and Human Development
https://www.nichd.nih.gov

Canadian Immunodeficiencies Patient Organization
http://www.cipo.ca

International Patient Organisation for Primary Immunodeficiencies
http://www.ipopi.org

REFERENCES

1. AIDS.gov. (2014). *Global HIV/AIDS overview.* Available at https://www.aids.gov/federal-resources/around-the-world/global-aids-overview
2. Immune Deficiency Foundation. (2016). *About primary immunodeficiencies.* Available at http://primaryimmune.org/about-primary-immunodeficiencies
3. Younger, E. M., Epland, K., Zampelli, A., & Hintermeyer, M. K. (2015). Primary immunodeficiency diseases: A primer for PCPs. *The Nurse Practitioner, 40*(2), 1–7.
4. AIDS.gov. (2010). Opportunistic infections and their relationship to HIV/AIDS. Available at https://www.aids.gov/hiv-aids-basics/staying-healthy-with-hiv-aids/potential-related-health-problems/opportunistic-infections
5. Chauveau, L., Puigdomenech, I., Ayinde, D., et al. (2015). HIV-2 infects resting $CD4^+$ T cells but not monocyte-derived dendritic cells. *Retrovirology, 12*(2), 1–13.
6. Centers for Disease Control and Prevention. (2015). *HIV basics: About HIV/AIDS.* Available at http://www.cdc.gov/hiv/basics/whatishiv.html
7. Dye, C., Boerma, T., Evans, D., et al. (2013). *The world health report 2013: Research for universal health coverage.* Geneva, Switzerland: World Health Organization.
8. Joint United Nations Programme on HIV/AIDS. (2013). *Global report: UNAIDS update on the global AIDS epidemic 2013.* Available at http://www.unaids.org/en/media/unaids/contentassets/documents/epidemiology/2013/gr2013/UNAIDS_Global_Report_2013_en.pdf
9. Centers for Disease Control and Prevention. (2016). *HIV in the United States: At a glance.* Available at http://www.cdc.gov/hiv/statistics/overview/ataglance.html
10. Centers for Disease Control and Prevention. (2015). *Care and prevention for people living with HIV.* Available at http://www.cdc.gov/nchhstp/newsroom/HIVFactSheets/Epidemic/Care.htm
11. Eremin, O., & Sewell, H. (Eds.). (2011). *Essential immunology for surgeons.* Oxford, UK: Oxford University Press.
12. Centers for Disease Control and Prevention. (2015). *HIV transmission.* Available at http://www.cdc.gov/hiv/basics/transmission.html
13. Jones, R. E., Lopez, K. H. (2014). *Human reproductive biology* (4th ed.). London, UK: Academic Press.
14. Centers for Disease Control and Prevention. (2013). *Prevention benefits of HIV treatment.* Available at http://www.cdc.gov/hiv/prevention/research/tap
15. American Red Cross. (n.d.). *Infectious disease testing.* Available at http://www.redcrossblood.org/learn-about-blood/bloodtesting#Human_Immunodeficiency_viruses_Types_1_and_2_HIV_1_2_Antibody_testing_1985_and_NAT_1999_
16. Reitz, M. S. (2011). Virology of HIV. In J. C. Hall, B. J. Hall, & C. J. Cockerell (Eds.), *HIV/AIDS in the post-HAART era: Manifestations, treatment, and epidemiology* (pp. 98–117). Shelton, CT: People's Medical Publishing House.
17. Stanford, J. F., & Stanford, C. W. (2011). An HIV vaccine: Is it possible? Are we getting closer? In J. C. Hall, B. J. Hall, & C. J. Cockerell (Eds.), *HIV/AIDS in the post-HAART era: Manifestations, treatment, and epidemiology* (pp. 938–965). Shelton, CT: People's Medical Publishing House.
18. Luzzi, G. A., Peto, T. E. A., Goulder, P., & Conlon, C. P. (2012). Viruses: HIV/AIDS. In D. A. Warrell, T. M. Cox, J. D. Firth, & E. Torok (Eds.), *Oxford textbook of medicine: Infection* (5th ed., pp. 226–250). Oxford, UK: Oxford University Press.
19. Centers for Disease Control and Prevention. (2014). Revised surveillance case definition for HIV infection—United States, 2014 recommendations and reports. *Morbidity and Mortality Weekly Report (MMWR), 63*(RR03), 1–10. Available at http://www.cdc.gov/mmwr/preview/mmwrhtml/rr6303a1.htm?s_cid=rr6303a1_e
20. Goldblatt, D., & Ramsay, M. (2012). Immunization. In D. A. Warrell, T. M. Cox, J. D. Firth, & E. Torok (Eds.), *Oxford textbook of medicine: Infection* (pp. 54–59). Oxford, UK: Oxford University Press.
21. Tan, I. L., Smith, B. R., von Geldern, G., Mateen, F. J., & McArthur, J. C. (2012). HIV-associated opportunistic infections of the CNS. *Lancet Neurology, 11*(7), 605–617.
22. Arts, E. J., & Hazuda, D. J. (2012). HIV-1 antiretroviral drug therapy. *Cold Spring Harbor Perspectives in Medicine, 2*(4), 1–23.
23. Greene, W. C., Peterlin, M., & Stremlau, M. H. (2012). Molecular biology of HIV: Implications for new therapies. In P. A. Volberding, W. C. Greene, J. Lange, J. Gallant, & N. Sewankambo (Eds.), *Sande's HIV/AIDS medicine: Medical management of AIDS* (2nd ed., pp. 25–44). Philadelphia, PA: Elsevier/Saunders.
24. Barbaro, G. (2011). Cardiovascular manifestations of HIV/AIDS. In J. C. Hall, B. J. Hall, & C. J. Cockerell (Eds.), *HIV/AIDS in the post-HAART era: Manifestations, treatment, and epidemiology* (pp. 240–253). Shelton, CT: People's Medical Publishing House.
25. Tungsiripat, M. (2013). *HIV for the primary care physician.* Available at http://www.clevelandclinicmeded.com/medicalpubs/diseasemanagement/infectious-disease/HIV-care/Default.htm
26. National Institute of Allergies and Infectious Diseases (2009). *More on how HIV causes AIDS.* Available at http://www.niaid.nih.gov/topics/HIVAIDS/Understanding/howHIVCausesAIDS/Pages/howhiv.aspx
27. van Manen, D., vant Wout, A. B., & Schuitemaker, H. (2012). Viral and host determinants of HIV-1 disease progression. In P. A. Volberding, W. C. Greene, J. Lange, J. Gallant, & N. Sewankambo (Eds.), *Sande's HIV/AIDS medicine: Medical management of AIDS* (2nd ed., pp. 59–76). Philadelphia, PA: Elsevier/Saunders.
28. Bell, S. K., Little, S. J., & Rosenberg, E. S. (2010). Clinical management of acute HIV infection: Best practice remains unknown. *Journal of Infectious Diseases, 202*(Suppl. 2), S278–S288.
29. Cooper, A., García, M., Petrovas, C., Yamamoto, T., Koup, R. A., & Nabel, G. J. (2013). HIV-1 causes CD4 cell death through DNA-dependent protein kinase during viral integration. *Nature, 498*(7454): 376–379.
30. Doitsh, G., Cavrois, M., Lassen, K. G., et al. (2010). Abortive HIV infection mediates CD4 T cell depletion and inflammation in human lymphoid tissue. *Cell, 143*, 789–801.
31. Cooper, A., García, M., Petrovas, C., Yamamoto, T., Koup, R. A., & Nabel, G. J. (2013). HIV-1 causes CD4 cell death through DNA-dependent protein kinase during viral integration. *Nature, 498*, 376–379.
32. Sainski, A. M., Dai, H., Natesampillai, S., et al. (2014). Casp8p41 generated by HIV protease kills CD4 T cells through direct Bak activation. *Journal of Cell Biology, 206*(7), 867–876.
33. Chalker, J. C., Andualem, T., Gitau, L. N., et al. (2010). Measuring adherence to antiretroviral treatment in resource-poor settings:

The feasibility of collecting routine data for key indicators. *BMC Health Services Research, 10*(1), 43.

34. Centers for Disease Control and Prevention. (2014). *HIV infection: Detection, counseling, and referral*. Available at http://www.cdc.gov/std/treatment/2010/hiv.htm
35. AIDSinfo. (2014). *Guidelines for the use of antiretroviral agents in HIV-1-infected adults and adolescents: Considerations for antiretroviral use in special patient populations*. Available at http://aidsinfo.nih.gov/guidelines/html/1/adult-and-adolescent-treatment-guidelines/20/acute-hiv-infection
36. AIDSinfo. (2014). *Guidelines for the use of antiretroviral agents in HIV-1-infected adults and adolescents: Initiating antiretroviral therapy in treatment-naïve patients*. Available at http://aidsinfo.nih.gov/guidelines/html/1/adult-and-adolescent-arv-guidelines/10/initiating-art-in-treatment-naive-patients
37. AIDSinfo. (2016). *HIV treatment: FDA-approved HIV medicines*. Available at https://aidsinfo.nih.gov/education-materials/fact-sheets/21/58/fda-approved-hiv-medicines
38. Waters, L., Scourfield, A., & Nelson, M. (2011). Treatment of HIV. In J. C. Hall, B. J. Hall, & C. J. Cockerell (Eds.), *HIV/AIDS in the post-HAART era: Manifestations, treatment, and epidemiology* (pp. 389–403). Shelton, CT: People's Medical Publishing House.
39. AIDSinfo. (2011). *Guidelines for the use of antiretroviral agents in HIV-1-infected adults and adolescents: Management of the treatment-experienced patient--Discontinuation or interruption of antiretroviral therapy*. Available at http://aidsinfo.nih.gov/guidelines/html/1/adult-and-adolescent-arv-guidelines/18/discontinuation-or-interruption-of-antiretroviral-therapy
40. AIDSinfo. (2014). *HIV treatment: Drug resistance*. Available at http://aidsinfo.nih.gov/education-materials/fact-sheets/21/56/drug-resistance
41. Oyanik, E. L., Napravnik, S., Hurt, C. B., et al. (2012). Prevalence of transmitted antiretroviral drug resistance differs between acutely and chronically HIV-infected patients. *Journal of Acquired Immune Deficiency Syndromes*, 61(2), 258–262.
42. AIDSinfo. (2014). *Guidelines for the use of antiretroviral agents in HIV-1-infected adults and adolescents: Cytomegalovirus*. Available at http://aidsinfo.nih.gov/guidelines/html/4/adult-and-adolescent-oi-prevention-and-treatment-guidelines/337/cmv
43. AIDSinfo. (2013). *Tuberculosis: Tuberculosis and HIV*. Available at. https://www.aids.gov/hiv-aids-basics/staying-healthy-with-hiv-aids/potential-related-health-problems/tuberculosis/index.html
44. Centers for Disease Control and Prevention. (2012). *Multidrug-resistant tuberculosis (MDR TB)*. Available at http://www.cdc.gov/tb/publications/factsheets/drtb/mdrtb.htm
45. Centers for Disease Control and Prevention. (2014). *Treatment of multidrug-resistant tuberculosis: Bedaquiline*. Available at http://www.cdc.gov/tb/publications/factsheets/treatment/bedaquiline.htm
46. National Cancer Institute. (2014). *Kaposi sarcoma treatment (PDQ®): Classic Kaposi sarcoma treatment*. Available at http://www.cancer.gov/cancertopics/pdq/treatment/kaposis/HealthProfessional/page3
47. Auwaerter, P. G. (2011). Epstein-Barr virus. In *Johns Hopkins HIV guide*. Available at http://www.hopkinsguides.com/hopkins/view/Johns_Hopkins_HIV_Guide/545067/all/Epstein_Barr_virus
48. Cai, Q., Chen, K., & Young, K. H. (2015). Epstein–Barr virus-positive T/NK-cell lymphoproliferative disorders. *Experimental & Molecular Medicine, 47*(1), e133.
49. Schütz, S. G., & Robinson-Papp J. (2013). HIV-related neuropathy: Current perspectives. *HIV/AIDS Research and Palliative Care, 5*, 243–251.
50. Loonam, C. R., & Mullen, A. (2012). Nutrition and the HIV-associated lipodystrophy syndrome. *Nutrition Research Reviews, 25*(2), 267–287.
51. National Institutes of Allergy and Infectious Diseases. (2015). *Primary immune deficiency diseases (PIDD)*. Available at http://www.niaid.nih.gov/topics/immunedeficiency/Pages/Default.aspx
52. Jeffrey Modell Foundation. (n.d.). *10 warning signs*. Available at http://www.info4pi.org/library/educational-materials/10-warning-signs

Chapter 16

Disorders of White Blood Cells

Eileen Hacker, Laurie Gaston, Kathy Lauer, and Matthew Sorenson

Chapter Outline and Learning Outcomes

16.1 Chapter Overview and Case Studies
Describe the basis of disorders of white blood cells and concepts related to those disorders.

16.2 Acute Myelogenous Leukemia
Identify the morphologic classification, etiology and pathogenesis, and clinical manifestations of acute myelogenous leukemia and approaches to diagnosis and treatment of the condition across the lifespan.

16.3 Acute Lymphocytic Leukemia
Identify the morphologic classification, etiology and pathogenesis, and clinical manifestations of acute lymphocytic leukemia and approaches to diagnosis and treatment of the condition across the lifespan.

16.4 Chronic Myelogenous Leukemia
Identify the morphologic classification, etiology and pathogenesis, and clinical manifestations of chronic myelogenous leukemia and approaches to diagnosis and treatment of the condition across the lifespan.

16.5 Chronic Lymphocytic Leukemia
Identify the morphologic classification, etiology and pathogenesis, and clinical manifestations of chronic lymphocytic leukemia and approaches to diagnosis and treatment of the condition across the lifespan.

16.6 Non-Hodgkin Lymphoma
Identify the morphologic classification, etiology and pathogenesis, and clinical manifestations of non-Hodgkin lymphoma and approaches to diagnosis and treatment of the condition across the lifespan.

16.7 Hodgkin Lymphoma
Identify the morphologic classification, etiology and pathogenesis, and clinical manifestations of Hodgkin lymphoma and approaches to diagnosis and treatment of the condition across the lifespan.

16.8 Multiple Myeloma
Identify the morphologic classification, etiology and pathogenesis, and clinical manifestations of multiple myeloma and approaches to diagnosis and treatment of the condition across the lifespan.

KEY TERMS

ABBREVIATIONS

ALL—acute lymphocytic leukemia
AML—acute myelogenous leukemia
CLL—chronic lymphocytic leukemia
CML—chronic myelogenous leukemia
HL—Hodgkin lymphoma
HRS—Hodgkin Reed-Sternberg
NHL—non-Hodgkin lymphoma

16.1 Chapter Overview and Case Studies

Hematologic (blood system) cancers are a group of malignancies that stem from genetically abnormal cells arising in the hematopoietic system (blood-making organs). Such malignancies develop as a consequence of one or more mutations in a single cell or a group of cells that result in immature and/or ineffective hematopoietic cells. The mutations may occur at any time during the process of maturation and differentiation and may affect any of the blood cell lines in the hematopoietic system. Like the various hematopoietic precursors, malignancies that arise in the hematopoietic system vary according to specific cell line of origin. The malignant cells may be located in the bone marrow, circulate through the bloodstream, and/or infiltrate particular organs and tissues, such as the lymphatic tissue.

The major hematologic malignancies reviewed in this chapter are the leukemias (acute myelogenous, acute lymphocytic, chronic myelogenous, and chronic lymphocytic), the lymphomas (Hodgkin lymphoma and non-Hodgkin lymphoma), and multiple myeloma. Although all of these malignancies arise in the hematopoietic system, their epidemiology, clinical manifestations, and treatment vary according to disease classification. This chapter provides the necessary background for understanding the general pathophysiology associated with hematologic malignancies and provides specific pathophysiologic information about the particular hematologic malignancies.

Leukemias and Lymphoma: An Introduction

Hematopoiesis is the process by which the cellular components of the blood are formed. All of the blood's cellular components are initially derived from multipotent hematopoietic stem cells. The multipotent stem cell is capable of self-renewal and can differentiate into any one of the 10 blood cell lines or lineages (erythrocytes, platelets, neutrophils, eosinophils, basophils, monocytes, T lymphocytes, B lymphocytes, natural killer cells, and dendritic cells).

The most common hematologic malignancies are leukemias and lymphomas. All hematologic malignancies are distinguished by cumulative genetic alterations in the DNA of cells that originate in the bone marrow or lymphatic tissue. The genetic abnormalities, which are potentially different for each malignancy, lead to altered functional ability and aberrant cell **proliferation** (unregulated cell growth). The terminology associated with the specific malignancy corresponds to the tissue of origin. **Leukemia** is the common name for hematologic malignances that originate in the bone marrow or blood. **Lymphoma** refers to hematologic malignancies that originate in the lymphatic tissues.

Hematologic malignancies represent a significant portion of the cancer burden in the United States. More than 820,000 people are living with leukemia, lymphoma, and other less common hematologic malignancies, such as multiple myeloma. Recent estimates suggest that over 162,020 people would be diagnosed with leukemia, lymphoma, or multiple myeloma in 2015, corresponding to approximately 9.7% of the 1,658,370 new cancer cases diagnosed in the United States.[1] An estimated 589,430 people were likely to succumb to cancer in 2015, and 56,630 (9.6%) of cancer-related deaths were estimated to result from leukemia, lymphoma, or multiple myeloma.

The hematologic malignancies are further divided into groups based on clinical and pathologic features. Leukemias are classified according to the underlying cell type (myelogenous or lymphocytic) and as acute or chronic depending on the degree of maturation or differentiation of the affected cell type and rate of aberrant cellular proliferation. Myelogenous or myeloid leukemia involves neoplastic changes (abnormal tissue growth) that occur in the myeloid cell line, affecting granulocytes, erythrocytes, megakaryocytes, or monocytes. Lymphocytic leukemia involves neoplastic changes that occur in the lymphoid cell line, affecting T lymphocytes and B lymphocytes. In both myelogenous leukemia and lymphocytic leukemia, the damaged DNA blocks normal differentiation and maturation of hematopoietic cells, resulting in an increased proliferation of nonfunctional or semifunctional hematopoietic cells.

In acute leukemia, blocks in early (precursor) hematopoietic cells render these cells less functional. Acute leukemia is characterized by the rapid proliferation of immature hematopoietic cells called blasts (**Figure 16.1** ■). In chronic

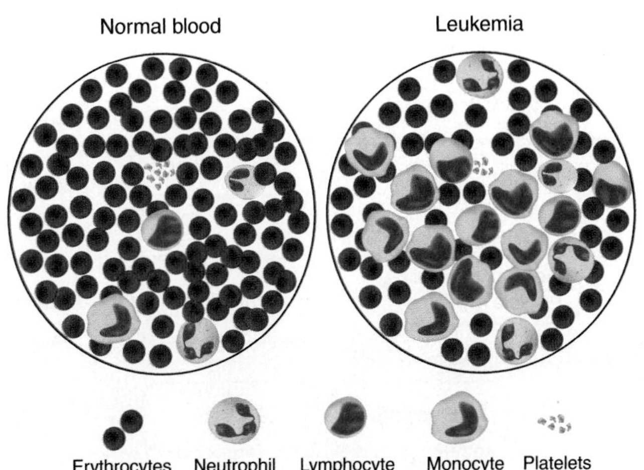

Figure 16.1 ■ Differences between normal blood and leukemia.

leukemia, there is a block in the later stages of maturation and differentiation of hematopoietic cells. The chronic leukemic cells more closely resemble normal cells and retain more of the functional properties of the underlying cell of origin. Chronic leukemia is characterized by the proliferation of cells that are more mature, though still abnormal. Based on these common divisions, four major types of leukemia emerge:

1. Acute myelogenous leukemia (AML)
2. Acute lymphocytic leukemia (ALL)
3. Chronic myelogenous leukemia (CML)
4. Chronic lymphocytic leukemia (CLL).

Lymphoma involves hematologic malignancies that originate in the lymphatic tissues. Two major classifications of lymphomas exist:

1. Hodgkin lymphoma
2. Non-Hodgkin lymphoma (NHL).

Hodgkin lymphoma, named after the British physician who first described the disease, is a specific type of lymphoma characterized by the presence of Reed-Sternberg cells. These cells are very large, malignant B lymphocytes. All other lymphomas are grouped together and classified as NHL. NHL is a broad category of lymphoid cancers that do not contain Reed-Sternberg cells. Classification of NHL is complex, with multiple staging systems available for use. Most of these staging or classification systems incorporate cell lineage, degree of cell maturation or differentiation, and location of the malignancy.

Multiple myeloma is a cancer involving a group of B cells known as plasma cells. These are B cells that produce large amounts of antibodies. The causes of multiple myeloma are not well understood, but obesity, toxin exposure, and substance abuse appear to play roles along with genetic influences.

Concepts Related to Disorders of White Blood Cells

Hematologic malignancies exert effects primarily through unregulated proliferation of certain cell types. This disruption in cellular regulation can occur from exposure to several environmental influences such as viruses, toxins, immunomodulatory or other medications, or exposure to radiation. Genetic variables also influence the proliferation of these cellular groups, leading to a disruption of cellular regulation. This chapter focuses on conditions characterized by the growth of cells that disrupt the function of other cells or body tissues. With leukemia and multiple myeloma, the proliferation of malignant cells disrupts the production of erythrocytes, neutrophils, and thrombocytes. This can then result in a loss of functional neutrophils, leading to infection and a disruption of thermoregulation. The loss of erythrocytes can lead to problems of oxygenation, which often manifest as anemia. A deficiency in thrombocytes can lead to coagulation issues and disrupt hemostasis. In multiple myeloma, heightened levels of calcium can occur in the bloodstream, leading to hypercalcemia, a disruption of fluid and electrolyte balance. The effects on bone cells can also manifest as pain. In lymphoma, the malignant cells are crowding together in the lymphatic system and can also cause cytopenia and coagulative issues, along with compression and damage to other tissues located near the affected lymph nodes (see **Figure 16.2** ■).

Case Studies

The following cases will be addressed throughout the chapter to assist in the application of chapter content to clinical situations that involve individuals with alterations of white blood cells.

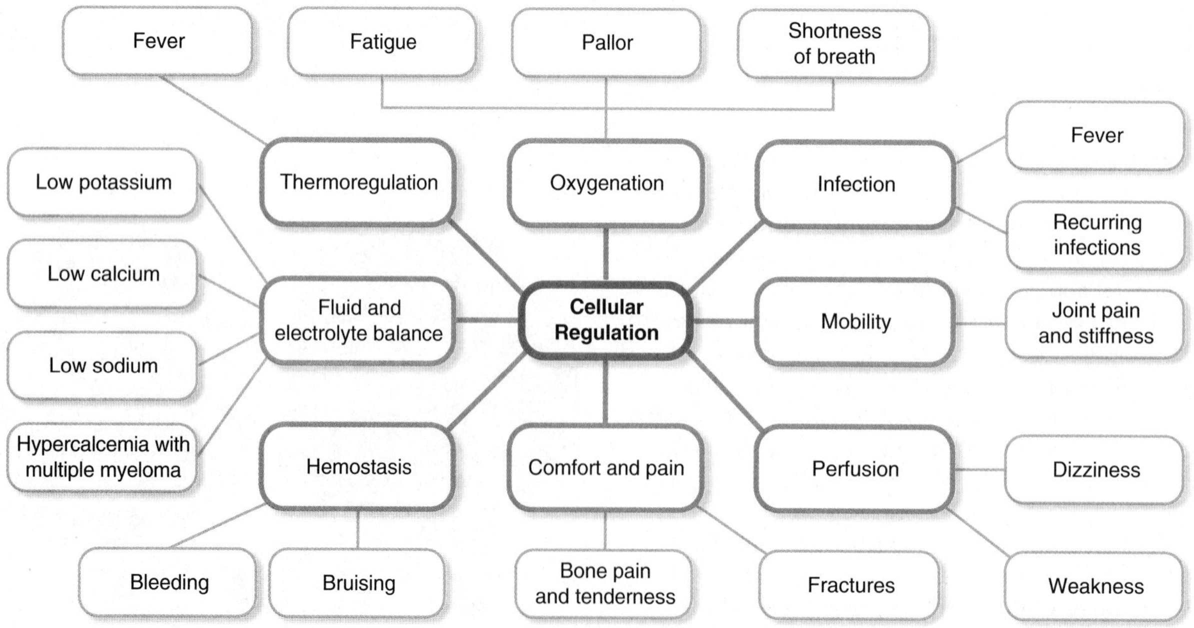

Figure 16.2 ■ Concepts related to disorders of white blood cells.

Tina McCarthy: Introduction

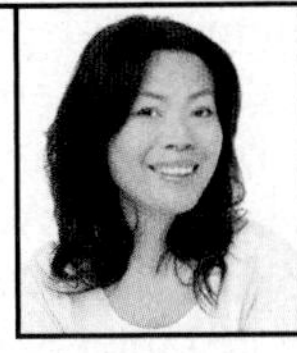

Tina McCarthy is a 46-year-old elementary school teacher. She is married and has three teenage boys. Ms. McCarthy is a dynamic member of the community, volunteering for local and state politicians' campaigns and participating as a member of a local charity board. He sons' varied activities also require her participation. Although she has always enjoyed her very active lifestyle, she has been feeling unusually fatigued for the past month. She recently lost 5 pounds, which was welcome but unintentional. She attributes the weight loss to increased activity and just forgetting to eat.

1. Why is Ms. McCarthy's complaint of fatigue worrisome?
2. Ms. McCarthy has experienced unintended weight loss. Why might this be a concern for her?

Tyler Johnson: Introduction

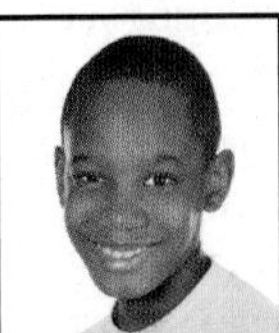

Tyler Johnson is a 10-year-old boy who is brought to the pediatrician by his parents for complaint of joint pain and a loss of appetite over the past 2 months. He plays soccer and reports that after even minor contact, he has a significant amount of bruising. Over the past month, Tyler's parents have noted a decrease in his energy level and say that he tires easily. His vital signs are pulse 100, respirations 20, temperature 101.3°F, blood pressure 128/68 mmHg.

1. Were Tyler's parents overreacting by bringing him to the pediatrician for evaluation? Why or why not?
2. Which of Tyler's vital signs and symptoms indicate the need for further testing?

Richard Geier: Introduction

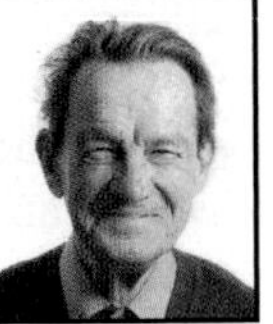

Richard Geier, a 77-year-old man, presents to his primary care physician's office after experiencing 2 weeks of night sweats that have required him to get up at night and change his pajamas. In addition, he reports fatigue, chills, and fevers. He thinks he might have a virus. A routine complete blood count (CBC) reveals a total WBC of 65,000/μL. The primary care physician repeats the CBC 4 weeks later, and leukocytosis is still present.

1. What is the rationale for the physician's decision to repeat the CBC?
2. Why are the symptoms of night sweats and fever worrisome?

Check Your Progress: Section 16.1

1. How do leukemia and lymphoma differ by tissue of origin?
2. Describe how Reed-Sternberg cells are used to differentiate between Hodgkin lymphoma and non-Hodgkin lymphoma.
3. Distinguish between acute leukemia and chronic leukemia.

16.2 Acute Myelogenous Leukemia

Acute myelogenous leukemia (AML) accounts for 30% of all new cases of leukemia. Recent estimates suggest that approximately 20,830 people were likely to be diagnosed with AML in 2015.[1] The incidence rates are expected to be slightly higher in males than females, with 12,730 expected new cases in males and 8100 cases in females.[1] AML strikes all age groups, although the incidence rates increase considerably in people ages 60 years and older. AML occurs most frequently in the sixth, seventh, and eighth decades of life. This malignancy is considered to be a serious, life-threatening disease; the 5-year relative survival rate based on data from 2005–2011 is 25.9% overall and greater than 65% for children under age 15 years.[2]

Etiology and Pathogenesis

While the exact cause of AML is unknown, some people who have been diagnosed with the disease exhibit one or more risk factors. It must be noted, however, that most of those diagnosed with AML show no evidence of risk factors, and the cause of AML in these cases remains unknown. The risk factors associated with AML include (1) chemotherapeutic treatment,[3,4] (2) ionizing radiation,[5,6] (3) long-term exposure to benzenes or other petroleum products,[7–9] and (4) smoking.[10] All of these factors are capable of inducing DNA damage through mutations, chromosome deletions, or translocations. A number of inherited genetic disorders are associated with AML, although AML itself is not considered to be an inherited disease. The increased risk of developing AML in these inherited disorders stems from the underlying defective DNA repair associated with the specific inherited disorder. Examples of these disorders include Bloom syndrome,[11] Fanconi anemia,[12] Down syndrome,[13] and Li-Fraumeni syndrome.[14]

Multiple variants of AML exist; therefore, a classification scheme to delineate the various types of AML must be used to help determine prognosis and treatment. The World Health Organization's classification system is most commonly used to provide more clinically and prognostically relevant information.[15] This classification system integrates morphology, cytogenetics, molecular genetics, and immunologic markers. The incidence of each type of AML and related neoplasms is as follows:

- Acute myeloid leukemia with recurrent genetic abnormalities: 11%
- Acute myeloid leukemia with myelodysplasia-related changes: 6%
- Therapy-related AML and myelodysplastic syndrome: 2%
- Acute myeloid leukemia, not otherwise specified: 81%.

CLINICAL POINT: For all cancers, the stage of the disease determines the treatment. Staging or classifying cancers, such as leukemias, serves a number or very important functions such as (1) helping the clinician to plan an appropriate treatment strategy, (2) providing some indication of prognosis, (3) facilitating communication between clinicians and across institutions, and (4) facilitating clinical research. A classification system also helps the patient understand the prognosis so that the patient and family can make the needed adjustments in their lives. ■

Like other neoplasms, AML develops after a series of mutations (deletions, inversions, or translocations) of genetic material in hematopoietic precursor cells that ultimately result in abnormal cellular proliferation. Leukemia is initiated by one or more mutations in a single cell. For the leukemia to fully develop and become clinically apparent, the transformed leukemic cell must be capable of dividing and passing on the genetic abnormalities to descendant cells. The mutations that result in hematologic neoplasms occur in a gene or genes that normally regulate cell proliferation, cell death, and cell repair. The genes that are involved in cellular division and proliferation include proto-oncogenes, tumor suppressor genes, and genes involved in apoptosis (programmed cell death). See **Box 16.1** for an explanation of genes involved in cellular division and proliferation.

Identifying the genetic mutations associated with AML and consequences of the mutation is an important area of continued investigation. Many defined genetic changes have been associated with AML.[15] For example, AML is associated with a balanced translocation (change in place) of the *RUNX1* gene normally found on chromosome 21 to the *RUNX1T1* gene found on chromosome 8, resulting in the *RUNX1-RUNX1T1* gene fusion protein.[16] This place change (noted scientifically as t(8;21)(q22;q22)), *RUNX1-RUNX1T1* is a common finding in adults with AML and one that confers a more favorable prognosis, meaning that patients who have this genetic situation have a better prognosis for the course of their AML.[16] This genetic translocation ultimately results in fusion proteins that cause changes to hematopoiesis.

Although the genetic mutations, deletions, and translocations affect different cellular pathways, together these changes alter the dynamic, highly regulated process of hematopoietic cell differentiation and maturation. Left unregulated, abnormal and immature hematopoietic cells accumulate in the bone marrow and peripheral blood, eventually crowding out other hematopoietic cells, such as other myelocytes, erythrocytes, and/or megakaryocytes. This crowding of the bone marrow with abnormal cells results in loss of function and eventually leads to **pancytopenia** (anemia, neutropenia, and thrombocytopenia) as the bone marrow is unable to produce sufficient numbers of normal hematopoietic cells. Pancytopenia may lead to anemia, infections, and bleeding. In addition, leukemic cells are capable of infiltrating other tissues, such as the oral mucosa and joints. Accumulation of leukemic cells in tissue and organs leads to site-specific changes. For instance, leukemic infiltration of the gingiva leads to gingival hypertrophy and bleeding.

Clinical Manifestations

A wide range of presenting signs and symptoms exist for AML, and these generally depend on the degree of pancytopenia. The clinical manifestations of AML are a direct consequence of ineffective hematopoietic cells and overcrowding of the hematopoietic system. Weakness and fatigue related to anemia are common complaints in people with AML. Unresolved fever and infection related to neutropenia may be present and are potentially life threatening, depending on the severity of the infection. Common infections include pneumonia, urinary tract infections, and upper respiratory infections. Individuals with AML may present with bleeding problems related to thrombocytopenia. This may present as ecchymoses, petechiae, epistaxis, bleeding from the gums, and menorrhagia in women. The severity of the symptoms ranges from mild bleeding to frank hemorrhaging, depending on the degree of thrombocytopenia. In addition, patients may complain of common constitutional symptoms, which are nonspecific symptoms that impact general well-being, such as fatigue, weight loss, and dyspnea. These symptoms have several potential causes and are tied to numerous disease states. Patients with AML who experience **leukocytosis** (an abnormally elevated white blood cell count) occasionally present with headache, diplopia, cranial nerve palsies, and mental status changes. Although not as commonly, AML infiltration and accumulation in tissues and organs may manifest as soft tissue tumors consisting of collections of leukemic cells (granulocytic sarcomas or chloromas) or gingival hypertrophy or skin infiltration (leukemic cutis).

Unfortunately, no one sign or symptom is universally present in all patients with AML. More often, a combination of symptoms is present at diagnosis. This lack of consistency in clinical presentation makes it difficult to pinpoint the onset of AML, as the threshold for seeking medical

Box 16.1
Genes Involved in Cellular Division and Proliferation

- Cancer is basically unregulated cellular growth; it is influenced by genetic variables that either inhibit or enhance cellular mutation and proliferation.
- Proto-oncogenes are the normal genes that stimulate cellular division and proliferation by encoding for proteins that stimulate cell growth. When proto-oncogenes mutate, they are known as oncogenes.
- Oncogenes allow cells to proliferate in an unregulated manner.
- Tumor suppressor genes "put the brakes on" cell growth by encoding for products that inhibit cellular proliferation. Mutations in tumor suppressor genes allow cellular proliferation to continue when it should be stopped.

Example:

Normal tumor suppressor genes allow cells with DNA damage to undergo repair to prevent the damaged cells from dividing further. Mutations to tumor suppressor genes disrupt the inhibition of cellular proliferations and allow cells with DNA damage to continue to divide. In essence, the "braking system" fails, and this results in uncontrolled cellular growth beyond the normal needs of the body.

advice varies from person to person. A thorough history and physical examination must be performed to develop a full appreciation of the problems associated with AML, as some problems may be clinically undetected by the patient. Particular attention should be given to a history of a hematologic disorder or cancer; exposure to radiation, chemicals, or viruses; and history of genetic abnormalities—all of which are known risk factors for AML. During the physical examination, it is important to identify any signs of infection, leukemic infiltration, anemia, or bleeding.

Tina McCarthy: Application

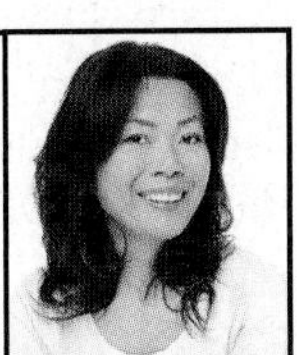

Ms. McCarthy has been feeling fatigued for the past month. She visits her primary healthcare provider to discuss a constellation of nonspecific symptoms. In addition to the fatigue, Ms. McCarthy complains of easy bruising. During the patient interview, the nurse notes that Ms. McCarthy has a history of chemotherapy for the treatment of breast cancer. On physical examination, multiple areas of ecchymosis are noted on all four extremities. Yesterday, she experienced a nosebleed for the first time since she was a child. A CBC with differential is ordered. The results indicate a normal white blood cell count with circulating leukemic blast cells. Ms. McCarthy is admitted the hospital for further testing.

3. What risk factors does Ms. McCarthy have that place her at risk for developing acute leukemia?
4. On the basis of Ms. McCarthy's nosebleed and areas of ecchymoses, which lab value is most likely to be abnormal?

Linking Pathophysiology to Diagnosis and Treatment

Restoring normal hematopoiesis is the primary goal of treatment for all AML subtypes, and systemic chemotherapy is the cornerstone of treatment. **Chemotherapy** is a general term used to describe drugs that arrest cellular proliferation by interfering with DNA synthesis and replication of both normal and malignant cells. With the exception of acute promyelocytic leukemia, all AML subtypes are treated in a similar fashion: induction therapy followed by consolidation therapy. Treatment is given in two or three phases: induction therapy followed by consolidation with or without a maintenance phase. Both induction and consolidation therapy involve chemotherapy. In some cases, the presence of other factors, such as the patient's age (older than 60 years) and treatment for relapsed or resistant AML, may influence treatment decisions. While an in-depth discussion linking all treatment options to all AML subtypes is beyond the scope of this chapter, there are several general principles pertaining to treating AML.

CLINICAL POINT: Chemotherapy (also known as antineoplastic agents or anticancer drugs) is administered to treat cancers, including leukemias and lymphoma. These drugs are given to arrest aberrant cellular proliferation. Chemotherapy affects normal as well as malignant cells, resulting in side effects that vary in intensity. ■

Although all AML subtypes are treated with systemic chemotherapy, the specific antineoplastic chemotherapy agents and dosages used vary from subtype to subtype. The purpose of induction chemotherapy is to reduce the leukemic cell burden to a level that is considered cytogenetically undetectable (from 10^{12} cells to 10^9 cells). Cancer, including hematologic malignancy, is generally considered detectable at levels above 10^9 cells. A complete remission is defined as the restoration of normal peripheral blood cell counts, maturation of all cell lines, and fewer than 5% blasts in the normocellular bone marrow. Induction chemotherapy is given to induce a complete remission. Inability to induce a complete remission in AML is considered to be a poor prognostic indicator.[17]

Although induction therapy substantially reduces the leukemic cell burden, it is generally assumed that residual disease still exists and that some leukemic cells (fewer than 10^9 cells) will have survived induction therapy. This minimal residual disease is the target of consolidation therapy. Consolidation therapy, consisting of one or more courses of high-dose chemotherapy and/or hematopoietic stem cell transplantation, is given to eradicate undetected leukemic cells so that a cure is possible. The drugs that are used for induction therapy can also be used for consolidation therapy. Current research focuses on linking specific genetic mutations with treatment strategies and prognosis.[18]

Both induction and consolidation therapy can be physically and psychologically challenging to patients during the period of marrow recovery. During this time of profound neutropenia, anemia, and thrombocytopenia, the risk for developing infection and bleeding increases. Patients frequently require support with appropriate antibiotics or antifungals as well as blood component therapy. Hematopoietic growth factors may be given in specific situations, such as febrile neutropenia, to hasten hematologic recovery by decreasing the duration of neutropenia following therapy, thus potentially limiting the number and severity of infections.[19] Improvements in supportive care, such as antibiotics, transfusion therapy, and growth factors, have improved the prognosis for AML. Supportive care particularly helps the patients who are at greatest risk for developing complications, such as very young children and older adults.

Tina McCarthy: Outcome

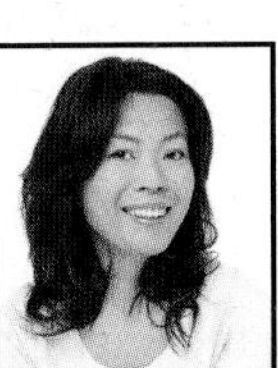

Ms. McCarthy undergoes a bone marrow aspiration, which reveals a hypercellular marrow with 94% blasts. Cytogenic evaluation of the leukemic cells indicates myeloid (marrow) origin with a balanced translocation of chromosomes 8 and 21, a common cytogenic (cell development) finding in people who are diagnosed with AML. Ms. McCarthy is admitted to the hospital to begin induction therapy with 7 + 3 therapy (7 days of continuous intravenous infusion of cytarabine combined with a short infusion of daunorubicin on days 1–3). Because of the toxicities associated with the high-dose chemotherapy, Ms. McCarthy is told to expect a potentially lengthy hospitalization. After hospitalization, she is discharged, and 6 months afterward she remains in remission.

5. What challenges might Ms. McCarthy and her family face during her treatment?
6. What challenges might Ms. McCarthy and her family face after her treatment is finished?

Check Your Progress: Section 16.2

1. Identify the risk factors for developing acute myelogenous leukemia (AML).
2. What role do oncogenes play in developing cancer?
3. What clinical manifestations are associated with pancytopenia?

16.3 Acute Lymphocytic Leukemia

Acute lymphocytic leukemia (ALL) accounts for 12% of all new cases of leukemia.[1] Approximately 6250 people were expected to be diagnosed with ALL in 2015; approximately two thirds of these were likely to be children.

Etiology and Pathogenesis

The incidence rates for ALL has gradually increased over the past 25 years, although the reason for this is unknown.[20] The incidence rate is expected to be slightly higher in females than in males, with 3100 expected new cases in males and 3150 in females in 2015. Although ALL can occur at any age, it is considered to be primarily a childhood malignancy, with most cases occurring in children 2–10 years of age.[21] In adults, the incidence rates begin to rise again after the age of 50. ALL is considered to be a serious, life-threatening disease in both children and adults, although the survival rates (particularly for children) are much higher for ALL than for AML. The 5-year survival rate for ALL exceeds 85% in children and 70% overall.[22]

Morphologic (change in shape), cytochemical (change in biochemical properties), cytogenetic (change in genetic properties), and immunologic (change in immunologic properties, such as surface proteins) features of the leukemic cells form the basis for classifying ALL. As in AML, the major classification scheme is the WHO system.[15] Lymphoid neoplasms are classified according to the cell of origin. Lymphoid leukemias present with blood and bone marrow involvement, while lymphomas present as a mass. It is important to note, however, that lymphoid leukemias occasionally present as a mass, while lymphomas may involve the blood and/or bone marrow and may progress to leukemia. The three general categories of the WHO classification are chronic lymphocytic leukemia and small lymphocytic lymphoma, precursor B-cell lymphoblastic leukemia and pre-B-cell lymphoblastic lymphoma, and pre-T-cell lymphoblastic leukemia and pre-T-cell lymphoblastic lymphoma.

In children, the subtypes of ALL are based on both laboratory and clinical features of the disease. A risk-based assessment is used to classify ALL, so treatment for ALL in children is based on cellular differentiation of the leukemic cells and prognostic variables.[23] Treatment is based on risk for recurrence; children receive enough therapy to place them into remission but as little therapy as possible to avoid the toxic effects of the drugs. For example, children with a more favorable prognosis using modest therapy are spared the more intensive regimens that are reserved for those with a less favorable prognosis. The prognostic variables for childhood ALL include (1) age at diagnosis, children between the ages of 1 and 9 years faring better than infants or older children[24]; (2) white blood cell count at diagnosis, as counts above 50,000/μL are indicative of a poorer prognosis[24]; (3) central nervous system (CNS) status at diagnosis, CNS involvement signifying greater risk for relapse[25]; (4) gender, girls faring better than boys (although this is not evident in all studies)[26,27]; and (5) race, survival rates for Caucasian children being slightly higher than those for African American and Hispanic children (although differences may be due to access to treatment).[28,29] Other variables that are used to assess risk for relapse and/or poorer prognosis include the leukemic cell characteristics such as morphology, immunophenotype, and cytogenetics (chromosome number, chromosome translocations, and other chromosomal abnormalities). ■

While the exact cause of ALL remains unknown, several genetic and nongenetic factors associated with increased risk of ALL have been identified. The nongenetic risk factors include prenatal exposure to x-rays and postnatal exposure to high doses of radiation for conditions such as tinea capitis and thymus enlargement.[30] A number of inherited genetic disorders are associated with ALL, although ALL is not by itself considered to be an inherited disease. As in AML, the increased risk of developing ALL in these inherited genetic disorder stems from the underlying defective DNA repair associated with the particular disorder. These disorders include Down syndrome,[31] neurofibromatosis,[32] Shwachman syndrome,[33] Bloom syndrome,[3] and ataxia telangiectasia.[35]

Like the other hematologic malignancies, ALL is considered to be a **clonal disease** (one in which all malignant cells derive from a single errant cell) that affects cells associated with lymphoid lineage. ALL develops after a series of mutations, deletions, or translocations of genetic material in hematopoietic lymphoid precursor cells that ultimately result in aberrant cellular proliferation (**Figure 16.3** ■). The initiation of ALL may begin with the transformation of one normal cell to a leukemic cell. ALL ultimately develops when the initially transformed leukemic cell divides and

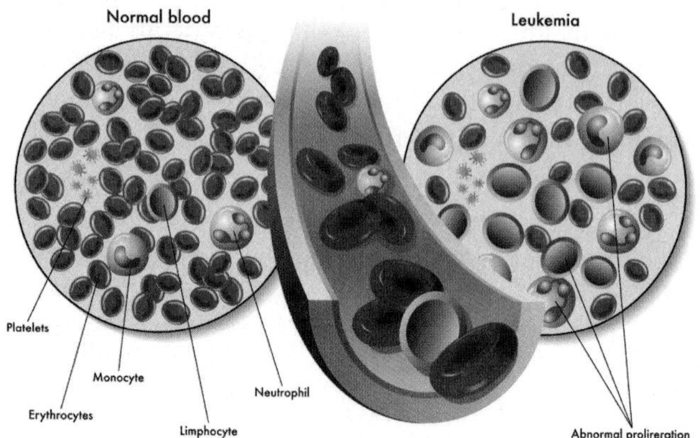

Figure 16.3 ■ The effects of acute lymphoblastic leukemia on bone marrow.

passes on the alterations in genetic material to descendant cells, or **progeny**, and these altered cells escape detection by the immune system.

Much progress has been made in understanding the common genetic alterations associated with the pathogenesis and prognosis of ALL. The type of genetic alteration may involve chromosomal translocations, deletions, inversions, and/or hyperdiploidy (more than 50 chromosomes), or hypodiploidy (fewer than 46 chromosomes). In ALL, these genetic alterations lead to leukomogenesis through one or more pathways, such as aberrant expression of proto-oncogenes or creation of fusion genes that encode for active kinases and transcription factors and affect cell growth trajectory.[36] A description of all genetic changes is beyond the scope of this chapter; however, several review articles address this topic thoroughly.[15,36–39] Some genetic alterations are more commonly seen in children than in adults and vice versa. This may account for at least some of the differences in prognosis between adults and children. The more common genetic alterations include t(9;22), seen primarily in adults; t(12;21), seen primarily in children; t(4;11), which is also present in some AML cases; and t(11q23), seen primarily in infants.[36]

While the genetic alterations vary among the subtypes of ALL, the underlying pathobiology is similar. The genetic alterations cause aberrant cellular proliferation of malignant, immature lymphocytes, and this disrupts the highly regulated process of cellular differentiation and maturation. Left unregulated, abnormal and immature hematopoietic cells accumulate in the bone marrow and infiltrate other organs. In addition to the loss of function in the malignant cells, an abnormal accumulation of ineffective cells crowds out the normal hematopoietic cells and eventually leads to problems with pancytopenia. In addition to overcrowding, leukemic cells associated with ALL are capable of infiltrating other tissues, such as the bones, lymph nodes, CNS, and testicles. Accumulation of leukemic cells in tissues and/or organs leads to site-specific changes. For instance, leukemic infiltration of the periosteum of the long bones may result in bone pain, especially in children.[40]

Clinical Manifestations

Early signs and symptoms of ALL are generally nonspecific and include fever, bleeding, bone pain, and lymphadenopathy, all commonly occurring signs and symptoms in a variety of medical conditions. When these problems persist despite treatment, the possibility of an underlying malignancy must be considered. These presenting signs and symptoms of ALL are a direct consequence of ineffective lymphoid cells, overcrowding of the bone marrow, and infiltration of leukemic cells into other organs. The degree of pancytopenia that is seen in ALL depends on the degree of marrow overcrowding. Infection related to neutropenia, weakness and fatigue related to anemia, and bleeding related to thrombocytopenia may be clinically evident on diagnosis in adults and children.

Children with ALL may present with additional signs and symptoms that are consistent with site-specific organ infiltration of leukemic cells, such as bone pain and enlarged lymph nodes. Bone pain in ALL may be caused by leukemic involvement of the periosteum or by aseptic necrosis related to bone marrow involvement. Unfortunately, bone pain is a common occurrence in children, particularly during adolescence. However, unresolved bone pain accompanied by limping and refusing to bear weight or in the context of other nonspecific complaints should be thoroughly investigated. On a rare occasion, ALL may present as testicular enlargement due to leukemic infiltration of the testes. Enlarged lymph nodes that are nontender, firm, and rubbery are a more common finding in people with ALL and suggest extramedullary (outside of the blood) leukemic spread. ■

Uncommonly, ALL may involve the CNS, causing headaches, vomiting, lethargy, and other symptoms associated with increased intracranial pressure. Some patients with ALL may present with a mediastinal mass, and as a result it may be difficult to differentiate ALL from NHL. Correctly diagnosing the patient is vital, as the treatment for ALL is different from that for NHL. Patients who present with a respiratory mass may develop respiratory distress due to the presence of the mass, which may cause narrowing of the trachea, pleural effusions, or superior vena cava syndrome. As is the case with AML, a thorough history and physical examination are necessary to develop a full appreciation of the problems associated with ALL, some of which may be clinically difficult to discern, particularly in children. During the physical examination, it is important to assess for signs of infection, leukemic infiltration, anemia, and bleeding. Appropriate tissue diagnosis for classifying leukemia is required, as the presenting signs and symptoms for ALL are similar to those for AML.

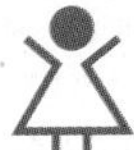

It is important to conduct a thorough investigation of vague, unresolved symptoms in children, particularly children who present with bone pain. ■

Tyler Johnson: Application

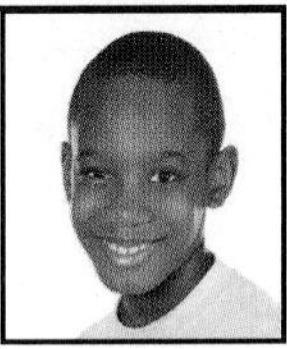

On physical examination, Tyler has adenopathy involving nodes of the anterior and posterior nuchal chains and the axillae. After consideration of physical examination findings and history, Tyler's healthcare provider orders laboratory panels (CBC, thyroid, chemistry). Findings include low hemoglobin and platelet levels along with an elevated white blood cell count. The healthcare provider recommends that Tyler be admitted to the hospital for a bone marrow biopsy to confirm acute lymphocytic leukemia.

3. Why is ALL difficult to recognize initially in children?
4. What are Tyler's risk factors for developing ALL?
5. What are the prognostic variables in children with ALL?

Linking Pathophysiology to Diagnosis and Treatment

As in treatment for AML, the goal of treatment for ALL is to eradicate the malignant immature lymphoid cells and restore normal hematopoiesis. Because ALL is a heterogeneous disease with multiple subtypes, treatment depends on the phenotype, genotype, and risk assessment for disease recurrence.[41] With the exception of the mature B-lymphocyte cell ALL subtype, induction therapy is given to induce a remission, followed by consolidation therapy to eliminate residual disease. In contrast to treatment for AML, however, therapy aimed at eliminating CNS disease is included as part of the therapeutic regimen for ALL, given the propensity for CNS involvement. The goal of induction therapy is to eradicate 99% of leukemic cells.[41] Although therapeutic goals for all ALL subtypes are similar, the intensity of the regimen, types of drugs used, and schedule of administration may differ depending on prognostic variables. Drugs that are commonly used in combination to induce a remission in ALL include glucocorticoids, vincristine, and asparaginase.[41] Complete remission rates of 98% for children and 85% for adults have been documented.[42,43]

Following restoration of normal hematopoiesis, intensification or consolidation therapy is given to eliminate any residual disease. Consolidation therapy, consisting of one or more courses of high-dose chemotherapy and/or hematopoietic stem cell transplantation, is given to eradicate undetected leukemic cells and potentially obtain a cure. Adults and children with ALL generally require treatment for at least 2 years after diagnosis to effectively improve overall survival.[44] The treatment strategies for ALL are quite effective, with high 5-year survival rates.

Tyler Johnson: Outcome

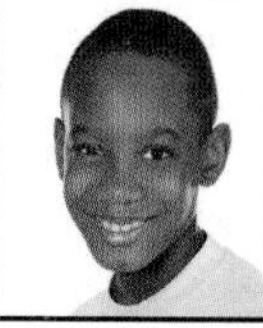

Although approximately 75% of children treated for ALL will enter long-term remission, Tyler has a risk factor that is tied to a slightly poorer prognosis (being an African American male). Therefore, after diagnostic confirmation of ALL, a combination of chemotherapeutic agents will be used as induction therapy in an attempt to induce remission. Patient and family teaching will focus on understanding the condition and the necessary precautions and maintenance therapy.

6. Although Tyler does not have signs of CNS involvement, therapy will also be aimed at eliminating CNS disease. What is the rationale for this?
7. What is the rationale for induction therapy followed by consolidation therapy in patients with ALL?

Check Your Progress: Section 16.3

1. How is risk-based assessment used in treatment decisions in children with ALL?
2. What are the nongenetic risk factors for ALL?
3. Describe the goal of consolidation therapy.

16.4 Chronic Myelogenous Leukemia

Chronic myelogenous leukemia (CML), a form of leukemia characterized by overproliferation of mature granulocytes, accounts for 12% of all leukemias, 2–3% occurring in children.[1] In 2015, an estimated 6660 new cases of CML were likely to be diagnosed, consisting of approximately 3530 males and 3130 females. Males are more likely to develop CML than are females, although the reason for this is unknown.[18] CML is primarily a disease of adulthood; the incidence increases dramatically in people over the age of 55 years.[18] The median age at diagnosis is 64 years. CML can be a life-threatening disease, particularly during the blast phase.[21] An estimated 1140 people were expected to die from CML in 2015.[1]

Staging systems for CML do not exist; instead, CML is classified according to phase (chronic, accelerated, or blast), which is based on the number of blast cells present in the blood and bone marrow.[45] In chronic phase CML, blast cells account for fewer than 10% of all cells in the blood or bone marrow. In accelerated phase CML, blast cells increase and account for 10–19% of all cells in the blood or marrow. During the blastic phase, blast cells account for over 20% of all cells in the blood or marrow (**Figure 16.4 ■**). The three phases represent the continuum of the CML disease process, the chronic phase being indicative of more stable disease and the blast phase representing more aggressive disease. Classifying CML in the appropriate phase is important for determining treatment strategies.

Etiology and Pathogenesis

There are very few known risk factors associated with developing CML. The only known environmental risk factor is exposure to high-dose radiation consistent with surviving an atomic bomb or nuclear reactor accident.[46] Like all other hematologic malignancies, CML is the direct result of a genetic alteration that results in aberrant cellular proliferation. CML is unique in that it was the first hematologic malignancy to be clearly linked to a specific genetic marker, which was discovered in 1960 by researchers Nowell and Hungerford.[47] CML arises when a well-known genetic alteration, the 9;22 translocation (Philadelphia chromosome), occurs at the stem cell level and results in overproduction of one or more myeloid elements in the bone marrow. Although the exact cause of the genetic translocation is not known, the result is increased myeloid cellular proliferation,

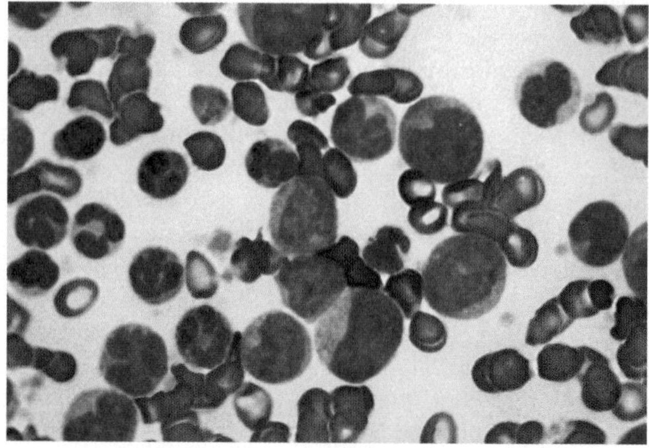

Figure 16.4 ■ Peripheral blood smear reveals histopathologic features of a blast crisis in a patient with CML.

consisting primarily of mature cells. This represents one of the main differences between AML and CML. The cells that are overproduced in AML consist of immature myeloid precursor cells, while the cells associated with CML are more mature. This constant proliferation or overproduction of cells causes cells to accumulate in the bone marrow and peripheral blood. In addition, clonal stem cells with the 9;22 translocation seed the spleen, resulting in splenomegaly.

Since Nowell and Hungerford's discovery of 9;22 translocation, much has been learned about the molecular pathogenesis of CML that results in aberrant cellular proliferation. This knowledge has aided in treatment of CML. Under normal circumstances, chromosomes 9 and 22 carry the *c-ABL* and *c-BCR* genes, respectively. It was originally hypothesized that this genetic alteration provided a growth advantage to the abnormal cells.[48] Much has been learned about the genetic alteration since that time. In the setting of CML, the translocation of these two chromosomes (9;22) results in the formation of a shortened chromosome 22 carrying the *BCR-ABL* fusion gene. The normal *c-ABL* gene codes for tyrosine kinase, an enzyme that is active in cellular proliferation. The fusion *BCR-ABL* gene displays constitutive tyrosine kinase activity, meaning that the gene is continuously active and does not require activation from other messenger proteins. Overproduction of this specific tyrosine kinase that is continuously active, the BCR-ABL fusion protein, results in the cell's oncogenic progression.[49] About 5% of patients with CML do not express the (9;22) translocation and are classified as having atypical or Philadelphia chromosome–negative CML.

Clinical Manifestations

Like other hematologic malignancies, the clinical manifestations of CML vary depending on the stage of the disease. Many people with CML are asymptomatic at diagnosis, and the disease is frequently found during routine blood work. The clinical manifestations of CML generally depend on the degree of overproduction of myeloid cells. The degree of myeloid overproduction at presentation varies. Approximately 52–72% of patients will present with a white blood cell count greater than 100,000/μL, 15–34% with platelet counts between 600,000 and 700,000/μL, and 45–62% with anemia. While some patients present with thrombocytosis (high platelet count), others may present with thrombocytopenia (decreased platelet count) caused by overcrowding of the marrow with other myeloid components. Accumulation of other myeloid cells, including basophils (basophilia) and eosinophils (eosinophilia), is present in almost all cases.[50]

Patients who are symptomatic may experience nonspecific as well as site-specific signs and symptoms. The degree of pancytopenia that is seen in CML depends on the degree of marrow overcrowding. Infection related to neutropenia, weakness and fatigue related to anemia, and bleeding related to thrombocytopenia may be present on diagnosis. Symptoms can also include excessive sweating or night sweats. Infiltration of the abnormal cells in the spleen can cause splenomegaly with abdominal pain, discomfort, early satiety, and upper left quadrant pain that is sometimes referred to the left shoulder. Acute gouty arthritis manifested as joint pain may also present at this time, caused by an overproduction of uric acid.[51]

The most important prognostic factor at diagnosis is identification of the phase of CML. More advanced CML cases can be much more challenging to treat. Better outcomes are found in people who stay in chronic phase CML than in those who progress to accelerated or blast phase.[45] Other poor prognostic indicators for patients with CML include older age, symptoms present at diagnosis, significant weight loss, hepatomegaly, splenomegaly, poor performance status, African American race, male, increased lactate dehydrogenase (LDH), and a complex cytogenetic profile.[52]

Linking Pathophysiology to Diagnosis and Treatment

Knowledge of the underlying pathophysiology of CML has led to substantial improvements in the treatment of CML. Therapeutic goals of CML treatment include achieving a hematologic response by normalizing the white blood cell count, eliminating immature myeloid cells, and eradicating signs and symptoms of the disease. Historically, available treatment options for CML included a number of different chemotherapeutic agents, including hydroxyurea, busulfan, and interferon-alfa (a biological modifier). Chemotherapy is given to arrest abnormal cellular proliferation. Given these treatments, a large percentage of patients achieved a hematologic remission (restoration of normal blood counts) and regression of symptoms. Few people, however, obtained a cytogenic remission, in which the 9;22 translocation reverted back to normal. The vast majority of people were not cured.

Drugs to address the genetic defect (specific inhibitors of the *BCR-ABL* gene) associated with CML has dramatically changed the treatment landscape for CML. These drugs, known as tyrosine kinase inhibitors, target the underlying genetic defect associated with CML (Philadelphia chromosome, t(9;22) to prevent aberrant proliferation of abnormal cells.

Check Your Progress: Section 16.4

1. Describe the classification system for chronic myelogenous leukemia.
2. What are the prognostic indicators for a poor outcome with CML?
3. Identify the therapeutic goals of CML treatment.

16.5 Chronic Lymphocytic Leukemia

Chronic lymphocytic leukemia (CLL), a form of leukemia characterized by the overproduction of B cells, is the most common type of lymphocytic leukemia, accounting for approximately 27% of all leukemia cases.[1] An estimated 14,620 new cases of CLL were likely to be diagnosed in 2015, consisting of approximately 8140 males and 6480 females.

Etiology and Pathogenesis

CLL is primarily a disease of older adults, the incidence increasing dramatically in people over the age of 50 years.[18] People as young as 30–39 years are being diagnosed with CLL, although this is less common. The incidence of CLL is highest among whites, while people of Asian descent have the lowest incidence rates.[21,53]

The classification systems that is most frequently used for staging CLL are the Rai (in the United States) and Binet (in Europe) staging systems.[54,55] Clinically, a modified version of the original Rai system is used that provides information related to overall survival. The Rai system divides CLL into five categories:

- ***Rai stage 0:*** Lymphocytosis and no enlargement of the lymph nodes, spleen, or liver, with near normal red blood cell and platelet counts.
- ***Rai stage I:*** Lymphocytosis plus enlarged lymph nodes. The spleen and liver are not enlarged, and the red blood cell and platelet counts are near normal.
- ***Rai stage II:*** Lymphocytosis plus an enlarged spleen (and possibly an enlarged liver), with or without enlarged lymph nodes. The red blood cell and platelet counts are near normal.
- ***Rai stage III:*** Lymphocytosis plus anemia (too few red blood cells), with or without enlarged lymph nodes, spleen, or liver. Platelet counts are near normal.
- ***Rai stage IV:*** Lymphocytosis plus thrombocytopenia (too few blood platelets), with or without anemia, enlarged lymph nodes, spleen, or liver.

The stages are separated into low-, intermediate-, and high-risk groups when determining treatment options:

- ***Low risk:*** Rai stage 0
- ***Intermediate risk:*** Combining Rai stages I and II
- ***High risk:*** Combining Rai stages III and IV.[56]

The Binet system classifies CLL according to the number of affected lymphoid tissues in an effort to better address prognostic indicators.[55] The areas of lymphoid tissue to be assessed include the axillary, cervical, and inguinal lymph nodes (unilateral or bilateral); the spleen; and the liver.

- ***Stage A:*** Assessment indicates fewer than three areas of involvement with no anemia or thrombocytopenia.
- ***Stage B:*** Assessment indicates three or more areas of enlarged lymphoid tissue with no anemia or thrombocytopenia.
- ***Stage C:*** Assessment indicates anemia (hemoglobin less than 10 g/dL) and/or thrombocytopenia (platelets less than 100,000/mm^3).

There is no known specific causative factor for CLL, although research is currently underway to identify occupational or environmental risks.[57] A link has now been identified in first-degree relatives with CLL or another B-lymphocytic disorder that may indicate a genetic predisposition in certain groups of patients.[58]

CLL is a chronic lymphoproliferative disorder involving the B-cell lymphocyte lineage. A disruption involving the B-cell lymphocyte differentiation pathway occurs, and these cells do not fully mature in terms of functional status. When viewed on a peripheral smear, the B lymphocytes are categorized as mature lymphocytes, but they are incompetent when it comes to full immune function.[59]

Like most other hematologic malignancies, CLL occurs as a result of a genetic alteration. However, the chromosomal abnormalities can be difficult to detect by using chromosomal analysis studies. Conventional cytogenetic testing requires the cells to be actively dividing in metaphase. The B-lymphocyte cells associated with CLL divide very slowly. As a result, the recommendation is to use fluorescence in situ hybridization (FISH) techniques to detect specific abnormalities in cells that are not dividing.[59] In a large database analysis of patients with CLL, trisomy 12 was the most common cytogenetic abnormality found; 15–20% of patients exhibited this chromosomal abnormality.[60] Structural abnormalities of chromosomes 11, 13, and 14 is the second most common find; these may occur alone or together with deletions or translocations of chromosome 13q14. The abnormalities seen on 13q may be associated with a more favorable outcome, while the abnormalities involving trisomy 12 tend to be associated with more advanced stages of disease and worse prognosis.[60] Other identified markers associated with CLL include *bcl-2*, a proto-oncogene, and *p53*, a tumor suppressor gene. *Bcl-2* is overexpressed in about 95% of patients with B-CLL. *Bcl-2* has been shown to suppress apoptosis (cell death), which is believed to prolong the life of involved cells.[61] About 10–47% of patients with CLL exhibit a *p53* gene mutation.[62] The *p53* gene, a tumor suppressor gene located on the short arm of chromosome 17, is inactivated by deletion or point mutation in many cancers.[63]

Clinical Manifestations

Approximately 25% of people with CLL are asymptomatic at diagnosis; the disease is frequently found during routine blood tests. The clinical manifestations of CLL are a direct consequence of the accumulation of lymphocytes in the lymphatic tissue. On physical examination, patients may present with lymphadenopathy, splenomegaly, and/or hepatomegaly (enlarged liver). Constitutional symptoms may be present and include fever greater than 100.5°F for 2 weeks without evidence of infection, night sweats without evidence of infection, unintentional weight loss that can be 10% of body weight in the preceding 6 months, and fatigue that interferes with the patient's ability to perform activities of daily living.[64] Other clinical findings may include anemia, thrombocytopenia, autoimmune hemolytic anemia, agranulocytosis, and hypogammaglobulinemia.[64]

Lymphocytosis is the hallmark sign of laboratory findings in CLL. Peripheral smear may show lymphocytes that appear flattened or smudged, called smudge cells. There may be nodular, interstitial, or diffuse patterns of bone marrow infiltration associated with CLL. The bone marrow aspirate may have normal to increased cellularity, and the lymphocytes will account for more than 30% of all nucleated cells. Bone marrow biopsy is not required to make the diagnosis but can be helpful in determining prognostic risk.[65] Blood chemistry results may show an elevation in LDH, beta 2 microglobulin, uric acid, and hepatic enzymes.[66]

Many patients with a variety of conditions, particularly infections, can present with leukocytosis; therefore, guidelines for diagnosing CLL have been proposed to delineate CLL from other conditions.[64] Diagnosis requires a persistent (more than 1 month) peripheral blood lymphocytosis (more than 5×10^9 cells/L) of mature-appearing lymphocytes in the absence of other causes and an immunophenotyping profile that is consistent with CLL (CD19, CD20 and CD79a, CD5, CD22, CD23, CD43, and CD11c markers as well as weak-intensity surface immunoglobulin [Ig], as shown by flow cytometry).

Richard Geier: Application

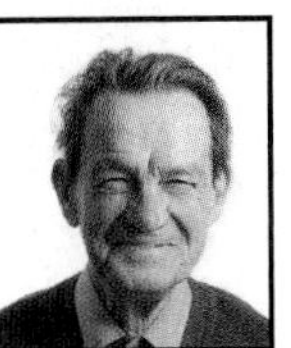

Mr. Geier is referred to a hematologist, who orders additional tests that reveal an elevated LDH of 300, an elevated beta 2-microglobulin, and smudge cells on the peripheral smear. Physical examination is remarkable only for small but palpable left axillary lymph nodes. A lymph node biopsy is performed, and peripheral blood is sent for flow cytometry. Diagnosis of CLL Rai stage 0–I is confirmed. Fludarabin chemotherapy will be started because of the presence of B symptoms.

3. Which examination findings place Mr. Geier at Rai stage 0–I?
4. What are Mr. Geier's risk factors for developing CLL?

Linking Pathophysiology to Diagnosis and Treatment

There is no known cure for CLL, although many advances in treating the disease have been made, leading to increased treatment options for patients. Treatment is determined by stage of the disease and is aimed at restoring normal lymphocyte counts. CLL generally progresses slowly, often with long periods of stability and occasional spontaneous remissions. Because the disease occurs primarily in older adults, follows an indolent course, and is not curable, a conservative approach to treatment is generally indicated. In patients with early-stage disease and without symptoms, watchful waiting is generally indicated. For patients with symptoms and/or more progressive disease, chemoimmunotherapy may be used. Chemotherapy is given to stop the cancer cells from progressing, and immunotherapy is used to stimulate the body's own defenses in fighting the disease. For patients who have clinically progressive disease that does not respond to other treatments, reduced-intensity allogeneic transplantation should be explored.

The progression of CLL varies. Predicting the disease course is difficult, as some patients have indolent disease for years, while others progress very rapidly and die within 1–2 years after diagnosis.[63] The clinical factors that best predict prognosis are the clinical stage, lymphocyte doubling time, and pattern of bone marrow infiltration.[67] The presence of other biological factors that have been identified to stratify prognosis in CLL include serum thymidine, serum beta 2 microglobulin, *p53* expression, mutational status of the *IgVH* gene, surface expression of CD38 and the cytoplasmic expression of *ZAP-70*.[68]

Richard Geier: Outcome

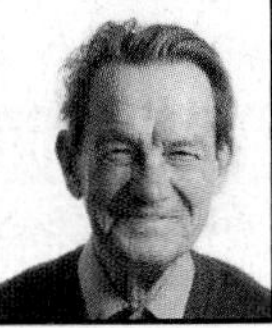

Mr. Geier was treated with a 5-day cycle of fludarabin. One week after treatment, his CBC reveals a white blood count of 4000/μL, a significant decrease from his pretreatment value. As a result of the significant decrease, he is given a nebulized treatment of pentamidine to help prevent the development of *Pneumocystis jiroveci* pneumonia. The hematologist recommends that Mr. Geier receive another treatment of pentamidine next month and advises him of special precautions that need to be taken if he happens to need a blood transfusion in the near future. At present, Mr. Geier is considered in remission, although he will be followed closely.

5. What is the most likely rationale for conservative treatment of CLL in Mr. Geier?
6. What factors determine Mr. Geier's prognosis?

Check Your Progress: Section 16.5

1. Identify the constitutional symptoms of CLL.
2. How is CLL differentiated from other conditions?
3. Describe the Binet staging system for CLL.

16.6 Non-Hodgkin Lymphoma

Non-Hodgkin lymphomas (NHLs) represent a heterogeneous group of malignancies that originate in the lymphatic system. Approximately 71,850 new cases of NHL were expected to be diagnosed in 2015, making this cancer the sixth most common in males and the fifth most common in females in the United States.[1] The incidence rates are higher in males than in females.

Etiology and Pathogenesis

NHL occurs in all age groups, including children, although the incidence rates are much higher in older individuals than in younger people. The incidence of NHL is highest in Americans of European descent, followed by Hispanics and African Americans. Approximately 19,790 individuals were expected to die from NHL in 2015.

The classification system of NHL lymphoma is complex because of the heterogeneous nature of diseases included under this umbrella term. Given the diverse nature of the disease, the importance of correctly diagnosing the patient cannot be underestimated, as the stage or classification of the disease determines treatment strategies. Although multiple classification systems for NHL have been used over the years, the updated Revised European American Lymphoma (REAL)/World Health Organization (WHO) classification is frequently cited.[69] The REAL/WHO classification system of lymphoid and leukemia neoplasms, presented in **Table 16.1** ■, classifies NHL on the basis of cell lineage (B cells versus T/NK cells) and the maturity level of the malignant cells (immature or blastic appearance versus a more mature stage of lymphoid differentiation).

Table 16.1 Updated REAL/WHO Classification of Lymphoid and Leukemia Neoplasms

B-cell Neoplasms	T-cell and Putative NK-cell Neoplasms
Precursor B-cell Neoplasm	**Precursor T-cell Neoplasm**
Precursor B-acute lymphoblastic leukemia/lymphoblastic lymphoma	Precursor T-acute lymphoblastic leukemia
Peripheral B-cell Neoplasms	**Peripheral T-cell and NK-cell Neoplasms**
1. B-cell CLL/small lymphocytic lymphoma	1. T-cell CLL/prolymphocytic leukemia
2. B-cell prolymphocytic leukemia	2. T-cell granular lymphocytic leukemia
3. Lymphoplasmacytic lymphoma/immunocytoma	3. Mycosis fungoides/Sézary syndrome
4. Mantle-cell lymphoma	4. Peripheral T-cell lymphoma, not otherwise characterized
5. Follicular lymphoma	5. Hepatosplenic gamma/delta T-cell lymphoma
6. Extranodal marginal zone B-cell lymphoma of mucosa-associated lymphatic tissue (MALT) type	6. Subcutaneous panniculitis-like T-cell lymphoma
7. Nodal marginal zone B-cell lymphoma (± monocytoid B-cells)	7. Angioimmunoblastic T-cell lymphoma
8. Splenic marginal zone lymphoma (± villous lymphocytes)	8. Extranodal T-/NK-cell lymphoma, nasal type
9. Hairy-cell leukemia	9. Enteropathy-type intestinal T-cell lymphoma
10. Plasmacytoma/plasma cell myeloma	10. Adult T-cell lymphoma/leukemia (human T-lymphotrophic virus [HTLV] 1+)
11. Diffuse large B-cell lymphoma	11. Anaplastic large cell lymphoma, primary systemic type
12. Burkitt lymphoma	12. Anaplastic large cell lymphoma, primary cutaneous type
	13. Aggressive NK-cell leukemia

SOURCE: Data from https://www.cancer.gov/types/lymphoma/hp/adult-nhl-treatment-pdq#cit/section_3.9

CLINICAL POINT: Non-Hodgkin lymphoma includes all lymphomas except Hodgkin lymphoma. ■

NHL may also be described in terms of the rate of cellular proliferation. The term *indolent* or *aggressive* may be used to differentiate the slower-growing tumors from tumors that proliferate at an accelerated rate. Indolent tumors, also called low-grade tumors, grow slowly and often do not result in discernible symptoms for patients at the time of diagnosis. Indolent lymphomas are frequently found accidentally in the course of a workup for another disorder. Aggressive tumors, by contrast, grow quickly, often causing symptoms that prompt the individual to seek medical attention. Indolent NHL accounts for approximately 40% of all cases of the disease, while aggressive NHL accounts for 60%.

The exact reasons for developing NHL are unknown, but at least some people who are diagnosed with the disease have one or more risk factors. As is the case in many hematologic malignancies, most people who are diagnosed with NHL do not exhibit any of the associated risk factors. Conversely, the vast majority of people who have one or more risk factors never progress to developing the disease. Risk factors common to NHL may be inherent to the host (host susceptibility) or to the environment. Risk factors that are inherent to the host include (1) weakened immune system, including patients treated with immunosuppressants following organ transplantation, those with a preexisting autoimmune disease, or those with an inherited immune deficiency disorder; (2) viral infections such as human immunodeficiency virus, Epstein-Barr virus (increased risk of Burkitt lymphoma in Africa), and human T-lymphotrophic virus Type 1; and (3) *Helicobacter pylori* associated with lymphoma of the stomach wall. Environmental factors such as exposure to pesticides, herbicides, wood preservatives, and other organic solvents have been implicated in the development of NHL.[70–73] Exposure to these chemicals may account for the increased incidence of the disease found in some occupations, such as farming. Again, it should be noted that the vast majority of people with identified risk factors associated with NHL never develop the disease.

The underlying pathophysiology of various NHL subtypes is as complex as the various staging systems. Like other neoplasms, malignant NHL cells undergo one or more genetic mutations over time that transform the cell from a normal cell to a malignant one. The mutations, in the form or translocations, additions, deletions, or inversions, affect the highly regulated process of cell proliferation, cell death, and/or cell repair, ultimately resulting in aberrant cellular proliferation. Although the genetic mutations, deletions, and translocations affect different cellular pathways, together these changes alter the dynamic, highly regulated process of hematopoietic cell differentiation and maturation.

Unlike leukemic cells, which reproduce primarily in the bone marrow and then circulate in the bloodstream, NHL cells tend to form solid tumors. The malignant cells congregate in the lymphoid tissue, causing destruction of the lymphatic tissue, such as the nodal architecture. NHL may arise from any of the lymphoid cells, including B cells, T cells, natural killer cells (NKCs), or NK-like cells.

Although the site of origin for NHL and lymphoid leukemia may differ, the diseases have some commonalities, including the same cell of origin. For instance, the malignant cell associated with B-cell small lymphocytic lymphoma (B-SLL) is identical to the cell involved in mature B-cell chronic lymphocytic leukemia (B-CLL). The difference relates to the stage of the disease, as 10% of patients present with only nodal involvement, a feature of B-CLL. Most patients with this type of malignancy have bone marrow and blood infiltration at diagnosis in the case of B-CLL.

Multiple genetic alterations are associated with NHL. Balanced, reciprocal translocation is the genetic hallmark of NHL genetic alterations, although the precise mechanism leading to the translocation is unknown. One of the most common features of the translocation is the proximity to known proto-oncogenes, ultimately resulting in proto-oncogene deregulation.[74] Other commonly occurring genetic alterations associated with NHL include inactivation of tumor suppressor genes (such as the *p53* tumor suppressor gene), unbalanced chromosomal abnormalities, and aberrant somatic hypermutation.[75] Somatic hypermutation is the normal programmed mutation of immunoglobulin genes in response to various antibodies, and aberrant somatic hypermutation involves malignant defects in the process that may occur in B-cell lymphomas.

Clinical Manifestations

NHLs constitute a diverse group of malignancies involving the immune system, each with different clinicopathologic features. As a result, the clinical manifestations of NHL vary and include generalized symptoms as well as site-specific signs and symptoms. NHLs originate primarily in the lymphatic system (lymph nodes, bone marrow, or spleen); however, the disease may begin in or spread to other organs (termed *extranodal disease*). Lymphadenopathy, or painless swelling of one or more lymph nodes (less than 1 centimeter), is the most common presenting sign of NHL. Enlargement of lymph nodes occurs as a direct result of infiltration of nodes with malignant lymphoma cells. Lymphadenopathy, particularly nodes that are painful and localized, is a common manifestation of inflammation, particularly during an infectious process, and the enlargement of nodes generally resolves with appropriate treatment. Conversely, nodes that are painless, have a rubbery consistency, and appear in more than one body region may be cause for concern, particularly if other signs and symptoms consistent with a malignant process are present. NHL rarely presents as localized disease; it commonly presents with multiple sites of involvement at diagnosis.

The signs and symptoms of extranodal disease are site-specific and depend on the organ or tissue that is involved. The most common site of extranodal disease is the gastrointestinal tract; patients often present with abdominal pain, swelling, and loss of appetite.[76] Other sites of extranodal involvement include the skin, liver, breast, bone, respiratory system, and oral cavity (**Figure 16.5** ■).[77–79] The clinical manifestation of extranodal disease varies extensively and depends primarily on the underlying pathology and the stage of the disease. For instance, cutaneous T-cell lymphoma may present as localized erythematous (red) patches of skin resembling an infectious process or may present as widespread disease with generalized erythroderma and pruritus.[78,80]

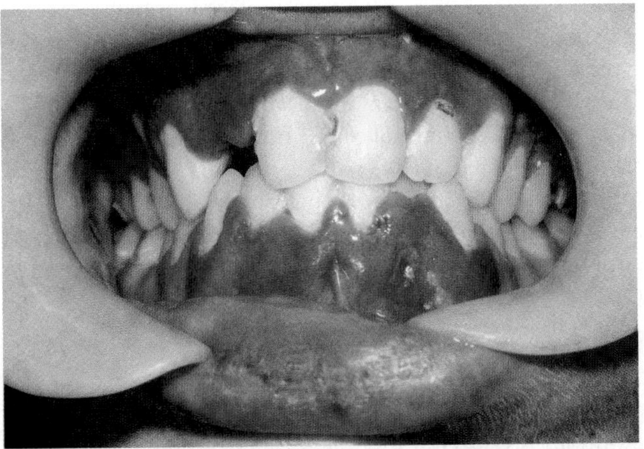

Figure 16.5 ■ Patient with mycosis fungoides, the most common type of cutaneous T-cell lymphoma.

At least some patients with NHL will present with constitutional symptoms. These include night sweats, unexplained fever, severe fatigue, weight loss, and appetite loss. The presence or absence of constitutional symptoms is included in the staging of NHL by indicating A for absence or B for presence. If the lymphoma involves the bone marrow, anemia may also be present, further contributing to fatigue. Unfortunately, no one sign or symptom is universally present in all cases of NHL, given the diversity of sites that may be involved and the underlying pathology. Typically, a combination of symptoms is present at diagnosis. This lack of consistency in clinical presentation makes it difficult for patients with signs and symptoms to determine when to seek medical attention. A thorough history and physical examination must be undertaken to begin to develop a full appreciation of the problems associated with NHL, some of which may be clinically undetectable by the patient.

Linking Pathophysiology to Diagnosis and Treatment

Treatment of NHL depends on a variety of factors, including underlying pathology, stage of the disease, whether the tumor is considered indolent or aggressive, expected prognosis, and individual characteristics such as age and comorbid conditions. Because of the wide range of potential factors that influence treatment choice and a growing understanding of the molecular biology and cellular behavior of the various NHL subtypes, treatment options continue to evolve. Common treatment modalities include surgery, chemotherapy, radiation therapy, immunotherapy, high-dose chemotherapy followed by autologous or allogeneic stem-cell transplantation, and even watchful waiting.

Surgery for NHL is generally reserved for biopsy at diagnosis, splenectomy to remove a spleen that has extensive malignant involvement, and/or surgical resection of tumors that are localized in the gastrointestinal cavity (primary gastrointestinal lymphoma). Radiation therapy refers to the therapeutic use of directed ionizing radiation to kill malignant cells by damaging the genetic material that controls cellular proliferation; therefore, it works best in cells that are dividing rapidly. In general, radiation therapy damages normal cells along with malignant cells. However, normal cells are better equipped to repair damaged DNA, while malignant cells are more likely to die. Radiation therapy is used to treat NHL in a local area. For instance, radiation therapy is used to treat nonbulky low-grade disease or bulky disease in more advanced stages or to control symptoms in the palliative setting. For instance, extensive gastrointestinal involvement may cause obstruction. In this case, radiation therapy may be given as a palliative treatment to kill as many malignant lymphoma cells as possible to relieve the obstruction.

Chemotherapy to arrest cellular proliferation of malignant lymphoma cells is the mainstay of treatment for many NHL subtypes. Chemotherapy drugs may be used singularly or in combination. For instance, low-grade or slow-growing NHL may be treated with only one drug. Intermediate- or high-grade NHLs that are considered fast-growing or aggressive are typically treated with combination chemotherapy. Because chemotherapy works best on cells that are actively dividing, chemotherapy for NHL is more effective for treating aggressive disease than indolent disease. In some cases of indolent disease without symptoms, watchful waiting, or waiting until symptoms appear, may be the treatment of choice.

One of the major drawbacks of chemotherapy is the lack of specificity. Chemotherapy targets rapidly dividing cells, both normal and malignant. Recently, treatment of NHL has focused on the use of therapy directed at the specific cells involved in the malignancy. Rituximab, a monoclonal antibody, is now considered part of standard treatment for B-cell NHL. Rituximab binds to a specific cell surface molecule (CD20) that is expressed on the surface of mature B cells and over 90% of cells involved in B-cell NHL.[81] Rituximab eliminates normal and malignant B cells from the body, providing the opportunity for regeneration of normal B cells.

Like other hematologic malignancies, additional therapy may be given for relapsed disease or disease that recurs. Salvage therapy consisting of combination chemotherapy may be given to induce another complete remission; however, remissions are short-lived, and the disease frequently recurs. Some patients may be eligible for high-dose chemotherapy following by bone- or stem-cell transplantation. This therapy, given for curative purposes, is associated with higher rates of severe toxicities.

Check Your Progress: Section 16.6

1. What is the difference between indolent and aggressive tumors in non-Hodgkin lymphoma?
2. What is the role of surgery in the treatment of NHL?
3. Describe the difference in lymphadenopathy caused by inflammation versus lymphadenopathy caused by NHL.

16.7 Hodgkin Lymphoma

Hodgkin lymphoma (HL) is a specialized form of lymphoma and represents about 11% of all lymphomas diagnosed in 2015.[1] The total number of estimated new cases of Hodgkin lymphoma in 2015 was forecast to be 9070. Hodgkin lymphoma has a very high cure rate; 75% of patients who are newly diagnosed can expect to be cured.[82] An estimated 20,940 people were expected to die from lymphoma in the United States in 2007, 1150 of them from Hodgkin lymphoma.[1]

The classification system that is most frequently used for staging HL is the Cotswolds modification of the Ann Arbor Staging System (**Table 16.2** ■).[83] Accurate staging is very important, as this guides treatment decisions. The staging system for HL is based on the number of sites involved, whether the involved lymph nodes are present on one or two sides of the diaphragm, whether the sites are considered bulky disease, the extent of extranodal involvement, and the presence or absence of constitutional symptoms. Computed tomography of the chest, abdomen, pelvis, and (if indicated) the neck and whole-body positron emission tomography should be done at the initial workup. If surgically accessible, a lymph node biopsy to obtain tissue is needed to confirm the diagnosis of HL. A bone marrow biopsy and aspirate is indicated in most cases; it helps to establish the extent of disease. Laboratory evaluation includes CBC, LDH, electrolyte evaluation, erythrocyte sedimentation rate, renal and liver function tests, and serum albumin.[84]

Table 16.2 Cotswolds Modification of the Ann Arbor Staging System for HL

Major Stage*	Criteria
I	Involvement of a single lymph node region or a single extranodal organ or site
II	Involvement of *two* or more lymph node regions on the same side of the diaphragm or localized involvement of an extranodal organ or site and *one* or more lymph node regions on the same side of the diaphragm
III	Involvement of the lymph node regions on both sides of the diaphragm, which may be accompanied by localized involvement of the extranodal organ or site involvement of the spleen or both
IV	Widespread involvement of *one* or more extranodal sites with or without associated lymph node involvement or isolated extranodal organ involvement with distant lymph node involvement

*Each stage may be subdivided into A or B according to the absence or presence of general symptoms. The so-called B symptoms may include any of the following: temperatures greater than 38°C (100.4°F), drenching night sweats, or the unexplained loss of more than 10% body weight in the previous 6 months. Bulky disease is defined as any lymph node *greater than* 10 centimeters in largest dimension or as a mediastinal mass whose largest diameter is greater than one third of the widest transverse diameter of the thorax on standard chest x-ray. Bulky disease is denoted by a subscript X.

SOURCE: Lister, T. A., Crowther, D., Sutcliffe, S. B., et al. (1989). Report of a committee convened to discuss the evaluation and staging of patients with Hodgkin's disease: Cotswolds meeting. *Journal of Clinical Oncology, 7*, 1630–1636.

HL is divided into two broad groups. The most common type of HL is classical, which includes nodular sclerosis, mixed cellularity, lymphocyte-rich, and lymphocyte-depleted subtypes. The second type, nonclassical HL, includes only the uncommon nodular lymphocyte-predominant subtype. HL subtypes are differentiated by morphology and phenotypic analysis of the Hodgkin Reed-Sternberg (HRS) cells. The HRS cells of classical HL do not have the phenotypes that are typical of normal cells.[85] Immunophenotypic analysis of classical HL shows surface markers that are positive for CD15 and CD30. Nodular lymphocyte-predominant HL is very rare and differs from classical HL in that the immunophenotype is positive for CD20 and is usually negative for CD15 and CD30.[86]

Etiology and Pathogenesis

The etiology of HL is unknown, but several risk factors have been identified: familial factors, viral exposures, and immune suppression.[84] HL is associated with a neoplastic process that affects the lymphocytes: B cells in most cases. There is a pathologic feature specific to HL that is not seen in any other type of lymphoma: the Reed-Sternberg cell. It is very important to make sure that when the Reed-Sternberg cell is identified, it is in the appropriate cellular environment of normal reactive lymphocytes, eosinophils, and histiocytes.[87]

Historically, HRS cells have been difficult to study, as there is usually a small number of these cells: less than 1% in the involved tissues. This is also why obtaining an adequate amount of specimen on biopsy is so critical to making the diagnosis. The main areas of interest in the pathogenesis in HL are the etiology of the HRS cells, the identity of the events relating to the transformation of HRS cells, and the nature of the signals that produce the characteristic tissue response.[88] A technique for establishing a B-cell origin for HRS cells in HL has been identified through polymerase chain reaction (PCR) analysis.[89]

Clinical Manifestations

HL occurs primarily in patients ages 20–30 years and patients over the age of 50 years. Patients may present with very obvious signs of disease or with nonspecific vague complaints. The asymptomatic sign may be an enlarged lymph node, which occurs in about 70% of cases. The most commonly involved site is the neck; 60–80% of patients have enlarged supraclavicular and/or cervical nodes. Enlarged lymph nodes in the axillae and the inguinal area are less common. Splenomegaly often occurs, and sometimes hepatomegaly is also present. Mediastinal masses are difficult to note on physical examination but may be present on initial presentation in up to 60% of cases. A mediastinal mass can cause retrosternal chest pain, cough, and shortness of breath. Systemic symptoms that are associated with HL include fevers, night sweats, fatigue, weight loss, alcohol-induced pain, and pruritus.[84]

Linking Pathophysiology to Diagnosis and Treatment

The main factors that determine the choice of therapy for patients with HL are the anatomic stage of disease and the presence of constitutional symptoms. Another prognostic factor that influences the choice of therapy is the presence of bulky disease, which is defined as a single site of disease 10 centimeters or greater in diameter.[84] Treatment for Hodgkin lymphoma generally entails combination chemotherapy with or without radiation.[90,91] There are multiple treatment regimens for Hodgkin lymphoma.

Monoclonal antibody therapy, such as rituximab, has been added to regimens in patients who have a CD20+ Hodgkin lymphoma.[92] Monoclonal antibody therapy works like a targeted therapy, going after only CD20+ cells instead of attacking healthy and unhealthy tissue as traditional chemotherapy does. This is a conjugated monoclonal antibody that is connected or joined with an isotope. It works to destroy an antibody that is present on B cells, but it also delivers radiation that causes a cross-fire effect, killing neighboring cells that might not express the CD20 antigen.[86] Radioimmunotherapy treatments are also available. Growth factor support is also important to help support neutrophil recovery and to keep patients on course with their treatment. Patients who do not respond to standard therapy or who relapse after chemotherapy and radiation should be given salvage therapy and then be considered for autologous stem-cell transplantation.

Check Your Progress: Section 16.7

1. Describe the criteria that are used for staging Hodgkin lymphoma using the Cotswolds Modification of the Ann Arbor Staging System.
2. What is an advantage of using monoclonal antibody therapy in the treatment of HL?
3. What are the risk factors for HL?

16.8 Multiple Myeloma

Multiple myeloma is a disease characterized by the proliferation of malignant plasma cells. It occurs primarily in individuals over age 60, and it occurs twice as often in Blacks as in Whites.[94]

Etiology and Pathogenesis

Risk factors for the development of multiple myeloma include toxin and hazardous chemical exposure (e.g., work as a firefighter), obesity, and possible genetic influences.[93] While research into this condition still needs to identify a precise mechanism, the literature points to several possibilities that are primarily associated with aneuploidy (an abnormal number of genes). The most common genetic variations appear to be associated with the inactivation of tumor-suppressing genes or the activation of genes known to be associated with B-cell proliferation. The translocation (rearrangement) of genetic sequences seems to lead to an activation of mechanisms that lead to an increase in the number of plasma cells that then move into the bone marrow.[94] The increased number of cells also leads to an increase in the production of monoclonal proteins. Each B cell tends to produce one form of antibody. In this case, the malignant B cells are producing excess amounts of one particular antibody or simply pieces of an antibody.

Clinical Manifestations

As plasma cells infiltrate into the bone marrow or other tissues, functional cell classes are displaced or have their maturation disrupted. This results in a number of changes in the bone marrow, and as seen with other conditions described in this chapter, the development of pancytopenia.

Anemia (normocytic or normochromic) is a common symptom of multiple myeloma, resulting from the infiltration of bone marrow by plasma cells. This process prevents the maturation of erythrocytes. Lacking an adequate number of red blood cells to carry oxygen can result in fatigue and pallor. The movement of plasma cells into the bone marrow can in turn lead to a loss of osteocytes and a resultant destruction of bone (**Figure 16.6** ■). This can manifest as pathologic fractures and bone pain. Bone pain is more commonly manifested in the chest or back, vertebral weakness being a common issue in patients with multiple myeloma.[95] This can result in a loss of height over time and the

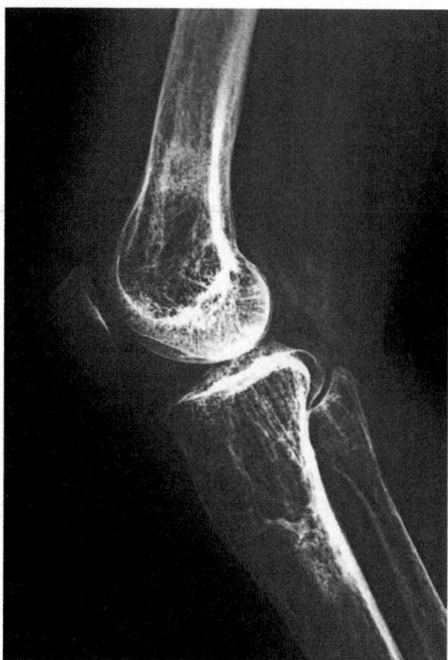

Figure 16.6 ■ X-ray of patient with multiple myeloma showing osteolytic lesions.

development of chronic lumbar pain. The resulting changes in the lumbar spine can lead to nerve compression and the development of radiculopathy. The destruction of bone cells results in the formation of bone lesions that are detectable on standard skeletal x-rays. In turn, the loss of bone cells can result in the release of calcium into the bloodstream. This hypercalcemia can result in confusion and other mental status changes and may have adverse effects on the kidney. Regardless of cause, hypercalcemia can result in the formation of renal stones and the development of renal failure. The heightened calcium level and the production of monoclonal proteins on the part of the plasma cells can result in elevated serum creatinine concentrations as a result of the strain placed on the renal system. Indeed, one of the first presenting symptoms in the hospital setting for a patient with multiple myeloma is renal insufficiency or failure.

In summary, anemia, bone pain, and apparent renal issues are considered warning indicators of the possible presence of multiple myeloma. A variety of laboratory diagnostic tests and a bone marrow biopsy are part of the diagnostic process.

Linking Pathophysiology to Diagnosis and Treatment

Treating multiple myeloma generally involves a combination of radiation and chemotherapy and often involves stem-cell transplantation. The precise treatment regimen varies in relation to the state of tumor growth and dissemination. A range of immunomodulatory medications and traditional chemotherapeutic agents are used in an attempt to reduce the number of malignant plasma cells. Research is underway to investigate more targeted therapies that could include nanoparticles and genetic agents. The process of disrupting the pathogenic process of multiple myeloma is combined with symptomatologic treatment.[94]

Anemia can be treated through a range of approaches from ferrous supplementation to transfusion of red blood cells. Agents that stimulate erythropoiesis may be incorporated into the treatment plan but can be somewhat controversial, since they cause an increase in clotting risk. Platelet transfusion may be utilized to treat thrombocytopenia, and prophylactic antibiotic therapy may be incorporated to aid in avoidance of infection due to neutropenia. At a minimum, the nurse should ensure that the patient is on infection precautions and monitor for bleeding. Rest periods should be incorporated into the treatment plan to aid the patient in managing the fatigue associated with anemia.

The movement of calcium out of the bone and into the circulation is treated through provision of hydration (to dilute the calcium concentration in the blood) and administration of a bisphosphonate to aid in strengthening of bone through effects on the activity of osteoclasts. Pathologic fractures often require either internal or external fixation. Braces may be applied to the patient's back and extremities to provide additional support and mitigate the development of fractures. Radiation and surgery may be necessary to address radiculopathy and lumbar spine issues.

Check Your Progress: Section 16.8

1. What are the risk factors for multiple myeloma?
2. Describe the process for the development of hypercalcemia in multiple myeloma.
3. What are the three conditions that are considered warning indicators of multiple myeloma?

CHAPTER SUMMARY

16.1 Chapter Overview and Case Studies

Describe the basis of disorders of white blood cells and concepts related to those disorders.

- Hematologic cancers are a group of malignancies that arise from abnormal cells in the hematopoietic system.
- Hematologic malignancies vary according to specific cell line of origin.
- Leukemia is the common name for hematologic malignances that originate in the bone marrow or blood.
- Lymphoma refers to hematologic malignancies that originate in the lymphatic tissues.
- Acute leukemia refers to blocks in early (precursor) hematopoietic cells, which render these cells less functional.
- Chronic leukemia refers to a block in the later stages of maturation and differentiation of hematopoietic cells.

- There are two major classifications of lymphomas: Hodgkin lymphoma and non-Hodgkin lymphoma.
- Hodgkin lymphoma is characterized by the presence of Reed-Sternberg cells.
- Non-Hodgkin lymphoma is a broad category of lymphoid cancers that do not contain Reed-Sternberg cells.

16.2 Acute Myelogenous Leukemia

Identify the morphologic classification, etiology and pathogenesis, and clinical manifestations of acute myelogenous leukemia and approaches to diagnosis and treatment of the condition across the lifespan.

- While the cause of acute myelogenous leukemia (AML) remains unknown, it appears associated with damage to DNA.
- AML associated risk factors include chemotherapy, ionizing radiation, long-term exposure to toxins, and smoking.
- Because of the presence of multiple variants of the AML, a classification needs to be used to help determine prognosis and treatment.
- The World Health Organization's classification system is the most commonly used classification method for AML.
- AML develops as a result of a series of mutations of genetic material in hematopoietic precursor cells that ultimately results in aberrant (abnormal) cellular proliferation.
- Genes that influence the process of mutation are referred to as proto-oncogenes and oncogenes.
- Proto-oncogenes are the normal genes that stimulate cellular division and proliferation.
- Oncogenes are mutated normal genes that allow cells to proliferate in an unregulated manner.
- The clinical manifestations of AML are a direct consequence of ineffective hematopoietic cells and overcrowding of the hematopoietic system.
- Weakness and fatigue related to anemia are common complaints in people with AML.
- Common infections include pneumonia, urinary tract infections, and upper respiratory infections.
- No one sign or symptom is universally present in all cases of AML. Typically, a combination of symptoms is generally present at diagnosis.
- Restoring normal hematopoiesis is the primary goal of treatment for all AML subtypes, and systemic chemotherapy is the cornerstone of treatment.

16.3 Acute Lymphocytic Leukemia

Identify the morphologic classification, etiology and pathogenesis, and clinical manifestations of acute lymphocytic leukemia and approaches to diagnosis and treatment of the condition across the lifespan.

- The presenting signs and symptoms of acute lymphocytic leukemia (ALL) are a direct consequence of ineffective lymphoid cells, overcrowding of the bone marrow, and infiltration of leukemic cells into other organs.
- Early signs and symptoms of ALL are generally nonspecific and include fever, bleeding, bone pain, and lymphadenopathy, all commonly occurring signs and symptoms in a variety of medical conditions.
- The treatment of ALL in children is very effective; approximately 90% of children survive at least 5 years.

16.4 Chronic Myelogenous Leukemia

Identify the morphologic classification, etiology and pathogenesis, and clinical manifestations of chronic myelogenous leukemia and approaches to diagnosis and treatment of the condition across the lifespan.

- Chronic myelogenous leukemia (CML) was the first hematologic malignancy to be clearly linked to a specific genetic marker (9;22 translocation), which was discovered in 1960 by researchers Nowell and Hungerford.
- Tyrosine kinase inhibitors, such as imatinib, are used as a targeted therapy directed at the underlying genetic defect associated with CML (Philadelphia chromosome, t(9;22)) to prevent aberrant proliferation of abnormal cells.

16.5 Chronic Lymphocytic Leukemia

Identify the morphologic classification, etiology and pathogenesis, and clinical manifestations of chronic lymphocytic leukemia and approaches to diagnosis and treatment of the condition across the lifespan.

- Chronic lymphocytic leukemia (CLL) is the most common type of leukemia, accounting for approximately 34% of all leukemia cases.
- The B lymphocytes that are involved in CLL are categorized as mature lymphocytes when viewed on a peripheral-blood smear, but they are incompetent when it comes to full immune function.
- There is no cure for CLL.

16.6 Non-Hodgkin Lymphoma

Identify the morphologic classification, etiology and pathogenesis, and clinical manifestations of non-Hodgkin lymphoma and approaches to diagnosis and treatment of the condition across the lifespan.

- Non-Hodgkin lymphoma (NHL) is a heterogeneous group of malignancies that originate in the lymphatic system.
- Constitutional symptoms frequently precede the diagnosis of NHL. These symptoms include night sweats, unexplained fever, severe fatigue, weight loss, and

appetite loss. The presence or absence of constitutional symptoms is included in the staging of NHL by indicating A for absence or B for presence.

- Treatment of NHL depends on a variety of factors, including underlying pathology, stage of the disease, whether the tumor is considered indolent or aggressive, expected prognosis and individual characteristics such as age and comorbid conditions.

16.7 Hodgkin Lymphoma

Identify the morphologic classification, etiology and pathogenesis, and clinical manifestations of Hodgkin lymphoma and approaches to diagnosis and treatment of the condition across the lifespan.

- Although the etiology of Hodgkin lymphoma (HL) is unknown, several risk factors have been identified, including familial factors, viral exposures, and immune suppression.
- HL is a neoplastic process associated most commonly with B lymphocytes. The specific cell involved is the Reed-Sternberg cell.
- The main factors that determine the choice of therapy for patients with HL include the anatomic stage of disease and the presence of constitutional symptoms. Another prognostic factor that influences the choice of therapy is the presence of bulky disease, which is defined as a single site of disease that is 10 centimeters or greater in diameter.

16.8 Multiple Myeloma

Identify the morphologic classification, etiology and pathogenesis, and clinical manifestations of multiple myeloma and approaches to diagnosis and treatment of the condition across the lifespan.

- Multiple myeloma is a disease characterized by the proliferation of malignant plasma cells.
- Malignant plasma cells come to displace other cells in the bone marrow and interfere with their function.
- As in other hematologic malignancies, pancytopenia is common.
- Bone cells are affected, resulting in pain and pathologic fractures.

REVIEW QUESTIONS

1. Which of the following conditions places a person at risk for developing chronic myelogenous leukemia?
   a. Living near a nuclear reactor accident
   b. Having a 20-pack-year history of smoking
   c. Having a sibling with CML
   d. Having received x-rays for sports injuries as a child

2. Which of the following is the most common presenting sign of non-Hodgkin lymphoma?
   a. Reed-Sternberg cells
   b. Bone pain
   c. Bleeding
   d. Enlarged lymph nodes

3. The client at stage III of the Cotswolds Modification of the Ann Arbor Staging System for Hodgkin lymphoma will exhibit which finding?
   a. A single involved lymph node
   b. Two involved lymph nodes on the same side of the diaphragm
   c. Involved lymph nodes on both sides of the diaphragm
   d. Widespread involvement of extranodal sites

4. Which of the following statements made by the parent of a child with acute lymphocytic leukemia demonstrates understanding of the treatment plan?
   a. "Induction therapy is a cure for ALL."
   b. "Consolidation therapy occurs if the disease returns."
   c. "Induction therapy is repeated until the disease is in remission."
   d. "Consolidation therapy eradicates the residual disease."

5. Which of the following clients is most at risk for developing chronic lymphocytic leukemia?
   a. A 70-year-old White man
   b. A 60-year-old Asian man
   c. A 40-year-old White man
   d. A 20-year-old Asian man

6. A client with acute myelogenous leukemia has pancytopenia. The nurse observes this client for which of the following conditions?
   a. Anemia, neutropenia, and thrombocytopenia
   b. Leukocytosis, polycythemia, and thrombocytopenia
   c. Anemia, neutropenia, and thrombocytosis
   d. Leukocytosis, thrombocytopenia, and polycythemia

7. Which of the following laboratory findings is most likely in the client with multiple myeloma?
   a. Hyperkalemia
   b. Hyponatremia
   c. Hypercalcemia
   d. Hypoglycemia

8. The nurse is admitting a client with a possible diagnosis of multiple myeloma. Which of the following findings would the nurse expect in this client?
   a. Chest pain
   b. Bone pain
   c. Joint pain
   d. Abdominal pain

ANSWERS

Answers to Review Questions can be found in Appendix A. Answers to Case Study and Check Your Progress questions are available on the faculty resources site. Please consult with your instructor.

RECOMMENDED WEBSITES

Hodgkin Disease (American Cancer Society)
https://www.cancer.org/cancer/hodgkin-lymphoma.html

Leukemia (American Cancer Society)
https://www.cancer.org/cancer/leukemia.html

Leukemia & Lymphoma Society
www.lls.org

Leukemia—Patient Version (National Cancer Institute)
https://www.cancer.gov/types/leukemia

Lymphoma—Patient Version (National Cancer Institute)
https://www.cancer.gov/types/lymphoma

Multiple Myeloma (American Cancer Society)
https://www.cancer.org/cancer/multiple-myeloma.html

Non-Hodgkin Lymphoma (Adults) (American Cancer Society)
https://www.cancer.org/cancer/non-hodgkin-lymphoma.html

Plasma Cell Neoplasms (Including Multiple Myeloma)—Patient Version (National Cancer Institute)
https://www.cancer.gov/types/myeloma

REFERENCES

1. Siegel, R. L., Miller, K. D., & Jemal, A. (2015). Cancer statistics, 2015. *CA: A Cancer Journal for Clinicians, 65*, 5–29.
2. Smith, M. A., Altekruse, S. F., Adamson, P. C., Reaman, G. H., & Seibel, N. L. (2014). Declining childhood and adolescent cancer mortality. *Cancer, 120*, 2497–2506.
3. Smith, R. E. (2003). Risk for the development of treatment-related acute myelocytic leukemia and myelodysplastic syndrome among patients with breast cancer: Review of the literature and the National Surgical Adjuvant Breast and Bowel Project experience. *Clinical Breast Cancer, 4*, 273–279.
4. Praga, C., Bergh, J., Bliss, J., et al. (2005). Risk of acute myeloid leukemia and myelodysplastic syndrome in trials of adjuvant epirubicin for early breast cancer: Correlation with doses of epirubicin and cyclophosphamide. *Journal of Clinical Oncology, 23*, 4179–4191.
5. Yoshinaga, S., Mabuchi, K., Sigurdson, AJ., Doody, M. M., & Ron, E. (2004). Cancer risks among radiologists and radiologic technologists: Review of epidemiologic studies. *Radiology, 233*, 313–321.
6. Bizzozero, O. J., Jr., Johnson, K. G., & Ciocco, A. (1996). Radiation-related leukemia in Hiroshima and Nagasaki, 1946–1964. I: Distribution, incidence and appearance time. *New England Journal of Medicine, 274*, 1095–1101.
7. Sorahan, T., Kinlen, L. J., & Doll, R. (2005). Cancer risks in a historical UK cohort of benzene exposed workers. *Occupational and Environmental Medicine, 62*, 231–236.
8. Kirkeleit, J., Riise, T., Bratveit, M., & Moen, B. E. (2008). Increased risk of acute myelogenous leukemia and multiple myeloma in a historical cohort of upstream petroleum workers exposed to crude oil. *Cancer Causes & Control, 19*, 13–23.
9. Stenehjem, J. S., Kjaerheim, K., Bratveit, M., et al. (2015). Benzene exposure and risk of lymphohaematopoietic cancers in 25000 offshore oil industry workers. *British Journal of Cancer, 112*, 1603–1612.
10. Musselman, J. R., Blair, C. K., Cerhan, J. R., Nguyen, P., Hirsch, B., & Ross, J. A. (2013). Risk of adult acute and chronic myeloid leukemia with cigarette smoking and cessation. *Cancer Epidemiology, 37*, 410–416.
11. Broberg, K., Hoglund, M., Gustafsson, C., et al. (2007). Genetic variant of the human homologous recombination-associated gene RMI1 (S455N) impacts the risk of AML/MDS and malignant melanoma. *Cancer Letters, 258*, 38–44.
12. Bochtler, T., Frohling, S., & Kramer, A. (2015). Role of chromosomal aberrations in clonal diversity and progression of acute myeloid leukemia. *Leukemia, 29*, 1243–1252.
13. Hasle, H., Clemmensen, I. H., & Mikkelsen, M. (2000). Risks of leukaemia and solid tumours in individuals with Down's syndrome. *Lancet, 355*, 165–169.
14. Anensen, N., Skavland, J., Stapnes, C., et al. (2006). Acute myelogenous leukemia in a patient with Li-Fraumeni syndrome treated with valproic acid, theophyllamine and all-trans retinoic acid: A case report. *Leukemia, 20*, 734–736.
15. Vardiman, J. W., Thiele, J., Arber, D. A., et al. (2009). The 2008 revision of the World Health Organization (WHO) classification of myeloid neoplasms and acute leukemia: Rationale and important changes. *Blood, 114*(5), 937–951.
16. Grimwade, D., Hills, R. K., Moorman, A. V., et al. (2010). Refinement of cytogenetic classification in acute myeloid leukemia: Determination of prognostic significance of rare recurring chromosomal abnormalities among 5876 younger adult patients treated in the United Kingdom Medical Research Council trials. *Blood, 116*, 354–365.
17. Yanada, M., Borthakur, G., Garcia-Manero, G., et al. (2008). Blood counts at time of complete remission provide additional independent prognostic information in acute myeloid leukemia. *Leukemia Research, 32*, 1505–1509.
18. Davis, C. D. (2008). Vitamin D and cancer: Current dilemmas and future research needs. *American Journal of Clinical Nutrition, 88*, 565S–559S.
19. Smith, T. J., Khatcheressian, J., Lyman, G. H., et al. (2006). 2006 update of recommendations for the use of white blood cell growth factors: An evidence-based clinical practice guideline. *Journal of Clinical Oncology, 2006;24*, 3187–3205.
20. Shah, A., & Coleman, M. P. (2007). Increasing incidence of childhood leukaemia: A controversy re-examined. *British Journal of Cancer, 97*, 1009–1012.
21. Ries, L., Melbert, D., Krapcho, M., et al. (2008). *SEER cancer statistics review, 1975–2005*. Bethesda, MD: National Cancer Institute. Available at https://seer.cancer.gov/archive/csr/1975_2005
22. Ward, E., DeSantis, C., Robbins, A., Kohler, B., & Jemal, A. (2014). Childhood and adolescent cancer statistics, 2014. *CA: A Cancer Journal for Clinicians, 64*, 83–103.
23. National Cancer Institute. (2017). *Childhood acute lymphoblastic leukemia treatment (PDQ®): Health professional version.*

Available at https://www.cancer.gov/types/leukemia/child-all-treatmen-pdq#section/all
24. Smith, M., Arthur, D., Camitta, B., et al. (1996). Uniform approach to risk classification and treatment assignment for children with acute lymphoblastic leukemia. *Journal of Clinical Oncology, 14*, 18–24.
25. Burger, B., Zimmermann, M., Mann, G., et al. (2003). Diagnostic cerebrospinal fluid examination in children with acute lymphoblastic leukemia: Significance of low leukocyte counts with blasts or traumatic lumbar puncture. *Journal of Clinical Oncology, 21*, 184–188.
26. Pui, C. H., Boyett, J. M., Relling, M. V., et al. (1999). Sex differences in prognosis for children with acute lymphoblastic leukemia. *Journal of Clinical Oncology, 17*, 818–824.
27. Pui, C. H., Sandlund, J. T., Pei, D., et al. (2004). Improved outcome for children with acute lymphoblastic leukemia: Results of Total Therapy Study XIIIB at St Jude Children's Research Hospital. *Blood, 104*, 2690–2966.
28. Pui, C. H., Sandlund, J. T., Pei, D., et al. (2003). Results of therapy for acute lymphoblastic leukemia in black and white children. *Jama, 290*, 2001–2007.
29. Bhatia S. (2004). Influence of race and socioeconomic status on outcome of children treated for childhood acute lymphoblastic leukemia. *Current Opinion in Pediatrics, 16*, 9–14.
30. Ross, J. A., Davies, S. M., Potter, J. D., & Robison, L. L. (1994). Epidemiology of childhood leukemia, with a focus on infants. *Epidemiologic Reviews, 16*, 243–272.
31. Whitlock, J. A. (2006). Down syndrome and acute lymphoblastic leukaemia. *British Journal of Haematology, 135*, 595–602.
32. Stiller, C. A., Chessells, J. M., & Fitchett, M. (1004). Neurofibromatosis and childhood leukaemia/lymphoma: A population-based UKCCSG study. *British Journal of Cancer, 70*, 969–972.
33. Woods, W. G., Roloff, J. S., Lukens, J. N., & Krivit, W. (1981). The occurrence of leukemia in patients with the Shwachman syndrome. *Journal of Pediatrics, 99*, 425–428.
34. Passarge, E. (1991). Bloom's syndrome: The German experience. *Annales de Genetique, 34*, 179–197.
35. Taylor, A. M., Metcalfe, J. A., Thick, J., & Mak, Y. F. (1996). Leukemia and lymphoma in ataxia telangiectasia. *Blood, 87*, 423–438.
36. Pui, C. H., Relling, M. V., & Downing, J. R. (2004). Acute lymphoblastic leukemia. *New England Journal of Medicine, 350*, 1535–1548.
37. Armstrong, S. A., & Look, A. T. (2005). Molecular genetics of acute lymphoblastic leukemia. *Journal of Clinical Oncology, 23*, 6306–6315.
38. Mullighan, C. G. (2013). Genomic characterization of childhood acute lymphoblastic leukemia. *Seminars in Hematology, 50*, 314–324.
39. Mullighan C. G. (2012). The molecular genetic makeup of acute lymphoblastic leukemia. *Hematology, 2012*(1), 389–396.
40. Sinigaglia, R., Gigante, C., Bisinella, G., Varotto, S., Zanesco, L., & Turra, S. (2008). Musculoskeletal manifestations in pediatric acute leukemia. *Journal of Pediatric Orthopedics, 28*, 20–28.
41. Pui, C. H., & Evans, W. E. (2006). Treatment of acute lymphoblastic leukemia. *New England Journal of Medicine, 354*, 166–178.
42. Vilmer, E., Suciu, S., Ferster, A., et al. (2000). Long-term results of three randomized trials (58831, 58832, 58881) in childhood acute lymphoblastic leukemia: A CLCG-EORTC report. Children Leukemia Cooperative Group. *Leukemia, 14*, 2257–2266.
43. Larson, R. A. (2004). The U.S. trials in adult acute lymphoblastic leukemia. *Annals of Hematology, 83*(Suppl. 1), S127–S128.
44. Arico, M., Baruchel, A., Bertrand, Y., et al. (2005). The seventh international childhood acute lymphoblastic leukemia workshop report: Palermo, Italy, January 29–30, 2005. *Leukemia, 19*, 1145–1152.
45. Cortes, J. E., Talpaz, M., O'Brien, S., et al. (2006). Staging of chronic myeloid leukemia in the imatinib era: An evaluation of the World Health Organization proposal. *Cancer, 106*, 1306–1315.
46. Brandt, L. (1985). Environmental factors and leukaemia. *Medical Oncology and Tumor Pharmacotherapy, 2*, 7–10.
47. Nowell, P. C., & Hungerford, D. A. (1960). Chromosome studies on normal and leukemic human leukocytes. *Journal of the National Cancer Institute, 25*, 85–109.
48. Rowley, J. D. (1973). Letter: A new consistent chromosomal abnormality in chronic myelogenous leukaemia identified by quinacrine fluorescence and Giemsa staining. *Nature, 243*, 290–293.
49. Ren, R. (2005). Mechanisms of BCR-ABL in the pathogenesis of chronic myelogenous leukaemia. *Nature Reviews, 5*, 172–183.
50. Lichtman, M. A., Kaushansky, D., Prchal J. T., Levin, M., Burns, L. J., & Armitage, J. O. (2017). *Williams manual of hematology* (9th ed.). New York, NY: McGraw-Hill.
51. Savage, D. G., Szydlo, R. M., & Goldman, J. M. (1997). Clinical features at diagnosis in 430 patients with chronic myeloid leukaemia seen at a referral centre over a 16-year period. *British Journal of Haematology, 96*, 111–116.
52. Savage, D. G., Szydlo, R. M., Chase, A., Apperley, J. F., & Goldman, J. M. (1997). Bone marrow transplantation for chronic myeloid leukaemia: The effects of differing criteria for defining chronic phase on probabilities of survival and relapse. *British Journal of Haematology, 99*, 30–35.
53. Gale, R. P., Cozen, W., Goodman, M. T., Wang, F. F., & Bernstein, L. (2000). Decreased chronic lymphocytic leukemia incidence in Asians in Los Angeles County. *Leukemia Research, 24*, 665–669.
54. Rai, K. R., Sawitsky, A., Cronkite, E. P., Chanana, A. D., Levy, R. N., & Pasternack, B. S. (1975). Clinical staging of chronic lymphocytic leukemia. *Blood, 46*, 219–234.
55. Binet, J. L., Auquier, A., Dighiero, G., et al. (1981). A new prognostic classification of chronic lymphocytic leukemia derived from a multivariate survival analysis. *Cancer, 48*, 198–206.
56. Rai, K. R., & Han, T. (1990). Prognostic factors and clinical staging in chronic lymphocytic leukemia. *Hematology/Oncology Clinics of North America, 4*, 447–456.
57. Zent, C. S., & Kay, N. E. (2007). Chronic lymphocytic leukemia: Biology and current treatment. *Current Oncology Reports, 9*, 345–352.
58. Goldin, L. R., & Caporaso, N. E. (2007). Family studies in chronic lymphocytic leukaemia and other lymphoproliferative tumours. *British Journal of Haematology, 139*, 774–779.
59. Inamdar, K. V., & Bueso-Ramos, C. E. (2007). Pathology of chronic lymphocytic leukemia: An update. *Annals of Diagnostic Pathology, 11*, 363–389.
60. Juliusson, G., Oscier, D. G., Fitchett, M., et al. (1990). Prognostic subgroups in B-cell chronic lymphocytic leukemia defined by specific chromosomal abnormalities. *New England Journal of Medicine, 323*, 720–724.
61. Hockenbery, D., Nunez, G., Milliman, C., Schreiber R. D., & Korsmeyer, S. J. (1990). Bcl-2 is an inner mitochondrial membrane protein that blocks programmed cell death. *Nature, 348*, 334–336.
62. Cordone, I., Masi, S., Mauro, F. R., et al. (1998). p53 expression in B-cell chronic lymphocytic leukemia: A marker of disease progression and poor prognosis. *Blood, 91*, 4342–4349.
63. Dohner, H., Stilgenbauer, S., Benner, A., et al. (2000). Genomic aberrations and survival in chronic lymphocytic leukemia. *New England Journal of Medicine, 343*, 1910–1916.
64. Cheson, B. D., Bennett, J. M., Grever, M., et al. (1996). National Cancer Institute-sponsored Working Group guidelines for chronic lymphocytic leukemia: Revised guidelines for diagnosis and treatment. *Blood, 87*, 4990–4997.
65. Lipshutz, M. D., Mir, R., Rai, K. R., & Sawitsky, A. (1980). Bone marrow biopsy and clinical staging in chronic lymphocytic leukemia. *Cancer, 46*, 1422–1427.
66. Keating, M. J., O'Brien, S., Albitar, M., et al. (2005). Early results of a chemoimmunotherapy regimen of fludarabine, cyclophosphamide, and rituximab as initial therapy for chronic lymphocytic leukemia. *Journal of Clinical Oncology, 23*, 4079–4088.
67. Montserrat, E., Sanchez-Bisono, J., Vinolas, N., & Rozman C. (1986). Lymphocyte doubling time in chronic lymphocytic leukaemia: Analysis of its prognostic significance. *British Journal of Haematology, 62*, 567–575.

68. Ghia, P., Ferreri, A. M., & Galigaris-Cappio, F. (2007). Chronic lymphocytic leukemia. *Critical Reviews in Oncology/Hematology, 64*, 234–246.
69. Pileri, S. A., Milani, M., Fraternali-Orcioni, G., & Sabattini, E. (1998). From the R.E.A.L. Classification to the upcoming WHO scheme: A step toward universal categorization of lymphoma entities? *Annals of Oncology, 9*, 607–612.
70. Steinmaus, C., Smith, A. H., Jones, R. M., & Smith, M. T. (2008). Meta-analysis of benzene exposure and non-Hodgkin lymphoma: Biases could mask an important association. *Occupational and Environmental Medicine, 65*, 371–378.
71. Zhang, Y., Sanjose, S. D., Bracci, P. M., et al. (2008). Personal use of hair dye and the risk of certain subtypes of non-Hodgkin lymphoma. *American Journal of Epidemiology, 167*, 1321–1331.
72. Boffetta, P., & de Vocht, F. (2007). Occupation and the risk of non-Hodgkin lymphoma. *Cancer Epidemiology, Biomarkers & Prevention, 16*, 369–372.
73. Fritschi, L., Benke, G., Hughes, A. M., et al. (2005). Risk of non-Hodgkin lymphoma associated with occupational exposure to solvents, metals, organic dusts and PCBs (Australia). *Cancer Causes & Control, 16*, 599–607.
74. Meijerink, J. P. (1997). t(14;18), a journey to eternity. *Leukemia, 11*, 2175–2187.
75. Halldorsdottir, A. M., Fruhwirth, M., Deutsch, A., et al. (2008). Quantifying the role of aberrant somatic hypermutation in transformation of follicular lymphoma. *Leukemia Research, 32*, 1015–1021.
76. Al-Akwaa, A. M., Siddiqui, N., & Al-Mofleh, I. A. (2004). Primary gastric lymphoma. *World Journal of Gastroenterology, 10*, 5–11.
77. Iida, T., Iwahashi, M., Nakamura, M., et al. (2007). Primary hepatic low-grade B-cell lymphoma of MALT-type associated with Helicobacter pylori infection. *Hepato-gastroenterology, 54*, 1898–1901.
78. Willemze, R., & Meijer, C. J. (2006). Classification of cutaneous T-cell lymphoma: From Alibert to WHO-EORTC. *Journal of Cutaneous Pathology, 33*(Suppl. 1), 18–26.
79. Demirci, H., Shields, C. L., Karatza, E. C., & Shields, J. A. (2008). Orbital lymphoproliferative tumors: Analysis of clinical features and systemic involvement in 160 cases. *Ophthalmology, 115*(9), 1626–1631.
80. Jayaraman, A. G., Cassarino, D., Advani, R., Kim, Y. H., Tsai, E., & Kohler, S. (2006). Cutaneous involvement by angioimmunoblastic T-cell lymphoma: A unique histologic presentation, mimicking an infectious etiology. *Journal of Cutaneous Pathology, 33*(Suppl. 2), 6–11.
81. Genentech. (2008). *Highlights of the prescribing information*. Available at http://www.gene.com/gene/products/information/pdf/rituxan-prescribing.pdf
82. Brenner, H., Gondos, A., & Pulte, D. (2008). Ongoing improvement in long-term survival of patients with Hodgkin disease at all ages and recent catch-up of older patients. *Blood, 111*, 2977–2983.
83. Lister, T. A., Crowther, D., Sutcliffe, S. B., et al. (1989). Report of a committee convened to discuss the evaluation and staging of patients with Hodgkin's disease: Cotswolds meeting. *Journal of Clinical Oncology, 7*, 1630–1636.
84. Ansell, S. M., & Armitage, J. O. (2006). Management of Hodgkin lymphoma. *Mayo Clinic Proceedings, 81*, 419–426.
85. Harris, N. L., Jaffe, E. S., Diebold, J., et al. (1999). World Health Organization classification of neoplastic diseases of the hematopoietic and lymphoid tissues: Report of the Clinical Advisory Committee meeting, Airlie House, Virginia, November 1997. *Journal of Clinical Oncology, 17*, 3835–3849.
86. Noonan, K. (2007). Introduction to B-cell disorders. *Clinical Journal of Oncology Nursing, 11*, 3–12.
87. Marafioti, T., Hummel, M., Foss, H. D., et al. (2000). Hodgkin and Reed-Sternberg cells represent an expansion of a single clone originating from a germinal center B-cell with functional immunoglobulin gene rearrangements but defective immunoglobulin transcription. *Blood, 95*, 1443–1450.
88. Kuppers, R., Schwering, I., Brauninger, A., Rajewsky, K., & Hansmann, M. L. (2002). Biology of Hodgkin's lymphoma. *Annals of Oncology, 13*(Suppl. 1), 11–18.
89. Re, D., Tyler, R. K., Behringer, K., & Diehl, V. (2005). From Hodgkin disease to Hodgkin lymphoma: Biologic insights and therapeutic potential. *Blood, 105*, 4553–4560.
90. Diehl, V., Engert, A., & Re, D. (2007). New strategies for the treatment of advanced-stage Hodgkin's lymphoma. *Hematology/Oncology Clinics of North America, 21*, 897–914.
91. Macdonald, D. A., & Connors, J. M. (2007). New strategies for the treatment of early stages of Hodgkin's lymphoma. *Hematology/Oncology Clinics of North America, 21*, 871–880.
92. Rehwald, U., Schulz, H., Reiser, M., et al. (2003). Treatment of relapsed CD20+ Hodgkin lymphoma with the monoclonal antibody rituximab is effective and well tolerated: Results of a phase 2 trial of the German Hodgkin Lymphoma Study Group. *Blood, 101*, 420–424.
93. Sergentanis, T. N., Zagouri, F., Tsilimidos, G., Tsagianni, A., Tseliou, M., Dimopoulos, M. A., & Psaltopoulou, T. (2015). Risk factors for multiple myeloma: A systematic review of meta-analyses. *Clinical Lymphoma, Myeloma & Leukemia, 15*(10), 563–577. e1-3. doi:10.1016/j.clml.2015.06.003.
94. Mutlu, P., Kiraz, Y., Gunduz, U., & Baran Y. (2015). An update on molecular biology and drug resistance mechanisms of multiple myeloma. *Critical Reviews in Oncology/Hematology, 96*(3), 413–424. doi:10.1016/j.critrevonc.2015.07.003
95. Rajkumar, S. W. (2017). Clinical features, laboratory manifestations, and diagnosis of multiple myeloma. *UpToDate*. Available at http://www.uptodate.com/contents/clinical-features-laboratory-manifestations-and-diagnosis-of-multiple-myeloma.

Unit VI
Disorders of Oxygenation

Injury or illness can impair or interrupt one or more of the processes that promote oxygenation, the process whereby humans transport oxygen we breathe to perfuse oxygen to tissues via oxygen-carrying red blood cells. The transfer of oxygen from the pulmonary system to the bloodstream takes place in the lungs, where alveoli exchange oxygen for carbon dioxide with the capillaries. Infections, neoplasms, acute inflammatory disorders, and chronic lung diseases can all contribute to impairment or interruption of oxygenation. For example:

- Restrictive lung disorders decrease the volume of airflow to the lungs by preventing expansion of the pulmonary structures and/or decreasing the compliance (elasticity) of the lungs or chest wall. Damage to the alveolar epithelium and capillaries may occur, causing ventilation and perfusion abnormalities and/or diffusion defects, which can cause hypoxemia (a decrease in arterial oxygen level).
- Inflammation characteristic of obstructive lung disorders contributes to dyspnea, defined as labored breathing or shortness of breath, a cardinal symptom of patients with asthma and chronic obstructive pulmonary disease (COPD). In addition to mucosal inflammation contributing to airway obstruction, constriction of bronchial smooth muscle may occur and be further exacerbated by an accumulation of mucus in the airway.
- Infectious respiratory disorders may cause impaired delivery of oxygen to the alveoli or alterations in intra-alveolar gas exchange.
- Respiratory failure is defined as an inadequate gas exchange that is demonstrated by hypoxemia with or without hypercapnia (increase in arterial carbon dioxide levels). Respiratory failure can result problems in any of the multiple neural pathways or systems that control respiration. These pathways and systems include the central nervous system that controls breathing patterns, peripheral nerves for sensory perception, and motor control of respiration, respiratory muscles, ventilation, gas exchange at the alveolar capillary wall, the cardiovascular system, and mitochondrial oxygenation.

Even mild cases of labored, difficult breathing can cause anxiety in patients and their families, especially for young children and their parents. Anxiety itself can be an invisible sign of dyspnea and an early indicator of hypoxia. In patients with chronic pulmonary disorders who have a high tolerance for symptom burden, anxiety may indicate unrelieved hypoxia even after treatment.[1,2] Assessment and monitoring of clients suspected of having a respiratory illness or pulmonary injury includes assessing for dyspnea and anxiety.

Any impairment or interruption in oxygenation increases the work of breathing and results in other organs (e.g., heart and kidneys) attempting to compensate in order to insure tissue perfusion and maintain homeostasis. *Work of breathing* refers to the energy it takes to accomplish the act of breathing. Lung compliance, airway patency and resistance, and the use of accessory muscles are factors that affect the work of breathing. The resulting increased metabolic demand experienced by individuals with chronic impairment or disruption in oxygenation exhibits in a number of ways over time. Early signs include irritability and fatigue. Later, patients experience difficulty maintaining a healthy weight, difficulty engaging in simple activities, compromised sleep, and gastroesophageal reflux, among others. Patients with disorders of oxygenation require patience, assistance in managing activities of daily living to reduce energy demands, prompt assessment of changes in status, and rest. Nurses who provide interventions to promote oxygenation and reduce metabolic demands will help ensure improved oxygenation and better clinical outcomes for their patients.[1,3]

References

1. Registered Nurses of Ontario. (2010). Nursing Care of Dyspnea: The 6th Vital Sign in Individuals with Chronic Obstructive Pulmonary Disease (COPD) Guideline supplement. Available from: http://rnao.ca/sites/rnao-ca/files/Nursing_Care_of_Dyspnea_-The_6th_Vital_Sign_in_Individuals_with_Chronic_Obstructive_Pulmonary_Disease.pdf
2. Doyle, G. R. & McCutcheon, J. A. (2015). *Clinical Procedures for Safer Care.* British Columbia Institute of Technology. Available from: https://opentextbc.ca/clinicalskills/chapter/5-3-causes-of-hypoxemia-2/
3. Bauldoff, G. S. (2012). When breathing is a burden: How to help patients with COPD. *American Nurse Today, 7*(8). Available from: https://www.americannursetoday.com/when-breathing-is-a-burden-how-to-help-patients-with-copd-2/

Neoplastic, Infectious, and Pulmonary Vascular Lung Disorders

- Malignant lung tumors
- Benign lung lesions
- Infectious diseases of the upper respiratory tract
- Infectious diseases of the lower respiratory tract
- Pulmonary vascular disorders

Work of Breathing

- ***Normal breathing:*** The energy expended to inhale and exhale uses about 5% of total body oxygen consumption

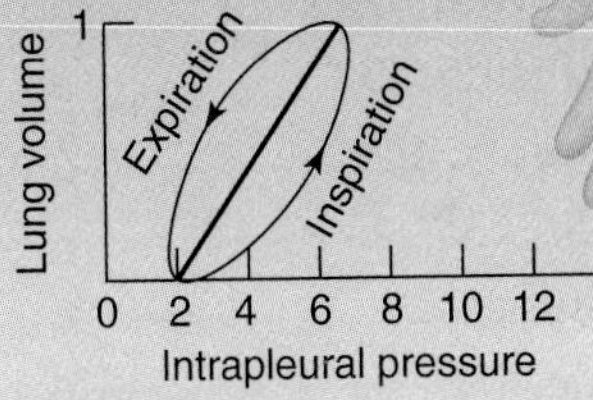

- ***Restrictive disease:*** It's harder to breath because of greater elastic force.

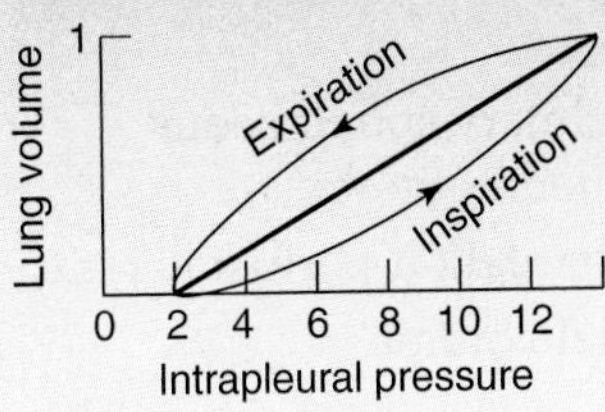

- ***Obstructive disease:*** It's harder to breath because airway resistance increases.

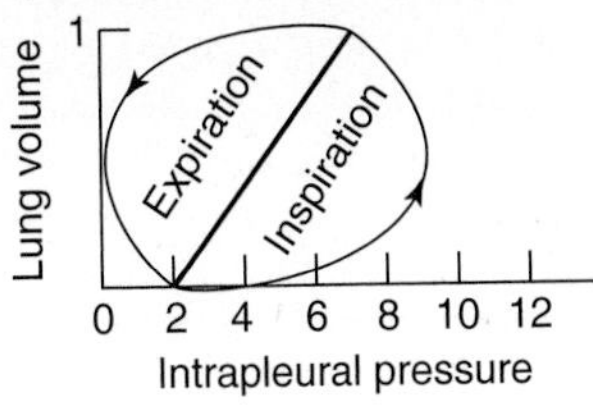

Restrictive Lung Disorders

- Disorders of pulmonary expansion
  - Aspiration
  - Atelectasis
  - Pneumothorax
  - Pleural effusion
  - Chest wall abnormalities
- Disorders of pulmonary compliance
  - Idiopathic pulmonary fibrosis
  - Sarcoidosis

Obstructive Lung Disease

- Alterations in respiratory structure and function
- Asthma
- Chronic obstructive pulmonary disease (COPD)
- Cystic fibrosis (CF)
- Bronchiectasis

Respiratory Failure

- Respiratory failure: Type I and Type II
- Disorders causing respiratory failure
  - Acute respiratory distress syndrome (ARDS)
  - Infant respiratory distress syndrome (IRDS)
  - Pulmonary edema
  - Advanced COPD

Chapter 17
Restrictive Lung Disorders

Nancy Pogue and Linda Blevins

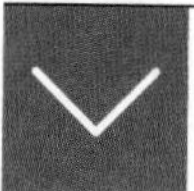

Chapter Outline and Learning Outcomes

17.1 Chapter Overview and Case Studies

Explain the factors that alter ventilation and oxygenation in restrictive lung disorders and concepts related to restrictive lung disorders.

17.2 Restrictive Lung Disorders of Pulmonary Expansion

Differentiate the causes, classification, underlying pathogenesis, and clinical manifestations of restrictive lung disorders that primarily limit pulmonary expansion and approaches to diagnosis and treatment of those conditions across the lifespan.

17.3 Restrictive Lung Disorders of Pulmonary Compliance

Differentiate the causes, classification, underlying pathogenesis, and clinical manifestations of restrictive lung disorders that primarily decrease pulmonary compliance and approaches to diagnosis and treatment of those conditions across the lifespan.

KEY TERMS

Aspiration, 427
Atelectasis, 428
Bleb, 429
Chylothorax, 432
Empyema, 432
Exudate, 432
Flail chest, 433
Hemothorax, 432
Idiopathic interstitial pneumonia (IIP), 434
Idiopathic pulmonary fibrosis (IPF), 434
Intercostal retraction, 429
Kyphoscoliosis, 433
Pectus carinatum, 433
Pectus excavatum, 433
Pleural effusion, 431
Pneumothorax, 429
Sarcoidosis, 435
Thoracentesis, 429
Transudate, 432

ABBREVIATIONS

DOE—dyspnea on exertion
DL_{CO}—carbon monoxide diffusing capacity in the lung
HRCT—high-resolution computed tomography
IIP—idiopathic interstitial pneumonias
IPF—idiopathic pulmonary fibrosis
PFTs—pulmonary function tests
PSP—primary spontaneous pneumothorax
V-Q—ventilation-perfusion ratio
VT—tidal volume

17.1 Chapter Overview and Case Studies

Restrictive lung disorders decrease the volume of airflow to the lungs by preventing expansion of the pulmonary structures and/or by decreasing the compliance (elasticity) of the lungs or chest wall. The restriction alters breathing patterns and can interfere with oxygenation. More muscle work is required for each breath to maintain adequate ventilation when airflow is restricted. In addition, many restrictive disorders damage the alveolar epithelium and capillaries, causing ventilation and perfusion abnormalities and/or diffusion defects, which can cause hypoxemia. The onset of the restriction can be acute (e.g., aspiration of gastric contents) or chronic (e.g., pulmonary fibrosis). In this chapter, we focus on the most commonly seen restrictive lung disorders, such as aspiration, pneumothorax, pleural effusion, chest wall abnormalities, idiopathic pulmonary fibrosis, and sarcoidosis. Some restrictive disorders, such as acute respiratory distress syndrome, are covered in other chapters. **Table 17.1** ■ lists some uncommon restrictive pulmonary disorders.

To help differentiate the etiologies of disorders discussed in this chapter, restrictive lung disorders are categorized on the basis of two primary disease manifestations: impaired lung expansion and decreased lung compliance.

Concepts Related to Restrictive Lung Disorders

Ultimately, all restrictive lung disorders can impair oxygenation. Because oxygen is essential to cellular function, decreased oxygenation can result in the destruction of cells and tissues. At the organ level, even limited periods of decreased oxygenation can cause numerous problems, including decreased cerebral perfusion and impaired cognition. Of course, at the organismal level, adequate oxygenation is essential to life. **Figure 17.1** ■ illustrates concepts related to restrictive lung disorders.

Altered Breathing Patterns

When chest expansion is difficult because of a stiff, noncompliant chest wall or stiff lungs, more muscle work is required for a normal breath, so the body conserves energy with shallow, rapid respirations. The problem with shallow breathing is that the anatomic dead space must be filled with each breath before any air reaches alveoli, so alveolar ventilation is limited. The anatomic dead space, which includes the conducting airways from the mouth or nose to the terminal bronchioles, averages approximately 150 mL of air. Because the individual with a restrictive lung disorder will conserve energy by breathing shallowly at a faster rate, tachypnea is a common symptom in these disorders. The calculations for alveolar ventilation are shown in Box 17.1.

Impaired Oxygenation

A pathophysiologic process can interfere with the volume and rate of airflow anywhere along the pathway from the nose or mouth to the terminal bronchioles, which house the alveoli. The decreased airflow can be caused by airway obstruction, decreased compliance of the lungs or chest wall, respiratory muscle weakness due to a neuromuscular disorder, medication-induced respiratory depression, disorders that increase the distance between alveoli and blood, or a combination of factors. The key factors in determining oxygen diffusion in restrictive lung disorders are the oxygen

Table 17.1 Uncommon Pulmonary Disorders with Unknown Etiologies

Disease	Pathophysiology	Characteristics	Diagnosis and Treatment
Bronchiolitis obliterans (not the same as BOOP)	Inflammation with bronchiole fibrosis that partially or completely obliterates airways. Associated with industrial inhalants.	Life-threatening nonreversible obstructive lung disease with fixed airways.	Lung biopsy for definitive diagnosis. Lung transplantation is often necessary.
Bronchiolitis obliterans organizing pneumonia (BOOP), a.k.a. cryptogenic organizing pneumonia (COP)	Inflammation of bronchioles, alveoli, and surrounding tissue with exudates that eventually undergo fibrosis. May be triggered by a variety of causes, including infections, organ transplantation, drugs, and toxic fumes.[1]	Manifestations include shortness of breath, cough, bilateral crackles, and lung opacities visible on CT scan.[1]	Clinically and radiologically resembles pneumonia, but the primary etiology involves activation of proinflammatory cytokines; therefore, corticosteroids are the preferred initial therapy. Although antibiotics may be included in the treatment regimen, most individuals recover with systemic corticosteroids.[1]
Pulmonary Langerhans cell histiocytosis (PLCH)	Smoke-related interstitial disease, a form of Langerhans histiocytosis that affects smokers	Pulmonary fibrosis or pulmonary hypertension may develop as complications	Some individuals recover after stopping smoking.
Chronic eosinophilic pneumonia	Eosinophils accumulate in the lung. Intrinsic etiology: autoimmune, cancer or idiopathic Extrinsic etiology: inhaled or ingested factors (e.g., drugs, bacterial or parasitic infections)	Cough, fever, increasing shortness of breath, and night sweats. Can progress rapidly to respiratory failure.	Increased eosinophils in blood and in bronchial lavage fluid or lung biopsy. Abnormal x-ray or CT scan. Treat cause, but systemic corticosteroids resolve symptoms.
Pulmonary alveolar proteinosis (PAP)	Interstitial infiltration and alveolar filling with surfactant phospholipids and proteins thought to be due to a defect in surfactant production or clearance	Four times more common in males, typically 20 to 50 years of age. Gradual onset with dry cough, progressive dyspnea, fatigue, malaise, and weight loss.	Can spontaneously resolve; fatal in about 10% of cases. Treatment depends on severity but often includes whole-lung lavage and systemic steroids.

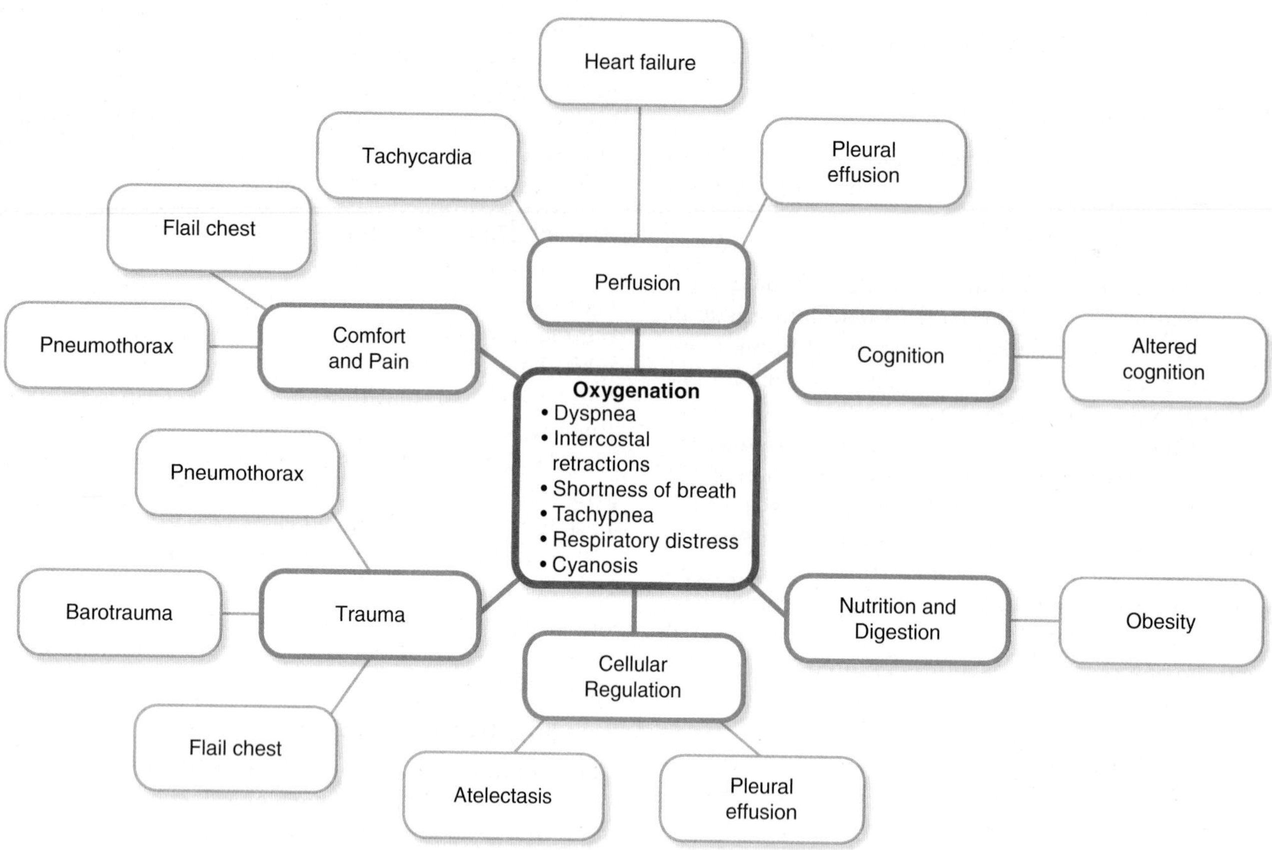

Figure 17.1 ■ Concepts related to restrictive lung disorders.

gradient (i.e., a low ventilation-perfusion [V-Q] ratio, and the length of the diffusion pathway).

Hypoxemia Due to Low Ventilation-Perfusion Ratios. If an individual cannot breathe deeply enough to replenish the alveolar oxygen gradient, less oxygen is available to diffuse into pulmonary blood, and hypoxemia results. The decreased ventilation causes a V-Q mismatch, and V-Q mismatch is the most common cause of hypoxemia. Ventilation/perfusion mismatches are discussed in detail in Chapter 18.

Box 17.1
Calculating Alveolar Ventilation

- When an adult inhales a normal tidal volume (VT) of 500 mL of air 12 times per minute, the minute volume is 12 × 500 mL = 6.0 L/min. To calculate alveolar ventilation, the dead space volume is subtracted from VT (500 mL − 150 mL dead space) for an alveolar ventilation of 350 mL per breath or (12 breaths × 350 mL) = 4.2 L/min.
- If the same adult is sedated after surgery and inhales only 350 mL of air in each breath 12 times per minute, the minute volume is decreased to (350 mL × 12 breaths) = 4.2 L/min, and the alveolar ventilation is decreased to (350 mL/breath − 150 ml dead space × 12 breaths/min) = 2.4 L/min, which is 1.8 L/min lower than normal.
- To achieve a normal alveolar ventilation of 4.2 L/min with shallow breaths (e.g., 200 mL/breath), the individual now needs to breathe about 21 times per minute (4200 mL/200 mL/breath = 21 breaths/min).

Hypoxemia Due to Diffusion Defects. The second key factor is the length of the diffusion pathway, which is determined by the thickness of the alveolar–capillary membrane. Normally, the diffusion pathway is very short and diffusion is rapid, but increased distance between the alveoli and blood markedly increases the diffusion time. The change in diffusion distance can occur acutely (e.g., pulmonary edema) or chronically with a more insidious onset (e.g., pulmonary fibrosis). With a gradual onset, an individual may initially maintain normal oxygenation at rest, but hypoxemia becomes evident with exercise. Even though the alveoli may be fully ventilated during exercise, insufficient diffusion of oxygen from the alveoli into the bloodstream produces hypoxemia. Examples of diseases that exhibit these diffusion defects are interstitial pulmonary fibrosis, connective tissue disease affecting the lung, and alveolar cell carcinoma (see **Figure 17.2** ■).

CLINICAL POINT: Inhaling 100% oxygen can correct the hypoxemia caused by a thickened alveolar–capillary membrane or hypoventilation but cannot correct hypoxemia caused by a venous-to-arterial shunt of blood. ■

The capacity of a gas to diffuse from the lung into capillary blood can be measured by the carbon monoxide

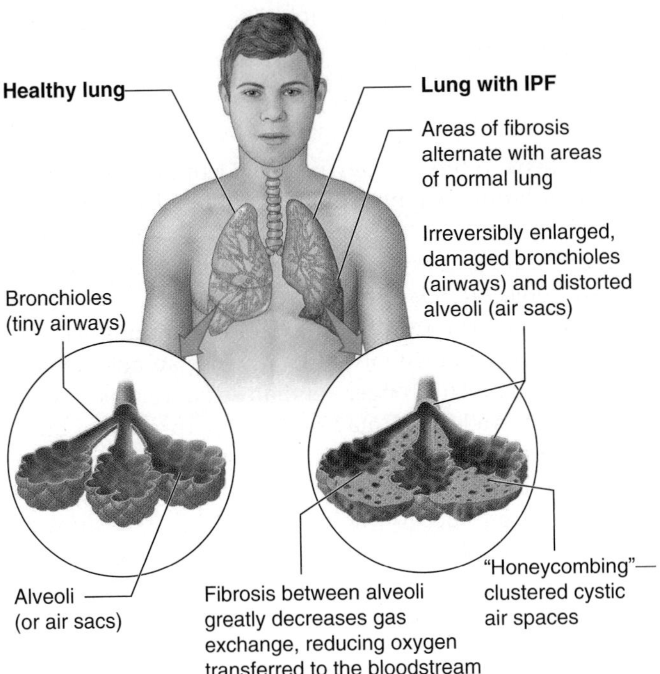

Figure 17.2 ■ Comparison of a healthy lung and a lung with interstitial pulmonary fibrosis.

diffusing capacity (DL_{CO}). The DL_{CO} measures the rate of uptake of a test gas, carbon monoxide (CO), compared to a gas that that does not cross the alveolar–capillary barrier. Measurement of DL_{CO} is indicated for obstructive and restrictive airway diseases and pulmonary vascular diseases.

Case Studies

The pathophysiology involved and the clinical significance of the symptoms experienced by the individuals in the following cases will be addressed throughout the chapter to assist in applying chapter content to clinical situations involving individuals with restrictive lung disorders.

Karla DeVry: Introduction

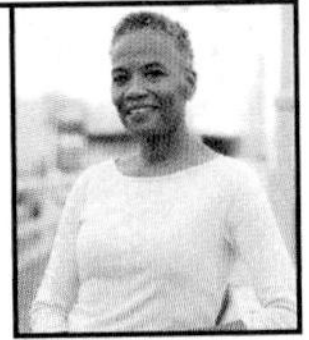

Karla DeVry, a 54-year-old accountant, was admitted to the hospital for evaluation of generalized abdominal pain. An exploratory laparoscopy revealed multiple abdominal adhesions, which likely formed subsequent to an open cholecystectomy (gallbladder removal) performed 15 years earlier. After surgical lysis of adhesions, Ms. DeVry is admitted to the hospital for recovery and observation. By her second postoperative day, Ms. DeVry's oxygen saturation has decreased from 98% on room air to 92% on 2 liters of oxygen per minute via nasal cannula. She rates her abdominal pain as a 6 on a scale of 0 to 10. She reports that the pain is "not too bad" as long as she does not move or cough.

1. What does the nurse consider to be the underlying reasons for the hypoxemia?
2. What is an appropriate nursing intervention to implement with Ms. DeVry?

Jacob Reinecker: Introduction

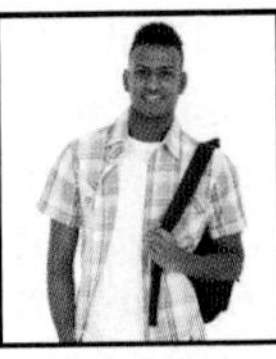

Jacob Reinecker, a healthy 22-year-old college student, was just admitted to the emergency department reporting that he has been "feeling out of breath" since he experienced a sudden, stabbing pain in his upper right chest when he was sitting in class. His vital signs include pulse of 102, respiratory rate of 24, no fever, and blood pressure of 140/86 mmHg, which is higher than his normal 110/70 mmHg. His oxygen saturation is 91% on room air. He has no history of respiratory problems, but 2 years ago he started smoking cigarettes to help him concentrate on his engineering studies. He is 6'2" tall and weighs 172 pounds (78.2 kg). His breath sounds are diminished over the apex of his right lung.

1. What diagnostic tests would provide useful information for Mr. Reinecker?
2. What additional information would the nurse seek from Mr. Reinecker?

Check Your Progress: Section 17.1

1. When there is decreased airflow to the lungs, how does the respiratory rate change?
2. What are possible causes of impaired oxygenation?
3. Why does a patient with pulmonary fibrosis experience exertional dyspnea?

17.2 Restrictive Lung Disorders of Pulmonary Expansion

This section focuses on disorders of oxygenation and ventilation that result from conditions that limit or prevent expansion of the pleura and the alveoli. Respiratory disorders caused by inadequate lung expansion may occur secondary to neurologic injuries, especially those that cause impaired diaphragmatic function. Chronic, progressive neuromuscular diseases that cause respiratory muscle weakness also may lead to restrictive lung disorders. Examples include multiple sclerosis, amyotrophic lateral sclerosis (ALS), and muscular dystrophy. Obesity also can contribute to diminished expansion of the pleura and alveoi, leading to development of a restrictive lung disorder.

The next sections will address several acute disorders of oxygenation and ventilation that may impair expansion of pulmonary structures, including aspiration, atelectasis, pulmonary edema, pneumothorax, and pleural effusion. Selected chest wall abnormalities that may cause restrictive lung disorders due to diminished lung expansion also will be discussed.

Aspiration

Aspiration is the entry of secretions or foreign material into the trachea and lungs. Aspiration of a foreign body that blocks the trachea causes a life-threatening emergency, while aspiration of a very small object may not cause immediate symptoms.

Etiology and Pathogenesis

Aspirating very small quantities of food or fluid is not unusual, and normally, the aspirate is quickly, reflexively coughed out. Food aspiration that completely obstructs the upper airway, causing the individual to collapse suddenly, is often termed a *café coronary*.

Among healthy individuals, children under 4 years of age are at highest risk of aspiration because they have no molar teeth and have a strong tendency to put things in their mouth. ■

Older adults are at increased risk of aspiration, particularly those who wear dentures and drink alcohol. The incidence of foreign body aspiration in older adults increases at the holidays. Neurologic impairment (e.g., decreased gag reflex, traumatic brain injury), impaired muscular control (e.g., stroke, dysphagia, nasogastric feeding tube), and decreased level of consciousness (e.g., general anesthetic, drug overdose) significantly increase the risk of aspiration. ■

In adults, a small foreign body is more likely to enter the more vertical right mainstem bronchus. However, in children younger than 15 years of age, the angles of the mainstem bronchi are similar, so objects may tend to enter either bronchus.

In children, food is the most frequently aspirated object (e.g., peanuts, popcorn, or hot dogs). Oily foods such as peanuts cause inflammation, which makes visualizing and removing the object more difficult. Additional objects that cause a high risk of aspiration include toy parts, pins, nails, and plastic materials. Morbidity increases when an object is not extracted within 24 hours. ■

Clinical Manifestations

Clinical presentation following aspiration depends on the degree of the individual's airway obstruction. Manifestations of partial airway obstruction include coughing, audible wheezing, and choking. Lung auscultation may reveal decreased breath sounds and localized wheezing on the affected side. Even in the absence of significant airway obstruction, complications of aspiration may include infection, hemoptysis, lung abscess, or pneumothorax.

Linking Pathophysiology to Diagnosis and Treatment

Definitive diagnosis and treatment of foreign body aspiration may require direct visualization and removal of the object through use of a laryngoscope or rigid bronchoscope. If bronchoscopy or laryngoscopy is not successful, a thoracotomy may be required, in which the surgeon opens the chest cavity to remove the foreign body. Arterial blood gas (ABG) analysis can be used to assess the effects of aspiration on oxygenation, but most objects are radiolucent and so cannot be seen on chest x-ray (CXR). Aspiration of vomited food or gastric secretions that block airways can cause a medical emergency or death. Even after the food and secretions have been cleared, the acidic gastric contents can cause an injury.

Atelectasis

Atelectasis refers to partial lung collapse or inadequate inflation of a portion of the lung. This term also may be used to refer specifically to alveolar collapse (**Figure 17.3** ■). Lung regions that are affected by atelectasis are subject to relatively low ventilation in comparison to perfusion. The resulting physiologic shunt decreases the total oxygen content of blood. Once an alveolus has collapsed, a much stronger ventilatory effort is required to reinflate it. Atelectasis may be primary (present at birth) or secondary (developed during the neonatal period or later). Risk factors for atelectasis include anesthesia, prolonged immobility including bedrest with minimal activity, shallow respirations, underlying lung disease, fractured ribs, aspiration of foreign bodies, and mucus plugging of airways.

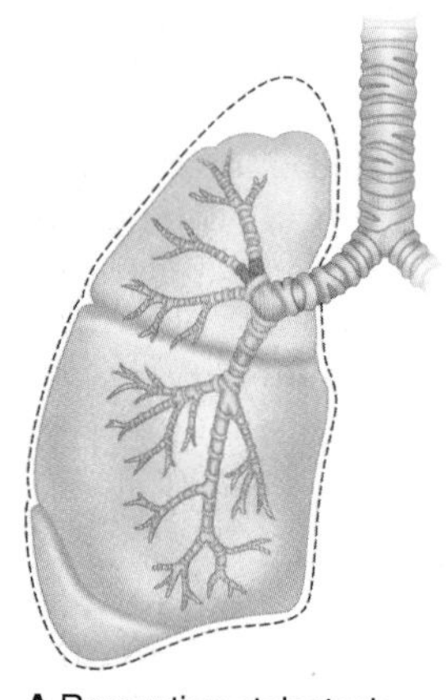

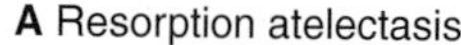

A Resorption atelectasis

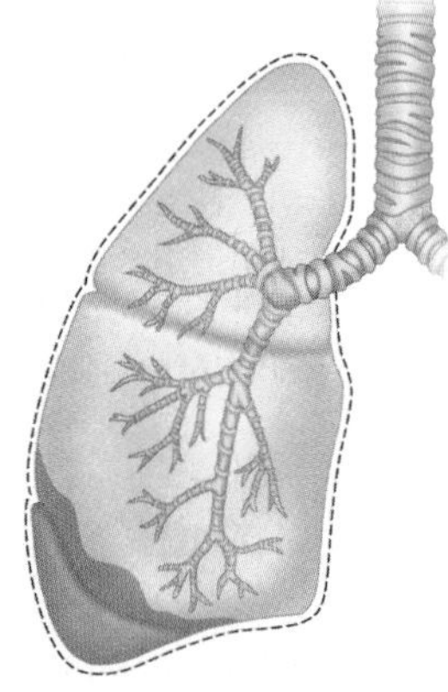

B Compression atelectasis

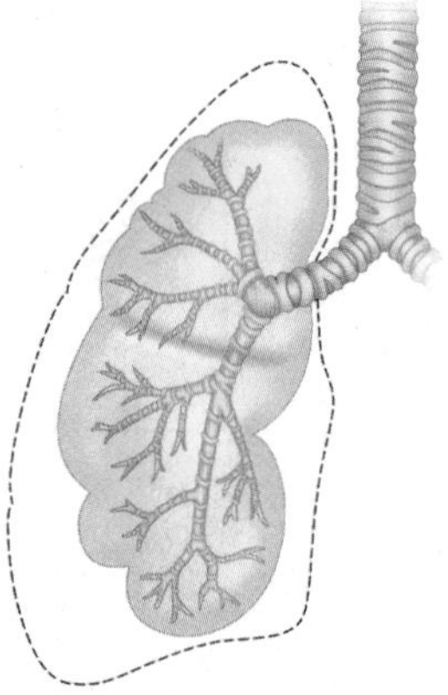

C Contraction atelectasis

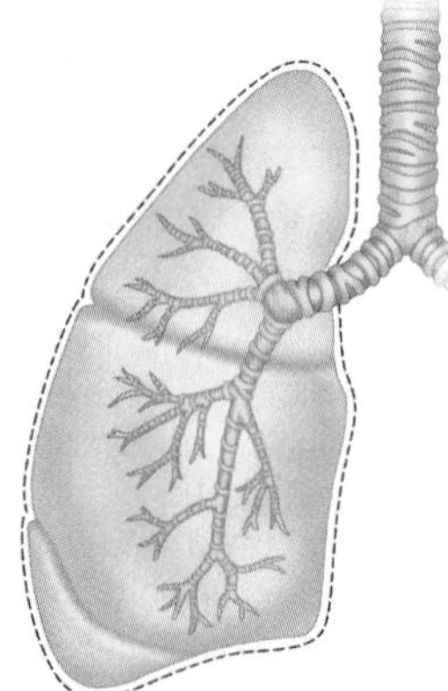

D Microatelectasis

Figure 17.3 ■ Forms of acquired atelectasis. **A.** Resorption atelectasis. **B.** Compression atelectasis, **C.** Contraction atelectasis. **D.** Microatelectasis. Dashed lines indicate the normal lung volume.

In premature infants, especially those who are born before 34 weeks' gestation, decreased surfactant production increases the risk for development of atelectasis. Surfactant reduces alveolar surface tension and helps to prevent alveolar collapse. Aspiration of blood or amniotic fluid that causes airway obstruction also may lead to atelectasis. ■

Etiology and Pathogenesis

There are four major types of atelectasis.

1. ***Resorption atelectasis.*** When airway obstruction occurs, gases trapped in the alveoli located distal to the obstruction may be absorbed by circulating blood without subsequent replacement by inhaled air. Resorption atelectasis can develop as a result. Most often, the associated obstruction is caused by excess mucus secretions. Additional causes include tumor-related bronchial compression and foreign body aspiration.
2. ***Compression atelectasis.*** Compression atelectasis occurs when an accumulation of exudates, fluid, air, or blood or a tumor in the pleural space mechanically collapses lung tissue.
3. ***Contraction atelectasis.*** Contraction atelectasis occurs when fibrotic changes in the lung or the pleura confine the lung and diminish lung expansion.
4. ***Microatelectasis.*** A less severe form of atelectasis, microatelectasis involves closure or collapse of the alveoli or respiratory microstructures to a degree that usually is undetectable on a CXR.[2]

Clinical Manifestations

The clinical presentation of atelectasis includes dyspnea, shortness of breath, tachypnea, tachycardia, and diminished chest expansion; a respiratory infection may follow. Cyanosis may be present. In very young children and thin adults who experience severe atelectasis, **intercostal retractions** (retraction of muscles between the ribs) may be visible during inspiration. On physical exam, breath sounds will be diminished or absent in the area of atelectasis.

Karla DeVry: Application

Ms. DeVry reports "a little" dyspnea on exertion. Lung auscultation reveals faint crackles in the lung bases bilaterally. Ms. DeVry's physician orders a CXR, which reveals scattered bibasilar atelectasis. The physician orders respiratory therapy, including monitored use of incentive spirometry. The frequency of administration of Ms. DeVry's pain medication is increased; by evening, she rates her pain as 3 on a scale of 0 to 10. She reports that she is able to cough and perform incentive spirometry without any significant increase in her abdominal pain. She is also regularly performing cough/deep breathing (CDB) exercises.

3. If the nurse calls the physician about Ms. DeVry's dyspnea on exertion, what patient information would the nurse anticipate that the physician may need?
4. What additional patient needs are created by the increased pain medication administration?

Linking Pathophysiology to Diagnosis and Treatment

The diagnosis of atelectasis is based on the clinical presentation, physical exam, and x-ray confirmation. Treatment is focused on the cause of the atelectasis and includes vigorous pulmonary toilet: deep breathing, coughing, and frequent changes of position. Atelectasis can often be prevented by vigorous pulmonary toilet.

Karla DeVry: Outcome

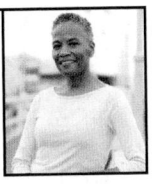

With her pain under control, Ms. DeVry is able to effectively complete respiratory therapy and pulmonary toilet activities without a significant increase in discomfort. Twenty-four hours after her diagnosis of atelectasis, lung auscultation reveals normal breath sounds in all fields. Ms. DeVry's physician orders a repeat CXR, which reveals normal pulmonary expansion with no apparent atelectasis. Ms. DeVry's oxygen saturation has increased to 98% on 2 L/min of oxygen via nasal cannula; on room air, her oxygen saturation is 97%. The physician discontinues Ms. DeVry's nasal oxygen, and her recovery proceeds without further complications. She is discharged to home on postoperative day 3.

5. What education does Ms. DeVry need prior to discharge?
6. What elements are essential for the nurse to assess and document prior to Ms. DeVry's discharge?

Pulmonary Edema

In pulmonary edema, fluid from pulmonary capillaries accumulates in the interstitial spaces and alveoli, causing severely compromised oxygenation to the point of being life-threatening. See Chapter 29 for a discussion of pulmonary edema.

Pneumothorax

Pneumothorax is the presence of air between the visceral and parietal pleurae that produces lung tissue compression, subsequently compromising lung function. Causes of pneumothorax include trauma, complications related to medical procedures, and chronic diseases.

Traumatic pneumothorax is most common during medical procedures such as **thoracentesis** (removal of fluid from the pleural space via a needle or a small catheter), biopsy, or chest surgery. This condition also may be caused by blunt force trauma to the chest wall that produces rib fractures and by penetrating chest wall injuries such as those caused by bullet or knife wounds.

Pneumothorax also may occur spontaneously and without any underlying disease. This is known as primary spontaneous pneumothorax (PSP). PSP most often occurs in tall, thin males (there is a 6:1 ratio males to females) between the ages of 20 and 40 years[3] who experience a ruptured congenital bleb. A **bleb** is a small, thin-walled, air-filled sac on the surface of the lung. In women, the incidence of PSP is increased 9 times by smoking; in men who smoke, the incidence is increased 22 times.[4] Recurrence is common. Secondary spontaneous pneumothorax usually is associated with asthma, emphysema, or tuberculosis but also may be caused by barotrauma related to positive pressure mechanical ventilation.

An open pneumothorax involves some form of chest wall defect that allows communication between the pleural cavity and the environment, such as a penetrating chest wound. With a closed pneumothorax, the chest wall is intact with no defects or open wounds. Both open and closed pneumothoraces are further classified as either a tension or a nontension pneumothorax (see **Figure 17.4** ■). In a tension pneumothorax, the lung or bronchial injury acts as a one-way valve, allowing air into the pleural space but preventing air from escaping during exhalation. As the air volume in the pleural space increases, the pressure collapses lung tissue and pushes the mediastinum toward the contralateral side. A tension pneumothorax is a medical emergency because the rapidly accumulating air compromises both ventilation and blood return to the heart and, when untreated, results in loss of consciousness and death. In a nontension pneumothorax, air in the pleural space can exit into alveoli or escape via the chest wall during exhalation.

Jacob Reinecker: Application

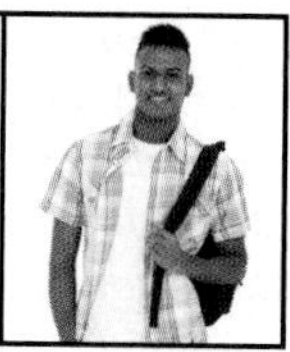

Mr. Reinecker reports continued shortness of breath, which worsens with activity. He reports no additional symptoms, including chest pain. Oxygen is administered at 4 L/min via face mask; Mr. Reinecker's oxygen saturation increases from 91% to 94%. A CXR reveals a 15% right pneumothorax with no shifting of the mediastinum. Mr. Reinecker is admitted to the hospital for further treatment and monitoring, including serial CXRs.

3. What are Mr. Reinecker's modifiable and nonmodifiable risk factors for a PSP?
4. What clinical findings would indicate that Mr. Reinecker's respiratory status is worsening?

Etiology and Pathogenesis

Pneumothorax occurs when air enters the normally negative pressure pleural space, partially collapsing the lung until the air pressures equilibrate or the pleural tear heals. A pneumothorax interferes with ventilation, causing a decrease in forced vital capacity and forced expiratory

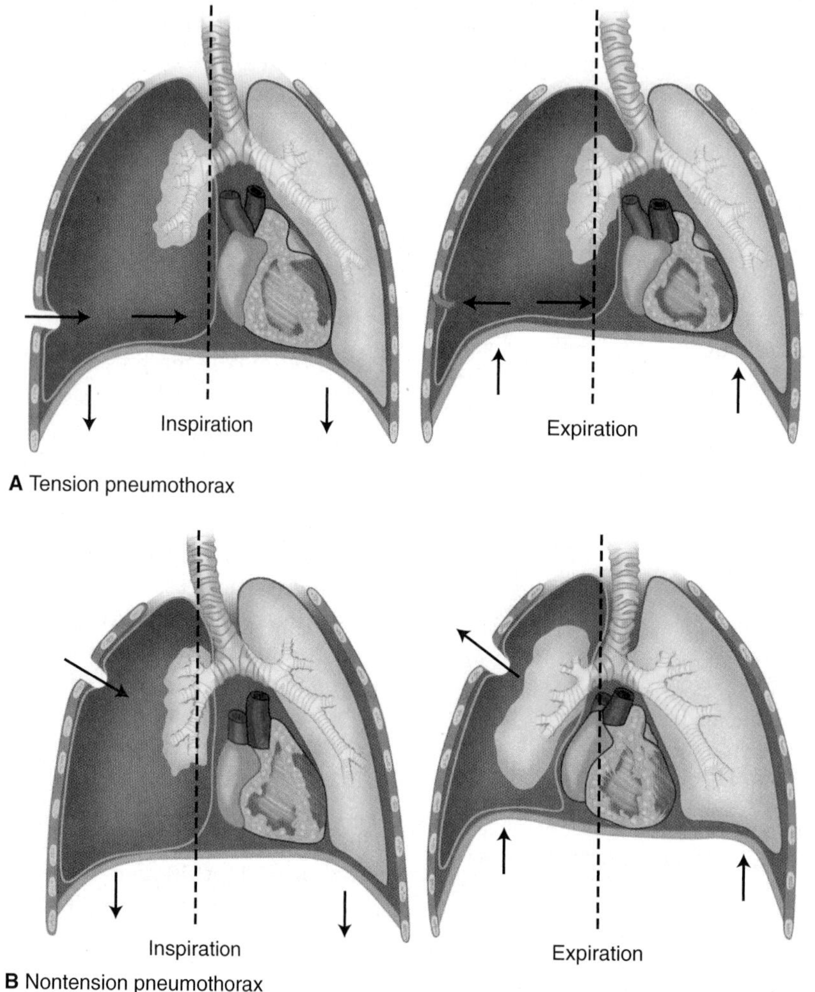

Figure 17.4 ■ Tension and nontension pneumothorax. **A.** In a tension pneumothorax, air enters the pleural space during inhalation but is blocked from exiting the pleural space during exhalation. As air accumulates, the mediastinum shifts toward the unaffected side, compressing the lung. **B.** In a nontension pneumothorax, air enters the pleural space with inhalation and can also exit the pleural space during exhalation.

volume in 1 second and impairs gas exchange. A large pneumothorax can compress the right atrium, compromising the blood return. When an open chest wound is greater than two thirds the size of the trachea, the intrapleural air limits normal ventilation and causes a shift in the mediastinum toward the unaffected (contralateral) side.

In spontaneous pneumothorax, there is a rupture of a small congenital bleb, usually in the lung apices. An adult can tolerate a small spontaneous pneumothorax fairly well, and over time, the air will be gradually absorbed into venous circulation because the partial pressure of gases in venous blood is lower than that in the pneumothorax.

Barotrauma is the overdistention and rupture of alveoli because of increased air pressure within the lungs. Barotrauma can occur with mechanical ventilation or with sudden changes in air pressure during scuba diving or flying at high altitudes.

Clinical Manifestations

The presentation varies with the size of the pneumothorax and whether it is a nontension or tension pneumothorax. When a small spontaneous pneumothorax involves less than 15% of the lung volume, up to 10% of individuals are asymptomatic or may not seek medical care. When the pneumothorax involves more than 40% of the lung, the presentation includes acute ipsilateral chest pain and dyspnea that is generally proportional to the size of the pneumothorax and may include cough. On physical exam, breath sounds may be diminished with hyperresonance (a drumlike quality) on percussion over the site of the pneumothorax, and the individual will be tachycardic, tachypneic, and possibly hypoxemic. With an open pneumothorax, there can be a "sucking" sound as air enters the pleural space.

The clinical presentation of a tension pneumothorax includes chest pain, dyspnea, anxiety, and rarely, acute epigastric pain. Physical exam reveals tachycardia, tachypnea, respiratory distress, and either ipsilateral adventitious breath sounds or no breath sounds over a large pneumothorax. Tachypnea and tachycardia are common, and cyanosis may be present with increasing hypoxemia.

Linking Pathophysiology to Diagnosis and Treatment

Diagnosis is made on the basis of the presenting symptoms, physical examination, and CXR or computerized tomography (CT) scan. On a posterior–anterior CXR, the visceral pleural border is evident, and there is a hyperlucent (black) area with an absence of lung markings between the chest wall and the pleural border. With a large tension pneumothorax, the diaphragm is lower on the affected side, and a mediastinal shift with tracheal deviation away from the pneumothorax may be evident with an increased expansion of the contralateral chest wall. A CT scan is a more sensitive test for diagnosing a smaller pneumothorax and in patients with blunt force trauma. In acute tension pneumothorax, the clinical presentation with hyperresonance and lack of breath sounds on the affected side can be adequate information for emergency treatment.

Appropriate treatment depends on the size of the pneumothorax. A larger pneumothorax is treated by insertion of a chest tube between the ribs into the intrapleural airspace. The distal end of the chest tube is submerged underwater, or a Heimlich valve is attached so that air can escape from the intrapleural space but no environmental air can enter. A small pneumothorax may be observed; the changes in the size of the pneumothorax can be documented by serial CXRs. Thoracostomy or thoracotomy (chest surgery) may be required for a traumatic pneumothorax.

CLINICAL POINT: Mediastinal shift and tracheal deviation usually are late signs of tension pneumothorax. Even when present, these manifestations may initially be subtle and difficult to identify. Prompt recognition of pneumothorax requires taking into account all aspects of the individual's condition, including recognizing tachycardia, tachypnea, and hypoxia, all of which commonly accompany tension pneumothorax. ■

Up to 50% of individuals with spontaneous pneumothorax have recurrence, but there are no long-term complications after appropriate therapy. Multiple recurring spontaneous pneumothoraces may be treated by pleurodesis, which promotes adhesion between pleural surfaces by insertion of an irritating substance into the pleural space or by mechanically roughing the pleural surfaces.

Jacob Reinecker: Outcome

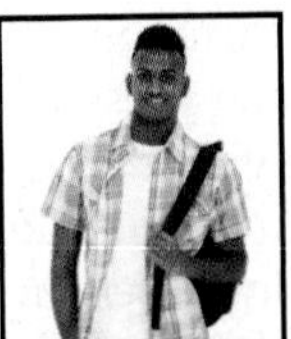

Six hours after admission, Mr. Reinecker reports that he is "breathing better now." A repeat CXR demonstrates a right-sided pneumothorax of less than 10%. Lung auscultation reveals mildly diminished breath sounds on the right side. He is able to maintain an oxygen saturation of 97% on room air. A final CXR performed 6 hours later reveals no abnormalities. Mr. Reinecker reports no symptoms of any kind, and his lung sounds are equal bilaterally. His oxygen saturation is 99% on room air. He is discharged from the hospital with instructions, including a recommendation to attend a smoking cessation class. Mr. Reinecker verbalizes understanding and agrees to set a goal of smoking cessation.

5. What factors contributed to Mr. Reinecker's recovery without an invasive procedure or surgery?
6. What information should be given to Mr. Reinecker about the cause of his chest pain and/or dyspnea?

Pleural Effusion

A **pleural effusion** is a collection of excess fluid in the pleural space. Pleural effusions develop when there is either an excess production of pleural fluid or a decrease in the drainage of the fluid. Excess pleural fluid is produced when an increased hydrostatic filtration force pushes excess fluid into the pleural space (e.g., heart failure or cirrhosis) or there is an increase in capillary permeability because of an inflammatory process or disease (e.g., tuberculosis, rheumatoid arthritis) or a more negative pleural pressure facilitates the accumulation of pleural fluid (e.g., atelectasis). Inadequate drainage of pleural fluid can occur when the lymphatic system is blocked (e.g., tumor) or when the plasma proteins are decreased so that adequate reabsorption does not occur. Pleural effusions are common after thoracic or high abdominal surgeries, and they may develop with inflammatory processes in the lungs (e.g., infections, rheumatoid arthritis) or inflammatory diseases such as pancreatitis.

Etiology and Pathogenesis

The volume and composition of pleural fluid are normally under tight control, and the fluid input is equal to its output. The systemic blood supply for the parietal pleura has higher hydrostatic forces that favor filtration of fluid into the pleural space. The visceral pleura is supplied by the pulmonary circulation, and the combination of its low hydrostatic pressure and the normal oncotic pressure of the pulmonary circulation favors absorption of pleural fluid. Under normal conditions, slightly more pleural fluid is filtered from the parietal pleura than is absorbed by the visceral pleura. The excess fluid is drained by the lymphatic system, so if the lymphatic system is blocked, pleural fluid accumulates. The normal volume of pleural fluid is less than 15 mL in an adult. It lubricates the pleural surfaces so that they slide smoothly during breathing, and it helps to couple the lungs to the chest wall.

When the filtration pressure is increased within the pulmonary or systemic circulation, more fluid enters the pleural space. In left ventricular failure, blood volume and pressure back up into the pulmonary circulation, increasing the hydrostatic filtration pressure. In cirrhosis, the pressure of ascites can force fluid back through the lymphatic system or through the defects in the diaphragm into the pleural space. With atelectasis, lung recoil is increased, making the intrapleural pressure more negative, so the pressure gradient between normal systemic blood pressure and intrapleural pressure is increased.

Characteristics of aspirated pleural fluid depend on the cause of the fluid accumulation. A transudate is serous, with low protein, but the chloride, sodium, specific gravity, and glucose are similar to those of plasma, while the bicarbonate content is higher, making the fluid slightly alkaline. A transudate contains only a few mesothelial cells that have sloughed off the pleura. An exudate contains a higher proportion of lactate dehydrogenase (LDH) compared to blood and increased protein that makes it look cloudy. A purulent exudate will contain pus with large numbers of neutrophils and other lymphocytes. A bacterial or mycotic infection will anaerobically metabolize glucose, so the glucose content and the pH will be low (acidic). See **Table 17.2** ■ for a summary of the characteristics of pleural effusion fluids.

Clinical Manifestations

Individuals with a small pleural effusion may be asymptomatic. A larger pleural effusion can cause shortness of breath and dyspnea because of decreased lung compliance, tachypnea because of shallow respirations and dullness to percussion over the effusion on the affected side.

Linking Pathophysiology to Diagnosis and Treatment

Small amounts of excess pleural fluid may be seen more readily on CT scan than on CXR. Gravity moves pleural fluid into the dependent pleural space; in an upright individual, 300 mL or more of fluid will be visible at the lung base(s) as the blunting of costophrenic angles. Once the fluid has been drained, by either thoracentesis or a chest tube, pleural fluid is analyzed (amylase, glucose, cell counts, and cultures) to determine the cause of the excess fluid.

Table 17.2 Characteristics of Pleural Effusion Fluid

Aspirate	Appearance	Characteristics	Pathophysiology	Etiology
Transudate	Straw-colored, clear pleural fluid	Serous with low protein; normal chloride, sodium, specific gravity and glucose; higher bicarbonate, making the fluid alkaline; few mesothelial cells	Increased filtration pressure or a more negative intrapleural pressure allows for accumulation of pleural fluid in the pleural space.	Noninflammatory processes, including heart failure, ascites, or atelectasis
Exudate	Cloudy and may have pus	Contains neutrophils and other leukocytes; large amount of protein; increased LDH compared to blood; low glucose and low pH (acidic)	Inflammatory process increases capillary permeability, allowing protein and excess fluid to filter into the pleural space; intrapleural proteins exert an osmotic force that opposes fluid absorption into capillaries in the visceral pleura.	Infection in the pleural space, cancer, pulmonary infarction, viral pleuritis (pleural inflammation)
Empyema	Yellow-green pus	Purulent exudate; may be loculated, meaning that it is confined into small pockets by fibrous tissue, or may extend to other regions of the lung.	Fibrous tissue that extends beyond localized areas can obliterate the pleural space or surround the lung limiting its expansion	Pneumonia, lung abscess, infected wound or sepsis
Hemothorax	Blood tinged to bloody	Blood in pleural fluid	Trauma (due to injury or surgery) causes blood to enter and collect within the pleural space.	Blunt force trauma, penetrating injury or thoracic surgery; hemothorax is present in about 25% of chest trauma cases, generally as a result of laceration of the lung or of a major thoracic vessel.
Chylothorax	Milky	Collection of lymphatic fluid with chylomicrons (fine fat particles) in the pleural space	Chylomicrons are absorbed from the GI tract and transported through the lymphatic system.	Blockage of the thoracic duct; thoracic duct damage due to intraoperative laceration or traumatic injury

The treatment depends on the cause of the effusion. Repeated pleural effusions may require pleurodesis, the scarring of the pleura so that no further fluid can accumulate. Pleurodesis is accomplished by inserting an irritating chemical into the pleural space or by roughing the visceral and parietal pleural surfaces in a surgical procedure.

Chest Wall Abnormalities

Restrictive lung disorders include conditions caused by chest wall abnormalities that limit or prevent expansion of the thoracic cavity to such a degree that lung expansion is impaired. Chest wall abnormalities that may cause a restrictive lung disorder include traumatic injuries, such as flail chest. Congenital conditions, such as pectus excavatum, pectus carinatum, and kyphoscoliosis, also may cause a restrictive lung disorder. An overview of each of these conditions is provided in the following sections.

Flail Chest

Flail chest is a complication of blunt chest trauma with multiple rib fractures that cause an unstable chest wall. Flail chest is associated with a mortality rate of approximately 10–15%.[5] The unstable section of the chest wall allows paradoxic movement during respirations: with inspiration, the unstable section of the chest wall moves inward, but during exhalation, the unstable section of the chest wall moves outward. These paradoxic movements of the chest wall limit ventilation and restrict lung volumes. The clinical presentation includes dyspnea, painful inhalation, unequal chest expansion, hypoventilation, and hypoxemia. Crepitus, a coarse crackling sensation caused by air in the subcutaneous tissues, from the trauma may be palpable. The standard treatment is to stabilize the chest wall with mechanical ventilation or with surgical fixation of the rib fractures. The surgical approach allows earlier discontinuation of mechanical ventilation. Pneumonia is a common complication.

Chest Wall Deformities

Congenital chest wall deformities such as pectus excavatum and pectus carinatum cause restrictions in chest wall movement (**Figure 17.5** ■). **Pectus excavatum,** also known as a sunken or funnel chest, gives a concave appearance to the anterior chest wall. With the rapid growth during adolescence, the abnormal growth of the sternum and four or five ribs on each side of the sternum becomes more obvious. Pectus excavatum usually causes a mild restrictive defect with exercise, but a major defect may require surgical repair.

In contrast, the congenital deformity **pectus carinatum,** also called pigeon chest, gives a convex appearance to the anterior chest wall. It can interfere with the compliance of the chest wall, although most patients with pectus carinatum are asymptomatic. Both pectus excavatum and pectus carinatum can be treated surgically.

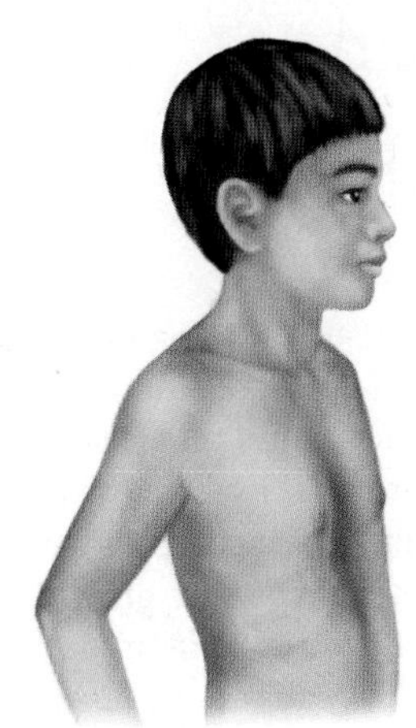

A Pectus excavatum

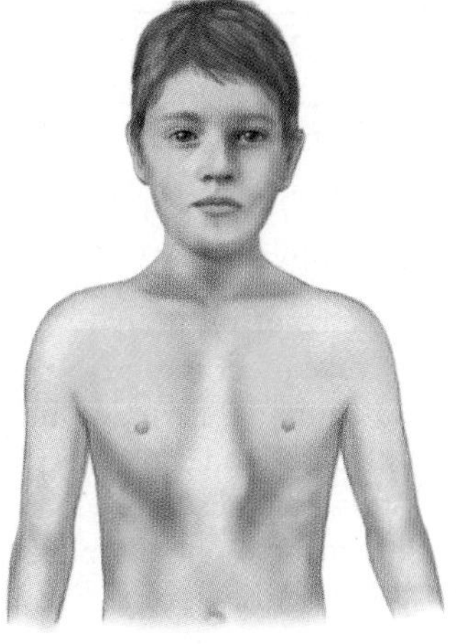

B Pectus carinatum

Figure 17.5 ■ Abnormal chest shape. **A.** In pectus excavatum (funnel chest), the lower portion of the sternum is depressed, decreasing the anteroposterior diameter. **B.** In pectus carinatum (pigeon chest), the sternum protrudes, increasing the anteroposterior diameter.

Kyphoscoliosis

Kyphoscoliosis is an abnormal progressive curvature of the spine. It combines an abnormal front-to-back curvature, which causes a dowager's hump, with a lateral curvature that leaves the shoulders or the hips uneven. Kyphoscoliosis can be a congenital defect with an abnormal formation of vertebra or ribs, or it can be caused by neuromuscular disease or the collapse of vertebrae because of osteoporosis. It can be idiopathic in adolescent girls. The curves get worse during growth spurts, and they impair the mobility of the chest wall and restrict lung volumes. Usual symptoms include backache or low back pain and fatigue, and in severe kyphoscoliosis, hypoxemia is common. Braces can be applied to children to slow or limit the curvature, but braces are ineffective for congenital scoliosis.

Acute Respiratory Distress Syndrome

Acute respiratory distress syndrome is massive inflammatory response with acute, diffuse, severe alveolar–capillary wall damage that results in progressive noncardiogenic pulmonary edema and respiratory failure. It is discussed in Chapter 20.

Check Your Progress: Section 17.2

1. Aspiration is suspected in an elderly patient. Where does the nurse expect to find abnormal breath sounds on auscultation?
2. The patient with cirrhosis of the liver is scheduled for a thoracentesis. What does the nurse anticipate will be the appearance of the aspirate obtained from this procedure?
3. How can the patient with osteoporosis of the spine develop hypoxemia?

17.3 Restrictive Lung Disorders of Pulmonary Compliance

Certain restrictive lung disorders cause stiffening or noncompliance of pulmonary structures. In particular, these conditions affect the interstitium and interalveolar septa. One category of restrictive lung disorders for which the primary dysfunction centers on decreased lung compliance is interstitial lung disease, which comprises a diverse group of more than 200 nonmalignant, noninfectious inflammatory conditions.[6] The various forms of interstitial lung disease cause fibrosis within the lung interstitium.

Idiopathic pulmonary fibrosis, which is discussed in this chapter, is both the most common and the most deadly type of interstitial lung disease. Although the cause of idiopathic pulmonary fibrosis is unknown, numerous known causes of other forms of interstitial lung disease have been identified. For example, interstitial lung disease has been linked to the following[7]:

- Use of pharmacologic agents, such as certain antibiotics, cardiac medications, and chemotherapy drugs
- Exposure to pollutants and toxins, including tobacco smoke, asbestos, silica dust, and radiation treatments
- Exposure to animal feces and bird droppings
- Occupational exposure to potentially hazardous substances, including those encountered during the course of mining, farming, and construction
- Medical conditions, including rheumatoid arthritis, scleroderma, and systemic lupus erythematosus.[7]

Sarcoidosis, which also is discussed in this chapter, is another form of interstitial lung disease.[7]

Idiopathic Pulmonary Fibrosis

Idiopathic pulmonary fibrosis (IPF) is a progressive, lethal disease that profoundly affects the individual's quality of life. It is the most common lung disease of unknown etiology and it presents a bleak outlook for survival and treatment options.

Forms of interstitial lung disease for which no cause is identifiable are categorized as **idiopathic interstitial pneumonias (IIPs)**. When discussing IIPs, the term "pneumonia" refers to inflammation, not infection. The clinical presentation, diagnostic data, and pathology of IIPs are similar but the effectiveness of treatment and the prognosis vary widely, so a surgical biopsy may be necessary. Of all disorders included among the IIPs, idiopathic pulmonary fibrosis is the most common and the most aggressive.[8]

Etiology and Pathogenesis

Idiopathic pulmonary fibrosis is a relatively rare disorder with an estimated prevalence in the United States of 14 to 63 cases per 100,000.[9] For an individual with IPF, the prognosis depends on several factors, in particular the presence of coexisting disease and the degree of functional lung impairment. With IPF, a greater degree of functional lung impairment is associated with a higher mortality rate.[10]

Individuals who are at increased risk for IPF include older adults, especially white males, who currently smoke or have a history of smoking.[11] Exposures to occupational or environmental toxins or radiation therapy and chemotherapy increase the risk for IPF. Chronic gastroesophageal reflux with aspiration of stomach contents and viral infections have also increased the risk for IPF in some studies.[12]

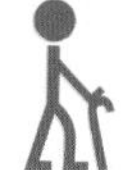

The incidence and prevalence of IPF increase with age. Most often, this disease is diagnosed in individuals who are age 60 years or older.[13] ■

IPF results from an aberrant repair of alveolar epithelial type II cells after repetitive injuries (**Figure 17.6** ■; see also, Figure 17.2). The cause of the injury to the alveolar epithelium is not known, and the aberrant repair process can occur with or without inflammation. With normal wound repair, epithelial cells restore the intact epithelium, and myofibroblasts undergo apoptosis; but in IPF, myofibroblasts accumulate, closely associated epithelial cells undergo apoptosis rather than restoring an intact epithelium, and the basement membrane is persistently degraded.[14] The persistence of

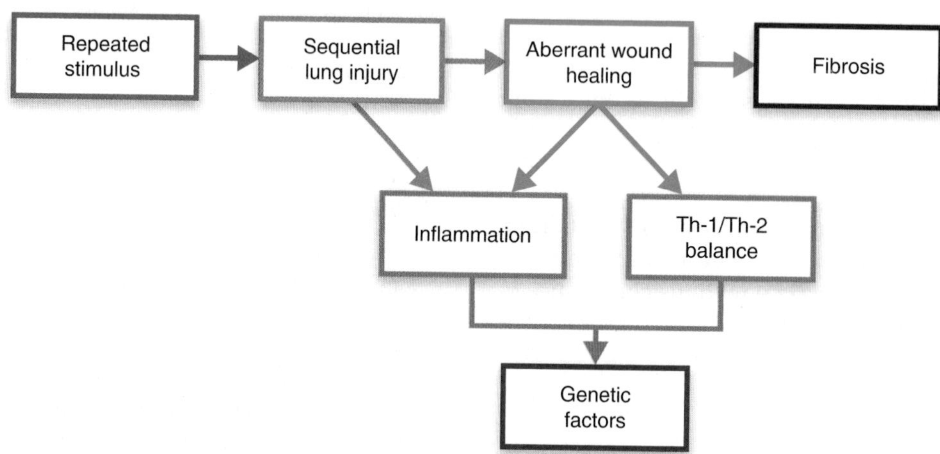

Figure 17.6 ■ Pathogenesis of idiopathic pulmonary fibrosis.

myofibroblast foci, considered areas of active fibrogenesis, is the histologic hallmark for IPF.

Genetics influences an individual's susceptibility to IPF. Approximately 8% of familial cases of IPF can be traced to one specific set of genes.[6] Other studies suggest that IPF may occur because of age-related cellular changes such as shortened telomeres and altered protein folding, which impair regeneration of the alveolar epithelium.[14] Recent epigenetic studies indicate that an imbalance or the presence of abnormal mediators results in paradoxic actions. For example, prostaglandin-E_2 (PGE_2) normally exhibits strong antifibrolytic properties, inducing apoptosis in fibroblasts, but in IPF, there is a diminished production of PGE_2 and it may be dysregulated.[8,15]

In earlier stages of the disease, there are areas of normal lung, areas with fibroblast foci, areas with some inflammatory infiltrate, and other fibrotic areas. The fibrosis decreases lung compliance, increasing the work of breathing, and the increased interstitial collagen increases the diffusion distance, compromising oxygenation of blood. As the disease progresses, the fibrotic areas are described as "honeycombed," and once the structural lung damage occurs, it is usually irreversible.[14]

Clinical Manifestations

Idiopathic pulmonary fibrosis usually has an insidious onset that begins with dyspnea on exertion (DOE) and/or a cough that produces very little sputum. Disease progression may occur in a steplike process, with periods of relative stability, then marked worsening of the disease with an acute exacerbation.[14] Deterioration of lung function can occur secondary to an infection, pulmonary embolism, pneumothorax, or heart failure.[16] Even at rest, individuals with IPF have rapid, shallow respirations to limit the work of ventilating stiff lungs. On physical examination, bibasilar inspiratory crackles (Velcro-like crackles) and clubbing of the distal fingers are commonly present.[16] Disease progression or acute exacerbation may cause increasing DOE, hypoxemia, and cyanosis. Heart failure and peripheral edema also may occur.[14]

Linking Pathophysiology to Diagnosis and Treatment

The diagnosis of IPF is a diagnosis of exclusion, as there are no specific tests for it, and is based on clinical evidence. Results of pulmonary function tests (PFTs) and CXR deteriorate with disease progression. Initially, PFTs may be normal or nearly so, with a decreased DL_{CO} as the fibrosis lengthens the oxygen diffusion pathway. Later, a restrictive impairment will be apparent on PFTs as well as a decreased PaO_2 and exercise capacity on the 6-minute walk. A CXR shows nonspecific diffuse reticular opacities, but high-resolution computed tomography (HRCT) is more sensitive and specific for IPF.[17]

Oxygen therapy is initially prescribed with exercise but increases to continuous O_2 therapy as the fibrosis increases. Currently, medications include anti-inflammatory agents (corticosteroids or steroid-sparing cytotoxic agents) without good evidence from controlled trials to support their use. Lung transplantation is recognized to prolong survival of individuals with advanced IPF; the posttransplant survival at 5 years is about 50–56%.[16]

Sarcoidosis

Fungal infections, tuberculosis, and sarcoidosis result in the formation of granulomas, which can cause restrictive lung disorders. This chapter will provide an overview of sarcoidosis. Fungal infections and tuberculosis are discussed in Chapter 19.

Sarcoidosis is a systemic disease of unknown origin that is characterized by formation of chronic noncaseating (solid) granulomas. Sarcoidosis most commonly affects the lungs, lymph nodes, skin, and eyes but can affect any tissue or organ in the body. It is more common in adults 20–40 years of age. The incidence of sarcoidosis is higher in African Americans (three times more frequent than in Caucasians), particularly African American women. The mortality rate for African Americans with sarcoidosis is 17 times higher than that for Caucasians. This disease is rare in Pacific Islanders and Asians.[18]

Impact of Current Research on Clinical Practice

GERD and IPF

Description: Gastroesophageal reflux disease (GERD), which is a risk factor for microaspiration, has been proposed as a potential risk factor for the development of idiopathic pulmonary fibrosis. In seeking to describe the relationship between chronic microaspiration and IPF, researchers explored biological and clinical rationales to support the link between these two conditions. Additionally, researchers reviewed available literature to help establish a scientific relationship between GERD and IPF. Particularly because no known cause for IPF has yet been identified, current approaches to IPF center on treating the condition rather than on preventing its occurrence. Should GERD-related microaspiration be identified as one cause of IPF, preventive measures for IPF might include a more aggressive approach to treating GERD.

Clinical Practice: Both human and animal data support the proposed relationship between GERD-related microaspiration and pulmonary fibrosis. Research also suggests that chronic microaspiration produces histologic changes in the lungs that are clinically consistent with interstitial pneumonia. Although further research is needed, results of the literature review suggest a need to consider IPF to be one potential consequence of GERD. Approaches to treatment of patients with GERD from the standpoint of preventing microaspiration may represent a practical means by which to prevent IPF.

Research Study:

Lee, J. S., Collard, H. R., & Raghu, G. (2010). Does chronic microaspiration cause idiopathic pulmonary fibrosis? *American Journal of Medicine*, *123*(4), 304–311.

Etiology and Pathogenesis

A genetic predisposition to sarcoidosis plus exposure to an unknown antigen triggers the granulomatous inflammation. An infectious cause has been suspected but never proven. There is an abnormal immune response with an exaggerated helper T cell lymphocyte response to the antigen, and large numbers of macrophages are recruited. Activation of B cell lymphocytes may lead to hyperglobulinemia (IgM).[19] Sarcoidosis is often a mild disease that is discovered incidentally on CXR; in the vast majority cases, the CXR of an individual with this disorder will demonstrate the presence of granulomas.[20] The typical granulomas that are visible on CXR are well-defined, bilateral hilar and paratracheal nodes that make the mediastinum look wider.

Clinical Manifestations

The most common symptoms, cough and dyspnea, are worse with exertion, but the clinical presentation may also involve the eyes; this disorder may cause symptoms that include reddened, sore, watery eyes.[18] Sarcoidosis also may cause discrete enlarged lymph nodes, or erythema nodosum. Erythema nodosum often brings the individual to medical attention because of the presence of reddish, painful nodules, usually located on the shin. The nodules are caused by inflammation in the fatty layer of the skin and usually resolve spontaneously over time. Integumentary changes, including skin ulceration and discoloration, also may occur on the scalp, face, and back.[18] When systemic symptoms are present, they can include fever, night sweats, malaise, fatigue, and weight loss.

Linking Pathophysiology to Diagnosis and Treatment

There are no laboratory tests for sarcoidosis; it is a diagnosis of exclusion. When sarcoidosis is asymptomatic, two thirds of cases resolve spontaneously, so no therapy is indicated. Acute symptomatic sarcoidosis is effectively treated with corticosteroids, and most patients have a good prognosis. Although sarcoidosis is rarely fatal, serious organ damage caused by sarcoidosis increases the risk for death.[18]

Check Your Progress: Section 17.3

1. Interstitial lung disease has been linked to what environmental or occupational exposures?
2. What factors influence the prognosis and mortality rates associated with idiopathic pulmonary fibrosis?
3. The incidence of sarcoidosis is highest in which groups of individuals?

CHAPTER SUMMARY

17.1 Chapter Overview and Case Studies

Explain the factors that alter ventilation and oxygenation in restrictive lung disorders and concepts related to restrictive lung disorders.

- Tachypnea is a common symptom of restrictive disorders because rapid shallow breathing saves energy.
- Key factors for oxygen diffusion in restrictive disorders are the oxygen gradient and the diffusion distance.
- A low ventilation-perfusion (V-Q) ratio is the most common cause of hypoxemia.
- Increasing diffusion distance greatly increases diffusion time and results in hypoxemia
- Carbon monoxide diffusing capacity (DL_{CO}) provides an objective measurement of the rate of uptake of gases from the alveoli into the blood.

17.2 Restrictive Lung Disorders of Pulmonary Expansion

Describe the causes, classification, underlying pathogenesis, and clinical manifestations of restrictive lung disorders that primarily limit pulmonary expansion and approaches to diagnosis and treatment of those conditions across the lifespan.

- Individuals at increased risk for aspiration have difficulty defending their airways because of age or pathologic conditions.
- Aspiration of a large foreign object causes coughing, wheezing, and choking. Small objects may not be clinically evident initially, but morbidity is increased if they are not removed within 24 hours.
- Aspirated objects can generally be seen and removed through a laryngoscope or rigid bronchoscope.
- Atelectasis is defined as a collapsed lung that is not fully expanded or re-expanded; risk factors include diminished ventilation, restriction of lung volume, and immobility.
- The four types of atelectasis are resorption atelectasis with airway obstruction; compression atelectasis with accumulation of air, fluid, or tumor in the pleural space; contraction atelectasis with fibrotic changes; and microatelectasis, which involves alveolar collapse that may be undetectable by x-ray.
- Atelectasis presents with dyspnea, tachypnea, tachycardia, and an increased work of breathing with diminished or absent breath sounds over the atelectasis. Treatment focuses on the cause of atelectasis and includes vigorous pulmonary toilet.
- Pneumothorax occurs when air collects between the visceral and parietal pleura, compressing lung tissue. It can occur spontaneously or secondary to barotraumas, chest trauma, or disease.
- In a tension pneumothorax, air enters but cannot leave the pleural space, so the enlarging pneumothorax compresses the lungs and heart, creating a medical emergency.

- A small pneumothorax may be asymptomatic; the loss over 40% of lung volume causes dyspnea, tachypnea, tachycardia, ipsilateral chest pain, and anxiety.
- The area over a large pneumothorax will not have breath sounds and will be hyperresonant on percussion; a chest tube is inserted into the intrapleural space to remove the air.
- A pleural effusion is a collection of excess fluid in the pleural space that develops when there is an increased production or decreased drainage of pleural fluid.
- Risk factors include thoracic and abdominal surgeries, inflammatory processes in the lung, atelectasis, blockage of lymphatic drainage, and decreased plasma proteins.
- Pleural fluid is classified as a transudate, exudate, empyema, hemothorax, or chylomicron effusions on the basis of the composition of the fluid.
- Pleural effusions are demonstrated by CXR or CT scan and can be drained with insertion of a chest tube. Pleurodesis may be required for recurrent pleural effusions.
- In resorption atelectasis, microatelectasis, and aspiration of a large foreign body, lung ventilation is compromised; with pneumothorax and pleural effusions, the expanded pleural space compresses lung tissue.
- Flail chest is a complication of blunt chest trauma with multiple ribs fractures that allows paradoxic chest wall movement with respirations that limits ventilation and requires treatment by stabilizing the chest wall.
- Pectus excavatum and pectus carinatum are congenital chest wall deformities that cause restrictive defects.
- Kyphoscoliosis is a progressive lateral and back-to-front curvature of the spine that limits chest mobility, impairing ventilation.

17.3 Restrictive Lung Disorders of Pulmonary Compliance

Describe the causes, classification, underlying pathogenesis, and clinical manifestations of restrictive lung disorders that primarily decrease pulmonary compliance and approaches to diagnosis and treatment of those conditions across the lifespan.

- Restrictive lung disorders that cause stiffening or noncompliance of pulmonary structures commonly affect the interstitium and interalveolar septa.
- Interstitial lung disease comprises a diverse group of more than 200 nonmalignant, noninfectious inflammatory conditions that cause fibrosis within the lung interstitium.
- Pharmacologic agents that are known to cause interstitial lung disease include certain antibiotics, cardiac medications, and chemotherapy drugs.
- Pollutants and toxins that are known to cause interstitial lung disease include cigarette smoke, asbestos, silica dust, and radiation treatments.
- Exposure to animal feces and bird droppings may cause interstitial lung disease.
- Occupations that increase an individual's risk for exposure to potentially hazardous substances increase the risk for developing interstitial lung disease; examples are mining, farming, and construction.
- Medical conditions that are linked to the development of interstitial lung disease include rheumatoid arthritis, scleroderma, systemic lupus erythematosus, and sarcoidosis.
- Idiopathic pulmonary fibrosis (IPF) is the most common and most deadly type of interstitial lung disease.
- IPF is a gradually progressive, lethal disorder caused by aberrant healing of alveolar type II cells that results in areas of fibroblast foci.
- Although the cause of IPF is unknown, it may have a genetic basis in some cases.
- Forms of interstitial lung disease for which no cause is identifiable are categorized as idiopathic interstitial pneumonias (IIPs).
- Sarcoidosis is a systemic disease of unknown origin that often causes noncaseating granulomas of the lung, most frequently in young African American women.
- Sarcoidosis is often asymptomatic, but individuals may have cough and dyspnea that worsens with exertion and responds well to corticosteroids.

REVIEW QUESTIONS

1. The nurse is preparing to assess a client who was newly admitted with a severe exacerbation of IPF. What abnormal assessment findings does the nurse anticipate may be present? (Select all that apply)
   a. Productive cough with excessive sputum production
   b. Inspiratory crackles noted upon auscultation
   c. Clubbing of the fingers
   d. Cardiac murmur
   e. Peripheral edema

2. What is the alveolar ventilation for an adult who inhales a normal tidal volume of air with a respiratory rate of 14 breaths per minute?
   a. 1.8 L/min
   b. 4.9 L/min
   c. 49 L/Min
   d. 21 L/min

3. A parent brings a 2-year-old into the emergency department with new-onset cough, which began in the past hour. No one in the household has been ill, and the child is afebrile. What additional information would be a priority for the nurse ask the parent?
   a. "What was your child doing before the coughing began?"
   b. "Has your child had their annual flu shot?"
   c. "Is there a family history of any lung disease?"
   d. "Does your child attend daycare?"
4. A patient has a chest tube present secondary to a large left-sided pneumothorax after sustaining multiple fractured ribs in a motor vehicle accident. What does the nurse expect to find on assessment of this client?
   a. Absent left-sided breath sounds in the left lower lobe of the lung
   b. Absent right-sided breath sounds in the right lower lobe of the lung
   c. Normal breath sounds throughout both lungs
   d. Equal movement of the chest with inspiration
5. When the nurse obtains the following information from a client with interstitial lung disease, which information is relevant to this condition? (Select all that apply.)
   a. A 5-year history of osteoarthritis
   b. Stopped smoking 1 year ago
   c. Currently owns a pet store
   d. Family history of diabetes
   e. History of bilateral mastectomy
6. The nurse is assessing a client who is suspected of having sarcoidosis. Which findings are pertinent? (Select all that apply.)
   a. Recent constipation
   b. Mild dyspnea on exertion
   c. Redness of the conjunctiva
   d. Intact skin that is lesion free
   e. Enlarged cervical lymph nodes
7. A family member is assisting an elderly client in eating lunch. Which observation by the nurse warrants immediate intervention by the nurse?
   a. The patient is lying supine in bed.
   b. The food has been cut into small pieces.
   c. The patient asks to drink after swallowing a bite of food.
   d. The patient's tray is located within the patient's reach.
8. What is the most likely appearance of pleural fluid removed by thoracentesis in the client with a pleural effusion secondary to lung cancer?
   a. Clear
   b. Straw-colored
   c. Blood-tinged
   d. Cloudy

ANSWERS

Answers to Review Questions can be found in Appendix A. Answers to Case Study and Check Your Progress questions are available on the faculty resources site. Please consult with your instructor.

RECOMMENDED WEBSITES

American Lung Association
http://www.lung.org

American Thoracic Society (ATS) Guidelines
https://www.thoracic.org/statements/index.php

Foundation for Sarcoidosis Research
http://www.stopsarcoidosis.org

National Heart, Lung, and Blood Institute
http://www.nhlbi.nih.gov

REFERENCES

1. Epler, G. R. (2011). Bronchiolitis obliterans organizing pneumonia, 25 years: A variety of causes, but what are the treatment options? *Expert Review of Respiratory Medicine, 5*(3), 353–361.
2. Marini, J. J., & Wheeler, A. P. (2010). *Critical care medicine: The essentials* (4th ed.). Philadelphia, PA: Lippincott Williams & Wilkins.
3. Lee, P. (2013). Primary spontaneous pneumothorax: To pleurodese or not? *Lancet*, 381(9874), 1252–1254.
4. Parrish, S., Browning, R. F., Turner, J. F., Jr., et al. (2014). The role for medical thoracoscopy in pneumothorax. *Journal of Thoracic Disease, 6*(Suppl 4), S383–S391.
5. Vana, P. G., Neubauer, D. C., & Luchette, F. A. (2014). Contemporary management of flail chest. *American Surgeon, 80*(6), 527–535.
6. Olson, A. L., Schwarz, M. I., Roman, J. (2010). Interstitial lung disease. In D. E. Schraufnage (Ed.), *Breathing in America: Diseases, progress, and hope*. New York, NY: American Thoracic Society, 99–108

7. Mayo Clinic. (2014). Interstitial lung disease: Causes. Retrieved from http://www.mayoclinic.org/diseases-conditions/interstitial-lung-disease/basics/causes/con-20024481
8. Eickelberg, O., & Selman, M. Update in diffuse parenchymal lung diseases 2009. (2010). *American Journal of Respiratory and Critical Care Medicine, 181*(9), 883–888.
9. Nalysnyk, L., Cid-Ruzafa, J., Rotella, P., & Esser, D. (2012). Incidence and prevalence of idiopathic pulmonary fibrosis: Review of the literature. *European Respiratory Review, 21*(126), 355–361.
10. King, T. E., Jr., Albera, C., Bradford, W. Z., et al. (2014). All-cause mortality rate in patients with idiopathic pulmonary fibrosis: Implications for the design and execution of clinical trials. *American Journal of Respiratory and Critical Care Medicine, 189*(7), 825–831.
11. Mayo Clinic. (2014). Interstitial lung disease: Risk factors. Retrieved from http://www.mayoclinic.org/diseases-conditions/interstitial-lung-disease/basics/risk-factors/con-20024481
12. Lee, J. S., Collard, H. R., & Raghu, G. (2010). Does chronic microaspiration cause idiopathic pulmonary fibrosis? *American Journal of Medicine, 123*(4), 304–311.
13. Selman, M., & Pardo, A. (2014). Revealing the pathogenic and aging-related mechanisms of the enigmatic idiopathic pulmonary fibrosis: An integral model. *American Journal of Respiratory and Critical Care Medicine, 189*(10), 1161–1172.
14. Harari, S., & Caminati, A. (2010). IPF: New insight on pathogenesis and treatment. *Allergy, 65*(5), 537–553.
15. Horowitz, J. C.,& Peters-Golden, M. (2010). Prostaglandin E2's new trick: "Decider" of differential alveolar cell life and death. *American Journal of Respiratory and Critical Care Medicine, 182*(1), 2–3.
16. Raghu, G., Collard, H. R., Egan, J. J., et al. (2011). An official ATS/ERS/JRS/ALAT statement: Idiopathic pulmonary fibrosis: Evidence-based guidelines for diagnosis and management. *American Journal of Respiratory and Critical Care Medicine, 183*(6), 788–824.
17. Sverzellati, N. (2013). Highlights of HRCT imaging in IPF. *Respiratory Research, 14*(Suppl. 1), S3.
18. American Lung Association. (2010). Sarcoidosis. In *State of lung disease in diverse communities 2010* (pp. 81–86). Chicago, IL: American Lung Association.
19. Patterson, K. C., Hogarth, K., Husain, A. N., Sperling, A. I., & Niewold, T. B. (2012). The clinical and immunologic features of pulmonary fibrosis in sarcoidosis. *Translation Reearch,. 160*(5), 321–331.
20. Greco, F. G., Spagnolo, P., Muri, M., et al. (2014). The value of chest radiograph and computed tomography in pulmonary sarcoidosis. *Sarcoidosis Vasculitis and Diffuse Lung Disease, 31*(2), 108–116.

Chapter 18

Obstructive Lung Disorders

Nancy Pogue and Linda Blevins

Chapter Outline and Learning Outcomes

18.1 Chapter Overview and Case Studies

Describe the common characteristics of obstructive lung disorders and explain their impact on other concepts and systems.

18.2 Alterations in Respiratory Structure and Function

Describe the alterations of the anatomic airway structure and pulmonary function present in individuals with obstructive lung disorders.

18.3 Asthma

Differentiate the causes, classification, underlying pathogenesis, and clinical manifestations of asthma and approaches to diagnosis and treatment of the condition across the lifespan.

18.4 Chronic Obstructive Pulmonary Disease

Differentiate the causes, classification, underlying pathogenesis, and clinical manifestations of chronic obstructive pulmonary disease and approaches to diagnosis and treatment of the condition.

18.5 Cystic Fibrosis

Differentiate the causes, classification, underlying pathogenesis, and clinical manifestations of cystic fibrosis and approaches to diagnosis and treatment of the condition across the lifespan.

18.6 Bronchiectasis

Differentiate the causes, classification, underlying pathogenesis, and clinical manifestations of bronchiectasis and approaches to diagnosis and treatment of the condition across the lifespan.

KEY TERMS

Air trapping, 443
Asthma, 445
Atopy, 445
Bronchiectasis, 459
Bronchoconstriction, 443
Bronchodilation, 443
Chronic bronchitis, 453
Chronic obstructive pulmonary disease (COPD), 441
Cystic fibrosis (CF), 457
Dyspnea, 441
Emphysema, 453
Hemoptysis, 454
Hypercapnia, 452
Hyperinflation, 452
Hyperreactivity, 445
Pulmonary acini, 454
Shortness of breath (SOB), 451
Trigger, 445
Wheeze, 448

ABBREVIATIONS

CF—cystic fibrosis
COPD—chronic obstructive pulmonary disease
DOE—dyspnea on exertion
FEV_1—forced expiratory volume in 1 second
FEV_1/FVC—ratio of the forced expiratory volume in the first one second to the forced vital capacity of the lungs
FRC—functional residual capacity
FVC—forced vital capacity
GOLD—Global Initiative for Chronic Obstructive Lung Disease
PFTs—pulmonary function tests
RV—residual volume
SOB—shortness of breath
TLC—total lung capacity
TV—tidal volume
VC—vital capacity

18.1 Chapter Overview and Case Studies

Obstructive lung disorders encompass a spectrum of disorders, including asthma, chronic bronchitis, emphysema, cystic fibrosis (CF), and bronchiectasis. **Chronic obstructive pulmonary disease (COPD)** is an umbrella term for progressive lung disorders such as chronic bronchitis and emphysema.. Inflammation has an important role in the development of obstructive lung disorders, and they share dyspnea as their common symptom. **Dyspnea** refers to difficulty breathing. Subjective descriptions of dyspnea by an individual who experiences it may include "heaviness," "air hunger," or "gasping."[1] Regardless of the specific obstructive disorder, common characteristics involving alterations in airway structure and pulmonary function are present.

Healthy People 2020, which was introduced by the U.S. Department of Health and Human Services in 2010, is a national health initiative that targets the achievement of enhancing quality of life and longevity by reducing the incidence of preventable illness, disability, injury, and premature mortality.[2] Both respiratory disease and tobacco use are included as topics in *Healthy People 2020*.

Concepts Related to Obstructive Lung Disorders

Common features of obstructive lung disorders include their ability to impair oxygenation and perfusion, which may lead to destruction of cells and tissues as well as subsequent organ dysfunction. Because oxygen is essential to life, impaired oxygenation affects practically every aspect of health. With regard to nutrition, the increased work of breathing associated with obstructive lung disorders leads to an increase in metabolic demand. In particular, the risk for undernutrition associated with COPD has been well documented.[3] **Figure 18.1** ■ illustrates concepts related to oxygenation in application to obstructive lung disorders.

Case Studies

The pathophysiology involved and the clinical significance of the symptoms experienced by the individuals in the following cases will be addressed throughout the chapter to assist in application of chapter content to clinical situations involving individuals with obstructive lung disorders.

Barbara Morgan: Introduction

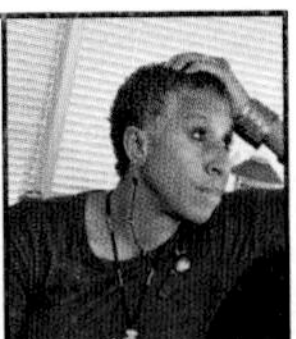

Barbara Morgan is a 57-year-old woman who is chief architect for a firm that remodels and restores historic buildings. Recently, Ms. Morgan saw her physician because of persistent congestion, dyspnea on exertion, wheezing that is worse at night, and an intermittent cough that produces thick white mucus that "strings."

1. What additional history would be useful to obtain at this time?
2. What physical assessment findings would be useful to obtain at this time?

Healthy People 2020

Respiratory Disease and Tobacco Use

Goal: "Promote respiratory health through better prevention, detection, treatment, and education efforts."[1]

Overview: Asthma and COPD are significant public health burdens. Specific methods of detection, intervention, and treatment exist that may reduce this burden and promote health.

Why are respiratory diseases important?

Currently in the United States, more than 23 million people have asthma. Approximately 13.6 million adults have been diagnosed with COPD, and it is estimated that an approximately equal number have not yet been diagnosed. The burden of respiratory diseases affects individuals and their families, schools, workplaces, neighborhoods, cities, and states. Because of the cost to the healthcare system, the burden of respiratory diseases also falls on society; it is paid for with higher health insurance rates, lost productivity, and tax dollars. Annual healthcare expenditures for asthma alone are estimated at $20.7 billion.

Objectives that address the reduction of respiratory disease and its effects include the following:

- Reduce asthma deaths.
- Reduce hospitalizations from asthma.
- Reduce emergency department (ED) visits for asthma.
- Reduce activity limitations among persons with current asthma.
- Reduce the proportion of persons with asthma who miss school or work days.
- Increase the proportion of persons with current asthma who receive formal patient education.
- Increase the proportion of persons with current asthma who receive appropriate asthma care according to National Asthma Education and Prevention Program (NAEPP) guidelines.
- Increase the number of states, territories, and the District of Columbia with a comprehensive asthma surveillance system for tracking asthma cases, illness, and disability at the state level.
- Reduce activity limitations among adults with chronic obstructive pulmonary disease (COPD).
- Reduce deaths from COPD among adults.
- Reduce hospitalizations for COPD.
- Reduce emergency department (ED) visits for COPD.[2]

References

1. Healthy People 2020. (2016). *Respiratory diseases: Overview*. Available at https://www.healthypeople.gov/2020/topics-objectives/topic/respiratory-diseases
2. Healthy People 2020. (2016). *Respiratory diseases: Objectives*. Available at https://www.healthypeople.gov/2020/topics-objectives/topic/respiratory-diseases

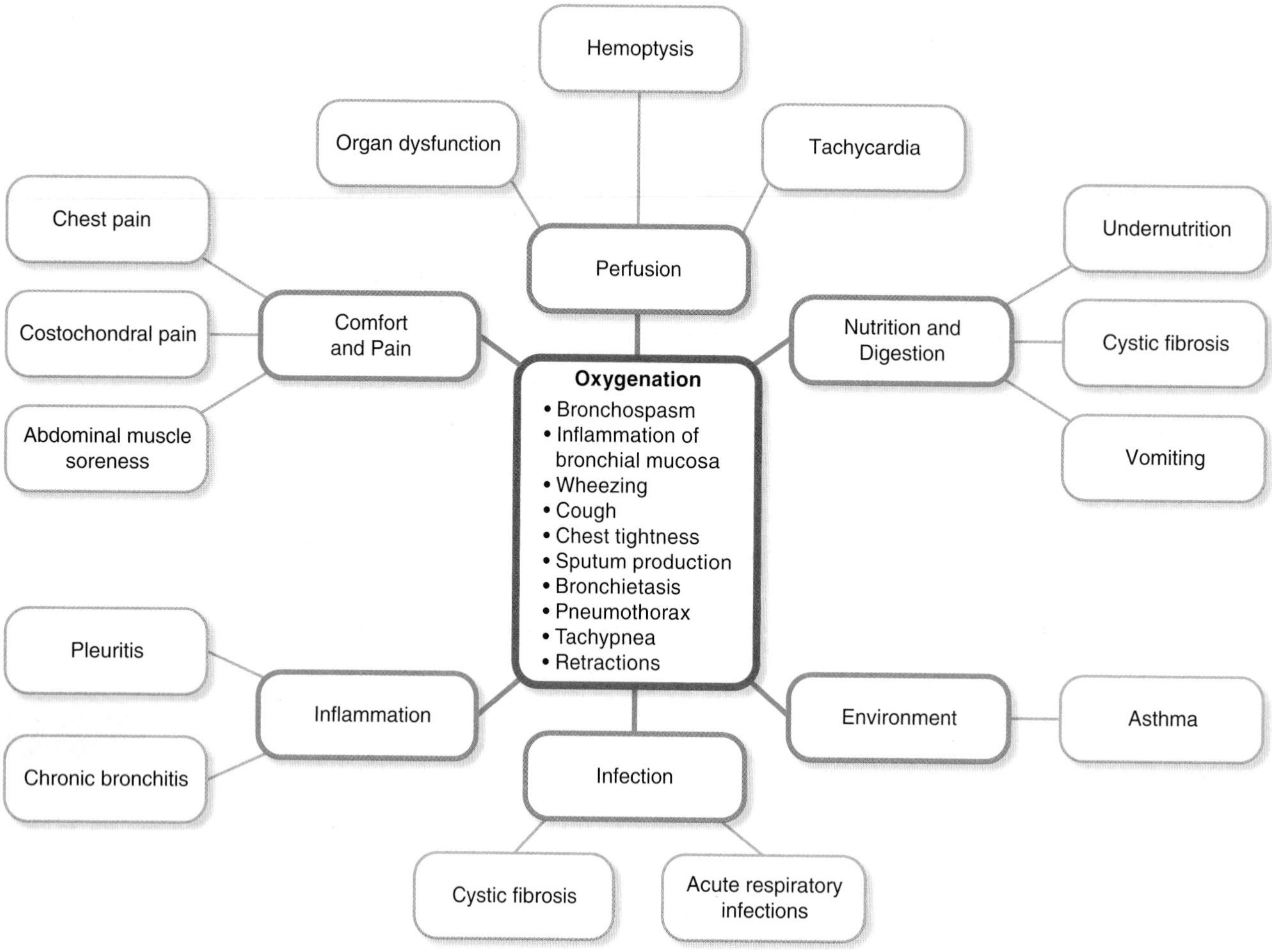

Hemoptysis
Organ dysfunction
Tachycardia
Chest pain
Perfusion
Undernutrition
Costochondral pain
Comfort and Pain
Nutrition and Digestion
Cystic fibrosis
Abdominal muscle soreness
Vomiting

Oxygenation
- Bronchospasm
- Inflammation of bronchial mucosa
- Wheezing
- Cough
- Chest tightness
- Sputum production
- Bronchietasis
- Pneumothorax
- Tachypnea
- Retractions

Pleuritis
Inflammation
Environment
Asthma
Chronic bronchitis
Infection
Cystic fibrosis
Acute respiratory infections

Figure 18.1 ■ Concepts related to obstructive lung diseases.

Jimmy Bley: Introduction

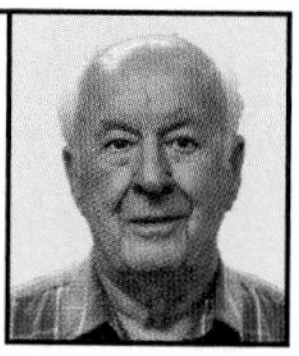

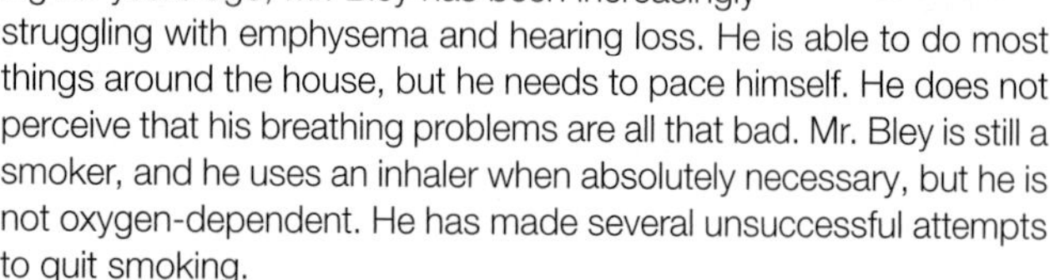

Jimmy Bley, an 84-year-old male, is a retired veteran who served as an electronics technician in the Army for his entire career. Since retiring 20 years ago, Mr. Bley has been increasingly struggling with emphysema and hearing loss. He is able to do most things around the house, but he needs to pace himself. He does not perceive that his breathing problems are all that bad. Mr. Bley is still a smoker, and he uses an inhaler when absolutely necessary, but he is not oxygen-dependent. He has made several unsuccessful attempts to quit smoking.

1. What question should the nurse ask about Mr. Bley's current practice of smoking?
2. What question should the nurse ask about Mr. Bley's use of an inhaler?

Check Your Progress: Section 18.1

1. What are some of the disorders included in the spectrum of obstructive lung disorders?
2. In addition to dyspnea what physiologic process is common to obstructive pulmonary diseases?
3. What is the goal of the *Healthy People 2020* initiative that relates to respiratory disease?

18.2 Alterations in Respiratory Structure and Function

Anatomic Airway Structure

Obstructive lung disorders include conditions for which exhalation is especially difficult. In obstructive lung disorders, airway obstruction occurs because of mucosal inflammation, loss of structural support for the small peripheral bronchi and bronchioles, and/or constriction of bronchial smooth muscles that can be exacerbated by an accumulation of mucus in airways. The trachea and large central airways have significant cartilage support, but the cartilage diminishes in more peripheral airways and disappears in the terminal bronchioles. Small bronchioles are attached to and supported by the surrounding lung tissue. The lung tissue consists of the functional pulmonary structures, including the alveoli, capillary endothelium, interstitial space, and tissues within the septa and around bronchi and bronchioles. The extracellular matrix provides elasticity and structural stability in normal lungs. The lung tissue tends to resist stretching during inhalation, so during exhalation, bronchioles are held open by the elastic recoil of the stretched tissue. In damaged lung tissue, the small bronchi

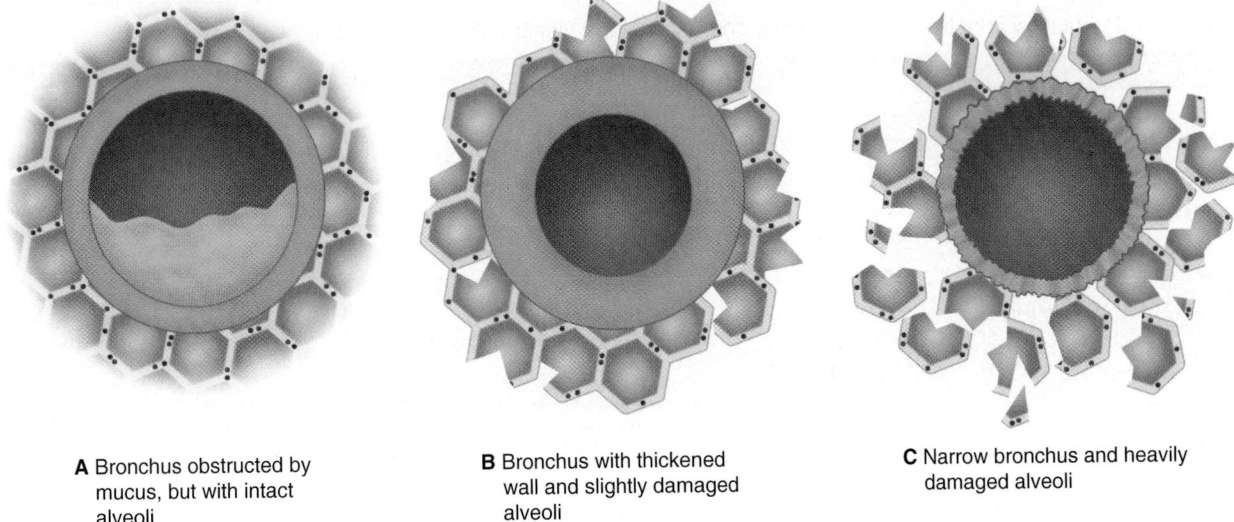

A Bronchus obstructed by mucus, but with intact alveoli
B Bronchus with thickened wall and slightly damaged alveoli
C Narrow bronchus and heavily damaged alveoli

Figure 18.2 ■ Mechanisms of airflow obstruction in COPD. **A**. Partial obstruction of the lumen by mucus secretions. **B**. Thickening of the airway wall due to bronchoconstriction, muscle hypertrophy, and fibrotic changes. **C**. Narrowing of the airway from lost radial traction secondary to deterioration of attachments to lung tissue.

and bronchioles are not supported by elastic recoil, and the result is airway obstruction that is worse during exhalation. This is the obstruction of COPD (**Figure 18.2** ■).

Smooth muscles spiral the inner surfaces of the bronchial and bronchiolar walls. When stimulated by acetylcholine from parasympathetic nerves, bronchial and bronchiolar smooth muscles contract, resulting in **bronchoconstriction** (narrowing of the airways). In contrast, sympathetic stimulation of pulmonary beta-2 adrenergic receptors by norepinephrine and epinephrine produces muscular relaxation and **bronchodilation** (widening of the bronchi and bronchioles). When smooth muscles become irritable or "twitchy" with inflammation, they constrict strongly but do not readily relax. With chest expansion during inhalation, inflamed airways are pulled open, and that helps to counteract the muscle contraction. But with exhalation, the thorax is smaller, and the effects of smooth muscle contraction become more dominant, so the airway obstruction is increased.

Airway obstruction decreases the airway diameter, which in turn increases the resistance to airflow and results in a slower speed of exhalation. For healthy individuals, the normal inspiratory to expiratory ratio (I:E ratio) is approximately 1:2, meaning that expiration takes approximately twice as long as inspiration. Individuals with an obstructive lung disease demonstrate a prolonged expiratory phase, with an I:E ratio of up to 1:5 or longer.[4] For these individuals, especially during exercise or activity, increased inspiratory volumes combined with exhalation through a constricted airway leads to **air trapping** in the lungs, which can impair ventilation and gas exchange and may produce lung hyperinflation.

Alterations in Pulmonary Function

Airway obstruction negatively affects the speed and volume of airflow during exhalation; these effects can be measured by pulmonary function tests (PFTs), which indicate the patterns of ventilatory airflow. To understand PFTs, it is important to understand the lung volumes that the tests measure and their approximate values in the "standard man." The measurement techniques that are commonly used for PFTs include spirometry, body plethysmography, and nitrogen washout. Spirometry, which measures airflow through the

Genetics and Genomics for Clinical Practice

Genomics in Obstructive Lung Disorders

Rita Kaspar

There are important genetic components in obstructive lung disorders, and tumors and genetic-environmental interactions strongly influence the expression of the disease phenotypes. "Epigenetics is the study of changes in gene transcription that are dependent on molecules that bind to DNA, rather than the sequence of DNA."[1] Epigenetic mechanisms that regulate gene expression depend on methylation, noncoding RNAs, and histone modification. Epigenetic regulation of gene expression occurs by turning on or turning off transcription of the specific DNA strands at specific times or in response to specific stimuli. The genetic–environmental interactions that regulate genetic expression also depend on the individual's age and state of health. The specific epigenetic mechanisms that influence the phenotype expression and how they can be influenced by factors such as diet, environmental exposure, and drugs are currently under study.[1]

Reference

1. Schwartz D. A. (2010). Epigenetics and environmental lung disease. *Proceedings of the American Thoracic Society*, 7(2), 123–125.

Table 18.1 Pulmonary Function Test Definitions and Values for a Healthy Young Adult Male

Measurement	Typical Value	Definition
Tidal volume (TV)	500 mL	Volume of air inhaled and exhaled during one cycle of normal quiet breathing
Inspiratory reserve volume (IRV)	3000 mL	After TV inhalation, IRV is the maximal volume of air that can be inhaled.
Inspiratory capacity (IC)	3500 mL	Maximal volume of air that can be inhaled after a normal exhalation (TV + IRV = IC)
Expiratory reserve volume (ERV)	1200 mL	After TV exhalation, ERV is the maximal volume of air that can be exhaled.
Residual volume (RV)	1300 mL	Volume of air remaining in the lung after a maximal exhalation
Functional residual capacity (FRC)	2500 mL	Volume of air remaining in the lung after a normal quiet exhalation. It is determined by the balance between the recoil of the chest wall and the recoil of the lung between breaths. (ERV + RV = FRC)
Vital capacity (VC)	4700 mL	The maximal amount of air that can be exhaled in a relaxed, nonforced manner after a maximal inhalation (TV + ERV + IRV = VC)
Total lung capacity (TLC)	6000 mL	Maximal volume of air in the lungs (RV + VC = TLC)
Forced expiratory volume in one second (FEV_1)	≥ 70% of VC	Volume of air exhaled in the first second of a forced maximal exhalation maneuver. It reflects airflow through large, medial bronchi.
FEV_1/ forced vital capacity (FVC)	≥ 70%	Calculated ratio for the speed of airflow during the first second to the total FVC; estimates the degree of airflow obstruction

mouth when nasal airflow is obstructed, is used clinically to measure the volume and speed of airflow during either a maximal inhalation or a maximal exhalation. Body plethysmography measures the total volume of air in the lungs or total lung capacity (TLC) and includes unevenly ventilated regions of the lungs. The nitrogen washout technique is an alternative method that is used to estimate TLC when body plethysmography is not available. For each PFT technique, there are reference values for each measurement, which are calculated values from lifetime nonsmokers without respiratory disorders or symptoms. The reference values are based on the individual's age, gender, height, weight, and race. **Table 18.1** lists some reference values for pulmonary function tests. A graphic representation of lung volumes is shown in **Figure 18.3**).

Check Your Progress: Section 18.2

1. What are the three causes of airway obstruction in a patient with an obstructive lung disorder?
2. How do norepinephrine, epinephrine, and acetylcholine affect the pulmonary musculature?
3. Why does a patient with an obstructive lung disorder experience impaired ventilation and gas exchange when physical activity is increased?

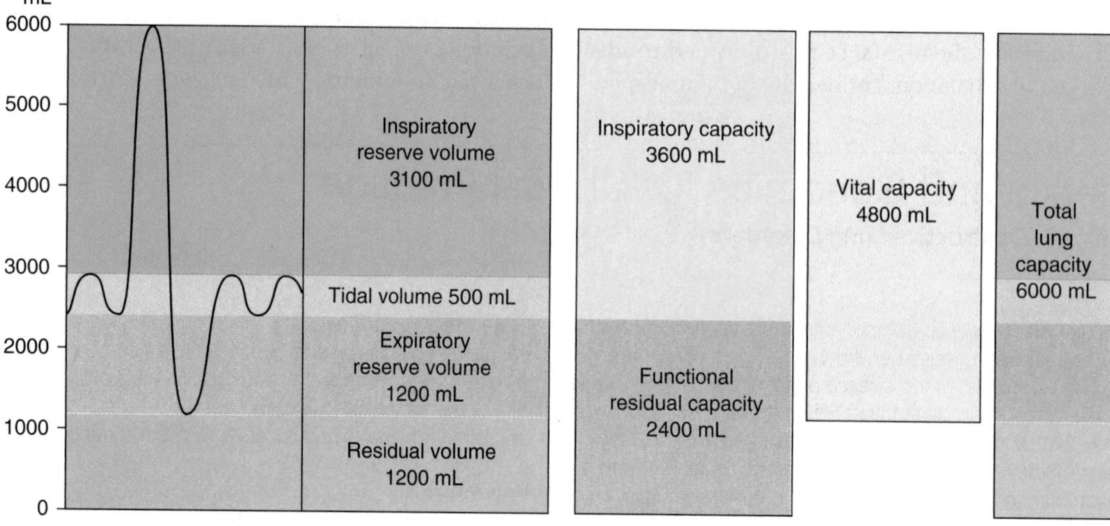

Figure 18.3 The relationship between lung volumes and capacities. Volumes (in milliliters) shown are for an average adult male.

18.3 Asthma

Asthma is a chronic inflammatory disorder of the airways characterized by recurrent episodes of reversible airway obstruction and hyperreactive airways. **Hyperreactivity** refers to an exaggerated response to a stimulus. The variable airflow obstruction is widespread but can reverse either spontaneously or with treatment.[5] During an asthma episode, inflammation causes wheezing, breathlessness, chest tightness, and cough, particularly at night and in the early morning. The primary immune cells that are involved in asthma are large numbers of eosinophils and $CD4^+$ T lymphocytes.

Etiology and Pathogenesis

The prevalence, morbidity, and mortality of asthma have increased since the 1980s in all ages, sex, and racial groups worldwide. The increase has been greatest in Western, industrialized nations, while asthma remains uncommon in children living in nonindustrialized, developing countries. The increased asthma prevalence in the Western world has occurred in spite of our improved understanding of the chronic inflammatory mechanisms in asthma and the availability of greatly improved treatment.

The patterns of asthma occurrence and severity in the United States. vary with age, sex, and race or ethnicity. In 2014, an estimated 22.6 million people in the United States were living with asthma.[6] Asthma prevalence in children under 18 years of age was 8.3%; for adults age 18 years and older, the prevalence of asthma was 7.0%.[6]

Among racial and ethnic groups, individuals of multiple race have the highest asthma prevalence (14.1%), while the lowest rates are found among Asians (5.2%).[7] Asthma prevalence is lower among Caucasians (7.7%) than among individuals of African American (11.2%) and American Indian or Alaska Native (9.4%) descent. The overall prevalence of asthma among Hispanics is 6.5%, with a higher prevalence among individuals of Puerto Rican (16.1%) descent than among those of Mexican (5.4%) descent.[7]

Risk Factors. Risk factors for developing asthma include the following:[8–10]

- *Genetic factors:* A parental or sibling history of asthma or **atopy** (the genetic predisposition toward developing allergies) is especially noteworthy.
- *History:* A history of severe respiratory syncytial virus infection requiring hospitalization may be an indicator of the genetic predisposition to asthma.
- *Gender:* Females after adolescence have an increased risk for asthma persisting into adulthood, while males are at increased risk before puberty. Some adult women have increased asthma severity with hormonal changes near the time of menstruation, but the reason for the sex-specific differences is not clear.
- *Obesity:* A high BMI is associated with severe asthma in women. Obesity may contribute to gastroesophageal reflux, which can precipitate asthma when gastric contents are aspirated into the lungs. Obesity also affects exercise and may alter the inflammatory response.
- *Exposure to allergens:* Cockroaches, smoke, and house dust mites are among the allergens that may, result in cytokine dysregulation that favors atopy (an allergic response).
- *Exposure to irritants:* Repeated exposures to a minor irritant may trigger asthma, but it can also be triggered by a single massive exposure.
- *Maternal smoking/environmental tobacco exposure:* Tobacco exposure is associated with wheezing and asthma severity in children.

Other proposed risk factors for the development of asthma include early childhood diet as a potential source of multiple allergens; low socioeconomic status, which also may be related to allergen exposure; low birth weight or premature birth; and infection.

Etiology. The etiology of asthma is not known. A genetic predisposition for asthma is necessary but not sufficient to cause asthma without an inciting stimulus, known as a **trigger**. Multiple genes were implicated in asthma susceptibility as a result of genetic mapping studies of families in isolated populations.[11] Whether the populations were isolated on the basis of their religion or geography, asthmatics all showed evidence for linkages by more than one gene, but there were also some novel regions that were expressed in only one of the isolated groups. So there are multiple genes that determine asthma susceptibility, and it is the exposure to environmental stimuli that influences the expression of the asthma phenotype.

Genetic alterations in asthmatics were reported for the arachidonic acid metabolic pathway for synthesis of leukotrienes, which are potent inflammatory mediators; variations in the expression of immunoglobin E (IgE); and polymorphisms in beta-2 receptors.[12] A polymorphism is a genetic variation that occurs in at least 1% of the population. More recent studies describe polymorphisms in asthma susceptibility genes that are related to airway hyperresponsiveness. Some of the genetic polymorphisms in asthma overlap with those for atopy, and they may reinforce each other. Asthma is more common in people with allergies, but allergies can occur independently from asthma, just as asthma can occur in people who do not have allergies.

Classification. There are multiple ways to classify asthma. For example, it may be classified on the basis of the presence or absence of its association with an allergic reaction. Allergic asthma, also called extrinsic or atopic asthma, is triggered by allergens that are external to the individual. Allergic asthma results in a type 1 hypersensitivity allergic reaction. Nonallergic asthma, sometimes called intrinsic or nonatopic asthma, is triggered by factors that do not produce a true allergic reaction. However, nonallergic asthma does generate an inflammatory response that involves IgE.

Asthma also may also be classified by its precipitating factor or trigger. See **Table 18.2** ■ for an overview of precipitating factors that may trigger an acute exacerbation of asthma.

Table 18.2 Precipitating Factors and Triggers of Asthma

Precipitating Factors	Description
Allergens	Allergic asthma (atopic asthma, which is precipitated by the inhalation of an allergen, is the most common type of asthma in children; it is also the best understood. In a classic type 1 hypersensitivity reaction, sensitized Th-2 type $CD4^+$ cells stimulate the development of IgE in response to a specific allergen such as cockroach feces, dust mites, pollens, or pet dander. This induction of the humoral Th-2 response is basic to the pathogenesis of allergic asthma.
Occupational stimuli	In some instances, stimuli in a work environment may provoke an asthmatic response. Weeks or years of exposure may precede the development of asthma. For these individuals, symptoms will abate when the individual is away from work (e.g., on days off and vacations) and worsen on return to the work environment. An IgE-mediated hypersensitivity allergic response is responsible for asthma in individuals exposed to organic dusts (e.g., bakers, animal handlers, weavers), inorganic dusts (e.g., metal salts), industrial chemicals, or pharmaceutical agents. In other instances, the offending agent can directly stimulate the autonomic nervous system or cause the production of mediators that result in bronchospasm.[13]
Infection	Viral infections cause bronchial inflammation, trigger bronchoconstriction, and can cause asthma to be expressed in susceptible individuals. In children under 2 years of age, respiratory syncytial virus is the usual cause for bronchiolitis, and it is a strong risk factor for asthma even into adolescence. In older children, rhinoviruses and parainfluenza viruses are the usual cause of respiratory infections. The viruses can activate airway epithelial cells to produce cytokines and chemokines to attract inflammatory cells. Neutrophils responding to a rhinoviral airway infection further induce inflammation, while the rhinoviruses damage respiratory epithelia and induce bronchoconstriction. Severe rhinoviral or influenza viral infections frequently cause a loss of asthma control in children and adults.[14]
Exercise	For some individuals, 10–15 minutes of physical exertion can induce asthma, possibly owing to an increase in loss of heat and water from the bronchial mucosa during deep breathing. The temperature and humidity of the ambient air influence the response; for example, an individual who exercises in cold, dry air is more likely to be symptomatic than is one who is exercising in warm, humid air.
Medications	Primarily in asthmatics, aspirin and nonsteroidal anti-inflammatory agents can trigger drug-induced bronchospasm by interrupting one arachidonic acid metabolic pathway that produces prostaglandins. As a result, the alternate pathway increases production of leukotrienes, the very potent mediators of inflammation and bronchospasm.
Air pollution	The pronounced air pollution that occurs with temperature inversions has been associated with bronchospasm in asthmatics and other people with chronic breathing problems. Ozone, sulfur dioxide, and nitrogen oxides are implicated in the development of bronchospasm.
Strong emotions	Strong emotions may either precipitate bronchospasm or increase asthma responsiveness. In either case, the proposed mechanism is vagal stimulation and acetylcholine release, which stimulates contraction of bronchial smooth muscle.

Barbara Morgan: Application

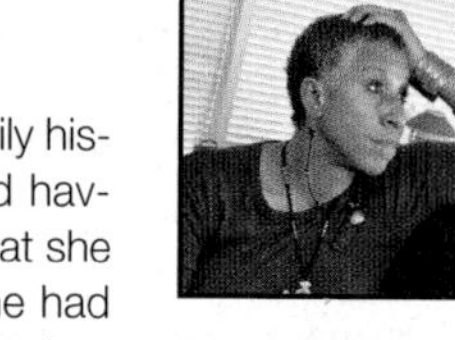

Ms. Morgan has a strong personal and family history of asthma and allergies. She reported having had asthma as a small child but says that she "outgrew" it. Ms. Morgan reported that she had not experienced dyspnea on exertion or a wheeze since childhood until she began working on restoring a historic building a month ago. Shortly after she began working inside the 120-year-old building, she noticed shortness of breath and wheezing when she was inside the building, especially when climbing stairs. She feels better and has fewer symptoms when she is away from her work site. Her brother was diagnosed with asthma as young child, and she remembers that her maternal grandfather had problems with his breathing. Ms. Morgan is 5 feet 4 inches tall and weighs 114 pounds. Her predicted peak flow is 430 L/min, but her actual peak flow is 385 L/min.

3. On the basis of Ms. Morgan's history, what is the most likely trigger for her asthma?
4. What does Ms. Morgan's actual peak flow value of 385 L/sec reflect?
5. Is Ms. Morgan's African American and Hispanic heritage significant in this case? If so, how?

Pathophysiology. Asthma is a disorder that is expressed in genetically susceptible individuals after exposure to diverse stimuli or triggers. Although the stimuli are diverse, they all cause a persistent inflammatory response in the airways that results in bronchial hyperreactivity. Asthma triggers are specific to the individual, so a stimulus that triggers symptoms in one asthmatic individual may not affect another. Table 18.2 summarizes the pathophysiology of asthma based on various triggers and precipitating factors. **Figure 18.4** ■ shows the pathogenesis of an acute asthma attack.

During a classic type 1 hypersensitivity reaction, exposure to a specific allergen leads sensitized Th-2 type $CD4^+$ cells to stimulate the development of IgE. This induction of the humoral (Th-2) response is basic to the pathogenesis of allergic asthma. The Th-2 subtype humoral immunity is predominant in infancy, but during normal growth and development, a shift is usually made to Th-2 cell–based immunity. In individuals with asthma, it may be that the immune system did not make the shift to cell-mediated immunity,[15] or a later stimulus (e.g., infection or bronchial inflammation) may have caused a dysregulation of the immune system.

In allergic asthma, the Th-2 subtype T lymphocytes release specific cytokines (interleukin [IL]-4, IL-5 and IL-13) that stimulate the synthesis of IgE, the activation of eosinophils, and the growth of mast cells. Eosinophils and Th-2 T lymphocytes are considered critical cells in both allergic and nonallergic asthma. Immunoglobulin E is important for maintaining the persistent inflammation of asthma, but other inflammatory cells may be equally important. The mechanisms are not known for asthma that does not exhibit eosinophilia, subepithelial fibrosis, and a poor response to corticosteroids.[16]

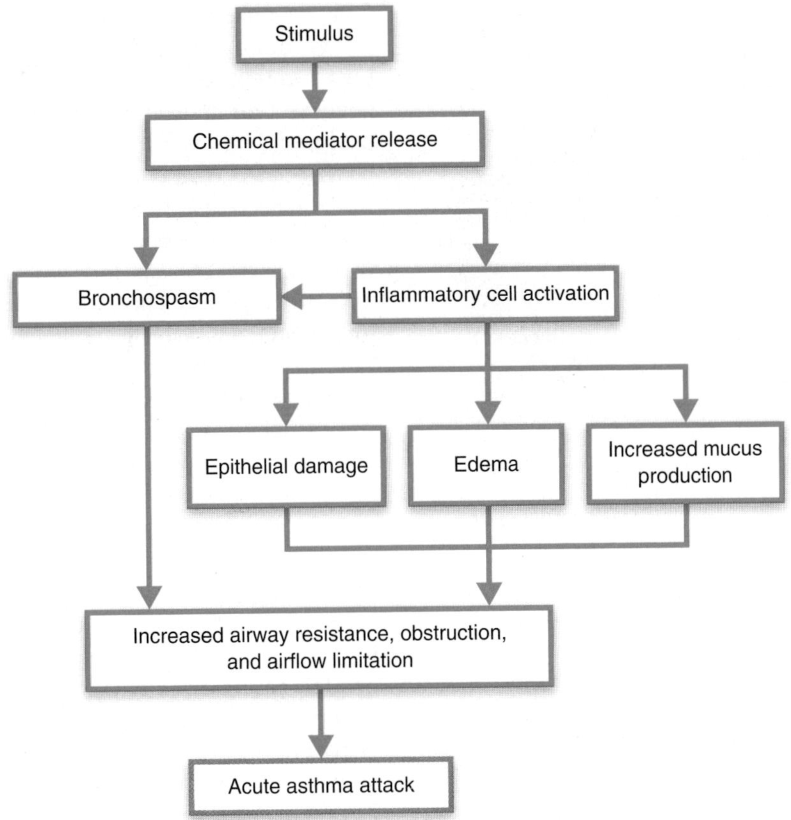

Figure 18.4 ■ Pathogenesis of an acute episode of asthma.

In the immediate phase of asthma, the inhaled allergens cross-link to IgE on the surface of a mast cell, initiating the allergic response by causing mast cells to degranulate. Mast cell granules release preformed histamine and other inflammatory mediators, including cytokines that strongly recruit eosinophils. Antigens also attach to Th-2 $CD4^+$ cells and possibly macrophages in the airway, which release inflammatory mediators such as bradykinin, leukotrienes, prostaglandins, thromboxane A2, and platelet-activating factor. The inflammatory mediators open tight junctions between mucosal epithelial cells, allowing antigens to flow into the submucosa, where they cross-link IgE on more mast cells, releasing even more inflammatory mediators and chemotactic factors. The increased vascular permeability causes edema and causes chemotactic factors to recruit more cells to the site of the inflammation. Mediators cause a reflex bronchoconstriction by stimulating subepithelial vagal nerve endings. Histamine alone can mediate bronchoconstriction, edema, mucus secretion, and itching. This immediate phase begins 30–60 minutes after inhalation of the trigger; it may be followed by a late phase 4–8 hours later.

In the late phase, the large numbers of eosinophils and some neutrophils that are recruited into the submucosa maintain and increase the bronchial inflammation. The neutrophils release more mediators and further damage the epithelial mucosa. The damaged epithelial cells stimulate mucosal nerve endings, causing further bronchoconstriction and mucus production. Activated eosinophils synthesize platelet-activating factor and leukotrienes, which are extremely potent inflammatory mediators. Activated eosinophils can maintain and amplify the inflammatory response without any additional antigen exposure, so eosinophilic infiltration is basic to the atopic asthma response (**Figure 18.5** ■).

Airway obstruction is increased during subsequent asthma episodes by structural changes caused by inflammation and bronchospasm. The increased exercise of bronchospasm causes hyperplasia and hypertrophy of bronchial smooth muscle cells. This gives bronchial smooth muscles an increased capacity for constriction, so bronchoconstriction in asthmatics narrows their airways more than it does in nonasthmatics. The number and size of submucosal mucus glands are increased, and they produce thick, sticky mucus. On expectoration into a tissue, the mucus "strings" as the tissue is removed from the mouth; there is little evidence of inflammatory cells in the tissue. As an asthma episode resolves, healing of inflamed airways occurs, with fibrosis under the basement membrane, which gives the appearance of a thickening of the basement membrane. Over long periods of time, the accumulation of fibrosis can cause the airways to become less responsive to bronchodilators.

Clinical Manifestations

Asthmatics with mild disease can be asymptomatic between asthma episodes. Asthmatics with persistent asthma have varying degrees of symptoms on a weekly or daily basis.

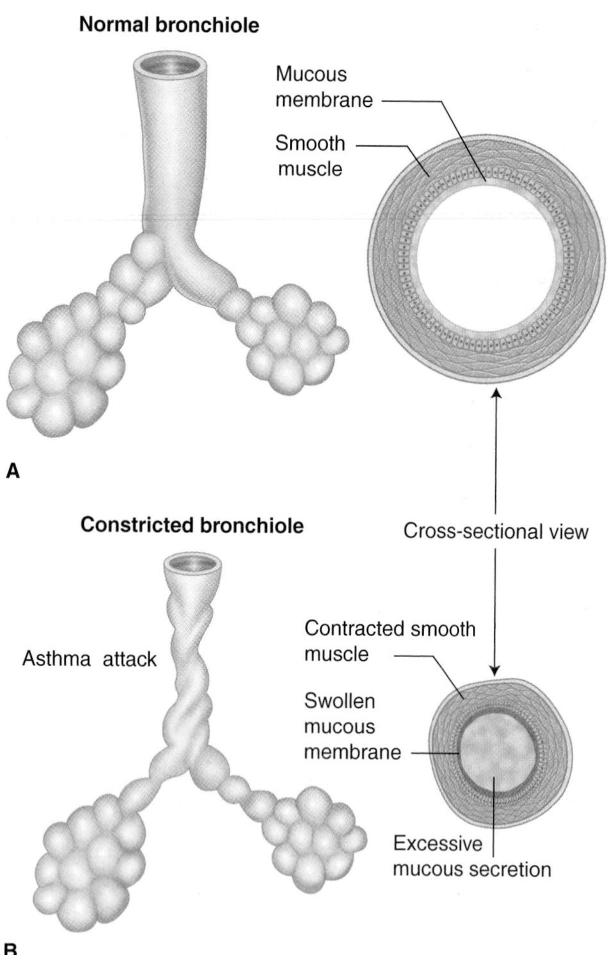

Figure 18.5 ■ Changes in bronchioles during an asthma attack. **A**. Normal bronchiole. **B**. In asthma attack.

The signs and symptoms of an asthma episode are related to the inflamed mucosa and bronchial hyperresponsiveness. Common manifestations include the following:

- Recurrent chest tightness and/or shortness of breath related to bronchospasm and inflammation of the bronchial mucosa, which narrow the airways
- Wheezing related to bronchospasm and mucus in the airways. Anything that interrupts the airflow though bronchial tubes causes an air vibration that is audible as a **wheeze**, which is similar to the noise made by blowing across the top of a glass bottle. Not all asthmatics wheeze; they may cough or have chest tightness instead.
- A cough that may be worse at night or in the early morning. The increased cough and wheeze at night are related to decreased serum cortisol levels and changes in breathing patterns. The cough may be a dry, hacking cough, or it may produce sputum. In cough-variant asthma, a cough may be the principal or only manifestation.[17]
- Production of thick, tenacious sputum that "strings." In severe asthma episodes, thick mucus can plug the very small airways.

Children who persistently wheezed from infancy through 6 years of age are more likely to have limitations of their lung function than are children who never or only intermittently wheezed, but the reasons for the limitations are not clear. Development of a wheeze may be associated with childhood anxiety, obesity or increased BMI, or sleep disordered breathing. Passive environmental smoke exposure is related more to airway size than to airway hyperreactivity and wheezing.[18] Children under 2 years of age who wheeze are more likely to have a respiratory syncytial viral bronchiolitis rather than allergic asthma. The bronchiolitis has the same clinical presentation as asthma, so asthma is not diagnosed in this age group unless specific factors associated with the development of persistent asthma are present. The factors are (a) key factor of recurrent wheezing defined as more than wheezing episodes in the past year; (b) major factors including eczema, airborne allergen sensitization, and maternal or paternal asthma; (c) minor factors including eosinophilia, wheezing apart from colds (crying, laughing, playing), food sensitivity, and increased IgE; and (d) other factors, including male gender, cesarean delivery, tobacco smoke exposure, and allergic rhinitis. The presence of one major factor and one or two minor factors in addition to recurrent wheezing is necessary to diagnose persistent asthma in children under 2 years of age.[19] ■

In severe asthma episodes, the increased work of breathing results in tachypnea and tachycardia. In infants and very thin adults, muscle retraction between the ribs is evidence of a very high level of effort to breathe. In chronic persistent asthma, young children and adults can have a loss of lung function as measured by PFTs, and adults may lose reversibility of their airflow obstruction. The fibrosis that occurs under the basement membrane of small airways with healing of the inflammation can result in fixed airways and a decreased responsiveness to beta-2 bronchodilators.

Maternal hypoxia from an asthma exacerbation poses the greatest risk to the fetus. There can be a decrease in intrauterine fetal growth when women have severe asthma, and the decreased growth is likely due to chronic mild hypoxia. ■

Asthma severity is the biologic intensity of the disease process measured clinically as the intensity of treatment needed to attain control and the number of exacerbations. Asthma severity is classified as mild intermittent asthma or mild, moderate, or severe persistent asthma based on daytime and nighttime symptoms, frequency of use of short-acting beta-2 agonists, activity limitations, lung function, and the risk for exacerbations.[12] Mild intermittent asthma may be asymptomatic between episodes, while untreated persistent asthma requires the use of bronchodilators more than twice a week (excluding pre-exercise use), causes nighttime awakenings more than twice per month, and interferes with daily activities. Classification of asthma severity and asthma control are separate and distinct concepts.[12] Asthma control is the degree to which asthma symptoms, functional impairments, and risks of untoward events are minimized and therapeutic goals are met.[12] It is possible to have severe disease but relief of asthma symptoms with appropriate medications, just as it is possible for patients with mild asthma to die with a severe exacerbation (**Table 18.3** ■).

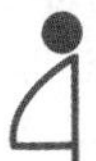

When women with asthma are pregnant, one third have improvements in their asthma, one third remain the same, and one third have worse asthma. ■

Linking Pathophysiology to Diagnosis and Treatment

An asthma diagnosis is based on a thorough medical history, physical examination, and PFTs. The individual's symptoms and a personal or family history of atopy and/or asthma may strongly suggest asthma. Laboratory test results that suggest asthma include an elevated sedimentation rate, indicating the presence of inflammation, and an increase in eosinophils. A good response to empiric treatment to reduce asthma symptoms also increases the suspicion of asthma. Confirmatory tests can include PFTs before and after administration of a bronchodilator to assess the reversibility of airway obstruction greater than 15% after inhalation of a beta-2 agonist. Other tests may be ordered to rule out other possible causes for the symptoms. One indication of diminished airflow that can be done in real time is called peak flow. The peak flow maneuver measures the maximal airflow through large airways when the individual exhales very strongly after a maximal inhalation. Asthmatic individuals can carry a peak flow meter to use when wheezing or chest tightness indicates reduced airflow.

The classic confirmatory test for asthma is a challenge test. During this test, the individual breathes dilute amounts of an irritating substance, such as methacholine or very cold air, to provoke airway obstruction and asthma symptoms. If exercise-induced asthma is suspected, the challenge test is an exercise test, generally with exercise on a cycle ergometer.

Assessment of exhaled nitrogen oxide is a biomarker for inflammation that can be useful to evaluate the effectiveness of treatment. Asthmatics exhale higher levels of nitrogen oxide than do control subjects matched by age, gender, and lung function, and levels are higher when asthma is not in good control.

Barbara Morgan: Application

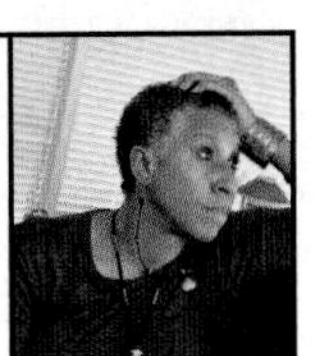

On her prebronchodilator and postbronchodilator PFTs, Ms. Morgan demonstrated an obstructive airflow pattern. As was noted previously, Ms. Morgan has a strong personal and family history. Additionally, her work involves exposure to older building structures, which are especially susceptible to indoor mold infestation. Further tests revealed that Ms. Morgan had an increased number of eosinophils and sedimentation rate of red blood cells on her complete blood count. Her FEV_1 was improved by 18% after she inhaled a beta-2 agonist bronchodilator. At 5 feet 4 inches tall and 114 pounds, Ms. Morgan had a predicted peak flow of 430 L/min, but her actual peak flow was 385 L/min. Considering her personal and family history of asthma, work-related exacerbation of signs and symptoms, decreased peak flow, obstructive pattern on PFTs, and laboratory reports, she was diagnosed with asthma.

6. What is the significance of Ms. Morgan report of "stringy" sputum?
7. What is the significance of the increased number of eosinophils and sedimentation rate of the red blood cells?
8. What can cause the nighttime cough that Ms. Morgan has experienced?

Table 18.3 The Classification of Asthma Severity

Components of Severity		Classification of Asthma Severity (Youths ≥ 12 years of age and adults)			
			Persistent		
		Intermittent	*Mild*	*Moderate*	*Severe*
Impairment Normal FEV_1/FVC 8–19 years: 85% 20–39 years: 80% 40–59 years: 75% 60–80 years: 70%	Symptoms	≤ 2 days/week	≥ 2 days/week but not daily	Daily	Throughout the day
	Nighttime awakenings	≤ 2/month	3–4×/month	> 1×/week but not nightly	Often 7×/week
	Short-acting beta-2 agonist use for symptom control (not prevent EIB)	≤ 2 days/week	> 2 days/week but not > 1×/day	Daily	Several times/day
	Interference with normal activity	None	Minor limitations	Some limitations	Extremely limited
	Lung function	Normal FEV_1 between exacerbations FEV_1 ≥ 80% predicted FEV_1/FVC normal	FEV_1 ≥ 80% predicted FEV_1/FVC normal	FEV_1 > 60% but < 80% predicted FEV_1/FVC reduced 5%	FEV_1 > 60% predicted FEV_1/FVC reduced 5%
Risk	Exacerbations requiring oral systemic corticosteroids	0–1/year	2/year	2/year	2/year
		Consider severity and interval since last exacerbation. Frequency and severity may fluctuate over time for patients in any severity category. Relative annual risk of exacerbations may be related to FEV_1.			

Goals of asthma management include reduction of impairments and asthma risks. Impairments are reduced when symptoms are prevented, a short-acting bronchodilator is needed not more than twice a week, PFTs are normal or nearly normal, and the individual can perform normal activities and is satisfied with the care received. The reduction of risk includes preventing exacerbations, emergency department visits, hospitalizations, and loss of lung function as well as minimizing the adverse effects of drug therapy.[12]

Among older adults, the dangers of asthma include an increased susceptibility to respiratory failure, even during a relatively mild asthma exacerbation. Additionally, controlling asthma may be more challenging in older adults because of the presence of comorbidities. ■

Components of asthma management include environmental control, asthma education for patients and families, and bronchodilator and anti-inflammatory medications (**Figure 18.6** ■). Environmental control to remove the stimuli that trigger asthma is tailored to an individual, since each person responds to different triggers. To actively participate in asthma management, asthmatics and their families need to learn about asthma, how to monitor it, and when to seek help. Usual medications include inhaled short- and long-acting bronchodilators, inhaled corticosteroids, combinations of bronchodilators and inhaled corticosteroids (anti-inflammatory), leukotriene receptor agonists (anti-inflammatory), antihistamines (anti-inflammatory), theophyllines (bronchodilator), mast cell stabilizers that reduce release of inflammatory mediators, and anti-IgE therapy to suppress inflammation. Asthmatics need a written asthma self-management plan that incorporates the appropriate elements for their care.

During pregnancy, the risks of any medication must always be balanced with the benefits to the mother and fetus. ■

The initial treatment for asthma is based on the assessment of asthma severity. Mild intermittent asthma is managed with the occasional use of a short-acting bronchodilator and treatment of respiratory infections with appropriate antibiotics and/or corticosteroids. The gold standard treatment for persistent asthma is inhaled corticosteroids.[20]

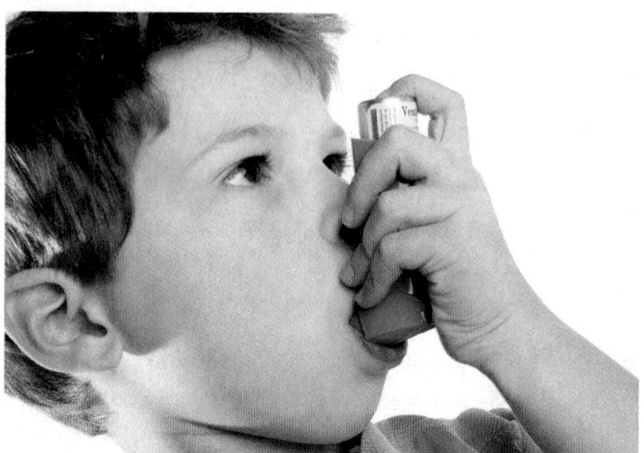

Figure 18.6 ■ Proper use of a metered-dose inhaler.

Although corticosteroids provide control, they do not alter the underlying disorder. In addition, a significant number of patients do not respond well to corticosteroids. The lack of response varies among individuals and may be due to an inflammatory response that is not as sensitive to corticosteroids. Corticosteroid-resistant asthma requires management with alternative anti-inflammatory therapy. This emphasizes the point that asthma is a heterogeneous group of disorders rather than a single entity. None of the currently available asthma therapy medications prevent lung remodeling. For further details, refer to the American Thoracic Society/European Respiratory Society Statement on Asthma Control and Exacerbations.[21]

Barbara Morgan: Outcome

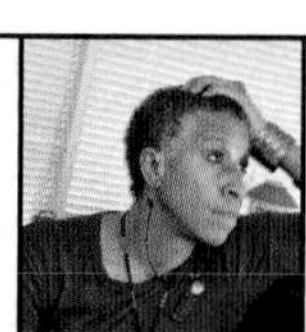

Ms. Morgan was started on a short-acting inhaled beta-2 agonist to control her acute asthma exacerbations. For long-term control, she was prescribed an inhaled corticosteroid. On the advice of her healthcare provider, Ms. Morgan sought to eliminate her exposure to potential environmental triggers such as mold. To do this, she transferred to a work position that did not require her to be inside the buildings that were under renovation by her firm. Within a week of the transfer, Ms. Morgan no longer experienced wheezing or dyspnea. Repeat PFTs revealed that her predicted peak flow had increased to 405 L/min. She maintained the inhaled corticosteroid regimen but no longer needed to use the short-acting inhaled beta-2 agonist. Ms. Morgan's healthcare provider advised her that she would probably be able to discontinue the inhaled corticosteroid in the near future.

9. What are the asthma outcome goals for the inhaled beta-2 agonist and the inhaled corticosteroid prescribed to Ms. Morgan?
10. What is the significance of the repeat PFTs and the predicted peak flow rate?

Check Your Progress: Section 18.3

1. How is asthma affected by pregnancy?
2. What is peak flow?
3. What types of medications are used to treat asthma?

18.4 Chronic Obstructive Pulmonary Disease

Chronic obstructive pulmonary disease (COPD) is the umbrella term used to describe progressive lung diseases including chronic bronchitis and emphysema. Because of their frequent coexistence in an individual, the symptoms and management strategies for these disorders often overlap. COPD is characterized by progressive airflow limitations that are not fully reversible. The airflow limitations are associated with an "enhanced chronic inflammatory response in the airways and the lung to noxious particles or gases" (p. 2).[1]

CLINICAL POINT: The 2017 GOLD Report states, "Emphysema, or destruction of the gas-exchanging surfaces of the lung (alveoli), is a pathologic term that is often (but incorrectly) used clinically and describes only one of several structural abnormalities present in patients with COPD."[1] Rather than addressing emphysema and chronic bronchitis as distinct subsets of COPD, the 2017 GOLD Report focuses on COPD as a primary disorder.[1] ■

COPD is the third leading cause of chronic morbidity and mortality in the United States[22] and is projected to become the third most prevalent cause of death in the world by 2020.[1] Cigarette smoking accounts for 90% of the cases of COPD in industrialized countries; COPD remains relatively rare in nonsmokers. COPD also is more prevalent among adults age 45 years of age and older.[22] Only an estimated 20% of smokers develop COPD, so additional factors such as genetics and/or inhalation of other irritants are involved.[23]

Etiology and Pathogenesis

In 2010, the cost of COPD in the United States was projected to be approximately $50 billion, which includes $20 billion in direct costs and $30 billion in indirect costs.[24] The cost of caring for COPD increases with the severity of the disorder. While COPD is considered a preventable and treatable disorder, in some patients, the extrapulmonary effects of COPD (e.g., weight loss) and comorbidities contribute to the severity of COPD and its effects on quality of life.[1]

The usual onset of COPD is gradual with slowly progressive symptoms of dyspnea and **shortness of breath (SOB)** (breathlessness). Diagnosis of COPD typically occurs among cigarette smokers between the ages of 50 and 60 years, by which point effects of the disorder are already moderately severe.

CLINICAL POINT: Long-term smoking causes an abnormal inflammatory response in the lungs that persists even after the individual stops smoking, so COPD occurs in former smokers as well as current smokers. ■

Risk Factors. The risk factors for developing COPD include the following:

- *Direct inhalation of tobacco smoke:* Smoking cigarettes, as well as smoking cigars or a pipe (including a water pipe)[1]
- *Environmental tobacco smoke:* Also known as secondhand smoke or passive smoking exposure
- *Genetics:* Variations in genetic codes affecting inflammation and lung remodeling that were found in smokers with COPD
- *Occupational exposures:* Prolonged, intense exposure to occupational dusts or chemicals (vapors, irritants and fumes) can cause COPD independent of smoking
- *Indoor air pollution:* Particularly when biomass fuels are used for heating and cooking in poorly ventilated dwellings[25]
- *Severe respiratory tract infections:* Maintain inflammation and produce exacerbations

Additional factors may influence the risk for developing COPD. There is an inverse relationship between COPD and socioeconomic status, that is, people with a low socioeconomic status have more COPD, though the reasons are not clear.[1] Unlike indoor pollution, outdoor air pollution has only a relatively small effect on the development of COPD.

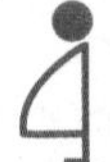

Maternal smoking during pregnancy may decrease fetal lung growth, and the decreased lung growth may increase the risk for COPD. ■

Etiology. The chronic airflow limitation of COPD is caused by an abnormal inflammatory response to inhaled particles and gases in the lungs. The slowly progressive chronic airway obstruction can occur in individuals exposed to toxic industrial inhalants and in those who have a history of numerous, severe respiratory infections, but the major cause of COPD is cigarette smoking. All smokers have evidence of inflammation and structural abnormalities in their airways, whether or not they have COPD, and there is evidence of cellular changes even with passive smoke exposure. However, because of the abnormal inflammatory response, the chronic inflammation continues and worsens as the disorder progresses rather than "burning out" as it does in other chronic inflammatory disorders. In advanced COPD, the inflammation extends to other organs such as the heart, blood vessels, and skeletal muscles.

For older adults, preexisting alterations in lung function combined with decreased tolerance for bronchoconstriction and hypoxia increase the risk of complications due to COPD, including mortality.[26] ■

Many people who smoke water pipes and hookahs believe that these forms of smoking are less harmful, owing to water's filtration of the smoke. However, this belief is false. Research suggests that the water pipe smoker's exposure to carbon monoxide (CO) is comparable to that experienced by cigarette smokers and can produce toxicity.[27] And compared to cigarette smoking, hookah smoking is associated with a higher incidence of both COPD and lung cancer.[28]

Classification. The Global Initiative for Chronic Obstructive Lung Disease (GOLD) was undertaken by the National Heart, Lung, and Blood Institute and the World Health Organization in an international effort to improve the diagnosis and management of COPD. In the GOLD classification of COPD, outlined in **Table 18.4** ■, there are four grades that describe the progressive severity of the disorder. Values necessary for grading via the GOLD classification system include forced vital capacity (FVC), which refers to the maximal amount of air that can be exhaled after a maximal inhalation; this maneuver requires forced effort during exhalation. FVC is similar to vital capacity (VC); however, VC is unforced and is performed in a relaxed manner, except near the end-inspiration and end-expiration.[29] In the GOLD classification system, all values for FVC and forced expiratory volumes are in 1-second (FEV_1) postbronchodilator values. The ratio of FEV_1 to FVC indicates how quickly an individual can forcefully exhale air. Normal values for FEV_1/FVC change with age but are 70% or more of the FVC, so most air is exhaled in the first 1 second.[1]

Table 18.4 Four Grades of COPD

Grade and Severity	Description
GOLD 1: mild COPD	• Mild airflow limitation ($FEV_1/FVC < 70\%$; $FEV_1 \geq 80\%$ of predicted) • Symptoms of chronic cough and sputum production may be present but are not always present. • At this stage, the individual may not be aware that lung function is abnormal.
GOLD 2: moderate COPD	• Worsening airflow limitations ($FEV_1/FVC < 70\%$; $50\% \leq FEV_1 < 80\%$ of predicted), with SOB typically developing on exertion, and cough and sputum production are sometimes also present. • This is the stage at which patients typically seek medical care because of chronic respiratory symptoms or an exacerbation of their disease.
GOLD 3: severe COPD	• Further worsening of airflow limitations ($FEV_1/FVC < 70\%$; $30\% \leq FEV_1 < 50\%$ of predicted), greater SOB, reduced exercise capacity, fatigue, and repeated exacerbations that almost always have an impact on patient's quality of life.
GOLD 4: very severe COPD	• Severe airflow limitations ($FEV_1/FVC < 70\%$; $FEV_1 < 30\%$ of predicted) or $FEV_1 < 50\%$ predicted plus chronic respiratory failure.

Source: Global Initiative for Chronic Obstructive Lung Disease. (2017). Pocket guide to COPD diagnosis, management, and prevention: 2017 report. GOLD Reports. Retrieved from http://goldcopd.org/wp-content/uploads/2016/12/wms-GOLD-2017-Pocket-Guide.pdf

Pathophysiology. Discussion of the pathophysiology of COPD is focused on the destructive effects of chronic inflammation, including structural remodeling of lung tissue. Additional hallmarks of COPD include fixed airway obstruction, alterations in vascular structure, destruction of pulmonary structures, and pulmonary hyperinflation.

The chronic inflammation of COPD occurs throughout the airways, lung tissue, and vasculature of the lung (**Figure 18.7** ■). Inhaled smoke attracts an increased numbers of activated macrophages, $CD8^+$ T lymphocytes, and neutrophils that release inflammatory mediators such as leukotrienes, IL-1, tumor necrosis factor alpha, and others that are capable of damaging lung structure. Interactions of multiple cytokines are involved in the recruitment, activation, and survival of inflammatory cells.[30] The inflammation is also supported by increased oxidative stress.[31] Peripheral airways less than 2 millimeters in internal diameter are the major site of COPD, and the repeated cycles of inflammation and healing cause structural remodeling. The increased collagen and formation of scar tissue in the basement membrane narrow the airways, increasing the resistance to airflow. The central airways with a internal diameter of 2–4 millimeters show evidence of inflammatory cell infiltration, and there is an increase in the number and size of mucus glands that are responsible for mucus hypersecretion.[1]

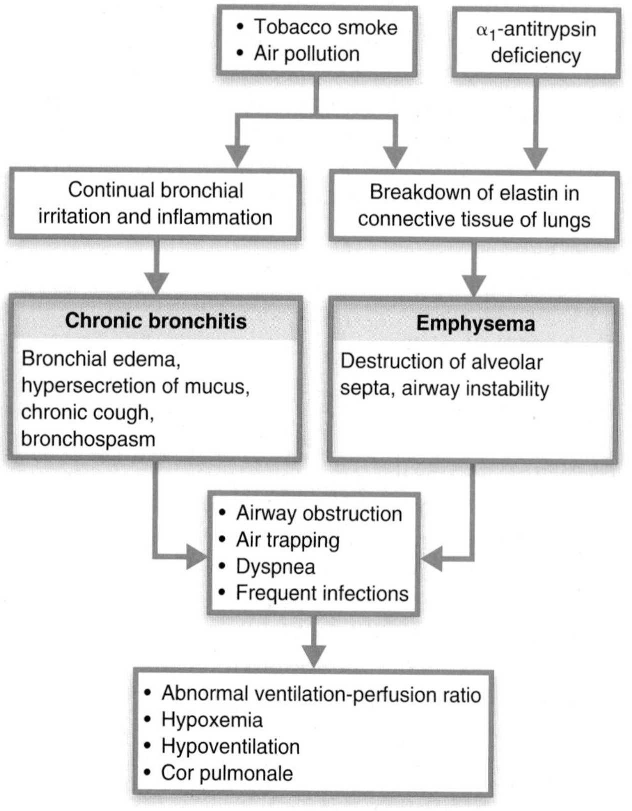

Figure 18.7 ■ Pathogenesis of chronic obstructive pulmonary disease.

Fixed airway obstruction narrows the airways, increasing resistance to airflow, so more energy and more work are required to achieve normal tidal volume (TV). Bronchospasms and mucus in the airways can cause additional narrowing, further increasing the work of breathing. Air trapping and impaired ventilation produce an increase in retained carbon dioxide, or **hypercapnia**.

Structural vascular changes also occur in the pulmonary vasculature in COPD. Vascular inflammatory changes begin in endothelium and progress as the vessel walls are infiltrated by inflammatory cells, proteoglycans, and collagen. This results in an increase in smooth muscle and thickening of the vessel intima, which is composed of the endothelium, subendothelial space, and basement membrane.

Approximately 80% of people with COPD experience pulmonary **hyperinflation**, which is overexpansion of the lungs due to air trapping. Hyperinflated lungs are the result of two mechanisms: dynamic hyperinflation, which occurs with the process of breathing, and static hyperinflation, which occurs when the lungs are at rest between breaths. Dynamic hyperinflation occurs when an inhalation occurs before a full exhalation is completed. The normal inspiratory to expiratory (I:E) ratio is approximately 1:2. For individuals with an obstructive lung disease, the expiratory phase is prolonged, producing an I:E ratio of up to 1:5 or more.[4] When the individual with COPD inhales a large breath with activity, then exhales for the same amount of time through a smaller fixed airway, only part of the inhaled volume is exhaled, and the remainder of the air is trapped in the lung. The trapped air increases the functional residual capacity (FRC), so the next inhalation intrudes into the inspiratory reserve. As this cycle repeats, the dynamic hyperinflation increases. Static hyperinflation occurs because of the loss of elastic recoil in the lungs, decreasing the force for exhalation. Either or both of these mechanisms can contribute to hyperinflation in an individual with COPD,[32] but it is the dynamic hyperinflation that has the strongest association with an individual's level of physical activity, regardless of the severity classification of COPD.[33]

The work of breathing is increased by hyperinflation and fixed airway obstruction and can be exacerbated by bronchospasm and mucus in the airways. More muscle work is required to ventilate hyperinflated lungs, so respiratory muscles require more oxygen. Airflow in the respiratory system is based on changes in air pressure as respiratory muscles change the size of the thorax. Inspiratory muscles increase the size of the thorax by moving the chest wall outward and the diaphragm downward. When a skeletal muscle, such as the diaphragm, is at its normal resting length, it can generate maximum tension. In hyperinflation, the inspiratory muscles are in a preshortened resting state, so respiratory muscles must work harder for an individual to inhale a normal volume of air.

The pathophysiologic alterations of COPD are compensated for by slowing and increasing the depth of respirations, using pursed lip exhalation, and coughing. Because the dead space (non–gas-exchanging airways) is filled with every breath, taking a deeper breath increases the proportion of air reaching the alveoli (alveolar ventilation). Deeper breaths allow a slower respiratory rate and a decrease in the energy required for the work of breathing. It is thought that pursed lip exhalation exerts a back pressure on small airways, helping to hold them open during exhalation. Prolonging the pursed lip exhalation time to approximately twice the inhalation time allows exhalation of inhaled air through narrowed airways, thus limiting air trapping. Individuals with COPD have a productive cough that increases in frequency over time because of increased mucus production and the decrease in the number and activity of cilia in people who smoke. Both mucus hypersecretion and ciliary damage make the mucociliary system less effective, so individuals with chronic bronchitis must cough to clear their lungs of mucus.

While chronic bronchitis and emphysema frequently coexist, discussion of these disorders typically includes distinguishing among pathologic changes that are most often associated with each individual disorder. In particular, hallmarks of chronic bronchitis include persistent, inflammation-induced narrowing of the airways, copious mucus production, and a chronic productive cough. In emphysema, characteristic changes involve damage to the lung parenchyma, destruction of gas-exchanging pulmonary surfaces (including the alveolar walls), and subsequent pulmonary hyperinflation.[1,34]

Chronic Bronchitis. In **chronic bronchitis**, inflammatory changes cause an increase in the thickness of the basement membrane and loss of structural support for small airways (**Figure 18.8** ■). The end result is airway fixation. Exposure to cigarette smoke and other noxious agents causes chronic irritation of the airways, leading to an increase in the number of goblet cells and an increase in the size of submucosal glands. Subsequently, the goblet cell proliferation and submucosal gland hypertrophy may cause an increase in mucus production.[1] In many cases, mucus hypersecretion leads to the development of a chronic cough. However, not every patient with COPD will develop symptomatic hypersecretion of mucus or the chronic cough that often accompanies this alteration.[1]

Emphysema. **Emphysema** is characterized by the irreversible loss of walls between alveoli with no evidence of fibrosis (**Figure 18.9** ■). Emphysema results in larger, baggier alveoli

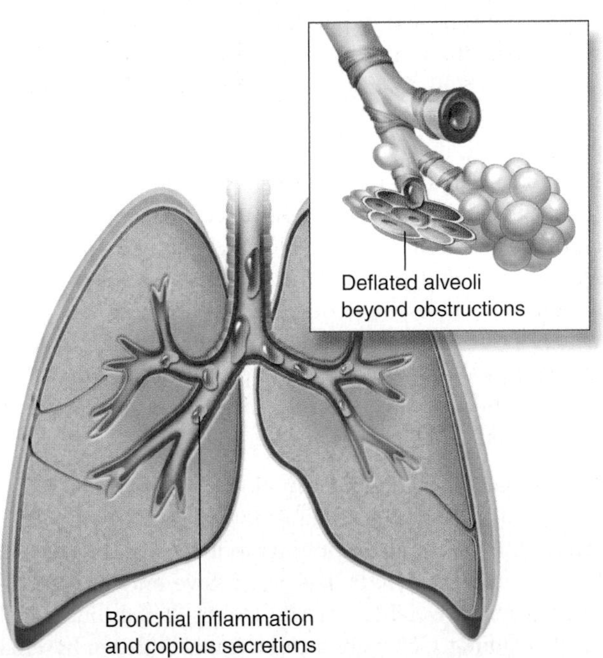

Figure 18.8 ■ Chronic bronchitis.

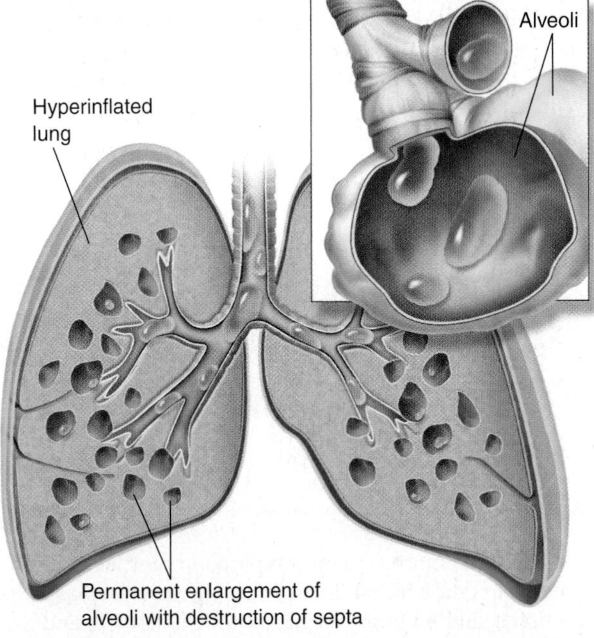

Figure 18.9 ■ Emphysema.

that lack sufficient elastic recoil to push air out during exhalation, resulting in a reduced airflow during exhalation. The loss of alveoli results in fewer walls available for diffusion of gases, affecting the PaO_2 in advanced COPD. Some degree of emphysema is found in approximately 50% of adults at autopsy, although most of them were not diagnosed with emphysema.

Cigarette smoking is the primary cause of emphysema, and it is implicated in the damage to the alveolar walls. Nicotine attracts macrophages and neutrophils and stimulates the release of elastase and proteases. Elastase is an enzyme that breaks down elastin, part of the supporting structure in the extracellular matrix. This breakdown of elastin is not balanced by elastin synthesis, so the elasticity of the alveolar walls is diminished. Proteases break down the lung tissue, and antiproteases, such as alpha-1 antitrypsin inhibit the excess destruction of the elastic elements in alveolar walls. Smoking inhibits alpha-1 antitrypsin activity, so its protective effects are lost. A rare genetic deficiency of alpha-1 antitrypsin occurs in about 1% of people with emphysema. It is more common in young adults under 40 years of age who develop emphysema, and the severity is increased when the affected individual smokes cigarettes.[35] In addition, oxygen radicals in smoke inactivate antiproteases, thus amplifying the effects of proteases. They may also enhance the inflammatory response.

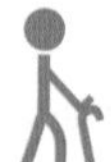

Oxidative stress may accelerate lung aging, leading to the pathogenesis of emphysema because aging lungs are less able to repair oxidative damage.[36] ■

The loss of lung tissue elasticity or recoil increases the time required for a full exhalation and increases FRC. Normally, if the chest wall is opened, lungs have a natural tendency to collapse (elastic recoil of the lungs pushing air out of the lungs), while the chest wall has a tendency to spring outward (elastic recoil of the chest wall). In the intact chest, the lung volume at the point of balance between lung and chest wall recoil is the FRC. The loss of lung tissue elasticity increases the volume of air in the lung required to counteract the recoil of the chest wall, thus increasing the FRC and residual volume (RV).[32]

Emphysema is classified according to the anatomic location of the damage. The two types of emphysema that cause airway obstruction are centriacinar emphysema, which typically involves the terminal and respiratory bronchioles in the upper portion of the lung and is most common in heavy cigarette smokers, and panacinar emphysema, which involves the entire acinus in the lower portions of the lung and is associated with alpha-1 antitrypsin deficiency (**Figure 18.10** ■).

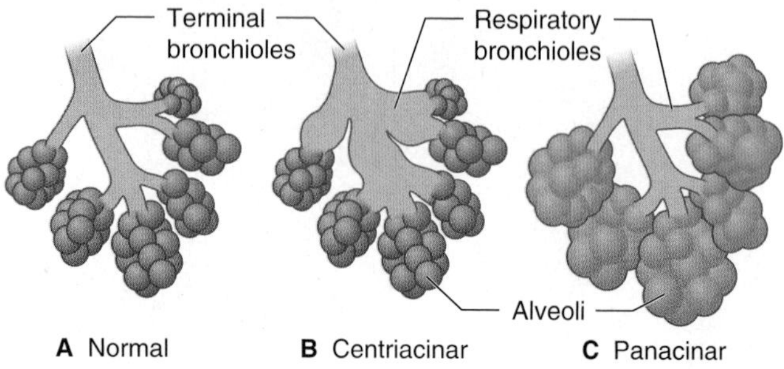

Figure 18.10 ■ Normal acini compared to centriacinar and panacinar emphysema. In centriacinar emphysema, destruction is limited to the terminal bronchioles (TB) and the respiratory bronchioles (RB). In panacinar emphysema, the alveoli (A) also are affected.

Clinical Manifestations

The clinical presentation of COPD at the time of diagnosis can vary depending on whether the cough and mucus production of chronic bronchitis are dominant or the structural pulmonary acini damage of emphysema is primary. **Pulmonary acini** refer to the functional units of the lung in which gas exchange occurs, specifically the respiratory bronchioles and their associated alveolar ducts and alveolar sacs. As COPD becomes advanced, differences in presentation become blurred. Note that cough and sputum production may precede the development of the airway limitations of COPD by many years, and not all individuals with cough and sputum production develop COPD.

Chronic Bronchitis. Chronic bronchitis is defined by a productive cough in the absence of a pulmonary infection on most days for 3 months in 2 consecutive years. Typically, individuals in their 50s with at least a 20 pack-year smoking history report a lingering productive cough in the winter the past 2 or 3 years even though they did not have a chest cold. Cigarette pack-years are calculated as the packs of cigarettes smoked each day times the years the individual smoked. Each pack contains 20 cigarettes, so an individual smoking 30 cigarettes daily for one year would have a 1.5 pack-year history of cigarette smoking.

The cough is worse in the morning, and the individual feels better after having coughed out the mucus. Later, the cough increases until it is present all year and mucus is expectorated throughout the day. The individual gradually notices or recalls SOB or dyspnea with activities that did not previously affect breathing. Dyspnea and SOB are exacerbated by bronchospasm; the effects of bronchoconstriction are more dominant during exhalation and add to dynamic hyperinflation.

Over time, as airway obstruction and resistance to airflow increase, the individual becomes progressively more dyspneic with SOB, limiting the choice of activities, dyspnea on exertion (DOE) can be exacerbated by the deconditioning effects of inactivity. Chronic bronchitis can progress to cor pulmonale and respiratory failure.

Individuals frequently experience respiratory infections that exacerbate symptoms of SOB, cough, wheezing, excess mucus, and possibly hemoptysis. **Hemoptysis** is defined as expectoration (coughing up) of blood from the airways as a result of an erosion through a pulmonary or bronchial blood vessel wall. Hemoptysis can occur with a severe bronchitis and is often the exacerbation that causes the individual to seek medical care.

Emphysema. The clinical presentation of emphysema is generally that of a smoker in his 60s who reports increased DOE but has little or no cough or sputum production unless he has a pulmonary infection. The SOB is progressive, and the individual may be losing weight primarily as a result of the increased work of breathing. Generally, the individual with emphysema can maintain oxygenation for a much longer period of time than someone presenting with chronic bronchitis.

Physical findings are similar for chronic bronchitis and emphysema: (a) The individual has a barrel chest, with an increased anterior–posterior diameter because of hyperinflation (**Figure 18.11** ■); (b) respiratory muscles in a partially contracted position with hyperinflation require more energy because they must do more work to move same amount of air; (c) accessory muscles are recruited to maintain ventilation; (d) soft distant breath sounds are heard with a prolonged exhalation; (e) if mucus hypersecretion or an infection is present, coarse rales may be heard as well; (f) signs of early hypoxemia may be subtle (e.g., clubbing of distal fingers), while a ruddy complexion indicates more severe hypoxemia with polycythemia; and (g) foot and ankle swelling may be present later in the day because of a decreased level of physical activity, but it usually resolves overnight.

Advanced COPD. In advanced COPD, distinctions between symptoms of chronic bronchitis and emphysema blur. Damage to bronchi, lung tissue, and pulmonary vasculature is widespread and results in reduced capacity for gas exchange and deterioration of pulmonary function. Air movement occurs by diffusion earlier in bronchioles, increasing the time needed for air to diffuse into acini, and ventilation–perfusion mismatch is common. Progressive

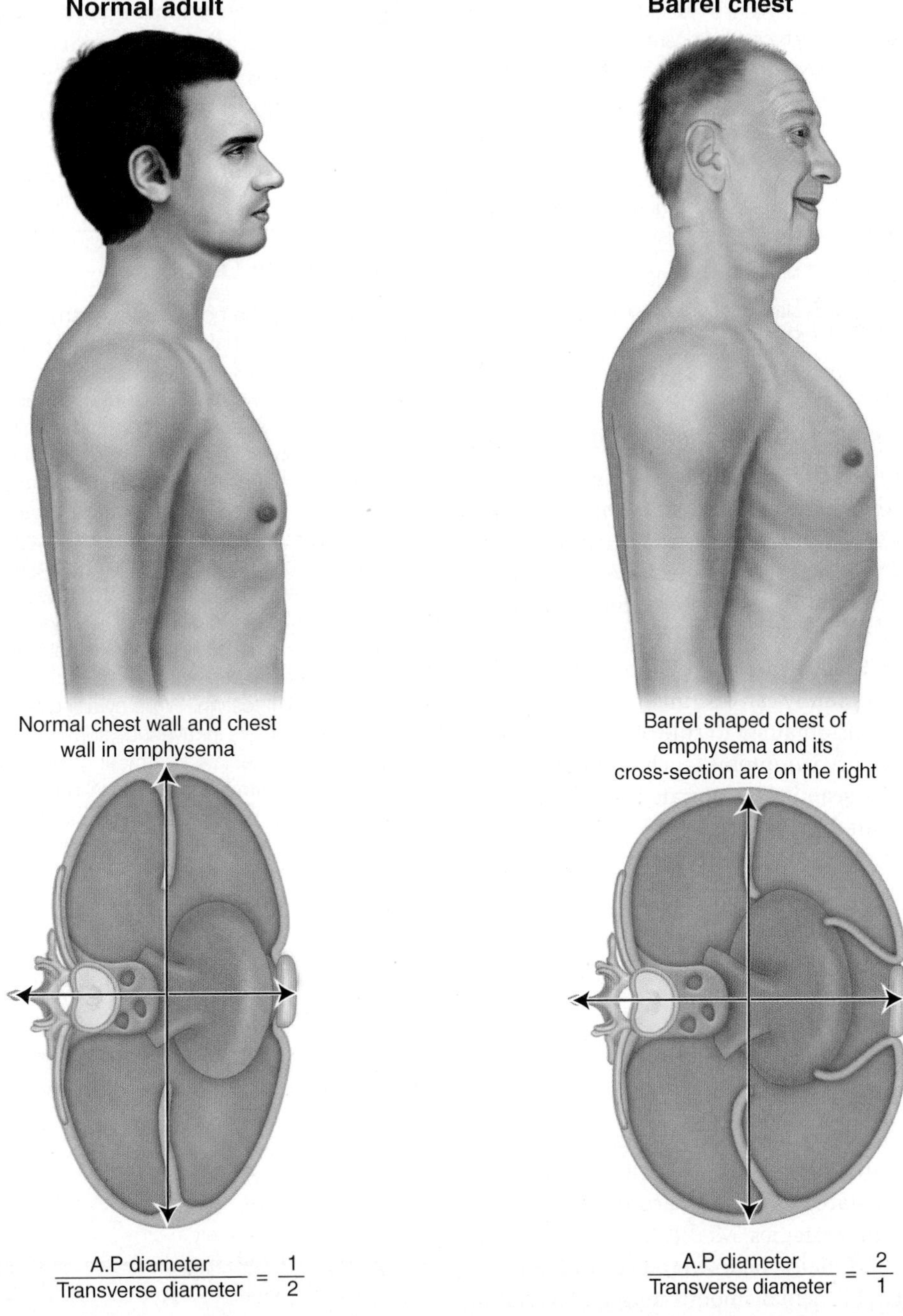

Figure 18.11 ■ Physical changes with hyperinflation. The thoracic changes associated with hyperinflation are evident on physical examination. A barrel chest is the result of the increased anterior–posterior diameter. Percussion reveals expanded lung tissue during exhalation, which pushes the diaphragm into a partially contracted position.

hypoxemia and hypoxia are accompanied by increasing symptoms of SOB and dyspnea. The individual's activities of daily living and quality of life are both severely impaired.

Jimmy Bley: Application

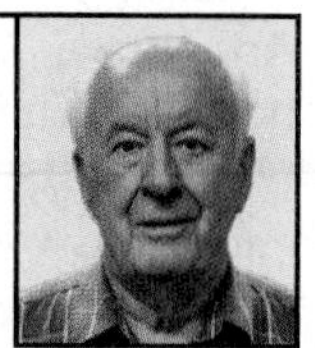

Mr. Bley has begun waking in the middle of the night with a persistent, productive cough. He finds himself needing his inhaler as soon as he is awake. Mr. Bley believes that he just has a bad cold. To help him sleep, he props himself up on several pillows. His wife sets up a humidifier in the room at night, which seems to help. For several days, Mr. Bley spends most of the day resting and taking over-the-counter antitussive medicine in an effort to treat this worsening cough and "cold." He is resistant to his wife's suggestion that he schedule an appointment with his healthcare provider. "It is just a cold," Mr. Bley tells her. However, after a week, Mr. Bley's condition worsens to such a degree that he is unable to walk to the bathroom because of to dyspnea. Despite the use of antitussive medication, he is coughing up copious amounts of thick, yellow mucus, and he admits to feeling chilled. At his wife's insistence, he agrees to seek medical treatment. Although he refuses her request to call an ambulance, he allows her to drive him to the emergency department.

3. What facts indicate that Mr. Bley does not have a cold?
4. According to the GOLD classification system, what degree of severity is Mr. Bley's COPD?
5. What is the significance of Mr. Bley's report of feeling chilled?

Linking Pathophysiology to Diagnosis and Treatment

Lung volumes on PFTs are compared to those of healthy people of the same age, gender, and size. On spirometry, individuals with COPD typically show a decrease in both the FVC and the FEV_1/FVC ratio, and the FEV_1 may be modestly improved (less than 15%) on postbronchodilator PFTs. The degree of abnormality on spirometry generally reflects the severity of the COPD as defined by the GOLD categories.[1] Body plethysmography can document changes in TLC and RV. A chest x-ray is obtained to rule out other possible causes of the respiratory symptoms, such as a lung tumor. A high-resolution CT scan is appropriate if lung reduction surgery is contemplated.

The management plan for an individual with COPD includes four components:

1. Assessment and monitoring of the disorder
2. Reducing risk factors
3. Managing stable COPD
4. Managing acute exacerbations.[1]

The critical risk reduction strategy is smoking cessation. Additionally, exposures to occupational and indoor and outdoor pollutants should be reduced or eliminated.

Management of stable COPD and acute exacerbations involves a number of strategies. Medications are typically a critical component. Inhaled beta-2 agonists and anticholinergic agents relax bronchial smooth muscle; fast-acting bronchodilators are used on an as-needed basis for the immediate relief of SOB, while long-acting bronchodilators are used preventively. Inhaled corticosteroids in relatively low doses can reduce the frequency of exacerbations and improve health status but do not alter the long-term decline in FEV_1. Inhaled corticosteroids are appropriate for patients with an FEV_1 less than 60% of predicted or patients who have repeated exacerbations. Use of some inhaled corticosteroids increases the risk for pneumonia with long-term use, but there is no defined recommended length of time for use.[1] Systemic corticosteroids may be needed for exacerbations. For patients with COPD, annual influenza and pneumococcal vaccines are recommended to help prevent serious lower respiratory tract infection and reduce mortality.[1] Antibiotics are recommended only for bacterial infections. Mucolytic agents may help to thin viscous sputum. Regular use of antitussives is not recommended. Additional management tools include oxygen therapy, patient and family education, pulmonary rehabilitation, and chest physiotherapy. For selected patients with severe COPD (stage 4), surgical intervention (e.g., lung transplantation) may be recommended, but lung reduction surgery is not recommended for general use.

Jimmy Bley: Outcome

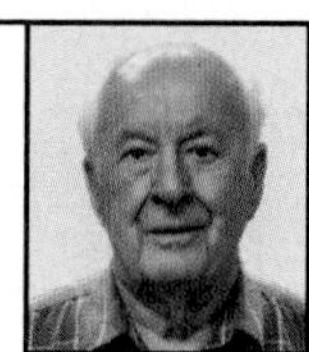

Upon arrival at the hospital emergency department, Mr. Bley is pale and sweating profusely, with labored respirations. His oxygen saturation is 83% on room air. His oral temperature is 101.6°F. He is rapidly triaged and admitted to the hospital. Initial treatment includes immediate administration of a nebulized inhaled beta-2 agonist and insertion of an intravenous access device for fluid administration. When asked about his recent intake of food and fluid, Mr. Bley tells the healthcare provider, "I haven't been eating or drinking much since I caught this cold. It's too much work to eat a meal." Laboratory tests include a chest x-ray, which reveals pneumonia. Mr. Bley's white blood cell count is elevated, indicating the presence of infection. Arterial blood gases reveal hypercapnia and respiratory acidosis. Blood samples are sent to the laboratory for culture and sensitivity (C&S) testing. While awaiting the C&S results, the healthcare provider orders intravenous administration of a broad-spectrum antibiotic for immediate treatment of Mr. Bley's pneumonia. Following 5 days of treatment for bacterial pneumonia, Mr. Bley's condition improves to the point at which he can be discharged to his home. Mr. Bley's discharge instructions include a course of oral antibiotics, scheduled use of his beta-2 agonist inhaler, and smoking cessation. In addition, the healthcare provider advises Mr. Bley to immediately discontinue use of any over-the-counter antitussive medication, as this class of medication inhibits the ability to expectorate mucus secretions and may lead to formation of a mucus plug, which can cause airway obstruction.

6. What immunizations would be beneficial to Mr. Bley?
7. What actions should be taken, given Mr. Bley's statement that "it's too much work to eat"?
8. What information about the oral antibiotics should Mr. Bley receive at discharge?

Check Your Progress: Section 18.4

1. What are risk factors for the development of COPD?
2. How does maternal smoking affect the fetus?
3. What pathophysiologic changes are the hallmarks of COPD?

18.5 Cystic Fibrosis

Cystic fibrosis (CF) is a recessive genetic disorder that inhibits sodium reabsorption in skin sweat ducts but enhances sodium transport across epithelial cells in the respiratory system, pancreas, bile ducts, and sperm ducts. Because it is a recessive disorder, the affected individual must inherit one defective cystic fibrosis gene from each parent for the disease to be expressed.

CLINICAL POINT: Known carriers of the cystic fibrosis gene who are planning to have children may benefit from genetic counseling. ■

CF is characterized by the inhibition of sodium reabsorption in skin sweat ducts with enhancement of sodium transport across epithelial cells in the respiratory system, pancreas, bile ducts, and sperm ducts. Critical complications of CF include obstruction of airway passages and pancreatic ducts by viscous mucus secretions.

CF is the most common lethal genetic disorder, with lifelong morbidity that primarily affects Caucasians. It is estimated that between 2% and 5% of Caucasians carry the gene for CF; it is uncommon in blacks and Asians. In the United States, CF is reported to be present in up to 1 of every 3500 births.[37] CF may be diagnosed at birth or years later. Approximately 10% of infants with CF are diagnosed shortly after birth because of meconium ileus, a bowel obstruction caused by impacted mucin.[38]

Etiology and Pathogenesis

The primary defect in CF is abnormal functioning of epithelial chloride channels, which is coded by the cystic fibrosis transmembrane conductance regulator (CFTR) gene on the long arm of chromosome 7. CF is the classic example of one gene–one disorder, but other genes may modify CF. There are many mutations of the CFTR gene that result in varying clinical presentations of CF, and the severity of the symptoms is related to the number and types of mutation. The CFTR gene regulates multiple other channel processes in addition to chloride; its regulation of the epithelial sodium channels is the most important in CF. Sodium is transported from luminal fluids in the renal tubules by the epithelial sodium channels.[39] There is also a defect in the submucosal glands that produce airway surface fluid, and the lack of surface fluid contributes to the dehydration of mucus secretions (**Figure 18.12** ■).[40]

The CFTR gene mutation has different effects in different tissues. In sweat glands, the reabsorption of sodium is inhibited, but sodium reabsorption is enhanced in epithelial exocrine cells in the respiratory system, pancreas, bile ducts, and sperm ducts.[41] Normally, the CFTR-regulated channel inhibits the transport of sodium from luminal fluid by the exocrine sodium channels, but in CF, the transport of sodium is increased. Water follows the reabsorbed sodium, decreasing the already low airway surface water content, leaving secretions dehydrated and sticky. The sticky mucus and intermittent airway obstruction in the lungs predispose the individual with CF to *Staphylococcus aureus* and *Pseudomonas aeruginosa* pulmonary infections and bronchiectasis. There is an exaggerated, ineffective immune response to the infections, and neutrophils contribute to further damage of the respiratory epithelia.[42] The

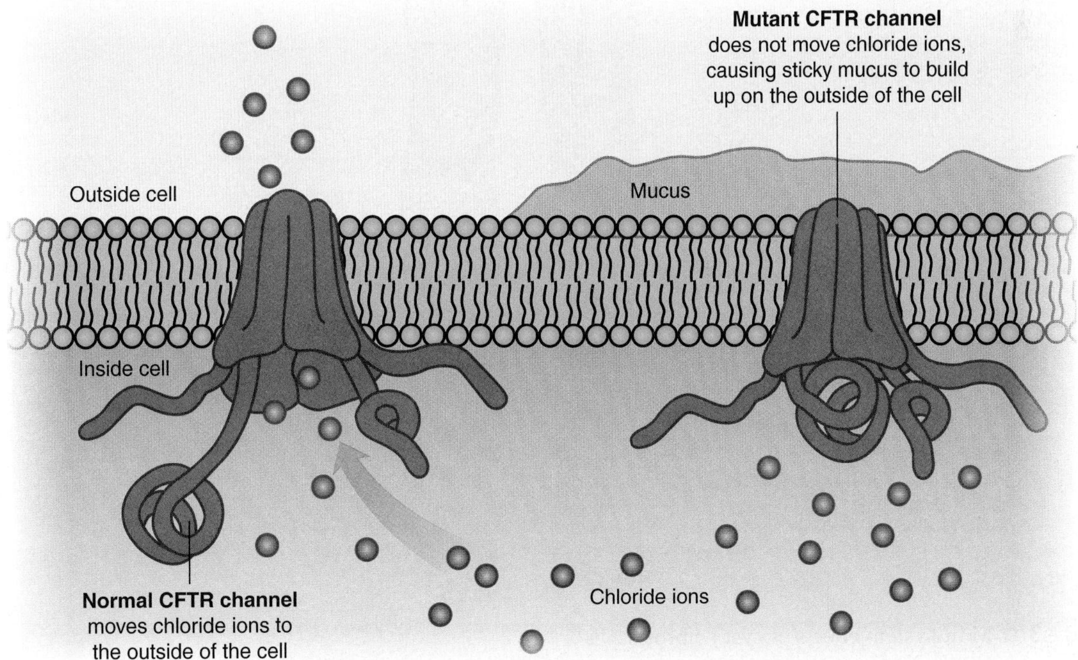

Figure 18.12 ■ Gene mutations in CF. A normal CTFR channel (left) moves chloride ions to the outside of the cell. A mutant CTFR channel (right) does not move chloride ions, causing a sticky mucus to build up on the outside of the cell.

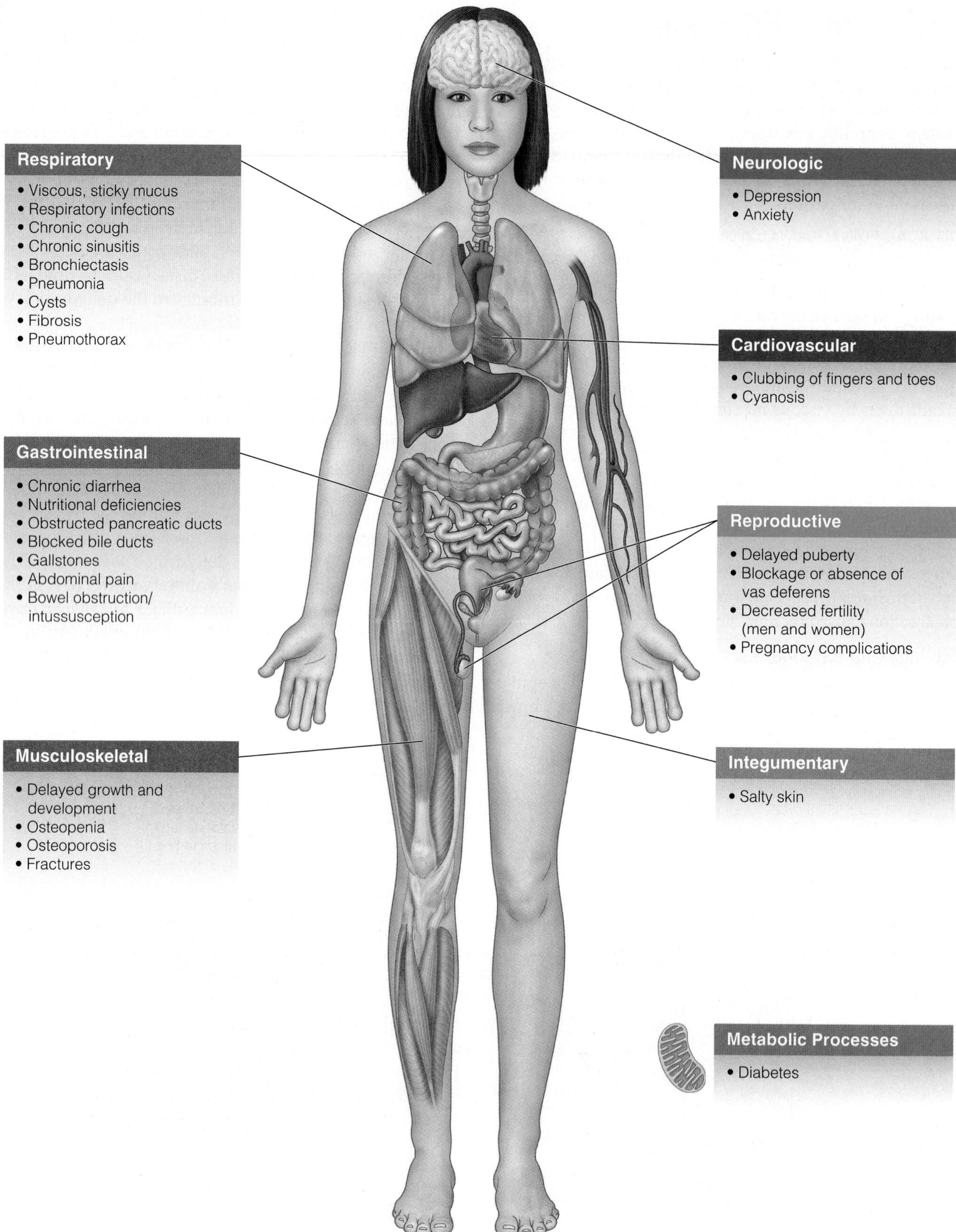

Figure 18.13 ■ Multisystem effects of cystic fibrosis.

toxin pyocyanin produced by *P. aeruginosa* interferes with macrophage clearance of apoptotic cells and induces oxidative stress that impairs host defenses and may contribute to lung damage.[40]

In the pancreas, dilated pancreatic ducts are filled with the sticky mucus, and the abnormal transport of bicarbonate contributes to the precipitation of mucin, the gel component of secretions, and the plugging of ducts. When pancreatic ducts are completely blocked, pancreatic cells that produced digestive enzymes atrophy; over time, bile ducts become blocked. The result is severe malabsorption, especially of fats and fat-soluble vitamins.

Clinical Manifestations

The clinical presentation of CF varies with the severity of the CFTR mutation from a mild to a severe disorder that is diagnosed anytime from birth to adulthood. When the CFTR gene is absent, there is a classic presentation of CF with pancreatic insufficiency, gastrointestinal symptoms, and thick pulmonary secretions with frequent infections and a chronic cough. Cystic fibrosis affects many body systems (**Figure 18.13** ■). The lack of pancreatic enzymes results in abdominal distention and large, foul-smelling stools that float because of their high fat content. Children have stunted growth, and individuals with CF tend to have a shortened lifespan. Sterility in men is common because of the viscous secretions in the sperm duct.

In the lungs, CF results in dehydrated airways and impaired mucociliary clearance. Individuals have problems clearing secretions from their lungs even with a strong cough because of the viscous secretions; this results in frequent infections and inflammation. Bronchiectasis, hemoptysis, and pneumothorax are common complications.[41]

Linking Pathophysiology to Diagnosis and Treatment

The diagnosis of CF is based on elevated sodium and chloride transport in skin sweat glands (sweat test); parents sometimes report that their infants with CF "taste salty." Genetic analysis can divide the CFTR gene mutations into one of six groups. A CFTR mutation should be suspected in people with idiopathic chronic pancreatitis, obstructive pulmonary disease, idiopathic bronchiectasis, and obstructive azoospermia.

The treatment of CF is largely symptomatic: treating infections, using supplements, and replacing pancreatic digestive enzymes. When individuals are chronically infected with *P. aeruginosa*, inhaled tobramycin and other antibiotics are recommended.[42] New therapies that are under study would leave the individual less susceptible to developing resistance and would potentially allow for a reduction in dosing frequency.[42]

Check Your Progress: Section 18.5

1. What is the percent chance of cystic fibrosis occurring in the offspring of two parents who both carry the recessive gene?
2. In cystic fibrosis, what causes the abnormal absorption of fats and fat-soluble vitamins?
3. What are potential complications associated with cystic fibrosis?

18.6 Bronchiectasis

Bronchiectasis is a disorder characterized by excessive mucus accumulation leading to irreversibly dilated bronchi that readily collapse, airway obstruction, and frequent infections. Congenital bronchiectasis affects infants and children. Acquired bronchiectasis, which is the most common form of this disease, affects children and adults.[43]

Etiology and Pathogenesis

Risk factors for bronchiectasis include (a) bronchial obstruction caused by lung tumors, aspiration of foreign bodies, impacted mucus, or atelectasis; (b) congenital or hereditary conditions, including problems such as a congenital weakness of the bronchial wall, CF, or an impaired immune condition; and (c) repeated infections that occur over many years, although a single severe infection with pertussis, tuberculosis, mycoplasmas, *Mycobacterium avium*, or a bacterial pneumonia can also cause bronchiectasis. Bronchiectasis is common in individuals with CF because of the very viscous sputum, which may easily grow *P. aeruginosa*.

Bronchiectasis is an acquired disorder that results when there is a blockage of airways and a chronic necrotizing infection that causes persistent airway dilation and thickening of bronchial walls. Bronchiectasis also occurs in individuals who do not have CF (as evidenced by a normal sweat test) but do have a mutation in CFTR function that alters the normal rates of ion transport. In another subgroup of individuals, other mutations may interfere with the function of epithelial sodium channels.[44] These mutations interfere with clearance of mucus from airways.

The abnormal dilation of bronchi and bronchioles results in peripheral airways that are up to four times their normal size. The areas of bronchiectasis are similar to the weakened, baggy area of a balloon that has been blown up too many times, and these areas can no longer force all the air out. The abnormally dilated bronchi can collapse during coughing episodes, trapping infected mucus in areas of bronchiectasis. Antibiotics clear the infection in other areas of the lung, but the infection recurs because the areas of bronchiectasis are still infected. Bronchiectasis occurs most commonly in the lower lobes bilaterally and the right middle lobe.

Clinical Manifestations

The classic signs and symptoms of bronchiectasis are a severe persistent cough with a daily production of tenacious, mucopurulent sputum that can persist over months or years. Patients cough so hard that they often report costochrondral pain, abdominal muscle soreness, vomiting, and urinary incontinence in women. Individuals frequently report a history of acute respiratory infections that were treated effectively with antibiotics, improved for a week or two, and then recurred. Other common symptoms include dyspnea, wheezing, pleuritis, chest pain, and "bad breath" or a "bad taste" in the mouth. An increase in the volume and darkness of sputum signals an acute exacerbation of bronchiectasis.

Hemoptysis occurs in about 25% of individuals with bronchiectasis. It can range from a small amount of blood streaking in sputum to fresh blood or clots without much visible mucus to loss of life-threatening amounts of blood. Massive hemoptysis is defined as coughing up 200–600 mL of blood within a 24-hour period. Large of amounts of hemoptysis are difficult to manage because there are no rigid structures to compress the bleeding vessel.

Linking Pathophysiology to Diagnosis and Treatment

In individuals with bronchiectasis, a bronchogram may reveal dilation of the bronchi and bronchioles. The definitive test for diagnosing bronchiectasis is a high-resolution computed tomography scan with thin sections that show the dilated bronchi. Bronchiectasis is strongly suspected on the basis of the patient history, sputum cultures, complete blood count, and an abnormal chest x-ray (**Figure 18.14** ■). An obstructive pattern is seen on PFTs with a low FEV_1 and FEV_1/FVC with either a normal or reduced FVC.

Treatment goals for bronchiectasis are the control or eradication of infection and improvement of bronchial hygiene. Strategies to control or eliminate infection include various regimens of antibiotics, often over long periods of time, as antibiotics do not readily reach areas of infection because of the damaged blood vessels and lung tissue in areas of bronchiectasis. Examples of medication strategies are daily oral antibiotics or oral antibiotics for 7–14 days each month. When *P. aeruginosa* is present in CF, an aerosolized antibiotic, such as tobramycin, reduces organisms in sputum and improves FEV_1.[45] Other medications may include bronchodilators and inhaled corticosteroids.

Bronchial hygiene is improved with chest physiotherapy three or four times each day when an active infection is present. Chest physiotherapy uses percussion or vibration to loosen the viscous mucus, followed by postural drainage to drain mucus into larger, intact bronchi so that it can be coughed out. Bronchial hygiene is important as a daily preventive measure even when the patient with bronchiectasis is asymptomatic.

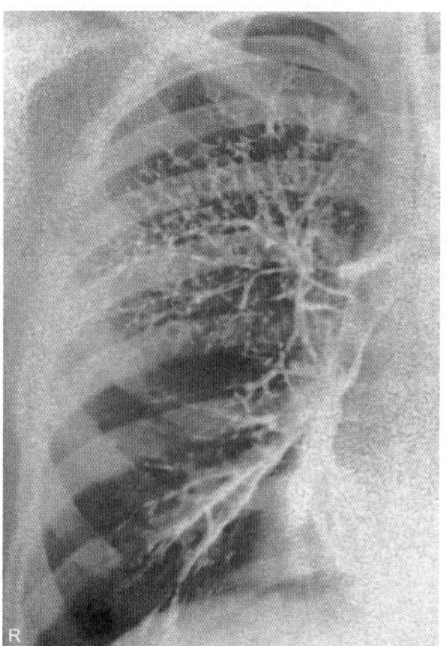

Figure 18.14 ■ Radiograph of bronchiectasis.

Check Your Progress: Section 18.6

1. What are three risk factors for the development of bronchiectasis?
2. Where does bronchiectasis most commonly occur?
3. How does chest physiotherapy assist in the treatment of bronchiectasis?

CHAPTER SUMMARY

18.1 Chapter Overview and Case Studies

Describe the common characteristics of obstructive lung disorders and explain their impact on other concepts and systems.

- Obstructive lung disorders encompass a spectrum of disorders, including asthma, chronic bronchitis, emphysema, cystic fibrosis, and bronchiectasis.
- Dyspnea, which is the subjective experience of difficulty breathing, is a common feature of obstructive lung disorders.
- Obstructive lung disorders impair oxygenation and perfusion.
- Inflammation plays a key role in the development of obstructive lung disorders.

18.2 Alterations in Respiratory Structure and Function

Describe the alterations of the anatomic airway structure and pulmonary function present in individuals with obstructive lung disorders.

- Airway obstruction, which is a hallmark of obstructive lung disorders, worsens during exhalation because of inflammation, the loss of support for small airways, bronchoconstriction and mucus in airways.
- Airway obstruction increases resistance to airflow resulting in a decreased volume and speed of airflow per unit of time.
- Pulmonary function tests used for assessment of obstructive lung disorders include spirometry, body plethysmography, and nitrogen washout.

18.3 Asthma

Differentiate the causes, classification, underlying pathogenesis, and clinical manifestations of asthma and approaches to diagnosis and treatment of the condition across the lifespan.

- Asthma classification may be based on clinical presentation, precipitating factors or triggers, or relationship to allergies.
- Common asthma triggers include allergies, infections, exercise, and medications.
- Asthma triggers are specific to an individual, but all result in persistent airway inflammation and bronchial hyperreactivity.

- Asthma is expressed clinically when a precipitating stimulus triggers expression of a genetic susceptibility for asthma.
- Allergic asthma, the most common type of asthma, is precipitating by the inhalation of an allergen that causes a type 1 hypersensitivity response.
- In recurrent asthma, airways are remodeled and bronchial smooth muscles hypertrophy, increasing their capacity for bronchoconstriction.
- Asthma severity is classified by the degree of biologic intensity and number of exacerbations.
- Asthma control is assessed by the degree to which asthma symptoms are relieved.
- Common asthma symptoms include chest tightness, shortness of breath, wheezing, and cough with or without the production of thick sputum. Classic confirmatory test are challenge tests performed with an irritating chemical, cold air, or exercise.
- The gold standard therapy for persistent asthma is the use of inhaled corticosteroids, but patients are not all equally responsive to corticosteroids.

18.4 Chronic Obstructive Pulmonary Disease

Differentiate the causes, classification, underlying pathogenesis, and clinical manifestations of chronic obstructive pulmonary disease and approaches to diagnosis and treatment of the condition.

- Chronic obstructive pulmonary disease is characterized by progressive airflow limitation caused by abnormal pulmonary inflammation secondary to inhalation of noxious substances.
- COPD includes chronic bronchitis and emphysema; often, individuals with COPD demonstrate manifestations that combine the two disorders.
- Hallmarks of chronic bronchitis include persistent, inflammation-induced narrowing of the airways, copious mucus production, and a chronic productive cough.
- Emphysema is associated with damage to the lung parenchyma, destruction of gas-exchanging pulmonary surfaces (including the alveolar walls), and subsequent pulmonary hyperinflation
- Smoking is the greatest risk factor for COPD. Exposure to secondhand smoke and exposure to environmental or occupational aerosolized particles increase the risk to a lesser degree.
- COPD is classified in four grades according to the progressive degree of airflow limitations, as measured by the FEV_1 and FEV_1/FVC and by symptoms.
- Fixed airway obstruction is caused by scarring that thickens the basement membranes, the increased number and size of mucus glands, and the loss of support for small airways.
- The airway obstruction of COPD is primarily the result of fixed airways that have an increased resistance to airflow, thus slowing the rate of airflow.
- Respiratory symptoms increase, and hypoxemia, hypercapnia, and activity limitations occur with disease progression.

18.5 Cystic Fibrosis

Differentiate the causes, classification, underlying pathogenesis, and clinical manifestations of cystic fibrosis and approaches to diagnosis and treatment of the condition across the lifespan.

- Cystic fibrosis is the most common lethal genetic disorder, with lifelong morbidity that primarily affects Caucasians. It is estimated that between 2% and 5% of Caucasians carry the gene for CF, but it is uncommon in blacks and Asians.
- CF is a recessive genetic disorder that affects the epithelial transport of fluids. Reabsorption of sodium is inhibited in the skin but enhanced in epithelial exocrine cells in the lung, pancreas, bile duct, and sperm ducts.
- Chloride transport is abnormal due to an abnormal epithelial chloride channel encoded by the cystic fibrosis transmembrane conductance regulator (CFTR) gene.
- CF is diagnosed by a skin sweat test.
- Clinical manifestations of CF include thick pulmonary secretions, frequent respiratory infections, chronic cough, abdominal distention, and large, fatty, foul-smelling stools.
- Treatment for CF includes symptomatic measure, such as antibiotic administration for treatment of secondary infections, vitamin supplements, and pancreatic digestive enzyme replacement.

18.6 Bronchiectasis

Differentiate the causes, classification, underlying pathogenesis, and clinical manifestations of bronchiectasis and approaches to diagnosis and treatment of the condition across the lifespan.

- Bronchiectasis occurs when there is airway blockage and an acute necrotizing infection or a mutation affecting epithelial ion transport.
- Abnormally dilated bronchi fill with infected mucus and do not empty with coughing, so respiratory infections frequently recur.
- Individuals with bronchiectasis have a hard cough that produces mucopurulent sputum over periods of weeks to months.
- A definitive diagnosis is made with a fine section CT scan that demonstrates the dilated bronchi.
- Treatment includes antibiotic regimens and bronchial hygiene.

REVIEW QUESTIONS

1. Which value would be useful in evaluation of airway obstruction in a client with obstructive lung disease?
   a. FEV_1
   b. VC
   c. FEV_1/FVC
   d. RV
   e. TLC
2. Which factors contribute to diminished expiratory airflow in individuals with obstructive lung disease? Select all that apply.
   a. Loss of elastic recoil in small airways
   b. Decreased distensibility of lung tissue
   c. Increased mucus secretion
   d. Decreased mucosal inflammation
   e. Bronchodilation
3. What is the primary reason for airway obstruction early in an allergic asthma attack?
   a. Severe bronchoconstriction
   b. Infiltration of the bronchi with inflammatory white blood cells
   c. Dilation and collapse of respiratory bronchioles
   d. Excessive mucous secretion
4. Which of the following are critical effector cells in both allergic and nonallergic asthma? Select all that apply.
   a. Basophils
   b. Plasma cells
   c. Eosinophils
   d. Neutrophils
   e. Th-2 T lymphocytes
5. Which of the following statements are true about CF? Select all that apply.
   a. CF severity relates to the number and types of CFTR gene mutations.
   b. CF is most common in Caucasians and uncommon in blacks and Asians.
   c. CF is caused by abnormal potassium channel transport.
   d. CF is not related to the development of bronchiectasis.
   e. CF affects the absorption of fats and fat-soluble vitamins.
6. Which intervention is important for improved bronchial hygiene for individuals with bronchiectasis?
   a. Use of an incentive spirometer to stimulate deep breathing
   b. Lifelong use of bronchodilators to open the airways
   c. Chest percussion and vibration to remove retained mucus
   d. Repeated bronchoscopy and bronchial washing
7. What is the reason for the assessment finding of increased anterior–posterior diameter of the chest in an individual with COPD?
   a. Hypoventilation
   b. Dilation of the bronchi
   c. Hyperinflation of the lungs
   d. Use of accessory muscles
8. Which assessment findings are expected in the individual with long-standing COPD? Select all that apply.
   a. Use of accessory respiratory muscles
   b. Prolonged expiratory phase
   c. Barrel chest
   d. Decreased respiratory rate
   e. Retained O_2

ANSWERS

Answers to Review Questions can be found in Appendix A. Answers to Case Study and Check Your Progress questions are available on the faculty resources site. Please consult with your instructor.

RECOMMENDED WEBSITES

Asthma

http://www.lung.org/lung-health-and-diseases/lung-disease-lookup/asthma

Bronchiectasis

http://www.lung.org/lung-health-and-diseases/lung-disease-lookup/bronchiectasis

COPD
http://www.lung.org/lung-health-and-diseases/lung-disease-lookup/copd

Cystic Fibrosis Foundation
https://www.cff.org

What Is COPD?
https://www.nhlbi.nih.gov/health/health-topics/topics/copd

REFERENCES

1. Global Initiative for Chronic Obstructive Lung Disease. (2017). *Global strategy for the diagnosis, management, and prevention of chronic obstructive pulmonary disease*. Available at http://goldcopd.org/gold-2017-global-strategy-diagnosis-management-prevention-copd/
2. Centers for Disease Control and Prevention. (2017). *Healthy people 2020*. Available at https://www.healthypeople.gov
3. Itoh, M., Tsuji, T., Nemoto, K., Nakamura, H., & Aoshiba, K. (2013). Undernutrition in patients with COPD and its treatment. *Nutrients, 5*(4), 1316–1335.
4. American Academy of Orthopedic Surgeons. (2011). *Emergency care and transportation of the sick and injured* (10th ed.). Burlington, MA: Jones & Bartlett Learning.
5. American College of Allergy, Asthma & Immunology. (2014). *Allergy symptoms: Asthma attack*. Available at http://acaai.org/asthma/symptoms/asthma-attack
6. Centers for Disease Control and Prevention. (2015). *Most recent asthma data*. Available at http://www.cdc.gov/asthma/most_recent_data.htm
7. Akinbami, L. J., Moorman, J. E., Bailey, C., et al. *Trends in asthma prevalence, health care use, and mortality in the United States, 2001–2010*. NCHS Data Brief 94. Hyattsville, MD: National Center for Health Statistics.
8. Romberg, K., Tufvesson, E., & Bjermer, L. (2014). Late-breaking abstract: Gender differences in asthma and allergies in relation to sports. *European Respiratory Journal, 44*(Suppl. 58), P3014.
9. Asthma and Allergy Foundation of America. (2001). *Asthma overview*. Available at http://www.aafa.org/display.cfm?id=8&cont=6
10. Choo, E. M., Hoyte, F. C. L., & Katial, R. H. (2014). Adult and pediatric asthma. In P. K. Vedanthan, H. S. Nelson, S.N. Agashe, P. A. Mahesh, & R. Katial R. (Eds.), *Textbook of allergy for the clinician* (pp. 135–142). Boca Raton, FL: CRC Press.
11. Bijanzadeh, M., Mahesh, P. A., & Ramachandra, N. B. (2011). An understanding of the genetic basis of asthma. *Indian Journal of Medical Research, 134*(2), 149–161.
12. Lang, D. M., Erzurum, S. C., & Kavu, M. (n.d.). *Asthma*. Available at http://www.clevelandclinicmeded.com/medicalpubs/diseasemanagement/allergy/bronchial-asthma.
13. Undem, B. J., & Taylor-Clark, T. (2014). Mechanisms underlying the neuronal-based symptoms of allergy. *Journal of Allergy and Clinical Immunology, 133*(6), 1521–1534.
14. Ernst, P., Amnon, A., & Suissa, S. (2013). Differences between asthmatics and nonasthmatics hospitalised with influenza A infection. *European Respiratory Journal, 41*, 772–774.
15. Simon, A. K., Hollander, G. A., & McMichael, A. (2015). Evolution of the immune system in humans from infancy to old age. *Proceedings of the Royal Society*. Retrieved from http://rspb.royalsocietypublishing.org/content/282/1821/20143085
16. Fahy, J. V. (2010). Identifying clinical phenotypes of asthma: Steps in the right direction. *American Journal of Respiratory and Critical Care Medicine, 181*(4), 296–297.
17. Niimi, A. (2011). Cough and asthma. *Current Respiratory Medicine Reviews, 7*(1), 47–54.
18. Wenzel, S. E., & Covar, R. (2006). Update in asthma 2005. *American Journal of Respiratory and Critical Care Medicine, 173*, 698–706.
19. Bukstein, D. A. (2007). *A chronic disease with serious consequences: Strategies for disease identification and lifetime management*. Chicago, IL: Chicago Asthma Consortium.
20. National Heart, Lung, and Blood Institute. (2014). *How is asthma treated and controlled?* Available at http://www.nhlbi.nih.gov/health/health-topics/topics/asthma/treatment
21. Chung, K. F., Wenzel, S. E., Brozek, J. L., et al. (2014). International ERS/ATS guidelines on definition, evaluation and treatment of severe asthma. *European Respiratory Journal, 43*(2), 343–373.
22. American Lung Association. (2014). *Chronic obstructive pulmonary disease (COPD) fact sheet*. Available at http://www.lung.org/lung-disease/copd/resources/facts-figures/COPD-Fact-Sheet.html
23. Mayo Clinic. (2014). *COPD: Causes*. Available at http://www.mayoclinic.org/diseases-conditions/copd/basics/causes/con-20032017
24. Guarascio, A. J., Ray, S. M., Finch, C. K., & Self, T. H. (2013). The clinical and economic burden of chronic obstructive pulmonary disease in the USA. *Journal of ClinicoEconomics and Outcomes Research, 5*, 235–245.
25. World Health Organization. (2014). *Household air pollution and health*. Fact sheet 292. Available at http://www.who.int/mediacentre/factsheets/fs292/en
26. Gooneratne, N. S., Patel, N. P., & Corcoran, A. (2010). Chronic obstructive pulmonary disease diagnosis and management in older adults. *Journal of the American Geriatrics Society, 58*(6), 1153–1162.
27. Lopez, J. R., Somsamouth, K., Mounivong, B., Sinclair, R., & Singh, P. N. (2012). Carbon monoxide levels in water pipe smokers in rural Laos PDR. *Tobacco Control, 21*(5), 517–518.
28. Leung, J. M, & Sin, D. D. (2014). Smoke and mirrors: The perils of water-pipe smoking and implications for Western countries. *Chest, 146*(4), 875–876.
29. Yuan, W., He, X., Xu, Q., Wang, H., & Casaburi, R. (2014). Increased difference between slow and forced vital capacity is associated with reduced exercise tolerance in COPD patients. *BMC Pulmonary Medicine, 14*(1), 16.
30. Barnes, P. J. (2009). The cytokine network in chronic obstructive pulmonary disease. *American Journal of Respiratory Cell and Molecular Biology, 41*(6), 631–638.
31. Maclay, J. D., Rabinovich, R. A., & MacNee, W. (2009). Update in chronic obstructive pulmonary disease 2008. *American Journal of Respiratory and Critical Care Medicine, 179*(7), 533–541.
32. Ferguson, G. T. (2006). Why does the lung hyperinflate? *Proceedings of the American Thoracic Society, 3*(2), 176–179.
33. Garcia-Rio, F., Lores, V., Mediano, O., Rojo, B., Hernanz, A., López-Collazo, E., & Alvarez-Sala, R. (2009). Daily physical activity in patients with chronic obstructive pulmonary disease is mainly associated with dynamic hyperinflation. *American Journal of Respiratory and Critical Care Medicine, 180*(6), 506–512.
34. U.S. Department of Health & Human Services, National Heart, Lung, and Blood Institute. (2013). *What is COPD?* Available at http://www.nhlbi.nih.gov/health/health-topics/topics/copd
35. Husain, A. N. (2010). The lung. In V. Kumar, A. K. Abbas, N. Fausto, & J. C. Aster (Eds.), *Robbins and Cotran pathologic basis*

of disease (8th ed., pp. 677–738). Philadelphia, PA: Saunders Elsevier.

36. Cosio, B. G., & Agusti, A. (2010). Update in chronic obstructive pulmonary disease 2009. *American Journal of Respiratory and Critical Care Medicine, 181*(7), 655–660.
37. World Health Organization. (n.d.). *Genes and human disease: Monogenic diseases.* Available at http://www.who.int/genomics/public/geneticdiseases/en/index2.html#CF
38. Rescorla, F. J., & Grosfeld, J. L. (2013). Meconium ileus. In L. Spitz & A. G. Koran (Eds.), *Operative pediatric surgery* (7th ed., pp. 433–444). Boca Raton, FL: CRC Press.
39. Subramanya, A. R., & Ellison, D. H. (2014). Distal convoluted tubule. *Clinical Journal of the American Society of Nephrology, 9*, 2147–2163.
40. Kreda, S. M., Davis, C. W., & Callaghan, M. C. (2012). CFTR, mucins, and mucus obstruction in cystic fibrosis. *Cold Spring Harbor Perspectives in Medicine, 2*(9), a009589.
41. Antunovic, S. S., Lukac, M., & Vujovic, D. (2013). Longitudinal cystic fibrosis care. *Clinical Pharmacology & Therapeutics, 93*(1), 86–97.
42. Akhand, S. S., Pettit, R. S., Gardner, T. E., & Anderson, G. G. (2014). New treatments in development for *Pseudomonas aeruginosa* infections in the lungs of individuals with cystic fibrosis. *Orphan Drugs: Research & Reviews, 4*, 71–81.
43. U.S. Department of Health & Human Services, National Heart, Lung, and Blood Institute. (2014). *What is bronchiectasis?* Available at http://www.nhlbi.nih.gov/health/health-topics/topics/brn
44. Bergin, D. A., Hurley, K., Mehta, A., et al. (2013). Airway inflammatory markers in individuals with cystic fibrosis and non-cystic fibrosis bronchiectasis. *Journal of Inflammation Research, 6*, 1–11. doi:10.2147/JIR.S40081.
45. Vendrell, M., Muñoz, G., & de Gracia, J. (2015). Evidence of inhaled tobramycin in non-cystic fibrosis bronchiectasis. *Open Respiratory Medicine Journal, 9*, 30–36.

Chapter 19

Neoplastic, Infectious, and Pulmonary Vascular Respiratory Disorders

Nancy Pogue and Linda Blevins

Chapter Outline and Learning Outcomes

19.1 Chapter Overview and Case Studies

Describe the primary considerations and concepts related to pulmonary vascular, neoplastic, and infectious respiratory disorders.

19.2 Malignant Lung Tumors

Differentiate the causes, classification, underlying pathogenesis, and clinical manifestations of malignant lung cancers and approaches to diagnosis and treatment of these conditions across the lifespan.

19.3 Benign Lung Lesions

Differentiate the causes, classification, underlying pathogenesis, and clinical manifestations of benign lung lesions and approaches to diagnosis and treatment of these conditions across the lifespan.

19.4 Infectious Diseases of the Upper Respiratory Tract

Differentiate the causes, classification, underlying pathogenesis, and clinical manifestations of upper respiratory tract infections and approaches to diagnosis and treatment of these conditions across the lifespan.

19.5 Infectious Diseases of the Lower Respiratory Tract

Differentiate the causes, classification, underlying pathogenesis, and clinical manifestations of lower respiratory tract infections and approaches to diagnosis and treatment of these conditions across the lifespan.

19.6 Pulmonary Vascular Disorders

Differentiate the causes, classification, underlying pathogenesis, and clinical manifestations of pulmonary vascular disorders and approaches to diagnosis and treatment of these conditions across the lifespan.

KEY TERMS

Acute bronchitis, 479
Adenocarcinoma, 469
Antigenicity, 481
Bacillus Calmette-Guérin (BCG), 474
Benign, 466
Blastomycosis, 475
Bronchiolitis, 479
Coccidioidomycosis, 475
Croup, 477
Embolism, 487
Embolus, 487
Egoghony, 478
Epiglottitis, 478
Goodpasture syndrome, 488
Healthcare-associated pneumonia (HCAP), 482
Histoplasmosis, 475
Hospital-acquired pneumonia (HAP), 481
Influenza, 480
Pertussis, 480
Pneumonia, 481
Pulmonary arterial hypertension (PAH), 486
Pulmonary embolism (PE), 487
Pulmonary granulomas, 471
Pulmonary hypertension (PH), 486
Rhinorrhea, 477
Tuberculosis (TB), 471
Upper respiratory tract infection (URI), 476
Ventilator-associated pneumonia (VAP), 482
Wegener granulomatosis, 488

ABBREVIATIONS

ANCA—antineutrophilic cytoplasmic antibody
BCG—bacillus Calmette-Guérin
CAP—community-acquired pneumonia
HAP—hospital-acquired pneumonia
HCAP—healthcare-associated pneumonia
HIV—human immunodeficiency virus
NSCLC—non–small cell lung cancer
PAH—pulmonary arterial hypertension
PE—pulmonary embolism
PH—pulmonary hypertension
SCLC—small cell lung cancer
TB—tuberculosis
URI—upper respiratory tract infection
VAP—ventilator-associated pneumonia

19.1 Chapter Overview and Case Studies

Pulmonary disorders include alterations caused by neoplastic growths, infectious diseases, abscesses, and vascular disorders. Neoplastic growths may be malignant or benign. Malignant growths are composed of cancerous cells that are capable of metastasizing (spreading) from the site of origin to other body sites or invading local body sites and causing tissue destruction.[1] **Benign** growths contain cells that are nonmalignant (noncancerous). Infectious diseases that serve as sources of pulmonary disorders include a variety of alterations that may affect the upper respiratory tract, the lower respiratory tract, or both. Pulmonary vascular disorders include alterations of blood flow within the lungs or blood flow to or from the pulmonary circuit.

Concepts Related to Pulmonary Disorders

Pulmonary vascular, neoplastic, and infectious respiratory disorders share the ability to significantly impair oxygenation. For example, infectious respiratory disorders may cause impaired delivery of oxygen to the alveoli or alterations in intralveolar gas exchange. Perfusion also is affected by respiratory disorders; pulmonary vascular disorders are characterized by alterations in blood flow within, to, or from the respiratory system. Malignant neoplasms are characterized by tumors that demonstrate cellular dysregulation. Specifically, malignant cells demonstrate rapid, unregulated cellular replication and destruction of local tissue in conjunction with cellular metastasis. Alterations that impair respiratory function affect the individual's ability to consume nutrition that is sufficient to meet metabolic demands. As a result, alterations in respiratory function are associated with inadequate nutrition. **Figure 19.1** ■ illustrates concepts related to oxygenation in application to pulmonary vascular, neoplastic, and infectious respiratory disorders.

Case Studies

The following cases will be addressed throughout the chapter to assist in application of chapter content to clinical situations that involve individuals with neoplastic, infectious, and pulmonary vascular disorders.

Carrilyn Proust: Introduction

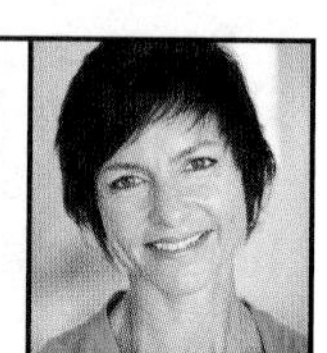

Carrilyn Proust, age 43, presents to her primary care provider's office complaining of a chronic, nonproductive cough and shortness of breath with even minor physical activities, such as climbing stairs. Ms. Proust was recently diagnosed with a viral upper respiratory tract infection, which was treated symptomatically. She suspects that her shortness of breath is secondary to her viral respiratory infection. She states that her primary concern is her chronic cough, which is preventing her from sleeping at night. She has been taking an over-the-counter cough suppressant, but she reports that this treatment is not effectively reducing her cough. She is afebrile and denies any recent history fever or chills. She reports that she has been "coughing so hard that sometimes blood comes up." Ms. Proust has a 20 pack-year history of cigarette smoking. She began smoking at age 21 and quit smoking at age 41. She denies allergies to any medications or foods. Her vital signs are within normal limits.

1. On the basis of Ms. Proust's history, describe the pathophysiologic mechanism of her shortness of breath.
2. What factor in Ms. Proust's history puts her at risk for a neoplastic respiratory disorder?

James Gerrity: Introduction

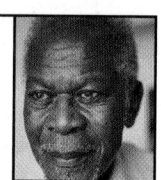

James Gerrity, age 72, has moderate emphysema and hearing loss. He has been married for 48 years to his wife, Olivia. Mr. Gerrity is a nonsmoker, but he worked for 40 years in an industrial factory, during which time he was routinely exposed to various chemicals. Mr. Gerrity's medications include an inhaled bronchodilator and an inhaled corticosteroid. Despite meticulous adherence to his medication regimen, Mr. Gerrity is very aware that his breathing has worsened and that he is using his inhaler much more frequently. Mrs. Gerrity hears an announcement on the radio that free flu shots are being offered at a local health clinic. She decides to receive the influenza vaccination, but Mr. Gerrity declines, explaining to his wife that he is certain the vaccine will only make him feel worse.

1. Which factor from Mr. Gerrity's work history is a risk factor for developing lung cancer?
2. On the basis of his history, what other possible risk factors for lung cancer does Mr. Gerrity have?

Check Your Progress: Section 19.1

1. Describe the difference between malignant and benign pulmonary growths.
2. How does having a pulmonary disorder affects a person's nutritional status?
3. Describe how perfusion is affected by a pulmonary disorder.

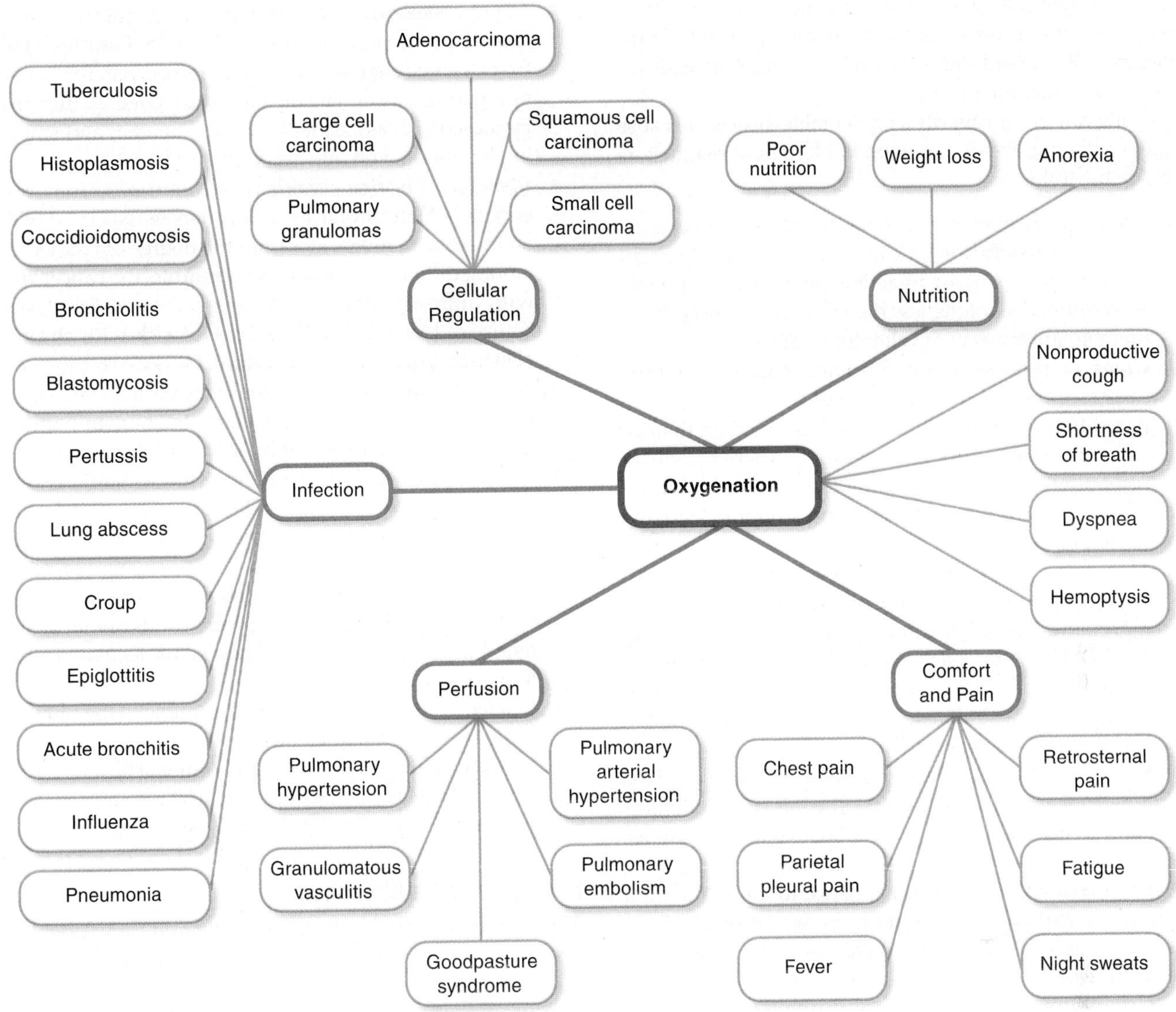

Figure 19.1 ■ Concepts related to pulmonary diseases.

19.2 Malignant Lung Tumors

Lung cancer is the leading cause of cancer death for both men and women in the United States.[2] Although the most commonly diagnosed cancers are prostate cancer in men and breast cancer in women, lung cancer causes more deaths than prostate, breast, and colorectal cancers combined.[3] Cigarette smoking is the primary risk factor for development of lung cancer, and there is a 15- to 20-year delay between smoking onset and the development of lung cancer.

In the 1950s, the first report was published that associated lung cancer and cigarette smoking. In 1964, the Surgeon General of the United States characterized cigarette smoking as the major cause of lung cancer.[4] Among adults in the United States, the cigarette smoking rate decreased from 20.9% in 2005 to 17.8% in 2013.[5]

Epidemiology and Risk Factors

Cigarette smoking is responsible for 85–90% of lung cancers. Current cigarette smokers are 15 times more likely to die from lung cancer than are lifelong nonsmokers. Compared to individuals who have never smoked, male smokers have a 23-fold increase in likelihood of developing lung cancer. Female smokers are 13 times more likely to develop lung cancer than are females who have never smoked.[3]

The American Cancer Society morbidity and mortality estimates for 2015 include approximately 221,200 new cases of lung cancer and 158,040 deaths from lung cancer.[6] Among individuals with lung cancer, the 5-year survival rate is significantly lower (17.8%) compared to the rates for many other forms of cancer, including prostate cancer (99.6%), breast cancer (90.5%), and colon cancer (65.4%).[3] Absence or presence of metastasis affects lung cancer survival rates. For individuals whose lung cancer is confined to the lungs, the 5-year survival rate is 54%. Conversely, metastasis of cancer from the lungs to other organs is associated with a

5-year survival rate of 4%.[3] Early diagnosis of lung cancer occurs in only an estimated 15% of cases; subsequently, more than 50% of individuals with lung cancer die within 1 year of the initial diagnosis.[3]

Lung cancer is primarily a preventable disorder because many of the risk factors are modifiable. These risk factors include the following:

- ***Smoking cigarettes.*** Smoking cigarettes is the most important risk factor for cancer. Eighty-seven percent of lung cancers occur in active smokers or in people who stopped smoking less than 5 years ago; only 2% of lifelong nonsmokers develop lung cancer.[7,8]
- ***Cigar or pipe smoking.*** Smoking cigars or a pipe increases the risk for lung cancer by 2–5 times compared to nonsmokers, but the risk is less than that for cigarette smokers. As with cigarettes, there is a dose–response relationship based on the amount and duration of cigar or pipe smoking, and stopping smoking decreases the risk for lung cancer.
- ***Marijuana and cocaine smoking.*** Emerging studies do not support the existence of a relationship between marijuana smoking, pulmonary damage, and lung cancer.[9] The pulmonary effects of cocaine smoking are not fully understood,[10] but the changes in the bronchial epithelium are similar to the premalignant epithelial changes seen in cigarette smokers.
- ***Secondhand smoke.*** Passive smoke exposure doubles lung cancer risk for exposures during childhood and adolescence and increases for spouses with the number of pack-years exposure.
- ***Occupational exposures.*** Exposure to environmental and occupational carcinogens increases the risk for lung cancer, and risks are greatly increased when the exposed individual also smokes cigarettes. The best-known risk factors are exposures to radon and asbestos. Other exposures related to lung cancer include polycyclic aromatic hydrocarbons, nickel, and arsenic, which can occur as contaminants in tobacco or in some industries.
- ***Genetic susceptibility.*** Genetic susceptibility is suggested by clusters of lung cancer in families, and first-degree relatives have an increased risk for developing lung cancer. The increased risk persists after any increased risk associated with age, gender, and smoking habits is taken into account.
- ***Presence of benign chronic lung conditions.*** The presence of benign chronic lung disorders is associated with an increase in lung cancer, but the degree of risk varies among different disorders; for example, the cancer risk with diffuse pulmonary fibrosis is increased 14 times compared to a 2–4 times increased risk with chronic obstructive pulmonary disease (COPD).
- ***Viral infections.*** Viral infections may participate in lung tumor carcinogenesis, particularly the human papillomavirus, which is present in 24.5% of lung cancers.
- ***Dietary factors.*** Epidemiologic studies suggest that low serum levels of antioxidants are associated with an increased risk for cancer. Diets containing foods with high levels of vitamin A and E and cruciferous vegetables (e.g., broccoli and cauliflower) were associated with a lower risk for lung cancer. Results are inconsistent, but drinking green tea may be protective against lung cancer.[11]
- ***Gender.*** Women may be more susceptible to the carcinogenic effects of smoking, possibly because of differences in DNA repair mechanisms and hormonal factors. In the United States, women younger than 50 years of age have a disproportionately high rate of lung cancer.

Etiology and Pathogenesis

The primary cause of lung cancer is cigarette smoking, the result of the carcinogenic character of multiple chemicals in cigarette smoke. The chemicals bind and mutate DNA (see the feature on Genetics and Genomics for Clinical Practice).[12] There is a linear relationship between the intensity of smoking and progressive epithelial changes. As in other cancers, exposure to carcinogens causes a stepwise

Genetics and Genomics for Clinical Practice

DNA Mutation in Lung Cancer

A variety of oncogenes (e.g., *MYC*, *KRAS*, *EGFR*, *c-MET*, and *cKIT*), deleted or mutated tumor suppressor genes such as *p53*, fusion genes such as *EML4-ALK*,[12] and activated signal transduction molecules have been associated with lung cancer. The pattern for specific genetic alterations varies with the type or subtype of lung cancer. For example, *KRAS* is most common genetic mutation in adenocarcinomas in women who smoke, while epidermal growth factor receptor gene (*EGFR*) occurs more commonly in adenocarcinomas in women who do not smoke and Asians; *p53* mutations occur most commonly in squamous cell carcinomas but also are present in small cell carcinomas.[12] The *EML4-ALK* fusion gene in non–small cell lung cancer does not exist with *EGFR* or *KRAS* mutations, and its presence identifies a subset of individuals with non–small cell lung cancer that will respond to ALK-targeted agents but not *EGFR* tyrosine kinase inhibitors.[12] The importance of this genetic research is that it will allow targeting of the specific sensitivities of a tumor with oncology medications that will interfere with tumor growth.[12,13]

CLINICAL POINT: Cigarette smoking has been directly linked to DNA mutations by a specific metabolite of benzo(a)pyrene in cigarette smoke that damages three specific loci on the *p53* tumor suppressor gene. The *p53* tumor suppressor gene mutations are present in approximately 60% of all lung cancers. Cigarette smoke contains over 200 carcinogens that act as initiators (polycyclic aromatic hydrocarbons), promoters (phenol derivatives), and contaminants such as radioactive elements, arsenic, nickel, molds, and additives. ■

accumulation of 10–20 genetic abnormalities that transform benign bronchial and alveolar cells into malignant tumors.

Approximately 10–15% of all lung cancers are classified as small cell lung cancer (SCLC).[14] Named because of the relatively small size of the cancer cells when viewed microscopically, SCLC may also be referred to as oat cell cancer, oat cell carcinoma, or small cell undifferentiated carcinoma. In many cases, SCLC originates in the bronchi. Because SCLC tends toward rapid growth and metastasis, this virulent form of cancer frequently has already spread to distant sites before it is identified.[14] SCLC is slightly more prevalent among men than among women.[15]

The vast majority of lung cancers—approximately 85–90%—are classified as non–small cell lung cancer (NSCLC). Non–small cell lung cancer comprises three primary subtypes: adenocarcinoma, squamous cell carcinoma, and large cell carcinoma.[14] Pathologists further classify adenocarcinomas and squamous cell carcinomas as either well-differentiated or poorly differentiated. Being well-differentiated means that the dividing cancer cells retain more of the normal features (e.g., size and shape of the cell and nuclei) but cell division is unregulated and faster than normal. In contrast, poorly differentiated cells retain enough histologic characteristics to be identified as adenocarcinoma or squamous cell carcinoma but have fewer normal cell features, so cell division is faster and the prognosis is worse.

Adenocarcinoma, which is the most common form of lung cancer, is more common in women than in men.[16] The incidence of adenocarcinoma has significantly increased in the past 20 years. It is hypothesized that the increase is related to filtered cigarettes and those with lower tar and nicotine, which allow smokers to inhale more deeply, increasing peripheral lung exposure to smoke. Squamous cell carcinoma is more common in men than in women and is most closely associated with cigarette smoking.

Large cell carcinoma, also referred to as undifferentiated tumors, is the least common form of NSCLC.[17]

Adenocarcinomas are glandular epithelial cancers. A single tumor frequently contains more than one cell subtype. Adenocarcinomas are the most common lung cancers in women and in nonsmokers, but the majority of adenocarcinomas occur in smokers. Adenocarcinomas occur primarily in the periphery of the lung and may initially present as a single nodule that does not cause pulmonary symptoms. Adenocarcinomas are relatively slow growing but metastasize widely and early by invading blood vessels or through lymphatic spread. Bronchioloalveolar cancers are a distinct subtype of adenocarcinomas that grow along preexisting alveolar walls without metastasizing or destroying the alveolar structure.

Squamous cell carcinoma occurs almost exclusively in cigarette smokers and are much more common in men than in women. Squamous cell carcinomas are also called epidermoid carcinomas because they originate in the bronchial epithelial mucosa and spread along the bronchial wall. The majority of squamous cell cancers originate medially in the chest at points of bronchial bifurcation, but peripheral squamous cell cancers are becoming more common. Central squamous cell cancers can spread to the adjacent lymph nodes and lung tissue; peripheral tumors can invade the chest wall. Squamous cell cancers are relatively slow growing and metastasize more slowly than other non–small cell cancers. Because of their central location, squamous cell carcinomas are more likely to obstruct bronchi. The blockage decreases mucus clearance, increasing the risk of infection and development of obstruction pneumonia. The central location also increases the probability of cancer cells being found in sputum.

Large cell carcinoma is a poorly differentiated epithelial cell cancer that cannot be histologically identified as squamous cell carcinoma, adenocarcinoma, or small cell carcinoma. Like adenocarcinoma, there are multiple subtypes of large cell carcinomas that often present as bulky, solitary tumors in the periphery of the lung. Large cell carcinomas tend to metastasize early and widely; 50% metastasize to the brain by the time cancer is diagnosed

Small cell lung cancer comprises aggressive, highly malignant, fast-growing tumors that metastasize early and widely into regional lymph nodes. In the past, small cell cancers were often called oat cell cancer because of their distinctive small cell size and appearance, but that terminology is no longer used. There is a very strong linear relationship between SCLC and smoking, and only 1% of SCLC occurs in nonsmokers. Small cell lung cancer can develop in major bronchi or in the periphery of the lung. Enlarging cancer in mediastinal lymph nodes can gradually impede blood return to the superior vena cava, causing the insidious development of a superior vena cava syndrome. In superior vena cava syndrome, there is a progressive blockage of blood return from the upper part of the body; blockage results in slowly developing signs such as distention of veins in the neck and chest wall, facial and upper extremity edema, and mental changes. When the individual lies down, the increased blood return to the heart may cause worsening of the signs and symptoms associated with vena cava syndrome. The severity of the symptoms depends on the location of the blockage and how quickly it occurs. The most common cause of vena cava syndrome is SCLC.

Clinical Manifestations

Most patients with lung cancer do not seek medical care until they after they become symptomatic. The most common symptom is a persistent cough with or without sputum production. Cough is not a specific symptom for lung cancers, and initially it is typically attributed to cigarette smoking, COPD, or a respiratory infection. Other common signs and symptoms of lung cancer are sputum streaked with blood, recurrent pneumonia or bronchitis, dyspnea, chest pain, hoarseness, and paraneoplastic syndromes.[18]

- Obstructive pneumonia occurs when lung cancer blocks bronchi, decreasing airflow and mucus clearance. The mucus distal to the blockage can become infected.
- Dyspnea may be due to a pleural effusion (an accumulation of fluid within the pleural space), which compresses

normal lung, resulting in shortness of breath. A pleural effusion may indicate that cancer has spread to the pleura.

- Chest pain varies with the lung cancer site. Mediastinal pain is generally dull and poorly localized. Retrosternal pain is poorly localized because pain receptors are limited to the peribronchial vagal afferent nerves, larger blood vessels, and mediastinum. Parietal pleural pain is more specifically localized and persistent.
- Hoarseness occurs if the recurrent laryngeal nerve is compressed or invaded by the tumor.
- Paraneoplastic syndromes generally occur with advanced lung cancer. Some tumors produce hormone analogs that cause symptoms of inappropriate neuroendocrine secretions or dysfunction in neurologic or connective tissue. For example, a squamous cell carcinoma may produce an analog of parathyroid hormone, resulting in increased serum calcium levels.

The systemic signs and symptoms include fatigue and weight loss. Weight loss is considered a negative prognostic sign.

When lung cancer is not discovered incidentally on a chest x-ray, the presenting symptoms that initiate the diagnostic workup may be an obstructive pneumonia with atelectasis, dyspnea associated with a pleural effusion, hemoptysis, pain, hoarseness, or a paraneoplastic syndrome.

Carrilyn Proust: Application

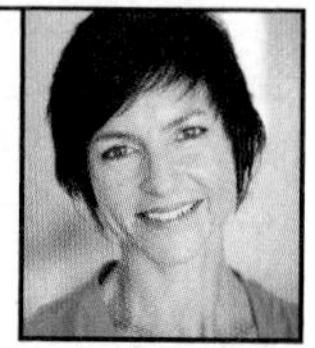

Ms. Proust's primary care provider orders a chest x-ray, which reveals a mass in the lower lobe of Ms. Proust's right lung. For further evaluation, the primary care provider schedules Ms. Proust for a pulmonary computed tomography (CT) scan. In addition, a sputum sample is collected for analysis. Ms. Proust's sputum sample contains a moderate amount of blood. Ms. Proust's CT reveals an abnormal mass approximately 1 centimeter in diameter in the lower lobe of her right lung. Cytology of her sputum sample reveals suspected malignant cells. Ms. Proust is referred to an oncologist for further evaluation and treatment.

3. On the basis of her gender, what type of lung cancer does Ms. Proust most likely have?
4. What finding in Ms. Proust's history and physical examination suggests that Ms. Proust does not have small cell carcinoma?

Linking Pathophysiology to Diagnosis and Treatment

Diagnostic tests for lung cancer include chest x-ray, computed tomography (CT), sputum cytology, and directly sampling cells from the tumor or pleural fluid. An abnormal chest x-ray often triggers the diagnostic workup for lung cancer.

- CT scan of the thorax is done to identify tumors larger than 1 cm in diameter and to better visualize tumors in the hilar or mediastinal area. The scan area is usually extended to include images of the liver, upper abdominal lymph nodes, and adrenal gland to assess for metastases.
- Cytologic analysis of freshly expectorated sputum looks for centrally located lung cancers.
- Bronchoscopy requires the insertion of a thin lighted tube through the nose or mouth, down the trachea to the area of concern in the lung. Any suspicious-appearing tissue can be lavaged (washed), brushed, or biopsied for cells for cytologic analysis.
- Needle aspiration requires insertion of a thin needle into a peripheral tumor. This technique is not used for central tumors or tumors near large blood vessels.
- Thoracentesis requires insertion of a large-gauge needle into the pleural space to remove fluid and cells for analysis.
- Mediastinoscopy is used to sample lymph nodes in the upper mediastinum. A small incision is made in the neck above the sternum, a thin lighted scope is inserted into the mediastinum, and suspicious nodes can be biopsied.

The appropriate treatment for non–small cell cancer depends on the clinical staging of the cancer at time of the diagnosis and on the individual's health status. Clinical staging is based on the tumor size (T), location of cancer in lymph nodes (N), and metastases (M) with a system developed by the American Joint Committee on Cancer (AJCC)[19] (**Figure 19.2**). Surgery alone may be the treatment of choice when NSCLC is localized with no regional lymph node involvement and no metastases (stages 0 and I).[20] However, for individuals with stage IB non–small cell cancer, additional treatment modalities, such as chemotherapy

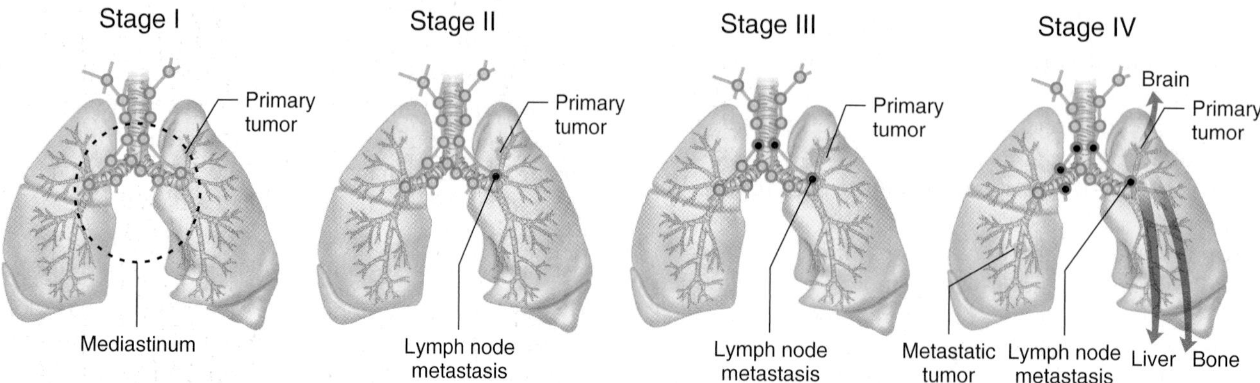

Figure 19.2 The staging system for lung cancers depends on tumor size (T), presence of cancer in lymph nodes (N), and metastases (M).

and radiation, may be included to reduce the risk of cancer recurrence.[20] For stage II through stage IV cancer, the inclusion of surgery as a treatment depends on a variety of factors, including the presence and extent of metastasis.[20] If surgery is performed, radiation and/or chemotherapy may be added to the treatment plan to help reduce the risk of cancer recurrence. A careful evaluation of the respiratory and cardiovascular status is necessary when surgery is considered for older adults.

For individuals whose treatment includes surgery, a second cancer staging may be conducted postoperatively. This pathologic staging takes into account the same criteria that are used for determining the clinical stage, with the addition of surgical findings related to factors including metastasis. But when it is available, the pathologic stage is likely to be more accurate than the clinical stage, as the pathologic stage uses the additional information that is obtained at surgery.

Because of the extraordinarily aggressive nature of SCLC, surgery typically is not indicated. Instead, treatment includes adjuvant therapies with multiple chemotherapeutic agents and radiation.[21] The survival for untreated SCLC is only 2–4 months, but SCLC is more sensitive to multiple chemotherapy regimens and radiation than are non–small cell cancers.[22]

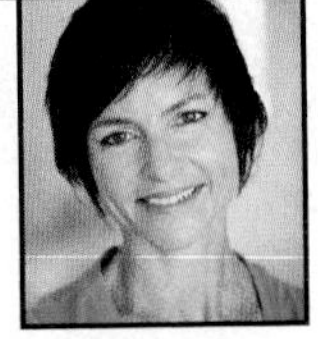

Carrilyn Proust: Outcome

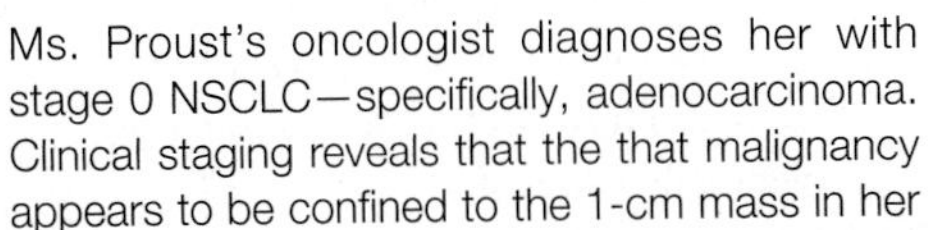

Ms. Proust's oncologist diagnoses her with stage 0 NSCLC—specifically, adenocarcinoma. Clinical staging reveals that the that malignancy appears to be confined to the 1-cm mass in her right lower lung field. No lymph node involvement or metastasis is identified. Ms. Proust undergoes uncomplicated surgical excision of the tumor. Postoperative pathologic staging reveals no apparent lymph node involvement or cancer metastasis. However, because of Mrs. Proust's smoking history and subsequent increased risk for cancer recurrence, radiation and chemotherapy are added to her treatment plan to help reduce her risk for cancer recurrence.

5. Discuss the rationale for pathologic staging in Ms. Proust's treatment.
6. Although Ms. Proust has a small tumor with no lymph node involvement or metastasis, explain the rationale for adding chemotherapy and radiation therapy to her surgical treatment.

Check Your Progress: Section 19.2

1. What are the clinical manifestations of superior vena cava syndrome?
2. Identify the three components of tumor staging.
3. Compare and contrast needle aspiration and thoracentesis in the diagnostic workup for lung cancer.

19.3 Benign Lung Lesions

While many lung tumors are malignant, benign masses often occur as granulomas. **Pulmonary granulomas** are small, localized collections of macrophages that form in response to an inhaled antigen that cannot be degraded or in response to an autoimmune disorder. When the antigen cannot be destroyed by neutrophils, macrophages phagocytose the antigen to prevent it from stimulating a chronic inflammatory response. The macrophages may fuse to form giant cells, and they are often surrounded by T lymphocytes. As the long-lived macrophages die, the slowly released antigen stimulates further inflammatory responses by monocytes and lymphocytes that maintain the granuloma as long as the individual has a healthy immune system.

Causes of pulmonary granulomas include bacterial infections (e.g., tuberculosis), fungal infections (e.g., histoplasmosis, coccidioidomycosis, or blastomycosis), inhalation of insoluble substances (e.g., dusts), or autoimmune disorders such as rheumatoid arthritis. In the case of sarcoidosis, the cause is not known. Tuberculosis and fungal infections of the lung are discussed here. Sarcoidosis is discussed in Chapter 26.

Tuberculosis

Tuberculosis (TB) is an infectious airborne bacterial disease caused by the organism *Mycobacterium tuberculosis*. Primarily, TB affects the lungs; however, organs and tissues may be affected as well. Tuberculosis has been dated in 6000-year-old Egyptian mummies, Indians of North American, the Mayans of Central America, and the Andeans of Peru. In Europe in the 17th century, 20% of the deaths in London were due to TB; by the mid-18th century, life expectancy was less than 40 years of age. During the 19th to the mid-20th century, industrialization spurred the development of cities and TB, and the "white plague" became epidemic. The discovery of the causative organism, *Mycobacterium tuberculosis*, was an important breakthrough, but tuberculosis is still a worldwide epidemic.

TB still represents a formidable challenge in terms of disease burden. Worldwide, in 2014, an estimated 9.6 million individuals were infected with TB. The global incidence of TB is higher among men (5.4 million) than women (3.2 million). Additionally, an estimated 1 million children are infected with TB globally. In 2014, TB killed an estimated 1.5 million individuals globally, 1.1 million of whom were HIV negative and 390,000 of whom who were HIV positive.[23] In the United States, 9421 new cases of TB were reported in 2014 (2.96 cases per 100,000), which represents a 1.5% decrease from 2013. The rate of TB cases in foreign-born individuals was 13 times greater than that among U.S.-born individuals.[24]

It is important to differentiate between a primary TB infection and the disease tuberculosis. A TB infection means that *M. tuberculosis* organisms have seeded areas in the lung but have not caused significant tissue damage; symptoms of fever and pleural effusion are infrequent. The disease TB means that clinically significant tissue damage has occurred and the infection is contagious. Approximately 3–4% of individuals with a primary TB infection become ill with the disease during the first year after their exposure. After the first year, up to 15% of those who have been exposed

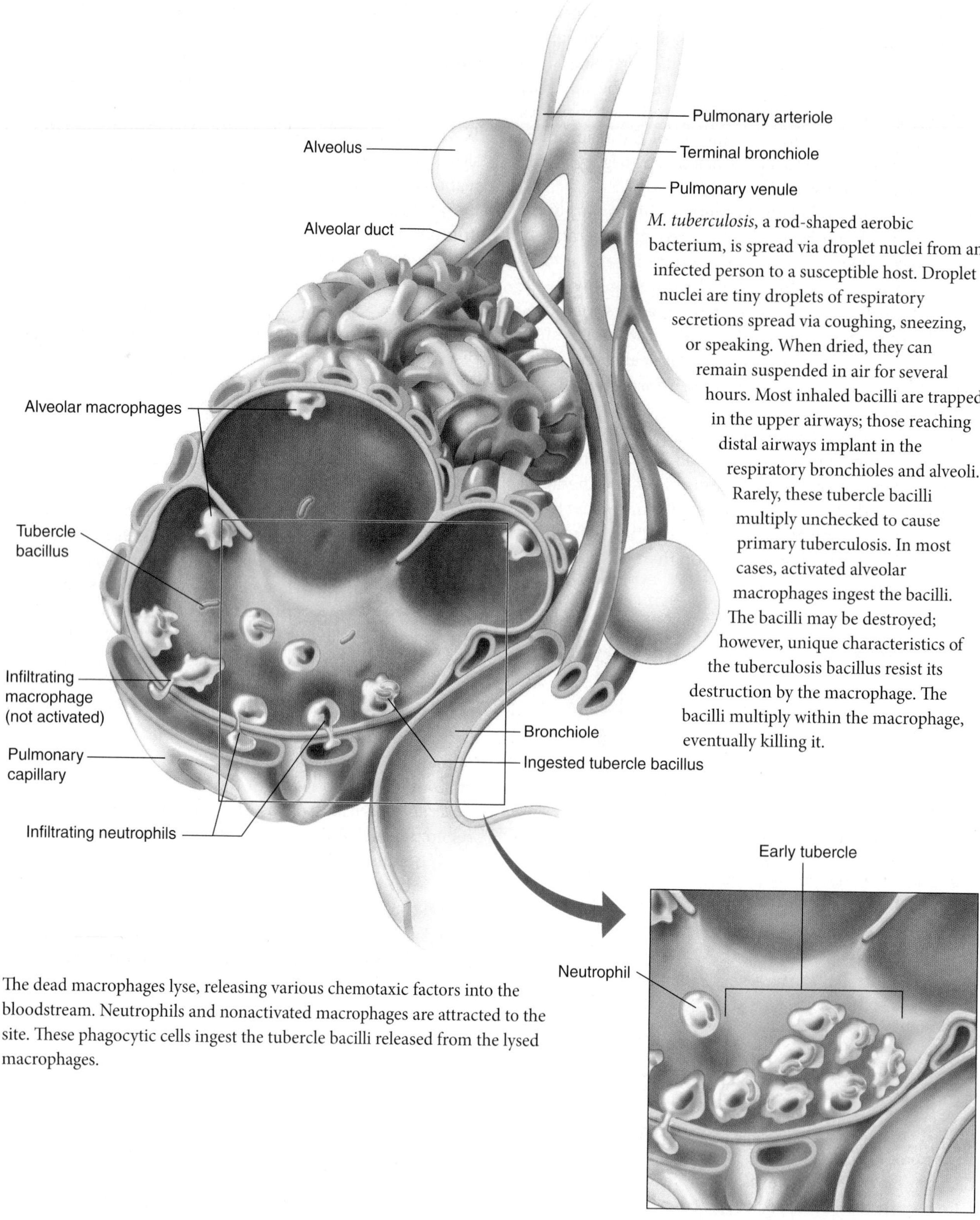

Pulmonary arteriole
Alveolus
Terminal bronchiole
Pulmonary venule
Alveolar duct
M. tuberculosis, a rod-shaped aerobic bacterium, is spread via droplet nuclei from an infected person to a susceptible host. Droplet nuclei are tiny droplets of respiratory secretions spread via coughing, sneezing, or speaking. When dried, they can remain suspended in air for several hours. Most inhaled bacilli are trapped in the upper airways; those reaching distal airways implant in the respiratory bronchioles and alveoli. Rarely, these tubercle bacilli multiply unchecked to cause primary tuberculosis. In most cases, activated alveolar macrophages ingest the bacilli. The bacilli may be destroyed; however, unique characteristics of the tuberculosis bacillus resist its destruction by the macrophage. The bacilli multiply within the macrophage, eventually killing it.
Alveolar macrophages
Tubercle bacillus
Infiltrating macrophage (not activated)
Bronchiole
Pulmonary capillary
Ingested tubercle bacillus
Infiltrating neutrophils
Early tubercle
Neutrophil
The dead macrophages lyse, releasing various chemotaxic factors into the bloodstream. Neutrophils and nonactivated macrophages are attracted to the site. These phagocytic cells ingest the tubercle bacilli released from the lysed macrophages.

(*Continued*)

Figure 19.3 ■ The pathogenesis of tuberculosis, illustrated.

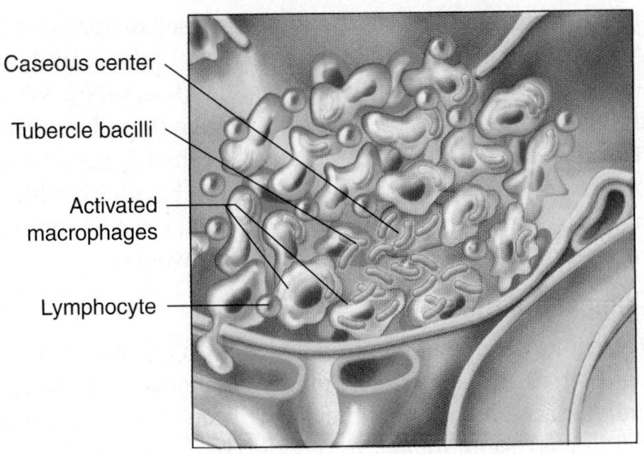

After several weeks, a delayed hypersensitivity response to bacterial antigens destroys many of the macrophages. Concurrently, a cell-mediated immune response activates additional macrophages, which ingest and destroy the bacilli. The lysed macrophages and bacilli are surrounded by a mass of live, activated macrophages and lymphocytes. Scar (granulomatous) tissue forms, encapsulating the primary lesion. Most lesions calcify and are visible on x-ray. These lesions may remain dormant for a year or more (in some cases, many years) before being reactivated to produce secondary or reactivation tuberculosis.

When the immune and macrophage-activating responses are weakened by age or disease (e.g., HIV disease), the tuberculosis bacilli continue to multiply within the lesion. The caseous material at the center of the lesion liquefies, and the lesion grows.

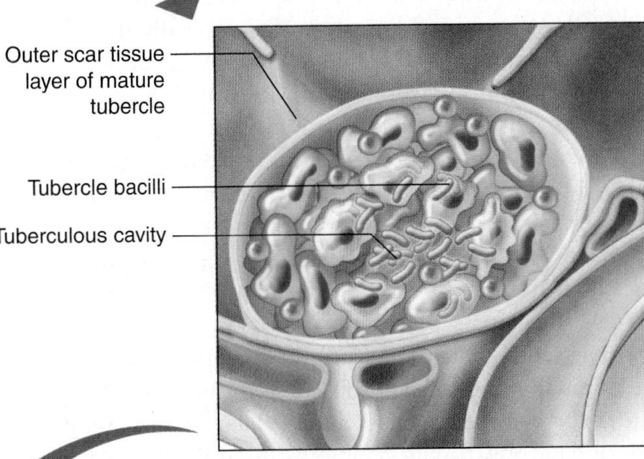

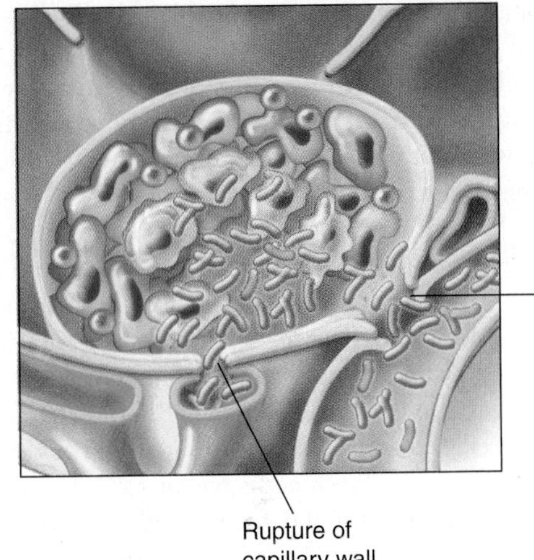

The enlarging lesion damages surrounding bronchial walls and blood vessels. Granulomatous tissue surrounding the lesion can erode into a bronchus, forming an air-filled cavity. Within this cavity, the bacilli multiply, spreading into the airways and the environment via infected sputum. Bacilli multiply, spreading into the airways and the environment via infected sputum. Bacilli also spread via the blood and within macrophages to regional lymph nodes, and from there to many organs and tissues. Resulting extrapulmonary lesions evolve in the same sequence as pulmonary lesions.

Figure 19.3 ■ *Continued*

become ill at some time in their lives. In the United States, primary risk factors for TB include the following:[25–27]

- HIV/AIDS
- Foreign immigration
- Low income, homelessness, and/or malnourishment
- Residing in crowded urban conditions
- Incarceration, which increases the risk of exposure to TB
- Ethnic minorities (e.g., Hispanics, African Americans, Asians)
- Old age
- Chronic disease (e.g., diabetes mellitus, chronic lung disease, Hodgkin disease, chronic renal failure, alcoholism, immunosuppression)
- Currently smoking cigarettes.

Etiology and Pathogenesis

In the United States, tuberculosis is primarily transmitted between an infected person and a susceptible person by inhalation of aerosolized droplets contaminated with *Mycobacterium tuberculosis.* The bacilli are slender, rod-shaped, acid-fast, aerobic organisms that travel in airflow directly to alveoli (**Figure 19.3** ■). *M. tuberculosis* grows best in well-ventilated regions of the lung, and the bacilli have a waxy capsule that is resistant to destruction and allows it to survive even in necrotic granulomas. Individuals with advanced pulmonary TB with evidence of cavitation (liquid necrosis of granulomas) on chest x-ray and acid-fast bacilli on sputum culture are the most infectious. Atypical mycobacterial infections, such as *M. kansasii* and *M. avian* complex (formerly *M. avium-intracellulare*) are opportunistic infections that occur predominantly in chronically ill individuals with compromised immune systems. In underdeveloped nations, oropharyngeal and intestinal TB can be contracted by drinking raw milk from tuberculous cows.

In a primary infection of an immune competent individual who has not previously been exposed to TB, *M. tuberculosis* primarily infects alveolar macrophages. It enters macrophages by endocytosis but blocks the fusion of phagosomes with lysosomes by multiple mechanisms (e.g., inhibition of calcium signals, blocking recruitment and assembly of proteins that mediate the fusion), so the replication of TB bacilli is initially unchecked. This seeds multiple sites, but in spite of the bacteremia, most individuals remain asymptomatic or have only flulike symptoms. As antigens drain to lymph nodes, T_H1 helper T cells are activated. After 3 weeks, the mature T_H1 helper T cells produce interferon-gamma, which stimulates macrophages to become bacteriocidal, containing the infection. Bacilli may be killed by the immune system; they may multiply, causing the disease TB; or they may become dormant, contained within granulomas.

The distinguishing characteristic of *M. tuberculosis* infections is the formation of a granuloma.[30] The development of a granuloma with an associated lymph node, called a Ghon complex, signals an immune response to the bacilli. This is a type IV hypersensitivity reaction mediated by T_H1 helper T cells. At this stage, the individual is infected but is not contagious. The infection usually heals without a trace or forms foci of caseous necrosis or leaves a scar with microcalcification that looks like a fibrocalcific node.[28] In a caseating granuloma, the tissue changes into a dry, cheeselike substance surrounded by a fibrous membrane. *M. tuberculosis* can remain latent in this dormant state for many years. Individuals with latent TB are not infectious. In contrast, active TB is symptomatic and communicable to other individuals. Active TB is progressive and can involve multiple tissues such as those of the central nervous system, gastrointestinal system, or genitourinary system in addition to the lungs.

Reactivation of latent TB (secondary TB) occurs when there is a decreased T-cell–mediated immunity in a previously sensitized host. Secondary TB is frequently localized to one or both apices of the lung because of the high oxygen content. Caseous necrosis occurs when inflammatory granulomas have an inadequate circulation and undergo necrosis, giving the granuloma a soft, white, cheeselike appearance. Any surviving TB bacilli in the periphery of the granuloma are released and multiply to cause the disease TB. When the granuloma center undergoes cavitation (liquid necrosis), it creates the air–fluid level that is seen in TB granulomas on chest x-rays. Cavitation indicates that bacilli have likely been disseminated into airways, where they can be communicated to other people via aerosolized droplets.

Clinical Manifestations

The clinical presentation of TB depends on whether an infection or the disease is present. Primary infections in most healthy individuals who have not previously been exposed to TB are self-limited asymptomatic infections. The classic symptoms of an active tuberculosis infection can include cough, weight loss and anorexia, fever, night sweats, dull aching chest pain, and hemoptysis, but about 20% of individuals may be asymptomatic (e.g., immunocompromised or older individuals).

In latent TB, the bacilli are initially walled off, and the individual is asymptomatic at first, but TB is activated when host immune defenses are weakened by aging or immunosuppression. Symptom onset is generally insidious, with systemic symptoms of malaise, anorexia, fever, and weight loss that are likely related to cytokines released by the inflammatory response. A low-grade fever appears in the late afternoon and then subsides, and night sweats occur. Increasing pulmonary involvement is indicated by increasing cough and sputum, and cavitation can result in hemoptysis. Pleuritic pain indicates an extension of the infection to the pleural surfaces. Extrapulmonary symptoms depend on the system that is involved.

Linking Pathophysiology to Diagnosis and Treatment

Diagnosis is suggested by the history, physical examination, and presence of consolidation or cavitations with air–fluid levels on chest x-ray. Among individuals with latent TB, sputum culture and chest x-ray may be negative. Individuals with active TB may demonstrate positive sputum cultures and a positive chest x-ray.[29]

To confirm the diagnosis, the TB bacilli must be identified, generally in acid-fast smears or sputum cultures; sputum smears have low sensitivity, so sputum cultures are needed in HIV disease.[30] Blood testing for TB may be conducted by using interferon-gamma release assays (IGRAs),[31] such as the QuantiFERON®–TB Gold In-Tube test or the T-SPOT®.TB test. IGRAs evaluate the individual's immune response to *M. tuberculosis* bacteria.[32]

Screening for TB often uses the Mantoux test, an intradermal injection of a purified protein derivative of *M. tuberculosis*; a positive reaction causes a palpable induration that peaks in 48–72 hours. A positive reaction indicates a cell-mediated hypersensitivity response to a previous exposure, but the size of the induration for a positive test varies with the health status of the person. The Mantoux test does not differentiate between infection and disease, and it can give false positives with atypical mycobacteria or vaccination with **bacillus Calmette-Guérin (BCG)** or false negatives in viral infections, sarcoidosis, malnutrition, Hodgkin disease, anergy, immunosuppression, and overwhelming TB disease.[33] Quanti

FERON-TB® has the advantage of being less subject to interpretation than the Mantoux test. The two tests measure different components of the cell-mediated immune response to TB, so they are not directly comparable.[31,33]

For individuals who convert to a positive TB test but do not have the disease, shorter courses and fewer drugs are prescribed for therapy. When individuals have the disease TB, a brief isolation period is necessary until sputum smears are negative.

At present, the U.S. Food and Drug Administration (FDA) has approved 10 medications for the treatment of TB.[33] For most patients with TB, one of four initial treatment protocols is used. At the core of each treatment regimen is a combination of four medications: isoniazid, rifampin, pyrazinamide, and ethambutol.[33] For each regimen, an initial 2-month treatment phase is followed by a continuation treatment phase of either 4 or 7 months in duration.[33]

Fluoroquinolone medications (e.g., levofloxacin, moxifloxacin, and gatifloxacin) also may be used to treat TB.[33] Although the fluoroquinolones are not FDA-approved for use in the treatment of TB, these medications are often used to treat individuals who are intolerant of first-line medications or for the treatment of drug-resistant TB.[33]

Throughout the world, particularly in developing nations, the TB vaccine BCG is among the most widely used vaccines. In children, BCG has been proven effective for prevention of disseminated TB,[34] which occurs when mycobacterium tuberculosis spreads to distant sites by way of the blood or the lymphatic system.[35] Additionally, BCG has been proven effective for preventing meningitis.[34] However, BCG is not useful in preventing primary TB infection; nor does this vaccine prevent reactivation of latent pulmonary infection. At present, research is limited with regard to determining the BCG vaccination's impact on preventing mycobacterium tuberculosis transmission.[34]

Fungal Infections

Dimorphic fungal infections are endemic to particular geographic areas and cause primary infections in both healthy and immunocompromised individuals. In healthy individuals, the infections are self-limited but in immunocompromised individuals, they can result in disseminated disease.

Etiology and Pathogenesis

Fungal infections are generally transmitted by inhalation of the fungal spores in dust or from bird droppings.

Histoplasmosis, caused by inhaling spores of *Histoplasma capsulatum*, is endemic to the Ohio, Missouri, and Mississippi valleys. It is also found in the St. Lawrence valley and along the Appalachian Mountains as well as in the Caribbean and Central and South America.

Coccidioidomycosis, also known as San Joaquin Valley fever, is caused by *Coccidioides immitis*, which is endemic in the soil in the southwestern United States but can be found throughout the world. It grows best in bird feces, and a significant proportion of the population has most likely been exposed to this organism.

Blastomycosis is caused by *Blastomyces dermatitidis*, an uncommon fungus that is found in Ohio, the Great Lakes region, and the Mississippi River valley.[36] Blastomycosis is common in dogs in endemic areas but also occurs in horses, cows, and bats. Infections in animals can serve as an indicator of human disease in areas of infections. The fungi cause a granulomatous inflammation, which results in formation of pulmonary granulomas of varying size within the parenchyma or nodes. In immune competent individuals, the granulomas heal with fibrosis and tend to calcify over time, but the fungus can persist in immunocompromised individuals, so it is possible for the infection to be reactivated at a later time.

Clinical Manifestations

In individuals with competent immune systems, primary infections are commonly asymptomatic and may be discovered as an incidental finding on chest x-ray, or the individual may report mild flulike symptoms. In contrast, immunocompromised individuals are generally symptomatic and often have widely disseminated disease before diagnosis. The usual pulmonary symptoms in immunocompromised individuals are those of cough and fever plus hemoptysis, dyspnea, and chest pain in more severe disease. The symptoms of disseminated disease are fever, weight loss, and hepatosplenomegaly. Disseminated blastomycosis can also present with a pseudoepitheliomatous hyperplasia that looks much like squamous cell carcinoma.[37]

Linking Pathophysiology to Diagnosis and Treatment

Diagnosis of an active infection is made primarily by identifying organisms in sputum or bone marrow or in a liver biopsy. Bronchoalveolar lavage fluid (fluid used to wash out the lung during bronchoscopy) can be analyzed by a direct smear or culture to reveal the organisms in the lung. Serology tests with increasing concentrations of antibodies to individual fungi are available; a reaction at low concentrations strongly suggests an infection, but the specificity and sensitivity of the test are low. A capsular antigen assay is available for detecting *Histoplasma* in the urine or serum, but no equivalent test is available for coccidioidomycosis or blastomycosis. A previous exposure to *Coccidioides* or *Histoplasma* can be confirmed by skin test, but no skin test exists for *Blastomyces*. On chest x-ray, a fungal infection can initially result in a lesion similar to a Ghon complex in tuberculosis that often calcifies at a later time.

Often, no treatment is indicated for asymptomatic patients. Symptomatic patients require therapy with oral itraconazole; amphotericin B is required for hospitalized immunocompromised individuals. Immunocompromised individuals may require long-term oral therapy to prevent relapse.

Lung Abscess

A lung abscess is usually a complication of a pulmonary infection that resulted in the destruction of pulmonary parenchyma with an accumulation of pus within the localized area. The most common cause of a lung abscess is aspiration; 90% are caused by aspiration of multiple anaerobic bacteria from the oropharynx. The risk for aspiration is greatly increased with a decreased level of consciousness and in a recumbent individual whose more vertical airways in the right lung provide more direct paths to the posterior segment of the upper lobe or the apical segments of the lower lobe. Lung abscess can also result from a necrotizing pneumonia, a bronchogenic carcinoma, or an infection in a distant site. Once pus begins to accumulate in localized, isolated pockets, it is surrounded and isolated by neutrophils and occasional fibroblasts.

Symptoms of a lung abscess are similar to those of bronchiectasis (which is discussed in Chapter 18) with a cough that produces foul-smelling sputum. Fevers, malaise, and hemoptysis are also common; over time, the person may lose weight and become anemic. Treatment includes antibiotics, and often surgical drainage is necessary.

Check Your Progress: Section 19.3

1. What is the difference between a TB infection and the disease tuberculosis?
2. Compare the differences in the presentations of fungal pulmonary infections in individuals with competent and incompetent immune systems.
3. What is the significance of a skin induration in the Mantoux skin test?

19.4 Infectious Diseases of the Upper Respiratory Tract

In the United States, respiratory viral infections are the most common cause of acute illness and outpatient physician visits. An **upper respiratory tract infections (URI)** is an acute infection of one or more structures of the upper respiratory tract, including the nose, paranasal sinuses, pharynx, larynx, trachea, and bronchi. Infections of the upper respiratory tract range in severity from mild self-limiting illnesses such as the common cold to life-threatening complications such as epiglottitis. The high prevalence of viral URIs is due to the large numbers of viruses, their ease of transmission, the incomplete immunity developed after viral infection that allows reinfection, and the ability of some viruses to mutate.

The incidence of URIs peaks in 4-year-old children, declines in teenagers, then increases again in parents of young children. Schoolchildren are the major reservoir for respiratory viruses; children become infected at school and bring the virus home to their families. In families, adults average between two and four respiratory viral infections each year, while preschool children have five to seven colds each year. Generally, the prevalence of respiratory viral infections declines in older adults, but the infections are associated with a higher mortality rate in frail or immunocompromised individuals. The high prevalence of URIs is expensive because of loss of productivity and the cost of treatment.

Individuals who are at increased risk for respiratory tract infections include those with the following characteristics:

- Very old or very young, who have less effective immune systems
- Malnourished, including alcoholics
- Exposed to cigarette smoke or other inhaled irritants that compromise mucociliary clearance and suppress the immune system
- Chronic illnesses such as COPD or cystic fibrosis
- Impaired immune status, either congenital (e.g., immotile cilia syndrome) or acquired (e.g., HIV, immunosuppressive therapy).

Etiology and Pathogenesis

Most respiratory infections are transmitted by social contact between humans. The primary mode of transmission varies with the type of pathogen. Small and some large aerosolized droplets can be transmitted by coughing or sneezing (e.g., tuberculosis, influenza, H1N1 virus), but most infections are transmitted by hand-to-hand contact or by an individual touching a fomite, an inanimate object that was contaminated with aerosolized droplets from an infected individual's cough or sneeze, then touching their face near the nose, eyes, or mouth.

Viral infections have strong seasonal patterns that depend on their ability to survive in the environment. Rhinoviruses lack protective lipid-containing envelopes and so are prevalent from spring to fall. Viruses with protective envelopes (e.g., influenza viruses, respiratory syncytial virus, and coronaviruses) are prevalent in the midwinter months. The incubation time varies for the different pathogens, with ranges of 1–21 days or even 4–6 weeks with the Epstein-Barr virus.

Respiratory tract infections occur when an individual is exposed to a particularly virulent pathogen or there is a breakdown in the normal respiratory defense mechanisms. The primary defense mechanisms of the upper respiratory tract include trapping inhaled particles in mucus, which the mucociliary system removes, a strong cough and the immune cells in tonsils and adenoid glands. As you inhale, your nose traps nearly all particles larger than 10 microns in aerodynamic diameter (particle size in moving air) and about half of particles 3 microns in aerodynamic diameter. In the upper respiratory tract, mucus is cleared from the nose and parasinuses by sneezing or blowing the nose and by cilia that move mucus toward the oropharynx. When the cilia do not function properly, mucus accumulates in sinuses, predisposing the individual to infections. Dental problems contribute substantially to bacterial infections in the mouth and in the upper and lower respiratory tract.

A cough can be instigated voluntarily or as a reflex stimulated by cough receptors located throughout the respiratory tract. A reflex cough can be stimulated by stretch receptors in the lung parenchyma and irritant receptors in the larynx and large airways to expel aspirated substances or in response to respiratory infections, irritation, or excess mucus.

Viruses in the upper respiratory tract usually cause acute, self-limiting infections that most often occur as colds, sore throat, sinusitis, and influenza. The nose is the most commonly infected part of upper respiratory system. Individuals are most contagious in the first 3 days of the infection, and spread may occur before the individual is aware of the illness. In children, viral infections commonly cause croup, laryngitis, colds, and influenza, but they can also result in complications such as otitis media, secondary bacterial infections, exacerbations of asthma, and epiglottis.

Respiratory bacterial infections can occur as primary or secondary infections. Examples of primary bacterial URIs are acute streptococcus pharyngitis (e.g., "strep throat" or tonsillitis), pertussis (whooping cough), and sinus infection. A secondary bacterial infection follows the onset of another infection, such as a bacterial pneumonia that follows influenza.

Clinical Manifestations

The usual clinical presentation of URIs is related to the inflammatory response to the invading pathogens and their toxins. Symptoms include a cough that may or may not be productive, localized mucosal edema with erythema, and mucus secretions. Rhinovirus and coronavirus infections inflict minor damage to the nasal mucosa that allows extracellular fluid to escape as **rhinorrhea** (a profuse, watery discharge from the nose). Fever is common in children with infections, but adults can be very ill with respiratory infections and have a normal or below-normal body temperature. A sore throat, myalgias, and malaise can add to the discomfort, but there are few findings on physical examination. When a URI extends into the lower respiratory tract, adventitious sounds such as wheezing or fine (Velcro-like) crackles may be present.

The common cold often begins with a sore or scratchy throat, nasal congestion and/or rhinorrhea, and sneezing, although symptoms may vary among individuals. Initially, the nasal symptoms predominate, followed by a cough, and the individual may have headache, hoarseness, and malaise. Young children with a rhinovirus will have a fever and lower respiratory tract symptoms, while 60% of older adults with viral infections will have a productive cough and wheeze as the infection extends into the lower respiratory tract.

Linking Pathophysiology to Diagnosis and Treatment

Management of URIs consists primarily of supportive measures to increase the individual's comfort as well as treating the specific cause of the infection. Supportive measures generally include rest, increased fluids to dilute respiratory secretions and replace fluid loss, and antipyretics for systemic symptoms. Warm saline gargles or lozenges can soothe a sore throat, and using humidifiers and saline nasal sprays may provide relief from nasal congestion. Over-the-counter medications include antipyretics, decongestants, antihistamines, and mucolytics to relieve specific symptoms. Prescription medications can include antibiotics for bacterial infections, antiviral agents, bronchodilators, and anti-inflammatory medications. Antiviral medications may be prescribed for individuals with impaired immune systems or serious underlying chronic diseases. When started within 48 hours of symptom onset, antiviral medications can shorten the length of a viral infection by 1– 2 days. Bronchodilators can relieve bronchospasm that is common with lower respiratory tract diseases. Oral or topical corticosteroids may be necessary to decrease the inflammation.

Croup

Croup (laryngotracheobronchitis) is an acute viral infection of the upper respiratory tract commonly caused by parainfluenza viruses that spread among children younger than 5 years of age in daycare centers, families, and hospitals.

Croup affects 5% of children each year. Its incidence peaks in the second year of life. Its prevalence is higher in males by nearly a 2:1 ratio. ■

Transmission occurs by direct contact with respiratory secretions or large aerosol droplets. Croup is often preceded by a mild URI. The virus causes an acute inflammation of the larynx and trachea (laryngotracheitis) with subglottal narrowing that obstructs breathing more during inhalation than exhalation because of the highly compliant airways of young children (**Figure 19.4** ■). The airway obstruction causes an inspiratory stridor (high pitched wheezy sound), brassy or barking cough, and hoarseness. Other symptoms include fever, dyspnea, and restlessness. Symptoms are generally worse during the night. The disease is usually self-limiting with symptoms improvement in 3–4 days, but the infection can extend into the lower respiratory tract, causing bronchiolitis, pneumonia, and respiratory failure. Treatment is supportive, including moisture and nebulized bronchodilators. Systemic glucocorticoids may be administered for severe illnesses.

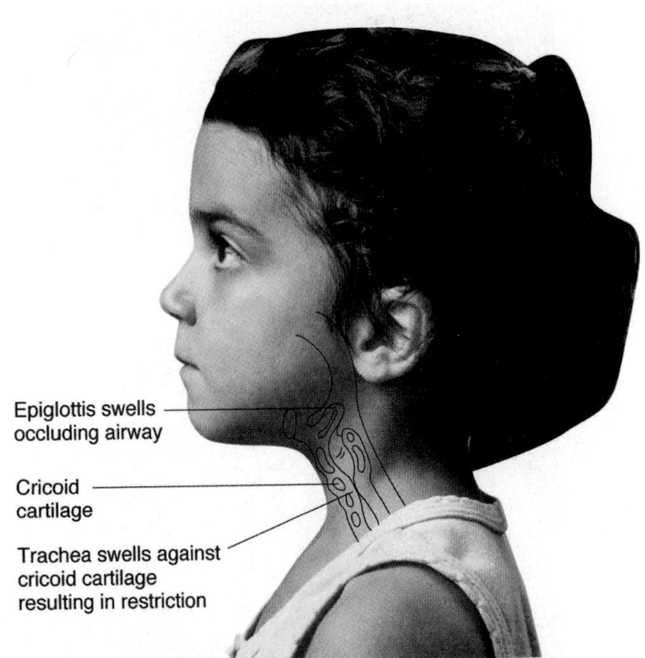
Epiglottis swells occluding airway
Cricoid cartilage
Trachea swells against cricoid cartilage resulting in restriction

Figure 19.4 ■ Airway changes with croup. There are two important changes in the upper airway with croup: The epiglottis swells, occluding the airway, and the trachea swells against the cricoid cartilage, causing restriction and narrowing the airway.

Epiglottitis

Epiglottitis is a rapidly progressive inflammation of the epiglottis and adjacent structures that is usually caused by bacterial infection, most commonly *Haemophilus influenzae* type b (Hib). The abrupt onset of severe inflammation results in edema that can obstruct the upper airway. In preschool children, epiglottitis peaks at 3 years of age, but the incidence has been decreased by routine infant vaccination.

Epiglottitis can occur in children after ingestion of very hot beverages (thermal injury) or corrosive liquids. ■

In adults, the incidence of epiglottitis is 0.97–3.1 per 100,000, and the mortality rate is 7.1%.[38] In addition to bacterial infections, thermal injuries sustained by way of smoking crack cocaine have been implicated as a cause of epiglottitis.[39]

Signs and symptoms of epiglottitis can include a sore throat, painful swallowing, a choking sensation, muffled speech and drooling, or difficulty swallowing liquids. With progressive upper airway obstruction, symptoms include stridor, dyspnea, and tachycardia.

CLINICAL POINT: To improve air intake, patients with severe respiratory distress will often refuse to lie down and instead will sit up, lean forward, and assume a tripod posture, often called a sniffing posture (**Figure 19.5** ■). Maintaining a patent airway is crucial and may require emergency medical intervention.[38] ■

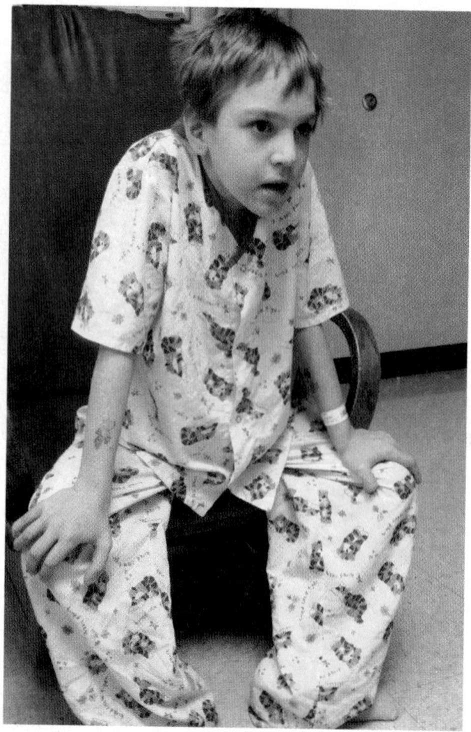

Figure 19.5 ■ This child with epiglottitis has assumed the tripod position in an attempt to keep his airway open.

Check Your Progress: Section 19.4

1. What is the most common cause of epiglottitis?
2. What are the characteristic clinical manifestations of croup caused by airway obstruction?
3. What is the focus of treatment for upper respiratory tract infections?

19.5 Infectious Diseases of the Lower Respiratory Tract

Lower respiratory tract infections range in severity from acute bronchitis to severe infections that destroy the lung parenchyma. These infections are caused by viruses, bacteria, and fungi. Their incidence and associated morbidity and mortality vary by season and by the individual's age and health status. For example, bronchiolitis triggered by a respiratory syncytial virus infection is most common in infants under 1 year old, while community-acquired pneumonia (CAP) is most likely to occur as a bacterial infection in adults. Primary bacterial infections occur more frequently in individuals with an underlying chronic lung disease, a compromised immune system, or an altered airway (e.g., endotracheal intubation or tracheostomy).

Additional risk factors for lower respiratory tract infections include the following:

- Altered level of consciousness, which predisposes to microaspiration of upper airway secretions or macroaspiration of gastric contents (e.g., postcerebral vascular accident, drug or alcohol overdose, postoperative sedation)
- Atelectasis postanesthesia for major surgery, particularly thoracic or abdominal surgery
- Mechanical ventilation via an artificial airway with endotracheal suctioning of accumulated secretions
- Impaired ventilation because of chest trauma, neuromuscular problems (e.g., Guillain-Barré syndrome), neural control (e.g., spinal cord injuries), or mechanical obstruction of a bronchus (e.g., foreign body or tumor)
- Metabolic alterations such as hypoxia, acidosis, or uremia
- Previous episode of pneumonia or chronic bronchitis
- Immotile cilia syndrome
- Acute respiratory injury due to inhalation of smoke or irritant gases (e.g., ozone, high levels of oxygen, nitrogen oxides, and sulfur dioxide) or toxic fumes (e.g., ammonia or chlorine released in industrial accidents).[40]

James Gerrity: Application

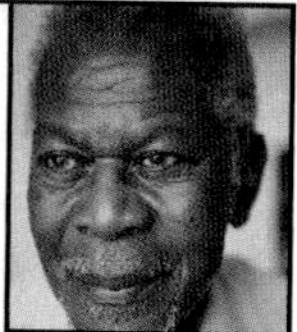

Mr. Gerrity continues to feel very tired and has a nagging cough. He gets short of breath very easily while doing chores. Over the weekend, he has so much difficulty mowing the lawn that he lets his son finish the job for him. He goes into the house, lies on the couch to watch TV, and naps off and on for the rest of the afternoon. Mrs. Gerrity encourages her husband to see his doctor, but he insists on waiting until his scheduled appointment, which is 3 weeks away. However, in less than a week, Mr. Gerrity feels significantly worse. He continues to have a persistent, productive cough. He develops a sore throat and rhinorrhea. He finds that he becomes short of breath much more easily than he normally would, and it takes him twice as long to shower and get dressed in the morning. His appetite has dropped off, and he has not been drinking as many fluids as he needs, partly because of the effort involved in eating and drinking.

Mr. Gerrity awakens in the middle of the night and is unable to catch his breath. He attempts to use his inhaled bronchodilator, but he can't move air well enough to take a deep breath and deliver medication to his lungs. He feels as though he is suffocating and becomes very anxious. Mrs. Gerrity insists on calling emergency medical services, and Mr. Gerrity is transported to the emergency center via ambulance.

3. Which factors in Mr. Gerrity's history place him at risk for a respiratory tract infection?
4. Which of Mr. Gerrity's symptoms suggest that he may have influenza?

Etiology and Pathogenesis

There is overlap between URIs and lower respiratory tract infections; some infections begin as URIs, then move to the lower respiratory tract. The thin mucus blanket in bronchi traps particles that range from 2 to 10 microns in aerodynamic diameter, and cilia move mucus toward the larynx to be either swallowed or coughed out when mucus production overwhelms the mucociliary system.

Alveolar macrophages are the major defense against inhaled microorganisms and other particles that reach alveoli. These macrophages roam alveoli and phagocytose particles less than 2 microns in diameter, then degrade microbes and foreign cells with hydrolases and enzymes such as lysozyme, collagenase, and beta-glucuronidase. Macrophages contain additional enzymes such as α_1 antitrypsin (a protease inhibitor) that control tissue breakdown, but the protection can be inhibited by tobacco smoke, hypoxia, excess alcohol intake, or immunosuppressant drugs or if the immune system is impaired (e.g., HIV disease).

Microaspirations of saliva and gastric contents introduce pathogens into the lungs when the cough reflex is impaired or absent. Individuals lose cough reflexes with anesthesia, loss of consciousness, or a loss of efferent neural control of chest wall and abdominal muscles (e.g., spinal cord injury, Guillain-Barré syndrome) or impaired strength of muscles needed to cough (e.g., amyotrophic lateral sclerosis). Normally, acidic gastric secretions destroy pathogens that have been swallowed by denaturing proteins, but when antacids or histamine 2 blockers are prescribed to limit the formation of stomach acid, the incidence of hospital-acquired pneumonias can increase.

Clinical Manifestations

Many of the signs and symptoms for lower respiratory tract infections, such as a cough, are nonspecific. The usual presentation of tracheobronchial infections include a sore, inflamed throat that can make swallowing painful and enlarged lymph nodes; these may be accompanied by a cough, malaise, and fever. The usual signs and symptoms of lung infections include a cough that may be dry or may produce mucoid or purulent sputum, wheezing, fine crackles on auscultation, malaise, and fever in some individuals. Additional information on epidemiology, signs and symptoms, and treatment will be presented as part of the discussions of specific diseases.

CLINICAL POINT: A change in the color of sputum is not specific for a bacterial infection. With bronchial inflammation, epithelial cells are sloughed off, and leukocytes responding to the infection release peroxidase, the enzyme responsible for the change in sputum color. ■

Acute Bronchitis

Acute bronchitis is a very common, self-limited lower respiratory tract inflammation, that is often referred to as a "chest cold." It is a primary reason for individuals to seek health care in the fall and winter. In otherwise healthy individuals, acute bronchitis can occur at the same time as a URI or follow one. Acute bronchitis is most often diagnosed in children younger than 5 years of age. In healthy individuals, the organisms that cause acute bronchitis are numerous viruses, particularly influenza viruses, and bacteria such as *Mycoplasma pneumoniae*, *Chlamydophila pneumoniae*, and *Bordetella pertussis*. In individuals with underlying immune deficiencies, chronic lung disease, tracheostomy or endotracheal tubes, and bacterial infections with *Streptococcus pneumoniae*, *Haemophilus influenzae*, or *Moraxella catarrhalis* are common. Noninfectious triggers for acute bronchitis include asthma, air pollutants, inhaling ammonia or other irritating substances, cannabis smoke, and tobacco smoke.

Acute bronchitis is characterized by bronchial inflammation with mucosal congestion and a cough that may produce sputum. The early symptoms are those of a URI, but the cough typically lasts 10–20 days and can persist much longer with pertussis. With a viral infection, the cough may be severe and prolonged but not produce much sputum. Sore throat with hoarseness, dyspnea, chest pain, and myalgias are common, and hemoptysis can occur with a severe acute bronchitis. Acute bronchitis often results in bronchial hyperreactivity, causing bronchospasm and wheezing with exposure to environmental triggers; the hyperreactivity can persist for 5–6 weeks. Acute bronchitis must be differentiated from exacerbations of COPD or bacterial pneumonia, which is always treated with antibiotics. Generally, no diagnostic tests are indicated, but if symptoms are prolonged, pneumonia can be differentiated from acute bronchitis by the consolidation (increased lung density) that is evident on chest x-ray in pneumonia.

Bronchiolitis

Bronchiolitis involves inflammation of the bronchioles, which are the smallest airway passages in the lungs. The prevalence of bronchiolitis is increased in winter and spring, and it is frequently preceded by a URI. It can be epidemic in nurseries, and there is an increased risk for bronchiolitis in premature infants and children with underlying pulmonary problems. Recurrent bronchiolitis may be due to underlying cystic fibrosis. Bronchiolitis can also occur in high-risk adults, such as cigarette smokers who are exposed to toxic fumes and develop a viral infection.

The incidence of bronchiolitis peaks in infants 2–6 months old; in 80% of cases, the child is younger than 1 year of age. ■

In most cases, the etiology of bronchiolitis is not clear, but an injury to the bronchiolar epithelium from an infection likely initiates the inflammatory process. Respiratory syncytial virus is the most common cause of bronchiolitis in children younger than 1 year of age,[41] but bronchiolitis can also be related to adenoviruses or measles infections.[42] Respiratory syncytial virus infections are highly contagious with transmission by aerosolized respiratory secretions; 10% of the droplets can cause infections up to 24 hours later.

Bronchiolitis results in the necrosis of the respiratory epithelium within the first 24 hours of the infection, and excess mucus production and submucosal swelling contribute to blockage of small airways. Recovery from the inflammation of bronchiolitis can result in bronchiolitis obliterans, which is characterized by fibrosis that narrows or obliterates small airways. Bronchiolitis obliterans is often accompanied by bronchiectasis and mucus plugging in adjacent airways.[43]

In small children, hyperinflation of alveoli distal to bronchioles occurs with the decreased bronchiole diameter during exhalation, increased airway resistance caused by bronchial edema, and airway mucus plugging. Atelectasis develops when small bronchioles are obstructed by mucus and desquamated cells (cells scaled off airways) and the remaining air is absorbed from the distal alveoli. Most healthy children recover, but in severe cases, respiratory failure with hypercapnea and cyanosis can develop and may be fatal. ■

The presentation of bronchiolitis varies with the age of the individual. In the early stages, infants may have subtle symptoms with increased fussiness and feeding problems. After 1–2 days, infants will have fever and tachypnea with shallow respirations in an effort to reduce the work of breathing. Infants have compliant chest walls, so sternal and intercostal retractions indicate that the infant is working hard to breathe and, coupled with hypoxemia, signal serious respiratory distress. Infants may also flare their nostrils in an attempt to decrease airway resistance. The initial symptoms of bronchiolitis in older children are those of a common cold with a cough and nasal discharge. Among older children and thin adults with stiffer chest walls, intercostal retractions also indicate a very effort strong to breathe. Symptoms of fine crackles and expiratory wheezing with deep breaths are similar to asthma symptoms, but asthma is uncommon in children under 2 years of age. A chest x-ray can confirm the presence of atelectasis. Therapy is supportive, focused on respiratory symptoms.

Pertussis

Pertussis (whooping cough) is a highly contagious respiratory infection that is usually caused by *Bordetella pertussis*. It has been controlled in children through pertussis vaccination but is increasingly common among adults as their immunity from childhood vaccination wanes. Pertussis is directly transmitted by inhalation of contaminated droplets or indirectly by touching fomites contaminated by secretions from a person in the acute stage of the illness. *B. pertussis* attaches to and damages ciliated respiratory epithelium. Pertussis in nonimmunized individuals causes an uncontrollable, spasmodic cough that ends in a loud, crowing, inspiratory whoop. The cough is so hard that the individual may vomit. The infection lasts about 6 weeks, but the cough can persist for 3–4 months. Other symptoms are myalgias and fever; later, sputum becomes progressively more tenacious, and pneumonia is a relatively common complication. Adults who have partial immunity will have symptoms that resemble those of a viral pneumonia rather than exhibiting the classic whooping cough.

Influenza

Influenza (flu) is a highly contagious viral infection that sweeps through a geographic region as an epidemic that lasts 6–8 weeks during the winter months. It infects 5–10% of adults and an even a higher percentage of children. Its short incubation period (1–4 days, with an average of 2 days) facilitates rapid spread among individuals. In influenza pandemics, a new viral strain or mutation is introduced that no one has immunity against, and it rapidly spreads worldwide as a serious illness. In 1918–1919, the Spanish influenza pandemic killed between 20 million and 40 million people worldwide and a half million individuals in the United States. It was the deadliest pandemic since the "black death" that occurred in the Middle Ages.

The emergence of H1N1 influenza A in 2009 resulted in the first worldwide pandemic in 40 years.[44,45] The Centers for Disease Control and Prevention (CDC) estimated that 22 million individuals were infected with the H1N1 virus between April and October 2009, with about 2500–6100 flu deaths in that period.[45] Hospitalizations were highest in children from birth to 4 years of age, and infections caused or contributed to 7.3% of deaths in the United States.[44] Although the H1N1 virus originated in pigs, it has since become a regular human influenza virus that circulates globally on a seasonal basis.[45]

Influenza with pneumonia is the eighth leading cause of death in the United States,[46] and individuals over 65 years of age and/or those with chronic cardiopulmonary diseases or diabetes are at increased risk for developing pneumonia or dying as a result of their infection. Individuals who are at high risk for influenza-related complications and severe disease include the following:

- Children under 5 years of age, especially those under the age of 2 years
- Pregnant women
- Individuals over 50 years of age
- Individuals of any age with chronic medical conditions such as cardiac or pulmonary disease or diabetes mellitus
- Individuals who live with or care for individuals at high risk (e.g., household contacts, healthcare workers).[47]

Etiology and Pathogenesis

Influenza viruses are highly contagious, causing upper and lower respiratory tract infections that can become pneumonia. Influenza virus type A is the most common cause of influenza and causes a more severe disease than type B or C. Other respiratory viruses such as respiratory syncytial virus, adenoviruses, or rhinoviruses can also cause flulike symptoms.

Influenza viruses are transmitted by inhalation of small aerosolized particles of virus-containing respiratory secretions. Large amounts of virus in respiratory secretions can be transmitted by coughing, talking, or sneezing or contact with contaminated hands or fomites. To initiate an infection, a surface glycoprotein of the influenza virus binds to glycoproteins on the surface of respiratory epithelial cells. After the virus replicates in the cell, the newly created viral particles are bound to the host cell until neuraminidase cleaves the links, freeing the new virus particles and preventing them from agglutinating in respiratory secretions.[48] The immune system responds to the surface glycoprotein structures of the viruses.

Influenza viruses are classic examples of viruses that frequently mutate or change their antigenicity to cause illness in individuals who had been immunized against influenza. **Antigenicity** is the ability to stimulate the formation of antibodies. Antigenic shifts are major changes in the surface glycoproteins. Type A influenza viruses in particular periodically change their antigenic properties. Major shifts in antigenicity are associated with epidemics and pandemics of influenza.

Influenza viral infections cause necrosis and desquamation of respiratory tract epithelial cells, leaving gaps between the underlying basal cells and allowing extracellular fluid to escape. The loss of ciliated cells results in a diffuse watery nasal discharge and necessitates coughing, sneezing, or blowing the nose to clear the mucus. The primary lymphocytic immune response produces an accumulation of active lymphocytes that release inflammatory mediators. Thus, influenza symptoms are the result of inflammatory mediators as well as the infection.

Clinical Manifestations

Influenza presents with a range of symptoms, from those of a common cold to an illness with primarily systemic symptoms. Influenza has an abrupt onset with nonspecific symptoms of fever, headache, myalgias, and severe malaise after 1–2 days of incubation. Photophobia and pain with eye movements can occur early in the illness. Respiratory symptoms of cough, sore throat, and often rhinorrhea are followed later by purulent sputum and fatigue. Uncomplicated influenza gradually improves over 2–5 days but can last longer. Some individuals experience a postinfluenza asthenia (postflu syndrome) with persistent symptoms of weakness and fatigue that can last for several weeks. The most serious complication is a viral pneumonia or secondary bacterial pneumonia. A combination bacterial–viral pneumonia also may occur after influenza infection.[49]

Linking Pathophysiology to Diagnosis and Treatment

Diagnosis is based on the symptoms and the presence of influenza in the geographic region. Though not usually necessary, a bronchoscopy reveals fiery red bronchi that remain hyperreactive for weeks after the infection has resolved.

Treatment is primarily supportive to alleviate symptoms and if initiated within the first 48 hours of symptom onset, antiviral therapy can shorten the duration of uncomplicated influenza by 1–2 days. Antiviral therapy cannot prevent serious complications such as pneumonia or an exacerbation of chronic diseases. A yearly influenza vaccine can attenuate or prevent symptoms of influenza and limit the risk for hospitalization and death. The CDC issues yearly recommendations for which individuals should receive influenza vaccines.

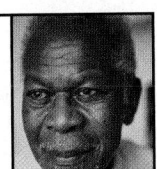

James Gerrity: Outcome

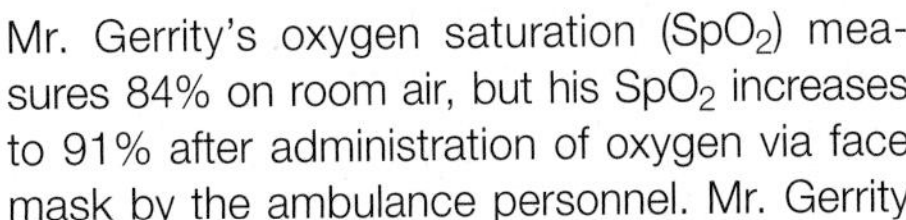

Mr. Gerrity's oxygen saturation (SpO_2) measures 84% on room air, but his SpO_2 increases to 91% after administration of oxygen via face mask by the ambulance personnel. Mr. Gerrity is transported to the nearest hospital emergency center, where he is evaluated by a primary care provider. Laboratory tests and diagnostics include a complete blood count (CBC); serum electrolytes; chest x-ray; sputum Gram stain, culture, and sensitivity; and arterial blood gases. Mr. Gerrity's CBC reveals an elevated white blood cell count, and his chest x-ray demonstrates diffuse, patchy infiltrates. His arterial blood gases suggest mild respiratory acidosis. Mr. Gerrity receives a nebulized albuterol treatment, after which he reports he is breathing "a little better." Mr. Gerrity's sputum Gram stain reveals the presence of both viral and bacterial organisms. Antibiotic therapy is initiated, and Mr. Gerrity is admitted to the hospital with a diagnosis of combination bacterial–viral pneumonia, which the primary care provider suspects began with a viral influenza infection.

5. On the basis of the location of exposure to the organism that caused Mr. Gerrity's pneumonia, what type of pneumonia does Mr. Gerrity have?
6. Compare the differences in treatment for bacterial pneumonia and viral pneumonia.

Pneumonia

Pneumonia is defined as an inflammation of the lung parenchyma that is typically characterized by lung consolidation with alveoli filled with exudate (**Figure 19.6** ■). Although it is often caused by an infection, other causes of the inflammation range from the inhalation of noxious fumes (e.g., chlorine, smoke inhalation) to aspiration of gastric contents or other substances such as mineral oil (lipoid pneumonia). This section focuses on pneumonia caused by infections.

Along with influenza, pneumonia is the eighth leading cause of death in the United States[46] and a major cause of morbidity. In 2009, the incidence of CAP was between 3 and 40 per 1000 inhabitants per year, and the rate increased with age. Between 40% and 60% of individuals with CAP were hospitalized, 10% of them in intensive care units, and the overall mortality rate was approximately 8–10%.[50]

As defined by the American Thoracic Society, **hospital-acquired pneumonia (HAP)** involves pneumonia

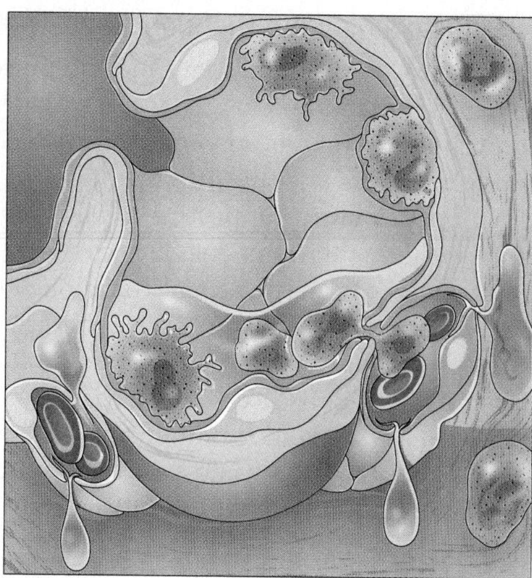

Figure 19.6 ■ In pneumonia, the inflammatory response causes fluid to accumulate in the alveoli and edema to form as alveolar capillaries dilate and allow fluid to leak into interstitial tissues.

that was not incubating at the time of hospital admission and develops 48 hours or more after hospital admission.[51] **Ventilator-associated pneumonia (VAP)** is pneumonia that develops more than 48–72 hours after tracheal intubation.[51] In 2009, the incidence of VAP was about 20%, with an approximate mortality rate of 30%.[50] Examples of **healthcare-associated pneumonia (HCAP)** include patients who were hospitalized in an acute care hospital for 2 or more days within 90 days of developing the infection, or who resided in a long-term care facility or nursing home at the time of infection. Patients who develop pneumonia within 30 days of receiving intravenous antibiotic medications, chemotherapy, or wound care are classified as having HAP, as are individuals who visited a hospital or hemodialysis clinic before the infection.[51]

The patterns of pneumonia occurrence vary with different organisms and the person's age, health status, and environment. In general, pneumonia is more common in winter than summer, in men than women, and in African Americans than Caucasians. *Streptococcus* pneumonia used to be called "the old person's friend" because it was such a common cause of death for older adults before the advent of antibiotics and *S. pneumoniae* vaccines, and pneumonia is still common among older adults with chronic diseases. In contrast, myocoplasma and *Chlamydia* pneumonias are spread by close contact (e.g., in dormitories, military camps) and are more frequent among young adults[52]; they cause less severe pulmonary symptoms but may have severe neurologic complications.[53] The influenza viral pneumonias range in severity from a mild disease with patchy infiltrates to a rapidly fatal infection, particularly in debilitated patients.

Many of the risk factors for pneumonia are the same as those for other respiratory tract infections, including the virulence of the pathogens, the age of the host, and the individual's health and immune status. Specifically, smoking, impairment in mucociliary clearance, loss or suppression of cough, chronic pulmonary disease, loss of splenic function, and pulmonary congestion and edema predispose individuals to pneumonia. In addition, one type of pneumonia (e.g., a viral pneumonia) may predispose the individual to developing another type (e.g., bacterial pneumonia), particularly if the individual is frail or debilitated.[54]

CLINICAL POINT: In VAP, the risks for infection were decreased by adequate oral and airway care, use of saline instillation with suctioning, a semirecumbent 45-degree position, and early tracheostomy in older adults.[50] ■

Pneumonias are generally classified by the location where the patient was exposed to the pathogen, the causative pathogen, or the location of the pathogen within the lung. Classification includes CAP that occurs in individuals living in the community versus healthcare-associated pneumonias that occur in hospitalized individuals. Opportunistic pneumonias occur in individuals with compromised immune systems. Zoonotic pneumonias occur when the infecting organism was transmitted from animals.

Traditionally, pneumonias were classified by their location within the lung. When the consolidation of lung tissue is patchy, the pneumonia is called *bronchopneumonia*. In lobar pneumonia, the consolidation is homogeneous and involves most of the entire lobe. Some of the same pathogens cause both lobar pneumonia and bronchopneumonia, and distinguishing between pneumonias anatomically on chest x-rays can be difficult, so pneumonias are more often classified by the causative pathogen or the setting in which the infection occurred.

Etiology and Pathogenesis

Pneumonia is more probable with a breakdown of the normal respiratory tract defense mechanisms, but it can occur with a very large exposure to an infectious pathogen or exposure to a highly virulent pathogen. Pneumonia is usually a primary infection caused by the microaspiration of pathogens into the respiratory tract. Other possible routes for infection include aspiration with vomiting or aerosol inhalation (primarily viruses, *Legionella pneumophila*, and *Mycobacterium tuberculosis*) or a secondary infection caused by a bloodborne pathogen that originated in distant infected site.

- ***Community-acquired pneumonia.*** CAP can be caused by bacteria or viruses, and bacterial pneumonias frequently follow URIs. Pathogens that cause CAPs are designated as typical or atypical (see **Table 19.1** ■). With typical pneumonias, there is an acute onset with chills, fever, and a productive cough with purulent sputum. With atypical pneumonias, the subacute onset is characterized by fever, moderate amounts of sputum, but no lung consolidation, since the inflammation is primarily in the septa and lung interstitium.[54] Traditionally, these designations were made on the basis of the clinical presentation of pneumonia as acute or subacute, but in older adults or immunocompromised individuals, the presentation of typical pneumonias is

Table 19.1 Pathogens of, Risk Factors for, and Characteristics of Pneumonias

Pathogen	Risk Factors and Specific Characteristics
Typical Community-Acquired Pneumonias	
Streptococcus pneumoniae (gram positive)	At risk: Underlying chronic disease (e.g., COPD), congenital or acquired immunodeficiency, decreased or absent splenic function Transmission by microaspiration from upper airway
Haemophilus influenzae (gram negative)	At risk: Chronic pulmonary disease (e.g., COPD, cystic fibrosis, bronchiectasis)
Moraxella catarrhalis	At risk: Older adults, COPD; causes otitis media in children
Staphylococcus aureus Methicillin-resistant *S. aureus* (MRSA)	At risk: Individuals with cystic fibrosis and older adults Secondary bacterial infection in healthy children and younger adults recovering from influenza or a viral respiratory infection MRSA may be associated with severe necrotizing pneumonia that can occur with influenza. Requires long, intensive therapy and can result in death.
Legionella pneumophila (mild form: Pontiac fever, a self-limiting URI)	At risk: Older adults who smoke cigarettes, or have chronic lung disease or illnesses associated with immunosuppression or are immunosuppressed Transmission via aerosol from contaminated water source (e.g., showers, whirlpool spas, decorative fountains, cooling towers, grocery story mist machines), not person to person
Enterobacteriaceae *Klebsiella pneumoniae* *Pseudomonas* spp.	At risk: Alcoholics and individuals with significant chronic disease (e.g., COPD, diabetes mellitus, immunosuppression) At risk: Patients with immunosuppression (e.g., transplant patients, HIV infection), structural lung abnormalities (e.g., cystic fibrosis, bronchietasis), burns, prolonged antibiotic therapy, urinary catheterization
Atypical Community-Acquired Pneumonias	
Mycoplasma pneumoniae	At risk: Healthy young adults (college students), school-aged children, military recruits,[55] cigarette smokers, families with infected member Extrapulmonary disease can include hemolysis, skin rash, joint involvement, and signs and symptoms of gastrointestinal, central nervous system, and heart disease that may be due to immune mechanisms rather than the direct effect of the organism.
Chlamydia psittaci *C. pneumoniae* *C. trachomatis*	At risk: Pet bird owners At risk: Older adults 65–79 years of age
Respiratory syncytial virus	At risk: Infants up to 1 year old
Influenza viruses	At risk: Adults with heart or lung disease, diabetes mellitus, renal disease, hemoglobinopathy, or immunosuppression; residents of nursing homes or chronic care facilities; and otherwise healthy individuals over age 65[47]
Adenoviruses	At risk: Military recruits
Parainfluenza virus	At risk: Children
Healthcare-Associated Pneumonias	
Staphylococcus aureus	At risk: Intubated individuals or those prone to aspiration
Enterobacteriaceae *Pseudomonas*	At risk: Hospitalized individuals with significant chronic diseases (e.g., chronic heart or lung disease, diabetes mellitus), malnourished, immunosuppressed individuals
Klebsiella, Serratia marcescens	At risk: Alcoholics, significant chronic disease
Escherichia coli	At risk: Bacteremia post gastrointestinal or genitourinary surgery, cancer patients on chemotherapy, chronic lung or heart disease
Pneumonias Caused by Opportunistic Pathogens	
Pneumocystis jiroveci	At risk: Immunocompromised by HIV disease or cytotoxic agents, malnourished
Mycobacterium avian complex (MAC) *M. avian* *M. intercellulare*	At risk: Immunocompromised, individuals with chronic lung disease, older women with lung infections and bronchiectasis who suppress a cough, allowing stagnation of secretions (a.k.a. Lady Windermere syndrome) (*M. avian* in HIV disease; *M. intercellulare* in COPD) Transmitted by inhalation and ingestion (translocation across GI mucosa)
Aspergillosis (fungal infection)	At risk: Immunosuppressed individuals (e.g., cytotoxic therapy or HIV infection), asthmatic patients with type I hypersensitivity reaction to aspergillosis (allergic bronchopulmonary aspergillosis)
Nocardia	At risk: Immunocompromised patients (e.g., lymphoma, neutropenia)
Candidiasis (invasive fungal)	At risk: Immunocompromised patients (e.g., HIV disease or cytotoxic suppression of the immune system)

(*Continued*)

Table 19.1 Pathogens of, Risk Factors for, and Characteristics of Pneumonias *Continued*

Pathogen	Risk Factors and Specific Characteristics
Acinetobacter spp.	At risk: Endotracheal intubation, mechanical ventilation for 48 hours or longer, treatment in an intensive care unit, recent major surgery, prior treatment with broad-spectrum antibiotics, alcoholism
C. neoformans Cryptococcosis	At risk: Immunocompromised, particularly in HIV infection or hematologic or lymphoid malignancies
Necrotizing Pneumonias and Lung Abscesses	
Anaerobic organisms (e.g., *Bacterioides* spp.)	At risk: Impaired consciousness (e.g., ETHOL, seizures, anesthetized patients), swallowing disorders, aspiration
Aerobic organisms including *Staphylococcus aureus, Klebsiella pneumonia, Streptococcus pyogenes*	As above in healthcare-associated pneumonias
Zoonotic Infections	
Sin Nombre virus (hantavirus pulmonary syndrome)	At risk: Humans in direct contact with infected rodents their urine or feces; virus has been found throughout the United States. Deadly disease causes an acute respiratory distress-like response rather than pneumonia because of the host response to the virus.
SARS-associated coronavirus (SARS-RoV)	At risk: Exposure to ill individuals Transmitted to humans from wild masked palm civets, which are eaten in China, then transmitted from human to human. Last case documented in 2004.[54]
Avian influenza A (H5N1) (strongly pathogenic strain)	At risk: Close exposure to poultry and wild birds, very rare person-to-person transmission. Similar to the influenza virus that caused the 1918 pandemic and frequently causes death in humans.[54]
Coxiella burnetti (Q fever)	At risk: Contact with cattle, sheep, and goats (primary reservoirs), especially during birthing. Can be transmitted by tick bite, but human-to-human transmission is rare.

muted. This classification of pneumonias is still useful because different antibiotic therapies are required for typical and atypical pathogens.

- ***Hospital-acquired pneumonia.*** HAP is common in individuals who have severe preexisting chronic diseases, are immunosuppressed, have invasive procedures, or have undergone a long course of antibiotic therapy. Additional factors that predispose hospitalized individuals to healthcare-associated pneumonias are (1) more virulent bacteria in a hospital environment that may be resistant to antibiotics; (2) risk of cross-contamination from an infected individual; (3) invasive procedures ranging from catheterization to surgery that interrupt normal defense mechanisms, leaving the individual more susceptible to infection; and (4) risk for bacterial contamination of respiratory care equipment. The most common pathogens are gram-negative enterobacteria and *Pseudomonas* spp.
- ***Opportunistic pneumonia.*** Opportunistic infections are caused by common organisms that do not cause illness in healthy individuals with intact immune systems. For example, the bacteria *Pseudomonas aeruginosa* is common in soil and water and on plant surfaces but causes pneumonia in debilitated, malnourished individuals or those with cystic fibrosis, while pneumonia caused by *Pneumocystis jiroveci*, also called PCP, is common in individuals with HIV disease. Fungal pneumonias can occur in immunocompromised individuals, particularly those with neutropenia or those on long-term immunosuppressive therapy or infected with HIV.
- ***Zoonotic infection.*** Zoonotic infections are caused by viruses that are transmitted from their usual animal reservoirs to humans. The danger of an epidemic exists if the virus mutates to allow transmission among humans. A mutation could occur if an individual with a transmissible human virus also is infected with a zoonitic virus. Humans would have no immunity to a newly mutated zoonitic virus, so it could spread rapidly, as happened with H1N1.
- ***Infections with bioterrorism potential.*** *Bacillus anthracis*, gram-positive bacillus spores known as anthrax, were used as a bioterrorism weapon in the United States in 2001. A powder containing anthrax was placed in letters and mailed through the U.S. postal service. It caused great concern because inhalation anthrax is the most deadly form of the disease. The incident caused more disruption and worry than illness, but an aerosolized form of anthrax as well as *Yersinia pestis* (plague), *Coxiella burnetii* (Q fever), and *Francisella tularensis* (tularemia) have the potential for use in bioterrorism.

Both innate and acquired immune mechanisms normally eliminate pathogens, but some pathogens have specific mechanisms to help them overcome the host's immune system, and these mechanisms may determine the virulence of the pathogens. Encapsulated bacteria such as *Streptococcus* resist phagocytosis; other bacteria such as *Microbacterium*, *Nocardia*, and *Legionella* resist destruction by phagocytes. Cilia are targeted by *Chlamydophila pneumoniae*, which produces a factor that inactivates cilia, while

Microplasma pneumoniae and viruses can shear cilia off of respiratory epithelia. Inactivating cilia reduces mucociliary clearance within hours of the onset of infection. *Streptococcus pneumoniae* and *Neisseria meningitidis* secrete proteases that inactivate immunoglobulin A.[56]

A typical bacterial pneumonia is characterized by a consolidation of lung tissue primarily by bacterial exudates within alveoli, but there is very little interstitial involvement (**Figure 19.7** ■). As alveoli fill with fluid and dying cells, primarily neutrophils, pus is formed. Tissue necrosis from the infection and lysosomal damage from dying lymphocytes contribute to the cellular debris. An alveolus filled with exudates has little or no oxygen available for gas exchange, so depending on the extent of the pneumonia, hypoxemia can result.

Viral pneumonia is characterized by interstitial pneumonitis with patchy inflammatory changes in the lung interstitium and septa. The thickened alveolar walls are infiltrated by mononuclear leukocytes, and inflammatory mediators can allow fluid to leak into alveoli. The thickened alveolar walls and alveolar fluid lengthen the route for diffusion, interfering with oxygenation of blood.

Clinical Manifestations

In immune competent individuals, the major clinical features of a typical pneumonia include an abrupt onset of a high fever, chills, and a productive cough with mucopurulent sputum. Reports of dyspnea are common, while hemoptysis, pleural pain, and a friction rub occur less frequently. Lung consolidation is indicated by bronchial breath sounds or **egophony** (increased resonance of voice sounds heard on auscultation) and tachypnea.

The presentation of atypical pneumonias is generally milder than that of typical pneumonias, but symptoms last longer. A fever lower than 102°F (38.9°C), fatigue, and muscle aches are common. Cough is common in viral pneumonias but not in other atypical pneumonias; in either case, there are relatively small amounts of sputum because the infection is primarily interstitial. Mycoplasma pneumonias can result in systemic symptoms such as anemia, rashes, or neurologic syndromes such as meningitis, myelitis, and encephalitis, but the mortality rate is usually low.[57] The interstitial processes can interfere with diffusion of oxygen and result in hypoxemia.

In older adults, many symptoms are blunted or absent. Older adults and individuals on corticosteroids are much less likely to have a fever, and symptoms tend to last longer. A worsening of chronic pulmonary disease can be the only feature seen in older adults. ■

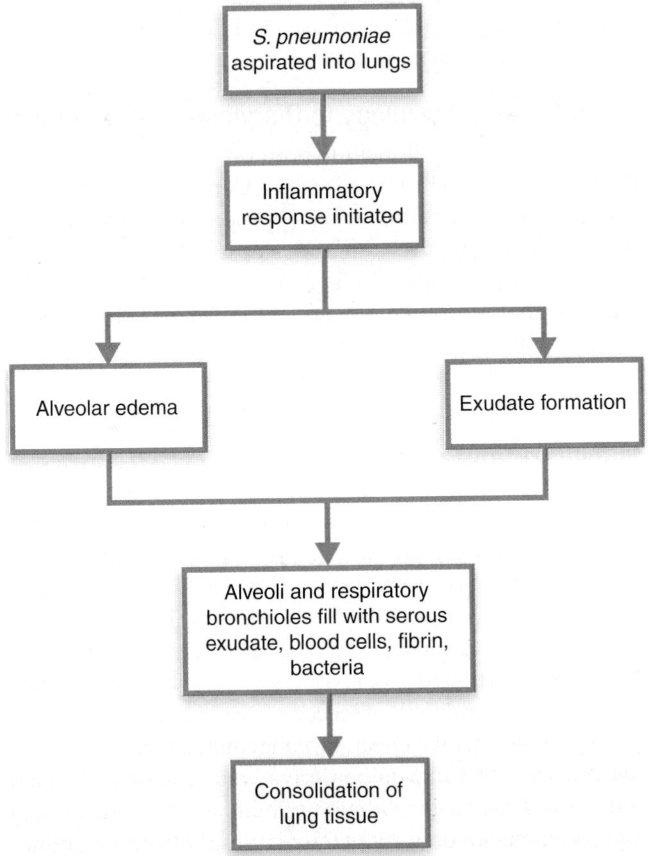

Figure 19.7 ■ The pathogenesis of pneumococcal pneumonia.

Linking Pathophysiology to Diagnosis and Treatment

The clinical presentation and physical examination can suggest the possibility of pneumonia, but a chest x-ray is needed to distinguish between pneumonia and acute bronchitis.[58] Bronchopneumonia is characterized by focal opacities scattered throughout the lung on the x-ray while the lobe will be well circumscribed in lobar pneumonia. Chest x-rays are not specific for differentiating between viral and bacterial pneumonias. CT scan is the gold standard for diagnosis, as it is more sensitive to infiltrates than a chest x-ray, but a CT scan is not routinely necessary.

Sputum analyses can be helpful in bacterial pneumonias. Sputum Gram stain can be correlated with culture results to help identify dominant or unsuspected pathogens. Sputum culture and sensitivities for bacterial pneumonia can be useful for drug-resistant or unusual pathogens, but it may not be possible to separate pathogens from colonizing bacteria.

Treatment of pneumonia depends on the severity of the pneumonia, the causative pathogen, and the health status of the individual. It includes supportive measures and administration of supplemental oxygen in more serious cases. The appropriate pharmaceutical treatment depends on the cause of the pneumonia and the presence of underlying chronic disease. Pneumonias that are treated with antibiotics specific for the bacteria can show quick and dramatic improvement; the individual may exhibit few clinical signs and symptoms after 48–72 hours. Hospitalization may be necessary in severe infections or for individuals who have multiple risk factors (e.g., chronically ill, immunocompromised) or require therapies that are not easily administered at home (e.g., cardiac monitoring, intravenous therapy). Viral pneumonias are treated with supportive measures but no antibiotics. Severe viral infections can be treated with antiviral medications such as acyclovir if these are started within 36 hours of symptom onset.

Check Your Progress: Section 19.5

1. What factors predispose individuals to hospital-acquired pneumonia?
2. Describe the primary pathologic difference between bacterial and viral pneumonia.
3. Describe the role of transmission of the influenza virus.

19.6 Pulmonary Vascular Disorders

This section discusses the major pulmonary vascular disorders that cause respiratory failure—pulmonary hypertension, pulmonary embolism, and pulmonary contusion—as well as two of the more uncommon diffuse pulmonary hemorrhage syndromes. These two pulmonary hemorrhage syndromes, Goodpasture syndrome and Wegener granulomatosis, are autoimmune disorders.

Pulmonary Hypertension

Pulmonary hypertension (PH), which is increased blood pressure in the pulmonary arteries, may represent a primary disease called pulmonary arterial hypertension, which is discussed later in this section. Alternatively, PH can occur secondary to other diseases processes such as advanced COPD, which is the usual presentation.

Etiology and Pathogenesis

When the cause of PH is secondary to another disease process, the PH is the result of an increased pulmonary blood flow and/or venous pressure, increased vascular resistance, or back pressure that results from left ventricular failure. The specific etiologies are as follows:

- Increased pulmonary blood flow occurs with left-to-right ventricular or atrial septal defects or with portal hypertension.
- Increased vascular resistance occurs with a locally mediated response to hypoxemia (e.g., COPD, sleep apnea); inflammatory disorders that narrow blood vessels and eventually destroy the pulmonary vascular bed (e.g., rheumatoid arthritis, scleroderma, systemic lupus erythematosus pulmonary thrombosis or embolisms; and lack of surfactant, which results in the persistent PH of the newborn.
- Back pressure from the left ventricular commonly occurs with left ventricular failure or mitral and aortic valve disease, but dilated cardiomyopathy or a pulmonary venous obstruction can also increase pulmonary blood volume and pressure.
- Drugs that can cause PH include stimulants such as cocaine and methamphetamines (either inhaled or intravenous), designer drugs such as "ice" or "euphoria," and prolonged use of appetite suppressants such as fenfluramine that increase extracellular serotonin.[59]

The endothelium of the normally low-pressure pulmonary vessels is damaged by the increased pressure or the injury produced by thrombi or emboli. The damaged endothelium decreases synthesis and release of the vasodilator nitric oxide and increases the accumulation of endothelin, a mediator of vasoconstriction and remodeling. The structural remodeling of pulmonary vessels narrows the vascular bed, increasing vascular resistance and PH.[59]

No matter what the cause of PH, the right ventricle must generate a higher pressure to pump blood returned from the systemic circulation through the pulmonary vascular system. The right heart hypertrophies to accommodate the increased load, then later dilates. The increased pulmonary arterial pressure further damages the vasculature, accelerating the injury process. Without appropriate therapy, the increased stress on the right heart eventually leads to right ventricular failure (cor pulmonale) and death.

Clinical Manifestations

In the early stages of PH, individuals report dyspnea on exertion, lethargy, and fatigue because the heart is not able to increase cardiac output with exercise. As the PH progresses to right ventricular failure, individuals may experience angina or syncope with exercise and develop edema as the right heart failure progresses. This results in symptoms of hepatic congestion (e.g., anorexia, abdominal pain, ascites) and jugular venous distention. Respiratory symptoms are not common but can include cough, hoarseness, or hemoptysis. Auscultation of the heart may reveal systolic ejection murmurs and/or an accented pulmonic component of the second heart sound.

Linking Pathophysiology to Diagnosis and Treatment

A careful history will include both prescription and illegal drugs as well as chronic diseases. Depending on the history and physical examination, appropriate diagnostic tests will vary with the probable cause of the PH. PH is treated with vasodilators, specifically prostacyclin and prostacyclin analogs, that are effective when administered either intravenously or by aerosolization.[60]

Pulmonary Arterial Hypertension

Pulmonary arterial hypertension (PAH) is a disease characterized by an increased pulmonary arterial resistance in the absence of left ventricular failure or chronic thromboembolism. It is a relatively rare disease that without treatment results in death. The prevalence of PAH in the general population is not known, and the estimated prevalence associated with specific etiologies for PAH varies widely. The etiology of PAH is either idiopathic or secondary to another disease such as systemic sclerosis and other connective tissue diseases, portal hypertension, HIV infection, congenital heart disease, and drugs such as fenfluramine derivatives or toxins. Affected individuals have a genetic susceptibility to PAH, but familial PAH accounts for only about 6% of cases.[61] The small pulmonary arteries are continually remodeled, causing a progressive increase in pulmonary resistance. Increased pulmonary vascular resistance leads to right ventricular enlargement and eventually to cor pulmonale. Right ventricular dysfunction is associated with a higher risk of death even with effective therapy.[61] The clinical presentation of PAH is similar to that for other causes of PH. New treatments for decreasing pulmonary vascular resistance include prostacyclin derivatives, endothelin receptor antagonists, and phosphodiesterase type-5 inhibitors. The diagnosis of PAH requires invasive hemodynamic monitoring to reveal a mean pulmonary artery pressure of 25 mmHg or more (3 standard deviations above normal) with a pulmonary capillary wedge pressure or left ventricular end-diastolic pressure of 15 mmHg or less.[62] Assessments of PAH also include tests such as the 6-minute walk and acute vasodilator challenges.[62]

Pulmonary Embolism

An **embolus** is a substance or object that travels via the bloodstream to a blood vessel and subsequently lodges in the blood vessel, creating a partial or complete obstruction of blood flow through the affected vessel. Emboli may comprise various substances, including a blood clot, fat globule, air bubble, bone fragment, or foreign matter, such as a tiny portion of an intravenous catheter. **Embolism** refers to a condition in which an embolus travels via the bloodstream and subsequently lodges in a blood vessel, creating a partial or complete obstruction of blood flow through the affected vessel. **Pulmonary embolism (PE)** occurs when an embolus is pumped from the right heart into progressively smaller pulmonary arteries until it wedges in a vessel that is too small for it to pass through. The PE blocks the blood flow, compromising the circulation to the area of the lung beyond the blockage, which can result in infarction of the distal lung.

The consequences of a PE depend on the size of the embolus, whether it spontaneously breaks up quickly, restoring circulation, or whether it is a larger clot that blocks off an area of lung that does not have adequate collateral circulation. In the United States, mortality from PE is estimated at 2–8% among individuals who receive treatment but increases to 30% in individuals who do not receive treatment.[63]

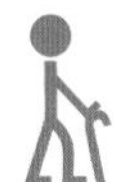

Deaths from PE occur in all age groups but increase with aging and are highest in older adults with comorbidities. ■

Individuals who are at increased risk for PE include the following:

- Individuals who have a prior history of deep vein thrombosis or PE or a family history of PE or deep vein thrombosis
- Individuals with prolonged immobilization (e.g., bedrest more than 3 days, long journeys sitting in a cramped position)
- Individuals who have recently had surgery (e.g., orthopedic, gynecologic, coronary bypass surgeries)
- Women during pregnancy and 6–12 weeks following delivery
- Women on oral contraceptive or hormonal replacement therapy, particularly cigarette smokers over 35 years of age
- Older adults, particularly those with comorbid conditions or dehydration
- Individuals with cardiovascular system disorders, including venous valve malfunction
- Individuals with active cancers (e.g., ovarian, pancreatic, lung) that produce substances that increase coagulability, the risk being further increased by chemotherapy
- Individuals with pathologic conditions (e.g., hypercoagulability, burns, HIV disease, drug abuse).

PE is more common among African Americans than Caucasians, and women are more likely to develop this condition than are men.[64]

Etiology and Pathogenesis

The origin of PE is usually an embolus that breaks off from a deep vein thrombosis and travels through the venous system to the right heart. Pulmonary embolism occurs when there is a loss of balance between the formation and lysis (disintegration) of microemboli. Microemboli propagate (increase), the accumulation of platelets and fibrin usually being in the region of venous valves in the legs unless the individual had a major trauma or recent procedure (e.g., surgery, indwelling venous catheter). Thrombus formation can result from venous stasis caused by dehydration, immobility, venous compression or the increased venous pressure of heart failure, injury to the intima, or hypercoagulability. Generally, there are multiple emboli rather than a single embolus.

Rarely, other substances cause PE. For example, fat emboli are formed from lipid droplets from the marrow of fractured long bones, and amniotic fluid can enter the bloodstream during delivery. Clumps of cancer cells or parasites can also form emboli. An air embolism is usually the result of a deep water diver's surfacing too quickly without exhaling freely (breath holding). The compressed air that divers breathe expands their lungs as they swim upward, and their overinflated lungs force air bubbles into the blood. Air embolism is a common cause of death among scuba divers. Air embolism can also occur if a large amount of air enters the blood during intravenous infusions.[65]

The pathophysiology that results from PE depends on the number and size of emboli, the number and size of pulmonary arteries that are blocked, and the status of the right ventricle. Pulmonary embolism results in the impairment of gas exchange because the emboli block the blood flow past ventilated alveoli and the increased vascular resistance causes PH. When major blood vessels are occluded, the sudden increase in pulmonary artery pressure and decrease in cardiac output can result in right ventricular failure or death.

Clinical Manifestations

The classic clinical presentation of PE is a triad of sudden shortness of breath or dyspnea that is not related to activity; hemoptysis; and chest pain that is worse with a deep breath, cough, eating, or bending. The chest pain is worse with exertion but does not go away with rest. With a smaller PE, most individuals are initially asymptomatic or have vague, nonspecific complaints. While dyspnea is a common complaint, the classic triad of hemoptysis, dyspnea, and chest pain is not specific and occurs in only about 20% of individuals with PE. Individuals often present for care with chest-related symptoms such as chest pain, shoulder pain, shortness of breath, or hemoptysis. The sudden onset of pleuritic pain is an important symptom in young, active individuals. With the loss of surfactant after the first 24–72 hours, a PE cannot be distinguished from pneumonia by clinical exam or on x-ray.

Linking Pathophysiology to Diagnosis and Treatment

Diagnostic tests for PE include CT scanning with contrast, lung ventilation/perfusion scanning, and pulmonary angiography.[66] Blood tests may include measurement of D-dimer, which is a fibrin protein fragment that is released during thrombus breakdown, as well as arterial blood gas analysis.[66,67]

Treatment of PE includes thrombolytic therapy to dissolve the clot, anticoagulation to prevent further clots, and oxygen supplementation. In chronic PE or if there are absolute contraindications to anticoagulation, an inferior vena cava filter can be inserted to prevent emboli from reaching the right heart and lung. The most important treatment is prevention with increased activity, compression hose and/or intermittent compression therapy, and early ambulation of individuals after surgery.

Initially, other disorders that cause similar symptoms, such as pneumonia, heart failure, ribs fractures, or pleurisy must be quickly eliminated. Finding evidence of a deep vein thrombosis using duplex ultrasound increases the index of suspicion for PE. A D-dimer serum test for fibrin fragments is sometimes used to rule out a diagnosis of PE when the individual is at low risk. Other tests, such as arterial blood gas analysis, document hypoxemia but are not specific.

Pulmonary Contusion

A pulmonary contusion is the most common, potentially lethal chest injury and in the United States generally occurs after motor vehicle accidents, but it can also occur with exposure to an explosion. Pulmonary contusion is more common in younger individuals, as older individuals have stiffer, thinner chest walls, and their ribs fracture with the force of the blow. A pulmonary contusion is the bruising of lung tissue from a shock wave of force, a propagation of a tissue disturbance that travels rapidly through the parenchyma. The initial force causes tissue rupture, and the injury worsens with tissue recoil, so the damage causes diffuse hemorrhage as well as interstitial and alveolar edema. Gas exchange is impaired, and the greater the pulmonary contusion, the greater the impairment of gas exchange. Respiratory failure develops over time, not immediately.

Alveolar Hemorrhage Syndromes

There is a group of collagen vascular diseases, such as Goodpasture syndrome and granulomatous vasculitis, that can result in alveolar hemorrahagic syndromes. Alveolar hemorrhagic syndromes are autoimmune disorders that affect the lungs and kidneys of relatively young Caucasian adults. A genetic susceptibility is suspected, but in each case, the etiology is unknown.

Goodpasture Syndrome

Goodpasture syndrome is an uncommon antiglomerular basement antibody disease that targets the lungs and kidneys. The antibodies initiate inflammation of the basement membranes of alveoli and renal glomeruli. The onset and disease progression are variable with initial nonspecific early symptoms such as cough, dyspnea, fatigue, hemoptysis, and burning on urination. In late stages, Goodpasture syndrome causes a necrotizing alveolar hemorrhage and a rapidly progressive glomerulonephritis. Because early symptoms are so vague, diagnosis is often delayed until late in the disease. Treatment includes immunosuppressant drugs combined with intensive plasmapheresis, a procedure of plasma exchange to remove circulating antibasement antibodies and inflammatory mediators. Kidney dialysis or transplantation may become necessary.

Wegener Granulomatosis

Wegener granulomatosis is a rare systemic vasculitis that restricts blood flow, causing damage that may be limited to the upper and lower respiratory tracts but can involve the kidneys and other organs. The clinical presentation and severity of symptoms vary widely. Early diagnosis and therapy may result in recovery, but without therapy, Wegener granulomatosis can be fatal. Antineutrophilic cytoplasmic antibodies (ANCAs) damage tissue and stimulate an inflammatory response by activating neutrophils. Neutrophil degranulation causes extensive damage to vessel walls, and the granulomas that develop around blood vessels damage normal tissue. The most common presenting symptoms are a persistent rhinorrhea or sinusitis that doesn't respond to usual treatment. The usual lower respiratory tract symptoms include cough, dyspnea, shortness of breath, and sometimes hemoptysis. Renal involvement may be evident only on urinalysis, or it can present as acute renal failure. Systemic symptoms are nonspecific. Diagnostic criteria for Wegener granulomatosis include evidence of granulomatous inflammation and vasculitis of small to medium-sized blood vessels in the lung or biopsy of the nasopharynx, skin, or kidneys when there is evidence of involvement. A positive ANCA test is suggestive but not conclusive evidence of Wegener granulomatosis. The treatment is long-term immunosuppression with cytotoxic agents, but long-term complications are common, and relapses occur in 20–40% of affected individuals.

Check Your Progress: Section 19.6

1. Explain the cause of right ventricular hypertrophy in the person with pulmonary hypertension.
2. What are the three classic manifestations of pulmonary embolism?
3. What laboratory blood test is useful in the diagnosis of pulmonary embolism?

CHAPTER SUMMARY

19.1 Chapter Overview and Case Studies

Describe the primary considerations and concepts related to pulmonary vascular, neoplastic, and infectious respiratory disorders.

- Pulmonary disorders include alterations caused by neoplastic growths, infectious diseases, abscesses, and vascular disorders.
- Neoplastic growths may be malignant or benign.
- Malignant growths are composed of cancerous cells that are capable of metastasizing (spreading) from the site of origin to other body sites or invading local body sites and causing tissue destruction.
- Benign growths contain cells that are nonmalignant (noncancerous). Infectious diseases that serve as sources of pulmonary disorders include a variety of alterations that may affect either the upper respiratory tract, the lower respiratory tract, or both.
- Pulmonary vascular disorders include alterations of blood flow within the lungs or to or from the pulmonary circuit.

19.2 Malignant Lung Cancer

Differentiate the causes, classification, underlying pathogenesis, and clinical manifestations of malignant lung cancers and approaches to diagnosis and treatment of these conditions across the lifespan.

- Cigarette smoking is the primary risk factor for lung cancer. There is a 15- to 20-year delay between starting smoking and development of lung cancer.
- Other smoke exposures (cigars, pipes, passive exposure) and exposures to environmental and occupational carcinogens (radon or asbestos) also increase the risk for lung cancer.
- Genetic susceptibility, benign chronic lung disorders, and diet contribute to lung cancer risk.
- Histologically, carcinomas are classified as adenocarcinoma, squamous cell carcinomas, and large cell carcinomas (all three of which are considered non–small cell carcinomas) and small cell carcinomas.
- Adenocarcinoma and squamous cell carcinomas are classified as differentiated (retaining more normal cell features, but cell division is unregulated) or undifferentiated (retaining enough features for identification, but cell division is faster and the prognosis is worse).
- Adenocarcinomas are glandular cancers, usually in the lung periphery. They grow slowly but can metastasize early because of invasion of blood vessels and lymphatics.
- Squamous cell carcinomas usually originate in medial bronchial mucosa at bronchial bifurcations and metastasize to adjacent lymph nodes and lung tissue.
- Large cell carcinomas often present as big, bulky solitary tumors in the lung periphery.
- Small cell carcinomas are aggressive, highly malignant, and fast-growing tumors that metastasize early and widely.
- Symptoms initiating a diagnostic workup include obstructive pneumonia, dyspnea with a pleural effusion, hemoptysis, pain, hoarseness, or a paraneoplastic disorder.
- Initial lung cancer symptoms are often nonspecific with a persistent cough that is attributed to another cause.
- Diagnostic tools include sputum cytologic analysis, CT scan of the thorax, bronchoscopy, fine needle aspiration, thoracentesis, and mediastinoscopy.

19.3 Benign Lung Lesions

Differentiate the causes, classification, underlying pathogenesis, and clinical manifestations of benign lung lesions and approaches to diagnosis and treatment of these conditions across the lifespan.

- Pulmonary granulomas are formed to control an inhaled antigen that cannot be digested or in response to an autoimmune inflammatory process.
- Macrophages engulf the antigen, and helper T cells surround the macrophages, preventing a chronic inflammatory response.
- As macrophages die, the exposed antigen stimulates a further granulomatous inflammatory response.
- Tuberculosis is caused by the rod-shaped aerobic *M. tuberculosis* bacillus, which is protected by a waxy capsule. Transmission is primarily through inhalation of infected droplets by a susceptible person.
- *M. tuberculosis* can remain latent and in a state of dormancy for years; individuals with latent TB are not infectious.
- Active TB is symptomatic and communicable to other individuals.
- Reactivation of latent TB (secondary TB) occurs when there is a decreased T-cell–mediated immunity in a previously sensitized host.
- Fungal infections in the lung are endemic to particular geographic areas: histoplasmosis and blastomycosis in the Midwest, the St. Lawrence valley, and along the Appalachian Mountains and coccidioidmycosis in the southwestern United States.
- Fungal infections are transmitted by inhalation of fungal spores in dust or from bird droppings and may be asymptomatic in healthy individuals.

- A lung abscess is usually a complication of a pulmonary infection that results in destruction of pulmonary parenchyma.

19.4 Infectious Diseases of the Upper Respiratory Tract

Differentiate the causes, classification, underlying pathogenesis, and clinical manifestations of upper respiratory tract infections and approaches to diagnosis and treatment of these conditions across the lifespan.

- Respiratory infections are the most common cause for physician visits in the United States, and schoolchildren are the major reservoir for viral illnesses.
- Risk for respiratory infections is increased in the very young, the very old, immunosuppressed individuals, and those with chronic diseases.
- Respiratory infections are usually viral, but bacterial infections can occur as primary or secondary infections, and transmission is usually by social contact.
- Clinical presentations vary depending on the location and severity of the infection and the age of the patient, but a cough and change in mucus are common.
- Epiglottitis involves rapidly progressive inflammation of the epiglottis and adjacent structures. Because of the high risk for airway obstruction, this condition requires immediate medical intervention.

19.5 Infectious Diseases of the Lower Respiratory Tract

Differentiate the causes, classification, underlying pathogenesis, and clinical manifestations of lower respiratory tract infections and approaches to diagnosis and treatment of these conditions across the lifespan.

- Risk factors for lower respiratory tract infections include altered levels of consciousness, mechanical ventilation, impairment of normal ventilation, and chronic diseases.
- Acute bronchitis is a common, self-limited lower respiratory tract infection characterized by bronchial inflammation with mucosal congestion and a cough.
- Bronchiolitis is an inflammation of the peripheral airways characterized by wheezing, hyperinflation, and atelectasis that is usually caused by respiratory syncytial virus in infants.
- Influenza is a highly contagious viral infection because the viruses, particularly type A, change their antigenicity by mutating surface glycoproteins.
- Croup and whooping cough are acute infections transmitted by contact with contaminated respiratory secretions.
- In croup, the laryngotracheitis obstructs breathing during inhalation, resulting in inspiratory stridor and a brassy or barking cough. Whooping cough is characterized by a hard, spasmodic cough that ends in a loud, crowing inspiratory whoop.
- Bacterial pneumonia is characterized by pulmonary tissue consolidated by bacterial exudates primarily within the alveoli with very little interstitial involvement.
- Viral pneumonia is characterized by interstitial involvement with patchy inflammatory changes in the lung alveolar walls and septa.
- Typical pneumonias present abruptly with fever, chills, and a cough that produces mucopurulent sputum. Symptoms are blunted in individuals with atypical pneumonia and in older adults.
- Hospital-acquired pneumonias are common when patients are chronically ill or immunosuppressed or have taken a long course of antibiotic therapy. Microaspiration of pathogens or particulates from the upper airway is the most common cause of pneumonia.

19.6 Pulmonary Vascular Disorders

Differentiate the causes, classification, underlying pathogenesis, and clinical manifestations of pulmonary vascular disorders and approaches to diagnosis and treatment of these conditions across the lifespan.

- PH can occur as a primary disease or secondarily as a result of an increased pulmonary blood flow and/or venous pressure, increased vascular resistance, or back pressure that results from left ventricular failure.
- The increased pressure further damages pulmonary endothelia, decreasing nitric oxide production, which causes vasodilation, and increasing endothelin, which causes vasoconstriction.
- Treatment is vasodilation with intravenous or aerosolized prostacyclin and prostacyclin analogs.
- PE occurs when a substance, usually an embolus, flows through the right heart to a point where it lodges in a pulmonary artery, blocking circulation to the distal lung tissue.
- Increased risk for PE is associated with immobility, recent surgery, contraceptive therapy in women, comorbid conditions in older adults, long bone fracture, cancer, parasites, and the perinatal period.
- PEs may be asymptomatic or cause vague complaints, but individuals often present with chest pain, shoulder pain, shortness of breath, or hemoptysis.
- Definitive diagnosis is made by demonstrating a blockage in the pulmonary vasculature with pulmonary

angiography or multidetector computed tomographic angiography (MDCTA) scans.

- Treatment of PE includes anticoagulation therapy and preventive measures and may include thrombolytic agents.
- Alveolar hemorrhagic syndromes are autoimmune disorders that affect the lungs and kidneys of young Caucasian adults.
- Goodpasture syndrome causes alveolar hemorrhage and a rapidly progressive glomerulonephritis because the autoantibodies target both pulmonary and renal basement membranes.
- Wegener granulomatosis is a systemic vasculitis that affects the upper and lower respiratory tracts and the kidneys.

REVIEW QUESTIONS

1. The public health nurse is preparing for the winter season of viral infections. Which of the following groups has the highest incidence of upper respiratory tract viral infections?
   a. Infants
   b. Preschool children
   c. Adolescents
   d. Young adults
2. Which of the following would the nurse expect to find in a client with active tuberculosis?
   a. A negative chest x-ray
   b. A nonreactive Mantoux test
   c. A positive sputum culture
   d. A positive needle aspiration
3. The nurse is caring for a child with epiglottitis. Which of the following is the best position in which to place the child?
   a. Lying flat on the back
   b. Lying on the left side with the head slightly elevated
   c. High Fowler position with the legs in a dependent position
   d. Sitting upright, leaning forward
4. The public health nurse is speaking to a community group about tuberculosis. Which of the following groups is most at risk for developing tuberculosis in the United States?
   a. Those living in a rural environment
   b. Those with HIV
   c. Those who immigrated a decade ago
   d. Those who quit smoking 5 years age
5. A 70-year-old female nonsmoker presents with cough, weight loss, and chest pain. Her chest x-ray shows a peripheral lung mass, and sputum cytology is positive for neoplastic cells. The nurse understands that this client most likely has what type of tumor?
   a. Adenocarcinoma
   b. Large cell carcinoma
   c. Squamous cell carcinoma
   d. Small cell carcinoma
6. The nurse is teaching a client about the influenza vaccine. Which of the following should the nurse include?
   a. A booster vaccine will be needed in 6 weeks.
   b. The vaccine provides lifelong immunity.
   c. The vaccination needs to be repeated every year.
   d. The vaccine is not needed if an individual has had influenza.
7. Which of the following is a lower respiratory manifestation of Wegener granulomatosis?
   a. Rhinorrhea and sinusitis
   b. A positive ANCA test
   c. Acute renal failure
   d. Shortness of breath
8. The nurse is caring for a client with HIV who has developed pneumonia. Which nursing action has the highest priority for this client?
   a. Providing oral care
   b. Encouraging proper nutrition
   c. Administering supplemental oxygen
   d. Assisting with hygiene

ANSWERS

Answers to Review Questions can be found in Appendix A. Answers to Case Study and Check Your Progress questions are available on the faculty resources site. Please consult with your instructor.

RECOMMENDED WEBSITES

Hospital-Acquired & Ventilator-Associated Pneumonia (HAP/VAP)
http://www.idsociety.org/Guidelines/Patient_Care/IDSA_Practice_Guidelines/Infections_by_Organ_System/Lower/Upper_Respiratory/Hospital-Acquired_Pneumonia_(HAP)

Hypersensitivity Pneumonitis
https://www.nhlbi.nih.gov/health/health-topics/topics/hp

Influenza
https://www.cdc.gov/flu/index.htm

Pneumonia
https://www.cdc.gov/pneumonia

Pneumoconioses
https://www.cdc.gov/niosh/topics/pneumoconioses

Tuberculosis
https://www.cdc.gov/tb

What Is Atelectasis?
https://www.nhlbi.nih.gov/health/health-topics/topics/atl

REFERENCES

1. National Library of Medicine. (2014). *Malignancy*. Available at https://www.nlm.nih.gov/medlineplus/ency/article/002253.htm
2. Centers for Disease Control and Prevention. (2015). *Lung cancer*. Available at http://www.cdc.gov/cancer/lung
3. American Lung Association. (2016). *Lung cancer fact sheet*. Available at http://www.lung.org/lung-health-and-diseases/lung-disease-lookup/lung-cancer/learn-about-lung-cancer/lung-cancer-fact-sheet.html
4. U. S. Surgeon Generals' Advisory Committee on Smoking and Health. (1964). *Smoking and health: Report of the Advisory Committee to the Surgeon General of the Public Health Service*. Washington, DC: U.S. Government Printing Office.
5. Centers for Disease Control and Prevention. (2014). *Adult cigarette smoking rate overall hits all-time low*. Available at http://www.cdc.gov/media/releases/2014/p1126-adult-smoking.html
6. American Lung Association Epidemiology and Statistics Unit Research and Program Services Division. (2014). *Trends in lung cancer morbidity and mortality*. Chicago, IL: American Lung Association.
7. Jha, P., Ramasundarahettige, C., Landsman, V., et al. (2013). 21st-century hazards of smoking and benefits of cessation in the United States. *New England Journal of Medicine, 368*(4), 341–350.
8. American Cancer Society. (2010). *Cancer facts & figures 2010*. Atlanta, GA: American Cancer Society.
9. Zhang, L. R., Morgenstern, H., Greenland, S., et al. (2015). Cannabis smoking and lung cancer risk: Pooled analysis in the International Lung Cancer Consortium. *International Journal of Cancer, 136*(4), 894–903.
10. Drent, M., Wijnen, P., & Bast, A. (2012). Interstitial lung damage due to cocaine abuse: Pathogenesis, pharmacogenomics and therapy. *Current Medicinal Chemistry, 19*(33), 5607–5611.
11. National Cancer Institute. (2015). *Tea and cancer prevention: Strengths and limits of the evidence*. Available at http://www.cancer.gov/about-cancer/causes-prevention/risk/diet/tea-fact-sheet
12. Sculier, J. P., Berghmans T., & Meert A. P. (2015). Update in lung cancer and mesothelioma 2009. *American Journal of Respiratory and Critical Care Medicine, 181*(8), 773–781.
13. Horn, L., & Pao, W. (2009). ENL4-ALK: Honing in on a new target in non-small-cell lung cancer. *Journal of Clinical Oncology, 27*(26), 4232–4235.
14. American Cancer Society. (2015). *What is small cell cancer?* Available at http://www.cancer.org/cancer/lungcancer-smallcell/detailedguide/small-cell-lung-cancer-what-is-small-cell-lung-cancer
15. U.S. National Library of Medicine. (2015). *Lung cancer: Small cell*. Available at https://www.nlm.nih.gov/medlineplus/ency/article/000122.htm
16. American Cancer Society. (2014). *What is non-small cell lung cancer?* Available at http://www.cancer.org/cancer/lungcancer-non-smallcell/detailedguide/non-small-cell-lung-cancer-what-is-non-small-cell-lung-cancer
17. Kelly, R., Gutierrez, M. E., & Giaccone, G. (2012). Non-small cell lung cancer. In J. Abraham, J. L. Gulley, & C. J. Allegra (Eds.), *Bethesda handbook of clinical oncology*. (3rd ed., pp. 35–45). Philadelphia, PA: Wolters Kluwer.
18. American Cancer Society. (2015). *Signs and symptoms of lung cancer*. Available at https://www.cancer.org/cancer/lung-cancer/prevention-and-early-detection/signs-and-symptoms
19. American Cancer Society. (2015). *Non-small cell lung cancer staging*. Available at https://www.cancer.org/cancer/non-small-cell-lung-cancer/detection-diagnosis-staging/staging
20. American Cancer Society. (2015). *Treatment choices by stage for non-small cell lung cancer, by stage*. Available at https://www.cancer.org/cancer/non-small-cell-lung-cancer/treating/by-stage
21. American Cancer Society. (2015). *Treating small cell lung cancer treated*. Available at https://www.cancer.org/small-cell-lung-cancer/treating
22. National Cancer Institute. (2015). *Small cell lung cancer treatment (PDQ®)—Professional version*. Available at https://www.cancer.gov/types/lung/hp/small-cell-lung-treatment-pdq#link/_6_toc
23. World Health Organization. (2015). *2015 global tuberculosis report* (20th ed.). Geneva, Switzerland: World Health Organization.
24. Centers for Disease Control and Prevention. (2015). *Tuberculosis (TB): Fact sheet*. Available at http://www.cdc.gov/tb/publications/factsheets/statistics/tbtrends.htm
25. Mayo Clinic. (2014). *Tuberculosis: Risk factors*. Available at http://www.mayoclinic.org/diseases-conditions/tuberculosis/basics/risk-factors/con-20021761
26. Centers for Disease Control and Prevention. (2010). *Immigrant and refugee health: Guidelines for screening for tuberculosis infection and disease during the domestic medical examination for newly arrived refugees*. Available at http://www.cdc.gov/immigrantrefugeehealth/guidelines/domestic/tuberculosis-guidelines.html
27. Centers for Disease Control and Prevention. (2013). *Tuberculosis (TB): Health disparities in TB*. Available at http://www.cdc.gov/tb/topic/populations/HealthDisparities/default.htm
28. Knechel, N. A. (2009). Tuberculosis: Pathophysiology, clinical features, and diagnosis. *Critical Care Nurse, 29*(2), 34–43.
29. Centers for Disease Control and Prevention. (2016). *Questions and answers about tuberculosis (TB) 2014*. Available at http://www.cdc.gov/tb/publications/faqs/pdfs/qa.pdf
30. Luetkemeyer, A. (2013). Tuberculosis and HIV: HIV in site knowledge base chapter. HIV InSite, University of California, San Francisco. Available at http://hivinsite.ucsf.edu/InSite?page=kb-05-01-06

31. Centers for Disease Control and Prevention. (2011). *Tuberculosis (TB): Fact sheets.* Available at http://www.cdc.gov/tb/publications/factsheets/testing/igra.htm
32. Centers for Disease Control and Prevention. (2014). *Tuberculosis (TB): Testing & diagnosis.* Available at http://www.cdc.gov/tb/topic/testing
33. Centers for Disease Control and Prevention. (2013). *Core curriculum on tuberculosis: What the clinician should know* (6th ed.). Atlanta, GA: National Center for HIV/AIDS, Viral Hepatitis, STD, and TB Prevention, Division of Tuberculosis Elimination.
34. World Health Organization. (n.d.). *Biologicals: BCG vaccine.* Available at http://www.who.int/biologicals/areas/vaccines/bcg/en
35. U.S. National Library of Medicine. (2013). *Disseminated tuberculosis.* Available at https://www.nlm.nih.gov/medlineplus/ency/article/000624.htm
36. Centers for Disease Control and Prevention. (2015). *Blastomycosis.* Available at http://www.cdc.gov/fungal/diseases/blastomycosis
37. Tan, K. B., Tan, S. H., Aw, D. C., et al. (2013). Simulators of squamous cell carcinoma of the skin: Diagnostic challenges on small biopsies and clinicopathological correlation. *Journal of Skin Cancer, 2013,* 1–10. doi:10.1155/2013/752864
38. Abdallah, C. (2012). Acute epiglottitis: Trends, diagnosis and management. *Saudi Journal of Anaesthesia, 6*(3), 279–281.
39. Chong, K., Dalawari, P., Walline, J., & Jang, T. B. (2013). Short answer question case series: Noisy breathing in an adult. *Emergency Medicine Journal,* 30(10), 861–862.
40. Aggarwal, S., Lam, A., Bolisetty, S., et al. (2016). Heme attenuation ameliorates irritant gas inhalation-induced acute lung injury. *Antioxidants & Redox Signaling, 24*(2), 99–112.
41. Centers for Disease Control and Prevention. (2014). *Respiratory syncytial virus infection (RSV).* Available at http://www.cdc.gov/rsv
42. American Academy of Pediatrics. (2015). *Respiratory syncytial virus (RSV).* Available at https://www.healthychildren.org/English/health-issues/conditions/chest-lungs/Pages/Respiratory-Syncytial-Virus-RSV.aspx
43. Cordier, J. F., Cottin, V., Khouatra, C., et al. (2013). Hypereosinophilic obliterative bronchiolitis: A distinct, unrecognised syndrome. *European Respiratory Journal, 41*(5), 1126–1134.
44. Centers for Disease Control and Prevention. (2010). Update: Influenza activity—United States, August 30, 2009–January 9, 2010. *MMWR, 59*(2),1–62.
45. Centers for Disease Control and Prevention. (2009). *CDC Estimates of 2009 H1N1 influenza cases, hospitalizations and deaths in the United States, April–October 17, 2009.* Available at http://www.cdc.gov/h1n1flu/estimates/April_October_17.htm
46. Centers for Disease Control and Prevention. (2016). *Deaths and mortality.* Available at http://www.cdc.gov/nchs/fastats/deaths.htm
47. Centers for Disease Control and Prevention. (2015). *Are you at high risk for serious illness from flu?* Available at http://www.cdc.gov/features/fluhighrisk
48. da Silva, D. V., Nordholm, J., Dou, D., Wang, H., Rossman, J. S., & Daniels, R. (2015). The influenza virus neuraminidase protein transmembrane and head domains have coevolved. *Journal of Virology, 89*(2), 1094–1104.
49. Metersky, M. L., Masterton, R. G., Lode, H., File, T. M., & Babinchak, T. (2012). Epidemiology, microbiology, and treatment considerations for bacterial pneumonia complicating influenza. *International Journal of Infectious Diseases, 16*(5), e321–e331.
50. Torres, A., & Rello, J. (2010). Update in community-acquired and nosocomial pneumonia 2009. *American Journal of Respiratory and Critical Care Medicine, 181*(8), 782–787.
51. American Thoracic Society, and Infectious Diseases Society of America. (2005). Guidelines for the management of adults with hospital-acquired, ventilator-associated, and healthcare-associated pneumonia. *American Journal of Respiratory and Critical Care Medicine, 171,* 388–416.
52. Centers for Disease Control and Prevention. (2014). *Mycoplasma pneumoniae infection.* Available at http://www.cdc.gov/pneumonia/atypical/mycoplasma
53. Chaudhry, R., Ghosh, A., & Chandolia, A. (2016). Pathogenesis of Mycoplasma pneumoniae: An update. *Indian Journal of Medical Microbiology, 34*(1), 7–16.
54. Husain, A. N. (2010). The lung. In V. Kumar et al. (Eds.), *Robbins and Cotran pathologic basis of disease* (pp. 677–738). Philadelphia, PA: Saunders Elsevier.
55. Sanchez, J. L., Cooper, M. J., Myers, C. A., et al. (2015). Respiratory infections in the US military: Recent experience and control. *Clinical Microbiology Reviews, 28*(3), 743–800.
56. Woof, J. (2013). Immunoglobulin A: Molecular mechanisms of function and role in immune defense. In F. Nimmerjahn (Ed.), *Molecular and cellular mechanisms of antibody activity* (pp. 31–60). New York, NY: Springer.
57. Beasley, M. B., Travis, W. D., & Rubin, E. (2007). The respiratory system. In R. Rubin & D. Strayer (Eds.), *Rubin's pathology* (pp. 483–548). Philadelphia, PA: Wolters Kluwer/Lippincott Williams & Wilkins.
58. Evertsen, J., Baumgardner, D. J., Regnery, A., & Banerjeeb, I. (2010). Diagnosis and management of pneumonia and bronchitis in outpatient primary care practices. *Primary Care Respiratory Journal, 19*(3), 237–241.
59. Montani, D., Seferian, A., Savale, L., Simonneau, G., & Humbert, M. (2013). Drug-induced pulmonary arterial hypertension: A recent outbreak. *European Respiratory Review, 22,* 244–250.
60. Ruan, C. H., Dixon, R. A., Willerson, J. T., & Ruan, K. H. (2010). Prostacyclin therapy for pulmonary arterial hypertension. *Texas Heart Institute Journal, 37*(4), 391–399.
61. Dweik, R. A., Heresi, G. A., Minai, O. A., & Tonelli, A. R. (2011). *Pulmonary hypertension.* Available at http://www.clevelandclinicmeded.com/medicalpubs/diseasemanagement/pulmonary/pulmonary-hypertension
62. Lai, Y. C., Potoka, K. C., Champion, H. C., Mora, A. L., & Gladwin, M. T. (2014). Pulmonary arterial hypertension: The clinical syndrome. *Circulation Research, 115*(1), 115–130.
63. Ozaki, A., & Bartholomew, J. R. (2012). *Venous thromboembolism (deep venous thrombosis & pulmonary embolism).* Available at http://www.clevelandclinicmeded.com/medicalpubs/diseasemanagement/cardiology/venous-thromboembolism
64. DeMonaco, N. A., Dang, Q., Kapoor, W. N., & Ragni, M. V. (2008). Pulmonary embolism incidence is increasing with use of spiral computed tomography. *American Journal of Medicine, 121*(7), 611–617.
65. Cook, L. S. (2013). Infusion-related air embolism. *Journal of Infusion Nursing, 36*(1), 26–36.
66. National Heart, Lung, and Blood Institute. (2011). *How is pulmonary embolism diagnosed?* Available at http://www.nhlbi.nih.gov/health/health-topics/topics/pe/diagnosis
67. Youssf, A. R. I., Ismail, M. F., ElGhamry, R., & Reyad, M. R. (2014). Diagnostic accuracy of D-dimer assay in suspected pulmonary embolism patients. *Egyptian Journal of Chest Diseases and Tuberculosis, 63*(2), 411–417.

Chapter 20

Respiratory Failure

Nancy Pogue and Laurie Quinn

Chapter Outline and Learning Outcomes

20.1 Chapter Overview and Case Studies

Define respiratory failure, and describe the concepts related to respiratory failure.

20.2 Respiratory Failure: Type I and Type II

Differentiate the causes, classification, underlying pathogenesis, and clinical manifestations of type I and type II respiratory failure and approaches to diagnosis and treatment of these conditions across the lifespan.

20.3 Disorders Causing Respiratory Failure

Differentiate the causes, classification, underlying pathogenesis, and clinical manifestations of disorders that cause respiratory failure and approaches to diagnosis and treatment of these conditions across the lifespan.

KEY TERMS

Acute respiratory distress syndrome (ARDS), 501
Advanced COPD, 507
Alveolar-arterial O_2 gradient (A-a gradient), 498
Colonization, 507
Hypercapnia, 495
Hypoventilation, 496
Hypoxemia, 495
Hypoxia, 499
Infant respiratory distress syndrome (IRDS), 505
Panic breathing, 508
Pulmonary edema, 496
Respiratory failure, 495
Type I respiratory failure, 495
Type II respiratory failure, 495

ABBREVIATIONS

A-a gradient—alveolar arterial O_2 gradient
ARDS—acute respiratory distress syndrome
FEV_1—total volume of air that can be forcefully exhaled in 1 second
FIO_2—fraction (percent) of inspired oxygen
FVC—total volume of air an individual can forcefully exhale
IRDS—infant respiratory distress syndrome
$PaCO_2$—partial pressure of carbon dioxide dissolved in arterial blood
PaO_2—partial pressure of oxygen dissolved in arterial blood
PAO_2—partial pressure of oxygen in alveolar gas
PEEP—positive end-expiratory pressure
SpO_2—peripheral capillary oxygen saturation
V-Q—ventilation-perfusion

20.1 Chapter Overview and Case Studies

Respiratory failure is defined as an inadequate gas exchange that is demonstrated by **hypoxemia** (decrease in arterial oxygen level) with or without **hypercapnia** (increase in arterial carbon dioxide levels). Respiratory failure has been grouped into two primary classifications. **Type I respiratory failure**, also called *hypoxemic respiratory failure*, is characterized by hypoxemia without hypercapnia and can result from any acute lung disease, such as pneumonia or acute respiratory distress syndrome (ARDS). **Type II respiratory failure**, also called *hypercapnic respiratory failure* or *ventilatory failure*, results from inadequate alveolar ventilation, causing an increased level of carbon dioxide in the blood (hypercapnia) with or without a low level of oxygen in the blood (hypoxemia). Type II respiratory failure can arise from pulmonary causes (e.g., chronic obstructive pulmonary disease), thoracic wall abnormalities (e.g., kyphoscoliosis), or central nervous system causes (e.g., coma). The morbidity and mortality associated with respiratory failure vary according to the underlying etiology and the individual's overall health status. This chapter focuses on the alterations in ventilation and perfusion that are associated with type I and type II respiratory failure.

Concepts Related to Respiratory Failure

Respiratory failure is an acute or chronic condition defined as an inability to oxygenate or ventilate to meet metabolic needs at a given time.[1] Acute respiratory failure is an immediate threat to life and can develop in minutes to hours; chronic respiratory failure develops over several days or longer. The clinical presentation of respiratory failure is often characterized by a variety of general, cardiac, respiratory and central nervous system (CNS) symptoms. Mechanisms associated with type I respiratory failure include lower inspired oxygen partial pressure, alveolar hypoventilation, diffusion impairment, ventilation-perfusion (V-Q) mismatch, and right-to-left shunt.[2] Mechanisms associated with type II respiratory failure include reduced alveolar ventilation for a given CO_2, increased CO_2 production secondary to increased metabolism (e.g., sepsis, fever), or decreased CO_2 excretion.[2] Treatment therapies are directed toward the specific type of respiratory failure. For individuals with persistent conditions that result in chronic respiratory failure, their nutritional status, sleep patterns, neurologic function, and ability to perform activities of daily living (including personal hygiene and basic safety considerations) can be affected. In turn, access to appropriate and timely healthcare, family and other support systems, and financial considerations have implications for patient outcomes. Selected concepts related to respiratory failure are shown in **Figure 20.1** ■.

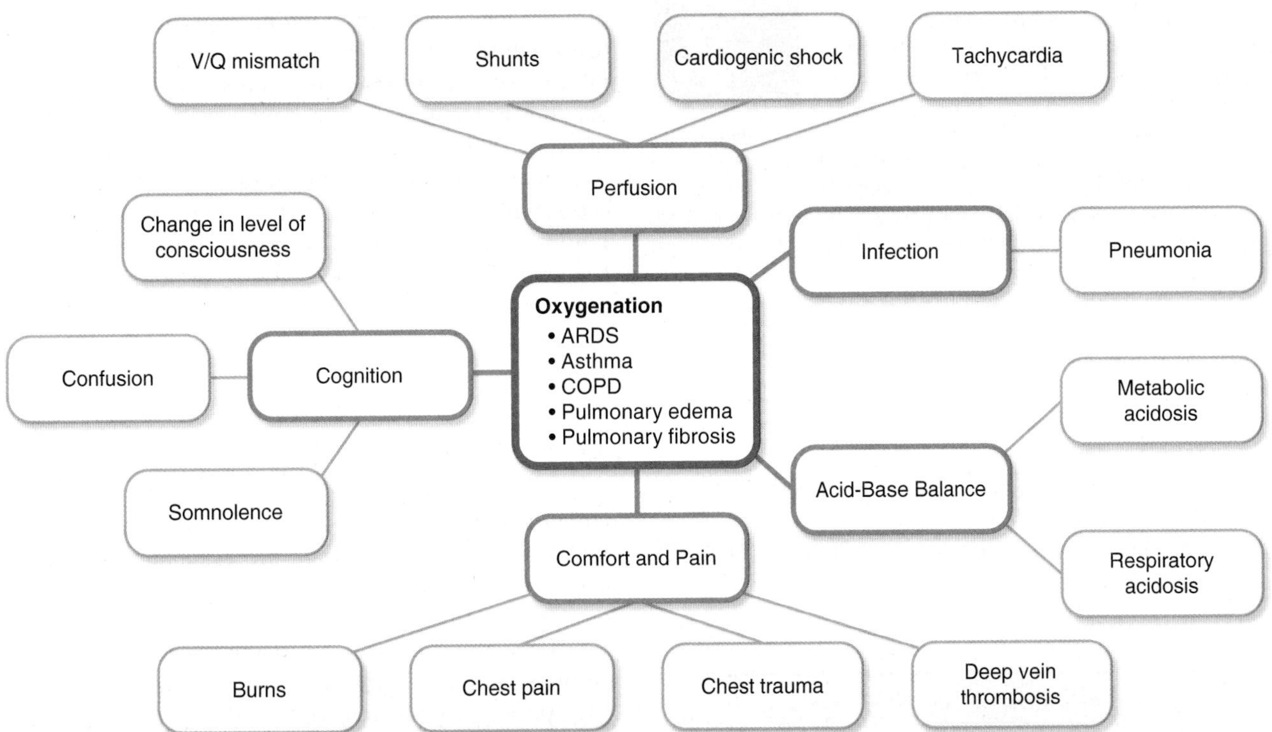

Figure 20.1 ■ Concepts related to respiratory failure.

Case Studies

The following cases are addressed throughout the chapter to assist in application of chapter content to clinical situations that involve individuals with respiratory failure.

Vanessa Toomey: Introduction

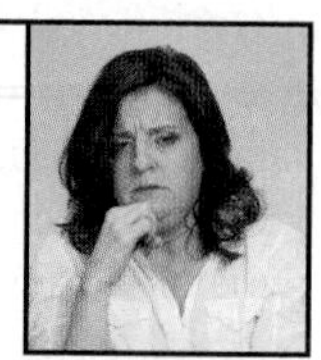

Vanessa Toomey is a 40-year-old woman who is obese. She is a financial consultant and travels frequently, flying from New York to San Francisco several times per month. The job is very stressful, and Ms. Toomey smokes one pack of cigarettes per day to "calm" her nerves. After a recent trip, she noticed pain and tenderness in her right calf that she treated with ibuprofen. After a subsequent flight from Chicago to New York, Ms. Toomey developed chest pain and shortness of breath. Her husband called an ambulance that took her to a local emergency department (ED). On admission to the ED, her vital signs were pulse 88, respirations 32, temperature 99°F, blood pressure 130/80. Radiography and spiral computed tomography (CT) scanning (a type of CT that is used often in the diagnosis of pulmonary emboli) demonstrated bilateral pulmonary emboli. A venous Doppler ultrasound of the lower legs revealed extensive deep vein thrombosis in Ms. Toomey's right lower leg. She is treated with supplemental oxygen and started on a regimen of anticoagulant therapy. After an overnight stay in the hospital, Ms. Toomey remains stable and is discharged with a scheduled appointment to visit her healthcare provider.

1. What type of respiratory failure is Ms. Toomey experiencing?
2. Explain how a pulmonary embolus causes this type of failure.

Drew Seligson: Introduction

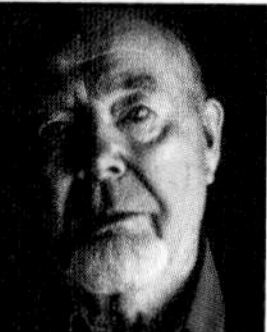

Drew Seligson, a 65-year-old man with chronic obstructive pulmonary disease (COPD), visits his pulmonologist complaining of a "chest cold" with increased shortness of breath, head and chest congestion, and a hard cough that produces thick, purulent tenacious sputum. His vital signs are pulse 105, respirations 26, temperature 101°F, blood pressure 150/90. The healthcare provider notes that Mr. Seligson has an audible expiratory wheezes and diminished breath sounds in both lower lobes on auscultation. Mr. Seligson is started on antibiotics, corticosteroids, and increased doses of his prescribed bronchodilators to treat infection and improve pulmonary function. Mr. Seligson leaves the pulmonologist's office accompanied by his daughter with instructions to call the next day if his symptoms worsen.

1. How is Mr. Seligson's respiratory failure different from Ms. Toomey's respiratory failure?
2. What is a similarity in Mr. Seligson's and Ms. Toomey's respiratory failure types?
3. Explain what role Mr. Seligson's temperature plays in a COPD exacerbation.

Check Your Progress: Section 20.1

1. Define type I respiratory failure.
2. Define type II respiratory failure.
3. Explain the importance of determining which type of respiratory failure a patient presents with.

20.2 Respiratory Failure: Type I and Type II

Type I respiratory failure is defined as severe hypoxemia characterized by the arterial oxygen level (PaO_2) less than 60 mmHg. Type II respiratory failure is characterized by hypercapnia as evidenced by $PaCO_2$ (partial pressure of carbon dioxide dissolved in arterial blood) greater than 50 mmHg pressure.[2]

Etiology and Pathogenesis of Type I Respiratory Failure

Type I respiratory failure is characterized by the presence of hypoxemia without hypercapnia. Hypoxemia is a PaO_2 less than 60 mmHg (8.0 kPa) with a normal or low partial pressure for carbon dioxide ($PaCO_2$). The reference value for a normal PaO_2 is greater than 80 mmHg (11 kPa), whereas a normal $PaCO_2$ is less than 45 mmHg (6.0 kPa). Hypoxemia can exist without hypercapnia because the more lipid-soluble CO_2 diffuses through a cell membrane about 20 times faster than O_2 even though their molecular weights are similar. This explains why many individuals maintain a normal $PaCO_2$ much longer than a normal PaO_2. A low $PaCO_2$ level can be the result of increased ventilatory efforts in response to hypoxemia; with hyperventilation, the individual exhales CO_2, decreasing alveolar CO_2 levels, which allows more CO_2 to diffuse into alveoli from blood.

The most common cause of type I respiratory failure is V-Q mismatch. This mismatch can occur in a wide array of pulmonary disorders, ranging from **pulmonary edema** (excess fluid in the lungs) to pneumonia. Type I respiratory failure also can be caused by any disorder that impairs oxygenation of blood by blocking airways, decreasing the level of oxygen in inspired air, shunting deoxygenated blood into oxygenated blood, impaired diffusion, inflammatory process, or fibrosis. Some individuals with type I respiratory failure progress to type II respiratory failure when more severe disease (e.g., asthma, COPD) or an infection affects their ventilation. See Box 20.1 for etiologies of type I respiratory failure.

Etiology and Pathogenesis of Type II Respiratory Failure

Type II respiratory failure is the result of **hypoventilation**, which is defined as inadequate alveolar ventilation, and V-Q mismatches. Any disease process that reduces breathing effort (e.g., neuromuscular diseases, drug overdose) or increases airway resistance (e.g., asthma), that severely decreases the available diffusion area (e.g., advanced emphysema) or greatly increases the diffusion distance (e.g., pulmonary fibrosis), or that alters the integrity of the chest wall (e.g., crushed chest) can result in type II failure. See Box 20.2 for etiologies of type II respiratory failure.

Acute type II respiratory failure develops over minutes to hours and results in an acidic pH that is below the normal range (7.35–7.45) because of the increased $PaCO_2$. There is

Box 20.1

Etiologies of Hypoxemic Respiratory Failure (Type I)

Aspiration (e.g., gastric contents)
Shunts
- Intracardiac shunt: atrial or venous septal defect
- Pulmonary shunt: flow of systemic venous blood to arterial blood

Inhalation of hypoxic gasses
Pneumonia
Pulmonary edema
- Cardiogenic shock
- Noncardiogenic shock

Pulmonary embolism
- Blood clot or fat embolism

Pulmonary hemorrhage
Chronic lung disease (less severe)
- Asthma

Pulmonary arterial hypertension
Pulmonary fibrosis
Abnormal desaturation of systemic venous blood
- Anemia

Abnormal lung tissue
- Burns
- Pulmonary contusion
- Lung tumors

Inflammation
- ARDS
- Acute irritant inhalation

Chlorine, dust, smoke

no time for renal compensation to occur. Increased CO_2 is acidic because in the presence of the enzyme carbonic anhydrase, CO_2 combines with water (H_2O) to form bicarbonate (HCO_3^+) and a free hydrogen ion (H^+). The production of free H^+ in blood explains why CO_2 is considered a volatile acid; the reaction reverses at the lungs and CO_2 is exhaled.

Compensated type II respiratory failure, which has been present for 3–5 days, allows time for the kidneys to compensate for the increased $PaCO_2$ by conserving and producing additional HCO_3^+ to buffer the increased H^+ and return the pH to normal limits. However, the pH remains on the acidic side of normal (below 7.4) because renal production of HCO_3 will never overcompensate for the acidemia. (For further explanation, see Chapter 9.)

Mechanisms Contributing to Type I Respiratory Failure

Multiple mechanisms contribute to the hypoxemia that occurs in type I respiratory failure. They include V-Q

Box 20.2

Etiologies of Hypercapnic Respiratory Failure (Type II)

Upper airway obstruction
- Acute epiglottitis
- Foreign body aspiration
- Sleep apnea (obesity/hypoventilation)

Reduced breathing effort (fatigue)
- ARDS
- Metabolic acidosis
- Drug suppression
- Legal and illicit narcotics
- Sedatives

Neuromuscular diseases/muscle weakness
- Post-polio syndrome
- Myasthenia gravis
- Myxedema
- Amyotrophic lateral sclerosis
- Guillain-Barré syndrome
- Muscular dystrophy

Altitude sickness
Severe airway disorders
- Asthma
- COPD
- Cystic fibrosis
- Emphysema

Nervous system injury
- High cervical spinal cord injury
- Head injury

Chest wall abnormalities
- Flail chest
- Kyphoscoliosis

Chest trauma
Pulmonary fibrosis

mismatches, diffusion impairments, shunting of systemic venous blood to the systemic arterial circulation, and inhalation of a hypoxic gas mixture.

Ventilation-Perfusion Mismatches

When alveolar ventilation is blocked or a shunt occurs, the deoxygenated blood added to oxygenated blood flowing to the left side of the heart results in a wider alveolar-arterial O_2 gradient and hypoxemia. The **alveolar-arterial O_2 gradient (A-a gradient)** compares the partial pressure of oxygen in alveolar gas (PAO_2) to the PaO_2, reflecting whether hypoxemia has an intrapulmonary or extrapulmonary cause. The normal A-a gradient is between 5 and 10 mmHg in young adult nonsmokers and increases by 1 mmHg for each decade of life. The normal A-a gradient for a 40-year-old nonsmoker should be less than 14 mmHg. The addition of systemic venous blood to oxygenated blood in the left heart increases the A-a gradient.

Diffusion Impairment

Diffusion is impaired when the alveolar oxygen pressure does not equilibrate with the pressure of oxygen dissolved in pulmonary capillary blood. This can be caused by any process that decreases the oxygen gradients (e.g., fills alveoli with fluid, causes alveoli to collapse, or blocks airways), lengthens the diffusion pathway (e.g., interstitial fibrosis), or limits the transit time for red blood cells to pass by alveoli.

Shunting of Systemic Venous Blood to the Systemic Arterial Circulation

Physiologic shunts or right-to-left shunts add systemic venous blood to oxygenated blood flowing into the left side of the heart. The term *shunt* refers to the percentage of deoxygenated blood that is mixed with oxygenated blood in the systemic arterial circulation. Examples of shunts include the following:

- ***Physiologic shunt.*** Systemic venous blood flowing past unventilated alveoli mixes with oxygenated blood from other regions of the lung (low V-Q).
- ***Right-to-left shunt.*** A right-to-left shunt occurs when systemic venous blood bypasses all alveoli and joins with oxygenated blood flowing into the left side of heart; this is also called a pulmonary shunt (**Figure 20.2** ■). An example is an arteriovenous shunt in the lungs. An intracardiac right-to-left shunt can occur when there is a congenital cardiac septal defect, when increasing right ventricular volumes and pressure open the foramen ovale, or when blood flows through abnormal vascular channels in the heart. A shunt that exceeds 30% results in hypoxemia, and increasing the fraction of inspired oxygen (FIO_2) to 100% cannot eliminate the lower PaO_2 because of the addition of deoxygenated shunted blood to oxygenated blood.

Inhalation of a Hypoxic Air Mixture

The inhalation of air with low oxygen levels can occur in fires or with exposure to high concentrations of toxic fumes or very low barometric pressures. In addition to limiting the availability of oxygen, the inflammatory response to smoke or toxic fume inhalation further interferes with the diffusion of oxygen. A hypoxic air mixture normally occurs at very high altitudes (elevations of 14,000 feet or higher) with mountain climbing or the loss of pressurization in an airplane. Exposure to low oxygen levels at high altitudes can cause symptoms of altitude sickness (headache and fatigue) that diminish when the individual returns to a lower elevation. However, with continued exposure to low barometric pressure, altitude sickness can progress to high altitude pulmonary edema. The accumulated fluid interferes with oxygenation and if left untreated can progress to respiratory failure and death.

Vanessa Toomey: Application

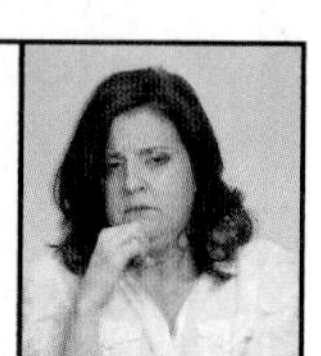

Ms. Toomey returns to work within 3–4 days. Because she continues to feel fine, she discontinues her anticoagulation therapy. Approximately 3 weeks later, the pain and tenderness in her right calf return, she has pain in her right groin, her pulse has become rapid, she feels faint, she has chest pain, and she is acutely short of breath. On admission to the emergency department, her vital signs are pulse 120, respirations 32, temperature 99.8°F, blood pressure 90/60. Because of the possibility of vascular compromise, she is admitted to the ICU, where intravenous fluids are started, and an echocardiography, electrocardiography (ECG), and ultrasounds of both her calves are performed. The echocardiogram is normal, and the ECG shows sinus tachycardia; however, an additional deep vein thrombosis is noted on her left calf. A repeat spiral CT is consistent with increased emboli. Fortunately, Ms. Toomey stabilizes and is transferred from the ICU to a medical unit after 2 days. Once again, she is discharged on anticoagulation therapy.

3. After reviewing Ms. Toomey's case, would you expect that she is hypoxic? Explain your answer.
4. Which mechanism has contributed to her condition?

Mechanisms Contributing to Type II Respiratory Failure

Type II hypercapnic respiratory failure results with inadequate alveolar ventilation. Normal ventilation removes CO_2 with exhalation and dilutes the remaining alveolar CO_2 with the inhalation of fresh air. With hypoventilation, inadequate amounts of O_2 are inhaled, and levels of CO_2 build up in alveoli. To maintain a diffusion gradient for CO_2, levels of arterial CO_2 ($PaCO_2$) must increase so that CO_2 will diffuse from blood into alveoli. Supplemental oxygen therapy can compensate for the hypoxemia but will not affect the hypercapnia.

There are several mechanisms that cause hypoventilation and result in V-Q inequalities and hypercapnia. The inability to generate adequate ventilation can result from a variety of factors such as CNS dysfunction, respiratory muscle dysfunction, or deformities of the chest wall or airways.

CLINICAL POINT: Exposure to low O_2 levels at high altitudes can cause symptoms of altitude sickness, such as headache and fatigue, which diminish when the individual returns to a lower elevation; but with continued exposure to low barometric pressures,

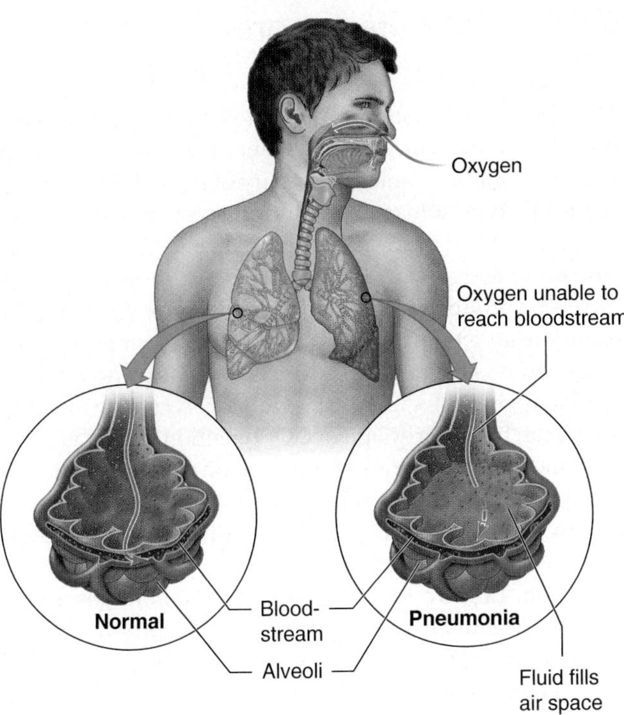

Figure 20.2 ■ In an intrapulmonary shunt, blood flows through the pulmonary capillaries without participating in gas exchange.

altitude sickness can progress to high-altitude pulmonary edema. The accumulated fluid interferes with oxygenation, and if untreated, it can progress to respiratory failure and death. ■

Altered Central Control of Ventilation

With normal ventilation, the CNS controls ventilation by coordinating information from sensors with the stimulation of respiratory muscles to contract. Increased CO_2 in the blood diffuses into cerebrospinal fluid (CSF), combines with water, and is converted to free hydrogen ions, lowering the CSF pH. The lower pH stimulates the respiratory centers in the medulla and pons to begin ventilation. The central respiratory drive can be depressed by prescription drugs (e.g., anesthesia, pain medications) and nonprescription drugs (e.g., heroin, crack cocaine), strokes, neoplasms, or trauma to brain regions that control respirations. Obesity can also be associated with an abnormal central respiratory drive as well as an increased work of breathing.

With the increased airway obstruction and uneven regional ventilation in advanced chronic obstructive pulmonary disease, the physiologic dead space and work of breathing are increased, particularly with chest hyperinflation, resulting in CO_2 retention. With constantly elevated levels of CO_2, there is a decreased chemical response to pH in the medulla, so chemoreceptors in the carotid and aortic bodies control respirations. Carotid and aortic bodies respond primarily to changes in PaO_2 in the range of 30–60 mmHg to stimulate breathing, but they also respond to increased CO_2 and decreased pH (more acidic pH) in arterial blood. The changes in $PaCO_2$ and pH increase the sensitivity of aortic and carotid bodies to the PaO_2.

Altered Neuromuscular Control of Ventilation

Interference with the peripheral neural control of respiratory muscles causes respiratory muscle weakness. The problem may be in the nerve or myelin covering or at the myoneural junction. When respiratory muscles cannot generate adequate negative pressure for normal ventilation, hypoventilation causes respiratory failure. Neuromuscular disorders that affect respiratory muscle strength include Guillain-Barré syndrome, myasthenia gravis, spinal cord injuries, post-polio syndrome, and amyotrophic lateral sclerosis. Respiratory weakness may be worse at night from fatigue and altered body position; the results are a reduced vital capacity and reduced expiratory reserve. Weak respiratory muscles cause a poor cough and often result in atelectasis and respiratory infections.

Altered Chest Wall Structure

An alteration in the chest wall structure can limit ventilation, resulting in hypercapnia. Severe kyphoscoliosis is a common chest wall deformity that limits ventilation by greatly decreasing chest compliance. A traumatic crushing injury to the chest with fractures of several ribs on one side of the thorax is called a flail chest. When flail chest occurs, the chest wall no longer provides a stable structure for respiratory muscles to contract against. With inhalation, the fractured area moves inward and then outward with exhalation, and hypoventilation results (**Figure 20.3** ■).

Altered Airway Structure

The airway structure can become altered from severe COPD or from sleep apnea. In COPD, the airway structure can become unstable with the dynamic airway compression and increased airway resistance during exhalation. In chronic obstructive sleep apnea, the neck and throat muscles relax when the individual reclines and falls asleep, allowing the tongue and soft palate to temporarily block the trachea during inhalation. The individual awakens enough to contract neck and throat muscles, breathe, and then fall back to sleep. With sleep apnea, there are multiple periods when the individual does not breathe for at least 10 seconds during the night and then awakens. The cycle repeats, leaving the individual seriously sleep deprived. Sleep apnea is most common in obese individuals who have thick necks. Obesity hypoventilation syndrome often accompanies sleep apnea. If left untreated, the vasoconstriction caused by alveolar **hypoxia** (inadequate oxygenation of tissues) strains the right heart, and right ventricular failure and cor pulmonale can result.

Drew Seligson: Application

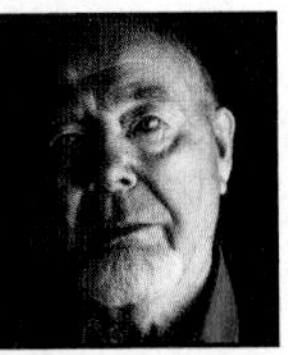

Mr. Seligson's chest x-ray is consistent with bilateral pneumonia, and he is treated with intravenous antibiotics. His condition continues to deteriorate with increasing PCO_2 (65 mmHg) and acidosis (pH 7.2). He also becomes increasingly lethargic. He is placed on mechanical ventilation. His condition remains critical for the following week. However, with resolution of his pneumonia, his arterial blood gases continue to improve, and he is removed from mechanical ventilation and placed on supplemental oxygen via nasal cannula at 1–2 L/min.

4. Discuss how Mr. Seligson developed the PCO_2 of 65 mmHg and acidosis (pH 7.2).
5. What role do the kidneys play in Mr. Seligson's improved blood gas results?

Research on the respiratory muscle strength of older adults with neurocognitive and neurodegenerative disorders is scarce. A small study found that adults with Parkinson disease and Alzheimer disease exhibited lower maximal inspiratory and expiratory pressures, indicating reduced respiratory muscle strength, putting them at increased risk for atelectasis and other pulmonary complications.[3] This suggests that early evaluation of respiratory health in these patients may be a helpful component of their overall assessment and treatment plan. ■

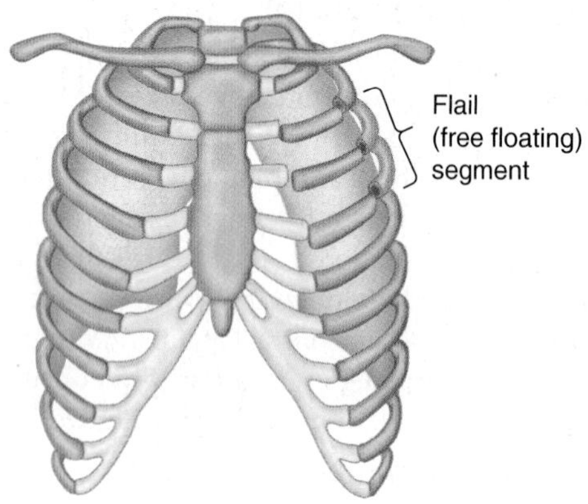

A Fracture pattern of flail chest

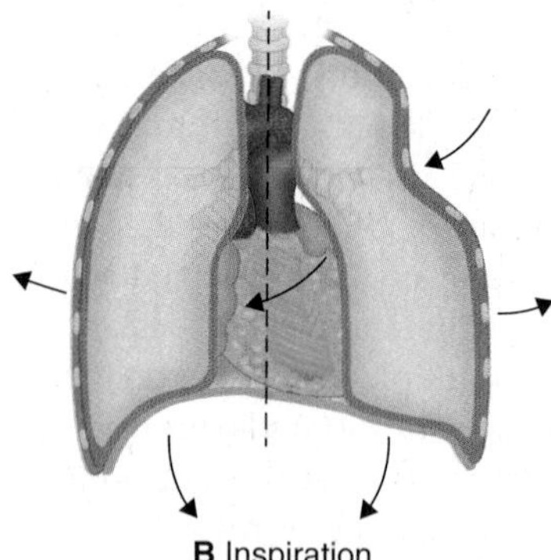

B Inspiration

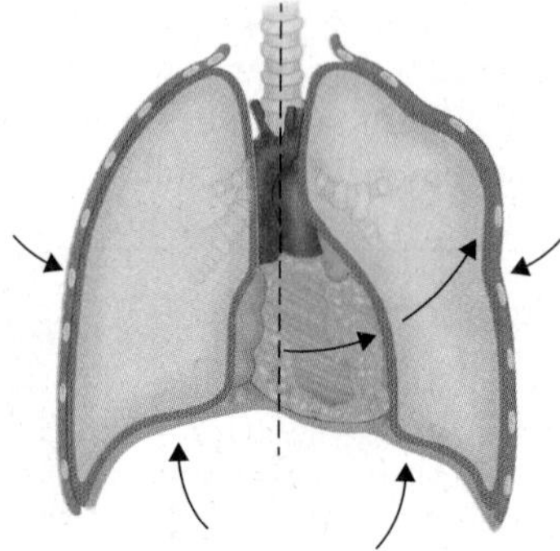

C Expiration

Figure 20.3 ■ Flail chest with paradoxical movement.

Clinical Manifestations of Respiratory Failure

The clinical presentation of respiratory failure varies according to the underlying cause, whether the respiratory failure is acute or chronic, and the severity of the failure. Common signs and symptoms include dyspnea, shortness of breath, wheezing, tachypnea, tachycardia, cyanosis, and nonspecific complaints such as chest pain. Depending on the cause of the respiratory failure, additional signs will vary. For example, an ineffective cough may be present with neuromuscular or skeletal defects, or chest abrasion and hemoptysis may present with chest contusion. A change in mental status can be an early sign of CO_2 retention, whereas confusion and somnolence are common with severe hypercapnia even when arterial oxygen concentrations are adequate.

In chronic type II respiratory failure, the persistently low levels of PaO_2 stimulate the kidneys to release erythropoietin. Erythropoietin stimulates the bone marrow to produce additional red blood cells (RBCs), producing polycythemia, which is defined as increased RBCs per volume of blood, which may give an individual a ruddy complexion. Polycythemia improves the total oxygen-carrying capacity of blood, although each RBC is not fully saturated. Polycythemia is usually accompanied by right ventricular hypertrophy, which can progress to right ventricular failure as it pumps blood against the increased pulmonary vascular resistance. Polycythemia increases blood viscosity, which increases the risk for clotting and stroke.[4]

Confirming Respiratory Failure

Arterial blood gases are critical to identifying respiratory failure. In type I respiratory failure, the PaO_2 is decreased; in type II respiratory failure, PaO_2 is decreased, and $PaCO_2$ increased to 50 mmHg or higher. In acute type II failure, the bicarbonate levels are decreased, and the pH is acidic, but in chronic type II failure with renal compensation, the bicarbonate levels are increased to maintain the pH within normal limits but less than 7.4. Other diagnostic tests vary with the cause of the respiratory failure.

Managing Respiratory Failure

The treatment of respiratory failure is focused on improving oxygenation and restoring normal ventilation. Hypoxemia represents an imminent threat to organ function and must be corrected before focusing on the underlying cause of the respiratory failure. There are a number of techniques to improve oxygenation. Three examples are described below:

- Providing supplemental oxygen to spontaneously breathing individuals can be achieved by increasing the FIO_2 with the use of a nasal cannula or by using various masks such as a simple plastic masks or a Venturi mask (a medical device that delivers a specific oxygen concentration to patients on controlled oxygen therapy with adjustable levels of FIO_2).

- Improving breathing can be accomplished by a variety of techniques such as using bronchodilators, altering positions in bed, and increasing expectoration of pulmonary secretions. Positioning an individual in a decubitus upright or prone position facilitates breathing. Prone positioning improves the functional residual capacity, drainage of secretions, and V-Q matching and may improve oxygenation.[5] Turning, coughing, and deep breathing are the simplest techniques for improving breathing. Turning the patient regularly rotates and maximizes lung zones to assist V-Q matching. Use of incentive spirometry assists in maximizing diffusion and improving alveolar surface area.[5] Percussion or vibration devices can be used to loosen thick, heavy secretions so that they can be coughed or suctioned out. Postural drainage requires the temporary positioning of an individual with the hips higher than the chest in an attempt to use gravity to drain secretions into larger airways and thus improve expectoration of pulmonary secretions.
- Mechanical ventilation is used to restore adequate gas exchange while reducing the work of breathing. Mechanical ventilation can be used to secure unprotected airways, reducing the risk of aspiration, to relieve respiratory muscle fatigue, and to correct gas exchange. Mechanical ventilation is most frequently used during surgical procedures. Outside of the operating room, mechanical ventilation is frequently employed in the management of pulmonary disorders that cause respiratory failure and in cardiopulmonary arrest.

Vanessa Toomey: Outcome

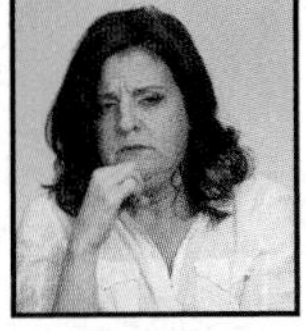

Ms. Toomey's most recent hospital stay has made her very cognizant of the risks of pulmonary emboli. She maintains her anticoagulation regimen, has increased her fluid intake, and moves around the airplane frequently while flying. She continues to work on smoking cessation and has made significant strides in this area.

5. In light of Ms. Toomey's experience, what teaching would be important to include for patients being discharged home after hospitalization for a pulmonary embolism?
6. Ms. Toomey moves around the airplane frequently while flying. What other nonpharmacologic actions could she take to reduce her risk of developing another pulmonary embolism?

Check Your Progress: Section 20.2

1. Explain the body's response to constantly elevated levels of CO_2.
2. Explain why a patient with rib fractures (not flail chest) is at an increased risk of developing type II respiratory failure.
3. Explain why the mechanical ventilator treatment for a patient may be different during the night than during the day.

20.3 Disorders Causing Respiratory Failure

Disorders that commonly cause respiratory failure include acute respiratory distress, pulmonary edema, and advanced COPD.

Acute Respiratory Distress Syndrome

Acute respiratory distress syndrome (ARDS) is a type of diffuse lung injury characterized by severe inflammation, leading to increased pulmonary vascular permeability, increased lung weight, and a loss of aerated lung tissue.[6] This current definition of ARDS was developed by an international consensus group and is known as the Berlin definition of ARDS.[6] Despite the fact that ARDS has been recognized for several decades, the exact pathophysiologic mechanisms remain unclear. ARDS remains a multisystem disorder originating in the lung and associated with high mortality. A recently published international, multicenter, prospective cohort study of patients undergoing invasive or noninvasive ventilation in intensive care units noted that hospital mortality rates were 34.9%, 40.3%, and 46.1% for patients with mild, moderate, and severe ARDS, respectively.[7]

Risk Factors

A number of risk factors are associated with the development of ARDS. All of these factors are associated with insults to the lung or vasculature such as pneumonia, aspiration, toxic inhalation, pulmonary contusion, near-drowning, sepsis, multiple blood transfusions, pancreatitis, and major trauma. Pneumonia and sepsis are the most common causes of ARDS.[7]

Etiology and Pathogenesis

In ARDS, a precipitating insult disrupts the integrity of alveolar and capillary walls and results in an acute, massive inflammatory response involving multiple cells and inflammatory mediators. The initial damage frequently involves the capillary endothelium. However, it can affect the alveolar epithelial cells, and eventually both are involved. The damage is not uniform throughout the lungs; some areas will be less affected, while others will be severely damaged. The progression of ARDS occurs in three overlapping and sequential phases: the exudative phase followed by a fibroproliferative phase and then a resolution phase. An illustrative overview of the pathogenesis of ARDS can be found in **Figure 20.4** ■.

Exudative Phase. The exudative phase develops 5–7 days after the initial injury and is characterized by damage to the alveolar–capillary membrane. The membrane has two distinct parts: the microvascular endothelium and the alveolar epithelium. Microvascular endothelial injury allows gaps to form between the endothelial cells, which increases their permeability, allowing alveolar flooding with protein-rich fluid.[7]

Additionally, injury to the microvascular endothelium may precipitate damage to the pulmonary vascular bed, decreasing perfusion to adequately ventilated areas of the lung.[7]

Alveolar macrophages rapidly synthesize inflammatory mediators in response to the damage. Examples of the mediators include interleukin 1 (IL-1) which recruits neutrophils, interleukin 8 (IL-8), and tumor necrosis factor plus a neutrophil activator. Neutrophilic inflammation plays an important role in ARDS because neutrophils release oxidants, proteases and platelet activating factor, which cause tissue damage, and inflammatory mediators that maintain the inflammatory response. Abnormal fibrinolysis and coagulation are present in ARDS and may contribute to the ongoing inflammation in the lung.

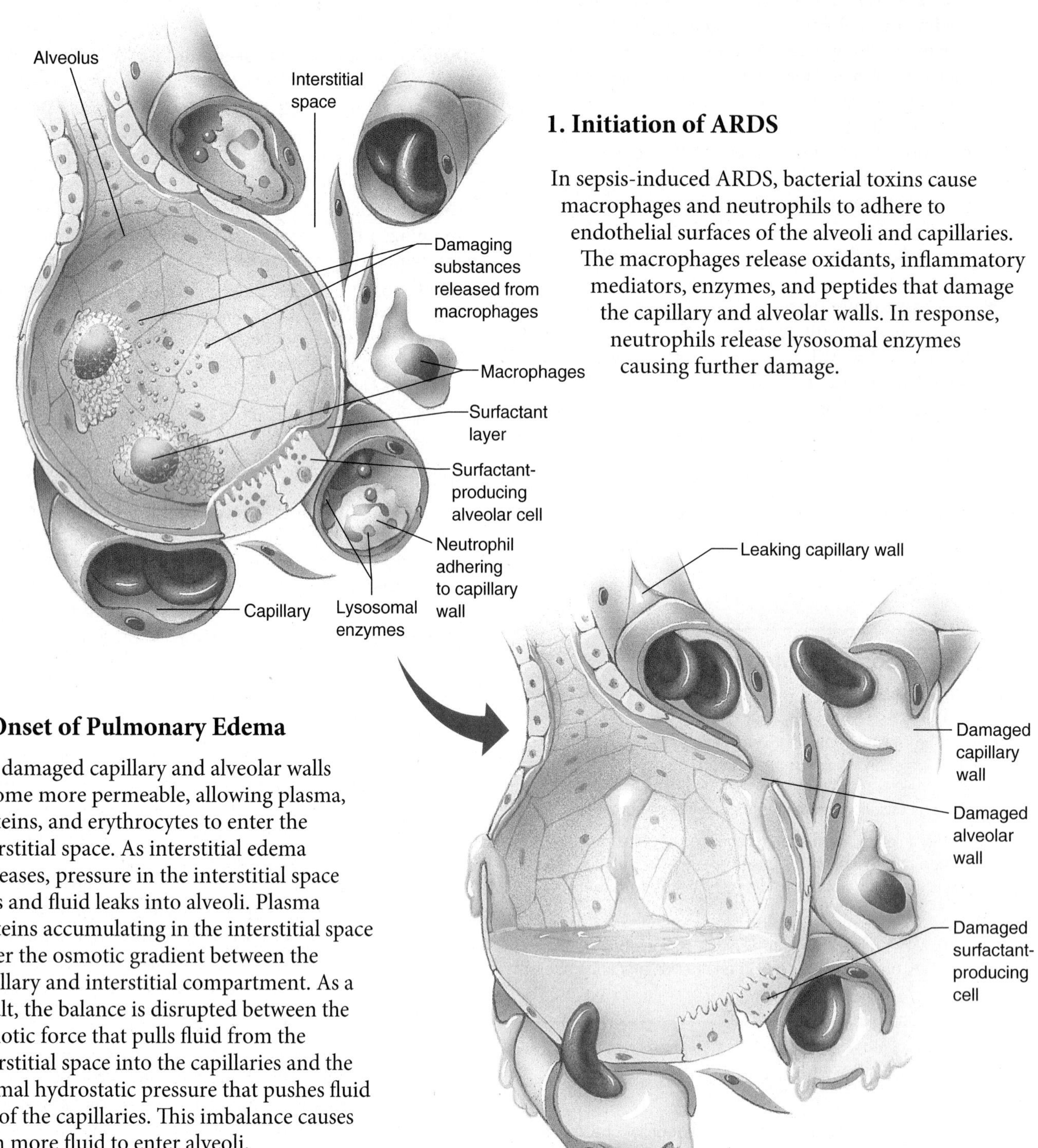
Alveolus
Interstitial space
1. Initiation of ARDS
In sepsis-induced ARDS, bacterial toxins cause macrophages and neutrophils to adhere to endothelial surfaces of the alveoli and capillaries. The macrophages release oxidants, inflammatory mediators, enzymes, and peptides that damage the capillary and alveolar walls. In response, neutrophils release lysosomal enzymes causing further damage.
Damaging substances released from macrophages
Macrophages
Surfactant layer
Surfactant-producing alveolar cell
Neutrophil adhering to capillary wall
Capillary
Lysosomal enzymes
Leaking capillary wall
2. Onset of Pulmonary Edema
The damaged capillary and alveolar walls become more permeable, allowing plasma, proteins, and erythrocytes to enter the interstitial space. As interstitial edema increases, pressure in the interstitial space rises and fluid leaks into alveoli. Plasma proteins accumulating in the interstitial space lower the osmotic gradient between the capillary and interstitial compartment. As a result, the balance is disrupted between the osmotic force that pulls fluid from the interstitial space into the capillaries and the normal hydrostatic pressure that pushes fluid out of the capillaries. This imbalance causes even more fluid to enter alveoli.
Damaged capillary wall
Damaged alveolar wall
Damaged surfactant-producing cell

Figure 20.4 ■ The pathophysiology of acute respiratory distress syndrome. Acute respiratory distress syndrome (ARDS) is a severe form of acute respiratory failure that occurs in response to pulmonary or systemic insults. ARDS is characterized by noncardiogenic pulmonary edema caused by inammatory damage to alveolar and capillary walls. Many disorders may precipitate ARDS, although sepsis is the most common.

During the exudative phase, type I and type II pneumocytes (alveolar epithelial cells) are irreversibly damaged. Normally, the thin, flat type I pneumocytes cover 95% of the alveolar wall and permit the rapid exchange of gases with pulmonary capillaries, while the larger and more plentiful type II pneumocytes cover just 5% of the alveolar wall. Type II pneumocytes produce surfactant to counteract alveolar surface tension (the tendency for

4. End-Stage ARDS

Fibrin and cell debris from necrotic cells combine to form hyaline membranes, which line the interior of the alveoli and further reduce alveolar compliance and gas exchange. Because CO_2 cannot diffuse across hyaline membranes, $PaCO_2$ levels now begin to rise while PaO_2 levels continue to fall. Rising $PaCO_2$ levels can lead to respiratory acidosis. Without respiratory support, respiratory failure will develop.
Even with aggressive treatment, almost 50% of clients with ARDS die.

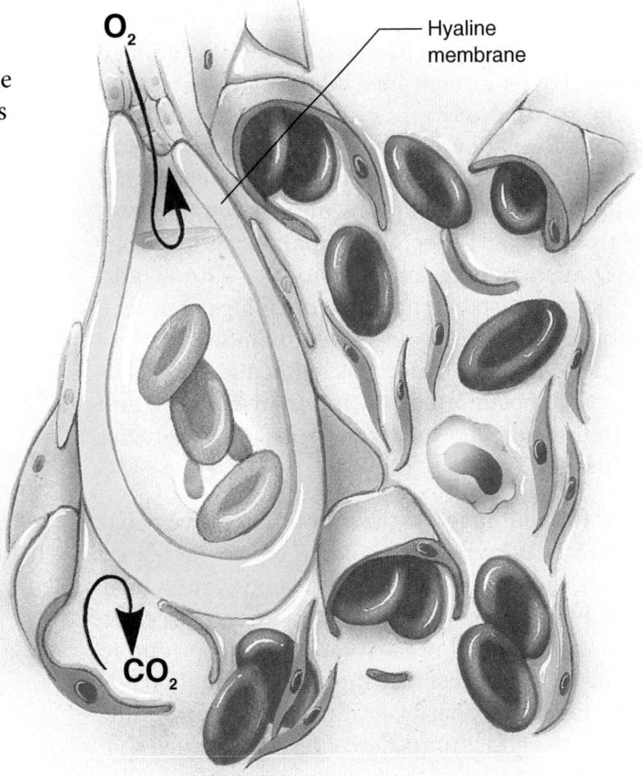

3. Alveolar Collapse

Protein-rich fluid accumulates in the alveoli, inactivating surfactant and damaging type II alveolar cells that produce surfactant. (Surfactant is important in maintaining alveolar compliance—the ability of tissue to stretch or distend.) As active surfactant is lost, the alveoli stiffen and collapse, leading to atelectasis, which increases breathing effort.

Decreased alveolar compliance, atelectasis, and fluid-filled alveoli interfere with gas exchange across the alveolar-capillary membrane. Blood oxygen (PaO_2) levels fall. Because carbon dioxide diffuses more readily than oxygen, however, blood carbon dioxide ($PaCO_2$) levels also fall initially as tachypnea causes more CO_2 to be expired.

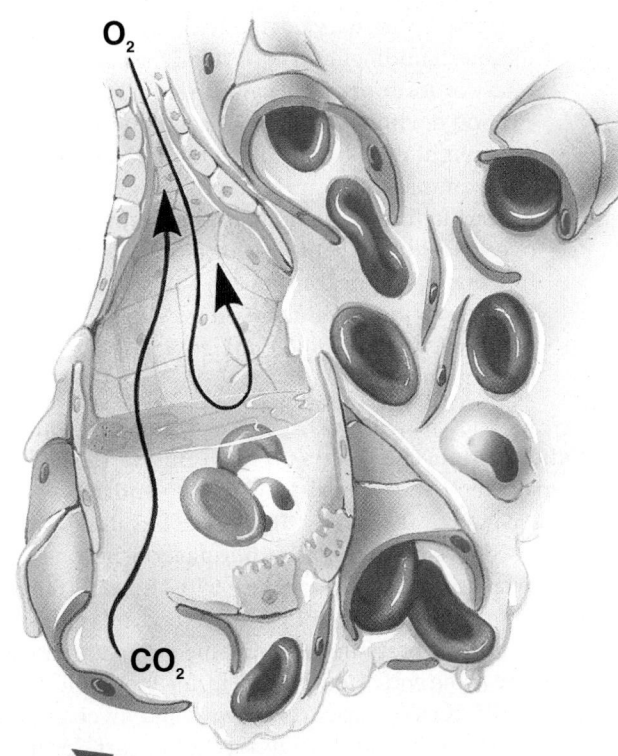

Figure 20.4 ■ Continued

smaller alveoli to collapse into larger alveoli) and repair alveolar epithelium when fragile type I cells are damaged. In ARDS, type I pneumocytes lose their ability to transport sodium and water. The diffusion of gases becomes disrupted. Type II pneumocytes cannot produce surfactant, and the combination of diffusion disruption and lack of surfactant causes alveoli to collapse. With the inflammation, pulmonary capillaries become congested, and their damaged endothelia allow proteins, fluid, and small hemorrhages to leak into interstitial spaces and alveoli. The cardiac output is often elevated, further increasing the formation of pulmonary edema. Proteins, fluid, and cellular debris collect within the alveoli and alveolar ducts to form a hyaline membrane, a hallmark of ARDS. The physiologic effects are impaired gas exchange due to V-Q mismatching and physiologic shunts, stiff lungs due to decreased compliance of collapsed alveoli and pulmonary edema, and increased pulmonary artery pressure due to hypoxic vasoconstriction and parenchymal destruction. Postmortem, the lungs are dark red and heavy, with little air, and the tissue looks more like liver than lung tissue.

Fibroproliferative Phase. As the fibroproliferative phase begins, there is persistent hypoxemia with increased physiologic dead space and reduced lung compliance. Marked proliferation of type II pneumocytes is seen in damaged areas, and pulmonary capillaries continue to be disrupted by microvascular thrombus formation. As the fibroproliferative phase continues, the neutrophilic inflammation resolves, production of reactive oxygen species stops, pulmonary edema is resorbed, and alveolar macrophages phagocytose the hyaline membrane. Myofibroblasts infiltrate the interstitium and began the early deposition of collagen. Overall, these changes result in the resolution of hypoxemia, a decrease in physiologic dead space, and improved lung compliance. The fibroproliferative phase lasts 2–3 weeks, after which the ARDS resolves in some individuals and progresses to the chronic phase in others.

Resolution Phase. In the resolution phase, diffuse pulmonary scarring alters the normal lung architecture in some individuals. Over time, the radiographic abnormalities may resolve, but microscopic fibrosis remains. Survivors tend to be young, and pulmonary function generally recovers gradually over 6 months to 1 year, but residual abnormalities (e.g., mild restriction or obstructive defect, low diffusing capacity, or impaired gas exchange with exercise) may remain.

Clinical Manifestations

The clinical presentation of ARDS is one of an acute onset of dyspnea and hypoxemia that worsens in spite of increasing levels of FIO_2.[8] Tachycardia and tachypnea are present as the individual works hard to generate higher pressures needed to breathe. Tachypnea initially causes respiratory alkalosis from hyperventilation; then respiratory acidosis occurs when ventilation is not adequate. Most individuals require mechanical ventilation. On physical exam, normal breath sounds give way to coarse crackles and signs of consolidation as the respiratory distress increases. There are diffuse, bilateral fluffy infiltrates on chest radiograph but no evidence of left ventricular failure; later, the progressive infiltrates "white out" the lung on chest x-ray. As pulmonary edema begins to resolve in the fibroproliferative phase, oxygenation improves, but most individuals still require mechanical ventilation because of their stiff lungs (low compliance), large physiologic dead space, and high minute ventilation requirements. This fibroproliferative phase may last for several weeks with the resolution occurring over several months.

Linking Pathophysiology to Diagnosis and Treatment

The diagnosis of ARDS is directed toward identifying the causes of ARDS that may respond to treatment, excluding conditions that are also present with acute hypoxemia, bilateral alveolar infiltrates, and respiratory distress.[8] One of the most challenging clinical issues is to differentiate between cardiogenic pulmonary edema and ARDS. Diagnostic tests used to differentiate between the two disorders often include the following:

- ***Brain natriuretic peptide.*** A plasma level of brain natriuretic peptide (BNP) below 100 pg/mL is suggestive of congestive heart disease; however, higher levels do not confirm heart failure, nor do these levels confirm ARDS.[9]
- ***Echocardiography.*** Many clinicians order transthoracic echocardiography as a first-line diagnostic test if cardiogenic pulmonary edema cannot be excluded based in clinical findings and BNP.[9] Evidence on echocardiography of aortic or mitral valve dysfunction or a reduced ejection fraction would make heart failure more likely. This might not be conclusive for a variety of reasons. For example, echocardiography may be inconclusive if heart failure is due to diastolic dysfunction or fluid overload due to acute renal failure, as the left heart function will appear normal.
- ***Pulmonary artery catheterization.*** An increased wedge pressure greater than 18 mmHg suggests that heart failure is involved.

Individuals with ARDS almost invariably require intubation and mechanical ventilation during their illness to manage the hypoxemia.[10] Mechanical ventilation supports oxygenation by decreasing the work of breathing, providing increased levels of FIO_2, recruiting atelectactic lung regions, and decreasing the venous return to the heart. Positive end-expiratory pressure (PEEP) is a method of ventilation in which airway pressure is maintained above atmospheric pressure at the end of exhalation during mechanical ventilation. PEEP further supports airways and alveolar patency but reduces venous return to the right heart. In turn, this decreases the hydrostatic pressure in the pulmonary circulation.

In spite of the advantages, mechanical ventilation in ARDS may induce significant lung injury due to barotraumas and alveolar overdistention. The lung injury in ARDS is heterogeneous, so less affected areas of the lung receive a larger portion of the tidal volume and become overinflated. Use of PEEP can increase alveolar overinflation, causing microvascular injury and increased pulmonary edema. In addition, neuromuscular blocking and sedative agents can cause prolonged depression of mental status and neuromuscular weakness. Ventilator-induced injuries can be minimized or avoided by using lung protective strategies. These include using a low tidal volume, using a low plateau pressure, having the pressure applied to small airways and alveoli measured during an inspiratory pause on the ventilator, and a nontoxic inspired oxygen level less than 60%. Additional supportive measures are required to maintain nutrition, mobility, and communication and to prevent healthcare-acquired infections that are important causes of increased morbidity and mortality in ARDS.[11]

Infant Respiratory Distress Syndrome

Respiratory distress syndrome in newborns is life threatening. Because the syndrome is primarily a disease of prematurity, prevalence rates are higher when premature birth rates are higher. The disorder affects 0.6–1% of newborns.[12]

Etiology and Pathogenesis

Infant respiratory distress syndrome (IRDS) arises from a deficiency of surfactant due to either the immature lung's inability to produce enough surfactant or a genetic mutation of the SP-B surfactant protein (**Figure 20.5** ■). Lack

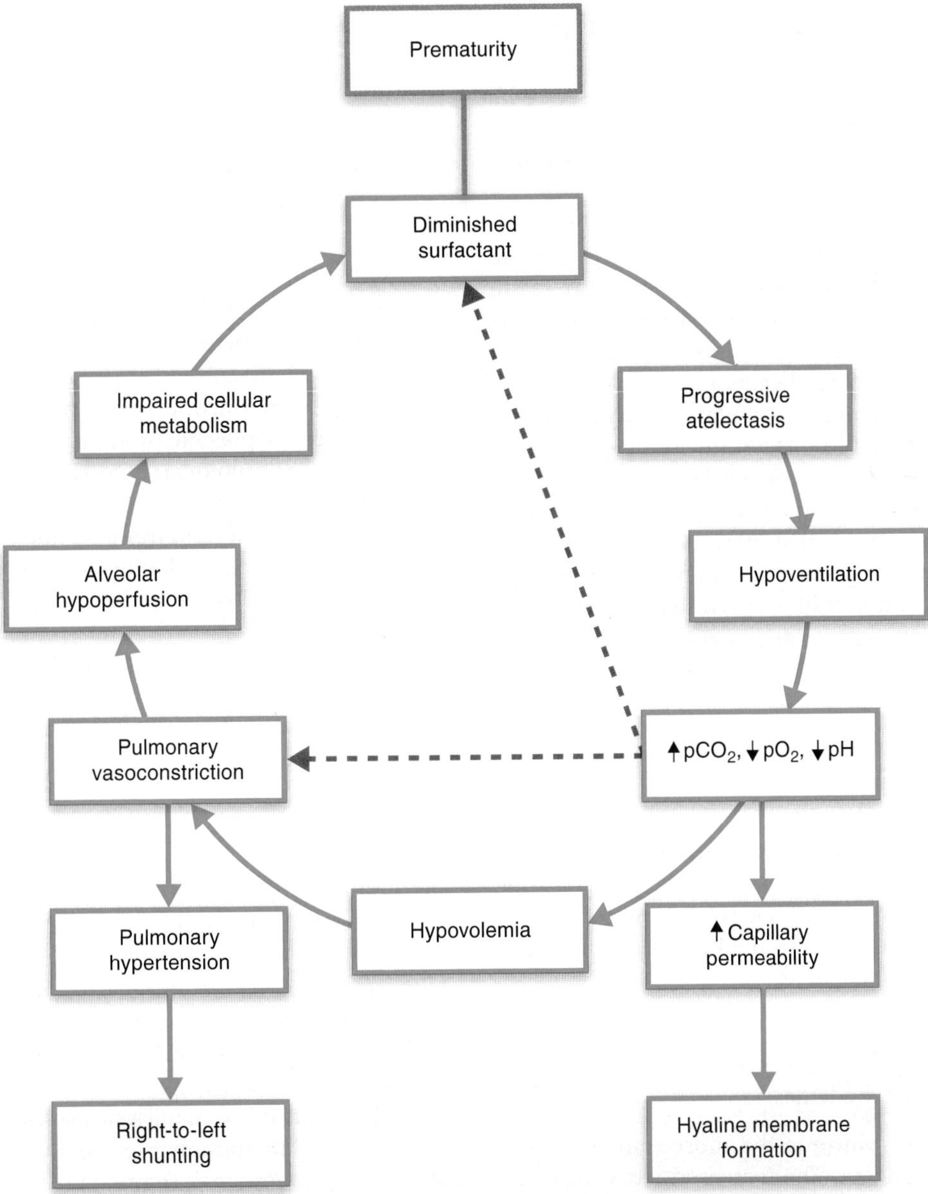

Figure 20.5 ■ The pathogenesis of infant respiratory distress syndrome.

of surfactant leads to high surface tension, which leads to instability of the lung at end-expiration, low lung volume, and decreased compliance.[12] The changes lead to hypoxia due to V-Q mismatch resulting from a variety of factors including atelectasis and intrapulmonary to extrapulmonary right-to-left shunts.[10] Surfactant deficiency also leads to inflammation in the lung and respiratory epithelial injury and worsening lung function; this can result in pulmonary edema and increased airway resistance. Abnormal absorption of fluid in the lung results in poor clearance of fluid from the lung, leading to edema that impairs gas exchange.[12]

Clinical Manifestations

Clinical manifestations of IRDS include obvious signs of respiratory distress such as nasal flaring, rapid breathing, shallow breathing, shortness of breath, and grunting with breathing. Other signs include cyanosis, apnea, and decreased urine output.

Linking Pathophysiology to Diagnosis and Treatment

In addition to clinical manifestations indicating acute respiratory distress, the newborn with IRDS will present with decreased oxygen and excess acid in the arterial blood gases report. A chest x-ray will show a "ground glass" appearance of the lungs.

The combination of surfactant therapy and mechanical ventilation with continuous positive airway pressure (CPAP) to prevent alveoli from collapsing has been a mainstay of treatment of IRDS since the 1990s. Typically, the newborn in distress breathes more easily within hours of surfactant therapy. Although there is a risk of bleeding into the lungs from surfactant replacement, complications are less likely and morbidity rates are much lower for newborns who receive timely therapy.[12] More recent clinical guidelines include some refinements. For extremely preterm infants (those younger than 30 weeks' gestation) with severe IRDS, surfactant therapy is not recommended until after initial stabilization with early initiation of CPAP.[12] Delivery of surfactant therapy and monitoring of newborns with IRDS require experienced providers with training and clinical expertise. ■

Pulmonary Edema

In pulmonary edema, fluid from pulmonary capillaries accumulates in the interstitial spaces and alveoli; the edema can severely compromise oxygenation to the point of being life threatening (**Figure 20.6** ■). The excess fluid exceeds the capacity of the capillaries to resorb fluid and the lymphatic system to drain it from the lung.

Etiology and Pathogenesis

There are four pathophysiologic mechanisms that cause the formation of pulmonary edema:

- Left ventricular failure is the most common cause of pulmonary edema. The increased left ventricular pressure is reflected back into the pulmonary capillary bed. The increased pulmonary capillary pressure (wedge pressure $\geq$ 20 mmHg) increases the hydrostatic drive for fluid to flow from the capillaries into the interstitial space. Pulmonary edema associated with left ventricular failure is referred to as *cardiogenic pulmonary edema*.[13]
- Decrease of oncotic pressure due to anemia or a decrease in plasma proteins can cause pulmonary edema. The pulmonary hydrostatic pressure is normal, but the oncotic pressure is not adequate to resorb normal amounts of fluid from the interstitial space.
- Capillary endothelial injury makes capillaries "leaky," so more fluid leaks into the interstitial space.
- Blockage of lymphatic drainage prevents the removal of excess fluid from the interstitial space. Normally, excess fluid in the lung interstitial space is collected at the periphery of acini to drain through the lymphatic system. Fluid moves through the lymphatics toward the hilar nodes and finally enters the brachiocephalic vein.

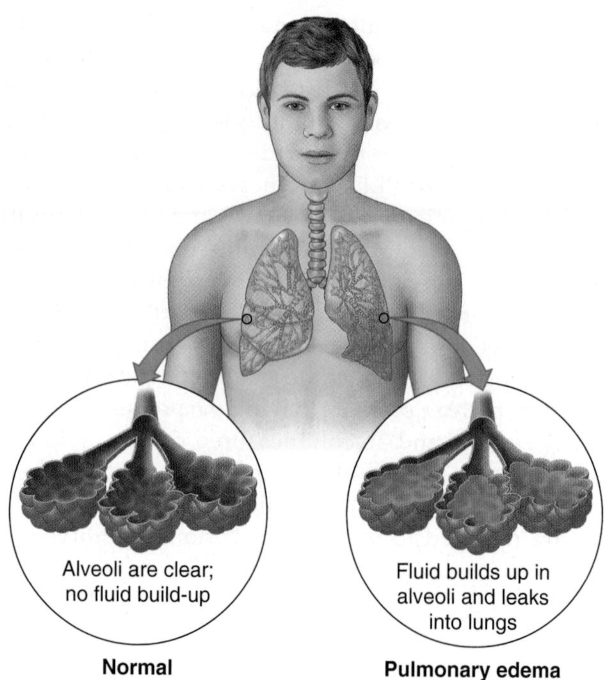

Figure 20.6 ■ With pulmonary edema, fluid accumulates in the alveoli and then leaks into the lungs.

Clinical Manifestations

The patient with acute pulmonary edema is dyspneic, anxious or distressed, diaphoretic, and sitting upright because of being unable to breathe lying flat (orthopnea). Tachycardia and tachypnea may be accompanied by sympathetically mediated hypertension. With severe pulmonary edema, signs include hypoxemia, hypercarbia, severe shortness of breath with an inability to talk in full sentences, and a cough that produces pink, frothy sputum from the fluid that has leaked into alveoli. The patient may complain of "air hunger" or have the sensation of drowning and may appear cyanotic. On initial physical examination, fine crackles are heard in the lung bases; as the pulmonary edema worsens, the crackles will progress toward the apices, and coarse crackles and wheezes may be present as well. On auscultation of the heart, an S_3 and accentuated pulmonic component of S_2 will be heard, and jugular distention reflects the congestion in the pulmonary bed. Patients with noncardiogenic pulmonary edema usually present with ARDS as a consequence or complication of an underlying pulmonary or systemic condition.[14]

Pulmonary edema during pregnancy is uncommon. Risk factors include administration of tocolytic agents (labor suppressants), underlying maternal cardiovascular disease, fluid overload, and preeclampsia.[15] ■

Linking Pathophysiology to Diagnosis and Treatment

Diagnostic tests include blood tests, assessment of cardiac status, and measurement of the pulmonary capillary wedge pressure. Blood tests include the following:

- Complete blood count with differential to identify severe anemia
- Serum albumin levels as albumin is the primary protein responsible for normal oncotic pressure
- Serum electrolytes to identify abnormalities from diuretic use
- Arterial blood gases to quantify hypoxemia and hypercarbia
- Plasma BNP to help differentiate between heart failure and pulmonary causes of dyspnea.

A chest x-ray may reveal fluid around the lung and evidence of an enlarged heart, which is also evident on echocardiogram. An elevated pulmonary wedge pressure that is greater than 18 mmHg indicates an increased left atrial pressure associated with heart failure and an increased pulmonary capillary permeability, which means that there is a greater hydrostatic pressure for filtration of fluid.[16]

Management of pulmonary edema usually includes administration of supplemental oxygen. Patients with cardiogenic pulmonary edema may require treatment for associated dysrhythmia or myocardial infarction. After initial management, treatment focuses on reducing pulmonary venous return and systemic vascular resistance.[16] Treatment of noncardiogenic pulmonary edema includes priority care for presenting clinical signs (see the earlier section on treatment of ARDS) and treatment of the underlying cause of the edema.

In children, pulmonary edema may result from a pulmonary contusion (bruising of the lung), causing capillaries to bleed into the alveoli. Initially, no symptoms may present; however, as blood and fluid accumulate, respiratory distress, crackles, fever, wheezing, and hemoptysis may develop. Therapy includes supplemental oxygen, fluid restrictions, pain management, and incentive spirometry. Severe injury to the lungs may require mechanical ventilation.[17] ■

Advanced COPD

In the GOLD classification system, the end stage of **advanced COPD** is stage 4, in which the forced expiratory volume in 1 second divided by the total volume of air the person can forcefully exhale (FEV_1/FVC) is less than 70%, the FEV_1 is less than 30% predicted, or the FEV_1 is less than 50% predicted with chronic respiratory failure (see Table 18.4). Individuals with end-stage COPD are at high risk for type II respiratory failure. COPD is the third leading cause of death in the United States, more than 11 million people being affected each year. More women than men die from COPD, in part because women are more vulnerable to lung damage from cigarette smoking.[18]

Etiology and Pathogenesis

In progressive COPD, distinctions between symptoms of chronic bronchitis and those of emphysema blur. Damage to bronchi, parenchyma, and pulmonary vasculature is widespread; the chronic airflow limitations of COPD reduce the capacity for gas exchange; and pulmonary function deteriorates. The primary damage in chronic bronchitis is to the small bronchi, so the effect on diffusion and the distribution of ventilation is greater and occurs earlier than when emphysematous changes dominate.

Damage to bronchioles increases the disruption of airflow, and hypoxemia occurs because of low alveolar ventilation that is uneven throughout the lung fields, resulting in V-Q mismatch. Type II respiratory failure can develop or worsen as hypercapnia can increase rapidly with exacerbations. In chronic hypercapnia, the renal conservation and production of bicarbonate compensate for the increased carbon dioxide levels and maintain the pH within normal levels.

Individuals with COPD are highly susceptible to infection, and frequent, severe infections further damage the small airways and cause a faster decline in lung function. Airways can become chronically colonized because smoking decreases the numbers and activity of macrophages and neutrophils. **Colonization** means that bacteria are present in the lung but do not cause illness. However, colonization of airways in stable COPD causes greater airway inflammation and increases inflammatory mediators. Pathogens often implicated in colonization include viruses (adenovirus, influenza, parainfluenza, coronavirus, and rhinoviruses), *Chlamydia pneumoniae*, *Pneumocystis jiroveci*, and bacterial pathogens such as *Haemophilus influenzae*, *Streptococcus pneumoniae*, and *Moraxella catarrhalis*.

In stage 4 COPD, pulmonary hypertension develops because of the localized pulmonary vasoconstriction in response to lower oxygen levels. The lower alveolar oxygen levels are diffuse, so vasoconstriction of pulmonary vessels is diffuse as well, but the right heart must pump the blood it receives into the pulmonary vascular bed. Initially, the right heart hypertrophies to generate the increased pressure needed to pump blood through the pulmonary vasculature. As pulmonary resistance and hypertension increase, more blood accumulates in the right ventricle, stretching the muscle fibers to increase the strength of contraction. Cor pulmonale (right heart failure) develops when the right ventricle is stretched or dilated to the point at which it can no longer effectively pump adequate blood through the pulmonary vasculature.

Clinical Manifestations

Acute Exacerbations. With acute exacerbations, symptoms are pronounced and are accompanied by deterioration of lung function. Acute exacerbations are characterized by increased dyspnea and/or cough, increased respiratory rate, and increased sputum volume or prevalence. The change in sputum is often an increased volume and a change in the character of the sputum (e.g., thicker consistency, darker color). The increased cough, dyspnea, and shortness of breath may be accompanied by muscle aches or fatigue, but body temperature may be normal or decreased. With pulmonary function tests, the FEV_1 and vital capacity will be decreased, but changes on chest radiograph will likely be lacking unless pneumonia is present. Other presenting manifestations include accessory muscle use, tachypnea, hypoxemia or hypercapnia above baseline, and failure to respond to current treatment regimen.[19] Exacerbations take a toll on the quality of life as well as morbidity and mortality of individuals with COPD.

Acute exacerbations are the most frequent cause of healthcare visits and hospitalizations for individuals with COPD. As the baseline FEV_1 deteriorates, individuals take longer to recover from exacerbations and might not return to their baseline level on pulmonary function tests or activities of daily living. Older individuals with mucus hypersecretion and a low FEV_1 are more likely to experience multiple exacerbations in a year. Severe exacerbations, particularly when other comorbidities are present (e.g., ischemic heart disease, heart failure, or diabetes mellitus), may result in acute respiratory failure, hospitalization, or death. Acute exacerbations are most often caused by bacterial or viral infections, but 16% of individuals with COPD who are hospitalized may have a pulmonary embolism.[20] Other causes of acute exacerbations include air pollution, smoke, occupational exposures, allergens, and unknown etiologies. Contributing factors have been identified as abnormal coordination of breathing with swallowing, gastroesophageal reflux disease, and defective macrophage phagocytosis of bacteria. Predictors of mortality include patient age, baseline dyspnea severity, previous need for long-term oxygen therapy, altered mental status, FEV_1 score, exercise capacity, and body mass index.[19]

CLINICAL POINT: The six-minute walk test is a helpful assessment tool for patients with cardiopulmonary disease that assesses functional exercise capacity. A distance less than 350 meters is associated with increased mortality for patients with COPD and chronic heart failure.[21] ■

Progression of COPD. The progressive hypoxemia and hypercapnia of advanced COPD are accompanied by increasing symptoms of shortness of breath and dyspnea until the individual is symptomatic at rest. Cough, mucus production, and wheeze may increase as well, and the individual may use pursed lip breathing to assist exhalation. Exhaling through pursed lips is thought to produce a back pressure that helps to support small airway patency during prolonged exhalation. Individuals often sit in a tripod position with their arms supported on chair arms or a table; the tripod position allows them to stabilize their shoulder girdle to better use accessory muscles for breathing. A ruddy complexion is evident when polycythemia is present. Physical activities become limited because of shortness of breath, increased cough, and wheeze with activity. As the COPD advances, retraction of inspiratory muscles between ribs may be seen in thin individuals with the increased work of breathing. The individual's activities of daily living and quality of life become severely impaired, and this limits the person's ability to continue to live at home without the care of a spouse or family member. With development of pulmonary hypertension and cor pulmonale, clinical signs will include cyanosis, ankle edema and edema in other dependent areas of the body, and an increase in the jugular venous pressure.

Tachypnea and polycythemia are compensatory responses seen in advanced COPD. Tachypnea is the result of hypoxemia and the increased oxygen demand of muscles of inspiration; hypoxemia drives an increase in the depth and frequency of respirations. With hyperinflation, the cost of breathing limits increased depth of respirations, so there is an increase in the respiratory rate. In addition, as individuals work harder to breathe, accessory muscles are recruited for inhalation, and they require additional oxygen for the work. The oxygen demand of inspiratory muscles can be greater than the increased ventilation, resulting in **panic breathing**, which is a fast, shallow, ineffective breathing pattern that results when the person has the sensation of air hunger. As individuals feel more panicky with their air hunger, they increase their respiratory rate and the oxygen demand of respiratory muscles, further exacerbating the problem.

Polycythemia is a consequence of hypoxemia as the kidneys increase production of erythropoietin to stimulate production of additional RBCs by the bone marrow. Even though each RBC is not fully saturated with oxygen, the total oxygen content of blood is increased. Unfortunately, polycythemia carries an increased risk for venous stasis, and coupled with the decreased level of physical activity, it puts individuals at risk for venous thrombosis, strokes, and myocardial infarctions.

Linking Pathophysiology to Diagnosis and Treatment

Treatment of advanced COPD is similar to treatment at earlier stages and includes bronchodilators and anti-inflammatory inhaled medications. During acute exacerbations, systemic corticosteroids prescribed for a period of 5–7 days can reduce hospital stays, improve symptoms, and accelerate the recovery of the FEV_1 and lung function. Suppression of inflammation may be important in preventing exacerbation recurrence.[21] Antibiotics can be used to prevent or treat a secondary bacterial infection, but their use in the absence of clinical signs of infection or pneumonia is controversial.

Exercise training programs may help patients to reduce the work of breathing and increase exercise capacity. Frequent, small, high-protein meals may assist in providing energy and preventing excess weight loss. Patients with stage 4 COPD should take steps to protect themselves from extreme temperatures, inclement weather, and poor air quality.[22]

Hypoxemia is characteristic of acute exacerbations, so supplemental oxygen is a critical part of the treatment because increasing the FIO_2 increases the concentration gradient for oxygen diffusion into the blood. Use of noninvasive positive pressure ventilation or mechanical ventilation may be necessary when hypercapnia results in a depressed mental state, profound acidemia, or cardiac arrhythmias. Long-term oxygen therapy is recommended, depending on the presence of severe resting hypoxemia ($PaO_2 \leq 55$ mmHg or peripheral capillary oxygen saturation (SpO_2) $\leq 88\%$) when the patient is stable.[21]

Drew Seligson: Outcome

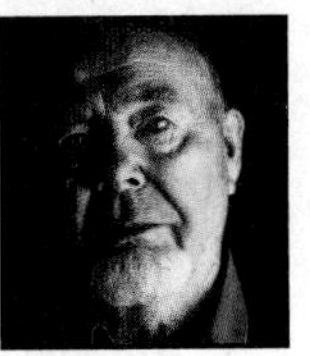

Mr. Seligson recovers slowly from his acute respiratory failure in the context of COPD. He is discharged when his arterial blood gases reflect his pre-pneumonia baseline. As a result of several factors, including immobilization from bedrest, Mr. Seligson is sent to a rehabilitation center for physical therapy. He is discharged after 2 weeks to his home with a plan for frequent visits from his daughter.

6. What teaching to reduce the risk of COPD exacerbations would be important to provide when Mr. Seligson is discharged home?
7. What do you think Mr. Seligson's baseline arterial blood gas results look like?

Check Your Progress: Section 20.3

1. When a patient with COPD begins panic breathing, how would you intervene?
2. Describe the mechanisms that contribute to the hypoxemia that occurs in type I respiratory failure.
3. Explain the importance of identifying whether respiratory failure is type I or type II.

CHAPTER SUMMARY

20.1 Chapter Overview and Case Studies

Define respiratory failure, and describe the concepts related to respiratory failure.

- Respiratory failure is defined as an inadequate gas exchange that is demonstrated by hypoxemia (decrease in arterial oxygen level) with or without hypercapnia (increase in arterial carbon dioxide levels).
- Type I respiratory failure, or hypoxemic respiratory failure, is characterized by hypoxemia without hypercapnia.
- Type II respiratory failure, sometimes referred to as hypercapnic respiratory failure or ventilatory respiratory failure, is characterized by hypoxemia with hypercapnia.
- Acute respiratory failure is an immediate threat to life due to the body's failure to provide oxygen to the tissues. The cardiac system, compensatory systems including acid–base balance, neurologic status, and fluid status are all implicated.

20.2 Respiratory Failure: Type I and Type II

Differentiate the causes, classification, underlying pathogenesis, and clinical manifestations of type I and type II respiratory failure and approaches to diagnosis and treatment of these conditions across the lifespan.

- In type I respiratory failure, the arterial oxygen level (PaO_2) is less than 60 mmHg (8.0 kPa) with a normal or low arterial level of carbon dioxide ($PaCO_2$). A low $PaCO_2$ occurs when the individual, hyperventilating in response to hypoxemia, "blows off" CO_2 with the increased alveolar ventilation.
- In type II failure, the PaO_2 is less than 60 mmHg (8 kPa), and the $PaCO_2$ is equal to or greater than 50 mmHg (6.7 kPa) pressure. Acute type II respiratory failure develops over minutes to hours and results in an acidic pH that is below the normal range because of the increased carbon dioxide (CO_2) with no time for renal compensation to occur.
- In contrast, compensated type II respiratory failure has been present for several days, allowing time for the kidneys to compensate for the increased CO_2. The kidneys conserve and produce additional bicarbonate to buffer the increased hydrogen ions and return the pH to within the normal limits.
- The most common cause of type I respiratory failure is ventilation–perfusion mismatch; it can also be caused by any disorder that impairs oxygenation of blood by blocking airways, decreasing the level of oxygen in inspired air, or shunting deoxygenated blood into oxygenated blood.
- Type I respiratory failure also results from impaired diffusion when the diffusion area is severely decreased (e.g., in advanced emphysema) or the oxygen diffusion pathway is lengthened by an accumulation of fluid, an inflammatory process, or fibrosis.
- Type II respiratory failure is the result of hypoventilation, defined as inadequate alveolar ventilation, and ventilation-perfusion (V-Q) mismatches.
- Mechanisms that contribute to the hypoxemia that occurs in type I respiratory failure include V-Q mismatches, diffusion impairments, shunting of systemic

venous blood to the systemic arterial circulation, and inhalation of a hypoxic gas mixture.

- Type II respiratory failure results from inadequate alveolar ventilation. Normal ventilation removes CO_2 with exhalation and dilutes the remaining alveolar CO_2 with the inhalation of fresh air. With hypoventilation, inadequate amounts of O_2 are inhaled, and levels of CO_2 build up in the alveoli. To maintain a diffusion gradient for CO_2, levels of arterial CO_2 ($PaCO_2$) must increase so that CO_2 will diffuse from blood into alveoli.
- The inadequate alveolar ventilation seen in type II respiratory failure can result from problems anywhere along the pathway from the central nervous system to the respiratory muscles or from deformities of the chest wall or airways.
- The clinical presentation of respiratory failure varies according to the underlying cause, whether the respiratory failure is acute or chronic, and the severity of the failure. Common signs and symptoms include dyspnea, shortness of breath, wheezing, tachypnea, tachycardia, cyanosis, and nonspecific complaints such as chest pain. Additional signs will vary according to the etiology.
- Treatment of respiratory failure is case specific and depends on the underlying cause.

20.3 Disorders Causing Respiratory Failure

Differentiate the causes, classification, underlying pathogenesis, and clinical manifestations of disorders that cause respiratory failure and approaches to diagnosis and treatment of these conditions across the lifespan.

- ARDS is a syndrome of acute, diffuse, severe inflammation with alveolar and capillary wall damage. Critical features of ARDS are an acute onset of dyspnea, progressive hypoxemia in spite of increasing FIO_2, and development of bilateral pulmonary infiltrates on chest x-ray with no evidence of left ventricular heart failure or pulmonary hypertension.
- A precipitating insult disrupts the integrity of alveolar and capillary walls and results in an acute, massive inflammatory response with neutrophils as an essential component. Mechanical ventilation is usually required, and diagnosis is based on the clinical presentation of an acute respiratory failure with bilateral fluffy infiltrates on chest x-ray.
- Pulmonary edema is the accumulation of fluid in the interstitial spaces and alveoli that exceeds the capacity for resorption into capillaries or drainage into lymphatics. The mechanisms that cause pulmonary edema are left ventricular failure, decreased oncotic pressure, capillary endothelial injury, and blockage of lymphatic drainage. Symptoms of pulmonary edema include dyspnea, orthopnea, tachypnea, and tachycardia.
- In advanced COPD, distinctions between chronic bronchitis and emphysema are blurred with widespread lung damage. Pulmonary function and the capacity for gas exchange are decreased, resulting in hypoxemia and hypercapnia. Tachypnea results when hypoxemia drives an increase in respiratory rate to increase oxygenation, and pulmonary hypertension occurs when reduced alveolar oxygen levels cause diffuse vasoconstriction. Diffuse pulmonary vasoconstriction increases the work of the right heart, which initially hypertrophies, then dilates, then fails. Erythropoietin is produced when the kidneys, sensing hypoxemia, stimulate the production of additional RBCs, resulting in polycythemia.
- Acute exacerbations of COPD triggered by infections or environmental or unknown etiologies are characterized by an acute increase in symptoms with a deterioration of lung function. Clinical presentation of acute exacerbations includes a marked change in sputum, increased cough and respiratory rate, and increased dyspnea.

REVIEW QUESTIONS

1. A 45-year-old male presents at the emergency department reporting that he had been smoking a cigarette that fell onto the couch. The couch was reported to have gone up in flames. The client reports that he ran out of the house without sustaining any burns. He is coughing and complains of feeling short of breath. The healthcare provider suspects which of the following?
   a. Respiratory failure type I with findings of PaO_2 55 mmHg and $PaCO_2$ 44 mmHg
   b. Respiratory failure type I with findings of PaO_2 77 mmHg and $PaCO_2$ 45 mmHg
   c. Respiratory type II with findings of PaO_2 55 mmHg and $PaCO_2$ 44 mmHg
   d. Respiratory type II with findings of 65 PaO_2 and $PaCO_2$ 45 mmHg
2. What findings would a healthcare provider expect when assessing a client with type II respiratory failure?
   a. Pulmonary edema, PaO_2 80 mmHg, $PaCO_2$ greater than 50 mmHg
   b. Pulmonary edema, PaO_2 less than 60 mmHg, $PaCO_2$ less than 45 mmHg
   c. Use of narcotics, pH 7.25, $PaCO_2$ 50 mmHg
   d. Use of narcotics, pH 7.45, $PaCO_2$ 45 mmHg

3. When you are mountain climbing with friends, one of your fellow climbers complains of a headache and feeling tired and weak. You conclude that your friend:
   a. is coming down with respiratory influenza.
   b. has an upper respiratory infection.
   c. has type I respiratory failure.
   d. has altitude sickness.

4. What findings would prove that a client with ARDS is responding to treatment? (Select all that apply.)
   a. Increased pulmonary pressure due to improved cardiac output
   b. Decreased ventilator pressure for breaths delivered
   c. Brain natriuretic peptide: A plasma level below 100 pg/mL
   d. Improved PaO_2 with provision of decreased levels of FIO_2
   e. Decreased heart rate

5. In providing care for infants with infant respiratory distress syndrome, which of the following infants should be treated with an initial stabilization with early initiation of CPAP?
   a. A 32-week gestation newborn with clear lung sounds
   b. A 28-week gestation newborn with "ground glass" appearance on x-ray
   c. A 34-week gestation newborn with nasal flaring and grunting respirations
   d. A 30-week gestation newborn with cyanosis and tachypnea

6. While caring for a postsurgical trauma client, the provider assesses bilateral crackles. The $PaCO_2$ is 60 mmHg, and the chest x-ray shows bilateral infiltrates. The provider is concerned that the client is developing:
   a. acute respiratory distress syndrome (ARDS).
   b. left ventricular failure.
   c. pneumonia.
   d. hypocapnia.

7. A healthcare provider assessing a client with a COPD recognizes that the client is losing weight. What would be an unexpected meal indicating that the client does not understand her diet recommendations?
   a. Chicken breast
   b. Spaghetti and marinara sauce
   c. Steak
   d. Peanut butter and celery

8. A healthcare provider working in a clinic setting is providing teaching for a nursing student about COPD. Which of the following statement is appropriate to include?
   a. Clients with chronic COPD commonly develop colonization causing chronic illnesses.
   b. Clients should be instructed to perform purse lipped breathing to prolong inspiration.
   c. Corticosteroids are contraindicated in advanced COPD.
   d. There is an increased risk for developing a deep vein thrombosis from the increased red blood cell production.

ANSWERS

Answers to Review Questions can be found in Appendix A. Answers to Case Study and Check Your Progress questions are available on the faculty resources site. Please consult with your instructor.

RECOMMENDED WEBSITES

American Lung Association
www.lung.org

American Thoracic Society
www.thoracic.org

Boston Children's Hospital
www.childrenshospital.org

CHEST: American College of Chest Physicians
www.chestnet.org

REFERENCES

1. Cutrer, W. B., Castro, D., Roy, K. M., & Turner, T. L. (2011). Use of an expert concept map as an advance organizer to improve understanding of respiratory failure. *Medical Teacher, 33*(12), 1018–1026.
2. Lamba, T. S., Sharara, R. S., Singh, A. C., & Balaan, M. (2016). Pathophysiology and classification of respiratory failure. *Critical Care Nursing Quarterly, 39*(2), 85–93.
3. Sanches, V. S., Santos, F. M., Fernandes, J. M., Santos, M. L. M., Muller, P. T., & Christofoletti, G. (2014). Neurodegenerative disorders increase decline in respiratory muscle strength in older adults. *Respiratory Care, 59*(12), 1838–1845.
4. Nabili, S.N. (2016). Polycythemia (elevated red blood cell count). *MedicineNet.* Retrieved from http://www.medicinenet.com/polycythemia_high_red_blood_cell_count/article.htm

5. Kaynar, A. M. (2016). Respiratory failure treatment & management. *Medscape*. Available at http://emedicine.medscape.com/article/167981-treatment
6. ARDS Definition Task Force, Ranieri, V. M., Rubenfeld, G. D., et al. (2012). Acute respiratory distress syndrome: The Berlin definition. *JAMA, 307*(23), 2526–2533.
7. Bellani, G., Laffey, J. G., Pham, T., et al. (2016). Epidemiology, patterns of care, and mortality for patients with acute respiratory distress syndrome in intensive care units in 50 countries. *JAMA, 315*(8), 788–800.
8. Siegel, M. D. (2016). Acute respiratory distress syndrome: Clinical features and diagnosis in adults. *UpToDate*. Available at https://www.uptodate.com/contents/acute-respiratory-distress-syndrome-clinical-features-and-diagnosis-in-adults
9. Harman, E. M. (2016). Acute respiratory distress syndrome workup. *Medscape*. Retrieved from http://emedicine.medscape.com/article/165139-workup#c6
10. Villar, J., Blanco, J., Anon, J. M., et al. (2011). The ALIEN study: Incidence and outcome of acute respiratory distress syndrome in the era of lung protective ventilation. *Intensive Care Medicine, 37*(12), 1932–1941.
11. Carlucci, M., Graf, N., Simmons, J. Q., & Corbridgem S. J. (2014). Effective management of ARDS. *Nurse Practioner, 39*(12), 35–40.
12. Martin R. (2017). Pathophysiology, clinical manifestations, and diagnosis of respiratory distress syndrome in the newborn. *UpToDate*. Available at www.uptodate.com/contents/pathophysiology-clinical-manifestations-and-diagnosis-of-respiratory-distress-syndrome-in-the-newborn?source=search_result&search=respiratory+distress+in+newborn&selectedTitle=2~150
13. Sovari, A. A. (2016). Cardiogenic pulmonary edema. *Medscape*. Available at http://emedicine.medscape.com/article/157452-overview
14. Khan, A. N. (2015). Noncardiogenic pulmonary edema imaging. *Medscape*. Available at http://emedicine.medscape.com/article/360932-overview
15. Farrar, J., & Sullivan, J. T. (2015). Pulmonary edema in pregnancy. In Pacheco, L. D., Saade, G. R., & Hankins, G. D. V. (Eds.), *Maternal medicine* (pp. 137–154). New York, NY: McGraw-Hill.
16. Brunner, S. (2017). Pulmonary edema: Causes, symptoms, and treatment. *MedicalNewsToday*. Available at http://www.medicalnewstoday.com/articles/167533.php
17. Purohit, P. (2016). Pediatric acute respiratory distress syndrome. *Medscape*. Available at http://emedicine.medscape.com/article/803573-overview
18. American Lung Association. (2013). Trends in COPD: Morbidity and mortality. Available at http://www.lung.org/assets/documents/research/copd-trend-report.pdf
19. Mosenifar, Z. (2017). Chronic obstructive pulmonary disease (COPD). *Medscape*. Available at http://emedicine.medscape.com/article/297664-overview
20. Alvea, F. E., Voets, L. W. L. M., Simons, S. O., de Mast, Q., van der Ven, A. J. A. M., & Heijdra, Y. F. (2016). Prevalence and localization of pulmonary embolism in unexplained acute exacerbations of COPD: A systematic review and meta-analysis. *Chest*, 151(3): 544-554.
21. American Thoracic Society. (2002). *ATS statement: Guidelines for the six-minute walk test*. Available at https://www.thoracic.org/statements/resources/pfet/sixminute.pdf
22. Han, M. K. (2017). Patient education: COPD treatments (beyond the basics). *UpToDate*. Available at https://www.uptodate.com/contents/chronic-obstructive-pulmonary-disease-copd-treatments-beyond-the-basics

Chapter 21

Disorders of Oxygen Transport

Matthew Sorenson

Chapter Outline and Learning Outcomes

21.1 Chapter Overview and Case Studies

Define anemia and discuss concepts related to the disorders of red blood cells.

21.2 Characteristics of Anemia

Describe the morphologic classification, etiology and pathogenesis, and clinical manifestations of anemia and approaches to diagnosis and treatment of the condition across the lifespan.

21.3 Nutritional Deficiency Anemias

Differentiate the causes, classification, underlying pathogenesis, and clinical manifestations of nutritional anemias and approaches to diagnosis and treatment of those conditions.

21.4 Hemolytic Anemia

Differentiate the causes, classification, underlying pathogenesis, and clinical manifestations of hemolytic anemias and approaches to diagnosis and treatment of these conditions.

21.5 Anemia of Chronic Disease

Differentiate the causes, classification, underlying pathogenesis, and clinical manifestations of anemia of chronic disease and approaches to diagnosis and treatment of the condition.

21.6 Polycythemia Vera

Differentiate the causes, classification, underlying pathogenesis, and clinical manifestations of polycythemia vera and approaches to diagnosis and treatment of the condition.

KEY TERMS

Anemia, 514
Anemia of chronic disease (ACD), 527
Aplastic anemia, 526
Erythrocytes, 514
Erythropoietin, 517
Femtoliter (fL), 515
Folate, 521
Folic acid, 515
Hematocrit (HCT), 515
Hemoglobin (Hb), 514
Hypochromic, 514
Iron, 514
Iron deficiency anemia, 520
Macrocytic, 515
Mean corpuscular hemoglobin (MCH), 515
Mean corpuscular volume (MCV), 515
Microcytic, 515
Normochromic, 515
Normocytic, 528
Polycythemia vera, 528
Sickle cell disease (SCD), 523
Thalassemia, 516

ABBREVIATIONS

ACD—anemia of chronic disease
fL—femtoliter
Hg—hemoglobin
HCT—hematocrit
MCH—mean corpuscular hemoglobin
MCHC—mean corpuscular hemoglobin concentration
MCV—mean corpuscular volume
RBC—red blood cell
RDW—red blood cell distribution width
SCD—sickle cell disease

21.1 Chapter Overview and Case Studies

Anemia is a common clinical condition characterized by a reduction in the number of **erythrocytes** (red blood cells) or a decline in the ability of erythrocytes to carry oxygen (**Figure 21.1** ■). Nutritional deficits can contribute to a lack of mature erythrocytes or even to a decrease in the body's ability to manufacture erythrocytes or to produce the necessary protein for oxygen to attach to. Globally, anemia is often associated with a deficiency of iron[1] and other nutritional deficits. **Iron** is a chemical element that plays an important role by forming complexes with molecular oxygen to create **hemoglobin (Hb)** and myoglobin. Blood loss from either traumatic or surgical causes can lead to a loss of erythrocytes, and a state of chronic inflammation can influence how the body uses iron. Regardless of cause, the loss of the ability of erythrocytes to carry oxygen ultimately results in tissue hypoxia. Anemia commonly results from another medical condition; potential causes range from genetic to traumatic to nutritional in nature.

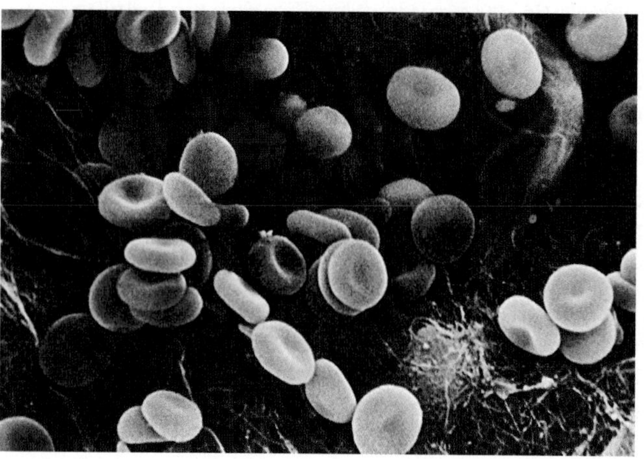

Figure 21.1 ■ Normal red blood cells have a slightly flattened, almost doughnut-like shape.

While anemia is a state of deficiency, in which the blood may lack the necessary number of red blood cells (RBCs), an excess of red blood cells may also exist, resulting in a condition known as polycythemia vera. This results in blood that is more viscous, which can lead to a decrease in the flow of blood that can also deprive organs of necessary oxygen.

Concepts Related to the Pathophysiology of Red Blood Cell Disorders

Anemia is ultimately a disorder of oxygenation. The ability of blood to carry oxygen can be disrupted through a loss of mature erythrocytes or the presence of genetic variation that prevents the formation of mature erythrocytes or hemoglobin. The presence of misshapen erythrocytes can cause the cells to clump together, leading to blockage or slowing of blood flow. This results in ischemia, which causes damage to tissues or organs, and an inability to carry oxygen manifests as hypoxia. In cases of excessive numbers of red blood cells, these cells cause the blood to become thicker, also reducing blood flow to organs and tissue. A concept map of the concepts related to the signs and symptoms of anemia is shown in **Figure 21.2** ■.

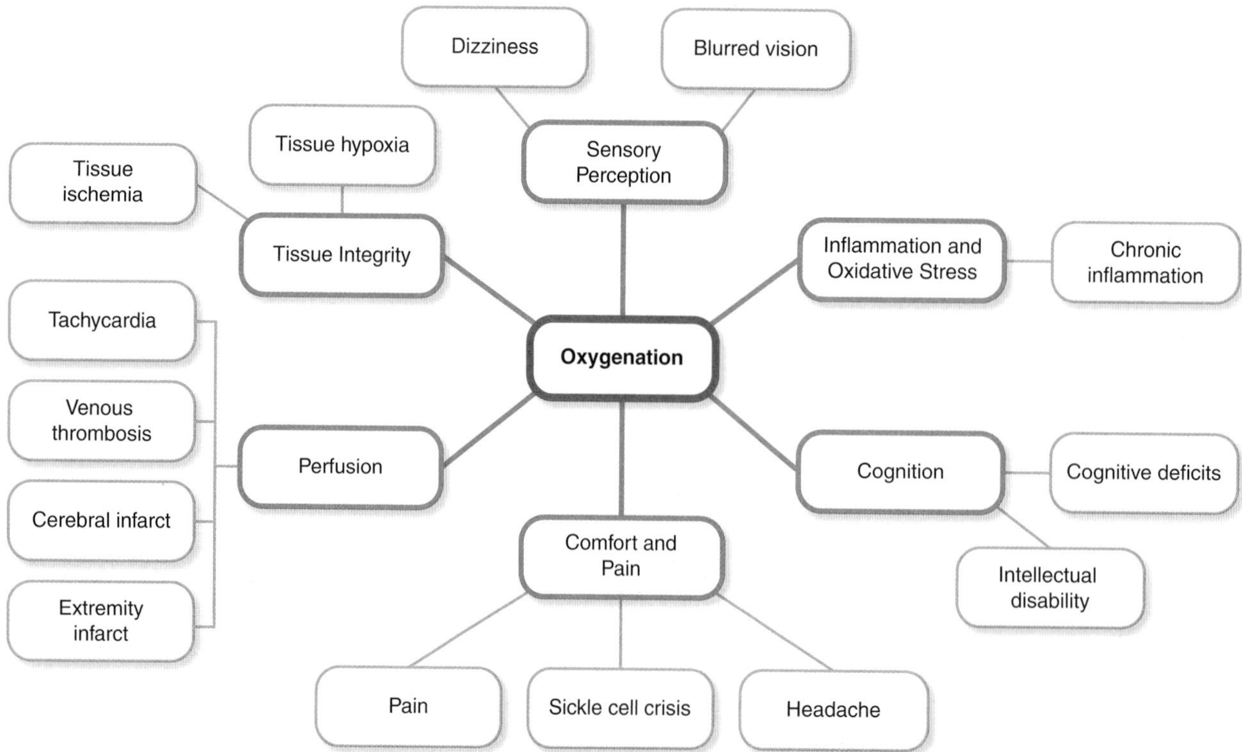

Figure 21.2 ■ Concepts related to the signs and symptoms of anemia.

Case Studies

The pathophysiology involved and the clinical significance of the symptoms experienced by the individuals in the following cases will be addressed throughout the chapter to assist in applying chapter content to clinical situations involving individuals with red blood cell disorders.

Etienne Ngeze: Introduction

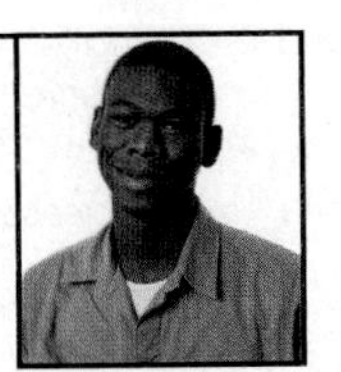

Etienne Ngeze, age 25, presents to the emergency department. Mr. Ngeze and his family emigrated from Rwanda to the United States in 1998. He was admitted to the hospital six times last year with abdominal pain, and he was most recently discharged 2 months ago. He is complaining of abdominal and bilateral lower extremity pain—his usual sites of pain—but also right-sided chest pain. Mr. Ngeze reports that he recently had a "bad cold" that lasted almost 6 weeks and complains that the cough has returned in the past week.

1. Given this patient's history of recurring pain, specifically in certain regions of the body, what is the likely underlying physiologic mechanism that is causing his bouts of pain?
2. Does this patient's ethnicity have any direct correlation with the underlying cause of his pain? Why or why not?

Charles Smith: Introduction

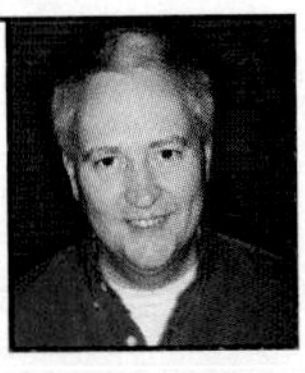

Charles Smith, age 68 presents with a chief complaint of fatigue over the past 2 months. He has a prior medical history of hypertension and type 2 diabetes mellitus, and he is being treated with two medications for hypertension and one for diabetes. He reports feeling easily tired during daily activities but better after resting. Walking more than one block often results in shortness of breath and palpitations. On physical examination, his heart rate is elevated with a strong character. In terms of general appearance, he appears pale.

1. With a chief complaint of fatigue over the past 2 months and difficulty with activities, what is the most likely to be the direct cause of this patient's condition?
2. Which physical symptoms and objective findings corroborate the presence of this condition?

Check Your Progress: Section 21.1

1. What are the defining characteristics of anemia?
2. What is the predominant concern in treating a patient who has anemia?

21.2 Characteristics of Anemia

Anemia can be identified through morphologic characteristics or on the basis of the condition's causing a loss or decreased carrying capacity of red blood cells. The etiology of anemia can be grouped into four broad categories: (1) a decrease in the production of erythrocytes, (2) a reduction in the survival time of erythrocytes, (3) a loss of erythrocytes due to either acute or chronic blood loss, and (4) functional changes in the structure of erythrocytes. Beyond the use of laboratory tests to classify anemia, a number of blood tests are also used to identify the cause or risk for anemia (see **Table 21.1** ■).

Classification of Anemia

The laboratory findings associated with anemia reflect the appearance of certain morphologic characteristics as outlined in **Table 21.2** ■. Morphologic characteristics reflect changes in either the size or the color of an erythrocyte. Color changes are noted through microscopic examination and relate to the ability of the erythrocyte to reflect light. After examination of the morphologic characteristics, attention is then paid to the etiology of anemia.[2]

Morphologic Classification

Changes in erythrocyte size are identified through a measurement referred to as **mean corpuscular volume (MVC)** that reflects the average erythrocyte size. This value is reported in **femtoliters (fL)**, a unit of measure equal to 1 mm^3, and has a normal range of 80–100 fL. The value is determined by dividing the relative **hematocrit (HCT)** (the proportion of red blood cells in a volume of blood) by the number of cells (see **Figure 21.3** ■).

An anemia can be classified as **microcytic** or **macrocytic**, indicating the presence of small or large erythrocytes, respectively. In microcytic anemia, cells are smaller than normal, generally as a result of lack of maturation time or lower levels of iron. Macrocytic anemia (also known as megaloblastic anemia) reflects cells that are larger than normal, generally because of a lack of certain nutrients necessary for successful deoxyribonucleic acid (DNA) replication. When cellular DNA cannot be successfully replicated at the right point of cell division, the cell cannot divide in a timely fashion, and a larger cell emerges from the bone marrow.

Cell color is determined through a measurement referred to as the **mean corpuscular hemoglobin (MCH)**, which is reported in picograms, with a normal range of 27–34 pg. This value is determined through dividing the total mass of hemoglobin by the number of red blood cells. The mass of hemoglobin contributes to the red color of erythrocytes as a result of the presence of iron. Cells with a lower amount of hemoglobin appear washed out and pale and are identified as **hypochromic**. Cells that resemble the normal cell color are referred to as **normochromic**. A normochromic anemia often reflects a decrease in the number of cells through blood loss or premature destruction of erythrocytes.[2]

Etiology and Pathogenesis

The production of red blood cells can be decreased because of a lack of necessary nutritional components for the synthesis of DNA, which leads to continued cell growth with a lack of appropriate cell division. The lack of vitamin B_{12} and **folic acid** (a B vitamin that is necessary for cell maturation and DNA repair) can lead to macrocytic anemia with a disruption of DNA synthesis. A lack of iron can disrupt

Table 21.1 Common Diagnostic and Laboratory Tests for Anemia

Test with Description, Rationale, and Normal Values	Expected Abnormality	Used to Diagnose
Nutritional Measures		
Ferritin	Increased or decreased	Increased values indicate hemolytic anemia Decreased values indicate iron deficiency anemia
Folate (folic acid)	Increased or decreased	Increased values indicate pernicious or vitamin B_{12} deficiency anemia Decreased values indicate hemolytic anemia
Iron	Increased or decreased	Increased values indicate aplastic, hemolytic, pernicious, or vitamin B_{12} deficiency anemia and thalassemia Decreased values indicate iron deficiency anemia
Transferrin	Increased	Increased values indicate iron deficiency anemia
Total iron binding capacity	Increased	Increased values indicate iron deficiency anemia Decreased values indicate hemolytic anemia
Vitamin B_{12}	Decreased	Decreased values indicate pernicious anemia or a lack of intrinsic factor
Red Blood Cell Measures		
RBC count	Low	Anemia
Hemoglobin	Decreased	Anemia
Hematocrit	Decreased	Hemolytic anemia
Mean corpuscular volume (MCV)	Increased or decreased	Increased values indicate larger RBCs (macrocytic) Decreased values indicate smaller RBCs (microcytic)
Mean corpuscular hemoglobin (MCH)	Decreased	Increased values indicate larger RBCs (macrocytic) Decreased values indicate hypochromic anemia
Mean corpuscular hemoglobin concentration (MCHC)	Increased or decreased	Indicates whether cells are hypochromic or hyperchromic
RBC distribution width (RDW)	Increased range	Elevated levels indicate significant variance in cell size often found in iron or folic acid deficiency anemia
Reticulocyte count	Provides an estimate of RBC production	Increased levels can be seen in hemolytic, iron deficiency, and megaloblastic anemia Decreased levels can indicate aplastic anemia or anemia of chronic disease
Genetic-Associated Measures		
Glucose-6-phosphate dehydrogenase	Increased or decreased	Increased levels can indicate pernicious anemia Reduced levels of the enzyme indicate a genetic deficiency
Sickle cell test	Positive	Positive findings indicate the presence of the sickle cell trait or sickle cell disease

Table 21.2 Laboratory Tests and Values Used in Classification of Anemia

Test	Abbreviation	Measures	Values
Hemoglobin	Hb	Protein in RBCs that binds to oxygen	12–17.4 g/dL
Hematocrit	HCT	Proportion of RBCs to total blood cell population	36–52%
Mean corpuscular hemoglobin	MCH	Average mass of hemoglobin per RBC	27–34 pg
Mean corpuscular hemoglobin concentration	MCHC	Concentration of hemoglobin in a select volume of packed RBCs	32–36 g/dL
Mean corpuscular volume	MCV	Average RBC size	80–100 fL
Red blood cell count	RBC	Number of RBCs	4.2–6.1 million cells/mcL
Red blood cell distribution width	RDW	Range of RBC sizes	11.5–14.5

NOTE: Values are a general estimation and may vary depending on the population.

the synthesis of hemoglobin, as is found in cases of iron deficiency anemia and **thalassemia** (a group of genetic disorders that affect hemoglobin). There can also be a reduction in the number of stem cells necessary for maturation, such as found with aplastic anemia. The administration of several classes of medications or the use of radiation in the treatment of cancer can also lead to the destruction of red blood cells and commonly results in anemia.[3]

The survival of erythrocytes can be adversely affected through a process of inflammation or through the presence of genetic influences. Red blood cells have a normal lifespan of 120 days. A decrease in the number of red blood cells

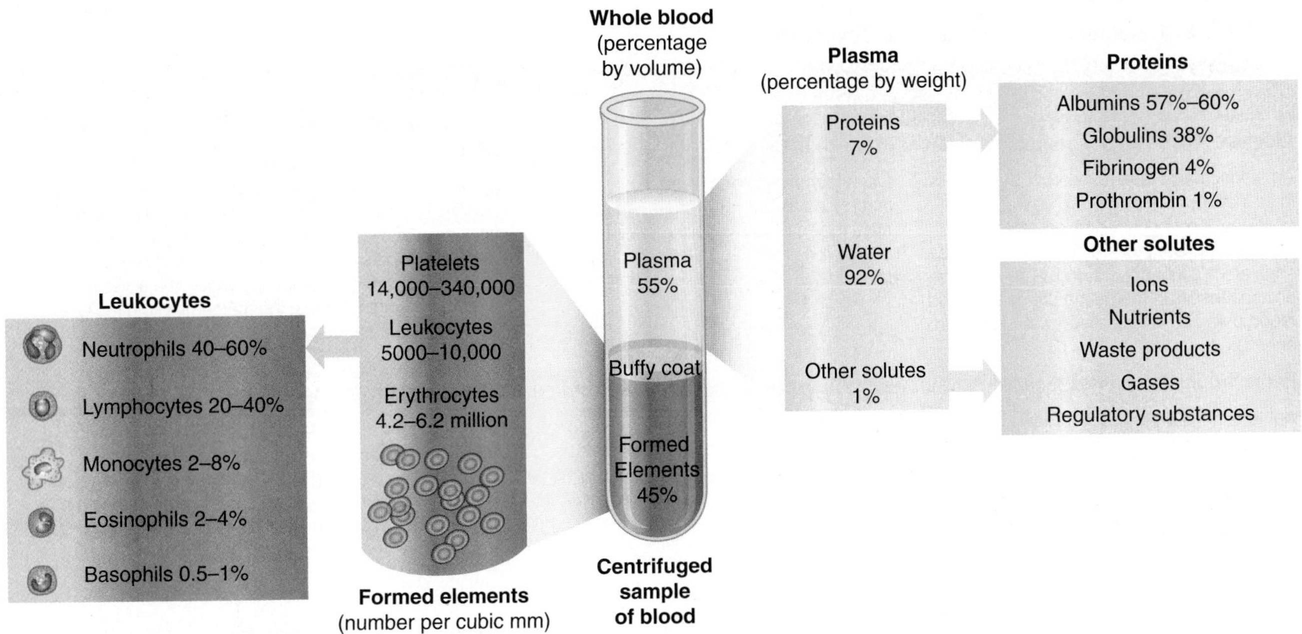

Figure 21.3 ■ Hematocrit and the components of blood.

will often stimulate erythropoiesis, which is the process of production or maturation of red blood cells. In general, the production of new red blood cells matches the process of cell destruction. Defects in the mechanism of red cell blood development will prevent the normal process of erythropoiesis and result in anemia, primarily as a result of the loss of cells through destruction without replacement. In anemia of chronic disease, there is a reduction in the number of erythrocytes along with a shortening of their lifespan, due to the presence of an immune mediator. In individuals with renal disease, there may be a lack in the production of a vital hormone that stimulates the release and maturation of red blood cells. This hormone, **erythropoietin**, is commonly provided in the clinical setting as a pharmacologic therapy to aid in the treatment of anemia. This process of premature destruction of red blood cells is commonly found in hemolytic anemia.[4]

The loss of erythrocytes through blood loss can be acute or chronic. Trauma patients and surgical patients often experience significant blood loss. This acute loss of blood can result in a state of anemia due to the loss of red blood cells. The replacement of blood volume by the use of plasma expanders or intravenous fluids does not replace missing red blood cells. In such cases, blood products are often given to replace the missing cells. Chronic blood loss is often found in individuals with iron deficiency anemia. A chronic gastrointestinal bleed (such as an ulcer), internal or external hemorrhoids, or a heavy menstrual flow can increase the loss of both iron necessary for the maturation of cells and the red blood cells themselves.

Functional changes in the structure of erythrocytes are found in sickle cell disease. In this condition, the red blood cells can appear normal while saturated with oxygen. On the release of oxygen, these cells collapse into a sickled shape. Genetic factors are the primary contributor to the development of this form of anemia and to the development of thalassemia.

Risk factors associated with anemia are several health issues the nurse is likely to encounter. These may be seen in (1) patients with nutritional deficits (iron and B vitamins), (2) patients with intestinal disorders preventing the ability to absorb nutrients, (3) patients with chronic health problems, (4) patients who are pregnant, (5) patients who are experiencing gastrointestinal bleeding, or (6) patients who have genetic risks such as those with sickle cell disease.

There are a number of other anemias that are relatively rare. Many of these syndromes or conditions are associated with mutations in genes necessary for the development of erythrocytes or can be acquired through exposure to certain medications. **Table 21.3** ■ provides a brief overview of selected rare red blood cell disorders.

Clinical Manifestations

The clinical manifestations of anemia occur because of a reduction in the ability of red blood cells to carry oxygen. Physiologically, there is an attempt to compensate for the reduction in oxygen through increases in both heart rate and cardiac output and a shunting of blood flow to vital organs such as the heart and brain. Pulmonary function is also increased through increased respiratory rate and hemodynamic changes in the ability of hemoglobin to bind oxygen. Anemia can be graded on the basis of the amount of hemoglobin in the circulation. More severe levels of anemia result in pallor of the skin and mucous membranes (**Figure 21.4** ■). Cyanosis may not be present, as its appearance reflects deoxygenated hemoglobin rather than a lack of hemoglobin saturated with oxygen. The presence of a headache, dizziness, or light-headedness can reflect the decrease in oxygen delivery to the brain. Compensatory cardiac mechanisms result in tachycardia and possibly ejection murmur. If the anemia is associated with blood loss, orthostatic hypotension may be found. Fatigue is also a common finding

Table 21.3 Additional Red Blood Cell Disorders

Etiology and Pathogenesis	Clinical Manifestations	Linking Pathophysiology to Diagnosis and Treatment
Aldolase A deficiency: A metabolic disorder in which there is a deficit of an enzyme (aldolase A)		
An autosomal recessive disorder that results in an inability to manufacture an enzyme (aldolase A) found in red blood cells and muscle that catalyzes fructose. While the reasons are not fully understood, a deficit in this enzyme results in the premature death of red blood cells and is associated with hemolytic anemia.	Often found in infancy when the infant is introduced to dietary fructose. An acidotic state may develop, resulting in tachypnea, and the child may appear icteric. Hypoglycemia can result in tremors or seizure activity.	Initial testing is a point-of-care test of the urine for sugar. Positive results are followed by more detailed metabolic screening of the urine. Blood results can indicate a decrease in plasma bicarbonate, which is being consumed in a compensatory attempt to counter the acidosis. Further treatment centers on treating the hemolytic anemia and avoiding dietary fructose.
Hemochromatosis: A genetic disorder that results in excessive accumulation of iron, leading to organ damage		
An autosomal recessive disorder on chromosome 6 that affects primarily males of Northern European descent (primary hemochromatosis). Inherited mutations in the HFE (hemochromatosis) gene lead to an extremely high rate of iron absorption. The excess iron then leads to production of large amounts of free radicals causing cellular damage.	Often asymptomatic. Can lead to liver damage, resulting in fatigue, diabetes mellitus, hyperpigmentation of the skin, and joint pain. Symptoms appear later in life and are often the result of long-term liver damage.	Symptoms usually develop in males between 30 and 50 years of age. First presentation is usually severe fatigue accompanied by joint pain. Laboratory tests show elevated serum iron levels and, in the presence of a possible familial history, can include testing for genetic mutations in the HFE gene.[5]
Myelodysplastic syndrome: A group of related conditions in which the production of all blood cell groups are impaired		
A syndrome of diseases closely related to aplastic anemia and leukemia. Often associated with genetic mutations that suppress the development of healthy cell populations in the bone marrow. Can be acquired through exposure to radiation and chemotherapeutic agents.	Patients are often asymptomatic. Generally found later in life when an explainable macrocytic anemia may be accompanied by thrombocytopenia and/or neutropenia. Generally, first signs are fatigue and malaise accompanied by signs of bleeding and infection.	Laboratory testing will reveal findings comparable with a macrocytic anemia in tandem with a reduction in the number of white blood cells and platelets. Bone marrow aspiration is used to obtain cells for genetic evaluation. These findings are then incorporated in classifying the form of disease.[6] Clinical management can involve transfusion of missing cell populations and preventive treatment for infection.
Sideroblastic anemia: A condition in which bone marrow is producing sideroblasts rather than erythrocytes		
Sideroblasts are erythrocyte precursor cells in which iron is found within the cytoplasm of the cell. In this relatively rare condition, iron is readily present but cannot be incorporated into hemoglobin. The disease can be inherited through genetic variation in genes responsible for the synthesis of heme. A less frequent form can be acquired through exposure to certain medications or toxins.	Can present during infancy or later in life. In infants, often associated with failure to thrive and cerebellar signs such as incoordination or ataxia. In adults, often presents first with fatigue, accompanied by hypothermia and visual disturbances. Diarrhea may exist along with muscular weakness.	History and physical assessment findings often lead to laboratory tests such as a complete blood count (CBC) and iron studies. A peripheral blood smear may display mature sideroblasts. Definite diagnosis is through bone marrow aspiration. Extracted cells are stained and evaluated. Clinical management generally begins with the administration of a B vitamin (pyridoxine). In pediatric patients, treatment may include bone marrow transplantation. In cases of acquired sideroblastic anemia, treatment is centered on removal of the possible causative toxin or medication. Transfusion may be used, along with pharmacology therapies designed to remove iron from the circulation.[7]

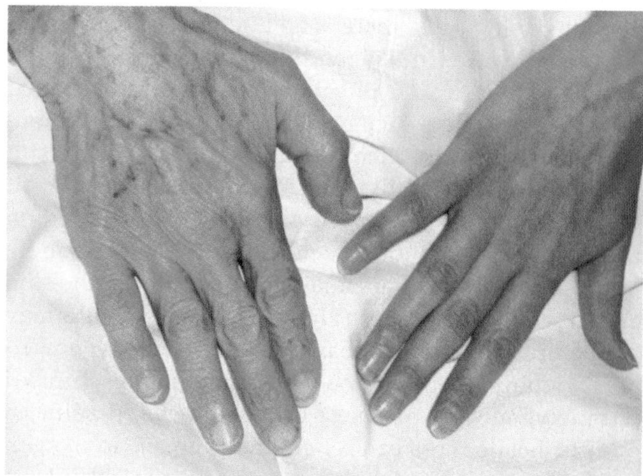

Figure 21.4 ■ The hands of an individual with anemia are paler than those of an individual with normal levels of hemoglobin and hematocrit.

in patients with anemia. The decreased level of oxygen can lead to muscle weakness and generalized fatigue.

Etienne Ngeze: Application

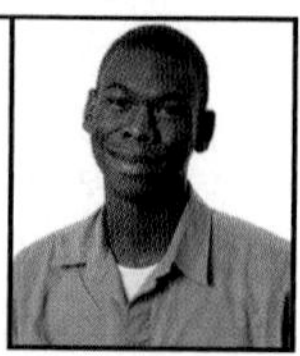

On examination, Mr. Ngeze's vital signs are pulse 100, respirations 28, temperature 101°F, blood pressure 126/74. His breathing is somewhat labored. His oxygen saturation is 92% on 2 L/min via nasal cannula. His conjunctiva, skin, and mucous membranes are pale and slightly jaundiced. He has decreased breath sounds at the right lung base. His heart rate and rhythm are regular, with grade II systolic ejection murmur. His abdomen, especially the left upper quadrant, and extremities are tender to palpation.

3. On the basis of Mr. Ngeze's clinical presentation, which objective findings would indicate that he may be experiencing the physiologic effects of anemia?
4. How does the appearance of slight jaundice correlate with the condition of anemia?

Charles Smith: Application

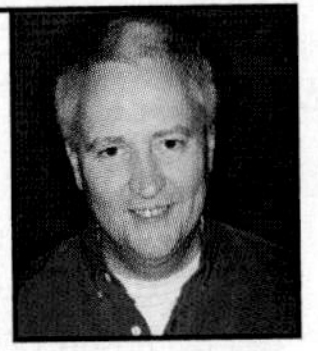

An evaluation of Mr. Smith begins with a thorough history and physical. Blood is drawn for laboratory tests to help identify the potential cause of anemia and to provide a direction for treatment. Because the clinical manifestations of anemia are often found in other medical conditions, a careful evaluation of the patient is necessary to aid in proper diagnosis.

3. Which laboratory tests would be beneficial in helping to determine the nutritional factors that are directly contributing to Mr. Smith's anemia?
4. Mr. Smith's laboratory results show that his MCH is 23 pg. What does this finding suggest?

Linking Pathophysiology to Diagnosis and Treatment

The initial signs and symptoms of anemia are often subtle and resemble those of other medical conditions. Clinically, anemia is identified through a detailed history and physical examination, which includes a complete blood count. Through the analysis of the complete blood count, a classification of the cause of anemia can be initiated, although additional testing is necessary to pinpoint a precise cause. There are several potential risk factors for the development of anemia, reflecting potential genetic causes as well as nutritional deficiencies that can lead to a lack of maturation on the part of red blood cells.

A major risk factor is the loss of blood through surgical interventions or the presence of other chronic disease states such as hemorrhoids or chronic gastrointestinal bleeding. In women, heavy menstruation can lead to anemia through the loss of blood. The body has an increased need for iron in these conditions, and a poor diet could easily exacerbate anemia during these times.

The presence of genetic deficits, such as the lack of intrinsic factor, can prevent the individual from absorbing vitamins (such as B_{12}) that are necessary for the maturation of blood cells. Other genetic variations, such as glucose-6-phosphate dehydrogenase deficiency, adversely affect blood cell maturation through the absence of a necessary metabolic enzyme involved in blood cell maturation. Other genetic conditions, such as thalassemia, directly influence the formation of hemoglobin itself. In cases of sickle cell disease, the cells actually become misshapen at points and are not only lacking in oxygen but also predisposed to clumping together and possibly blocking blood flow within vessels.

Clinically, the risk for anemia and its manifestations can vary.

CLINICAL POINT: During several stages of life, such as pregnancy and older age, it is important to monitor the dietary intake of iron and other nutrients. Otherwise, a nutritional deficiency can quickly result in anemia. ■

In newborn infants, the presence of an Rh incompatibility can place the infant at risk for hemolytic anemia. Rh factor is a protein that appears on the surface of red blood cells. In the case of an incompatibility, maternal antibodies travel across the placental barrier and initiate a process of immune-mediated attack on the red blood cells of the infant. The maternal antibodies are treating the red blood cells of the infant as a foreign antigen. This presents as both a pregnancy and a pediatric consideration. ■

With pregnancy, there is a state of fluid retention resulting in increased blood volume. The increased blood volume can then result in a dilutional anemia. The increase in fluid volume decreases the relative concentration of red blood cells and can lead to complications if untreated. There is also an increased loss of iron during pregnancy, and a poor diet can lead to a lack of adequate nutritional intake, resulting in a nutritional anemia. ■

In older adults, there is often a decrease in the overall amounts of hemoglobin and hematocrit,[8] often as a result of nutritional deficits and reduced fluid intake. This can place the older adult at risk for developing anemia, particularly in conjunction with the development of slow gastrointestinal bleeding, which is a leading cause of anemia in the elderly. ■

In summary, the evaluation of anemia begins with an examination of the laboratory and diagnostic tests to determine the potential cause. For anemia associated with blood loss, the replacement of blood volume may be combined with blood transfusions to replace missing red blood cells. When the cause is related to a lack of iron or vitamin B_{12}, replacement of those nutrients is indicated. The presence of sickle cell trait reflects a potential for risk that requires careful education of the individual to help avoid situations that may precipitate a sickle cell crisis. Clinically, iron supplementation is often combined with other nutritional augmentation to ensure that older adults have adequate stores of these nutrients to help prevent the development or worsening of anemia. Stimulatory factors can be given through injection to help encourage the maturation of red blood cells in order to increase the relative number.

Check Your Progress: Section 21.2

1. What role does vitamin B_{12} play in the formation of red blood cells?
2. How does aplastic anemia ultimately affect the hemoglobin count?
3. List the four broad categories of the etiology of anemia.

21.3 Nutritional Deficiency Anemias

Several nutrients are necessary for the successful maturation and proliferation of red blood cells. Some of these nutrients are stored in the body; others require continual replacement through the diet. The lack of iron and vitamin B_{12} can lead to the development of anemia through effects on cell maturation. The absence of these nutrients can be reliably determined through evaluation of blood tests and cell characteristics.

Impact of Current Research on Clinical Practice

Identifying Disease Risk and Possible Outcome

Description: In a study of 101 patients with myelodysplastic disorders, a means of highlighting the types of cells present in the system known as flow cytometry was used. This technique uses select markers present on all cells to identify the type of cells that are present in the circulation. By using this technique in combination with other methods of disease identification, it is possible to identify what kind of precursor cells are present in the circulation and help to determine whether a certain cell makeup is associated with poorer outcomes for the patient.

Clinical Practice: Myelodysplastic syndromes are a group of hematologic diseases that often result in severe anemia. These disorders are known to be associated with a variety of genetic variations, some of which are very rare, that lead to a decrease in the cells produced by marrow. The results from the study indicate that using this technique in combination with other clinical assessments can help to distinguish the patients who may have a poorer prognosis and can aid in verifying the diagnosis. This approach may be useful in clinical settings to ensure appropriate diagnosis and identify those patients most at risk. Having this information ahead of time will allow for more effective planning of care and early treatment.

Research Study:

Reis-Alves, S. C., Traina, F., Harada, G., Campos, P. M., Saad, S. T. O., Metze, K., & Lorand-Metze, I. (2013). Immunophenotyping in myelodysplastic syndromes can add prognostic information to well-established and new clinical scores. *PLoS One*, *8*(12), e81048. doi: 10.1371/journal.pone.0081048

Iron Deficiency

Iron is a necessary element in the function of several metabolic mechanisms. In particular, iron is a major component of hemoglobin and is responsible for the binding of oxygen. Deficits in iron level can then result in a reduction of the ability to bind oxygen. After consumption, iron is absorbed through the small intestine by multiple pathways. Iron deficiency anemia occurs when the blood lacks adequate healthy red blood cells as a result of a lack of iron.

Etiology and Pathogenesis

Iron deficiency anemia can occur through either a reduction in dietary iron or a loss of iron (**Figure 21.5** ■). A reduction in dietary iron can occur through malabsorption of iron through the gastrointestinal tract or through reduced dietary intake. The loss of iron most commonly occurs through hemorrhage, menstrual blood loss in females, and gastrointestinal bleeding in males and females.

Reduced intake or usability of iron contributes to a state of anemia that is found in approximately 20–30% of the global population. Iron is lost continually through sweat and other bodily elimination processes. This necessitates a consistent resupply of iron through the diet. In terms of hemorrhage, 2 mL of whole blood contains 1 mg of iron. Even a minor hemorrhagic state can then induce a significant loss of iron. The primary means of chronic blood loss are gastrointestinal bleeding and loss through the genitourinary system. As the individual ages, a process of chronic minor blood loss can develop through gastrointestinal ulcers or the development of hemorrhoids. This loss of blood may not appear immediately significant, but in conjunction with other medical issues, it can lead to an insidious onset of iron deficiency anemia. (See Nutrition in Clinical Practice.)

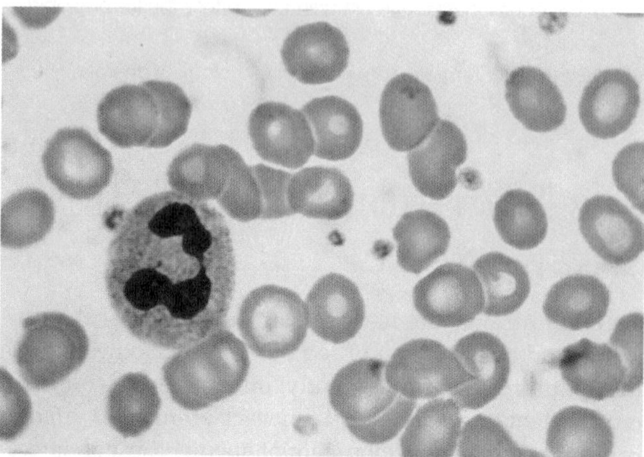

Figure 21.5 ■ In iron deficiency anemia, the erythrocytes are paler and often misshapen in comparison with normal erythrocytes.

The presence of gastrointestinal disorders and their treatment can significantly influence the acidity of the stomach. The pH of the gastrointestinal tract significantly influences the absorption of iron. At normal pH, ferrous iron is oxidized into the ferric form. A lower gastric pH enhances the absorption of ferric iron. A higher gastric pH can significantly reduce the absorption of iron. The administration of gastrointestinal agents, such as proton pump inhibitors and histamine blockers, can influence the pH of the stomach and reduce the absorption of iron.

Iron deficiency anemia is characterized at first by a gradual reduction in hematocrit and hemoglobin. As the loss of iron becomes more significant, the development of erythrocytes is affected, and the cells become microcytic in nature and hypochromic.

Cobalamin Deficiency

Cobalamin (vitamin B_{12}) is a water-soluble vitamin that is necessary for cell metabolism. All cobalamin is obtained through dietary sources, particularly foods derived from animal sources. Once consumed, cobalamin becomes bound to a protein secreted by gastric partial cells, known as intrinsic factor. The complex formed between cobalamin and intrinsic factor then travels through the intestine and is absorbed. After absorption, cobalamin is carried in the plasma and stored in the liver. Intrinsic factor is therefore a necessary step in the utilization of cobalamin; changes in the release or absorption of this factor can have adverse effects on red blood cell function.

Impact of Nutrition in Clinical Practice

Dietary Considerations of Iron Deficiency Anemia

Joanne Kouba

Nutritional anemias result from sustained inadequacies of nutrients that are key to red blood cell production. Iron, vitamin B_{12}, and folic acid are the primary nutrients involved. The Dietary Reference Intakes (DRIs) are a set of nutrient recommendations that include the Recommended Dietary Allowances (RDAs) established by the Institute of Medicine by gender, age, and other life situations. The RDA for iron varies considerably from 8 mg/day for adult men to 27 mg/day for pregnant women.[1]

Both heme and nonheme food sources may contribute to dietary iron intake. Beef, pork, lamb, and poultry provide heme iron sources from hemoglobin in animal tissues. This source of dietary iron is better absorbed (15–35%) than nonheme iron (2–20%).[2] However, most of the iron that Americans consume is the nonheme form from iron-fortified cereals, iron-fortified infant formulas, legumes, and leafy greens.[2] It should be noted that iron bioavailability from breast milk is excellent. Nonheme iron absorption is enhanced by animal protein and a rich source of vitamin C at the same meal. However, this can be decreased by ingestion of tannins (a compound in tea), phytates (in whole grains), and calcium. The following table summarizes the iron content of some common foods.[2]

Iron Content of Selected Foods[2]

Food	Serving Size	Iron (mg/serving)	% Daily Value
Ready-to-eat cereal, iron fortified	3/4 cup	18.0	100
Lentils, boiled	1 cup	6.6	35
Beef, chuck	3 oz	3.2	20
Spinach, boiled	1/2	3.2	20
Chicken, breast	3 oz	1.1	6
Whole wheat bread	1 slice	0.9	6

Excess intake of iron, like that of many other elements, can be toxic. The DRIs contains a category known as the tolerable upper limit (TUL), which indicates the level at which chronic intake, if exceeded, may be dangerous. The TUL for iron ranges from 40 mg/day for healthy infants older than 7 months of age to 45 mg/day for adults.[2] For this reason, care should be taken to keep supplemental sources of iron tightly capped and away from children. However, higher doses may be advised to treat deficiency states.

A recent analysis of data from the Women's Health Initiative found the prevalence of anemia to be 5.5% in the cohort of 93,676 postmenopausal women.[3] Women with anemia had lower intakes of glucose, protein, folate, vitamin B_{12}, iron, vitamin C, and red meat than women without anemia. In addition, those whose diets were deficient in three or more nutrients had a 44% increased risk for anemia compared to those with adequate nutrient intakes.[3] While the authors noted that the exact amount of anemia attributable to dietary factors could not be determined, inadequate nutrient intake is linked to anemia in postmenopausal women, a group that is not usually considered to be at risk for this condition. In addition, they urge clinicians to carefully evaluate anemia in this population, including assessment of dietary quality for iron, folate, and vitamin B_{12}.

References

1. Institute of Medicine. Food and Nutrition Board. (2001). *Dietary reference intakes for vitamin A, vitamin K, arsenic, boron, chromium, copper, iodine, iron, manganese, molybdenum, nickel, silicon, vanadium and zinc*. Washington, DC: National Academies Press.
2. National Institutes of Health. (2016). *Iron: Dietary supplement fact sheet*. Retrieved from Office of Dietary Supplements website: https://ods.od.nih.gov/factsheets/Iron-HealthProfessional
3. Thomson C. A., Stanaway J. D., Neuhouser M. L., et al. (2011). Nutrient intake and anemia risk in the Women's Health Initiative observational study. *Journal of the American Dietetic Association, 111*, 532–541.

Etiology and Pathogenesis

Cobalamin plays an essential role in the synthesis of DNA within red blood cells. Without cobalamin, the synthesis of DNA is disrupted, leading to a cell that cannot divide but continues to grow. Cobalamin deficiency then results in a macrocytic condition with misshapen erythrocytes.

In pernicious anemia, an autoimmune-mediated process leads to a loss of gastric parietal cells. The loss of these cells then leads to a decrease in the secretion of intrinsic factor, with resultant anemia through an inability to properly absorb cobalamin. The autoimmune response can also contribute to weakening of the intestinal wall. Other potential contributing factors include the administration of medications that influence partial cell function; these include gastrointestinal agents, such as histamine receptor antagonists, and proton pump inhibitors. Diseases of the bowel, such as celiac disease, gastritis, or Crohn disease, can also adversely affect the absorption of cobalamin. The disease generally develops over a significant period of time, often taking several months until symptoms appear.[9]

Folic Acid Deficiency

Folic acid, which is obtained primarily through the consumption of fruits and leafy green vegetables, is a necessary component in the synthesis and repair of DNA. Folic acid works in conjunction with cobalamin, and in its absence, a macrocytic anemia can result. After consumption, folic acid is converted into an active form known as tetrahydrofolic acid (THFA). This active form then interacts with other vitamins (niacin, cobalamin, and vitamin C) and is involved in the synthesis of red blood cell DNA (**Figure 21.6** ■) and formation of the heme component of hemoglobin.[10]

Etiology and Pathogenesis

As with cobalamin, folic acid is stored in the liver in sufficient amounts to cover physiologic needs for approximately 3 months; this accounts for a more chronic, insidious presentation. Medications that antagonize **folate** (a B vitamin that is essential for maintenance of DNA) can contribute to the development of anemia. These medications are commonly used in the treatment of cancer or serve as antibiotics.

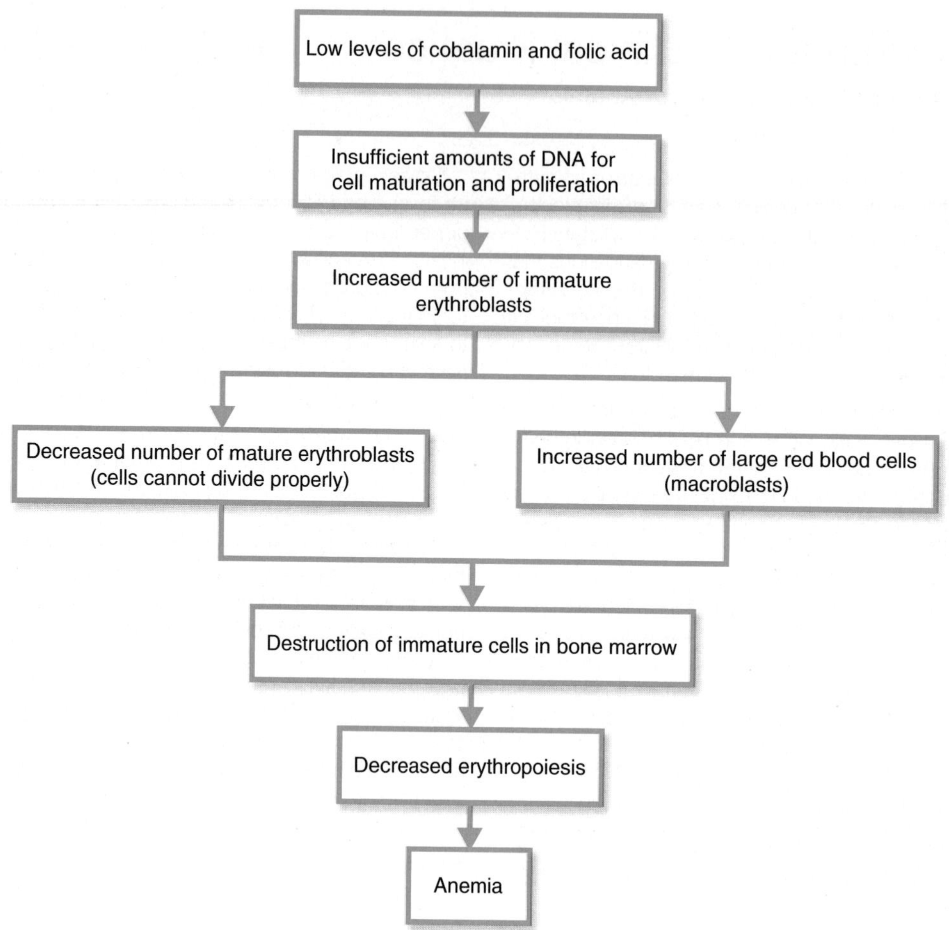

Figure 21.6 ■ The role of folate and cobalamin in erythrocyte maturation and DNA synthesis.

CLINICAL POINT: Folic acid requirements are increased in pregnant women and women who are breastfeeding. These requirements can place these individuals at increased risk for the development of folic acid deficiency. ■

Linking Pathophysiology to Diagnosis and Treatment of Nutritional Anemias

The treatment of anemia depends to an extent on the severity of the anemia. When the cause of anemia is nutritional, treatment is twofold. The first step is providing supplementation to address the nutritional deficiency that is contributing to the development of anemia. The patient's diet should be evaluated to determine the missing components. Dietary supplements are then given in the form of B vitamins, folic acid, or iron to correct the deficiency. Then the lack of red blood cells could be addressed through the administration of red blood cells to rectify decreased hematocrit and hemoglobin or through the administration of pharmacologic agents to increase the number of red blood cells. Issues that may contribute to a nutritional deficiency, such as a lack of income or the use of alcohol, should also be evaluated and addressed. Alcohol abuse can contribute to a loss of several B vitamins that are necessary for erythrocyte maturation and function.

Check Your Progress: Section 21.3

1. How does chronic blood loss through gastrointestinal bleeding eventually lead to iron deficiency anemia?
2. What is the role of gastric parietal cells in ensuring that the body receives enough vitamin B_{12} for RBC production?
3. A deficiency in folic acid can result in which potential outcome?

21.4 Hemolytic Anemias

Hemolytic anemia begins with the destruction or hemolysis of red blood cells. This can occur through a process of physical trauma and stress to cells, as is seen in sickle cell disease, or a disruption in the formation of hemoglobin (as in thalassemia) or through an immune-mediated process (as in transfusion reactions, autoimmune reactions). Hemolytic anemia has signs and symptoms similar to those of other forms of anemia but includes jaundice. Bilirubin is released through the process of hemolysis and contributes to the development of jaundice seen in patients with hemolytic anemia.[11]

Hemolytic anemia can result from an autoimmune process in which antibodies are produced that then target red blood cells. These autoimmune reactions can occur in individuals with other autoimmune diseases or can be stimulated through the administration of selected medications.

Furthermore, certain viral infections can lead to a disruption of the red blood cell, eliciting a state of anemia.

Sickle Cell Disease

Sickle cell disease (SCD) is a cluster of autosomal recessive disorders that results in misshapen forms of hemoglobin that resemble a sickle or crescent in shape (**Figure 21.7** ■). The genetic mutation results in a structural change in the beta-globin gene in which glutamic acid is exchanged for the amino acid valine. This change in structure prevents hemoglobin from forming an appropriate shape. Sickle cell disease occurs when an individual has inherited a mutated form of hemoglobin referred to as hemoglobin S (HbS) from both parents. When a mutated form is inherited from one parent and a normal copy (hemoglobin A) is inherited from the other, this is referred to as sickle cell trait[12] (**Figure 21.8** ■).

Etiology and Pathogenesis

The beta-globin gene, found on chromosome 11, is responsible for the structure of hemoglobin. When the gene is damaged, the structure of hemoglobin cannot bind oxygen effectively. In sickle cells, the hemoglobin can bind oxygen, but when oxygen is released, the cell collapses into a sickle shape (**Figure 21.9** ■). These cells are more rigid and less pliable than normal erythrocytes. Because of their rigid and hooked shape, these cells are more prone to grouping

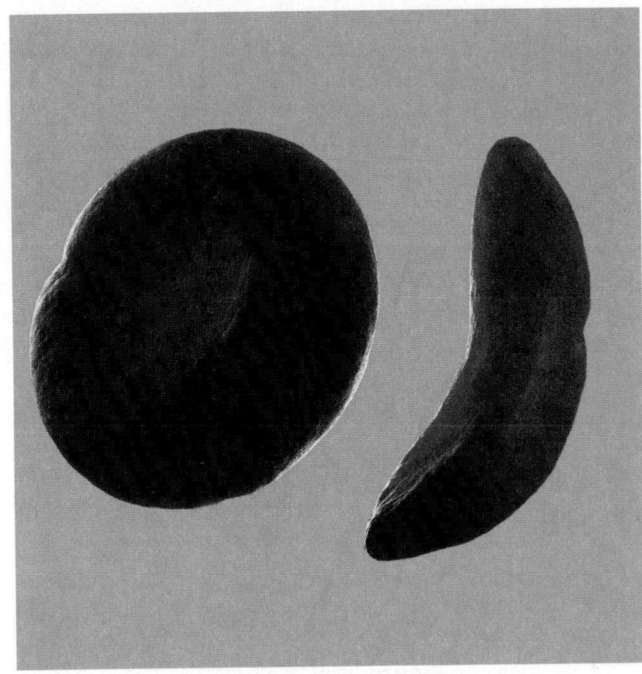

Figure 21.7 ■ Sickle cells have a characteristic shape once oxygen has been released from the cell. This allows for the identification of the condition through microscopic evaluation of the blood.

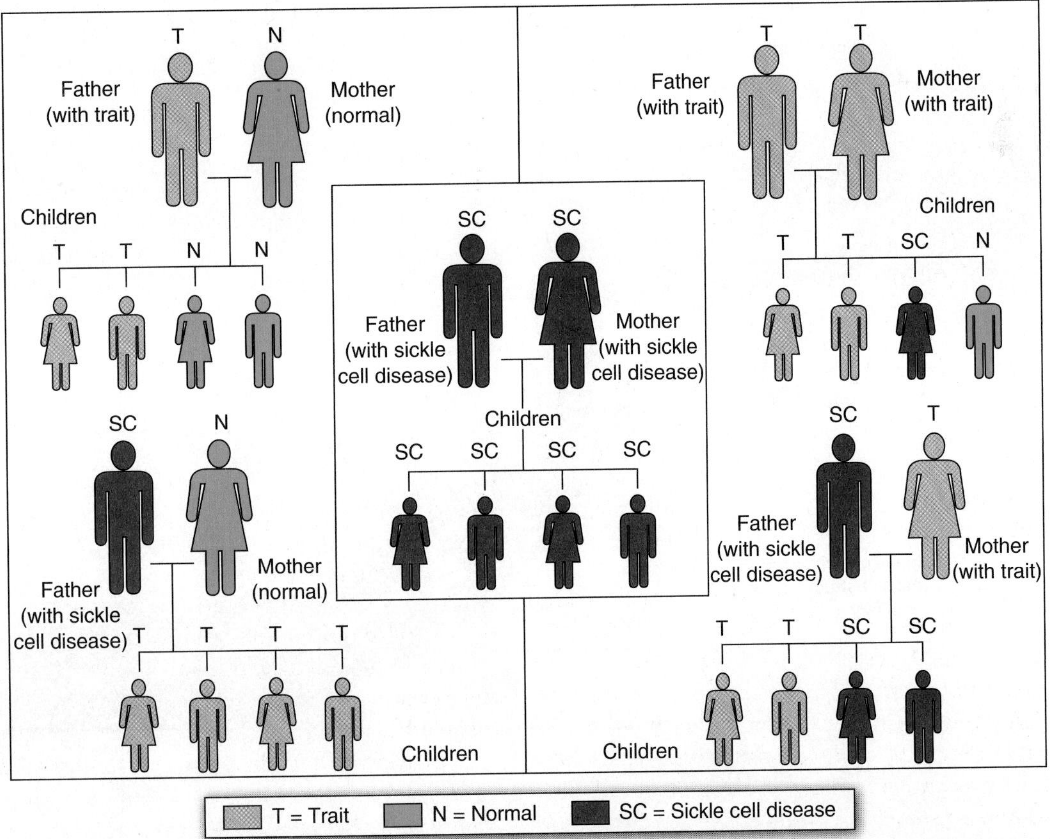

Figure 21.8 ■ Genetic transmission of sickle cell trait and disease.

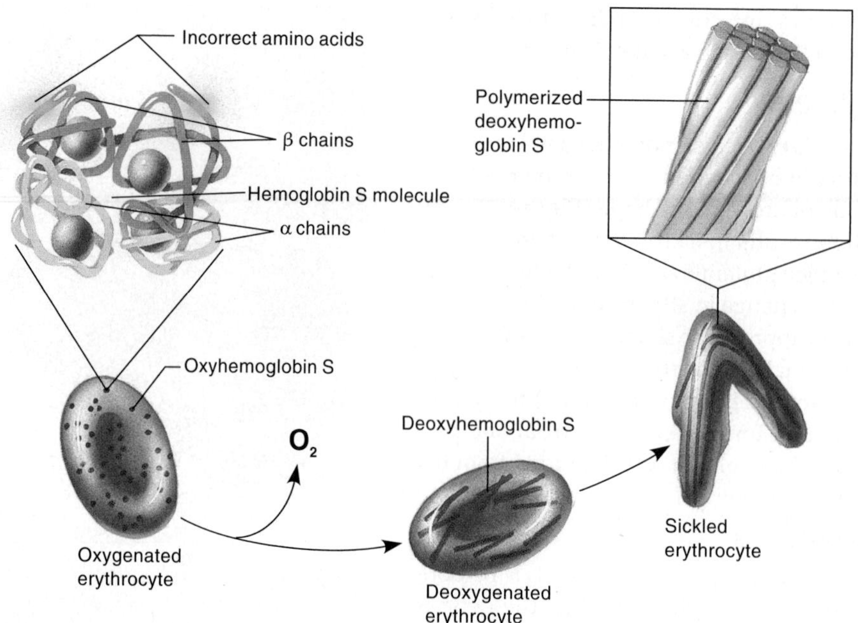

Figure 21.9 ■ Sickle cell disease is caused by an inherited autosomal recessive defect in hemoglobin synthesis.

or clumping together. When this occurs, the flow of blood can become obstructed, and hypoxia can result from decreased flow (**Figure 21.10** ■). This is referred to as vaso-occlusive phenomenon, and it can produce a state of crisis in those with sickle cell disease.

When the sickle cell takes up oxygen, it can return to a more normative shape. When it releases the oxygen, the cell becomes misshapen again. This repeated process of cell stress contributes to the significantly shortened lifespan of sickle cells. While most red blood cells have a lifespan of 120 days, those found in sickle cell disease have a lifespan of between 10 and 20 days. The cells are then hemolyzed, with resultant anemia as cells are destroyed faster than the body can produce more red blood cells. The

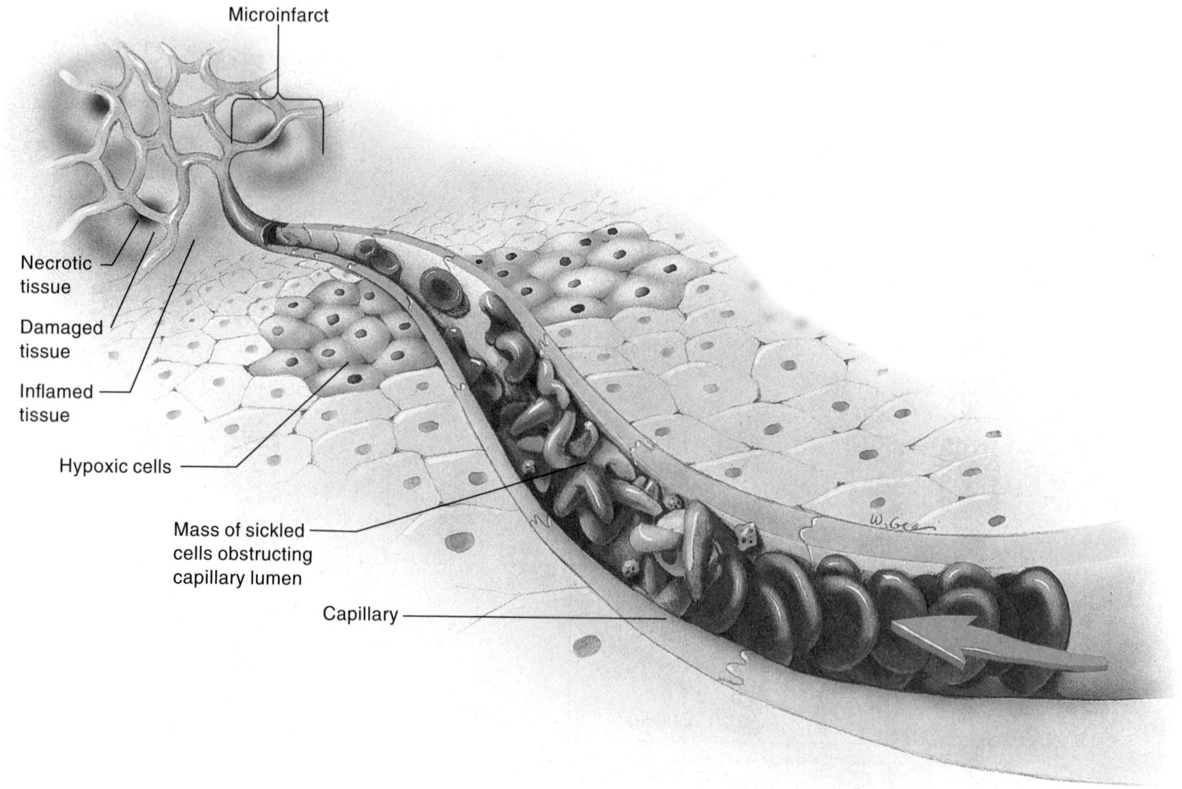

Figure 21.10 ■ Sickle cell disease is characterized by episodes of acute painful crises that are triggered by conditions that cause high oxygen demand.

need to continually produce more erythrocytes also leads to a chronic state of inflammation as inflammatory mediators are released in a compensatory response to stimulate the production of more red blood cells.[9]

The sickle cells can also group together within the lung or brain, contributing to pulmonary obstruction and potentially stroke. The spleen is often a site of damage, as the clumped together complexes of cells congregate there. Over time, a vaso-occlusive phenomenon occurs within the spleen, leading to scarring and atrophy.

Clinical Manifestations

The hypoxia that can result from groups of sickle cells clumping together and obstructing blood flow often causes tissue ischemia. The ischemia can lead to the development of a significant level of pain that can manifest anywhere in the body. The back, chest, and extremities are the most common pain sites. The pain is accompanied by other signs of ischemic damage, such as swelling, tenderness, a rapid respiratory rate and hypertension. The presence of anemia, chronic tissue hypoxia, and tissue damage can result in several significant complications (see **Figure 21.11** ■).

Linking Pathophysiology to Diagnosis and Treatment

Treatment of SCD involves prevention, screening, supportive care, disease-modifying strategies, and curative procedures. Genetic analysis, prenatal counseling, and multidisciplinary strategies are available for individuals with sickle cell trait and those at risk for the development of SCD.

Supportive care for individuals with SCD includes avoidance of risk factors and maintenance of adequate hydration and oxygen to decrease the risk of hemoglobin polymerization. Blood transfusion may be needed in some situations. Transfusion is not only beneficial in the raising of hemoglobin levels; it also provides a significant increase in the relative percentage of normal hemoglobin. At times, a procedure known as erythrocytapheresis may be performed, in which red blood cells are exchanged with the intent of replacing damaged cells with cells free from the mutated form of hemoglobin (HbS) found in sickle cell disease. In addition, because of the inevitable occurrence of vaso-occlusive crisis and the pain it entails, chronic pain management is a major component of treatment. Often, this involves the use of opioid analgesics and the accompanying risk of dependence, tolerance, and addiction.

The nature of SCD requires the need for transfusions but also heightens the risk of complications from multiple transfusions. The misshapen hemoglobin causes stress within the erythrocyte, contributing to the release of chemically active molecules referred to as reactive oxygen species that play an important role in oxidative stress. These can lead to the damage and destruction of cell membranes. Repeated transfusions can lead to a state of iron overload, which contributes further to oxidative cell stress.

The only disease-modifying therapy that has been approved for the treatment of SCD is hydroxyurea. Hydroxyurea is a cytotoxic drug that stimulates the formation of normal hemoglobin and reduces the production of HbS. The effect of the drug is related to its ability to bind metals; it inhibits ribonucleic reductase by binding its two iron molecules, inactivating a critical tyrosyl radical and decreasing production of RBCs containing an increased level of HbS. This in turn reduces the amount of sickling and is a potent modifier of disease activity.

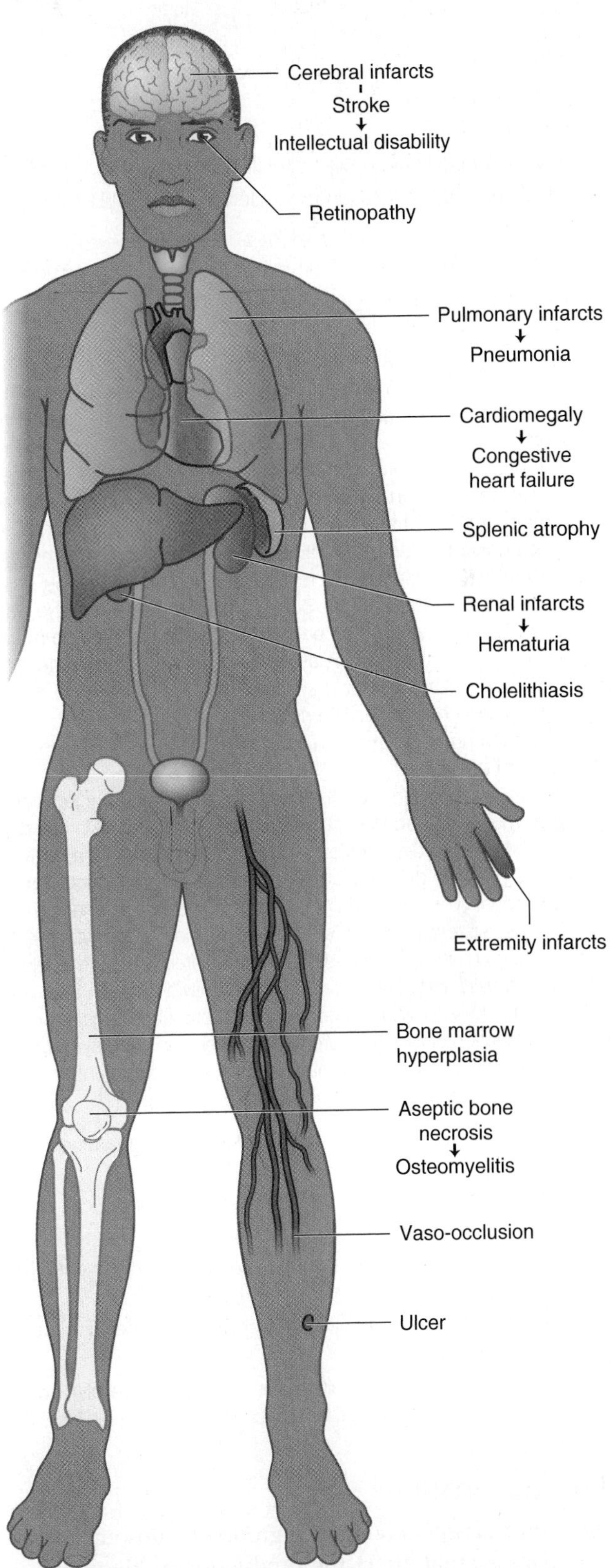

Figure 21.11 ■ Manifestations and complications associated with sickle cell disease.

Etienne Ngeze: Outcome

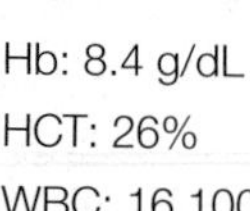

Mr. Ngeze has been admitted to the hospital. His laboratory findings include the following:

Hb: 8.4 g/dL

HCT: 26%

WBC: 16,100

Reticulocytes: 3%

Platelets: 475,000

Sickle and target cells and Howell–Jolly bodies present on PBS

LFTs: hyperbilirubinemia (unconjugated); increased LDH

Absent haptoglobin

Hemoglobin electrophoresis shows 90% HbS, 8% HbF, and no HbA

CXR: infiltrate right lower lung field

These findings indicate reduced hemoglobin and hematocrit in conjunction with elevation in the numbers of white blood cells and platelets. The findings support the presence of anemia along with infection. The elevated reticulocyte count indicates an increase in the number of immature erythrocytes, a finding that reflects anemia. Such an elevation indicates increased activity on the part of bone marrow in an attempt to compensate for the lack of mature red blood cells. The lack of haptoglobin helps to identify hemolytic anemia, and the presence of Howell–Jolly bodies and sickle cells indicate that the cause is sickle cell disease. Taken as a whole, the laboratory findings confirm the presence of sickle cell disease along with infection. Infection often is associated with the development of sickle cell crisis. This patient presented with abdominal pain along with right-sided chest pain. The right-sided chest pain could reflect underlying pneumonia, while the abdominal pain is a component of his standard pain crisis.

Treatment would include the use of supplemental oxygen along with pain management. Pain crisis in individuals with sickle cell disease is often tied to dehydration, and fluid supplementation is given to address possible dehydration. Pain management would start with acetaminophen for mild pain and progress to opioid therapy for moderate to severe pain levels. Transfusion may be considered to correct the low hemoglobin and hematocrit. Often, elevated levels of white blood cells and platelets are found in individuals with SCD and reflect an underlying inflammatory state. These elevations may not require correction unless they are tied to other signs and symptoms. Such patients require close monitoring for the development of other complications and to ensure effective treatment of pain.[13]

5. Why would a patient with sickle cell disease display tachycardia?
6. What can contribute to the elevated white blood cell count found in this patient?
7. The patient's platelet count is elevated. Why would this occur?
8. Would altitude affect the individual with sickle cell disease? If so, in what way?
9. In the patient's laboratory results, the presence of Howell–Jolly bodies is noted. What are they?

Thalassemia

The term *thalassemia* refers to a group of autosomal recessive diseases that affect the production of hemoglobin. There is an increased incidence of thalassemia in individuals from the Mediterranean area and parts of Asia.

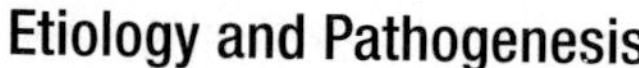

Etiology and Pathogenesis

In thalassemia, there is a defect in production of one or more of the globin chains. Hemoglobin comprises four protein chains: a set of two alpha chains and two beta chains. Thalassemia is referred to either alpha-thalassemia or beta-thalassemia, indicating which chains of hemoglobin are disrupted. In beta-thalassemia, a mutation of a gene on chromosome 11 is the causative agent, while in alpha-thalassemia, the mutation occurs on chromosome 16. Ultimately, there is a disruption of hemoglobin synthesis, resulting in a microcytic and hypochromic anemia. (See Genetics and Genomics for Clinical Practice.)

Clinical Manifestations

In thalassemia, the genetic effects often result in other defects being present at birth. Growth retardation and cognitive deficits can occur, thalassemia often being identified early in infancy. As with other hemolytic anemias, jaundice can also be present owing to the premature destruction of red blood cells. The cells are subject to early death because of the defective structure of hemoglobin and unstable cell membranes. The death of cells stimulates the production of more red blood cells in the bone marrow, and the immaturity of the cells can result in their remaining within the marrow. The accumulation of immature cells in the bone marrow can influence the production of other cells and enlarge the bone (**Figure 21.12** ■).

Aplastic Anemia

The term *aplastic* refers to a decrease in all cell populations produced by the bone marrow. This includes erythrocytes, leukocytes, and platelets. **Aplastic anemia** occurs when the body stops producing enough new blood cells. It is often associated with genetic causes but also can be acquired though viral exposure or the administration of drugs or toxins. Aplastic anemia is relatively rare, and in a high percentage of cases, a cause cannot be identified.

Etiology and Pathogenesis

The primary mechanism is an immune-mediated attack on the bone marrow. Activated T cells lead to a process of apoptosis (programmed cell death) within the bone marrow. These apoptotic processes result in a relative depletion of both immature and stem cell populations within the bone marrow.[14] Individuals with aplastic anemia are also at risk for the development of infection and bleeding as a result of the loss of lymphocytes and thrombocytes along with erythrocytes.

In terms of clinical evaluation, decreases in the white blood cell and platelet counts are found concomitant with a reduction in hemoglobin and the number of red blood cells. This condition is then classified as a normocytic, normochromic anemia in that the size and relative color of red blood cells are not changed.

Genetics and Genomics for Clinical Practice

Genetics and Red Blood Cells

Rita Kaspar

The development and growth of red blood cells are heavily influenced by genetic factors.[1] Most of the encoding of hemoglobin involves a cluster of genes located on chromosome 16. Adult hemoglobin consists of protein subunits referred to as alpha-globin and beta-globin, which are encoded by the gene *HBB* (hemoglobin-beta). There are numerous variations that can occur in the *HBB* gene, the most common of which leads to the manufacture of an abnormal form of hemoglobin (HbS) that replaces the normal adult hemoglobin. This is the mechanism behind sickle cell disease. Changes in the structure of beta-globin are associated with sickle cell disease, while the absence of the beta unit is associated with a form of beta-thalassemia. Fetal hemoglobin is formed through the influence of two gamma-globin genes (*HBG1* and *HBG2*). Normally, fetal hemoglobin is replaced by adult hemoglobin after birth. Changes in the structure of *HBG2* (hemoglobin subunit gamma 2) can lead to continued production of the gamma globins into adulthood, which replace normal adult hemoglobin.[2] This is often found in cases of beta-thalassemia. In cases of alpha-thalassemia, variation is often found in the ability to manufacture hemoglobin through mutations in genes that encode for hemoglobin proteins: HBA1 (hemoglobin, alpha 1) and HBA2 (hemoglobin, alpha 2). Mutations in either HBA1 or HBA2 are associated with alpha-thalassemia.[3]

References

1. van der Harst, P., Zhang, W., Mateo Leach, I., et al. (2012). Seventy-five genetic loci influencing the human red blood cell. *Nature, 492*(7429), 369–375.
2. Alter, B. P., Rosenberg, P. S., Day T., et al. (2013). Genetic regulation of fetal haemoglobin in inherited bone marrow failure syndromes. *British Journal of Haematology, 162*(4), 542–546.
3. Vichinsky, E. P. (2013). Clinical manifestations of alpha-thalassemia. *Cold Spring Harbor Perspectives in Medicine, 3*(5), a011742. Retrieved from http://perspectivesinmedicine.cshlp.org/content/3/5/a011742.abstract

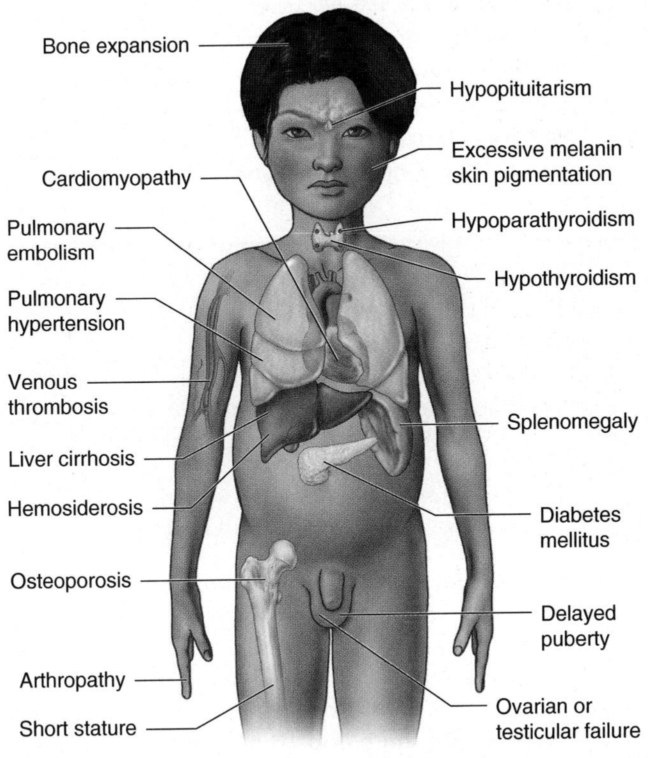

Figure 21.12 ■ Manifestations and complications associated with thalassemia major.

Linking Pathophysiology to Diagnosis and Treatment of Hemolytic Anemias

As with the treatment of nutritional anemia, treatment of hemolytic anemia begins with a determination of severity. The hematocrit and hemoglobin levels are monitored along with other indicators of the morphologic characteristics of anemia. On the basis of the severity of the anemia, blood transfusion may be used to replace missing erythrocytes and enhance the delivery of oxygen to tissue. Iron supplementation may not be indicated, as the destruction of red blood cells can lead to a reutilization of iron released from destroyed cells. The list of patient medications should be evaluated for the presence of medications that are known to be associated with hemolytic anemia. Alternatives can then be explored with the prescribing physician and the pharmacy.

Sickle cell disease is often treated from several different angles. Hydroxyurea may be given to infants and children to stimulate the production of hemoglobin. Blood transfusions may be used to compensate for the lack of an adequate number of red blood cells. Stem cell transplantation may be used to enhance the ability of the bone marrow to provide an adequate supply of red blood cells.

Check Your Progress: Section 21.4

1. What is the underlying cause of pain in patients with sickle cell disease?
2. In thalassemia, what clinical finding is most often seen in relation to the premature destruction of red blood cells?
3. What is the primary mechanism in aplastic anemia?

21.5 Anemia of Chronic Disease

Anemia of chronic disease (ACD) is also known as anemia of chronic inflammation. It is found in patients with chronic disease, being associated with inflammatory or infectious processes such as infection, chronic immune activation, or malignancy. The release of immune-mediating proteins known as cytokines can lead to an increase in the uptake and retention of iron, particularly in macrophages. This diverts iron from being able to contribute to the development of hemoglobin and can block oxygen binding. The red blood cells in ACD are normochromic (not paler than usual), **normocytic** (the cell size is within the normative range), and hypoproliferative (the number of RBCs is reduced). The disease process can therefore interact with treatments that can influence the bone marrow or hasten the destruction of red blood cells. Cancer patients receiving immunosuppression and radiation treatments are at increased risk.

Etiology and Pathogenesis

The pathogenesis of ACD lies within a defensive response of the body. Iron is a necessary nutrient for bacterial growth. In ACD, the body is attempting to reduce the available iron to deprive bacteria of this necessary nutrient. This is achieved through an inflammatory process that can be triggered by the presence of a bacterial infection. A hormone named hepcidin is needed to move iron out of macrophages, which are immune cells that store necessary reserves of iron. The release of hepcidin prevents iron from being released by macrophages, reducing the level in the bloodstream. This process not only denies bacteria the iron necessary for growth but also prevents other cells of the body from getting necessary iron.[15]

Clinical Manifestations

The anemia found in individuals with ACD is generally mild; the patient may feel tired with some shortness of breath, as there is not enough oxygen for bodily tissues. In general, the signs and symptoms of ACD are no different from those of other forms of anemia, and the patient may not even exhibit significant symptomatology.

Linking Pathophysiology to Diagnosis and Treatment

ACD is normochromic and normocytic, as the maturation of red blood cells has not been influenced. The number of cells released is often decreased because of an inability to utilize iron as a result of the reduction in the concentration of iron in the bloodstream. One of the major markers of this disease is a decrease in serum iron level accompanied by a drop in transferrin saturation. Ferritin is a protein that the body uses to aid in the storing of iron. Serum levels of ferritin rise as the body stores iron. These findings are thought to indicate the inhibition of iron release on the part of macrophages.[15,16]

In general, treatment is focused on the chronic condition that contributed to the development of inflammation rather than on simply resolving the ACD. Often, parenteral iron supplementation is used along with the administration of erythropoietin. It has been suggested that the ACD is simply an adaptive response, and as long as it remains mild, treatment may not be required.[13]

Charles Smith: Outcome

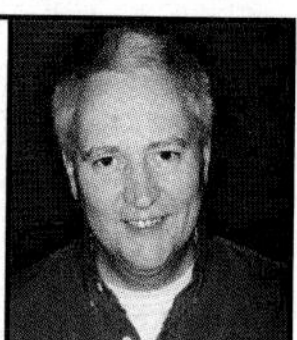

Mr. Smith has been admitted to the hospital. His laboratory findings include the following:

RBC: 3.5 million cells/mcL

Hb: 8.5 g/dL

HCT: 30.2%

MCV: 100 fL

MCH: 25

The relative number of red blood cells is decreased, as are hemoglobin and hematocrit. The MCV is within the normal range, indicating cells of the appropriate size, while the MCH is slightly decreased. These characteristics fit within the parameters of a normocytic anemia, and would fit with anemia of chronic disease. The presence of impaired renal function should be considered, given the patient's history of hypertension and diabetes, which could lead to a reduction in the release of erythropoietin.

On the basis of Mr. Smith's symptoms, consideration would be given to possible transfusion of red blood cells. Further evaluation would be done to help pinpoint potential causes and rule out the possibility of chronic gastrointestinal bleeding.

5. What are some potential limitations to relying solely on hematocrit as a measure of anemia?
6. Why is fatigue associated with anemia?
7. How could a higher altitude influence anemia?
8. Can anemia contribute to peripheral neuropathy (a loss of sensation in the hands or feet)?
9. Why would a patient with renal disease be at risk for anemia?

Check Your Progress: Section 21.5

1. How does the function of hepcidin affect the body's ability to manufacture red blood cells in ACD?
2. What laboratory test findings are typically found with ACD?
3. What is the focus of treatment for ACD?

21.6 Polycythemia Vera

Anemia represents a decrease in the number of red blood cells or the ability of the cells to carry oxygen. By contrast, an excess of red blood cells can result in a condition known as polycythemia. In polycythemia, the high concentration of red blood cells makes the blood more viscous. Increased viscosity prevents the blood from flowing efficiently through the body, leading to end organ ischemia. **Polycythemia vera** is a disorder of the bone marrow in which too many red blood cells are produced; white blood cells and platelets may increase as well.

Etiology and Pathogenesis

Polycythemia is classified as being either primary or secondary. In primary or absolute polycythemia, there is an increase in the production of erythrocytes on the part of bone marrow. *Polycythemia vera* is a term referring to a primary polycythemia that is often identified as a myeloproliferative condition. *Myelogenous* is a term referring to cells produced in the bone marrow. A myeloproliferative condition is therefore one in which there is an increase in the cell classes emerging from the bone marrow. Secondary polycythemia results from genetic modifications related to the production of erythropoietin, a hormone that regulates the production of red blood cells.[17]

Clinical Manifestations

The clinical manifestations of polycythemia vera reflect the increased blood viscosity and blood volume that result from the increased number of red blood cells. The patient will often complain of a headache, dizziness, and blurred vision associated with the increased blood volume. The increased preload can also manifest in hypertension. The increased thickness of the blood places the patient at an increased risk for the development of thrombi, or blood clots.

Linking Pathophysiology to Diagnosis and Treatment

Evaluation of polycythemia begins with an examination of laboratory values. The RBC count will be increased, along with a hematocrit that is often over 70. There may be a corresponding increase in the number of platelets and white blood cells in individuals with myeloproliferative conditions. Iron counts are often decreased, owing to consumption of iron in the increased production of erythrocytes.

Treatment involves the use of anticoagulation to prevent the development of thrombi. Therapeutic erythropheresis (also known as blood-letting) is often employed to reduce the number of red blood cells and to dilute the concentration within the bloodstream. In certain situations, chemotherapeutic approaches may be used to suppress the production of cells within the bone marrow for a period of time.[17]

Check Your Progress: Section 21.6

1. In polycythemia, what is the resulting effect of the increased number of erythrocytes produced by bone marrow?
2. How does primary polycythemia differ from secondary polycythemia?
3. What major complication can develop from untreated polycythemia?

CHAPTER SUMMARY

21.1 Chapter Overview and Case Studies

Define anemia and discuss concepts related to the disorders of red blood cells.

- Anemia is a common clinical condition characterized by a reduction in the number of erythrocytes (red blood cells) or a decline in the ability of erythrocytes to carry oxygen.
- Deficits in select B vitamins or iron are common causes of anemia.
- Iron attaches to hemoglobin and serves to bind oxygen.
- Anemia is ultimately a loss of oxygen in tissue.

21.2 Characteristics of Anemia

Describe the morphologic classification, etiology and pathogenesis, and clinical manifestations of anemia and approaches to treatment of the condition across the lifespan.

- Anemia is classified through an evaluation of the cell size or appearance of red blood cells. Smaller cells carry less hemoglobin.
- Microcytic anemia involves cells that are smaller, generally as a result of lack of maturation time or to lower levels of iron.
- Macrocytic anemia involves larger cells, generally as a result of a lack of certain nutrients necessary for successful deoxyribonucleic acid (DNA) replication.
- Changes in cell shape occur in sickle cell disease, when the cell collapses and forms a crescent shape.
- The most common clinical manifestation of anemia is fatigue.
- Chronic anemia can lead to a state of hypoxia in which organs are deprived of necessary oxygen.

21.3 Nutritional Deficiency Anemias

Differentiate the causes, classification, underlying pathogenesis, and clinical manifestations of nutritional anemias and approaches to treatment of those conditions.

- The lack of iron and cobalamin (vitamin B_{12}) can lead to the development of anemia through effects on cell maturation.
- These nutrients are necessary for cell maturation. The lack of them leads to larger cells with a pale appearance.
- Iron deficiency anemia can occur through the lack of an adequate diet or through chronic blood loss, as in GI bleeding.
- Reduced intake or usability of iron contributes to a state of anemia that is found in approximately 20–30% of the global population.
- The treatment of anemia can involve blood transfusion to replace missing cells and nutritional supplementation to replace necessary nutrients.

21.4 Hemolytic Anemias

Differentiate the causes, classification, underlying pathogenesis, and clinical manifestations of hemolytic anemias and approaches to treatment of these conditions.

- Hemolytic anemia refers to the destruction or hemolysis of red blood cells.
- The major etiologic causes of hemolytic anemia are genetic.
- Sickle cell disease is a cluster of autosomal recessive disorders that results in a misshapen form of hemoglobin that resembles a sickle or crescent in shape.
- Thalassemia refers to a group of autosomal recessive diseases that affect the production of hemoglobin.

21.5 Anemia of Chronic Disease

Differentiate the causes, classification, underlying pathogenesis, and clinical manifestations of anemia of chronic disease and approaches to treatment of the condition.

- Anemia of chronic disease is a condition of inflammation.
- The process of inflammation is associated with the release of immune proteins that play a role in uptake and retention of iron.
- In ACD, iron is taken up into macrophages, which diverts it from being able to play a role in the binding of oxygen.
- ACD is normochromic, normocytic, and hypoproliferative.

21.6 Polycythemia Vera

Differentiate the causes, classification, underlying pathogenesis, and clinical manifestations of polycythemia vera and approaches to treatment of the condition.

- In anemia, there is an inability of red blood cells to carry enough oxygen to organs.
- One of the potential causes of anemia is a lack of red blood cells or a large number of immature red blood cells.
- Polycythemia vera is characterized by an increase in the number of red blood cells.
- The increase in the concentration of red blood cells in the bloodstream leads to blood that is more viscous. As a result, blood flow to tissue and organs is decreased, leading to ischemia.

REVIEW QUESTIONS

1. Regardless of the cause, the most significant impact of anemia on the body's ability to function properly is the development of:
   a. free radicals.
   b. tissue hypoxia.
   c. electrolyte imbalances.
   d. fluid shifts.
2. A 62-year-old client presents to his primary care physician with chief complaints of fatigue, shortness of breath, and difficulty with exertion. The physician orders two laboratory tests: a complete blood count and iron studies. The results show a decreased RBC count and low serum iron levels, but all other lab values are within normal range. What anemia does this most likely indicate?
   a. Pernicious anemia
   b. Sickle cell disease
   c. Polycythemia vera
   d. Iron deficiency anemia
3. One of the most important strategies in helping clients with sickle cell disease (SCD) to prevent episodes of crisis is to remind them to:
   a. take their prescribed corticosteroids.
   b. exercise at least 3 days a week for 30 minutes each time.
   c. maintain adequate hydration.
   d. eat more green leafy vegetables.
4. In performing a complete blood count (CBC) for a patient with aplastic anemia, which of the findings below would be expected with this condition?
   a. Increased RBCs, increased WBCs, decreased platelets
   b. Decreased RBCs, decreased WBCs, decreased platelets
   c. Increased RBCs, decreased WBCs, increased platelets
   d. Decreased RBCs, increased WBCs, increased platelets
5. Which vital nutrient is required for the proper synthesis of red blood cell DNA and the formation of the heme component of hemoglobin?
   a. Folic acid
   b. Thiamine
   c. Chromium
   d. Zinc
6. In anemia of chronic disease (ACD), which of the following morphologic classifications is NOT associated with this condition?
   a. Normochromic
   b. Hyperproliferative
   c. Normocytic
   d. Hypoproliferative

7. A 72-year-old client with a known diagnosis of iron deficiency anemia asks her primary care nurse how to modify her diet to boost her iron level. She is already on oral iron supplementation. Which of the following food combinations would help to meet the client's dietary needs?
   a. Raisins, nuts, legumes, and enriched bread
   b. Fish, cranberries, oranges, and oatmeal
   c. Lean meats, carrots, kale, and pumpernickel bread
   d. Lentils, chuck beef, spinach, and whole wheat bread

8. What determines the effectiveness of therapeutic erythropheresis for a client with polycythemia vera?
   a. There is an increase in the platelet count.
   b. There is a decrease in the mean corpuscular hemoglobin level.
   c. There is a decrease in the red blood cell count.
   d. There is an increase in the white blood cell count.

ANSWERS

Answers to Review Questions can be found in Appendix A. Answers to Case Study and Check Your Progress questions are available on the faculty resources site. Please consult with your instructor.

RECOMMENDED WEBSITES

American Society of Hematology
http://www.hematology.org

Aplastic Anemia & MDS International Foundation
http://www.aamds.org

Association of Pediatric Hematology/Oncology Nurses
http://www.aphon.org

Centers for Disease Control—Nutrition for Everyone
http://www.cdc.gov/nutrition/everyone/basics/vitamins/iron.html

Cooley's Anemia Foundation
http://www.thalassemia.org/

Pernicious Anaemia Society
http://www.pernicious-anaemia-society.org/

REFERENCES

1. World Health Organization. (2011). *Worldwide prevalence of anaemia 1993–2005: WHO global database on anaemia.* Geneva: World Health Organization.
2. Kee, J. L. (2014). *Laboratory and diagnostic tests with nursing implications.* (9th ed.). Hoboken, NJ: Pearson Education.
3. Young, N. S. (2013). Current concepts in the pathophysiolgy and treatment of aplastic anemia. *Hematology*, 2013, 76–81. doi: 10.1182/asheducation-2013.1.76
4. Panwar, B., & Gutierrez, O. M. (2016). Disorders of iron metabolism and anema in chronic kidney disease. *Seminars in Nephrology, 36*(4), 252–261.
5. Salgia, R. J., & Brown, K. (2015). Diagnosis and management of hereditary hemochromatosis. *Clinics in Liver Disease, 19*(1), 187–198.
6. Giagoundis, A., & Haase, D. (2013). Morphology, cytogenetics and classification of MDS. *Best Practice and Research: Clinical Haematology, 26*(4), 337–353.
7. Swerdlow, S. H., Campo, E., Harris, N. L., et al. (Eds.). (2008). *WHO classification of tumours of haematopoietic and lymphoid tissues* (4th ed.). Geneva: IARC Press.
8. Rohrig, R. (2016). Anemia in the frail, elderly patient. *Clinical Interventions in Aging 11*, 319–326. doi: 10.2147/CIA.S90727
9. Bizzaro, N., & Antico, A. (2014). Diagnosis and classification of pernicious anemia. *Autoimmunity Reviews 13*(4–5), 565–568.
10. Nazki, F. H., Sameer, A. S., & Ganaie, B. A. (2014). Folate: Metabolism, genes, polymorphisms and the associated diseases. *Gene 533*(1), 11–20.
11. Bass, G. F., Tuscano, E. T., & Tuscano, J. M. (2014). Diagnosis and classification of autoimmune hemolytic anemia. *Autoimmunity Reviews, 13*(4–5), 560–564.
12. Costa, F. F., & Conran, N. (Eds.). (2016). *Sickle cell anemia.* New York: Springer.
13. Wang, W. C. (2013). Sickle cell anemia and other sickling syndromes. In J. P. Greer, J. Foerster, G. M. Rodgers, F. Paraskevas, B. Glader, D. A. Arber, & R. T. Means, (Eds.), *Wintrobe's clinical hematology* (13th ed.). Philadelphia: Lippincott Williams & Wilkins.
14. Schrier, S. L. (2017). Aplastic anemia: Pathogenesis; clinical manifestations; and diagnosis. In: UpToDate. Post. T. W. (Ed), Retrieved from UpToDate: http://www.uptodate.com/contents/aplastic-anemia-pathogenesis-clinical-manifestations-and-diagnosis
15. Prakash, D. (2012). Anemia in the ICU: Anemia of chronic disease versus anemia of acute illness. *Critical Care Clinics, 28*(3), 333–343, v.
16. Nemeth, E., & Ganz, T. (2014). Anemia of inflammation. *Hematology/Oncology Clinics of North America, 28*(4), 671–681. doi: 10.1016/j.hoc.2014.04.005
17. Tefferi, A. (2012). Polycythemia vera and essential thrombocythemia: 2012 update on diagnosis, risk stratification, and management. *American Journal of Hematology, 87*(3), 285–293. doi: 10.1002/ajh.23135

Unit VII
Disorders of Perfusion

Perfusion is the process by which oxygenated blood is transferred from the arteries to organs and tissues, ensuring adequate oxygenation of vessels necessary to maintain function. In healthy individuals, these processes are automatic. For example, due to autoregulation, the brain has the ability to maintain relatively constant blood flow despite changes in perfusion pressure, and therefore is able to maintain cognition. Altered mental status is an early symptom of decreased cerebral blood flow. Without adequate cerebral blood flow, energy-dependent brain processes cease, leading to irreversible brain injury. Adequate cerebral blood flow or intracranial regulation must be maintained to ensure adequate cerebral perfusion pressure.

Impairment in tissue perfusion results when the blood supply to a site increases or decreases beyond the normal limits due to pathological processes resulting from illness, defect, or injury. Impairment or disruption to perfusion can occur at any time in the life span, and occasionally the etiology may stem from prenatal incident or injury. For example, structural heart defects (SHDs) are a group of structural abnormalities that occur during gestation resulting in abnormal blood flow through the heart in the postnatal period. Of these, congenital heart defect may be the most well known, as it affects approximately 40,000 infants each year.

There are many disease processes that can alter profusion. Among them is coronary artery disease (CAD), the most common type of cardiac disease in the United States.[1] CAD is sometimes used interchangeably with coronary heart disease (CHD) to describe the buildup of plaque, which are made up of cholesterol (fatty) deposits, in the coronary arteries in a pathologic process called atherosclerosis that leads to reduced blood flow to the myocardium. CHD includes diagnoses that result from CAD such as angina pectoris, acute coronary syndrome (ACS), silent myocardial ischemia, and myocardial infarction (MI).

Regardless of the defect, illness, or injury that is causing impaired perfusion, without treatment, failure to perfuse tissues can result in loss of function and, if the degree of impairment is significant enough, loss of life through the onset of shock or sudden cardiac failure (cardiac arrest). Shock is a clinical syndrome characterized by an acute circulatory failure with inadequate or inappropriately distributed tissue perfusion resulting in generalized cellular hypoxia and end-organ dysfunction.

Nursing care of clients with altered perfusion requires ongoing assessment and careful monitoring of vital signs, capillary refill and conjunctiva, and level of consciousness, as well as the ability to recognize quickly when the client has a change in status. Even small changes in clinical presentation, such as a slight alteration in mental status as mentioned earlier, can signal significant changes in perfusion. These changes include increased anxiety and anger, both of which have been reported by patients shortly before cardiac events such as shock or ventricular tachycardia.[2] For patients with chronic cardiac conditions, management of stress and stressful life events is closely linked to quality of life.[3] Further, long-term stress responses such as anxiety and negative affect increase the risk for cardiovascular events and mortality. Nurses working with patients with alterations in perfusion should assess stress levels and support systems, provide emotional support, and provide referrals to helpful resources in an effort to try to assist patients with managing stress.[3]

References

1. Centers for Disease Control and Prevention. (2015). Coronary artery disease. Retrieved from https://www.cdc.gov/heartdisease/coronary_ad.htm
2. Peacock, J. & Whang, W. (2013). Psychological distress and arrhythmia: Risk prediction and potential modifiers. *Progressive Cardiovascular Disorders*, *55*(6), 582–89.
3. Staniute, M., Brozaitiene, J., & Bunevicius, R. (2013). Effects of social support and stressful life events on health-related quality of life in coronary artery disease patients. *Journal of Cardiovascular Nursing*, *28*(1), 83–89.

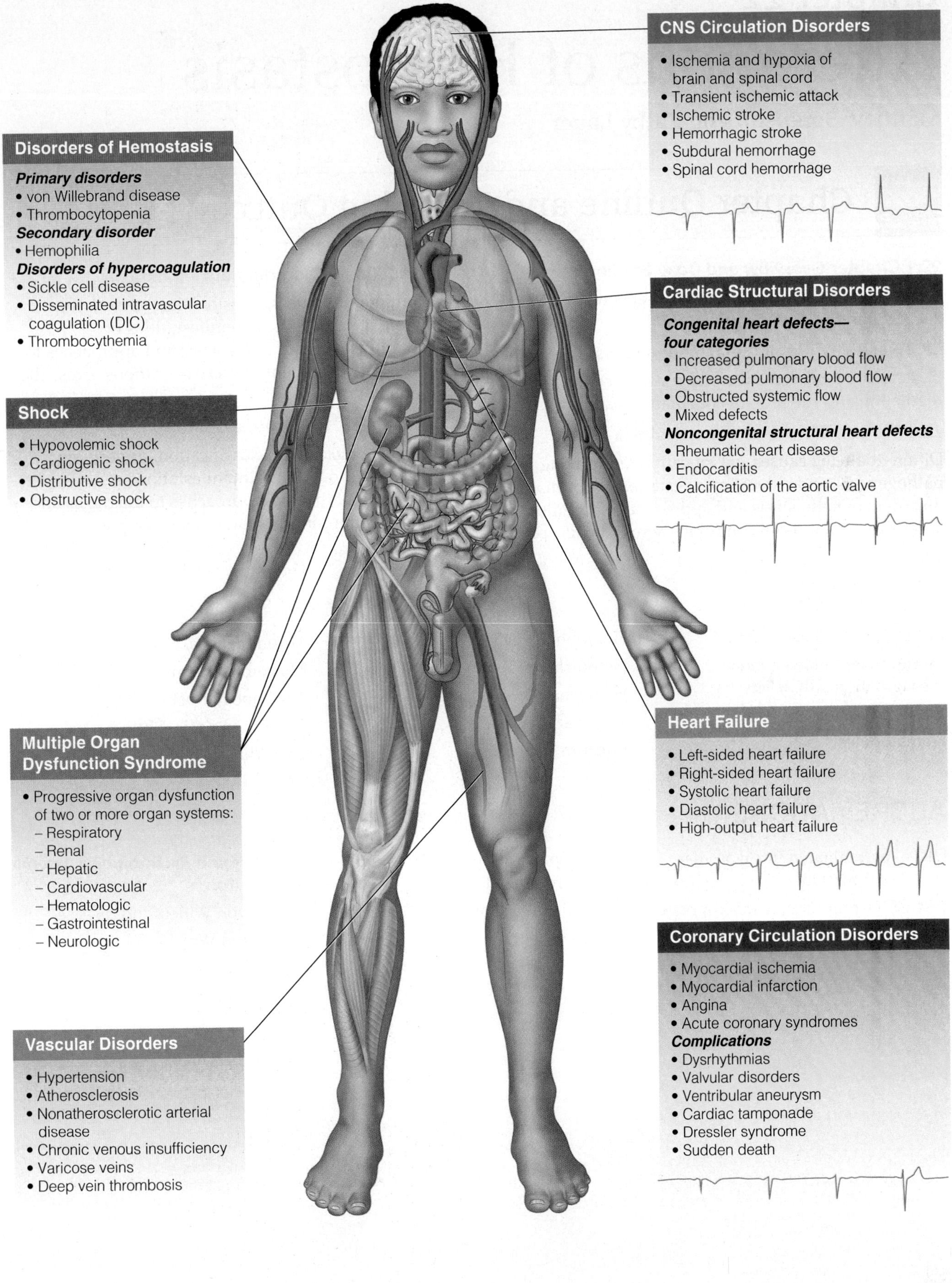

Disorders of Hemostasis

Primary disorders
- von Willebrand disease
- Thrombocytopenia

Secondary disorder
- Hemophilia

Disorders of hypercoagulation
- Sickle cell disease
- Disseminated intravascular coagulation (DIC)
- Thrombocythemia

Shock

- Hypovolemic shock
- Cardiogenic shock
- Distributive shock
- Obstructive shock

Multiple Organ Dysfunction Syndrome

- Progressive organ dysfunction of two or more organ systems:
  - Respiratory
  - Renal
  - Hepatic
  - Cardiovascular
  - Hematologic
  - Gastrointestinal
  - Neurologic

Vascular Disorders

- Hypertension
- Atherosclerosis
- Nonatherosclerotic arterial disease
- Chronic venous insufficiency
- Varicose veins
- Deep vein thrombosis

CNS Circulation Disorders

- Ischemia and hypoxia of brain and spinal cord
- Transient ischemic attack
- Ischemic stroke
- Hemorrhagic stroke
- Subdural hemorrhage
- Spinal cord hemorrhage

Cardiac Structural Disorders

Congenital heart defects—four categories
- Increased pulmonary blood flow
- Decreased pulmonary blood flow
- Obstructed systemic flow
- Mixed defects

Noncongenital structural heart defects
- Rheumatic heart disease
- Endocarditis
- Calcification of the aortic valve

Heart Failure

- Left-sided heart failure
- Right-sided heart failure
- Systolic heart failure
- Diastolic heart failure
- High-output heart failure

Coronary Circulation Disorders

- Myocardial ischemia
- Myocardial infarction
- Angina
- Acute coronary syndromes

Complications
- Dysrhythmias
- Valvular disorders
- Ventribular aneurysm
- Cardiac tamponade
- Dressler syndrome
- Sudden death

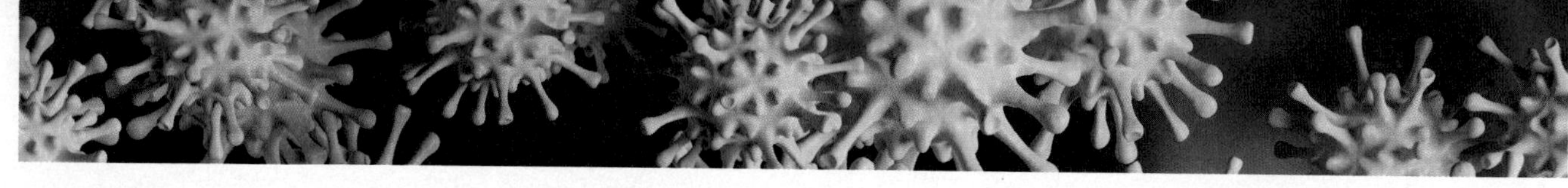

Chapter 22
Alterations of Hemostasis

Matthew Sorenson and Kathy Lauer

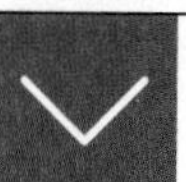

Chapter Outline and Learning Outcomes

22.1 Chapter Overview and Case Studies
Define hemostasis, and discuss concepts related to coagulation.

22.2 Review of Hemostatic Mechanisms
Describe major mechanisms involved in cellular regulation and function of coagulation pathways.

22.3 Primary Disorders of Hemostasis
Differentiate the causes, classification, underlying pathogenesis, and clinical manifestations of primary disorders of hemostasis and approaches to diagnosis and treatment of those conditions across the lifespan.

22.4 Secondary Disorders of Hemostasis
Differentiate the causes, classification, underlying pathogenesis, and clinical manifestations of secondary disorders of hemostasis and approaches to diagnosis and treatment of these conditions across the lifespan.

22.5 Issues of Hypercoagulopathy
Differentiate the causes, classification, underlying pathogenesis, and clinical manifestations of hypercoagulopathy and approaches to diagnosis and treatment of the condition across the lifespan.

KEY TERMS

Bleeding precautions, 535
Disseminated intravascular coagulation (DIC), 546
Ecchymosis, 535
Hematopoiesis, 539
Hemophilia, 545
Hemorrhage, 535
Hemostasis, 535
Megakaryocytopoiesis, 539
Purpura, 545
Thrombocytes, 535
Thrombocythemia, 535
Thrombocytopenia, 535
Thrombopoiesis, 539
von Willebrand disease (vWD), 539

ABBREVIATIONS

DIC—disseminated intravascular coagulation
GM-CSF—granulocyte macrophage colony-stimulating factor
HIT—heparin-induced thrombocytopenia
ITP—idiopathic thrombocytopenic purpura
TTP—thrombotic thrombocytopenia purpura
vWD—von Willebrand disease
vWF—von Willebrand factor

22.1 Chapter Overview and Case Studies

Hemostasis is a term that refers to cessation of blood flow, particularly through the action of coagulation (clotting) mechanisms. The term **hemorrhage** refers to copious bleeding, which can be outside of the skin (as from a laceration) or in the skin, which is called **Ecchymoses,** or bruising. Disorders of hemostasis are ultimately conditions related to excessive coagulation or excessive bleeding. Disruptions of hemostasis can occur at any point in the process of coagulation. Often, a lack of certain genes will lead to a loss of necessary factors that enable **thrombocytes**, also known as platelets, to adhere to binding sites or can even influence the number of thrombocytes themselves.[1]

Another way to view hemostasis is as a set of reactions leading to formation of a blood clot when a blood vessel is injured or damaged. This process has three primary steps or phases (**Figure 22.1** ■):

1. *Vascular phase.* Injury to a blood vessel causes a reactive constriction or spasm of the blood vessel. Afterward, platelets are activated and travel to the site of injury.
2. *Aggregation phase.* The platelets begin to clump together to form a dam or plug.
3. *Coagulation phase.* Platelets release immune proteins and other factors, leading to the formation of fibrin, which forms a layer over the platelet plug to help stop blood loss.

A common alternative approach to the naming of these phases is as follows:

1. Initiation
2. Amplification
3. Propagation.[2]

This nomenclature is seeing greater use in the literature and is often used in describing the release of clotting factors and platelet activation. In such a model, the first stage begins with vessel injury and the release of tissue factor. Tissue factor then stimulates the release of thrombin, which in turn activates a clotting factor referred to as factor IX. Factor IX then further propagates clotting through binding of platelets and results in clot formation.

Regardless of phrasing, the phases of hemostasis involve a complex interaction between thrombocytes, inflammatory mediators, and other factors associated with the breakdown of blood clots. With disorders of hemostasis, there can be a loss of necessary coagulation factors to prevent the formation of fibrin, loss of a factor necessary to help platelets adhere to one another, or changes in the number and functional ability of platelets.[2] The purpose of this chapter is to review conditions in which the process of coagulation is disrupted to the point of placing the individual at risk for obstruction of blood flow leading to tissue and organ damage or resulting in the loss of blood through bleeding.

Primary and Secondary Disorders of Hemostasis

Several classification schemes are used in discussing hemostasis. In one of the most common, disorders of hemostasis are referred to as either primary or secondary. Primary disorders of hemostasis are associated with abnormalities in the number or function of platelets. A reduction in the number of platelets is referred to as **thrombocytopenia** and can lead to spontaneous bleeding. Disruptions in the functional ability of platelets are seen in conditions such as von Willebrand disease, in which a lack of a certain factor prevents platelets from adhering to the site of injury, preventing the formation of a blood clot. Secondary disorders of hemostasis are associated with a lack of, or reduction in, factors tied to coagulation. For example, a genetic lack of factor VIII leads to hemophilia. Liver disease can lead to secondary disorders, as the majority of proteins involved in coagulation are synthesized in the liver. A number of clotting factors require vitamin K in order to function properly. Dietary deficiency or excess of this vitamin can then influence clotting. Warfarin, a common anticoagulant, influences vitamin K, restricting the function of several clotting factors.

In another method of classification, alterations of hemostasis are considered hereditary or acquired. The hereditary disorders include von Willebrand disease (although there is an acquired form as well) and hemophilia. The acquired disorders include issues related to vitamin K utilization and liver disease. Included among acquired disorders of coagulation would be the therapeutic use of anticoagulant drugs. Regardless of formal classification, the concern is excessive bleeding or, on rare occasions, the possibility of excessive clotting. When an excess of platelets can lead to spontaneous blood clot formation, it is referred to as **thrombocythemia**.

CLINICAL POINT: Patients who are at risk of excessive bleeding need to be educated about their condition and provided with instructions about preventing bleeding. These are commonly called **bleeding precautions,** and include such recommendations as using a soft toothbrush, wearing shoes at all times, avoiding contact sports, and using stool softeners to prevent straining. ■

Concepts Related to Disorders of Hemostasis

Many disorders of hemostasis are associated with genetic defects that prevent the maturation of thrombocytes or can influence the ability of platelets to adhere to the site of injury. These disruptions of cellular regulation then involve hemostatic mechanisms. In turn, several products of the immune system are involved in the regulation of coagulation and hemostasis. Many proteins that are involved in immunologic defense also play a role in clotting pathways, and thrombocytes secrete a primary chemoattractant protein (interleukin 8) that draws immune cells to the site of injury. Selected concepts related to disorders of hemostasis are shown in **Figure 22.2** ■.

Vascular Phase

The **vascular phase** of hemostasis lasts for roughly 30 minutes after the injury occurs. It is dominated by the response of the endothelial cells and the contraction, or **vascular spasm**, of smooth muscle of the vessel walls.

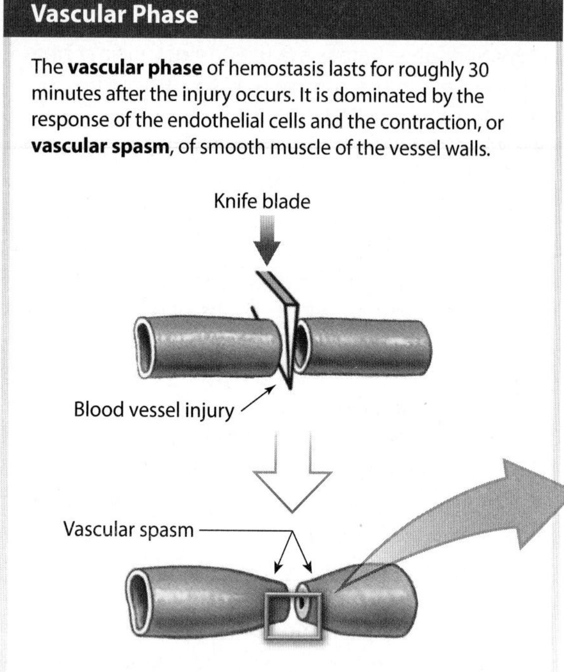

Events of the Vascular Phase

- The endothelial cells contract and expose the underlying basement membrane to the bloodstream.
- The endothelial cells begin releasing chemical factors and local hormones. Endothelial cells also release **endothelins**, peptide hormones that (1) stimulate smooth muscle contraction and promote vascular spasms and (2) stimulate the division of endothelial cells, smooth muscle cells, and fibroblasts to accelerate the repair process.
- The endothelial plasma membranes become "sticky." A tear in the wall of a small artery or vein may be partially sealed off by the attachment of endothelial cells on either side of the break. In small capillaries, endothelial cells on opposite sides of the vessel may stick together and prevent blood flow along the damaged vessel. The stickiness also aids the attachment of platelets as the platelet phase gets under way.

Platelet Phase

The **platelet phase** of hemostasis begins with the attachment of platelets to sticky endothelial surfaces, the basement membrane, exposed collagen fibers, and each other.

Release of chemicals (ADP, PDGF, Ca^{2+}, platelet factors)
Plasma in vessel lumen
Platelet aggregation
Endothelium
Platelet adhesion to damaged vessel
Basement membrane
Vessel wall
Platelet plug may form
Contracted smooth muscle cells
Interstitial fluid
Cut edge of vessel wall

Chemicals Released by Activated Platelets

- Adenosine diphosphate (ADP), which stimulates platelet aggregation and secretion
- Several chemicals that stimulate vascular spasms
- **Platelet factors**, proteins that play a role in blood clotting
- **Platelet-derived growth factor (PDGF)**, a peptide that promotes vessel repair
- Calcium ions (Ca^{2+}), which are required for platelet aggregation and in several steps in the clotting process

Figure 22.1 ■ Phases of clot formation.

SOURCE: MARTINI, FREDERIC H.; OBER, WILLIAM C.; NATH, JUDI L.; BARTHOLOMEW, EDWIN F.; PETTI, KEVIN, VISUAL ANATOMY & PHYSIOLOGY (SUBSCRIPTION), 2nd Ed., ©2015. Reprinted and Electronically reproduced by permission of Pearson Education, Inc., New York, NY.

Coagulation Phase

The **coagulation** (cō-ag-ū-LĀ-shun) **phase** of hemostasis does not start until 30 seconds or more after vessel damage. **Coagulation**, or blood clotting, involves intertwined cascades called the extrinsic, intrinsic, and common pathways. These pathways lead to the conversion of circulating fibrinogen (a soluble protein) into **fibrin** (an insoluble protein). As the fibrin network grows, blood cells and additional platelets become trapped, forming a **blood clot** that seals off the damaged portion of the vessel. **Procoagulants** (clotting factors) in the plasma play a key role in this phase. Essential clotting factors include Ca^{2+} and 11 different proteins (identified by Roman numerals). Many clotting factors are **proenzymes** (inactive enzymes), which, when converted to active enzymes, direct essential reactions in the clotting response. The activation of one proenzyme commonly creates a **cascade**, or chain reaction of successive events.

Common Pathway

The **common pathway** begins when enzymes from either the extrinsic or intrinsic pathway activate factor X. Activated factor X activates a complex called prothrombin activator. Prothrombin activator converts the proenzyme **prothrombin** into the enzyme **thrombin** (THROM-bin). Thrombin then completes the clotting process by converting fibrinogen to fibrin.

Extrinsic Pathway

The **extrinsic pathway** begins with the release of **tissue factor** (factor III) by damaged endothelial cells or peripheral tissues. The greater the damage, the more tissue factor is released, and the faster clotting occurs. Tissue factor then combines with Ca^{2+} and another clotting factor to form an enzyme complex capable of activating factor X, the first step in the common pathway.

Intrinsic Pathway

The **intrinsic pathway** begins with the activation of proenzymes exposed to collagen fibers at the injury site. This pathway proceeds with the assistance of **PF-3**, a platelet factor released by aggregating platelets. After a series of linked reactions, activated clotting factors combine to form an enzyme complex capable of activating factor X.

Thrombin from the common pathway also speeds up clotting by stimulating additional tissue factor formation and platelet factor release. This is a positive feedback loop (see Module 1.18).

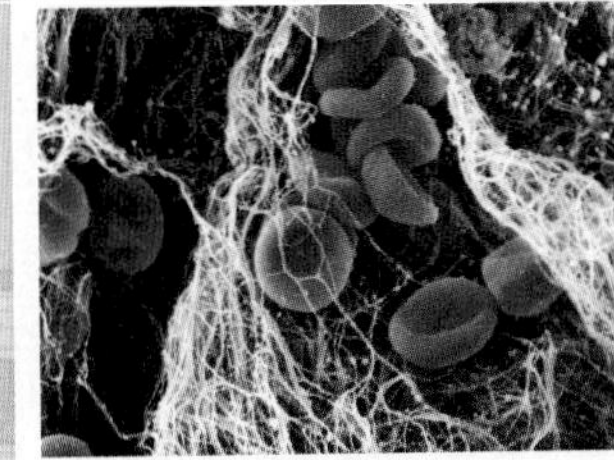

Blood clot containing trapped RBCs SEM × 1200

Clot Retraction

Once the fibrin meshwork has formed, platelets and red blood cells stick to the fibrin strands. The platelets then contract, and the entire clot begins to undergo **clot retraction**, a process that continues over a period of 30–60 minutes and pulls the cut edges together.

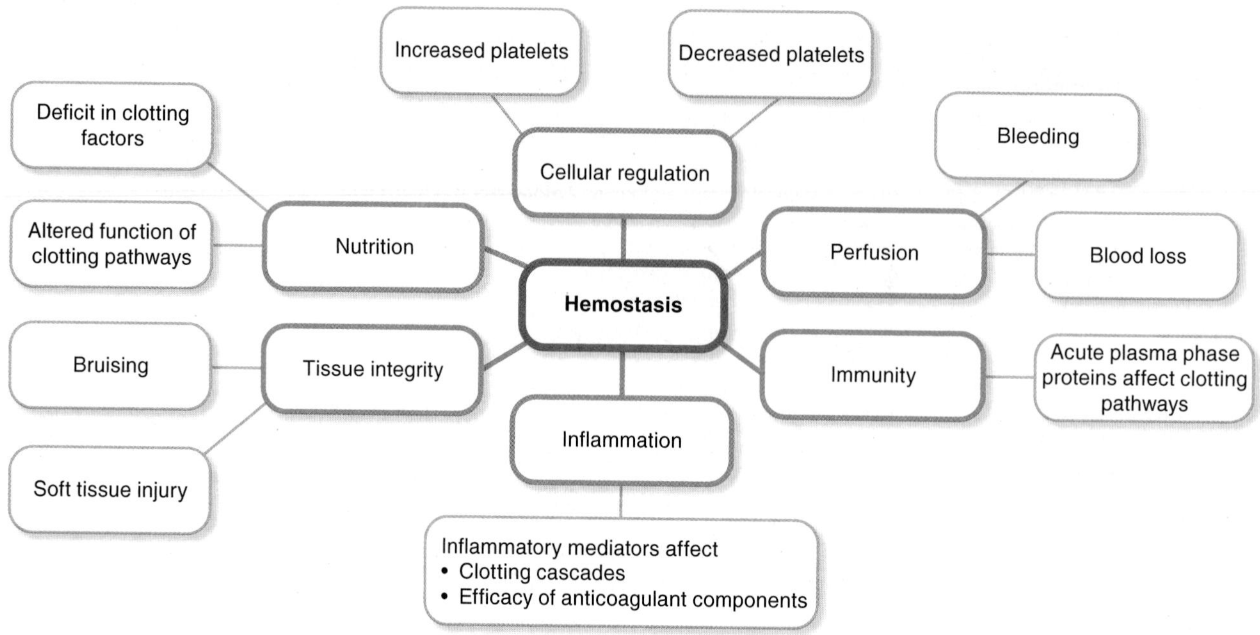

Figure 22.2 ■ Concepts related to disorders of hemostasis.

Case Studies

The following cases are addressed throughout the chapter to assist in the application of chapter content to clinical situations that involve individuals with disorders of hemostasis.

Brayden Grey: Introduction

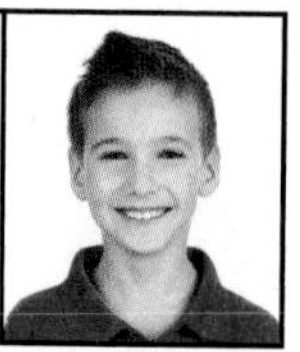

Brayden Grey is an 8-year-old boy who has recently begun to participate in a soccer program. After falling in practice today, he seems to have a significant number of bruises along his torso and both legs. He has no significant medical history, although his parents report that he seems to experience frequent nosebleeds, which they have attributed to the climate in which they live. Because the bruising seems to be significant in relationship to the injury he experienced, Brayden's parents have brought him to the emergency department for evaluation.

1. What term is used to refer to bleeding under the skin caused from trauma or direct injury?
2. If Brayden has a disorder of hemostasis, what would be the significance of frequent episodes of epistaxis (nosebleed)?

Francis Jenkins: Introduction

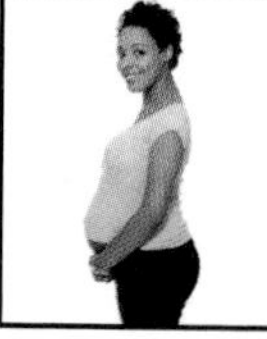

Francis Jenkins, age 36, presents to the emergency department. She is 22 weeks pregnant with her second child. This morning she experienced a sudden onset of abdominal pain with slight vaginal bleeding. Her past medical history is significant for hypertension. Ms. Jenkins is admitted to the hospital for observation and testing.

1. What immediate education should the nurse provide to Ms. Jenkins?
2. Since the immune system is involved in the process of coagulation and hemostasis, how might those processes be affected by pregnancy?

Check Your Progress: Section 22.1

1. Describe the concept of disorders of hemostasis.
2. What is thrombocytopenia?
3. What organ disease can contribute to bleeding disorders?

22.2 Review of Hemostatic Mechanisms

The blood, a specialized type of connective tissue, is made up of two main components: plasma (the liquid portion) and blood cells (the formed elements). Plasma accounts for approximately 55% of the total blood volume. Much of the plasma volume (approximately 91%) is water, and approximately 8% is plasma proteins, including albumin, coagulation factors, immunoglobulins, and complement. The remaining 1% is composed of a number of substances, including nutrients, electrolytes, vitamins, hormones, waste products, drugs, and dissolved gases such as oxygen and carbon dioxide.[3]

The second component, blood cells, includes red blood cells or erythrocytes, white blood cells or leukocytes, and platelets or thrombocytes or megakaryocytes. Leukocytes comprise a number of subpopulations of white blood cells, including monocytes, macrophages, granulocytes, B lymphocytes, and T lymphocytes.[3]

Hematopoietic stem cells are not fundamentally committed to a particular developmental pathway (i.e., self-renewal, differentiation, or apoptosis). It is their genetic programming and microenvironment that mediate the final decision. Hematopoietic stem cell development, maturation, proliferation, lineage commitment, and survival depend on a complex interplay among a number of transcription factors, receptors, growth factors, and cytokines. For example, growth factors, such as erythropoietin and granulocyte macrophage colony stimulating factor (GM-CSF) and cytokines, such as interleukin 3 (IL-3) and interleukin 6 (IL-6), create an environment that sustains **hematopoiesis** (the process behind the formation of blood cells) by permitting viability or preventing cell death. In addition, the expression and concentration of both positive and negative transcription factors influence what lineage the HSC will follow. Many of the growth factors and cytokines have little specificity in that they act on one or more cell lines.[3]

The development of all blood cells begins with a hematopoietic stem cell. From there, the proliferation and differentiation of blood cells are influenced by a number of different growth factors and other immune mediators that lead to the hematopoietic stem cell being divided in two different cells: the lymphoid precursor and the myeloid precursor. The common myeloid progenitor or stem cell can then differentiate into erythrocytes, granulocytes, monocytes, or megakaryocytes. The megakaryocyte is a large cell in the bone marrow that is responsible for the production of thrombocytes, also known as platelets. One megakaryocyte can produce thousands of thrombocytes. The formation of thrombocytes is referred to as **megakaryocytopoiesis** or **thrombopoiesis**, reflecting their emergence from megakaryocytes. The megakaryocyte is the earliest identifiable cell in the pathway to platelet production. Platelets are small, anucleated blood cells produced in the bone marrow from megakaryocytes, which are large polypoid cells derived from hematopoietic stem cells (**Figure 22.3** ■).[3]

Thrombopoiesis is regulated by a variety of cytokines and growth factors, including thrombopoietin, IL-3, IL-6, IL-11, and GM-CSF. Thrombopoietin is the most important protein in the production of platelets. Platelets have receptors for this protein, which increases as platelet numbers decrease and decreases as platelet numbers increase. Thrombopoietin stimulates proliferation of progenitor cells and supports differentiation of the megakaryocyte. IL-3 is needed to support the early development of progenitor cells such as the burst forming unit, the megakaryocyte; IL-6 acts in synergy with thrombopoietin to increase numbers of megakaryocytes; and IL-11 is elevated in response to low platelet levels in the blood and stimulates platelet production by acting on both the early progenitor cells and in the development of the megakaryocytes.[3]

Hemostasis is then a complex interplay of a number of clotting factors and components of the immune system (**Table 22.1** ■). There are two main pathways involved in coagulation: intrinsic and extrinsic. The pathways share certain factors, and the shared components are referred to as the common pathway (see Figure 22.1).

An injury to tissue often results in the release of blood from vessels. The presence of blood outside the standard circulating system stimulates the release of tissue factor from cells that are normally not directly in contact with circulating blood, such as fibroblasts (which surround blood vessels) or smooth muscle cells. The release of tissue factor activates the extrinsic pathway. This factor is so noted for the ability to activate the extrinsic pathways that several authors have begun to refer to the extrinsic pathway as the tissue factor pathway. Other factors such as von Willebrand factor then aid platelets in binding the site of injury. The intrinsic pathway can be activated by the actions of the extrinsic particularly through platelet activation, but can also be activated through damage in the vascular system (see Figure 22.1). The main protein involved in the pathway is thrombin, which transforms fibrinogen to fibrin.[1,2]

The release of thrombin induces the release of other mediators such as tissue factor pathway inhibitor, which then limit the coagulation process. At this point, sufficient thrombin is usually present to initiate the intrinsic pathway, which takes over the role of manufacturing fibrin. Fibrin itself provides the necessary structure to form a mesh layer, which forms a blood clot. The formation of a clot is then influenced by plasmin-mediated fibrinolysis, resulting in the formation of D-dimers and other components that lead to the breakdown and degradation of fibrin.[1,2] Through the evaluation of several of these clotting factors, it is then possible to determine the relative efficacy of the clotting system in the individual (**Table 22.2** ■ and **Table 22.3** ■).

Check Your Progress: Section 22.2

1. As what does the blood cell begin in the bone marrow?
2. What are the main pathways involving coagulation?
3. What does the nurse suspect with a positive D-dimer test?

22.3 Primary Disorders of Hemostasis

Primary disorders of hemostasis are centered on platelet function and binding, along with considerations related to integrity of vascular endothelial cells. Primary disorders of hemostasis are often associated with genetic deficits. Clinically, these disorders manifest with spontaneous or mild contact bruising, spontaneous bleeding from mucous membranes, and excessive blood loss after trauma.

von Willebrand Disease

One of the main glycoproteins involved in hemostasis is von Willebrand factor. This factor aids in protein binding, allowing platelets to adhere to points of injury. Defects in the genetic expression of this protein lead to the most common bleeding disorder with a genetic cause known as **von Willebrand disease (vWD)**.[4]

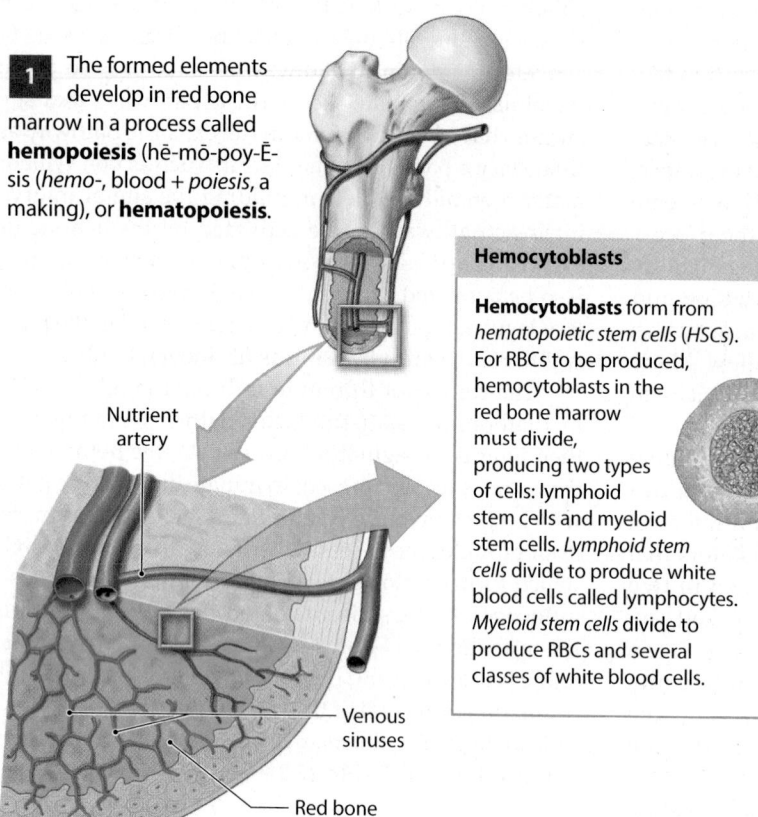

1 The formed elements develop in red bone marrow in a process called **hemopoiesis** (hē-mō-poy-Ē-sis (*hemo-*, blood + *poiesis*, a making), or **hematopoiesis**.

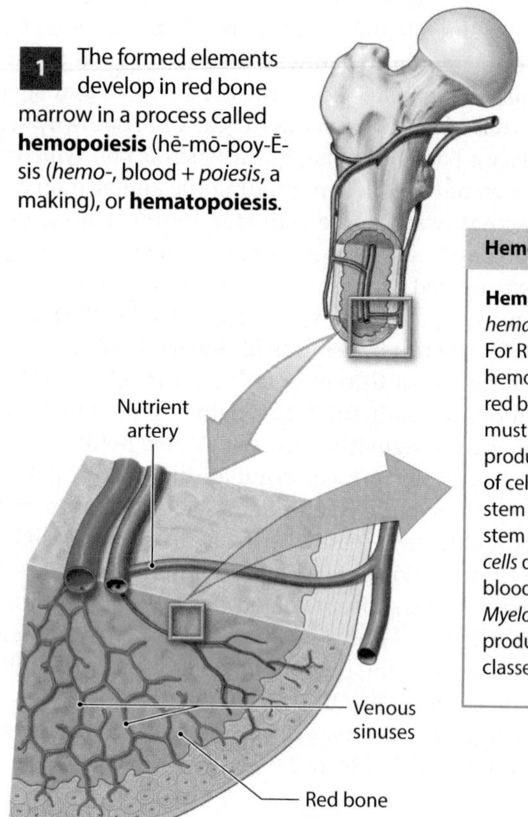

Hemocytoblasts

Hemocytoblasts form from *hematopoietic stem cells (HSCs)*. For RBCs to be produced, hemocytoblasts in the red bone marrow must divide, producing two types of cells: lymphoid stem cells and myeloid stem cells. *Lymphoid stem cells* divide to produce white blood cells called lymphocytes. *Myeloid stem cells* divide to produce RBCs and several classes of white blood cells.

Lymphoid Stem Cells

Lymphoid stem cells are responsible for the production of *lymphocytes*, which are cells that function in the immune response. These stem cells originate in the red bone marrow. Some remain there, whereas others migrate to **lymphoid tissues**, including the thymus, spleen, and lymph nodes. Lymphocytes are then produced in these organs as well as in the red bone marrow.

Colony-stimulating factors are hormones released by activated lymphocytes and other cells during an immune response to stimulate blood cell formation.

Stimulation

Myeloid Stem Cells

Myeloid stem cells are stem cells in red bone marrow that divide to give rise to all types of formed elements other than lymphocytes.

2 The term *formed elements* is appropriate because platelets are cell fragments rather than specialized cells. The flowchart above describes the origin of platelets from megakaryocytes. The table below summarizes important information about platelets.

Structure and Function of Platelets

Appearance in a Stained Blood Smear	Abundance (Average Number per µL)	Function	Remarks
Platelets are flattened discs that appear round when viewed from above and appear spindle shaped in section or in a blood smear.	350,000 (range: 150,000–500,000)	Platelets clump together and stick to damaged vessel walls, and they release chemicals that stimulate blood clotting.	Platelets are continuously replaced. Each platelet circulates for 9–12 days before being removed by phagocytes, mainly in the spleen.

Figure 22.3 ■ Development of thrombocytes.

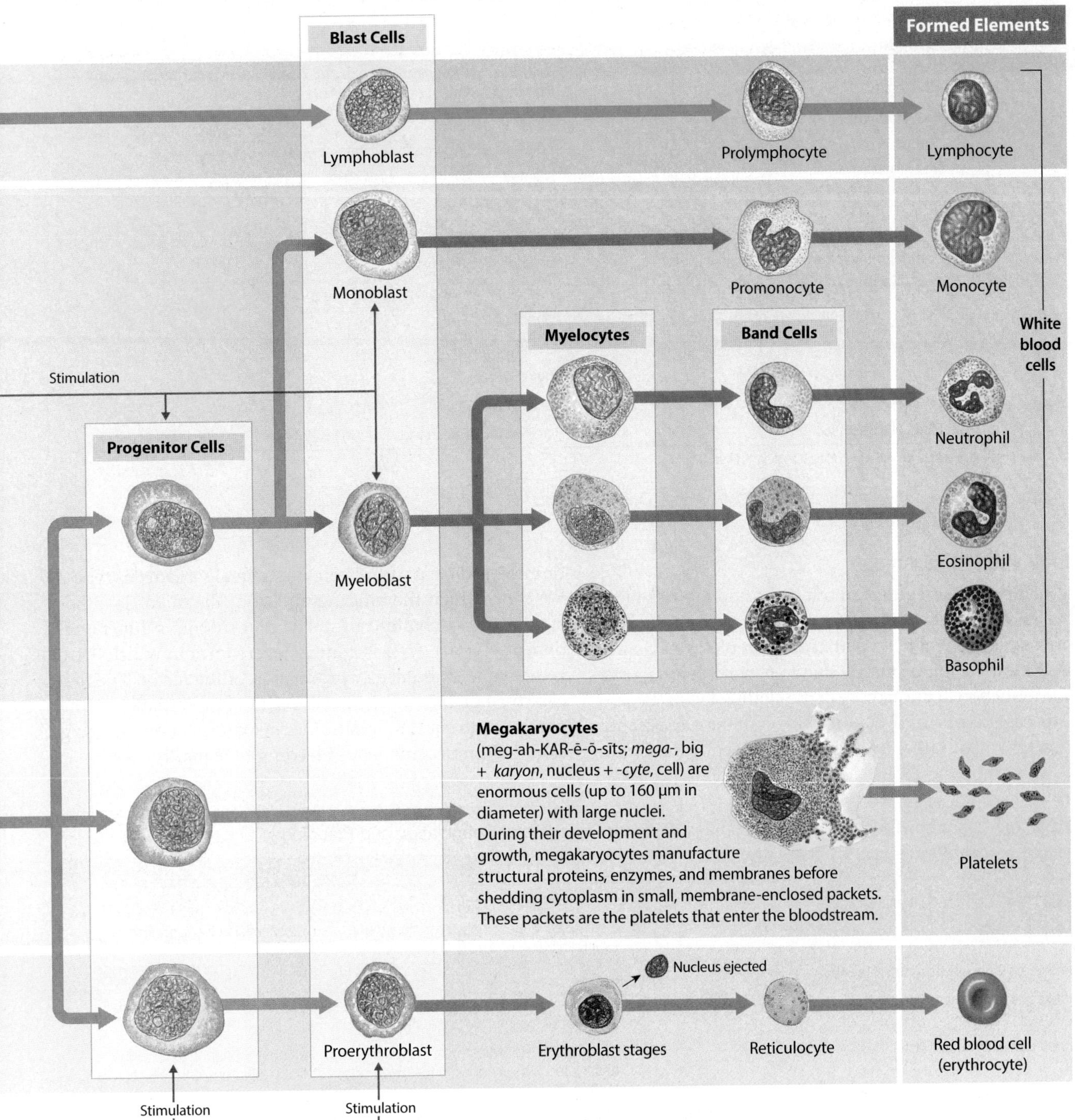

Erythropoietin (EPO) is released into the plasma when peripheral tissues, especially the kidneys, are exposed to low oxygen concentrations. The state of low tissue oxygen levels is called **hypoxia** (hī-POKS-ē-uh; *hypo-*, below + *oxy-*, presence of oxygen). Erythropoietin is released (1) during anemia; (2) when blood flow to the kidneys decreases; (3) when the oxygen content of air in the lungs decreases due to disease or high altitude; and (4) when the respiratory surfaces of the lungs are damaged. Once in the bloodstream, EPO is carried to areas of red bone marrow, where it stimulates stem cells and developing RBCs.

Table 22.1 Blood Clotting Factors

Factor	Name	Function or Pathway
I	Fibrinogen	Common pathway; converted to fibrin
II	Prothrombin	Common pathway; converted to thrombin
III	Thromboplastin	Activates extrinsic pathway; catalyzes conversion of thrombin
IV	Calcium ions	Needed for all steps of coagulation
V	Proaccelerin	Common pathway
VI*		
VII	Serum prothrombin conversion accelerator	Both intrinsic and extrinsic pathways
VIII	Antihemophilic factor	Intrinsic pathway
IX	Plasma prothrombin component	Intrinsic pathway
X	Stuart factor	Common pathway
XI	Plasma prothrombin antecedent	Intrinsic pathway
XII	Hageman factor	Intrinsic pathway
XIII	Fibrin stabilizing factor	Cross-links fibrin strands to form insoluble clot

*Term no longer used; this substance is believed to be the same as factor V.

Etiology and Pathogenesis

Von Willebrand disease affects both males and females with a prevalence estimated as high as 1% of the population. The disease results from either a partial or a complete deficiency in the clotting factor, primarily due to genetic defects, or a relative reduction in the efficacy of the clotting factor. Type 1 vWD disease occurs in 70–80% of all cases of the disease and is characterized by either a failure to manufacture the factor or increased clearance. There are several variants of type 2 vWD, in which the binding ability of the factor is either significantly enhanced or delayed, resulting in functional deficits. Type 3 vWD is a more severe form in which there is a complete absence of production of the factor. The disease type greatly influences the clinical presentation of the patient, with substantial variance in manifestations, ranging from mild mucocutaneous bleeding to hemarthroses.[4]

Table 22.2 Common Diagnostic and Laboratory Tests for Disorders of Coagulation and Bleeding

Test	Expected Abnormality	Used to Diagnose
Nutritional Measures		
Vitamin B12	Decreased	Decreased values imply a deficiency of a vitamin essential in the formation of several clotting factors.
Measures of Coagulation and Bleeding		
Activated coagulation time	Increased	Measures number of seconds for clotting of whole blood on exposure to an activator of the intrinsic pathway.
Activated partial thromboplastin time (aPTT)	Increased	Increased levels indicate prolonged bleeding. Particularly prolonged bleeding is associated with changes in the levels of select clotting factors, primarily factors II, V, IX, X, XI, and XII.
D-dimer	Increased	D-dimer is a product of fibrin degradation that is present after blood clots are broken down. An elevated result may imply the presence of significant clotting propensity. Elevated levels can also be found in a number of other medical conditions and states.
International normalized ratio (INR)	Increased	Often used as a measure of the therapeutic effectiveness of warfarin, a common oral anticoagulant.
Partial thromboplastin time (PTT)	Decreased	Increased levels indicate prolonged bleeding. Particularly prolonged bleeding is associated with changes in the levels of select clotting factors, primarily factors II, V, IX, X, XI, and XII.
Prothrombin time (PT)	Increased	Increased levels indicate prolonged bleeding. Examines factors II (prothrombin), V, VII, X, and fibrinogen.
Genetic Associated Measures		
Factor assays	Decreased	Each of the primary factors involved in the clotting pathways can be evaluated to determine level. Decreased levels imply a lack of the factor that may be associated with genetic variations.
von Willebrand factor antigen	Decreased	Measures for the presence of a factor released from endothelium and activated platelets that aids platelet adhesion.

Table 22.3 Laboratory Tests and Values Used in Evaluation of Coagulation

Test	Measures	Values
D-dimer	A fragment of fibrin degradation.	< 0.5 ug/mL
Activated partial thromboplastin time (aPTT)	Measures the same parameters as PTT but with the addition of a clotting activator to enhance the speed of clotting. This results in a test that is seen as more sensitive.	30–40 seconds
Factor assays	Measure the level of each factor in the clotting cascade to determine concentration. Common factors evaluated: factors II, V, VII, VIII, IX, X, and XI.	Varies according to factor evaluated
Fibrinogen	Measures the presence of a soluble protein necessary for formation of fibrin.	150–400 mg/dL
International normalized ratio (INR)	Calculated from prothrombin time, providing a normalized ratio allowing for cross-laboratory comparison.	0.8–1.2
Partial thromboplastin time (PTT)	Measures the effectiveness of factors I (fibrinogen), II (prothrombin), V, VIII, IX, X, XI, and XII.	60–70 seconds
Platelets	Cells necessary for clot formation.	150,000–400,000/mm^3
Prothrombin time (PT)	Measures the functional ability of the extrinsic clotting pathway. Examines factors II (prothrombin), V, VII, and X and fibrinogen.	9.5–13.5 seconds
Vitamin K	A vitamin essential to formation of several clotting factors.	0.2–3.2 ng/mL
von Willebrand factor antigen (factor VIII-R antigen)	A factor released from endothelium and activated platelets. Aids in platelet adhesion.	Ranges depend on age and blood type. Newborn: 60–230% Adult: 60–200%

Note: Values are a general estimation and may vary depending on the population.

Brayden Grey: Application

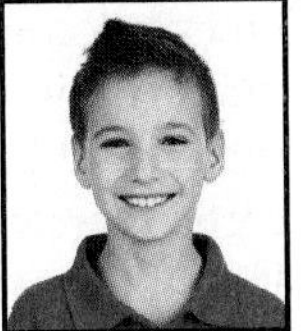

Brayden is alert and oriented in all spheres. Physical examination of the lower abdomen and bilateral lower extremities reveals significant bruising. Brayden denies suffering any other trauma during practice, reporting that "I just tripped." He denies contact with another player. On abdominal percussion, his spleen appears enlarged, and bowel sounds are present in all four quadrants. Vital signs are pulse 94, respirations 12, temperature 99.0ºF (oral), and blood pressure 100/60.

3. What lab work is likely to be ordered for Brayden?
4. What should the nurse explain about von Willebrand disease to Brayden's parents?

Clinical Manifestations

Diagnosis of vWD is often difficult, owing the variability in clinical signs and symptoms among the different types. Also, because von Willebrand factor (vWF) is an acute-phase reactant, its level can increase with stress, exercise, acute inflammatory processes, pregnancy, and menses. The presence of vWF even varies with blood type, which may help in diagnosis. Levels of vWF antigen appear 25% more in individuals with the AB blood type, and levels of vWF antigen are 25% lower with the O blood type.[4]

Patients with type 1 vWD are often asymptomatic for long periods of time, without overt evidence of a clotting disorder. Often, the disease becomes apparent when the individual is having diagnostic testing for other conditions or has emergent surgery in which excessive bleeding occurs postoperatively. In type 3 vWD, the presentation is similar to that of hemophilia, with life-threatening clinical manifestations and internal bleeding.[4]

Linking Pathophysiology to Diagnosis and Treatment

There are two treatment options for spontaneous bleeding episodes: desmopressin (DDAVP) and transfusion with plasma-derived vWF products. Desmopressin is used for individuals with type 1 vWD and a subset of type 2 vWD. Desmopressin increases vWF levels twofold to fourfold and generates a similar increase in factor VIII activity. The major adverse effects of DDAVP are facial flushing, headache, tachycardia, and hyponatremia. For individuals with type 3 vWD and those with type 2 in whom DDAVP is ineffective or contraindicated, plasma concentrates of factor VIII and vWF are used.[4]

Brayden Grey: Outcome

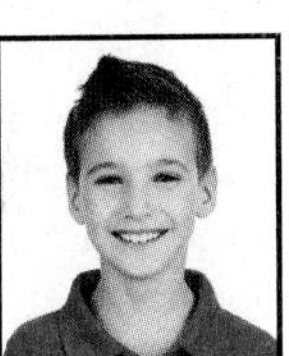

Laboratory assessments are ordered for Braden, and the findings include the following:

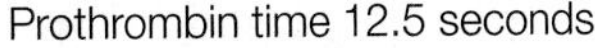

Prothrombin time 12.5 seconds

Activated partial thromboplastin time 60 seconds

Hemoglobin 12.8 g/dL

Hematocrit 35%

vWF antigen 52%

The findings indicate a slight decrease in hemoglobin and hematocrit for his age. This could be related to the bruising recently sustained in response to mild trauma or to Brayden's recurrent epistaxis. Either way, the history of easy bruising in conjunction with frequent episodes of epistaxis is suggestive of von Willebrand disease. The slight decrease in aPTT value indicates the possibility of prolonged bleeding. It is not uncommon to note a PT result within the expected range while the aPTT demonstrates an increase. The vWF antigen is at the lower end of the range, and such a decrease is consistent with type 2 disease. Confirmation of these findings requires further diagnostic testing, which will include genetic analysis and evaluation of other clotting factors. In the meantime, Brayden's parents are educated on the need for Brayden to wear a medical alert bracelet to provide necessary information in case of an emergency. Brayden and his parents are also advised of the importance of his engaging in a pattern of regular noncontact-based activity.

5. What symptoms should the nurse explain to Brayden and his parents about his possible diagnosis?
6. What instructions should the nurse provide to Brayden and his parents on discharge?

Thrombocytopenia

Thrombocytopenia is defined as a decrease in the number of circulating blood platelets and is the most common cause of abnormal bleeding. The normal range of circulating platelets is approximately 150,000–450,000/μL. An increased risk of bleeding rarely occurs until there are fewer than 80,000–100,000/μL, and there is a particularly high risk of spontaneous bleeding once the count drops below 10,000/μL. In general, however, there is not a close relationship between the number of platelets and the severity of bleeding.[5]

Etiology and Pathogenesis

Thrombocytopenia can result from four pathophysiologic processes: artifact; deficient production; increased destruction, consumption, or both; or abnormal distribution or pooling.

Pseudothrombocytopenia. Thrombocytopenia due to an artifact is referred to as pseudothrombocytopenia or false thrombocytopenia. The usual cause is platelet clumping secondary to the use of an anticoagulant called ethylenediaminetetraacetic acid that results in incorrect counting of platelets. This occurs in about 1 in 1000 cases and generally has no clinical significance.[5]

Deficient Platelet Production. Deficient production of platelets results from processes that affect the bone marrow and produce marrow aplasia. Bone marrow replacement, congenital disease, or chemical injury can cause marrow aplasia. Bone marrow replacement occurs when large abnormal cells compress and displace normal thrombocytes (e.g., leukemia, lymphoma, myelofibrous disease, granulomatous disease, metastatic neoplasms). Thrombocyte hypoplasia can also result from congenital abnormalities. Chemical injury may result from exposure of the marrow to toxic chemicals (e.g., benzene, insecticides), medications (e.g., anticonvulsants, tranquilizers, thiazide diuretics, cancer chemotherapy), or alcohol. Drug-induced thrombocytopenia is most commonly caused by heparin. Heparin-induced thrombocytopenia (HIT) occurs primarily in hospitalized individuals.

CLINICAL POINT: Individuals who are taking low-molecular-weight forms of heparin (e.g., enoxaparin and tinzaparin) are still at risk for the development of HIT. ■

There are two types of HIT. Type 1 HIT involves a modest transient decrease in platelet count within the first 2–3 days after initiation of heparin therapy. Platelet counts return to normal spontaneously even if the drug is continued. This type is generally of no clinical significance. Type 2 HIT, also called heparin-induced thrombocytopenic thrombosis or white clot syndrome, is less common; it is seen in 0.3–0.5% of individuals treated with unfractionated heparin. It is caused by antibodies to platelet factor 4 on the heparin complex. It is seen about 4–14 days after initiation of heparin therapy but may be seen earlier in individuals with previous exposure to heparin.[5]

Chemotherapy-associated thrombocytopenia is associated with decreases in other cell lines as well. With most chemotherapeutic agents, the nadir for the platelet count occurs 7–10 days after treatment, with recovery in 2–3 weeks. Platelet transfusions may be required occasionally, along with dose adjustment for future cycles.[5]

Increased Destruction and/or Consumption of Platelets. Increased destruction of platelets is the mechanism involved in immune thrombocytopenic purpura (ITP). This is a relatively common autoimmune disease and involves destruction of platelets by antiplatelet antibodies, resulting in decreased platelet survival rate. The antibodies are frequently immunoglobulin G (IgG), and they are directed against platelet antigens. The spleen is the major site of platelet destruction. Those affected are frequently young adult females. A severe thrombocytopenia results without anemia or leukopenia. In adults, this is typically a chronic disease that can remit and relapse over time, as is characteristic of other autoimmune disorders. Therapy is initiated on an individual basis, considering platelet counts, presence of hemorrhage, and lifestyle-related bleeding risk. Initial therapy is corticosteroids, in particular, short pulses of dexamethasone. If a rapid platelet increase is needed, intravenous immunoglobulin infusion or anti-RhD antibodies may be administered. Anti-RhD antibodies are used only in individuals who are RhD^+ and have an intact spleen. Splenectomy is still considered the gold standard treatment for chronic ITP. Other therapies include danazol, cytoxan, azathioprine, rituximab, and autologous BM transplant.[6]

Thrombotic thrombocytopenia purpura (TTP) is a relatively uncommon but life-threatening type of thrombocytopenia. The disorder may be idiopathic or secondary in association with *E. coli* O157-H7 diarrhea, HIV, certain drugs (e.g., ticlopidine, clopidogrel, quinine, cyclosporine, mitomycin A, cisplatin), pregnancy, bone marrow transplantation, or metastatic neoplasms. The pathophysiologic basis for TTP appears to be a deficiency or absence of a protease called ADAMTS13. This protease normally breaks down the vWF multimer if it begins to unfold in the absence of vessel injury. The vWF multimer, at the time of vessel injury, unfolds to provide a platform for platelet aggregation and the formation of a platelet plug. If the vWF multimer begins to unfold without vessel injury, platelet thromboses can form; ADAMTS13 prevents this phenomenon.[6]

Abnormal Distribution or Pooling of Platelets. Uncomplicated splenomegaly or hypersplenism may lead to thrombocytopenia by inducing a reversible pooling of up to 90% of the total body platelets. This is an exaggeration of normal splenic pooling, in which approximately 30% of the total body platelets are in the spleen at any one time. Survival of platelets in the spleen may be normal or moderately reduced. Thus, the total platelet pool could be unaffected even though venous blood shows only 20% of normal.

Platelet production is usually normal. Splenic pooling is not associated with increased platelet production, so it seems that the total platelet pool, not platelet concentration, is responsible for the feedback regulation of platelet production.

The most common problem causing splenic pooling is chronic liver disease with portal hypertension and congestive splenomegaly, in which moderate thrombocytopenia is the rule, with platelet counts rarely below 40,000/μL. This type of thrombocytopenia with untreated splenomegaly is usually not clinically significant, and no treatment is needed. If it is associated with chronic liver disease, bleeding manifestations are related to underlying coagulation deficits due to a decrease in the synthesis of coagulation proteins.[7]

Clinical Manifestations

The bleeding associated with thrombocytopenia is usually mucocutaneous in nature—on the skin in the form of tiny pinprick hemorrhages called **purpura** or bruises called ecchymoses that may occur after relatively minor trauma. Bleeding from the nose (epistaxis) and from the gums is also quite common. More serious hemorrhage can occur in the retina of the eye, leading to blindness and potentially fatal spontaneous bleeding in the brain (intracranial) or from the mucosal lining of the GI tract.[5]

Five clinical manifestations of TTP, referred to as the pentad of TTP, are (1) microangiopathic hemolytic anemia, (2) thrombocytopenia, (3) renal insufficiency, (4) fever, and (5) mental status changes that can wax and wane (e.g., confusion, headache, fatigue, seizures, strokelike syndrome). The thrombocytopenia can be severe, with platelet counts as low as 20,000/mL. Not all five clinical manifestations are always seen; the complete pentad is found in only about 40% of individuals and is a late finding that is associated with a poor outcome.[5]

Linking Pathophysiology to Diagnosis and Treatment

The main risk in thrombocytopenia is bleeding. In cases of significant blood loss, emergent care involves plasma exchange (plasmapheresis), which is the cornerstone of therapy for TTP. This therapy is designed to aid in reducing the concentration of autoimmune antibodies in the plasma and slowing the destruction of platelets. If plasma exchange is not immediately available, an infusion of fresh frozen plasma may be given. Intravenous administration of plasma is designed to help restore the necessary concentrations of ADAMTS13, an enzyme that cleaves vWF. Corticosteroids, dipyridamole, and aspirin have been used but are of questionable value.[5]

Check Your Progress: Section 22.3

1. The nurse is caring for a patient who has an IV infusion of heparin with a low platelet count. What should the nurse suspect?
2. What is the normal range of circulating platelets?

22.4 Secondary Disorders of Hemostasis

Secondary disorders of hemostasis are those associated with deficits in the formation or function of coagulation factors. Among these conditions is hemophilia, an inherited condition. An acquired issue is a deficiency in levels of vitamin K, an important constituent element of several clotting factors. Clinically, the manifestations of secondary disorders are similar to those seen in primary disorders of hemostasis. Some sources place von Willebrand disease in the category of secondary disorders even though the effects influence platelet adhesion.

Hemophilia

Hemophilia is a hereditary genetic bleeding disorder resulting from the loss of select clotting factors. There are two main forms of hemophilia; hemophilia A results from a lack of factor VIII, and hemophilia B results from a deficiency in factor IX. These disorders result from chromosomal abnormalities in which a nonfunctioning form of the related gene is produced. There are acquired forms of hemophilia that may result from autoimmune disorders, pregnancy, or cancer. The clinical manifestation of all forms of hemophilia is bleeding resulting from an inability to clot.[8]

Etiology and Pathogenesis

The incidence of hemophilia A is about 1 in 50,000 male births, and the incidence of hemophilia B is about 1 in 30,000 male births. The genes for both factor VIII and factor XI are on the X chromosome; therefore, the disorder primarily affects males, although females may be symptomatic carriers. All female offspring of affected males are carriers. Carrier females have a 50% chance of passing the affected chromosome to their male offspring. Acquired hemophilia is associated with the development of factor VIII and factor IX inhibitors.[9]

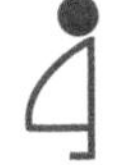

Women with a familial history of hemophilia have the option of having prenatal testing to determine diagnosis of heritable bleeding disorders prior to birth. ■

Treatment advances have helped to ensure the possibility of a normal lifespan for individuals with bleeding disorders. This requires additional assessment considerations for the older adult with a bleeding disorder. Prophylactic therapy early in life will often prevent the development of joint and liver disease later on, but such approaches are newer strategies. Older adults may still be at risk for a number of complications, so they require additional assessment and consideration. ■

Clinical Manifestations

Often in male infants with hemophilia, the typical presentation is excessive bleeding after circumcision. Later presentation in infancy can include severe mucosal bleeding from tongue or gum injuries and prominent bruising over both the trunk and the extremities. ■

In infants with hemophilia, the classic manifestations of severe bleeding—soft tissue bleeding and hemarthroses—typically do not begin until the child becomes ambulatory, usually after the first birthday. Diagnostically, individuals with hemophilia usually have prolonged PTT, with normal PT, platelet counts, and bleeding time or platelet function assay testing. Diagnosis is confirmed by the analysis of factor VIII or factor IX activity.[9]

Linking Pathophysiology to Diagnosis and Treatment

Treatment of hemophilia involves episodic or prophylactic administration of factor VIII or factor XI concentrates, much of which is eventually home-based. Because of concerns about transfusion-transmitted diseases, most individuals with hemophilia are now treated with recombinant-derived factor VIII or factor XI concentrates.[10] Factor VIII concentrates increase factor VIII approximately 2% per 1 IU/kg infused and factor IX concentrates increase factor IX approximately 0.8% per 1 IU/kg infused. Target factor replacement is a 50% correction of plasma values for most hemorrhages, but with major hemorrhages (head, neck, abdominal, and intracranial), the goal is for 100% correction.

Following factor VIII concentrate treatment, up to 30% of patients develop inhibitors to the factor, usually within the first 50 exposures. In hemophilia B, approximately 1–3% of patients develop inhibitors. Serious complications can arise if inhibitors emerge during surgery or treatment. Individuals can be treated with bypassing agents such as rFVIIa or activated prothrombin complex concentrates.[10]

> **Check Your Progress: Section 22.4**
>
> 1. What is the definition of hemophilia?
> 2. When is the most common time for hemophilia to be suspected in children?
> 3. What diagnostic lab tests would the nurse anticipate for a patient suspected of having hemophilia?

22.5 Issues of Hypercoagulopathy

Hypercoagulability and Sickle Cell Disease

The focus here is on the specific issues of hypercoagulability in sickle cell disease. Sickle cell disease is discussed in more detail in Chapter 21.

Etiology and Pathogenesis

The etiology of hypercoagulability in sickle cell disease is complex and not well understood. In sickle cell disease, nearly every aspect of hemostasis, including platelet function and procoagulant, anticoagulant, and fibrinolytic systems, is altered. Pathophysiologic abnormalities identified in sickle cell disease include but are not limited to (a) increased thrombin levels; (b) abnormal activation of fibrinogen; (c) decreased anticoagulant proteins; (d) abnormal platelet activation; (e) increased tissue factor levels; (f) decreased protein C and S activity; (g) abnormal expression of anionic, negatively charged glycolipids such as phosphatidylserine on the surface of sickled red blood cells; (i) elevated levels of procoagulant, prothrombotic, tissue factor–inducing antiphospholipid antibodies (especially IgG against phosphatidylserine); (j) moderate thrombocytosis characteristic of older children and adults; and (k) increased levels of young platelets being generated because of diminished or absent splenic function and splenic sequestration. Fetal hemoglobin provides protection from abnormal clotting because it decreases phosphatidylserine expression on the surface of the red blood cell and reduces thrombin generation.[11]

Clinical Manifestations

The hypoxia that can result from groups of sickle cells clumping together and obstructing blood flow often results in tissue ischemia, which can lead to the development of a significant level of pain in the back, chest, and extremities. The pain is accompanied by other signs of ischemic damage, such as swelling, tenderness, a rapid respiratory rate, and hypertension. The presence of anemia, chronic tissue hypoxia, and tissue damage can result in several significant complications. Thrombosis is an important aspect of the clinical spectrum of sickle cell disease (e.g., clinical and silent strokes) and occurs frequently. The outcomes of hypercoagulability in terms of neurologic complications such as stroke may occur, but thrombi in the pulmonary system and those associated with avascular necrosis in large joints and leg ulcers are also causes of increased morbidity and mortality.

Linking Pathophysiology to Diagnosis and Treatment

Individuals with sickle cell disease have an increased concentration of thrombin with a corresponding loss of anticoagulant proteins. Therapeutic approaches include the use of pharmacologic treatments designed to reduce platelet binding and inhibit platelet activation.

Disseminated Intravascular Coagulation

Disseminated intravascular coagulation (DIC) is a life-threatening condition in which the proteins that control clotting become overactive. As clotting factors are consumed, a number of small clots are formed, which can disrupt the blood supply to organs or cause serious spontaneous bleeding, and the individual faces an increased risk of hemorrhage. Clinical manifestations include issues associated with tissue and organ ischemia and bleeding.

Pregnancy should be considered a time of high risk for the development of DIC, which can occur as a result of a number of complications associated with pregnancy and delivery.[12] ■

Etiology and Pathogenesis

Several medical conditions are known to trigger DIC, including sepsis, shock, and trauma. Damage to blood vessels and tissue and inflammation can lead to an increase in the concentration of a protein known as tissue factor. This factor is involved in the activation of coagulation through the extrinsic pathway and stimulates the production of thrombin.[13]

With DIC, there is then a systematic activation of clotting mechanism, and a significant increase is seen in the production of thrombin such that compensatory hemostatic mechanisms may become unable to cope with the sudden increase, leading to the activation of factors V, VIII, and IX. Thrombin also enhances platelet aggregation through activation of receptors located on the surface of thrombocytes.[13]

The systemic activation of coagulation pathways also results in an inability to remove fibrin effectively, primarily because of an increase in levels of plasminogen activator inhibitor type 1. Fibrin in turn is activated by the presence of thrombin. The increase in these two clotting components initiates the formation of numerous small blood clots in the circulation and organs. These clots interfere with the flow of blood, leading to tissue ischemia. As clotting components are consumed, the individual is suddenly at increased risk of hemorrhage due to an inability to stop the loss of blood.

Francis Jenkins: Application

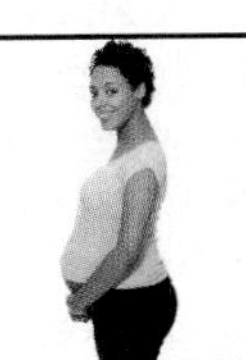

A nursing assessment is performed when Ms. Jenkins is admitted to the unit. While taking an oral temperature, the nurse notes blood on the thermometer. On further inspection, blood is also seen on the surface of Ms. Jenkins's gums and tongue. Vital signs are pulse 100, respirations 22, temperature 101.2°F (oral), blood pressure 88/56. After taking the blood pressure, the nurse notes the appearance of petechiae on Ms. Jenkins's upper arm where the blood pressure cuff had been located. Ms. Jenkins appears lethargic but is arousable.

3. What type of precautions should the nurse take with Ms. Jenkins?
4. What are petechiae?

Clinical Manifestations

With the formation of numerous clots, organ dysfunction is often found. Renal and hepatic dysfunction are not uncommon, and patients are at risk for the development of deep vein thrombosis and pulmonary embolism. While it may take time for renal and hepatic manifestations to become apparent, assessing for the signs of a deep vein thrombosis or pulmonary embolism is critical. The patient may experience dyspnea, hemoptysis, and shortness of breath. Tachycardia and hypotension may also be readily apparent. It is crucial to monitor for signs of bleeding such as hematuria, hematemesis, and overt hemorrhage from sites tied to injury or intravascular access.[13]

Linking Pathophysiology to Diagnosis and Treatment

Diagnostically, as clotting factors are consumed in the patient with DIC, there are often low platelet and fibrinogen levels. There is a prolongation of PT and aPTT results, with an elevation in D-dimer values. These findings are consistent with prolongation of bleeding as a result of the consumption of clotting factors. In clinical practice settings, scoring systems are often available for estimating the risk for development of DIC. Nursing interventions will focus on evaluation of vital signs, assessment of intake and output, and monitoring circulatory status for either the obstruction of blood flow or the presence of hemorrhage. Platelets and other blood factors may be administered to aid in the restoration of clotting mechanisms; in some situations, anticoagulation may be used during the clotting phase of DIC. The administration of anticoagulant therapy is not universal and is debated in some settings. Ultimately, the primary focus will be on attempting to determine the underlying cause for initiation of DIC.[13]

Francis Jenkins: Outcome

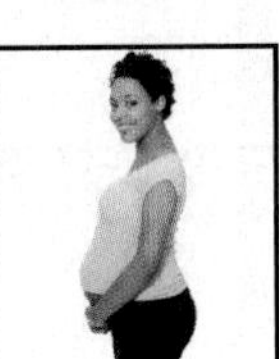

Immediate laboratory assessments are ordered for Ms. Jenkins. Findings include the following:

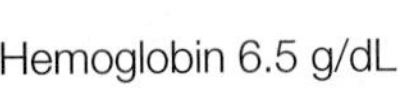

Hemoglobin 6.5 g/dL

Hematocrit 21%

Platelets 90,000

Prothrombin time 16 seconds

D-dimer 0.8 μg/mL (elevated)

The findings indicate a decrease in the number of platelets in conjunction with decreased hemoglobin and hematocrit values, suggesting the presence of blood loss. While a slight decrease may be expected as a result of significant vaginal bleeding, the values are below anticipated values. The prothrombin time is elevated, indicating a risk for bleeding. The elevated D-dimer supports ongoing activation of the hemostatic system, with heightened values indicating increased degradation of fibrin. Taken in combination with the decreased platelet levels, this indicates that Ms. Jenkins is at significant risk for the development of DIC, as the normal mechanisms to aid in clot formation are reduced in the presence of findings that indicate increased fibrin breakdown.

Treatment for Ms. Jenkins focuses on continuous monitoring of vital signs and neurologic assessment. All intravenous access sites require frequent evaluation for bleeding. Her intake and output are closely monitored, and all output is assessed for the presence of blood. The nurse prepares for the administration of intravenous fluids and possible administration of plasma and platelets. The primary focus of care is on the prevention of hypovolemic shock.

As a result of early identification of DIC, intravenous access is secured, and fluid resuscitation is initiated to help support blood pressure. Ms. Jenkins is found to have placental abruption requiring surgical intervention. Given that the fetus is only at 22 weeks gestational age, the respiratory system is not fully developed. An emergency cesarean delivery is performed. The baby girl, named Hope, weighs 1 pound at birth. She is taken to the neonatal intensive care unit, and after 7 days on a ventilator, she dies. Mrs. Jenkins makes a full recovery but mourns the death of her baby girl.

5. What assessments should the nurse do while caring for Ms. Jenkins?
6. What are the findings that led to the diagnosis of DIC?

Thrombocythemia

Thrombocythemia is a condition characterized by higher than expected numbers of thrombocytes. Typically, this is defined as an elevated platelet count greater than 600,00/μL. This condition is often referred to as *essential thrombocythemia*.

Impact of Current Research on Clinical Practice

Sequential Analysis of 18 Genes in Polycythemia Vera and Essential Thrombocythemia Reveals an Association between Mutational Status and Clinical Outcome

Description: Luque and colleagues performed genetic analysis of 18 select genes in 50 individuals with essential thrombocythemia or polycythemia vera. The genes that were selected were involved in a signaling pathway (janus kinase) that is crucial for the production and development of cells from hematopoietic stem cells. The purpose of the study was to determine whether certain genetic variations were tied to clinical outcomes. It was found that more than one genetic mutation in one of the genes studied was likely to lead to disease progression in either of the two disease states.

Clinical Practice: The ability to identify genetic mutations tied to a particular disease could help to identify people who are at risk for disease progression or eventually help to identify possible therapeutic agents. Ongoing research is looking at genetic therapies for a variety of differing disease states. If a genetic profile can be identified in a particular disease state, it could allow for early identification and more targeted treatment.

Research Study:

Luque Paz, D., Chauveau, A., Boyer, F., et al. (2017). Sequential analysis of 18 genes in polycythemia vera and essential thrombocythemia reveals an association between mutational status and clinical outcome. *Genes Chromosomes & Cancer, 56*(5), 354–362.

Etiology and Pathogenesis

The cause of thrombocythemia is not well understood. Cases of thrombocythemia are often associated with infection and other inflammatory states. Immunologic activation appears to stimulate the production of platelets through the release of a series of inflammatory mediators. It is speculated that this excess of cellular proliferative and maturational components results in an increase in the number of platelets. The increase in the number of platelets can then overwhelm the necessary concentration of vWF, leaving platelets unable to adhere to one another and initiating the clotting cascade.[14]

Clinical Manifestations

Thrombocythemia has some of the same hallmarks as DIC. The individual may experience the development of thrombi accompanied by headache and visual disturbances. The possibility of hemorrhage also exists, depending on the concentration of other clotting factors. Thrombocythemia is not commonly seen as a life-threatening condition.[14]

Linking Pathophysiology to Diagnosis and Treatment

The diagnosis of thrombocythemia is often one of exclusion. The number of red blood cells is often within expected parameters, while a small increase may be seen in the concentration of lymphocytes. Biologic agents may be used to reduce the number of platelets and, in emergent situations, are used in combination with plasma exchange (plasmapheresis). Low doses of anticoagulants may be administered, depending on the levels of other clotting components.[14] Research is under way to determine whether particular genetic variations are tied to clinical outcomes (see the Impact of Current Research on Clinical Practice).[15]

Check Your Progress: Section 22.5

1. What are some of the most common symptoms of sickle cell disease?
2. On a cellular level, what is lacking in the blood related to sickle cell disease?
3. The nurse is caring for a patient in sickle cell crisis. What critical assessments should the nurse be conducting? Why?

CHAPTER SUMMARY

22.1 Chapter Overview and Case Studies

Define hemostasis, and discuss concepts related to coagulation.

- Hemostasis is the cessation of blood flow, particularly through the action of clotting mechanisms.
- Disorders of hemostasis are related to excessive coagulation or excessive bleeding.
- Hemostatic disruptions can occur at any point during the process of coagulation.
- Clot formation has three phases: vascular (initiation), aggregation (amplification), and coagulation (propagation).
- Tissue factor is a protein that has an essential role in hemostasis. Tissue factor stimulates the release of thrombin, which leads to the release of other factors, ultimately resulting in clot formation.
- Primary disorders of hemostasis are associated with abnormalities in the number or function of platelets.
- Secondary disorders of hemostasis are associated with a lack of, or reduction in, factors tied to coagulation.

22.2 Review of Hemostatic Mechanisms

Describe major mechanisms involved in cellular regulation and function of coagulation pathways.

- Hematopoietic stem cells divide into two different cells: lymphoid precursor cells and myeloid precursor cells.
- Myeloid stem cells differentiate into erythrocytes, granulocytes, monocytes, and megakaryocytes.
- The megakaryocyte is a large cell in the bone marrow that is responsible for the production of thrombocytes, also known as platelets.
- Thrombopoiesis results in the production of blood platelets, which are small, anucleated blood cells produced in the bone marrow from megakaryocytes.
- Thrombopoiesis is well regulated by a variety of cytokines and growth factors, including thrombopoietin.
- Thrombopoietin stimulates the proliferation of platelets and functions in an inverse relationship with the number of platelets.
- The clotting pathway has two major arms: intrinsic and extrinsic. These arms share certain factors that participate in a process referred to as the common pathway.
- Vessel injury leads to the release of tissue factor, which in turn activates the extrinsic pathway.
- The intrinsic pathway is activated through the actions of the extrinsic pathway, particularly through platelet activation but also through damage in the vascular system.
- Thrombin alters the structure of fibrinogen, transforming it into fibrin.
- Fibrin provides a meshlike framework on which platelets can begin to clump.

22.3 Primary Disorders of Hemostasis

Differentiate the causes, classification, underlying pathogenesis, and clinical manifestations of primary disorders of hemostasis and approaches to diagnosis and treatment of those conditions across the lifespan.

- Primary disorders of hemostasis are centered on platelet function and binding, along with considerations related to integrity of vascular endothelial cells.
- von Willebrand disease is the most common genetic bleeding disorder. von Willebrand factor is required for the formation of the platelet plug. The primary clinical manifestation of von Willebrand disease is an inability to clot, which can result in hemorrhage.
- There are three forms of von Willebrand disease. Type 1 is the most frequent and least severe; type 2 can result in some bleeding issues; and type 3 can result in significant blood loss due to a complete loss of the clotting factor.
- Thrombocytopenia, defined as a decrease in the number of circulating blood platelets, is the most common cause of abnormal bleeding.
- Thrombocytopenia can result from four pathophysiologic processes: (a) artifact; (b) deficient production; (c) increased destruction, consumption, or both; or (d) abnormal distribution or pooling.
- There are two types of heparin-induced thrombocytopenia (HIT). Type 1 HIT involves a modest transient decrease in platelet count within the first 2–3 days after initiation of heparin therapy. Platelet counts return to normal spontaneously even if the drug is continued. Type 2 HIT places the individual at the risk for the development of thrombi.
- Increased destruction of platelets is the mechanism involved in immune thrombocytopenic purpura (ITP) and thrombotic thrombocytopenic purpura (TTP). ITP is a relatively common autoimmune disease and involves destruction of platelets by antiplatelet antibodies, resulting in decreased platelet survival rate.

22.4 Secondary Disorders of Hemostasis

Differentiate the causes, classification, underlying pathogenesis, and clinical manifestations of secondary disorders of hemostasis and approaches to diagnosis and treatment of these conditions across the lifespan.

- Secondary disorders of hemostasis are associated with deficits in the formation or function of coagulation factors.
- An acquired secondary issue of hemostasis is a deficiency in levels of vitamin K, an important constituent element of several clotting factors.
- Hemophilia is a hereditary genetic bleeding disorder that results from the loss of select clotting factors. There are two main forms of hemophilia; hemophilia A results from a lack of factor VIII, and hemophilia B results from a deficiency in factor IX.
- Acquired forms of hemophilia result from autoimmune disease, cancer, or pregnancy.
- Hemophilia can result in significant bleeding into soft tissues or joints.
- Prophylactic treatment can often aid in avoiding serious complications of hemophilia later in life and is centered on intravenous administration of the missing clotting factor.

22.5 Issues of Hypercoagulopathy

Differentiate the causes, classification, underlying pathogenesis, and clinical manifestations of hypercoagulopathy and approaches to diagnosis and treatment of the condition across the lifespan.

- Sickle cell disease affects not only the shape of blood cells but also the clotting pathways.
- Sickle cell disease is tied to increased levels of thrombin, increased activity on the part of platelets, and a decrease in the proteins that serve as anticoagulants. This leaves the individual at risk for the development of thrombi.
- Disseminated intravascular coagulation (DIC) is a life-threatening condition associated with sepsis, pregnancy, and traumatic injury.
- In DIC, clotting factors are consumed and a number of small clots are formed, which can disrupt the blood supply to organs or cause serious spontaneous bleeding. Clinical manifestations of DIC include difficulty in breathing, hemoptysis, and often tachycardia. The individual with DIC requires monitoring for blood loss and the signs of organ failure as a result of ischemic damage.
- Thrombocythemia is a condition characterized by increased platelet production, resulting in higher than expected numbers of thrombocytes.
- The individual with thrombocythemia is at an increased risk for the development of blood clots.

REVIEW QUESTIONS

1. The nurse is discussing the clotting process with a student nurse. Which explanation is correct in explaining the vascular phase?
   a. "In the vascular phase, injury to a blood vessel causes a reactive constriction or spasm of the blood vessel, and then platelets are activated and travel to the site of injury."
   b. "In the vascular phase, no injury to the blood vessel is present, but constriction or spasm occurs, and then platelets are activated."
   c. "In the vascular phase, the platelets begin to clump together to form a dam or plug, and then platelets are deactivated that travel to the site."
   d. "In the vascular phase, the immune proteins and other factors are released by platelets, leading to the formation of fibrin, which forms a layer over the platelet plug to help stop blood loss."

2. Which clotting factor is missing in hemophilia A?
   a. Factor I
   b. Factor III
   c. Factor VI
   d. Factor VIII

3. Which vitamin is helpful in clotting?
   a. Vitamin A
   b. Vitamin B
   c. Vitamin D
   d. Vitamin K

4. A student is explaining the D-dimer test to a client's family. Which response by a family member demonstrates understanding of the test?
   a. "My father has to have this lab test to determine whether he has a bleeding problem."
   b. "My father needs this x-ray to show whether he has bleeding in his left chest wall."
   c. "My father need this lab test to show whether he has a possible blood clotting problem."
   d. "My father is having this test to show whether he has internal bleeding and where it is."

5. A nurse is caring for a client who currently is being infused with a heparin IV drip. What lab work would the nurse anticipate being ordered daily by the provider?
   a. Fibrin level
   b. D-dimer
   c. PT and CBC
   d. aPTT

6. Which conditions are commonly associated with DIC? (Select all that apply.)
   a. Sepsis
   b. Pregnancy
   c. Trauma
   d. Stroke
   e. Diabetes

7. The nurse is caring for a newborn after circumcision. The bandage was changed at 0800, and when the nurse checks it again at 0805, it is saturated with bright red fluid. What should the nurse suspect?
   a. Hemophilia
   b. Thrombocytopenia
   c. DIC
   d. Sickle cell disease

8. The nurse is discussing the possible causes of thrombocytopenia with the client in an outpatient clinic who is being seen for low platelet count. Which statement made by the client demonstrates a need for further discussion?
   a. "I might have cancer of the blood because my platelets are too low."
   b. "I might have hemophilia because my platelets are so low right now."
   c. "Leukemia and lymphoma are two possible causes of a low platelet count."
   d. "Because I work with chemicals, this could be the reason for the low platelet count."

ANSWERS

Answers to Review Questions can be found in Appendix A. Answers to Case Study and Check Your Progress questions are available on the faculty resources site. Please consult with your instructor.

RECOMMENDED WEBSITES

American Society of Hematology
http://www.hematology.org

Cleveland Clinic Center for Continuing Education: Bleeding Disorders
http://www.clevelandclinicmeded.com/medicalpubs/diseasemanagement/hematology-oncology/bleeding-disorders

U.S. National Library of Medicine: Hemophilia
https://ghr.nlm.nih.gov/condition/hemophilia

REFERENCES

1. Versteeg, H. H., Heemskerk, J. W. M., Levi, M., & Reitsma, P. H. (2013). New fundamentals in hemostasis. *Physiological Reviews, 93*(1), 327–358. doi:10.1152/physrev.00016.2011
2. Katrancha, E. D., & Gonzalez, L. S., III. (2014). Trauma-induced coagulopathy. *Critical Care Nurse, 34*(4), 54–63.
3. Bain, B. J. (2015). *Blood cells: A practical guide* (5th ed.). Hoboken, NJ: Wiley-Blackwell.
4. Castaman, G., Goodeve, A., & Eikenboom, J. (2013). Principles of care for the diagnosis and treatment of von Willebrand disease. *Haematologica, 98*, 667–674.
5. Sekhon, S. S., & Roy, V. (2006). Thrombocytopenia in adults: A practical approach to evaluation and management. *Southern Medical Journal, 99*(5), 491–498.
6. Scully, M., Hunt, B. J., Benjamin, S., et al. (2012). Guidelines on the diagnosis and management of thrombotic thrombocytopenic purpura and other thrombotic microangiopathies. *British Journal of Haematology, 158*(3), 323–335.
7. Mitchell, O., Feldman, D. M., Diakow, M., & Sigal, S. H. (2016). The pathophysiology of thrombocytopenia in chronic liver disease. *Hepatic Medicine, 8*, 39–50.
8. Srivastava, A., Brewer, A. K., Mauser-Bunschoten, E. P., et al. (2013). Guidelines for the management of hemophilia. *Haemophilia, 19*(1), e1–e47.
9. Franchini, M., & Mannucci, P. M. (2012). Past, present and future of hemophilia: A narrative review. *Orphanet Journal of Rare Diseases, 7*, 24. doi:10.1186/1750-1172-7-24
10. Peyvandi, F., Garagiola, I., & Young, G. (2016). The past and future of haemophilia: Diagnosis, treatments and its complications. *Lancet, 388*(10040), 9–15.
11. Noubouossie, D., Key, N. S., & Ataga, K. I. (2016). Coagulation abnormalities of sickle cell disease: Relationship with clinical outcomes and the effect of disease modifying therapies. *Blood Reviews, 30*(4), 245–256.
12. Erez, O., Mastrolia, S. A., & Thachil, J. (2016). Disseminated intravascular coagulation in pregnancy: Insights in pathphysiology, diagnosis, and management. *Obstetric Anesthesia Digest, 213*(3), 452–463.
13. Levi, M., & van der Poll, T. (2013). Disseminated intravascular coagulation: A review for the internist. *Internal and Emergency Medicine, 8*(1), 23–32.
14. Tefferi, A. (2013). Polycythemia vera and essential thrombocythemia: 2013 update on diagnosis, risk-stratification, and management. *American Journal of Hematology, 88*(6), 507–516.
15. Luque Paz, D., Chauveau, A., Boyer, F., et al. (2017). Sequential analysis of 18 genes in polycythemia vera and essential thrombocythemia reveals an association between mutational status and clinical outcome. *Genes Chromosomes & Cancer, 56*(5), 354–362.

Chapter 23

Vascular Disorders

Suzanne DeYoung and Michael P. Adams

Chapter Outline and Learning Outcomes

23.1 Chapter Overview and Case Studies

Describe normal arterial and venous circulation, peripheral vascular diseases, and concepts related to alterations in vascular health.

23.2 Peripheral Arterial Disease

Differentiate the causes, classification, underlying pathogenesis, and clinical manifestations of peripheral arterial disease and approaches to diagnosis and treatment of these conditions across the lifespan.

23.3 Chronic Venous Disease

Differentiate the causes, classification, underlying pathogenesis, and clinical manifestations of chronic venous disease and approaches to diagnosis and treatment of these conditions across the lifespan.

23.4 Hypertension

Differentiate the causes, classification, underlying pathogenesis, and clinical manifestations of hypertension and approaches to diagnosis and treatment of this condition across the lifespan.

KEY TERMS

Aneurysm, 556
Angioplasty, 558
Arterial dissection, 557
Arteriosclerosis, 555
Atheroma, 555
Atherosclerosis, 555
Chronic venous disease (CVD), 559
Chronic venous insufficiency (CVI), 560
Claudication, 556
Deep vein thrombosis (DVT), 561
Essential (primary) hypertension, 563
High-density lipoproteins (HDLs), 555
Hyperlipidemia, 555
Hypertension (HTN), 562
Hypertensive crisis, 565
Hypertensive urgency, 565
Infarction, 556
Leg ulcers, 560
Low-density lipoproteins (LDLs), 555
Nonatherosclerotic peripheral arterial disease (NAPAD), 558
Peripheral artery disease (PAD), 553
Peripheral vascular disease (PVD), 553
Plaque, 555
Raynaud disease, 559
Secondary hypertension, 563
Thoracic outlet syndrome (TOS), 558
Thromboembolism, 561
Varicose veins, 560
Vulnerable plaque, 556

ABBREVIATIONS

ABI—ankle–brachial index
ACE—angiotensin-converting enzyme
ARB—angiotensin receptor blocker
CAD—coronary artery disease
CCB—calcium channel blocker
CVD—chronic venous disease
CVI—chronic venous insufficiency
DVT—deep vein thrombosis
HDL—high-density lipoprotein
HTN—hypertension
LDL—low-density lipoprotein
MI—myocardial infarction
NAPAD—nonatherosclerotic peripheral arterial disease
PAD—peripheral arterial disease
PVD—peripheral vascular disease
RAAS—renin-angiotensin-aldosterone system
TLC—therapeutic lifestyle change
TOS—thoracic outlet syndrome

23.1 Chapter Overview and Case Studies

All cells need a continuous supply of nutrients to perform their physiologic tasks. Furthermore, all cells create metabolic waste, which must be removed to maintain adequate function. Failure to provide nutrients or remove waste can result in tissue ischemia or necrosis. Perfusion, the passage of blood through the circulatory system, is therefore a critical concept that affects all body cells and tissues. This chapter examines diseases of the vascular system that affect perfusion. Chapter 24 examines the role of the heart in perfusion.

The vascular system consists of a series of vessels that transport blood. Arteries carry oxygen-rich blood away from the heart to the other parts of the body, where they branch into tiny capillaries, which deliver the oxygen and other nutrients to organs and tissues. In the capillaries, the tissues return carbon dioxide and other wastes to the blood, which is carried back to the heart. Although the vascular system may appear to be simple, remember that the tissues of the body are absolutely dependent on this system for their survival. Lack of sufficient blood flow may result in hypoxia and a buildup of waste products that can cause acute or chronic organ damage.

Arteries and veins are composed of three layers, called tunicas. The inner layer, the tunica intima consists of a single layer of epithelium that provides an extremely smooth surface for efficient blood transport. Disruptions to this smooth surface, such as tearing or lipid accumulation, may affect blood flow. The middle layer, the tunica media, consists of vascular smooth muscle, which provides a method for vessels to change the diameter of their lumens. The diameter affects the dynamic resistance to blood flow, which is responsible for systemic blood pressure. Changing the diameter of the lumen directs more blood to specific areas when needed, such as the digestive tract following a meal. Arteries contain a thick tunica media and thus are the primary means of changing resistance in the vascular system. The thin-walled veins contain only small amounts of smooth muscle, have low pressure, and contribute little to systemic blood pressure. The third vessel layer, the tunica externa (or adventitia), contains connective tissue that anchors the blood vessels to surrounding organs and tissues. Capillaries contain only one layer: the tunica intima.

Perfusion may be divided into two broad categories: central and local. Central perfusion is blood flow pumped by the heart to the entire vascular system. It is determined primarily by the cardiac output (milliliters of blood pumped per minute) and blood pressure. Pathologic processes of central perfusion such as shock or hypertension affect the entire body. Local perfusion (or microvascular perfusion) is the volume of blood flowing through a specific tissue. This volume changes dynamically with activities such as digestion, sleep, or exercise. Local perfusion is controlled by capillaries serving the specific region. Pathologic processes of local perfusion such as a blocked blood vessel or edema affect specific tissues rather than the entire body.

The study of vascular system pathophysiology is usually divided into conditions that affect arteries and those that affect veins. **Peripheral vascular disease (PVD)** is a general term referring to conditions affecting circulation in the tissues other than the brain or heart. If the condition affects the *arteries*, the term **peripheral artery disease (PAD)** is used. PAD is usually caused by arteriosclerosis, which is the most common chronic arterial disorder. Common types of PVD that affect *veins* include chronic venous insufficiency, deep vein thrombosis, leg ulcers, and varicose veins. Hypertension is also discussed in this chapter because it is often caused by arterial disease.

Risk factors for PVD are similar to those for other cardiovascular diseases. These include smoking, hypertension, coronary heart disease, high cholesterol, diabetes, family history of vascular disease, obesity, and sedentary lifestyle. PVD primarily affects adults over age 50. Men are affected more often than women.[1]

Concepts Related to Vascular Disorders

A number of concepts and systems affect and are affected by impaired perfusion, including, cognition, comfort and pain, fluids and electrolytes, acid–base balance, nutrition. and oxygenation.

Cognition can be affected by atherosclerosis or blood clots in vessels serving the brain. Clinical signs or symptoms of ischemia can be seen when cerebral perfusion pressure drops below the lower limit for brain function. Altered mental status is an early symptom of decreased cerebral blood flow. Without adequate cerebral blood flow, energy-dependent brain processes cease, leading to irreversible brain injury.

Impaired tissue perfusion results when the blood supply to a site of injury is diminished. Comfort can be a concern, as pain is a common symptom of vascular disorders. Local redness and edema of extremities, especially the legs, result when peripheral vascular disease impairs blood return to the heart. Fluids and electrolytes may not reach peripheral tissues when circulation is impaired. Inadequate fluid distribution may lead to multiple organ failure.

Respiratory gases are transported by red blood cells; therefore, adequate pulmonary ventilation, diffusion, and perfusion are essential for gas exchange to occur. The process of perfusion pumps blood to and from the lungs by way of the pulmonary circuit of the cardiovascular system. Blood clots in vessels serving the lungs will affect oxygenation of the blood and subsequently the tissues. Inadequate lung perfusion may lead to acid–base imbalances. Selected concepts related to vascular disorders are mapped in **Figure 23.1** ■.

Case Studies

The following cases are addressed throughout the chapter to assist in application of chapter content to clinical situations that involve individuals with disorders of vascularization.

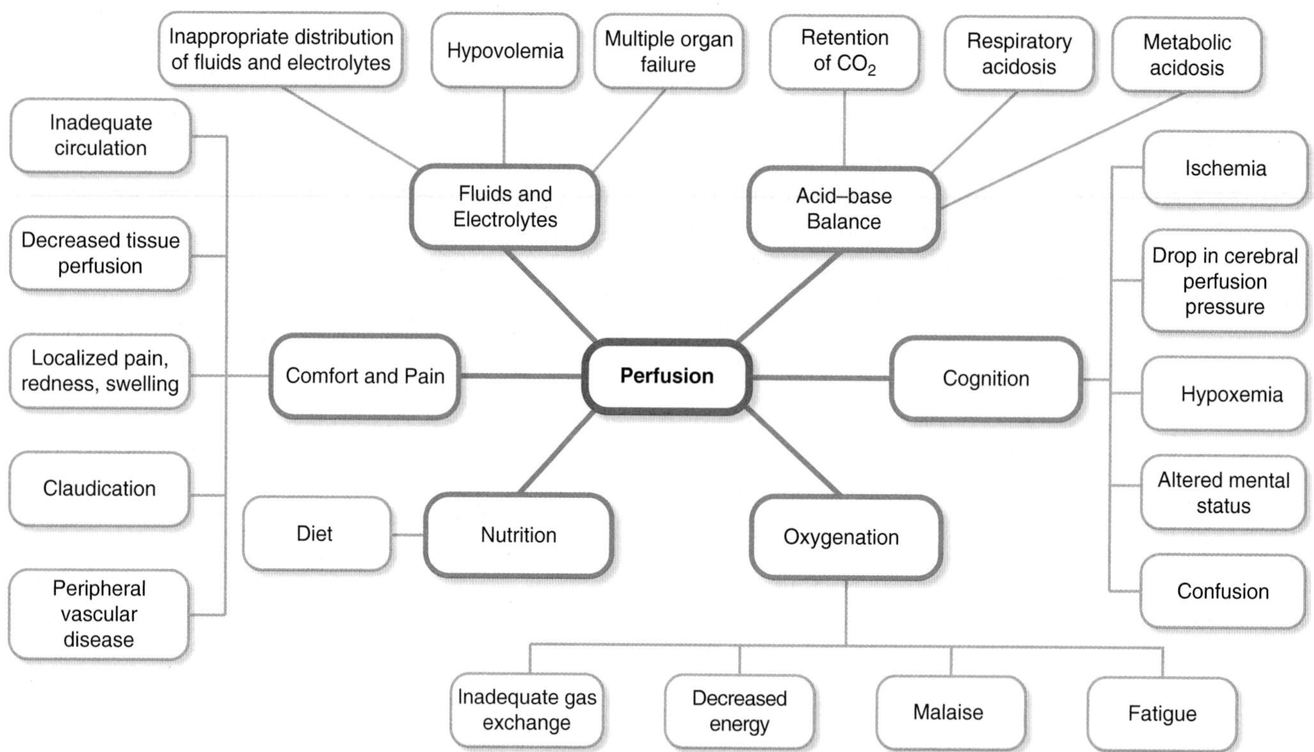

Figure 23.1 ■ Concepts related to vascular disorders.

Daniel Covington: Introduction

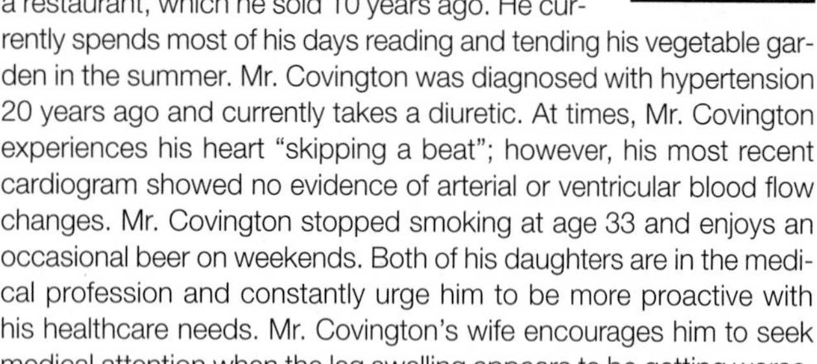

Daniel Covington, a 75-year-old male, noticed that his lower legs began to swell after he sat for long periods of time. Mr. Covington used to own a restaurant, which he sold 10 years ago. He currently spends most of his days reading and tending his vegetable garden in the summer. Mr. Covington was diagnosed with hypertension 20 years ago and currently takes a diuretic. At times, Mr. Covington experiences his heart "skipping a beat"; however, his most recent cardiogram showed no evidence of arterial or ventricular blood flow changes. Mr. Covington stopped smoking at age 33 and enjoys an occasional beer on weekends. Both of his daughters are in the medical profession and constantly urge him to be more proactive with his healthcare needs. Mr. Covington's wife encourages him to seek medical attention when the leg swelling appears to be getting worse.

1. What are Mr. Covington's risk factors for the development of peripheral arterial disease?
2. Which type of perfusion dysfunction is Mr. Covington experiencing?
3. What is the pathologic process resulting in Mr. Covington's leg swelling?

Aadila Shakoor: Introduction

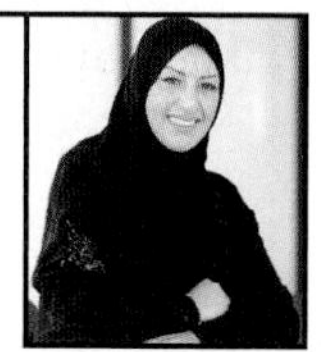

Aadila Shakoor, age 34, arrived in the United States from Lebanon a week ago, having received a work-related visa to work at NASA as a physicist. She is slowly getting used to the warm Texas climate. This morning while getting dressed, Dr. Shakoor feels pain in her right lower leg. She notices that the lower leg is swollen and warm to the touch. On arrival at work, Dr. Shakoor asks to see the facility nurse to discuss the leg swelling. The nurse notes that the pulses in Dr. Shakoor's right foot are diminished and her lower leg is becoming more edematous. Dr. Shakoor is transported to the local emergency department for evaluation and treatment.

1. What might be a reason for Dr. Shakoor's leg swelling?
2. What caused the pulses in Dr. Shakoor's right leg to be diminished?
3. Why did the nurse have Dr. Shakoor transported to the local emergency department?

Emilio Suarez: Introduction

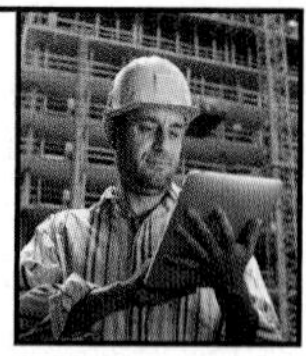

Emilio Suarez is a 48-year-old male who has just been hired to work with a major contractor to build a multi-office complex. Before starting the job, Mr. Suarez arrives for his pre-employment physical, at which his blood pressure is found to be 168/90 mmHg. Mr. Suarez's heart rate is 90 beats per minute, and he has a BMI of 30. The clinic physician prescribes a diuretic and clears Mr. Suarez for employment only after he agrees to have his blood pressure checked weekly at the work site infirmary.

1. What could be contributing to Mr. Suarez's high blood pressure?
2. For what other risk factors for hypertension should Mr. Suarez be assessed?

Check Your Progress: Section 23.1

1. What are the two major categories of perfusion?
2. List three risk factors for peripheral vascular disease.
3. List two peripheral vascular diseases that affect the veins.

23.2 Peripheral Arterial Disease

Arteriosclerosis

The most common PAD is **arteriosclerosis**, the thickening, loss of elasticity, and calcification of the walls of arteries. Healthy blood vessels are very elastic, which allows for rapid changes in cardiac output and blood pressure that are required for activities such as physical exercise. With aging, arteries begin to calcify and lose their elasticity. Arteriosclerosis prevents rapid vascular changes in blood pressure. **Atherosclerosis** is a form of arteriosclerosis caused by a buildup of **plaque**, which is made up of cholesterol, calcium, and other substances that harden on arterial walls, causing them to narrow. The two terms, *arteriosclerosis* and *atherosclerosis* are sometimes used interchangeably.

Etiology and Pathogenesis

While the exact etiology of atherosclerosis is unknown, risk factors associated with the disorder are well documented. Risk factors include both genetic and lifestyle components. The genetic nature of atherosclerosis is evidenced by people who inherit familial hypercholesterolemia, a condition in which the blood contains extremely high levels of cholesterol. People with homozygous familial hypercholesterolemia develop severe cardiovascular disease in childhood and often die by their mid-30s.[2]

Lifestyle factors associated with atherosclerosis are similar to those for related cardiovascular diseases. These factors include smoking, hypertension, heart disease, high levels of cholesterol and LDLs, diabetes, obesity, advanced age, and physical inactivity. Most lifestyle risk factors may be controlled by healthy dietary habits, regular exercise, and proper medical management.

CLINICAL POINT: Nurses are instrumental in educating patients about their risk for vascular disorders and teaching patients measures to reduce their risks. ■

Because atherosclerosis is essentially a result of a buildup of plaque containing primarily cholesterol, the pathogenesis of the disorder requires an understanding of lipid metabolism and transport. Several terms are used to describe lipid disorders. *Dyslipidemia* is a general term referring to abnormally high or low lipid levels in the blood. The most common form of dyslipidemia is **hyperlipidemia**, which is defined as an elevated level of blood lipids. More specific terms include *hypercholesterolemia* (high blood cholesterol levels) and *hypertriglyceridemia* (high blood triglyceride levels). When medication is used to treat a lipid disorder, the specific drug depends on the type of lipid that is elevated.

Because lipids are not soluble in plasma, they are carried as part of complexes called lipoproteins, which consist of various amounts of cholesterol, triglycerides, and phospholipid bound to the carrier protein. These lipoproteins are classified on the basis of their size and composition as high density, low density, or very low density. **Low-density lipoproteins (LDLs)** are the primary carriers of cholesterol. Elevated levels of LDL promote atherosclerosis because LDL deposits cholesterol on arterial walls. (LDL can also be considered a mnemonic for "less desirable lipoproteins.") In contrast, **high-density lipoproteins (HDLs)** help to clear cholesterol from the arteries, transporting it to the liver for excretion. (HDL can also be considered a mnemonic for "highly desirable lipoproteins.") HDL levels of 60 mg/dL or more have a protective effect, reducing the risk of atherosclerosis, whereas HDL levels below 40 mg/dL for men and below 50 mg/dL for women are associated with an increased risk for CAD.[3] A therapeutic goal is to maximize HDL levels and minimize the levels of LDL.

In addition to LDL and HDL, triglyceride levels are an important risk factor for cardiovascular disease. Triglycerides contain three fatty acids bound to glycerol and are used for fat storage and energy use by the body. Almost all triglycerides are transported to adipose tissue for storage by very-low-density lipoproteins (VLDL). Through a series of steps, the VLDLs are transformed into LDL molecules after the triglycerides have been transported to adipose tissue. **Table 23.1** ■ lists desirable and high-risk levels for total cholesterol, LDL cholesterol, and triglycerides.

Atherosclerosis begins when endothelial cells are damaged. When LDL cholesterol reaches the damaged endothelium, white blood cells attack the LDL, and plaque begins to form (**Figure 23.2** ■). The region of plaque, called an **atheroma**, consists of calcium, macrophages, lipids, and fibrous connective tissue. Depending on various factors such as the presence of associated risk factors, especially hyperlipidemia, the atheroma may grow slowly or rapidly.

The presence of T cells, monocytes, and macrophages at the site of plaque formation creates a chronic inflammatory response. As a consequence of chronic inflammation, growth factors are released from platelets, macrophages, and endothelial cells that stimulate the proliferation of smooth muscle cells. The smooth muscle cells secrete extracellular matrix, which tends to stabilize the plaque. Over many years, the continued inflammation and proliferation

Table 23.1 Classification of Serum Cholesterol and Triglyceride Values

	Total Cholesterol (mg/dL)	Low-Density Lipoprotein Cholesterol (mg/dL)	Triglycerides (mg/dL)
Optimal		< 100	
Desirable	< 200	100–129	< 150
Borderline high risk	200–239	130–159	150–199
High risk	≥ 240	160–189	200–499
Very high risk		≥ 190	≥ 500

SOURCES: Data from Cleveland Clinic. (2013). *What do cholesterol numbers mean?* Retrieved from https://my.clevelandclinic.org/health/diseases_conditions/hic_Cholesterol/hic_what_do_cholesterol_numbers_mean; Mayo Clinic. (2016a). *High cholesterol: Diagnosis.* Retrieved from http://www.mayoclinic.org/diseases-conditions/high-blood-cholesterol/diagnosis-treatment/diagnosis/dxc-20181913.; National Heart, Lung, and Blood Institute (NHLBI). (2014). *How is high blood cholesterol diagnosed?* Retrieved from https://www.nhlbi.nih.gov/health/health-topics/topics/hbc/diagnosis.

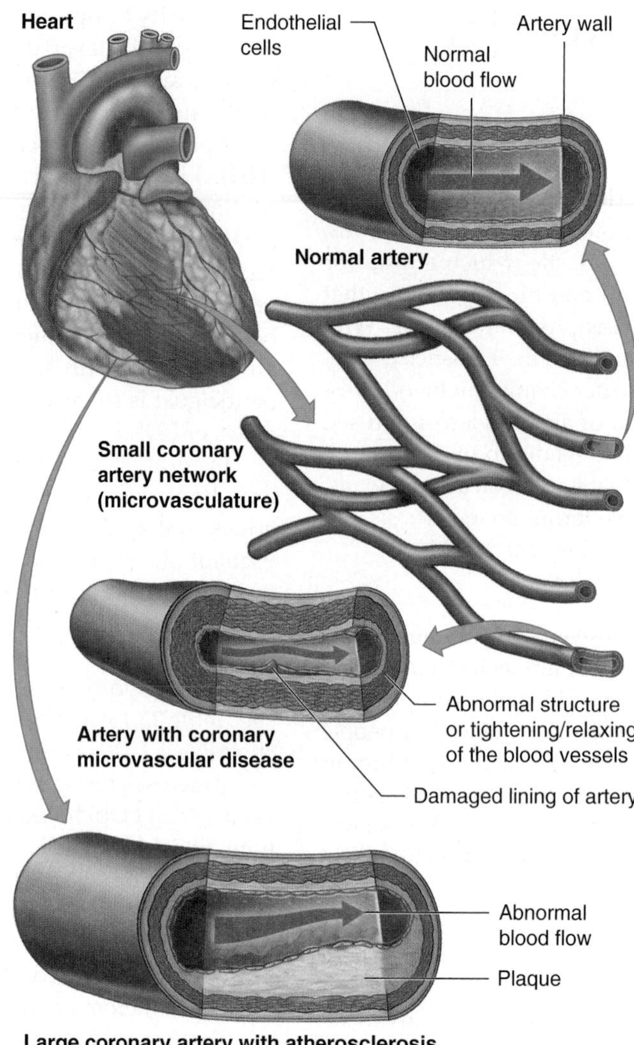

Figure 23.2 ■ Atherosclerosis begins when endothelial cells are damaged. When LDL cholesterol reaches the damaged endothelium, white blood cells attack the LDL, and plaque begins to form.

enlarge the atheroma, which may eventually intrude on the vessel lumen and impair circulation.[4] In addition to growing larger, atheromas commonly undergo calcification over time.

Clinical Manifestations

The three major consequences of atherosclerosis are myocardial infarction, stroke, and PAD. These consequences are the result of either atherosclerotic stenosis or plaque rupture.

Atherosclerotic stenosis is the partial or complete blockage of an artery due to atherosclerotic plaque. If the plaque is found in the carotid arteries, it is referred to as carotid artery disease, which can lead to stroke. Plaque located in the heart is identified as coronary artery disease (CAD). CAD can cause ischemia of the myocardium, resulting in angina and possibly a myocardial infarction (MI). Stenosis of vessels serving the kidneys may result in chronic kidney disease. Stenosis of vessels in the extremities causes PVD. When blood flow to skeletal muscle is insufficient, the patient may experience **claudication**, a cramping muscle pain in the region of the narrowing. At first, claudication may be intermittent and occur only during exercise, but it may progress to pain even when at rest.[5]

Plaque rupture is usually followed by thrombosis (blood clot) and possibly **infarction**, which is complete obstruction of a vessel. Thrombosis is responsible for acute life-threatening or disabling conditions such as MI, pulmonary embolism, and stroke. Some types of plaque are more likely to rupture than others. Stable plaque contains a thick fibrous cap that protects the atheroma from shearing forces within the artery. **Vulnerable plaque** has more inflammation and a thinner fibrous cap, which makes it more susceptible to rupture with subsequent thrombi formation. Not all plaque ruptures are fatal; some are small, and the thrombi do not cause clinically significant events.

Other manifestations of atherosclerosis include arterial aneurysms, arterial dissection, and acute arterial occlusion (**Figure 23.3** ■). An **aneurysm** is the bulging of a weak arterial wall, of which plaque and hypertension make up a primary cause. Aneurysms occur throughout the body,

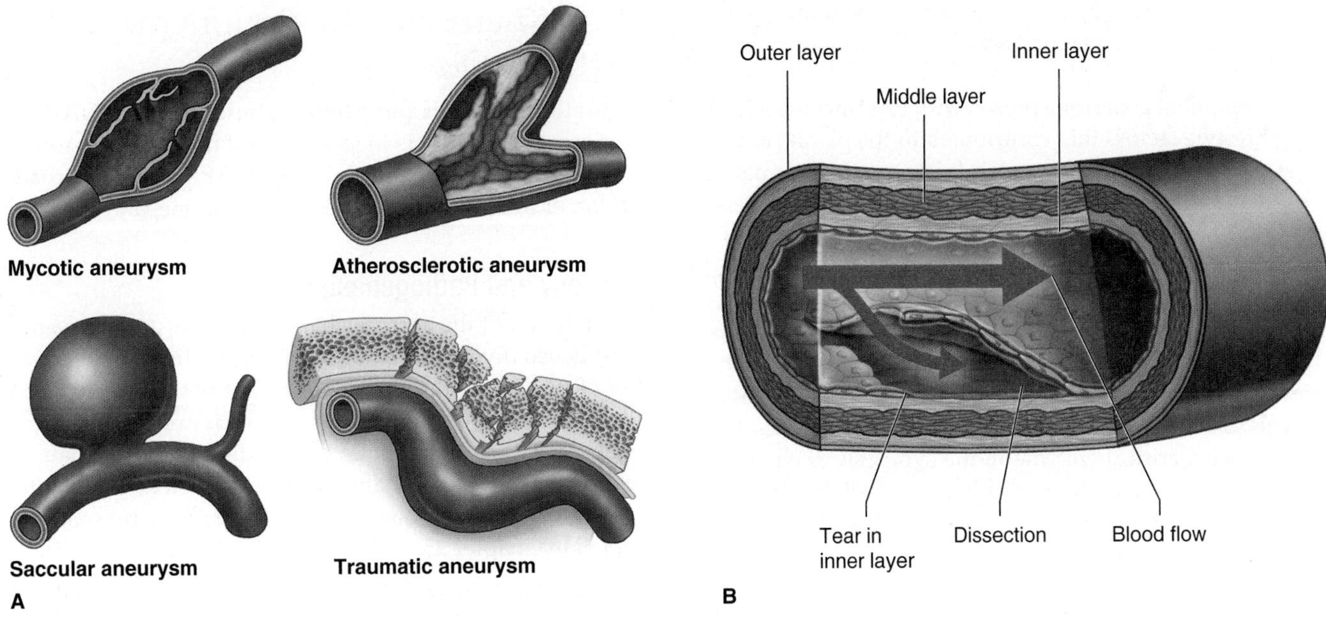

Figure 23.3 ■ Arterial abnormalities. **A.** Various types of aneurysms. **B.** Arterial dissection and clot formation.

but they are more serious in some areas than in others.[6] Of major concern are brain, eye, popliteal, and abdominal aortic aneurysms. Depending on the location, aneurysms may or may not cause any signs or symptoms. Aneurysms in the brain may cause headaches, dilated pupils, visual changes, and left or right facial weakness or numbness. Eye aneurysms are not noticed unless they cause a loss of vision. Popliteal aneurysms may be more noticeable because of their location and the shape of the artery involved. Abdominal aortic aneurysms are medical emergencies that may or may not cause clinical symptoms. The rupture of an aortic aneurysm has a high mortality rate.

Arterial dissection is caused by a tear in the tunica intima in which the blood vessel splits and blood goes between the inner and outer layers, separating or dissecting the walls of the vessel. It is unclear what leads to the splitting, but trauma, heredity, cocaine use, pregnancy, and hypertension are associated risk factors. The damage and severity depend on the size of the split. Arterial dissection is considered an emergency because it can lead to arterial obstruction or emboli that may cause a stroke, MI, or renal failure.[7]

Daniel Covington: Application

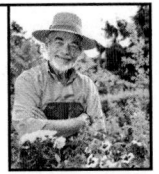

At the insistence of his wife and daughters, Mr. Covington sees his primary care physician for evaluation of his lower leg edema. The physical examination finds good popliteal, dorsalis pedis, and posterior tibial pulses. Edema is +2 on the left anterior lower leg and +1 on the right anterior lower leg. The skin is slightly reddened and easily blanched. Mr. Covington's blood pressure is 148/88 mmHg, and his BMI is 28.5. Blood samples are drawn for serum cholesterol and triglyceride levels. Mr. Covington is given a prescription for an additional antihypertensive medication and instructions to begin a low-fat, 1800-calorie diet. A follow-up appointment is scheduled for 2 weeks from now, at which time the laboratory values will be available.

At the appointment 2 weeks later, Mr. Covington learns that his total cholesterol level is 210 mg/dL, his LDL level is 140 mg/dL, and his triglyceride level is 160 mg/dL. He has lost several pounds during the 2 weeks, bringing his BMI to 28.1. Diet teaching is reinforced, and he is strongly urged to begin a walking program of 10 minutes per day, increasing at the rate of 1 minute per day each week. The primary care provider schedules an appointment to see Mr. Covington again in 3 months.

4. What could be the reason why Mr. Covington's amount of edema is different on each leg?
5. What do Mr. Covington's laboratory results indicate?
6. Why is a walking program prescribed for Mr. Covington?

Linking Pathophysiology to Diagnosis and Treatment

Diagnosis of PAD and atherosclerosis is accomplished by a thorough physical examination and several diagnostic tests. Checking pulses in the extremities is used to detect unequal blood flow. Listening with a stethoscope over certain arteries may help to detect a bruit, a whooshing sound that occurs as blood tumbles over and around areas of plaque buildup. A laboratory workup is necessary to identify existing risk factors for atherosclerosis such as hyperlipidemia or diabetes. If cardiac involvement is suspected, a treadmill test with echocardiography may be ordered to detect abnormal increases in heart rate and blood pressure, shortness of breath, or angina. If renal involvement is suspected, kidney function tests may be ordered.

A simple test used to help diagnose PAD is the ankle–brachial index (ABI). The ABI compares the blood pressure in the arms with the blood pressure in the ankles. An abnormal reading may indicate that circulation in the legs is diminished.

Several types of imaging are useful in detecting atherosclerosis. Ultrasonography is a noninvasive method that is used to detect and measure the degree of plaque in major arteries of the neck and limbs. Angiography is a medical imaging procedure that injects a contrast medium (dye) into arteries to identify plaque and other abnormalities such as aneurysms.

Treatment goals for a person with PAD include addressing lifestyle factors that contributed to the plaque and surgery to open occluded arteries. It is essential that patients understand the critical importance of changing lifestyle habits. This includes controlling blood glucose levels, managing high blood pressure, maintaining optimal weight, engaging in a regular program of physical activity, and eating a healthy diet. Medications may be necessary to manage blood pressure and to lower blood glucose and cholesterol levels. The primary medications used to lower cholesterol levels are called statins. Statins such as atorvastatin (Lipitor) block a critical enzyme in the synthesis of cholesterol in the liver and can dramatically lower LDL levels. Statins have been shown to reduce the risk of MI and stroke.[8]

If severe plaque is identified in a critical artery, such as one serving a major organ, the vessel must be reopened to prevent infarction. **Angioplasty** with stent placement is the minimally invasive procedure usually employed for this purpose. A balloon-tipped catheter is placed into an artery and advanced to the area of blockage. The balloon is inflated, pressing the plaque against the arterial wall. Once opened, the balloon is deflated, and a small wire mesh tube called a stent is placed in the vessel to keep it from narrowing or closing again. Drug-eluting stents are coated with an anti-inflammatory medication such as everolimus that reduces the risk of inflammation and scar formation around the stent. Following stent placement, most patients receive an antiplatelet medication such as clopidogrel (Plavix) and aspirin for about 12 months or longer to prevent clots from forming on the stent.

Daniel Covington: Outcome

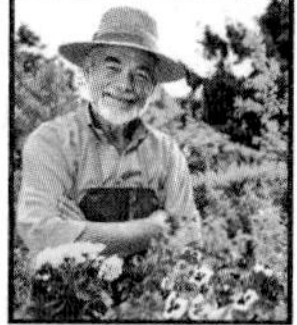

Mr. Covington returns to the primary care physician for a 3-month evaluation. His blood pressure is 130/78 mmHg, and his BMI is 26.5. However, the leg edema persists. Mr. Covington is scheduled for an ultrasound of the bilateral lower extremities in a few days. In the meantime, he is encouraged by the results and reports walking for 20-minute periods every day without needing to stop and rest. Follow-up cholesterol and triglyceride samples are drawn.

A few days later, the ultrasound is performed. This test reveals the arterial blood flow of both lower extremities to be at 70%. An angiogram is not required at this time, but Mr. Covington is informed that it might be required in the future. Follow-up laboratory values show that his total cholesterol is now 190 mg/dL, his LDL level is 120 mg/dL, and his triglyceride level is 140 mg/dL. Mr. Covington is instructed to continue to take the prescribed medication, continue the walking program to achieve 30 minutes per day, and strive to reach a BMI below 24.9. Another appointment is scheduled to occur in 3 months.

7. Why was the ultrasound performed first?
8. Why is Mr. Covington instructed to continue to lose weight?
9. What is the importance of Mr. Covington continuing a walking program?
10. What would determine whether Mr. Covington needs an angiogram in the future?

Nonatherosclerotic Peripheral Arterial Disease

Nonatherosclerotic peripheral arterial disease (NAPAD) is a group of disorders in which blood flow is decreased for reasons other than plaque buildup. NAPADs include coarctation of the aorta, thoracic outlet syndrome, and Raynaud disease.

Etiology and Pathogenesis

Coarctation of the aorta is characterized by a narrow aorta and is usually identified at birth. Depending on the severity of the defect, the symptoms might not be evident until the individual reaches an age at which exertion produces symptoms. Treatment options include surgery to repair the coarctation or balloon angioplasty with stent to open the narrowed vessel.[9] Coarctation of the aorta is presented in detail in Chapter 25.

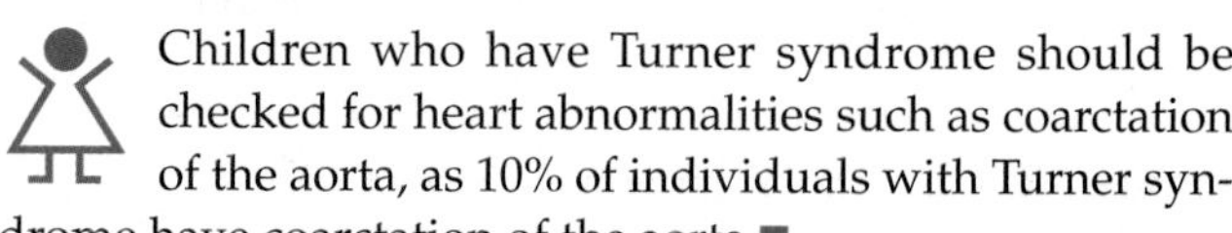

Children who have Turner syndrome should be checked for heart abnormalities such as coarctation of the aorta, as 10% of individuals with Turner syndrome have coarctation of the aorta.■

Another NAPAD is **thoracic outlet syndrome (TOS)**. The thoracic outlet starts at the base of the neck and goes behind the clavicle, over the first rib, and down the arm (**Figure 23.4** ■). This area houses blood vessels and nerves that travel to the arms and fingers. If the path is narrowed, it can restrict the flow of blood and nerve function. For some individuals, the problem happens periodically; for others, it is a continuous problem. One of the main causes of TOS is the upper body meeting resistance on a frequent basis. Resistance can come in the form of excess muscle tissue from heavy labor or lifting weights. Obesity, excess fluid due to pregnancy, and even slouching can also cause

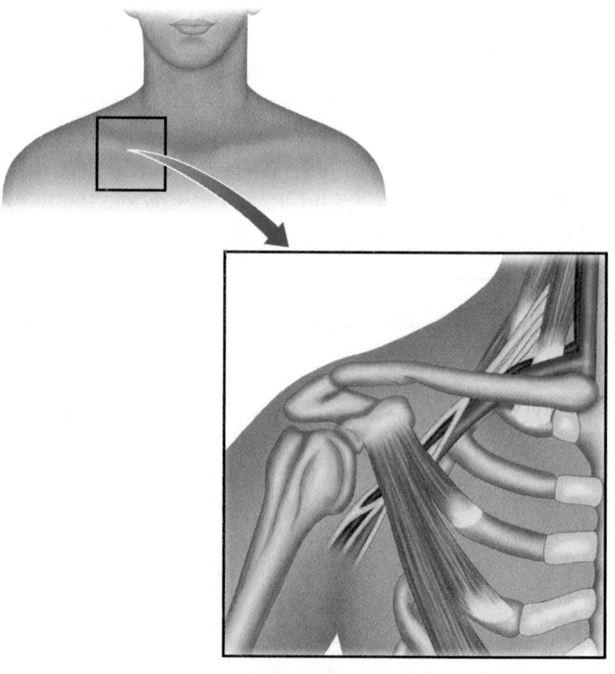

Figure 23.4 ■ The location of the thoracic outlet.

the thoracic outlet space to become constricted. Treatment for TOS includes analgesics for pain and physical therapy to stretch the shoulder muscles, open the outlet, and promote range of motion. In severe cases, surgery may be necessary to relieve compression on nerves and blood vessels.[10]

Raynaud disease is a condition characterized by attacks of vasospasm in the small arteries and arterioles in the fingers (**Figure 23.5** ■). Less frequently, Raynaud disease may affect the toes, ears, nose, lips, and areola. Raynaud attacks are often triggered by cold weather and emotional stress. The two types of Raynaud disease are primary (having no underlying cause) and secondary (caused by another condition). The etiology of primary Raynaud disease is unknown. The primary form begins at a younger age (between ages 15 and 30), and up to half of the patients have a close relative with the disorder, suggesting a hereditary component.[11] Secondary Raynaud (called Raynaud syndrome or Raynaud phenomenon) is often associated with connective diseases such as scleroderma, systemic lupus erythematosus, or rheumatoid arthritis. Diseases that affect arterial function, such as atherosclerosis, can also cause vasospasms. Medications such as beta blockers, antimigraine drugs, sinus decongestants, and chemotherapy agents can cause blood vessels to constrict. Smoking has a direct effect on blood vessels, increasing the risk for Raynaud disease.

Clinical Manifestations

Clinical manifestations of NAPADs depend on the location and severity of the decreased blood flow. Clinical manifestations of coarctation of the aorta depend on the severity of the deformity and how quickly the symptoms manifest (see Chapter 25).

With TOS, the symptoms are related to poor blood flow or decreased nerve function. Not only will there be symptoms distal from the outlet, there will also be ramifications in the neck and shoulder area. These symptoms are in relation to blood backing up and nerves being pinched. The stretching of the blood vessels and dysfunctional nerves lead to pain. The extremity itself may be discolored, may tingle, and may feel weak. The degree of compaction of the thoracic outlet space dictates the severity of symptoms.

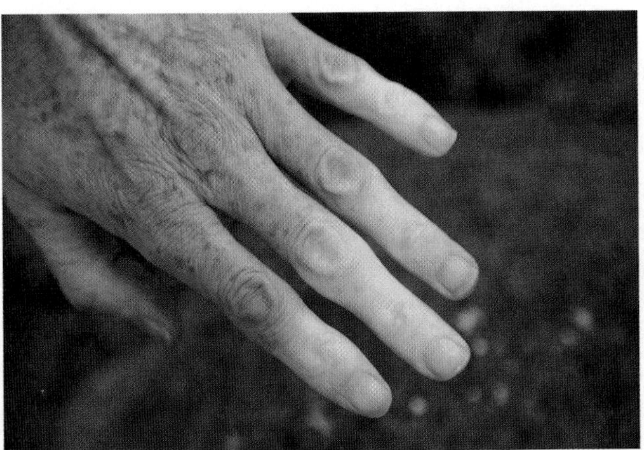

Figure 23.5 ■ Hands of a patient during a Raynaud attack.

Raynaud disease often presents with skin devoid of color or taking on an ashy white appearance. Sluggish blood flow to the region causes the skin to become blue as a result of cyanosis. Symptoms include numbness, tingling, a burning sensation, and, in severe cases, signs of tissue ischemia.[12] Ischemia may result in ulceration or tissue necrosis.

Linking Pathophysiology to Diagnosis and Treatment

Coarctation of the aorta causes the blood to back up into the left ventricle and can lead to heart failure. Because the blood is backed up, the blood pressure in the upper extremities is usually higher than that in the lower extremities. If the healthcare provider suspects coarctation of the aorta, the blood pressure may be taken on the arms and the legs. See Chapter 25 for details of diagnosing and treating coarctation of the aorta. TOS can be diagnosed on the basis of the patient's symptoms as verbalized to the healthcare provider, who can then try to stimulate or exacerbate symptoms. The healthcare provider performs the Adson maneuver (movement of the shoulder joint) to help identify the cause of pain and decreased blood flow and may also manipulate the neck and arm. If the symptoms warrant further testing, it may include measures to monitor blood flow. The treatment for TOS usually involves physical therapy to widen the thoracic outlet and allow the nerves and blood vessels to function normally.

Most individuals with Raynaud disease do not seek medical attention because the events are not severe and symptoms can be improved by simple lifestyle adjustments such as avoidance of cold or wearing protective clothing in cold climates.[11] Other ways to avoid triggers may include stopping smoking or discontinuing medications that exacerbate vasospasms. Drugs that may trigger Raynaud disease include medications for migraines and those for attention-deficit/hyperactivity disorder. Treatment for secondary Raynaud disease addresses the underlying connective tissue problems such as taking anti-inflammatory medications. The primary pharmacologic treatment for Raynaud disease is a calcium channel blocker such as nifedipine, which dilates arterioles. Nifedipine is also used to treat angina and hypertension.

Check Your Progress: Section 23.2

1. List ways to address modifiable risk factors in the development of atherosclerosis.
2. List three diseases for which atherosclerosis is a major risk factor.
3. Which type of arterial aneurysm has the potential for high mortality?

23.3 Chronic Venous Disease

Peripheral vascular disease may affect arteries or veins. When a chronic vascular condition affects veins, it is called **chronic venous disease (CVD)**. The most common cause of CVD is chronic venous insufficiency.

Chronic Venous Insufficiency

Chronic venous insufficiency (CVI) is a disorder in which the veins are unable to return adequate blood to the heart (**Figure 23.6** ■). It is a long-term disorder that most commonly occurs as a result of blood clots in the deep veins of the legs, a condition called deep vein thrombosis. CVI may also be caused by ruptured valves, a condition called varicose veins. In a person with CVI, blood pools in the veins, causing stasis, instead of returning to the heart.

Etiology and Pathogenesis

The etiology of CVI is unclear, but the conditions associated with the disorder are well documented. They include genetic predisposition, gender (the disorder is more common in women), pregnancy, age over 50 years, smoking, lack of physical activity, obesity, and occupations requiring long periods of standing or sitting. Use of oral contraceptives is an additional risk factor in young women.[13]

The central problem in CVI begins with the low pressure that is normally present in the venous system. With such low pressure, blood sometimes has difficulty moving from the legs to the heart, especially when the person is standing. Venous blood flow is assisted by the squeezing of skeletal muscles surrounding the veins, especially the calf muscles, and the presence of valves. The valves open as blood surges forward and close when the blood attempts to move backward. However, venous valves are unable to withstand high pressure. Because veins have only a thin layer of smooth muscle, they are easily stretched when faced with edema, inflammation, or pooling of blood in the legs. Given enough time and elevated pressure, the pooling effect can lead to a rupturing of the valves as well as clot formation.

Clinical Manifestations

General symptoms occurring with CVI include leg cramps and pain that worsens on standing, edema of the leg or ankle, thickening or discoloration of the skin on the calves, and heaviness or weakness in the legs. Three conditions that are closely associated with CVI are chronic leg ulcers, varicose veins, and deep vein thrombosis.

Chronic Leg Ulcers. CVI is the most common cause of chronic **leg ulcers**, which are sores on the skin that persist for more than 6 weeks and take several months or longer to heal. (**Figure 23.7** ■). Other causes include arterial disease and neuropathy. Venous ulcers are usually located from the mid-calf to just below the malleoli; arterial ulcers occur more commonly on the toes, heels, and pressure points on the foot. Severe ulcers may lead to a complete loss of epidermis and extend to portions of the dermis and subcutaneous tissue. Once the skin breaks down, resident bacteria that live on the skin, such as *Staphylococcus*, can infect the open wound.

Leg ulcers affect about 3–5% of individuals between 60 and 80 years of age. Women tend to be more prone to leg ulcers than are men. Some of the contributing risk factors are obesity; leg injuries that cause vein damage; deep vein thrombosis, which can cause increased pressures within the veins; and phlebitis, which is swelling of a vein or veins.[14]

Varicose Veins. Closely associated with CVI, **varicose veins** are veins that have become enlarged and twisted because of the rupture of valves (**Figure 23.8** ■). Spider veins are a milder form of the condition that affect superficial veins. Varicose veins appear bulging and blue in color and primarily affect the legs, although other areas may be affected. Pain and aching associated with varicose veins may be related to tissue lacking sufficient oxygen and nutrients. Varicose veins are prone to inflammation, called superficial thrombophlebitis. The affected leg may feel heavy as a result of the inability of the veins to drain oxygen- and nutrient-depleted blood to make way for freshly oxygenated and nutrient-filled blood.[15] The lack of oxygen and nutrients can also lead to cramping. As blood pools and the veins leak, the legs swell, the skin begins to stretch, and some of the tissue dies, causing dry, cracked skin. As the outer layer of skin dries and cracks, this leads to more pain and itching. As veins give way to pressures and rupture, the individual may experience bruising.

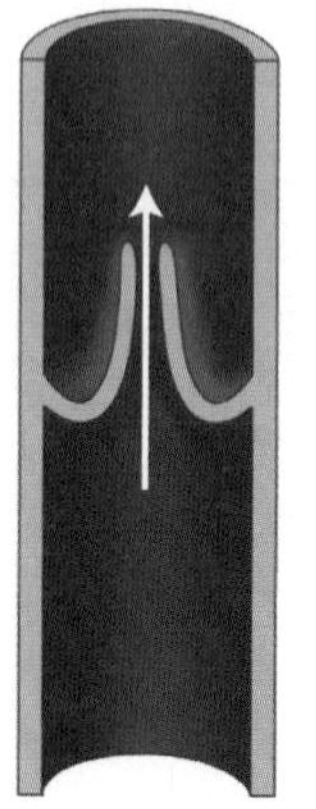

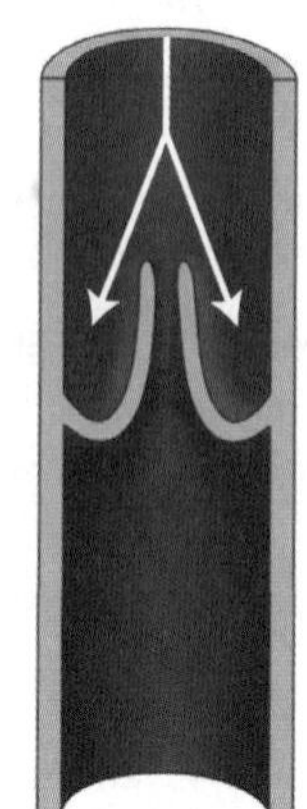

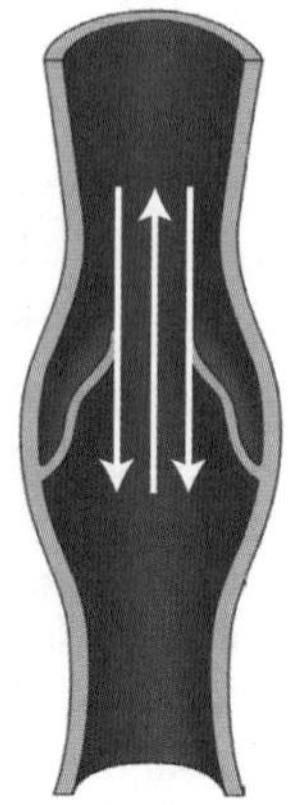

Figure 23.6 ■ Vein abnormalities. **A.** Normal venous valve during dilation of the heart. **B.** Normal venous valve during contraction of the heart. **C.** Damaged valve that leaks.

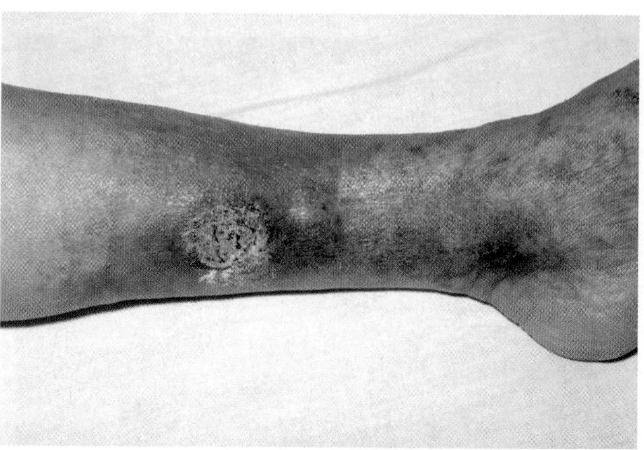

Figure 23.7 ■ A patient with chronic venous insufficiency. Note the discoloration of the ankle and the stasis ulcer.

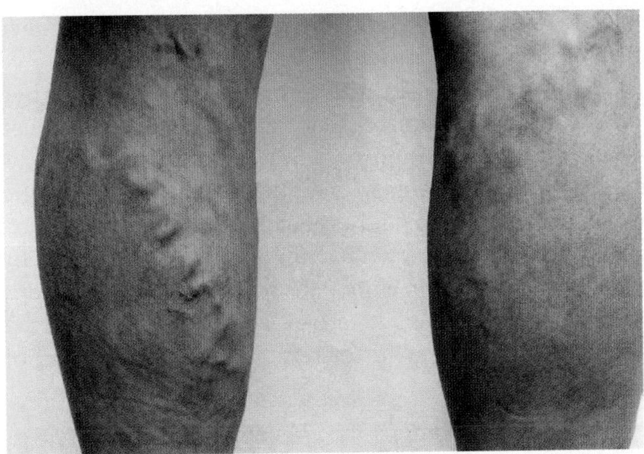

Figure 23.8 ■ A patient with varicose veins.

Telangiectasia, or reddened-purplish clusters of veins, are also a sign of venous pressures changes.

Although varicose veins most commonly occur in the legs, they may occur in other locations. For example, esophageal varices are dilated veins in the esophagus or proximal stomach that occur as a result of portal hypertension. Portal hypertension occurs in the hepatic portal vein and is often seen in advanced stages of hepatic cirrhosis. Rupture of these varices can cause massive gastrointestinal bleeding.[16]

Deep Vein Thrombosis. A third condition closely associated with CVI is **deep vein thrombosis (DVT)**, which occurs when a thrombus (blood clot) occurs in a vein deep in the body (**Figure 23.9** ■). The thrombus may become an embolism that can travel to the heart, lungs, brain, or other vital organs of the body. **Thromboembolism** occurs when the embolism blocks a blood vessel. Depending on where the embolism lodges, it could cause lasting physical problems or even lead to death.[17]

In a person with CVI, the ruptured valves lead to a slowing of venous blood flow (stasis) and inflammation of the endothelium. Platelets and neutrophils are attracted to the site and become activated. This creates an environment that promotes blood coagulation and thrombosis.[18]

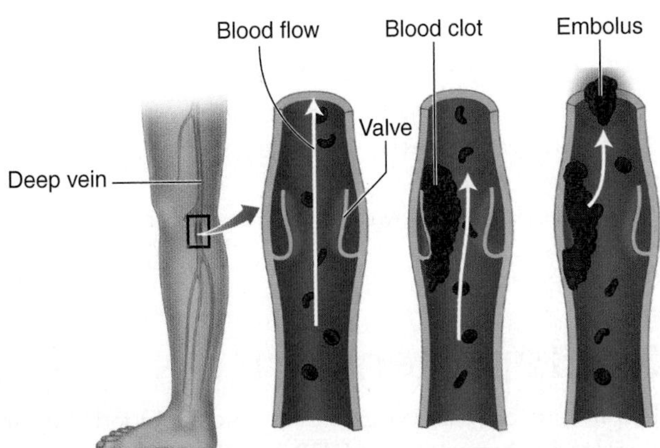

Figure 23.9 ■ Development of deep vein thrombosis.

Risk factors for the development of DVT are primarily the same as those for CVI, and the two disorders often occur concurrently.

A DVT usually manifests first through swelling and pain, although a significant percentage of DVTs are asymptomatic.[19] The pain is due to blood backing up in the vein and causing increased pressure on the lower aspect of the vein. As the pressure builds, fluid starts to leak out of the swollen veins, causing edema and additional pain. The area may become reddened, hard, and warm as a result of blood backing up in the area. If an embolus breaks free of the vein, other symptoms will be noted in the area in which the blood is compromised. If the embolus lodges in vessels that serve the heart, symptoms may include chest pain, shortness of breath, diaphoresis, and other symptoms of an MI. If the clot lands in a lung vessel, symptoms may include sudden shortness of breath, pain with breathing, increased heart rate, coughing that may include blood in the mucus, dizziness, fatigue, and anxiety. If the embolus is located in the brain, symptoms of stroke will manifest. Strokes are discussed in Chapter 27.

Aadila Shakoor: Application

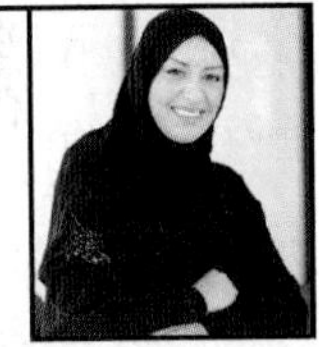

At the emergency department, Dr. Shakoor is taken immediately to an examination room. She rates her pain as a 7 on a scale from 1 to 10 and has a blood sample drawn for a D-dimer test. While waiting for the results, Dr. Shakoor mentions that the flight from Lebanon to Texas took 12 hours. She was able to get up and move around two times during the flight and noticed that her right calf was starting to feel "tight" with walking. The last several days at work, Dr. Shakoor has been in planning meetings and walked only during breaks, at lunchtime, and to the transportation stop. She has not experienced any shortness of breath, coughing, or chest pain. Her vital signs are pulse 72, respirations 14, blood pressure 118/70 mmHg, and her temperature is within normal limits. The right calf is 4 cm larger in diameter than the left calf. The skin over the right leg is warm to the touch and reddened.

4. Why was a D-dimer test done?
5. What is the significance of Dr. Shakoor's vital signs?
6. Why is Dr. Shakoor experiencing limb pain?

Linking Pathophysiology to Diagnosis and Treatment

CVI and its associated disorders of leg ulcers, varicose veins, and DVT are diagnosed primarily by assessing for the symptoms noted above during a physical examination. Imaging studies such as ultrasound or venography may be employed to better define the pathology. Venography is an x-ray procedure that injects contrast media into a vein to examine for blood clots.

During the physical examination, the healthcare provider assesses for triggers that may have prompted the venous disease. For example, is the patient taking oral contraceptives that may have increased her risk for DVT? If the patient is taking anticoagulant medications, is the dose correct? If the dose is too low, thrombi can form. Is the person employed in an occupation that involves constant standing? If so, can the person take breaks to raise the legs?

If a DVT is suspected, a D-dimer test may be ordered. A positive D-dimer test indicates the presence of abnormally high amounts of fibrin degradation products in the blood. This suggests that a high level of clot formation and breakdown is occurring.[20] The D-dimer test is not done during pregnancy or after surgery, trauma, recent MI, or other physical conditions that would initiate the D-dimer response. The D-dimer results must be correlated with other clinical findings because a high level of false positives may occur in older adults and in people with rheumatoid arthritis.

It is easier to prevent chronic venous disease than to treat it. Preventive measures for varicose veins include exercise and wearing compression (support) hosiery. Maintaining a healthy weight is important for all types of venous disease because obesity increases the pressure in the veins and makes it harder to return blood to the heart. Exercise is important, as good muscle tone decreases blood pooling in the veins. Although some situations and occupations require standing or sitting in one location for long periods of time, tightening and releasing the leg muscles can increase circulation and prevent blood pooling. Smokers should be encouraged to stop smoking.

Pregnancy is a major risk factor for varicose veins, which may occur in the vulva as well as the legs. Pregnant women should take opportunities to elevate their legs, change position frequently, and wear compression socks or support pantyhose as preventive measures.[21] ■

Surgical interventions for CVI include sclerotherapy, a procedure in which the physician injects a solution into a varicose vein that causes it to close, become scar tissue, and eventually fade. New veins, called collaterals, will form around the treated area to maintain venous function in the region. Another way to destroy varicose veins is by using lasers. Laser treatment of spider veins is a simple procedure performed on the surface of the skin. When deeper veins require intervention, radiofrequency or laser ablation may be used to destroy the vein. These methods require entry into the deep vein. If veins are too large for these methods, surgical procedures include the tying off the affected vein (ligation) and removing the vein in a procedure called vein stripping.[22]

No medications are currently available to reverse CVI. If the patient has a history of DVT, anticoagulant drugs are prescribed for prevention. These become especially important when a person is bedridden or expects to be recumbent for an extended time after an accident or surgical procedure. Traditional anticoagulants to prevent DVT and emboli include warfarin (Coumadin), which is given orally, and heparin, which is given intravenously. However, newer generations of anticoagulants have produced safer drugs that are equally effective. The American College of Chest Physicians now recommends 3-month therapy with dabigatran (Pradaxa), rivaroxaban (Xarelto), apixaban (Eliquis), or edoxaban (Savaysa) as initial treatment for venous thromboembolism.[23] Like all anticoagulants, these medications do not dissolve existing thrombi, but they do prevent existing ones from enlarging and new ones from forming.

Some patients continue to develop DVT even after venous surgery or anticoagulant therapy. Also, some people are unable to take anticoagulants because these medications are contraindicated in conditions such as hemorrhagic stroke, severe trauma, and pregnancy and after major surgery. In these patients, a filter can be placed in the inferior vena cava (IVC) to trap emboli that could travel to the heart, lungs, or brain.[24] Some filters are placed permanently in the IVC; others are designed for removal once the danger of emboli has passed.

The risk of venous thromboembolism during pregnancy is about 5 times greater than the risk for nonpregnant women. In the third trimester, the enlarged uterus can press on iliac veins and the IVC, further increasing the risk of venous thromboembolism. Because anticoagulants are contraindicated when childbirth is near, the use of a removable IVC filter has been found to be a safe alternative for preventing emboli in high-risk pregnant women.[25] ■

Aadila Shakoor: Outcome

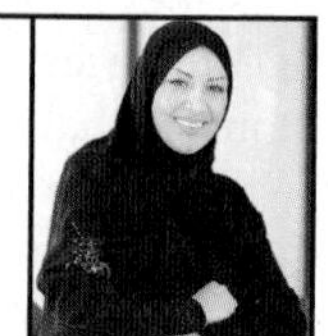

Dr. Shakoor's D-dimer test is positive, and she is admitted to the hospital for heparin therapy as treatment for a deep vein thrombosis of the right lower leg. Once in the room, Dr. Shakoor is started on an infusion of heparin 5000-unit bolus to be followed by 1500 units per hour. Her right leg is elevated, and she is prescribed bedrest.

On the second day of heparin therapy, Dr. Shakoor's right leg circumference is 0.5 cm larger than the left. Warfarin is prescribed, and after 3 days, Dr. Shakoor is discharged. She is instructed to continue on the warfarin and have blood tests done weekly. She is also instructed to wear antiembolism stockings and to perform leg and foot pumping exercises every hour when she must sit for extended periods of time. Dr. Shakoor has a follow-up appointment with the primary care physician in 3 weeks.

7. Why was Dr. Shakoor started on heparin therapy?
8. Why was Dr. Shakoor started on warfarin?
9. What is the significance of Dr. Shakoor wearing antiembolism stockings?
10. Why should Dr. Shakoor perform exercises when she must sit for long periods of time?

Check Your Progress: Section 23.3

1. Describe the pathophysiology of chronic leg ulcer.
2. What lifestyle changes may become necessary in the management of CVD?
3. List three diseases for which chronic venous insufficiency is a major risk factor.

23.4 Hypertension

When atherosclerosis progressively blocks blood flow in major arteries, **hypertension (HTN)**, or high blood pressure, may result. The primary concern about HTN is the serious consequences that result when the condition remains undiagnosed or untreated for many years. HTN is a contributing cause in the majority of people who experience their first stroke or first heart attack or who have heart failure.[26]

Elevated blood pressure is defined as systolic blood pressure above between 120 and 129 mmHg and diastolic blood pressure less than 80 mmHg.

The blood pressure measured by a conventional cuff over the brachial artery estimates *systemic* arterial pressure. *Local* HTN may occur in specific organs. For example, portal HTN often occurs in vessels serving the liver in people with advanced hepatic disease. Pulmonary HTN may occur in patients with left-sided heart failure.

Etiology and Pathogenesis

Hypertension creates excess pressure on arterial walls. For a visual example of this pressure, imagine a long, skinny balloon (the type used in making balloon animals) attached to a garden hose and filled with water. Once the balloon is full but not ready to burst, this can be considered "normal" pressure. If more water is slowly added to the balloon, the water starts to cause "high pressure" inside the balloon. The excess water is pushing outward from the inside of the balloon. If the balloon sits for a while with the maximum amount of water it can hold without immediately popping, there is a good chance that a weak area will develop in the balloon and eventually cause it to rupture. In this overfilled state, the balloon is very fragile, and minor stresses may cause it to burst. If even more water is added and the pressure increases, the balloon will break immediately. Now think of the water as blood and the balloon as an artery. The same principle applies to the arteries as to the balloon.

Over time, the arterial wall may thicken as a result of arteriosclerosis. The arteries then lose their elasticity and are unable to constrict and dilate properly. Plaque begins to build up on the arterial endothelium, and the lumen narrows. High pressure pushing against the narrowed, stiff walls may cause pieces of plaque to break off, resulting in an embolism.

Table 23.2 ■ shows the 2017 guidelines for classifying blood pressure values.[27] It also helps healthcare providers decide on treatment. For example, a person who has elevated blood pressure generally can manage the disease without medication by implementing positive lifestyle changes such as a healthier diet, increased physical exercise, and weight management. A person with stage 1 or stage 2 HTN has a clear risk for experiencing health consequences from the disorder, and lifestyle changes *combined* with antihypertensive medications are usually prescribed. The higher the blood pressure, the more aggressive will be the management of the disease, such as prescribing higher doses or several different medications for the HTN. In addition, people with a concurrent medical condition such as diabetes, kidney disease, or heart disease will likely require more aggressive management of HTN.

HTN that does not have a known cause is called **essential** or **primary hypertension**. If there is an identifiable cause, it is categorized as **secondary hypertension**. Essential hypertension is thought to account for about 90% of the cases diagnosed and has been associated with a large number of factors, including genetics, age, race, diet (especially sodium intake), smoking, alcohol consumption, and a sedentary lifestyle. Hyperthyroidism and chronic kidney disease are conditions associated with secondary HTN. Tumors of the adrenal gland that secrete large amounts of catecholamines are another cause of secondary HTN. For a patient with secondary HTN, the goal is to remove the underlying cause.

Table 23.2 Categories of Blood Pressure

Category	Definition (mmHg)	Examples (mmHg)
Normal	Less than 120/80	112/75 119/79
Elevated	Systolic from 120 – 129 ***and*** diastolic less than 80	125/72 129/79
Stage 1 hypertension	Systolic from 130 – 139 ***or*** diastolic from 80 - 89	130/79 129/80
Stage 2 hypertension	Systolic at least 140 ***or*** diastolic at least 90	135/90 140/85
Hypertensive crisis	Systolic over 180 ***and/or*** diastolic over 120	180/90 165/120

SOURCE: Data from American Heart Association. (2017c). *Understanding blood pressure readings.* Retrieved from http://www.heart.org/HEARTORG/Conditions/HighBloodPressure/GettheFactsAboutHighBloodPressure/Understanding-Blood-Pressure-Readings_UCM_301764_Article.jsp#.WMmGVhg-leo; Mayo Clinic. (2017c). *High Blood Pressure (Hypertension).* Retrieved from http://www.mayoclinic.org/diseases-conditions/high-blood-pressure/in-depth/blood-pressure/art-20050982

Although many factors affect blood pressure, they may be divided into two types: hormonal and nervous. When these hormonal and nervous factors are disrupted, chronic HTN may result. The pharmacologic treatment of HTN is targeted at returning these factors to homeostasis. **Figure 23.10** ■ illustrates hormonal and nervous factors affecting blood pressure.

When the kidneys detect hypotension or low sodium, the juxtaglomerular cells release renin into the bloodstream. Renin converts angiotensinogen to angiotensin I. When angiotensin I passes through the lungs, it is converted to angiotensin II by angiotensin-converting enzyme (ACE). Angiotensin II is a potent vasoconstrictor that returns blood pressure back to normal. Angiotensin II also causes the release of aldosterone from the adrenal glands. Aldosterone helps the body to retain sodium, which increases blood volume and raises blood pressure. This is known as the renin-angiotensin-aldosterone system (RAAS). Additional details about the RAAS may be found in Chapter 8.

Disruption of the RAAS homeostatic mechanism can lead to HTN, primarily through the presence of angiotensin II. In addition to being a potent vasodilator, angiotensin II affects the growth and maturation of adipocytes (fat cells). Adipocytes release a variety of hormones that regulate energy balance, including adiponectin, which has both anti-inflammatory and anti-plaque properties that offer a degree of cardiovascular protection. Plasma adiponectin levels are low in patients with HTN. When adiponectin levels increase, the risk for HTN diminishes.[28]

Disruption of the RAAS mechanism may also contribute to the close link between HTN and obesity. Obesity leads to increased expression of angiotensin II in adipocytes, especially in visceral fat, and a reduced level of plasma adiponectin. It appears that adiponectin may be a key molecule linking obesity to HTN as well as to the metabolic syndrome.[29]

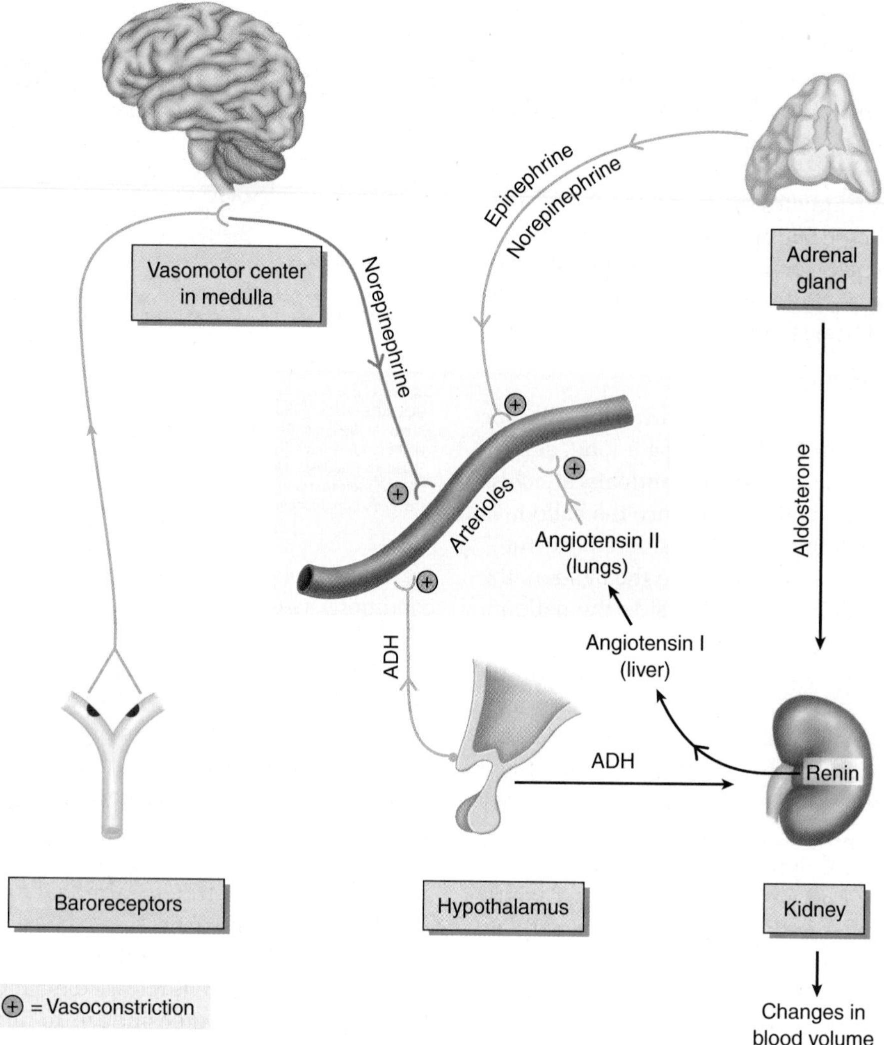

Figure 23.10 ■ Hormonal and nervous factors influencing blood pressure.

Endothelial dysfunction is likely an additional contributor to the development of HTN. The endothelium is more than a single layer of cells lining blood vessels. It is a highly active organ that is able to regulate local blood pressure through the release of vasoactive substances. For example, the endothelium releases nitric oxide (NO), which acts as a vasodilator, anti-inflammatory agent, and antiplatelet agent when a vessel is damaged or experiencing constriction. Risk factors such as smoking, aging, and HTN have all been associated with reduced the amounts of NO in the endothelium.[30]

In addition to hormones, the sympathetic nervous system (SNS) has a role in the development of HTN. In people with HTN, there is an increase in SNS activity, although the exact mechanism is unclear. Activation of the SNS initiates the fight-or-flight response, which causes increased heart rate, increased blood flow, and retention of renal sodium. Norepinephrine activates alpha-adrenergic receptors in arterial smooth muscle to raise blood pressure. Epinephrine acts on both adrenergic and beta receptors, promoting increased vasoconstriction. Activation of beta receptors increases heart rate and cardiac workload, as well as enhancing renin release.

Consuming large amounts of alcohol can cause hypertension by both hormonal and nervous mechanisms. Alcohol appears to activate the RAAS and cause a prolonged elevation of plasma renin and angiotensin II. The angiotensin II constricts the arteries and depletes the vessel of NO, a natural vasodilator. The SNS is also activated after consumption of alcohol, causing the fight-or-flight response and elevated blood pressure. Reducing alcohol consumption can lower both systolic and diastolic pressure. Other mechanisms are likely to be involved in the pathogenesis of alcohol-related hypertension.[31]

Lifestyle factors such as increased stress, high salt intake, lack of physical exercise, and obesity also contribute to a higher SNS activity.[32] Increases in norepinephrine and epinephrine are frequently seen in individuals with a family history of HTN, a finding that suggests a genetic relationship. The fact that ethnic groups differ in their susceptibility to HTN also suggests a genetic component to the disease.[33] African Americans have the highest rate of HTN among ethnic groups. Caucasians (non-Hispanic White) are less likely to have high blood pressure than are non-Hispanic Blacks (**Figure 23.11** ■). Asians are less likely to have HTN than are non-Hispanic Blacks and non-Hispanic Whites. Non-Hispanic Black men tend to have higher blood pressure than do non-Hispanic Black women.

Clinical Manifestations

The consequences of chronic HTN occur over many years or even decades. During most of this time, the person with HTN has no overt symptoms of the disorder. Indeed, HTN usually goes undetected until identified by a healthcare provider, often during a routine physical examination. Symptoms such as dizziness, nosebleeds, headache, facial flushing, and blood spots in the eyes are rare until blood pressure is extremely high.[34]

It is important to understand that although the condition may be asymptomatic, damage is progressively occurring to nearly all organ systems, especially the blood vessels, brain, heart, and kidneys. By the time it is diagnosed, some of the tissue damage caused by chronic HTN may be irreversible. The long-term consequences of chronic HTN are serious and even fatal. These include stroke, heart failure, MI, chronic kidney disease, vision loss, and erectile dysfunction. At age 50, total life expectancy is increased 5 years or more for people who have normal blood pressure compared to those with HTN.[26]

A **hypertensive crisis** is a relatively rare condition that occurs when systolic pressure exceeds 180 and/or diastolic pressure exceeds 120 mmHg. It was formerly called *malignant hypertension* or *hypertensive emergency*.[35] Organ damage from extreme HTN occurs primarily in the cardiovascular system, kidneys, or brain. Aggressive treatment within minutes or hours is required to prevent additional organ damage. In a related condition, **hypertensive urgency**, the patient presents with severe HTN without evidence of organ damage.

The most common symptoms of hypertensive crisis are chest pain and dyspnea. The increased workload on the heart may cause acute left heart failure with pulmonary edema, often accompanied by myocardial ischemia or infarction. Renal function is diminished, and blood or protein may be found in the urine. Acute renal failure may occur. In the brain, thrombotic or hemorrhagic stroke may occur. The capillaries in the brain become leaky, producing hypertensive encephalopathy (edema of the brain), with symptoms of headache, paralysis, seizures, or coma. Retinal hemorrhages and edema of the retina (papilledema) are signs of severe HTN.[36]

The most common cause of hypertensive crisis is untreated or poorly controlled primary HTN. However, there are a large number of possible secondary causes of hypertensive crisis, including renovascular hypertension, pheochromocytoma, cocaine use, eclampsia or preeclampsia, head injuries, meningitis, and hyperthyroidism or thyroid storm.

Emilio Suarez: Application

A week after starting work, Mr. Suarez reports to the work site infirmary as directed. His blood pressure is 166/92 mmHg, and he asks whether feeling chest heaviness is a part of the high blood pressure. Mr. Suarez admits that he has not been taking the medication as prescribed because it makes him have to "go to

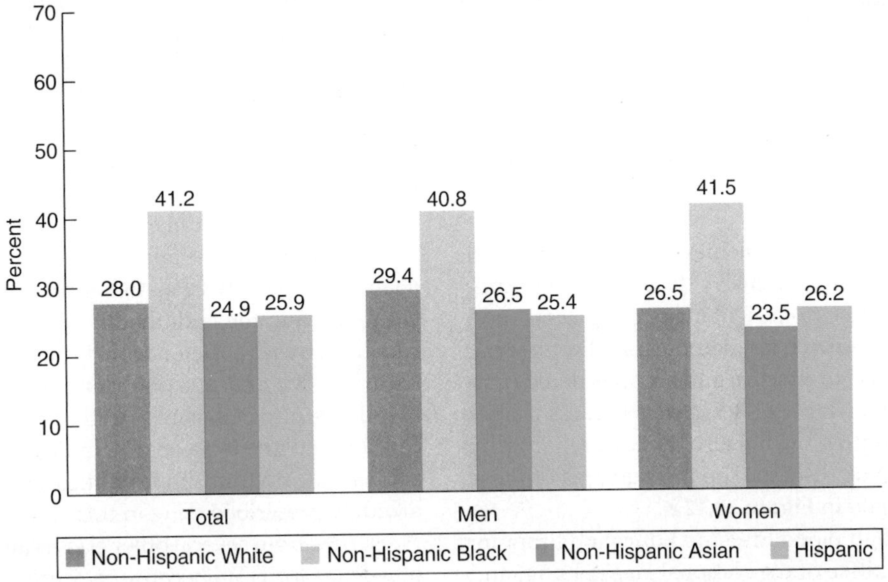

Figure 23.11 ■ Prevalence of hypertension among adults age 18 and over by sex, race, and Hispanic origin: United States, 2011–2014.

SOURCE: CDC/NCHS, National Health and Nutrition Examination Survey, 2011–2014. Retrieved from http://www.cdc.gov/nchs/images/databriefs/201-250/db220_fig2.png

the bathroom" frequently while at work. The onsite physician prescribes 12-lead electrocardiography and tells Mr. Suarez to begin a 1 gram low-sodium diet immediately. Mr. Suarez is also directed take his medication as prescribed, to stop smoking, and to ingest no alcohol before returning in 2 weeks for another blood pressure evaluation.

3. Why was 12-lead electrocardiography prescribed for Mr. Suarez?
4. Why wasn't Mr. Suarez's medication adjusted?
5. Why was Mr. Suarez instructed to ingest no alcohol?
6. Why was Mr. Suarez prescribed a 1-gram sodium diet

Linking Pathophysiology to Diagnosis and Treatment

Blood pressure is easily measured by using an inflatable cuff and a pressure-measuring gauge. A single measurement taken during a routine office visit is not sufficient for a diagnosis of HTN. Blood pressure readings taken in a healthcare setting may be artificially high because the patient experiences fight-or-flight symptoms around medical workers, a phenomenon called *white coat hypertension*. Blood pressure can also be temporarily elevated by physical activity, mental excitement or nervousness, pain, tobacco use, ingestion of caffeinated food or beverages, and the position of the body. A person being evaluated for HTN should be rechecked several times. If unable to go to the office on a regular basis, the person may record readings taken at home and report values to the healthcare provider. Most pharmacies also have blood pressure checking devices.

The first step in treating chronic HTN is to implement therapeutic lifestyle changes (TLCs). Minor to moderate HTN may respond to TLCs without the need for medications. These TLCs are the same as those for other cardiovascular disorders, so the person may experience multiple benefits. TLCs include the following:

- Restrict sodium consumption
- Limit alcohol consumption
- Stop smoking
- Maintain an optimal weight
- Reduce intake of saturated fat and cholesterol, and increase consumption of fruits and vegetables
- Increase physical activity
- Reduce stress levels.

If TLCs are not enough to achieve the desired blood pressure reduction, antihypertensive drugs are used. Antihypertensive drugs come from eight major drug classes and several minor ones. Research has demonstrated some drug classes are safer and more effective and are considered first-line drugs, as shown in **Table 23.3** ■. Drugs in these classes not only lower blood pressure but also can lower morbidity and mortality from the disease. The mechanisms of these medications are shown in **Figure 23.12** ■.

The National High Blood Pressure Education Program Coordinating Committee of the National Heart, Lung, and Blood Institute at the National Institutes of Health have established guidelines for the treatment of HTN. In 2013, the Eighth Joint National Committee significantly revised the HTN guidelines on the basis of the latest research.[37]

Table 23.3 Drug Classes Used to Treat Hypertension

Type	Class
First-line drugs	Angiotensin-converting enzyme (ACE) inhibitors Angiotensin receptor blockers (ARBs) Calcium channel blockers (CCBs) Thiazide diuretics
Second-line drugs	Adrenergic blockers Centrally acting drugs Direct-acting vasodilators Direct renin inhibitors

SOURCE: Holland, L. N., Adams, M. P., & Brice, J. (2019). *Core concepts in pharmacology* (5th ed., Table 19.1, p. 299). Hoboken, NJ: Pearson.

For many decades, diuretics, especially the thiazide class, were the preferred drugs for the initial treatment of HTN. Diuretics lower blood pressure by increasing urine output and reducing blood volume. They are safe and effective medications that are still widely prescribed. Hydrochlorothiazide is the most widely prescribed diuretic. However, with the discovery of the importance of the RAAS in controlling blood pressure, medications were developed to block aspects of this pathway in hypertensive patients. Drugs blocking the RAAS have become first-line drugs in treating both HTN and heart failure.[8] The primary medications in this class block angiotensin-converting enzyme (ACE). Blocking ACE reduces the formation of angiotensin II, resulting in less vasoconstriction and less SNS activation, thus lowering blood pressure. The blocking of angiotensin II also lowers aldosterone secretion, which in turn allows more sodium to be excreted. The increase in sodium excretion results in decreased arterial wall pressure. About ten ACE inhibitors are available to treat HTN. Lisinopril (Prinivil) is a widely prescribed medication in this drug class.

Two other classes of antihypertensives block parts of RAAS. Angiotensin receptor blockers (ARBs) affect receptors for angiotensin II in the adrenal gland and arteriolar smooth muscle. These drugs do not alter the formation of angiotensin II, but instead block its action on target tissues. About eight ARBs are available, of which Losartan (Cozaar) is widely prescribed. The third class that affect the RAAS are called direct renin inhibitors. Stopping the action of renin will prevent the formation of angiotensin I, thus stopping the RAAS. Aliskirin (Tekurna) is an example of a direct renin inhibitor.

Another first-line antihypertensive class is the calcium channel blockers (CCBs). CCBs decrease the amount of calcium entering the endothelium. The decreased amount of calcium entering the endothelium slows the heart's electrical activity and relaxes arteriolar smooth muscle in the blood vessels. CCBs are effective in treating a number of cardiovascular conditions, including HTN, angina pectoris, and cardiac rhythm abnormalities. Diltiazem (Cardizem) is a widely prescribed drug in this class.

Drugs from several other classes are considered alternative drugs for HTN because they are less effective or cause more adverse effects than first-line drugs.[8] Once considered first-line drugs, beta-adrenergic blockers (beta blockers) inhibit activation of the SNS. Levels of norepinephrine and epinephrine are reduced, dampening the effects of the

Alpha$_2$ agonists
Decrease sympathetic impulses from the CNS to the heart and arterioles, causing vasodilation
Brain
Arterioles
α_2
Alpha$_1$ blockers
Inhibit sympathetic activation in arterioles, causing vasodilation
Sympathetic nervous system
α_1
Direct vasodilators
Act on the smooth muscle of arterioles, causing vasodilation
Beta blockers
Decrease the heart rate and myocardial contractility, reducing cardiac output
β_1
Ca^{2+}
Calcium channel blockers
Block calcium ion channels in arterial smooth muscle, causing vasodilation
Heart
Angiotensin receptor blockers
Prevent angiotensin II from reaching its receptors, causing vasodilation
Angiotensin II
Renin
Kidney
ACE inhibitors
Block formation of angiotensin II, causing vasodilation, and block aldosterone secretion, decreasing fluid volume
Diuretics
Increase urine output and decrease fluid volume
⊖ = Inhibitory effect causing vasodilation

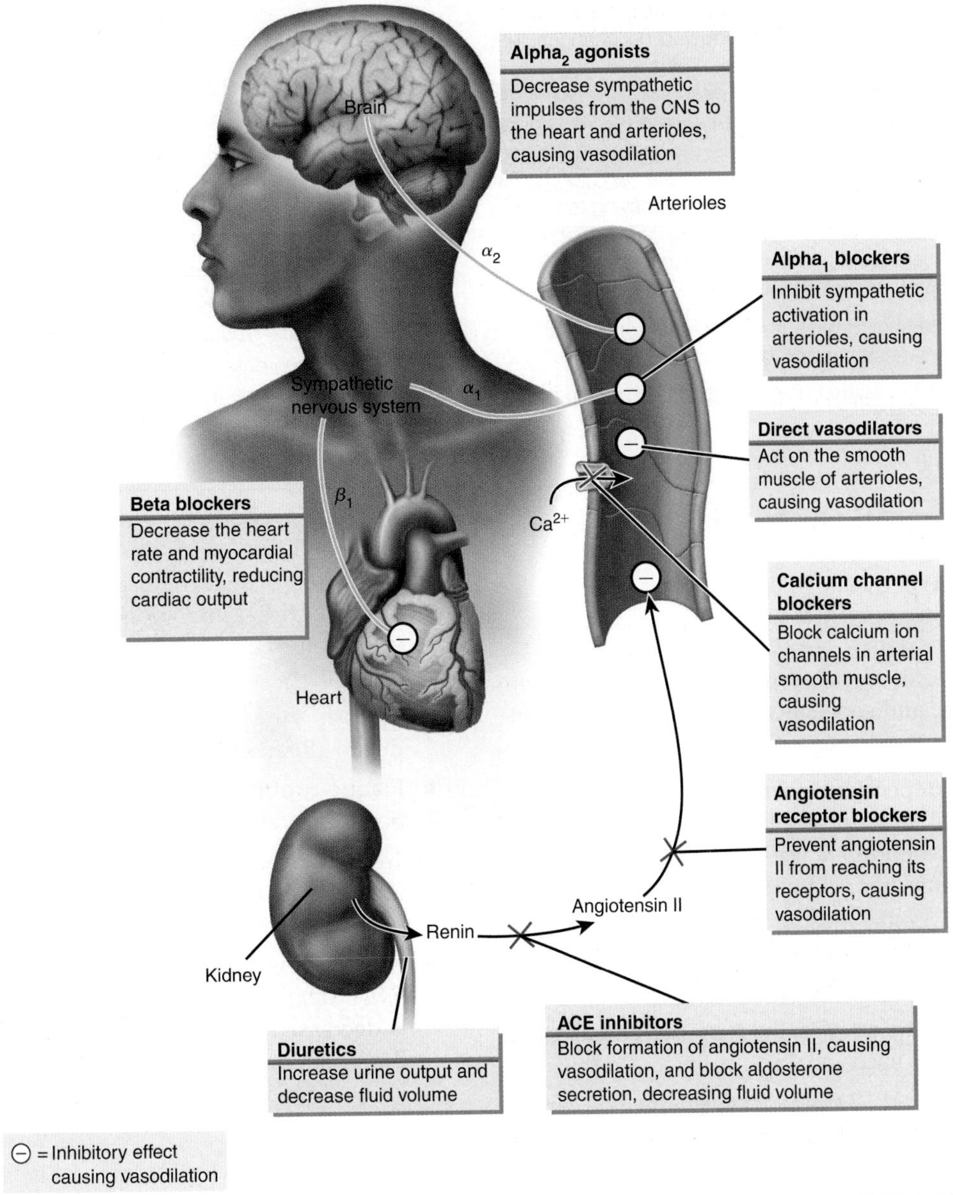

Figure 23.12 ■ Mechanism of action of antihypertensive drugs.

fight-or-flight response. The blood vessels remain relaxed, sugar levels remain normal, and renin is not released.

It is common practice in treating HTN to use drugs from two or more classes, often combined into a single pill. For example, Zestorectic combines a diuretic (hydrochlorothiazide) with an ACE inhibitor (lisinopril). Using two drugs allows for lower doses of each drug and a reduced potential for adverse effects. A greater reduction in blood pressure may also be obtained by combining two drugs that attack the HTN by different mechanisms of action.

When a person arrives at the emergency department with a HTN-E, the blood pressure must be reduced as quickly and as safely as possible to prevent additional target-organ damage. Reductions in blood pressure are made gradually over a 12- to 24-hour period. Lowering blood pressure too quickly can result in lack of perfusion to vital organs. Intravenous antihypertensives are used for hypertensive crisis because they act immediately and can be precisely controlled. A first-line drug for hypertensive crisis is nitroprusside (Nitropress).

Emilio Suarez: Outcome

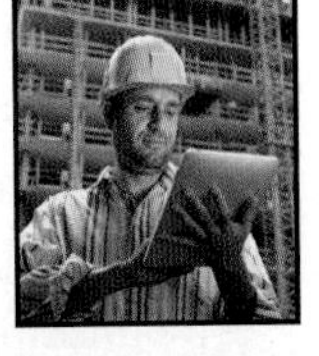

After 2 weeks, Mr. Suarez arrives for his scheduled appointment. His blood pressure is 162/88 mmHg, and his BMI is 29.6. Mr. Suarez states that he has been taking the prescribed number of doses of medication each day but has adjusted the times so that he wasn't "running to the bathroom" every 15 minutes. Mr. Suarez admits to having a cigarette after lunch each day and several over the weekend. He reports having stayed away from all alcohol for the full 2 weeks and has asked his spouse to stop adding salt to the foods prepared at home. Mr. Suarez had 12-lead electrocardiography completed a week ago, which showed no changes. Mr. Suarez reports that the chest heaviness has "gone away."

Because Mr. Suarez's blood pressure is still elevated, he is prescribed an ACE inhibitor in addition to the diuretic. He is given teaching material on smoking cessation techniques and is again asked to refrain from all alcoholic beverages until the next blood pressure check in 2 weeks. Mr. Suarez is upset about having to take an additional medication but is encouraged when he learns that weight reduction, smoking cessation, and low to no alcohol intake will help bring his blood pressure under control.

7. What question should have been asked before the current blood pressure measurement was made?
8. What else can Mr. Suarez be instructed to do to help control his blood pressure?
9. Why was an ACE inhibitor medication prescribed for Mr. Suarez?
10. Why is it important for Mr. Suarez to take both medications as prescribed?

Check Your Progress: Section 23.4

1. What is the mechanism of action of ARBs?
2. A rapidly acting hypotensive agent such as nitroprusside is used to quickly reduce blood pressure to prevent what?
3. Hypertension due to pheochromocytoma and renal disease is classified as what?

CHAPTER SUMMARY

23.1 Chapter Overview and Case Studies

Describe normal arterial and venous circulation, peripheral vascular diseases, and concepts related alterations in vascular health.

- Tissues are dependent on the vascular system for survival. Lack of sufficient blood flow may result in hypoxia and a buildup of waste products that can cause acute or chronic organ damage
- Peripheral vascular disease (PVD) is a general term referring to conditions that affect circulation in tissues other than the brain or heart.
- If PVD affects the arteries, the term peripheral artery disease (PAD) is used.
- Common types of PVD that affect veins include chronic venous insufficiency, deep vein thrombosis, leg ulcers, and varicose veins.
- Risk factors for PVD include smoking, hypertension, coronary heart disease, high cholesterol, diabetes, family history of vascular disease, obesity, and sedentary lifestyle. PVD primarily affects adults over age 50 and men are affected more often than women.

23.2 Peripheral Arterial Disease

Differentiate the causes, classification, underlying pathogenesis, and clinical manifestations of peripheral arterial disease and approaches to diagnosis and treatment of these conditions across the lifespan.

- Arteriosclerosis is a thickening, loss of elasticity, and calcification of the walls of arteries.
- Atherosclerosis is a form of arteriosclerosis caused by a buildup of plaque, which is composed of cholesterol deposits.
- PAD has both genetic and lifestyle causes.
- Plaque buildup is the result of hyperlipidemia, excess cholesterol, and high levels of LDL.
- The three primary consequences of atherosclerosis are myocardial infarction, stroke, and PAD. They are the result of either atherosclerotic stenosis or plaque rupture.
- Stenosis is the partial or complete blockage of an artery due to atherosclerotic plaque.
- Plaque rupture is often followed by thrombosis and possibly infarction.
- Treatment goals for a person with PAD include addressing lifestyle factors that contributed to the plaque and surgery to open occluded arteries.
- Nonatherosclerotic peripheral arterial disease (NAPAD) is a group of disorders in which blood flow is decreased for reasons other than plaque buildup. Examples include coarctation of the aorta, thoracic outlet syndrome, and Raynaud disease.

23.3 Chronic Venous Disease

Differentiate the causes, classification, underlying pathogenesis, and clinical manifestations of chronic venous disease and approaches to diagnosis and treatment of these conditions across the lifespan.

- When a chronic vascular condition affects veins, it is called chronic venous disease (CVD). The most common cause of CVD is chronic venous insufficiency (CVI).
- CVI is a disorder in which the veins are unable to return adequate blood to the heart. Conditions closely associated with CVI are chronic leg ulcers, varicose veins, and deep vein thrombosis.
- Leg ulcers are sores on the skin that persist for more than 6 weeks and take several months or longer to heal.
- Varicose veins are veins that have become enlarged and twisted as a result of the rupture of valves.
- A deep vein thrombosis (DVT) is a thrombus or blood clot occurs in a vein deep in the body.

23.4 Hypertension

Differentiate the causes, classification, underlying pathogenesis, and clinical manifestations of hypertension and approaches to diagnosis and treatment of this condition across the lifespan.

- HTN is a consistent elevation of blood pressure above 120 mmHg systolic and less than 80 mmHg diastolic.
- HTN that does not have a known cause is called essential or primary hypertension. If there is an identifiable cause, it is categorized as secondary hypertension.
- The primary hormones regulating blood pressure are part of the renin-angiotensin-aldosterone system (RAAS).
- Disruption of the RAAS homeostatic mechanism can lead to HTN, primarily through the production of angiotensin II.
- The consequences of chronic HTN occur over many years, during which the person with HTN exhibits no overt symptoms.
- The long-term consequences of chronic HTN include stroke, heart failure, MI, chronic kidney disease, vision loss, and erectile dysfunction.
- Antihypertensive drugs come from eight major drug classes. Research has demonstrated that some drug classes are safer and more effective and are considered first-line drugs. First-line drug classes include ACE inhibitors, angiotensin receptor blockers, calcium channel blockers, and thiazide diuretics.

REVIEW QUESTIONS

1. A nurse takes a client's blood pressure, which reads 160/95 mmHg. Which of the following would the nurse ask the client to change to manage the hypertension?
   a. Add more salt to the diet
   b. Drink red wine
   c. Use less salt
   d. Drink lots of water

2. A client presents at a clinic complaining of pain in his calf when he goes on a walk. He also complains of a tingling sensation in his feet. What is the client possibly suffering from?
   a. Peripheral vascular disease
   b. Varicose veins
   c. Raynaud disease
   d. Deep vein thrombosis (DVT)

3. Thrombophlebitis is inflammation of the vein accompanied by blood clot. What are the risk factors for thrombophlebitis?
   a. Hypertension, hypercoagulability, and an autoimmune disease
   b. Varicose vein, blood stasis, and hypercoagulability
   c. 20 year-old client, history of renal disease, and hypercoagulability
   d. Heart failure, hypercoagulability, and atherosclerosis

4. What is the major predisposing risk factor for developing atherosclerosis?
   a. Male gender
   b. Aging
   c. Family history of premature coronary heart disease
   d. Hypercholesterolemia and dyslipidemia

5. A 65-year-old female client is complaining to the nurse about the ugly varicose veins on her leg. Which of the following would the nurse include in telling the client about nonsurgical treatment options of her condition?
   a. Sclerotherapy
   b. Vein stripping
   c. Surgical ligation
   d. Leg elevation

6. What are the risk factors for primary hypertension?
   a. Intake of potassium and aging
   b. Family history and renal disease
   c. Obesity and type 2 diabetes mellitus
   d. Excessive sodium intake and sedentary lifestyle

7. A nurse is a preceptor to a nursing student who wants to know about the renin-angiotensin-aldosterone system (RAAS) and the control of blood pressure. How does aldosterone influence blood pressure?
   a. Decreases sodium and water reabsorption by the kidney tubules
   b. Induces vasocontriction and increases blood pressure
   c. Causes vasodilation and decreases blood pressure
   d. Increases sodium and water reabsorption by the kidney tubules

8. The nurse tells the 60-year-old client that he was receiving lisinopril for the treatment of hypertension. The nurse knows that lisinopril belongs to a group of drugs called angiotensin-converting enzyme (ACE) inhibitors. What is their mechanism of action in lowering blood pressure?
   a. Block angiotensin receptors
   b. Block the conversion of angiotensin I to angiotensin II
   c. Inhibit the release of renin
   d. Block the activation of angiotensinogen to angiotensin I

ANSWERS

Answers to Review Questions can be found in Appendix A. Answers to Case Study and Check Your Progress questions are available on the faculty resources site. Please consult with your instructor.

RECOMMENDED WEBSITES

American Heart Association
http://www.heart.org

American College of Cardiology
http://www.acc.org/latest-in-cardiology/articles/2017/11/08/11/47/mon-5pm-bp-guideline-aha-2017

Mayo Clinic: High Blood Pressure (Hypertension)
http://www.mayoclinic.org/diseases-conditions/high-blood-pressure/basics/definition/con-20019580

National Heart, Lung, and Blood Institute
https://www.nhlbi.nih.gov/

REFERENCES

1. Johns Hopkins Medicine. (n.d.). *Peripheral vascular disease*. Retrieved from http://www.hopkinsmedicine.org/healthlibrary/conditions/cardiovascular_diseases/peripheral_vascular_disease_85,P00236
2. Mose, J. (2017). Familial hypercholesterolemia. *Medscape*. Available at http://emedicine.medscape.com/article/121298-overview
3. Cleveland Clinic. (2013). *What do cholesterol numbers mean?* Available at https://my.clevelandclinic.org/health/diseases_conditions/hic_Cholesterol/hic_what_do_cholesterol_numbers_mean
4. Falk, E. (2006). Pathogenesis of atherosclerosis. *Journal of the American College of Cardiology*, *47*(8), C7–C12. doi:10.1016/j.jacc.2005.09.068
5. Mayo Clinic (2015). *Claudication*. Available at http://www.mayoclinic.org/diseases-conditions/claudication/basics/definition/con-20033581
6. American Heart Association. (2017). *Types of aneurysms*. Available at http://www.heart.org/HEARTORG/Conditions/VascularHealth/AorticAneurysm/Types-of-Aneurysms_UCM_454436_Article.jsp#.WM21tRg-KFA
7. Mancini, M. C. (2016). Aortic dissection. *Medscape*. Available at http://emedicine.medscape.com/article/2062452-overview
8. Adams, M. P., & Urban, C. Q. (2019). *Pharmacology: Connections to nursing practice*. Hoboken, NJ: Pearson Education.
9. Mayo Clinic. (2017). *Coarctation of the aorta*. Available at http://www.mayoclinic.org/diseases-conditions/coarctation-of-the-aorta/basics/definition/con-20031772?p=1
10. Mayo Clinic. (2017). *Thoracic outlet syndrome*. Available at http://www.mayoclinic.org/diseases-conditions/thoracic-outlet-syndrome/home/ovc-20237878
11. Wigley, F. M., & Flavahan, N. A. (2016). Raynaud's phenomenon. *New England Journal of Medicine*, *375*(6), 556–565. doi:10.1056/NEJMra1507638
12. Mayo Clinic. (2015). *Raynaud's disease*. Available at http://www.mayoclinic.org/diseases-conditions/raynauds-disease/basics/definition/con-20022916
13. Weiss, R. (2016). Venous insufficiency. *Medscape*. Available at http://emedicine.medscape.com/article/1085412-overview
14. Agale, S. V. (2013). Chronic leg ulcers: Epidemiology, aetiopathogenesis and management. *Ulcers*, *2013*, Article 413604, doi.org/10.1155/2013/413604. Available at https://www.hindawi.com/journals/ulcers/2013/413604
15. Atta, H. M. (2012). Varicose veins: Role of mechanotransduction of venous hypertension. *International Journal of Vascular Medicine*, *2012*, Article 538627. Available at https://www.hindawi.com/journals/ijvm/2012/538627
16. Ansari, P. (2016). Varices. *Merck manual: Professional version*. Available at http://www.merckmanuals.com/professional/gastrointestinal-disorders/gi-bleeding/varices
17. Mayo Clinic. (2014). *Deep vein thrombosis (DVT)*. Available at http://www.mayoclinic.org/diseases-conditions/deep-vein-thrombosis/basics/definition/con-20031922?p=1
18. Brenner, B. E. (2016). Deep vein thrombosis. *Medscape*. Available at http://emedicine.medscape.com/article/1911303-overview#a4
19. Centers for Disease Control and Prevention. (2017). *Venous thromboembolism (blood clots)*. Available at https://www.cdc.gov/ncbddd/dvt/facts.html
20. American Association for Clinical Chemistry. (2017). *D-dimer*. Available at https://labtestsonline.org/understanding/analytes/d-dimer/tab/test
21. Mayo Clinic. (2013). *Pregnancy week by week*. Available at http://www.mayoclinic.org/healthy-lifestyle/pregnancy-week-by-week/expert-blog/varicose-veins-and-pregnancy/bgp-20055799
22. U. S. Department of Health and Human Services. (2017). *Varicose veins and spider veins*. Available at https://www.womenshealth.gov/publications/our-publications/fact-sheet/varicose-spider-veins.html#K
23. Kearon, C., Akl, E. A., Ornelas, J., et al. (2016). Antithrombotic therapy for VTE disease: CHEST guideline and expert panel report. *CHEST Journal*, *149*(2), 315–352. doi:10.1016/j.chest.2015.11.026
24. Puppala, S. (2017). Inferior vena cava filter placement. *Medscape*. Available at http://emedicine.medscape.com/article/1377859-overview?pa=X6NVLJ%2B08xQ8Cq6uOQQAN1qJIj2NCMaAes3m2B9smO41qRV3SUBwY3MqNlXcTEap8SIvl8zjYv73GUyW5rsbWA%3D%3D
25. DeYoung, E., & Minocha, J. (2016). Inferior vena cava filters: Guidelines, best practice, and expanding indications. *Seminars in Interventional Radiology*, *33*(2), 65–70. doi:10.1055/s-0036-1581088.
26. American Heart Association. (2017). *Consequences of high blood pressure*. Available at http://www.heart.org/HEARTORG/Conditions/HighBloodPressure/Avoid-the-Consequences-of-High-Blood-Pressure-Infographic_UCM_464643_Article.jsp
27. American College of Cardiology. (2017). New ACC/AHA high blood pressure guidelines lower definition of hypertension. Retrieved from http://www.acc.org/latest-in-cardiology/articles/2017/11/08/11/47/mon-5pm-bp-guideline-aha-2017
28. Kim, D. H., Kim, C., Ding, E. L., Townsend, M. K., & Lipsitz, L. A. (2013). Adiponectin levels and the risk of hypertension. *Hypertension*, *65*, 27–32. doi:10.1161/HYPERTENSIONAHA.113.01453
29. Iwashima, Y., Horio, T., & Kawano, Y. (2010). Role of adiponectin in obesity, hypertension, and metabolic syndrome. *Current Hypertension Reviews*, *6*(2), 110–117. doi:10.2174/157340210791171029
30. Bleakley, C., Hamilton, P. K., Pumb, R., Harbinson, M., & McVeigh, G. E. (2015). Endothelial function in hypertension: Victim or culprit? *Journal of Clinical Hypertension*, *17*(8), 651–654.

31. Husain, K., Ansari, R. A., & Ferder, L. (2014). Alcohol-induced hypertension: Mechanism and prevention. *World Journal of Cardiology*, *6*(5), 245. doi:10.4330/wjc.v6.i5.245
32. Bolívar, J. J. (2013). Essential hypertension: An approach to its etiology and neurogenic pathophysiology. *International Journal of Hypertension*, *2013*, Article 547809. doi.org/10.1155/2013/547809
33. Nwankwo, T., Yoon, S. S., Burt, V., & Gu, Q. (2013). Hypertension among adults in the United States: National Health and Nutrition Examination Survey, 2011–2012. *NCHS Data Brief*, *133*, 1–8. Available at https://www.cdc.gov/nchs/products/databriefs/db133.htm
34. American Heart Association. (2017). *What are the symptoms of high blood pressure*? Available at http://www.heart.org/HEARTORG/Conditions/HighBloodPressure/UnderstandSymptomsRisks/What-are-the-Symptoms-of-High-Blood-Pressure_UCM_301871_Article.jsp#.WMwn-Bg-Ieo
35. Stafford, E. E., Wsill, K. K., & Brooks-Gumbert, A. N. (2012). Management of hypertensive urgency and emergency. *Clinician Review*, *22*, 20–25. Available at https://scholar.google.com/scholar?q=%22Management+of+Hypertensive+Urgency+and+Emergency%22&btnG=&hl=en&as_sdt=0%2C10
36. Bakris, G. L. (2016). Hypertensive emergencies. *Merck manual: Professional version*. Available at http://www.merckmanuals.com/professional/cardiovascular-disorders/hypertension/hypertensive-emergencies
37. James, P. A., Oparil, S., Carter, B. L., et al. (2014). 2014 Evidence-based guideline for the management of high blood pressure in adults: Report from the panel members appointed to the Eighth Joint National Committee (JNC 8). *JAMA*, *311*, 507–520. doi:10.1001/jama.2013.284427

Chapter 24
Coronary Circulation Disorders

Jori Reigle

Chapter Outline and Learning Outcomes

24.1 Chapter Overview and Case Studies

Describe coronary artery disease, acute coronary syndromes, and concepts related to disorders of coronary circulation.

24.2 Epidemiology and Risk Factors Related to Coronary Artery Disease

Outline the epidemiology and risk factors related to coronary artery disease as well as methods of preventing coronary artery disease.

24.3 Pathophysiology, Diagnosis, and Treatment of Coronary Artery Disease

Outline the pathophysiology, diagnosis, and treatment of coronary artery disease.

24.4 Myocardial Ischemia and Infarction

Differentiate the causes, classification, underlying pathogenesis, and clinical manifestations of myocardial ischemia and infarction and approaches to diagnosis and treatment of these conditions across the lifespan.

24.5 Specific Acute Coronary Syndromes

Differentiate the causes, classification, underlying pathogenesis, and clinical manifestations of specific acute coronary syndromes and approaches to diagnosis and treatment of these conditions across the lifespan.

24.6 Complications of Acute Coronary Syndromes

Differentiate the causes, classification, underlying pathogenesis, and clinical manifestations of complications of acute coronary syndromes and approaches to diagnosis and treatment of these conditions across the lifespan.

24.7 Valvular Disorders

Differentiate the causes, classification, underlying pathogenesis, and clinical manifestations of valvular disorders and approaches to diagnosis and treatment of these conditions across the lifespan.

KEY TERMS

Absolute refractory period, 594
Acute coronary syndrome (ACS), 588
Aneurysm, 577
Angina, 573
Atherosclerosis, 573
Atrial fibrillation, 591
Automaticity, 594
Autoregulation, 582
Bradycardia, 592
Cardiac output (CO), 583
Cardiac tamponade, 602
Cardiovascular disease (CVD), 573
Claudication, 573
Coronary angiogram, 580
Coronary artery disease (CAD), 573
Coronary collateral circulation, 576
Coronary heart disease (CHD), 573
Coronary microvascular disease, 588
Coronary perfusion pressure, 582
Dressler syndrome, 601
Dysrhythmia, 580
Embolus, 591
Ideal cardiovascular health, 575
Myocardial infarction (MI), 573
Myocardial ischemia, 573
Non–ST-segment elevation acute coronary syndrome (NSTE-ACS), 588
Non–ST-segment elevation myocardial infarction (NSTEMI), 589
Pericarditis, 601
Stable angina, 585
Stroke volume (SV), 583
ST-segment elevation myocardial infarction (STEMI), 591
Tachycardia, 582
Thrombosis, 577
Unstable angina, 589
Valvular disorder, 603
Vasospasm, 577
Ventricular aneurysm, 601
Ventricular septal rupture, 601

ABBREVIATIONS

ACE—angiotensin-converting enzyme
ACS—acute coronary syndrome
AED—automated external defibrillator
ARB—angiotensin II receptor blockers
ASCVD—atherosclerotic cardiovascular disease
AV—atrioventricular node
BNP—B-type natriuretic peptide
CABG—coronary artery bypass grafting
CAD—coronary artery disease
CCB—calcium channel blocker
CHD—coronary heart disease
CK-MB—creatine kinase-MB
CO—cardiac output
CPR—cardiopulmonary resuscitation
CRP—C-reactive protein
CVD—cardiovascular disease
EC—endothelial cell
ECG—electrocardiogram
HDL—high-density lipoprotein
HR—heart rate
ICD—implantable cardioverter defibrillator
IHD—ischemic heart disease
IFN-γ—interferon-γ
LAD—left anterior descending artery
LBBB—left bundle branch block
LDL—low-density lipoprotein
LCA—left main coronary artery
MCP-1—monocyte chemoattractant protein 1
MI—myocardial infarction
MVD—coronary microvascular disease
NSTE-ACS—non-ST-segment elevation acute coronary syndrome
NSTEMI—non-ST-segment elevation myocardial infarction
oxLDL—oxidized low-density lipoprotein
PAC—premature atrial contraction
PCI—percutaneous coronary intervention
PSVT—paroxysmal supraventricular tachycardia
PVC—premature ventricular contraction
RBBB—right bundle branch block
RCA—right coronary artery
SA—sinoatrial node
SMC—smooth muscle cell
STEMI—ST-segment elevation myocardial infarction
SV—stroke volume
TEE—transesophageal echocardiography
TTE—transthoracic echocardiography
VCAM-1—vascular cell adhesion molecule 1
VF—ventricular fibrillation
VT—ventricular tachycardia

24.1 Chapter Overview and Case Studies

The coronary circulation is the blood flow to and from the heart muscle (myocardium) through the coronary arteries and cardiac veins. Problems with coronary circulation arise when blood flow to the myocardium is reduced as a result of conditions such as **coronary artery disease (CAD)**, which leads to reduced supplies of oxygen and nutrients. The term *coronary artery disease* is sometimes used interchangeably with **coronary heart disease (CHD)** to describe the buildup of plaque, which is made up of cholesterol (fatty) deposits, in the coronary arteries in a pathologic process called **atherosclerosis** that leads to reduced blood flow to the myocardium. CHD includes diagnoses that result from CAD, such as angina pectoris, acute coronary syndrome (ACS), silent myocardial ischemia, and myocardial infarction (MI).[1] **Angina**, or angina pectoris, describes the chest pain (*pectoris* means "chest"), discomfort, pressure, and squeezing symptoms of CAD when the heart is not receiving enough perfusion of blood.

Cardiovascular disease (CVD) is the pathologic process, commonly atherosclerosis, that causes disease of the heart and coronary and systemic circulation. CVD includes diagnoses such as stroke, transient ischemic attack (TIA), **claudication** (leg pain that is induced by exercise, typically caused by decreased arterial blood flow), and limb ischemia in addition to heart-related angina pectoris, myocardial ischemia, and myocardial infarction.[1] Ischemia is a temporary deficiency of blood flow to tissue, and **myocardial ischemia** is the restriction of blood supply to heart muscles tissues, causing a shortage of oxygen and nutrients needed for cellular function and survival. A **myocardial infarction (MI)** results when an area of tissue death, or necrosis, related to obstructed blood flow to the myocardium occurs; an MI is commonly caused by atherosclerosis leading to a thromboembolism, in which a thrombus (blood clot) is carried through the blood vessel and becomes dislodged (embolism).

Concepts Related to Coronary Circulation Disorders

A number of concepts and systems affect and are affected by adequate or impaired coronary circulation, including, but not limited to, cognition, pain, fluids and electrolytes, and oxygenation (**Figure 24.1** ■).

As a result of autoregulation, the brain has the ability to maintain relatively constant blood flow despite changes in perfusion pressure and therefore is able to maintain cognition. Clinical signs or symptoms of ischemia can be seen when the cerebral perfusion pressure drops below the lower limit of autoregulation. Altered mental status is an early symptom of decreased cerebral blood flow.

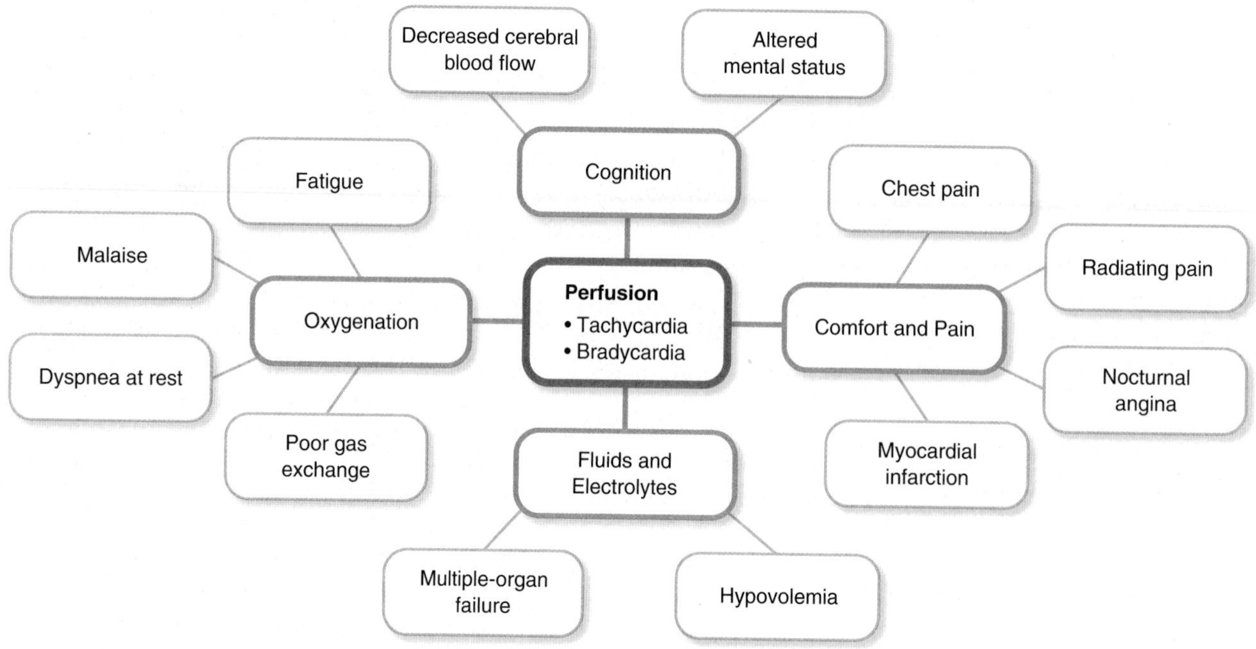

Figure 24.1 ■ Concepts related to coronary circulation disorders.

The heart generates enough cardiac output to transport and distribute blood to the body's tissues. Impaired tissue perfusion results when the blood flow to the site of injury is present but decreased. Comfort can be a concern, as pain is a common symptom.

Inadequate fluid resuscitation may lead to multiple organ failure and death due to fluid and electrolyte imbalances. Hypovolemia causes a decrease in extracellular fluid. In severe cases, inadequate tissue perfusion may occur. A loss of volume causes an inappropriate redistribution of body fluids and electrolytes via passive transport.

Without adequate cerebral blood flow, energy-dependent brain processes cease, leading to irreversible brain injury. Adequate cerebral blood flow or intracranial regulation must be maintained to ensure adequate cerebral perfusion pressure.

Respiratory gases are transported with the assistance of red blood cells, resulting in oxygenation by means of internal respiration. Ventilation, diffusion, and perfusion are essential for gas exchange to occur. The process of perfusion pumps bloods from the cardiovascular system to the lungs.

Case Studies

The following cases will be addressed throughout the chapter to assist in application of chapter content to clinical situations that involve patients with coronary circulation disorders.

Mary Kate Scot: Introduction

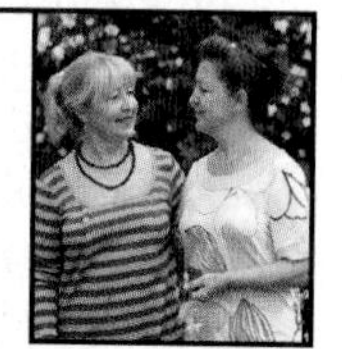

Mary Kate Scot is a 62-year-old woman. On a Saturday evening, she feels nauseated and thinks she must have eaten something that upset her stomach. By Sunday morning, she is having trouble breathing, and she dials 9-1-1. She is taken by ambulance to the nearest hospital emergency department (ED). On the basis of her history and clinical symptoms, the ED staff begin a diagnostic workup for an MI and consult the cardiologist who is on call. Ms. Scot feels confused and hears voices around her, but she cannot really understand or respond to her surroundings. She thought she knew the symptoms of a heart attack, but like many other people, she did not understand that vague symptoms like nausea/vomiting, back or jaw pain, and shortness of breath, particularly in women, may be signs of an MI.

1. What symptoms did Ms. Scot start with that led to her calling 9-1-1?
2. What are the signs of a myocardial infarction for a woman that are often overlooked?

Maggie Craig: Introduction

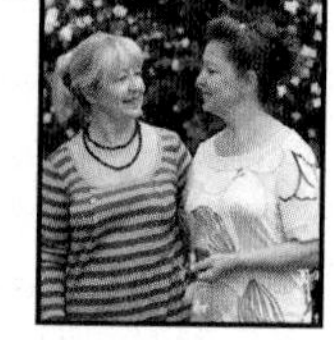

Mary Kate Scot has an older sister, Maggie Craig, who has always been physically active, eats a heart-healthy diet, and has no known medical problems. Ms. Craig decides to get checked out after her sister's experience. Though Ms. Craig has no overt signs of cardiac disease, her healthcare provider is concerned enough to refer her to a cardiologist for a workup.

CLINICAL POINT: Maggie Craig does not know yet that the choice to be evaluated will save her life. "Biologically related first-degree relatives (siblings, offspring, and parents) share roughly 50% of their genetic variation with one another," according to the American Heart Association.[2] ■

1. Why would the physician refer Ms. Craig to see a cardiologist?
2. Does Ms. Craig have any signs of cardiovascular disease at this time?

Check Your Progress: Section 24.1

1. What happens to the heart in coronary artery disease?
2. What types of diagnoses can a patient have with cardiovascular disease?
3. What causes myocardial infarction?

24.2 Epidemiology and Risk Factors Related to Coronary Artery Disease

Epidemiology

More than one in three adults in the United States have one or more types of CVD, which include MI, hypertension, stroke, and/or heart failure. CVD is the major leading cause of death internationally, and CHD is the leading major cause of death in the United States, accounting for more deaths than all cancer types combined.[2] Nearly 1.5 million deaths are related to CVD; an average of one CVD-related death occurs every 40 seconds.[2] More women than men and more Blacks than Whites or Hispanics die from CHD.

Risk Factors

Death and disability in the United States and throughout the world are most often caused by lifestyle-related risk factors that are modifiable.[2] Major modifiable risk factors that contribute to a risk of CAD include smoking and tobacco use, lack of physical activity, poor nutrition, overweight, obesity, hypertension, dyslipidemias, insulin resistance, and metabolic syndrome. Other modifiable risk factors are sleep apnea, stress, depression, heavy alcohol use, and air pollution.[3,4] Studies have found that people who are lonely and socially isolated are at an increased risk for CAD and that deficiencies in social relationships are comparable in degree of risk to that of previously recognized risk factors such as anxiety and job strain.[5] Infections have been associated with CAD[6] as well as periodontal disease possibly related to shared risk factors and inflammatory processes, but more research is needed to determine causation.[7] In women, preeclampsia during pregnancy has been linked[4]; recently, endometriosis[8] and migraines[9] have been linked to an increased risk of CAD in women.

Nonmodifiable risk factors include family history, age of more than 45 years in men and more than 55 years in women, race, and ethnicity.[10] Family history has been associated with an increased risk of developing CAD; however, its predictive value should be viewed in terms of degree of risk, in that risk is increased when more than one sibling develops CAD.[3,11] Some genetic testing is available to determine risk factors for CAD, and continued research has identified more and more loci with the goal of integrating the genetic information as part of risk assessment scores.[12] This would allow more predictive power, especially for asymptomatic individuals, to recommend specific preventive measures.[12]

Emerging research continues to look at factors such as inflammation that increase the risk of CAD. C-reactive protein (CRP) is a biomarker and mediator of the inflammatory process in the development of atherosclerosis.[13,14] Proinflammatory cytokines, which are small proteins that are important for cell signaling, influence hepatocytes (liver cells) to synthesize CRP.[13] An elevated plasma or serum CRP level is strongly associated with atherosclerosis and CAD and is predictive of cardiovascular events such as MI, stroke, peripheral artery disease, and sudden cardiac death.[13] Recent research has looked at using inflammatory biomarkers for risk stratification and treatment of affected patients, including those who may not have been identified by lipid level assessment alone.[13] Other risk factors that are evaluated through laboratory results include elevated plasma levels of lipoprotein(a), which is made up of protein and fat molecules and carries cholesterol in the blood. Levels of lipoprotein(a) are highly genetically determined, and hyperlipoproteinemia is a risk factor for CAD.[10,15]

The presence of other medical conditions such as end-stage renal disease, chronic inflammatory conditions such as lupus and rheumatoid arthritis, and HIV and its treatment with highly active antiretroviral therapy (HAART) may contribute to the development of CAD.[10] As is often the case with pathophysiologic disorders, both modifiable and nonmodifiable risk factors are involved in development of CAD and other coronary circulation disorders discussed in this chapter, making the precise risk factors and etiology difficulty to determine.

Prevention

CAD can be prevented by having **ideal cardiovascular health**, which the American Heart Association (AHA) defines as being without cardiovascular disease and having ideal levels, rather than poor or intermediate levels, of "Life's Simple 7" health indicators, or modifiable risk factors.[2] The seven indicators are blood pressure, physical activity, cholesterol, diet, weight, smoking status, and blood glucose level.[2] The Life's Simple 7 serves as a template to achieve heart-healthy living by providing targets for lifestyle modifications and evidence-based treatments. Lifestyle modifications such as physical activity have been shown to lower risk factors for CAD, such as CRP inflammatory markers,[13] resulting in decreased risk for MI, stroke, and vascular death.[16] A healthy diet includes low sodium intake, whole grains, and plenty of fruits and vegetables; such a diet also contributes to a healthy weight. Medications such as antihypertensives to control blood pressure, statins to lower cholesterol levels, and insulin to control blood glucose may be used to prevent the development of CAD.

Measurements to determine the range of cardiovascular health and guide treatment are shown in **Figure 24.2** ■. Increasing evidence shows that targeting Life's Simple 7 risk factors prevents CAD, thereby improving cardiovascular and brain health, and leads to less age-related decline in cognitive factors such as brain processing speed.[17]

Check Your Progress: Section 24.2

1. What are the four types of cardiovascular disease?
2. What are the modifiable risk factors for CVD?
3. What are some of the medical conditions that can contribute to CAD?

Life's Simple 7	Poor	Intermediate	Ideal
Blood Pressure			
Adults >20 years of age	SBP ≥140 or DBP ≥90 mm Hg	SBP120-139 or DBP 80-89 mm Hg or treated to goal	<120/<80 mm Hg
Children 8-19 years of age	>95th percentile	90th-95th percentile or SBP ≥120 or DBP ≥80 mm Hg	<90th percentile
Physical Activity			
Adults > 20 years of age	None	1-149 min/wk mod or 1-74 min/wk vig or 1-149 min/wk mod + vig	150+ min/wk mod or 75+ min/wk vig or 150+ min/wk mod + vig
Children 12-19 years of age	None	>0 and <60 min of mod or vig every day	60+ min of mod or vig every day
Cholesterol			
Adults >20 years of age	≥240 mg/dL	200-239 mg/dL or treated to goal	<170 mg/dL
Children 6-19 years of age	≥200 mg/dL	170-199 mg/dL	
Healthy Diet			
Adults >20 years of age	0-1 components	2-3 components	4-5 components
Children 5-19 years of age	0-1 components	2-3 components	4-5 components
Healthy Weight			
Adults > 20 years of age	≥30 kg/m²	25-29.9 kg/m2	<25 kg/m²
Children 2-19 years of age	>95th percentile	85th-95th percentile	<85th percentile
Smoking Status			
Adults >20 years of age	Current Smoker	Former ≤ 12 mos	Never/quit ≥ 12 mos
Children (12–19)	Tried prior 30 days		
Blood Glucose			
Adults >20 years of age	126 mg/dL or more	100-125 mg/dL or treated to goal	Less than 100 mg/dL
Children 12-19 years of age	126 mg/dL or more	100-125 mg/dL	Less than 100 mg/dL

Figure 24.2 ■ The American Heart Association's "Life's Simple 7" measurements to determine poor, intermediate, and ideal cardiovascular health and guide prevention and treatment.

24.3 Pathophysiology, Diagnosis, and Treatment of Coronary Artery Disease

Pathophysiology of CAD

Coronary arteries are blood vessels that deliver the necessary supplies of oxygen and nutrients required by myocardial cells to function and survive. Most blood flow to the myocardium is delivered during ventricular diastole (filling), when the ventricles, the lower chambers of the heart, fill with blood from the atria, the upper chambers, and the microcirculation (flow through small vessels entering the myocardium) is not compressed by contraction, as it is during systole.[18]

The left main coronary artery (LCA) and the right coronary artery (RCA) are the two main muscular-walled arteries that originate from the base of the aorta and branch across the epicardium, which is the outer surface of the heart and inner layer of the pericardium, before entering the myocardium and the endocardium (**Figure 24.3** ■). The coronary arteries then deliver blood to the arterioles, which are composed mostly of smooth muscle tissue that decreases blood flow through vasoconstriction and increases blood flow through vasodilation, and ultimately to the capillary network that envelops the cardiomyocytes (cardiac muscle cells).[18]

The LCA supplies the left atrium, left ventricle, interventricular septum (between the left and right ventricles), and atrioventricular (AV) bundles.[19] The LCA branches into the left anterior descending artery (LAD) and left circumflex artery.[18] The LAD, also known as the anterior interventricular artery, supplies blood to both left and right ventricles and the interventricular septum.[19] The left circumflex artery branches into the obtuse marginal artery to supply the left ventricle lateral wall and the atrial circumflex artery to supply the left atrium.[19] Disruption in the supply of blood through the LAD can be critical, and occlusion of the LAD is sometimes called the "widow maker."

The RCA supplies the right atrium, right ventricle, interventricular septum, and sinoatrial (SA) and AV nodes. The SA and AV nodes are essential for maintaining the cardiac conduction system. The RCA branches into the right marginal artery that supplies the right ventricle and also branches into the posterior descending artery to supply blood to the interventricular septum, alongside the LAD artery, as well as the posterior heart and papillary muscle.

Insufficient blood supply to the heart may trigger the development of **coronary collateral circulation**, in which collateral vessels anastomose (branch) to reroute blood flow.[20] Coronary collateral circulation was once believed to develop in the presence of myocardial ischemia. However, the process of coronary collateral circulation has been observed in people without CAD.[20] Therefore, the

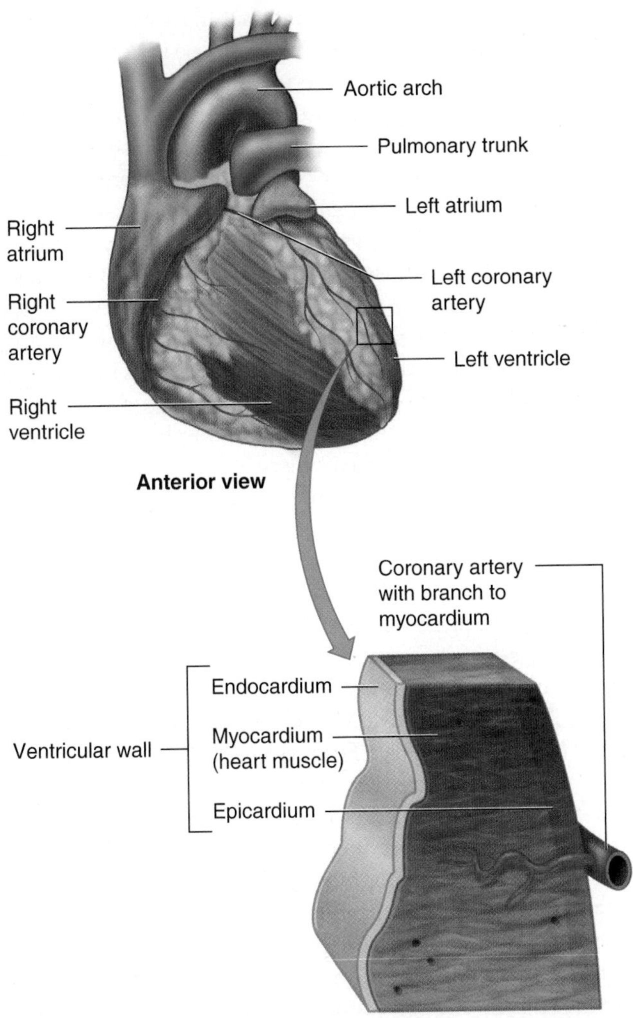

Figure 24.3 ■ Coronary circulation is the movement of blood through blood vessels of the heart muscle. The left main coronary artery (LCA) and the right coronary artery (RCA) are the two main coronary muscular-walled arteries that originate from the base of the aorta and branch the layers of the heart wall to deliver blood to the heart muscle.

pathophysiologic triggers are not fully understood, but their presence serves to preserve function by enabling an alternative route for delivery of blood to the myocardium.[20]

The normal artery is composed of two major cell types, which are both essential for normal vascular homeostasis: endothelial cells (ECs) and smooth muscle cells (SMCs). The endothelium lines the vessels of the entire circulatory system, including the coronary arteries, arterioles, and capillaries as well as the lymphatic system. ECs play a major role in regulation of blood flow by maintaining both an anticoagulant and a procoagulant surface as well as fibrinolytic mechanisms in the presence of thrombus formation to promote blood flow.[21,22] Endothelial dysfunction occurs with a shift from normal anti-inflammatory and antithrombotic (inhibiting clot formation) state with appropriate vasoconstriction and vasodilation of the endothelium toward a proinflammatory, prothrombotic (promoting blood clot formation) state of reduced vasodilation.[22] Problems with the vascular endothelium related to genetics and/or lifestyle factors precede CAD and other major diseases because they lead to atherosclerosis and possible arterial thrombosis, which obstruct blood flow in an artery.[22] **Thrombosis** is the process of formation of a blood clot (thrombus) that obstructs blood flow to organs depending on where it forms; when formed in a coronary artery, the blockage can cause a MI.

ECs that will make up the inner layer of arteries form during embryogenesis. Cells that make up other arterial wall components arise from bone marrow after birth in addition to formation during embryogenesis.[21] Endothelial progenitor cells derived from the bone marrow may facilitate vascular repair through endothelial regeneration. Research to understand the mechanism of endothelial regeneration is ongoing in order to develop treatments.[23]

SMCs contract to decrease blood flow and dilate to increase blood flow and are a target for many therapies to treat CVDs.[21] SMCs have a role in synthesizing arterial extracellular matrix, which provide structure and support and promote normal vascular homeostasis. However, SMCs also play a role in the development of atherosclerosis as well as disruption of atheromatous plaque resulting in decreased blood flow.[21] Atheromatous plaque, or atheroma, is often described as fatty deposits. Problems also arise when vasospasms occur as a result of abnormal SMC contraction in atherosclerotic arteries.[21] A **vasospasm** is a spasm (sudden constriction) of a blood vessel that decreases the vessel's diameter and consequently decreases blood flow.

The blood vessel wall is a three-layered structure that is composed of the tunica intima (inner layer), tunica media (middle layer), and tunica adventitia (external layer) (**Figure 24.4** ■). The tunica intima is made up of ECs; the tunica media is made up of SMCs; and the tunica adventitia is made up of collagen, fibroblasts, and mast cells.[21] The walls of blood vessels may be thicker or thinner depending on the presence of all or some of these layers. Coronary arteries are considered medium-sized or muscular arteries and are thicker than veins in order to bear higher pressure and pulsatile flow from the heart's contraction.[18]

Atherosclerosis is characterized by the deposition of lesions on the intima called atheromas, or atheromatous plaques, leading to narrowing and reduced blood flow. These lesions may mechanically obstruct flow because they may protrude into the vessel and rupture, leading to thrombosis and decreased blood flow; or they may weaken the intima and form an aneurysm. An **aneurysm** is a localized, blood-filled, balloon-like bulge in the wall of a blood vessel. Atherosclerosis can affect all arteries in the body and may be called atherosclerotic cardiovascular disease (ASCVD) or its specific associated disease named by location. ASCVD is a diffuse condition because it often involves the entire arterial circulation. *Carotid artery disease* is atherosclerosis of the carotid arteries that deliver blood to the brain. This occlusion can lead to stroke. *Renal artery stenosis* is atherosclerosis affecting the renal arteries and their occlusion can lead to hypertension or kidney disease. *Peripheral artery disease* is atherosclerosis

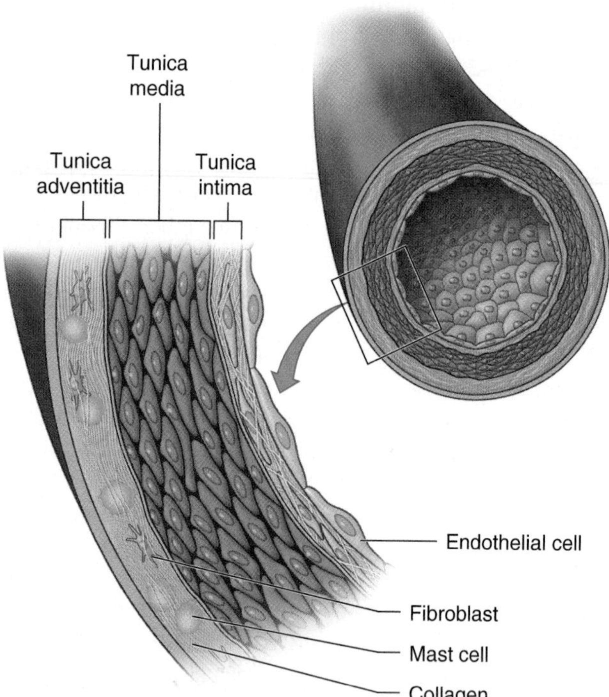

Figure 24.4 ■ The blood vessel wall has three layers: the tunica intima (made of endothelia cells [ECs]), tunica media (made of smooth muscle cells [SMCs]), and tunica adventitia (made of fibroblasts, mast cells, and collagen).

affecting blood flow in the upper or lower extremities and can cause a person to experience numbness, pain, or tingling related to lack of oxygen from decreased blood flow. CAD is named because it relates to atherosclerosis leading to reduced blood flow through the coronary arteries to the myocardium. Atherosclerosis may be asymptomatic ("silent"), or it may cause obvious symptoms of ischemia such as MI, stroke, kidney disease, or limb ischemia when plaque causes narrowing of the arteries and leads to inadequate blood flow or when plaque ruptures leading to thrombosis.

The first steps of atherosclerosis involve the accumulation of small particles of low-density lipoprotein (LDL) cholesterol in the tunica intima (**Figure 24.5** ■). Genetics as well as lifestyle factors such as an atherogenic diet, which is a diet that is high in cholesterol and saturated fat, may lead to an accumulation and aggregation of lipoproteins.[21] LDLs are susceptible to modifications such as oxidation in the presence of free oxygen radicals related to risk factors such as smoking, diabetes, and hypertension. Oxidized LDLs (oxLDL) induce cytokines, which are small protein molecules important in cell signaling that lead to the increased expression of adhesion molecules that attract, attach, and direct migration of leukocytes (white blood cells) into the intima.[21] Monocytes, a large phagocytic type of leukocyte, and T cells, lymphocytes with roles in cell-mediated immunity, are attracted to cytokines such as vascular cell adhesion molecule 1 (VCAM-1).[21] Chemoattractant cytokines, in response to oxLDL, such as monocyte chemoattractant protein 1 (MCP-1) direct the migration of monocytes into the intima of the arterial wall.[21] Interferon-γ (IFN-γ) is a cytokine that induces many genes expressed in macrophages, including those that encode chemoattractant cytokines that recruit T cells.[21]

The endothelium expresses anti-inflammatory factors such as nitric oxide (NO) in the presence of shear stress, which is stress from laminar blood flow (concentric layers of blood that flow down the length of a blood vessel in parallel formation). NO is a vasodilator produced by endothelial nitric oxide synthase that increases blood flow; it also has anti-inflammatory actions, expression of VCAM-1 and MCP-1 to prevent plasma lipoprotein entry, monocyte and T-cell attachment, and migration into the arterial intima.[21] In contrast to laminar flow, turbulent flow is disturbed, irregular flow in which development of atherosclerotic plaque is more likely. Free radicals can disrupt NO balance, causing disrupted endothelial signaling, resulting in increased permeability, which allows substances such as toxins and CRP to cross into the intima and further damage the blood vessels.[22]

Inside the arterial wall, monocytes differentiate into macrophages that engulf modified lipoprotein particles, such as oxLDL, to become foam cells. The process of internalizing lipids is mediated by scavenger receptors. Uptake by macrophages is increased by CRP, which enhances the macrophages' ability to form foam cells.[13] Foam cells are reservoirs for excess lipid, and a fatty streak describes the lesion that results from their replication and accumulation.[21] Foam cells release proinflammatory mediators such as cytokines and chemokines to enhance lesion development through innate immunity.[21] Innate immunity is nonspecific, whereas adaptive immunity describes an antigen-specific process to amplify the inflammatory process and lesion progression into an atheroma. Antigen-presenting cells, which include macrophages, dendritic cells, or ECs, present antigens to T cells in the intima that secrete more proinflammatory cytokines.[21] These proinflammatory cytokines, such as IFN-γ and tumor necrosis factor alpha (TNF-α), also have roles in plaque disruption and thrombosis in addition to generating an inflammatory state.

SMCs move from the media into the intima and replicate and accumulate in the developing atheroma as the fatty streak becomes a fibrous fatty lesion.[21] In the presence of SMC replication, which appears to occur in bursts, or "crises," there is also SMC apoptosis (cell death), which is triggered by inflammatory cytokines as well as T cells that enter the intima.[21] Extracellular lipids accumulate when released by apoptotic cells into a central lipid-rich core. Normally, the extracellular matrix is produced and destroyed by the SMCs in a balance that maintains the artery. However in the developing atheroma, SMCs synthesize extracellular matrix macromolecules that include collagens, proteoglycans, and elastin fibers in excessive amounts when stimulated by platelet-derived growth factor and other factors.[21] The result is a fibrous cap surrounding a lipid-rich core with apoptotic cells and their debris that protrudes into the blood vessel lumen, narrowing it and disrupting laminar blood flow, leading to turbulent flow. Stenosis (narrowing) of more than 60% of the diameter of the vessel can cause limitation of blood flow, especially in times of increased demand.[21] Additionally concerning is that dysfunctional endothelium leads to instability of the atheroma with potential plaque rupture and

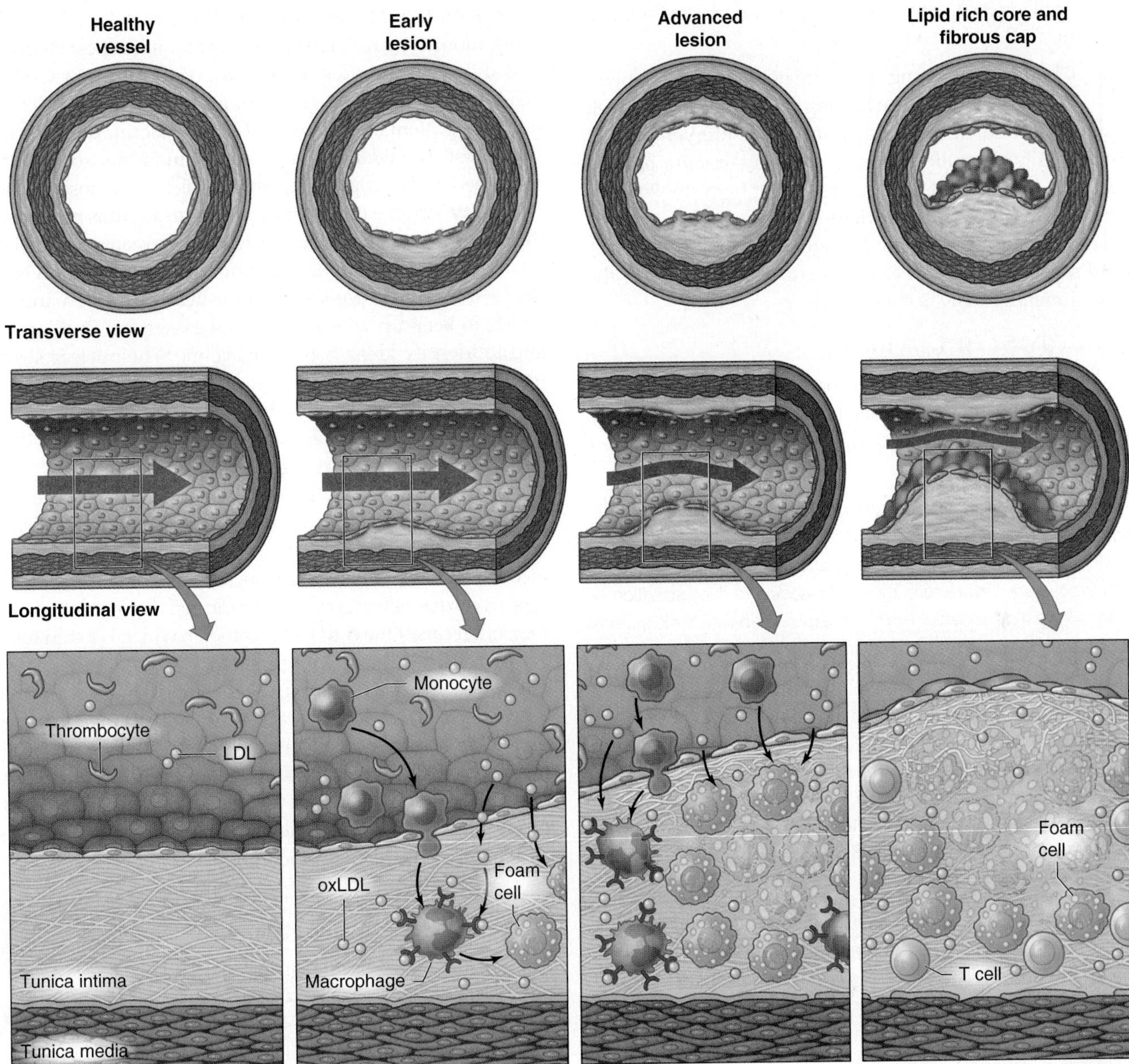

Figure 24.5 ■ *Microscopic view:* Lipoprotein particles (LDL) accumulate in the arterial intima, which become oxidized by free radicals into oxLDL. Monocytes and T cells attach and migrate into the intima. Monocytes differentiate into macrophages that engulf modified lipoprotein particles, such as oxLDLs, to become foam cells mediated by scavenger receptors. Foam cells replicate, and a fatty streak develops. Antigen-presenting cells present antigens to T cells in the intima. SMCs migrate, divide, and accumulate in the developing atheroma and die triggered by inflammatory cytokines. Extracellular lipids accumulate when released by apoptotic macrophages into a central lipid-rich core surrounded by a fibrous cap.

Longitudinal and transverse views: The development of atherosclerotic plaque protruding into the vessel lumen leads to narrowed artery, which disrupts laminar flow, thereby reducing blood delivery to distal tissue. Progressive narrowing of the coronary artery occurs as the atherosclerotic plaque builds up and decreased blood flow results in insufficient supply to distal tissues such as the myocardium.

thrombosis. Subsequent and repetitive cycles of rupture and healing with fibrous tissue formation further occlude the blood vessel, and it is the plaque disruptions with healing that are typically implicated in the cause of sudden cardiac death.[21]

The development of atherosclerosis can occur over many years. Fatty streak regression and return of a functioning endothelium may occur; however, the mechanisms involved in this regression are not understood, so treatment is controversial. The treatment paradigms that are under study include short-term aggressive statin therapy followed by periodic use to lower LDL and regress early atherosclerosis.[24] Additionally, the presence of high-density lipoprotein (HDL) exerts anti-inflammatory actions and allows for the uptake of cholesterol from the lipid-laden macrophages in the developing atheroma, also known as reverse cholesterol transport.[21] However, despite evidence of the strong inverse relationship between HDL levels and cardiovascular risk, research is lacking in showing that treatments such as niacin (or nicotinic acid) supplements to increase HDL will reduce cardiovascular events.[21]

4 Children and young adults are not immune to atherosclerosis, which is the leading cause of death in developed and developing countries.[24] Interventions to promote a healthy lifestyle such as maintaining a healthy weight and blood pressure and abstaining from smoking are necessary to prevent atherosclerosis or to regress developed and developing atheromas at any age before they cause CAD. More research is needed to identify the mechanisms in the development of CAD in children. ■

Diagnosis of CAD

The diagnosis of CAD is based on a collection of information gathered from risk factors, family and medical history, symptoms, the physical examination, and diagnostic test results and procedures.

CLINICAL POINT: A risk assessment is an important first step in screening for CAD or any CVDs. However, risk prediction is an imperfect science, and current algorithms do not incorporate accumulated long-term exposure to risk factors; thus, they leading to overestimation or underestimation of risk estimates.[25] The expansion of electronic medical records, which allows the ability to incorporate cumulative exposures over a person's lifetime, will strengthen estimates of future risk for a cardiovascular event if incorporated in risk prediction algorithms.[25] ■

Tests used for diagnosing CAD include blood tests, an electrocardiogram (ECG), an echocardiogram, and, if indicated, a coronary arteriogram. Blood tests include a lipid profile, and lipoprotein(a) testing has recently been added because hyperlipoproteinemia, which is highly heritable, has been linked to CVD.

CLINICAL POINT: Laboratory measurements such as the lipid profile are important in diagnosis of dyslipidemia and associated CVD. The fasting lipid profile assesses for abnormalities of four lipid biomarkers: elevated levels of total cholesterol, LDL, and triglycerides and low levels of HDL. ■

CRP is tested by using high-sensitivity assays and indicates the body's inflammatory process related to atherosclerosis. CRP testing in combination with lipid profile screening allows the identification of patients who might benefit from primary prevention in the presence of normal blood cholesterol levels as many studies direct attention to the role of inflammation as a major cause of altered endothelium and atherosclerosis.[13] Blood tests for diabetes or kidney disease may also determine the presence of coexisting diseases that are linked to atherosclerosis.

An ECG is used to assess and record the heart's electrical activity and show the presence of dysrhythmias related to CVDs. A **dysrhythmia** is an abnormal heart rhythm that can be irregularly slow or fast, also known as an arrhythmia. Irregularities on the ECG may indicate cardiac abnormalities such as ventricular hypertrophy, which is enlargement and thickening of the ventricle walls, or delays in conduction, which signal a delay in the signal to the heart to contract.[26]

Stress tests may be performed to determine whether the heart is receiving adequate blood flow or is affected by lack of perfusion present in CAD. An exercise stress test requires the person to walk on a treadmill or ride a bicycle while being monitored for signs and symptoms of chest discomfort, dyspnea (shortness of breath), or dizziness as well as ECG or vital sign changes. A pharmacologic stress test is used for patients who are unable to undergo the exercise stress test. Medications such as dobutamine, sometimes combined with atropine, dipryridamole, or adenosine, may be used to increase the workload of the heart, thus increasing the need for oxygen similarly to the requirements of exercise.

Echocardiography uses sound waves to create a video image that can be used to monitor heart perfusion and its ability to keep up with the stress of exercise or medication and to identify areas that are ischemic. The nuclear stress test uses single-photon emission computed tomography (SPECT) and injected radioactive tracer (technetium or thallium) to record x-ray images to identify ischemic areas during exercise or pharmacologically induced stress.[3]

A **coronary angiography**, also known as coronary arteriography, is an invasive procedure that is usually used to confirm the diagnosis of CAD after noninvasive tests have been inconclusive.[3] It can be diagnostic or interventional and is a type of cardiac catheterization performed in a special laboratory, often called the cath lab. A catheter, which is a thin tube, is inserted into a blood vessel, usually through the radial or femoral artery, and moved up to the large coronary arteries, where dye is injected and x-ray images are captured to determine the presence and extent of coronary artery narrowing. If interventional, the procedure is called a percutaneous coronary intervention (PCI), also known as angioplasty, in which procedures are used to unblock narrowed coronary arteries and reestablish adequate blood flow.

Maggie Craig: Application

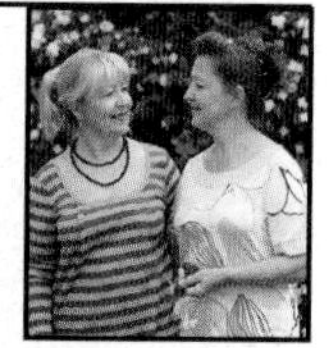

The cardiologist decides that although Ms. Craig has no apparent symptoms of heart disease, she is a candidate for a coronary angiography because of her family history. The coronary angiography is performed, and it shows that Ms. Craig's LAD is occluded such that eight or nine stents will be needed to maintain patency and adequately deliver blood. The angiogram also showed that the RCA has some blockages to blood flow.

3. What is the nonmodifiable risk factor that affects Ms. Craig and ultimately leads to her having a diagnostic procedure?
4. What did Ms. Craig's coronary angiogram show?

Treatment of CAD

Treatment for CAD does not necessarily mean medication. Changes in lifestyles, including the Life Simple 7 health indicators, correlate with improvement in cardiovascular health. Lifestyle modifications (physical activity, heart-healthy diet, tobacco avoidance, and healthy weight) remain crucial in both prevention and treatment of CVDs.[27] Some studies suggest that a Mediterranean diet is associated with lower cardiovascular mortality rate.[28] An international study found that consuming a high proportion of healthy foods such as fruit, vegetables, legumes, whole grains, fish, moderate alcohol, and little meat may be more important than avoiding the unhealthy foods typical of Western diets after CAD has occurred.[28] Unfortunately, fewer than 1% of adults in the United States eat an ideal healthy diet that is low in sodium and low in saturated and trans fats.[2]

Hypertension is treated with lifestyle modifications and medications (see Chapter 23 for a discussion of hypertension). Angiotensin-converting enzyme (ACE) inhibitors have benefits in addition to lowering blood pressure; these include inhibiting the progression of atherosclerotic lesions, plaque rupture, and thrombosis as well as improving endothelial function.[21] Beta blockers also appear to inhibit the progression of atherosclerosis with effects on endothelial function similar to those of angiotensin II receptor blockers (ARBs),[29] calcium channel blockers (CCBs), and diuretics; however, the beneficial effects of beta blockers are lower than those of ACE inhibitors.[30]

Guidelines suggest lipid-lowering therapy as a primary prevention strategy for individuals older than 21 years who have LDL levels of 190 mg/dL or higher, regardless of their level of short-term risk, because this level indicates a high lifetime atherosclerotic cardiovascular risk.[31] Statins are the recommended lipid-lowering drugs for individuals with increased LDL levels as well as those who present with clinically diagnosed ASCVD and individuals 40–75 years old with diabetes and LDL levels of 70–189mg/dL. Statins are also recommended as primary prevention for individuals 40–75 years old without diabetes but with a higher atherosclerotic cardiovascular risk and LDL levels of 70–189 mg/dL.[31] Research is being conducted to develop and study medications to lower increased levels of lipoprotein(a) that are genetically determined, because diet and lifestyle changes do not appear to lower levels.[15] Lipoprotein apheresis includes procedures to remove lipoproteins that contribute to atherosclerosis from circulation in patients with hyperlipoproteinemia with maximally tolerated lipid-lowering medication, and its use appears to effectively lower the incidence of cardiovascular events in those at risk.[32]

Patients coping with CVDs are likely to experience anxiety related to their disease as well as symptoms of depression and anger.[33] Many seek professional help (e.g., counseling) or the support of family, friends, or their church to manage these feelings.

CLINICAL POINT: Addressing loneliness and social isolation should be done through a multitude of interventions focused on a group level, such as education programs, or an individual level, such as cognitive–behavioral therapy. However, research is needed to evaluate the outcomes of these interventions.[5] ■

Check Your Progress: Section 24.3

1. What are the three coronary arteries that provide blood to the heart?
2. Which coronary arteries provide blood flow to the muscular wall?
3. What triggers the development of coronary collateral circulation?

24.4 Myocardial Ischemia and Infarction

Cell and Tissue Features

The coronary arteries supply the myocardium with blood to meet oxygen and nutrient demands. When oxygen exchange is insufficient, coronary arteries are capable of vasodilation to increase blood flow to meet demand. However, in the presence of atherosclerosis, complications arise as a result of narrowed coronary arteries and decreased blood flow. Growth of the atherosclerotic plaque does not occur linearly but instead is described as occurring in crises, in which periods of no progression alternate with periods of rapid lesion progression.[21] The process may develop over many decades during which the person is asymptomatic until blood flow obstruction causes significant areas of ischemia from lack of oxygen and nutrient supply. Subsequent acute infarction, or tissue death known as necrosis, most often results from plaque rupture and thrombosis. Repetitive cycles of plaque rupture and nonfatal thrombus leads to subsequent healing with SMC proliferation and matrix deposition to form fibrous tissue that further constricts flow.

Most atherosclerotic plaque rupture involves a fracture in its fibrous cap, but a second mechanism has been described that involves superficial erosion of the intima, which is not fully understood but appears to affect more women than men and may cause sudden cardiac death.[21] Fibrous cap rupture occurs because of several mechanisms that represent endothelial dysfunction. SMCs affected by IFN-γ derived from T cells are unable to synthesize collagen at the same time that platelet-derived growth factor is increasing SMC synthesis of collagen necessary to maintain extracellular matrix of the fibrous cap; as a result, there is an imbalance of maintenance and repair.[21] Additionally, because of apoptosis, there are fewer SMCs, further weakening and thinning the fibrous cap. Thin fibrous caps are prone to rupture, and this can precipitate a fatal MI.[21] The extracellular matrix may also be degraded by enzymes such as matrix metalloproteinases that are overexpressed by the macrophages in the atheroma.[21]

Rupture exposes the lipid-rich core and its thrombogenic material to the blood, which activates the clotting cascade and triggers thrombosis on top of the ruptured atherosclerotic plaque (see **Figure 24.6** ■).[21] Thrombogenic material such as collagen and von Willebrand factor interact with glycoprotein receptors on platelets, resulting in platelet adhesion to the site of blood vessel injury.[21] Platelets are activated by the interaction and release adenosine diphosphate and thromboxane A_2, which further activate and recruit surrounding platelets.[21] Activated platelets change shape and express glycoprotein IIb/IIIa receptors on their surface and bind adhesive proteins such as von Willebrand factor and fibrinogen as well as stimulating thrombin formation on their surface, which leads to platelet aggregation and coagulation.[34] Thrombin is a clotting enzyme that converts fibrinogen in the blood into fibrin, which weaves the aggregating platelets into a platelet–fibrin thrombus.[21] The clinical consequence of thrombosis depends on the amounts of tissue

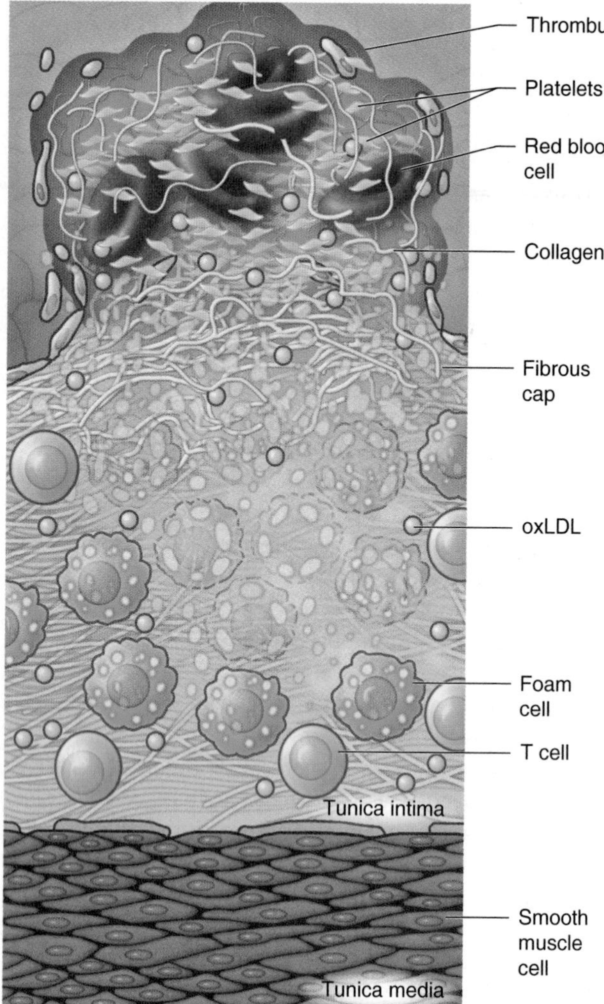

Figure 24.6 ■ Thrombus formation and atherosclerotic plaque rupture have clinical consequences related to amount and interaction of tissue factors in the lipid-rich core (solid state of plaque) exposed and the amount of fibrinogen and fibrinolysis inhibitors in the blood (fluid phase).

factors in the plaque, the levels of fibrinogen and fibrinolysis inhibitors in the blood, and their interaction.[21] An occlusive thrombus can cause acute coronary thrombosis in a coronary artery, leading to a potentially fatal MI.

Disruption of coronary blood flow can cause major problems resulting from an imbalance among oxygen supply, demand, and consumption. This balance is key to the production of sufficient arterial pressure to perfuse both systemic and coronary circulation. During systole, the aortic valve is opened, and aortic pressure forces blood through systemic circulation, while the diameter of coronary microvessels is reduced and the coronary artery flow is reduced. Diastole marks aortic valve closure and relaxation of ventricles as blood is delivered through the coronary arteries to the myocardium. **Coronary perfusion pressure** is the pressure of blood through coronary circulation as a result of the pressure gradient between the aortic pressure and the right atrial pressure. Perfusion to the subendocardial muscle, situated between the myocardium and endocardium, is favored during diastole.[21] Recall that the endocardium is the innermost layer of tissue that lines the atria, ventricles, and heart valves and that the myocardium is the muscular wall that is responsible for heart contraction (see Figure 24.3).

Myocardial oxygen demand and consumption are determined by heart rate, systolic pressure (pressure on arteries during contraction), and left ventricular contractility (strength of contraction).[21] Increases in these determinants lead to proportional increases in coronary blood flow and oxygen delivery under normal conditions. When determinants of oxygen consumption are constant, **autoregulation** is the phenomenon that maintains the constant regulation of coronary blood flow through the myocardium despite changes in coronary perfusion pressure.[21] Changes in vessels, such as vasodilation, lead to increased blood flow to meet increased metabolic demands or a drop in coronary perfusion pressure that caused the decreased blood flow. These changes are stimulated by pathways involving substances such as endothelium-dependent hyperpolarizing factor, NO, and prostacyclins.[21] Endothelium-dependent hyperpolarizing factor changes the cell membrane potential to make it more negative (hyperpolarized) by opening the SMC potassium (K^+) channels that are activated by calcium (Ca^{2+}), which leads to vascular smooth muscle relaxation and artery dilation.[21] NO and prostacyclins also induce vascular relaxation and dilation.[22] Constriction inducing factors include endothelium-dependent factors such as endothelins[21]; however, dysfunction of these endothelium-dependent pathways occurs in atherosclerosis, leading to needs for increased blood flow not being met because the effects of vasodilation are reduced.[35]

Injury may range from reversible to irreversible effects when blood flow is decreased or completely blocked, resulting in hypoxia (oxygen deprivation) of the myocardial cells (see Chapter 10 for a discussion of cellular effects of hypoxia). Myocardial cell injury is reversible when the blood supply is compromised for a 10- to 15-minute period. The heart muscle will be injured, but it can recover normal function. Occlusion of the blood supply through the coronary arteries for 20 minutes or more may lead to death of myocardial fibers and irreversible injury; however, the exact length of time to irreversible tissue injury depends on the presence of coronary collateral circulation (see **Figure 24.7** ■).[21] Additionally, factors that lead to increased myocardial oxygen requirements such as hypotension (low blood pressure), coronary vasospasm, and **tachycardia** (abnormal rapid heart rate, generally more than 100 beats per minute) may accelerate the time to irreversible injury. Additionally, factors that lower oxygen delivery such as hypotension and anemia, which is marked by reduced red blood cells and therefore reduced oxygen-carrying capacity, also accelerate the time to irreversible injury. Irreversible injury progresses in a wavelike fashion from the subendocardium to the subepicardium.[36] The inner third wall of the left ventricle is irreversibly damaged after 60 minutes of coronary artery occlusion; damage is expanded to the subepicardium after 3 hours; and transmural ischemia results in transmural infarction after 3–6 hours.[36]

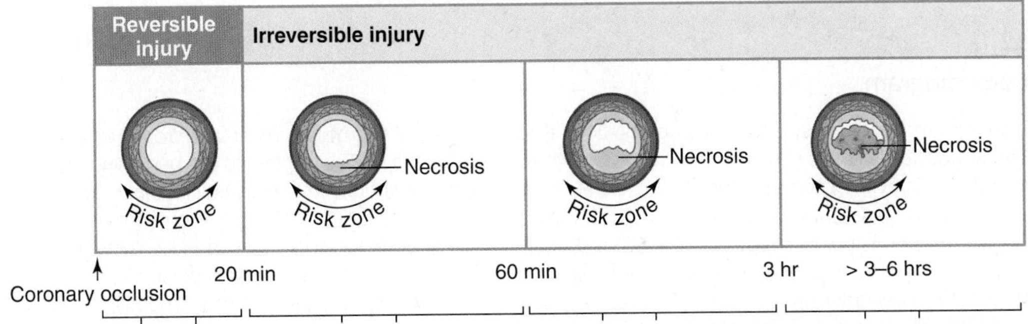

Figure 24.7 ■ Myocardial cell injury is reversible when the blood supply is compromised as a result of coronary artery occlusion for less than 20 minutes. Irreversible injury progresses in a wavelike fashion from the subendocardium to the subepicardium. The inner third wall of the left ventricle is irreversibly damaged after 60 minutes of coronary artery occlusion. Damage is expanded to the subepicardium between 60 minutes and 3 hours. The transmural extent of infarction occurs between 3 and 6 hours.

A person may experience brief periods of ischemia on a daily basis without its resulting in myocardial necrosis.[36] Myocardial cells that are ischemic have reduced contractility, leading to decreased cardiac output. **Cardiac output (CO)** is the amount of blood pumped from the left or right ventricle; it is determined by stroke volume (SV) and heart rate (HR) as represented by the equation $CO = SV \times HR$. **Stroke volume (SV)** is the amount of blood pumped from the ventricle during one contraction measured in milliliters per heartbeat. Recall that CO is determined by heart rate, contractility, preload, and afterload. Preload is amount of volume, and therefore stretch, in the right or left ventricle at the end of diastole. Afterload is the pressure, or force, that the heart has to contract against to eject blood from the ventricle during systole. CO is measured in liters per minute and is related to tissue perfusion. When cardiac output is decreased, further problems of ischemia may develop, such as reduced systemic blood perfusion.

The Cardiac Conduction System

Ischemia disrupts the cardiac conduction system, which disrupts the electrical charge transmission via cardiac muscle fibers throughout myocardial tissue and affects the heart's ability to contract and perfuse systemic and coronary circulation. Recall that the main structures of the cardiac conduction system are the SA and AV nodes, bundle of His, left and right bundle branches, and Purkinje fibers and that an electrical impulse travels through these structures, creating an electrical current that can be captured on an ECG or cardiac monitor. These are depicted in **Figure 24.8** ■ and discussed with their relationship to the ECG in Box 24.1.

The Ischemic Cascade

The progression from ischemia to infarction can be thought of as an ischemic cascade in which coronary occlusion from problems such as atherosclerotic plaque disruption and

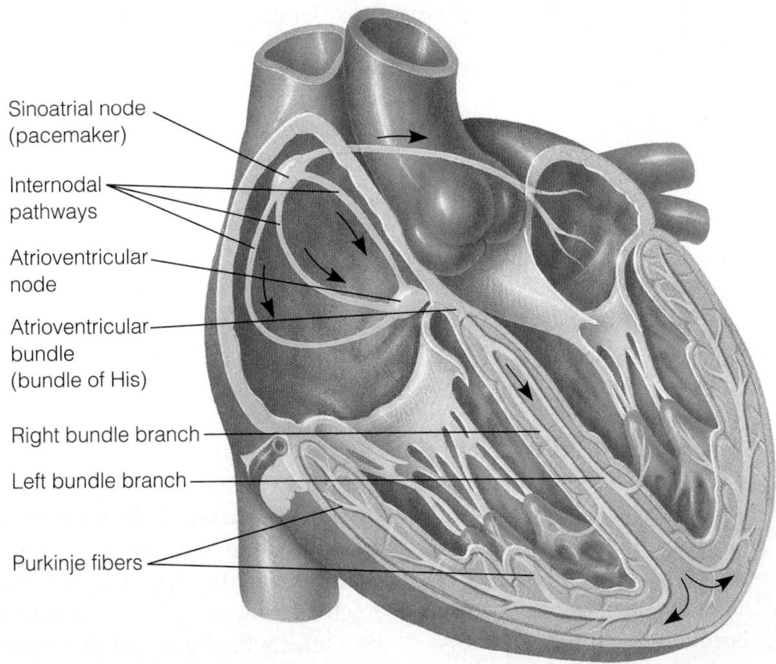

Figure 24.8 ■ The cardiac conduction system.

Box 24.1

The Electrocardiogram

The electrocardiogram (ECG) is used to assess and record the heart's electrical activity and show the presence of dysrhythmias related to CVD. An ECG of normal sinus rhythm is shown in **Figure 24.9**. The SA node is the inherent cardiac pacemaker that normally generates an impulse at a rate of 60–100 beats per minute.[18] The P wave represents atrial depolarization and contraction when the impulse is generated in or near the SA node. The AV node is a gatekeeper that delays the signal transmission traveling from the atria to the ventricles to ensure that the atria contract before the ventricles,[18] displayed by the P wave occurring before the QRS complex, which represents ventricular depolarization and contraction. The autonomic nervous system, which also controls blood pressure, is responsible for the rate of SA node firing, or electrical impulse generation.[18] The PR interval begins at the end of the P wave and ends at the beginning of the QRS complex and normally has a 120- to 200-millisecond duration (0.12–0.20 second) in most adults.[21] The PR interval often reflects the time of conduction through the AV node, between atrial and ventricle activation.[21] The QRS complex is typically less than 120 milliseconds ($\leq$ 0.12 second), and women typically have a shorter QRS than men.[21]

The ST segment is measured from the J point, which is at the end of the QRS complex, to the beginning of the T wave. The ST segment is normally nearly isoelectric. However, in the presence of acute severe ischemia, ST-segment changes such as elevation or depression are early and consistent ECG findings.[21] The T wave reflects ventricular repolarization of the cardiac action potential, and changes from its smooth, rounded shape occur in the presence of myocardial ischemia or electrolyte imbalances.[37] The U wave follows and is usually in the same direction as the T wave on the ECG tracing.[21] The pathophysiologic basis of the U wave is not fully understood but is thought to be related to late repolarization of the Purkinje fibers.[21] The QT interval is measured from the beginning of the QRS complex to the end of the T wave and reflects the total duration of the ventricular action potential, which is essentially the time of activation and recovery of the ventricles.[21] The formula to measure the QT intervals, which are rate-dependent and decrease as heart increase, results in the correct QT interval (QTc), and its equation components are measure in seconds.[21] The equation is $QTc = QT/\sqrt{RR}$, where RR is the interval between two R waves).[21]

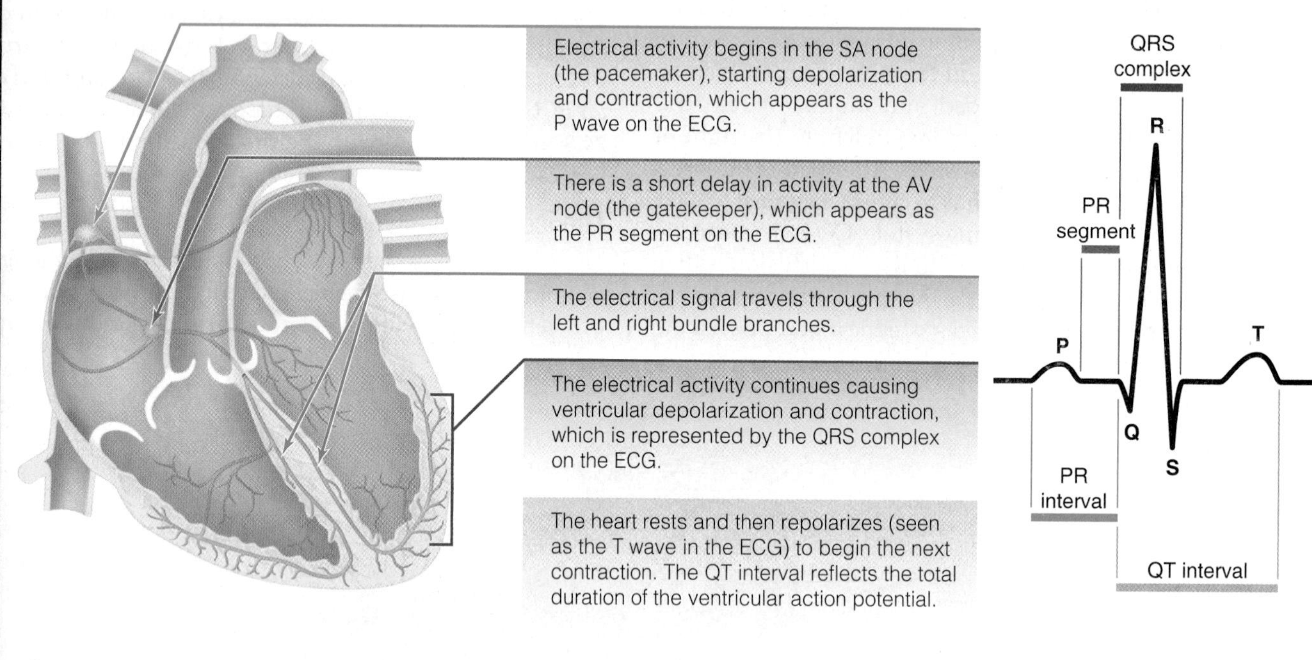

Electrical activity begins in the SA node (the pacemaker), starting depolarization and contraction, which appears as the P wave on the ECG.
There is a short delay in activity at the AV node (the gatekeeper), which appears as the PR segment on the ECG.
The electrical signal travels through the left and right bundle branches.
The electrical activity continues causing ventricular depolarization and contraction, which is represented by the QRS complex on the ECG.
The heart rests and then repolarizes (seen as the T wave in the ECG) to begin the next contraction. The QT interval reflects the total duration of the ventricular action potential.
QRS complex
R
PR segment
P
T
Q
S
PR interval
QT interval

Figure 24.9 ■ Normal sinus rhythm.

thrombosis initiates the steps (**Figure 24.10**).[38] Occlusion of the coronary artery leading to perfusion abnormalities and resultant ischemia is the first step of the ischemic cascade.

Cardiac conduction relies on electrolyte balance, particularly of Ca^{2+}, K^{+}, and Na^{+}. Myocardial relaxation normally occurs when Ca^{2+} is pumped out of the cardiomyocytes or into the sarcoplasmic reticulum in a process that requires adenosine triphosphate (ATP).[38] When oxygen is not available, aerobic metabolism switches to anaerobic metabolism, which results in an imbalance of ATP production and consumption and subsequent impaired cardiomyocyte relaxation.[38] Regional diastolic dysfunction results from impaired myocardial relaxation.[38] Ca^{2+} and lactic acid accumulate, affecting the cardiomyocyte's ability to contract, leading to systolic dysfunction.[38] Diastolic dysfunction affects the heart's ability to relax and fill with blood, and systolic dysfunction affects the heart's ability to contract and perfuse coronary and systemic circulation, resulting

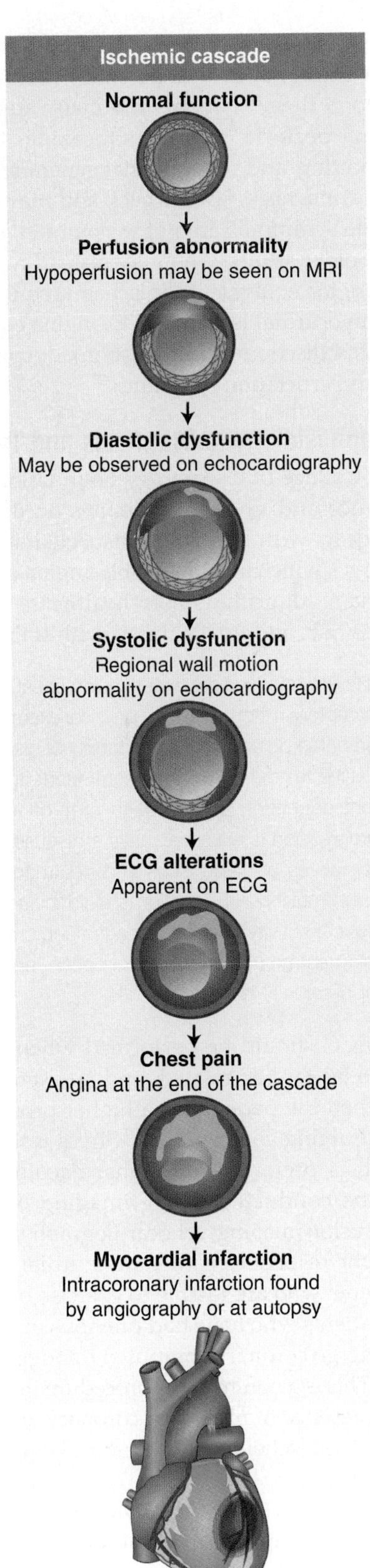
Ischemic cascade
Normal function
Perfusion abnormality
Hypoperfusion may be seen on MRI
Diastolic dysfunction
May be observed on echocardiography
Systolic dysfunction
Regional wall motion abnormality on echocardiography
ECG alterations
Apparent on ECG
Chest pain
Angina at the end of the cascade
Myocardial infarction
Intracoronary infarction found by angiography or at autopsy

Figure 24.10 ■ Ischemic cascade is initiated when coronary artery occlusion and subsequent decrease in coronary blood flow cause a blood perfusion abnormality and result in transmural ischemia. Impaired cardiomyocyte relaxation causes diastolic dysfunction, and impaired cardiomyocyte contraction leads to regional systolic dysfunction. Diastolic dysfunction affects the heart's ability to relax and fill with blood, and systolic dysfunction decreases cardiomyocyte contraction and ability to perfuse circulation. As ischemia from occlusion or spasm persists, ECG changes occur as a result of the systolic and diastolic injury currents, and the patient experiences clinical symptoms such as angina pectoris. If ischemia persists long enough without reperfusion, cardiomyocytes die, and the tissue is infarcted.

in ECG changes. Waste products of anaerobic metabolism such as lactic acid accumulate, causing the person to experience typical angina symptoms by stimulating the cardiac nerves that fuse with nerves traveling toward the outside of the chest, arms, neck, jaw, shoulders, and back, generating pain.[38]

The ECG is key in diagnosing both acute and chronic coronary syndromes. ECG abnormalities depend on the time of ischemia, including whether it is an acute process or a developing chronic process; the extent of the ischemia, such as its size and transmural location; and whether there are any other underlying abnormalities, such as dysrhythmias.[21] The early and consistent ECG abnormality that occurs in acute ischemic processes is deviation of the ST segment from the isoelectric line.[21] Under normal conditions, the ST segment is isoelectric as a result of the plateau phase of the ventricular action potential as the transmembrane voltage stays at approximately the same potential in all cardiomyocytes.[21,38] However, the process of ischemia reduces the resting membrane potential, which shortens the action potential and decreases the amplitude of the action potential plateau phase.[21,38] The resulting voltage gradient between the normal cells and ischemic cells causes an injury current between the normal zone and ischemic zones on the myocardium, reflected by deviation of the ST segment (**Figure 24.11** ■).[21,38] Subendocardial injury involves the inner layer, not the full thickness, of the affected ventricle and causes ST-segment depression (**Figure 24.12A** ■). Transmural (epicardial) injury affects the outer ventricular layer as it extends from the subendocardium to the epicardium and causes ST elevation with the presence of ST-segment depression in other leads (Figure 24.12B).[38] Eventually, if the ischemia is severe and perfusion of blood flow is not restored, cardiomyocytes distal to the occluded coronary artery are irreversibly injured and die, and the tissue is considered necrotic, or infarcted.

Stable Angina

Stable angina is considered a chronic form of ischemic heart disease (IHD). IHD is also referred to as CHD; however, to assume that IHD is synonymous with CAD is overly simplistic and does not account for other causes of myocardial ischemia.[21]

Etiology and Pathogenesis

Stable angina usually occurs with increased myocardial oxygen demand and reduced blood flow during exertion or emotional stress, commonly caused by atherosclerosis. Other causes of gradual narrowing of arteries that are commonly implicated in stable angina are endothelial dysfunction, coronary microvascular disease (MVD), and vasospasms.[21] Obstructive CAD from atherosclerotic plaque

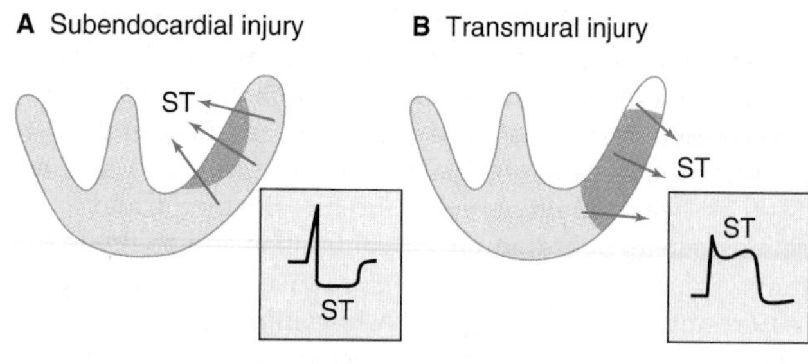

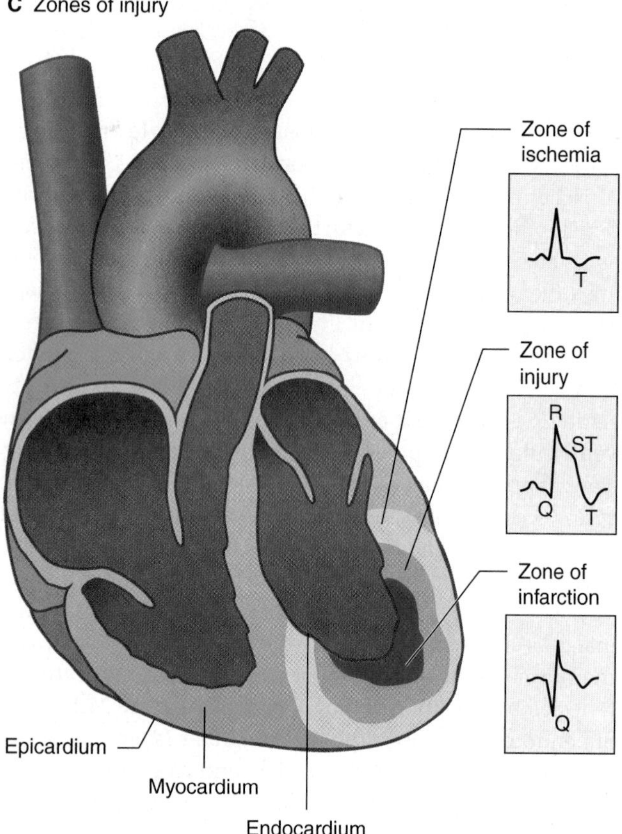

Figure 24.11 ■ ECG changes depend on many factors, including the time, location, and extent of ischemia and the presence of other abnormalities. **A.** Subendocardial injury is characterized by ST-segment depression. **B.** Transmural (epicardial) injury extends from the endocardium to epicardium and is characterized by ST-segment elevation. **C.** Zones of injury include areas of ischemia, injury, and infarction.

that causes narrowing of more than 60% of the diameter of the artery leads to flow limitations and produces symptoms of chronic stable angina in the presence of increased myocardial demand.[21] However, ischemia and subsequent angina pectoris can occur in patients who are experiencing extreme myocardial oxygen demand in the presence of no underlying obstructive CAD, as in the presence of aortic valve disease.

Clinical Manifestations of Stable Angina

Chest discomfort is typically the main symptom of stable angina; it is usually related to exertion and often resolves with rest or short-acting nitroglycerin, an antianginal agent.[21] Exertion may include physical activity or mental or emotional stress. The pain may also manifest as postprandial (after eating) angina as a result of redistribution of coronary blood flow.[21] Patients use many adjectives to describe angina pectoris, such as squeezing, tightness, crushing, suffocating, and pressure that generally occurs in the shoulders, arms, neck, jaw, or back and may radiate.[39] However, vague symptoms are not uncommon, especially in women and older adults, who may instead report what are known as angina equivalents or ischemic equivalents as symptoms of myocardial ischemia.[21,40] Angina equivalents include epigastric discomfort (indigestion), dyspnea, faintness, fatigue, and eructation (belching).[21]

Linking Pathophysiology to Diagnosis and Treatment

The American College of Cardiology Foundation and the AHA[41,42] produce and update guidelines on diagnosing and treating adults with known or suspected stable ischemic heart disease, which includes stable angina or low-risk unstable angina.[40] Algorithms help healthcare providers diagnose, assess risk, and treat patients with stable angina.

CLINICAL POINT: Patients who are experiencing chest pain should have a review of symptom history, focused physical examination, and risk factor assessment to determine the probability of disease before additional noninvasive testing, which is recommended, or invasive testing.[21,40] Patient education about health promotion and CAD prevention and progression is essential, as is a discussion of risks, benefits, and alternatives of diagnostics and treatment proposed with shared decision making.[40] Education should include diabetes management, physical activity, weight management, smoking cessation, psychologic treatment, alcohol consumption, and exposure to air pollution if applicable.[40] ■

A resting ECG should be performed when the chest pain appears to be cardiac-related, and an exercise stress ECG is used when the patient has a higher probability of CAD and no disabling comorbidity.[40] Stress testing using exercise, which is preferred, or a pharmacologic stress test may also be conducted, using imaging by nuclear myocardial perfusion imaging, echocardiography, or cardiovascular magnetic resonance (CMR) myocardial perfusion imaging.[40] Patients who are unable to exercise or undergo other tests or patients who have had previous inconclusive results may undergo coronary computed tomography (CT) angiography.[40] This is a noninvasive procedure that helps to determine the presence of narrowed coronary arteries and resultant myocardial ischemia; it is preferred over invasive coronary angiography.

Guidelines include risk factor modification and recommendations on follow-up and medical therapy to prevent MI and death, such as the use of an antiplatelet agent such as aspirin. Beta blockers may be used as initial therapy for relief of symptoms, and CCBs or a long-acting nitrate is used when beta blockers are contraindicated or not tolerated by the patient.[40] Other medications such as ACE inhibitors may be considered for patients with comorbidities such as diabetes, hypertension, chronic kidney disease, and/or left ventricle dysfunction.[40] ARBs are used for these patients when ACE inhibitors are not tolerated.[40]

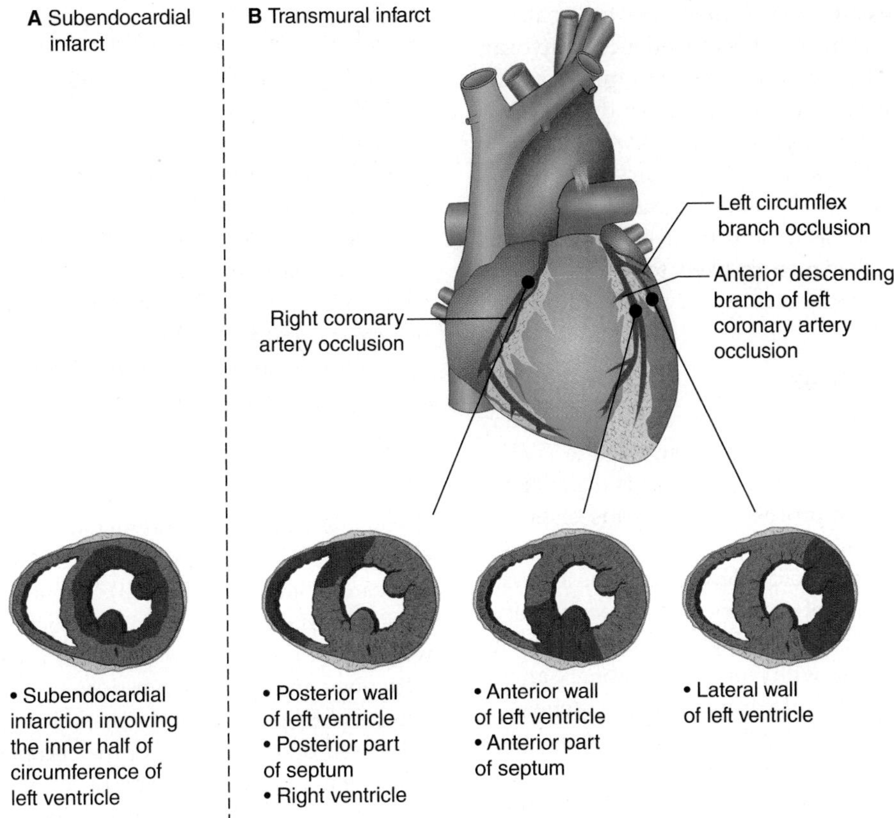

Figure 24.12 ■ **A.** Subendocardial injury involves the inner layer, not the full thickness, of the affected ventricle and causes ST-segment depression. **B.** Transmural (epicardial) injury affects the outer ventricular layer as it extends from the subendocardium to the epicardium and causes ST elevation with the presence of ST-segment depression in other leads.

The resolution of angina pectoris with rest or the use of short-acting nitroglycerin can be diagnostic and treatment for stable angina.[21] Short-acting nitroglycerin is a nitrate that may be administered as a sublingual tablet or spray. Nitrates stimulate vasodilation of blood vessels; increase the epicardial coronary diameter, which is commonly implicated in stable angina; improve coronary collateral blood flow; and impair platelet aggregation.[35]

CLINICAL POINT: As prophylactic treatment, short-acting nitroglycerin may allow the patient who is experiencing stable angina to improve exercise tolerance and quality of life.[35] If relief is not achieved after more than 5–10 minutes, the symptoms of angina pectoris are likely not related to myocardial ischemia or are caused by severe ischemia, such as an acute MI.[21] ■

Silent Ischemia

Many people may live with widespread coronary artery obstruction but never experience the typical symptoms of angina pectoris.[21] Episodes of silent ischemia are estimated to be present in one third of patients who are treated for angina, a higher prevalence being likely for patients with diabetes.[21]

Etiology and Pathogenesis

The pathogenesis for silent ischemia is unclear but is thought to be related to a defective anginal warning system as a result of problems in peripheral and central neural processing of pain.[21]

Clinical Manifestations

The usual symptom of chest pain may not always be present in the patient who is experiencing IHD. ST-segment depression may or may not be evident on ambulatory electrocardiographic recording.

Linking Pathophysiology to Diagnosis and Treatment

Together, the use of ambulatory electrocardiographic monitoring and SPECT may complement each other to help identify silent ischemia.[21] Management of asymptomatic ischemia should be similar to management of symptomatic ischemia because it is likely that the prognosis is similar.[21] Management to reduce or eliminate episodes of silent ischemia may include the same medical therapies, such as nitrates, beta blockers, and CCBs, that are used to reduce or eliminate episodes of symptomatic ischemia.[21] Coronary angiography and revascularization may also be considered as invasive management strategies. Lipid-lowering therapy should be considered as secondary prevention.

Coronary Microvascular Disease

Patients who present with angina pectoris but have no obvious associated cardiac or systemic disease have traditionally been diagnosed with cardiac syndrome X.[42] These patients may have no visible atherosclerosis or evidence of myocardial ischemia evident on coronary angiography,[21] owing to the presence of coronary microvascular dysfunction. **Coronary microvascular dysfunction** involves damage to the walls and inner linings of small coronary arteries that can lead to narrowing, spasms, and decreased blood flow. MVD can also be known as nonobstructive coronary heart disease. More women than men are likely to be affected, and women are at greater risk for a major adverse cardiovascular event such as a MI.[42]

Etiology and Pathogenesis

The cause of MVD is not clearly understood, which may be partly why the literature does not clearly define MVD.[42] In fact, it is not clear whether the pain that is experienced is caused by an ischemic process or other causes such as endothelial and microvascular dysfunction, coronary vasospasms, or myocardial metabolism problems.[21] The iPOWER study used measurements of coronary flow velocity reserve by transthoracic Doppler echocardiography in women who presented with angina but with a previous coronary angiogram showing no significant coronary artery stenosis.[43] Women with impaired coronary flow velocity reserve possibly explained by MVD had significantly more history of CAD risk factors, such as hypertension, diabetes mellitus, smoking, low HDL cholesterol, and elevated heart rate.[43]

Clinical Manifestations

Angina in the absence of myocardial ischemia caused by coronary artery obstruction is characteristic of MVD and is often difficult to differentiate from angina caused by ischemia-related epicardial coronary artery obstruction.[42] Angina without the presence of obstruction may occur in up to 30% of patients who undergo a coronary angiography to assess for cause of angina.[42]

Linking Pathophysiology to Diagnosis and Treatment

Diagnosis of MVD is difficult because standard tests used to diagnose CAD do not detect MVD and some tests such as the coronary angiography appear to show clear, nonatherosclerotic coronary arteries in women. MVD is the possible explanation for the presence of angina with no evidence of obstructive CAD on coronary angiography.[43] Noninvasive techniques such as transthoracic Doppler echocardiography, SPECT scan, and CMR myocardial perfusion imaging may help to improve identification of MVD.[42,43] More research is needed on a standardized definition of MVD[42] as well as diagnostics and treatment for symptoms and prognosis of MVD.[43]

Check Your Progress: Section 24.4

1. What is coronary perfusion pressure?
2. What is the phenomenon that maintains the constant regulation of coronary blood flow through the myocardium despite changes in coronary perfusion pressure?
3. What are the factors that lead to increased myocardial oxygen requirements?

24.5 Specific Acute Coronary Syndromes

In the United States, one person has an acute coronary event approximately every 34 seconds, and one person dies from an event approximately every 1 minute and 24 seconds.[2] Each year, approximately 635,000 people in the U.S. have a new coronary attack, defined as first hospitalized MI or death related to CAD, and approximately 300,000 have a recurrent event.[2]

Acute coronary syndrome (ACS) is an acute form of CAD. ACS encompasses any cluster of clinical signs and symptoms that are related to acute myocardial ischemia and infarction. The types of ACS are non–ST-segment elevation acute coronary syndrome (NSTE-ACS), which formerly was known as unstable angina; non–ST-segment elevation myocardial infarction (NSTEMI); and ST-segment elevation myocardial infarction (STEMI).[34] An acute MI includes diagnosis of NSTEMI and STEMI in which necrosis is involved, whereas NSTE-ACS, or unstable angina, accelerates in frequency and severity but does not result in myocardial necrosis.[2] Regardless of the specific type of ACS, therapy is focused on reperfusion of the coronary arteries through an ischemia-guided strategy or invasive PCI.[34] The AHA and American College of Cardiology (AHA/ACC) produce a task force that presents guidelines and updates that are evidence-based for the management of patients who present with ACS.

Pathogenesis of ACS

It is well established that patients with CAD have an increased risk of developing ACS; however, specific causes that trigger ACS events are still being explored. The pathophysiology of all types of ACS is shared. CAD most commonly progresses to its acute form, ACS, when atherosclerotic plaque ruptures, which is the stimulus for thrombogenesis and blood flow obstruction. The progression from asymptomatic atherosclerotic plaque to thrombosis in relation to the resulting clinical conditions is shown in **Figure 24.13** ■ and discussed in the previous section. Plaque rupture can also cause the artery walls to constrict, which results in vasospasm and additional artery narrowing and ischemia distal to the area.

The sudden imbalance of myocardial oxygen consumption, which is the amount of oxygen consumed by the heart, and the myocardial demand, which is the amount of energy required, is the hallmark of ACS. There are other causes for increased demand, such as exercise, valvular disorders, and increased heart rate and blood pressure from other causes; however, the presence of atherosclerosis is a common cause.

Non–ST-Segment Elevation Acute Coronary Syndrome

Non–ST-segment elevation acute coronary syndrome (NSTE-ACS) encompasses NSTEMI and unstable angina as a condition characterized by the clinical signs and symptoms

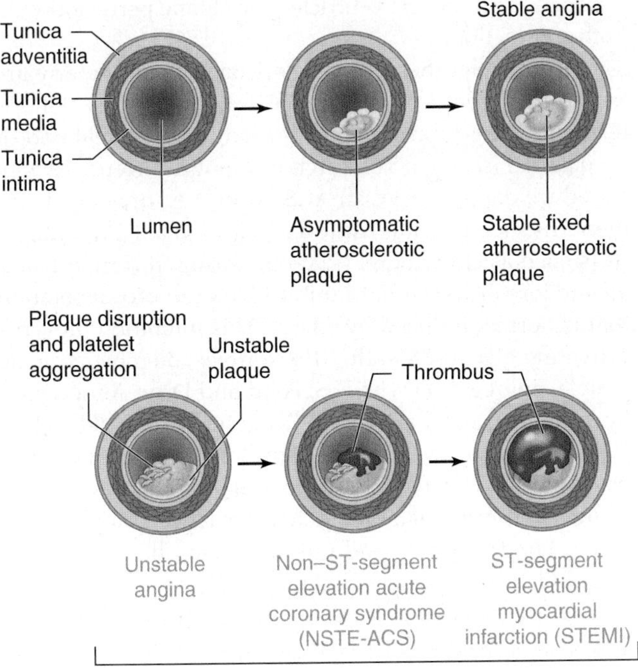

Figure 24.13 ■ The progression from clean coronary artery to asymptomatic atherosclerotic plaque to stable plaque leading to plaque disruption and thrombosis in relation to the resulting clinical conditions.

of myocardial ischemia in the absence of ST-segment elevation on ECG. The use of the term NSTE-ACS emphasizes that there is a continuum of disorders between acute myocardial ischemia and infarction.[44] Management of NSTE-ACS is similar to that of NSTEMI, as the two conditions are indistinguishable in their presentation.[44,45] **Unstable angina** is chest discomfort or pain related to lack of blood flow through coronary arteries and subsequent myocardial ischemia that is less predictable than stable angina and may occur at rest. **Non–ST-segment elevation myocardial infarction (NSTEMI)** is a condition characterized by clinical signs and symptoms of myocardial ischemia in the absence of ST elevation on ECG but the presence of elevated biomarkers of necrosis; it is considered an acute MI. The treatment for low-risk unstable angina along with stable angina was discussed previously; here, high-risk unstable angina and NSTEMI are discussed under the umbrella term NSTE-ACS.

Etiology and Pathogenesis

The major differences between unstable angina and NSTEMI are the degree of ischemia that results and whether the damage is significant enough to release biomarkers indicating myocardial necrosis (diagnostic for acute MI).[34] Pathogenesis of NSTE-ACS involves the process of atherosclerotic plaque rupture, coronary artery vasoconstriction, and myocardial oxygen demand and supply imbalance. Gradual narrowing of epicardial coronary arteries continues with evolving atherosclerosis but can also occur with post-stent restenosis, which is recurrence of artery narrowing.[21] Coagulation cascade activation occurs after atherosclerotic plaque rupture and may cause the platelet and fibrin thrombus to embolize (break free) and obstruct the coronary artery (see **Figure 24.14** ■). Vasoconstriction increases coronary vascular resistance and may result from spasms such as those that occur in Prinzmetal angina, release of vasoconstrictors such as thromboxane by platelets, MVD, or an adrenergic stimulus such as the systemic response to cold or certain illicit drugs (e.g., cocaine, amphetamines). Prinzmetal angina, or vasospastic angina, results in transmural ischemia and left ventricle dysfunction; its precise mechanism is unclear, given that it occurs in obstructed as well as normal coronary arteries. The major risk factor for vasospastic angina is cigarette smoking; it may also be triggered by stress, hyperventilation, cold, and exertion.[44] Myocardial oxygen supply and demand imbalances occur in cases of decreased supply, as in patients with anemia and hypotension or increased demand of stress, tachycardia, fever, and hyperthyroidism.[21]

Clinical Manifestations

The presentation of unstable angina and that of NSTEMI are similar; they largely vary in severity depending on the degree of ischemia. Often, the term *possible ACS* is used during initial presentation and evaluation.[46] Chest pain described as pressure and heaviness is similar to stable angina but typically more severe, and its duration is more than 20 minutes.[21] Pain may radiate to the left arm, left shoulder, neck, or jaw and may occur in the absence of exertion while the person is at rest.[21] Angina equivalents without chest pain, such as dyspnea or indigestion, more often occur in women, older adults, and patients with other chronic disease. Nocturnal angina (chest pain at night while asleep) or pleuritic chest pain may present but may be unrelated, which confounds the diagnosis of ACS.[21]

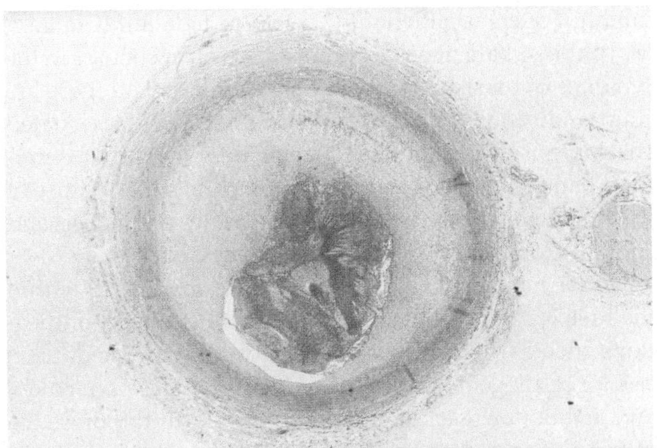

Figure 24.14 ■ A hematoxylin and eosin stain is used to show a coronary artery narrowed by atherosclerotic plaque and acute coronary thrombosis and embolization, in which a platelet–fibrin thrombus broke free and lodged, obstructing the coronary artery.

Linking Pathophysiology to Diagnosis and Treatment

Patients who present with signs and symptoms of NSTE-ACS such as chest pain, severe dyspnea, syncope or pre-syncope episode (fainting, sudden loss of consciousness), and/or palpitations need emergency medical services.[44] NSTE-ACS conditions are characterized by the clinical signs and symptoms of myocardial ischemia in the absence of ST-elevation on ECG, which is diagnostic for STEMI. A 12-lead ECG should be performed and analyzed within 10 minutes of presentation. ST-segment depression, transient ST elevation, or T-wave inversion may be present on the ECG of a patient who is experiencing NSTE-ACS.[46] The ECG may be performed en route to the emergency department by paramedic services and transferred electronically to the receiving facility to expedite care; cardiac monitoring should continue. Serial cardiac troponins are drawn immediately and then 3 and 6 hours after presentation or symptom onset if the event occurs in a hospital facility. Additional troponins may be drawn beyond the 6-hour mark. Myoglobin and creatine kinase-MB (CK-MB) may be included but are not cardiac-specific or diagnostic for ACS.[44] However, CK-MB is useful in determining noncardiac muscle injury as a differential diagnosis when its level is elevated and levels of troponins are not. The presence of elevated biomarkers indicating significant myocardial necrosis is diagnostic for NSTEMI, and the absence of biomarkers confirms the diagnosis of unstable angina.[46] B-type natriuretic peptide (BNP) gives information on the patient's prognosis, as its level increases with worsening heart function.[44] A fasting lipid profile may also be obtained within the first 24 hours.[44]

Supplemental oxygen should be applied, and short-acting sublingual nitroglycerin (in a dose of 0.3–0.4 mg) should be administered under the patient's tongue every 5 minutes for up to three doses. If ischemic chest pain continues, intravenous nitroglycerin may be considered, especially in the presence of hypertension.[44] However, nitrates (sublingual nitroglycerin or intravenous) are contraindicated if the patient has recently used a phosphodiesterase inhibitor such as sildenafil (Viagra) or tadalafil (Cialis).[44] Morphine sulfate may be administered intravenously in the presence of persistent ischemic chest pain unless there are contraindications such as hypotension. Non–enteric-coated chewable aspirin should be given at presentation of symptoms and continued throughout the patient's life because of its antiplatelet function in preventing future thrombosis and coronary artery occlusion.

Oral, not intravenous, beta blockers are initiated within the first 24 hours if the patient does not have contraindications such as signs of heart failure or low cardiac output, risk for cardiogenic shock, heart block without a pacemaker, and asthma or reactive airway disease.[44] In the presence of beta-blocker contraindications, calcium channel blockers may be used.[44] High-intensity statin therapy is started or continued, if not contraindicated, to lower cholesterol. Other medications to be considered include ACE inhibitors and ARBs, especially in the presence of HF and low left ventricular ejection fraction,[44] which is the amount of blood pumped from the left ventricle to systemic perfusion with each contraction.

Antiplatelet therapy and anticoagulation therapy are key to treatment options. Antiplatelet therapy is a short-term and long-term approach to reduce the likelihood of myocardial ischemia or infarction event recurrence as well as reduce damage from an ACS event.[34] Antiplatelet treatments include first-line aspirin in addition to $P2Y_{12}$ antagonists such as clopidogrel (Plavix), Prasugrel (Effient), and Ticagrelor (Brilinta) that inhibit $P2Y_{12}$ receptor activation that is normal induced by ADP.[34] This inhibition prevents activating glycoprotein IIb/IIIa complex, thereby reducing platelet aggregation. The U.S. Food and Drug Administration (FDA) recently approved Ticagrelor; its special feature is the increase in levels of adenosine locally to improve coronary artery blood flow.[34] Anticoagulation therapy options include low-molecular-weight heparin (enoxaparin), Bivalirudin, Fondaparinux, and unfractionated heparin, which are administered per hospital protocols.

Invasive strategies for diagnosis and treatment are considered. Risks and benefits are weighed in the decision to use an ischemia-guided strategy with medical therapy as previously discussed and/or perform an invasive strategy immediately or later. These strategies include PCI or coronary artery bypass grafting (CABG).

CLINICAL POINT: PCI is performed in a special laboratory that is often referred to as a cath lab. Balloon angioplasty (also called percutaneous transluminal coronary angioplasty) is performed by a cardiologist to open the narrowed artery, and usually a stent is placed to keep the artery open (**Figure 24.15** ■). However, gradual narrowing of coronary arteries can occur, leading to post-stent restenosis. Drug-eluting stents are used to release medication that inhibits surrounding tissue growth. ■

The goal of CABG is complete revascularization to improve myocardial blood flow through bypassing all occluded coronary arteries; this will relieve angina as well as prolong and improve the patient's quality of life.[35] An artery or vein is taken from the chest, arm, or leg, and one

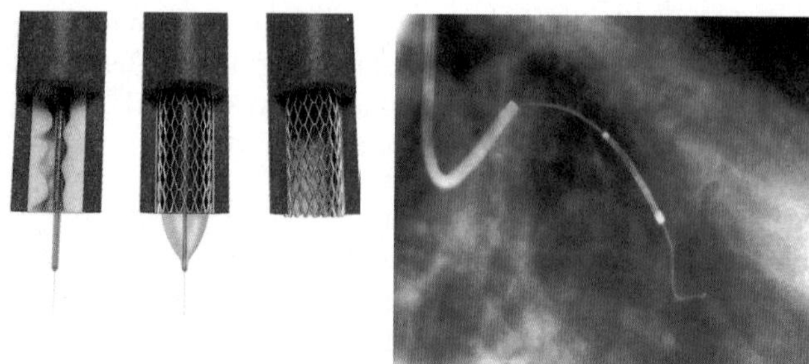

Figure 24.15 ■ In PCI, a catheter is inserted through the radial or femoral artery to the coronary arteries to locate the blockage by using dye and x-ray images. Then a catheter with an attached balloon is inflated to widen the culprit coronary artery. Typically, a stent is implanted to reestablish and maintain blood flow and to prevent restenosis.

end is sewn from the aorta to an area on the diseased coronary artery that is distal to the occlusion. A CABG may be performed through open heart surgery or minimally invasive surgery using smaller incisions or even robotics.

Given the current demographic trends of an increasing population of older adults (> 75 years old) and given that ACS incidence increases with age, older patients present challenges for providing optimal medical care. In the older adult with NSTE-ACS, there is difficulty in diagnosis due to atypical symptoms, confounding noncardiac symptoms, and comorbidities. Additionally, older adults are at a higher risk for polypharmacy and possible adverse drug–drug interactions. The approach in treatment of the older adult presenting with NSTE-ACS should be similar to the recommended ischemia-guided therapy or invasive strategies used for younger patients.[21] ■

Mary Kate Scot: Outcome

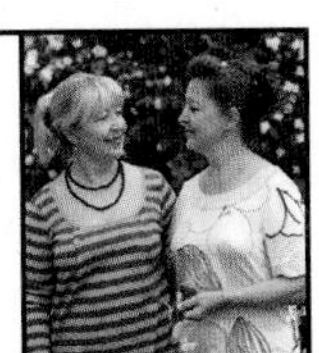

In the ambulance, the paramedics administer aspirin and sublingual nitroglycerin to Ms. Scot. Although confused when she arrives at the ED, Ms. Scot is able to follow commands and safely take clopidogrel as IV heparin is started and she is prepared to go to the cardiac catheterization lab. The ECG shows ST-segment depression in the anterior leads, and troponins are elevated, but vital signs and other lab values remain normal. PCI is performed with a drug-eluting stent, and Ms. Scot is continued on aspirin, clopidogrel, and beta-blocker therapy at discharge. If she had delayed seeking medical attention longer, she could have developed a deadly MI.

3. What initial medications are given to Ms. Scot for a potential MI?
4. What procedure was done to determine whether Ms. Scot was having an MI?

ST-Segment Elevation Myocardial Infarction

ST-segment elevation myocardial infarction (STEMI) is a more precise definition of the common term heart attack, where "STE" refers to the ECG tracing of ST-segment elevation and "MI" refers to myocardial infarction. It is a very serious condition that requires rapid recognition, reperfusion treatment, and management to prevent death.

Etiology and Pathogenesis

Recall that the disruption of atherosclerotic plaque leads to platelet activation and aggregation and thrombosis that disrupts blood flow and ultimately leads to an imbalance of myocardial oxygen supply and demand. Ultimately, if severe and persistent, myocardial necrosis and infarction result and are complete within approximately 6 hours unless reperfusion strategies are successful or sufficient collateral circulation is present.[21] STEMI is a state of heightened inflammation with prothrombotic components.[47] Imbalances of clot-dissolving enzymes such as tissue plasminogen activator (tPA) and their inhibitors such as plasminogen activator inhibitor-1 may increase a person's risk for MI as a result of the imbalance of clotting and clot breakdown.[10]

Myocardial infarction is typically the consequence of advanced atherosclerosis; however, nonobstructive CAD may also be the cause of a MI. Nonobstructive CAD is atherosclerotic plaque that is not expected to disrupt blood flow and cause clinical symptoms of angina and may be characterized as insignificant when observed on coronary angiogram.[48] The stenosis, or narrowing, is 20% or more but less than 50% in the LAD and 20% or more but less than 70% in any other epicardial coronary artery.[48] Historically, obstructive CAD has been targeted in disease management, but studies are recognizing the role of nonobstructive plaque rupture and subsequent occlusion rather than occlusive plaque as the pathogenesis for most MIs.[48]

The risk of an MI was observed in a study of U.S. veterans who were mostly male without previous CAD events and who had a coronary angiogram. The study found that a significantly increased risk for both nonobstructive and obstructive CAD with a greater 1-year risk of MI and all-cause mortality in participants with nonobstructive CAD.[48] It is not uncommon for the patient presenting with a STEMI to have more than one coronary artery obstructed, known as multivessel CAD. Multivessel CAD is the stage of atherosclerosis in which two or three or more coronary arteries, which can be nonculprit vessels, are severely affected by unstable plaque that may lead to future major adverse cardiac events.[47]

Traditional risk factors of CAD are similar for ACS events, including STEMI. Additionally, some studies have found risk factors that are specific triggers for an ACS event. Short-term exposure to ambient fine particulate matter air pollution increases the risk of an ACS event, including NSTE-ACS but particularly a STEMI, for patients with diseased coronary arteries evidenced by coronary angiography.[49]

It is important to understand that other causes and their associated risk factors may lead to myocardial injury and subsequent MI. For example, spasms associated with Prinzmetal angina (coronary artery vasospasm) in the presence of normal coronary arteries, contusions related to trauma to coronary arteries, cocaine abuse, aortic insufficiencies such as stenosis, and hematologic problems such as hypercoagulability may cause an MI.[21] An **embolus** is a mass in the bloodstream that may be a blood clot, foreign material such as air or a gas bubble, a fat droplet, or a clump of bacteria. An embolus may occur as a result of **atrial fibrillation**, a dysrhythmia that may cause pooling and clotting of blood and the risk of embolization if the clot breaks free and obstructs an artery. A person may experience an MI as a complication of a diagnostic coronary angiogram. Recall that the presence of decreased perfusion to the myocardium, which can occur secondary to a multitude of problems such as hypotension during shock related to sepsis or hemorrhage, and the presence of increased oxygen demands, which can occur during tachycardia, stress, and aortic stenosis, can lead to ischemia and subsequent infarction.[21]

Clinical Manifestations

The obstructed blood flow in a coronary artery and lack of oxygen and nutrients required by the myocardium, resulting in ischemia and subsequent tissue infarction, produce clinical signs and symptoms, ST-segment elevation on ECG, and elevated cardiac biomarkers that are characteristic of a STEMI. Recall that nerve endings that are ischemic will cause pain due to the accumulation of metabolites as a result of anaerobic processes used to generate ATP; however, pain will not arise from fully necrotic myocardium. Symptoms of STEMI include classic chest pain and possibly dyspnea at rest or with minimal exertion. The person may also experience general malaise and fatigue. The classic chest pain may be described as tightness, crushing, squeezing, and stabbing or like a heavy weight sitting across the chest but also can be described as indigestion (an angina equivalent). Pain may radiate to the shoulders, neck, and jaw and down the left arm, causing tingling in the left wrist, hand, and fingers.[21] Other symptoms may include cold sweat (diaphoresis), dizziness, weakness, a feeling of rapid or fluttering heart (palpitations), altered mental status, or a feeling of impending doom. Patients may feel lightheaded, or faint or may actually have syncope, in which they temporarily lose consciousness, commonly as a result of a drop in blood pressure. Vital signs assessed may include a heart rate reflecting tachycardia or **bradycardia**, which is an abnormally slow heart rate that is lower than the normal resting rate, generally less than 60 beats per minute in an adult. The pulse may be regular or irregular depending on the underlying cardiac rhythm. The patient may be hypertensive or hypotensive, and the respiratory rate and temperature may be elevated. The presence of S1 and S2 may be normal, but additional heart sounds such as a third heart sound (S3) may be diagnostic for possible severe left ventricular dysfunction.[21] A systolic murmur may be audible and related to mitral regurgitation, possibly from mitral valve dysfunction or tricuspid regurgitation related to right ventricular dysfunction.[21] Patients may also present with a pericardial friction rub.

Women are more likely to be older at the time of a STEMI than men, and women are twice as likely as men to die from a STEMI, according a Yale-led study of the global effect of gender disparities of STEMI care and outcomes.[50] There was a mean delay of 5.3 minutes from hospital presentation to coronary reperfusion ("door to balloon" time).[50] Disparities may result from the differences in risk factors between men and women such as older age at time of event as well as lack of awareness and knowledge of signs and symptoms of a STEMI, such as the presence of angina equivalents.[50] ■

Linking Pathophysiology to Diagnosis and Treatment

Diagnosis of STEMI is a combination of assessing characteristic symptoms, ECG (refer to Figure 24.11), and labs such as cardiac biomarkers that reflect necrosis of the myocardium. The universal definition for acute myocardial infarction requires new ST-segment elevation at the J point in two of the 12 leads on an ECG with additional criteria for specific height (≥ 0.1 mV in all leads except V2 and V3) and cut points related to gender and age with ST-segment depression and T-wave changes in two other leads.[41] The 12-lead ECG remains an essential component of diagnosis and should be performed within 10 minutes of presentation. It may be performed prehospital by paramedics. The leads that display the ECG abnormalities help to determine the location of the myocardium involved. However, ST-segment and T-wave abnormalities can be nonspecific and affected by factors such as time, location, and extent of infarction as well as the person's age, presence of conduction abnormalities such as dysrhythmias, electrolyte imbalances, and administration of cardioactive drugs, which limit its usefulness.[21] Transmural (epicardial) injury affects the full-thickness ventricular layer and causes ST-segment elevation with the presence of ST-segment depression in other leads. ST-segment elevation can also be associated with pericarditis, acute myocarditis (inflammation of heart muscle), hypothermia, and certain cardiac tumors.[38] Some patients will exhibit evidence of a heart block; others may develop Q waves, indicating necrosis. It can be a clinical challenge to diagnose a STEMI, and the ECG alone is not sufficient because ST-segment abnormalities may be present in other conditions. Portable bedside echocardiography may be helpful to support diagnosis and to assess and identify possible development of heart failure and mechanical complications of an MI.[21]

As in management of patients who present with NSTE-ACS, cardiac troponins should be drawn immediately at presentation and then 3 and 6 hours later; they are diagnostic if there is a rise and/or fall in which at least one level measure exceeds the 99th percentile upper reference limit.[41] Myoglobin and CK-MB levels may be tested in addition to CRP, BNP, and serum lipid levels. CRP as a marker of inflammation rises substantially as a result of cardiomyocyte necrosis in a STEMI and is associated with risk of heart failure or death.[21] Other labs may include a complete blood cell count, which might indicate elevation in white blood cells (leukocytosis), low red blood cells (anemia), and baseline platelet count, which is important to determine before administration of certain medications, such as heparin.

Researchers are studying diagnostic protocols to identify patients who present with clinical manifestations of ACS, such as chest pain, and are appropriate for early emergency department discharge because their condition is not immediately life threatening.[51]

CLINICAL POINT: One diagnostic protocol for identifying patients whose condition is not immediately life threatening uses a strategy of identifying individuals older than 65 years with no known CAD history, ECG with no signs of ischemia, and high-sensitivity cardiac troponin levels that are below the limit of detection at time of presentation and 4–14 hours later.[51] The FDA has not approved high-sensitivity cardiac troponin for use in the United States; however, its use may be very beneficial in combination with other clinical predictive instruments to identify low-risk individuals and save costs and burden associated with unnecessary tests and treatment.[51] ■

The goal of STEMI management is timely reperfusion to return blood flow and function of cardiomyocytes using medical therapy, PCI, or CABG. Management depends on the capabilities of the hospital where the person makes first medical contact. Timely PCI in the patient with a STEMI is preferred and will improve the patient's chance of survival more than medical therapy when performed by a physician who is experienced and when the patient is cared for in a unit that is proficient in PCI care. Proficient cardiac-related care is often found in hospitals with designated coronary care units, where highly trained nurses have the skills and ability to recognize and initiate the treatments needed.[21] According to the ACCF/AHA guidelines for STEMI, if a patient is first seen in a PCI-capable hospital, the goal for time from arrival hospital to device deployment, or "door to balloon," in the cath lab is 90 minutes or less. If first seen at a non-PCI-capable hospital, the patient should be transferred quickly so that the time from door to balloon is no more than 120 minutes.[52] Unless it is contraindicated, the patient who arrives at non-PCI-capable hospital with a STEMI should be administered fibrinolytic therapy if the transfer is expected to cause a delay of more than 120 minutes for door to balloon.[52] If medical therapy is chosen as the reperfusion strategy, it should be administered within 30 minutes ("door to drug") of the patient's arrival at the hospital.[52] A small number of patients undergo urgent CABG instead of PCI.

Aspirin, which is used in initial management of ACS presentation, is similarly used on STEMI presentation. Other antiplatelet therapies include the $P2Y_{12}$ antagonists such as clopidogrel, prasugrel, and ticagrelor. Anticoagulation agents such as unfractionated heparin and low-molecular-weight heparin are important regardless of whether a fibrinolytic or PCI reperfusion strategy is used, and the choice of which agents to use depends on the patient and the strategy that is used. Interventions to restore the balance of myocardial oxygen supply and demand include those previously discussed for NSTE-ACS; they include oxygen, nitrates, beta blockers, ACE inhibitors or ARBs, CCBs, and high-intensity statins. Ischemic pain management includes a wide variety of analgesics, but morphine remains the drug of choice.

Current treatment strategies differ in approach depending on whether all diseased but noninfarct arteries, characterized by nonculprit lesions, are completely revascularized at time of hospitalization for a STEMI or whether only the culprit vessel is fixed with either a plan for later revascularization or use of medical therapy.[47] Studies report fewer major adverse cardiac events, revascularization due to recurrent ischemia, or repeat PCI when complete revascularization of all diseased coronary arteries at time of hospitalization or staged (planned later) revascularization of all diseased arteries is performed in comparison to treating only the culprit lesion.[47] A rationale for fixing only the culprit lesion rather than complete revascularization of noninfarct arteries is the idea that "less is more" because of the risk for MI during procedure.[47] Procedural time and exposure to contrast are higher in complete or staged revascularization, but the number of times vascular access is needed, anticoagulant-related bleeding complications, and resulting hospitalization costs should be lower. More studies are needed to determine the indications and appropriate timing for revascularization of noninfarct arteries,[52] including reassessment of the current guidelines suggesting evidence of harm in complete revascularization of noninfarct vessels.[47]

Patients remain at high risk for having a recurrent major adverse cardiac event after an ACS event. Research is ongoing for treatments that target the inflammatory process. The p38 mitogen-activated protein kinase (MAPK) participates in several phases of atherosclerosis, plaque destabilization, and thrombosis. The LATITUDE-TIMI 60 trial was designed to test the efficacy and safety of losmapimod, an inhibitor of p38 MAPK.[53] Losmapimod is an oral medication that was tested in patients who were hospitalized with a NSTEMI or STEMI compared to placebo with the endpoint of cardiovascular death, MI, or severe recurrent ischemia that required urgent coronary artery revascularization.[53] Unfortunately, the use of losmapimod compared to placebo did not result in reduction of major ischemic cardiovascular events, and further research in identifying treatment is needed.[54]

The effects of a STEMI turn the myocardium into fibrotic tissue that is unable to move and pump blood at full capacity or regenerate itself effectively.[55] As the least regenerative organ in the body, the injured heart may develop chronic heart failure. Chronic heart failure has a low survival rate; treatment is palliative care, complete organ transplant, or insertion of a mechanical assist device.[55] Research has been done on transplanting nearly every cell type into the injured myocardium as a means to regenerate the heart. Most recently, human stem cell–derived cardiomyocytes have been shown to be a promising cell type.[55]

Maggie Craig: Outcome

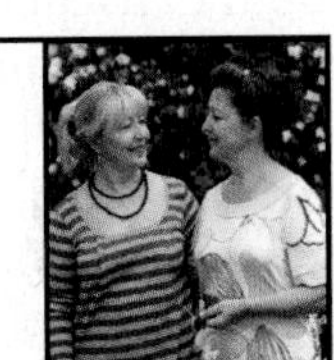

Maggie Craig and her family discuss the risk and benefits with the interventional cardiologist and decide that Ms. Craig should undergo CABG to treat the occlusions of her LAD and RCA. The CAD is extensive, and Ms. Craig is at risk for a deadly acute MI, especially because of the involvement of the LAD. She is referred to a cardiac surgeon who specializes in minimally invasive robotically assisted CABG. The surgery is performed, and Ms. Craig is discharged after 2 days and prescribed lifetime aspirin as well as clopidogrel, rosuvastatin, metoprolol, and short-term furosemide. She is referred to cardiac rehabilitation and is able to return to normal activities of daily life 2 weeks later, thanks to her timely diagnosis and treatment.

5. Why does Ms. Craig need to have a CABG?
6. Why are the listed medications prescribed for Ms. Craig on discharge?

Check Your Progress: Section 24.5

1. What are the three types of acute coronary syndrome (ACS)?
2. How would you describe unstable angina?
3. What condition, considered an acute MI, is characterized by clinical signs and symptoms similar to those of myocardial ischemia in the absence of ST elevation on ECG but the presence of elevated biomarkers of necrosis?

24.6 Complications of Acute Coronary Syndromes

Dysrhythmic, inflammatory, embolic, and mechanical complications may follow an ACS event. Inflammatory complications include pericarditis and Dressler syndrome. Embolic events include thromboembolism in the peripheral or central nervous system such as a stroke (see Chapter 27). Mechanical complications include mitral regurgitation, ventricular aneurysm and rupture, heart failure (see Chapter 26), and cardiogenic shock. Cardiogenic shock is caused by the obstruction of blood flow, resulting in decreased cardiac output and body tissue metabolic needs not being met (see Chapter 28 for a discussion of cardiogenic shock). Circulatory failure as a result of mechanical complications or severe left ventricular dysfunction causes most fatalities related to ACS.

Dysrhythmias and Sudden Cardiac Death

Each year, approximately 325,000 individuals in the United States suffer an out-of-hospital cardiac arrest; slightly over 10% survive who are treated by emergency medical services. If the arrest was witnessed, approximately 31% survive.[2] Every year, roughly 200,000 people in the United States experience a cardiac arrest in a hospital.[2]

Cardiac arrest is characterized by abrupt loss of cardiac function. A clear relationship exists between sudden cardiac death and CHD as a result of cardiac arrest.[1] Death rates from CHD and CVD appear to be declining in the United States and many developed countries. However, it is concerning that there is a projected increase in CHD mortality in developing areas such as China, India, sub-Saharan Africa, the Middle East, and Latin America as a result of social and economic changes that have led to an increase of life expectancy, adaptation to Westernized diets, physical inactivity, and increases in smoking.[1] It is expected that CVDs will be the major cause of morbidity and mortality in most developing countries worldwide by the year 2020.[56] Possible reasons for the decrease in mortality from CHD in adults 25–84 years old in the United States include improvements in initial treatment of ACS, secondary preventive measures, heart failure therapy, and use of revascularization in chronic cases of angina.[1]

Etiology and Pathogenesis

Sudden cardiac death frequently results from an acute MI when plaque ruptures, leading to thrombosis that completely occludes the coronary artery with subsequent lack of blood flow and death of myocardium, inducing a fatal ventricular dysrhythmia. CAD and its consequences account for about 80% of sudden cardiac deaths in Western countries; nonischemic coronary circulation disorders cause about 10–15%.[21] The causes of acute MI may also be the result of a dysrhythmia such as emboli related to atrial fibrillation.

Dysfunction of the autonomic nervous system may lead to the development of dysrhythmias as a result of increased automaticity of the myocardium and conduction systems as well as the damaged myocardium becoming susceptible to reentrant circuits due to disturbance of refractory periods.[57] **Automaticity** is the ability of specialized myocardial cells, or pacemaker cells, to generate an electrical impulse (depolarize) to regulate the heart rate in accordance to the body's needs. The **absolute refractory period** is the time after the firing of a nerve fiber during which the nerve fiber cannot be stimulated, regardless of the strength of the stimulus applied. Abnormal refractory periods related to disease can cause dysrhythmias. The most serious dysrhythmia is ventricular fibrillation (VF), and the risk of occurrence is greatest in the first hour of an acute MI.[57]

Ninety percent of people who have an acute MI experience a cardiac dysrhythmia during or after the MI, and 25% experience the dysrhythmia in the first 24 hours, occurrence being more likely with a STEMI than with a NSTEMI. [57] Dysrhythmia development is more likely if hypoxia or an electrolyte imbalance, such as low potassium (hypokalemia) and/or low magnesium (hypomagnesemia), is present.[57]

Recall that cardiac conduction requires a balance of electrolytes, and the presence of ischemia can have electrophysiologic consequences when there is inappropriate Ca^{2+} entry and K^+ exit from the cardiomyocyte. Acidosis, shortened transmembrane potentials, increased automaticity of tissues, and reentry (cycling of electrical impulses) occur, leading to clinical symptoms and dysrhythmias.[21] However, serum electrolyte disturbances in an acute MI have not been extensively studied, and insufficient information is available about their related prognosis.[58] Low sodium (hyponatremia) and hypokalemia have been associated as indicators of an acute MI, and it appears that a rise in their values is indicative of clinical improvement.[58] Low Mg^{2+} levels are associated with increased CHD mortality risks and sudden cardiac death, but the mechanism is unclear.[59] Low Mg^{2+} is associated with inflammation and endothelial dysfunction related to CHD but also has a role in cardiomyocyte electrical stability and is associated with dysrhythmias as well as QT prolongation, which is a risk factor for sudden cardiac death.[59] Hypercalcemia (excess calcium) shortens the QT interval; if severe, it can cause VF. Recall that the QT interval reflects the time between the start of the ventricular depolarization to the end of ventricular repolarization, or the total duration of the ventricular action potential, which is essentially the time of activation and recovery of the ventricles.[21]

Dysrhythmias may occur during an acute MI or as a result of reperfusion treatments. Peri-infarction (around the area of myocardial ischemia or infarction) dysrhythmias are classified into categories, including supraventricular tachydysrhythmias, accelerated junctional rhythms, ventricular dysrhythmias, intraventricular blocks, and bradydysrhythmias (see **Table 24.1** ■).

Supraventricular tachydysrhythmias include sinus tachycardia, premature atrial contractions (PACs), paroxysmal supraventricular tachycardia (PSVT), atrial flutter, and atrial fibrillation. PACs often occur prior to the onset of PSVT, atrial flutter or atrial fibrillation. Of these, PSVT and

Table 24.1 Characteristics of Selected Cardiac Rhythms and Dysrhythmias

Rhythm/ECG Appearance and Characteristics	Pathogenesis and Management
Normal sinus rhythm (NSR) Rate: 60–100 bpm Rhythm: regular P:QRS: 1:1 PR interval: 0.12–0.20 sec QRS complex: 0.6–0.10 sec	*Pathogenesis:* NSR is normal and set by the SA node, the inherent pacemaker, generating and transmitting an electrical impulse to the atria and ventricles. *Management:* None; normal heart rhythm.
Sinus dysrhythmia 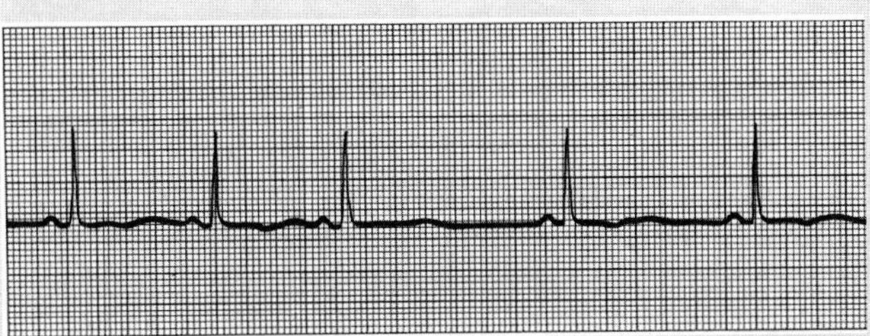 Rate: 60–100 bpm Rhythm: irregular, varying with respirations P:QRS: 1:1 PR interval: 0.12–0.20 sec QRS complex: 0.6–0.10 sec	*Pathogenesis:* Heart rate increases with inspiration and is normal and indicates a healthy heart; whereas absence of heart rate changes with breathing may be related to cardiac and/or nervous system problems. *Management:* Generally none; considered a normal rhythm in the very young and very old.
Supraventricular Tachydysrhythmias	
Sinus tachycardia 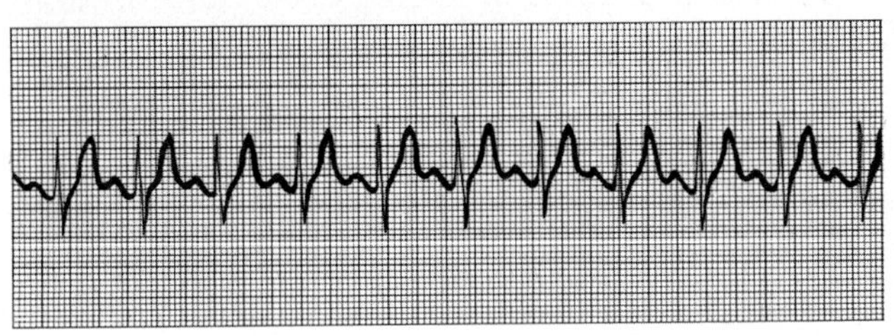 Rate: 101–150 bpm Rhythm: regular P:QRS: 1:1 (with very fast rates, P wave may be hidden in preceding T wave) PR interval: 0.12–0.20 sec QRS complex: 0.6–0.10 sec	*Pathogenesis:* Enhanced sympathetic stimulation causing SA node to fire at a rapid but regular rate. Some causes include pain, anxiety, heart failure, hypovolemia (decreased blood volume), hypoxia, anemia, pericarditis, and pulmonary embolism. *Management:* Treated only if symptomatic or patient is at risk for myocardial damage. Treat underlying cause (i.e., hypovolemia, fever, pain). Beta-blockers or verapamil may be used.
Premature atrial contractions (PACs) 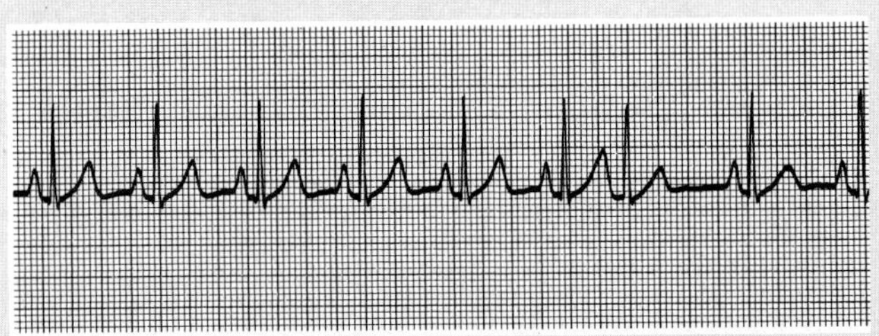 Rate: variable Rhythm: irregular, with normal rhythm interrupted by early beats arising in the atria P:QRS: 1:1 PR interval: 0.12–0.20 sec, but may be prolonged QRS complex: 0.6–0.10 sec	*Pathogenesis:* Ectopic focus in atria generates an electrical impulse before the SA node begins to fire causing an early heartbeat. Causes include certain medications, tension, tobacco, alcohol, and caffeine, as well as some disease-related causes such as infection (i.e., pericarditis), inflammation, myocardial ischemia. *Management:* Usually require no treatment. Advise to reduce alcohol and caffeine intake, to reduce stress, and to stop smoking. Beta-blocker may be prescribed.

(*Continued*)

Table 24.1 Characteristics of Selected Cardiac Rhythms and Dysrhythmias *Continued*

Rhythm/ECG Appearance and Characteristics	Pathogenesis and Management
Paroxysmal supraventricular tachycardia (PSVT) 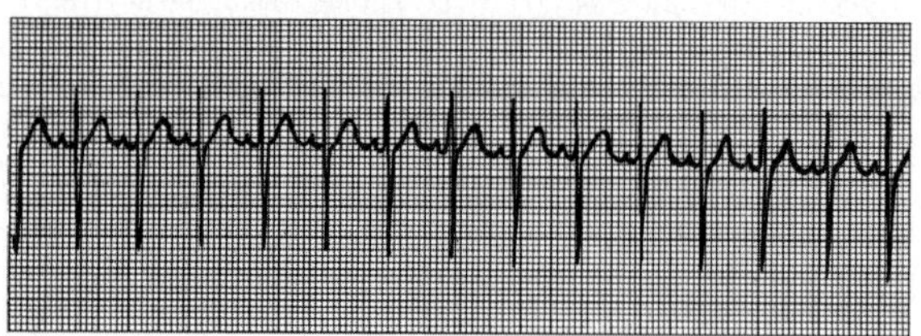 Rate: 100–280 bpm (usually 150–200 bpm) Rhythm: regular P:QRS: P waves often not identifiable PR interval: not measured QRS complex: 0.6–0.10 sec	*Pathogenesis:* Cycling of an electrical impulse through the myocardium that has been recently stimulated. *Management:* Treat if symptomatic. Treatment may include vagal maneuvers (Valsalva, carotid sinus massage), oxygen therapy, adenosine or a beta-blocker, temporary pacing, or synchronized electrical cardioversion.
Atrial flutter 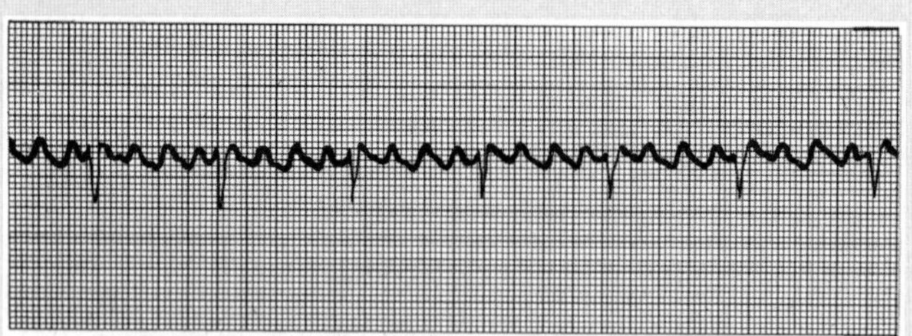 Rate: atrial, 240–360 bpm; ventricular rate depends on degree of atrioventricular block and usually is < 150 bpm Rhythm: atrial, regular; ventricular, usually regular P:QRS: 2:1, 4:1, 6:1; may vary PR interval: not measured QRS complex: 0.6–0.10 sec	*Pathogenesis:* Cycling of an electrical impulse through the recently stimulated myocardium with increased sympathetic stimulation of the atria. *Management:* Medications to slow ventricular response, such as a beta-blocker or calcium-channel blocker, followed by a class I antidysrhythmic agent (Na channel blocker) or class III (K channel blocker such as amiodarone); synchronized electrical cardioversion.
Atrial fibrillation 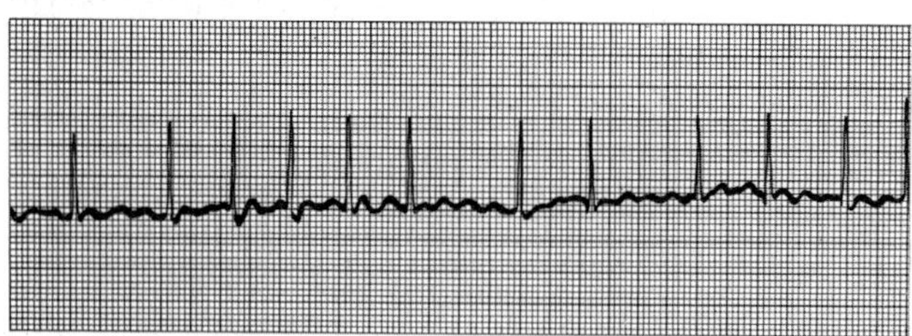 Rate: atrial, 300–600 bpm (too rapid to count); ventricular, 100–180 bpm in untreated clients Rhythm: irregularly irregular P:QRS: variable PR interval: not measured QRS complex: 0.06–0.10 sec	*Pathogenesis:* Complex pathogenesis with various mechanisms including impulse generation from a ectopic focus, a group of cells outside of SA node, and cycling of electrical impulses which cause rapid firing rates and quivering of the atria. *Management:* Immediate electrical cardioversion if client's condition is unstable; medications to reduce ventricular response rate: metoprolol, diltiazem, or digoxin; anticoagulant therapy to reduce risk of clot formation (deep vein thrombosis and/or pulmonary embolism) and stroke.
Accelerated Junctional Rhythms	
Junctional rhythms 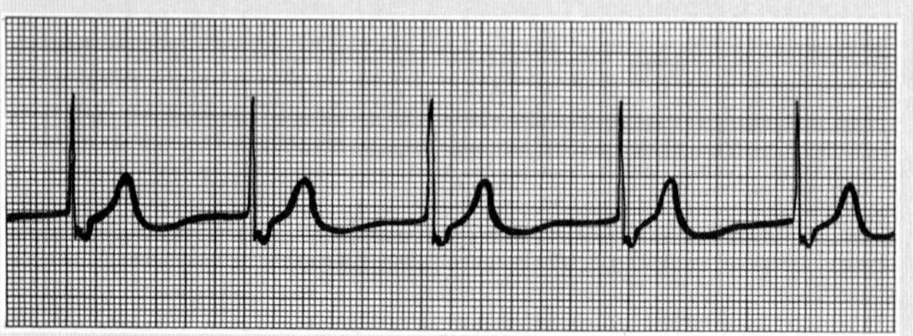 Rate: 40–60 bpm; junctional bradycardia < 40 bpm; junctional escape rhythm 40–60; accelerated junctional rhythm 60–100 bpm; junctional tachycardia, 60–140 bpm Rhythm: regular P:QRS: P waves may be absent, inverted and immediately preceding or succeeding QRS complex, or hidden in QRS complex PR interval: < 0.10 sec if present QRS complex: 0.06–0.10 sec	*Pathogenesis:* Increased automaticity of AV junction tissue and escape rhythm that causes firing at a rate that supersedes the SA node and is common in clients with inferior MI. *Management:* Treatment is directed at the cause of myocardial ischemia if symptomatic.

Rhythm/ECG Appearance and Characteristics	Pathogenesis and Management
Ventricular Dysrhythmias	
Premature ventricular contractions (PVCs) 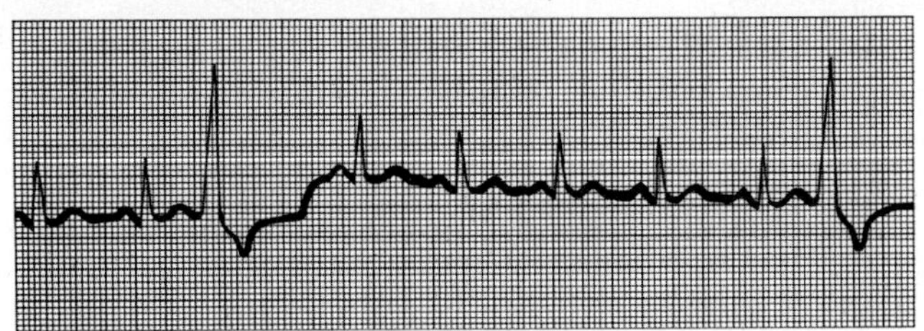 Rate: variable Rhythm: irregular, with PVC interrupting underlying rhythm and followed by a compensatory pause P:QRS: no P wave noted before PVC PR interval: absent with PVC QRS complex: wide (> 0.12 sec) and bizarre in appearance; differs from normal QRS complex	*Pathogenesis:* Ectopic focus in ventricle generates an electrical impulse before the SA node causing an early heartbeat. Causes may be related to heart disease or certain medications, tobacco, alcohol and caffeine. *Management:* Treat if symptomatic or in presence of severe heart disease. Advise against stimulant use (caffeine, nicotine). Beta-blockers or class I or III antidysrhythmic agents may be used in clients with severe heart disease who are symptomatic but prophylactic suppression of PVCs once thought to prevent impending ventricular dysrhythmias is no longer recommended.
Ventricular tachycardia (VT, V tach) 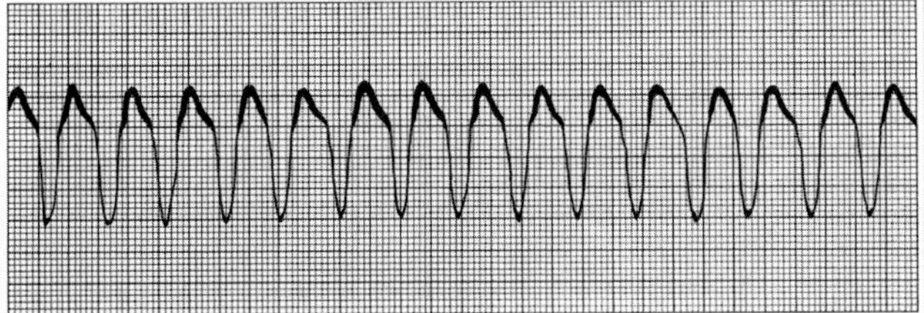 Rate: 100–250 bpm Rhythm: regular P:QRS: P waves usually not identifiable PR interval: not measured QRS complex: ≥ 0.12 sec; bizarre shape	*Pathogenesis:* Interaction of factors including increased automaticity leading to disorders of impulse formation and conduction problems such as cycling of electrical impulses. May occur during or following MI related to myocardial ischemia and electrolyte disturbances. *Management:* Treat if VT is sustained, symptomatic, or associated with heart disease. Treatment includes direct current unsynchronized cardioversion or intravenous procainamide or a class III antidysrhythmic agent (amiodarone is drug of choice) if hemodynamic instability accompanies; surgical ablation or antitachycardia pacing with an implanted cardioverter–defibrillator for repeated episodes. If no pulse, treat as ventricular fibrillation. Begin CPR, if needed and follow advanced cardiac life support algorithm.
Ventricular fibrillation (VF, V fib) 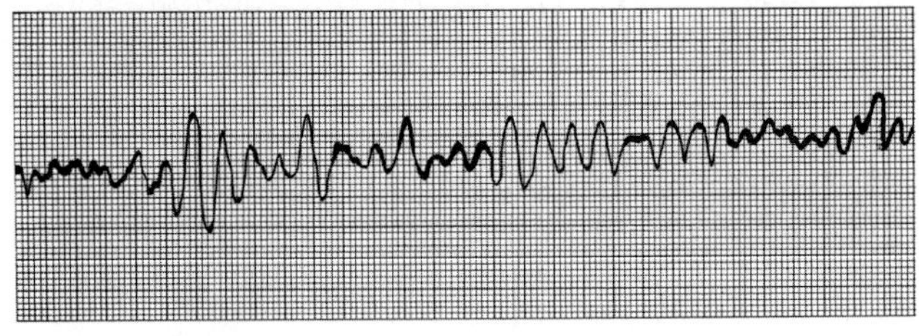 Rate: too rapid to count Rhythm: grossly irregular P:QRS: no identifiable P waves PR interval: none QRS: bizarre, varying in shape and direction	*Pathogenesis:* Terminal event of severe CAD and subsequent ACS events. Can also occur as a result of certain antiarrhythmic medications, hypoxia, ischemia, atrial fibrillation with rapid ventricular rate, cardioversion, or improperly grounded electrical equipment. *Management:* Immediate unsynchronized defibrillation to restore rhythm of inherent pacemaker. Intravenous antiarrhythmics (amiodarone and lidocaine) help defibrillation as well and prevent recurrent episode of ventricular fibrillation. Early use of beta-blockers reduces episodes as well as sudden cardiac death.
Accelerated idioventricular rhythm 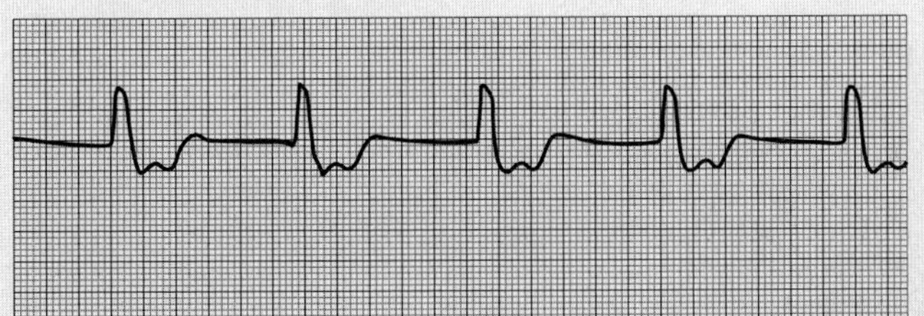 Rate: 50–110 bpm Rhythm: regular or irregular; alternates with period of NSR P:QRS: P waves may or may not be identified PR interval: none QRS complex: wide, > 0.10 sec	*Pathogenesis:* Ectopic focus in ventricle takes over as pacemaker or structural damage and depressed automaticity of the SA or AV node. In client with heart disease including acute MI or as a reperfusion dysrhythmia following ACS treatment. *Management:* Treatment with temporary pacing or atropine to increase the sinus rate and suppress accelerated idioventricular rhythm is indicated if client has sustained abnormal rhythm and/or presence of hypotension and symptoms of myocardial ischemia.

(*Continued*)

Table 24.1 Characteristics of Selected Cardiac Rhythms and Dysrhythmias *Continued*

Rhythm/ECG Appearance and Characteristics	Pathogenesis and Management
Bradydysrhythmias	
Sinus bradycardia 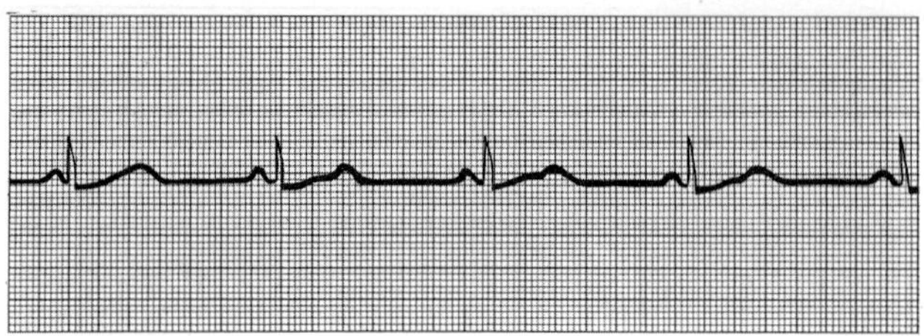 Rate: < 60 bpm Rhythm: regular P:QRS: 1:1 PR interval: 0.12–0.20 sec QRS complex: 0.6–0.10 sec	*Pathogenesis:* Increased vagal or sympathetic tone causing SA node to generate impulses at slower rate. Also can be caused by side effects of medication or problems of the SA node. Common arrhythmia in clients with MI. *Management:* Treated only if symptomatic because CO inadequate and/or in concurrence with MI because of risk of further decrease of CO, hypotension and other dysrhythmias. Can occur in healthy young adults and athletes. Intravenous atropine or isoproterenol, and/or pacemaker therapy may be used. Dopamine, epinephrine, and/or dobutamine may also be used if other interventions fail to increase HR.
First-degree AV block 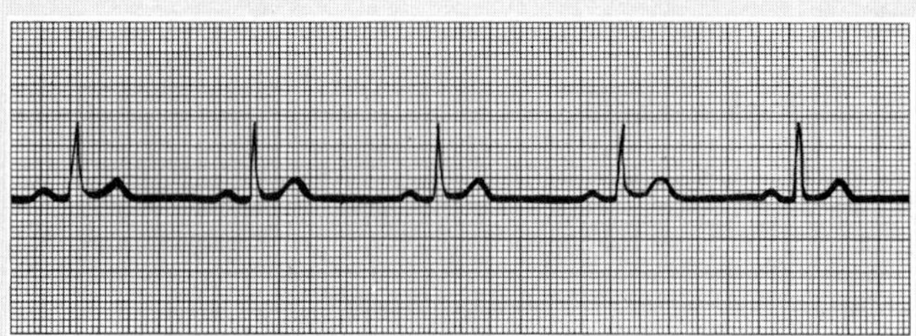 Rate: usually 60–100 bpm Rhythm: regular P:QRS: 1:1 PR interval: > 0.20 sec QRS complex: 0.06–0.10 sec	*Pathogenesis:* Conduction disturbance at AV node or above the bundle of His which can occur with MI. Other causes include medications such as CCBs and beta blockers. *Management:* None required unless associated with hemodynamic compromise. Continuous cardiac monitoring advised.
Second-degree AV block (Mobitz Type I, Wenckebach) 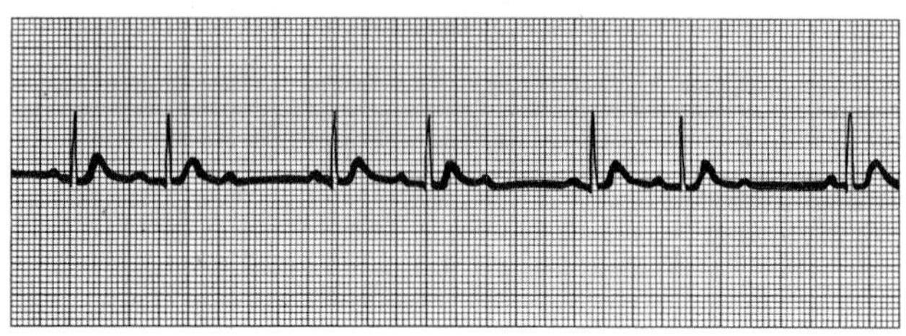 Rate: 60–100 bpm Rhythm: atrial, regular; ventricular, irregular P:QRS: 1:1 until P wave blocked with no subsequent QRS complex PR interval: progressively lengthens in a regular pattern QRS complex: 0.06–0.10 sec; sudden absence of QRS complex	*Pathogenesis:* Some atrial impulses are blocked from reaching ventricles at level of AV node next to the bundle of His causing progressive slowing of heartbeat until it is skipped; indicated by lengthening of the PR interval until the P wave is completely blocked and there is a skipped heartbeat (missing QRS complex). *Management:* Cardiac monitoring and observation; rarely progresses to a higher degree of block or requires treatment if perfusion is adequate. Can occur in normal healthy children and athletes. Atropine or pacing used if HR inadequate for perfusion.
Second-degree AV block (Mobitz Type II) 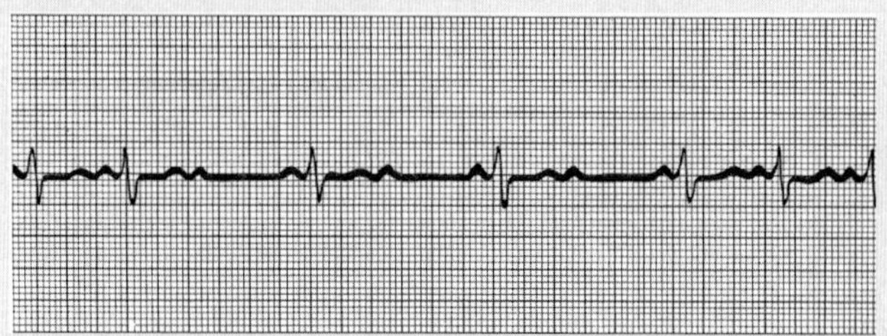 Rate: atrial, 60–100 bpm; ventricular, < 60 bpm Rhythm: atrial, regular; ventricular, irregular P:QRS: typically 2:1, may vary PR interval: constant PR interval for each conducted QRS complex QRS complex: 0.06–0.10 sec	*Pathogenesis:* Some atrial impulses reach the ventricles but some do not due to failure of conduction system at the level of the bundle of His and Purkinje fiber system (His-Purkinje system) indicated by skipped heartbeat (missing QRS complex) causing a more severe prognosis. *Management:* Immediate treatment with atropine or pacing because often progresses to complete heart block with approximately 80% mortality rate. Atropine should be used with caution if MI suspected because could worsen block; pacemaker therapy such as a permanent demand pacemaker is ultimately placed.

Rhythm/ECG Appearance and Characteristics	Pathogenesis and Management
Third-degree AV block (complete heart block) 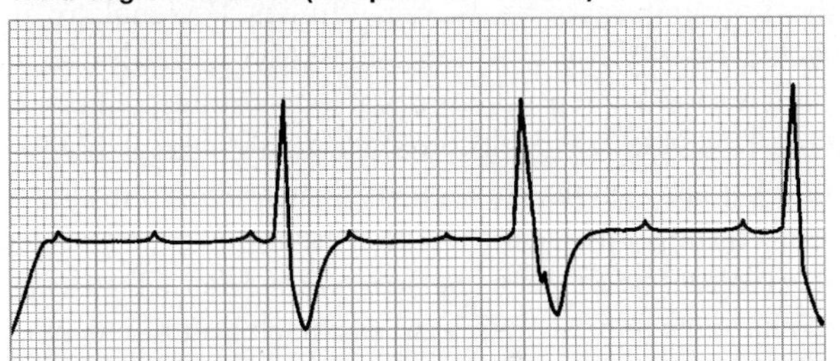 Rate: atrial, 60–100 bpm; ventricular, 15–60 bpm Rhythm: atrial, regular; ventricular, regular P:QRS: no relationship between P waves and QRS complexes; independent rhythms PR interval: not measured QRS complex: 0.06–0.10 sec if junctional escape rhythm; > 0.12 sec if ventricular escape rhythm	*Pathogenesis:* Complete atrial impulse conduction blockage at level of AV node, bundle of His, or Purkinje system that usually develops gradually from a first-degree or second-degree block. *Management:* Immediate pacemaker therapy and/or atropine because high risk of mortality. Atropine used with caution because potential risk of worsening block. Survivors of third-degree AV block will receive a permanent pacemaker.

SOURCES: LeMone, P., Burke, K. M., Bauldoff, G., & Gubrud, P. (2015). *Medical surgical nursing* (6th Ed.). Hoboken, NJ: Pearson Education; Kondur A, Afonso L, Hari P. Complications of Myocardial Infarction. 2014; http://emedicine.medscape.com/article/164924.overview - a1. Accessed April 4, 2016; Mann DL, Zipes DP, Libby P, Bonow RO, Braunwald E. Braunwald's heart disease : a textbook of cardiovascular medicine. Tenth edition. ed. Philadelpher, PA: Elsevier; 2015: https://www.clinicalkey.com/dura/browse/bookChapter/3-s2.0-C2012001143X.

atrial flutter are less common in patients with acute MI.[57] Atrial fibrillation is the most common dysrhythmia, causing atria to beat at a rapid, irregular rate, which can lead to pooling and clotting of blood and subsequent emboli that may cause MI or stroke and increase the risk of mortality. Atrial fibrillation occurs in about 10–15% of patients with acute MI.[57] Atrial fibrillation has a complex pathogenesis, but its occurrence during the first few hours of an acute MI is often related to left ventricular failure, ischemia in the atria, infarction of the right ventricle, or possibly pericarditis.[57]

Ventricular dysrhythmias include premature ventricular contractions (PVCs), ventricular tachycardia (VT), VF, and accelerated idioventricular rhythm. These dysrhythmias are caused by electrical instability that may be related to electrolyte imbalances.[21] Other causes may be cardiomyopathies (heart muscle disease) related to ischemia such as severe CAD or nonischemic causes, structural problems, or heart failure affecting the ability of the ventricle to pump adequately. Pulseless VT or VF are serious dysrhythmias because the heart is not pumping out any blood, leading to cardiac arrest. In the past, it was believed that frequent PVCs were a warning dysrhythmia for serious ventricular dysrhythmias. However, development of VF often occurs without previous rhythms of frequent PVCs, but it can be preceded by sustained VT.[57] Accelerated idioventricular rhythms are seen in about 20% of patients with acute MI[57] but also occur after successful reperfusion using fibrinolytic therapy.[21]

Bradydysrhythmias include sinus bradycardia, first-degree AV block, second-degree AV block, and third-degree (complete) AV block. Second-degree AV blocks are divided into Mobitz type I (also known as Wenckebach), which is commonly associated with an inferior MI, and Mobitz type II, which is commonly associated with an anterior wall MI.[57] A third-degree block may occur with both an anterior or inferior MI and is the most concerning of the blocks, often occurring suddenly and with a high mortality rate.[57]

Other peri-infarction dysrhythmias, not featured in Table 24.1, include intraventricular blocks such as a right bundle branch block (RBBB) or left bundle branch block (LBBB). An impulse conducted through the bundle of His passes through three fascicles (bundles of structures): the anterior division of the left bundle, the posterior division of the left bundle, and the right bundle.[57] Electrical conduction abnormalities in one or more of these fascicles is observed in about 15% of patients with acute MI.[57] A LBBB results from conduction delay or block from any of the several intraventricular conduction system sites, including the left main bundle branch, and is more likely to appear in the patient with heart failure or left ventricular hypertrophy (enlargement) than in the patient with heart disease.[21] However, its presence is correlated with more extensive disease and reduced survival rates.[21] RBBB results from conduction delay that occurs in any part of the right-sided intraventricular conduction system, commonly in the right bundle branch, which receives most of its blood supply from the LAD and therefore is compromised in acute MI and suggestive of a large infarct area. [21] The patient with an acute MI and new RBBB development is likely to have an increased risk of death related to cardiogenic shock owing to the size of the myocardial infarction.[57] However, RBBB may be a normal finding, unrelated to heart disease and an associated increased risk of mortality.[21]

Mortality from dysrhythmias is related to their systemic effects as a result of inadequate blood flow to meet the body's needs. The heart rate may be too fast to allow sufficient ventricular filling, too slow to allow sufficient perfusion, or absent as in pulseless VT or VF. Eventually, cardiac arrest occurs, characterized by sudden loss of consciousness from inadequate blood flow to the cerebrum because of failure of the heart to pump, and the heart stops, indicated by asystole, or a flatline, on the cardiac monitor.

Clinical Manifestations

Prodromal symptoms of sudden cardiac death may include angina, dyspnea, weakness, fatigue, palpitations related to dysrhythmias, syncope, and possibly other vague complaints.[21] Symptoms more specific to heart disease that occur within hours or minutes of cardiac arrest may include those related to dysrhythmias, ischemia, and heart failure.[21]

The person may feel that the heart is skipping a beat or beating hard and fast, which may lead to seeking treatment; however, many people in this situation observe no symptoms of a present dysrhythmia. Individuals who are experiencing cardiac arrest may be unconscious and nonresponsive, may display abnormal or no breathing, and/or may be pulseless. The patient's presentation determines acuity and guides diagnosis and treatment.

Linking Pathophysiology to Diagnosis and Treatment

An ECG and continuous cardiac monitoring are used to assess and record the heart's electrical activity and to determine whether dysrhythmias are present. In the nonacute situation, exercise and stress testing may be used to induce supraventricular dysrhythmia and tachydysrhythmia or sometimes bradydysrhythmias[21] Long-term ECG recording may be used as a noninvasive method to assess the frequency and type of dysrhythmias and to compare with the patient's symptoms and response to antiarrhythmic treatments.[21] Options for long-term recordings include the Holter monitor, event recorders, and implantable loop recorders. The Holter monitor provides a 24- to 48-hour recording of the patient's rhythm; a computer scans the recording to identify abnormalities and correlate with symptomatic events.[21] When longer-term monitoring is necessary, an event recorder may be used to record the cardiac rhythm over a period of 30 days. The event recorder requires the patient to push the event button, which the patient might not be able to do, depending on the patient's condition.[21] Patients with infrequent symptoms may benefit from an implantable loop recorder that is inserted under the skin on the left chest to record patient-activated symptomatic events and computer-identified abnormalities such as slow or fast heart rate.[21] Recent FDA approval of the Zio Patch, which is a wire-free monitor that is worn as a lightweight adhesive patch, allows long-term monitoring over 14 days. The Zio Patch has been found to detect more events than the Holter monitor, does not require implantation, and is less bulky.[60]

Invasive electrophysiologic studies may be used to identify patients who are at risk for sudden cardiac death.[21] Multipolar catheter electrodes are entered into the venous or arterial system and positioned at sites within the heart to record abnormal cardiac rhythms.[21] Electrophysiologic studies are diagnostic and may be therapeutic when used to terminate tachycardia by administering an electroshock.[21]

Patients who are predisposed to sudden cardiac death need identification of risk factors and prevention and treatment that targets and reduces underlying causes. Antiarrhythmics may be used to treat dysrhythmias, and anticoagulants prevent clots and related complications. An integrated approach using nurse-based, physician-supervised care may be beneficial to overall cardiovascular morbidity and mortality.[61] For example, a study that examined the use of a focused clinic for the management of atrial fibrillation showed an improvement in adherence to atrial fibrillation guidelines, including oral anticoagulants, and a decrease in major cardiovascular events.[61]

Devices such as pacemakers and implantable cardioverter-defibrillators (ICDs) may be used in addition to medication therapy to treat dysrhythmias. Pacemakers are indicated mainly for symptomatic bradydysrhythmias or for patients with asymptomatic bradydysrhythmia if development to serious or symptomatic dysrhythmia is likely.[21] Pacemakers are single, dual, or triple chambered and may be used in the short term for acute situations or implanted permanently. The FDA has approved the Micra Transcatheter Pacing system, which is a 1-inch self-contained wire-free single-chamber pacemaker that is implanted in the right ventricle to control the heartbeat.[62] The leadless pacing system meets prespecified safety and efficacy goals according to a study in which 99.2% of participants had successful device implantation. Ideally, this system will eliminate problems with traditional pacemakers that have wired leads.[63]

ICD implantation has been associated with reduced mortality in patients who are at high risk for sudden cardiac death. However, the surgically placed device has contraindications, such as active infection.[64] For these patients, the wearable cardioverter–defibrillator vest is a temporary treatment option that requires no surgical operation until the contraindications have been treated and resolved.[64] Time to defibrillation must be immediate, and neither the ICD nor the wearable life vest depends on a second person to defibrillate.[64]

In the acute situation, assessment and basic life support are the initial steps performed in accordance to the AHA guidelines for cardiopulmonary resuscitation (CPR) and emergency cardiovascular care. Trained professionals and laypeople can carry out activities to resuscitate the patient in cardiac arrest to prevent death, using the acronym *CAB*, which stands for compressions, airway, and breathing. The goal is keeping the central nervous system, heart, and other vital organs viable until return of spontaneous circulation can be achieved.[21] Automated external defibrillators (AED) in the community increase the likelihood of survival when first responders are able to defibrillate shockable rhythms (pulseless VT, VF). The next step in resuscitation is advanced cardiac life support; the goals are a return of spontaneous circulation restoration of a cardiac rhythm that is hemodynamically stable, improved breathing, and maintenance of restored circulation.[21] Defibrillation using an AED or manual monophasic or biphasic device must be timely and must be alternated with pharmacotherapy in patients with persistent or recurrent VT or VF in a drug–shock–drug–shock rhythm simultaneous with CPR.[21] The AHA guidelines provide algorithms to determine steps, including pharmacotherapy for treating patients who are experiencing sudden cardiac arrest from pulseless VT or VF, pulseless electrical activity, and asystole as well as bradycardia and tachycardia with a pulse. The patient may be intubated to achieve ventilation. Postresuscitation care is determined by the cause of cardiac arrest.

Eighty percent of patients who experience cardiac arrest have IHD, and therapy is directed at preventing ischemia by reducing myocardial oxygen demand and increasing supply as well as treating left ventricular dysfunction.[21] Treatments previously discussed to reperfuse blocked coronary arteries must occur quickly to avoid hemodynamic compromise such as hypotension, which causes an additional increase in myocardial oxygen requirements and further complications.[57] Management should also include the treatment of electrolyte disturbances.

Ventricular Aneurysm and Rupture

Myocardial rupture related to the ischemia associated with an acute MI may involve the free walls of the left or right ventricle, the ventricular septum, and/or the left ventricle papillary muscle. Other causes of rupture besides acute MI may include blunt or penetrating trauma, abscesses related to infective endocarditis (infection and inflammation of heart valves or endocardium), and rarely autoimmune diseases or tumors.[65] Complications may involve acute mitral regurgitation and cardiac tamponade.

Ventricular Aneurysm

A **ventricular aneurysm** is a defect in the left or sometimes right ventricle wall in which there is bulging outward during both systole and diastole, usually as a result of a MI. The wall is usually weak and consists of a thin, fibrous scar. Risk factors for a left ventricular aneurysm include female sex, LAD artery occlusion, usually CAD of one vessel without collateral circulation, and no history of angina.[57] A third or fourth heart sound may be present on physical examination, and the apical impulse may be displaced to left of the midclavicular line. A systolic murmur may be auscultated related to coexisting mitral regurgitation. ECG is characterized by evidence of ST elevation related to the history of an ACS episode, usually a large anterior MI.[66] Typically, imaging such as transthoracic echocardiography (TTE) is used to identify the characteristic abnormal wall motion.[66] Aneurysmectomy (surgical removal of the aneurysm) might be performed if the patient is already undergoing CABG or other valve surgery. Otherwise, treatment of ventricular aneurysm is related to its complications, which may include heart failure, dysrhythmias, thromboembolism, and rarely ventricular rupture.[66] ACE inhibitors might be used to reduce afterload due left ventricular enlargement, antianginals to treat ischemic chest pain, and anticoagulation in the presence of left ventricular mural (on the wall) thrombus, which is also a common cause of acute MI or severe left ventricular dysfunction.[66]

Ventricular Septal Rupture

A **ventricular septal rupture** is a type of ventricular septal defect in which there is an abnormal opening between the left and right ventricles causing oxygenated blood (from the left ventricle) to mix with deoxygenated blood (from the right ventricle) as a result of left-to-right shunting. It is a rare but lethal complication that most often occurs in the first 24 hours of an acute MI but also can occur 3–5 days later or, less commonly, up to 2 weeks later.[57] Usually, the cause is complete coronary artery occlusion with little collateral circulation of either the LAD, the posterior descending branch of the RCA, or the circumflex artery.[67] A patient with an acute MI who does not receive reperfusion therapy is at risk for coagulation necrosis, in which neutrophils move to the necrotic area, undergo apoptosis, and release lytic enzymes that cause cell rupture and further myocardial necrosis, which thin and weaken the septum until it ruptures.[57] Poor septal collateral circulation is a risk factor in addition to older age, female sex, extensive area of infarct, and right ventricle involvement.[57] A patient who is experiencing ventricular septal rupture may present with symptoms of left and right ventricular failure, recurring chest pain, shortness of breath, and hypotension. A new, loud, and harsh holosystolic murmur may be auscultated, after which the patient may suddenly deteriorate into heart failure and often cardiogenic shock in the first 24 hours or few days of an acute MI.[57,67] ST-segment elevation and Q waves on some leads may be present on the ECG related to a large anterior MI, which is more commonly the cause of ventricular septal rupture than is an inferior MI.[57]

Echocardiography with Doppler imaging is used to identify the rupture and its site, its size, and the presence of left-to-right shunting. Cardiac catheterization confirms the diagnosis, degree of shunting, and extent of CAD.[57,67] Cardiac catheterization helps to determine anatomy of coronary arteries and extent of disease, but surgical intervention to remove necrotic tissue and patch the opening must be performed emergently because 90% of patients who are treated without surgery die.[67] Hemodynamic stabilization is essential during preparation for surgery, using medication and an intra-aortic balloon pump if necessary.[57] A percutaneous approach for closing a ventricular septal rupture is an alternative to CABG; however, it is not yet available in many institutions.[57]

Pericarditis and Dressler Syndrome

Etiology and Pathogenesis

Pericarditis is swelling and inflammation of the pericardium, the thin double-layered sac surrounding the heart, as a result of injury such as an acute MI, infection, inflammatory disorder, trauma, cancer, or congenital causes. The incidence of pericarditis after MI is 10%, and it may occur within 24–96 hours after the MI as a result of the inflammation of pericardial tissue over the necrotic area of the myocardium; the incidence of pericarditis that occurs later (2–8 weeks) is 1–3% (**Figure 24.16** ■).[68] **Dressler syndrome**, also known as post-MI syndrome, is the late pericarditis and possibly has an autoimmune pathogenesis.[57]

Clinical Manifestations

Pericarditis often causes pleuritic chest pain as irritated layers rub against one another. The pain is worse with deep inspiration, coughing, swallowing, or lying in supine position and may radiate. However, patients with early pericarditis may be asymptomatic. A pericardial friction rub may be auscultated on physical examination.[68]

Linking Pathophysiology to Diagnosis and Treatment

ECG changes include ST-segment elevation in all or most of the leads with upright or inverted T waves. Echocardiography or CT scan may display a pericardial effusion, or fluid in the pericardial cavity (**Figure 24.17** ■).[68] The patient who is experiencing pericarditis or Dressler syndrome should be hospitalized for management and observation of possible cardiac tamponade.[57] Aspirin in a dose of 650 mg every 4 to

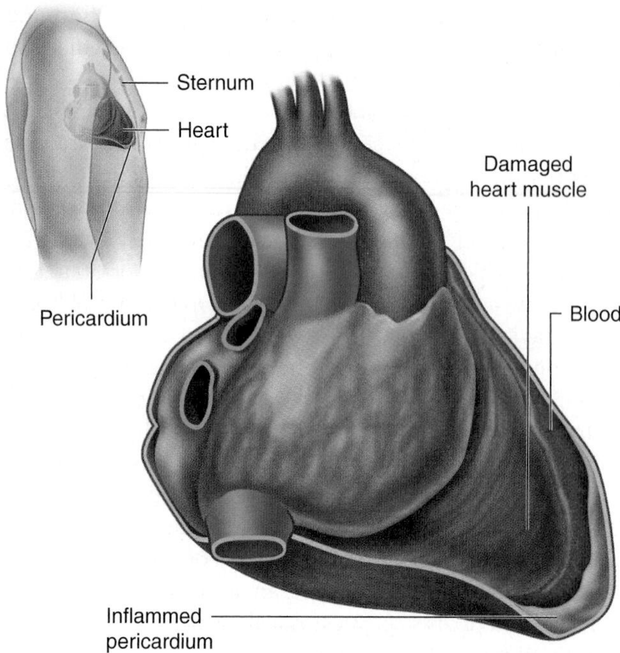

Figure 24.16 ■ Pericarditis is swelling and inflammation of the pericardium when injury to the heart causes blood to be present in the pericardium. Inflammation may occur over the necrotic area of the myocardium as a result of an ACS event.

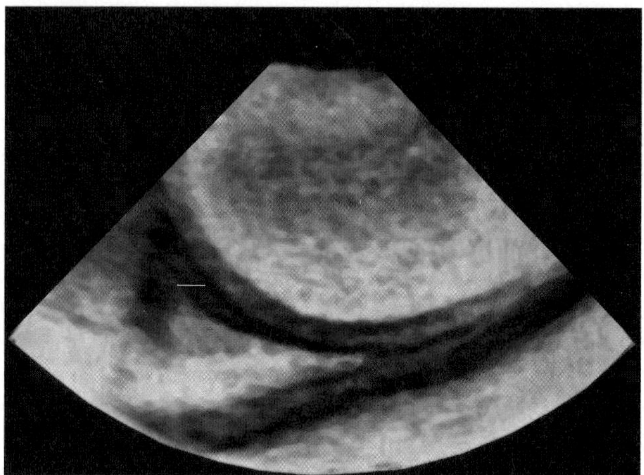

Figure 24.17 ■ A CT image displays a large pericardial effusion that is causing flattening of the ventricles and may cause cardiac tamponade because the compression on the heart impairs its function.

6 hours is prescribed for at least 4 weeks to reduce inflammation and treat pain. Colchicine, an anti-inflammatory agent, might be added if aspirin alone is not effective. Corticosteroids and other nonsteroidal anti-inflammatory drug (NSAID) use is determined on an individual basis, although aspirin is preferred.[68]

Cardiac Tamponade

Cardiac tamponade is a life-threatening condition of increased pericardial pressure as a result of blood or fluid buildup between the myocardium and the pericardium (**Figure 24.18** ■).

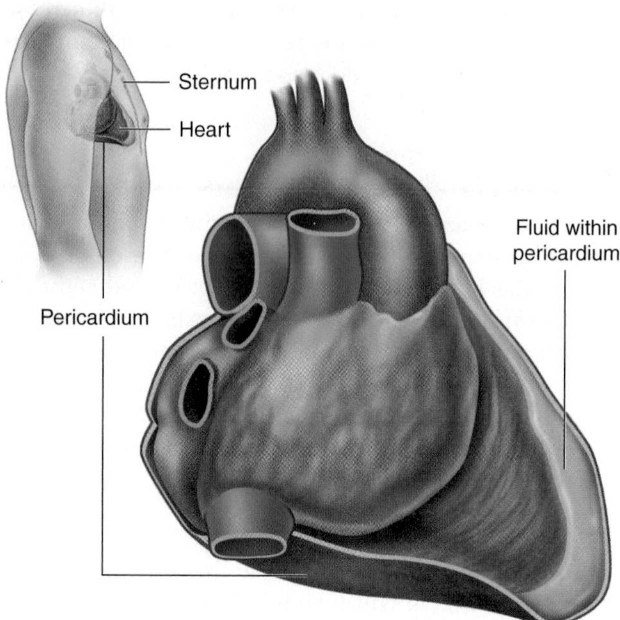

Figure 24.18 ■ Cardiac tamponade is a life-threatening condition because of impaired ventricular filling and subsequent insufficient systemic and pulmonary perfusion as a result of compression from increased pressure from blood or fluid buildup between myocardium and pericardium.

Etiology and Pathogenesis

Cardiac tamponade results from pericardial fluid accumulation (pericardial effusion) that may have causes related to MI but also can be caused by trauma, infection, cancer, medication side effects, heart failure, radiation, pericarditis (but rarely Dressler syndrome), inflammatory disease, PCI, or recent cardiac surgery.[69] As the fluid accumulates, there is a rise in pericardial pressure as well as the left- and right-sided atrial and ventricular pressures.[21] The pericardial pressure increases more than the central venous pressure,[69] which is the pressure in the vena cava near the right atrium that reflects that the amount of blood returning to the heart and the heart's pumping ability to deliver blood reflected by cardiac output. Impaired venous return and subsequent reduced cardiac output and arterial hypoperfusion of vital organs result.

Clinical Manifestations

Systemic and pulmonary hypoperfusion symptoms that are shared with other diseases may be present; these include dyspnea, edema, oliguria (low urine output), jugular venous distention, tachypnea, and tachycardia as a compensatory mechanism to maintain cardiac output.[69] If pericardial fluid accumulates rapidly, the patient will present with hypotension, whereas if the accumulation is slow, the patient may compensate and present with edema.[69] Pulsus paradoxus is a characteristic finding of cardiac tamponade in which there is an abnormal decrease of more than 10 mmHg in systolic blood pressure during inspiration.[21] Pulsus paradoxus is measured by using a stethoscope and manual sphygmomanometer to estimate hemodynamic impairment associated with pericardial effusion, which is more detrimental if the pericardial effusion is evolving rapidly.[69]

Linking Pathophysiology to Diagnosis and Treatment

History and imaging such as echocardiography, CT scan, or MRI findings confirm the presence of cardiac tamponade, and the patient should be examined for pulsus paradoxus. Prompt surgical treatment is needed. Consideration of the size and location as well as the patient's hemodynamic status is used in deciding how to treat cardiac tamponade.[69] Fluid is removed by pericardiocentesis, which is needle aspiration by percutaneous approach, or surgical pericardiostomy, which is the creation of a pericardial window (opening) into the pericardium.[69] The fluid should be removed slowly to avoid complications such as pulmonary edema (fluid in lungs) and may be analyzed to help identify the cause of tamponade.[21]

Check Your Progress: Section 24.6

1. What occurs with sudden cardiac death?
2. Which arrhythmia consists of an irregular atrial heart rate?
3. What symptoms may be present in a patient presenting to the emergency department in cardiac arrest?

24.7 Valvular Disorders

Valvular disorders include problems that disrupt blood flow through the atria and ventricles as a result of abnormal functioning of one or more of the four heart valves such as stenosis, regurgitation, or prolapse. The disorder may also be known as heart valve disease or valvular heart disease (see **Table 24.2** ■).

Etiology and Pathogenesis

The heart has four valves: the mitral and tricuspid valves (the atrioventricular valves), which control blood flow from the atria to the ventricles, and the aortic and pulmonic valves (the semilunar valves), which control blood flow out of the ventricles to the rest of the body and to the lungs, respectively. Three layers of extracellular matrix, including collagens, proteoglycans, and elastin, given the biomechanical support of the valve leaflets (cusps) to open for proper flow through the heart and closure to prevent backflow.[70] Causes of valvular disorders may be related to CAD and ACS and are usually age-related, inherited, or congenital (present from birth). Age-related changes include calcific valve changes, in which calcium deposits form on the valves of the heart, which can lead to narrowing (stenosis). Rheumatic fever is a possible cause that has become less common in the United States and Europe since the 1970s[71] but is still of concern in developing countries.[21] Valvular disorders are an increasing health issue, especially among the aging population; echocardiographic or radiologic evidence of calcific aortic valve stenosis is present in almost one third of older adults.[70] Increased risk of valvular disorders is associated with age, gender, tobacco use, high cholesterol levels, hypertension, and diabetes.[70]

Mitral Regurgitation as a Complication of Myocardial Infarction

A common mechanical complication of acute MI is mitral regurgitation, which has several mechanisms of cause (see Table 24.2). The mitral valve apparatus includes the mitral valve leaflet, the chordae tendinae (which attach the papillary muscles to the mitral valve), and the mitral annulus (fibrous ring attached to leaflet). Abnormalities of any of part of the apparatus may cause mitral regurgitation.[21] Papillary muscle rupture is a common mechanism leading to mitral regurgitation because of leaflet flapping (flailing) or prolapse, but chordae tendinae rupture can also be a cause.[57] The anterior portion of the papillary muscle receives blood from the LAD and left circumflex artery; therefore, an infarct of these coronary arteries will disrupt the muscle function and its role in supporting most of the mitral leaflet. Risk factors include older age, female sex, large infarct size, heart failure, and history of ACS and/or recurrent ischemic multivessel CAD.[57] Severe acute mitral regurgitation from papillary muscle or chordae tendinae rupture is a serious concern because it leads to hemodynamic deterioration and possible cardiogenic shock. To avoid death, rapid assessment and diagnosis are needed, followed by stabilization and immediate surgical intervention.[57]

Mild to moderate mitral regurgitation usually causes no apparent symptoms; acute severe mitral regurgitation symptoms include shortness of breath, fatigue, new holosystolic murmur, symptoms of flash pulmonary edema (respiratory distress related to fluid accumulation in the lungs), and shock.[57] Patients should receive diuretics and vasodilators (nitroprusside, nitroglycerin) to reduce afterload and achieve hemodynamic stability until surgical intervention involving mitral valve repair or replacement can be performed.[57] If the patient is hemodynamically compromised, an intra-aortic balloon pump may be necessary to improve myocardial oxygen perfusion and cardiac output until surgery can be performed.[57]

Linking Pathophysiology to Diagnosis and Treatment

Individuals with valvular disorders often do not recognize the effects because of the slow, progressive nature of this type of disorder. Diagnosis may be based on incidental findings on chest x-ray or other noninvasive testing or as a result of auscultation of a heart murmur during a physical examination.[71] TTE is the standard diagnostic test used for initial evaluation and as follow-up for the patient with known or suspected valvular disorder to determine cause, severity, hemodynamic effects, prognosis, and timing of interventions.[71] Transesophageal echocardiography (TEE) may also be used to determine the best treatment of a valvular disorder.[71] No effective nonsurgical therapies have been approved for valvular heart disease; therefore, surgical interventions are the treatment of choice.[70] Coexisting diseases such as CAD, hypertension, high cholesterol, and diabetes should be treated with lifestyle changes and appropriate medications. Aortic valve replacement for aortic stenosis is the primary treatment[70] and accounts for approximately two thirds of heart valve operations.[21] Mitral regurgitation, which is the most prevalent valvular disorder in the United States,[72] is treated with mitral valve surgery. Mitral stenosis is often

Table 24.2 Valvular Disorders

Valvular Disorder: Type and Definition	Etiology, Pathogenesis, and Clinical Manifestations	Diagnosis and Treatment
Aortic Valve Disease		
Aortic stenosis Obstruction of left ventricular flow to the aorta due to narrowing above or below the level of the aortic valve	• Age-related or congenital bicuspid aortic valve disease calcification (calcium accumulation); bicuspid aortic valve disease is a congenital defect where the aortic valve has two leaflets instead of three, which causes valvular dysfunction and backflow • Less commonly caused by rheumatic heart disease (inflammation and scarring from autoimmune reaction to rheumatic fever) or severe atherosclerosis of aorta or aortic valve • Systolic heart murmur on physical exam • Symptoms associated with degree of stenosis and related to left ventricular outflow obstruction problems such as angina due to myocardial ischemia, syncope, and heart failure	*ECG:* left ventricular hypertrophy noted in 85% of patients with aortic stenosis *Chest x-ray:* sometimes shows heavy calcification or aortic dilation *TTE:* test of choice to determine valve anatomy and severity of calcification and determine need for surgical intervention *Doppler echocardiography:* useful to follow disease severity and predict clinical outcome Cardiac catheterization: less often used but can be helpful to diagnose CAD • Aortic valve replacement because no medical therapy exists. Transcatheter aortic valve implant is less invasive alternative to surgical placement. • Treatment of coexisting diseases (hypertension, diabetes mellitus, CAD).
Aortic regurgitation Incompetence of aortic valve causing a backflow of blood into left ventricle resulting in increased left ventricular volume and pressure overload	• Aortic valve leaflet (flap) and aortic root abnormalities • Causes include infection such as infective endocarditis, aortic dissection, trauma to ascending aorta, uncontrolled hypertension, and inflammation from certain autoimmune diseases • Diastolic or systolic heart murmur on physical exam; symptoms usually tolerated for years and present when reduced cardiac reserve and myocardial ischemia (e.g. fatigue, angina, dyspnea) develops as a result of left ventricular dysfunction and cardiomegaly (heart enlargement) occur	*ECG:* may or may not show evidence of left ventricular hypertrophy *Chest x-ray:* possible pulmonary hypertension, pulmonary edema *Echocardiography (TEE or TTE):* to identify cause and measure left ventricular function such as ejection fraction, which is a measurement of how well blood is pumped from left ventricle. • Surgical intervention (aortic valve replacement) even if patient is asymptomatic when left ventricular dysfunction is severe because of problems associated with low cardiac output and should not be delayed especially if hypotension, pulmonary edema or evidence of low perfusion. • Vasodilators to improve cardiac output while patient prepared for surgery. • Treatment of coexisting diseases (aortic dissection, infective endocarditis, hypertension, left ventricular dysfunction).
Mitral Valve Disease		
Mitral stenosis Narrowing of mitral valve opening causing obstructed blood flow from left atrium to left ventricle	• Most common cause is rheumatic heart disease with possible multivalve (aortic, tricuspid) involvement • Calcification, infective endocarditis, autoimmune diseases such as systemic lupus erythematosus or rheumatoid arthritis • Elevated left atrial pressures lead to enlargement, which places patient at risk for atrial fibrillation and arterial thromboembolism; elevated pulmonary venous pressures may cause pulmonary congestion, pulmonary edema and lead to pulmonary hypertension, heart failure (right-sided) • Diastolic heart murmur and opening snap on physical exam • Dyspnea, fatigue, decrease exercise tolerance, hemoptysis (coughing up blood), chest pain, palpitations related to common coexisting atrial fibrillation or heart failure • Patients usually present ≥ 20 years after rheumatic fever occurrence	*ECG:* left atrial enlargement, atrial fibrillation and/or right ventricular hypertrophy *Chest x-ray:* left atrium enlargement, possible cardiomegaly, enlarged pulmonary arteries and congestion related to pulmonary hypertension *TTE*: diagnose and determine stenosis and hemodynamic severity *TEE:* performed before percutaneous mitral balloon commissurotomy where a catheter with a balloon is inflated to open the stenotic valve *Exercise Doppler echocardiography:* determines pulmonary artery pressures Cardiac catheterization: helpful if discrepancy between symptoms and ECG • Invasive options include: percutaneous mitral balloon commissurotomy, surgical mitral commissurotomy and mitral valve replacement to repair diseased valve. • Treatment of coexisting disease and complications: diuretics for pulmonary congestion, antiarrhythmics for atrial fibrillation and anticoagulants to decrease risk of clots, prophylactic treatment for rheumatic fever.
Mitral regurgitation Incomplete mitral valve closure causing a backflow (leakage) from the left ventricle into the left atrium during systole (contraction)	• Structural or functional abnormalities of the mitral valve apparatus or left ventricle related to rheumatic heart disease, infective endocarditis, CAD including acute MI, cardiomyopathy (heart muscle disease) • Volume overload in left ventricle leads to increased left atrial and pulmonary venous pressures and possible pulmonary congestion, pulmonary edema; enlarged left atria may lead to development of atrial fibrillation and arterial thromboembolism	*ECG:* left atrial enlargement, atrial fibrillation and/or right ventricular hypertrophy *Chest x-ray:* left atrium enlargement, possible cardiomegaly *TTE:* diagnose/determine cause and severity *Cardiac MRI:* assess left and right ventricle volumes, function

Table 24.2 Valvular Disorders *Continued*

Valvular Disorder: Type and Definition	Etiology, Pathogenesis, and Clinical Manifestations	Diagnosis and Treatment
	• Eventually, patient may develop pulmonary hypertension and heart failure (right-sided) • Systolic heart murmur, apical pulse displacement if ventricle enlarged, and possible third heart sound on physical exam • Usually asymptomatic if chronic disease for years whereas patient usually symptomatic (dyspnea, fatigue, new holosystolic murmur, palpitations, symptoms of shock or flash pulmonary edema) if acute	Additional invasive (cardiac catheterization) or noninvasive imaging (e.g. stress echocardiography, PET, computed tomography angiograpy) to determine cause and/or myocardial viability to guide treatment. • In acute disease, diuretics, vasodilators (nitroprusside, nitroglycerin) and possibly intra-aortic balloon pump to maintain perfusion and achieve hemodynamic stabilization until mitral valve repair or replacement surgery, which should be performed immediately to avoid death. • Transcatheter mitral valve repair: less invasive method as alternative for clients unable to undergo surgery to repair mitral valve
Mitral valve prolapse Non–life-threatening condition where the mitral valve leaflets bulge (prolapse) back into the left atrium during systole; sometimes leads to mitral valve regurgitation	• Classified according to its many causes that may or may not be genetic. • Most patients with mitral valve prolapse have normal mitral valve leaflets with or without mitral regurgitation • Usually asymptomatic and may remain so throughout life • Possible systolic-click murmur (related to mitral regurgitation) noted on physical exam	*ECG and chest x-ray:* unremarkable *TTE:* most important test to diagnose based on whether one or both of mitral valve leaflets are displaced into the left atrium during systole • Treatment not usually needed because mitral valve prolapse is usually benign
Tricuspid Valve Disease		
Tricuspid stenosis Narrowing of tricuspid valve that opens between the right atria and ventricle Generally also with mitral and/or aortic valve disorders, usually mitral stenosis	• Commonly caused by rheumatic heart disease and other unusual causes that are congenital or related to infection or tumor • Symptoms related to low cardiac output such as fatigue, hepatomegaly, ascites, anasarca because of decreased venous return to the heart • Symptoms of coexisting mitral stenosis or other valvular disorders may be present which confound diagnosis	*ECG:* right atrial enlargement *Chest x-ray:* cardiomegaly, right atrial enlargement and left atrial enlargement possible *Echocardiography:* leaflet thickening and decreased movement and reduce tricuspid opening diameter *Cardiac catheterization:* dye injection shows leaflet thickening and decreased mobility but has been typically replaced by noninvasive Doppler assessment to determine severity • Surgical intervention if severe and in the presence of coexisting valvular diseases. • Diuresis by medication and sodium restriction as well as treatment of coexisting disease (dysrhythmias)
Tricuspid regurgitation Incomplete tricuspid valve closure causing leakage from the right ventricle into the left atrium during systole	• Commonly caused by right ventricle dilation as a complication of right ventricular failure and its causes • May be related to right ventricular hypertension as a result of a mitral valve disorder, right ventricle infarction, congenital heart disease or pulmonary hypertension • Usually asymptomatic unless presence of pulmonary hypertension causing decreased cardiac output and symptoms of right-sided heart failure (ascites, hepatomegaly, edema, neck pulsation related to jugular venous distention, weakness, fatigue)	*ECG:* usually nonspecific and may show RBBB, Q waves or atrial fibrillation *Chest x-ray:* cardiomegaly, ascites, pleural effusion possible *Echocardiography:* determine severity, pulmonary arterial pressure and right ventricular function as well as dilation of tricuspid annulus, right atrium and ventricle if cause of tricuspid regurgitation • Treatment not usually necessary in absence of pulmonary hypertension. Tricuspid regurgitation with pulmonary hypertension requires surgical intervention because it is associated with heart failure and mortality.

SOURCES: Collier P, Phelan D, Griffin BP. (2014). Mitral Valve Disease: Stenosis and Regurgitation. Retrieved from http://www.clevelandclinicmeded.com/medicalpubs/diseasemanagement/cardiology/mitral-valve-disease/; Mann DL, Zipes DP, Libby P, Bonow RO, Braunwald E. (2015). Braunwald's heart disease : a textbook of cardiovascular medicine. Tenth edition. ed. Philadelpher, PA: Elservier; Nishimura RA, Otto CM, Bonow RO, et al. (2014). AHA/ACC guideline for the management of patients with valvular heart disease: a report of the American College of Cardiology/American Heart Association Task Force on Practice Guidelines. *J Am Coll Cardiol.* 2014;63(22):e57-185; Novaro GM. Aortic Valve Disease. (2014). Retrieved from http://www.clevelandclinicmeded.com/medicalpubs/diseasemanagement/cardiology/aortic-valve-disease/; Zeng YI, Sun R, Li X, Liu M, Chen S, Zhang P. (2016). Pathophysiology of valvular heart disease. Exp Ther Med. 11(4):1184-1188.

treated with a percutaneous approach.[21] Treatment models are changing toward a multidisciplinary approach that includes the invasive and noninvasive cardiologist, surgeons, and nurses who are knowledgeable about valvular disorders, organized as heart valve clinics or heart valve center of excellence.[21]

Pregnant women with mitral stenosis are at risk of pulmonary edema and atrial fibrillation related to increased pressure in the left atrium and pulmonary artery due to increased plasma volume, increased heart rate, and decreased afterload.[73] Pregnancy places the woman at an increased risk of worsening mitral stenosis and clinical decompensation.[73] Women with severe mitral stenosis should receive prepregnancy counseling about treatments and should be monitored at a heart valve clinic during pregnancy.[73] Appropriate medical therapy should be administered for coexisting diseases and complications, such as anticoagulation to prevent thromboembolism, beta blockers for cardiac rhythm control, and diuretics to reduce left atrial pressures.[73] Patients with mitral regurgitation usually tolerate changes related to pregnancy better. However, all patients with suspected or known valvular disorders should be managed by a heart valve clinic. ■

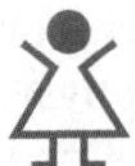

Children may be born with a congenital heart defect, which is the most common type of birth defect and may be critical or may cause no symptoms and have a good prognosis. Some examples of congenital heart defects are septal defects of the ventricles or atria, narrowing of heart valves, and a combination of defects. Tetralogy of Fallot is a complex heart defect that involves pulmonary valve stenosis, a large ventricular septal defect, an overriding aorta causing deoxygenated blood from the right ventricle to flow directly into the aorta instead of the pulmonary artery, and right ventricular hypertrophy, in which the right ventricle is thicker and must work harder to contract. Infants and children with simple ventricular septal defects are usually asymptomatic and have an excellent long-term prognosis,[67] whereas a ventricular septal defect as part of the complex disease process of tetralogy of Fallot requires open heart surgery, typically during the first year of life.[74] Prenatal sonography (image from ultrasound) and pulse oximetry screening during the first few days of an infant's life are methods to identify congenital heart disease and appropriately treat and avoid mortality related to late diagnosis of critical congenital heart disease.[75] ■

Check Your Progress: Section 24.7

1. What is commonly caused by right ventricle dilation as a complication of right ventricular failure and its causes, possibly related to right ventricular hypertension as a result of a mitral valve disorder, right ventricle infarction, congenital heart disease, or pulmonary hypertension?
2. Which is the most prevalent valvular disorder in the United States?
3. If a patient has severe mitral regurgitation, what will the patient be placed on as a result of being hemodynamically unstable?

CHAPTER SUMMARY

24.1 Chapter Overview and Case Studies

Describe coronary artery disease, acute coronary syndromes, and concepts related to disorders of coronary circulation.

- Coronary circulation is the blood flow to and from the heart muscle (myocardium) through the coronary arteries and cardiac veins. Problems with coronary circulation arise when blood flow to the myocardium is reduced as a result of conditions such as coronary artery disease (CAD), which leads to reduced supplies of oxygen and nutrients.
- Cardiovascular disease (CVD) is the pathologic process, commonly atherosclerosis, that causes disease of the heart and coronary and systemic circulation. CVD includes diagnoses such as stroke, transient ischemic attack (TIA), claudication (leg pain), and limb ischemia in addition to heart-related angina pectoris, myocardial ischemia, and myocardial infarction (heart attack).
- Patients with CVD may have alterations in cognition, comfort, fluids and electrolytes, and oxygenation.

24.2 Epidemiology and Risk Factors Related to Coronary Artery Disease

Outline the epidemiology and risk factors related to coronary artery disease as well as methods of preventing coronary artery disease.

- More than one in three adults in the United States have one or more types of CVDs, which include MI, hypertension, stroke, and/or heart failure.
- Major modifiable risk factors that contribute to a risk of CAD include smoking and tobacco use, lack of physical activity, poor nutrition that may lead to a defined overweight or obese status, unhealthy blood cholesterol and lipid levels, hypertension, insulin resistance, diabetes, metabolic syndrome, and family history (genetics).
- Nonmodifiable risk factors include family history, age of more than 45 years in men and more than 55 years in women, race, and ethnicity.
- The "Life's Simple 7" health indicators serve as a template to achieve heart-healthy living; increasing evidence shows that such lifestyle modifications improve cardiovascular and brain health.

24.3 Pathophysiology, Diagnosis, and Treatment of Coronary Artery Disease

Outline the pathophysiology, diagnosis, and treatment of coronary artery disease.

- The left main coronary artery (LCA) and the right coronary artery (RCA) are the two main coronary muscular-walled arteries that originate from the base of the aorta and branch across the epicardium before entering the myocardium and the endocardium.
- Insufficient blood supply to the heart may trigger the development of coronary collateral circulation.
- A thrombus is a blood clot that obstructs blood flow to organs. Depending on where it forms and when it forms in a coronary artery, the blockage can cause MI.
- Atherosclerosis is characterized by the deposition of lesions on the intima called atheromas, or atheromatous plaques, leading to narrowing and reduced blood flow.
- A coronary angiogram, also known as coronary angiography or arteriography, is an invasive procedure that is used to confirm the diagnosis of CAD after noninvasive tests have been inconclusive.

- Hypertension is treated with lifestyle modifications and medications. The general goal for most adults older than 20 years old is to attain less than 120 mmHg systolic and less than 80 mmHg diastolic blood pressure.

24.4 Myocardial Ischemia and Infarction

Differentiate the causes, classification, underlying pathogenesis, and clinical manifestations of myocardial ischemia and infarction and approaches to diagnosis and treatment of these conditions across the lifespan.

- The coronary arteries sufficiently supply the myocardium with blood to meet oxygen and nutrient demands under normal conditions.
- In the presence of atherosclerosis, complications arise as a result of narrowed coronary arteries and decreased blood flow. Most atherosclerotic plaque rupture involves a fracture in its fibrous cap, but a second mechanism has been described that involves superficial erosion of the intima.
- Injury may range from reversible to irreversible effects when blood flow is decreased or completely blocked, resulting in hypoxia of the myocardial cells.
- Myocardial cells that are ischemic have reduced contractility, leading to decreased cardiac output. Ischemia disrupts the cardiac conduction system, which disrupts the electrical charge transmission via cardiac muscle fibers throughout myocardial tissue, affecting the heart's ability to contract and perfuse systemic and coronary circulation.
- The progression from ischemia to infarction can be thought of as an ischemic cascade in which coronary occlusion from problems such as atherosclerotic plaque disruption and thrombosis initiates the steps.
- Stable angina usually occurs with increased myocardial oxygen demand and reduced blood flow during exertion or emotional stress, commonly caused by atherosclerosis.
- Episodes of silent ischemia are possibly present in one third of patients treated for angina with a higher prevalence likely for patients with diabetes.
- Coronary microvascular dysfunction involves damage to the walls and inner linings of small coronary arteries that can lead to narrowing, spasms, and decreased blood flow.

24.5 Specific Acute Coronary Syndromes

Differentiate the causes, classification, underlying pathogenesis, and clinical manifestations of specific acute coronary syndromes and approaches to diagnosis and treatment of these conditions across the lifespan.

- ACS is an acute form of CAD. ACS encompasses any cluster of clinical signs and symptoms that are related to acute myocardial ischemia and infarction.
- Non–ST-segment elevation acute coronary syndrome encompasses NSTEMI and unstable angina as a condition characterized by the clinical signs and symptoms of myocardial ischemia in the absence of ST-segment elevation on ECG.
- STEMI is a more precise definition of the common term *heart attack*, since "STE" refers to the ECG tracing of ST-segment elevation and "MI" refers to myocardial infarction. It is a very serious condition that requires rapid recognition, reperfusion treatment, and management to prevent death.

24.6 Complications of Acute Coronary Syndromes

Differentiate the causes, classification, underlying pathogenesis, and clinical manifestations of complications of acute coronary syndromes and approaches to diagnosis and treatment of these conditions across the lifespan.

- Cardiac arrest is characterized by abrupt loss of cardiac function. A clear relationship exists between sudden cardiac death and CHD as a result of cardiac arrest. Sudden cardiac death frequently results from an acute MI when plaque ruptures, leading to thrombosis that completely occludes the coronary artery with subsequent lack of blood flow and death of myocardium inducing a fatal ventricular dysrhythmia.
- Dysrhythmias may occur during an acute MI or as a result of reperfusion treatments. Supraventricular tachydysrhythmias include sinus tachycardia, premature atrial contractions (PACs), paroxysmal supraventricular tachycardia (PSVT), atrial flutter, and atrial fibrillation. PACs often occur before the onset of PSVT, atrial flutter, or atrial fibrillation. Ventricular dysrhythmias include premature ventricular contractions (PVCs), ventricular tachycardia, ventricular fibrillation, and accelerated idioventricular rhythm. Bradydysrhythmias include sinus bradycardia, first-degree AV block, second-degree AV block, and third-degree (complete) AV block.
- A ventricular aneurysm is a defect in the left or sometimes the right ventricle wall in which there is bulging outward during both systole and diastole, usually as a result of a MI. The wall is usually weak and consists of a thin, fibrous scar. A ventricular septal rupture is a type of ventricular septal defect in which there is an abnormal opening between the left and right ventricles, causing oxygenated blood (from the left ventricle) to mix with deoxygenated blood (from the right ventricle) as a result of left-to-right shunting.
- Pericarditis is swelling and inflammation of the pericardium, the thin double-layered sac surrounding the

heart, as a result of injury such as an acute MI, infection, inflammatory disorder, trauma, cancer, or congenital causes. Dressler syndrome, also known as post-MI syndrome, is the late pericarditis that occurs about 2–3 weeks after a MI with an unknown pathogenesis that is considered to be autoimmune.

- Cardiac tamponade is a life-threatening condition of increased pericardial pressure as a result of blood or fluid buildup between the myocardium and the pericardium.

24.7 Valvular Disorders

Differentiate the causes, classification, underlying pathogenesis, and clinical manifestations of valvular disorders and approaches to diagnosis and treatment of these conditions across the lifespan.

- Valvular disorders include problems that disrupt flow through atria and ventricles of the heart as a result of abnormal functioning of one or more of the four heart valves. These disorders include stenosis, regurgitation, and prolapse.

REVIEW QUESTIONS

1. Which of the following diagnoses would be appropriate for a client who is having leg pain while walking?
   a. Stroke
   b. Myocardial infarction
   c. Claudication
   d. Heart failure
2. According to the American Heart Association, there are seven modifiable risk factors. Which of the following is a modifiable risk factor? (Select all that apply.)
   a. Physical activity
   b. Blood pressure
   c. Diastolic heart failure
   d. Stroke
3. You are a nurse caring for a client who has been diagnosed with CAD. Which of the following procedures is used to diagnose the client?
   a. Coronary arteriogram
   b. Family history
   c. Symptoms
   d. Physical examination
4. What part of the cardiac conduction system is considered the pacemaker?
   a. The right ventricle
   b. The AV node
   c. The SA node
   d. The bundle branch
5. Which of the following symptoms indicate that a male client is having a STEMI? (Select all that apply.)
   a. Jaw pain
   b. Crushing pain
   c. Indigestion
   d. Flulike symptoms
6. You are a nurse educating a client about a procedure that may be used to identify whether the client is at risk for sudden cardiac death. Which procedure is this?
   a. Coronary angiogram
   b. ECG
   c. Electrophysiologic study
   d. Coronary arteriogram
7. Which of the following is not a valve in the heart?
   a. Tricuspid
   b. Aortic
   c. Mitral
   d. Vesicoureteral
8. Which of the following is not a risk factor for mitral regurgitation?
   a. Old age
   b. Male sex
   c. Heart failure
   d. History of ACS

ANSWERS

Answers to Review Questions can be found in Appendix A. Answers to Case Study and Check Your Progress questions are available on the faculty resources site. Please consult with your instructor.

RECOMMENDED WEBSITES

Assessing Cardiovascular Risk: Systematic Evidence Review from the Risk Assessment Work Group
https://www.nhlbi.nih.gov/health-pro/guidelines/in-develop/cardiovascular-risk-reduction/risk-assessment

Cardiovascular Disease (30-Year Risk)
https://www.framinghamheartstudy.org/risk-functions/cardiovascular-disease/30-year-risk.php#

Cardiac Conduction System
https://medlineplus.gov/ency/anatomyvideos/000021.htm

Hands-Only CPR
http://cpr.heart.org/AHAECC/CPRAndECC/Programs/HandsOnlyCPR/UCM_473196_Hands-Only-CPR.jsp

My Life Check - Life's Simple 7
http://www.heart.org/HEARTORG/Conditions/My-Life-Check---Lifes-Simple-7_UCM_471453_Article.jsp#.VvWmfceYei4

Resources for Health Professionals
https://www.nhlbi.nih.gov/health-pro/resources#heart

Watch, Learn, and Live: American Heart Association's Interactive Cardiovascular Library
http://watchlearnlive.heart.org/CVML_Player.php

REFERENCES

1. Wilson, P., & Douglas, P. (2015). Epidemiology of coronary heart disease. *UpToDate*. Available at http://www.uptodate.com/contents/epidemiology-of-coronary-heart-disease
2. Mozaffarian, D., Benjamin, E. J., Go, A. S., et al. (2015). Heart disease and stroke statistics—2015 update: A report from the American Heart Association. *Circulation, 131*(4), e29–e322.
3. Stone, P. H. (2013). *Diagnosis: Coronary artery disease.* Harvard Medical School Special Health Report. Cambridge, MA: Harvard Health Publications.
4. National Heart, Lung, and Blood Institute. (2016). *Who is at risk for coronary heart disease?* Available at http://www.nhlbi.nih.gov/health/health-topics/topics/cad/atrisk
5. Valtorta, N. K., Kanaan, M., Gilbody, S., Ronzi, S., & Hanratty, B. (2016). Loneliness and social isolation as risk factors for coronary heart disease and stroke: Systematic review and meta-analysis of longitudinal observational studies. *Heart, 102*(13), 987–989.
6. Vafaeimanesh, J., Hejazi, S. F., Damanpak, V., Vahedian, M., Sattari, M., & Seyyedmajidi, M. (2014). Association of Helicobacter pylori infection with coronary artery disease: Is Helicobacter pylori a risk factor? *Scientific World Journal, 2014*, 6.
7. Vedin, O., Hagström, E., Gallup, D., et al. (2015). Periodontal disease in patients with chronic coronary heart disease: Prevalence and association with cardiovascular risk factors. *European Journal of Preventive Cardiology, 22*(6), 771–778.
8. Mu, F., Rich-Edwards, J., Rimm, E. B., Spiegelman, D,. & Missmer, S. A. (2016). Endometriosis and risk of coronary heart disease. *Circulation: Cardiovascular Quality and Outcomes, 9*, 257–264.
9. Kurth, T., Winter, A. C., Eliassen, A. H., et al. (2016). Migraine and risk of cardiovascular disease in women: Prospective cohort study. *BMJ, 353*, i2610.
10. Boudi, F. (2016). Risk factors for coronary artery disease. *Medscape*. Available at http://emedicine.medscape.com/article/164163-overview.
11. Zöller, B., Li, X., Sundquist, J., & Sundquist, K. (2012). Multiplex sibling history of coronary heart disease is a strong risk factor for coronary heart disease. *European Heart Journal, 33*(22), 2849–2855.
12. Deloukas, P., Kanoni, S., Willenborg, C., et al. (2013). Large-scale association analysis identifies new risk loci for coronary artery disease. *Nature Genetics, 45*(1), 25–33.
13. Shrivastava, A., Singh, H., Raizada, A., & Singh, S. (2014). C-reactive protein, inflammation and coronary heart disease. *Egyptian Heart Journal, 67*(2), 89–97.
14. Morrow, D. (2016). C-reactive protein in cardiovascular disease. *UpToDate*. Available at http://www.uptodate.com/contents/c-reactive-protein-in-cardiovascular-disease
15. Stein, E. A., & Raal, F. (2016). Future directions to establish lipoprotein(a) as a treatment for atherosclerotic cardiovascular disease. *Cardiovascular Drugs and Therapy, 30*(1), 101–108.
16. Dong, C., Rundek, T., Wright, C. B., Anwar, Z., Elkind, M. S., & Sacco, R. L. (2012). Ideal cardiovascular health predicts lower risks of myocardial infarction, stroke, and vascular death across whites, blacks, and Hispanics: The northern Manhattan study. *Circulation, 125*(24), 2975–2984.
17. Gardener, H., Wright, C. B., Dong, C., et al. (2016). Ideal cardiovascular health and cognitive aging in the Northern Manhattan study. *Journal of the American Heart Association, 4*(3), e002731.
18. Kumar, V., Abbas, A. K., & Aster, J. C. (2015). *Robbins and Cotran pathologic basis of disease* (9th ed.). Philadelphia, PA: Elsevier.
19. Mancini, M. C. (2015). Heart anatomy. *Medscape*. Available at http://emedicine.medscape.com/article/905502-overview
20. Klugherz, B., & Kolanksy, D. (2016). Coronary collateral circulation. *UpToDate*. Available at http://www.uptodate.com/contents/coronary-collateral-circulation
21. Mann, DL., Zipes, D. P., Libby, P., Bonow, R. O., & Braunwald, E. (2015). *Braunwald's heart disease: A textbook of cardiovascular medicine* (10th ed.). Philadelphia, PA: Elsevier.
22. Rajendra, P., Rengarajan, T., Thangavel J., et al. (2013). The vascular endothelium and human disease. *International Journal of Biological Sciences, 9*(10), 1057–1069.
23. Zhang, M., Malik, A. B., & Rehman, J. (2014). Endothelial progenitor cells and vascular repair. *Current Opinion in Hematology, 21*(3), 224–228.
24. Robinson, J. G., & Gidding, S. S. (2014). Curing atherosclerosis should be the next major cardiovascular prevention goal. *Journal of the American College of Cardiology, 63*(25, Pt. A), 2779–2785.
25. Leening, M. J., Berry, J. D., & Allen, N. B. (2016). Lifetime perspectives on primary prevention of atherosclerotic cardiovascular disease. *JAMA, 315*(14), 1449–1450.
26. Wallace, M. L., Ricco, J. A., & Barrett, B. (2014). Screening strategies for cardiovascular disease in asymptomatic adults. *Primary Care, 41*(2), 371–397.
27. Ritchey, M. D., Wall, H. K., Gillespie, C., George, M. G., & Jamal, A. (2014). Million hearts: Prevalence of leading cardiovascular disease risk factors—United States, 2005–2012. *Morbidity and Mortality Weekly Report (MMWR), 63*(21), 462–467.
28. Stewart, R. A., Wallentin, L., Benatar, J., et al. (2016). Dietary patterns and the risk of major adverse cardiovascular events in a global study of high-risk patients with stable coronary heart disease. *European Heart Journal, 37*(25), 1993–2001.
29. Clarke, R., Bennett, D. A., Parish, S., et al. (2012). Homocysteine and coronary heart disease: Meta-analysis of *MTHFR* case-control studies, avoiding publication bias. *PLoS Medicine, 9*(2), e1001177.
30. Peller, M., Ozierański, K., Balsam, P., Grabowski, M., Filipiak, K. J., & Opolski, G. (2015). Influence of beta-blockers on endothelial function: A meta-analysis of randomized controlled trials. *Cardiology Journal, 22*(6), 708–716.

31. Stone, N. J., Robinson, J. G., Lichtenstein, A. H., et al. (2014). 2013 ACC/AHA guideline on the treatment of blood cholesterol to reduce atherosclerotic cardiovascular risk in adults: A report of the American College of Cardiology/American Heart Association Task Force on Practice Guidelines. *Circulation, 129*(25, Suppl. 2), S1–S45.
32. Leebmann, J., Roeseler, E., Julius, U., et al. (2013). Lipoprotein apheresis in patients with maximally tolerated lipid-lowering therapy, lipoprotein(a)-hyperlipoproteinemia, and progressive cardiovascular disease: Prospective observational multicenter study. *Circulation, 128*(24), 256–2576.
33. Ginting, H., Näring, G., Kwakkenbos, L., & Becker, E. S. (2015). Spirituality and negative emotions in individuals with coronary heart disease. *Journal of Cardiovascular Nursing, 30*(6), 537–545.
34. Bobadilla, R. V. (2016). Acute coronary syndrome: Focus on antiplatelet therapy. *Critical Care Nurse, 36*(1), 15–27.
35. Boden, W. E., Padala, S. K., Cabral, K. P., Buschmann, I. R., & Sidhu, M. S. (2015). Role of short-acting nitroglycerin in the management of ischemic heart disease. *Drug Design, Development and Therapy, 9*, 4793–4805.
36. Kloner, R. A., & Jennings, R. B. (2001). Consequences of brief ischemia: Stunning, preconditioning, and their clinical implications: Part 2. *Circulation, 104*(25), 3158–3167.
37. LeMone, P., Burke, K., Bauldoff, G., & Gubrud, P. (2015). *Medical-surgical nursing: Critical thinking in patient care.* Upper Saddle River, NJ: Pearson.
38. Engblom, H, & Strauss, D. G. (2011). Electrocardiography of ischemic heart disease. In O. Pahlm & G. S. Wagner (Eds.), *Multimodal cardiovascular imaging: Principles and clinical applications* (ch. 7). New York, NY: McGraw-Hill.
39. Centers for Disease Control and Prevention. (2015). Other conditions related to heart disease. Available at http://www.cdc.gov/heartdisease/other_conditions.htm
40. Fihn, S. D., Gardin, J. M., Abrams, J., et al. (2012). 2012 ACCF/AHA/ACP/AATS/PCNA/SCAI/STS guideline for the diagnosis and management of patients with stable ischemic heart disease: A report of the American College of Cardiology Foundation/American Heart Association Task Force on Practice Guidelines, and the American College of Physicians, American Association for Thoracic Surgery, Preventive Cardiovascular Nurses Association, Society for Cardiovascular Angiography and Interventions, and Society of Thoracic Surgeons. *Journal of the American College of Cardiology, 60*(24), e44–e164.
41. Thygesen, K., Alpert, J. S., Jaffe, A. S., et al. (2012). Third universal definition of myocardial infarction. *Journal of the American College of Cardiology, 60*(16), 1581–1598.
42. Löffler, A. I., & Bourque, J. M. (2016). Coronary microvascular dysfunction, microvascular angina, and management. *Current Cardiology Reports, 18*(1), 1.
43. Mygind, N. D., Michelsen, M. M., Pena, A., et al. (2016). Coronary microvascular function and cardiovascular risk factors in women with angina pectoris and no obstructive coronary artery disease: The iPOWER study. *Journal of the American Heart Association, 4*(3), e003064.
44. Amsterdam, E. A., Wenger, N. K., Brindis, R. G., et al. (2014). 2014 AHA/ACC guideline for the management of patients with non-ST-elevation acute coronary syndromes: Executive summary: A report of the American College of Cardiology/American Heart Association Task Force on Practice Guidelines. *Circulation, 130*(25), 2354–2394.
45. Amsterdam, E. A., & Wenger, N. K. (2015). The 2014 American College of Cardiology ACC/American Heart Association guideline for the management of patients with non-ST-elevation acute coronary syndromes: Ten contemporary recommendations to aid clinicians in optimizing patient outcomes. *Clinical Cardiology, 38*(2), 121–123.
46. Amsterdam, E. A., Wenger, N. K., Brindis, R. G., et al. (2014). 2014 AHA/ACC guideline for the management of patients with non-ST-elevation acute coronary syndromes: A report of the American College of Cardiology/American Heart Association Task Force on Practice Guidelines. *Journal of the American College of Cardiology, 64*(24), e139–e228.
47. Bajaj, N. S., Kalra, R., Aggarwal, H., et al. (2015). Comparison of approaches to revascularization in patients with multivessel coronary artery disease presenting with st-segment elevation myocardial infarction: Meta-analyses of randomized control trials. *Journal of the American Heart Association, 4*(12), e002540.
48. Maddox, T. M., Stanislawski, M. A., Grunwald, G. K., et al. (2014). Nonobstructive coronary artery disease and risk of myocardial infarction. *JAMA, 312*(17), 1754–1763.
49. Pope, C. A., Muhlestein, J. B., Anderson, J. L., et al. (2015). Short-term exposure to fine particulate matter air pollution is preferentially associated with the risk of ST-segment elevation acute coronary events. *Journal of the American Heart Association, 4*(12), e002506.
50. Kashef, Z. (2016). Gender gap in death from heart attack is global, Yale-led study finds. *YaleNews*. Available at http://news.yale.edu/2016/04/04/gender-gap-death-heart-attack-global-yale-led-study-finds
51. Fanaroff, A. C., Schulteis, R. D., Pieper, K. S., Rao, S. V., & Newby, L. K. (2015). Simplified predictive instrument to rule out acute coronary syndromes in a high-risk population. *Journal of the American Heart Association, 4*(12), e002351.
52. O'Gara, P. T., Kushner, F. G., Ascheim, D. D., et al. (2013). 2013 ACCF/AHA guideline for the management of ST-elevation myocardial infarction: Executive summary: A report of the American College of Cardiology Foundation/American Heart Association Task Force on Practice Guidelines: Developed in collaboration with the American College of Emergency Physicians and Society for Cardiovascular Angiography and Interventions. *Catheterization and Cardiovascular Interventions, 82*(1), E1–E27.
53. O'Donoghue, M. L., Glaser, R., Aylward, P. E., et al. (2015). Rationale and design of the losmapimod to inhibit p38 MAP kinase as a therapeutic target and modify outcomes after an acute coronary syndrome trial. *American Heart Journal, 169*(5), 622–630.e626.
54. O'Donoghue, M. L., Glaser, R., Cavender, M. A., et al. (2016). Effect of losmapimod on cardiovascular outcomes in patients hospitalized with acute myocardial infarction: A randomized clinical trial. *JAMA, 315*(15), 1591–1599.
55. Gerbin, K. A., & Murry, C. E. (2015). The winding road to regenerating the human heart. *Cardiovascular Pathology, 24*(3), 133–140.
56. Celermajer, D. S., Chow, C. K., Marijon, E., Anstey, N. M., & Woo, K. S. (2012). Cardiovascular disease in the developing world: Prevalences, patterns, and the potential of early disease detection. *Journal of the American College of Cardiology, 60*(14), 1207–1216.
57. Kondur, A., Afonso, L., & Hari, P. (2014). Complications of myocardial infarction. *Medscape*. Available at http://emedicine.medscape.com/article/164924.overview
58. Wali, V., & Yatiraj, S. (2014). Study of serum sodium and potassium in acute myocardial infarction. *Journal of Clinical and Diagnostic Research, 8*(11), CC07–CC09.
59. Kieboom, B. C., Niemeijer, M. N., Leening, M. J., et al. (2016). Serum magnesium and the risk of death from coronary heart disease and sudden cardiac death. *Journal of the American Heart Association, 5*(1), e002707.
60. Barrett, P. M., Komatireddy, R., Haaser, S., et al. (2014). Comparison of 24-hour Holter monitoring with 14-day novel adhesive patch electrocardiographic monitoring. *American Journal of Medicine, 127*(1), 95.e11–e97.
61. Carter, L., Gardner, M., Magee, K., et al. (2016). An integrated management approach to atrial fibrillation. *Journal of the American Heart Association, 5*(1), e002950.
62. U.S. Department of Health and Human Services. (2016). *Recently-approved devices*. Available at https://www.fda.gov/MedicalDevices/ProductsandMedicalProcedures/DeviceApprovalsandClearances/Recently-ApprovedDevices/default.htm

63. Reynolds, D., Duray, G. Z., Omar, R., et al. (2016). A leadless intracardiac transcatheter pacing system. *New England Journal of Medicine, 374*(6), 533–541.
64. Piccini, J. P., Allen, L. A., Kudenchuk, P. J., et al. (2016). Wearable cardioverter-defibrillator therapy for the prevention of sudden cardiac death: A science advisory from the American Heart Association. *Circulation, 133*(17), 1715–1727.
65. Shirani, J., Alaeddini, J., & Brofferio, A. (2014). Myocardial rupture. *Medscape*. Available at http://emedicine.medscape.com/article/156455-overview
66. Shapira, O. M. (2016). Left ventricular aneurysm and pseudoaneurysm following acute myocardial infarction. *UptoDate*. Available at http://www.uptodate.com/contents/left-ventricular-aneurysm-and-pseudoaneurysm-following-acute-myocardial-infarction
67. Bhimji, S. (2015). Post infarction ventricular septal rupture. *Medscape*. Available at http://emedicine.medscape.com/article/428240-overview
68. Grasso, A. W., & Brener, S. J. (2014). Complications of acute myocardial infarction. *Disease Management*. Available at http://www.clevelandclinicmeded.com/medicalpubs/diseasemanagement/cardiology/complications-of-acute-myocardial-infarction
69. Schiavone, W. A. (2013). Cardiac tamponade: 12 pearls in diagnosis and management. *Cleveland Clinic Journal of Medicine, 80*(2), 109–116.
70. Zeng, Y. I., Sun, R., Li, X., Liu, M., Chen, S., & Zhang, P. (2016). Pathophysiology of valvular heart disease. *Experimental and Therapeutic Medicine, 11*(4), 1184–1188.
71. Nishimura, R. A., Otto, C. M., Bonow, R. O., et al. (2014). 2014 AHA/ACC guideline for the management of patients with valvular heart disease: A report of the American College of Cardiology/American Heart Association Task Force on Practice Guidelines. *Journal of the American College of Cardiology, 63*(22), e57–e185.
72. Vesely, M. R., Benitez, R. M., Robinson, S. W., Collins, J. A., Dawood, M. Y., & Gammie, J. S. (2015). Surgical and transcatheter mitral valve repair for severe chronic mitral regurgitation: A review of clinical indications and patient assessment. *Journal of the American Heart Association, 4*(12), e002424.
73. Collier, P., Phelan, D., & Griffin B. P. (2014). Mitral valve disease: Stenosis and regurgitation. *Disease Management*. Available at http://www.clevelandclinicmeded.com/medicalpubs/diseasemanagement/cardiology/mitral-valve-disease
74. Ali, N. (2015). Tetralogy of Fallot. *Journal of the American Academy of Phyisican Assistants, 28*(6), 65–66.
75. Harold, J. G. (2014). Cardiology patient page: Screening for critical congenital heart disease in newborns. *Circulation, 130*(9), e79–e81.

Chapter 25
Cardiac Structural Disorders

Laura Robbins-Frank and Dawna Martich

Chapter Outline and Learning Outcomes

25.1 Overview and Case Studies

Discuss the statistics related to structural heart defects, the impact of the environment on their etiology, and concepts related to structural heart defects.

25.2 Structure of the Pediatric Cardiovascular System

Outline the structure of the pediatric cardiovascular system.

25.3 Prenatal and Postnatal Hemodynamics

Describe prenatal and postnatal hemodynamics and the screening used to detect critical congenital heart defects in newborns.

25.4 Genetics and Genomics of Critical Congenital Heart Defects

Differentiate the relationships among genetic factors, clinical features, and outcomes in individuals with congenital heart defects.

25.5 Congenital Heart Defects

Differentiate the causes, classification, underlying pathogenesis, and clinical manifestations of the four categories of congenital heart defects.

25.6 Linking Pathophysiology to Diagnosis and Treatment of Critical Congenital Heart Defects

Link the pathophysiology of congenital heart defects to the diagnosis and treatment of the disorders in infants.

25.7 Linking Pathophysiology to Diagnosis and Treatment of Adult Congenital Heart Disorders

Link the pathophysiology of congenital heart disorders to the diagnosis and treatment of the disorders in adults.

25.8 Noncongenital Structural Heart Defects

Differentiate the causes, classification, underlying pathogenesis, and clinical manifestations of noncongenital structural heart defects.

25.9 Linking Pathophysiology to Diagnosis and Treatment of Noncongenital Structural Heart Defects

Link the pathophysiology of noncongenital structural heart defects to the diagnosis and treatment of the disorders.

KEY TERMS

Adult congenital heart disorder (ACHD), 629
Atrial septal defect (ASD), 620
Coarctation of the aorta (COA), 624
Congenital heart defects (CHDs), 613
Critical congenital heart disease (CCHD), 616
Decreased pulmonary blood flow defects, 623
Hypoplastic left heart syndrome (HLHS), 625
Increased pulmonary blood flow defects, 619
Mixed blood flow defects, 626
Obstructed systemic blood flow defects, 624
Patent ductus arteriosus (PDA), 622
Pulmonary stenosis (PS), 624
Structural heart defects (SHDs), 613
Tetralogy of Fallot (TOF), 623
Total anomalous pulmonary venous return (TAPVR), 626
Transposition of the great arteries (TGA), 626
Ventricular septal defect (VSD), 620

ABBREVIATIONS

ACHD—adult congenital heart disorder
ASD—atrial septal defect
CCHD—critical congenital heart disorder
CHD—congenital heart defect
COA—coarctation of the aorta
HLHS—hypoplastic left heart syndrome
PDA—patent ductus arteriosus
PS—pulmonary stenosis
RHD—rheumatic heart disease
SHD—structural heart defect
TAPVR—total anomalous venous return
TGA—transposition of the great arteries
TOF—tetralogy of Fallot
VSD—ventricular septal defect

25.1 Chapter Overview and Case Studies

Structural heart defects (SHDs) are a group of structural abnormalities that occur during gestation and result in abnormal blood flow through the heart in the postnatal period. **Congenital heart defects (CHDs)** are grouped into the category of congenital heart disease, which was defined in a classic paper in 1971 a "gross structural abnormality of the heart or intrathoracic great vessels that is actually or potentially of functional significance."[1] The incidence of CHD appears to have increased in recent years. According to Hoffman and Kaplan, the probable reasons for this apparent increase are multifactorial.[2] Studies before the 1980s discussed only infants with severe CHD who were referred to cardiac centers; pediatricians had little interest in these defects, as they did not manage these patients in their practices; cardiac surgery had not yet reached the advanced techniques that are now available; echocardiography was not sophisticated enough to diagnose such defects; cardiac catheterization was the main diagnostic test available to these patients; and cardiac surgeons were reluctant to perform this procedure on this population.[2] The increased incidence that is seen in the literature today is attributed mainly to the improved diagnostic abilities of echocardiography in both the prenatal and postnatal periods.

According to the Centers for Disease Control and Prevention (CDC), 1% of infants born annually are diagnosed with a congenital heart defect, resulting in approximately 40,000 infants with CHD each year.[3] Of this number, 25% have a critical congenital heart defect that will require surgical intervention during the first year of life, often in the first few months of life. The CDC reports that CHDs are the leading cause of birth defect–associated deaths in the infant population younger than 1 year of age. The CDC statistics show that the survival rate for infants diagnosed with a noncritical CHD is 97% in the first year and 95% up to age 18 years.[3] These survival rates are presenting the medical community with a new patient population, adults with CHD, which is resulting in a new morbidity classification.

It has been determined that these heart defects develop during the embryonic period of cardiac development, mainly in weeks 6–9. Since the defect develops in utero during gestation, it is called a congenital defect in contrast to an inherited defect.

In the mid 20th century, it was the accepted medical theory that CHD occurred in isolation and that the incidence was relatively low. Beginning in the late 1960s, as more infants with CHD were diagnosed, this theory moved toward a multifactorial etiology. Since then, many theories have been proposed, and it commonly accepted now that the development of CHD is indeed multifactorial, a combination of environment and genetics. The genetic implications, which were overlooked in the past, are now at the forefront of CHD incidence research. In the 21st century, it is important to investigate underlying genetic patterns, such as deletions, duplications, or mutations, as there may be other important organ involvement and increased reproductive risks that the family needs to consider, as well as prognostic information for clinical outcomes. As genetic research proceeds, more information will become available about the possible underlying genetic involvement as well as tests for diagnostic purposes.

The environmental contributions to CHD include but are not limited to fetal exposure to drugs, such as antiepileptics, antipsychotics, antidepressants, and anticoagulants; alcohol; cigarette smoking; and secondhand smoke. Additionally, maternal conditions such as viral infections, metabolic disorders such as diabetes mellitus or phenylketonuria, and increased maternal age may all affect the development of CHD.

Concepts Related to Cardiac Structural Disorders

Even though the major concept affected by SHDs is perfusion, the changes in heart structure also affect oxygenation, nutrition, fluid balance, and energy. The environment and exposure to infections may have precipitated the development of the SHD. See **Figure 25.1** ■ for additional information about the concept structure and links to symptoms. These concepts will be addressed throughout the chapter.

Case Studies

The following cases will be addressed throughout the chapter to assist in application of chapter content to clinical situations that involve individuals with structural heart disorders.

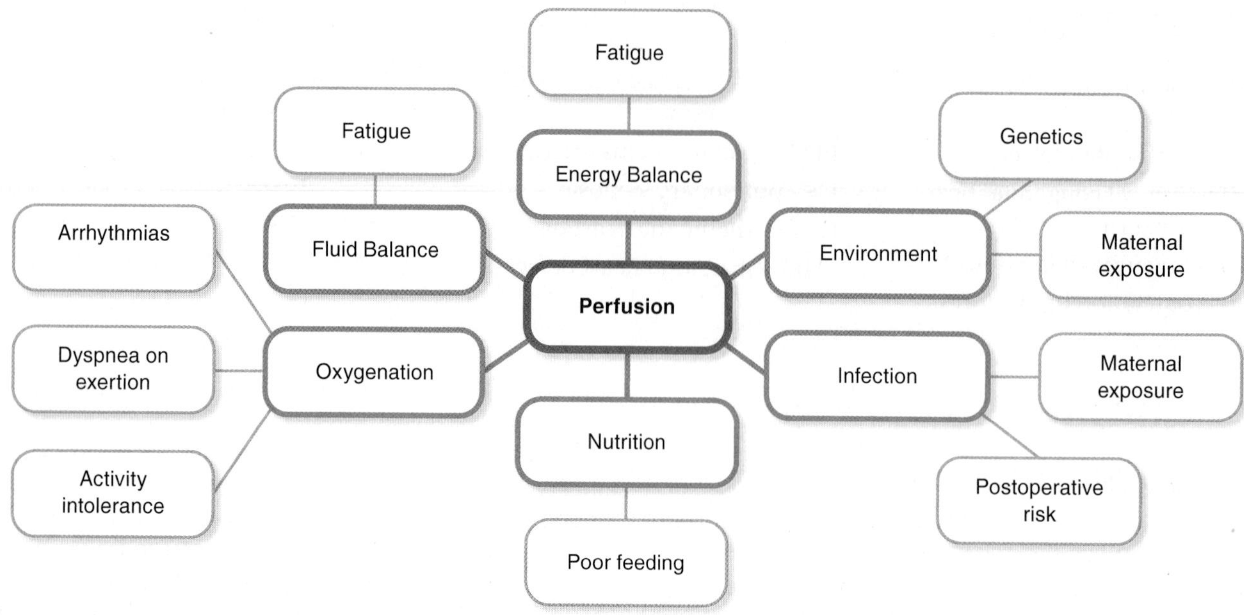

Figure 25.1 ■ Concepts related to structural heart defects.

Connor Whelan: Introduction

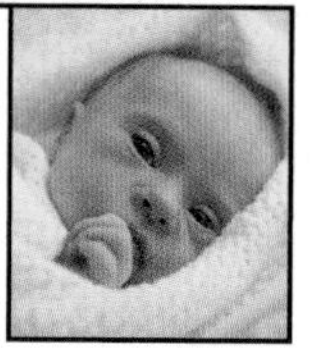

Connor Whelan was born at 38 weeks' gestation after an uneventful pregnancy and delivery. Connor weighed 3.2 kg (7 pounds) at birth. He had an Apgar score of 6 at 1 minute with points taken off for muscle tone and cry; his 5-minute Apgar score was 8 with points taken off for muscle tone. These scores were not worrisome to the neonatologist, as Connor had a prenatal diagnosis of Down syndrome based on the alpha-fetoprotein (AFP) test done at 16 weeks' gestation and findings suggestive of Down syndrome on the level 2 prenatal ultrasound. Connor's parents express their desire to keep Connor with them and room in. In the delivery room, Connor's vital signs were pulse 150, respirations 70, blood pressure 50/35 on his left leg, SpO_2 94% on room air on his right hand.

1. Interpret the vital signs for Connor using these guidelines for expected vital signs for a newborn: pulse 120–160, respirations 40–60, temperature 36.5–37.5°C, blood pressure 60–70/31–45, $SpO_2 > 90\%$

Geraldine McNamara: Introduction

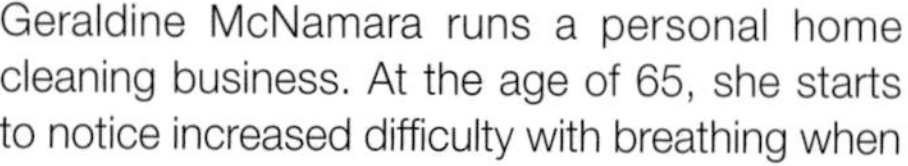

Geraldine McNamara runs a personal home cleaning business. At the age of 65, she starts to notice increased difficulty with breathing when she is performing routine housecleaning chores. Because Mrs. McNamara smoked for over 40 years, she attributes her shortness of breath to years of smoking. Within a few months, Mrs. McNamara decides to retire and turns the business over to her daughters. During her most recent visit with her healthcare provider, Mrs. McNamara mentions the increasing shortness of breath with walking and performing light chores around the house. In addition, she notes that since retiring, her ankles have been swollen nearly every day, making wearing shoes uncomfortable.

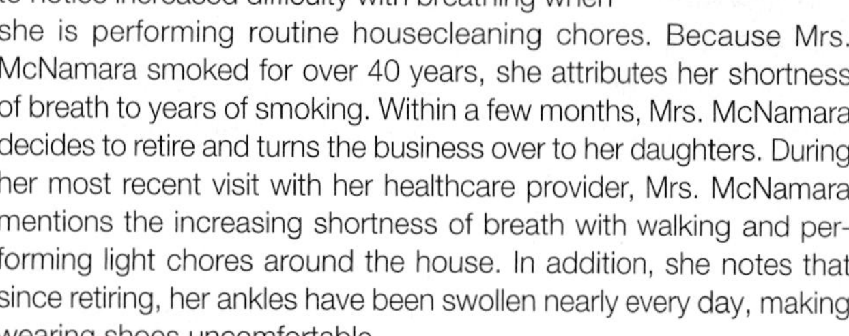

1. What symptoms is Mrs. McNamara experiencing that are worrisome for someone her age?

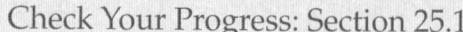

Check Your Progress: Section 25.1

1. The incidence of CHD seems to have risen in recent years. This can be attributed to what factor(s)?
2. Why is CHD considered a congenital defect rather than an inherited defect?
3. What factors contribute to the development of CHD in children?

25.2 Structure of the Pediatric Cardiovascular System

Differentiation of the four chambers of the heart begins in the sixth week of gestation and is completed by the ninth week. The mother might not even know that she is pregnant while this complex system is developing; this situation can contribute to the environmental exposures that can have a deleterious impact on the structural outcome of heart development.

Once implantation of the embryo has occurred, around the 12th day of human development, the cells begin to undergo mitosis, resulting in differentiation of cell types. By the 17th day of human development, the primary heart field has developed. The human heart is the first organ to fully develop and function in utero. On day 26 of human development, the neural tube forms after neurulation is complete. The cephalocaudal and lateral folding on day 20 result in development of the bilateral endocardial tubes into the ventral midline of the embryo. The fusion of the heart

Age (in weeks)								
1	2	3	4	5	6	7	8	9
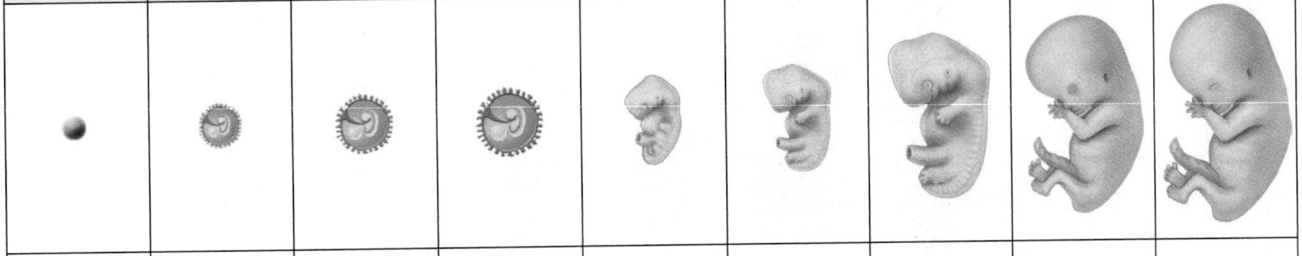								
Zygote cleaves; blastocyst implants	Two-layered embryo forms	Neural tube begins to form	Neural tube closes; heart beats; gill grooves, tail, and arm buds form	Incipient eye parts form	External ear and webbed fingers form; tail and gill grooves start to disappear	Webbed toes and eyelids form; bones begin to harden; back straightens	Arms bend at elbow; fingers are distinct; genitalia begin to differentiate	Major parts of brain are present; toes separate
					Heart defects develop			

Figure 25.2 ■ At the end of 9 weeks gestation, the main cardiac structures are developed, and any defects have already occurred.

tube occurs on days 21 and 22, leading to the first "heart" beat on day 22. Weeks 3–4 end with the looping of the heart tube and the accretion of the cells from the primary and secondary heart fields. In addition, the proepicardial cells line the outer layer of the heart tube, which will eventually form into the epicardium and coronary vasculature. By the end of the sixth week of gestation, the cardiac neural crest has migrated through the aortic arches and has entered the outflow tract of the heart, which is completed by the ninth week, resulting in the completion of the ventricular septation. Further differentiation of the four chambers continues until birth, but by the end of 9 weeks' gestation, the main structures are developed, and any structural defects have already occurred (**Figure 25.2** ■).[4]

Check Your Progress: Section 25.2

1. Why can the environment have such a deleterious impact on the developing fetus?
2. When is the first heartbeat detectable?
3. During which gestational period do the structural defects mainly occur?

25.3 Prenatal and Postnatal Hemodynamics

In the fetus, oxygenated blood enters through the umbilical vein and travels to the heart via the ductus venosus bypassing the liver. It then combines with deoxygenated blood in the inferior vena cava, mixes with deoxygenated blood in the superior vena cava, and then empties into the right atrium. This blood then shunts through the foramen ovale from the right atrium to the left atrium as a result of the high right atrial pressures and the lower left atrial pressures. From the left atrium, the blood travels to the left ventricle for ejection through the aorta to the body. Some blood does travel from the right atrium to the right ventricle via the pulmonary trunk; however, this blood is shunted across the ductus arteriosus to the aorta as a result of the very high pulmonary pressures. Blood then circulates throughout the fetal body and returns via the umbilical arteries to the placenta, where it becomes reoxygenated and reenters the fetal circulation via the umbilical vein (**Figure 25.3** ■).

At birth, the infant takes its first breath, which quickly reduces the pulmonary pressures as the pulmonary vasculature dilates in response to the change in the partial pressure of oxygen. Pulmonary blood flow increases as this pulmonary pressure decreases, as does the blood flow to the left atrium as the left atrial pressure increases. After the umbilical cord has been cut, systemic vascular resistance increases in response to the decrease in the right atrial pressures. As the pressure increases in the left atrium, the foramen ovale closes shortly after birth. The ductus arteriosus should begin to close within 10–15 hours after birth, with permanent closure resulting by 21 days of life (**Figure 25.4** ■). The conditions in which the ductus arteriosus remains open include low saturations, decreased pulmonary blood flow, and pulmonary pressures that remain elevated after birth. Cardiac assessment during the neonatal period often identifies symptoms of a CHD.

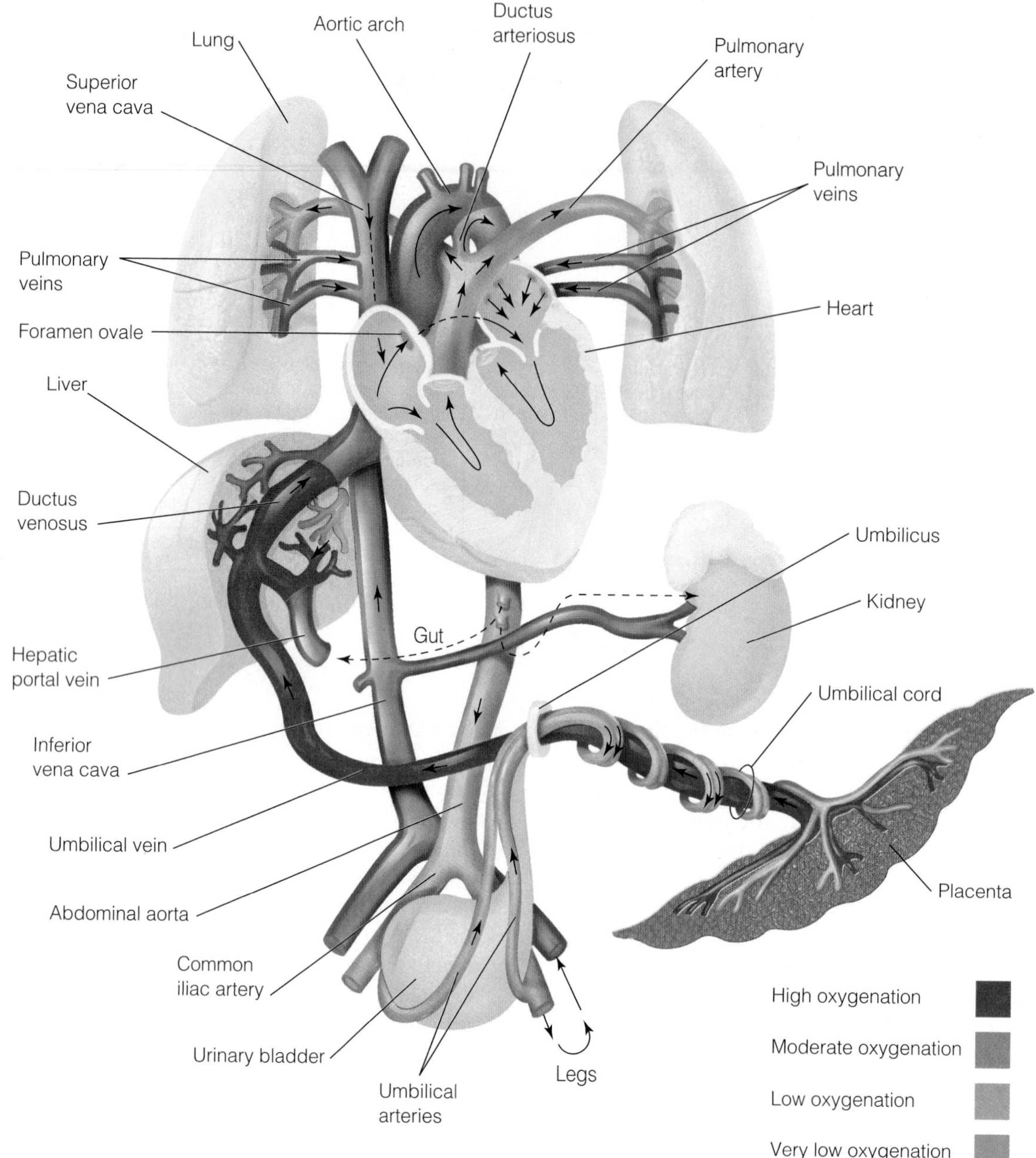

Figure 25.3 ■ Fetal circulation. Blood leaves the placenta and enters the fetus through the umbilical vein. After circulating through the fetus, the blood returns to the placenta through the umbilical arteries. The ductus venosus, the foramen ovale, and the ductus arteriosus allow the blood to bypass the fetal liver and lungs.

Critical congenital heart disease (CCHD) is a term used to refer to a group of serious congenital heart defects that usually require surgical correction within the first year of life. In September 2011, the U.S. Secretary of Health and Human Services publicly recommended that routine screening of newborns for CCHD be added to the current state-mandated newborn screenings.[5] The American Academy of Pediatrics publicly supported this recommendation in their January 2012 Policy Statement "Endorsement of Health and Human Services Recommendation for Pulse Oximetry Screening for Critical Congenital Heart Disease."[6] As of early 2017, 49 of 50 states had enacted legislation mandating routine screening of newborns for CCHD. Idaho was the only state that had yet to enact legislation and had no plans to implement it as part of the official newborn screening program.

CCHD screening should take place in the first 24–48 hours of life. It consists of a preductal and a postductal pulse oximeter reading; both sites are monitored for 5 minutes, and then the reading is recorded. A negative CCHD screening, or a pass, would include pulse oximeter readings of greater than 95% on room air on the right hand (preductal) and either foot (postductal) or less than a 3% difference between the preductal and postductal readings. A positive CCHD screening or a fail would be SpO_2 of 90–94% in the hand and foot or a hand–foot absolute difference greater than

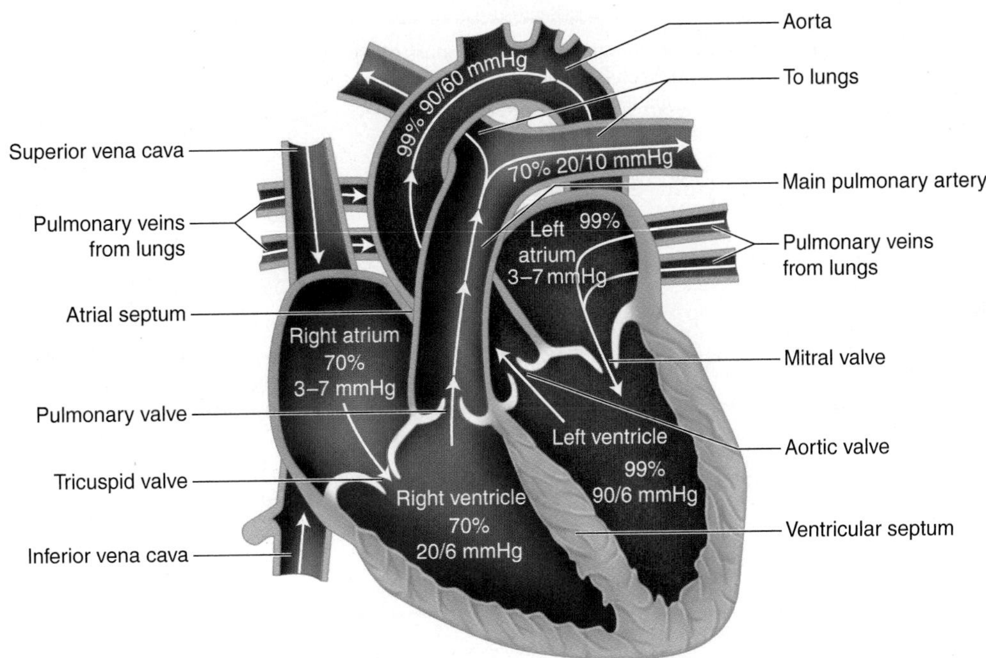

Figure 25.4 ■ Anatomy of the normal heart, direction of blood flow, and the normal pressure gradients and oxygen saturation levels in the heart chambers and great arteries. The right ventricle has a lower pressure during systole than the left ventricle because less pressure is needed to pump blood to the lungs than to the rest of the body.

3%. If the first CCHD screening results in a fail, also known as a positive result, the test is repeated after 1 hour up to three times. A confirmed positive result, that is, SpO_2 of less than 90% in hand or foot or three repeated positive screens, results in referral of the infant for echocardiography and further medical evaluation.[7] **Figure 25.5** ■ illustrates this process.

Connor Whelan: Application

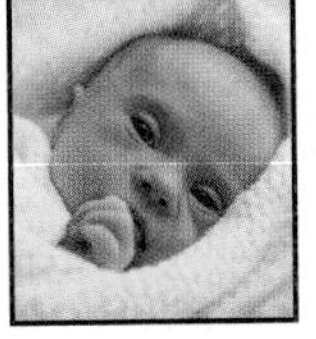

Connor's mother attempts to breastfeed him in the delivery room, but Connor has difficulty latching on and feeding. During this breastfeeding attempt, the labor and delivery nurse notes that Connor's respiratory rate increases significantly to 100 breaths per minute, and his saturations dropped to 90%. The nurse suggests that Ms. Whelan offer a bottle when Connor has difficulty latching and feeding. Connor and his mother are transferred to the postpartum floor. At 24 hours of age, Connor is examined in his mother's postpartum room by the newborn nursery nurse, who notes the following vital signs: pulse 200, respirations 84, temperature 36.4°C, blood pressure 50/30, SpO_2 93% on room air on his right hand.

2. Which vital sign is the most worrisome for the nurse in interpreting Connor's 24-hour vital signs?

Check Your Progress: Section 25.3

1. What is the purpose of the CCHD pulse oximeter screening in the first 48 hours of life?
2. What results of the CCHD pulse oximeter screening are considered suspicious for a CCHD?

25.4 Genetics and Genomics of Critical Congenital Heart Defects

In 2009, the Pediatric Cardiac Genomics Consortium, which is funded by the National Heart Lung and Blood Institute (NHLBI), created the Congenital Heart Disease Genetic Network Study (CHD GENES) to investigate relationships between genetic factors, clinical features, and outcomes in CHD.[8] Through population-based studies around the world, the CHD GENES study has concluded that epidemiologic evidence clearly indicates a very strong genetic role in the pathogenesis of CCHD. While the causes of CCHD are not clearly understood, genomic defects that cannot be readily detected with karyotyping are increasingly understood to have a role in CHD.[8] Additionally, through further research of isolated defects and syndromes, numerous gene mutations have been identified in the development of CCHD. The CHD GENES study will continue to work toward identifying the influence of genetics on the clinical outcomes and enabling development of new therapies and possibly approaches for prevention, such as newborn genetic screening. Another overarching goal is to look at how genetic variants affect neurodevelopmental outcomes of infants born with CCHD. The NHLBI has identified neurodevelopment as a critical mediator of quality of life and school success for children with CCHD. According to the NHLBI, up to 50% of children with complex CHD have neurodevelopmental abnormalities.[8]

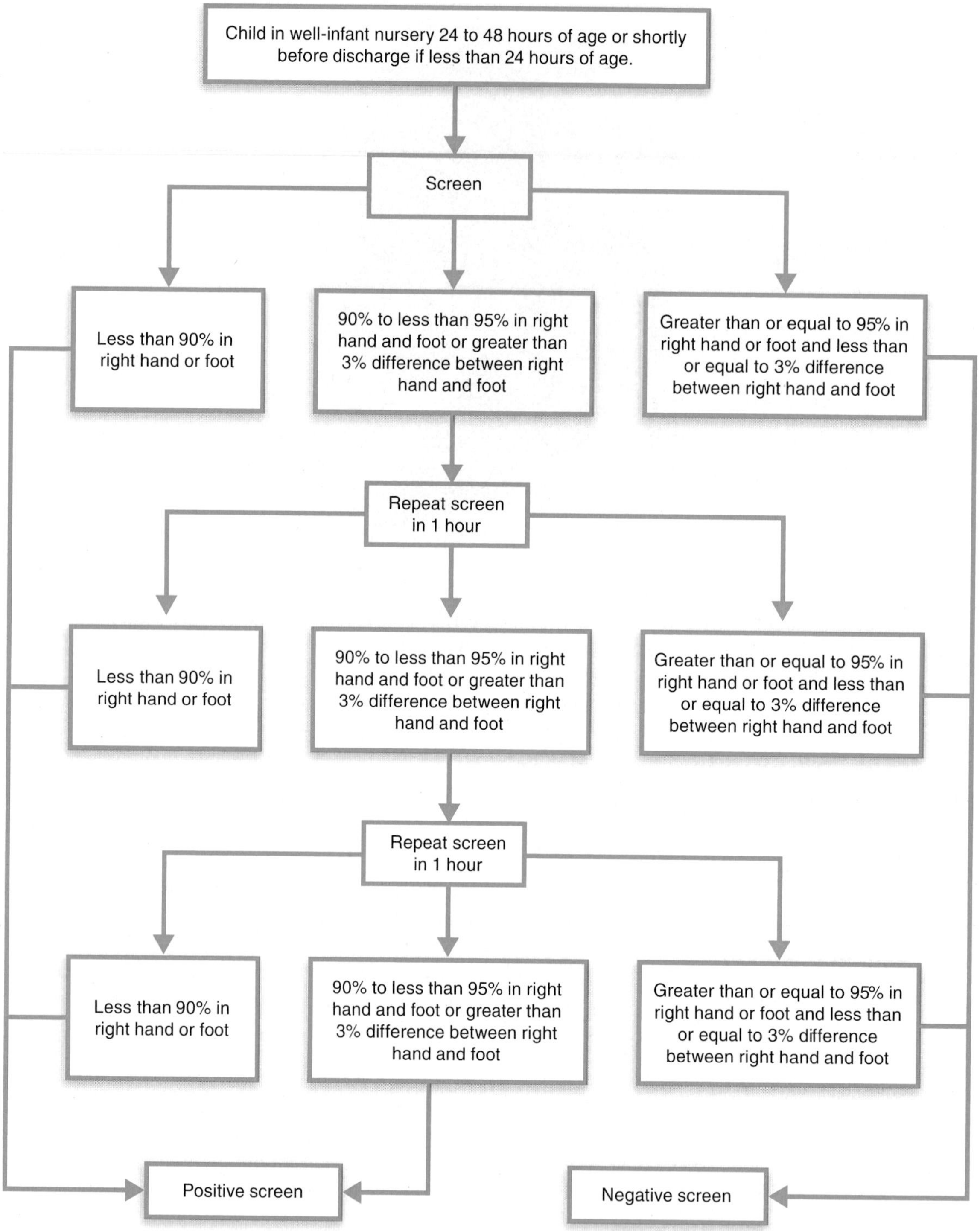

Child in well-infant nursery 24 to 48 hours of age or shortly before discharge if less than 24 hours of age.

Screen

Less than 90% in right hand or foot

90% to less than 95% in right hand and foot or greater than 3% difference between right hand and foot

Greater than or equal to 95% in right hand or foot and less than or equal to 3% difference between right hand and foot

Repeat screen in 1 hour

Less than 90% in right hand or foot

90% to less than 95% in right hand and foot or greater than 3% difference between right hand and foot

Greater than or equal to 95% in right hand or foot and less than or equal to 3% difference between right hand and foot

Repeat screen in 1 hour

Less than 90% in right hand or foot

90% to less than 95% in right hand and foot or greater than 3% difference between right hand and foot

Greater than or equal to 95% in right hand or foot and less than or equal to 3% difference between right hand and foot

Positive screen

Negative screen

Figure 25.5 ■ Algorithm for screening newborns for critical congenital heart defects.

SOURCE: Medscape, Pediatric Nursing ©2013 Jannetts Publications, Inc.

Connor Whelan: Application

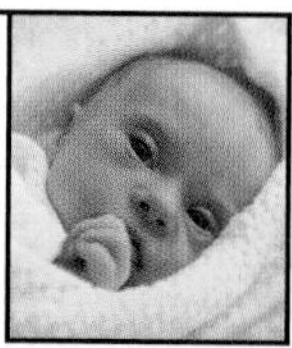

Crackles are heard in all Connor's lung fields on auscultation, and a soft murmur is appreciated. Bowel sounds are present and active in all quadrants. Color is mottled, and lower extremities are cool to the touch. Pulses are palpated and graded as 1+, nonbounding. The nurse assesses mild to moderate intercostal retractions and nasal flaring. The nurse calls the pediatrician and reports these assessment findings. The pediatrician orders a neonatal consult. The neonatologist comes to the newborn nursery, assesses Connor, and orders an arterial blood gas (ABG). A neonatal nurse comes to the newborn nursery to draw blood for the ABG. The results are as follows: pH 7.39, PaO_2 50 mmHg, $PaCO_2$ 36 mmHg, HCO_3 24 mEq/L, BE 0.

3. Interpret Connor's ABG results, and explain what is happening in his body.
4. Which assessment findings indicate that Connor might have a cardiac problem?

Check Your Progress: Section 25.4

1. The purpose of the CHD GENES study is to investigate relationships between genetic factors, clinical features, and outcomes in CCHD. Why is this important?
2. Alterations in perfusion can affect neurodevelopment. Why is the NHLBI concerned about this in children with CCHDs?

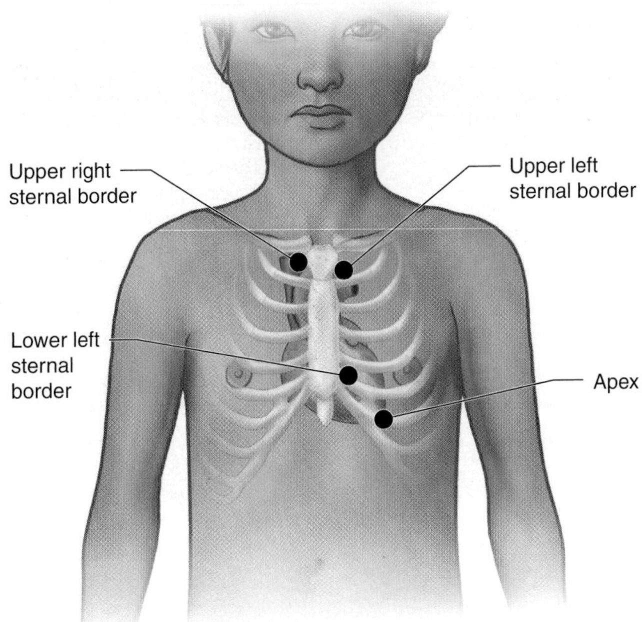

Figure 25.6 ■ Locations of heart murmurs.

25.5 Congenital Heart Defects

Alterations in the structure of the heart chambers, valves, or major vessels can all lead to the development of congenital heart defects (CHDs). These changes affect blood flow, oxygenation, and fluid balance, creating immediate or long-term manifestations.

Pathophysiology of Altered Blood Flow

In assessing a newborn in the first hours of life, it is not unusual to auscultate a murmur. A murmur indicates turbulent blood flow through a valve or congenital heart defect such as a ventricular septal defect or a ductus arteriosus. The intensity of the murmur directly correlates with the size of the defect through which the blood is flowing.

CLINICAL POINT: The larger the defect, the softer the murmur; the smaller the defect, the louder the murmur. ■

Murmurs are graded on a six-point scale to indicate intensity and pitch. A grade 1 murmur is barely audible, a grade 2 murmur is louder, and a grade 3 murmur is loud but not accompanied by a thrill. A grade 4 murmur is loud and associated with a palpable thrill. A grade 5 murmur is associated with a thrill, and the murmur can be heard with the stethoscope partially off the chest. A grade 6 murmur is audible without a stethoscope. All murmurs louder than grade 3 are considered pathologic and require further evaluation by a pediatric cardiologist. The location and intensity of the murmur are an important consideration for diagnosis (**Figure 25.6** ■).

CHDs are classified into one of four pathologic classifications. Previously, congenital heart defects were grouped according to whether or not they caused cyanosis. This type of classification can be misleading in interpreting clinical symptoms. Now, congenital heart defects are classified as follows:

1. Increased pulmonary blood flow
2. Decreased pulmonary blood flow
3. Obstructed blood flow
4. Mixed blood flow.

Table 25.1 ■ places each congenital heart defect into one of the pathologic categories and identifies where a murmur would most likely be auscultated. Diagnosis of a CCHD begins with the identification of the clinical signs and symptoms; then electrocardiography (ECG), echocardiography, and a chest x-ray are performed. The echocardiography is the most reliable diagnostic tool, and the chest x-ray can identify increased pulmonary blood flow as well as possible chamber hypertrophy.

Increased Pulmonary Blood Flow Defects

Increased pulmonary blood flow defects are the most common type of CCHD and include four different types of defects, all of which increase the blood flow to the pulmonary system. The left side of the heart has higher pressures in both the atria and the ventricles than the right side does. Because of this pressure gradient, when there is an opening between the right and left sides of the heart, as in an atrial septal defect, a ventricular septal defect, or a patent ductus arteriosus, blood naturally flows from an area of high pressure (the left side) to an area of lower pressure (the right side), resulting in an increased amount of blood moving through the pulmonary system. This movement of blood is called a shunt; when the blood moves from the left side (high pressure) to the right side (lower pressure), it is referred to as a left-to-right shunt. A murmur is heard on auscultation, and the intensity of the murmur is directly related to the turbulence of the blood flow through the defect and the size of the defect.

Table 25.1 Categories of Critical Congenital Heart Defects

Pathophysiologic Category	Congenital Cardiac Defects in Category	Location of Murmur	Clinical Manifestations
Increased pulmonary blood flow	Patent ductus arteriosus Atrial septal defect Ventricular septal defect Atrioventricular canal	Upper left sternal border Upper left sternal border Lower left sternal border Upper and lower left sternal border	Dyspnea Tachypnea Tachycardia Murmur Congestive heart failure Diaphoresis Periorbital edema Increased metabolic rate Feeding difficulties Failure to thrive Lethargy Risk for frequent respiratory infections
Decreased pulmonary blood flow	Pulmonary stenosis Tetralogy of Fallot, Pulmonary atresia Tricuspid atresia	Upper left sternal border Multiple locations Upper left sternal border Lower left sternal border	Cyanosis shortly after birth unresponsive to supplemental O_2 Dyspnea Murmur Difficulty feeding Failure to thrive Mottled skin Hypercyanotic spells Polycythemia
Obstructed systemic flow	Coarctation of the aorta Aortic stenosis Hypoplastic left heart syndrome Mitral stenosis Interrupted aortic arch	Posterior Upper right sternal border Upper left sternal border Apex Lower left sternal border	Diminished pulses Poor color Delayed capillary refill time Decreased urine output Congestive heart failure with pulmonary edema
Mixed defects	Transposition of great arteries Total anomalous pulmonary venous return Truncus arteriosus Double-outlet right ventricle	Dependent on associated defects for all of these defects	Cyanosis Poor weight gain Pulmonary congestion Congestive heart failure with increased shunting

Atrial Septal Defect

An **atrial septal defect (ASD)** is a hole in the wall (septum) between the atria that allows oxygenated blood from the left atrium to flow (shunt) to the right atrium, whereupon it moves through the tricuspid valve to the right ventricle and on to the pulmonary system (**Figure 25.7** ■). See **Table 25.1** for clinical signs and symptoms of an ASD. Treatment can be either a closed heart or open heart procedure. The closed heart procedure utilizes cardiac catheterization and the insertion of a synthetic patch on the atrial septum, closing the defect. The open heart procedure involves surgery and putting the patient on cardiac bypass during the procedure. The repair is made by affixing a synthetic patch to the septum, thereby closing the septal defect and preventing further left-to-right shunting. The size, location, and impact of the defect determine the type of procedure for closure. Once either of these procedures has been performed, the volume of blood moving to the pulmonary system decreases, resulting in a decrease in pulmonary congestion and an improvement in symptoms.

Without treatment, complications can ensue. One of the complications results from the increased volume of blood flow to the lungs, which can result in pulmonary hypertension. When this occurs, the right ventricle may become hypertrophic because of the increased pulmonary pressure it is pumping against. The long-term result of this is right-sided congestive heart failure (CHF).

Ventricular Septal Defect

A **ventricular septal defect (VSD)** is a hole in the wall (septum) between the ventricles. VSDs accounts for 25–30% of all CCHDs (**Figure 25.8** ■). As with the atrial pressures, the left ventricular pressure is higher than the right ventricular pressure; therefore, a left-to-right shunt occurs through a small to medium-sized defect (restrictive), and a murmur is heard as discussed earlier in the chapter. In a large VSD, the pressures are nearly equal; therefore, the shunting is both from left to right and from right to left. See **Table 25.1** for signs and symptoms of a VSD. If the left-to-right shunt is large, pulmonary hypertension gradually develops, and the flow across the shunt decreases. If the pulmonary vascular resistance exceeds the systemic vascular resistance, the direction of the shunt reverses, and cyanosis develops after a few years (Eisenmenger syndrome).[9]

Treatment of a VSD depends on the clinical course. In a large VSD that results in pulmonary congestions. a surgical repair is necessary along with medical management. Medical management of the VSD is aimed at reducing afterload. Afterload is the resistance the heart must overcome to eject the volume of blood from the ventricle and is expressed as

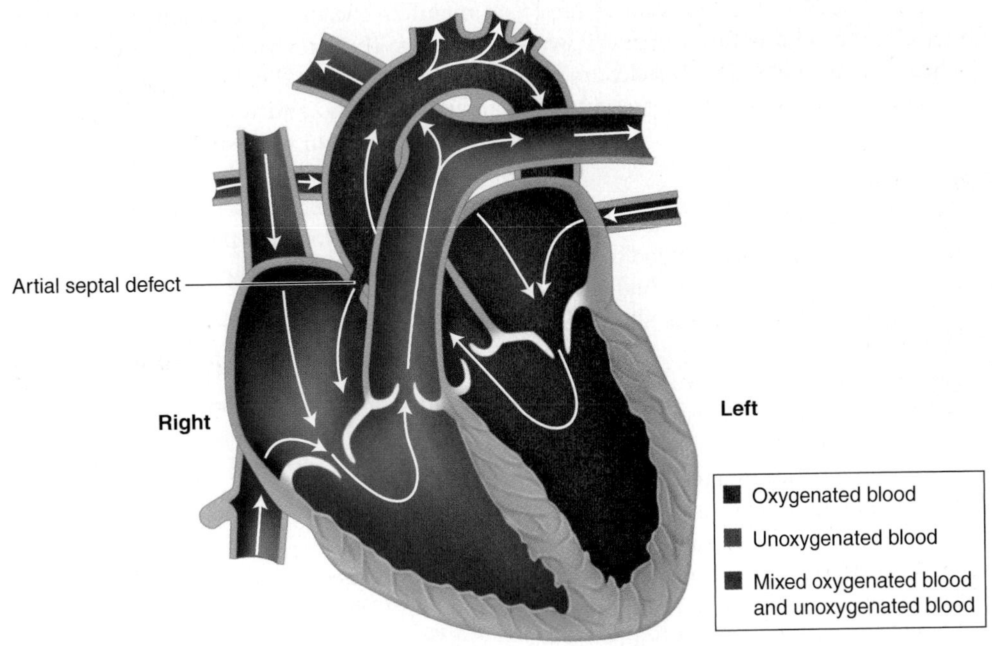

Figure 25.7 ■ In ASD, there is a hole in the wall (septum) of the atria that allows oxygenated blood from the left atrium to flow to the right atrium, whereupon it moves through the tricuspid valve to the right ventricle and on to the pulmonary system.

total peripheral resistance. Medical management includes a diuretic to help decrease pulmonary volume; an afterload-reducing agent such as an ACE inhibitor or aldosterone receptor blocker, and possibly digoxin, a cardiac glycoside agent that improves contractility of the ventricle. Surgical repair consists of an open heart procedure during which the patient is placed on cardiac bypass and the defect is repaired by using a synthetic patch. Surgical repair is indicated if the VSD is not closing on its own or is causing congestive heart failure and/or the child is not thriving. In these situations,

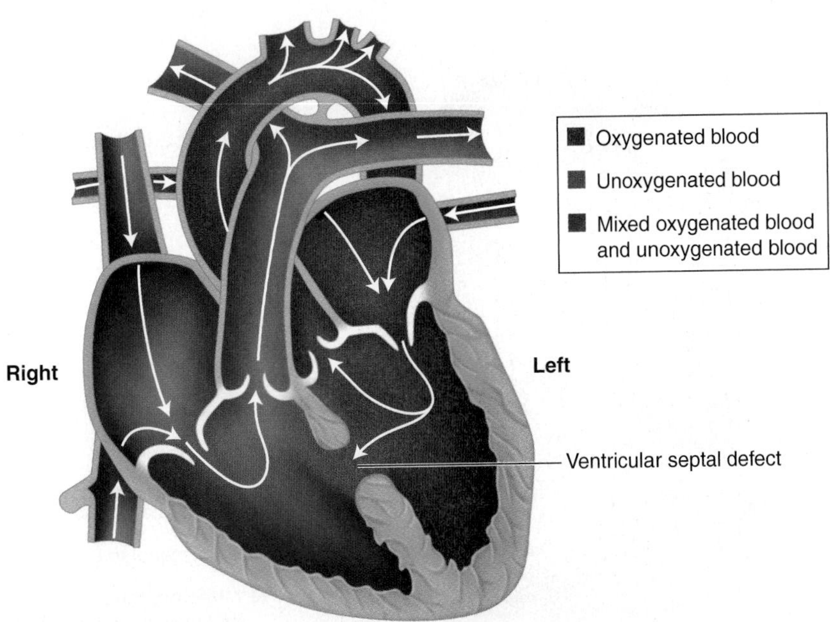

Figure 25.8 ■ In small- or medium-sized VSDs, the left ventricular pressure is higher than the right ventricle pressure, so a left-to-right shunt occurs. In large VSDs, the pressures are nearly equal, so the shunting is both from left to right and from right to left.

surgical repair is recommended in the first year of life to prevent complications. If the child is thriving and is well maintained on medical management, the VSD closure will occur later, depending on the child's clinical presentation on follow-up.

Patent Ductus Arteriosus

A **patent ductus arteriosus (PDA)** is a CHD in which the connection that is present in utero allowing blood to bypass the lungs after right ventricular ejection due to high pulmonary pressures remains open and continues to shunt blood to the aorta (**Figure 25.9** ■). PDA accounts for 5–10% of all CCHD. There is a higher incidence in premature infants and those with trisomy 21, and there is a 2:1 female:male incidence.[10] This in utero connection of the main left pulmonary artery to the aortic arch is maintained as a result of low oxygen tensions and high circulating levels of prostaglandin E2 (PGE2). Once the infant has taken the first breaths after birth, production of PGE2 decreases, and oxygen tensions rise as the pulmonary pressures fall. These changes result in the closure of the ductus over the first 48 hours of life, leaving only the fibrous ligament known as the ligamentum arteriosum. If the ductus fails to close in the first 48 hours of life, there is a left-to-right shunt across the ductus that returns blood to the pulmonary circulation. See **Table 25.1** for clinical manifestations of a PDA.

Treatment of the PDA can be medical management and/or surgical intervention. In premature infants, medical management is the first course of action and consists of administration of a nonsteroidal anti-inflammatory agent (NSAID) such as indomethacin or ibuprofen. These NSAIDs inhibit prostaglandin production, which is necessary to maintain the PDA postnatally. In addition to these medications, fluid restriction and oxygen administration are added to the medical management of the preterm infant with hemodynamically clinically significant PDA. If the medications fail to close the PDA or the infant is term and hemodynamically symptomatic, surgical intervention is necessary. In most cases, a closed heart procedure known as a catheter closure is performed. In some cases, open heart closure may be necessary.[11]

Connor Whelan: Outcome

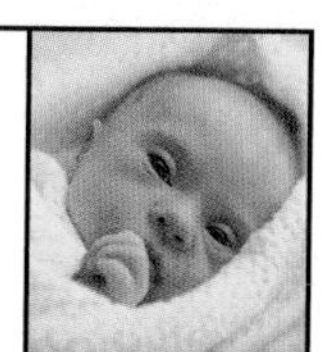

Connor's mother is concerned that he seems to struggle to eat and falls asleep within 10 minutes of trying to feed. The newborn nursery nurse calls the pediatrician, who orders a CCHD pulse oximetry screening to be completed.

The nurse places a pulse oximeter probe on Connor's right hand to assess the preductal value and another probe on Connor's left foot to assess the postductal value. At 5 minutes, the nurse records a preductal SpO_2 of 94% and a postductal SpO_2 of 89%. According to the algorithm, this is considered a positive screen, since there is a greater than 3% difference between the preductal and postductal readings. The CCHD screening protocol guides the nurse to repeat the screening in 1 hour. The second screening also results in a positive screen, the difference between the preductal and postductal readings remaining greater than 3%. The nurse notifies the pediatrician, who orders that Connor be admitted to the neonatal intensive care unit for further workup, assessment, and management. She also orders a cardiology consult.

The cardiologist performs an echocardiogram on Connor and diagnoses an atrial and ventricular septal defect. The cardiologist orders furosemide 1 mg/kg every 12 hours to manage the increased pulmonary congestion from the increased pulmonary blood flow. She

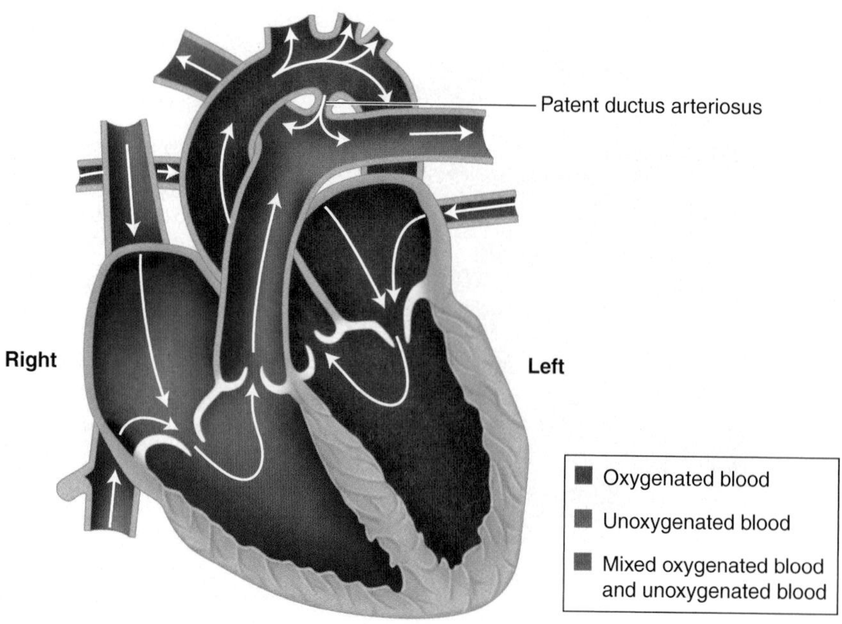

Figure 25.9 ■ In PDA, the connection that is present in utero allowing blood to bypass the lungs after right ventricular ejection due to high pulmonary pressures remains open after birth and continues to shunt blood to the aorta.

also orders lanoxin 5 μg/kg once daily to improve left ventricular cardiac output.

5. Why is Connor's pulse oximeter screening considered positive?
6. How will the drug furosemide help Connor's symptoms?
7. How will the drug lanoxin help Connor's symptoms?

Decreased Pulmonary Blood Flow Defects

Decreased pulmonary blood flow defects are those in which obstruction to pulmonary blood flow decreases the flow of blood to pulmonary circulation, which increases pressure on the right side of the heart. Disorders of decreased pulmonary blood flow include tetralogy of Fallot, pulmonary stenosis, pulmonary atresia, and tricuspid atresia. Of these four defects, Tetraology of Fallot accounts for 10% of all CCHDs and is the most common cause of cyanotic heart disease,[12] while pulmonary stenosis accounts for 8–12% of all CCHD and is the second most common cause of cyanotic heart disease.[13] This discussion will focus on these two defects in particular.

Tetralogy of Fallot

Tetralogy of Fallot (TOF) is a compilation of four defects: a VSD; pulmonary stenosis, also known as right ventricular outflow tract obstruction; right ventricular hypertrophy; and an overriding aorta (**Figure 25.10** ■). Each of the individual defects affects the infant's hemodynamic status, and when all are present at once, they create a state of cyanosis, especially in the absence of the ductus arteriosus. TOF can be considered a ductal-dependent cardiac lesion. The PS is the cause of the right ventricular hypertrophy. Because of the PS, the deoxygenated blood returned from the body is not able to move to the lungs and instead moves from the area of high concentration, the right ventricle, to the area of low concentration, the left ventricle, via right-to-left shunting through the VSD. Thus, the cardiac output volume ejected from the left ventricle consists predominantly of unoxygenated blood, resulting in systemic cyanosis. See **Table 25.1** for clinical signs and symptoms of TOF.

Treatment of TOF is performed in stages. While awaiting repair, infants with TOF have hypercyanotic spells, also known as Tet spells, when crying or with exertion. During a Tet spell, the infants pull their knees up to their chest, the effect being a reduction of systemic venous return and an increase in systemic vascular pressure. This compensatory movement helps to decrease the cyanosis for the time being. The current treatment recommendation is corrective repair early in infancy. If cyanosis is a major problem for the infant, the infant may be maintained on prostaglandins to keep the ductus arteriosus open, thereby improving pulmonary blood flow. The surgical repair occurs under cardiopulmonary bypass and involves closure of the VSD, resection of the stenotic areas, and relief of the right ventricular outflow tract obstruction. Staged procedures may be performed to

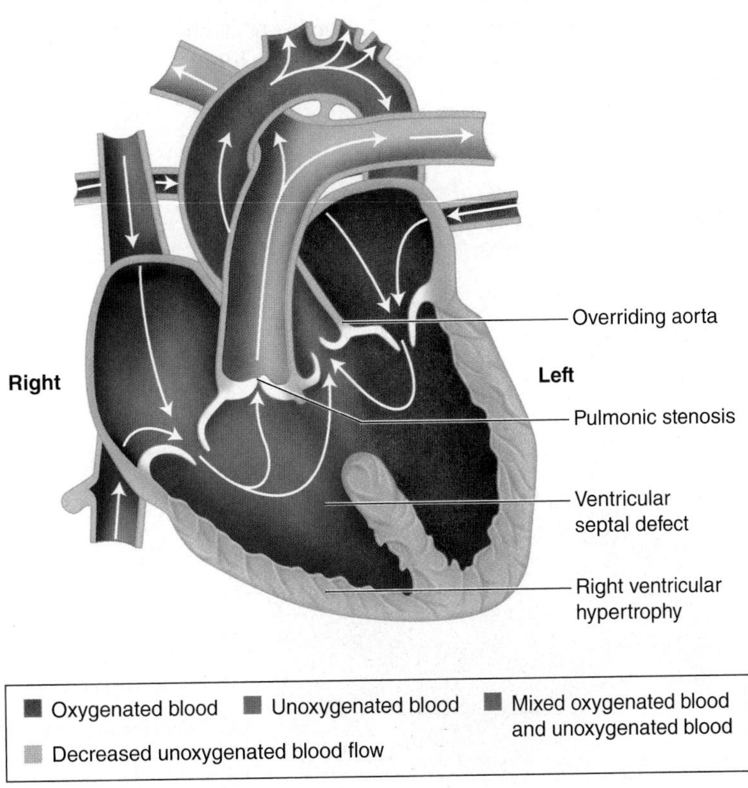

Figure 25.10 ■ Tetralogy of Fallot is a compilation of four defects: a ventricular septal defect, pulmonary stenosis, right ventricular hypertrophy, and an overriding aorta.

increase stability and survivability. The first staged procedure is the establishment of pulmonary blood flow independent of ductal patency via a Blalock-Taussig shunt.[12] The primary corrective as well as staged repair postoperative survival rates are 90–95% at 20 years of age.

Pulmonary Stenosis

Pulmonary stenosis (PS) is the narrowing of the pulmonary valve resulting in decreased pulmonary blood flow (**Figure 25.11** ■). PS can occur alone or in combination with other CHD such as TOF. PS can be valvar, subvalvar, or supravalvar and is also known as right ventricular outflow tract obstruction. In PS, the most commonly seen feature is a dome-shaped pulmonary valve that is the result of fused pulmonary valve leaflets. Because of the PS, the right ventricle has varying degrees of hypertrophy that may or may not be physiologically significant. This hypertrophy is necessary to maintaining some degree of pulmonary blood flow. Additionally, the pulmonary artery tends to be dilated, and this is thought to be due to the pressure of the blood flow that is ejected through the stenotic valve during right ventricular contraction. Depending on the degree of stenosis, infants with PS may require their ductus arteriosus to be kept open with a prostaglandin infusion. See **Table 25.1** for clinical signs and symptoms of PS. Infants with slight to mild stenosis are followed and treated medically. Infants with moderate to severe stenosis as determined by the valvar pressure gradient require surgical intervention. The pressure gradient is the measurement of the force of blood flow across the valve or vessel length.[14]

Surgical correction is determined on the basis of the pressure gradient. For a moderate pressure gradient, pulmonary balloon valvuloplasty is performed. For severe pressure gradients, a pulmonary valvotomy is the procedure of choice for repairing the valve. Postprocedure and postoperative follow-up is required at 1, 6, and 12 months and yearly after that.[15] Restenosis is the most common problem found during the first 2 years after the procedure. Treatment of restenosis is redilation of the pulmonary valve. A recent study documented only a 2% rate of restenosis, but long-term follow-up indicated late onset pulmonary regurgitation developing in 89% of patients.[15]

Obstructed Systemic Blood Flow Defects

Obstructed systemic blood flow defects are defects in which pulmonary blood flow is obstructed, resulting in little or no blood reaching the lungs to be oxygenated. Infants born with cardiac defects that obstruct the outflow of blood to the periphery are often cyanotic. These defects include coarctation of the aorta, aortic stenosis (a narrowing of the aortic valve opening), hypoplastic left heart syndrome, mitral stenosis (a narrowing of the mitral valve), and interrupted aortic arch (an uncommon genetic disorder that occurs in association with nonrestrictive ventricular septal defect and ductus arteriosus). Infants born with a left outflow tract obstruction most commonly have coarctation of the aorta or hypoplastic left heart syndrome or HLHS.

Coarctation of the Aorta

Coarctation of the aorta (COA) is the narrowing of the aorta, usually around the area of the arch and most commonly in the thoracic area (**Figure 25.12** ■). It is a fairly common CCHD, accounting for 5–8% of the CCHDs diagnosed in infancy.[16] The degree of constriction determines

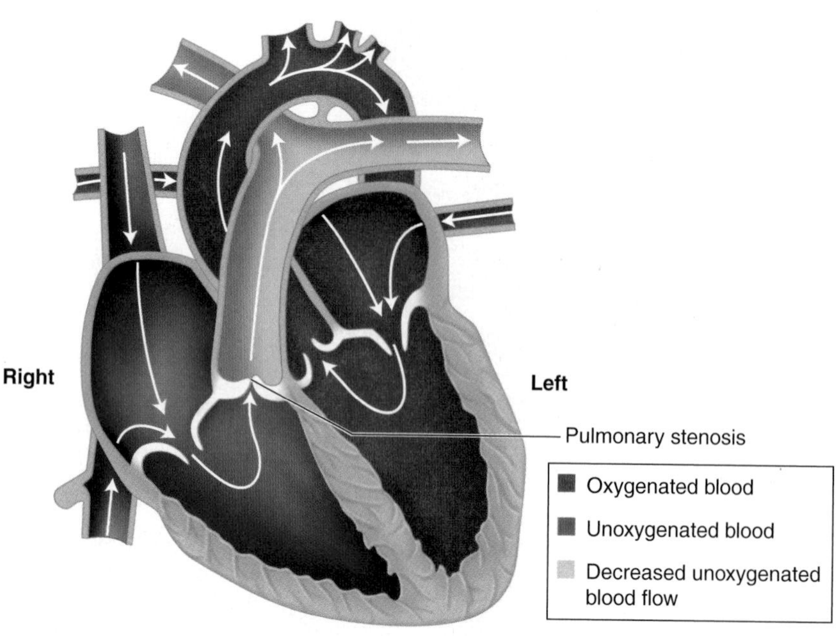

Figure 25.11 ■ PS is the narrowing of the pulmonary valve resulting in decreased pulmonary blood flow.

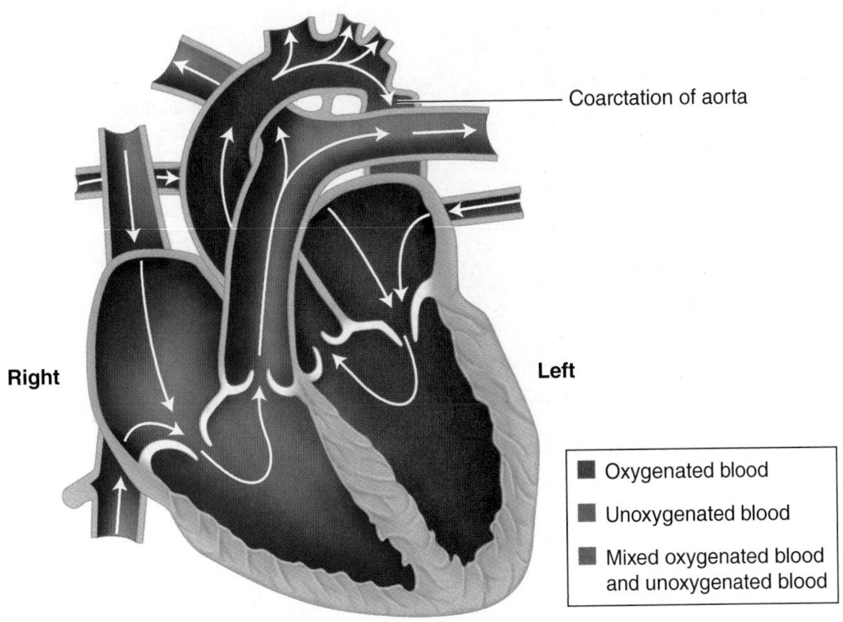

Figure 25.12 ■ In COA, the aorta narrows, usually around the area of the arch, most commonly in the thoracic area.

the extent of the infant's symptoms. A mild constriction might not be diagnosed until adolescence during a growth spurt. The more severely the aorta is constricted, the more symptoms of congestive heart failure the infant will present with. See **Table 25.1** for signs and symptoms of COA. The infant will have high left ventricular pressures and low systemic pressures, especially in the legs, where the pressures are usually 10–15% higher than those in the upper extremities. Additionally, once the ductus arteriosus closes, the left ventricular pressure will rise sharply. This dramatic increase in left ventricular pressure can result in the opening of the foramen ovale, which will result in a left-to-right shunt, causing right atrial and ventricular congestion and possibly resulting in hypertrophy. If the foramen ovale does not open, pulmonary congestion will result, and the infant will present with symptoms of pulmonary overload.

Initially, infants with COA are treated symptomatically. Diuretics are used to ease pulmonary congestion, and a continuous infusion of prostaglandins is started to maintain the patency of the ductus arteriosus to allow for systemic circulation. Inotropic infusions such as dopamine and dobutamine may be initiated to maintain renal perfusion in the lowered systemic perfusion state. Once the infant is medically stable, surgical intervention is considered. A balloon angioplasty with the placement of aortic stents is the procedure of choice in mild COA. For more severe COA, other surgical procedures are undertaken depending on the infant's anatomy. The most commonly reported procedure in the literature is an aortic resection with an end-to-end anastomosis; the second most common procedure is a subclavian flap aortoplasty. Positive postoperative outcomes were achieved most often in infants who were older than 3 months of age and younger than 1 year.[16] The mortality rate cited in the literature after an extensive review of published cases and results was 0.73%. There is a concern about postoperative aneurysm development at the site of the anastomosis resulting in recoarctation.

Hypoplastic Left Heart Syndrome

Hypoplastic left heart syndrome (HLHS) is a condition in which the left side of the heart does not fully develop during gestation, including many or all of the left side structures such as the left ventricle, mitral valve, aortic valve, and ascending portion of the aorta (**Figure 25.13** ■). An ASD is also present in many infants. Infants who are born with HLHS require the ductus arteriosus to remain patent. Therefore, these infants require a prostaglandin infusion to allow for any oxygenated systemic blood flow. According to the CDC, 960 infants are born annually with HLHS, accounting for 4.8% of the CCHDs.[3] Infants present fairly soon after birth with the symptoms of HLHS as identified in **Table 25.1**.

Treatment begins with a prostaglandin infusion to maintain the ductus arteriosus. Then several staged repairs are needed to bypass the underdeveloped left side of the heart and to establish systemic blood flow. The first staged repair is the Norwood procedure. This repair establishes the right ventricle as the main pumping chamber of the heart that will supply blood to both the lungs and the periphery. The second staged repair is the bidirectional Glenn shunt, which is usually performed about 6 months after the Norwood procedure and is done to direct half of the returning blood directly to the lungs, bypassing the ventricle. The third and final staged repair is the Fontan procedure, which

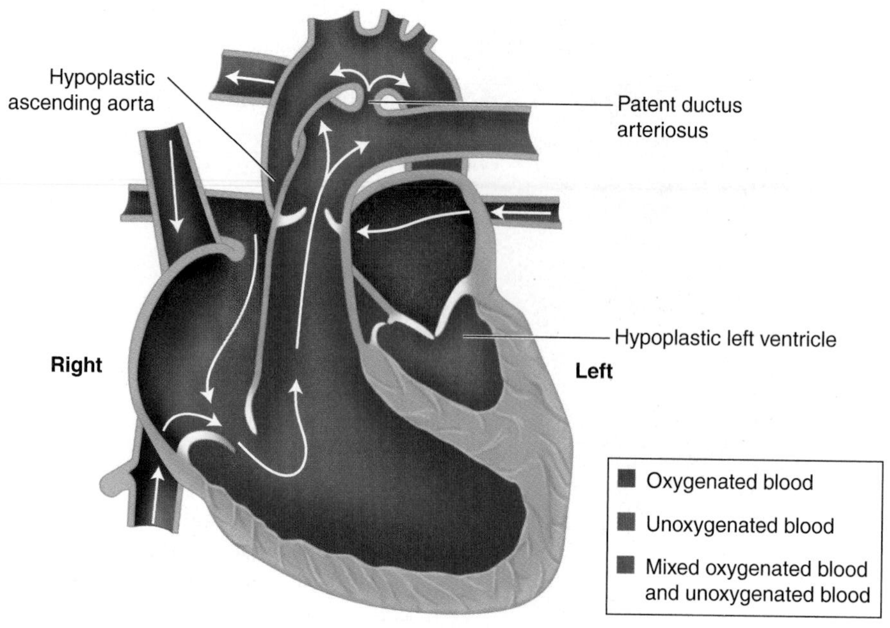

Figure 25.13 ■ In HLHS, the left side of the heart does not fully develop during gestation and includes many or all of the left side structures such as the left ventricle, mitral valve, aortic valve, and ascending portion of the aorta.

results in all the returning deoxygenated blood being sent directly, albeit passively, to the lungs, bypassing the ventricle altogether, thereby creating, in effect, a right and a left side of the heart all on the right side. While these staged surgical procedures improve the systemic perfusion, they are not curative, and these children will have lifelong complications and may require a heart transplant. The overall 5-year survivability after all three staged repairs is approximately 70%, with significant risks for postoperative complications such as acidosis, CHF, renal failure, liver failure, necrotizing enterocolitis, sepsis, pericardial or pleural effusion, phrenic or recurrent laryngeal nerve damage, stroke, coarctation of the aorta, and death.[17]

Mixed Blood Flow Defects

Mixed blood flow defects are those in which oxygenated and deoxygenated blood become mixed because of the structural defect, resulting in either increased or decreased pulmonary blood flow or obstructed systemic flow. These lesions are typically fairly complex and include transposition of the great arteries (TGA), total anomalous pulmonary venous return (TAPVR), truncus arteriosus (TA), and double-outlet right ventricle. TGA and TAPVR will be discussed as the examples of mixed defects.

Transposition of the Great Arteries

Transposition of the great arteries (TGA) occurs when the pulmonary artery arises from the left ventricle (in the normal heart, it arises it from the right ventricle) and the aorta arises from the right ventricle (it normally arises from the left ventricle) (**Figure 25.14** ■). When this occurs, the pulmonary and cardiac circulations are parallel rather than serial. Deoxygenated blood is returned to the right side and pumped out the aorta to the periphery, and oxygenated blood continually loops from the left ventricle to the lungs. The infant's presentation will depend on the associated defects, such as the presence of an ASD or VSD. If either is present, there is mixing of blood, and cyanosis is not as prominent. If an ASD or VSD is absent, patency of the ductus arteriosus is necessary. See **Table 25.1** for clinical symptoms of TGA.

Surgery is the only treatment for TGA and is performed early in the infant's life. The surgeon literally performs an arterial switch, thereby reestablishing the correct pulmonary and cardiac circulation. Postoperative survivability is very high, greater than 90%.[18]

Total Anomalous Pulmonary Venous Return

Total anomalous pulmonary venous return (TAPVR) occurs when the pulmonary veins drain into the right side of the heart instead of the left side, as normally occurs (**Figure 25.15** ■). There are three ways in which this anomaly occurs: supracardiac, cardiac, and infracardiac. In the supracardiac TAPVR, an abnormal connection occurs above the heart in which the pulmonary veins connect to the superior vena cava. In cardiac TAPVR, the anomalous vessels converge behind the heart and empty into the right atrium. Infracardiac TAPVR pulmonary veins form an abnormal connection below the heart, the inferior vena cava thereby delivering oxygen-rich blood back to the right atrium. The infant is cyanotic and often has a VSD in addition to TAPVR, which assists in delivering a small fraction of oxygenated blood to the periphery. See **Table 25.1** for signs and symptoms of TAPVR.[19]

Infants with TAPVR require surgery to correct the CHD after stabilization with prostaglandin to maintain the ductus arteriosus to allow for oxygenated blood to be pumped to the periphery. Surgical repair redirects the pulmonary veins to the left ventricle, reestablishing oxygenated blood flow to the periphery. The postoperative prognosis is greater than 90% in infants with two ventricles but drops to less than 60% in infants with only one ventricle and a more complex presentation of TAPVR.

Check Your Progress: Section 25.5

1. Explain the terms *preductal* and *postductal*.
2. What does a murmur indicate?
3. What are important considerations related to the murmur in the diagnosis of CCHD?

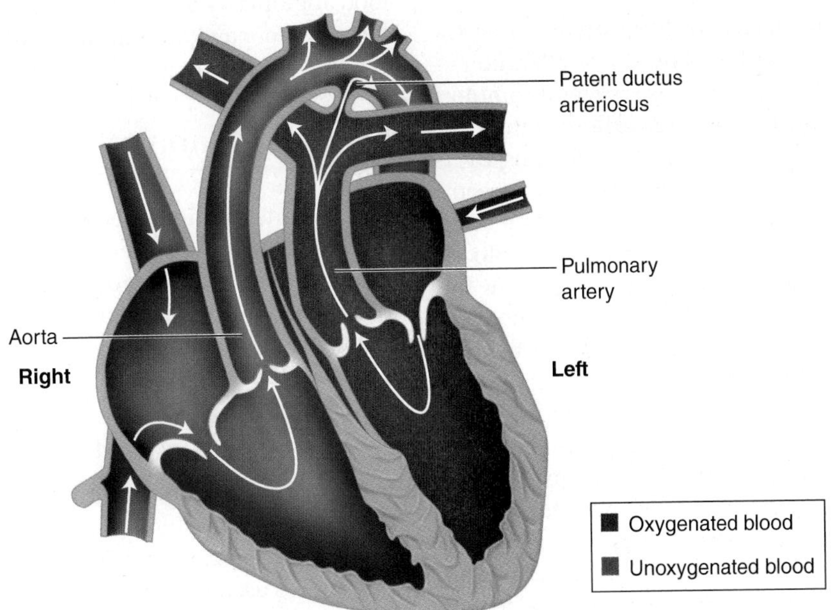

Figure 25.14 ■ In TGA, the pulmonary artery, which in the normal heart should arise from the right ventricle and provide blood flow to the lungs, actually arises from the left ventricle, and the aorta, which normally arises from the left ventricle and provides blood flow to the body, arises from the right ventricle.

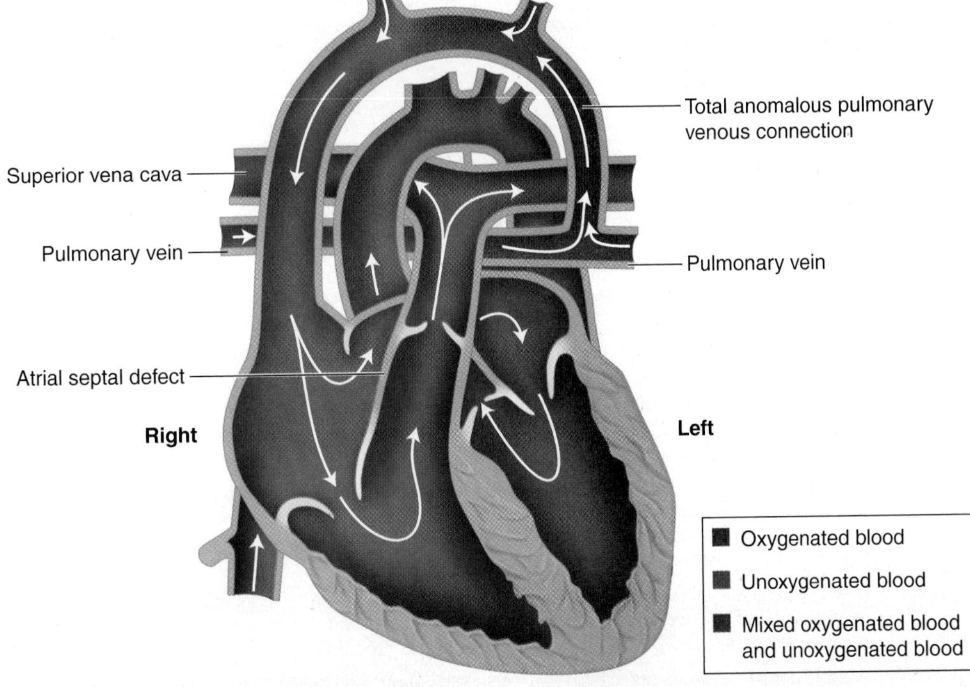

Figure 25.15 ■ Total anomalous pulmonary venous return occurs when the pulmonary veins drain into the right side of the heart instead of the left side, as normally occurs.

25.6 Linking Pathophysiology to Diagnosis and Treatment of Critical Congenital Heart Defects

Critical congenital heart defects result in an abnormality of cardiac and/or pulmonary blood flow. This alteration in cardiac or pulmonary blood flow causes several common signs and symptoms. Most infants, regardless of the type of CCHD, experience a degree of dyspnea, feeding difficulties, and fatigue. Additional symptoms relate directly to the abnormality in blood flow. The dyspnea is related to the decreased oxygen saturation of the infant's blood. The low arterial saturation results in an increase in the infant's respiratory rate, leading to tachypnea that worsens with exertion such as crying or feeding. Poor feeding is a common symptom related to the infant's increased work of breathing and tachypnea. Cyanosis is present in infants who have CCHD that involves decreased pulmonary blood flow, obstructive blood flow, or mixed blood flow. Many infants do not present as symptomatic in the hours immediately after birth; this is because of the presence of the ductus arteriosus. The ductus arteriosus allows for blood to be shunted to the periphery in defects of decreased pulmonary blood flow and obstructed blood flow. As was previously discussed, the ductus arteriosus normally closes within the first 48 hours of life, and many infants are discharged home before the ductus has closed completely and therefore may be asymptomatic until it closes completely. Hence, the implementation of the pulse oximetry screening before discharge and full closure of the ductus. Most infants with CCHD also have a murmur that is specific to the defect. Murmurs are adventitious heart sounds that indicate abnormal turbulent blood flow, often as a result of blood flow in an abnormal directions such as from a ventricle to an atrium or across the atrial or ventricular septa. Sometimes, this abnormal movement, also called shunting, is necessary for the well-being of the infant as the ductus arteriosus closes or is created via a balloon angioplasty to promote improved blood flow. Symptoms are managed medically until surgical interventions can be performed.

Medical Management

All infants with a CCHD are managed medically before surgical intervention. Medication such as diuretics, prostaglandins, antihypertensives, cardiac glycosides, and inotropes in addition to respiratory support are very common in all infants with CCHD. **Table 25.2** ■ highlights the most common medications used to treat infants with CCHD.

Surgical Intervention

If conservative treatment through medications is not effective to improve perfusion and oxygenation, surgical intervention may be indicated. **Table 25.3** ■ outlines the surgical procedures used to treat CHD.

Outcomes

The prognosis for long-term survivability for infants diagnosed with CCHD depends on many factors, including age at time of diagnosis, presenting symptoms, and whether it is critical or noncritical CHD. According to the CDC, 97% of infants born with noncritical CHD will survive to 1 year of age, and 95% will survive to 18 years

Table 25.2 Medications Used to Treat CHD

Medication Classification	Mechanism of Action	Indication
Loop diuretics	Prevent the reabsorption of Na^+ and Cl^- in the loop of Henle	Pulmonary congestion
Potassium-sparing diuretics	Inhibit the actions of aldosterone in the distal tubule and collecting ducts	Pulmonary congestion as an adjunct to loop diuretic to prevent excessive K^+ losses
Cardiac glycosides	Inhibit Na^+-K^+-ATPase in myocardial cells, resulting in the accumulation of Na^+ in the myocardial cell, which in turn causes the release of Ca^+ ions into the myocardial fibrils, which increase the force of contractility, thereby producing a positive inotropic, negative chronotropic and neutral dromotropic response	Decreased cardiac output Decreased ventricular function
ACE inhibitors	Inhibit conversion of angiotensin I to angiotensin II, resulting in a decrease in systemic pressure, resulting in decreased cardiac afterload and increased cardiac output. Also dilates veins which decrease preload, thereby decreasing pulmonary congestion.	High pressures systemically and/or centrally
Beta adrenergic antagonists	Inhibit sympathetic stimulation of cardiac beta receptors, resulting in decreased heart rate, reduction in blood pressure, and decreased cardiac workload	Decreased cardiac output, increased pressures
Inotropes	Activate adrenergic receptors, causing an increase heart rate and force of cardiac contraction, resulting in an increase in cardiac output and an increase in blood pressure.	Heart failure and shock
Prostaglandins	Dilate ductus arteriosus	Ductal dependent lesions

Table 25.3 Surgical Interventions Used to Treat CHD

Procedure	Purpose	Description
Balloon atrial septostomy: Rashkind or with transatrial needle puncture and balloon dilation	Palliative for TGA	Creates a larger defect (at the foramen ovale) between atria to increase blood mixing.
Balloon dilation procedure	Corrective for PS and MS; palliative for AS, COA	A deflated balloon is inserted and inflated to open a narrowed valve or blood vessel. A stent may be inserted to keep the vessel (e.g., ductus arteriosus).
Device closure	Corrective for PDA, ASD, VSD	Closure of ductus arteriosus by an umbrella or coil device and closure of a septal defect by a septal occluder.
Aorta end-to-end anastomosis	Corrective for COA	Resection of the narrowed section of the aorta and connection of the proximal and distal sections.
Blalock-Taussig shunt, modified	Palliative for TOF, single ventricle lesions with pulmonary outflow obstruction	Creation of aortopulmonary conduit (from the brachiocephalic artery to pulmonary artery) to increase pulmonary blood flow.
Damus-Kaye-Stansel: pulmonary artery-to-aortic anastomosis	Corrective for TGA, complex single ventricle defects	Pulmonary artery is cut in two, with the proximal section attached to the ascending aorta; the distal section is sewn over, and a shunt is created between the systemic circulation and the pulmonary artery to send blood to the lungs.
Jatene (arterial switch)	Corrective for TGA	Aorta and pulmonary arteries are transected and reattached to the opposite stumps; coronary arteries are moved to new aorta area.
Fontan	Palliative for HLHS, single ventricle defects	Creation of a conduit between inferior vena cava and pulmonary artery to increase pulmonary blood flow—total right heart bypass. The single ventricle assumes responsibility for the systemic circulation and ejects blood into the aorta.
Glenn or bidirectional Glenn	Palliative for HLHS, single ventricle defects	Superior vena cava connected to right pulmonary artery along with closure of aortopulmonary shunt. Systemic venous blood from the head is sent directly to the lungs without ventricular pumping.
Norwood	Palliative for aortic hypoplasia, single ventricle defects (e.g., HLHS)	Atrial septectomy, anastomosis of the main pulmonary artery to the aorta, and an arterial-pulmonary shunt (e.g., modified Blalock-Taussig shunt).
Patch aortoplasty	Corrective for COA	Insertion of a Dacron patch or opened left subclavian vein to expand the lumen of the aorta.
Pulmonary artery banding	Palliative for VSD, AV canal, single ventricle defects	Placement of constricting band around pulmonary artery to reduce pulmonary blood flow and pressure to lung blood vessels.
Subclavian flap aortoplasty	Corrective for COA	Division of the distal subclavian artery and insertion of a flap into the aorta through the coarcted segment.
Transplantation	Corrective for HLHS, complex defects, cardiomyopathies	Replacement of diseased heart with donor heart.

AS = aortic stenosis, ASD = atrial septal defect, AV = atrioventricular defect, COA = coarctation of the aorta, HLHS = hypoplastic left heart syndrome, MS = mitral stenosis, PDA = patent ductus arteriosus, PS = pulmonary stenosis, TOF = tetralogy of Fallot, TGA = transposition of the great arteries, VSD = ventricular septal defect.

SOURCE: Based on Ball, J. W., Bindler, R. C., & Cowen, K. J. (2017). *Principles of pediatric nursing* (7th ed.), Table 21-4, pages 523–524. Hoboken, NJ: Pearson Education.

of age. Infants born with CCHD have a 75% 1-year survivability prognosis and a 69% survivability rate to age 18.[3] The implementation of CCHD screening nationwide has improved the rate of early diagnosis, which should improve long-term outcomes.

Check Your Progress: Section 25.6

1. Why does a child with an increased pulmonary blood flow CCHD present with tachypnea and tachycardia?
2. Which symptom indicates a possible decreased pulmonary blood flow CCHD shortly after birth?
3. When an infant has an obstructed systemic flow CCHD, why does the infant have diminished pulses?
4. What does it mean when a child has a mixed CCHD?

25.7 Linking Pathophysiology to Diagnosis and Treatment of Adult Congenital Heart Disorders

Adult congenital heart disorders (ACHD) are common in that approximately 1 out of 150 adults have some form of defect in the structure of the heart.[20] The incidence of identified ACHD has been increasing. In 1968, the number of cases was 118,000, but by 2010, the number had increased to 273,000. It is estimated that the number of individuals with ACHD will level off around the year 2050.[21] These defects may have been identified at birth and the adult may have been medically managed throughout life, or the defect may go undiagnosed until symptoms occured or until diagnostic testing performed for another health problem revealed the presence of the defect.

ACHDs can be categorized as being caused by a shunt, stenosis, or a cyanotic or acyanotic complex problem. Shunt disorders occur within the heart structure and are often diagnosed in an individual with an enlarged right heart, arrhythmia, and pulmonary hypertension. The most common shunt disorder is an ASD. In severe cases of ASD, the adult has pulmonary hypertension, atrial fibrillation, and a stiff left ventricle, all of which increase the risk for an embolic stroke. The second most common ACHD is PDA, which can also lead to the development of pulmonary hypertension in the adult.

Adults may also experience manifestations of a patent foramen ovale (PFO). If not diagnosed at birth, it may be found during diagnostic testing for a stroke, transient ischemic attack, or deep vein thrombosis.

Two major ACHDs are caused by stenotic lesions. The first is PS, which can lead to right ventricular hypertrophy, heart failure, and arrhythmias in the adult. The second is COA. This lesion often goes undiagnosed unless the adult is having diagnostic testing for systemic hypertension. Even after repair, the adult may continue to have upper extremity hypertension.

The last category of ACHD disorders is considered complex and is divided into acyanotic and cyanotic lesions. Both types occur during fetal development but are not discovered until adulthood. The major acyanotic complex lesion is transposition of the great arteries. Two types can occur in the adult. The first is dextrotransposition of the great arteries (d-TGA); the second is levotransposition of the great arteries (l-TGA). In either case, the ventricles and major arteries are either switched or incorrectly attached to major vessels, leading to valve dysfunction, heart failure, or heart block.

The first cyanotic complex disorder of ASHD is TOF. Adults who are diagnosed with this disorder have a physiologically established balance between the pulmonary vessels and a ventricular septal defect; otherwise, this disorder is diagnosed in childhood.

In Ebstein anomaly, the tricuspid valve forms within the right ventricle, and the right ventricle is underdeveloped. The normal conduction pathways are altered, and these adults often have Wolff-Parkinson-White syndrome. Additional findings in adults with this anomaly include an ASD or a PFO.

The final cyanotic complex disorder is Eisenmenger syndrome. In this syndrome, an intracardiac shunt causes pulmonary hypertension that can be so severe that right-sided heart pressure exceeds systemic pressures. Providing oxygen does not improve the status of these adults, who often experience a rapid deterioration in status in the event of an atrial or ventricular arrhythmia or any health problem that causes hypotension. Additional adverse effects of the disorder include hemoptysis (coughing up blood), which can be life threatening; an elevated red blood cell count from chronic hypoxia; and acute renal failure caused by proteinuria, decreased glomerular filtration rate, and elevated uric acid levels.

ACHD can also be caused by malformation of the aortic valve. Instead of the valve having three leaflets, one, two, or four may be formed. Alterations in this structure can cause aortic stenosis or dilate the aortic root.

Diagnostic Tests

Because the structural defect was not diagnosed at birth, diagnostic testing is needed to investigate the reason for a new onset of symptoms such as a murmur, fixed or split heart sound, breathlessness, fatigue, pulmonary edema, lower extremity edema, lower extremity fatigue, exacerbation of cyanosis with exercise, general activity intolerance, and nail clubbing. Diagnostic tests that are often prescribed for these adults include electrocardiography, chest x-ray, echocardiography, CT or MRI scanning of the chest, and cardiac catheterization.

Treatment

Treatment of the adult with ACHD depends on the severity of the symptoms and whether the adult was diagnosed at birth or as an adult.

Nonsurgical

Conservative treatment for an adult diagnosed with an ASCD begins with teaching about actions to prevent the development of heart failure, primarily weight management, exercise, control of blood pressure, smoking cessation, and routine evaluation of laboratory data. Because studies have shown that adults with ASCS are more prone to developing metabolic syndrome, teaching should also focus on the prevention of this disorder.[22]

Medications

Medications for the adult with a structural disorder are prescribed for symptom management and to prevent or manage the development of heart failure. Typical medications prescribed include the following:

- Anticoagulants
- Angiotensin-converting enzyme inhibitors
- Angiotensin receptor blockers
- Spironolactone
- Beta blockers
- Digoxin
- Diuretics.

Surgical

Surgical treatment depends on the disorder. For an ASD, percutaneous closure may be indicated. Percutaneous closure may also be prescribed for PDA. Surgical ligation is another option. For the adult with pulmonary valve stenosis, percutaneous balloon valvuloplasty has been the surgical procedure of choice.

For the adult with COA, surgical approaches that may be considered include resection with end-to end anastomosis, interposition grafting, subclavian-to-distal-aorta

Impact of Current Research on Clinical Practice

Improving Heart Disease Knowledge and Research Participation in Adults with Congenital Heart Disease

Description: Valente and other researchers for the Alliance for Adult Research in Congenital Cardiology (AARCC) and the Adult Congenital Heart Association (ACHA) conducted the Health, Education and Access Research (HEART-ACHD) trial to identify the gaps in care on entering adulthood and the barriers that ACHD clients experience.[23] Nine hundred twenty-two clients with ACHD were surveyed in efforts to learn why the clients were not participating in lifelong cardiac care after being diagnosed with the CHD. The participants were introduced to the ACHD website and were asked to complete a questionnaire that focused on knowledge about heart disease. A follow-up survey was conducted 3 months later that asked the participants to identify gaps and barriers to ongoing cardiac care. Understanding why clients with ACHD are not following up with cardiac care after entering adulthood should help to reduce emergency department visits and hospitalizations.

Clinical Practice: The follow-up survey revealed that the participants were better able to name the heart condition and had a better understanding of exercise, symptoms of a heart problem, reasons for testing, birth control options, and pregnancy safety. The participants also had a better understanding of medical research and participation in research studies. The results from this study demonstrate that future efforts on education and research would be helpful to improve ongoing cardiac care and improved health for the population with ACHD.

Research Study:

Valente, A. M., Landzberg, M .J., Gianola, A., Harmon, A. J., Cook, S., Ting, J. G., Stout, K., Kuehl, K., Khairy, P., Kay, J. D., Earing, M., Houser, L., Broberg, C., Milliren, C., Opotowsky, A. R., Webb, G., Verstappen, A., & Gurvitz, M. for the Alliance for Adult Research in Congenital Cardiology (AARCC) Investigators and the Adult Congenital Heart Association (ACHA). (2013). Improving heart disease knowledge and research participation in adults with congenital heart disease (The Health, Education and Access Research Trial: HEART-ACHD). *International Journal of Cardiology, 168*, 3236–3240.

bypass, and prosthetic patch aortoplasty. If recoarctation occurs after surgery, angioplasty and stenting would be the procedure of choice.

Valve replacement is indicated to repair TOF in the adult with a significant decline in activity tolerance and right ventricular function. For adults who have been diagnosed with Ebstein anomaly, tricuspid valve replacement is indicated. For adults with transposition of the great vessels, cardiac transplantation may be considered if heart failure is severe.

Individuals with ACHDs require lifelong follow-up, although many do not regularly see their specialist (see Impact of Current Research on Clinical Practice).

Geraldine McNamara: Application

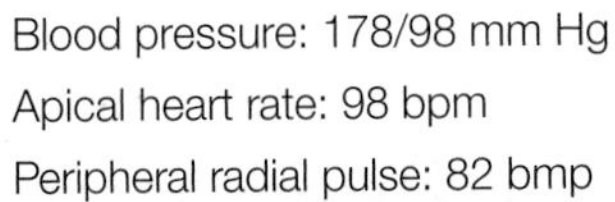

During the healthcare provider's examination of Mrs. McNamara, additional information collected includes the following:

Blood pressure: 178/98 mm Hg

Apical heart rate: 98 bpm

Peripheral radial pulse: 82 bmp

Murmur noted at the upper left sternal border.

Mrs. McNamara is referred to a cardiologist, who examines her within a few days. During the examination, the cardiologist asks about childhood illnesses, immunizations, and hospitalizations. Mrs. McNamara is unable to recall having had any illness that required hospitalization, antibiotics, or long-term rest at home. The cardiologist is concerned about the atrial fibrillation and murmur. Prescribed diagnostic tests include electrocardiography, echocardiography, chest x-ray, and CT scanning of the chest. Within a few days, the cardiologist contacts Mrs. McNamara to schedule a cardiac catheterization.

2. Interpret Mrs. McNamara's vital signs on the basis of these reference ranges: pulse 60–80, respirations 12–20, blood pressure < 120/< 80 mmHg.

Check Your Progress: Section 25.7

1. In an adult who was not diagnosed with a CCHD at birth, what symptoms might be present that may indicate an ACHD?
2. Which tests are included in diagnostic testing of an adult for CHD?
3. What medications that can be prescribed for an adult with CHD are the same as those used to treat children with CCHD?

25.8 Noncongenital Structural Heart Defects

Noncongenital structural heart defects (SHDs) are those that are occur from causes other than congenital ones. The main noncongenital structural heart defects include valvular changes caused by rheumatic heart disease, endocarditis, and calcification of the valves.

Rheumatic Heart Disease

Rheumatic heart disease (RHD) is a term used to describe changes to the cardiac valves that occur after repeated exposure to group A beta-hemolytic streptococcus. A single exposure to the bacterium does not typically cause valvular changes; however, with repeated attacks, the valve leaflets become deformed, rigid, and shortened.

Manifestations of RHD depend on the affected valve and the type of damage. **Table 25.4** ■ differentiates the changes that occur within the mitral and aortic valves in RHD.

Table 25.4 Valvular Changes Caused by Rheumatic Heart Disease

Valve Disorder	Pathophysiology	Clinical Manifestations
Mitral stenosis	Narrowing of the valve obstructs blood flow from the left atrium into the left ventricle during diastole. Valve leaflets stiffen, fuse, and calcify. Leads to left atrial hypertrophy, increased pulmonary pressures Increased pulmonary pressure leads to right ventricular hypertrophy and heart failure.	Dyspnea on exertion, cough, hemoptysis. Right heart failure: jugular vein distention; hepatomegaly, ascites, peripheral edema. Loud S1, split S2, and mitral opening snap.
Mitral regurgitation	Blood flows back into the left atrium during diastole, increasing left atrial volume. Leads to dilated left atrium and further dislocation of the valve leaflets.	Fatigue, weakness, dyspnea on exertion, orthopnea. Left heart failure: pulmonary congestion, edema. Loud high-pitched rumbling murmur.
Aortic stenosis	Blood flow obstructed from left ventricle into the aorta during systole. Associated with mitral valve deformity. Leaflets become fibrotic, calcify, and cause rigidity and scarring. Left ventricle hypertrophies, increasing cardiac workload, leading to possible ischemia.	Left heart failure: dyspnea on exertion, angina pectoris, syncope. Harsh systolic murmur. S3 and S4 heart sounds. Untreated: sudden cardiac death.
Aortic regurgitation	Backflow of blood from the aorta to the left ventricle during diastole. Valve leaflets thicken, contract, and calcify. Preload is increased along with pulmonary congestion. Right-sided heart failure is common.	Palpitations when recumbent; throbbing neck arteries, head bob, dizziness, exercise intolerance, fatigue, dyspnea on exertion, angina at night. Murmur heard on diastole. S3 and S4 may be present. Apical pulse displaced to the left.

Endocarditis

Endocarditis is an inflammation of the heart caused by pathogens that enter the bloodstream and colonize the valve structures. Individuals who have previous heart valve damage or prosthetic valve devices are more prone to developing this disorder. Any of the valves may be damaged from the infection and inflammation.

In this disorder, bacteria colonize the valve leaflets but are then covered by phagocytes, fibrin, and platelets. Over time, the bacteria, fibrin, and platelets break off, creating microemboli, which enter the general circulation.

Manifestations of endocarditis include general malaise, fatigue, chills, fever, arthralgias, anorexia, and splenomegaly. Symptoms caused by microemboli include microhemorrhages, petechiae, Osler nodes (small red painful growths on the finger and toe pads), Janeway lesions (small nonpainful purple lesions on the palms of the hands and soles of the feet), and Roth spots (small white spots seen on the retinas).

Calcification of the Aortic Valve

Although calcification can occur with any of the cardiac valves, the aortic valve is the most prone to this health problem. In the absence of another cardiac disorder that can affect valve structure, calcification of the aortic valve has been linked to atherosclerosis. Causes of atherosclerosis include smoking, elevated cholesterol and triglycerides, diabetes mellitus, and chronic kidney disease.[24] Thickening of the aortic valve from calcium deposits leads to the development of aortic stenosis. (See **Table 25.4** for the pathophysiologic changes of aortic stenosis and clinical manifestations.)

Geraldine McNamara: Outcome

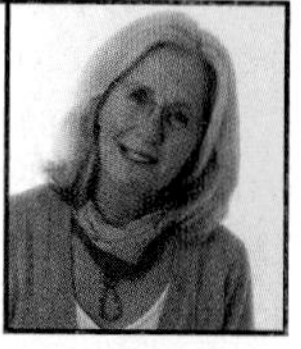

The cardiac catheterization reveals an atrial septal defect that most likely was not diagnosed at birth. This defect would explain the deficit between apical and radial pulse rates caused by atrial fibrillation and the murmur located at the upper left sternal border. Mrs. McNamara is scheduled for a percutaneous closure of the ASD in 1 week. Postoperatively, she continues to experience atrial fibrillation and requires long-term anticoagulation. The shortness of breath and lower-extremity edema have improved, and Mrs. McNamara is participating in a daily walking program to maintain muscle strength and improve stamina.

3. How did an undiagnosed ASD contribute to Mrs. McNamara's symptoms of shortness of breath, edema in the lower extremities, and activity intolerance?

Check Your Progress: Section 25.8

1. What is a noncongenital heart defect?
2. In mitral valve stenosis, blood flow from the left atrium to the left ventricle is obstructed. How does this cause shortness of breath on exertion?
3. How does endocarditis develop?

25.9 Linking Pathophysiology to Diagnosis and Treatment of Noncongenital Structural Heart Defects

Diagnostic Tests

Tests that are used to diagnose valve damage caused by RHD, endocarditis, and calcification include electrocardiography, echocardiography, chest x-ray, exercise tolerance testing, and cardiac catheterization. For endocarditis, additional testing through blood cultures is done to identify the offending microorganism.

Treatment

The treatment for noncongenital SHDs includes medications and surgical interventions. Medications to treat valvular dysfunction caused by RHD focus on symptom management and prevention or treatment of heart failure. These medications include diuretics, ACE, and vasodilators to reduce preload and afterload. Digoxin may be prescribed to maintain cardiac output.

For the client with endocarditis, antibiotic therapy is started as soon as the offending organism is identified. Depending on cardiac function, additional medications may be required to maintain cardiac output.

Depending on the reason for calcification of the aortic valve, medications may include those used to prevent or treat heart failure and those used to address elevated blood lipid levels.

Surgical treatment for RHD includes either valvuloplasty or valve replacement. Valvuloplasty may be done either to open a fused valve (open commissurotomy) or to repair a narrowed valve (annuloplasty).

Valve replacement is indicated when valve dysfunction cannot be repaired by any other route. Replacement can be through either a mechanical or a biologic valve. Mechanical valves require lifelong anticoagulation and are associated with an increased risk of thromboembolism. There is an audible click, and infections are more difficult to treat with this type of valve replacement. Biologic valves are provided from a pig, calf, or human cadaver. This type of replacement does not require long-term anticoagulation. Infections are much easier to treat, and there is a low risk of thromboembolism. This type of valve replacement often requires frequent replacement.

For endocarditis, valve replacement may be indicated if antibiotic therapy is not successful in removing or reducing large vegetation from the valve leaflets. Individuals with aortic calcification may need valvuloplasty or valve replacement surgery, depending on the severity of the symptoms.

Check Your Progress: Section 25.9

1. How does the reduction in preload and/or afterload improve cardiac function in patients with noncongenital heart defects?
2. What medications are used in the treatment of endocarditis?
3. In valve replacement surgery, where do the new valves come from and what is the difference between mechanical and biologic valves?

CHAPTER SUMMARY

25.1 Chapter Overview and Case Studies

Discuss the statistics related to structural heart defects, the impact of the environment on their etiology, and concepts related to structural heart defects.

- According to the CDC, CHDs are the leading cause of birth-defect associated deaths in the infant population less than 1 year of age.
- Environmental impact on the development of CHDs include fetal exposure to drugs, alcohol, cigarette smoke, secondhand cigarette smoke, and maternal conditions.
- Concepts related to SHDs include perfusion, oxygenation, fluid balance, nutrition, environment, and infection.

25.2 Structure of the Pediatric Cardiovascular System

Outline the structure of the pediatric cardiovascular system.

- Because the mother may not be aware of being pregnant, exposure to environmental conditions may negatively affect the development of the heart during weeks 6–9 of gestation.
- The main structures of the heart are fully formed by week 9 of gestation, making this the first organ to fully develop and function in utero.
- The first embryonic heart beat occurs on day 22 of gestation.

25.3 Prenatal and Postnatal Hemodynamics

Describe prenatal and postnatal hemodynamics and the screening used to detect critical congenital heart defects in newborns.

- In the fetus, oxygenated blood enters through the umbilical vein, enters the general fetal circulation after bypassing the liver, and returns to the placenta via the umbilical arteries.
- The first breath at birth causes an increase in pulmonary pressures, which facilitates the closure of the foramen ovale. The ductus arteriosus closes by day 21 after birth. Because of this delay, cardiac assessments during the neonatal period may indicate manifestations of CHD.

25.4 Genetics and Genomics of Critical Congenital Heart Defects

Differentiate the relationships among genetic factors, clinical features, and outcomes in individuals with congenital heart defects.

- Through the CHD GENES study, there is evidence to support a strong genetic role in the development of CCHD.
- Numerous gene mutations have been identified in the development of CCHD. This information will help to determine the use of genetics in identifying new therapies and treatments for CCHD.
- This research will help with understanding the role of neurodevelopment in children with CCHD.

25.5 Congenital Heart Defects

Differentiate the causes, classification, underlying pathogenesis, and clinical manifestations of the four categories of congenital heart defects.

- CHDs are classified as being caused by increasing pulmonary blood flow, decreasing pulmonary blood flow, obstructing blood flow, or mixing the blood flow.
- CHDs that increase pulmonary blood flow include patent ductus arteriosus, atrial septal defect, ventricular septal defect, and atrioventricular canal.
- CHDs that decrease pulmonary blood flow include pulmonary stenosis, tetralogy of Fallot, pulmonary atresia, and tricuspid atresia.
- Disorders that obstruct systemic flow include coarctation of aorta, aortic stenosis, hypoplastic left heart syndrome, mitral stenosis, and interrupted aortic arch.
- CHDs classified as mixed defects include transposition of the great arteries, total anomalous pulmonary venous return, truncus arteriosus, and double-outlet right ventricle.

25.6 Linking Pathophysiology to Diagnosis and Treatment of CHD

Link the pathophysiology of congenital heart defects to the diagnosis and treatment of the disorders in infants.

- Symptoms that are commonly associated with CCHD include dyspnea, feeding difficulties, and fatigue. A murmur specific to the anomaly is also present.
- Medical management of CCHD includes medications such as loop and potassium-sparing diuretics, cardiac glycosides, ACE inhibitors, beta adrenergic antagonists, inotropes, and prostaglandins.
- Surgical intervention for CCHDs include balloon atrial septostomy or dilation, device closure, end-to-end anastomoses, modified shunting procedures, patches, banding, aortoplasty, and transplantation.

25.7 Linking Pathophysiology to Diagnosis and Treatment of Adult Congenital Heart Disorders

Link the pathophysiology of congenital heart disorders to the diagnosis and treatment of the disorders in adults.

- The incidence of ACHD has been increasing and is expected to level off by the year 2050.
- ACHD disorders can be classified as being caused by a shunt, stenosis, or a complex condition that affects oxygenation.
- Diagnostic tests for ACHD include electrocardiography, chest x-ray, echocardiography, CT or MRI scanning of the chest, and cardiac catheterization.
- Conservative treatment of ACHD focuses on teaching to prevent the development of heart failure. Medication therapy includes diuretics, anticoagulants, ACE inhibitors, beta blockers, and digoxin.
- Surgical treatment depends on the disorder and can include percutaneous closure, end-to-end anastomoses, grafting, aortoplasty, and valve replacement.

25.8 Noncongenital Structural Heart Defects

Differentiate the causes, classification, underlying pathogenesis, and clinical manifestations of noncongenital structural heart defects.

- The major noncongenital SHDs are the result of RHD, endocarditis, or calcification of the aortic valve. These disease processes affect the mitral and aortic valves, causing either valvular stenosis or regurgitation.

25.9 Linking Pathophysiology to Diagnosis and Treatment of Noncongenital Structural Heart Defects

Link the pathophysiology of noncongenital structural heart defects to the diagnosis and treatment of the disorders.

- After diagnosing through the use of electrocardiography, echocardiogram, radiology studies, and cardiac catheterization, medication or surgical treatment is prescribed.
- Medications to treat valvular dysfunction caused by RHD focus on symptom management and prevention or treatment of heart failure. Antibiotics are used to treat endocarditis, and medication treatment for aortic valve calcification focuses on the prevention of heart failure and treat the underlying cause of atherosclerosis.
- Surgical treatment for noncongenital SHDs includes either valvuloplasty or valve replacement. Mechanical or biologic valves may be used.

REVIEW QUESTIONS

1. Fluid balance is an important concept in increased pulmonary blood flow CCHD because of which pathophysiologic impact on the infant?
   a. Tachypnea
   b. Hypertension
   c. Bradycardia
   d. Diminished pulses

2. A child with a decreased pulmonary blood flow CCHD would most likely have what symptoms? (Select all that apply.)
   a. Pulmonary congestion
   b. Cyanosis unresponsive to oxygen
   c. Murmur
   d. Diaphoresis
   e. Polycythemia

3. The research related to genetic and genomic factors in CCHD in relation to neurodevelopment is important for what main reason?
   a. Neurodevelopment is not associated with IQ.
   b. Neurodevelopment is associated with quality of life and school success.
   c. Neurodevelopment has no known association with children who have CCHD.
   d. Neurodevelopment abnormalities occur in fewer than 25% of children with CCHD.

4. Medical management of infants and children with CCHD includes which regimens?
   a. Medications only with surgery as a last resort
   b. Surgery only with medications only after a successful surgery
   c. A combination of medications and surgery dependent on the defect
   d. Medications only unless the family requests surgery for correction

5. Why does conservative treatment of ACHD focus on the prevention of heart failure?
   a. Heart failure increases the risk for cardiac hypertrophy, dysrhythmias, and symptoms that affect daily life.
   b. Heart failure is usually the cause of the ACHD and cannot be prevented.
   c. Heart failure is preventable in ACHD only through surgery.
   d. Heart failure in ACHD decreases the risk for other complications such as metabolic syndrome.

6. Rheumatic heart disease can include mitral regurgitation. A nurse would suspect mitral regurgitation if the patient presented with which symptoms?
   a. Hemoptysis
   b. Pulmonary congestion
   c. Angina pectoris
   d. Displaced apical pulse

7. For adults with endocarditis, when would a valve replacement be indicated?
   a. For all adults with endocarditis
   b. When antibiotic therapy fails completely
   c. When the symptoms become too debilitating for the patient
   d. When antibiotic therapy is not successful in reducing large vegetation

8. The purpose of long-term anticoagulation therapy in mechanical valve replacement is to
   a. prevent thromboembolism.
   b. normalize platelet counts.
   c. treat infection.
   d. prevent polycythemia.

ANSWERS

Answers to Review Questions can be found in Appendix A. Answers to Case Study and Check Your Progress questions are available on the faculty resources site. Please consult with your instructor.

RECOMMENDED WEBSITES

Adult Congenital Heart Association
https://www.achaheart.org

Alliance for Adult Research in Congenital Cardiology (AARCC)
http://www.aarcc.net

REFERENCES

1. Mitchell, S. C., Korones, S. B., & Berendes, H. W. (1971). Congenital heart disease in 56,109 births: Incidence and natural history. *Circulation, 43*, 323–332
2. Hoffmann, J. I., & Kaplan, S. (2002). The incidence of congenital heart disease. *Journal of the American College of Cardiology, 39*(12), 1890–1900.
3. Centers for Disease Control and Prevention. (2016). *Congenital heart defects (CHD)*. Available at http://www.cdc.gov/ncbddd/heartdefects/data.html
4. Martinsen, B. J., & Lohr, J. L. (2009). Cardiac development. In P. A. Iaizzo (Ed.), *Handbook of cardiac anatomy, physiology, and devices* (2nd ed., pp. 23–32). New York, NY: Springer.
5. Newborn Foundation. (2016). *Impact*. Available at http://www.newbornfoundation.org/impact
6. American Academy of Pediatrics. (2012). Endorsement of Health and Human Services recommendation for pulse oximetry screening for critical congenital heart disease. *Pediatrics, 129*(1). Available at http://pediatrics.aappublications.org/content/129/1/190
7. Kemper, A. R., Mahle, W. T., Martin, G. R., Cooley, W. C., Kumar, P., Morrow, R., Kelm, K., Pearson, G. D., Glidewell, J., Grosse, S. D., & Howell, R. R. (2011). Strategies for implementing screening for critical congenital heart disease. *Pediatrics, 128*(5). Available at http://pediatrics.aappublications.org/content/128/5/e1259
8. Pediatric Cardiac Genomics Consortium et al. (2013). The Congenital Heart Disease Genetic Network Study: Rationale, design, and early results. *Circulation Research, 112*, 698–706.
9. Ball, J. W., Bindler, R. C., & Cowen, K. (2015). *Principles of pediatric care: Caring for children*. Hoboken, NJ: Pearson Education.
10. Khalid, O. M., & Busse, J. (2011). Patent ductus arteriosus. In R. Abdulla (Ed.), *Heart diseases in children: A pediatrician's guide* (pp. 113–121). New York, NY: Springer.
11. Mancini, M. C. (2016). Patent ductus arteriosus surgery. *Medscape*. Available at http://emedicine.medscape.com/article/904895-overview
12. Bhimji, S. (2016). Tetralogy of Fallot. *Medscape*. Available at http://emedicine.medscape.com/article/2035949-overview#a7
13. Lowenthal, M. A. (2016). Pulmonic valvular stenosis. *Medscape*. Available at http://emedicine.medscape.com/article/759890-overview#a6
14. Klabunde, R. E. (2014). *Cardiovascular physiology concepts*. Available at http://www.cvphysiology.com/Hemodynamics/H010.htm
15. Syamasundar Rao, P. (2016). Valvular pulmonary stenosis treatment & management. *Medscape*. Available at http://emedicine.medscape.com/article/891729-treatment#d7
16. Syamasundar Rao, P. (2016). Coarctation of the aorta. *Medscape*. Available at http://emedicine.medscape.com/article/895502-overview
17. Syamasundar Rao, P. (2016). Pediatric hypoplastic left heart syndrome. *Medscape*. Available at http://emedicine.medscape.com/article/890196-overview#a2
18. Charpie, J. R. (2016). Transposition of the great arteries. *Medscape*. Available at http://emedicine.medscape.com/article/900574-overview
19. Wilson, A. D. (2016). Total anomalous pulmonary venous connection. *Medscape*. Available at http://emedicine.medscape.com/article/899491-overview
20. Cleveland Clinic. (2016). *About adult congenital heart disease*. Available at http://my.clevelandclinic.org/services/heart/disorders/congenital-heart
21. Benziger, C. P., Stout, K., Zaragoza-Macias, E., Bertozzi-Villa, A., & Flaxman, A. D. (2015). Projected growth of the adult congenital heart disease population in the United States to 2050: An integrative systems modeling approach. *Population Health Metrics, 13*, 29.
22. Krasuski, R. A. (2010). Congenital heart disease in the adult. *Disease Management*. Available at http://www.clevelandclinicmeded.com/medicalpubs/diseasemanagement/cardiology/congenital-heart-disease-in-the-adult/#bib8
23. Valente, A. M., Landzberg, M. J., Gianola, A., Harmon, A. J., Cook, S., Ting, J. G., Stout, K., Kuehl, K., Khairy, P., Kay, J. D., Earing, M., Houser, L., Broberg, C., Milliren, C., Opotowsky, A. R., Webb, G., Verstappen, A., & Gurvitz, M. for the Alliance for Adult Research in Congenital Cardiology (AARCC) Investigators and the Adult Congenital Heart Association (ACHA). Improving heart disease knowledge and research participation in adults with congenital heart disease (The Health, Education and Access Research Trial: HEART-ACHD). *International Journal of Cardiology, 168*, 3236–3240.
24. Mohler, E. R., Kaplan, F. S., & Pignolo, R. J. (2012). Boning-up on aortic valve calcification. *Journal of the American College of Cardiology, 60*(19). Available at http://content.onlinejacc.org/article.aspx?articleid=1377007

Chapter 26
Heart Failure

Cathy Murks

Chapter Outline and Learning Outcomes

26.1 Chapter Overview and Case Studies
Describe the prevalence of heart failure and concepts related to heart failure.

26.2 Classification and Staging of Heart Failure
Outline the classification and staging of heart failure.

26.3 Systolic Heart Failure (Heart Failure with Reduced Ejection Fraction)
Differentiate the causes, classification, underlying pathogenesis, and clinical manifestations of systolic heart failure and approaches to diagnosis and treatment of this condition across the lifespan.

26.4 Diastolic Heart Failure (Heart Failure with Preserved Ejection Fraction)
Differentiate the causes, classification, underlying pathogenesis, and clinical manifestations of diastolic heart failure and approaches to diagnosis and treatment of this condition across the lifespan.

26.5 Left-Sided Heart Failure
Differentiate the causes, classification, underlying pathogenesis, and clinical manifestations of left-sided heart failure and approaches to diagnosis and treatment of this condition across the lifespan.

26.6 Right-Sided Heart Failure
Differentiate the causes, classification, underlying pathogenesis, and clinical manifestations of right-sided heart failure and approaches to diagnosis and treatment of this condition across the lifespan.

26.7 High-Output Heart Failure
Differentiate the causes, classification, underlying pathogenesis, and clinical manifestations of high-output heart failure and approaches to diagnosis and treatment of this condition across the lifespan.

KEY TERMS

ABBREVIATIONS

ACE—angiotensin-converting enzyme
ADHF—acute decompensated heart failure
ARB—angiotensin receptor blocker
BNP—brain natriuretic peptide
CO—cardiac output
EF—ejection fraction
HF—heart failure
HFpEF—heart failure with preserved ejection fraction
HR—heart rate
LVAD—left ventricular assist device
PAC—pulmonary artery catheter
RAAS—renin-angiotensin-aldosterone system
SNS—sympathetic nervous system
SV—stroke volume
SVR—systemic vascular resistance

26.1 Chapter Overview and Case Studies

Heart failure (HF) is a condition caused by an inability of the heart to pump an adequate amount of blood to meet the body's metabolic needs. This can be caused either by a problem with muscular contraction, causing decreased ejection of the blood out of the heart; by a problem with muscular relaxation, thereby not allowing the heart to fill adequately with blood prior to contraction; or a combination of the two. People with HF may suffer from fatigue, shortness of breath, inability to exercise, swelling of the extremities, or even death.

Heart failure is a critical public health concern. There are approximately 5.1 million people in the United States with HF, and more than 650,000 new cases are diagnosed annually. There are more than one million hospitalizations for HF every year and an additional 1.8 million outpatient visits. The total cost for HF care is over $30 million per year. Mortality for HF is also high, with 50% of individuals with succumbing to this disease within 5 years of diagnosis.[1]

The lifetime risk of developing HF in a 40-year-old person is 20%, but the risk increases as the person ages. The annual rate per 1000 population of new HF events for a Caucasian male is 15.2. That rate increases to 31.7 for ages 75–84 and to 65.2 for people ages 85 and over. ■

Heart failure is a complex phenomenon that manifests itself in volume overload and fatigue, which occurs in response to a cascade of compensatory mechanisms set into motion by decreased **cardiac output (CO)**, or the amount of blood pumped out of the heart in liters per minute. In response to decreased CO, the renin-angiotensin-aldosterone system (RAAS) and the sympathetic nervous system (SNS) are activated. Ideally, these compensatory mechanisms will maintain adequate CO. However, in a prolonged state, such as the one that exists in HF, these mechanisms actually further exacerbate the HF syndrome by causing fluid retention, vasoconstriction, and direct myocardial stimulation.[2]

HF has many causes, such as disorders of the heart muscle itself, the pericardium or the outer layer of the heart, the blood supply to the heart, the valves of the heart, or even abnormalities of the blood vessels leading out of the heart. Regardless of the cause, people with HF experience a complex set of physiologic responses that ultimately lead to the symptomatology of the HF syndrome.

Concepts Related to Heart Failure

As was noted in the classic article by Mann and Bristow,[3] the conceptual framework for the development of HF is based on the following processes: initial cardiac injury, compensatory mechanisms, secondary damage, and cardiac decompensation. HF is a progressive disorder that begins after an initial injury, such as a myocardial infarction or cardiomyopathy, that damages the myocardium. The initial cardiac injury results in the loss of functioning cardiac myocytes or interferes with the ability of the myocardium to generate sufficient force.[3] As a result, the heart cannot contract normally, and the pumping capacity of the heart is reduced. The compensatory adaptive mechanisms that are activated after the reduction in the cardiac pumping capacity are initially able to maintain left ventricular function within a range that preserves or slightly reduces the functional capacity of the patient.[3] These neurohormonal responses include activation of the SNS, the RAAS, and inflammatory mediators. The SNS and the RAAS are responsible for maintaining CO through increased retention of sodium and water, increased contractility, and peripheral arterial vasoconstriction.[4] The inflammatory mediators are responsible for cardiac repair and remodeling. With longer duration of HF, however, these compensatory mechanisms become maladaptive, leading to secondary end-organ damage within the ventricle, worsening left ventricular remodeling, and cardiac decompensation (**Figure 26.1** ■).

Case Studies

The following cases are addressed throughout the chapter to assist in application of chapter content to clinical situations that involve individuals with HF.

Michael O'Malley: Introduction

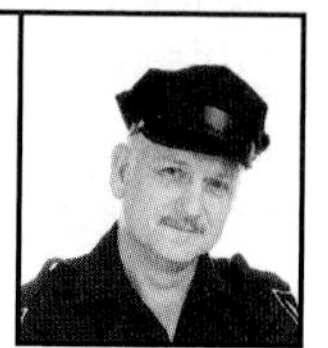

Michael O'Malley, age 49, lives in Staten Island, New York, with his wife, Sharon. He has been a New York City police office for 25 years. The O'Malleys have two sons, 20 and 16 years of age, and a daughter, 18 years of age. Mr. O'Malley has always taken pride in the fact that he is athletic, working out 3 days a week at the gym and playing softball in the police league. Overall, Mr. O'Malley is physically fit. However, despite his exercise routine, he continues to smoke two packs of cigarettes a day and drinks several beers on the weekends when he is off duty. He weighs 220 pounds, is 72 inches tall, and has a BMI of 29.8.

Mr. O'Malley thrives while working the midnight shift; in fact, he prefers it. For many years while his children were small, working the night shift made it possible for him to attend school plays, baseball games, and other activities in which his children were involved. He adapted to working this shift, and even now, when his children are nearly grown, he continues to work the midnight shift. He typically relies on fast food for lunch during his work hours. His wife, a nurse at a hospital near their home, works on the orthopedic unit. She enjoys her work and often works extra shifts to help defray the costs of college for their oldest son. Mr. O'Malley also frequently works overtime, leaving very little time for the two of them as a couple.

As an officer with the NYPD, Mr. O'Malley was an emergency responder to the World Trade Center on September 11, 2001. He quickly sprinted up several floors of the north tower before being called to evacuate because the south tower had collapsed. He developed a chronic cough from dust exposure during the collapse, but over the course of several years, the cough dissipated. Happy to be alive when many of his fellow officers had perished, he did not complain about his cough and never sought medical treatment.

1. What was the initial cardiac injury that Mr. O'Malley suffered?
2. What are three habits that Mr. O'Malley has that can negatively affect his heart?

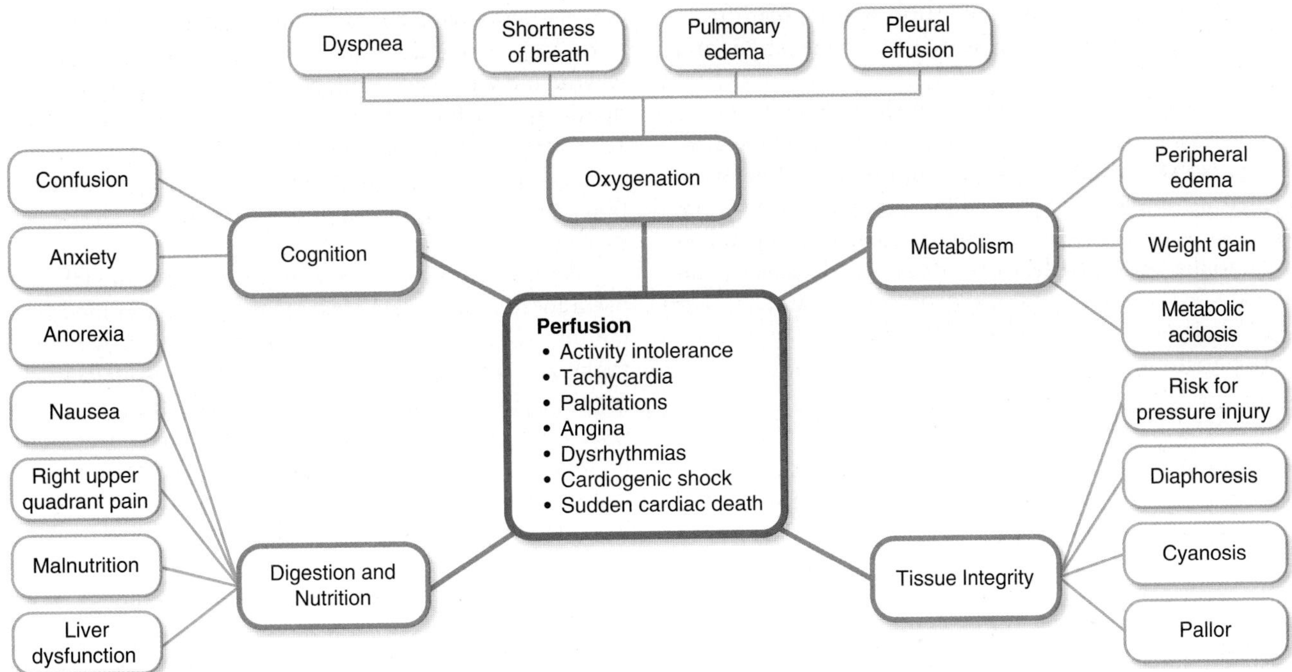

Figure 26.1 ■ Concepts related to heart failure.

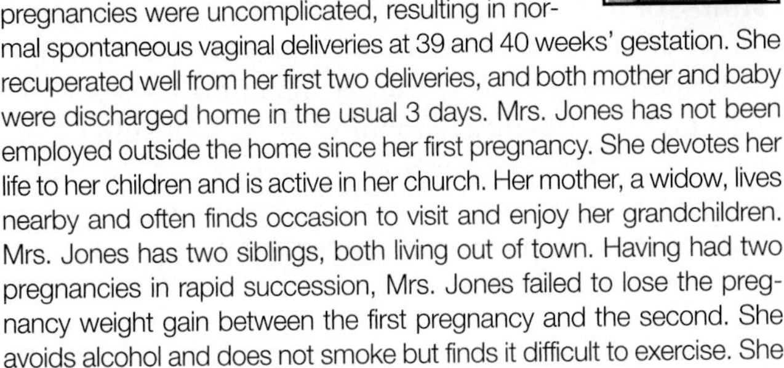

Felicia Jones: Introduction

Felicia Jones is a 25-year-old pregnant woman. She is married to Barry, a salesman at a new car dealership. This is her third pregnancy. Her first two pregnancies were uncomplicated, resulting in normal spontaneous vaginal deliveries at 39 and 40 weeks' gestation. She recuperated well from her first two deliveries, and both mother and baby were discharged home in the usual 3 days. Mrs. Jones has not been employed outside the home since her first pregnancy. She devotes her life to her children and is active in her church. Her mother, a widow, lives nearby and often finds occasion to visit and enjoy her grandchildren. Mrs. Jones has two siblings, both living out of town. Having had two pregnancies in rapid succession, Mrs. Jones failed to lose the pregnancy weight gain between the first pregnancy and the second. She avoids alcohol and does not smoke but finds it difficult to exercise. She weighs 220 pounds, is 65 inches tall, and has a BMI of 36.6.

1. What could cause Mrs. Jones to have heart failure?
2. What is one activity that Mrs. Jones could start doing to help with congestive heart failure?

Check Your Progress: Section 26.1

1. What systems are activated in response to decreased cardiac output?
2. Outline the development and progress of heart failure.
3. What role does cardiac output play in heart failure?

26.2 Classification and Staging of Heart Failure

Clinicians have sought to define and clearly describe or classify HF for many years. These categories reflect the heart chamber that is affected, the type of HF, the clinical sequelae, and the type and timing of symptoms. Despite the descriptions, it is difficult to make these designations clear and distinct, as we will see in the following sections.

Left-Sided versus Right-Sided Failure

The heart is a complex pump that is responsible for maintaining blood flow to the systemic circulation (left atrium and ventricle) and the lungs (right atrium and ventricle). Although the right and left ventricles are different in many ways, they rely on each other to function.

Left-sided HF can be caused by many things, but it typically causes volume overload and venous congestion in the lungs, leading to fatigue and shortness of breath. As circulating blood volume increases in response to sodium and water retention, pulmonary venous congestion ensues, and the patient develops dyspnea.

The right ventricle depends on the left ventricle for about one third to one half of the strength of muscular contraction, as it shares one wall of its chamber with the left ventricle.[5] The right ventricle, however, is a lower-pressure system, as the blood pressure in the pulmonary circuit is about one quarter of the blood pressure in the systemic circuit. The right ventricle therefore has a lower muscle mass and thinner walls than the left ventricle. This is an important difference, as the right ventricle is more vulnerable to volume overload states than the left ventricle.[6]

Right ventricular failure may occur as a result of left ventricular failure. When the left ventricle fails, pulmonary venous congestion increases the work of the right ventricle, which must generate more force to overcome the increased pressure from venous congestion. As venous congestion progresses backwards in the circulatory system, systemic venous congestion occurs, leading to elevated jugular venous pressure, liver congestion, and peripheral edema.

On the other hand, the left ventricle depends on the right ventricle to provide left ventricular filling. In the presence of isolated right ventricular failure, the left ventricle is filled incompletely, as the failing right ventricle cannot pump sufficient blood through the pulmonary vascular bed and into the left ventricle. CO is ultimately decreased, and HF may occur.[6] This interdependence of the right and left ventricle is only one example of the difficulty in making finite classifications in HF.

Systolic versus Diastolic Failure

Systolic and diastolic HF, at least outwardly, seem very different and easily discernible from one another. Although HF is typically due to reduced CO, the cause of the reduced CO is not always a matter of reduced contractility. A weakened or diseased heart muscle that is unable to contract effectively will lead to reduced **stroke volume (SV)**, the amount of blood pumped out of the heart with each beat in milliliters, and therefore reduced CO. **Ejection fraction (EF)** is a measurement of the percentage of blood ejected from the left ventricle with each contraction. Systolic HF is referred to as heart failure with reduced ejection fraction. However, the amount of blood present in the ventricle at the end of diastole, or preload, is also important. In patients with diastolic HF, or HF with preserved ejection fraction, heart muscle contractility is preserved or only slightly impaired but cardiac muscle relaxation is impaired, leading to impaired ventricular filling, decreased preload, and therefore reduced CO. This impaired filling becomes even more of an issue as the heart rate increases and as ventricular diastolic filling time is shortened, thereby leading to even lower SV.[7]

High-Output versus Low-Output Failure

Most of the time, HF occurs because the heart is incapable of pumping enough blood to meet the cells' need for oxygen and nutrients. For any number of reasons, the CO is reduced, leading to decreased tissue perfusion and setting into motion the neurohormonal consequences described earlier. This can be described as low-output HF but is typically referred to simply as HF.

By contrast, there is a condition known as high-output HF. Simply put, in this type of HF, the HF syndrome exists even though the heart is pumping a large amount of blood, more than 8 liters per minute. This condition is usually seen when there is vasodilation of the systemic blood vessels and blood pressure is decreased. When the blood pressure decreases, the SNS is activated, and the neurohormonal effects of HF emerge. Therefore, even though the CO is elevated, the HF syndrome exists.[8]

Acute versus Chronic Heart Failure

Heart failure is typically a chronic disease that requires patients to participate in managing specific aspects of their care. Patients with HF must take medications, adhere to a low-salt diet, monitor their symptoms, monitor their weight and vital signs, and, perhaps most important, make decisions about actions on the basis of their health status. There may be many barriers to these aspects of self-care, such as financial, social, cognitive, or motivational limitations, but self-care is an important aspect of chronic HF management.[9]

Patients with chronic HF may develop acute HF or, to use a more appropriate term, acute decompensated heart failure (ADHF). This is a condition manifested by worsening of HF symptoms to a level such that hospitalization is required. In a patient with stable chronic HF, any stress, such as infection, could result in decompensation. Similarly, dietary indiscretion, medication nonadherence, or poor decision making (failure to act on symptoms, for example), high blood pressure, myocardial ischemia, alcohol intake, or various endocrine disorders may also precipitate ADHF.[10] As patients approach the end stages of their illness, ADHF may be more frequent, and the precipitating events may become more subtle or even nonexistent. Acute decompensated HF may range from simple volume overload to cardiogenic shock. Patients with ADHF usually require hospitalization, and the underlying cause of the exacerbation must be identified and treated.

However, acute HF can be an isolated event without a prior history of HF. These patients typically have had a rapid progression to critical illness, and they may have suffered myocardial infarction, sudden cardiac death, myocarditis, or drug toxicity. Many patients in this group will recover from the acute illness but must be take inotropic medications, which affect contraction of the heart muscle, or be given mechanical support. Others will suffer from chronic HF if they recover from the acute event. Treatment of acute HF is aimed mostly at resolving the underlying cause of HF and providing supportive therapy until the condition can be reversed.

New York Heart Association: Staging by Symptoms

The New York Heart Association (NYHA) developed a system for classifying patients with heart disease that was based on functional capacity, that is, the type of activity a person could perform before being limited by symptoms of their disease. Patients are classified according to four levels of exertion: no symptoms, symptoms that occur with normal physical activity, symptoms that occur with less than normal physical activity, and symptoms that occur at rest. In this classification system, the higher the number, the more severe is the burden of disease or the smaller is the amount of exercise that can be performed comfortably. This system was developed initially in 1928 and had been revised several times since then; the most recent revision was published in 1994.[11] Descriptions of the classes include:

- **Class I:** Individuals with heart disease that does not affect their daily activities.

- **Class II:** Individuals with cardiac disease who are comfortable when resting, but results in slight limitations of activity.
- **Class III:** Individuals with heart disease that markedly limits their physical activity although they are still comfortable at rest.
- **Class IV:** Individuals with cardiac disease who experience symptoms with any level of activity and even sometimes at rest.

One of the criticisms of the NYHA classification system is that it is subjective and prone to individual bias. Another issue is that of defining just what constitutes normal activity. Is it walking three blocks or two? Is it washing and dressing in the morning or walking to the bathroom from the bedroom?

Despite these limitations, NYHA classification has proven to be effective in predicting mortality in both men and women with HF,[12] and it continues to be used to define medical necessity for interventions and inclusion in clinical trials.[10]

ACC and AHA: Staging and Managing Chronic Heart Failure

While the NYHA classification describes the severity of symptom burden in HF, the American College of Cardiology (ACC)/American Heart Association (AHA) HF classification system describes the movement of a patient with HF or the potential for developing HF through the evolution of the disease. The stages begin with risk factors or the physical substrate for the development of HF and advance through increasing severity of the disease to end-stage disease. In addition to describing the disease syndrome, the ACC/AHA guidelines for the management of HF describe treatment modalities targeted at specific stages in the continuum. The ACC/AHA stages of HF are described in **Table 26.1** ■.

For example, patients in ACC/AHA stage A HF are at risk for the development of HF but do not yet have heart disease. These patients would include those with hypertension, diabetes, obesity, smoking, genetics, or even elevated lipid levels. A 50-year-old obese male with diabetes would be in stage A HF. Interventions for patients in this stage include lifestyle modification or therapies designed to manage the underlying disorder.[10]

Table 26.1 ACC/AHA Stages of Heart Failure

Stage	Description
Stage A	At high risk for HF but without structural heart disease or symptoms of HF
Stage B	Structural heart disease but without signs or symptoms of HF
Stage C	Structural heart disease with prior or current symptoms of HF
Stage D	Refractory HF requiring specialized interventions

SOURCE: Yancy, C. W., Jessup, M., Bozkurt, B., et al. (2013). ACCF/AHA guideline for the management of heart failure. *Journal of the American College of Cardiology, 62*(16), e147–239. doi:10.1016/j.jacc.2013.05.019

Patients in stage B HF have heart disease but have yet to develop symptoms. Patients with left ventricular dysfunction might not have yet developed edema or dyspnea but would be classified as being in stage B HF. Finding an individual in stage B HF is a difficult task. Medical interventions for patients in this stage include angiotensin-converting enzyme (ACE) inhibitors, angiotensin receptor blockers (ARBs), blood pressure control, or beta blockers if there is a history of myocardial infarction.[10]

Patients in stage C HF are those with heart disease who have developed HF symptoms such as dyspnea, fatigue, or edema. The symptoms may come and go, depending on treatment, but patients with HF who have reached stage C cannot return to an earlier stage, as they have already had symptoms. However, their NYHA classification may change depending on their symptom burden. Targeted interventions for patients in this stage include the interventions noted for stage B above with the addition of diuretics, aldosterone blockers, or vasodilators such as isosorbide and hydralazine.[10]

Stage D HF includes patients with severe HF who require more than standard medical therapy to maintain life. These patients typically have a high symptom burden and must stop to rest with minimal exertion, such as shaving or dressing. They often develop renal dysfunction or hypotension. Often, medication doses must be reduced, and patients may lose weight. Interventions for patients in this stage include heart transplantation, left ventricular assist devices (LVADs), or continuous intravenous inotropes. Most frequently, these patients are classified in NYHA class IV or advanced NYHA class III.[10]

Killip Classification: Based on Heart's Hemodynamic Ability

The Killip Classification was developed by Killip and Kimball in 1967 to delineate the severity of myocardial infarction as it relates to the presence of HF or HF symptoms during the cardiac event. As described in their classic article, the Killip classification places patients into one of four classes based on the severity of HF symptoms that may occur as a result of depression of heart muscle function.[13] The Killip classification is listed in **Table 26.2** ■.

The higher the Killip class, the more severe is the burden of HF. In their study of 250 patients, those with a myocardial infarction and higher Killip classes, or more severe left ventricular dysfunction, had higher mortality rates than those with lower Killip classes.[13]

Although this scale was initially published in 1967, it remains clinically relevant today. Many other scales have been developed to predict survival after myocardial infarction. Three of these scales—the Thrombolysis in Myocardial Infarction Risk Score for ST-Elevation Myocardial Infarction (TIMI-RS), the Global Registry of Acute Coronary Events (GRACE-RS), and the Controlled Abciximab and Device Investigation to Lower Late Angioplasty Complications Risk Score (CADILLAC-RS)—use the Killip classification as one of the variables to determine risk of death after myocardial infarction.[14]

Table 26.2 Killip Classification

Killip Class*	Description
Class I	No heart failure. No clinical signs of cardiac decompensation
Class II	Heart failure. Diagnostic criteria include rales, S3 gallop and venous hypertension
Class III	Severe heart failure. Frank pulmonary edema
Class IV	Cardiogenic shock. Signs include hypotension (systolic blood pressure of ≤90 mmHg) and evidence of peripheral vasoconstriction such as oliguria, cyanosis, and diaphoresis. Heart failure, often with pulmonary edema, has been present in a majority of these patients.

* Note that the original classification used A, B, C, D.

SOURCE: Killip, T., & Kimball, J. T. (1967). Treatment of myocardial infarction in a coronary care unit: A two year experience with 250 patients. *American Journal of Cardiology, 20*, 457–464.

Check Your Progress: Section 26.2

1. Does systolic heart failure show reduced or preserved ejection fraction?
2. What is another name for acute heart failure? How does it manifest?
3. What classification system is used to stage the symptoms of heart failure? Why is it used?

26.3 Systolic Heart Failure (Heart Failure with Reduced Ejection Fraction)

Systolic heart failure is a condition in which the contraction of the heart muscle is impaired. It can affect the right side of the heart, the left side of the heart, or both sides of the heart. When the heart muscle function is impaired, CO is decreased, and blood pressure typically drops, setting many compensatory mechanisms into motion. This type of HF is called heart failure with reduced ejection fraction, as the characteristic HF in such patients is associated with a reduced ejection fraction.

Etiology and Pathogenesis

Dilated cardiomyopathy, a weakening of the heart muscle itself, is frequently a cause of systolic HF. Dilated cardiomyopathy may be idiopathic (unknown cause), ischemic (related to coronary artery disease), or familial (related to genetics). There may be other causes of systolic HF, such as coronary artery disease with myocardial infarction, or metabolic causes, such as diabetes, thyroid disease, or other hormonal abnormalities. Systolic HF may also be due to the effect of toxins to the heart, such as alcohol or cocaine, certain types of chemotherapy, or even nutritional deficiencies. Chronically elevated heart rates may also cause cardiomyopathy. The myocardium may develop inflammation or infection such as that seen in viral myocarditis or giant cell myocarditis. Obesity may cause dilated cardiomyopathy, as can AIDS or even extreme stress. There may also be diseases in which substances such as iron, proteins, or inflammatory cells are found in the heart muscle, leading to systolic HF.[10]

Heart failure may be related to a pregnancy and manifest itself during the pregnancy or shortly after delivery. In particular, peripartum cardiomyopathy is a type of pregnancy-related HF that usually develops during the last month of pregnancy and can occur up to 6 months after the end of pregnancy.[15] The pathophysiology of peripartum cardiomyopathy is not clear but may be related to a variety of factors including traditional CVD risk factors (e.g., diabetes, hypertension, dyslipidemia); pregnancy-related factors (e.g., age, number of pregnancies); oxidative stress; inflammation; viruses; autoimmunity; and possibly genetic susceptibility.[15] ■

Heart failure in children is associated with significant morbidity and mortality, placing a significant burden on the affected children and their families. Pediatric HF is a complex disorder that can occur in children as a result of a variety of diseases such as cardiomyopathies, myocarditis, and congenital heart disease. Two features may differentiate pediatric from adult HF. First, there is the possible coexistence of structural congenital heart defects, with simultaneous pulmonary overcirculation and systemic underperfusion.[16] This can occur when the pulmonary and systemic circulations are linked in parallel by structure abnormalities such as an intracardiac shunt or a patent arterial duct.[16] Additionally, the symptoms complexities may change over time, as during periods of growth and development.[16] ■

In thinking about systolic HF or even HF in general, it is important to remember several principles relating to the normal function of the heart. One of these concepts is CO, the amount of blood measured in liters per minute that the heart pumps out to the circulation. Normal CO is 4–6 L/min.[17–19] However, a normal CO for a 75-kilogram individual might not be sufficient to meet the demands of a 150-kilogram person. **Cardiac index** refers to the value obtained when the cardiac output is divided by the body surface area. A normal cardiac index is 2.5–4.3 L/min/m^2.[18]

CO can be measured with a catheter inserted into the pulmonary artery, by determining oxygen consumption, by echocardiography, or by other noninvasive imaging. It is determined by heart rate (HR) and stroke volume (SV) or by the simple equation

$$CO = HR \times SV$$

In words, the amount of blood pumped out of the heart with each beat in milliliters multiplied by the heart rate in beats per minute equals the CO in liters per minute.

Many things can affect HR and SV, thereby influencing CO. For example, faster heart rates typically increase CO, and slower heart rates typically decrease CO. Heart rate can be increased by stress, stimulant drugs, thyroid disease, abnormal cardiac rhythms, anemia, or hypovolemia.

Conversely, HR can be decreased by specific drugs, such as beta blockers or digoxin, cardiac rhythm abnormalities, or certain endocrine disorders, effectively reducing CO. However, a very fast HR may actually cause decreased CO because diastolic filling time is reduced, which reduces the amount of blood present in the ventricle for ejection.

Heart rate is only one factor in the equation; the other is SV, which is affected by preload, afterload, and contractility.

Preload is the amount of blood in the ventricle before contraction, at the end of diastole. It is affected by overall body fluid volume, venous return to the heart, and EF. If venous return is impaired or the individual is hypovolemic, preload is reduced and SV decreases. In the case of EF, which is the volume of blood the heart pumps out during a beat divided by the volume of blood in the ventricle when filled, reduction in EF means that more blood is present in the ventricle from the previous beat for the next beat, thereby increasing preload. Preload can also be increased by augmenting venous return to the heart, endocrine disorders, or fluid administration.

Afterload is the amount of pressure the heart needs to generate to pump blood out of the ventricle. Generally speaking, blood flows from areas of higher pressure to areas of lower pressure, so for the heart to pump blood out of the ventricle into the respective circulation, the ventricle must contract strongly enough to overcome the blood pressure in that system. For the right ventricle, this system is the pulmonary artery and pulmonary vascular bed; for the left ventricle, this system is the aorta and systemic circulation. However, it is also important to consider the effect of the pulmonary and aortic valves on afterload, as the ventricle must also generate enough pressure to open these valves during systole. Stenosis (narrowing) of these valves will also increase afterload. Reducing afterload typically allows the heart to work more efficiently, decreasing the amount of pressure it must generate with muscular contraction to eject blood.

Contractility is the strength of muscular contraction in the heart muscle. Greater contractility typically leads to increasing stroke volume, and lesser contractility typically leads to lower stroke volume. Keeping in mind the determinants of CO and the principles associated with them will provide the basis for a better understanding of the pathophysiology of this complicated disorder. **Figure 26.2** ■ displays the determinants of CO.

While it is easy to define these constructs in theory, there is some interdependence between them.

CLINICAL POINT: Generally speaking, increasing preload (or increasing cardiomyocyte stretch) produces an increase in the strength of ventricular contraction. This is known as the Frank-Starling law.[2] However, in cardiomyocytes with depressed function, increasing stretch might not result in increasing contractility but may result in no change in contractility or even depressed contractility. In a patient with HF, volume overload may increase preload, which in turn can actually decrease myocardial contractility. Similarly, an increasing heart rate may actually decrease ventricular filling time, leading to decreased stroke volume and CO. ■

Still another important concept is **systemic vascular resistance (SVR)**, the resistance to forward flow of blood generated by the blood vessels in the systemic circulation. It is calculated by taking into account the mean arterial blood pressure, the right atrial pressure, and the CO. Normal SVR is 800–1200 dynes-sec/cm^5.[17–19] The lower the SVR, the lower is the pressure needed to produce forward flow of blood through the vascular system. Conversely, the higher the SVR, the more difficult it is for the heart to provide forward flow.

Preload and afterload can be measured by the use of a pulmonary artery catheter (PAC). In this procedure, a small catheter is inserted into the jugular vein and advanced through the right atrium and right ventricle of the heart and into the pulmonary artery. Travel through the heart and vessel is assisted by the inflation of a small balloon at the tip of the catheter, (**Figure 26.3** ■) allowing it to move forward with

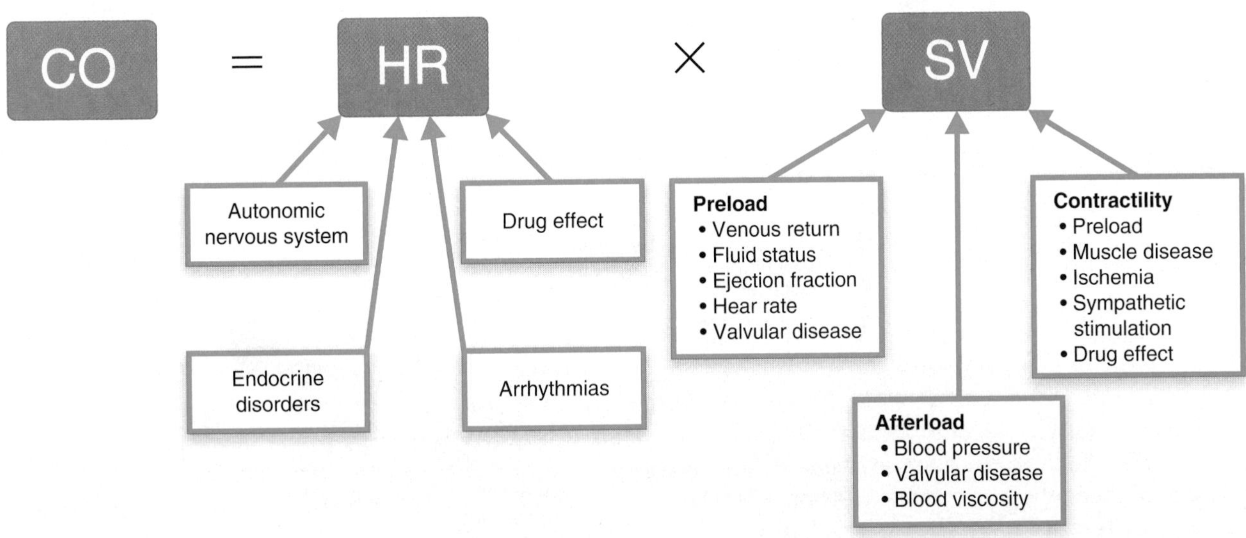

Figure 26.2 ■ Determinants of cardiac output: CO = cardiac output, HR = heart rate, SV = stroke volume.

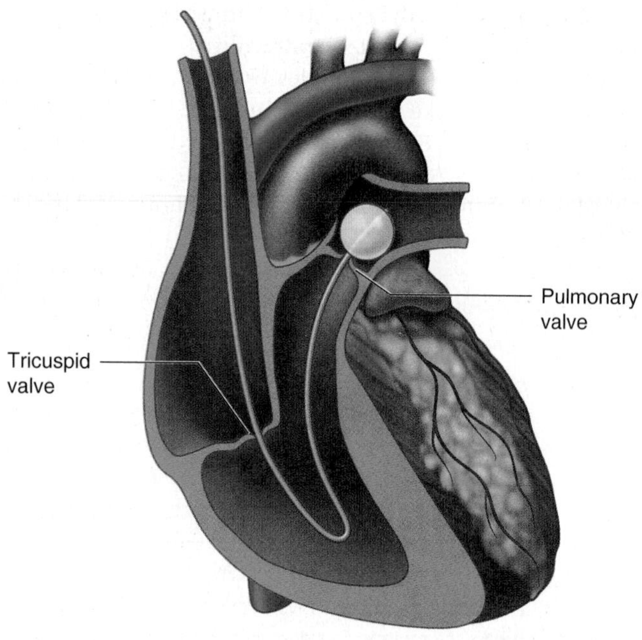

Figure 26.3 ■ Balloon inflation of a pulmonary artery catheter.

blood flow. The tip of the catheter is connected with pressurized tubing and a pressure transducer so that pressure in the pulmonary artery can be measured. Another port that is open to the right atrium measures pressure there (**Figure 26.4** ■).

Although the heart is divided into four chambers, during diastole while the **atrioventricular valves** (the valves between the atria and the ventricles) are open, the right side of the heart and the left side of the heart are each effectively one chamber on each side. In the absence of significant valve pathology, preload of the right atrium is preload of the right ventricle while the tricuspid valve is open, and preload of the left atrium is preload of the left ventricle while the mitral valve is open. As the volume of blood in the right atrium, or right atrial preload, increases, the right atrial pressure increases. Right atrial pressure is measured directly by the proximal port of the PAC. To measure the left atrial pressure, however, the balloon tip at the end of the catheter is inflated, occluding the pulmonary artery for a short period of time. Theoretically, the contribution of pressure behind the balloon is negated, and only the forward pressure of the balloon is measured, or the left atrial pressure. As the volume of blood in the left atrium increases, left atrial preload increases, left atrial pressure also rises. For a listing of normal hemodynamic pressures, see **Table 26.3** ■.

CO can be measured by injecting a small amount of fluid into the right atrial port of the PAC. CO is then calculated by measuring the time it takes for this fluid to travel from the right atrium to the pulmonary artery. Elapsed time is determined by sensing temperature changes in the blood as it mixes with the fluid injected into the right atrial port and travels to a temperature sensor on the pulmonary artery end of the catheter. The elapsed time is used in a set of calculations to determine CO. This is known as the thermodilution technique.

Regardless of the cause, as CO decreases, the body responds in an attempt to maintain enough CO to meet its metabolic needs. But even before these responses occur, decreased EF results in increased ventricular preload. As less blood is ejected from the ventricle during systole, there is more blood present in the ventricle for the subsequent cardiac contraction, and preload is increased. Cardiac muscle cells are stretched in response to increased preload. When the heart muscle function is normal, contractility increases in response to increased cardiac muscle stretch. However, when contractility is decreased, increasing muscle stretch does not necessarily lead to increasing contractility. As a

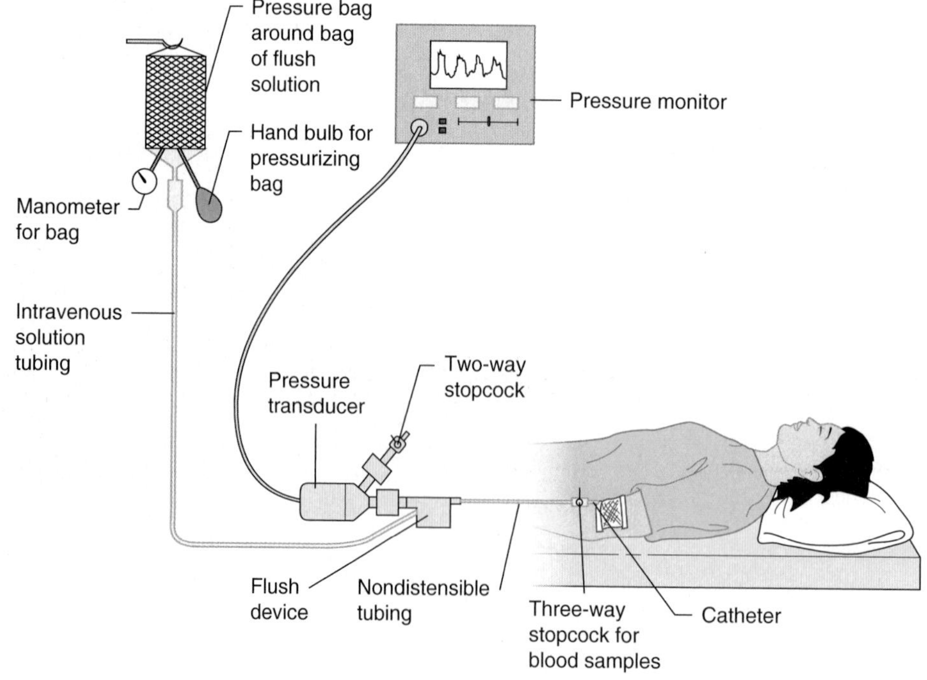

Figure 26.4 ■ A hemodynamic monitoring setup.

Table 26.3 Normal Pulmonary Pressures

Pressure	Normal Range
Right atrial pressure	2–8 mmHg*
Right ventricular pressure	15–30/0–8 mmHg*
Pulmonary artery systolic	15–30 mmHg*
Pulmonary artery diastolic	8–15 mmHg*
Pulmonary artery wedge	4–12 mmHg*
Cardiac output	4–8 L/min
Cardiac index	2.5–4.3 L/min/m*
Stroke volume	50–100*
Systolic vascular resistance	800–1200 dynes-sec/cm^2
Pulmonary vascular resistance	< 250 dynes-sec/cm^{2*}

* Represents high and low extremes from sources.

SOURCES: Lough, M. E. (2016). *Hemodynamic monitoring: Evolving technologies & clinical practice*. New York, NY: Elsevier; Miller, L. R. (2014). Hemodynamic monitoring. In S. Burns (Ed.), *AACN essentials of critical care nursing* (3rd ed., pp. 69–118). New York, NY: McGraw-Hill; Edwards Lifesciences. (2009). *Normal hemodynamic parameters and laboratory values*. Available at http://ht.edwards.com/scin/edwards/sitecollectionimages/edwards/products/presep/ar04313hemodynpocketcard.pdf

matter of fact, contractility typically remains the same or even may decrease in response to this stretch.[2]

In addition to the mechanical responses to reduced CO, there is a set of chemical responses known as the neurohormonal response. As the blood pressure drops, the SNS releases epinephrine and norepinephrine in an effort to maintain normal blood pressure. These two neurotransmitters directly affect the heart, causing increased heart rate and contractility through their effect on beta-1 receptors. The peripheral blood vessels respond with constriction and increased blood pressure by virtue of their effect on alpha receptors.[2] Although both of these measures are intended to increase CO, they may actually serve to further reduce cardiac contractility in systolic HF. For example, peripheral vasoconstriction increases afterload and further depresses CO as the weakened heart muscle struggles to generate the pressure required to exceed this increased resistance to ejection. Increasing peripheral vasoconstriction also increases venous return to the heart, further increasing preload.

Not only does the SNS affect the heart via epinephrine and norepinephrine, it also influences the activation of the RAAS. When blood flow to the kidneys is reduced, the kidneys respond by releasing renin. Sympathetic activation also acts directly on the kidneys to contribute to renin release. Renin promotes conversion of angiotensinogen to angiotensin I in the liver. ACE then mediates the conversion of angiotensin I to angiotensin II in the lungs. Angiotensin II works to provoke peripheral vasoconstriction and the release of aldosterone and antidiuretic hormone.[2,20,21] Aldosterone is released by the adrenal glands and causes resorption of sodium in the kidneys, leading to increased sodium and water retention. Finally, vasopressin, also called antidiuretic hormone, is released from the pituitary gland in response to decreased blood pressure. Vasopressin causes further vasoconstriction and water retention (**Figure 26.5** ■).[2,21] This

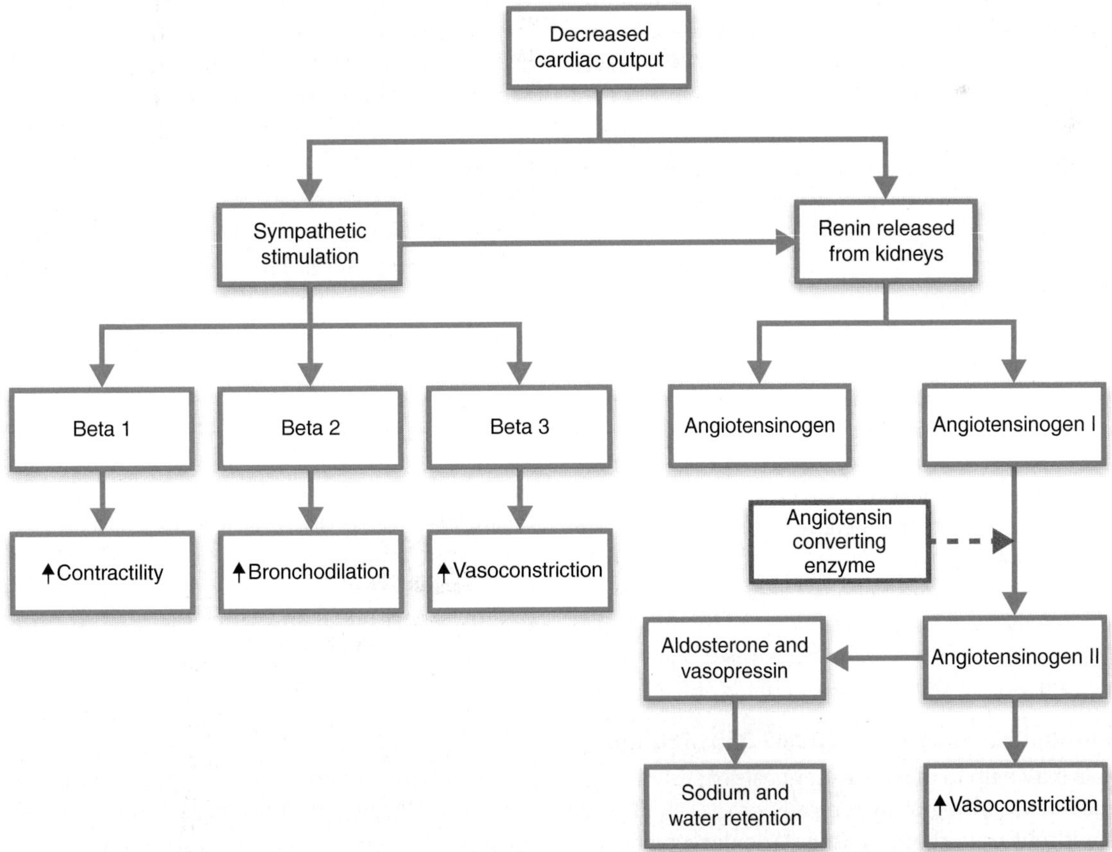

Figure 26.5 ■ Neurohormonal axis in heart failure.

neurohormonal response is beneficial in acute phases, as CO is increased; however, it is deleterious in chronic states.

It is easy to see that most of the natural responses to reduced CO serve to worsen the HF syndrome in people with decreased myocardial contractility.[2] Increasing afterload via vasoconstriction provoked by the SNS, vasopressin release, or the RAAS makes a struggling heart work harder to eject blood. Increased sodium and water retention provoked by the RAAS leads to increased preload, which under normal conditions would increase contractility. However, in the presence of already reduced contractility, increased preload may further impair contractility and reduce CO.

Not only does the neurohormonal response worsen the HF syndrome, it also leads to physical changes to the heart itself. Initially, under the stress of trying to increase CO, the left ventricle of the heart becomes less elongated and more rounded. The ventricular walls hypertrophy (thicken). In chronic HF states, however, the process continues, and the ventricle enlarges and becomes more and more rounded. There is muscle fibrosis and eventually muscle cell death as the ventricular walls are subjected to increasing levels of stress. Under normal circumstances, the right and left ventricles contract in a coordinated fashion, but as the ventricles dilate, this coordination is lost, leading to decreased efficiency of the heart as a pump.[2] Angiotensin II contributes to this phenomenon by promoting cardiac muscle cell hypertrophy.[21] This process is known as **cardiac remodeling**, and reversing this phenomenon has been the subject of many studies.[22]

On the other hand, there are bodily responses that are thought to be beneficial in HF. As the heart muscle in the atria and ventricles stretch, hormones known as the natriuretic peptides are released.

CLINICAL POINT: Substances known as brain natriuretic peptide (BNP), atrial natriuretic peptide, and c-type natriuretic peptide cause vasodilation and sodium and water excretion and limit the release of renin, aldosterone, and vasopressin.[2] ■

Clinical Manifestations

Symptoms of HF depend on the ventricle affected, but generally speaking, there is a lack of effective circulation forward to the ventricle and a backup of blood behind the ventricle affected. The patient may develop fatigue, sleep disturbances, weight loss, anorexia, and dyspnea. Depression and cognitive dysfunction is also common.[10,23] Clinicians may appreciate peripheral edema, diminished distal pulses, hypotension, tachycardia, and narrow pulse pressure. Pulmonary edema and hepatic congestion may also develop, manifesting in cough, frothy sputum, and right upper quadrant tenderness or pain. See **Figure 26.6** ■ for a depiction of the multisystem effects of HF

Linking Pathophysiology to Diagnosis and Treatment

Various tests may help to make the diagnosis of systolic HF. Transthoracic echocardiography typically reveals an EF less than 40% without or without ventricular enlargement.[2] A chest x-ray may show an enlarged cardiac shadow or evidence of pulmonary vascular congestion.

CLINICAL POINT: Serum BNP may be useful in determining HF as the cause of dyspnea, as BNP is elevated in volume overload.[10] ■

Pulmonary artery catheterization may be helpful in making the diagnosis of systolic HF and in determining the treatment. Typically, patients with systolic HF have elevated right atrial pressures, pulmonary artery pressures, and pulmonary arterial wedge pressures, owing to the fluid retention and venous hypertension. CO and index may also be reduced. Because of the effects of the RAAS, there may be an increase in SVR. Targeted therapies such as increasing diuresis or afterload reduction may be advised on the basis of the results of this procedure. Biopsy of the heart muscle and coronary arteriography may be done to determine the underlying cause of HF and guide treatment.[10]

Treatment of systolic HF is aimed at reducing symptoms by decreasing fluid retention and counteracting the neurohormonal effects of HF. ACE inhibitors are considered first-line therapy in the treatment of systolic HF.

CLINICAL POINT: ACE inhibitors block the conversion of angiotensin I to angiotensin II, thereby decreasing vasoconstriction and reducing afterload. ■

The major side effects of ACE inhibitors are a cough that can be very troublesome to patients and angioedema, which may be life threatening. In patients who are unable to tolerate ACE inhibitors, ARBs may be used. Angiotensin receptor blockers block the effects of angiotensin II, also decreasing vasoconstriction and reducing afterload. Angioedema and cough are typically not seen with ARBs, so ARBs are often used in place of ACE inhibitors in patients who experience these side effects. ACE inhibitors and ARBs should be used with caution for patients with elevated serum potassium, elevated creatinine, or low blood pressure. They are started at low doses and titrated upwards slowly, with careful monitoring of renal function and serum electrolytes.[10,21]

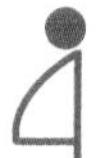

ACE inhibitors should not be used by patients who are pregnant or breastfeeding. ■

Other medications are used to treat systolic HF. Beta blockers are used in the treatment of systolic HF to block the effects of beta-adrenergic stimulation on the heart and blood vessels. Blocking the beta receptors helps to reduce vasoconstriction and heart rates, reducing blood pressure and allowing more time for ventricular filling.[2] Beta blockers may be given once or twice a day and are started at low doses and titrated upwards slowly. Beta blockers should be used with caution for patients with pulmonary disease or slow heart rates, and clinicians should be attentive to HF exacerbation, low blood pressure or heart rates, and decreased energy as side effects of this therapy.[10]

Vasodilators, such as hydralazine and nitrates, directly relax vascular smooth muscle, leading to vasodilation. Nitrates typically affect the venous system, reducing preload; hydralazine typically affects the arterial system, reducing afterload. Hydralazine is dosed three times daily, and it may be difficult for patients to adhere to this schedule. Long-acting nitrates can be dosed daily, but short-acting nitrates

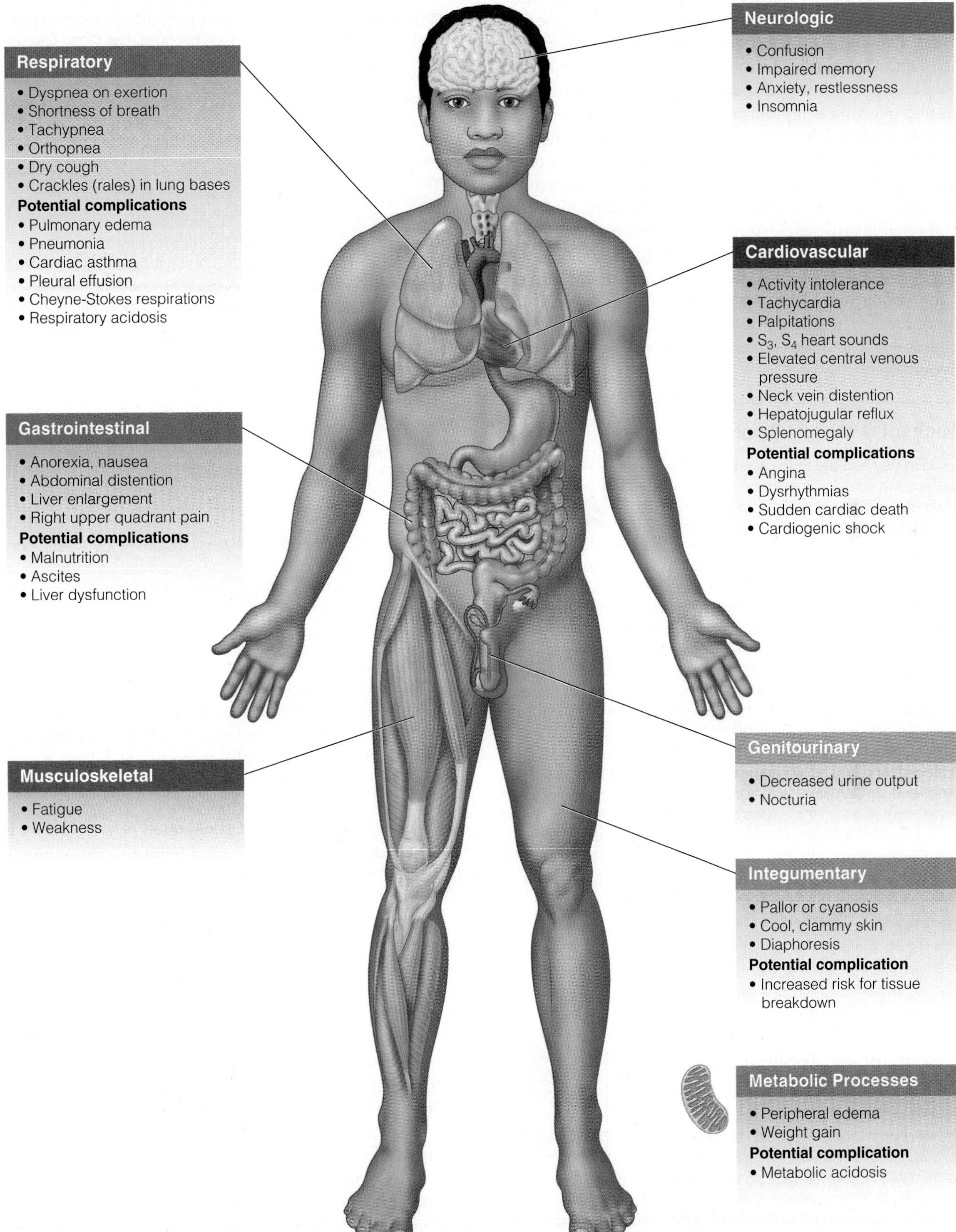
Neurologic
• Confusion
• Impaired memory
• Anxiety, restlessness
• Insomnia
Respiratory
• Dyspnea on exertion
• Shortness of breath
• Tachypnea
• Orthopnea
• Dry cough
• Crackles (rales) in lung bases
Potential complications
• Pulmonary edema
• Pneumonia
• Cardiac asthma
• Pleural effusion
• Cheyne-Stokes respirations
• Respiratory acidosis
Cardiovascular
• Activity intolerance
• Tachycardia
• Palpitations
• S_3, S_4 heart sounds
• Elevated central venous pressure
• Neck vein distention
• Hepatojugular reflux
• Splenomegaly
Potential complications
• Angina
• Dysrhythmias
• Sudden cardiac death
• Cardiogenic shock
Gastrointestinal
• Anorexia, nausea
• Abdominal distention
• Liver enlargement
• Right upper quadrant pain
Potential complications
• Malnutrition
• Ascites
• Liver dysfunction
Genitourinary
• Decreased urine output
• Nocturia
Musculoskeletal
• Fatigue
• Weakness
Integumentary
• Pallor or cyanosis
• Cool, clammy skin
• Diaphoresis
Potential complication
• Increased risk for tissue breakdown
Metabolic Processes
• Peripheral edema
• Weight gain
Potential complication
• Metabolic acidosis

Figure 26.6 ■ Multisystem effects of heart failure.

are also dosed three times daily. Nitrates may cause headaches that may be intolerable to patients. Hydralazine may cause flushing, dizziness, headaches, and palpitations.[10,21]

Diuretics, such as the loop diuretic furosemide, reduce sodium resorption in the kidneys, thereby promoting diuresis and relieving symptoms related to congestion. Aldosterone blockers, such as spironolactone, inhibit the effects of aldosterone, thereby preventing sodium and water retention. Loop diuretics may cause dehydration; electrolyte abnormalities, particularly potassium depletion; dizziness; and renal insufficiency. Aldosterone blockers help to prevent potassium wasting but may exacerbate renal insufficiency and therefore must be used cautiously for patients with renal insufficiency. Serum electrolyte and renal function studies should be routinely performed for patients taking these medications, and clinicians should watch for hyperkalemia.[10]

Michael O'Malley: Application

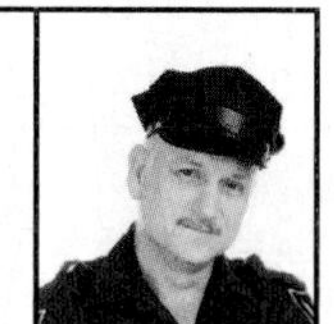

Mr. O'Malley is called to the scene of a domestic dispute. On arrival at the scene, he notices that the wife had several fresh bruises to her face and what appear to be fingerprints around her neck. She states that her husband has just left but said he would be back. Out of the corner of his eye, Mr. O'Malley notices an adult male running from the scene, and he gives chase. He runs after the subject for several blocks, finally catching up to him in a dead-end alley. Although trapped, the man fights with Mr. O'Malley, who has called for backup. After several minutes of intense wrestling, Mr. O'Malley finally succeeds in restraining the subject just as backup arrives.

About 30 minutes later, while filling out paperwork, Mr. O'Malley begins to feel a fullness in his chest, followed by pressure and tightness. He gets dizzy, stands up, and falls to the ground. Another officer present in the office feels for a pulse, but there is none. CPR is started, and when the paramedics arrive, Mr. O'Malley is defibrillated, and sinus rhythm is restored. He is taken to the emergency department and then the cardiac catheterization lab. A stent is placed in his left anterior descending artery. A pulmonary artery catheter is placed, after which the cardiac output is 3.5 and the cardiac index is 1.5. An intra-aortic balloon pump is placed, and milrinone, a phosphodiesterase 3 inhibitor used to treat HF, is started.

3. What type of HF is Mr. O'Malley experiencing, and what can cause it?
4. What are some of the factors that may have caused Mr. O'Malley to experience systolic HF?

Felicia Jones: Application

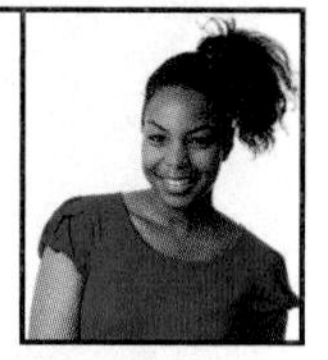

Mrs. Jones's third pregnancy is very different from the others. During the 26th week of pregnancy, she develops influenza and has to spend several days in bed. Even after she recuperates, she feels as though she never quite regains the stamina and energy level she had earlier in her pregnancy. She finds that she is dyspneic on exertion while caring for her two daughters, ages 3 and 2. Carrying laundry up the stairs is nearly impossible. She is constantly fatigued, and she begins to lose weight despite being in advanced stages of pregnancy. She finds herself enlisting the help of her mother more and more often for what she considers routine tasks that she should be fully capable of doing. This depresses her, but she explains it away, thinking that she is older and three pregnancies have taken a toll on her.

Mrs. Jones begin to develop lower extremity edema. Her obstetrician performs testing for pre-eclampsia. Her nonstress test is negative, and she does not have protein in her urine. Her blood pressure is normal, and her obstetrician is fairly certain that Mrs. Jones does not have pre-eclampsia. She is told to rest, keep her legs elevated, and reduce the salt in her diet. Several weeks pass. Mrs. Jones's weight is now increasing, but her lower extremity edema is getting worse. Her energy level is poor, and she is tired all the time. When she develops acute shortness of breath, she goes to the emergency department.

A chest x-ray demonstrates a large cardiac shadow and pulmonary edema. A stat echocardiogram is ordered. Her left ventricular EF is severely decreased to 20%. IV diuretics are initiated, and Mrs. Jones is admitted to the coronary care unit. She is at 38 weeks' gestation. Special precautions are taken because of her state of advanced pregnancy. Exposure to radiation is kept to a minimum. Her cardiologists and obstetricians develop a plan for monitoring and delivery. Because of the stress of delivery and the fluid shifts that are anticipated, a cesarean birth is proposed, which Mrs. Jones refuses. The experts reconvene and decide to optimize Mrs. Jones's fluid status with diuretics, begin afterload reduction with hydralazine, a vasodilator, and to keep Mrs. Jones in the intensive care unit until delivery. At the first sign of labor, a pulmonary artery catheter will be placed, and Mrs. Jones agrees that in the event of acute decompensation, a cesarean delivery will be done.

3. What early signs and symptoms of systolic HF does Mrs. Jones experience?
4. What late signs and symptoms of systolic HF does Mrs. Jones experience?

Patients with HF should participate in self-care activities to maintain their relative health and to manage their disease. Specific tasks include monitoring their HF symptoms, their weight, and their vital signs. Patient should adhere to their medication regimen and visit their healthcare provider as requested. Patients are also expected to follow a low-sodium diet and avoid alcohol, and they may be instructed to limit their fluid intake. Routine exercise and smoking cessation are also advised. If fluid retention or weight gain is noticed, patients may be instructed to take an extra dose of diuretic or at least notify their healthcare provider so that adjustments can be made to the medication regimen.[9]

To manage their disease effectively, patients should receive education about it and how to care for themselves. Social support is an important part of the self-care process, and significant others should be included in the education. Specifically, patients should be informed of the syndrome of HF, symptoms of exacerbation, what to do if symptoms are noted, and what sort of response to expect from interventions. Patients should also receive education specific to their medications, diet, and exercise requirements.[10] Patients with systolic HF may have difficulty paying attention or remembering this education, as these patients often have cognitive difficulties. Some studies have demonstrated that patients with cognitive difficulty have a limited ability to participate in their self-care.[24] Appropriately written condition-specific educational materials should be provided routinely. Patients should be carefully prepared for discharge to home after a hospital stay, and close follow-up must be scheduled.

In addition to medical therapy, treatment modalities for patients with HF include implantable

Impact of Current Research on Clinical Practice

Nurse Staffing Levels Associated with 30-Day Readmission Rates in Adults with Heart Failure

Description: In this retrospective observational study, data on nurse staffing ratios from 661 hospitals participating in the 2013 *U.S. News & World Report* annual Best Hospitals survey was compared to 30-day readmission rates for patients admitted to the hospital with HF who were 65 years of age or older and had Medicare as a payor. Hospitals with nurse staffing ratios greater than 1.5 nurses per patient had lower 30-day readmission rates than those with nurse staffing ratios equal to or less than 1.5 nurses per patient.

Clinical Practice: Numerous studies have supported the hypothesis that patient outcomes are improved with better nurse staffing ratios. This study supported the idea that for patients admitted with HF, higher nurse staffing is associated with decreased 30-day readmission rates. Although this study did not examine the specific reasons for the lower readmission rates, it is possible that increased nurse staffing ratios enable nurses to facilitate better discharge planning, provide more discharge education and/or better involve family and significant others in the education, provide more complete patient assessments, and contribute more overall to the team management of HF.

Research Study:

Giuliana, K. K., Danesh, V., & Funk, M. (2015). The relationship between nurse staffing and 30-day readmission for adults with heart failure. *Journal of Nursing Administration, 46*(1), 25–29. doi:10.1097/NNA0000000000000289

cardioverter-defibrillators, biventricular pacemakers, LVADs, or even cardiac transplantation. Implantable cardioverter-defibrillators are devices designed to restore normal heart rhythm if life-threatening rhythms are detected. They are advised in the prevention of sudden cardiac death in patients whose EF is less than 35%.[10]

Cardiac resynchronization therapy with biventricular pacemakers is another option. As the ventricle dilates, abnormalities in the spread of electrical impulses may occur, and the right and left ventricles might not contract simultaneously as they do in the normal state. Biventricular pacemakers provide a nearly simultaneous pacing impulse to both the right and left ventricles. Implantation of this type of pacemaker requires the insertion of an extra pacemaker lead in the coronary sinus on the left ventricle. Biventricular pacemakers may improve cardiac function by synchronizing the contraction of the right and left ventricles, mimicking normal cardiac function, and decreasing mitral valve regurgitation.[10]

LVADs are implanted pumps that support the heart, draining blood from the left ventricle and pumping it into the ascending aorta. They are implanted in either the chest or the abdomen, and a tube (called the driveline) exits the skin, providing a source of power to the motorized portion of the device (**Figure 26.7** ■).

LVADs can be used as destination therapy or as a bridge to transplantation. Patients who receive destination therapy LVADs are not candidates for heart transplantation and will likely have the LVAD until their death. Bridge-to-transplantation LVAD recipients have their LVAD in place until a suitable heart donor is identified, at which time they undergo cardiac transplantation (**Figure 26.8** ■).

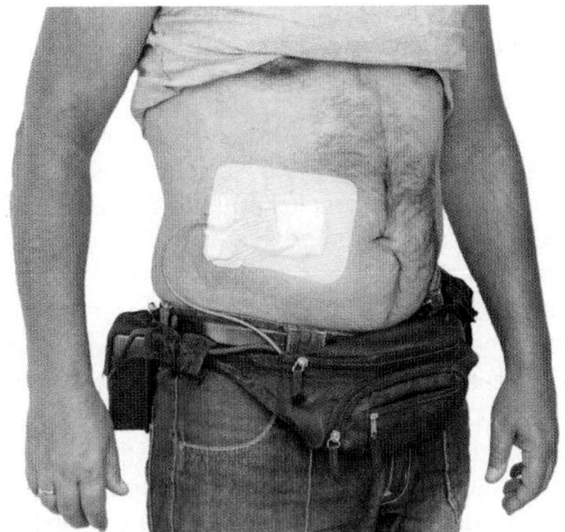

Figure 26.7 ■ Left ventricular assist device.

Michael O'Malley: Application

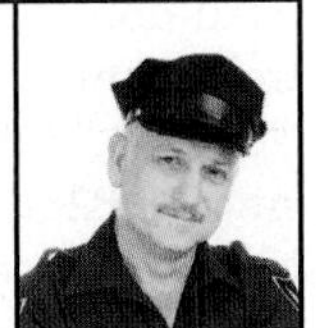

Over the course of the next several days, Mr. O'Malley's condition stabilizes. The balloon pump is weaned and removed. An echocardiogram reveals an EF of 25%, and lisinopril, which is an ACE inhibitor, and carvedilol, which is a beta blocker, are started. Mr. O'Malley is eventually weaned off the milrinone. His EF remains low, less than 30%. An implantable cardioverter-defibrillator is placed for primary prevention of sudden cardiac death. Mr. O'Malley is discharged home after 7 days.

Mr. O'Malley elects to retire on medical disability from his job, which has been his identity for many years. At first, many of his fellow officers come by frequently to visit, but after a few months, the visits become few and far between. Mr. O'Malley stops smoking and no longer drinks alcohol on weekends. He attends a cardiac rehabilitation program for 3 months and then begins a self-directed exercise program. He learns his medications and monitors his weight, blood pressure, and pulse rate. Mrs. O'Malley continues to work full time and continues to pick up extra shifts, since Mr. O'Malley's retirement and disability benefits do not cover the loss of his salary. Mr. O'Malley soon begins to experience depression and isolation, and after not smoking for several months, he begins smoking again. He gradually stops exercising and begins to gain weight.

A year later, Mr. O'Malley notices that his pants are getting tighter and tighter and his shoes no longer fit as well as they did. He complains to his wife that he has no energy and wonders whether he is coming down with a cold or the flu. Then he begins to wake up in the middle of the night gasping for breath. He develops lower extremity edema and progressively more fatigue. He goes to see his cardiologist, who performs an echocardiogram. Mr. O'Malley's EF is now 15%.

Mr. O'Malley is admitted to the hospital for diuresis and medication titration. A pulmonary artery catheter is inserted. His pulmonary artery pressures are elevated, and his CO is decreased. He is again placed on milrinone, and aggressive diuresis is begun.

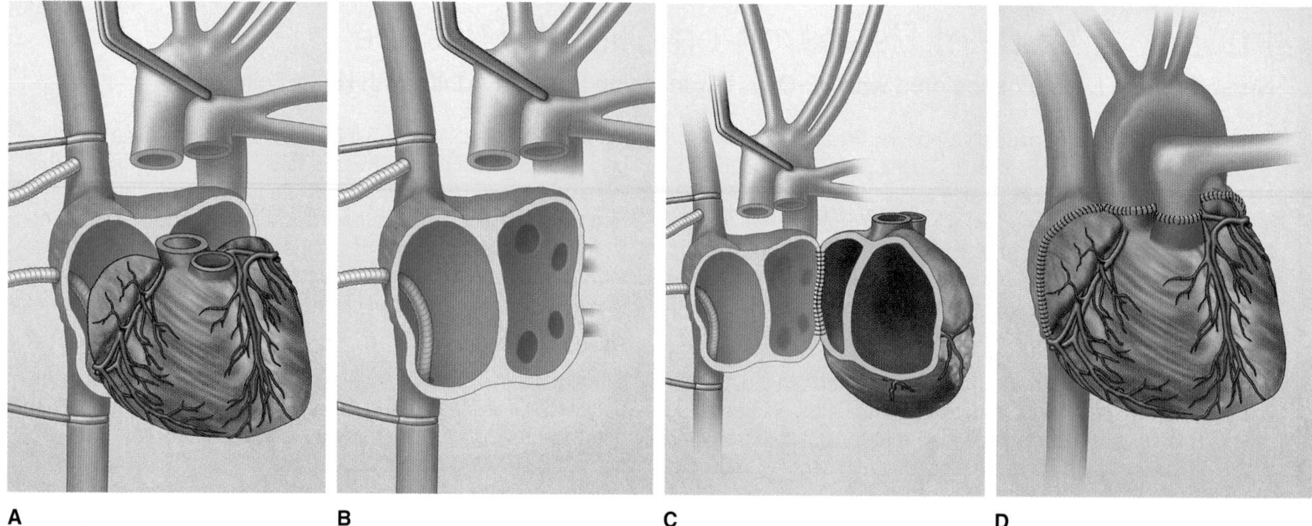

Figure 26.8 ■ Cardiac transplantation. **A.** The heart is removed, leaving the posterior walls of the atria intact, **B. C.** The donor heart is anastomosed to the atrial walls, atrial septum, and great vessels. **D.** The final result.

Mrs. O'Malley is worried. She requests family medical leave from her employer and calls their oldest son home from college. She spends a lot of time at the hospital and feels a sense of impending doom about the future, with good reason. The reports from Mr. O'Malley's doctors are not good, and every day seems to bring another obstacle to be overcome.

Mr. O'Malley suffers some kidney failure following diuresis. His milrinone is increased, and his renal function stabilizes. Once his fluid status has improved, attempts to wean the balloon pump are unsuccessful. The injury to his lungs suffered during the September 11 attacks is now apparent, and a pulmonary workup is performed. Ultimately, it is decided that he requires placement of a left ventricular assist device (LVAD).

5. Mr. O'Malley was started on a medication regimen and had what surgical intervention to prevent sudden cardiac death?
6. What are a few self-care activities that Mr. O'Malley did to decrease exacerbations?

Felicia Jones: Application

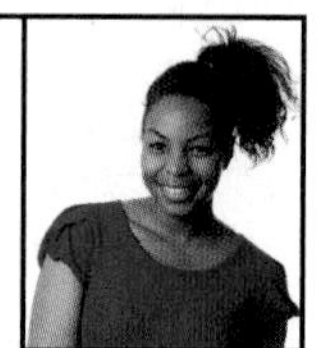

At 40 weeks' gestation, Mrs. Jones goes into labor 3 days before her due date. The PAC is placed as directed, and she is carefully monitored. After 8 hours of labor, a healthy 7 pound, 3 ounce baby boy is born, and Mrs. and Mr. Jones name him Jamie. She agrees to start medical therapy for HF immediately after delivery, even though it means that she cannot breastfeed because the medications would have damaging effects on her baby. She is started on metoprolol, a beta blocker; lisinopril; spironolactone; and furosemide, a loop diuretic. She is followed closely by her cardiologists, and her symptoms stabilize. She is advised to avoid further pregnancies.

Mrs. Jones remains on medical therapy for several months, and her EF eventually improves to normal. Her beta blockers are decreased and finally terminated, but she remains on lisinopril. She feels normal and is able to fully participate in caring for her children. She returns to choir singing and even starts taking classes at the local community college.

During the following year, Mr. Jones loses his job at the car dealership. He is able to find another job as a security guard, but the pay is lower. To help make ends meet, Mrs. Jones takes a job at a school cafeteria, as her two older daughters are now in school all day. Her mother watches Jamie while Mr. and Mrs. Jones are at work. After 6 months, Mr. Jones is able to find another job with a pay increase large enough that Mrs. Jones can quit her job. She is happy to stay home once again, and her HF symptoms remain stable. She continues on her ACE inhibitor and visits her cardiologist regularly. Then, to her cardiologist's dismay, Mrs. Jones becomes pregnant again.

Mrs. Jones is advised to terminate the pregnancy, but she refuses. Her ACE inhibitor is discontinued, and hydralazine is started. Her spironolactone is also discontinued, and she ultimately requires potassium supplementation. With careful monitoring and sodium management, her condition remains stable, but her EF deteriorates, at first to 30%, then to 20%. She delivers a healthy baby boy and has her fallopian tubes ligated.

Mrs. Jones is placed back on standard HF medical therapy, but her EF does not improve. She develops mitral regurgitation and pulmonary hypertension. She soon begins to notice increasing lower extremity edema and decreasing appetite. She feels full after eating a small amount of food and is unable to eat an entire meal. Her medications are continually adjusted, and her diuretic regimen requires increasing doses. With her low EF, the cardiologist decides to implant an implantable cardioverter-defibrillator. Mrs. Jones's QRS complex is wide so a biventricular implantable cardioverter-defibrillator/pacemaker is placed.

5. What medication therapy was Mrs. Jones put on after delivery of Jamie to manage her HF?
6. What surgical intervention was needed for Mrs. Jones in light of her decline in EF?

Heart transplantation can be a viable option in the surgical treatment of systolic HF. Cardiac transplantation involves the removal of most of the diseased heart and replacement with a healthy normal heart from a brain-dead donor (see Figure 26.8). Survival rates after cardiac transplantation are better than those with advanced HF; 82% of patients who have received heart transplantation since 1982 survived 1 year, and 69% survived 5 years. There has been a considerable improvement in survival in recent years (2009–2013), with the 1-year survival rate improving to 86%.[25] Despite this promising outcome, heart transplantation is not without its problems. Infection and rejection are always a concern for individuals with this lifesaving therapy. Patients who receive a heart transplantation must take antirejection medications for the rest of their lives. These medications reduce the natural ability to fight infection, rendering patients more susceptible to illness. Patients may experience other complications, such as hypertension, diabetes, osteoporosis, or even malignancies during their life with their new heart.

Michael O'Malley: Outcome

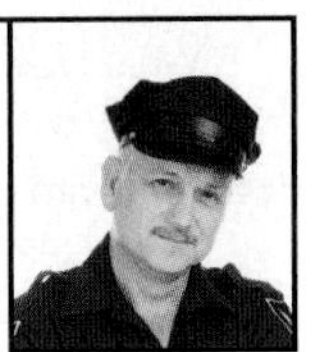

The LVAD surgery is successful, and Mr. O'Malley recuperates quickly. Still unable to work, he begins to cook and help more with the housework. He volunteers at the local library, reading to preschool-age children. He suffers a few complications related to the LVAD, including a driveline infection. He has regular visits with the LVAD team, and things are going well for a change. After 6 months, his care team decides that Mr. O'Malley is now a candidate for heart transplantation. His pulmonary function has improved, and he has stopped smoking. He is listed for a donor heart and receives his transplant 2 months later.

7. What is one complication that Mr. O'Malley faced after receiving the LVAD?
8. What two events occurred that allowed Mr. O'Malley to be placed on a donor list for a heart transplant?

Felicia Jones: Outcome

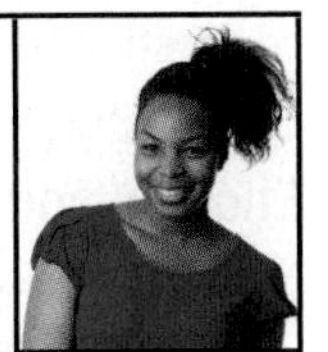

After placement of the biventricular implantable cardioverter-defibrillator/pacemaker, Mrs. Jones feels better almost instantly. Her physical endurance improves, and her lower extremity edema decreases. She is maintained on evidence-based medical therapy and remains stable, NYHA class I. She exercises regularly and follows a low-sodium diet. Her BMI is 25. She avoids alcohol. She sees her doctor every 6 months. She weighs herself every morning, notifying her doctor if she notices a weight gain over 2 pounds. She monitors her blood pressure and heart rate. Her husband remains an important source of support. Although he works full-time to support his family financially, he is attentive to Mrs. Jones and perceptive about her condition. He encourages her to maintain her active lifestyle and to continue her self-care activities. Mr. Jones is able to adjust his work schedule so that he can accompany his wife to her doctor visits.

7. What are some of the self-care activities that Mrs. Jones is doing to decrease HF exacerbations?
8. What does Mr. Jones do to provide support to Mrs. Jones?

Check Your Progress: Section 26.3

1. What is the difference between cardiac output and cardiac index?
2. What is one test that can be helpful in making the diagnosis of systolic HF and determining the treatment?
3. What are the most common medications used to treat systolic HF, and how do they work?

26.4 Diastolic Heart Failure (Heart Failure with Preserved Ejection Fraction)

Not all forms of HF are caused by cardiac muscle weakness and decreased contractility. A form of HF commonly known as **diastolic heart failure** is seen in patients with normal contractility of the heart but abnormal relaxation of the heart. This type of HF is called heart failure with preserved ejection fraction (HFpEF), as these patients have HF in the presence of a normal EF.

Etiology and Pathogenesis

In HFpEF, there are signs and symptoms of HF, normal left ventricular EF, and difficulty with ventricular relaxation that causes decreased filling of the ventricle during diastole.[10] This failure in relaxation of the heart muscle can be due to stiffness of the heart muscle cells themselves or in the complex set of proteins and connective tissues of the myocardium. It may also be due to abnormal electrolyte movement into and out of the myocardial cells causing failure of the heart muscle to completely relax after contraction.[7,26] HFpEF can also be seen in systemic diseases that cause deposits of proteins, collagen, or other materials in the heart muscle or in disease of the pericardium.[27] Decreased filling of the ventricle (decreased preload) due to ventricular stiffness leads to decreased CO and potentially HF.

Heart failure with preserved ejection fraction can be seen particularly in individuals with hypertension, aging, or diabetes, in which the arterial walls stiffen, causing stiffening of the ventricular walls of the heart also.[26] ■

Although HFpEF is termed *diastolic HF*, there is still some aspect of systolic heart function that is relevant. Left ventricular EF may be normal in these individuals at rest, but during exercise or at other times of increased demand, myocardial contractility may remain the same or even worsen. Additionally, there is concern that EF is not truly preserved but rather is effectively reduced, owing to changes in myocyte structure and function in the ventricle that are not appreciated on typical echocardiograms.[7,26]

Up to 50–55% of individuals with HF may have HFpEF. While there is no direct cause, HFpEF has been linked to many other disorders, such as obesity, hypertension, metabolic syndrome, diabetes, chronic kidney disease, chronic obstructive pulmonary disease, multiple myeloma, and amyloid heart disease. The exact mechanism linking these diseases with HFpEF is not known.[27]

Clinical Manifestations

Patients with HFpEF typically experience symptoms similar to those of systolic HF. Decreased CO activates the RAAS as detailed above, leading to fluid retention, pulmonary and hepatic congestion, and dyspnea. Because of the normal EF, patients with HFpEF typically experience dyspnea only with exercise, as CO may not be sufficient during increased demand.[7] The kidneys are particularly susceptible to the hemodynamic effects of HFpEF, and fluid retention is very problematic. The exact mechanism may be due to decreased CO, the effects of RAAS activation, or pressure exerted on the kidneys by fluid overload itself. Patients with HFpEF typically experience more fluid retention in the abdominal area than in the lower extremities. Patients may describe bloating and early satiety. Regardless of the cause, renal insufficiency in HFpEF increases both long- and short-term mortality rates.[26]

Linking Pathophysiology to Diagnosis and Treatment

Although it is a prevalent condition, there is no accepted diagnosis for HFpEF. According to the American College of Cardiology/American Heart Association Guidelines, the diagnosis of HFpEF is one of symptoms of HF without reduced ejection fraction.[10] Perhaps some of the difficulty in reaching consensus on the diagnosis of HFpEF is due to the varying nature of the etiology. Patients may have an underlying problem with relaxation, ventricular stiffness, myocyte stiffness, vascular stiffness, or a mismatch between systemic demands and what a stiff myocardium may provide. Therefore, diagnosis of HFpEF is largely a diagnosis of exclusion, that is, the patient has HF symptoms in the absence of reduced EF with or without evidence of impaired ventricular relaxation.

Treatment of HFpEF is equally challenging. No therapy has been shown to improve survival in patients with HfpEF.[28] Clinical trials have not shown benefit in treating HFpEF with standard therapies such as ACE inhibitors or beta blockers. There was some interest in the use of sildenafil to promote vascular relaxation; however, no survival benefit was found in randomized trials.[26] In a recent study, aldosterone was used to treat 3445 patients with HFpEF. Although there was no survival benefit, patients treated with spironolactone were hospitalized for HF less than were those not treated with spironolactone.[29] Diuretics may be used cautiously to treat volume overload. However, excessive use of diuretics or rapid volume removal may lead to dizziness and syncope as preload drops, and CO may be affected.

Several new medical therapies are being investigated for the treatment of HFpEF. Ivabradine acts on the sinus node of the heart to reduce heart rate, allowing more time for ventricular filling. This may be particularly important for patients with HfpEF, as diastolic filling is compromised. Neprilysin is a protease that breaks down natriuretic peptides, rendering them ineffective. LCZ696, a neprilyisin inhibitor, is being investigated in these patients as well. It is proposed that inhibiting neprilyisin in these patients will reduce afterload, promote diuresis, and improve diastolic function.[28]

Despite the lack of data to support effective medical therapy, medical experts have advised that patients with HFpEF should be treated according to guidelines for their underlying disease. Controlling the associated disease, such as hypertension, diabetes, and obesity, is advised. Sodium restriction may reduce fluid retention and in itself may be effective in reducing the symptom burden in HFpEF. Smoking cessation is recommended.[10] An exercise program may improve symptoms in patients with exercise-induced dyspnea as well as promoting weight loss in individuals for whom weight loss is advised.[28] Strict control of blood pressure and blood glucose should also be achieved.

Check Your Progress: Section 26.4

1. What type of HF is seen in patients with normal contractility of the heart but abnormal relaxation of the heart?
2. What are the most common medications used to treat diastolic HF?
3. What percentage of individuals with heart failure have HfpEF?

26.5 Left-Sided Heart Failure

Left-sided heart failure is a condition in which the left side of the heart is unable to pump blood sufficient to meet the needs of the body. In this condition, there is a lack of forward flow of blood to the aorta and the systemic circulation. CO is therefore decreased. There is also increased venous congestion in the lungs as blood begins to back up into the pulmonary vessels.

Etiology and Pathogenesis

Many things can cause left-sided HF. Any one of the number of causes of systolic HF, such as cardiomyopathy, coronary artery disease, alcohol or cocaine abuse, or even hypertension may cause left-sided HF. Left-sided HF may be caused by HFpEF and any of its associated conditions or may present as a combination of both systolic HF and HFpEF, further complicating management.

Clinical Manifestations

As left ventricular output decreases, regardless of the cause, blood pressure typically falls. As with systolic HF, the cardiac muscle initially enlarges or hypertrophies, and the heart rate increases in response to stimulation of the SNS due to the decreased CO. Eventually, the RAAS is activated, leading to increasing preload and afterload. As left ventricular preload increases, pressure is increased in the organs immediately preceding the left ventricle in the circulatory circuit, or the lungs (**Figure 26.9** ■). Pulmonary venous pressure increases, leading to **paroxysmal nocturnal dyspnea** (sudden shortness of breath while sleeping). Patients may have a cough and orthopnea (difficulty breathing while lying flat). Rales may develop. There may be extra heart sounds, such as gallop rhythms or murmurs. As left ventricular preload increases, pulmonary edema may develop, causing the patient to cough up frothy blood-tinged sputum.

However, pulmonary venous congestion is only half of the syndrome. Reduced CO leads to decreased tissue perfusion and hypotension and may also cause fatigue, decreased

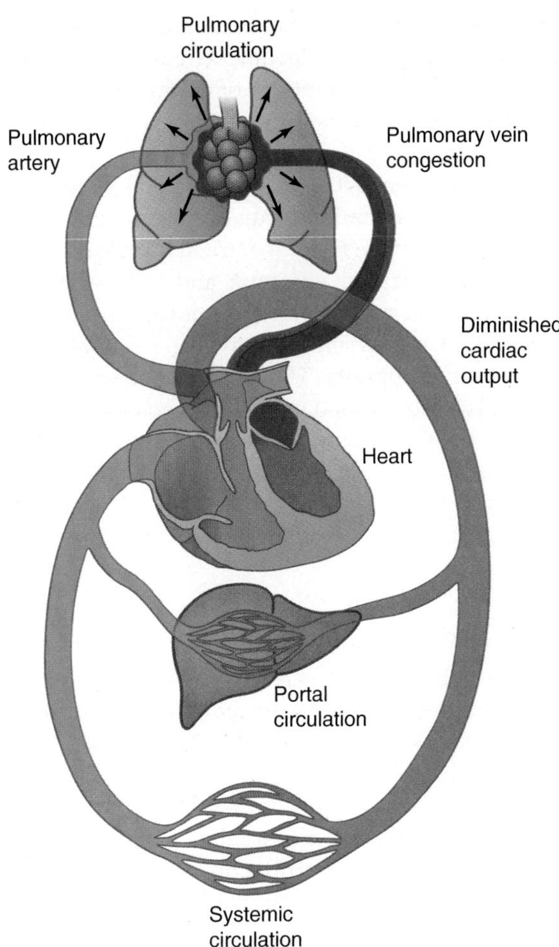

Figure 26.9 ■ The hemodynamic effects of left-sided heart failure.

urine output, and exercise intolerance. There may be dizziness and syncope. In addition to paroxysmal nocturnal dyspnea, patients may have difficulty falling asleep or staying asleep. The amplitude of distal pulses may be decreased, and skin temperature may be tepid or cool. Blood pressure is reduced, and tachycardia may develop. Patients with left-sided HF may lose weight despite consuming enough calories.

Linking Pathophysiology to Diagnosis and Treatment

The diagnosis and treatment of left-sided HF are similar to the diagnosis and treatment of systolic HF. Echocardiograms may reveal reduced left ventricular EF or, in the case of HFpEF, normal EF. Valve abnormalities may be seen, particularly mitral or tricuspid valve regurgitation. Pulmonary artery catheterization demonstrates elevated left ventricular preload and reduced CO. Laboratory examinations such as renal function panels and BNP can be used as well.[2]

As in systolic HF, treatment is aimed at reversing the effects of the body's natural responses to the HF syndrome. Fluid retention is alleviated by the use of diuretics. The RAAS is blocked by the use of ACE inhibitors or ARBs. Beta blockers are used to block the effects of the sympathetic stimulation. Aldosterone antagonists are used to block sodium and water retention.[2,10,21] Patients are also encouraged to participate in self-care activities such as weighing themselves, monitoring their symptoms, and limiting their sodium intake. In addition to standard medical therapy, treatment of left-sided HF should include management of associated disorders such as diabetes and hypertension. Patients should be instructed to exercise as tolerated and to lose weight if necessary. Patients should also be instructed to stop smoking and to avoid alcohol.[9,10] Surgical options for left-sided HF are similar to those for systolic HF, including implantable cardioverter-defibrillators, biventricular pacemakers, LVADs, or even cardiac transplantation.

Check Your Progress: Section 26.5

1. What is paroxysmal nocturnal dyspnea?
2. What are some of the surgical options for treating left-sided HF?
3. What are some of the causes of systolic HF? How can they complicate management of the condition?

26.6 Right-Sided Heart Failure

Right-sided heart failure is a condition in which the right side of the heart is unable to pump blood sufficient to meet the needs of the body. In this condition, there is a lack of forward flow of blood through the lungs to the left ventricle. This leads to decreased left ventricular preload and therefore reduced CO. Similarly, there is a backup of blood through the venous circulation to the liver, the mesentery, and the periphery (**Figure 26.10** ■).

Etiology and Pathogenesis

Right-sided HF can be caused by many conditions but is typically caused by left-sided HF.[5,10] As left ventricular function decreases, left ventricular preload increases, and pulmonary congestion ensues. The right ventricle, which typically is responsible for pumping against the lower afterload of the pulmonary circulation, struggles to exceed the afterload caused by this pulmonary congestion.

Left-sided HF is not the only cause of increased right ventricular afterload. Increased right ventricular afterload may also be caused by pulmonary embolus, sickle cell crisis, or stenosis (narrowing) of the pulmonary or mitral valve. In pulmonary embolus or sickle cell crisis, clotting of blood in the pulmonary arteries or capillary beds increases right ventricular afterload, leading to right-sided HF. Similarly, in pulmonary valve or mitral valve stenosis, narrowing of the valve adds to right ventricular afterload, as the right ventricle must exert greater pressure to eject blood smaller orifices. Right ventricular failure may also be caused by any of the conditions that cause left ventricular failure, as described above.[5]

Increased afterload can also lead to right ventricular failure in the presence of pulmonary hypertension. In pulmonary hypertension, changes in the structure of the pulmonary arteries increase the blood pressure in the lungs.

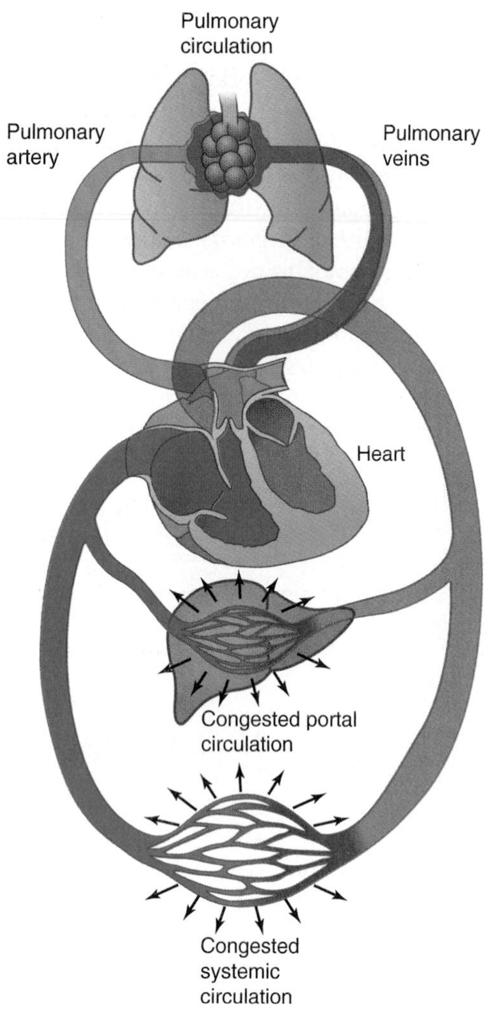

Figure 26.10 ■ The hemodynamic effects of right-sided heart failure.

Pulmonary hypertension can be related to specific drugs, scleroderma, lung disease, or pulmonary thrombosis, or it can be idiopathic, with no known cause.[5] Regardless of the cause, in the case of increased right ventricular afterload, the right ventricle responds by enlargement, but right ventricular contractility is soon impaired. The right ventricle begins to dilate, and right ventricular failure soon follows.[6]

Yet another cause of right ventricular failure may be ischemia or myocardial infarction. In the setting of ischemia or infarction, right ventricular contractility may be primarily reduced, leading to right ventricular failure. This may be seen in combination with left ventricular failure in the case of diffuse coronary artery disease or alone in the case of isolated coronary artery disease.

Clinical Manifestations

As in left-sided HF, activation of the RAAS due to reduced CO leads to sodium and water retention. It is often difficult to separate the symptoms of right-sided HF from those of left-sided HF, but by keeping in mind the function of the right ventricle, it is easier to tease out the differences.

The right ventricle is responsible for pumping blood through the pulmonary capillary bed to be oxygenated and from there to the left ventricle for pumping blood to the systemic circulation. In right ventricular failure, the left ventricle is inadequately filled, leading to reduced CO. Patients may exhibit signs and symptoms of reduced CO, including cool extremities, poor distal pulses, fatigue, exercise intolerance, and syncope.

Reduced CO leads to activation of the RAAS and SNS. Sodium and water retention occur, leading to right ventricular dilation and elevated right ventricular preload. Patients may complain of nausea, vomiting, and early satiety as the liver enlarges and causes pressure on the stomach. Similarly, edema of the mesentery may also cause abdominal pain and lack of appetite. There may be elevated jugular venous pressure, distended neck veins, peripheral edema in the legs or even the back in a recumbent patient, ascites, and hepatomegaly. The right upper quadrant of the abdomen may become tender as the liver enlarges and swells. There may be elevations in the liver enzymes, as liver function may become impaired.

Linking Pathophysiology to Diagnosis and Treatment

Right ventricular function can be measured noninvasively by cardiac magnetic resonance imaging. While transthoracic echocardiography is more widely performed, it is difficult to quantify right ventricular EF by echocardiography alone.[5] On standard transthoracic echocardiography, the right ventricle may appear dilated and weakly contractile. Despite their inability to quantify right ventricular EF, echocardiography may provide a clue to the etiology of right ventricular failure, as in mitral or pulmonic stenosis.

Pulmonary artery catheterization may be used. Typically, right atrial pressure is elevated and CO is reduced. In the case of increased right ventricular afterload, **pulmonary vascular resistance** may be increased.[5] Similar to SVR, pulmonary vascular resistance is the resistance to flow of blood generated by the blood vessels in the pulmonary circulation. It is calculated by taking into account the mean pulmonary artery pressure, the pulmonary capillary wedge pressure, and the CO. Insertion of a PAC may also help to determine an etiology for right ventricular failure, as in the case of pulmonary valve stenosis. In this condition, there is a difference in pressure between the right ventricle and the pulmonary artery due to narrowing of the valve itself.

Treatment of right ventricular failure depends on the underlying cause. Treatment of left ventricular failure will generally help to reduce right ventricular afterload and improve right ventricular failure. Adherence to a low-sodium diet will lessen fluid retention. Excess volume may be removed with diuretics and is effective in reducing venous congestion and alleviating peripheral edema, hepatomegaly, and mesenteric edema. Direct-acting pulmonary vasodilators such as prostacyclin can be used for patients with normal left ventricular function and idiopathic pulmonary hypertension but not for patients with reduced left ventricular function.[6] Severe right ventricular failure may require support with intravenous inotropes. In the case of right ventricular failure caused by pulmonary embolus, support of the right ventricle with inotropes during anticoagulation may be necessary.[5]

Surgical treatment of right ventricular failure is similar to that of left-sided HF and may involve replacement of pulmonary or mitral valves, right ventricular assist device placement, or even cardiac transplantation.

Check Your Progress: Section 26.6

1. What happens to the cardiac output in patients with right-sided HF?
2. What are the most common manifestations of right-sided HF?
3. What are the treatment options for patients with right-sided HF?

26.7 High-Output Heart Failure

Generally speaking, when the term *heart failure* is used, clinicians are referring to the clinical condition caused by reduced CO. However, clinical HF can exist in the presence of increased CO. This condition is called high-output HF, and it is typically present when CO is greater than 8 liters per minute or cardiac index is greater than 3.9 liters per minute per meter squared.[8]

Etiology and Pathogenesis

High-output HF is marked by an unusually low SVR and an elevated CO. This is typically caused by either dilation of the vascular bed or an abnormal connection between one or more arteries and one or more veins (arteriovenous fistula). Vasodilation can be caused by anemia, severe hyperthyroidism, sepsis syndrome, pregnancy, obesity, liver disease, elevated carbon dioxide levels, fever, exercise, or stress.[8,30] Systemic shunting, such as that caused by an arteriovenous fistula, can be caused by Paget disease, multiple myeloma, liver disease, or an artificially created fistula such as one created for dialysis. Regardless of the underlying cause, systemic blood pressure drops despite a normal or even high CO, and the sympathetic nervous system and the RAAS are activated, causing sodium and water retention, edema, and pulmonary congestion, as seen in low-output HF.[8]

A number of things can cause a decrease in SVR. In an effort to maintain adequate tissue oxygenation, anemia leads to vasodilation of the peripheral circulation due to the effect of nitric oxide. Nitric oxide, which is released as a result of anemia, causes arteriolar vasodilation, reducing SVR. Low blood viscosity, as seen in anemia, may also reduce the SVR, since blood viscosity also affects the resistance to systemic blood flow.[8]

Hyperthyroidism is a condition in which the thyroid gland produces an abnormally high level of thyroid hormone. Initially, this produces an increase in heart rate and preload and a resultant rise in CO. However, thyroid hormone also acts directly to promote vasodilation and to increase the production of nitric oxide, further increasing vasodilation.[31] As SVR decreases, so does systemic blood pressure, causing the activation of the RAAS. The resulting increase in sodium and water retention leads to HF in the setting of high CO. Eventually, chronic activation of the sympathetic nervous system and the RAAS leads to cardiac enlargement, ventricular remodeling, and the HF syndrome.

Finally, in sepsis, which is a systemic inflammatory response to an infection, there is profound vasodilation due to the release of a number of substances including interleukin 2, interleukin 6, interleukin 8, tumor necrosis factor alpha, and perhaps even endotoxins from invading bacteria. This profound vasodilation leads to low blood pressure and the resultant neurohormonal effects.[8]

Pregnancy, liver disease, elevated carbon dioxide levels, fever, and even exercise may induce high-output HF through vasodilation and the resultant lowering of SVR.[8] ■

Arteriovenous shunting may also cause decreased afterload. Arteriovenous fistulas shunt blood from a high-pressure arterial circuit to a low-pressure venous circuit. Regardless of the cause, arteriovenous fistulas shunt blood directly from the arterial circuit to the venous circuit, bypassing the capillary circulation. Removing the effect of the high pressure capillary circulation reduces SVR. CO increases, blood pressure decreases and the neurohormonal response to hypotension ensues.[30] Paget disease also causes arteriovenous shunting as a result of increase in blood flow in the bone and the area surrounding the bone. Multiple myeloma achieves reduction in SVR by a similar mechanism.[8] Arteriovenous fistulas may be congenital, iatrogenic, caused by trauma, or formed surgically as in the case of dialysis access.

Clinical Manifestations

As with systolic HF, activation of the RAAS causes sodium and water retention. Patients with high-output HF develop signs of volume overload such as hepatic congestion, elevated jugular venous pressure, and peripheral edema. Patients may also experience fatigue and dyspnea. The heart rate is typically normal but may be elevated in the case of high-output HF due to thyroid disease.[8]

CLINICAL POINT: Unlike patients with systolic HF, patients with high-output HF are typically warm with strong distal pulses. ■

Linking Pathophysiology to Diagnosis and Treatment

Treatment of high-output HF is aimed at treating the cause of the vasodilation, control of symptoms, and support of vital functions.[8] In the case of anemia, for example, treating the anemia and replacing blood volume may reverse the vasodilation. Similarly, treatment of hyperthyroidism with corticosteroids, methimizole, or propothiouricil will help to reverse the high-output state. In hyperthyroid states specifically, it may be necessary to control the heart rate with beta-blocker therapy. Control of the infection in sepsis with antibiotics and fluid administration to augment blood pressure may also be helpful.

High-output HF due to arteriovenous fistulas may be reversed by controlling the shunt between the arterial and venous beds. In the case of a dialysis fistula, this may include placing a band on the fistula itself to reduce blood flow. In severe cases, the fistula may need to be ligated or removed completely. It may be necessary to consider alternative methods of dialysis, such as catheter-based access or even peritoneal dialysis.[30]

Unlike systolic HF, treatment with vasodilators is not recommended in high-output HF, since the underlying cause of high-output HF is vasodilation. Similarly, excessive use of diuretics and rapid fluid removal may exacerbate the underlying process. In addition to treatment of the underlying cause, sodium and fluid restriction and careful use of diuretics may be effective in reducing volume overload and venous congestion.[8]

Supportive care may be necessary during treatment of the underlying condition. Medications that act directly on the alpha-adrenergic receptors causing vasoconstriction may be useful in supporting blood pressure.[8] These medications, such as ephedrine, norepinephrine, and phenylephrine, cause profound vasoconstriction and may lead to hypoperfusion of vital organs such as the liver, mesentery, and kidneys. They also require an intravenous catheter and intensive care monitoring and therefore are not practical for long-term use.

Aside from treating the underlying cause of high-output HF, controlling the symptoms, and supporting the individual acutely, there is little evidence to support other treatment options for high-output HF.

Check Your Progress: Section 26.7

1. What are some of the most common manifestations of high-output HF?
2. What are the causes of high-output HF?
3. What are some common treatments for patients with high-output HF?

CHAPTER SUMMARY

26.1 Chapter Overview and Case Studies

Describe the prevalence of heart failure and concepts related to heart failure.

- Heart failure is a critical public health concern, with more than 650,000 new cases diagnosed annually
- Fifty percent of all patients diagnosed with HF die within 5 years of diagnosis
- Patients with HF generally suffer from shortness of breath, swelling of the extremities, and fatigue
- Reduced cardiac output causes a complex set of responses that further worsen the heart failure syndrome

26.2 Classification and Staging of Heart Failure

Outline the classification and staging of heart failure.

- Heart failure may affect the right ventricle, the left ventricle, or both ventricles.
- Heart failure may be due to difficulty with contraction or relaxation of the ventricle.
- Heart failure may be a chronic condition, have acute decompensations, or be an acute condition causing critical illness or even death.
- Heart failure may be seen in patients with high cardiac output.
- There are various schemas to categorize HF, such as the NYHA class, the Killip Class, and the ACC/AHA stages of HF.

26.3 Systolic Heart Failure (Heart Failure with Reduced Ejection Fraction)

Differentiate the causes, classification, underlying pathogenesis, and clinical manifestations of systolic heart failure and approaches to diagnosis and treatment of this condition across the lifespan.

- In systolic HF, cardiac output is decreased.
- Cardiac output is decreased as a result of decreased contractility of the heart.
- Cardiac output is determined by heart rate and stroke volume.
- Stroke volume is determined by preload, afterload, and contractility.
- The sympathetic nervous system and the renin-angiotensin-aldosterone system (RAAS) are activated, causing the HF syndrome.
- Symptoms of systolic HF include dyspnea, pulmonary edema, weight loss, fatigue and dizziness.
- Treatment of systolic HF includes angiotensin-converting enzyme (ACE) inhibitors, angiotensin receptor blockers (ARBs), diuretics, aldosterone antagonists, and beta blockers.
- Implantable cardioverter-defibrillators or biventricular pacemakers may be used.
- Surgical therapy for systolic HF includes left ventricular assist device placement or cardiac transplantation.

26.4 Diastolic Heart Failure (Heart Failure with Preserved Ejection Fraction)

Differentiate the causes, classification, underlying pathogenesis, and clinical manifestations of diastolic heart failure and approaches to diagnosis and treatment of this condition across the lifespan.

- In diastolic HF, cardiac output is decreased.
- Diastolic HF is also called heart failure with preserved ejection fraction.
- Cardiac output is decreased as a result of decreased relaxation of the heart.
- The sympathetic nervous system and the RAAS are activated, causing the HF syndrome.
- Symptoms of HF include abdominal swelling and bloating and renal dysfunction.
- Treatment of diastolic HF is difficult, with no accepted therapy.
- Diuretics may be used cautiously.

26.5 Left-Sided Heart Failure

Differentiate the causes, classification, underlying pathogenesis, and clinical manifestations of left-sided heart failure and approaches to diagnosis and treatment of this condition across the lifespan.

- In left-sided HF, cardiac output of the left ventricle is decreased.
- Cardiac output is decreased as a result of decreased contractility of the left ventricle of the heart.
- The sympathetic nervous system and the RAAS are activated, causing the HF syndrome.
- Symptoms of left-sided HF include dizziness, syncope, fatigue, and shortness of breath.
- Treatment of left-sided HF is similar to that of systolic heart failure.

26.6 Right-Sided Heart Failure

Differentiate the causes, classification, underlying pathogenesis, and clinical manifestations of right-sided heart failure and approaches to diagnosis and treatment of this condition across the lifespan

- In right-sided HF, cardiac output of the right ventricle is decreased.
- Cardiac output is decreased as a result of decreased contractility of the right ventricle of the heart.
- The sympathetic nervous system and the RAAS are activated, causing the HF syndrome.
- Symptoms of right-sided HF include peripheral edema, abdominal bloating, fatigue, and dizziness.
- Treatment of right-sided HF is difficult. Diuretics may be used cautiously.
- Surgical therapy options include insertion of right ventricular assist devices and cardiac transplantation.

26.7 High-Output Heart Failure

Differentiate the causes, classification, underlying pathogenesis, and clinical manifestations of high-output heart failure and approaches to diagnosis and treatment of this condition across the lifespan.

- In high-output HF, cardiac output is increased, but systemic vascular resistance is low.
- High-output HF is caused by vasodilation or systemic shunting.
- Symptoms of high-output HF include shortness of breath and edema.
- Unlike patients with HF, patients with high-output heart failure are warm and have strong distal pulses.
- Treatment of high-output HF is based on treating the cause.
- ACE inhibitors and ARBs are not used to treat high-output HF.
- Vasoconstricting agents may be used to increase systemic vascular resistance in high-output HF.

REVIEW QUESTIONS

1. Which statement is *true* about the neurohormonal responses?
   a. The SNS is responsible for maintaining CO by decreasing sodium and water retention.
   b. The RAAS is the only neurohormonal response that maintains the CO.
   c. The inflammatory mediators are responsible only for cardiac repair.
   d. The compensatory mechanisms lead to secondary end-organ damage.

2. Which of the following describes stroke volume?
   a. The measurement of the percentage of blood ejected from the left ventricle with each contraction
   b. The amount of blood pumped out of the heart with each beat in milliliters
   c. A low-pressure system
   d. A high-pressure system

3. The nurse is educating a client on the treatment options for heart failure. Which of the following is a treatment option?
   a. Pacemaker insertion
   b. Coronary artery bypass graft
   c. Left ventricular assist device implantation
   d. Left heart catheterization
4. Which of the following are ways to reduce the symptoms of diastolic heart failure? (Select all that apply.)
   a. Smoking cessation
   b. Exercise program
   c. Control blood pressure
   d. Control diabetes
5. The nurse is educating the client on self-care activities. Which of the following is considered a self-care activity for the patient to perform at home?
   a. Medication management
   b. Monitoring of daily weights
   c. Blood pressure management
   d. Diabetes management
6. You are the nurse caring for a client with right-sided heart failure. What symptoms would you expect to see? (Select all that apply.)
   a. Peripheral edema
   b. Abdominal bloating
   c. Syncope
   d. Fatigue
7. You are the nurse caring for a client with high-output heart failure. Which of the following medications would you question? (Select all that apply.)
   a. ACE inhibitors
   b. Beta blockers
   c. ARBs
   d. Diuretics
8. You are a nurse getting a report for a client with heart failure. The report states that the client has an unusually low SVR and an elevated CO. What type of heart failure does the client have?
   a. Left-sided HF
   b. Diastolic HF
   c. High-output HF
   d. Systolic HF

ANSWERS

Answers to Review Questions can be found in Appendix A. Answers to Case Study and Check Your Progress questions are available on the faculty resources site. Please consult with your instructor.

RECOMMENDED WEBSITES

American Association of Heart Failure Nurses
http://www.aahfn.org

American Heart Association
http://www.heart.org

Centers for Disease Control and Prevention: Heart Disease
https://www.cdc.gov/heartdisease

Heart Failure Fact Sheet
http://www.cdc.gov/dhdsp/data_statistics/fact_sheets/docs/fs_heart_failure.pdf

Heart Failure Online
http://www.heartfailure.org

REFERENCES

1. Go, A. S., Mozaffarian, D., Roger, V. L., et al., for the American Heart Association Statistics Committee and Stroke Statistics Subcommittee. (2013). Heart disease and stroke statistics—2013 update: A report from the American Heart Association. *Circulation, 127*, e6–e245. doi:10.1161/CIR.0b013e31828124ad
2. Kemp, C. D., & Conte, J. V. (2012). The pathophysiology of heart failure. *Cardiovascular Pathology, 21*, 365–371. doi:10.1016/j.carpath.201.11.007
3. Mann, D. L., & Bristow, M. R. (2005). Mechanisms and models in heart failure: The biomechanical model and beyond. *Circulation, 111*(21), 2837–2849.
4. Rathi, S., & Deedwania, P. C. (2012). The epidemiology and pathophysiology of heart failure. *Medical Clinics of North America, 96*(5), 881–890.
5. Ryan, J. J., & Tedford, R. J. (2015). Diagnosing and treating the failing right heart. *Current Opinion in Cardiology, 30*(3), 292–300. doi:10.1097/HCO.0000000000000164
6. Voelkel, N. F., Quaife, R. A., Leinwand, L. A., et al. (2006). Right ventricular function and failure: Report of a National Heart, Lung and Blood Institute Working Group on Cellular and Molecular Mechanisms of Right Heart Failure. *Circulation, 114*, 1883–1891. doi:10.1161/CIRCULATIONAHA.106.632208
7. Borlaug, B. A., & Paulus, W. J. (2011). Heart failure with preserved ejection fraction: Pathophysiology, diagnosis and treatment. *European Heart Journal, 32*, 670–679. doi:10.1093/eurheartj/ehq426
8. Mehta, P. A., & Dubrey, S. W. (2009). High output heart failure. *QJM: An International Journal of Medicine, 102*, 235–241. doi:10.1093/qjmed/hcn147
9. Riegel, B., Moser, D. K., Anker, S. D., et al. (2009). Promoting self-care in persons with heart failure: A scientific statement from the American Heart Association. *Circulation, 120*, 1141–1163. doi:10.1161/CIRCULATIONAHA.109.192628

10. Yancy, C. W., Jessup, M., Bozkurt, B., et al. (2013). 2013 ACCF/AHA guideline for the management of heart failure. *Journal of the American College of Cardiology, 62*(16), e147–e239. doi:10.1016/j.jacc.2013.05.019
11. American Heart Association. (1994). 1994 revisions to classification of functional capacity and objective assessment of patients with heart disease. *Circulation, 90*, 644–645.
12. Chyu, J., Fonarow, G. C., Tseng, H., & Horwich, T. B. (2013). Four-variable risk model in men and women with heart failure. *Circulation: Heart Failure, 7*, 88–95. doi:10.1161/CIRCHEARTFAILURE.113.000404
13. Killip, T., & Kimball, J. T. (1967). Treatment of myocardial infarction in a coronary care unit: A two year experience with 250 patients. *American Journal of Cardiology, 20*, 457–464.
14. Scruth, E. A., Page, K., Cheng, E., Campbell, M., & Worrall-Carter, L. (2012). Risk determination after acute myocardial infarction: Review of 3 clinical risk prediction tools. *Clinical Nurse Specialist, 26*(1), 35–41. doi:0.097/NUR.0b013e31823bfafc
15. Sliwa, K., Hilfiker-Kleiner, D., Petrie, M. C., Mebazaa, A., Pieske, B., Buchmann, E., Regitz-Zagrosek, V., Schaufelberger, M., Tavazzi, L., Veldhuisen, D. J., Watkins, H., Shah, A. J., Seferovic, P. M., Elkayam, U, .Pankuweit, S., Papp, Z., Mouquet, F., & McMurray, J. J. (2010). Current state of knowledge on aetiology, diagnosis, management, and therapy of peripartum cardiomyopathy: A position statement from the Heart Failure Association of the European Society of Cardiology Working Group on Peripartum Cardiomyopathy. *European Journal of Heart Failure, 12*(8), 767–778.
16. Kantor, P. F, Lougheed, J., Dancea, A., et al. (2013). Presentation, diagnosis, and medical management of heart failure in children: Canadian Cardiovascular Society guidelines. *Canadian Journal of Cardiology, 29*(12), 1535–1552.
17. Lough, M. E. (2016). *Hemodynamic monitoring: Evolving technologies & clinical practice*. New York, NY: Elsevier.
18. Miller, L. R., (2014). Hemodynamic monitoring. In S. Burns (Ed.), *AACN essentials of critical care nursing* (3rd ed., pp. 69–118). New York, NY: McGraw-Hill.
19. Edwards Lifesciences. (2009) *Normal hemodynamic parameters and laboratory values*. Available at http://ht.edwards.com/scin/edwards/sitecollectionimages/edwards/products/presep/ar04313hemodynpocketcard.pdf
20. O'Donovan, K. (2015). Aldosterone antagonists in heart failure with reduced ejection fraction. *Nurse Prescribing, 13*(5), 242–248. Available at http://content.ebscohost.com.proxy.uchicago.edu/ContentServer.asp?T=P&P=AN&K=103798261&S=R&D=rzh&EbscoContent=dGJyMMvl7ESeqa44zOX0OLCmr02ep69Ss6q4TbKWxWXS&ContentCustomer=dGJyMPGut1C3r7ZMuePfgeyx44Dt6fIA
21. Paul, S., & Page, R. L. (2016). Foundations of pharmacotherapy for heart failure with reduced ejection fraction: Evidence meets practice. *Journal of Cardiovascular Nursing, 31*(2), 101–103. doi:10.1097/JCN.0000000000000284
22. Saraon, T., & Katz, S. D. (2015). Reverse remodeling in systolic heart failure. *Cardiology in Review, 23*(4), 173–181. doi:10.1097/CRD.0000000000000068
23. Pressler, S. J., Subramanian, U., Kareken, D., et al. (2010). Cognitive deficits in heart failure. *Nursing Research, 59*(2), 127–139. doi:10.1097/NNR.06013e3181d1a747
24. Cameron, J., Worrall-Carter, L., Page, K., Riegel, B., Lo, S. K., & Stewart, S. (2010). Does cognitive impairment predict poor self-care in patients with heart failure? *European Journal of Heart Failure, 12*, 508–515. doi:10.1093/eurjhf/hfq042
25. Lund, L. H., Edwards, L. B., Kucheryavaya, A. Y., et al. (2015). The Registry of the International Society for Heart and Lung Transplant: Thirty-second official adult heart transplantation report—2015: Focus theme: Early graft failure. *Journal of Heart and Lung Transplantation, 34*(10), 1244–1254.
26. Sharma, K., & Kass, D. A. (2014). Heart failure with preserved ejection fraction: Mechanisms, clinical features and therapies. *Circulation: Research, 115*, 79–96. doi:10.1161/CIRCRESEAHA.115.302922
27. Jumean, M., & Konstam, M. A. (2015). Heart failure with preserved ejection fraction: What's in a name? *Cardiology in Review, 23*(4), 161–167. doi:10.1097/CRD.0000000000000057
28. Tannenbaum, S., & Sayer, G. (2015). Advances in the pathophysiology and treatment of heart failure with preserved ejection fraction. *Current Opinion in Cardiology, 30*(30), 250–258. doi:10.1097/HCO.0000000000000163
29. Pitt, B., Pfeffer, M. A., Assmann, S. F., et al. (2014). Spironolactone for heart failure with preserved ejection fraction. *New England Journal of Medicine, 370*, 1383–1392.
30. Wasse, H., & Singapuri, S. (2012). High-output heart failure: How to define it, when to treat it and how to treat it. *Seminars in Nephrology, 32*(6), 551–557. doi:10.1016/jsemnephrol.2012.10.006
31. Biondi, B. (2012). Mechanisms in endocrinology: Heart failure and thyroid dysfunction. *European Journal of Endocrinology, 167*(5), 609–618. doi:10.1530/EJE-12-0627

Chapter 27

Disorders of Circulation Within the CNS

Angela Starkweather

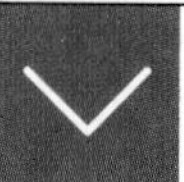

Chapter Outline and Learning Outcomes

27.1 Chapter Overview and Case Studies

Describe the function of the central nervous system and concepts related to disorders of circulation within the central nervous system.

27.2 Vascular Supply of the Central Nervous System

Outline the vascular supply of the brain and spinal cord.

27.3 Production and Circulation of Cerebrospinal Fluid

Distinguish the normal flow of cerebrospinal fluid through the brain and spinal cord in contrast with the circulation of blood.

27.4 Blood–Brain Barrier

Summarize the protective role of the blood–brain barrier.

27.5 Cerebral Autoregulation

Predict the influence of cerebral autoregulation on the blood vessels that supply the central nervous system.

27.6 Ischemia and Hypoxia of the Central Nervous System

Explain the cellular events that follow from ischemia and hypoxia of the brain and spinal cord.

27.7 Transient Ischemic Attack

Differentiate the causes, classification, underlying pathogenesis, and clinical manifestations of transient ischemic attack and approaches to diagnosis and treatment of this condition across the lifespan.

27.8 Ischemic and Hemorrhagic Stroke

Differentiate the causes, classification, underlying pathogenesis, and clinical manifestations of ischemic and hemorrhagic strokes and approaches to diagnosis and treatment of these conditions across the lifespan.

27.9 Subdural and Spinal Cord Hemorrhage

Differentiate the causes, classification, underlying pathogenesis, and clinical manifestations of subdural and spinal cord hemorrhage and approaches to diagnosis and treatment of these conditions across the lifespan.

KEY TERMS

Aneurysm, 672
Arteriovenous malformation (AVM), 672
Blood–brain barrier, 665
Cerebral autoregulation, 666
Cerebral blood flow, 666
Cerebrospinal fluid (CSF), 664
Delayed cerebral ischemia (DCI), 673
Hematoma, 661
Hemorrhagic stroke, 672
Hydrocephalus, 664
Intracranial pressure, 667
Ischemia, 661
Ischemic stroke, 671
Stroke, 671
Transient ischemic attack (TIA), 670

ABBREVIATIONS

AVM—arteriovenous malformation
CBF—cerebral blood flow
CPP—cerebral perfusion pressure
CSF—cerebrospinal fluid
CVR—cerebrovascular resistance
DCI—delayed cerebral ischemia
NPH—normal pressure hydrocephalus
TIA—transient ischemic attack

27.1 Chapter Overview and Case Studies

The brain and the spinal cord are the major components of the central nervous system (CNS) and act synergistically to detect, transmit, and analyze sensory information and generate signals to autonomic and motor pathways that orchestrate visceral and endocrine functions, coordination, and movement. This chapter highlights the importance of maintaining adequate circulation to tissues of the CNS, which rely heavily on receiving constant perfusion from cardiac output. The pathophysiology of blood circulation and the production and flow of cerebrospinal fluid through the CNS are reviewed. Cerebral autoregulation and the blood–brain barrier protect the tissues in the CNS but can become dysfunctional with exposure to chronic high blood pressure, trauma, infection, metabolic disorders, and medications. Understanding the major diseases that directly influence circulation within the CNS and the associated neurologic impairments that follow requires knowledge of molecular and biochemical processes and of functional neuroanatomy.

The major disorders of circulation within the CNS are transient ischemic attack, ischemic and hemorrhagic stroke, and subdural and spinal cord hemorrhage. These are discussed in this chapter along with approaches to treatment that aim to deter or reduce neurologic injury. These conditions result from a lack of oxygen or disruption of blood flow. A transient ischemic attack is a brief appearance of symptoms that resemble those of a stroke. A stroke (also known as a brain attack) is an enduring disruption of speech, motor, communication, and cognitive deficits, while hemorrhage into tissue of the brain or spinal cord results in compression of surrounding tissue, resulting in lasting deficits that depend on the location. Less common disorders of circulation within the CNS are presented in **Table 27.1** ■. Advances in understanding the pathogenesis of circulatory disorders of the CNS are leading to new diagnostic and therapeutic modalities with the goal of preventing the occurrence and improving functional outcomes of these potentially devastating events.

Concepts Related to Disorders of Circulation Within the CNS

The major concepts concerning disorders of circulation within the brain revolve around a lack of oxygen and the possibility of increased pressure within the skull (**Figure 27.1** ■). Obstructed blood vessels or a drop in blood flow to the brain can result in **ischemia**, a lack of oxygen and glucose that leads to tissue damage. This is one of the main mechanisms underlying stroke. The other major means of injury is increasing pressure within the skull, from bleeding into tissue (**hematoma**) or from excessive production of cerebral spinal fluid. Blockage of the duct system that conveys cerebral spinal fluid can also result in increasing pressure within the brain. The increased pressure compresses tissue and blood vessels, causing tissue injury and ischemia. The bleeding into the brain or lack of oxygen initiates compensatory mechanisms that lead to vessel dilation and other metabolic changes that can worsen intracranial pressure.

Table 27.1 Less Common Disorders of Circulation Within the Central Nervous System

Disorder	Description
Carotid or vertebral artery dissection	A separation of the layers of the artery wall supplying oxygen-carrying blood to the brain and/or spinal cord. Symptoms include headache and neck pain, Horner syndrome (triad of miosis, partial ptosis, and anhidrosis), and transient vision loss (amaurosis fugax).
Cerebral venous sinus thrombosis	The presence of a thrombosis (blood clot) in the dural venous sinuses that drain blood from the brain. Symptoms may include headache, abnormal vision, or any symptoms of stroke.
Fibromuscular dysplasia	A condition that causes narrowing (stenosis) and enlargement of the medium-sized arteries. It can lead to high blood pressure or arterial dissection and most commonly appears in the arteries leading to the kidneys.
Moyamoya disease	A rare, progressive cerebrovascular disorder caused by blocked arteries at the base of the brain in the basal ganglia. It most often affects children but can occur in adults and tends to be familial, so it may be an inherited genetic disorder. Moyamoya disease leads to recurrent TIAs and stroke.
Vascular dementia	A condition that is caused by reduced blood flow to the brain resulting in cognitive impairments. It occurs from narrowing and blockage of the small blood vessels deep in the brain and is associated with high blood pressure. It is likely an inherited disorder.
Vasculitis	A condition causing inflammation of blood vessels that can cause thickening, weakening, narrowing, and scarring. Also known as arteritis, it can be so severe that it leads to ischemia of tissues and organs.
Vein of Galen malformations	A type of arteriovenous fistula involving the vein of Galen, a large vein deep in the brain. The fistula is formed during early prenatal development and is often identified during ultrasound in late pregnancy. It can result in increased head circumference, hydrocephalus, and heart failure.

Case Studies

The following cases will be addressed throughout the chapter to assist in application of chapter content to clinical situations that involve individuals with disorders of circulation within the CNS.

Norma James: Introduction

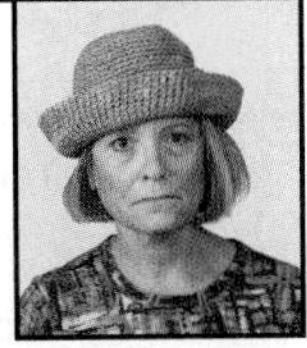

Norma James is a 65-year-old widow with a history of type 2 diabetes, atrial fibrillation, and hypertension. She wakes up one morning with her right arm feeling numb. She goes about her morning routine and decides to return to bed. When she again wakes up, her right arm feels heavy, as does her right leg. While concerned about these symptoms, she does not immediately seek assistance. Later in the day, a neighbor notes that Mrs. James's words are slurred and that she is not making sense. She is also unable to walk. Her neighbor decides to call 9-1-1 to get Mrs. James transported to the emergency department.

1. What is the most likely cause of the symptoms Mrs. James is experiencing?
2. What risk factors increase the likelihood of a CNS circulation disorder for Mrs. James?
3. Why is it unlikely that Mrs. James is having a transient ischemic attack?

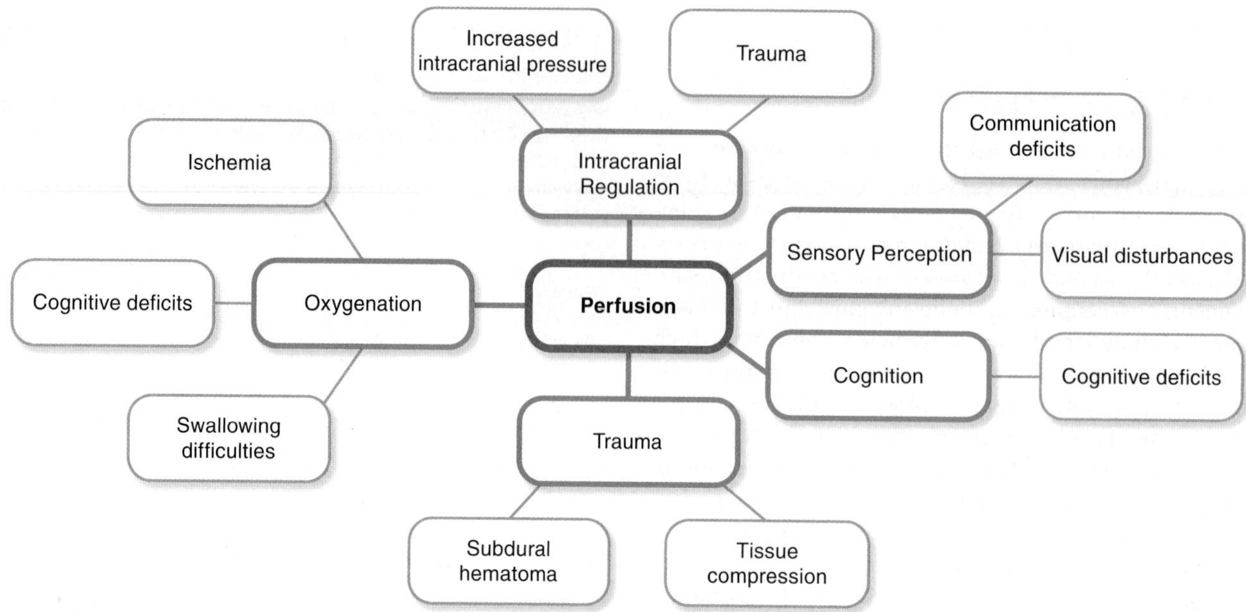

Figure 27.1 ■ Concepts related to disorders of circulation in the CNS.

Abigail Martin: Introduction

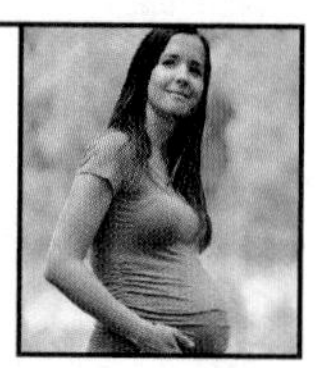

Abigail Martin, a 34-year-old woman, is 37 weeks pregnant when she experiences the "worst headache of her life" and blindness in her left eye while on a picnic with her husband. Her husband quickly drives her to the emergency department, where she suddenly develops nuchal rigidity, expressive aphasia, and somnolence. She is gravida 2 para 1 and denies any complications with her pregnancy up to this point. She does not smoke, drink alcohol, or use illicit drugs. On arrival, her blood pressure is 145/85 mmHg with a heart rate of 84 beats per minute. Clinical and ultrasound evaluations demonstrate an active fetus, gestational age compatible with the date of amenorrhea, and fetal heartbeats of 140 beats per minute. CT angiography of Ms. Martin's brain detects signs of subarachnoid hemorrhage due to rupture of an ophthalmic segment aneurysm in the internal carotid artery.

1. What risk factors does Ms. Martin have for cerebral aneurysm rupture?
2. What symptoms indicate a subarachnoid hemorrhage?
3. What is the reason for experiencing a headache with subarachnoid hemorrhage?

Check Your Progress: Section 27.1

1. In addition to cerebral autoregulation, which structure protects the tissues of the CNS?
2. What is the primary difference between a transient ischemic attack and a stroke?
3. What is one of the main mechanisms underlying stroke?

27.2 Vascular Supply of the Central Nervous System

The CNS contains an eloquent vascular network that maintains perfusion throughout the brain and spinal cord. Although the brain weighs only 2.5% of total body mass, it receives approximately 15% of cardiac output, which is used to supply adequate oxygen and nutrients to cells of the CNS.[1] This resource-intensive system does not require an even distribution in the supply of oxygen and nutrients; rather, some tissue types have a higher dependency on a constant supply of oxygen than others. Although the white matter of the CNS makes up 60% of brain mass, it uses only 6% of cerebral oxygen, whereas the gray matter of the brain utilizes 94% of cerebral oxygen, owing to its high metabolic demand.[2]

Two pairs of large arteries that branch off from the aorta supply a constant flow of blood to the brain and spinal cord: the right and left internal carotid arteries, which branch from the common carotid arteries, and the right and left vertebral arteries, which arise from the subclavian arteries (**Figure 27.2** ■). The internal carotid arteries branch off within the cranium to form two major cerebral arteries: the anterior and middle cerebral arteries.[3] The vertebral arteries and 10 medullary arteries that arise from segmental branches of the aorta provide vascularization of the spinal cord. The right and left vertebral arteries join at the level of the pons on the surface of the brainstem to form the basilar artery.

Within the brain, the basilar artery joins the blood supply from the internal carotids in an arterial ring called the circle of Willis at the base of the brain.[3] From this ring, several branches arise, including the posterior cerebral arteries and two bridging arteries: the anterior and posterior communicating arteries (**Figure 27.3** ■). The circulatory pattern created by the circle of Willis, which conjoins the two major sources of cerebral vascular supply, improves the likelihood of ensuring vascular supply to the brain tissues if one of the major arteries becomes occluded.

The two internal carotid arteries and their branches comprise the anterior circulation of the brain.[1] The internal carotids pass through the cavernous sinus, or carotid siphon, and give rise to the ophthalmic arteries, which divide to form the anterior choroidal branches, which follow the optic tract posteriorly. The internal carotids then divide into the middle cerebral and anterior cerebral arteries. Both the anterior and middle cerebral arteries give rise to branches that supply the cortex as well as branches that supply the deep structures of the brain, including the basal ganglia, thalamus, and internal capsule. The anterior cerebral arteries enter the fissure separating the left and right hemispheres to supply the medial and superior surface of the cortex; the middle cerebral artery traverses the fissure to supply the lateral part of the cerebral cortex.[3]

The posterior circulation of the brain comprises arterial branches arising from the posterior cerebral, basilar, and vertebral arteries, which supply the posterior cortex, midbrain, and brainstem. The basilar artery ends as the posterior cerebral arteries that supply the medial temporal lobes and most of the occipital lobe and the superior cerebellar artery. Within the brainstem, the anterior inferior cerebellar artery and posterior inferior cerebellar artery supply distinct regions of the medulla and pons. Because of their location, these arteries are especially common sites of occlusion, which results in functional deficits of cranial nerve, somatic sensory, and motor function.[4]

The venous drainage of the brain travels through bridging veins on the brain surface into sinuses that are tunnels in the dura (**Figure 27.4** ■). The superior sagittal sinus is one of the largest sinuses and is located where the falx cerebri attaches to the dura over the skull.[2] The great cerebral vein of Galen is an important vein that drains the deep structures of the brain. The dural venous sinuses receive blood from the microcirculation of the brain as well as cerebrospinal fluid from the subarachnoid space, which ultimately flows into the internal jugular vein.[3]

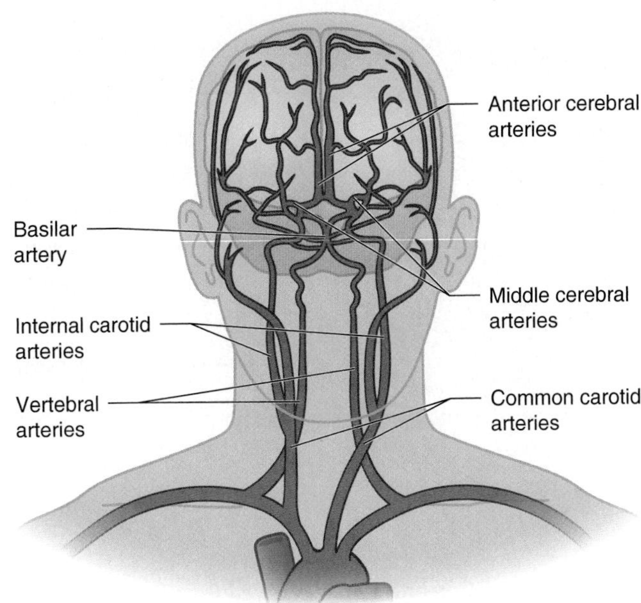

Figure 27.2 ■ Arterial circulation of the CNS. The right and left internal carotid arteries branch from the common carotid arteries and travel into the brain, where they branch off into the right and left middle cerebral arteries and the right and left anterior cerebral arteries. The right and left vertebral arteries branch from the subclavian arteries and travel to the back of the brain, where they merge to form the basilar artery.

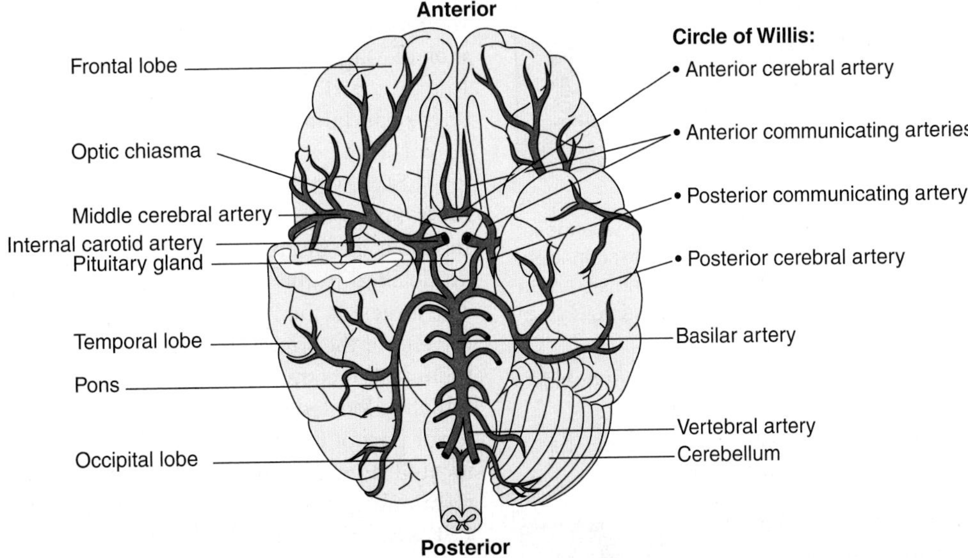

Figure 27.3 ■ Located at the base of the brain is the circle of Willis, composed of a network of arteries. In the distal portion is the posterior communicating artery. In the middle portion is the superior cerebellar artery and the anterior inferior cerebellar artery. In the proximal portion is the posterior inferior cerebellar artery and the anterior spinal artery.

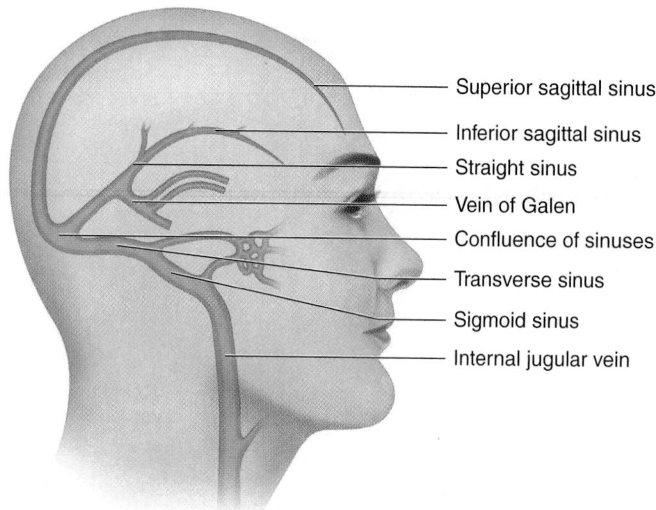

Figure 27.4 ■ Cerebral sinuses viewed from the right side of the brain. Venous drainage flows through sinuses that traverse across the outer edges of the brain in the superior sagittal sinus and the deep structures of the brain in the vein of Galen. Venous blood drains into the internal jugular vein.

CLINICAL POINT: Changes in neurologic function can be caused by a wide range of metabolic, infectious, or vascular events. Any time there is a progression of neurologic impairment, especially on one side of the body, a vascular etiology should be highly suspected. A hemorrhage or interruption in blood flow at any point between the heart and the brain can lead to alterations in neurologic function, which is why a computed tomography (CT) scan of the brain is initially used to identify the presence of hemorrhage. When no hemorrhage is present on the initial brain CT scan, the patient is assumed to have an ischemic event and may be treated accordingly until additional diagnostic tests can be undertaken.[4] ■

Norma James: Application

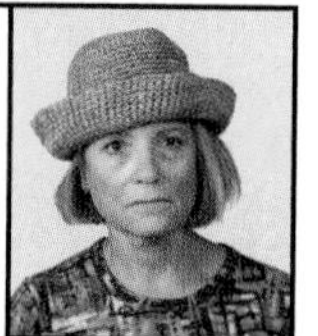

Mrs. James displayed right arm weakness that quickly progressed to right arm and leg weakness. On arrival at the emergency department, her blood pressure is 195/98 mmHg, and her heart rate is 90 with normal sinus rhythm. Her blood glucose is tested to determine whether this could explain her weakness; it is slightly elevated at 137 mg/dL. On physical examination, a right facial droop is noted along with right hemiparesis and a positive Babinski reflex. A CT scan of her brain shows no sign of hemorrhage.

4. An occlusion to which cerebral artery would interrupt blood flow to the lateral part of the cerebral cortex?
5. Because the CT scan does not show hemorrhage, what is the most likely cause of Mrs. James's symptoms?

Abigail Martin: Application

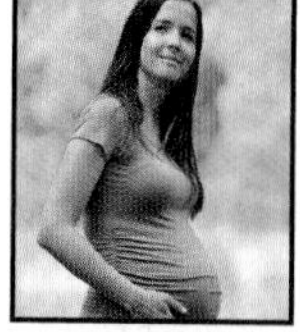

Ms. Martin is in her third trimester of pregnancy, a time when blood volume and cardiac output increase along with alterations in prostaglandin metabolism and consequent vascular intima hyperplasia that can weaken the wall of the arteries, resulting in an aneurysm. Increased hemodynamic stress and hormonal changes can contribute to the development and rupture of cerebral aneurysms.

4. What is a cerebral aneurysm?
5. What occurs after a cerebral aneurysm ruptures?
6. Ms. Martin's aneurysm involved her ophthalmic artery, which divides into what branch that follows the optic nerve posteriorly?

Check Your Progress: Section 27.2

1. High metabolic demand is characteristic of which type of brain matter?
2. The internal carotid arteries branch off into which two main arteries within the brain?
3. What is the name of the arterial ring located at the base of the brain that is formed by the joining of the basilar arteries with the internal carotid arteries?

27.3 Production and Circulation of Cerebrospinal Fluid

The brain actively produces **cerebrospinal fluid (CSF)** in the choroid plexi, which are located in the ventricles (**Figure 27.5** ■). CSF normally has half the glucose concentration of peripheral blood and contains few cells and a low concentration of protein.[2] CSF produced in the ventricles flows into the third ventricle via the foramen of Monro. A narrow cerebral aqueduct located in the core of the midbrain connects the third ventricle to the fourth ventricle. CSF flows from the fourth ventricle to the subarachnoid space via the foramen of Magendie and two lateral foramina of Luschka. The fourth ventricle also connects with the tiny central canal of the caudal medulla, allowing CSF to flow to the sacral spinal cord.[3]

CSF flows in the subarachnoid space surrounding the brain and spinal cord, providing buoyancy and nourishment for the brain.[2] Collections of CSF, known as cisterns, are located in the brain and spinal cord (see Figure 27.5). The largest is the lumbar cistern, which is located between the end of the spinal cord and the thecal sac. Other cisterns include the cisterna magna (cerebellomedullary cistern), which is located between the dorsal medulla and the posterior part of the cerebellum; the superior cistern, which is located dorsal to the midbrain; and the cistern of lamina terminalis, which is located rostral to the third ventricle. CSF is resorbed into the venous dural sinuses via the arachnoid villi. Conditions that impair the flow of CSF through the ventricles or disrupt the ability of the arachnoid villi to resorb CSF can result in **hydrocephalus**, an excessive accumulation of CSF in the brain that can cause increased pressure within the skull.

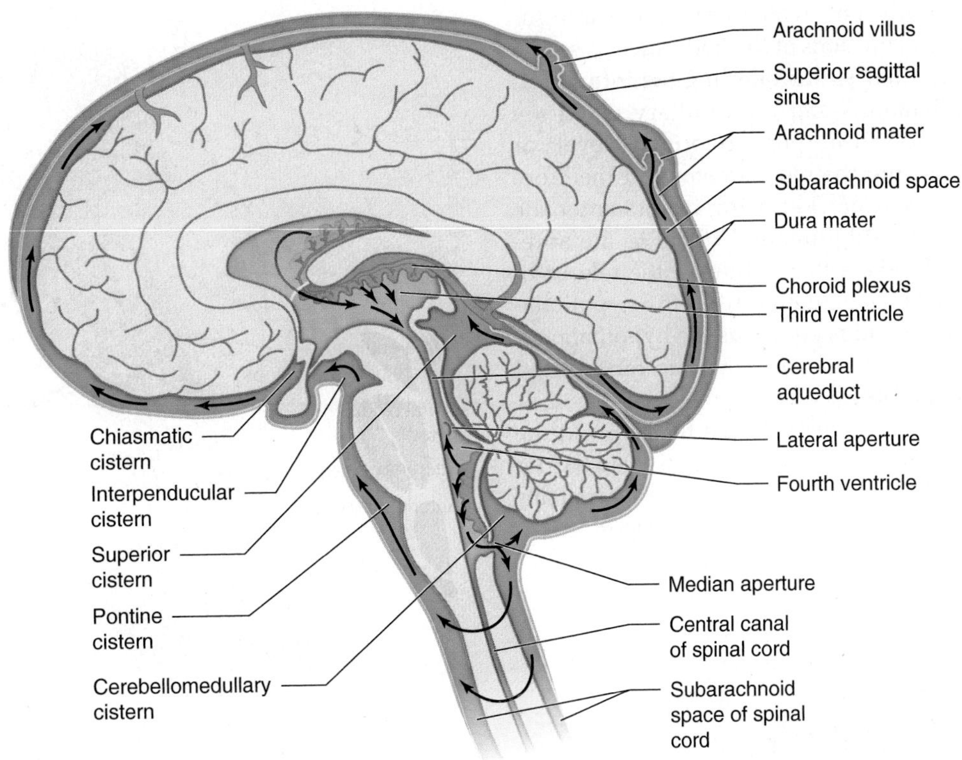

Figure 27.5 ■ CSF, shown here in blue, is formed in the choroid plexi of the ventricles. The CSF flows throughout the ventricles of the brain and into the outer surface and subarachnoid space of the brain and spinal cord and then collects within cisterns in the brain and spinal cord.

Norma James: Application

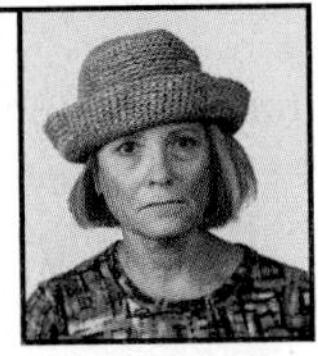

Mrs. James is diagnosed with an ischemic stroke and will be closely monitored in the intensive care unit to track any changes in her neurologic function. This will help to determine whether the area of infarction is growing. Areas of infarction that develop around the brainstem, such as cerebellar infarction, can lead to compression of brain tissue and obstructive hydrocephalus.

6. What signs would be present if the area of infarction continued to grow?
7. What complication would you expect to occur as a result of hydrocephalus?

Abigail Martin: Application

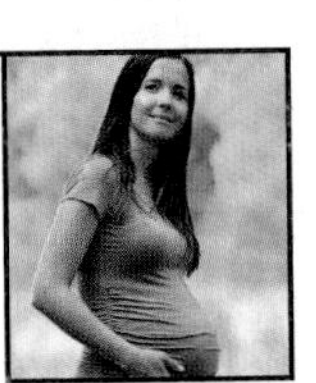

Ms. Martin undergoes an emergency cesarean delivery that results in no complications for her or the newborn. Ms. Martin remains under sedation and mechanical ventilation in the intensive care unit and is receiving constant management of her hemodynamic status. Serial CTs of her brain are obtained to monitor for the development of hydrocephalus, as the blood in the subarachnoid space can block the arachnoid villi and deter the resorption of CSF.

7. Why is it important to manage Ms. Martin's hemodynamic status?
8. An increasing size of the ventricles on head CT would be a sign of what condition?

Check Your Progress: Section 27.3

1. What structure of the brain produces cerebrospinal fluid?
2. What is the structure through which CSF flows from the ventricles to the third ventricle?
3. Where does the CSF flow when it travels from the fourth ventricle through the foramen of Magendie and two lateral foramina of Luschka?

27.4 Blood–Brain Barrier

The **blood–brain barrier** is composed of specialized endothelium in the brain capillaries that permits selective entry of substances into the brain (**Figure 27.6** ■). The brain capillary endothelium includes tight junctions between endothelial cells, few pinocytotic vesicles, no fenestra, and high amounts of metabolic activity involved in active transport.[1] Highly lipophilic substances are able to cross the membrane directly and enter the brain, and water can cross the membrane by simple diffusion.[2] Most nutrients cross the barrier by facilitated diffusion through mechanisms that couple the movement of the nutrient with movement of an ion that is moving down its concentration gradient (see Figure 27.6).

There are areas of the brain that lack a blood–brain barrier, including the subfornical organ and the area postrema of the brainstem, which are responsible for sensing the internal conditions of the body such as serum osmolarity.[1] The capillaries surrounding the infundibulum of the hypothalamus and the pituitary gland are regions that are involved in sensing hormone levels or releasing hormones into the bloodstream and therefore lack a blood–brain barrier.[2] Releasing factors enter the capillaries of the infundibulum and travel to the anterior pituitary gland, where they influence the release of trophic hormones. This circulation from the hypothalamus to the pituitary gland is known as the hypothalamo-hypophyseal portal system and contains fenestrated capillaries (**Figure 27.7** ■).

Because there is no barrier between the CSF and the brain, the epithelium of the choroid plexus creates a barrier between the CSF and blood circulation. This barrier contains tight junctions between cells and specific transport mechanisms for nutrient passage and electrolyte regulation.[1]

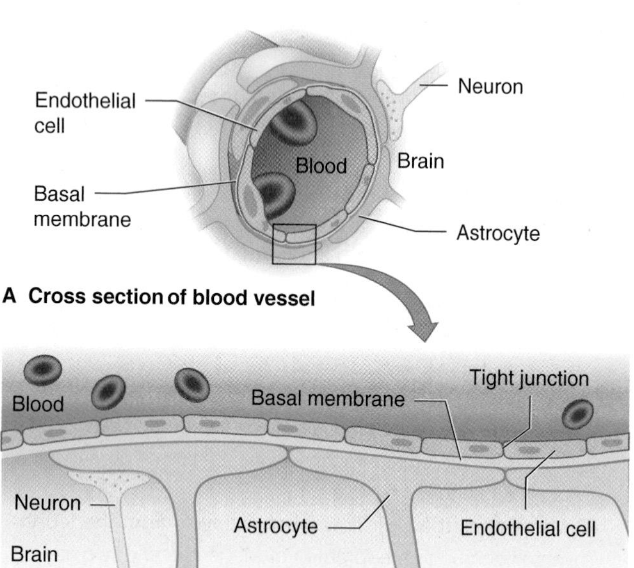

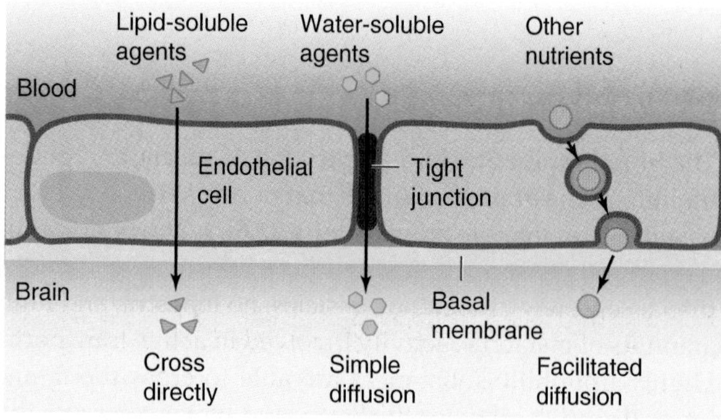

Figure 27.6 ■ The blood–brain barrier is composed of specialized endothelial cells in brain capillaries that permit selective entry of substances into the brain. Water, oxygen, and glucose pass freely across the blood–brain barrier from the blood to the brain tissue.

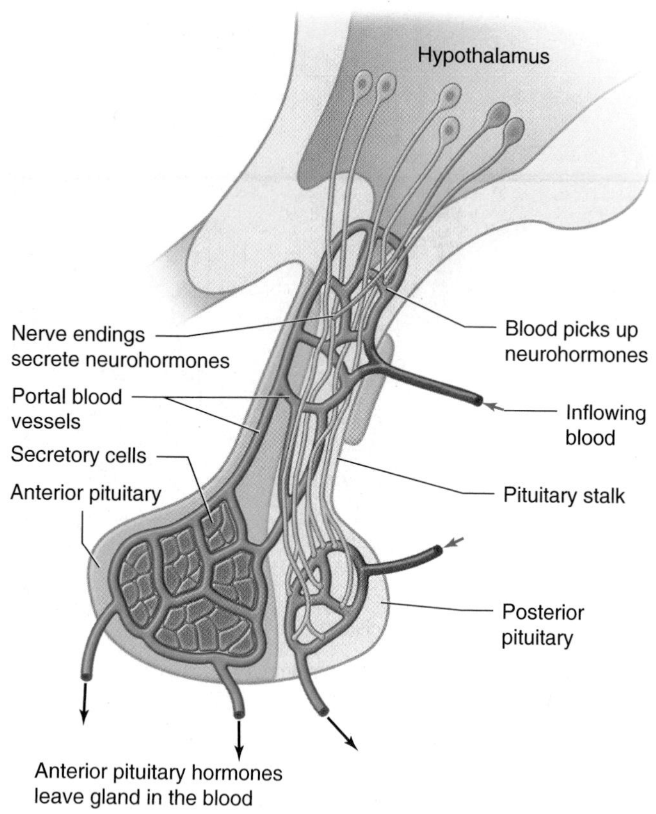

Figure 27.7 ■ The hypothalamo-hypophyseal portal system. Hormones produced and secreted by the hypothalamus enter the bloodstream through fenestrated capillaries.

Tanycytes, which are specialized glial cells that are present between areas of the brain with and without blood–brain barriers, prevent substances from moving between these brain regions.

Check Your Progress: Section 27.4

1. What types of substances are able to directly cross the blood–brain barrier?
2. Why do some areas of the brain lack a blood–brain barrier?
3. What are the specialized glial cells that are present between areas of the brain with and without blood–brain barriers?

27.5 Cerebral Autoregulation

Cerebral autoregulation is critically important for providing a steady flow of oxygen and nutrients to brain cells and removing metabolic wastes.[3] Cerebral autoregulation maintains blood flow to the brain and spinal cord despite wide fluctuations in mean arterial pressure. **Cerebral blood flow** (the blood supply to the brain in a given time) is closely matched to metabolic needs, and the arteries respond to metabolic factors such as pH, carbon dioxide, and oxygen

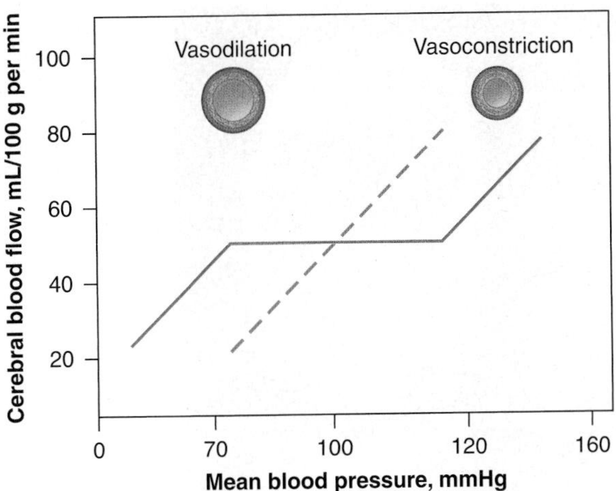

Figure 27.8 ■ Cerebral blood flow is closely matched to metabolic needs, and the arteries respond to metabolic factors such as pH, carbon dioxide, and oxygen by either relaxing or contracting. With low mean arterial pressure as indicated by the dotted line, vasodilation occurs, allowing more blood flow to the cerebral tissues. As mean arterial pressure rises, vasoconstriction occurs. This autoregulatory response helps to maintain a constant cerebral perfusion pressure as seen by the solid line.

by either relaxing or contracting (**Figure 27.8** ■). When blood pressure rises, the cerebral capillaries constrict, preventing a significant rise in blood flow, whereas the capillaries dilate to allow more blood flow to circulate when mean arterial blood pressure falls or brain metabolism increases. In the presence of severe hypotension or malignant hypertension, autoregulation is no longer effective. Severe hypotension predisposes the brain tissue to ischemia, whereas malignant hypertension can result in damage to the endothelium and the blood–brain barrier.

The partial pressure of carbon dioxide ($PaCO_2$) in arterial blood influences cerebral autoregulation more significantly than the partial pressure of oxygen (PaO_2) does.[2] Cerebral blood flow increases or decreases briskly in response to changes in $PaCO_2$; cerebral vessels constrict as $PaCO_2$ levels fall and dilate to increase blood flow when $PaCO_2$ levels rise. This autoregulatory response can cause detrimental increases in cerebral blood flow when respiratory compromise leads to hypercapnia. The cerebral vessels dilate in response to hypercapnia and can allow excessive cerebral blood volume that exacerbates cerebral edema. Hyperventilation to reduce $PaCO_2$ causes the arteries to dilate, which can reduce intracranial pressure but also increases the risk of ischemia.

Autoregulatory mechanisms fail as there is a loss of matching between the oxygen supply and demand of tissues in the CNS. Increased neuronal activity with excessive release of catecholamines and excitatory amino acids drives up oxygen demand. Effort to reduce the release of excitatory neurotransmitters through sedation, pain management, and rest may be beneficial. Hypothermia is also used to reduce the metabolic demands of brain tissue after injury and to prevent further impairment of blood flow or ischemia. Other methods to maintain functional autoregulation include treating increased intracranial pressure, reducing cerebral edema, removing mass lesions or space-occupying tumors, or hemorrhage from the brain or spinal cord.

Intracranial pressure is the pressure exerted by the contents of the cranium: brain tissue, blood, and CSF. The Monro-Kellie hypothesis describes the compensatory relationship in response to changes in volume of any of the three components.[3] If there is a slight increase in any one of the components, such as a cranial tumor growing in the brain cortex, it can be offset by a reduction in volume of the other two—in this example, blood flow and CSF. This is known as cerebral compliance, the ability to accommodate changes in volume without a significant rise in intracranial pressure. However, because the skull creates a closed compartment, compliance is limited to accommodation of only small volumes, whereas moderate to severe changes in volume result in significant increases in intracranial pressure. Brain tissue does not have the ability to reduce volume to compensate for expansions in the volume of CSF or blood. However, the cerebral vessels can constrict to reduce the volume of blood, and the CSF compartment can shunt blood to the spinal cord or increase resorption. In addition to mass lesions, cytotoxic and vasogenic edema as well as hydrocephalus are common causes of increased intracranial pressure.

In infants and young children, increased intracranial pressure can manifest as an increase in head circumference because the bones of the skull have not yet fused. At these ages, the skull can expand to accommodate the increased volume within the cranium. ■

Injured brain tissue is susceptible to cytotoxic edema, which occurs in the intracellular compartment when ischemic tissue swells because of cellular energy failure. Without adequate amounts of adenosine triphosphate (ATP), Na^+ ions are allowed to accumulate in the cell and create an osmotic force that pulls water inside the cell.[2] In addition, fluid can accumulate in the interstitial compartment between cells through extravasation of protein, electrolytes, and fluid in the intracellular space. This type of edema, known as vasogenic edema, results from increased capillary pressure, damage to the capillary endothelium, or sudden increases in the vascular pressure beyond the limits of autoregulation. Clearance of brain tissue swelling resolves with absorption into the CSF system.

Hydrocephalus, an excessive accumulation of CSF in the cranial vault, is another cause of increased intracranial pressure (**Figure 27.9** ■). As CSF accumulates in the ventricles or other regions of the brain, it compresses surrounding cerebral brain structures. Hydrocephalus can occur from lesions that obstruct the flow of CSF from the ventricles or due to problems with resorption, as when residual blood from a subarachnoid hemorrhage clogs the arachnoid villi.

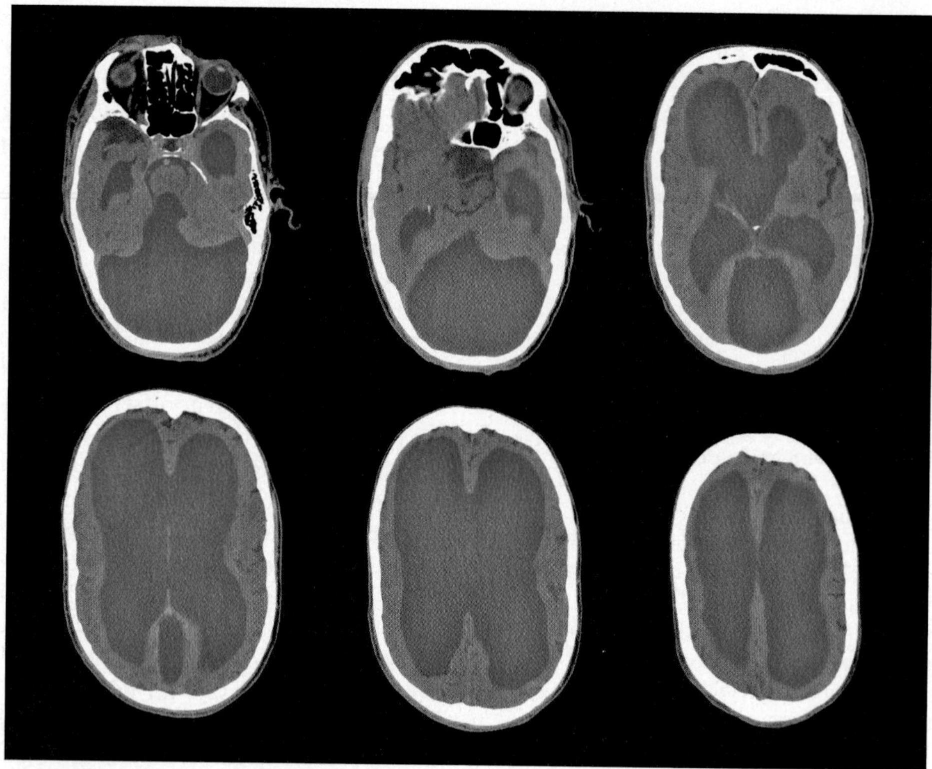

Figure 27.9 ■ A CT scan showing severe hydrocephalus in a 67-year-old man. The ventricular system (highlighted in blue) is dilated with CSF.

Normal pressure hydrocephalus (NPH) is an abnormal accumulation of CSF in the ventricles or cavities that places pressure on the brain tissue. While it can result from a blockage in the normal flow of CSF, such as from a tumor, infection, or subarachnoid hemorrhage, it can also develop when none of these factors are present. NPH can develop at any age but is most common in older adults. Symptoms of NPH include progressive mental impairment and dementia, instability particularly with walking, and bladder incontinence. A variety of tests are used to diagnose NPH, including a head CT scan, magnetic resonance imaging (MRI), lumbar puncture, intracranial monitoring, and neuropsychologic testing. Treatment for NPH may entail placement of a ventriculoperitoneal shunt, a catheter that is placed in the ventricles of the brain to drain CSF into the abdomen, where it is resorbed as part of the normal circulatory process. ■

Norma James: Application

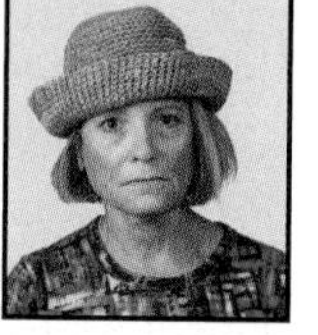

Mrs. James was diagnosed with an ischemic stroke. Pathologic changes in remote areas of the brain can contribute to chronic deficits after ischemic stroke. These changes are caused by a compromised blood–brain barrier, a condition known as diaschisis, which allows harmful substances to enter the brain. Diaschisis can lead to microvascular damage in areas outside of the ischemic region, adding to the long-term deficits experienced by patients with ischemic stroke.

Cerebral autoregulation normally maintains a constant flow of blood to the tissues of the brain in a range of 50–150 mmHg. However, under the increased stress of chronic hypertension, the threshold to which autoregulatory mechanisms respond increases to approximately 100–250 mmHg; thus, cerebral hypertension with resulting increased intracranial pressure may ensue, adding to the risk of cytotoxic and vasogenic edema. On the other hand, maintaining adequate perfusion is critically important, and the person's body is acclimated to a higher blood pressure threshold. Therefore, unless the person has a comorbid cardiac condition or other process that requires a reduction in blood pressure, maintaining a higher blood pressure is safer than drastically reducing it.

8. What comorbid conditions is Mrs. James at risk for?
9. According to the Monro-Kellie hypothesis, swelling of Mrs. James's brain tissue or an increase in blood flow would cause a compensatory decrease in which contents?

Abigail Martin: Application

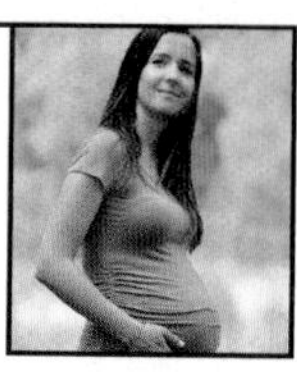

The additional blood in Ms. Martin's cranial vault due to the ruptured aneurysm may increase intracranial pressure if she does not have adequate cerebral compliance. To compensate for the blood that is now in her subarachnoid space, her body may respond by diverting CSF from the ventricles into the spinal cord. However, because the spinal cord can hold only a small amount of additional CSF, there is a limit to this compensatory response. Ms. Martin's management in the intensive care unit will entail continuous monitoring of her mean arterial pressure and mechanical ventilation, which are important interventions for maintaining adequate perfusion and oxygenation. Because increased intracranial pressure can become life threatening, a ventriculostomy may be surgically placed to monitor intracranial pressure with or without an external ventricular drain to allow the drainage of CSF.

9. If a ventriculostomy is placed with an external ventricular drain for Ms. Martin, what is the therapeutic goal for draining the CSF?
10. In draining CSF, why is it important to continuously monitor mean arterial pressure?

Check Your Progress: Section 27.5

1. When cerebral blood pressure rises, what is the compensatory response of the cerebral capillaries?
2. When the $PaCO_2$ level rises in the blood, what is the compensatory response of the cerebral vessels?
3. What is an important risk to consider in using hyperventilation to decrease intracranial pressure?

27.6 Ischemia and Hypoxia of the Central Nervous System

The brain normally receives approximately 750 milliliters of blood per minute, or 15% of the cardiac output, and uses 20% of the body's oxygen consumption.[1] Cerebral blood flow (CBF), the supply of blood to the brain in a given time, is influenced by autoregulation, blood viscosity, cerebral vascular resistance (CVR), and cerebral perfusion pressure (CPP). CBF is equal to CPP divided by CVR, as represented by the equation $CBF = CPP/CVR$. CVR is typically low but fluctuates in response to intracranial pressure. In a normotensive patients, the CBF is maintained at approximately 50 milliliters per 100 grams of brain tissue per minute if the CPP is in the range of 60–160 mmHg.

Brain ischemia occurs when the supply of blood or extraction of oxygen and nutrients is insufficient to meet the metabolic demands of the brain tissue. Hypoxia is a deficiency of oxygen at the cellular level resulting from ischemia or hypoxemia, a state of decreased blood oxygenation. Ischemia and hypoxia often occur simultaneously when brain tissue is damaged, whether the damage is due to stroke, trauma, or infection. Neurologic dysfunction occurs rapidly during ischemia and hypoxia because neurons depend on readily accessible sources of glucose to produce ATP and the amount of ATP that can be produced through anaerobic metabolism is restricted as a result of to lack of stored glycogen.

Mitochondrial dysfunction caused by a deficiency of cellular oxygen is a critical event leading to infarction and tissue death. Without enough oxygen, the transport proteins and cytochromes that normally accept electrons from the mitochondrial electron transport chain are reduced and cannot accept electrons from the Krebs (tricarboxylic acid) cycle. To compensate for the lack of oxygen and energy deficiency, anaerobic glycolytic pathways are initiated. Glycolysis produces pyruvate, a by-product that is converted to lactate with the release of hydrogen ions (H^+). A buildup of hydrogen ions leads to cellular acidosis and loss of neuronal integrity.

Energy deprivation and loss of ion homeostasis caused by ischemia cause inability of the cells to maintain a negative membrane potential. Most of the ATP used by neurons is directed toward maintaining the ion gradients across the plasma membrane; the sodium–potassium pumps consume 75% of the ATP. Anoxic depolarization causes potassium to leave the cell and sodium, chloride, and calcium to enter. Thus, the cells depolarize and open the voltage-gated calcium channels, thereby releasing excitatory amino acids into the extracellular space. The release and accumulation of excitatory amino acids, most specifically glutamate, in the extracellular space lead to cell death (apoptosis).[2]

Normally, glutamate is released at excitatory synapses, and levels in the extracellular spaces are tightly regulated by sodium-dependent reuptake systems in neurons and glia. Glutamate is further detoxified in glia by conversion to glutamine via the ATP-dependent enzyme glutamine synthetase. Glutamine released by glia is then taken up by neurons and repackaged into synaptic vesicles for subsequent release. However, ischemia deprives the brain tissue of the oxygen and glucose required to maintain normal transmembrane ion gradients and conversion of glutamate to glutamine in glia. This leads to accumulation of intracellular Na^+ and collapse of the transmembrane Na^+ gradient, which in turn inhibits glutamate uptake and promotes accumulation of extracellular glutamate. The high level of extracellular glutamate stimulates glutamate receptors on surrounding neurons, causing entry of Ca^{2+} and Na^+, which depolarizes these neurons and stimulates additional Ca^{2+} influx through voltage-gated channels.

These events lead to a massive entry of calcium into the cell, which is transmitted to the matrix of mitochondria by calcium channels on the inner mitochondrial membrane. Exposure to toxic levels of excitatory neurotransmitters and release of calcium from the endoplasmic reticulum leads to mitochondrial calcium overload and activation of apoptosis. In particular, the neurons that are directly affected by the ischemic event die from energy deprivation while neurons at the edge of the ischemic region die from excessive stimulation of glutamate receptors.

With cerebral hemorrhage in sepsis, immune cells are activated, which can cause leakage of the blood–brain barrier, allowing leukocytes to enter the brain (see Figure 27.6). Pro-inflammatory cytokine released from cells of the blood–brain barrier, astrocytes, and glia activate leukocytes and other immune cells to move into the brain tissue, contributing to brain inflammation. Neutrophils, vascular endothelium, and activated microglia increase the release of reactive oxygen species and stimulate activation of the nitric oxide/nitric oxide synthetase pathway, resulting in mitochondrial dysfunction and eventually apoptosis.

Norma James: Application

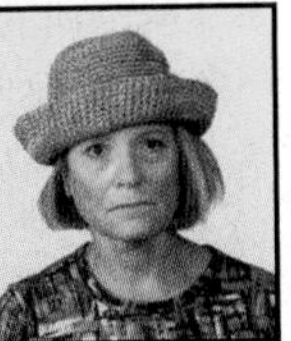

The main focus of treatment for Mrs. James is to preserve tissue in the ischemic penumbra, the area of tissue surrounding the infarction where perfusion is decreased. The penumbra can be

Impact of Current Research on Clinical Practice

Evidence for Benefits of Cerebrovascular Assessment

Description: Results from a longitudinal study demonstrated the benefit of evaluating cerebrovascular circulation and cognitive function in older adults. This study examined cognitive performance measured by the Mini–Mental Status Examination (MMSE) over a 3-year period in subjects with bilateral asymptomatic severe internal carotid artery stenosis. The study involved 159 subjects with severe internal carotid artery stenosis and measured intima–media thickness (IMT) as well as a transcranial Doppler-based breath-holding index test to evaluate cerebral hemodynamics. The investigators found that pathologic values of IMT did not influence the risk of MMSE score change. However, the risk of decreasing MMSE score increased progressively from patients with bilaterally normal breath-holding index to those with unilaterally abnormal breath-holding index, reaching the highest risk in patients with bilaterally abnormal breath-holding index.

Clinical Impact: These findings suggests that cognitive deterioration is due to hypoperfusion of the brain caused by atherosclerosis of the internal carotids. The authors suggest that earlier and more aggressive treatment of internal carotid atherosclerosis may be indicated even in asymptomatic individuals to prevent cognitive deterioration caused by hypoperfusion.

Research Study:

Buratti, L., Balucani, C., Viticchi, G., Falsetti, L., Altamura, C., Avitabile, E., Provinciali, L., Vernieri, F., & Silvestrini, M. (2014). Cognitive deterioration in bilateral asymptomatic severe carotid stenosis. *Stroke, 45,* 2072–2077.

preserved by restoring blood flow and optimizing collateral flow. Recanalization strategies aim to establish revascularization so that cells of the penumbra can be rescued before irreversible damage occurs. Recanalization is performed through the administration of intravenous recombinant tissue-type plasminogen activator (rt-PA) or intra-arterial approaches that directly inject rt-PA at the site of ischemia.

10. The accumulation of which excitatory neurotransmitter can damage neurons that are at the edge of the ischemic region?

Abigail Martin: Application

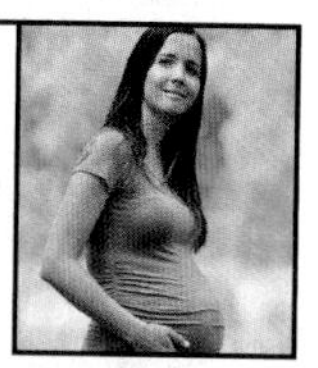

Ms. Martin's care will focus on detecting and treating increased intracranial pressure caused by the hemorrhage. Following subarachnoid hemorrhage, cerebral vasospasm can occur, resulting in ischemic regions of the brain. This typically occurs several days after the initial event, so continuous observation for signs and symptoms of cerebral vasospasm is important. Transcranial Doppler and serial CT scans of the brain are performed to evaluate for cerebral vasospasm, edema, and hydrocephalus.

11. If Ms. Martin's head is turned to the side, her cerebral vascular resistance increases. What does a rise in the cerebral vascular resistance do to the cerebral blood flow?
12. Cerebral vasospasm raises the cerebral vascular resistance. What would you expect to see if Ms. Martin has cerebral vasospasm?

Check Your Progress: Section 27.6

1. To compensate for the lack of oxygen and energy deficiency during ischemia, which pathways are initiated that produce the by-product pyruvate?
2. Neurons that are directly affected by ischemia die as a result of which mechanism?
3. Leakage of the blood–brain barrier during sepsis allows which type of cell to enter the brain?

27.7 Transient Ischemic Attack

A **transient ischemic attack (TIA)** is a temporary episode of neurologic dysfunction caused by focal brain, spinal cord, or retinal ischemia without acute infarction.[5] Approximately 33% of people who have a TIA go on to have a stroke within 1 year.

Etiology and Pathogenesis

The origins of a TIA are the same as those of an ischemic stroke. A TIA occurs as a result of a clot that blocks the supply of blood to a region of the brain. However, because it is transient, it does not cause permanent tissue damage or infarction. The most likely reason for a TIA is a buildup of fatty deposits on arterial walls known as atherosclerosis. There are many risk factors for TIA and stroke, most of which are modifiable and can be controlled with lifestyle choices (**Table 27.2** ■).

Clinical Manifestations

Signs and symptoms of TIA are temporary and do not cause permanent neurologic injury or deficits. The signs and symptoms depend on the area of the brain affected but can include facial drooping, arm or leg weakness especially on one side of the body, speech difficulty or sudden trouble seeing in one or both eyes, difficulty walking with dizziness, lack of balance or coordination, or severe headache without a known cause.

Linking Pathophysiology to Diagnosis and Treatment

Although there is controversy about the need for hospitalization for TIA, all patients who have experienced a TIA should receive urgent evaluation, risk stratification, and initiation of stroke prevention therapy.[5] The National Stroke Association consensus guidelines recommend considering hospitalization if the first TIA occurred within the previous

Table 27.2 Modifiable and Nonmodifiable Risk Factors of Transient Ischemic Attacks and Stroke

Factor	Description
Nonmodifiable Risk Factors	
Age	Risk increases with age, particularly after age 55.
Family history	Risk is greater if immediate family members have a history of TIA or stroke.
Prior TIA or stroke	A person with a history of TIA is 10 times more likely to have a stroke; the risk of recurrent stroke is 24% in women and 42% in men within 5 years of the first stroke.
Race	African Americans are at greater risk of dying from stroke.
Sex	Men are at higher risk of TIA, but more than half of stroke deaths occur in women.
Sickle cell disease	Stroke is a frequent complication of sickle cell disease.
Modifiable Risk Factors	
Cardiovascular disease	Including heart failure, defects, infection or abnormal rhythm.
Carotid artery disease	Atherosclerotic blood vessels from the heart to the brain can cause blockage or result in emboli.
Diabetes	Diabetes increases atherosclerosis and the speed with which it develops.
Excess weight	A body mass index of 25 or higher or a waist circumference greater than 35 inches in women and 40 inches in men.
High blood pressure	Risk increases with blood pressure higher than 110/75 mmHg.
High cholesterol	Eating less saturated fat and trans fat may reduce plaques in the arteries.
High levels of homocysteine	Elevated levels of this amino acid causes arteries to thicken and scar, thereby increasing the risk of clots.
Peripheral artery disease	A disorder associated with increased risk of clots.
Cigarette smoking	Elevates blood pressure, risk of clots and atherosclerosis.
Heavy drinking	Elevates blood pressure, cholesterol, and the risk of heart failure.
Use of illicit drugs	Elevates blood pressure and the risk of heart failure.
Physical inactivity	Increases the risk of excess weight, high blood pressure, high cholesterol, diabetes, and atherosclerosis.
Poor nutrition	Increases the risk of excess weight, high blood pressure, high cholesterol, diabetes, and atherosclerosis.
Use of birth control pills	Increases the risk of atherosclerosis and blood clot formation.

24–48 hours to facilitate possible treatment with recombinant tissue plasminogen activator (rt-PA) and other medical management for recurrent symptoms.[4]

Initial assessment is aimed at excluding conditions that can mimic TIA, including hypoglycemia, seizure, or intracranial hemorrhage.[5] A fingerstick blood glucose test is performed on presentation, and blood is drawn for serum electrolyte levels, complete blood count, and coagulation studies. A 12-lead electrocardiography is performed to evaluate for arrhythmias or evidence of ischemia. Brain imaging is recommended with either a noncontrast CT or an MRI with diffusion-weighted imaging. Vessel imaging using CT angiography or magnetic resonance angiography can identify a stenosis or occlusion that may warrant intervention. Carotid Doppler ultrasonography of the neck can be used to identify occlusions of the internal carotids that may require surgical or endovascular therapy.

Check Your Progress: Section 27.7

1. What percentage of people who have a transient ischemic attack have a stroke within 1 year?
2. What is a major cause of transient ischemic attack?
3. A person with a past history of transient ischemic attack is how much more likely to have a stroke compared with a person without a history of transient ischemic attack?

27.8 Ischemic and Hemorrhagic Stroke

Stroke occurs when there is an interruption in the supply of blood to a region of the brain or bleeding of a vessel that results in an area of brain tissue damage or infarction.[2] Stroke is the leading cause of long-term disability and the third leading cause of death in the United States.[4] There are two types of stroke: ischemic and hemorrhagic. Approximately 87% of strokes are ischemic, and 13% are hemorrhagic. Patients with ischemic stroke often present with focal neurologic deficits that are caused by damage to the area of brain supplied by the affected vessel. Hemorrhagic stroke often causes symptoms associated with elevated intracranial pressure. The rate of mortality is higher with hemorrhagic stroke.

Etiology and Pathogenesis

Ischemic Stroke. An **ischemic stroke** may involve partial or complete occlusion of cerebral blood flow to an area of the brain due to a thrombus or embolus (**Figure 27.10** ■). Several vascular disorders can lead to cerebral ischemia, the most common being atherosclerosis. Atherosclerosis develops from injury to vascular endothelial cells by mechanical, biochemical and/or inflammatory insults (see Figure 24.5 in Chapter 24). Monocytes and lymphocytes that migrate to the vessel attach to the area of injury along the wall of

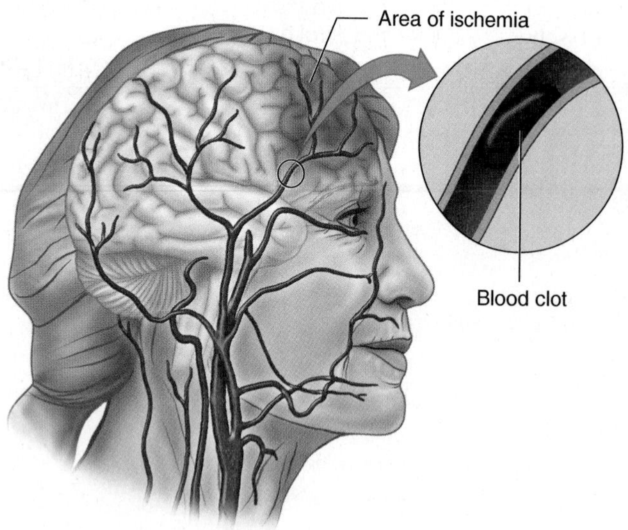

Figure 27.10 ■ ***Ischemic stroke.*** Decreased or blocked blood flow can occur from thrombus formation or an embolus, leading to ischemia and necrosis of brain tissue.

the vessel and stimulate proliferation of smooth muscle cells and fibroblasts, leading to the formation of a fibrous plaque.[3] The damaged endothelial cells also cause aggregation and activation of platelets that secrete growth factors, leading to further proliferation of smooth muscle and fibroblasts. As an atherosclerotic plaque forms and enlarges on the vessel wall, it begins to reduce the amount of blood that can travel through the vessel. Over time, the plaque can fully occlude blood from reaching the brain tissue, leading to an ischemic stroke, or the plaque may rupture, releasing emboli.

Cardiac disorders including mural thrombus, rheumatic heart disease, arrhythmias, endocarditis, mitral valve prolapse, atrial myxoma, and the presence of prosthetic heart valves can increase the risk of stroke. In addition, hematologic disorders such as thrombocytosis, polycythemia, sickle cell disease, leukocytosis, and hypercoagulable states can increase the risk of ischemia.

Thrombotic strokes caused by occlusion of a vessel as a result of the buildup of plaque along the vessel wall are more common and usually involve the internal carotid, middle cerebral, or basilar artery.[3] Embolic strokes occur as a result of a moving clot that can form in anywhere in the body. Most cerebral embolisms are of cardiac origin, usually caused by atrial fibrillation or breakage of an atherosclerotic plaque from a carotid artery, which lodges in a cerebral vessel. Emboli that pass through the carotid arteries commonly occlude the middle cerebral artery, which carries more than 80% of blood flow to the cerebral hemisphere. Emboli that travel to the vertebral or basilar arteries can lodge at the apex of the basilar artery or in the posterior cerebral arteries. Lacunar strokes develop from occlusion in the deeper vessels of the brain.

Hemorrhagic Stroke. A **hemorrhagic stroke** involves bleeding into the brain from a burst blood vessel (**Figure 27.11** ■).[6] A hemorrhagic stroke is intracerebral when a vessel bleeds into the brain tissue, intraventricular when it bleeds into the ventricles, or extracerebral when a vessel bleeds into the membranes surrounding the brain. An intracerebral hemorrhage (also called an intraparenchymal hemorrhage) occurs in the brain tissue or parenchyma, most often in the basal ganglia or thalamus, and is commonly associated with long-standing hypertension.[7] A subarachnoid hemorrhage occurs under the arachnoid membrane and above the pia mater. Cerebral aneurysms and arteriovenous malformations are two structural abnormalities that can cause a hemorrhagic stroke. Approximately 85% of subarachnoid hemorrhages are caused by a cerebral aneurysm.[7]

An **aneurysm** is an abnormal bulge along the vessel wall that fills with blood and is caused by a weak or thin area of the vessel wall. The aneurysm can cause symptoms when it puts pressure on the brain tissue or surrounding nerves or when it leaks or ruptures, causing a hemorrhage. Aneurysms can occur anywhere in the brain or spinal cord but are most likely to form along regions of bifurcation, where vessels branch off, and along the circle of Willis. They can be congenital, from an abnormality when the vessel is formed, or may be associated with genetic diseases, including connective tissue disorders or polycystic kidney disease. Aneurysms can also form as a result of trauma, high blood pressure, atherosclerosis, tumors, or infection.

Arteriovenous malformations (AVMs) are a tangle of abnormal or poorly formed blood vessels, including arteries

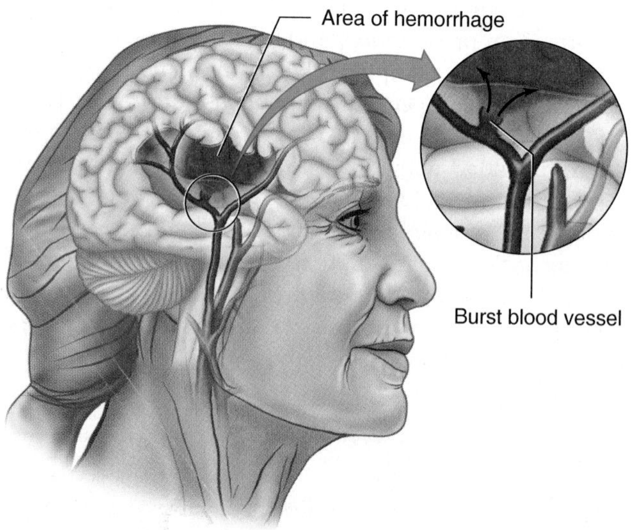

Figure 27.11 ■ ***Hemorrhagic stroke.*** Bleeding into the brain from a burst blood vessel, often caused by an aneurysm, can lead to necrosis of brain tissue.

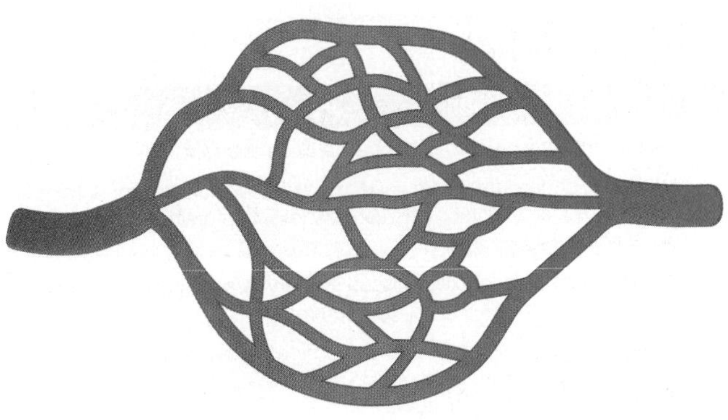

A Normal connection

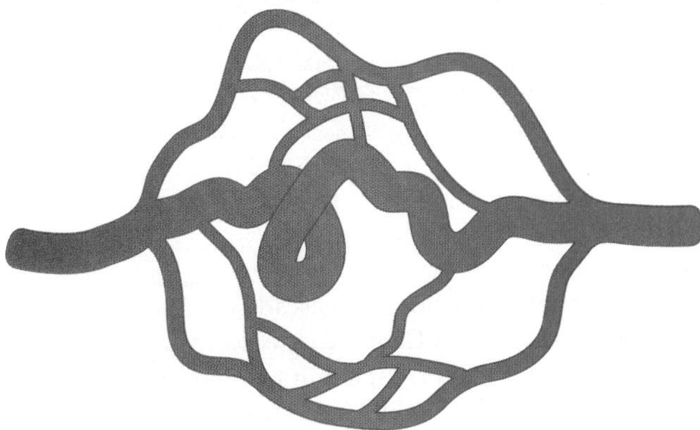

B Arteriovenous malformation

Figure 27.12 ■ **A**. Arteries and veins normally connect via capillary beds. **B**. In AVM, arteries and veins connect directly without intervening capillaries.

and veins (**Figure 27.12** ■). AVMs can occur anywhere in the body and have a higher risk of bleeding than normal vessels. Brain AVMs carry a substantial risk when bleeding occurs. Dural AVMs are located on the covering of the brain and are an acquired disorder, most often due to an injury. The turbulent blood flow through the AVM can cause cerebral bruits, and as the AVM enlarges over time, it can irritate the surrounding brain tissue, leading to headaches or seizure. Left untreated, AVMs can rupture, causing an intracerebral, subarachnoid, or spinal hemorrhage.

Clinical Manifestations

Stroke is characterized by the sudden onset of a focal neurologic deficit that persists for at least 24 hours and is due to a reduction or occlusion of cerebral circulation or rupture of blood vessels. The focal signs and symptoms of stroke depend on the area of brain or spinal cord affected by the hemorrhage or lack of blood supply (**Table 27.3** ■).

Linking Pathophysiology to Diagnosis and Treatment

Ischemic Stroke. Treatment for ischemic stroke focuses on restoring blood flow and reducing the area of infarction as much as possible. Although infarction, or brain tissue death, cannot be reversed, the tissue surrounding the infarction, called the penumbra, can be salvaged if perfusion is restored in a timely manner. In the acute period of stroke, supplemental oxygen is used to improve oxygenation, glycemic control is maintained within a normal range, and blood pressure is managed to provide adequate cerebral perfusion. For patients who are not candidates to receive fibrinolytic therapy, permitting moderate hypertension is recommended. Antihypertensive therapy may be used in these patients when the blood pressure is higher than 220/120 mmHg, but care must be taken not to lower the blood pressure too quickly. A reasonable goal is to lower the blood pressure by 15% over the first 24 hours after the onset of stroke.

Aspirin 325 mg orally given within 24–48 hours of ischemic stroke onset provides a modest benefit in ischemic stroke outcomes and may reduce the risk of recurrent stroke. Hypothermia has become a standard of care for patients who survive cardiac arrest from ventricular tachycardia or ventricular fibrillation; however, its role in the early treatment of ischemic stroke has not been demonstrated.

Norma James: Outcome

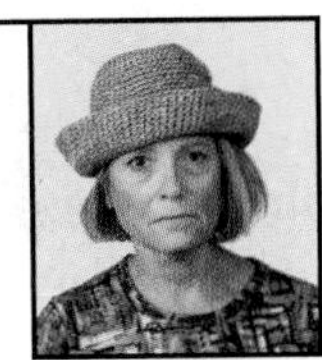

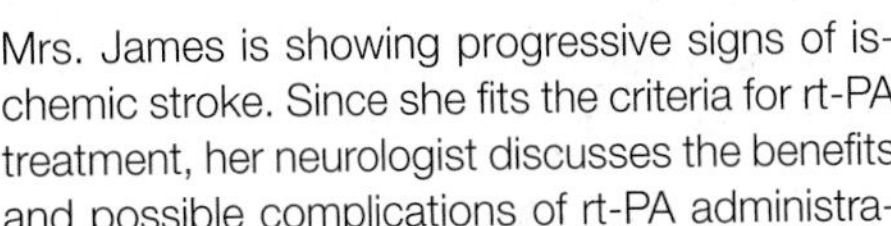

Mrs. James is showing progressive signs of ischemic stroke. Since she fits the criteria for rt-PA treatment, her neurologist discusses the benefits and possible complications of rt-PA administration as well as other therapeutic options. Mrs. James consents to treatment with intravenous rt-PA. Afterward, she has some swallowing difficulty along with mobility restrictions. During her hospital stay, she becomes depressed, which complicates her course of treatment. After a course of rehabilitation, she is discharged home with her son and visiting healthcare providers to coordinate care in the home.

11. What is the therapeutic goal of rt-PA administration for is-chemic stroke?

Hemorrhagic Stroke. When hemorrhagic stroke is identified on CT scan of the brain, the priority of care depends on adequate ventilation and management of blood pressure.[8] Osmotic diuretics may be used to decrease intracranial pressure. Glucose levels should be monitored, and normoglycemia should be maintained. Supratentorial intracranial hemorrhage may benefit from surgical evacuation; both lobar and cerebellar hemorrhages treated with craniotomy have shown improved outcomes. For aneurysmal subarachnoid hemorrhage, a craniotomy with aneurysm clipping may be performed to block the flow of blood from entering the aneurysm (**Figure 27.13** ■). Endovascular therapy with coil embolization has been used successfully as an alternative to surgical clipping of the aneurysm.

Delayed cerebral ischemia remains the single most important cause of morbidity and mortality in patients who survive aneurysmal subarachnoid hemorrhage. **Delayed cerebral ischemia (DCI)** is a clinical syndrome of focal neurologic deficits, cognitive deficits, or both that occurs in approximately 30% of patient during the initial 3–14 days following hemorrhage. Early brain injury that occurs during the first 72 hours after the initial bleed can lead to cortical spreading depression, spontaneous waves

Table 27.3 Vascular Territories and Focal Signs and Symptoms of Ischemic Stroke

Artery	Territory	Signs and Symptoms
Anterior cerebral	Medial frontal and parietal cortex, anterior corpus callosum	Paresis and sensory loss of contralateral leg and foot
Middle cerebral	Lateral frontal, parietal, occipital, and temporal cortex; caudate, putamen, internal capsule	Aphasia (if stroke affects dominant hemisphere), neglect (nondominant hemisphere), contralateral hemisensory loss, homonymous hemianopia, hemiparesis
Vertebral	Medulla, lower cerebellum	Ipsilateral cerebellar ataxia, crossed sensory loss, nystagmus, vertigo, dysarthria, dysphagia, Horner syndrome
Basilar	Lower midbrain, pons, upper and mid cerebellum	Hemiparesis or quadriparesis, hemi or crossed sensory loss, nystagmus, vertigo, diplopia, gaze palsies, dysarthria, ipsilateral cerebellar ataxia, Horner syndrome, coma
Posterior cerebral	Proximal: upper midbrain, thalamus	Contralateral hemiparesis, sensory loss, ataxia, third nerve palsy, vertical gaze palsy, hemiballismus, choreoathetosis, impaired consciousness
	Distal: medial occipital and temporal cortex, posterior corpus callosum	Contralateral homonymous hemianopia, dyslexia without agraphia, visual hallucinations and distortions, memory defect, cortical blindness (if bilateral occlusion)

of depolarization across the cerebral tissue that is followed by profound hypoperfusion of the cortex due to vasoconstriction. In addition, microthrombosis can occur with DCI as a result of activation of the coagulation cascade and impairment of the fibrinolytic cascade resulting in the formation of microemboli. Cerebral vasospasm, a complication of subarachnoid hemorrhage that can induce rebleeding, may be treated with balloon angioplasty to open up the affected vessel. Ventriculostomy, placement of an intraventricular catheter for monitoring and drainage of CSF, is often used in the setting of obstructive hydrocephalus. However, ventriculostomy is associated with an increased risk of infection.

Figure 27.13 ■ Cerebral aneurysm clipping. A craniotomy, or opening of the skull, must be performed to access the aneurysm. Once the aneurysm is reached, a clip that resembles a paper clip is placed around the neck of the aneurysm to stop blood from flowing into the aneurysm. Residual blood is evacuated during the procedure.

Abigail Martin: Outcome

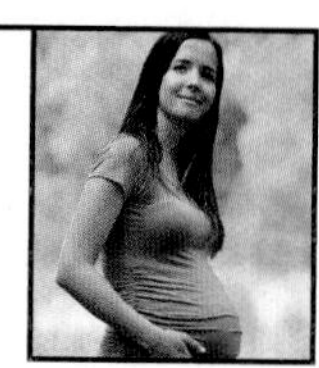

Ms. Martin is taken to the neurointerventional radiology suite for coiling of the ophthalmic aneurysm. This entails placing a catheter in her femoral artery and threading it to the area of the aneurysm. Small metal threads are then placed in the body of the aneurysm to block the flow of blood into the aneurysm. Ms. Martin is transferred to the intensive care unit after the procedure for close monitoring. She receives nimodipine, serial neurologic examinations, and scheduled transcranial Doppler exams to detect any delayed cerebral ischemia. When she is awake and alert, she is evaluated for extubation. She is monitored in the intensive care unit for 14 days from the time of the initial bleed.

13. What is the most significant risk factor for Ms. Martin after receiving treatment for a cerebral aneurysm?

Check Your Progress: Section 27.8

1. Most strokes are of which type?
2. The risk of death is highest with which type of stroke?
3. What type of cerebral vascular disorder is characterized as a tangle of abnormal or poorly formed arteries and veins?

27.9 Subdural and Spinal Cord Hemorrhage

Subdural Hemorrhage

A subdural hematoma is bleeding from the bridging veins below the inner layer of the dura, between the dura mater and arachnoid membrane (**Figure 27.14** ■). Because a subdural hematoma does not directly occlude a cerebral vessel that leads to brain tissue, it is not considered to be a stroke. However, it can become large enough to cause a stroke, and it can have other negative effects.

Etiology and Pathogenesis

A subdural hematoma most commonly develops as a result of trauma in which there is a high-speed impact to the skull, but subdural hematomas can also occur spontaneously. The diagnosis of acute subdural hematoma is made when the bleeding is identified immediately after an injury. Left untreated, the expanding mass can compress brain tissue and lead to brain herniation. In contrast, chronic subdural hematoma is commonly associated with brain atrophy. As the brain shrinks from the skull, the tension placed on the bridging veins can make them more vulnerable to bleeding.

Child abuse or shaken baby syndrome can result in subdural hematoma, retinal hemorrhages, and cerebral edema. This occurs when an infant or child's head is shaken violently with or without deceleration. Because very young children do not have well-developed neck muscles to support the head, shearing of the nerve cell bodies and bridging veins can occur, resulting in hemorrhage. ■

Coagulopathy or medical anticoagulation as well as chronic alcoholism can increase the risk of sustaining a subdural hematoma even with seemingly innocuous head injuries. Patients with these conditions who sustain a fall should be carefully assessed to identify the onset of neurologic deficits associated with subdural hematoma. ■

Clinical Manifestations

Symptoms of subdural hemorrhage include headache, confusion, changes in behavior, dizziness, nausea and vomiting, lethargy or excessive drowsiness, weakness, apathy, and seizures. People may vary widely in their symptoms of subdural hemorrhage. In addition to the size of the hemorrhage, the age of the patient and other medical conditions can affect their response.

Linking Pathophysiology to Diagnosis and Treatment

Once a subdural hematoma has been identified on CT scan of the brain, surgical treatment must be considered.[2] Adequate ventilation and management of the patient's blood pressure should be priorities before surgery. A patient with coagulopathy or one who is receiving anticoagulant medication should be transfused with fresh frozen plasma, platelets, or both to maintain prothrombin time within the reference range and platelet count above 100,000. The effects

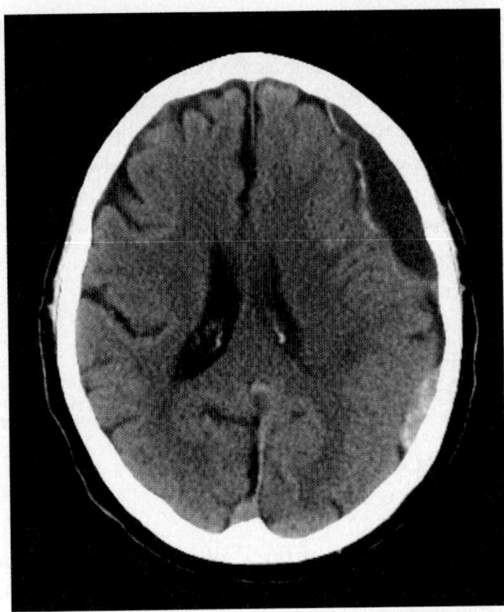

Figure 27.14 ■ CT scan of older adult with a subdural hematoma (highlighted in red).

of heparin may need to be reversed with protamine, and patients receiving warfarin are given vitamin K to reverse its effects. Standard treatment for acute subdural hematoma includes emergent decompression when there is a midline shift of 5 millimeters or more.[3] Surgery has also been recommended for acute subdural hematomas exceeding 1 centimeter in thickness. For uncomplicated chronic subdural hematoma, a burr hole craniostomy may provide the most efficient method of surgical drainage.

Spinal Cord Hemorrhage

Etiology and Pathogenesis

Hemorrhage of the spinal cord is rare but may occur with trauma, vascular malformation, or bleeding disorders and may be epidural, subdural, subarachnoid, or intramedullary in origin. Intramedullary hemorrhage (hematomyelia) is bleeding in the white and gray matter of the spinal cord. Epidural spinal cord hemorrhage and subdural spinal cord hemorrhage cause compression of the spinal cord. Spinal cord hemorrhage presents as sudden severe back pain, headache, neck stiffness, and photosensitivity and can lead to irreversible myelopathy with sensory loss below the level of the bleed. Depending on the location of hemorrhage, it can cause hemiparesis, paraparesis, or tetraplegia.

Clinical Manifestations

Patients with spinal cord hemorrhage typically present with sudden, severe, localized back pain with or without radiculopathy. If the hemorrhage is intramedullary, the patient may experience hemiparesis, paraparesis, or quadriparesis; sensory loss below the lesion; and loss of sphincter control. A patient with spinal subarachnoid hemorrhage may have headache, neck stiffness, and photosensitivity. An epidural hemorrhage or subdural hemorrhage of the spinal cord is usually associated with the same symptoms as an intermedullary hemorrhage.

Linking Pathophysiology to Diagnosis and Treatment

Surgical decompression may be performed for spinal subdural hemorrhage or epidural hemorrhage to salvage the spinal cord.[2] Treatment of spinal subarachnoid hemorrhage consists of surgical resection or catheter-based interventional techniques such as embolization and coiling for spinal angiomas. Focal radiation therapy, with gamma knife or cold photon knife, is also a consideration with spinal arteriovenous malformations.

Check Your Progress: Section 27.9

1. A subdural hematoma is an accumulation of blood between which two membranes?
2. A patient with subdural hematoma who is taking warfarin would likely have which therapeutic agent prescribed to reverse the effects of warfarin?
3. What is the term used to describe bleeding in the white and gray matter of the spinal cord?

CHAPTER SUMMARY

27.1 Chapter Overview and Case Studies

Describe the function of the central nervous system and concepts related to disorders of circulation within the central nervous system.

- The brain and the spinal cord are the major components of the central nervous system.
- The tissues of the CNS rely heavily on receiving constant perfusion.
- Cerebral autoregulation and the blood–brain barrier function to protect the tissues within the central nervous system.
- Transient ischemic attack (TIA) is a brief appearance of symptoms that resemble a stroke and generally resolve within 24 hours.
- A cerebrovascular accident, or stroke, is an enduring disruption of speech, motor, communication accompanied by cognitive deficits.
- The major concepts concerning disorders of circulation within the brain revolve around a lack of oxygen and the possibility of increased pressure within the skull.

27.2 Vascular Supply of the Central Nervous System

Outline the vascular supply of the brain and spinal cord.

- Cerebral circulation is maintained by two sets of arteries: the right and left internal carotid arteries, which branch from the common carotid arteries, and the right and left vertebral arteries, which arise from the subclavian arteries.
- The internal carotid arteries branch off within the cranium to form two major cerebral arteries, the anterior and middle cerebral arteries, while the vertebral arteries join to form the basilar artery.
- The vascular supply from the internal carotids and basilar arteries join to form the circle of Willis at the base of the brain.
- The venous drainage of the brain travels through bridging veins on the brain surface into sinuses, which empty into the internal jugular vein.
- Spinal cord circulation is maintained by the vertebral arteries that branch to form the anterior spinal artery and posterior spinal arteries
- The anterior spinal artery travels down the anterior median fissure of the spinal cord; the posterior spinal arteries travel longitudinally down the posterior aspect of the spinal cord.
- A plexus of small arteries on the surface of the cord called the arterial vasocorona creates a connection between the anterior and posterior spinal arteries.

27.3 Production and Circulation of Cerebrospinal Fluid

Distinguish the normal flow of cerebrospinal fluid through the brain and spinal cord in contrast with the circulation of blood.

- Cerebrospinal fluid is produced in the choroid plexi of the ventricles and flows through the ventricular system of the brain and through the subarachnoid space surrounding the brain and spinal cord.
- Cerebrospinal fluid is resorbed into the venous dural sinuses via arachnoid villi.
- Hydrocephalus can develop when there is a blockage in the flow of cerebrospinal fluid through the ventricles of the brain or when the CSF cannot be resorbed by the arachnoid villi.

27.4 Blood–Brain Barrier

Summarize the protective role of the blood–brain barrier.

- The blood–brain barrier is composed of specialized endothelium present in brain capillaries that permits selective entry of substances into the brain
- Regions of the brain that lack a blood–brain barrier have fenestrated capillaries or tanycytes to prevent the movement of molecules between the brain and circulation.

27.5 Cerebral Autoregulation

Predict the influence of cerebral autoregulation on the blood vessels that supply the central nervous system.

- Cerebral autoregulation is an important protective mechanism that maintains a steady flow of blood to the brain and spinal cord despite wide variations in mean arterial pressure.
- When blood pressure rises, the cerebral capillaries constrict to prevent a significant rise in blood flow; when blood pressure falls, the capillaries dilate to allow more blood flow to circulate.
- Cerebral vessels constrict as $PaCO_2$ levels fall and dilate to increase blood flow when $PaCO_2$ levels rise.
- Intracranial pressure is the pressure exerted by the contents of the cranium: brain tissue, blood, and cerebrospinal fluid.
- The Monro-Kellie hypothesis describes the compensatory relationship that maintains cerebral compliance in response to changes in volume of the three components.

27.6 Ischemia and Hypoxia of the Central Nervous System

Explain the cellular events that follow from ischemia and hypoxia of the brain and spinal cord.

- Ischemia and hypoxia occur simultaneously when there is decreased blood flow or blockage of blood flow to regions of the brain or spinal cord.
- Mitochondrial dysfunction caused by a deficiency of cellular oxygen is a critical event leading to infarction and tissue death in the brain and spinal cord.
- Energy deprivation and loss of ion homeostasis caused by ischemia causes inability of the cells to maintain a negative membrane potential, while the accumulation of excitatory amino acids in the extracellular space and influx of calcium ion leads to apoptosis.

27.7 Transient Ischemic Attack

Differentiate the causes, classification, underlying pathogenesis, and clinical manifestations of transient ischemic attack and approaches to diagnosis and treatment of this condition across the lifespan.

- A transient ischemic attack (TIA) is a temporary episode of neurologic dysfunction caused by focal brain, spinal cord, or retinal ischemia without acute infarction.
- The risk factors for TIA and stroke are the same.
- Up to 33% of patients who experience a TIA will have a stroke in the following year.

27.8 Ischemic and Hemorrhagic Stroke

Differentiate the causes, classification, underlying pathogenesis, and clinical manifestations of ischemic and hemorrhagic strokes and approaches to diagnosis and treatment of these conditions across the lifespan.

- Stroke occurs when there is an interruption in the supply of blood to a region of the brain or bleeding of a vessel that results in an area of brain tissue damage or infarction.
- An ischemic stroke may involve partial or complete occlusion of cerebral blood flow to an area of the brain due to a thrombus or embolus. For ischemic stroke, the goal of treatment is restoration of blood flow to minimize the area of infarction and neurologic deficits by salvaging the penumbra with fibrinolytics or other methods to reestablish blood flow.
- A hemorrhagic stroke involves bleeding from a burst blood vessel and is described by location as intracerebral, intraventricular, or subarachnoid. For hemorrhagic stroke, the goal of treatment is preventing further bleeding, managing increased intracranial pressure, and reducing cerebral edema. Surgical management is often indicated. Most cases of subarachnoid hemorrhage are caused by a ruptured cerebral aneurysm, which is treated with surgical clipping or coiling or embolization.

27.9 Subdural and Spinal Cord Hemorrhage

Differentiate the causes, classification, underlying pathogenesis, and clinical manifestations of subdural and spinal cord hemorrhages and approaches to diagnosis and treatment of these conditions across the lifespan.

- A subdural hematoma is bleeding from the bridging veins below the inner layer of the dura, between the dura mater and arachnoid membrane. Subdural hematomas typically require surgical evacuation.
- Hemorrhage of the spinal cord is rare but can occur with trauma, vascular malformation, or bleeding disorders.
- As with the brain, hemorrhage may occur between any of the meningeal layers.
- Intramedullary hemorrhage (hematomyelia) is bleeding in the white and gray matter of the spinal cord.
- Epidural and subdural spinal cord hemorrhage causes compression of the spinal cord.
- Spinal cord hemorrhage presents as sudden, severe back pain, headache, neck stiffness, and photosensitivity and can lead to irreversible sensory loss below the level of the bleed.

REVIEW QUESTIONS

1. What pair of arteries arise from the segmental branches of the aorta and vascularize the spinal cord?
   a. External carotids
   b. Circle of Willis
   c. Vertebrals
   d. Internal carotids
2. A 68-year-old African American male with a past history of hypertension treated with hydrochlorothiazide presents to the emergency department stating that he has the worst headache of his life. On presentation, his pupils are slightly sluggish, he has dysarthria, and his right arm and leg are weak. What should the nurse prioritize for this patient?
   a. Prepare him for evaluation by the speech therapist.
   b. Get him prepared for a head CT.
   c. Determine whether he is able to swallow safely.
   d. Perform a vision test with the Snellen chart.
3. A 70-year-old right-handed female with a history of atrial fibrillation presents to the emergency department with new onset of aphasia and right-sided hemiplegia. On the basis of her symptoms, in which vessel is the occlusion occurring?
   a. Right posterior cerebral artery
   b. Basilar artery
   c. Left anterior cerebral artery
   d. Left middle cerebral artery
4. A 34-year-old female presents with headache, nausea, and vomiting. On head CT, there is a tumor occluding the third ventricle. Because of the occlusion, the cerebrospinal fluid is unable to pass through to the fourth ventricle via which route?
   a. Foramen of Monro
   b. Foramina of Luschka
   c. Foramen of Magendie
   d. Great cerebral vein of Galen
5. A 55-year-old African American male with a past history of transient ischemic attack presents to the emergency department with new onset of right-sided hemiplegia. He already has oxygen being delivered by nasal cannula, and a CT of the head has been ordered to evaluate for hemorrhagic stroke. What would the next priority be for this patient?
   a. Administer a calcium channel blocker.
   b. Give one ampule of 50% dextrose stat.
   c. Start an intravenous infusion of phenytoin.
   d. Take a finger stick to measure his blood glucose.
6. A 60-year-old Caucasian female is being treated for stroke in the intensive care unit. She is having episodes of hypotension. What fluid does the nurse anticipate would be ordered for this patient to prevent cytotoxic and vasogenic edema?
   a. Dextrose 5% in water (D5W)
   b. 0.45% sodium chloride (0.45% NS)
   c. 0.9% sodium chloride (0.9% NS)
   d. Dextrose 2.5% in water (D2.5%W)
7. While a heparin infusion is being administered to a patient for treatment of deep vein thrombosis of her left leg, she suddenly develops a left facial droop and weakness of her arm. What immediate therapy would the nurse anticipate for this patient?
   a. Intubation with mechanical ventilation
   b. Administration of protamine as a reversal agent
   c. Infusion of one ampule of D50
   d. ECG to determine the source of cardiac arrhythmia
8. A patient with a subarachnoid hemorrhage is being managed in the intensive care unit after undergoing cerebral coiling of a cerebral aneurysm 4 days ago. For the nurse, the focus of therapy turns to preventing which condition?
   a. Delayed cerebral ischemia
   b. Hydrocephalus
   c. Diabetes insipidus
   d. Subdural hematoma

ANSWERS

Answers to Review Questions can be found in Appendix A. Answers to Case Study and Check Your Progress questions are available on the faculty resources site. Please consult with your instructor.

RECOMMENDED WEBSITES

American Stroke Association
www.strokeassociation.org

Brain Injury Association of America
www.biausa.org

Brain Trauma Foundation
www.braintrauma.org

Moyamoya
www.moya-moya.com

National Stroke Association
www.stroke.org

REFERENCES

1. Hammer, G. D., & McPhee, S. J. (2014). *Pathophysiology of disease: An introduction to clinical medicine* (7th ed.). New York, NY: McGraw-Hill.
2. Schuenke, M., Schulte, E., Schumacher, U., Ross, L. M., Lamperti, E. D., & Voll M. (2010). *Head and neuroanatomy (Thieme atlas of anatomy)*. New York, NY: Thieme.
3. Waxman, S. G. (2014). *Clinical neuroanatomy* (27th ed.). New York, NY: McGraw-Hill.
4. Jauch, E. C., Saver, J. L, Adams, H. P., Bruno, A., Connors, J. J., Demaerschalk, B. M., et al. (2013). Guidelines for the early management of patients with acute ischemic stroke: A guideline for healthcare professionals from the American Heart Association/American Stroke Association. *Stroke, 44*, 870–947.
5. Kernan, W. N., Ovbiagele, B., Black, H. R., Bravata, D. M., Chimwitz, M. I., Ezekowitz, M. D., et al. (2014). Guidelines for the prevention of stroke in patients with stroke and transient ischemic attack. *Stroke, 45*, 2160–2236.
6. Caprio, F. Z., & Prabhakaran, S. (2013). Advances in imaging of intracranial atherosclerotic disease and implications for treatment. *Current Treatment Options in Cardiovascular Medicine, 15*(3), 335–347.
7. Connolly, E. S., Rabinstein, A. A., Carhuapoma, J. R., Derdyn, C. P., Dion, J., Higashida, R. T., et al. (2012). Guidelines for the management of aneurysmal subarachnoid hemorrhage: A guideline for healthcare professionals from the American Heart Association/American Stroke Association. *Stroke, 243*, 1711–1737.
8. Naranjo, D., Arkuszewski, M., Rudzinski, W., Melhem, E. R., & Krejza, J. (2013). Brain ischemia in patients with intracranial hemorrhage: Pathophysiologic reasoning for aggressive diagnostic management. *Neuroradiology Journal, 26*(6), 610–628.

Chapter 28

Shock and Multiple Organ Dysfunction Syndrome

Immaculata Igbo

Chapter Outline and Learning Outcomes

KEY TERMS

ABBREVIATIONS

MODS—multiple organ dysfunction syndrome
NO—nitric oxide
RAAS—renin-angiotensin-aldosterone system
SOFA—Sequential Organ Failure Assessment

28.1 Chapter Overview and Case Studies

Shock is a clinical syndrome characterized by acute circulatory failure with inadequate or inappropriately distributed tissue perfusion resulting in generalized cellular hypoxia and end-organ dysfunction.[1] It can be simplified as a condition in which there is inadequate perfusion to meet the metabolic needs of the cells. There is an imbalance between oxygen supplied and the oxygen demands of the cells. The resulting hypoxia subjects the tissues to anaerobic metabolism and lactic acid generation, which is damaging to the cells. Furthermore, the hypoperfusion can trigger both inflammatory and clotting cascades. The hypoxic vascular endothelial cells activate white blood cells, which bind to the endothelium and release damaging substances (e.g., reactive O_2 species) and inflammatory mediators (cytokines, leukotrienes). Some of these mediators bind to cell surface receptors, leading to the production of additional cytokines and nitric oxide (NO), a potent vasodilator. Excess NO is converted to peroxynitrite, a free radical that damages mitochondria and decreases ATP production. Thus, while there is evidence of cellular hypermetabolism (increase in ATP needs), there is decreased coupling of O_2 consumption and ATP production.

Types of shock are named according to the underlying cause:

- Shock caused by obstruction of blood flow is *obstructive shock.*
- Failure of the heart to pump is *cardiogenic shock.*
- Abnormal redistribution of blood is *distributive shock.*
- Low blood volume is *hypovolemic shock.*
- Shock due to inflammatory vascular response to infection is *septic shock* or *anaphylactic shock.*

The form of shock encountered by the nurse varies across practice settings. For example, septic shock, which is a type of distributive shock, is the most common in intensive care settings, while obstructive shock is less common.[2] Regardless of practice setting, the common characteristic of all types of shock is the development of acute circulatory failure resulting in hypotension and inadequate tissue perfusion to meet the metabolic needs of the cells. The four possible circulatory alterations leading to shock include heart failure, low blood volume in circulation, redistribution of extracellular fluid (ECF) to extravascular sites, and obstruction of blood flow. These alterations and their impact on circulatory function can be summarized by using the following equation:

$$\text{Blood pressure} = \text{cardiac output} \times \text{systemic vascular resistance.}$$

Cardiac output is the product of stroke volume and heart rate, so factors that affect blood or ECF volume, cardiac filling, contractility, and rate will affect cardiac output. These include factors that decrease blood volume (hemorrhage, diarrhea, vomiting, and burns); cardiac filling (cardiac tamponade, pulmonary edema, tension pneumothorax); cardiac contractility (heart failure, myocardial infarction, cardiac arrhythmia); and heart rate (decreased sympathetic outflow).

The fall in systemic vascular resistance is caused by an extensive increase in systemic vascular dilation and permeability leading to loss of fluid into the interstitial space. This fluid redistribution leaves a low circulating blood volume that is inadequate to perfuse vital organs. This happens with systemic inflammatory reactions associated with sepsis, anaphylactic reactions, neurologic injury such as spinal cord injury, and liver failure.

Shock is a condition that often occurs in patients in critical care, affecting about one third of patients in intensive care settings.[1] A diagnosis of shock is based on changes in clinical, hemodynamic, and biochemical data. Clinically, systemic arterial hypotension is usually present, with systolic arterial pressure less than 90 mmHg or mean arterial pressure less than 70 mmHg in adults. This is often accompanied by tachycardia. Clinical signs of tissue hypoperfusion are evident in cold, clammy skin as a result of vasoconstriction and cyanosis. Renal output also decreases because of the hypoperfusion manifested in oliguria (urine output of < 0.5 mL/kg of body weight per hour). Another impact of hypoperfusion on neurologic function is altered mental state, obtundation, disorientation, and confusion. Biochemical alteration as a result of shock is hyperlactatemia, indicating abnormal cellular oxygen metabolism. The normal blood lactate level is approximately 1 mmol/L, but the level is increased (> 1.5 mmol/L) in acute circulatory failure.[2] Evidence of hypercoagulability is also present.

Aging has been found to increase the risk of mortality in cases of circulatory shock, regardless of the cause of the shock.[3] ■

Concepts Related to Shock

Whatever its cause, shock is ultimately a deficit of fluid in the circulatory system. The loss of fluid results in compensatory responses that strain the cardiovascular system. The loss of fluid results in an increased heart rate along with increased sympathetic stimulation in an attempt to increase cardiac contraction to maintain adequate cardiac output. The skin becomes cool and clammy as a result of vasoconstriction, designed to increase the amount of fluid in circulation. As the individual becomes hypotensive, the development of tissue hypoxia releases further mediators, which are intended to enhance cardiac output, including the shunting of fluid away from organs. Ultimately, as the reduction of circulating volume continues, the left ventricle fails, resulting in cardiovascular collapse. (See **Figure 28.1** ■).

Case Studies

The following cases are addressed throughout the chapter to assist in application of chapter content to clinical situations that involve individuals with shock and multiple organ system dysfunction.

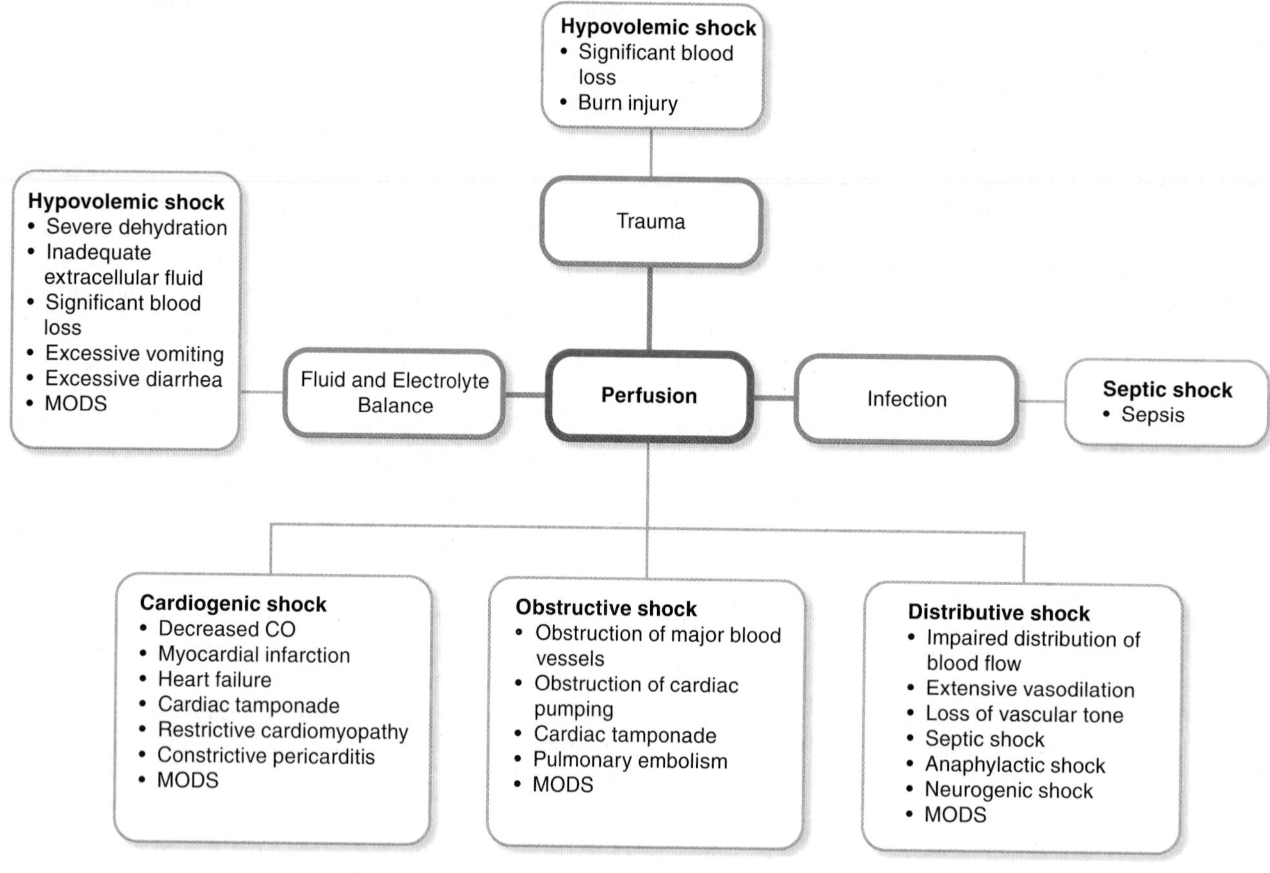

Figure 28.1 Concepts related to shock and multiple organ dysfunction syndrome.

Jimmy Bley: Introduction

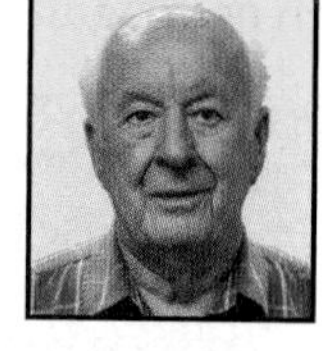

Jimmy Bley is an 85-year-old male with moderate emphysema and hearing loss. He has been married for 61 years. Mr. Bley considers himself healthy and describes his emphysema as "not that bad." Recently, his episodes of shortness of breath have interfered with activities more than usual, and he has made efforts on two occasions to stop smoking but without success. Mr. Bley is aware that his breathing has worsened and that he is using his inhaler much more frequently. He refused to get the flu vaccine. Mr. Bley is taken to the emergency department complaining of breathlessness that did not respond to his use of the inhaler.

1. What is one independent risk factor for circulatory shock in this case?
2. Why was Mr. Bley taken to the emergency department?

Betty Williams: Introduction

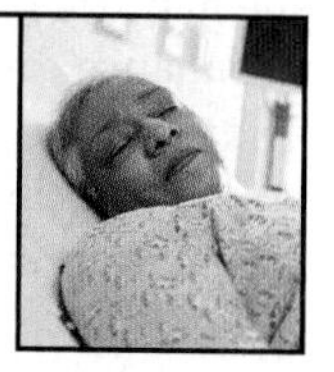

Betty Williams, age 65, is accompanied by her daughter, Felicia, to the emergency department. Felicia reports that she went to visit her mother and found Ms. Williams on the floor, incoherent (disoriented), with cold, clammy skin, so she called 9-1-1. Ms. Williams has a history of a previous heart attack, hypertension, diabetes mellitus, and chronic renal failure. A year ago, Ms. Williams presented with dyspnea and orthopnea accompanied by bilateral pedal edema. She was admitted with the diagnosis of heart failure.

1. What sign does Ms. Williams present with at the emergency department that indicates a deficit of fluid in the circulatory system?
2. What type of perfusion is evident when a patient has cold, clammy skin?

Check Your Progress: Section 28.1

1. What is the product of stroke volume and heart rate?
2. What is the most common form of shock?
3. What type of perfusion is evidenced by altered mental state, obtundation, disorientation, and confusion?

28.2 Pathophysiology of Shock

Hemodynamics of Shock

Hemodynamics deals with the forces the heart has to respond to in order to maintain blood flow through the cardiovascular system and supply oxygen to all tissues. Four factors influence circulation: blood volume, systemic vascular tone, heart rate, and force of contraction. Blood pressure and vascular resistance affect blood flow. Shock is a complication that follows several life-threatening conditions as a result of decreased circulating blood volume, heart failure, collapse of vasculature, or obstruction of blood flow. This creates an imbalance between oxygen needed by the cells and oxygen supplied. Shock is failure of the circulatory system to maintain adequate tissue perfusion to support cellular metabolic needs, which, if not well managed, can lead to multiple organ dysfunction syndrome (MODS).[4] The resulting hypoxia and decreased oxygen delivery to cells shift the metabolism to anaerobic metabolism with increased production of lactic acid (**Figure 28.2** ■). Serum level of lactate increases with shock, and this correlates with the patient outcome.[2]

Categories of Shock

There are four broad categories of shock:

- Hypovolemic shock (rapid blood or other ECF fluid loss)
- Cardiogenic shock (failure of the heart to maintain adequate cardiac output, as in heart failure)[5]
- Distributive shock (abnormal redistribution of blood), which includes septic shock
- Obstructive shock (obstruction of blood flow).[6]

Each is named on the basis of the etiology, but the general outcome is the same: poor tissue perfusion. The four types are illustrated in **Figure 28.3** ■, and each is explored in detail in the following sections.

Stages of Shock

There are three stages of shock: stage I (early, reversible, compensated or nonprogressive shock), stage II (intermediate or progressive shock), and stage III (refractory or irreversible shock). The multisystem effects of the three stages of shock are shown in **Figure 28.4** ■.

Stage 1: Early, Reversible, or Compensated Shock

In **stage I shock**, a number of compensatory systems are activated to maintain or restore perfusion when low blood

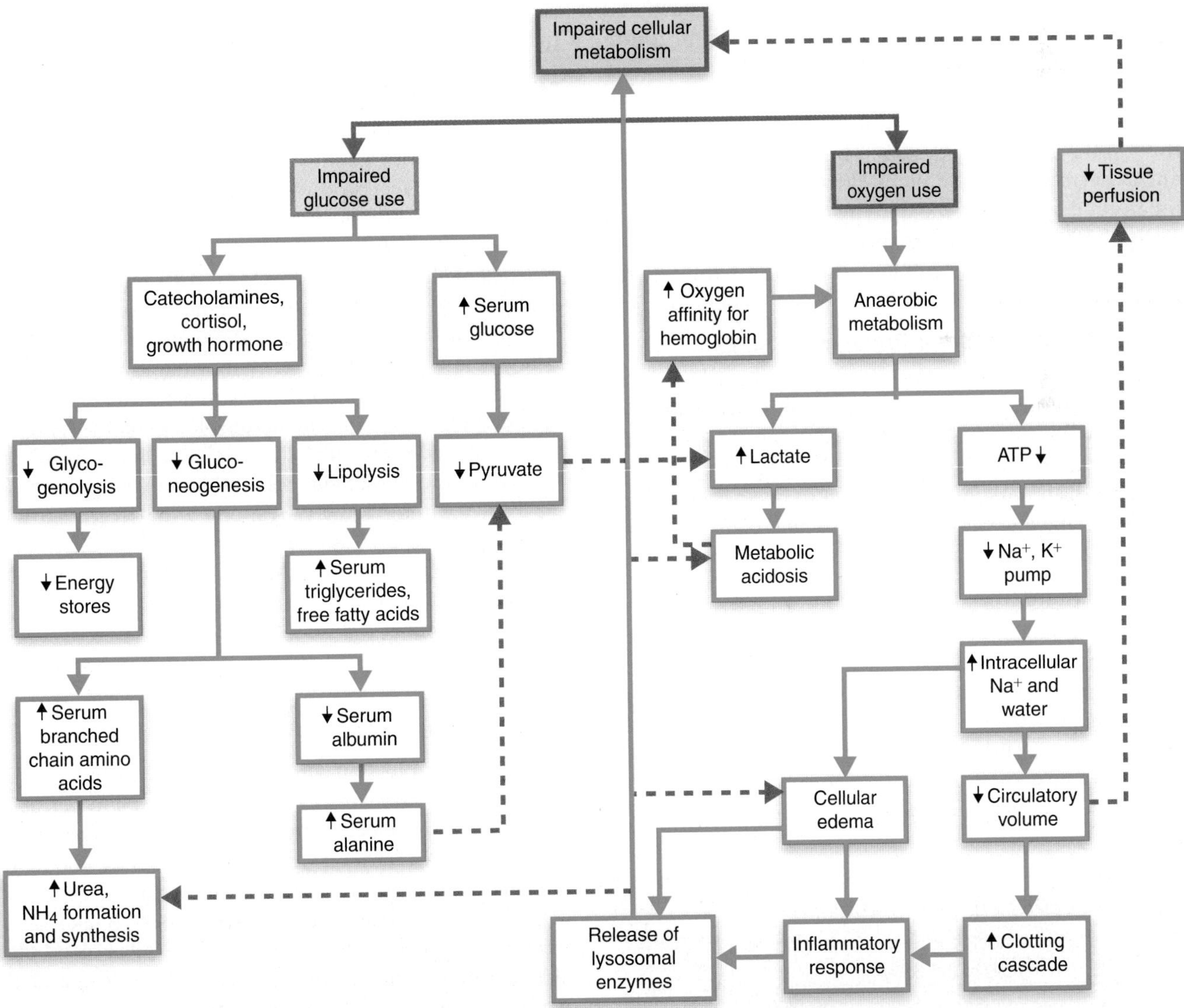

Figure 28.2 ■ Metabolic modifications within shock. ATP = adenosine triphosphate, K^+ = potassium ion, Na^+ = sodium ion, NH_4 = ammonium.

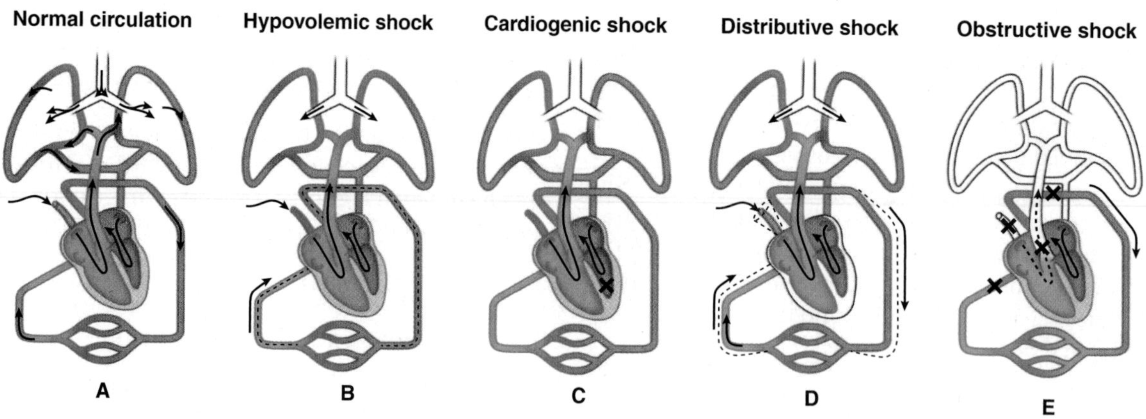

Figure 28.3 Compare **A** normal circulation with **B** hypovolemic shock, **C** cardiogenic shock, **D** distributive shock, and **E** obstructive shock.

flow is initially detected. The baroreceptors respond to the low blood pressure by stimulating the cardiovascular center in the brain to increase sympathetic outflow to the heart and blood vessels. The heart rate then increases and the blood vessels constrict as a result of increased sympathetic stimulation. The kidney responds to poor perfusion by activating the renin-angiotensin-aldosterone system (RAAS), which works to resorb sodium and water and maintain adequate fluid in the circulatory system. This compensatory mechanism helps to maintain blood flow to the most essential organs and systems in the body with minimal symptoms. The patient in this stage of shock has a strong chance of recovery with proper treatment. (Refer to Chapter 45 for more information on the RAAS.)

Stage II: Intermediate or Progressive Shock

In **stage II shock**, the compensatory mechanisms begin to fail. The resulting decrease in perfusion leads to cellular hypoxia with accompanying hypoxic tissue injuries. The patient will experience neurologic changes such as confusion and disorientation, angina due to decreased oxygen delivery to the myocardium, and muscular pain. This stage is reversible if appropriate treatment is instituted promptly.

Stage III: Refractory or Irreversible Shock

In **stage III shock**, poor perfusion has persisted for long enough that it begins to take a permanent toll on the body's organs and tissues. The heart's functioning continues to decline, and the kidneys usually shut down completely. Cells in organs and tissues throughout the body are injured as a result of hypoxia and cell death. The endpoint of stage III shock is the patient's death due to multiple organ dysfunction.

> **Check Your Progress: Section 28.2**
>
> 1. What stage of shock begins to take a permanent toll on the organs and tissues of the body?
> 2. What category of shock includes rapid blood or other ECF fluid loss?
> 3. If shock is not well managed, what can it lead to?

28.3 Hypovolemic Shock

Hypovolemic shock, which is also called hemorrhagic shock, is a life-threatening condition that occurs when a patient loses more than 15% of the body's fluids.

Etiology and Pathogenesis

Hypovolemic shock occurs when there is rapid or excessive loss of significant amount of whole blood as in trauma, internal bleeding from a ruptured ectopic pregnancy or gastrointestinal lesions, or loss of other body fluids (from diarrhea, vomiting, diaphoresis, severe burns, or diuresis as occurs in diabetes mellitus and diabetes insipidus), edema, or severe dehydration. This may lead to hemodynamic instability, decreases in tissue perfusion and oxygen delivery, cellular hypoxia, and organ damage. Hemorrhagic shock can lead to death, and the primary goals of management are to stop the bleeding and restore circulating blood volume.[7] A loss of 15% body fluid will result in hypovolemic shock. As in other types of shock, the skin is cool and clammy with decreased capillary refill; the kidneys respond with decreased urine output (oliguria of < 0.5 mL/kg/h); and changes in mental functioning such as disorientation and confusion result. Blood laboratory testing will also confirm the presence of hyperlactatemia of > 2 mEq/L.

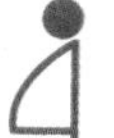

Postpartum hemorrhage, which can lead to hypovolemic shock, is a major cause of maternal death around the world.[7]

The body's response to hypovolemia includes initial compensatory mechanisms to address the fall in perfusion pressure and to maintain cardiac output. These mechanisms are hematologic, cardiovascular, renal, and neuroendocrine. Hematologic response includes the clotting of blood in the coagulation process to end further blood loss. It takes about 24 hours for the thrombus to mature. The fall in blood pressure stimulates increased sympathetic outflow and the release of epinephrine and norepinephrine (catecholamines) from the adrenal medulla and sympathetic nerve ending to increase systemic vascular resistance and heart rate while decreasing vagal (parasympathetic) outflow. These two

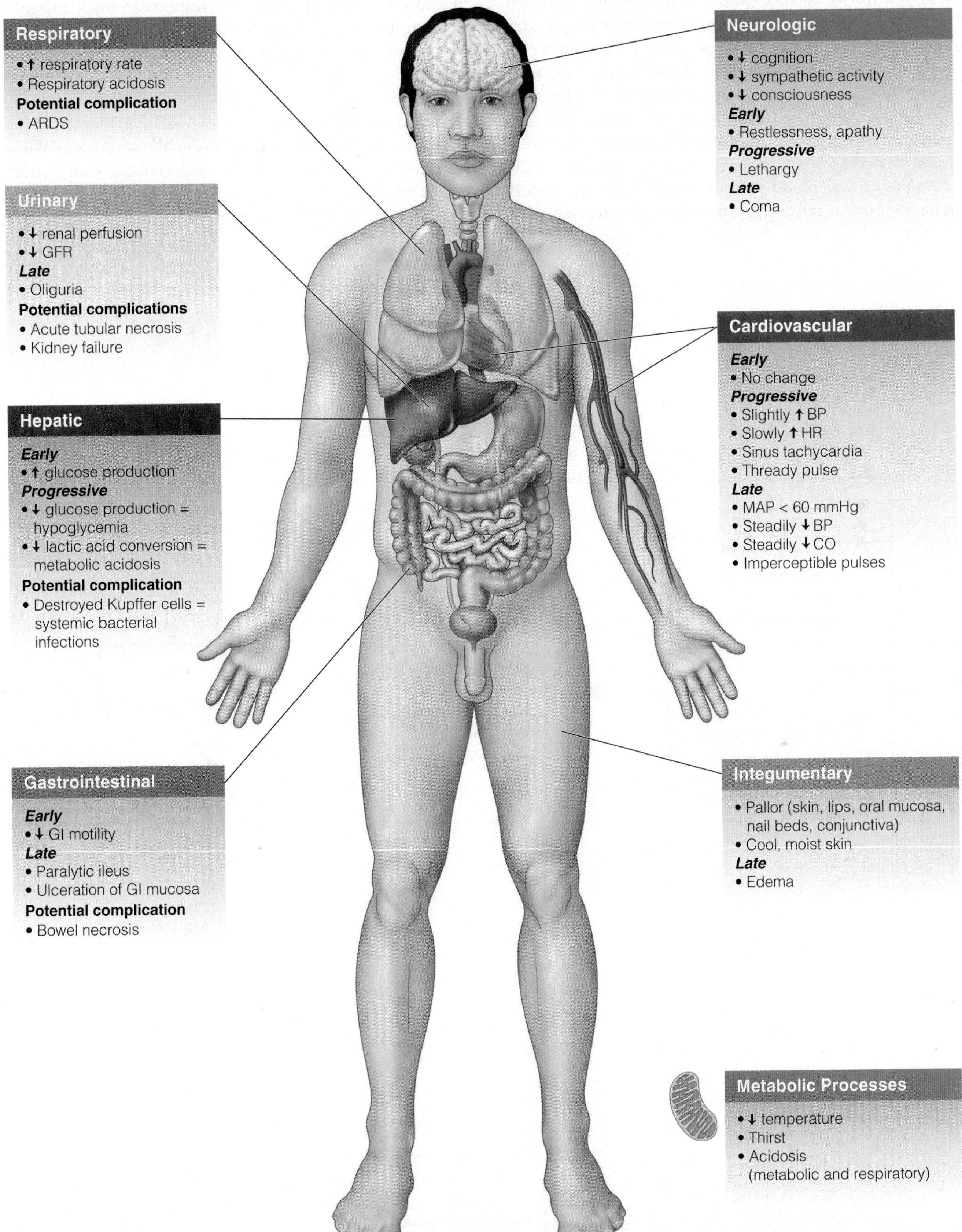

Respiratory
• ↑ respiratory rate
• Respiratory acidosis
Potential complication
• ARDS
Urinary
• ↓ renal perfusion
• ↓ GFR
Late
• Oliguria
Potential complications
• Acute tubular necrosis
• Kidney failure
Hepatic
Early
• ↑ glucose production
Progressive
• ↓ glucose production = hypoglycemia
• ↓ lactic acid conversion = metabolic acidosis
Potential complication
• Destroyed Kupffer cells = systemic bacterial infections
Gastrointestinal
Early
• ↓ GI motility
Late
• Paralytic ileus
• Ulceration of GI mucosa
Potential complication
• Bowel necrosis
Neurologic
• ↓ cognition
• ↓ sympathetic activity
• ↓ consciousness
Early
• Restlessness, apathy
Progressive
• Lethargy
Late
• Coma
Cardiovascular
Early
• No change
Progressive
• Slightly ↑ BP
• Slowly ↑ HR
• Sinus tachycardia
• Thready pulse
Late
• MAP < 60 mmHg
• Steadily ↓ BP
• Steadily ↓ CO
• Imperceptible pulses
Integumentary
• Pallor (skin, lips, oral mucosa, nail beds, conjunctiva)
• Cool, moist skin
Late
• Edema
Metabolic Processes
• ↓ temperature
• Thirst
• Acidosis (metabolic and respiratory)

Figure 28.4 ■ Multisystem effects of early, progressive, and late shock.

changes improve cardiac output and perfusion pressure. The kidney responds to the decrease in perfusion pressure by releasing renin in the activation of the RAAS. Angiotensin II from this system stimulates aldosterone release from the adrenal cortex. Aldosterone increases the renal resorption of sodium, followed by water, leading to an increase in circulating intravascular fluid volume. Angiotensin II also causes vasoconstriction, thus increasing peripheral vascular resistance and blood pressure (**Figure 28.5** ■). Antidiuretic hormone is released by the posterior pituitary gland in response to the input from the osmoreceptors to increase the permeability of the collecting tubules of the nephron to water leading to water resorption. The cardiovascular system also shunts blood to vital organs that require large amounts of oxygen, such as the brain, heart, and kidneys, while decreasing blood flow to less vital organs such as the skin, muscle tissue, and gastrointestinal tract. This explains the delay in capillary refill and cold, clammy skin characteristic of shock. The overall impact of these compensatory mechanisms is maintenance of both cardiac output and

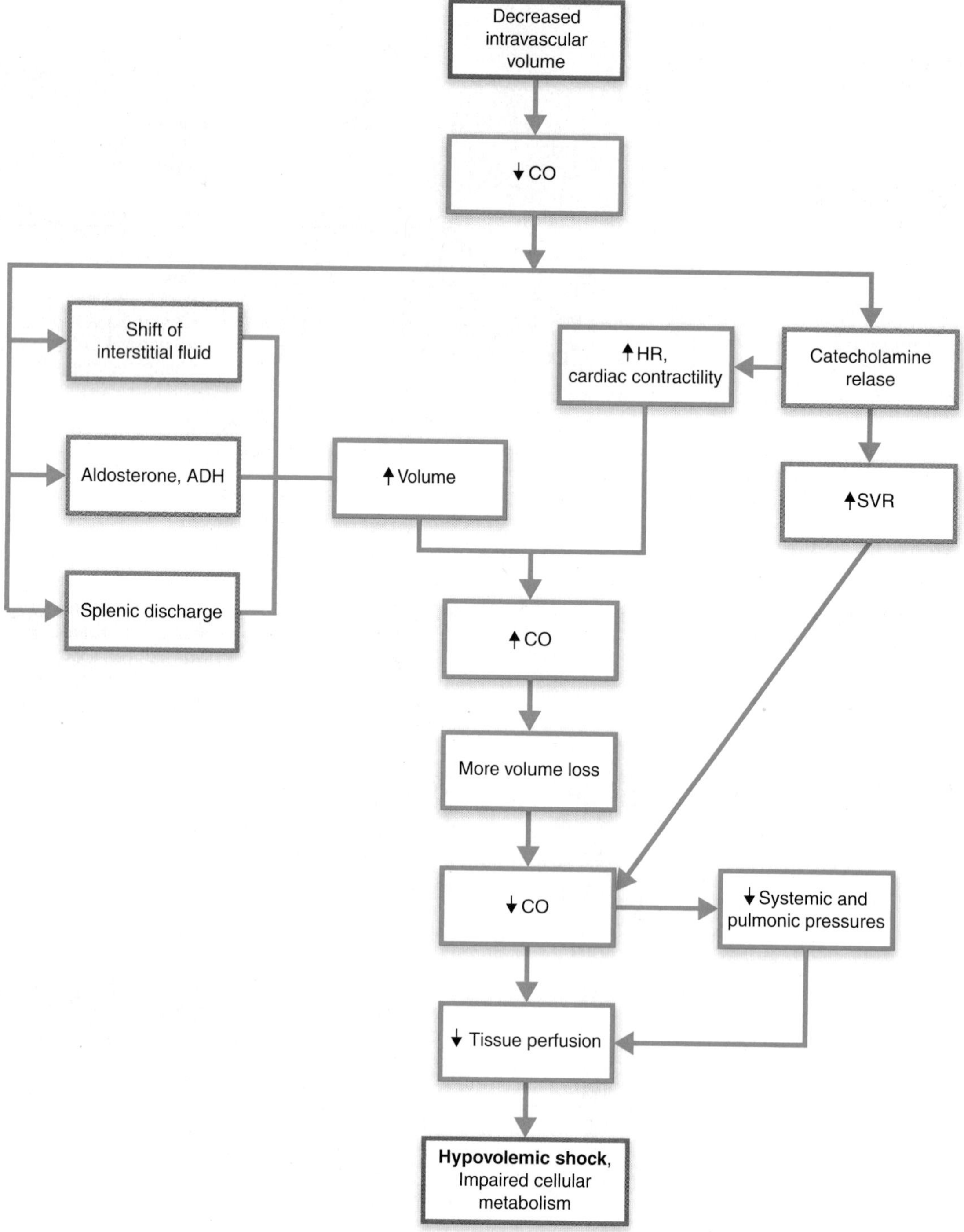

Figure 28.5 ■ The pathogenesis of hypovolemic shock. ADH = antidiuretic hormone, CO = cardiac output, HR = heart rate, SVR = systemic vascular resistance.

blood pressure. There is also mobilization of blood stored in the liver and abdominal large veins (about 350 mL) into circulation when needed. These mechanisms in addition to therapeutic fluid correction can reverse the progression of the shock. If this resuscitation fails because of continued ECF loss, multiple organ damage and failure may occur.

Clinical Manifestations

The patient's history is important in the diagnosis and appropriate clinical workup for hypovolemic shock. Frequent measurements of heart rate and blood pressure are essential to assess the patient's status. Hypotension in an adult is defined as a systolic blood pressure of 90 mmHg or less and is consistent with depleted intravascular volume. Depleted intravascular volume is also suggested by orthostatic or postural hypotension. The American Autonomic Society and the American Academy of Neurology define orthostatic hypotension as a systolic blood pressure decrease of at least 20 mmHg or a diastolic blood pressure decrease of at least 10 mmHg within 3 minutes after standing up. Some experts also consider an increase in pulse rate greater than 15 beats/min with positional change to be a sign of orthostatic hypotension.

The American College of Surgeons developed a practical classification scheme, based on the patient's presentation, for estimating the amount of blood that has been lost (**Table 28.1** ■).[8]

In this classification system, the blood loss and the severity of the clinical characteristics increase with the class. Heart rate, tachypnea, capillary refill time, and degree of oliguria increase with the class. In class IV, mental function becomes severely impaired, progressing from agitation and anxiety to confusion and loss of consciousness.

Standard laboratory tests for patients with possible hypovolemic shock include the following:

- Complete blood count
- Determination of serum electrolyte concentrations
- Determination of blood glucose level
- Arterial blood gas determinations
- Prothrombin time and partial thromboplastin time to detect a clotting disorder
- Hemoglobin and hematocrit to determine the severity of blood loss or hemoconcentration due to dehydration
- Serum lactate concentration and arterial pH to detect metabolic acidosis.

Estimated blood volume differs according to age. It is 7% in adults, 8–9% in children, and 9–10% in infants.[9] ■

Hypovolemic shock signs and symptoms include the following:

- Rapid breathing
- Severe shortness of breath
- Sudden, rapid heartbeat (tachycardia)
- Loss of consciousness
- Weak pulse
- Sweating
- Pale skin
- Cold hands or feet
- Urinating less than normal or not at all.

Linking Pathophysiology to Diagnosis and Treatment

There are three primary objectives for managing the patient with hypovolemic shock:

1. Maximize oxygen delivery by ensuring adequate ventilation and oxygen saturation of the blood and by restoring blood flow.
2. Prevent further fluid loss.
3. Replace lost fluids.

Effective treatment depends on prompt evaluation of the patient and an accurate assessment of the cause of fluid loss. Initial therapy consists of basic life support: airway maintenance, high-flow supplemental oxygen assistance, cardiopulmonary resuscitation if necessary, intravenous access, and fluid resuscitation to restore filling pressure. Cardiac monitoring can detect a cardiac arrhythmia that is treatable with standard advanced life-support protocols. A central venous line is placed for hemodynamic pressure measurements. Central lines are useful for administering medications, measuring central venous oxygen saturation, and monitoring the effects of fluid resuscitation or vasopressor medications. Treatment is directed at maintaining a central venous pressure of 8–12 mmHg, a mean arterial

Table 28.1 Classification of Hemorrhage

	Class			
Parameter	**I**	**II**	**III**	**IV**
Blood loss (mL)	< 750	750–1500	1500–2000	> 2000
Blood loss (%)	$< 15\%$	15–30%	30–40%	$> 40\%$
Pulse rate (beats/min)	< 100	> 100	> 120	> 140
Blood pressure	Normal	Decreased	Decreased	Decreased
Respiratory rate (breaths/min)	14–20	20–30	30–40	> 35
Urine output (mL/h)	> 30	20–30	5–15	Negligible
CNS symptoms	Normal	Anxious	Confused	Lethargic

SOURCE: Data from American College of Surgeons. (2017). *Advanced trauma life support* (10th ed.). Chicago, IL: American College of Surgeons.

blood pressure of 65–90 mmHg, and central venous oxygen saturation greater than 70%.

Control of further fluid loss frequently depends on the source of bleeding. External bleeding is controlled with direct pressure and various other techniques. Internal bleeding requires surgical intervention. Long bone fractures are treated with traction to decrease blood loss. In patients with gastrointestinal bleeding, intravenous vasopressin and H_2 (i.e., histamine receptor-2) blocking agents have been used. Infusions of somatostatin or octreotide have been shown to reduce gastrointestinal bleeding from esophageal varices and peptic ulcers. Virtually all cases of acute gynecologic bleeding that cause hypovolemia require surgery.

Current recommendations include aggressive fluid resuscitation for all patients with clinical manifestations of hypovolemic shock, regardless of the underlying cause. The patient's response is assessed after administration of 1–2 liters of a crystalloid, either isotonic saline or lactated Ringer's solution.

Blood products are indicated in hemorrhagic shock. Preferably, type-specific or type O-negative packed red blood cells are given to maintain a hematocrit above 30%. Whole blood provides both intravascular volume and clotting factors.

Plasma expanders (e.g., dextran and albumin) remain in the circulation longer than crystalloids and do not necessitate blood typing. These medications increase intravascular blood volume by increasing the intravascular osmotic pressure. However, plasma expanders must be used with caution, as they may induce serious allergic reactions, including anaphylactic shock. Oxygen-carrying synthetic plasma expanders, known as *artificial blood*, are being used in some trauma centers to effectively treat hypovolemic shock.

Pharmacotherapy may include the administration of calcium, sodium bicarbonate (if arterial pH $\leq$ 7.20), and vasopressor drugs. Vasopressor agents are best given only when hypotension persists after volume deficits have been corrected. Dopamine, which produces a more favorable array of positive actions on the heart and arterioles than many other vasopressors, is often used in the treatment of severe and prolonged shock. When administered in low doses (2–3 μg/kg/min), dopamine increases heart rate and cardiac contractility; increases blood flow to the kidneys, liver, and other abdominal organs; and maintains vasoconstriction in the skin and skeletal muscles.

The use of sedation, anxiolytic agents, and pain medications is tailored for each individual case. When acute renal insufficiency becomes a complication of hypovolemic shock, urgent hemodialysis or continuous hemofiltration may be indicated for maintenance of fluid and electrolyte balance.

Check Your Progress: Section 28.3

1. What is another name for the life-threatening condition of hypovolemic shock?
2. Pharmacotherapy may include the administration of calcium, sodium bicarbonate, and what other drug?
3. How many classes of hemorrhage are there in the American College of Surgeons classification scheme?

28.4 Cardiogenic Shock

Myocardial damage can result in the heart's being unable to contract effectively or in restricted filling of the ventricles such that output is significantly reduced. When the heart is unable to circulate an adequate amount of blood, hypoxic damage to the organs can result. This state is referred to as **cardiogenic shock**.

Etiology and Pathogenesis

Cardiogenic shock is a sudden onset of decreased cardiac output and tissue hypoxia without evidence of intravascular fluid loss associated with a large myocardial infarction and heart failure. Cardiogenic shock is due to failure of the cardiac pump related to loss of myocardial function and contractility resulting in elevations of diastolic filling pressures and volumes. Recent studies support that microcirculatory changes in the myocardium contribute to the decrease in cardiac output in cardiogenic shock and that measures to improve the microcirculation can improve the patient outcome.[5] Cardiogenic shock has also been defined by using the hemodynamic changes associated with it: persistent hypotension (systolic blood pressure less than 80–90 mmHg or mean arterial pressure 30 mmHg lower than baseline) with severe reduction in the cardiac index (less than 1.8 L/min/m^2 without support or less than 2.0–2.2 L/min/m^2 with support) and adequate or elevated filling pressures.[2,5]

Cardiogenic shock is the number one cause of in-hospital mortality from Q-wave myocardial infarction. It requires at least 40% loss of functional myocardium. It usually involves obstruction of the left main or left anterior descending coronary artery and affects 8–20% of patients with myocardial infarction, with a mortality rate of 70–90%.

Other causes of cardiogenic shock are left heart failure, blunt cardiac trauma, myocarditis, hypertrophic cardiomyopathy, valvular failure (stenotic or regurgitant), sustained cardiac dysrhythmia (bradycardia, tachycardia), ventricular or septal ruptures, massive pulmonary embolism, drug cardiotoxicity (calcium channel blockers, anthracyclines), and pericardial infections.

Cardiogenic shock caused by acute myocardial infarction shows a progressive decrease in coronary perfusion pressure, increased myocardial oxygen demand, and hypoxia. This cycle contributes to a decrease in myocardial contractility and stroke volume and an increase in end-systolic volume. The weak heart pumps less blood, and the pressure increases in the left ventricle, causing an increase in pulmonary pressure and pulmonary edema. Furthermore, hypoperfusion of the myocardium and other cells increases anaerobic metabolism of the cells and the production of lactic acid. The resulting acidosis and hypoxia disrupt cellular activities and maintenance of membrane integrity, causing lysosomal breakdown, mitochondrial swelling, disruption of nuclear envelopes, activation of inflammatory cascades, and oxidative stress. Microcirculatory function also deteriorates during cardiogenic shock.[10]

Compensatory mechanisms involving the sympathetic nervous system, the RAAS, and the ADH system attempt to correct the hypotension and poor perfusion of essential organs such as the brain, kidney, and liver. This results in increased fluid retention, heart rate, and contractility, further increasing cardiac oxygen and nutrient demand. The compensatory changes only worsen the state of the heart, leading to shock and impaired tissue metabolism (**Figure 28.6** ■).

Betty Williams: Application

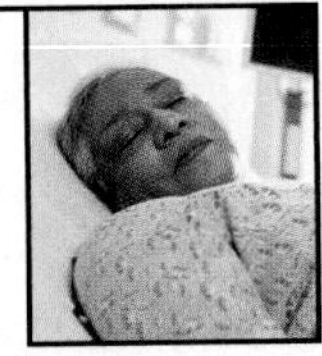

On arrival at the emergency department, Ms. Williams is cyanotic and tachycardic (heart rate 105 beats/min) with low pulse pressure. Her blood pressure is 97/60. Heart sounds are low and distant, and on chest examination, she has crackles. She is admitted to the intensive care unit with the diagnosis of cardiogenic shock. A cardiac catheterization is performed and reveals an ejection fraction of 30%.

3. What hemodynamic changes are evident in Ms. Williams?
4. What is one cause of cardiogenic shock that is evidenced by the results from the cardiac catheterization?

Clinical Manifestations

Clinical manifestations of cardiogenic shock include the following:

- The patient is generally cyanotic with cool skin and mottled extremities (as a result of poor tissue perfusion).

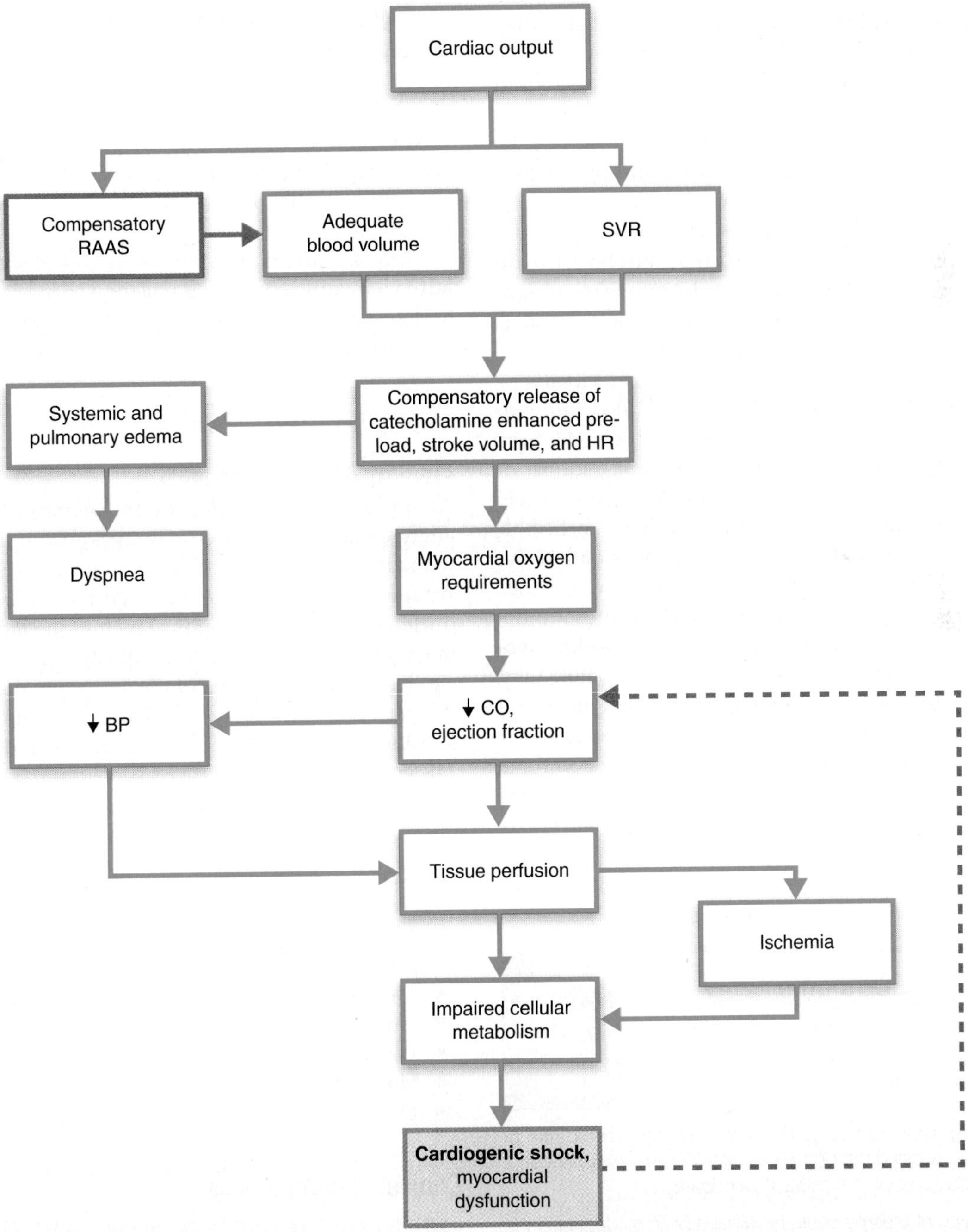

Cardiac output

Compensatory RAAS

Adequate blood volume

SVR

Systemic and pulmonary edema

Compensatory release of catecholamine enhanced preload, stroke volume, and HR

Dyspnea

Myocardial oxygen requirements

↓ BP

↓ CO, ejection fraction

Tissue perfusion

Ischemia

Impaired cellular metabolism

Cardiogenic shock, myocardial dysfunction

Figure 28.6 ■ The pathogenesis of cardiogenic shock. ADH = antidiuretic hormone, BP = blood pressure, CO = cardiac output, HR = heart rate, RAAS = renin-angiotensin-aldosterone system, SVR = systemic vascular resistance.

- The patient has rapid and faint peripheral pulses that may be irregular if the patient has cardiac arrhythmia.
- The pulse pressure is low and tachycardic.
- Heart sounds are low and distant.
- The patient may have peripheral edema and jugular distension (as a result of right-sided heart failure).
- The patient may have crackles in the lungs (associated with left-sided heart failure).

Linking Pathophysiology to Diagnosis and Treatment

The first and most important step is to identify the cause of the cardiogenic shock so that treatment can be initiated to address it. A patent airway must be maintained, and mechanical ventilation must be readily available if the patient develops respiratory distress. Some patients may present with more than one kind of shock, such as hypovolemic shock with cardiogenic shock. In that case, fluid resuscitation will be initiated unless there is pulmonary edema. Patients will have hypotension as a result of the failure of the heart to pump enough blood (low cardiac output) and low perfusion pressure. This is modified by giving inotropic agents (drugs that improve cardiac contractility). Coronary vasodilators such as nitroglycerin are given to dilate the coronary arteries and improve blood supply to the myocardium. When fluid overload is present, as manifested by pulmonary edema and the presence of crackles, diuretic therapy is instituted. Thrombolytic therapy or coronary artery revascularization improves blood flow to the myocardium. Monitoring and correction of acid–base and electrolyte imbalances is also important because of their impact on cellular function and especially on cardiac function. Other interventions, such as an intra-aortic balloon pump, are directed at reducing the workload of the heart. Surgical interventions include valvular or ventricular septal repairs if valvular failure or septal ruptures are the underlying cause of the cardiogenic shock. If cardiac dysrhythmia is implicated, pacemakers and defibrillators may be implanted to assist in maintaining cardiac rhythm. The mortality rate is substantially better for cardiogenic shock than for other types of shock because surgical interventions can correct most of the underlying coronary vascular lesions The American College of Cardiology/American Heart Association guidelines for myocardial infarction now recommend emergency revascularization for patients younger than 75 years with cardiogenic shock.[11]

Betty Williams: Outcome

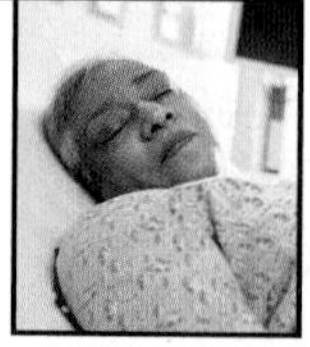

Ms. Williams and her daughter are informed that Ms. Williams has a reduced ejection fraction along with a prior history of heart failure. She is encouraged to consider revascularization procedures that may improve her quality of life and reduce the risk of mortality. While awaiting the procedure, Ms. Williams experiences a pulmonary embolism, which results in her death.

5. What type of therapy could have been used to decrease the risk of the pulmonary embolism?
6. What type of emergency procedure is now recommended for patients younger than 75 years of age with cardiogenic shock?

Check Your Progress: Section 28.4

1. What is the number one cause of in-hospital mortality from Q-wave myocardial infarction?
2. A clinical manifestation of cardiogenic shock includes what type of peripheral pulses?
3. Patients may have crackles in the lungs associated with what type of heart failure?

28.5. Distributive Shock

Distributive shock results in impaired distribution of blood flow due to extensive vasodilation and loss of vascular tone. Septic shock, anaphylactic shock, and neurogenic shock are the different types of distributive shock. Septic shock is the most common form of distributive shock, resulting in 40% of deaths in patients diagnosed with shock. Septic shock resulting from sepsis causes the most noncardiac deaths in intensive care unit (ICU) patients in the United States.[12]

Other causes of distributive shock include anaphylaxis, adrenal insufficiency, drug reactions, hepatic insufficiency, and systemic inflammatory response syndrome due to a noninfectious inflammatory condition such as burns.

Anaphylactic Shock

Etiology and Pathogenesis

Anaphylaxis is an acute, life-threatening, IgE-mediated allergic reaction that occurs on reexposure in individuals who are sensitive to an allergen or antigen (**Figure 28.7** ■). **Anaphylactic shock** occurs when the antibody IgE produced by plasma cells binds to membrane receptors on the mast cells and basophils. Subsequent exposure to the antigen results in the binding of the antigen to the antibody on the mast cells, leading to the release of histamine and other substances of anaphylaxis (leukotrienes and bradykinin). These mediators cause increased vascular permeability through vasodilation as well as bronchoconstriction.

Anaphylaxis is typically triggered by the following:

- Drugs (e.g., β-lactam antibiotics, insulin, radio dyes, streptokinase, allergen extracts)
- Foods (e.g., peanuts, eggs, seafood, sulfite-containing food additives)
- Proteins (e.g., tetanus antitoxin, blood transfusions)
- Animal or insect venoms
- Latex
- Heavy metal poisoning
- Occasionally, exercise and exposure to cold temperature.

Clinical Manifestations

Symptoms of anaphylactic shock can include stridor, tachycardia, dyspnea, wheezing, coughing, edema, laryngospasm, bronchoconstriction, angioedema, urticaria, pruritus, hives, gastrointestinal cramps, and hypotension.

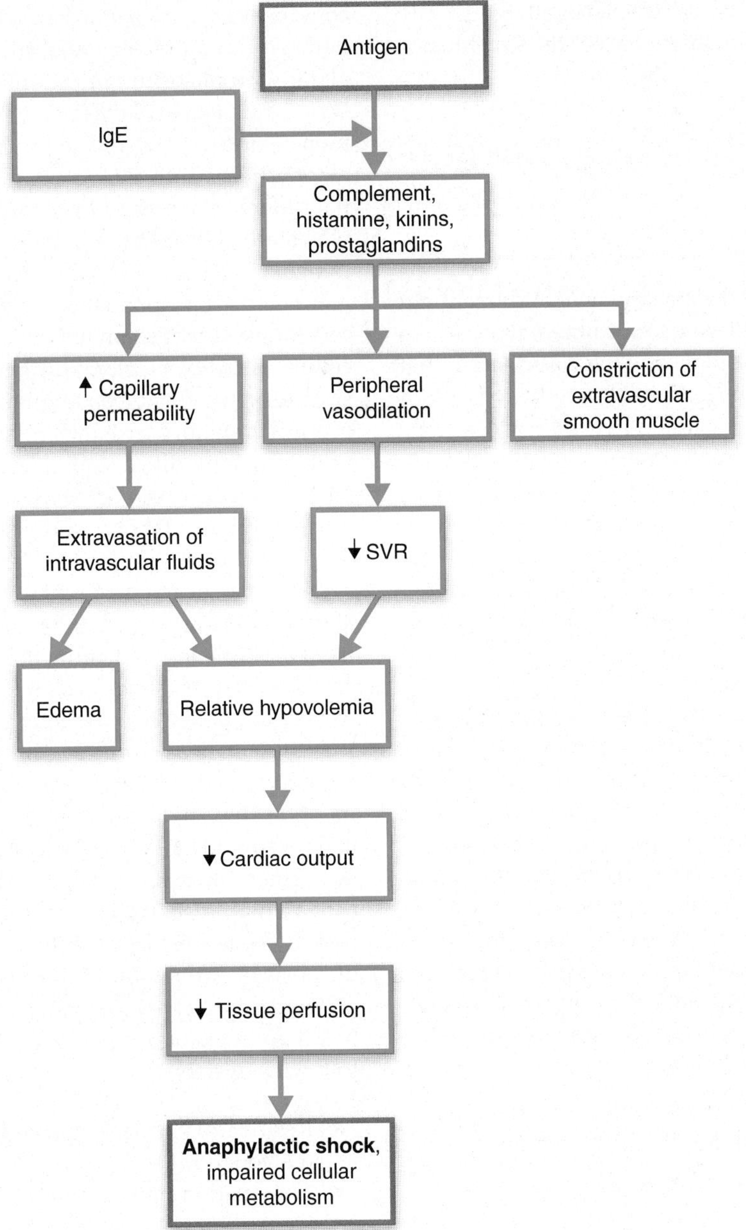

Figure 28.7 ■ The pathogenesis of anaphylactic shock. SVR = systemic vascular resistance.

Linking Pathophysiology to Diagnosis and Treatment

Interaction of antigen with IgE on basophils and mast cells triggers the release of histamine, leukotrienes, and other mediators that cause diffuse nonvascular smooth muscle contraction, resulting in bronchoconstriction and respiratory difficulty, vomiting, or diarrhea, but with vasodilation causing increased vascular permeability and ECF leakage into the intestinal space (urticarial or angioedema).

To ensure oxygenation, a patent airway is maintained by either tracheostomy, endotracheal intubation, or mechanical ventilation. Bronchospasm and upper airway edema may require inhaled or injected beta agonists such as albuterol and epinephrine and anti-inflammatory agents such as corticosteroids. Diphenhydramine is given to reduce allergic reactions. Persistent hypotension requires intravenous fluid expanders and vasopressors (dopamine) to support blood pressure.

Diagnosis is clinical. Anaphylaxis should be suspected if any of the following suddenly occur without explanation:

- Shock
- Respiratory symptoms (e.g., dyspnea, stridor, wheezing)
- Two or more other manifestations of possible anaphylaxis (e.g., angioedema, rhinorrhea, gastrointestinal symptoms).

The cause of anaphylaxis is usually easily recognized on the basis of the patient's history. If healthcare workers have unexplained anaphylactic symptoms, latex allergy should be considered. Treatment for anaphylactic shock includes:

- Epinephrine given immediately
- Sometimes intubation
- Intravenous fluids and sometimes vasopressors for persistent hypotension
- Antihistamines
- Inhaled beta agonists for bronchoconstriction.

Epinephrine is vital to the management and treatment of anaphylaxis and should be given immediately. It can relieve the bronchospasm and reduce the vasodilation that is responsible for the pathogenesis of anaphylaxis. Both pediatric and adult patients with known allergic reactions should carry on their person a prefilled epinephrine autoinjector (Epi-Pen or Adrenaclick) for immediate injection as needed. It can be given subcutaneously, intramuscularly, or intravenously in patients with cardiovascular collapse or severe airway constriction. Other routes of administration include sublingually and through an endotracheal tube. Patients who have wheezing that is unresponsive to epinephrine should be given oxygen.

Intravenous epinephrine often reverses the hypotension, but when this is unsuccessful, dopamine (vasopressor) can be added in conjunction with intravenous fluid. Both histamine receptor blockers (H_1 and H_2) and steroidal anti-inflammatory drugs such as methylprednisolone are useful in reducing the inflammatory reaction in the center of anaphylaxis and anaphylactic shock. Patients who have had an anaphylactic reaction to insect stings, foods, or other known substances should wear a medic alert bracelet and carry on their person a prefilled epinephrine syringe (containing 0.3 mg for adults and 0.15 mg for children) for prompt self-treatment after exposure.

The most common agents that cause anaphylactic reaction in children are food (e.g., legumes, nuts, fish, shellfish, cow's milk, eggs), hymenoptera (i.e., bee or wasp) stings, and medications (particularly penicillins).[13] ■

CLINICAL POINT: Anaphylactoid reactions are similar to anaphylaxis in clinical manifestations and treatment. The major difference is that anaphylactoid reactions do not involve IgE and do not require prior sensitization. ■

Septic Shock

Etiology and Pathogenesis

Septic shock is defined as life threatening organ dysfunction caused by a dysregulated host response to infection (**Figure 28.8** ■).[14,15] This is the revised definition of septic shock by the Third International Consensus Definitions for Sepsis and Septic Shock. This new definition highlights the nonhomeostatic host response to infection as the core pathophysiology of sepsis, the potential lethality it presents, and the need for urgent recognition and treatment. Earlier definitions of sepsis and septic shock were based heavily on the assumption that it was an excessive inflammatory response of the body to infection. Current research and international consensus recognize that sepsis involves early activation of both pro-inflammatory and anti-inflammatory responses, along with major modifications in nonimmunologic pathways such as cardiovascular, neuronal, autonomic, hormonal, bioenergetic, metabolic, and coagulation pathways, all of which contribute to the outcome. There are individual differences in the clinical and biological presentations, which are affected by age and comorbidities, among other things.

The body responds to the infecting microorganism in several ways that ultimately overwhelm the immunologic, cellular, cardiovascular, and hematologic systems.[16] Sepsis is now recognized as involving early activation of both pro-inflammatory and anti-inflammatory responses, along with major modifications in nonimmunologic pathways such as cardiovascular, neuronal, autonomic, hormonal, bioenergetic, metabolic, and coagulation pathways.[17] The Sepsis Definitions Task Force defined septic shock as a subset of sepsis in which circulatory, cellular, and metabolic abnormalities are associated with a greater risk of mortality from multiple organ dysfunction than is the case with sepsis alone.[1] Septic shock accounts for 40% of deaths in out-of-hospital patients, those in emergency departments, and those in general hospitals. Clinically, a number of assessment tools and algorithms are used to guide patient assessment for the risk or presence of sepsis. Once such measure is the **Sequential Organ Failure Assessment (SOFA)**. This assessment measure evaluates the different systems (cardiovascular, respiratory, coagulation, renal, hepatic, neurologic) believed to be involved in the pathogenic process of sepsis or influenced by the resultant organ failure. The SOFA places the patient into four potential categories of risk based upon relative organ function. The SOFA evaluates the following systems:

- Respiratory status through evaluation of arterial oxygenation
- Coagulation status through evaluation of platelet count
- Hepatic status through evaluation of bilirubin level
- Cardiovascular status through evaluation of blood pressure
- Neurologic status through calculation of Glasgow Coma Scale ratings
- Renal status through evaluation of urinary output and creatinine.

Evaluating these systems provides a measure of organ function and a means of predicting potential mortality and can guide clinical intervention. For example, patients with septic shock are dependent on vasopressin to maintain a mean arterial pressure of 65 mmHg and have a serum lactate level greater than 2 mmol/L in the absence of hypovolemia. The patient's age, underlying comorbidities, concurrent injuries (including surgery), and medications and the source of infection increase the complexity of diagnosis and treatment of septic shock.[18] An international study of a large database highlights that sepsis remains a major health problem worldwide, associated with high mortality rates in all countries.[19]

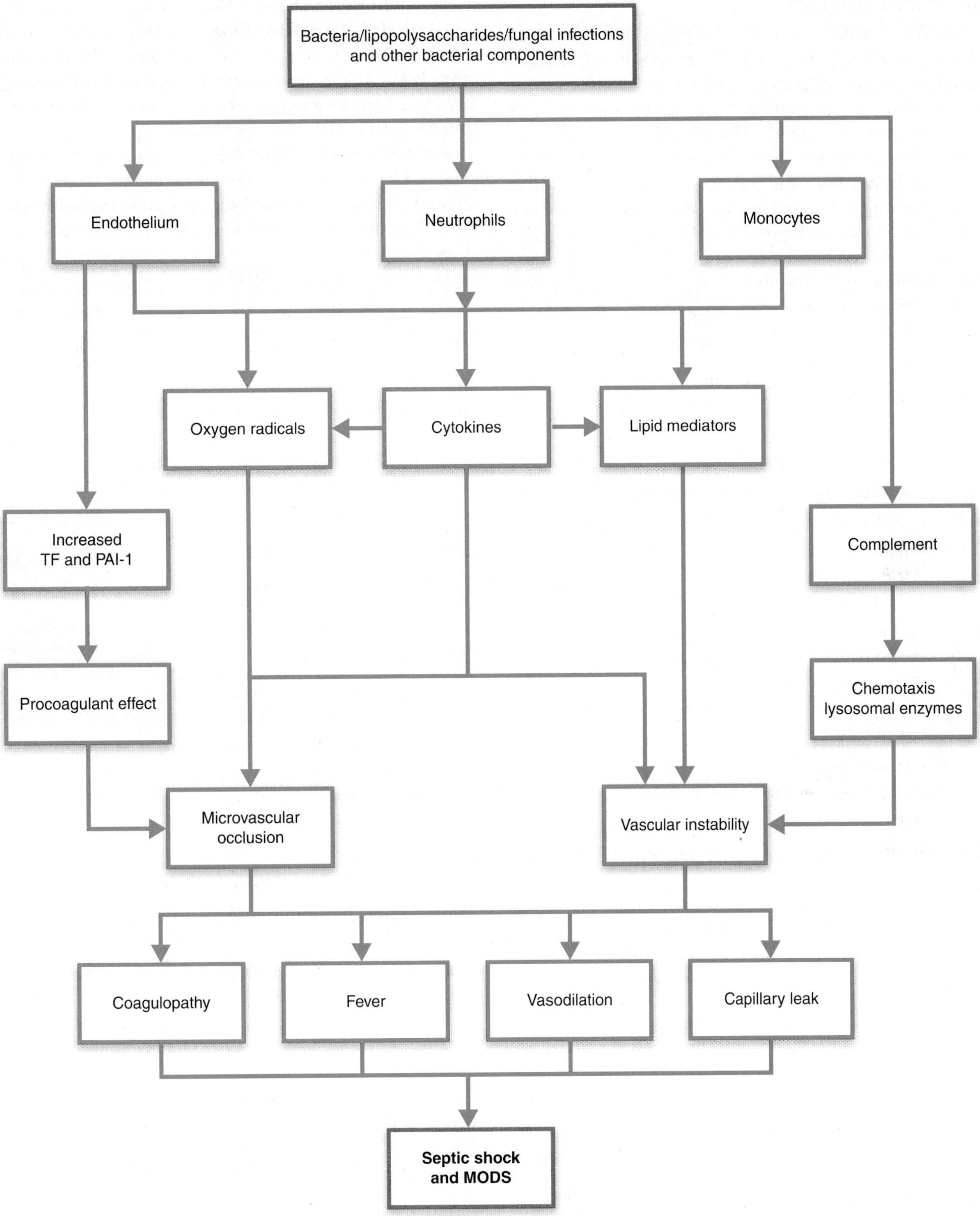

Bacteria/lipopolysaccharides/fungal infections and other bacterial components

Endothelium

Neutrophils

Monocytes

Oxygen radicals

Cytokines

Lipid mediators

Increased TF and PAI-1

Complement

Procoagulant effect

Chemotaxis lysosomal enzymes

Microvascular occlusion

Vascular instability

Coagulopathy

Fever

Vasodilation

Capillary leak

Septic shock and MODS

Figure 28.8 ■ The pathogenesis of septic shock. PAI-1 = type 1 plasminogen activator inhibitor.

Jimmy Bley: Application

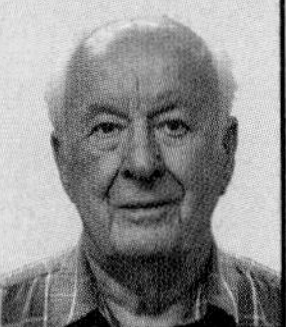

Mr. Bley is diagnosed with pneumonia and acute respiratory failure and is admitted to the ICU, requiring intubation and mechanical ventilation. He suffers from delirium during the acute illness.

Mr. Bley is found to have developed sepsis, and his blood pressure has dropped significantly. He remains on a ventilator, is receiving medications to maintain his blood pressure, and is on multiple antibiotics.

3. What type of shock is Mr. Bley experiencing?
4. What type of medication is used to maintain Mr. Bley's blood pressure?

Clinical Manifestations

A clinical or bedside diagnosis of septic shock utilizes the **qSOFA** (short for "quick SOFA") criteria, which include altered mentation (Glasgow Coma Scale < 10), systolic blood pressure of 100 mmHg or less, and respiratory rate of 22/min or greater, to identify adult patients with suspected infection who are likely to have poor outcomes.[14,20] Developed by Seymour and colleagues,[20] qSOFA is useful in the ICU because it does not require laboratory tests and can be assessed quickly and repeatedly. The task force suggests that qSOFA criteria be used to prompt clinicians to investigate further for organ dysfunction and to begin appropriate therapy with frequent monitoring as needed. The criteria in qSOFA include the following:

- Whether the patient is in the ICU
- Respiratory rate ≥ 22/min
- Altered mentation
- Systolic blood pressure ≤ 100 mmHg.

Linking Pathophysiology to Diagnosis and Treatment

Treatment for patients with septic shock includes the following:

- Perfusion restored with intravenous fluids and sometimes vasopressors
- O_2 support
- Broad-spectrum antibiotics to treat infection
- Infection source control
- Sometimes other supportive measures (e.g., corticosteroids, insulin).

Patients with septic shock should be treated in an ICU. The following should be monitored hourly:

- Central venous pressure, pulmonary capillary wedge pressure, or central venous oxygen saturation
- Pulse oximetry
- Arterial blood gases to assist in maintaining blood gases and pH within reasonable limits
- Blood glucose, lactate, and electrolyte levels
- Renal function as assessed by urine output per hour.

Urine output, a good indicator of renal perfusion, should be measured, usually with an indwelling catheter. The onset of oliguria (e.g., less than about 0.5 mL/kg/h) or anuria or a rising creatinine level may signal impending renal failure.

In neonates, sepsis is due to infection acquired during the neonatal period. Healthcare-associated infections in pediatric patients in the ICU include primarily bloodstream infections and pneumonia. Neonatal sepsis occurs in approximately 2 per 1000 live births.[21] The highest rates occur in the following circumstances:

- Maternal fever greater than 38°C
- Low-birth-weight infants
- Infants with depressed function at birth as manifested by a low Apgar score
- Infants with maternal perinatal risk factors (e.g., low socioeconomic status, poor maternal nutrition, poor prenatal care, premature rupture of membranes).

Neonatal sepsis can be early onset (within 3 days of birth) or late onset (after 3 days). Early-onset sepsis usually results from organisms acquired intrapartum, and symptoms appear within 6 hours of birth. Late-onset sepsis is usually acquired from the environment and is more likely in preterm infants, particularly those with prolonged hospitalization, use of intravenous catheters, or both. Such infections can be reduced by proper hand hygiene by healthcare professionals and aseptic or sterile techniques during procedures such as catheter insertion and changing of ventilator tubings.[21] ■

Incidence of severe sepsis in older adults in the United States is 26.2 cases per 1000, compared to 3 cases per 1000 in the younger population, according to the study by Angus and van der Poll.[16] Predisposing factors in older adults include comorbidities and frequent and prolonged hospitalizations resulting from decreased immunity. Aging is an independent factor that increases the risk of death in patients with sepsis, increasing morbidity and mortality in older patients and associated with rapid progression of sepsis to severe sepsis and septic shock.[4] ■

Jimmy Bley: Outcome

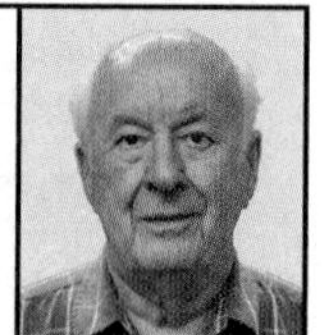

Mr. Bley responds to the antibiotic therapy and is discharged. During hospitalization, a degree of myocardial damage was found that resulted from the sepsis. The myocardial damage in conjunction with his existing emphysema necessitates close monitoring of Mr. Bley's cardiovascular and respiratory function over the next several months. He is placed on continuous cardiac monitoring on initial discharge.

5. What damage occurred as a result of the sepsis Mr. Bley experienced?
6. What two systems need to be monitored closely after Mr. Bley is discharged?

Neurogenic Shock

Etiology and Pathogenesis

Neurogenic shock is caused by blockage of the sympathetic nervous system outflow to the intrathoracic sympathetic chain. It can be caused by any factor/condition that increases parasympathetic stimulation (**Figure 28.9** ■). Neurogenic shock tends to occur more commonly in spinal cord injuries above T6, secondary to the disruption of the sympathetic outflow from T1–L2 and to unopposed vagal (parasympathetic) tone. The higher the spinal cord injury, the more severe is the neurogenic shock and the more extensive is neurologic peripheral manifestation. This kind of shock is characterized by a decrease in vascular resistance (arterial and venous) and loss of vascular capacitance with associated vascular dilation and bradycardia in the absence of hypovolemia.[22] In contrast, hypovolemic shock tends to be accompanied by tachycardia.

Other causes of neurogenic shock are brain injury, barbiturate overdose, hypoglycemia, medications, severe pain, spinal anesthesia, and vasomotor center depression. Decreased glucose and oxygen to the medulla can result in neurogenic shock. Enterovirus 71 (EV71) is implicated in a widespread outbreak of hand-foot-and-mouth disease, and

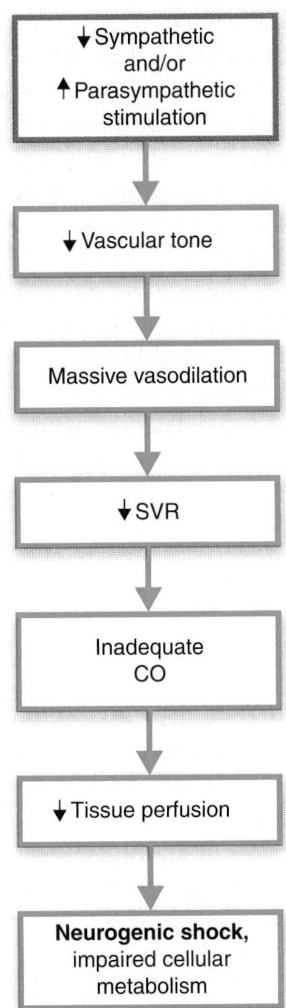

Figure 28.9 The pathogenesis of neurogenic shock. CO = cardiac output, SVR = systemic vascular resistance.

neurogenic shock with pulmonary edema is a fatal complication of EV71 infection.[23] Other types of shock would have hypotension with tachycardia, particularly at the earlier stage. Neurogenic shock needs to be differentiated from spinal shock and hypovolemic shock. Spinal shock is response of the spinal cord to a spinal cord injury. It involves temporary loss of reflex function below the level of injury and resolves gradually over 4 to weeks. Hypovolemic shock tends to be associated with tachycardia.

Clinical Manifestations

Neurogenic shock is manifested by the triad of systolic hypotension, bradycardia, and hypothermia. The blockage of sympathetic outflow results in bradycardia and vascular dilation. Blood pools in the peripheral vessels, causing a decrease in venous return and cardiac output. Both of these contribute to hypoperfusion of organs. Flaccid paralysis below the level of injury, poikilothermia, and priapism are other clinical manifestations that result from the neurologic disruption.

Linking Pathophysiology to Diagnosis and Treatment

Neurogenic shock is treated, like most shocks, with careful fluid replenishment and vasopressors to stabilize blood pressure. In addition, care is taken to avoid any further spinal or brain injury that might cause permanent damage; this is done by stabilizing the spine and neck. Airway patency is established, and oxygen therapy is started. Corticosteroids are given to decrease spinal cord edema, and atropine is given to increase the heart rate. Neurologic assessment is done regularly to monitor for any changes. The signs and symptoms of neurologic shock improve or diminish as the spinal cord swelling decreases.

Check Your Progress: Section 28.5

1. What type of shock is defined as life-threatening organ dysfunction caused by a dysregulated host response to infection?
2. What type of shock occurs when the antibody IgE produced by plasma cells binds to membrane receptors on the mast cells and basophils?
3. How is neurogenic shock treated?

28.6 Obstructive Shock

Obstructive shock is a life-threatening condition caused by an obstruction of blood flow to the body's organs. Obstructive shock shares a number of features with cardiogenic shock, and the end point is a collapse of circulatory function, as in cardiogenic shock.

Etiology and Pathogenesis

Obstructive shock is diagnosed when acute circulatory failure occurs as a result of obstruction of blood supply to central vessels of systems or pulmonary circulation, causing the clinical symptoms of shock. Obstructive shock is rare, accounting for 2% of ICU cases involving shock.[6] It is accompanied by disturbances of consciousness, centralization, oliguria, hypotension, and tachycardia. Among the causes of obstructive shock is a pulmonary embolism that results in right ventricular failure. Nonpulmonary causes include cardiac tamponade and tension pneumothorax, which results in impaired diastolic filling and decreases cardiac output.

Clinical Manifestations

The clinical symptoms of obstructive shock include disturbances of consciousness, oliguria, hypotension, and tachycardia. Obstructive shock manifests clinically with decreased cardiac function and circulatory failure.

Linking Pathophysiology to Diagnosis and Treatment

Treatment of obstructive shock must be well aimed to address the cause as quickly as possible because of the high potential for fatality. The treatment for obstructive shock following pneumothorax includes decreasing chest tension or pressure on the heart by needle thoracotomy and pericardiocentesis for pericardial effusion or cardiac tamponade. For obstructive shock due to pulmonary emboli, surgical removal of the block or the use of a thrombolytic agent is recommended.

Check Your Progress: Section 28.6

1. What are two causes of nonpulmonary obstructive shock?.
2. The clinical signs of obstructive shock include hypotension, tachycardia, disturbance of consciousness, and what else?
3. Obstructive shock and what other form of shock end in a collapse of circulatory function?

28.7 Multiple Organ Dysfunction Syndrome

Multiple organ dysfunction syndrome (MODS) is characterized by progressive organ dysfunction of two or more organ systems in a patient who is critically ill. Homeostasis in such a patient cannot be maintained without intervention.

Etiology and Pathogenesis

Common risk factors for MODS include infection, inflammation, acute lung injury, burn, multiple trauma, ischemia, intoxication (drug reactions), and iatrogenic factors (e.g., blood transfusion). In MODS, the vascular derangement from hypoperfusion, hypermetabolic state in the presence of hypoxia, hyperinflammation, hypercoagulation, hyperlactemia, acidosis, and dysregulated immune response all combine to cause tissue injury and multiple organ failure. MODS is most commonly caused by septic shock due to failure of homeostasis or dysregulation of organ function. Severity of organ dysfunction has been assessed with various scoring systems that quantify abnormalities according to clinical findings, laboratory data, or therapeutic interventions. The predominant score in current use is the SOFA, which was outlined in Table 28.2. A higher SOFA score is associated with an increased probability of mortality. The score grades abnormality by organ system and is used as guide for clinical interventions. However, laboratory variables—namely, PaO_2, platelet count, creatinine level, and bilirubin level—are needed for full computation. Other organ failure scoring systems exist, but none is used commonly. The patient outcome for MODS depends on the severity of the underlying organ dysfunction as it relates to the number of failing organs and/or the organ dysfunction score of the specific organ or organs. Risk factors for MODs include infection, inflammation, injury, ischemia, immune reactions, iatrogenic factors, intoxication, and idiopathic factors.[24]

Clinical Manifestations

MODS can have variable clinical manifestations, as the primary characteristic is failure of organ function across two or more systems. Six primary systems are considered emblematic of MODS: respiratory, renal, hepatic, cardiovascular, gastrointestinal, and neurologic. Assessment can then focus on evaluating the function of these systems on the basis of laboratory data or symptomatology. Renal and hepatic function are generally evaluated by using serum creatinine or bilirubin levels. Hematologic manifestations are mostly commonly related to thrombocytopenia. Cardiovascular function will generally manifest through changes in blood pressure and the heart. Changes in responsiveness or level of consciousness reflect the neurologic issues found in those with MODS. In general, assessment will focus on Glasgow Coma scale scores. Gastrointestinal manifestations are often associated more with issues with organs located in the abdominal cavity. Tenderness on palpation accompanied by palpable masses can indicate an enlarged organ demonstrating pathologic changes.

Linking Pathophysiology to Diagnosis and Treatment

Progression in MODS is prevented by optimizing hemodynamic, metabolic, and immunologic function and minimizing iatrogenic injury. Hemodynamic support includes fluid resuscitation using volume expanders (e.g., blood, normal saline, lactated Ringer solution), inotropic agents (dopamine, epinephrine), vasoactive agents, and mechanical ventilation. Metabolic support is highly important for critically ill patients, and protein-rich nutrition has been shown to support the hypermetabolic needs of such patients, resulting in a better outcome.[25] To address immunologic support, treatment must address infection with targeted antibiotics.

Check Your Progress: Section 28.7

1. How many organ systems need to be involved for a diagnosis of MODS?
2. Changes in responsiveness or level of consciousness are reflective of what kind of issue found in patients with MODS.
3. Common risk factors for MODS include infection, inflammation, burn, multiple trauma, ischemia, intoxication (drug reactions), and iatrogenic factors (e.g., blood transfusion), and what else?

CHAPTER SUMMARY

28.1 Chapter Overview and Case Studies

Describe the prevalence of shock, its multisystem effects on the body, and concepts related to shock.

- Circulatory shock occurs in about 10% of patients admitted to the ICU.
- The overall impact of shock is seen in decreased cardiac output and organ hypoperfusion.
- Certain forms of shock such as distributive can result in significant vasodilation leading to a reduction in circulatory blood volume resulting in hypotension.
- Hypotension is a significant manifestation regardless of the form of shock.
- As a result of decreased circulatory volume, compensatory responses elicit an increase in respiratory rate as an attempt to enhance tissue oxygenation.

28.2 Pathophysiology of Shock

Outline the pathophysiology, categories, and stages of shock.

- The pathophysiology of shock involves circulatory collapse, vasodilation, and decrease in cardiac output, leading to poor organ perfusion.
- The categories of shock are cardiogenic shock, hypovolemic shock, distributive shock, and obstructive shock.
- The causes of shock are different from one type to another and could result from cardiac failure; inadequate ECF volume from hemorrhage or severe dehydration; extensive vasodilation presenting as relative inadequate ECF volume due to anaphylaxis or sepsis; and obstruction of blood flow due to thrombosis.
- There are three stages of shock. Stage I is reversible or compensatory shock, stage II is progressive or intermediate shock, and stage III is irreversible shock.

28.3 Hypovolemic Shock

Differentiate the causes, classification, underlying pathogenesis, and clinical manifestations of hypovolemic shock and approaches to diagnosis and treatment of this condition across the lifespan.

- Hypovolemic shock results from significant loss of blood and/or ECF fluid.
- Risk factors for hypovolemic shock include trauma or accidents, ruptured ectopic pregnancy, excessive or protracted vomiting and diarrhea, severe burns, excessive sweating, and inadequate fluid intake.
- Clinical signs of hypovolemic shock include hypotension, cool and clammy skin, oliguria, hyperlactatemia, and changes in mental status.
- Treatment for hypovolemic shock includes fluid resuscitation to restore filling pressure and packed red blood cells in cases of hemorrhagic shock.

28.4 Cardiogenic Shock

Differentiate the causes, classification, underlying pathogenesis, and clinical manifestations of cardiogenic shock and approaches to diagnosis and treatment of this condition across the lifespan.

- Cardiogenic shock results from decreased cardiac output that cannot meet tissue metabolic needs. Causes include myocardial infarction, heart failure, cardiac tamponade, restrictive cardiomyopathy, and constrictive pericarditis.
- Myocardial infarction causes a decrease in coronary perfusion pressure and hypoxia, leading to a decrease in myocardial contractility and stroke volume.
- An increase in left ventricular pressure causes an increase in pulmonary pressure and pulmonary edema.
- Treatment for cardiogenic shock includes inotropic agents such as dopamine to increase cardiac contractility, vasodilators to reduce left ventricular workload, diuretics to reduce preload, and thrombolytic therapy to improve coronary artery blood flow.

28.5 Distributive Shock

Differentiate the causes, classification, underlying pathogenesis, and clinical manifestations of distributive shock and approaches to diagnosis and treatment of these conditions across the lifespan.

- Distributive shock results in impaired distribution of blood flow due to extensive vasodilation and loss of vascular tone.
- Septic shock, anaphylactic shock, and neurogenic shock are the different types of distributive shock. Septic shock is the most common type.
- Treatment of distributive shock is directed at eliminating the infection and restoring and maintaining blood pressure.

28.6 Obstructive Shock

Differentiate the causes, classification, underlying pathogenesis, and clinical manifestations of obstructive shock and approaches to diagnosis and treatment of this condition across the lifespan.

- Obstructive shock occurs as a result of obstruction of major blood vessels or obstruction of the cardiac pumping action. Cardiac tamponade and pulmonary embolism can result in obstructive shock.
- Clinical manifestations of obstructive shock include disturbances of consciousness, oliguria, hypotension, and tachycardia.

28.7 Multiple Organ Dysfunction Syndrome

Differentiate the causes, classification, underlying pathogenesis, and clinical manifestations of multiple organ dysfunction syndrome and approaches to diagnosis and treatment of this condition across the lifespan.

- Multiple organ dysfunction syndrome (MODS) is a process that can be caused by circulatory shock but is most commonly caused by septic shock due to failure of homeostasis or dysregulation of organ function.
- In MODS, the vascular derangement from hypoperfusion, a hypermetabolic state in the presence of hypoxia, hyperinflammation, hypercoagulation, hyperlactemia, acidosis, and a dysregulated immune response all combine to cause tissue injury and multiple organ failure.
- The predominant score in current use for clinical assessment of MODS is the Sequential Organ Failure Assessment (SOFA). This tool scores or grades organ abnormalities in respiratory, hematologic, liver, cardiovascular, renal, and nervous systems. A higher score indicates an increasing probability of mortality.

REVIEW QUESTIONS

1. Which stage of shock is considered progressive or intermediate?
   a. Stage I
   b. Stage II
   c. Stage III
   d. Stage IV
2. Multiple organ dysfunction syndrome is most commonly caused by what type of shock?
   a. Anaphylactic
   b. Cardiogenic
   c. Septic
   d. Distributive
3. Cardiac tamponade and pulmonary embolism can result in what type of shock?
   a. Obstructive
   b. Cardiogenic
   c. Hemorrhagic
   d. Hypovolemic
4. What is the most common type of distributive shock?
   a. Septic
   b. Cardiogenic
   c. Obstructive
   d. Distributive
5. In what kind of shock does the treatment include fluid resuscitation to restore filling pressure?
   a. Hemorrhagic
   b. Cardiogenic
   c. Anaphylactic
   d. Hypovolemic
6. What type of shock is manifested by the triad of systolic hypotension, bradycardia, and hypothermia?
   a. Distributive
   b. Neurogenic
   c. Septic
   d. Anaphylactic
7. What drug is vital to the management and treatment of anaphylactic shock and should be given immediately?
   a. Epinephrine
   b. Norepinephrine
   c. Antidepressants
   d. Inotropic agents
8. Blood pressure equals systemic vascular resistance times what?
   a. Mean arterial pressure
   b. Respiratory rate
   c. Cardiac output
   d. Vascular resistance

ANSWERS

Answers to Review Questions can be found in Appendix A. Answers to Case Study and Check Your Progress questions are available on the faculty resources site. Please consult with your instructor.

RECOMMENDED WEBSITES

American College of Chest Physicians
http://www.chestnet.org

American College of Emergency Physicians
http://www.acep.org

American Heart Association
http://www.heart.org

Society of Critical Care Medicine
http://www.sccm.org

REFERENCES

1. Shankar-Hari, M., Philips, G. S., Levy, M. L., et al., for the Sepsis Definitions Taskforce. (2016). Developing a new definition and assessing new clinical criteria for septic shock for the Third International Consensus Definitions for Sepsis and Septic Shock (Sepsis 3). *JAMA, 315*(8), 775–787.
2. Vincent, J.-L., & De Backer, D. (2013). Circulatory shock. *New England Journal of Medicine, 369*, 1726–1734. doi:10.1056/NEJMra1208943
3. Biston, P., Aldecoa, C., Devriendt, J., Madl, C., Chochrad, D., Vincent, J. L., & De Backer, D. (2014). Outcome of elderly patients with circulatory failure. *Intensive Care Medicine, 40*(1), 50–46. Available at https://www.ncbi.nlm.nih.gov/pubmed/24132383
4. Asada, T., & Doi, K. (2016). Hypothesis concerning the pathogenesis of multiple organ dysfunction syndrome. *Critical Care Medicine, 44*(5), 314.
5. Ashruf, J. F., Bruining, H. A., & Ince, C. (2013). New insights into the pathophysiology of cardiogenic shock: The role of the microcirculation. *Current Opinion in Critical Care, 19*(5), 381–386.

6. Pich, H., & Heller, A. R. (2015). Obstructive shock. *Anaesthetist, 64*(5), 405–419.
7. Pacagnella, R. C., Souza, J. P., Durocher, J., Perel, P., Blum, J., Winikoff, B., & Gülmezoglu, A. M. (2013). A systematic review of the relationship between blood loss and clinical signs. *PLoS ONE, 8*(3), e57594. doi:10.1371/journal.pone.0057594
8. American College of Surgeons. (2017). *Advanced trauma life support* (10th ed.). Chicago: American College of Surgeons.
9. Gutierrez, G., Reines, H. D., & Wulf-Gutierrez, M. E. (2004). Clinical review: Hemorrhagic shock. *Critical Care, 8*(5), 373–381.
10. Knotzer, H., & Pajk, W. (2014). The right target at the right time: The microcirculation in circulatory shock. *Critical Care Medicine, 42*(2), 482–483.
11. Amsterdam, E. A., Wenger, N. K., Brindis, R. G., et al. (2014). 2014 AHA/ACC guidelines for the management of patients with non–ST-elevation acute coronary syndromes. *Journal of the American College of Cardiology, 64*(24), e139–e228. Available at http://content.onlinejacc.org/article.aspx?articleid=1910085
12. Mayr, F. B., Yende, S., & Angus, D. C. (2014). Epidemiology of severe sepsis. *Virulence, 5*(1), 4–11. Available at http://www.ncbi.nlm.nih.gov/pmc/articles/PMC3916382
13. Goldman, R. D. (2013). Acute treatment of anaphylaxis in children. *Canadian Family Physician, 59*(7), 740–74114.
14. Singer, M., Deutschman, C. S., Seymour, C., et al. (2016). The Third International Consensus Definitions for Sepsis and Septic Shock (Sepsis-3). *JAMA, 315*(8), 801–810. Available at http://jama.jamanetwork.com/article.aspx?articleid=2492881
15. Abraham, E. (2016). New definitions for sepsis and septic shock: Continuing evolution but with much still to be done. *JAMA, 315*(8), 757.
16. Angus, D.C., & van der Poll, T. (2013). Severe sepsis and septic shock. *New England Journal of Med*icine, *369*(9), 840–851.
17. King, E. G., Bauzá. G. J., Mella, J. R., & Remick, D. J. (2014). Pathophysiologic mechanisms in septic shock. *Laboratory Investigation, 94*, 4–12; doi:10.1038/labinvest.2013.110
18. Iskander, K. N., Osuchowski, M. F., Stearns-Kurosawa, D. J., et al. (2013). Sepsis: Multiple abnormalities, heterogeneous responses, and evolving understanding. *Physiological Reviews, 93*(3), 1247–1288.
19. Vincent, J.-L., Marshall, J. C., Namendys-Silva, S. A., et al. (2014). ICON Investigators. Assessment of the worldwide burden of critical illness: The Intensive Care Over Nations (ICON) audit. *Lancet Respiratory Medicine, 2*(5), 380–386.
20. Seymour, C. W., Liu, V. X., Iwashyna, T. J., et al. (2016). Assessment of clinical criteria for sepsis: For the Third International Consensus Definitions for Sepsis and Septic Shock (Sepsis-3). *JAMA, 315*(8), 762–774.
21. Anderson-Berry, A. L. (2015). Neonatal sepsis. *Medscape*. Available at http://emedicine.medscape.com/article/978352-overview
22. Summers, R. L., Baker, S. D., Sterling, S. A., Porter, J. M., & Jones, A. E. (2013). Characterization of the spectrum of hemodynamic profiles in trauma patients with acute neurogenic shock. *Journal of Critical Care, 28*(4), 531.e1–531.e5. doi:10.1016/j.jcrc.2013.02.002
23. Wang, S. M., & Liu, C. C. (2014). Update of enterovirus 71 infection: Epidemiology, pathogenesis and vaccine. *Expert Review of Anti-Infective Therapy, 12*(4), 447–456.
24. Al-Khafaji, A. H. (2017). Multiple organ dysfunction syndrome in sepsis. *Medscape*. Available at http://emedicine.medscape.com/article/169640-overview
25. Weijs, P. (2016). Protein delivery in critical illness. *Current Opinions in Critical Care,* 22(4), 279–411.

Unit VIII

Disorders of Mood and Cognition

Chapter 29
Emotional Regulation and Mood

Chapter 30
Neurodevelopment and Neurocognition

Mood and cognition are closely linked and have clear impact on individual functioning. Both depressed mood and cognitive impairment are associated with poor psychosocial functioning, and the presence of an anxiety disorder in adolescents is associated with poor psychosocial outcomes and functioning later in life.[1,2] Aspects of psychosocial functioning include communication, interpreting others' behaviors, choices regarding and control of one's own behaviors, and ability to manage activities of daily living, among others.

Self-care is an aspect of psychosocial functioning that is frequently impacted by changes in mood and cognition. When self-care is impaired related to an increased level of anxiety, a depressive or manic state, or as a result of cognitive or developmental impairment, whether transient or progressive, the burden of care in both inpatient and outpatient settings increases. Patients need greater assistance with hygiene, activities of daily living, and adhering to medications and other treatments.

Individuals with alterations of mood, development, or cognition are at greater risk for comorbid illnesses ranging from substance use to general medical illnesses such as lung or heart disease. For example, patients with depressive and bipolar disorders experience both greater frequency of comorbid illness as well as greater burdens related to illness than do their mentally healthy peers. Although this may, to some extent, be related to the interference in functioning brought on by the nature of their mental illness, recent research indicates that these individuals may experience greater underlying pathologies than individuals who are in good mental health.[3]

Similarly, individuals with neurocognitive disorders often experience psychiatric symptoms. For example, patients with Parkinson disease often manifest symptoms such as depression and apathy. Studies suggest there may be some overlap of symptoms, and it can be difficult to distinguish the underlying causality of psychiatric manifestations in patients with Parkinson disease and other progressive neurocognitive disorders.[4]

While there are many implications for the nursing care of individuals with disorders of emotional regulation, cognition, and development, care priorities will need to include:

- Careful physical and mental assessments. Establish a baseline at the first healthcare interaction and monitor for changes from baseline at following interactions. This includes assessing for pain and finding ways to accurately assess pain in individuals with communication impairments.
- Medication reconciliation at each healthcare interaction. For example, a primary care provider may not understand the implications of prescribing certain medications, such as corticosteroids and opiates, to patients with bipolar disorder. Similarly, older adults with neurocognitive disorders may experience paradoxical effects of some psychotropic medications, including medications to assist with sleep.
- Assessment of supports and resources at each healthcare interaction. Particularly as adolescents with mental illness or developmental delays approach age 18 and begin to "age out" of public support programs, nurses will need to assess how to help these patients meet their ongoing needs after high school.
- Tailoring patient education according to anxiety level and/or degree of cognitive or developmental impairment.

References

1. Rock, P. L., Roiser, J. P., Riedel, W. J., & Blackwell, A. D. (2015). Cognitive impairment in depression: a systematic review and meta-analysis. *Psychological Medicine, 44*(10), 2029–2040.
2. Essau, C. A., Lewinsohn, P. M., Olaya, B., & Seeley, J. R. (2014). Anxiety disorders in adolescents and psychosocial outcomes and age 30. *Journal of Affective Disorders, 163,* 125–132.
3. Forty, L., Ulanova, A., Jones, L., Jones, I., Gordon-Smith, K., Fraser, C., . . . Craddock, N. (2014). Comorbid medical illness in bipolar disorder. *British Journal of Psychiatry, 205*(6), 465–472.
4. Aarsland, D., Taylor, J. P. & Weintraub, M. D. (2014). Psychiatric issues in cognitive impairment. *Movement Disorders, 29*(5) 651–662.

Psychosis
- Delusions
- Hallucinations
- Altered thought processes
- Loss of executive function
- Flat affect
- Memory, attention deficits

Dementia
- Slow onset, progressive course
- Loss of memory, abstract thinking
- Depression, apathy
- Increasing need for assistance with ADLs
- Loss of motor function (early in Parkinson disease; late in Alzheimer disease)

Depression
- Sadness, crying
- Emptiness, despondency
- ↓ Energy
- Pain
- Apathy
- Psychomotor agitation or retardation
- Sleep disturbance
- Suicidality

Delirium
- Sudden, acute onset
- Acute confusion
- Loss of consciousness
- Delusions, hallucinations
- Relieved by treating underlying illness

Anxiety
- Worry
- Irritability
- Difficulty concentrating
- Chest pain
- Diaphoresis
- Dyspnea
- ↑ Pulse, blood pressure

Neurodevelopmental Impairments
- Inattentive or restrictive behaviors
- Poor impulse control
- Communication deficits
- Social functioning impairments
- Sensory impairments

Mania
- Hyperactivity, hypersexuality
- Euphoria
- Sleep, appetite disturbances
- Paranoia
- Psychosis
- Lack of insight

Disorders of Neurodevelopment and Neurocognition
- Schizophrenia
- Neurocognitive disorders
  - Dementia
  - Delirium
- Neurodevelopmental disorders
  - Attention-deficit/hyperactivity disorder (ADHD)
  - Autism spectrum disorder (ASD)
  - Fetal alcohol syndrome (FAS)

Disorders of Emotional Regulation and Mood
- Anxiety
- Major depressive disorder
- Persistent depressive disorder
- Peripartum depression
- Bipolar I disorder
- Bipolar II disorder
- Clyclothymia

Chapter 29

Emotional Regulation and Mood

Matthew Sorenson and Kathy Lauer

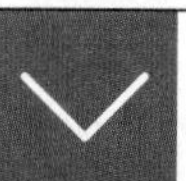

Chapter Outline and Learning Outcomes

29.1 Chapter Overview and Case Studies

Define emotional regulation, and discuss concepts related to anxiety and depression.

29.2 Anxiety

Describe the etiology, pathogenesis, and clinical manifestations of anxiety and approaches to diagnosis and treatment of the condition across the lifespan.

29.3 Depression

Describe the etiology, pathogenesis, and clinical manifestations of depression and approaches to diagnosis and treatment of the condition across the lifespan.

29.4 Bipolar Disorders

Describe the etiology, pathogenesis, and clinical manifestations of bipolar disorders and approaches to diagnosis and treatment of these conditions across the lifespan.

KEY TERMS

Anxiety, 704
Bipolar disorders, 722
Bipolar I disorder, 722
Bipolar II disorder, 722
Cognitive-behavioral therapy (CBT), 712
Conditioned response, 708
Conditioned stimulus, 707
Consolidation, 706
Cyclothymic disorder, 723
Depression, 713
Dopamine (DA), 714
Dysthymia, 713
Extinction, 709
Fear-centered anxiety disorder, 705
Gamma-aminobutyric acid (GABA), 709
Generalized anxiety disorder (GAD), 704
Hypomania, 722
Major depressive disorder (MDD), 713
Major depressive episode, 720
Mania, 722
Norepinephrine (NE), 714
Panic disorder, 705
Persistent depressive disorder, 713
Premenstrual dysphoric disorder, 713
Rapid cycling, 722
Reconsolidation, 706
Selective serotonin reuptake inhibitor (SSRI), 706
Serotonin (5-HT), 714
Social anxiety disorder (SAD), 704
Worry-centered anxiety disorders, 705

ABBREVIATIONS

5-HT—5-hydroxytryptamine (serotonin)
ACC—anterior cingulate cortex
ACTH—adrenocorticotropin hormone
BDNF—brain-derived neurotrophic factor
BZDs—benzodiazepines
CBT—cognitive-behavioral therapy
COMT—catechol-O-methyltransferase
CRF—corticotropin-releasing factor
CRH—corticotropin-releasing hormone
DA—dopamine
GABA—gamma-aminobutyric acid

Abbreviations are continued on the next page.

GAD—generalized anxiety disorder
HPA axis—hypothalamic-pituitary-adrenal axis
LCSPT—limbic-cortical-striatal-pallidal-thalamic
MAO—monoamine oxidase
MDD—major depressive disorder
NE—norepinephrine
NMDA—N-methyl-D-aspartic acid
SAD—social anxiety disorder
SNRI—selective norepinephrine reuptake inhibitor
SSRI—selective serotonin reuptake inhibitor

29.1 Chapter Overview and Case Studies

Emotional regulation is the ability to manage emotional responses to environmental stimuli that are perceived as aversive or negative. When these responses disrupt daily functioning, the individual could experience anxiety or a mood disorder. The most common mood disorders are centered on states of depression.

Depression is a pervasive mental illness that touches all parts of society, regardless of age, race, gender, or socioeconomic status. It is a debilitating condition that creates a serious negative impact on functioning and interpersonal relationships. In most cases, depression is treated successfully with pharmacologic and nonpharmacologic therapies. However, if an individual can see no other resolution but suicide, depression can be a fatal illness.[1]

Anxiety is an emotion that helps individuals adapt to a perceived challenge or threat. Unfortunately, anxiety can also create sustained apprehension such that the individual develops avoidance patterns as a means of coping with distress. For instance, before a test, students are likely to experience mild anxiety due to performance expectations or fear of the unknown. This anxiety generally passes when the test is completed. However, some individuals experience an incapacitating sense of dread without any apparent stimulus. They may then cope by avoiding any situation that might generate such feelings. This avoidance can severely limit their social interaction, social relationships, and, in some instances, opportunities for growth. At this point, these individuals may develop feelings of anxiety in social situations or feelings of panic.[1]

The bipolar disorders are a group of mood disorders characterized by manic, hypomanic, and depressive episodes. These episodes represent periods of fluctuation between two poles: depression and mania. The pathophysiology of depression is best understood in terms of the action of specific neurotransmitters and intracellular mechanisms that alter gene expression, as well as how these mechanisms compromise neuronal growth.[2] An important component of the pathophysiology of depression is the body's stress response system. It is both affected by depression and, when in a hypersensitive state, thought to play a pivotal role in exacerbating many symptoms of depression.[3] Finally, the pathophysiology of depression is associated with the manner in which neurons generate and transmit impulses. Variance in the rate of neuronal discharge can be tied to the primary symptoms of depression and treatment response.

Certain brain mechanisms are also major players in the development of anxiety, primarily in the parts of the brain associated with threat and fear. Perceiving a stimulus as a threat activates sympathetic responses, and the classification of anxiety is primarily based on signs and symptoms that reflect sympathetic nervous system activation. Neurotransmitters associated with autonomic responses such as norepinephrine (NE), dopamine (DA), and serotonin are tied into the pathogenesis of anxiety disorders with the regulation of gamma-aminobutyric acid (GABA) playing a role in the treatment process.

Concepts Related to Emotional Regulation

Emotional regulation integrates several bodily systems in determining emotional responses to environmental stimuli. The neurotransmitters associated with anxiety and depressive states are also tied into immunologic responses and inflammation. Immunologic disruptions or genetic dysregulation could then predispose an individual to the development of depression or anxiety. In turn, emotional states influence immunologic responses, placing the individual at the risk for disease.

Concepts related to emotional regulation are found in **Figure 29.1** ■. The individual is presented with stimuli or events through interaction with the surrounding environment. If a response engenders a state of stress, the person then needs to cope with emerging stress. If coping mechanisms fail, the individual is at risk for the development of maladaptive emotional responses such as depression. These emotional states manifest clinically through the expression of bodily symptoms such as tachycardia or changes in sleep pattern.

Case Studies

The following cases are addressed throughout the chapter to assist in application of chapter content to clinical situations that involve individuals with disorders of emotional regulation.

Alice Parry: Introduction

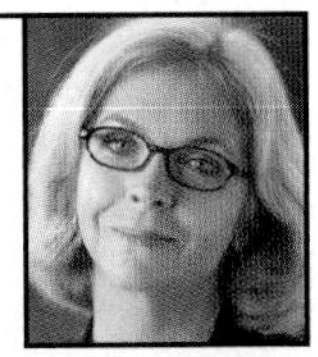

Alice Parry is a woman in her mid-50s who arrives for outpatient treatment at the local community mental health center. She says that approximately 2 years ago, in the summer, she began to have problems sleeping and was increasingly irritable at home and her job. As summer moved into autumn, she found herself feeling sad and no longer enjoying life. Her mood may brighten with highly pleasurable events but quickly returns to sad and depressed. She believes that her peers at work are seeing her as a different person, and, hurt by their response, she has begun to skip days at the office.

Ms. Parry reports that her early 50s were a difficult time. Her two children were away at college, and her husband was laid off

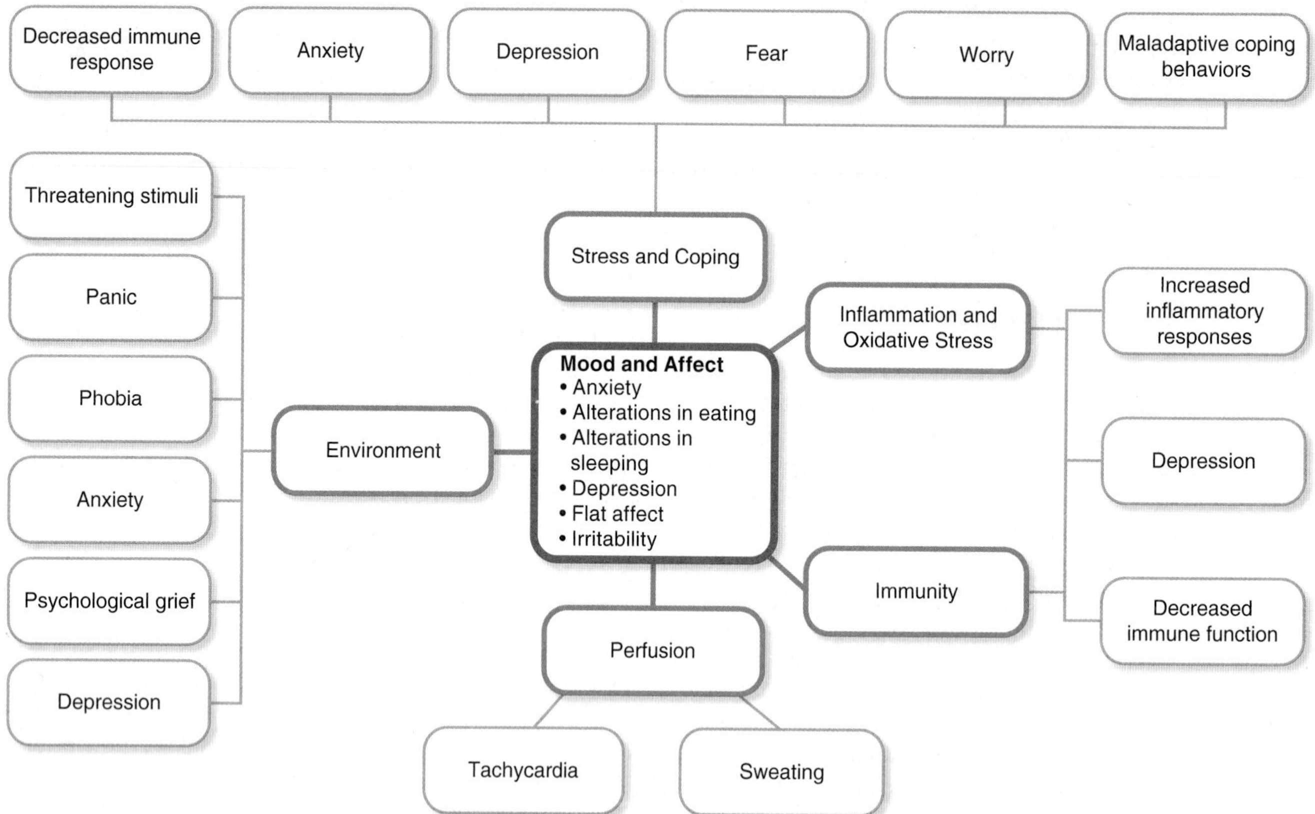

Figure 29.1 ■ Concepts related to emotional regulation.

from work. The financial strain of these two situations created stress in their marriage. She depicts the majority of her life as fortunate and fulfilling but notes that lately she finds herself ruminating more on the recent negative events in her life. She has passing thoughts of suicide but denies any suicide attempts or plan.

1. What has been Ms. Parry's mood over the last couple years?
2. What are the two major events that occurred in Ms. Parry's life recently that affected her mood?

Jasmine Mercado: Introduction

Jasmine Mercado, age 20, is attending a community college. One day when caught in traffic on the way home, she experiences a sudden sense of fear and dread. Her heart begins to beat very strongly, and she experiences shortness of breath. As the event progresses, Ms. Mercado develops a sense that she is going to die. Her mother insists that Ms. Mercado be seen in the emergency department (ED). Once there, she begins to feel a bit more in control. The ED physician informs Ms. Mercado that she has been having symptoms consistent with a panic attack.

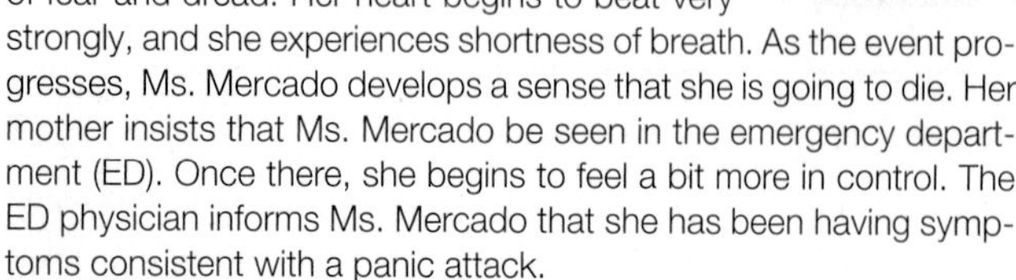

Over the next several days, Ms. Mercado becomes apprehensive if she experiences any trace of the symptoms that signal that a panic attack might be beginning. However, relaxation exercises help her to decrease the initial panic and she believes that she is getting the panic attacks under control.

1. What symptoms did Ms. Mercado experience that led her to be seen in the emergency department?
2. What does Ms. Mercado do to decrease her initial panic with the attacks?

Check Your Progress: Section 29.1

1. What is an emotion that helps individuals adapt to a perceived challenge or threat?
2. What is emotional regulation?
3. What is a debilitating condition that has a serious negative impact on functioning and interpersonal relationships?

29.2 Anxiety

Anxiety is a state of apprehension mixed with fear or worry that occurs in response to a real or perceived threat. This state of apprehension initiates somatic responses including palpitations, sweating, rapid breathing, or nausea. While fear responses can be adaptive, prompting alertness for potential danger, these responses can become associated with stimuli that are generally considered benign. There is then a difference between anxiety or fear in response to a perceived threat and anxiety or fear that becomes a sustained response to a variety of nonthreatening stimuli.[4] There are many types of anxiety disorders, including the following:

- **Generalized anxiety disorder (GAD)** is a state of excessive worrying that interferes with daily function.
- **Social anxiety disorder (SAD)** is a condition characterized by periods of significant fear resulting from a

feeling of being judged that leads to significant impairment of daily functioning.
- **Panic disorder** is a condition characterized by sudden episodes of intense fear that often results in increased sympathetic function.

Excessive anxiety is thought to affect approximately 40 million individuals in the United States each year between the ages of 18 and 54.[5] The prevalence rates and patterns vary among the specific anxiety disorders. For instance, GAD affects approximately 6.8 million adults each year in the United States with an adult lifetime prevalence of 3.6–7.7.[6] SAD is thought to affect 15 million Americans yearly with a lifetime prevalence of 13%; it affects women more than men, and most individuals with SAD seem to experience onset before 18 years of age.[4] Panic disorder affects some 6 million Americans yearly, in twice as many women as men, and has an adult lifetime prevalence rate of 2.0–5.9%.[7]

Ultimately, the expression of anxiety involves a degree of uncertainty and/or fear. One way of thinking about **fear-centered anxiety disorders**, such as panic disorder and social anxiety disorder, is that they may occur following a situation that the mind associates with overwhelming negative consequences. The mediating neural structures that should be able to process a presenting threat are functioning suboptimally. The **worry-centered anxiety disorders**, such as GAD, are also thought to involve functional disruptions in neuronal circuitry. In the case of GAD, this would be increased activity on the part of the cortical-striatal-thalamic pathway. This section focuses on the neural structures that play a role in anxiety, how these neural structures misfire or underperform during anxiety states, and the neurochemicals that are thought to sustain the malfunction. The mechanisms underlying the fear circuitry and the role of stress in priming particular neuronal systems for hyperresponsivity will be highlighted, as this situation can perpetuate anxiety and lead to other mental disorders.

The Etiology and Pathogenesis of Anxiety

The risk for the development of anxiety disorders is associated with genetic, familial, and environmental factors (**Figure 29.2** ■). These factors are sometimes depicted as three sets of vulnerabilities. First, anxiety disorders appear to be familial; this means that these disorders appear with greater frequency in affected families, which implies a genetic component. Research demonstrates that having a first-degree relative with an anxiety disorder increases the risk of developing such a disorder.[8] One of the main avenues of research investigation involves specific genes that are believed to be tied to genetic vulnerability for the development of anxiety. Variations of the 5-hydroxytryptophan (5-HT) transporter gene (*SLC6A4*) seem to be related to hyperreactivity of the amygdala, a part of the brain involved in emotional reactions.

Familial influences operate beyond genetic influences passed on to the child. A parent who is anxious models anxious responses and is more likely to transmit a negative, dangerous, or unrealistic depiction of events. The parent also may reinforce fearful behavior. Genetics may also influence temperament; anxious children are often depicted as having traits such as nervousness or behavioral inhibition. From an early age, anxious children display a fearful tendency, shyness, and an aversion to novelty. Such a temperament is thought to be a predisposition for the avoidance behavior that accompanies several anxiety disorders, particularly social anxiety disorder.[9]

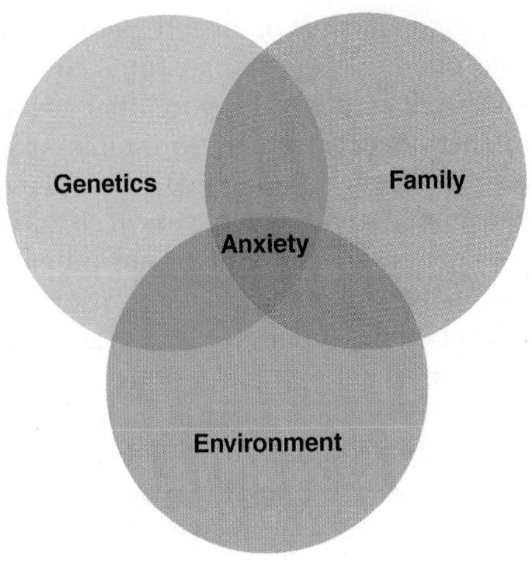

Figure 29.2 ■ Factors contributing to anxiety include genetics, family, and the environment.

Finally, there are environmental risk factors for anxiety disorders, including negative and stressful life events, socioeconomic status, and culture. Negative and stressful life events are seen as risk factors for panic disorder and generalized anxiety disorder.[1] Socioeconomic status may also play a role in the expression of and risk for anxiety disorders. Life conditions such as poverty are seen to contribute to the incidence of anxiety disorders; individuals with low income who are uninsured have a rate of anxiety disorders three times higher than that of the general population. Low occupational prestige and low educational achievement also place individuals at risk for anxiety disorders.[10]

One of the most prevalent comorbidities with anxiety is depression.[1] The reason for the overlap between anxiety disorders and depression is unclear. Theories purporting to explain the relationship include a shared genetic vulnerability, a similar disturbance in neurotransmitter transmission and regulation, and/or anxious hyperarousal leading to depletion of 5-HT (5-hydroxytryptamine, also known as serotonin) and depression.

Anxiety disorders are comorbid with several medical conditions.[1] Important comorbidities include panic disorder with respiratory disease, vestibular dysfunction, thyroid problems, and cardiac disease. GAD is associated with chronic pain, medically unexplained somatic symptoms, and sleep disorders.

CLINICAL POINT: The nurse will encounter individuals with pain or in respiratory distress the etiology of which might not be explained by physical findings. The nurse should consider the possibility of an underlying anxiety disorder and assess for anxiety symptoms. ■

Most etiologic models of anxiety depict genetics and environment operating in complex interactive ways. For example, research evidence supports that approximately one third of the variance found in twin studies of social anxiety disorder is genetically inherited, while the other two thirds results from the environment in which the individual is reared.[11] Genetics also contributes to an individual's temperament, as in the case of social anxiety disorder, in which behavioral inhibition is thought to lead to an increased tendency to develop anxiety.

There is considerable interest in the possibility that a particular genetic vulnerability exists for anxiety disorders. Several lines of research point to a variation of the 5-HT transporter gene (*SLC6A4*) called *5-HTTLPR*. The 5-HT transporter gene has received particular attention, since 5-HT-enhancing drugs, the **selective serotonin reuptake inhibitors (SSRIs)**, are used widely for the treatment of anxiety. Understanding the genetic vulnerability in a key 5-HT transporter may explain the relationship between SSRIs and their mechanism of action in anxiety. Current evidence points toward one variant of *5-HTTLPR*, a short allele, which is associated with a reduction in 5-HT transporter protein and inadequate response to SSRIs.[12] Understanding such genetic vulnerabilities is considered an essential step toward both treatment and prevention of anxiety disorders.

Classic Fear Conditioning and Anxiety

Anxiety can be viewed in terms of fear conditioning. However, in anxiety, the fear response becomes more generalized. With anxiety, an individual's increased awareness and sustained attention to potential threat increases arousal and biases risk assessment. One explanation for how a fear response becomes anxiety is through two processes termed *consolidation* and *reconsolidation*. These processes are based on a preliminary process involving how human beings come to label an event or object as threatening. The process of **consolidation** occurs largely in the amygdala, where memories of fearful stimuli are stored. Through a process in the amygdala involving two calcium receptors, the N-methyl-D-aspartic acid (NMDA) and voltage-gated calcium channels, a single fearful event becomes stored as a long-term memory. This molecular mechanism, called long-term potentiation, is thought to involve protein synthesis and is outlined in **Figure 29.3** ■.

The process by which an older memory is activated and once again consolidated or reinforced is called **reconsolidation.** It is believed that when an internal or external event cues recall of a fear memory, that memory becomes part of a new experience. When this new fear experience is consolidated into long-term memory, it serves to make the fear memory even stronger. In effect, anxious responses beget

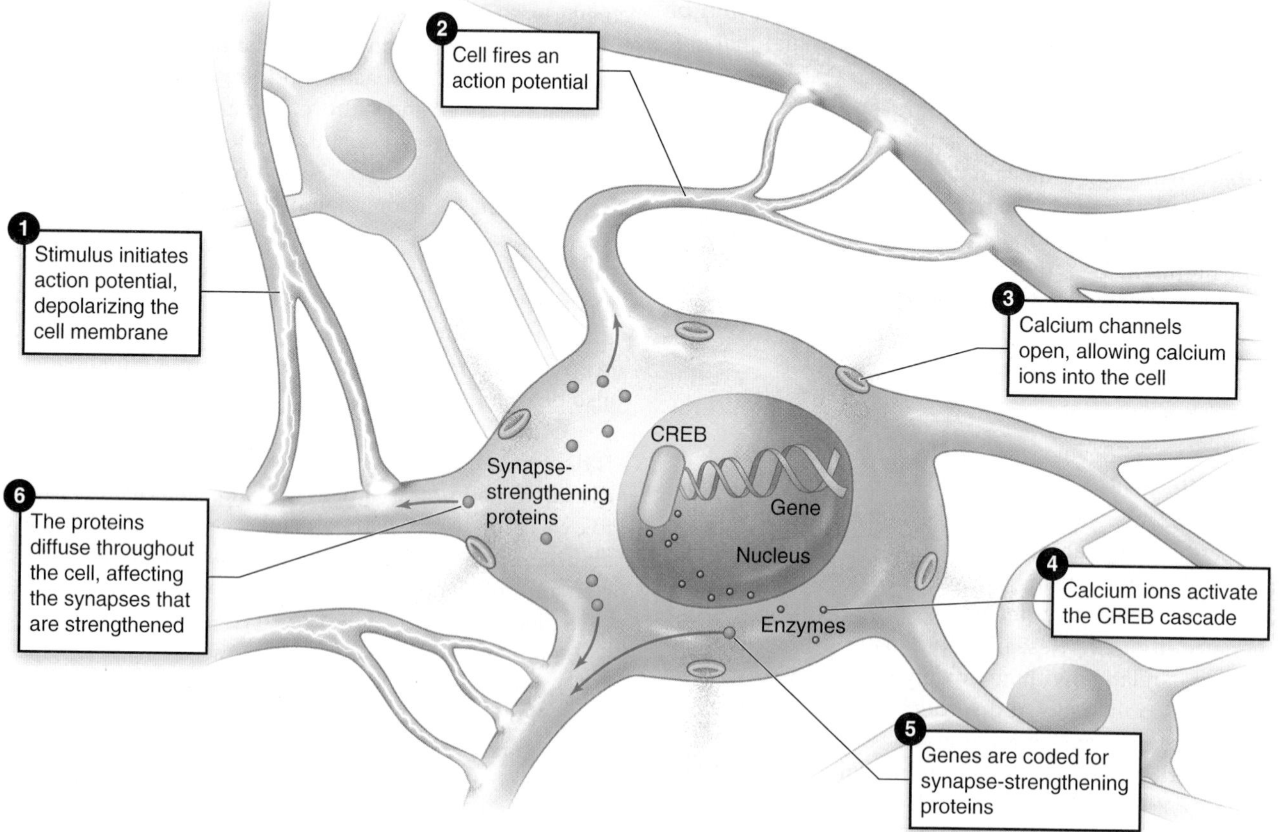

Figure 29.3 ■ The construction of long-term memories. A stimulus initiates an action potential (1 and 2), which opens voltage-sensitive calcium channels and allows calcium ions to accumulate in the cell (3). This increase in intracellular calcium activates the cAMP response element binding factor (CREB) cascade (4), which leads to activation of genes that code for synapse-strengthening proteins (5 and 6).

strong anxiety responses; the neuronal circuits strengthen with each successive firing. Researchers designing new medications to treat anxiety believe that the reconsolidation process may present an opportunity to disrupt the chemicals and receptors involved in the process and thus prevent traumatic and anxiety-producing memories from strengthening.[13]

To further understand anxiety, this section addresses the specific neural structures that are thought to be involved in this type of fear conditioning and consolidation, how humans come to extinguish a fear response, and the type of learning and mechanisms involved when extinction is weak and individuals have difficulty relearning new, less fearful associations. Fear conditioning, consolidation, and extinction pathways are carefully examined to highlight specific neural structures in the pathway and their supposed role in the fear conditioning process.

The Role of Neuroanatomic Pathways in Anxiety

Less is known about the neurocircuitry of anxiety than that of depression. This is in part because the number of neuroimaging studies focused on anxiety is not as extensive as the number of studies focused on mood disorders. Because it is difficult to induce severe anxiety during imaging studies, many of the anxiety studies are conducted in animal laboratories. These studies attempt to isolate the fear circuitry and, where applicable, place the findings in the context of human physiology.

Considering the differing age of onset and gender distributions of the various anxiety disorders, the basic pathways and neuronal structures that are thought to be involved in fear conditioning hold true for many anxiety disorders; however, there are also unique neural circuitries underlying specific disorders. Owing to the volume of studies, more is known about the neurocircuitry of panic disorders and less about disorders such as phobias. However, the basics of fear conditioning provide a good foundation to explain the pathophysiology of anxiety.

The fear conditioning pathway begins with stimuli that trigger apprehensions, either external stimuli that are picked up by sensory organs or internal stimuli that arise from thoughts or bodily sensations. This is called the **conditioned stimulus**. Once this sensory information reaches the filtering thalamus, it travels by two different routes. An incoming stimulus is first read by the thalamus and then sent through two routes in the brain (**Figure 29.4** ■). Along the first route, the stimulus goes directly from the thalamus to the amygdala without stopping along the way for any conscious thought that might attenuate the fear response. If the amygdala labels the stimulus as a possible threat, it sends a message to the hypothalamus, which alerts several areas of the body to get ready for danger.

At the same time, the thalamus sends a nerve impulse down a second route. This nerve impulse terminates in the visual cortex and provides some additional information about the visual stimulus. For instance, the mind asks, "Does this really represent a threat?" The visual cortex then feeds this information into the amygdala and interior parts of the cortex (medial prefrontal cortex and the insula), which in turn influence the strength of the amygdala firing. Thus, there are two pathways through which the brain registers fear. The amygdala is thought to have three important roles in the response to stimuli. First, it confers significance on the stimuli that come from the thalamus or the hypothalamus. Second, it holds "emotional memories." As new stimuli come into the brain, they may be similar to previous stimuli or emotion events the amygdala is storing. Thus, the preliminary threat assessment of a stimulus (e.g., a thought, event, or sensation) occurs in the amygdala. Third, the amygdala has extensive projections to motor areas and areas of the brainstem that control autonomic responses (e.g., heart rate, breathing). Once a stimulus is "read" as potentially dangerous, the amygdala fires off signals to ready the body for fight or flight. Luckily, lest we jump at every stimulus that smacks of potential danger,

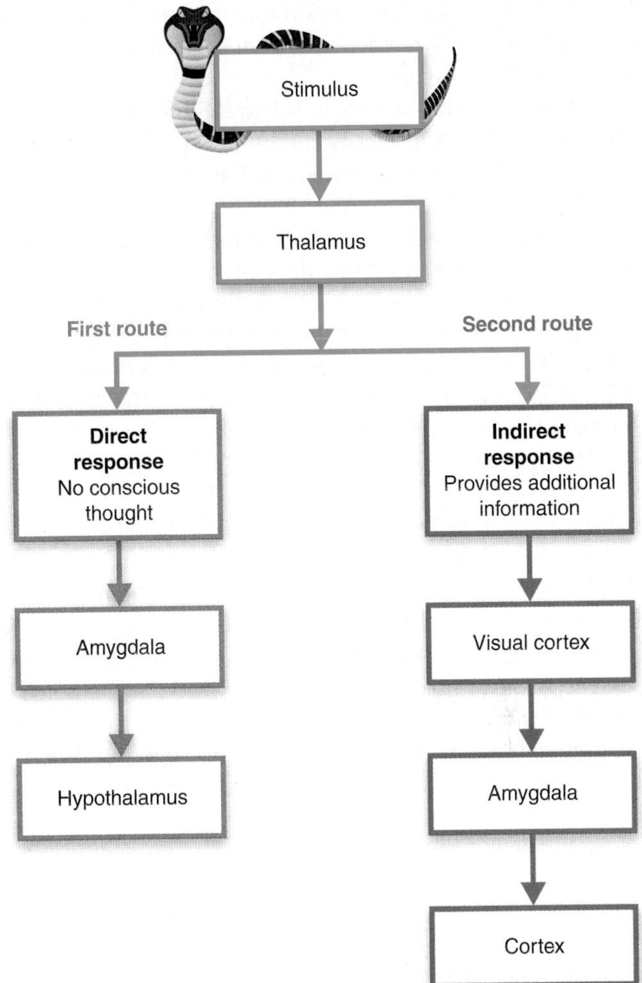

Figure 29.4 ■ A stimulus entering through the eyes travels to the thalamus. From the thalamus, the sensory impulse can be transmitted directly to the amygdala, resulting in a fear response. The sensory impulse may also be transmitted to the amygdala by a somewhat longer and less direct route through the visual cortex. This second pathway provides more information about the stimulus and may attenuate the fear response generated by the amygdala.

the amygdala also receives information about the stimulus from cortical areas that (depending on the information) may attenuate the threat alert.

The amygdala's ability to integrate information from other brain areas is also critical in reducing a fear response once the stimulus dissipates. When the amygdala assesses danger, it quickly retrieves data from other brain areas. One key bit of information is the individual's past associations with the event. For example, suppose a child climbs over a fence into a neighbor's backyard and realizes that there is no exit from the yard except through the neighbor's house. The child then encounters the neighbor's vicious guard dog. If this happens on more than one occasion, the stimulus (an empty yard) becomes associated with the appearance of a dangerous dog—a process called *fear learning*. It may be that years later, when cutting though a yard, the now-grown child experiences a feeling of apprehension; this is called a **conditioned response**. Here, the similarities around the sense of place may create a sense of apprehension and trigger the amygdala to retrieve the previous association.

In clinical disorders such as phobia, there appear to be several pathophysiologic mechanisms at work. In addition to amygdala hyperarousal, there are flaws in the mechanisms that prevent the brain from making quick, intense associations between a stimulus and fear response as well as disturbances in the neuronal circuits that help the brain learn new associations and thus extinguish fears. Everyone develops fears, but as time passes or with new information, these fears diminish or are forgotten. Part of the reason that individuals do not hold onto every childhood fear is that with repeated presentation of a condition stimulus (a deserted yard) and no accompanying unconditioned stimulus (a vicious dog), the amygdala will form new associations about walking through back yards. These new associations will eventually be retrieved when the individual is in a deserted yard, and the individual will not experience apprehension. The original conditioned response has undergone the process of extinction. Note that the first fear association is still lurking somewhere in the amygdala, but new associations that do not connect deserted yards with vicious dogs take prominence.

While it is not exactly clear which parts of the amygdala are involved in extinction, it is believed that the lateral nucleus of the amygdala plays a role, primarily by blocking the synaptic flow through other parts of the amygdala that are generating a fear response. Understanding exactly how fear learning is overridden or partially erased by new associations (extinction) is key to treatments aimed at helping individuals rid themselves of traumatic memories.

When there is damage to the hippocampus, there are deficits in forming memories around the emotional context of a stimulus. This has two important ramifications. First, the individual may have problems processing new situations and making decisions about how to deal with challenges. Second, the volume loss results in less efficient self-limiting mechanisms on the stress response system. We will return to the complex relationship between stress and anxiety later in the chapter during a review of the neurotransmitters and hormones involved in anxiety.

Prefrontal Cortex. The frontal cortex occupies a large portion of the brain and is roughly segmented into several functional areas. The prefrontal cortex is situated right in front of the premotor strip. Several regions of the prefrontal cortex are involved in the fear circuitry. Under normal circumstances, the medial section of the prefrontal cortex registers and assigns meaning to the emotions generated by our body or the amygdala. Another part, the orbital prefrontal cortex, is responsible for weighing action on the basis of potential reward and helps the individual to adjust to changing circumstances. Another section, the anterior cingulate cortex (ACC), is responsible for balancing emotion and thought and controlling attention. It is believed that the ACC also is involved in the ability to focus attention on important events. The ACC is where emotional or fearful stimuli are appraised; thus, it is key to regulating the amygdala's response.

As was discussed above, the prefrontal cortex plays a critical role in fear learning. It receives information from the visual cortex about the presenting threat and this information is relayed to the amygdala. Of particular importance are the orbital region and the ventrolateral area of the cortex, which adjust behavior on the basis of emotional, motivational, or social cues. The medial section also alerts the amygdala once danger has passed or the meaning of a potentially dangerous stimulus has changed. The medial prefrontal cortex is also a player in fear extinction in that signals from this area are capable of disrupting the amygdala's conditioned stimulus–response patterns. A key element of extinction is the ability to adjust response once a threat has changed. Therefore, a poorly integrated or slow-firing medial prefrontal cortex would disrupt this basic extinction mechanism.

Caudate Nucleus. The prefrontal cortex and its component parts seem to play specific roles in anxiety disorders that involve hyperactivity in the cortical-striatal-thalamic tract. The loop begins when the individual has a sense of unease, the caudate nucleus is pushing the individual to do something about the unease, the orbitofrontal cortical interpretation is that something is wrong, and the ACC is stimulated to keep attention on the apprehension. The initiating culprit seems to be the caudate nucleus, which is not working well enough to filter stimuli coming in from the thalamus. Recent research regarding dysfunction in the caudate and putamen (the striatum) may help to explain the underlying pathophysiology of SAD.[14] Striatal dysfunction explains key behaviors common to the experience of SAD. First, it explains the tendency to see the negative wherever it may appear; this is referred to as *negative information-processing bias*. The striatum, specifically the caudate, is the part of the brain that orchestrates action–reward sequencing; it drives behavior based on the recall of past successful outcomes. Research suggests that a poorly functioning caudate would impair this recall, perhaps creating a focus on the negative aspects of social interactions rather than the potential reward.[14] These sensations and cognitions could lead individuals to believe that they are unable to deal with social situations. Isolating neural circuitry has implications for treatment. The overarching hope is that the knowledge of the pathophysiology and neural circuitry will improve treatment methods, both nonpharmacologic and psychopharmacologic.

Neurochemical and Neurotransmitter Components

The overfiring or underfunctioning of any neuronal structure (amygdala, hippocampus, or prefrontal cortex) is prompted by or initiates the flow of particular neurotransmitters. For instance, a sense of apprehension that prompts amygdala firing of a conditioned response will initiate an increase in the flow of norepinephrine (NE). Neurotransmitter systems involved in anxiety disorders include NE, 5-HT, and, to a lesser extent, DA. Anxiety involves threat, which produces stress and therefore alerts the hypothalamic-pituitary-adrenal (HPA) axis, thus recruiting corticotropin-releasing hormone (CRH), adrenocorticotropin hormone (ACTH), and cortisol. (Refer to Figure 11.8 in Chapter 11 for more information on the HPA axis.) Finally, transmissions through key brain structures that result in neuronal excitement and/or inhibition involve the amino acid neurotransmitters gamma-aminobutyric acid and glutamate. The following discussion outlines how each of these substances is thought to be involved in fear learning and extinction and selected anxiety disorders.

GABA-BZD-Receptor System. **Gamma-aminobutyric acid (GABA)** is a primary inhibitory amino acid neurotransmitter that is widely distributed in the central nervous system (CNS). The mind–body response to stress offers a platform for explaining how GABA operates in the CNS. When the mind or body senses threat, the HPA axis is set in motion, secreting hormones to prepare the body for fight or flight. The key hormone is CRH, which initiates a cascade activation of other hormones in the stress system. Lest the system mount too large or too sustained a stress response, GABA steps in, countering the action of CRH, especially in the hypothalamic region.

Under normal circumstances, both GABA and its partner, naturally occurring benzodiazepines (BZDs), are also circulating in the neural system, maintaining mind–body homeostasis. As with the other major neurotransmitters, GABA exerts its effects at the cellular level. GABA has three dedicated receptors. The most important for this discussion is GABA-A, or the GABA-BZD receptor. It is helpful to think of this as a "coupled" receptor that has binding sites for both GABA and BZD compounds. When the receptor is stimulated, it causes an increase of chloride ions, which causes membrane hyperpolarization and neuronal inhibition, making the neuron less excitable. Research suggests that many anxiety disorders may be caused by either GABA deficiencies or problems in this receptor system. These receptor system problems may involve either a deficiency, reduced receptor density, or an insufficient sensitivity to BZD compounds.[15]

As was noted earlier, glutamate, an excitatory amino acid neurotransmitter, is the immediate precursor to GABA. Like GABA, glutamate can be found in almost every area of the brain and thus has a myriad of actions in the CNS. Of particular concern in anxiety disorders is the action of glutamate on the NMDA receptor. Glutamate is an agonist of the NMDA receptor, and along with several secondary messengers, it increases neuronal firing. Glutamate release increases when an individual experiences stress. When glutamate is released at the NMDA receptor site, the ion channel opens, and calcium enters the cell. If too much glutamate is released and too much calcium enters the cell, an excitatory condition is created that is thought to be related to panic disorder.

The action of glutamate at the NMDA receptor is essential to the formation of long-term extinction memories. **Extinction** is the process in which a new association forms between a conditioned stimulus and a conditioned response. The process involves the stimulus being repeatedly presented in the absence of the unconditioned stimulus; this stimulus is thought to originally produce the fear response. The process of extinction learning is key to cognitive treatments for anxiety and can be boosted with drugs that are agonists at NMDA receptors.

Norepinephrine. The molecular composition of these neurotransmitters remains the same in the case of anxiety disorders, with distinct differences in their functional role. When the body enters into a stressful or anxious state, NE function increases. As a result, NE increases in key regions associated with anxiety, particularly the locus coeruleus, limbic regions, and cerebral cortex. Recall that the locus coeruleus is the primary site of NE synthesis; projections from the locus coeruleus to the frontal-cortical areas are responsible for approximately 70% of the NE pathways. In the case of anxiety, the increase in NE brings results in the down-regulation of its autoreceptor (alpha-2), which is thought to mediate increased sympathetic autonomic arousal (e.g., increased heart rate, increased blood pressure). Panic disorder provides a good illustration of how treatments for anxiety operate on the assumption of NE hyperactivity. Panic disorder is marked by symptoms of NE-mediated sympathetic hyperarousal, including a pounding heart, sweating, trembling, shortness of breath, nausea, and light-headedness. While the actual neurobiological mechanisms of panic disorder are unclear, the associated NE-mediated hyperarousal symptoms have pointed researchers to a relationship between NE and the BDZ receptors.[16] As was explained above, the BDZ receptor is linked to the GABA receptor and together with it, when stimulated, produces an inhibitory or calming effect on the CNS. The GABA-BDZ receptor complex also inhibits activation of the locus coeruleus, a key area for NE activation. Thus, the overproduction of NE and the accompanying anxiety may represent a situation in which too little GABA is available to inhibit the locus coeruleus firing.

Therefore, it is not surprising that one of the first-line, immediate treatments for panic disorder involves fast-acting BDZs such as lorazepam. The take-home point is that medications that increase circulating levels of benzodiazepines have a downstream effect on NE and thus on the autonomic manifestations of anxiety.

CLINICAL POINT: Individuals who use alcohol or opiates are using agents that are known to decrease locus coeruleus firing. These individuals may be self-medicating, in part to address anxiety symptoms. When individuals present with substance use, nurses should consider the possibility that they are self-medicating to reduce feelings of anxiety and should query them about a history of anxiety disorders. ■

Serotonin. The neurotransmitter 5-HT also plays a role in neural firing that creates anxiety states. One line of evidence for the involvement of 5-HT in the pathophysiology of anxiety disorders is the fact that 5-HT-enhancing drugs such as SSRIs are effective agents in the treatment of anxiety, particularly SAD. Exactly why increasing 5-HT levels decrease the rise of anxiety is unclear. It may be that increased 5-HT levels inhibit the firing of key structures in the fear learning circuitry, mainly via its action between raphe nuclei (a source of 5-HT neurons) and the periaqueductal gray area (a descending pathway of the CNS). Alternatively, it may be related to the activity of 5-HT_{1A} receptors in the subgenual area of the prefrontal cortex, which seems to be a "crosswalk" between the amygdala and the prefrontal cortex and controls amygdala reactivity.

Another reason it is difficult to isolate the therapeutic mechanism of 5-HT is because it does not by itself drive any behavior; rather, 5-HT and NE modulate many behaviors in combination or by indirect regulation of another neurotransmitter. For example, the action of 5-HT that may relate to fear learning occurs through effects on NE and DA, which in turn affects anxiety. SAD provides a good illustration of the possible interplay between NE and 5-HT pathways. Recall that when a person is presented with a threat, the amygdala fires in many directions. One route is to the paraventricular nucleus of the hypothalamus, which in turn sends neural impulses to the locus coeruleus. In essence, this increases NE in the frontal part of the brain, and the individual experiences increased autonomic activity. One possibility is that via its connection to the locus coeruleus, 5-HT holds the release of NE in check; but in depression or anxiety, with diminished 5-HT, firing in the NE pathways increases, thereby increasing threat and arousal.

Dopamine. A final monoamine neurotransmitter implicated in anxiety is DA. As with 5-HT, the role of DA in anxiety disorders is not entirely clear. It has been observed that acute stress increases DA release and turnover, especially in the medial prefrontal cortex.[17] But the role of this increase is unclear in panic disorder and SAD. Speculation is that the common pathway may involve impairment in the DA reward pathways. In studying phobic responses, researchers suspect that the disorder may be associated with a poorly functioning caudate nucleus which also suggests the presence of low striatal DA.[18]

The HPA Axis

The HPA axis is a unique response system that comes into play when an individual is confronted by a threatening stimulus. In response to stress, the body primes itself for fight or flight with an immediate sympathetic discharge from the autonomic nervous system that increases the heart rate and blood pressure. The body also mounts a stress response through the HPA axis. This response is initiated by a quick relay from the thalamus, which reads the potential threat in the stimulus, to the amygdala, which registers the warning and sends out messages to other brain regions, especially the paraventricular nucleus of the hypothalamus. In any of the anxiety disorders in which there is excessive or prolonged activation of amygdala threat signaling, there is a danger that the HPA axis becomes activated too long or too often.

CRH is the key hormone that initiates the HPA stress cascade. It is released from the paraventricular nucleus of the hypothalamus and travels to the anterior pituitary. The anterior pituitary, in turn, releases ACTH which stimulates the adrenal glands and results in glucocorticoid production. Glucocorticoids (e.g., cortisol) act to provide the body with the needed energy for the fight ahead, mainly by increasing the availability of glucose, fatty acids, and amino acids and by decreasing insulin resistance. CRH also influences all monoamine neurotransmitters throughout the brain, especially the GABA system and the NE circuits that serve to increase arousal and attention.

The particular role of CRH in anxiety is based largely on animal models. Mice exposed to various types of stress-inducing situations were found to have increases in the amount of circulating CRH. These increases correlate with anxiogenic-like behaviors in the mice. Many organs in the brain have CRH-producing neurons; thus, increased CRH has widespread effects. When stimulated, CRH-producing neurons in the amygdala increase fear-related behaviors.[19] In most individuals, once the acute stressor has been removed, the system "rights" itself via signaling in the CRH glucocorticoid receptors.

Jasmine Mercado: Application

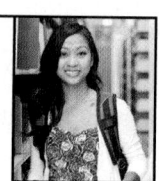

Several weeks after the initial event, Ms. Mercado finds herself in traffic on the way home and begins to experience symptoms similar to those that characterized the initial panic attack. She begins to feel her apprehension rising. She tries the breathing exercises, but they are ineffective, and the anxiety continues to build. She finally pulls off the road and calls her mother to bring her lorazepam, a medication she was prescribed to take as needed. She holds on for 20 minutes until her mother arrives. Although the panic attack subsides, Ms. Mercado formulates a plan to avoid being caught in traffic. She begins to organize her life around reducing the risk of feeling trapped with no escape route. Ms. Mercado has not followed up at the clinic, thinking that she can "tough out" the attacks. She also does not want to be labeled as someone with an emotional problem. However, Ms. Mercado realizes that she needs more help to deal with the paralysis that the anticipation of panic attacks has brought into her life.

3. What is the effect of lorazepam?
4. Was Ms. Mercado's second panic attack a result of consolidation or reconsolidation?

Clinical Manifestations and Diagnosis of Anxiety

Several conditions fall under the umbrella of anxiety disorders. Selected anxiety disorders from the American

Psychiatric Association's *Diagnostic and Statistical Manual of Mental Disorders*, Fifth Edition (DSM-5), are summarized in **Table 29.1** ■.[1]

The assessment of anxiety disorders in children and adolescents is complicated by several factors. First, all children have fears. While listening to the child's worries, the clinician must differentiate between the normal fears of childhood and fears whose persistence and intensity are such that they interfere with normal functioning. Second, in a clinical assessment interview, children and adolescents might not report their fears or anxieties. They may be embarrassed, or they may have normalized living with their fears. ■

Linking Pathophysiology to Treatment of Anxiety

Treatments for anxiety disorders involve psychopharmacology and nonpharmacologic therapies either alone or in combination.

Pharmacologic Therapy

Medications are an important component of treatment of anxiety disorders, either alone or in combination with cognitive-behavioral therapy (CBT). The first-line choice for the psychopharmacologic treatment of anxiety disorders is SSRIs or selective norepinephrine reuptake inhibitors (SNRIs), not only because they are effective, but also because of their safety and side effect profiles. SSRIs inhibit the reuptake of 5-HT, thereby increasing the amount of neurotransmitter in the synapse. Because of the interconnections within the monoamine system, increasing 5-HT also increases plasma levels of NE and DA. SNRIs directly increase both 5-HT and NE and have demonstrated efficacy, particularly in the treatment of GAD. Other antidepressants such as tricyclics and monoamine oxidase inhibitors are also effective agents for anxiety disorders, but they have less desirable side effect profiles.

It is not entirely clear how agents that increase 5-HT and other related monoamines (DA and NE) effectively reduce anxiety symptoms. At the most basic level, 5-HT pathways innervate several of the key structures involved in anxiety disorders, such as the amygdala, hippocampus, thalamus, and hypothalamus. Increasing 5-HT in these pathways is thought to expedite avoidance behavior and control fight-or-flight stress responses. But increasing 5-HT in the synapse is actually anxiogenic. Thus, the therapeutic response to SSRIs appears to be related to the effect of increasing plasma levels of 5-HT on stress adaptation mechanisms, including enhancing the steady state messenger RNAs (mRNAs) for the mineralocorticoid (MR-1) and glucocorticoid (GR-II) receptors and brain-derived neurotrophic factor (BDNF), while decreasing mRNA expression for CRH. 131 The most widely used SSRI is paroxetine (Paxil), which is approved for all major anxiety disorders. Sertraline (Zoloft) is also frequently prescribed and is approved for use in all anxiety disorders except GAD.

An older form of treatment for anxiety disorders is the benzodiazepines. The benzodiazepines have the advantage of rapid onset of action, but the distinct disadvantage of physiologic dependency that can develop with long-term administration. Although benzodiazepines are considered a second-line treatment, alprazolam (Xanax) is the most prescribed agent for the treatment of anxiety disorders. The duration of action of benzodiazepines is short, so the medications must be taken several times throughout the day. They can cause sedation, ataxia, and cognitive impairments, so individuals must be educated on the need to curtail particularly dangerous activities (e.g., driving) while taking the medications.

Finally, there is considerable research demonstrating the effectiveness of combination therapy, that is,

Table 29.1 Major Anxiety Disorders and Defining Features

Anxiety Disorder	Distinguishing Features
Panic disorder with/or without agoraphobia	• Recurrent, unexpected episodes of panic marked by palpitations, sweating, trembling, shortness of breath, chest pain, nausea, dizziness, feelings of unreality, fears of dying or "going crazy." • Panic attacks may be accompanied by a marked avoidance of any situation that is seen as inescapable or in which there is no help in the event of an attack (agoraphobia). This agoraphobia may or may not be a feature of an individual suffering from panic attacks.
Specific phobia	• Unreasonable or excessive, persistent fear that is cued by either the presence of, or anticipation of, specific objects or situations (e.g., heights, animals, flying). The phobic situation is avoided or endured with intense distress.
Social anxiety disorder	• Fear generated by social or performance situations in which the individual experiences being exposed to the unfamiliar or scrutiny. The feared situations are avoided or endured with intense distress.
Generalized anxiety disorder	• Excessive worry about any number of events that is difficult to control. The worry generates restlessness, fatigue, difficulty concentrating, irritability, tension, and sleep disturbance. These symptoms cause clinically significant distress.
Other anxiety disorders: a. Anxiety due to a medical condition b. Substance-induced anxiety disorder c. Anxiety disorder not otherwise specified	• These disorders are marked by predominant anxiety, panic, or obsessions and compulsions. But in (a) the anxiety is a direct physiologic consequence of a general medical condition, while in (b) the anxiety symptoms occur during or within 1 month of substance intoxication or withdrawal. In both disorders, the anxiety does not occur during a course of delirium. Finally, there are (c) anxiety disorders in which there is clinically significant anxiety that does not meet the criteria for a specific anxiety or depressive disorder.

SOURCE: Data from American Psychiatric Association. (2013). *Diagnostic and statistical manual of mental disorders* (5th ed.). Washington, DC: American Psychiatric Association; Sadock, B. J., Sadock, V. A., & Ruiz, P. (2014). *Synopsis of psychiatry, behavioral sciences/clinical psychiatry.* Philadelphia, PA: Wolters Kluwer Health; Potter, M. L., & Moller, M. D. (2016). *Psychiatric–mental health nursing: From suffering to hope.* Hoboken, NJ: Pearson.

medications plus psychotherapy. Overall, there does not appear to be a single definitive answer to the question of the superiority of combination therapies. Rather, the most effective combination of treatments differs between different anxiety disorders.

Nonpharmacologic Therapies

Many of the anxiety disorders are mediated by a hyperactive or hyperresponsive amygdala; one that is firing too often, too quickly, or too intensely. When the amygdala engages in any of these patterns, we count on the higher-level functioning portions of the brain, particularly parts of the prefrontal cortex, to provide additional pertinent information to the amygdala about the presenting threat. Also important is input from the hippocampus about the context of the current threat and its similarity to the one that generated the first conditioned response. Threat also triggers activity in the HPA axis. As the threat subsides, it is necessary to turn down the alarm system. This is usually accomplished by the activity of its own self-regulating receptors. For the anxious individual, these modulating factors might not be working well enough or the amygdala firing might be overpowering, in which case a cycle of apprehension, worry, dread, and accompanying autonomic reactions overwhelm the anxious individual's psyche. These responses may be so distressing that the individual begins to arrange life to avoid the perceived stimulus that initiates the anxiety.

At the most basic level, therapy for anxiety disorders works by either decreasing the amygdala response or by calling up stronger prefrontal cortical controls. For example, fear may begin with an initial impulse originating from the thalamus and traveling to the amygdala, which projects another cluster of impulses that signal threat to the rest of the body. A basic tenet of the neuroscience of psychotherapy is that experience sculpts certain portions of the brain's neural networks. Scientists believe that during therapy, the enriched cognitive and/or emotional environment promotes the development of new synapses and richer connectivity.[20] For instance, in **cognitive-behavioral therapy (CBT)**, the anxious individual learns to identify and challenge the fearful automatic and catastrophic thoughts. This is seen as boosting cortical processing circuits and at the same time dampening subcortical activation.

During cognitive restructuring, individuals are taught to identify automatic and faulty assumptions connected with their sensation of anxiety. In cognitive therapy, individuals learn how to identify these automatic thoughts, evaluate their accuracy, and then practice alternative, more realistic ways of thinking about their responses to the situation. The field of CBT for anxiety disorders continues to expand and is becoming increasingly sophisticated.

Anxiety disorder therapies often include a form of exposure therapy, in which the a simulation or image of the threatening stimulus is presented but the individuals are taught not to remove themselves or to respond in their habitual manner. For example, the individual with panic disorder thinks about a situation that generates panic and learns to relax and breathe in response. Individuals with SAD may begin by constructing a list of situations that generate fear or may role play reading a script while imagining themselves before an audience. They are taught to experience the fear fully yet also experience remaining safe. In doing so, the association is loosened between the stimulus and the anticipation of aversive consequences. The process is akin to extinction, "teaching" the amygdala a new association—one that involves a once-feared stimulus but now is associated with safety.

Therapies for anxiety disorders also include progressive muscle relaxation, psychoeducation aimed at reattribution of symptoms, and cognitive approaches that focus on automatic thoughts and schemas. Psychoeducation focuses on teaching individuals about anxiety symptoms, especially autonomic manifestations. They learn that a racing heart and hyperventilation are part of the body's response to their thoughts and not a sign of an impending medical disaster. This approach is essential in panic disorder, in which the bodily sensations of anxiety are so exaggerated that they become the feared cues that can set off another panic attack. Helping individuals understand the mechanisms of these bodily cues is the precursor to exposure work, which involves the systematic relearning of safety in response to a phobic cue.

CLINICAL POINT: Most patients benefit from a combination of pharmacologic and nonpharmacologic therapy. ■

Jasmine Mercado: Outcome

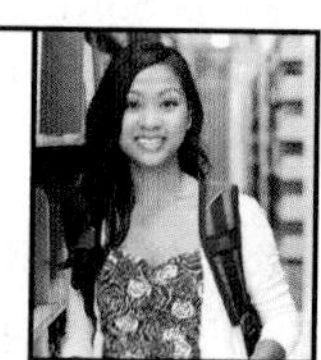

At the college counseling center, Ms. Mercado begins to talk about her sense of panic and learns that anticipatory anxiety can sometimes trigger a panic attack. Together, she and the nurse practitioner set goals for treatment and establish a schedule for sessions so that she can learn cognitive-behavioral techniques to deal with her growing pattern of avoidance. They discuss the use of more long-term medications to deal with the anxiety but decide to wait and see whether the CBT will alleviate the anticipatory anxiety and avoidance. Two months later, Ms. Mercado has not experienced any more panic attacks and has regained a sense of control with the help of CBT and relaxation work. She continues to check in at the clinic, especially when stress is building, but essentially has learned to deal with signs of impending anxiety. She has also begun to study yoga. By practicing daily meditation and attuning to the sensations of her inner body, she has found that her stress response has lessened and she has begun to live a more balanced life.

5. What techniques was Ms. Mercado encouraged to use to deal with the anticipatory anxiety?
6. What other activity has Ms. Mercado begun to help live a more balanced life?

Check Your Progress: Section 29.2

1. What are the three factors that put an individual at risk for the development of anxiety?
2. What type of education focuses on teaching individuals about anxiety symptoms, especially autonomic manifestations?
3. What anxiety disorder presents as excessive worry about events that are difficult to control?

29.3 Depression

Depression is a serious, life-threatening, often lifelong disorder. The World Health Organization reports that depression is the leading cause of disability, affecting 300 million people worldwide.[21]

Depression is a mood disorder in which the individual has persistent feelings of sadness and lack of interest in life. It has several subtypes that are categorized by their severity, duration, and symptom clusters (**Table 29.2** ■). While everyone has felt depressed at one time or another, **major depressive disorder (MDD)** is a clinical syndrome characterized by the presence of one or more depressive episodes of 2 weeks or longer over an individual's lifetime. Symptoms of MDD include depressed mood, significantly less interest in activities, changes in weight and sleep patterns, and feelings of worthlessness or guilt.[1] **Persistent depressive disorder,** also called **dysthymia,** is a depressed mood (feeling sad or down) that occurs on more days than not for at least 2 years. **Premenstrual dysphoric disorder** is a severe form of PMS (premenstrual syndrome) in which typical premenstrual symptoms appear but are so severe that they affect the woman's mental health, resulting in depression or anxiety. Other types of depression include substance or medication-induced depression and depression due to another medical disorder.

Table 29.2 Classification and Symptoms of Depression

Type of Depression	Symptoms
Major depressive disorder	At least five symptoms must be present from this list every day during the same 2-week period: • Depressed mood • Markedly diminished interest or pleasure in usual activities • Significant weight loss • Insomnia or hypersomnia • Psychomotor changes (increased or decreased) • Fatigue • Feelings of worthlessness or guilt • Diminished ability to think or concentrate • Recurrent thoughts of death or suicide
Persistent depressive disorder, dysthymia	Includes daily symptoms of depressed mood occurring for a period of at least 2 years. Two additional symptoms must be present from the following list: • Increased or decreased appetite • Sleeping too much or too little • Fatigue or low energy • Low self-esteem • Difficulty making decisions • Feelings of hopelessness
Premenstrual dysphoric disorder	At least five of the following symptoms are present in the week before the period starts, improve a few days after the period starts, and are minimal or completely disappear the week after the period ends: • Mood swings • Irritability • Depressed mood • Anxiety • Lack of interest in usual activities • Difficulty concentrating • Overeating • Too little or too much sleep • Feeling overwhelmed • Physical symptoms such as breast tenderness, bloating, joint pain

SOURCE: Data from American Psychiatric Association. (2013). *Diagnostic and statistical manual of mental disorders* (5th ed.). Washington, DC: American Psychiatric Association Publishing.

CLINICAL POINT: Even mild forms of depression create dysfunction and can lead to a more severe form of depression with an increased risk of greater dysfunction and suicide.[22] ■

Depression in older adults is underrecognized. It is estimated that 1–5% of community-dwelling older adults and approximately 13.5% of hospitalized older adults suffer from depression. Depression is not a normal part of aging and is a major risk factor for suicide in older adults.[23] ■

The Etiology and Pathogenesis of Depression

The etiology of depression is multifactorial. While having a family history of depression creates a particular risk for individuals, depressive episodes also occur on the heels of stress or medical illness and, at times, without apparent precipitants. Depressive symptoms present in several clusters, partially reflecting variations in which neuronal circuits are involved. As the broad array of symptoms suggests, depression is not just feeling "low"; it is a disturbance that can increase pain sensitivity, disrupt sleep, and affect memory and concentration. In addition, depressed individuals do not necessarily feel sluggish and low but can be anxious and have a jumpy or jittery sensation.

Young children are at significant risk for depression. and almost half of cases of depression begin in the teen years.[24] ■

MDD is a highly comorbid disorder that can occur in the context of chronic medical illnesses. Depression may be a cause and/or a consequence of illnesses such as cardiovascular and cerebrovascular disorders, HIV/AIDS, cancer, and epilepsy. MDD also appears to have a bidirectional association with Alzheimer disease and Parkinson disease.[25]

Little is known about the etiology of MDD, but there appears to be a genetic component to its development. Twin and adoption studies have determined that first-degree relatives of people with MDD have a 2–3 times greater risk of developing MDD than do people in the general population. However, genetics alone cannot explain the development of MDD.

Understanding the pathophysiology of depression helps nurses recognize mood disorders, particularly when individuals present with subthreshold symptoms such as concerns around mood, sleep, and energy. Understanding the pathophysiology also helps nurses to understand the connection between seemingly disparate symptoms, such as deceased pain tolerance and depressed mood. Finally, knowledge of the pathophysiology of mood disorders provides a conceptual bridge between depression and the medical conditions that sometimes precede it, such as diabetes, myocardial infarctions, and several neurologic disorders including cerebrovascular accidents.

The brain creates states of mind. For example, incoming stimuli may trigger an emotion, which is "read" for its significance and then compared to past experiences with similar emotion event memory tracks. With such an occurrence, key parts of the brain and their underlying neuronal networks synchronize in a split second so that the individual can process a situation and experience its accompanying sensation. This process may be derailed in individuals with depression because key neural networks are not firing with enough frequency or strength to bring energy and blood flow to the key processing regions of the brain. Parts of the brain may be reduced in volume, and that, together with faulty connectivity, establishes firing patterns that create a depressed state of mind.

For instance, neural impulses travel from the locus coeruleus to the frontal lobe across a pathway that utilizes the neurotransmitter NE (also known as the noradrenergic pathway). This pathway is thought to mediate attention and concentration (**Figure 29.5** ■). Neural impulses traveling along this pathway help individuals process information. Given a smiling face as a stimulus, an individual will usually focus on the smile and perk up. Facilitating that neuronal action is the NE flow to the orbitofrontal and prefrontal regions. At the same time, neural impulses from the orbitofrontal cortex travel to the amygdala to read the valance on the face, determining whether it is a happy or sad expression. Perhaps the individual goes back to his memory store (located roughly in the hippocampus) to determine whether he knows this person. As the neuronal firing progresses, the smiling face may unconsciously generate an affective state of mild pleasure in the person who sees it.

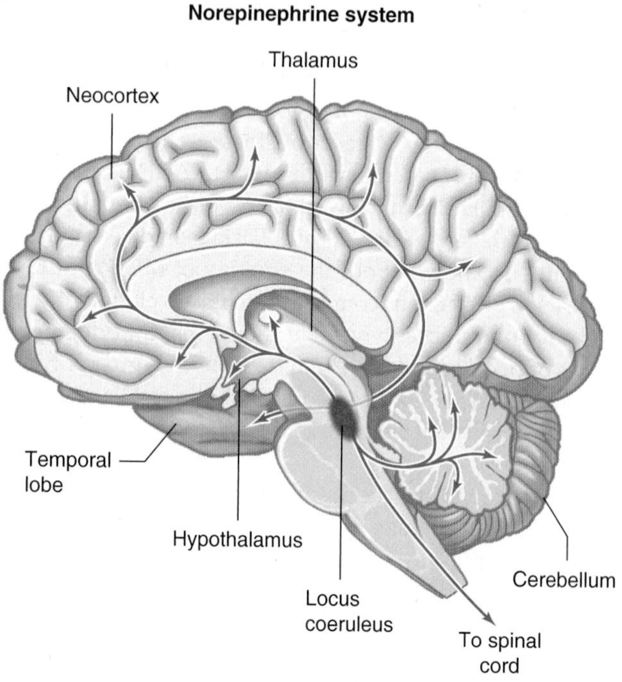

Conversely, in depression, the noradrenergic neurons may not be firing strongly, and the affected individual does not attend outward; specifically, he might not attend to happy facial expressions. Thus, he does not read or process the potential significance of that smiling face. It may be that the neurons in the orbitofrontal and prefrontal cortex are not firing well, or it may be that the affect registers as not significant when it is sent back for a second read to the amygdala and medial area of the prefrontal cortex. Often in depression, a negative bias resides that colors the potential reward of stimuli and therefore how strongly they are read. In this instance, the neural mechanisms that filter information become so biased in favor of negative information that the individual with depression is less likely to attend to positive information; hence, that smiling face is likely disregarded. As a result of this complex neural activation pattern, the individual's affective state of mind maintains a low, negative mood.

The search for a neurobiologic explanation of depression has continued for over 50 years, with differing explanations being proposed over the decades. Each theory of depression added a new piece of information to the neurologic puzzle. As scientists moved from one theory to the next, they built more complex models of how various systems of the brain interacted during a depressive episode. The first theories of depression centered on imbalances and/or dysregulation in monoamine neurotransmitters and their receptors. The next theory focused on intracellular gene transcription and how depression may cause neurons that nourish the cells to die out. More recent explanatory theories have focused on key systems dealing with stress responses and the injury/inflammatory process and how both might influence the onset of depression. To understand the pathophysiology of depression, we start at the most basic level: monoamine neurotransmitters.

Figure 29.5 ■ The norepinephrine (NE) system with emphasis on the pathway to the orbitofrontal complex (OFC) and prefrontal cortex (PFC). The OFC registers incoming stimuli such as facial expressions. The PFC also reads incoming stimuli.

The Role of Neurotransmitters in Depression

In the 1960s, researchers first proposed the so-called monoamine theory of depression. This theory posited that depression was the result of imbalances in the monoamine system of neurotransmitters, particularly **serotonin (5-HT)**, **norepinephrine (NE)**, and **dopamine (DA)**. However, in the ensuing decades, the seemingly simple causal link between depression and neurotransmitter levels became complicated when research revealed the role of receptor levels, receptor alterations, and gene transcription in response to antidepressant medication. Doubts were also cast on the monoamine theory when medications designed to increase levels of these neurotransmitters proved ineffective in decreasing depressive symptoms in more than half of depressed individuals treated with these antidepressant drugs. Current thinking is that depression is most likely the result of complicated reactions between stress (including medical illnesses) and genetic vulnerability. It is also recognized that environmental factors and life events may play a role in the onset of a depressive episode.

However, the actions of monoamines are still considered to be a critical link in the regulation of multiple neural systems, and during depressive episodes, their actions produce changes in mood, cognition, and behavior. Much goes on at the cellular level as receptors, transporters, and membrane gates all affect the balance in the level of circulating neurotransmitters. The actions and interactions of all these elements can become quite complex and, at this point, are not fully understood by researchers in the field. But because understanding depression involves understanding how these monoamine pathways coordinate activity in several regions of the brain, the pathophysiology of depression often begins here. For purposes of discussion, first the neurochemical system changes in depression will be outlined, and then the alterations in the anatomic system will be explored with a focus on changes that are typically seen in depression.

Evidence suggests that three major monoamine neurotransmitters are tied to different aspects of depression. It appears that serotonin transmission regulates obsessions and compulsions; dopamine transmission mainly regulates motivation, pleasure, and reward; and norepinephrine regulates alertness and energy.[26]

But the model becomes a bit more complex once it incorporates how the actions of neurotransmitters combine to produce an effect. For instance, serotonin and norepinephrine together regulate mood, emotions, pain, and cognitive functions (**Figure 29.6** ■).

CLINICAL POINT: Understanding the target behaviors or functions regulated by neurotransmitters becomes particularly important for nurses who may be educating individuals on the actions of antidepressant medications and on why a particular medication might help with particular symptoms. ■

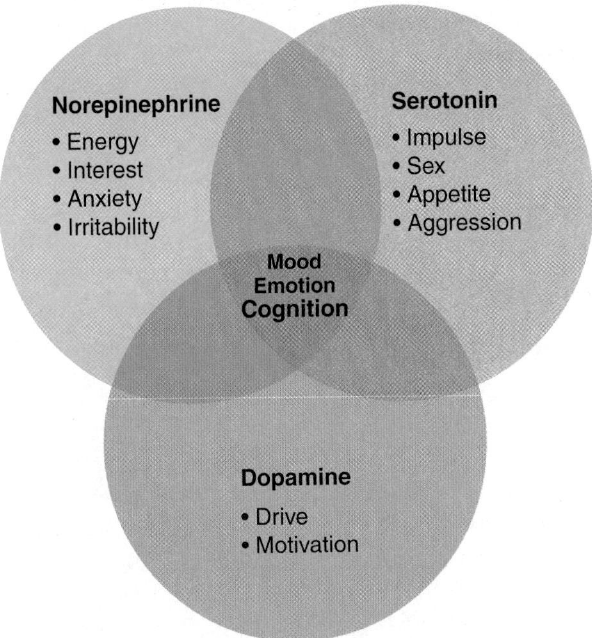

Figure 29.6 ■ The complex interplay of three neurotransmitters: norepinephrine, serotonin, and dopamine.

Understanding the role of neurotransmission in depression requires examining the separate actions of norepinephrine, serotonin, and dopamine, which are the three major players in the monoamine system; how their actions maintain mood and function; and how their availability can be linked to symptoms of depression.

Norepinephrine. At the most basic level, NE is seen as the neurotransmitter responsible for interest and energy. It is also an intermediary neurotransmitter that, when working in parallel with dopamine, is critical in the maintenance of a sense of hope and purpose in life. Research has found an association between NE and depressed mood by examining the activation of NE neurons and their axonal projections that originate in the locus coeruleus and end in the amygdala, an area of the brain that attaches significance to emotions. In the amygdala, NE acts as an inhibitory neurotransmitter; therefore, a deficiency of NE results in overactivity, potentially resulting in the overreading of and overattending to negative emotions.[26]

Norepinephrine is synthesized in a stepwise fashion from its precursor neuroprotein, tyrosine. The take-home lesson from this array of reactions and intermediary enzymes is that a deficit of any component of the pathway at any stage of the synthesis process will limit the amount of NE that is produced. For example, the lack of the final precursor, dopamine, will limit the relative amount of NE. This becomes of particular interest in illnesses such as Parkinson disease, which is marked by dopamine deficiency and, not surprisingly, often characterized by a comorbid depression.

NE neurons fire throughout the brain at a steady rate. Of prime importance is the amount of NE in the neuronal synapse, which is primarily controlled by three mechanisms. The first control mechanism is the presence of a presynaptic alpha-2 (α_2) autoreceptor. This autoreceptor binds NE released from the nerve terminal and subsequently modulates further NE release from that neuron. The second control mechanism is the presence of a transporter, a pumplike mechanism on the presynaptic membrane that carries NE back into the presynaptic neuron. The final mechanism involves enzymes in the neuronal cell body that metabolize any excess NE released into the synaptic cleft and transported back into the cell. In the case of NE, the two enzymes are monoamine oxidase (MAO), particularly MAO-A, and catechol-O-methyltransferase (COMT). Because little COMT is found in monoaminergic neurons, MAO-A is the critical enzyme in the biotransformation of NE.

It is not only the amount of NE in the synaptic cleft that determines postsynaptic neuronal firing but also the behavior of its receptors, which are located on both the presynaptic and postsynaptic neuronal membranes. The NE receptors are subdivided into two categories: alpha (α_1, α_2) and beta (β_1, β_2, β_3). The important presynaptic receptor is α_2, the autoreceptor. Stimulation of this autoreceptor is thought to inhibit neurotransmitter release. For example, when there is too much NE in a synapse, stimulation of these receptors results in a decrease in the release of NE from storage vesicles. This regulatory system is important. For example, if the release of NE did not have a braking mechanism, postsynaptic neuronal firing might occur at too high a rate, which is thought to occur in panic disorders. On the postsynaptic side are α_1 and β receptors that, when stimulated, bring about an increase in K^+ conductance and eventually firing of the postsynaptic neuron.

NE neurons project to several areas of the brain and affect the cortex (higher learning), amygdala (emotions), hippocampus (memory), and thalamus and hypothalamus (**Figure 29.7** ■). Each pathway mediates a different function, such as maintaining mood, attention, and emotional regulation. Most NE neurons originate in the locus coeruleus, which is thought to control how individuals focus attention, particularly the balance of outward focus versus monitoring the internal body state. Projections from the locus coeruleus to the prefrontal region of the brain control attention and the shifting of attention, via a firing in the postsynaptic α_2. NE is thought to control mood by firing along a tract that again goes to the prefrontal region of the brain, but in this instance, NE stimulates postsynaptic β_1 receptors. Finally, low projection of NE from the locus coeruleus to the limbic areas is thought to be involved in presentation of apathy, fatigue, and psychomotor retardation (motor slowing). These of course match up with many of the cardinal symptoms of depression listed in Table 29.2.

This is a simple depiction of the role of NE in depression. The pathophysiology ultimately involves the synchrony of all key neurotransmitters in interaction with various parts of the brain. For instance, NE firing patterns in particular locations of the brain are dependent on the action of serotonin (5-HT). In animal studies, when the 5-HT neuron is intentionally damaged, NE firing is increased. Alternately, the presynaptic NE heteroreceptors that sit on the serotonin neuron, when occupied, can turn off 5-HT release. These insights have clinical relevance for treatment with antidepressants. It may be that using a medication that boosts the level of a single neurotransmitter, such as 5-HT, will not be as effective as a combination drug that works on increasing levels of both 5-HT and NE.

The proposed action of NE in depression is also complicated because in some regions of the brain, NE creates an inhibitory action on brain function. As a result, decreased NE (as is thought to occur in some depressions) leads to increased activity. The underlying explanation is that an overactive amygdala colors stimuli with a negative emotional valence; the lateral prefrontal section of the brain pulls up and holds on to negative memories to support the attribution; an overactive ACC, a master organ of recognizing internal states, "locks on" to that sense of sadness; and the thalamus stimulates the amygdala and keeps this circuit of negative thought going. This linkage, known also as the limbic-thalamic-cortical tract, is considered one branch of the larger limbic-cortical-striatal circuit that is thought to play a critical role in the response of depressed clients to therapy and medication.

Serotonin. Serotonin (5-HT) is the neurotransmitter that mediates positive mood, optimism, and impulsivity. Its role in depression came to light when the linkage between depression and NE was established and it was determined that serotonin is essential to keep NE at its appropriate level. The linkage between 5-HT and depression was bolstered by the effectiveness of SSRIs, whose primary aim was to boost 5-HT levels.

Most serotonin neurons originate in the dorsal raphe nuclei in the pons and upper brainstem and then project widely to several areas of the brain, including the prefrontal cortex, limbic system, basal ganglia, hypothalamus, and brainstem sleep centers (**Figure 29.8** ■). These pathways

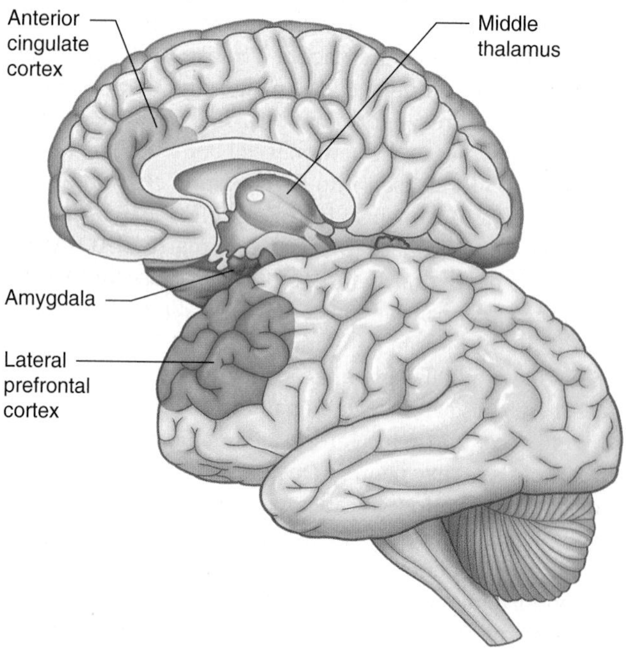

Figure 29.7 ■ The areas of the brain that are thought to be overactive in depression.

Serotonin system

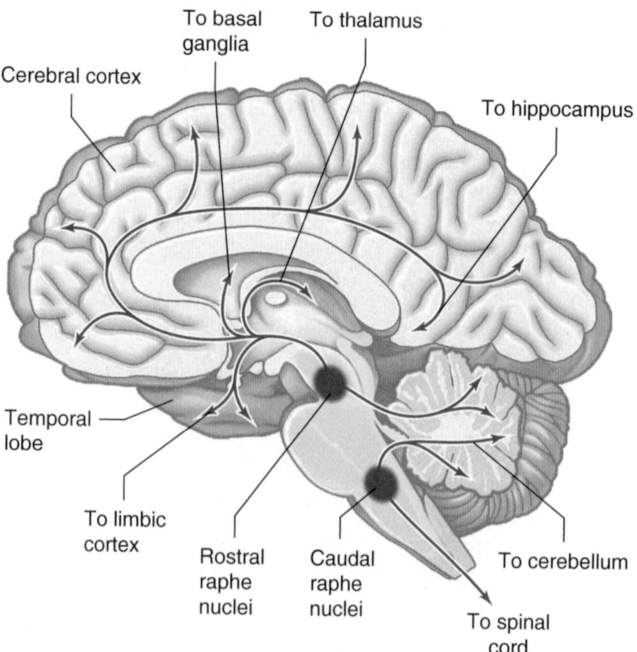

Figure 29.8 ■ The serotonin (5-HT) pathways. Note the extensive connections to all parts of the forebrain, midbrain, and cerebellum.

are thought to mediate specific functions. For instance, the serotonin pathway to the prefrontal cortex is important in maintaining mood. The serotonin pathways to the hippocampus, septum, and amygdala perform inhibitory functions, and similar to NE, low 5-HT results in overactivity in these areas. For instance, since the amygdala is responsible for assigning significance to emotion and regulating the intensity of feelings, it makes sense that the inhibitory action of 5-HT keeps this mechanism in check and a lack of 5-HT allows negative emotions to run wild.

Serotonin also plays a role in the pathways that control many somatic functions. The 5-HT pathway to the hypothalamus is thought to regulate appetite, and the pathway to the brainstem is thought to regulate sleep. Additional 5-HT receptors in these systems may also regulate gastrointestinal function and participate in the sexual response system. The wide reach of serotonin pathways and their accompanying functions correlate with many of the primary symptoms of depression, thus making 5-HT dysfunction a prime candidate in the etiology of depression.

On the cellular level, 5-HT is released into the synaptic cleft on axon firing. There, similar to NE, the amount of 5-HT present is determined by reuptake by a 5-HT transporter as well as enzymatic destruction both in the presynaptic neuron and in the synaptic cleft. What is not destroyed or transported back into the presynaptic neuron is free to bind to one of the 14 subtypes of 5-HT receptors grouped into seven families. These receptors exert diverse actions; some are inhibitory, and some are excitatory. The receptors that are most relevant to the study of mood disorders were identified as 5-HT_{1A}, 5-HT_2, 5-HT_4, 5-HT_6, and 5-HT_7. It is the uptake of 5-HT by these receptors that is thought to ultimately regulate mood, pain, sleep, and body temperature.[2] Balance in the 5-HT_{1A} and 5-HT_{2A} receptors is seen to be critical in maintaining mood.

CLINICAL POINT: Understanding the action of neurotransmitters and stress is important for more than mental illness. The interaction of stress, cortisol, and depression has implications for several medical conditions that have a relationship with depression (e.g., diabetes, cardiac disorders, decreased bone mineral density). For the specific disorders that are comorbid with depression, treating the depression may be critical to prevention of these stress-related disorders. Treating existing comorbid depression may also lessen pain and organ sensations that accompany the primary disorder. ■

Dopamine. Dopamine is derived from the same neuroprotein as NE but does not go through the final conversion by dopamine beta-hydroxylase (**Figure 29.9** ■). If a DA receptor is present on the presynaptic neuron, it acts as an autoreceptor, and when stimulated, it halts the release of DA. Similar to NE, DA is controlled by a presynaptic pump that sweeps excess DA back into the neuron and by enzymatic destruction either intracellularly by MAO or in the synapse by COMT. Dopamine also has its own army of receptors that control its transmission. The most important for this discussion are the dopamine receptors D_1 through D_5.

Evidence for the role of DA in depression is not entirely clear. Interest in the neurotransmitter grew with the realization that patients with DA dysfunction, such as patients with Parkinson disease, frequently exhibit a comorbid depression. These individuals experience a marked improvement in mood when given levodopa for their Parkinson disease. Additional evidence supporting the role of dopamine in depression includes the findings that medications that boost DA by blocking its reuptake have antidepressant effects and that drugs that curtail DA can create a syndrome that resembles depression.[26] Several areas of the brain innervated by dopamine projections are implicated in depression, especially those from the ventral tegmental area (VTA) to the orbital prefrontal cortex (mesocortical), striatum, and ACC. As was noted earlier in the chapter, depression can be categorized by the prevalent symptom presentation as well as additional symptom patterns, such as melancholic or psychotic. It is thought that a DA deficiency is at work in individuals presenting with melancholic depression and depression with psychotic features. But the connection is a bit complicated because of the interaction of DA, NE, and 5-HT. For instance, antidepressant medications that boost NE and 5-HT also boost dopamine, primarily by preventing dopamine reuptake in NE neurons. As is illustrated in **Figure 29.10** ■, there is considerable overlap in the 5-HT and DA pathways. Therefore, isolating one neurotransmitter as a "cause" of a particular type of depression is difficult.

Of particular interest in depression is a DA pathway associated with the dopamine reward system, a pathway that travels from the VTA toward the nucleus accumbens (NAc). Using mood enhancing drugs, researchers

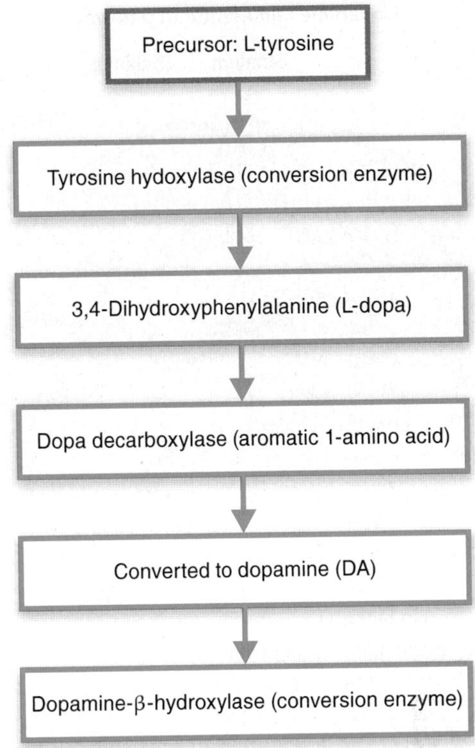

Figure 29.9 ■ The synthesis of dopamine (DA).

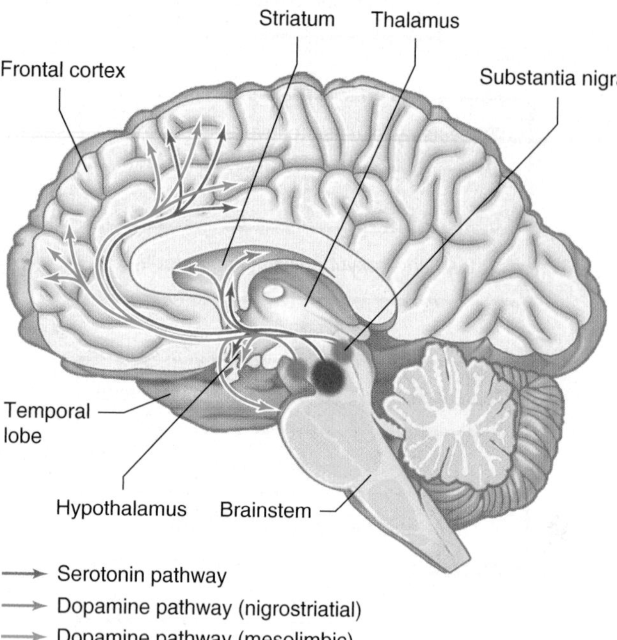

Figure 29.10 The dopamine and serotonin pathways, illustrating the dual overlapping innervations to the frontal areas, accounting for their dual effects on mood and cognition.

demonstrated that substances that prompt a DA release in this area result in euphoria, and a DA deficiency is thought to be related to anhedonia, defined as the inability to experience pleasure from what would be considered normally pleasurable events.[26] The pathways from the VTA travel not only to the NAc but also to the prefrontal area of the brain and the amygdala. In the face of a rewarding stimulus, the ventromedial prefrontal cortex reads the context of the stimulus and what might be the possible outcomes of the reward. The amygdala attaches significance to the cue that suggests reward. For instance, when a candy bar is seen, the amygdala triggers the association between pleasure and eating sweets that has developed over time.

The flow of DA through the mesolimbic pathway becomes more complex when one considers that DA neurons receive inputs and transmit outputs to not only the prefrontal area but also to the hippocampus. This suggests a complex interaction of several brain systems, and how they interact in depression is not yet fully understood. Researchers studying depression think that so much attention has been paid to the role of NE and 5-HT that the role of dopamine has been overlooked.

Stress and HPA Axis Dysfunction in Depression

Another important system implicated in the pathophysiology of depression is the stress response system. It may be that a key to the pathophysiology of several subtypes of depression involves an interaction between the HPA axis and the 5-HT/NE systems. The HPA axis response system is designed to prime the body for fight or flight. Classically, its action is initiated when an individual senses a threat in her environment. This threatening stimulus reaches the thalamus, where it is quickly sent to the amygdala, which registers the warning and sends messages to other brain regions (especially the hypothalamus) to prepare the body for the possibility of fight or flight. This quick response system generates an immediate response in the brain and body that does not involve thinking or processing in its cortical regions.[27]

As individuals continue to take in information on the threatening situation, the hippocampus comes into play. It processes the information and past associations that are relevant to the situation. If what the person recalls is also associated with fear, the brain can upregulate the amygdala response as well as stimulating a more general bodily response. In this instance, the HPA axis begins a familiar chain of hormone excretion to prepare the body for what it might be about to face.[27]

To understand how stress and depression intermingle, one begins with a key hormone in the stress cascade, the corticotropin-releasing factor (CRF), released from the paraventricular nucleus of the hypothalamus. It is this hormone that makes its way to the anterior pituitary, which in turn releases ACTH. The ACTH stimulates the adrenal glands, and glucocorticoids are produced. To provide the body energy for the fight or flight ahead, glucocorticoids (mainly cortisol in humans) act to increase the synthesis of lipids and proteins and decrease insulin resistance.[28] The CRF system also activates the NE circuit, which serves to increase arousal and attention.

While useful in the short term, overstimulation of the HPA axis can damage the body if the adrenals continue to produce cortisol. Luckily, a negative feedback system exists, so when cortisol reaches a certain level, receptors in the pituitary, hypothalamus, and hippocampus turn the system off. This is the essential work of the mineralocorticoid (MR-1) and glucocorticoid (GR-II) receptors.[28] Unfortunately, when circumstances generate continual stress, especially in early infant life, the brain may create a toxic neurochemical environment, killing off or desensitizing those receptors.[28] In that case, the CRF and NE systems rest on an unresponsive feedback loop that may be hypersensitive to stress or remain hyperactive in the face of minimal threat.

The CRF and HPA axis system is linked to depression in several ways. For decades, it was recognized that depressed patients demonstrated increased cortisol levels and did not suppress cortisol secretion following the administration of dexamethasone.[28] This is particularly true of individuals with a melancholic depression, which is a depression particularly marked by low mood and loss of pleasure. Along with high levels of cortisol, individuals with depression display higher levels of CRF in the cerebrospinal fluid and increased CRF receptors in the frontal cortex. It became clear that while CRF is a key link in the HPA axis stress response chain, it has additional functions, owing to the presence of CRF receptors and signaling devices in the amygdala and cortical regions of the brain.[28]

In depressed individuals, the HPA axis system in a sense turns in on itself because of excessive stimulation of the system and problems with self-limiting receptors. In particular, cells in the hippocampus appear to stop growing, and the organ suffers volume loss. The reason for the cell loss is not exactly clear. It may be caused by a decrease in the production of neurotrophic factor required for cell nourishment and thus decreasing neurogenesis. It may also be due to the persistent high cortisol levels that, along with the decrease of its regulating receptors, results in high circulating glutamate that causes cell death.[28]

In either case, hippocampal atrophy has profound effects on its functions. The hippocampus regulates the HPA axis, so there is decreased restraint on the very system generating the problem. As demonstrated in animal research, damage to the hippocampus results in deficits in learning and memory formation. This can result in an inability to form memories related to the emotional context of a stressor.[28] The hippocampus is also involved in mood and emotion via inputs to the prefrontal and cingulate cortex and amygdala.

Neuroanatomic Changes and Depression

In depression, there is an interaction between the identified neurochemistry and certain neuroanatomic structures that are believed to be involved in the disorder. For instance, researchers demonstrated that when individuals with depression are asked to perform tests that require focused concentration, a reduction in the activation of parts of the prefrontal cortex and anterior cingulated is observed. Individuals recruit these areas of the brain to attend, block interference, and perform working memory tasks.[29] Recall that the prefrontal cortex receives innervations through NE, 5-HT, and DA neurons. Therefore, it is reasonable that depression would affect the activity in these regions. The following discussion highlights the key changes in several brain structures, the pathophysiology of which can be tied to depressive symptoms and medication response.

Late-life depression often presents in the context of medical and neurologic disorders, such as cardiovascular disorders, dementia, and stroke. The pathophysiology of late-onset depression is particularly marked by changes in the frontostriatal pathway. Anatomic studies suggest some volume loss there and in caudate structures. Older adults with such frontostriatal changes present with executive dysfunction, increased feelings of apathy, and psychomotor retardation.[30,31] ■

To begin exploring these changes, certain parts of the brain will be discussed separately along with their assumed role in the pathophysiology of mood disorders.

Frontal Cortex. The frontal cortex is an area of the brain with numerous functions (**Figure 29.11** ■). It is most often thought to be involved in executive functions such as planning and problem solving. The lateral frontal cortex is the seat of self-willed action, agency, and aliveness. All of these functions are compromised in depression. Depression also affects the upper temporal parietal region, which mediates how individuals attend to situations outside of themselves. A perceived lack of agency and a focus on the interior world result when these areas are understimulated. The medial frontal cortex (Figure 29.11, orange area) is thought to influence how one attends and assigns significance to stimuli and also contains a pathway to block emotional interference. Emotional suppression is key to maintaining focus and to the function of a working memory. The ACC (Figure 29.11, green area) is thought to be the part of the brain that helps individuals lock onto and focus on situations. The ventral lateral cortex (pink area) is thought to help individuals suppress their emotions. Finally, the area of the frontal cortex directly behind the eyes and nose, the orbitofrontal cortex (Figure 29.11, turquoise area) has an important integrative function because it receives input from many areas of the brain. The orbitofrontal cortex also helps individuals deal with the unexpected and adjust to changing circumstances. Two areas of the frontal cortex (the orbitofrontal cortex and medial frontal cortex) are considered key to depression because they receive projections from the limbic region, which is critical to experiencing and reading emotions.[32]

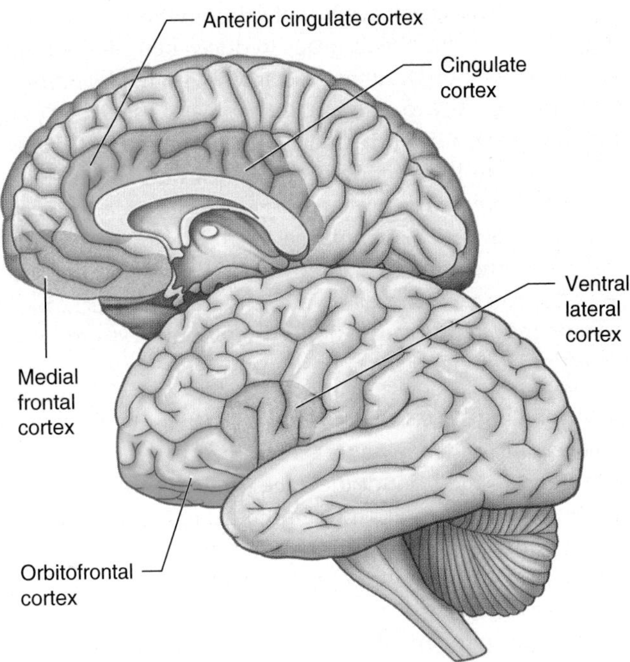

Figure 29.11 ■ Five key sections of the frontal cortex that are tied to depressive symptoms and medication response: the orbitofrontal cortex, ventral lateral cortex, medial frontal cortex, cingulate cortex, and anterior cingulate cortex.

In postmortem studies, individuals with depression have reduced numbers of cells that provide growth-producing nourishment (BDNF) to the glial cells in several areas of the frontal cortex. Researchers believe that glial cells provide many essential services to neurons and that a reduction in their numbers in depression is significant and may be the underlying mechanism for reduced neuronal density in the prefrontal cortex. Functional studies also attest to abnormalities in these areas, which are thought to be indicative of the state effects of the illness.[32]

Of special interest is the area lying ventral to the corpus callosum. This area is called the subgenual prefrontal cortex. This area was shown to have reduced functional activity and in some studies reduced neuronal density in depressed individuals, especially those who have a close family relative with the disorder. Reduced neuronal activity in this area is thought to be associated with the inability to respond viscerally to emotional stimuli and accompanying mood alteration in individuals with depression. Reduced cell activity in this section of the cortex may also be connected to increased neuronal firing in the amygdala. Recent evidence has demonstrated that when the subgenual area underfires, the amygdala overfires.[32] Thus, when the subgenual cortex does not keep the amygdala in check, individuals may both overrespond to emotional stimuli and have a greater visceral response to stress.

Anterior Cingulate Cortex. Another area of the brain that has been implicated in depression is the ACC. The ACC lies above and to the front of the knee (or genu) of the corpus callosum. It is situated between the frontal cortex with its dorsal portion connected to the prefrontal executive function areas and is thought to significantly influence cognitive controls and reward-based decision making. The more ventral portion (perigenual) projects downward to the limbic system and is involved with emotional control (processing emotional information, controlling the valence of emotions, affecting motivation, and ultimately regulating autonomic and endocrine functions).[33] Research supports some volume loss as well as functional alterations in the ACC during major depression.[33] Because the ACC is an important way station for controlling the balance of thinking and processing emotions, improvement in its functioning may be critical in the response to antidepressant treatment.

Basal Ganglia. In the face of depression, the basal ganglia undergo some structural changes and several functional changes. In depression research, the basal ganglia are now viewed in the context of the interconnections among key areas in the limbic-cortical-striatal-pallidal-thalamic (LCSPT) tract.[34] The LCSPT tract includes brain structures involved in cognitive activity and emotional regulation and its functioning depends on the neuronal release of NE, DA, and 5-HT. The LCSPT tract conducts neuronal impulses and energy from the front of the brain, the striatum (caudate and putamen), and the globus pallidus to the limbic and subcortical areas.

Depending on their connectivity, the basal ganglia play a different role in controlling thought, emotion, and somatic responses. Orchestrating negative thoughts and feelings is believed to be a function of various structures located along the top of the brain—the dorsal tract of the LCSPT tract. It is composed of prefrontal cortex, the dorsal ACC, and the inferior parietal lobe. This tract also connects with the basal ganglia. Functional imaging techniques demonstrated that this dorsal section of the LCSPT tract is hypoactive during depression.[34] These structures are heavily innervated by NE. Lack of NE or dysfunction of these monoamine pathways may be at the heart of the NE-linked depressive symptoms such as impaired cognition, fatigue, psychomotor retardation, and apathy.[35] The ventral tract of the LCSPT tract includes the ventral striatum or other parts of the basal ganglia. As was described earlier, in depression, this tract may be overactive, keeping negative thoughts and their significance in attention. The basal ganglia, a component of both of these tracts, demonstrate lower cerebral blood flow with depression, but they also demonstrate improvement with medication.

Hippocampus. Of particular interest in depression research are reductions in hippocampal volume associated with affective disorders. The hippocampus plays an important role in learning and memory. As was discussed above, excessive, prolonged stress and the accompanying overactivation of the HPA axis plays a role in the damage to hippocampal neurons. This damage is thought to occur because of excess cortisol as well as the effects of stress-related damage to BNDF genes and resultant glial cell loss.[36] As is often the case, when results across brain imaging studies are compared, findings are mixed. But there seems a clear indication of hippocampal volume loss in depression, particularly among individuals who have problems with declarative and recollection memory.

Amygdala. In investigations of hippocampal and amygdala volume loss during depression, there is significant variation in reported results. Much depends on how one measures and defines the boundaries of the two organs, which are highly interconnected. However, studies of the amygdala demonstrate that amygdala function is increased in depression, and in some reports, the volume increases.[37] The amygdala is an important player in the limbic-thalamic-cortical circuit of the LCSPT tract, particularly its connections to the medial prefrontal cortex. The overactivity that is seen in depression appears to contribute to the proclivity of depressed individuals to pick up on negative or aversive emotional meaning. An overactive amygdala might also drive ruminations because of its involvement in stirring up negative memories.

The few neuroimaging studies of children with depression have small sample sizes but do suggest that there may be changes in frontal lobe and amygdala volume.[38] Evidence demonstrates that depressed children and adults more than likely differ in their biological correlates; depressed children exhibit less HPA axis hyperactivity as well as increased (versus decreased) activity in raphe neurons.[38] ■

Clinical Manifestations and Diagnosis of Depression

The DSM-5 distinguishes between a major depressive episode and major depressive disorder.[39] A **major depressive episode** lasts for 2 weeks and includes one of the two major symptoms of depressed mood (anhedonia) and at least four additional symptoms from the list in Table 29.2. These symptoms must be new or different and persist for most of the day nearly every day. The diagnosis of major depressive disorder (MDD) is assigned when there is evidence of one or more instances of a major depressive episode without a history of manic, mixed, or hypomanic episodes. (These episodes are discussed in the following section on bipolar disorders.) Defining features of the current depressive episode may be described by using a variety of specifiers, such as mild; moderate; severe with and without psychotic features; chronic, with catatonic, melancholic, or atypical features; and with postpartum onset.

Persistent depressive disorder, also called *dysthymia,* is characterized by the combination of chronicity and milder depressive symptoms. Dysthymia is diagnosed when an individual has a depressed mood most of the day and for more days than not over 2 years. Two symptoms from the following list are required along with depressed mood:[39]

- Poor appetite or overeating
- Insomnia or hypersomnia
- Lower energy or fatigue
- Low self-esteem
- Poor concentration, or difficulty making decisions
- Feelings of hopelessness.

Chronic depression is major depression that lasts 2 years or longer with no more than a 2-month period of remission. Chronic depression overlaps with dysthymia, and the majority of individuals diagnosed with dysthymiaexperiencing exacerbations meeting the criteria for MDD at some point in their lives (see Table 29.2).

4 Pregnancy and the postpartum period are times of particular risk for depression. While evidence to support the biological basis for the increased risk is scant, it is thought that the rapid decline of estrogen in the postpartum period contributes to the onset of depression. The estrogen–serotonin interaction in depression has not yet been fully explained, but evidence suggests that estrogen is also useful in treatment of perimenopausal depression. This benefit is thought to be associated with estrogen's promotion of cortical 5-HT_{2A} binding.[40] ■

Alice Parry: Application

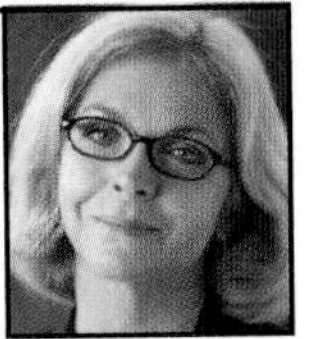

Ms. Parry reports impairment both at work and at home. At work, she is more irritable. Along with her depressed mood, Ms. Parry gets upset when her coworkers react negatively to her irritability. Ms. Parry's response is to avoid work. At home, she also reports more irritability in conjunction with sadness, hypersomnia, anhedonia, weight gain, suicidal ideation, and fixation on negative events in the past.

3. What other symptom did Ms. Parry experience at work that impaired her relationships?
4. Is Ms. Parry manifesting symptoms of major depressive disorder or persistent depressive disorder?

Linking Pathophysiology to Treatment of Depression

Treatments for depression involve psychopharmacology and nonpharmacologic therapies either alone or in combination. While pharmacologic therapy is most widely used, there is increasing evidence that psychotherapy, particularly CBT, is effective with or even instead of medication.[41]

The primary pharmacologic agents used to treat depression are antidepressants (**Table 29.3** ■). The most widely used antidepressant medications affect one or more of the major neurotransmitters (NE, DA, and/or 5-HT). The first antidepressant mediations were called the tricyclic antidepressants because of the three rings of atoms in their chemical structure. Their primary aim was to boost levels of NE at the synapse by inhibiting NE reuptake. As was detailed previously, NE deficiencies are one of the main putative causes of depression. Drugs that increase NE at the synapse were found to be effective in improving mood and are particularly effective in individuals with melancholic depression.[20] Unfortunately, the tricyclics also block histaminergic, muscarinic, and cholinergic receptors, resulting in side effects such as weight gain, drowsiness, urinary retention, dry mouth, and constipation.

A second class of antidepressants, MAO inhibitors, has a different mechanism of action that results in an increase in synaptic levels of NE and 5-HT. There are two types of MAO inhibitors: MAO-A and MAO-B. Because MAO-B inhibitors result in an increase in NE levels, increased blood pressure is an anticipated side effect. If MAO inhibitors are taken in combination with foods that contain the NE precursor tyramine, then serious hypertension, cerebral hemorrhage, myocardial infarction, and death may ensue. Tyramine is contained in foods such as aged cheeses, sausage, nuts, wine, and processed meats. Newer forms of

Table 29.3 Major Classes of Antidepressant Medications and Their Actions

Drug Class	Examples	Action
Tricyclics	Amitriptyline Desipramine Imipramine Nortriptyline	Blocks the reuptake pumps for NE, 5-HT, and to some extent DA, thus increasing the synaptic supply of NE and 5-HT.
MAO inhibitors (MAOs)	Isocarboxazid Phenelzine Tranylcypromine	Inhibits and binds to the MAO enzyme, which destroys its ability to destroy a monoamine neurotransporter, thus increasing NE. Irreversible.
Selective serotonin reuptake inhibitors (SSRIs)	Citalopram Escitalopram Fluoxetine Fluvoxamine Paroxetine Sertraline	Selectively blocks 5-HT reuptake, with far less influence on the uptake of NE.
Selective norepinephrine reuptake inhibitors (SNRIs)	Reboxetine	Selectively inhibit the reuptake of NE with less blockage of alpha-1, and muscarinic cholinergic receptors.
Norepinephrine and dopamine reuptake inhibitors	Bupropion	Enhances transmission of NE and DA with little effect on 5-HT.
Norepinephrine and specific serotonin antagonists	Mirtazapine Nefazodone Trazodone	Blocks both 5-HT_{2A} and alpha-2 receptors.
Serotonin and norepinephrine reuptake inhibitors (SNRIs)	Venlafaxine Duloxetine	Inhibits reuptake of both NE and 5-HT.

MAO inhibitors, reversible inhibitors of MAO-A, contain a component that continues to metabolize amines consumed in foods such as cheese, thus averting dangerous increases in blood pressure.

Partly in response to the drawbacks of tricyclics and irreversible MAO inhibitors and partly in recognition of the role of 5-HT in depression, the selective serotonin reuptake inhibitors were developed. As the name implies, SSRIs inhibit the reuptake of 5-HT and thus boost the level of the neurotransmitter at the synapse. Because of the interconnections of the monoamine system, they also increase plasma levels of NE and DA.[20] It may be that the antidepressant effects of SSRIs occur because of their ability to initiate an intracellular cascade that leads not only to receptor synthesis but also to BDNF production.[20] Thus, while the SSRIs are successful in treating depression and increases in 5-HT ameliorate many symptoms of depression, it remains unknown whether disruption in the monoamine system alone results in depressive symptoms.[20]

Alice Parry: Outcome

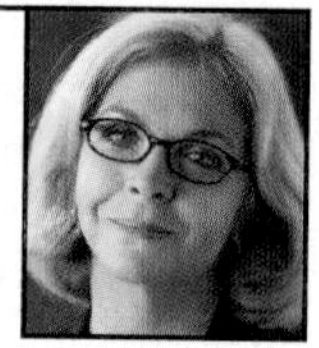

Ms. Parry's history reveals that both her father and a maternal aunt suffered from depression. Her physical examination is unremarkable, thyroid functions and ECG are normal. Her lipid profile is slightly elevated.

Following a discussion with the advanced practice nurse (APN), an antidepressant is initiated. Ms. Parry also agrees to a 10-week trial of cognitive-behavioral therapy, a new regime to improve her sleep hygiene and increase her exercise, and a diet that includes freshwater fish. The APN explained that Ms. Parry appears to be experiencing symptoms consistent with a type of major depression with atypical features. This type of depression, while responsive to antidepressants, may also improve with cognitive treatment as well as complementary therapies.

5. What symptoms did Ms. Parry experience that led to a diagnosis of major depression?
6. Why did the APN suggest both medication and cognitive-behavioral therapy for Ms. Parry?

Check Your Progress: Section 29.3

1. What disorder is characterized by a depressed mood that occurs on more days than not and occurs for most of the day for a period of 2 years or more?
2. What is a clinical syndrome characterized by the presence of one or more depressive episodes of 2 weeks or longer over an individual's lifetime?
3. What is the neurotransmitter that mediates positive mood, optimism, and impulsivity?

29.4 Bipolar Disorders

The **bipolar disorders** are a group of mood disorders characterized by manic, hypomanic, and depressive episodes. These episodes represent periods of fluctuation between two poles: depression and mania. Cyclothymic disorder, a related disorder, is characterized by alternating periods of hypomanic and depressive symptoms that are not significant enough to meet the criteria for hypomania or depression. Although less than 2% of the population is diagnosed with bipolar disorders, these types of disorders can have a tremendous impact on the people closest to the individual with the disorder.[39]

Bipolar I disorder consists of one or more manic or mixed episodes, and the course of illness is usually accompanied by major depressive episodes. **Bipolar II disorder** consists of one or more major depressive episodes accompanied by at least one hypomanic episode.

Mania and Hypomania

Mania is characterized by an abnormal and persistently elevated, expansive, or irritable mood and increased energy (or activity) present for most of the time, nearly every day, or a week or more and accompanied by other symptoms such as flight of ideas (rapidly changing, fragmented thoughts), pressured speech patterns, and increasing goal-directed activities. Psychotic symptoms such as delusions or hallucinations may be a feature of severe mania.

Hypomania is less extreme in presentation than mania. Typically, the individual experiencing hypomania does not experience impairment in function or need hospitalization. Psychosis does not occur. Despite feelings of euphoria during episodes of hypomania, the individual might not be aware that a change has occurred. Family members and coworkers, however, are aware of both mood and behavior changes.

Although manic episodes may begin to occur at any age, most people with bipolar disorders experience onset around age 18.[39] Onset of mania often occurs following an emotional trigger. In addition to feelings of euphoria, mania is characterized by bursts of activity that may alternate with periods of irritability if someone or something prevents the individual from maintaining or completing activities. Other characteristics of manic episodes include an increase in sexual behaviors, including wearing provocative clothes and makeup, and grandiosity. Individuals experiencing mania will deny any difficulty and typically refuse attempts at treatment.

Depressive Episodes

A diagnosis of bipolar disorder does not always mean that manic or hypomanic behaviors will be manifested in the current episode of illness. Bipolar I disorder and bipolar II disorder are characterized by periods of mania or hypomania alternating with major depressive episodes.

Mixed Features

The DSM-5 recognizes certain specifiers for bipolar and related disorders. These include the specifier "with mixed features," which recognizes that depressive episodes may occur and be accompanied by symptoms of mania or hypomania; and manic or hypomanic episodes may occur and be accompanied by symptoms characteristic of depressive episodes.[39]

Rapid Cycling

In bipolar disorder with **rapid cycling**, the individual experiences four or more depressive and/or manic episodes within 12 months. Each episode must be of appropriate duration (at least 1 week for manic or hypomanic episodes, 2 weeks for depressive episodes), and there must be either a period of remission in between the episodes or a switch to the opposite mood.[39]

Cyclothymic Disorder

Cyclothymic disorder is characterized by reoccurring episodes of hypomanic symptoms alternating with episodes of symptoms of depression that do not meet the criteria for diagnosis of a full episode of either hypomania or major depression. The symptoms must occur over a period of 2 or more years (1 year for children and adolescents) for a diagnosis to be made, and the symptoms must not be able to be explained by any other psychiatric disorder.[39]

The Etiology and Pathogenesis of Bipolar Disorders

No definitive cause or specific pathophysiology has been identified for bipolar spectrum disorders. Rather, they are thought to arise from a complex combination of genetic, physiologic, environmental, and psychosocial factors. Studies have not found significant evidence that bipolar disorder is localized to a specific area of the brain. However, studies in adults have found that the prefrontal cortex tends to be smaller and have decreased functioning in people who have been diagnosed with bipolar disorder.[42]

Immunologic abnormalities, including unusual patterns of inflammation and glial cell activation, may contribute to the pathophysiology of mania and bipolar disorder.[43] Mitochondrial dysfunction and oxidative stress also may be involved in bipolar disorder.[44,45] Children of parents with bipolar disorders have a 4–15% risk of having a bipolar disorder. Stressful life events (especially suicide of a family member); sleep cycle disruptions; family or caregivers with high expressed emotion; and an emotionally overinvolved, hostile, and critical communication pattern are factors associated with heritability. Bipolar disorders, schizophrenia, and major depressive disorders share biological susceptibility and inheritance patterns. Several genes and loci that may be associated with bipolar disorders, including glycogen synthase kinase-3β, have been discovered.[46]

Although family history remains the strongest predictor of bipolar disorders, among adolescents with depressive disorders, the presence of a disruptive disorder (such as oppositional-defiant disorder or intermittent explosive disorder) increases the likelihood of a diagnosis of bipolar disorder in adulthood.[47]

Clinical Manifestations and Diagnosis of Bipolar Disorders

For mania to be diagnosed, manifestations must occur daily, for most of the day, or a week or more, or less if hospitalization is required. Key aspects of mania include flight of ideas (racing thoughts), psychomotor agitation, pressured speech (rapid talking that may be insensible), altered sleep patterns, grandiosity (exaggerated sense of self-worth), and risky behaviors.[39] At least one manic episode is necessary to diagnose bipolar disorder type I. At least one hypomanic episode is necessary to diagnose bipolar disorder type II.

Children with bipolar disorders present with mood changes (such as being overly silly or joyful when that is unusual for the child) and behavioral changes (such as sleeping little but not feeling tired, and talking a lot and having racing thoughts).[48] Some children may exhibit lengthy, violent temper tantrums. Older children may take on multiple tasks simultaneously and develop grandiose plans for their projects.[39] Children must be assessed on the basis of their personal baseline because children of the same age may be at different developmental stages. Taking into consideration the different developmental stages, it is difficult to define "normal" and "abnormal."

The average onset of the first episode of mania, hypomania, or major depression is approximately 18, and the lifetime prevalence of bipolar disorders in adolescents is 0–3%.[39,49] Treatment for adolescents will follow the same guidelines as are used for children. Because teenagers commonly show mood changes, including changes in sleeping and eating patterns, it is important not to confuse typical mood swings with bipolar disorder. ■

Studies suggest that women who have been diagnosed with bipolar disorder are 5–10 times more likely to experience an episode during pregnancy than when not pregnant. Because stopping medications can worsen symptoms, some healthcare providers will slowly taper the woman off medications, decrease the dose, or change the medication when the woman learns that she is pregnant.[50] ■

Onset of bipolar disorder may occur at any time during life, including in the 60s or 70s.[39] As with any clients, first episodes of manic symptoms that present during midlife or late life indicate a need to perform medical testing to verify that there is no medical or substance-related etiology. Treatment will be the same for older adults as for younger adults, although doses of medications may be lower. Older adults are also prone to experience more side effects and toxicity, so they must be monitored very closely. For example, lithium is contraindicated in older clients with kidney disease and should be used cautiously in clients with thyroid disease. ■

Linking Pathophysiology to Treatment of Bipolar Disorders

For decades, lithium was the treatment of choice for mania, but its narrow therapeutic index and extensive side effect profile combined with the fact it takes up to 3 weeks to achieve its full effect often result in poor adherence by patients. Increasingly, atypical antipsychotics such as olanzapine, risperidone, and aripiprazole are being used to treat mania. Their demonstrated efficacy and lower side effect profile make them attractive for the initial management of acute mania. It is believed they block $5H2_2$ and D_2 receptors. They may be used in combination with lithium or anticonvulsants. Anticonvulsants have been found to be helpful in treating mania, possibly through modulation of GABA at presynaptic and postsynaptic nerve terminals.

Pregnant women should not take these medications except under the care of a healthcare provider and following a thorough discussion of the risks and benefits of continuing to take the medications. ■

CLINICAL POINT: Serum lithium levels should be determined before beginning lithium therapy, then should be carefully monitored once therapy has begun. Note also that what is considered a therapeutic level for one patient might produce toxic effects in another patient. Accordingly, individual response to specific lithium doses must be carefully documented.[51] For example, individuals of Asian descent may respond to lower doses and blood levels of lithium and therefore may experience toxicity at lower dosages than Caucasian patients will.[52] It is important to monitor therapeutic effects as well as side effects. ■

Nursing interventions include monitoring clients for adverse side effects of antipsychotic medications. These include extrapyramidal effects such as Parkinson-like symptoms (e.g., rigidity, tremor, or "pill rolling" movements of the fingers); dystonia, which is abnormal tonic contractions of the muscles (muscle spasms); and akathisia (subjective need to move, "jumping out of my skin"). Extrapyramidal symptoms should be reported and are usually treated by administration of an anticholinergic medication such as benztropine, diphenhydramine, or trihexyphenidyl. Acute dystonic reactions may be severe and require immediate medical intervention. These side effects can be distressing to the client. The nurse must reassure the client and explain what is occurring.

Bipolar disorder carries the highest risk suicide of any mental illness.[53] Nurses should conduct a suicide assessment at each healthcare interaction.

Check Your Progress: Section 29.4

1. Which bipolar disorder consists of one or more manic or mixed episodes, usually alternating with major depressive episodes?
2. What manifestations do bipolar disorders have in children?
3. What is the most common age of onset for bipolar disorders and what is the overall age range in which the condition is diagnosed?

CHAPTER SUMMARY

29.1 Chapter Overview and Case Studies

Define emotional regulation, and discuss concepts related to anxiety and depression.

- Emotional regulation is the ability to manage emotional responses to environmental stimuli that are perceived as aversive or negative.
- Disruption of emotional regulation can lead to the development of anxiety or depression.
- Anxiety and depression are normative emotional experiences that can be considered disorders when they affect social or personal functioning.
- Anxiety is an emotion that helps individuals adapt to a perceived challenge or threat.
- Anxiety-induced avoidance can severely limit social interaction and relationships.
- The pathophysiology of depression is best understood in terms of the action of specific neurotransmitters and intracellular mechanisms that alter gene expression, as well as how these mechanisms compromise neuronal growth.
- Certain brain mechanisms are also major players in the development of anxiety, primarily the parts of the brain associated with threat and fear.
- Perceiving a stimulus as a threat activates sympathetic responses, and the classification of anxiety is primarily based on signs and symptoms reflecting sympathetic nervous system activation. Neurotransmitters associated with autonomic responses such as norepinephrine, dopamine, and serotonin are tied to the pathogenesis of anxiety disorders, and the regulation of gamma-aminobutyric acid plays a role in the treatment process.

29.2 Anxiety

Describe the etiology, pathogenesis, and clinical manifestations of anxiety and approaches to diagnosis and treatment of the condition across the lifespan.

- Anxiety or fear is an emotion that helps individuals adapt to a perceived challenge or threat.
- Anxiety disorders occur when individuals experience an incapacitating sense of dread without any apparent threatening stimulus. These individuals cope by avoiding situations that generate these feelings, and this avoidance can severely limit social interaction, social relationships, and, in some instances, opportunities for growth.
- A variety of neuronal structures, neurotransmitters, neurochemicals, and hormones are posited to participate in the development of anxiety disorders, although

the exact nature of these components varies in relation to specific disorders.

- The development of anxiety disorders can be viewed in terms of classic fear conditioning, utilizing two processes called consolidation and reconsolidation, which underlie the formation of long-term memory development and reinforcement.
- The amygdala is thought to have three important roles in the response to stimuli. First, it confers significance on the stimuli that come from the thalamus or the hypothalamus. Second, it holds emotional memories and provides a preliminary threat assessment of a stimulus. Third, it has extensive projections to motor areas and areas of the brainstem that control autonomic responses (e.g., heart rate, breathing). Once a stimulus has been read as potentially dangerous, the amygdala fires off signals to ready the body for fight or flight. The amygdala also receives information about the stimulus from cortical areas that (depending on the information) may attenuate the threat alert.
- The hippocampus acts as a braking system on the HPA axis hormones, which play a role in the processing of threatening stimuli. Prolonged stress and prolonged activation of the HPA axis may result in hippocampal volume loss. The hippocampus is a critical structure for the formation of new memories, and volume loss may result in deficits in forming memories around the emotional context of a stimulus.
- Different areas in the prefrontal cortex function in the fear circuitry pathway, These areas register and assign meaning to the emotions generated by our body or the amygdala, weigh actions on the basis of potential reward and help the individual to adjust to changing circumstances, balance emotion and thought, control attention, and/or lock attention on important events.
- Disturbances with the caudate nucleus may affect the development of some anxiety disorders. The caudate nucleus orchestrates action–reward sequencing and drives behavior on the basis of the recall of past successful outcomes. A poorly functioning caudate would impair this recall, perhaps creating a focus on the negative aspects of a situation rather than the potential reward.
- The involvement of numerous neural structures in the pathophysiology of anxiety disorders is correlated with the involvement of a number of neurotransmitters, neurochemicals, and hormones. These include norepinephrine, serotonin, dopamine, GABA-benzodiazepine, glutamate, and HPA axis hormones.
- The GABA-benzodiazepine system is inhibitory within the CNS and functions through dedicated receptors. The role of this system in anxiety disorders is thought to be related either to GABA deficiencies or to a deficiency or decreased sensitivity of the receptors to BZD compounds.
- Norepinephrine function increases in key areas of the brain associated with anxiety when individuals enter stressful or anxious states. In these situations, the increased NE results in downregulation of its autoreceptor and the increased autonomic arousal (e.g., increased heart rate and blood pressure) that is characteristic of selected anxiety disorders.
- Decreased levels of serotonin are associated with attenuation of anxiety states. Although the mechanism involved is unclear, increased stress levels are correlated with increased turnover of 5-HT and subsequent depletion that may stimulate anxiety pathways.
- The hypothalamic-pituitary-adrenal (HPA) axis hormones, especially corticotropin-releasing hormone (CRH), are suspects in the pathophysiology of anxiety disorders. When stimulated, CRH-producing neurons in the amygdala increase fear-related behaviors. The relationship between CRH and cortisol levels with PTSD may be related to persistent stress that damages the hippocampus, an organ necessary for extinction; dysfunction at the level of the glucocorticoid receptors; or decreased hippocampal volume.

29.3 Depression

Describe the etiology, pathogenesis, and clinical manifestations of depression and approaches to diagnosis and treatment of the condition across the lifespan.

- Depression is a chronic, systemic mood disorder that can cause or result from comorbid medical disorders.
- Many theories have been posited to explain the neurobiological basis for depression, including monoamine theory, receptor dysregulation theory, intracellular gene transcription theory, stress and HPA axis dysfunction theory, neurotrophic theory, and inflammatory process theory.
- The monoamine theory of depression proposes that deficiencies of monoamine neurotransmitters such as norepinephrine, serotonin, and dopamine are responsible for depression.
- Each of the monoamines is related in a particular way to the mood alterations in depression. Serotonin transmission regulates obsessions and compulsions; dopamine transmission mainly regulates motivation, pleasure, and reward; and norepinephrine transmission regulates alertness and energy.
- Several aspects of neurotransmission involving monoamines may be related to the development of depression and relate to the monoamine deficiency theory, the receptor dysregulation theory, and the altered intracellular dynamics theory. These aspects include the amount of neurotransmitter released at the synaptic cleft; the removal of excess monoamine neurotransmitters from the synaptic cleft; the response, potentially dysregulatory, of monoamine receptors on both the

presynaptic and postsynaptic neurons; the targets of monoamine pathways in the brain (cortex, amygdala, hippocampus, thalamus, and hypothalamus); the interrelationships among the cellular effects of monoamine neurotransmitters; and the potential effects of monoamines on the intracellular dynamics of target cells.

- Overactivation of the hypothalamic-pituitary-adrenal axis in the context of continual stressful or threatening situations is posited as a potential cause of depression. The excessive secretion of cortisol and ensuing desensitization of receptors for mineralocorticoids and glucocorticoids that turn off the stress response can lead to a feedback loop that is hypersensitive to even minimal stress. Individuals with certain types of depression demonstrate increased cortisol levels. The excessive cortisol secretion appears to have a negative effect on the hippocampus, resulting in profound atrophy. The hippocampus is thought to mediate memory formation, learning, mood, and emotions.
- Depression is found to be associated with increased inflammatory markers called cytokines. This increase in immune response appears to be most obvious with males with a history of early life stress. The cytokines activate the HPA axis and demonstrate restrictive effects on the precursors of serotonin.
- Depression is increasingly associated with a variety of medical disorders, including cardiovascular disorders, hypertension, osteoporosis, and diabetes. The shared underlying pathophysiology may be related to chronic stress, HPA axis dysregulation, heightened inflammatory response, and/or hyperactivity of the sympathetic nervous system.
- Neuroanatomic (structural) abnormalities are also reported in individuals with depression. There is probably a relationship between the anatomic and physiologic changes noted in individuals with depression.
- The frontal and temporal lobes, basal ganglia, and limbic system are known to influence many aspects of emotion, mood, and associated behaviors. These key areas of the brain, therefore, are thought to play a prominent role in mood dysfunction. Depressed individuals demonstrate tissue loss in these areas.
- In correlation with the prominence and longevity of the monoamine deficiency theory and the monoamine receptor dysregulation theory, the primary treatment for depression currently is pharmacologic and involves an ever-expanding armamentarium of antidepressants.

29.4 Bipolar Disorders

Describe the etiology, pathogenesis, and clinical manifestations of bipolar disorders and approaches to diagnosis and treatment of these conditions across the lifespan.

- Bipolar disorders are a group of mood disorders that are characterized by manic, hypomanic, and depressive episodes.
- Bipolar I disorder consists of one or more manic or mixed episodes.
- Bipolar II disorder consists of one or more major depressive episodes accompanied by at least one hypomanic episode.
- Mania is an abnormal and persistently elevated, expansive, or irritable mood and increased energy (or activity) present for most of the time, nearly every day, or a week or more.
- Mania is also associated with several other symptoms such as pressured speech, increased participation in goal-directed activities, and a pattern of thinking that is often fragmented and moves from one topic to another incessantly.
- Cyclothymic disorder is characterized by recurring episodes of hypomanic symptoms alternating with episodes of symptoms of depression that do not meet the criteria for diagnosis of a full episode of either hypomania or major depression over a period of 2 or more years.
- No definitive cause or specific pathophysiology has been identified for bipolar spectrum disorders.
- Genetic and other factors are believed to interact in a complex fashion in the pathogenesis of bipolar disorders. Immunologic abnormalities, including unusual patterns of inflammation and glial cell activation, may contribute to disease pathogenesis. Lithium was the mainstay of treatment for many years. Over the past decade, anticonvulsants and antipsychotics have seen increased use.

REVIEW QUESTIONS

1. What type of regulation is the ability to manage emotional responses to environmental stimuli perceived as aversive or negative?
   a. Aversive
   b. Negative
   c. Emotional
   d. Depressive
2. What disorders occur when individuals experience an incapacitating sense of dread without any apparent threatening stimulus?
   a. Depression
   b. Anxiety
   c. GAD
   d. Bipolar
3. What is thought to have three important roles in the response to stimuli?
   a. Amygdala
   b. Cortex
   c. Thalamus
   d. Hypothalamus

4. What theory of depression proposes that deficiencies of monoamine neurotransmitters such as norepinephrine, serotonin, and dopamine are responsible for depression?
   a. Serotonin
   b. Dopamine
   c. Norepinephrine
   d. Monoamine
5. Overactivation of what axis in the context of continual stressful or threatening situations is posited as a potential cause of depression?
   a. Cortex
   b. Cortisol
   c. Hypothalamic-pituitary-adrenal
   d. Antidepressants
6. Nursing interventions while working with a client with depression include an awareness of the need to monitor for adverse side effects tied to which of the following categories of pharmacologic therapies:
   a. Antipsychotics.
   b. MAO inhibitors.
   c. Selective serotonin reuptake inhibitors (SSRIs).
   d. Anticholinergics.
7. Lithium is most likely to be a contraindicated therapy in which group of clients with kidney disease?
   a. Asian
   b. Children
   c. Older
   d. Pregnant
8. Which of the following disorders is characterized by recurring episodes of hypomanic symptoms alternating with episodes of symptoms of depression that do not meet the criteria for diagnosis of a full episode of either hypomania or major depression?
   a. Cyclothymic
   b. Bipolar
   c. Anxiety
   d. Depression

ANSWERS

Answers to Review Questions can be found in Appendix A. Answers to Case Study and Check Your Progress questions are available on the faculty resources site. Please consult with your instructor.

RECOMMENDED WEBSITES

American Psychological Association: Anxiety
http://www.apa.org/topics/anxiety/index.aspx

Anxiety and Depression Association of America
https://www.adaa.org

National Alliance on Mentally Illness
https://www.nami.org

National Institute of Mental Health: Anxiety Disorders
https://www.nimh.nih.gov/health/topics/anxiety-disorders/index.shtml

National Institute of Mental Health: Depression
https://www.nimh.nih.gov/health/topics/depression/index.shtml

REFERENCES

1. American Psychiatric Association. (2013). *Desk reference to the diagnostic criteria from DSM-5*. Arlington, VA: American Psychiatric Association Publishing.
2. Benson, C., et al. (2015). Biogenic amines and the amino acids GABA and glutamate: Relationships with pain and depression. *Modern Trends in Pharmacopsychiatry, 30*, 67–79.
3. Duman, R. S. (2014). Neurobiology of stress, depression, and rapid acting antidepressants: Remodeling synaptic connections. *Depression and Anxiety, 31*(4), 291–296.
4. American Psychiatric Association. (2016). *Anxiety disorders: DSM-5 selections*. Arlington, VA: American Psychiatric Association Publishing.
5. National Institute of Mental Health, National Institutes of Health. (2017). *Generalized anxiety disorder among adults*. Available at https://www.nimh.nih.gov/health/statistics/prevalence/generalized-anxiety-disorder-among-adults.shtml
6. Anxiety and Depression Association of America. (2017). *Generalized anxiety disorder*. Available at https://www.adaa.org/understanding-anxiety/generalized-anxiety-disorder-gad
7. National Institute of Mental Health. (2017). *Panic disorder among adults*. Available at https://www.nimh.nih.gov/health/statistics/prevalence/panic-disorder-among-adults.shtml
8. Shimada-Sugimoto, M., Otowa, T., & Hettma, J. M. (2015). Genetics of anxiety disorders: Genetic epidemiology and molecular studies in humans. *PCN Frontier Review, 69*(7), 388–401.
9. Hansen Lagattuta, K. (Ed.). (2014). *Contributions to Human Development*: Vol. 26: *Children and emotion: New insights into developmental affective sciences* (pp. 42–56). Davis, CA: Karger.

10. World Health Organization & Calouste Gulbenkian Foundation. (2014). *Social determinants of mental health*. Geneva, Switzerland: World Health Organization.
11. Isomura, K., Boman, M., Rück, C., Serlachius, E., Larsson, H., Lichtenstein, P., & Mataix-Cols, D. (2015). Population-based, multi-generational family clustering study of social anxiety disorder and avoidant personality disorder. *Psychological Medicine, 45*(8), 1581–1589. doi:10.1017/S0033291714002116
12. Plieger, T., Montag, C., Felten, A., & Reuter, M. (2014). The serotonin transporter polymorphism (5-HTTLPR) and personality: Response style as a new endophenotype for anxiety. *International Journal of Neuropsychopharmacology, 17*(6): 851–858. doi:10.1017/S1461145713001776
13. Farach, F. J., Pruitt, L. P., Jun, J. J., Jerud, A. B., Zoellner, L. A., & Roy-Byrne, P. P. (2012). Pharmacological treatment of anxiety disorders: Current treatments and future directions. *Journal of Anxiety Disorders, 26*(8), 833–843.
14. Frick, A., Åhs, F., Engman, J., Jonasson, M., Alaie, I., Björkstrand, J., Frans, Ö., Faria, V., Linnman, C., Appel, L., Wahlstedt, K., Lubberink, M., Fredrikson, M., & Furmark, T. (2015). Serotonin synthesis and reuptake in social anxiety disorder: A positron emission tomography study. *JAMA Psychiatry, 72*(8), 794–802.
15. Nuss, P. (2015). Anxiety disorders and GABA neurotransmission: A disturbance of modulation. *Neuropsychiatric Disease and Treatment, 11*, 165–175. doi:10.2147/NDT.S58841
16. Olivier, J. D. A, Vinkers, C. H., & Olivier, B. (2013). The role of the serotonergic and GABA system in translational approaches in drug discovery for anxiety disorders. *Frontiers in Pharmacology, 4*, 74. doi:10.3389/fphar.2013.00074
17. Belujon, P., & Grace, A. A. (2011). Hippocampus, amygdala, and stress: Interacting systems that affect susceptibility to addiction. *Annals of the New York Academy of Sciences, 1216*, 114–121. doi:10.1111/j.1749-6632.2010.05896.x
18. Nikolaus, S., Antke, C., Beu, M., et al. (2011). Cortical GABA, striatal dopamine and midbrain serotonin as the key players in compulsive and anxiety disorders: Results from in vivo imaging studies. *Reviews in the Neurosciences, 21*(2), 119–140.
19. Maras, P. M., & Baram, T. Z. (2012). Sculpting the hippocampus from within: Stress, spines, and CRH. *Trends in Neurosciences, 35*(5), 315–324.
20. Anderson, I. A., & McAllister-Williams, R. H. (2016). *Fundamentals of clinical psychopharmacology* (4th ed.). Boca Raton, FL: CRC Press.
21. World Health Organization. (2017). *Media center: Depression*. Available at http://www.who.int/mediacentre/factsheets/fs369/en
22. Nanayakkara, S., Misch, D., Chang, L. and Henry, D. (2013). Depression and exposure to suicide predict suicide attempt. *Depression and Anxiety, 30*, 991–996. doi:10.1002/da.22143
23. Centers for Disease Control and Prevention. (2017). *Depression is not a normal part of growing older*. Available at https://www.cdc.gov/aging/mentalhealth/depression.htm
24. Kessler, R. C., & Bromet, E. J. (2013). The epidemiology of depression across cultures. *Annual Review of Public Health, 34*, 119–138.
25. Alzahrani, H., & Venneri, A. (2015). Cognitive and neuroanatomical correlates of neuropsychiatric symptoms in Parkinson's disease: A systematic review. *Journal of Neurological Science, 356*(1–2), 32–44.
26. Hamon, M., & Blier, P. (2013). Monoamine neurocircuitry in depression and strategies for new treatments. *Progress in Neuro-Psychopharmacology and Biological Psychiatry, 45*(1), 54–63.
27. Gold, P. W. (2015). The organization of the stress system and its dysregulation in depressive illness. *Molecular Psychiatry, 20*(1), 32–47.
28. Gold, P. W., Machado-Vieira, R., & Pavlatou, M. G. (2015). Clinical and biochemical manifestations of depression: Relation to the neurobiology of stress. *Neural Plasticity, 2015*, Article ID 581976. doi:10.1155/2015/581976
29. Bianchi, R., & Laurent, E. (2016). Altered short-term plasticity within the working memory neural network: Is it neuroticism or is it depression? *Human Brain Mapping, 37*(4), 1512–1513.
30. Rock, P. L., Roiser, J. P., Riedel, W. J., & Blackwell, A. D. (2014). Cognitive impairment in depression: A systematic review and meta-analysis. *Psychological Medicine, 44*(10), 2029–2040.
31. Leyhe, T., et al. (2017). A common challenge in older adults: Classification, overlap, and therapy of depression and dementia. *Alzheimer's & Dementia, 13*(1), 59–71.
32. Goodwin, G. M. (2016). Neuroanatomy of cognition in major depressive disorder. In R. S. McIntyre & D. S. Cha (Eds.), *Cognitive impairment in major depressive disorder: Clinical relevance, biological substrates, and treatment opportunities* (pp. 60–68). Cambridge, UK: Cambridge University Press.
33. Webb, C. A., Weber, M., Mundy, E. A., & Killgore, W. D. S. (2014). Reduced gray matter volume in the anterior cingulate, orbitofrontal cortex and thalamus as a function of mild depressive symptoms: A voxel-based morphometric analysis. *Psychological Medicine, 44*(13), 2833–2843. doi:10.1017/S0033291714000348
34. Gunaydin, L. A., & Kreitzer, A. C. (2016). Cortico-basal ganglia circuit function in psychiatric disease. *Annual Review of Psychology, 78*, 327–350.
35. Moylan, S., Maes, M., Wray, N. R., & Berk, M. (2013). The neuroprogressive nature of major depressive disorder: Pathways to disease evolution and resistance, and therapeutic implications. *Molecular Psychiatry, 18*(5), 595–606. doi:10.1038/mp.2012.33.
36. Yu, H., & Chen, Z. (2011). The role of BDNF in depression on the basis of its location in the neural circuitry. *Acta Pharmacologica Sinica, 32*, 3–11.
37. Zhong, M., Wang, X., Xiao, J., Yi, J., Zhu, X., Liao, J., Wang, W., & Yao, S. (2011). Amygdala hyperactivation and prefrontal hypoactivation in subjects with cognitive vulnerability to depression, *Biological Psychology, 88*(2–3), 233–242.
38. Hulvershorn, L. A., Cullen, K., & Anand, A. (2011). Toward dysfunctional connectivity: A review of neuroimaging findings in pediatric major depressive disorder. *Brain Imaging and Behavior, 5*(4), 307–328. doi:10.1007/s11682-011-9134-3
39. American Psychiatric Association. (2015). *Diagnostic and statistical manual of mental disorders* (5th ed.). Washington, DC: American Psychiatric Association Publishing.
40. Schiller, C. E., Meltzer-Brody, S., & Rubinow, D. R. (2015). The role of reproductive hormones in postpartum depression. *CNS Spectrums, 20*(1), 48–59. doi:10.1017/S1092852914000480
41. Halverson, J.L. (2015). Cognitive behavioral therapy for depression medication. Medscape. Retrieved from http://emedicine.medscape.com/article/2094696-medication
42. Phelps, J. (2014). *Chapter 2: Brain differences in bipolar*. Available at http://psycheducation.org/the-biologic-basis-of-bipolar-disorder/1035-2
43. Stertz, L., Magalhaes, P. V. S., & Kapczinski, F. (2012). Is bipolar disorder an inflammatory condition? The relevance of microglial activation. *Current Opinion in Psychiatry, 26*, 19–26.
44. Andreazza, A. C., Wang, J. F., Salmasi, F., Shao, L., & Young, L. T. (2013). Specific subcellular changes in oxidative stress in prefrontal cortex from patients with bipolar disorder. *Journal of Neurochemistry, 127*, 552–561.
45. Morris, G., & Berk, M. (2015). The many roads to mitochondrial dysfunction in neuroimmune and neuropsychiatric disorders. *BMC Medicine, 13*, 68.
46. Price, A. L., & Marzani-Nissen, G. R. (2012). Bipolar disorder: A review. *American Family Physician, 85*(5), 483–493. Available at http://www.aafp.org/afp/2012/0301/p483.html
47. Paaren, A., Bohman, H., von Knorring, L., Olsson, G., von Knorring, A.-L., & Jonsson, U. (2014). Early risk factors for adult bipolar disorder in adolescents with mood disorders: A 15-year follow-up of a community sample. *BMC Psychiatry, 14*, 363. Available at https://bmcpsychiatry.biomedcentral.com/articles/10.1186/s12888-014-0363-z
48. American Academy of Child and Adolescent Psychiatry. (2015). *Bipolar disorder in children and teens*. Available at http://www

.aacap.org/AACAP/Families_and_Youth/Facts_for_Families/FFF-Guide/Bipolar-Disorder-In-Children-And-Teens-038.aspx

49. National Institute of Mental Health. (2013b). *Bipolar disorder among children*. Available at http://www.nimh.nih.gov/statistics/1BIPOLAR_CHILD.shtml
50. Freeland, K. N., & Shealy, K. M. (2013). Toolbox: Psychotropic use in pregnancy and lactation. *Mental Health Clinician, 3*(2) 45–57.
51. Machado-Vieira, R., Zanetti, M. V., De Sousa, R. T., Soeiro de Souza, M. G., Moreno, R. A., Busatto, G. F., & Gattaz, W. F. (2014). Lithium efficacy in bipolar depression with flexible dosing: A six-week, open-label, proof-of-concept study. *Experimental and Therapeutic Medicine, 8*, 1205–1208.
52. Yeung, T., & Cheng, D. (2012). Mood disorders in Asians. In E. C. Chang (Ed.), *Handbook of adult psychopathology in Asians: Theory, diagnosis, and treatment* (pp. 108–142). New York, NY: Oxford University Press.
53. da Silva Costa, L., et al. (2015). Risk factors for suicide in bipolar disorder: A systematic review. *Journal of Affective Disorders, 170*, 237–254. Available at http://www.jad-journal.com/article/S0165-0327(14)00548-5/abstract?cc=y=

Chapter 30

Neurocognitive and Neurodevelopmental Disorders

Cynthia Parkman

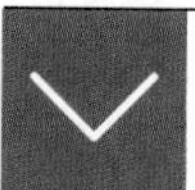

Chapter Outline and Learning Outcomes

30.1 Chapter Overview and Case Studies

Describe normal development and cognition, the range of disorders that affect development, and concepts related to those disorders.

30.2 Pathophysiology of Neurocognitive and Neurodevelopmental Disorders

Differentiate the causes, classification, underlying pathogenesis, and mechanisms related to development of neurocognitive and neurodevelopmental disorders across the lifespan.

30.3 Schizophrenia

Differentiate the causes, classification, underlying pathogenesis, and clinical manifestations of schizophrenia and approaches to diagnosis and treatment of this condition across the lifespan.

30.4 Neurocognitive Disorders

Differentiate the causes, classification, underlying pathogenesis, and clinical manifestations of neurocognitive disorders and approaches to diagnosis and treatment of these conditions across the lifespan.

30.5 Genetic Neurodevelopmental Disorders

Differentiate the genetics and genomics, classification, underlying pathogenesis, and clinical manifestations of neurodevelopmental disorders and approaches to diagnosis and treatment of these conditions across the lifespan.

KEY TERMS

Alzheimer disease (AD), 738
Attention-deficit/hyperactivity disorder (ADHD), 740
Autism spectrum disorder (ASD), 741
Cognition, 731
Delirium, 739
Dementia, 737
Development, 731
Down syndrome (DS), 742
Fetal alcohol syndrome disorders (FASD), 743
Neurocognitive disorders (NCDs), 731
Neurodevelopmental disorders, 731
Psychosis, 735
Schizophrenia, 735
Vascular dementia, 738

ABBREVIATIONS

AD—Alzheimer disease
ADHD—attention-deficit/hyperactivity disorder
ASD—autism spectrum disorder
DS—Down syndrome
FASD—fetal alcohol spectrum disorder
FTD—formal thought disorder
NCD—neurocognitive disorder

30.1 Chapter Overview and Case Studies

Normal development and cognition begin with maternal health, including adequate maternal nutrition; regular prenatal care; and avoidance of alcohol, nicotine, and other substances during pregnancy. A healthy baby born at or near term is likely to meet milestones normal for age at predictable intervals between birth and 5 months. **Cognition** is the way in which people acquire, store, learn, use and communication information. **Development** involves the ability to adapt to the environment and refers to behavioral aspects of growth such as talking, walking, and running. Growth and development, including cognitive development, generally occur in stages, beginning with simple tasks, such as grasping, and moving on toward more complex tasks, such as feeding oneself with utensils. Alterations in these areas that are severe and chronic may rise to the level of being a neurocognitive or neurodevelopmental disorder. It is beyond the scope of this text to discuss cognition and development in full, but the basics are covered in this chapter as they relate to pathophysiology.

Neurocognitive disorders (NCDs) are disorders whose primary features are cognitive impairments. The NCDs include delirium and the various forms of dementia. NCDs may be further characterized as mild or major.[1] This chapter provides an overview of delirium and the two most prevalent forms of dementia: Alzheimer disease and vascular dementia. It also provides an overview of psychosis, a severe clinical manifestation of disturbed thought processes that may occur with an illness or as an adverse effect of a recreational or prescription medication, and schizophrenia, a serious mental illness characterized by altered thought processes.

Neurodevelopmental disorders are impairments of brain function that occur as the brain develops and usually manifest before a child enters kindergarten. Neurodevelopmental disorders may affect children across several domains, including language, coordination, attention, and behavior. Although a number of neurodevelopmental disorders have been identified, this chapter focuses specifically on attention-deficit/hyperactivity disorder and autism spectrum disorder. Two other disorders that are identified in early childhood, Down syndrome and fetal alcohol syndrome, are also discussed.

Concepts Related to Neurocognitive and Neurodevelopmental Disorders

Cognitive function and other systems tend to be interdependent, so determining the extent to which other concepts or systems are involved can be complicated. For example, cerebral perfusion is necessary for normal cognitive functioning but depends on an adequate intake of oxygen and the osmotic pressure needed to maintain adequate blood flow. Any condition that impairs cerebral perfusion will result in inflammation and metabolic changes that further impair cognition. Even subtle variations in perfusion can result in acute alterations in cognitive function, such as delirium. Older adults are more sensitive to these changes, owing to diminished functional reserves.[2] Possible causes of diminished cerebral tissue perfusion include (but are not limited to) cerebral edema, cerebral vascular accidents, spasms or compression of cerebral vessels, hypotension, and shock. Chronic cerebral hypoperfusion from decreased cardiac output and vascular changes have been implicated in Alzheimer disease and other chronic and degenerative neurologic disorders.[3]

Cerebral perfusion and cognitive integrity depend on normal gas exchange. Decreased oxygenation leads to respiratory acidosis, in which levels of carbon dioxide increase and vasodilation of blood vessels occurs, resulting in increased intracranial pressure. Symptoms of acute oxygen deprivation include headaches, confusion, and irritability. Hypoxia and hypoxemia can both trigger delirium, especially if a respiratory or other infection is present or if the patient has other risk factors for delirium. Chronic and subtle mechanisms involved in decreased oxygen supply to the brain (as seen in chronic obstructive pulmonary disease and anemia) can negatively affect the neurochemical signaling and synaptic plasticity necessary for normal cognitive development and function.[4]

Fluid and electrolyte balance is also necessary to maintain adequate perfusion and to support cellular function in the brain. A change in mental status, memory, or attention is often an early sign of dehydration in older adults. Cerebral cells are the first to be affected by the shift from the vascular to the intracellular space that occurs as a result of fluid volume excess. Early signs of cerebral edema include headache, nausea and vomiting, and changes in mental status.[5]

Brain function depends on complex metabolic processes to meet the energy needs of neuronal cells and maintain the synthesis and function of neurochemicals in cognition. Any alteration in the normal glucose supply or an excess or deficiency of other metabolic products can result in either acute or chronic cognitive dysfunction.[6] Both hypoglycemia and hyperglycemic ketoacidosis can result in confusion, hallucinations, and changes in consciousness. Infection, inflammation, and alterations in thermoregulation increase overall metabolic demands and can precipitate changes in cognitive function.

Inflammation appears to play a key role in altered cognitive function. Stress, infection, surgery, and cancer all result in an inflammatory response and the release of cytokines. Inflammation can occur in the brain and central nervous system as a direct result of trauma, cerebral infarction, or bacterial, viral, fungi, or prion infections. Peripheral inflammation (outside of the central nervous system) causes a cascade of physiologic events that alter glutamate, serotonin, dopamine, and acetylcholine systems considered central in cognition, with implications for an array of affective, cognitive, and behavioral responses.[7] Initially, these changes are adaptive, enabling individuals to conserve energy necessary for healing. However, chronic or persistent inflammation can lead to irreversible neuronal changes. Both aging and chronic inflammation also appear to lead to increased sensitivity of the microglia to the effects of inflammation, partly explaining why older adults experience exaggerated changes in cognition in response to illness and infection. Recent research also demonstrates that some individuals with cognitive disorders such as Alzheimer disease and schizophrenia have higher levels of proteins associated with inflammatory response to illness and infection.[8]

Substances such as alcohol, illicit drugs, and some pharmaceuticals can affect cognitive function. Immediate consequences of alcohol intoxication include confusion, decreased attention, impaired judgment, loss of inhibition, disorientation, hallucinations, and memory loss. Chronic alcohol abuse can lead to hematologic changes that can limit oxygenation to the brain and lead to encephalopathy. Older adults are at a higher risk of permanent cognitive changes as a result of excessive alcohol consumption.[9]

Permanent brain injury caused by trauma or acute oxygenation deprivation is a common source of cognitive pathophysiology. Cognitive disorders such as schizophrenia and learning disabilities are associated with both obvious and subtle anatomic differences in brain development and structure as well as developmental delays. A map of concepts related to disorders of neurodevelopment and neurocognition is shown in **Figure 30.1** ■.

Case Studies

The following case studies will be addressed throughout the chapter to assist in application of chapter content to clinical situations that involve individuals with neurocognitive and neurodevelopmental disorders.

Anthony Martin: Introduction

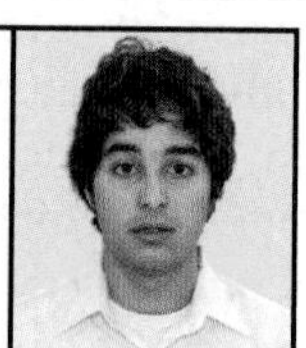

Anthony Martin is a 17-year-old high school senior. He lives with his parents, Helen and Gil Martin, and two siblings, Tracie and Kristina. He gets along with his family but still feels somewhat isolated. His parents are not aware that Anthony feels this way. They perceive him to be a quiet, serious child. He tends not to interact much with family members and prefers to isolate himself in his bedroom. Although Anthony is an excellent student with a 3.9 GPA, he does not participate in any school-related activities except science fairs. He has few friends and rarely socializes because he is more comfortable being alone. Many of the kids at school consider him to be weird, but he is never teased or bullied. For the most part, he just blends in with the other students. His typical routine involves going to school, coming home, and working part-time. Three nights a week, Anthony bags groceries at the local grocery store. He gets along well with his coworkers. In fact, the cashiers (who tend to be middle-aged women) like it when Anthony works because he is very polite and doesn't horse around. Anthony is in excellent health and, with the exception of dental examinations, has not needed health-related care since entering high school.

1. What social manifestations does Anthony exhibit that could be a cause for concern?
2. What, if any, cognitive factors might be a cause for concern in Anthony?

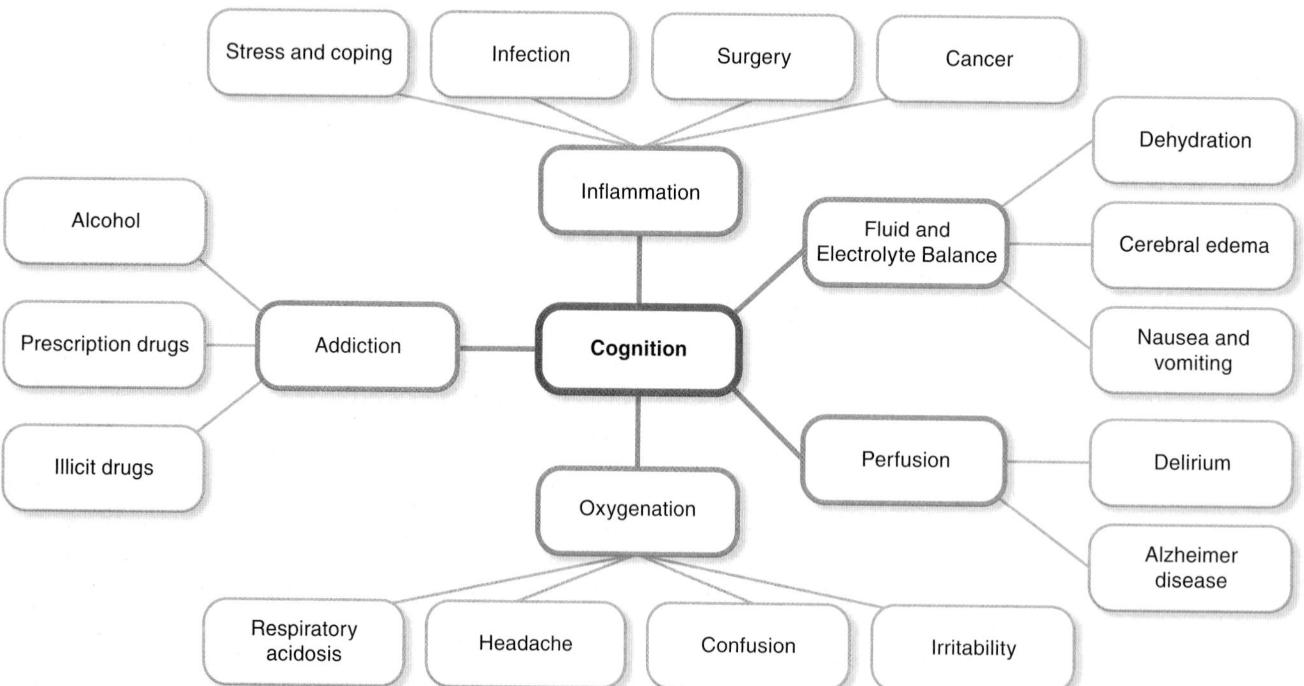

Figure 30.1 ■ Concepts related to neurocognitive and neurodevelopmental disorders.

Lydia Ocampo: Introduction

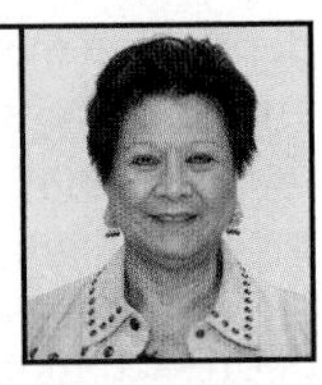

Lydia Ocampo, age 69, has been married to her husband Danilo for 51 years. Their only child, Emilio, was killed at age 22 in an automobile accident. His death devastated Mrs. Ocampo, but over time, she adjusted and coped with the loss. Mrs. Ocampo was born and raised in the Philippines and came to the United States with her husband when she was 18. Lydia has a 77-year-old sister who is still alive, but her other eight brothers and sisters have passed away. She has several nieces and nephews still living in the Philippines, whom Mr. and Mrs. Ocampo have not seen in years, and one grand-niece who is attending college in the United States. Mr. and Mrs. Ocampo have no relatives nearby. Mrs. Ocampo's overall physical health is good, and her only known condition is Alzheimer disease. She has had dementia for several years. Her husband is her caregiver, and she benefits from the consistent routine that he provides. She rarely socializes and spends most of her time at home. She is fully ambulatory and feeds, dresses, and toilets herself. She is often confused and is easily distracted. This morning, Mr. Ocampo places her clothes on the bed so that she can get dressed to go to the store with him. She puts on one shoe and then goes to the closet to find another shoe. She ends up wearing a brown slip-on shoe and a blue sandal. While Mrs. Ocampo is walking in the store with her husband, he asks her about the shoes, and she is surprised to see that they don't match.

1. On the basis of her history, does Mrs. Ocampo suffer from a neurodevelopmental or neurocognitive disorder?
2. What is the correlation between cerebral perfusion and Alzheimer disease?

Jason Riley: Introduction

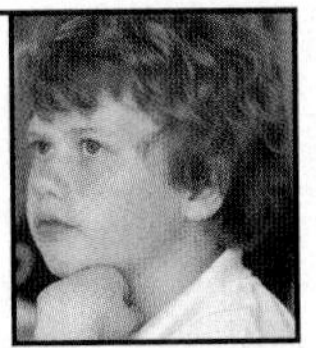

Jason Riley is a 10-year-old boy with a history of academic and behavioral problems at school. His mother has been trying to get help for him for some time but with no success. Jason has had problems in school for the past 3 years. Teachers report that he has difficulty staying on task and will not follow directions. Although Jason made some progress last year with his fourth-grade teacher, his grades this year have been consistently poor. His mother tries to help him with homework after school or in the evenings, but these sessions frequently turn into battles. It takes Jason hours to complete fairly simple assignments, resulting in a great deal of frustration for him and his mother. The fact that he frequently comes home from school with headaches further aggravates the situation. In addition to problems with academics, Jason has problems with social interactions. His teachers at school find him to be disruptive in the classroom. During the past year, he has frequently been sent to the principal's office for misbehaving. He is often teased at school. Most of his time at home is spent watching TV and playing video games. It is determined that he is nearsighted, and after an eye examination, he gets glasses, but this doesn't resolve the problems at school.

1. On the basis of Jason's history, is it more likely that he suffers from a neurocognitive disorder or a neurodevelopmental disorder?
2. Describe the behavioral aspects of development in children.

Check Your Progress: Section 30.1

1. What is an early cognitive sign of dehydration in older adults?
2. What is the difference between neurodevelopmental disorders and neurocognitive disorders?
3. What are the cognitive signs and symptoms of acute oxygen deprivation?

30.2 Pathophysiology of Neurocognitive and Neurodevelopmental Disorders

The pathophysiology of neurocognitive and neurodevelopmental disorders varies by disorder but often results from a combination of factors. Two overarching factors are maternal health and genetics. Although how these affect specific disorders can vary, maternal health during pregnancy and early childhood and genetic expression in environmental circumstances are implicated in many cases.

Maternal Health and Neurodevelopment

The circumstances surrounding a birth, during both the prenatal and postnatal periods, may have a profound influence on a person's neurodevelopment and neurocognition. The choices a woman makes during pregnancy can have serious, long-term consequences for both herself and her child.

Both active and passive smoking and the use of alcohol (in even small and moderate amounts) during pregnancy are recognized as significant issues from both clinical and public health perspectives.[10] Maternal smoking during pregnancy is associated with significant infant morbidity and mortality, and there is evidence that it increases disease risk.[11] For example, smoking during pregnancy is associated with increased prevalence of asthma among adolescents.[12] Recent studies have continued to show some relationship between active and passive maternal smoking and children's psychomotor development. However, this relationship is not straightforward. The association appears mostly for measures of academic achievements and behavioral problems that require further attention. The results of the studies on low or moderate exposure to alcohol during pregnancy are not fully conclusive, but some of them suggest that consumption of alcohol during pregnancy may adversely affect children's intelligence quotient (IQ), mental health, memory, and verbal or visual performance.[10]

Because any effects on fetal and infant brain development have consequences for the person's entire life, prenatal developmental issues need to be identified and understood at an early stage. According to the concept of fetal programming, fetal stress, among other factors, can permanently change fetal brain development and cause diseases in later life.[13]

One of the most important mechanisms related to neurocognitive development is maternal and early childhood nutrition. Developmental potential is the "ability to think, learn, remember, relate, and articulate ideas appropriate to age and level of maturity." Worldwide, 39% of children under age 5 years do not attain their developmental potential.[14] Appropriate maternal nutrition and breastfeeding support neurocognitive development through pregnancy and the first 6 months of life.

Numerous studies focusing on the positive effects of breastfeeding on various aspects of children's development can be found in the healthcare literature. This interest arises because breastfeeding is a modifiable health behavior that, it has been suggested, has the potential to enhance the baby's physical, emotional, and cognitive development.[15] Regarding the link between breastfeeding and cognition, "the debate centers around whether it is breast milk augmenting neurological development that is responsible for the cognitive advantages of breastfed children"[15] or whether these children simply had a more advantaged childhood environment that was correlated with higher academic achievement. That breastfeeding is so strongly related to socioeconomic status reinforces the need for health promotion campaigns to target socially disadvantaged groups to reduce social inequalities in health and optimize children's potential.[15]

CLINICAL POINT: Early assessment of maternal body mass index can highlight issues of undernutrition before a woman becomes pregnant or at the start of pregnancy. Women who are underweight may benefit from a full assessment and teaching related to nutrition and diet that is tailored to their individual needs, habits, schedules, and cultural beliefs and practices. ■

Diseases present in a pregnant female can influence her child's neurodevelopment. For example, one study compared the neurodevelopment of HIV-infected infants in combination with antiretroviral therapy with that of HIV-exposed uninfected infants.[16] This study suggested that HIV-positive infants are delayed when compared to exposed but uninfected infants. Antiretroviral therapy may help to prevent further developmental delays; however, it does not reverse the neurologic damage that is already present.[16] There is a need for therapists to be involved in pediatric HIV clinical services to provide early developmental screening as well as rehabilitative services to children in need.

Maternal mental health also has been linked to infant and child development. Some factors that affect maternal mental health are family and social supports, including the quality of the partner relationship; interpersonal violence; coping strategies; and physical health during pregnancy.[14] More recently, studies are focusing on the role of maternal depression, which is increasingly found to be a risk factor for poor child development. In particular, maternal depression may be associated with increased prevalence for attention-deficit/hyperactivity disorder and oppositional defiant disorder as well as lower levels of social engagement and empathy. Apter-Levy, Feldman, Vakart, Ebstein, and Feldman found that family members of chronically depressed mothers experienced dysfunction in their oxytocin systems. Oxytocin is a neuropeptide synthesized in the hypothalamus. Linked to social engagement, plasma oxytocin levels are lower in individuals with severe depression, and this can negatively affect a mother's ability to engage with her baby. Healthy mother–infant engagement promotes healthy infant brain activity, and reduced or impaired mother–infant engagement may affect the infant's ability to synthesize oxytocin.[17] Further, Apter-Levy and colleagues found that children of depressed mothers were more 4 times more likely to be diagnosed with a mental disorder on entry to school than were children of mothers with no history of depression.[17]

CLINICAL POINT: Screening for depression and assessment of risk factors should be done early in the pregnancy. Nurses should encourage women who are at risk to seek professional mental health care.[18] ■

Genetics and Neurocognition

A large body of evidence supports the role of genetics in the development of neurocognitive and neurodevelopmental disorders, but the genes that are implicated and their degree of involvement vary widely among disorders, as well as among individuals. In the cases of neurodevelopmental disorders and schizophrenia, maternal health is often a contributing factor, as are other environmental influences.

Both autism spectrum disorder (ASD) and intellectual disability have large genetic components. More than 800 ASD predisposition genes have been identified, and many of these implicate functional pathways related to synaptic organization and activity, chromatin remodeling, and wnt signaling during development.[19,20]

Advanced paternal age plays a role in the development of disorders such as autism, schizophrenia, and bipolar disorder. It is also thought to affect neurodevelopment generally. This may be a result of copy error mutations that occur as spermatogonial cells replicate across years in the life of the adult male, resulting in de novo mutations that may increase the risk for gene mutations in children.[21]

Genetic mutation of the amyloid precursor protein gene and two presenilin genes (*PSEN1* and *PSEN2*) has been found in familial patterns of Alzheimer disease (AD), but these mutations are rare and are more likely to occur in individuals with very early onset AD (i.e., onset in the 30s). In contrast, more than 20 gene variants have been identified that are linked to increased risk for late-onset AD. For example, apolipoprotein E has the greatest known effect, and it is also thought to play a role in the development of vascular dementia. In general, gene variants that affect risk for Alzheimer disease are genes linked to fat metabolism and transport in cells as well as genes linked to inflammation and immunity.[22]

Schizophrenia has long been recognized as an illness of multifactorial etiology. More specifically, both susceptibility and resilience to psychosis involve bidirectional interactions of biological and environmental factors.[23]

Psychosis

Psychosis is a symptom rather than a disorder. An individual with psychosis experiences abnormal thought processes that interfere significantly with perceptions of reality. These altered thought processes are usually manifested in odd or disturbed speech or behaviors. Psychosis may be associated with an underlying illness or may be substance induced. Psychosis is one of the hallmark features of schizophrenia; it may also be triggered by trauma or traumatic brain injury. Psychosis may be seen in individuals with severe peripartum depression, bipolar disorder, thyroid disorder, stroke, HIV, Parkinson disease, and Alzheimer disease, although it is not a core manifestation of any of these conditions.[24]

Of great concern is that delay between the onset of a first episode of psychosis and receipt of treatment has been well documented; the mean duration of untreated psychosis (DUP) ranges between 364 and 721 days in different studies.[25] Longer DUP has been consistently shown to predict poorer outcome; some studies suggest that the first 6 months of treatment delay is a critical period beyond which treatment response and recovery are impaired.[25] Awareness of the impact of this delay is critical for healthcare practitioners. Individuals who present with or report psychotic episodes require a full medical and neurologic assessment, including toxicology screenings. An immediate screening for suicidal ideation and self-injurious behavior is also necessary. If a medical diagnosis cannot be given, the individual should be referred to a qualified mental health provider for further evaluation. Pregnant or postpartum women who exhibit or report psychotic episodes require an immediate psychologic evaluation.

Millions of children are born to parents who are affected by psychosis. Often the cognitive dysfunctions exhibited by parents are later detectable in their children. In addition, childhood maltreatment increases the risk of psychosis later in life through unknown mechanisms.[26] Child abuse may predate psychotic experience in youths, and at least 40% of patients with psychosis retrospectively report personal exposure to abuse or neglect in childhood.[26] ■

Check Your Progress: Section 30.2

1. Describe the rationale for public health campaigns targeting breastfeeding in low socioeconomic groups.
2. How does maternal depression affect child development?
3. Explain why prompt recognition and treatment of psychosis are critical.

30.3 Schizophrenia

Schizophrenia is long-term mental disorder involving a breakdown in the relationships between thought, emotion, and behavior, leading to faulty perception, inappropriate actions and feelings, withdrawal from reality and personal relationships into fantasy and delusion, hallucinations, and a sense of mental fragmentation. *Delusions* are fixed beliefs that are not based in reality; for example, an individual who experiences delusions of grandeur may believe that a local fair or public event is being held in his honor. *Hallucinations* are perceptions that occur without an external stimulus, such as hearing voices that are not present.

Etiology and Pathogenesis

Schizophrenia affects approximately 1% of the world's population, and the prevalence rates are similar across all cultures and ethnicities.[27] Individuals with schizophrenia exhibit vast variability in presentation, illness trajectory, and response to treatment. This give further credence to the research findings that interactions of genetic, physiologic, and environmental factors contribute to the development of this disorder.[27]

Recent research also highlights an overlap in the genetic influences of schizophrenia and other neurodevelopmental disorders, such as autism.[28–30] Known pathologic mechanisms associated with schizophrenia include neurotransmitter abnormalities and impairments in immune function. The relationship between these mechanisms is complex, and it is not always clear which alterations are a cause of or a consequence of the disease. For example, alterations in the dopaminergic system have been implicated, in part because antipsychotic medications block the D2 receptors norepinephrine and serotonin and because gamma-aminobutyric acid and acetylcholine neurotransmitter systems are also believed to be involved. Nicotinic acetylcholine receptors appear to be diminished in the hippocampus of individuals with schizophrenia, resulting in disturbances in inhibitory gateways. It has been proposed that nicotine stimulates these receptors, providing temporary relief of symptoms of schizophrenia.[31] Research also implicates dysregulation in the N-methyl-D-aspartate subclass of glutamate receptors in the disease.[32–34]

Individuals with schizophrenia have increased levels of cytokines, especially during periods of acute psychosis or relapse.[35] It is possible that additional insults such as illness and stress overwhelm an already compromised neuroimmune system, resulting in an exacerbation of cognitive dysfunction.[36,37]

Some researchers argue that biological characteristics that are present shortly after conception and during the early stages of neurodevelopment may predispose the individual to serious mental illness. During brain development from the embryonic stage, neuronal malformation may occur, which can result in abnormal synaptic connections. This deviation in synaptic connections has been implicated in the development of schizophrenia.

A population-based study of 51,000 participants used retrospective data to investigate the associations between childhood infections and adult schizophrenia. This study found that subjects who had been hospitalized more than twice in the first 3 years of life for treatment of infections had an 80% increased risk of developing schizophrenia.[37]

Some researchers have suggested that the risk of developing schizophrenia increases with urban living. However, it is unclear whether factors specific to urban environments, such as greater exposure to pollutants and infections, and social circumstances cause schizophrenia or whether people with schizophrenia migrate to more densely populated areas seeking anonymity and cheaper living.[27] Childhood trauma is a nonhereditary factor that is intimately related to the development of schizophrenia in adulthood.[38]

Clinical Manifestations

The symptoms of schizophrenia constitute a devastating, serious, and persistent syndrome that can affect all aspects of life, including decreasing length of life through increased suicidality and other health consequences.[39] Cognitive impairment is prevalent in schizophrenia, but substantial minorities of the patient population perform within normal limits on many standard measures.[40] Schizophrenia is characterized by an array of cognitive disturbances. Formal thought disorder (FTD) is a term that refers to altered thought processes that are expressed as a disruption of speech. FTD is characteristic of schizophrenia. Symptoms of FTD include pressured or distracted speech that exhibits as rapid, often tangential speech with an extreme sense of urgency; poverty of speech, which is an absence of spontaneous speech; loose associations, in which the individual's ideas seem unrelated to the topic at hand or take another direction altogether; and word salad, speech that consists of meaningless phrases and words that are made up (neologisms), random, or not connected to each other or the current topic.[1,41]

Individuals with schizophrenia also experience social withdrawal, abnormal movements, memory and attention deficits, loss of executive function, and *avolition*, a reduced ability to engage in goal-directed behavior, making schizophrenia particularly hard to treat. Symptoms of schizophrenia may be characterized as positive, negative, or cognitive[1] (**Figure 30.2**).

Anthony Martin: Application

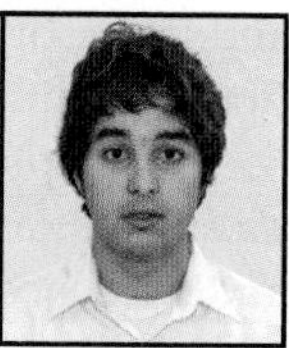

Anthony moves out of his family home and into college housing. He has a psychotic episode that requires hospitalization and is diagnosed with schizophrenia. He tries to go back to school but has a second episode and drops out of college. He moves back home.

3. What are the symptoms of formal thought disorder (FTD) that Anthony and other people with schizophrenia may display?
4. In addition to FTD, what manifestations may make it difficult for Anthony to be successful in college?

Linking Pathophysiology to Diagnosis and Treatment

The predictors and determinants of daily functioning and, ultimately, recovery from schizophrenia are of substantial interest to patients and clinical researchers. A number of key factors have been identified as predictors of functioning in the early course of schizophrenia, which generally parallel the factors found to predict functioning in chronic schizophrenia patients.[42] The authors of the study provide evidence that supports attempts to reduce negative symptoms and improve cognitive functions, as they are proximal influences on daily functioning.[42] Pharmacologic interventions have so far had limited effectiveness for improving negative symptoms or cognitive deficits. However, cognitive enhancement approaches have been effective in improving cognition to a moderate degree.

For an individual to be diagnosed with schizophrenia, clinical signs of the disorder must persist for at least 6 months.[1] Once seen as a disorder of premature and progressive deterioration, schizophrenia is now seen as a disorder that affects the individual episodically and from which many, if not most, patients will recover substantially with appropriate treatment and supports. Recovery involves the development of new meaning and purpose in one's life as one grows beyond the catastrophic effects of mental illness.[43] Lack of clinical insight has been accepted as one of the most important features of schizophrenia. *Insight* can be defined as the awareness of having a mental disorder, of specific symptoms and their attribution to the disorder, of social consequences, and of need for treatment. Tailored interventions are being considered that assist people in functioning in situations that are

Positive Symptoms	Negative Symptoms	Cognitive Symptoms
Additions to normal experiences:	Diminished affects and behaviors:	• Memory deficits
• Delusions	• Flat or blunted affect	• Attention deficits
• Hallucinations	• Thought blocking	• Language difficulties
• Abnormal movements	• Avolition	• Loss of executive function
• Formal thought disorder	• Poverty of speech	
	• Social withdrawal	

Figure 30.2 The symptoms of schizophrenia spectrum disorders are categorized as positive, negative, or cognitive.

important to them (as defined by them) and useful to challenge their illness and also help them to feel better. A determination of whether such efforts demonstrate outcomes that are superior to the gains from traditional, clinic-based cognitive and psychosocial rehabilitation efforts will help in efforts to provide the most effective treatment of schizophrenia.[43]

As important as tailored interventions for the individual is family psychoeducation. Living with or caring for an individual with schizophrenia can be difficult and puts a number of burdens on caregivers, including psychologic and financial ones. Interventions that provide education and promote coping among family members, especially when conducted over several months, can reduce the risk for relapse and rehospitalization for patients.[44,45]

Anthony Martin: Outcome

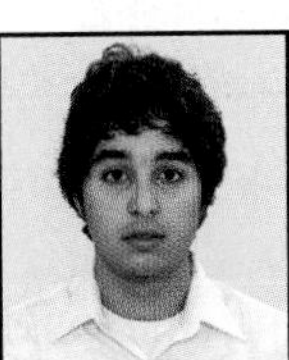

Anthony is in outpatient treatment but is not compliant with his medications. He makes a suicide attempt, is hospitalized again, and undergoes more outpatient treatment. Eventually, he leaves home after constant fighting with his parents and becomes homeless.

5. What family intervention could help Anthony reduce his risk for rehospitalization?
6. Describe the course of schizophrenia that Anthony should expect over his lifetime.

Check Your Progress: Section 30.3

1. Compare the difference between delusions and hallucinations in the person with schizophrenia.
2. What is the proposed role of nicotine in the treatment of schizophrenia?
3. Describe embryonic factors that may lead to the development of schizophrenia.

30.4 Neurocognitive Disorders

The neurocognitive disorders discussed here are dementia and delirium. In differentiating dementia from delirium, it is also necessary to consider depression, as they share some features but are very different in onset, illness trajectory, and treatment considerations. Delirium is an acute disturbance in cognition with a rapid onset that may last between hours and days, depending on how long it takes to resolve the underlying illness causing the delirium. Acute confusion is the hallmark manifestation, although mood swings, delusions, and hallucinations may also occur. **Dementia** is a chronic or persistent disorder of the mental processes caused by brain disease or injury and marked by memory disorders, personality changes, and impaired reasoning. It has a slow, progressive onset with initial manifestations including impairments in abstract thinking and memory loss. Depression and apathy may be seen during the course of the illness. In contrast, depression is variable in onset, typically episodic in nature, with core symptoms of persistent sadness, anxiety, impairment in concentration, and fatigue. Recovery from depression is possible with treatment.

Dementia

Aging populations and associated increases in the prevalence of dementia are of increasing concern worldwide. Countries are exploring national strategies to address dementia care and support services in relation to government and third party recommendations.[46] In developed regions of the world in particular, populations are aging, with a third estimated to be aged 60 years and over by 2050.[47]

Etiology and Pathogenesis

The primary determinants for diagnosis of dementia are clinical manifestation and the progressive nature of the illness. A number of illnesses as well as head trauma can cause dementia, and the pathogenesis of dementia varies depending on etiology. The most prevalent causes of dementia are

Healthy People 2020

Dementias, Including Alzheimer Disease

Goal: Reduce the morbidity and costs associated with, and maintain or enhance the quality of life for, persons with dementia, including Alzheimer disease.

Overview: Dementia affects an individual's health, quality of life, and ability to live independently. It can diminish a person's ability to effectively:

- Manage medications and medical conditions
- Make financial decisions
- Drive a car or use appliances and tools safely
- Avoid physical injury
- Maintain social relationships
- Carry out activities of daily living, such as bathing or dressing.

Objectives:

DIA-1 Increase the proportion of adults aged 65 years and older with diagnosed Alzheimer disease and other dementias, or their caregivers, who are aware of the diagnosis.

DIA-2 Reduce the proportion of preventable hospitalizations in adults aged 65 years and older with diagnosed Alzheimer disease and other dementias.

Reference

1. HealthyPeople 2020. (2017). *Dementias, including Alzheimer's disease.* Available at https://www.healthypeople.gov/2020/topics-objectives/topic/dementias-including-alzheimers-disease

Alzheimer disease and vascular dementia; Alzheimer disease accounts for more than 50% of diagnoses of dementia.[48]

Although the causes of **Alzheimer disease (AD)** are still under investigation, a buildup of plaques consisting of beta amyloid, a protein in the brain, as well as tangles of another protein, tau, interfere with neuronal transport and eventually the cortex thins and the brain gradually shrinks. (**Figure 30.3** ■). There is evidence of neuronal cell damage and death in the brain, which may result from interference from the plaques and tangles (**Figure 30.4** ■). Acetylcholine is also thought to play a role, as this enzyme is essential to many of the functions that deteriorate in individuals with AD.[1,48]

Vascular dementia, often referred to as *vascular cognitive impairment*, is associated with changes in thinking following a series of small strokes. Vascular changes in the brain can be present alongside other types of dementia.[48]

Clinical Manifestations

Dementia of any kind is characterized by a slow, progressive deterioration of cognitive functioning. Initial manifestations vary by etiology. For example, individuals with AD exhibit memory lapses in the early stages, forgetting familiar words and losing everyday objects. With vascular dementia, episodes of impaired judgment and planning or organization tend to be the first indications there is anything wrong.[48] Regardless of the type of dementia, individuals experience increasing cognitive impairments over a course of years and are eventually unable to care for themselves or communicate. Progressive changes in mobility also occur.

The majority (80%) of people with dementia in the United States are cared for in the community by approximately 15 million unpaid, informal caregivers. Informal caregivers are usually spouses, other family members, or friends who assume a critical role in the provision of dementia care.[49] Caregivers of individuals with dementia may initiate formal dementia evaluations, manage patient symptoms, provide emotional and financial support, and monitor the effects of care management strategies.

Caregivers are concerned that older patients with dementia and delirium may receive suboptimal hospital care. This is of particular concern to clinicians as well as patients and families because one third of beds in a typical hospital are occupied by older confused people, and the most common causes of confusion are delirium and dementia.[50]

Lydia Ocampo: Application

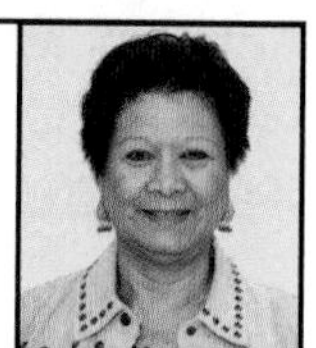

Mrs. Ocampo falls and breaks her hip in and is admitted to the hospital for an open reduction internal fixation. Her confusion escalates at the hospital. There are also issues in managing her postoperative pain, nausea, infection, and anemia. Mrs. Ocampo is transferred to a rehabilitation hospital for continued care. She receives appropriate care, but she continues to be more confused than she was before her fall. A niece comes from the Philippines to help Mr. Ocampo with Lydia's care when she is discharged home.

3. What caregiver roles may the Ocampos' niece assume?
4. How may Alzheimer disease affect Mrs. Ocampo's quality of life?

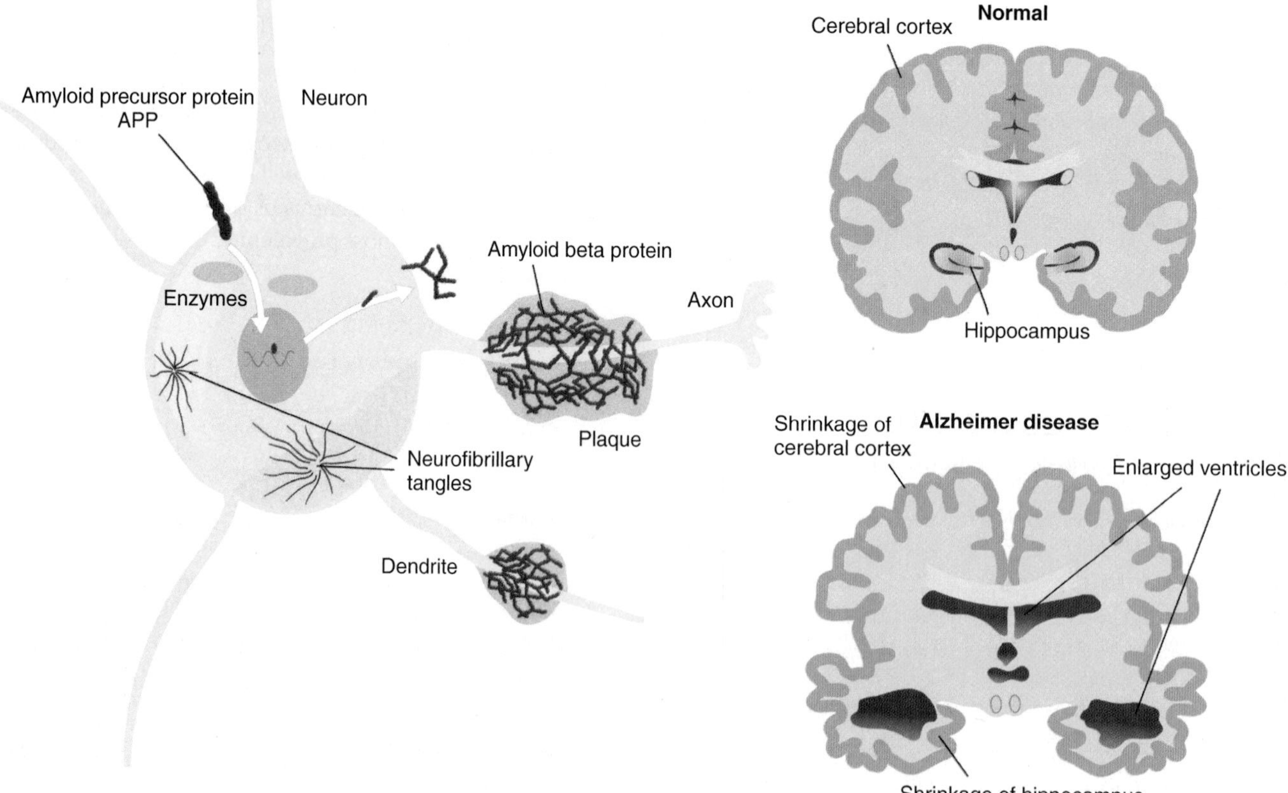

Figure 30.3 ■ In Alzheimer disease, a buildup of beta amyloid interferes with neuronal transport. Eventually the cerebral cortex thins and the brain shrinks, starting with hippocampus.

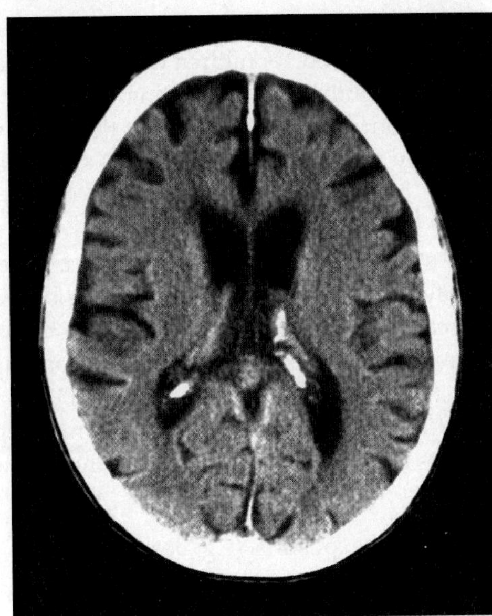

Figure 30.4 ■ CT scan of an 84-year-old man with Alzheimer disease. Note the atrophy of the brain.

Linking Pathophysiology to Diagnosis and Treatment

A complete physical and neurologic examination is necessary to determine the likely etiology, assess clinical manifestations and level of impairment, and recommend a treatment plan. Early interventions include regular monitoring to compare health and cognitive status to baseline; reinforcing orientation to person, time, and place at each contact; recommending that patients establish advance directives and discuss their illness and care with their families; and breaking instructions into simple steps and alternating activities with rest to prevent fatigue. Individuals will need greater levels of care as their disease progresses.[41] Routines, including consistency of caregivers, can provide additional support to the patient with dementia. Pharmacologic interventions are available, but these can only delay progression of symptoms. There is no cure for dementia of any kind at this time.

Lydia Ocampo: Outcome

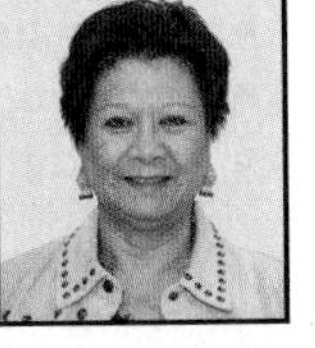

After her husband dies of heart failure, Mrs. Ocampo is placed in a nursing home. She has no visitors. She gradually declines, owing to lack of mobility and poor nutrition. She becomes confined to bed, does not eat, becomes incontinent, and develops a pressure injury.

5. What interventions may help to improve Mrs. Ocampo's nutrition?
6. What consults should be ordered for Mrs. Ocampo?

Delirium

A multitude of terms are used to describe delirium, including encephalopathy, acute brain failure, acute confusional state, and postoperative or intensive care unit psychosis. **Delirium** is an acute state of confusion caused by underlying illness or injury. To correct delirium and return the individual to baseline, it is essential to determine the causal mechanism of the delirium.

Etiology and Pathogenesis

Delirium can occur in the hospital environment as an effect of certain therapies and the surrounding unfamiliar environment. In addition, older adults are at risk for delirium during heat waves or extreme heat events. Older adults are more vulnerable to heat-related mortality, so the changing population structure may be leading to an increased health burden from heat.[51] Extreme heat is associated with increased hospital admissions, particularly for renal causes, among older adults in the United States. Common causes of delirium, regardless of age, include infection (especially respiratory and urinary infections) and dehydration. In children, some additional etiologies of delirium are high fevers, sepsis, chemotherapy, closed head injuries, and hypoxia. Common causes of delirium among adolescents and adults include substance use, overdose, or withdrawal; head injury; neoplasm; autoimmune disorders; and exposure to an environmental toxin.[41] However, in young people and younger adults, multiple insults are more likely to precipitate onset of delirium than any single factor.[52] In older adults, delirium is more likely to arise from a combination of factors that increase risk. For example, the older adult with dementia who develops dehydration and a urinary tract infection is at greater risk than the healthy older adult.[53] Selected precipitants of delirium in older adults include drug toxicity or adverse effects, urinary retention, stroke, acute myocardial or pulmonary events, and use of anticholinergic medications.[41] Uncontrolled pain and use of physical restraints may also cause delirium.[53]

Clinical Manifestations

Delirium is defined as a relatively acute decline in cognitions that fluctuates over hours or days. In addition to acute confusion, manifestations of delirium include inattention and perceptual disturbances. Individuals may alternate between hyperactive states (exemplified by restlessness and agitation) and hypoactive states (characterized by drowsiness or lethargy).[53,54]

Linking Pathophysiology to Diagnosis and Treatment

When delirium is diagnosed or suspected, a complete physical and neurologic assessment, including lab work, is necessary to determine and treat the underlying cause. No cause for delirium can be found in a small percentage of patients despite every effort. Components of delirium management include supportive therapy and pharmacologic management. Fluid and nutrition should be given carefully because the patient may be unwilling or physically unable to maintain a balanced intake. For the patient who is suspected of having alcohol toxicity or alcohol withdrawal, therapy should include multivitamins, especially thiamine.[55]

Reorientation techniques or memory cues such as a calendar, clocks, and family photos may be helpful. The environment should be stable, quiet, and well lit. One study showed that a reduction of sound during the night by providing earplugs to patients in the intensive care unit decreased the risk of delirium by 53% and improved the self-reported sleep perception of patients for 48 hours.[55] Family members and staff should explain proceedings to the patient at every opportunity, reinforce orientation, and reassure the patient. Support from a familiar nurse and family members should be encouraged.

Sensory deficits should be corrected, if necessary, with eyeglasses and hearing aids. Physical restraints should be avoided. Delirious patients may pull out intravenous lines, may climb out of bed, and may not be compliant. Perceptual problems lead to agitation, fear, combative behavior, and wandering. Severely delirious patients benefit from constant observation, which may be cost effective for these patients and help to avoid the use of physical restraints, which can exacerbate or extend the delirium. These patients should never be left alone or unattended.[55]

CLINICAL POINT: Because the behavioral manifestations of delirium can be distressing to both clinicians and caregivers, antipsychotics have become increasingly used in the treatment of delirium. However, the use of antipsychotics in this manner may be considered a form of chemical restraint rather than an actual treatment. Although antipsychotics may be warranted for the patient with severe agitation that may lead to a risk of harm to self or others or for the patient with active psychosis, there is insufficient evidence to support the use of antipsychotics as a general treatment for delirium. This is particularly true in treating older adult patients, who are at much greater risk of adverse drug effects than are young adults.[56] Dementia patients in particular may experience a paradoxic effect from psychotropic medications, such as a benzodiazepine causing rage instead of sedation. ■

Check Your Progress: Section 30.4

1. Explain the clinical differences between delirium and dementia.
2. Describe the pathophysiology of Alzheimer disease.
3. What are the concerns about using antipsychotics in the treatment of delirium?

30.5 Genetic Neurodevelopmental Disorders

The genetic neurodevelopmental disorders include attention-deficit/hyperactivity disorder, autism spectrum disorder, Down syndrome, and fetal alcohol syndrome. Each topic is discussed below.

Attention-Deficit/Hyperactivity Disorder

Attention-deficit/hyperactivity disorder (ADHD) is one of the most common neurodevelopmental disorders of childhood. It is usually first diagnosed in childhood and often lasts into adulthood.[57] Children with ADHD may have trouble paying attention and controlling impulsive behaviors (acting without thinking about what the result will be) or may be overly active.[58]

Etiology and Pathogenesis

Scientists are studying causes and risk factors in an effort to find better ways to manage and reduce the risk for developing ADHD. The causes and risk factors for ADHD are unknown, but current research shows that genetics plays an important role. Recent studies of twins link genes with ADHD.

In addition to genetics, scientists are studying other possible causes and risk factors, including the following:

- Brain injury
- Environmental exposures (e.g., lead)
- Alcohol and tobacco use during pregnancy
- Premature delivery
- Low birth weight.

Research does not support the popularly held views that ADHD is caused by eating too much sugar, watching too much television, improper parenting, or social and environmental factors such as poverty or family chaos. Of course, these and other factors may affect symptom severity or illness trajectory, especially in certain individuals, but the evidence is not strong enough to conclude that they are the main causes of ADHD.[58]

Clinical Manifestations

While it is normal for children to have trouble focusing and behaving from time to time, children with ADHD do not grow out of these behaviors. The symptoms continue and can cause difficulty at school, at home, or with friends. A child with ADHD might:

- daydream a lot
- forget or lose things a lot
- squirm or fidget
- talk too much
- make careless mistakes or take unnecessary risks
- have a hard time resisting temptation
- have trouble taking turns
- have difficulty getting along with others.

There are three types of ADHD, depending on which types of symptoms are strongest in the individual:

- ***Predominantly inattentive presentation.*** It is hard for the individual to organize or finish a task, pay attention to details, or follow instructions or conversations. The person is easily distracted or forgets details of daily routines.
- ***Predominantly hyperactive–impulsive presentation.*** The person fidgets and talks a lot. It is hard to sit still for long (e.g., for a meal or while doing homework). Smaller children may run, jump, or climb constantly. The individual feels restless and has trouble with impulsivity. Someone who is impulsive may interrupt others a lot, grab things from people, or speak at inappropriate times. It is hard for the person to wait their

turn or listen to directions. A person with impulsiveness may have more accidents and injuries than others.

- ***Combined presentation.*** Symptoms of the above two types are equally present in the person.[58]

Because symptoms can change over time, the presentation may change over time as well.

Jason Riley: Application

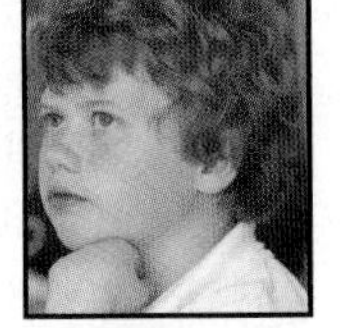

Jason's problems at school continue. He gets into fights frequently and does poorly academically. He is referred to a neuropsychologist, who diagnoses Jason with ADHD. Jason starts taking Ritalin, and an individualized education plan IEP is developed at school.

3. On the basis of his manifestations, Jason is most likely afflicted with which of the three types of ADHD?
4. How should the nurse respond if Jason's parents ask whether their parenting skills, the environment, or diet could have caused Jason's ADHD?

Linking Pathophysiology to Diagnosis and Treatment

Determining whether a child has ADHD is a multistep process. There is no single test to diagnose the disorder, and many other problems, such as anxiety, depression, and certain types of learning disabilities, can have similar symptoms. One step of the process involves having a medical examination, including hearing and vision tests, to rule out other problems with similar manifestations. Another part of the process may include a checklist for rating ADHD symptoms and taking a history of the child from parents, teachers, and sometimes the child.

In most cases, ADHD is best treated with a combination of behavior therapy and medication. For children age 5 years and under with ADHD, behavior therapy is recommended as the first line of treatment. No single treatment is the answer for every child, and good treatment plans will include close monitoring, follow-ups, and any changes in treatment that are found to be needed along the way.[58]

Studies in the last decade have demonstrated that ADHD continues to impair function into adulthood and responds to pharmacotherapy. Owing to age-specific changes in roles and challenges, it is possible that presentation and response to intervention may differ between older and younger adults. By definition, ADHD requires impairment in functioning due to ADHD traits.[59] Impacts on academic, occupational, and social functioning are well documented in younger adults, but hallmarks of functional impairment in older adults can be presumed to have different patterns in the years beyond school and work roles.

ADHD in older adults is a virtually unexplored area. The manifestations of ADHD among older adults are becoming of increasing interest because more adults over the age of 50 are seeking assessment for ADHD.[60] The population of people older than 65 years of age in the United States is expected to grow from 43.1 million to 88.5 million between 2012 and 2050. ADHD will be one of many psychiatric contributors to morbidity in this aging population.[59]

In treating older adult patients with ADHD, it is essential to provide good support based on knowledge and understanding of how ADHD symptoms have affected health, quality of life, and function through the lifespan. Individualized therapy for each patient should be recommended to balance the risk–benefit ratio when pharmacotherapy is considered to be a possible treatment. ■

Jason Riley: Outcome

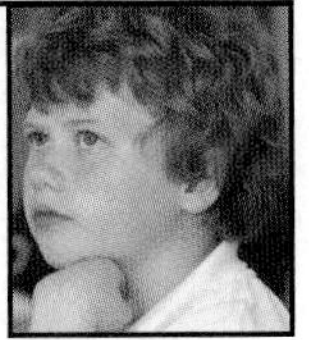

After adjusting to new medication and the IEP, Jason slowing begins to make academic progress, and his social skills improve. He also makes a couple of friends.

5. Describe the progression of ADHD that Jason can expect as he becomes a young adult.
6. Describe the progression of ADHD that Jason can expect as he becomes an older adult.

Autism Spectrum Disorder

Autism spectrum disorder (ASD) is characterized by deficits in communication and social interaction and by restricted and repetitive patterns of behavior that are not better explained by another medical or psychiatric diagnosis. Symptoms cause marked impairment and many challenges for the individual and caregivers, making it difficult for the individual to form and maintain relationships.[1,61] The word *spectrum* recognizes that the degree and nature of the impairment ranges along the continuum and that presenting symptoms can vary among individuals. There is often nothing about how people with ASD look that sets them apart from other people, but they may communicate, interact, behave, and learn in ways that are different from those of most people. The learning, thinking, and problem-solving abilities of people with ASD occur across a spectrum or continuum. Some individuals with ASD need a lot of help in their daily lives; others need less. A diagnosis of ASD now includes several conditions that used to be diagnosed separately: autistic disorder, pervasive developmental disorder not otherwise specified, and Asperger syndrome. These conditions are now all categorized as autism spectrum disorder.

Etiology and Pathogenesis

Research has yet to identify a distinct etiology and pathogenesis for autism spectrum disorder. Maternal health, genetics, and paternal age are thought to play a role. Researchers continue to examine multiple paths of inquiry to try to identify specific etiologies and biomarkers that might shed more light on this challenging disorder. For example, the presence of atopic disease in either mother or infant has a strong correlation with risk for ASD. Atopic diseases involve activation of the mast cell, which plays a role in inflammation. Inflammatory processes in the brain appear to be altered in individuals with ASD.[62] What is known is that, despite multiple studies, no known link between vaccines and autism spectrum disorder has been found.[63,64]

It is now widely recognized that ASD has a strong genetic component, is characterized by cognitive impairments in theory of mind (i.e., social understanding ability) and executive function (i.e., flexibility of thought) and weak central coherence (i.e., a tendency toward piecemeal processing). The difficulty in developing a full understanding of autism spectrum disorder can be partially explained by the lack of information on how it develops over time and the role of sociocultural factors in its development.[65]

Clinical Manifestations

ASD is characterized by a series of deficits in social interaction and communication and restricted, repetitive, and stereotyped behavior patterns.[66] In addition, in a high percentage of cases, ASD is associated with anxiety disorders. Children with ASD may not always be identified by preschool age, but some of their behavioral problems may nonetheless prompt a referral for behavioral intervention.[67]

Linking Pathophysiology to Diagnosis and Treatment

Diagnosing ASD can be difficult, since there is no medical test, such as a blood test, to diagnose the disorder. Doctors look at the child's behavior and development to make a diagnosis.

There is currently no cure for ASD. There are a variety of specific interventions for young children with ASD that are designed to control disruptive behaviors, improve school success, and increase social interactions. These interventions include such techniques as discrete trial training, comprehensive behavioral treatment, joint attention intervention, and self-management.[65] In addition to the stress of raising a child diagnosed with a disability, it is not uncommon for immigrant families to confront culture-related stress or adaptation issues. Additional issues for immigrant children and their families are likely to exist, including language barriers, cultural differences, and the lack of reliable and validated measures in the family's primary language. Immigrants who are referred to health care services may have more limited knowledge about how to navigate health care systems, further complicating their ability to get access to appropriate services.[66]

Down Syndrome

Down syndrome (DS) is the most common chromosomal condition associated with intellectual disability and other serious morbidity.[67] In developed countries, maternal age has been rising since the 1980s, with an increase in the number of pregnancies of a fetus with DS. Whether this has led to a higher number of live born children with DS depends on the extent to which pregnant women use antenatal testing and selective termination of pregnancies when the fetus is found to have DS. In this respect, there are clear differences. DS is usually an unexpected diagnosis at birth, based initially on typical clinical features. Recognizing these features may be difficult because not all features of DS need to be present in every case or can be subtle.[67] The diagnosis can be delayed when infants are not routinely examined by someone who is experienced in recognition of DS; this may happen, for instance, in home deliveries.

Etiology and Pathogenesis

Down syndrome is the most common genetic cause for intellectual disability, yet the pathophysiology of cognitive impairment in Down syndrome is unknown. Down syndrome occurs in 9.0 to 11.8 per 10,000 live births and is associated with impairments in language, cognition, learning, and memory.[68] Although clinical features of Down syndrome and the DNA sequence of chromosome 21 have been characterized, few neuroimaging studies have characterized the pathophysiology of neurologic deficits in Down syndrome. Early structural MRI reports suggested that total intracranial volume is smaller in Down syndrome, the greatest volumetric differences occurring in the cerebellum, brainstem and frontal lobes.[68]

Clinical Manifestations

DS is one of the most common and recognizable conditions associated with learning disability, and approximately 2.7 of 1000 pregnancies are affected.[69] Certain facial characteristics, short stature as the child grows, dysmorphism, growth delays, and hearing problems are common clinical manifestations of DS. The experience of receiving a diagnosis of DS for their child and the care around that time can be an emotional experience. In England and Wales, all pregnant women are offered prenatal screening tests for DS through the NHS. Midwives are tasked with providing balanced and accurate information about DS to enable pregnant women to make informed choices about screening and subsequent decisions, including continuation or termination of pregnancy.[70]

Linking Pathophysiology to Diagnosis and Treatment

There is no known cure for DS. Young children with DS typically experience delays in certain areas of development. Early childhood interventions such as physical therapy, occupational therapy, and speech therapy may be necessary to help children with DS make gains in development that will increase their independence. In addition to speech and language therapy, family interventions such as the use of sign language and visual cues can help family members and young children with DS communicate during the child's early stages of development.[71]

CLINICAL POINT: Adults with DS are at increased risk for a number of conditions, including sensory losses, hypothyroidism, obstructive sleep apnea, osteoarthritis and osteoporosis, cervical spine issues, and Alzheimer disease. Although they may require care from a number of specialists, it is essential that these patients have a complete medical examination regularly that includes a full review of medications (**Figure 30.5**). For individuals with Down syndrome, medications should be added one at a time and be prescribed at the lowest therapeutic level, with dosages increased slowly as needed.[72]

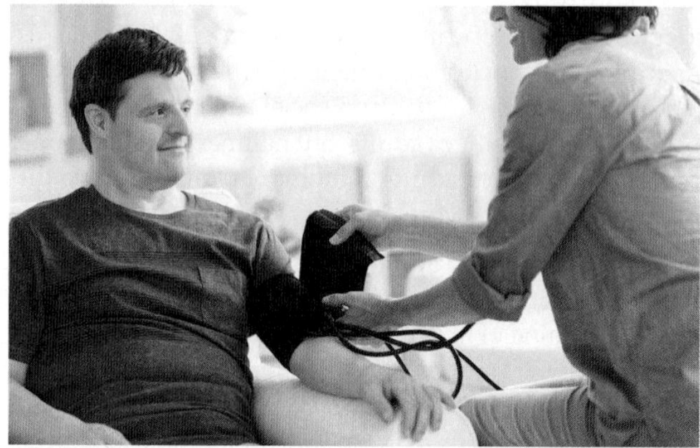

Figure 30.5 An adult man with Down syndrome at his regular checkup.

Fetal Alcohol Syndrome

Prenatal alcohol exposure can cause a number of physical, behavioral, cognitive, and neural impairments, collectively known as **fetal alcohol spectrum disorders (FASD)**.[73] Alcohol consumption during pregnancy can interfere with both embryonic and fetal development, producing a wide range of outcomes that fall under the rubric of FASD. FASD is the nondiagnostic umbrella term that is used to refer to the full range of effects that can occur as a result of prenatal alcohol exposure.

Etiology and Pathogenesis

Alcohol abuse during pregnancy is associated with health problems for both mother and fetus. Among possible harms to the fetus caused by alcohol consumption during pregnancy, the fetal alcohol syndrome (FAS) is considered to be the most severe of the FASDs, characterized by birth-induced morphologic injury and developmental disabilites.[74]

Clinical Manifestations

The typical clinical presentation of FAS includes a deficiency in the weight and height growth before and after birth, abnormalities in the neurodevelopment of the nervous central system, and a series of typical facial abnormalities, including small palpebral fissures, a thin upper lip, and a smooth philtrum (**Figure 30.6** ■).[73]

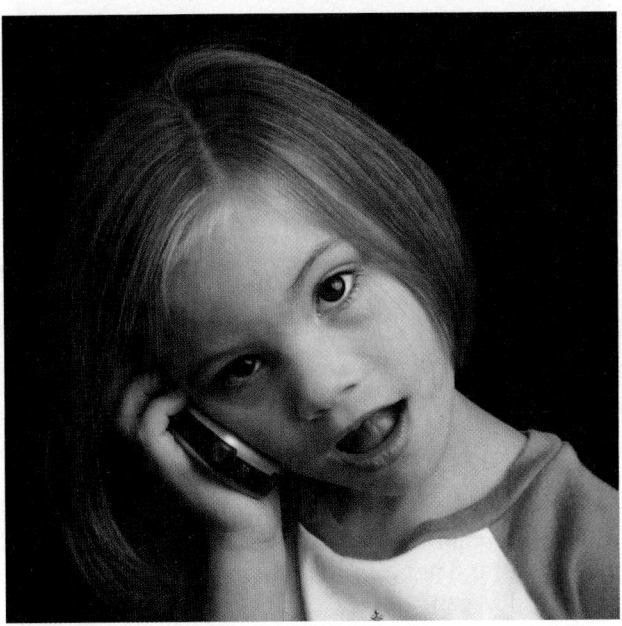

Figure 30.6 ■ A child with fetal alcohol syndrome.

Linking Pathophysiology to Diagnosis and Treatment

The routine use of objective, validated, and highly specific markers of prenatal alcohol exposure would help to improve FASD identification, which currently is hampered by a lack of good information. A recent study found that only 33% of the mothers of children given a diagnosis of FAS provided information about their alcohol consumption.[75] In addition, a large number of children with FASD are in adoptive situations or foster care, and little knowledge of their alcohol exposure may be available. Other novel FASD diagnostic techniques include ways to identify potential at-risk individuals on the basis of subtle, subclinical facial features.[75] In particular, researchers have developed a computerized method for detecting facial features using three-dimensional facial imaging and computer-based dense-surface modeling.[76]

Check Your Progress: Section 30.5

1. Describe the clinical presentation of a person with predominantly hyperactive–impulsive presentation of ADHD.
2. What is the meaning of the word *spectrum* in the diagnosis of autism spectrum disorder?
3. Why are fetal alcohol spectrum disorders (FASDs) difficult to identify?

CHAPTER SUMMARY

30.1 Chapter Overview and Case Studies

Describe normal development and cognition, the range of disorders that affect development, and concepts related to those disorders.

- Neurocognitive disorders (NCDs) are disorders whose primary features are cognitive impairments. The NCDs include delirium and the various forms of dementia. Neurodevelopmental disorders occur as the brain develops and usually manifest before a child enters kindergarten. Neurodevelopmental disorders may affect children across a number of domains, including language, coordination, attention, and behavior.
- Cerebral perfusion, respiratory health, fluid and electrolyte status, inflammatory processes, substance use, and trauma can, independently or in concert, affect developmental and cognitive processes.

30.2 Pathophysiology of Neurocognitive and Neurodevelopmental Disorders

Differentiate the causes, classification, underlying pathogenesis, and mechanisms related to development of neurocognitive and neurodevelopmental disorders across the lifespan.

- Issues of maternal health, such as prenatal nutrition, the presence of illness during pregnancy, and maternal depression can increase a child's risk for neurodevelopmental and other disorders.
- Interplay among genetics and environment has implications for both neurocognitive and neurodevelopmental disorders.
- Psychosis, characterized by altered thought processes often manifesting in odd or disturbed behaviors, is a symptom rather than a disorder. Psychosis may result from illness or trauma or as a response to a substance. It is a hallmark symptom of schizophrenia.

30.3 Schizophrenia

Differentiate the causes, classification, underlying pathogenesis, and clinical manifestations of schizophrenia and approaches to diagnosis and treatment of this condition across the lifespan.

- Schizophrenia is a form of severe mental illness with vast variability in presentation, response to treatment, and illness trajectory, suggesting that there is not one cause but many interacting factors that contribute to its development.
- Although the etiology of schizophrenia is still largely unknown, a combination of genetics, physiologic processes, and environmental risk factors is believed to predispose individuals to development of this disorder.[14]

30.4 Neurocognitive Disorders

Differentiate the causes, classification, underlying pathogenesis, and clinical manifestations of neurocognitive disorders and approaches to diagnosis and treatment of these conditions across the lifespan.

- An aging population and an associated increase in the prevalence of dementia are of increasing concern worldwide. Alzheimer disease and related forms of dementia are predominant, incurable conditions marked by prolonged and progressive cognitive, functional, and behavioral impairments.
- Delirium is an acute state of confusion resulting from illness or injury. Typically, its etiology is multifactorial, and treatment of one or more underlying causes can return the patient to baseline.

30.5 Genetic Neurodevelopmental Disorders

Differentiate the genetics and genomics, classification, underlying pathogenesis, and clinical manifestations of neurodevelopmental disorders and approaches to diagnosis and treatment of these conditions across the lifespan.

- The genetic neurodevelopmental disorders include attention-deficit/hyperactivity disorder, autism spectrum disorder, Down syndrome, and fetal alcohol syndrome.
- Attention-deficit/hyperactivity disorder (ADHD) is one of the most common neurodevelopmental disorders of childhood. It is usually first diagnosed in childhood and often lasts into adulthood. Children with ADHD may have trouble paying attention, may have difficulty controlling impulsive behaviors (acting without thinking about what the result will be), or may be overly active.[28]
- ADHD in older adults is a virtually unexplored area. The manifestation of ADHD among older adults has become a topic of interest because of the increasing number of adults aged 50 years and older who are seeking assessment for ADHD.[30]
- Autism spectrum disorder (ASD) is a developmental disability that can cause significant social, communication, and behavioral challenges. There is often nothing about how people with ASD look that sets them apart from other people, but they may communicate, interact, behave, and learn in ways that are different from those of most other people.
- Down syndrome is the most common chromosomal condition associated with intellectual disability and other serious morbidity.[35]
- Prenatal alcohol exposure can cause a number of physical, behavioral, cognitive, and neural impairments, collectively known as fetal alcohol spectrum disorders.[39] Alcohol consumption during pregnancy can interfere with both embryonic and fetal development, producing a wide range of outcomes that fall under the rubric of fetal alcohol spectrum disorders.

REVIEW QUESTIONS

1. Which of the following statements by a client with schizophrenia indicates to the nurse that the client is having a delusion?
   a. "I am the President of the United States."
   b. "I hear the President telling me to leave the hospital."
   c. "I see lions hiding in the corners of my room."
   d. "I smell palm trees and the ocean in my room."

2. The nurse is admitting a client with a diagnosis of schizophrenia. When asked about his living situation, the client responds with unrecognizable words that the nurse cannot understand. Which term describes this speech pattern?
   a. Poverty of speech
   b. Pressured speech
   c. Loose associations
   d. Word salad

3. When assessing an older client for early signs of dehydration, the nurse would expect to find:
   a. nausea and vomiting.
   b. a change in mental status.
   c. difficulty breathing.
   d. headache.

4. Which statement made by a pregnant woman requires follow-up?
   a. "I should stay away from people who are smoking."
   b. "Small amounts of alcohol are safe after the first trimester."
   c. "Breastfeeding is good for my baby's development."
   d. "My nutrition affects my baby's health."

5. An assessment of a client with delirium will most likely reveal:
   a. a fast onset of signs and symptoms.
   b. signs and symptoms that will take several months to resolve.
   c. impairment in abstract thinking.
   d. depression and apathy.

6. Which of the following statements made by a woman who is acting as caregiver to her husband with dementia would require more teaching?
   a. "I manage and pay all the bills that he used to take care of."
   b. "I orient him to his surroundings when he needs it."
   c. "I help him with his meals."
   d. "I adjust his medications depending on how he is feeling."

7. The nurse is teaching the parents of a child with possible ADHD about the diagnostic process. Which of the following would the nurse tell the parents?
   a. "A medical examination is needed to confirm the diagnosis."
   b. "Other similar disorders need to be ruled out."
   c. "Hearing and vision tests can confirm the diagnosis."
   d. "Genetic screening will be necessary."

8. The nurse assessing a child with fetal alcohol syndrome is likely to observe which of the following features?
   a. A smooth philtrum
   b. A thick upper lip
   c. Normal height and height
   d. A normal neurologic assessment

ANSWERS

Answers to Review Questions can be found in Appendix A. Answers to Case Study and Check Your Progress questions are available on the faculty resources site. Please consult with your instructor.

RECOMMENDED WEBSITES

Autism Speaks
https://www.autismspeaks.org

Dementia.org
https://www.dementia.org

National Alliance on Mental Illness
http://www.nami.org

Schizophrenia Basics
https://www.nimh.nih.gov/health/publications/schizophrenia-basics/index.shtml

What Is ADHD?
http://kidshealth.org/en/parents/adhd.html

REFERENCES

1. American Psychiatric Association. (2013). *Diagnostic and statistical manual of mental disorders* (5th ed.). Washington, D.C.: American Psychiatric Association.
2. Wan, M., & Chase, J. M. (2017). Delirium in older adults: diagnosis, prevention, and treatment. *British Columbia Medical Journal, 59*(3), 165–170. Retrieved from http://www.bcmj.org/articles/delirium-older-adults-diagnosis-prevention-and-treatment
3. Alosco, M. L., Gunstad, J., Jerskey, B. A., Xu, X., Clark, U. S., Hassenstab, J., Cole, D. M., Walsh, E. G., Labbe, D. R., Hoge, R., Cohen, R. A., & Sweet, L. H. (2013). The adverse effects of reduced cerebral perfusion on cognition and brain structure in older adults with cardiovascular disease. *Brain and Behavior, 3*(6), 626–636.
4. Lages, Y. M., Nascimento, J. M., Lemos, G. A., Galina, A., Castilho, L. R., & Rehen, S. K. (2015). Low oxygen alters mitochondrial function and response to oxidative stress in human progenitor cells. *PeerJ, 10*. Retrieved from https://www.ncbi.nlm.nih.gov/pubmed/26713239.
5. McCance, K. L, & Huether S. E. (2014). *Pathophysiology: The biologic basis for disease in adults and children.* London, UK: Mosby.
6. González-Reyes, R. E., Aliev, G., Ávila-Rodrigues, M., & Barreto, G. E. (2016). Alterations in glucose metabolism on cognition: A possible link between diabetes and dementia. *Current Pharmaceutical Design, 22*(7), 812–818.
7. Benros, M. E., Sørensen, H. J., Nielsen, P. R., Nordentoft, M., Mortensen, P. B., & Petersen, L (2015). The association between infections and general cognitive ability in young men: A nationwide study. *PLoS ONE, 10*(5), e0124005. doi:10.1371/journal.pone.0124005

8. Maier, S. F., & Watkins, L. (2012). *Consequences of the inflamed brain*. Available at http://www.dana.org/Publications/ReportOnProgress/Consequences_of_the_Inflamed_Brain/
9. Kim, J. W., Lee, D. Y., Lee, B. C., Jung, M. H., Kim, H., Choi, Y. S., & Choi, I. G. (2012). Alcohol and cognition in the elderly: A review. *Psychiatry investigation, 9*(1), 8–16.
10. Polanska, K., Jurewicz, J., & Hanke, W. (2015). Smoking and alcohol drinking during pregnancy as the risk factors for poor child neurodevelopment. *International Journal of Occupational Medicine and Environmental Health, 28*(3), 419–443.
11. Markunas, C. A., Xu, Z., Harlid, S., Wade, P. A., Lie, R. T., Taylor, J. A., & Wilcox, J. A. (2014). Identification of DNA methylation changes in newborns related to smoking and pregnancy. *Environmental Health Perspectives, 122*(10), 1147–153.
12. Hollams, E. M., de Klerk, N. H., Holt, P. G., & Sly, P. D. (2014). Persistent effects of maternal smoking during pregnancy on lung function and asthma in adolescents. *American Journal of Respiratory and Clinical Care Medicine, 189*(4), 401–405.
13. Hoyer, D., Tetschke, F., Jaekel, S., Nowack, S., Witte, O. W., Ekkehard Schleußner, & Schneider, U. (2013). Fetal functional brain age assessed from universal developmental indices obtained from neuro-vegetative activity patterns. *PLoS ONE, 8*(9), e74431. doi:10.1371/journal.pone.0074431
14. Aboud, F. E., & Yousafzai, A. K. (2016). Very early childhood development. In R. E. Black, R. Laximarayan, M. Temmerman, & N. Walker (Eds.), *Reproductive, maternal, newborn, and child health: Disease control priorities* (Vol. 2, 3rd ed., pp. 241–260. Washington, DC: The International Bank for Reconstruction and Development/The World Bank. Available at https://www.ncbi.nlm.nih.gov/books/NBK361924/
15. McCrory, C., & Murray, A. (2012). The effect of breastfeeding on neuro-development in infancy. *Maternal and Child Health Journal, 17*(9), 1680–1688. doi:10.1007/s10995-012-1182-9
16. Whitehead, N., Potterton, J., & Coovadia, A. (2014). The neurodevelopment of HIV-infected infants on HAART compared to HIV-exposed but uninfected infants. *AIDS Care, 26*(4), 497–504.
17. Apter-Levy, Y., Feldman, M., Vakart, A., Ebstein, R. P., & Feldman, R. (2013). Impact of maternal depression across the first 6 years of life on the child's mental health, social engagement, and empathy: The moderating role of oxytocin. *American Journal of Psychiatry, 170*, 1161–1168
18. Yazici, E., Kirkan, T., Aslan, P., Aydin, N., & Yazici, A. (2015). *Untreated depression in the first trimester of pregnancy leads to postpartum depression: High rates from a natural follow-up study*. Available at http://www.ncbi.nlm.nih.gov/pmc/articles/PMC4344179/
19. Yin, J., & Schaaf, C. P. (2016). Autism genetics: An overview. *Prenatal Diagnosis, 37*(1), 14–30. do:10.1002/pd.4942
20. Krumm, N., O'Roak, B. J., Shendure, J., & Eichler, E. E. (2014). A de novo convergence of autism genetics and molecular neuroscience. *Trends in Neuroscience, 37*(2), 95–105.
21. Frans, E. M., Sandlin, S., & Reichenberg, A. (2016). Autism risk across generations: A population-based study of advancing grandpaternal and paternal age. *JAMA Psychiatry, 70*(5), 516–521.
22. Alzheimer's Society. (2016). *Genetics and dementia*. Available at https://www.alzheimers.org.uk/factsheet/405
23. Walder, D. J., Faraone, S. V., Glatt, S. J., Tsuang, M. T., & Seidman, L. J. (2014). Genetic liability, prenatal health, stress and family environment: Risk factors in the Harvard Adolescent Family High Risk for Schizophrenia Study. *Schizophrenia Research, 157*(1–3), 142–148.
24. National Association of Mental Illness. (2016). *Early psychosis and psychosis*. Available at http://www.nami.org/earlypsychosis
25. Connor, C., Birchwood, M., Freemantle, N., Palmer, C., Channa, S., Barker, C., Patterson, P., & Singh, S. (2016). Don't turn your back on the symptoms of psychosis: The results of a proof-of-principle, quasi-experimental intervention to reduce duration of untreated psychosis. *BMC Psychiatry, 16*, 127.
26. Bertholot, N., Paccalet, T., Gilvert, E., Moreau, I., Merette, C., Gingras, N., Roleau, N., & Maziade, M. (2015). Childhood abuse and neglect may induce deficits in cognitive precursors of psychosis in high-risk children. *Journal of Psychiatry and Neuroscience, 40*(5), 336–342.
27. Cunningham, C., & Peters, K. (2014). Aetiology of schizophrenia and implications for nursing practice: A literature review. *Issues in Mental Health Nursing, 35*, 732–738.
28. De Lacey, N., & King, B. H. (2013). Revisiting the relationship between autism and schizophrenia: Toward an integrated neurobiology. *Annual Review of Clinical Psychology, 9*, 555–587.
29. Hommer, R. E., & Swedo, S. E. (2015). Schizophrenia and autism: Related disorders. *Schizophrenia Bulletin, 41*(2), 313–314.
30. Radeloff, D., Ciaramidaro, A., Siniatchkin, M., Hainz, D., Schlitt, S., Weber, B., Poustka, F., Boite, S., Walter, H., & Freitag, C. M. (2014). Structural alterations of the social brain: A comparison between schizophrenia and autism. *PLOSOne, 9*(9), e106539.
31. Mackowick, K. M., Barr, M. S., Wing, V. C., Rabin, R. A., Ouellet-Plamondon, C., & George, T. P. (2014). Neurocognitive endophenotypes in schizophrenia: Modulation by nicotinic receptor systems. *Progress in Neuro-Psychopharmacology and Biological Psychiatry, 52*, 79–85.
32. Frankenburg, F. (2017). Schizophrenia. *Medscape*. Available at http://emedicine.medscape.com/article/288259-overview#a3
33. Hu, W., MacDonald, M. L., Elswick, D. E., & Sweet, R. A. (2015). The glutamate hypothesis of schizophrenia: Evidence from human brain tissue studies. *Annals of the New York Academy of Sciences, 1338*(1), 38–57.
34. Moghaddam, B., & Javitt, D. (2012). From revolution to evolution: The glutamate hypothesis of schizophrenia and its implication for treatment. *Neuropsychopharmacology, 37*(1), 4–15.
35. Kirkpatrick, B., & Miller, B. J. (2013). Inflammation and schizophrenia. *Schizophrenia Bulletin, 39*(6), 1174–1179.
36. Fineberg, A. M., & Ellman, L. M. (2013). Inflammatory cytokines and neurological and neurocognitive alterations in the course of schizophrenia. *Biological Psychiatry, 73*(10), 951–966.
37. Liang, W., & Chikritzhs, T. (2012). Early childhood infections and risk of schizophrenia. *Psychiatry Research, 200*(2–3), 214–217.
38. Alvarez, M., Masramon, H., Pena, C., Pont, M., Gourdier, C., Roura-Poch, P., & Arrufat, F. (2015). Cumulative effects of childhood traumas: Polytraumatization, dissociation, and schizophrenia. *Community Mental Health Journal, 51*, 54–62.
39. MacDonald, A. (2015). Schizophrenia: Presentation, affect and cognition, pathophysiology, and etiology. In P. Blaney, R. Krueger, & T. Millon (Eds.), *Oxford textbook of psychopathology* (3rd ed., pp. 333–352). New York, NY: Oxford University Press.
40. Heinrichs, R., Pinnock, F., Muharib, E., Hartman, L., Goldberg, J., & McDermid, S. (2015). Neurocognitive normality in schizophrenia revisited. *Schizophrenia Research: Cognition, 2*(4), 227–232.
41. Potter, M. J., & Moller, M. D. (2016). *Psychiatric-mental health nursing: From suffering to hope*. New York, NY: Pearson.
42. Ventura, J., Subotnik, K., Ered, A., Gretchen-Doorly, D., Hellemann, G., Vaskinn, A., & Nuechterlein, K. The relationship of attitudinal beliefs to negative symptoms, neurocognition, and daily functioning in recent-onset schizophrenia. *Schizophrenia Bulletin, 40*(6), 1308–1318.
43. Giusti, L., Ussorio, D., Tosone, A., Di Venanzio, C., Bianchini, V., Necozione, S., Casacchia, M., & Roncone, R. (2015). Is personal recovery in schizophrenia predicted by low cognitive insight? *Community Mental Health Journal, 51*(1), 30–37. doi:10.1007/s10597-014-9767-y
44. Pitschel-Walz, G., Leucht, S., Bauml, J., Kissling, W., & Engel, R. R. (2004). The effect of family interventions on relapse and rehospitalization in schizophrenia: A meta-analysis. *Focus: A Journal of Lifelong Learning in Psychiatry, 2*(1), 78–94.
45. Harvey, C., & O'Hanlon, B. (2013). Family psycho-education for people with schizophrenia and other psychotic disorders and their families. *Australia and New Zealand Journal of Psychiatry, 47*, 516–520.

46. Sutcliffe, C., Roe, B., Jasper, R., Jolley, D., & Challis, D. (2015). People with dementia and carers' experiences of dementia care and services: Outcomes of a focus group study. *Dementia, 14*(6), 769–787.
47. World Health Organization. (2012). *Patterns of dementia globally*. Available at http://www.who.int/gho/publications/world_health_statistics/2012/en/
48. Alzheimer's Association. (2016). *Types of dementia*. Available at http://www.alz.org/dementia/types-of-dementia.asp#alzheimers
49. Alzheimer's Association. (2016). *What is dementia?* Available at http://www.alz.org/what-is-dementia.asp
50. Teodorzuk, A., Mukaetova-Ladinska, E., Corbett, S., & Welfare, M. (2015). Deconstructing dementia and delirium hospital practice: Using cultural historical activity theory to inform education approaches. *Advances in Health Science Education, 20*, 745–764.
51. Gronlund, C., Zanobetti, A., Schwartz, J., Wellenius, G., & O'Neill, M. (2014). Heat, heat waves, and hospital admissions among the elderly in the United States, 1992–2006. *Environmental Health Perspectives, 122*(11), 1187–1192.
52. Inouye, S. K., Westendorp, R. G. J., & Sacynski, J. S. (2014). Delirium in elderly people. *Lancet, 383*(9920), 911–922.
53. Bull, M. J., Boaz., L., & Jerme, M. (2016). Educating family caregivers for older adults about delirium. *Worldviews on Evidence-Based Nursing, 13*(3), 232–240.
54. Ranganath, K., Murthy, S., & Swetha, M. (2015). Study of delirium and its subtypes in medically ill hospitalized patients. *Cognitive Neuroscience*, e-Poster session 17.
55. Alagiakrishnan, K. (2016). *Delirium treatment & management*. Available at http://emedicine.medscape.com/article/288890-treatment
56. Inouye, S. K., Marcantonio, E. R., & Metzger, E. D. (2014). Doing damage in delirium: The hazards of antipsychotic treatment in elderly persons. *Lancet Psychiatry, 1*(4), 312–315.
57. Weusten, L., Heijnen-Kohl, M., Ellison, J., & van Alphen, S. (2014). Interference of attention-deficit hyperactivity disorder in an older adult with a severe personality disorder and dermatillomania. *International Psychogeriatrics, 26*(2), 341–343.
58. Centers for Disease Control and Prevention. (2016). *Attention-deficit/hyperactivity disorder (ADHD)*. Available at https://www.cdc.gov/ncbddd/adhd/facts.html
59. Goodman, D., Mitchell, S., Rhodewalt, L., & Surman, C. (2016). Clinical presentation, diagnosis, and treatment of attention-deficit hyperactivity disorder (ADHD) in older adults: A review of the evidence and its implications for clinical care. *Drugs & Aging, 33*, 27–36.
60. Lopez, B. (2015). Beyond modularisation: The need of a socio-neuro- constructionist model of autism. *Journal of Autism and Developmental Disorders, 45*, 31–41.
61. Torgerson, T., Gjervan, B., Lensing, M., & Rasmussen, K. (2016). Optimal management of ADHD in older adults. *Neuropsychiatric Disease and Treatment, 12*, 79–87.
62. Theoharides, T. C., Tsillioni, I., Patel, A. B., & Doyle, R. (2016). Atopic diseases and inflammation of the brain in the pathogenesis of ASD. *Translational Psychiatry, 6*(e844). Available at http://www.nature.com/tp/journal/v6/n6/abs/tp201677a.html
63. Mayo Clinic. (2014). *Autism spectrum disorder*. Available at http://www.mayoclinic.org/diseases-conditions/autism-spectrum-disorder/basics/causes/con-20021148
64. Stefano, F., Price, C. S., & Weintraub, E. S. (2013). Increasing exposure to antibody-stimulating proteins and polysaccharides in vaccines is not associated with risk of autism. *Journal of Pediatrics, 163*(2), 561–567.
65. Bermudez, M., Sanchez, J., del Sol, M., & Sevilla, F. (2015). Parents-perceived and self-perceived anxiety in children with autism spectrum disorder. *Educational Research & Reviews, 10*(18), 2531–2538.
66. Frey, A., et al. (2015). First step to success: Applications to preschoolers at risk of developing autism spectrum disorders. *Education and Training in Autism and Developmental Disabilities, 50*(4), 397–407.
67. De Groot-van der Mooren, M., Gemke, R., Cornel, M., & Weijerman, M. (2014). Neonatal diagnosis of Down syndrome in the Netherlands: Suspicion and communication with parents. *Journal of Intellectual Disability Research, 58*(10), 953–961.
68. Anderson, J. S., Nielsen, J. A., Ferguson, M. A., Burback, M. C., Cox, E. T., Dai, L., Gerig, G., Edgin, J. O., & Korenberg, J. R. (2013). Abnormal brain synchrony in Down syndrome. *NeuroImage: Clinical, 2*, 703–715.
69. Morris, J., & Springett, A. (2014). *The National Down Syndrome Cytogenetic Register for England and Wales: 2013 annual report*. London, U.K.: National Down Syndrome Cytogenetic Register.
70. Bryant, L., Puri, S., Dix, L., & Ahmed, S. (2016). Tell it right, start it right: An evaluation of training for health professionals about Down syndrome. *British Journal of Midwifery, 24*(2), 110–126.
71. National Down Syndrome Society. (2012). *Speech and language therapy for infants, toddlers, and young children*. Available at http://www.ndss.org/Resources/Therapies-Development/Speech-Language-Therapy/Speech-Language-Therapy-for-Infants-Toddlers-Young-Children/
72. Moran, J. (n.d.). *Aging and Down syndrome: A health and well-being handbook*. New York, NY: National Down Syndrome Society.
73. Murawski, N., Moore, E., Thomas, J., & Riley, E. (2015). Advances in diagnosis and treatment of fetal alcohol spectrum disorders. *Alcohol Research*, online.
74. Esper, L., & Furtado, E. (2014). Identifying maternal risk factors associated with fetal alcohol spectrum disorders: A systematic review. *European Child & Adolescent Psychiatry, 23*, 877–889.
75. May, P., et al. (2013). Maternal alcohol consumption producing fetal alcohol spectrum disorders (FASD): Quantity, frequency, and timing of drinking. *Drug and Alcohol Dependence, 133*(2), 502–512.
76. National Institute on Alcohol Abuse and Alcoholism. (2013). #3-D image analysis promises to improve detection of children affected by prenatal alcohol. *Research News*. Retrieved from https://www.niaaa.nih.gov/research/niaaa-research-highlights/3-d-image-analysis

Unit IX
Disorders of Sensory Perception and Thermoregulation

Sensory disorders, pain, and altered thermoregulation may appear to have little in common at first glance, but they all share the following characteristics:

- Subjective symptoms are initially reported by the patient. These symptoms are then confirmed or, occasionally, contradicted by clinical markers.
- Alterations in any of these areas can signal an increased risk for altered homeostasis and/or increased risk for injury.
- All subjective reports of discomfort must be considered seriously.

The five senses—vision, hearing, touch, smell, and taste—are essential for growth, development, and survival. Normal sensory function enables or affects nearly every human activity, from reading a book to alerting someone to smoke from a fire. Alterations in any aspect of sensory perception can affect an individual's ability to receive, process, and communicate information and can increase the individual's risk for illness or injury. In addition, any of these alterations may affect an individual's ability to participate in a treatment plan or necessitate interventions or accommodations to the treatment plan in order to ensure best outcomes. For example, older adults with vision impairment, especially those with multiple recent hospital admissions, are more likely to require community services such as home health nursing.[1]

Uncontrolled pain is associated with poor patient satisfaction, unplanned hospital readmissions, prolonged recovery from illness or surgery, exacerbation of unrelated disease states or organ dysfunction, excessive loss of work time, and long-term disability. Pain is a prevalent manifestation: Worldwide, it is estimated that 1 in 5 adults suffer from acute or chronic pain or a combination of both.[2] According to the Joint Commission over 76 million people in the United States suffer from acute or chronic pain.[3]

The usual range of core body temperature is called normothermia. The normal range for adults is between 36° and 38.5°C (96.8° and 101.3°F). A body temperature of 38.5°C (101.3°F) and above is called *hyperthermia* or, in lay terms, fever. Heat-related injuries may occur with even moderate increases in temperatures. Heat-related illnesses or injuries include *heat exhaustion* and *heat stroke*.

Hypothermia is a core body temperature below 35°C (95°F). Temperatures of 28°C (82.4°F) or lower can cause cell, tissue, and organ destruction. This can be caused by one or a combination of three mechanisms described in Chapter 33.

Disorders of sensory perception occur across the lifespan, but they may not be diagnosed immediately. Pain also occurs throughout the lifespan, with clinical manifestations varying in newborns and children who are too young to verbally express feelings of pain. Newborns and infants, young children, and older adults are at greatest risk for hyper- and hypothermia, as are individuals who spend time in extreme climates, such as construction workers and rescue personnel. Pathophysiology, clinical manifestations, and treatment for these various disorders are described in the chapters that follow.

References

1. Hong, T., Mitchell, P., Burlutsky, G., Fong, S., Rochtchina, E., & Wang, J. J. (2013). Visual impairment and subsequent use of support services among older people: Longitudinal findings from the Blue Mountains Eye Study. *American Journal Ophthalmology, 156*(2), 393–399.
2. Fong, A., & Schug, S.A. (2014). Pathophysiology of pain: A practical primer. *Plastic and Reconstructive Surgery, 134*(4S-2):8S–14S.
3. The Joint Commission. (2017). *Pain management*. Retrieved from http://www.jointcommission.org/pain_management/

Hearing, Balance, and Vision Disorders

- Conductive hearing loss disorders
- Sensorineural hearing loss disorders
- Vertigo and other disruptions in balance
- Vision disorders

Vision Loss

- Refractive errors
- Amblyopia and strabismus
- Cataracts
- Glaucoma
- Retinopathy
- Macular degeneration

Hearing Loss

- Conductive hearing loss disorders
  - Outer ear disorders
  - Otitis media
  - Otosclerosis
- Sensorineural hearing loss disorders
  - Presbycusis
  - Ménière disease
  - Ototoxicity
  - Noise-induced hearing loss
  - Genetic hearing loss

Disorders of Thermoregulation

- Hyperthermia
  - Heat stroke
  - Heat exhaustion
  - Fever
- Normothermia
- Hypothermia
  - Mild
  - Moderate
  - Severe

Pain, Neuropathy, and Headache

- Acute pain
- Chronic pain
- Neuropathic pain
- Headache
- Other pain syndromes
  - Central pain syndrome
  - Myofascial pain syndrome
  - Fibromyalgia
  - Psychogenic pain
  - Persistent postsurgical pain

Types of Pain

- Central
- Myofascial
- Neuropathic
- Phantom
- Psychogenic
- Radicular
- Somatic
- Vascular
- Visceral

Types of Headache

- Tension type
- Migraine
- Cluster

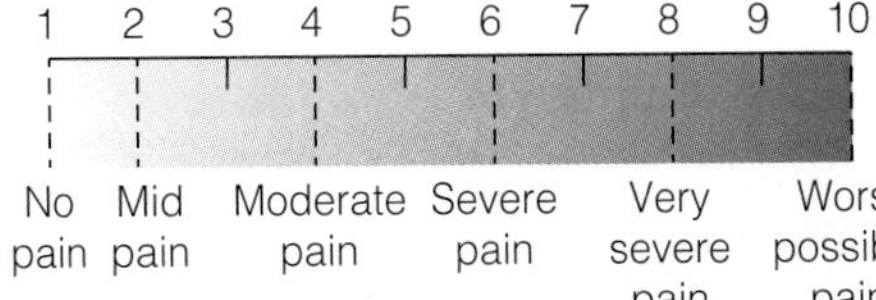

Chapter 31

Disorders of Hearing, Balance, and Vision

Patricia McCarthy, Amy K. Winston, and Matthew W. Gifford

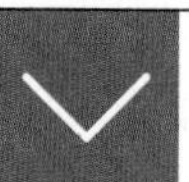

Chapter Outline and Learning Outcomes

31.1 Chapter Overview and Case Studies

Describe disorders of sensation and concepts related to disorders of hearing, vision, and balance.

31.2 Basic Anatomy and Physiology of Hearing and Balance

Describe the auditory and vestibular pathways, and identify critical peripheral and central structures involved in processing hearing and balance information.

31.3 Conductive Hearing Loss Disorders

Differentiate the causes, classification, underlying pathogenesis, and clinical manifestations of conductive hearing loss and approaches to treatment of those conditions across the lifespan.

31.4 Sensorineural Hearing Loss Disorders

Differentiate the causes, classification, underlying pathogenesis, and clinical manifestations of sensorineural hearing loss and approaches to treatment of those conditions across the lifepan.

31.5 Basic Anatomy and Physiology of Vision

Describe the visual pathway, and identify critical peripheral and central structures involved in processing visual information.

31.6 External Eye Disorders

Differentiate the causes, classification, underlying pathogenesis, and clinical manifestations of external eye pathologies and approaches to treatment of those conditions across the lifespan.

31.7 Vision Disorders

Differentiate the causes, classification, underlying pathogenesis, and clinical manifestations of vision pathologies and approaches to treatment of those conditions across the lifespan.

31.8 Nystagmus

Differentiate the causes, classification, underlying pathogenesis, and clinical manifestations of nystagmus and related approaches to treatment across the lifespan.

KEY TERMS

Acoustic trauma, 762
Acute otitis media (AOM), 757
Amblyopia, 769
Aminoglycoside antibiotics, 762
Assistive listening device, 760
Astigmatism, 769
Cataract, 769
Chronic otitis media (COM), 757
Closed-angle glaucoma, 770
Cochlear implant, 761
Cochleotoxic, 761
Conductive hearing loss, 755
Conjunctivitis, 767
Corneal abrasion, 768
Diabetic retinopathy, 771
Dry macular degeneration, 771
Endolymph, 754
Glaucoma, 770
Hearing aid, 760
Hordeolum, 767
Hyperopia, 769
Macular degeneration, 771
Ménière disease, 760
Middle ear effusion, 757
Mixed hearing loss, 759
Myopia, 769
Noise-induced hearing loss (NIHL), 762
Nonproliferative diabetic retinopathy, 771
Nonsyndromic genetic hearing loss, 764
Nystagmus, 772
Open-angle glaucoma, 770
Osseointegrated hearing implants, 759
Otitis media (OM), 757

Key Terms continue on next page.

Otolith, 755
Otosclerosis, 758
Ototoxic, 761
Perilymph, 754
Permanent threshold shift (PTS), 763
Platinum-based medications, 762
Presbycusis, 759
Presbyopia, 769
Pressure equalization (PE) tubes, 758
Proliferative diabetic retinopathy (PDR), 771
Pterygium, 768
Retinopathy, 771
Semicircular canals, 755
Sensorineural hearing loss, 759
Stapedectomy, 759
Strabismus, 769
Stye, 767
Syndromic hearing loss, 764
Temporary threshold shift (TTS), 762
Tinnitus, 759
Vertigo, 755
Vestibulotoxic, 761
Wet macular degeneration, 772

ABBREVIATIONS

AOM—acute otitis media
COM—chronic otitis media
IOP—intraocular pressure
NIHL—noise-induced hearing loss
OM—otitis media
PDR—proliferative diabetic retinopathy
PE—pressure equalization
PTS—permanent threshold shift
TM—tympanic membrane
TTS—temporary threshold shift

31.1 Chapter Overview and Case Studies

We are constantly interacting with our environment—tasting, touching, smelling, hearing, and feeling the world around us. But how are we able to experience these different sensations? The human body has specialized sensory organs designed to take in various stimuli from the environment. Unique receptors within the sensory organs respond to these inputs and initiate the transformation of this information into neural impulses that can ultimately be interpreted at a cortical level, allowing us to experience and interpret our world (**Figure 31.1** ■).

This chapter discusses the anatomy, physiology, and pathophysiology of two of these special sensory organs: the eye and the ear. Structures within the ear enable us to hear and interpret the sounds around us and provide information about the position and movement of the head in space. The shape and color of our

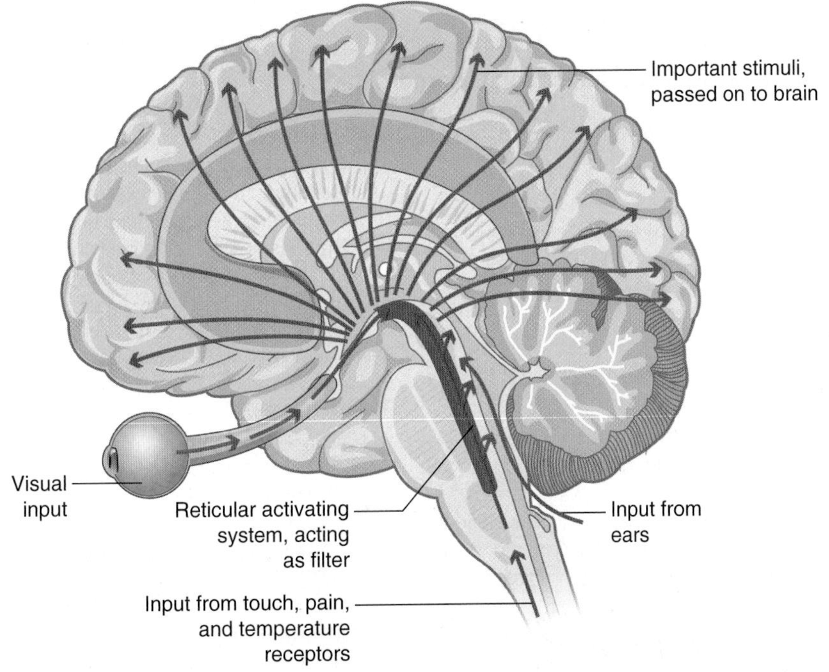

Figure 31.1 ■ The nerve impulses run along the ascending sensory tracts to reach the reticular activating system; then certain impulses reach the cerebral cortex, where they are perceived.

environment—conveyed in light energy—is captured by special receptors within the eye, allowing us to see the world. Impairments in the structures of the ear and eye or the related neural pathways alter the information that is available to our cortex to process and thus alter our ability to perceive and experience the world around us. Disease, aging, medications, environmental factors, and genetics are just some of the factors that can result in permanent or temporary problems with hearing or vision. Identification and assessment of hearing and vision changes can help to direct appropriate medical and rehabilitative interventions, which may directly restore lost sensory capacity or provide management strategies or tools to alleviate the negative effects of these sensory changes on quality of life.

Concepts Related to Disorders of Hearing, Balance, and Vision

Individuals who experience disorders of hearing, balance, and vision are likely to have issues in development or other areas that negatively affect their overall quality of life. For example, children born with hearing or vision deficits may experience developmental, communication, or mobility delays. Adults who lose their vision or hearing may experience problems with mobility, nutrition, stress and coping, mood and affect, and increased susceptibility to environmental issues. Selected concepts related to disorders of hearing, balance, and vision are shown in **Figure 31.2** ■.

Case Studies

The following cases are addressed throughout the chapter to assist in application of chapter content to clinical situations that involve individuals with disorders of hearing, balance, and vision.

Mateo Ramirez: Introduction

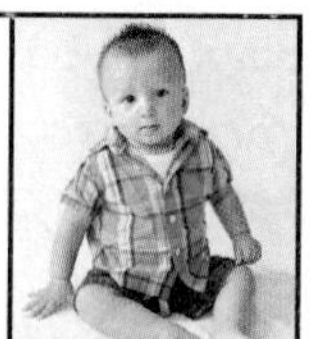

The parents of Mateo Ramirez, an 8-month-old boy, report that Mateo has been irritable, fussy, and waking in the middle of the night. Furthermore, he has stopped babbling and appears out of sorts. He had a slight head cold recently, but it seemed to resolve, so his parents did not seek medical care.

1. What are the *Healthy People 2020* recommendations for hearing screening in children?
2. Why is hearing important in growth and development?

Greg Seitz: Introduction

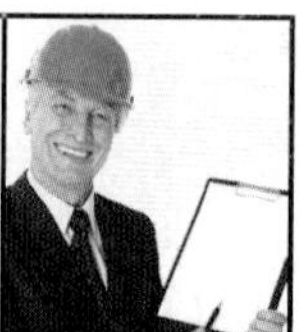

Greg Seitz, age 49, works in construction and also does part-time lawn work, which involves lawn mowers and leaf blowers. He is a veteran of the Gulf War and is married with three children. Although he has no complaints about his hearing, his wife reports that Mr. Seitz's hearing loss is interfering significantly with family communication.

1. What factors could contribute to Mr. Seitz's hearing loss?
2. According to *Healthy People 2020*, what interventions can be done to prevent or decrease the risk of hearing loss?

Healthy People 2020

Hearing and Other Sensory or Communication Disorders

Goal: "Reduce the prevalence and severity of disorders of hearing and balance; smell and taste; and voice, speech, and language."[1]

Overview: At least 1 in 6 Americans currently has a sensory or communication impairment or disorder. Even when these disorders are temporary or mild, they can affect physical and mental health. An impaired ability to communicate with others or maintain good balance can lead many people to feel socially isolated, have unmet health needs, and have limited success in school or on the job.

Why Hearing Loss Reduction Is Important: The effects of hearing loss on a child's speech, language, and psychosocial and academic achievement have been well documented.[2] In adults and older adults, hearing loss can have significant effects on quality of life.[3] Therefore, prevention, identification, diagnosis, and treatment of hearing loss are essential for communication and well-being of individuals of all ages.

Objectives: There are 15 specific *Healthy People 2020* objectives related to hearing, tinnitus, and balance in infants, children, and adults. Following are some examples of these objectives related to hearing:

- Increase the proportion of newborns who are screened for hearing loss by no later than age 1 month, have audiologic evaluation by age 3 months, and are enrolled in appropriate intervention services no later than age 6 months.
- Decrease otitis media in children and adolescents.
- Increase the number of persons who are referred by their primary care physician or other health care provider for hearing evaluation and treatment.
- Increase the use of hearing protection devices.

References

1. Healthy People. (2017). *Topics and objectives: Hearing and other sensory or communication disorders*. Available at http://www.healthypeople.gov/2020/topicsobjectives2020/ebr.aspx?topicId=20
2. Blamey, P. J., Sarant, J. Z., Paatsch, L. E. et al. (2001). Relationships among speech perception, production, language, hearing loss, and age in children with impaired hearing. *Journal of Speech, Language, and Hearing Research,* 44(2): 264–285.(2001).
3. McCarthy, P., & Schau, N. (2008). Adult audiologic rehabilitation: A review of contemporary practices. *Contemporary Issues in Communication Science and Disorders,* 35: 166–177.

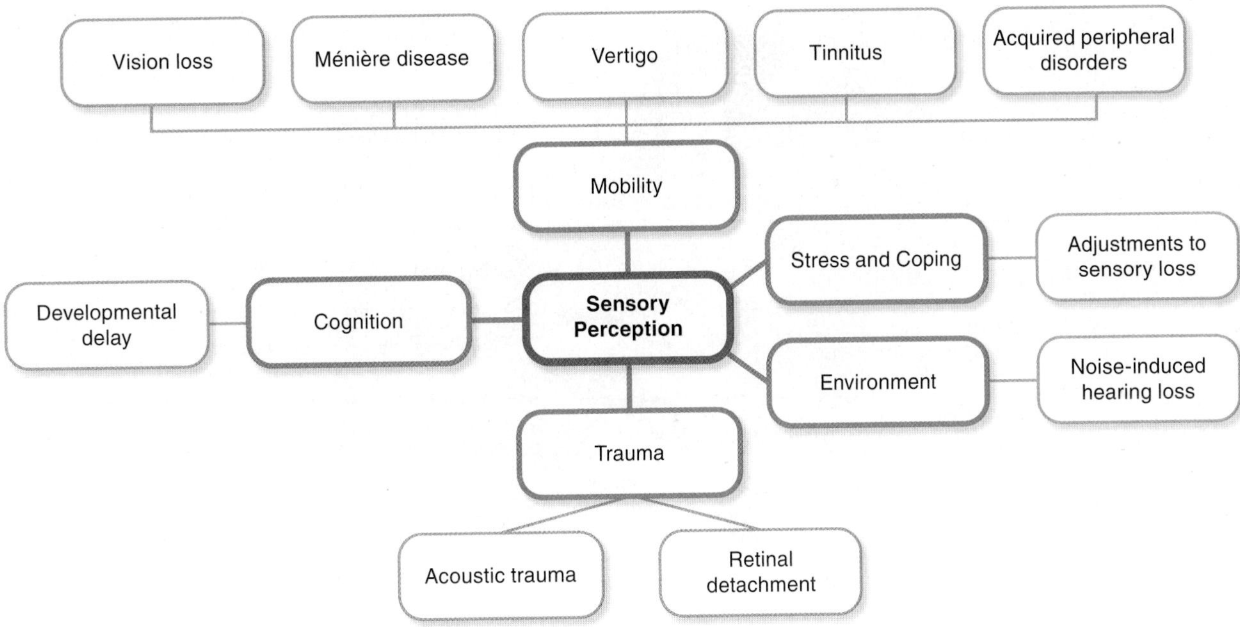

Figure 31.2 ■ Concepts related to disorders of hearing, vision, and balance.

Sam Park: Introduction

Sam Park is a financial analyst with a high-powered, stressful job that requires reading stock reports and newspapers. When in his late forties, he noticed some difficult visualizing small print. Now at 68 years of age, he is avoiding business

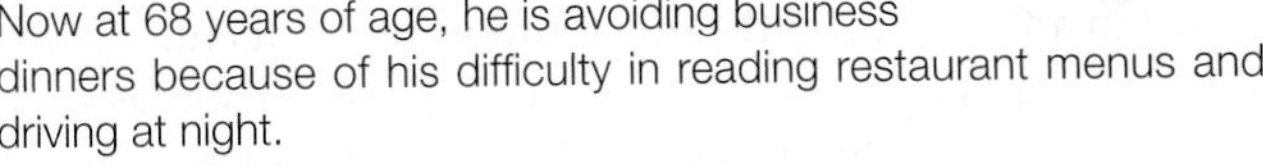

dinners because of his difficulty in reading restaurant menus and driving at night.

1. Why could there be a change in Mr. Park's vision?
2. What consequence is Mr. Park experiencing as a result of his vision changes?

Check Your Progress: Section 31.1

1. Why are vision and hearing important?
2. Describe why hearing and other sensory or communication disorders are part of *Healthy People 2020* objectives.

31.2 Basic Anatomy and Physiology of Hearing and Balance

The Auditory System

Hearing involves an amazing and complex series of energy transmissions and transformations mediated by the peripheral and central auditory system structures. In this system, sound waves, which are pressure waves that travel through the air, are captured and transformed into neural impulses that can be perceived by the brain. The structure and function of the auditory system structures are designed so that the characteristics of the sound itself, including pitch, loudness, and timing characteristics, are preserved at each step, allowing the brain to perceive the sound accurately (**Figure 31.3** ■).

Pathologies of the auditory system disrupt the normal sound transmission process and result in hearing loss. There are three types of hearing loss: sensorineural, conductive, and mixed; the location(s) of the pathology will determine the type of hearing loss that is present. The degree of hearing loss can vary depending on the cause and type of hearing loss involved. As will be discussed later in this chapter, the rehabilitative options for hearing loss differ depending on the degree and type of the loss.

The Peripheral Auditory System

Outer Ear. The outer ear comprises two structures: the auricle, or pinna, and the external auditory canal. The auricle, which consists primarily of cartilage, functions in sound collection, transmission, and localization. Sound pressure waves are collected by the auricle and directed into the external auditory canal. The position of the auricle on the side of the head also generates important cues about the timing and intensity of sounds that help us to localize them in our environment. The ear canal is a curved tube that is approximately 2–3 cm long in an adult. The ear canal ends at the tympanic membrane (TM), or eardrum, which forms the lateral wall of the middle ear. This canal is lined with hairs and specialized sweat glands that secrete a waxy substance; this waxy secretion combines with natural oils to produce cerumen (earwax). Together, cerumen and hairs in the ear canal help to protect the rest of the hearing system from dust and debris. The auricle and external auditory canal work together to shape the sounds that we hear, naturally filtering out some low-pitched sounds and increasing

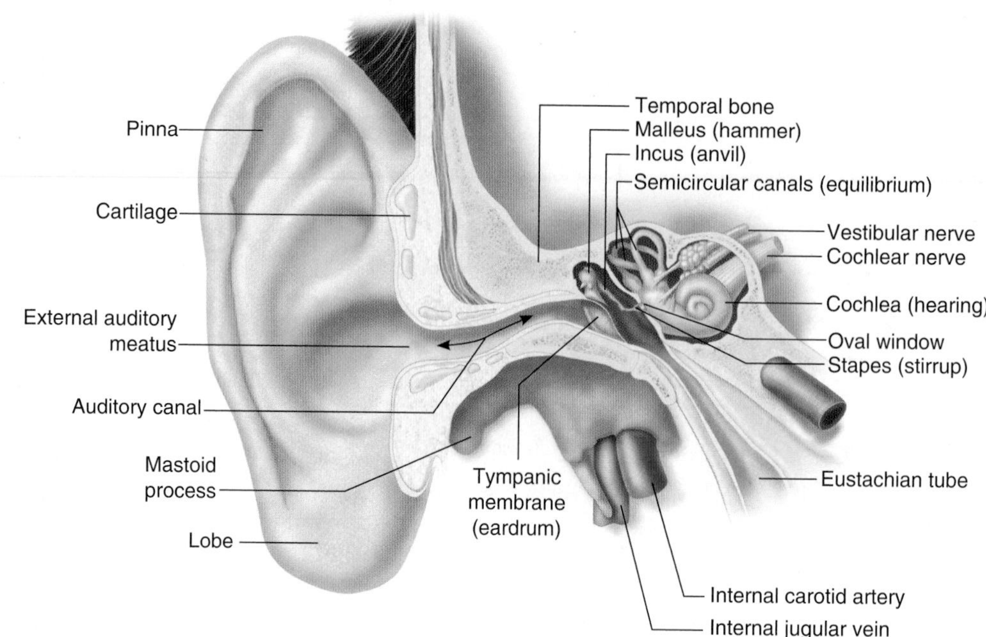

Figure 31.3 ■ Structures of the outer ear, middle ear, and inner ear.

the volume of higher-pitched sounds that are particularly important for speech perception.

Middle Ear. The middle ear is an enclosed, bony space with the tympanic membrane as the lateral, or outermost, wall. The tympanic membrane is a strong, flexible membrane that functions as a sound receptor and transmitter. Sound pressure waves travel down the external auditory canal and strike the tympanic membrane, causing it to vibrate. These vibrations are then transmitted to a chain of three small bones—the ossicles—that lie in the middle ear cavity. The largest and heaviest of these three bones, the malleus, is attached to the tympanic membrane; vibrations from the tympanic membrane travel down this chain of bones, from the malleus to the incus, and then to the stapes. The end of the stapes, the stapes footplate, is attached to another membrane, the oval window, which leads into the fluid-filled inner ear. The most important function of the middle ear structures is that of impedance matching. In moving from the outer ear to the inner ear, sound energy must move from air to fluid. Sound waves travel easily through air, but they do not travel readily through fluid. Natural amplification mechanisms in the middle ear increase the sound energy to overcome this difference so that the characteristics of the incoming sound are maintained in the inner ear. A moderate hearing loss would result without this critical middle ear function.

Inner Ear. The inner ear system includes the components of the peripheral balance system and the essential organ of hearing, the cochlea. All of the inner ear components are housed together in the bony labyrinth, a system of canals in the temporal bone. Within this system of bony canals is a fluid-filled membranous labyrinth.

The cochlea is a snail-shaped structure that turns 2.75 times around the modiolus, a central bony pillar. Within the cochlea, the membranous labyrinth has three distinct, parallel canals: the scala vestibuli, scala media, and scala tympani. The scala vestibuli and scala tympani are bounded by the walls of the bony labyrinth; these canals are filled with a fluid called **perilymph**, which is very high in sodium and ionically very similar to cerebrospinal fluid. The scala vestibuli and scala tympani are continuous, communicating through an opening at the top, or apex, of the cochlea called the helicotrema. The oval window, where the stapes footplate lies, opens into the scala vestibuli. A second membrane, the round window, lies at the end of the scala tympani. These two membranes serve as pressure "windows" that allow for the movement of fluid within these membranous tubes.

Between these two ducts lies the scala media, filled with **endolymph**, which is very high in potassium. The scala media houses the organ of Corti, the sensory system of hearing. The organ of Corti is bounded by two important membranes: the basilar membrane, on which the organ of Corti lies, and the gelatinous tectorial membrane, which lies at the top of the organ of Corti. The two sensory cells of hearing—outer hair cells and inner hair cells—lie within the organ of Corti. Stereocilia from both types of hair cells project into the overlying tectorial membrane.

The cochlea has two primary functions: to encode the frequency and intensity of the incoming sound and to transform mechanical energy from the middle ear into neural impulses. Movement of the stapes footplate displaces fluid in the membranous labyrinth and causes the basilar membrane to vibrate up and down. The basilar membrane is tonotopically organized, meaning that it vibrates to specific pitches of sound at different locations along its length. Movement of the basilar membrane causes the hair cell stereocilia to shear as they are moved relative to the tectorial membrane in which they are embedded, depolarizing both the outer and inner hair cells. The depolarized outer hair cells begin to contract and expand, exacerbating the initial movement of the basilar membrane and causing additional stimulation of the inner hair cells. Depolarization of the inner hair cells triggers a neural impulse in the auditory sensory nerve fibers that lie at their base.

The Central Auditory System

The neural impulse that is triggered by the action of the inner hair cell travels along the auditory portion of the vestibulocochlear nerve (cranial nerve VIII), which exits the cochlea through the internal auditory canal. This neural signal then travels through multiple nuclei in the brainstem before proceeding to the thalamus and finally to the primary auditory cortex, Heschl's gyrus, in the temporal lobe. Both this ascending auditory pathway and Heschl's gyrus itself maintain the tonotopic organization present in the cochlea, allowing for identification and characterization of the incoming sounds.

The Peripheral Balance System

In addition to housing the cochlea, the bony labyrinth of the inner ear contains the sensory organs of the peripheral balance system: the three paired **semicircular canals** (horizontal, posterior, and anterior) and the two **otolith** organs: the utricle and the saccule (**Figure 31.4** ■). The semicircular canals are sensitive to head movement; they provide information to the cerebellum about the velocity and direction of head motion and direct reflexive, compensatory changes in eye position that help us maintain clear vision when the head is in motion. The utricle and saccule are sensitive to linear acceleration and changes in head position relative to gravity, and they send information to the cerebellum about the position of the head as we move forward and backward or up and down in space.

Like the cochlea, the sensory organs of balance contain specialized hair cells, type I and type II, which are sensitive to changes in the movement of fluids within the membranous labyrinth. These cells trigger neural responses that travel along the vestibular portion of cranial nerve VIII to the cerebellum and ultimately to the cerebral cortex for processing.

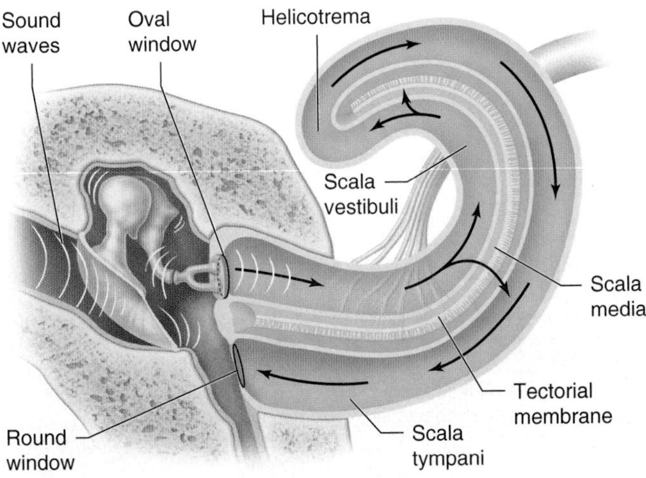

Figure 31.4 ■ Anatomy of the cochlea.

Certain diseases or conditions—including some viral or bacterial infections, temporal bone fractures, and benign tumors—can disrupt the normal function of the sensory cells in the peripheral balance system and/or transmission of that information along the vestibulocochlear nerve. This loss of peripheral balance function can result in **vertigo**, which is a false sensation of rotation of oneself or one's environment that may be accompanied by intense nausea and vomiting. In some cases, a peripheral balance disorder may generate feelings of unsteadiness and/or visual blurring, particularly with head movement. Factors such as disease or trauma that affect normal balance function can also affect hearing sensitivity; one such disorder, Ménière disease, is discussed later in this chapter.

Vertigo and other disruptions in balance can also result from central disorders that affect the transmission, processing, and/or integration of the different inputs to the balance system, which include the eyes, joints, and muscles in addition to the peripheral balance system structures. Central vestibular problems may develop from conditions such as cerebrovascular disease or multiple sclerosis. Finally, some medications, including anticonvulsant drugs, can affect balance by suppressing or altering the normal response of either the peripheral or central balance structures. Other medications can cause permanent damage to the sensory cells in the peripheral balance system. These medications are identified later in this chapter in the discussion of ototoxicity.

Check Your Progress: Section 31.2

1. Name and describe the two functions of the cochlea.
2. List the three main parts of the ear and the subparts of each main part.
3. Describe how the inner ear provides information about balance to the brain.

31.3 Conductive Hearing Loss Disorders

Problems that affect the outer and middle ear system structures prevent sound from traveling normally to the inner ear. The result is a **conductive hearing loss**. A conductive hearing loss reflects an audibility problem. Loss of the natural acoustic benefits of the outer ear and/or the impedance matching of the middle ear structures reduces the intensity (volume) of the sound that reaches the inner ear. So although sounds can be processed normally in the inner ear, they are no longer as loud as they should be when they reach that part of the auditory system.

Outer Ear Disorders

The outer ear is susceptible to a number of pathologies ranging from insect bites to inflammation to trauma to skin cancers. Fortunately, most outer ear pathologies are highly treatable, and many do not involve hearing loss; congenital outer ear malformations are the primary exception. Table 31.1 ■

Table 31.1 Common Outer Ear Disorders

Description	Incidence	Effect on Hearing	Treatment
Cerumen Impaction			
• Wax blockage in the ear canal causing a complete obstruction • May have sudden onset due to wax shifting • Attempt to clean or remove may push wax deeper into the canal	• Estimates suggest higher incidence in children, aging population and individuals with cognitive impairments	• Can cause conductive loss or no hearing loss • Mild to moderate degree depending on severity of impaction	• Cerumen softener • Irrigation or removal with instruments such as wax loops • Suction sometimes needed
Collapsed Ear Canal			
• Ear canal cannot support itself because of flaccid cartilage • Collapses and closes off the external portion of the auditory pathway • May be caused by headphones used in audiologic testing	• Most frequently seen in infant and aging populations	• May cause increased hearing thresholds at high frequencies	• Use of inserts to avoid collapsing canal during hearing testing
External Otitis			
• Infection (bacterial or fungal) of the external ear • May include discomfort in ear canal or auricle • Symptoms: erythema, swelling of canal with discharge, pain and inflammation • Causes: moisture, trauma, water with bacteria, high temperature, mechanical removal of cerumen, foreign objects • Canal usually red and swollen • Difficult to see TM	• 4 in every 1000 people in the United States • Increase in the summer months ("swimmers ear")	• Possible temporary conductive hearing loss depending on condition of ear canal • Hearing returns to normal after infection dissipates	• Topical aural medications to stop infection • Corticosteroid for inflammation • Oral antibiotics reserved for severe case • Antibiotic eardrops may be prescribed
Stenosis of Ear Canal			
• Narrowing of the external ear canal • Considered a mild form of atresia • Congenital or canal could narrow over time owing to chronic inflammation, prior surgery, scar tissue buildup in the canal • May cause increased ear infections and a higher chance of cerumen impaction	• Estimates not available	• Conductive hearing loss with severe cases of stenosis • Hearing may be normal	• Treatment depends on degree of stenosis • Surgery can widen canal, remove excess tissue or built-up scar tissue • If due to osteoma (bone growth), the surgeon may chisel away bone to widen the canal
Microtia			
• Very small or underdeveloped auricle • Bilateral or unilateral • Commonly associated with atresia • Four grades: 1. Slightly smaller ear with identifiable structures 2. Partial or hemi ear with closed off canal producing conductive loss 3. Absence of external ear with small peanut vestigial structure (most common) 4. Anotia, or complete absence of ear	• Occurs in 1 in every 10,000 births.	• Conductive loss may be present • Severity of hearing loss depends on status of ear canal • If no ear canal, air conduction sound not an option for hearing	• Baha® or Ponto® best option if conductive hearing loss • Reconstruction surgery of auricle • Plastic implant may be created • Full ear prosthesis may be used
Anotia			
• Total absence of the auricle • Occurs most often with a narrowing or absence of the ear canal • Considered the most severe form of microtia	• Occurs in 2.82 cases per 10,000 births • More common on the right ear in males • Approximately 10% occur bilaterally	• If ear canal is present, conductive loss will be less but still be impaired • If ear canal is closed, degree of conductive loss will increase • Inner ear function will be normal	• Traditional ear-level hearing aids are not an option • Baha®, Ponto® or bone conduction hearing aid is best option if conductive hearing loss • Reconstruction surgery can form auricle

Atresia			
• Absence of the external ear canal • Often accompanied by abnormalities of the ossicles and the external ear • Usually due to underdevelopment of the external ear	• Occurs in about 1 per 5000–20,000 births	• Conductive hearing loss may be mild to moderate	• Baha®, Ponto® or bone conduction hearing aid is best hearing option
Skin Cancer			
• UV rays cause 90% of skin cancers • Auricles exposed to sun, particularly in men • Most typical type is basal cell carcinoma • May develop on any part of the ear	• Ears are third most common location for basal cell carcinomas	• If limited to the auricle, no hearing loss • Lesion may be identified by audiologist during hearing testing	• Biopsy, surgical removal of the damaged cells • Further treatment if melanoma

describes the most common outer ear pathologies, incidence, effect on hearing and treatment.

Otitis Media

Otitis media (OM) is an inflammation of the middle ear space often associated with Eustachian tube dysfunction that is commonly diagnosed in children. Middle ear infections are not as common in adolescents, teenagers, and adults, but they can be seen in conjunction with Eustachian tube dysfunction.

It has been estimated that approximately 60% of infants experience one ear infection before 1 year of age.[1] Predisposing risk factors for OM include secondhand cigarette smoke, age younger than 2 years, drinking from a bottle while lying down, and daycare attendance.[2] Anatomic abnormalities of the palate, such as those seen in cleft palate and Down syndrome, increase a child's risk for ear infections, as does chronic hypersensitivity.[3] ■

Etiology and Pathogenesis

Otitis media is an inflammation of the middle ear space often associated with Eustachian tube dysfunction (**Figure 31.5** ■).

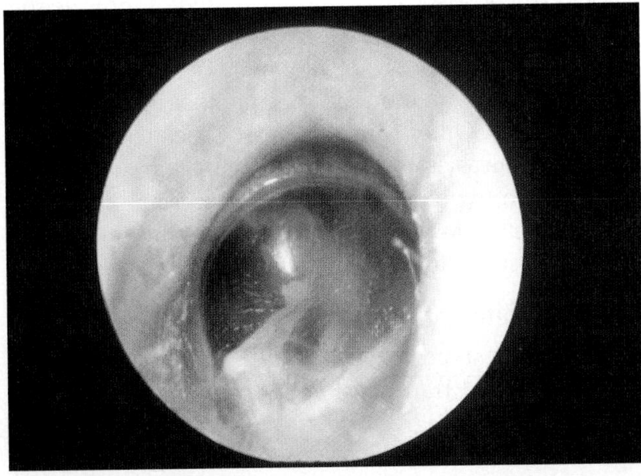

Figure 31.5 ■ Otitis media.

The Eustachian tube, a narrow tube that connects the middle ear to the back of the throat, acts as a pressure-equalizing valve for the middle ear by opening and closing with talking, swallowing, and yawning. Infants are at particular risk of OM because of their short, horizontal Eustachian tubes.[3]

Clinical Manifestations

OM can begin with coldlike symptoms and/or upper respiratory problems that can cause the Eustachian tube to become obstructed and unable to properly ventilate the middle ear space. If the mucosa of the middle ear space does not have sufficient oxygen to absorb, the tympanic membrane can become retracted, resulting in negative middle ear pressure often accompanied by the development of serous fluid. A number of terms are used to describe various types of OM. The American Academy of Pediatrics and the updated American Academy of Family Physicians Clinical Practice Guideline define **acute otitis media (AOM)** as inflammation of the middle ear with acute onset with moderate to severe bulging of the TM and **middle ear effusion** (serous or mucoid fluid).[4] The tympanic membrane can rupture, resulting in immediate pain relief and a possible purulent discharge.[3,4] Although conductive hearing loss can be associated with AOM, given its relatively short duration, the hearing loss is typically temporary. Medical management of AOM includes antibiotics as the initial therapy. *Recurrent AOM* is defined as three or more episodes of AOM in 6 months or four or more episodes in a 12-month period if there has been at least one episode in the previous 6 months. Factors that increase risk of recurrence include male gender, passive exposure to smoking, and winter season.[4]

Acute otitis media most commonly occurs in children and may be associated with the sudden onset of ear pain. Infants and younger children may demonstrate irritability, crying, and ear tugging. Subtle changes in the TM may be difficult to discern, or cerumen may cloud the TM, making differential diagnosis difficult.[4] ■

Chronic otitis media (COM) involves a consistently infected middle ear, typically longer than 6 weeks, with persistent effusion in the middle ear space.[5] COM is associated with damage to middle ear structures, including tympanic membrane perforations, atrophy, erosion of the middle ear ossicles, and cholesteatoma. Typical conductive loss associated with COM ranges from mild to moderately severe loss, depending on the severity of the infection.

Because COM is rarely associated with pain, it can go undetected in children. ■

Mateo Ramirez: Application

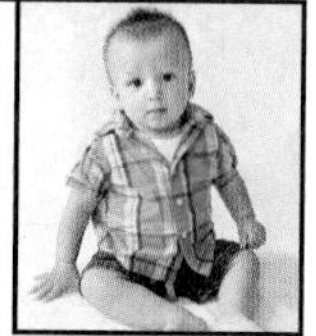

Mateo subsequently woke up in the middle of the night crying. He seemed to sleep better after this episode, but his parents followed up with an appointment with his pediatrician. The parents report seeing a discharge on Mateo's crib sheets after the episode. The pediatrician prescribes antibiotics for acute otitis media. Mateo appears to respond well, and the earlier behavioral symptoms resolve.

3. Why is Mateo at a higher risk of OM?
4. Why did Mateo sleep better after his parents noticed a discharge on his crib sheets?

Linking Pathophysiology to Diagnosis and Treatment

Treatment of COM depends on its advancement. Uncomplicated COM is treated with topical antibiotics and/or steroids and frequent cleaning of the ear canal.[5] Surgical intervention and/or systemic antibiotics may be required for more severe cases. Middle ear ventilation tubes, also called **pressure equalization (PE) tubes**, are hollow cylinders made of plastic or metal. They are inserted during surgery to allow normal aeration of the middle ear space until the Eustachian tube is functional.

Recurrent AOM is of particular concern in infants and toddlers because of the risk of hearing loss and its effects on speech and language development. Children diagnosed with recurrent AOM are often treated with prophylactic antibiotics and followed with serial hearing evaluations. ■

Once otitis media has been resolved successfully, hearing thresholds should return to normal levels. Chronic otitis media and its sequelae can produce a residual conductive hearing loss that may require hearing aids. Sensorineural hearing loss can develop with long-term COM that does damage the cochlea.

All children with fluid in the ear or OM experience some hearing loss. The hearing of children who experience recurrent infections, COM, or hearing loss that lasts more than 6 weeks should be evaluated by a professional.[6] ■

Mateo Ramirez: Outcome

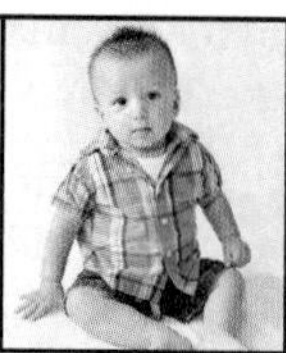

Although the initial episode of AOM resolved quickly, Mateo was diagnosed with AOM twice more over the next 2 months. At this point, his parents were quick to recognize the symptoms and followed up with their pediatrician. After the third bout of AOM, Mateo is referred to a pediatric otologist. Mateo is assessed by both the otologist and an audiologist and diagnosed with recurrent AOM and mild bilateral conductive hearing loss. He is treated with prophylactic antibiotics, and his hearing thresholds improve to within normal limits with serial audiometric testing. The parents are informed that PE tubes are an option if the AOM develops into COM. Mateo is at risk for delayed speech and language development because of the frequency of OM and his decreased babbling during these episodes. However, because Mateo had early identification, assessment, and treatment, his prognosis for normally developing speech and language is good.

5. Why did Mateo have some hearing loss?
6. What do PE tubes do?

Otosclerosis

Otosclerosis involves abnormal bone growth in the middle ear space. Otosclerosis affects more than three million Americans, and most cases are thought to be inherited. Middle-aged Caucasian women are at greatest risk.[7] Hearing loss is typically bilateral, slowly progressive, and conductive in nature, but it can be mixed if the otic capsule of the cochlea is involved. Onset usually begins when individuals are in their 20s, although only 10–15% of affected people experience symptoms.[8]

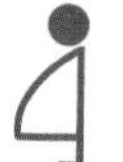

Pregnancy has been associated with acceleration in otosclerosis.[9] ■

Etiology and Pathogenesis

The otosclerosis disease process involves alternating bone resorption and formation.[8,9] Initially, an abnormal sponge-like process (otospongiosis) invades the otic capsule, followed by bone hardening called otosclerosis. The anterior oval window and the stapes footplate are most commonly affected, although otosclerosis can invade the round window and cochlea as well.

Otosclerosis tends to occur more often in certain families and consequently is considered to have a genetic component. Otosclerosis is generally thought to be inherited as an autosomal dominant condition with reduced penetrance.[8] Genetic association and other studies indicate that the transforming growth factor beta 1 (TGF-beta 1) is very likely associated with the development of otosclerosis.[10]

Viral factors are thought to be another possible cause of otosclerosis. Other causal factors associated with otosclerosis are measles and autoimmune system disorders. It has also been hypothesized that otosclerosis is caused by genetic transmission with a viral trigger. At this point, there is no consensus as to the etiology of otosclerosis.[8,10]

Clinical Manifestations

Fixation of the stapes footplate in the oval window interferes with sound transmission resulting in a conductive hearing loss. The degree of loss depends on the extent of the disease process and can range from mild to moderately severe. Speech recognition remains intact if the hearing loss is purely conductive; however, if cochlear structures are involved, a sensorineural component may contribute to a mixed hearing loss. Speech recognition ability could then be reduced, depending on the extent of cochlear involvement.

Tinnitus, the subjective experience of hearing a noise such as ringing, buzzing, or hissing in the head or ears in the absence of any external noise, is a common symptom among individuals with otosclerosis. Dizziness and/or imbalance and aural fullness are also common complaints.[7] The ability to hear better in a noisy environment, known as paracusis Willisii, is also commonly reported.

Linking Pathophysiology to Diagnosis and Treatment

Because of the slow progression of otosclerosis, diagnosis may be delayed until the hearing loss begins to interfere with communication. Patient history, otoscopy, audiologic results, and radiologic studies are key to the diagnosis of otosclerosis. Audiologic assessment includes pure tone audiometry, which often reveals the Carhart notch, an elevation of bone conduction thresholds of approximately 5 dB at 500 Hz, 10 dB at 1000 Hz, 15 dB at 2000 Hz, and 5 dB at 4000 Hz. Tympanometric results are consistent with the stiff middle ear system seen in otosclerosis. High-resolution CT scans can confirm, localize, and determine the size of clinically suspected foci of otosclerosis.[7]

Treatment of otosclerosis depends on the severity of the hearing loss and symptoms. If the patient is experiencing minimal symptoms, no intervention may be in order other than annual hearing tests to monitor hearing loss. However, once the individual reports significant symptoms, treatment options include surgery, medications, and hearing aids.

Surgical procedures have been used in the treatment of otosclerosis for the past 50 years. **Stapedectomy** involves removal of diseased bone and attachment of a prosthetic stapes in its place.[7] A similar surgical option, stapedotomy, avoids removal of the entire stapes footplate; it involves creation of a small hole in the fixed stapes footplate and insertion of a piston-like prosthesis. In rare cases, surgery can worsen the hearing loss and/or cause dizziness.

Hearing aids are another treatment option. They have overall high success rates for individuals with mild otosclerosis.

CLINICAL POINT: In some cases, hearing aids represent the best option, because the amplification they provide can effectively compensate for the impaired sound transmission inherent in the conductive hearing loss. **Osseointegrated hearing implants** such as the Baha© or Ponto© represent a relatively new option for individuals with otosclerosis. These osseointegrated hearing implants are surgically implanted and use bone conduction of sound to stimulate the inner ear, thus bypassing the conductive component of the hearing loss caused by otosclerosis. ■

Fluoride, calcium, and vitamin D have been used as treatments for otosclerosis, although the efficacy of these interventions has not yet been proven.[9] Because otosclerosis is progressive and may get worse without treatment, patients are advised to have regular evaluations by an otolaryngologist and audiologist.

Check Your Progress: Section 31.3

1. Describe two conditions of the outer ear that can lead to conductive hearing loss.
2. Why is the outer ear important for hearing?
3. How does OM differ from COM?

31.4 Sensorineural Hearing Loss Disorders

Damage to the structures of the inner ear, including the central auditory pathway and the inner and outer hair cells, results in a **sensorineural hearing loss**. In sensorineural hearing loss, sound is transmitted normally to the cochlea, but the characteristics of the incoming sound—including the frequency and intensity—can no longer be accurately processed and/or transmitted to the auditory cortex. Some individuals may have a **mixed hearing loss**, which means that their hearing loss has both conductive and sensorineural components.

Presbycusis

Hearing loss due to aging is commonly referred to as **presbycusis**, a term derived from the Greek word *presbys*, meaning "old," and *akouein*, meaning "to hear." Presbycusis is the most common form of hearing loss, affecting 25–30% of Americans age 65–74 years and as many as 50% of people age 75 and older.[11]

Etiology and Pathogenesis

Aging changes occur throughout the auditory system from the outer ear to the auditory cortex. Age-related changes to the outer and middle ear do not result in hearing loss. However, the inner ear and auditory pathway are vulnerable to structural aging changes that can result in sensorineural hearing loss.

The mainstay of research in this area remains the classic temporal bone histologic studies. Schuknecht described four types of presbycusis in humans[11–13]:

- *Sensory presbycusis.* This type mainly involves atrophy with loss of sensory hair cells and supporting cells in the organ of Corti. This process originates in the basal turn of the cochlea and slowly progresses toward the apex.
- *Neural presbycusis.* This is typified by loss of afferent neurons in the cochlea and central neural pathways. Schuknecht estimated that some 2100 neurons are lost in every decade of life. However, the loss is not noticeable until almost 90% of the approximately 35,000 neurons are gone.
- *Metabolic, or strial, presbycusis.* This type results from atrophy of the stria vascularis, which is responsible for the health and biochemical balance of the cochlea.
- *Mechanical, or cochlear conductive, presbycusis.* This type results from thickening of the basilar membrane and organ of Corti of the cochlea.

Schuknecht correlated hearing loss with each of these types of presbycusis, but he later demonstrated that individuals with presbycusis typically cannot be separated by specific types but may have mixtures of these pathologic types, termed *mixed presbycusis*.[11,14] Furthermore, presbycusis typically develops simultaneously at multiple sites in individuals, making it difficult to associate specific clinical symptoms or signs with specific anatomic locations.[11]

There is no widely accepted etiology of presbycusis. Many aging adults present with a variety of factors that can contribute to hearing loss, including heredity, noise exposure, environmental factors, and history of ear pathologies. Current research is focused on finding underlying genetic causes that may lead to or predispose aging individuals to presbycusis.

Clinical Manifestations

Presbycusis is characterized by a progressive decrease in hearing thresholds and decreased ability to understand speech, particularly in noisy environments. Some individuals may have more difficulty understanding rapidly spoken words.[11] Audiograms of individuals with presbycusis are typically bilateral, sloping, and sensorineural.[15] Mean audiometric thresholds as a function of age show decreased high-frequency hearing loss as compared to lower frequencies. Men typically have poorer hearing thresholds than women, but these changes may be due to other factors, such as noise exposure. Although speech understanding in quiet remains stable with age, older listeners experience greater difficulty understanding comfortably loud speech in the presence of background noise.

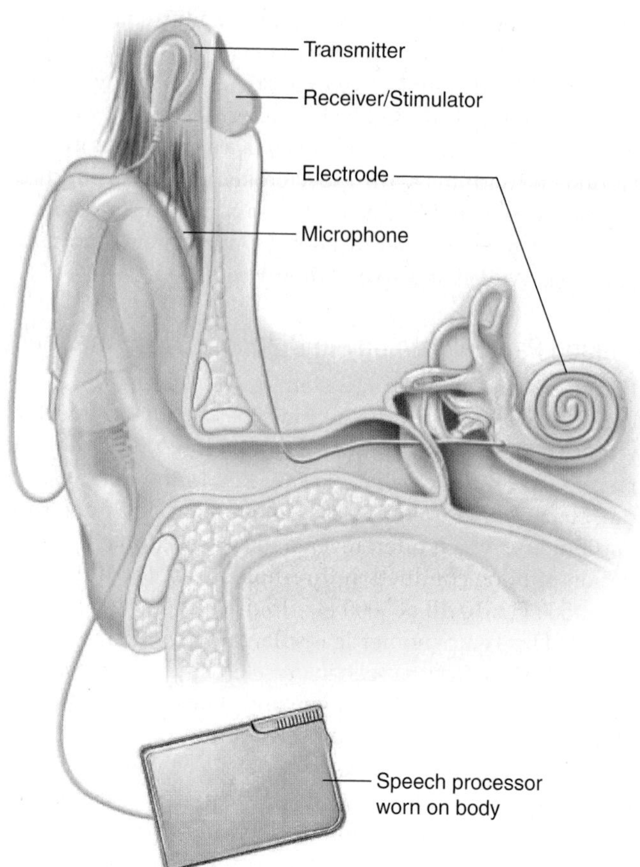

Figure 31.6 ■ A cochlear implant.

Linking Pathophysiology to Diagnosis and Treatment

Diagnosis of presbycusis is typically made on the basis of exclusion to rule out such etiologic factors as noise exposure, ototoxicity, diabetes, and autoimmune hearing loss. A careful history and complete audiologic assessment by an audiologist contribute to this diagnosis. However, a combination of factors may contribute to the presenting audiometric profile for an aging individual.

Amplification in the form of **hearing aids** (small devices that fit in or on the ear to amplify sound) and assistive listening technology is key to management of presbycusis. Binaural hearing aids are typically recommended for bilateral hearing loss. Hearing aid features are based on the individual's audiometric profile as well as lifestyle needs, vision, cognition, quality of life, and environmental factors. **Assistive listening devices** include amplified telephones and televisions as well smoke detectors and other warning and listening devices. Success with amplification depends on a personalized, comprehensive rehabilitation plan that involves the person's family and communication partners. Some patients with presbycusis may benefit from cochlear implants[11] (**Figure 31.6** ■).

Ménière Disease

Etiology and Pathogenesis

Ménière disease is an inner ear disorder that manifests with both auditory and vestibular symptoms. Excess endolymph within the membranous labyrinth of the inner ear system is thought to be the underlying cause. In a normally functioning ear, endolymph is continually produced and resorbed. In Ménière disease, this normal production and/or resorption process is disrupted, resulting in the buildup of excess endolymph—and thus extreme pressure—within the membranous labyrinth. This extreme pressure causes the membranous labyrinth to become distended, resulting in impairment of the sensory cells and support structures of the peripheral hearing and balance systems. Patients experience recurrent symptomatic episodes due to fluctuations in this pressure. There is some evidence that Ménière disease runs in families; this suggests a possible genetic component to the disorder.[16] Other theories about the etiology of Ménière disease include viral and autoimmune etiologies as well as the possibility that constriction of blood vessels is involved.[17]

Clinical Manifestations

The classic symptoms of Ménière disease include intense vertigo with accompanying nausea and vomiting, tinnitus, a feeling of pressure or fullness in the ear, and fluctuating hearing loss. Patients may present with any combination of greater or lesser degrees of these symptoms.

CLINICAL POINT: In the early stages of Ménière disease, the hearing loss primarily involves low-pitched sounds and can fluctuate dramatically, falling suddenly during a Ménière episode and then recovering to normal or near normal sensitivity levels immediately afterward. As the disease progresses, the hearing no longer recovers fully after an episode, and the hearing loss expands to include high-pitched sounds. Speech comprehension is severely impaired in these patients. ■

Ménière disease occurs in episodes that may last from a few minutes to 24 hours.[18] Some patients are completely symptom free between attacks; others experience persistent imbalance and/or low-intensity tinnitus. The frequency of symptomatic episodes can vary dramatically from person to person. In some individuals, months or even years pass between Ménière attacks, while others have recurrences with much greater frequency. The progression of the disease also varies considerably. In some Ménière sufferers, the frequency of the episodes and the intensity of the presenting symptoms increase as the disease progresses; many of these individuals eventually lose most of their usable hearing and may be plagued by persistent tinnitus and vertigo. Other patients, while still suffering recurrent episodes, may experience no real progression in their symptoms over time. While Ménière disease can involve both ears, the disease affects only one ear in most individuals. The average age at onset is between 40 and 60 years of age, and approximately 615,000 Americans are affected.[17]

Linking Pathophysiology to Diagnosis and Treatment

Diagnosis of Ménière disease is typically made on the basis of clinical presentation, including the presence of characteristic symptoms and the episodic nature of attacks. Diagnostic testing can provide important data to inform the diagnosis of Ménière disease. Specifically, audiologic evaluation, electrocochleography (a method for recording electrical potentials of the cochlea), electronystagmography (a test that records involuntary movements of the eye), andvideonystagmography (a technology for testing inner ear and central motor control functions) can be used to evaluate and document the patient's audiologic and vestibular function. If the patient is asymptomatic and in the early stages of the disease, these tests will likely be normal. As the disease progresses, a characteristic pattern of hearing and balance test results will begin to emerge to support the Ménière diagnosis. Additional tests and imaging studies are typically used to rule out alternative diagnoses that may present with similar symptoms, such as vestibular schwannoma or autoimmune inner ear disease.

There is no known cure for Ménière disease, but medical and surgical interventions are available to help patients cope with the symptoms. Antinausea, antiemetic, and vestibular suppressant medications are generally prescribed to help Ménière sufferers manage their severe vertiginous symptoms. Longer-term medical management is designed to decrease the intensity of symptoms and reduce the frequency of attacks. Adherence to a strict low-salt diet has been found to effectively reduce the intensity of symptoms in some patients by reducing fluid and pressure in the ear.[17] Avoidance of any possible triggering allergens would be included in any medical management plan. If dietary modifications prove insufficient, diuretic medications may be prescribed in an attempt to reduce the volume of endolymph and thus lower the pressure in the membranous labyrinth.

Ultimately, if a patient's vertigo cannot be effectively controlled through medical management, surgical intervention may be considered. Surgical decompression of the endolymphatic sac is one approach. If the vertigo is deemed intractable, peripheral vestibular function on the impaired side may be obliterated by sectioning the vestibular nerve or infusing gentamicin, a vestibulotoxic medication, into the labyrinth to destroy the vestibular sensory cells. However, gentamycin carries an increased risk of hearing loss. Because of this, some providers may choose to inject a corticosteroid instead.[17] Pressure pulse treatment is a new intervention by which pressure pulses of air are transmitted to the middle ear by way of a device that fits onto the outer ear. The air pressure may prevent dizziness by acting on endolymphatic fluid.[17]

Hearing aids or other rehabilitative interventions can help to ameliorate communication problems in patients with Ménière disease. If a patient's hearing loss is so severe that traditional hearing aids are deemed inappropriate, a **cochlear implant** (a device implanted in the cochlea to stimulate it to cause hearing) for severe bilateral hearing impairment or an osseointegrated hearing implant such as Baha© or Ponto© for single-sided deafness may be considered.

Ototoxicity

Virtually every medication in use in healthcare today has potential negative side effects—some minor and some severe. Certain medications are known to be **ototoxic**; that is, they can damage the sensory cells of the inner ear. The use of ototoxic drugs can result in hearing loss and/or balance problems in certain individuals.

Ototoxic medications are of two types, depending on their primary site of effect. **Cochleotoxic** medications damage the sensory cells of the cochlea, resulting in sensorineural hearing loss. The hearing loss associated with use of cochleotoxic medications is usually bilateral and typically affects hearing in the high frequencies first. With continued use, this hearing loss can spread to affect hearing for mid- and low-pitched sounds as well. Tinnitus is a common secondary side effect of cochleotoxic medications. In some patients, the development of tinnitus is the first sign of medication-related cochlear damage.

Vestibulotoxic medications damage the sensory cells of the peripheral balance system, including those in the semicircular canals, utricle, and saccule. As with cochleotoxic medications, effects from vestibulotoxic medications are typically bilateral. Changes to the balance system resulting from ototoxic medications tend to be gradual. Given this, while a small percentage of patients may experience vertigo, an intense illusory sensation of movement or spinning, the majority suffer from blurred vision and unsteadiness, particularly with head movement.[19,20]

Ototoxic Medications

Ototoxic medications can result in varying degrees of permanent or temporary changes in sensory function. The extent to which a given individual is adversely affected depends on many variables, including the person's age, coexisting medical conditions, genetic predisposition, the drug in use, and drug dosage and schedule. Two of the most widely used groups of ototoxic medications associated with permanent changes in function are aminoglycoside antibiotics and platinum-based antineoplastic (chemotherapy) medications. **Aminoglycoside antibiotics** are used to treat infections caused by gram-negative bacteria and are administered either intramuscularly or intravenously. Among these drugs, kanamycin, amikacin, and neomycin are considered to be primarily cochleotoxic. Gentamicin, another aminoglycoside antibiotic, is known to be highly vestibulotoxic. The vestibulotoxic characteristics of gentamicin have led to its use in the treatment of cases of intractable vertigo, as can occur with Ménière disease. In these cases, gentamicin is administered to intentionally destroy peripheral sensory cells of balance.

Platinum-based medications—specifically cisplatin and carboplatin—are among the most widely used chemotherapy drugs. They are a primary course of treatment for many different types of cancer, including cancers of the head and neck, ovarian cancer, and bone cancers such as osteosarcoma. Cisplatin is known to be highly cochleotoxic; it is believed to damage the function of the outer hair cells of the cochlea in particular, resulting in a loss of both hearing sensitivity and frequency specificity. Carboplatin, although considered to be relatively less cochleotoxic than cisplatin, can cause damage to the inner hair cells of the cochlea in some individuals, resulting in sound distortion and decreased speech recognition abilities.

In higher doses, loop diuretics and salicylates may cause tinnitus and hearing loss.[19]

Ototoxic Monitoring and Cautions

Patients who are preparing to begin treatment with a known ototoxic agent should undergo testing to establish a baseline measure of hearing and balance function.

CLINICAL POINT: Once treatment is initiated, a regular schedule of repeat testing can then be used to document any changes in hearing or balance relative to the baseline measure. Reported changes can, in some cases, direct modifications to the patient's ongoing plan of care. Because some ototoxic medications are known to have long-term effects, this testing should ideally continue for at least one year after completion of treatment. ■

Patient education on avoidance of potentially ototoxic medications is essential. Patients with hearing loss need to be evaluated for the necessity of hearing aids or other assistive devices to help ensure safety, communication, and continued engagement in regular work and activities. Vestibular rehabilitation therapy can help patients regain posture and balance.[19,21]

Noise-Induced Hearing Loss

The world is a noisy place, and more and more attention is being given to the potential effects of this continuous barrage of noise on our overall health and, in particular, on our hearing. Exposure to excessive noise can damage hearing. But how much noise is too much noise? There is a relationship between the intensity of a sound and the duration of exposure one can safely have. The National Institute for Occupational Safety and Health (NIOSH) promotes an allowable exposure limit of 8 hours per day for an 85-dB sound and applies a reduction in that time exposure limit as the intensity of the sound increases above 85 dB.[22] Following NIOSH calculations, time exposure is cut in half for each 3-dB increase in the noise intensity (a doubling of the energy). **Noise-induced hearing loss (NIHL)**, then, can result either from prolonged exposure to a high-intensity noise, such as a jackhammer or leafblower, or from a single exposure to a brief but intense impulse sound, such as a gunshot close to the ear or a fireworks explosion. **Table 31.2** ■ outlines the decibel levels of some common sounds.

Etiology and Pathogenesis

Acoustic Trauma. The damage to hearing that results from exposure to an intense impulse noise is known as **acoustic trauma**. An impulse sound such as an explosion can exceed 120–150 dB; consider this relative to 30–40 dB for a whisper and 55–60 dB for a normal conversation. The high noise levels involved in acoustic trauma typically exceed the elastic limits of the basilar and tectorial membranes in the cochlea and can tear these structures apart, resulting in complete destruction of the organ of Corti. In some cases, high noise levels may also cause separation or fracture of the ossicular chain.

Chronic NIHL. Hearing loss that develops from repeated, prolonged exposure to a loud noise progresses through two distinct stages. Individuals who are exposed to a moderately loud noise for a period of time may first experience a temporary loss of hearing known as a **temporary threshold shift (TTS)**, followed by a recovery of hearing if no repeated exposure occurs. A TTS may occur, for example, after a rock concert, with complete hearing recovery within the hours or days following the concert. In addition to incurring a

Table 31.2 Decibel Levels of Everyday Sounds

Category	Decibel Level	Examples
Faint	20–30	Leaves rustling in a breeze, quiet library, whisper
Moderate	50	Moderate rainfall
	60	Dishwasher, clothes dryer, normal conversation
Very loud	70	Alarm clock, vacuum cleaner
	80–90	Hair dryer, food processor
Extremely loud	90	Passing motorcycle
	106	Snowblower, gas-powered lawn mower, sporting event
Painful	120	Siren
	124	Maximum volume of MP3 ear buds, MRI scanner
	140	Jet engine, firearms

SOURCES: Based on American Speech-Language-Hearing Association. (2015). *Noise*. Available at http://www.asha.org/public/hearing/Noise; Center for Hearing, Speech and Language. (2014). *How loud is it?* Available at http://www.chsl.org/soundchart.php; Centers for Disease Control and Prevention. (2013). *Noise and hearing loss prevention*. Available at http://www.cdc.gov/niosh/topics/noise/noisemeter.html

loss of hearing sensitivity, individuals with TTS may also develop tinnitus. In the majority of TTS cases, this tinnitus goes away as hearing thresholds recover. With repeated exposure to an offending noise, the hearing fails to recover completely between exposures and then does not recover at all; at this point, the TTS become a **permanent threshold shift (PTS)**.

Damage from chronic exposure to excessively loud sounds initially occurs in the outer hair cells of the cochlea. Noise exposure triggers ionic changes in these cells that cause the stereocilia to lose their integrity and become misshapen, diminishing their ability to function normally. With continued exposure, the outer hair cells themselves degenerate, followed by degeneration of the inner hair cells and cochlear support cells. As the cochlear damage progresses, the hearing loss becomes more severe, and speech intelligibility worsens.

Clinical Manifestations

Acoustic Trauma. The main symptom of acoustic trauma is (usually sudden) hearing loss, although tinnitus may signal its onset.[23] The hearing loss is usually sensorineural (or has a significant sensorineural component) but can be conductive if the ossicular chain or tympanic membrane is damaged. Hearing loss from acoustic trauma is typically evident to some degree across all frequencies of hearing, although the configuration of the hearing loss varies depending on the sound source.

Chronic NIHL. As a result of the natural sound-shaping function of the outer ear, hearing loss from noise exposure most often presents as a hearing loss "notch" at about 4000 Hz, with a recovery to better hearing at higher and lower frequencies. With continued exposure to that noise source, the hearing loss typically then begins to progress to higher frequencies and then to flatten out as it finally involves the lower frequencies. This hearing loss can be bilateral, but it may or may not be symmetric, depending on the type of noise and the relative position of the noise source to the ears.

In some cases of NIHL, the change in hearing is so gradual that it goes undetected until identified during a formal hearing test. In other cases, the hearing loss may first come to light when an individual begins to notice that he can hear other people speak but often struggles to understand certain words. In addition, with continued noise exposure and progression to a PTS, tinnitus commonly increases and becomes permanent.

Greg Seitz: Application

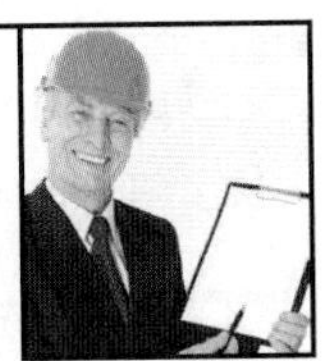

Mr. Seitz experienced hearing loss caused by repeated gunfire while serving in the military during the Gulf War. However, his hearing difficulties caused him only minor communication problems, so he sought no follow-up. Once he was discharged, Mr. Seitz's employment in construction and lawn maintenance work involved repeated exposure to occupational noise. However, because the NIHL was so gradual, he did not associate it with the hearing loss he experienced with military service, nor was he aware of the permanent damage to his hearing that was occurring. His wife recognized that his gradually increasing hearing loss was interfering with Mr. Seitz's ability to understand conversational speech both with her and with their young children. Although Mr. Seitz initially denied that he had significant hearing loss, with his wife's encouragement, he scheduled an audiologic assessment.

3. What type of hearing loss is Mr. Seitz suffering from?
4. How does this type of hearing loss occur?

Linking Pathophysiology to Diagnosis and Treatment

Diagnosis of noise-induced hearing loss is made on the basis of patient history and audiometric test findings. The presence of a noise "notch" along with a report of excessive noise exposure supports the likely diagnosis of NIHL. Note, however, that even when NIHL is suspected, it is not always possible to rule out other known contributors to hearing loss that may be present, including medical conditions, genetic factors, and age-related hearing changes.

Appropriate rehabilitative intervention for NIHL depends on its stage and progression. In most cases, amplification and/or assistive listening devices can provide access to critical speech sounds and improve communication abilities. Regardless of the severity of the hearing loss, treatment should always include education on noise-related changes in hearing, including possible progression, and the critical importance of properly fitting hearing protection. Counseling and assistance with coping with the loss of hearing may be helpful. Note that education and hearing protection are also the keys to the *prevention* of NIHL. As described in the Impact of Current Research on Clinical Practice box, exciting new research may provide the key to preventing NIHL in the future.

Greg Seitz: Outcome

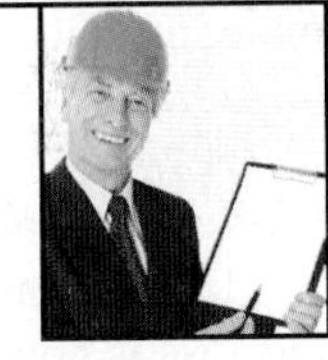

The history taken prior to assessment will include questions regarding the use of protective devices (ear plugs, for example), during occupational activities. It is also important to conduct a physical examination including assessment of the head. Often in cases of noise-induced hearing loss, the physical examination is unremarkable as is the case with Mr. Seitz. The audiologic assessment will explore whether the hearing loss experienced by Mr. Seitz is specific for conversational speech. In such cases, this would reflect a loss of ability to hear selective frequencies rather than a global reduction in hearing ability.

The audiologic assessment indicates that Mr. Seitz has noise-induced hearing loss related to occupational exposure. Hearing loss compatible with the occupational history of Mr. Seitz is generally a symmetrical sensorineural loss.

5. What interventions need to be implemented to protect the remaining hearing capability of Mr. Seitz?
6. What factors need to be considered in discussing the use of adaptive hearing devices?

Genetic Hearing Loss

Statistics from the National Institute on Deafness and Other Communication Disorders indicate that approximately 2–3 of every 1000 children in the United States are born with some degree of hearing loss.[24]

Impact of Current Research on Clinical Practice

Preventing Noise-Induced Hearing Loss

Description: Exciting new research is being conducted to develop otoprotective agents that would prevent hearing loss and tinnitus resulting from noise exposure. Promising results are emerging from studies using pharmacologic agents administered both before and after potentially damaging noise exposure. For example, in animal studies, D-methionine (D-met) administered up to 5 hours after noise exposure provided significant protection from permanent hearing threshold shift and noise-related outer hair cell loss.[1,2] Campbell and colleagues are now conducting phase 3 clinical trials to establish the efficacy of D-met an NIHL prevention agent.[3] Other lines of research are investigating the efficacy of D-met as an otoprotective agent for cisplatin, carboplatin, and aminoglycoside antibiotics.

Clinical Practice: Together, these promising lines of research are opening new paths for possible hearing loss prevention.

Research Studies:

1. Campbell, K. C. M., Meech, R. P., Klemens, J. J., et al. (2007). Prevention of noise- and drug-induced hearing loss with D-methionine. *Hearing Research*, *226*(1–2), 92–103.
2. Campbell, K. C. M. (2009). *Emerging pharmacologic treatments for hearing loss and tinnitus.* Available at http://www.asha.org/Publications/leader/2009/090526/f090526b.htm
3. National Institutes of Health. (2017). *Phase 3 clinical trial: D-methionine to reduce noise-induced hearing loss (NIHL).* Available at https://clinicaltrials.gov/ct2/show/NCT02903355

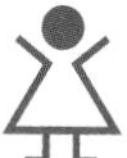

Congenital hearing loss is one of the most common birth defects. Inherited genetic defects play a role in approximately 60% of cases of deafness in infants.[25] ■

Etiology and Pathogenesis

Genetic hearing loss results from a mutation an individual's genetic code. Genes direct the building of the many different proteins that make up the human body; a mutation in any part of the genetic code will disrupt the production of the related proteins, changing their structure and altering or preventing their normal function. Changes in certain proteins alter normal auditory system function, resulting in hearing loss. Depending on the protein(s) involved, genetic hearing loss can be sensorineural, conductive, or mixed, and it can affect one ear only (unilateral) or both ears (bilateral). The degree of hearing loss also varies depending on the type and location of the genetic mutation, and the hearing loss can be stable or progressive.

In some cases, the genetic mutation that results in hearing loss is spontaneous, meaning that it is unique to the individual and is not present in any form in the parents. The majority of genetic mutations, however, are inherited. More than 50% of hearing loss that is diagnosed before the onset of language development is autosomal recessive and nonsyndromic.[26]

Clinical Manifestations

There are two categories of genetic hearing loss: syndromic and nonsyndromic. In **nonsyndromic genetic hearing loss**, the specific genetic alteration causes hearing loss only, with no other physical changes in the individual. In contrast, **syndromic hearing loss** is accompanied by a pattern of other clinical abnormalities. Of genetic-based hearing losses, approximately 70% are nonsyndromic, and 30% are syndromic.

Nonsyndromic Hearing Loss. Over 100 genes have been linked to nonsyndromic hearing loss.[27] One of the primary genes involved in nonsyndromic hearing loss is the *Cx26* gene (located on chromosome 13), which is responsible for producing the connexin 26 protein. There are over 90 mutations of the *Cx26* gene that are known to cause hearing loss,[28] the majority of which are inherited in an autosomal recessive pattern. The connexin 26 protein is involved in the formation of channels through the plasma membranes of many types of cells, including the supporting cells in the cochlea. When the connexin 26 protein is abnormal, transmission of potassium ions between these cells is disrupted, resulting in a sensorineural hearing loss. The most common of these *Cx26* genetic mutations is the 35delG mutation. Individuals with a 35delG mutation typically have a severe-to-profound high-frequency hearing loss.

Syndromic Hearing Loss. Researchers have identified over 400 syndromes that involve hearing loss.[25] In each case, hearing loss is but one of the physical abnormalities that result from the causal genetic mutation. With some disorders, the presentation of specific physical characteristics may help physicians identify the syndrome and the potential for associated hearing loss in an infant. The specific pattern of inheritance differs across syndromes, but within a syndrome, it is possible for individuals to demonstrate variable expression of the disorder. With variable expression, individuals with the same syndrome can demonstrate different degrees of severity of their symptoms. Four syndromic hearing loss types are described in **Table 31.3** ■.

Linking Pathophysiology to Diagnosis and Treatment

Individuals with syndromic hearing loss are often initially identified from the characteristic pattern of physical attributes related to the syndrome. However, both syndromic and nonsyndromic hearing loss can be definitively diagnosed only through genetic testing.

Today, newborn hearing screening programs are identifying children with hearing loss at a very young age. Given this, the importance of genetic testing in infants with hearing loss is growing. Genetic testing can help to direct further diagnostic testing, treatment, and rehabilitative intervention; and genetic counseling can inform families not only about the nature and progression of a disorder but also about recurrence risk related to a specific inheritance pattern. ■

Table 31.3 Syndromic Hearing Loss

Syndrome	Etiology and Epidemiology	Clinical Manifestations
Waardenburg	Autosomal dominant. Incidence rate is estimated at 1 in 4000 births.[27]	Individuals often suffer from bilateral or unilateral sensorineural hearing loss. Other characteristic features include a white forelock of hair, different colored eyes (heterochromia), premature graying of the hair, partial albinism, and widely spaced eyes. High variability in the expression of the pigmentation and craniofacial abnormalities.
Treacher-Collins	Autosomal dominant	Significant craniofacial anomalies are the hallmark. Individuals present with malformed or absent auricles and narrow or absent external auditory canals. Other abnormalities include cleft palate, downward slanting eyes, abnormally small mandible (lower jaw bone), small malar (cheek) bone, and teeth alignment problems. The primary type of hearing loss is conductive, but sensorineural loss can occur in some individuals.
Usher	Autosomal recessive. There are three distinct subtypes of Usher syndrome, which are characterized by the degree of hearing loss and extent of vestibular system involvement. All three subtypes include a progressive decline in vision leading to blindness.	Characterized by the presence of progressive sensorineural hearing loss and retinitis pigmentosa, a progressive eye disease involving the retina. Some individuals also suffer from balance problems. The hearing loss is bilateral and can vary in severity from moderate to profound. The vestibular system function may be normal, entirely absent, or partially impaired.
Jervell and Lange-Nielsen	Autosomal recessive. Characterized by heart defect and profound sensorineural hearing loss.	Individuals have an abnormality in the heart's electrical activity, called a long QT, that can result in heart arrhythmia, fainting episodes, and even sudden death.

Treatment for genetic hearing loss varies depending on the degree and nature of the hearing loss. Regular audiologic monitoring should be performed when progressive hearing loss is a concern. Traditional hearing aids or a cochlear implant could be appropriate for individuals with sensorineural hearing loss. Patients with conductive hearing loss would more likely benefit from a traditional hearing aid, a bone-conducted hearing aid, or an osseointegrated hearing implant.

Check Your Progress: Section 31.4

1. How does conductive hearing loss differ from sensorineural hearing loss?
2. Name and describe the four types of presbycusis.
3. Name two ways in which medication can be ototoxic.

31.5 Basic Anatomy and Physiology of Vision

Vision is the process of transforming light energy (electromagnetic radiation) into neural impulses that can be perceived and interpreted by the central nervous system (see Figure 31.1). The human visual system is composed of unique peripheral structures designed to admit this light energy and focus it onto specialized sensory receptors in the eye known as photoreceptor cells. These sensory receptors initiate a transformation of the light information into neural impulses that then travel along the optic nerve to the central nervous system for processing and interpretation. Together, these structures provide us not only with images of our environment but also with the color, shading, depth, and clarity that make up what we know as our visual world.

The Visual System

The human eye is made up of two chambers—anterior and posterior—and several tissue layers (**Figure 31.7**). The front "wall" of the anterior chamber is the cornea, the transparent dome on the front of the eye. The back "wall" of the anterior chamber is the iris, the colored ring of spongy tissue with a hole, the pupil, in the center. The anterior chamber contains a clear fluid, called the aqueous humor, which nourishes the cornea and lens of the eye. The aqueous humor drains through the trabecular meshwork, which forms the 360-degree border where the iris meets the cornea. The juncture where the cornea meets the sclera, the tough connective tissue that is the white part of the eye, is the boundary of the posterior chamber within the eye. Directly behind the pupil is the lens of the eye, which is suspended by fibers called zonules. The zonules are connected to the ciliary body, an annular ring of muscle fibers and connective tissue that can contract to control the tension on the lens, allowing for accommodation, or focusing. The ciliary body also produces aqueous humor, which flows through the pupil into the anterior chamber. The posterior chamber contains a gel-like mass called the vitreous humor.

The inside of the posterior chamber is lined with the retina, a thin, transparent nerve layer that leaves the back of the eye via the optic nerve. The retina is made up of 10 layers. These layers (from innermost to outermost) are the internal limiting membrane, nerve fiber layer, ganglion cell layer, inner plexiform layer, inner nuclear layer, outer

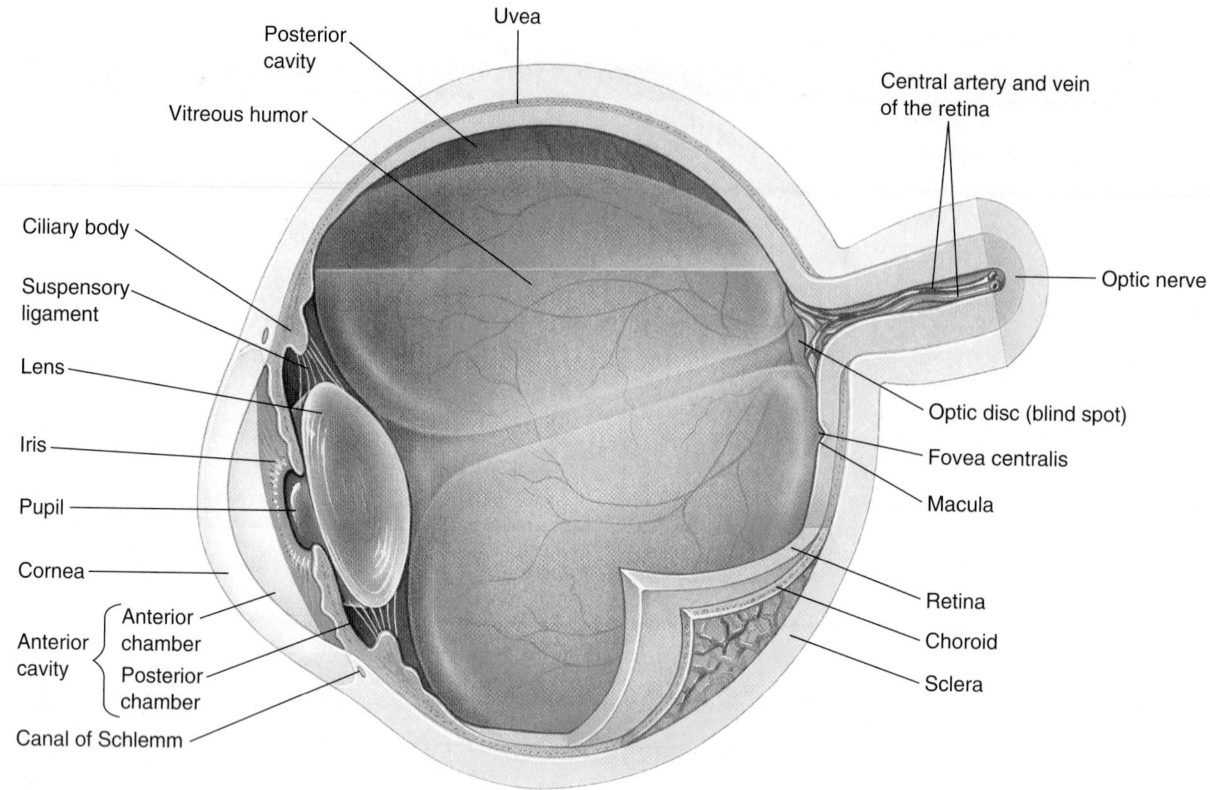

Figure 31.7 ■ Internal structures of the eye.

plexiform layer, outer nuclear, external limiting layer, photoreceptor layer, and retinal pigment epithelium. The photoreceptor layer contains the rods and cones of the retina. Rods function in dim lighting conditions and are responsible for the perception of black and white. Cones function in brightly lit conditions and are responsible for color vision. The macula is a small area on the retina with a high concentration of cones; it provides central vision. Retinal areas outside of the macula provide peripheral vision and are responsible for the visual inputs necessary to achieve binocular depth perception.

Underneath the retina is the choroid, a spongy vascular layer that nourishes the retina and delivers arteries and nerves to the entire eye. On the outside of the choroid and retina is the sclera, which envelops the entire eye. Each eye has six extraocular muscles that form tight adhesions to the sclera and are responsible for eye movement.

The Visual Pathway

Light entering the eye passes first through the cornea across the anterior chamber and then through the pupil (**Figure 31.8** ■). Once light has passed through the pupil,

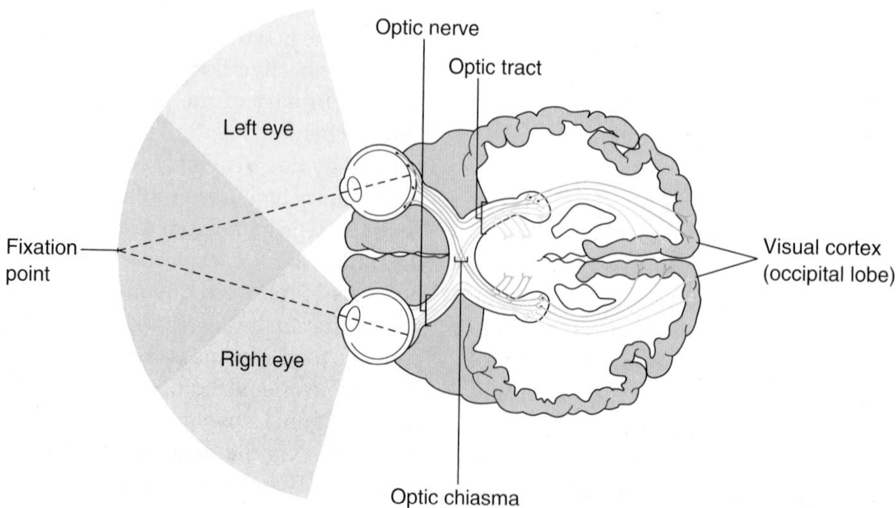

Figure 31.8 ■ The visual fields of the eye and the visual pathways to the brain.

it travels through the lens; it is there that the image is inverted. The inverted light then lands on the retina, initiating a cascade of biochemical and electrical events that ultimately trigger an action potential in the retinal ganglion cells, the axons of which form the optic nerve. The optic nerve exits the back of the eye at a region known as the optic disc.

The neural pathway for visual information is dictated by the visual field in which an image is located and the resulting retinal field onto which the image falls. For example, an image that is to the left of center as you look forward will be in the left visual field, and this image will fall on the right side of each retina. This means that the image will fall on the temporal portion of the retina—the side nearer the temple—of the right eye and the nasal portion of the retina—the side nearer the nose—of the left eye. The opposite is true for an image in the right visual field. Neural signals triggered by light landing on the nasal portion of the retina criss-cross at the optic chiasm, which is located at the base of the hypothalamus of the brain and above the pituitary gland. Past the optic chiasm, then, neural information from each eye generated by the left visual field is traveling via the right optic tract, and neural information generated by the right visual field is traveling via the left optic tract. The optic tract terminates in the lateral geniculate nucleus of the thalamus, which serves as a relay center in the ascending visual pathway. From the lateral geniculate nucleus, the neural impulses travel via optic radiations to the visual cortex in the occipital lobe of the brain, where the impulses are translated as vision.

Visual acuity is clarity or sharpness of vision and is measured in terms of how clear a person's vision is at a specific distance from the object of interest. Normal vision is represented as 20/20, which means that an individual can see clearly from 20 feet away an object that should normally be visible from that distance. For example, an individual with 20/50 vision must be within 20 feet to see an object clearly that a person with normal vision can see clearly at a distance of 50 feet. The Snellen eye chart, which contains a series of letters or letters and numbers of graduated sizes, is commonly used to measure visual acuity.

Check Your Progress: Section 31.5

1. Describe the parts of the eye.
2. Describe the visual pathway.
3. What is visual acuity?

31.6 External Eye Disorders

The external structures of the eye, including the eyelid, cornea, and conjunctiva, are susceptible to injury and infection. Although most of these problems are easily treated, some can lead to temporary or permanent changes in vision if not addressed medically.

Hordeolum (Stye)

A **hordeolum**, or **stye**, is a tender, red, often pus-filled bump that develops along the edge of the eyelid (**Figure 31.9** ■). This bump often grow in size over the course of 2–3 days before rupturing. Styes result from a bacterial infection in oil glands found at the base of an eyelash. Styes are usually found on the outside of the eyelid but can develop on the inside of the lid as well. Although they are painful and may cause eyelid swelling and excessive tearing, styes are generally harmless and typically resolve in a week without treatment. Periodic application of a warm, moist washcloth may be recommended to ease discomfort.

Conjunctivitis (Pinkeye)

The conjunctiva is a thin membrane that covers the sclera and lines the inner surface of the eyelid. Inflammation of the conjunctiva causes **conjunctivitis**, also known as pinkeye. Symptoms of conjunctivitis include redness, discharge, itching, and burning of the eyes; increased tearing; blurred vision; and light sensitivity. There are several different causes of conjunctivitis, the most common being bacterial infection, viral infection, and exposure to environmental irritants and allergens. Treatment for conjunctivitis is specific to the identified cause.

Viral conjunctivitis and bacterial conjunctivitis are highly contagious. Patients with infectious conjunctivitis should be counseled to avoid touching their eyes, to wash their hands frequently, and to wash bedding and towels frequently to avoid spreading and reinfection. Individuals who wear contact lenses should be directed to discontinue use and wear glasses until the infection has resolved.

Viral Conjunctivitis

Viral conjunctivitis, which is typically unilateral on presentation, is the most common cause of conjunctivitis overall. Between 65% and 90% of cases of viral conjunctivitis are caused by adenoviruses, while the herpes simplex virus is believed to be responsible for up to 4.8% of cases.[29] Most cases of viral conjunctivitis typically resolve in 7–21 days without treatment, though supportive care in the form of

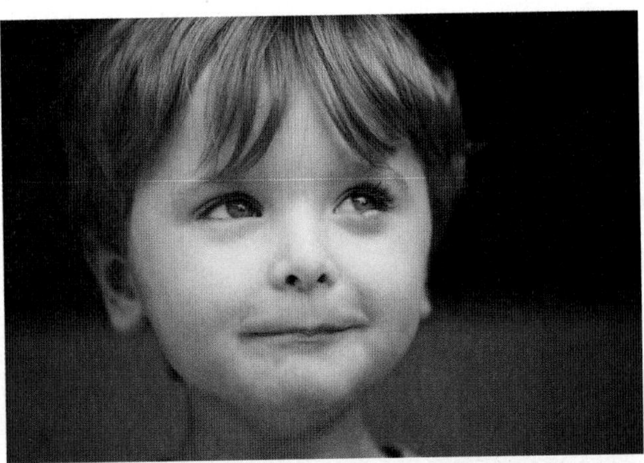

Figure 31.9 ■ Child with a hordeolum (stye) on the lower lid of his left eye.

eyedrops, cold compresses, and topical antihistamines may be used to alleviate symptoms.[29,30]

Bacterial Conjunctivitis

Bacterial conjunctivitis is the second most common cause of conjunctivitis and the most common cause of this disorder in children. When left untreated, bacterial conjunctivitis typically resolves within 1 week, but symptoms may persist for as long as 3 weeks.[30] Use of topical antibiotics may be prescribed to shorten the duration of the infection in some cases.

Children with bacterial conjunctivitis should be removed from school and/or daycare settings until their healthcare provider indicates that they are no longer contagious. Caregivers and teachers should be notified so that appropriate steps can be taken to thoroughly clean shared surfaces, thereby reducing the risk of spreading bacterial conjunctivitis to other children. ■

Allergic Conjunctivitis

Unlike conjunctivitis of bacterial and viral origin, allergic conjunctivitis is not contagious. The duration of allergic conjunctivitis is directly related to the level of ongoing exposure to the allergen, which may include pollen or animal dander, among others.[29] With that, the first step in treatment involves removing or limiting exposure to the identified irritant. A sterile saline solution can be used to dilute the allergen and remove it from the eye. Oral and topical medications (antihistamines, corticosteroids, etc.) can be prescribed to reduce the allergic response and speed recovery.[29]

Pterygium

A **pterygium** is a benign growth that develops on the conjunctiva. It is often wedge shaped and can extend to the cornea in some cases. The precise cause of a pterygium is not known, but individuals with high levels of exposure to ultraviolet light, wind, and/or airborne irritants such as smoke, sand, and pollen are believed to be at higher risk of developing this growth.[31] The majority of people with a pterygium experience no symptoms and therefore require no treatment. In some cases, the growth is removed because it is deemed unsightly, begins to interfere with vision, or becomes large enough to cause the person to sense that there is a foreign body in the eye.

Corneal Abrasion

A **corneal abrasion** is a scratch or cut that causes a defect on the surface of the cornea. Corneal abrasions can result from getting a foreign body in the eye, such as sand or dirt; rubbing the eye too aggressively; being poked in the eye; or getting an irritating chemical in the eye. Symptoms of a corneal abrasion include eye redness, tearing, eye pain that worsens when the eye is opened and closed, blurred vision, and light sensitivity. The cornea is important for both protection and visual acuity, so corneal abrasions should be treated to prevent additional damage. If a chemical or foreign body is involved, the eye should be flushed liberally with water or a sterile saline solution. Topical antibiotics and anti-inflammatory medications may be prescribed to reduce pain and swelling and to lower the possibility of a secondary bacterial infection.[32] Because a corneal abrasion can progress to an ulcer if improperly treated, close follow-up is necessary.[33]

Check Your Progress: Section 31.6

1. What teaching should be presented to patients who have viral of bacterial conjunctivitis to prevent spread of the disease?
2. What are some signs and symptoms of a corneal abrasion?
3. Why is it important to treat corneal abrasions?

31.7 Vision Disorders

Changes in or loss of vision may result from any condition that alters the structure and/or function of any component in the visual pathway. For example, a disorder of the lens can alter the amount of light that is let into the eye or even change the way that light is focused onto the macula. Conditions in which the eye has an abnormal position or abnormal connections to the brain can reduce the amount of usable information that the brain receives from the eye. Disorders of the visual system can be congenital or age related or may even develop secondary to other medical conditions.

Color Blindness

The perception of colors requires the use of cones, specialized receptor cells in the retina. There are three types of cones—red, green, and blue—that together allow us to see a full spectrum of colors. A deficiency in any or all of these types of cones results in color blindness. Red/green color blindness is the most common form of the disorder, followed by blue/yellow color blindness. Individuals with red/green or blue/yellow color blindness can see some color but may not be able to distinguish between complementary colors.[34] Achromotopsia, the most severe form of color blindness, is rare; sufferers see the world only in shades of black, white, and gray and have decreased vision and light sensitivity.[35]

Color blindness can be congenital or acquired. Congenital color blindness is one of the most common inherited vision disorders, with prevalence as high as 8% in males and 0.5% in females.[36,37] Congenital color blindness typically affects both eyes and encompasses the entire visual field. In contrast, acquired color blindness, which can present as a complication of diabetes or sickle cell disease, may affect one or both eyes and may involve only a portion of the visual field.[36,37] Currently, there is no treatment for congenital color blindness, though use of special filtered glasses or contact lenses can help some color-blind individuals to better distinguish between colors when in bright light. In addition, smartphone applications have been developed to assist color-blind users in identifying colors in photos. Acquired color blindness may resolve with treatment for the underlying cause.

Refractive Errors

A refractive error is any condition in which the eye is unable to focus light onto the macula. Common refractive errors include myopia, hyperopia, astigmatism, and presbyopia. **Myopia**, or nearsightedness, is caused by an eye that has a long axial length. Light entering a "long eye" focuses short of the retina, making distant objects blurry while leaving vision for near objects unaffected. Myopia is typically treated with concave glasses, which help to curve the light properly onto the retina, contact lenses, or laser surgery. **Hyperopia**, or farsightedness, results when an eye has a short axial length, causing light to focus "behind" the retina. Individuals with hyperopia have difficulty seeing near objects clearly but can see objects at distance relatively well. Hyperopia is treated with convex glasses, contacts, or laser surgery.

In **astigmatism**, the eye has an elliptical shape rather than a spherical shape; as a result, light focuses on two different points in the eye. Astigmatic refractive errors can make objects both far away and up close appear blurry. Toric (two-curvature) glasses or contact lenses are used to treat astigmatism. Laser surgery is also a treatment option. **Presbyopia** is a condition that develops when the ciliary muscle that controls the shape of the lens is no longer able to function properly, resulting in a decline in the accommodative (focusing) ability of the eye. Presbyopia, which is slowly progressive, results in difficulty viewing objects, such as reading materials, at close range. Glasses with convex lenses can effectively treat presbyopia. There are currently no known preventive measures for any of these refractive errors.

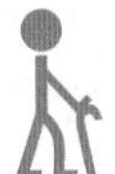

Presbyopia is caused by natural age-related changes in the eye and often begins to occur around 40 years of age. ■

Sam Park: Application

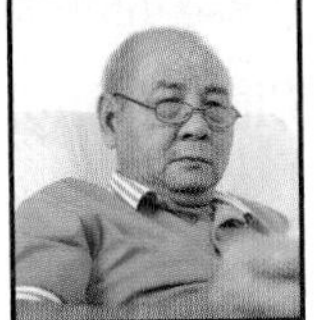

Sam Park reported having had increasing difficulty reading the daily newspaper and restaurant menus starting at about 48 years of age. Initially, he purchased over-the-counter "reading glasses" from his local drugstore. Over the next few years, reading small print became increasingly difficult. This prompted Mr. Park to be evaluated by an optometrist and be fitted with the appropriate prescription eyeglasses.

3. What type of refractory error does Mr. Park probably suffer from?
4. Why do glasses help Mr. Park see better?

Amblyopia and Strabismus

Amblyopia is a condition in which one or both eyes cannot see clearly despite corrective lenses and a normal, healthy ocular appearance. Amblyopia occurs most commonly in the pediatric population, presenting as refractive amblyopia.[38] In refractive amblyopia, one eye has normal vision, and the other eye has a high refractive error that goes untreated. In this condition, the side of the visual cortex that does not get a clear image from the corresponding eye during childhood development will never develop normal vision. Amblyopic eyes appear normal and healthy despite the fact that the "wiring" to the brain was interrupted during the person's formative years. Strabismus and congenital cataracts can also cause amblyopia, as both of these conditions prevent light from reaching the retina clearly. Amblyopia can be diagnosed at a regular ophthalmologic exam. Treatment for amblyopia involves correction of the refractive error and occlusion (patching) therapy.

CLINICAL POINT: It is important to treat amblyopia as early as possible. Very often, amblyopia is first diagnosed in adolescence or adulthood, at which point therapy has no effect. ■

Strabismus is a condition in which one or both eyes turn in, out, up, or down. When the eyes are misaligned, the brain suppresses, or "turns off," one eye to prevent double vision. Therapeutic intervention usually involves treating any identified refractive error along with occlusion therapy, vision therapy, prisms in glasses if necessary, and surgery to straighten the eyes.

Strabismus is common in newborns or can manifest within the first several years of life (**Figure 31.10** ■).[39] Symptoms of strabismus in children include head turning or tilting, closing one eye, headaches, and poor coordination. Treatment for strabismus should be initiated as early as possible to prevent amblyopia. The prognosis is good if strabismus is treated before the age of 24 months. ■

Cataracts

Etiology, Pathogenesis, and Clinical Manifestations

A **cataract** is a cloudy or opaque discoloration of the otherwise clear lens. Symptoms of cataracts are very gradual in onset, occurring over a course of years, and entail a

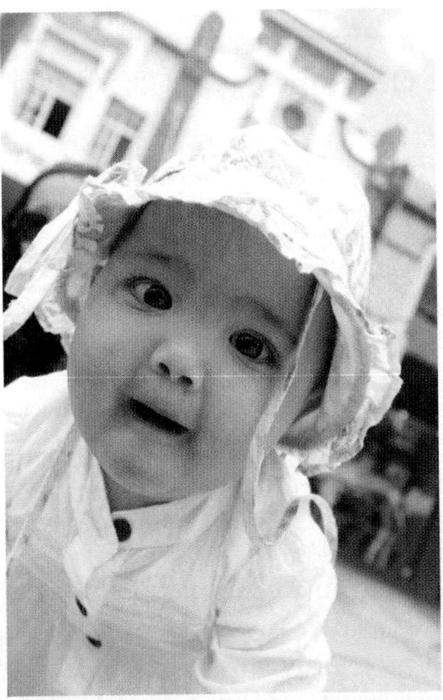

Figure 31.10 ■ An infant, 10 months old, with strabismus.

slow decrease in acuity, clouding or blurry vision, dulling of color perception, and increasing difficulty with night vision. Cataract formation can be stimulated by age-related changes, trauma, congenital anomalies, systemic disease, and pharmacologic triggers. These conditions along with ultraviolet light exposure can lead to the development of free radicals in the lens, which precipitates the formation of cataracts.

Age-related cataracts typically develop later in life. It is estimated that half of all Americans 80 years or older have had some sign of cataract.[40] ■

Linking Pathophysiology to Diagnosis and Treatment

Cataracts are diagnosed through ophthalmologic exam using a low-power microscope (slit lamp). Although cataracts are virtually impossible to prevent, limiting exposure to ultraviolet light has been shown to slow their progression. When eyesight decreases to the point at which quality of life is diminished (the person is unable to drive, read, take part in hobbies, etc.), cataract extraction is necessary.

Cataract surgery is a routine outpatient procedure. In this surgery, a small incision is made in the sclera, through which a phacoemulsifier is placed. This device uses ultrasonic vibrations to break apart the lens so that it can be drawn out of the eye. An artificial lens is then placed inside the capsule from which the natural lens was removed. Some cataract patients develop a secondary cataract, called an after-cataract, after lens replacement surgery. In this condition, the lens capsule itself becomes cloudy.[40]

To address after-cataracts, a procedure known as a capsulotomy is performed in which an yttrium-aluminum-garnet (YAG) laser is used to make an opening in the capsule. Cataracts do not return after a YAG capsulotomy. Although performed millions of times a year, cataract surgery does have inherent risks and complications, two of which are infection and macular edema (see the discussion of retinopathy below).

Sam Park: Outcome

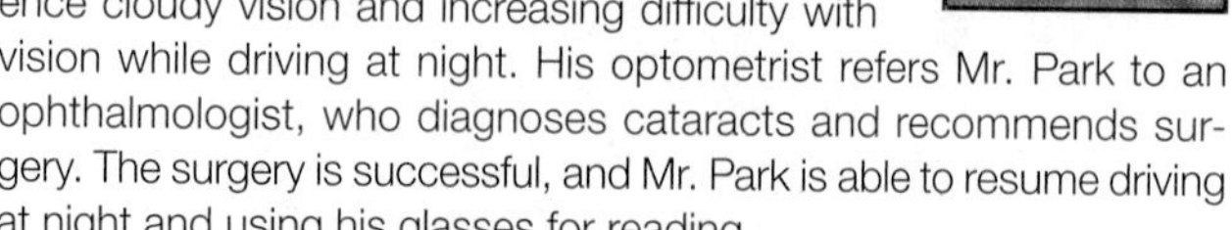

Mr. Park continued to wear glasses for reading as the result of his diagnosis of presbyopia. However, by his mid-sixties, he has begun to experience cloudy vision and increasing difficulty with vision while driving at night. His optometrist refers Mr. Park to an ophthalmologist, who diagnoses cataracts and recommends surgery. The surgery is successful, and Mr. Park is able to resume driving at night and using his glasses for reading.

5. What is a cataract?
6. How are cataracts treated?

Glaucoma

Glaucoma is a group of diseases characterized by an increase in intraocular pressure (IOP) leading to a slow, painless, and progressive loss of vision. The IOP elevates when too much aqueous humor is produced or if the aqueous humor in the anterior chamber does not drain through the trabecular meshwork (the angle where the iris meets the cornea) at a sufficient rate. Over time, this increase in IOP can cause compression to the retinal blood supply and irreversible damage to the retina and optic nerve, leading to blindness. Risk factors for glaucoma include age greater than 40 years, family history, African or Hispanic heritage, need for corrective lenses, previous history of eye injury, thinning of the optic nerve, and systemic health issues such as diabetes.[41] Glaucoma comes in several basic forms: primary open-angle glaucoma, closed-angle or narrow-angle glaucoma, low-tension glaucoma, and pigmentary glaucoma. Open-angle and closed-angle glaucoma are described below.

Open-Angle Glaucoma

Open-angle glaucoma is the most commonly diagnosed form of glaucoma. The etiology of this disorder remains unclear. In this condition, the trabecular meshwork channels are open, but the aqueous humor does not drain fast enough, perhaps owing to partially blocked channels within the meshwork. Excess aqueous humor production is another cause of elevated IOP in open-angle glaucoma. Open-angle glaucoma is particularly difficult to treat because there are no symptoms or warning signs during the early stages of the disease. The peripheral vision is affected first, but these changes often go unnoticed because central vision is not involved. Once damage has been done to the optic nerve, it cannot be reversed. If glaucoma goes undiagnosed or untreated, the vision loss gradually affects the central portion of the patient's vision. Glaucoma can be diagnosed through a routine eye exam. During examination, the IOP is measured, and the optic nerves and visual fields are evaluated. Medical management is directed toward reducing the IOP with the use of eyedrops that either lower the production of aqueous humor (prostaglandins, cholinergics) or increase the outflow of aqueous humor (beta blockers, alpha agonists, and carbonic anhydrase inhibitors).

Closed-Angle, or Narrow-Angle, Glaucoma

Usually treated as an emergency, **closed-angle glaucoma**, also called *narrow-angle glaucoma*, occurs when the angle between the iris and cornea is blocked. When this occurs, the outflow of aqueous humor is essentially halted, causing a rapid and extreme elevation in IOP. Symptoms of closed-angle glaucoma include a dilated pupil that does not react to light, a "steamy" looking cornea, redness, and pain. Vomiting and blurred vision in the form of halos and glare around lights may also occur. Closed-angle glaucoma is much rarer than open-angle glaucoma and often occurs after application of dilating eyedrops in an ophthalmologic examination. When the pupil dilates, it crowds the angle and causes a disruption of aqueous humor outflow. Diagnosis of closed-angle glaucoma entails measuring the IOP and pupils. Treatment to lower the IOP through the use of miotic eyedrops, carbonic anhydrase inhibitors, and acetazolamide works in many cases. In other cases, an iridectomy is performed, in which a laser is used to make an opening through the iris to drain the aqueous humor away from the anterior chamber.

Retinopathy

Retinopathy is broadly defined as any disorder of, or damage to, the retina. Retinopathies can result from diabetes, hypertension, or trauma. Because the retina is the nerve layer that lines the inside of the eye, damage to it results in vision loss in the corresponding visual field.

Diabetic Retinopathy

Diabetic retinopathy occurs in individuals with diabetes when blood vessels in the retina change. There are two types of diabetic retinopathy. **Nonproliferative diabetic retinopathy** occurs when blood glucose levels are elevated for a prolonged period. Over time, the walls of the retinal blood vessels weaken and begin to leak blood and fluid—a condition known as a microaneurysm. As the disease progresses, the small vessels in the retina shut down, causing fluid to leak into the macula and the space between the nerve fiber layers. The resulting macular edema, or swelling, causes a decrease in vision. Ocular manifestations of diabetes are thought to occur in 80% of people who have had diabetes for 10 years or more.[42]

As the disease advances, **proliferative diabetic retinopathy (PDR)** develops. At this stage in the disease, tiny new vessels grow from the retina into the vitreous humor, clouding vision. In severe PDR, the presence of new vessels can also signal proliferation of fibrovascular tissue, creating traction on the retina. This can ultimately lead to retinal detachments and blindness. The new vessel growth can also extend toward the front of the eye into the iris angle. When this occurs, the outflow of aqueous humor is disrupted, resulting in elevated IOP, a condition called neovascular glaucoma.

Diagnosis of diabetic retinopathy is made through ophthalmologic examination by looking at the retina. There is no cure for diabetic retinopathy, but treatments are available to slow the progression of the disease. Fluorescein angiography can be used to locate blood vessels that may be leaking in the retina. In this procedure, fluorescein dye is injected into one arm, and sequential photos of the retina are then taken. Once the leaking vessels have been identified, a laser is used to coagulate, or seal, them. Other laser treatments include panretinal photocoagulation, a technique in which 50–100 laser "burns" are made 360 degrees around the peripheral retina. The goal of this procedure is to destroy large areas of the retina so that it requires less oxygen. Reducing the retinal oxygen requirement diminishes the growth of dangerous new blood vessels. When macular edema is present, triamcinolone, a steroid, can be injected into the vitreous humor to reduce swelling. Disadvantages of triamcinolone treatment include the necessary frequency of the injections (every 3–6 months) and the fact that prolonged steroid use has significant side effects, including cataracts and glaucoma.

Retinal Detachment

When the retina separates from the underlying structures, vision is lost in the corresponding visual field. Retinal detachments occur more often in people with significant myopia because their axial length can stretch the retina. Retinal detachment can also occur secondary to cataract surgery, PDR, and trauma.

There are three basic types of retinal detachment: rhegmatogenous, exudative, and tractional. Rhegmatogenous detachments, the most common type, involve a tear in the retina.[43] Fluid from the vitreous humor moves into the tear and causes the retina to peel away from the underlying structures. Exudative, or serous, detachments are less common and occur when fluid from the underlying structures pushes into the retina and causes the retina to separate. Finally, a tractional detachment often results from PDR when new blood vessel growth into the vitreous humor triggers scarring that tugs the retina away from the underlying structures.

Symptoms of retinal detachments can be a sudden onset of floaters in the vision, flashes of light, and a veil falling over the vision. A retinal detachment is usually considered an emergency situation. If caught early enough by a dilated eye examination and optical coherence tomography, it can be effectively treated with laser surgery. The goal of laser surgery is to "tack down" the area of detachment to prevent it from further detachment, which can lead to blindness. Another common surgery for retinal detachment, known as a scleral buckle, involves sewing a piece of silicone onto the outside of the sclera to push it up to the detached portion of retina.

Macular Degeneration

Macular degeneration, also called age-related macular degeneration, is a condition in which the macula (the central part of the retina) degenerates, resulting in distortion or loss of central vision. It occurs most often in older adults. There are two forms of macular degeneration: dry and wet.

Individuals over age 45 should have a complete eye exam every 2–4 years. Those with age-related macular degeneration should check their vision daily and notify their ophthalmologist of any changes in their vision. ■

There are a number of forms of juvenile macular degeneration, the most common of which is Stargardt disease.[44] It is caused by a mutated form of the *abca4* gene. ■

Dry Macular Degeneration

Dry macular degeneration is the more common and less severe type of this disorder. Dry macular degeneration symptoms are a blurry or "wavy" central vision with normal peripheral vision. Diagnosis of dry macular degeneration is made through ophthalmologic exam using fluorescein angiography to localize areas that have leaked fluid or become ischemic. Optical coherence tomography, a newer and less invasive technique than fluorescein angiography, may also be used in diagnosis. In this procedure, an infrared light is passed across the retina, and a detailed digital image is produced of each layer of the retina. Results are then reviewed for yellowish dots around the macula, called drusen, which can be an early sign of macular degeneration. However, the presence of drusen is not always correlated with vision loss; it is not until atrophy of the photoreceptor layer below the macula occurs that vision declines. Because the macula is responsible for most of our useful acuity (the majority of visual cortex is used to process macular signals), a very apparent and destructive decline in vision results, resulting in difficulty reading, driving, and viewing detailed images such as photographs.

Wet Macular Degeneration

Wet macular degeneration is the more severe form of the disease and represents about 10–15% of cases.[45] In wet macular degeneration, new blood vessels from the underlying retinal layer, called Bruch's membrane, grow around the macula and cause bleeding, scarring, and photoreceptor atrophy. The onset of this disorder is very swift, and the damage is irreversible. Fortunately, drug therapy with anti–vascular endothelial growth factor medications has proven to stimulate the regression of neovascularization and to slow the damage to vision caused by macular degeneration.[46]

> **Check Your Progress: Section 31.7**
>
> 1. Name two types of glaucoma, and explain how each type is treated.
> 2. Describe the two types of diabetic retinopathy, and explain how they affect vision.
> 3. List the symptoms of retinal detachment, and explain why this is an emergency situation.

31.8 Nystagmus

Nystagmus is a rapid, involuntary eye movement. Rarely, nystagmus develops secondary to a visual system disorder; more commonly, it is due to an acquired pathology in the peripheral or central vestibular system. In nystagmus, the eyes drift in one direction to the end of the orbit and then move, or jerk, quickly in the opposite direction. The nystagmus is named for this corrective "jerk" phase. For example, in a right-beating nystagmus, the eyes drift leftward and then jerk back rightward. The direction of the nystagmus can be horizontal, vertical, oblique, or rotary. It may be present when the eyes are open, when they are closed, or in both conditions.

Latent Nystagmus

Latent nystagmus is a rare form of nystagmus that it associated with lack of binocular vision. It develops in some individuals with amblyopia and strabismus and is present from infancy. This nystagmus is not present when both eyes are open but becomes visible when one eye is covered. Latent nystagmus is horizontal in nature, but the direction of the nystagmus can change and is always directed away from the eye that is covered. For example, if the right eye is covered, a leftward-beating nystagmus is present; if the left eye is covered, the nystagmus reverses and beats to the right.

Congenital Nystagmus

Congenital nystagmus is most commonly horizontal and fixed in direction. It is typically faster when the eyes are open than when the eyes are closed. In some patients, the direction of the nystagmus changes depending on the orientation of their gaze. In others, the congenital nystagmus may lack a "jerk" phase and thus presents as an apparent pendular oscillation of the eyes. Some individuals with congenital nystagmus have a null point—a specific eye and/or head position that reduces the velocity of the nystagmus. Individuals with congenital nystagmus may also have a visual system abnormality, such as strabismus and hyperopia.[47]

Acquired Nystagmus

Acquired nystagmus develops secondary to a pathology in the peripheral and/or central vestibular system. Characteristics of the nystagmus typically indicate the general site of lesion as peripheral or central.

Peripheral Nystagmus

Peripheral nystagmus develops due to disruption of the normal function of the sensory cells in the peripheral balance system—typically on one side only—and/or in the transmission of that information along the vestibulocochlear nerve. Peripheral nystagmus is primarily horizontal in direction and is faster when the eyes are closed and slower when the eyes are open.

Peripheral nystagmus results from inaccurate inputs to the vestibulo-ocular reflex. This reflex pathway receives inputs from the three semicircular canals and is responsible for corrective eye movements that allow us to maintain clear vision during movement. Peripheral nystagmus typically resolves over time as the cerebellum "resets" to reflect the change sensory input.

CLINICAL POINT: Vestibular therapy can speed recovery from an acquired peripheral disorder. This treatment, which requires the patient to move the head, eyes, and body in specific ways, reduces the velocity of nystagmus when the patient is in motion and ultimately helps to relieve the sensation of dizziness with movement. ■

Central Nystagmus

Central nystagmus can be vertical, rotary, horizontal, or oblique, and it may be faster when the eyes are open than when they are closed. In some cases of central nystagmus, the eye movements are disconjugate, meaning that the eyes move in different directions rather than moving together. Central acquired nystagmus most commonly develops after an insult to the central components of the vestibular system, typically the cerebellum or brainstem. For example, this nystagmus can result from cerebellar degeneration or brainstem stroke. Central nystagmus may also develop secondary to prolonged use of some centrally acting medications. For example, long-term lithium use may result in a down-beating nystagmus in which the eyes drift upward and then jerks downward. Depending on the site of lesion, central nystagmus may resolve. or it may be permanent. Medications may be useful in slowing central nystagmus, and thus improving visual acuity, in some patients.[48]

Check Your Progress: Section 31.8

1. Describe central nystagmus, and explain how it usually develops.
2. Describe nystagmus, and explain how it is named.
3. Describe the vestibulo-ocular reflex, and explain what it does.

CHAPTER SUMMARY

31.1 Chapter Overview and Case Studies

Describe disorders of sensation and concepts related to disorders of hearing, vision, and balance.

- The human body has specialized sensory organs designed to take in various stimuli from the environment.
- Unique receptors in the sensory organs respond to these inputs and initiate the transformation of this information into neural impulses that can ultimately be interpreted at a cortical level, allowing us to experience and interpret our world.
- Concepts related to disorders of sensation include mobility, mood and affect, stress and coping, and nutrition. Children with disorders of sensation may experience developmental delays.

31.2 Basic Anatomy and Physiology of Hearing and Balance

Describe the auditory and vestibular pathways, and identify critical peripheral and central structures involved in processing hearing and balance information.

- The outer ear, comprising the auricle and the external auditory canal, collects sound waves and directs them to the middle ear. The most important function of the middle ear (the tympanic membrane and ossicles) is impedance matching. The middle ear structures transform the sound wave energy into vibratory energy.
- The organ of Corti, the sensory system of hearing, is located in the scala media within the cochlea. The cochlea encodes the frequency and intensity of the incoming sound and transforms it into neural impulses.
- The neural impulse from the cochlea travels along cranial nerve VIII through the brainstem and then ascends to primary auditory cortex (Heschl's gyrus) in the temporal lobe.
- The five sensory organs of the peripheral vestibular system (three semicircular canals, utricle, and saccule) are located in the bony labyrinth of the inner ear. The semicircular canals respond to angular acceleration; the utricle and saccule are sensitive to linear acceleration and provide information about the position of the head relative to gravity.

31.3 Conductive Hearing Loss Disorders

Differentiate the causes, classification, underlying pathogenesis, and clinical manifestations of conductive hearing loss and approaches to treatment of those conditions.

- Congenital outer ear pathologies include malformation, underdevelopment, or complete lack of development of the auricle and/or the external ear canal. Hearing loss depends on whether the middle ear is accessible for sound conduction.
- Otitis media (OM) is an inflammation of the middle ear space often associated with Eustachian tube dysfunction that can cause conductive hearing loss. OM can be acute or chronic. Treatment of otitis media depends on the severity and frequency but can include antibiotics, steroids and/or surgery.
- Otosclerosis involves abnormal bone growth in the middle ear. The resulting hearing loss is typically bilateral, slowly progressive, and primarily conductive. Stapedectomy is the most common surgery for otosclerosis.

31.4 Sensorineural Hearing Loss Disorders

Differentiate the causes, classification, underlying pathogenesis, and clinical manifestations of sensorineural hearing loss and approaches to treatment of those conditions across the lifespan.

- Presbycusis (hearing loss due to aging) is the most common form of hearing loss. It is characterized by a progressive sensorineural hearing loss (typically bilateral) in the high frequencies and a decreased ability to understand speech, particularly in noisy environments.
- Ménière disease is an inner ear disorder that is believed to result from excess endolymph in the membranous labyrinth of the inner ear system. It is characterized by

episodic attacks of hearing loss, tinnitus, vertigo, and aural fullness that may last from minutes to hours.

- Cochleotoxic medications, such as cisplatin, carboplatin, and certain aminoglycoside antibiotics, damage the inner and outer hair cells of the cochlea, resulting in a high-frequency sensorineural hearing loss that is typically bilateral. Vestibulotoxic medications, such as gentamicin, damage the type I and type II hair cells of the peripheral balance system, resulting in imbalance and blurred vision with head movement.
- Noise-induced hearing loss (NIHL) can result from exposure to a brief but intense sound (acoustic trauma) or prolonged exposure to high-intensity sounds (chronic NIHL). The resultant hearing loss is typically sensorineural but may be conductive or mixed if middle ear structures are damaged.
- Genetic-based hearing loss may be syndromic or nonsyndromic. Syndromic hearing loss results from a genetic mutation that also causes a pattern of other clinical abnormalities (e.g., heart problems, craniofacial anomalies, vision problems). In nonsyndromic genetic hearing loss, the specific genetic alteration causes hearing loss only, with no other physical changes in the individual. Most cases of genetic-based hearing loss are nonsyndromic.

31.5 Basic Anatomy and Physiology of Vision

Describe the visual pathway, and identify critical peripheral and central structures involved in processing visual information.

- Vision is the process of transforming light energy (electromagnetic radiation) into neural impulses that can be perceived and interpreted by the central nervous system.
- The front "wall" of the anterior chamber of the eye is the cornea, the transparent dome on the front of the eye. The back "wall" of the anterior chamber is the iris, the colored ring of spongy tissue with the pupil in the center. The anterior chamber contains a clear fluid, called the aqueous humor, which is responsible for nourishment of the cornea and lens.
- The posterior chamber is lined with the retina, a thin, transparent nerve layer that leaves the back of the eye via the optic nerve. The retina is made up of 10 layers.
- The photoreceptor layer of the retina contains the rods and cones. Rods function in dim lighting conditions and are responsible for the perception of black and white. Cones function in brightly lit conditions and are responsible for color vision.
- The macula is a small area on the retina with a high concentration of cones providing central vision. Retinal areas outside of the macula provide peripheral vision and binocular depth perception.
- The sclera, the white of the eye, envelops the entire eye. Each eye has six extraocular muscles that form tight adhesions to the sclera and are responsible for eye movement.
- Visual acuity is measured in terms of clarity of vision at a specific distance from the object of interest. Normal vision is represented as 20/20, meaning that from 20 feet away, an individual can see clearly an object that should normally be visible from that distance.

31.6 External Eye Disorders

Differentiate the causes, classification, underlying pathogenesis, and clinical manifestations of external eye pathologies and approaches to treatment of those conditions across the lifespan.

- A stye is a red, pus-filled bump that develops along the edge of the eyelid and develops from a bacterial infection. Styes can be painful but are harmless and typically resolve without intervention.
- Conjunctivitis, or pinkeye, is an inflammation of the conjunctiva that causes eye redness, discharge, itching, and burning. It can result from a viral or bacterial infection, or it may develop as part of an allergic reaction. Bacterial conjunctivitis is highly contagious, so precautions should be taken to prevent reinfection and spreading the infection to other people. Symptoms may be treated to reduce discomfort, but conjunctivitis typically resolves in 1–3 weeks without intervention.
- Pterygium is a benign, wedge-shaped growth on the conjunctiva that is thought to develop secondary to extended exposure to wind, airborne irritants, and/or ultraviolet light. Most cases of pterygium require no intervention, though treatment may be required if the growth interferes with vision.
- A corneal abrasion is a scratch or cut on the surface of the cornea. It can develop after getting a foreign body or chemical in the eye, rubbing the eye too hard, or getting poked in the eye. Symptoms of a corneal abrasion include blurred vision, excessive tearing, and eye redness. Corneal abrasions should be treated to avoid further damage to the cornea.

31.7 Vision Disorders

Differentiate the causes, classification, underlying pathogenesis, and clinical manifestations of vision pathologies and approaches to treatment of those conditions across the lifespan.

- Color blindness results from a deficiency in the cones of the retina that can be congenital or acquired. Individuals with color blindness can typically see some color but are unable to distinguish complementary colors. Congenital color blindness is the most common inherited visual disorder and occurs more commonly in males. Acquired color blindness can develop as a complication from diabetes or sickle cell anemia.
- A refractive error is any condition in which the eye is unable to focus light onto the macula. In myopia (nearsightedness), distant objects are blurry; in hyperopia

(farsightedness), near objects cannot be seen clearly. Astigmatism is characterized by an eye with an elliptical shape, causing light to focus on two different points in the eye and resulting in blurred vision for both near and far objects. Presbyopia, a slowly progressive decline in the focusing ability of the eye associated with aging, is characterized by difficulty viewing objects at close range.

- In amblyopia, one or both eyes cannot see clearly despite normal ocular appearance and corrective lenses. Strabismus is a condition in which one or both eyes turns in, out, up, or down; it is common in newborns or manifested within the first several years of life.
- Cataracts are cloudy or opaque discolorations of the lens. They are very gradual in onset and cause a slow decline in acuity and a dulling of color perception. Cataract formation can be stimulated by age-related changes, trauma, congenital anomalies, systemic disease, and pharmacologic triggers.
- Glaucoma is a group of diseases that lead to a slow, painless, and progressive loss of vision caused by an increase in intraocular pressure (IOP). Over time, increased IOP can cause compression to the retinal blood supply and irreversible damage to the retina and optic nerve, leading to blindness.
- Retinopathy involves any disorder of, or damage to, the retina. Retinopathies can result from diabetes, hypertension, or trauma. Nonproliferative diabetic retinopathy occurs when blood glucose levels are elevated for a prolonged period. Retinal detachment is separation of the retina from underlying structures resulting in vision loss in the corresponding field.
- Macular degeneration occurs most often in the elderly population and is seen in two forms: dry and wet.

31.8 Nystagmus

Differentiate the causes, classification, underlying pathogenesis, and clinical manifestations of nystagmus and related approaches to treatment across the lifespan.

- Nystagmus is a rapid, involuntary eye movement; it can be congenital or acquired. Nystagmus most often develops as a result of a lesion in the peripheral or central vestibular system, but it can occur secondary to a visual system disorder.
- Latent nystagmus develops in some individuals with amblyopia and strabismus. This direction-changing nystagmus is visible when one eye is covered. It is horizontal in direction and always beats away from the eye that is covered.
- Congenital nystagmus is most often horizontal and is fixed in direction. This eye movement is typically faster when the eyes are open and slower when the eyes are closed. Most individuals with congenital nystagmus have a specific head or eye position—a null point—in which their nystagmus is reduced.
- A lesion in the peripheral vestibular system causes acquired peripheral nystagmus. This nystagmus is primarily horizontal and is faster with the eyes closed. It reflects an abnormal input to the vestibulo-ocular reflex.
- Central acquired nystagmus is nystagmus that develops following insult to the central vestibular system, typically the cerebellum or brainstem, or from long-term use of certain medications. Central acquired nystagmus can beat in any direction (horizontal, vertical, or rotary) and may be faster when the eyes are open than when they are closed. In some cases, medications may be used to control central nystagmus.

REVIEW QUESTIONS

1. Treatment of otitis media may include which of the following? Select all that apply.
   a. PE tubes
   b. Stapedectomy
   c. Prophylactic antibiotics
   d. Surgery
   e. Watchful waiting
2. What are the primary functions of the cochlea? Select all that apply.
   a. To encode the frequency and intensity of incoming sound
   b. To transmit vibratory sound energy to the ossicular chain
   c. To detect changes in head position relative to gravity
   d. To transform mechanical energy from the middle ear into neural impulses
   e. To maintain balance
3. Which of the following disorders can result from the use of vestibulotoxic medications?
   a. Conductive hearing loss
   b. Sensorineural hearing loss
   c. Imbalance
   d. Tinnitus
4. The first symptom of glaucoma is usually:
   a. no symptoms until vision is compromised.
   b. pain with eye movements due to elevated eye pressure.
   c. headaches.
   d. flashes and floaters.
5. A mixed hearing loss is characterized in the following way. Select all that apply.
   a. It has both sensorineural and conductive components.
   b. It reflects damage to the auditory cortex.

c. It reflects damage to both inner and middle ear system structures.
d. It is caused by damage to the auricle.
e. It is caused by damage to the external canal.

6. What are the hallmark symptoms of Ménière disease? Select all that apply.
   a. Fluctuating sensorineural hearing loss
   b. Vertigo
   c. Fluctuating conductive hearing loss
   d. Tinnitus
   e. Vision changes

7. A corneal abrasion can result from which of the following? Select all that apply.
   a. A chemical irritant in the eye
   b. Sand in the eye
   c. Pollen
   d. A bacterial infection
   e. Rubbing the eye too aggressively

8. Which of the following are true about color blindness? Select all that apply.
   a. Color blindness results from an abnormality in the rods of the retina.
   b. Acquired color blindness can develop as a complication from diabetes.
   c. Red/green color blindness is the most common form of this disorder.
   d. Sufferers are unable to see any color.
   e. Congenital color blindness is most common in males.

ANSWERS

Answers to Review Questions can be found in Appendix A. Answers to Case Study and Check Your Progress questions are available on the faculty resources site. Please consult with your instructor.

RECOMMENDED WEBSITES

American Academy of Audiology
https://www.audiology.org

American Speech-Language-Hearing Association
http://www.asha.org

Centers for Disease Control and Prevention: Hearing Loss in Children
https://www.cdc.gov/ncbddd/hearingloss

National Eye Institute
https://www.nei.nih.gov

REFERENCES

1. University of Maryland Medical Center. (2016). *Otitis media.* Available at http://umm.edu/health/medical/altmed/condition/otitis-media
2. Centers for Disease Control and Prevention. (2017). *Ear infection.* Available at https://www.cdc.gov/getsmart/community/for-patients/common-illnesses/ear-infection.html
3. Waseem, M. (2016). *Otitis media.* Available at http://emedicine.medscape.com/article/994656-overview#a4
4. Lieberthal, A. S., Carroll, A. E., Chonmaitree, T., et al. (2013). The diagnosis and management of acute otitis media: The American Academy of Pediatrics Clinical Guideline. *Pediatrics, 131*(3). Available at http://pediatrics.aappublications.org/content/131/3/e964
5. Miaymoto, R. T. (2017). *Otitis media (chronic).* Available at http://www.merckmanuals.com/professional/ear,-nose,-and-throat-disorders/middle-ear-and-tympanic-membrane-disorders/otitis-media-chronic
6. American Academy of Otolaryngology–Head and Neck Surgery. (2016). *Middle ear infection (chronic otitis media) and hearing loss.* Available at http://www.entnet.org/content/middle-ear-infection-chronic-otitis-media-and-hearing-loss
7. National Institute on Deafness and Other Communication Disorders. (2015). *Otosclerosis.* Available at https://www.nidcd.nih.gov/health/otosclerosis
8. Kutz, J. W. (2015). *Pediatric otosclerosis.* Available at http://emedicine.medscape.com/article/994891-overview
9. Hain, T. C., & Micco, A. (2012). *Otosclerosis.* Available at http://american-hearing.org/disorders/otosclerosis
10. Thys, M. van Camp, G. (2009). Genetics of otosclerosis. *Otologic Neurology, 30*(8), 1021–1032.
11. Roland, P. S. (2015). *Presbycusis.* Available at http://reference.medscape.com/article/855989-overview#a6
12. Schuknecht, H. F. (1964). Further observations on the pathology of presbycusis. *Archives of Otolaryngology, 80,* 369–382.
13. Schuknecht, H. F., & Kirchner, J. C. (1974). Cochlear otosclerosis: Fact or fantasy? *Laryngoscope, 84*(5), 766–782.
14. Schuknecht, H. F., & Gacek, M. R. (1993). Cochlear pathology in presbycusis. *Annals of Otology, Rhinology, and Laryngology, 102,* 1–16.
15. Academy of Doctors of Audiology. (n.d.). *Practice resources: Hearing disorders and audiogram interpretation.* Available at http://www.audiologist.org/_resources/documents/diabetes/Hearing%20Disorders%20and%20Audiogram%20Interpretation.pdf
16. Frykholm, C., Larsen, H. C., Dahl, N., Klar, J., Rask-Andersen, H., & Friberg, U. (2006). Familial Meniere's disease in five generations. *Otology and Neurotology,* 27(5): 681–686.
17. National Institute on Deafness and Other Communication Disorders. (2017). *Meniere's disease.* Available at https://www.nidcd.nih.gov/health/menieres-disease
18. Meniere's Society. (2013). *Meniere's disease.* Available at http://www.menieres.org.uk/information-and-support/symptoms-and-conditions/menieres-disease
19. Mudd, P. A. (2016). *Ototoxicity.* Available at http://emedicine.medscape.com/article/857679-overview#a4
20. Black, F. O., Pesznecker, S., & Stalling, V. (2004). Permanent gentamicin vestibulotoxicity. *Otology & Neurology, 25,* 559–569.

21. Zapanta, P. E. (2016). *Vestibular rehabilitation*. Available at http://emedicine.medscape.com/article/883878-overview
22. National Institute for Occupational Safety and Health. (2014). *Occupational noise exposure: Revised criteria 1998*. Available at https://www.cdc.gov/niosh/docs/98-126/pdfs/98-126.pdf
23. Stoltzfus, S. & Boskey, E. (2015). *Acoustic trauma*. Available at http://www.healthline.com/health/acoustic-trauma#Overview1
24. National Institute on Deafness and Other Communication Disorders. (2016). *Quick statistics on hearing*. Available at https://www.nidcd.nih.gov/health/statistics/quick-statistics-hearing
25. American Academy of Otolaryngology–Head and Neck Surgery. (2017). *Genes and hearing loss*. Available at http://www.entnet.org/content/genes-and-hearing-loss
26. Smith, R. J. H., Shearer, A. E., Hildebrand, M. S., & Van Camp, G. (2014). Deafness and hereditary hearing loss overview. In R. A. Pagan, M. P. Adam, H. H. Ardinger, et al.(Eds.), *Gene reviews*. Seattle, WA: University of Washington. Available at https://www.ncbi.nlm.nih.gov/books/NBK1434
27. Centre for Genetics Education. (2007). *Deafness and hearing loss: Genetic aspects*. Available at http://www.genetics.com.au/factsheet/fs60.asp
28. Francis, S. P., & Cunningham, L. L. (2010). The connection between connexins and hearing loss. *Audiology Today, 22*(6), 72.
29. Azari, A. A., & Barney, N. P. (2013). Conjunctivitis: A systematic review of diagnosis and treatment. *JAMA, 310*(160), 1721–1729.
30. Centers for Disease Control and Prevention. (2016). *Conjunctivitis (pink eye)*. Available at http://www.cdc.gov/conjunctivitis/about/treatment.html
31. Boyd, K. (2017). *What is a pinguecula and a pterygium (surfer's eye)?* Available at https://www.aao.org/eye-health/diseases/pinguecula-pterygium
32. Wipperman, J. L., & Dorsch, J. N. (2013). Evaluation and management of corneal abrasions. *American Family Physician, 87*(2), 114–120.
33. Verma, A. (2016). *Corneal abrasion treatment and management*. Available at http://emedicine.medscape.com/article/1195402-treatment#d16
34. National Eye Institute. (2015). *Facts about color blindness*. Available at https://nei.nih.gov/health/color_blindness/facts_about
35. America Association for Pediatric Ophthalmology and Strabismus. (2015). *Achromatopsia*. Available at https://www.aapos.org/terms/conditions/10
36. Simunovic, M. P. (2010). Colour vision deficiency. *Eye, 24*(5), 747–755.
37. Simunovic, M. P. (2016). Acquired color vision deficiency. *Survey of Ophthalmology, 61*(2), 132–155.
38. National Eye Institute. (2013). *Facts about amblyopia*. Available at https://nei.nih.gov/health/amblyopia/amblyopia_guide
39. American Optometric Association. (2017). *Strabismus (crossed eyes)*. Available at http://www.aoa.org/patients-and-public/eye-and-vision-problems/glossary-of-eye-and-vision-conditions/strabismus?sso=y
40. National Eye Institute. (2015). *Facts about cataract*. Available at https://nei.nih.gov/health/cataract/cataract_facts
41. Boyd, K. (2017). *Who is at risk for glaucoma?* Available at https://www.aao.org/eye-health/diseases/glaucoma-risk
42. Mayo Clinic. (2016). *Retinal diseases*. Available at http://www.mayoclinic.org/diseases-conditions/retinal-diseases/basics/definition/con-
43. Wu, L. (2017). *Rhegmatogenous retinal detachment*. Available at http://emedicine.medscape.com/article/1224737-overview
44. Boyd, K. (2015). *Juvenile macular degeneration*. Available at https://www.aao.org/eye-health/diseases/juvenile-macular-degeneration
45. American Macular Degeneration Foundation. (2011). *"Wet" macular degeneration*. Available at http://www.macular.org/wet.html.
46. Prall, F. R. (2017). *Exudative (wet) age-related macular degeneration (AMD) treatment & management*. Available at http://emedicine.medscape.com/article/1226030-treatment
47. American Association for Pediatric Ophthalmology and Strabismus. (2016). *Nystagmus*. Available at https://www.aapos.org/terms/conditions/80
48. Strupp, M., Thurtell, M. J., Shaikh, A. G., Brandt, T., Zee, D. S., & Lee, R. J. (2011). Pharmacotherapy of vestibular and ocular motor disorders, including nystagmus. *Journal of Neurology, 258*, 1207–1222.

Chapter 32
Pain, Neuropathy, and Headache

Bernadette Roche

Chapter Outline and Learning Outcomes

32.1 Chapter Overview and Case Studies

Define pain, and discuss concepts related to pain.

32.2 Neuroanatomy of Pain

Outline the four parts of the pain pathway, and explain the significance of pain threshold and tolerance.

32.3 Assessment of Pain

Discuss the components of a thorough assessment of pain.

32.4 Acute Pain

Differentiate the causes, classification, underlying pathogenesis, and clinical manifestations of acute pain and approaches to treatment of acute pain across the lifespan.

32.5 Chronic Pain

Differentiate the causes, classification, underlying pathogenesis, and clinical manifestations of chronic pain and approaches to treatment of chronic pain across the lifespan.

32.6 Neuropathic Pain

Differentiate the causes, classification, underlying pathogenesis, and clinical manifestations of neuropathic pain and approaches to treatment of neuropathic pain.

32.7 Headache

Differentiate the causes, classification, underlying pathogenesis, and clinical manifestations of headaches and approaches to treatment of headaches across the lifespan.

32.8 Other Pain Syndromes

Differentiate the causes, classification, underlying pathogenesis, and clinical manifestations of selected other pain syndromes and approaches to treatment of these syndromes across the lifespan.

32.9 Pain Assessment and Management in Nonverbal or Cognitively Impaired Patients

Compare and contrast the assessment and treatment of pain in nonverbal or cognitively impaired patients across the lifespan.

KEY TERMS

Acute pain, 781
Allodynia, 783
Aura, 801
Breakthrough pain, 790
Central pain, 786
Central pain syndrome (CPS), 803
Chronic pain, 781
Cluster headache (CH), 801
Complex regional pain syndrome (CRPS), 798
Diabetic peripheral neuropathy (DPN), 794
Ephaptic crosstalk, 794
Fibromyalgia (FM), 803
First-order neuron, 783
Gamma-aminobutyric acid (GABA), 785
Glutamate, 784
Herpes zoster (HZ), 797
Hyperalgesia, 783
Migraine headache (MH), 800
Modulation, 781
Myofascial pain syndrome, 803
Neuralgia, 793
Neuritis, 793
Neuropathic pain, 788
Neuropathy, 793
Nociceptive-specific (NS) neuron, 784
Nociceptive pain, 780
Nociceptor, 781
Nonnociceptive pain, 781
Pain, 779
Pain threshold, 786
Pain tolerance, 787
Paresthesia, 793
Perception, 781
Peripheral neuropathy, 793

Key Terms continue on next page.

Persistent postsurgical pain (PPSP), 804
Phantom limb pain (PLP), 795
Phantom sensations, 797
Postherpetic neuralgia (PHN), 797
Psychogenic pain, 789
Radicular pain, 788
Radiculopathy, 793
Referred pain, 784
Second-order neuron, 784
Somatic pain, 788
Stump pain, 795
Sudomotor, 794
Telescoping, 799
Tension type headache (TTH), 799
Third-order neuron, 785
Transduction, 781
Transmission, 781
Trigeminal neuralgia (TN), 796
Vascular pain, 789
Visceral pain, 788
Wide dynamic range (WDR) neuron, 784
Wind-up, 794

ABBREVIATIONS

CGRP—calcitonin gene-related peptide
CH—cluster headache
CPS—central pain syndrome
CRPS—complex regional pain syndrome
DPN—diabetic peripheral neuropathy
DRG—dorsal root ganglion
FM—fibromyalgia
HZ—herpes zoster
GABA—gamma-aminobutyric acid
MH—migraine headache
NS—nociceptive-specific
NMDA—N-methyl-D-aspartate
PHN—postherpetic neuralgia
PLP—phantom limb pain
PPSP—persistent postsurgical pain
SCS—spinal cord stimulation
TENS—transcutaneous electrical nerve stimulation
TN—trigeminal neuralgia
TTH—tension type headache
VZV—varicella zoster virus
VIP—vasoactive intestinal peptide
WDR—wide dynamic range

32.1 Chapter Overview and Case Studies

The word *pain* is derived from the Latin "peona," which means a punishment from God. According to the International Association for the Study of Pain (IASP), **pain** is "an unpleasant sensory and emotional experience associated with actual or potential tissue damage, or described in terms of such damage."[1] Clinically, pain is subjectively defined as whatever the patient reports experiencing whenever it occurs. Pain is affected by the patient's age, developmental level, cognitive and communication skills, and level of fear and anxiety. It is also affected by the patient's prior pain experiences and cultural beliefs. Pain can be both a symptom of trauma or inflammation (acute pain) and a disease in itself (neuropathic pain). It is estimated that one in five adults worldwide suffer from acute or chronic pain or a combination of the two.[2] According to the Joint Commission, over 76 million people in the United States suffer from acute or chronic pain.[3] In addition to unnecessary suffering, uncontrolled pain is associated with poor patient satisfaction, unplanned hospital readmissions, prolonged recovery from illness or surgery, exacerbation of unrelated disease states or organ dysfunction, excessive loss of work time, and long-term disability. The Patient Protection and Affordable Care Act of 2010 identified pain as a public health problem. The Joint Commission has developed pain standards for ambulatory care facilities, behavioral health care organizations, home care settings, hospitals, office-based surgery practices, and nursing care centers.[3] These standards require screening of all patients or residents for pain during their initial assessment and, if clinically indicated, during ongoing, periodic reassessments. This chapter discusses the neuroanatomy of pain, assessment of pain, acute pain, chronic pain syndromes, headaches, miscellaneous chronic pain syndromes, and therapeutic interventions for the management of acute and chronic pain. It also includes an overview of the assessment and management of pain in the pediatric and geriatric patient populations.

Concepts Related to Pain

The physiologic response to pain initiates a stress response, which consists of hormonal and metabolic changes that are mediated by the hypothalamic–pituitary–adrenal (HPA) axis and sympathetic nervous system. The coordinated neuroendocrine response induces a catabolic state to meet the increased tissue demand for oxygen and energy substrates. Sympathetic stimulation of the cardiovascular system and respiratory system increases oxygen delivery and organ perfusion. Increased secretion of adrenocorticotropic hormone, cortisol, catecholamines, glucagon, and growth hormone inhibit insulin release, increase glycogenolysis, and stimulate metabolism of proteins and fat; the net effect is increased plasma glucose, proteins, and free fatty acids. Aldosterone and vasopressin, also known as antidiuretic hormone, stimulate water and water retention by the kidneys to support cardiovascular homeostasis. However, this stress response can have negative effects. The resultant hypertension and tachycardia increases oxygen consumption of the myocardium. Hyperglycemia, negative nitrogen state, and immunosuppression can impair wound healing. Pain also stimulates a hypercoagulable state, which increases the risk of deep vein thrombosis and pulmonary embolism (**Figure 32.1** ■).

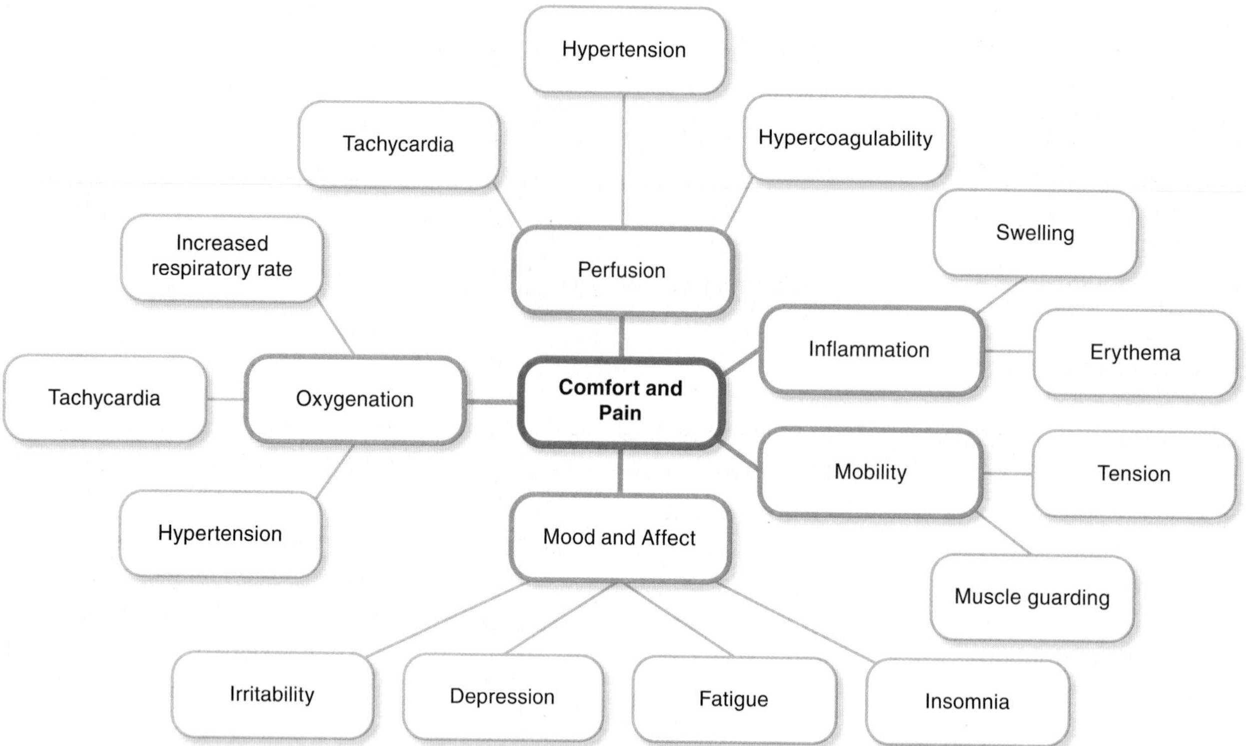

Figure 32.1 ■ Concepts related to pain.

Case Studies

The pathophysiology involved and the clinical significance of the symptoms experienced by the individuals in the following cases will be addressed throughout the chapter to assist in application of chapter content to clinical situations involving individual with acute and chronic pain.

Chelsea Collins: Introduction

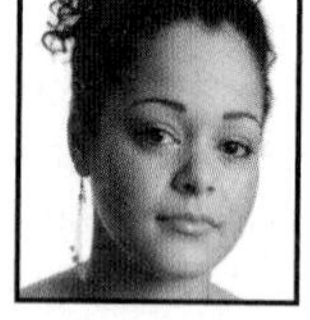

Chelsea Collins, age 24, is admitted to the emergency department with complaints of abdominal pain. The pain started over 16 hours earlier and has increased in intensity. Ms. Collins also complains of nausea and vomiting for the past 4 hours. She denies any abdominal trauma. Her last menstrual period was 8 days ago.

1. According to The Joint Commission's pain standards, when should Ms. Collins be assessed for pain?
2. Describe the process that may increase Ms. Collin's plasma glucose level.

Pam Allen: Introduction

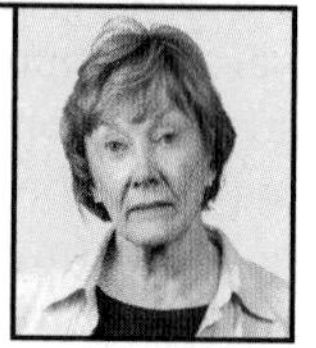

Pam Allen is a 66-year-old woman who was diagnosed with colorectal cancer a year ago. She was treated with chemotherapy along with radiation, and she felt good on completion of the treatment. On follow-up, her cancer is found to have metastasized to her liver and pancreas. After a discussion with her family, Ms. Allen chooses to enroll in hospice care.

1. It is likely that as Ms. Allen's cancer progresses, she will experience pain. Clinically, how is pain defined?
2. What factors may affect Ms. Allen's experience of pain?

Eduardo Torres: Introduction

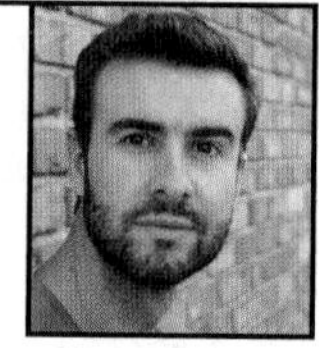

Eduardo Torres is a 35-year-old construction worker who 2 months ago underwent a left above-the-knee amputation after a motorcycle crash. The stump has healed, but Mr. Torres is complaining of pain in the stump and states that he feels pain in his missing leg.

1. Describe the sympathetic response to pain on the cardiovascular and respiratory systems that Mr. Torres may experience.
2. Explain negative effects of the stress response that Mr. Torres may experience.

Check Your Progress: Section 32.1

1. Differentiate acute pain and neuropathic pain.
2. What are some of the consequences of uncontrolled pain?
3. Why is it important that a nurse accept a patient's level of pain as described by the patient?

32.2 Neuroanatomy of Pain

Pain can be described as nociceptive or nonnociceptive. **Nociceptive pain** is a physiologic response to heat, cold, vibration, stretch, or chemicals released from damaged cells that may cause tissue damage.[1] It serves a protective biological purpose in the prevention of additional or continuing tissue trauma. In contrast, **neuropathetic** is a result of nerve cell dysfunction in the peripheral nervous system (PNS) and/or the central nervous system (CNS). There are two categories or forms of nociceptive pain: somatic and visceral. Somatic pain is an aching, throbbing, or dull pain arising from the skin, muscles, and joints that is usually discrete and intense. Visceral pain is a squeezing, cramping, dull, and deep pain originating in a bodily organ that is often poorly localized to the affected organ and commonly associated with referred patterns of pain.

Pain can also be categorized along a continuum of duration and may be diagnosed as either acute or chronic pain. **Acute pain** can last from hours to weeks and is associated with acute tissue damage or trauma, inflammation, a surgical procedure, or a brief disease process. It serves as a physiologic warning that something is wrong.[2] In contrast, chronic pain increases in intensity over time and persists for months or years. **Chronic pain** may occur after resolution of an acute injury or inflammation; it is also associated with other chronic diseases such as diabetes mellitus or cancer. The different types of pain are listed in **Table 32.1** ■.

Pain involves the transduction, transmission, modulation, and perception of a noxious stimulus (**Figure 32.2** ■). **Transduction** is the conversion of a noxious thermal, mechanical, or chemical stimulus into a nerve impulse. **Transmission** involves the transfer of a noxious peripheral stimulus to the CNS. **Modulation** involves peripheral and central neurotransmitters and other substances that enhance or dampen the transduction and transmission of a noxious stimulus. The final stage, **perception**, is the cognitive appreciation of a noxious stimulus. It involves the somatosensory cortex and limbic structures and includes the subjective, sensory, and emotional aspects of pain.

Transduction of Pain

Specialized sensory (afferent) neurons are responsible for the detection of a noxious thermal, mechanical, or chemical stimuli (**Figure 32.3** ■). Their free peripheral endings, called **nociceptors**, are widely distributed in the body, are responsive to a variety of noxious stimuli, and are responsible for the transduction of a noxious stimulus into a nerve impulse. Somatic nociceptors respond to thermal, mechanical, or chemical stimuli. In contrast, visceral nociceptors are stimulated by inflammation, ischemia, dilation, stretch, and spasm.

Two types of afferent nociceptive fibers with voltage-gated sodium channels are responsible for transmission of a noxious stimulus to the CNS: the A-delta (Aδ) and C fibers. The large myelinated Aδ fibers have a low stimulation threshold and a fast conduction velocity. There are two types of Aδ nociceptors. Type I are high-threshold mechanical nociceptors that respond to both chemical and mechanical stimuli. They have a high threshold for thermal stimuli but will respond to lower temperatures with continued stimuli or in the presence of tissue injury. They are responsible for the "first" or "fast" pain of a mechanical

Table 32.1 Types of Pain

Type of Pain	Description and Location	Examples
Central	Results from damage or injury to nerve conduction pathways in the central nervous system. Pain can appear in an area associated with the cause of injury, with a great deal of variance in severity and duration.	Epilepsy Parkinson disease Stroke
Myofascial	Pain of the skeletal muscle and surrounding fascia usually a result of chronic overuse or acute muscle injury. Characterized by trigger points (highly sensitive areas in the muscle that are painful to touch) and referred pain. Myofascial pain affects the muscles head, neck, shoulder and arm, and back and hip.	Plantar fasciitis Tension headache
Neuropathic	Pain without obvious injury or protracted pain that persists for months or years after the initial injury. Resulting from CNS or PNS dysfunction.	Carpal tunnel syndrome Diabetic neuropathy Postherpetic neuralgia Trigeminal neuralgia
Phantom	Pain associated with a missing body part or a surgically removed limb. Believed to result from damaged or dysfunctional nerve pathways at the site of injury.	Phantom limb pain. Pain after loss of an eye. Pain perceptions following a complete spinal cord injury.
Psychogenic	Physical pain with psychologic causes such as stress or anxiety	Stress-induced headache Facial or lower back pain following an emotional situation.
Radicular pain	Pain caused by inflammation or compression of a spinal nerve root. The pain follows the sensory distribution of the affected nerve.	Cervical radicular pain Lumbar radiculopathy
Somatic	Pain that rises from the skin, ligaments, muscles, bones, or joints, as result of an acute injury or chronic degenerative disease	Burns Arthritis Fracture
Vascular	Pain associated with dilation or constriction of blood vessels	Chest pain as with angina pectoris or myocardial infarction Lower extremity pain associated with peripheral artery disease Migraine headache
Visceral	Pain originating from inflammation or obstruction of internal organs	Appendicitis Gallbladder disease Kidney stones

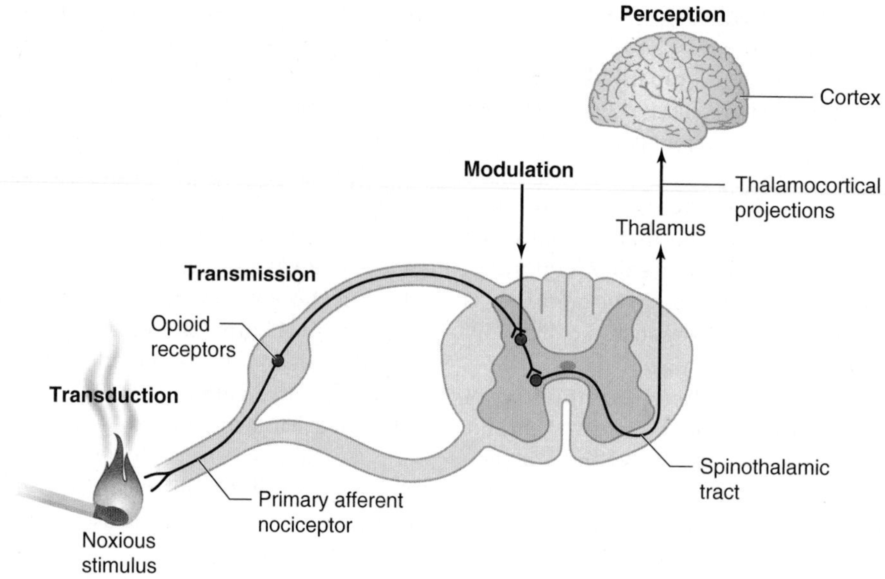

Figure 32.2 ■ The pain pathway.

stimulus—a short, well-localized, stabbing sensation that is proportional to the stimulus. "Fast" pain starts abruptly and ends when stimulus is removed. Type II Aδ nociceptors have a low heat threshold and a high mechanical threshold; they are responsible for the conduction of "fast" pain in response to a noxious heat stimulus.[4] In contrast to the Aδ nociceptors, the smaller unmyelinated, polymodal, mechano-heat–responsive C nociceptors have a slow conduction velocity and respond to mechanical and heat stimuli. Some C fibers are heat and chemical sensitive only but can develop mechanical sensitivity in the presence of tissue injury. C fibers are responsible for conducting the "second" or "slow" pain, a throbbing, burning, aching sensation that is poorly localized and not specifically related to a stimulus. **Table 32.2** ■ provides a comparison of the Aδ and C fibers with sensory (Aβ), motor (Aα), and autonomic (B and sympathetic nerve) fibers.

Once the threshold of the fibers has been reached, an action potential is generated, and the nociceptor transduces the thermal, mechanical, or chemical stimulus into electrical energy that carries the noxious stimulus into the CNS, ultimately leading to the conscious perception of pain. Nociceptors show no adaptation and depolarize in proportion to the intensity and frequency of the stimulus; the greater the stimulus, the greater is the transduction of the stimulus into a nerve impulse. Activation of voltage-gated sodium and potassium channels on the Aδ and C fibers is necessary for the generation and conduction of the action potential. Activation of voltage-gated calcium channels is responsible for central and peripheral release

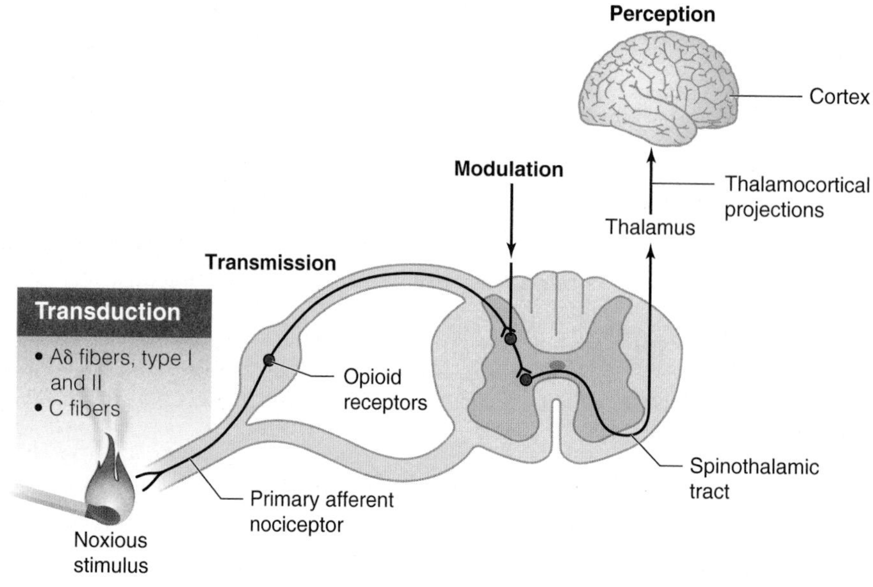

Figure 32.3 ■ Transduction of pain.

Table 32.2 Classification of Nerve Fibers

Fiber	Diameter (microns)	Myelination	Conduction Velocity (m/sec)	Function
A-alpha (Aα)	12–20	Myelinated	70–120	Responsible for proprioception, the appreciation of the spatial position of the body, and transmission of impulses from the ventral horn of the spinal cord that produce muscle movement.
A-beta (Aβ)	5–12	Myelinated	30–70	Responsible for the transmission of touch and pressure from the periphery of the body or internal viscera to the dorsal horn of the spinal cord.
A-delta (Aδ)	2–5	Myelinated	15–30	Responsible for transmission of "first" or "fast" pain to the dorsal horn of the spinal cord
B	< 3	Lightly myelinated	3–15	Responsible for transmission of parasympathetic and sympathetic impulses from the brain and spinal cord to the postganglionic fibers.
C	0.4–1.2	Unmyelinated	0.5–2.3	"Second" or "slow" pain; diffuse, aching.
Sympathetic	0.3–1.3	Unmyelinated	0.7–2.3	Responsible for sympathetic stimulation of the heart blood vessel, smooth muscle, viscera, and glands.

of neurotransmitters necessary for the transmission of pain or mediation of neurogenic inflammation.[4] In C fibers, upregulation of calcium (Ca^{2+}) channels may play a role in injury-evoked **hyperalgesia** (an exagerated and prolonged response to pain) and **allodynia** (a perception of pain from a stimulus that does not usually cause pain). Peripheral sensitization can result from inflammation- or trauma-triggered changes in the chemical environment of the free endings of the nociceptor. In response to tissue injury, endogenous inflammatory chemical mediators are released from mast cells, macrophages, platelets, neutrophils, endothelial cells, and fibroblasts (**Figure 32.4** ■). These mediators include potassium (K^+), serotonin, bradykinin, histamine, cytokines, nitric oxide, peptides such as substance P, calcitonin gene-related peptide (CGRP), bradykinin, prostaglandins, thromboxanes, leukotrienes, cytokines, and chemokines. The resulting "inflammatory soup" increases the excitability and sensitivity of the nociceptors.[2] Antidromic (conduction in the opposite direction of normal) release of substance P and

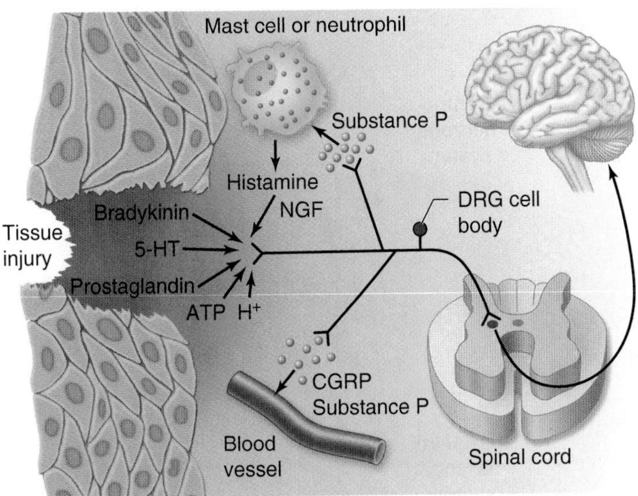

Figure 32.4 ■ Peripheral nociception. In response to tissue injury, endogenous inflammatory chemical mediators are released from mast cells, macrophages, platelets, neutrophils, endothelial cells, and fibroblasts.

glutamate from the nociceptor also increases the excitability of the nociceptor. Damage to peripheral nociceptors can result in spontaneous depolarization or altered conduction.

The cell bodies of trunk and limb Aδ and C afferents are located in the dorsal root ganglion (DRG); the trigeminal ganglion contains the cell bodies of Aδ and C afferents that innervate the face. Unlike other neurons that have an axonal branch and a dendritic branch, Aδ and C afferents have both a peripheral branch and a central axonal branch that innervate their peripheral target and the spinal cord, respectively. Consequently, proteins synthesized by the DRG or the trigeminal ganglion are released by both their spinal and peripheral terminals, and nerve fibers can send and receive message between the two locations.[4]

Transmission of Pain

Transmission is the next step in the transfer of a noxious peripheral stimulus to the CNS (**Figure 32.5** ■). The dorsal horn of the spinal cord is the relay center for nociceptive and sensory input. Activation of the dorsal horn depends on the intensity of the noxious stimulus, the release of excitatory or inhibitory neurotransmitters, and activation of descending and segmental inhibitory neurons. The gray matter of the spinal cord is divided into 10 layers called the Rexed laminae (**Figure 32.6** ■). The dorsal horn (sensory) contains laminae I–VI; lamina I is also called the marginal layer, lamina II is called the substantia gelatinosa, and laminae III–VI are known as the nucleus proprius. The ventral horn (motor) contains laminae VII–IX, and lamina X surrounds the central canal.

Three types of neurons are involved in the transmission of pain: the first-, second-, and third-order neurons (**Figure 32.7** ■). The **first-order neurons**, Aδ and C fibers, synapse with second-order neurons and interneurons in laminae I, II, and V of the dorsal horn. The Aδ fibers synapse directly with second-order neurons in laminae I and V; C fibers synapse in laminae I and II, primarily with interneurons that synapse in turn with second-order neurons.[2] First-order neurons also synapse in the dorsal horn with sympathetic fibers and ventral motor nuclei. A-beta

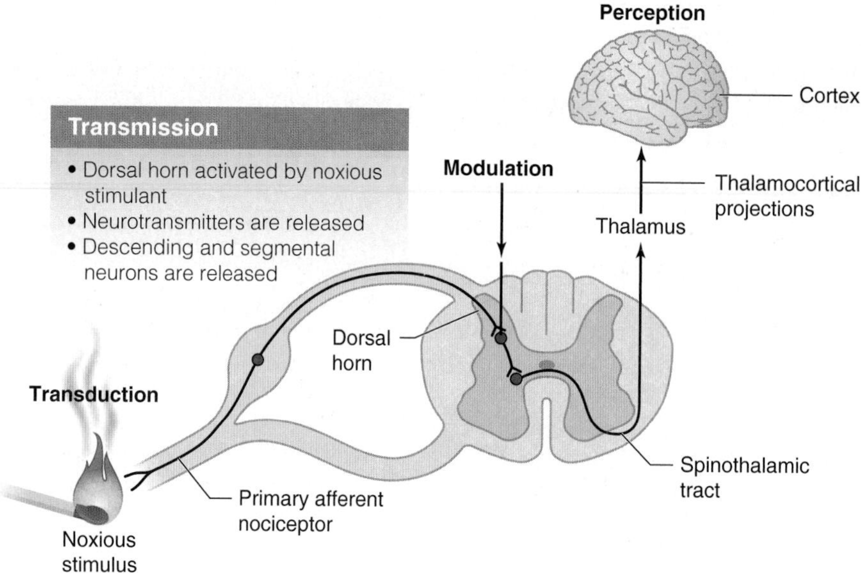

Figure 32.5 ■ Transmission of pain.

(Aβ) fibers, sensory afferents involved in the transmission of touch, terminate in laminae III–VI and may be involved in the transmission of chronic pain.[2]

Second-order neurons have their cell bodies in the dorsal horn. They are classified as **nociceptive-specific (NS) neurons** (lamina I), which have small receptive fields and respond only to nociceptive stimuli, or **wide dynamic range (WDR) neurons** (lamina V), which have complex receptive fields and respond to nociceptive and nonnociceptive (tactile) input received directly from Aδ and Aβ fibers and indirectly from C fibers. The WDR neurons also receive input from the viscera; the resultant convergence of the somatic and visceral input is responsible for **referred pain** patterns of visceral inflammation or injury in which the visceral pain is perceived as originating from a somatic site.

Excitatory neurotransmitters in the dorsal horn include glutamate, aspartate, vasoactive intestinal peptide (VIP), substance P, cholecystokinin, and CGRP. The predominant excitatory neurotransmitter is **glutamate**, which initially binds to the α-amino-3-hydroxy-5-methyl-4-isoxazolepropionic acid receptor, which mediates fast synaptic transmission between first-order and second-order neurons. With increasing intensity of the stimuli, glutamine activates the N-methyl-D-aspartate (NMDA) receptor, which leads to continuing excitability of the second-order neuron.[2] The subsequent Ca^{2+} influx increases sensitivity to glutamate and exacerbates the response to noxious stimuli resulting in primary hyperalgesia. Continuing C fiber input increases the response of WDR neurons, a process known as "wind-up" and appears to be related to activation of the NMDA receptor. Inhibitory neurotransmitters in the dorsal

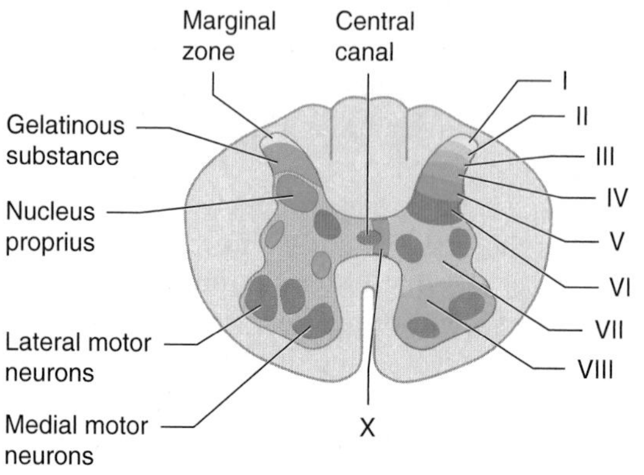

Figure 32.6 ■ The gray matter of the spinal cord is divided into 10 layers called Rexed laminae.

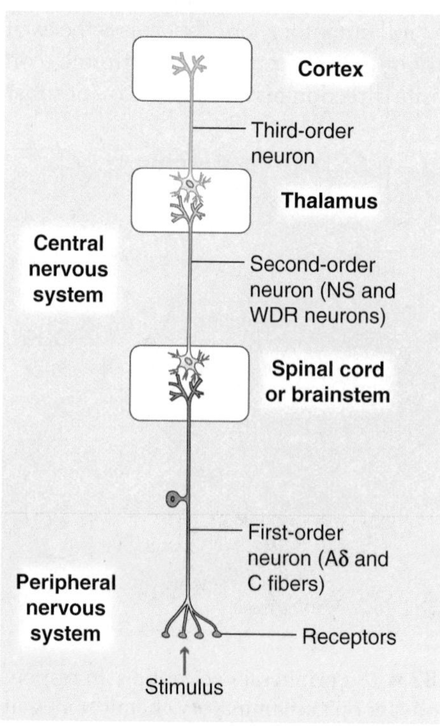

Figure 32.7 ■ First-, second-, and third-order neurons.

horn include two amino acids, gamma-amino butyric acid (GABA), and glycine.

Ascending tracts, composed of second-order NS and WDR neurons, are responsible for the transmission of noxious stimuli within the CNS (**Figure 32.8** ■). Second-order NS and WDR neurons in the dorsal horn cross to the contralateral anterior spinal cord and ascend to the thalamus via the spinothalamic tract (STT), the spinoreticular tract (SRT), and the spinomesencephalic tract (SMT). The majority of the STT and SRT axons crosses close to their level of origin and participate in multiple components of pain. The lateral STT synapses with third-order neurons in the posterior thalamus and is involved with discriminative functions such as location, intensity, and duration of noxious stimuli. **Third-order neurons** transmit noxious impulses from the thalamus to the primary somatosensory areas for perception of pain. The medial STT synapses with third-order neurons in the medial thalamus; their collaterals synapse with third-order neurons in the periaqueductal gray matter, hypothalamus, and reticular formation in the midbrain.

The medial STT is responsible for stimulation of the autonomic nervous system and the emotional or unpleasant associations with noxious stimuli. The SRT terminates in the reticular formation of the medulla and pons and is responsible for the aversive responses to pain and possible control of the descending tract. Other tracts such as the spinocervical tract and the dorsal columns are also believed to be involved in the transmission of pain, as some patients can still perceive pain after ablation of the STT, SRT, and SMT. The third-order neurons project from the thalamus and midbrain to the somatosensory cortex for perception and localization of the pain; they also project to the limbic system, which is associated with the behavior, emotion, and memory of pain.[2] Some second-order neurons pass to the anterior and anterolateral horns of the spinal cord to initiate spinal reflexes that result in reflex withdrawal, increased muscle tone, inhibition of phrenic nerve function, and decreased gastrointestinal motility.

The descending tracts arise in the somatosensory cortex and terminate in laminae I and II of the dorsal horn (see Figure 32.8). On the way, they synapse in the periaqueductal gray matter, nucleus raphe magna, and medullary reticular formation. The primary neurotransmitters of the descending tracts are norepinephrine and serotonin. The descending tracts stimulate inhibitory neurons in the dorsal horn to release inhibitory neurotransmitters, primarily **Gamma-aminobutyric acid (GABA)** and glycine, which prevent activation of third-order neurons. GABA is the predominant inhibitory neurotransmitter in the CNS; it binds to the $GABA_A$ and $GABA_B$ receptors. The descending tracts also stimulate the release of supraspinal and spinal endogenous opioids (endorphins, dynorphins, and enkephalins).

Modulation of Pain

Nociceptive transmission is modified through a number of peripheral, spinal, and supraspinal influences (**Figure 32.9** ■). In the periphery, injured tissues release substance P and glutamate, which directly activates nociceptors. Potassium, hydrogen ions, lactic acid, acetylcholine, serotonin, bradykinin, histamine, prostaglandins released from injured cells, local mast cells, plasma, and platelets sensitize and excite nociceptors and mediate inflammation. This peripheral sensitization results in primary hyperalgesia, in which a reduced stimulus intensity can activate nociceptors. Primary hyperalgesia decreases as healing reduces the amount of the sensitizing substances.[2] In the spinal cord, neurotransmitters released in the dorsal horn modulate spinal transmission. Excitatory transmitters include glutamate, substance P, aspartate, neuropeptide Y, neurokinin A, galanin, VIP, and CGRP (**Table 32.3** ■).

The descending tracts provide supraspinal modulation of pain through the release of inhibitory neurotransmitters

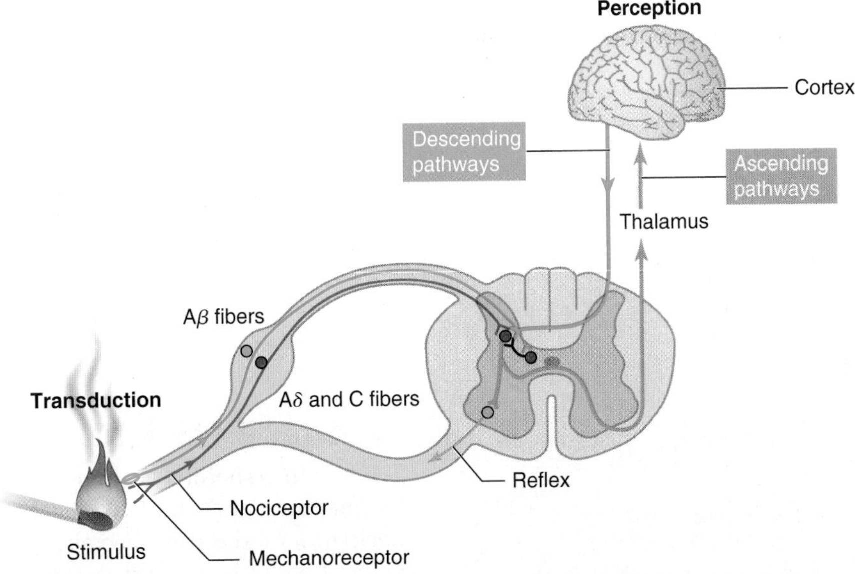

Figure 32.8 ■ Ascending (blue) and descending (green) pathways of pain transmission.

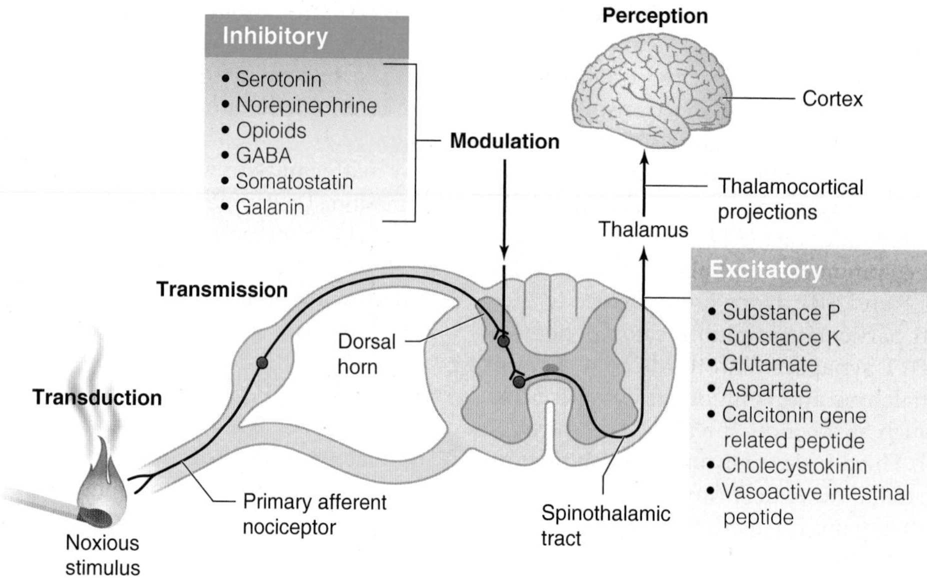

Figure 32.9 ■ Modulation of pain.

and peptides that act presynaptically on first-order neurons and postsynaptically on second-order neurons to decrease synaptic transmission between the two neurons. Inhibitory substances that decrease transmission of peripheral noxious stimuli include glycine, dopamine, GABA, norepinephrine, adenosine, beta endorphins, acetylcholine, somatostatin, serotonin, and magnesium (Mg^{2+}) (see Table 32.3) Glial cells, especially microglia and astrocytes, are found throughout the CNS, where they function as macrophages. When a peripheral nerve is injured, glial cells accumulate in the dorsal horn in the terminal lamina of the injured nerve. They release proinflammatory cytokines (tumor necrosis factor, interleukin 1, and interleukin 6), glutamate, and nitric oxide, which directly activate first-order and second-order neurons in the dorsal horn and favor the development of persistent **central pain** (regional pain that is caused by a primary lesion or dysfunction of the central nervous system and persists after resolution of the initial inflammation or trauma). Peripheral nerve injury also activates glial cells in the brainstem that decrease the effectiveness of the inhibitory function of the descending tracts. Central sensitization is a result of increased excitability of the dorsal horn that results in an amplification of the noxious stimulus. Excessive or continued activation of the dorsal horn results in an abnormal response to sensory input and secondary hyperalgesia, an increased peripheral sensitivity beyond the site of the injury.[2] Increased glutamate release or decreased reuptake, changes in NMDA sensitivity, decreased GABA or glycine release, damage to inhibitory interneurons in the dorsal horn, and continued glial cell activation can all contribute to central sensitization.

Table 32.3 Substances That Modulate the Transmission of Noxious Stimuli in the Dorsal Horn

Type of Transmitter	Substances
Excitatory	Glutamate Substance P Aspartate Neuropeptide Y Neurokinin A Galanin Vasoactive intestinal peptide Cholecystokinin CGRP
Inhibitory	GABA Glycine Dopamine Norepinephrine Adenosine Beta endorphins Acetylcholine Somatostatin Serotonin Magnesium (Mg^{2+})

Perception of Pain

Sensory information from the thalamus, reticular formation, and limbic system is transmitted by third-order neurons to the somatosensory cortex, where it is perceived as pain and alerts the individual to a real or potential internal or external injury (**Figure 32.10** ■). The perception of pain is influenced by emotional or psychologic stress, cultural and religious beliefs, and prior experience with pain.

CLINICAL POINT: Pain is a subjective experience, and perception of pain can be accurately described only by the individual who is experiencing the pain. ■

Pain Threshold and Tolerance

The **pain threshold** is the minimum intensity of a noxious thermal, mechanical, or chemical stimulus that activates nociceptors and is perceived as painful. While the intensity of the stimulus is an external event, the threshold is the perception of the patient. Pain thresholds are modulated in the

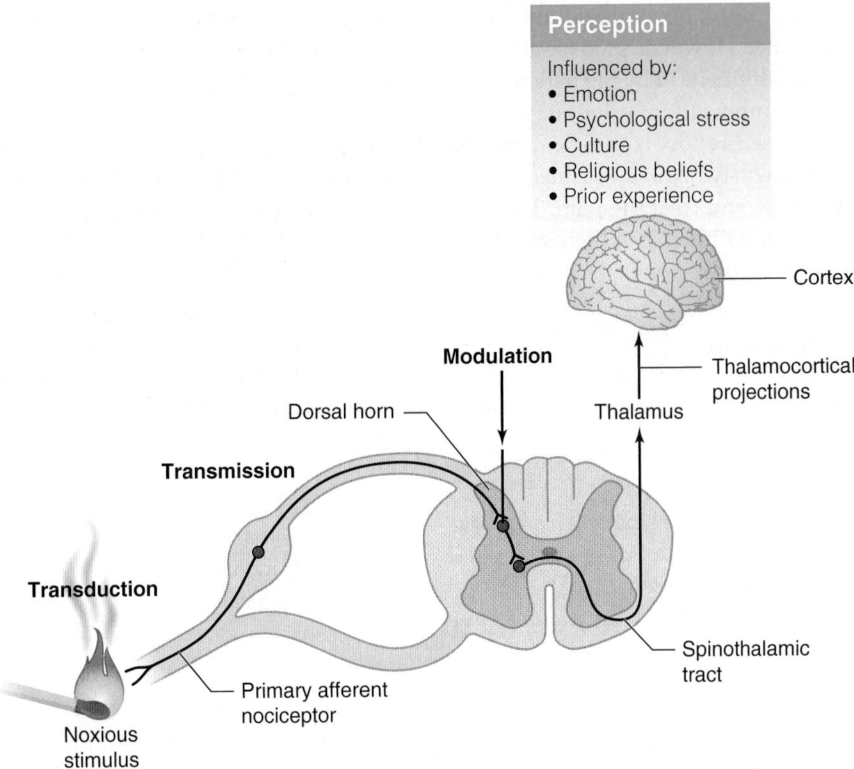

Figure 32.10 ■ Perception of pain.

periphery through increased release of chemical mediators that increase or decrease the threshold of nociceptors. Likewise, excitatory or inhibitory neurotransmitters in the CNS increase or decrease the threshold of second- and third-order neurons in the dorsal horn and thalamus. Sensitization, an increased excitability of neurons, occurs when the pain threshold is lowered and there is increased responsiveness of the neuron. This produces hyperalgesia and allodynia. Peripheral sensitization is a result of a decreased threshold and increased responsiveness of the peripheral nociceptors. Central sensitization is a result of increased excitability of neurons in the CNS, and normal inputs begin to produce abnormal responses. Central sensitization is usually triggered by increased activity of peripheral nociceptors in response to trauma or inflammation that alters the synaptic connections between the first- and second-order neurons in the dorsal horn. With sensitization, low-threshold sensory fibers responsive to light touch can activate neurons in the dorsal horn that normally respond only to noxious stimuli. As a consequence, an innocuous stimulus can produce a pain that is perceived as originating in the periphery but is actually due to abnormal sensory processing in the CNS. Central sensitization is responsible for tactile allodynia and secondary hyperalgesia.

Pain tolerance is the amount of pain an individual can take or tolerate; it is affected by the person's gender, age, culture, emotional state, and physical activity. Tolerance can be increased by activation of large somatic fibers that prevent the transmission of pain. In 1965, the gate control theory of pain of Ronald Melzack and Patrick Wall proposed that nonpainful input closes a "pain gate" to painful input in the dorsal horn and prevents the transmission of pain to the CNS. When there is no input from Aδ and C fibers, inhibitory interneurons in the dorsal horn block activation of the second-order neurons, effectively closing the pain gate. In contrast, activation of Aδ and C fibers will block the inhibitory interneuron and allow activation of the second-order neuron, effectively opening the pain gate and allowing the ascending transmission of pain. Input from large somatic nerve fibers also activates the inhibitory interneurons and prevents the smaller pain fibers from activating the second-order neuron. Therefore, nonnoxious input, such as rubbing an injured body part, can decrease the transmission of pain. This is the proposed mechanism of action for transcutaneous electrical nerve stimulation (TENS) and spinal cord stimulation (SCS).

Check Your Progress: Section 32.2

1. Describe the differences between nociceptive and neuropathic pain.
2. What is the role of type I Aδ nociceptors?
3. Using the gate control theory, describe how nonnoxious input, such as TENS, can reduce pain.

32.3 Assessment of Pain

In 1996, the American Pain Society introduced the concept of pain as the "fifth vital sign," and in 2001, the Joint Commission required pain assessment in all accredited facilities.[3]

Like other vital signs, pain must be assessed and documented in an objective manner. However, pain is subjective, and the perception of pain is influenced by the patient's age, cognition, culture, and communication or language skills. Although the individual's self-report is the most reliable indicator of pain, a comprehensive pain assessment is necessary to accurately diagnose and treat the pain. This may include using the mnemonic **OPQRST**, which stands for assessing the following factors of the pain:

Onset
Provocative and palliative factors
Quality
Region or radiation
Severity
Timing.

Associated physical symptoms such as nausea, vomiting, constipation, confusion, urinary retention, and muscle weakness should also be assessed. Assessment of the impact of the pain on the patient's quality of life (recreational activities, relationships, and work), sleep, mood, and stress level is also important. A variation on OPQRST, the mnemonic **OPQRSTUV**, may also be used. It includes the patient

Understanding the cause of the pain and the
Values the patient assigns to relief of the pain.

The mnemonic **OPQRST-AAA** includes three additional assessments:

Aggravating or alleviating factors
Associated symptoms
Attributions or adaptations.

The factors of OPQRST are expanded below, and sample questions that can be used to elicit answers from the patient during the assessment are outlined in **Table 32.4** ■.

CLINICAL POINT: Recognizing and managing pain in patients is a priority of care for all healthcare professionals. It is important to remember that a patient in pain should always be believed. Pain is whatever the person experiencing the pain says it is. ■

Onset

The onset of pain may be acute, or the pain may gradually increase in severity and duration. Acute pain is associated with acute tissue injury or inflammation. Patients can easily recall the onset of acute pain that is associated with a traumatic injury such as a fall. Pain that is a result of tissue inflammation and visceral inflammation or obstruction is characterized by a gradual onset that increases in duration, frequency, and severity. Patients may have difficulty identifying exactly when the pain started.

Provocative or Palliative Factors

Provocative factors that increase or trigger pain include movement, position, food ingestion, and certain activities such as walking or bending. Palliative factors that lessen pain include the supine position, rest, analgesics, and fasting.

Quality

Patients use a variety of words to describe the quality of their pain, including *sharp, dull, stabbing, burning, crushing, throbbing, nauseating, shooting, twisting*, and *stretching*. The quality of pain is frequently associated with the location or source of the pain.

- **Somatic pain** is associated with damage to the skin, soft tissues, ligaments, muscles, bones, and joints. It is an aching, throbbing, or dull pain that is well localized to the area of inflammation or trauma and is frequently associated with a traumatic event.
- **Visceral pain** is internal, arising from the organs or the blood vessels, which lack significant sensory innervation. Nociceptors in the viscera are stimulated by inflammation, ischemia, dilation, stretch, and spasm, and visceral pain is described as squeezing, pressure, cramping, distention, and dull.
- **Neuropathic pain** is due to peripheral or central damage or dysfunction of first-order neurons and is described as burning, shooting, tingling, radiating, lancinating, or numbing.
- **Radicular pain**, a type of neuropathic pain, is caused by inflammation or compression of a spinal nerve root and is frequently associated with a herniated intervertebral disc and spinal stenosis. The pain is steady and dull, radiates along the sensory distribution of the nerve, and is frequently accompanied by weakness, numbness, tingling, or loss of reflexes in the affected limb.

Table 32.4 OPQRST Mnemonic for Assessment of Pain

OPQRST Mnemonic	Assessment	Sample Questions
Onset	Acute or gradual onset	• When did the pain start? • What were you doing when the pain started?
Provocative and palliative factors	Increased or decreased pain	• What makes the pain worse? • What makes the pain better?
Quality	Description of pain	• How would you describe the pain? What does your pain feel like?
Region or radiation	Anatomic location of the pain	• Can you point to the site of your pain? • Has the pain moved or changed location?
Severity	Pain intensity	• Is this the worst pain you have ever experienced? • On a scale of 0 to 10, how bad is your pain?
Timing	Onset, duration, frequency	• When is your pain the worst? • How long does the pain last?

- **Vascular pain** is a result of severe peripheral artery disease or vascular vasospasm in response to cold and/or increased activity of the SNS. Claudication refers to ischemic muscular pain and cramping in an extremity that is triggered by muscle activity.

Region and Radiation

The location of pain is an important part of the assessment process, as it will help to identify the site and the possible cause of the pain. The location of somatic pain is easily identified by the patient and often visible to the observer. The location of visceral, neuropathic, and radicular pain may be more readily identified by referring or radiating patterns. Referred pain is a result of convergence of visceral and somatic sensory neurons in the dorsal horn; the CNS interprets the perceived pain as arising in the somatic dermatome that converges with the visceral afferents in the dorsal horn. Consequently, visceral pain is "referred" to another distant area of the body. **Psychogenic pain** is caused by emotional or mental stress; it is not associated with any somatic or visceral inflammation or trauma but may present as referred pain.

Severity

It is essential to quantify the severity of the pain so that appropriate therapeutic interventions are implemented. Pain perception and expected behavior in response to pain depend on the age of the patient (**Table 32.5** ■). Pain scales, based on self-report and/or observational (behavioral) or physiologic data, are used to quantify the severity of the pain. Self-reported pain scales allow the patient to accurately rate the intensity or severity of their pain (**Figure 32.11** ■). Several pain scales are currently used for assessing acute pain. The most commonly used is the visual analog scale (VAS); in using the VAS, patients rate their pain by indicating a position along a continuous line between two end points of no pain to very severe pain. In using the verbal numeric scale (VNS), patients verbally rate their pain on a scale of 0 (no pain) to 10 (most intense pain imaginable). The McGill Pain Questionnaire (MPQ), which lists 78 pain descriptor items categorized into 20 subclasses, is a multidimensional pain questionnaire that measures the sensory, affective, and evaluative aspects of chronic pain. A shorter form, the MPQ (SF-MPQ), includes 15 descriptors (11 sensory, 4 affective), which are rated on an intensity scale of 0 to 3.[5]

Timing

It is important to assess the timing, frequency, and duration of the pain. Pain can be intermittent and frequently stimulated by a specific movement or behavior. Pain can be constant but with severity that varies over time. The timing of pain may be worse at different times of the day, before or after meals, or after periods of exercise. The pain may also occur randomly or be seasonal in nature. Stable pain is

Table 32.5 Influence of Age on Pain Perception and Behavior

Developmental Stage	Response to Pain
Infant	Exhibits body rigidity or thrashing. Exhibits facial expression of pain. Cries inconsolably. Exhibits hypersensitivity or irritability. Has poor oral intake. Is unable to sleep.
Toddler and preschooler	May describe pain through basic words or gestures. May be verbally aggressive. May cry intensely. Exhibits physical resistance by pushing away painful stimulus. Guards painful area of body. May see pain as punishment. May request emotional support from parent.
School-age child	Should be able to accurately describe their pain. Attempts to be brave in response to pain. May exhibit stalling behaviors. Exhibits muscle rigidity and other behaviors in anticipation of pain. May revert to earlier developmental stage with persistent or severe pain.
Adolescent	May deny pain in the presence of peers. Exhibits changes in sleep patterns or appetite. Exhibits body control. May regress to an earlier developmental stage in the presence of a trusted adult.
Adult	May exhibit gender-specific behaviors learned as a child. May ignore pain in order to be a "good" client. May ignore pain to prevent appearing weak. May deny pain for fear that the condition has worsened.
Older adult	Pain may result from multiple conditions. May view pain as being inherent to aging. May have increased pain threshold in comparison to younger adults. Manifestations of pain may include decreased energy level, loss of appetite, and general lethargy. May deny pain to prevent becoming dependent on others.

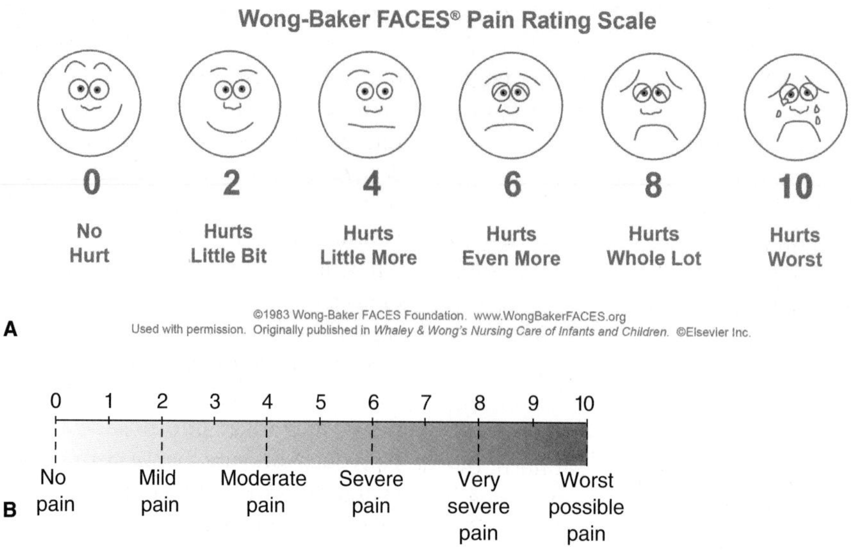

Wong-Baker FACES® Pain Rating Scale

0	2	4	6	8	10
No Hurt	Hurts Little Bit	Hurts Little More	Hurts Even More	Hurts Whole Lot	Hurts Worst

A

0 1 2 3 4 5 6 7 8 9 10

No pain | Mild pain | Moderate pain | Severe pain | Very severe pain | Worst possible pain

B

Figure 32.11 ■ Examples of visual pain scales. **A.** The Wong-Baker FACES pain rating scale is useful with children and whenever there is a language barrier. **B.** A numeric rating scale from 0 to 10 can be used verbally, or a patient can point to the appropriate pain level.

constant with little variation in severity. **Breakthrough pain** occurs when a patient with continuous stable pain has a sudden and transient exacerbation or flare-up of intense pain.

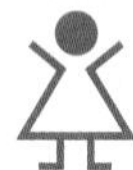

The visual analog scale is useful in determining pain in young children. ■

Chelsea Collins: Application

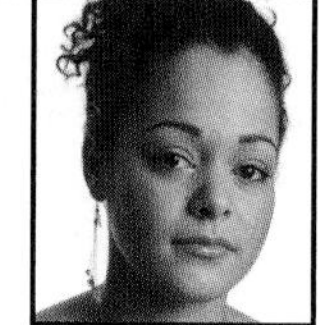

On examination, Ms. Collins reports a pain level of 8 on a scale of 0–10. Her vital signs are pulse 100, respirations 24, temperature 99°F, blood pressure 116/68. She previously denied abdominal injury or trauma, along with any significant previous medical history. Her pain is located in the upper quadrants of the abdomen with a primarily central presentation. She describes it as gnawing. Bowel sounds are hyperactive across all quadrants. Mild epigastric tenderness is noted on light palpation of the abdomen.

3. What associated physical symptoms of pain is Ms. Collins experiencing?
4. Describe the intensity of Ms. Collins's pain using the numeric rating scale.

Pam Allen: Application

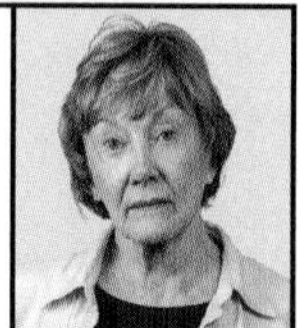

A hospice nurse meets with Ms. Allen and her family for an intake interview. Ms. Allen reports a loss of appetite along with feeling bloated or full. She significantly reduced her fluid intake over the past 48 hours because she felt bloated. She reports her pain as a 7 on a scale of 0–10 and says that it is partly alleviated by sitting and leaning forward. The pain is generalized across the abdomen, and Ms. Allen refuses palpation of the abdomen. Before referral, her physician prescribed a 100 mcg fentanyl patch.

3. What factors should be included in the routine assessment of Ms. Allen's pain?
4. On the basis of Ms. Allen's history and clinical manifestations, name one type of pain that she may be experiencing.

Eduardo Torres: Application

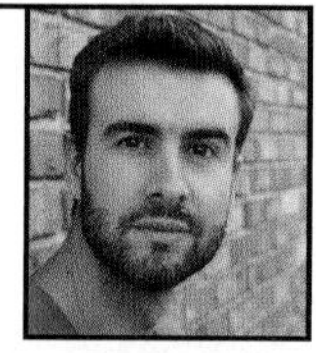

Mr. Torres reports a pain rating of 6 on a scale of 0 to 10. He describes the pain as burning and achy and says that it is greater when he is tired. He also describes a sensation of feeling his missing leg moving and of the sense that he could touch his missing toes.

3. How should the nurse respond when Mr. Torres asks whether the nurse believes that he has pain in his amputated limb?
4. Give an example of how the nurse would document Mr. Torres's pain using onset, location, radiation, quality (character) and intensity (severity), exacerbating and relieving factors, and associated physical symptoms.

Check Your Progress: Section 32.3

1. Compare and contrast somatic and visceral pain.
2. Which is the most useful pain scale to use with young children?
3. Describe the response of an infant to pain.

32.4 Acute Pain

Acute pain has a sudden onset and is associated with acute or potential trauma to somatic or visceral tissue. Acute pain occurs a short time after the injury; the pain is transient, sharp, and localized to the site of the injury or inflammation. The duration and intensity of the pain diminish as tissue healing occurs. Physiologic responses to acute pain involve many signs and symptoms, some of which are listed in **Table 32.6** ■. A thorough history and physical

Table 32.6 Physiologic Response to Acute Pain

Concept	Signs and Symptoms
Oxygenation	Increased respirations Pallor
Perfusion	Increased blood pressure Increased pulse
Digestion and endocrine regulation	Nausea Vomiting Diarrhea Loss of appetite Increased glucose
Mobility	Increased muscle tension Avoidance of movement
Mood, sleep, and behavior	Anxiety Restlessness Insomnia Grimacing, moaning, crying

examination of the patient are necessary to determine the source and cause of the pain.

Somatic Pain

Somatic pain is a result of inflammation or trauma to the skin, soft tissues, ligaments, skeletal muscles, bones, or joints. The onset of the pain is sudden and usually related to a specific time and activity, such as a fall. The intensity and duration of the pain is related to the degree of tissue trauma. The location of the pain can be readily identified by the patient and examined by the healthcare provider.

Visceral Pain

Visceral pain may be a result of organ inflammation, spasm, dilation, mechanical obstruction, or impaired blood supply. It can have a gradual or sudden onset and is described with vague terms such as squeezing, pressure, cramping, and distention with a dull quality. The exact source of visceral pain is difficult to pinpoint, as the pain is frequently referred to a distant site of the body as a result of visceral and somatic convergence in the dorsal horn. The CNS interprets the pain as arising in the somatic dermatome that converges with the visceral nociceptor in the dorsal horn. Examples of common referral patterns are included in **Figure 32.12** ■. Acute visceral pain is frequently accompanied by nausea, vomiting, diarrhea, and loss of appetite.

Treatment of Acute Pain

Multimodal pain management of acute pain includes the use of two or more agents with different mechanisms of action. Initially introduced to reduce the use of opioids and avoid their adverse side effects, multimodal pain management in fact provides better pain control.[6] Commonly used drugs in multimodal pain management include opioids, nonopioids, and a variety of adjuvant analgesics that target different parts of the PNS and CNS pain pathways. Advantages include improved analgesia due to synergistic or additive effects between the agents, reduced doses of each analgesic, and decreased incidence and severity of side effects.[6] Although developed as a framework for the management of cancer-related pain, the World Health Organization's (WHO) three-step analgesic ladder provides guidance for the management of acute pain (**Figure 32.13** ■).[7]

1. In the first step of the ladder, the pain is initially managed with nonopioids such as nonsteroidal anti-inflammatory drugs (NSAIDs) (e.g., ibuprofen, naproxen, ketorolac), COX-2 selective inhibitor (celecoxib), acetaminophen, and aspirin. Adjuvant medications, including steroids, anxiolytics, antidepressants, hypnotics, and anticonvulsants, are administered to treat related signs and symptoms of the trauma or disease.
2. In the second step, a weak opioid such as codeine, dihydrocodeine, or tramadol is added to the nonopioid with or without adjuvant medications.
3. For persistent or escalating pain, the addition of a strong opioid such as morphine is included in the third step. Other opioid options include fentanyl, buprenorphine oxymorphone, oxycodone, hydromorphone, and methadone.

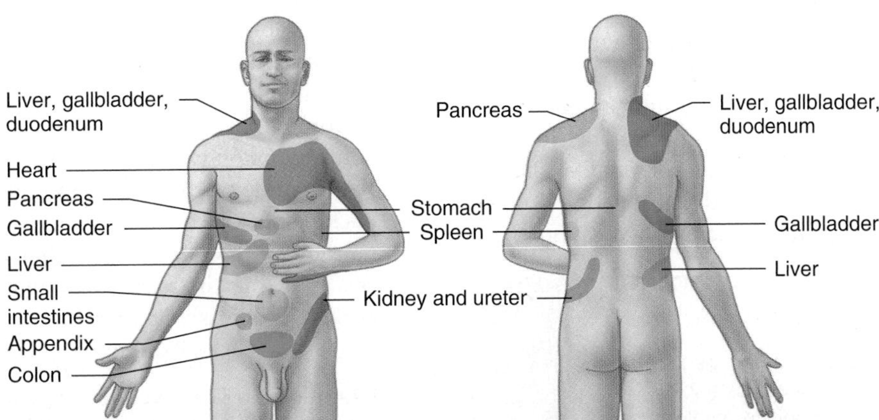

Figure 32.12 ■ Referred pain is the result of the convergence of sensory nerves from certain areas of the body before they enter the brain for interpretation. For example, a toothache may be felt in the ear, pain from inflammation of the diaphragm may be felt in the shoulder, and pain from ischemia of the heart muscle (angina) may be felt in the left arm.

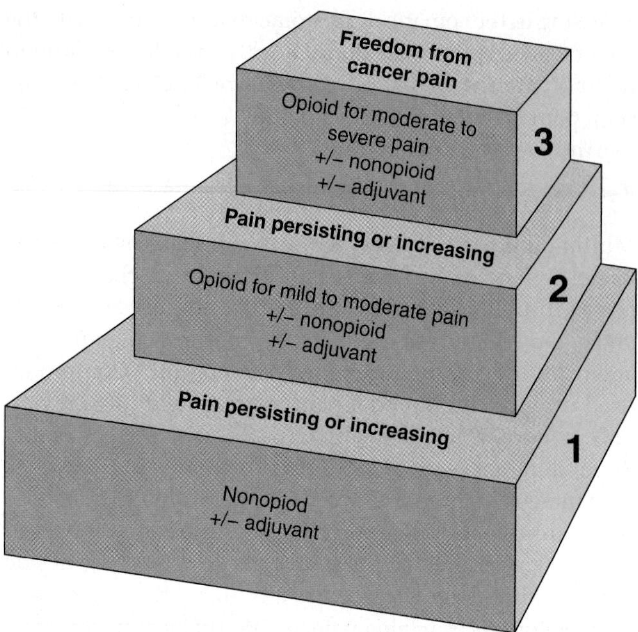

Figure 32.13 ■ The WHO three-step analgesic ladder.

Because acute pain can be intense, its initial management usually starts at the third step of the WHO ladder with gradual movement down the ladder during the recovery phase. To maintain a pain-free state, the WHO recommends that medications be administered around the clock, usually every 3–6 hours rather than on demand.[7] According to the WHO, administration of the right dose of the right drug at the right time is economical and provides effective pain relief in 80–90% of patients.[7] Patient-controlled analgesia (PCA) is an intravenous system that allows patients to press a button and administer their own pain medication. PCA provides more effective pain relief than intermittent nurse-administered intermittent intravenous or intramuscular medication and is associated with increased patient satisfaction.[8]

Breakthrough pain is characterized as a sudden and temporary increase in the severity of pain over and above a preexisting baseline pain level in a patient with an established stable analgesic regimen. Breakthrough pain may occur with increased physical activity but can also occur randomly and suddenly without warning. The duration is short, but several episodes can occur in one day. Breakthrough pain should be treated with short-acting opioids along with continuation of longer-acting medications.

Chelsea Collins: Outcome

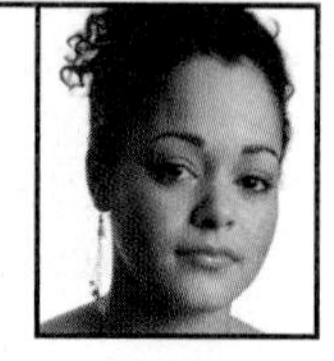

Ms. Collins is presenting with acute visceral abdominal pain. On the basis of her history, the pain suggests gastritis, a condition involving inflammation of the stomach lining. Such acute abdominal pain can be related to medication or substance consumption along with the eating of infected foods. The inflammation of the stomach lining causes pressure on nerve fibers, resulting in pain. Verification of the diagnosis would involve imaging of the abdomen, collection of blood samples to evaluate organ function and assess for the presence of bacteria, and an analysis of cardiovascular function to rule out potential cardiac etiology. Collecting a detailed dietary history over the 24- to 48-hour period before symptom development can aid in identifying potential causes.

Treatment would focus on the underlying condition and use of therapies to reduce acid levels in the stomach. Antacids, proton pump inhibitors, and histamine receptor blocking agents would all be considered as part of first-line treatment. In cases of such abdominal pain, opioids would be avoided because of the suppressing effects this class of medication can have on gastrointestinal function.

5. Why is the exact source of visceral pain often difficult to pinpoint?
6. What are common causes of visceral pain?

Check Your Progress: Section 32.4

1. What are the advantages of multimodal pain management?
2. Describe the management of pain in the first step of the three-step analgesic ladder.
3. What type of pain scheduling is most effective in relieving pain?

32.5 Chronic Pain

Chronic pain is defined as any pain that lasts longer than 12 weeks or longer than expected for healing to take place. According to the Institute of Medicine, approximately 100 million adults in the United States suffer from chronic pain at an annual national cost of $560 billion to 635 billion.[9] Although it may initially be associated with an injury or disease, chronic pain does not serve to warn of an actual or potential health threat. Many times, there is no clear cause for the pain.

CLINICAL POINT: Chronic pain is frequently accompanied by fatigue, insomnia, disturbed sleep patterns, decreased appetite, reduced muscle flexibility and strength, immobility, and depression. ■

Chronic pain has three main categories:

- Chronic recurrent pain is characterized by repeated and intense episodes of pain separated by pain-free periods. A common example of chronic recurrent pain is migraine headaches.
- Chronic intractable benign pain is characterized by continuous pain but with varying levels of intensity. An example of chronic benign pain is continuing low back pain.
- Chronic progressive pain is characterized by continuous pain that increases in intensity. An example of chronic progressive pain is cancer pain that worsens as the disease nears its terminal phase.

Chronic pain is a severe biological condition with profound emotional and cognitive effects. It is affected by a variety of biological, behavioral, environmental, and societal factors. Its onset, severity, duration, and response to treatment vary among patients, making it difficult to find a specific treatment plan. Because of its associated emotional, psychologic, and physical effects, chronic pain is best managed by an interdisciplinary team that includes primary care physicians, pain specialists, advanced practice nurses, physical therapists, psychologists, and dietitians.[10] The goal of chronic pain management is pain reduction, not pain elimination, and improved quality of life. The WHO pain ladder is appropriate for the management of chronic pain (see Figure 32.13). In contrast to acute pain, management of chronic pain starts at the first step and advances slowly up the ladder. Breakthrough pain can occur randomly and suddenly; it needs to be treated with shorter-acting opioids while longer-acting medications continue to be used for the chronic pain. For chronic or escalating unrelieved pain, a fourth step of the WHO analgesic ladder adds interventional treatments, which include nerve blocks, spinal and epidural local anesthetics, opioids, alpha-2 agonists, TENS, SCS, deep brain stimulation, radiofrequency ablation, or chemical neurolysis.

Chronic neuropathic pain is covered in the next section.

Pam Allen: Outcome

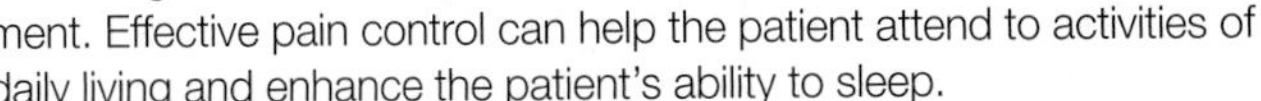

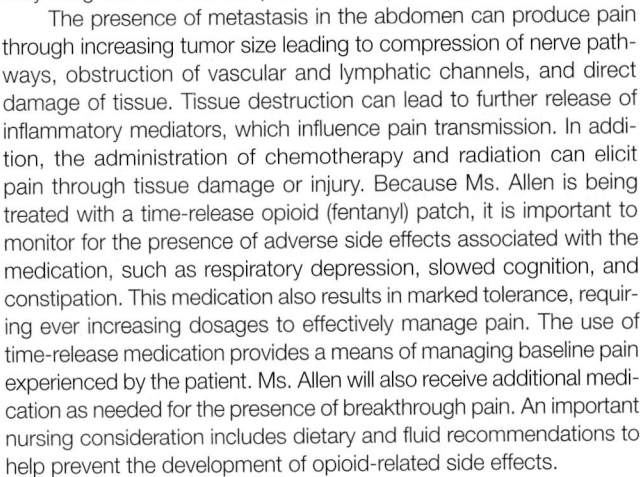

Ms. Allen's referral to a hospice provider indicates the her cancer is not curable. The focus of hospice is on enhancing the quality of the patient's remaining life, which may include pain management. Effective pain control can help the patient attend to activities of daily living and enhance the patient's ability to sleep.

The presence of metastasis in the abdomen can produce pain through increasing tumor size leading to compression of nerve pathways, obstruction of vascular and lymphatic channels, and direct damage of tissue. Tissue destruction can lead to further release of inflammatory mediators, which influence pain transmission. In addition, the administration of chemotherapy and radiation can elicit pain through tissue damage or injury. Because Ms. Allen is being treated with a time-release opioid (fentanyl) patch, it is important to monitor for the presence of adverse side effects associated with the medication, such as respiratory depression, slowed cognition, and constipation. This medication also results in marked tolerance, requiring ever increasing dosages to effectively manage pain. The use of time-release medication provides a means of managing baseline pain experienced by the patient. Ms. Allen will also receive additional medication as needed for the presence of breakthrough pain. An important nursing consideration includes dietary and fluid recommendations to help prevent the development of opioid-related side effects.

5. How can Ms. Allen's breakthrough pain best be managed?
6. Identify members of the interdisciplinary team needed to best manage Ms. Allen's cancer pain.

Check Your Progress: Section 32.5

1. Compare the three types of chronic pain.
2. Describe the fourth step of the WHO analgesic ladder used in the treatment of chronic pain.
3. Define chronic pain.

32.6 Neuropathic Pain

Neuritis is inflammation of a nerve. **Neuralgia** is pain that follows the distribution of a nerve. **Radiculopathy** refers to pain or the loss of sensory and/or motor function as a result of impaired conduction block in a spinal nerve or its roots. **Neuropathy** is a disease or disorder of the PNS and/or CNS. Peripheral neuropathies include motor, sensory, and autonomic fiber lesions or dysfunction. Central neuropathies are a result of injury, stroke, disease, or congenital conditions in the brain and/or spinal cord. An estimated 20 million people in the United States have a **peripheral neuropathy** (constant or intermittent burning, aching, or lancinating limb pain due to lesions or dysfunction of peripheral nerves).

Etiology and Pathogenesis

Neuropathies can occur in a large number of unrelated conditions. These include traumatic injuries or surgical procedures that partially or completely sever, crush, compress, or stretch a peripheral nerve; repetitive stress that leads to nerve entrapment; metabolic and endocrine disorders including diabetes, hypothyroidism, and acromegaly; autoimmune diseases including Sjögren syndrome, lupus, rheumatoid arthritis, Guillain-Barré syndrome, and chronic inflammatory demyelinating polyneuropathy; chemotherapeutic agents and radiation; viral and bacterial infections by the herpes varicella zoster virus, Epstein-Barr virus, West Nile virus, cytomegalovirus, human immunodeficiency virus (HIV), and the bacterium *Borrelia burgdorferi*; nutritional deficiencies including vitamin B12 thiamine, and folate; heavy alcohol consumption; and environmental exposure to lead, mercury, or arsenic.

Neuropathic pain is a pathologic disorder that occurs without obvious tissue injury or disease and serves no protective biological function. It can also be protracted pain that persists for months or years after an initial tissue injury or surgical procedure. A disease in itself, neuropathic pain is due to a lesion or disease of the somatosensory nervous system. The pathophysiology is complex; the damage or dysfunction in the PNS and/or CNS can be a result of trauma, ischemia, infection, or metabolic abnormalities.

Clinical Manifestations

Symptoms include **paresthesias**, which are described as a numbness, tingling, or pricking sensation. Allodynia occurs when an area of the body becomes abnormally sensitive and pain results from an innocuous stimulus such as light touch. Allodynia is associated with sensitization of peripheral nociceptors in the skin resulting in hyperalgesia. Descriptors of neuropathic pain include burning, electric shock, shooting, numbness, and severe throbbing. It can occur spontaneously or be trigged by a nonnoxious stimulus. Other sensory features of neuropathic pain include the following:

- *Hypoalgesia:* Diminished pain response to a normally painful tactile and/or thermal stimulus
- *Dysesthesia:* Unpleasant sensation
- *Hyperesthesia:* Increased sensitivity to tactile or thermal stimulation
- *Hypoesthesia:* Decreased sensitivity to tactile or thermal stimulation.

Neuroplasticity in the PNS and CNS is characteristic of neuropathic pain. Lesions or damage of the primary sensory neurons result in an increased number of abnormal sodium channels that are capable of spontaneous or ectopic depolarization. The ectopic activity causes generation of spontaneous pain with recruitment of immediate neighboring noninjured neurons. When a peripheral nerve is damaged, there is a loss of sensory input to the dorsal horn, which can lead to central changes. In the dorsal horn, upregulation of excitatory neurotransmitters such as glutamate and/or downregulation of inhibitory neurotransmitters such as GABA can result in increased neurotransmission. For example, increased glutamate in the dorsal horn is associated with destruction of the inhibitory interneurons, responsible for inhibiting transmission between first- and second-order neurons. Repetitive input to the dorsal horn from C fibers acting on NMDA receptors results in **wind-up**, in which the second-order neurons are sensitized and remain activated long after the input from the C fiber has ceased. Release of inflammatory cytokines from central glial cells may also play a role in neuropathic pain.[1] Some neuropathic pain syndromes are sensitive to stimulation of the SNS. Following a nerve injury, there is an increased growth of alpha-adrenoreceptors on nociceptors that have an exaggerated response to both systemic catecholamines and norepinephrine released from postganglionic sympathetic terminals. Sympathetically mediated pain syndrome is associated with vasomotor and **sudomotor** changes in the area innervated by the damaged nerve. In addition, sympathetic nerves (B fibers) can spout into the dorsal horn laminae that are normally occupied by Aδ and C fibers and activate ascending pain tracts.

Linking Pathophysiology to Diagnosis and Treatment

Neuropathic pain is a result of a complex interaction of genetic, physiologic, and psychologic factors that affect the transduction, transmission, modulation, and perception of a noxious stimulus. Consequently, a multidisciplinary pain management team that includes physicians, nurses, mental health professionals, physical therapists, dietitians, and social workers is considered the gold standard.[10]

Neuropathic pain is often difficult to control and responds poorly to opioids. Antidepressants and anticonvulsant medications tend to be the most effective medications for neuropathic pain.[11] These include tricyclic antidepressants (TCAs), which inhibit the reuptake of norepinephrine and serotonin, and serotonin-norepinephrine reuptake inhibitors (SNRIs). The efficacy of these medications is independent of their antidepressant effects and related to their modulation of descending inhibitory activity in the dorsal horn.

Anticonvulsants such as pregabalin and gabapentin stabilize peripheral sodium channels and reduce ectopic activity and ephaptic crosstalk between adjacent fibers. **Ephaptic crosstalk** is the depolarization of a demyelinated neuron from electrical potentials that jump from adjacent nerve fibers. They also stabilize central calcium channels and decrease the release of excitatory neurotransmitters. Second-line therapy includes tramadol, a weak opioid that also inhibits central norepinephrine reuptake. Cannabinoids such as tetrahydrocannabinol and cannabidiol are effective in refractory neuropathic pain with allodynia. Topical medications such as lidocaine (a local anesthetic that stabilizes sodium channels and reduces ectopic depolarizations), capsaicin (a member of the vanilloid family that binds to the vanilloid receptor subtype 1 on Aδ and C nociceptors and inhibits nociception for an extended period of time), and botulinum toxin type may be useful for focal muscle hyperactivity.[11] Acupuncture, massage, and herbal medications may also be effective in the treatment of some neuropathic pain syndromes. Surgical intervention should be considered only for compression or entrapment neuropathies such as carpal tunnel syndrome of the wrist. Neuropathic pain syndromes include diabetic peripheral neuropathy, phantom limb pain, trigeminal neuralgia, postherpetic neuralgia, and complex regional pain syndrome.

Diabetic Peripheral Neuropathy

Diabetic peripheral neuropathy (DPN), the most frequent form of peripheral neuropathy, is a common complication of diabetes characterized by a progressive loss of nerve fibers in both the autonomic and peripheral nervous systems. Approximately 60–70% of people with diabetes have some form of neuropathy.[12] Diabetic neuropathy is associated with 50–75% of nontraumatic limb amputations. Sensorimotor neuropathy or distal symmetric polyneuropathy is the most common type of DPN, affecting approximately 50% of people with diabetes.[13–15] Although diabetic neuropathy commonly results in paresthesia, it manifests as pain in 7.5–25% of diabetic patients.

Etiology and Pathogenesis

Diabetic neuropathy is a microvascular complication of diabetes caused by high blood glucose and decreased blood flow. It is characterized by the progressive loss of nerve fibers due to ischemia of nerve trunks, nociceptor sensitization, and damage to the Aδ and C fibers. Centrally, wind-up of the WDR neurons in lamina V results in central sensitization and expansion of the receptive field and allodynia. The incidence of diabetic neuropathy can be drastically reduced by good glucose control of vascular risk factors, hyperlipidemia, hypertriglyceridemia, and hypertension[15]

Clinical Manifestations

Pain and paresthesia are usually symmetric and start in the feet with gradual progression up the legs, followed by involvement of the fingers, hands, and arms.[14] A dying-back pattern is characteristic of DPN and classically progresses in a symmetric stocking–glove pattern. It is characterized by sharp, burning, aching, and tingling pain; cold sensations; numbness; and allodynia.[15,16] Associated clinical findings include vasomotor changes such as pallor, cyanosis, and mottling. The pain of DPN is more severe at night, and motor manifestations appear as the disease progresses.

Linking Pathophysiology to Diagnosis and Treatment

The most effective medications for treating DPN are the TCAs, which inhibit the reuptake of norepinephrine and serotonin. Decreased reuptake of serotonin and norepinephrine in the descending tracts inhibits the transmission of pain impulse. Anticonvulsants bind to the calcium channel and prevent release of excitatory neurotransmitters in the dorsal horn; pregabalin is approved by the FDA for DPN. Dextromethorphan, an NMDA antagonist, may also be effective in blocking the action of excitatory neurotransmitters in the dorsal horn. Mexiletine, an oral analog of lidocaine, exerts an analgesic effect through stabilization of sodium channels in peripheral nerves. Capsaicin cream or spray may also be effective, but several weeks of use may be required for it to exert a therapeutic effect. Although they are not a first-line treatment, opioids continue to be prescribed for over 50% of patient with DPN.[17] For DPN pain that is unresponsive to antidepressants and anticonvulsants, opioids such as tramadol, a weak opioid analgesic with serotonergic properties, or controlled-release oxycodone may be necessary for refractory pain. Because of their negative effect on the kidney, NSAIDs should be used with caution in diabetic patients who have impaired renal function.

Percutaneous electrical nerve stimulation, using acupuncture-like needles in the affected extremity, is effective in some patients. Use of a TENS unit activates cutaneous sensory fibers and increases the release of inhibitory neurotransmitters in the dorsal horn.[18] For refractory DPN pain, SCS electrodes in the epidural space stimulate Aß fibers in the dorsal column and cause orthodromic (conduction in the normal direction) supraspinal stimulation and antidromic (conduction in the opposite direction) spinal or segmental stimulation.[19] Hyperexcitability of dorsal horn WDR neurons is suppressed with SCS; it may also increase levels of GABA and serotonin and decrease release of glutamate and aspartate. Paresthesia, painless tingling or numbness, skin crawling, or itching is associated with SCS.[20]

Phantom Limb Pain

Loss of a limb can result in stump pain, phantom sensations, telescoping, or phantom pain. **Stump pain** is acute nociceptive pain at the site of amputation that generally resolves as the stump heals. **Phantom sensations**, feelings other than pain in the missing body part, include sensations of movement, numbness, or twitching. **Telescoping** is the sensation that the distal part of the missing limb is gradually approaching the limb stump. **Phantom limb pain (PLP)** is pain that is perceived to be coming from a limb or body part that has been removed or amputated. Most commonly associated with limb amputations, it can also occur after surgical removal of other body parts, such as the breast, penis, rectum, eye, and tongue. The incidence of PLP in people with amputations ranges from 42.2% to 78.8%.[21] Over 1.6 million individuals in the United States have lost a limb, usually as a result of trauma or surgical amputation for diabetes, cancer, or chronic vascular disease.[22,23] The number of traumatic amputations of more than one limb has increased since the start of the Iraq and Afghanistan wars. Risk factors for PLP include female gender, upper extremity amputations, bilateral lower limb amputations, presence of pain in the limb before amputation, persistent pain in the remaining portion of the limb or stump, anxiety, and depression.

Etiology and Pathogenesis

Like other neuropathic pains, PLP does not have a protective function and is related to both PNS and CNS dysfunction. Peripheral and central neuroplasticity, that is, dynamic changes in the neural pathways and synapses secondary to the amputation, is responsible for PLP. In the periphery, surgical or traumatic loss of a limb induces retrograde degeneration of afferent neurons and peripheral sensitization, resulting in a lower threshold for activation of nociceptors. Neuromas may sprout in the stump that have an increased sensitivity to mechanical and chemical stimuli, resulting in abnormal spontaneous ectopic discharges.[24] The DRG may also be a source of new ectopic activity and increasing afferent input to the dorsal horn. Peripheral nerve injury can lead to the degeneration of C fibers in the dorsal horn of the spinal cord. In the dorsal horn, Aß fibers (low-threshold mechanoreceptors), which normally synapse in lamina III, branch into laminae I and II, where thermal or tactile stimuli are perceived as high-intensity noxious stimuli (hyperalgesia). There may also be a reduction in the number and/or activity of the inhibitory interneurons in the dorsal horn. Maladaptive cortical plasticity induced by loss of input from the missing limb may also be the source of the PLP.[25] Almost all patients with amputations experience cortical remapping. When the area of the sensory cortex associated with the amputated limb no longer receives sensory information from the limb, the sensory cortex is remapped to associate with another area of the body; stimulation of the second area is perceived as phantom pain. Magnetic resonance imaging (MRI) and positron emission tomography of the brain areas associated with the missing limb show activity during acute PLP.

Clinical Manifestations

The onset of PLP is rapid, occurring in the first few days after the body part is amputated. However, in some patients, onset of PLP may be delayed for months or years. The pain is described as shooting, stabbing, squeezing, throbbing, or burning and often affects the part of the limb farthest from the body, such as the foot of an amputated leg. The duration of symptoms is unpredictable, resolving in months in some people and persisting for decades in others. If the PLP persists for longer than 6 months, the prognosis for improvement is poor.

Linking Pathophysiology to Diagnosis and Treatment

The most successful pharmacologic treatments for PLP include TCAs, anticonvulsants, and local anesthetics.[26] The TCAs exert a central analgesic effect through inhibition of serotonin and norepinephrine reuptake; the SNRIs, such as duloxetine, and selective serotonin reuptake inhibitors, such as fluoxetine, have shown mixed results in the treatment of PLP. The anticonvulsants, especially gabapentin have demonstrated efficacy in the management of PLP. Sodium channels blockers, that is, local anesthetics such as lidocaine, and NMDA receptors blockers such as ketamine appear to be more effective if administered before or shortly after the amputation. Acetaminophen and NSAIDs can decrease nociception in both the PNS and the CNS. Opioids can also be used for the treatment of PLP and may be beneficial in reducing cortical remapping. Tramadol, a weak opioid agonist, also blocks the reuptake of norepinephrine and serotonin.

The area of the brain involved in PLP, the posterior parietal cortex, is located on the side opposite that of the amputated limb. With transcranial magnetic stimulation, an external electromagnetic coil on the scalp delivers electric currents that decrease activity in this area and reduce PLP with long-lasting analgesic effects. The delivery of electrical current through TENS produces analgesia through activation of large-diameter afferent fibers. Once hyperalgesia has developed, TENS is effective when applied to either the contralateral or the ipsilateral limb.[18]

In mirror box therapy, a form of visual feedback therapy, the patient watches the movement of the intact limb in a mirror placed between the patient's arms or legs and perceives the phantom limb as moving in a similar manner (**Figure 32.14** ■). Mirror neurons in the brain are activated and enable sensations of touch or movement in the phantom limb. The perception of movement in the phantom limb modulates the sensory input and blocks perception of PLP. Neuroimaging studies have shown correlations between cortical reorganization following mirror box therapy and self-reported patient pain scores.[23,24]

Other noninvasive interventions for treatment of PLP include acupuncture, hypnosis, and biofeedback. Myoelectric prosthetics, artificial limbs that are controlled with electrical signals generated by the patient's muscle contractions, are associated with decreased cortical remapping and decreased PLP.[24] Motor cortex stimulation is effective in over 50% of patients with PLP. Upper limb PLP responds better to motor cortex stimulation, owing to the large representation of the upper limbs on the motor cortex.[24] With SCS, electrodes are placed in the epidural space corresponding to the source of the PLP. Surgical revision for stump pain is indicated only when localized pathology is identified. A reduced incidence of PLP is associated with the use of postoperative nerve blocks following limb amputation.[21]

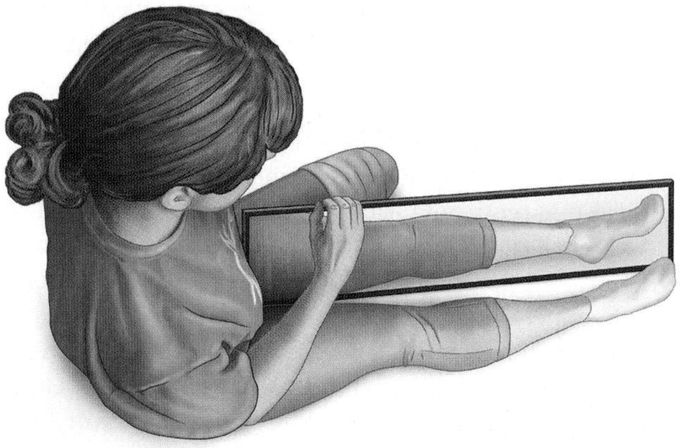

Figure 32.14 ■ Mirror box therapy for phantom limb pain.

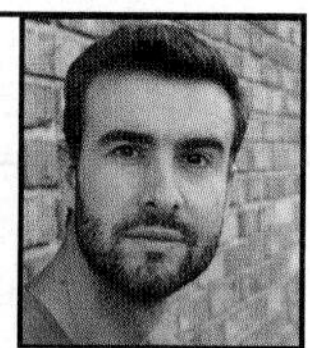

Eduardo Torres: Outcome

Mr. Torres is experiencing phantom limb pain (PLP). The presence of pain in the stump area can trigger the experience of PLP through several potential pathways. The regeneration of injured peripheral nerves can lead to the development of neuromas, which are highly sensitive to mechanical stimuli. Therefore, movement or manipulation of the stump area may trigger the development of PLP. Also, the loss of a limb leads to a process of spatial reorganization in the central nervous system. This lack of tactile and other input from the area of the missing extremity triggers the development of pain in the cerebral cortex. Use of a mirror box may be of benefit for this patient because visual feedback can help to compensate for the lack of sensory input from the missing extremity.

Treatment of PLP relies less on opioid and other standard pharmacologic approaches. Instead, tricyclic antidepressants and anticonvulsant medications such as gabapentin can be effective in managing PLP. It is possible that over time, the severity and frequency of pain associated with a missing extremity may fade, leading to a decrease in the use of therapies.

5. Describe the difference between phantom sensations and phantom limb pain.
6. Describe the process of cortical remapping in a patient with a missing limb.

Trigeminal Neuralgia

Trigeminal neuralgia (TN), formerly known as tic douloureux, is a severe chronic pain syndrome that affects the trigeminal nerve. The trigeminal nerve, the fifth and largest cranial nerve, has three branches. The ophthalmic branch (V1) supplies sensation to the scalp, forehead, and front of the head; the maxillary branch (V2) supplies sensation to the cheek, upper jaw, top lip, teeth, and gums; and the mandibular branch (V3) supplies both sensory and motor innervation to the lower jaw, teeth and gums, and bottom lip. More than one nerve branch can be affected by the disorder. The incidence is higher in females and rarely seen before the age of 40 years.[27,28]

Etiology and Pathogenesis

The pathophysiology of TN involves segmental demyelination of trigeminal sensory fibers in the nerve root or the brainstem. In most patients with TN, the demyelination is due to chronic compression of the nerve root at or near its exit from the pons by vascular abnormalities or tumors.[27,28] In approximately 85% of patients with TN, the trigeminal root is compressed by a loop of artery or vein as it exits the brainstem, usually the superior cerebellar artery.[28] Compression of the nerve root leads to segmental demyelination and ephaptic communication from nearby sensory fibers where neuronal impulses "jump" from one nerve to another without a neurochemical synapse. Ephaptic crosstalk between the demyelinated trigeminal nerve and nearby sensory nerves results in stimulation of the trigeminal nerve.[28] The damaged fibers also generate impulses automatically at ectopic pacemaker sites on the demyelinated

Impact of Current Research on Clinical Practice

Internet-Delivered Self-Help for Chronic Pain

Description: Interest in internet-based strategies for managing disease has increased greatly over the past several years. In a study of 69 adolescents with chronic pain, a guided internet-based intervention was used in an attempt to aid these patients. A cognitive–behavioral therapy intervention was delivered through a series of internet-based modules. There was a significant amount of attrition during the study, indicating that providing such therapies only over the internet can be difficult. The study did show that the intervention produced a reduction in pain behaviors and improved sleep while improving quality of life.

Clinical Practice: The use of alternative therapies such as guided imagery, breathing techniques, and cognitive–behavioral therapies are common strategies used in the management of pain. These strategies attempt to reframe the thought process of individuals with chronic pain to improve their awareness of coping strategies and bodily sensations. By making the patient more aware of positive coping strategies, pain control can be improved. Also, such strategies decrease sympathetic stimulation, which mediates pain perceptions and transmission. Through such influence, pain management is thought to be more effective. While there were problems keeping patients involved in this study, it demonstrated that internet-based technologies may be a helpful addition in the management of pain.

Research Study:

Voerman, J. S., Remerie, S., Westendorp, T., Timman, R., Busschbach, J., Passchier, J., & de Klerk, C. (2015). Effects of a guided internet-delivered self-help intervention for adolescents with chronic pain. *Journal of Pain, 6*(11), 1115–1126. doi:10.1016/j.jpain.2015.07.011

sections. Ectopic pacemakers also demonstrate aftercharge, prolonged spontaneous firing when triggered by an external stimulus. Demyelination of nerves that occurs with multiple sclerosis may also be responsible for TN. The diagnosis of TN is based on history, identification of pain triggers, and lack of neurologic findings. An MRI may demonstrate vascular compression of the nerve root.[27]

Clinical Manifestations

With TN, extreme, sudden burning or shocklike paroxysms of facial pain occur spontaneously or in response to nonnoxious tactile stimulation of a trigger point on the face or the mouth or motor activities such as chewing, speaking, yawning, eating, or brushing the teeth.[28] The pain is unilateral, typically affecting the V2 and V3 branches.[27] TN can last from a few seconds to as long as 2 minutes per episode, and attacks can occur in quick succession for up to 2 hours.

Linking Pathophysiology to Diagnosis and Treatment

Anticonvulsants are the primary medication used to treat TN although lamictil is also used. Carbamazepine, the drug of choice, blocks sodium channels, inhibits spontaneous generation of ectopic nerve impulses and reduces the transmissions of ephaptic impulses. Other anticonvulsants may be used if the side effects of carbamazepine cannot be tolerated; these include oxcarbazepine, topiramate, gabapentin, pregabalin, clonazepam, phenytoin, lamotrigine, and valproic acid.[27,28] Baclofen, a GABA agonist that blocks the excitation of second-order neurons, may also be effective.

Surgical interventions for TN include microvascular decompressions of the trigeminal nerve root and trigeminal nerve ablation. Microvascular decompression, especially of the superior cerebellar artery, can provide long-term pain relief and is not associated with sensory loss to the face. Open trigeminal rhizotomy involves partial resection of the trigeminal nerve just past its exit from the pons; it is most effective for V3 compression but is associated with some degree of permanent facial numbness.[28] Ablative procedures, radiofrequency, and chemical rhizolysis are less effective for long-term relief of TN and are associated with major sensory loss and motor weakness.[28] Gamma knife stereotactic radiosurgery targets the nerve root as it exits the pons and destroys the fibers responsible for the pain. Anesthesia dolorosa is a deafferentiation pain caused by damage to the trigeminal nerve. It can occur after surgery and is characterized by numbness and constant, severe burning pain. It is treated with TCA with varying success.

Postherpetic Neuralgia

According to the Centers for Disease Control and Prevention (CDC), an estimated 1 million individuals in the United States develop herpes zoster, commonly known as shingles, each year, and 30% of individuals will develop herpes zoster, commonly known as shingles, in their lifetime.[29] **Herpes zoster (HZ)** is caused by the varicella zoster virus (VZV); initial VZV infection usually occurs in childhood and causes varicella (chicken pox). Over 95% of the world's population has the VZV, and 50% of them will develop HZ by the age of 85 years.[30] Those aged 60 years and older have a higher risk of developing HZ, and the CDC recommends that this population receive the vaccine for shingles (Zostavax) even if they had chickenpox as a child.[29] **Postherpetic neuralgia (PHN)** is a painful peripheral neuralgia that is a sequela of HZ infection. In patients with PHN, the pain associated with the initial HZ infection continues past 1 month.

Etiology and Pathogenesis

Following the initial VZV infection, cell-mediated immunity prevents reactivation of the virus, and it lies dormant in the DRG. The VZV is reactivated when the immune system is suppressed by aging or disease. The reactivated virus travels anterograde to the skin to cause zoster and retrograde to the CNS to produce meningoencephalitis, myelitis, and stroke.[30,31]

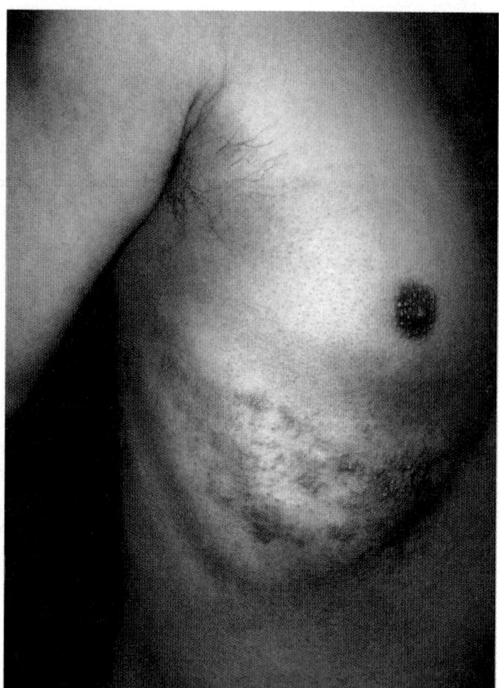

Figure 32.15 ■ An outbreak of shingles on the torso.

Clinical Manifestations and Treatment of Herpes Zoster

Acute HZ causes a painful unilateral rash with vesicular eruptions in one or more dermatomes corresponding to the DRG that is harboring the VZV (**Figure 32.15** ■). The thoracic dermatomes innervated by the T_1–L_2 ganglia and the ophthalmic branch of the trigeminal nerve (V1) are most frequently affected. Before the rash appears, pain, itching, or tingling may be present in the area where the rash will develop; headache and fever frequently accompany the rash. The HZ vesicles typically dry up in 7–10 days and clear within 2–4 weeks.

Antiviral medications, including acyclovir, valacyclovir, and famciclovir, administered within 72 hours of vesicular eruption can shorten the duration and severity of HZ. Acetaminophen, aspirin, NSAIDs, or tramadol may be used to control the pain of acute HZ. Corticosteroids may be beneficial in combination with antivirals in patients over age 50 years who have moderate to severe pain. Sympathetic blocks are effective for pain relief if administered within 2 weeks of the first symptoms.

Clinical Manifestations and Treatment of Postherpetic Neuralgia

PHN is described as a burning, itching pain with periods of lancinating pain (pain with piercing or stabbing sensations). The risk of PHN increases with age; 80% of PHN occurs after the age of 50 years.[30] Individuals with compromised immune systems and those taking immunosuppressive medications are at increased risk for development of PHN. The pathophysiology of PHN is complex and includes hyperesthesia and allodynia in the affected dermatomes. There is increased spontaneous activity of peripheral and central nociceptors, destruction of large myelinated fibers associated with modulation of nociceptive stimuli in the dorsal horn, and reorganization of central connections, all of which contribute to the hyperalgesia of PHN. Allodynia is caused by formation of new connections involving central pain transmission neurons.

There is no reliable predictor of the progression from HZ to PHN. The TCAs are the most frequently used medication for PHN. Their blockade of serotonin and norepinephrine reuptake in the CNS effectively inhibits nociception transmission. Anticonvulsants such as gabapentin and pregabalin appear to be effective and have been approved by the FDA for treatment of PHN.[32,33] Capsaicin cream and lidocaine patches are also approved by the FDA for PHN.[33] Baclofen, a GABA derivative may be effective for cases refractory to TCAs. Most analgesics, including opioids, are ineffective in PHN. Intercostal nerve blocks may be beneficial for thoracic PHN. Sympathetic nerve blocks are usually unsuccessful unless performed early. Neurolytic blocks may be considered for refractory severe PHN.

Complex Regional Pain Syndrome

Complex regional pain syndrome (CRPS) is a neuropathic pain disorder that affects one of the upper or lower limbs after an injury or trauma and is associated with significant dysfunction of both the PNS and CNS.

Etiology and Pathogenesis

Two types of CRPS have been identified.[34] Type I (CRPS-I), formerly called *reflex sympathetic dystrophy*, occurs without detectable nerve trauma but is frequently associated with an initiating limb trauma, including fracture, sprain, laceration, soft tissue injury, limb immobilization, burn, and surgery. Intra-articular fractures and ankle fractures and dislocations appear to be risk factors for CRPS.[34] A seemingly innocuous event such as vaccination may be the cause of a later CRPS.[35] Type II (CRPS-II), formerly called *causalgia*, is associated with injury to major peripheral nerves, such as a high-velocity injury to a large nerve from a gunshot. It most frequently affects the brachial plexus, median nerve, and tibial division of the sciatic nerve. Ninety percent of patients have a history of trauma to the extremity. Differential diagnosis of the remaining 10% includes arthritic syndromes, Lyme disease, muscle diseases, vascular disorders, or peripheral polyneuropathies. The highest incidence of CRPS occurs in females and individuals over the age of 40 years. CRPS is rare under the age of 10 years.

The pathophysiology of CRPS is complex and multifactorial. It is hypothesized that the traumatic injury damages the myelin layer of peripheral nerves and allows ephaptic crosstalk from adjacent nerve fibers. Persistent sensory input from low-threshold Aβ mechanoreceptors and polymodal C fibers causes WDR sensitization in the dorsal horn, resulting in hyperalgesia. Abnormal proliferation of Aβ fibers into lamina II in the dorsal horn results in a painful perception of nonnoxious stimuli such as light touch or pressure or temperature change. There is an increase in the number of adrenergic receptors on Aδ and C fibers distant from the site of nerve injury, and the nerve becomes sensitive to circulating catecholamines. The sympathetically maintained pain component of CRPS is supported clinically by the presence of abnormal skin temperature, skin color, and sweating in the affected limb. The pain of CRPS is exacerbated by increased sympathetic tone, including stimuli that initiate a sympathetic response, such as a sudden loud noise or flash of light and increased anxiety.

Clinical Manifestations

Only the distal extremities are affected by CRPS, irrespective of the location of the nerve trauma.[36] The constellation of nonspecific symptoms of CRPS can delay a timely diagnosis of the disease. Both types of CRPS cause allodynia. The pain can be severe and may spread to involve the entire limb, resulting in widespread muscle hyperalgesia.[37] Typically, patients with CRPS-I will seek treatment 4–8 weeks after the limb trauma; patients with severe pain in the first week are at heightened risk of the disease. Symptoms of CRPS-II have an immediate onset after the nerve injury and include severe burning, crushing, or stabbing pain.[36] Associated symptoms of CRPS include constant or intermittent temperature changes in blood flow as evidenced by skin color, edema of the affected limb, abnormal sudomotor activity in the painful region, and tropic changes in the hair and nails. Bones undergo excess resorption, resulting in osteopenia and osteoporosis. Patients with CRPS exhibit neglect-like symptoms, in which they must concentrate on the affected limb to use it.[36] The perception of body symmetry is impaired in the dark, and the affected limb is perceived as larger. This abnormal sensory perception is attributed to cortical remapping similar to that which occurs with PLP.[36] Anxiety, depression, and reduced physical activity can accompany CRPS and contribute to a reduced quality of life.[38]

CRPS symptoms vary in severity and duration. Both types require the exclusion of any other condition that might account for the pain and dysfunction. A history of trauma or surgery, physical examination, and the response to sympathetic nerve block can help to confirm the diagnosis. Most cases are mild, and individuals recover gradually with time. In more severe cases, the individual may not recover and may have long-term disability.

Linking Pathophysiology to Diagnosis and Treatment

Treatment of CRPS is multimodal with an emphasis on early diagnosis and treatment and a focus on functional restoration of the sensory motor cortex. A positive response to a sympathetic block, as evidenced by a reduction in pain and improvement in motor function, temperature, and color of the limb, confirms the diagnosis of CRPS. The presence of allodynia and hypoesthesia is associated with a poor response to sympathetic blocks.[39] Several medications have been shown to be effective in CRPS, especially if used early in the disease. These include NSAIDs such as ibuprofen and naproxen; corticosteroids such as prednisolone and methylprednisolone; anticonvulsants such as gabapentin and pregabalin; antidepressants such as amitriptyline, nortriptyline, and duloxetine; botulinum toxin injections; NMDA receptor antagonists such as dextromethorphan and ketamine; nasal calcitonin, especially for deep bone pain; and topical medications, including lidocaine and capsaicin. Intrathecal baclofen, a presynaptic and postsynaptic GABA agonist, possesses analgesic properties; it appears to be effective early in the disease.[40] Opioids are considered second- or third-line agents. Methadone, because of its antagonism of the NMDA receptor, may have advantages over other opioids.[41]

A peripheral nerve block is indicated for pain related to a single peripheral nerve; sympathetic blocks are necessary for trauma to a nerve trunk. Sympathetic blocks with antiarrhythmic agents and local anesthetics are 90% successful if initiated early. For upper extremities, a cervicothoracic sympathetic block of the stellate ganglion is performed at C6 or C7 For lower extremities, a block of the lumbar sympathetic chain is performed at L2. The blocks are continued until symptoms are minimal or there is no further progression of benefit. Mirror box therapy is also effective in restoring the physiologic brain circuits of the somatosensory cortex by teaching the brain that the limb where pain is being felt is actually pain free (see Figure 32.14). Physical therapy is necessary to improve blood flow and lessen the circulatory symptoms of the disorder. In addition, improved strength and flexibility of the affected limb may prevent or reverse changes in the CNS, including cortical remapping. A TENS unit may be necessary for patients with refractory pain; SCS is effective for lower limb CRPS. In advanced cases, a surgical sympathectomy may be the only option for relief of SMP pain.

Check Your Progress: Section 32.6

1. Describe the classic pattern of pain in diabetic peripheral neuropathy (DPN).
2. How does mirror box therapy reduce phantom limb pain PLP?
3. Identify the cranial nerve affected by trigeminal neuralgia, its branches, and their distribution pattern.

32.7 Headache

Headache, a pain in the head, scalp, or neck, is the most common form of pain. In the United States, headache is the fifth leading cause of visits to the emergency department; 1.2% of outpatient visits are due to headaches.[42] A chronic daily headache is a general term for frequent headaches of long duration, usually 4 hours or more. The most common types of headaches are tension type headaches, migraine headaches, and cluster headaches.[42,43]

Tension Type Headache

The most common type of headache is **tension type headache (TTH)**, a pericranial myofascial pain. It is estimated that 30–80% of adults in the United States suffer from TTH once or twice a month, while 3% suffer from chronic daily TTH. There is an increased incidence of TTH in females.

Etiology and Pathogenesis

The pain of TTH is caused by excessive contraction, ischemia, and inflammation of neck and scalp muscles. The increased muscle tension may be exacerbated by emotional stress, inadequate rest, and poor posture. Pain tolerance is decreased in individuals with chronic TTH. They also have a generalized hyperalgesia, possibly due to central sensitization of second- or third-order neurons or decreased supraspinal inhibition of the dorsal horn.[44]

Clinical Manifestations

Tension type headaches are characterized by a constant, bilateral, dull, nonthrobbing bandlike pain around the head, especially at the temples or the back of the head and neck. Episodic TTH occurs fewer than 15 days per month and can last from 30 minutes to several days. Episodic TTH usually begins gradually and often occurs in the middle of the day. Chronic TTH is a daily or continuous headache with variable pain intensity throughout the day.

Linking Pathophysiology to Diagnosis and Treatment

Episodic TTH usually responds to aspirin, acetaminophen, or NSAIDs. However, excessive or daily use of these medications can cause an analgesic rebound headache. A TCA such as amitriptyline is often effective in the management of chronic TTH and associated with reduced severity and frequency. Other preventive and treatment interventions for chronic TTH include stress management, counseling, and biofeedback.

Migraine Headache

The word *migraine* is derived from the Greek *hemikrania*, meaning "half of the cranium." **Migraine headache (MH)** is a chronic, complex neurovascular disorder characterized by episodic exacerbations of unilateral throbbing head pain and a number of associated neurologic symptoms. An estimated 16% of the world's population, including over 35 million individuals in the United States, suffer from MH.[45,46] In the United States, migraine headaches are associated with an annual expense of $4.275 billion for outpatient costs, emergency department visits, and inpatient hospitalizations.[46–48] Approximately 75% of migraine sufferers are female, and migraines account for 64% of severe headaches in females. Migraines occur in both adults and children.

The peak incidence of MH occurs at 5 years of age in males and at 12–13 years of age in females. The peak incidence of MH without aura peaks at 10–11 years of age in males and at 14–17 years of age in females. ■

Migraine frequency and severity decrease after the age of 40 years except in perimenopausal females. There is a strong genetic component to migraines, as is evidenced by twin studies and population-based studies, which reveal a 70% increased incidence in first-degree relatives.[44,49]

Etiology and Pathogenesis

Migraine headaches were historically thought to be vascular in origin and caused by cerebral vasoconstriction followed by a period of rebound vasodilation. The current neurovascular theory of MHs describes a complex pathophysiology that is neurogenic in nature with secondary changes in cerebral perfusion. MH is a primary complex, genetic disorder that involves an altered brain excitability that activates the trigeminalovascular system.[45,50] Cerebral cortex hyperexcitability, especially in the occipital cortex, has been demonstrated on MRIs of individuals with MH. Cortical spreading depression, a wave of neuronal excitation, spreads across the cortical gray matter at a rate of 3–5 mm/min followed by a suppression of neuronal activity that can last several minutes.[44] Fibers from the trigeminal nerve innervate cerebral vessels, and the cortical spreading depression waves activate the trigeminal nociceptors in the affected hemisphere, stimulating them to release pain-producing peptides, including CGRP, substance P, VIP, and neurokinin A. Activation of the trigeminalovascular system also results in cerebral vasodilation. This pattern of cortical spreading depression has been speculated to be the mechanism underlying the presence of aura in migraine headache.[44] An **aura** is a change in perception that may precede the development of migraine. The aura may develop in any sense modality (vision, olfactory, or auditory).

MH also involves peripheral and central sensitization, a reduction in pain threshold, and an increase in responsiveness of the peripheral and central afferent neurons involved in the transduction and transmission of pain.[50] Peripheral sensitization of first-order trigeminal neurons is responsible for the throbbing unilateral pain.[51] Sensitization of second- and third-order neurons is responsible for the cutaneous allodynia that accompanies MH. The majority of patients have cephalic allodynia, scalp pain, and tenderness that is aggravated by brushing or washing their hair or lying supine. Scalp allodynia is ipsilateral to the headache and within the receptive field of the trigeminal nerve; it is attributed to sensitization of second-order neurons. Extracephalic cutaneous allodynia involves the upper and lower extremities; truncal allodynia is less common. It is believed that extracephalic allodynia and hyperalgesia are mediated by sensitized third-order thalamic neurons that process nociceptive information from the cranial meninges and sensory information from the skin of the body and limbs. Most patients can identify several factors that can trigger MH. These include dietary triggers such as alcohol; caffeine; chocolate; aspartame; monosodium glutamate (MSG); peanuts; and tyramine, which is found in aged cheese, smoked or cured meats, nuts, and wine vinegars. MH can also be triggered by hormonal changes during menstruation; environmental factors such as bright lights, odors, and altitudes; and physical activities such as sexual intercourse and sports.[52] There is even a positive correlation between the incidence of MH and environmental factors such as high temperature and low humidity.[53] Increased psychologic stress, sudden feelings of anxiety or happiness, and a change in sleep patterns have also been associated with acute onset of MH.

Clinical Manifestations

Patients with MH can present with any of the following symptoms: a throbbing or pulsatile unilateral headache (frontal or ocular) that lasts anywhere from 4 to 72 hours, nausea and vomiting, and sensitivity to light (photophobia) and sound (phonophobia). In many patients, the headache is preceded by premonitory or prodromic symptoms that last less than 24 hours. These include fatigue, excessive yawning, fluid retention, sensory hypersensitivity, mood changes, and increased appetite and thirst. Over 30% of migraines are accompanied by an **aura**, a reversible focal neurologic symptom that generally precedes the headache.[45] It is a result of cortical spreading depression and gradually develops over 10–20 minutes, lasting less than 60 minutes. There is usually a short latent period between the aura and the onset of the headache. The most common aura is a defect in the visual field, either a partial loss of vision or a blind spot. Sensory auras, the second most common type of aura, occur in 40% of patients and include unilateral paresthesia and numbness of the face and limbs. Motor auras, feelings of heaviness in the limbs and speech disturbances, occur in 18% of patients and usually accompany sensory auras. Patients also complain of cranial or cervical muscle tenderness and overall muscle weakness (hemiplegic migraine). Postdromal symptoms can be present for up to 24 hours after the headache and include muscle weakness of pain, irritability, euphoria, or extreme fatigue.

Linking Pathophysiology to Diagnosis and Treatment

According to the International Headache Society, diagnostic criteria for MH include five or more headaches lasting 4–72 hours with at least two of the following characteristics:

- Unilateral location
- Pulsatile nature
- Moderate to severe pain
- Aggravation by physical activity
- Accompanied by nausea and/or vomiting or photophobia and phonophobia.[54]

Neuroimaging studies are not necessary in patients who meet the diagnostic criteria for MH, but they may be performed for a differential diagnosis of other conditions that can cause severe headache, including cerebral aneurysms, intracranial hemorrhage, space-occupying lesions, cerebral venous thrombosis, meningitis, congenital cerebral defects such as Chiari malformation, or carbon monoxide poisoning.

Treatment of MH is twofold and includes prophylactic and acute abortive therapy. Prophylactic therapy to reduce the frequency, severity, or duration of acute migraine headaches is indicated for the following conditions: MH that occurs more than twice monthly, headaches that last longer than 24 hours, and overuse or ineffective use of abortive medications. Preventive drugs include anticonvulsants (topiramate and valproic acid), tricyclic antidepressants (amitriptyline nortriptyline), and antihypertensives (beta blockers, propranolol, timolol). The 5-HT2 antagonist methyseride is also used for prevention of migraine. Botulinum toxin A injections to the scalp and temple can be used in patients who do not respond to at least three preventive medications. A TENS device for prophylactic stimulation of the trigeminal nerve can be used for 20 minutes a day on the forehead and over the ears.

In addition to rest in a dark, quite room, the choice of abortive medications for MH depends on the severity of the pain and associated symptoms. For mild to moderate pain, analgesics alone or in combination with other compounds may be effective if administered within 15 minutes of the onset of pain. These include acetaminophen, NSAIDs, and narcotics such as oxycodone. For severe pain, the use of triptans and ergot alkaloids are indicated; opioids and dopamine antagonists such as prochlorperazine may also be necessary for severe headache. Triptans are the most commonly ordered medication for treatment of MH, accounting for approximately 80% of prescriptions. Triptans are selective serotonin agonists, acting at the 5-hydroxytryptamine 1B/1D/1F receptors of cerebral blood vessels. They can be administered orally, nasally, subcutaneously, or intramuscular; a sumatriptan transdermal patch received FDA approval in 2013. These are most effective when applied early in the attack before allodynia gets established, and can be repeated once in 2 hours. Longer-acting triptans, such as frovatriptan and naratriptan, may be used for several days for management of a menstrual-related MH. Combined products, such as Treximet, contain a triptan and an NSAID. Ergot alkaloids are nonselective 5-HT1 receptor agonists; they include ergotamine and dihydroergotamine. Both drugs are also alpha-adrenergic and dopaminergic antagonists. To prevent development of a rebound headache, abortive medications should be limited to 2–3 days per week. Status migrainosus, an attack lasting longer than 72 hours and unresponsive to triptans, frequently requires emergency care that includes intravenous valproate or dihydroergotamine and narcotics. Current studies with subcutaneous botulinum toxin reveal that it inhibits peripheral release of CGRP, glutamate, and substance P, primarily reducing peripheral sensitization that in turn reduces central sensitization.[50]

Nonpharmacologic therapy includes the use of transcranial magnetic stimulation (TMS), which was approved by the FDA in 2013 for use in adults. In TMS, a pulse of magnetic energy is applied to the occipital cortex. TMS can be used once daily after the onset of pain. Surgical avulsion of the zygomaticotemporal branch of the trigeminal nerve is associated with a reduction in the frequency, duration, and severity of MH.[46]

Cluster Headache

A **cluster headache (CH)** is a unilateral severe pain with associated with ipsilateral cranial autonomic symptoms. Although they are the least common of all headaches, cluster headaches are among the most painful. They can occur at any age but are most common in adolescence and middle age; 80% occur in males.

Etiology and Pathogenesis

The exact cause of CH is unknown. Because blood vessel dilation follows the pain and does not precede it, the cause of CH is believed to originate in the brain. The abnormalities may lie in the hypothalamus, the part of the brain that regulates the biologic or circadian rhythms of the body. The trigeminal nerve, the chief sensory nerve of the face, is also

Impact of Nutrition in Clinical Practice

Migraine Headaches and Nutritional Factors

Joanne Kouba

Identification and avoidance of precipitating factors constitute the ideal prevention for migraine headaches. Migraine sufferers often examine environmental exposures, including food and dietary components, as triggers for their headaches. While the concept seems simple, the evaluation of this relationship is not, resulting in limited, evidence-based recommendations.

The usual suspects as food triggers of MH include processed, fermented, pickled, and marinated foods. These are often high in MSG, histamine (seafood), tyramine (aged cheese, red wine, smoked fish), and nitrates (salami, bacon).[1] In a review of 45 articles on the topic, Rockett and colleagues evaluated the link between migraines and 30 potential dietary triggers; the results were inconclusive, owing to a lack of high-quality studies.[2] Study limitations included likely reporting bias, retrospective nature resulting in questionable recall regarding timing of food intake and the onset of migraines, and small sample size. However, frequently reported dietary triggers were noted. Few clinical trials with control groups have been conducted related to this topic.

Fasting or skipping meals was the most commonly reported and most significant dietary factor linked to migraines, with a reported frequency of 40–82%. Inadequate fluid intake, independent of meals and fasting, was found to be associated with increased frequency of migraine reports in three of the four studies reviewed. Participants in one intervention study reported resolution of headache after early ingestion of fluids.[2]

Extremes of body mass index are associated with migraine chronicity and/or severity. For obese individuals, this may be mediated through the inflammatory and prothrombotic states.[1] The direction of the association is not completely understood, and it may operate in both directions. The inflammatory neuropeptides orexin A and B are involved in regulation of food metabolism and pain with antinociceptive (antipain) properties. Migraine headaches may reduce orexin and impair hypothalamic function, pain modulation, and physical activity, resulting in weight gain with augmented inflammatory activity. A cycle of sedentary behavior, weight gain and a heightened pro-inflammatory response for the migraine sufferer can be compounded by medication adverse effects.

As major components of vascular, immune cell, myelin and neuronal cell membranes, omega-6 and omega-3 fatty acids are involved in pain-related pathways.[3] In the three studies in Rockett and colleagues' review that evaluated lipid intake, all reported an association between fatty or oily foods and migraines.[2] In another clinical trial with 67 individuals who suffered from chronic daily migraine headaches, Ramsden and colleagues tested two 12-week, food-based interventions based on lipid intake.[3] The high omega-3/low omega-6 diet was hypothesized to improve headache outcomes as a result of antinociceptive properties and improved metabolism of omega-3 eicosapentaenoic and docosahexaenoic fatty acids. The other group received a low omega-6 diet. Linoleic and arachidonic, which are omega-6 fatty acids, are considered to be pronociceptive and contribute to the pathogenesis of headaches. Study participants in the high omega-3/low omega-6 intervention experienced greater improvements in migraine headache impact score, headache days per month, and headache hours per day than did the low omega-6 group. In addition, greater increases in antinociceptive biochemical markers were noted with the high omega-3/low omega-6 group. Alterations in lipid profile show promise in headache management.

A frequency of about 30% was reported in regard to the link between alcohol (including red wine) and migraines, though reports were inconsistent and mixed. There may be an interaction between alcohol and some other foods, such as cheese, chocolate, and citrus fruit, that increases alcohol's potential as a migraine trigger.[2] Many of us have experienced the temporary "brain freeze" that comes with a large gulp of a frozen beverage or quickly eating a frozen dessert. However, the data conflict as to whether this is a migraine-precipitating factor beyond the typical and temporary cold-induced headache. Citrus fruits, milk, cheese, and chocolate have all been evaluated in these studies with low frequencies and/or inconsistent reports of association.[2]

Additional trials are underway to evaluate the effectiveness of weight management and lipid alternations.[1,3] Prudent advice for migraine sufferers related to diet should encourage a healthy body, a consistent meal pattern with adequate fluids, reducing intake of foods that are high in pro-inflammatory omega-6 fatty acids (e.g., processed lunch meats and peanut butter), encouraging foods high in omega-3 fatty acids (e.g., flaxseed and salmon), and being mindful of individual dietary triggers.[1,2,3]

References

1. Finkel, A. G., Yerry, J. A., & Mann, D. (2013). Dietary considerations in migraine management: Does a consistent diet improve migraine? *Current Pain and Headache Reports, 17*, 373–380.

2. Rockett, F. C., Oliveira, V. R., Casto, K., Chaves, M. L. F., Perla, A., & Perry, I. D. S. (2012) Dietary aspects of migraine trigger factors. *Nutrition Reviews, 70*(6), 337–356.

3. Ramsden, C. E., Faurot, K. R., Zamora, D., Suchindran, C. M., MacIntosh, B. A., Gaylord, S., Ringel, A., Hibbeln, J. R., Feldstein, A. R., Mori, T. A., Baden, A., Lynch, C., Coble, R., Mas, E., Palsson, O., Barrow, D. A., & Mann, J. D. (2013). Targeted alteration of dietary n-3 and n-6 fatty acids for the treatment of chronic headaches: A randomized trial. *Pain, 154*, 2441–2451.

involved, as it is responsible for eye pain associated with CH. The trigeminal nerve also stimulates the parasympathetic autonomic system, which is responsible for the eye tearing and redness and nasal congestion.

Clinical Manifestations

Cluster headaches generally last 15 minutes to 3 hours and can occur several times a day. The great majority of patients with CH have episodic headaches that occur regularly for 1 week up to 1 year, separated by long pain-free periods. Between 10% and 20% of patients with CH have chronic, continuous headaches. Triggers for CH include alcohol, cigarette smoke, hot weather, high altitudes, bright light, physical exertion, and foods that are high in nitrites. Symptoms of CH include a sudden onset of a severe unilateral pain that is piercing or burning in nature and located behind or around the eye. The pain is strongest in the first 10–15 minutes and spreads to the forehead, jaw, upper teeth, temples, nostrils, shoulder, or neck. Associated ipsilateral symptoms include excessive tearing of the eye, a swollen or droopy eyelid, pupillary constriction, nasal congestion, forehead or facial sweating, and agitation. Cluster headaches have a circadian pattern and tend to occur at the same time of day, usually in the early evening and early morning, with a peak between midnight and 3:00 a.m. Patients can experience one to eight attacks per day during a 6- to 12-week cluster cycle with remissions lasting up to 1 year.

Linking Pathophysiology to Diagnosis and Treatment

Treatment of an acute CH includes subcutaneous or nasal triptans, dihydroergotamine, and 100% oxygen. Occipital nerve blocks with a local anesthetic and a corticosteroid may also be beneficial. Preventive measures include avoidance of known triggers and administration of antidepressants, anticonvulsants, intranasal capsaicin or lidocaine, or verapamil.[55,56]

Check Your Progress: Section 32.7

1. Explain the pathophysiology of pain in tension type headaches.
2. What dietary guidelines may be given to reduce or avoid migraine headaches?
3. List common triggers for cluster headaches.

32.8 Other Pain Syndromes

There are a number of other pain syndromes associated with numerous disease states and conditions. The manifestation of pain is the primary symptoms across these syndromes that are tied to insult or injury to the central nervous system or muscles of the face.

Central Pain Syndrome

Central pain syndrome (CPS) is a result of damage to or dysfunction of the CNS, including the brain, brainstem, and spinal cord. Causes include cerebral vascular accidents (stroke), brain and spinal cord tumors, epilepsy, multiple sclerosis, CNS infections, aneurysms, Parkinson disease, and head and spinal cord trauma. The pain may begin shortly after the injury or may be delayed for months, especially after a stroke. The intensity and location of pain depend on the CNS injury. The pain can be referred to any part of the body but is most severe in the feet and hands. The pain is constant; moderate to severe in intensity; and aggravated by movement, touch, temperature change (especially cold), emotions, and stress. It is frequently described as burning and accompanied by a "pins and needles" sensation. Sensory loss may also occur in the areas affected by the pain. Thalamic pain is an example of CPS; it occurs after a stroke in the lateroposterior thalamus, and symptoms include contralateral intracranial pain and sensory loss. Severe facial pain without sensory loss may also occur.[51] In addition to opioids, treatment for CPS includes tricyclic antidepressants such as nortriptyline and anticonvulsants such as gabapentin. Deep brain stimulation of the periventricular gray matter, the periaqueductal gray matter, and/or the sensory thalamus may be necessary for CPS that is refractory to pharmacologic interventions. Use of deep brain stimulation is associated with increased secretion of endogenous opioids and the inhibitory neurotransmitter GABA. Motor cortex stimulation is an alternative and less invasive treatment. It is associated with intracortical GABA release, reduction of the thalamic hyperactivity, and increased release of endogenous opioids.

Myofascial Pain Syndrome

Myofascial pain syndrome is a regional pain syndrome characterized by discrete trigger point localized areas of deep muscle tenderness or hyperirritability and a pattern of referred pain that may be localized or remote from the trigger point. The onset is heralded by an acute muscle injury that results in sustained or repeated muscle contractions. There is an inadequate blood flow for the level of contraction; the resulting depletion of adenosine triphosphate, which is necessary for muscle relaxation, causes the muscle to remain taut and rigid. Local release of prostaglandins, bradykinin, and serotonin causes increased activation of nociceptors. Central sensitization results in hyperalgesia, allodynia, and referred pain. Symptoms of myofascial pain include a taut or hard muscle band, a twitch or local contraction of muscle band on stimulation, restricted range of motion, and referred pain. Palpation of the taut muscle reproduces pain. The most common trigger point is on the upper scapula with radiation to the occiput, shoulder, medial arm, and anterior chest wall. Trigger points of the piriformis muscle, which overlies the sciatic nerve, produces sciatic irritation, which can mimic S_1 radiculopathy.

Treatment of myofascial pain includes NSAIDs, muscle relaxants, and physical therapy for trigger point compression or stretch. Topical vapocoolants, such as ethyl chloride, and injection of local anesthetics or botulinum cause a reflex muscle relaxation. Dry needling, the introduction of a needle without solution into the muscle band, and acupuncture are also effective in relieving the spasm. Persistent myofascial pain may require the use of TENS.

Fibromyalgia

Fibromyalgia (FM) is the most common cause of widespread musculoskeletal pain, with an incidence of 1–5%, including more than 6 million patients in the United States; it is 3–4 times more common in females.[57,58] Pain sensitivity in females is affected by the menstrual cycle. FM usually starts in middle adulthood but can occur in teens and adolescents.[59] There is also an increased incidence of obesity and insulin resistance in patients with FM. An idiopathic functional disorder, FM is characterized by chronic widespread pain lasting longer than 3 months, nonrestorative sleep patterns, fatigue, and cognitive impairment. Neuroendocrine abnormalities, including decreased secretion of cortisol, growth hormone, and thyroid hormone, can be seen with FM. Some component of the pain appears to be sympathetically mediated and sensitive to catecholamines.[60]

Unlike the specific regional trigger points of myofascial pain, FM is associated with widespread areas of tenderness distributed symmetrically on the trunk and proximal limbs. Eighteen symmetric tender points (nine pairs) have been identified that are sensitive to tactile stimulation, although there is no evidence of gross muscle pathology. They include the neck, back, chest, elbows, hips, buttocks, and knees (**Figure 32.16**). Current research supports the involvement of central sensitization in FM, including wind-up of the NMDA receptor in the dorsal horn and sensitization of the sensory cortex.[61] Other central pain or inflammatory disorders associated with FM include ulcerative colitis, irritable bowel syndrome, migraine headache, temporomandibular disorder, vulvodynia, restless leg syndrome, chronic pelvic pain, and myofascial pain syndrome.[58,60,61] These comorbidities may share a common etiology, a result of viscerosomatic convergence in the dorsal horn or thalamus. A genetic component cannot be ruled out; patients with FM may have abnormal nociceptive pathways that predispose them to chronic pain syndromes. There is an eightfold risk of FM in first-degree relatives.[58] Symptoms of FM are exacerbated by physical or emotional trauma, and stress.

The diagnosis of FM is one of exclusion; there are no laboratory or imaging tests for the disorder. However, studies have demonstrated increased cortical activity in key pain-processing areas of the brain in patients with FM in response to painful and nonpainful thermal stimuli.[62,63] Diagnostic criteria include a 3-month duration of widespread pain, presence and severity of pain in 7 of the 18 trigger points, fatigue, and absence of other disorders that could explain the pain.

The FDA has approved three drugs for the treatment of FM: two serotonin–norepinephrine reuptake inhibitors (duloxetine and milnacipran) and one anticonvulsant (pregabalin). Tricyclic antidepressants may also be effective. Acetaminophen and NSAIDs are effective for acute pain flare-ups. Tramadol, a weak opioid, is effective because it also inhibits the reuptake of norepinephrine and serotonin. Intravenous ketamine can be used as a diagnostic test to identify patients who may benefit from an oral NMDA receptor antagonist such as dextromethorphan. Sodium oxybate (a precursor of GABA, the main central inhibitory neurotransmitter), which the FDA has approved as a drug for narcolepsy and excessive daytime sleepiness, may also be effective s in FM.[63]

Although the use of opioids is not recommended in FM, approximately 80% of patients with FM receive opioid therapy. Opioid-induced hyperalgesia, a result of central sensitization primarily due to a reduction of a nociceptive threshold in the ascending pathways, can cause greater pain sensitivity. Opioid-induced hyperalgesia presents as persistent pain in response to opioid administration; the intensity of the pain increases with increasing doses of opioids and continues with ongoing opioid administration.[58] Physical therapy and exercise can improve a number of the symptoms of FM, including disrupted sleep patterns and mental and physical fatigue.[60,61,63] Cognitive–behavioral therapy is also associated with decreased FM pain.[63] Acupuncture, biofeedback, and chiropractic and massage therapy may be beneficial for some patients.

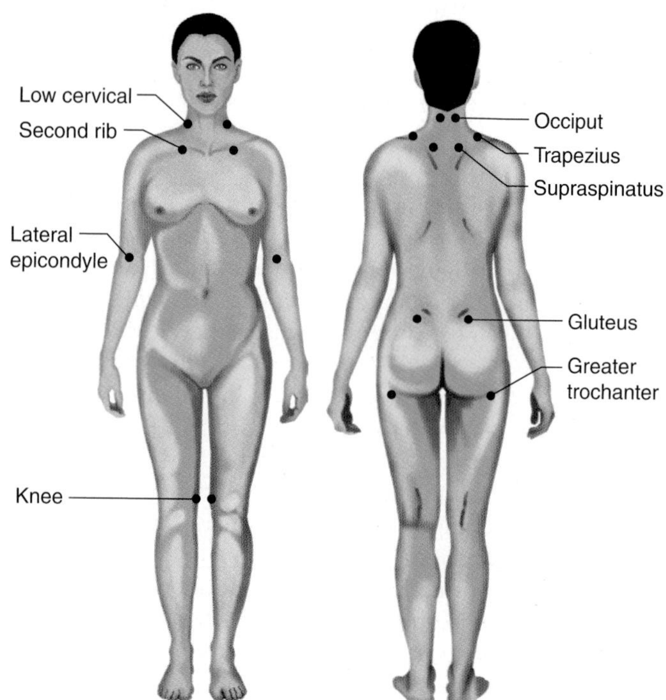

Figure 32.16 The locations of 18 paired tender points in fibromyalgia.

Psychogenic Pain

Psychogenic pain is an older term that describes both short- and long-term episodes of pain that occur as the result of some underlying psychologic disorder, rather than a response to an immediate physical injury. Historically attributed to psychologic factors, psychogenic pain is now believed to be due to CNS dysfunction and is influenced by psychologic factors. Symptoms are vague and include headache, muscle pain, and gastrointestinal distress. For example, nonspecific (or psychogenic) chest pain syndrome commonly occurs in individuals under the age of 50. These patients typically experience symptoms that include chest wall pain as well as radiating arm and neck pain. Although some patients mistake these symptoms as the early warning signs of a heart attack, in most cases, chest pain syndrome arises from an underlying anxiety and/or panic disorder. Treatment options for psychogenic pain include antidepressants, nonopioid analgesics, and psychotherapy.

Persistent Postsurgical Pain

Persistent postsurgical pain (PPSP) is defined as pain that persists more for than 2 months after a surgical procedure and cannot be attributed to other causes. Over 40 million people undergo surgery annually in the United States.[64] PPSP is underdiagnosed, but it is estimated to affect 10–50% of the surgical population. In relatively minor surgical procedures, such an inguinal hernia repairs, the incidence is 2–10%.[65,66] The surgical procedures that are associated with highest incidence of PPSP are amputations, thoracotomies, mastectomies, inguinal hernia repairs, coronary bypass, cesarean sections, and repeat surgeries.[64,67] Risk factors for PPSP include preoperative pain lasting longer than 1 month, repeat surgeries, female gender, and surgical approach. Severe preoperative and postoperative pain is a strong predictor of PPSP.[64] Additional risk factors include thoracic surgery in patients over 60 years of age, prolonged duration of postoperative chest tube drainage, and preexisting hypertension.[68]

Animal research has identified the importance of descending endogenous noradrenergic signaling in the prevention of PPSP.[65] Preventive strategies include the use of regional anesthesia for operative procedures and intraoperative use of NMDA receptor antagonists such as ketamine and anticonvulsants such as gabapentin. Multimodal postoperative pain management, which includes opioids, acetaminophen, NSAIDs, regional anesthesia, nerve blocks, short-term ketamine, and gabapentin, is indicated for optimum management of persistent postoperative pain.[64]

Check Your Progress: Section 32.8

1. What conditions may cause central pain syndrome?
2. How does the pain of fibromyalgia differ from myofascial pain?
3. How is fibromyalgia diagnosed?

32.9 Pain Assessment and Management in Nonverbal or Cognitively Impaired Patients

The gold standard of pain assessment is a patient's self-report; patients' pain is whatever they say it is. The majority of pain tools rely on a verbal self-report of pain, but they are inappropriate for use with nonverbal or cognitively impaired patients, including children, cognitively impaired adults, and older adults with dementia. Consequently, pain in those populations tends to be underassessed and undertreated.

Pediatric Considerations

Acute nociceptive pain in a child is a result of tissue trauma as a consequence of illness, injury, or medical procedure. Studies of neuropathic pain in infants, children, and adolescents are lacking, but neuropathic pain can occur in children as a result of a nerve injury caused by HIV infection, nerve entrapment or compression by a space-occupying lesion such as a tumor, postoperative neuroma, or traumatic or surgical limb amputation. Cancer treatments, including chemotherapy and radiation, may cause persistent neuropathic pain. Children also suffer from congenital degenerative peripheral neuropathies and inflammatory neuropathies, such as Guillain-Barré syndrome. Idiopathic pain, such as recurrent abdominal pain with no identifiable etiology, occurs in children. However, DPN, PHN, and TN are rare in children.

Untreated pediatric pain is associated with long-term physical and psychologic sequelae that can influence the child's response to future traumatic incidents or medical procedures. Long-term consequences of untreated pediatric pain include increased anxiety during medical or surgical procedures, lowering of the pain threshold and sensitization, and reduced effectiveness of analgesics. Neonates undergo a number of routine painful procedures after birth. Neonates who experience repeated painful needle punctures in the first 24 hours of life are at risk for developing hyperalgesia.[69] Classic studies of neonatal circumcision performed without anesthesia show that it is associated with a greater pain response to routine immunizations 4 and 6 months later as a result of a lowered pain threshold.[69,70] ■

Pediatric Pain Assessment

The Joint Commission requires pain assessment and management of pain in patients of all ages.[3] Pain is subjective, and self-reported VAS or NRS pain scales are not appropriate for young children who cannot communicate verbally because of their age or developmental status. Behavioral indicators of acute pediatric pain include facial expression, body movement or posture, crying, groaning, and inability to be consoled (**Figure 32.17** ■). Behaviors associated with chronic pain include abnormal posture, fear of being moved, lack of facial expression, loss of appetite, lack of interest in surroundings, sleep disturbances, undue quietness, increased irritability, and anger. Children may deny that they have pain because they fear a painful treatment such as an intramuscular injection.

There are a number of pain assessment scales for neonates and children.[71,72] Assessment scales for pain in children younger than 1 year of age include the Neonatal Infants Pain Scale (NIPS), which assesses facial expression, cry, breathing pattern, muscle state of arms and legs, and state of arousal, and the Face, Legs, Activity, Crying, Consolability (FLACC) scale. The Premature Infant Pain Profile Revised (PIPP-R) includes assessment of three facial actions of a premature infant (brow bulge, eye squeeze, and nasolabial furrow); two physiologic responses (heart rate and oxygen saturation); gestational age; and behavioral state before the painful event. The CRIES observational assessment tool for children younger than 3 years old can also be utilized for pain assessment of older developmentally disabled children. It assesses crying, oxygen requirement, increased vital signs, facial expression, and sleep. For children over the age of 3 years, the Wong-Baker FACES (see Figure 32.11) or the Bieri-Modified scale is used for pain assessment.[73] Both scales have six cartoon faces with increasing levels of stress or hurt, from no hurt to worst hurt. The VAS or NRS can be utilized for pain assessment in older children and adolescents. ■

Pediatric Pain Management

Nonpharmacologic methods of pain relief, such as oral sucrose, breastfeeding, and swaddling, are effective in reducing pain in both premature infants and neonates undergoing routine painful procedures such as heel lancing for blood samples.[69,72] The WHO recommends a two-step approach for treatment of pediatric pain.

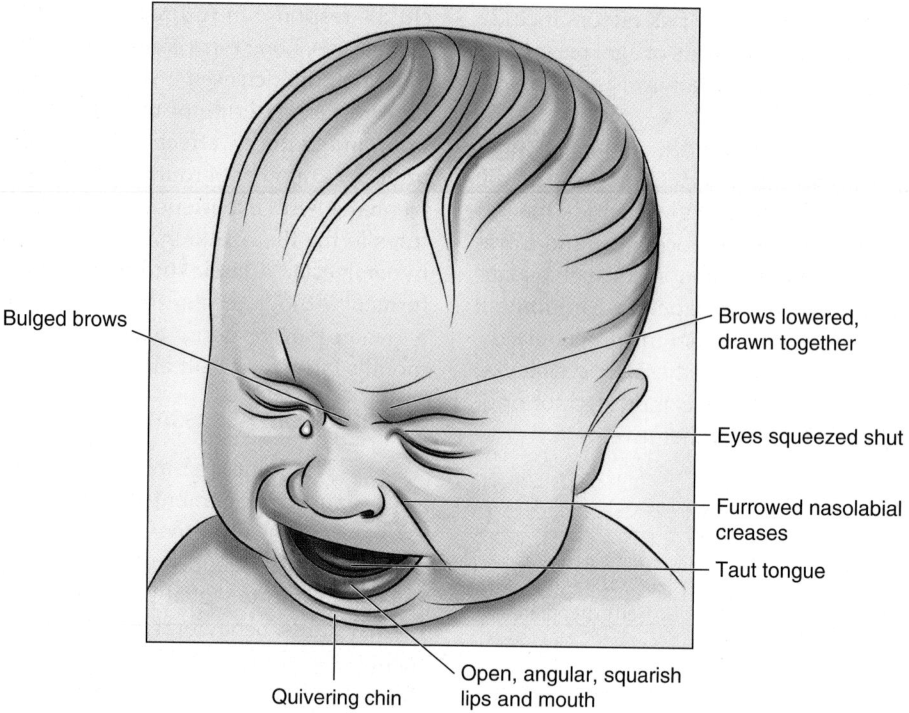

Figure 32.17 ■ Characteristic facial responses of an infant to pain include bulged brow, eyes squeezed shut, furrowed nasolabial creases, open lips, stretched mouth, taut tongue, and quivering chin.

For infants younger than 3 months of age, acetaminophen is recommended for mild to moderate pain. For infants older than 3 months of age, acetaminophen and ibuprofen are the medicines of choice.[74]

Administration of a strong opioid, preferably morphine, is indicated for the treatment of moderate to severe pain. Codeine is not recommended for control of pediatric pain. Codeine is a prodrug that is converted to an active metabolite, morphine, by the enzyme CYP2D6. Fetal CYP2D6 activity is less than 1% of adult values and less than 25% of the adult values in children below the age of 5 years. Consequently, the analgesic effect of codeine is essentially absent in neonates and young children. In addition, up to 30% of the U.S. population are poor metabolizers of codeine; the drug is ineffective in these patients. Conversely, some individuals can metabolize codeine quickly and are at risk of opioid toxicity.

Analgesic dosing must be based on the age and weight of the patient. Other considerations include health and nutrition status and concomitant administration of drugs with synergistic actions. Analgesics should be administered to children by the simplest, most effective, and least painful route; oral formulations are the most convenient and usually the least expensive route of administration. Because of associated pain, the intramuscular route of injection should be avoided.

Rectal administration has an unreliable bioavailability. The WHO recommends that analgesics be administered to pediatric patients at regular intervals with the addition of rescue doses for intermittent and breakthrough pain.[74] Intravenous patient-controlled analgesia is effective for children who can understand directions for pushing a button to take away their pain.[75] Parent- or nurse-controlled analgesia may also be an option for some patients. Regional anesthesia, spinal, epidural, and caudal blocks in combination with general anesthesia can provide significant postoperative pain relief.[75] Adjuvant medicines may be coadministered with analgesics to enhance pain relief. However, there is no evidence to support the use of antidepressants, anticonvulsants, bisphosphonates, corticosteroids, or local anesthetics for the management of neuropathic pain in children.[74] ■

Geriatric Considerations

Individuals older than 65 years of age make up the fastest-growing segment of the world's population. In the United States, older adults account for 12.8% of the population; 14% of this group are 85 years or older.[76] Older adults are more likely to experience pain, both acute and chronic, than are younger individuals, but pain in older adults tends to be undertreated. Contributing to the undertreatment of pain are the myth that pain is a normal consequence of aging, nonadherence with expensive chronic pain medications by economically challenged patients, poor memory or recall of pain triggers and response to treatment, and unacceptable adverse side effects. Older adults with moderate to severe dementia are especially vulnerable to the underassessment and undertreatment of pain. ■

Geriatric Pain Assessment

Pain assessment in older adults can be challenging. The American Geriatrics Society recommends assessment of six behavioral domains: facial expressions, verbalizations/vocalizations, body movements, interpersonal interactions, activity patterns and routines, and mental status.[66] Facial expressions are an easily observed, nonverbal behavioral indicator of pain in older adults.[77] The VAS and the NRS are appropriate pain assessment tools for older patients who have intact cognitive and verbal skills. However, some older adults report difficulty in understanding the scales. The McGill Pain Questionnaire is effective for older adults because it assesses multiple components of pain. Originally developed for use with children, the Wong-Baker FACES scale or the Bieri-Modified scale can be used for assessment of pain in older adults. Each includes six facial expressions with increasing degrees of pain. With the pain thermometer, patients identify the intensity of their pain on a diagram of a thermometer that has increasing levels of pain. Both the visual faces scales and the pain thermometer can also be used for older adults with mild to moderate cognitive impairments or verbal impairment.

The Pain Assessment Checklist for Seniors with Limited Ability to Communicate (PACSLAC), a 60-item tool, can be used for older adults who have a limited ability to communicate.[78] It includes assessment of four behaviors that may be pain-related: facial expression, activity/body movement, social/personality/mood, and physiologic changes/eating and sleeping changes/vocal behaviors. The shorter 31-item PACSLAC-II has also proven to be a reliable and valid tool for the differentiation of pain and pain-free states in older adults.[79]

Dementia is a progressive disease that includes disturbances of higher cortical functions including memory, cognition, comprehension, language, orientation, and judgment. Alzheimer disease is the most common form of dementia; other types include vascular dementia, frontotemporal dementia, and Lewy body dementia. It is estimated that 35 million people worldwide, including 5% of people over the age of 65 years, suffer from dementia.[80] Assessing pain, especially neuropathic pain, in confused patients or patients with severe dementia is difficult because they cannot reliably communicate their pain. Behaviors indicative of pain in these patients include guarding of a body part, reluctance to be moved, decreased mobility, crying or wincing when touched, insomnia, restlessness, vocalizations, irritability, and decreased appetite. The Pain Assessment in Advanced Dementia (PAINAD) is used to assess pain in older patients with dementia or other cognitive impairments.[81] Patients are observed for five behaviors: respiratory status, negative vocalization, facial expression, body language, and consolability. The total score ranges from 0 to 10 points; scores of 1–3 indicate mild pain, scores of 4–6 indicate moderate pain, and scores of 7–10 are associated with severe pain. However, atypical behavioral responses to pain have been observed in patients with Alzheimer disease. For example, patients with excessive movement and vocalization may become quiet and withdrawn when they are in pain. ■

Geriatric Pain Management

Older adults appear to have an increased pain threshold, a consequence of aging.[76] They also have increased sensitivity to most drugs because of altered pharmacokinetics, including changes in volumes of distribution and protein binding, and decreased organ function, especially the liver and kidneys, which are responsible for drug biotransformation and elimination. Older adults are also at increased risk for adverse drug effects. The WHO three-step analgesic ladder (see Figure 32.13) is appropriate for pain management in older adults.[7] Acetaminophen is the first choice for mild to moderate pain; NSAIDs may be added for uncontrolled pain. Weak opioids (codeine, hydrocodone, and oxycodone) may be used in combination with acetaminophen for moderate to severe pain, and morphine is indicated for severe refractory pain. Adjunctive drugs include antidepressants, anticonvulsants, local anesthetics, NMDA agonists, calcitonin, baclofen, and topical creams. Because of the propensity of older adults to suffer from adverse side effects, therapy with these agents should begin with the lowest possible dose and be titrated slowly to achieve the desired therapeutic effects. ■

Check Your Progress: Section 32.9

1. How is pain assessed in premature infants?
2. What is the rationale for not administering codeine to pediatric patients?
3. How is pain assessed in older adults who have a limited ability to communicate?

CHAPTER SUMMARY

32.1 Chapter Overview and Case Studies

Define pain, and discuss concepts related to pain.

- Pain is unpleasant sensory experience resulting from tissue damage.
- The sensory experience leading to pain is mediated by emotional state and in turn can heavily influence mood and affect.
- Approximately 20% of all people worldwide suffer from acute or chronic pain.
- The experience of pain can lead to strong sympathetic activation resulting in increased heart rate, a change in the force of cardiac contraction, and increased respiratory rate.

32.2 Neuroanatomy of Pain

Outline the four parts of the pain pathway, and explain the significance of pain threshold and tolerance.

- Pain can be described as nociceptive or nonnociceptive.
- Nociceptive pain is a physiologic response to heat, cold, vibration, stretch, or chemicals released from damaged cells. This response can be referred to as somatic or visceral.
- Somatic pain is an aching, throbbing, or dull pain arising from the skin, muscles, and joints that is usually discrete and intense in character.
- Visceral pain is a squeezing, cramping, dull, and deep pain originating in a bodily organ that is often poorly localized to the affected organ and commonly associated with referred patterns of pain.
- Neuropathic pain is a result of nerve cell dysfunction in the peripheral nervous system (PNS) and/or the central nervous system (CNS).
- Acute pain serves as a physiologic warning that something is wrong.
- Chronic pain may occur after resolution of an acute injury or inflammation. It is also associated with other chronic diseases such as diabetes mellitus or cancer.
- Pain transduction is the conversion of a noxious thermal, mechanical, or chemical stimulus into a nerve impulse.
- Pain transmission involves the transfer of a noxious stimulus to the CNS.
- Three types of neurons are involved in the transmission of pain: first-, second-, and third-order neurons.
- The first-order neurons serve as the communication pathway between pain receptors in the skin and tissue and the spinal cord and brainstem.
- Second-order neurons rely the nerve impulse from the spinal cord and brainstem to the thalamus.
- Third-order neurons transmit noxious impulses from the thalamus to the primary somatosensory areas of the brain, resulting in perception of pain.
- Pain modulation involves peripheral and central neurotransmitters and other substances that enhance or dampen the transduction and transmission of a noxious stimulus.
- Pain perception is a stage of cognitive awareness of a noxious stimulus.
- The pain threshold is the minimum intensity of a noxious stimulus to be perceived as painful.
- Pain tolerance is the amount of pain an individual can take or tolerate. It is affected by gender, age, culture, emotional state, and physical activity.

32.3 Assessment of Pain

Discuss the components of a throughout assessment of pain.

- Pain can be considered the fifth vital sign.
- Pain can be assessed by using the mnemonic OPQRST.
- Location of pain is often determined in respect to specific patterns.
- Somatic pain is associated with damage to the skin, soft tissues, ligaments, muscles, bones sand joints. It is an aching, throbbing, or dull pain that is well localized to the area of inflammation or trauma and is frequently associated with a traumatic event.
- Visceral pain is internal, arising from the organs or the blood vessels, which lack significant sensory innervation. Nociceptors in the viscera are stimulated by inflammation, ischemia, dilation, stretch, and spasm, and visceral pain is described as squeezing, pressure, cramping, distention, and dull. It is difficult to pinpoint the exact source of the pain; frequently the pain is referred to another, distant area of the body.
- Referred pain is a result of convergence of visceral and somatic sensory neurons in the dorsal horn. The CNS interprets the perceived pain as arising in the somatic dermatome that converges with the visceral afferents in the dorsal horn.
- Neuropathic pain is due to peripheral or central damage or dysfunction of first-order neurons and is described as burning, shooting, tingling, radiating, lancinating, or numbing.
- Radicular pain, a type of neuropathic pain, is caused by inflammation or compression of a spinal nerve root and is frequently associated with a herniated intervertebral disc and spinal stenosis.
- Vascular pain is a result of severe vasospasm, usually in response to cold and/or increased activity of the sympathetic nervous system.
- Psychogenic pain is caused by emotional or mental stress and is not associated with any somatic or visceral inflammation or trauma.
- Breakthrough pain is a transient exacerbation or flare-up of pain in an individual with continuous stable pain.
- Pain scales are based on self-report and/or observational (behavioral) or physiologic data.

32.4 Acute Pain

Differentiate the causes, classification, underlying pathogenesis, and clinical manifestations of acute pain and approaches to treatment of acute pain across the lifespan.

- Acute pain has a sudden onset and is associated with acute or potential trauma to somatic or visceral tissue.
- Somatic pain usually has a readily identifiable location with a sudden onset and is related to a specific time and activity.
- Visceral pain can have a gradual or sudden onset and is often described in vague terms such as squeezing, pressure, cramping, and distention with a dull quality.

- The exact source of visceral pain is difficult to pinpoint, as the pain is frequently referred to a distant site of the body as a result of visceral and somatic convergence.
- Multimodal pain management of acute pain includes the use of two or more agents with different mechanisms of action.
- The three-step analgesic ladder provides guidance for the management of acute pain.
- In the first step, pain is initially managed with nonopioids such as nonsteroidal anti-inflammatory drugs.
- In the second step, a weak opioid such as codeine, dihydrocodeine, or tramadol is added to the nonopioid with or without adjuvant medications.
- In the third step, a strong opioid such as morphine is included.

32.5 Chronic Pain

Differentiate the causes, classification, underlying pathogenesis, and clinical manifestations of chronic pain and approaches to treatment of chronic pain across the lifespan.

- Chronic pain is defined as any pain that lasts longer than 12 weeks or longer than expected for healing to take place.
- Chronic pain is frequently accompanied by fatigue, insomnia, disturbed sleep patterns, decreased appetite, reduced muscle flexibility and strength, immobility, and depression.
- There are three main categories of chronic pain.
- Chronic recurrent pain is characterized by repeated and intense episodes of pain separated by pain-free periods.
- Chronic intractable benign pain is characterized by continuous pain but with varying levels of intensity.
- Chronic progressive pain is characterized by continuous pain that increases in intensity.
- The goal of chronic pain management is pain reduction, not pain elimination, and improved quality of life.

32.6 Neuropathic Pain

Differentiate the causes, classification, underlying pathogenesis, and clinical manifestations of neuropathic pain and approaches to treatment of neuropathic pain.

- Neuropathic pain is a pathologic disorder that occurs without obvious tissue injury or disease and serves no protective biological function. It can also be protracted pain that persists for months or years after an initial tissue injury or surgical procedure.
- Peripheral neuropathies include motor, sensory, and autonomic fiber lesions or dysfunction. Central neuropathies are a result of injury, stroke, disease, or congenital conditions in the brain and/or spinal cord.
- Symptoms of neuropathic pain include paresthesias, described as a numbness, tingling, or pricking sensation.
- Neuroplasticity in the PNS and CNS is characteristic of neuropathic pain. Lesions or damage of the primary sensory neurons result in an increased number of abnormal sodium channels that are capable of spontaneous or ectopic depolarization. The ectopic activity causes generation of spontaneous pain with recruitment of immediate neighboring noninjured neurons.
- Repetitive input to the dorsal horn from C fibers acting on NMDA receptors results in wind-up, in which the second-order neurons are sensitized and remain activated long after the input from the C fiber has ceased.
- Neuropathic pain is often difficult to control and responds poorly to opioids. Antidepressant and anticonvulsant medications tend to be the most effective medications for neuropathic pain. These medications stabilize peripheral sodium channels and reduce ectopic activity and ephaptic crosstalk between adjacent fibers.
- Diabetic peripheral neuropathy is the most common form of peripheral neuropathy and a common complication of diabetes characterized by a progressive loss of nerve fibers in both the autonomic and peripheral nervous systems.
- Diabetic neuropathy is a microvascular complication of diabetes caused by high blood glucose and decreased blood flow. It is characterized by the progressive loss of nerve fibers due to ischemia of nerve trunks.
- Phantom limb pain is pain that is perceived to be coming from a limb or body part that has been removed or amputated.
- In the periphery, surgical or traumatic loss of a limb induces retrograde degeneration of afferent neurons and peripheral sensitization resulting in a lower threshold for activation of nociceptors. Neuromas may sprout in the stump that have an increased sensitivity to mechanical and chemical stimuli that can result in abnormal spontaneous ectopic discharges.
- When the area of the sensory cortex associated with the amputated limb no longer receives sensory information from the limb, the sensory cortex is remapped to associate with another area of the body. When the second area is stimulated, it is perceived as phantom pain.
- CRPS is hypothesized to emerge from damage to peripheral myelin allowing for ephaptic crosstalk from adjacent nerve fibers. CRPS pain is exacerbated by increased sympathetic tone, including stimuli that initiate a sympathetic response such as a sudden loud noise or flash of light and increased anxiety.

32.7 Headache

Differentiate the causes, classification, underlying pathogenesis, and clinical manifestations of headaches and approaches to treatment of headaches across the lifespan.

- Headache is the most common form of pain. The most common types of headaches are tension type headache, migraine headache, and cluster headache.
- The most common type of headache is tension type headache, which is caused by excessive contraction, ischemia, and inflammation of neck and scalp muscles.
- The increased muscle tension tied to tension headache may be exacerbated by emotional stress, inadequate rest, and poor posture.
- Individuals with chronic tension headache have a generalized hyperalgesia, possibly due to central sensitization of second- or third-order neurons or decreased supraspinal inhibition of the dorsal horn.
- Migraine headache is a chronic, complex neurovascular disorder characterized by episodic exacerbations of unilateral throbbing head pain and a number of associated neurologic symptoms.
- Migraine headaches were historically thought to be vascular in origin and caused by cerebral vasoconstriction followed by a period of rebound vasodilation.
- Migraine headache is initiated through a pattern of cerebral cortex hyperexcitability, with cortical spreading depression followed by a suppression of neuronal activity.
- Cortical spreading depression has been speculated to be the mechanism underlying the presence of aura in migraine headache.
- There is usually a triggering factor such as dietary triggers (alcohol, caffeine, chocolate, aspartame, monosodium glutamate, peanuts, and tyramine); hormonal changes during menstruation; environmental factors such as bright lights, odors, and altitudes; and physical activities such as sexual intercourse and sports.
- Treatment of migraine headache is twofold and includes prophylactic and acute abortive therapy. Prophylactic therapy to reduce the frequency, severity, or duration of acute migraine headaches is indicated for migraine headaches that occur more than twice monthly, headaches that last longer than 24 hours, and overuse or ineffective use of abortive medications.
- Triptans are selective serotonin agonists, acting at the 5-hydroxytryptamine 1B/1D/1F receptors of cerebral blood vessels, and are the most commonly ordered medication for treatment of migraine.
- A cluster headache is a unilateral severe pain with associated with ipsilateral cranial autonomic symptoms.
- The exact cause of cluster headaches is unknown but is speculated to be associated with the release of histamine in the hypothalamus.

32.8 Other Pain Syndromes

Differentiate the causes, classification, underlying pathogenesis, and clinical manifestations of selected other pain syndromes and approaches to treatment of these syndromes across the lifespan.

- Central pain syndrome (CPS) is a result of damage to or dysfunction of the CNS, including the brain, brainstem, and spinal cord.
- CPS-related pain may begin shortly after injury or be delayed for months, especially after a stroke. The intensity and location of pain depend on the CNS injury.
- Myofascial pain syndrome is a regional pain syndrome characterized by discrete trigger point localized areas of deep muscle tenderness or hyperirritability and a pattern of referred pain.
- Fibromyalgia is the most common cause of widespread musculoskeletal pain.
- An idiopathic functional disorder, fibromyalgia is characterized by chronic widespread pain lasting longer than 3 months, nonrestorative sleep patterns, fatigue, and cognitive impairment.
- Fibromyalgia is believed to be caused by central sensitization, including wind-up of the NMDA receptor in the dorsal horn and sensitization of the sensory cortex.
- Three medications are approved for the treatment of fibromyalgia: two serotonin-norepinephrine reuptake inhibitors (duloxetine and milnacipran) and one anticonvulsant (pregabalin).

32.9 Pain Assessment and Management in Nonverbal or Cognitively Impaired Patients

Compare and contrast the assessment and treatment of pain in nonverbal or cognitively impaired patients across the lifespan.

- The gold standard of pain assessment is patient self-report, but most pain tools rely on a verbal self-report and are inappropriate for use with nonverbal or cognitively impaired patients.
- Acute nociceptive pain in children is a result of tissue trauma as a consequence of illness, injury, or medical procedure.
- Untreated pediatric pain is associated with long-term physical and psychologic sequelae that can influence the child's response to future traumatic or medical procedures.
- Older adults are most likely to experience pain, both acute and chronic, but pain in this population tends to be undertreated.
- Older adults with moderate to severe dementia are especially vulnerable to the underassessment and undertreatment of pain.
- For both pediatric and geriatric populations, assessment of behavioral and physiologic pain symptomatology is important.

REVIEW QUESTIONS

1. The nurse is assessing the pain level of an older adult with dementia. Which of the following would the nurse most assess using the Pain Assessment in Advanced Dementia scale?
   a. Respiratory status, cardiovascular status, facial expression
   b. Breathing pattern, state of arousal facial expression
   c. Muscle state of arms and legs, body language, respiratory status
   d. Consolability, negative vocalization, facial expression

2. The nurse teaches the client with a history of migraine headaches that triggers may include:
   a. dim lighting.
   b. foods with tyramine.
   c. decaffeinated coffee.
   d. low temperatures.

3. A client with myocardial infarction tells the nurse that he is having pain in his left shoulder. The nurse explains that this pain is called:
   a. visceral pain.
   b. neuropathic pain.
   c. somatic pain.
   d. referred pain.

4. The nurse asks the client to point to a position along a line that represents his level of pain. Which of the following tools is the nurse using to assess the client's level of pain?
   a. Verbal numeric scale
   b. Wong-Baker FACES scale
   c. McGill Pain Questionnaire
   d. Visual analog scale

5. Which of the following vital signs would the nurse expect to assess in the client with acute pain?
   a. Respirations 26, blood pressure 160/92, pallor
   b. Pulse 120, respirations 16, flushed face
   c. Pulse 94, blood pressure 82/60, pallor
   d. Pulse 60, respirations 16, flushed face

6. The nurse is caring for a client in acute pain. Which of the following actions by the nurse would be expected at the first step of the WHO three-step analgesic ladder?
   a. Administration of a weak opioid
   b. Administration of a strong opioid
   c. Administration of a nonsteroidal anti-inflammatory drug
   d. Administration of an adjuvant drug

7. The nurse notes that a client has pain along the distribution of a nerve. The nurse documents this pain as:
   a. neuralgia.
   b. neuritis.
   c. radiculopathy.
   d. paresthesia.

8. Which statement by a client with an above-the-knee amputation indicates that she understands the discharge instructions?
   a. "Phantom leg pain is all in my head."
   b. "I can take my prescribed analgesic for phantom limb pain."
   c. "Phantom limb pain should not last more than 6 weeks."
   d. "Phantom limb pain is a complication that requires immediate treatment."

ANSWERS

Answers to Review Questions can be found in Appendix A. Answers to Case Study and Check Your Progress questions are available on the faculty resources site. Please consult with your instructor.

RECOMMENDED WEBSITES

International Association for the Study of Pain
https://www.iasp-pain.org

Pain Management Nursing
http://www.painmanagementnursing.org

WHO's Cancer Pain Ladder for Adults
http://www.who.int/cancer/palliative/painladder/en

REFERENCES

1. International Association for the Study of Pain. (2015). *IASP taxonomy*. Available at http://www.iasp-pain.org/Taxonomy
2. Fong, A., & Schug, S. A. (2014). Pathophysiology of pain: A practical primer. *Plastic and Reconstructive Surgery*, 134(4S-2), 8S–14S
3. Joint Commission. (2015). *Facts about pain management*. Available at http://www.jointcommission.org/pain_management
4. Basbaum, A. I., Bautista, D. M., Scherrer, G., & Julius, D. (2009). Cellular and molecular mechanisms of pain. *Cell, 139*(2), 267–284. doi: 10.1016/j.cell.2009.09.028.
5. Dansie, E. J., & Turk, D. C. (2013). Assessment of adults with chronic pain. *British Journal of Anaesthesia, 111*(1), 19–25. doi:10.1093/bja/aet124
6. Lamplot, J. D., Wagner, E. R., & Manning, D. W. (2014). Multimodal pain management in total joint arthroplasty: A prospective randomized controlled trial. *Journal of Arthroplasty, 29*(2), 329–334. doi:10.1016/j.arth.2013.06.005
7. World Health Organization. (2016). *WHO's cancer pain ladder for adults*. Available at http://www.who.int/cancer/palliative/painladder/en
8. Rahman, N. H. N. A., & DeSilva, T. (2012). The effectiveness of patient control analgesia in the treatment of acute traumatic pain in the emergency department: A randomized controlled trial. *European Journal of Emergency Medicine, 19*(4), 241–245. doi:10.1097/MEJ.0b013e32834bfc17
9. Pizzo, P. A., & Clark, N. M. (2012). Alleviating suffering 101: Pain relief in the United States. *New England Journal of Medicine, 366*, 197–199.
10. Kaiser, U., Arnold, B., Pfingsten, M., Nagel, B., Lutz, J., & Sabatowski, R. (2013). Multidisciplinary pain management programs. *Journal of Pain Research, 6*, 355–358. doi:10.2147/JPR.S40512
11. Attal, N., & Bouhassira, D. (2015). Pharmacotherapy of neuropathic pain: Which drugs, which treatment algorithms? *Pain, 156*, S104–S114.
12. Khalil, H. (2013). Painful diabetic neuropathy management. *International Journal of Evidence-Based Healthcare, 11*, 77–79.
13. Griebeler, M. L., Morey-Vargas, O. L., Brito, J. P., et al (2014). Pharmacologic interventions for painful diabetic neuropathy: An umbrella systematic review and comparative effectiveness network meta-analysis. *Annals of Internal Medicine, 161*(9), 639–649. doi:10.7326/M14-0511
14. Tesfave, S. T., Boulton, A. J. M., & Dickenson, A. H. (2013). Mechanisms and management of diabetic painful distal symmetrical polyneuropathy. *Diabetes Care, 36*, 2456–2465.
15. Russell, J. W., & Zilliox, L. (2014). Diabetic neuropathies. *Continuum, 20*(5), 1226–1240. doi:10.1212/01.CON.0000455884.29545.d2
16. Zilliox, L., & Russell, J. W. (2011). Treatment of diabetic sensory polyneuropathy. *Current Treatment Options in Neurology, 13*(2), 143–159. doi:10.1007/s11940-011-0113-1
17. Patil, P. R., Wolfe, J., Said, Q., Thomas, J., & Martin, B. C. (2015). Opioid use in the management of diabetic peripheral neuropathy (DPN) in a large commercially insured population. *Clinical Journal of Pain, 31*(5), 414–424.
18. DeSantana, J. M., Walsh, D. M., Vance, C., Rakel, B. A., & Sluka, K. A. (2008). Effectiveness of transcutaneous electrical nerve stimulation for treatment of hyperalgesia and pain. *Current Rheumatology Reports, 10*(6), 492–499.
19. deVos, C. C., Meier, K., Zaalberg, P. B., et al. (2014). Spinal cord stimulation in patients with painful diabetic neuropathy: A multicentre randomized clinical trial. *Pain, 155*, 2426–2431.
20. Slavin, K. V., Vaisman, J., Pollack, K. L., et al. (2013). Treatment of chronic, intractable pain with a conventional implantable pulse generator: A meta-analysis of 4 clinical studies. *Clinical Journal of Pain, 29*(1), 78–85. doi:10.1097/AJP.0b013e318247309a
21. Borghi, B., D'Addabbo, M., White, P. F., et al. (2010). The use of prolonged peripheral neural blockade after lower extremity amputation: The effect on symptoms associated with phantom limb syndrome. *Anesthesia & Analgesia, 111*(5), 1308–1315.
22. McCormick, Z., Chang-Chien, G., Marshall, B., Huang, M., & Harden, R. N. (2013). Phantom limb pain: A systematic neuroanatomical-based review of pharmacologic treatment. *Pain Medicine, 15*(2), 292–305. doi:10.1111/pme.12283
23. Vaso, A., Haim-Moshe, A., Gjika, A., Zahaj, S., Zhurda, T., Vyshka, G., & Devor, M. (2014). Peripheral nervous system origin of phantom limb pain. *Pain, 155*(7), 1384–1391. doi:10.1016/j.pain.2014.04.018
24. Knotkova1, H., Cruciani, R. A., Tronnier, V. M., & Rasche, R. (2012). Current and future options for the management of phantom-limb pain. *Journal of Pain Research, 5*, 39–49.
25. Vaso, A., Adahan, H. M., Gjika, A., et al. (2014). Peripheral nervous origin of phantom limb pain. *Pain, 155*, 1384–1391.
26. Alviar, M. J., Hale, T., & Dungca, M. (2016). Pharmacologic interventions for treating phantom limb pain. *Cochrane Database of Systematic Reviews*. doi:10.1002/14651858.CD006380.pub3
27. Bennetto, L., Patel, N. K., & Fuller, G. (2007). Trigeminal neuralgia and its management. *BMJ, 334*, 201–205.
28. Zakrzewska, J. M., & Linskey, M. E. (2014). Trigeminal neuralgia. *BMJ, 348*, g474. doi:10.1136/bmj.g474
29. Centers for Disease Control and Prevention. (2014). *About shingles*. Available at http://www.cdc.gov/shingles/about/index.html
30. Nagel, M. A., & Gilden, D. (2014). Neurological complications of varicella zoster virus reactivation. *Current Opinion in Neurology, 27*(3), 356–360. doi:10.1097/WCO.0000000000000092
31. Breuer, J., Pacou, M., Gautier, G., & Brown, M. M. (2014). Herpes zoster as a risk factor for stroke and TIA: A retrospective cohort study in the UK. *Neurology, 83*(2), e27–e33. doi:10.1212/WNL.0000000000000584
32. Markley, H. G., Edwin, D. D., Kareht, S., & Sweeney, M. (2015). Real-world experience with once daily gabapentin for the treatment of postherpetic neuralgia (PHN). *Clinical Journal of Pain, 31*(1), 58–65.
33. Wilson, D. D. (2014). Herpes zoster: A rash demanding careful evaluation. *Nurse Practitioner, 39*(5), 31–36.
34. Geertzen, J. H. B., Bodde, M. I., van Den Dungen, J. J. A., Dijkstra, P. U., & den Dunnen, W. F. A. (2015). Peripheral nerve pathology in patients with severely affected complex regional pain syndrome type 1. *International Journal of Rehabilitation Research, 38*(2), 121–130. doi:10.1097/MRR.0000000000000096
35. Al-Nesf, M. A., & Abdulaziz, H. M. (2014). Complex regional pain syndrome type 1 following tetanus toxoid injection. *Journal of Clinical Rheumatology, 20*(1), 49–50.
36. Birklein, F., & Schlereth, T. (2015). Complex regional pain syndrome: Significant progress in understanding. *Pain, 156*(4, S1), S94–S103.
37. Van Rooijen, D. E., Marinus, J., & van Hilten, J. J. (2013). Muscle hyperalgesia is widespread in patients with complex regional pain syndrome. *Pain, 154*, 2745–2749. doi:10.1016/j.jpain.2014.10.010
38. Van Velzen, G. A. J., Perez, R. S. G. M., van Gestel, M. A., et al. (2014). Health-related quality of life in 975 patients with complex pain syndrome type 1. *Journal of Pain, 155*, 629–634.
39. Van Eijs, F., Geurts, J., van Kleef, M., et al. (2012). Predictors of pain relieving response to sympathetic blockade in complex regional pain syndrome type 1. *Anesthesiology, 116*, 113–121.

40. Van der Plas, A. A., van Rijn, M. A., Marinus, J., Putter, H., & van Hilten, J. J. (2013). Efficacy of intrathecal baclofen on different pain qualities in complex regional pain syndrome. *Anesthesia & Analgesia, 116*(1), 211–215.
41. Murakami, M., Kosharskyy, B., Gritsenko, K., & Shaparin, N. (2015). Complex regional pain syndrome: Update and review of management. *Topics in Pain Management, 30*(7), 1–8.
42. Smitherman, T. A., Burch, R., Sheikh, H., & Loder, E. (2013). The prevalence, impact, and treatment of migraine and severe headaches in the United States: a review of statistics from national surveillance studies. *Headache, 53*(3), 427–436. doi:10.1111/head.12074
43. International Headache Society. (2013). *The international classification of headache disorders* (3rd ed.). London, UK: Sage.
44. Ashina, S., Bendtsen, L., & Ashina, M. (2012). Pathophysiology of migraine and tension type headaches. *Techniques in Regional Anesthesia and Pain Management, 16*(1), 14–18.
45. Noseda, R., & Burstein, R. (2013). Migraine pathophysiology: Anatomy of the trigeminovascular pathway and associated neurological symptoms, CSD, sensitization and modulation of pain. *Pain, 154*(Suppl. 1), S44–S53.
46. Kurlander, D. E., Punjabi, A., Liu, M. T., Sattar, A., & Guyuron, B. (2014). In-depth review of symptoms, triggers, and treatment of temporal migraine headaches. *Plastic and Reconstructive Surgery, 133*(4), 897–903.
47. Messali, A., Sanderson, J. C., Blumenfeld, A. M., Goadsby, P. J., Buse, D. C., Varon, S. F., & Stokes, M., Lipton, R. B. (2016). Direct and indirect costs of chronic and episodic migraine in the United States: A web-based survey. *Headache, 56*, 306–322. doi:10.1111/head.12755
48. Buse, D. C., & Lipton, R. B. (2013). Global perspectives on the burden of episodic and chronic migraine. *Cephalalgia, 33*(11), 885–890.
49. Burstein, R., Noseda, R., & Borsook, D. (2015). Migraine: multiple processes, complex pathophysiology. *Journal of Neuroscience, 35*(17), 6619–6629. doi:10.1523/JNEUROSCI.0373-15.2015
50. Paemeleire, K., Louis, P., Magis, D., et al. (2015). Diagnosis, pathophysiology and management of chronic migraine: A proposal of the Belgian Headache Society. *Acta Neurologica Belgica, 115*, 1. doi:10.1007/s13760-014-0313-z
51. Burstein, R., Jakubowski, M., Garcia-Nicas, E., et al. (2010). Thalamic sensitization transforms localized pain into widespread allodynia. *Annals of Neurology, 68*(1), 81–91.
52. Silva-Neto, R. P., Peres, M. F. P., & Yalenca, M. M. (2014). Odorant substances that trigger headaches in migraine patients. *Cephalalgia, 34*(1), 14–21.
53. Yilmaz, M., Gurger, M., Atescelik, M., Yildiz, M., & Gurbuz, S. (2015). Meteorologic parameters and migraine headache: ED study. *American Journal of Emergency Medicine, 33*(3), 409–413.
54. Headache Classification Committee of the International Headache Society. (2013). The International Classification of Headache Disorders, 3rd edition (beta version). *Cephalalgia, 33*(9), 629–808. doi:10.1177/0333102413485658
55. Francis, G. J., Becker, W. J., & Pringsheim, T. M. (2010). Acute and preventive pharmacologic treatment of cluster headache. *Neurology, 75*(5), 463–473.
56. Robbins, M. S., Starling, A. J., Pringsheim, T. M., Becker, W. J., & Schwedt, T. J. (2016). Treatment of cluster headache: The American Headache Society evidence-based guidelines. *Headache, 56*, 1093–1106. doi:10.1111/head.12866
57. Oaklander, A. L., Herzoz, Z. D., Downs, H. M., & Klein, M. M. (2013). Objective evidence that small-fiber polyneuropathy underlies some illnesses currently labeled as fibromyalgia. *Pain, 154*(11), 2310–2316. doi:10.1016/j.pain
58. Painter, J. T., & Crofford, L. J. (2013). Chronic opioid use in fibromyalgia syndrome: A clinical review. *Journal of Clinical Rheumatology, 19*(2), 72–77. doi:10.1097/RHU.0b013e3182863447
59. Crayne, C. B., Gomez, R., & Gedalia, A. (2015). A 14-year old with diffuse musculoskeletal pain. *Clinical Pediatrics, 54*(3), 299–301. doi:10.1177/0009922814553423
60. Larson, A. A., Pardo, J. V., & Pasley, J. D. (2014). Review of overlap between thermoregulation and pain modulation in fibromyalgia. *Clinical Journal of Pain, 30*(6), 544–555. doi:10.1097/AJP.0b013e3182a0e383
61. Martinez, J. E. (2014). Fibromyalgia and the old dilemma: Theory vs. practice. *Psychology & Neuroscience, 7*(1), 9–14. doi:10.3922/j.psns.2014.1.03
62. Albrecht, P. J., & Rice, F. L. (2016). Fibromyalgia pathology and environmental influences on afflictions with medically unexplained symptoms. *Reviews on Environmental Health, 31*(2), 281–294. doi:10.1515/reveh-2015-0040
63. Clauw, D. J. (2014). Fibromyalgia: A clinical review. *JAMA, 311*(15), 1547–1555. doi:10.1001/jama.2014.3266
64. Van deVen, T., & Hsia, H. L. J. (2012). Causes and prevention of chronic postsurgical pain. *Current Opinion in Critical Care, 18*(4), 366–371. doi:10.1097/MCC.0b013e3283557a7f
65. Peters, C. M., Hayashida, K. I., Suto, T., Houle, T. T., Ashenbrenner, C. A., Martin, T. J., & Eisenach, J. C. (2015). Individual differences in acute pain-induces endogenous analgesia predict time to resolution of postoperative pain in the rat. *Anesthesiology, 122*(4), 895–907.
66. Lints-Martindale, A. C., Hadjistavropoulos, T., Lix, M., & Thorpe, L. (2012). A comparative investigation of observational pain assessment tools for older adults with dementia. *Clinical Journal of Pain, 28*(3), 226–237. doi:10.1097/AJP.0b013e3182290d90
67. Reddi, D., & Curran, N. (2014). Chronic pain after surgery: Pathophysiology, risk factors and prevention, *Postgraduate Medical Journal, 90*(1062), 222–227.
68. Peng, Z., Li, H., Zhang, C., Qian, X., Feng, Z., & Zhu, S. (2014). A retrospective study of chronic post-surgical pain following thoracic surgery: Prevalence, risk factors, incidence of neuropathic component, and impact on quality of life. *PLoS One, 9*(2). doi:10.1371/journal.pone.0090014
69. Taddio, A., Shah, V., Atenafu, E., & Katz, J. (2009). Influence of repeated painful procedures and sucrose analgesia on the development of hyperalgesia in newborn infants. *Pain, 144*(1–2), 43–48. doi:10.1016/j.pain
70. Taddio, A., Katz, J., Ilersich, A. L., & Koren, G. (1997). Effect of neonatal circumcision on pain response during subsequent routine vaccination. *Lancet, 349*(9052), 599–603.
71. Chang, J., Versloot, J., Fashler, S. R., McCrystal, K. N., & Graig, K. D. (2015). Pain assessment in children: Validity of facial expression items in observational pain scales. *Clinical Journal of Pain, 31*(3), 189–197. doi:10.1097/AJP.0000000000000103
72. Cordero, M. J., Villar, N. M., & Garcia, I. G. (2015). Evaluation of pain in healthy newborns and in newborns with developmental problems. *Pain Management Nursing, 16*(3), 267–272. doi:10.1016/j.pmn.2014.08.001
73. Garra, G., Singer, A. J., Domingo, A., & Thode, B. C. (2013). The Wong-Baker pain FACES scale measures pain, not fear. *Pediatric Emergency Care, 29*, 17–20. doi:10.1097/PEC.0b013e31827b2299
74. World Health Organization. (2012). WHO guidelines on the pharmacological treatment of persisting pain in children with medical illnesses. Available at http://whqlibdoc.who.int/publications/2012/9789241548120_Guidelines.pdf?ua=1
75. Verghese, S. T., & Hannallah, R. S. (2010). Acute pain management in children. *Journal of Pain Research, 3*, 105–123.
76. Kaye, A. D., Baluch, A., & Scott, J. T. (2010). Pain management in the elderly population: A review. *Ochsner Journal, 10*(3), 179–187.
77. Oosterman, J. M., Zwakhalen, S., Sampson, E. L., & Kunz, M. (2016). The use of facial expressions for pain assessment purposes in dementia: A narrative review. *Neurodegenerative Disease Management, 6*(2), 119–131.
78. Fuchs-Lacelle, S., & Hadjistavropoulos, T. (2004). Development and preliminary validation of the pain assessment checklist for

seniors with limited ability to communicate (PACSLAC). *Pain Management Nursing, 5*(1), 37–49.

79. Chan, S., Hadjistavropoulos, T., Williams, J., & Lints-Martindale, A. (2014). Evidence-based development and initial validation of the pain assessment checklist for seniors with limited ability to communicate-II (PACSLAC-II). *Clinical Journal of Pain, 30*(9), 816–824. doi:10.1097/AJP.0000000000000039

80. Achterbergg, W. P., Pieper, M. J. C., van Dalen-Kok, A. H., et al. (2013). Pain management in patients with dementia. *Clinical Interventions in Aging, 8*, 1471–1482. doi:10.2147/CIA.S36739

81. Warden, V. (n.d.) Pain Assessment in Advanced Dementia scale (PAINAD). Available at https://www.mdcalc.com/pain-assessment-advanced-dementia-scale-painad

Chapter 33

Disorders of Thermoregulation

Barbara J. Holtzclaw

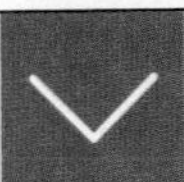

Chapter Outline and Learning Outcomes

33.1 Chapter Overview and Case Studies

Explain the history and importance of monitoring body temperature and the concepts related to thermoregulation.

33.2 Body Temperature Regulation

Describe how changes in body temperature involve both physics and physiologic factors.

33.3 Thermoregulatory Processes and Control Mechanisms

Explain the sensory inputs and effectors of thermoregulatory responses as complex, separate, but interacting responses with both autonomic and behavioral components.

33.4 Hypothermia

Differentiate the causes, classification, underlying pathogenesis, and clinical manifestations of hypothermia and frostbite and approaches to treatment of those conditions, and explain the rationale for therapeutic hypothermia.

33.5 Fever

Differentiate the causes, underlying pathogenesis, clinical manifestations, benefits and adverse effects of fever and approaches to its treatment.

33.6 Hyperthermia

Differentiate the causes, underlying pathogenesis, and clinical manifestations of disorders causing hyperthermia and treatment approaches for those disorders.

KEY TERMS

Accidental hypothermia, 823
Chill phase, 830
Defervescence phase, 831
Eccrine sweat, 820
Fever, 829
Frostbite, 828
Heat exhaustion, 832
Heat stress, 832
Heat stroke, 832
Hyperthermia, 832
Hypothermia, 822
Iatrogenic hypothermia, 823
Inadvertent hypothermia, 823
Malignant hyperthermia, 833
Neuroleptic malignant syndrome, 833
Normothermia, 816
Plateau phase, 830
Poikilothermia, 820
Pyrogen, 829
Rhabdomyolysis, 832
Shivering, 820
Therapeutic hypothermia, 823
Thermoeffector responses, 820
Thermoeffector threshold zone, 819
Thermoneutral zone, 818
Thermoreceptors, 819
Thermoregulation, 818

ABBREVIATIONS

BMR—basal metabolic rate
CPB—cardiopulmonary bypass

33.1 Chapter Overview and Case Studies

Concern about disorders in body temperature has occupied nurses for all of the profession's history; the invention of the thermometer increased the preoccupation with monitoring and recording the rise and fall of this important vital sign. It is remarkable that much of the scientific understanding of the underlying dynamics of temperature regulation emerged only during the last quarter of the 20th century. Not all of these scientific discoveries were suggested in the laboratory. Survival of hypothermic victims produced evidence that cooling preserves cells but presents other hazards. Advances in anesthetic agents subjected genetically susceptible patients to newly identified type of hyperthermia. Air and space travel posed situations of temperature extremes that required research, while technologic discoveries enlightened temperature monitoring and environmental control. Discoveries of the molecular mechanisms of fever that were beneficial as well as worrisome led to more rational treatment of fever. Research and mapping of neuroregulatory centers and feedback circuits that affect thermoregulation were scientific breakthroughs with which nurses and other caregivers must become familiar to plan and test appropriate interventions.

The usual range of core body temperature is called **normothermia**. As shown in **Figure 33.1** ■, the normal range for adults is between 36°C and 38.5°C (between 96.8°F and 101.3°F). This chapter focuses on the physical, physiologic, and behavioral homeostatic mechanisms that maintain the stable core body temperature required for optimal cell function. Disorders of body temperature regulation, such as hypothermia, fever, and hyperthermia, are addressed.

Concepts Related to Thermoregulation

Infectious and inflammatory processes can cause fever, and as seen in heat-related injuries, uncontrolled hyperthermia can quickly result in dehydration. Both hyperthermia and hypothermia can affect patient comfort levels. The concept of thermoregulation extends to individuals who are at risk for hypothermia and hyperthermia on the basis of age and developmental factors that may increase their risk for injury due to environmental extremes. Individuals diagnosed with a neurocognitive disorder such as dementia or with a severe mental illness may have a diminished ability to detect environmental changes, which may increase their risk for weather-related injuries. Individuals who are homeless or living in substandard housing are also vulnerable to injuries caused by extreme temperatures. Thermoregulation is an important public health concept for which communities, cities, municipalities, and states can develop and promote initiatives to minimize the effects of extreme temperatures on people who do not have the means to alter their environment for their own safety. **Figure 33.2** ■ shows some of the concepts related to thermoregulation.

Thermoregulation	Temperature °C	Temperature °F
Hyperthermia	41.2	106.1
Heat stroke >41.1°C, 106°F	41.0	105.8
	40.8	105.4
	40.6	105.1
	39.2	102.6
	39.0	102.2
Heat exhaustion 38.3–38.9°C, 101–102°F	38.8	101.8
Fever >38.5°C, 101.4°F	38.6	101.5
Normothermia 36–38.5°C, 96.8–101.3°F	38.4	101.1
	38.2	100.8
	37.4	99.3
	37.2	99.0
	37.0	98.6
	36.8	98.2
	36.6	97.9
	36.4	97.5
	35.4	95.7
	35.2	95.4
Mild hypothermia 32–35°C, 89.6–95°F	35.0	95.0
	34.8	94.6
	34.6	94.3
	34.4	93.9
	34.2	93.6
	34.0	93.2
	32.8	91.0
	32.6	90.7
	32.4	90.3
	32.2	90.0
	32.0	89.6
	31.2	88.2
	31.0	87.8
Moderate hypothermia 28–32°C, 82.4–89.6°F	30.8	87.4
	30.6	87.1
	30.4	86.7
	30.2	86.4
	30.0	86.0
	29.8	85.6
	28.2	82.8
	28.0	82.4
Severe hypothermia below 28°C, 82.4°F	27.8	82.0
	27.6	81.7
	27.4	81.3
	27.2	81.0
	27.0	80.6

Figure 33.1 ■ Terms used to describe alterations in body temperature (oral measurements) and ranges in Celsius and Fahrenheit scales. The wavy lines in the temperature columns reflect where temperatures were skipped.

Case Studies

The following cases are addressed throughout the chapter to assist in application of chapter content to clinical situations that involve individuals with altered body temperature.

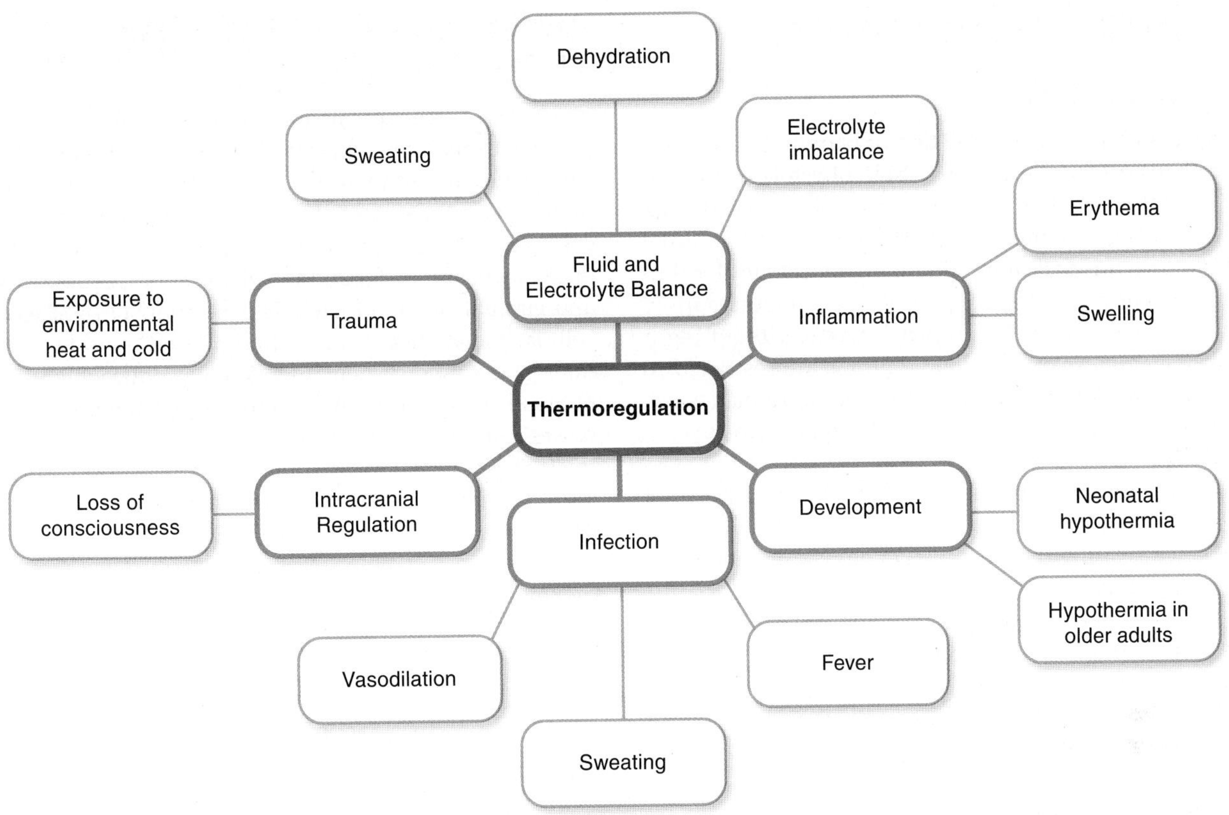

Figure 33.2 ■ Concepts related to thermoregulation.

Dylan Shubert: Introduction

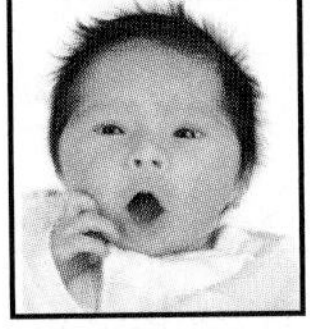

Dylan Shubert is a 5-day old newborn. His parents notice that Dylan seems cool to the touch with decreased muscle tone. They bring him to the emergency department for evaluation. His mother reports that Dylan has been reluctant to feed and seems to be breathing faster. His parents report that they have been putting him in a bassinette near a window.

1. The usual range of core body temperature is referred to as what?
2. Given the information provided, what type of temperature regulation issue might Dylan be experiencing?

Alexandra Holloway: Introduction

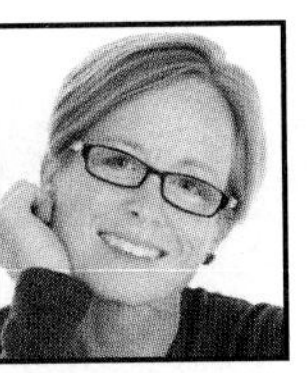

Alexandra Holloway, a 59-year-old woman, lives an active life. She is married with three children, is a retired accountant, and has been in good health most of her life. She became ill this morning after a family potluck dinner yesterday and now complains of nausea, pain over her right lower abdomen, and a feeling of malaise. Her husband becomes concerned when he finds her having severe shaking chills and experiencing more abdominal pain. He calls the family physician, who advises Mr. Holloway to take her the emergency department.

1. Severe shaking chills can be a symptom of what thermoregulation disorder?
2. Which of Mrs. Holloway's symptoms might be severe enough in combination that going to the emergency department would be important?

Robert Warfield: Introduction

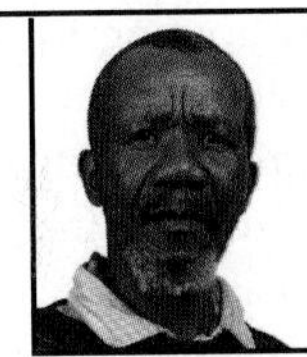

Robert Warfield, age 84, lives alone. A friend was worried that the heat and 88% humidity that day might be too much for Mr. Warfield to tolerate. When she could not reach him by phone, she called 9-1-1. The first responders report that Mr. Warfield's house is like an oven, there is no air conditioning, and a tiny electric fan provides no relief from the heat. They estimate that the room temperature is over 37.7°C (100°F). Mr. Warfield is unconscious and unresponsive, and he appears to be having a mild seizure. In the field, the paramedics apply ice packs for external cooling of the head. They start intravenous fluid and electrolyte replacement to support Mr. Warfield's vital functions.

1. Given the case information, what thermoregulation disorder might Mr. Warfield be experiencing? Provide your rationale, and define the specific condition.
2. What factor or factors put Mr. Warfield at higher risk for sensitivity to thermoregulation changes?

Check Your Progress: Section 33.1

1. What is normothermia?
2. What discovery led to more rational treatment of fever?
3. What vulnerable populations are at risk for hypothermia and hyperthermia?

33.2 Body Temperature Regulation

The dynamic process of regulating of body temperature is called **thermoregulation**. Remarkable physiologic mechanisms maintain stable body temperatures despite very high or very low environmental temperatures. Stable internal temperatures are critical in optimizing biochemical, cellular, and kinetic processes that produce a continuous supply of heat, which can reach dangerous levels without regulation. Thus, internal body temperatures are restricted to a relatively narrow range that varies no more than 1.5°C before compensatory warming or cooling mechanisms are stimulated.

When core body temperatures are stable and do not require any regulatory changes in heat production or heat loss, they are in the **thermoneutral zone**. Maintaining the thermoneutral zone involves a dynamic balance that must constantly respond to both physical and physiologic challenges that commonly occur. These challenges can push body temperatures beyond the limits of the thermoneutral zone and set into motion a delicately balanced system of thermoeffector responses. Because the process of thermoregulation involves both the physical and biologic mechanisms that control heat transfer, it is important to review both physics and physiology as factors in maintaining thermal balance.

The Nature of Heat: Physics in Action

Following the laws of thermodynamics, heat flows along a temperature gradient from warmer to cooler regions. As a result, body heat is continually lost from deeper, warmer regions of the body to the circulating blood that is delivered to skin surfaces. Ultimately, the heat is then transferred to the environment through conduction, convection, radiation, and evaporation. These are principles of physics that are directly related to the body's physiologic efficacy in regulating heat loss (**Table 33.1** ■). Heat exchange from the skin to the surrounding air is dramatically influenced by the environment.

Active Processes to Maintain Thermal Balance

Physiologic mechanisms must interact with principles of physics to maintain thermal balance. The body's chemical, enzymatic, and immune functions depend on the maintenance of stable and optimal body temperatures in constantly changing conditions. These conditions are influenced by heat transfer and the physical properties of tissue and circulating blood. Heat is continuously produced by cellular metabolism, combustion of food, muscle contractions, and, to some extent, the friction produced by the flow of blood against vessel walls. Physiologic and physical processes combine to either conserve heat within, or promote the transfer of heat away from, the body's most vulnerable regions. Even anatomic features, such as tissue thickness and proximity of blood vessels to one another, affect heat transfer as regional blood flow is diverted closer to or farther away from the body surface.

Check Your Progress: Section 33.2

1. What are the principles of physics that are directly related to the body's physiologic efficacy in regulating heat loss?
2. What condition dramatically influences the heat exchange from the skin to the surrounding air?
3. How is heat continuously produced in the body?

33.3 Thermoregulatory Processes and Control Mechanisms

Thermoregulation is not accomplished by a single physiologic system but rather by interactions involving multiple body systems. Thermal balance in the body is controlled by the central nervous system and maintained by a negative feedback loop similar to the thermostat that controls the temperature in your home.

Table 33.1 Mechanisms of Heat Transfer

Mechanism of Heat Transfer	Definition/Examples
Conductive heat loss	The transfer of heat from warmer skin to colder surfaces such as examining tables, bed linens, or examining instruments
Conductive heat gain	The transfer of heat from warmer surfaces to the skin
Convective heat loss	The transfer of heat that is promoted by currents from fans, air conditioning, or drafty conditions that rapidly remove heat from the skin
Convective heat gain	The transfer of heat that is promoted when heaters or warming blankets use forced air movement to restore heat to the skin
Radiant heat loss	The transfer of heat that involves an electromagnetic energy exchange between two objects of different temperatures, again from warmer to cooler areas; because body temperatures are warmer than ambient conditions, heat is radiated to the air, even through windows
Radiant heat gain	Heat transfer to the body from exposure to rays of the sun, heat-producing lights, or reflected light from snow or water
Evaporative heat loss	Heat loss when a liquid on the skin, such as sweat, vaporizes. Evaporative heat loss is effective only when the environmental humidity is relatively low and convective flow keeps the air moisture concentration low. The larger the evaporative area and the more dilute the sweat, the more effective sweating will be in increasing heat loss

Thermoregulatory Feedback System

Figure 33.3 ■ is a simplified diagram of the components of the thermoregulatory feedback system.

Thermoeffector Threshold Zone

Beginning at the top of Figure 33.3 at point 1, you can see the **thermoeffector threshold zone**. This zone defines the acceptable core temperature range of 36–38.5°C. A set point mechanism, like a home thermostat, is thought to keep core temperature levels within this range. The upper and lower levels of the thermoeffector threshold zone that affect the set point range are not fixed limitations. This means they can be influenced by fever, acclimatization, and periodic and systemic physiologic processes.[1] As long as core temperatures remain within the set range, a steady state exists in which no compensatory mechanisms either increase or decrease the temperature.

Central and Peripheral Thermoreceptors

Moving clockwise in Figure 33.3 to point 2, you can see that this feedback system depends on both peripheral and central sensors that monitor the core temperature. These sensors are called **thermoreceptors**.

Central Thermoreceptors. Most central thermoreceptors are warm-sensitive. That is, they are activated by temperatures that could overheat delicate neuroregulatory cells. This makes central sensory receptors critical to the initiation of overheating responses. However, research in the past decade shows that defensive responses to both cold and heat are triggered by changes in the activity of warm-sensitive neurons.[2] Cold-sensitive central thermoreceptors are less numerous. Sensitivity to rising heat undoubtedly has some survival benefit. Overheating is physiologically more dangerous to survival than cooling because the potential breakdown of the structure of proteins can cause permanent brain damage when brain temperatures rise only a few degrees above normal.[3] This condition is typical of hyperthermia, in which damaged thermosensitive neurons become unable to signal cooling thermoeffectors, so temperatures continue to rise even higher.

Thermoreceptors, especially the heat-sensitive central thermoreceptors, not only function to monitor core temperatures but are also affected by them. The central thermoreceptors depend on an optimal temperature range to function properly. Low body temperatures in the range of 32–35°C depress the central nervous system and lead

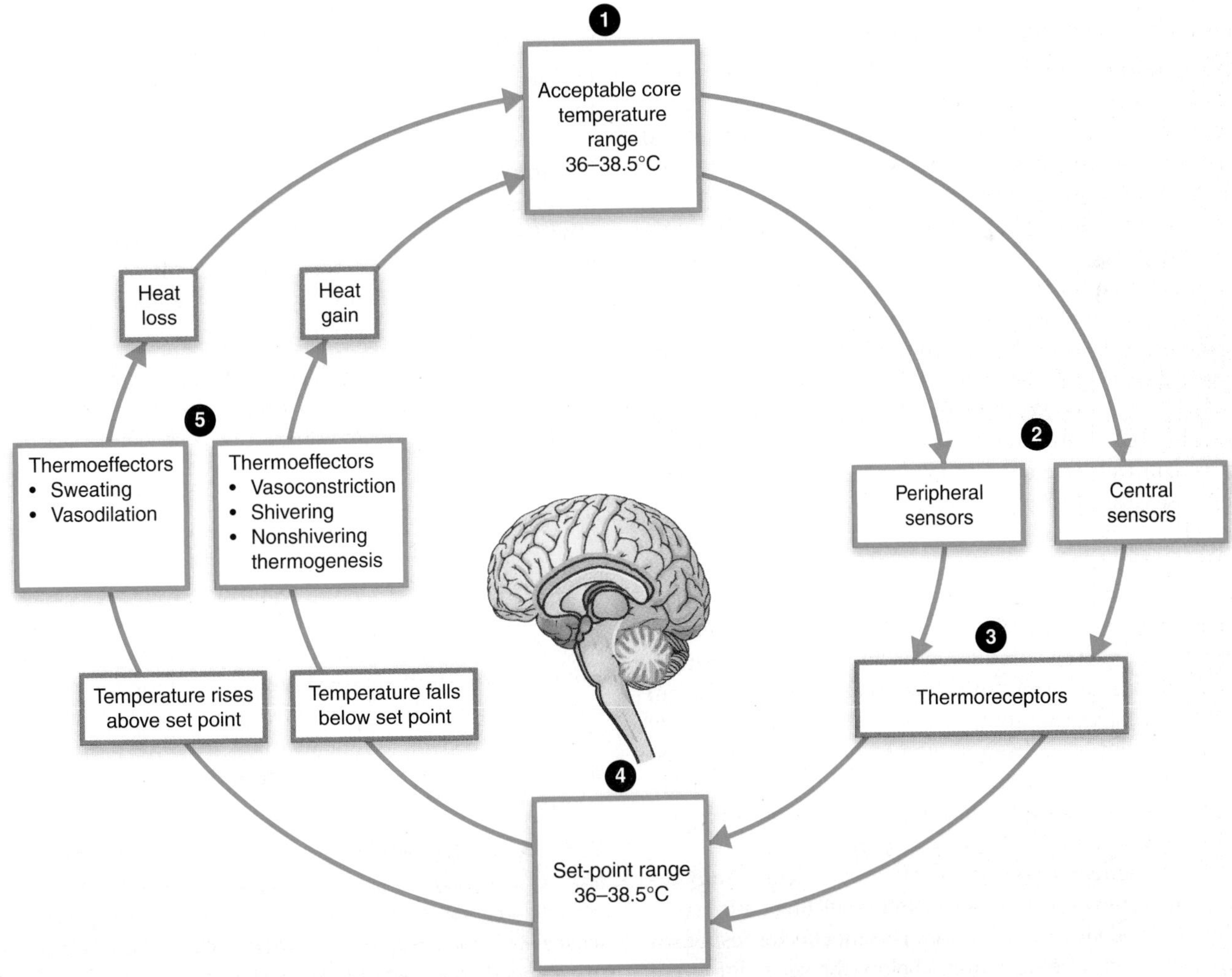

Figure 33.3 ■ The components of the thermoregulatory feedback system.

to a condition of disrupted body temperature regulation called **poikilothermia**. The poikilothermic individual loses the ability to maintain internal body temperature within the thermoeffector threshold zone. Without central thermoregulatory control, the individual's core temperature will continue to fall below 30.8°C, accompanied by apnea, coma, coagulation defects, cardiac dysrhythmias, and cardiac arrest leading to death.[4] Hyperthermia in conditions where injury or overheating affects the brain's thermoregulatory centers also can cause poikilothermia.[5] When core temperatures rise beyond 41.2°C and heat loss mechanisms and body water reserves are exhausted, permanent neural damage, coma, and death can result.[6]

Peripheral Thermoreceptors. Peripheral thermoreceptors exist near the surface of the body in the skin and the oral and urogenital mucosa. In contrast to central thermosensitive receptors, most peripheral thermoreceptors are cold-sensitive, making them more responsive in stimulating cold-defense mechanisms and making a person seek warmth. Cutaneous cold sensors are located just beneath the skin, while the less common warm sensors are located deeper in the dermis.[3] Although warm-sensitive signals from the periphery are also integrated with those from central receptors, they are less influential in triggering heat-defense responses.[3]

Physiologic Thermoeffector Responses

Let's continue around the feedback loop in Figure 33.3. As was noted previously, thermal balance operates via a negative feedback loop. We have seen that both central and peripheral sensors monitor core temperatures. Integrated information from both types of thermoreceptors (as seen at point 3 in Figure 33.3) is then transmitted to the hypothalamus, where it is compared to the set point range of the thermoeffector threshold zone (point 4 in Figure 33.3). If the core temperature is maintained within the threshold zone, no regulatory action is required. If, however, the core temperature is rises above or falls below the set point range, mechanisms that are can stabilize or restore thermal balance are activated. These mechanisms are called thermoeffector responses (see point 5 in Figure 33.3). **Thermoeffector responses** are involuntary responses to heat and cold stimuli that combine both physiologic and physical processes to either conserve heat within, or promote the transfer of heat away, from the body's most vulnerable regions.[1] The complex and interactive pathways that provide regulatory information for the stimulation or inhibition of thermoeffector responses are not simple one-track routes for all input and feedback. Instead, they are complex thermoregulatory pathways that have been shown to have their own distinct thermoeffector loops. Neuroscientists have not fully mapped out which thermoreceptors in which body regions stimulate which thermoeffector responses.[3]

Thermoeffector responses activated by core temperatures above the set point range include sweating and vasodilation of blood vessels in the skin. Thermoeffector responses activated by core temperatures below the set point range include shivering, vasoconstriction of blood vessels in the skin, and nonshivering heat production in brown adipose tissue. Neurons providing these effects receive signals from cells in the medulla of the brainstem and are governed by neurons in regions of the hypothalamus and midbrain and possibly the pons. As thermoeffector responses are activated, heat is lost or gained, and core temperatures return to within the set point range.

Sweating. Thermoregulatory sweat is secreted from millions of eccrine sweat glands that cover most of the body.[7,8] **Eccrine sweat** is a clear, odorless, and dilute solution that differs from the less abundant, thicker, and odorous apocrine sweat from underarms and other hairy locations. Evaporative heat loss is essential for survival when the environment is warmer than the skin temperature. It is the evaporation of sweat that promotes cooling of skin surfaces and makes it effective as a heat-defense thermoeffector.[8] Thus, the inability to sweat can lead to dangerously high core temperatures and can be life threatening in warm climates or during febrile illness. The precise pathway from the brain to the sweat gland is not entirely understood, but the efferent signals are thought to travel from the preoptic hypothalamus through the pons and medullary raphe to the intermediolateral region of the spinal cord. Sweat glands are innervated through sympathetic postganglionic fibers that combine with peripheral nerves and become entwined around the tissue surrounding sweat glands.[8] Normally, sympathetic postganglionic fibers utilize norepinephrine to effect neural activity at their target organs. However, the sympathetic postganglionic nerves innervating sweat glands consist of numerous cholinergic terminals that utilize acetylcholine instead of norepinephrine as their terminal neurotransmitter.[8] These peculiarities in sweat gland innervation mean that sweating can be stimulated by stimulation of sympathetic postganglionic fibers or by drugs, such as pilocarpine, that stimulate parasympathetic activity.

CLINICAL POINT: The importance of eccrine sweating as a cooling mechanism is apparent in individuals with hypohidrotic ectodermal dysplasia (a rare genetic condition characterized by a reduced ability to sweat) or other conditions with impaired or abnormal sweat gland function.[9] ■

Shivering. The primary thermoeffector response to generate heat is **shivering**. This involuntary motor activity generates heat by the friction produced as a result of aerobic muscle contractions. Peripheral thermoreceptors that detect a drop in core temperature below the set point range transmit signals to the primary shivering center in the posterior hypothalamus. Subsequently, efferent impulses from the primary shivering center descend through pathways in the brainstem and spinal cord, resulting in skeletal muscle contractions.[10,11]

CLINICAL POINT: Although shivering creates considerable heat, it tends to be energy inefficient in cold environments. This is because, although the oxygen consumption required for shivering increases the metabolic rate threefold to fivefold over the resting rate, shivering muscle contractions actually promote heat loss by increasing blood flow to the skin, perfusing cooler vascular regions, and creating convective currents through movement.[10] ■

Nonshivering Heat Production. Generation of heat from brown adipose tissue occurs from effects of uncoupling protein 1 in the mitochondria, resulting in the release of energy in the form of heat. Nonshivering thermogenesis is of relatively less importance in an adult than in infants; infants have large deposits of brown adipose tissue and depend heavily on this mechanism for survival.[12] Because brown adipose tissue is prominent in the newborn infant, its presence was earlier thought to be a leftover embryonic mechanism before the infant was able to initiate shivering activity. It is now acknowledged that nonshivering thermogenesis is an acquired mechanism that developed to meet the need for heat production.[12] The fact that small islets of brown adipose tissue are found in the white fat of adults suggests that there may be some rudimentary thermogenic potential that may come into play during adaptation to cold conditions or increased sympathetic stimuli.[12,13]

Vasoconstriction and Vasodilation of Blood Vessels in the Skin. Vasomotor responses, both vasoconstriction and vasodilation, are mediated by two different sympathetic nervous system branches: adrenergic vasoconstrictor nerves and cholinergic vasodilator nerves.[14,15] Nerves that cause vasodilation are not active in normothermia but cause up to 90% of vasodilation that occurs with warming. Signals from the vasomotor center trigger vasoconstriction or vasodilation to adjust circulation closer to or farther away from skin surfaces. As a result, heat is either conserved or lost from the skin to the environment. Vasodilator control of skin circulation is the primary thermoeffector response for promoting heat loss during heat stress from exercise or environmental temperature.[14] Vasoconstrictor control of skin circulation is the primary thermoeffector response for promoting heat conservation. It is achieved by the action of sympathetic norepinephrine on alpha$_1$- and alpha$_2$-receptors on the vascular smooth muscle of cutaneous arterioles.[15] This change in perfusion is readily observed in flushing of the skin when an individual is warm and pallor when the individual is cold.

Behavioral Thermoeffector Responses

In addition to physiologic mechanisms that maintain thermal balance, several behavioral mechanisms are recognized in humans. Heat generation resulting from increased voluntary skeletal muscle activity is a behavioral thermoeffector mechanism that occurs when individuals rub their hands together or pat their arms to get warm. Cognitively intact individuals recognize the need to seek shelter, adjust what they wear, or adapt their surroundings as environmental temperatures change. They conserve heat by hugging their extremities close to their body and wrapping up in warmer clothing. Infants, older adults, individuals impaired by drugs or alcohol, or those who are unable to perform behavioral thermoeffector activities are especially vulnerable to alterations in body temperature. Each year, incapacitated older adults, cognitively impaired individuals, and homeless people living on the streets die from hypothermia because they find themselves in locations with inadequate heating. Likewise, the heat takes a toll on individuals without air conditioning who are fearful of living with windows open and on victims of exposure. Drug and alcohol intoxication incapacitates behavioral survival in both hot and cold environments, in addition to the physiologic effects these substances have on thermoregulation.

The neonate has few behavioral responses for protection against passive heat loss at birth and is at added risk because of the sharp temperature gradients between the infant and the cool delivery room. Without active heat replacement, the infant will lose heat rapidly through radiation, conduction, convection, and evaporation. Because of musculoskeletal and neurologic immaturity, the newborn is not yet equipped to generate heat by movement or shivering. The full-term neonate depends on nonshivering thermogenesis by increased fat oxidation from brown adipose tissue, which at room temperature has a metabolic cost of about 150 kcal/min.[16,17] A preterm infant lacks minimal insulation from body fat and has not developed brown adipose tissue deposits until 28 weeks of gestation.[12] Therefore, for neonates, the behavioral responsibilities for survival and thermal balance rest with caregivers to provide warmth, ensure oxygenation for infant breathing, and support heat conservation. For preterm infants, who are not able to use nonshivering thermogenesis, the need for warmth is on a par with that for oxygenation. When the neonate's temperature falls below 36.5°C, hypothermia occurs.[16,17] ■

The older adult is susceptible to extremes of both heat and cold. Research findings show that adults over age 65 have a lower resting metabolic rate and metabolic response to generate heat under cold stress.[18] When tested in mildly colder conditions in a comparative study with younger adults, older adults had a lower vasoconstrictor response. They also had lower mean body mass and lower metabolic rate throughout the study,[18] resulting in lower core temperatures, which makes the older adult particularly vulnerable to severely cold temperatures. Older adults with chronic diseases may also be taking medications that further reduce vascular or behavioral compensatory responses to cold stress. ■

While the dangers of heat loss and hypothermia mandate that people who care for older adults be vigilant for this occurrence, the risk factors for heat stress during heat extremes pose an equally dangerous threat. Individuals over age 60 are reported to be the most severely affected by heat. Sadly, those who are in long-term care, are confined to bed, or live alone have the highest rates of heat-related death and injury. Reviews of research literature find a complex variety of physiologic factors that increase the risk for heat stress in older adults, including decreases in sweating, skin perfusion, and cardiovascular function. The major cause of morbidity and heat-related illness is clearly lack of access to a cooler environment.[19] This includes lack of cooling devices, decreased mobility and transportation to seek cooler surroundings, and lack of contact with people who are willing to monitor and assist the older person.

The usual behavioral thermoregulation activities of adjusting environmental temperature or adding more clothing may be impaired by developmental, physical, social, or economic conditions. These examples show that some individuals and some situations call for family and friend caregivers to be in contact with the individuals who are at risk. At the same time, the public at large needs to understand the hazards associated with water sports, ice and snow activities, and athletic exertion that increases the risk of exposure to temperature extremes. Likewise, ancient approaches to cool down fevers, warm up hypothermic individuals, or manage hyperthermia should be reevaluated on a foundation that includes emerging research as well as a sound understanding of the principles of thermoregulation.[4,20]

CLINICAL POINT: Nurses have both a direct care responsibility and an indirect opportunity to inform families and community members about the dangers of extreme thermal environments for vulnerable populations such as infants, older adults, and chronically ill people. Preventing injury or death in extremely hot or cold temperatures is often a matter of ensuring supervision and providing basic necessities to heat, cool, or ventilate the person's home. However, there is a general community unawareness of the susceptibility and impaired compensatory response to heat and cold in these vulnerable populations. ■

Community-dwelling older adults, especially those with mild cognitive impairment, are particularly vulnerable. They may accidentally lock themselves out of their house while going outside to empty the trash or pick up the mail during severely cold weather. If a neighbor is not home or it is too far to walk for help, they may develop hypothermia and further confusion. If they are not discovered before mild hypothermia occurs, they may become unconscious and may not be found until the next day. ■

Circadian Oscillations in Body Temperature

The rise and fall of body temperature have fascinated scientists since the advent of thermometers. The first publication of circadian patterns was published in 1871 by German physician Carl R. A. Wunderlich.[21] His observations that normal body temperatures were highest in the early evening (from 4 p.m. to 9 p.m.) and lowest in the early morning (from 2 a.m. to 8 a.m.) are consistent with current research. However, it was not until the middle of the 20th century that these physiologic variations were considered to be more complicated than homeostatic defenses of a narrow thermoneutral set point range. Discoveries in chronobiology during the 1960s revealed an endogenous (built-in) circadian mechanism controlling body temperature.[22] These variations in core temperature persisted even when subjects were deprived of environmental cues of light, noise, or awareness of time. As circadian rhythms of temperature and other bodily functions were studied further, the existence of biologic clocks, or endogenous regulators, became known. Today, these regulators of cyclic physiologic activities are well accepted, but huge areas of discovery remain in locating where and how they act.

Core body temperature remains a powerful indicator of circadian synchrony among most body systems and is one of the most commonly studied circadian variables. Like all circadian rhythms, core temperatures are endogenously generated oscillations that persist when environmental stimuli are removed, have a persistent pattern that does not change despite a wide range of physiologic temperatures, and can be synchronized or reset by a periodic environmental signal (e.g., a shift in daily light–dark cycle).[22]

CLINICAL POINT: The tendency for body temperatures to rise and fall at different times of the day or night may reflect circadian, homeostatic, or pyrogenic influences that are often indistinct. For most of medical history, clinicians have tried to use patterns of temperature oscillation to diagnose specific illnesses or infection. A few disorders, such as Alzheimer disease, Parkinson disease, and Huntington disease appear to cause circadian rhythm dysfunction that may have influences on sleep and nocturnal behavioral.[23,24] A few infections, such as miliary tuberculosis, have shown morning temperature elevations to have predictive diagnostic significance.[25] However, results of attempts to link night sweats or fever patterns to a specific disorder have been disappointing because such variations often reflect levels of specific cytokines rather than a particular disease or infection.[22] ■

Check Your Progress: Section 33.3

1. What is poikilothermia?
2. What is thermoregulatory sweating, and how does it affect the body?
3. Describe behavioral thermoeffector heat-conserving responses that cognitively intact individuals can use when there is a change in environmental temperature.

33.4 Hypothermia

Hypothermia is a condition of mild to profound heat loss in which the body is unable to maintain even the lowest limits of core temperature set point range required for metabolic, enzymatic, and other physiologic functions. The term is often used imprecisely to describe any lower than normal temperature, and even authorities do not entirely agree on standardized ranges of temperatures that can be used to assess levels of hypothermia.[26,27] Contributing to the lack of standardization in staging hypothermia are differences in the risk potential in different populations.

Among neonates, fatality is correlated with severity of hypothermia, using the World Health Organization Classification.[28] Newborns with skin temperatures in the 36°C to 36.4°C range are considered mildly hypothermic. Preterm infants with low birthweight, birth asphyxia and associated illness such as sepsis, and respiratory distress are categorized to a higher stage of hypothermia because these infants are more vulnerable to its effects. At the same time, these features reflect a vulnerability and high potential for central heat loss from the infant's circulation through the skin to the cooler ambient air, cold surfaces, and bed linen. Because the neonate's skin is thin on the upper abdomen and has superficial vasculature that does not vasoconstrict, thermistors can be adhered to the abdominal skin to get a representative measure of core temperature. ■

Dylan Shubert: Application

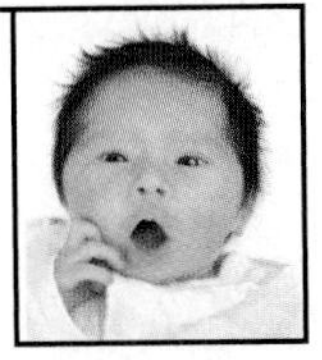

On his arrival at the emergency department, Dylan's vital signs are pulse 130, respirations 60, temperature 35.6°C (96.08°F), blood pressure 60/30. On examination, pallor is evident across the torso with slight circumoral cyanosis. These signs and symptoms are compatible with moderate hypothermia, and Dylan is admitted for observation and warming.

3. Generally, a 5-day-old infant with a working thermoregulatory feedback system would present within what acceptable range of core temperature?
4. Why might the nurse find pallor and circumoral cyanosis during her assessment of Dylan?

Accidental and Therapeutic Hypothermia

The term **accidental hypothermia** is used to designate situations in which an unintended fall in core temperature to hypothermic levels occurs. A systematic review of literature showed that the term *accidental hypothermia* was used most often to describe a situation outside the hospital, typically in association with exposure to cold or traumatic conditions.[28] This same review found that the term **inadvertent hypothermia** was used to refer to unintended heat loss in homes or institutional settings and often included vulnerable infants, ill individuals, or those with impaired thermoregulation. The term **iatrogenic hypothermia** or *nosocomial hypothermia* was used to designate the inadvertent heat loss associated with anesthesia, convective air flow, or evaporation of solutions from the skin during treatments.

Therapeutic hypothermia is the deliberate lowering of the body temperature to decrease the oxygen requirements of vital tissue, particularly those of the brain and heart. It has been most widely studied in hypothermic cardiac bypass surgery and ischemic disorders of the brain. Mild hypothermia (32–35°C) to protect neurons during ischemia was explored as early as the 1950s, particularly in situations in which surgery or trauma involving the brain induces edema.[29,30]

Etiology and Pathogenesis

It is not clinically useful to define hypothermia in terms of absolute body temperatures because the usual range and significance of a specific temperature vary with the age and condition of the individual. Instead, different groups of clinicians and rescue professionals have staged and developed standards of care for dealing with hypothermia. In perioperative or hemodialysis clinical settings, the need to assess hypothermia occurs frequently, either to prevent its occurrence or to monitor its effects when cooling is used as a therapeutic approach.[31–33] The American Society of Peri-Anesthesia Nursing defines hypothermia as a core temperature less than 36°C.[32,34] But clinicians in the field who rescue victims of severe accidental injury, avalanche, or near drowning must often deal with profoundly deep levels of hypothermia without having the monitoring and survival devices found in hospitals. To plan treatment, they seek criteria to specifically distinguish between levels of severity. The related recommendations and precautions for each level help to ensure that experts and volunteers in rescue follow the same guidelines. Among the experts, there remain a few inconsistencies in temperature ranges for hypothermia levels and medical approaches for individuals with severe hypothermia, but **Table 33.2** ■ reflects growing agreement on emergency treatments. In 2010, the European Resuscitation Council adopted the Swiss staging system.[35] They also caution that consciousness in a person after trauma or exposure to cold environments can be affected by causes other than hypothermia. For example, head injury, asphyxia, and intoxication from drugs or alcohol are frequently associated with accidents in snow or icy water.

CLINICAL POINT: Hypothermia is a potentially lethal complication of inadvertent heat loss. It can occur in many situations that may be unfamiliar to caregivers. Media coverage of accidental cold exposure when individuals are lost in the snow or at sea or experience near drowning in cold water has familiarized the public with the danger of hypothermia in extremely low temperatures. Less familiar to the public and health professionals alike are the risks of hypothermia that exist in milder temperatures when physiologic or behavioral thermoregulatory mechanisms are impaired. ■

Advanced age, lean body mass, and poor cardiovascular health are major risk factors that affect tolerance to temperature extremes. Healthy adults who usually maintain a core temperature of 36–38.5°C, may find a dive into an icy lake in celebration of winter a brisk but survivable lark if they get out quickly and warm up. Compensatory vasoconstriction, shivering, a rise in metabolic rate, protective insulation from body fat, and behavioral responses may not even cause a change in core temperature. However, a variety of conditions termed *cold shock* that are caused by sudden immersion in cold water can affect cognition, cause a gasp reflex and inability to hold one's breath, and quickly lead to the onset of hypothermia.[36] As in most strategies to treat thermal events, time is of the essence in preventing death or permanent injury.

An older adult who falls on a tile floor or pavement loses heat quickly and can become hypothermic even when in a temperate environment. Disturbing news that two U.S. deaths of older adults from hypothermia occurred in presumably supervised nursing home settings should alert caregivers that risk for vulnerable patients is not confined to extremes in environmental temperature.[37,38] ■

The paralyzed patient is at risk for hypothermia in mild temperature conditions as a result of the inability to move about, add bedcovers, or adjust the room temperature. Core temperatures of individuals with high spinal cord injury can vary with environmental conditions and may increase the risk for hypothermia.[39] When communication is impaired by a stroke, caregivers may attribute hypothermia-related slurred speech and loss of coordination to existing

Table 33.2 Different Classifications of Hypothermia Based on Core Temperature Ranges

Swiss Hypothermia Staging System				Danzl's Classification		Emergency Treatment	Support and Transfer
Stage	**Shivering**	**LOC**	**Temperature range**	**Classification**	**Temperature range**		
I	Yes	Conscious	32–35°C	Mild	34–35°C	• Encourage active movement • Give warm oral fluids • Insulate body	• Move to nearest emergency facility
II	No	Impaired	28–32°C	Moderate	30–34°C	• Gently remove from site and immobilize • Insulate entire body • Apply heat packs to trunk • Administer O_2 • Establish IV line	• Do not delay transport • If circulation is stable, move to hospital with active rewarming resources • If circulation is unstable, move to hospital with ECMO or CPB
III	No	Unconscious	24–28°C	Severe (deep)	17–30°C	• Previous actions plus upper airway support • Hypothermia slows drug metabolism • Avoid depolarizing paralytic agents (such as succinylcholine) • Limited use of vasopressors or other life-support drugs that could induce dysrhythmias	• Do not delay transport • If circulation is stable, move to hospital with active rewarming resource • If circulation is unstable, move to hospital with ECMO or CPB
IV	No	0 vital signs	< 24°C	Profound	< 17°C	• Add CPR to above actions • Avoid excessive attempts to defibrillate	• Move to hospital with ECMO or CPB

CPB = cardiopulmonary bypass, CPR = cardiopulmonary resuscitation, ECMO = extracorporeal membrane oxygenation, LOC = level of consciousness.

SOURCE: Data from Brugger, H., Durrer, B., Elsensohn, F., Paal, P., Strapazzon, G., Winterberger, E., Zafren, K., Boyd, J., & Icar, M. Resuscitation of avalanche victims: Evidence-based guidelines of the International Commission for Mountain Emergency Medicine (ICAR MEDCOM): Intended for physicians and other advanced life support personnel. *Resuscitation*, *84*(5), 539–546; Danzl, D. F., & Pozos, R. S. (1994). Accidental hypothermia. *New England Journal of Medicine*, *331*(26), 1756–1760.

musculoskeletal impairment. Individuals with hypothyroidism generate less heat from metabolic processes and are at higher risk of hypothermia in cool surroundings. Those with diabetes are also at risk because they are less able to compensate for the insulin resistance that accompanies hypothermia.[40] Hypothermia is a frequent complication of vehicular accidents or other traumatic injuries and plays a role in the so-called lethal triad of hypothermia, acidosis, and disrupted coagulation, which often result in death.[41] In addition to the immediate hazards of hypothermia, there is clear evidence that incidents of accidental hypothermia are associated with immunosuppression and increased likelihood of infection.[42,43] **Figure 33.4** ■ illustrates some of the many effects of hypothermia on the human body.

A number of drugs, including anesthesia, analgesics, narcotics, tranquilizers, and vasodilators, promote heat loss and raise the risk for hypothermia. Alcohol intoxication not only alters judgment about cold exposure, but is also accompanied by vasodilation and hypoglycemia.[44] Cannabis lowers the thermoregulatory set point limit that induces hypothermia,[45] and hypothermia often complicates heroin overdose.[46] Drugs such as the phenothiazines affect central hypothalamic activity and autonomic responses and promote hypothermia. Many psychotropic drugs (serotonin-2 antagonists, $alpha_1$ receptor–blocking agents, haloperidol, lithium, benzodiazepines, and tricyclic antidepressants) also increase the risk for hypothermia.[47]

CLINICAL POINT: Standards of care in perioperative and newborn care have been developed to reduce the threat of inadvertent heat loss. In both settings, radiant heat, polyethylene wraps, and warmed surroundings have been used to maintain the thermal balance of infants with impaired or undeveloped thermoregulatory capacity.[48] ■

Babies who are born en route to a hospital are at high risk of hypothermia and may need treatment during transport by emergency vehicles.[49] Low-birth-weight neonates are particularly at risk for several reasons. Their thin skin and subcutaneous tissue provide poor insulation from heat loss, and their flaccid positions do little to conserve heat. They have lower amounts of brown adipose tissue deposits, which are therefore less able to support nonshivering thermogenesis.[16] In addition, the metabolic activity required to convert brown adipose tissue into heat requires extra oxygen, so the cold-stressed infant often experiences respiratory distress when exposed to unwarmed environmental air. ■

Therapeutic hypothermia is increasingly used in field survival approaches for stroke, heart attack, traumatic brain injury, and heat stroke.[5] Hypothermic temperatures were found to reduce both swelling and neuronal O_2 demand, leading to improved survival outcomes.[50] Techniques vary with the specific disorder and organs at risk. They include cooling at the recovery scene or in transport with an IV bolus of ice-cold saline, endovascular cooling catheters, and newly developed surface cooling devices. While therapeutic

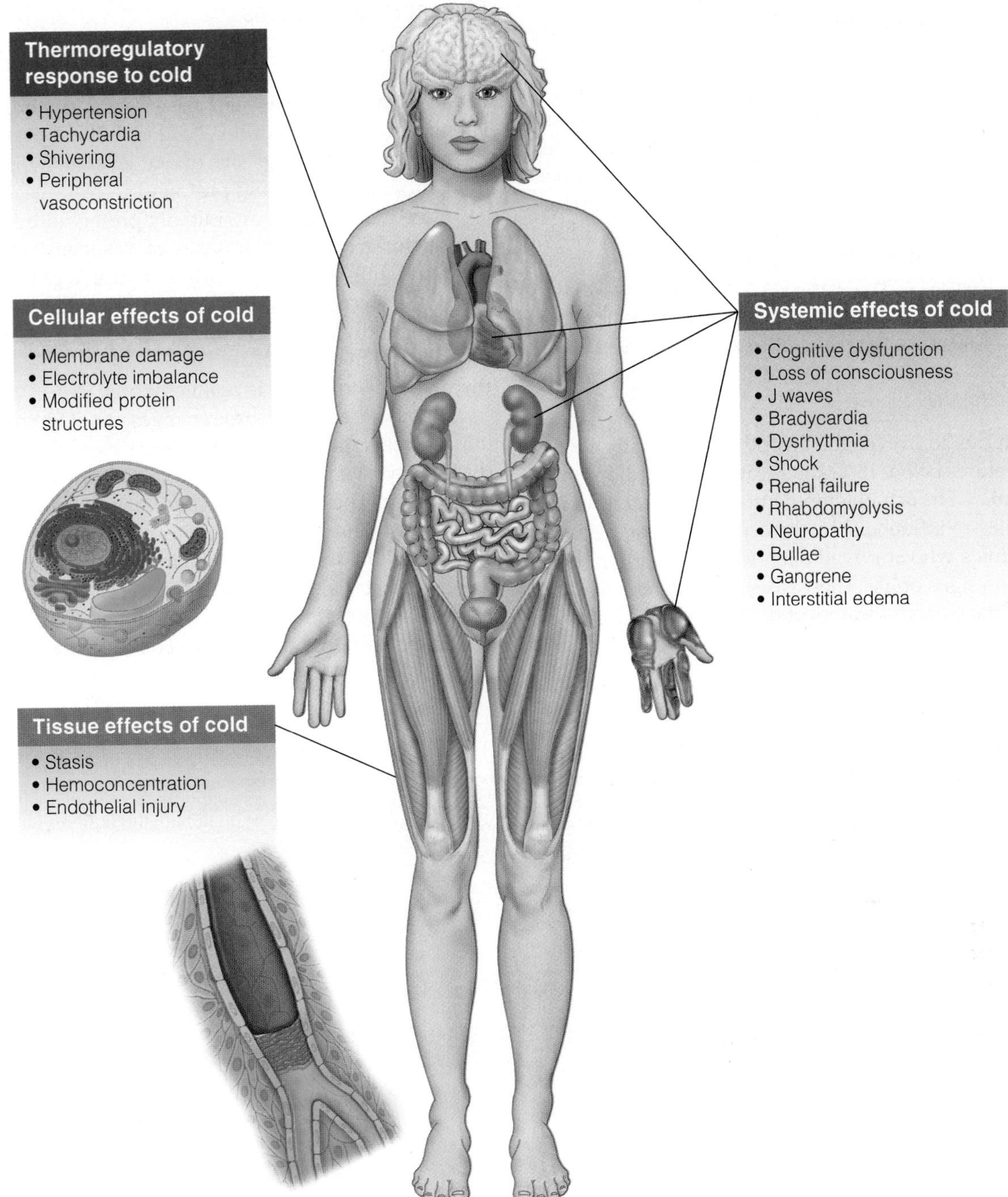

Figure 33.4 ■ Cold-induced injuries such as hypothermia and frostbite lead to thermoregulatory response (e.g., shivering, increased sympathetic activity), cellular and tissue effects (e.g., membrane damage, electrolyte imbalance, endothelial injury, thrombosis), and systemic effects (e.g., shock, arrhythmia, neuromuscular dysfunction).

hypothermia offers cellular protection in situations of cardiac arrest and open heart or brain surgery, it is accompanied by the same systemic changes and potential hazards as are seen in accidental hypothermia; that is, the individual becomes poikilothermic and unable to control body temperature from drifting downward.

The difference in survival between therapeutic and accidental hypothermia is the ability to monitor and support cardiopulmonary and cardiac electrical function with drugs and mechanical means when necessary. Despite this benefit, close surveillance is required during and after the procedure for signs of cardiac irritability and dysrhythmias during rewarming stages. Shivering after anesthesia and neuromuscular blocking agents have worn off poses a severe metabolic toll and energy expenditure. The increased demand for O_2 may be poorly tolerated by the individual after cardiac or neurologic surgery. Shivering suppression by the analgesic medication meperidine is not always effective, particularly when the individual has been cooled to hypothermic levels by cardiopulmonary bypass (CPB).[51]

CLINICAL POINT: Experts in rescuing victims of hypothermia say that because of primitive conditions or lack of monitoring equipment in the field, it is often impossible to get accurate core temperatures Therefore, they rely on associated signs to determine the severity of hypothermia. The Commission for Mountain Emergency Medicine bases its classification on decline of general body function combined with core temperatures: (1) mild hypothermia (32–35°C) designates an individual who is still conscious and able to move about; (2) moderate hypothermia (28–32°C) is reserved for an individual with altered consciousness, inability to shiver, and abnormal cardiac rhythms; (3) severe hypothermia (< 28°C) is used to describe an individual who has become unconscious and progresses from ventricular fibrillation to asystole; (4) apparent death (24–15°C) describes an individual who shows no usual signs of life but who might possibly be resuscitated with cardiopulmonary support. ■

Death due to irreversible hypothermia usually occurs at temperatures below 15°C and is caused by cardiopulmonary failure.[36] The actual temperatures that are considered irreversible are influenced by the occasional case histories of individuals who survived deep to profound hypothermia with no signs of life. These cases serve to remind clinicians that the usual indicators of death cannot be assumed in these conditions.

Clinical Manifestations

As body temperatures decline, the systemic effects of hypothermia are seen in four areas: core temperature decline, metabolic and acid–base changes, respiratory and cardiovascular signs, and neurologic signs. **Table 33.3** ■ outlines these systemic effects for each of four levels of hypothermia: mild, moderate, deep, and profound.[4]

Core temperatures are initially preserved by the thermoeffector warming responses of vasoconstriction and shivering, but the brain's central control is gradually lost with each succeeding stage. By the moderate hypothermia stage, the individual is confused and no longer perceiving the cold and may actually begin undressing. In deep hypothermia, the individual is poikilothermic.

Metabolic and acid–base changes in mild hypothermia initially reflect responses to the rising basal metabolic rate (BMR), hyperventilation-induced respiratory alkalosis, and hypocapnia. The renal tubules become resistant to arginine vasopressin and diuresis depletes both water and potassium, resulting in hypokalemia, increased thickness of the blood, and stasis of blood flow. Onset of moderate hypothermia suppresses BMR and respiration, inducing a progressive respiratory acidosis. Decreased renal blood flow

Table 33.3 Multisystem Effects of Hypothermia

Metabolism and Acid–Base Alterations	Respiratory and Perfusion Alterations	Sensory Perception, Cognition, and Intracranial Regulation Alterations
Mild hypothermia: Core temperature 32–35°C		
• Increased BMR, 3–5 times normal • Respiratory-induced alkalosis and hypocapnia • Cold-induced diuresis from ADH resistance • Increased blood viscosity • Increased potassium excretion leading to hypokalemia	• Hyperventilation • Increased VO_{2max} • Peripheral vasoconstriction • Increased BP, HR, and CO • Cyanosis • Intravascular sludging and coagulopathy	• Sensation of cold • Agitation • Clumsiness • Dysarthria • Confusion • Disorientation • Vigorous shivering
Moderate hypothermia: Core temperature 28–32°C		
• Decreased BMR • Progressive respiratory acidosis • Fluid shifts to third space • Decreased renal blood flow • Decreased tubular capacity for H^+ ion secretion leading to metabolic acidosis and hyperkalemia • Glycemic autoregulation impaired	• Shallow respirations • Decreased VO_{2max} • At 30°C, there is a 50% fall in VO_{2max} and VCO_2 • BP may be undetectable • ECG may show J waves and premature ventricular beats • At 32°C, prolonged asystole with decreases in HR, CO, and cerebral blood flow • Atrial and ventricular dysrhythmias can lead to a 50% decrease in HR and CO	• Stupor • Delirium • No shivering • Exaggerated tendon reflex and hyperactivity • At 30°C, paradoxical undressing and burrowing activity may occur • Muscle rigidity
Deep hypothermia: Core temperature 17–28°C		
• Progressive worsening of acidosis • Shivering-induced lactic acidosis contributes to accumulating CO_2 from respiratory failure	• Erythema and edema • Pulse is undetectable • Decreased stroke volume • ECG shows decreased cardiac conduction • At 27–30°C, there is cardiac irritability and increased risk of arrhythmias • Below 27°C, atrial fibrillation is common • Ventricular fibrillation may cause death • Below 25°C, apnea	• Loss of thermoregulation • Absent muscle reflexes • At 26°C, muscle rigidity is absent • Decreased nerve conduction • Decreased reflexes • Pupils fixed and dilated • At 19°C, loss of brain activity with flat EEG waves
Profound hypothermia: Core temperature less than 17°C		
• Respiratory and metabolic acidosis • Hyperkalemia • Decreased renal blood flow	• At 10°C, QRS complex disappears on ECG while P waves may remain visible • Asystole	• Absent neurologic reflexes • Absent muscular activity • Appearance of death

BMR = basal metabolic rate, BP = blood pressure, CO = cardiac output, ECG = electrocardiogram, EEG = electroencephalogram, HR = heart rate.

results in decreased hydrogen ion and potassium excretion, leading to metabolic acidosis and hyperkalemia. Control of blood glucose levels is impaired. In deep hypothermia, respiratory acidosis progresses. Renal failure worsens, and associated metabolic acidosis progresses. Lactic acidosis develops from shivering.

Respiratory and cardiovascular signs in mild hypothermia are usually caused by warming responses of vasoconstriction to conserve heat and hyperventilation to provide O_2 to shivering muscles. Increased sympathetic nervous system stimulation raises heart rate, blood pressure, and cardiac output. Moderate hypothermia suppresses respiratory drive and vasomotor activity, leading to a fall in cardiac output, heart rate, and blood pressure. The myocardium becomes irritable and cardiac dysrhythmias can occur. Osborne waves (**Figure 33.5** ■), which are also called J waves because its deflection creates an inverted dome after the QRS complex in the electrocardiogram, occur in about 80% of hypothermic individuals, although it can be seen in other cardiac conditions in individuals who are not hypothermic.[52]

Neurologic signs of mild hypothermia begin with a strong sensation of heat loss, agitation, and neurobehavioral responses to generate heat. As hypothermia progresses, the individual becomes clumsy, confused, and disoriented. In moderate hypothermia, stupor and delirium develop, and shivering subsides. There are exaggerated tendon reflexes, muscle rigidity, and hyperactivity. Bizarre undressing behaviors while outdoors or even in snow and burrowing under furniture have also been noted.[53] In deep hypothermia, thermoregulatory responses are absent, and the individual is poikilothermic. At the lowest temperatures, the pupils become fixed and dilated. Because hypothermia effectively slows metabolic processes and lowers O_2 requirements for cell survival, induced or therapeutic hypothermia has increasingly been adopted as an adjunct to treatment.[54] One important factor to remember about hypothermia, whether incidental, accidental, or therapeutic, is its ability to render the individual poikilothermic. Therefore, when temperatures drop from the initial cooling, they will continue to drop if the person's temperature is not controlled externally.

Linking Pathophysiology to Diagnosis and Treatment

Among the issues in diagnosing and treating accidental hypothermia are those about whether to institute cardiopulmonary resuscitation before or after transport to a medical facility. The primary factor in this decision is based on weighing the metabolically induced oxygen debt from hypoxia and shivering with the irritability of the extremely cold myocardium. Cardiac irritability constitutes one of the most serious hazards of treatment, and the risk for dysrhythmia increases in a specific range of core temperatures. Raising the core temperature of a severely hypothermic person to 28°C, may actually induce temperature-related irritability of the heart because atrial fibrillation occurs at 28°C.[4] As the patient rewarms to 30°C, accumulations of pooled lactic acid enter the circulation and produce acidosis. In addition, ventricular fibrillation related to cardiac hyperirritability during hypothermia is triggered by rough handling or vagal stimulation associated with cardiopulmonary resuscitation that involves chest compression. Similar risks occur with intubation and associated airway trauma. The decision to transport is therefore a crucial step in emergency care of hypothermia. If the victim manifests signs of moderate to profound hypothermia, transport is crucial, and the

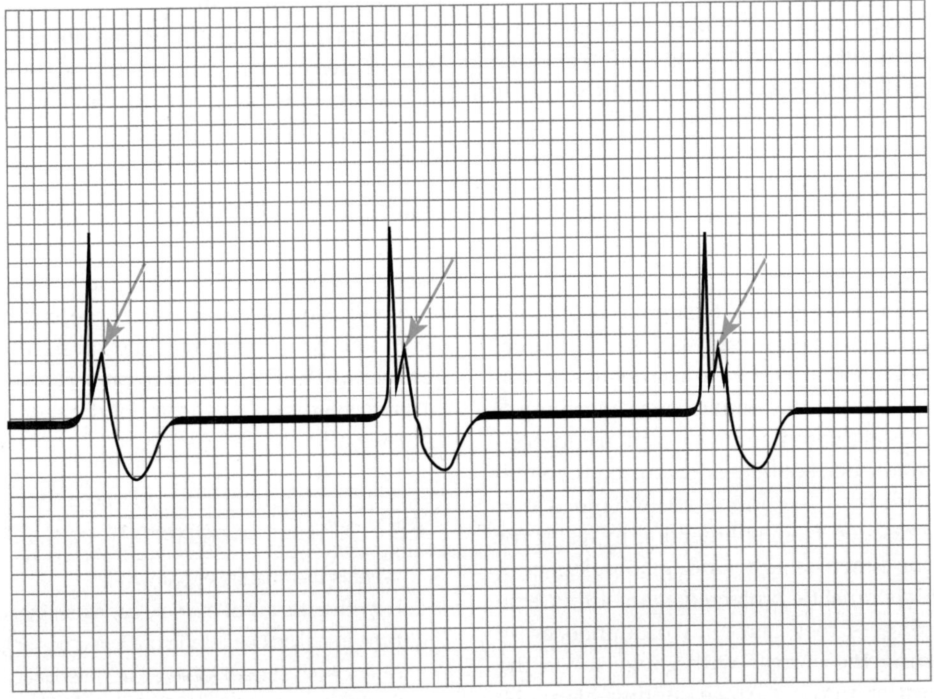

Figure 33.5 ■ ECG showing Osborne waves, also known as J waves.

profoundly hypothermic person will need the technologic benefit of CPB, which is available at a well-equipped emergency center. During transport, gentle handling and warm dry clothing are needed. If warming is indicated, the basic preliminary approach involves warm fluid infusions and warm humidified air. As forced air-warming devices, electric resistive heating devices, or radiant heated beds become available, they should be employed.

CLINICAL POINT: It is crucial to call emergency services when an individual is found in cold surroundings and is hypothermic and nonresponsive. Attempts to warm, intubate, or otherwise stimulate the person may induce dysrhythmias or ventricular fibrillation. Emergency responders should be ready to give cardiorespiratory support if these complications occur.[36] ■

Dylan Shubert: Outcome

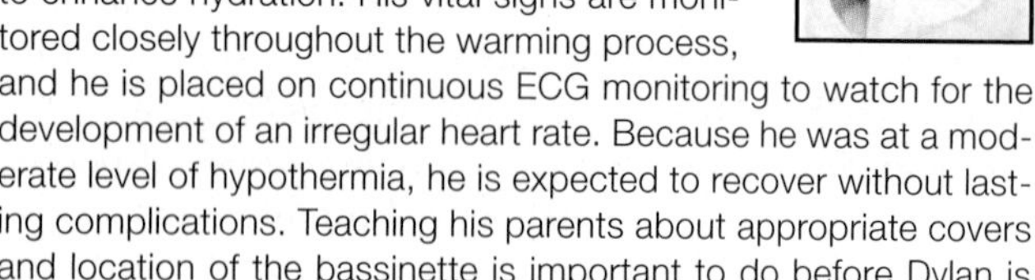

Dylan is placed in a warming incubator to counter hypothermia and provided intravenous fluids to enhance hydration. His vital signs are monitored closely throughout the warming process, and he is placed on continuous ECG monitoring to watch for the development of an irregular heart rate. Because he was at a moderate level of hypothermia, he is expected to recover without lasting complications. Teaching his parents about appropriate covers and location of the bassinette is important to do before Dylan is discharged.

5. Dylan's hypothermia would most likely be classified as what type?
6. Dylan's parents will be taught why putting the bassinette by the window can result in convective heat loss. Define convective heat loss.

Frostbite

Etiology and Pathogenesis

Frostbite is a familiar phenomenon that most people associate with exposure to freezing temperatures. In this situation, frozen extracellular fluids form ice crystals that injure and disrupt the osmotic gradient across cell membranes, causing water to move from the cells into the extracellular fluid. This increases the concentration of electrolytes in the cells, which initiates cell death.[55] As temperatures fall further, intracellular fluids freeze, and their expansion mechanically destroys cells.[56]

However, frostbite is not limited to situations of freezing temperature and is more reasonably defined as a spectrum of injury severities that range from irreversible cell death of tissue to reversible conditions from rewarming.[45] Frostbite-like injuries are common in the military in nonfreezing temperatures when soldiers are required to march for long periods with their feet immersed in cold water, in people who are rescued from submersion in water for extended periods, and increasingly among homeless people.[55, 57–59] Individuals must be protected against this type of tissue injury to fingers, toes, and bony prominences by wrapping or padding these areas with gauze when the person is placed on or under surface cooling blankets. Frostbite-like injury can occur at temperatures above freezing and is partially explained by the involvement of two mechanisms leading to tissue injury: cell death from cold exposure and tissue necrosis from progressive dermal ischemia.

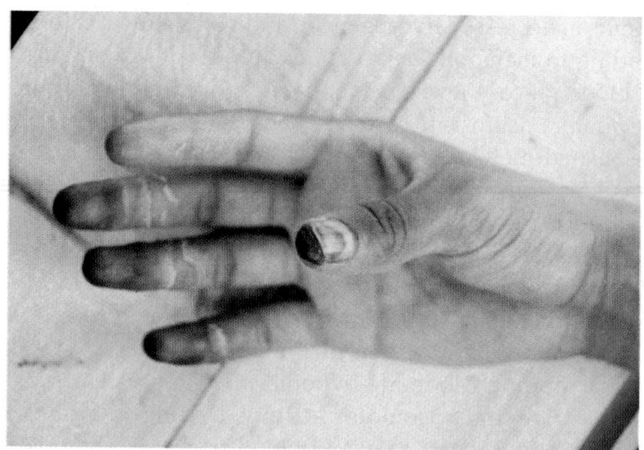

Figure 33.6 ■ Frostbite on fingers after 2 weeks. White, waxy skin turns black as the top layer comes off.

Physiologic responses to tissue cooling are alternate vasoconstriction and vasodilation that leads to cycles of thaw and refreezing that promote progressive thrombosis. Anticoagulants such as heparin and efforts to promote vasodilation with drugs or sympathetic stimulation are not always successful, so other factors may be involved in the progressive dermal ischemia. The similarity of frostbite to burn injury raises the possibility that the same mediators are involved (e.g., prostaglandins, thromboxanes, bradykinin, histamines).[55]

Clinical Manifestations

Like burns, frostbite can be classified by degree of injury. First-degree frostbite appears as hard white plaque; second-degree frostbite has clear fluid in superficial blisters; and third-degree frostbite presents with purple fluid in deep blisters with discolored skin (**Figure 33.6** ■).[56]

Linking Pathophysiology to Diagnosis and Treatment

The diagnosis of frostbite is based on the appearance of the skin and a history of exposure to cold. Treatment is based on reperfusion of viable tissue, keeping the frostbitten area clean, and preventing mechanical injury. Hyperbaric oxygen therapy has been used to preserve fingers and toes with variable success, and thrombolytic therapy is employed to improve affected circulation.[60]

Check Your Progress: Section 33.4

1. What is therapeutic hypothermia?
2. Hypothermia is not the only condition that can lead to alterations in consciousness in cold weather or cold water immersion. Name at least three other potential causes.
3. Explain how frostbite is diagnosed and treated.

33.5 Fever

One of the most prevalent deviations in body temperature, **fever** is defined as an elevation of body temperature due to an increase in core temperature set point. Unfortunately, this definition has led caregivers and the public to view fever in terms of its thermal consequence alone. Failure to recognize that the elevated body temperature in fever is an effect rather than the cause of febrile illness leads caregivers to erroneously try to cool down the febrile patient. Fear of fever is likely the result of centuries of tradition and lack of information about what actually causes fever to occur. Fever is a systemic host response to potentially harmful antigens that is generated in part to the vasoconstriction and shivering during fever's preliminary phase. By attempting to cool the body when the elevated set point is already sensing a chill, these measures promote further shivering and generate more heat.

Research in the past few decades not only has elucidated the molecular mechanisms of fever, but also has identified specific immunologic benefits from the rising temperature.[61,62] Of course, it is not always obvious whether the rising temperature is due to fever or one of the hyperthermias that require artificial cooling. For that reason, better understanding of fever's clinical manifestations, interventions that support beneficial responses, and vigilant monitoring of rising temperatures are essential. As a metabolically active process, fever requires supportive fluids, calories, and oxygen. Cooling the patient is counterproductive because it promotes shivering, raises oxygen consumption, and causes physical distress.[63] Vasoconstriction during this phase can cause patients to complain of numbness in their fingers and toes.

Etiology and Pathogenesis

Another misunderstood factor related to fever reflects unawareness that the temperature is regulated by hypothalamic control in response to an elevated thermoregulatory set point. The set point elevation is caused by a pyrogen that causes the body to release a cascade of pro-inflammatory mediators that affect temperature and cause malaise, aches, and a sick feeling. These symptoms are not due to the rising temperature.

CLINICAL POINT: Because thermoregulation is intact in a person with fever, cooling the body will trigger compensatory shivering and vasoconstriction and will raise core temperatures even higher.[20] ■

Fever should not be referred to as, or confused with, hyperthermia, which is a condition in which body temperature is unregulated.

Contrary to popular belief, fever is not directly produced by infectious disease or foreign substances associated with the febrile response. Fevers of bacterial, fungal, and viral origin and those caused by foreign bodies, blood transfusions, and immune responses are only indirectly generated by pyrogens. A **pyrogen** is any agent that causes fever. Even injury, inflammation, necrosis, and stress only indirectly cause the febrile response. These are exogenous pyrogens and elicit a systemic host response that causes the individual's own cells to release pro-inflammatory substances that produce a cascade of biochemical, immune, and autonomic reactions (**Figure 33.7** ■).

Fever is induced by pro-inflammatory cytokines that act as endogenous pyrogens. Cytokines are immunoregulatory proteins produced by phagocytes, fibroblasts, and endothelial cells. The cytokines most closely linked with fever are interleukin 1 (IL-1), interleukin 6 (IL-6), and tumor necrosis factor alpha (TNF-α).[62] Prostaglandin E_2 is the key fever mediator thought to be responsible for shifting the set point upward, regardless of the source of the pyrogen.[64]

Body temperature elevation is only one of the physiologic and acute phase effects of the febrile response. Fever is catabolic, with IL-1, IL-2, and TNF-α leading to protein breakdown and contributing to negative nitrogen balance and anemia. Catabolism is promoted by disrupted lipid metabolism and gluconeogenesis. Among the most distressing consequences for the febrile individual are muscle aches, headache, and feelings of malaise, which are not related to temperature elevations but instead are attributable to the molecular activities of circulating pro-inflammatory cytokines.[29]

Despite these seemingly negative responses, the febrile response brings about molecular, cellular, and subjective responses that are believed to have survival benefit by enhancing leukocyte mobility, stimulating bactericidal and antitumor activity, and transforming lymphocytes.[62,65,66] Higher core temperature ranges during fever not only are optimal for antimicrobial host defenses, but also are accompanied by changes in trace mineral levels (declines in serum iron and zinc levels and an increase in copper levels) that suggest survival benefits.[62,65] The lower serum iron level inhibits bacterial replication but only at febrile temperature levels.[67] Finally, even the feelings of fatigue, loss of appetite, and lethargy associated with fever are thought to have some survival benefit by decreasing energy expenditure needed for physical activity and food metabolism.[68]

In fever, thermoregulatory responses are functional but are operating at higher temperature limits; the upper limits of the thermoeffector threshold zone are reset to a higher core temperature. In fact, there is considerable evidence that the body produces several endogenous antipyretics called cryogens that include steroid hormones, neuropeptides, cytokines, and other molecules.[62] Evolving science from the past quarter of a century demonstrates the power of these endogenous cryogens to keep the elevation of body temperature during fever from exceeding a safe upper limit.[62,66]

CLINICAL POINT: Realization that there are endogenous physiologic factors working to maintain temperatures within safe ranges should not give caregivers a casual disregard for the brain's sensitivity to high core temperatures. Cautious surveillance of rising temperatures and constant attention to the possibility of conditions leading to hyperthermia are always prudent. ■

Clinical Manifestations

Evidence of intact thermoregulatory function during fever is manifested by warming and cooling responses as the set point rises and falls, from initial chills and shivering

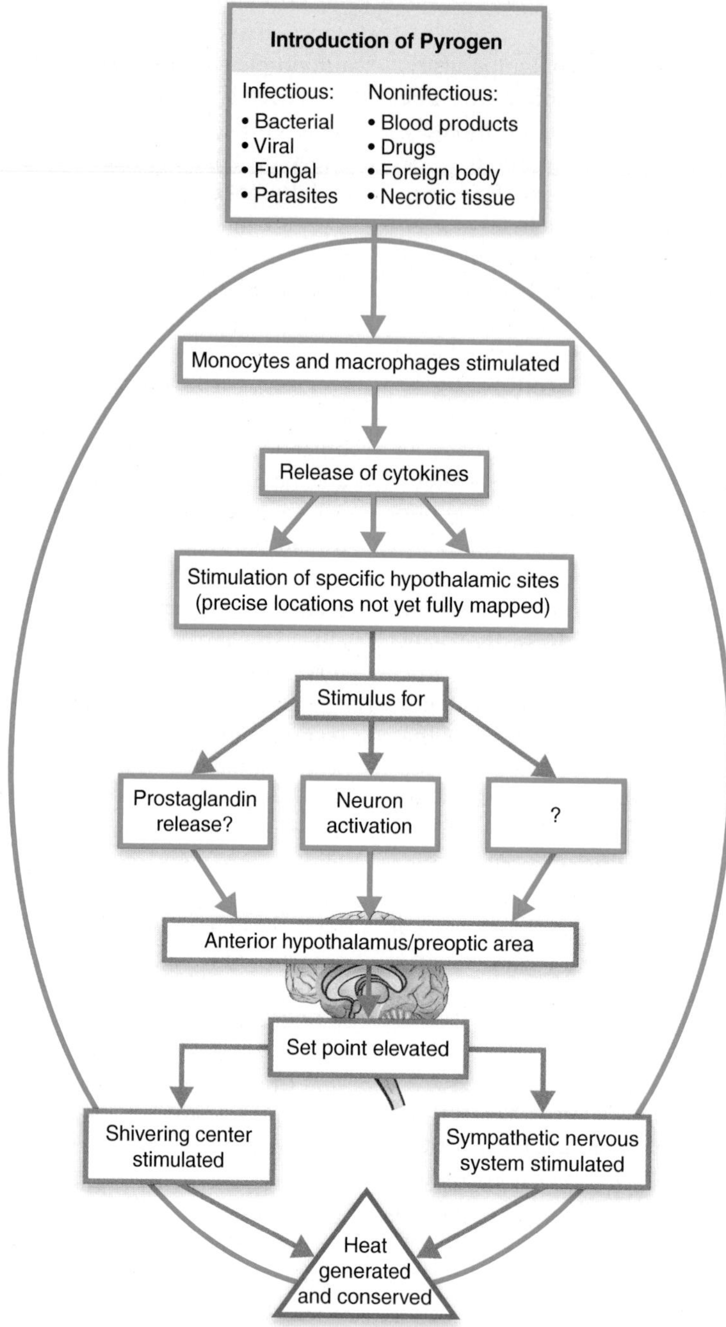

Figure 33.7 ■ Cytokine release and fever. At the molecular level, cytokines induce a regulated rise in body temperature. This means that thermoregulatory mechanisms work but at a higher level. While the precise mechanisms are still not all known, cytokines are thought to stimulate specific sites in the hypothalamus that initiate prostaglandin release and neuron activation in the preoptic area of the anterior hypothalamus. ? = other mechanisms are currently being studied.

until febrile core temperatures are reached, to sweating and diaphoresis when cytokine levels fall. The temperature elevations that accompany fever occur in three distinct phases (**Figure 33.8** ■). The familiar **chill phase** is marked by mild to severe shivering, vasoconstriction, and an uncomfortable sense of cold. Thermoregulatory responses in the chill phase generate and conserve heat to adjust the body temperature to the new higher set point. The **plateau phase** occurs when body temperature reaches the new set point and thermoregulatory warming responses are no

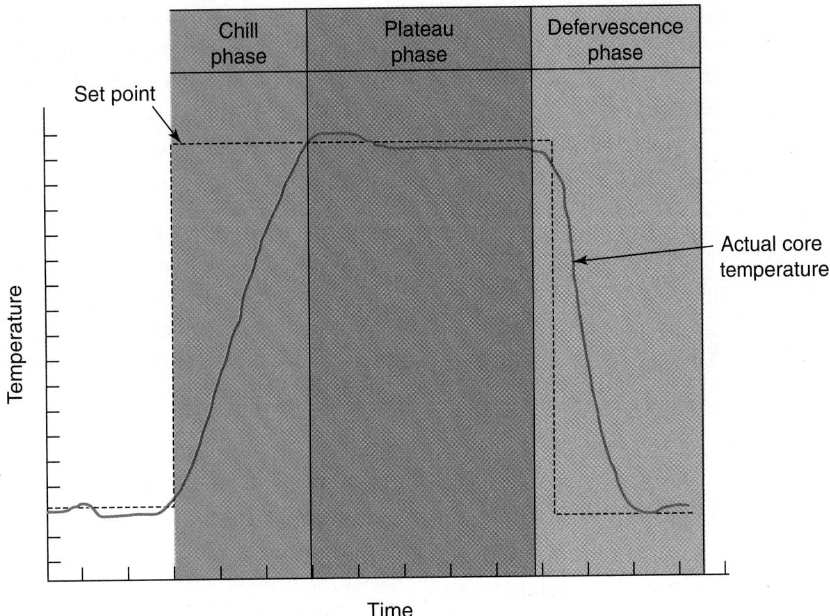

Figure 33.8 ■ The three phases of fever. This schematic shows the typical febrile episode, which is typified by three phases and closely associated with cytokine levels. When they rise, they induce the chill phase, causing the body temperature to rise to the new thermoneutral range. Even when the core temperature is 38.5°C, if the set point moves higher, the person will shiver and feel cold. This is the phase in which febrile shivering is most likely to occur. The plateau phase follows, in which chills stop and the warm body temperature is not particularly distressful. When the cytokine levels fall, so does the set point level, and the warm body temperature becomes unbearably hot. The patient kicks off the covers but is still sensitive to abrupt temperature changes. A draft or cool bath may elicit more shivering.

longer stimulated. The **defervescence phase** occurs when the pyrogen level subsides, the set point stabilizes to lower levels, and febrile temperatures feel uncomfortably hot. Sweating becomes profuse, and the individual complains of feeling hot.

Alexandra Holloway: Application

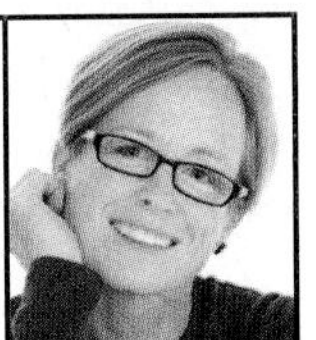

On admission to the emergency department, Mrs. Holloway tells the healthcare provider that she thinks she is having a reaction to something she ate at the potluck dinner. Her temperature is 38.9°C (102°F), but she is still shaking and feeling chilled. Her symptoms included rebound abdominal tenderness and rigidity, fever, confusion, dyspnea, and muscle aches. The healthcare provider orders comprehensive laboratory testing and finds that Mrs. Holloway's blood count is elevated to 20,000/mm^3 (normal: 5,000–10,000/mm^3). The healthcare provider determines that Mrs. Holloway is suffering from acute appendicitis.

3. Why might Mrs. Holloway's healthcare provider have ordered a comprehensive blood count?
4. Describe the three phases of temperature elevation that accompany fever.

Linking the Pathophysiology to Treatment

The simplified roadmap shown in Figure 33.3 is designed to help caregivers predict responses to heat loss and heat gain. These expected responses should underlie interventions for fever. As was previously discussed, to maintain the narrow thermoneutral set point range of about half a degree higher or lower than 38.5°C, thermoreceptors are constantly monitoring the internal body temperature. The external body temperature is monitored by neurons in the skin. In fever, the pyrogen elevates the set point, so existing temperatures are sensed as too cool. This is why the first noticeable symptoms at the onset of fever are a chill and vasoconstriction; shivering is triggered to warm the body. Vigorous shivering or shaking chills are promoted by cooling the febrile individual and will further elevate the temperature by shivering thermogenesis.[63] While it is tempting to cool the individual when temperatures rise to febrile levels and individuals begin to sweat, caution is advised. Cutaneous neurons remain highly sensitive to heat loss during fever, and rapid cooling, drafts, or applications of cold can cause shivering to resume.[69]

Alexandra Holloway: Outcome

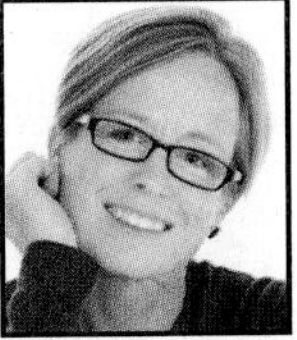

Mrs. Holloway is scheduled for a laparoscopic appendectomy. The surgery is uneventful, and the inflamed appendix is removed. A single dose of antibiotic is administered prophylactically, and Mrs. Holloway's temperature returns to normal within 24 hours after surgery. She is discharged home the day after the surgery.

5. After surgery, Mrs. Holloway's temperature returned to normal within 24 hours. What should normal be for her?
6. What is the rationale for prescribing only a single antibiotic dose for Mrs. Holloway after surgery?

Check Your Progress: Section 33.5

1. As fever is a metabolically active process, what interventions does it require?
2. Why is cooling a patient with a fever counterproductive?
3. Name at least three consequences of fever that are distressing to the individual.

33.6 Hyperthermia

Hyperthermia is a potentially lethal condition that should not be confused with fever. Unlike fever's regulated rise in temperature, **hyperthermia** involves dysfunctional thermoregulatory mechanisms and an unregulated temperature elevation. This hypermetabolic state is most frequently caused by exertional heat illness, exertional **rhabdomyolysis** (a breakdown of muscle tissue that releases damaging toxic intracellular substances into circulating blood), or malignant hyperthermia.[70] Occasionally, individuals with direct damage to thermoregulatory control centers in the brain develop hyperthermia. However, aggressive therapies in these cases often make it difficult to determine whether the origin of the temperature rise was hyperthermia or fever from underlying sepsis.

Etiology and Pathogenesis

Heat stress is defined as the point at which the net heat load to which a person is exposed begins to overcome the body's means of controlling it. Heat stress is associated with several conditions known as heat-related illnesses. Heat-related illnesses may begin with excessive sweating, tachypnea, and tachycardia and may progress along a continuum of severity of heat cramps, heat edema, syncope, heat exhaustion, and heat stroke.[71]

These conditions are common among military troops, athletes, and hikers who engage in excessive physical activity under hot humid conditions. Each year, there are numerous cases of exertional heat-related illness reported during marathons, football workouts, and basic military training.[71–73] Heat-related illnesses also occur to sedentary individuals who engage in physical exertion in warm weather. Individuals who are unable to cool their environmental temperature in hot weather, for physical or financial reasons, are at risk for heat stress.

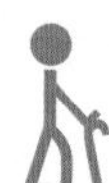

The risk for heat stress increases with age in older adults who reside in warm climates without air conditioning, particularly if they are not well hydrated.[74] ■

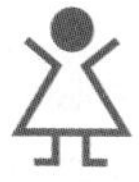

Full-term infants have limited ability to adapt to warmth by vasodilation and cannot cope physiologically with the intense heat in summer if they are left unattended for even a few minutes in a closed, parked automobile. Deaths from this cause are documented each year despite warnings in the media. Overheating a wrapped infant in a warm room, with artificial bedwarmers, and even in a hospital incubator with faulty controls,[75] are causes of death tied to heat stress in infants. ■

Clinical Manifestations

The clinical manifestations associated with heat-related illnesses increase in severity along the heat stress continuum. They range from excessive sweating, tachypnea, and tachycardia at the least severe end of the continuum to heat stroke at the most severe end of the continuum.

Heat exhaustion begins with malaise, headache, and nausea. While this disorder is a milder form of heat-related illness than heat stroke, it is considered to be on the same continuum. If the core temperature is under 38.9°C and individuals are treated early with fluid and electrolyte replacement, a cool environment, rest, and close surveillance, symptoms of heat exhaustion may resolve within 20–30 minutes.[71] If symptoms do not resolve, or neurologic impairment occurs, the individual should be considered and treated as a victim of heat stroke. Water depletion, sodium depletion, or both are common in heat exhaustion and may lead to circulatory collapse. Hyponatremia may occur when the individual overhydrates by drinking copious amounts of water without electrolytes. Hyponatremia-related CNS symptoms, such as dizziness and confusion, can progress to seizures and death.[71]

Heat stroke is an uncompensated conflict between homeostatic thermoregulatory drives to lose heat by increasing skin blood flow and cardiovascular drives to maintain blood pressure.[65] Loss of thermoregulatory control in heat exhaustion or heat shock can allow core temperatures to rise to levels above 41.2°C, at which neural damage, coma, and death result from protein catabolism, rhabdomyolysis, microthrombi, and coagulative necrosis of vital tissues, cerebral edema, confusion, and convulsions.[61] Physiologic changes caused by hyperthermia have been demonstrated by cellular studies in animals.[66] Neural polyribosomes begin to break down at temperatures between 40°C and 42°C, and irreversible destruction of cerebral mitochondria begins at 41.2°C.

Robert Warfield: Application

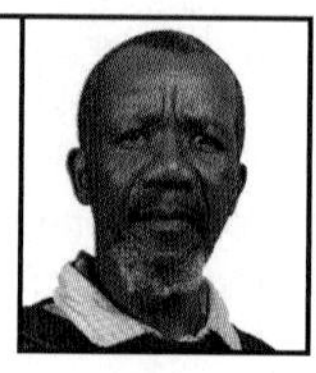

On admission to the emergency department, Mr. Warfield is unconscious, and his vital signs are pulse 156, respirations 46, rectal temperature 40°C (104°F), blood pressure 72/48 His skin is dry and hot to the touch, and his respirations are labored. A plan is instituted to reduce Mr. Warfield's core temperature by at least 0.2°C/min to approximately 39°C, with care not to induce cooling too suddenly so as to avoid iatrogenic hypothermia.

Because Mr. Warfield's admission temperature is 40°C, neurologic system signs and symptoms are expected. Mr. Warfield has poor skin turgor on physical examination as well as other indications of hypovolemia (tachycardia, tachypnea, and hypotension), which may be related to poor fluid intake. It is determined that Mr. Warfield has mild heart failure, for which he is taking diuretics, which might account for an increased renal fluid loss. The high heat, humidity, and lack of air circulation along with his hypovolemia and absence of sweating suggest hyperthermia. Subsequent comprehensive laboratory testing and imaging studies are able to rule out cardiac, endocrine, and infectious causes of his symptoms.

3. What is iatrogenic hypothermia?
4. Why is it important to make sure that Mr. Warfield's core temperature does not rise above 41.2°C?

Linking Pathophysiology to Diagnosis and Treatment

The pathophysiology and symptoms of heat exhaustion are a reflection of the severe depletion of body water and resulting loss of circulating fluid volume. It frequently is the result of overexertion in a hot environment. The patient may manifest heavy sweating, excessive thirst, nausea, bradycardia, weakness, and dizziness. Temperatures rise to 38.9°C or greater. In heat exhaustion, the pathology can be viewed as an overtaxing of a functional thermoregulatory system in a hot environment. If heat exhaustion is not adequately treated and body temperature is not lowered, it can progress to heat stroke.

Heat stroke has many of the same symptoms of nausea, bradycardia, and weakness as heat exhaustion, but it can also occur if other conditions impair the body's thermoregulatory cooling functions in a hot environment. Confusion, anxiety, or loss of consciousness occurs as the body temperature rises. Unlike the clammy, drenched skin of the heat exhaustion victim, heat stroke is characterized by a decrease in sweating and hot, flushed, dry skin. Body temperatures can rise above 41°C, and convulsions and delirium can occur at 41.2°C. At 41.2°C, serious brain damage can be expected, and death will be preceded by cardiorespiratory collapse.

Robert Warfield: Outcome

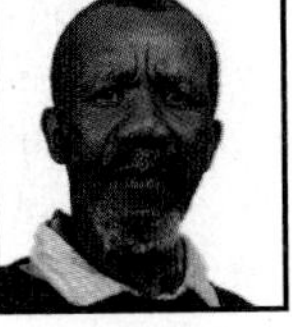

The plan for cooling Mr. Warfield was started in the field by the paramedics, who applied ice packs to Mr. Warfield's head and started IV fluids and electrolytes. In the emergency department, treatment is continued. Mr. Warfield's clothes are removed, and ice packs are applied to the axillae and groin, while the rest of his body is sprayed with water, and a fan is placed to blow across his body, allowing the heat to evaporate. A temperature-sensing Foley catheter is placed to monitor temperature continuously and track urine output.

Once Mr. Warfield's temperature reaches 39°C, the active external cooling is halted to prevent overshooting, which might have resulted in iatrogenic hypothermia.

Mr. Warfield is kept in the hospital overnight to ensure his stability. Social services are called to help Mr. Warfield and ensure that his home is adequately cooled. Before discharge, Mr. Warfield is educated about hyperthermia and encouraged to drink fluids regularly (not just when he is thirsty), to use his fan, to seek a cooler place (such as a library or shopping mall) if he feels overheated, and to work with social services to obtain air conditioning or new housing.

5. Mr. Warfield's discharge diagnosis was hyperthermia. Explain why the diagnosis was not heat stroke.
6. Appropriate education about thermoregulation protection will be very important for Mr. Warfield to receive and understand before he is discharged home. Name two geriatric considerations that apply to Mr. Warfield.

Malignant Hyperthermia

Malignant hyperthermia is a rare, life-threatening hypermetabolic crisis that can occur when a genetically susceptible individual is exposed to an anesthetic agent that has adrenergic, anticholinergic, serotonergic, and antidopaminergic properties.[76] Volatile inhalational anesthetic gases (e.g., ether, halothane, isoflurane) and succinylcholine, a depolarizing neuromuscular blocker, can trigger the response.[77] The earliest signs are muscle rigidity, tachycardia, and elevated body temperature that usually occurs as a rapidly rising hyperthermia above 38.5°C.

The reaction is caused by a mutation in the type 1 ryanodine receptor (*RYR1*) gene. This mutation is transmitted in an autosomal dominant pattern and causes the intracellular Ca^{2+} release channel in skeletal muscle to react when a susceptible individual receives inhalation anesthetics or depolarizing muscle relaxants.[70,76,78] In each of these conditions, there are similar characteristics leading to uncontrolled heat production: (1) high demands for adenosine triphosphate (ATP); (2) rapid oxidative, chemical, and kinetic activity in muscles; and (3) pathologic elevations of intracellular calcium.[70] The rise in calcium levels in the cytoplasm results in skeletal muscle contraction, which accelerates heat production. The resulting rise in heat gain overwhelms compensatory cooling responses, so temperatures rise quickly above the normal set point limits. The ATP in skeletal muscle is depleted, and increased lactate production produces lactic acidosis.[76] Rhabdomyolysis can occur in any situation in which there is muscle breakdown, such as crush injuries and muscle necrosis, but it can also be a serious outcome of severe exertion, such as marathon running, calisthenics, or heat stroke. The myoglobin released from muscle breakdown is metabolized, and these metabolic by-products are potentially nephrotoxic compounds that damage kidneys and lead to acute renal failure from tubular necrosis.[70,79]

Although the disorder is considered rare, individuals with a family history and possible inherited malignant hyperthermia susceptibility should be tested. The true prevalence of malignant hyperthermia is probably underestimated because affected people may never have been tested or may have experienced mild undiagnosed reactions.[77]

Neuroleptic Malignant Syndrome

Neuroleptic malignant syndrome is a rare but life-threatening reaction linked to neuroleptic antipsychotic drug or tranquilizer use. The most commonly prescribed antipsychotic drugs in this category block neurotransmission of dopamine; they include haloperidol, chlorpromazine, fluphenazine, perphenazine, and quetiapine.[80] The familial incidence of neuroleptic malignant syndrome suggests that the central dopamine deficiency that underlies the disorder may be a genetic factor. However, with rare incidence, small samples for research, and only partial polymorphisms showing influence, there are still no strongly predictive genetic tests.[81] Patients being treated for antipsychotic disorders are primary recipients of neuroleptic drugs, so awareness of the symptoms of neuroleptic malignant syndrome should be raised among care providers. However, other patients receive neuroleptic drugs for anesthetic analgesia or asthma treatment, which widens the need for awareness of neuroleptic malignant syndrome across practice settings.[82–84] The tetrad of neuroleptic malignant syndrome consists of intractable hyperthermia, muscular rigidity, autonomic dysfunction, and altered consciousness. If two of these four symptoms occur over 1–3 days, neuroleptic malignant syndrome should be suspected. Laboratory findings include elevated serum creatine kinase and leukocytosis. Neuroleptic malignant syndrome is difficult to diagnose because of its similarities to other symptoms and syndromes experienced by individuals who are prescribed neuroleptic drugs. When a suspected case occurs, other drug-related disorders with similar symptoms must be ruled out. These include malignant hyperthermia, malignant catatonia, and serotonin syndrome.[80,82,83,85,86]

Check Your Progress: Section 33.6

1. What is malignant hyperthermia?
2. What are the earliest signs of malignant hyperthermia?
3. Describe neuroleptic malignant syndrome.

CHAPTER SUMMARY

33.1 Chapter Overview and Case Studies

Explain the history and importance of monitoring body temperature and the concepts related to thermoregulation.

- After the invention of the thermometer, the healthcare profession became increasingly preoccupied with monitoring and recording the rise and fall of body temperature.
- Discoveries of the molecular mechanisms of fever that were beneficial as well as worrisome led to more rational treatment of fever.
- Infectious and inflammatory processes can cause fever, and uncontrolled hyperthermia, as seen in heat-related injuries, can quickly result in dehydration.
- Both hyperthermia and hypothermia can affect patients' comfort levels. The concept of thermoregulation extends to those who are at risk for hypothermia and hyperthermia because of age and developmental factors that may increase risk for injury due to environmental extremes.
- Thermoregulation is an important public health concept for which communities, cities, municipalities, and states can develop and promote initiatives to minimize the effects of extreme temperatures on people who do not have the means to alter their environment for their own safety.

33.2 Body Temperature Regulation

Describe how changes in body temperature involve both physics and physiologic factors.

- Regulation of body temperature, called thermoregulation, depends on critical physiologic mechanisms to stabilize core body temperatures within a precisely defined range to optimize cell function and prevent dangerous levels of heat gain or heat loss.
- Principles of physics, called thermodynamics, form the basis for heat transfer from the body into the surrounding environment or from the surrounding environment into the body. These include conductive, convective, and radiant heat gain and heat loss and evaporative heat loss.

33.3 Thermoregulatory Processes and Control Mechanisms

Explain the sensory inputs and effectors of thermoregulatory responses as complex, separate, but interacting responses with both autonomic and behavioral components.

- A negative feedback system is an essential component in thermoregulation.
- This feedback system includes a normal set point range for core body temperature, central and peripheral sensors that constantly monitor the temperature, a hypothalamic system for comparing actual with established set point temperatures, and physiologic and behavioral responses aimed at adjusting core temperatures up or down.
- Mechanisms to promote heat loss and reduce core temperature include sweating and vasodilation. Mechanisms to promote heat gain and raise core temperature include shivering, nonshivering thermogenesis, and vasoconstriction.
- Behavioral responses, including rubbing the hands together to generate heat, seeking shelter from extreme environmental temperatures, and adjusting the amount and nature of clothing, are important in maintaining stable core body temperatures.
- Studies of circadian oscillations in humans show that they are regulated by an endogenous regulator, or "biological clock," that runs on its own. While the circadian rhythm can be phase shifted, as occurs when night workers must adjust sleep and wake cycles, there appear to be physiologic consequences to health that are still under study. Thermal balance is believed to be a function of both homeostatic and circadian modulation, although it is not certain whether they are integrated or separate processes.

33.4 Hypothermia

Differentiate the causes, classification, underlying pathogenesis, and clinical manifestations of hypothermia and frostbite and approaches to treatment of those conditions, and explain the rationale for therapeutic hypothermia.

- Hypothermia is a condition in which the body is unable to maintain the lower limits of the core temperature set point range that are required for optimal metabolic, enzymatic, and other physiologic functions.
- Hypothermia can be classified by specific core body temperatures and/or severity.
- Different types of hypothermia, based on etiology, include accidental, inadvertent, iatrogenic, and therapeutic. Regardless of the cause, rewarming is the most critical component of treatment. If not done carefully, rewarming can result in life-threatening cardiopulmonary dysfunction.
- Hypothermia is not always the result of extremely low environmental temperatures; it can occur in low-birth-weight infants, ill individuals with lean body mass, or older adults who are unable to generate or conserve heat.
- The systemic effects of hypothermia increase in severity as core temperature drops and primarily result in metabolic, acid–base, respiratory, cardiovascular, and neurologic alterations.
- Transport to a hospital with cardiopulmonary bypass facilities is needed to revive a severely hypothermic individual because of the potential for respiratory arrest and dysrhythmias during rewarming.
- Therapeutic hypothermia limits the harmful effects of cerebral hypoxia by slowing cerebral metabolism. This prevents death of cerebral cells and reduces cerebral edema.
- The mechanical injury of frostbite is similar in several ways to that of burns. Improvement in tissue injury is largely a factor of improved circulation to the affected areas.
- Prevention of frostbite injury to fingers, toes, and bony prominences with insulation is necessary when an individual is treated with hypothermia-inducing therapies that reduce circulation to these body regions.

33.5 Fever

Differentiate the causes, underlying pathogenesis, clinical manifestations, benefits and adverse effects of fever and approaches to its treatment.

- Fever is a commonly occurring alteration in body temperature that is an effect rather than the cause of febrile illness. Unlike hyperthermia, fever is a regulated temperature elevation that occurs in response to an elevated thermoregulatory set point.
- Fever results from the release of pro-inflammatory cytokines such as interleukin-1 (IL-1), interleukin-6 (IL-6), and tumor necrosis factor alpha (TNF-α) from phagocytes, fibroblasts, and endothelial cells. These cytokines act as endogenous pyrogens.
- Fever seems to confer a survival benefit by enhancing leukocyte mobility, stimulating bactericidal and antitumor activity, and transforming lymphocytes. Furthermore, the higher core temperature is optimal for antimicrobial host defenses; fever lowers serum iron levels that inhibit bacterial replication; and associated symptoms such as fatigue, anorexia, and lethargy decrease energy expenditure needed for physical activity and food metabolism.
- The elevated core temperature that accompanies fever occurs in three distinct phases: the chill phase, the plateau phase, and the defervescence phase.
- The thermoregulatory feedback system incorporates predictable responses to heat loss and heat gain. These expected responses should underlie interventions in fever.

33.6 Hyperthermia

Differentiate the causes, underlying pathogenesis, and clinical manifestations of disorders causing hyperthermia and treatment approaches for those disorders.

- Elevations in core body temperature include fever, hyperthermia, and malignant hyperthermia.
- Hyperthermia is a potentially lethal condition that, unlike fever, involves a disruption in thermoregulation and an unregulated temperature elevation. Heat-related illnesses progress along a continuum of severity from heat cramps to heat stroke.
- Hyperthermia is usually related to excessive physical activity in hot, humid conditions, sometimes combined with excessive exertional muscle tissue catabolism (e.g., marathons). Hyperthermia can also occur in sedentary individuals who engage in physical exertion in warm weather and in those who are unable to cool their environment in hot weather. Older adults and newborns are high-risk populations.
- The clinical manifestations associated with hyperthermia increase in severity along the continuum of heat-related illnesses, ranging from excessive sweating, tachypnea, and tachycardia at the least severe end of the continuum to circulatory collapse, seizures, and death at the most severe end of the continuum.
- Malignant hyperthermia involves high demands for ATP; rapid oxidative, chemical, and kinetic activity in muscles; and pathologic elevations of intracellular calcium. These abnormalities result in uncontrolled heat production.
- Malignant hyperthermia is caused by a mutation in the type 1 ryanodine receptor (*RYR1*) gene that is transmitted in an autosomal dominant pattern and induces an increase in intracellular calcium in skeletal muscle. The increased calcium activates destructive cytoplasmic

and nuclear enzymes and leads to cell death. In addition, the myoglobin released from muscle breakdown is metabolized, and these metabolic by-products are potentially nephrotoxic compounds that damage kidneys and lead to acute renal failure from tubular necrosis.

- Neuroleptic malignant syndrome should be suspected when an individual develops muscular rigidity, fluctuating blood pressure, elevated body temperature, and a decline in consciousness soon after the start or increase in dosage of a neuroleptic drug such as thioridazine, haloperidol, chlorpromazine, fluphenazine, perphenazine, or quetiapine.
- Factors common to malignant hyperthermia and neuroleptic malignant syndrome are the potential for rhabdomyolysis and the release of toxic substances from the resulting muscle injury. Both conditions constitute a medical emergency and can be lethal.

REVIEW QUESTIONS

1. The nurse is educating a parent about the best place to set up an infant's crib in the home. The nurse knows that because body temperatures are warmer than ambient conditions, heat is radiated to the air, even through windows. This knowledge is based on what mechanism of heat transfer?
   a. Conductive heat loss
   b. Radiant heat loss
   c. Evaporation
   d. Convective heat loss

2. During assessment, the client tells the nurse, "I never sweat, no matter what I do." The nurse knows that the inability to sweat can lead to what type of complication?
   a. Lowered core body temperature
   b. No complications
   c. Dangerously high core temperature
   d. Poikilothermia

3. During high heat extremes, which group of people are at the highest risk for developing serious thermoregulation disorders?
   a. Children under 5 years of age
   b. Infants
   c. Young athletes and marathon runners
   d. People over 60 years of age

4. A nurse is talking with a 20-year-old client who has just landed his first job as a full-time ski instructor in Colorado and has presented for the required job history and physical exam. During the history, the client admits to "almost daily" use of alcohol and cannabis. The nurse recognizes that he will need to educate the client about his admitted alcohol and cannabis use related to what accurate information?
   a. The legal drinking age in Colorado is 22 years, so the client will not be eligible to purchase alcohol.
   b. Alcohol and cannabis promote heat loss and increase the risk for hypothermia.
   c. Cannabis is an illegal drug in all 50 states.
   d. Alcohol and cannabis impair the ability to think critically and make accurate decisions, which is not a good trait for a ski instructor.

5. The nurse is assessing a client who presents with shallow respirations, exaggerated tendon reflex, hyperactivity, delirium, atrial and ventricular dysrhythmias on ECG, and some muscle rigidity. The client's core temperature is 33°C, and there is no shivering. The nurse believes that the most likely diagnosis is which of the following?
   a. Moderate hypothermia
   b. Poikilothermia
   c. Atrial fibrillation
   d. Frostbite

6. Which objective findings might the nurse expect to assess in a client with second-degree frostbite?
   a. Reddened or pinkish discoloration of the hands and feet
   b. Purple fluid in blisters with discolored skin
   c. Hard white plaque on the affected areas of the body
   d. Clear fluid in superficial blisters of the affected area

7. After diagnosis, the nurse educates the client with frostbite about the evidence-based treatment options. The goal of treatment is based on which of the following principles?
   a. Reperfusion of viable tissue
   b. Returning the core body temperature to normal
   c. Increasing prostaglandin production
   d. Debriding necrotic tissue

8. Malignant hyperthermia involves which of the following characteristics leading to uncontrolled heat production?
   a. Fluctuating blood pressure
   b. Low demand for ATP
   c. Pathologic elevations of intracellular calcium
   d. Excessive sweating

ANSWERS

Answers to Review Questions can be found in Appendix A. Answers to Case Study and Check Your Progress questions are available on the faculty resources site. Please consult with your instructor.

RECOMMENDED WEBSITES

American Red Cross Heat Wave Safety
http://www.redcross.org/get-help/how-to-prepare-for-emergencies/types-of-emergencies/heat-wave-safety

American Society of PeriAnesthesia Nurses: Normothermia Clinical Guideline
http://www.aspan.org/Clinical-Practice/Clinical-Guidelines/Normothermia

Centers for Disease Control and Prevention: Extreme Heat
https://www.cdc.gov/disasters/extremeheat/index.html

Federal Emergency Management Agency: Extreme Heat Fact Sheet
https://www.fema.gov/media-library/assets/documents/12364

Malignant Hyperthermia Association of the United States
https://www.mhaus.org

National Institute for Occupational Safety and Health: Heat Stress
https://www.cdc.gov/niosh/topics/heatstress

REFERENCES

1. Commission for Thermal Physiology of the International Union of Physiological Sciences. (2001). *Glossary of terms for thermal physiology* (3rd ed.). Available at http://www.or.org/pdf/ThermalPhysiologyGlossary.pdf
2. Nakamura, K., & Morrison, S. F. (2010). A thermosensory pathway mediating heat-defense responses. *Proceedings of the National Academy of Sciences, 107*(19), 8848–8853.
3. Romanovsky, A. A. (2007). Thermoregulation: Some concepts have changed—Functional architecture of the thermoregulatory system. *American Journal of Physiology-Regulatory, Integrative and Comparative Physiology, 292*(1), R37–R46.
4. Holtzclaw, B. J. (2008). Managing inadvertent and accidental hypothermia. *Online Journal of Clinical Innovations, 10*, 1–58.
5. Broessner, G., Beer, R., Franz, G., Lackner, P., Engelhardt, K., Brenneis, C., Pfausler, B., & Schmutzhard, E. (2005). Case report: Severe heat stroke with multiple organ dysfunction-a novel intravascular treatment approach. *Critical Care, 9*(5), R498–501.
6. Holtzclaw, B. J. (2003). Monitoring body temperature. In V. Carrieri-Kohlman, A. Lindsey, & C. West (Eds.), *Pathophysiological phenomena in nursing* (3rd ed., pp. 15–34). Philadelphia, PA: W.B. Saunders.
7. Shibasaki, M., Wilson, T. E., & Crandall, C. G. (2006). Neural control and mechanisms of eccrine sweating during heat stress and exercise. *Journal of Applied Physiology, 100*(5), 1692–1701.
8. Shibasaki, M., & Crandall, C. G. (2010). Mechanisms and controllers of eccrine sweating in humans. *Frontiers in Bioscience, 2*, 685–696.
9. Blüschke, G., Nüsken, K.-D., & Schneider, H. (2010). Prevalence and prevention of severe complications of hypohidrotic ectodermal dysplasia in infancy. *Early Human Development, 86*(7), 397–399.
10. Holtzclaw, B. J. (2004). Shivering in acutely ill vulnerable populations. *AACN Advanced Critical Care, 15*(2), 267–279.
11. Nagashima, K., Nakai, S., Tanaka, M., & Kanosue, K. (2000). Neuronal circuitries involved in thermoregulation. *Autonomic Neuroscience, 85*(1–3), 18–25.
12. Cannon, B., & Nedergaard, J. (2004). Brown adipose tissue: Function and physiological significance. *Physiological Reviews, 84*(1), 277–359.
13. Virtanen, K. A., Lidell, M. E., Orava, J., Heglind, M., Westergren, R., Niemi, T., Taittonen, M., Laine, J., Savisto, N.-J., & Enerbäck, S. (2009). Functional brown adipose tissue in healthy adults. *New England Journal of Medicine, 360*(15), 1518–1525.
14. Charkoudian, N. (2010). Mechanisms and modifiers of reflex induced cutaneous vasodilation and vasoconstriction in humans. *Journal of Applied Physiology, 109*(4), 1221–1228.
15. Kellogg, D. (2006). In vivo mechanisms of cutaneous vasodilation and vasoconstriction in humans during thermoregulatory challenges. *Journal of Applied Physiology, 100*(5), 1709–1718.
16. Çınar, N. D., & Filiz, T. M. (2006). Neonatal thermoregulation. *Journal of Neonatal Nursing, 12*(2), 69–74.
17. Soll, R. (2008). Heat loss prevention in neonates. *Journal of Perinatology, 28*, S57–S59.
18. DeGroot, D. W., & Kenney, W. L. (2007). Impaired defense of core temperature in aged humans during mild cold stress. *American Journal of Physiology-Regulatory, Integrative and Comparative Physiology, 292*(1), R103–R108.
19. Kenny, G. P., Yardley, J., Brown, C., Sigal, R. J., & Jay, O. (2010). Heat stress in older individuals and patients with common chronic diseases. *Canadian Medical Association Journal, 182*(10), 1053–1060.
20. Holtzclaw, B. J. (2002). Use of thermoregulatory principles in patient care: Fever management. *Online Journal of Clinical Innovations, 5*(5), 1–64.
21. Mackowiak, P. A., & Worden, G. (1994). Carl Reinhold August Wunderlich and the evolution of clinical thermometry. *Clinical Infectious Diseases, 18*(3), 458–467.
22. Holtzclaw, B. J. (2001). Circadian rhythmicity and homeostatic stability in thermoregulation. *Biological Research for Nursing, 2*(4), 221–235.
23. Videnovic, A., Lazar, A. S., Barker, R. A., & Overeem, S. (2014). 'The clocks that time us'": Circadian rhythms in neurodegenerative disorders. *Nature Reviews Neurology, 10*(12), 683–693.
24. Volicer, L., Harper, D. G., Manning, B. C., Goldstein, R., & Satlin, A. (2001). Sundowning and circadian rhythms in Alzheimer's disease. *American Journal of Psychiatry, 158*(5), 704–711.
25. Cunha, B. A., Krakakis, J., & McDermott, B. P. (2009). Fever of unknown origin (FUO) caused by miliary tuberculosis: Diagnostic significance of morning temperature spikes. *Heart & Lung, 38*(1), 77–82.
26. Brown, D. J. A., Brugger, H., Boyd, J., & Paal, P. (2012). Accidental hypothermia. *New England Journal of Medicine, 367*(20), 1930–1938.

27. Durrer, B., Brugger, H., & Syme, D. (2003). The medical on-site treatment of hypothermia: ICAR-MEDCOM recommendation. *High Altitude Medicine & Biology*, *4*(1), 99–103.
28. Mathur, N. B., Krishnamurthy, S., & Mishra, T. K. (2005). Evaluation of WHO classification of hypothermia in sick extramural neonates as predictor of fatality. *Journal of Tropical Pediatrics*, *51*(6), 341–345.
29. Jacobs, S. E., & Tarnow-Mordi, W. O. (2010). Therapeutic hypothermia for newborn infants with hypoxic–ischaemic encephalopathy. *Journal of Paediatrics and Child Health*, *46*(10), 568–576.
30. Suehiro, E., Koizumi, H., Fujisawa, H., Fujita, M., Kaneko, T., Oda, Y., Yamashita, S., Tsuruta, R., Maekawa, T., & Suzuki, M. (2015). Diverse effects of hypothermia therapy in patients with severe traumatic brain injury based on the computed tomography classification of the traumatic coma data bank. *Journal of Neurotrauma*, *32*(5), 353–358.
31. Rickard, C. M., Couchman, B. A., Hughes, M., & McGrail, M. R. (2004). Preventing hypothermia during continuous veno-venous haemodiafiltration: A randomized controlled trial. *Journal of Advanced Nursing*, *47*(4), 393–400.
32. Berry, D., Wick, C., & Magons, P. (2008). A clinical evaluation of the cost and time effectiveness of the ASPAN hypothermia guideline. *Journal of PeriAnesthesia Nursing*, *23*(1), 24–35.
33. Jones, S. (2004). Heat loss and continuous renal replacement therapy. *AACN Advanced Critical Care*, *15*(2), 223–230.
34. Hooper, V. D., Chard, R., Clifford, T., Fetzer, S., Fossum, S., Godden, B., Robertez, E. A., Noble, K. A., O'Brien, D., & Odom-Forren, J. (2010). ASPAN's evidence-based clinical practice guideline for the promotion of perioperative normothermia. *Journal of PeriAnesthesia Nursing*, *25*(6), 346–365.
35. Brugger, H., Durrer, B., Elsensohn, F., Paal, P., Strapazzon, G., Winterberger, E., Zafren, K., Boyd, J., & Icar, M. (2013). Resuscitation of avalanche victims: Evidence-based guidelines of the International Commission for Mountain Emergency Medicine (ICAR MEDCOM): Intended for physicians and other advanced life support personnel. *Resuscitation*, *84*(5), 539–546.
36. Giesbrecht, G. G. (2000). Cold stress, near drowning and accidental hypothermia: A review. *Aviation, Space, and Environmental Medicine*, *71*(7), 733–752.
37. Dharmarajan, T., Manalo, M., Manalac, M., & Kanagala, M. (2002). Hypothermia in the nursing home: Adverse outcomes in two older men. *Journal of the American Medical Directors Association*, *3*(2), S35–S38.
38. Dharmarajan, T., & Widjaja, D. (2007). Hypothermia in the geriatric population. *Aging Health*, *3*(6), 735–741.
39. Khan, S., Plummer, M., Robertez-Arizala, A., & Banovac, K. (2007). Hypothermia in patients with chronic spinal cord injury. *Journal of Spinal Cord Medicine*, *30*(1), 27.
40. Polderman, K. H., & Herold, I. (2009). Therapeutic hypothermia and controlled normothermia in the intensive care unit: Practical considerations, side effects, and cooling methods. *Critical Care Medicine*, *37*(3), 1101–1120.
41. Tsuei, B. J., & Kearney, P. A. (2004). Hypothermia in the trauma patient. *Injury*, *35*(1), 7–15.
42. Fairchild, K. D., Singh, I. S., Patel, S., Drysdale, B. E., Viscardi, R. M., Hester, L., Lazusky, H. M., & Hasday, J. D. (2004). Hypothermia prolongs activation of NF-κB and augments generation of inflammatory cytokines. *American Journal of Physiology-Cell Physiology*, *287*(2), C422–C431.
43. Russwurm, S., Stonans, I., Schwerter, K., Stonane, E., Meissner, W., & Reinhart, K. (2002). Direct influence of mild hypothermia on cytokine expression and release in cultures of human peripheral blood mononuclear cells. *Journal of Interferon & Cytokine Research*, *22*(2), 215–221.
44. Fitzgerald, F. T. (1980). Hypoglycemia and accidental hypothermia in an alcoholic population. *Western Journal of Medicine*, *133*(2), 105.
45. Bonfils, P. K., Reith, J., Hasseldam, H., & Johansen, F. F. (2006). Estimation of the hypothermic component in neuroprotection provided by cannabinoids following cerebral ischemia. *Neurochemistry International*, *49*(5), 508–518.
46. Boyd, J., Kuisma, M., Alaspää, A., Vuori, E., Repo, J., & Randell, T. (2006). Outcome after heroin overdose and cardiopulmonary resuscitation. *Acta Anaesthesiologica Scandinavica*, *50*(9), 1120–1124.
47. Cuddy, M. L. S. (2004). The effects of drugs on thermoregulation. *AACN Advanced Critical Care*, *15*(2), 238–253.
48. Simon, P., Dannaway, D., Bright, B., Krous, L., Wlodaver, A., Burks, B., Thi, C., Milam, J., & Escobedo, M. (2011). Thermal defense of extremely low gestational age newborns during resuscitation: exothermic mattresses vs polyethylene wrap. *Journal of Perinatology*, *31*(1), 33–37.
49. Wyckoff, M. H., & Perlman, J. M. (2004). Effective ventilation and temperature control are vital to outborn resuscitation. *Prehospital Emergency Care*, *8*(2), 191–195.
50. Els, T., Oehm, E., Voigt, S., Klisch, J., Hetzel, A., & Kassubek, J. (2006). Safety and therapeutical benefit of hemicraniectomy combined with mild hypothermia in comparison with hemicraniectomy alone in patients with malignant ischemic stroke. *Cerebrovascular Diseases*, *21*(1–2), 79–85.
51. Holtzclaw, B. J. Postoperative shivering after cardiac surgery: A review. (1986). *Heart & Lung*, *15*(3), 292–302.
52. Kanna, B., & Wani, S. (2003). Giant J wave on 12-lead electrocardiogram in hypothermia. *Annals of Noninvasive Electrocardiology*, *8*(3), 262–265.
53. Rothschild, M., & Schneider, V. (1995). "Terminal burrowing behaviour": A phenomenon of lethal hypothermia. *International Journal of Legal Medicine*, *107*(5), 250–256.
54. Zeitzer, M. B. (2005). Inducing hypothermia to decrease neurological deficit: Literature review. *Journal of Advanced Nursing*, *52*(2), 189–199.
55. Murphy, J. V., Banwell, P. E., Roberts, A. H., & McGrouther, D. A. (2000). Frostbite: pathogenesis and treatment. *Journal of Trauma and Acute Care Surgery*, *48*(1), 171.
56. Mccauley, R. L., Hing, D. N., Robson, M. C., & Heggers, J. P. (1983). Frostbite injuries: A rational approach based on the pathophysiology. *Journal of Trauma and Acute Care Surgery*, *23*(2), 143–147.
57. Long, W. B., Edlich, R., Winters, K. L., & Britt, L. (2005). Cold injuries. *Journal of Long-term Effects of Medical Implants*, *15*(1), 67–78.
58. Patel, N. N., & Patel, D. N. (2008). Frostbite. *American Journal of Medicine*, *121*(9), 765–766.
59. Biem, J., Koehncke, N., Classen, D., & Dosman, J. (2003). Out of the cold: Management of hypothermia and frostbite. *Canadian Medical Association Journal*, *168*(3), 305–311.
60. Bruen, K. J., Ballard, J. R., Morris, S. E., Cochran, A., Edelman, L. S., & Saffle, J. R. (2007). Reduction of the incidence of amputation in frostbite injury with thrombolytic therapy. *Archives of Surgery*, *142*(6), 546–553.
61. Kluger, M. J., Kozak, W., Conn, C. A., Leon, L. R., & Soszynski, D. (1996). The adaptive value of fever. *Infectious Disease Clinics of North America*, *10*(1), 1–20.
62. Kozak, W., Kluger, M. J., Tesfaigzi, J., Kozak, A., Mayfield, K. P., Wachulec, M., & Dokladny, K. (2009). Molecular mechanisms of fever and endogenous antipyresis. *Annals of the New York Academy of Sciences*, *917*(1), 121–134.
63. Holtzclaw, B. J. (1992). The febrile response in critical care: State of the science. *Heart & Lung*, *21*(5), 482–501.
64. Ivanov, A. I., & Romanovsky, A. A. (2004). Prostaglandin E2 as a mediator of fever: Synthesis and catabolism. *Frontiers in Bioscience*, *9*(1–3), 1977–1983.
65. Kluger, M., Bartfai, T., & Dinarello, C. (Eds.). (1998). *Molecular mechanisms of fever*. New York, NY: New York Academy of Sciences.
66. Kluger, M., Kozak, W., Leon, L., Soszynski, D., & Conn, C. (1995). Cytokines and fever. *Neuroimmunomodulation*, *2*(4), 216–223.
67. Kluger, M., & Rothenburg, B. (1979). Fever and reduced iron: Their interaction as a host defense response to bacterial infection. *Science*, *203*(4378), 374–376.

68. Lennie, T. (1999). Anorexia in response to acute illness. *Heart Lung, 28*(6), 386–401.
69. Rowsey, P. J. (1997). Applied pathophysiology: Pathophysiology of fever. Part 2: Relooking at cooling interventions. *DCCN: Dimensions of Critical Care Nursing, 16*(5), 251–256.
70. Muldoon, S., Deuster, P., Voelkel, M., Capacchione, J., & Bunger, R. (2008). Exertional heat illness, exertional rhabdomyolysis, and malignant hyperthermia: Is there a link? *Current Sports Medicine Reports, 7*(2), 74–80.
71. Glazer, J. L. (2005). Management of heatstroke and heat exhaustion. *American Family Physician, 71*(11), 2133–2140.
72. Kenefick, R. W., Sawka, M. N. (2007). Heat exhaustion and dehydration as causes of marathon collapse. *Sports Medicine, 37*(4–5), 378–381.
73. Sawka, M. N., Latzka, W. A., Montain, S. J., Cadarette, B. S., Kolka, M. A., Kraning, K. K., & Gonzalez, R. R. (2001). Physiologic tolerance to uncompensable heat: Intermittent exercise, field vs laboratory. *Medicine and Science in Sports and Exercise, 33*(3), 422–430.
74. Vassallo, M., Gera, K. N., & Allen, S. (1995). Factors associated with high risk of marginal hyperthermia in elderly patients living in an institution. *Postgraduate Medical Journal, 71*(834), 213–216.
75. Fineschi, V., D'Errico, S., Neri, M., Panarese, F., Ricci, P. A., & Turillazzi, E. (2005). Heat stroke in an incubator: An immunohistochemical study in a fatal case. *International Journal of Legal Medicine, 119*(2), 94–97.
76. McAllen, K. J., & Schwartzm D. R. (2010). Adverse drug reactions resulting in hyperthermia in the intensive care unit. *Critical Care Medicine, 38*, S244–S252.
77. Litman, R. S., & Rosenberg, H. (2005). Malignant hyperthermia: Update on susceptibility testing. *JAMA, 293*(23), 2918–2924.
78. Wappler, F. (2010). Anesthesia for patients with a history of malignant hyperthermia. *Current Opinion in Anesthesiology, 23*(3), 417–422.
79. Sauret, J. M., Marinides, G., & Wang, G. K. (2002). Rhabdomyolysis. *American Family Physician, 65*(5), 907–912.
80. Tomasi, G., Portal, B., Franciscatto, L., Klein, B., Passos, G., Cristovam, R., & Schilling, L. (2015). Neuroleptic malignant syndrome induced by quetiapine. *Journal of the Neurological Sciences, 357*, e453.
81. Mihara, K., Kondo, T., Suzuki, A., Yasui-Furukori, N., Ono, S., Sano, A., Koshiro, K., Otani, K., & Kaneko, S. (2003). Relationship between functional dopamine D2 and D3 receptors gene polymorphisms and neuroleptic malignant syndrome. *American Journal of Medical Genetics, Part B: Neuropsychiatric Genetics, 117*(1), 57–60.
82. Davis, S. (2015). Neuroleptic malignant syndrome: A pathophysiological dilemma. *MSN Student Scholarship*, Otterbein University. Available at http://digitalcommons.otterbein.edu/cgi/viewcontent.cgi?article=1119&context=stu_msn
83. Pandey, S., Singh, M., Singh, K., Sandhu, S., & Hussain, A. (2012). Neuroleptic malignant syndrome: A rare post operative complication. *Indian Hernia Society Newsletter, 6*(2), 28.
84. Portel, L., Hilbert, G., Gruson, D., Favier, J. C., Gbikpi-Benissan, G., & Cardinaud, J. P. (1999). Malignant hyperthermia and neuroleptic malignant syndrome in a patient during treatment for acute asthma. *Acta Anaesthesiologica Scandinavica, 43*(1), 107–110.
85. Adnet, P., Lestavel, P., & Krivosic-Horber, R. (2000). Neuroleptic malignant syndrome. *British Journal of Anaesthesia, 85*(1), 129–135.
86. Strawn, J. R., Keck, P. E., Jr., & Caroff, S. N. (2007). Neuroleptic malignant syndrome. *American Journal of Psychiatry, 164*(6), 870.

Unit X

Disorders of Mobility

The ability to move freely is central to an individual's independence. Disorders of mobility typically restrict movement, with the extent of restriction depending, in part, on the severity and nature of the disorder, the individual's ability to access appropriate treatment and assistive devices, and the individual's own resilience. If the disorder causes additional impairments, such as the dementia that some patients with Parkinson disease exhibit, then the individual will experience even greater limitations to independent functioning, and require more and more assistance with activities of daily living (ADLs) as the illness progresses. Mobility may be further limited if the individual has a co-occurring condition such as obesity or COPD. Individuals with limited mobility or independence are at greater risk for social isolation, falls, and abuse and neglect.

Chronic, degenerative neurologic disorders are associated with tremendous social, financial, economic, and healthcare-related costs. For example, approximately one million people in the U.S. are living with Parkinson disease, with a combined economic burden estimated at $25 billion annually.[1] As individuals with degenerative disorders progress in their illness, many require part-time or full-time help to remain in their homes, further adding to their economic burden. In 2015, the average national cost of a paid caregiver working in the home was $20 per hour, with state averages ranging between $15 and $26 per hour.[2]

Acute disorders of mobility are often associated with acute onset due to an accident. Examples include ankle and knee injuries as the result of sports and leisure activities. Repetitive motion injuries, also called repetitive stress injuries, are injuries to soft tissues such as muscles and tendons. These injuries occur as a result of repeating an activity over time and can be temporary or permanent. Tissues can become compressed, which prevents the flow of blood to the tissues, and inflamed and painful.[3] In some cases, repetitive motion injuries can lead to a tearing of tissue. A classic example is the torn rotator cuff that some baseball and softball pitchers experience.

All disorders of mobility can result in pain, so pain assessment is critical at each healthcare interaction. Like degenerative disorders, chronic musculoskeletal disorders can result in impaired mobility, reduced independence, and increased social isolation. Similarly, the economic burden associated with these disorders is also considerable. For example, individuals with rheumatoid arthritis (or their insurance plans) can pay up to $30,000 for medications annually. Nationwide, the cost of arthritis care is estimated to be $9.3 billion by 2020.[4]

Care of individuals with musculoskeletal disorders is often collaborative. General nursing activities will include assessment of motor function, assessment of fall risk, assessment of ability to perform ADLs, pain assessment, patient education, and facilitating referrals. Referrals to the following may be necessary depending on assessment results and orders by the treating healthcare provider:

- Physical therapy, to assist with movement and gross motor function
- Occupational therapy, to assist with fine motor function and ADLs
- Speech therapy, to assist with oral motor and speech and language processing (sometimes necessary for patients with degenerative disorders)
- Assistive technology providers, to help with fitting crutches, braces, walkers, and other devices
- Mental health providers, to help with coping with loss of motor function
- Nonprofit providers and support groups who can assist with transportation and other supports that can reduce social isolation.

References

1. Parkinson's Disease Foundation. (2017). Statistics on Parkinson's. Retrieved from http://www.pdf.org/en/parkinson_statistics
2. Paying for Senior Care. (2015). Elder care costs by type of care. Retrieved from https://www.payingforseniorcare.com/longtermcare/costs.html
3. Johns Hopkins Medicine. (n.d.). Repetitive motion injury. Retrieved fromhttp://www.hopkinsmedicine.org/healthlibrary/conditions/physical_medicine_and_rehabilitation/repetitive_motion_injury_85,P01176/
4. RheumatoidArthritis.org. (2016). Rheumatoid arthritis treatment costs. Retrieved from https://www.rheumatoidarthritis.org/treatment/costs/

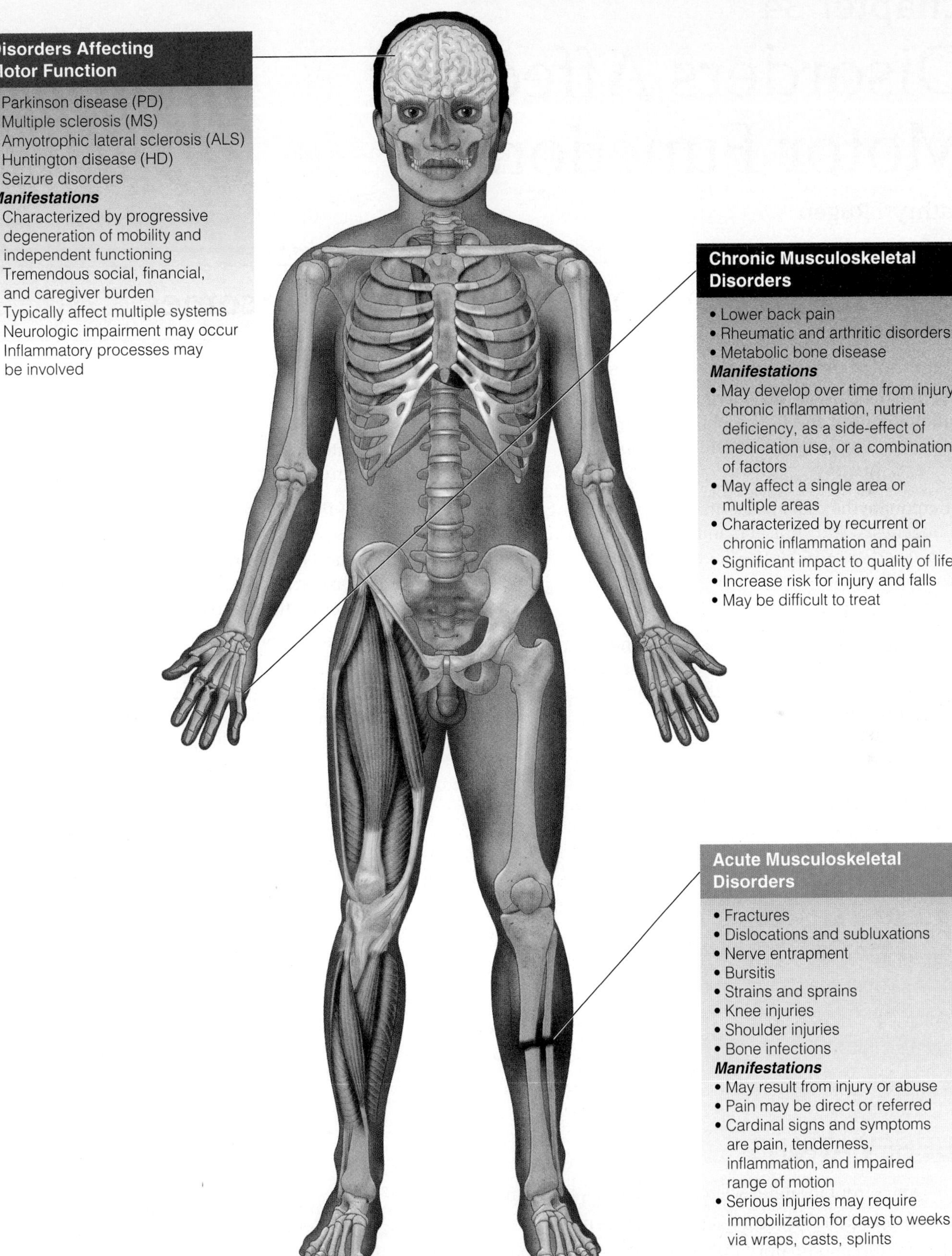
Disorders Affecting Motor Function
• Parkinson disease (PD)
• Multiple sclerosis (MS)
• Amyotrophic lateral sclerosis (ALS)
• Huntington disease (HD)
• Seizure disorders
Manifestations
• Characterized by progressive degeneration of mobility and independent functioning
• Tremendous social, financial, and caregiver burden
• Typically affect multiple systems
• Neurologic impairment may occur
• Inflammatory processes may be involved
Chronic Musculoskeletal Disorders
• Lower back pain
• Rheumatic and arthritic disorders
• Metabolic bone disease
Manifestations
• May develop over time from injury, chronic inflammation, nutrient deficiency, as a side-effect of medication use, or a combination of factors
• May affect a single area or multiple areas
• Characterized by recurrent or chronic inflammation and pain
• Significant impact to quality of life
• Increase risk for injury and falls
• May be difficult to treat
Acute Musculoskeletal Disorders
• Fractures
• Dislocations and subluxations
• Nerve entrapment
• Bursitis
• Strains and sprains
• Knee injuries
• Shoulder injuries
• Bone infections
Manifestations
• May result from injury or abuse
• Pain may be direct or referred
• Cardinal signs and symptoms are pain, tenderness, inflammation, and impaired range of motion
• Serious injuries may require immobilization for days to weeks via wraps, casts, splints

Chapter 34

Disorders Affecting Motor Function

Kathryn Rugen

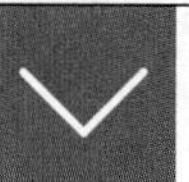

Chapter Outline and Learning Outcomes

34.1 Chapter Overview and Case Studies

Describe the chronic, degenerative neurologic disorders of motor control and how mobility dysfunction is experienced by individuals with the disorders.

34.2 Parkinson Disease

Differentiate the causes, classification, underlying pathogenesis, and clinical manifestations of Parkinson disease and approaches to diagnosis and treatment of the condition.

34.3 Multiple Sclerosis

Differentiate the causes, classification, underlying pathogenesis, and clinical manifestations of multiple sclerosis and approaches to diagnosis and treatment of the condition across the lifespan.

34.4 Amyotrophic Lateral Sclerosis

Differentiate the causes, classification, underlying pathogenesis, and clinical manifestations of amyotrophic lateral sclerosis and approaches to diagnosis and treatment of the condition.

34.5 Huntington Disease

Differentiate the causes, classification, underlying pathogenesis, and clinical manifestations of Huntington disease and approaches to diagnosis and treatment of the condition across the lifespan.

34.6 Seizure Disorders

Differentiate the causes, classification, underlying pathogenesis, and clinical manifestations of seizure disorders and approaches to diagnosis and treatment of these conditions across the lifespan.

KEY TERMS

Absence seizure, 857
Amyotrophic lateral sclerosis (ALS), 853
Aura, 857
Clonic phase, 858
Demyelination, 849
Epilepsy, 856
Excitotoxicity, 853
Febrile seizures, 856
Generalized seizure, 856
Huntington disease (HD), 854
Intractable seizure, 857
Mitochondrial dysfunction, 846
Multiple sclerosis (MS), 848
Neurodegenerative, 844
Oxidative stress, 846
Parkinson disease (PD), 844
Parkinsonism, 844
Partial seizure, 856
Plaques, 849
Postictal period, 858
Proteolytic stress, 845
Postural instability, 846
Seizure, 856
Status epilepticus, 857
Tonic–clonic seizure, 857
Tonic phase, 857

ABBREVIATIONS

ALS—amyotrophic lateral sclerosis
HD—Huntington disease
IMT—immunomodulatory therapy
LMN—lower motor neuron
MS—multiple sclerosis
PD—Parkinson disease
SN—substantia nigra
UMN—upper motor neuron
UPS—ubiquitin–proteasomal system

34.1 Chapter Overview and Case Studies

Chronic degenerative neurologic disorders are associated with tremendous social, financial, economic, and healthcare-related costs. They can afflict individuals across the lifespan and occur worldwide, although some occur most often at an older age or in certain geographic areas. Most of these disorders are often labeled *movement disorders*; however, they are typically multisystem disorders in which the nonmotor manifestations are as serious and disabling as the motor manifestations. Most of these degenerative disorders have unknown etiologies, but genetic and environmental risk factors have been identified. A wide array of chronic degenerative movement disorders exists. Three common movement disorders—Parkinson disease, multiple sclerosis, and amyotrophic lateral sclerosis—are addressed in this chapter.

Other disorders that are discussed in this chapter include Huntington disease, which presents genetic, ethical, and family planning issues that are critical for the people who may have this heredity disease, and seizures, which are periods of abnormal electrical discharges in the brain that may cause involuntary movement and/or behavior and sensory alterations. There are many other disorders that affect motor function, some of which are quite rare. Relatively common ones include benign essential tremor, Lewy body disease, and Tourette syndrome. Restless leg syndrome, which affects primarily older adults, is covered in Chapter 7.

Concepts Related to Disorders of Motor Control

The musculoskeletal system comprises the bones and joints of the skeletal system and the muscles, ligaments, tendons, and cartilage of the muscular system. The skeletal and muscular systems work together to support body weight, control movements, and provide stability. Some musculoskeletal structures, such as the rib cage and skull, provide protection for other organs, including the heart, lungs, and brain. The musculoskeletal system allows the performance of gross movement, such as walking, and fine movement, such as writing.

The musculoskeletal system works in tandem with the circulatory and nervous systems. The bones store nutrients and produce white and red blood cells. Subsequently, the blood provides oxygen, calcium, and other nutrients to strengthen bones and transports electrolytes that are needed for muscle movement. Similarly, nerves innervate the muscles to provide the electrical stimulus needed to initiate contraction. Coordinating all movement is the central nervous system (CNS). Thus, many issues related to mobility are associated with dysregulation or dysfunction of CNS pathways.

Most people take mobility for granted until a disease or injury restricts their freedom of movement. Because the musculoskeletal system is interconnected, injury to one structure can impair the function of other structures as well.

Alterations in musculoskeletal integrity have a detrimental effect on the individual's ability to perform activities of daily living, communicate, and participate in recreational activities (**Figure 34.1** ■). Impaired mobility is a common

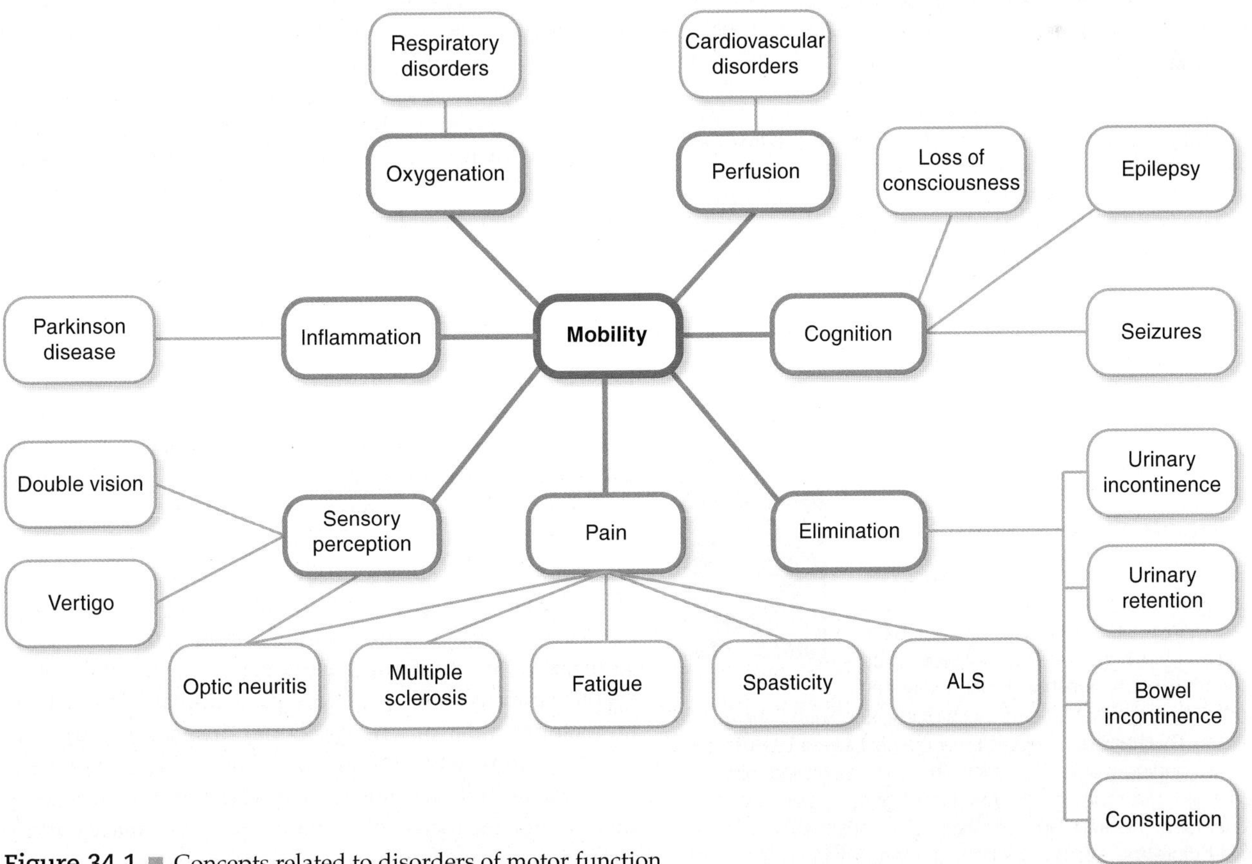

Figure 34.1 ■ Concepts related to disorders of motor function.

source of frustration and pain for people with musculoskeletal dysfunction or injury.

Conditions that may limit mobility include pain, fatigue, respiratory disorders, cardiovascular disease, nervous system disorders, and musculoskeletal diseases or injuries. Patients with a prolonged decrease in mobility may develop an inability to cope and may benefit from counseling.

Case Studies

The following cases will be addressed throughout the chapter to assist in application of chapter content to clinical situations that involve individuals with movement disorders.

Matthew Horn: Introduction

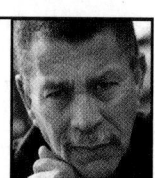

Matthew Horn is a 62-year-old architect. He is seeing his primary care provider for his annual checkup with his wife present. He complains that in the past 6 months, he has noticed shaking in his right hand that occurs when he is watching TV or "just sitting around doing nothing" and occasionally when he is walking. The shaking happens once in a while and seems to disappear when he is drawing or otherwise actively using his hand. But he states that the shaking seems worse when he is really stressed at work to meet a deadline. His wife says that she has never noticed the shaking. Mr. Horn also thinks that he has weakness in his hands and states that his "manual dexterity has gotten bad" in performing such daily tasks as buttoning his shirt, tying his shoes, or double clicking his computer mouse. He attributes this to arthritis.

On physical examination, a resting tremor is noted in Mr. Horn's right hand while his hands are at rest in his lap. In examining each extremity, the healthcare provider notes that the speed, amplitude, and rhythm of finger tapping, hand gripping, pronating, and supinating hand movements and toe and heel tapping are slow and show a decrease in amplitude. Mr. Horn is also very slow to get up out of the chair. On gait observation, a tremor in his right hand is present. Rigidity is not present in passive range of motion of the extremities. However, a decrease in arm swing with walking is present.

The healthcare provider tells the Horns that she is highly suspicious of Parkinson disease owing to the presence of a resting tremor, bradykinesia (slowness in movement), and some mild rigidity as seen with decreased arm swing when walking. She refers Mr. Horn to a neurologist for further evaluation and treatment options.

1. On the basis of Mr. Horn's history, which findings suggest that he has Parkinson disease?
2. What is the pathophysiologic mechanism that accounts for Mr. Horn's symptoms?

Susan Harris: Introduction

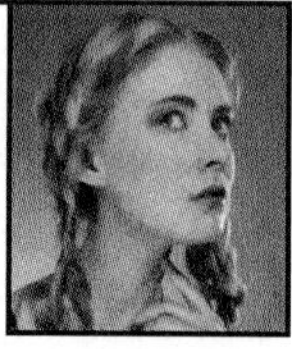

Susan Harris is a 28-year-old schoolteacher. She is of Scandinavian descent and has lived in St. Paul, Minnesota, all her life. She has been having pain in her right eye that is worse when she moves her eyes, and her visual acuity has decreased. She says that "everything is blurry, and I can't see as far as I used to." This has been occurring for the past several weeks and seems to be getting worse. She thinks she may be having migraine headaches like her roommate's. Ms. Harris goes to see her nurse practitioner for a checkup. She tells the nurse practitioner that about 2 months before the eye pain began, she was having a "pins and needles" sensation in her left arm that was sometimes very painful, but it seems to be going away, and then the eye pain started.

On physical examination, her right eye visual acuity is 20/100, the left eye visual acuity is 20/20, and the right peripheral visual field is decreased. The ophthalmologic exam reveals swelling of the disc. Horizontal and vertical gaze nystagmus is seen in both eyes, and Ms. Harris experiences pain during the eye movement exam. Her motor exam is normal, and strength in the four extremities is 5/5. There is a decrease in the vibratory and position sense in her left arm. The deep tendon reflexes are hyperreflexic throughout, and there is Babinski reflex on the right foot. The nurse practitioner tells Ms. Harris that she has an abnormal neurologic exam that warrants an urgent MRI scan with contrast and a referral to a neurologist.

1. What are Ms. Harris's risk factors for multiple sclerosis?
2. Explain the interaction between ethnicity and geographic location in the occurrence of multiple sclerosis.

Check Your Progress: Section 34.1

1. Explain the functions of the musculoskeletal system.
2. How does the musculoskeletal system interact with other body systems?
3. What are some of the psychosocial effects of musculoskeletal system impairment?

34.2 Parkinson Disease

Parkinson disease (PD) was first described in 1817 by physician James Parkinson. It is an idiopathic, chronic, progressive degenerative disorder of the CNS. The classic motor symptoms associated with the disorder correlate well with disruption in the function of the basal ganglia as a result of a decrease in the amount of the neurotransmitter dopamine. Traditionally, PD was considered a movement disorder. However, now it is widely accepted that PD is a complex condition with diverse clinical features that include motor, nonmotor, and neuropsychiatric manifestations.

There are many **neurodegenerative** disorders that display signs and symptoms that are collectively known as **parkinsonism** (tremors, bradykinesia, rigidity, and postural instability). These disorders include Lewy body dementia, late-stage Alzheimer disease, corticobasal degeneration, multiple-system atrophy, spinocerebellar ataxia, and progressive supranuclear palsy. A wide array of conditions can cause secondary parkinsonism. These include head trauma; toxins including manganese, cyanide, and carbon monoxide; metabolic disorders, including hypoparathyroidism and chronic liver failure; infections, including encephalitis, HIV/AIDS, and neurosyphilis; and multiple strokes in the basal ganglia region of the brain. The most common cause of secondary parkinsonism is use of certain drugs, most often atypical antipsychotic (e.g., reserpine) and antiemetic (e.g., metoclopramide, prochlorperizine) drugs. Parkinsonism resulting from some of these secondary causes is reversible when the underlying cause is removed. For the purposes of this chapter, the focus will be on idiopathic primary parkinsonism, commonly known as Parkinson disease.

Parkinson disease affects around 1% of the population and increases with age up to a prevalence of 5% in the 80-year-old population.[1] According to the National Institutes of Health, Parkinson disease affects approximately 500,000 people in the United States.[2] About 50,000 new cases are diagnosed each year. PD usually affects individuals over the age of 50, and the likelihood of acquiring PD increases with age. PD is the second most common neurodegenerative disorder, after Alzheimer disease.[3] The total direct and indirect costs to the nation exceed $6 billion annually.[2] PD has a significant personal and public health burden, which is expected to increase as the population ages. Therefore, it is imperative that we advance the understanding of the disease through research and improve treatment options.

Etiology and Pathogenesis

In approximately 90% of cases, PD is idiopathic (due to an unknown cause); the other 10% of cases have a genetic cause. Risk factors for the development of PD include increased age; male gender; environmental exposures to pesticides, metals, and compounds such as manganese, lead, copper, iron, zinc, and aluminum; family history of PD; and genetic factors if age at onset is younger than 50 years.[4] Cigarette smoking, caffeine intake, and high levels of urate in the blood are inversely related to the risk of PD.[4] Age is the most significant risk factor. There is little difference in incidence between men and women before 60 years of age. After 60 years of age, however, males are affected approximately 1.5 times more often than females, and this difference becomes greater as the age at onset gets older.[1] Genetic mutation of several genes, including *LRRK2*, *PARK2*, and *SNCA*, has been linked to PD.[2] People with early-onset or juvenile PD are more likely to have a genetic mutation than are those with late-age onset.

The most prominent pathophysiologic abnormality associated with PD is the progressive depletion of the presynaptic neurotransmitter dopamine in the basal ganglia, specifically in the substantia nigra (SN) and the pathways to the corpus striatum (caudate and putamen) (**Figure 34.2** ■). The depletion of dopaminergic neurons that connect the SN to the cholinergic neurons in the corpus striatum results in abnormal nerve-firing patterns that cause increased inhibition of the thalamus and reduced excitatory input to the motor cortex due to the imbalance of dopamine and acetylcholine. This imbalance results in the classic clinical manifestations seen in PD: bradykinesia, tremor, and rigidity. At the time of onset of symptoms of PD, about 60% of the neurons in the SN have been depleted.[5]

Although the exact pathogenesis of PD remains uncertain, it appears that the disappearance of dopaminergic neurons in the SN is likely due to a number of potentially interrelated pathogenic mechanisms of neurodegeneration. Suspects include proteolytic stress, oxidative stress, mitochondrial dysfunction, and inflammation.

Proteolytic Stress. In the course of a lifetime, intracellular proteins become mutated, damaged, misfolded, senescent, or otherwise unwanted. These proteins must be removed to maintain cell survival and are normally removed by the ubiquitin–proteasomal system (UPS). A balance between

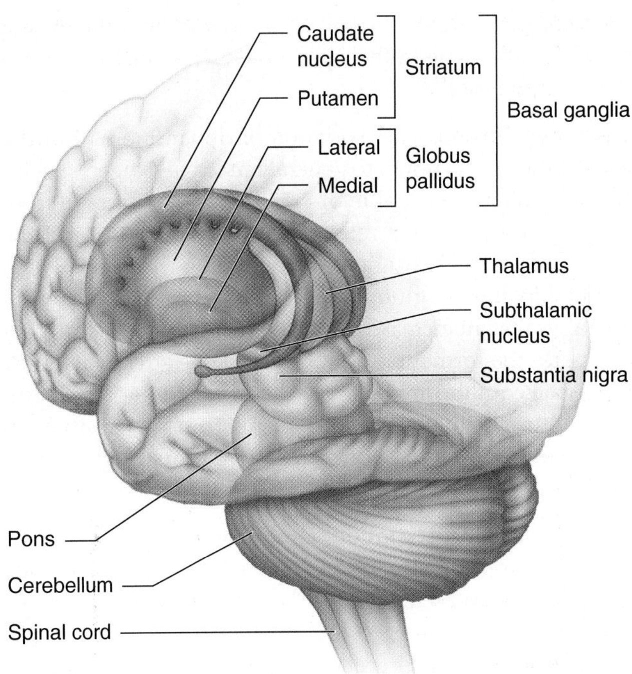

Figure 34.2 ■ Main connections of the basal ganglia.

the synthesis and clearance of unwanted proteins is normally maintained within the cell. If this balance is upset by excess formation of unwanted proteins or impaired protein degradation, the proteins accumulate and aggregate. These protein aggregates can interfere with normal UPS function, impair critical cellular processes (axonal transport, synaptic plasticity, and neurotransmission), and induce cytotoxicity. This is the origin of **proteolytic stress**. Neurons may be especially likely to accumulate abnormal proteins, as neurons do not regenerate. Abnormal protein-filled structures called inclusions or Lewy bodies are typical, but not universal, findings on autopsy of individuals with PD (**Figure 34.3** ■). Lewy bodies contain an oxidatively modified protein called alpha-synuclein. This is a naturally unfolded protein that is vulnerable to misfolding and aggregation. The accumulation of alpha-synuclein interferes with transmission of nerve signals or other important neuronal functions. Several herbicides or pesticides have been found to cause

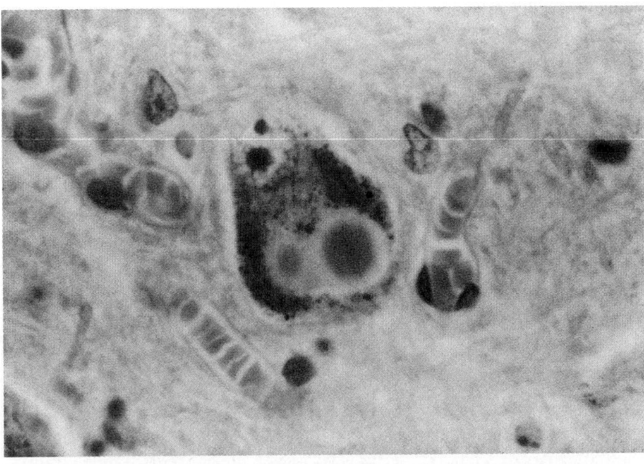

Figure 34.3 ■ Lewy bodies seen in Parkinson disease.

misfolding or aggregation of alpha-synuclein; this finding may partially explain their potential as risk factors for the development of PD.

Oxidative Stress. The oxidation of dopamine within the cells of the SN is known to generate reactive oxygen species (ROS), which are capable of creating a state of **oxidative stress**. The theory of a relationship between ROS and the pathogenesis of PD originated from autopsy results, which found depletion of glutathione, an antioxidant in the brain, and a significant increase in levels of iron, a pro-oxidant that promotes the formation of ROS. Oxidative stress can occur when the equilibrium between the production of ROS and the ability of protective mechanisms to scavenge them is disrupted. Aging is a strong risk factor for oxidative stress and the development of PD.

Mitochondrial Dysfunction. A **mitochondrial dysfunction** theory is supported by the fact that mitochondrial complex activity is decreased by 30–40%, which disrupts calcium homeostasis and induces endoplasmic reticulum stress, which in turn results in cell damage.

Inflammation. Inflammation as a pathogenic mechanism in PD is most commonly linked to the activation of microglia. Microglia are the resident immune cells in the brain. They are usually in a resting state but can be activated by direct stimulation from environmental toxins or endogenous proteins and neuronal damage. However, microglia can become overactivated and induce significant and highly detrimental neurotoxic effects by the excess production of neurotoxic factors such as superoxide, nitric oxide, and tumor necrosis factor alpha. The toxic effects associated with microgliosis tend to be progressive, and activated microglia are present in large numbers in neurodegenerative diseases.

Clinical Manifestations

The onset of PD is insidious. The progression of clinical manifestations may occur over 10–30 years or more, although some individuals may deteriorate more rapidly. Deterioration is not linear. The nature, severity, and impact of the signs and symptoms vary among individuals and may also vary within an individual over the course of the disorder. Early signs are frequently overlooked and are often ascribed to normal aging changes.

CLINICAL POINT: One hallmark of PD is that motor manifestations are unilateral, although they typically become bilateral in the later stages of the disorder. ■

Motor Features of PD. Tremor is the most visible sign of PD (**Figure 34.4** ■). Approximately 85% of individuals with PD display a supination–pronation, or "pill-rolling," resting tremor of the hand. In 75% of people with PD, it is first presenting motor feature. The tremor disappears with action and during sleep but worsens with walking or excitement. In the early phase of PD, tremor usually involves the hand, although it may eventually affect all four limbs. Tremor also affects the lips, chin, jaw, tongue, and legs; it rarely involves the head, neck, or voice.

Rigidity results from increased muscle stiffness and tone. It is usually accompanied by cogwheeling (slight hesitations during movement that cause a stop-and-go effect) caused by alternating contraction and relaxation of muscles, with passive range of motion. Rigidity often begins on one side, the same side as the tremor; it can affect any body part and can be manifested as decreased arm swing with walking.

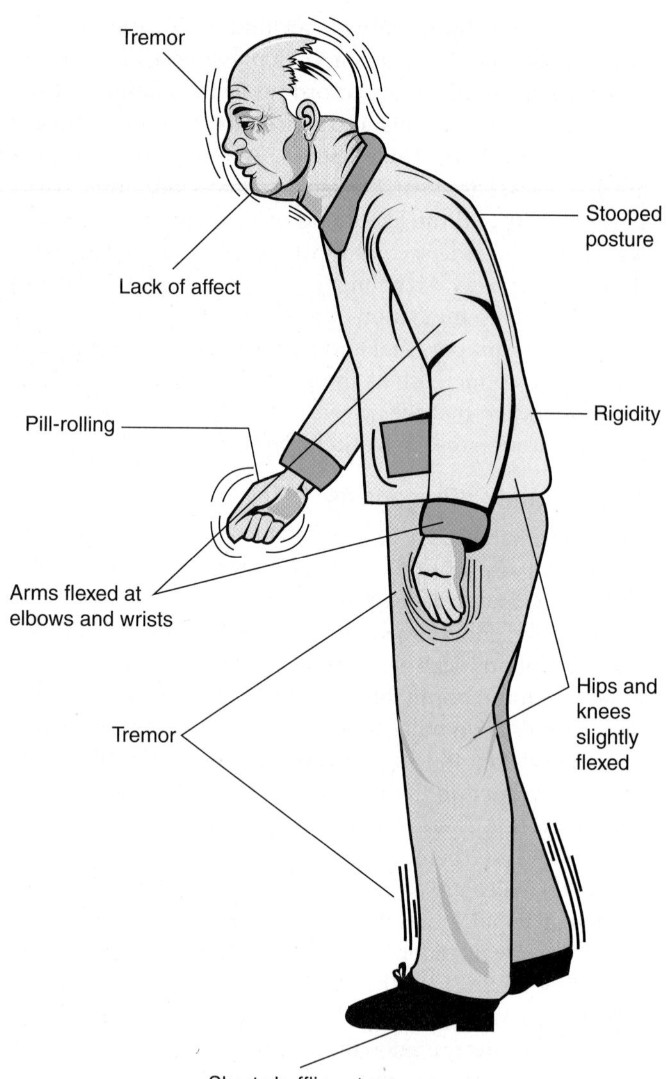

Figure 34.4 ■ The classic motor symptoms of Parkinson disease.

Bradykinesia is reflected in a slowing down of voluntary muscle activity. Walking is characterized by a shuffling gait, short steps and steppage height, and turning en bloc. Festination, an acceleration while walking in an effort to "catch up," results from flexed posture and postural instability. An extreme form of bradykinesia is called *freezing of gait*. Freezing of gait is a sudden and transient inability to move and is associated with an increase in falls. Other manifestations of bradykinesia can be seen in a loss of facial movement leading to a fixed stare with reduced eye blinking. Bradykinesia is the most disabling feature of PD, as it affects all aspects of daily life.

Postural instability, a feeling of imbalance, occurs as a result of the loss of postural reflexes and appears late in the disease progression. Of the classic motor symptoms of PD, it is the least responsive to treatment.

CLINICAL POINT: Bradykinesia plus one other of the cardinal symptoms (tremor or rigidity) must be present to make the diagnosis of PD. The diagnosis of PD is based on the patient's medical history and a thorough neurologic examination. There are no tests that confirm the diagnosis. ■

Nonmotor Features of PD. A number of nonmotor manifestations are also significant components of PD and may present earlier or later in the course of the disorder. Nonmotor manifestations result from widespread involvement of the brainstem, olfactory lobe, thalamus, and diverse cortical structures. The nonmotor symptoms can include fatigue, sleep disturbances, olfactory dysfunction, pain, and autonomic dysfunction (e.g., orthostatic hypotension, constipation, urinary retention, sexual dysfunction). Neuropsychiatric symptoms can include cognitive dysfunction, dementia, psychosis, hallucinations, mood disorders, depression, and anxiety.

Stages of PD. The Hoehn and Yahr Staging of Parkinson's Disease Scale is used to measure disease progression and monitor response to treatment (**Table 34.1** ■). This scale identifies five stages of disease progression, ranging from stage 0 (no signs of disease) to stage 5 (wheelchair bound or bedridden unless assisted). Another commonly used scale, the Unified Parkinson's Disease Rating Scale, is a more complex and comprehensive scale.

Matthew Horn: Application

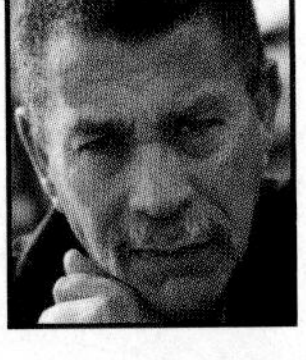

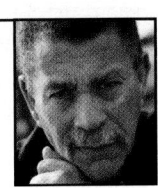

Mr. Horn sees the neurologist, Dr. Thomas. Dr. Thomas concurs with the neurologic findings of resting tremor, bradykinesia, and some mild rigidity as found by the primary care provider. On further questioning, Mr. Horn states that he is depressed and not interested in socializing or even going to work, which is very unusual for him. When asked about his sleep, he admits that he has insomnia and says when he does sleep, the dreams he remembers are "wild." Lately, he has experienced some constipation and is having some difficulty urinating, and he states that he cannot empty his bladder completely and feels that he always needs "to go." Mr. Horn has never smoked and does not drink coffee. He is diagnosed with Parkinson disease at Hoehn and Yahr Stage 1 with both motor and nonmotor symptoms. The nonmotor symptoms are mild depression, sleep disturbances, and autonomic dysfunction (constipation and urinary retention).

3. Identify the signs and symptoms that place Mr. Horn at stage 1 of the Hoehn and Yahr Staging of Parkinson Disease Scale.
4. What neuropsychiatric symptoms does Mr. Horn display?

Table 34.1 Hoehn and Yahr Staging of Parkinson Disease Scale

Stage	Parkinson Disease Symptoms
Stage 1	• Signs and symptoms on one side only • Symptoms mild • Symptoms inconvenient but not disabling • Usually presents with tremor of one limb • Friends have noticed changes in posture, locomotion, and facial expression
Stage 2	• Symptoms bilateral • Minimal disability • Posture and gait affected
Stage 3	• Significant slowing of body movements • Early impairment of equilibrium on walking or standing • Generalized dysfunction that is moderately severe
Stage 4	• Severe symptoms • Can still walk to a limited extent • Rigidity and bradykinesia • No longer able to live alone • Tremor may be less than in earlier stages
Stage 5	• Cachectic stage • Invalidism • Cannot stand or walk • Requires constant care

SOURCE: Data from Hoehn, M. M., & Yahr, M. D. (1967). Parkinsonism: Onset, progression, and mortality. *Neurology, 17*, 427.

Linking Pathophysiology to Diagnosis and Treatment

Unfortunately, despite intensive investigation and research, no current therapy prevents PD, halts its progression, or restores lost function. Treatment is individualized and is based on the individual's signs and symptoms, age, stage of disease, and degree of functional disability. Pharmacologic replenishment with dopaminergic drugs is the most common treatment. Other treatment options that are used in selected cases include ablation surgery, deep brain stimulation, and complementary and supportive therapies. The use of stem cell therapy, gene therapy, or neuroprotective agents remains experimental.

Levodopa is the most effective drug for the symptomatic treatment of PD, especially for bradykinesia, and it is often the drug of first choice. Other drugs that are used in the treatment of PD are dopamine agonists, anticholinergic agents, amantadine, monoamine oxidase inhibitors, and catechol-O-methyltransferase inhibitors. Although not all clinical features improve with the drug therapy, it has benefitted millions of patients in terms of improved quality of life, reduced disability, prolonged employability, and reduced mortality (**Figure 34.5** ■). In most cases, however, chronic drug therapy is associated with serious adverse effects, which can include confusion, hallucinations, psychosis, orthostatic hypotension, motor fluctuations, and involuntary movements called dyskinesias.

Matthew Horn: Outcome

At his initial visit with the neurologist, Mr. Horn is started on a low dose of carbidopa-levodopa. The neurologist explains that the levodopa will help to replenish dopamine in Mr. Horn's brain and that carbidopa is combined to block the levodopa conversion into dopamine by the liver so that it can get into the brain to work. At his 6-month follow-up visit with Dr. Thomas, Mr. Horn shows improvement in his motor symptoms but not his sleep abnormalities. His positive response to levodopa further supports the diagnosis of PD. Dr. Thomas recommends routine exercise and refers Mr. Horn to a physical therapist to help with balance, flexibility, and strength. Dr. Thomas also recommends a high-fiber diet with adequate hydration to help manage constipation and suggests that Mr. Horn avoid high-fat meals because fat slows gastric emptying and interferes with medication absorption.

5. Mr. Horn shows improvement in his motor symptoms while taking carbidopa-levodopa. How does this help to confirm the diagnosis of Parkinson disease?
6. What serious adverse effects can occur with long-term drug therapy for Parkinson disease?

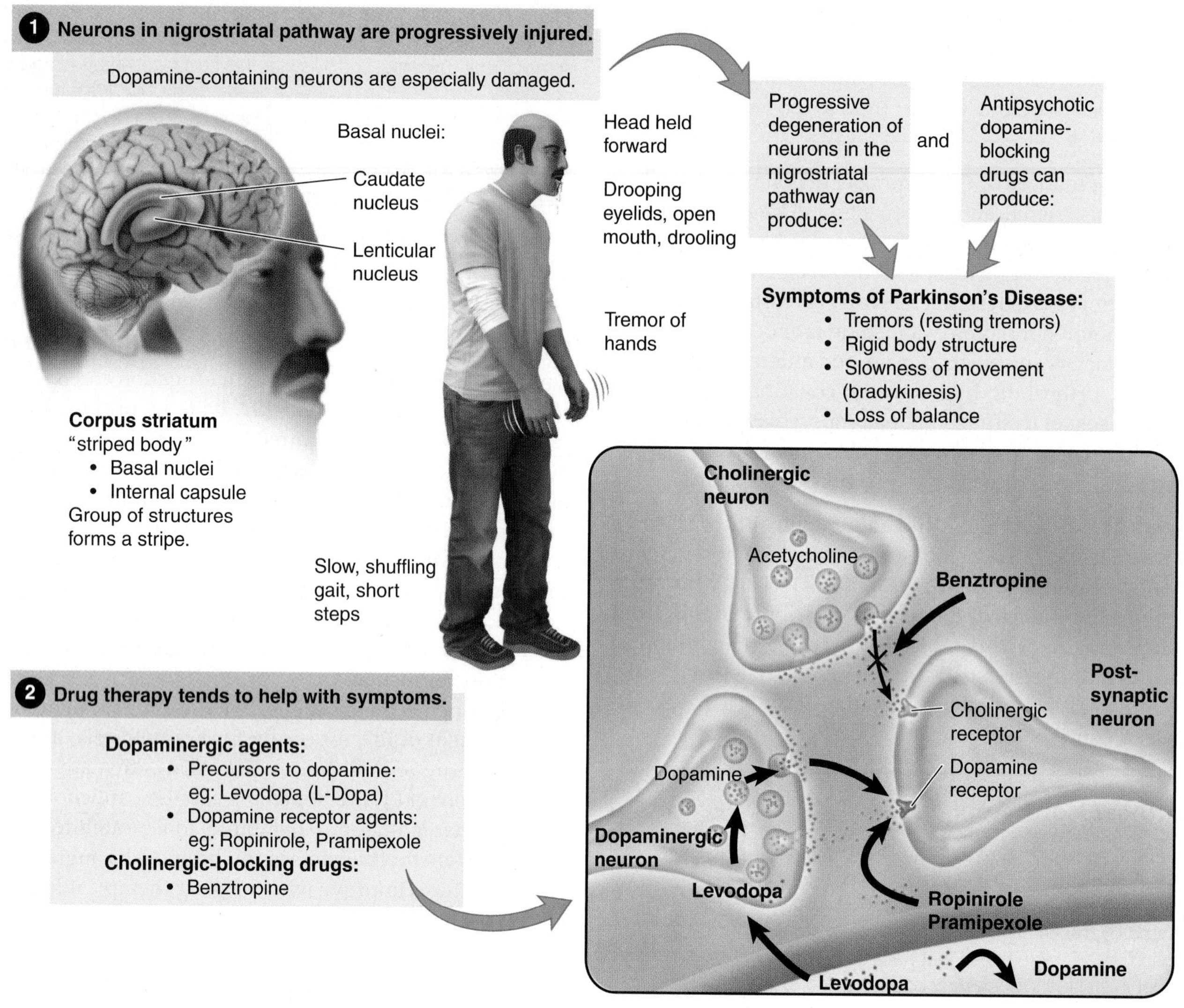

Figure 34.5 ■ Pharmacotherapy for Parkinson disease.

Check Your Progress: Section 34.2

1. What are the risk factors for developing Parkinson disease?
2. Explain the role of oxidative stress in the development of Parkinson disease.
3. What is the predominant concern in a patient with freezing of gait?

34.3 Multiple Sclerosis

Multiple sclerosis (MS) is a chronic, inflammatory, demyelinating and axonal degenerative disorder of the CNS. It is generally thought to be an inflammatory autoimmune disease. MS lesions can arise anywhere in the CNS; they are commonly seen in the periventricular white matter of the brain, optic nerve, cerebellum, and spinal cord. MS is a heterogeneous disease with a highly variable age at onset and clinical presentation. Disease progression ranges from benign and relatively stable to devastating with rapid deterioration and early death.

According to the National Multiple Sclerosis Society, approximately 2.3 million individuals worldwide have MS.[6] Because diagnosing MS is challenging, the incidence of the disease is difficult to determine. The risk factors for MS are related to age, gender, ethnicity, geography related to latitude, and genetics. Most people with MS are diagnosed between the ages of 20 and 50. MS is at least 2–3 times more common in women than in men; this suggests that hormones may play a role in the susceptibility to MS. MS occurs in most ethnic groups but is more common in Caucasians of northern European descent. MS is more common in areas farther from the equator; however, in some groups living far from the equator, such as the Inuits of Canada, MS is extremely rare. Therefore, ethnicity and geography must interact in some way that is not well understood. Moving from an area of high risk for MS to an area of low risk appears to have protective factors for individuals who move before 15 years of age. For those who move later in life, relocation is not a protective factor. Therefore, it appears that environmental exposure makes individuals susceptible to developing MS. Genetic factors are thought to play an important role in the development of MS, as the disease clusters within families. There is a 2.5–5% risk of developing MS if a first-degree relative, such as a parent or sibling, has the disorder. The risk increases to 25% if an identical twin has MS.[6]

Etiology and Pathogenesis

As in most other degenerative disorders of the nervous system, the exact cause of MS remains unknown. A widely accepted theory is that MS is caused by an autoimmune reaction. It is likely that multiple factors, such as viral infections, environmental factors, and genetic predisposition, act in concert as triggers for disease development.

MS is characterized by lesions that develop at different times and in different locations throughout the CNS. They typically occur in the periventricular white matter, optic nerve, brainstem, and cerebellum. These lesions are called **plaques**, and they vary in size from 1–2 millimeters to several centimeters. Plaques are the manifestations of pathologic processes, including inflammation, demyelination, degeneration, and gliosis or scar formation. A trigger sets off an inflammatory process, and the protective blood–brain barrier is disrupted. Inflammatory T cells, B cells, and macrophages enter the brain and attack myelin. Myelin coats the axon of the neuron and increases conduction velocity, allowing for salutary conduction from nodes of Ranvier to another with depolarization, thereby enabling fast conduction velocities (**Figure 34.6** ■). In MS, **demyelination** (damage to the myelin sheath) causes conduction blocks and dysfunction of the sodium and potassium channels, which are important in neuron depolarization and impulse transmission.

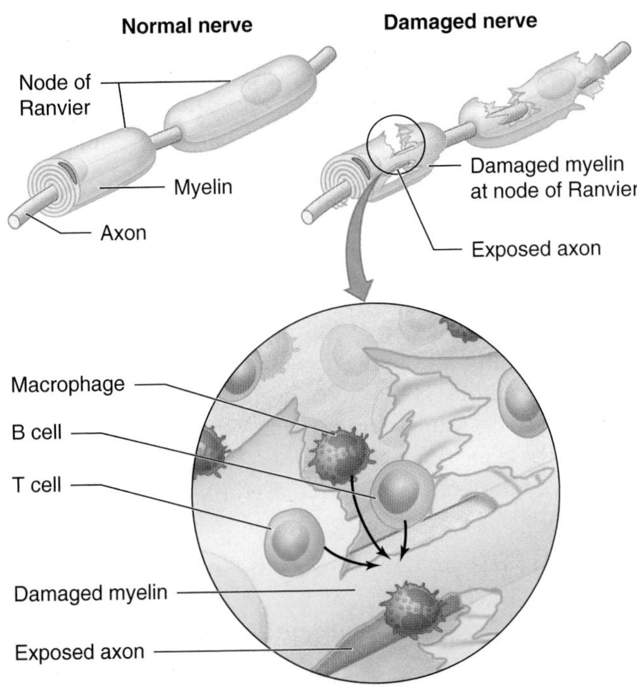

Figure 34.6 ■ Pathogenesis of demyelination in multiple sclerosis.

This demyelination will eventually cause axonal degeneration. Both white matter and gray matter brain atrophy can be seen in early stages of MS, but gray matter atrophy can increase rapidly and is directly related to the individual's cognitive functioning. Neuroaxonal degeneration and cortical demyelination are the most likely cause of gray matter atrophy in MS.[7]

Clinical Manifestations

Multiple sclerosis is classified principally by the clinical course at onset. The first presentation of MS is often a clinically isolated syndrome that exhibits characteristics of a demyelinating disease but has not yet met the MS diagnostic criteria. MS evolves as short-term episodes of neurologic deficit that resolve completely or leave a residual deficit. There are three types of progression of MS:

- Relapsing-remitting multiple sclerosis (RRMS) accounts for 85–90% of cases at onset. Patients with RRMS will remain stable or nearly stable for 10–20 years but can then transition from RRMS to secondary progressive multiple sclerosis.
- Secondary progressive multiple sclerosis (SPMS) is characterized by a gradual worsening with or without occasional relapses, minor remissions, and plateaus.
- Primary progressive multiple sclerosis (PPMS) is characterized by progressive deficits from the onset of the disease with occasional plateaus, temporary improvements, or acute relapses. PPMS accounts for approximately 10% of MS cases.

The progression of the three types of MS is shown in **Figure 34.7** ■.

It was once thought that getting MS at an older age and being male was associated with worse disease outcomes. However, research has demonstrated that this is not accurate.[8] In fact, there is evidence that the worsening of symptoms in people with MS is slowing.[8,9]

There are no clinical features that are unique to MS, but some are highly characteristic of the disease. These include sensory symptoms in the extremities or face, visual loss, double vision, weakness, vertigo, gait and balance disturbances, bladder problems, and pain. Bilateral internuclear ophthalmoplegia can be distinctive for MS. Internuclear ophthalmoplegia involves abnormal horizontal ocular movement with lost or delayed adduction and horizontal nystagmus of the abducting eye and vertical nystagmus on upward gaze. Many individuals can have multiple symptoms at onset. Fatigue and cognitive dysfunctions are other very common signs and symptoms that can occur with MS. See **Figure 34.8** ■ for other common symptoms.

CLINICAL POINT: Individuals with MS may experience temporary worsening of symptoms when the weather is very hot and humid, when they have a fever, or when they get overheated from exercising, sunbathing, or taking a hot shower or using a hot tub. They may experience blurred vision, called Uhthoff sign. The symptoms resolve as the body temperature returns to normal. ■

A Relapsing-Remitting MS (RRMS) — Most common form of MS, characterized by clearly defined acute attacks with full recovery.

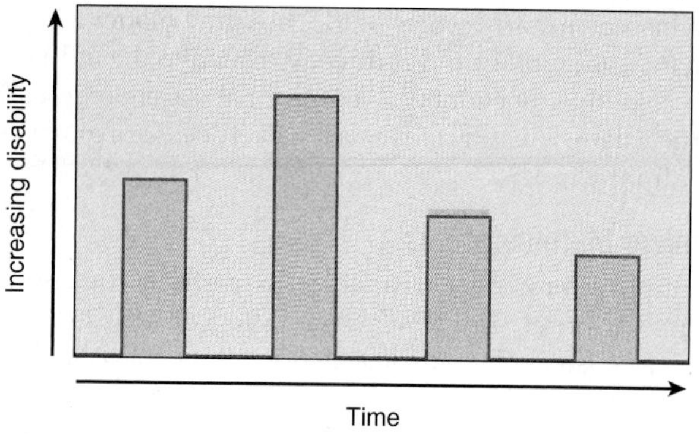

B Primary Progressive MS (PPMS) — Characterized by progression of disability from onset, with or without occasional plateaus and temporary minor improvements.

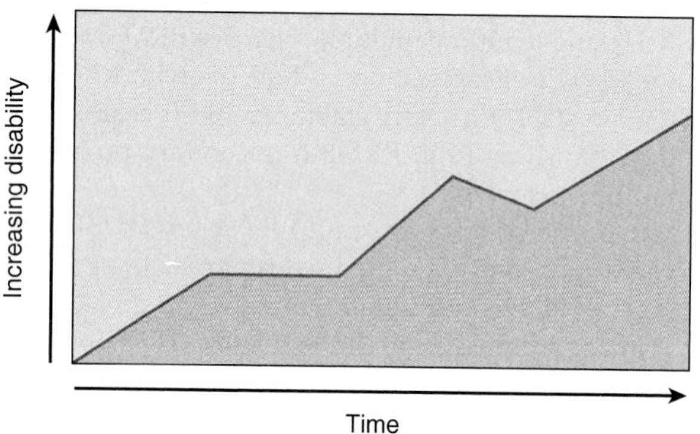

C Secondary–Progressive MS (SPMS) — Begins with initial RRMS disease course, followed by progression of disability with occasional relapses and minor remissions/plateaus.

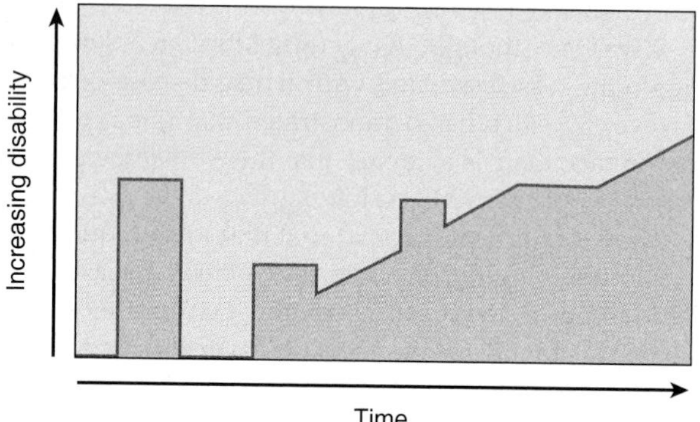

Figure 34.7 ■ Disease course in multiple sclerosis.

Susan Harris: Application

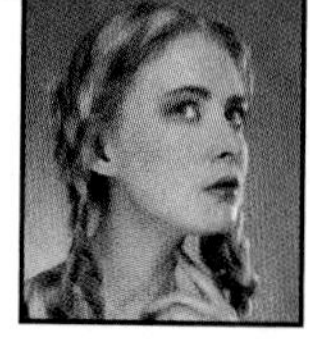

Ms. Harris has an MRI with gadolinium contrast and goes to see the neurologist. The neurologist, Dr. Sanchez, examines Ms. Harris and finds that she has impaired visual acuity bilaterally and diplopia (double vision), and her eye movements demonstrate vertical and horizontal nystagmus in both eyes, consistent with internuclear ophthalmoplegia. The decreased vibratory and position sense in her left arm resolved shortly after she saw the nurse practitioner. Dr. Sanchez tells Ms. Harris that her MRI shows that she has inflammation around her optic nerve, called optic neuritis, which is responsible for her vision problems and plaque in the posterior aspect of her cervical spinal cord, which is responsible for her sensory impairments that have now resolved. Dr. Sanchez states that this is consistent with criteria for MS: two distinct lesions (dissemination in space) in the brain that have occurred over a several-month time period (dissemination in time). He classifies the type of MS as relapsing-remitting and tells Ms. Harris that her visual problems will most likely resolve. He is going to start her on a medication called Avonex, which is given weekly as an intramuscular injection. Dr. Sanchez tells Ms. Harris that it also important that she abstain from sexual intercourse or use an effective method of birth control. She also needs to avoid exposure to saunas and hot tubs, and to avoid overheating in general, as this may worsen her symptoms temporarily.

3. What type of progression of disease can Ms. Harris expect with relapsing-remitting MS?
4. Describe specific activities that Ms. Harris should avoid that may cause overheating.

Linking Pathophysiology to Diagnosis and Treatment

MS is primarily diagnosed clinically by the demonstration of a CNS lesion disseminated in time and space. MRI with gadolinium contrast is the test of choice to support the diagnosis of MS and can reveal the characteristic lesions of demyelination, or plaque (**Figure 34.9** ■).

The McDonald criteria include specific MRI evidence used for diagnosing MS (see **Table 34.2** ■).[10]

There are multiple conditions that have presenting symptoms similar to those of MS and should be considered in the differential diagnosis. The main differential diagnoses for MS include, but are not limited to, migraine with visual disturbances, carpal tunnel syndrome, neurosyphilis, sarcoidosis, transverse myelitis, spinal cord tumor, vasculitis, and stroke. Other tests that may be used in diagnosing MS include blood tests to rule out infections, endocrine abnormalities, vitamin B12 deficiency, and collagen diseases; evoked potentials that record the timing of the CNS response to various stimuli, which could be visual, auditory, or sensory; electroencephalography (EEG); and lumbar puncture, which shows oligoclonal bands and immunoglobulins in cases of MS. Lumbar puncture is not routinely used, owing to the high sensitivity and specificity of MRI.

MS is treated with immunomodulatory therapy (IMT) for the underlying immune disorder and therapies to relieve or limit other symptoms. IMT is used to reduce the frequency and severity of MS attacks, to slow the progress of disability, and to decrease the accumulation of CNS plaque. Several IMTs that have been approved by the U.S. Food and Drug Administration (FDA) for RRMS are on the market; these include, but not limited to, interferon beta-1a (Avonex), interferon beta-1b (Betaseron), and natalizumab (Tysabri).

IMT has an FDA category C warning for possible teratogenicity that can have adverse effects on fertility, pregnancy outcomes, and breastfed infants. IMT should be discontinued before pregnancy. If MS relapse occurs during pregnancy, the woman can be treated safely with a short course of corticosteroids after the first trimester.[11] ■

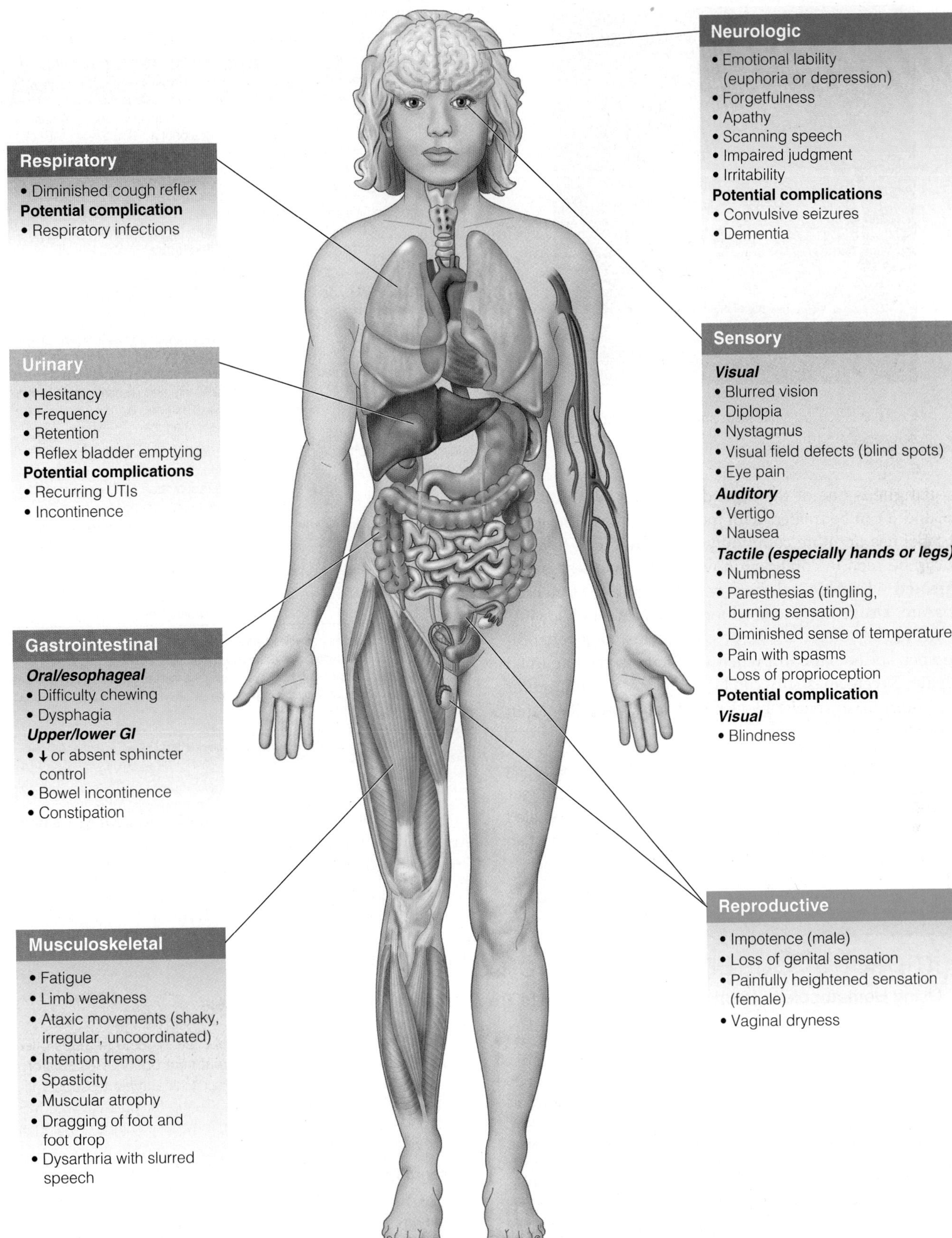

Neurologic
• Emotional lability (euphoria or depression)
• Forgetfulness
• Apathy
• Scanning speech
• Impaired judgment
• Irritability
Potential complications
• Convulsive seizures
• Dementia
Respiratory
• Diminished cough reflex
Potential complication
• Respiratory infections
Urinary
• Hesitancy
• Frequency
• Retention
• Reflex bladder emptying
Potential complications
• Recurring UTIs
• Incontinence
Sensory
Visual
• Blurred vision
• Diplopia
• Nystagmus
• Visual field defects (blind spots)
• Eye pain
Auditory
• Vertigo
• Nausea
Tactile (especially hands or legs)
• Numbness
• Paresthesias (tingling, burning sensation)
• Diminished sense of temperature
• Pain with spasms
• Loss of proprioception
Potential complication
Visual
• Blindness
Gastrointestinal
Oral/esophageal
• Difficulty chewing
• Dysphagia
Upper/lower GI
• ↓ or absent sphincter control
• Bowel incontinence
• Constipation
Reproductive
• Impotence (male)
• Loss of genital sensation
• Painfully heightened sensation (female)
• Vaginal dryness
Musculoskeletal
• Fatigue
• Limb weakness
• Ataxic movements (shaky, irregular, uncoordinated)
• Intention tremors
• Spasticity
• Muscular atrophy
• Dragging of foot and foot drop
• Dysarthria with slurred speech

Figure 34.8 ■ Multisystem effects of multiple sclerosis.

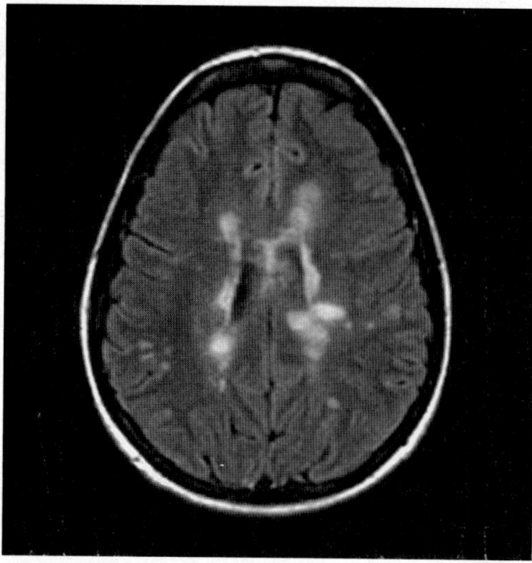

Figure 34.9 ■ MRI scan showing multiple sclerosis plaques.

Table 34.2 2010 McDonald Criteria for MS Diagnosis

Clinical Presentation	Additional Data Needed for MS Diagnosis
Two or more attacks Objective clinical evidence of two or more lesions with reasonable historical evidence of a prior attack	None; clinical evidence will suffice. Additional evidence (e.g., MRI of brain) is desirable but must be consistent with MS.
Two or more attacks Objective clinical evidence of one lesion	Dissemination in space demonstrated by MRI or await further clinical attack implicating a different site.
One attack Objective clinical evidence of two or more lesions	Dissemination in time demonstrated by MRI or second clinical attack.
One attack Objective clinical evidence of one lesion (clinically isolated syndrome)	Dissemination in space demonstrated by MRI or await a second clinical attack implicating a different CNS site and dissemination in time, demonstrated by MRI or a second clinical attack.
Insidious neurologic progression suggestive of MS	1 year of disease progression and dissemination in space, demonstrated by two of the following: • One or more T2 lesions in the brain in regions characteristic of MS • Two or more T2 focal lesions in the spinal cord • Positive CNS.

NOTE: An attack is defined as a neurologic disturbance of the kind see in MS. It can be documented by subjective report or objective observation, but it must last for at least 24 hours. Pseudo-attacks and single paroxysmal episodes must be excluded. To be considered separate attacks, at least 30 days must elapse between the onset of one event and the onset of another.

SOURCE: Polman, C. H., Reingold, S. C., Banwell, B., Clanet, M., Cohen, J. A., Filippi, M., et al. (2011). Diagnostic criteria for multiple sclerosis: 2010 revisions to the McDonald criteria. *Annals of Neurology*, 69(2), 292–302.

Fatigue is one of the most debilitating symptoms of MS, and it can be treated with the drug Amantadine as an off-label use or, more commonly, with modafinil. Spasticity can be seen in conjunction with motor weakness and is treated with physical therapy and a routine stretching program. Drugs that are used for the treatment of spasticity include baclofen with the possible inclusion of benzodiazepines and gabapentin when spasticity is accompanied by pain. Severe spasticity can be treated by intramuscular botulinum toxin, nerve blocks, and intrathecal baclofen pump placement.

CLINICAL POINT: The use of live attenuated virus vaccines, such as herpes zoster vaccine for protection from shingles, is not recommended for individuals with MS, particularly those being treated with IMT. The live virus in the vaccine can trigger the onset of an MS attack. ■

The use of stem cell transplantation to treat MS is being studied. See the Impact of Current Research on Clinical Practice feature.

Impact of Current Research on Clinical Practice

Using Hematopoietic Stem Cell Transplantation to Treat Patients with Multiple Sclerosis

Description: Burt and colleagues studied 123 patients with RRMS and 28 patients with SPMS who received peripheral blood stem cells transplants between 2003 and 2014. Expanded Disability Status Scale scores improved significantly from pretransplantation to 2 years posttransplantation. Also seen was a significant improvement in quality of life, a decrease in MS lesion volume on MRI, and an increase in progression-free periods. This study has several limitations: It was conducted at a single institution, treatment was done for compassionate reasons, neurologic improvement may have been part of continuing recovery, patients were followed for only 4 years, and it was an observational study. However, the findings were associated with significant and sustained improvement in neurologic disability, function, quality of life, and MS lesion volume in comparison to recent pharmacology studies. Randomized controlled trials are warranted.

Clinical Practice: Stem cell transplantation could perhaps offer patients with MS a potential new treatment option. Results from this study warrant future randomized clinical trials to substantiate its uses as a treatment option. Caring for patients with MS undergoing stem cell transplantation may pose unique challenges for the nurse.

Research Study:

Burt, R. K., Balabanov, R., Han, X., Sharrack, B., Morgan, A., & Quigley, K. (2015). Association of nonmyeloablative hematopoietic stem cell transplantation with neurologic disability in patients with relapsing-remitting multiple sclerosis *Journal of the American Medical Association, 312*(3), 275–284.

Susan Harris: Outcome

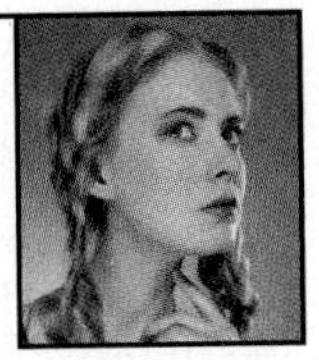

It has been 2 years since Ms. Harris was diagnosed with MS. She comes to see Dr. Sanchez for her regularly scheduled visit and complains that she has some new weakness in her right leg but says that it is not too bad. Dr. Sanchez tells her that her most recent MRI shows another brain lesion in her left frontal lobe that is causing her right leg weakness, but he tells her that she is doing well, since that is the only attack she has had since being diagnosed, so the Avonex is working well to decrease the frequency and severity of the MS attacks.

He asks her about symptoms of depression, suicidal ideation, and allergic reaction, since they are all side effects of Avonex. Ms. Harris tells Dr. Sanchez that she has none of these symptoms and is very excited that she will be getting married in 2 months and she really wants to start a family. Dr. Sanchez says that it would be a good idea to continue taking birth control pills and Avonex for the next 2 months so that the stress of the wedding plans does not cause another attack and she does not become pregnant during that time. He also says that she should schedule another appointment after the wedding to discuss stopping Avonex and how pregnancy can affect a woman with MS.

5. How does Ms. Harris's treatment for MS affect her family planning decisions?
6. What treatment goals can Ms. Harris expect with immunomodulatory therapy (IMT)?

Check Your Progress: Section 34.3

1. Describe the criteria for an MS attack.
2. Explain why live attenuated virus should not be administered to a person with MS.
3. How is spasticity in the person with MS treated pharmacologically?

34.4 Amyotrophic Lateral Sclerosis

Amyotrophic lateral sclerosis (ALS) is a progressive neurodegenerative disease that causes weakness, disability, and death within 3–5 years. ALS is also known as Lou Gehrig's disease, for the famous baseball player who died from the disease. The cause of ALS is unknown. In ALS, both upper motor neurons, found in the corticospinal tract, and lower motor neurons, found in the anterior horn cells of the spinal cord, are affected by neurodegeneration. The motor deficits are the most devastating feature, but nonmotor deficits also occur.

More than 12,000 people in the United States have ALS, and 7000 new cases are diagnosed each year. ALS is one of the most common neuromuscular diseases worldwide and affects all races and ethnicities. It is more common in Caucasian males and in people age 60–69 years but can occur at younger ages. About 90–95% of ALS cases are sporadic or idiopathic; that is, the disease occurs at random with no clear associated risk factors. About 5–10% of cases are inherited, and most of these follow an autosomal dominant inheritance pattern in which a genetic mutation is inherited from one parent. The children of a parent with an autosomal dominant mutation have a 50% chance of inheriting the gene and developing ALS.[12] The only recognized risk factors for ALS are age and family history. There is some evidence suggesting that cigarette smoking may be a risk factor. There is weaker and conflicting evidence on other possible risk factors, including military service in the Gulf War, exposure to heavy metals such as lead and mercury, heavy manual labor, repetitive muscle use, and trauma.

Etiology and Pathogenesis

No direct mechanism or cause for ALS has been determined. It falls into the category of a neuronal degenerative disease; however, its specificity in its attack on motor neurons is similar to that of a prion disease (misfolded protein derangement with spread) or malignancy (DNA change). In ALS, motor axons die by Wallerian degeneration, larger motor neurons being affected to a greater extent. This degeneration occurs in the CNS (corticospinal and corticobulbar pathways) and peripheral nervous system (motor neurons in the anterior horn of the spinal cord and the motor nuclei of the lower brainstem). Certain motor neurons are spared until late in the disease, including motor neurons for ocular motility, parasympathetic sacral spinal cord neurons that innervate the bowel and bladder sphincters, and the posterior column of the spinal cord, which is responsible for various sensory functions.

Pathways that lead to axonal degeneration and cell death can be mediated by various factors, which are not mutually exclusive. These include oxidative stress; aggregation of abnormal superoxide dismutase proteins causing mitochondrial dysfunction; defect of axonal transport by protein aggregates or mutant neurofilament proteins; abnormal growth factor expression; **excitotoxicity** due to defective glutamate uptake into astrocytes, as excitotoxins are thought to precipitate neuronal death by triggering excess calcium influx into motor neurons; caspase-mediated cell death (apoptosis); and glial cell pathology.

Research on familial cases of ALS has shown that mutations in the copper/zinc superoxide dismutase 1 (*SOD1*) gene causes oxidative damage to proteins and in turn causes glutamate excitotoxicity. This finding paved the way for the development of riluzole (Rilutek), the only treatment that has been shown to extend life in ALS, albeit for only 2–3 months.

Clinical Manifestations

ALS has an insidious onset of slowly progressive, painless weakness in one or more body parts. The clinical hallmark of ALS is the presence of upper motor neuron (UMN) and lower motor neuron (LMN) signs and symptoms. UMN manifestations are slowness of movement, stiffness, incoordination, hyperreflexia, and spasticity due to involvement of the motor neuron in the frontal lobe of the cerebrum and the axons that traverse through the midbrain, the brainstem, and the lateral corticospinal tract of the spinal cord.

UMN symptoms seen in the hand are poor manual dexterity, such as difficulty buttoning clothes or tying shoes; leg UMN symptoms manifest as poor balance, slow, stiff gait, and spasms. LMN manifestations include weakness and muscle atrophy in the extremities, fasciculations (muscle twitches), and cramps due to involvement of the motor neurons in the anterior horn cells. In most individuals with ALS, symptoms begin with extremity involvement. As the disease advances, muscle atrophy and spasticity are severe. In approximately 20%, initial symptoms are of bulbar dysfunction, including dysarthria, dysphagia, and hoarse voice, which can be caused by either UMN or LMN involvement. UMN dysphagia results in slow, uncoordinated contractions of the swallowing muscles, while LMN dysphagia is due to tongue weakness that disrupts the oral phase of swallowing. Progression of bulbar symptoms leads to poor nutrition and dehydration and to choking on food or on the person's own secretions and aspiration. ALS patients can also develop frontotemporal executive dysfunction (poor insight and inability to plan) without overt dementia, and the cognitive impairment may be subtle. Patients with ALS usually succumb to respiratory failure due to aspiration pneumonia and/or respiratory muscle weakness.

Linking Pathophysiology to Diagnosis and Treatment

The diagnosis of ALS is based primarily on clinical manifestations. A definitive diagnosis of ALS may be difficult to determine early in the disease because many other diseases have similar manifestations. Disease entities such as stroke, brain or spinal cord tumor, radiculopathies and neuropathies, acute viral infection involving motor neurons (West Nile, herpes zoster), heavy metal poisoning, and vasculitis need to be excluded. The diagnostic workup for ALS can include electromyography and nerve conduction studies, MRI or CT scan of the brain and spinal cord, muscle or nerve biopsy, genetic testing for various gene mutations, and blood tests for a wide variety of abnormalities, including vitamin B12 and folate, HIV, thyroid function, syphilis, and Lyme disease.

CLINICAL POINT: Patients with ALS should have serial assessments of their respiratory function every 3 months starting at the time of diagnosis. Pulmonary function tests help the medical team to understand the pace of disease progression and to plan for the right intervention at the right time. A decrease in vital capacity to 50% of predicted value is associated with development of respiratory symptoms such as development of pneumonia, while a vital capacity of 25–30% of predicted value is associated with respiratory failure and sudden death. ■

The World Federation of Neurology has developed a diagnostic algorithm that combines clinical and electrophysiologic findings. The degree of certainty of the diagnosis of ALS increases with the number of regions of the body that demonstrate UMN and LMN signs. The regions are bulbar (muscles of the face, mouth, and throat), cervical (muscles of the head, neck, shoulders, upper back, and arms, including muscles of respiration), thoracic (muscles of the chest, abdomen, and middle portion of the spinal muscles), and lumbosacral (muscles of the lower back, groin, and legs). The presence of at least three body regions demonstrating UMN and LMN signs is clinically definitive of ALS.

ALS is incurable and fatal. There is a median survival of 3 years, although treatment can extend the length of survival and improve the patient's quality of life. The most effective predictor of life expectancy is the rate of disease progression. A system of stages or milestones has been proposed that standardizes the mean time from onset to diagnosis and from onset to death through the course of ALS (see **Table 34.3** ■).[13]

The glutamate pathway antagonist riluzole (Rilutek) is the only FDA-approved medication that has shown efficacy in extending life in ALS patients by 2–3 months. In addition to riluzole, the American Academy of Neurology recommends the use of noninvasive ventilation and percutaneous endoscopic gastrostomy tube placement and feeding to extend life.[14] A wide variety of medications may be used to relieve the symptoms associated with ALS and to maximize the patient's remaining function. These medications include muscle relaxants for spasticity, pain medications, antidepressant and antianxiety medications, anticholinergic medications for sialorrhea (drooling), and medications for cognitive dysfunction. A multidisciplinary approach to care from neurologists, nurse care managers, dietitians, social workers, and physical, occupational, speech–language, and respiratory therapists can improve survival and quality of life. As ALS progresses, early involvement of hospice and palliative care services is important.

Table 34.3 Stages of Amyotrophic Lateral Sclerosis

Stage	Description
Stage 1	Symptom onset (involvement of the first body region)
Stage 2A	Diagnosis (35% of the way through the disease course)
Stage 2B	Involvement of a second body region (38% of the way through the disease course)
Stage 3	Involvement of a third body region (61% of the way through the disease course)
Stage 4A	Need for gastrostomy/feeding tube (77% of the way through the disease course)
Stage 4B	Need for noninvasive ventilation (80% of the way through the disease course)

SOURCE: Roche, J. C., Rojas-Garcia, R., Scott, M. K., Scotton, W., Ellis, C. E., et al. (2012). A proposed staging system for amyotrophic lateral sclerosis. *Brain, 135*, 847–852.

Check Your Progress: Section 34.4

1. What are the recognized risk factors for ALS?
2. What are the hallmark manifestations of ALS?
3. How is ALS clinically diagnosed?

34.5 Huntington Disease

Huntington disease (HD) is named for George Huntington, who published the first accurate and comprehensive account of the disorder in 1872. HD is a progressive, incurable, neurodegenerative disease of the brain that causes uncontrolled, involuntary movements; dementia; and behavior changes. It is an autosomal dominant inherited disease in which a child of a parent with HD has a 50% chance of inheriting the gene mutation that causes the disease.

The estimated prevalence of HD is 3–7 per 100,000 people of European ancestry. HD occurs worldwide and in all ethnic groups; however, it is less common in people of Japanese, Chinese, and African descent.[15] A few isolated populations in Venezuela and the islands of Mauritius and Tasmania have an unusually high prevalence of HD, which is thought to be the result of the founder effect (reduced genetic diversity when a population is descended from a small number of ancestors).

Onset of symptoms usually occurs at 35–44 years of age. Onset in people younger than 10 years or older than 70 years of age is rare. The duration of the disease course varies, with a mean of approximately 19 years. Most people survive 10–25 years after the onset of symptoms. The primary causes of death are pneumonia and cardiovascular disease.

Etiology and Pathogenesis

Mutation in the huntington gene (*HTT*) on the short arm of chromosome 4 causes HD. The HTT gene encodes for a protein called huntingtin. Its exact role is unknown, but it is important for neuronal function. In HD, the *HTT* mutation involves the DNA segment CAG (cytosine, adenine, and guanine) trinucleotide repeat. Normally, the CAG segment is repeated 10–35 times within the gene; in patients with HD, the CAG segment is repeated 36–120 times. Individuals with more than 40 CAG repeats almost always develop HD. The higher the number of CAG repeats, the earlier the onset of HD symptoms can occur, possibly with more rapid than usual onset. The CAG repeat leads to huntingtin accumulation and formation of inclusion in the cell nucleus, which alters transcription and transport and leads to neuronal cell death. Several mechanisms of neuronal cell death have been proposed for HD, including excitotoxicity, oxidative stress, impaired metabolism, and apoptosis.

The most striking pathology in HD occurs within the striatum, particularly gross atrophy in the caudate nucleus and putamen accompanied by selective neuronal loss and gliosis. Marked neuronal loss is also seen in the cerebral cortex; other areas in the midbrain and cerebellum show varying degrees of atrophy. The brain will shrink in volume up to 40% early in HD (**Figure 34.10** ■). Numerous biochemical defects also occur, including impaired glucose metabolism, excessive dopamine, disturbances in concentrations of GABA, acetylcholine, choline acetyltransferase, and norepinephrine.

A system for grading the severity of HD is based on the extent of gross striatal pathology, neuronal loss, and gliosis (see **Table 34.4** ■).

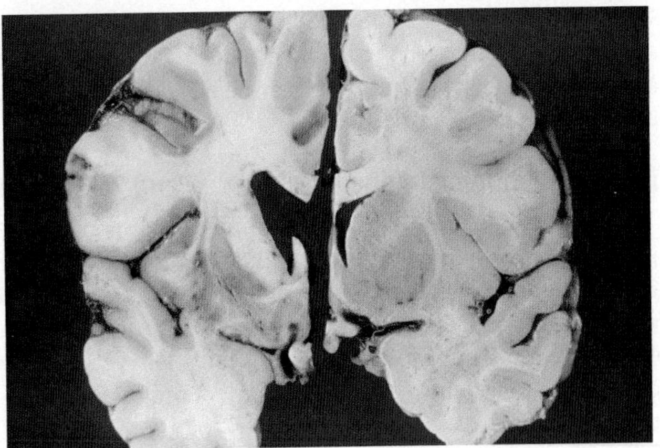

Figure 34.10 ■ Caudate atrophy seen in Huntington disease.

Table 34.4 Grading for Severity of Huntington Disease

Grade	Pathology
Grade 0	There is no detectable histologic neuropathology and no gross striatal atrophy in the presence of clinical manifestations and positive family history.
Grade 1	Neuropathologic changes can be detected microscopically but without gross atrophy.
Grade 2	Striatal atrophy is present, but the caudate nucleus remains convex.
Grade 3	Striatal atrophy is more severe, and the caudate nucleus is flat.
Grade 4	Striatal atrophy is most severe, and the medial surface of the caudate nucleus is concave.

SOURCE: Data from Vonsattel, J. P., Myers, R. H., Stevens, T. J., Ferrante, R. J., Bird, E. D., & Richardson, E. P., Jr. (1985). Neuropathological classification of Huntington's disease. *Journal of Neuropathology and Experimental Neurology, 44*(6), 559–577.

Clinical Manifestations

The clinical manifestations of HD are involuntary movements, cognitive impairment, and behavioral changes, any or all being present in varying degrees. The most common movement disorder is chorea, which is derived from the Greek word meaning "to dance." As defined by the World Federation of Neurology, chorea is a state of excessive spontaneous movements that are irregularly timed, randomly distributed, and abrupt. Mild chorea appears as fidgetiness; severe chorea can be an uncontrolled flailing of extremities, called *ballism*, which hinders normal functioning. As HD progresses, chorea is replaced with parkinsonian features of rigidity, bradykinesia, and postural instability. In advanced or late disease, individuals can develop akinetic–rigid syndrome, with minimal or no chorea. Dysarthria, dysphagia, abnormal eye movements, tics, and myoclonus can also be seen in individuals with HD.

Short-term memory loss is seen early in the disease, then impaired intellectual function, and eventual progression to dementia, but the rate of progression is variable. This pattern of progression corresponds with the syndrome of subcortical dementia and is reflective of frontal–subcortical circuitry dysfunction.

A wide range of psychiatric manifestations can be seen in HD, including depression, obsessive–compulsive disorder, psychosis, and mania consistent with bipolar disorder. The behavioral changes that are common in HD are irritability, moodiness, untidiness, antisocial behavior, and apathy or loss of interest. These manifestations are seen early in the disease.

CLINICAL POINT: The incidence of suicide is increased in individuals with HD in comparison to the general public. It is important to assess the patient for depressed mood and suicidal ideations early and throughout the disease course. ■

Linking Pathophysiology to Diagnosis and Treatment

The diagnosis of HD can be determined by a genetically proven family history and clinical presentation. Genetic testing, which is available commercially, tests for the CAG repeat number. Genetic testing should be performed at a center recommended by the Huntington's Disease Society of America that follows a strict protocol of pretest and post-test counseling.

For individuals with HD who want to have a child who does not have the HD gene, there are some options. Genetic diagnostic testing can be used with in vitro fertilization to ensure that the fertilized egg does not have the abnormal gene. If the woman is already pregnant, a chorionic villus biopsy can be performed at 10–11 weeks or amniocentesis at 14–18 weeks to test the fetus for the HD gene. ■

MRI or CT scan can be used to measure brain atrophy. Referral to a neurologist who specializes in HD, neuropsychologic testing, and psychiatric evaluation are important early considerations.

There is no cure for HD, and there are no medications or therapies that can delay the onset of HD symptoms or prevent disease progression. Treatment options are focused on reducing the symptoms of HD and improving the patient's quality of life. Indicators to initiate treatment for chorea symptoms include physical injury and interference with function and activities such as work and sleep.[15] Tetrabenazine is the only FDA-approved medication for HD chorea. If chorea is accompanied by depression or psychosis, antidepressant or antipsychotic medications should be considered as the first choice. If parkinsonian features are present, individuals may benefit from levodopa or dopamine agonist medications.[16] Ablative surgical procedures and fetal cell transplantation have been performed to treat HD, but minimal data support these procedures, and they remain experimental.

Check Your Progress: Section 34.5

1. What is the correlation between CAG segment repeats and the development of Huntington disease?
2. What are the three categories of clinical manifestations of Huntington disease?
3. Describe the progression of movement impairment in the person with Huntington disease.

34.6 Seizure Disorders

Seizure activity represents abnormal electrical discharges within the brain that result in involuntary movement and/or behavior and sensory alterations. The involuntary movements may encompass the entire body or just certain muscle groups, such as those of one arm. The classic presentation of seizure activity in the media is of an individual falling to the ground and shaking. This pattern of involuntary movement is what most individuals consider seizure activity. However, seizure activity can manifest as changes in the level of consciousness, behavior, or sensory perception.

It is estimated that 2.2 million people in the United States are affected with seizure disorders. Seizures can occur in any age group but tend to occur more often in older adults and children. Recurrent seizure activity as a result of central nervous system disorder or disruption is referred to as **epilepsy**.[17,18]

Etiology and Pathogenesis

Some seizures may be caused by underlying pathologic conditions such as infection, electrolyte imbalance, trauma, hypoglycemia, endocrine dysfunction, or tumors. Other seizures are idiopathic.

Febrile seizures usually occur in children as the result of a rapid temperature rise above 102.2°F (39°C, rectal), often in association with an acute illness. Most febrile seizures present as generalized seizures and last only a few minutes. Sometimes the fever can occur a few hours after the seizure. No evidence of intracranial infection or other definitive cause is found. Febrile seizures usually occur in children between the ages of 6 months and 5 years old, peaking in incidence during the second year of life. Infants and toddlers have a lower seizure threshold than adults and therefore are more susceptible to seizures caused by minor stimuli such as fevers. There is often a family history of febrile seizures. Children who have one febrile seizure have a 40% chance of experiencing more febrile seizures, especially if a relatively low temperature accompanied the seizure, the first febrile seizure occurred before the age of 18 months, or the seizure was the first sign of an illness.[19]

Partial seizures (also known as *focal seizures*) occur when abnormal electrical activity is contained within a limited area of the brain. These seizures are referred to as partial seizures because the electrical activity resulting in a seizure may occur only within one lobe or hemisphere of the brain, in comparison to generalized seizures. In generalized seizures, the abnormal electrical activity tends to involve both brain hemispheres. Partial seizures tend to be divided into two categories: simple and complex. A simple partial seizure may result in a loss of motor control without affecting memory or awareness. Complex partial seizures may or may not influence awareness but often lead to behavior changes or memory impairment. The individual may display repetitive behaviors without awareness, such as lip smacking or flipping a light switch over and over again. A partial seizure could progress into a generalized seizure.

Generalized seizures are caused by abnormal electrical discharges that originate from both hemispheres of the brain. Types of generalized seizures include tonic–clonic, absence, and status epilepticus. Generalized seizures are associated with a loss of awareness or consciousness and may manifest in the traditional pattern of muscle stiffness and twitching as often depicted in the media.[20]

Intractable seizures are those that are refractory, that is, they continue to occur even with optimal medical management. The individual with intractable seizures should be referred to care environments that specialize in dealing with seizure activity, such as an epilepsy center.

The lifetime prevalence of epilepsy in children is 10 per 1000 (1%), with 6 per 1000 (0.6%) reporting a currently active seizure disorder. Prevalence is higher in low-income families and in older male children.[21] In addition, about 1.8% of adults age 18 years and older have had a seizure disorder, with 1% reporting a currently active seizure disorder.[22] Other risk factors include being an infant who is small for gestational age, the presence of underlying neurologic conditions, brain tumor or infection of the brain, stroke, cerebral palsy, autism spectrum disorder, family history, or abuse of drugs.[23] ■

Clinical Manifestations

Seizure activity can result in a number of different clinical manifestations depending on the area of the brain in which the abnormal electrical activity occurs. Manifestations typically include a loss of conscious awareness of the environment and varying patterns of muscular rigidity and relaxation (see **Table 34.5** ■). A change in sensation or perception may precede the seizure activity. This sensory or perceptual disturbance is referred to as an **aura**. The aura is often considering a warning sign of impending seizure activity and often precedes seizure activity restricted to a particular region of the brain. The advent of an aura gives the individual the opportunity to lie down or take other precautions to avoid injury that may result from seizure activity, such as falling or the striking of parts of the body against hard surfaces.

Tonic–clonic seizures are the most common seizure type in children, characterized by alternating repetitive tonic–clonic activity. ■

The patterns of generalized seizures occur in certain phases, which are referred to as tonic, clonic, and postictal.

- The initial **tonic phase** is characterized by muscular rigidity and a sudden loss of consciousness. The individual will fall and may display a pattern in which the head and feet bend backwards with the body arched forward. Muscles are rigid, with the arms and legs extended and the jaw clenched. Pupils are fixed and dilated. This pattern of muscular rigidity increases metabolic demands, increasing the need for glucose and oxygen. However, the individual may be unable to breathe because of the muscular rigidity, and

Table 34.5 Types of Seizures

Type and Etiology	Manifestations	Therapies
Focal Seizures		
Simple partial seizure Involves activation of one restricted part of one cerebral hemisphere	Patient does not lose awareness/consciousness. Recurrent muscle contractions of the face or one side of the body occur. Sensory manifestations such as tingling or numbness may occur.	Antiseizure medications Gamma knife surgery Vagal nerve stimulation
Complex partial seizure Usually originates in the temporal lobe and involves activation of one restricted part of one cerebral hemisphere	Usually preceded by an aura. Lasts 30 seconds to 2 minutes. Impaired consciousness for several hours. Amnesia following seizure is common.	Antiseizure medications Resection of epileptogenic focus Vagal nerve stimulation
Generalized Seizures		
Absence seizure Involves both hemispheres of the brain and deeper brain structures such as the brainstem, thalamus, and basal ganglia	Patient has sudden, brief cessation of all motor activity. Blank stare and unresponsive to the environment usually for 5–10 seconds but can last as long as 30 seconds. LOC is impaired. More common in children. Frequency ranges from occasional to several hundred per day.	Antiseizure medications
Tonic–clonic seizure Most common type of seizure seen in adults	No aura or warning. Sudden loss of consciousness. Tonic and clonic phases.	Antiseizure medications, especially valproic acid, phenytoin, or carbamazepine Diazepam, lorazepam, or phenobarbital may be administered during seizure to limit length of seizure.
Status epilepticus Seizures may be any type but most often are generalized tonic–clonic.	Involves continuous seizure activity, with only short periods of calm between intense and persistent seizures. Patient is in great danger of hypoxia, hypoglycemia, hyperthermia, acidosis, and exhaustion if seizure activity is not halted.	Medical emergency Establish and maintain airway Administer 50% glucose Administer diazepam or lorazepam IV; repeat every 10 minutes until seizure activity stops. Administer antiseizure medications such as phenytoin or fosphenytoin. Phenobarbital may also be administered. IV general anesthesia with propofol may be used as a last resort if seizure activity does not cease.

the resultant hypoxia leads to skin pallor and cyanosis. Commonly, urinary incontinence can be noted; there may also be bowel incontinence. This phase typically lasts 15–60 seconds.

- During the **clonic phase**, the patient experiences alternating periods of muscular contraction and relaxation in all extremities. Hyperventilation occurs, the eyes roll back, and the patient may froth at the mouth. This phase varies in length from 60 to 90 seconds and subsides gradually.
- In the **postictal period**, which also varies in length, the patient's level of consciousness is decreased, and the patient is often sleepy but can be aroused. Breathing is quiet and relaxed. The patient will regain consciousness gradually and may be confused or disoriented and may have a headache, muscle aches, or fatigue. The patient may sleep for several hours after the seizure.

Status epilepticus is a life-threatening condition characterized by enhanced and sustained electrical activity. Within the brain, seizure activity is maintained by a pattern of increased neuronal excitation with reduced inhibition. If the pattern of excitation continues, it may result in unremitting seizure activity or a pattern of recurrent activity that does not allow the individual the opportunity to recover. Generally, recurrent activity over a period of 30 minutes is sufficient to qualify as status epilepticus. Alternatively, a seizure that continues for longer than 5 minutes is unlikely to cease activity without intervention and also meets the standard. The administration of agents that enhance inhibitory neurotransmitter activity, such as gamma-aminobutyric acid, is part of the pharmaceutical interventions used for status epilepticus.

Linking Pathophysiology to Diagnosis and Treatment

Laboratory tests that may be ordered for patients experiencing seizures include a complete blood cell count, blood chemistry, urine culture, and lumbar puncture. An EEG is usually ordered on the first occurrence of seizure activity and can be performed under conditions that lower the seizure threshold, such as sleep deprivation, hyperventilation, or exposure to flashing lights. An EEG is often performed at a follow-up visit between seizures. A lead level, toxicology screening, and radiologic tests such as a CT scan or MRI and angiography may be performed to identify cerebral lesions or metabolic disorders in the brain. If the patient is taking any anticonvulsants, the serum drug level is monitored regularly.

If drug therapy is ineffective and the patient continues to have seizure activity that interferes with daily life, surgical intervention may be considered (see Table 34.5). Antiseizure drugs can reduce or control most seizure activity. The goals of medication administration are to protect the patient from harm and to reduce or prevent seizure activity without impairing cognitive function or producing undesirable side effects. The lowest possible dose of a single medication that will control the patient's seizures is prescribed to start. However, there is often a trial involving several different pharmacologic therapies to determine which is most effective in controlling the seizure activity. In some cases, a combination of drugs may be needed to manage the patient's seizures.

Children whose seizures continue to occur despite medical management should be referred to an epilepsy center for other potential treatments, such as vagal nerve stimulation, a ketogenic diet, or surgery. ■

Every year, approximately 20,000 women with a seizure disorder give birth. With proper care, these women can have healthy pregnancies and healthy babies. Most healthcare providers believe that the risk of fetal birth defects associated with antiseizure medications is minor in comparison to the potential complications associated with a tonic–clonic seizure during pregnancy. If the pregnant woman has a seizure during pregnancy, it can result in injury to the woman and fetus due to a fall, or it can result in decreased oxygen to the fetus, preterm labor, or preterm birth.[24] ■

Approximately 1.1% of older adults on Medicare have epilepsy; the highest rate occurs in African Americans.[25] Epilepsy in older adults is often caused by stroke, Alzheimer disease, heart disease, tumors, and injuries from falls. However, approximately half of the seizures seen in older adults are cryptogenic, meaning their cause cannot be identified.[23] Epilepsy in older adults can threaten their independence and quality of life by increasing their risk for falls and fractures, forcing driving restrictions, increasing social isolation and depression, and causing low self-esteem and loss of employment.[26]

The manifestations of seizures in older adults are often different from those in children and younger adults. Older adults more frequently have simple or complex partial seizures rather than the classic tonic–clonic seizures. Older adults often present with a blank stare, brief unresponsiveness, language difficulties, confusion, and automatisms such as lip smacking. The postictal phase is also longer in older adults, sometimes lasting up to 2 weeks, with symptoms such as sleepiness and confusion. Older adults with epilepsy have a higher mortality rate than older adults without epilepsy.[26] ■

Check Your Progress: Section 34.6

1. Who is most at risk for febrile seizures?
2. What are the characteristics of a simple partial seizure?
3. What is the mechanism that produces hypoxia during a seizure?

CHAPTER SUMMARY

34.1 Chapter Overview and Case Studies

Describe the chronic, degenerative neurologic disorders of motor control and how mobility dysfunction is experienced by individuals with the disorders.

- Degenerative motor disorders are associated with tremendous social, financial, economic, and healthcare-related costs.
- Movement disorders are multisystem disorders, and the nonmotor manifestations are as serious and disabling as the motor symptoms.
- Most movement disorders have unknown etiologies; however, some genetic and environmental risk factors have been identified.
- Concepts related to disorders of motor function include mobility, perfusion, oxygenation, cognition, pain, and stress and coping.

34.2 Parkinson Disease

Differentiate the causes, classification, underlying pathogenesis, and clinical manifestations of Parkinson disease and approaches to diagnosis and treatment of the condition.

- Parkinson disease (PD) is a chronic, degenerative, and progressive disorder of the central nervous system characterized by both motor and nonmotor clinical manifestations.
- The onset of PD is insidious, and the presentation is variable. Onset of the disease usually occurs after the age of 50.
- The most apparent pathophysiologic abnormality is the progressive disappearance of dopaminergic neurons in the substantia nigra. This leads to a deficiency of dopamine in the corpus striatum of the basal ganglia and affects motor function.
- The disappearance of dopaminergic neurons in the SN is likely due to a number of potentially interrelated pathogenic mechanisms. Potential suspects include proteolytic stress, oxidative stress, mitochondrial dysfunction, inflammation, and excitotoxicity.
- Motor features of PD include tremor, rigidity, bradykinesia, and postural instability. Nonmotor features include autonomic abnormalities; cognitive, affective, and behavioral impairments; and sleep disturbances
- No current therapy prevents PD, halts its progression, or restores lost function. Pharmacologic therapy involves replenishment of dopamine.

34.3 Multiple Sclerosis

Differentiate the causes, classification, underlying pathogenesis, and clinical manifestations of multiple sclerosis and approaches to diagnosis and treatment of the condition across the lifespan.

- MS is a chronic, inflammatory, demyelinating and axonal degenerative disorder of the CNS. It thought to be an inflammatory autoimmune disease.
- MS lesions are commonly seen in the periventricular white matter of the brain, optic nerve, cerebellum, and spinal cord.
- Most people with MS are diagnosed between the ages of 20 and 50 years. MS is 2–3 times more common in women than in men, more common in Caucasians of northern European descent, and seen more often in areas farther from the equator.
- MS plaques are caused by inflammation, demyelination, degeneration, and gliosis or scar formation. Brain atrophy can begin early in the disease process.
- Clinical features include sensory symptoms in the extremities or face, visual loss, double vision, weakness, vertigo, gait and balance disturbances, bladder problems, and pain.
- MS is diagnosed primarily through the use of MRI, which shows the characteristic lesions of MS.
- MS is treated with immunomodulatory therapy (IMT) to reduce the frequency and severity of attacks, slow the progress of disability, and decrease the accumulation of plaque. IMT has an FDA category C warning for possible teratogenicity.

34.4 Amyotrophic Lateral Sclerosis

Differentiate the causes, classification, underlying pathogenesis, and clinical manifestations of amyotrophic lateral sclerosis and approaches to diagnosis and treatment of the condition.

- Amytrophic lateral sclerosis is an incurable progressive neurodegenerative disease that causes weakness, disability and eventual death in 3–5 years.
- ALS is more common in Caucasian males and in individuals aged 60–69 years but can occur at younger ages.
- ALS has no known cause. Pathways that lead to axonal degeneration and cell death can be mediated by oxidative stress, mitochondrial dysfunction, defect of axonal transport abnormal growth factor, excitotoxicity due to defective glutamate uptake, and caspase-mediated cell death (apoptosis).
- ALS has upper motor neuron (UMN) and lower motor neuron (LMN) signs and symptoms, which include slowness of movement, stiffness, incoordination, hyperreflexia, spasticity, poor manual dexterity, poor balance, weakness and muscle atrophy dysarthria, dysphagia, and hoarse voice.

- The diagnosis of ALS is based on clinical manifestations and exclusion of other disease entities that have similar manifestations.
- Riluzole (Rilutek) is the only FDA-approved medication for treatment of ALS. Noninvasive ventilation, percutaneous endoscopic gastrostomy tube placement and feeding, medications to relieve symptoms, and multidisciplinary care are recommended.

34.5 Huntington Disease

Differentiate the causes, classification, underlying pathogenesis, and clinical manifestations of Huntington disease and approaches to diagnosis and treatment of the condition across the lifespan.

- Huntington disease is a progressive, incurable, autosomal dominant neurodegenerative disease of the brain that causes uncontrolled, involuntary movements, dementia, and behavioral changes.
- Onset of symptoms of HD usually occur at 35–44 years of age. Most people with HD survive 10–25 years, and the primary causes of death are pneumonia and cardiovascular disease.
- Mutation in the huntington gene (*HTT*) causes HD; the CAG segment is repeated 36–120 times, which leads to huntingtin accumulation.
- The most striking pathology in HD is gross atrophy in the caudate nucleus and putamen; the brain will shrink up to 40% early in HD.
- Diagnosis can be determined by a genetically proven family history and clinical presentation.
- There is no cure for HD, and there are no medications or therapies that delay the onset of symptoms or prevent disease progression. Treatment is geared toward reducing the symptoms and improving quality of life. Tetrabenazine is the only FDA-approved medication for HD chorea.

34.6 Seizure Disorders

Differentiate the causes, classification, underlying pathogenesis, and clinical manifestations of seizure disorders and approaches to diagnosis and treatment of these conditions across the lifespan.

- Seizure activity results from abnormal electrical discharges within the brain resulting in involuntary movement and/or behavior and sensory alterations.
- Seizure activity may result from by underlying pathologic conditions such as infection, electrolyte imbalance, trauma, hypoglycemia, endocrine dysfunction, or tumors. Other seizures are idiopathic.
- Febrile seizures usually occur in children as the result of a rapid temperature rise above 102.2°F (39°C, rectal).
- Febrile seizures tend to present as generalized seizures and last only a few minutes.
- Infants and toddlers have a lower seizure threshold than adults and therefore are more susceptible to seizures caused by minor stimuli such as fevers.
- Partial seizures (also known as focal seizures) occur when abnormal electrical activity is contained within a limited area of the brain. These seizures are referred to as partial seizures, in that the electrical activity resulting in a seizure may occur only within one lobe or hemisphere of the brain.
- Generalized seizures involve abnormal electrical discharge across both brain hemispheres.
- Intractable seizures are those that are refractory; that is, they continue to occur even with optimal medical management. The individual with intractable seizures should be referred to care environments that specialize in dealing with seizure activity, such as an epilepsy center.
- Seizure manifestations typically include a loss of conscious awareness of the environment and varying patterns of muscular rigidity and relaxation.
- The tonic phase of a seizure is characterized by a sudden loss of consciousness and muscular rigidity.
- The clonic phase of a seizure reflects periods of alternating muscular contraction and relaxation in all extremities.
- The postictal phase of a seizure is best viewed as a period of recovery, in which the individual is often lethargic but rousable.
- Status epilepticus is a life-threatening emergency characterized by periods of unremitting or recurrent activity within a short span of time.
- Laboratory tests that may be ordered for patients who are experiencing seizures include a complete blood cell count, blood chemistry, urine culture, EEG, and lumbar puncture.

REVIEW QUESTIONS

1. Which of the following people is most likely to develop Parkinson disease?
   a. A 20-year-old man
   b. A 30-year-old woman
   c. A 65-year-old man
   d. A 65-year-old woman
2. Which of the following should the nurse recognize as the first presenting motor feature in the majority of people with Parkinson disease?
   a. Fatigue
   b. Dementia
   c. Pill-rolling tremor
   d. Cogwheeling

3. A patient reports that before his seizures, he sees flashing lights. The nurse explains that this visual disturbance is known as which of the following?
   a. Postictal state
   b. Retinal detachment
   c. Status epilepticus
   d. Aura
4. The nurse is providing education to a couple. The husband was found to have the gene for Huntington disease, but the wife was not. Which statement made by the wife requires follow-up by the nurse? Select all that apply.
   a. All our children will inherit the gene for Huntington disease.
   b. Each of our children will have a 50% chance of inheriting the gene mutation.
   c. 50% of our children will inherit the gene for Huntington disease.
   d. Only our male children will inherit the gene for Huntington disease.
5. Which of the following should the nurse include when teaching a patient with multiple sclerosis about ways to avoid fatigue on hot and humid days?
   a. Rest in an air-conditioned room.
   b. Take a hot bath or shower.
   c. Drink plenty of fluids.
   d. Exercise regularly.
6. The nurse is developing a care plan for a patient with amyotrophic lateral sclerosis. Which of the following should be given the highest priority?
   a. Altered nutrition
   b. Impaired mobility
   c. Self-care deficits
   d. Ineffective breathing
7. The nurse is caring for a patient with absence seizures. During a seizure, the nurse is most likely to observe which of the following?
   a. Loss of consciousness preceded by an aura
   b. No loss of consciousness with muscle contractions on one side of the body
   c. A loss of consciousness and muscle rigidity
   d. A loss of consciousness without a change in muscle activity
8. The nurse is assessing a patient with amyotrophic lateral sclerosis. Which of the following does the nurse assess as a lower motor neuron finding?
   a. Slow movement
   b. Stiff gait
   c. Incoordination
   d. Fasciculations

ANSWERS

Answers to Review Questions can be found in Appendix A. Answers to Case Study and Check Your Progress questions are available on the faculty resources site. Please consult with your instructor.

RECOMMENDED WEBSITES

ALS Association
http://alsa.org

American Parkinson Disease Association
https://www.apdaparkinson.org

Huntington's Disease Society of America
http://www.hdsa.org

Les Turner ALS Foundation
http://lesturnerals.org

The Michael J. Fox Foundation for Parkinson's Research
https://www.michaeljfox.org

Multiple Sclerosis Association of America
http://mymsaa.org

Multiple Sclerosis Foundation
https://msfocus.org

National Institute of Neurological Disorders and Stroke
https://www.ninds.nih.gov

National Multiple Sclerosis Society
http://nationalmssociety.org

National Parkinson Foundation
http://parkinson.org

REFERENCES

1. de Lau, L. M., & Breteler, M. M. (2006). Epidemiology of Parkinson's disease. *Lancet Neurology, 5*, 525–535.
2. National Institute of Neurological Disorders and Stroke. (2014). *Parkinson's disease: Challenges, progress, and promise*. Available at http://www.ninds.nih.gov/disorders/parkinsons_disease/parkinsons_research.htm#basics
3. Lin, M. K., & Farrer, M. J. (2014). Genetics and genomics of Parkinson's disease, *Genome Medicine, 6*(48), 1–16.
4. Pan-Montojo, F., & Reichmann, H. (2014). Considerations on the role of environmental toxins in idiopathic Parkinson's disease pathophysiology. *Translational Neurodegeneration*, 3(10), 1–13.

5. Hornykiewicz, O. (2006). The discovery of dopamine deficiency in the parkinsonian brain. *Journal of Neural Transmission Supplement, 70*, 9.
6. National Multiple Sclerosis Society. (2015). *What is MS?* Available at http://www.nationalmssociety.org
7. Popescu, V., Klaver, R., Voorn, P., et al. (2015). What drives MRI-measured cortical atrophy in multiple sclerosis? *Multiple Sclerosis, 21*(10), 1–11.
8. Tremlett, H., Paty, D., & Devonshire V. (2006). Disability progression in multiple sclerosis is slower than previously reported. *Neurology, 66*(2), 172–177.
9. Tremlett, H., Zhao, Y., Rieckmann, P., & Hutchinson, M. (2010). New perspectives in the natural history of multiple sclerosis. *Neurology, 74*(24), 2004–2015.
10. Polman, C. H., Reingold, S. C., Banwell, B., et al. (2011). Diagnostic criteria for multiple sclerosis: 2010 revisions to the McDonald criteria. *Annals of Neurology, 69*(2), 292–302.
11. Cree, B. A. (2013). Update on reproductive safety of current and emerging disease-modifying therapies for multiple sclerosis, *Multiple Sclerosis, 19*(7), 835–843.
12. National Institute of Neurological Disorders and Stroke. (2015). *Amyotrophic lateral sclerosis (ALS) fact sheet*. Available at http://www.ninds.nih.gov/disorders/amyotrophiclateralsclerosis/detail_ALS.htm
13. Roche, J. C., Rojas-Garcia, R., Scott, M. K., Scotton, W., Ellis, C. E., et al. (2012). A proposed staging system for amyotrophic lateral sclerosis. *Brain, 135*, 847–852. Available at http://www.ncbi.nlm.nih.gov/pmc/articles/PMC3286327/
14. Miller, R. G., Jackson, C. E., Kasarskis, E. J., et al. (2009). Practice parameter update: The care of the patient with amyotrophic lateral sclerosis: Drug, nutritional, and respiratory therapies (an evidence based review). Report of the Quality Standards Subcommittee of the American Academy of Neurology. *Neurology, 73*, 1218–1226.
15. Genetics Home Reference. (2015). *Huntington disease*. Available at http://ghr.nlm.nih.gov/condition/huntington-disease
16. Burgunder, J. M., Guttman, M., Perlman, S., Goodman, N., van Kammen, D. P., Goodman, L. (2011). An international survey-based algorithm for the pharmacologic treatment of chorea in Huntington's disease. *PLoS Currents, 3*, RRN1260.
17. Epilepsy Foundation. (2014). *Epilepsy statistics*. Available at http://www.epilepsy.com/learn/epilepsy-statistics
18. National Institutes of Health. (2016). *Seizures*. Available at http://www.nlm.nih.gov/medlineplus/seizures.html
19. National Institute of Neurological Disorders and Stroke. (2015). *Febrile seizures fact sheet*. Available at http://www.ninds.nih.gov/disorders/febrile_seizures/detail_febrile_seizures.htm
20. Mayo Clinic. (2015). *Epilepsy*. Available at http://www.mayoclinic.org/diseases-conditions/epilepsy/home/ovc-20117206
21. Russ, S. A., Larson, K., & Halfon, N. (2012). A national profile of childhood epilepsy and seizure disorder. *Pediatrics, 129*(2), 256–264.
22. Centers for Disease Control and Prevention. (2016). *Epilepsy fast facts*. Available at http://www.cdc.gov/epilepsy/basics/fast-facts.htm
23. Epilepsy Foundation. (2014). *What are the risk factors?* Available at http://www.epilepsy.com/learn/epilepsy-101/what-are-risk-factors
24. American College of Obstetricians and Gynecologists. (2013). *Seizure disorders in pregnancy*. Available at http://www.acog.org/~/media/For%20Patients/faq129.pdf
25. Faught, E., Richman, J., Martin, R., Funkhouser, E., Foushee, R., Kratt, P., Kim, Y., Clements, K., Cohen, N., Adoboe, D., Knowlton, R., & Pisu, M. (2012). Incidence and prevalence of epilepsy among older US Medicare beneficiaries. *Neurology, 78*(7), 448–453.
26. Austin, J., & Abdulla, A. (2013). Identifying and managing epilepsy in older adults. *Nursing Times*. Available at http://www.nursingtimes.net/clinical-archive/neurology/identifying-and-managing-epilepsy-in-older-adults/5053730.fullarticle

Chapter 35

Acute Musculoskeletal Disorders

Dawna Martich

Chapter Outline and Learning Outcomes

35.1 Chapter Overview and Case Studies

Describe the normal musculoskeletal function and concepts related to acute disorders of musculoskeletal function.

35.2 Fractures

Differentiate the causes, classification, underlying pathogenesis, and clinical manifestations of fractures and approaches to diagnosis and treatment of these conditions across the lifespan.

35.3 Dislocations and Subluxations

Differentiate the causes, classification, underlying pathogenesis, and clinical manifestations of dislocations and subluxations and approaches to diagnosis and treatment of these conditions across the lifespan.

35.4 Nerve Entrapment

Differentiate the causes, classification, underlying pathogenesis, and clinical manifestations of nerve entrapment and approaches to diagnosis and treatment of these conditions across the lifespan.

35.5 Bursitis

Differentiate the causes, classification, underlying pathogenesis, and clinical manifestations of bursitis and approaches to diagnosis and treatment of these conditions across the lifespan.

35.6 Strains and Sprains

Differentiate the causes, classification, underlying pathogenesis, and clinical manifestations of strains and sprains and approaches to diagnosis and treatment of these conditions across the lifespan.

35.7 Knee Injuries

Differentiate the causes, classification, underlying pathogenesis, and clinical manifestations of knee injuries and approaches to diagnosis and treatment of these conditions across the lifespan.

35.8 Shoulder Injuries

Differentiate the causes, classification, underlying pathogenesis, and clinical manifestations of shoulder injuries and approaches to diagnosis and treatment of these conditions across the lifespan.

35.9 Bone Infections and Tumors

Differentiate the causes, classification, underlying pathogenesis, and clinical manifestations of bone infections and tumors and approaches to diagnosis and treatment of these conditions across the lifespan.

KEY TERMS

ABBREVIATIONS

ACL—anterior cruciate ligament
FES—fat embolism syndrome
ORIF—open reduction internal fixation
POLICE—protection, optimal loading, ice, compression, elevation
RICE—rest, ice, compression, elevation
ROM—range of motion

35.1 Chapter Overview and Case Studies

The musculoskeletal system is the scaffolding of the human body. Given the wide array of bones, muscles, and joints, any injuries, infections, and disease processes can hinder maximum motor function. This chapter focuses on the most commonly occurring acute musculoskeletal disorders.

Acute musculoskeletal injuries can occur in anyone, at any age. The most frequently reported injuries in children are strains and sprains, dislocations, and fractures,[1,2] whereas fractures of the hip, distal radius, and vertebrae occur most often in people over age 65.[3] See **Table 35.1** for the most common acute musculoskeletal conditions.

Concepts Related to Acute Musculoskeletal Disorders

The concepts related to acute musculoskeletal disorders include comfort and pain, infection, inflammation and oxidative stress, cellular regulation, and mobility. Although the primary concept is mobility, comfort is affected by all disorders of the musculoskeletal system. See **Figure 35.1** for more information.

Table 35.1 Common Acute Musculoskeletal Conditions

Anatomic Area	Common Acute Musculoskeletal Conditions
Shoulder	• Dislocation • Rotator cuff injury
Elbow	• Dislocation • Bursitis
Wrist	• Fracture • Carpal tunnel syndrome
Hand	• Fractured finger
Back	• Slipped disc • Muscle strain/sprain
Abdomen	• Fractured pelvis
Upper leg	• Fractured hip • Dislocated hip • Fractured femur
Knee	• Anterior cruciate ligament injury/tear • Meniscus injuries
Lower leg	• Fractured tibia
Ankle	• Ankle sprain or strain

Case Studies

The following cases are addressed throughout the chapter to assist in application of chapter content to clinical situations that involve individuals with acute musculoskeletal disorders.

Lydia Ocampo: Introduction

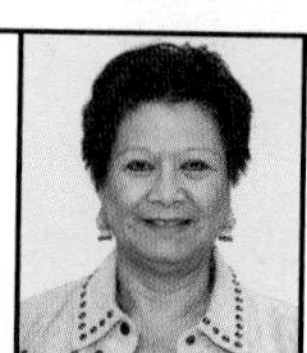

Lydia Ocampo, age 69, has Alzheimer disease. She is originally from the Philippines and has been married to Danilo for 51 years. He is her primary caregiver in the home. Mrs. Ocampo has periodic urinary incontinence, she wanders, and she frequently forgets how to perform personal care activities and routine tasks in the kitchen. One night, Mrs. Ocampo slips and falls in the bathroom, fracturing her left hip.

1. What type of acute musculoskeletal injuries are the most common at Mrs. Ocampo's age?
2. What common concepts are related to Mrs. Ocampo's acute musculoskeletal injury?

Jeannine Cartwright: Introduction

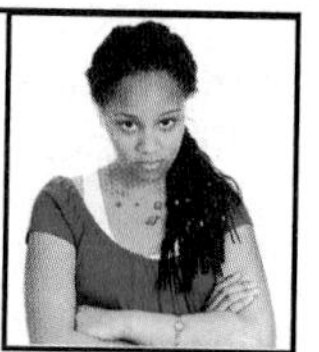

Jeannine Cartwright is a 16-year-old female who plays on the girls' soccer team at her high school. During practice one afternoon, Jeannine is going for the ball and feels a pop in her right knee. She immediately falls to the ground and grips the knee with both hands. Emergency medical services transport Jeannine to the local hospital, where she is diagnosed with an anterior cruciate ligament (ACL) tear.

1. What type of acute musculoskeletal injury is most common in adolescents such as Ms. Cartwright?
2. What other common type of acute musculoskeletal injury to the knee may occur?

Check Your Progress: Section 35.1

1. What are the most frequently reported acute musculoskeletal injuries in children?
2. Identify two common acute musculoskeletal injuries of the wrist.
3. Dislocation may commonly occur in which joints?

35.2 Fractures

A **fracture** is a break in a bone that occurs as a result of an increase in energy, more than the bone can tolerate. Fractures can be caused by either direct or indirect force. With

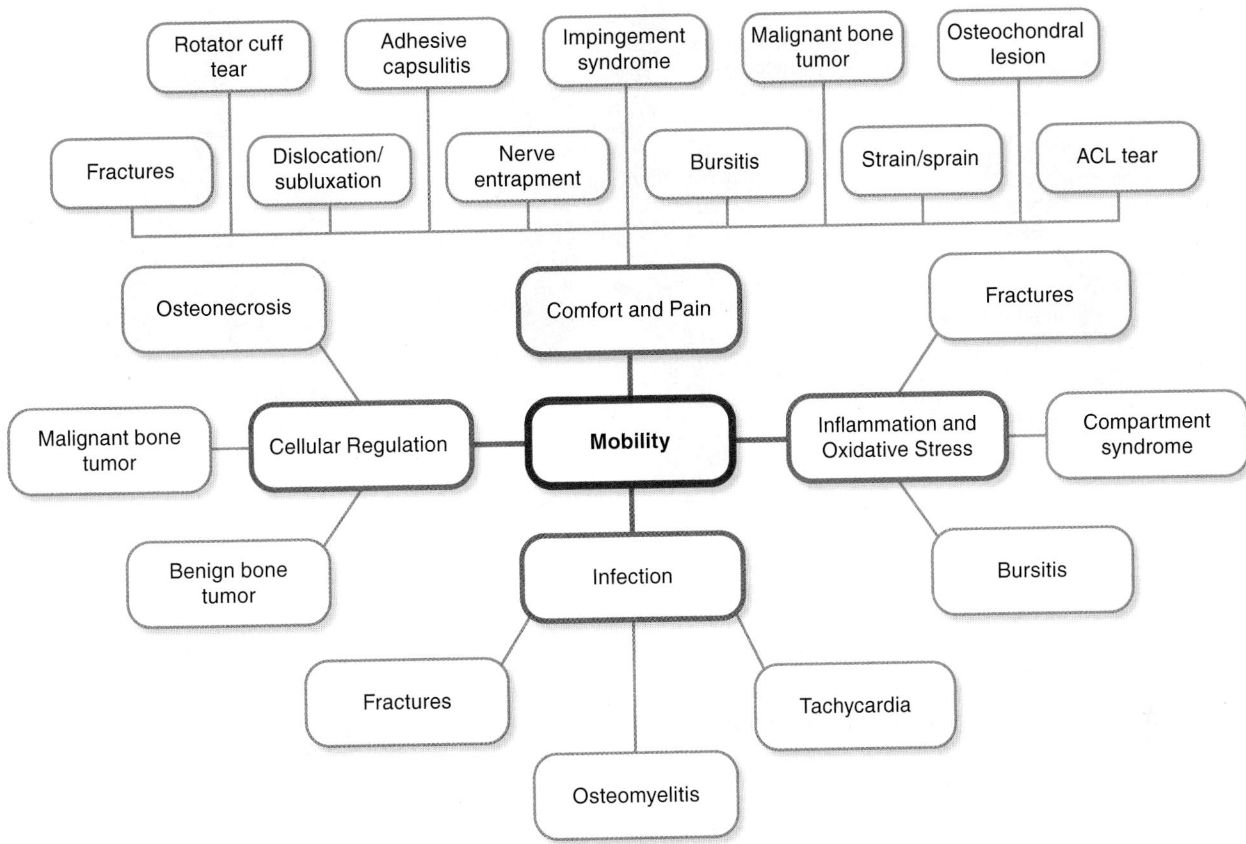

Figure 35.1 ■ Concepts related to acute musculoskeletal disorders.

direct force, the bone is exposed to energy near to or directly over the bone area that breaks. With indirect force, the bone is exposed to energy, however the break occurs at the location of bone weakness.[4] Besides being caused by direct impact, a fracture can be caused by compression, torsion, or a pathologic condition.

The primary risk factors associated with bone fractures are age, presence of bone disease, and poor nutrition. Younger patients are more likely to sustain fractures related to sports injuries; older patients are at higher risk of fractures related to falls and disease. Bone diseases that decrease the strength of the bone, such as osteoporosis, osteogenesis imperfecta, and bone cancer, increase the patient's risk of bone fracture. Inadequate intake of vitamin D, calcium, and phosphorus also contributes to poor bone strength. Lifestyle habits, such as participation in dangerous activities, can also increase the risk of fracture.

In children, fractures can be caused by direct trauma while engaging in play or sports. Fractures occur often in children because their bones are less dense. However, one cause of fractures in children is child abuse. This should be considered if a type of fracture is unlikely considering the child's age and the reported circumstances of the injury, such as a fractured femur in an infant.[2] ■

Fractures in older adults occur as a result of trauma or a fall. The bone that is most commonly fractured in all adults is the rib. However, hip fractures are seen most often in older adults (**Figure 35.2** ■). Additional fractures common in the adult population include fractures of the humerus and the wrist (Colles fracture). Fractures of the humerus, wrist, and hip most likely result from a fall and may be associated with osteoporosis.[4] ■

Classification of Fractures

Fractures are classified and described in many ways. **Figure 35.3** ■ illustrates many of the descriptive terms used for fractures.

Etiology and Pathogenesis

A fracture can be caused by either direct or indirect force. In direct force, the energy that is focused on one area of the bone is not dispersed and cannot be absorbed. In response, the bone fractures. In a fracture caused by indirect force, the bone is weakened and breaks away from the energy focus.

Clinical Manifestations

The most common manifestation of a fracture is pain. This pain is caused by direct tissue trauma, muscle spasms, and nerve compression. Additional manifestations

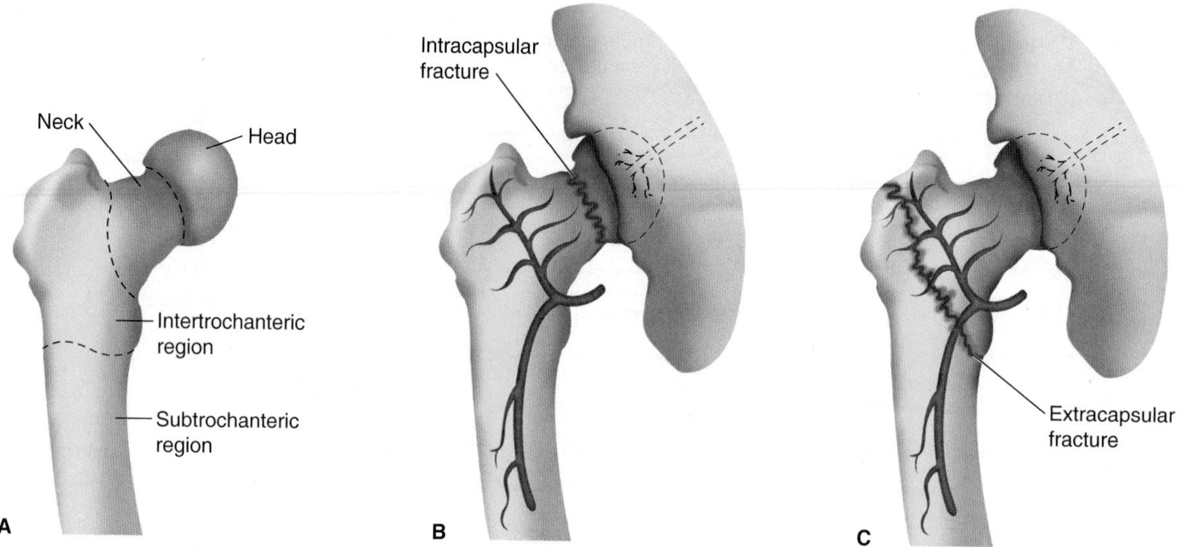

Figure 35.2 Regions of hip fractures: **A.** Femur head, neck, and trochanter. **B.** Intracapsular fracture along the femur head and neck. **C.** Extracapsular fracture along the trochanteric region.

associated with a fracture include deformity, edema, numbness, muscle spasms, bleeding that causes skin bruising and possible hypovolemia, depending on the fracture site, and crepitus.[4]

Linking Pathophysiology to Diagnosis and Treatment

The approaches used to treat a fracture will depend on the type of fracture and whether surgical intervention is required to rejoin the bone ends or fragments. Healing time is related to the size of the bone. Phalanges typically heal in about 3 weeks, whereas femur fractures take about 12 weeks.[5]

Healing of Fractures

Healing of fractures occurs either through indirect or direct approaches.

Indirect Healing

Indirect healing of a fractured bone progresses through three stages: inflammatory, reparative, and remodeling (**Figure 35.4**).[6]

1. ***Inflammatory stage.*** In the reactive or inflammatory phase, damage to the bone, blood vessels, and surrounding tissues causes bleeding and the formation of a hematoma around the injury. Inflammatory cells, mainly macrophages and neutrophils, then enter the wound and degrade debris and bacteria in the area. This phase usually lasts until osteoblasts and endothelial cells begin to proliferate at the fracture site, usually a few days.
2. ***Reparative stage.*** In the reparative phase, fibroblasts, osteoblasts, and chondroblasts begin to secrete collagen to form fibrocartilage, which develops into a soft callus that joins the fractured bone. Endothelial cells begin to form blood vessels in the damaged area. Once the soft callus has formed, it is replaced by woven bone through endochondral ossification, which forms a hard callus. This woven bone is immature bone with a random collagen and bone structure. The reparative phase usually lasts 6–8 weeks for relatively simple fractures.
3. ***Remodeling stage.*** In the remodeling phase, woven bone is replaced by highly organized lamellar bone. Lamellar bone is stronger and more compact with better blood circulation in comparison to woven bone. Because bones are being continually remodeled, bone fractures usually heal without a scar. However, it may be several years before the bone returns to its original strength.

A bone that fractures and undergoes normal healing is called a **union**. If the bone does not heal properly, it may be classified as a nonunion, a delayed union, or a malunion. A **nonunion** is a fracture that shows no clinically significant progress toward complete healing for at least 3 months according to x-rays. This may occur at any point along the healing process. A **delayed union** occurs when the healing process takes significantly longer than expected. A **malunion** occurs when the bone fragments join in a position that is not anatomically correct. Nonunions and malunions may need to be corrected surgically.

Direct Healing

Direct healing involves the use of a surgical procedure to realign the bone. This healing approach is most often used for fractures that have common long-term complications or those that are severely comminuted and the vascularity of the bone is threatened.

Surgical procedures used for direct healing include external fixation, or the application of a device placed

Closed

- Bone breaks but skin remains intact.
- Also called a simple fracture.

Open

- Bone breaks and protrudes through the skin; increased risk of osteomyelitis,
- Also called a compound fracture.

Complete

- Fracture involves the entire width of the bone.

Greenstick

- Bone fragments are still partially joined.
- Also called an incomplete fracture.
- Occurs commonly in children.

Comminuted

- Bone fragments into many pieces.
- Common in individuals with brittle bones, such as patients with osteogenesis imperfecta.

Impacted

- The two ends of the bone are forced together.
- Also called a buckle fracture.
- Often seen with children's arm and hip fractures.

Oblique

- Fracture occurs diagonal to the bone's axis.

Transverse

- Fracture occurs at a right angle to the bone's axis.

Linear

- Fracture occurs parallel to the bone's axis.

Displaced

- Broken ends of bones move out of correct anatomical alignment.
- Also called an unstable fracture.
- Requires immediate attention to prevent further damage.

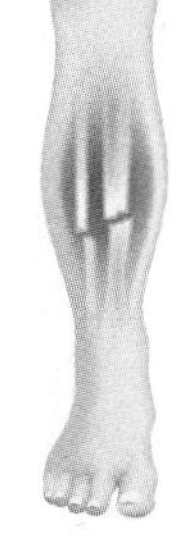

Nondisplaced

- Broken ends of bones remain aligned.
- Also called a stable fracture.

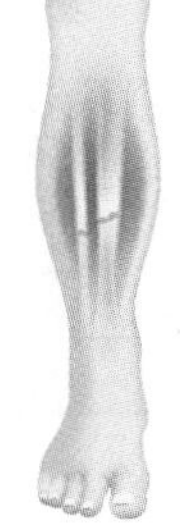

Avulsion

- A fragment of bone is separated from the rest of the bone.
- May also involve displacement of surrounding tissues.

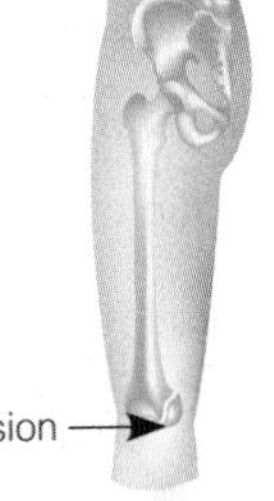

Stress

- Caused by small repetitive forces on the bone.
- Often caused by participation in sports or exercise.

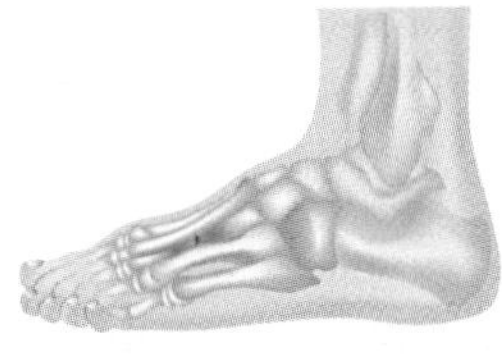

Spiral

- Fracture spirals around the bone.
- Occurs as the result of a twisting force, often during sports.
- Occurs commonly in children.

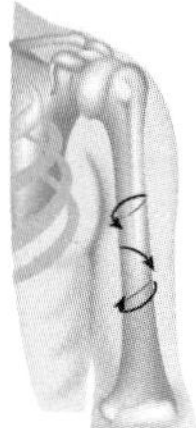

Depression

- Bone is forced inward.
- Occurs commonly in skull fractures.

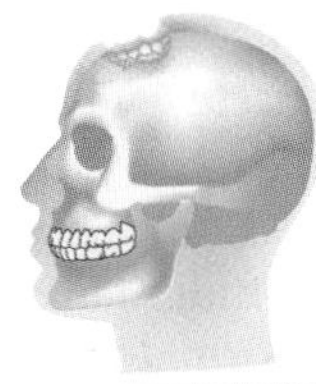

Pathologic

- Caused by a disease that weakens the bone such as osteoporosis, bone cancer, and osteogenesis imperfecta.

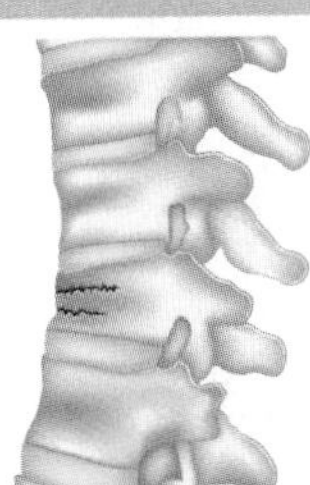

Compression

- Bone is crushed; occurs most commonly in vertebrae.
- Common in patients with osteoporosis.

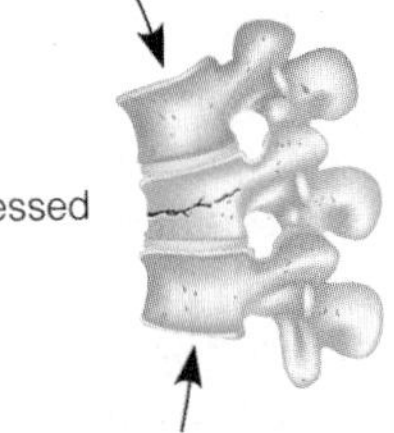

Figure 35.3 ■ Common fractures.

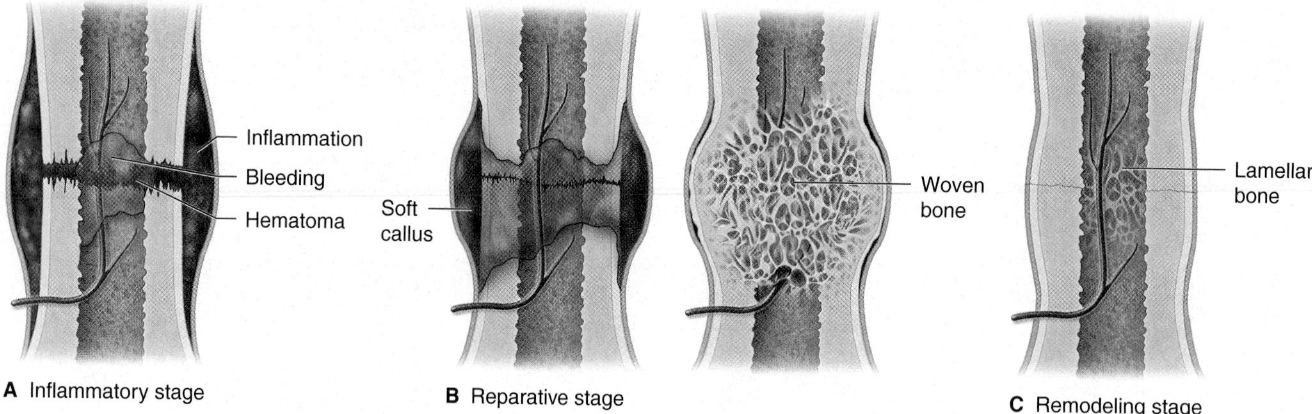

Figure 35.4 ■ The three phases of bone healing.

over and attached to the bone through external pins (**Figure 35.5** ■). These pins are placed above and below the fracture line to stabilize the fracture. Internal fixation is the term used to describe a procedure called an open reduction and internal fixation (ORIF). With this procedure the bone is realigned or reduced and held into place with nails, screws, plates, or pins (**Figure 35.6** ■). This approach is most commonly used to directly heal fractures of the extremities and hip.

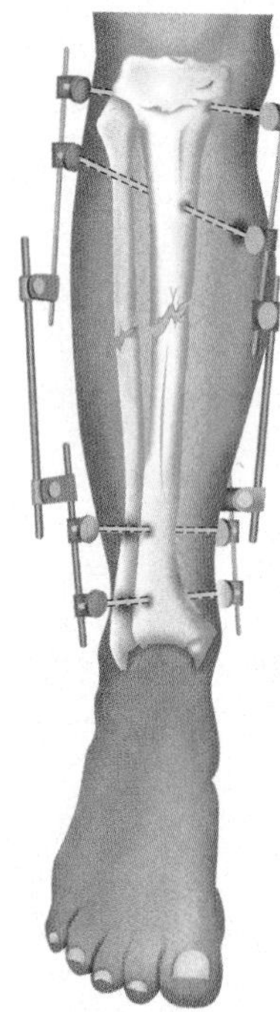

Figure 35.5 ■ In external fixation, pins are placed through the bone above and below the fracture site to immobilize the bone. External fixation rods hold the pins in place.

Lydia Ocampo: Application

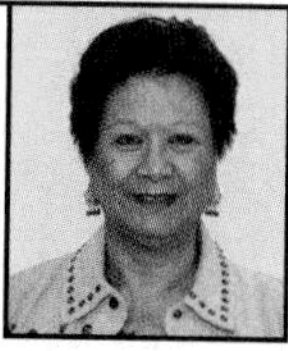

On arrival at the emergency department, Mrs. Ocampo is in severe pain. An x-ray of her hip shows a complete fracture below the left greater trochanter of the femur. An ORIF is performed the next morning to stabilize the joint.

3. In addition to her severe pain, what clinical manifestations may Mrs. Ocampo experience as a result of her hip fracture?
4. Describe the procedure of ORIF that Mrs. Ocampo will undergo to stabilize her hip joint.

Closed Reduction

Closed reduction occurs when the bone is repositioned externally. After the bone and fragments are realigned, the bone is stabilized through the use of traction or a cast. Traction applies a straightening or pulling force on the bone to maintain normal alignment and bone integrity (**Figure 35.7** ■). Casting is the application of a rigid device intended to immobilize the fractured bone and promote healing (**Figure 35.8** ■).

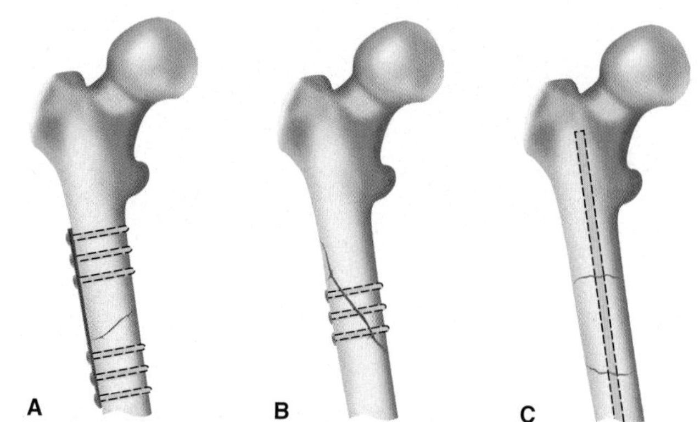

Figure 35.6 ■ Internal fixation hardware is entirely within the body. **A.** Fixation of a short oblique fracture using a plate and screws above and below the fracture. **B.** Fixation of a long oblique fracture using screws through the fracture site. **C.** Fixation of segmental fracture using a medullary nail.

Complications

Complications from a fracture can occur because of an infection from the fracture itself or from a surgical procedure performed to correct the fracture. Additional complications seen in fractures include compartment syndrome, fracture blisters, and fat embolism syndrome (FES).

Infection

Impaired skin integrity as a result of an open fracture or surgical correction of a fracture increases the risk of

Line of pull
Footplate
A
B

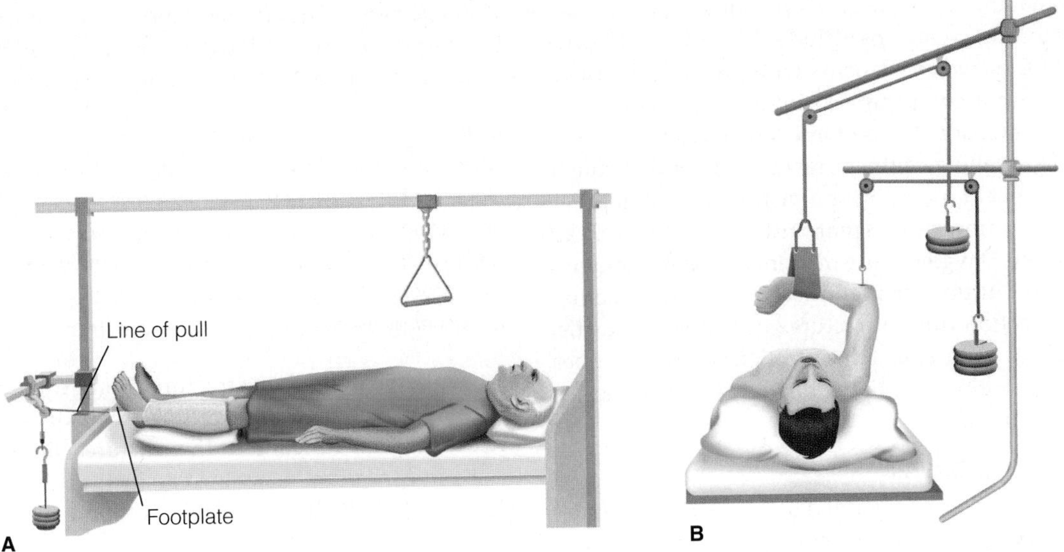

Figure 35.7 ■ Traction is the application of a pulling force to maintain bone alignment during fracture healing. Different fractures require different types of traction. **A.** Skin traction applies force to the soft tissues through a pulley system attached to the bed, such as Buck traction shown here for stabilization of the knee and hip. **B.** Skeletal traction applies force directly to the bone, such as the traction used here for a humerus fracture.

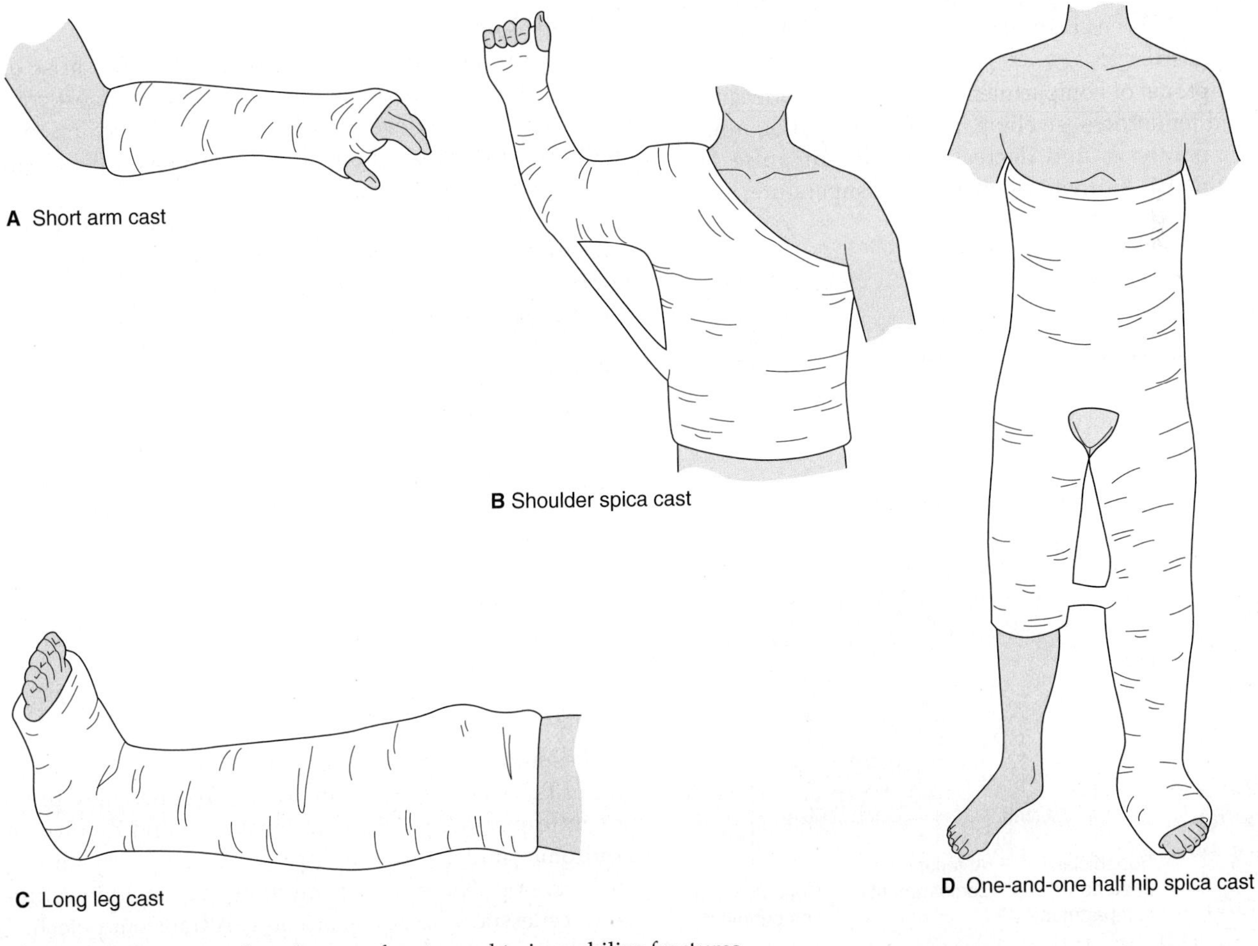

A Short arm cast
B Shoulder spica cast
C Long leg cast
D One-and-one half hip spica cast

Figure 35.8 ■ Examples of types of casts used to immobilize fractures.

bacterial contamination and development of an infection. Common infecting organisms include *Pseudomonas, Staphylococcus*, and *Clostridium*. Patients with greater soft tissue damage or with a compromised immune system are at higher risk of infection. Signs of infection include warmth, redness, pain, swelling, stiffness, fever, chills, and purulent drainage. Treatment includes administration of antibiotics according to the infecting agent and proper hygiene of the infection site. Hygiene care may include debridement, drainage, and culture for identification of the infecting organism. Infection due to fractures can cause cellulitis, osteomyelitis, or gangrene. If the infection is severe or does not respond to antibiotics, tissue death may occur, necessitating amputation.

Compartment Syndrome

Individual muscles are surrounded by fascia, and the muscle tissue, nerves, and blood vessels in the fascia are part of a compartment. Fasciae are designed to hold the muscle in place; therefore, they do not expand, and pressure can build up within the compartment. Compartment syndrome occurs when edema and swelling cause increased pressure in a muscle compartment, leading to decreased blood flow and possibly muscle and nerve damage (**Figure 35.9** ■).[7] Decreased blood flow leads to dilation of the blood vessels, causing more edema and stimulating a cycle of continually increasing pressure in the limb. If ischemia to the compartment continues for a significant length of time, the muscles and nerves may die, and the limb might need to be amputated.

Symptoms of compartment syndrome include severe pain and tenderness, swelling, paresthesia, pallor, numbness or paralysis, and decreased or absent pulse and **poikilothermia** (normalization to room temperature) in the distal portion of the affected limb. Compartment syndrome is most common in the lower leg and forearm, but it can also occur in the hand, foot, thigh, and upper arm.

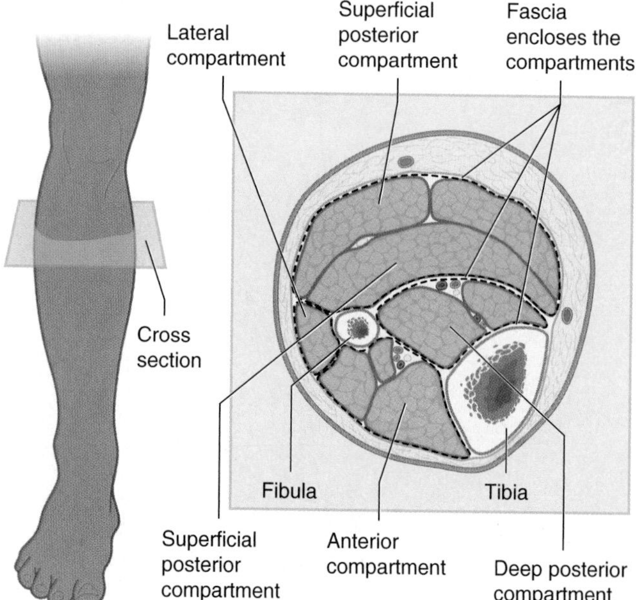

Figure 35.9 ■ Compartment syndrome.

CLINICAL POINT: Compartment syndrome should be suspected when complaints of pain and swelling are disproportionate to negative x-ray findings. It can result from a fracture, a muscle bruise, a crush injury, or a bandage that is too tight, such as a cast. Compartment syndrome is a medical emergency. The first step in treatment is to remove a tight cast. If internal pressure is causing the symptoms, it is generally treated by surgery to relieve the pressure.[8] ■

Patients with a bone fracture in an extremity should be regularly evaluated for swelling, pain, discoloration, and neurovascular function in the fractured limb. Methods to prevent compartment syndrome include elevation and ice to reduce swelling and delaying casting until the swelling is gone.

Compartment syndrome can lead to many complications, including paralysis, the need for amputation, or a Volkmann contracture. A **Volkmann contracture** is a deformity of the wrist, hand, and fingers caused by ischemia to the forearm, usually as a result of compartment syndrome. Ischemia in the forearm causes the nerves and muscles to become scarred and shortened, forcing the joint to be permanently bent.[9] A Volkmann contracture is common after elbow injuries, especially in children.

Fracture Blisters

Fracture blisters are tense vesicles or bullae that arise on swollen skin directly overlying a fracture. The most common areas for the development of these blisters are over the tibia, ankle, and elbow. In most instances, the blister appears within 24–48 hours after the fracture. Although the blisters contain sterile fluid, they can contribute to infection after fracture stabilization surgery. If the blister ruptures, normal skin flora can colonize the blister area and lead to the development of a skin infection.

Fat Embolism Syndrome

Fat embolism may occur in conjunction with closed long bone or pelvic fractures. Fat emboli released from the bone marrow enter the bloodstream and become trapped in the pulmonary and dermal capillaries. In most patients, release of fat from the bone marrow after a fracture produces no symptoms. Patients who experience release of large amounts of fat, as many as 90% of major trauma victims, may experience a fat embolism.

CLINICAL POINT: Although FES is rare, multiple systems may be affected, and there are high morbidity and mortality rates.[10] ■

Respiratory consequences are typically the first symptom of FES to occur. In severe cases, dyspnea may progress to respiratory failure with tachypnea and hypoxia. A syndrome similar to acute respiratory distress syndrome may develop. Neurologic symptoms may include confusion, restlessness, seizures, or coma. A transient petechial rash usually covers the upper anterior trunk, arms, and neck as well as the buccal mucosa and conjunctiva. Other symptoms may include Purtscher retinopathy (sudden loss of vision that is most often associated with traumatic injury) and mild fever.

Treatment of FES is supportive and includes oxygen administration; approximately 50% of patients will require mechanical ventilation. Neurologic symptoms usually resolve with adequate oxygenation, and the petechial rash disappears spontaneously within a week. Prophylactic treatment with corticosteroids and early immobilization of the injury may reduce the risk of FES. FES is rarely seen in children under the age of 10.

Lydia Ocampo: Outcome

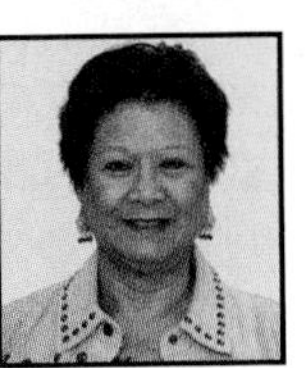

On the third postoperative day, Mrs. Ocampo begins to run a low-grade fever. Throughout her hospital stay, she has been mildly confused, and she has made repeated attempts to get out bed. Mrs. Ocampo's confusion has made it challenging to keep her safe. The surgical wound site is reddened and is seeping purulent drainage. The wound culture report identifies the infecting microorganism as *Staphylococcus aureus*, and antibiotics are prescribed as treatment.

Within a few days, the wound drainage decreases, and Mrs. Ocampo begins physical therapy sessions. She is able to transfer from a sitting to a standing position and ambulate a few steps with the aid of a walker. Mrs. Ocampo is scheduled for transfer to a rehabilitation facility to continue her recovery.

5. What clinical manifestations did Mrs. Ocampo display that suggested she had an infection?
6. What are Mrs. Ocampo's risk factors for infection?

Check Your Progress: Section 35.2

1. Describe the process of closed reduction.
2. Why is compartment syndrome dangerous?
3. How does fat embolism syndrome occur?

35.3 Dislocations and Subluxations

A **dislocation** is an injury in which the ends of the bones are moved out of the normal position and attachment to the joint is lost. When the bones of a joint remain in partial contact, a **subluxation** has occurred.

Etiology and Pathogenesis

Dislocations and subluxations most commonly occur after a trauma such as a fall or direct blow to the joint. These injuries are seen often in contact sports such as football and after falls that occur during skiing.

Clinical Manifestations

The most common manifestations of dislocations and subluxations include pain, limb or joint deformity, and altered mobility of the affected joint.

Linking Pathophysiology to Diagnosis and Treatment

Treatment of both dislocation and subluxation is done by reducing the joint with manual traction (closed reduction). If this fails, an open reduction is required to realign the joint and prevent neurovascular injury. Dislocations or subluxations of the shoulder can be managed by closed reduction and short-term immobilization. Injuries of this type to the hip require immediate reduction to prevent necrosis of the femoral head. Bedrest is required for several days after a closed reduction of the hip.[4]

Check Your Progress: Section 35.3

1. What is the difference between a dislocation and a subluxation?
2. Describe the common clinical manifestations of dislocations and subluxations.
3. Why does dislocation or subluxation of the hip require immediate reduction?

35.4 Nerve Entrapment

Nerve entrapment is a type of neuropathy that causes nerve damage and muscle weakness or atrophy. The body areas that are most prone to developing entrapment are places where the nerves pass over rigid areas or through narrow canals (see **Table 35.2** ■). Of the various nerve entrapment syndromes, one of the most commonly occurring is carpal tunnel.

Carpal Tunnel Syndrome and Cubital Tunnel Syndrome

Carpal tunnel syndrome gets its name from irritation of the nerves that pass through the carpal tunnel, which is the tunnel through which the flexor tendons and median nerve pass between the wrist and the hand (**Figure 35.10** ■). Cubital tunnel syndrome is entrapment of the ulnar nerve at the elbow.

Etiology and Pathogenesis

Often referred to as a repetitive use injury, carpal tunnel syndrome is most often caused by an action where the hands are used such as for computer work, needlepoint,

Table 35.2 Locations for Nerve Entrapment

Body Area	Condition
Forearm, wrists, hands	• Carpal tunnel syndrome • Ulnar tunnel syndrome
Pudendal nerve	• Pelvis
Spine	• Slipped disc • Herniated disc • Spinal stenosis • Spondylolisthesis

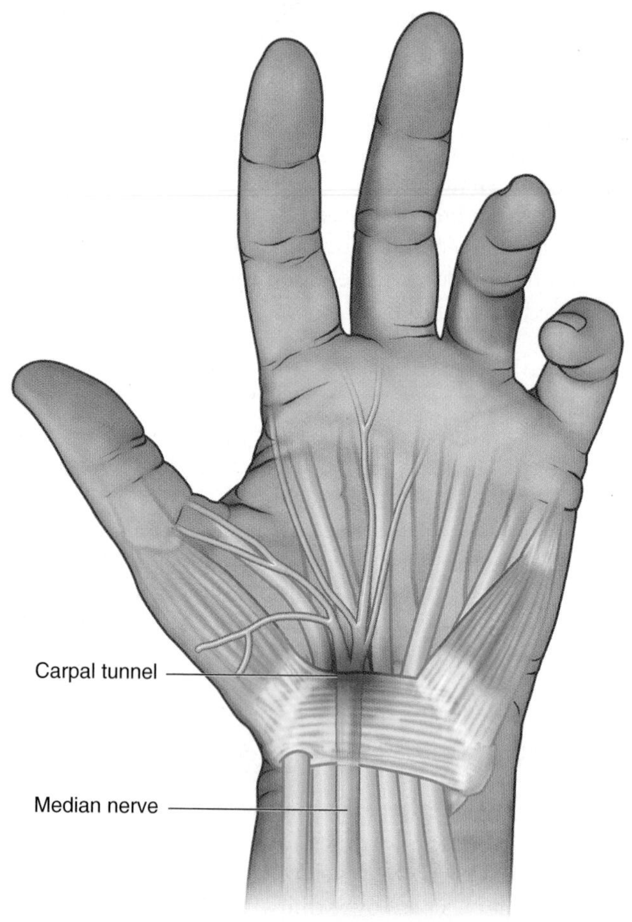

Figure 35.10 ■ Carpal tunnel syndrome.

or the use of a jackhammer. In this syndrome, the median nerve becomes compressed by inflammation and swelling of the synovial lining of the tendon sheaths.[4]

Clinical Manifestations

At first, the patient may experience numbness and tingling of the thumb, index finger, and lateral ventral surface of the middle finger. Over time, the numbness and tingling become more acute during sleep and are alleviated by shaking or rubbing the hand and wrist. If the syndrome is left untreated, the hand can become weak, altering the patient's ability to use the hand to perform common activities such as holding eating utensils.

Linking Pathophysiology to Diagnosis and Treatment

Diagnosing carpal tunnel syndrome begins with a review of the patient's current symptoms. The wrists and hands are examined for motion, sensation, tenderness, swelling, and warmth. The Tinsel test is positive for the disorder if the patient experiences tingling in the fingers when the median nerve is tapped. The Phalen maneuver is positive if the patient experiences tingling or numbness of the fingers when the wrists are flexed. In some situations, nerve conduction studies might be performed along with ultrasound to validate the size of the median nerve.

Treatment of carpal tunnel syndrome is at first conservative and accomplished with splinting and application of ice or heat. If numbness and reduced motor function continue, surgery is recommended to enlarge the tunnel to take pressure off the compressed nerve.

Check Your Progress: Section 35.4

1. Describe the conservative treatment of carpal tunnel syndrome.
2. Describe the progression of symptoms in carpal tunnel syndrome.
3. Distinguish between the Tinsel test and Phalen maneuver in diagnosing carpal tunnel syndrome.

35.5 Bursitis

Bursae are enclosed fluid-filled sacs that act as cushions between muscles, tendons, and bony prominences. Inflammation of a bursa results in **bursitis**. The most common body areas for bursitis to occur are the shoulders, hips, knees, and elbows.

Etiology and Pathogenesis

Bursitis is commonly caused by overuse of a joint or direct trauma to a joint. Constant friction between the bursa and musculoskeletal tissue around the sac causes inflammation, irritation, and edema.

Clinical Manifestations

Clinical manifestations of bursitis include tenderness of the area around the sac and pain with extension and flexion of the joint. The skin area over the bursa is warm, red, and swollen.

Linking Pathophysiology to Diagnosis and Treatment

Reduction of pain and inflammation is the priority when treating bursitis. The patient may be prescribed rest, compression, elevation, and nonsteroidal anti-inflammatory drugs (NSAIDs). If the inflammation is acute, ice may be recommended. However, if the inflammation is chronic, ice will not be beneficial. Once the initial pain is reduced, gentle stretching and strengthening exercises are recommended. If the inflammation continues after conservative treatment, a corticosteroid injection may be prescribed. If the condition continues beyond 6–12 months, arthroscopic surgery may be indicated to repair tissue damage and relieve pressure on the bursa. If the condition is caused by an infection, antibiotics are prescribed.[11]

Check Your Progress: Section 35.5

1. What is bursitis?
2. What is the cause of bursitis?
3. What is the treatment of bursitis?

35.6 Strains and Sprains

A **strain** is an injury to a muscle or a muscle–tendon unit caused by overstretching. A **sprain** occurs when the ligaments around a joint are stretched or torn. Strains and sprains are among the most commonly reported injuries, accounting for about 50% of all work-related injuries. The lower back and neck are the most common sites for muscle strains. The ankle is the most common area for a sprain.

Etiology and Pathogenesis

A strain occurs when the muscle is forced to extend beyond capacity. Microscopic tears develop in the muscle tissue, leading to an acute injury. Bending from the waist to lift a heavy object can cause strains to the lower back and hamstring muscles. Sprain injuries commonly occur when oppositional forces cause the ligament to overstretch and tear. Besides the ankle, a common site for sprains is the knee.

Clinical Manifestations

A strain causes immediate pain, reduced range of motion (ROM), muscle spasms, edema, and muscle weakness. If the muscle is partially or completely torn, bleeding, swelling, and bruising occur. With a sprain, ROM is severely hindered. The patient may report feeling a "pop" or "rip" when the injury occurs. Additional manifestations include bruising, pain, and immediate swelling. Pain is exacerbated with movement.

Linking Pathophysiology to Diagnosis and Treatment

Traditional treatment has been through the use of RICE:

Rest
Ice
Compression
Elevation.

However, the treatment approach is changing. See the Impact of Current Research feature on treating strains and sprains.

Until research proves otherwise, traditional treatment for strains and sprains includes NSAIDs, casts, splints, immobilizers, or slings. Surgery may be required for severe injuries. Physical therapy may be prescribed to facilitate joint mobility and return to normal function. The amount of time required for healing depends on the severity of the injury and can range from 1 to 2 months for mild injuries and up to a year for those that are more severe.

Check Your Progress: Section 35.6

1. Distinguish between a strain and a sprain.
2. What are the clinical manifestations of strains and sprains?
3. What is the traditional treatment for strains and sprains?

35.7 Knee Injuries

The knee is the joint that connects the femur with the tibia through four major ligaments (**Figure 35.11** ■). Because of the location and function, the knee is particularly vulnerable

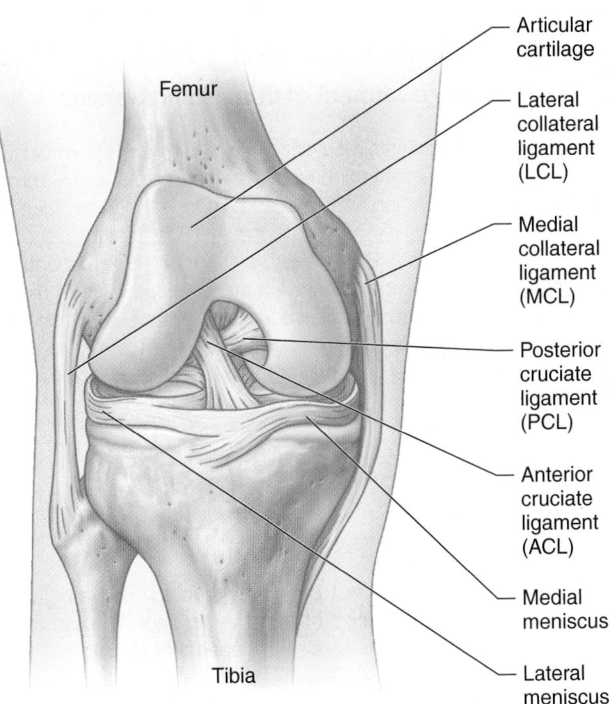

Figure 35.11 ■ Anatomy of the knee.

to injuries, tears, and dislocations. Knee injuries are most closely associated with sports activities that can lead to falls or twisting of the lower extremity.

A knee injury occurs when a particular ligament holding together a part of the knee joint is stressed, strained, or torn. The anterior cruciate ligament (ACL) is the most common site for a knee injury. Less common but equally painful knee injuries include a tear of the meniscus and osteochondral lesions.

Anterior Cruciate Ligament Injuries

The ACL connects the femur to the tibia. Injuries to this ligament average 150,000 to 200,000 each year and can cost up to half a million dollars in medical expenses. The sports that cause the most ACL injuries include basketball, soccer, skiing, and football. Even though these sports are played predominantly by men, women are at a higher risk for an ACL injury. This type of injury occurs most often in people between the ages of 15 and 45, and approximately 1 in every 1700 people will experience an ACL injury in their lifetime.[12]

Etiology and Pathogenesis

Most ACL injuries occur when the individual is decelerating while running. This is considered a noncontact injury and may also occur in twisting or jumping. Direct contact ACL injuries occur most often in sports such as football. Depending on the activity, the tear might be down the middle of the ligament, or the ligament may be torn completely from the femur.

Clinical Manifestations

At the time of an injury, the patient typically reports intense pain and a feeling that the knee "popped" and "gave out." Swelling may begin immediately or develop over the next few hours.

Impact of Current Research on Clinical Practice

Altering the Treatment of Strains and Sprains

Description: Patients recovering from strains and sprains who are prescribed rest might experience more problems, since immobility reduces circulation and can cause muscles, nerves, ligaments, and tendons to weaken from disuse. In 1994, a study conducted at Oregon Health & Science University found that patients who engaged in early mobilization of a strain or sprain injury returned to work sooner and experienced less pain than did those whose injury was immobilized with a splint or cast.[1] In 2012, an editorial in the *British Journal of Sports Medicine* suggested replacing RICE with **POLICE**[2]:

Protection
Optimal **L**oading
Ice
Compression
Elevation.

The use of ice has not been well studied. Some individuals respond well to application of ice; others do not. The use of compression and elevation has also not been well studied.

Clinical Practice: Leading sports medicine providers agree that until additional research on treatment is done, the best approach is to implement RICE until the person can be seen by a healthcare provider.[3]

Research Studies:

1. Eiff, M. P., Smith, A. T., & Smith, G. E. (1994). Early mobilization versus immobilization in the treatment of lateral ankle sprains. *American Journal of Sports Medicine*, 22(1), 83–88. Available at https://www.ncbi.nlm.nih.gov/pubmed/8129116
2. Bleakley, C. M., Glasgow, P., & MacAuley, D. C. (2011). Editorial: PRICE needs updating, should we call the POLICE? *British Journal of Sports Medicine, 46*(4). Available at http://bjsm.bmj.com/content/46/4/220
3. Harrison, L. (2014). Treating sprains and strains: Are you doing it wrong? *Healthline News*. Available at http://www.healthline.com/health-news/rice-method-for-sports-injuries-not-best-practice-040314#

Linking Pathophysiology to Diagnosis and Treatment

Diagnosis of an ACL injury is made after an x-ray and MRI of the joint. Treatment of this injury begins with the application of ice, elevating the extremity, and oral pain medication such as NSAIDs. The patient will be non-weight bearing on the extremity until the swelling subsides. Physical therapy is prescribed to improve joint mobility and muscle tone. If symptoms persist, the patient might need surgery to repair the torn ligament.[13]

Jeannine Cartwright: Outcome

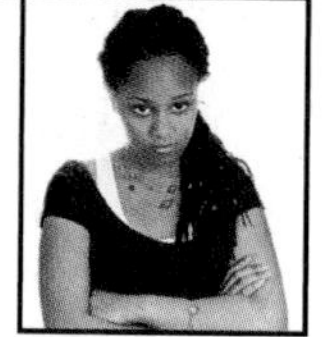

While waiting for a knee x-ray, Ms. Cartwright is given an ice pack for her knee along with an NSAID pain medication. The findings from the x-ray are unclear, so an MRI is ordered, which will be done within a few hours. The knee is edematous. Elevation on two pillows and the pain medication have reduced Ms. Cartwright's discomfort.

The results of the MRI show a midline tear of Ms. Cartwright's ACL. Because she will not be able to bear weight on the leg for a week, she is fitted with crutches and instructed on their use before being sent home with her mother. Ms. Cartwright has an appointment with the outpatient physical therapy department in 1 week. At home, she is instructed to keep the leg elevated, apply ice, and continue taking the NSAID medication. A follow-up appointment at the orthopedic clinic in 2 weeks is scheduled.

3. How does an ACL injury, such as Ms. Cartwright's, occur?
4. What are the clinical manifestations of an ACL tear?
5. What is the treatment plan for Ms. Cartwright's ACL tear?

Meniscus Injuries

The meniscus is a piece of cartilage located between the femur and tibia (see Figure 35.11). Each knee has two menisci. This cartilage can be injured in performing any activity that places pressure on the knee it or causes to rotate.

Etiology and Pathogenesis

During participation in football, tennis, basketball, or soccer, the knee can be exposed to a forced twist or rotation. This can also occur in moving from a squatting to a standing position.

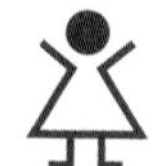

More children are being diagnosed with meniscus injuries primarily because of increased participation in team sports. Boston Children's Hospital estimates that more than 500,000 meniscal tears take place in the United States each year.[14] ■

Meniscus injuries are common in older patients with osteoarthritis because the cartilage is drier and prone to separation with activities that place stress on the knee joint. ■

Clinical Manifestations

At the time of injury, the patient may hear a popping sound at the knee joint. Additional manifestations that indicate a meniscus injury include pain when the knee is touched, edema, restricted mobility of the joint, a feeling that the knee is "locking up" or not moving smoothly, and a feeling that the knee is weak or "buckling." Continuing to hear a popping sound when the knee is moved could indicate that a piece of the cartilage is loose.

Linking Pathophysiology to Diagnosis and Treatment

Immediately after sustaining an injury to the knee, the patient should apply ice to the knee, elevate the extremity, and take an NSAID while seeking medical attention. The healthcare provider will place the knee through various ROM positions to assess for a popping sound, which indicates a meniscus tear. Further diagnostic testing includes knee x-ray, MRI, and ultrasound. MRIs have successfully diagnosed a meniscus tear approximately 77% of the time, and ultrasound is often used to check for cartilage fragments.[14]

Treatment of a torn meniscus includes rest, no weight bearing, an elastic bandage, NSAIDs, and crutches. Physical therapy may be prescribed to assist with joint mobility and muscle strength. It takes approximately 1–3 months for a meniscus tear to heal. If the injury continues to produce pain with walking after this period of time, arthroscopic surgery may be prescribed to repair the torn area of the meniscus. Recovery after this surgery takes approximately 6 weeks.

Osteochondral Lesions

An osteochondral lesion is one that occurs at the end of the bone. For the knee, this lesion would be at the end of the femur or the tibia. This injury is more common in adolescents and young adults and can occur in the ankle and elbow as well as the knee.[15]

Etiology and Pathogenesis

The lesion can range from a small crack on the surface to a large chunk of the bone breaking off. Reasons for occurrence of this lesion include lack of blood supply to the affected area, direct trauma to the joint, repetitive use, and heredity. The lesion can be graded by surface area, shape, and depth.[16]

Clinical Manifestations

Manifestations of an osteochondral lesion include pain with weight bearing, swelling, tenderness over the area, limited mobility, and occasional "locking" of the knee. An injury that affects the entire width and depth of the bone end results in a loose body.

Linking Pathophysiology to Diagnosis and Treatment

Treatment begins conservatively with NSAIDs and the use of growth hormone for younger patients. Additional approaches include weight loss, rest, ice, using assistive devices to walk, and physical therapy. Nutritional supplements such as glucosamine and chondroitin, calcium, and vitamins are also recommended.

If pain and joint instability continue, arthroscopic surgery may be indicated to remove loose bone fragments, realign the bones with the cartilage, maximize function, and prevent the development of osteoarthritis.[16]

Check Your Progress: Section 35.7

1. Why are older adults prone to meniscus injuries?
2. Describe the clinical manifestations that are characteristic of a meniscus injury.
3. What is the etiology of osteochondral lesions?

35.8 Shoulder Injuries

The shoulder is particularly prone to injury because of the degree of motion and position in the body. The injuries that are most common to the shoulder include rotator cuff tears, adhesive capsulitis (frozen shoulder), and nerve impingement leading to bursitis.[4]

Rotator Cuff Tears

The shoulder is supported in the joint by four muscles, called the rotator cuff. If these muscles become injured or worn out, a tendon supporting one or several of the muscles rips or tears from the bone (**Figure 35.12**). The people who are most prone to rotator cuff injuries are those who perform repeated overhead motions, such as painters, carpenters, and anyone who plays baseball or tennis. The frequency of experiencing a rotator cuff injury increases with age.

Etiology and Pathogenesis

The rotator cuff is made up of a group of shoulder muscles and tendons that connect the humerus to the scapula. The tendons hold the bones together, while the muscles provide movement. Frequent use can cause the tendons to become inflamed or an acute injury, such as a fall on the shoulder or an attempt to break a fall with an outstretched hand, can jar one or more of the tendons, leading to a microscopic or complete tear.

Clinical Manifestations

The pain of a rotator cuff tear can be acute if caused by a direct blow or other injury. Microscopic tears caused by repeated use most often begin as a dull ache in the joint. The ache or pain is intensified when laying on the shoulder and may disturb sleeping. Changes in function may begin as a weakness when raising the arm to comb the hair or perform other routine functions. Over time, limited ROM progresses to an inability to reach behind the back.

Linking Pathophysiology to Diagnosis and Treatment

Diagnosis of a rotator cuff tear begins with evaluation of the patient's shoulder joint ROM. If pain and weakness occur when the patient moves the arm but it can be moved fully with passive ROM, a rotator cuff tear should be suspected. Testing for a rotator cuff tear usually begins with an x-ray of the shoulder to rule out other causes for the weakness and pain. Additional diagnostic tests include a CT scan or MRI of the shoulder, an ultrasound, or an arthrogram. In an arthrogram, x-rays of the shoulder are taken after contrast medium is injected into the shoulder. Leaking of the medium out of the shoulder joint validates the diagnosis of a rotator cuff tear.

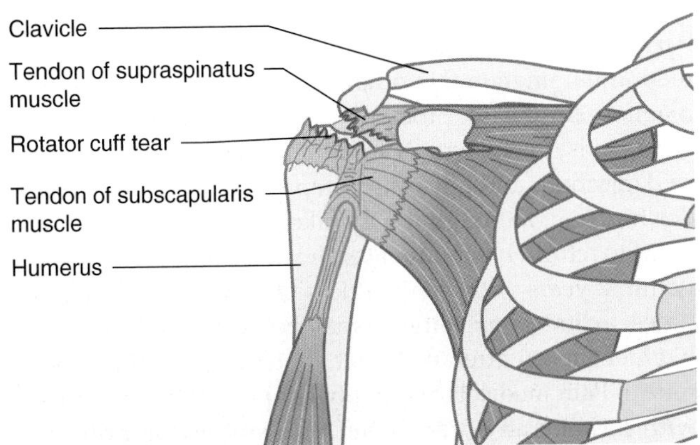

Figure 35.12 Rotator cuff tear.

Treatment of a rotator cuff tear begins conservatively with rest, application of cold or heat to the area, NSAIDs, and possible electrical stimulation of the joint muscles. Cortisone injections may be prescribed to help reduce acute tendon inflammation.

Surgery might be indicated for a patient with an injury taking longer than 6–12 months to heal that is accompanied by severe arm weakness and loss of shoulder function or when an acute injury has caused a large tendon tear. Procedures to repair the tear include open or arthroscopic approaches. Arm and shoulder immobilization occurs for the first 4–6 weeks after surgery and may include passive exercising. Active exercising begins during the next 4–6 weeks and progresses until full or maximum shoulder ROM and arm function return.[17]

Adhesive Capsulitis

Adhesive capsulitis, or frozen shoulder, is an acute inflammation of the ligaments in the shoulder joint. The capsule of the shoulder joint has ligaments that hold the shoulder bones together to form the joint. When the capsule becomes inflamed, the shoulder bones are unable to move freely in the joint.

Etiology, Pathogenesis, and Clinical Manifestations

At times, there is no known reason for a frozen shoulder. However, this health problem has been seen in patients with cervical disc disease of the neck or diabetes, after open heart surgery, and in those experiencing changes in hormone levels such as in menopause. Frozen shoulder has also been seen in individuals who have experienced an acute shoulder injury or who are recovering from surgical repair of another shoulder problem.

Inflammation of the shoulder ligaments causes pain and a loss of shoulder motion. Because movement exacerbates the pain, the person begins to limit arm and shoulder movements. This self-imposed immobility of the shoulder leads to stiffness, more pain, and continued loss of motion. Eventually, the patient is unable to move the arm above the head or behind the back.

Linking Pathophysiology to Diagnosis and Treatment

The diagnosis of frozen shoulder is suspected when the patient is unable to freely move the shoulder joint. A shoulder x-ray may be done to rule out another disease process. An MRI might be considered to estimate and diagnose ligament inflammation. No other imaging studies are used to diagnose this health problem.

Pain is treated with NSAIDs and steroid injections. Steroid injections and physical therapy help to improve shoulder function, although it may take up to 9 months for full ROM to return. If left untreated, frozen shoulder can resolve within 2 years with minimal loss of shoulder function. At times, arthroscopic surgery may be performed to cut the ligament in an attempt to get shoulder joint function to return. Pain medication and physical therapy are included with postoperative care. Even with surgery and physical therapy, a patient may continue to experience shoulder pain and stiffness.[18]

Impingement Syndrome

Impingement syndrome of the shoulder occurs when the tendons of the shoulder muscles are trapped under the acromion, a part of the shoulder blade. Consistent impingement can lead to the development of rotator cuff tendinitis.[19]

Etiology, Pathogenesis, and Clinical Manifestations

Impingement syndrome occurs when the rotator cuff tendon becomes trapped at the top of the shoulder and scrapes against the bone. Pain occurs when the arm is raised above the head and may be described as a persistent ache that is worse at night. This syndrome is seen after an acute shoulder injury or in people who use their arm for repeated movement, such as baseball pitchers. It also has been diagnosed in people with no obvious cause other than advancing age.

Additional reasons for the development of impingement syndrome include the development of bone spurs, calcium deposits or inflammation of the rotator cuff tendon, or shoulder bursitis.[20]

Manifestations of impingement syndrome include pain when raising the arms above the head and difficulty moving the arms behind the back. The shoulder is noticeably weaker, with limited ROM.

Linking Pathophysiology to Diagnosis and Treatment

The diagnosis of impingement syndrome is made when pain is immediately relieved after an anesthetic is injected into the space below the acromion. Additional diagnostic testing may include x-rays to assess for arthritis, bone spurs, or a rotator cuff tear.

Treatment for impingement syndrome includes the application of ice, NSAIDs, and physical therapy. At first, moving the arms over the head is avoided to help the tendon heal. Then progressive exercising is used to strengthen the muscles and maintain joint flexibility. For ongoing pain, steroid injections may be used to reduce tendon inflammation. Shoulder pain that continues after conservative treatment may be treated with arthroscopic surgery to widen the subacromial space. Postoperative care after surgery includes pain management and progressive physical therapy to ensure shoulder muscle strength and joint mobility.[20]

Check Your Progress: Section 35.8

1. What is the initial step in diagnosing a rotator cuff tear?
2. Describe the clinical manifestations of frozen shoulder.
3. How is diagnosis of impingement syndrome made?

35.9 Bone Infections and Tumors

Additional injury or pathology can occur to the bones themselves. This section focuses on osteomyelitis (bone infection), osteonecrosis, and bone tumors. Bone tumors can be benign or malignant or can develop as a result of metastatic bone disease.

Osteomyelitis

A bone infection, or **osteomyelitis**, can occur after a penetrating wound, as a result of a blood infection or bacteremia, or from skin breakdown. These infections are also seen after joint replacement and internal fixation surgeries. Although osteomyelitis can occur at any age, it is seen most frequently in people over the age of 50. It may be an acute, subacute, or chronic infection.

Etiology and Pathogenesis

In osteomyelitis, an offending microorganisms, such as bacteria, fungi, parasites, or viruses, lodge and multiply in the bone. The most common cause is an infection from the *Staphylococcus aureus* bacteria. The microorganism causes inflammation and an immune response with the formation of pus, edema, and vascular congestion. Canals within the bone permit the infection to move to other bone areas, which could potentially disrupt blood supply to the bone tissue. If the infection is left untreated, ischemia and necrosis will occur.

Osteomyelitis can also occur if an infection from another body area is carried to a bone through the blood supply. This is often seen in older patients, patients with sickle cell disease, and patients who engage in intravenous substance abuse. Individuals with a chronic health problems such as diabetes are prone to developing osteomyelitis from an infected foot wound. A postoperative joint replacement that becomes infected can also cause osteomyelitis and is considered the most common cause of the bone infection in adults.[4]

Clinical Manifestations

Manifestations of osteomyelitis can be local or systemic. Local indications of a bone infection include bone pain, drainage and ulceration at the site, swelling, redness, warmth, and localized tenderness. Lymph node swelling, fever with chills, general malaise, tachycardia, nausea, vomiting, and anorexia are manifestations of a systemic bone infection.

Linking Pathophysiology to Diagnosis and Treatment

Osteomyelitis is diagnosed after bone x-rays, a bone scan, and an MRI show evidence of an abscess or bone changes. An elevated white blood cell count and altered sedimentation rate help to confirm the presence of an infection, along with blood cultures and bone biopsy/tissue samples.

When osteomyelitis is suspected, treatment begins with a broad-spectrum antibiotic until bone and blood culture results confirm the offending microorganism and the antibiotic most applicable for treatment is identified. Parenteral antibiotic therapy may continue for 4–6 weeks. Depending on the microorganism and the patient's overall health status, oral medication may be prescribed.

In cases of severe ischemia, surgery is required to debride necrotic areas and is the primary treatment for chronic osteomyelitis. For some patients, drainage tubes are inserted in the bone canals and used for direct antibiotic irrigation. If extensive amounts of bone tissue are excised, further treatment may include a procedure to fill the dead tissue space with the muscle adjacent to the affected bone.[4]

Osteonecrosis

When the blood supply to the bone is altered, the area is prone to developing necrosis. Other names for **osteonecrosis** are avascular necrosis, aseptic necrosis, or ischemic necrosis. It most often affects the bones of the lower extremities but can also occur in the shoulders. More than one area can experience osteonecrosis at the same time.

Etiology and Pathogenesis

Normally, new bone constantly replaces old bone. But if blood flow to a joint is reduced, bone breakdown occurs faster than replacement bone is made. Over time, the bone in the joints breaks down, leading to pain and alterations in joint mobility. Although this health problem can occur in anyone at any age, it is most commonly seen in people between the ages of 30 and 50 years.

Risk factors for the development of osteonecrosis include long-term use of steroids, heavy alcohol intake, and direct injury to the bone or joint. The people who are most prone to developing this health problem are those who are undergoing chemotherapy or radiation or who have had an organ transplantation. Osteonecrosis is seen most often in patients with cancer, systemic lupus erythematosus, HIV, gout, vasculitis, osteoarthritis, osteoporosis, and sickle cell disease. However, some individuals with no known health problem or risk factor can develop the disorder.

Clinical Manifestations

The disorder may begin insidiously and have no symptoms. In time the patient may begin to experience pain when pressure or weight is applied to the affected joint. As the necrosis progresses pain increases and joint pain at rest occurs. Breakdown of the bone at a joint may render the limb unusable, affecting the patient's ability to walk. The onset of the disease process to complete loss of limb function may take months to over a year.

Linking Pathophysiology to Diagnosis and Treatment

The diagnosis of osteonecrosis will be made after a physical examination and diagnostic tests confirm necrosis of a joint. Testing used to aid in the diagnosis include x-rays, MRI or CT scan, a bone scan, bone biopsy, and a measurement of bone pressure.

Treatment of osteonecrosis is focused on interventions to prevent joint breakdown. Without treatment, the limb may become unusable within 2 years. Conservative treatment includes the use of NSAIDs, avoiding weight bearing, ROM exercises, and electrical stimulation. If conservative treatment does not stop disease progression, surgery may be indicated sooner rather than later. Most people with the disorder will need surgery at some point in time. Procedures used to treat osteonecrosis include core decompression surgery to reduce bone pressure and increase bone blood flow, an osteotomy to reshape the bone, a bone graft, or a total joint replacement.[21]

Benign Bone Tumors

A benign tumor is an abnormal growth of normal tissue that does not metastasize or interfere with normal body organ function. The sites for most benign bone tumors include the femur, tibia, humerus, and pelvis. Some benign tumors can also develop in the spine.

Etiology, Pathogenesis, and Clinical Manifestations

Benign bone tumors occur in children and young adults up to age 30. The vast majority of benign tumors are affected by growth hormones and stop growing when the child's bones stop growing.

These tumors can be of various types, including endochondromas, osteochondromas, nonossifying fibromas, chondroblastomas, osteoid osteomas, osteoblastomas, periosteal chondromas, giant cell tumors, and chondromyxoid fibromas.

Manifestations of a benign bone tumor may begin as a lump associated with an ache or pain in the area. At times, these tumors are diagnosed after a tumor weakens the bone and causes a fracture.

Linking Pathophysiology to Diagnosis and Treatment

Treatment of a benign bone tumor depends on its type, size, and location and the age of the patient. For some patients, the tumor heals when the fracture heals. Others stop growing when the amount of growth hormone slows with body maturity. If a benign bone tumor is found during a routine x-ray scan, watchful waiting may be the approach of choice.

Surgery is often needed to remove the tumor and provides the remaining bone with space and nutrients to rebuild healthy bone tissue. For patients with an osteoblastoma, spinal deformity and paralysis can result. Treatment for this type of tumor includes surgery, physical therapy, and pain management. If an osteoid osteoma is diagnosed, this small bone tumor that primarily affects the spine in adolescents, may require surgery to support the spinal structure.[22]

Malignant Bone Tumors

The incidence of malignant primary bone tumors is rare, and they account for fewer than 0.2% of all cancers in adults. Unfortunately, these tumors grow fast and metastasize quickly.

Etiology and Pathogenesis

Primary malignant bone tumors come from bone tissue including cartilage, bone cells, collagen, and bone marrow. See **Table 35.3** ■ for more information about primary malignant bone tumors.

The exact etiology of a primary malignant bone tumor is unknown; however, it is possible that these tumors are potentiated during periods of high bone growth or bone overstimulation by another disease. Radiation and bone marrow transplantation increases the risk for the development of these tumors.

A primary malignant bone tumor causes **osteolysis**, or bone breakdown. This leads to bone weakening and fractures. The surface of the bone changes to permit the contours of the growing tumor. Further, the tumor destroys adjacent bone tissue, promoting bone resorption and interfering with the bone blood supply.

Clinical Manifestations

Clinical manifestations of a primary malignant bone tumor depend on the location. For the upper and lower extremities and the pelvis, the patient experiences deep bone pain that is worse at night or at rest and is associated with muscle weakness and atrophy. For tumors that affect the ends of the bones, the skin over the mass may be warm and erythematous and associated with a fever. The bone mass is described as a lump that can be palpated through the skin and may affect normal bone function or cause a fracture.

Linking Pathophysiology to Diagnosis and Treatment

The diagnosis of a primary malignant bone tumor is made after x-rays, CT scans, and an MRI. Radiographic examination shows a characteristic "moth-eaten" pattern. The mass has ill-defined borders that cannot be distinguished from normal bone tissue. A bone biopsy confirms the type of tumor cell. Additional tests performed to diagnose these tumors include alkaline phosphatase and calcium levels, which are both elevated in the presence of a bone tumor.

Treatment options for a primary malignant bone tumor include surgery, chemotherapy, and radiation. Surgery may be done to either completely excise the tumor or amputate the limb. Chemotherapy is provided before surgery to shrink the tumor. Chemotherapy may be provided after surgery to prevent metastasis. Most primary malignant bone tumors are resistant to radiation, but it may be prescribed if the tumor type is found to be sensitive to the therapy.[4]

Metastatic Bone Disease

Metastatic bone disease occurs when a cancer in another body site migrates to a bone. The most common metastatic bone tumors originate from the prostate, thyroid, lung, kidney, and breast.

Etiology and Pathogenesis

Metastatic bone disease most often affects older people and occurs when cancer cells from a tumor or other site break away and travel to a bone, where the cells grow and

Table 35.3 Primary Malignant Bone Tumors

Tissue Type	Type of Tumor	Affected Bone	Incidence
Bone	Osteosarcoma Ewing sarcoma	Femur, tibia, humerus Shaft of long bones, flat bones	Adolescents, young adults, males more than females Adolescents and young adults
Cartilage	Chondrosarcoma	Pelvis, scapula, shaft of long bones	Adults and older adults
Bone marrow	Multiple myeloma	Multiple sites	Considered a hematologic cancer

multiply. The metastasis to the bone comes from another primary site and is not referred to as bone cancer. Although it can occur in any bone, metastasis most commonly occurs in the spine, pelvis, and thigh. Finding bone metastasis or being diagnosed with bone metastasis may be the first sign that a patient has cancer. Metastasis to the bone can occur at any time during and after treatment for cancer in another area. It is not clear why some cancers spread to bone whereas other cancers spread to soft tissue or major organs such as the liver or pancreas.

Clinical Manifestations

Metastatic bone disease does not always cause symptoms. The individual may have no indications that cancer has invaded a bone. However, when they do occur, the primary manifestations include bone pain, fractures, changes in urinary and bowel continence, and limb weakness. Laboratory values that support metastatic bone disease include an elevated calcium level, which causes nausea, vomiting, constipation, and confusion.

Linking Pathophysiology to Diagnosis and Treatment

Diagnosis of metastatic bone disease includes x-rays, CT scans, an MRI, and blood tests. A bone or positron emission tomography scan is used to determine the area and extent of bone affected. Increased areas of uptake usually indicate areas of metastasis.

Treatment for metastatic bone disease depends on the primary cancer site. Radiation may be prescribed to relieve pain and prevent fractures. Chemotherapy helps to prevent the need for surgery or radiation and may also be used to prevent fractures.[23]

Check Your Progress: Section 35.9

1. Compare the local and systemic manifestations of osteomyelitis.
2. Identify risk factors for the development of osteonecrosis.
3. What population is most at risk for benign bone tumors?

CHAPTER SUMMARY

35.1 Chapter Overview and Case Studies

Describe the normal musculoskeletal function and concepts related to acute disorders of musculoskeletal function.

- The musculoskeletal system is the scaffolding of the human body.
- Injuries, infections, and disease processes can hinder maximum motor function.
- Musculoskeletal injuries can occur to anyone at any age.
- The most frequently reported injuries in children are strains, sprains, dislocations, and fractures.

35.2 Fractures

Differentiate the causes, classification, underlying pathogenesis, and clinical manifestations of fractures and approaches to diagnosis and treatment of these conditions across the lifespan.

- Fractures can be caused by direct or indirect force.
- Fractures can occur from compression, torsion, or a pathologic condition.
- Risk factors for fractures include age, nutrition, and bone disease.
- Younger patients are more prone to fractures related to sports injuries. In additional to falls, older patients have more bone diseases that weaken bone integrity, which contribute to fractures.
- Fractures can be classified as closed, open, complete, greenstick, comminuted, impacted, oblique, transverse, linear, displaced, nondisplaced, avulsion, stress, spiral, depression, pathologic, or compression.
- The most common clinical manifestations of a fracture are pain and altered mobility and function.
- Treatment of a fracture includes immobility through casting or traction or external or internal fixation.
- Fractures heal through indirect or direct healing. Indirect healing has three stages: inflammatory, reparative, and remodeling. Direct healing requires a surgical procedure to realign the bone.
- Complications associated with fractures include infection, compartment syndrome, fracture blister, or FES.

35.3 Dislocations and Subluxations

Differentiate the causes, classification, underlying pathogenesis, and clinical manifestations of dislocations and subluxations and approaches to diagnosis and treatment of these conditions across the lifespan.

- A dislocation occurs when the ends of bones are moved out of normal position, losing attachment to a joint. A subluxation is a partial dislocation.
- Dislocations and subluxations most often occur after a fall or trauma to a joint.
- Clinical manifestations of a dislocation or subluxation include pain, limb or joint deformity, and altered mobility and function.
- Treatment of both dislocation and subluxation begins with manual traction. Surgery may be required to realign the bones of the joint and prevent neurovascular injury.

35.4 Nerve Entrapment

Differentiate the causes, classification, underlying pathogenesis, and clinical manifestations of nerve entrapment and approaches to diagnosis and treatment of these conditions across the lifespan.

- Nerve entrapment is a type of neuropathy that causes nerve damage and muscle weakness or atrophy.
- Common areas for nerve entrapment to occur include the forearm, wrist, hand, pelvis, and spine.
- Carpal tunnel syndrome is the most common type of nerve entrapment. This injury is often caused by repetitive use and causes median nerve compression.
- Early manifestations of carpal tunnel syndrome include numbness and tingling of the thumb, index finger, and lateral ventral surface of the middle finger. Later signs of this syndrome include hand numbness and tingling during sleep.
- Treatment includes splinting and application of heat or ice. Surgery may be indicated to enlarge the tunnel and take pressure off of the compressed nerve.

35.5 Bursitis

Differentiate the causes, classification, underlying pathogenesis, and clinical manifestations of bursitis and approaches to diagnosis and treatment of these conditions across the lifespan.

- Bursitis is the inflammation of the fluid-filled sac that cushions muscles, tendons, and bony prominences.
- The most common areas for bursitis are the shoulders, hips, knees, and elbows.
- Bursitis is most commonly caused by overuse or direct joint trauma, which leads to joint tenderness and pain with joint extension and flexion. The skin over the area may be warm, red, and swollen.
- Treatment of bursitis includes NSAIDs, ice during the acute phase of the disorder, gentle stretching, and exercise. Steroid injections are indicated if conservative treatment is ineffective. Surgery may be prescribed to repair damaged tissue and relieve pressure on the bursa.

35.6 Strains and Sprains

Differentiate the causes, classification, underlying pathogenesis, and clinical manifestations of strains and sprains and approaches to diagnosis and treatment of these conditions across the lifespan.

- A strain is an injury to a muscle or muscle–tendon unit caused by overstretching. A sprain is an injury caused by stretched or torn ligaments. These are the most commonly reported injuries.
- A strain causes microscopic tears in muscle tissue. Sprains occur when oppositional forces cause a ligament to overstretch and tear.
- Strains cause immediate pain, change in function, muscle spasms, edema, and weakness. Sprains cause severely limited ROM, bruising, pain, and swelling.
- Traditional treatment for strains and sprains includes rest, ice, compression, and elevation, although studies have shown that rest might adversely affect mobility after recovery. Additional treatment includes NSAIDs, casts, splints, immobilizers, or slings. Physical therapy helps with joint mobility and function. Surgery may be required for severe injuries.

35.7 Knee Injuries

Differentiate the causes, classification, underlying pathogenesis, and clinical manifestations of knee injuries and approaches to diagnosis and treatment of these conditions across the lifespan.

- The knee is prone to injuries, tears, and dislocations. The ACL is the most common site for a knee injury. Other common injuries include a torn meniscus and osteochondral lesions.
- ACL injuries are more likely to occur during participation in sports. The tear might be down the middle of the ligament or the ligament may be completely torn from the femur. The injury causes intense pain, swelling, and a feeling that the knee has "popped." Treatment includes ice, elevation, and NSAIDs. The patient should not bear weight on the extremity. Surgery may be required to repair the torn ligament.
- The meniscus, or cartilage between the femur and tibia, can be injured by any activity that causes knee rotation. This injury causes popping of the knee joint, pain on touch, swelling, restricted function, and a buckling sensation. Treatment includes immediate application of ice, elevation, NSAIDs, compression, and no weight bearing on the extremity. Surgery may be required to repair the tear.
- Osteochondral lesions occur at the ends of bones and can range from a small crack to a large area of bone breaking off. Manifestations include pain with weight bearing, swelling, tenderness, altered function, and possible locking of the knee. Treatment includes NSAIDs, weight loss, rest, ice, crutches, and physical therapy. Surgery may be required to remove bone fragments.

35.8 Shoulder Injuries

Differentiate the causes, classification, underlying pathogenesis, and clinical manifestations of shoulder injuries and approaches to diagnosis and treatment of these conditions across the lifespan.

- The most common shoulder injuries include rotator cuff tears, adhesive capsulitis, and nerve impingement.
- A rotator cuff injury occurs when a tendon supporting a shoulder muscle rips or tears from the bone. Manifestations of this injury include a dull ache, arm weakness, and limited ROM. Treatment begins with rest,

application of heat or cold, and NSAIDs. Cortisone injections and surgery may be required.

- Adhesive capsulitis is an acute inflammation of the ligaments in the shoulder joint. Inflammation of the ligaments causes pain, stiffness, and loss of shoulder function that is exacerbated by self-imposed immobility. Treatment includes NSAIDs, steroid injections, and physical therapy. If left untreated, the condition may spontaneously resolve after 2 years.
- Impingement syndrome occurs when the shoulder tendons are trapped under the shoulder blade. Manifestations include pain when raising the arm above the head and limited mobility. Treatment includes ice, NSAIDs, and physical therapy. Steroid injections and surgery may be required if the condition continues.

35.9 Bone Infections and Tumors

Differentiate the causes, classification, underlying pathogenesis, and clinical manifestations of bone infections and tumors and approaches to diagnosis and treatment of these conditions across the lifespan.

- Injury and pathology that occur to bones include osteomyelitis, osteonecrosis, and tumors.
- Osteomyelitis is an infection of the bone caused by bacteria, fungi, parasites, or viruses leading to pus formation, edema, and vascular congestion. Local manifestations include pain, drainage, ulceration, swelling, redness, warmth, and tenderness. Systemic manifestations include lymph node enlargement, fever, chills, malaise, tachycardia, nausea, vomiting, and anorexia. Treatment includes long-term antibiotic therapy. Surgery may be required to debride the necrotic bone tissue and promote healing.
- Osteonecrosis is the death of bone tissue caused by a reduction in blood supply to the bone. It causes bone to break down faster than it can be replaced. Clinical manifestations include pain and immobility that can progress to complete loss of limb function. Treatment begins with NSAIDs, no weight bearing, ROM exercises, and electrical stimulation. Surgery will be required to restore bone and limb function at some point in time.
- Bone tumors can be benign, malignant, or metastatic. Benign tumors cause pain and a possible fracture. Treatment of a benign tumor may include watchful waiting or surgery.
- Malignant bone tumors are rare in the adult population but cause bone breakdown, weakness, and fractures. Manifestations include bone pain, muscle weakness, and atrophy. Treatment includes surgery, chemotherapy, and radiation.
- Metastatic bone disease occurs when cancer from another body location migrates to a bone. This bone disease does not always cause symptoms. The most common manifestations are bone pain, fractures, changes in urinary and bowel continence, and limb weakness. Treatment depends on the primary cancer site and can include radiation, chemotherapy, and surgery.

REVIEW QUESTIONS

1. Which of the following laboratory results would the nurse expect to see in a client with a primary malignant bone tumor?
   a. Reduced serum alkaline phosphatase, reduced serum calcium
   b. Reduced serum alkaline phosphatase, elevated serum calcium
   c. Elevated serum alkaline phosphatase, reduced serum calcium
   d. Elevated serum alkaline phosphatase, elevated serum calcium
2. Which of the following postoperative clients is most likely to develop a fat embolism?
   a. A client with a collarbone fracture
   b. A client with a pelvic fracture
   c. A client with a rib fracture
   d. A client with an ankle fracture
3. Which of the following assessment findings suggests local manifestations of osteomyelitis?
   a. Enlarged lymph nodes
   b. Fever with chills
   c. General malaise
   d. Drainage and ulceration
4. A client with a positive Phalen maneuver will exhibit:
   a. tingling in fingers when the wrist is flexed.
   b. tingling in fingers when the wrist is extended.
   c. tingling in fingers when the ulna nerve is tapped.
   d. tingling in fingers when the median nerve is tapped.
5. What action by the nurse is a priority when a client with an arm cast complains of increasing pain despite receiving opioid medications?
   a. Performing neurovascular checks every 2 hours
   b. Increasing the dose of opioid as ordered
   c. Notifying the orthopedist immediately
   d. Elevating the limb
6. Which of the following clients is most at risk for developing osteonecrosis?
   a. A 10-year-old boy taking steroids for asthma
   b. A 25-year-old woman on short-term steroids for acute bronchitis

c. A 45-year-old woman with systemic lupus erythematosus
d. A 30-year-old woman who has approximately three alcoholic drinks per month

7. A client with bursitis in the elbow will most likely report:
a. pain at rest.
b. pain with movement of the joint.
c. crepitus over the joint.
d. reduced range of motion.

8. A client in the emergency department with a painful ankle reports feeling a "rip" while running. The nurse observes bruising and swelling of the ankle and is unable to assess range of motion because the client feels severe pain with movement. The nurse determines that the client most likely has experienced:
a. an ankle sprain.
b. an ankle strain.
c. an ankle dislocation.
d. an ankle fracture.

ANSWERS

Answers to Review Questions can be found in Appendix A. Answers to Case Study and Check Your Progress questions are available on the faculty resources site. Please consult with your instructor.

RECOMMENDED WEBSITES

National Institute of Arthritis and Musculoskeletal and Skin Diseases
https://www.niams.nih.gov

NIH Osteoporosis and Related Bone Diseases National Resource Center
https://www.niams.nih.gov/Health_Info/Bone/default.asp

REFERENCES

1. National Institute of Arthritis and Musculoskeletal and Skin Diseases. (2013). Preventing musculoskeletal sports injuries in youth: A guide for parents. *Sports Injuries.* Available at http://www.niams.nih.gov/Health_Info/Sports_Injuries/child_sports_injuries.asp#most
2. Ball, J. W., Bindler, R. C., Cowen, K., & Shaw, M. (2017). *Principles of pediatric nursing: Caring for children* (7th ed.). Hoboken, NJ: Pearson Education.
3. Huether, S. E., McCance, K. L., Brashers, V. L., & Rote, N. S. (2017). *Understanding pathophysiology* (6th ed.). St. Louis, MO: Elsevier.
4. LeMone, P., Burke, K. M., Bauldoff, G., & Gubrud, P. (2015). *Medical surgical nursing* (6th ed.). Hoboken, NJ: Pearson Education.
5. Schubert, R. (n.d.) *Fracture healing.* Available at http://radiopaedia.org/articles/fracture-healing
6. Gerber, R. (2015). *Healing bone fractures: Your body's do-it yourself remodeling process.* Available at http://www.dignityhealth.org/cm/content/pages/healing-bone-fractures-your-bodys-do-it-yourself-remodeling-process.asp
7. Vorvick, L. J., Ma, C. B., & Zieve, D. (2012). Compartment syndrome. *PubMed Health.* Available at http://www.ncbi.nlm.nih.gov/pubmedhealth/PMH0002204
8. Medline Plus. (2014). *Compartment syndrome.* Available at https://www.nlm.nih.gov/medlineplus/ency/article/001224.htm
9. Vorvick, L. J., Ma, C. B., & Zieve, D. (2012). Volkmann's ischemic contracture. *PubMed Health.* Available at http://www.ncbi.nlm.nih.gov/pubmedhealth/PMH0002201.
10. Bulauitan, C. S. (2015). *Fat embolism: Background.* Available at http://emedicine.medscape.com/article/460524-overview
11. National Institute of Arthritis and Musculoskeletal and Skin Diseases. (2016). *Bursitis and tendonitis.* Available at https://www.niams.nih.gov/Health_Info/Bursitis/default.asp
12. Health Research Funding. (2014). *14 Extraordinary ACL injury statistics.* Available at http://healthresearchfunding.org/acl-injury-statistics
13. Medline Plus. (2016). *Anterior cruciate ligament (ACL) injury.* Available at https://medlineplus.gov/ency/article/001074.htm
14. Healthline. (2015). *Meniscus tear of the knee.* Available at http://www.healthline.com/health/meniscus-tears#Overview1
15. UW Health Sports Medicine Clinic. (2017). *Osteochondral injuries.* Available at http://www.uwhealth.org/sports-medicine/clinic/osteochondral-injuries/10110
16. Falah, M., Nierenberg, G., Soudry, M., Hayden, M., & Volpin, G. (2010). Treatment of articular cartilage lesions of the knee. *International Orthopedics, 34*(5), 621–630. Available at https://www.ncbi.nlm.nih.gov/pmc/articles/PMC2903160
17. Medline Plus. (2016). *Rotator cuff injuries.* Available at https://medlineplus.gov/rotatorcuffinjuries.html
18. Medline Plus. (2017). *Frozen shoulder.* Available at https://medlineplus.gov/ency/article/000455.htm
19. Medline Plus. (2017). *Impingement syndrome.* Available at https://medlineplus.gov/ency/imagepages/19614.htm
20. NHS Choices. (2015). *Impingement syndrome.* Available at http://www.nhs.uk/conditions/impingement-syndrome/Pages/Impingement-syndrome.aspx
21. National Institute of Arthritis and Musculoskeletal and Skin Diseases. (2014). *What is osteonecrosis?* Available at https://www.niams.nih.gov/Health_Info/Osteonecrosis/osteonecrosis_ff.asp
22. Cedars Sinai. (2016). *Bone tumors (benign).* Available at https://www.cedars-sinai.edu/Patients/Health-Conditions/Bone-Tumors-Benign.aspx
23. Medline Plus. (2016). *Bone tumor.* Available at https://medlineplus.gov/ency/article/001230.htm

Chapter 36

Chronic Musculoskeletal Disorders

Dawna Martich

Chapter Outline and Learning Outcomes

36.1 Chapter Overview and Case Studies

Describe the wide-ranging prevalence and etiology of chronic musculoskeletal disorders and concepts related to these disorders.

36.2 Lower Back Pain

Differentiate the causes, classification, underlying pathogenesis, and clinical manifestations of lower back pain and approaches to diagnosis and treatment of these conditions across the lifespan.

36.3 Rheumatic and Arthritic Disorders

Differentiate the causes, classification, underlying pathogenesis, and clinical manifestations of rheumatic and arthritic disorders and approaches to diagnosis and treatment of these conditions across the lifespan.

36.4 Metabolic Bone Disease

Differentiate the causes, classification, underlying pathogenesis, and clinical manifestations of metabolic bone disease and approaches to diagnosis and treatment of these conditions across the lifespan.

KEY TERMS

Adam forward bend test, 890
Cauda equina, 887
Crepitus, 891
Dextroscoliosis, 890
Discectomy, 888
Effusion, 891
Enthesitis, 894
Gout, 892
Herniated (ruptured) disc, 886
Intervertebral disc degeneration, 886
Juvenile dermatomyositis (JDM), 891
Juvenile idiopathic arthritis (JIA), 896
Kyphoscoliosis, 890
Kyphosis, 889
Laminectomy, 887
Laminotomy, 887
Levoconvex, 890
Lordosis, 889
Lower back pain, 885
Osteoarthritis (OA), 891
Osteocalcin level, 898
Osteomalacia, 897
Osteopenia, 897
Osteoporosis, 898
Paget disease, 898
Pannus, 894
Rheumatoid arthritis (RA), 893
Rotoscoliosis, 890
Sciatica, 886
Scoliometer, 890
Scoliosis, 889
Spinal fusion, 888
Spinal stenosis, 888
Spondyloarthropathies, 894

ABBREVIATIONS

CCP—cyclic citrullinated peptide
CES—cauda equina syndrome
DEXA—dual-energy x-ray absorptiometry
DMARDs—disease-modifying antirheumatic drugs
JIA—juvenile idiopathic arthritis
JDM—juvenile dermatomyositis
OA—osteoarthritis
PTH—parathyroid hormone
RA—rheumatoid arthritis
RF—rheumatoid factor

36.1 Chapter Overview and Case Studies

Chronic musculoskeletal disorders are those that persist despite treatment for an injury or that develop as a part of a pathologic condition. The number of such conditions is quite large; this chapter focuses on those that affect the most people. In some cases, a chronic musculoskeletal condition is the result of lifestyle choices, employment, or strenuous recreational activity. In other cases, an individual has a genetic predisposition to developing the disorder.

These health problems can affect the bones, muscles, and joints and may begin with an acute ailment; for example, tendinitis, bursitis, or repetitive strains or sprains may lead to the development of osteoarthritis in the joint. Regardless of the cause, chronic musculoskeletal disorders affect the person's physical, psychologic, and possibly socioeconomic status. One of the goals of *Healthy People 2020* is to prevent illness and disability related to arthritis, osteoporosis, and chronic back problems.

Concepts Related to Chronic Musculoskeletal Disorders

The concepts related to chronic musculoskeletal disorders are similar to those for acute musculoskeletal disorders and include mobility, inflammation and oxidative stress, immunity, comfort and pain, stress and coping, and sensory perception. In addition, individuals with chronic musculoskeletal disorders may have issues with mood and affect, specifically depression and/or anxiety, because of the difficulties of living with a chronic, painful condition. See **Figure 36.1** ■ for a map of concepts related to chronic musculoskeletal disorders.

Case Studies

The following cases are addressed throughout the chapter to assist in application of chapter content to clinical situations that involve individuals with chronic disorders of musculoskeletal function.

Kevin Anderson: Introduction

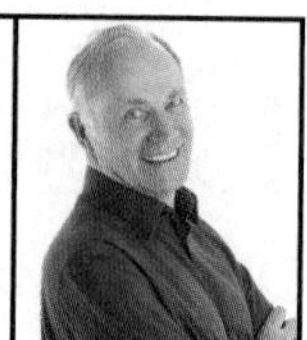

Kevin Anderson, age 56, comes to the emergency department (ED) complaining of back pain of 5 days' duration. The pain is located in the lower lumbar region. There is no radiculopathy. The patient reports having participated in a paddle ball game 1 week before his visit to the ED. The game is part of Mr. Anderson's normal activity routine. He is assessed by the ED healthcare provider. Plain x-rays are obtained that are read as normal. No laboratory studies are done. The diagnosis is lumbar strain. Mr. Anderson is given a prescription for a muscle relaxant with instructions to follow up with his family healthcare provider if the pain does not improve.

1. According to *Healthy People 2020*, what is the objective of care for individuals suffering from chronic back problems, such as Mr. Anderson?
2. What is the probable cause of Mr. Anderson's back pain?

Cecelia Bley: Introduction

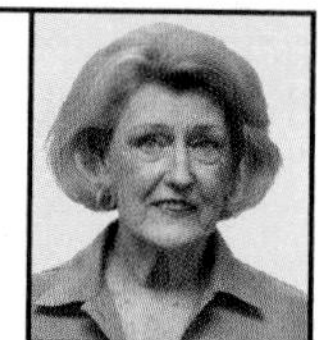

Cecelia Bley is 83 years old and has been experiencing increasing joint stiffness and pain that is more noticeable in the morning. She enjoys gardening and painting as hobbies. After a period of time and urging from her daughter, Ms. Bley sees her primary care healthcare provider because of significant joint pain after a day of gardening. The healthcare provider prescribes x-rays and laboratory

Healthy People 2020

Arthritis, Osteoporosis, and Chronic Back Conditions

Arthritis, osteoporosis, and chronic back conditions affect how a person will be able to function later in life. The pain and disability associated with each condition may prevent employment, activities of daily living and decrease the quality of life. Obesity, smoking, lack of physical activity, and poor diet play a role in these major health problems. Education related to developing healthy habits is important to changing these disease processes. The objectives are detailed below:

Arthritis

- Reduce the mean level of joint pain among adults with doctor-diagnosed arthritis
- Reduce the proportion of adults with doctor-diagnosed arthritis who experience a limitation in activity due to arthritis or joint symptoms.
- Reduce the proportion of adults with doctor-diagnosed arthritis who find it "very difficult" to perform specific joint-related activities.
- Reduce the proportion of adults with doctor-diagnosed arthritis who have difficulty in performing two or more personal care activities, thereby preserving independence.
- Reduce the proportion of adults with doctor-diagnosed arthritis who report serious psychologic distress.
- Reduce the impact of doctor-diagnosed arthritis on employment in the working-aged population.
- Increase the proportion of adults with doctor-diagnosed arthritis who receive health care provider counseling.
- Increase the proportion of adults with doctor-diagnosed arthritis who have had effective, evidence-based arthritis education as an integral part of the management of their condition.
- Increase the proportion of adults with chronic joint symptoms who have seen a health care provider for their symptoms.

Osteoporosis

- Reduce the proportion of adults with osteoporosis.
- Reduce hip fractures among older adults.

Chronic Back Conditions

- Reduce activity limitation due to chronic back conditions.

Reference

1. Healthy People 2020. (2017). *2020 topics & objectives: Arthritis, osteoporosis, and chronic back conditions*. Available at http://www.healthypeople.gov/2020/topicsobjectives2020/overview.aspx?topicId=3

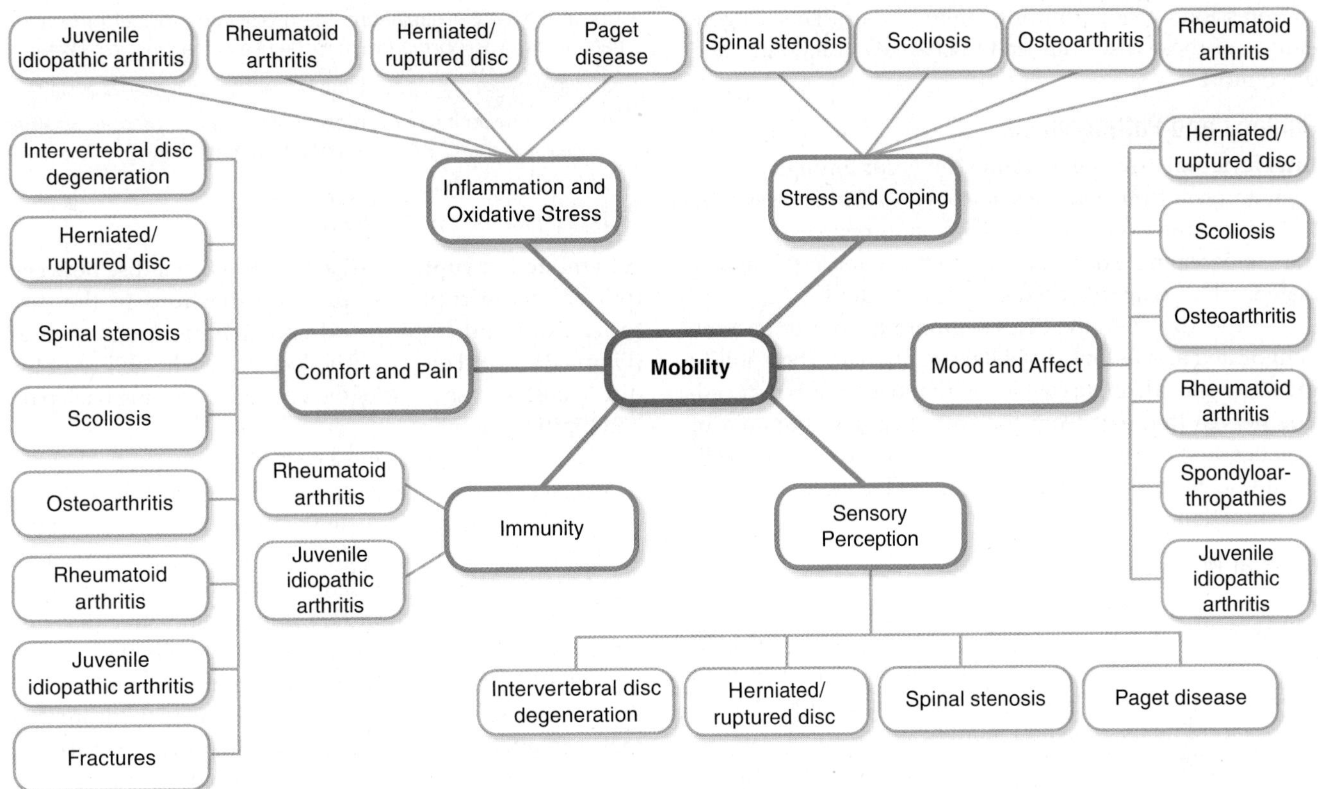

Figure 36.1 ■ Concepts related to musculoskeletal dysfunction.

work, which confirm that Ms. Bley has osteoarthritis. She is told to use over-the-counter acetaminophen, ibuprofen, and glucosamine and is advised to increase the period of rest between activities and to avoid strenuous movement of her knee and hip joints.

1. Which of Ms. Bley's symptoms are suggestive of a chronic musculoskeletal disorder?
2. How might osteoarthritis affect Ms. Bley's quality of life?

Check Your Progress: Section 36.1

1. What is a chronic musculoskeletal disorder?
2. In what way can a chronic musculoskeletal condition affect a person?
3. What are two *Healthy People 2020* goals for osteoporosis?

36.2 Lower Back Pain

Lower back pain is a common occurrence for most people; approximately 80% of adults experience this disorder at some time during their life.[1] Back pain is one of the most common medical problems in the United States. Approximately one in four adults suffers at least 1 day of back pain within a 3-month period.[2] Back problems are associated with decreased quality of life, including decreased mobility, increased pain and frustration, and loss of work hours. Although patients usually attribute back pain to a specific injury, back problems often result from years of improper bending, lifting, and standing, with one incident triggering an acute event.

Back problems are linked to certain lifestyle habits, including bad posture, low fitness level, smoking, athletic injuries, and occupational risk factors. Even children are susceptible to back pain as a result of carrying heavy backpacks. Diseases that contribute to back problems include degenerative disorders (e.g., spondylosis, spinal stenosis, osteoporosis), systemic disorders (e.g., osteomyelitis, osteoporosis, neoplasms), referred pain (e.g., gastrointestinal or genitourinary disorders, abdominal aortic aneurysms, hip pathology), and other disorders such as fibromyalgia and post–Lyme disease syndrome. Pregnancy is also a major cause of back pain, resulting from changes in posture to compensate for increasing anterior weight.

Overview of Lower Back Pain

Long-term back problems are often associated with chronic back pain. While patients may describe other problems, such as stiffness and a feeling of weakness in the back, back pain is most often the precipitating factor that leads the patient to seek treatment.

Disease processes that cause chronic back problems include sprains, strains, degenerative disorders such as spinal stenosis, and spinal deformities. Each of these areas is discussed in this chapter, and treatment options are outlined.

Intervertebral Disc Degeneration

Intervertebral discs are pads of fibrocartilage that are located between the spinal vertebrae. These discs help to prevent compression of the spinal cord and resist spinal compression while permitting limited movements. Degeneration of these discs can lead to changes in mobility and discomfort.

Etiology and Pathogenesis

Intervertebral disc degeneration can occur through normal wear and tear from activities or from an arthritic condition. It is more common in older people and primarily affects the lumbar spine. There is evidence that intervertebral disc degeneration is an inherited genetic disorder.[3]

In this disorder, the discs begin to dry out or become dehydrated and to look like a flat tire on a car. Their ability to serve as an adequate cushion with movement is reduced. The nerves that exit from the spinal cord at the area of degeneration can become compressed and swell. The swelling and compression create pain and alter motor and sensory function.

Clinical Manifestations

The most common manifestation of intervertebral disc degeneration is pain in the back that may spread to the buttocks and upper thighs. Additionally, the patient may experience numbness and tingling in the leg or foot. Sitting may exacerbate the pain and numbness.

Linking Pathophysiology to Diagnosis and Treatment

Diagnosis of intervertebral disc degeneration begins with a physical examination to assess for the location on the spine that is affected. This examination includes current motor function, muscle strength, sensory status, reflexes, and location of the pain. Tests used to diagnose this health problem include spinal x-rays and magnetic resonance imaging (MRI). X-rays are used to determine the amount of space between the discs and the integrity of the vertebral bones. An MRI shows the impact of the disc degeneration on the nerves and ligaments.

Treatment for intervertebral disc degeneration usually begins with medications such as aspirin and nonsteroidal anti-inflammatory drugs (NSAIDs) and periods of rest. These rest periods should be limited to a few hours a day, since prolonged rest weakens the back muscles. Physical therapy may be prescribed to help the patient with exercises to strengthen the core muscles and prevent back strain. A back brace may be suggested along with heat or ice, massage, ultrasound, and electrical stimulation. If the pain persists, the patient may be prescribed a narcotic analgesic. Other medications that may be used to help reduce the pain of intervertebral disc degeneration include muscle relaxants and antidepressants. If these approaches fail to bring pain relief, a nerve block with steroid injections may be considered.

Kevin Anderson: Application

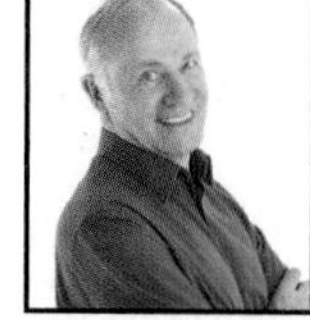

One week after his visit to the emergency department, Mr. Anderson goes to see his family healthcare provider because of ongoing and increasing back pain. The healthcare provider reviews a copy of the emergency department report and completes another assessment. No laboratory studies are performed. The diagnosis at this time is continued lumbar strain, and the healthcare provider prescribes a narcotic medication in addition to the use of the muscle relaxant.

3. How might back pain affect Mr. Anderson's quality of life?
4. How should the nurse respond if Mr. Anderson asks whether physical therapy might help with his back strain?

Herniated or Ruptured Disc

A **herniated or ruptured disc** occurs when a disc between two vertebrae ruptures, allowing the fluid in the disc to leak out and impinge on and irritate nearby nerves (**Figure 36.2** ■). This causes a decrease in the ability of the disc to cushion the joints of the vertebrae, causing back pain and limiting mobility.

Herniated discs are most common between the ages of 30 and 50 years, because discs naturally degenerate with age. Other risk factors for herniated discs include excess weight; regular heavy lifting, bending, and twisting; previous back problems; and smoking.[2] Genetic factors such as male gender, tall height, bone disorders, and degenerative disc disorders also contribute to increased risk of herniated discs.

A herniated disc in the lumbar region may cause a condition called **sciatica.** Pressure on one or more of the lumbar roots can affect the sciatic nerve, leading to pain, burning, tingling, and numbness that radiates from the buttock into the leg and foot. Usually sciatica affects only one side of the body, and it may be more severe when the person is standing, walking, or sitting.

Etiology and Pathogenesis

Loss of fluid within the disc shrinks the disc, increases the risk of microscopic tears, decreases the disc's ability to absorb shock, and increases the risk of herniation. Because of the structure of the vertebral column and the pressure of body weight on the spine, herniation occurs most frequently at C5–C6, C6–C7, L4–L5, and L5–S1. Herniation of a thoracic disc is a medical emergency that can result in paralysis. Herniation may occur gradually because of degenerative changes such as osteoarthritis or ankylosing spondylitis, or it may occur abruptly as a result of trauma such as lifting a heavy object or a being in a motor vehicle crash.

Intervertebral discs lie between adjacent bones of the vertebral column. The outer layer is composed of strong fibrocartilage; the inner layer contains loose fibers in a mucoprotein gel. These discs provide cushioning, shock absorption, and support for the vertebrae during movement. Herniation occurs when the inner layer seeps through a compromised outer layer.

Clinical Manifestations

Abrupt herniation is associated with nerve root compression, severe pain, and muscle spasms. Gradual herniation usually results in a slow onset of pain and may be associated with neurologic symptoms such as weakness or tingling. If herniation occurs centrally rather than posterolaterally, it can put pressure on the spinal cord.

Clinical manifestations of a herniated disc will depend on the severity and location of the herniation. If the herniated disc is not compressing a nerve, the patient may be

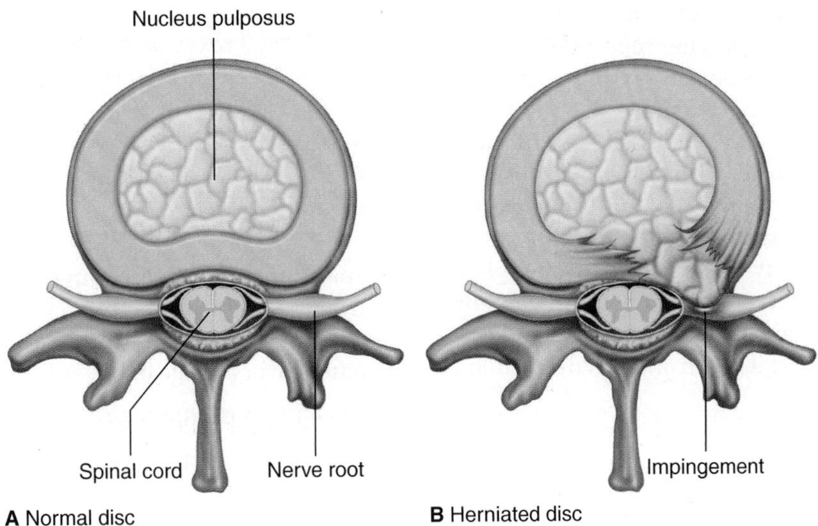

Figure 36.2 ■ **A.** Normal intervertebral disc. **B.** Herniated intervertebral disc. The herniated nucleus pulposus impinges on the nerve root causing irritation.

asymptomatic. If nerve compression is present, clinical manifestations may include pain in the lower back, buttocks, thigh, and leg; numbness or tingling; and muscle weakness. If a disc leaks, it may irritate the nerves and cause pain. The location of the symptoms depends on the area innervated by the compressed nerve.[4,5] Sciatica may also be aggravated by sneezing or coughing.

Other symptoms associated with lumbar disc herniation include a forward tilt to the trunk when standing and changes in mobility, motor function, and knee and ankle reflexes. Spinal changes may include lumbar lordosis or scoliosis of the lumbar spine. Some patients may experience muscle spasms and problems with sexual function.

The spinal cord does not extend through the entire spinal canal; rather, at approximately L1–L2, it branches into a bundle of free-flowing nerve roots. This portion of the spinal cord is called the **cauda equina**, which means "horse's tail" in Latin, describing its appearance. Compression of the nerve roots of the cauda equina can lead to cauda equina syndrome (CES), which may result in permanent neurologic impairment, including urinary incontinence and paralysis. Causes of CES include massive lumbar disc herniation, spinal stenosis, epidural hematoma, epidural abscess, and trauma.[6] CES is a medical emergency.[7] Immediate surgery should be performed to relieve pressure on the nerves.

Herniation of the cervical discs can result in numbness, tingling, muscle spasms, and weakness in the areas serviced by the affected nerves. A stiff neck is also a common feature of cervical disc herniation. In addition, neck and shoulder pain that shoots into the arm or fingers is likely present. The location and intensity of pain may depend on the movement of the neck and area of herniation.[8] If a cervical disc compresses the spinal cord instead of a nerve root, symptoms in the lower body may be similar to those seen with lumbar disc herniation.

Linking Pathophysiology to Diagnosis and Treatment

A health history and physical examination is completed first when diagnosing a herniated disc. Mobility test such as straight-leg raises, gait, reflexes, and muscle strength are performed at this time. Diagnostic tests include a computed tomography (CT) scan, MRI, or myelography in addition to nerve conduction studies and blood tests to measure for the presence of inflammation, infection, or arthritis.[9]

Treatment of a herniated disc begins with NSAIDs to reduce pain and swelling. If the patient is experiencing neurologic problems such as numbness or sciatica, additional medications may include opioids for severe pain and antispasmodics to reduce muscle spasms. Medications used to treat neuropathic pain, such as gabapentin (Neurontin), pregabalin (Lyrica), and duloxetine (Cymbalta), may also be useful for reducing pain related to nerve damage and have milder side effects than those of opioids. Tramadol (Ultram), which is a centrally acting opiate receptor agonist, may be used to treat moderate to severe pain. Epidural injection of cortisone or corticosteroids or anesthetics may also help to reduce pain and inflammation.[9] If severe pain and neurologic symptoms are still present after 1–2 months, surgery may be considered. Nonpharmacologic treatment options for individuals with herniated discs include hot or cold packs and mild, low-impact exercise to help strengthen the back.

Surgical treatment of a herniated disc is reserved for the most severe cases, in which patients do not respond to other therapies. Other indications for spinal surgery include progressive leg weakness or numbness, loss of normal bowel and bladder functions, difficulty standing or walking, and back and leg pain that limits normal activity.[8] The type of surgery that is chosen depends on the location of the disc and the integrity of the spinal column. The possible surgical treatments of a herniated disc include the following:

- A **laminectomy** is performed to remove the lamina, or the part of the vertebra that covers the spinal canal. This enlarges the spinal canal and relieves pressure on the associated nerves. During a **laminotomy**, which is a similar procedure, only a portion of the lamina is removed. A laminectomy or laminotomy is often performed in conjunction with other procedures, such as a discectomy or spinal fusion.

- A **discectomy** is performed to remove all or part of the herniated disc. Muscles and other tissues are dissected away from the spine to allow for surgical exposure of the ruptured disc. After removal of the disc, surrounding structures are returned to their natural positions. A microdiscectomy may be performed if there is no need for surgical intervention on bones, ligaments, or muscles. Compared to a discectomy, microdiscectomy requires a smaller incision and less disruption of tissues.
- **Spinal fusion** is performed to join two or more vertebrae together using bone grafts, screws, and rods. This prevents motion between the two vertebrae and reduces pain. Bone grafts are usually taken from the hip or pelvis. Tissue rejection may occur if donor bone is used. After spinal fusion, the fused area is immobile. Spinal fusion can be performed on the anterior spine by an incision in the patient's abdomen or on the posterior side by an incision in the patient's back.
- During artificial disc surgery, a herniated disc is replaced with an artificial disc, similar to a traditional hip or knee replacement. This may be done as an alternative to spinal fusion to maintain flexibility of the spinal joint.
- Newer technology has allowed the use of laser surgery to treat herniated discs. During laser surgery, the surgeon inserts a needle into the disc and delivers laser energy to vaporize the tissue in the disc. This reduces the size of the disc and relieves pressure on the nerves.

Herniated discs are rare in children, although they have become more common and are often caused by trauma. Children with herniated discs do not necessarily experience back pain. Symptoms may include sciatica, numbness, tingling, or weakness in one or both legs. Treatment begins with physical therapy. If that is not effective, a discectomy may be necessary. Children often recover from this surgery better than adults, returning to school and activities quickly.[10] ■

Nearly half of women report back pain during pregnancy. Approximately 70% of the women with back pain during pregnancy reported that the pain was severe, and about 9% reported complete disability related to the pain. A herniated disc is rare, however, occurring in about 1 in 10,000 pregnancies.[11] Most often, the symptoms resolve after delivery. ■

Kevin Anderson: Outcome

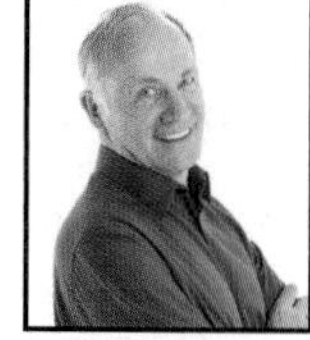

A few days after the office visit to his healthcare provider, Mr. Anderson is awakened from sleep by severe pain down his right leg. His foot is tingling and occasionally becomes numb when he gets up and walks around. Mr. Anderson's healthcare provider orders an MRI, which shows a herniated disc at level L1–L2. Mr. Anderson is prescribed physical therapy, which is to include heat application and mild lower back exercises. His medication is changed to tramadol (Ultram). After 3 weeks of therapy and medication, Mr. Anderson's symptoms subside, and he is able sit at work without back or leg pain and numbness.

5. What manifestations of sciatica does Mr. Anderson display?
6. Why was tramadol (Ultram) prescribed?

Spinal Stenosis

Spinal stenosis is a narrowing of the spinal column. This narrowing places pressure on the spinal cord, leading to symptoms similar to nerve compression. It is most common in adults over the age of 50.

Etiology and Pathogenesis

Spinal stenosis most often occurs from vertebral bone degeneration that occurs with aging. With aging, the ligaments of the spine thicken and calcify leading to the development of bone spurs on the vertebrae. Although it is seen in both men and women over the age of 50, it can occur in younger people who have sustained a spinal injury or who have congenital narrowing of the spinal canal.[12]

Clinical Manifestations

Some people have spinal stenosis and experience no symptoms. For others, narrowing of the spinal canal causes slow progressive manifestations such as numbness, weakness, cramping, or general pain that corresponds with the affected spinal segment. If the narrowed area places pressure on a nerve root, pain may radiate down an arm or a leg. Flexing the lower back helps to relieve the symptoms by enlarging the spinal spaces. Individuals who have more severe stenosis can experience bowel and bladder dysfunction and loss of motor and sensory control of the foot.[12]

Linking Pathophysiology to Diagnosis and Treatment

Diagnosis of spinal stenosis begins with a medical history and physical examination to determine the degree of mobility and sensory changes and presence of pain. Testing for this health problem includes spinal x-rays, an MRI, and a CT scan. Myelography may be performed to identify the spinal cord areas being compressed by the narrowed canal.

Treatment of spinal stenosis begins with NSAIDs and may progress to steroid injections or nerve blocks. Physical therapy will be prescribed to maintain normal spine function and motion and to strengthen the core abdominal and back muscles. For some patients, swimming or bicycling is prescribed. A lumbar brace may be suggested for patients with weakened abdominal muscles or for older patients in whom several areas of the spinal canal are affected with the disorder. Alternative therapies for spinal stenosis include chiropractic treatments and acupuncture.

Surgery may be indicated for individuals with severe narrowing and progressively worsening symptoms. Types of procedures used for spinal stenosis include decompressive laminectomy or spinal fusion. The patient may experience a period of relief; however, the degenerative process may continue, causing ongoing pain or mobility and sensory changes to continue after surgery.[12]

Skeletal Irregularities

There are three major types of skeletal irregularities: lordosis, kyphosis, and scoliosis (**Figure 36.3** ■). In **lordosis,** the spinal column is more concave; it is seen frequently in individuals who are pregnant or obese. Lordosis in pregnancy resolves after delivery. Lordosis caused by obesity improves with weight loss. In either case, lordosis is not treated. **Kyphosis,** which is common in older adults, is characterized by a spinal column that is convex.

Lordosis in pregnancy is caused by a change in the pelvic muscles and ligaments in response to the growth of the fetus. After delivery, these muscles and ligaments return to their normal anatomic position, and the appearance of lordosis resolves. ■

Kyphosis is a deformity that changes the shape of the vertebrae in the upper back. It is more common in older adults because they are prone to health problems such as osteoporosis, disc degeneration, and cancer of the spine and they may be more likely to have had cancer treatments such as radiation and chemotherapy. There is no treatment for kyphosis, but surgery might be needed if disc herniation or spinal cord compression occurs. ■

Scoliosis is a lateral, or sideways, curve of the spine; it can be C shaped or S shaped. It is often diagnosed during the growth spurt just before puberty. Most cases of scoliosis are mild, but severe scoliosis can cause a rotation of the spine, leading to deformities and disability.

Scoliosis

Etiology and Pathogenesis

Adolescents are at greatest risk of developing scoliosis as they go through a growth spurt just before puberty, usually between the ages of 9 and 15. Girls are more likely to progress to a greater curvature than boys are.[13] ■

Other risk factors for developing scoliosis include having a neuromuscular disorder such as cerebral palsy or muscular dystrophy and having a family history of scoliosis; about 30% of individuals with scoliosis are found to have a family history of the disorder.[14]

Most causes for scoliosis are unknown (idiopathic). It is most often diagnosed between the age of 10 years and the time of growth completion.[14] Congenital scoliosis occurs when the individual is born with a curved spine. This usually results from incomplete formation or separation of the vertebrae, and it can be associated with other health issues such as heart and kidney problems. Neuromuscular scoliosis occurs when a medical condition that affects the nerves and muscles, such as cerebral palsy, muscular dystrophy, or spinal cord injury, leads to sideways curvature of the spine.

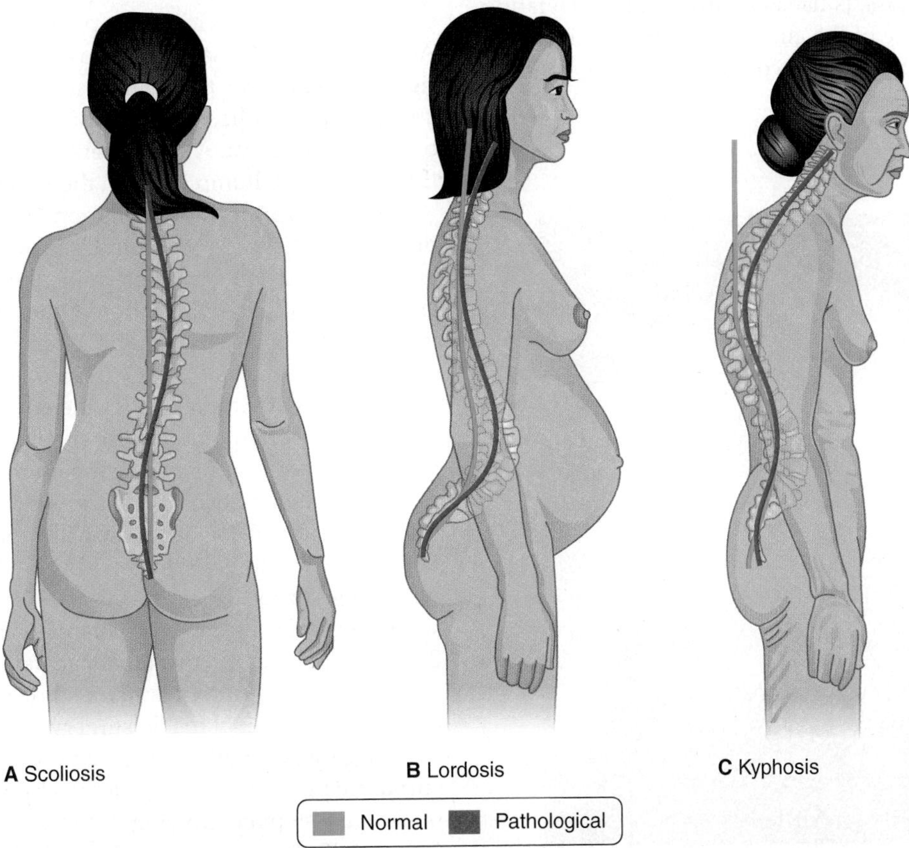

Figure 36.3 ■ Skeletal irregularities include **A.** scoliosis, which occurs mostly during adolescence. **B.** Lordosis, which occurs mostly in pregnant women and obese individuals. **C.** Kyphosis, which occurs mostly in older adults. All three conditions occur in men as well as women. Normal curves are shown in blue; pathologic curves are shown in red.

The most common curve pattern is a right thoracic curve, or **dextroscoliosis**. Other curve patterns include **kyphoscoliosis**, or a combination of outward and lateral spine curvature; **rotoscoliosis**, or curvature of the vertebral column turned on its axis; and **levoconvex**, or curvature of the spine to the left and thoracolumbar scoliosis, or a curvature related to both the thoracic and lumbar regions of the spine.[15] The lateral curvature of the spine causes several structural changes to the skeleton. As the curve worsens, the vertebrae rotate, causing a twisting of the spine. The ribs on the inside of the curve are forced closer together, and the ribs on the outside of the curve are spread farther apart. This causes formation of the typical rib hump. Similarly, the spinal disc spaces are narrowed on the inside curve and wider on the outside of the curve. This creates an asymmetric vertebral canal that may cause additional complications such as paresthesia.

A small degree of sideways curvature is found in many individuals (**Figure 36.4** ■). Scoliosis is diagnosed if the sideways curvature measures more than 10 degrees.[16] Mild scoliosis reflects a curve between 10 and 20 degrees, moderate scoliosis is a curve between 20 and 40 degrees, and severe scoliosis is a curve over 40 degrees. Scoliosis can be classified as either structural or nonstructural. Nonstructural scoliosis occurs as the spine bends to compensate for poor posture, differences in leg length, presence of tumors, adaptation to pain, or other physical conditions. Nonstructural scoliosis is usually corrected by alleviating the underlying cause of the curve. Structural scoliosis is a more severe form that involves deformities of the bones in the spinal column.

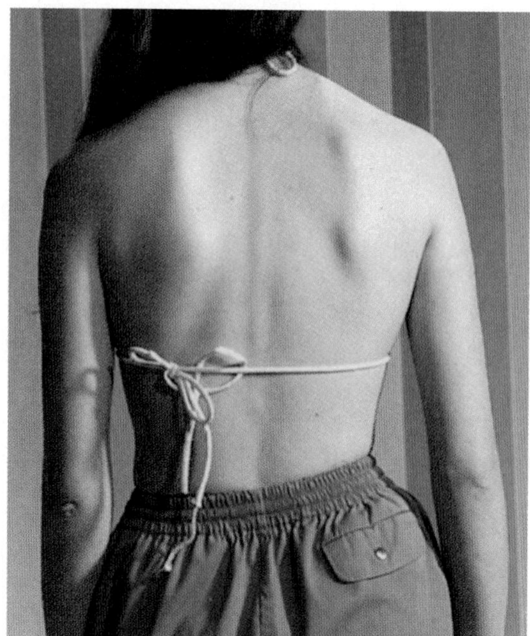

Figure 36.4 ■ A child may have varying degrees of scoliosis. Clothes that fit at an angle, such as this girl's shorts, and anatomic asymmetry of the back indicate spinal irregularities.

Clinical Manifestations

Common manifestations of scoliosis include a spinal curvature to one side, uneven hips or shoulders, differences in leg length, tiredness of the spine, a prominent shoulder blade, and a rib bump. Although not common, back pain may accompany scoliosis. Severe scoliosis may cause heart and lung problems such as difficulty breathing and pneumonia; compression of nerve roots may cause paralysis. Curvature of more than 100 degrees may increase mortality rates.

Mild curves of scoliosis (less than 20 degrees) often do not progress and do not need treatment. Moderate and severe curves (20 degrees to over 100 degrees) require treatment, especially if the curve continues to progress. Curves usually progress only 0.5–1 degree per year or less in adults.

Scoliosis curves often worsen as the child grows; progression of curvature dramatically slows when the child stops growing. For girls, this is usually 2 years after the start of menstruation. For boys, growth usually stops in the late teens or early 20s. ■

Linking Pathophysiology to Diagnosis and Treatment

Most schools require scoliosis screenings for children between the ages of 10 and 15 years. One of the primary screening tests for scoliosis is the **Adam forward bend test**, in which the individual leans forward at the waist with the arms hanging straight down. This allows the clinician to see the spine more clearly. In patients with scoliosis, the Adam test often causes an obvious rib hump, usually on the right side. However, the Adam test may be negative in some patients with scoliosis, so it should never be used as the only diagnostic test. A **scoliometer** can be used to measure the patient's rib hump when in the Adam position.

X-rays are the most common imaging test used to definitively diagnose scoliosis. Using an x-ray of the spine, healthcare providers can determine the angle of the curve and degree of vertical rotation. Other imaging tests may include MRIs, CT scans, and bone scans.

Usually, scoliosis is not treated with medication. If needed, patients can take over-the-counter (OTC) analgesics, such as acetaminophen, for mild pain. Pain associated with severe scoliosis or spinal surgery may require stronger pain medications, such as prescription NSAIDs or opioids.

Nonpharmacologic therapy will depend on the angle of the spinal curvature viewed on frontal plane x-ray. Patients with angles of 15–25 degrees may be treated conservatively with physical therapy. For patients with angles between 20 and 40 degrees, medical management includes wearing a brace. Patients with great than 40-degree angles may be considered for spinal fusion surgery.

Surgery is usually performed only on patients whose curvature progression is not slowed by bracing and whose bones have stopped growing. If curve progression is severe (at least 45 degrees) before the child has stopped growing, surgeons may insert a rod that can be adjusted in length as the child grows; adjustments usually occur every 6 months.[13] Scoliosis surgery involves spinal fusion combined with inserting metal rods on either side of the spine, which are held together by hooks, screws, and wires until the bone heals. Surgery can correct the lateral curvature of the spine, but it often does not correct the abnormal rotation of the spine. After surgery, most patients will not require long-term therapy or postoperative casting but will be fitted for a brace and will need to limit activities for 6–8 months. Because spinal surgery involves fusion of the spine, the patient will need to learn to perform simple tasks without bending or twisting the torso.

Although most types of scoliosis are diagnosed in childhood and adolescence, myopathic deformity and secondary scoliosis may develop in adulthood. Treatment of scoliosis in adults begins with conservative measures similar to those used for adolescents: physical therapy, exercise, and braces. Surgery is considered as a last resort. As patients with idiopathic adult scoliosis age, they are more likely to experience chronic or acute back pain than are patients without idiopathic adult scoliosis.[17] ■

Check Your Progress: Section 36.2

1. What is the function of intervertebral discs?
2. Distinguish between the clinical manifestations of abrupt herniation and those of gradual herniation.
3. What is the role of physical therapy in spinal stenosis?

36.3 Rheumatic and Arthritic Disorders

There are more than 100 rheumatic diseases, including degenerative conditions such as osteoarthritis and inflammatory conditions such as rheumatoid arthritis. Rheumatic diseases are caused by an immune system dysfunction. Degenerative conditions, such as osteoarthritis, are caused by body wear and tear. Some rare rheumatic and arthritic conditions include polymyositis, an inflammatory disease of the muscle, and **juvenile dermatomyositis (JDM)**, an inflammatory disease that causes muscle weakness and a skin rash on the eyelids and knuckles that affects an estimated 3,000–5,000 children between the ages of 5 and 10 years in the United States.[18] This section focuses on osteoarthritis, rheumatoid arthritis, spondyloarthropathies, and juvenile idiopathic arthritis.

Osteoarthritis

Osteoarthritis (OA) is the most common form of arthritis, affecting 50% of the world's population ages 65 years and older.[19] OA develops as wear and tear on the joints breaks down the cartilage in the joint, causing bone to rub on bone. It is the most common cause of disability in older adults and can affect any joint in the body, especially the hands, knees, and hips.

The greatest risk factor for OA is older age. OA rarely occurs in individuals under the age of 40, but at least 80% of individuals over age 55 have some x-ray evidence of the disorder. ■

Sixty percent of individuals with arthritis are women.[20] Men usually develop OA in the hip, knees, and spine; women usually develop OA in the hip, knees, and hands. Jobs that require hard labor, heavy lifting, bending, or repetitive motion are linked to increased rates of OA. Obesity also increases the risk of developing OA because the added weight increases stress on weight-bearing joints, causing the joints to wear down more quickly.

Certain medical conditions may increase an individual's risk of developing OA. For example, individuals born with malformed joints (bow legs, unequal leg length) or defective cartilage have an increased risk of developing OA. In addition, diseases such as diabetes, hypothyroidism, gout, and Paget disease increase the risk of developing OA. Joint injuries from sports, accidents, or repetitive use also increase the risk of OA.[20]

Etiology and Pathogenesis

Osteoarthritis can be classified as either idiopathic or secondary. Idiopathic OA has no identifiable cause, but most researchers believe that it is caused by both mechanical and molecular factors. Idiopathic OA can be further divided into localized or generalized. Localized OA affects one or two joints; generalized OA affects three or more joints. Secondary OA is caused by an underlying condition, such as injury; congenital malformation; metabolic, endocrine, or neuropathic disease; or other medical cause.

In healthy joints, the slick surface of articular cartilage covers the ends of bones, allowing the bones to glide over each other without friction during movement of the joint. Cartilage also absorbs shock from physical movement. As an individual ages, the cartilage begins to break down, becoming rough and eventually wearing away, allowing the bones to rub against each other. Bone spurs (particles that break off the joint irritate the synovial tissue) cause the pain, stiffness, inflammation, and swelling that are characteristic of OA (**Figure 36.5** ■).

As OA progresses, slowly developing changes occur to the joint's synovium, subchondral bone, and cartilage. As changes to the joint occur, the joint no longer moves smoothly, causing mobility problems. OA typically involves the weight-bearing joints of the hips and knees, the digits of the hands and big toe, and the cervical and lumbar spine.

Clinical Manifestations

Osteoarthritis begins with mild symptoms and progressively worsens over time. Symptoms of OA vary depending on the joint affected and individual factors. Some patients with visible joint degeneration on x-ray have no associated symptoms in the affected joint. However, many patients with OA develop pain associated with joint degeneration; this pain is usually worsened by activity and relieved by rest. Pain and stiffness are also associated with prolonged inactivity, such as sleeping at night or taking a long car ride. Other symptoms include tenderness to the touch, swelling related to excess fluid in the joint (**effusion**), crackling or grating of the joint (**crepitus**) due to rough surfaces rubbing against each other, and bone spurs that contribute to joint

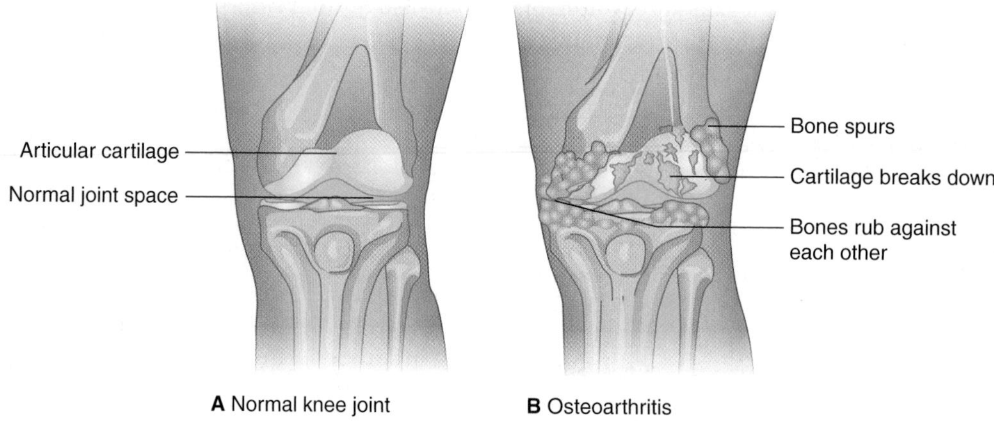

Figure 36.5 ■ **A.** Normal knee joint. **B.** Joint degeneration with OA.

swelling (**Figure 36.6** ■). This joint damage typically causes the joint to have a decreased range of motion.

Treatment aims to reduce pain, improve function of the affected joint, and slow disease progression. Osteoarthritis can lead to a host of complications as the severity of the condition worsens. Joint pain and degeneration, stiffness, an unsteady gait, and effects of medications all increase the risk of falling, which may cause fractures and additional mobility limitations. As physical limitations increase, the patient may experience a decreased ability to perform activities of daily living. As the individual is less able to perform work responsibilities, she may develop financial difficulties related to the cost of treatment and lost wages. As the disability persists, the individual may develop anxiety, depression, and feelings of helplessness. Both the physical disability and the associated mood disorder may lead the individual to have difficulty participating in social and family activities.

Cecelia Bley: Application

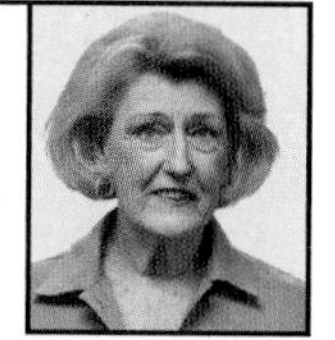

Ms. Bley has been resting between activities and has limited the amount of time she spends working in her garden because of the strenuous movement required of the knees and hips. After attending a grandchild's soccer game on a chilly day, Ms. Bley experiences prolonged knee, hip, and hand pain. Unfortunately, OTC ibuprofen and glucosamine have not helped with pain management, and Ms. Bley schedules another appointment with her healthcare provider.

3. What is Ms. Bley's greatest risk factor for osteoarthritis?
4. Do Ms. Bley's symptoms appear to be following the typical course of osteoarthritis?

Linking Pathophysiology to Diagnosis and Treatment

In addition to a medical history and physical examination, several tests can be used to help diagnose OA and track the disease's course. The most commonly used diagnostic test is an x-ray of the affected joint, but other tests may include an MRI, ultrasound, blood tests, and joint fluid analysis. An x-ray can reveal a narrowing of the space between bones in the joint, indicating a lack of cartilage. However, x-rays may not show signs of OA until significant cartilage loss has occurred. An x-ray may also show bone spurs or other bone damage. MRI and ultrasound produce more detailed images of the bone and soft tissues, including cartilage, ligaments, and tendons. This is a more sensitive way to determine the extent of joint damage.

Although no blood test is available that can conclusively identify OA, blood tests can help to rule out other causes of joint pain, such as rheumatoid arthritis. Joint fluid analysis is used to detect inflammation and the presence of bacteria (infection) or uric acid crystals (**gout**).

Management of OA begins with medications and nonpharmacologic approaches. Many OTC medications are effective for treatment of mild to moderate osteoarthritis pain. Acetaminophen (Tylenol) is usually suggested as a first-line therapy because most patients tolerate it well. However, acetaminophen can produce liver toxicity if taken in high doses or by patients with chronic liver disease or

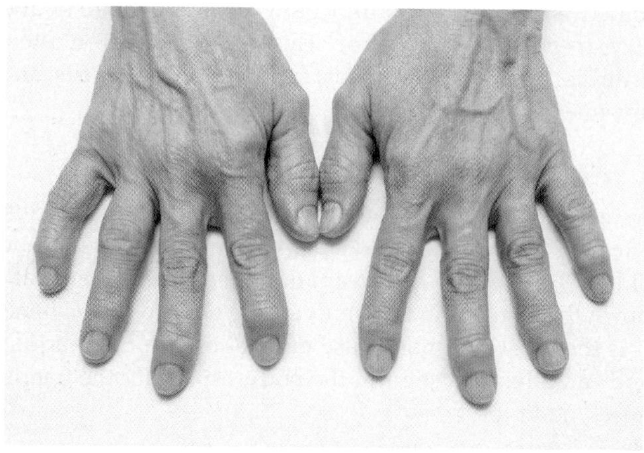

Figure 36.6 ■ Typical interphalangeal joint changes associated with OA.

excessive alcohol intake. Ibuprofen (Advil, Motrin) and naproxen (Aleve) are NSAIDs that treat both pain and inflammation. Stronger NSAIDs are available by prescription, including the COX-2 inhibitor celecoxib (Celebrex). NSAIDs are generally well tolerated, but they can produce cardiovascular and gastrointestinal effects. For patients with severe OA pain, opioid analgesics such as codeine, tramadol, or hydrocodone may be prescribed. However, opioids carry the risk of tolerance and addiction, so they should be prescribed only as a last resort.

Topical analgesic creams, rubs, and sprays may also be prescribed for patients with OA. These drugs are applied directly to the skin surrounding the joint. They work by stimulating nerve endings, depleting the neurotransmitter called substance P, or blocking prostaglandins to decrease pain signals received by the brain. Examples include capsaicin cream (Capzasin, Zostrix), diclofenac gel (Voltaren), salicylates (Aspercreme, Bengay), and menthol (Icy Hot, Biofreeze).

Cortisone injections may also be administered for treatment of OA pain. The corticosteroid medication is injected directly into the joint to reduce inflammation and pain. Because frequent use of corticosteroids can cause joint damage, cortisone injections are limited to three to four injections per year for weight-bearing joints.

One of the newest treatments for OA is hyaluronic acid injections into the affected joint. The Impact of Current Research feature compares the use of corticosteroid and hyaluronic acid injections for relief of OA.

In addition to treating pain with analgesics and injections, nonpharmacologic treatment for OA includes heat and cold application; use of assistive technology; weight reduction; rest; and education about the disease, exercise, and coping techniques.

Patients with severe arthritis that is not well managed by medication and nonpharmacologic interventions may be candidates for surgery. Depending on the joint and extent of damage, several options are available for surgery: arthroscopy, joint resurfacing, joint irrigation, osteotomy, joint fusion, and arthroplasty. The purpose of surgery is to remove damage, relieve pain, and restore function of the joint.

Cecelia Bley: Outcome

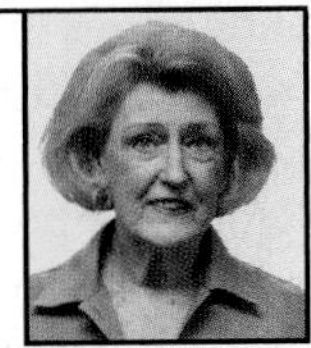

Because of Ms. Bley's progressively worsening symptoms, her healthcare provider prescribes tramadol and a topical analgesic cream. Ms. Bley is also encouraged to apply heat to painful joints and is given a referral for home care to have a home safety assessment completed. The home care nurse recommends installing grab bars in the bathroom near the shower and commode. In addition, hand rails need to be installed in all stairwells in Ms. Bley's home.

The healthcare provider suggests that Ms. Bley participate in an arthritis swimming exercise class that is conducted at the community center twice a week. Ms. Bley has another appointment with the healthcare provider in 2 months as a follow-up. She is provided with information on joint replacement surgery, but she does not want to consider that as an option at this time.

5. Why did the healthcare provider recommend a swimming class for Mrs. Bley?
6. What other treatments might be considered before surgery is considered?

Rheumatoid Arthritis

Rheumatoid arthritis (RA) is a chronic systemic autoimmune disorder (a disease caused by abnormal, overactive functioning of the immune system that produces a response against the body's own cells and tissues, normally resulting in damage to the tissues). RA causes inflammation of connective tissue, primarily in the joints.[21]

Etiology and Pathogenesis

RA is the most common form of autoimmune arthritis, affecting 1–2% of the worldwide population and all races of people. RA affects three times as many women as men, and while the typical age of onset is between 40 and 60 years, this disease strikes people of all ages.[22,23] Approximately 10% of patients diagnosed with RA experience long-term remission within 1 year. Following the onset of RA, an estimated 60% of individuals whose disease does not enter remission within approximately 10 years will be disabled to the extent of being unable to maintain employment.[24]

The cause of RA is unknown. Genetic, environmental, hormonal, and immunologic factors are thought to be involved. Infectious agents, such as bacteria, mycoplasmas,

Impact of Current Research on Clinical Practice

Hyaluronic Acid or Corticosteroid Injections for the Treatment of OA of the Knee

Description: The purpose of the study was to evaluate the therapeutic effect of intra-articular hyaluronic acid in comparison to corticosteroids for knee OA. One hundred and forty patients with knee OA being treated for 3 months were randomly assigned to receive an intra-articular injection of either hyaluronic acid or a corticosteroid. The mean age of the patients in the corticosteroid group was 57 ±1.9 years, and in that in the hyaluronic acid group was 58.5 ±8.3 years.

Clinical Practice: The hyaluronic acid injection was determined to be more effective in managing the pain of OA than the corticosteroid injections. As a result of this study, clinicians may consider administering hyaluronic acid every 3 months instead of the routine corticosteroid injection that needs to be repeated every 2 months.

Research Study:

Askari, A., Gholami, T., NaghiZadeh, M. M., Farjam, M., & Shahabfard, Z. (2016). Hyaluronic acid compared with corticosteroid injections for the treatment of osteoarthritis of the knee: A randomized control trial. *SpringerPlus, 5,* 442. doi:10.1186/s40064-016-2020-0 and viruses (especially Epstein-Barr virus), may play a role in initiating the autoimmune processes in RA. Genetic factors are believed to account for 50% of the risk of developing RA, and approximately 60% of patients in the United States with the disease have been found to carry a specific genetic marker of the human leukocyte antigen (HLA)-DR4 cluster.[25]

RA is believed to be caused by exposure to an antigen that causes an unexpected response. Instead of responding normally by creating antibodies, the body believes that normal tissue is foreign and begins to attack the tissues. The antibodies that wage this attack include rheumatoid factor (RF) and anti–cyclic citrullinated peptide antibodies.

The antibodies in RA bind with other proteins and tissues and create immune complexes that cause an inflammatory response in synovial and other musculoskeletal tissues. The body senses this inflammation and sends white blood cells to the joint tissue, which release enzymes that cause further joint tissue degradation. The combination of inflammation and immune response harms the synovial membranes. In response, these membranes become hyperactive and form new tissue called **pannus**. This tissue covers joint cartilage and produces enzymes that encourage additional tissue damage. Added to the immune complexes, the body activates osteoclasts, which cause underlying bone to demineralize.

Clinical Manifestations

Joint manifestations of RA include joint swelling, stiffness, warmth, tenderness, and pain. This involves more than one joint and is bilateral, or affecting both sides and same body joints. The joints of the fingers, wrists, knees, ankles, and toes are most frequently affected. Stiffness is more acute in the morning although it can occur with inactivity during the day or after strenuous activity. The joints feel "boggy" or spongelike when palpated. If the RA is not treated, the joints become deformed, including ulnar deviation of the fingers, Swan-neck deformity of the proximal interphalangeal joint, and a boutonniere deformity caused by extension of the distal interphalangeal joint (**Figure 36.7** ■).

Additional manifestations of RA are systemic and include fatigue, anorexia, weight loss, weakness, and a low-grade fever. Rheumatoid nodules may develop in subcutaneous tissue that is prone to pressure, such as the forearm, elbow, joints of the hands, and the toes. Other manifestations can include pleural effusion, vasculitis, pericarditis, and an enlarged spleen (**Figure 36.8** ■).

Linking Pathophysiology to Diagnosis and Treatment

Diagnostic tests are used to identify RA and to rule out other forms of arthritis and connective tissue disorders. In approximately 25–35% of patients with RA, the complete blood count reveals a mild anemia. The white blood cell (WBC) and platelet counts are usually normal; however, the inflammatory response may lead to an increase in both these components. Certain subgroups of patients may also demonstrate a decreased WBC count. More than 70% of patients with RA test positive for RF. However, a more specific marker for this condition is antibodies to cyclic citrullinated peptide (CCP). The anti-CCP test detects these antibodies and may yield positive results even years before RA symptoms emerge. Blood tests also include the erythrocyte sedimentation rate

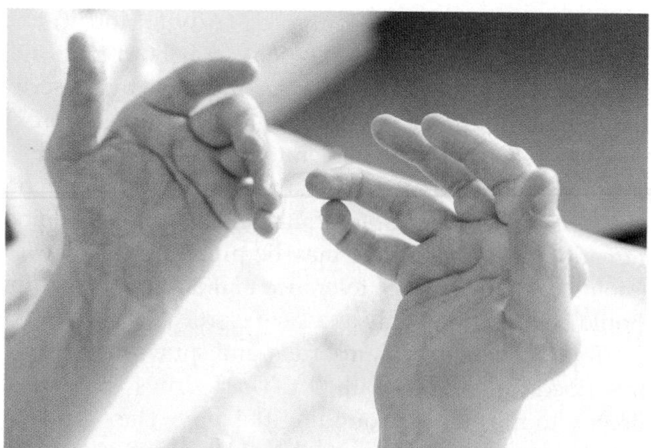

Figure 36.7 ■ Hand deformities associated with RA.

(ESR), which typically is elevated with RA, and C-reactive protein, which is a nonspecific indicator of inflammation.[26] In the earliest stages of RA, when bone damage is not yet apparent, x-rays are not of great use for diagnosis but may be used to rule out other disease processes and to monitor disease progression. Examination of the synovial fluid will demonstrate changes associated with inflammation, including increased turbidity (cloudiness), decreased viscosity, and increased protein and WBC levels.

Treatment of RA is largely through pharmacologic measures. The four general approaches used in the pharmacologic management of RA are (1) NSAIDs for reduction of inflammation and pain; (2) low-dose oral corticosteroids for reduction of inflammation and pain, as well as for slowing disease progression; (3) disease-modifying antirheumatic drugs (DMARDs) to relieve disease-related symptoms and to slow disease progression; and (4) intra-articular steroid injection administration for localized relief of pain and inflammation.

Nonpharmacologic approaches to the treatment of RA include rest and exercise, physical and occupational therapy, application of heat and cold, use of assistive devices and splints, nutritional supplementation, and complementary approaches such as acupuncture and hydrotherapy.

Spondyloarthropathies

Spondyloarthropathies are a group of diseases that affect the joints and include ankylosing spondylitis, reactive arthritis, psoriatic arthritis and enteropathic arthritis or joint problems that occur with inflammatory bowel disease. They can occur in both children and adults and usually involve the sacroiliac joint and **enthesitis**, or inflammation of the areas around the sites where the ligaments and tendons attach to the bone in the knee, foot, or hip.

Etiology and Pathogenesis

Spondyloarthropathies are linked by their association with the HLA-B27 gene and by the presence of enthesitis as the basic pathologic lesion. Ankylosing spondylitis is more likely to run in families than other forms of rheumatic disease.

The HLA-B27 gene is believed to initiate an inflammatory reaction that targets the body tendons and ligaments. Chronic inflammation leads to shortening and stiffening of these structures.

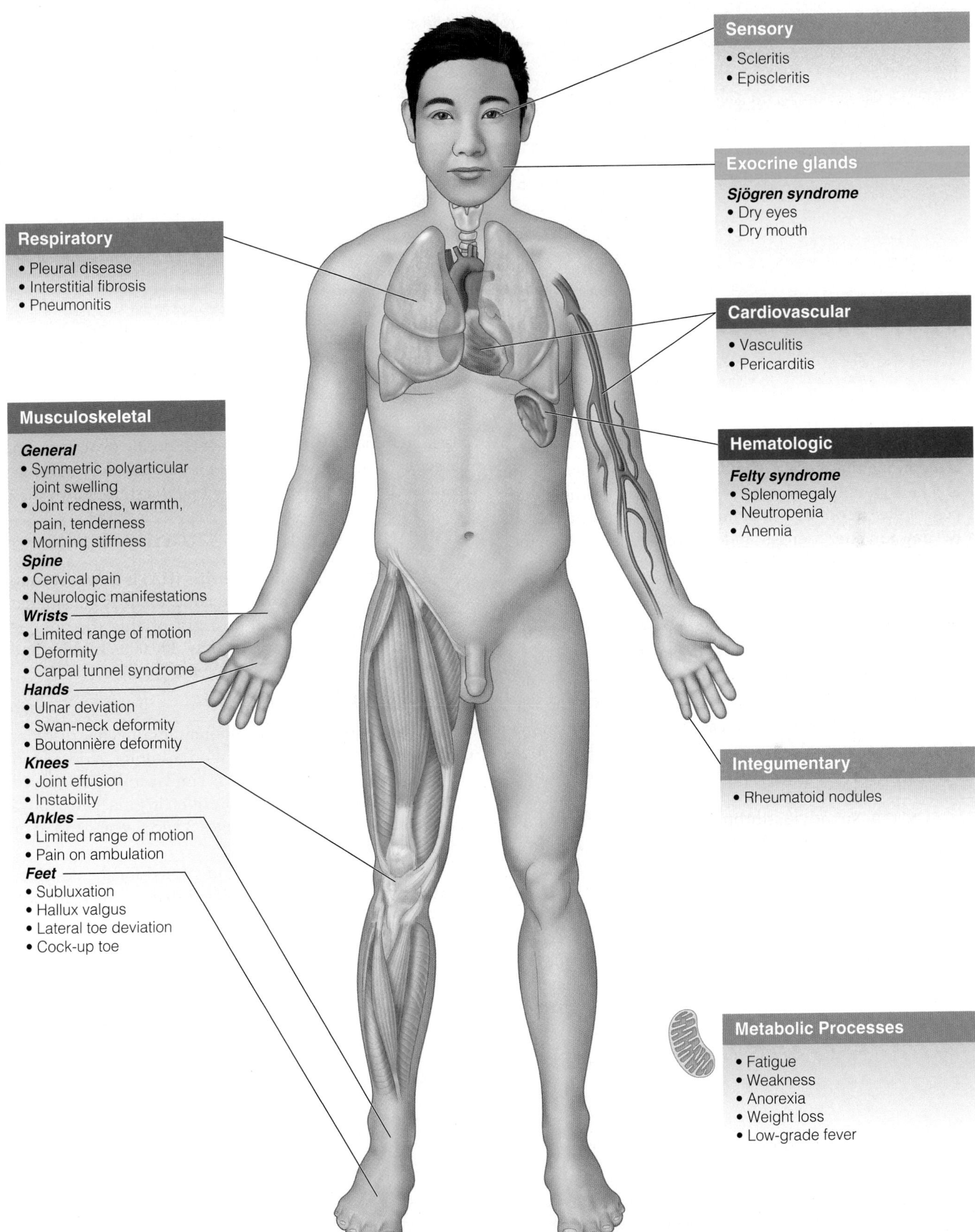
Sensory
• Scleritis
• Episcleritis
Exocrine glands
Sjögren syndrome
• Dry eyes
• Dry mouth
Respiratory
• Pleural disease
• Interstitial fibrosis
• Pneumonitis
Cardiovascular
• Vasculitis
• Pericarditis
Musculoskeletal
General
• Symmetric polyarticular joint swelling
• Joint redness, warmth, pain, tenderness
• Morning stiffness
Spine
• Cervical pain
• Neurologic manifestations
Wrists
• Limited range of motion
• Deformity
• Carpal tunnel syndrome
Hands
• Ulnar deviation
• Swan-neck deformity
• Boutonnière deformity
Knees
• Joint effusion
• Instability
Ankles
• Limited range of motion
• Pain on ambulation
Feet
• Subluxation
• Hallux valgus
• Lateral toe deviation
• Cock-up toe
Hematologic
Felty syndrome
• Splenomegaly
• Neutropenia
• Anemia
Integumentary
• Rheumatoid nodules
Metabolic Processes
• Fatigue
• Weakness
• Anorexia
• Weight loss
• Low-grade fever

Figure 36.8 ■ Multisystem effects of rheumatoid arthritis.

Table 36.1 Manifestations of Spondyloarthropathies across the Lifespan

Disease Process	Manifestations in Adults	Manifestations in Children
Ankylosing spondylitis	• Stiffness • Low back pain that moves to the upper back • Spinal joints fuse (**Figure 36.9** ■) • May affect hips, chest wall, and heels	• Symptoms begin in the hips, knees, heels, or great toe before moving to the spine
Reactive arthritis	• Pain, swelling, inflammation of the sacroiliac joint • Swelling of fingers and toes • Fever, weight loss, and skin rash	• Affects joints of the lower leg
Psoriatic arthritis	• Scaly red patches on the skin followed by symptoms of arthritis • Pitting or thickening and yellowing of the finger and toe nails • Affects hips and sacroiliac joint • Edematous toes and fingers	• Red, scaly skin that may or may not be in the joint areas • Pitted and yellowed toe and finger nails • Red and inflamed skin over the joint area • Stiffness, swelling, and pain in the joint
Enteropathic arthritis	• Arthritis symptoms occur with bowel flare • Affects knees, hips, ankles, and elbows	• Arthritis symptoms appear before intestinal inflammation

Clinical Manifestations

General manifestations of spondyloarthropathies include low back pain that may affect the buttocks, morning stiffness of the back or neck that improves during the course of the day and after exercise, and generalized fatigue.[27] Other manifestations are associated with a specific disease process as identified in **Table 36.1** ■.

Linking Pathophysiology to Diagnosis and Treatment

Diagnosis of a spondyloarthropathy begins with a history and complete physical examination. Laboratory tests that measure inflammation levels may be prescribed along with x-rays and an MRI of body areas experiencing inflammation. The symptoms of a specific type of spondyloarthropathy are used to guide whether further diagnostic testing is required before diagnosis.

Overall, spondyloarthropathies are considered mild nuisance disorders and might not be diagnosed. However, in some individuals, spinal stiffness and fusion can lead to significant issues with daily activities. The goals of treatment are to relieve pain and stiffness and to maintain posture. This is accomplished with NSAIDs and stretching exercises. Additional approaches to relieve the symptoms include heat for stiffness, ice for swelling, ultrasound, massage therapy, electrical stimulators, weight reduction, and, in extreme cases, surgery for joint replacement. Specific treatments are based on the therapy prescribed for inflammatory bowel or psoriasis that accompanies the spondyloarthropathy.

Juvenile Idiopathic Arthritis

Juvenile idiopathic arthritis (JIA) is the most common type of arthritis in children. It is considered idiopathic, since the origin of this disorder is unknown. It affects approximately 300,000 children and adolescents in the United States.[28] ■

Etiology and Pathogenesis

JIA is a chronic inflammatory autoimmune juvenile disorder characterized by joint inflammation resulting in decreased mobility, swelling, and pain. It is similar to RA diagnosed in adults. JIA occurs slightly more often in girls than in boys and typically occurs between ages 3 and 6 years and at or around puberty.

There is no specific reason identified for the development of JIA. Research has indicated that a genetic marker needs to be present before a trigger, such as a virus, starting the disease process. The manifestations of arthritis, including intra-articular swelling and synovitis, develop as part of the autoinflammatory or autoimmune process, causing the immune system to attack healthy tissue.

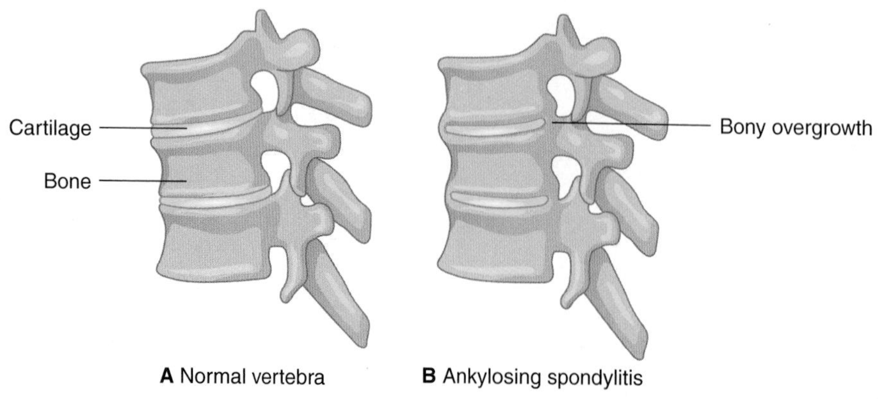

Figure 36.9 ■ **A.** Normal vertebra. **B.** Ankylosing spondylitis.

Clinical Manifestations

There are six different types of JIA, as detailed in **Table 36.2** ■.

Linking Pathophysiology to Diagnosis and Treatment

The diagnosis of JIA begins with a history and physical examination. The child may have difficulty walking or a rash, which serve as clues to the type of JIA. Additional testing will include ESR, antinuclear antibody testing, RF, and anti-CCP antibody level. Joint and bone x-rays will be done, in addition to possible CT scans, MRI, ultrasound, and nuclear studies to help identify changes. An arthrocentesis and synovial biopsy may also be performed.

Treatment of JIA is focused on reducing pain, improving mobility, and supporting developmental growth. Approaches include pharmacologic therapy with NSAIDs, DMARDs, biologic agents, or intra-articular and oral corticosteroids. Physical and occupational therapy will be prescribed. The child may need additional interventions to support nutrition, psychosocial development, and school performance. Surgical procedures that may be considered for extreme cases include joint replacement, synovectomy, osteotomy, and arthrodesis.[29]

Check Your Progress: Section 36.3

1. What is the difference between idiopathic and secondary osteoarthritis?
2. What is the role of inflammation in the development of rheumatoid arthritis?
3. What is the role of inflammation in the development of spondylarthopathies?

Table 36.2 Types of Juvenile Idiopathic Arthritis

Type	Manifestations
Systemic	Inflammation in one or more joints High fever lasting > 2 weeks Skin rash Inflammation of the heart or lungs Anemia Enlarged lymph nodes, liver or spleen
Oligoarticular	Inflammation of the knees, ankles, and elbows Associated with uveitis (chronic eye inflammation)
Polyarticular	Inflammation in five or more joints of the fingers, hands, hips, knees, and jaw Can resemble adults' rheumatoid arthritis
Psoriatic	Associated with psoriasis, which may begin years before joint symptoms Pain, swelling in one or more joints Affects wrists, knees, ankles, and toes
Enthesitis-related	Tenderness at the bone–tendon or bone–ligament junction Affects the hips, knees, and feet More common in males between the ages of 8 and 15 years Associated with the HLA-B27 gene
Undifferentiated	Involves symptoms of two or more types

36.4 Metabolic Bone Disease

Metabolic bone diseases are those that alter bone strength. These diseases occur because of insufficient or poorly metabolized calcium, phosphorus, and vitamin D. The most prevalent metabolic bone disease is osteoporosis. Osteoporosis may be confused with osteomalacia; however, the processes differ. Osteoporosis is a weakening of bone that has already been formed, whereas **osteomalacia** is a softening of the bones during the building process. Other common metabolic bone diseases that are of importance include osteopenia and Paget disease.

Osteopenia

Osteopenia is a term used to describe a decrease in bone density. This disorder can lead to fractures. Not all people with osteopenia need extensive treatment; however, actions should be taken to strengthen the bone. Although osteopenia can occur in men, women are more prone to developing osteopenia because of hormonal changes during menopause.

Etiology and Pathogenesis

As people age, bone resorption (breakdown) is greater than formation. This reduces the density of the bone and leads to bone weakness, which increases the risk of fractures. The most common reasons for the development of osteopenia are as follows:

- Chronic eating disorders or issues with metabolism that alter the intake and absorption of vitamins and minerals needed for bone growth and strength
- History of having chemotherapy or taking glucocorticoids for other health problems
- Radiation exposure
- Family history of low bone density
- Being white or of Asian descent
- Thin body structure
- Engaging in only limited physical activity, smoking, drinking cola-based beverages, and having a high intake of alcohol.

Clinical Manifestations

Osteopenia causes no clinical manifestations. The only time it may be detected is during a routine diagnostic test or at the time of a spontaneous fracture. However, pain does not always occur at the time of a fracture in a person with osteopenia. The lack of symptoms and limited pain with fractures contribute to the number of people who have the disorder that is undiagnosed.

Linking Pathophysiology to Diagnosis and Treatment

The main diagnostic test for osteopenia is the dual-energy X-ray absorptiometry (DEXA) scan. This scan is recommended for all women over the age of 65 to screen for osteoporosis. The results may indicate that the individual's bone density is low, though not at the level of osteoporosis. This scan may also be prescribed for any adult who sustains a fracture as a measure to diagnose osteopenia as a possible cause.

Osteopenia is treated by addressing the patient's risk factors. Diet therapy includes increasing the intake of calcium and vitamin D. The patient is encouraged to increase weight-bearing exercises, since bone forms in response to stress. Smoking cessation and reduction of cola-based and alcoholic beverages are other actions to slow the loss of bone. Medications are not routinely prescribed for osteopenia but are considered as options should the disease process progress and additional bone loss occurs.[30]

Osteoporosis

Osteoporosis is the most commonly diagnosed metabolic bone disorder. It is caused by low bone density that occurs because of low intake of nutrients for bone growth or an increase in bone resorption that naturally occurs with aging. Osteoporosis causes weak bones that increase the risk of fractures.

Etiology and Pathogenesis

More than 53 million people in the United States have osteoporosis or are at risk for developing it. Osteoporosis is more common in non-Hispanic white women, although it can affect older people of any race or either sex.[31]

There are two types of osteoporosis: primary and secondary. Primary osteoporosis may be either type 1, which is associated with menopause, or type 2, which is associated with decreasing bone formation that accompanies the aging process. Type 1 osteoporosis has been linked to estrogen deficiency resulting in increased calcium resorption from bone as the lack of estrogen renders the body more sensitive to parathyroid hormone (PTH). Type 2 osteoporosis typically results as the kidneys lose their ability to process vitamin D, causing decreased calcium absorption, which in turn increases sensitivity to PTH and bone resorption.[32]

Secondary osteoporosis occurs as the result of a disease process or a deficiency or as an effect of a drug. Renal hypercalciuria is one of the more common causes of secondary osteoporosis and is treated with thiazide diuretics. Many patients with primary osteoporosis also have one or more secondary factors, such as Cushing syndrome, adrenal insufficiency, calcium deficiency, or diabetes mellitus.[32] Medications that increase risk for osteoporosis include heparin, antiretroviral therapy, selective serotonin reuptake inhibitors, lithium, furosemide, glucocorticoids, and some chemotherapeutic agents.

Osteoporosis is believed to be caused by an imbalance between bone resorption and bone formation. Once peak bone mass has been reached, which occurs around the age of 30, the amount of bone resorption begins to increase. The amount of bone resorption will be heightened with a diet low in calcium and low vitamin D intake; this leads to weakening of the bone structure. Bone resorption is influenced by estrogen and testosterone levels. In women, bone resorption is accelerated after menopause. In men, the bone loss is subtler but still occurs.

Clinical Manifestations

The most common manifestations of osteoporosis are loss of height; progressive curvature of the spine; low back pain; and fractures of the forearm, spine, or hip. The patient may develop a progressive "buffalo hump" or "dowager hump" between the shoulder blades. Osteoporosis is often called a silent disease, because bone loss occurs without symptoms; the problem may not become apparent until the patient has a fracture or radiologic studies reveal the condition.

Linking Pathophysiology to Diagnosis and Treatment

The test that is used to definitively diagnosis the disorder is the DEXA scan that measures bone density in the hip or lumbar spine. Even so, osteoporosis may not be diagnosed until the patient sustains a fracture. A serum bone G1a (osteocalcin) level may be taken. The **osteocalcin level** test measures osteoclastic activity and helps to determine bone turnover. It is not used as an indication of disease severity.

Treatment of osteoporosis is focused on preventing fractures. This is achieved through nutritional support, exercise, and measures to prevent falls. In addition to calcium and vitamin D supplements, medications used to treat osteoporosis include bisphosphonates, PTH, estrogen, and calcitonin.[31]

Paget Disease

Paget disease is a metabolic disorder that causes select bones to overgrow and become weak. The bones most often affected include the skull, spine, pelvis, and femur. It can occur in more than one bone in the body, but it does not affect every bone in the body.

Etiology and Pathogenesis

Paget disease affects approximately one million people in the United States. It is most frequently diagnosed in older people of Northern European descent. The incidence of the disorder is higher in men than in women.

In this disorder, bone resorption is faster than bone formation. The body compensates by accelerating the creation of new bone; however, this new tissue is weak, brittle, and easily fractured. Paget disease is believed to be a genetic disorder initiated by an environmental factor, such a virus.

Clinical Manifestations

The vast majority of people with Paget disease are unaware of having the disorder. Others may have mild or more exaggerated symptoms that depend on the bone affected. General manifestations of Paget disease include pain, an enlarged or several enlarged bones, fractures, or damaged joint cartilage. People with disease in the femurs may have bowed legs. If the disease is present in the vertebrae, the spine may be curved. If the disorder affects the bones of the skull then headaches, hearing loss, and a large head size may be the major clinical manifestations. In general, symptoms of the disorder progress slowly, and the disease does not metastasize to other body areas.

Linking Pathophysiology to Diagnosis and Treatment

A person may be unaware of having Paget disease until a fracture occurs. At this time, the disorder may be diagnosed with x-rays and blood tests such as bone-specific alkaline phosphatase level, which is elevated in people with the disorder, and a bone scan, which is used to identify the affected bones. Depending on the bone or bones that are affected, Paget disease can contribute to the development of arthritis, deafness, heart disease, kidney stones, neuropathic pain, bone cancer, poor dentition, and vision changes.

The goals of treatment for Paget disease are to strengthen the bone, prevent fractures, and reduce the development of complications. Medications used for the disorder include bisphosphonates and calcitonin. Nutritional support includes calcium and vitamin D supplements. Exercise is recommended to maintain healthy bones, maintain a healthy weight, and prevent fractures. Surgery may be indicated to repair fractures, correct bone malformations, or replace arthritic joints.[33]

Check Your Progress: Section 36.4

1. Why are many people with osteopenia undiagnosed?
2. What is the difference between type 1 and type 2 osteoporosis?
3. Describe the pathophysiology of Paget disease.

CHAPTER SUMMARY

36.1 Chapter Overview and Case Studies

Describe the wide-ranging prevalence and etiology of chronic musculoskeletal disorders and concepts related to these disorders.

- Chronic musculoskeletal disorders persist despite treatment for an injury or develop as a part of a pathologic condition.
- These disorders can develop as a result of lifestyle choices, employment, or strenuous recreational activity. They may have a genetic link.
- These health problems can affect the bones, muscles, and joints and may begin with an acute ailment.
- Chronic musculoskeletal disorders can affect the person's physical, psychologic, and possible socioeconomic status.
- These disorders relate to the concepts of mobility, inflammation and oxidative stress, immunity, comfort/pain, stress and coping, and sensory perception.

36.2 Lower Back Pain

Differentiate the causes, classification, underlying pathogenesis, and clinical manifestations of lower back pain and approaches to diagnosis and treatment of these conditions across the lifespan.

- Back pain is one of the most common medical problems in the United States.
- Lower back pain can be caused by degenerative disc changes, a herniated disc, inflammation, or a spinal deformity.
- Lifestyle and habits can contribute to the development of low back pain.
- Intervertebral disc degeneration can occur through normal body wear and tear or as the result of an arthritic condition. It causes back pain that may radiate to the buttocks or thighs. Treatment includes NSAIDs, rest, physical therapy, back bracing, or injections with a steroid or analgesic.
- A herniated or ruptured disc permits the fluid within vertebral disc to be released into the disc space and adjacent tissues. This causes nerve irritation, pain, muscle spasms, and motor and sensory changes. Treatment includes NSAIDs, antispasmodics, medications to treat neuropathic pain, nerve blocks, and possible surgery.
- Spinal stenosis is a narrowing of the spinal column. This causes pressure on the spinal cord and creates symptoms similar to nerve compression. Manifestations include numbness, weakness, cramping, generalized pain, or pain that radiates down an arm or a leg. Treatment includes NSAIDs, steroid or analgesic injections, physical therapy, bracing, and possible surgery.
- Skeletal irregularities include lordosis, kyphosis, and scoliosis. Most causes for scoliosis are unknown. Besides involving an alteration in spinal structure, additional symptoms of scoliosis include uneven leg length, spinal fatigue, and back pain. Treatment includes exercises, bracing, and possible surgery. Lordosis, where the spinal column is more concave; it is seen frequently in individuals who are pregnant or obese. Kyphosis, which is common in older adults, is characterized by a spinal column that is convex.

36.3 Rheumatic and Arthritic Disorders

Differentiate the causes, classification, underlying pathogenesis, and clinical manifestations of rheumatic and arthritic disorders and approaches to diagnosis and treatment of these conditions across the lifespan.

- Arthritis and rheumatic disorders include osteoarthritis, rheumatoid arthritis, spondyloarthropathies, and juvenile rheumatoid arthritis.
- Osteoarthritis is the most common form of arthritis and causes the most disabilities in older adults. It can occur from no identified cause or as a symptom of an underlying condition. Manifestations of osteoarthritis include joint pain, stiffness, tenderness, effusion, and crepitus. Treatment includes NSAIDs, topical analgesics, steroid injections, and complementary approaches. Surgery may be required to smooth the joint surface or replace the damaged joint.
- Rheumatoid arthritis is a chronic systemic autoimmune disorder that causes inflammation of connective tissue in the joints. Clinical manifestations include joint swelling, stiffness, warmth, tenderness, and pain. The joints may feel boggy or sponge-like. Patients with this disorder are at risk for joint deformities, primarily of the fingers. Treatment includes pharmacologic approaches, rest, exercise, application of heat or cold, use of assistive devices, and other complementary approaches.

- Spondyloarthropathies are diseases that cause inflammation and structural changes of the bones. They are associated with the HLA-B27 gene. Manifestations of these disorders include back pain, stiffness, and generalized fatigue. Treatment may be conservative, with NSAIDs and stretching exercises. Joint replacement surgery may be required for extreme cases.
- Juvenile idiopathic arthritis is the most common type of arthritis in children. The cause is unknown; however, it leads to changes in mobility and joint swelling and pain. Treatment includes NSAIDs, DMARDs, other medications, physical therapy, and possible joint replacement surgery.

36.4 Metabolic Bone Disease

Differentiate the causes, classification, underlying pathogenesis, and clinical manifestations of metabolic bone disease and approaches to diagnosis and treatment of these conditions across the lifespan.

- Metabolic bone diseases alter bone strength and occur because of insufficient or poorly metabolized calcium, phosphorus, and vitamin D. The most prevalent metabolic bone disease is osteoporosis. Other common metabolic bone diseases that are of importance include osteopenia and Paget disease.
- Osteopenia is a change in bone density that occurs when bone resorption occurs faster than bone generation. It causes no clinical manifestations unless a fracture occurs. Treatment of ostopenia includes diet therapy, calcium and vitamin D supplementation, weight bearing exercises, smoking cessation, and reducing the intake of cola-based and alcoholic beverages.
- Osteoporosis is caused by a low intake of bone-supporting nutrients or an increase in bone resorption. It causes weak bones that are prone to fracture. Manifestations of this disorder include a loss of height, curvature of the spine, low back pain, and fractures. Treatment includes medication, nutritional supplements, exercise, and measures to prevent falls.
- Paget disease is a metabolic disorder that causes bone resorption faster than bone formation. Manifestations can range from no symptoms to pain, enlarged bones, fractures, or damaged cartilage. Treatment includes medication, nutritional supplements, exercise, and efforts to prevent fractures. Surgery may be required to correct bone malformations or replace affected joints.

REVIEW QUESTIONS

1. Which of the following statements indicates to the nurse that a client with rheumatoid arthritis understands discharge instructions?
   a. "I will be cured with treatment and RA will not affect my ability to work."
   b. "I will have periods of remissions and flare-ups."
   c. "I can completely control the disease with medications."
   d. "Surgery can cure the disease."
2. The nurse explains to the patient with rheumatoid arthritis that the goal of disease-modifying antirheumatic drugs (DMARDs) is to:
   a. reduce inflammation.
   b. control anemia.
   c. increase synovial viscosity.
   d. slow disease progression.
3. An assessment of a client with osteopenia is most likely to reveal:
   a. curvature of the spine.
   b. bowed legs.
   c. joint swelling.
   d. no clinical manifestations.
4. During the physical assessment of a child with oligoarticular juvenile idiopathic arthritis, the nurse is most likely to observe which of the following?
   a. High-fever
   b. Skin rash
   c. Inflammation of the knees
   d. Enlarged lymph nodes
5. When performing the Adam forward bent test, the nurse asks the child to:
   a. lean forward at the waist with arms hanging down.
   b. lean forward at the waist with hands clasped behind the back.
   c. lean forward at the waist with arms reaching forward.
   d. lean forward at the waist with hands on the hips.
6. The nurse assesses that a child has a right thoracic curve. The nurse documents this conditions as:
   a. levoconvex.
   b. rotoscoliosis.
   c. dextroscoliosis.
   d. kyphoscoliosis.
7. Which findings would the nurse expect to assess in a patient with a gradual herniated disc at L4–L5?
   a. Slow onset of pain, tingling
   b. Severe pain, muscle spasms
   c. Urinary incontinence, paralysis
   d. Bowel incontinence, loss of feeling
8. Which of the following statements should the nurse make to the pregnant woman experiencing back pain?
   a. "Your back pain will probably go away after delivery."
   b. "Labor will cause disc compression."
   c. "You will require a cesarean section."
   d. "The back pain will be a continual problem for you."

ANSWERS

Answers to Review Questions can be found in Appendix A. Answers to Case Study and Check Your Progress questions are available on the faculty resources site. Please consult with your instructor.

RECOMMENDED WEBSITES

Arthritis Foundation
http://www.arthritis.org

Arthritis Foundation: Kids Get Arthritis Too
http://www.kidsgetarthritistoo.org

National Institute of Health Osteoporosis and Related Bone Diseases National Resource Center
https://www.niams.nih.gov/Health_Info/Bone

National Osteoporosis Foundations
https://www.nof.org

REFERENCES

1. National Institute of Neurological Disorders and Stroke. (2014). *Low back pain fact sheet*. Available at https://www.ninds.nih.gov/Disorders/Patient-Caregiver-Education/Fact-Sheets/Low-Back-Pain-Fact-Sheet
2. National Institute of Arthritis and Musculoskeletal and Skin Diseases. (2016). *Handout on health: Back pain*. Available at http://www.niams.nih.gov/health_info/Back_Pain/default.asp
3. Adams, M. A., & Roughley, P. J. (2006). What is intervertebral disc degeneration, and what causes it? *Spine, 31*(18), 2151–2161. Available at http://www.medscape.com/viewarticle/543611_8
4. Mayo Clinic. (2014) *Herniated disk: Tests and diagnosis*. Available at http://www.mayoclinic.org/diseases-conditions/herniated-disk/basics/tests-diagnosis/con-20029957
5. University of Maryland Medical Center. (2014). *Herniated disk*. Available at http://umm.edu/health/medical/ency/articles/herniated-disk
6. Schiel, W. C. (2016). *Cauda equina syndrome*. Available at http://www.medicinenet.com/cauda_equina_syndrome/article.htm
7. Mayo Clinic. (2014). *Spinal cord injury*. Available at http://www.mayoclinic.org/diseases-conditions/spinal-cord-injury/basics/risk-factors/con-20023837
8. American Association of Neurological Surgeons. (2016). *Herniated disc*. Available at http://www.aans.org/patient%20information/conditions%20and%20treatments/herniated%20disc.aspx
9. Mayo Clinic. (2014) *Herniated disk: Tests and diagnosis*. Available at http://www.mayoclinic.org/diseases-conditions/herniated-disk/basics/tests-diagnosis/con-20029957
10. Children's Healthcare of Atlanta. (2016). *Herniated disc*. Available at https://www.choa.org/medical-services/neurosciences/herniated-disc
11. Matthews, L. J., McConda, D. B., Lalli, T. A. J., & Daffner, S. D. (2015). Orthostetrics: Management of orthopedic conditions in the pregnant patient. *Orthopedics (Online), 38*(10), e874–e880. doi:10.3928/01477447-20151002-53
12. National Institute of Arthritis and Musculoskeletal and Skin Diseases. (2016). *Spinal stenosis*. Available at https://www.niams.nih.gov/health_info/spinal_stenosis/\#spine_b
13. Mayo Clinic. (2016). *Scoliosis*. Available at http://www.mayoclinic.org/diseases-conditions/scoliosis/home/ovc-20193685
14. American Academy of Orthopaedic Surgeons. (2015). *Idiopathic scoliosis in children and adolescents*. Available at http://orthoinfo.aaos.org/topic.cfm?topic=A00353
15. Davis, C. P. (2016). Scoliosis. *Medicine Net*. Available at http://www.medicinenet.com/scoliosis/article.htm
16. Mehlman, C. T. (2012). Idiopathic scoliosis. *Medscape Reference*. Available at http://emedicine.medscape.com/article/1265794-overview
17. Scoliosis Research Society. (n.d.). *Idiopathic scoliosis: Adult*. Available at http://www.srs.org/patients-and-families/conditions-and-treatments/adults/scoliosis
18. Arthritis Foundation. (n.d.). *Juvenile dermatomyositis*. Available at http://www.arthritis.org/about-arthritis/types/juvenile-dermatomyositis-jd
19. Musumeci, G, Szychlinska, M. A., & Mobasheri, A. (2015). Age-related degeneration of articular cartilage in the pathogenesis of osteoarthritis: Molecular markers of senescent chondrocytes. *Histology and Histopathology, 30*, 1–12. Available at http://www.hh.um.es
20. Centers for Disease Control and Prevention. (2016). *Arthritis*. Available at http://www.cdc.gov/arthritis/index.htm
21. Centers for Disease Control and Prevention. (2016). *Rheumatoid arthritis*. Available at http://www.cdc.gov/arthritis/basics/rheumatoid.htm
22. American College of Rheumatology. (2016). *Rheumatoid arthritis*. Available at http://www.rheumatology.org/practice/clinical/patients/diseases_and_conditions/ra.asp
23. Mayo Clinic. (2016). *Diseases and conditions: Rheumatoid arthritis*. Available at http://www.mayoclinic.org/diseases-conditions/rheumatoid-arthritis/home/ovc-20197388
24. Ruffing, V., & Bingham, C. O. (2012). *Rheumatoid arthritis signs and symptoms*. Available at http://www.hopkinsarthritis.org/arthritis-info/rheumatoid-arthritis/ra-symptoms
25. Smith, H. R. (2016). Rheumatoid arthritis. *Medscape*. Available at http://emedicine.medscape.com/article/331715-overview\#a4
26. National Institute of Arthritis and Musculoskeletal Skin Diseases. (2014). *Handout on health: Rheumatoid arthritis*. Available at http://www.niams.nih.gov/Health_Info/Rheumatic_Disease/default.asp
27. Dartmouth-Hitchcock. (2016). *Spondyloarthropathies*. Available at https://www.dartmouth-hitchcock.org/medical-information/health_encyclopedia/hw87580spec
28. Arthritis Foundation. (n.d.). *What is juvenile idiopathic arthritis?* Available at http://www.arthritis.org/about-arthritis/types/juvenile-idiopathic-arthritis-jia/what-is-juvenile-idiopathic-arthritis.php
29. Sherry, D. D. (2016). Juvenile idiopathic arthritis. *Medscape*. Available at http://emedicine.medscape.com/article/1007276-overview
30. Romito, K. (2015). Osteopenia overview. *WebMD*. Available at http://www.webmd.com/osteoporosis/tc/osteopenia-overview\#1
31. National Institute of Health Osteoporosis and Related Bone Diseases National Resource Center. (2016). *Handout on health: Osteoporosis*. Available at https://www.niams.nih.gov/Health_Info/Bone/Osteoporosis/osteoporosis_hoh.asp
32. Bethel, M., Lohr, K. M., Carbone, L. D., & Machua, W. (2016). Osteoporosis. *Medscape: Drugs & Diseases*. Available at http://emedicine.medscape.com/article/330598-overview\#a4
33. National Institute of Health Osteoporosis and Related Bone Diseases National Resource Center. (2014). *What is Paget's disease of bone?* Available at https://www.niams.nih.gov/Health_Info/Bone/Pagets/pagets_disease_ff.asp

Unit XI
Disorders of Endocrine Regulation

Disorders of endocrine regulation can disrupt homeostasis individually or in combination with factors such as stress, infection, and/or changes in fluid and electrolyte balance. Hormones regulate the narrow range of plasma glucose concentrations, assist in the maintenance of blood pressure, drive sexual development and functioning, and help regulate immune and inflammatory responses, among others. Hormones also play a role in the regulation of anxiety and mood. For example, repeated chronic stress results in hyperactivity of the hypothalamic-pituitary-adrenal (HPA) axis, resulting in increased release of hormones such as cortisol.[1]

Although many factors play a role in endocrine health and pathophysiology, one area of increasing interest is that of endocrine-disruptor chemicals (EDCs). EDCs include, but are not limited to, bisphenol-A (BPA), phthalates, tribulytin, and pesticides. EDCs are associated with a number of disorders of endocrine and hormone dysregulation, including obesity, type 2 diabetes mellitus, reproductive cancers in women, and prostate cancer in men. There is also evidence that prenatal exposure to thyroid disruptors can cause cognitive deficits in children. Because exposure can occur through a variety of sources (e.g., soil, water, air, manufactured products such as plastics and pesticides, and foods), it can be challenging to both confirm exposure and trace it to its source.[2]

Endocrine disorders can develop and manifest over time, as in the case of Addison disease and type 2 diabetes, or manifest as an acute crisis, as in acute adrenal failure (Addisonian crisis) or diabetic ketoacidosis (DKA). In some cases, as that of Addison disease, clinical manifestations may resemble those of other illnesses and careful assessment is necessary to differentiate an endocrine disorder from other etiologies. More severe cases may be more easily differentiated but still require careful assessment and, likely, ongoing monitoring and patient education to manage the disorder and prevent another acute crisis.

References

1. Potter, M. L., & Moller, M. D. (2015). *Psychiatric–Mental Health Nursing: From Suffering to Hope.* Hoboken, NJ: Pearson Education.
2. Gore, A. C., Chappell, V. A., Fenton, S. E., Flaws, J. A., Nadal, A., Prins, G. S., Tappari, J., & Zoeller, R. T. (2015). EDC-2: The Endocrine Society's second scientific statement on EDCs. *Endocrine Review, 36*(6) E1-E150 and 593-602 (Executive Summary).

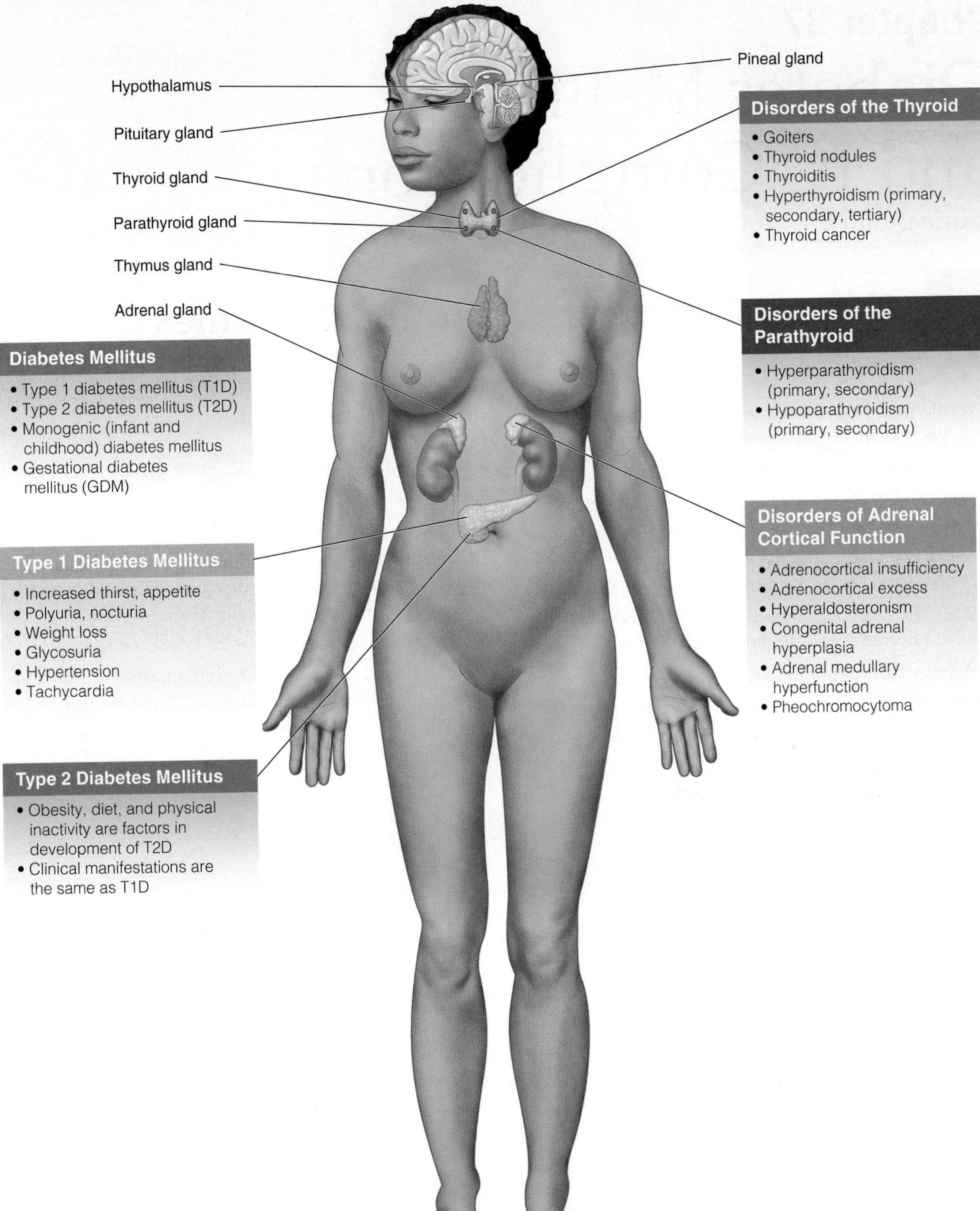

Pineal gland
Hypothalamus
Pituitary gland
Thyroid gland
Parathyroid gland
Thymus gland
Adrenal gland
Disorders of the Thyroid
• Goiters
• Thyroid nodules
• Thyroiditis
• Hyperthyroidism (primary, secondary, tertiary)
• Thyroid cancer
Disorders of the Parathyroid
• Hyperparathyroidism (primary, secondary)
• Hypoparathyroidism (primary, secondary)
Diabetes Mellitus
• Type 1 diabetes mellitus (T1D)
• Type 2 diabetes mellitus (T2D)
• Monogenic (infant and childhood) diabetes mellitus
• Gestational diabetes mellitus (GDM)
Disorders of Adrenal Cortical Function
• Adrenocortical insufficiency
• Adrenocortical excess
• Hyperaldosteronism
• Congenital adrenal hyperplasia
• Adrenal medullary hyperfunction
• Pheochromocytoma
Type 1 Diabetes Mellitus
• Increased thirst, appetite
• Polyuria, nocturia
• Weight loss
• Glycosuria
• Hypertension
• Tachycardia
Type 2 Diabetes Mellitus
• Obesity, diet, and physical inactivity are factors in development of T2D
• Clinical manifestations are the same as T1D

Chapter 37

Diabetes Mellitus and Its Complications

Laurie Quinn

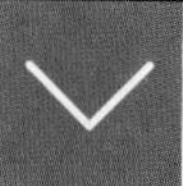

Chapter Outline and Learning Outcomes

37.1 Chapter Overview and Case Studies

Describe the epidemiology of diabetes mellitus and concepts related to diabetes mellitus.

37.2 Classification of Diabetes Mellitus and Prediabetes

Compare and contrast the four categories of diabetes mellitus.

37.3 Maintenance of Normal Blood Glucose Levels

Identify the hormones and biochemical processes involved in fuel substrate metabolism.

37.4 Type 1 Diabetes Mellitus

Differentiate the causes and underlying pathogenesis of type 1 diabetes mellitus.

37.5 Type 2 Diabetes Mellitus

Differentiate the causes and underlying pathogenesis of type 2 diabetes mellitus.

37.6 Clinical Manifestations of and Diagnostic Criteria for Diabetes Mellitus

Describe the clinical manifestations of type 1 and type 2 diabetes mellitus, gestational diabetes mellitus, and prediabetes.

37.7 Acute Complications of Diabetes Mellitus

Differentiate the causes, underlying pathogenesis, and clinical manifestations of acute complications of diabetes mellitus across the lifespan.

37.8 Chronic Complications of Diabetes Mellitus

Differentiate the causes, underlying pathogenesis, and clinical manifestations of chronic complications of diabetes mellitus.

KEY TERMS

Anabolism, 911
Autoantibody, 913
Catabolism, 910
Counterregulatory hormones, 910
Diabetes mellitus (DM), 905
Diabetic ketoacidosis (DKA), 918
Gestational diabetes mellitus (GDM), 908
Gluconeogenesis, 909
Glucosuria, 917
Glycogen, 909
Glycogenolysis, 909
Glycolysis, 908
Hemoglobin A1C, 908
Honeymoon period, 913
Hyperglycemia, 906
Hyperglycemic hyperosmolar syndrome (HHS), 921
Hypoglycemia, 918
Impaired fasting glucose (IFG), 908
Impaired glucose tolerance (IGT), 908
Insulin resistance, 909
Ketogenesis, 909
Ketonemia, 919
Ketonuria, 920
Kussmaul respirations, 919
Lipemia, 919
Lipolysis, 909
Macrovascular disease, 924
Maturity-onset diabetes of the young (MODY), 908
Microvascular disease, 924
Neonatal diabetes mellitus (NDM), 908
Nephropathy, 927
Neuropathy, 927
Nocturia, 917
Polydipsia, 916
Polyphagia, 916
Polyuria, 916
Prediabetes, 908
Retinopathy, 926
Type 1 diabetes mellitus (TID), 907
Type 2 diabetes mellitus (T2D), 907

ABBREVIATIONS

Acetyl-CoA—acetyl-coenzyme A
AGE—advanced glycation end product
CHO—carbohydrate
DKA—diabetic ketoacidosis
DM—diabetes mellitus
FFA—free fatty acids
GDM—gestational diabetes mellitus
GFR—glomerular filtration rate
HHS—hyperglycemic hyperosmolar syndrome
HLA—human leukocyte antigen
IFG—impaired fasting glucose
IGT—impaired glucose tolerance
MODY—maturity-onset diabetes of the young
NDM—neonatal diabetes mellitus
OGTT—oral glucose tolerance test
PKC—protein kinase C
T1D—type 1 diabetes mellitus
T2D—type 2 diabetes mellitus

37.1 Chapter Overview and Case Studies

Diabetes mellitus (DM) is general term for a group of disorders in which the body's ability to produce or respond to the hormone insulin is impaired; this affects its ability to use the energy in food. It is a major public health problem that affects approximately 29.1 million people in the United States, or 9.3% of the U.S. population. Of this number approximately, 8.1 million people remain undiagnosed.[1] In 2013, an estimated 382 million people worldwide had DM; this number is expected to increase to 592 million by 2035.[2] Diabetes mellitus is the seventh leading cause of death in the United States; it is the leading cause of kidney failure, nontraumatic lower-limb amputations, and new cases of blindness among U.S. adults, and it remains a major cause of heart disease and stroke.[1]

The treatment and prevention of DM are high-priority goals among public health initiatives, as is noted in the *Healthy People 2020* objectives (see the feature). An understanding of the pathogenesis of DM is essential for meeting these goals.

This chapter provides a general overview of the classifications of DM, followed by a discussion of relevant concepts in endocrinology and metabolism that provide context for understanding the progression and development of DM. The chapter progresses to discussion of the risk factors, etiology, and pathophysiology of the two major forms of DM, as well as signs and symptoms, diagnostic criteria, and relevant laboratory testing. This is followed by discussion of the acute and chronic complications of type 1 DM (T1D) and type 2 DM (T2D).

Concepts Related to Diabetes Mellitus and Its Complications

The three primary components involved in the pathophysiology of DM include a relative or absolute insulin deficiency, insulin resistance, and hyperglycemia. People with

Healthy People 2020

Diabetes Mellitus

The prevention and treatment of DM require aggressive public health initiatives. *Healthy People 2020* contains several objectives related to the prevention and treatment of DM. The major objectives are as follows:

- Reduce the annual number of new cases of diagnosed DM in the population.
- Reduce the death rate among the population with DM (all-cause mortality).
- Reduce the DM death rate (diabetes-related mortality).
- Reduce the rate of lower-extremity amputations in individuals with diagnosed DM.
- Improve glycemic control among the population with diagnosed DM.
- Improve lipid control among individuals with diagnosed DM.
- Increase the proportion of the population with diagnosed DM whose blood pressure is under control.
- Increase the proportion of individuals with diagnosed DM who have at least an annual dental examination.
- Increase the proportion of adults with diagnosed DM who have at least an annual foot examination.
- Increase the proportion of adults with diagnosed DM who have an annual dilated eye examination.
- Increase the proportion of adults with diagnosed DM who have a hemoglobin A1C measurement at least twice a year.
- Increase the proportion of individuals with diagnosed DM who obtain an annual urinary microalbumin measurement.
- Increase the proportion of adults with diagnosed DM who perform self-blood glucose-monitoring at least once daily.
- Increase the proportion of individuals with diagnosed DM who receive formal DM education.
- Increase the proportion of individuals with DM whose condition has been diagnosed.
- Increase prevention behaviors in individuals at high risk for DM with prediabetes.

These extensive objectives underline the importance of ameliorating DM and it complications, as this disorder exacts huge personal social and economic burdens.

Reference

1. Data from HealthyPeople.gov (2017). 2020 Topics & Objectives: Diabetes. Retrieved from http://www.healthypeople.gov/2020/topicsobjectives 2020/overview.aspx?topicid=8

T1D have an almost complete lack of insulin secretion, and the insulin deficiency is considered total or absolute. People with T2D have a relative insulin deficiency (i.e., the insulin secretion is too low in relation to the blood glucose level) and insulin resistance (i.e., the endogenous insulin is unable to produce its biological response). The relative or absolute loss of insulin production and insulin resistance result in **hyperglycemia** (high blood glucose). The hyperglycemia leads to a number of acute symptoms (e.g., increased thirst, increased urination, and weight loss), while the combination of hyperglycemia and the absolute or relative insulin deficiency can lead to acute metabolic emergencies. Additionally, the hyperglycemia, insulin resistance, and insulin deficiency can lead to chronic complications, particularly affecting the eyes, kidneys, nerves, heart, and blood vessels. Individuals who have DM may develop cardiovascular disease, peripheral neuropathies, or nephropathy. They will also likely be prone to infections and have difficulty with wound healing (see **Figure 37.1** ■).

Diabetes mellitus is a progressive disease, and various physiologic changes throughout the lifespan affect the progression of DM. The potential for DM-related complications increases with the duration of DM, while comorbidities increase with age. ■

Case Studies

The following cases featuring patients with the four major types of DM are addressed throughout the chapter to assist in applying chapter content to clinical situations that involve individuals with DM.

Melissa Bailey: Introduction

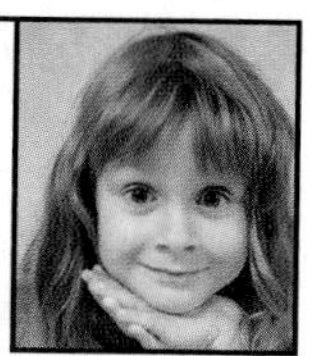

Melissa Bailey, age 5, is brought to her pediatrician's office by her mother. Melissa had a bout of "flu" 2 weeks before the visit. Her mother is concerned because Melissa does not seem to be recovering. In addition, her mother reports that Melissa is thirsty most of the time, has a poor appetite, urinates frequently, and is unusually fatigued. On the morning before the visit, Melissa complained of abdominal pain, and her mother noted a fruity odor to Melissa's breath. Her normal weight was 30 kg; however, at the pediatrician's office, a 3-kg weight loss was noted. Her blood glucose level was 250 mg/dL.

1. What did Melissa's blood glucose level indicate?
2. What symptoms are noted that relate to Melissa's current blood sugar level?
3. What are possible reasons for Melissa's hyperglycemia?

Norma James: Introduction

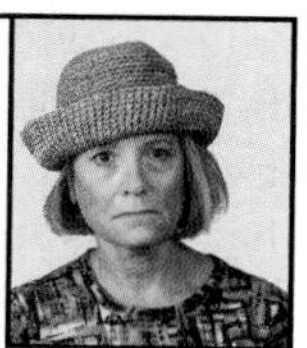

Norma James is 65 years old and was diagnosed with T2D several years ago following a 1-month history of weight loss (4.5 kg), polyuria, polydipsia, and polyphagia. In addition, she has a history of hypertension and atrial fibrillation.

1. Among the three primary concepts involved in DM, which ones are potentially affecting Ms. James's blood glucose level?
2. Considering Ms. James's age, explain possible factors that may contribute to the progression of DM. What comorbidities does Ms. James have?
3. What happens to DM-related complications during the duration of DM in older adult patients?

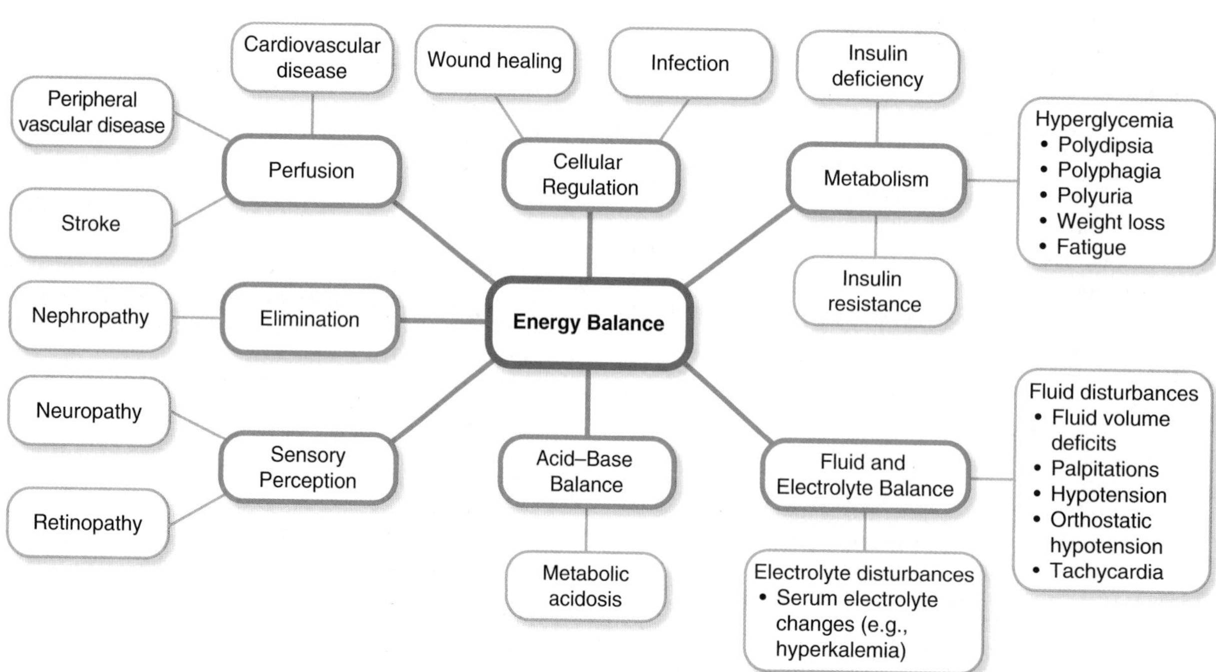

Figure 37.1 ■ The primary concept related to diabetes mellitus is energy balance. Related concepts, disorders and symptoms are shown in the middle and outer rings.

Rosa Garcia: Introduction

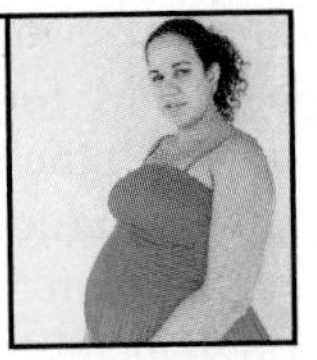

Rosa Garcia, is 36 years old, overweight, and pregnant with her third child. Her history shows that her two previous children weighed more than 9 pounds at birth and that both newborns had hypoglycemia during the initial 24 hours of life. Ms. Garcia has no history of any type of DM. Her fasting blood glucose at 24 weeks gestation is 99 mg/dL.

1. What are major concerns that you should consider for Ms. Garcia?
2. Is Ms. Garcia at risk for developing type 2 diabetes mellitus if her hyperglycemia is prolonged and is left untreated?
3. What is the child Ms. Garcia is expecting likely to develop once born?

Isaiah Coleman: Introduction

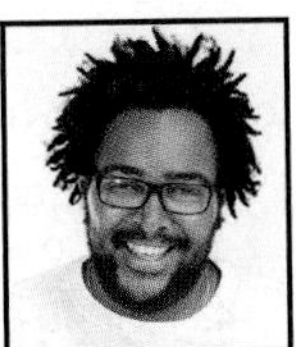

Isaiah Coleman is 40 years old and obese. He is undergoing a routine yearly examination. He has no physical complaints; however, the results of his diagnostic workup indicate that he has an elevated fasting glucose level (106 mg/dL), hypertension, and hyperlipidemia. A fasting blood glucose level on a second occasion is also elevated (110 mg/dL). The occupational health nurse notes that Mr. Coleman's hemoglobin A1C is 6.2%.

1. What chronic complications can Mr. Coleman develop over time as his diabetes progresses?
2. How often should Mr. Coleman have his Hg A1C measurement done, according to the *Healthy People 2020* objectives?

Check Your Progress: Section 37.1

1. What are known diseases that are caused by diabetes mellitus (DM)?
2. What are the high-priority public health initiatives in regard to diabetes mellitus as noted in the *Healthy People 2020* objectives?
3. Describe the three primary components of DM—relative/absolute insulin deficiency, insulin resistance, and hyperglycemia—in relation to T1D and T2D.
4. What is the effect of relative/absolute insulin deficiency and insulin resistance to the blood glucose level?

37.2 Classification of Diabetes Mellitus and Prediabetes

Diabetes mellitus is not a single disease. It is a group of metabolic disorders characterized by hyperglycemia (high blood glucose level), resulting from defects in insulin secretion, insulin action, or both.[3] There are four clinical classifications of DM and two categories of increased risk for developing DM. The clinical classifications include type 1 diabetes mellitus (T1D), type 2 diabetes mellitus (T2D), other specific types of DM, and gestational diabetes mellitus (GDM). Categories associated with increased risk of DM include impaired fasting glucose and impaired glucose tolerance. The introductory case studies exemplify the different clinical presentations of these classifications.

Type 1 diabetes mellitus is an autoimmune condition that results in the pancreas being unable to make insulin. It was previously called *juvenile diabetes* and *insulin-dependent diabetes* and it comprises 5% of all DM cases in adults.[3] T1D is associated with destruction of the pancreatic beta cells, which secrete insulin. In the vast majority of people with T1D, an autoimmune process mediates this destruction. However, a small subgroup of people have an idiopathic (occurring spontaneously from an unknown cause) destruction of pancreatic beta cells. Because people with T1D produce almost no insulin, they require pharmacologic insulin therapy for survival. T1D can occur at any age but is frequently diagnosed before 30 years of age; however, there is an adult form of autoimmune T1D that is termed *latent autoimmune DM in adults*.[4]

Melissa Bailey: Application

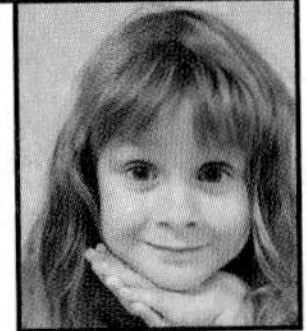

Melissa has classic symptoms of hyperglycemia along with a blood glucose level that is over 200 mg/dL. Her age, clinical symptoms, and blood glucose level clearly suggest a diagnosis of T1D. In particular, the increased thirst, frequent urination, and abdominal pain and a fruity odor to her breath suggest that she is experiencing diabetic ketoacidosis, a medical emergency, so she is brought to the emergency department.

4. Describe the action of pancreatic beta cells in Melissa's blood glucose level.
5. Considering Melissa's presentation, what hormone is required to decrease her blood glucose level or treat the diabetic ketoacidosis?
6. In Melissa's case, what process mediates the destruction of pancreatic beta cells?

Type 2 diabetes mellitus, previously called *adult-onset diabetes* and *noninsulin-dependent diabetes*, accounts for approximately 90–95% of cases of DM.[1] This type of DM is associated with insulin resistance and defects in insulin secretion. T2D typically is diagnosed in adulthood but is now occurring more frequently at younger ages. Individuals with T2D are not dependent on exogenous insulin to sustain life; however, they may need insulin therapy and/or oral and other injectable medications to control hyperglycemia.

Norma James: Application

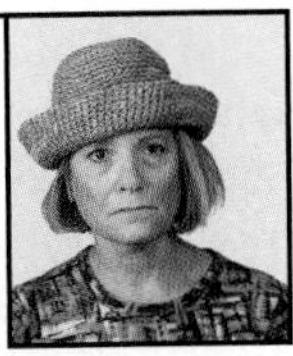

Ms. James has T2D that is treated with an oral glucose-lowering medication. She is taught how to test her blood glucose level using a portable glucose monitor. Additionally, she attends classes on nutrition and on integrating exercise into her daily schedule.

4. What is the insulin mechanism of action in T2D?
5. What treatment will help to control Ms. James's hyperglycemia?
6. Is Ms. James's pancreas still producing insulin?

Other specific types of diabetes mellitus can result from certain specific genetic conditions (e.g., monogenic forms of DM), surgery (e.g., pancreatectomy), drugs (e.g., corticosteroids), infections (e.g., congenital rubella), and other illness. The initial diagnosis and clinical presentation of the DM in these groups vary with the underlying disorder. Monogenic DM comprises 1–5% of all cases of childhood DM.[5] The monogenic forms of DM mellitus result from a single-gene mutation, whereas T1D and T2D result from polygenic (multiple gene) defects. The two main forms of monogenic DM are **neonatal diabetes mellitus (NDM)** and **maturity-onset diabetes of the young (MODY)**. NDM first occurs in newborns and young infants. MODY usually first occurs in children or adolescents and is characterized by mild hyperglycemia.[5]

Gestational diabetes mellitus (GDM) refers to a condition in which the onset of DM is first diagnosed during pregnancy. The prevalence of GDM ranges from 2–10% of all pregnancies.[6] Individuals who have been diagnosed with GDM need dietary treatment and possibly oral medications or exogenous insulin to control hyperglycemia.[7] Hyperglycemia during pregnancy can result in fetal and maternal complications. GDM resolves after childbirth; however, women with GDM have a 35–60% chance of developing DM in the 10–20 years following the pregnancy.[6] Risk factors for GDM include previous GDM, advanced maternal age, obesity, family history of DM, and racial/ethnic origin (African American, Hispanic/Latino American, and American Indian).

4 The risk of GDM increases with age and requires combinations of dietary adjustments, insulin treatment, and/or oral medications for the woman to maintain normoglycemia to prevent maternal and fetal complications. ■

Rosa Garcia: Application

Ms. Garcia is diagnosed with GDM and begins treatment with insulin injections. She is taught how to use a portable glucose monitor and is provided a strict schedule of glucose testing before and after meals. Additionally, she attends classes on nutrition and on incorporating physical activity into her lifestyle.

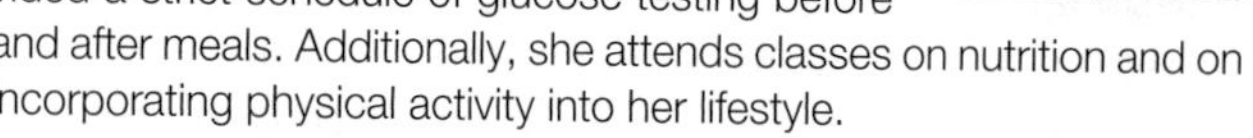

4. What are risk factors associated with Ms. Garcia's GDM?
5. Discuss complications associated with hyperglycemia during pregnancy.
6. What management needs to be considered to prevent GDM complications in both the mother and the fetus?

Prediabetes is a term that is used to identify people who are at increased risk for developing DM. An estimated 86 million U.S. adults aged 20 or over have prediabetes.[1] The two types of abnormal glucose intolerance that are included in the classification of prediabetes are impaired fasting glucose and impaired glucose tolerance. People with prediabetes have impaired fasting glucose, impaired glucose tolerance, or both. **Impaired fasting glucose (IFG)** is a condition in which the fasting blood glucose level or **hemoglobin A1C** (a measure of glucose control over the previous 3 months) is higher than normal but not diagnostic of DM. **Impaired glucose tolerance (IGT)** is a condition in which the blood glucose level 2 hours after an oral glucose load (during an oral glucose tolerance test [OGTT]) is higher than normal but not diagnostic of DM. People with prediabetes have an increased risk of DM (primarily T2D), cardiovascular disease, and stroke. However, the abnormal blood glucose levels associated with prediabetes often can be normalized with dietary modification, weight loss, and physical activity.

Isaiah Coleman: Application

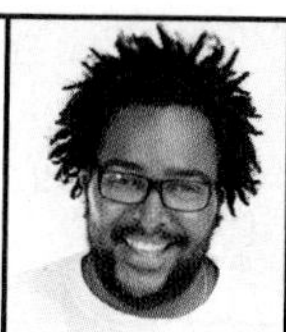

Mr. Coleman has been diagnosed with prediabetes. The main focus of his treatment is weight loss. He begins an aggressive weight loss and exercise program. He is committed to both of these treatments to prevent the onset of T2D.

3. What appropriate assessments may have been done on Mr. Coleman to verify the diagnosis of prediabetes?
4. Is it possible to normalize Mr. Coleman's prediabetes condition? What actions may be done to alter his present condition?

Check Your Progress: Section 37.2

1. What are the four categories of diabetes?
2. Compare and contrast the four categories of diabetes.
3. Describe prediabetes.
4. What are the ways in which prediabetes can be diagnosed?

37.3 Maintenance of Normal Blood Glucose Levels

Glucose is an obligate fuel for the brain and central nervous system. The brain cannot synthesize or store glucose and requires a continuous supply of glucose from the arterial circulation. Plasma glucose concentrations are maintained within a narrow range that is achieved by a balance between glucose entry into the circulation from the liver, intestinal absorption, and glucose uptake into the peripheral sites, such as adipose tissue and skeletal muscle. This process is regulated by a network of hormones (e.g., insulin, glucagon, catecholamines, cortisol, growth hormone, glucagon-like peptide 1, and gastric inhibitory polypeptide), neural signals, and substrates (e.g., carbohydrates, fats, proteins).

Important Terminology in Fuel Metabolism

Central to an understanding of glucose metabolism is knowledge of the following concepts: glycolysis, glycogen, glycogenolysis, gluconeogenesis, lipolysis, ketogenesis, and insulin resistance. The relationship between hormones associated with these concepts is outlined in (**Table 37.1** ■).

Glycolysis, the breakdown of carbohydrate (CHO), is central to all the metabolic pathways of CHO metabolism.

Table 37.1 Primary Hormones of Fuel Metabolism and Metabolic Effects

	Insulin	Glucagon	Cortisol	Growth Hormone	Epinephrine/ Norepinephrine
Glycolysis	Increased	Decreased			
Glycogenolysis	Decreased	Increased			Increased
Gluconeogenesis	Decreased	Increased	Increased	Increased	Increased
Lipolysis	Decreased	Increased	Increased	Increased	Increased
Ketogenesis	Decreased	Increased			
Protein synthesis	Increased		Decreased	Increased	
Insulin resistance		Increased	Increased	Increased	Increased

All body tissues use the glycolytic pathway for the breakdown of glucose to provide energy (in the form of adenosine triphosphate [ATP]). Glycolysis can occur under aerobic or anaerobic conditions. Aerobic glycolysis occurs in cells with mitochondria and an adequate supply of oxygen; the end product of aerobic glycolysis is pyruvate. Anaerobic glycolysis occurs in cells with no mitochondria (e.g., red blood cells) or cells that are deprived of oxygen; the end product of anaerobic glycolysis is lactic acid.

Glycogen is the storage form of glucose, which is located primarily in skeletal muscle and the liver. In skeletal muscle, glycogen mostly acts as a fuel reserve for use in the synthesis of ATP during muscle contraction. In the liver, glycogen mostly acts as a fuel reserve used to maintain blood glucose concentrations, especially during fasting.

Glycogenolysis is the process through which liver and muscle glycogen are converted to glucose.

Gluconeogenesis is the formation of glucose or glycogen from non-CHO sources. The process of gluconeogenesis requires a coordinated supply of precursors from muscle and adipose tissue to the liver and the kidneys (to lesser extent), where they can be converted to glucose or glycogen. Precursors such as pyruvate, alanine, glutamine, and other amino acids may be mobilized from muscle to the liver, where they can be converted to glucose or glycogen. Additionally, the glycerol component of triglycerides can be a precursor for gluconeogenesis.

Fatty acids are stored primarily in the form of triglycerides and serve as the body's main fuel reserve. **Lipolysis** is the process through which triglycerides (composed of a glycerol backbone with three fatty acids attached) are hydrolyzed (a chemical process in which a molecule is cleaved into two parts by the addition of a molecule of water) to fatty acids and glycerol. Triglycerides are stored primarily in adipose tissue and to a lesser extent in muscle. The hydrolysis of triglycerides results in the mobilization of fatty acids and glycerol into the bloodstream. Subsequently, fatty acids can be oxidized for energy; glycerol can be used in the process of glycolysis, gluconeogenesis, and again in the production of triglycerides.

Ketogenesis is the production of ketones, which are important sources of energy for peripheral tissues such as muscle. Liver mitochondria have the ability to convert acetyl coenzyme A (acetyl-CoA), which is derived from fatty acid oxidation, to ketone bodies, which include acetoacetate, 3-hydroxybutyrate (previously termed β-hydroxybutyrate), and acetate. The two functional ketone bodies are acetoacetate and 3-hydroxybutyrate, which are transported in the blood to peripheral tissues for oxidation by the tricarboxylic acid (TCA) cycle. In peripheral tissues with mitochondria, 3-hydroxybutyrate can be oxidized to acetoacetate. Subsequently, acetoacetate can be converted to acetyl-CoA and used for energy production in the TCA cycle.

Insulin resistance is defined as the inability of either endogenous or exogenous insulin to achieve its biological response in its target tissues.

Hormones of the Endocrine Pancreas

The pancreas, located in the posterior portion of the upper abdomen, consists of a head, body, and tail (**Figure 37.2** ■). Structurally, the pancreas is divided into the exocrine and endocrine sections, which make up 80% and 20%, respectively, of the entire organ. The exocrine pancreas is primarily composed of small glands called acini; the endocrine pancreas is made up of small cells called islets of Langerhans

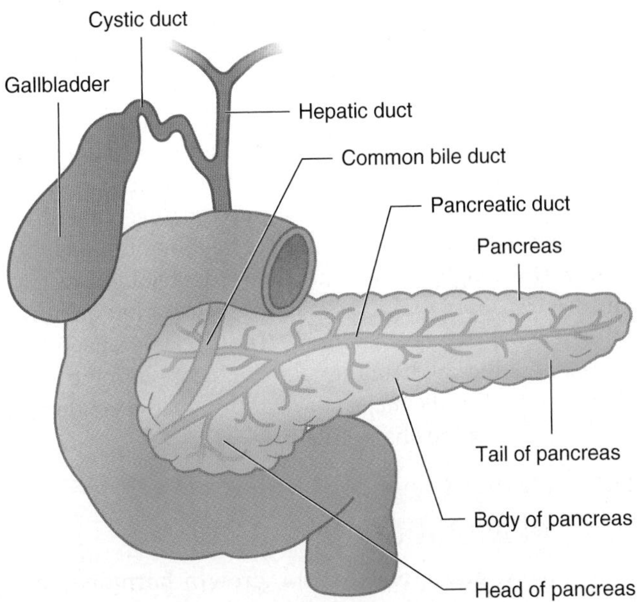

Figure 37.2 ■ Structure of the pancreas.

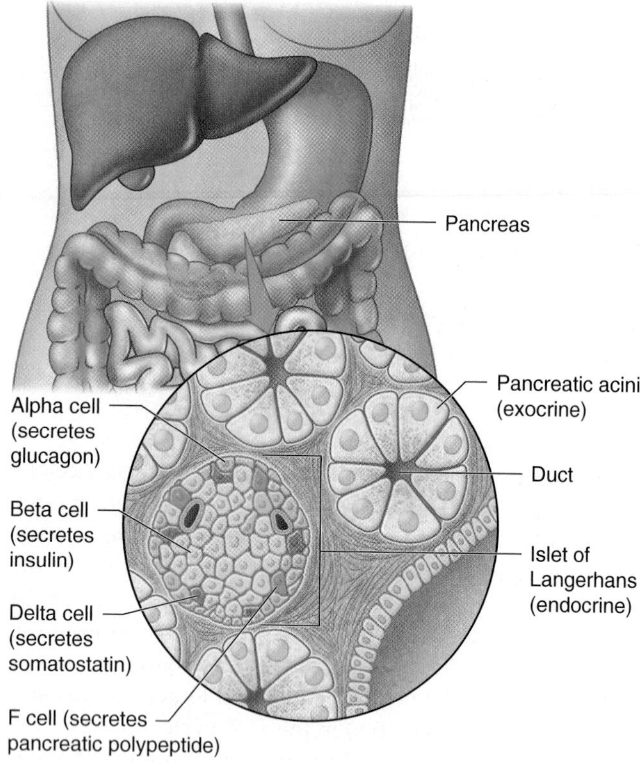

Figure 37.3 ■ Islet cells in the pancreas.

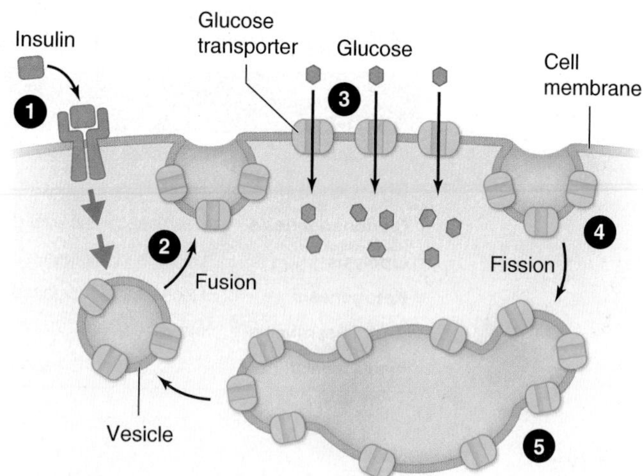

Figure 37.4 ■ The four steps in insulin-sensitive glucose transport: (1) Insulin binds to its receptor in the cell membrane. (2) Activated receptor promotes recruitment of glucose transporter from the intracellular pool to the cell membrane. (3) Glucose transporters increase insulin-mediated uptake of glucose into the cell. (4) When insulin levels decrease, glucose transporters move from the cell membrane to the intracellular storage pool, where they can be recycled.

(**Figure 37.3** ■). These islet cells are distributed throughout the pancreas and are divided into the alpha cells, beta cells, delta cells, and F cells. The alpha cells secrete glucagon; the beta cells secrete insulin; the delta cells secrete somatostatin; and the F cells secrete pancreatic polypeptide.

The effects of insulin are most prominent in the liver, adipose tissue, and muscle. The primary functions of insulin include the synthesis of glycogen in liver and muscle, the synthesis of protein in liver and muscle, and the synthesis of triglycerides in adipose tissue and, to a smaller extent, in muscle. In addition, insulin is necessary for glycolysis and glucose transport into insulin-sensitive tissues, such as muscle. Most important, insulin suppresses gluconeogenesis, glycogenolysis, and lipolysis.

The binding of insulin with its cell membrane receptor results in a cascade of reactions and consequences. One of the most important results is enhanced glucose transport into various insulin-sensitive tissues, including skeletal muscle and adipose tissue. Insulin enhances this transport through the recruitment of the insulin-sensitive glucose transporter GLUT-4 (**Figure 37.4** ■) from an intracellular pool to the cell membrane. The GLUT-4 transporters increase insulin-mediated uptake of glucose into the cells. Skeletal muscle is the major site of insulin-mediated glucose disposal during the absorptive state.

Endocrine Hormones Involved in Fuel Metabolism

Collectively, glucagon, cortisol, growth hormone, epinephrine, and norepinephrine are referred to as **counterregulatory hormones** because their actions oppose the effects of insulin. The primary functions of glucagon, secreted from pancreatic alpha cells, include hepatic gluconeogenesis, glycogenolysis, lipolysis, and ketogenesis. Cortisol is a hormone secreted by the adrenal cortex. This hormone causes protein **catabolism** (breakdown) and lipolysis, which provide precursors for gluconeogenesis and ketogenesis. Growth hormone, secreted by the anterior pituitary, causes lipolysis and also provides precursors for gluconeogenesis and ketogenesis. The catecholamines are epinephrine and norepinephrine. Of the two catecholamines, epinephrine has the greatest role in fuel metabolism. This hormone primarily is secreted by the adrenal medulla and is associated with glycogenolysis, gluconeogenesis, and lipolysis.

Growth hormone, released during puberty, is a counterregulatory hormone that opposes the effects of insulin. As a result, insulin needs during adolescence increase markedly. ■

Normal Fuel Metabolism

Metabolic processes involved in fuel metabolism revolve around absorptive (fed) and postabsorptive (fasted) states. These are described below.

Postabsorptive State

The primary goal of fuel metabolism during the postabsorptive state or fasting state is to provide glucose for the brain and nervous tissue. There is a higher ratio of glucagon to insulin during this time. Hepatic glycogenolysis and gluconeogenesis increase plasma glucose levels. Muscle oxidizes free fatty acids (FFAs), released from adipose tissue lipolysis, for energy (**Figure 37.5** ■).

Absorptive State

Following ingestion of CHO, insulin levels rise and stimulate glucose uptake into insulin-sensitive tissues, primarily muscle. Insulin is a hormone that results in **anabolism** (building tissue); it is the primary hormone during the absorptive state. Glucagon levels decrease, so there is a higher ratio of insulin to glucagon. Glucose is the primary oxidative fuel for all tissues during the absorptive state. Glucose in excess of the oxidative needs of the major tissues is stored as glycogen or lipids (**Figure 37.6** ■).

Starvation

If fasting continues past 10–12 hours, insulin remains suppressed, glucagon levels remain elevated, and the principal source of hepatic glucose production is gluconeogenesis. The muscles oxidize FFAs, released from adipose tissue lipolysis, for energy. In addition, the brain begins to oxidize ketones for energy (**Figure 37.7** ■).

Eating disorders, particularly in children and adolescents with T1D, can lead to uncontrolled DM and accelerated development of diabetic complications. ■

Fuel Metabolism in Diabetes Mellitus

A number of metabolic derangements are associated with DM. In T1D, there is a near complete loss of insulin production; in T2D, there is decreased insulin production and insulin resistance. The abnormalities of fuel metabolism associated with DM result from a deficiency in insulin and an increase in glucagon and other counter-regulatory hormones. These hormonal abnormalities most profoundly affect the muscle, liver, and adipose tissue. Hyperglycemia results from decreased glucose transport into insulin-sensitive tissues (e.g., skeletal muscle), hepatic gluconeogenesis, and hepatic and muscle glycogenolysis. In T1D, the increased mobilization of FFAs from adipose tissue leads to increased hepatic synthesis of ketone bodies and can result in the acute complication of diabetic ketoacidosis

Figure 37.5 ■ ***Postabsorptive state:*** Fuel metabolism during an overnight fast. After approximately 12 hours of starvation, insulin concentrations have returned to basal levels, and glucose (G) entering the circulation is derived from both hepatic glycogen and gluconeogenesis. Free fatty acids (FFAs) produced from adipocyte lipolysis have become a principal fuel for skeletal muscle. AA = amino acids.

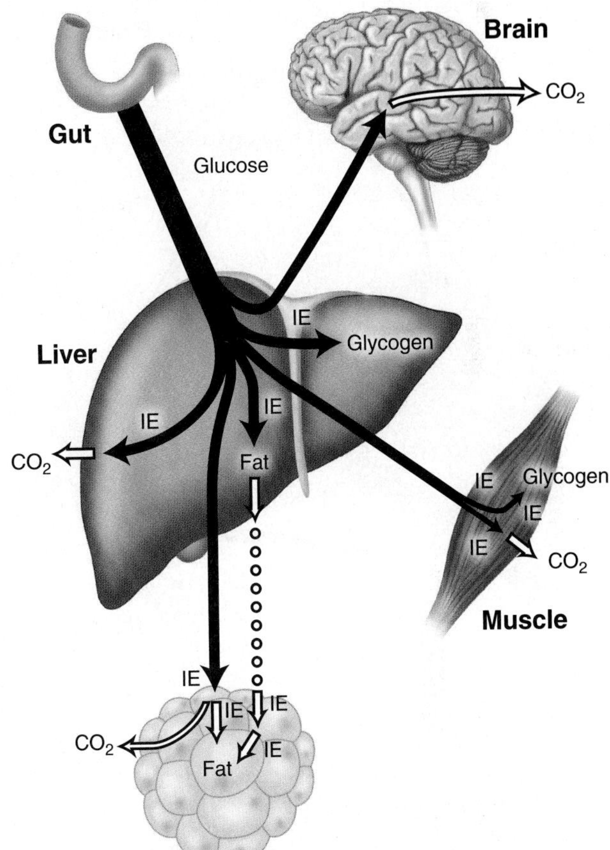

Figure 37.6 ■ ***Absorptive state:*** Fuel metabolism during a carbohydrate meal. Soon after the ingestion of carbohydrate, insulin levels rise and stimulate the uptake of glucose. Glucose is the main oxidative fuel of all major tissues at this time. Glucose that is present in excess of the oxidative needs of tissues is stored as glycogen. IE = insulin effects.

(DKA). In T2D, the amount of FFAs that are converted to ketone bodies is usually not sufficient for the development of DKA. Ultimately, these abnormalities lead to clinical symptoms, which are described later in the chapter.

Growth and development are delayed in children with chronically uncontrolled DM. When the blood glucose level is chronically elevated, food substrates cannot be stored or utilized appropriately. Children with chronically uncontrolled DM may present with a fatty liver and stunted growth. ■

Check Your Progress: Section 37.3

1. What are the hormones of the endocrine pancreas? What is the function of each?
2. What are the major processes involved in fuel metabolism? Define each.
3. What are the primary hormones of fuel metabolism? What is the function of each?
4. What are the primary bodily structures involved in fuel metabolism?
5. How is fuel metabolism altered in diabetes mellitus?

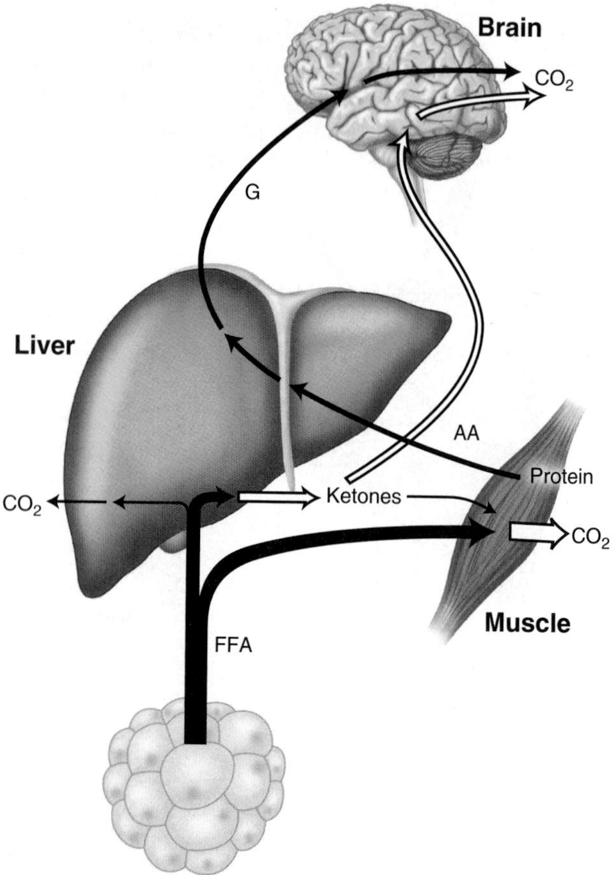

Figure 37.7 ■ ***Starvation:*** Fuel metabolism during prolonged starvation. As fasting continues, insulin levels remain suppressed, and the principal source of hepatic glucose (G) production is gluconeogenesis. Skeletal muscle continues to use free fatty acids (FFAs) for fuel but also uses ketone bodies produced in the liver. Ketone bodies may be used by the brain. AA = amino acids.

37.4 Type 1 Diabetes Mellitus

There is currently a worldwide epidemic of T1D. The most comprehensive epidemiologic study to date has reported that the global incidence of T1D is increasing by 2.8% annually.[8] The incidence rates vary from fewer than 5 to more than 40 per 100,000 persons, the highest rates being in northern latitudes; Finland has one of the highest rates T1D in the world.[9] The most common form of T1D is T-cell-mediated autoimmune destruction of the pancreatic beta cell, leading to loss of insulin production.[9]

Etiology of Type 1 Diabetes Mellitus

The etiology of T1D is complex and appears to result from an interaction among genetics, environment, and autoimmunity.

Genetics

A familial predisposition to T1D does exist; however, the exact mode of genetic inheritance remains unclear. The risk of developing T1D is approximately 0.4% in the general population; while children with an affected family member have a 5% risk of developing T1D by age 20. This risk changes on the basis of the specific relative(s) affected. Those with an affected sibling have a 7% risk of developing T1D; those with an affected father have a 5% risk; those with an affected mother have a 3% risk; and those with multiple affected first-degree relatives have a 20% risk. The risk of developing T1D increases dramatically among identical twins.[10] If one twin is affected, the unaffected monozygotic twin has a 50% of developing T1D[10]; this increases to approximately 65–70% if the affected twin developed T1D under 5 years of age.[11] This risk is 19% in a dizygotic twin.[11] The risk of developing T1D increases among siblings of individuals affected with T1D.

Genetic susceptibility to the development of T1D is associated with the human leukocyte antigen (HLA) genes that lie in the major histocompatibility complex region on the short arm of chromosome 6. This area is currently called the IDDM1 locus.[9] The inheritance of particular HLA alleles (e.g., HLA DR/4, DQA1* 0301-DQB1* 0302, and DQA1* 0501-DQB1*0201) accounts for over 50% of the genetic susceptibility for T1D. However, the inheritance of other HLA alleles (e.g., DQA1* 0102-DQB1*1401) are protective against the development of T1D.[9]

Environment

A triggering event in individuals who are at risk for T1D initiates a series of autoimmune events ending in pancreatic beta-cell destruction. Various environmental triggers have been proposed, but no single factor has been consistently associated with initiating T1D. Some of the possibilities are viral infections, dietary factors, and toxins.[9]

Viruses

For many years, researchers have suspected an association between the development of T1D and viral infection; however this relationship has never been firmly established. The relationship between viruses and T1D is appearing more and more complex as viruses appear to be associated with both increased and decreased risk of T1D. The hygiene hypothesis suggests that exposures to microbes in early childhood stimulate immunoregulatory mechanisms that control autoimmune reactions and decrease risk of T1D; the triggering hypothesis suggests that specific microbes damage insulin-producing cells and increase the risk of T1D.[12] Certain viruses, particularly enteroviruses, are currently the primary candidates for increased risk of T1D. Enteroviruses have been shown to cause T1D in animals, have been associated with increased risk of T1D in epidemiologic studies, and have been detected in the pancreas of T1D patients.[12] The possible protective effect of microbes in the development of T1D has been studied in animal models and in epidemiologic studies. Certain enteral microbes (e.g. hepatitis A virus and *Helicobacter pylori*) and emerging patterns of gut microbiota have been associated with low risk of T1D.[12]

Dietary Factors

It has been hypothesized that early exposure to complex foreign proteins increases the risk of T1D in predisposed individuals. Of the possible dietary etiologic factors, cow's milk proteins have received the most attention. A large-scale, prospective, randomized, international intervention trial titled the Trial to Reduce IDDM in the Genetically at Risk (TRIGR) was designed to answer this question in infants who are genetically susceptible to developing T1D.[13] The results of this study so far do not support the role of cow's milk in increasing T1D risk. Among infants who are at risk for T1D, the use of a hydrolyzed formula (cow's milk proteins that were split into small peptides) when compared with a conventional formula (intact cow's milk proteins) did not reduce the incidence of diabetes-associated autoantibodies after 7 years.[14]

Autoimmunity

Several circulating **autoantibodies** (antibodies that are active against tissues, cells, or cell components of the individual who produce the antibodies) to pancreatic beta-cell components have been identified in people with T1D. These autoantibodies include cytoplasmic ICAs, insulin autoantibodies, antibodies directed against the enzyme glutamic acid decarboxylase, and antibodies against islet tyrosine phosphatase (i.e., IA-2 and IA-2α).[15] These autoantibodies can serve as markers of an ongoing autoimmune process, especially in individuals who are genetically susceptible to T1D.

Pathogenesis of Type 1 Diabetes Mellitus

Researchers are working on understanding the pathogenesis of developing T1D. The proposed scheme for the development of T1D is detailed in **Figure 37.8** ■. Environmental factors trigger an immune response that leads to the development of islet cell autoantibodies (ICAs), insulin autoantibodies, and other islet cell antigens, such as glutamic acid decarboxylase. These antibodies are markers of a progressive loss of pancreatic beta-cell mass. As Figure 37.8 illustrates, when the beta-cell mass is reduced by 80–90%, insulin production is markedly impaired, and overt T1D develops. A period of endogenous insulin secretory recovery, called the **honeymoon period**, follows for up to 1 year. Eventually, however, insulin production ceases.

The question remains as to how an environmental trigger actually initiates the cascade of events leading to pancreatic beta-cell dysfunction. Two theories have been proposed. The first theory is that an environmental trigger, such as a virus, induces tissue damage and inflammation. As a result, beta-cell antigens are released, and lymphocytes

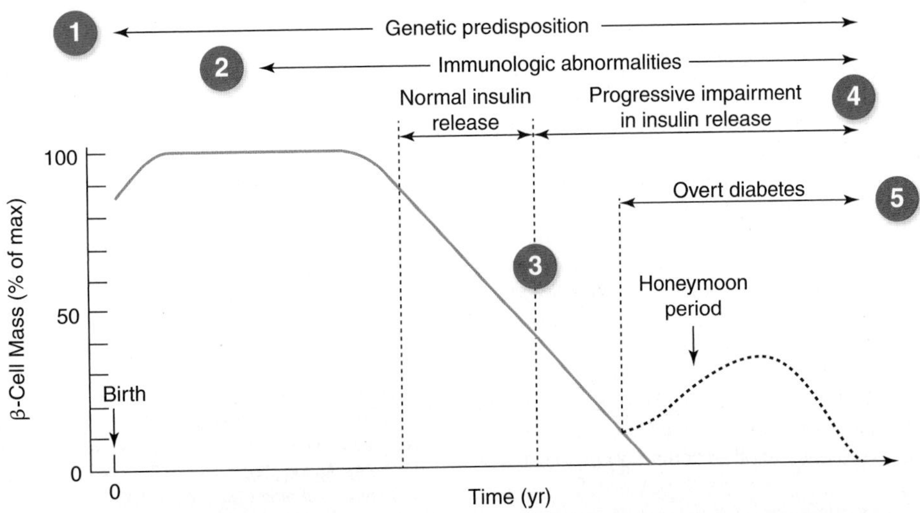

Figure 37.8 ■ Proposed scheme in the development of T1D. The process leading to the development of T1D is thought to occur over a period of time in the following stages: (1) genetic predisposition, (2) triggering of autoimmunity, (3) development of antibodies (insulitis and beta-cell injury are present), (4) loss of the initial (first-phase) insulin response to glucose challenge (an impairments in glucose tolerance is present), and (5) overt T1D.

and additional inflammatory leukocytes are activated and recruited to the tissue. The second proposed theory is termed *molecular mimicry* and has been used to explain several autoimmune diseases. According to the molecular mimicry hypothesis, a susceptible host encounters an environmental trigger, such as a virus, with antigens that are immunologically similar to those of the host but differ enough to induce an immune response when presented to T cells. Subsequently, the tolerance to autoantigens breaks down, and the immune response that is generated cross-reacts with host structures to cause tissue damage and disease.

Check Your Progress: Section 37.4

1. What are the primary factors involved in the development of T1D?
2. What is the proposed sequence of events leading to T1D?
3. What country has the highest T1D occurrence?

37.5 Type 2 Diabetes Mellitus

Type 2 diabetes mellitus, the most common form of DM, is a heterogeneous disorder that results from the interaction of genetic susceptibility and environmental factors. This disorder is characterized by decreased liver, muscle, and adipose tissue sensitivity to insulin and a defect in insulin secretion from the pancreatic beta cell.

Etiology of Type 2 Diabetes Mellitus

Several factors are associated with the development of T2D.

Genetics

The genetic heritability of T2D is stronger than that for T1D and is estimated to account for 40–80% of disease susceptibility.[11] People with T2D often have a family history of the disorder. In the general population, the risk of developing T2D is approximately 3%.[11] The concordance rate among monozygotic twins, dizygotic twins, and siblings is approximately 90%, 10%, and 10%, respectively. Having a mother with T2D presents a T2D risk of approximately 15–20%, while having a father with T2D elicits a T2D risk of 15%.[11] If both parents have T2D, the risk increases to 75%. Type 2 diabetes is a polygenic disorder; no single gene explains its inheritance.[11] Over the past decade, the use of genome-wide association studies have successfully identified 40 genetic loci associated with T2D; this information has the potential to allow for greater T2D prediction and personalized treatment.[16] See the Genetics and Genomics for Clinical Practice feature.

Ethnicity

Diabetes disproportionately affects minority populations; 7.6% of non-Hispanic Whites, 9.0% of Asian Americans, 12.8% of Hispanics/Latinos, 13.2% of non-Hispanic Blacks, and 15.9% of American Indians/Alaskan Natives have diagnosed DM.[17]

Data from populations whose origins are a mixture of different ethnic groups with varying risks for T2D have provided indirect evidence that there is a genetic predisposition to this disease. Many Hispanics living in the southwestern United States share genes with Native Americans, such as the Pima Indians, and with Caucasians, who are at much lower risk for developing DM. A study of Mexican Americans indicated that the prevalence of T2D in this group is associated with the proportion of Native American genes in

Genetics and Genomics for Clinical Practice

Genetics and Diabetes Management

Rita Kaspar

Type 2 diabetes mellitus is an extremely common condition in the United States. Current approches to treatment include lifestyle modifications and a number of antidiabetics, such as metformin, sulfonylureas, and insulin.[1] Despite the wide use and established validation of recommended guidelines, considerable drug response variation exists among patients. Genetically, the C allele of a single nucleotide polymorphism, rs8192675, in the intron of Solute Carrier Family 2 Member 2 (SLC2A2), an important glucose transporter gene, has been found to contribute to a genetic defect in glucose metabolism and therefore a higher baseline glycated hemoglobin (HbA1C, an indicator of average blood glucose over a period of time). A recent landmark study revealed that in treating carriers of C allele at rs8192675, the use of metformin resulted in better glycemic control as defined by higher net HbA1C reduction, in comparison to sulfonylureas,[2] another commonly used class of antidiabetic.

Debates are ongoing regarding whether or not to perform genomic screening procedures before initiating treatment to determine the most effective drug to treat each diabetic individual. Genomic screening involves additional cost, while inexpensive blood tests such as HbA1C monitoring can easily serve as a treatment response indicator. However, using HbA1C as a tool for treatment response monitoring requires many months of time, which may be followed by many rounds of drug changes. Also controversial is whether existing financial resources should be redirected toward developing genomic screening techniques or toward offering innovative educational programs on nutrition and exercise to help patients with type 2 diabetes maintain glycemic control. What do you think?

References

1. Nathan, D. M., Buse, J. B., Davidson, M. B., Ferrannini, E., Holman, R. R., Sherwin, R., & Zinman, B. (2009). Medical management of hyperglycemia in type 2 diabetes: A consensus algorithm for the initiation and adjustment of therapy: A consensus statement of the American Diabetes Association and the European Association for the Study of Diabetes. *Diabetes Care*, *32*(1), 193–203. http://doi.org.proxy.lib.ohio-state.edu/10.2337/dc08-9025

2. Zhou, K. K. (2016). *Nature genetics: Variation in the glucose transporter gene SLC2A2 is associated with glycemic response to metformin.* Bethesda, MD: Genetics Society of America. doi:10.1038/ng.3632

this population.[18] Although this study is dated, its results are still relevant to understanding the etiology of DM.

Obesity

A Westernized lifestyle, including high-calorie diets and reduced physical activity, is linked to the global increase in both T2D and obesity. Although total body obesity has long been established as a risk factor for T2D, the role of central obesity (obesity centered on the trunk) has gained prominence as a risk factor for T2D. Central body obesity appears to be a prognostic marker for glucose intolerance, hyperinsulinemia, and hypertriglyceridemia. In addition, the development of metabolic syndrome is associated with increased risk of T2D.[15] Chapter 5 details the role of obesity in the development of chronic diseases, including T2D.

Physical Inactivity

A number of classic epidemiologic studies during the past few decades have demonstrated that high levels of physical activity protect against the development of T2D.[19–21] One of the most important intervention studies delineating the role of exercise in the prevention of DM was the Diabetes Prevention Program. In this study, 3234 adults with elevated fasting and postprandial plasma glucose concentrations (i.e., individuals with prediabetes) were randomized into three groups: placebo, medication metformin (an oral hypoglycemic medication), or a lifestyle modification program.[22] The lifestyle intervention program reduced the incidence of T2D by 58%, and metformin reduced the incidence by 31% when compared with placebo. The study concluded that to prevent one case of DM during a 3-year period, 6.9 individuals would have to participate in the lifestyle intervention program, and 13.9 would have to receive metformin. Therefore, the lifestyle intervention was more effective than the metformin.

Urbanization

When certain populations migrate from rural to urban settings, their incidence of T2D increases. Because urbanization is associated with changes in diet, physical activity, socioeconomic activity, and obesity, the risk of T2D increases. The best example is the Pima Indians of the southwestern United States, who have a greater than 50% chance of developing T2D in their lifetime but whose relatives in Mexico have a very low risk of DM.[23]

Socioeconomic Status

Socioeconomic status is associated with the development of T2D. Individuals in the lowest socioeconomic brackets have the highest risk of T2D.[24] In addition, lower levels of education also are inversely related to T2D risk.[25]

Intrauterine Environment

Intrauterine factors may increase the risk of T2D. For example, low birth weight has been associated with increasing insulin resistance and DM in the offspring.[11] Conversely, infants of women with DM often have a high birth weight and are at increased risk of DM.[11] Research in the role of intrauterine environment and DM is ongoing and important in understanding the fetal origins of DM.

At any age, pregnancy in a woman with DM is associated with significant maternal and fetal risks, especially if the mother does not have excellent glucose control before gestation. ■

Pathogenesis of Type 2 Diabetes Mellitus

The development of T2D follows a typically evolving course, which can be divided broadly into three stages.

In the first stage, likely genetic factors influence both insulin sensitivity and insulin secretion. For example, environmental factors such as obesity and physical inactivity may decrease insulin sensitivity or increase insulin resistance. At this stage, although there is an underlying defect in insulin secretion, the pancreatic beta cell can produce a high level of insulin, and compensatory hyperinsulinemia maintains normal blood glucose levels (**Figure 37.9** ■).

In the second stage, insulin resistance increases further, and this compensatory hyperinsulinemia becomes insufficient to maintain normal glucose homeostasis. Under conditions of insulin resistance, visceral adipose tissue is very sensitive to the effects of catecholamines and associated with enhanced lipolysis. This leads to increased FFA production and mobilization, exacerbating insulin resistance in liver and muscle. In addition, impairments in insulin-mediated glucose uptake, particularly at the muscle, become evident. Insulin-mediated glucose transport into skeletal muscle, the major target for glucose disposal, becomes impaired. Fasting plasma glucose levels remain normal, but postprandial plasma glucose levels rise (**Figure 37.10** ■).

In the third stage, insulin resistance increases further. The restraining effects of insulin on hepatic glucose

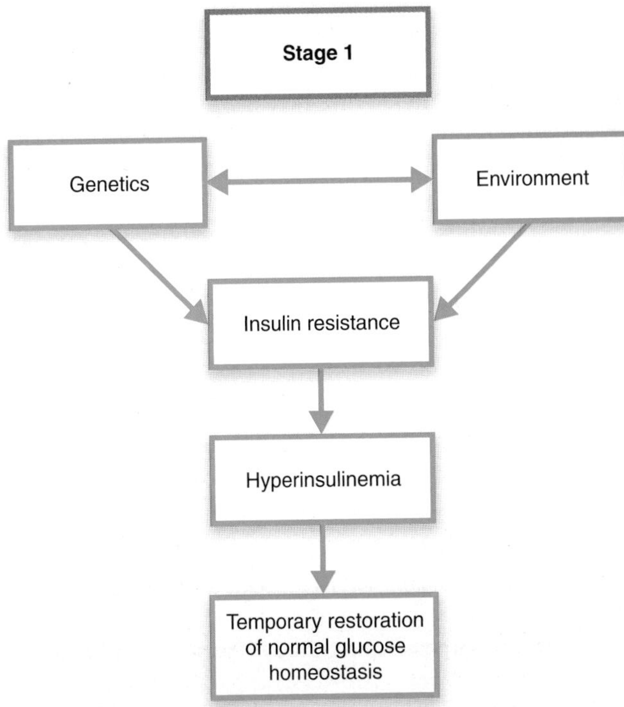

Figure 37.9 ■ Stage 1 in the development of T2D.

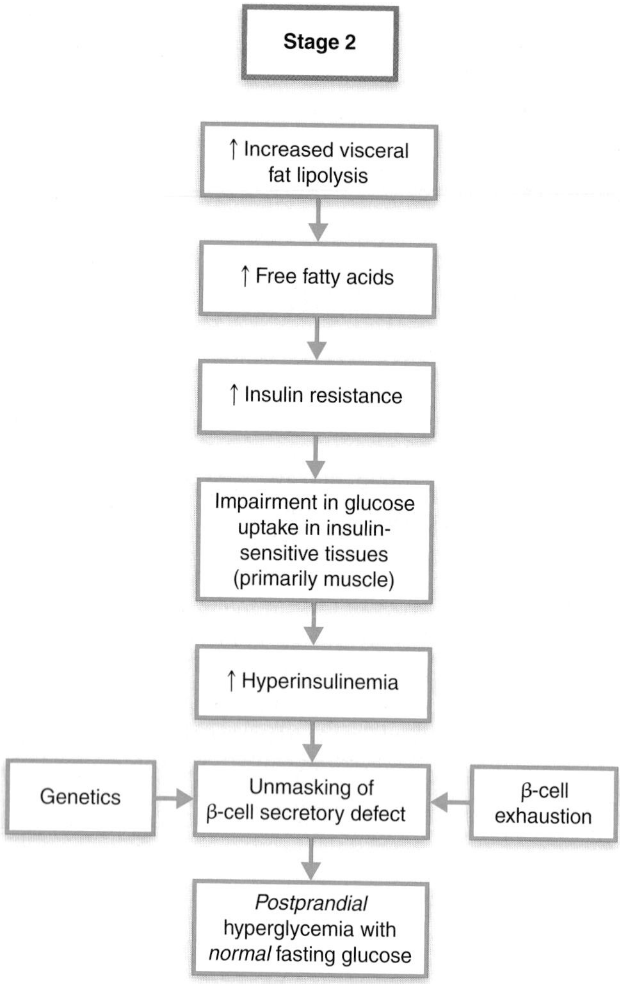

Figure 37.10 ■ Stage 2 in the development of T2D.

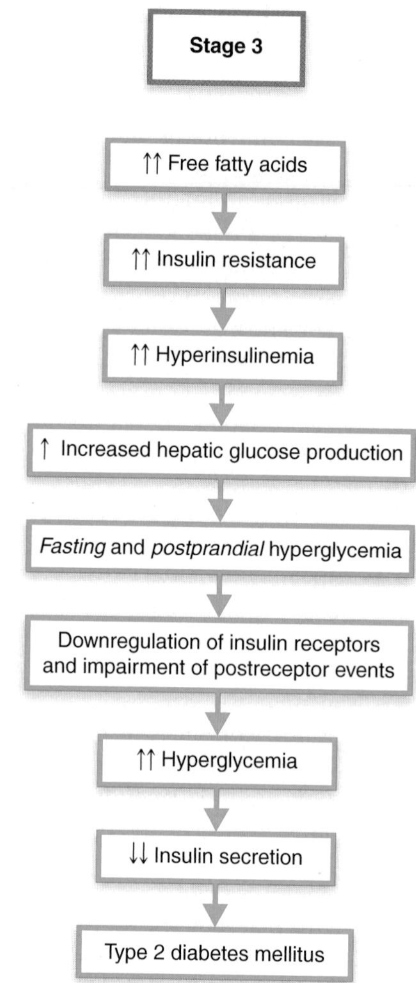

Figure 37.11 ■ Stage 3 in the development of T2D.

production become impaired, and plasma glucose levels increase. In addition, effects of worsening hyperglycemia on the pancreatic beta cell become toxic, and insulin secretion subsequently declines. With increasing insulin resistance, FFA production and mobilization become even greater. The increased FFAs lead to subsequent increases in insulin resistance. Fasting and postprandial hyperglycemia result from increased insulin resistance, unrestrained hepatic glucose production, and glucose toxicity (**Figure 37.11** ■).

Menses in adolescent and adult women is often accompanied by hyperglycemia and increased insulin needs each month. The reasons for these increased insulin requirements are not certain; however, this consideration poses significant management challenges for women with DM. ■

Check Your Progress: Section 37.5

1. What are the different factors associated with the development of T2D?
2. Which factor is considered the highest predisposing factor in the development of T2D?
3. Which ethnicity has the highest incidence of DM?
4. Discuss the stages of T2D pathogenesis.

37.6 Clinical Manifestations of and Diagnostic Criteria for Diabetes Mellitus

Clinical Manifestations of Diabetes Mellitus

Diabetes mellitus has numerous clinical signs and symptoms, which are primarily related to hyperglycemia and ketosis. The symptoms that are primarily related to hyperglycemia are discussed below. The clinical signs and symptoms of ketosis are discussed in Section 37.7.

The following are common signs and symptoms of T1D and T2D:

- ***Polydipsia*** (increased thirst) is a compensatory response to dehydration and volume depletion.
- ***Polyphagia*** (increased appetite) results from the significant calories that are lost through the urine.
- ***Polyuria*** (increased urination) is associated with the presence of glucose in the renal tubules leading to an osmotic diuresis.

- *Weight loss* occurs through dehydration, volume depletion, and loss of calories in the urine.
- *Nocturia* is frequent urination at night in response to polyuria.
- *Glucosuria* (excretion of glucose in the urine) occurs when blood glucose levels exceed the renal threshold for reabsorption of glucose.
- *Hypotension* (decreased blood pressure) results from dehydration and volume depletion.
- *Tachycardia* (increased heart rate) also results from dehydration and volume depletion.
- *Fatigue* is most likely related to alterations in CHO, protein, and lipid metabolism; however, the causes are not completely clear.

Although people with GDM can have these clinical symptoms if their blood glucose is elevated, most people with GDM do not exhibit any signs and symptoms. In general, people with prediabetes do not exhibit any signs and symptoms.

Diagnostic Criteria for Diabetes Mellitus

The diagnostic criteria for diabetes, prediabetes, and GDM are detailed below.

Type 1 and Type 2 Diabetes Mellitus in the Nonpregnant Adult

The diagnosis of DM in nonpregnant adults should be restricted to those who have one of the following[26]:

- *A1C ≥ 6.5%.* The *A1C* test result reflects your average blood glucose level for the past 2 to 3 months.
- *Symptoms of diabetes plus casual plasma glucose concentration ≥ 200 mg/dL.* The classic symptoms of DM include polyuria, polydipsia, and unexplained weight loss. Casual refers to any time of day without regard to time since last meal.
- *Fasting plasma glucose ≥ 126 mg/dL.* The classic symptoms of DM include polyuria, polydipsia, and unexplained weight loss. Casual refers to any time of day without regard to time since last meal. In the absence of unequivocal hyperglycemia with acute metabolic decompensation, these criteria should be confirmed by repeat testing on a different day.
- *2 hour plasma glucose ≥ 200 mg/dL during an oral glucose tolerance test.* The test should be performed by using a glucose load containing the equivalent of 75 grams of anhydrous glucose dissolved in water. The OGTT measures the body's ability to metabolize glucose. Blood glucose levels are measured before and periodically after ingesting 75 grams of glucose. In this case, the glucose level is measured at 2 hours following ingestion of glucose.

Gestational Diabetes Mellitus

GDM carries an increased risk for both the mother and the infant. The Hyperglycemia and Adverse Pregnancy Outcomes study,[27] a large-scale multinational epidemiologic study, demonstrated that the risk of adverse maternal, fetal, and neonatal outcomes continuously increases as a function of maternal blood glucose levels at 24–28 weeks, even within ranges that were previously considered normal for pregnancy. The most recent diagnostic criteria for the development of GDM are outlined in **Box 37.1**.

Rose Garcia's fasting blood glucose during the OGTT at this time is greater than 92 mg/dL, which is diagnostic of GDM. There are factors in her history that suggest that she may previously have had undetected GDM. These include the

Box 37.1
Screening for and Diagnosis of Gestational Diabetes Mellitus

One-Step Strategy

- Perform a 75-gram OGTT, with fasting plasma glucose measurements following at 1 and 2 hours, at 24–28 weeks of gestation in women not previously diagnosed with DM.

The diagnosis of GDM is made when any of the following plasma glucose values are met or exceeded:

- Fasting: 92 mg/dL
- 1 hour: 180 mg/dL
- 2 hours: 153 mg/dL.

Two-Step Strategy

- **Step 1:** Perform a nonfasting 50-g glucose load test with plasma glucose measurements at 1 hour, at 24–28 weeks of gestation in women not previously diagnosed with diabetes.
- If the plasma glucose level measured 1 hour following the glucose load is ≥ 140 mg/dL,* practitioners follow-up with a 100-gram OGTT.
- **Step 2:** A fasting 100-gram OGTT should be performed.

The diagnosis of GDM is made if at least two of the following four plasma glucose levels are met or exceeded. In general, practitioners choose one of the following sets of criteria:

Criteria 1[1]	*Criteria 2*[2]
Fasting 95 mg/dL	105 mg/dL
1 hr 180 mg/dL	190 mg/dL
2 hr 155 mg/dL	165 mg/dL
3 hr 140 mg/dL	145 mg/dL

The American Congress of Obstetricians and Gynecologists recommends a threshold of 135 mg/dL in women from high-risk ethnic populations with higher prevalence of GDM; others recommend a threshold of 130 mg/dL.[3]

References

1. Carpenter, M. W., & Coustan, D. R. (1982). Criteria for screening tests for gestational diabetes. *American Journal of Obstetrics and Gynecology, 144*, 768–73.
2. American Diabetes Association. (1979). Classification and diagnosis of diabetes mellitus and other categories of glucose intolerance. National Diabetes Data Group. *Diabetes, 28*, 1039–1057.
3. American Diabetes Association. (2015). Classification and diagnosis of diabetes. *Diabetes Care, 38*(Suppl.), S8–S16.

birth of two children with a birth weight over 9 pounds and the neonatal hypoglycemia.[28] Infants of mothers with GDM may develop hyperinsulinemia in response to their mother's blood glucose during the pregnancy. These infants may have periods of **hypoglycemia** (low serum glucose level) shortly after birth because of increased insulin levels (in response to their mother's blood glucose in their blood).

Rosa Garcia: Outcome

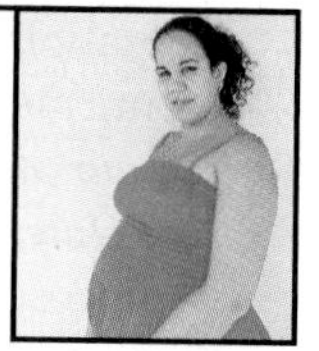

Ms. Garcia maintains normal blood glucose levels throughout her pregnancy through the use of insulin and nutrition therapy. In addition, she has worked with an exercise physiologist to guide her on individualized and appropriate exercise during pregnancy. Ms. Garcia delivers a normal weight infant with no complications such as hypoglycemia.

7. What factors may have contributed to the normal symptoms of the newborn?

Prediabetes

The diagnostic criteria for prediabetes are as follows[26]:

- ***Impaired fasting glucose.*** Fasting plasma glucose of 100–125 mg/dL
- ***Impaired glucose tolerance:*** 2-hour plasma glucose during the OGTT of 140–199 mg/dL
- ***Elevated A1C:*** 5.7–6.4%

Isaiah Coleman: Outcome

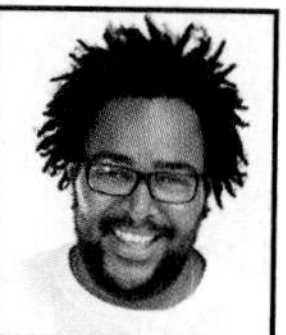

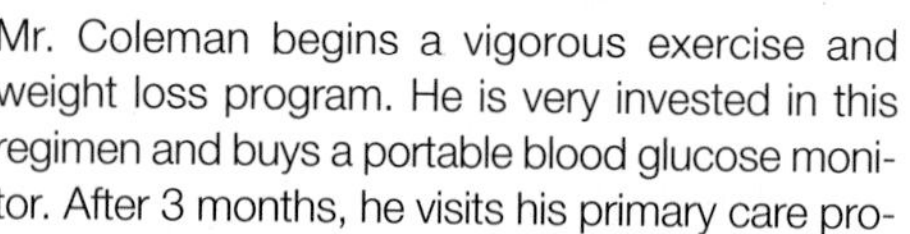

Mr. Coleman begins a vigorous exercise and weight loss program. He is very invested in this regimen and buys a portable blood glucose monitor. After 3 months, he visits his primary care provider. He has lost 4.5 kg. His fasting blood glucose is 101 mg/dL. He tells his healthcare provider that he has noticed that his blood glucose is consistently elevated a few hours after meals. The healthcare provider orders an OGTT and notes that Mr. Coleman's blood glucose is 155 mg/dL 2 hours after he drinks 75 grams of a glucose solution. Additionally, his A1C is 5.8%. His healthcare provider notes that although Mr. Coleman still has prediabetes, his metabolic status has improved. After 3 more months and a weight loss of an additional 10 pounds, Mr. Coleman's values normalize (fasting plasma glucose [95 mg/dL]; A1C [5.4%]; 2-hour post-glucose [120 mg/dL]). His healthcare provider tells him that he no longer has prediabetes but needs to maintain his current treatment plan.

5. Discuss the results of Mr. Coleman's tests the first time he lost weight.
6. What factors contributed to Mr. Coleman's resolution of prediabetes?
7. What does the A1C 5.4 result from Mr. Coleman's blood test indicate?

Check Your Progress: Section 37.6

1. What are the common signs and symptoms of T1D and T2D? Describe each.
2. List the diagnostic criteria for DM.
3. List the diagnostic criteria for prediabetes.

37.7 Acute Complications of Diabetes Mellitus

Diabetes mellitus is associated with a number of life-threatening and debilitating acute and chronic complications. The acute complications include diabetic ketoacidosis, hyperglycemic hyperosmolar syndrome, and hypoglycemia.

Acute complications are associated with increased morbidity and mortality in older adults. Longer duration of DM is associated with increased complications and severe comorbidities. ■

Diabetes mellitus complications increase with duration of disease. Women who are pregnant and have a longstanding history of DM, associated complications, or both usually require care from healthcare teams who specialize in high-risk pregnancy. ■

Diabetic Ketoacidosis

Diabetic ketoacidosis (DKA) is one of the most serious complications of DM and is most commonly associated with T1D. DKA is a state of absolute or relative insulin deficiency that is typically characterized by hyperglycemia, metabolic acidosis, and ketonemia. The most common causes of DKA are underlying infection, disruption of insulin treatment, and new onset of T1D.

Etiology and Pathogenesis

One of the best ways to understand the pathophysiology of DKA is to explore the independent effects of insulin deficiency and counterregulatory hormones on CHO and fat metabolism and to discuss how these processes are interrelated.

Insulin Deficiency and CHO Metabolism. The effects of insulin deficiency on CHO metabolism are illustrated in **Figure 37.12** ■. An absolute or relative insulin deficiency results in decreased glucose utilization by the peripheral tissues, particularly muscle and adipose tissue. Hyperglycemia occurs as a result of decreased glucose transport, hepatic and muscle glycogenolysis, and hepatic gluconeogenesis. Glycosuria and osmotic diuresis occur when blood glucose levels exceed the renal threshold. This results in an osmotic diuresis caused by the presence of certain substances, such as glucose, in the kidney tubules. An osmotic diuresis results in volume depletion and a reduced glomerular filtration rate (GFR). Such reductions in GFR cause decreased renal excretion of glucose, further increasing the hyperglycemia.

Adults with an intact thirst mechanism and normal renal function may initially become only mildly hyperglycemic during DKA because the kidneys are able to excrete some of the filtered glucose load. Adults without intact thirst mechanisms (e.g., following a stroke) may not be able to compensate for their fluid loss and may become severely hyperglycemic. The loss of water and electrolytes leads to dehydration and hemoconcentration. There is a marked reduction in circulating blood volume, leading to peripheral circulatory failure progressing to shock, hypotension, and

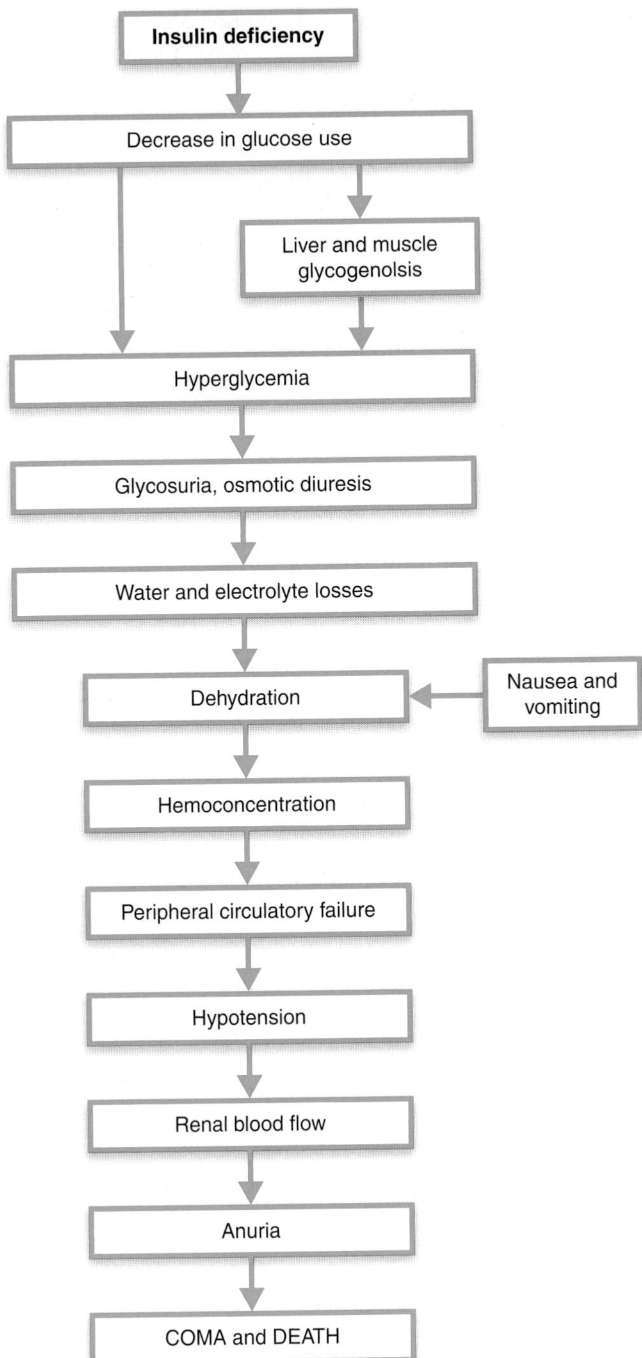

Figure 37.12 ■ Effects of insulin deficiency on carbohydrate metabolism.

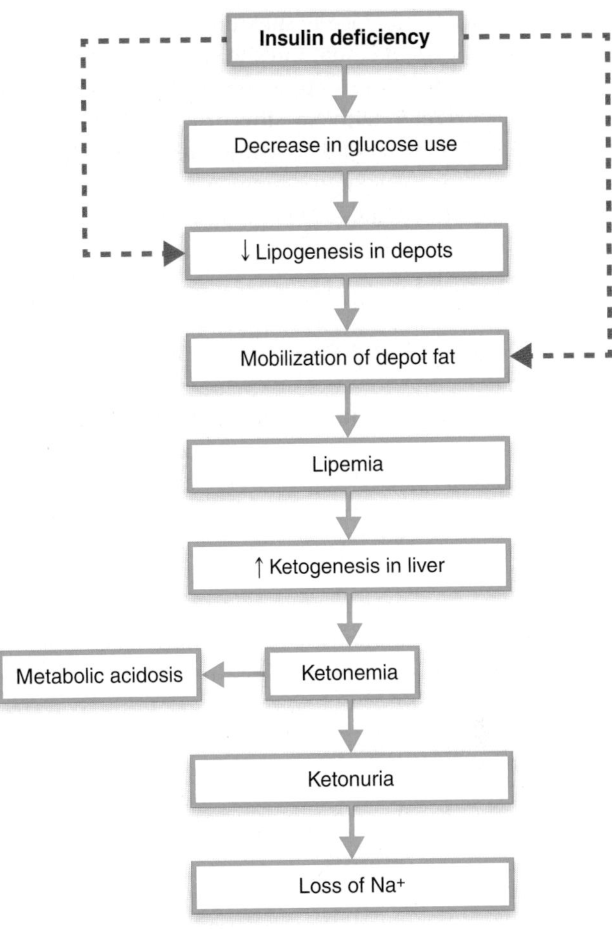

Figure 37.13 ■ Effects of insulin deficiency on fat metabolism.

anuria (inability of the kidneys to produce urine). In addition, there is generalized tissue anoxia (absence of oxygen supply to an organ), with a shift to anaerobic metabolism (oxidation of substrates in the absence of oxygen), resulting in increasing concentrations of lactic acid in the blood. Coma and death eventually result after the development of peripheral circulatory failure.

The potential for dehydration increases with age, especially in individuals who cannot easily access fluids or who lack intact thirst mechanisms (e.g., following stroke). ■

Insulin Deficiency and Fat Metabolism. The effects of insulin deficiency on fat metabolism are illustrated in **Figure 37.13** ■. Insulin deficiency and decreased glucose utilization by adipose tissue result in mobilization of depot fat in the blood. There is a generalized **lipemia** (excess lipids in the blood). A secondary hypertriglyceridemia (excess triglycerides in the blood) occurs as free FFAs are synthesized in the liver into very low-density lipoproteins (LDLs). The liver is flooded with FFAs, which are oxidized as far as the acetyl-CoA stage. Acetyl-CoA is converted in the mitochondria to acetoacetate, which is spontaneously decarboxylated (loses a carboxyl group) to acetone or converted to 3-hydroxybutyrate.

The ketone bodies that are produced during DKA include acetoacetate, 3-hydroxybutyrate, and acetone. Acetoacetate and 3-hydroxybutyrate are strong organic acids that dissociate readily and account for the acidosis in DKA.[29] Acetone does not dissociate readily and does not contribute to acidosis but is excreted slowly by the lungs. Ketones are buffered after release from the liver, decreasing the body's buffering capacity.[29] The developing **ketonemia** (excess ketones in the blood) leads to progressive metabolic acidosis, which in turn initiates the characteristic deep and rapid respirations accompanied by an acetone odor to the breath (**Kussmaul respirations**). These Kussmaul respirations are a compensatory response to metabolic acidosis, designed to reduce CO_2. As the renal threshold for ketone reabsorption is exceeded, ketones appear in the urine (**ketonuria**). Ketones are excreted with Na^+; this process contributes to a net Na^+ loss. Severe metabolic acidosis results in depression of the respiratory vasomotor center, compromised cardiovascular output, and reduced vascular tone. This may result in cardiovascular collapse with the generation of lactic acid, which adds to the existing acidosis.

Insulin Deficiency and Protein Metabolism. The effects of insulin deficiency on protein metabolism are illustrated in **Figure 37.14** ■. Insulin deficiency results in decreased protein synthesis and promotes overall protein catabolism (breakdown), particularly in muscle. This catabolism results in a net loss of nitrogen from the body, which can be manifested in elevated levels of blood urea nitrogen (BUN). This is accompanied by a net loss of K^+, particularly from muscle protein breakdown. Progressive dehydration also results in protein catabolism, and additional K^+ is subsequently lost in the urine. The final result is a net loss of body K^+ stores.

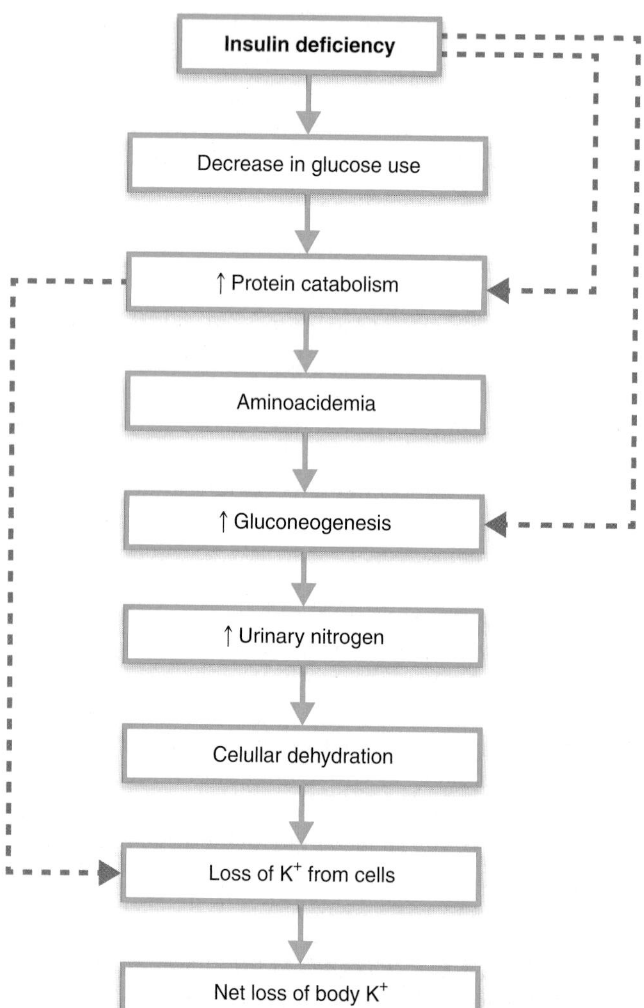

Figure 37.14 ■ Effects of insulin deficiency on protein metabolism.

Precipitating Factors. The most common precipitating factor in the development of DKA is infection.[30] Other precipitating factors include new-onset T1D and omission or reduction in the current insulin dose. For example, when patients are unable to afford their medications, they may omit their insulin injections or inject lower than prescribed doses. Eating disorders in adolescents with T1D are also associated with DKA, as such patients may withhold insulin injections to lose weight.[31] When patients with T1D or insulin-requiring T2D develop other medical conditions (e.g., pancreatitis, myocardial infarction), the physiologic stress of such conditions usually requires an increase in overall exogenous insulin doses. If the insulin dose is not increased, DKA may develop.

Clinical Manifestations

The signs and symptoms of DKA include the following:

- Polyuria resulting from a hyperglycemia-induced osmotic diuresis.
- Polyphagia resulting from the inability to appropriately metabolize energy substrates. As the metabolic acidosis progresses, however, polyphagia is generally replaced by anorexia (loss of appetite), owing to the appetite-suppressing effects of ketones.
- Polydipsia is a compensatory response to fluid volume depletion.
- Weight loss results from fluid volume depletion and altered CHO, protein, and lipid metabolism.
- Fatigue likely occurs in response to altered CHO, protein, and lipid metabolism, especially protein catabolism.
- Blurred vision occurs in response to hyperglycemia, as fluid accumulates in the lens of the eye, causing refractory changes.
- Hypotension, tachycardia, and poor skin turgor result from fluid volume depletion. As the metabolic acidosis and volume depletion progress, orthostatic hypotension occurs.
- Cardiac arrhythmias result primarily from electrolyte disturbances, such as abnormal serum K^+ levels.
- Nausea and vomiting are thought to result from the accumulation of serum ketones.
- Abdominal pain is frequently present in DKA. The cause of this pain has not been determined, but it may be related to a decrease in total body K^+ stores.
- Kussmaul respirations (deep rapid respirations) are a compensatory mechanism to decrease $PaCO_2$.
- The red, flushed face that is seen in concert with Kussmaul respirations is due to the increased levels of $PaCO_2$, which have a vasodilating effect.
- Decreased mental status and coma in DKA are primarily due to fluid volume depletion and serum hyperosmolality.

Linking Pathophysiology to Diagnosis and Treatment

The diagnosis of DKA is based on laboratory criteria that reflect hyperglycemia, ketosis, and metabolic acidosis, particularly these three: (1) plasma glucose greater than

250 mg/dL, (2) presence of ketones in serum or urine, and (3) presence of acidosis (serum bicarbonate $<$ 18 mEq/L and/or an arterial pH $<$ 7.3 and an elevated anion gap).[30]

The general treatment of DKA involves support measures to prevent cardiac, pulmonary, and neurologic decompensation; intravenous insulin therapy to reduce hyperglycemia and correct the acidosis; intravenous fluids correct the fluid volume deficits; and intravenous electrolyte replacements to correct electrolyte disturbances.

CLINICAL POINT: DKA presents special problems in the pediatric and geriatric populations. For example, toddlers and elderly people may not be able to access fluids readily in response to thirst and can develop significant fluid volume deficits quickly. Mortality from DKA increases with age. Cerebral edema is a possible complication of DKA. Although the exact cause of DKA is unknown, a number of theories have been proposed. The most popular of these include the cytotoxic and vasogenic theories. The cytotoxic theory suggests that brain cells become hypertonic. The vasogenic hypothesis suggests that during DKA, there is a disruption of vascular permeability in the blood–brain barrier, which contributes to the cerebral edema.[32] ■

Melissa Bailey: Outcome

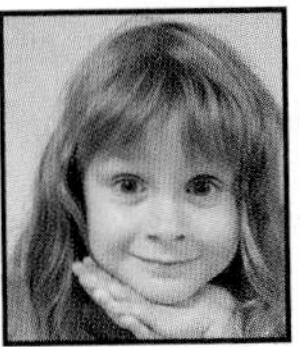

Melissa Bailey presented to the emergency department with an episode of the "flu" from which she is not recovering appropriately. She has polyuria, polyphagia, and weight loss, which are classic signs of hyperglycemia. The signs are substantiated by a random blood glucose level of 250 mg/dL. She recently developed generalized anorexia abdominal pain, and her breath has an acetone odor. These signs and symptoms are consistent with a diagnosis of DKA. On further evaluation in the emergency department, the healthcare provider notes that Melissa is dehydrated, has Kussmaul respirations, and has a deteriorating mental status. On further workup, her arterial blood pH is 7.1, reflecting metabolic acidosis and elevated K^+. The diagnosis of T1D and DKA is substantiated with hyperglycemia, dehydration, fluid and electrolyte imbalances, and a metabolic acidosis. Melissa is hospitalized for several days, during which time she is provided with supportive care and is given intravenous insulin and fluids and electrolyte replacements as appropriate. Her response to therapy is closely monitored. As she recovers from the DKA, Melissa and her mother are taught insulin injection techniques and blood glucose monitoring and receive dietary instructions. Melissa and her mother are introduced to insulin pump therapy, which provides continuous basal insulin levels with a calculated insulin bolus before meals and snacks They decide that they will adopt this method at a later date. Melissa is discharged with a follow-up appointment within a week.

7. What may have caused Melissa's dehydration?
8. Why did Melissa experience weight loss?
9. Explain Melissa's DKA symptoms.
10. What laboratory criteria verified the diagnosis of Melissa's DKA?

Hyperglycemic Hyperosmolar Syndrome

Hyperglycemic hyperosmolar syndrome (HHS) was first described in the 1950s with published reports of patients presenting to emergency departments with severe hyperglycemia and coma but without ketosis.

Etiology and Pathogenesis

Individuals who have IGT or T2D are most vulnerable to developing HHS. HHS is associated with conditions that are known to impair insulin action or insulin secretion or both, especially if ready access to fluids is not available. Therefore, infirm, neglected, very young, very old, institutionalized, and mentally deficient patients who cannot recognize their thirst or express their need for water are often at risk. In addition, this syndrome is seen in patients with excessive unreplaced fluid losses secondary to massive glycosuric diuresis and following gastrointestinal fluid losses and a limited fluid intake. More commonly, patients present with a significant diuresis that is associated with severe hyperglycemia and hyperosmolarity. In this case, the hyperglycemia is likely initiated by prednisone therapy.

The pathophysiology of HHS, detailed in **Figure 37.15** ■, is similar to that of DKA; however, there are some underlying differences. HHS usually occurs in individuals with suboptimally treated or undiagnosed IGT or T2D. The development of the hyperglycemia is initiated by factors (e.g., stress and medications) that increase insulin resistance and/or decrease insulin secretion. In HHS, blood glucose levels are increased by factors that cause insulin resistance and/or insulin secretion. As in DKA, HHS is associated with glycosuria, an osmotic diuresis, and urinary electrolyte losses. The osmotic diuresis can lead to dehydration, severe volume depletion, shock, coma, and possibly death. A number of factors, such as vomiting and diarrhea, may also contribute to the degree of dehydration. A significant reduction in GFR from dehydration and volume depletion results in an inability to dispose of some of the excess glucose through the kidneys; this further potentiates hyperglycemia. Metabolic acidosis does not develop, presumably because the underlying plasma insulin levels are sufficient to inhibit unrestrained lipolysis and the subsequent formation of ketones. HHS may evolve over a period of days to weeks, leading to more profound hyperglycemia, dehydration, and hyperosmolality than are seen in DKA.

Clinical Manifestations

As was noted previously, the clinical signs and symptoms of DKA are primarily associated with hyperglycemia, fluid volume deficits, electrolyte disturbances, metabolic acidosis, and ketosis. Patients with HHS do not have clinical signs and symptoms related to metabolic acidosis and ketosis; however, the other clinical signs and symptoms related to hyperglycemia (fluid volume deficits and electrolyte imbalances) are often present. In HHS, the hyperglycemia, dehydration, and serum hyperosmolality are usually much more severe than in DKA. In addition to the clinical signs and symptoms detailed in DKA, the following may be present in HHS:

- Neurologic symptoms such as hemiparesis, seizures, and coma result from cerebral dehydration.
- Vascular thrombosis results from severe dehydration, with HHS patients at greater risk cause of the severity of dehydration and hyperosmolality.

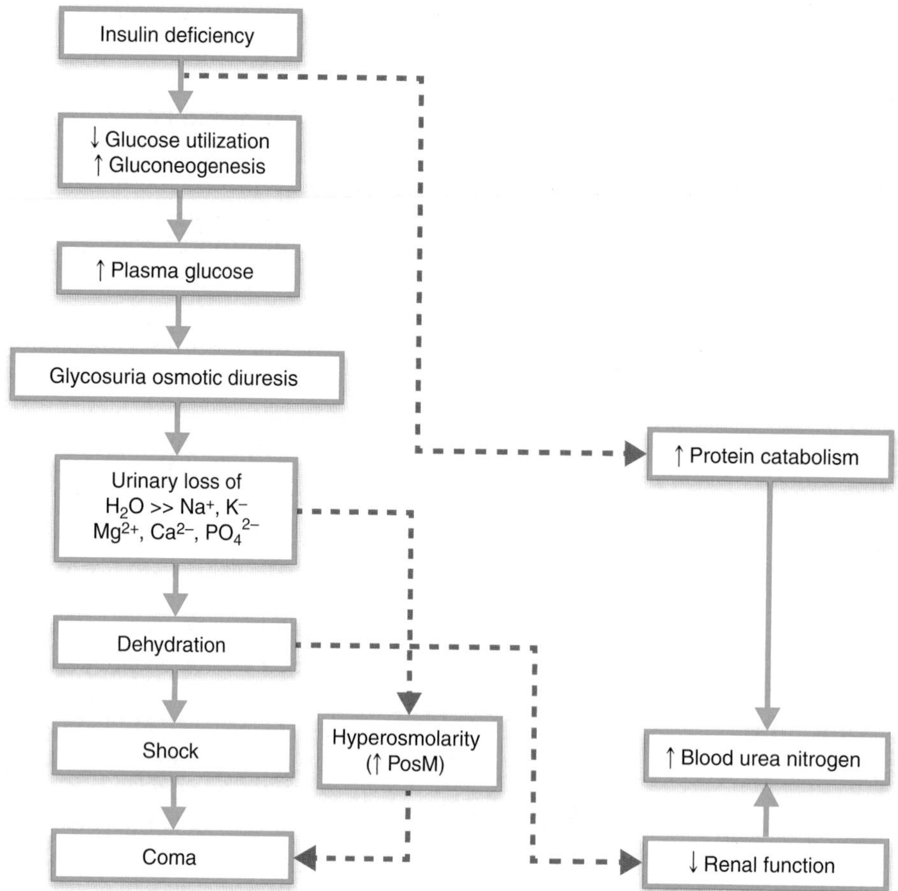

Figure 37.15 ■ Hyperglycemic hyperosmolar syndrome.

Linking Pathophysiology to Diagnosis and Treatment

The diagnostic features of HHS include (1) a plasma glucose level of 600 mg/dL or more, (2) effective serum osmolality of 320 mOsm/kg or more, (3) profound dehydration (typically 8–12 L) with elevated BUN:creatinine ratio, (4) a bicarbonate level greater than 18 mEq/L, and (5) alteration in consciousness.[33]

Treatment of HHS involves support measures to prevent cardiac, pulmonary, and neurologic decompensation; intravenous insulin therapy to reduce hyperglycemia; intravenous fluids correct the fluid volume deficits; and intravenous electrolyte replacements to correct electrolyte disturbances.

CLINICAL POINT: HHS has been considered a disease of the elderly and infirm, rarely occurring in children and adolescents. With the increased prevalence of DM in children and adolescents, HHS is becoming more likely to occur in pediatric populations. There have been increasing numbers of case reports of children and adolescents with DM developing HHS.[34] Providers need to have a heightened awareness of this condition so that treatment can be initiated early. ■

Hypoglycemia

Hypoglycemia is a medical emergency that is characterized by decreased blood glucose levels (< 60 mg/dL) and associated with a variety of autonomic nervous system (ANS) and neuroglycopenic symptoms.

Etiology and Pathogenesis

Glucose is the obligate fuel for the brain and central nervous system. The brain is unable to synthesize or store glucose and must rely on circulating plasma blood glucose. In nondiabetic subjects, the normal plasma blood glucose level is maintained through the complex interplay among insulin, glucagon, and other counterregulatory hormones. In nondiabetic patients, plasma insulin levels decline as blood glucose levels decline; plasma insulin levels increase as blood glucose increases. However, in patients who are being treated with insulin or insulin secretagogues, plasma insulin levels and blood glucose may not decline appropriately with lower blood glucose levels. The counterregulatory hormones such as glucagon, epinephrine, cortisol, and growth hormone increase in an attempt to correct the hypoglycemia. Normal glucose counterregulation in response to hypoglycemia is diagrammed in **Figure 37.16** ■. Hypoglycemia results when glucose utilization is greater than glucose production.

Hypoglycemia is primarily a complication of T1D and insulin-treated T2D. Hypoglycemia can also occur with oral hypoglycemic medications that stimulate endogenous insulin secretion (e.g., sulfonylureas, meglitinides). In normal physiology, a decline in blood glucose levels is paralleled by a decline in endogenous insulin secretion and an increase in counterregulatory hormones. This process leads to increased blood glucose levels. When patients are treated with exogenous insulin and (to a lesser extent) selected oral hypoglycemic

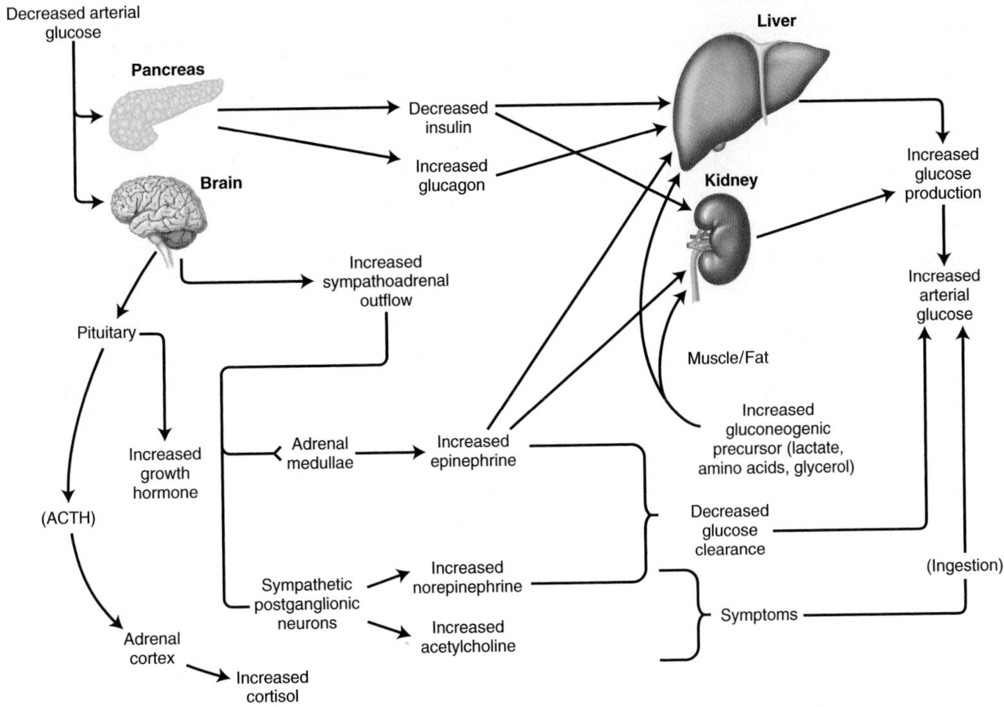

Figure 37.16 ■ Counterregulatory response to hypoglycemia.

SOURCE: Bilous, R. W., Donnelly, R., & Williams ,G. (2010). (4th ed.). Hoboken, NJ: Wiley-Blackwell.)

medications, the glucose-stimulated decline in plasma insulin levels is impaired. There is an inappropriately high plasma insulin level in relation to the prevailing blood glucose level; this causes hypoglycemia. Precipitating factors of hypoglycemia in diabetic patients (treated with exogenous insulin or selected oral hypoglycemic medications) include factors that increase exogenous or endogenous insulin in relation to plasma glucose. Some of these factors include an incorrect amount (too much) or type of insulin (e.g., rapid-acting instead of long-acting), missing meals and snacks, and exercise.

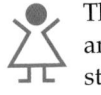
The potential for hypoglycemia in infants, toddlers, and younger children is increased as a result of struggles over food intake, which are common at these ages. For example, a toddler's refusal to eat following administration of insulin may place the child at risk for hypoglycemia. ■

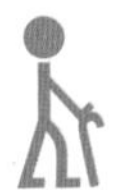
The potential for hypoglycemia in older adults increases as a result of several factors (e.g., change in taste perception, satiety, defective counterregulation). ■

Clinical Manifestations

Hypoglycemia is associated with a number of symptoms that are generally grouped into two major categories: those related to the ANS and those related to neuroglycopenia (decreased glucose to the brain and nervous tissues). These are listed in **Table 37.2** ■. ANS symptoms prompt individuals to eat and thus raise the blood glucose level; these symptoms are subdivided into adrenergic (e.g., tremors, palpitations, nervousness, anxiety) and cholinergic (e.g., sweating and hunger) categories. The neuroglycopenic symptoms result from glucose deprivation to the central nervous system and include irritability, confusion, drowsiness, weakness, difficulty speaking, unresponsiveness, unconsciousness, seizures, and coma.

Table 37.2 Physiologic Responses to Hypoglycemia

Autonomic Nervous System Symptoms	Neuroglycopenic Symptoms
Sweating	Difficulty speaking
Palpitations	Incoordination
Tremors	Visual disturbances
Hunger	Atypical behavior
	Drowsiness
	Confusion
	Seizures
	Coma

In hypoglycemia unawareness, there is a loss of ANS symptoms during a hypoglycemic event. These symptoms are crucial because they prompt individuals to consume food to raise the blood glucose. In the absence of these symptoms, patients may progress rapidly to severe hypoglycemia. Hypoglycemia unawareness results from altered counterregulation, particularly decreased glucagon response to hypoglycemia and deficient epinephrine response. Patients with hypoglycemic unawareness develop neuroglycopenic symptoms without warning and are at significant risk for injury.

Linking Pathophysiology to Diagnosis and Treatment

The symptoms of hypoglycemia clearly mimic the underlying pathophysiologic process with both ANS symptoms (e.g., shaking and diaphoresis) and neuroglycopenia (e.g., behavioral changes). When people with hypoglycemia are treated with glucose and the blood glucose is normalized, these symptoms should resolve.

Check Your Progress: Section 37.7

1. What are the symptoms of hypoglycemia?
2. How do the symptoms of the ANS differ from those related to neuroglycopenia?
3. How are these symptoms altered in hypoglycemic unawareness?
4. What are the signs and symptoms of DKA?
5. What are the signs and symptoms of HHS?

37.8 Chronic Complications of Diabetes Mellitus

The chronic complications of DM include **microvascular diseases** (diseases of smaller vasculature, including retinopathy, nephropathy, and neuropathy) and **macrovascular diseases** (diseases of large vasculature, including accelerated development of all forms of cerebrovascular disease, stroke, and peripheral vascular disease).

Proposed Pathogenesis of Microvascular Complications

The classic Diabetes Control and Complications Trial (DCCT)[35] and the United Kingdom Prospective Diabetes Study (UKPDS)[36] identified hyperglycemia as the primary factor in the development of the microvascular complication of DM. The microvascular changes include retinopathy (eye disease), neuropathy (nerve disease), and nephropathy (kidney disease). The tissue-damaging effect of hyperglycemia occurs primarily in capillary endothelial cells in the retina, mesangial cells of the renal glomerulus, and neurons and Schwann cells in the peripheral nerves.[37] These cells become the target of hyperglycemia because they are not able to reduce the transport of glucose inside the cell when they are exposed to hyperglycemia, so their internal glucose concentration stays constant. The development of these complications has been the focus of ongoing research. There appear to be four major processes involved; these involve increased flux through the polyol pathway, intracellular production of advanced glycation end product precursors, protein kinase C activation, and increased hexosamine pathway activity. A general review of each of these processes is provided below.

Increased Glucose Flux Through the Polyol Pathway

Unlike many tissues (such as muscle) that depend on insulin for glucose transport, cells in the retina, kidney, and nervous tissue do not require insulin to transport glucose across the cell membrane. The polyol pathway is a biochemical pathway (**Figure 37.17** ■) that, under conditions of normoglycemia, allows for the metabolism of a small amount of glucose. Under conditions of hyperglycemia, however, significantly more glucose enters this pathway. The general theory as to how increased glucose flux through this pathway may contribute to complications is illustrated in Figure 37.17.

Aldose reductase is one of the primary enzymes in this pathway. The primary function of aldose reductase is to reduce toxic aldehydes (highly reactive organic compounds) in the cell to inactive alcohols. When the glucose concentration in the cell becomes too high, aldose reductase reduces glucose to sorbitol, which is later oxidized to fructose. In this process, aldose reductase consumes a cofactor, nicotinamide adenine dinucleotide phosphate, which is used for regenerating a critical intracellular antioxidant, reduced glutathione. This inability to regenerate reduced glutathione increases the person's susceptibility to intracellular oxidative stress.[37]

Intracellular Production of Advanced Glycation End Product Precursors

Chronic hyperglycemia results in the development of advanced glycation end products (AGEs). Glycation refers to the nonenzymatic binding of a sugar molecule, such as

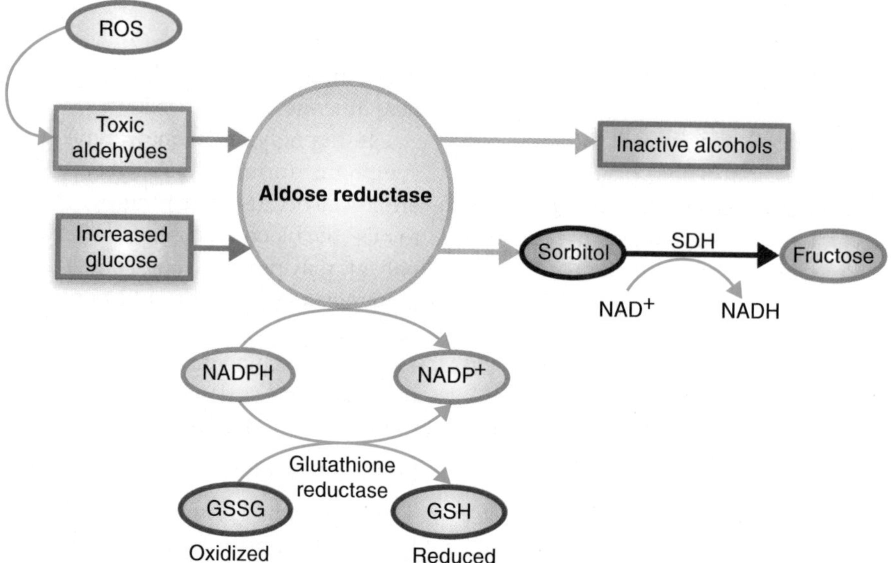

Figure 37.17 ■ Increased glucose flux through the polyol pathway. GSH = glutathione; GSSG = oxidized glutathione; NAD+ = nicotinamide adenine dinucleotide, oxidized; NADH = nicotinamide adenine dinucleotide, reduced; NAP+ = nicotinamide adenine dinucleotide phosphate, oxidized; NADPH = nicotinamide adenine dinucleotide phosphate, reduced; ROS = reactive oxygen species; SDH = sorbitol dehydrogenase.

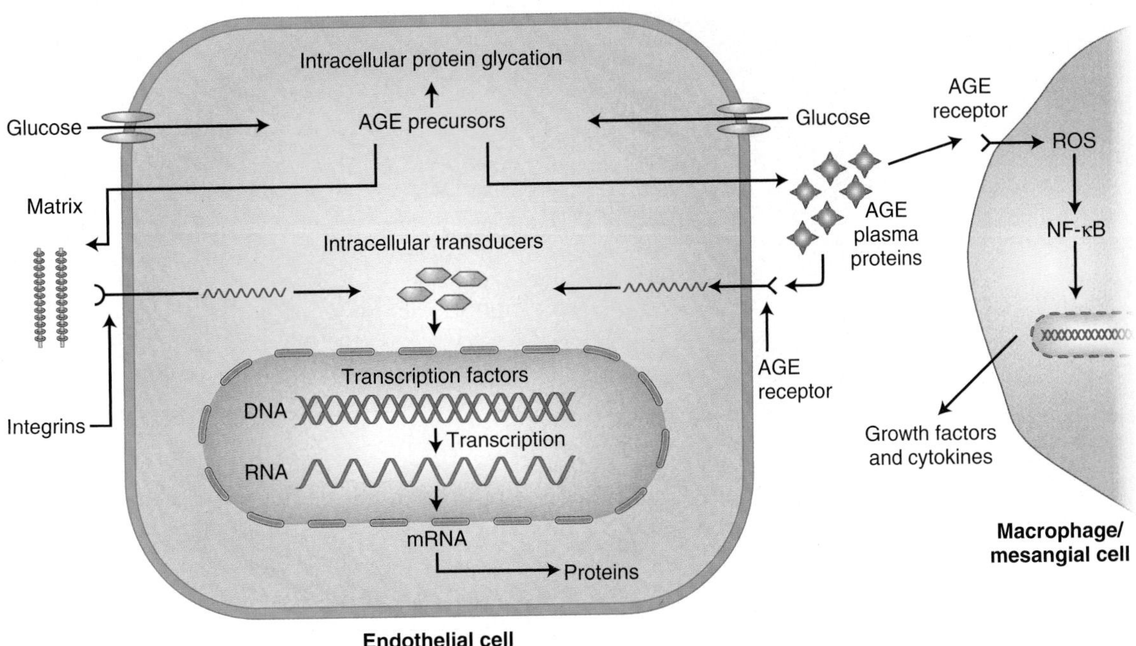

Figure 37.18 ■ Intracellular production of advanced glycation end product precursors.

fructose or glucose, to a protein or lipid molecule. The binding of glucose to a protein results in alterations in the protein structure, in turn resulting in the development of irreversible AGEs. These AGEs appear to damage cells by three mechanisms (**Figure 37.18** ■): (1) alteration of intracellular proteins that are essential in the regulation of gene transcription; (2) diffusion from the cell of AGE precursors that modify nearby extracellular matrix molecules such that signaling between the matrix and the cell is altered, leading to cellular dysfunction; and (3) diffusion of AGE precursors from the cell and subsequent alteration of circulating proteins in the blood, such as albumin. These modified circulating proteins bind to AGE receptors and activate them, thereby causing the production of inflammatory cytokines and growth factors, which contribute to vascular dysfunction.

Protein Kinase Cs

Protein kinase Cs (PKCs) are a family of protein kinases, most of which are activated by the lipid second messenger system diacylglycerol. When PKC is activated by intracellular hyperglycemia, it appears to initiate a variety of effects on gene expression, leading to a variety of pathogenic abnormalities, such as basement membrane thickening, blood flow abnormalities, increased vascular permeability, angiogenesis, decreased fibrinolysis, and vascular occlusion (**Figure 37.19** ■).

Increased Hexosamine Biosynthetic Pathway Activity

Most of glucose is metabolized through glycolysis. However, in conditions of hyperglycemia, some of the fructose-6-phosphate (an intermediate in the pathway) is channeled into the hexosamine pathway. This pathway eventually produces a biochemical compound called uridine diphosphate (UDP) N-acetyl glucosamine, which attaches to serine and threonine residues of transcription factors. This attachment results in biochemical changes (e.g., increased expression

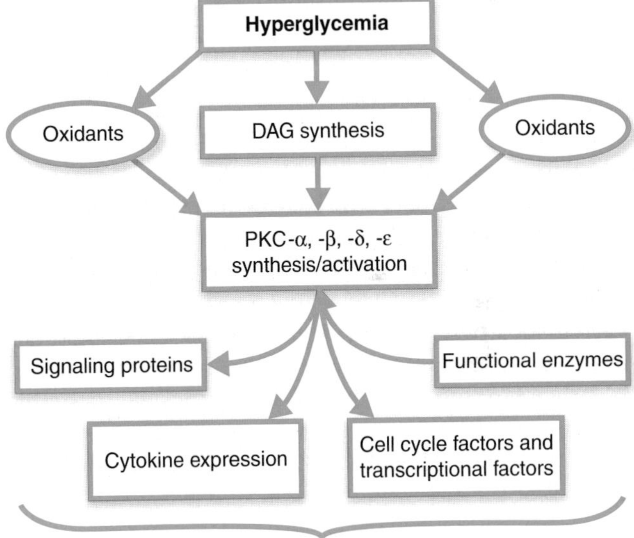

Figure 37.19 ■ Protein kinase C. DAG = diacylglycerol.

of transforming growth factor-1 and plasminogen activator inhibitor-1) that are implicated in the development of complications (**Figure 37.20** ■).

Integration of the Four Causative Mechanisms in the Development of Microvascular Disease

A theory uniting all of the previously described pathogenic mechanisms (i.e., increased flux through the polyol pathway, intracellular production of AGE precursors, PKC activation, and increased hexosamine pathway activity) has been developed. Although this theory was published in 2005, it remains relevant today.[37] The common thread among all of these processes is overproduction of superoxide by the mitochondrial electron transport chain. In summary,

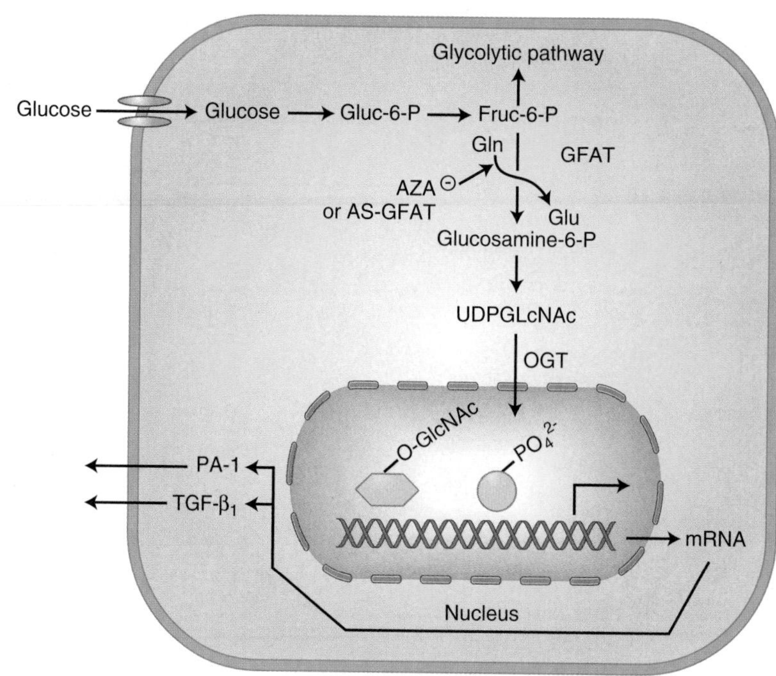

Figure 37.20 ■ Increased hexosamine biosynthetic pathway activity. AS-GFAT = antisense to GFAT; AZA = azaserine; Fruc-6-P = fructose-6-phosphate; GFAT = glutamine fructose-6-phosphate aminotransferase; Gln = glutamine; Gluc-6-P = glucose-6-phosphate; O-GlcNAc = O-linked *N*-acetylglucosamine; OGT = O-linked *N*-acetylglucosamine transferase; TGF = transforming growth factor; UDP-GLcNAc = uridine diphosphate *N*-acetylglucosamine.

when intracellular hyperglycemia develops in target cells of DM complications, such as those in the retina, kidney, and peripheral nerves, there is an increase in mitochondrial production of reactive oxygen species (ROS). The ROS causes strand breaks in nuclear DNA. In response to these breaks, an enzyme, poly(ADP-ribose) polymerase (PARP), is activated to repair these breaks. The increase in PARP modifies glyceraldehyde-3-phosphate dehydrogenase (GAPDH), an important enzyme in glycolysis and gluconeogenesis. This decreases GAPDH's activity, which activates the polyol pathway, increases the production of AGE precursors, and activates PKC and the hexosamine pathway.

Retinopathy

Retinopathy (disease of the retina that results in loss of vision) is a major cause of blindness and visual disturbances. In fact, DM is the leading cause of new cases of blindness among adults aged 20–74 years.[6] Diabetic retinopathy involves damage to the blood vessels in the retina, which can result in a variety of pathophysiologic changes, including the formation of microaneurysms (pouchlike dilation of terminal retinal capillaries), excessive vascular permeability, vascular occlusion, neovascularization (proliferation of new blood vessels), fibrous tissue on the retina, contraction of the fibrous tissues, and new vessels on the vitreous.

Etiology and Pathogenesis

The primary contributors to visual impairment are excessive vascular occlusion or vascular permeability. These precipitating events lead to macular edema, neovascularization, and fibrous tissue proliferation, which can result in vitreous hemorrhage. Vitreous hemorrhages are associated with the development of more severe forms of diabetic retinopathy, while the neovascularization and fibrous tissue proliferation are associated with retinal distortion and detachment. Each of these processes can result in visual loss. The classification of diabetic retinopathy is based on the severity of the retinal microvascular changes and the presence of retinal neovascularization.

Retinopathy can be divided into pre-retinopathy, nonproliferative retinopathy, and proliferative retinopathy. Normally, the retinal veins are approximately 1.5 times the size of the retinal arteries. In pre-retinopathy, the major retinal veins grow to approximately 2–3 times the size of the arteries. In nonproliferative or background retinopathy, microaneurysms appear as small red dots on the retina. These small aneurysms are outpouchings of the retinal capillaries and are often referred to as *dot and blot hemorrhages*. These hemorrhages usually do not cause visual impairment; however, they may be associated with the development of diabetic macular edema and may progress to proliferative retinopathy. Proliferative retinopathy is characterized by neovascularization of the retinal surface. These vessels can bleed into the vitreous or preretinal space and cause visual loss. A diagram of diabetic retinopathy is presented in **Figure 37.21** ■.

Clinical Manifestations

The development and progression of retinopathy generally depend on the duration of DM and overall glucose control. As was noted in the DCCT,[34] optimal glucose control decreases development and progression of retinopathy. Macular edema is associated with hypertension; therefore, well-controlled blood pressure reduces the likelihood of development of macular edema.

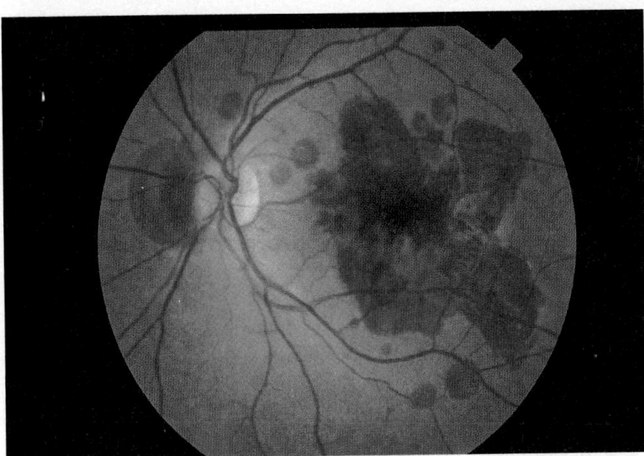

Figure 37.21 ■ Damaged blood vessels in the retina of an individual with diabetic retinopathy.

Not only the retina, but also the lens and vitreous can suffer ocular complications associated with DM. Glucose concentrations equilibrate between the lens and the surrounding aqueous humor; this leads to shifts in water, altering the shape of the eye and causing temporary blurring of vision and refractory changes. These changes resolve with normalization of blood glucose levels, but the process may take up to a month. In addition, in the patient with DM, the lens is more prone to cataract formation. In particular, the more common "senile" cataracts develop at a younger age among individuals with DM.

Linking Pathophysiology to Diagnosis and Treatment

Depending on the severity of the retinopathy and associated complications, there are a variety of treatments to prevent blindness. Initially, however, retinopathy may be asymptomatic. This is why routine eye examinations are part of the standard of care for individuals with DM. The loss of vision associated with proliferative retinopathy and macular edema can be reduced by laser photocoagulation if patients at risk are identified in an expedient manner. Unfortunately, the progressive nature of proliferative retinopathy may lead to blindness despite treatments.

Nephropathy

DM is also the leading cause of **nephropathy** (damage to the kidneys), accounting for 44% of new cases in 2008.[6] Diabetic nephropathy is a clinical syndrome characterized by proteinuria, hypertension, edema, and renal insufficiency occurring in patients with long-standing DM (usually more than 10 years' duration).

Etiology and Pathogenesis

Nephropathy is characterized by three classes of renal histopathologic changes: glomerulosclerosis, structural vascular changes (primarily in the small arterioles), and tubulointerstitial disease. The most characteristic feature of diabetic nephropathy is glomerular damage characterized by renal mesangial expansion and basement membrane thickening leading to diffuse scarring of the glomeruli.

The usual course of diabetic nephropathy is insidious, and it progresses through several stages. The first evidence of diabetic nephropathy is the development of elevated microalbuminuria (> 30 mg albumin/24 hours). As the nephropathy progresses, there is an increase in proteinuria (> 300 mg albumin/24 hours), which coincides with the development of hypertension. Nephrotic-range proteinuria develops, GFR decreases, and serum creatinine increases. Eventually, end-stage renal disease occurs.

Clinical Manifestations

The development of diabetic nephropathy is often asymptomatic, and it is detected on routine laboratory screening tests. The development of diabetic nephropathy largely depends on the duration of disease and glucose control. The first sign of developing nephropathy is the presence of microalbuminuria.

Linking Pathophysiology to Diagnosis and Treatment

Microalbuminuria should prompt the healthcare provider to aggressively treat even minor elevations in blood pressure to preserve renal function. In particular, angiotensin-converting enzyme inhibitors and angiotensin receptor blockers are most beneficial in delaying the progression of nephropathy in patients with DM and microalbuminuria. If diabetic nephropathy leads to kidney failure, renal replacement therapy can be provided by hemodialysis, continuous ambulatory peritoneal dialysis, and kidney transplantation.

Neuropathy

Neuropathy is damage to nerves. Diabetic neuropathy is the nerve damage caused by DM.

Etiology and Pathogenesis

The pathogenesis of diabetic neuropathy is highly complex, involving several mechanisms. The prevailing theory suggests that chronic hyperglycemia increases polyol pathway activity. As a result, fructose and sorbitol accumulate in nerves, damaging them by unknown mechanisms. This is accompanied by decreased myoinositol uptake and inhibition of Na^+/K^+ ATPase. This results in a variety of pathologic conditions, including Na^+ retention, edema, myelin swelling, and nerve degeneration.

Clinical Manifestations

Diabetic neuropathy can affect any area of the body and exists primarily as autonomic neuropathies, distal symmetric polyneuropathies, and mononeuropathies.

- *Autonomic neuropathy* can affect all aspects of autonomic functioning, particularly those involving the cardiovascular, gastrointestinal, and genitourinary systems.
- *Cardiovascular autonomic neuropathy* is associated with a variety of clinical manifestations, most particularly resting tachycardia (more than 100 beats per minute) and orthostasis (a decrease in systolic blood pressure greater than 20 mmHg on standing).[38] Patients may complain of dizziness or weakness, nausea, vomiting, and syncope when they rise quickly.
- *Gastrointestinal disturbances* are common in DM and may include esophageal disturbances, gastroparesis, diarrhea, and fecal incontinence.[38] Gastroparesis is characterized by the impaired transit of food from the stomach to the duodenum in the absence of

a mechanical obstruction. This condition is characterized by early satiety, nausea, vomiting, and abdominal discomfort. These symptoms are often accompanied by fluctuations in blood glucose levels due to delayed gastric emptying or retention of food products.

- *Diabetic diarrhea* is characterized by the frequent passage of loose stools occurring primarily after meals and during the night. Some patients have alternating periods of diarrhea and constipation. The cause of the diarrhea is unknown, and diagnosis is made after other causes of diarrhea (e.g., infection) are excluded.
- *Neurogenic bladder and sexual dysfunction* may occur because diabetic autonomic neuropathy is associated with genitourinary tract disturbances. These may include bladder and and/or sexual dysfunction. Neurogenic bladder is characterized by a pattern of frequent, small voiding and incontinence leading to urinary retention.[38] In males, diabetic neuropathy may result in the loss of penile erection and/or retrograde ejaculation.
- *Symmetric distal polyneuropathy* is most commonly seen in the legs, feet, and hands. Although symmetric distal polyneuropathy is predominantly associated with sensory loss, motor and autonomic nerve fibers can be affected. As the name implies, it usually appears first in the distal portions of the extremities, moving proximally in a "stocking–glove" distribution, encompassing both sensory and motor nerve damage and affecting both limbs. Clinical symptoms associated with sensory nerve damage may include numbness, pain, burning, tingling, and eventual partial or total loss of sensation. The pain associated with symmetric distal polyneuropathy is first felt distally, in the lower legs, and usually worsens at night. The pain can be persistent or intermittent, occurring over periods of weeks or months. This pain is usually described as an aching or burning. Eventually, there is loss of protective sensation and increased risk of lower limb and foot injuries, including ulcers. Most diabetic lower-extremity amputations in individuals with DM originate from the combination of diabetic foot ulcers, peripheral arterial disease, peripheral vascular disease, peripheral neuropathy, minor trauma, deformity, increased plantar pressures, and infection contributing to the development and progression of these ulcers.
- *Mononeuropathies* tend to be abrupt and painful in isolated cranial or peripheral nerves or in multiple isolated nerves. Vascular occlusion and ischemia are thought to be implicated in the development of these asymmetric focal neuropathies.[15] The third nerve is the most common cranial nerve involved in mononeuropathy, which is characterized by ipsilateral headache, ptosis (weakening of the eyelid), and ophthalmoplegia (weakening of one or more muscles supporting the eye).

Linking Pathophysiology to Diagnosis and Treatment

Diabetic neuropathy may have diverse clinical presentations, and there are a number of treatments, which depend on the underlying type of neuropathy and associated complications. Regardless of the type of neuropathy, optimal glucose control is needed to prevent and slow the progression of diabetic neuropathy.

Norma James: Outcome

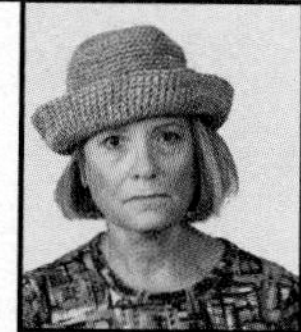

Ms. James has bilateral peripheral neuropathy that affects her lower extremities. Although it had initially caused severe pain, the neuropathy has now progressed to numbness in both lower extremities. Ms. James notices a skin ulcer on her right ankle that has been present for several weeks; she begins to place "wound butter" on the ulcer, on the recommendation of a cashier at a convenience store. The ulcer becomes infected, requiring dressing changes by a visiting nurse and a 10-day course of antibiotics. The ulcer does heal; however, Ms. James's nurse practitioner outlines a plan of care on DM management, emphasizing good foot care practices.

7. Explain the type of neuropathy Ms. James is experiencing.
8. What contributed to the worsening symptom of Ms. James's right ankle ulcer?
9. What were the signs and symptoms of diabetic neuropathy Ms. James experienced?
10. Apart from the medical treatment administered, what factor is important to prevent the progression of diabetic neuropathy?

Proposed Pathogenesis of Macrovascular Complications

As was noted previously, the causal link between DM and microvascular complications is hyperglycemia. The causal link between DM and macrovascular complications is not as clear. The macrovascular complications include aggressive and accelerated rates of stroke, cardiovascular disease, and peripheral vascular disease.

The primary theory of pathogenesis suggests that the macrovascular complications are mediated by both hyperglycemia and insulin resistance. Insulin resistance is associated with increased release of FFAs, which causes an atherogenic lipid and lipoprotein profile, which is characterized by reduced high-density lipoprotein (HDL); increased triglycerides; and increased small, dense LDLs. In addition to the lipoprotein abnormalities, FFA flux increases from adipocytes into arterial endothelial cells. This increased flux results in increased FFA oxidation by the mitochondria and overproduction of ROS. As with hyperglycemia, this FFA-induced increase in ROS activates the same damaging pathways, the polyol pathway, the hexosamine pathway, and PKC and causes increased production of AGE precursors. Atherosclerotic macrovascular disease occurs more frequently in patients with DM and is associated with an increased incidence in all major forms of large-vessel disease.

Refer to Chapter 23 for more information on peripheral vascular disease Refer to Chapter 27 for more information on stroke.

Check Your Progress: Section 37.8

1. What are the major chronic complications of DM?
2. What are macrovascular and microvascular complications?
3. What are the fundamental pathways implicated in the development of these complications?
4. What are the effects of these complications on physical functioning?

CHAPTER SUMMARY

37.1 Chapter Overview and Case Studies

Describe the epidemiology of diabetes mellitus and concepts related to diabetes mellitus.

- Diabetes mellitus affects approximately 29.1 million people in the United States, or 9.3% of the of the U.S. population.
- In 2013, an estimated 382 million people worldwide had DM; this number is expected to increase to 592 million by 2035.
- Diabetes mellitus is the leading cause of kidney failure, nontraumatic lower-limb amputations, and new cases of blindness among U.S. adults; and it remains a major cause of heart disease and stroke.

37.2 Classification of Diabetes Mellitus and Prediabetes

Compare and contrast the four categories of diabetes mellitus.

- There are four clinical classifications of DM and two categories of increased risk for developing DM.
- The clinical classifications are T1D, T2D, other specific types, and GDM.
- Categories associated with increased risk of DM are IFG and IGT, which are referred to as prediabetes.

37.3 Maintenance of Normal Blood Glucose Levels

Identify the hormones and biochemical processes involved in fuel substrate metabolism.

- Plasma glucose concentrations are maintained within a narrow range that is achieved through a balance between glucose entry into the circulation from the liver, intestinal absorption, and glucose uptake into the peripheral sites, such as adipose tissue and skeletal muscle.
- This process is regulated by a network of hormones (e.g., insulin, glucagon, catecholamines, cortisol, growth hormone, glucagon-like peptide 1, and gastric inhibitory polypeptide), neural signals, and substrates (e.g., carbohydrates, fats, and proteins).

37.4 Type 1 Diabetes Mellitus

Differentiate the causes and underlying pathogenesis of type 1 diabetes mellitus.

- Type 1 diabetes mellitus results from an autoimmune destruction of the pancreatic beta cells.
- The etiology of T1D is complex and appears to result from an interaction among genetics, environment, and autoimmunity.
- A familial predisposition to T1D does exist; however, the exact mode of genetic inheritance remains unclear.
- A triggering event in individuals who are at risk for type T1D initiates a series of autoimmune events ending in pancreatic beta-cell destruction.
- Various environmental triggers have been proposed, but no single factor has been consistently associated with initiating T1D. Some of the possibilities include viral infections, dietary factors, and toxins.

37.5 Type 2 Diabetes Mellitus

Differentiate the causes and underlying pathogenesis of type 2 diabetes mellitus.

- People with T2D have a relative insulin deficiency and insulin resistance
- There is genetic heritability of T2D, which is estimated to account for 40–80% of disease susceptibility.
- Other major factors associated with the development with T2D include ethnicity, obesity, and physical inactivity.

37.6 Clinical Manifestations of and Diagnostic Criteria for Diabetes Mellitus

Describe the clinical manifestations of type 1 and type 2 diabetes mellitus, gestational diabetes mellitus, and prediabetes.

- The primary clinical manifestations of all types of DM include those related to hyperglycemia (e.g., polyuria, polydipsia, and polyphagia)
- Severe metabolic decompensation in DKA and HHS is associated with a variety of other clinical manifestations.
- Gestational diabetes mellitus is generally asymptomatic; however, the clinical manifestations of hyperglycemia may occur if the blood glucose remains elevated.
- Prediabetes is an asymptomatic condition.

37.7 Acute Complications of Diabetes Mellitus

Differentiate the causes, underlying pathogenesis, and clinical manifestations of acute complications of diabetes mellitus across the lifespan.

- DKA is an acute medical emergency that is primarily associated with T1D. HHS is a medical emergency that is primarily associated with T2D.

- The most common precipitating factor in the development of both DKA and HHS is infection.
- The laboratory values associated with DKA may include those related to hyperglycemia (increased serum blood glucose; increased serum BUN, creatinine, total protein, hematocrit, hemoglobin, and urine or serum osmolality), metabolic acidosis (decreased arterial pH and increased anion gap), and ketosis (increased serum and urinary ketones).
- The laboratory tests are very similar for DKA and HHS. In HHS, there is no metabolic acidosis; therefore, the bicarbonate and arterial pH are normal, and serum and urinary ketones are negative.
- The clinical signs and symptoms of DKA are primarily associated with hyperglycemia (e.g., polyuria, polydipsia); fluid volume deficits (e.g., hypotension); electrolyte disturbances (e.g., abnormal cardiac rhythms); and metabolic acidosis and ketosis (e.g., Kussmaul respirations) or combinations of factors (e.g., increased osmolality serum and worsening metabolic acidosis are associated with decreasing mental status).
- The clinical signs and symptoms of HHS are primarily associated with hyperglycemia, severe fluid volume deficits (e.g., orthostatic hypotension), electrolyte disturbances (e.g., abnormal cardiac rhythms), and hyperosmolality (e.g., neurologic change, venous thrombosis).
- Hypoglycemia is an acute complication that is associated with a number of autonomic (e.g., tremors) and neuroglycopenic (e.g., confusion) symptoms.
- People with DM can develop hypoglycemic unawareness, a condition in which they are not able to feel autonomic symptoms, such as tremors.

37.8 Chronic Complications of Diabetes Mellitus

Differentiate the causes, underlying pathogenesis, and clinical manifestations of chronic complications of diabetes mellitus.

- The chronic complications of DM are those related to microvascular (retinopathy, nephropathy, and neuropathy) and macrovascular disease (cardiovascular disease, peripheral vascular disease, and stroke).
- The clinical manifestations are diverse and related to the system or systems that are affected.
- There appear to be four major processes involved in the development of chronic DM complications. These involve increased flux through the polyol pathway, intracellular production of advanced glycation end product precursors, protein kinase C activation, and increased hexosamine pathway activity.
- These pathophysiologic processes appear to be initiated by hyperglycemia with other pathophysiologic processes, such as abnormal lipids, contributing.
- The development and progression of DM complications can be reduced through maintaining normal blood glucose levels. However, treatment plans also include therapies directed toward normalizing blood pressure and serum lipids.

REVIEW QUESTIONS

1. Which of the following is the primary concept involving the pathophysiology of diabetes mellitus, which is described as insulin secretion that is too low in relation to the blood glucose level?
   a. Absolute insulin deficiency
   b. Relative insulin deficiency
   c. Insulin resistance
   d. Hyperglycemia
2. Which type of diabetes mellitus is associated with the destruction of pancreatic beta cells, which secrete insulin?
   a. Type 1 diabetes mellitus
   b. Type 2 diabetes mellitus
   c. Gestational diabetes mellitus
   d. Other specific types of diabetes mellitus
3. What is the mechanism in fuel metabolism that involves formation of glucose or glycogen from non-CHO sources?
   a. Lipolysis
   b. Glycogenolysis
   c. Ketogenesis
   d. Gluconeogenesis
4. Which of the following is not a factor that results in T1D?
   a. Genetics
   b. Obesity
   c. Environment
   d. Autoimmunity
5. In which stage of T2D does insulin resistance increase further, fasting plasma glucose levels may remain normal, but postprandial plasma glucose levels rise?
   a. First stage
   b. Second stage
   c. Third stage
   d. None of the above
6. How can the diagnosis of DM in individuals who are not pregnant be verified?
   a. Symptoms of diabetes plus casual plasma glucose concentration $\geq$ 125 mg/dL
   b. 2 hour plasma glucose $\geq$ 300 mg/dL during an oral glucose tolerance test.
   c. A1C $\geq$ 6.5%
   d. Fasting plasma glucose $\geq$ 250 mg/dL

7. Which of the following are clinical manifestations of DKA? (Select all that apply.)
   a. Polyuria
   b. Weight loss
   c. Kussmaul respirations
   d. Fluid overload
   e. Cardiac arrhythmias

8. Which condition is described as visual impairment caused by excessive vascular occlusion or vascular permeability?
   a. Retinal detachment
   b. Retinopathy
   c. Glaucoma
   d. Cataract

ANSWERS

Answers to Review Questions can be found in Appendix A. Answers to Case Study and Check Your Progress questions are available on the faculty resources site. Please consult with your instructor.

RECOMMENDED WEBSITES

American Association of Diabetes Educators
www.diabeteseducator.org

American Diabetes Association (ADA)
www.diabetes.org

National Institute of Diabetes and Digestive and Kidney Diseases
www.niddk.nih.gov

JRDF (formerly the Juvenile Diabetes Research Foundation)
www.jdrf.org

REFERENCES

1. Centers for Disease Control Prevention. (2014). *National diabetes statistics report: Estimates of diabetes and its burden in the United States, 2014.* Atlanta, GA: U.S. Department of Health and Human Services, Centers for Disease Control and Prevention.
2. Guariguata, L., Whiting, D., Hambleton, I., Beagley, J., Linnenkamp, U., & Shaw, J. (2014). Global estimates of diabetes prevalence for 2013 and projections for 2035. *Diabetes Research and Clinical Practice, 103,* 137–149.
3. American Diabetes Association. (2014). Diagnosis and classification of diabetes mellitus. *Diabetes Care,* 37(Suppl. 1), S81–S90.
4. Nambam, B., Aggarwal, S., & Jain, A. (2010). Latent autoimmune diabetes in adults: A distinct but heterogeneous clinical entity. *World Journal of Diabetes, 1,* 111–115.
5. National Diabetes Information Clearinghouse. (2014). *Monogenic forms of diabetes: National diabetes mellitus and maturity-onset diabetes of the young.* Bethesda, MD: U.S. Department of Health and Human Services, National Institutes of Health 2014.
6. Centers for Disease Control and Prevention. (2011). *National diabetes fact sheet: National estimates and general information on diabetes and prediabetes in the United States.* Atlanta, GA: U.S. Department of Health and Human Services, Centers for Disease Control and Prevention 2011;201.
7. Barbour, L. A. (2014). Unresolved controversies in gestational diabetes: Implications on maternal and infant health. *Current Opinion in Endocrinology, Diabetes, and Obesity, 21,* 264–270.
8. WHO Multinational Project for Childhood Diabetes (DIAMOND) Research Group. (2006). Incidence and trends of childhood Type 1 diabetes worldwide 1990–1999. *Diabetic Medicine, 23,* 857–866.
9. Bilous, R. W., Donnelly, R., & Williams, G. (2010). *Handbook of diabetes* (4th ed.). Hoboken, NJ: Wiley-Blackwell.
10. Bonifacio, E., & Ziegler, A. G. (2010). Advances in the prediction and natural history of type 1 diabetes. *Endocrinology and Metabolism Clinics of North America, 39,* 513–525.
11. Holt, R. I. G., & Hanley, N. A. (2012). *Essential endocrinology and diabetes* (6th ed.). Chichester, UK: Wiley-Blackwell.
12. Kondrashova, A., & Hyoty, H. (2014). Role of viruses and other microbes in the pathogenesis of type 1 diabetes. *International Reviews of Immunology,* 33, 284–295.
13. Akerblom, H. K., Krischer, J., Virtanen, S. M., et al. (2011). The Trial to Reduce IDDM in the Genetically at Risk (TRIGR) study: Recruitment, intervention and follow-up. *Diabetologia, 54,* 627–633.
14. Knip, M., Akerblom, H. K., Becker, D., et al. (2014). Hydrolyzed infant formula and early beta-cell autoimmunity: A randomized clinical trial. *JAMA, 311,* 2279–2287.
15. Funk, J. (2010). Disorders of the endocrine pancreas. In S. McPhee & G. D. Hammer (Eds.), *Pathophysiology of disease: An introduction to clinical medicine* (6th ed., pp. 497–522). New York, NY: Lange Medical Books/McGraw-Hill.
16. Imamura, M., & Maeda, S. (2011). Genetics of type 2 diabetes: The GWAS era and future perspectives [Review]. *Endocrine Journal, 58,* 723–739.
17. American Diabetes Association. (2014). *Statistics about diabetes.* Retrieved from http://www.diabetes.org/diabetes-basics/statistics.
18. Gardner, L. I., Jr., Stern M. P., Haffner S. M., et al. (1984). Prevalence of diabetes in Mexican Americans: Relationship to percent of gene pool derived from native American sources. *Diabetes, 33,* 86–92.
19. Manson, J. E., Stampfer, M., Colditz, G., et al. (1991). Physical activity and incidence of non-insulin-dependent diabetes mellitus in women. *Lancet, 338,* 774–778.
20. Helmrich, S. P., Ragland, D. R., Leung, R. W., & Paffenbarger, R. S. Jr. (1991). Physical activity and reduced occurrence of non-insulin-dependent diabetes mellitus. *New England Journal of Medicine, 325,* 147–152.
21. Hu, F. B., Manson, J. E., Stampfer, M. J., et al. (2001). Diet, lifestyle, and the risk of type 2 diabetes mellitus in women. *New England Journal of Medicine, 345,* 790–797.
22. Knowler, W. C., Fowler, S. E., Hamman, R. F., et al. (2009). 10-year follow-up of diabetes incidence and weight loss in the Diabetes Prevention Program Outcomes Study. *Lancet, 374,* 1677–1186.

23. Esparza-Romero, J., Valencia, M. E., Martinez, M. E., Ravussin, E., Schulz, L. O., & Bennett, P. H. (2010). Differences in insulin resistance in Mexican and U.S. Pima Indians with normal glucose tolerance. *Journal of Clinical Endocrinology & Metabolism, 95,* E358–E362.
24. Krishnan, S., Cozier, Y. C, Rosenberg, L., & Palmer, J. R. (2010). Socioeconomic status and incidence of type 2 diabetes: Results from the Black Women's Health Study. *American Journal of Epidemiology, 171,* 564–570.
25. Dinca-Panaitescu, S., Dinca-Panaitescu, M., Bryant, T., Daiski, I., Pilkington, B., & Raphael, D. (2011). Diabetes prevalence and income: Results of the Canadian Community Health Survey. *Health Policy, 99,* 116–123.
26. American Diabetes Association. (2015). Classification and diagnosis of diabetes. *Diabetes Care, 38*(Suppl.), S8–S16.
27. Catalano, P. M., McIntyre, H. D., Cruickshank, J. K., et al. (2012). The Hyperglycemia and Adverse Pregnancy Outcome Study associations of GDM and obesity with pregnancy outcomes. *Diabetes Care, 35,* 780–786.
28. Nolan C. J. (2011). Controversies in gestational diabetes. *Best Practice & Research Clinical Obstetrics & Gynaecology, 25,* 37–49.
29. Joslin E. P., & Kahn C. R. (2005). *Joslin's diabetes mellitus* (14th ed.). Philadelphia, PA: Lippincott Williams & Willkins.
30. Maletkovic, J., & Drexler, A. (2013). Diabetic ketoacidosis and hyperglycemic hyperosmolar state. *Endocrinology and Metabolism Clinics of North America, 42,* 677–695.
31. Larranaga, A., Docet, M. F., & Garcia-Mayor, R. V. (2011). Disordered eating behaviors in type 1 diabetic patients. *World Journal of Diabetes, 2,* 189–195.
32. Tasker, R. C., & Acerini, C. L. (2014). Cerebral edema in children with diabetic ketoacidosis: Vasogenic rather than cellular? *Pediatric Diabetes, 15,* 261–270.
33. Corwell, B., Knight, B., Olivieri, L., & Willis, G. C. (2014). Current diagnosis and treatment of hyperglycemic emergencies. *Emergency Medical Clinics of North America, 32,* 437–452.
34. Bagdure, D., Rewers, A., Campagna, E., & Sills, M. R. (2013). Epidemiology of hyperosmolar hyperglycemic syndrome in children hospitalized in USA. *Pediatric Diabetes, 14,* 18–24.
35. Diabetes Control and Complications Trial Research Group. (1993). The effect of intensive treatment of diabetes on the development and progression of long-term complications in insulin-dependent diabetes mellitus. *New England Journal of Medicine, 329,* 977–986.
36. Turner, R., Holman, R., Cull, C., et al. (1998). Intensive blood-glucose control with sulphonylureas or insulin compared with conventional treatment and risk of complications in patients with type 2 diabetes (UKPDS 33). *Lancet, 352,* 837–853.
37. Brownlee, M. (2005). The pathobiology of diabetic complications: A unifying mechanism. *Diabetes, 54,* 1615–1625.
38. American Diabetes Association. (2011). Standards of medical care in diabetes: 2011. *Diabetes Care, 34*(Suppl. 1), S11–S61.

Chapter 38

Thyroid, Parathyroid, and Adrenal Disorders

Laurie Quinn

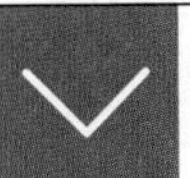

Chapter Outline and Learning Outcomes

38.1 Chapter Overview and Case Studies

Define hormones and concepts related to thyroid and adrenal regulation.

38.2 Mechanisms of Hormonal Alterations in Thyroid and Adrenal Disease

Outline the mechanisms of hormonal alterations, including hormone excess, hormone deficiency, and levels of hormone dysfunction across the lifespan.

38.3 Disorders of the Thyroid

Differentiate the causes, classification, underlying pathogenesis, and clinical manifestations of disorders of the thyroid across the lifespan.

38.4 Disorders of the Parathyroid

Differentiate the causes, classification, underlying pathogenesis, and clinical manifestations of disorders of the parathyroid across the lifespan.

38.5 Disorders of Adrenocortical Function

Differentiate the causes, classification, underlying pathogenesis, and clinical manifestations of disorders of adrenocortical function across the lifespan.

KEY TERMS

Acropachy, 939
Addison disease, 944
Adenoma, 937
Congenital adrenal hyperplasia (CAH), 948
Cushing disease, 946
Cushing syndrome, 946
Dermopathy, 939
Differentiated cancers, 941
Euthyroid, 935
Exophthalmos, 938
Goiter, 936
Graves disease, 938
Hashimoto thyroiditis, 940
Hyperthyroidism, 938
Hypothyroidism, 936
Ophthalmopathy, 939
Pheochromocytoma, 948
Pretibial myxedema, 938
Primary hyperaldosteronism, 947
Primary hypothyroidism, 940
Secondary adrenal insufficiency, 945
Secondary hyperaldosteronism, 947
Tetany, 943
Thyroiditis, 938
Thyroid nodule, 937
Thyroid scintigraphy, 938
Thyroid storm, 939
Thyrotoxicosis, 939
Undifferentiated cancer, 941

ABBREVIATIONS

ACTH—adrenocorticotropic hormone
CKD—chronic kidney disease
CRH—corticotropin-releasing hormone
MEN—multiple endocrine neoplasia
MTC—medullary thyroid cancer
PTH—parathyroid hormone
PTU—propylthiouracil
T3—triiodothyronine
T4—thyroxine
TRAb—TSH receptor antibodies
TRH—thyrotropin-releasing hormone
TSH—thyroid-stimulating hormone

38.1 Chapter Overview and Case Studies

The endocrine system is essential to the regulation of the body. Through hormones secreted by its glands, the endocrine system regulates functions such as growth, reproduction, metabolism, and fluid and electrolyte balance. Disorders of the endocrine system result primarily from either too much or too little production of hormones. These alterations in hormone levels affect many functions, including activity and exercise, nutrition and metabolism, elimination, sexuality and reproduction, and the ability to cope with stress. The locations of the endocrine glands are shown in **Figure 38.1** ■.

Concepts Related to Endocrine Regulation

All major organ systems and physiologic processes such as growth, homeostasis, regulation of energy, and reproduction are regulated by the endocrine system and its interaction with other body systems (e.g., the central nervous system). More specifically, the endocrine system is involved in sodium and water balance; control of blood pressure and blood volume; regulation of energy balance, including fluid mobilization, utilization, and storage; coordination of hemodynamic and metabolic counterregulatory responses to stress; and reproduction, growth, and development.[1] The thyroid, parathyroid, and adrenal glands are intimately involved in endocrine function, supporting these processes. A map of concepts related to disorders of the endocrine system is shown in **Figure 38.2** ■.

Figure 38.1 ■ Location of the endocrine glands in the male and female bodies.

Case Studies

The following cases are addressed throughout the chapter to assist in application of chapter content to clinical situations that involve individuals with disorders of thyroid and adrenal function.

Beatrice Diaz: Introduction

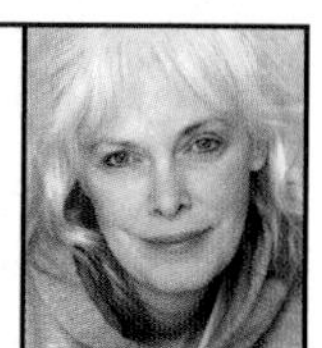

Beatrice Diaz is a 55-year-old woman who has been in her usual state of health until 6 years ago, when she developed bilateral exophthalmos (forward displacement or "bulging" of the eyeball). She reports to her ophthalmologist for her annual examination, and he refers her to an endocrinologist. When her history is taken, she reports that she has lost 20 pounds over the past 3 months in spite of an increased appetite. She has noted an increase in her neck size, as she is no longer able to button the top button on her shirts. The endocrinologist notes that the skin on Ms. Diaz's shins bilaterally is thickened with an orange peel appearance. She is hyperreflexic and has a fine tremor of both hands. She has thinning hair and temporal balding and reports that she has developed palpitations along with feelings of nervousness and anxiety. She attributes her feelings of anxiety to increased pressures and demands at work over the previous year. In addition, she reports heat intolerance that has developed over the past 3 months.

1. What are two abnormal physical symptoms that Ms. Diaz is experiencing?
2. What are two abnormal physical signs that were found during the physical examination?

Reginald Owens: Introduction

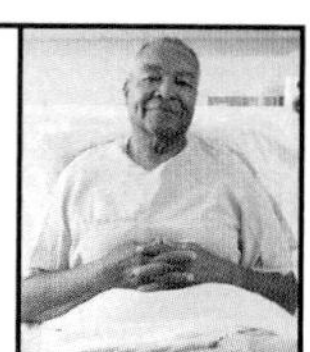

Reginald Owens is a 65-year-old male with a 40-year history of type 1 diabetes and hypothyroidism caused by Hashimoto thyroiditis. He recently noticed that he has increased lethargy, anorexia, weight loss, and lightheadedness on arising. He has had an increased number of hypoglycemic events and has needed to call the paramedics for hypoglycemic treatments twice over the previous month. He has been having increased difficulty carrying out activities of daily living because of his symptoms, so he makes an appointment to see his endocrinologist.

1. Name two symptoms of endocrine dysfunction from which Mr. Owens is suffering.
2. Name the life-threatening symptom Mr. Owens has experienced.
3. What are two endocrine diseases Mr. Owens suffers from?

Check Your Progress: Section 38.1

1. What functions are affected by alterations in hormone levels?
2. List five processes the endocrine system regulates.
3. What three glands are intimately involved in endocrine function?

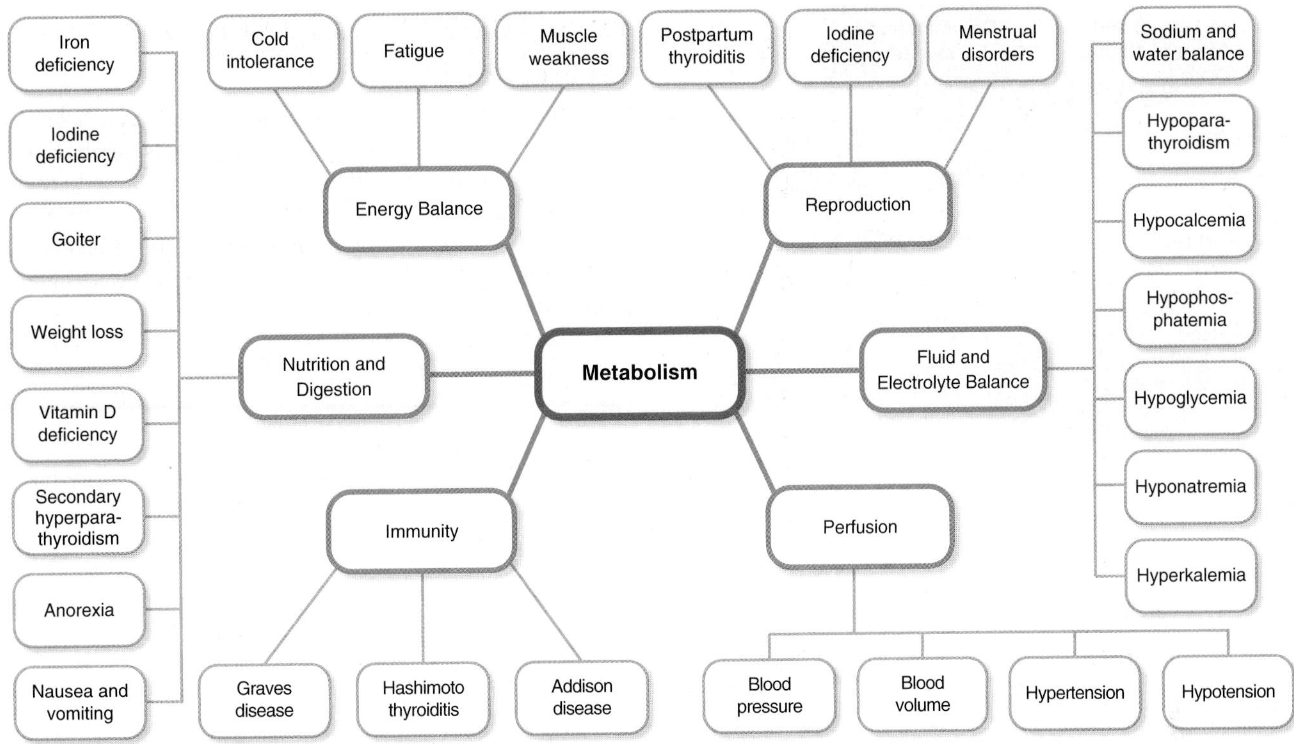

Figure 38.2 ■ Concepts related to endocrine regulation.

38.2 Mechanisms of Hormonal Alterations in Thyroid and Adrenal Disease

The thyroid gland consists of a right and a left lobe connected by a thin isthmus and located anterolateral to the trachea (**Figure 38.3** ■). The normal thyroid gland is soft in consistency, is highly vascularized, and weighs approximately 12–20 grams. The functional unit of the thyroid gland is the thyroid follicle, which contains colloid composed of thyroglobulin, a protein that is essential for the synthesis of thyroid hormones. The thyroid gland produces two primary hormones: triiodothyronine (T3) and thyroxine (T4). Parafollicular cells called C cells are scattered throughout the thyroid gland and secrete a hormone called calcitonin. Thyroid hormones have multiple and diverse effects and are needed for maturation and differentiation; fetal and neonatal brain development; and neurologic function, growth, and metabolism. In addition, thyroid hormone has effects on sympathetic nervous system function, skeletal muscle, cardiovascular function, and reproduction.

Regulation of Thyroid Function

Thyroid function is regulated by the hypothalamic–anterior pituitary–thyroid gland axis. **Euthyroid** is the term used to describe normal function of the thyroid. Thyroid-releasing hormone (TRH) is released from the hypothalamus, thyroid-stimulating hormone (TSH) is released from the anterior pituitary, and T3 and T4 are released from the thyroid gland. TRH stimulates secretion of TSH, which stimulates secretion of T3 and T4. The appropriate secretion of hormones along the hypothalamic–anterior pituitary–thyroid axis is regulated by negative feedback. This feedback loop is detailed in **Figure 38.4** ■.

Hormone Excess and Deficiency

Thyroid hormone dysfunction usually results in hormone excess or hormone deficiency. Two autoimmune thyroid diseases provide specific examples. Graves disease can

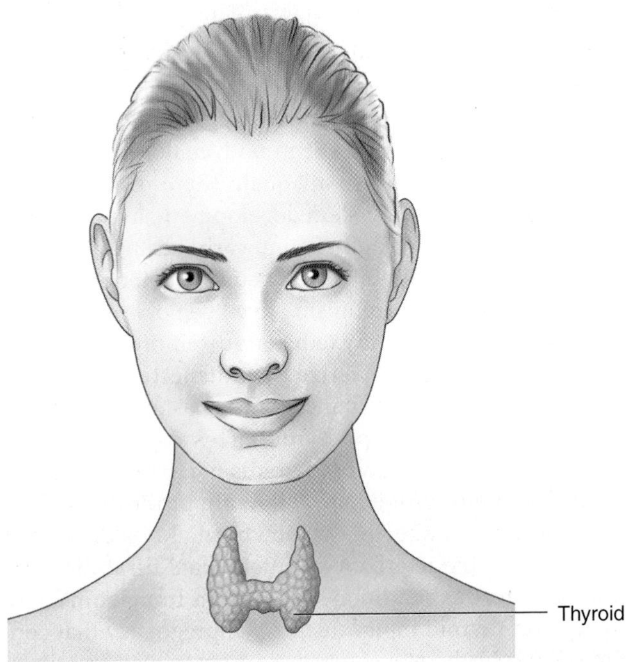

Figure 38.3 ■ The thyroid gland.

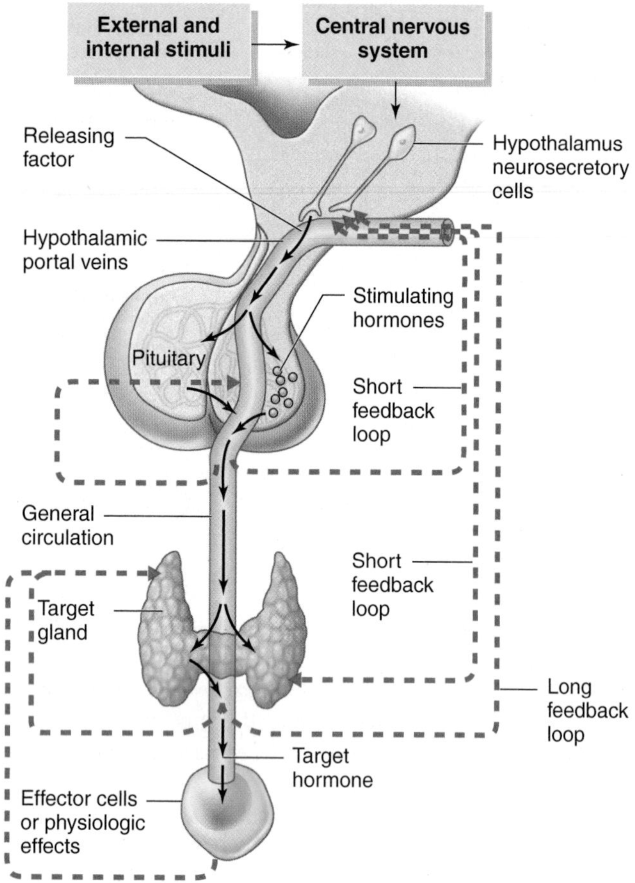

Figure 38.4 ■ General feedback loop.

precipitate hyperthyroidism and causes inflammation of the eyes and orbital tissues and inflammation and thickening of the skin on the shins. Hashimoto thyroiditis can precipitate **hypothyroidism** (disorders characterized by a less than normal amount of thyroid hormones). Selected manifestations of Hashimoto thyroiditis include dry, cold skin; goiter; weight gain; and hair loss. These two disorders are discussed in detail later in this chapter.

Iodine is essential for the synthesis of thyroid hormones; optimal maternal iodine intake is essential for fetal development. Severe iodine deficiency during pregnancy can result in both maternal and fetal hypothyroidism. Because adequate thyroid hormone is necessary for nervous system development, hypothyroidism during fetal development and early postnatal life can lead to intellectual disability and neurologic abnormalities. Two classic forms of cretinism have been described: neurologic cretinism and myxedematous cretinism. Neurologic cretinism is characterized by intellectual disability, deaf-mutism, gait disturbances, and spasticity; however, the infants are not hypothyroid. This condition likely results from maternal hypothyroidism during early pregnancy but a euthyroid state following birth due to adequate iodine intake in the newborn. Myxedematous cretinism is characterized by intellectual disability and short stature; this condition likely results from iodine deficiency and thyroid injury during late pregnancy that continues after birth.[2] ■

Levels of Thyroid Hormone Dysfunction

Because the thyroid gland is regulated by the hypothalamic–anterior pituitary–target gland axis, levels of thyroidal dysfunction can occur at the thyroid (primary disease), anterior pituitary (secondary disease), and hypothalamus (tertiary disease). Dysfunction at any of these levels can result in thyroid disease, particularly hyperthyroidism and hypothyroidism.

Check Your Progress: Section 38.2

1. Name at least three systems on which the thyroid gland has an effect.
2. Describe the feedback loop of the thyroid gland.
3. What are the three levels of dysfunction that can occur for the thyroid gland?

38.3 Disorders of the Thyroid

According the American Thyroid Association, an estimated 20 million people in the United States have some form of thyroid disease, and more than 12% of the U.S. population will develop a thyroid condition during their lifetime. Women are 5–8 times more likely than men to have thyroid problems, and one woman in eight will develop a thyroid disorder during her lifetime. Additionally, up to 60% of people with thyroid disease are unaware of their condition, placing them at risk for other chronic conditions such as cardiovascular disease.[3]

Goiters

A **goiter** is an abnormal growth of the thyroid gland that can be nodular or diffuse and may be associated with normal, decreased, or increased thyroid hormone production. The clinical manifestations vary with thyroid function and with the size and location of the goiter. Specific types of goiters are detailed below and discussed throughout the chapter.

- **Nontoxic Diffuse Goiters.** These goiters, often called "simple" goiters, are defined as diffuse thyroid enlargement that are not associated with overt hyperthyroidism or hypothyroidism and do not result from cysts, inflammation, or neoplasia.
- **Nontoxic Multinodular Goiters.** These goiters are initially diffuse but eventually become nodular as some thyroid follicles proliferate more than others and larger nodules undergo hemorrhage, cystic changes, and calcification. People with nontoxic multinodular goiters have normal serum TSH concentrations. In these individuals, the thyroid enlargement is probably caused by several growth factors, in addition to TSH, that affect the thyroid follicles.[4]

- **Endemic Goiter.** Globally, one of the most common causes of goiter is iodine deficiency.[4] In patients with iodine deficiency, the most common cause of goiter is an increase in TSH secretion. Individuals with long-standing endemic goiters may undergo nodular changes with sequelae described above.
- **Chronic Autoimmune (Hashimoto) Thyroiditis.** Hashimoto thyroiditis is the most common cause of hypothyroidism. In this disorder, an increase in TSH secretion is the predominant cause of goiter.
- **Toxic Multinodular Goiter (Graves Disease).** Graves disease is the most common cause of hyperthyroidism. In patients with Graves disease, TSH receptor antibodies (TRAb) stimulate the TSH receptor to cause thyroid growth, goiter formation, and excessive secretion of thyroid hormones (**Figure 38.5** ■).

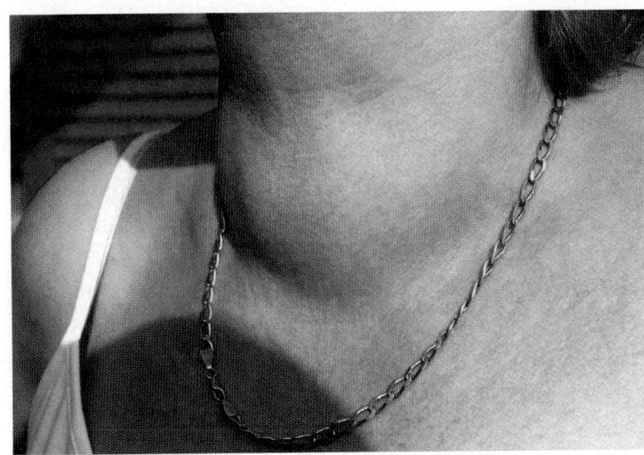

Figure 38.5 ■ Toxic multinodular goiter. The formation and growth of numerous nodules in the thyroid gland cause the characteristic massive enlargement of the neck.

Etiology and Pathogenesis

The most common cause of goiter worldwide is iodine deficiency. Because iodine deficiency is generally not a problem in the United States, multinodular goiter, Hashimoto thyroiditis, and Graves disease are more common causes of goiter. Additionally, tumors, thyroiditis, and infiltrative disease can be uncommon causes of goiters.

Beatrice Diaz: Application

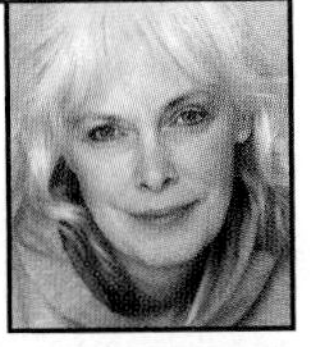

Suspecting thyroid dysfunction, the endocrinologist orders thyroid function tests. Results of the tests include undetectable TSH and elevated T3 and T4. On the basis of clinical and laboratory findings, the endocrinologist diagnoses Ms. Diaz with Graves disease and orders propylthiouracil (PTU), a medication to decrease the synthesis of thyroid hormone. The plan is to reevaluate her status in approximately 6 weeks and decide on radioactive iodine^{131} ablation therapy or thyroidectomy to permanently treat her Graves disease.

Ms. Diaz's symptoms resolve within a month. Feeling better, she does not renew her prescription for PTU. Approximately 2 weeks later, she notes a recurrence of diaphoresis, palpitations, tremors, hyperreflexia, heat intolerance, and feelings of anxiety and nervousness. She also notes dyspnea on exertion and weakness of the muscles in her shoulders and thighs. She is admitted to the hospital for observation to evaluate for possible cardiac arrhythmias. She is placed on PTU again and begins radioactive iodine^{131} ablation therapy. She develops a transient thyroiditis that resolves without complications. Her thyroid function tests are monitored for 2 years, after which time she is lost to follow-up.

3. What is Graves disease?
4. What is PTU, and how does it work?

Clinical Manifestations

The majority of goiters are asymptomatic. Clinical manifestations of goiters are associated with the type of thyroidal dysfunction (e.g., hypothyroidism or hyperthyroidism) and the growth rate of the goiter. One of the risks of long-standing goiters is obstruction due to progressive compression of the trachea or a sudden increase in size from a nodular hemorrhage.[4]

Linking Pathophysiology to Diagnosis and Treatment

The diagnosis of goiter is usually made on the basis of physical examination through palpation of the thyroid gland and surrounding structures for size, symmetry, texture (e.g., smoothness), and the presence of nodules. In addition, the neck is assessed for masses or cervical adenopathy. These findings are corroborated with clinical symptoms and biochemical testing. If the TSH level is below normal, serum T4 and serum total T3 should also be measured to evaluate for hyperthyroidism. If serum TSH is above normal, free T4 should be measured to evaluate for hypothyroidism.

Thyroid Nodules

The term **thyroid nodule** refers to an abnormal growth of thyroid cells that forms a lump within the thyroid gland. These nodules are often asymptomatic and detected by the patient but may be revealed during physical examination or a radiologic procedure such as carotid ultrasonography. The discovery of a thyroid nodule necessitates a diagnostic workup, particularly to exclude cancer.

Etiology and Pathogenesis

The majority of thyroid nodules are benign. Multinodular goiter, Hashimoto thyroiditis, and follicular **adenomas** (benign tumors) are the primary causes of benign thyroid nodules. Approximately 5–15% of all thyroid nodules are malignant; age, gender, radiation exposure, and family history contribute to this incidence.[5]

Clinical Manifestations

Most thyroid nodules are asymptomatic. An autonomous hyperfunctioning nodule that secretes excessive amounts of T3 and T4 is associated with hyperthyroidism and related clinical signs and symptoms. Obstructive symptoms, cervical lymphadenopathy, vocal cord paralysis, and the presence of a hard fixed mass are suggestive of a malignancy.[5]

Linking Pathophysiology to Diagnosis and Treatment

The initial workup of a thyroid nodule includes a history and physical examination, measurement of serum TSH, and a thyroid ultrasound. A subnormal TSH suggests that hyperthyroidism may be present, resulting from an autonomous hyperfunctioning nodule. These nodules secrete T3 and T4 independent of hypothalamic–anterior pituitary regulation. A **thyroid scintigraphy** (thyroid scan) is a nuclear medicine procedure that visually identifies the functional status (hyperfunctioning or hypofunctioning) of thyroid tissue on the basis of the selective uptake of various radionuclides. Patients with normal or elevated TSH may be candidates for thyroid fine-needle aspiration cytology biopsy.[5] In this procedure, a needle is inserted into the thyroid nodule, and tissue is extracted. The tissue is examined by a cytopathologist and classified as benign, nondiagnostic or unsatisfactory, malignancy or suspicious for malignancy, or atypical or follicular neoplasm.[6]

Thyroiditis

Thyroiditis encompasses a group of disorders characterized by inflammation of the thyroid gland that can result in hyperthyroidism, hypothyroidism, or a nontoxic euthyroid goiter.[6] The classification system for categorizing thyroiditis is controversial; however, the specific disorders reflect the range of thyroiditis and include Hashimoto thyroiditis, painless thyroiditis, postpartum thyroiditis, subacute thyroiditis (de Quervain thyroiditis) and acute infectious thyroiditis.

Etiology, Pathogenesis, and Clinical Manifestations

- ***Hashimoto thyroiditis,*** a form of autoimmune thyroid disease, is discussed later in the chapter.
- ***Subacute thyroiditis*** is generally associated with transient hyperthyroidism following an acute release of stored T3 and T4 and followed by transient hypothyroidism and then recovery. Occasionally, hypothyroidism may become permanent. Subacute thyroiditis may follow an upper respiratory infection. Clinical manifestations include a tender, painful, and minimally enlarged thyroid.
- ***Painless thyroiditis,*** also known as *silent thyroiditis* and *lymphocytic thyroiditis with spontaneously resolving hyperthyroidism,* follows a pattern of transient hyperthyroidism, followed occasionally by hypothyroidism, and then recovery. This disorder accounts for 1–5% of cases of hyperthyroidism and is considered a variant form Hashimoto thyroiditis. Clinical manifestations include mild hyperthyroidism of short duration and minimal or no thyroid enlargement without Graves ophthalmopathy or pretibial myxedema.[7]
- ***Postpartum thyroiditis*** is an autoimmune disorder that is most common during the first 6 months of the postpartum period[6] and is associated with an infiltrative process in the thyroid gland. The thyroid may be normal or slightly enlarged without tenderness or pain and is characterized by transient hyperthyroidism followed by hypothyroidism. The hyperthyroidism results from follicular damage and acute release of stored T3 and T4 by a lymphocytic infiltrate.[6] Concentrations of antithyroid antibodies (e.g., antithyroglobulin or thyroid peroxidase antibodies) are higher in postpartum thyroiditis than in painless thyroiditis.[7]
- ***Infectious thyroiditis*** is an infection of the thyroid gland associated with acute and chronic symptomatology. Although rare, the infection can be caused by a variety of organisms and may occur in immunocompromised or debilitated individuals and older adults. Acute infectious thyroiditis is associated with sudden onset of neck pain, thyroid tenderness, fever, chills, dysphagia, and neck swelling. A unilateral neck mass may be present. The diagnosis can be made through fine-needle aspiration and culture; the infection is then treated with appropriate antibiotics.

Linking Pathophysiology to Diagnosis and Treatment

Although the biochemical manifestations of thyroiditis vary according to etiology, most thyroid disorders share the feature of inflammation. Some patients may experience pain and tenderness of the thyroid and surrounding structures; some may be asymptomatic. Treatments are aimed toward normalizing thyroid levels, if indicated.

Primary Hyperthyroidism

Hyperthyroidism, also referred to as *thyrotoxicosis*, is the synthesis and release of excessive quantities of thyroid hormone. The most common causes of primary hyperthyroidism are Graves disease and toxic multinodular goiter. These and other causes of primary hyperthyroidism are discussed below.

Etiology and Pathogenesis

Graves disease is an autoimmune thyroid disease that is associated with hyperthyroidism along with one or more of the following conditions: goiter, **exophthalmos** (a forward displacement or "bulging" of the eyeball), and **pretibial myxedema** (thickening of the skin over the pretibial area) (**Figure 38.6** ■). In Graves disease, TRAb bind receptors on the thyroid follicular cells, causing growth of the thyroid gland and hypersecretion of T3 and T4. In addition, the

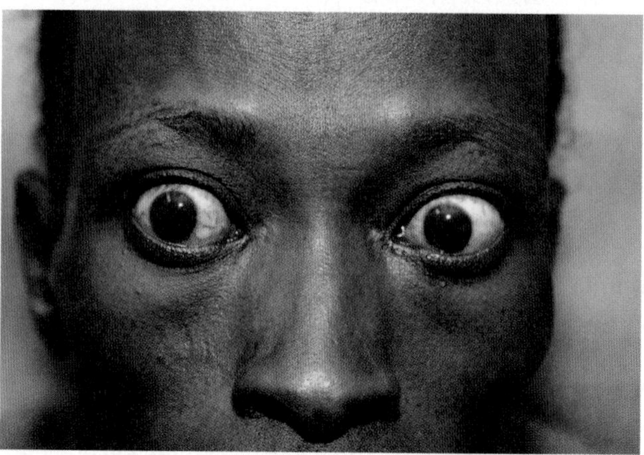

Figure 38.6 ■ Exophthalmos in a patient with Graves disease. The disease causes edema of the far deposits behind the eyes and inflammation of the extraocular muscles. The accumulating pressure forces the eyes outward from their orbits.

presence of excessive amounts of T3 and T4 causes suppression of TSH.[8]

- *Multinodular goiters* may result in hyperthyroidism if one of the nodules becomes autonomous or independent from TSH regulation and excretes excessive amounts of T3 and T4. This usually occurs in patients with long-standing multinodular goiter.
- *Toxic adenomas* are associated with autonomous hypersecretion of T3 and T4 from a functioning adenoma. The pathologic process begins as a small functioning nodule that increases in size to produce excessive amounts of T3 and T4. The endogenous secretion of TSH is suppressed.
- *Iodine-induced hyperthyroidism* may occasionally occur in patients with autonomous functioning thyroid adenomas after treatment with high doses of iodine. This can occur following certain drug therapies (e.g., amiodarone) or iodinated contrast agents used during diagnostic radiography.
- *Thyrotoxicosis factitia* is a psychoneurotic disorder in which the patient has ingested large quantities of T4 hormone replacement (e.g., levothyroxine), usually for the purposes of losing weight.

Clinical Manifestations

Clinical signs associated with hyperthyroidism include tachycardia, atrial fibrillation, fine tremors, goiter, warm moist skin, proximal muscle weakness, hyperreflexia, eye changes such as lid lag or retraction, stare, and hair loss. Clinical symptoms of hyperthyroidism include anxiety, heat intolerance, dyspnea on exertion, palpitations, palmar erythema, weakness and fatigue, weight loss with increased appetite, and diarrhea. There are a number of clinical manifestations that are more specific to Graves disease; these include a firm diffuse goiter and a thrill or bruit on the thyroid gland, reflecting increased vascularity of the gland. **Ophthalmopathy** is often present in patients with Graves disease and is characterized by eye changes, including lid lag and retraction, periorbital edema, exophthalmos, diplopia, corneal involvement, and visual loss. Thyroid **dermopathy** may be present and manifested as a noninflamed, indurated plaque with a deep pink or purple color and an orange-peel appearance. This is frequently seen on the anterior and lateral aspects of the lower leg, where it is referred to as pretibial myxedema. Thyroid **acropachy** refers to a form of soft tissue swelling and clubbing in hands and fingers found in Graves disease.

Older adults with hyperthyroidism may present with symptoms of fatigue and weight loss but without the symptoms of hyperactivity, tremor, and sympathetic overactivity. This is a condition called apathetic thyrotoxicosis. This hypermetabolic rate is also associated with profound myopathy, especially in the quadriceps, and with atrial fibrillation. ■

CLINICAL POINT: **Thyrotoxicosis** (also called **thyroid storm** is a life-threatening condition characterized by an exacerbation of all of the signs and symptoms of hyperthyroidism. Thyroid storm may occur in a patient with a history of Graves disease who has discontinued the antithyroid medication or in a patient who has undiagnosed hyperthyroidism. The patient may present with a fever (with a temperature less than 104°F), diaphoresis, tachycardia, atrial fibrillation, nausea, vomiting, diarrhea, tremors, agitation, and delirium. ■

Beatrice Diaz: Application

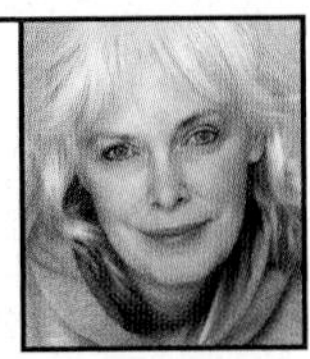

Approximately 5 years after treatment, Ms. Diaz is brought to the emergency department by her daughter, who states that Ms. Diaz has been complaining of depression, fatigue, tiredness, and lack of energy and has recently become very lethargic. On physical examination, Ms. Diaz has delayed deep tendon reflexes, periorbital edema, and hair loss. Her temperature is 97.2°F, and her chest x-ray reveals bilateral pneumonia. She reports a 30-pound weight gain in the past year. Suspecting thyroid dysfunction, the attending physician orders thyroid function tests, which reveal an increased TSH and decreased T3 and T4. Ms. Diaz is diagnosed with hypothyroidism and started on levothyroxine for thyroid replacement therapy. An appointment is made for follow-up.

5. Why does Ms. Diaz now have hypothyroidism?
6. Why is there an increase in TSH and a decrease in T3 and T4?

Linking Pathophysiology to Diagnosis and Treatment

A combination of a suppressed serum TSH with an elevated serum free thyroxine (FT4) confirms the diagnosis of hyperthyroidism. Laboratory markers for Graves disease include an elevated serum FT4 and an undetectable serum TSH; however, the presence of thyroid peroxidase antibodies helps to confirm the diagnosis. A small number of patients have a normal FT4 but an elevated serum free triiodothyronine (FT3) in combination with a suppressed TSH. This condition is referred to as T3 thyrotoxicosis.[6]

A radioactive iodine uptake (RAIU) test may be used to help differentiate the etiology of hyperthyroidism. The RAIU measures the percentage of radioactivity in the thyroid after the administration of oral radioactive iodine. A high RAIU reading usually indicates hyperthyroidism, as seen in Graves disease or toxic nodular goiter. A radionuclide scan (I^{123}) can be used to help differentiate between Graves disease and hyperthyroidism from other causes, such as toxic multinodular goiter. In Graves disease, the concentration of the radionuclide tracer is intense and more uniformly distributed throughout the thyroid, whereas there is more discrete concentration of the tracer, with suppression of thyroidal tissue around the nodules.[9]

Pregnant women with Graves disease are treated with antithyroid drugs, such as propylthiouricil (PTU) and methimazole, throughout most of pregnancy. Because these medications cross the placental barrier, the dosage is kept to the minimum needed to control symptoms. Methimazole is associated with rare teratogenic effects. General recommendations advise limiting PTU to the first trimester and then switching to methimazole. Radioactive iodine is absolutely contraindicated during pregnancy because it crosses the placenta freely and may cause injury to the fetal thyroid.[9] ■

Beatrice Diaz: Outcome

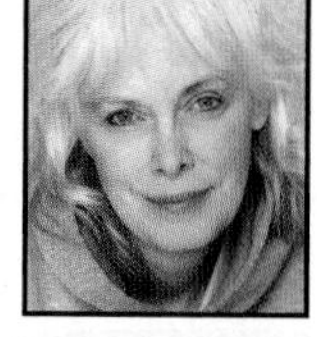

Ms. Diaz's daughter becomes increasingly concerned about her mother's health and makes a plan to ensure that her mother will attend scheduled medical appointments and refill all prescriptions. Ms. Diaz's symptoms resolve with levothyroxine therapy.

7. What is levothyroxine therapy?
8. Why is it important that Ms. Diaz follow all the recommendations made by her doctor?

Secondary Hyperthyroidism

Secondary causes of hyperthyroidism are rare; however, one cause of secondary hyperthyroidism may be a TSH-secreting pituitary adenoma. TSH-induced hyperthyroidism is a very rare cause of overt hyperthyroidism. These patients have normal or high serum TSH despite high FT4 and FT3 concentrations.[10]

Etiology and Pathogenesis

TSH-secreting adenomas secrete biologically active TSH in autonomous fashion and have normal or high serum TSH despite high serum FT4 and FT3 concentrations.[10]

Clinical Manifestations

The majority of patients with secondary hyperthyroidism have symptoms of hyperthyroidism as described previously. A tumor mass that is increasing in size may cause symptoms related to obstruction (e.g., visual disturbances related to obstruction of optic chiasm) and symptoms related to possible cosecretion of other hormones such as growth hormone and prolactin.[10]

Linking Pathophysiology to Diagnosis and Treatment

A TSH-secreting pituitary adenoma should be suspected in hyperthyroid patients with diffuse goiter without signs and symptoms of Graves disease, who have high (and sometimes normal) serum free T4 and T3 concentrations and elevated serum TSH concentrations in the presence of headache or clinical features of concomitant hypersecretion of other pituitary hormones. An MRI may help to confirm the existence of a pituitary adenoma.

Primary Hypothyroidism

Primary hypothyroidism results from inadequate production of thyroid hormones and is one of the most common endocrine disorders worldwide. It can result in destruction or injury to the thyroid gland (e.g., surgical, irradiation, autoimmune); inhibition of thyroid hormone synthesis (e.g., dietary iodine deficiency, enzymatic defects, antithyroid drugs); hypothalamic or pituitary disorders; or resistance to thyroid hormone. Primary hypothyroidism may be transient or permanent.[11]

Etiology and Pathogenesis

In areas of the world where iodine intake is sufficient, the major cause of hypothyroidism is Hashimoto thyroiditis.[11] **Hashimoto thyroiditis** is an immunologic disease characterized by the development of autoantibodies, particularly directed toward thyroglobulin, resulting in lymphocytic infiltration and fibrosis of the thyroidal tissue. This leads to diminished production of T3 and T4 and the development of hypothyroidism. Hashimoto thyroiditis usually presents with a goiter or enlargement of the thyroid gland. Initially, the patient may be euthyroid or have mild hypothyroidism. As the hypothyroidism progresses, the patient may exhibit signs and symptoms of hypothyroidism.

Clinical Manifestations

Clinical symptoms of Hashimoto thyroiditis include weakness, fatigue, lethargy, somnolence, mental slowness, muscle soreness, cold intolerance, and mood changes (e.g., depression). Clinical signs of Hashimoto thyroiditis include goiter, dry cold skin, hair loss, weight gain, constipation, delay in the relaxation phase of deep tendon reflexes, and sinus bradycardia.

Linking Pathophysiology to Diagnosis and Treatment

Hypothyroidism typically can be diagnosed by measuring the serum FT4 and TSH concentrations. The patient is likely to have an elevated serum TSH and a reduced serum FT4. Testing for thyroid autoantibodies (antithyroid peroxidase antibodies and antithyroglobulin antibodies and measuring serum FT4 and TSH concentrations are usually sufficient to confirm the diagnosis of Hashimoto thyroiditis. Initially, the patient may present with a mildly elevated TSH and normal FT4. When the disease progresses to overt hypothyroidism, the patient will present with decreased serum FT4 and elevated TSH.

Secondary and Tertiary Hypothyroidism

Secondary hypothyroidism is caused by TSH deficiency, and tertiary hypothyroidism is caused by TRH deficiency. Secondary and tertiary hypothyroidism are exceedingly rare; fewer than 1% of hypothyroid patients have one of these particular types.[12]

Etiology and Pathogenesis

Secondary hypothyroidism can be caused by conditions that cause injury to the anterior pituitary gland, such as pituitary and nonpituitary tumors, infiltrative diseases, postpartum pituitary necrosis (Sheehan syndrome), and trauma. TSH deficiency also may occur together with other pituitary hormone deficiencies. Tertiary hypothyroidism can be caused by any disorder that damages the hypothalamus or interferes with hypothalamic–pituitary portal blood flow, as such damage may decrease TRH delivery to the anterior pituitary. Hypothalamic damage can occur from tumors, trauma, radiation therapy, or infiltrative diseases. Like TSH deficiency, TRH deficiency can occur alone or in combination with other hormonal deficiencies.[12]

Clinical Manifestations

The clinical manifestations of secondary hypothyroidism are similar to those of primary hypothyroidism; however, if the damage to the pituitary or hypothalamus results in decreased TSH or TRH, the release of other hormones (e.g., growth hormone) may decrease, resulting in a variety of clinical manifestations unrelated to thyroid function.

The clinical manifestations of tertiary hypothyroidism include coarseness and thinning of hair, cold intolerance, weight gain, joint pain, muscle weakness, fatigue and depression, menstrual disorders, and dry skin.

Linking Pathophysiology to Diagnosis and Treatment

Because there is a deficiency of TSH and TRH in secondary and tertiary hypothyroidism, respectively, these disorders cannot be distinguished by biochemical tests. Any patients with suspected TSH or TRH deficiency should undergo MRI evaluation of the hypothalamus and pituitary to identify the possible hormone deficiency.

Thyroid Cancer

The American Cancer Society estimates approximately 56,870 new cases of thyroid cancer and approximately 2010 deaths from thyroid cancer for the year 2017, the preponderance of which were expected to be among women.[13] The major types of thyroid cancer are papillary, follicular, medullary, and anaplastic thyroid cancer.

Etiology and Pathogenesis

Papillary and follicular cancers arise from follicular cells and are referred to as **differentiated cancers**. These cancers are composed of more mature cells and maintain many properties of normal thyroid gland. They tend to be less aggressive than **undifferentiated cancers**, which are composed of immature cells, as in aplastic thyroid cancer.

Papillary thyroid cancer is the most common type of thyroid cancer, making up about 70–80% of all thyroid cancers in the United States. This type of thyroid cancer can occur at any age and tends to grow slowly, and there is often lymphatic spread to the cervical nodes in the neck.[14]

Follicular thyroid cancer makes up about 10–15% of all thyroid cancers in the United States.[14] Follicular cancer is an aggressive cancer that can spread to lymph nodes in the neck; however, this type of cancer is more likely than papillary cancer to spread to distant organs, particularly the lung.[14]

Medullary thyroid cancer (MTC) accounts for 1–2% of thyroid cancers in the United States.[15] MTC is different from other types of thyroid cancers in that it originates from the parafollicular C cells of the thyroid gland, which make a hormone called calcitonin. MTC can spread to lymph nodes and to other organs. MTC can be inherited into up to 25% of cases. When inherited, MTC can be associated with other endocrine disorders called multiple endocrine neoplasia (MEN) 2A or 2B.[15] For example, patients with MEN 2A may have MTC and tumors of adrenal or parathyroid glands. Patients with MEN 2B may have MTC, adrenal tumors, and neuromas in the lining of the mouth or gastrointestinal tract. Patients with an inherited form of MTC often have a mutation in the *RET* proto-oncogene, that can be determined by blood work. If patients do not have the *RET* proto-oncogene, they are said to have sporadic MTC, the etiology of which is unknown.[15]

Anaplastic thyroid cancers are undifferentiated tumors of the thyroid follicular epithelium. They are extremely aggressive, with a disease-specific mortality near 100%.[16]

Clinical Manifestations

Thyroid cancer typically presents as a thyroid nodule. Characteristics that suggest that the nodule may be cancerous are a rapid nodular growth, the nodule's being fixed to the surrounding tissues, new onset hoarseness or vocal cord paralysis, or the presence of cervical lymphadenopathy on the same side as the mass.[15]

Linking Pathophysiology to Diagnosis and Treatment

The initial treatment of papillary and follicular cancer is total thyroidectomy. If the patient is at high risk for recurrence of papillary cancer or has follicular cancer, thyroid remnant ablation therapy is performed. In this procedure, radioactive iodine (I^{131}) is given to destroy any residual thyroid tissue that may have metastasized or may have the potential to become malignant. Patients are then treated with levothyroxine in levels sufficient to suppress TSH, a trophic and growth-producing hormone.[17]

Patients with MTC are treated with total thyroidectomy. Radioactive iodine is not useful in the treatment of MTC. Serum calcitonin levels are used to monitor the patient for recurrence. Levothyroxine is used to maintain TSH levels in a normal range.[17] The treatment of anaplastic thyroid carcinoma includes surgical resection, radiation therapy, and chemotherapy.

Check Your Progress: Section 38.3

1. What is Hashimoto thyroiditis, and what symptoms would you expect a patient to present with?
2. What are the causes of secondary and tertiary hypothyroidism and why do these occur?
3. Why is an MRI of the hypothalamus and pituitary needed to determine secondary from tertiary hypothyroidism?

38.4 Disorders of the Parathyroid

Parathyroid hormone (PTH) is secreted from four parathyroid glands located adjacent to the thyroid gland (**Figure 38.7** ■). PTH is the most important mediator in the regulation of calcium and phosphate physiology. Involved in this feedback loop are PTH, vitamin D (1,25-(OH)2D), and calcitonin (**Figure 38.8** ■). The target organs include the intestinal mucosa, kidney, and bone. The primary effect of PTH is to maintain the normal serum calcium concentration. PTH has direct effects on the kidney and bone. In the kidney, PTH promotes calcium reabsorption in the distal tubule and the medullary thick ascending limb of the loop of Henle. PTH stimulates the release of calcium from a rapidly exchangeable pool of calcium in bone. These processes act together to maintain normal serum calcium concentrations. The effect of PTH on the intestinal mucosa is indirect; PTH stimulates the production of the vitamin D metabolite 1,25-(OH)2D, which increases the intestinal absorption of calcium.[18]

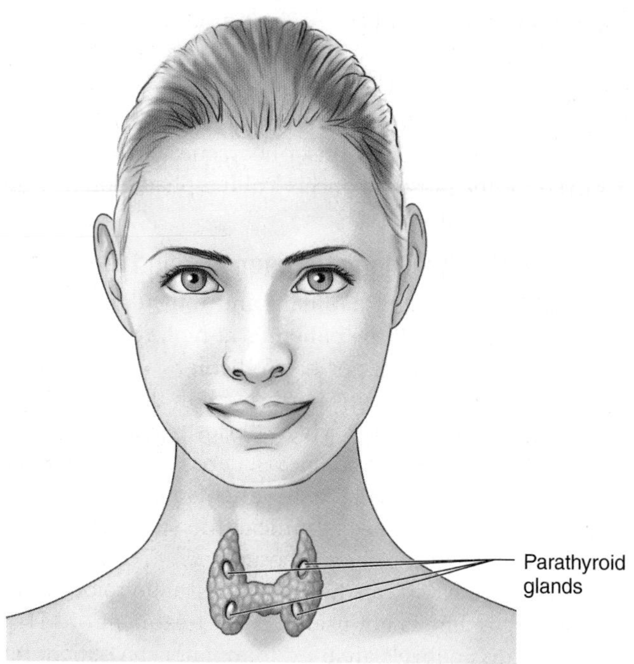

Figure 38.7 ■ The parathyroid glands.

Primary, Secondary, and Tertiary Hyperparathyroidism

Etiology and Pathogenesis

Primary hyperparathyroidism is a generalized disorder of calcium, phosphate, and bone metabolism resulting from an increased secretion of PTH. The main causes of primary hyperparathyroidism include adenomas, hyperplasia, and carcinomas.

Secondary hyperparathyroidism refers to a diffuse hyperplasia of the parathyroid glands due to a cause external to the parathyroid glands. Chronic kidney disease (CKD) contributes to the development of secondary hyperparathyroidism. In CKD, there is decreased production of the active vitamin D metabolite 1,25-(OH)2D, which is essential for the intestinal absorption of calcium. This results in increased secretion of PTH and hyperplasia of the parathyroid glands. Individuals who are deficient in 1,25-(OH)2D, regardless of the cause, can develop secondary hyperparathyroidism.

Tertiary hyperparathyroidism occurs in the setting of chronic secondary hyperparathyroidism. The parathyroid

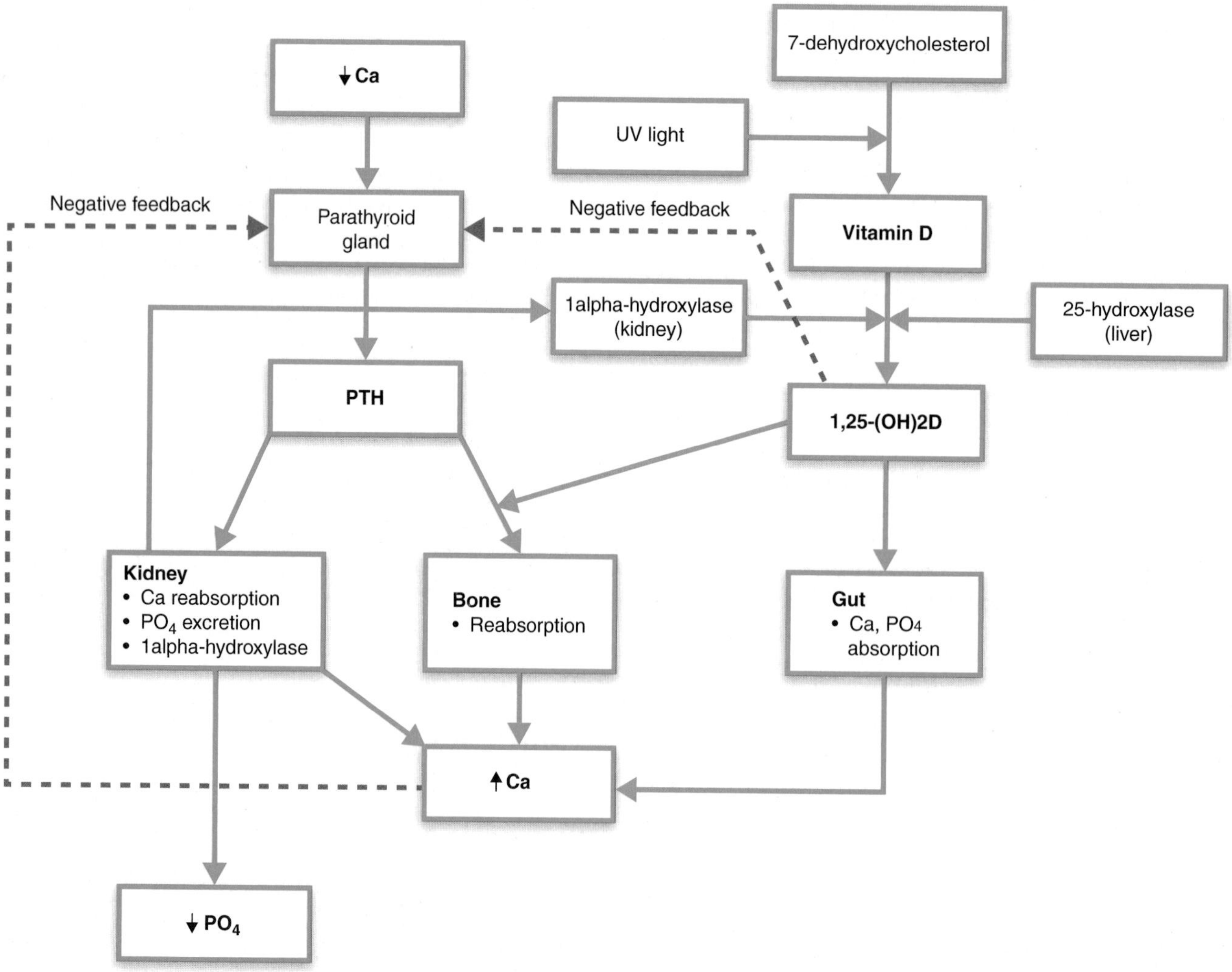

Figure 38.8 ■ The regulation of calcium and phosphate occurs in a negative feedback loop.

glands become hyperplastic, but correction of the causative factor does not result in correction of the hyperplasia, and the parathyroid glands continue to produce excessive sustained release of PTH.

Clinical Manifestations

Primary hyperparathyroidism may present in a variety of ways. Most patients are diagnosed when routine blood work reveals an elevated serum calcium and subsequent diagnostic workup indicates primary hyperparathyroidism. Patients may exhibit systemic signs and symptoms, including weakness, fatigue, weight loss; neuropsychiatric and neuromuscular manifestations, such as depression, poor concentration, memory changes, peripheral sensory neuropathy, motor neuropathy, and proximal and generalized muscle weakness; cardiac signs, such as hypertension and shortened QT; renal manifestations, such as stones, polyuria, and metabolic acidosis; skeletal challenges, such as pathologic fractures or osteopenia; and gastrointestinal signs and symptoms, such as those associated with peptic ulcer disease.

Secondary hyperparathyroidism due to severe vitamin D deficiency may be associated with osteomalacia resulting from abnormal mineralization of the bone. Renal osteodystrophy is a bone disorder that develops in part from secondary hyperparathyroidism in CKD.

Tertiary hyperparathyroidism may occur in individuals with a history of secondary hyperparathyroidism if glandular hyperfunction and increased serum PTH and calcium levels continue following correction of the underlying etiology.[18]

Linking Pathophysiology to Diagnosis and Treatment

The measurement of serum PTH with a simultaneous measurement of serum calcium helps to establish the diagnosis of primary hyperparathyroidism. In patients with normal kidney function, elevated serum PTH and elevated serum calcium levels are usually diagnostic of primary hyperparathyroidism. Additionally, studies may be performed to assess possible target-organ damage from primary hyperparathyroidism, such as radiologic studies (e.g., spine films). Skeletal abnormalities such as osteopenia and osteoporosis may support the diagnosis of primary hyperparathyroidism.

Patients with secondary hyperparathyroidism may have normal or decreased serum calcium levels. Serum phosphate may be reduced; urinary calcium may be low; and 1,25-$(OH)_2D$ levels may be deficient. These patients will often have an underlying disorder that may contribute to the secondary hyperparathyroidism.

The main indication for treatment is persistent hypercalcemia and/or an increased PTH level. The primary treatment is surgery. The purpose of surgical treatment is to reduce the parathyroid mass and cell number and thus normalize the serum calcium concentration.

Hypoparathyroidism

Etiology and Pathogenesis

Hypoparathyroidism refers to decreased production of PTH. The primary causes of hypoparathyroidism are surgical, autoimmune, familial, or idiopathic. The most common cause is surgery on the neck (e.g., thyroidectomy, parathyroidectomy, cancer surgery) that results in destruction or removal of the parathyroid glands.

CLINICAL POINT: Precipitating causes of PTH-deficient hypocalcemia occurs after surgery for resection of parathyroid adenomas, malignancy, or hyperplasia of the parathyroid glandular tissue. Following resection of the adenoma, it may take 1–2 days for the calcium and PTH levels to return to normal. ■

Clinical Manifestations

Hypoparathyroidism is characterized by hypocalcemia and hypophosphatemia. The hypocalcemia is due to the loss of PTH-stimulated calcium resorption at the kidney and the ability to produce active vitamin D (1,25-$(OH)_2D$); the hypophosphatemia is due to the loss of the phosphaturic effect of PTH. Hypocalcemia is characterized by increased neuromuscular excitability. Patients may complain of numbness and tingling sensations in the perioral area or in the fingers and toes. Muscle cramps in the back and lower extremities are common.

Tetany refers to a constellation of symptoms caused by hypocalcemia and is characterized by painful carpal spasms and laryngeal stridor. The presence of latent tetany may be demonstrated through the use of Chvostek sign and Trousseau sign. Chvostek sign can be elicited by tapping on the facial nerve anterior to the ear. Twitching in the ipsilateral facial muscle is considered a positive test. Trousseau sign can be demonstrated by inflating the blood pressure cuff above the systolic blood pressure and holding for 3 minutes. In individuals who have hypocalcemia, this results in painful carpal muscle contractions and spasms.

Linking Pathophysiology to Diagnosis and Treatment

In hypoparathyroidism, serum calcium levels are decreased, and serum phosphate is increased. Serum PTH levels may be inappropriately low, normal, or undetectable; however, the normal levels are inappropriately low in relation to the level of calcium.[19]

Check Your Progress: Section 38.4

1. What is the primary purpose of the parathyroid gland?
2. Name the direct and indirect organs in which PTH works directly and indirectly. What does PTH do in each organ?
3. What are five signs and symptoms of hyperparathyroidism?

38.5 Disorders of Adrenocortical Function

The adrenal glands are bilateral structures located on the superior poles of each kidney and consist of two major divisions: the adrenal medulla and the adrenal cortex (**Figure 38.9** ■). The adrenal cortex is divided into three layers. The inner layer is the zona reticularis; the middle layer is the zona fasciculata; and the outer layer is the zona glomerulosa. The zona glomerulosa produces aldosterone, a mineralocorticoid. The primary function of aldosterone is in the distal nephron, where it promotes Na^+

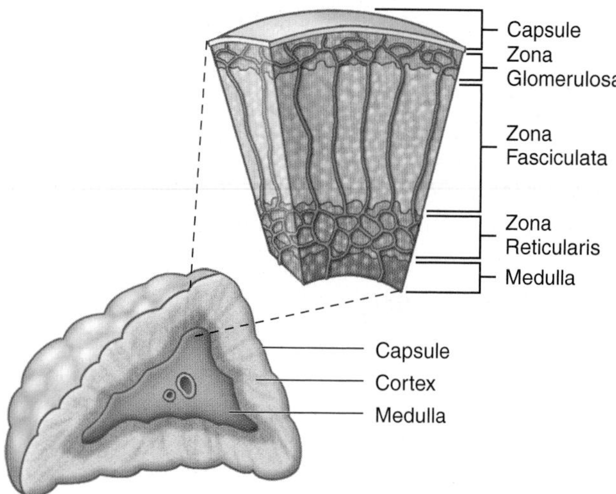

Figure 38.9 ■ The layers of the adrenal gland include the zona reticularis, the zona fasciculata, and the zona glomerulosa.

and water resorption and K^+ and H^+ excretion. The zona fasciculata produces glucocorticoids, primarily cortisol, which have diverse effects on a variety of tissues. Cortisol increases gluconeogenesis and lipolysis, decreases protein synthesis, inhibits bone formation and stimulates bone resorption, suppresses the immune system and is a potent anti-inflammatory, stimulates red blood cell production, and alters mood and behavior. Cortisol is necessary for the integrity of the gastrointestinal tract; it is also necessary for the vascular response to catecholamines.[20]

The zona reticularis produces the androgen precursors dehydroepiandrosterone (DHEA), DHEA-sulfate, and androstenedione. These are converted peripherally to active androgens, providing approximately 50% of circulating androgens in women. They promote pubic and axillary hair growth in women but have little effect on men.

The adrenal medulla is part of the sympathetic nervous system. The major secretory products of the adrenal medulla are the catecholamines, epinephrine, norepinephrine, and a small amount of dopamine. In humans, approximately 90% of circulating epinephrine is produced in the adrenal medulla. In general, the release of catecholamines increases heart rate, cardiac output, and vasoconstriction, resulting in increased blood pressure. In addition, catecholamines have effects on extravascular smooth muscle in a variety of tissues. These include contraction and relaxation of the uterine myometrium, relaxation of intestinal and bladder smooth muscle, contraction of smooth muscle in the bladder and intestinal sphincters, relaxation of tracheal smooth muscle, and papillary dilation. Catecholamines also have effects on metabolism, stimulating gluconeogenesis, glycogenolysis, and lipolysis.

Corticotropin-releasing hormone (CRH), which is secreted by the hypothalamus, causes the secretion of adrenocorticotropic hormone (ACTH) from the anterior pituitary. ACTH is a trophic hormone that is responsible for the development of the adrenal cortex. Additionally, ACTH stimulates the release of glucocorticoids, mineralocorticoids, and androgens from the adrenal cortex.[20] This hypothalamic–anterior pituitary–adrenocortical axis is maintained through negative feedback. (For a review of the HPA axis, x-ref to Figure 11.8 in Chapter 11.) The zona glomerulosa is controlled by the renin-angiotensin-aldosterone system (RAAS). (For a review of the RAAS, refer to Figure 8.9 in Chapter 8.)

Reginald Owens: Application

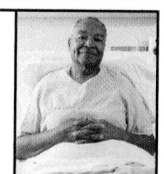

Mr. Owens visits the endocrinologist, who reviews his medical history and clinical signs and symptoms in detail. The endocrinologist notes increased pigmentation in light-exposed areas, pressure points, and the buccal mucosa. Mr. Owens's vital signs are pulse 100, respirations 20, blood pressure 90/50 mmHg. Orthostatic changes in blood pressure are noted when Mr. Owens moves from lying to a standing position. Laboratory values are significant for dehydration, and thyroid function is normal. Suspecting adrenal dysfunction, the endocrinologist orders an ACTH challenge test that reveals primary adrenal insufficiency. Mr. Owens is placed on prednisone and fludrocortisone for cortisol and mineralocorticoids, respectively. His symptoms resolve, and he is maintained on a stable dose of these medications. In addition, he is given instructions to contact his endocrinologist in the event of any other stressful event or acute illness.

4. Why did the endocrinologist prescribe prednisone and fludrocortisone?
5. Why was dehydration present in Mr. Owens's laboratory values?

Primary Adrenocortical Insufficiency

The are a number of causes of primary adrenocortical insuffiency. The most prominent cause is **Addison disease**, a rare autoimmune disorder affecting approximately 0.01% of people in the United States.[21] The disease is named for Thomas Addison, the English physician and scientist who, in the mid-1800s, originally described the symptoms that are characteristic of adrenal insufficiency. Onset of symptoms usually occurs between the third and fifth decades of life, and the disease is more commonly diagnosed in women than in men. Tuberculosis involving the adrenal cortex is a less common cause of primary adrenal insufficiency; other less common causes are HIV, AIDs, sarcoidosis, radiation therapy, adrenal hemorrhage, and infarction.

Etiology and Pathogenesis

Primary adrenal insufficiency is caused by dysfunction of the adrenal cortex, resulting in deficiency of adrenocortical hormones (e.g., mineralocorticoids, androgens, glucocorticoids). In primary adrenal insufficiency, gradual destruction of the adrenal cortex may occur as a result of autoimmune, tuberculosis, or other infiltrative processes, resulting in decreased secretion of adrenocortical hormones. The basal glucocorticoid level may be normal but cannot increase in response to physiologic stresses, such as trauma, surgery, or infection. With further destruction of the adrenal cortex, there is progressive loss of glucocorticoids, mineralocorticoids, and androgens, and the clinical signs and symptoms of primary adrenal insufficiency become apparent. The decreased cortisol level leads to increased release of ACTH from the anterior pituitary via negative feedback mechanisms.[21]

The etiology of primary adrenal insufficiency is diverse, but the vast majority of cases in developed countries result from autoimmune destruction of adrenal cortex (Addison disease). Autoantibodies to 21-hydroxylase are found in most cases. The 21-hydroxylase enzyme is required for synthesis of aldosterone and cortisol from cholesterol. The addition of a hydroxyl group to the 21 carbon position on progesterone produces 11-deoxycorticosterone. Without proper functioning of this enzyme, deficiencies of cortisol and aldosterone develop. Destruction of the adrenal gland results in decreased secretion of the hormones secreted by the adrenal gland. As was noted previously, the adrenal cortex is made up of three zones, each of which secretes specific hormones. Insufficient production of these hormones, particularly cortisol, results in increased ACTH production and secretion via negative feedback mechanisms from the anterior pituitary gland.[21]

CLINICAL POINT: Acute adrenocortical insufficiency (adrenal crisis) is a life-threatening complication characterized by dehydration, fever, hyponatremia, hyperkalemia, vascular collapse, and death. This crisis occurs in patients with chronic adrenocortical insufficiency and is often precipitated by physiologic stressors, such as trauma or infection.[22] ■

Reginald Owens: Application

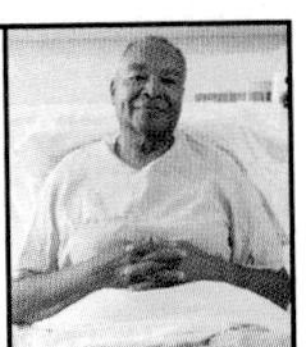

Mr. Owens is stabilized on his medication regimen. He develops a respiratory infection while traveling overseas and decides to wait until he returns home to seek treatment. He develops nausea, vomiting, abdominal pain, and diarrhea on the plane home and proceeds directly to the emergency department (ED) after arriving home from the airport. In the ED, he is diagnosed with pneumonia and acute adrenal insufficiency. He begins antibiotic treatment for pneumonia and is given intravenous glucose and fluids for hypoglycemia and dehydration. Because he continues to have nausea and vomiting, he is provided with intravenous forms of cortisol with mineralocorticoid activity. His symptoms begin to resolve. However, in view of his underlying type 1 diabetes, he is admitted to a hospital unit for observation.

6. What are the causes of acute adrenal insufficiency?
7. Why did this occur?

Clinical Manifestations and Treatment

The signs and symptoms of primary adrenocortical insufficiency are related to decreased production of glucocorticoids (e.g., cortisol), mineralocorticoids (e.g., aldosterone), and androgens. These signs and symptoms may include fatigue, weakness, weight loss, anorexia, nausea, vomiting, abdominal pain, diarrhea, constipation, hypotension, dehydration, hypoglycemia, hyponatremia, hyperkalemia, and acidosis. Primary adrenocortical insufficiency is characterized by pigmentation changes such as freckling; diffuse darkening of skin; creases of the hands, knuckles, and areola; and bluish-black patches on mucous membranes.[21,23] Most of the signs and symptoms are due to lack of production of cortisol and aldosterone; the pigmentation changes are related to increased levels of ACTH. Other, less common symptoms include dizziness, myalgia, hyponatremia, hyperkalemia, elevated serum creatinine levels, and salt craving.[21]

Treatment for primary adrenocortical insufficiency includes intravenous injections of hydrocortisone, saline solution, and glucose for hypoglycemia and dehydration.

Reginald Owens: Outcome

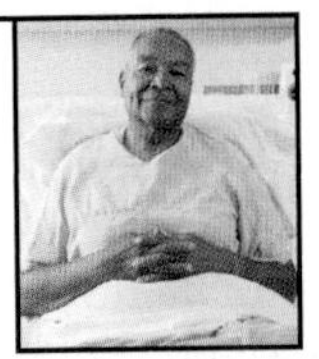

Mr. Owens returns home after a 1-day admission to the hospital. The discharge nurse meets with Mr. Owens and his family to review the need for changes in cortisol and mineralocorticoid coverage during times of physiologic stress, such as trauma or infection. Mr. Owens feels confident that he will consult with healthcare providers in the future when under stressful circumstances.

8. What signs and symptoms of adrenal insufficiency should the nurse teach Mr. Owens and his family?
9. Why should Mr. Owens consult his healthcare provider in times of stress?

Secondary Adrenocortical Insufficiency

Secondary adrenocortical insufficiency may be caused by hypothalamic-pituitary disease or suppression of the hypothalamic-pituitary axis. One of the most common causes of this suppression is the use of exogenous corticosteroids (e.g., prednisone).[24]

Etiology and Pathogenesis

Secondary adrenal insufficiency is caused by dysfunction of the anterior pituitary leading to loss of ACTH production resulting in deficiency of adrenocortical hormones. Secondary adrenocortical insufficiency can occur after surgery or damage to the pituitary (e.g., removal of the pituitary, pituitary infarction). However, a major cause of secondary adrenocortical insufficiency is chronic exogenous glucocorticoid therapy. Many patients are treated with exogenous glucocorticoids (e.g., prednisone) for a number of chronic disorders. These medications increase the serum concentration of cortisol and suppress ACTH secretion from the anterior pituitary via negative feedback principles. Patients who have used glucocorticoids for extended periods of time are warned that abrupt discontinuation of glucocorticoids can result in life-threatening adrenocortical crisis. Such medications should be discontinued gradually under the guidance of the person's healthcare practitioner.[24]

Clinical Manifestations

The clinical signs and symptoms of primary and secondary adrenal insufficiency are similar; however, there are a few exceptions. In secondary adrenocortical insufficiency, the pigmentation changes are not present because ACTH is not increased. Because the zona glomerulosa is regulated by the RAAS, mineralocorticoids are still produced; therefore, hypokalemia is not present, and hypotension is less prominent.

Linking Pathophysiology to Diagnosis and Treatment

The laboratory abnormalities associated with adrenocortical insufficiency are related to the type (primary or secondary) and nature (acute versus chronic) of the insufficiency. The general laboratory approach to the diagnosis of adrenal insufficiency can be complex. Because urinary and basal plasma levels of adrenocortical hormones may be normal in partial adrenocortical insufficiency, provocative tests of adrenocortical function are necessary to establish the diagnosis of adrenocortical insufficiency and to differentiate between primary and secondary dysfunction.[23]

When there is clinical suspicion of adrenal insufficiency, one must determine whether the disorder is caused by inadequate functioning of the adrenal cortex or by inadequate secretion of ACTH. Diagnostic tests include basic metabolic panels and early morning (8:00–9:00 a.m.) cortisol levels. Hyponatremia and hyperkalemia, due to low serum mineralocorticoid levels, and low serum cortisol levels would be expected for Addison disease. A positive test for 21-hydroxylase antibody confirms the cause as Addison disease.[21]

The rapid ACTH stimulation test assesses adrenocortical function and helps to differentiate between primary and secondary adrenal insufficiency. In the rapid ACTH test, a dose of synthetic ACTH is injected, and plasma cortisol levels are drawn at specific predetermined times. A subnormal rise in cortisol in response to ACTH stimulation indicates primary adrenocortical insufficiency.

Plasma ACTH levels also can help to differentiate between primary and secondary disease. Elevated levels of ACTH are associated with primary adrenocortical insufficiency; inappropriately normal or low levels are associated with secondary adrenocortical insufficiency. A normal response to the ACTH stimulation test excludes primary adrenocortical insufficiency; however, this does not exclude individuals with partial secondary adrenocortical insufficiency who may produce sufficient ACTH to maintain cortisol levels. In this case, insulin-induced hypoglycemia may be used to test the hypothalamic–anterior pituitary–adrenocortical axis. Insulin-induced hypoglycemia should result in a stress response associated with increases in plasma ACTH, serum cortisol, growth hormone, prolactin, and activation of the sympathetic nervous system.[25]

Patients with adrenocortical insufficiency are treated with specific hormone replacement regimens to correct the glucocorticoid and mineralocorticoid deficiencies. The primary medication of choice is hydrocortisone (cortisol). Treatment includes lifelong replacement of glucocorticoids, mineralocorticoids, and androgens for men. The levels of these hormones need to be monitored closely to avoid symptoms of hormonal excess.[21]

In an adrenal crisis, the primary treatment is directed toward replacing glucocorticoids and sodium and water deficits. This involves intravenous infusions of hydrocortisone, normal saline, and vasopressor medications (e.g., dopamine) if necessary. The high doses of hydrocortisone needed during treatment of adrenal crisis usually provide sufficient mineralocorticoid replacement. Electrolyte levels should be measured to assist in determining adjustments to drug dosages.

Cushing Syndrome

Cushing syndrome is a clinical condition that results from chronic exposure to excess glucocorticoids; this can be the result of exogenous pharmacologic doses of corticosteroids or an endogenous source of cortisol.[26] Cushing syndrome is generally classified as ACTH-dependent (80%) or ACTH-independent (20%).[26]

ACTH-dependent Cushing syndrome that results from pituitary corticotropic adenoma is referred to as **Cushing disease** (**Figure 38.10**). This disorder affects more women than men, accounts for approximately 65–70% of the cases of hypercortisolism, and is most commonly diagnosed in the second to fourth decades.[26–28] Other causes of ACTH-dependent Cushing syndrome include ectopic ACTH secretion from a nonpituitary tumor (10–15%), ectopic secretion of CRH (< 1%), and iatrogenic administration of ACTH (< 1%).[29]

Etiology and Pathogenesis

Cushing syndrome develops over a period of years. Excessive secretion of ACTH by the pituitary adenoma results in excessive stimulation of the adrenal cortex, leading to adrenal cortical hyperplasia and the excessive production of glucocorticoids. The secretion of ACTH from a nonpituitary tumor (e.g., bronchogenic carcinoma) also can lead to bilateral adrenocortical hyperplasia and excessive production of glucocorticoids. CRH secretion from the hypothalamus can cause hyperplasia of the pituitary corticotrophs, bilateral hypersecretion of ACTH, and excessive production of glucocorticoids.[25]

Clinical Manifestations

Clinical manifestations of Cushing syndrome vary widely and are due to excessive levels of cortisol. They include the following:

- Progressive redistribution of fat in the abdomen (central obesity), face (moon facies), and neck (supraclavicular fat pads) and exophthalmos (retro-orbital fat deposition)
- Dermatologic manifestations such as skin atrophy, fragile skin that is easily bruised, striae (purple and red

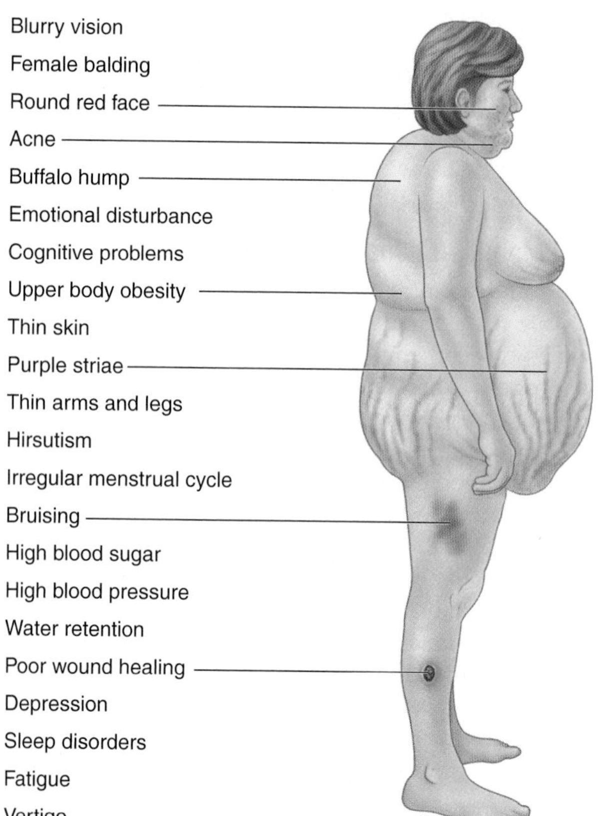

Figure 38.10 Characteristic features of a patient with Cushing disease.

stretch marks) from stretching over fragile skin, and hyperpigmentation (from ectopic ACTH secretion)

- Metabolic complications, such as impaired glucose tolerance from cortisol-stimulated gluconeogenesis and insulin resistance and hypertension from complex, not clearly defined mechanisms
- Reproductive changes such as menstrual abnormalities, hirsutism, and acne associated with increased virilization from adrenal androgens
- Musculoskeletal changes such as proximal muscle myopathy associated with the catabolic effects of glucocorticoids, osteoporosis from decreased bone formation, increased bone reabsorption (breakdown), and reduced intestinal and renal calcium resorption
- Neuropsychiatric changes such as labile mood, agitated depression, anxiety, impaired memory, and impaired cognition.[25]

Linking Pathophysiology to Diagnosis and Treatment

Determining a diagnosis of Cushing syndrome includes establishing the presence of hypercortisolism, determining whether the hypercortisolism is ACTH-dependent or ACTH-independent, and determining the source of the ACTH in the ACTH-dependent form.[25]

Examples of tests used to determine the presence of hypercortisolism include a 24-hour urinary free cortisol, a 1-mg overnight dexamethasone suppression test, and/or a 2 mg/day low-dose dexamethasone suppression test.[25] The suppression tests are based on the premise that dexamethasone, a pharmacologic corticosteroid preparation, will provide negative feedback to the pituitary gland to suppress the ACTH secretion. Therefore, nonsuppression of ACTH indicates hypercortisolism.

Once the presence of hypercortisolism has been established, the differentiation between ACTH-independent and ACTH-dependent Cushing syndrome can be supported through diagnostic tests such as serum ACTH and cortisol levels. For example, undetectable or low levels of ACTH and high levels of serum cortisol would support a diagnosis of ACTH-independent hypercortisolism. An MRI of the adrenal glands would then be indicated to assess for adrenocortical masses that might be the source of hypercortisolism.

An elevated ACTH level indicates that the hypercortisolism is ACTH-dependent. In this case, the healthcare provider must assess whether the source of the ACTH is Cushing disease or ectopic ACTH secretion. A procedure used to differentiate between these is the high-dose dexamethasone suppression test. This test is based on the fact that high doses of glucocorticoid partially suppress ACTH secretion from most ACTH-secreting pituitary tumors, whereas most nonpituitary tumors associated with ectopic ACTH production are resistant to feedback inhibition. In addition, inferior petrosal sinus sampling, an invasive procedure that samples ACTH in the blood draining the pituitary to peripheral levels of ACTH, may be performed. Assessing the gradient between the pituitary and peripheral ACTH may be helpful when the source of ACTH production (pituitary versus ectopic) is not clear.

The treatment of hypercortisolism depends on the source. Primary treatment of Cushing disease involves resection of the ACTH-secreting tumor. After removal, the individual will require lifetime replacement of glucocorticoids. Radiotherapy is a secondary option for patients who cannot have surgery or if the tumor was not completely removed with surgery.[26]

Iatrogenic Cushing syndrome, caused by pharmacologic therapy, can be treated with *gradual* withdrawal of medications. This gradual withdrawal is necessary because chronic use of pharmacologic glucocorticoid preparations suppress ACTH secretion, and sudden discontinuation of these medications can result in adrenal insufficiency. ACTH-independent Cushing syndrome, demonstrated by CT or MRI imaging, may be treated with bilateral or unilateral adrenalectomy, as indicated. The source of ectopic ACTH production needs to be identified. ACTH-secreting tumors are resected when possible; however, if metastatic disease is present, patients may need to be treated medically with medications that interfere with production of adrenocortical hormones (e.g., ketoconazole).

Primary Hyperaldosteronism

There are two major disorders of excess production of aldosterone: primary hyperaldosteronism and secondary hyperaldosteronism. **Primary hyperaldosteronism** or *Conn syndrome* is referred to as renin-independent hyperaldosteronism. **Secondary hyperaldosteronism** is referred to as renin-dependent hyperaldosteronism.[30] In primary hyperaldosteronism, the cause of excess aldosterone production resides within the adrenal cortex; in secondary hyperaldosteronism, the cause resides external to the adrenal cortex. Primary hyperaldosteronism primarily results from an aldosterone-producing adenoma or bilateral adrenocortical hyperplasia; secondary hyperaldosteronism occurs when aldosterone is stimulated by excess secretion of renin by the juxtaglomerular apparatus of the kidney. Secondary hyperaldosteronism is a response to hypovolemia as seen in renovascular hypertension and with diuretic therapy.[30]

Etiology and Pathogenesis

The synthesis and release of mineralocorticoids are regulated by the RAAS. Renin is an enzyme produced by the juxtaglomerular cells of the kidney; these cells are sensitive to changes in both blood volume and plasma sodium concentration. In the presence of hypovolemia or hyponatremia, the juxtaglomerular cells secrete renin, which acts on angiotensinogen to form angiotensin I. Angiotensin I is converted to angiotensin II by angiotensin-converting enzyme. Angiotensin II stimulates the release of aldosterone from the zona glomerulosa. In addition to the RAAS, the zona glomerulosa is controlled to a lesser degree by potassium and ACTH.

Clinical Manifestations

Patients with primary hyperaldosteronism generally present with hypertension, muscle weakness, polydipsia, polyuria, headaches, and fatigue.[30] The hypertension is often long-standing and refractory to multiple medications. The diagnosis of primary hyperaldosteronism is suspected in any patient with unexplained hypokalemia or hypokalemia while on diuretic therapy despite potassium supplementation. Other biochemical abnormalities may include hypernatremia, alkalosis, and hypochloremia. The two major biochemical tests used to diagnose primary hyperaldosteronism measure the plasma aldosterone concentration and the plasma renin activity.[30] Elevated plasma and urine aldosterone levels with suppressed plasma renin activity assist in confirming the diagnosis. Failure to suppress plasma aldosterone with oral or intravenous salt loading also supports the diagnosis of primary hyperaldosteronism. Following the biochemical diagnosis, localization of the adenoma or bilateral hyperplasia can be confirmed through imaging studies such as adrenal MRI or CT.

Linking Pathophysiology to Diagnosis and Treatment

Primary hyperaldosteronism caused by an adenoma is usually treated by surgical removal of the adenoma. If the underlying cause is bilateral hyperplasia, surgery is indicated only if the hypokalemia cannot be controlled with medical treatment. The medical treatment involves the administration of an aldosterone antagonist (e.g., spironolactone).[30] The hypertension and hypokalemia associated with primary hyperaldosteronism are usually controlled with daily doses of spironolactone. Treatment of secondary hyperaldosteronism depends on the cause. For example, one of the causes of secondary hyperaldosteronism is renal artery stenosis, which results in decreased renal perfusion; therefore, correction of this problem is indicated.

Congenital Adrenal Hyperplasia

Congenital adrenal hyperplasia (CAH) is an autosomal recessive disorder. The genes that encode for this disorder are programmed within the adrenal steroid biosynthetic pathway and lead to impaired cortisol biosynthesis and an increase in ACTH via negative feedback mechanisms (**Figure 38.11** ■). These high levels of ACTH induce hyperplastic changes of the impaired adrenocortical tissue and increased production of virilizing steroids with minimal or no increase in the production of cortisol.[31] CAH exists in a variety of phenotypical presentations. A severe form of CAH presents with no aldosterone production and is characterized by salt-wasting; another form presents with aldosterone production and virilization. Together, these are referred to as classic CAH.

Etiology and Pathogenesis

Approximately 95% of cases of CAH are due to 21-hydroxylase deficiency, and 5–8% are due to 11β hydroxylase deficiency.[31] Cortisol deficiency is central to the pathogenesis of CAH, and the severity of the clinical presentation results from mutations in genes encoding for enzymes in the pathway, such as 21-hydroxylase. Three fourths of patients with classic CAH are considered "salt wasters."[31] These individuals produce no 21-hydroxylase activity and produce insufficient aldosterone for sodium retention. The remaining patients produce low amounts of aldosterone and do not waste sodium; however, they are virilized and are known as "simple virilizers."[31] Individuals with classic 21-hydroxylase deficiency are at risk for adrenal insufficiency without exogenous glucocorticoid administration.[31]

Clinical Manifestations

Female infants with classic CAH may present with ambiguous genitalia at birth. In such instances, the external genitalia cannot be identified as male or female at birth. Males present with precocious puberty; females present with hirsutism, menstrual irregularities, and infertility.

Linking Pathophysiology to Diagnosis and Treatment

Classic CAH is a highly complex disease. Because cortisol deficiency is the central deficiency, all individuals need glucocorticoid replacement.[32] This restores normal negative feedback to the anterior pituitary on ACTH production and assists in minimizing androgen overproduction.[32] Mineralocorticoids may be supplemented as indicated but are necessary for "salt wasters."

Adrenal Medullary Hyperfunction: Pheochromocytoma

Pheochromocytomas are neuroendocrine tumors that arise from catecholamine-producing chromaffin cells.

Etiology and Pathogenesis

In general, pheochromocytomas are catecholamine-producing tumors located in adrenal or extra-adrenal sites (e.g., retroperitoneal, pelvis, and thorax). Although the majority of these tumors have no defined cause, there is increasing evidence that approximately one fourth of patients with

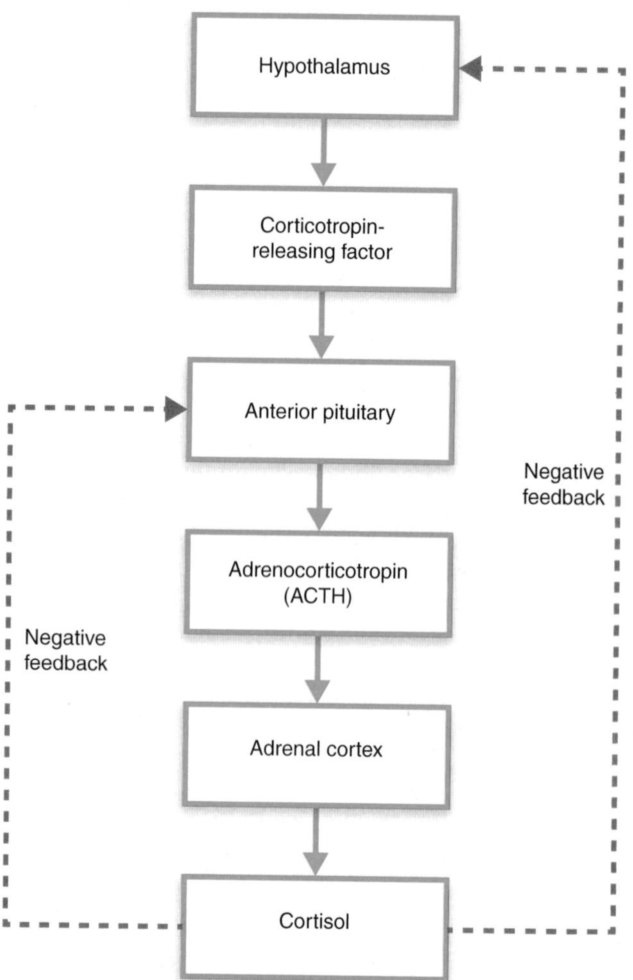

Figure 38.11 ■ The adrenal steroid biosynthetic pathway.

pheochromocytoma carry a germ line mutation consistent with a familial or genetic syndrome. Additionally, pheochromocytomas are sometimes part of MEN syndromes.[32]

Clinical Manifestations

The clinical signs and symptoms of pheochromocytoma are variable and related to the hypersecretion of catecholamines. The clinical features include headaches, excessive sweating, palpitations, tachycardia, sustained and paroxysmal hypertension, anxiety, and panic attacks. The most predominant symptom is hypertension, which may be episodic or sustained. A catecholamine crisis may lead to heart failure, pulmonary edema, arrhythmias, and intracranial hemorrhage. The duration of the episodic hormone release is variable, generally lasting less than an hour, and is characterized by palpitations and tachycardia. These episodes may be precipitated by a number of factors, including surgery, pregnancy, and medications (e.g., tricyclic antidepressants).

Linking Pathophysiology to Diagnosis and Treatment

The diagnosis of pheochromocytoma is based on evidence of catecholamine excess through biochemical testing and localization of the tumor by imaging. These include measurement of plasma and urinary catecholamines and their methylated metabolites: metanephrines. A 24-hour urine collection for fractionated catecholamines, fractionated metanephrines, and dopamine can be done. A variety of methods have been used to localize the tumors, including CT (with contrast) and MRI scanning. Other scanning tests may include radioactive tracers (e.g., I^{31} or iodine-123-metaiodobenzylguanidine).[32]

The complete removal of the tumor is the primary goal of treatment for pheochromocytoma. The patients must be adequately prepared for surgery to avoid effects of excess catecholamines during surgery (e.g., hypertensive crisis). Alpha-adrenergic blockers (e.g., phenoxybenzamine) should be initiated for approximately 10–15 days before surgery. Beta blockers may be added after alpha blockade for control of hypertension. Other antihypertensive medications (e.g., calcium channel blockers or angiotensin-converting enzymes) may be used if blood pressure is difficult to control with phenoxybenzamine alone.

Check Your Progress: Section 38.5

1. Describe the components of the adrenal gland and what each component produces.
2. What would be expected in the treatment of an adrenal crisis?
3. What is a pheochromocytoma, what does it do, what are some of the signs and symptoms, and what can occur in a catecholamine crisis?

CHAPTER SUMMARY

38.1 Chapter Overview and Case Studies

Define hormones and concepts related to endocrine regulation.

- The endocrine system is essential to the regulation of the body.
- The endocrine system regulates functions such as growth, reproduction, metabolism, and fluid and electrolyte balance.
- These alterations in hormone levels affect many functions, including activity and exercise, nutrition and metabolism, elimination, sexuality and reproduction, and the ability to cope with stress.

38.2 Mechanisms of Hormonal Alterations in Thyroid and Adrenal Disease

Outline the mechanisms of hormonal alterations, including hormone excess, hormone deficiency, and levels of hormone dysfunction across the lifespan.

- Disorders of the endocrine system result primarily from either too much or too little production of hormones.
- Normal thyroid and adrenal gland function is dependent on an appropriately functioning hypothalamic–pituitary–target gland access that is guided by negative feedback principles
- Normal parathyroid function is dependent on appropriate hormone–substrate feedback and negative feedback principles.
- Primary dysfunction occurs at the level of target gland. Secondary dysfunction occurs at the level of the anterior pituitary. Tertiary dysfunction occurs at the level of the hypothalamus.

38.3 Disorders of the Thyroid

Differentiate the causes, classification, underlying pathogenesis, and clinical manifestations of disorders of the thyroid across the lifespan.

- Thyroid disorders are exceedingly prevalent in the overall population.
- Thyroid disorders are associated with structural and inflammatory changes in the thyroid.
- Thyroid disorders are characterized primarily by hypofunction and hyperfunction of the thyroid gland.
- Hypothyroidism is associated with decreased metabolic activity.
- The predominant form of hypothyroidism is Hashimoto thyroiditis.
- Hyperthyroidism is associated with increased metabolic activity.
- The predominant form of hyperthyroidism is Graves disease.

38.4 Disorders of the Parathyroid

Differentiate the causes, classification, underlying pathogenesis, and clinical manifestations of disorders of the parathyroid across the lifespan.

- Normal parathyroid function is essential for appropriate calcium and phosphorus metabolism.
- Primary hyperthyroidism results from adenomas or hyperplasia of the parathyroid glands.
- Secondary forms of hyperthyroidism can result from chronic stimulation of the parathyroid glands from disorders that result in calcium deficiency (e.g., renal failure).
- Hypoparathyroidism can result in loss of calcium and phosphorus metabolism.

38.5 Disorders of Adrenocortical Function

Differentiate the causes, classification, underlying pathogenesis, and clinical manifestations of disorders of adrenocortical function across the lifespan.

- The adrenal gland is a highly complex organ consisting of the adrenal cortex and adrenal medulla.
- The adrenal cortex is divided into three layers that produce and secrete a predominant hormone: the adrenal glomerulosa (mineralocorticoids), adrenal fasciculata (glucocorticoids), and reticularis (androgens).
- Adrenocortical disorders are characterized primarily by hypofunction and hyperfunction of the adrenal cortex and are the result of primary (adrenal cortex), secondary (anterior pituitary), or hypothalamic dysfunction.
- Addison disease is the primary disorder associated with adrenal insufficiency.
- Cushing syndrome involves a clinical constellation of symptoms associated with hypercortisolism.
- Primary hyperaldosteronism, or Conn disease, is a disorder of excessive aldosterone production.
- Congenital adrenal hyperplasia is an autosomal recessive disorder in which genes encoding enzymes in the adrenal steroid biosynthetic pathway are impaired, resulting in alterations in the production of glucocorticoids, mineralocorticoids, and androgens.
- Pheochromocytomas are catecholamine-producing tumors located in adrenal or extra-adrenal sites.

REVIEW QUESTIONS

1. Chronic kidney disease can contribute to the development of which disorder?
   a. Primary hyperparathyroidism
   b. Secondary hyperparathyroidism
   c. Primary adrenal insufficiency
   d. Secondary adrenal insufficiency
2. Latent tetany can be demonstrated by which set of signs?
   a. Holman and Trousseau signs
   b. Chvostek and Markle signs
   c. Holman and Chvostek signs
   d. Chvostek and Trousseau signs
3. To confirm Hashimoto thyroiditis, the nurse would expect to see which of the following laboratory results?
   a. Decreased TSH and decreased FT4
   b. Elevated TSH and elevated FT4
   c. Elevated TSH and decreased FT4
   d. Decreased TSH and elevated FT4
4. Which of the following can secrete ACTH?
   a. Bronchogenic carcinoma
   b. Thyroid carcinoma
   c. Parathyroidoma
   d. Pheochromocytoma
5. A client presents to the hospital with central obesity, striae, impaired glucose tolerance, proximal muscle myopathy, and impaired memory. The nurse suspects which of the following conditions?
   a. Hashimoto thyroiditis
   b. Toxic adenoma
   c. Cushing syndrome
   d. Graves disease
6. The adrenal medulla is part of the
   a. peripheral nervous system.
   b. central nervous system.
   c. sympathetic nervous system.
   d. parasympathetic nervous system.
7. Which system regulates the release of mineralocorticoids?
   a. ANS
   b. RAAS
   c. HPA
   d. TABB
8. What is the primary deficiency in CAH?
   a. Cortisol
   b. Thyroxine
   c. Calcitonin
   d. Triiodothyronine

ANSWERS

Answers to Review Questions can be found in Appendix A. Answers to Case Study and Check Your Progress questions are available on the faculty resources site. Please consult with your instructor.

RECOMMENDED WEBSITES

American Thyroid Association
https://www.thyroid.org

Congenital Adrenal Hyperplasia
https://rarediseases.info.nih.gov/diseases/1467/congenital-adrenal-hyperplasia

Endocrine Diseases
https://www.niddk.nih.gov/health-information/endocrine-diseases/adrenal-insufficiency-addisons-disease

REFERENCES

1. Molina, P. E. (2013). *Endocrine physiology* (3rd ed.). New York, NY: McGraw-Hill Medical.
2. Vitti, P. (2017). Iodine deficiency disorders. *UpToDate.* Available at https://www.uptodate.com/contents/iodine-deficiency-disorders
3. American Thyroid Association. (2017a). *General information/press room.* Available at http://www.thyroid.org/media-main/about-hypothyroidism
4. Ross, D. (2015). Overview of thyroid nodule formation. *UpToDate.* Available at https://www.uptodate.com/contents/overview-of-thyroid-nodule-formation
5. Ross, D. (2017). Clinical presentation and evaluation of goiter in adults. *UpToDate.* Available at http://www.uptodate.com/contents/clinical-presentation-and-evaluation-of-goiter-in-adults
6. Clutter, W. E. (2013). Hyperthyroidism. In J. B. McGill, W. E. Clutter, & T. J. Baranski (Eds.), *Washington manual endocrinology subspecialty consult* (pp. 52–60). Baltimore, MD: Lippincott Williams & Wilkins.
7. Burman, K. D. (2017). *Overview of thyroiditis.* Available at https://www.uptodate.com/contents/overview-of-thyroiditis
8. Holt, R., & Hanley, N. (2013). *Essential endocrinology and diabetes.* Hoboken, NJ: John Wiley & Sons.
9. Cooper, D., & Ladenson, P. (2011). The thyroid gland. In D. Gardner & D. Shoback (Eds.), *Greenspan's basic and clinical endocrinology* (pp. 163–226). New York, NY: McGraw-Hill.
10. Weiss, R. E., & Refetoff, S. (2017). *TSH-secreting pituitary adenomas.* Available at https://www.uptodate.com/contents/tsh-secreting-pituitary-adenomas
11. Almandoz, J. P., & Gharib, H. (2012). Hypothyroidism: Etiology, diagnosis, and management. *Medical Clinics of North America, 96*(2), 203–221. doi:10.1016/j.mcna.2012.01.005
12. Ross, D. S. (2017). Disorders that cause hypothyroidism. *UpToDate.* Available at https://www.uptodate.com/contents/disorders-that-cause-hypothyroidism
13. American Cancer Society. (2017). *Key statistics for thyroid cancer.* Available at https://www.cancer.org/cancer/thyroid-cancer/about/key-statistics.html
14. American Thyroid Association. (2017). *Thyroid cancer.* Available at http://www.thyroid.org/wp-content/uploads/patients/brochures/ThyroidCancer_brochure.pdf?pdf=Thyroid-Cancer-Brochure
15. American Thyroid Association. (2017). *Medullary thyroid cancer.* Available at http://www.thyroid.org/wp-content/uploads/patients/brochures/medullary-thyroid-cancer-brochure.pdf?pdf=Medullary-Thyroid-Cancer-Brochure
16. Tuttle, R. M., & Sherman, E. J. (2017). Anaplastic thyroid cancer. *UpToDate.* Available at https://www.uptodate.com/contents/anaplastic-thyroid-cancer
17. Clutter, W. E. (2013). Euthyroid goiter and thyroid nodules. In J. B. McGill, W. E. Clutter, & T. J. Baranski (Eds.), *Washington manual endocrinology subspecialty consult* (pp. 46–51). Baltimore, MD: Lippincott Williams & Wilkins.
18. Essig, G. F. (2016). Parathyroid physiology. *Medscape.* Available at http://emedicine.medscape.com/article/874690-overview
19. Shoback, D., Sellmeyer, D., & Bikle, D. (2011). Metabolic bone disease. In D. G. Gardner & D. Shoback (Eds.), *Greenspan's basic and clinical endocrinology* (pp. 237–284). New York, NY: McGraw-Hill Medical.
20. U.S. National Library of Medicine. (2017). Adrenal gland disorders. *MedlinePlus.* Available at https://medlineplus.gov/adrenalglanddisorders.html
21. Michels, A., & Michels, N. (2014). Addison disease: Early detection and treatment principles. *American Family Physician, 89*(7), 563–568.
22. Kirkland, L. (2017). Adrenal crisis. *Medscape.* Available at http://emedicine.medscape.com/article/116716-overview
23. Melmed, S., Polonsky, K. S., Larsen, P. R., & Kronenberg, H. M. (2016). *Williams textbook of endocrinology* (13th ed.). Philadelphia, PA: Elsevier.
24. Nieman, L. K. (2017). Causes of secondary and tertiary adrenal insufficiency in adults. *UpToDate.* Available at http://www.uptodate.com/contents/causes-of-secondary-and-tertiary-adrenal-insufficiency-in-adults
25. Goodwin, S., & Silverstein, J. (2013). Cushing's syndrome. In J. B. McGill, W. E. Clutter, & T. J. Baranski (Eds.), *Washington manual endocrinology subspecialty consult* (pp. 98–107). Baltimore, MD: Lippincott Williams & Wilkins.
26. Lacroix, A., Feelders, R. A., Stratakis, C. A., & Nieman, L. K. (2015). Cushing's syndrome. *Lancet, 386*(9996), 913–927. doi:10.1016/S0140-6736(14)61375-1
27. Else, T., Hammer, G., & McPhee, S. (2010). Disorders of the adrenal cortex. In S. J. McPhee & G. D. Hammer (Eds.), *Pathophysiology of disease: An introduction to clinical medicine* (6th ed., pp. 571–601). New York, NY: McGraw-Hill Lange.
28. Raff, H., Sharma, S. T., & Nieman, L. K. (2014). Physiological basis for the etiology, diagnosis, and treatment of adrenal disorders: Cushing syndrome, adrenal insufficiency, and congenital adrenal hyperplasia. *Comprehensive Physiology, 4*(2), 739–769.
29. Nieman, L. K. (2017). Causes of secondary and tertiary adrenal insufficiency in adults. *UpToDate.* Available at http://www.uptodate.com/contents/causes-of-secondary-and-tertiary-adrenal-insufficiency-in-adults
30. Johnson, M., & Baranski, T. J. (2013). Conn's syndrome. In J. B. McGill, W. E. Clutter, & T. J. Baranski (Eds.), *Washington manual endocrinology subspecialty consult* (pp. 89–97). Baltimore, MD: Lippincott Williams & Wilkins.
31. Dunai, J. & Carmichael, K. (2013). Adult congenital adrenal hyperplasia. In J. McGill, W. E. Clutter, & Baranski (Eds.), *Washington manual endocrinology subspecialty consult* (pp. 84–88). Baltimore, MD: Lippincott Williams & Wilkins.
32. Joshi, P. M., & Fisher, S. J. (2013). Pheochromocytoma. In J. B. McGill, W. E. Clutter, & T. J. Baranski (Eds.), *Washington manual endocrinology subspecialty consult* (pp. 108–120). Baltimore, MD: Lippincott Williams & Wilkins.

Unit XII
Altered Tissue Integrity

The term *tissue integrity* typically applies to the skin and mucous membranes. Alterations in tissue integrity can range from minor, such as the scratches from brush or tree limbs associated with playing outdoors, to more complicated alterations such as psoriasis, a chronic inflammatory skin disorder, or pressure injuries that develop as a result of unrelieved pressure to an area of the skin, or even life-threatening infections. The etiology of alterations to tissue integrity is as varied as the types of alterations. Herpes simplex virus 2 is spread through sexual contact; vitiligo is a multifactorial disorder involving genetic and environmental elements; and cellulitis is an infection that can occur via a break in the skin. Wounds may occur as a result of accident, an act of violence, or as a result of a surgical procedure.

Regardless of the nature of the alteration or its etiology, all but the most minor impairments in tissue integrity require prompt assessment and care to prevent worsening of the condition, increased discomfort or embarrassment, and, in some cases, life-altering or life-threatening sequelae. Nursing assessment of the patient with an alteration in skin integrity includes explaining any procedures or tests in advance; assessing for use of medications or complementary therapies that may affect skin integrity or test results; and monitoring and documenting any procedures and tests and their results.[1]

Nursing care of the patient with alterations in tissue integrity varies according to the nature of the disorder and the extent of the alteration. For example, nursing care of an infant with diaper rash is very different from care of the patient having a basal cell carcinoma removed, which is very different from care of the patient just out of surgery. However, some general guidelines regarding patient teaching will apply in most cases[1]:

- Practice thorough hand hygiene
- Avoid sharing personal hygiene products
- Know and look for manifestations of infection
- Call the healthcare provider if signs of infection occur or if pain increases or the condition worsens
- Avoid scratching or picking the skin
- Apply topical medications or take oral medications as prescribed.

References

1. Lemone, P., Burke, K., Bauldoff, G., & Gubrud, P. (2014). *Medical-Surgical Nursing: Clinical Reasoning in Patient Care* (6th ed.). Hoboken, NJ: Pearson Education.

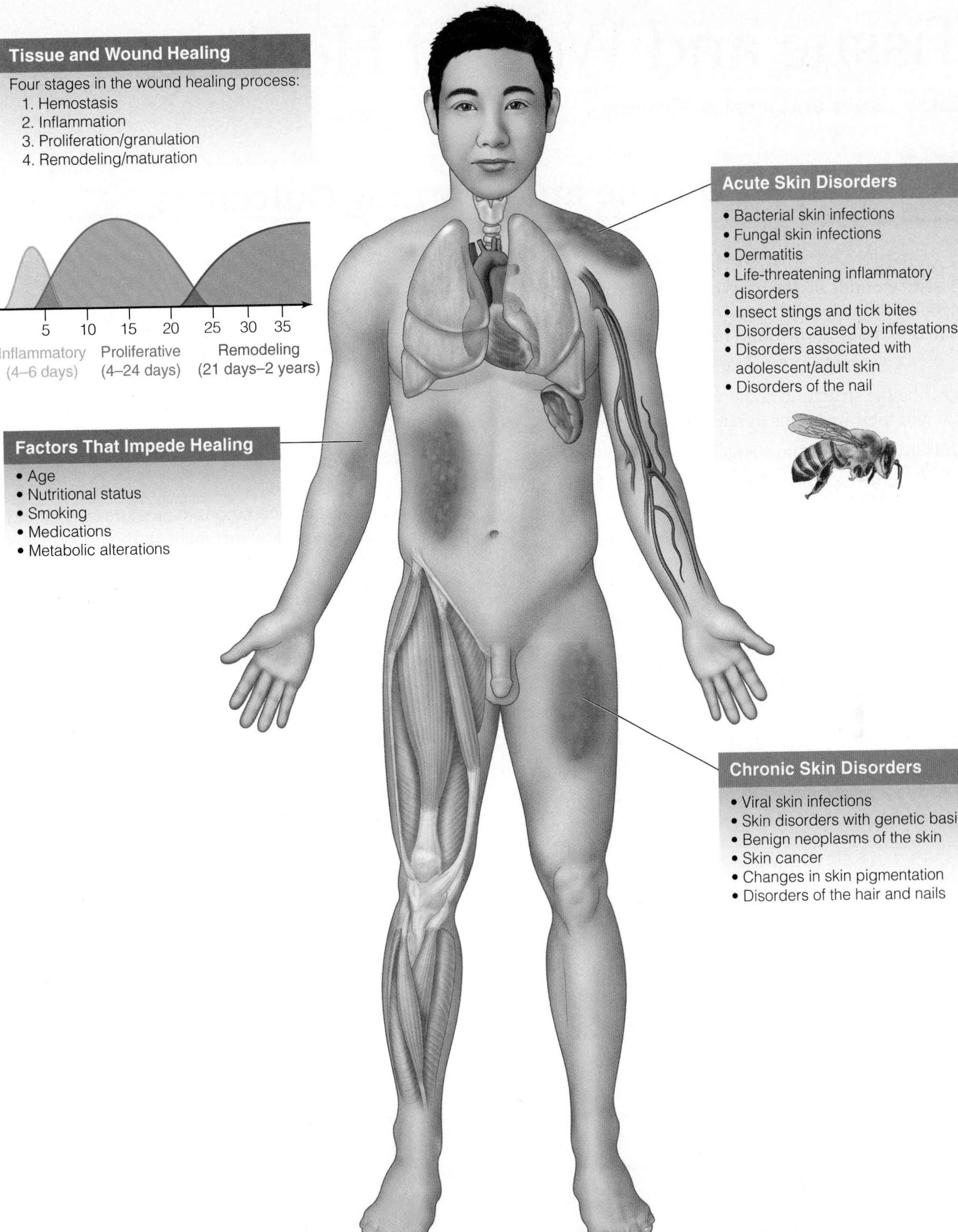
Tissue and Wound Healing
Four stages in the wound healing process:
1. Hemostasis
2. Inflammation
3. Proliferation/granulation
4. Remodeling/maturation
5
10
15
20
25
30
35
Inflammatory (4–6 days)
Proliferative (4–24 days)
Remodeling (21 days–2 years)
Factors That Impede Healing
• Age
• Nutritional status
• Smoking
• Medications
• Metabolic alterations
Acute Skin Disorders
• Bacterial skin infections
• Fungal skin infections
• Dermatitis
• Life-threatening inflammatory disorders
• Insect stings and tick bites
• Disorders caused by infestations
• Disorders associated with adolescent/adult skin
• Disorders of the nail
Chronic Skin Disorders
• Viral skin infections
• Skin disorders with genetic basis
• Benign neoplasms of the skin
• Skin cancer
• Changes in skin pigmentation
• Disorders of the hair and nails

Chapter 39
Tissue and Wound Healing

Kathy Lauer and Jessica Simmons

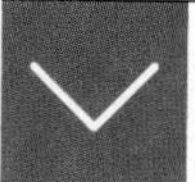

Chapter Outline and Learning Outcomes

39.1 Chapter Overview and Case Studies

Classify wounds on the basis of acute/chronic and partial/full thickness criteria and describe concepts related to tissue and wound healing.

39.2 The Structure of the Skin

Describe the structural components of each layer of skin and their functions in maintaining homeostasis.

39.3 Cutaneous Wound Healing

Differentiate the types of cutaneous wound healing by intention and the phases of wound healing.

39.4 Factors Impeding Wound Healing

Analyze the impact of local and systemic factors on wound healing.

39.5 Spectrum of Wound Healing

Compare the mechanisms of the continuum of wound healing, from scarless fetal wound healing to abnormal wound healing.

39.6 Pressure Injuries

Differentiate the causes, classification, underlying pathogenesis, and clinical manifestations of pressure injuries and approaches to diagnosis and treatment for these conditions.

KEY TERMS

Angiogenesis, 967
Apoptosis, 958
Collagen, 959
Contracture, 974
Cytokine, 955
Debridement, 976
Dendritic (Langerhans) cells, 958
Dermal papillae, 958
Dermis, 958
Elastin, 959
Epidermis, 957
Eschar, 976
Extracellular matrix (ECM), 959
Evisceration, 974
Fibroblasts, 967
Full thickness wound, 955
Glycosaminoglycans (GAGs) , 960
Granulation tissue, 967
Growth factor, 963
Hemostasis, 963
Hyaluronan, 960
Hypertrophic scar, 974
Hypodermis, 959
Integrins, 961
Keloid, 973
Keratinization, 957
Keratinocyte, 957
Laminin, 959
Maceration, 976
Melanocyte, 957
Partial thickness wound, 955
Pressure injury, 975
Primary intention, 961
Reepithelialization, 955
Secondary intention, 961
Shearing forces, 975
Stratum basale, 957
Stratum corneum, 958
Stratum granulosum, 958
Stratum lucidum, 958
Stratum spinosum, 957
Tertiary intention, 962
Wound, 955

ABBREVIATIONS

CSF—colony-stimulating factor
DEJ—dermal–epidermal junction
ECM—extracellular matrix
EGF—epidermal growth factor
FGF—fibroblast growth factor
GAG—glycosaminoglycan
GM-CSF—granulocyte macrophage colony-stimulating factor
IGF—insulin-like growth factor
IL—interleukin
IFN—interferon
KGF—keratinocyte growth factor
PDGF—platelet-derived growth factor
PMN—polymorphonuclear neutrophil
TGF—transforming growth factor
TNF—tumor necrosis factor
VEGF—vascular endothelial growth factor

39.1 Chapter Overview and Case Studies

The human body has a remarkable ability to heal itself after suffering a wound or injury. A **wound** may be defined as an injury that disrupts the normal structure and function of a tissue or organ. Healthcare providers often care for patients in various stages of the wound healing process from the initial injury to the repair, which may continue for several months. A firm grasp of the wound healing process is important for providing effective care.

Concepts Related to Tissue and Wound Healing

A simple means of classifying wounds is based on whether they are acute or chronic and whether they are partial thickness or full thickness. An acute wound is one that occurs suddenly or over a brief period of time. Acute wounds result from physical trauma, such as lacerations, abrasions, and burns, or from medical interventions such as surgical repair. An acute wound typically heals in an organized and timely manner, resulting in the restoration of structural and functional integrity, often within a 4- to 6-week period.

A chronic wound is one that occurs over a relatively long period of time. An acute wound that does not heal properly may become a chronic wound as the result of a prolonged state of inflammation. Chronic wounds do not proceed through the stages of healing in an organized and timely manner, and they often result in some degree of impairment of structural and functional integrity in the tissue.

Wounds may also be described as partial or full thickness on the basis of the depth of the injury. A **partial thickness wound** is one in which damage extends through the epidermis while all or a portion the dermis remains intact. Partial thickness wounds are predominantly repaired by **reepithelialization**, a process whereby epithelial cells migrate to the area and replicate by mitosis. A **full thickness wound** is one involving extension of damage through the epidermis and the entire thickness of the dermis, with possible extension into subcutaneous tissue, muscle, and bone.[1] Repair of a full thickness wound is quite complex and may result in considerable scar formation.

The phenomenon of wound healing, also referred to as tissue repair, is a dynamic and complex yet somewhat predictable process. The process of healing in cutaneous wounds has been studied extensively. Because most organs in the body are capable of tissue repair in a manner similar to that in the skin, cutaneous wound healing is used as the prototype in this chapter.

The wound healing process proceeds in four sequential, overlapping phases:

1. Hemostasis
2. Inflammation
3. Proliferation/granulation
4. Remodeling/maturation.

Each phase of the process is directed by cells that secrete chemical mediators that direct the healing process. These cells include neutrophils, macrophages, lymphocytes, platelets, keratinocytes, fibroblasts, and endothelial cells. The chemical mediators include a significant number of growth factors and **cytokines**, substances secreted by cells that help cells to communicate with each other and coordinate the healing process. The profile of cell types and chemical mediators at the site of injury changes as the healing processes unfolds.

Although many wounds heal without complications, a variety of local and systemic factors can impede wound healing. Lifestyle risk factors (e.g., obesity, smoking) and environmental risk factors (e.g., medications, radiation, exposure to heat) influence the success of wound healing. Nutritional deficits and inadequate hydration status place an individual at risk through the loss of skin turgor and necessary vitamins necessary for proper wound healing. The individual who has lost mobility because of a stroke or chronic disease (e.g., multiple sclerosis, spinal cord injury) is more prone to experience pressure in sensitive areas, such as bony prominences. Increased pressure in these areas restricts blood flow, resulting in ischemic damage and tissue necrosis, manifesting as pressure injuries. A lack of adequate perfusion to distal extremities can cause arterial or venous ulceration. Furthermore, wounds sometimes result in a lack of skin integrity, placing the individual at risk for development of infection, which can complicate the healing process. Selected concepts related to tissue and wound healing are shown in **Figure 39.1** ■.

Case Studies

To reinforce important clinical concepts regarding tissue and wound healing, the following cases will be addressed throughout the chapter to assist in application of chapter content to clinical situations involving wound healing.

Helen Baker: Introduction

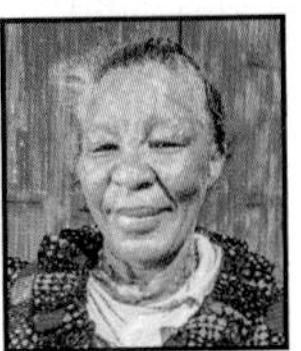

Helen Baker is 80 years old and lives in a nursing home. She is taken to the emergency department (ED) with altered mental status. Mrs. Baker has a history of dementia as well as Crohn disease and is taking prednisone. Within the past 3 days, her activity has been declining, and she is staying in bed. Her food intake has decreased to less than 25% of her meals. This morning, she was nonverbal with an elevated temperature of 38.7°C (101.6°F). Upon arrival at the ED, Mrs. Baker is incontinent of urine and stool. While providing incontinence care, the healthcare provider notes a dressing over Mrs. Baker's sacrum. The provider removes the dressing and notes a 4 cm × 4 cm × 0.5 cm wound with red cobblestone-like tissue in the wound bed. A small amount of serous drainage is noted on the dressing. The surrounding skin is intact with no erythema, induration, or fluctuance.

1. On the basis of her history, which findings increase Mrs. Baker's risk for poor wound healing?
2. Which of Mrs. Baker's physical findings support the presence of a partial thickness wound?

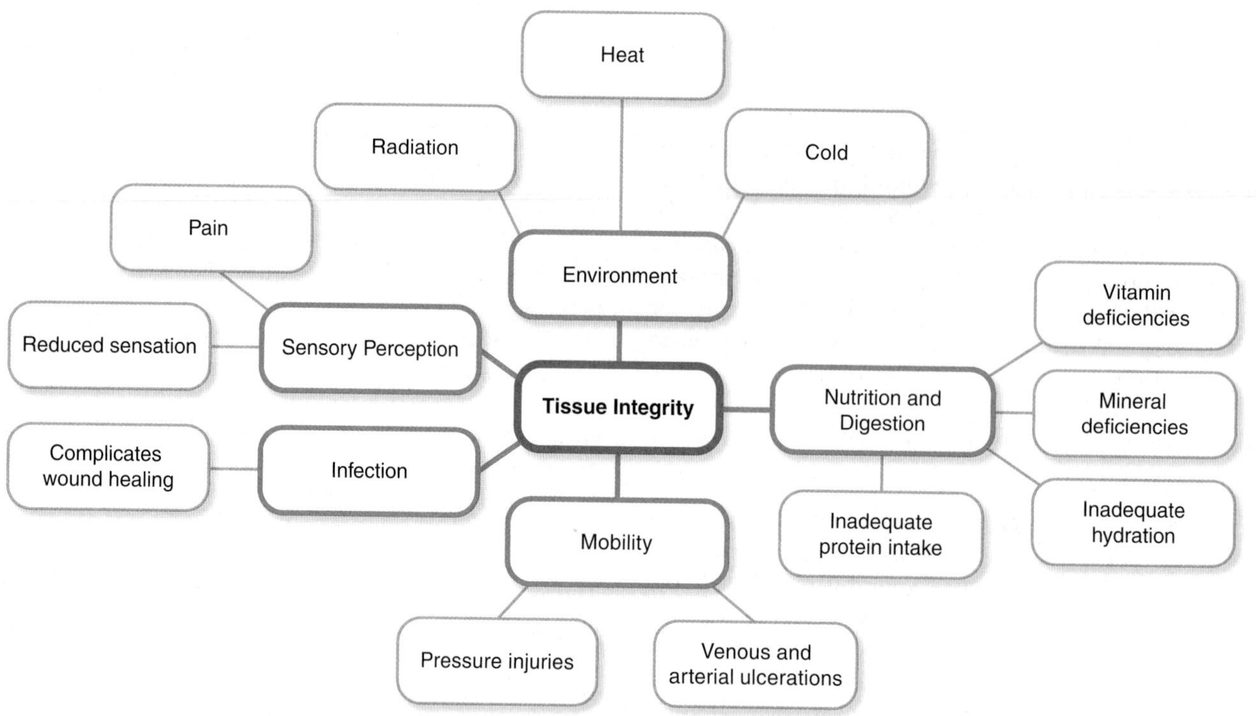

Figure 39.1 ■ Concepts related to tissue and wound healing.

Maria King: Introduction

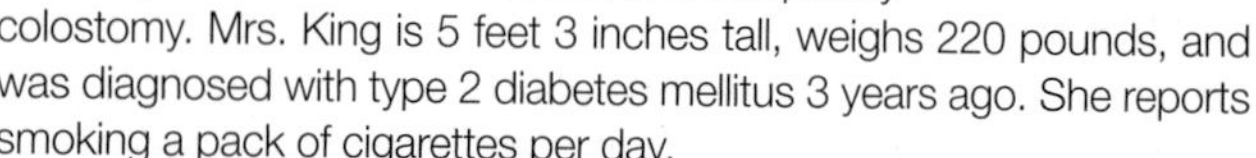

Maria King, age 56, was diagnosed with a large polyp in her descending colon that showed severe dysplasia on biopsy. She was admitted to the hospital for a colon resection and temporary colostomy. Mrs. King is 5 feet 3 inches tall, weighs 220 pounds, and was diagnosed with type 2 diabetes mellitus 3 years ago. She reports smoking a pack of cigarettes per day.

After surgery, she had a midline incision approximated with staples and a drain placed in the inferior portion of the incision. Ms. King had moderate serosanguineous output from the drain, which decreased significantly by the third postoperative day. On auscultation of the chest immediately after surgery and for the first 2 days postoperatively, Ms. King had coarse crackles in both lung fields that cleared with vigorous coughing, hourly use of an incentive spirometer, and frequent reminders and coaching by the nurses.

Ms. King was discharged on the fifth postoperative day. At that time, her drain had been removed, and she had minimal incisional drainage. However, the discharge nurse noted redness around the lower two thirds of the incision and a superficial 2-cm-long separation of her incision at midpoint.

Ms. King has returned to the surgeon's office on the tenth postoperative day for staple removal. The surgeon notes that Ms. King has a frequent and productive cough. When questioned, Ms. King admits to resuming her preoperative smoking habit. On inspection of the incision, the surgeon notes several areas of what appear to be partial dermal separation. On removal of the staples, dehiscence of the wound is apparent in the lower half of the incision, and a large amount of dark serosanguineous drainage is expressed. The entire lower half of the incision is opened down to the fascial layer, which is found to be intact.

1. On the basis of Ms. King's clinical presentation on her postoperative visit with her surgeon, what factors may be affecting her wound healing?
2. Which observations indicate that Ms. King's wound healing is impaired?

Check Your Progress: Section 39.1

1. What are the stages of wound healing?
2. Explain the differences between a partial thickness wound and a full thickness wound.
3. What factors negatively affect wound healing?

39.2 The Structure of the Skin

The skin is the largest organ in the body, comprising 1.2–2.2 square meters, weighing 4–5 kilograms (9–11 pounds), and accounting for 7% of total body weight.[2] Important functions of the skin include the following:

- It provides a waterproof barrier that serves as a first line of defense to prevent entry of harmful environmental stressors, such as microorganisms, ultraviolet radiation, toxins, or dirt into the body.
- It minimizes excessive water loss.
- It maintains effective thermoregulation.
- It contains receptors for somatic sensations, including touch, pain, and temperature.
- It participates in the metabolism and activation of the vitamin D in the skin when exposed to ultraviolet light.

Skin in different regions of the body varies in thickness, pigment, and distribution. Its normal thickness can vary from about 1.5–4.0 mm.[2] The differences are based on the functions required of specific regions. For example, the skin is very thick in areas of the body that are exposed to high levels of friction, such as the soles of the feet.

Skin is divided into two layers: the epidermis and the dermis. The layers are separated by a thin layer of connective tissue called the basement membrane.

The Epidermis

The **epidermis** is the visible, upper layer of skin. It is composed of multiple layers of stratified squamous epithelial cells called **keratinocytes**.[3] Keratinocytes in the deepest layer of the epidermis can be columnar or cuboidal, but they become flatter as they progress toward the skin surface (**Figure 39.2** ■). Other cells that are present in the epidermis, but in much smaller numbers, are melanocytes, T lymphocytes, dendritic (Langerhans) cells, and tactile (Merkel) cells These cells have important specialized functions that contribute to epidermal homeostasis and repair.[4] Although the epidermis is avascular and contains no lymphatic vessels, it is sustained by nutrients from the blood vessels in the dermis that diffuse though the basement membrane.

As they migrate from the basal layer to the skin surface, keratinocytes synthesize large amounts of keratin, a water-insoluble protein. By the time they reach the surface, all the cytoplasm has been replaced by keratin, and the cells are dry, scaly, and dead. This process, which takes approximately 3–5 weeks, is called **keratinization**. Keratinization gives the outer layers of the epidermis a tough, horny quality that provides protection for the underlying basal layers, which contain the stem cells needed for keratinocyte regeneration.

The epidermis comprises three to five layers: the stratum basale, stratum spinosum, stratum granulosum, stratum lucidum, and stratum corneum. (**Figure 39.3** ■).

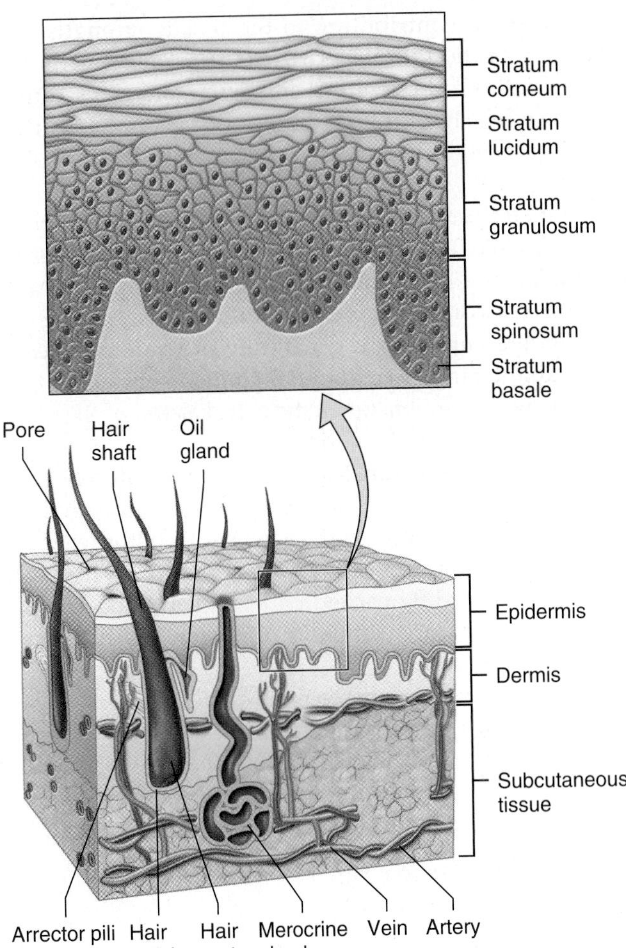

Figure 39.3 ■ The epidermal layers of human skin.

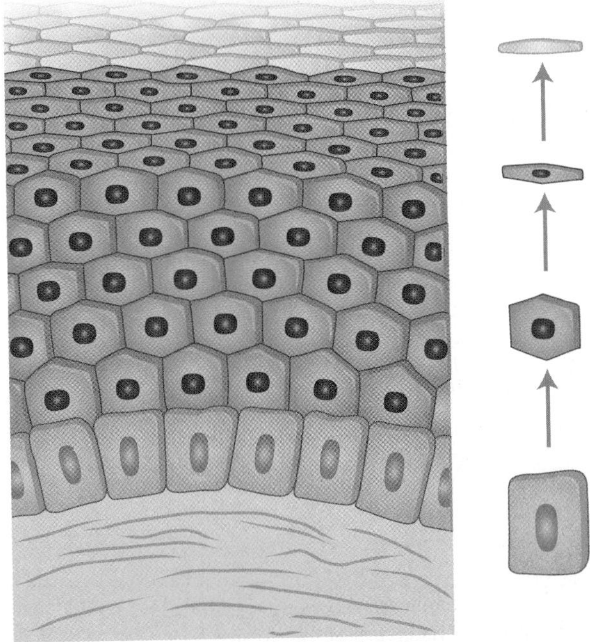

Figure 39.2 ■ Basal cells are originally cuboidal or columnar. As the cells migrate toward the surface layers of skin, their shape changes as they flatten.

The number varies because thick skin (such as the soles of the feet) has more layers than thin skin.

The **stratum basale** is the deepest layer of the epidermis. It consists of a single row of stem cells that will replace keratinocytes lost on the skin surface. The new keratinocytes are nourished by the blood supply from the dermis. However, as the new cells migrate farther from the stratum basale, they receive less nourishment, resulting in cellular death. Because the skin is continually exposed to environmental stressors, the epidermis must be constantly regenerated by keratinocyte stem cells in the stratum basale. The stratum basale contains three types of cells: keratinocytes, melanocytes, and tactile (Merkel) cells. **Melanocytes** produce a dark pigment called melanin that is phagocytized by the keratinocytes, where it provides protection from ultraviolet rays from the sun. Light-skinned and dark-skinned individuals have the same number of melanocytes, but in darker skin and freckles, each melanocyte produces more melanin. Tactile cells are sensory mechanoreceptors for touch. The stratum basale is separated from the dermis by the basement membrane.

The **stratum spinosum** (spiny layer) contains several layers of keratinocytes. As new keratinocytes move into the stratum spinosum, they lose their ability to divide. The rounder and spiky-shaped cells in this layer draw adjacent cells together, contributing to the tensile strength and flexibility of the skin. **Dendritic (Langerhans) cells** are present in both the stratum spinosum and the stratum granulosum. These cells are types of macrophages that engulf pathogenic microorganisms entering from the skin surface.

The **stratum granulosum** (granular layer), which is less developed in thin skin, contains 3–5 layers of flattened keratinocytes. In the stratum granulosum, keratinohyalin granules dehydrate and break up the nucleus, causing the cells undergo an orderly, genetically programmed death called **apoptosis**. These granules contain substances that combine with components of the cytoskeleton of the keratinocyte and convert them to keratin.

The **stratum lucidum** (clear layer) is a translucent zone above the stratum granulosum that is present only in thick skin located in the palms of the hands, soles of the feet, and corresponding surfaces of the fingers and toes. This layer contains clear, tightly packed flattened keratinocytes that are composed of large amounts of keratin and thickened plasma membranes.

The **stratum corneum** consists of 15–30 layers of flattened, keratinized squamous cells that are dead, dry, and flaky. The cytoplasm in these cells has been completely replaced by keratin, making the cell membrane thick and resistant to water and most chemicals. Thick skin typically has a thicker stratum corneum than thin skin does.[3,5]

The Dermis

The **dermis** is the layer of skin just below the epidermis. It is much thicker than the epidermis, and its depth varies according to factors such as age and anatomical location. The dermis provides most of the strength of the skin and contains plentiful blood vessels that provide nutrients and oxygen for both the dermis and the epidermis. The dermis also serves as a storage area for water and electrolytes. Skin appendages, including sweat glands, sebaceous glands, hair follicles, and nail roots are also present in the dermis. However, these appendages are derived from the epidermis and contain keratinocyte stem cells that have the potential to regenerate. Partial thickness wounds reepithelialize in part from the stem cells derived from these dermal appendages. The dermis also contains sensory receptors for pain, touch, and temperature as well as smooth and skeletal muscle cells.

The dermis has two layers: a superficial papillary layer and a thicker, deeper reticular layer. The papillary layer comprises approximately 20% of the dermis and is composed of loosely and irregularly organized connective tissue, including predominantly type III collagenous fibers, type I collagenous fibers, and elastic fibers as well as the blood vessels and nerve endings that supply the epidermis (**Figure 39.4** ■). The papillary layer also contains cells typical of connective tissue, including fibroblasts, macrophages, plasma cells, mast cells, endothelial cells, and adipose cells. The open meshwork of cells and fibers in this layer allows space for white blood cells and defensive substances to move around, thus providing defense against microorganisms attempting to enter the vascular system in the dermis. The papillary layer projects upward and interdigitates with ridges in the epidermis, forming structures called **dermal papillae**.[6] The dermal ridges on the fingertips comprise fingerprints. Fibrils of type VII collagen extend from the basement membrane into the papillary layer, where they either terminate or loop back into the basement membrane. These collagenous anchors help to "glue" the epidermis to the dermis.

The deeper reticular layer that makes up 80% of the dermis is composed of dense connective tissue, which is

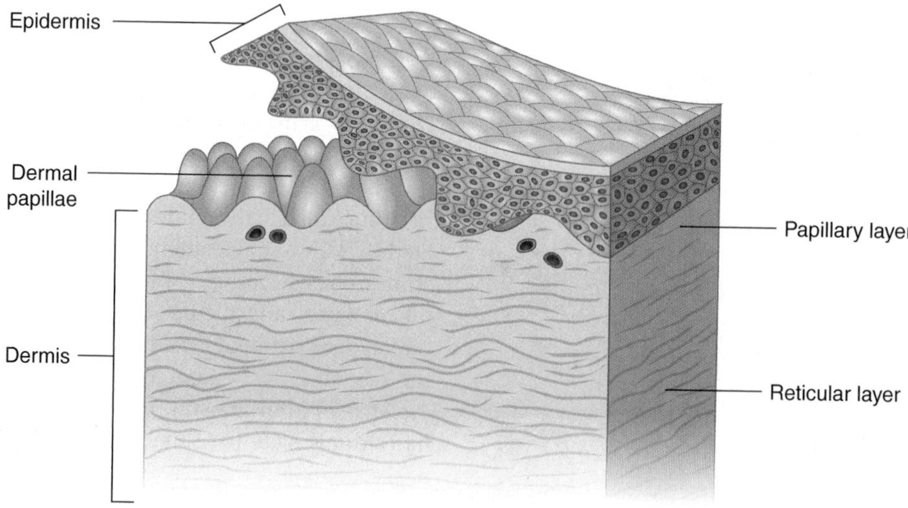

Figure 39.4 ■ Micrograph illustrating the epidermis and dermis as well as the dermal papillae interdigitating with the rete ridges of the epidermis. The layers of the dermis are separated by the rete subpapillare. The papillary dermis consists of loosely organized connective tissue with vessel and nerve endings that supply the epidermis. The reticular dermis is composed of dense connective tissue that is responsible for the thickness of the skin.

responsible for the majority of the skin thickness. This layer contains predominantly type I collagenous fibers as well as type III collagenous fibers and elastic fibers. There is no clear demarcation between the papillary and reticular layers; the primary difference in the collagen and elastic fibers found in each layer is the gradual change in size of the fibers. Unlike the papillary layer, collagenous fibers in the dermis are more highly organized into thick bundles that lie parallel to the skin surface, forming tension lines. The reticular layer contains fewer cells than the papillary layer.

The layer below the dermis, the subcutaneous layer or **hypodermis**, contains two primary structures: fat and fascia. The hypodermis is a major storage area for adipose tissue. The hypodermal fat anchors the skin to underlying structures and serves as a shock absorber to protect deeper tissues and organs from injury.[6]

The Dermal–Epidermal Junction

The boundary between the epidermis and dermis, the dermal–epidermal junction (DEJ), is referred to as a *basement membrane zone.* The DEJ underlies the basal layer of keratinocytes and separates the epidermis from the dermis while simultaneously binding the two layers of skin together to minimize slippage or separation (**Figure 39.5** ■). Additionally, the DEJ functions as a barrier to protect against the passage of chemicals or pathogens into the body as well as water and electrolytes out of the body.[7] An intact DEJ provides a framework on which regenerating cells can migrate and restore the architecture of the tissue.[4]

The Extracellular Matrix

The extracellular space of the dermis is filled with **extracellular matrix (ECM)**, sometimes referred to as the *ground substance*, which is essential for tissue growth and wound healing. As in most connective tissues, the ECM of the dermis is secreted largely by fibroblasts.

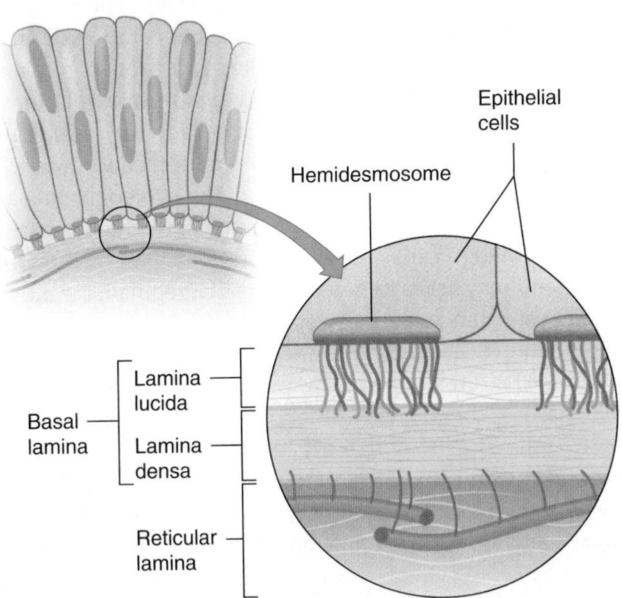

Figure 39.5 ■ Illustration of the dermal–epidermal junction layers and their use of hemidesmosomes to anchor the epidermal and dermal layers together.

The ECM provides a framework that promotes the structural integrity of the body by helping it to withstand compressive forces. The ECM acts as a scaffold that facilitates cell adhesion and migration through the matrix. Most cells in the dermis, to proliferate and survive, must attach to the ECM and spread out over it. The ECM accounts for much of the tensile strength, elasticity, and compressibility of the skin. At the same time, the ECM provides a medium for the rapid diffusion of nutrients, metabolites, chemical mediators, and hormones between the blood and tissue cells.

Three main classes of substances make up the extracellular matrix of the skin (**Figure 39.6** ■):

1. Fibrous structural proteins, including collagen and elastin
2. Adhesive glycoproteins such as laminin, fibronectin, and vitronectin
3. Polysaccharide chains called glycosaminoglycans (GAGs), which are usually bound to protein as proteoglycans.[4,8] The proteoglycans include heparan sulfate, chondroitin sulfate, and dermatan sulfate.

Fibrous Structural Proteins of the ECM

Collagen. Collagen is the most abundant protein in the human body and in the ECM. There are about 16 types of collagen, but the matrix of the dermis is composed primarily of types I, III, and V. Cross-linking of collagen chains provides great strength and stability. Hydration in the dermis is maintained by collagen's strong water-binding capabilities (**Figure 39.7** ■).

Elastin. The protein **elastin** is the primary structural component of elastic fibers of connective tissue found in tissues such as skin, lungs, and blood vessels. These molecules are synthesized by fibroblasts and smooth muscle cells of blood vessels. In contrast to collagen fibers, elastic fibers are loosely arranged in all directions, allowing this tissue to coil and recoil like a spring.

Elastic fibers tend to calcify with age, and the elasticity of the skin deteriorates. Elastic fibers are absent from mature scar or fibrotic tissue, accounting for its lack of elasticity. ■

Adhesive Glycoproteins of the ECM

Laminin. Laminin is a large glycoprotein that is located almost exclusively within the basement membrane. It provides a sticky surface that facilitates the attachment of basement membrane to the epidermal cells above as well as to components of the ECM below.

Fibronectin. Fibronectin is a glycoprotein that helps cells attach to the ECM and acts as a guide for cell migration through the matrix. Fibronectin plays an important role in cell adhesion and communication signals between cells and the ECM.

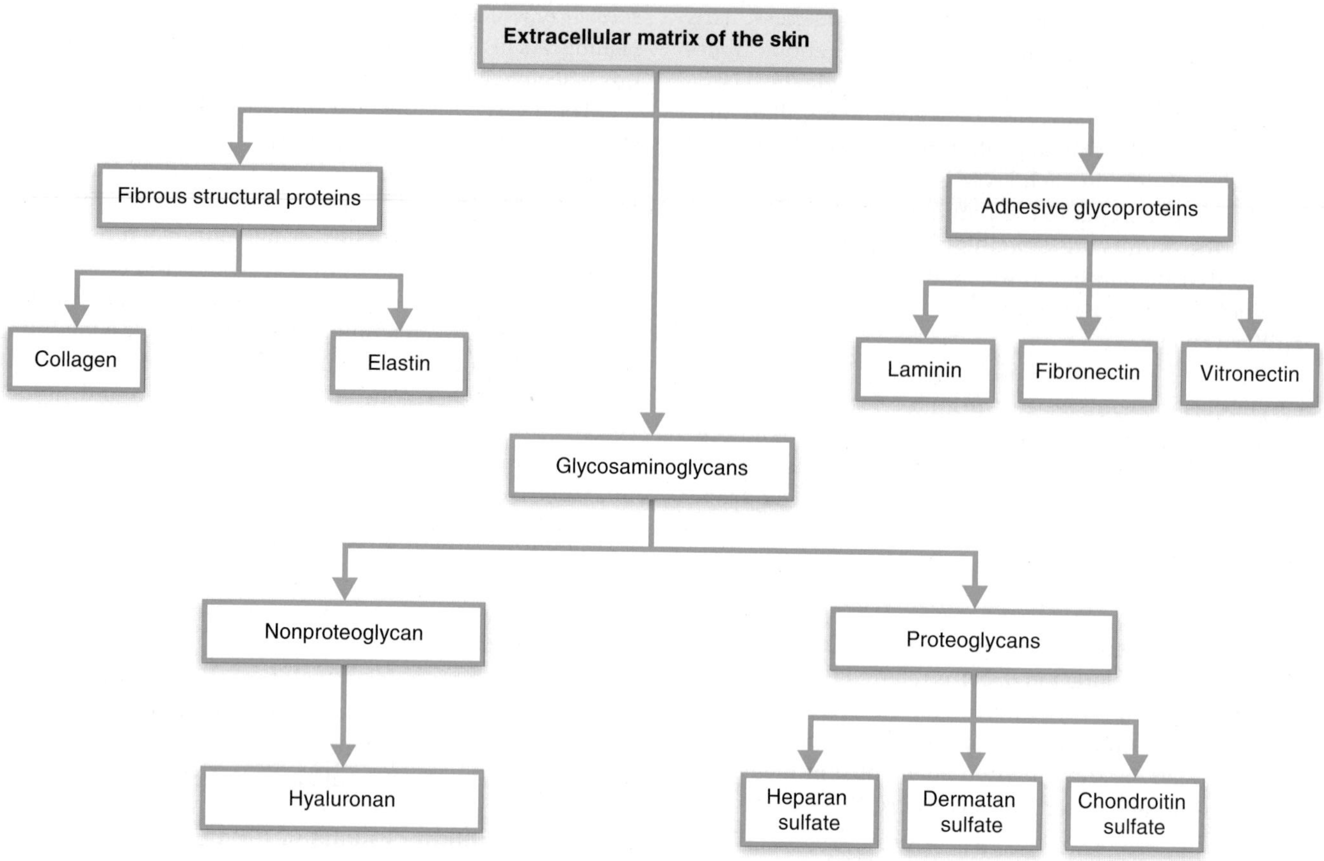

- **Extracellular matrix of the skin**
  - Fibrous structural proteins
    - Collagen
    - Elastin
  - Glycosaminoglycans
    - Nonproteoglycan
      - Hyaluronan
    - Proteoglycans
      - Heparan sulfate
      - Dermatan sulfate
      - Chondroitin sulfate
  - Adhesive glycoproteins
    - Laminin
    - Fibronectin
    - Vitronectin

Figure 39.6 ■ Components of the extracellular matrix.

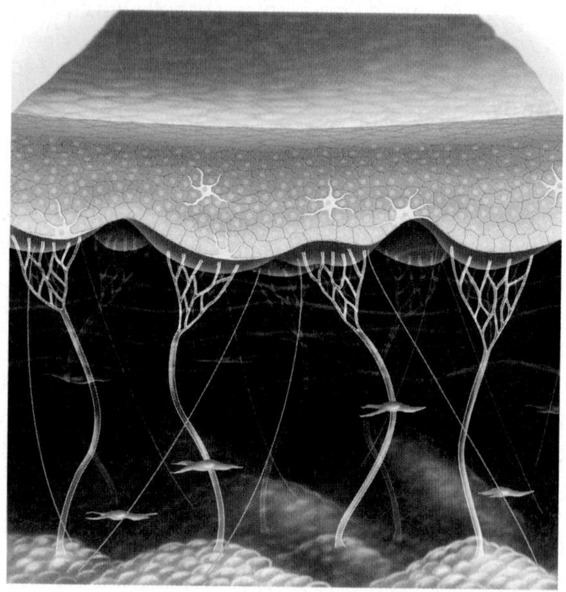

Figure 39.7 ■ The dermis and the components that give the skin its elasticity: collagen fibrils (white vertical fibers), elastic fibers (elastin, horizontal fibers), reticular fibers (single vertical fibers), and fibroblasts (horizontal cells).

Vitronectin. Vitronectin is a glycoprotein found in plasma and in the ECM of certain tissues such as bone. In plasma, vitronectin plays a role in hemostasis. This molecule mediates cell–matrix interactions in the skin similarly to the function of fibronectin.

Glycosaminoglycans of the ECM

Glycosaminoglycans (GAGs) are polysaccharides that are highly polar and attract water to the ECM. The influx of water determines the dermal volume and compressibility.

The majority of GAGs are linked to a protein core and are called proteoglycans. Proteoglycans form a gelatinous substance that fills spaces between cells in the ECM. This allows ions, hormones, chemical mediators, and nutrients to move freely through the matrix. The proteoglycans act as shock absorbers, protecting the body from compressive forces. Proteoglycans are also found in the basement membrane and may act as two-way filters that regulate the movement of substances between epidermal cells and the matrix. Modulation of cell signaling and the inflammatory response may also be functions of ECM proteoglycans.[39]

Hyaluronan (hyalouronic acid) is a type of GAG abundant in the ECM that is produced in large amounts during wound healing (see **Figure 39.6**). Like the proteoglycans, hyaluronan makes the ECM viscous, promoting cell migration by physically stretching and enlarging the surface area of the ECM.[10] Hyaluronan is the substance that lubricates synovial joints. It was recently identified as a factor that may be associated with scarless fetal wound healing, as it is present in larger amounts in fetal tissues than in scar-forming adult tissues[10]

Cell–Matrix and Cell–Cell Interaction

Tissues have established a complex system for enabling cell-to-cell communication and cell-to-ECM communication. This communication is essential if cells are to respond to internal and external changes in their environment. **Integrins** are the best-studied and most prominent family of receptors involved in this elaborate communication network. Remarkably, integrins are able to transmit information bidirectionally: from intracellular to extracellular and from extracellular to intracellular. As transmembrane receptors, integrins bind extracellular substances, a process that ultimately results in a cascade of events within the receiving cell that responds to the external environment. The integrin receptors also serve as adhesion molecules that facilitate cell maintenance and repair.

Cytokines and growth factors are essential components for this cell-to-cell and cell-to-ECM cross-talk.[9] This communication underlies the ability of epidermal cells to influence the location and structure of the ECM as well as the ability of the ECM to influence keratinocyte growth, mitosis, proliferation, apoptosis, and/or death.[11]

Check Your Progress: Section 39.2

1. What are five important functions of the skin?
2. What are the functions of the extracellular matrix?
3. Why are cell-to-cell communication and cell-to-ECM communication important processes in the body?

39.3 Cutaneous Wound Healing

Types of Wound Healing

Most wounds heal uneventfully. Uncomplicated wound healing can occur by primary intention, secondary intention, or tertiary intention, depending on the following:

- The type of injury
- The extent of tissue loss
- The presence of infection, necrotic tissue, or secondary tissue breakdown
- The type of cells involved.

The healing process is very similar in primary, secondary, and tertiary intention, but the amount of granulation tissue, the length of healing time, and the amount of scar formation vary (**Figure 39.8** ■).

Primary Intention

Wound healing by **primary intention** (primary closure) typically occurs after surgical closure of a wound. It may also occur in wounds that involve minimal loss of tissue, that are not infected or contaminated, and in which the edges of the wound can be approximated and closed (**Figure 39.8A**). Closure can be achieved by suture, staple, butterfly closure, or fibrin glue, which is a type of "superglue" for the skin.

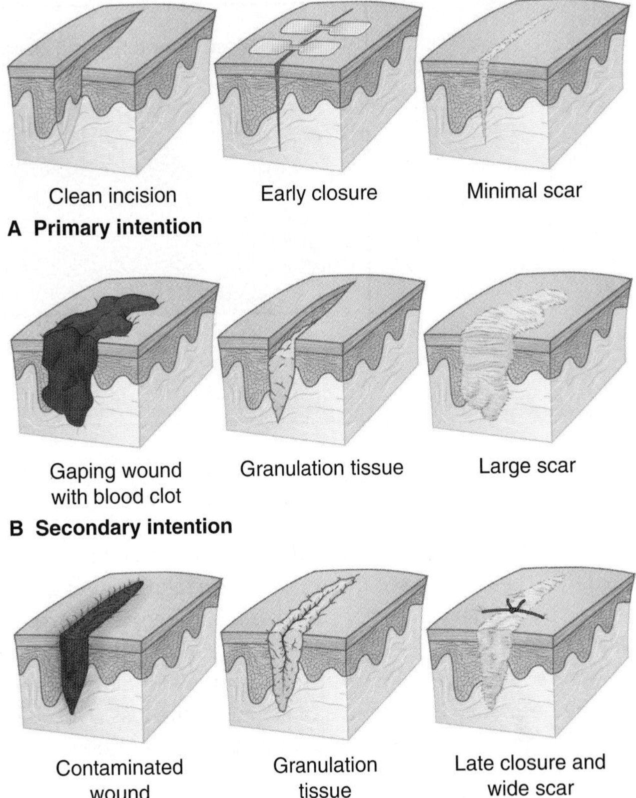

Figure 39.8 ■ Wound healing by intention. **A.** Primary intention. **B.** Secondary intention. **C.** Tertiary intention.

The two principal events during healing by primary intention are repair and regeneration. Repair is the formation of new ECM to replace what was damaged or lost (repair); regeneration is reepithelialization. Because the tissue defect is minimal, little granulation tissue is needed to fill the dead space. Epidermal cells undergo rapid mitosis, regenerate, and cover the wound. Because epithelium migrates over the suture line, wound healing is completed with minimal scarring, and normal tissue structure and function are restored. The process is completed in approximately 5–21 days, which is much faster than the healing of open wounds.

Secondary Intention

Wound healing by **secondary intention** (secondary or spontaneous closure) occurs when a full thickness wound is allowed to heal without a closure attempt (**Figure 39.8B**). Reasons for leaving a wound open to heal through secondary intention include the following:

- The size of the tissue injury or the wide irregular wound margins prevent approximation of the wound edges.
- A large amount of exudate is present.
- Infection, tissue necrosis, or contamination of the wound is present.[7]

As the body attempts to close the wound, a large amount of granulation tissue is generated. The primary mechanism underlying healing by secondary intention is contraction of the wound by myofibroblasts interacting with

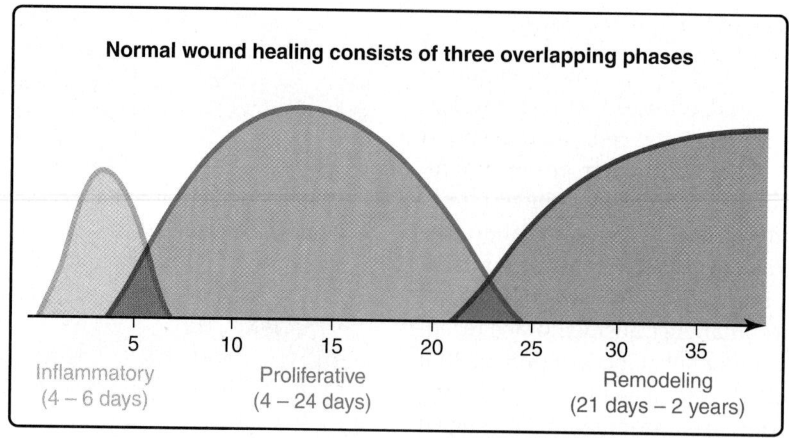

Figure 39.9 ■ Timeline for the inflammatory, proliferative, and remodeling phases of wound healing.

the ECM. Because more connective tissue is needed to fill the defect, healing by secondary intention takes longer than healing by primary intention, and the resulting scar is larger. Natural regeneration of the epidermis overlying the wound is possible; however, skin grafting or other skin substitutes may be necessary in instances of severe tissue loss. The risk for infection is greater than that in primary intention.

Tertiary Intention

Wound healing by **tertiary intention**, sometimes referred to as delayed primary closure, occurs when wound closure is delayed (**Figure 39.8C**). This type of healing is a combination of primary intention and secondary intention. In some cases, a contaminated wound is cleaned and left open for several days for drainage of exudate and is observed to ensure that no infection is present. The center of the wound fills with granulation tissue, and the wound edges are subsequently approximated.[7] In general, the degree of scarring will be greater than that in primary intention but less than that in secondary intention.

Helen Baker: Application

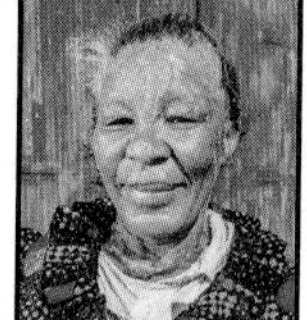

Mrs. Baker's wound has been left to heal by secondary intention because of the amount of tissue loss and inability to approximate margins. As a result, a larger amount of granulation tissue will be required to heal this wound.

3. What findings may have led to the surgeon's decision to leave Mrs. Baker's incision open to heal by secondary intention?
4. How does healing by secondary intention increase the risk for infection?
5. What conditions are required for a wound to heal by primary intention?

Phases of Wound Healing

Whether a wound heals by primary, secondary, or tertiary intention, the healing process involves a complex progression of events that overlap in time and activity. For example, physiologic events such as wound contraction may begin in one phase but then continue into the next. Wound healing may be conceptualized as occurring in four phases: hemostasis, inflammatory, proliferative, and remodeling (**Figure 39.9** ■). The extent and duration of these phases vary according to the type and nature of the wound.

For effective wound healing to occur, communication must occur between the ECM and surrounding cells. This communication is facilitated by an array of chemical mediators that drive the physiologic events that are characteristic of each phase of the wound healing process. Each step is regulated either directly or indirectly by these mediators, which include cytokines, growth factors, proteases, and amines as well as structural and adhesion proteins, GAGs, and proteoglycans.[12] Some of these mediators are derived from inflammatory and resident cells, including neutrophils, macrophages, lymphocytes, platelets, keratinocytes, fibroblasts, and endothelial cells. Others mediators are substances that are found in plasma, such as fibrinogen and thrombin.

Cytokines and growth factors are two of the most important classes of mediators in the wound healing process. In the literature, the term *growth factor* is frequently subsumed under the term *cytokine*; in this chapter, the terms are used separately. During the wound healing process, the biological effects of cytokines and growth factors on target cells and their interactions with other mediators are highly complex, constantly interactive, and exquisitely coordinated.[13]

Almost every type of cell in the skin participates in the production of cytokines and growth factors to some extent. Cytokines are small proteins or glycoproteins, primarily secreted by cells of the immune system such as neutrophils, monocytes, macrophages, and lymphocytes. Common groups of the cytokine family are interleukins (IL), interferons (IFN), tumor necrosis factors (TNF), and colony-stimulating factors (CSF). Cytokines modulate the wound healing process in a number of ways, including the following:

- Initiation of cell chemotaxis, activation, differentiation, and proliferation of inflammatory cells
- Production of growth factors and cytokines from inflammatory cells
- Stimulation of the expression of growth factors for fibroblasts, endothelial cells, and keratinocytes
- Development of the ECM
- Coordination of intercellular communication.[12]

Growth factors are proteins that have the ability to stimulate the growth, division, or differentiation of other cells. They are secreted by a variety of cells in a wound and are named for either the cell of origin (e.g., platelet-derived growth factor [PDGF]) or the target cell (e.g., epidermal growth factor [EGF]).[7] They are also grouped into families that have similar structures and functions. Like cytokines, growth factors control activities of other cells by regulating intercellular communication.

Although not a growth factor or cytokine, nitric oxide is a mediator that is critical to wound healing.[13] Nitric oxide is a reactive oxygen species or free radical. Its role in the wound healing process may be direct (e.g., by participating in bacterial killing) or indirect (e.g., by modulating cytokine and growth factor activity that affects vascular reactivity and cellular activity).[13]

The profile of chemical mediators at the injury site during each phase of the healing process is critical to ensure successful wound closure. This profile changes as healing progresses. The timing and concentration of cytokines and growth factors, as well as the relationship of these factors to that of other mediators, are quite complex and influence the success or failure of wound closure.

The phases of wound healing are described in the following sections. Reference to chemical mediators associated with wound healing are made throughout the chapter. These chemical mediators are outlined in **Tables 39.1** ■, **39.2** ■, and **39.3** ■.

Inflammatory Phase

The first phase of wound healing is acute inflammation. The goal of the inflammatory phase is to minimize tissue damage, prevent additional tissue injury, and prepare the wound for healing and regeneration. The inflammatory response functions to stop bleeding, break down damaged extracellular matrix, recruit phagocytic cells, and remove injurious agents and debris from the wound bed.[14]

Hemostasis. Hemostasis, the first step in the inflammatory phase, controls hemorrhage and maintains vascular integrity. Two physiologic processes are involved: formation of a platelet plug and generation of a fibrin-based clot.

Immediately following injury, a brief but intense period of vasoconstriction at the site of injury reduces the vessel diameter and slows blood loss. Narrowing of the blood vessel lumen brings the endothelial surfaces into contact

Table 39.1 Source of Selected Growth Factors and Cytokines Active in Wound Healing

		Source							
Family	**Member**	**Platelet**	**Neutrophil**	**Macrophage**	**Lymphocyte**	**Fibroblast**	**Endothelium**	**Keratinocyte**	**Mast Cell**
Growth Factors									
Platelet-derived growth factor	PDGF (AA, AB, CC, DD)	X		X		X	X	X	
	VEGF (A, B, C, D, E)	X		X		X	X	X	
Epidermal growth factor	EGF	X		X				X	
	TGFα	X		X				X	
Fibroblast growth factor	FGF 1–6, 39.9			X	X	X	X		
	KGF (1–2)		X			X		X	
Transforming growth factor	TGFβ (1–3)	X		X	X	X	X	X	
Insulin-like growth factor	IGF (1–6)	X		X		X		X	
Cytokines									
Interleukin-1 (IL-1)			X	X				X	
Interleukin-2 (IL-2)					X				
Interleukin-4 (IL-4)					X				X
Interleukin-6 (IL-6)			X	X		X		X	
Interleukin-8 (IL-8)				X		X		X	
Interleukin-10 (IL-10)				X				X	
TNFα, TNFβ			X	X					
IFN-γ				X	X				
Granulocyte macrophage colony-stimulating factor (GM-CSF)			X	X					

SOURCES: Bryant, R., & Nix, D. (2012). *Acute & chronic wounds: Current management concepts* (4th ed.). St Louis, MO: Elsevier Health Sciences. Reinke, J., & Sorg, H. (2012). Wound repair and regeneration. *European Surgical Research, 49*(1), 35–43. Olczyk, P., Mencner, L., & Komosinska-Vassev, K. (2014). The role of the extracellular matrix components in cutaneous wound healing. *BioMed Research International*. doi:10.1155/2014/747584. Rodero, M., & Khosrotehrani, K. (2010). Skin wound healing modulation by macrophages. *International Journal of Clinical and Experimental Pathology, 3*(7), 643–653. Mohd, J., Yussof, S., Omar, E., et al. (2012). Cellular events and biomarkers of wound healing. *Indian Journal of Plastic Surgery, 45*(2), 220–228.

Table 39.2 Function of Selected Growth Factors Active in Wound Healing

Growth Factor	Function
Platelet-derived growth factor (PDGF)	Neutrophil, monocyte, macrophage, and fibroblast chemotaxis; fibroblast proliferation; stimulates angiogenesis; ECM deposition; collagen synthesis
Vascular endothelial growth factor (VEGF)	Angiogenesis
Epidermal growth factor (EGF)	Keratinocyte and fibroblast proliferation; keratinocyte migration; ECM deposition
Transforming growth factor-alpha (TGFα)	Activate endothelial cells promoting angiogenesis; fibroblast chemotaxis
Fibroblast growth factor (FGF)	Angiogenesis; fibroblast chemotaxis, proliferation, and migration; keratinocyte proliferation and migration; ECM deposition
Keratinocyte growth factor (KGF)	Keratinocyte proliferation
Transforming growth factor-beta (TGFβ)	Neutrophil, monocyte, and fibroblast chemotaxis; ECM deposition; collagen synthesis; keratinocyte proliferation; wound contraction; maturation of epithelial cell layers
Insulin-like growth factor (IGF)	Fibroblast chemotaxis, activation, and proliferation; keratinocyte proliferation; endothelial cell activation; angiogenesis; ECM deposition

SOURCES: Bryant, R., & & Nix, D. (2012). *Acute & chronic wounds: Current management concepts* (4th ed.). St Louis, MO: Elsevier Health Sciences. Schultz, G., Davidson, J., Kirsner, R., et al. (2011). Dynamic reciprocity in the wound microenvironment. *Wound Repair and Regeneration, 19*(2), 134–148. Olczyk, P., Mencner, L., & Komosinska-Vassev, K. (2014). The role of the extracellular matrix components in cutaneous wound healing. *BioMed Research International*. doi:10.1155/2014/747584. Mohd, J, Yussof, S.., Omar, E., et al. (2012). Cellular events and biomarkers of wound healing. *Indian Journal of Plastic Surgery, 45*(2), 220–228.

Table 39.3 Function of Selected Cytokines Active in Wound Healing

Cytokine	Function
Interleukin-1 (IL-1)	Enhances TNFα and IFNγ; activates granulocytes and endothelial cells; increases fibroblast and keratinocyte proliferation; increases collagen synthesis; stimulates hematopoiesis; chemotaxis for keratinocytes, fibroblasts, and endothelial cells
Interleukin-2 (IL-2)	Activates macrophages and T cells; stimulates differentiation of activated B cells; stimulates proliferation of activated B and T cells; upregulates fibroblast activation
Interleukin-4 (IL-4)	Inhibits fibroblast proliferation and collagen synthesis; downregulates cytokine expression
Interleukin-6 (IL-6)	Released in response to IL-1; inhibits extracellular matrix breakdown during proliferative phase; induces neutrophil infiltration and fibroblast proliferation; induces keratinocyte migration and proliferation
Interleukin-8 (IL-8)	Enhances neutrophil and macrophage adherence, chemotaxis, and secretion; promotes keratinocyte maturation
Interleukin-10 (IL-10)	Downregulates proinflammatory cytokine expression; inhibits neutrophil and macrophage activation and infiltration
Interferon gamma (IFN-γ)	Attracts and activates granulocytes; slows collagen synthesis and cross-linking; stimulates collagenase production
Tumor necrosis factor alpha (TNFα)	Stimulates expression of growth factors for macrophages; facilitates collagen synthesis; induces matrix metalloproteinase (MMP) transcription
Granulocyte-macrophage colony-stimulating factor (GM-CSF)	Activates granulocytes and macrophages; stimulates granulation tissue formation

SOURCES: Bryant, R., & Nix, D. (2012). *Acute & chronic wounds: Current management concepts* (4th ed.). St Louis, MO: Elsevier Health Sciences. Sussman, C., & Bates-Jensen, B. (2012). *Wound care: A collaborative practice manual* (4th ed.). Philadelphia, PA: Lippincott Williams & Wilkins. Mohd, J., Yussof, S., Omar, E., et al. (2012). Cellular events and biomarkers of wound healing. *Indian Journal of Plastic Surgery, 45*(2), 220–228.

with one another. This leads to increased stickiness of these surfaces, causing the severed ends of the blood vessel to adhere to one another.

Platelet Adhesion, Platelet Activation, and the Platelet Plug. Normally, an intact endothelium provides a mechanical barrier that prevents the blood from contacting the underlying extracellular matrix. However, when the endothelial lining is disrupted and blood contacts collagen in the ECM, platelets release clotting factors that activate platelets and promote their adherence to the injured site.[15]

Platelet adhesion and activation is mediated primarily by von Willebrand factor,[5] an adhesive glycoprotein synthesized by endothelial cells and platelets. The binding of von Willebrand factor to the collagen in the ECM provides the initial capture of platelets from the rapidly moving blood.

Platelet activation results in the development of a platelet plug at the injury site that stops the leak until a more substantial barrier, the fibrin clot, can develop.

CLINICAL POINT: Drugs such as abciximab (ReoPro), tirofiban (Aggrastat), and eptifibatide (Integrilin) are glycoprotein IIb/IIIa receptor antagonists that reversibly block these receptors, preventing cross-linking and aggregation of platelets and thus decreasing the likelihood of clot formation.[16] ■

Platelets are storehouses for chemical mediators. Activated platelets at the injury site release an abundance of vasoactive substances, cytokines, growth factors, adhesion molecules, digestive enzymes, and other molecules. These granular components participate in all phases of the wound healing process. They initiate wound closure, support additional platelet adhesion and activation, attract phagocytic cells to the wound site, initiate reepithelialization and wound contraction, participate in ECM deposition and degradation, and stimulate angiogenesis.[14,15]

Two important mediators released from activated platelets are PDGF and transforming growth factor beta (TGFβ). PDGF attracts repair cells, such as fibroblasts, neutrophils, and macrophages. The macrophages then secrete mediators including PDGF, fibroblast growth factor (FGF), TNFα, and IL-1.[7,8] These mediators enhance fibroblast chemotaxis and increase collagen formation. These two mediators, then, ensure rapid debridement and response by matrix producing cells and bridging the inflammatory and proliferative phases of wound healing.

The Fibrin Clot. The activated platelets initiate a series of events leading to the coagulation cascade (**Figure 39.10** ■). Progression through the cascade ultimately culminates in the cleavage of prothrombin to produce thrombin.[2] Thrombin, in addition to amplifying further platelet activation, cleaves fibrinogen in the platelet plug to form fibrin. The fibrin strands infiltrate the platelet plug, become cross-linked, and provide stability to the clot. In addition, the ability of fibrin to contract results in clot retraction.

Patients who take anticoagulants such as heparin, warfarin (Coumadin), or Plavix are at a higher risk for bleeding.[16] ■

The final structure of the fibrin-based clot contains platelets embedded among cross-linked fibrin fibers and is rich in fibronectin and hyaluronan; neutrophils, macrophages, and red blood cells also become ensnared in the clot. The resulting clot, in addition to its critical hemostatic role, acts as a barrier against contamination of the wound from invading microorganisms until reepithelialization occurs.[14]

The fibrin-based clot provides an early blueprint for wound healing that is referred to as the provisional matrix. The provisional matrix forms a scaffolding across the wound space to hold damaged tissues together and provide a temporary framework for wound healing. The fibronectin provides an adhesive foothold for leukocytes, keratinocytes, endothelial cells, and fibroblasts migrating through the clot. The hyaluronan expands the matrix to provide a larger space for migrating cells. The provisional matrix also serves as a protein reservoir by binding cytokines and growth factors, increasing their concentration, and amplifying the effects of inflammatory cells at the wound site.

At the same time that hemostasis is proceeding, an inflammatory exudate seeps out of the wound bed. As it dries over the provisional matrix, it forms a scab (eschar) that contracts, pulling the wound edges closer together and preventing

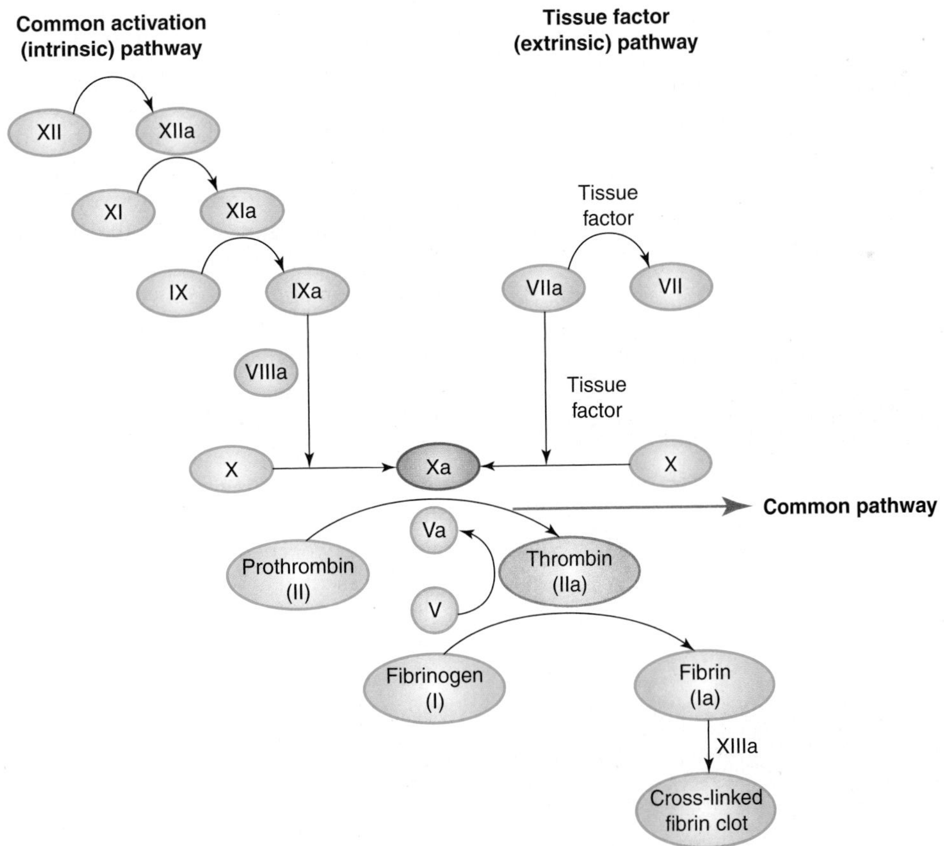

Figure 39.10 ■ The coagulation cascade. When the endothelium is damaged, tissue factor (TF) is exposed to the bloodstream and binds factor VIIa, which is an activated form of factor VII. The TF–VIIa complex enables subsequent activation of factor X and prothrombin, after which small amounts of thrombin activate the factor XI–IX feedback loop on the platelet surface. Factor IXa will then activate additional factor X. Simultaneously, the trace amounts of thrombin will then activate factors VIII (cofactor to factor IX) and V (cofactor to factor X), dramatically enhancing catalytic activity of factors IX and X. Finally, thrombin (factor IIa) activation leads to fibrin deposition. In parallel, local polyphosphate (polyP) release by activated platelets may additionally stimulate activation of factor XII, factor V, and factor FXI and inhibit clot lysis.

surface microorganisms from penetrating the wound bed. This scab provides a natural "dressing" for the surface of the wound while repair and regeneration occur underneath.[15]

CLINICAL POINT: Absence of bleeding and subsequent hemostasis can have a significant impact on wound healing. This is evident in wounds that heal by secondary intention, as bleeding and hemostasis do not occur. It is thought that one of the benefits of surgical debridement of these wounds is to activate clot formation and the release of growth factors to restart the repair process. ■

Recruitment of Phagocytic Cells and Wound Debridement. Once hemostasis has been achieved, the inflammatory phase of wound healing is choreographed by the activities and secretions of blood platelets, mast cells, neutrophils, and macrophages (**Figure 39.11** ■). These cells not only maintain and amplify the inflammatory response but also prepare the wound for granulation tissue formation in the proliferative phase. For the first 24–48 hours after initiation of the inflammatory process, polymorphonuclear neutrophils (PMNs) are the primary phagocytic cells present in the wound. PMNs migrate out of vessels to the injured area within minutes after injury via margination, which involves adhering to the endothelial cells lining the capillaries in the wound bed, and diapedesis, in which the neutrophils squeeze though the dilated capillaries.[2,15] They are attracted to the injury through chemotaxis by inflammatory mediators secreted from platelets as well as bacterial products and fibrinolytic products. Once at the wound site, PMNs secrete lysosomal enzymes along with reactive oxygen species, which debride the wound bed, breaking down and removing necrotic tissue, bacteria, and foreign material.

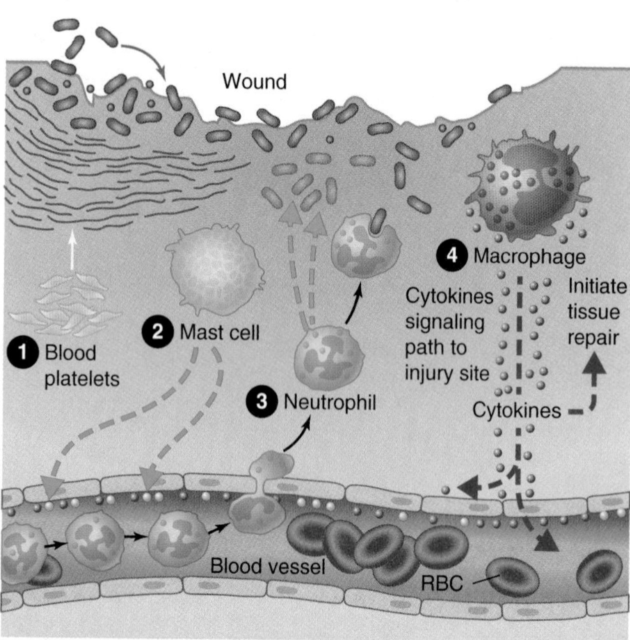

Figure 39.11 ■ The inflammatory response. 1. Platelets release blood-clotting proteins at the wound site. 2. Mast cells secrete factors that mediate dilation and constriction of blood vessels. 3. Neutrophils secrete factors that kill/degrade pathogens. Neutrohils and macrophages secrete factors that remove pathogens by phagocytosis. 4. Macrophages secrete cytokines that attract immune system cells.

In addition to phagocytosis, neutrophils participate in the initiation of angiogenesis, help to degrade the ECM and facilitate cell migration, and increase the infiltration of macrophages, fibroblasts, endothelial cells, and keratinocytes into the wound bed. These actions are mediated by proinflammatory cytokines, growth factors (see **Tables 39.1**, **39.2**, and **39.3**), and adhesion molecules. The length of time that neutrophils are active is short lived, and monocytes and macrophages soon take over the primary phagocytic function.[14]

The second wave of cells arriving at the wound site is composed of monocytes, macrophages, and T lymphocytes. Monocytes arrive at the wound site shortly after the neutrophils. Monocytes bind to integrin receptors in the ECM and immediately differentiate into tissue macrophages. Monocytes and macrophages are attracted to the injury site by a variety of chemical mediators, including PDGF, TGFα, TGFβ, IGF, VEGF, and degraded components of the ECM.[1]

Macrophages play two roles in wound healing: phagocytosis and the release of chemical mediators that stimulate, augment, and maintain the healing process.[8] Although the phagocytic role of the macrophages is similar to that of the neutrophils, it is more complex. The numbers of macrophages peak at approximately 48–96 hours, and they remain at the wound site longer. Macrophages are effective phagocytic cells that constantly monitor the wound area, ingesting bacteria as well as dead tissue and neutrophils. They produce reactive oxygen species, proteases, collagenases, and elastase to assist in antimicrobial activity and breaking down damaged or destroyed cells and ECM. At the same time, macrophages secrete inhibitors for these proteolytic enzymes to minimize healthy tissue damage. Thus, the wound bed is cleaned out and prepared for healing, and resident cells needed for cell proliferation are able to move into the wound. Healing cannot continue until the necrotic debris, foreign material, and cellular debris have been lysed and removed.

Macrophages also mediate the transition from the inflammatory phase of wound healing to the proliferative phase and upregulate wound repair systems that eventually move the healing process forward into the remodeling phase. Their major role in this transition is the release of a wide variety of chemical mediators that coordinate activities that are essential to wound healing, including recruiting and activating additional macrophages; stimulating ECM deposition by recruiting and activating fibroblasts; stimulating differentiation of fibroblasts into myofibroblasts; promoting angiogenesis by stimulating endothelial cell proliferation; and influencing reepithelialization (see **Tables 39.2** and **39.3**).[9] In this way, macrophages maintain and amplify the wound healing signals produced earlier by platelets and neutrophils. Overall, macrophages are the most important producer of cytokines and growth factors that amplify the inflammatory response and upregulate wound repair systems.[12]

Proliferative Phase

In the proliferative phase, the wound healing is guided toward tissue repair. Fibroblasts, endothelial cells, and keratinocytes are the cells responsible for the events of the proliferative phase: collagen deposition, angiogenesis, and reepithelialization. These events depend heavily on the process of cell migration. Cell migration is a dynamic process that involves coordinated changes in the cell cytoskeleton that allows detachment from basement membrane, neighboring cells, and ECM components; adhesion to components of the ECM: and forward movement through the ECM.

Granulation Tissue. Granulation tissue is a mass of new connective tissue that forms on the surface of a healing wound. Granulation tissue serves as a foundation for the collagen-based matrix that will eventually replace the fibrin-based provisional matrix. The amount of granulation tissue that is generated depends on the extent of the injury. In wounds that heal by primary intention, the tissue loss is minimal, so little granulation tissue is produced. On the other hand, in wounds that heal by secondary or tertiary intention, the tissue defect is greater, and the amount of granulation tissue needed is larger.

The synthesis of granulation tissue begins approximately 3–5 days after injury and overlaps the inflammatory phase. The fibrin-based provisional matrix is replaced by the addition of new collagen and elastin fibers and proteoglycans. The rapid proliferation of cells and the generation of a new matrix requires oxygen and nutrients. Thus, angiogenesis begins, endothelial cells migrate into the wound bed, and new and leaky capillaries are formed. These immature and leaky capillaries are responsible for the reddened, knobby, and moist or cobblestone-like appearance of granulation tissue (**Figure 39.12** ■).[12]

Fibroblasts and Myofibroblasts. Fibroblasts are one of the last cell types to enter the wound and are key to the proliferative phase of wound healing. These cells produce collagen and adhesive proteins for the new ECM. By 48–72 hours after injury, fibroblasts migrate into the wound space.

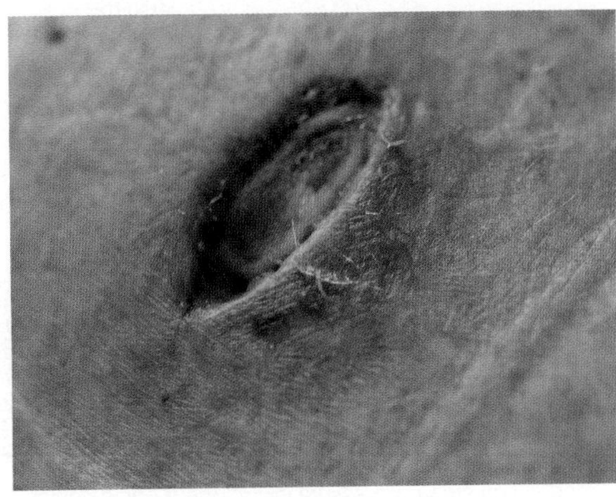

Figure 39.12 ■ Granulation tissue in a wound bed.

The first fibroblasts in the wound area differentiate into myofibroblasts. Myofibroblasts are fibroblasts that have acquired characteristics of smooth muscle cells.[14] They intermingle with collagen bundles and growth factors to promote wound contraction.[9] Subsequently, the myofibroblasts disappear from the wound bed, possibly through apoptosis at the end of this phase.[7] Collagen production becomes significant approximately 1 week after injury.

Endothelial Cells. Endothelial cells are responsible for new vessel growth within the wound bed. The formation of new blood vessels within a tissue is called **angiogenesis** but may also be referred to as *neovascularization*.[7] The growth of new capillaries in a wound typically occurs as capillary buds or sprouts arise from preexisting capillary venules adjacent to the wound (**Figure 39.13** ■).

The creation of new blood vessels in the wound bed is critical to provide oxygen and nutrients to the developing

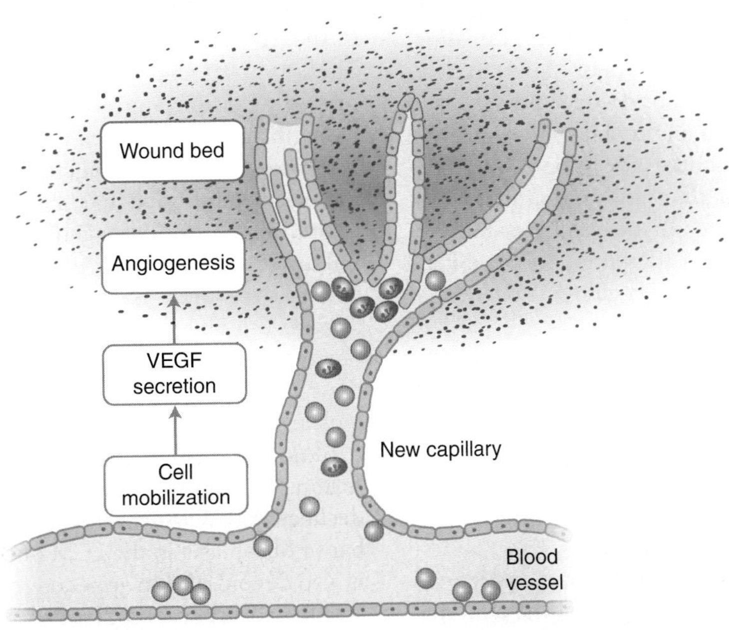

Figure 39.13 ■ Vascular endothelial growth factors mediating growth of new capillaries (angiogenesis).

granulation tissue. In 2–3 days after wounding, new capillary buds or sprouts extend into the wound space. The successful progression of angiogenesis is proportional to the amount of perfusion and the oxygen tension in the wound.[3] Growth factors and other molecules stimulate and regulate angiogenesis, including VEGF, FGF, TGFβ, TNFα, and PDGF.

Helen Baker: Application

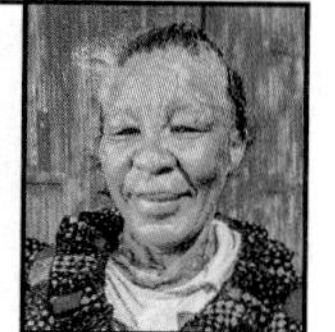

While Mrs. Baker is in the ED, the nurse accesses and reviews her electronic medical records and notes that Mrs. Baker has been seen at a local wound clinic affiliated with the hospital for a nonhealing sacral stage 4 pressure injury. The progress notes from the wound clinic indicate that Mrs. Baker's wound was originally 8 cm × 8 cm × 3 cm with 70% devitalized tissue, 20% pink nongranulating tissue, and 10% bone found in the wound bed. The wound was sharp debrided to remove the necrotic tissue and treated with negative pressure wound therapy. Once the wound bed was free from necrotic debris, the wound was able to move toward tissue repair. This marks the proliferative phase. After the wound decreased in size and filled in, the negative pressure wound therapy was discontinued, and an adhesive foam dressing was used. Myofibroblasts played a key role in the reduction in Mrs. Baker's wound size. Fibroblasts generate the ground substance for the new ECM to fill in the wound. Angiogenesis begins with endothelial cells migrating into the wound bed forming leaky capillary sprouts. The new tissue found in the wound bed is granulating tissue.

6. In the proliferative phase, how would the nurse expect Mrs. Baker's wound to appear?
7. Before the proliferative phase began, what role did platelet activation play in the inflammatory phase of Mrs. Baker's wound healing?
8. How do myofibroblasts aid in the healing of Mrs. Baker's wound?

Reepithelialization. Reepithelialization is the process of regeneration of keratinocytes that will provide a protective barrier for the wound bed lying underneath the scab. Overlapping the inflammatory phase of wound healing, reepithelialization begins within hours of injury. In healing by primary intention, the wound edges are apposed (placed against each other), and minimal reepithelialization is required. In healing by secondary or tertiary intention, the extent of tissue injury determines the amount of reepithelialization. There are wounds that exceed the ability of keratinocytes to regenerate over the entire surface of the wound. In these cases, another type of wound covering or skin graft must be used.

Reepithelialization requires keratinocyte stem cells primarily from the stratum basale at the wound edges. If the basement membrane is intact, reepithelialization occurs more quickly. If the basement membrane is not intact, it must first be repaired.

Remodeling Phase

Remodeling is the final phase of wound healing, and it overlaps with the proliferative phase. The goal of the remodeling phase is to restore the structural and functional integrity of the skin. However, the dermal matrix is not regenerated as is the epidermis; it is mended. Slowly, the granulation tissue laid down in the provisional matrix is replaced with a more stable collagen-based matrix. Although collagen deposition into the matrix began in the proliferative phase, it continues in the remodeling phase. The outcome of this dermal repair process is scar or fibrotic tissue. Scar tissue collagen is not structurally organized in the same manner as collagen in uninjured tissue; while unwounded dermis has a reticular or netlike collagen arrangement, in scar tissue, collagen fibers are in a parallel orientation along stress lines.[7,14] In the end, the dermal repair, though rapid and efficient, is not functionally or aesthetically perfect, as it cannot completely restore the quality structure of uninjured tissue.

Several events occur during the remodeling phase, including wound contraction, decline in the fibroblast population leading to decreased collagen synthesis with a corresponding increase in collagen breakdown, and decreased angiogenesis.

Wound contraction is a mechanical force exerted by cells that cause a reduction in wound size, leading to closure.[4] It begins about 4–5 days after injury, during the early proliferative phase, and continues for about 2 weeks. This process is mediated, at least in part, by contractile myofibroblasts. Myofibroblasts adhere to one another as well as to the wound edges, so when they contract, the entire granulating wound bed contracts. Wound contraction continues even after reepithelialization.[12]

Continuous turnover of collagen in the matrix occurs during the remodeling phase. Initially, collagen production exceeds destruction. Approximately 3 weeks after the wounding, when the collagen content is maximal, the net production of collagen declines and the degradation of collagen increases. Although synthesis and breakdown continue to occur, there is no net increase in collagen content during this phase.

Qualitatively, the type of collagen fiber also changes. Initially, type III collagen was synthesized in large amounts in the granulation tissue during the proliferative phase. These type III collagen fibrils were laid down randomly, providing large amounts of collagen but little tensile strength.[14] During the remodeling phase, type III collagen is replaced by type I collagen, and the ratio of type I to type III becomes similar to that of intact connective tissue. These type I fibrils are rearranged, and there is increased cross-linking of collagen molecules, maximizing tensile strength against stress and shear forces on the skin.[15] Approximately 3 weeks after injury, when collagen content is maximal, the newly epithelialized skin wound has only about 20–25% of the tensile strength of uninjured tissue. By 6 months, the tensile strength is maximal at about 75–80%.[14]

As the scar matures, the capillary density decreases, turning the scar from pink to white.[14] Cellular content also declines. As collagen production begins to decline, the number of fibroblasts in the ECM decreases. Mature scar tissue is also devoid of skin appendages such as hair follicles and sweat and sebaceous glands.[7] Maturation of scar tissue continues for a minimum of 1 year after the original injury. Thus, despite the external appearance of stasis, the wound

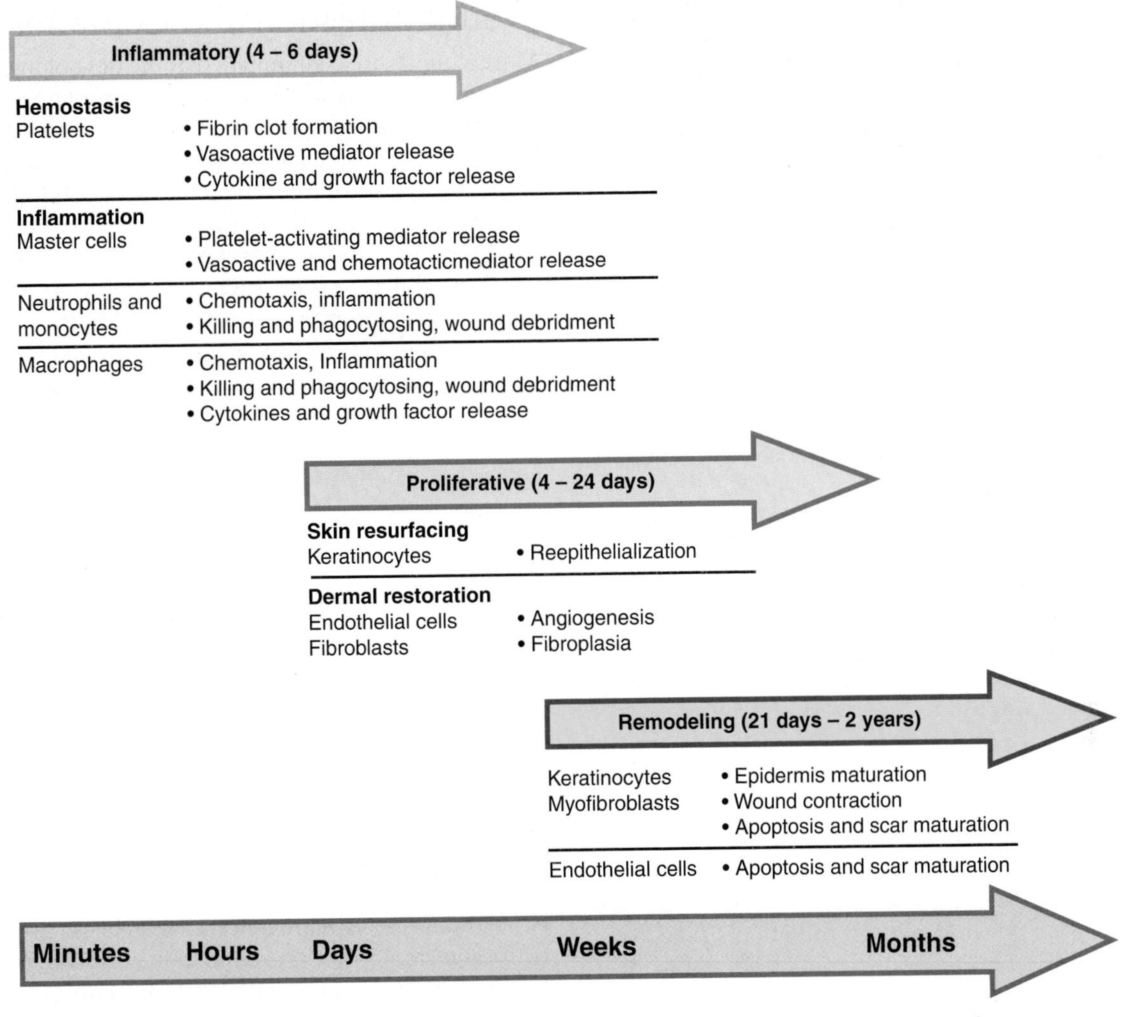

Figure 39.14 ■ The stages of wound healing with cellular involvement.

healing process continues for a significant period of time. The major events, cell types, and ECM components that are involved in the wound healing process are summarized in **Figure 39.14** ■.

Check Your Progress: Section 39.3

1. What is the goal of the remodeling phase of wound healing?
2. What is the process that occurs in the remodeling phase?
3. How does collagen fiber orientation in uninjured skin differ from that in healed skin?

39.4 Factors Impeding Wound Healing

Although most wounds heal uneventfully, numerous factors can negatively affect healing (**Table 39.4** ■). While some of these factors will eventually resolve with appropriate wound care, others will lead to chronic, nonhealing wounds. This section presents five of the most important factors affecting would healing.

Blood Flow and Hypoxia

Blood flow to the injury site is one of the most important factors affecting the healing process. Hypoxia can significantly delay or even stop the wound healing process. Killing of bacteria, collagen deposition, angiogenesis, and reepithelialization directly depend on the oxygen tension in the wound bed. Because of the initial disruption of the vascular supply and ischemia that occur with many injuries, early hypoxia of the wound bed is expected. Hypoxia is greatest at the center of the wound and diminishes toward the edges.

Table 39.4 Local and Systemic Factors That Impede Wound Healing

Local	Systemic
Blood flow and hypoxia Infection Infection and contamination (necrotic tissue, foreign exogenous material, endogenous material) Radiation exposure Movement/tension Desiccation Excessive edema Denervation	Advanced age Malnutrition Nutritional status (vitamins A, C, E, and K; minerals zinc, magnesium, copper, and iron) Immune deficiency Smoking Medications (corticosteroids, antineoplastics) Metabolic status (diabetes mellitus)

Hypoxia is reported to be the leading cause of wound infection.[4] This is because oxygen is required for optimal phagocytic cell function during the inflammatory phase, and the presence of oxygen in the wound results in an improvement of host immune defenses against microbial infection. Paradoxically, because inflammatory cells consume a large amount of oxygen for the production of reactive oxygen species, wound hypoxia can be amplified by infection.

In addition to its deleterious effect on inflammatory cells, hypoxia inhibits fibroblast activity and collagen deposition in the matrix.[4] The rate of collagen production is directly related to the oxygen tension in the wound. Fibroblasts cannot produce collagen without mature blood vessels to deliver oxygen, but new blood vessels fail to mature without a strong collagen matrix.

The presence of hypoxia acts as a powerful stimulus for angiogenesis within the wound bed during the proliferative phase. Angiogenesis results in the reestablishment of oxygen and nutrient supply to the wound. However, if hypoxia of the wound bed persists in spite of revascularization, necrosis of tissue will result, and wound healing will be impeded (**Figure 39.15** ■). A protracted period of hypoxia, resulting from a prolonged decrease in arterial or venous flow to the wound, can result in chronic, nonhealing wounds, as in the case of foot ulcers in people with diabetes and pressure injuries in patients who are bedridden.

Lastly, reepithelialization of the wound is impeded by hypoxia. Reepithelialization can occur only when the wound has been covered with granulation tissue, This requires the production of collagen and the development of new blood vessels in the wound, both of which are oxygen-dependent processes.[17]

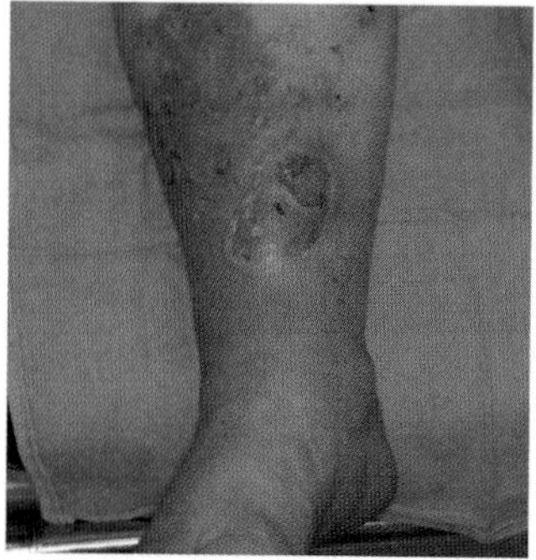

A Arterial ulcer

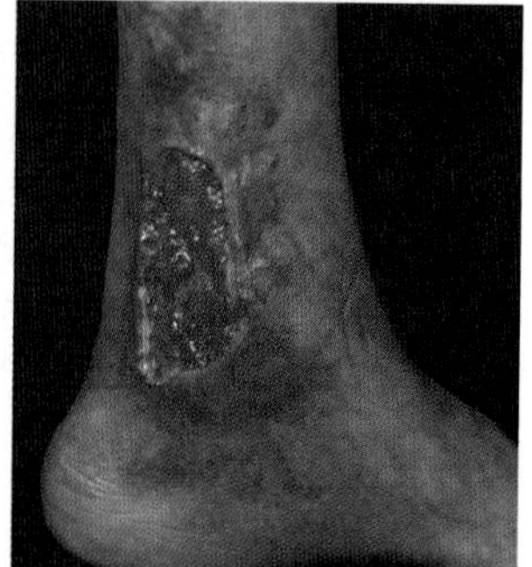

B Venous ulcer

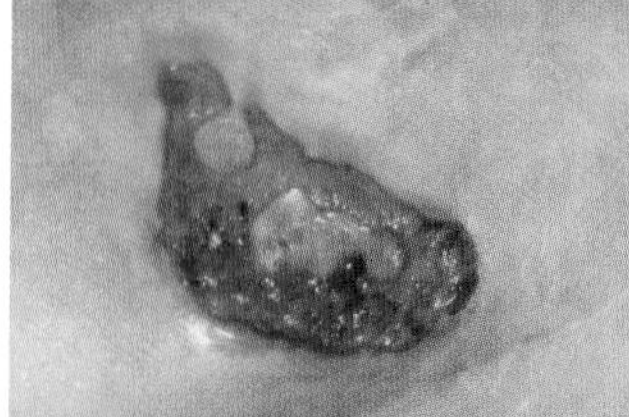

C Pressure injury

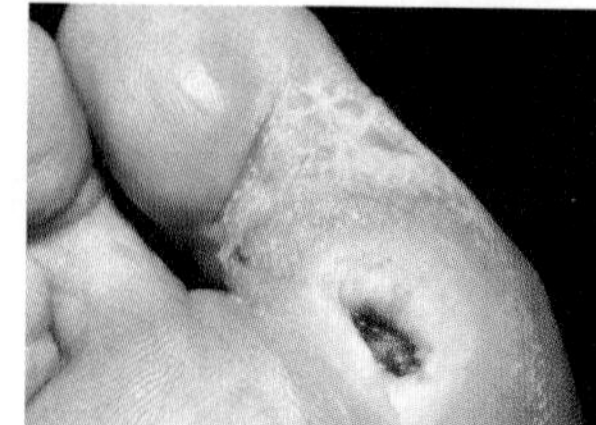

D Diabetic foot ulcer

Figure 39.15 ■ Examples of poorly healing wounds caused by hypoxia. **A.** Arterial ulcer. **B.** Venous ulcer. **C.** Pressure injury. **D.** Diabetic foot ulcer.

Wound Infection and Contamination

Most wounds are contaminated at the time of injury, and it is the responsibility of host defenses to contain the infection. However, badly contaminated wounds may overwhelm host defenses, especially if the wound contains foreign bodies such as dirt, glass, wood, or metal. Infection limits the ability of neutrophils to phagocytize bacteria and is the most common cause of delayed healing.

Technical aspects of surgical wound handling and closure can affect the occurrence of wound infection. The use of inappropriate suture material increases the likelihood of foreign body reaction leading to infection. Additional risk factors include a break in asepsis, duration of surgery or "open time," a spill of intestinal contents into the peritoneum, and failure to properly prepare the skin preoperatively.

The presence of infection stimulates complement activation and exaggerates and prolongs the inflammatory phase, causing failure to heal. The presence of excessive exudate, inflammatory cells, necrotic tissue, and microorganisms in the wound interferes with the preparation of the wound bed for collagen deposition, reepithelialization, and contraction.[15]

Tissue damage caused by infection may be extensive if it is allowed to proceed for a prolonged period. Microorganisms compete with undamaged cells for oxygen and nutrients that are in short supply early in wound healing.

In the context of factors impeding wound healing, the term *contamination* refers to necrotic tissue, foreign, exogenous material, or endogenous substances. Any necrotic or foreign material that remains in a wound will delay healing. Necrotic tissue acts as a mechanical barrier to reepithelialization and deposition of granulation tissue in the wound. Necrotic material provides a nidus for the initiation and maintenance of infection and prolongs the inflammatory phase. Necrotic tissue also releases endotoxins that may inhibit the migration of fibroblasts and keratinocytes, thus impairing reepithelialization and collagen formation. To speed wound healing, necrotic material must be debrided.

Foreign or exogenous material enters the wound from the environment. For example, when cloth is carried into a wound by a penetrating object, such as a bullet or knife, or when a wound is exposed to dirt or contaminated water, wound healing is delayed. In addition, the foreign material acts as a continuing stimulus for infection and inflammation.[15] Like necrotic material, foreign material can act as a mechanical barrier that blocks the entry of fibroblasts, endothelial cells, and keratinocytes into the wound matrix, resulting in impairment of reepithelialization and granulation tissue formation.

In some situations, wound healing is impaired by contamination with substances generated within the body itself or endogenous substances. Examples include contamination of the sterile peritoneal cavity with intestinal fluids, as occurs when the appendix ruptures before it can be removed, or traumatic injury to the bowel that leads to leakage of intestinal contents into the peritoneal cavity.[18]

Nutritional Status

Nutritional status plays a major role in successful wound healing. Wound healing is an anabolic process of tissue building that requires energy expenditure and adequate nutritional resources

Carbohydrates and fats are essential macronutrients in areas of cellular regeneration as are found in healing wounds. A negative nitrogen balance affects wound healing in a number of ways. Both B- and T-lymphocyte immune responses are blunted, the inflammatory response is depressed, bacterial phagocytosis and killing are attenuated, and the probability of delayed wound healing and wound infection are increased Furthermore, angiogenesis is diminished, collagen synthesis and cross-linking are decreased, tensile strength and stability are attenuated, and matrix formation and remodeling are reduced.

Multiple vitamins and minerals are required for successful wound healing.[15] Vitamin and mineral deficiencies are commonly associated with chronic, nonhealing wounds in ill individuals who are nutritionally debilitated. Whereas vitamin deficiencies affect wound healing directly, mineral deficiencies affect intracellular activities by serving as cofactors or participants in enzyme systems needed for healing to occur.[14]

Vitamin A Deficiency

Vitamin A deficiency has the potential to negatively affect reepithelialization and impair the deposition of collagen and fibronectin, thus decreasing the formation of granulation tissue and adversely affecting the tensile strength and stability of the healing wound. Vitamin A deficiency also impedes the inflammatory process and impairs white blood cell function, resulting in impaired debridement of the wound bed, reduced antimicrobial activity, and decreased secretion of cytokines and growth factors that contribute to the initiation and successful continuation of the wound healing process. The development of new capillaries in the wound bed is also impeded by vitamin A deficiency.[19]

Vitamin C Deficiency

A deficiency of vitamin C is most common in older adults, chronic alcohol and drug abusers, smokers, individuals after major trauma, and malnourished individuals.[9,] Vitamin C deficiency affects all phases of wound healing. It leads to retardation of the inflammatory process, resulting in reduction in inflammatory cell function and decrease in proinflammatory complement activity. Vitamin C deficiency inhibits collagen secretion by fibroblasts and decreases cross-linking, resulting in decreased tensile strength and wound stability. Another result of vitamin C deficiency is decreased ability to wall off bacteria and localize infection, resulting in an increased susceptibility to infection. Vitamin C deficiency also decreases angiogenesis, resulting in prolonged hypoxia within the wound bed and impairment of granulation tissue formation.

Vitamin E Deficiency

Vitamin E deficiency is most common in individuals with fat malabsorption.[19] Vitamin E acts as an antioxidant that limits lipid peroxidation, maintains and stabilizes the cell membrane, and protects against oxidative injury associated with prolonged or overwhelming inflammation.[18] However, supplementation remains controversial; some reports indicate that vitamin E inhibits collagen synthesis, thus impeding the proliferative phase of wound healing and decreasing excess scar formation.

Vitamin K Deficiency

Vitamin K is required for synthesis of four coagulation factors: II, VII, IX, and X. Vitamin K deficiency affects hemostasis and formation of the fibrin clot. As a result, hemorrhage, impaired wound healing, and infection may occur.

Zinc Deficiency

Zinc is a trace mineral that serves as a cofactor in RNA and DNA polymerase and is thus involved in DNA synthesis, protein synthesis, and cell proliferation and growth, all essential in facilitating optimal wound healing.[19] Zinc deficiency leads to decreased fibroblast proliferation and collagen synthesis as well as epidermal cell proliferation.[14] Thus, decreased wound strength and stability and a delay in reepithelialization can result. Zinc deficiency is seen in older adults, chronic alcohol abusers, individuals with malabsorptive disorders, and individuals with an increased need for zinc, such as pregnant women and children during growth spurts.

Magnesium, Copper, and Iron Deficiencies

Magnesium, copper, and iron are coenzymes that are required for protein synthesis and cellular proliferation for normal wound healing. In particular, these minerals are critical in collagen synthesis and cross-linking, and deficiencies impair wound tensile strength and stability. Iron is also required for oxygen transport in the hemoglobin molecule, and severe deficiencies can impair oxygen delivery to cells and tissues and result in wound hypoxia.

Medications

Certain medications can affect wound and tissue healing. For example, use of immunosuppressant medications or corticosteroids can greatly influence immunologic mechanisms involved in tissue repair and healing. Medications affecting blood flow may also influence wound healing by altering perfusion of the wound bed.

Corticosteroids

Corticosteroids are hormones given for a large number of diseases, including asthma, rheumatoid arthritis, allergies, and shock.[16] These hormones promote the breakdown of carbohydrates, fats, and proteins. This nutrient breakdown can impair the anabolic processes needed for cell growth and proliferation during wound healing. Corticosteroids also exert a powerful anti-inflammatory action that may impede the inflammatory phase of wound healing. Corticosteroids normally affect wound healing only when they are taken in high doses over a prolonged period of time. Negative effects may include reduced phagocytosis, reduction in fibroblast proliferation and collagen synthesis, and decreased angiogenesis.[15] These actions lead to prolonged wound hypoxia, increased susceptibility to wound infection, reduced granulation tissue formation, decreased wound tensile strength and stability, increased incidence of wound dehiscence, and reduced wound contraction.[15]

Antineoplastic Drugs

Antineoplastic drugs are those used to treat cancer. Many antineoplastic drugs are quite toxic to human cells and can interrupt the mitotic cycle of rapidly proliferating cells in the healing wound such as keratinocytes, fibroblasts, and endothelial cells. Many are potent immunosuppressants that diminish the production of leukocytes, erythrocytes, and platelets, all of which are critical to wound healing. As a result, reepithelialization, granulation tissue formation, and angiogenesis are impaired. In addition, the negative effects of antineoplastic drugs on wound healing may be compounded in that malignancies themselves can deplete nutrients and inhibit wound healing directly.

Metabolic Status

A detailed discussion of the many disease conditions associated with impaired wound healing is beyond the scope of this chapter. Diabetes mellitus is used as a prototype for this category.

Diabetes Mellitus

Diabetes mellitus is a condition in which the body has insufficient insulin, a reduced sensitivity to insulin (insulin resistance), or both. The persistent hyperglycemia that occurs with untreated diabetes causes serious chronic macrovascular disease that is a major cause of impaired tissue repair at all stages of wound healing.[20] The altered macrovascular function accelerates atherosclerosis, causing tissue ischemia and hypoxia. The increased microvascular disease results in profound thickening of the basement membranes, which underlies the development of diabetic lesions in the kidneys, eyes, and nervous system. With impaired perfusion, granulocyte function and chemotaxis are impaired, resulting in a reduced ability to fight infection. Sensory neuropathy reduces pain sensation, causing a lack of ability to feel problems, such as infections, associated with wound healing.

Helen Baker: Application

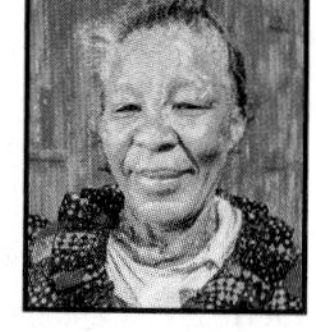

The results of a wound culture obtained in the ED show moderate amounts of *Staphylococcus aureus* and few *Escherichia coli*. Because this wound shows no other clinical signs of infection, it is contaminated and likely colonized. The wound's location over the sacrum in conjunction with Mrs. Baker's incontinence means that there is a high risk for contamination and infection of the wound. While Mrs. Baker's advanced age may slow the wound healing process, her comorbidities may play a larger role in impeding her wound healing. Mrs. Baker is taking a corticosteroid to manage her Crohn disease. With her decrease in food intake as well as malabsorption associated with Crohn disease, Mrs. Baker may be malnourished.

9. On the basis of Mrs. Baker's history, identify factors that increase her risk of wound infection?
10. Because of her poor intake and absorption of nutrients, what role may a vitamin C deficiency play in Mrs. Baker's wound healing?
11. Describe the relationship between incontinence and wound healing.

Check Your Progress: Section 39.4

1. How does a deficiency in vitamin K affect wound healing?
2. Why are patients who are receiving chemotherapy prone to abnormal wound healing?
3. How does a negative nitrogen balance affect wound healing?

39.5 Spectrum of Wound Healing

The spectrum of wound healing involves several considerations; some are lifespan specific, and others reflect elements of the healing process. In terms of a dynamic spectrum, a wound can heal without scarring or demonstrate significantly delayed healing. Scarring can result in contractures, or hypertrophy can manifest. It is therefore important to understand issues that can arise at either end of the wound healing spectrum.

Scarless Fetal Wound Healing

Little was known about fetal wound healing until the advent of intrauterine surgery. At that time, it was discovered that cutaneous wounds in a fetus younger than 24 weeks of gestation, referred to as an early-gestation fetus, healed with little or no scarring.[6,7] This discovery was the impetus for an explosion of research targeting the physiologic mechanisms underlying this phenomenon. But although a great deal more is now known about tissue repair during fetal life, the multifactorial nature of scarless fetal healing is still not well understood.

Two characteristics of scarless fetal healing of cutaneous wounds are consistently demonstrated in the literature; much of this research was done using animal models. Cutaneous wound healing with minimal or no scarring is related to the gestational age of the fetus and the size of the wound. As the gestational age of the fetus increases, healing proceeds from no scar to barely visible to faint mark to obvious scar.[21] Thus, gestational age is positively correlated with the extent of scarring. For scarless healing to result, the gestational age at time of surgery must decrease as the size

Table 39.5 Differences Between Fetal Scarless and Adult Scar-Forming Wound Healing

Fetal Factors	Adult Factors
Amniotic fluid, sterile environment	Dry, contaminated environment
Rapid reepithelialization	Slow reepithelialization
Less differentiated skin	Fully differentiated skin
Predominant form of TGFβ is $TGF\beta_3$ (antiscarring properties)	Predominant form of TGFβ is $TGF\beta_1$ (scar-forming properties)
Platelets: less degranulation of active cytokines	Platelets: potent degranulation of active cytokines
Faster fibroblast migration	Slower fibroblast migration
High proportion of type III collagen	High proportion of type I collagen
Minimal inflammatory response	Intense inflammatory response

SOURCES: Satish, L., & Kathju, S. (2010). Cellular and molecular characteristics of scarless versus fibrotic wound healing. *Dermatology Research and Practice*. doi:10.1155/2010/790234. Rolfe, K., & Grobbelaar, A. (2012). A review of fetal scarless healing. *ISRN Dermatology*. doi:10.5402/2012/698034. Namazi, M., Fallahzadeh, M., & Schwartz, R. (2011). Strategies for prevention of scars: What can we learn from fetal skin? *International Journal of Dermatology, 50*(1), 85–93.

of the wound increases. Thus, different degrees of wounding at the same gestational age may or may not result in a scar.

The physiologic mechanisms underlying the phenomenon of scarless fetal cutaneous wound healing are unclear. However, the voluminous research on this subject revealed anatomical and physiologic differences between scarless fetal wound healing and scar-forming adult wound healing (**Table 39.5** ■). These differences include, but are not limited to, the four mentioned here.

First, the likelihood of scar development during fetal wound healing is associated with an increasing inflammatory response. Scarless fetal wounds heal with minimal inflammation.[7,22] The weak inflammatory response in scarless healing is thought to be related to the diminished function of early fetal neutrophils, macrophages, and platelets. Apparently, as the immune system matures and the inflammatory response strengthens, the likelihood of fetal scar formation increases. Second, the collagenous structure of the ECM after wound repair appears to differ between scarless fetal wounds and scar-forming adult wounds.[22] Unlike the collagenous architecture of the ECM in adult wounds after remodeling, the collagenous architecture in scarless fetal wounds contains less collagen and more hyaluronan. In addition, the pattern of collagen in fetal scarless healing is reticular as opposed to the bundled pattern in adults. As the gestational age increases, the collagen profile becomes more and more like that of an adult, and scar production increases. These differences are thought to be related to a difference in phenotypic characteristics between adult and fetal fibroblasts. Third, the appearance of fetal scarring occurs in close proximity to the appearance of myofibroblasts in the wound.[6] Finally, scarless fetal wounds manifest a different cytokine and growth factor profile from that of scar-forming adult wounds.[6,22]

Cutaneous fetal wounds tend to heal not only without a scar but also more rapidly than adult wounds. Studies of fetal wound healing in bone demonstrated the same regenerative qualities as those seen in the skin. However, observations of fetal wound healing in other tissues failed to show the same scarless healing pattern.

Abnormal Wound Healing

Excessive Wound Healing

Scarring is a natural result of the body's attempt to repair an area of epithelial skin loss. Enormous individual variation exists in the degree and quality of scar formation. Excessive wound healing involves abnormally high connective tissue deposition that results in altered tissue structure and function.[7] Excessive wound healing may manifest as fibrosis or contracture.

Fibrosis. Fibrosis is the replacement of normal tissue elements with excessive, nonfunctional collagen or scar tissue, resulting in the destruction of the normal tissue architecture and composition. The excessive accumulation of collagen at the wound site involves excess synthesis and/or delayed degradation.[15] It is likely, however, that the etiology of the exaggerated scar tissue formation is multifactorial, involving processes in all stages of wound healing. Many clinical problems can result from the fibrotic process, including keloids, hypertrophic scars, adhesions, strictures, and liver cirrhosis. Only keloids and hypertrophic scars are discussed in this section.

Keloids. Keloids are lesions characterized by an excess of dermal scar or fibrotic tissue. They typically occur in individuals under the age of 30 and those who have darker-pigmented skin. Wounds associated with trauma, burns, and areas of tension are more likely to develop keloids. Keloids are raised above the level of the surrounding skin; in some cases, they may be disfiguring.[7] They extend beyond the boundary of the original injury into the surrounding tissue, resulting in a scar that is larger than the original wound (**Figure 39.16** ■).[23] Keloids usually appear from 6 months to 1 year after wounding. They tend

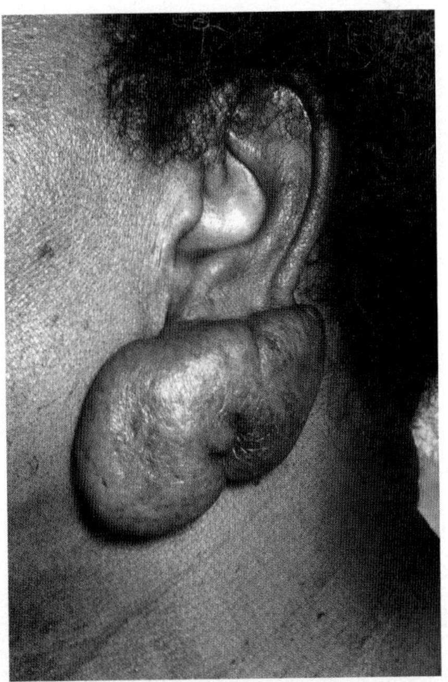

Figure 39.16 ■ Keloid scars occur most often in areas of high melanocyte concentrations such as above the clavicles, arms, and face.

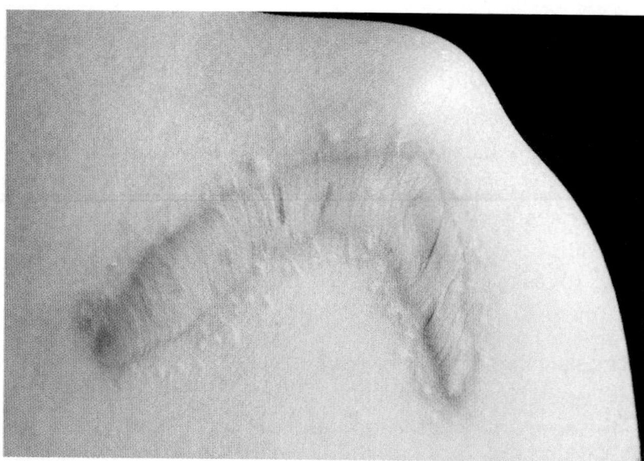

Figure 39.17 ■ A hypertrophic scar from a knee wound.

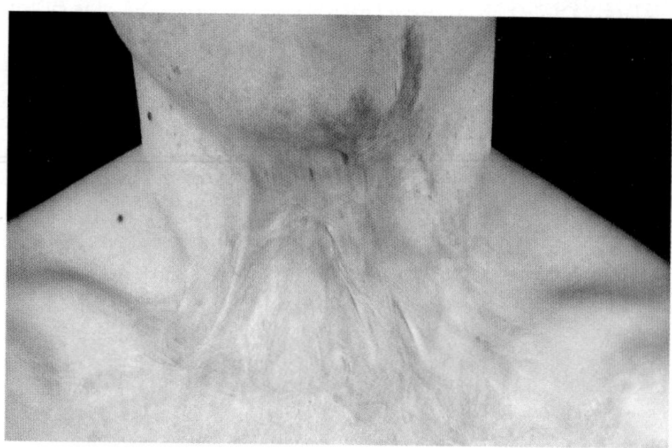

Figure 39.18 ■ Severe contractures from burn wounds.

to grow over time, do not regress spontaneously, and almost always recur after simple excision.[23]

Hypertrophic Scars. Like keloids, **hypertrophic scars** are characterized by an excess of fibrotic tissue; they are more likely to be associated with wounds associated with trauma and burns and are raised above the level of the surrounding skin. However, unlike keloids, hypertrophic scars grow within the boundaries of the original injury and often regress spontaneously (**Figure 39.17** ■).[15,23] Hypertrophic scars develop within the first month after wounding, and their appearance is thought to be related the time spent in the inflammatory phase, especially if that is longer than 3 weeks. Hypertrophic scars are often located in wounds on the trunk and those that cross flexor surfaces such as in the extremities. Hypertrophic scars may be pruritic and edematous but are often less painful than keloids.[23]

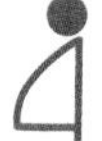

Hormone triggers and mechanical tension of the abdomen during pregnancy are factors that may increase the risk for keloid or hypertrophic scarring. ■

Contractures. **Contractures** result from an abnormal exaggeration of the normal process of wound contraction; shrinking scars severely deform the wound and surrounding tissues and reduce mobility. These are areas in which the scar tissue crosses joints or skin creases at right angles. Contractures are commonly seen in the healing of severe burns and may compromise the mobility of involved joints (**Figure 39.18** ■).

Deficient Wound Healing

Deficient wound healing is characterized by insufficient deposition of dermal connective tissue matrix, resulting in weakening of the tissue to a point of wound failure. Wound dehiscence and chronic, nonhealing wounds are examples of deficient wound healing.

Wound Dehiscence. There are two types of wound dehiscence: extrafascial and fascial. Extrafascial wound dehiscence is the partial or complete separation of the outer layers of a sutured wound, usually an abdominal incision while the underlying fascial layer remains intact. Fascial wound dehiscence, often referred to as **evisceration**, is separation of the fascial layers. In an abdominal wound, this disruption of the fascia allows extrusion of the intestines and omentum upward onto the abdominal wall. Wound dehiscence is associated with a much higher rate of complication and death.

The risk of wound dehiscence usually involves the handling of the involved tissue during surgery, as well as the suturing technique (e.g., too close to the wound edge, too far apart, or under too much tension), and/or factors specific to the individual. Three factors that are commonly associated

Impact of Current Research on Clinical Practice

Evidence for Negative Pressure Wound Therapy for Incisional Wound Care

Description: Results from a randomized control trial demonstrated the benefits of negative pressure wound therapy (NPWT) for patients with high-risk surgical incisions. The study involved 249 patients with high-risk lower extremity fractures who were randomly assigned to receive either NPWT or standard postoperative dressings. Each group had similar Injury Severity Scores. The group of patients who received NPWT had fewer postoperative infections in comparison to those who received standard postoperative dressings. Additionally, there were fewer cases of wound dehiscence in those who were treated with NPWT than in patients who received standard postoperative dressings. While the mechanism of action of NPWT is not completely understood, prior research supports the hypothesis that NPWT is associated with increased microvascular blood flow through capillary blood vessels, reduction of edema, and stretching of the cells, leading to tissue growth and expansion.

Clinical Practice: The findings indicate that prophylactic NPWT treatment of high-risk wounds before their failure may be an effective treatment strategy.

Research Study:

Stannard, J., Volgas, D., McGwin, G., et al. (2013). Incisional negative pressure wound therapy after high-risk lower extremity fractures. *Journal of Orthopaedic Trauma, 26*(1), 37–42.

with wound dehiscence are diabetes mellitus, high-dose corticosteroid use, and infection.[24] Sepsis is associated with a rate of wound dehiscence approaching 50%. Some additional individual factors that favor dehiscence are increased mechanical strain on the wound, age greater than 65 years, dehydration, malnutrition, hypoproteinemia, malignancy, and obesity.[24]

The incidence of dehiscence peaks at approximately 5–9 days after surgery. In the current health care environment, this high-risk time often occurs after discharge from the hospital. Clinical manifestations of impending wound disruption include noticeable signs of infection, absence of a healing ridge by the fifth to ninth postoperative day, seroma or hematoma formation, and an increase in serous discharge.[18] In some instances, individuals may report that they felt something "give way or pop."

Maria King: Application

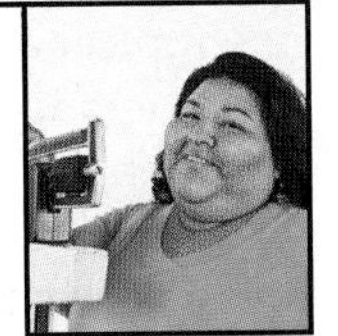

Ms. King suffered extrafascial wound dehiscence, as the fascia was found to be intact. Her wound dehiscence was beginning on her fifth postoperative day, which was also her discharge day; the dehiscence progressed after discharge to home. The nurse noted redness in the lower two thirds of Ms. King's incision on discharge. Ms. King reported no other signs and symptoms while at home. The expression of dark serosanguineous drainage by the surgeon on the tenth postoperative day indicates the presence of a hematoma in the wound. Ms. King's history of type 2 diabetes mellitus is a major risk factor for dehiscence. She also has additional risk factors, including obesity and frequent coughing postoperatively caused by smoking.

3. What are the differences between extrafascial and fascial wound healing?
4. What clinical manifestations of a wound dehiscence did Ms. King display?

Chronic Nonhealing Wounds. Chronic nonhealing wounds are a heterogeneous collection of skin lesions that either do not proceed through the healing process in an organized and timely manner to produce structural and functional integrity or progress appropriately through the healing process but cannot maintain structural and functional integrity. They are sometimes characterized as wounds that do not heal within 3 months of onset.[11] Most frequently, there is arrest in the inflammatory phase. All chronic wounds harbor bacteria, and their chronicity relates directly to the high bacterial concentrations in the wound. As a result, these wounds contain an overabundance of neutrophils and an imbalance between neutrophilic proteolytic enzymes and their inhibitors.[25] Proteolytic enzymes such as collagenase and elastase, as well as neutrophil and macrophage-derived reactive oxygen species, destroy ECM and growth factors and damage healing tissues. They also contain increased levels of inflammatory mediators, including IL-1, IL-6, and TNFα, that are not present in normally healing wounds.[25] This results in chronic inflammation, necrosis, and fibrosis. An abnormal profile of other cytokines and growth factors exists in chronic wounds in which levels may be abnormally elevated or depressed. Examples of chronic wounds include diabetic ulcers, venous stasis ulcers, pressure injuries (as shown in **Figure 39.15**), atherosclerotic ulcers, and severe burns.[20]

Maria King: Outcome

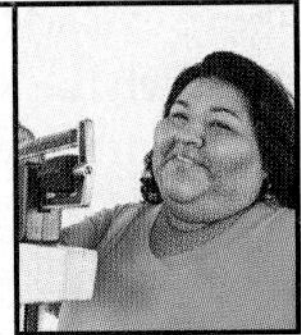

Ms. King's wound is dressed and left to heal by secondary intention. Because of her continued smoking and her comorbidities of diabetes and obesity, she exhibits a delay in wound healing.

5. Why should Ms. King expect a pronged period of healing?
6. How does Ms. King's diabetes affect her wound healing?

Check Your Progress: Section 39.5

1. What role does gestational age play in fetal scar formation?
2. Describe the characteristics of collagen in fetal scarless tissue versus that of scars of the adult.
3. How do keloids differ from hypertrophic scars?

39.6 Pressure Injuries

A **pressure injury** is a localized ischemic lesion of the skin and underlying tissue, usually over a bony prominence, caused by external pressure that impairs the flow of blood and lymph. Pressure injuries are a significant health issue, especially for hospitalized patients, residents of nursing homes, and older adults. Pressure injuries are preventable.[26] As of 2008, the Centers for Medicare and Medicaid Services will not pay for additional costs incurred for hospital-acquired pressure injuries.[27]

Etiology and Pathogenesis

Immobility can result from a number of different disease states or injuries. Regardless of cause, immobility can result in several complications. One of the main is the development of pressure-related injury. An individual with intact sensation becomes aware of numbness or pain in a pressure site and seeks to change position. When the person does not have the ability to sense pressure or lacks the capacity to move to alleviate pressure, blood flow to the site can become slowed or obstructed.

Initially, pressure can result in redness (reactive hyperemia), but as the blockage of blood flow continues, platelets begin to aggregate in the area of pooled blood and can form small clots known as microthrombi. These thrombi can further obstruct the flow of blood to the pressure site, leading to tissue ischemia. Immobility also predisposes the individual to **shearing forces**, which occur when an immobile individual is turned or repositioned and tissue layers slide in opposition to one another. Shearing forces can result in tearing of the skin and damage to underlying tissue.

Although a pressure injury may develop in anyone, the three most important risk factors are immobility or inactivity, poor perfusion (including diabetes), and skin status.[28] Any significant reduction in an individual's ability to move and reposition himself or an extremity places the individual at increased risk for the development of a pressure injury. Poor nutritional status over time leads to a loss of muscle and lean tissue, removing tissue that could aid in mitigating the effects of immobility. Skin status is influenced by aging and the presence of moisture. Moisture trapped against the skin can lead to **maceration**, a form of overhydration of cells in which the skin softens and breaks down, and sloughing, in which a layer of tissue or skin may slide, particularly in response to shearing forces.

Patients who are at risk should be assessed regularly for development of pressure injuries.[29]

Several age-related changes put older patients at increased risk for pressure-related injury. The loss of muscle mass, thinning of the outer layers of the skin, and decreased blood flow to the outer layers of skin and tissue place older adults at risk.

Clinical Manifestations

Pressure injuries can manifest in different ways depending on their severity. This variation is attributed to the soft tissue, muscle, and skin resisting pressure to differing degrees. Muscle is generally the least resistant to pressure and will become necrotic before the skin breaks down. In addition, pressure is not distributed equally from a bony prominence, where it is greatest, to the overlying skin. Pressure decreases gradually from the bony area toward the periphery, and a small area of skin breakdown might not be representative of what lies underneath.[30]

Pressure injuries range from discoloration to blisters or areas of denuded superficial skin to deep tissue damage with necrosis. As a result, pressure injuries are graded or staged to classify the degree of tissue damage. The stages and clinical manifestations of pressure injuries developed by the National Pressure Ulcer Advisory Panel are listed in **Table 39.6**.[31]

Linking Pathophysiology to Diagnosis and Treatment

The primary objective for the patient who is at risk for developing pressure injury is prevention. Members of the healthcare team should assess patients for ulcer development regularly and reposition patients according to an established schedule. In repositioning, the proper technique is essential to prevent injuries related to shear. Pressure-relieving devices should be used in placing patients on any support surface.[27,32] If ulcers develop, they should be regularly assessed to ensure that they do not advance to a more severe stage. The patient and family members should be taught how to protect and treat ulcers and how to assess for stage changes.

Diagnostic tests are conducted to determine whether a secondary infection is present and to differentiate the cause of the pressure injury. White blood cell counts can be used to indicate the degree of inflammation or invasive infection. Evaluation of the erythrocyte sedimentation rate is useful in determining the presence of osteomyelitis. Laboratory studies that evaluate nutritional parameters (albumin, prealbumin, transferrin, serum protein) should be used to assess a patient's nutritional status, as adequate nutrition is needed for wound healing. Other laboratory studies such as urine, stool, or blood cultures may be required if indicated by specific patient situations.[30] If the pressure injury is deep or appears infected, drainage or biopsied tissue is cultured to determine the causative organism.

Nonviable tissue must be removed from a wound before the wound can be staged or heal.[30] Surgical **debridement** (removal of necrotic material) may be necessary if the pressure injury is deep, if subcutaneous tissues are involved, or if **eschar** (a scab or dry crust consisting of dried plasma proteins and dead cells that forms over skin damaged by burns, infections, or excoriations) has formed over the ulcer, preventing healing by granulation.

Autolytic debridement may be used to treat pressure injuries. In autolytic debridement, dressings that contain wound moisture, such as hydrocolloid and clear absorbent acrylic dressings, trap the wound drainage against the eschar. The body's own enzymes in the drainage break down the necrotic tissue. Although this method takes longer than the other three, it is the most selective and therefore causes the least damage to healthy surrounding and healing tissues. Large wounds may require skin grafting for complete closure.

Topical and systemic antibiotics specific to the infectious organism should eradicate any infection present. Additionally, a variety of topical products promote healing. For pressure injuries that are clean and granulating, dressings that maintain moisture are typically used, such as hydrocolloid and transparent film dressings. In addition to maintaining moisture, these dressings protect the wound from friction and bacterial colonization. Dressings may be impregnated with substances that offer microbial benefits, such as silver sulfadiazine and medical-grade honey. For deep, exudative wounds, alginate, foam, and iodine dressings may be preferable. The type of dressing that is used changes over time as the wound either heals or worsens.[30]

Helen Baker: Outcome

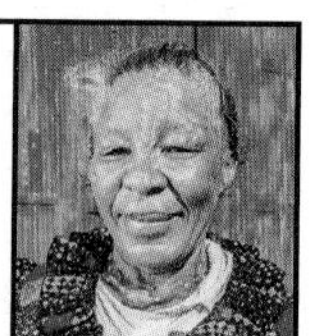

Mrs. Baker is admitted to the hospital for urosepsis and is placed on IV antibiotics. While she is in the hospital, a registered dietitian is consulted and provides recommendations for improving Mrs. Baker's nourishment to promote wound healing. The wound is evaluated by the nurse practitioner from the wound clinic, and an adhesive foam dressing is prescribed to keep the wound covered to protect it from contamination and to provide a moist wound healing environment. A plan is made to place Mrs. Baker on a pressure redistribution surface with a turning schedule to reduce pressure, one of the underlying causes of this wound, and frequent checks for incontinence. During her hospitalization, follow-up wound checks are made, and her wound continues to decrease in size. The wound care treatment plans made in the hospital will be continued post discharge back to the nursing home with anticipation that the wound will eventually reepithelialize and mature into a scar.

12. Mrs. Baker receives a dressing to keep her wound moist. What is the benefit of a moist wound environment?
13. How does the redistribution of pressure promote wound healing in Mrs. Baker?

Check Your Progress: Section 39.6

1. Why do pressure-related injuries occur?
2. Where do pressure injuries usually occur?
3. What stage of pressure injury shows full thickness skin loss and muscle exposure.

Table 39.6 Pressure Injury Staging

Stage	Description
Stage 1	
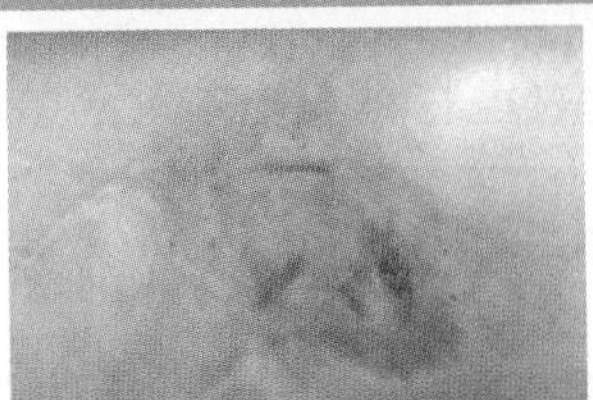	Nonblanchable erythema of intact skin, the heralding lesion of skin ulceration. Usually occurs in a localized area over a bony prominence. Identification of stage 1 pressure injuries may be difficult in patients with darkly pigmented skin. *Note:* Affected areas may be painful and a different temperature and consistency than surrounding skin.
Stage 2	
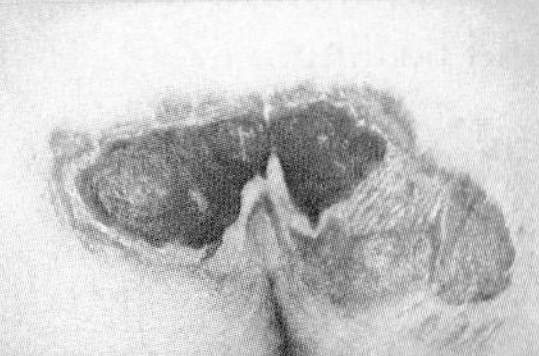	Partial thickness skin loss involving the dermis. Presents as a shallow open ulcer with a viable pink or red moist wound bed; granulation tissue, eschar (dead tissue) not present; may also present an intact or open serum-filled blister. *Note:* Skin tears, tape burns, incontinence-associated dermatitis, maceration, and excoriation are not included in this classification.
Stage 3	
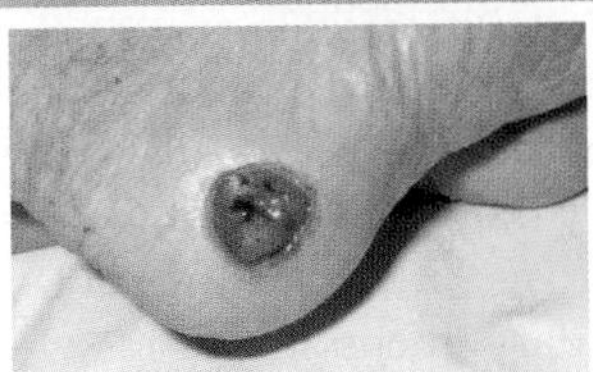	Full thickness skin loss involving damage or necrosis of subcutaneous tissue; adipose tissue is visible within the ulcer; granulation and rolled wound edges are often present; bone, tendon, and muscle are not exposed. The ulcer presents clinically as a deep crater with or without undermining and tunneling of adjacent tissue; slough and/or eschar may be present. *Note:* The depth of a stage 3 pressure injury varies by anatomic location. In areas without adipose tissue, the ulcer may be very shallow. The presence of slough or eschar that obscures the extent of tissue loss makes this an unstageable pressure injury.
Stage 4	
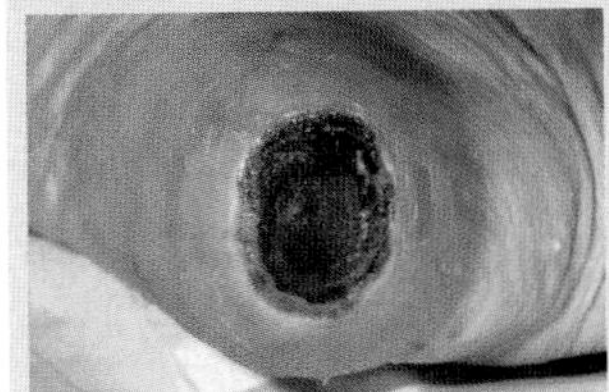	Full thickness skin loss with extensive tissue damage and necrosis. Fascia, muscle, ligament, cartilage, tendon, and/or bone are exposed and directly palpable; slough or eschar may be present. Undermining and tunneling and rolled wound edges are usually present. *Note:* The depth of a stage 4 pressure injury can vary by anatomic location, and injuries can extend into muscle and supporting structures (including fascia, tendons, or joint capsules), increasing the likelihood of osteomyelitis. The presence of slough or eschar that obscures the extent of tissue loss makes this an unstageable pressure injury.
Unstageable	
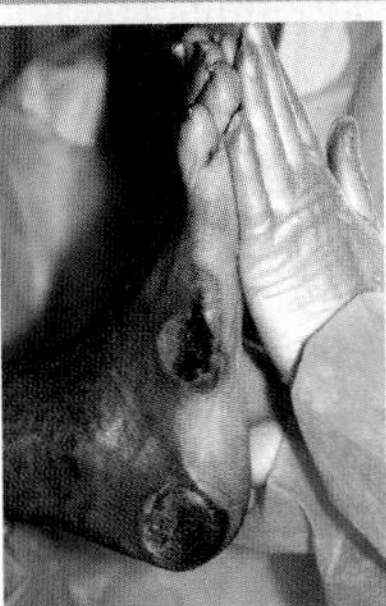	Full thickness tissue loss with depth completely obscured by slough or eschar in the wound bed. The depth of the wound cannot be determined until the slough or eschar is removed; once it has been removed, the injury will be classified as stage 3 or 4. *Note:* Stable eschar on the heels serves as a natural biological cover and should not be removed.
Deep tissue injury	
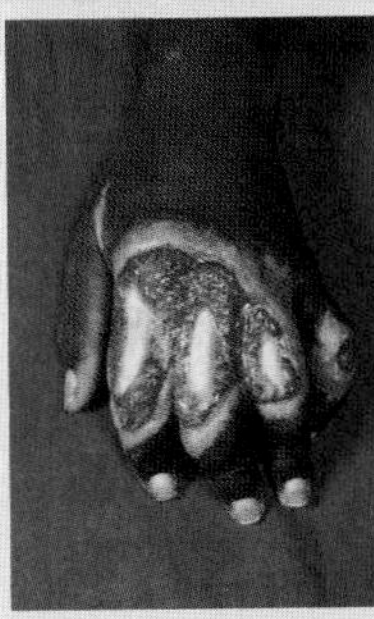	Intact or nonintact skin with localized, nonblanchable, maroon, deep red or purple discoloration or blood-filled blister. Indicates damage to underlying soft tissue from pressure or shear. May rapidly evolve into a thin blister over a dark wound bed or may develop thin eschar. May be difficult to detect in patients with darkly pigmented skin. *Note:* Discoloration or blister may be preceded by painful tissue that is of a different temperature and consistency than surrounding skin.

SOURCE: Adapted from National Pressure Ulcer Advisory Panel. (2016). *NPUAP pressure injury stages*. Available at http://www.npuap.org/resources/educational-and-clinical-resources/npuap-pressure-injury-stages.

CHAPTER SUMMARY

39.1 Chapter Overview and Case Studies

Classify wounds on the basis of acute/chronic and partial/full thickness criteria and discuss concepts related to tissue and wound healing.

- Acute wounds move through the healing process in a timely and organized manner.
- Chronic wounds fail to proceed through phases of wound healing in a timely and organized manner, instead entering into a prolonged state of inflammation.
- Partial thickness wounds involve lost or destroyed epidermis and partial dermis and are able to heal by reepithelialization.
- Full thickness wounds include damage or destruction of the epidermis and the entire thickness of the dermis, possibly extending to subcutaneous tissue, muscle, and bone.
- Concepts related to tissue and wound healing include mobility, nutrition, perfusion, and trauma.

39.2 The Structure of the Skin

Describe the structural components of each layer of skin and their functions in maintaining homeostasis.

- The skin is the largest organ in the body.
- Skin varies in thickness and is thicker in areas that are exposed to higher amounts of friction and shear.
- Skin is composed of two layers: the epidermis, which is the superficial layer, and dermis, which is the deep connective tissue layer.
- The epidermis is composed almost exclusively of keratinocytes with a smattering of melanocytes and tactile (Merkel cells). The epidermis contains no blood vessels and derives its nourishment from the dermis.
- The upper layers of the epidermis are dead or dying, giving the skin a thick, horny quality that is resistant to environmental stressors.
- The tissues of the body are composed of cells and a ground substance called the extracellular matrix (ECM), which is the largest component of the dermis and accounts for the tensile strength, elasticity, and compressibility of the skin.
- ECM components include water, fibrous structural proteins, adhesive glycoproteins, polysaccharides called glycosaminoglycans (GAGs), and a combination of GAGs and a protein core called proteoglycans.
- The fibrous structural proteins in the ECM are collagen and elastin. These proteins provide structure to the matrix and a blueprint for cells migrating through the matrix. Collagen is the most abundant protein in the ECM and imparts strength to the skin. Elastin imparts the ability to recoil after stretching.
- The GAGs attract large amounts of water, resulting in significant tissue swelling known as skin turgor. The gel-like nature of GAGs allows these substances to act as a fill between fibers and cells in the matrix. This fill also acts as a filter for ions, hormones, nutrients, and other substances before they enter the epidermis.

39.3 Cutaneous Wound Healing

Differentiate the types of cutaneous wound healing by intention and the phases of wound healing.

- Wound healing can occur by primary, secondary, or tertiary intention.
- Healing by primary intention occurs when the edges of the wound can be brought together. Characteristics include minimal tissue loss, absence of infection or contamination, and minimal scarring results.
- Healing by secondary intention occurs when the edges of the wound cannot be brought together because of the magnitude of tissue loss or the presence of infection, contamination, tissue necrosis, or a large amount of exudate. Healing by secondary intention takes longer than healing by primary intention, and the resulting scar is larger.
- Healing by tertiary intention or delayed primary intention occurs when wound closure is delayed and the subsequent primary closure brings two granulating surfaces together. This type of healing may occur or when a contaminated wound is left open until infection resolves and is then closed.
- The wound healing process comprises three phases: inflammatory, proliferative, and remodeling. The successful initiation, maintenance, and completion of all phases depend on the presence of a multitude of cytokines, growth factors, and bioamines and a large number of other protein and nonprotein molecules.
- The inflammatory phase, which is critical to the initiation of wound healing, functions to stop the bleeding, degrade damaged extracellular matrix, recruit phagocytic cells, and remove injurious agents, foreign material, and necrotic debris.
- The proliferative phase involves the generation of granulation tissue to replace the provisional matrix and the reepithelialization of the wound surface.
- The final phase of wound healing, the remodeling phase, encompasses wound contraction, decreased collagen synthesis, increased collagen breakdown, rearrangement of collagen fibers, decreased angiogenesis, and decline in the fibroblast population.
- The tensile strength of the wound increases during remodeling to approximately 75–80% that of uninjured tissue. This is accomplished primarily by quantitative and qualitative changes in collagen. Collagen synthesis

peaks during this phase and is followed by increasing collagen breakdown. Type I collagen predominates, replacing type III. Collagen fibers are also rearranged in a systematic manner, lining up along the lines of tension in the wound.

- During the remodeling phase, angiogenesis decreases and the capillary density within the wound declines, accounting for the pale white color of the maturing scar tissue.

39.4 Factors Impeding Wound Healing

Analyze the impact of local and systemic factors on wound healing.

- Although most wounds heal without complication, a number of local and systemic factors can impede wound healing.
- Local factors that may result in delayed wound closure include hypoxia, wound infection, contamination, radiation exposure, movement or tension, desiccation, excessive edema, and denervation.
- Systemic factors that may result in delayed wound closure include advanced age, malnutrition, micronutrient deficiency, immune deficiency, smoking, drugs, and disease (e.g., diabetes mellitus, severe anemia, coagulopathies, genetic connective tissue disorders, obesity).

39.5 Spectrum of Wound Healing

Compare the mechanisms of the continuum of wound healing from scarless fetal wound healing to abnormal wound healing.

- Fetuses younger than 24 weeks, gestation are able to heal cutaneous wounds with minimal or no scarring. As gestational age increases, scar formation becomes more likely.
- Anatomic and physiologic differences exist between scarless fetal wound healing and scar-forming adult wound healing. There appears to be less inflammation, a different ECM collagenous architecture, a lack of myofibroblasts, and a different cytokine and growth factor profile in fetal healing than in adult healing.
- Abnormalities of wound healing include fibrosis (e.g., keloids and hypertrophic scars) and contractures.
- Keloids contain an excess of collagen, grow into surrounding tissues, and result in a scar that is larger than the original wound. Collagen deposition exceeds degradation. Cytokines and growth factors responsible for fibroblast proliferation show increased activity; there are few myofibroblasts.
- Like keloids, hypertrophic scars contain excessive fibrotic tissue but grow within the bounds of the original wound. Although hypertrophic scars contain an overabundance of collagen, similar to keloids, they contain a large number of myofibroblasts.
- Contractures represent an exaggeration of normally occurring wound contraction and result in severe deformity of the wound and surrounding tissues. They often occur in areas where the wound crosses joints or skin creases at a right angle. Contractures are commonly seen after severe burn injuries.
- Wound dehiscence may be extrafascial or fascial. Extrafascial wound dehiscence involves separation of the layers of the skin and subcutaneous fat but no disruption of the underlying fascia. Fascial wound dehiscence, or evisceration, involves disruption of the layers of the skin, subcutaneous fat, and underlying fascia. In an abdominal wound with fascial wound dehiscence, the intestine is able to protrude onto the abdominal wall. Wound dehiscence is associated with a much higher rate of complication and death.
- Chronic nonhealing wounds do not progress through the orderly and timely repair process to produce structural and functional integrity, or they have proceeded through the repair process without establishing a sustained anatomic and functional result. Examples of chronic wounds are diabetic ulcers, venous stasis ulcers, pressure injuries, atherosclerotic ulcers, and severe burns.
- All chronic wounds harbor bacteria, and their chronic nature relates to the high bacterial concentrations in the wound. The resulting influx of phagocytic cells and their secretions result in chronic inflammation. These wounds therefore contain an overabundance of neutrophils and an imbalance between neutrophilic proteolytic enzymes and their inhibitors, which results in chronic inflammation.

39.6 Pressure Injuries

Differentiate the causes, classification, underlying pathogenesis, and clinical manifestations of pressure injuries and approaches to diagnosis and treatment for these conditions.

- Pressure-related injury can result from unrelieved pressure restricting blood flow, leading to tissue hypoxia and ischemia.
- Older adults are at increased risk because of reductions in thickness of skin layers, muscle mass, and sensation.
- There are several categories or grades of pressure injury that reflect the degree of injury. The first stage differs from normal redness caused by pressure in that the tissue will not blanch with additional pressure.
- An injury in which the extent cannot be fully determined visually because of eschar or slough is referred to as unstageable.
- Frequent repositioning is the most effective means of preventing the development of pressure-related injury.
- Nonsurgical techniques are available to aid in wound debridement and protection of skin around the area of injury.
- A major concern is the development of infection through a wound emerging from pressure-related injury.

REVIEW QUESTIONS

1. The nurse is caring for a chronically ill patient with a long-standing wound. The nurse explains to the patient that a diet rich in which of the following vitamins is necessary for wound healing?
   a. A, C, E, and K
   b. A, B, C, and E
   c. A, C, D, and K
   d. B, C, E, and K

2. When assessing an abdominal wound, the nurse observes a loop of intestine protruding through the incision. What action should the nurse take?
   a. Redress the wound and assess it again in 4 hours.
   b. Leave the wound open and place the patient on bedrest.
   c. Cover the wound with a moist sterile dressing and call the surgeon.
   d. Redress the wound and tell the patient to avoid strain on the incision.

3. The nurse is caring for a patient with a right ischial pressure injury. In which of the following positions should the nurse position the patient?
   a. On the back in bed
   b. On either side in bed
   c. Seated upright in a chair
   d. Reclining in a chair

4. The nurse is assessing the wound healing of a patient at his follow-up appointment 2 weeks after a total hip replacement. Which of the following wound appearances would the nurse expect to see?
   a. A gap between the edges of the wound
   b. Granulation tissue in the wound bed
   c. Hematoma formation
   d. Wound edges well approximated

5. The nurse is assessing the skin of a patient with a sacral pressure injury who was admitted from home. The nurse assesses that the wound is healing by secondary intention when which of the following is observed?
   a. A large amount of granulation tissue
   b. Hematoma formation
   c. A minimal amount of exudate
   d. Abscess formation

6. Which of the following systemic factors places a patient at risk for impaired wound healing?
   a. Low body mass index
   b. Young age
   c. Vitamin B deficiency
   d. Diabetes mellitus

7. Which of the following patients is likely to experience the most scarless wound healing?
   a. A newborn
   b. A fetus at 22 weeks, gestation
   c. A teenager
   d. A young adult

8. The nurse is teaching a postoperative patient about wound healing. Which of the following statements made by the patient indicates that the patient requires more education?
   a. "My scar will be stronger than my injured tissue."
   b. "A normal scar is raised above the level of the surrounding skin."
   c. "A maturing scar will be pale white in color."
   d. "It is normal for the wound to be open in the first few weeks of healing."

ANSWERS

Answers to Review Questions can be found in Appendix A. Answers to Case Study and Check Your Progress questions are available on the faculty resources site. Please consult with your instructor.

RECOMMENDED WEBSITES

European Tissue Repair Society
http://www.etrs.org

National Pressure Ulcer Advisory Panel
http://www.npuap.org

Wound Healing Society
http://woundheal.org

REFERENCES

1. Hess, C. (2013). *Clinical guide to skin and wound care* (7th ed.). Ambler, PA: Lippincott Williams & Wilkins.
2. Marieb, E., & Hoehn, K. (2016). *Human anatomy & physiology* (10th ed.). Hoboken, NJ: Pearson.
3. Yip, W. L. (2015). Influence of oxygen on wound healing. *International Wound Journal, 12*(6), 620–624.
4. Dauwe, P. B., Pulikkottil, B. J., Lavery, L., Stuzin, J. M., & Rohrich, R. J. (2014). Does hyperbaric oxygen therapy work in facilitating acute wound healing: A systematic review. *Plastic and Reconstructive Surgery, 133*(2), 208e–215e.
5. Gawaz, M., & Vogel, S. (2013). Platelets in tissue repair: Control of apoptosis and interactions with regenerative cells. *Blood, 122*(15), 2550–2554.
6. Satish, L., & Kathju, S. (2010). Cellular and molecular characteristics of scarless versus fibrotic wound healing. *Dermatology Research and Practice*. doi:10.1155/2010/790234.
7. Eming, S. A., Martin, P., & Tomic-Canic, M. (2014). Wound repair and regeneration: Mechanisms, signaling, and translation. *Science Translational Medicine, 6*(265), 265sr6–265sr6.
8. Sindrilaru, A., & Scharffetter-Kochanek, K. (2013). Disclosure of the culprits: Macrophages—Versatile regulators of wound healing. *Advances in Wound Care, 2*(7), 357–368.
9. Schultz, G., Davidson, J., Kirsner, R., et al. (2011). Dynamic reciprocity in the wound microenvironment. *Wound Repair and Regeneration, 19*(2), 134–148.
10. Griffiths, C., Barker, J., Bleiker, T., Chalmers, R., & Creamer, D. (2016). *Rook's textbook of dermatology* (9th ed.). West Sussex, UK: Wiley-Blackwell.
11. Werdin, F., Tennenhaus, M., Schaller, H., & Rennekampff, H. (2009). Evidence-based management strategies for treatment of chronic wounds. *Eplasty, 9*, e19.
12. Olczyk, P., Mencner, L., & Komosinska-Vassev, K. (2014). The role of the extracellular matrix components in cutaneous wound healing. *BioMed Research International*. doi:10.1155/2014/747584.
13. Bernatchez, S., Menon, V., Stoffel, J., et al. (2013). Nitric oxide levels in wound fluid may reflect the healing trajectory. *Wound Repair and Regeneration, 21*(3), 410–417.
14. Sussman C, & Bates-Jensen B. (2012). *Wound care: A collaborative practice manual* (4th ed.). Philadelphia, PA: Lippincott Williams & Wilkins.
15. Bryant R. A., & Nix, D. P. (2016). *Acute & chronic wounds: Current management concepts* (5th ed.). St Louis, MO: Elsevier Health Science.
16. Adams, M., & Urban, C. (2016). *Pharmacology: Connections to nursing practice* (3rd ed.). Hoboken, NJ: Pearson.
17. Ross, C., Alston, M., Bickenbach, J., & Aykin-Burns, N. (2011). Oxygen tension changes the rate of migration of human skin keratinocytes in an age-related manner. *Experimental Dermatology, 20*(1), 58–63.
18. Yokoe, D. S., Anderson, D. J., Berenholtz, S. M., et al. (2014). A compendium of strategies to prevent healthcare-associated infections in acute care hospitals: 2014 updates. *American Journal of Infection Control, 42*(8), 820–828.
19. Quain, A. M., & Khardori, N. M. (2015). Nutrition in wound care management: A comprehensive overview. *Wounds: A Compendium of Clinical Research and Practice, 27*(12), 327.
20. Greer, N., Foman, N. A., MacDonald, R., Dorrian, J., Fitzgerald, P., Rutks, I., & Wilt, T. J. (2013). Advanced wound care therapies for nonhealing diabetic, venous, and arterial ulcers: A systematic review. *Annals of Internal Medicine, 159*(8), 532–542.
21. Walmsley, G. G., Maan, Z. N., Wong, V. W., et al. (2015). Scarless wound healing: Chasing the holy grail. *Plastic and Reconstructive Surgery, 135*(3), 907–917.
22. Rolfe, K., & Grobbelaar, A. (2012). A review of fetal scarless healing. *ISRN Dermatology*. doi:10.5402/2012/698034.
23. Andrews, J. P., Marttala, J., Macarak, E., Rosenbloom, J., & Uitto, J. (2016). Keloids: The paradigm of skin fibrosis—Pathomechanisms and treatment. *Matrix Biology, 51*, 37–46.
24. Sandy-Hodgetts, K., Carville, K., & Leslie, G. D. (2015). Determining risk factors for surgical wound dehiscence: A literature review. *International Wound Journal, 12*(3), 265–275.
25. Mckelvey, K., Xue, M., Whitmont, K., et al. (2012). Potential anti-inflammatory treatments for chronic wounds. *Wound Practice & Research, 20*(2), 86.
26. Agency for Healthcare Research and Quality. (2014). *Preventing pressure ulcers in hospitals*. Available at https://www.ahrq.gov/professionals/systems/hospital/pressureulcertoolkit/index.html
27. Joint Commission. (2016). Preventing pressure injuries. *QuickSafety*. Available at https://www.jointcommission.org/assets/1/23/Quick_Safety_Issue_25_July_20161.PDF
28. Coleman, S., Gorecki, C., Nelson, E. A., Closs, S. J., et al. (2013). Patient risk factors for pressure ulcer development: Systematic review. *International Journal of Nursing Studies, 50*(7), 974–1003.
29. Moore, Z. E., & Cowman, S. (2014). Risk assessment tools for the prevention of pressure ulcers. *Cochrane Database System Review, 5*(2): CD006471. doi:0.1002/14651858.CD006471.pub3
30. Kirman, C. N. (2016). Pressure ulcers and wound care. *Medscape*. Available at http://emedicine.medscape.com/article/190115-overview#a4
31. National Pressure Ulcer Advisory Panel. (2016). *NPUAP pressure injury stages*. Available at http://www.npuap.org/resources/educational-and-clinical-resources/npuap-pressure-injury-stages
32. McInnes, E., Jammali-Blasi, A., Bell-Syer, S. E. M., Dumville, J. C., Middleton, V., & Cullum, N. (2015). Support surfaces for pressure ulcer prevention. *Cochrane Database of Systematic Reviews, 5*: CD001735. doi:10.1002/14651858.CD001735.pub5

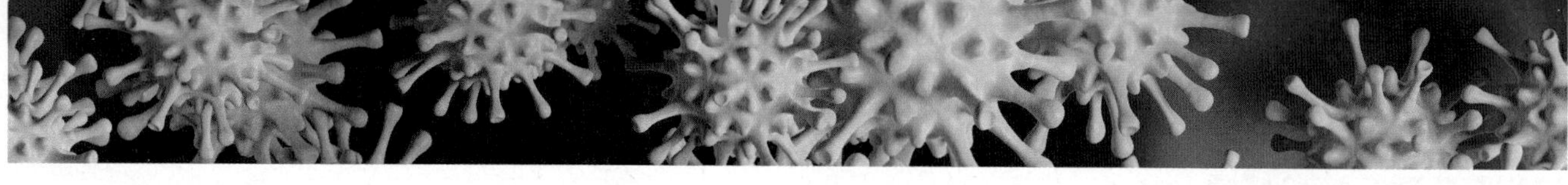

Chapter 40
Acute Skin Disorders

Karen Hill

Chapter Outline and Learning Outcomes

40.1 Chapter Overview and Case Studies

Differentiate acute from chronic skin conditions, and describe concepts related to acute disorders of the skin.

40.2 Bacterial Skin Infections

Differentiate the causes, classification, underlying pathogenesis, and clinical manifestations of bacterial skin infections and approaches to diagnosis and treatment of these conditions across the lifespan.

40.3 Fungal Skin Infections

Differentiate the causes, classification, underlying pathogenesis, and clinical manifestations of fungal skin infections and approaches to diagnosis and treatment of these conditions across the lifespan.

40.4 Dermatitis

Differentiate the causes, classification, underlying pathogenesis, and clinical manifestations of dermatitis and approaches to diagnosis and treatment of these conditions across the lifespan.

40.5 Life-threatening Inflammatory Disorders

Differentiate the causes, classification, underlying pathogenesis, and clinical manifestations of life-threatening inflammatory disorders and approaches to diagnosis and treatment of these conditions across the lifespan.

40.6 Stings and Bites

Differentiate the causes, classification, underlying pathogenesis, and clinical manifestations of insect stings and bites and approaches to diagnosis and treatment of these conditions across the lifespan.

40.7 Disorders Caused by Infestations

Differentiate the causes, classification, underlying pathogenesis, and clinical manifestations of disorders caused by infestations and approaches to diagnosis and treatment of these conditions across the lifespan.

40.8 Disorders Associated with Adolescent/Adult Skin

Differentiate the causes, classification, underlying pathogenesis, and clinical manifestations of disorders associated with adolescent/adult skin and approaches to diagnosis and treatment of these conditions across the lifespan.

40.9 Disorders of the Nail

Differentiate the causes, classification, underlying pathogenesis, and clinical manifestations of disorders of the nail and approaches to diagnosis and treatment of these conditions across the lifespan.

KEY TERMS

Acne vulgaris, 1002
Brittle nails, 1004
Bulla, 985
Candidiasis, 989
Carbuncle, 987
Cellulitis, 984
Contact dermatitis, 991
Exfoliative dermatitis (ED), 992
Folliculitis, 986
Furuncle, 987
Impetigo, 986
Lichen planus (LP), 994
Necrotizing fasciitis (NF), 995
Pediculosis, 999
Rosacea, 1003
Scabies, 1000
Seborrheic dermatitis (SD), 992
Stevens-Johnson syndrome (SJS), 996
Tinea, 990
Tinea corporis, 990
Tinea cruris, 990
Tinea pedis, 990
Toxic epidermal necrolysis (TEN), 996
Urticaria, 993
Vesicles, 985

ABBREVIATIONS

ED—exfoliative dermatitis
LP—lichen planus
MRSA—methicillin-resistant *Staphylococcus aureus*
NF—necrotizing fasciitis
SD—seborrheic dermatitis
SJS—Stevens-Johnson syndrome
TEN—toxic epidermal necrolysis

40.1 Chapter Overview and Case Studies

Unlike chronic skin conditions and disorders that are usually long-term and relapsing, acute skin conditions are short-term and respond readily to treatment. In this chapter, acute skin conditions are the focus. Selected acute skin disorders included in this chapter may be caused by bacterial or fungal infections, contact with an offending organism, or contact with an allergen. Acute skin conditions associated with parasites and insects, medications, and disorders of the nail are also included. Acute skin conditions that may become chronic, depending on the individual and whether treatment is sought, include acne, cellulitis, exfoliated skin, furuncles, impetigo, nail fungus, nail loss, tick bites, tinea, and urticaria. In addition to infectious skin problems, life-threatening inflammatory disorders are discussed.

Concepts Related to Acute Skin Disorders

Most acute skin disorders are not serious, but a few can be life threatening. Many cause pain because the first layer of the skin has been damaged, injured, or punctured and nerve endings right under the first layer of skin are stimulated. If untreated, some skin disorders caused by infections can develop into more serious disorders.

The primary responsibility of the immune system and intact skin are to protect the body from microorganisms or antigens. When there is a break in the skin, impaired tissue integrity can lead to an immune response. Conversely, the immune response that occurs as a result of allergic reactions and inflammation can lead to lack of tissue integrity. For example, when an individual encounters an allergen, an allergic reaction may occur, which may result in contact dermatitis; the resulting discomfort may lead to scratching that leads to impaired skin integrity. When inflammation occurs as a result of an immune response, scars or abscesses may form. If healing is slow or impaired, these breaks in the skin can lead to infection.

Infection is the invasion of body tissue by microorganisms that have the potential to cause illness. Microorganisms grow on intact skin and can enter the body through many portals. Most microorganisms on the skin are harmless; however, if their growth is unchecked or if they enter the body through breaks in the skin, even normally harmless microorganisms can cause disease. These problems are further compounded if the immune system is compromised.

Patients with alterations in mobility may be at an increased risk for impaired skin integrity and subsequently an infection due to pressure injuries. Areas of the skin and bony protuberances that are subjected to prolonged pressure may cause the skin to break down and lessen skin integrity. Essentially, this pressure reduces blood flow to that area of skin, causing the skin to break open or die. The weight of the body pressing down on areas such as the buttocks, shoulders, and elbows of bedridden patients can lead to ulcerations.

Perfusion plays an important role in tissue integrity by delivering oxygen and nutrients to the organs and tissues of the body. When blood flow is decreased, interrupted, or not occurring at all, oxygen and nutrients cannot be supplied. If perfusion to organs or tissue is decreased for an extended period, irreversible damage or necrosis may occur. Specific disease processes such as diabetes mellitus and coronary artery disease can affect tissue perfusion. All patients should be routinely assessed for adequate tissue perfusion, and patients who have been identified as being at increased risk should be assessed more frequently.

Nutrition is needed to maintain tissue integrity. In addition, adequate nutrition is required for proper healing and recovery. Patients who are at risk for or have impaired tissue integrity should have their nutritional intake monitored, especially protein, to ensure that it is appropriate for their body's demands.

Alterations in tissue integrity can affect a patient's perception of self. This can be related to the patient's body image or functional ability caused by damage to an area from a wound. Concepts related to acute skin disorders are shown in **Figure 40.1** ■.

Case Studies

The following cases are addressed throughout the chapter to assist in application of chapter content to clinical situations that involve individuals with acute skin disorders.

Stacy May: Introduction

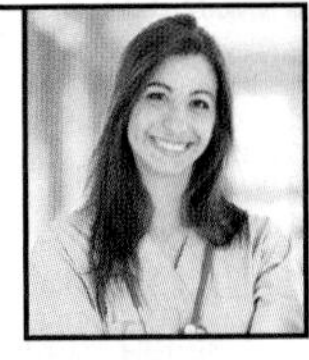

Stacy May, age 23, has just started her first job at a hospital, working 7 a.m. to 7 p.m. as a nursing assistant. On her first day, she worked with other assistants and learns where things are and the routine of the shift. She assisted with baths, toiletry, passing trays, and taking vital signs. On her second day, Ms. May has her own case load of three patients who require full care, including feeding, bathing, turning, and toileting. She follows the hospital's policy of wearing gloves as well as washing her hands or using hand sanitizer when she enters each patient's room. Around 1:00 p.m., Ms. May goes to her charge nurse and reports that her hands are burning. They appear red, and they itch intensely, though she does not have a rash. Ms. May is not aware of having any allergies, and this has never happened to her before.

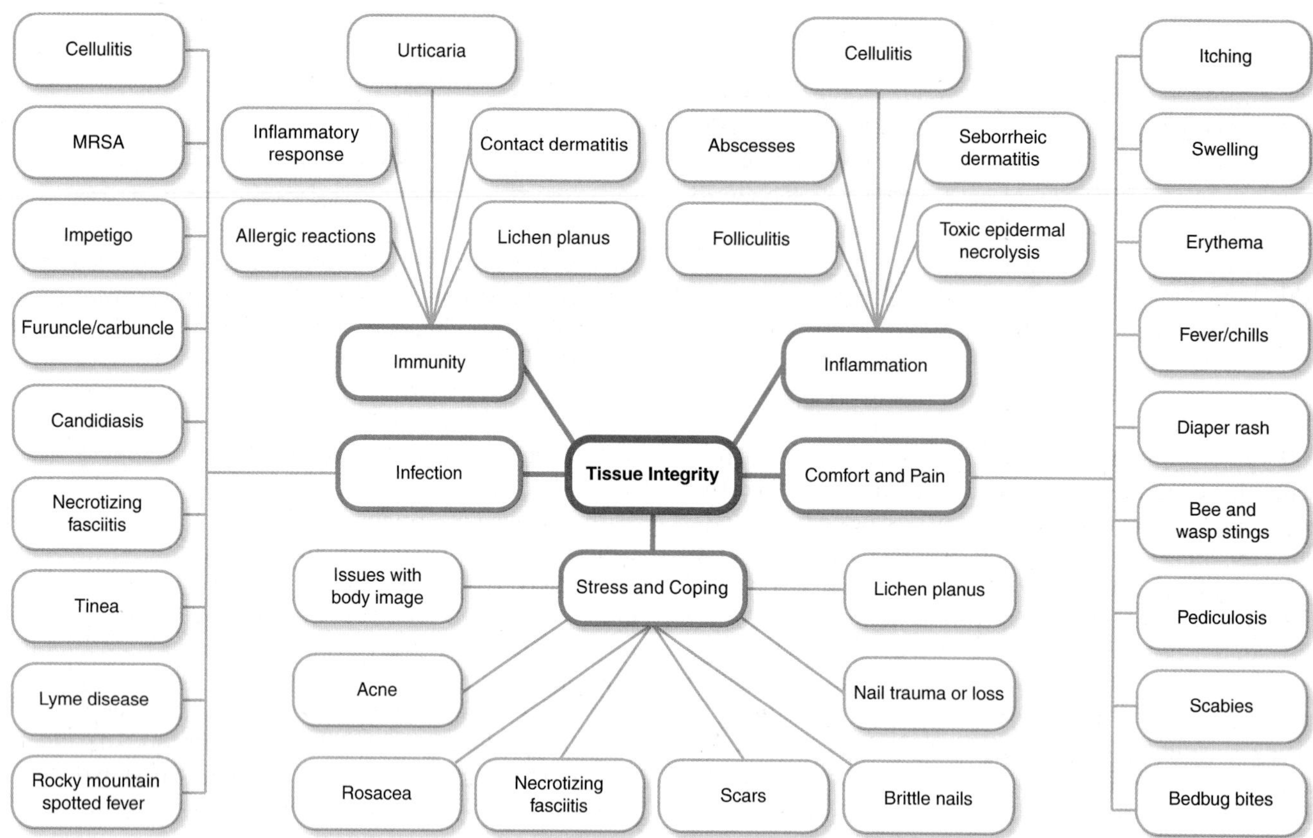

Figure 40.1 ■ Concepts related to acute skin disorders.

1. On the basis of Ms. May's recent occupational history, what new exposures may have precipitated the symptoms she is experiencing on her hands?
2. The symptoms don't appear until Ms. May's second day of work. Does this timeline support your initial thoughts about the reason for her skin reaction?

Marc McMann: Introduction

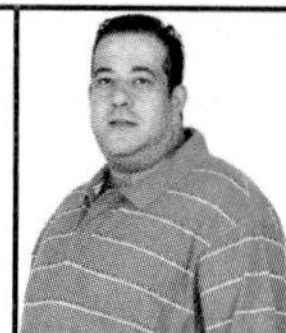

Marc McMann is a 32-year-old construction worker who weighs 350 pounds. He typically goes to another state for a month at a time to work and comes home for a month. While away, he stays in motels. He has been experiencing pain and discomfort in the groin area of his left leg and inner thigh. He has noticed that the area is swollen, the skin is red, and there is a foul odor from a discharge. He does not remember injuring his leg and does not know what is causing the severe pain. He does not want to go to the hospital until he returns home after working his month in another state. When he comes home, he immediately goes to the emergency department in immense pain that he rates a 10/10. The drainage is soaking through his clothing, and the left leg is twice the size of the right leg. The odor has increased and is foul smelling with a yellowish discharge. The skin appears irritated and is red, warm, and painful to touch. The healthcare provider orders a complete blood count (CBC), culture of the discharge, an IV, application of a dressing, an antibiotic, and diluaded. Mr. McMann is admitted to the hospital about 10:00 p.m., and his primary care provider is notified.

1. On the basis of the information given, is Mr. McMann at risk for a condition that might predispose him to skin infection?
2. In Mr. McMann's lifestyle, are there potential exposures that would contribute to bacterial skin infection?

Check Your Progress: Section 40.1

1. Why is impaired mobility associated with an increased risk of different types of skin breakdown?
2. List three acute skin disorders that may become chronic if not treated appropriately.
3. Why does protein nutritional deficiency create a risk for reduced skin integrity?

40.2 Bacterial Skin Infections

The most common organism that causes acute bacterial skin infections is *Staphylococcus aureus* (*S. aureus*). Although methicillin-resistant *Staphylococcus aureus* (MRSA) and *Streptococcus* (strep) can be causative agents, *S. aureus* is by far the most common. The focus of this section is on the most common acute bacterial skin infections, including those causing cellulitis, impetigo, folliculitis, furuncles, and carbuncles.

Cellulitis

Cellulitis is diffuse painful inflammation of the skin and subcutaneous layers. It is one of the most common skin infections. *S. aureus* is the cause of about 50–60% of the cases, 20% are isolated to MRSA, and 10% are both *S. aureus* and strep. The people who are most at risk for developing cellulitis include athletes, children, men who have sex with men, military recruits, prisoners, residents of long-term care facilities, intravenous drug users, and individuals who have had prior MRSA exposure. In addition, individuals who are immunosuppressed, who have chronic liver or kidney disease, or who sustain animal or human bites are at higher risk.[1] Cellulitis can involve part of the skin but most commonly involves the extremities. The inflammation can spread to other parts of the body, but it cannot spread to other individuals.[2]

CLINICAL POINT: Cellulitis is usually under the first layer of the skin but can become systemic if left untreated. Systemic cellulitis can be life threatening, involving the lymph nodes and contaminating the blood.[2] ■

Etiology and Pathogenesis

Cellulitis is most commonly caused as a result of a break in the skin from an injury such as a scrape, wound, puncture, or burn. Conditions such as athlete's foot can cause swelling and allow bacteria to enter. Other skin conditions may allow the organisms to enter the skin even when there is no injury.

Many bacteria can cause cellulitis. The most common are *Streptococcus* and *Staphylococcus* species. Most commonly today, the organism is MRSA. This strain is less resistant to common antibiotics used in the past. *Streptococcus* produces an enzyme that causes the inflammation to spread quickly through the skin. The enzyme hinders the ability of the inflammation to be confined. *Staphylococcus* appears more readily as open wounds and pus-filled pockets (abscesses).[3]

The body's own immune system will initiate the inflammatory response and may be responsible for some of the signs and symptoms as well as those caused by the bacteria. Heavy neutrophil infiltrate occurs with later stages showing lymphocytes and histiocytes. The spreading factor, a substance produced by the causative organism, breaks down the fibrin network and other barriers that normally keep the bacteria localized.[4]

In older adults, various factors increase the risk for cellulitis. Diminished skin perfusion from impaired circulation, impaired mobility, and diminished immune function create a situation in which a simple skin breakdown can develop into a serious infection. The primary concern with cellulitis among older adults is the use of antibiotics that may be hard on their systems, especially if they have renal or liver disease. Older adults may need additional help at home to care for the affected area. ■

Clinical Manifestations

Cellulitis manifests as a painful, red, swollen area of the skin that is hot and tender to touch. (**Figure 40.2** ■). Some individuals may run a fever and have chills. The symptoms are usually on only one side of the body. Various presenting lesions including **vesicles** (small sacs of fluid) and **bullae** (large blisters), and plaques may occur with *Staphylococcus* infections. Other, less common symptoms include tachycardia, hypotension, confusion, and headache. If the infection spreads, lymphadenitis (enlarged and tender lymph nodes) and lymphangitis (inflammation of a lymph node) may occur.

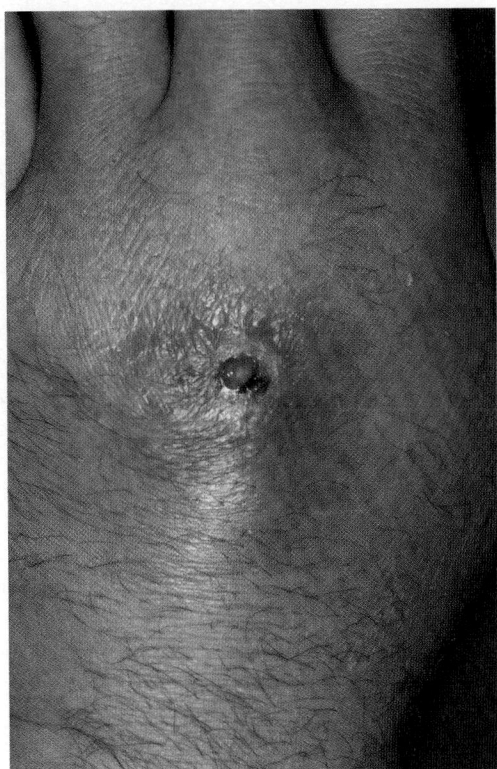

Figure 40.2 ■ Hand of a 52-year-old man with cellulitis and MRSA.

Linking Pathophysiology to Diagnosis and Treatment

Diagnosis of cellulitis is usually done by physical examination of presenting manifestations, although many other conditions have similar symptoms. A culture, complete blood count (CBC), sedimentation rate, and C-reactive protein may be ordered. These lab tests are not specific to cellulitis, but they may help the healthcare provider to rule out necrotizing fasciitis. Imaging studies are not diagnostic of cellulitis but may be used to rule out other serious conditions with similar symptoms.[1] Patients with more systemic symptoms such as fever, chills, and blisters may be hospitalized for treatment.

The goal of treatment for cellulitis is to manage and prevent the spread of the infection. The initial plan of treatment may be a topical antibiotic ointment or oral antibiotic medication. If the patient develops systemic symptoms or has open lesions, intravenous antibiotics may be prescribed. Multiple furuncles and carbuncles are treated with cloxacillin (a penicillinase-resistant penicillin) and the cephalosporins. For MRSA, antimicrobial treatment includes trimethoprim-sulfamethoxazole, minocycline, doxycycline, or clindamycin. Repeated infections may require mupirocin ointment. Pain medication is usually needed for those with severe cases. Low-dose opioids may be required if acetaminophen or nonsteroidal anti-inflammatory (NSAID) agents are not helpful. In the event of a fever, acetaminophen or ibuprofen can be used. Teaching should include good hand hygiene, cleaning open lesions, changing and discarding dressings, and identification of worsening infection. In addition, good nutrition, cleanliness at home, compliance with the medications and/or dressings and taking the full prescribed amount of the antibiotic should be emphasized.[4,5]

CLINICAL POINT: Because cellulitis is right under the skin where the nerve endings are, pain management should be a priority until the antibiotic decreases the infection. ■

Impetigo

Impetigo is an acute, highly contagious skin infection that is most common in children but can occur in adults. Impetigo is a common childhood skin condition when a wound or injury to the skin becomes infected. It is highly contagious and therefore spreads quickly. Impetigo is more common in hot, humid climates. There are two forms of impetigo: bullous and nonbullous. The nonbullous form is the most common in children, accounting for about 70% of the cases. Nonbullous impetigo is also known as impetigo contagiosa and is the most common skin condition in children. It accounts for 10% of cutaneous problems seen in healthcare offices and clinics. Bullous impetigo is more contagious than nonbullous impetigo. Common impetigo is usually a result of a wound or injury, or it can be a secondary skin condition from a preexisting injury, known as impetiginous dermatitis.[6]

CLINICAL POINT: The nurse should teach the patient's parents that impetigo is highly contagious. The child's contact with other children in the home or school or with playmates might need to be limited until the condition has resolved. ■

Etiology and Pathogenesis

Group A strep and *Staphylococcus aureus* (staph) are the usual bacteria that cause impetigo. Any break in the skin can lead to impetigo if not treated. A break in the skin may be from a cut, scrape, insect bite, or even microscopic scrapes that may not be visible.[6]

The bacteria enter the skin and create a blister filled with pus that will eventually burst and leave a crust. The bullous form causes larger blisters, and staph is the usual organism of infection. The nonbullous form causes smaller blisters. The organisms cannot colonize on intact skin. With a break in the skin, the organisms colonize, and colonization is facilitated by high temperature, humidity, preexisting skin disorders, young age, or recent antibiotic treatment. Common reasons for disruption of the skin that can allow impetigo to grow are scratching, infections (varicella, herpes simplex), infestations (scabies, pediculosis), thermal burns, surgery, trauma, puncture wounds, insect bites, cuts and even irritation from a runny nose.[6]

Transmission of the bacteria that cause impetigo is usually rapid and must be treated quickly. Transmission occurs by scratching, touching the infected area, or touching a surface that the infected area has touched. Bedsheets, towels, and clothing are common ways through which the infection can spread.

Clinical Manifestations

Typical manifestations of impetigo include red pimples, fluid-filled blisters, and an oozing rash with yellow crusts (**Figure 40.3** ■). These symptoms are most frequently on the face, around the mouth and nose, or on skin that is not covered by clothing. The infecting bacteria lives under the crust and in the blisters.

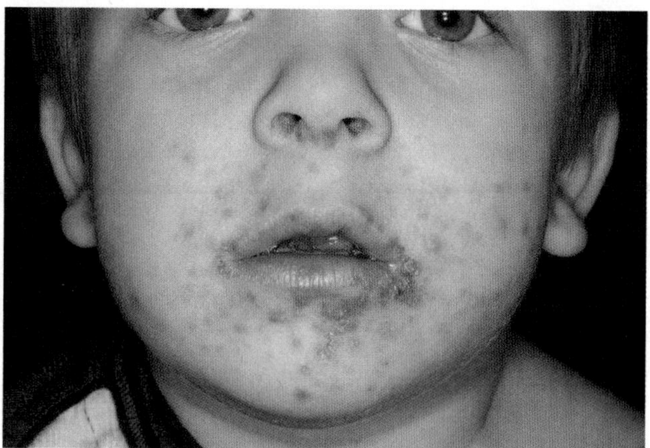

Figure 40.3 ■ A child with a rash from impetigo.

A common place for infants to have impetigo is around the diaper area. The rash, which may cause severe itching and be painful, can appear red and round. If it is severe, the child may have fever, feel weak, and experience pain and swelling.[7] ■

Linking Pathophysiology to Diagnosis and Treatment

Diagnosis of impetigo is usually done by physical examination along with signs and symptoms. If needed, a culture will be done to determine the causative organism or organisms. Topical over-the-counter (OTC) ointments are not usually effective. Prescription ointments such as mupirocin may be ordered to rub on the rash. An ointment may be the only treatment necessary for nonbullous impetigo. For more severe cases, oral forms of antibiotics are ordered; penicillin or cephalosporin is the usual antibiotic of choice. If the patient cannot take penicillin, then erythromycin, clarithromycin, or azithromycin may be ordered. If the impetigo is caused by MRSA, clindamycin or trimethoprim-sulfamethoxazole may be ordered.[6]

The patient's family should be taught that the infection is contagious and that precautions need to be taken. Good hand hygiene, use of antibacterial soap and water, and use of a separate washcloth and hand towel are necessary. Adults with impetigo should avoid shaving the area where the blisters are located. Airflow is needed for healing; therefore, loose dressings may be used. Sores should be covered until they are healed, and good hand hygiene should be used after the sores are dressed.

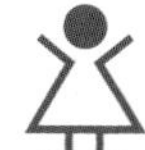

Children's fingernails should be kept trimmed, and children should be taught to avoid scratching.[7] ■

Folliculitis

Folliculitis is an inflammation of the hair follicle. This disorder is rarely reported, as it is seen in clinics and healthcare providers' offices or patients do not seek medical treatment for it. Epidemiology shows that folliculitis occurs more in males and affects all races and all ages. Folliculitis can be confined to the follicle of the hair (superficial folliculitis) or may extend deeper into the dermis surrounding the follicle of hair (deep folliculitis).[8] Conditions that make patients more prone to folliculitis are immunosuppressive disorders, diabetes mellitus, long-term use of antibiotics, being overweight, hot and humid temperatures, occlusive clothing or dressings, use of epidermal growth factor receptor (EGFR) inhibitors, and frequent shaving of heavy beards.[8] The type of folliculitis that occurs in association with EGFR receptor inhibitors shows acne eruption in 50–100% of the patients and depends on the dose prescribed. Folliculitis is seen more often in individuals who use hot tubs, whirlpool baths, and public swimming pools.[4]

There are several types of folliculitis. Pseudofolliculitis barbae occurs when beard hair curls and reenters the skin. There is no infection, but there may be inflammation. Hot tub folliculitis is seen in people who use hot tubs frequently. The area under a bathing suit is where the condition may manifest. Gram-negative folliculitis occurs as a result of long-term antibiotic use.[9] A stye is a folliculitis on the eyelid. Folliculitis, no matter the type, is usually not serious. It is seen in healthy people, is benign, and usually resolves on its own.

Etiology and Pathogenesis

Folliculitis can be caused by an infection from bacteria, a virus, fungi, or a parasite. It can also be noninfectious and be caused by trauma, inflammation, or damaged or blocked follicles. Two other causes of folliculitis are the EGFR receptor inhibitors and autoimmune diseases. The most common organism causing folliculitis is *S. aureus*.[9,10]

CLINICAL POINT: *Candida albicans* and *Pseudomonas aeruginosa* have been noted to cause folliculitis. A newer finding in folliculitis is the presence of MRSA.[11] ■

The infection begins at the follicle opening and follows the follicle downward. Enzymes are released by the bacteria along with chemical agents that cause an inflammation.[4] The bacteria can also enter through a small scrape or opening in the skin. Risk factors include crowded conditions, poor hygiene, nasal passages with *S. aureus*, and chronic skin conditions.[9] Infected hairs easily fall out or are removed. Complications include permanent hair loss, plaques (large, itchy patches of skin), recurring skin infections, scarring or dark spots, and furuncles.[11]

Clinical Manifestations

Signs and symptoms of folliculitis include pruritus, burning, or mild discomfort. Multiple small papules and pustules present with a red base that has a single hair follicle through the center (**Figure 40.4** ■). The hair may or may not be visible. Each looks like a tiny red or white-headed pimple and may be single or many. They itch and may be slightly painful. Each affected hair follicle swells into pus-filled pimples. As these pimples break open, they will crust over. Follicles on the scalp, face, chest, back, buttocks, and legs can be involved. A small swollen lump or mass can even occur.[9,11]

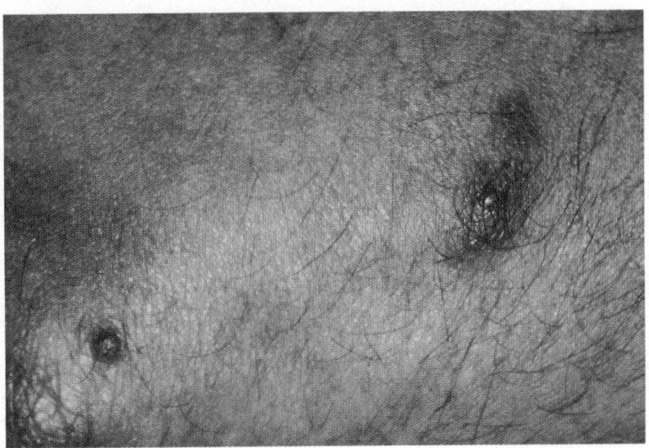

Figure 40.4 ■ Folliculitis.

Linking Pathophysiology to Diagnosis and Treatment

The healthcare provider will assess the signs and symptoms of folliculitis. There are usually no diagnostic tests performed. Rarely, a culture will be done to determine the causative organism if the condition does not improve. Most cases require no treatment, resolving in 7–10 days. If treatment is needed, it will consist of treating the infection or fungus and reducing the inflammation. Oral antibiotics are usually not prescribed unless the condition is severe. An antibiotic cream such as mupirocin or fusidic acid is used to treat the bacterial infection. Corticosteroid creams and occasionally oral corticosteroids may be ordered. OTC benzoyl peroxide may also be recommended along with good hygiene with an antibacterial soap. Other recommendations may be hot, moist compresses or a moisturizer (emollient) to soothe the skin. Hot tub folliculitis usually heals on its own. Measures for proper chlorination should be taken to prevent further infection in the water.[9-11] Laser hair removal or light therapy with a medicated cream has been used for individuals whose folliculitis does not respond to conventional treatment or does not improve.[11,12]

Furuncles and Carbuncles

A **furuncle** is an extension of folliculitis and is usually referred to as a boil. **Carbuncles** are a cluster of infected hair follicles. Patients with either of these conditions may be seen by their primary care provider for treatment or hospitalized if their condition is severe. Furuncles and carbuncles are more common in teens and young adults, although children and older adults have been seen in the emergency department. An active furuncle or carbuncle is contagious because *S. aureus* is the primary cause. When a person has more than one carbuncle, it is called carbunculosis; more than one furuncle is furunculosis.[13]

Etiology and Pathogenesis

The primary causative agent for furuncles and carbuncles is *S. aureus*, although MRSA has been cultured. The body's immune system triggers an inflammatory reaction in the underlying and surrounding connective tissue to the organism. Risk factors include obesity, immunosuppressive conditions, poor hygiene, *S. aureus* nasal congestion, carriers of MRSA, close contact with other people who have these conditions, crowded conditions, trauma to the skin, areas of excessive moisture or perspiration, hot and humid climates, and possibly diabetes or kidney diseases. Long-term steroid use can depress the natural immune system and make an individual more susceptible. In addition, malnutrition, drug addiction, and living in a college dorm or any situation in which towels and washcloths are shared create the means of acquiring or spreading the organism.[4,13,14]

A furuncle starts as folliculitis or infection of a sebaceous gland, and the infection spreads down the hair shaft through the wall of the follicle and into the dermis. It is usually a deep nodule surrounding a hair follicle that turns into a cyst within days. The cyst is filled with sanguineous pus and may abscess, leading to necrosis.[4] They are common on the neck, breasts, armpits, face, buttocks, and areas exposed to friction. They are uncomfortable and may be painful when closely attached to underlying structures (e.g., on the nose, ear, or finger).[13]

A carbuncle is a cluster of furuncles that forms a firm mass involving the deeper tissues with multiple openings to the skin surface, essentially a cluster of boils. The cluster coalesces to form one large lesion that drains through multiple tracts and involves the subcutaneous tissue and the lower dermis.[4] These masses filled with pus, dead tissue, and fluid must drain before healing can occur. Sometimes the mass is too deep to drain on its own. A sterile abscess can turn into a hard, solid lesion as it scars. Carbuncles are found most frequently on the back of the neck, upper back, and inner thighs.[4,13,14]

Both furuncles and carbuncles are highly contagious because of the causative organism and the ease of spread when they are draining. Outbreaks may occur in families when one member has the infection and it spreads to other family members by direct contact.[14]

Clinical Manifestations

The symptoms of furuncles and carbuncles are similar. The area is firm, red, and painful (**Figure 40.5** ■). The mass of a carbuncle is swollen and extremely painful. Purulent drainage is seen in both conditions. The healthcare provider might have to open the area to allow the copious amount of drainage to flow and the pain to ease. The furuncle may be firm or fluctuant, the carbuncle will be firm, and both will be tender. The size of the mass may as small as a pea or as large as a golf ball. The tips of the mass may be white or yellow with an erythematous base that will crust when draining. Individuals with carbuncles may generally feel unwell, experience malaise, and run a fever. Pruritus may occur in a carbuncle before it starts to drain.[4,13,14] Complications include scarring, MRSA, sepsis, cellulitis, gas-containing abscesses, and necrotizing fasciitis.[14]

Linking Pathophysiology to Diagnosis and Treatment

Diagnosis of furuncles and carbuncles is usually done by physical examination and a culture to determine the organism in order to prescribe the correct antibiotic. Treatment involves moist heat, usually oral antibiotics, and incision of the lesion once the point comes to a head. The head of the furuncle may open and drain spontaneously, but antibiotic treatment is still recommended. carbuncles usually require an incision by a healthcare provider. Proper dressing after the incision has drained is required. If the carbuncle is deep, packing with iodoform gauze in the area is necessary. If the carbuncle is extremely deep, the healthcare provider may recommend intravenous antibiotics. Antibiotics used include first-generation cephalosporins, flucloxacillin, erythromycin (or clarithromycin if penicillin is contraindicated), and clindamycin.[13,14] Acetaminophen or ibuprofen may be used if fever is present or for pain. If pain is severe, a low-dose opioid may be prescribed. Universal precautions should be taken in dealing with the area and in disposal of the dressings. All equipment should be disinfected.

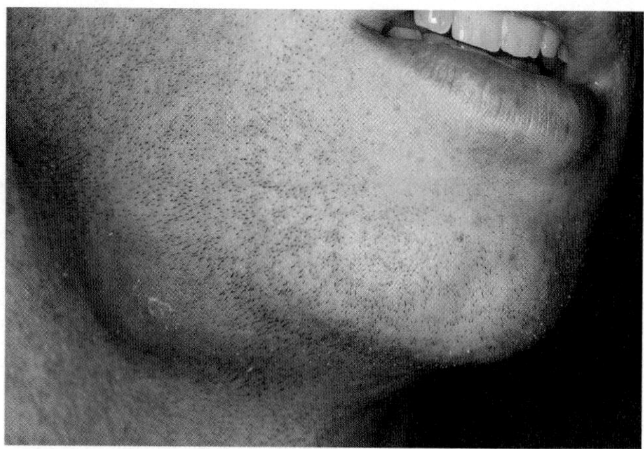

Figure 40.5 ■ A red and painful furuncle caused by *S. aureus* or MRSA.

Teaching the patient and family should include how to clean and redress the area and destroy the old dressing material, the importance of avoiding contact with the drainage, good hand hygiene with antibacterial soap, and how to disinfect linens and clothing with very hot water. Squeezing and pinching the pimple area should be avoided. Most of these masses will heal within 2–3 weeks.[14]

Mothers of infants or toddlers who develop a boil on their buttocks while in diapers may find it hard to contain the infection. It can be difficult to get toddlers to avoid scratching and rubbing the painful area Secure dressings along with good hygiene for the child and mother are necessary. ■

Check Your Progress: Section 40.2

1. Why is pain control a priority in management of cellulitis?
2. What structure of the eye is involved in the development of a stye?
3. How is furunculosis different from folliculitis?

40.3 Fungal Skin Infections

The common causes of most acute fungal skin infections are *Candida albicans* and yeast. Fungal infections are usually not serious and can be treated by using OTC or prescription medications. Many of these disorders are highly contagious, and proper hygiene should be taught. The focus for this section will be the most common acute fungal skin infections, including candidiasis and tinea.

Candidiasis

Candidiasis is an infection of the skin or mucous membranes with any species of *Candida*. There are over 20 *Candida* species that can cause infections in the human, but *Candida albicans* is the most common. *Candida albicans* is a yeast-like fungus that most often causes superficial cutaneous infections. Candidiasis can occur in the mouth, throat, lungs, vagina, folds of the skin, or bowel. It can invade the bloodstream or be passed on to a fetus in the birth canal. Candidiasis is usually a secondary infection.

CLINICAL POINT: A new form of Candida, *Candida aureus*, has been cultured in hospitalized patients and is unresponsive to antifungals. The Centers for Disease Control and Prevention (CDC) has issued warnings to healthcare personnel about this new form of *Candida* that has been reported in the United States and nine other countries.[15] ■

Etiology and Pathogenesis

Candida is part of the normal flora of the skin and mucous membranes. In certain circumstances, as when there are warmth, moisture, and breaks in the epidermis, an infection may start. Because candidiasis can occur in many places of the body, many names are associated with this fungal infection:

- Infection of the oral cavity is called *thrush*.
- In the vagina, it is called *vulvovaginitis* or *yeast infection*.
- In the diaper area, it is called a *diaper rash*.
- In the glans and prepuce of penis, it is called *balanitis*.
- In the nail folds, it is called *paronychia*.
- In the bloodstream, it is called *invasive candidiasis*.
- In the ear, it is called *swimmer's ear*.

In addition, the scalp, axillae, umbilical area, area under the breasts, and perineal area can be involved. Once *Candida* has infiltrated the skin, it is an opportunistic pathogen, and multiplication is rapid. Candidiasis is more prevalent and serious than it has been in the past. Most healthcare providers will see at least one person who has candidiasis some place on the body on a daily basis. About 70% of women will get a vaginal yeast infection at some point in their life. and 90% of HIV/AIDS patients will develop candidiasis.[15]

Although usually associated with humans, *Candida* has been found on food, countertops, ventilators, air-conditioning vents, floors, and medical personnel in the hospital setting. Areas of highest concern in the hospital are intensive care units (adult, neonatal, and pediatric) as well as medical and surgical units.[16]

CLINICAL POINT: Candidiasis is one of the most common healthcare-associated infections. Good hand hygiene with soap and water is recommended rather than just using hand sanitizer. ■

Candidiasis is normally not life threatening, but it can become so if the organism gains access to the bloodstream. If candidiasis becomes life threatening, 45% of patients will die. This is especially true for individuals who are immunosuppressed, have neutropenia, are taking certain antibiotics, or are being treated for cancer. Other risk factors include poor hygiene, extensive antibiotic or corticosteroid use, chemotherapy drugs, surgery, poorly cleaned dentures, obesity, low birth weight infants, burns, prolonged hospitalization, invasive procedures (intravenous lines, Foley catheters, chest ports, etc.), mechanical ventilation, and organ transplants.[16,17]

Clinical Manifestations

Symptoms of candidiasis are site specific. Thrush causes a white covering of the tongue and may include the buccal area and roof of the mouth and may proceed into the throat (**Figure 40.6** ■). Complaints of a sore throat and cracking of the corners of the mouth may also be seen with thrush. Vaginal yeast infection causes excessive itching; a foul odor; and a thick, white vaginal discharge. In balanitis, flattened pustules, edema, burning, and tenderness of the penis are common. Diaper rash manifests as dark red patches in the folds of the skin and yellow, fluid-filled spots that can break open and become flaky are seen. Once the infection has become invasive, fever and chills may manifest.[16,17]

CLINICAL POINT: Individuals who are taking strong or long-term antibiotics or who have an immunosuppressive condition are more likely to develop thrush. Checking the mouth using a penlight is essential. If the nurse suspects thrush but is not sure, use of a tongue blade is recommended. If the white material on the tongue cannot be scraped off with a tongue blade, it is usually thrush. ■

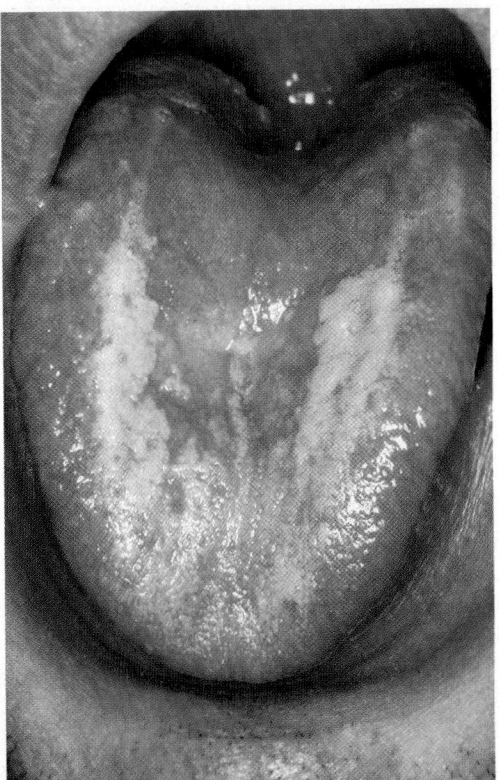

Figure 40.6 ■ Candidiasis (oral thrush) in an adult.

Linking Pathophysiology to Diagnosis and Treatment

Diagnosis of candidiasis is usually made through physical examination. A skin scraping may be taken and examined for the presence of *Candida*. For invasive candidiasis, blood cultures may be ordered. Antifungal drugs in the forms of creams, shampoos, vaginal suppositories, and oral tablets are usually recommended regardless of the location of the candidiasis. For thrush, nystatin is often the drug of choice, used as a swish and swallow or swish and spit. Other antifungals include miconazole for vaginal infections; undecylenic acid for diaper rash; and ketoconazole, fluconazole, and amphotericin B for invasive candidiasis. Most treatments last from 2–3 days to 2 weeks. Complementary therapies include probiotics, yogurt, honey, and vitamins E, C, and B complex. Herbal products such as tea tree oils, Echinacea, pomegranate, and garlic are time-honored treatments but should be used with the consultation of a healthcare provider. Herbal products can depress the immune system if used for an extended period of time or too often.[18]

Bottle-fed infants may get candidiasis if the nipples, bottles, and pacifiers have not been sterilized. OTC sterilizers are available, or the bottles can be boiled in hot water for about 10 minutes. Breastfed infants can also contract thrush and then pass it to their mother, so both mother and baby should be treated. ■

Older adults who use disposable briefs are highly prone to candidiasis, especially if the garments are not changed as often as they should be. Severe cases of candidiasis from the moisture of disposable briefs may benefit from leaving the brief open on top of a waterproof pad. Also, providing privacy but exposing the area to air can prove beneficial. Dentures that are not properly cleaned and soaked can be another root of candidiasis in older adults. ■

Tinea

Tinea is a contagious infection by different types of fungus that can occur on any part of the body and are named by location. These infections are superficial and called dermatophytoses. Tinea is also known as ringworm because it sometimes takes on a circular pattern that resembles a worm chasing its tail; however, worms are not involved in any of these infections. The most common forms are the following:

- Tinea capitis, found on the scalp (most common in children)
- Tinea faciei, found on the face
- **Tinea corporis,** found on the trunk and extremities
- **Tinea cruris,** found in the groin (jock itch)
- Tinea manuum, found on the hands
- **Tinea pedis,** found on the feet (athlete's foot)
- Tinea unguium, or onychomycosis, found on the nails
- Tinea versicolor, found on many parts of the body, often on the back, caused by yeast (a type of fungus). This type is more common in teens and young adults and is the only form that is not contagious.[4,19,20]

Etiology and Pathogenesis

Tinea infections are highly contagious and are spread by direct contact, most often when an individual touches another person who is infected. Warm, damp environments are the ideal habitat for the fungus to grow. It can spread on moist surfaces, such as floors of locker rooms and public showers, and through pets. Sweating, weak immune system, oily skin or hair, and shared clothing, linen, towels, or hairbrushes can facilitate the spread of the fungus. The incubation period for tinea is not well known.[19,20]

There are a variety of organisms that cause the different tinea diseases. *Trichophyton rubrum, T. tonsurans,* and *Microsporum canis* are the most common dermatophytes, in that order. These dermatophytes infect the superficial layers of the skin, and there is a 1- to 3-week incubation period, after which the dermatophytes invade peripherally. Cell-mediated immunity usually eliminates dermatophytes. Tinea infections are common in all age groups.[19,20]

Clinical Manifestations

Tinea corporis begins as a scaly plaque with erythema that may worsen rapidly. Crust, papules, vesicles and bullae may develop also. With tinea corporis, the same symptoms appear, but as new patches emerge, the center of the older patches will clear up. Slight itching, dry and brittle hair, and bald patches will be seen in tinea capitis. In tinea pedis, the skin becomes soft, white and peels away, especially between the toes; itching, unpleasant odor and blistering may also occur (**Figure 40.7** ■). This may be in both feet or just one. In tinea versicolor, the skin produces yellow or fawn-colored patches. The acidic bleach from the yeast causes the change in color of the skin. Most tinea infections have a 70–100% cure rate.[21]

Linking Pathophysiology to Diagnosis and Treatment

Diagnosis of tinea infection may be done in several different ways, including potassium hydroxide (KOH) examination of skin scrapings, fungal culture, polymerase chain reaction assay, skin biopsy, or use of a blue-green fluorescence during a Wood light examination. In some cases, just a physical examination is needed to determine the type of infection.[19-21]

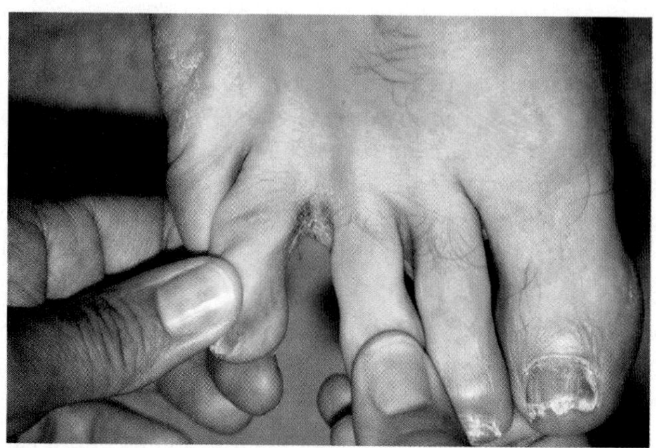

Figure 40.7 ■ Tinea pedis (athlete's foot) in an adult.

Treatment of tinea infection can involve OTC medications or prescription medications that are usually more costly. OTC creams such as Lamisil-AT and Micatin AF are useful for tinea pedis, tinea cruris, and tinea corporis. Stronger oral prescriptions that may work faster and are administered less often include griseofulvin, terbinafine, itraconazole, and fluconazole. Occasionally, selenium sulfide shampoo for tinea capitis, and corticosteroids (prednisone) may be recommended.[19-21]

Check Your Progress Section 40.3

1. In what circumstances does *Candida*, part of the normal flora of the skin, become problematic?
2. What types of diagnostic testing are done to confirm fungal infections of the skin?
3. Sometimes people refer to tinea infections as ringworm. What is the name of the worm that causes the infection?

40.4 Dermatitis

Dermatitis is an inflammation of the skin that may be from an irritant, systemic disease, or hypersusceptability. Dermatitis can be acute or chronic. Urticaria and lichen planus are skin disorders that are often caused by an autoimmune response. The most classic symptoms of most of skin inflammation are erythema, lesions, and itchy skin. The focus of this section is on contact dermatitis, seborrheic dermatitis, exfoliative dermatitis, urticaria, and lichen planus.

Contact Dermatitis

Contact dermatitis is inflammation and irritation of the skin caused by contact with an irritant or allergen. The irritant may be plants (poison ivy, poison oak, or poison sumac), drugs, corrosives, acids, alkalis, latex, soaps, perfumes, deodorants, materials (tape, elastic, latex), or innocuous compounds (hair dye, metals, rubber, cosmetics). In addition, flowers, herbs, fruits, and vegetables may cause contact dermatitis. Some individuals have hypersensitivity to many agents and materials that can cause contact dermatitis. Contact dermatitis is usually easily remedied, but recurrent exposure or the lack of identifying the cause can cause relapsing dermatitis. How bad the dermatitis can be may depend on the allergen or the dose of an irritant.[22]

Etiology and Pathogenesis

Irritant contact dermatitis accounts for 80% of all cases.[23] Allergic contact dermatitis is the result of an immune response to a subsequent exposure. Upon the first exposure, no symptoms are experienced. The second exposure triggers the immune reaction and is due to a cellular-mediated response by T lymphocytes. The lymphocytes enable the body to recognize allergens. The initial response is a release of IgE, which releases histamine, serotonin, and heparin. This release is the usual cause of the symptoms experienced and occurs in 24–48 hours unless it is a type I reaction such as anaphylactic shock. With irritant contact dermatitis, no allergen is needed. Contact with an irritant on first exposure can damage or irritate the skin. Typically, contact dermatitis, regardless of cause, is a type IV hypersensitivity reaction. The latest concern in healthcare is allergy to latex, which can cause a contact dermatitis. It is estimated that 8–12% of healthcare workers are allergic to latex (**Figure 40.8** ■).[24]

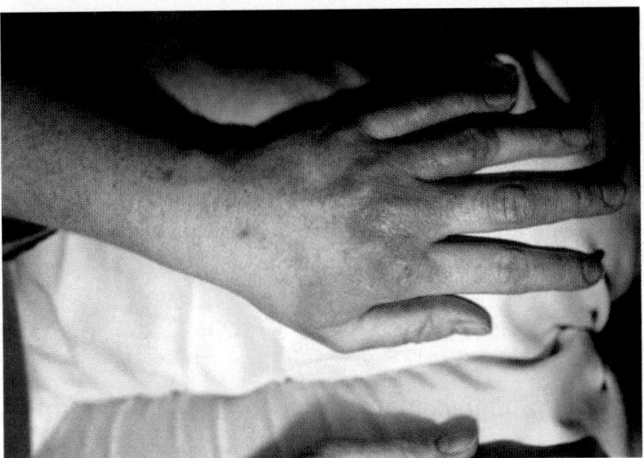

Figure 40.8 ■ Latex allergy (contact dermatitis) from gloves. Nurses are cautioned to be alert for this allergy.

Clinical Manifestations

Symptoms of contact dermatitis vary from hyperemia, itching, and various skin lesions to gangrene and sloughing. Eruptions in the skin become vesicular or pustular and may burn as well as itch. With allergic contact dermatitis, a rash or bumps do not appear for 1–2 days after exposure. In irritant contact dermatitis, a red rash appears immediately, and the skin may be more painful than itchy. The skin may produce vesicles that can weep or hives, which are itchy welts. Some reactions take up to 4 weeks to resolve. Frequent or constant scratching can cause breaks in the skin and edema. The inflammation can range from erythema to blistering and ulceration. The most common of all the symptoms is pruritus. The hands and legs are the most common part of the body affected, but any part of the body can be affected.[22-24]

CLINICAL POINT: Unfortunately, sometimes the initial reaction is so severe as to cause anaphylaxis, in which case the symptoms are system-wide (respiratory, cardiovascular, gastrointestinal), immediate, and may be life-threatening. Symptoms include vomiting, shortness of breath, drop in blood pressure, elevated heart rate, and airway edema. If these physical reactions are severe, the combination may be life threatening and require immediate medical care to support respiratory and cardiovascular function. Thus for any suspected allergic condition, an assessment should be made to rule out anaphylaxis. ■

Stacy May: Application

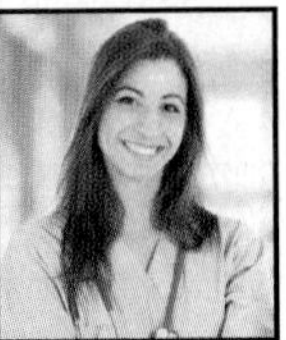

Ms. May is sent to the emergency department to be examined. Her vital signs are all within normal limits. She is not having any shortness of breath or palpitations, she swallows well, and no swelling is noted except on her hands. While in the emergency department, she begins to show slight signs of a rash on both hands. The healthcare provider orders blood work and gives Ms. May an antihistamine and intravenous corticosteroid. Her lab results show elevated IgE, and she is diagnosed with contact dermatitis. The healthcare provider suspects that Ms. May is allergic to latex and refers her to an allergist to have testing done for allergies.

3. Why is Ms. May tested for IgE elevation as part of her emergency department evaluation?
4. Why does the emergency department provider assess Ms. May for changes in vital signs as well as respiratory symptoms and airway edema?

Linking Pathophysiology to Diagnosis and Treatment

A full examination and history may be needed to distinguish allergic contact dermatitis from irritant contact dermatitis. When home agents are suspected, the "use" test may be done. A small amount of a household agent is applied to the skin far from the original area affected. Patch testing may require direct application of chemicals to the skin using special occlusive dressings for 48–72 hours. The patch test is usually given by an allergy specialist to try to reproduce the eruption. A skin biopsy is usually the last resort. Treatment should be sought if the symptoms do not go away, symptoms worsen, or the rash becomes more widespread or affects the face or genitals. If signs of infection occur, a visit to a healthcare provider is definitely needed.[22-24]

An essential part of treatment for contact dermatitis is to determine the cause and avoid it. Home remedies and OTC medications may work. Steroid creams, anti-itch ointments, diphenhydramine cream or oral pill, and calamine lotions may help with some of the symptoms. Other options are applying cool, moist cloths; soaking in lukewarm water with a baking soda or oatmeal bath product; trimming nails to avoid scratching; and covering the area with a bandage to avoid scratching. Herbal remedies include witch hazel cream and St. John's wort. If these do not work, the patient should see a healthcare provider. The healthcare provider may order systemic corticosteroids for 2 weeks, topical immunomodulators, medicated shampoo, topical calcineurin inhibitors such as pimecrolimus and tacrolimus, and antibiotics if an infection occurs. Teaching should include good hand hygiene, avoiding dry, cracked skin from harsh soap. Emollients to avoid dryness are also recommended if frequent hand washing is required where the patient works.[22-24]

Stacy May: Outcome

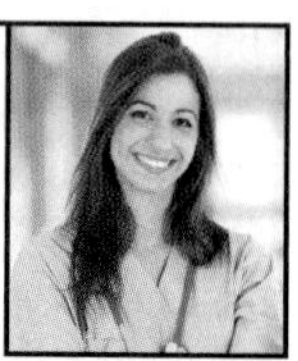

Ms. May is sent home from the emergency department with instructions to take diphenhydramine and is given a prescription for a 5-day steroid pack. She stays home from work for 2 days, after which her hands are no longer red, itching, or swollen. She visits an allergist and has testing done. Ms. May shows a severe reaction to latex and is informed that she should avoid using any products with latex. A list of products with latex are given to her, and she is prescribed an epinephrine autoinjector to carry with her at all times. She notifies her supervisor at work and asks whether she will be able to return to work. Ms. May's supervisor informs her that latex-free gloves and products will be provided for her.

5. Why is it important for Ms. May to carry an epinephrine autoinjector with her at all times?
6. At this time, what important patient education should Ms. May receive from the healthcare provider?

Seborrheic and Exfoliative Dermatitis

Seborrheic dermatitis (SD) is a chronic skin inflammation with exacerbations and remissions. It typically involves the scalp, eyebrows, eyelids, ear canals, nasolabial folds, axillae, or trunk. It is called cradle cap in infants, dandruff in adults, and seborrheic eczema and seborrheic psoriasis (**Figure 40.9** ■). **Exfoliative dermatitis (ED)** is a widespread skin inflammation that is caused by preexisting skin disorders, drugs, cancer, or unknown causes.[4,25,26]

Etiology and Pathogenesis

Seborrheic dermatitis is a papulosquamous disorder on the sebum glands of the body. In addition to sebum, SD has been linked to immunologic abnormalities involving *Malassezia* (a group of yeasts). SD ranges from mild dandruff to exfoliative erythroderma. Worldwide, there is a prevalence of SD in 3–5% of the population, with dandruff estimated to occur in 15–20% of the population.[25] SD is commonly aggravated by changes in humidity, seasons, trauma such as scratching, or stress. It may worsen in those with Parkinson disease or AIDS. Normal levels of *Malassezia* cause an abnormal immune response. Helper T cells and antibody titers are decreased. The *Malassezia* may activate the alternative complement pathway.

Exfoliative dermatitis is widespread erythema and scaling of the skin and affects at least 90% of the body surface area. Approximately 25% of patients with ED have no identifiable underlying cause. Bacterial superinfections can complicate ED. The pathogenesis varies with the underlying disorder, but common to all conditions is an increased rate of skin turnover. The decreased transit time for the

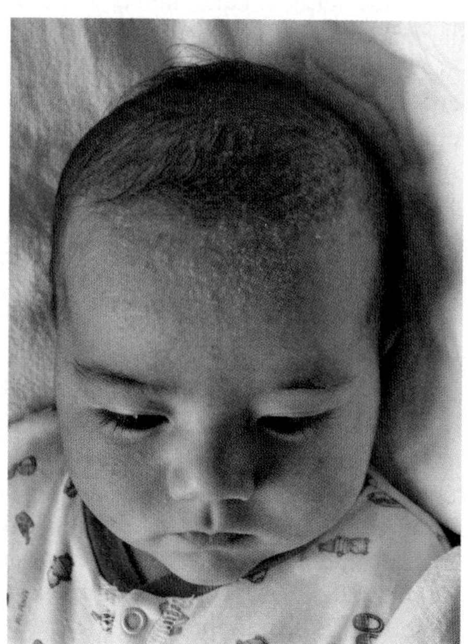

Figure 40.9 ■ Seborrheic dermatitis (cradle cap) in an infant.

epidermis results in impaired skin barrier protection and damaged skin. Since the skin barrier function is already impaired, the other pathogenesis is increased blood flow, which causes insensible fluid loss. ED occurs in all races and is more common in males, with an average age at onset of 52–60 years.[26] Complications of the generalized form include debilitation, dehydration, and secondary infection.

CLINICAL POINT: The increased rate at which normal epidermis is turned over increases in ED. Therefore, the exfoliated scales contain material that the skin normally retains (proteins, amino acids, and nucleic acids), and the result may be a negative nitrogen balance. The insensible fluid loss along with the nitrogen level should be monitored. ■

Clinical Manifestations

Seborrheic dermatitis is characterized by rounded, irregular or circular lesions covered with yellow or brown-gray greasy scales that may flake off. Itching is common, especially of the scalp. Most of the scales and skin will have a greasy appearance.[4,25,26]

Exfoliative dermatitis is erythematous and scaly. The erythema will be in patches but later spreads and involves all or nearly all of the body. Other symptoms include pruritus, malaise, and chills. The skin will slough, and widespread sloughing leads to abnormal thermoregulation, nutritional deficiencies, increased metabolic rate, and hypovolemia. The sloughing of exfoliated (peeling) skin can lead to debilitation, dehydration, and secondary infection. Local effects include loss of hair and nails. Systemic effects include lymphadenopathy, hepatomegaly, eosinophilia, and depression because of cosmetic changes.[4,25,26]

Linking Pathophysiology to Diagnosis and Treatment

In SD, the diagnosis is usually made based on the intermittent and recurring severity and by the distribution of involvement on examination. A skin biopsy and fungal culture to rule out other similar conditions may be needed. For ED, the diagnosis usually requires a referral to a dermatologist and a skin biopsy.[25,26] For SD, topical corticosteroids are discouraged except for acute flares because they can cause a rebound effect. The involvement of the skin responds to ketoconazole, naftifine, or ciclopirox creams and gels. Calcineurin inhibitors, sulfur or sulfonamide combinations, or propylene glycol are alternatives. Combination therapy is often indicated. Dandruff shampoos containing salicylic acid, selenium, sulfur, or zinc are effective when the scalp is involved. For ED, most patients require hospitalization to treat dehydration, urticaria, fever, and insensible fluid losses. Previous medications should be discontinued until the cause has been determined and a dermatologist has been consulted. Intravenous therapy, antibiotic administration, bland emollients for fluid losses, systemic or topical corticosteroid therapy or immunosuppressants, and antihistamines for pruritus may be ordered. Nonadherent dressings are used to control the weeping to decrease damage to newly formed skin.[25,26]

Urticaria

Urticaria, also known as hives, is welts on the skin that often itch (**Figure 40.10** ■). Hives vary in size and may join together to form one large welt on any part of the body. Acute hives may appear and go away within 24 hours or last for less than 6 weeks. Chronic hives last more than 6 weeks. Hives that occur deep under the skin are known as angioedema, acute episodes that often involve the lips, eyes, and face.[27]

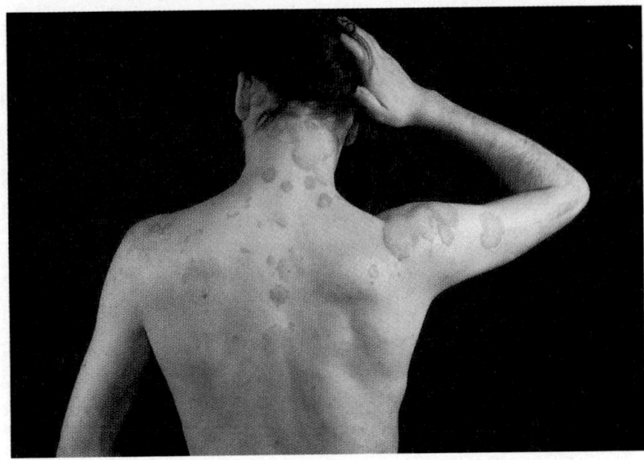

Figure 40.10 ■ Urticaria (hives) on the back on an individual with many welts, some of which are joined together.

Etiology and Pathogenesis

Hives will occur at least once in a lifetime in 10–20% of the population and are more common in women than men. A specific etiology can be identified in about 50% of acute urticaria. Acute urticaria is more common (70%) than chronic urticaria. Causes of urticaria can be numerous, including reactions to drugs, contact with allergens (e.g., dust mite feces), ingesting or inhaling allergens, exposure to water (aquagenic), emotional stimuli (anxiety, stress), physical stimuli (cold, exercise, heat, sunlight, pressure), infections (all types), insect bites, transfusion reactions, and some medical conditions. Acute urticaria occurs more commonly in children and young adults. Hives can occur within minutes or may be delayed for up to 2 hours.[28]

The immunoglobulin E (IgE) initiates a release of histamine, bradykinin, leukotrienes, and prostaglandins from a mast cell in the skin. These vasoactive substances cause extravasation of plasma into the dermis of the skin, leading to the characteristic raised lesion. The activation of the histamine receptors leads to itching and increased capillary permeability, which can lead to swelling. A type I, II, or III reaction can result in hives. Occasionally, the cause is unknown, as an allergy can develop without warning to a previously encountered allergen.[29]

Clinical Manifestations

Urticaria appears as a vascular reaction of the skin and is characterized by a sudden eruption of pale wheals or papules that cause severe itching. Some individuals have burning or stinging. The wheals will appear, then disappear, and move around. The swellings are well demarcated and vary in size. The skin is not broken, and there is no scarring or trace of the wheal once it disappears.[27-29] Any signs of stridor, wheezing, or other respiratory problems or angioedema (swelling of the face, lips or tongue) are concerning, and medical treatment should be sought.

Linking Pathophysiology to Diagnosis and Treatment

Urticaria usually goes away on its own, and no testing is needed. If urticaria recurs, an IgE level and eosinophil count may be ordered, especially if the cause is thought to be an allergen. Scratch or intradermal tests for allergy testing by a dermatologist may be recommended. A skin biopsy may be done if the hives last longer than normal or the cause is unknown. Treatment usually begins with trying to determine the cause and avoiding it so that further episodes do not occur. If needed, OTC treatment is usually effective. Treatment may include antihistamines, calamine lotion or cortisone creams for itching, and topical emollients and aluminum acetate for drying of the skin. Wet dressings and oatmeal baths may aid in easing the discomfort. Newer antihistamines such as certirizine, fexofenadine, desloratadine, and levocetirizine allow fewer doses per day and are nonsedating. Antihistamines such as diphenhydramine, hydroxyzine, or doxepin may be more useful at night because of their sedating side effect. If an oral steroid is needed, a short-term dose pack is recommended.[27-29]

Lichen Planus

Lichen planus (LP) is an inflammatory disorder of the skin, mouth, nails, scalp, and mucous membranes. It can also affect the external genitals. It is not contagious and may occur in people of any age, race, or culture. It most often affects middle-aged adults and affects men and women equally, though women are more susceptible to the oral form. The condition can disfigure the fingernails and toenails. It is usually easy to cure and not serious, although rarely, it may be more painful and more serious than usual. One in five individuals will have another breakout, and LP can intermittently occur over the years.[30]

Etiology and Pathogenesis

The exact cause of LP is unknown. It may be caused by the allergic or autoimmune response of the body. In an autoimmune response, the body recognizes self as non-self and mistakenly attacks the cells of the skin and mucous membranes. It is not clear why the body decides to initiate a self-attack. The same mechanism that occurs in an allergic reaction occurs with LP. Patients should get to know the trigger or risk factor that seems to cause the LP in their case. An area of the skin or nail where a former trauma occurred could cause LP. Risk factors include having another family member with LP, a viral infection such as hepatitis C, and certain allergens. Common allergens include medications (antibiotics, diuretics, antihypertensives, NSAIDs, and cardiac and arthritic drugs); flu vaccine; and gold, arsenic, or iodine compounds. Stress, genetics, tick bites, and autoimmune diseases may also trigger the disease. Oral LP can be caused by products used in dental procedures. The condition is not harmful but may take up to 18 months to clear up. About half of patients with oral symptoms will also have the skin form of LP.[30]

Clinical Manifestations

The onset of symptoms of LP can be slow or quick. Symptoms depend on the location of the LP. However, the usual symptom is a rash with few to many flat-topped, firm, reddish to purple bumps with symmetrical sides and sharp borders. Thin white streaks or stretch marks (Wickham striae) can be seen if the bumps are examined closely. The bumps are darker on the legs. The bumps may be shiny or scaly and can blister, break open, and crust. On the skin, the inner wrists, forearms, legs, and back are most involved. Itching is usually present and can be mild to severe. On the scalp, itching, redness, irritation, and possible hair loss may occur. If LP occurs on the nails, a lengthwise ridge can be seen on the nails, which become brittle and come off (temporarily or permanently). White patches that have a lacy appearance will appear on the sides of the mouth or tongue and on the gums. Oral lesions may appear and be nonpainful or burn (**Figure 40.11** ■). They can complicate eating if the lesion ulcerates and becomes painful. Some people report a metallic taste in the mouth. Genital LP causes bright red sores that may be uncomfortable but are otherwise not painful. Scarring and painful sex may occur with genital LP. Vaginal LP is much harder to treat. Over time, the bumps may become dark and fade, but scarring can occur.[30]

Linking Pathophysiology to Diagnosis and Treatment

Diagnosis of LP is usually done by a skin biopsy. A dentist can usually identify LP in the mouth. Lab work may be ordered to rule out similar diseases. A test for hepatitis C may be needed to determine whether that is the trigger. A dermatologist should be consulted. Treatment might not be needed, and the condition may clear on its own, but there is no cure for LP. If treatment is needed for the symptoms, it may consist of oral antihistamines, corticosteroids, or retinoic acid (a form of vitamin A). An injection of a corticosteroid may be used. In addition, corticosteroid or retinoic creams may be recommended. The first treatment choice is a prescription steroid cream. A type of ultraviolet light treatment (PUVA therapy) can clear the skin. Topical calcineurin inhibitors can be particularly helpful in managing lichen planus of mucous membranes. Immune response medicines such as tacrolimus

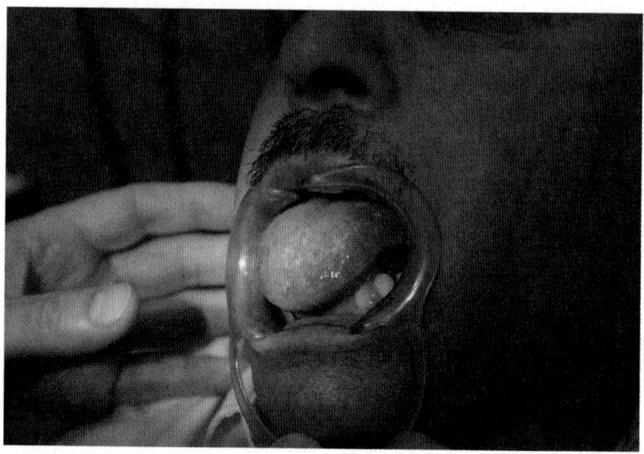

Figure 40.11 ■ White patches and oral lesions of lichen planus from a tick bite.

(Protopic) and pimecrolimus (Elidel) can suppress the body's own immune system. Home remedies include soaking in an oatmeal bath, avoiding scratching, and cool compresses.[30]

Pregnant women, women who could become pregnant, and breastfeeding mothers should not take retinol, which has been associated with birth defects. For these patients, the healthcare provider will opt for a different treatment.[31] ■

Check Your Progress: Section 40.4

1. Why does the treatment regimen for exfoliative dermatitis involve discontinuing all previous medications?
2. Why is it important to assess the patient's hydration status in exfoliative dermatitis?
3. What are the common causes of urticarial reactions?

40.5 Life-threatening Inflammatory Disorders

Life-threatening inflammatory disorders are conditions that involve the skin, usually result in shedding exposing the individual to infection, and harbor many complications. These disorders can be considerably long-term in healing or even fatal. The earlier the treatment in these disorders, the better the outcome and chances of survival. These disorders are extremely painful, often systemic and involve destruction of the skin along with many complications. The focus of this section is on necrotizing fasciitis, Stevens-Johnson syndrome, and toxic epidermal necrolysis.

Necrotizing Fasciitis

Necrotizing fasciitis (NF) is a rare but deadly disease that is also known as the "flesh-eating disorder." It is a rapidly spreading infection that can be caused by different bacteria. It usually starts from a wound or an existing infection and can lead to necrosis of the tissue. It spreads beyond the existing area of infection. Every year, between 600 and 700 cases are diagnosed in the United States, and 25–30% of those result in death. About 20–30% of cases occur in individuals with diabetes, about 30% occur in alcoholics, and the rest occur in healthy, young individuals. NF usually involves the extremities and perineum.[32,33]

Etiology, Pathogenesis, and Clinical Manifestations

Necrotizing fasciitis is usually caused by a mixture of aerobic and anaerobic organisms that affect the subcutaneous tissue and the fascia, including group A streptococci (e.g., *Streptococcus pyogenes*), *Escherichia coli (E. coli)*, and *Bacteroides* sp. Other organisms that are responsible for NF include *S. aureus, Clostridium, Peptostreptococcus, Proteus, Pseudomonas*, and *Klebsiella*. Community-acquired MRSA and contaminated saltwater with a *Vibrio* species have also been associated with NF.[32,33]

A contagious ulcer, a wound from trauma, or an untreated skin infection can be the start of NF. A complication of surgery, perirectal abscess or periurethreal gland infection often leads to perineal NF. Widespread occlusion of small subcutaneous vessels is caused by NF, leading to tissue ischemia, infarction, and necrosis. How fast the NF spreads is directly proportional to the thickness of the subcutaneous skin.

Typical symptoms include skin tissue that becomes red, hot, swollen, and malodorous (depending on the organism). The symptoms mimic cellulitis, but the pain is more severe and unrelenting. Septicemia and gangrene set in quickly causing necrosis of the skin.

Marc McMann: Application

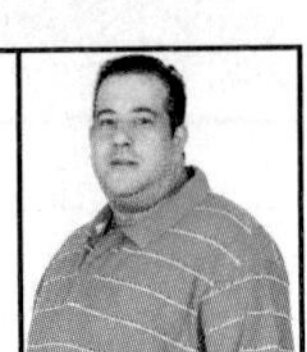

The nurse who admits Mr. McMann notices the foul odor and asks him about his pain. He states that the medicine given to him in the emergency department has not given him any relief. His vital signs are as follows: pulse 110 and regular, respirations 25, temperature 102.6°F, and blood pressure 165/90 mmHg. An assessment reveals that the area of infection is extremely edematous; the skin is taut, red, and warm; and the discharge has already soaked through the dressing applied in the emergency department. Mr. McMann is given acetaminophen with codeine at 11:00 p.m., and the nurse reports the findings to the charge nurse. The CBC results come back with a white blood cell (WBC) of 25.2 and neutrophils of 13,000/mm^3. His glucose level is 250, and an Accu-Chek test gives a reading of 300. Mr. McMann states that he has been urinating a lot and is very hungry. He is sweating profusely and is agitated and unable to get comfortable. The charge nurse calls Mr. McMann's healthcare provider, who orders more diluaded, and Mr. McMann is transferred to the intensive care unit.

3. What clinical condition is suggested by Mr. McMann's symptoms of increased urination and hunger as well as his blood chemistry results?
4. Why are Mr. McMann's WBC and neutrophil levels elevated?

Linking Pathophysiology to Diagnosis and Treatment

Patients with NF are acutely ill and need immediate attention before necrosis begins.

Antibiotics, dressing changes, possibly surgical debridement, and pain control are the essential interventions. Surgical debridement means removing all the superficial tissue from the fascia, including amputation of limbs if necessary (**Figure 40.12** ■). The use of hyperbaric oxygen therapy has proven to be beneficial.

Although NF is rare in children, healthcare providers who work with children need to be aware that it is a possibility. ■

Marc McMann: Outcome

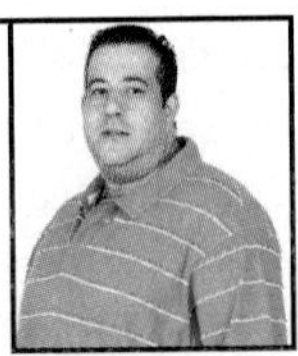

The day after Mr. McMann is admitted the intensive care unit and is tested for necrotizing fasciitis, diabetes, and hypertension. He is placed in isolation. He then undergoes surgery for debridement of the left groin area and inner thigh. The area is cultured and returns positive for necrotizing fasciitis. Further tests are done to determine whether Mr. McMann also has MRSA. That culture returns positive also. The healthcare provider orders a 5-hour GTT, and Mr. McMann is diagnosed with type 2 diabetes. He is placed on insulin, an antihypertensive agent, and antibiotics and is given vacuum-assisted

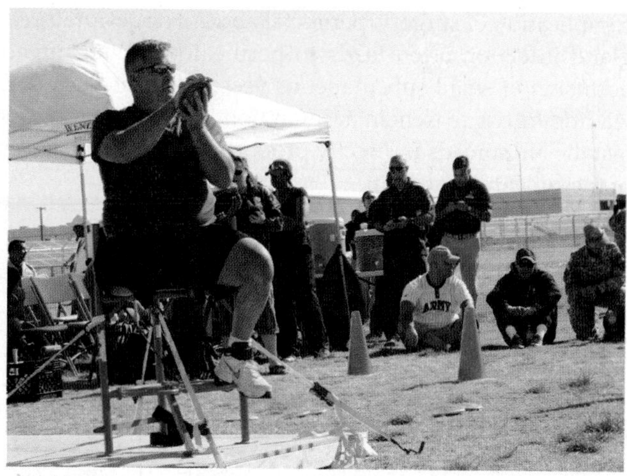

Figure 40.12 ■ First Lt. Christopher Parks, a physician assistant in the U.S. Army, competes in the discus event of the Army Trials. Around 80 wounded or injured soldiers and veterans competed in the event. Lt. Parks's right leg was amputated in 2014 because of an infection from necrotizing fasciitis.

wound therapy. After a month, Mr. McMann is transferred to the medicine unit. He has a positive attitude about caring for his diabetes and hypertension. A dietitian visits to discuss his food intake and the nurse educates him about his insulin injections along with his other medications. He is sent home a month later with stable glucose values and normal BP levels. He continues with wound care and physical therapy and makes a full recovery.

5. Why is Mr. McMann placed in isolation as part of his treatment plan?
6. Because of Mr. McMann's long hospital stay and the type of care he requires, what type of emotional support might he need?

Stevens-Johnson Syndrome

Stevens-Johnson syndrome (SJS) is a rare disorder of the skin and mucous membranes in which cell death causes the epidermis to separate from the dermis. It is on the opposite end of a continuum from toxic epidermal necrolysis (TEN) in that it is considered to be a milder form of the same disease. The difference between the two is the amount of body surface area affected. In SJS, less than 10% of the body surface area is involved. It is highly unpredictable, and more than half of the cases are idiopathic. Risk factors that increase susceptibility to SJS are viral infections, weakened immune system, a previous history of SJS, or family history of SJS.[34,35]

Etiology, Pathogenesis, and Clinical Manifestations

SJS can be caused by more than 200 medications such as antigout medications, pain relievers, NSAIDs, antibiotics, anticonvulsants, and antipsychotics. Infectious causes include herpes simplex or herpes zoster, pneumonia, HIV and AIDS, hepatitis, coxsackie viral infections, influenza, mumps, and many bacterial infections. In children, Epstein-Barr virus and enteroviruses have been identified with SJS.[34,35] SJS is a delayed hypersensitive (allergic) reaction. One explanation is that it occurs in people who are slow acetylators, that is, people who do not detoxify reactive drug metabolites. These drug metabolites have direct toxic effects and render host tissue as antigenic. With the presence of an antigen, the inflammatory reaction of the body triggers T-lymphocyte responses. Disintegration and death of the skin cells cause the separation of the epidermis from the dermis. The inflammatory process leads to extensive epidermal necrolysis.[34,35]

Early symptoms of SJS include flulike symptoms that occur several days before the rash appears. A symmetric burning rash beginning on the face and the upper part of the torso spreads within hours to days. The skin is painful and looks burned, with peeling, blistering, and hives. Lesions that form are cutaneous, with the appearance of a target and red and purple coloration. The core lesion is surrounded by macular erythema that later ruptures, sheds, and may become susceptible to infection. The trunk is the most common area of the body affected, but the lesions may occur in the palms, soles, dorsum of the hands, genitals, nose, mouth, and extensor surfaces. The mucosa, eyelids, conjunctiva, and cornea may also be involved, along with swelling of the tongue and face.[34,35]

Linking Pathophysiology to Diagnosis and Treatment

Diagnosis usually involves a physical examination, CBC with CD4+ and CD8+ T lymphocytes, electrolytes, kidney function studies, and possibly other specific tests (interleukins, C-reactive protein, and tissue necrosis factor). An ocular examination is usually essential. Skin, urine, wound, and blood cultures are taken to monitor for infections and possible sepsis. A chest x-ray, bronchoscopy, esophagogastroduodenoscopy, and colonoscopy may be needed.The initial treatment begins with stopping all nonessential medications that could be the cause of the SJS. Supportive care includes fluid replacement, nutrition, and wound and eye care. Medications that may be required for comfort and care are pain medications, antihistamines for itching, antibiotics to control infection (or treat cultured organisms), and topical steroids to reduce inflammation.[34,35]

Toxic Epidermal Necrolysis

Toxic epidermal necrolysis (TEN) is an inflammation of the skin caused by a poison resulting in necrosis and dissolving of the tissue. It is an idiosyncratic dermatologic disorder that is commonly caused by medications or other metabolites. Although similar to SJS, TEN is more extensive. TEN with spots is widespread with detachment of the epidermis and erosion involving more than 30% of the body surface area (BSA). TEN without spots is also widespread with erythema but no lesions and involves more than 10% of the BSA. TEN is considered more severe but less common than SJS. Both disorders are more common in women and occur more often in HIV-positive individuals. All age groups are involved; infections are the primary cause for pediatric patients.[36,37]

Etiology, Pathogenesis, and Clinical Manifestations

Antibiotics and anticonvulsants by systemic or topical application usually cause the drug reaction. Drugs include sulfa drugs, antibiotics, anticonvulsants, and some drugs used for gout. Other etiologies include bacterial infection (mycoplasma, herpes simplex, and cytomegalovirus) malignancy, graft-versus-host disease, and vaccinations. TEN is thought to be an immune-related cytotoxic reaction intended to destroy keratinocytes that announce a foreign antigen. It is a delayed hypersensitivity reaction to an initial exposure, and there will be a rapid reaction with repeated exposure. Keratinocyte apoptosis (programmed cell death) leads to cell changes and death because of biochemical reactions. The increased cell death differentiates TEN from SJS, which is known more for necrosis. The numbers of inflammatory T cells are low, however, and do not explain the massive destruction or the cell death.[36,37]

TEN begins about 1–3 weeks after the start of a new drug with flulike symptoms. Then a rash develops over the face, the neck, the trunk, and eventually the entire body, including the soles of the feet and palms of the hand. The major manifestation is large blisters in the center of the rash with a thin membrane that can rupture easily. Once ruptured, the skin peels off in large quantities, leaving these areas painful and bleeding. Because the disorder can affect the entire body, symptoms are numerous and related to the area of the body involved. The large amount of skin shedding leaves the individual susceptible to infection and life-threatening sepsis. Age, extent of epidermal involvement, and serum urea level are usually considered the most important factors to consider for prognosis.[36]

Linking Pathophysiology to Diagnosis and Treatment

A thorough history is needed, including when the suspected drug was started and the time between the initial dose and the onset of symptoms. Diagnosis is made by the amount of body-surface area affected and whether widespread purpuric macules or flat atypical targets are seen or no macules at all. A predictive test that is done early is serum granulysin, which will be elevated in TEN. Skin biopsies and blood testing help to confirm whether the diagnosis is SJS or TEN. Treatment includes immediate discontinuation of the offending drug or treating the infection. Supportive care is used for management of nutrition, fluids, temperature, urinary and bowel function, musculoskeletal function, and skin and wound care. Other treatments may include topical antiseptics with dressings to the skin, daily assessment by an eye doctor with antiseptic ointments, mouthwashes and an oral topical anesthetic, antibiotics, corticosteroids, and pain medications.[36,37]

Check Your Progress: Section 40.5

1. Why is an ocular examination essential in cases of Stevens-Johnson syndrome?
2. What healthcare conditions and medications are associated with development of Stevens-Johnson syndrome or toxic epidermal necrolysis?
3. What unusual area of the body may demonstrate a rash in cases of Stevens-Johnson syndrome or toxic epidermal necrolysis?

40.6 Stings and Bites

Stings from bees and wasps are often more annoying than dangerous, but any of them can cause anaphylaxis if the victim is allergic to the venom. Ticks carry diseases that can be severe. Usually, at-home treatment for these stings and bites will be enough. If they are more severe, medical treatment should be sought.

Bee and Wasp Stings

Various types of bee and wasp stings include those of vespids (yellow jackets, hornets, and wasps) and apids (bumblebees, Africanized "killer" bees, and honeybees). The female of each species has a stinging apparatus in the abdomen that includes a sac containing a large amount of venom (about 50 μg) and a barbed stinger. The insect may inject between 2 and 15 μg with one sting. A bee can sting only one time because the stinger detaches and the insect dies. After the stinger is detached from the insect, venom will continue to be injected; therefore, stingers should be removed from the victim immediately. Wasps, by contrast, can sting multiple times because the stinger does not detach. The venoms are chemically different but have similar results.[38,39]

Etiology and Pathogenesis

The venoms of both bees and wasps contain mixtures of chemicals. The venom causes the human body to release histamine and produces a hives-like reaction. Wasp venom contains enzymes that break down cell membranes and neurotransmitters (acetylcholine and serotonin), which inflame the nerve endings. Bee stings are half melittin, a toxin that is powerful and works by arousing an enzyme that causes inflammation. Both bee venom and wasp venom contain hyaluronidase, which causes the venom to spread.[38,39]

Clinical Manifestations

Most common reactions to bee and wasp stings are mild and include swelling, redness, itching, and mild pain. Blisters may occur, but are not common. The pain and swelling may last hours to days. Occasionally, more severe anaphylactic reactions may occur, especially if an individual is allergic to the insect sting. These can include shortness of breath, more intense swelling (may include face, lips, and eyes), tachycardia, hives, dizziness, nausea and vomiting. These symptoms are considered an emergency and urgent care should be sought.[38,39]

Linking Pathophysiology to Diagnosis and Treatment

The first treatment for a bee or wasp sting is to remove the stinger. At home, a cool compress applied immediately to the site of the sting is helpful. The area should be washed with water only. The victim should be told to avoid trying to scratch or rub the bite area. Oral and topical antihistamines will help to reduce swelling and itching, and a simple nonsteroidal analgesic will help with the pain. OTC creams designated for bites or stings contain a local anesthetic and may relieve some of the pain. A corticosteroid cream can be used to relieve some of the itching and swelling.[38,39]

About 10% of people have adverse reactions to insect bites. If the victim is allergic, anaphylaxis requires emergency management. Victims with a known allergy to bee and wasp stings should use their autoinjector (Adrenaclick or EpiPen), which contains epinephrine. If victims do not know of an allergy or do not have access to an autoinjector, they should be taken to the emergency department. Vital signs are monitored, and an examination for life-threatening symptoms is performed. Adrenaline is the drug of choice for severe symptoms, and advanced life support may be needed.[38,39]

Tick Bites

Ticks are arachnids that are common in the United States and live in grass, trees, shrubbery, and leaf piles. Humans are commonly bitten, but ticks are also attracted to furry animals. Ticks can move from outdoors to indoors via pets and humans. Ticks can be as small as a poppy seed. Ticks are blood-sucking animals that embed their head into the skin and grow as they suck blood. Ticks are different shades of brown to black. As they engorge on the blood and become full, they may turn a greenish-blue color. The most common time for tick bites is early spring to late summer. In the United States, ticks are more common east of the Rocky Mountains and along the Pacific coast in California. Ticks are either hard or soft, and this helps to determine the symptoms they cause. Hard ticks feed for days to weeks; soft ticks usually feed and leave. Risk factors for tick bites include outdoor activities, camping, hiking, walking, and contact with animals. Although most ticks are usually harmless, they can harbor diseases that can affect humans (**Table 40.1** ■).[40,41]

Etiology and Pathogenesis

Ticks are parasites that can cause dermatologic disease as a result of their bite or act as vectors of other diseases. The skin conditions can be acute or chronic and usually result from the physical trauma, salivary secretions, toxins, excretions, body parts, or scratching by the bitten victim. Ticks like warm areas, so they often migrate to the armpits, groin, or hair. Tick-borne diseases include bacterial infections, rickettsial infections, and viral diseases (see Table 40.1).[40,41]

Children are especially susceptible to tick bites because they play outside. Prevention includes checking the child's skin and hair after playing outside. Check clothing, as ticks can be on clothing when they enter a building. Long sleeves and long pants with socks should be worn when in wooded areas. Tucking the shirt into the pants and the pants into the sock helps to prevent the possibility of a tick bite. Use of an insect repellant with at least 10–20% DEET in children older than 2 years of age can also help.[42] ■

Clinical Manifestations

Most tick bites are harmless and do not cause any signs or symptoms. Common symptoms of tick bites for victims who are allergic to ticks include a red area that forms at the site of the bite, swelling, blisters, mild to severe itching, pain at the site, a rash, and a burning sensation. Some ticks cause purpura (bruising) and ulceration. Soft ticks may cause necrotic ulcers and pain. Over days or months, the lesions from the bite may cause a granuloma or nodules made up of inflammatory cells. Temporary hair loss and infection of the skin from *S. aureus* may occur. Symptoms of a severe allergic reaction include hives; swelling of the throat, mouth, lips, and tongue; and trouble breathing.[40-42]

Most of the diseases carried by ticks cause flulike symptoms with fever, headache, nausea, vomiting, and muscle aches. Other symptoms caused by diseases carried by ticks include rash over the entire body, stiffness in the neck, chills, and swollen lymph nodes. Tick paralysis is rare but can occur and usually subsides within 24 hours. Symptoms of tick paralysis resemble those of Guillain-Barré syndrome or botulism and are caused by a toxin in the tick's saliva.[40-42]

A red bump with a ringed red rash that resembles a bulls-eye is typical of Lyme disease (**Figure 40.13** ■). Common symptoms of Lyme disease include fever, headache,

Table 40.1 Selected Human Diseases Transmitted by Tick Bite

Disease	Carriers	Geographic Region in U.S.
Anaplasmosis	Blacklegged tick (*Ixodes scapularis*) Western blacklegged tick (*Ixodes pacificus*)	Northeast and upper Midwest Pacific coast
Babesiosis	Blacklegged tick (*Ixodes scapularis*)	Northeast and upper Midwest
Colorado tick fever	Rocky Mountain wood tick (*Dermacentor andersoni*)	Rocky Mountain states at elevations above 4000 feet
Ehrlichiosis	Lone star tick (*Ambylomma americanum*)	South central and eastern United States
Lyme disease	Blacklegged tick (*Ixodes scapularis*) Western blacklegged tick (*Ixodes pacificus*)	Northeast and upper Midwest Pacific coast
Rocky Mountain spotted fever (RMSF)	American dog tick (*Dermacentor variabilis*) Rocky Mountain wood tick (*Dermacentor andersoni*) Brown dog tick (*Rhipicephalus sangunineus*)	South central and eastern United States
Southern tick-associated rash illness (STARI)	Lone star tick (*Ambylomma americanum*)	Southeastern and eastern United States
Tularemia	American dog tick (*Dermacentor variabilis*) Wood tick (*Dermacentor andersoni*) Lone star tick (*Amblyomma americanum*).	Throughout the United States

SOURCE: Data from Centers for Disease Control and Prevention. (2016). *Tickborne diseases of the United States*. Available at https://www.cdc.gov/ticks/diseases

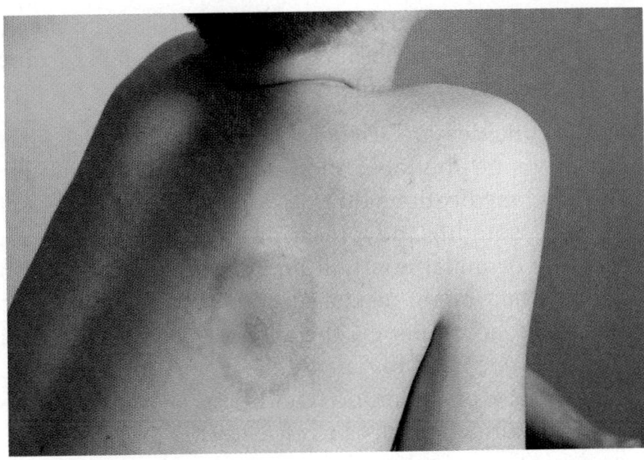

Figure 40.13 ■ A child with a classic bull's-eye rash from Lyme disease.

fatigue, and a skin rash called erythema migrans.[43] Red dots on the ankles and wrists are typical in Rocky Mountain spotted fever (RMSF).[44] Other early symptoms of RMSF usually occur about 5–14 days after the tick bite and may include fever, nausea, vomiting, muscle pain, loss of appetite, and headache. Because the symptoms of Lyme disease and RMSF are general, both can be misdiagnosed until more severe symptoms occur. If left untreated, these diseases can become systemic and involve multiple organs.[43,44]

Linking Pathophysiology to Diagnosis and Treatment

The first treatment for a tick bite is to remove the tick by using tweezers close to the skin with a steady upward pull until the tick lets go. Avoid twisting or rocking back and forth to remove the tick. The site of the bite and the hands of the person removing the tick should be washed with soap and water. The bite can be swabbed with alcohol. Never use heat to try to remove the tick; heat causes the tick to burrow further into the skin. If the tick is removed but the head stays in the skin, it will usually fall out in several days. Any signs of infection or symptoms of severe disease require medical treatment from a healthcare provider.

If the tick is still present, a skin biopsy helps with diagnosis of the type of tick. If the tick has fallen off, diagnosis may be difficult. Topical antihistamines and corticosteroids help with the itching. Calamine lotion for itching and benzocaine spray (such as Solarcaine) can provide local anesthetic effects. Use of an ice pack for the first 6 hours applied 20 minutes on and 20 minutes off will assist with swelling and pain.[40-44] If severe symptoms are present, tests may be ordered to rule out a specific disease carried by ticks.

In the acute stage of Lyme disease, individuals are treated with oral antibiotics such as doxycycline, amoxicillin, or cefuroxime axetil. If Lyme disease is treated early, recovery is usually rapid and complete. However, the condition can last for 6 months and is then considered chronic Lyme disease.[43] In RMSF, the first-line treatment of choice for adults and children of all ages is doxycycline. The antibiotic should be started immediately, as the disease can be fatal in 8 days without treatment. Use of other antibiotics is associated with a high risk of a fatal outcome.[44]

Check Your Progress: Section 40.6

1. What measures are recommended to prevent tick bites?
2. What are the infectious syndromes that may occur as a result of tick bite?
3. Wasp and bee stings usually cause minor symptoms. Why do they cause serious symptoms in some individuals?

40.7 Disorders Caused by Infestations

Bites and infestations from parasites such as lice, scabies, and bedbugs cause uncomfortable annoying symptoms that can resemble each other. For most of the bites, itching is the most common symptom, and OTC medications can be used to alleviate the problem. More serious side effects can occur, such as an infection or anaphylaxis, but these are rare. Treating the individual and the environment are the biggest challenges.

Pediculosis

Pediculosis is an infestation of the hairy parts of the body or clothing with the eggs, larvae, or adults of lice. These parasitic insects can be found on the head, body, or pubic areas:

- Pediculosis humanus capitis is head lice.
- Pediculosis humanus corporis is body lice.
- Pthiriasis is pubic lice.

Pubic lice are usually transmitted by intimate contact or possibly caught by using blankets, towels, sheets, or clothing of people who have pubic lice. Body lice are usually acquired through close contact with people, poor hygiene, or overcrowding.[45-47]

Head lice are most commonly found in preschool or elementary school–age children. Approximately 6–12 million infestations of head lice occur each year among children 3–11 years old.[47,48] ■

Etiology and Pathogenesis

In the United States, anyone of any age can become infested with lice (**Figure 40.14** ■). The infestation can be transmitted to household members and caretakers. There is evidence that girls get head lice more commonly than boys, and head lice infestation is much less common in African Americans than in people of other races.[46] The lice found in the United States have claws that allow for better gripping. Head lice are not known to cause diseases and may be asymptomatic with the exception of itching. Body lice can spread disease and are bigger in size. Body lice are found worldwide and occur in people of all races. In the United States, body lice occur more often in the homeless population, transient people, or those who do not often bathe and change into clean clothing. The diseases transmitted by body lice include typhus and louse-borne relapsing fever. Although typically limited to the hair of the pubic area, pubic lice can be found on eyebrows, eyelashes, beards, mustache, chest,

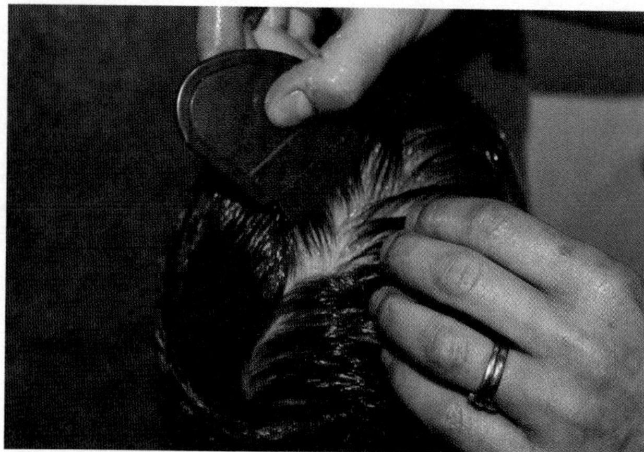

Figure 40.14 ■ A child with nits from a lice infestation.

and armpits. Pubic lice do not carry diseases but can cause secondary bacterial infections.

The life cycle of lice has three stages: egg, nymph, and adult. Nits are the eggs of head lice. Nits are hard to see and often look like dandruff. The female lays nits at the base of the hair shaft near the scalp. In about a week, they hatch and release nymphs. The nymph is small, about the size of a pinhead. In about a week, the nymph matures three times and becomes an adult. An adult louse has six legs with claws and is grayish-white. Female lice are larger than males. Lice can live up to 30 days on the head. They feed on blood several time daily and die within 1–2 days if there is no blood supply.[46]

Clinical Manifestations

The most common symptom of pediculosis is pruritus, which is caused by an allergic reaction to the louse bites. The first infestation may not cause symptoms and it often takes 4–6 weeks for itching to occur. Other symptoms include feeling something moving in the hair, and irritability, sleeplessness and sores from scratching. These sores can become infected. When body lice are long-standing, the heaviest bitten area of the skin can thicken and darken, especially in the mid-section of the body. Body lice are usually in the crevices and skinfolds of the body. Pubic lice can also cause low-grade fever, lack of energy, and pale bluish spots near the bites.[45]

Linking Pathophysiology to Diagnosis and Treatment

Diagnosis of pediculosis is usually made at home by the individual. The symptoms and the appearance of nits are usually the initial steps in diagnosis. A live louse and/or a viable nit can be examined under a microscope for identification. Cellulose tape applied over an infected area can pick up lice to help identify them. A Wood lamp will reveal yellow-green fluorescence of lice and nits. If needed, dermoscopy can be used to identify the lice. An infestation with pubic lice is considered a sexually transmitted infection, and 25% of individuals with pubic lice typically have another sexually transmitted infection. Screening of individuals with pubic lice includes HIV, syphilis, gonorrhea, chlamydia, genital herpes, and trichomonas.

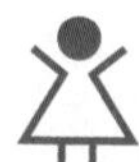

Pubic lice found on the head, eyelashes, or eyebrows of children may be an indication of sexual exposure or abuse and should be followed up.[46] ■

Pediculicides are used to rid the hair of lice. The instructions on the label should be followed carefully. If the OTC medications do not work, medical treatment should be sought, and prescription medications such as lindane or malathion will be ordered. Children with extra-long hair might need a second bottle. The nit comb that usually accompanies the OTC medications should be the only one used to remove the nits. After treatment, a cream rinse or shampoo/conditioner should not be used. The hair should not be rewashed for 1–2 days after treatment. The hair should be combed with the nit comb every 2–3 days. If the lice are not dead or moving slowly 8–12 hours after treatment, a professional should be seen. Retreatment is usually recommended in 7–10 days after the first OTC treatment.

The infested individual should change clothing after treatment. All individuals in the home should be checked for potential lice and treated if lice are found. The clothing and bed linens of the infected person should be washed in hot water and dried with the hot cycle for at least 20 minutes. Anything nonwashable (e.g., certain fabrics, stuffed animals, cloth toys) should be placed in a sealed plastic bag for 2 weeks, enough time to kill the lice. Combs and brushes should be soaked with rubbing alcohol, Lysol or washed with soap and hot water, then placed in a bag and left in the freezer for 2 days. Vacuuming the floor and furniture is recommended. If lice are found on eyelashes, petroleum jelly applied 3 times a day for several days can help in plucking the nits using a tweezers. The petroleum jelly works by suffocating the lice, and OTC lice treatments should not be used around the eyes. For body lice, a pediculicide is usually not necessary.[47]

Unfortunately, in the United States there is an increase in drug-resistant lice. After routine treatment for head lice, the response to treatment should be evident upon examination of the scalp. The lice should be dead or at least moving very slowly. If not, this may indicate treatment resistance and other types of drug therapy may be necessary that will require a prescription from a healthcare provider and follow-up to confirm cure.

CLINICAL POINT: Treatment with lindane or prescription medications is not recommended for children under 2 years old, pregnant or breastfeeding women, older adults, and individuals with immunosuppressive disorders. A healthcare provider should be seen to obtain recommendations for treatment.[46] ■

Scabies

Scabies is an intense pruritic rash caused by a parasitic mite that burrows in the skin. The microscopic mite, which is called *Sarcoptes scabei*, has eight legs and cannot be seen on the skin. Scabies is extremely contagious and spreads quickly through physical contact. Scabies acquired the name the "seven-year-itch" because it can come and go in 7-year cycles. There are millions of cases of scabies each year. It occurs worldwide and affects people of all ages, races, and income levels. Crusted scabies, also called Norwegian scabies, is a more severe form of the disease.[49,50]

Etiology and Pathogenesis

Transmission of scabies is by close contact with an infected person. Sexual contact is the most common form of transmission, especially in young adults. Children and therefore mothers are susceptible as well. Scabies crawl, burrowing under the skin, leaving eggs, and living off the hosts for 23–26 hours. They cause a rash on the skin that appears as small red bumps and blisters, but not every bump is a mite. Scabies burrow under the skin, making it appear as thin gray, brown, or red lines in the affected area. Folds of the skin, fingers, wrists, backs of the elbows, knees, around the waist and umbilicus, axillary folds, areas around the nipples, sides and backs of the feet, genital area and the buttocks are where scabies are usually found.[49,50]

A more serious form of scabies, called Norwegian scabies or crusting scabies, causes crusting. The crusted scabies are filled with mites that can fall off. Therefore, the crust can provide food and protection for the mites. After mating, the male mite dies and the female scabies mite burrows into the outside layers of the skin. There she will lay up to three eggs each day for her lifetime.[51]

Residents of nursing homes and extended living facilities are particularly susceptible to scabies. Although the symptoms are the same in older adults, diagnosis of scabies may be delayed, causing a rapid spread of the infestation. Treatment is the same as for other age groups, although toxicity of the medications should be considered in older adults.[49,52] ■

Clinical Manifestations

Symptoms of scabies might not occur until 4–6 weeks after transmission. The most common symptom is a rash and itching that is more intense at night, interrupting sleep. The rash is a hypersensitivity reaction that occurs after infestation and can have various appearances: pimple appearing, erythematous papules, dermatitis, erythema, vesicles, crusting, sores from scratching, nodules, and raised tracks (**Figure 40.15** ■).[49,50]

Linking Pathophysiology to Diagnosis and Treatment

Diagnosis of scabies usually includes examination by a healthcare provider, who looks for the characteristic burrows. A scraping from the skin is taken to be examined under a microscope to look for mites or eggs. Another method is to remove a mite with a needle from the end of the burrow and examine it under a microscope. Skin biopsy can be done but is usually not necessary. Crusted scabies will cause IgE elevation and eosinophilia.[51]

Treatment is usually recommended by a dermatologist and typically requires one dose; however, widespread scabies may require two or three doses.[52] Everyone who lives with the infested person and all recent sexual partners should be treated. Medicines include 5% permethrin cream (the most common treatment and safe for children 1 month old and pregnant women), 25% benzyl benzoate lotion, 10% sulfur ointment, 10% crotamiton cream, and 1% lindane lotion. The cream should be applied all over the body and on the face and scalp of young children. The prescription is applied at bedtime and washed off in the morning. The treatment is often repeated in 1 week. Oral medicine for stronger cases of scabies includes ivermectin, which is safe for children and immunosuppressed patients. An antihistamine to help with the itching, an antibiotic for any infection, and a steroid cream for the swelling and redness may be helpful.[49-52]

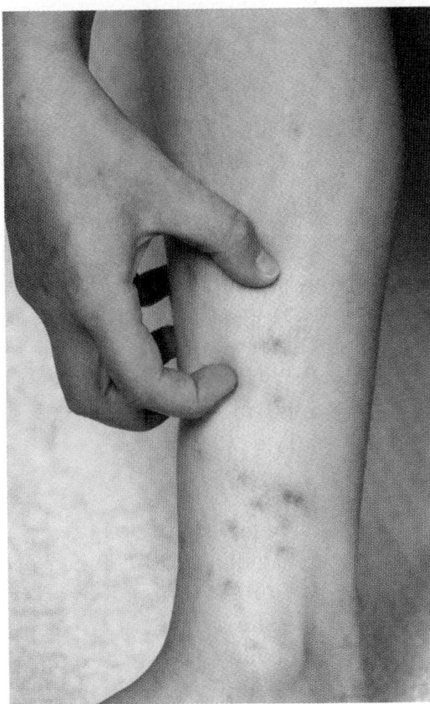

Figure 40.15 ■ Raised tracks and rash from scabies.

CLINICAL POINT: Treatment with lindane is not recommended for children under 2 years old, pregnant or breastfeeding women, individuals with immunosuppressive disorders, and older adults. The healthcare provider will recommend other treatments.[53] ■

Bedbug Bites

Bedbugs (*Cimex lectularius*) are ectoparasites, that is, they are capable of living outside of the host, which in this case are humans and birds. The common bedbug is small, oval, flat, and reddish-brown in color. They are blood-sucking insects that are more a pest than a risk. Bedbugs are increasing around the world, occurring in places where they were not formerly found. Increasingly, bedbugs are being found in places with a high rate of turnover in human guests such as hotels, hospitals, dormitories, cruise ships, jails, and homeless shelters. The place does not have to be unsanitary to have bedbugs. They generally live in or near mattresses, box springs, headboards, and bed frames, usually within 8 feet of where humans sleep. Females will lay eggs in cracks of furniture or upholstery, and newborns will occur in 4–5 days. Bedbugs affect people of all races and ages.[54]

Etiology and Pathogenesis

Bedbug infestations have been increasing in recent years worldwide and in the United States, partly because of resistance to the treatment. They are wingless and depend on humans to carry them from place to place. They also travel via luggage, furniture, clothing, and used mattresses. They are most active at night and feed off victims while they are sleeping, especially at early dawn. They feed off the human every 5–10 days. They pierce the skin and inject saliva that contains anticoagulants, anesthetics, proteases, and kinins. The anesthetics account for why most people do not feel the bites. After feeding, the bedbug returns to its warm hiding place. Bedbugs are annoying, but they are not dangerous and usually do not carry deadly diseases.[54]

Clinical Manifestations

Some individuals have no symptoms after a bedbug bite; others do. It can also be hard to distinguish bedbug bites from the bites of other insects. Typical symptoms are redness around the site with a darker red spot in the middle, stinging, and itching. The bites can be flat welts or raised bumps and usually are occur clusters or a linear pattern (**Figure 40.16** ■). The parts of the body bitten that are usually bitten are the face, neck, arms, and hands. Worst-case symptoms include an allergic reaction that becomes systemic, scarring, skin infection, insomnia, and anxiety.[54]

Linking Pathophysiology to Diagnosis and Treatment

Diagnosis of bedbug bites does not require blood work or imaging and is done by physical examination and history. It helps with the diagnosis if the patient brings in an actual bedbug (in a sealed plastic bag) or a picture of what they have seen when bitten. Typical treatment that can be done at home includes taking an antihistamine for itching, applying ice packs to reduce scratching, and applying an antiseptic cream or lotion if an infection begins. If signs of anaphylaxis occur, immediate medical treatment is needed.

Treatment for the home to get rid of bedbugs includes placing the legs of the bed in paraffin oil or water, tucking sheets and blankets in so they are not on the floor, removing clutter, vacuuming and steam cleaning all mattresses and box springs, and placing infested clothing or bedding in the dryer for 10–20 minutes on medium to high heat or laundering the items using hot water. A bedbug-proof mattress encasement can prevent an infestation. The home might need to be treated by a pest control professional.[54]

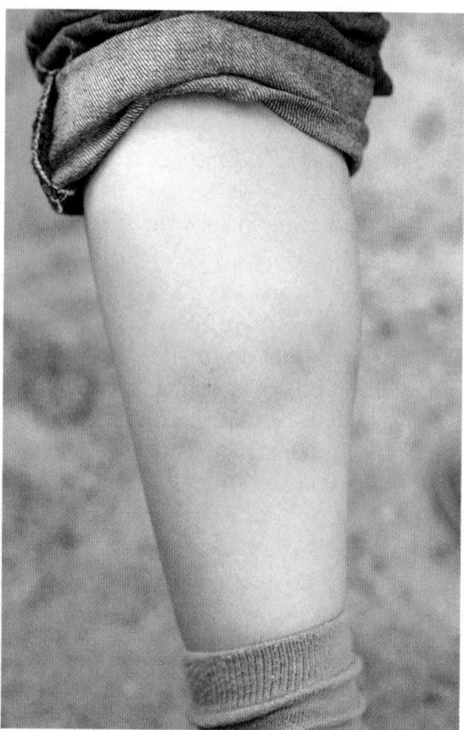

Figure 40.16 ■ A cluster of raised, red bedbug bites.

Check Your Progress: Section 40.7

1. Why is it important to screen for sexually transmitted infections (STIs) in individuals diagnosed with pubic lice?
2. Why should a healthcare provider be seen if the lice are not dead or moving slowly 8–12 hours after treatment?
3. What serious diseases are transmitted by bedbugs?

40.8 Disorders Associated with Adolescent/ Adult Skin

Acne vulgaris is a common acne that typically occurs in adolescents. Rosacea is a chronic rash on the face. Rosacea is not really an acne, although the symptoms are similar. Both of these conditions can be treated by a healthcare provider and usually require topical medications.

Acne Vulgaris

Acne vulgaris (often called just acne) is the formation of comedones, papules, pustules, nodules, or cysts when hair follicles and sebaceous glands become inflamed because of obstruction. It most often affects adolescents, but most people have some form of acne during their lifetime. It is the most common skin condition in the United States. In adolescence, acne is more common in males. In adulthood, women have acne vulgaris more often than men. Acne is common in North American whites, African Americans, and people in the Mediterranean region.[55]

Etiology and Pathogenesis

Acne can be inflammatory, noninflammatory, or a combination of the two. Noninflammatory acne is impacted plugs within follicles. These comedones are open (blackheads) or closed (whiteheads). When comedones are closed, this leads to inflammatory acne. Inflammatory acne happens when *Propionibacterium acnes* inhabits the closed comedones and causes an inflammatory reaction. Closed comedones can rupture into the dermis and produce papules.[55]

The pathophysiology behind acne is multifaceted, and genetics can play a major role. The interaction of four factors usually accounts for acne: release of multiple inflammatory mediators into the skin, follicular hyperproliferation and plugging of the follicle, excess production of sebum, and colonization of follicles by *P. acnes*. Other causes can be attributed to high hormone (androgen) levels in puberty, growth hormone, insulin-like growth factor, and corticotropin-releasing hormones especially in stressful times.[55] Other triggers include hormonal changes in pregnancy, cosmetics, lotions that are occlusive, and sweating. Acne may disappear in the summer months because the sunlight has anti-inflammatory effects. Drugs such as corticosteroids, phenytoin, and isoniazid can worsen acne. Acne most often affects the face but may spread to the chest, neck, and back.[55]

Clinical Manifestations

Acne is graded as mild, moderate, or severe. The grading depends on the number of comedones and inflammatory lesions and the total lesion count. It is common for different lesion types to be apparent at the same time. Closed comedones (whiteheads) are flesh-colored palpable lesions; open comedones (blackheads) are similar but have a dark center. Red lesions called papules (often deep) and pustules (superficial) may appear. Large, deep nodules and cysts, which may be painful, may also be seen in acne vulgaris. Severe acne can lead to permanent physical scarring, which can create emotional distress for the patient.[55]

Linking Pathophysiology to Diagnosis and Treatment

Physical examination by a healthcare provider is usually enough to determine the severity and any contributing factors (hormonal, drug-related, etc.). For women with dysmenorrhea or hirsutism, laboratory tests may be indicated for hormonal evaluation. If the acne does not clear up, a culture of the skin lesion may be needed.

Treatment includes medications, diet therapy, and procedures. Medications used for acne are retinoid-like agents, antibiotics, selective aldosterone antagonists, estrogen/progestin combination oral contraceptive pills, and OTC acne products. Diet therapy aims at avoiding junk foods and eating foods with a low glycemic index. Procedures include manual extraction of comedones, intralesional steroid injection, and superficial peels.[55]

CLINICAL POINT: Sun sensitivity may be a side effect of many of the prescription retinoid-like agents for acne. Individuals taking these medications should avoid long periods of time in the sun or use extra sun protection.[55] ■

Rosacea

Rosacea is a chronic rash that is distinct from acne but was previously called acne rosacea. It involves the central part of the face and is characterized by its red color. It affects people 30–60 years of age with fair skin and blue eyes. Individuals with Celtic and Scandinavian ancestry are prone to rosacea. It may be recurring, persistent, or transient. There is no cure for rosacea, but the symptoms can be controlled.[56,57]

Etiology and Pathogenesis

The cause of rosacea is unknown, but certain risk factors, hereditary factors, and environmental factors may account for outbreaks. Hygiene has nothing to do with this disorder. An increase in blood flow to the surface of the skin can be triggered by hot drinks, spicy foods, alcohol, temperature extremes, sunlight or wind, emotions, exercise, cosmetics, and vasodilating drugs. Risk factors include being female, being fair skinned, being over age 30, smoking, and having a family history of rosacea. Some theories about the cause of rosacea include genetics, chronic exposure to UV rays, high levels of cathelicidins (skin's normal defense), enzymes such as collagenase and elastase, hair follicle mites, and infection with *Helicobacter pylori*. A seborrheic dermatitis often coexists with rosacea that makes the skin condition even more sensitive.[56,57]

Clinical Manifestations

The most common symptoms of rosacea are facial redness where small blood vessels on the nose and cheeks become visible because of swelling (telangiectasia). Other common symptoms include swollen red bumps (appearance of pimples that are hot and tender and contain pus), eye problems (dryness, irritation, swelling, reddened eyelids, styes, conjunctivitis), and an enlarged nose (thickening of the skin on the nose) (**Figure 40.17** ■). Other characteristics of rosacea are frequent blushing; dry, flaky skin; and burning or stinging in reaction to make-up, sunscreens, or other facial creams. In addition to the physical symptoms, patients may suffer from frustration, embarrassment, worry, low self-esteem, work-related problems, anxiety, and depression.[56,57]

Linking Pathophysiology to Diagnosis and Treatment

A clinical diagnosis of rosacea can usually be made by examination. If there are signs of a chronic inflammation, a skin biopsy may be taken. The patient may be referred to a dermatologist to rule similar conditions, and a referral to ophthalmologist is needed if the eye is involved. Treatment involves a combination of skin care and prescriptions. Medications include brimonidine (Mirvaso), azelaic acid, and metronidazole for the redness and pimples; oral antibiotics

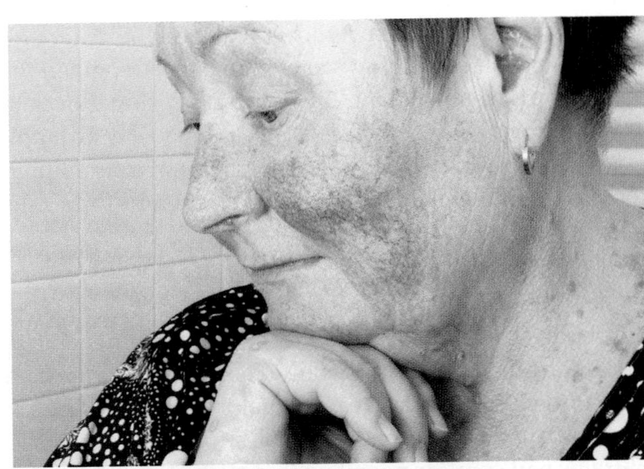

Figure 40.17 ■ A woman with a red face rash characteristic of rosacea.

if inflammation occurs; and isotretinoin (an oral acne drug) for severe rosacea. For treating the enlarged vessels, laser therapy, dermabrasion, intense pulsed light therapy, and electrosurgery have been used. Alternative therapies include colloidal silver, emu oil, laurelwood, and oregano oil. Plastic surgery to reshape the nose may be needed for thickening of the nose. Other recommendations are gentle massage, avoiding oil-based facial creams and sunscreens, avoiding topical steroids, and using a cool face cloth.[56,57]

Check Your Progress: Section 40.8

1. What is a potential complication of severe acne vulgaris?
2. What are the potential complications of severe rosacea?
3. For patients on retinoid-type acne medications, what patient education is important?

40.9 Disorders of the Nail

Nail disorders can be caused by a variety of factors and are usually not life threatening.

Brittle Nails

Brittle nails mean that the nails are not hard and instead easily crack, chip, split, or peel. Onychoschizia refers to brittle or soft nails with splitting. This condition is more common in women.[58]

Brittle nails can be a sign of aging, long-term use of nail polish, exposure to moist conditions (dishwashing, swimming), or dryness. Some diseases such as hyperthyroidism, hypothyroidism, lichen planus, nail psoriasis, reactive arthritis, and iron deficiency anemia can cause brittle nails. Chemotherapy can also cause brittle nails as well as a fungal nail infection. Cleaning fluids, chemicals in detergents, and acetone removers may be a cause of brittle nails.[58]

Symptoms include nails that bend easily, split with little effort, and may crack if used on something hard. Nail color remains the same. There are no specific tests for brittle nails. To prevent nails from splitting if brittle, keep the nails short and avoid nail polish remover with acetone. Although clear nail polish containing protein can help strengthen the nails, the problem is taking the polish off. Using gloves to avoid getting nails wet will also help, as will using an emollient after washing or bathing. The vitamin biotin in high doses is recommended, but it may take 6 months for results to be seen.[58]

Nail Infections

Onychomycosis (*tinea unguium*), is a common fungal infection of the fingernails and toenails. The toenails are affected more often. Anyone can get a fungal infection of the nail, but they are most common in males, people with a nail injury or nail surgery, people with diabetes, anyone with a weakened immune system or blood circulatory problems, and those with athlete's foot.[59]

Fungal nail infections are common among adults over 65 years of age. Older adults are at the highest risk partly because they have poorer circulation and their nails grow more slowly and thicken as they age. Periodic checkups with a podiatrist may be recommended.[60] ■

CLINICAL POINT: When toenails become thick in an individual with diabetes, the nurse should refer the patient to a podiatrist to have the nails trimmed. In some long-term nursing care facilities, a podiatrist comes monthly to assess residents who need nail care. The nurse should assess whether the shoes the individual is wearing are too narrow at the toe area or pay attention if the individual complains of toe pain and have the healthcare provider recommend specific shoes. ■

Etiology and Pathogenesis

Different types of fungi (*Tinea unguium*, yeasts, *Candida albicans*, or molds) can cause a fungal nail infection. These organisms live in the environment. Small cracks in the nail or surrounding skin allow the organisms to enter, and an infection ensues. Onycholysis is a fungal infection that causes the nail to separate from the nail bed. Fungi live in warm, moist, dark environments. Toenails are confined to this environment within shoes. Risk factors for fungal nail infections include heavy perspiration, working in a humid or moist environment, wearing socks and shoes without ventilation, living with someone who has a fungal nail infection, walking barefoot in damp areas, and athlete's foot (a fungal infection of the feet that can spread to the toenails). Professional manicures or pedicures can result in a nail infection if the salon does not disinfect the tools.[59,60]

Clinical Manifestations

The first symptom of a fungal infection of the nail is usually a white or yellow spot under the tip of the fingernail or toenail. As the infection increases, the nail may turn colors (yellow, green, or black), appear dull, become distorted in shape, and thicken. There may be scaling under the nail, with flaky white patches and pits that crumble at the edges. Fungal nail infections usually affect only one toe but can affect more than one. Symptoms may be mild, and the patient may even asymptomatic. If the nail infection is symptomatic, there may be pain and odor, and the nail can be completely destroyed. If the infection starts near the nail plate, the cuticle may be swollen and red.[59,60]

Linking Pathophysiology to Diagnosis and Treatment

Nail infections need to be diagnosed by a podiatrist or healthcare professional because they can mimic other disorders. A nail scraping will be taken and examined microscopically. If necessary, the scraping will be sent off for analysis. Nail clippings from the crumbling part of the nail may be taken also. Nail infections are often difficult to cure. It may take months to a year for the infection to be cured, and it may reappear. Treatment might include an oral antifungal (e.g., terbinafine, fluconazole), a topical antifungal, medicated nail polish (ciclopirox), and antifungal cream. If the infection is severe, the nail may be removed. Other methods that have more recently been tried are laser and light-based therapies. Ultrasound has been used with success to deliver the antifungal drug to the nail plate.[59,60]

CLINICAL POINT: Antifungal treatment for the nails should be given as directed and usually every day for a month. Skipping days can interfere with the effectiveness of the treatment. ■

Nail Trauma or Loss

Nail trauma is injury to the nail caused by various means that may result in deformities or loss of the nail (total removal of the nail). This usually includes the nail, nail bed, and cuticle and the skin around the nail. An injury can be a cut, a torn nail, a nail that has been smashed, or a nail that has been brushed or torn from the skin. Typical causes are crush injuries (from an automobile accident, machinery, or playing a sport), smashing the nail in a door, catching the nail on something causing it to rip, hitting the nail with a hammer or heavy object, or cutting the nail with a knife. An injury that damages the soft tissue under the nail plate can leave permanent deformity of the nail. Other injuries include an ingrown toenail, a broken toe, a subungual hematoma, a tumor of the nail, artificial nails, an improper manicure, or even nail biting. Nail injuries can be complex wounds to fix and may leave permanent deformity.[61,62]

Etiology and Pathogenesis

Nail injuries such as crushing or smashing can lead to a subungual hematoma, which is a collection of blood under the nail. Typically, this is red or purple in color and will fade over weeks. Pressure will build under the nail from the blood and may require introducing a hole in the nail to allow the blood to escape. Any fracture or crushing injury can cause the nail to lift completely from the nail bed. In this case, seeking treatment, such as removal of the nail, at an emergency department is best. A nail laceration can lead to part of the nail being removed and leaves the nail mangled in appearance. An amputation of a fingertip may involve all or part of the nail bed. Individuals with diabetes, circulatory problems, or AIDS and those on chemotherapy have poor healing and increased risk of infection when a nail injury occurs.[61,62]

Clinical Manifestations

Symptoms of nail injuries include throbbing pain, bleeding underneath the nail or around the nail, swelling, warmth, red streaks leading from the finger or toe, signs of infection (redness, fever, or drainage), and being able to lift all or part of the nail.[61,62]

Linking Pathophysiology to Diagnosis and Treatment

Diagnosis of a nail injury begins with a thorough history and physical examination by a healthcare provider. Most nail injuries are best managed in the emergency department. Depending on the cause, the nail may be treated with a dressing after the bleeding has been stopped. Any jewelry on the finger or toe should be removed immediately. Stitches may be used for lacerations, and the nail may be partially or completely removed after an anesthetic has been applied. An antibiotic may be prescribed to prevent infection and a mild pain reliever may be given. The healthcare provider may recommend elevation, ice, and soaking for the toe, especially if the toenail was removed. It may take 3–6 months for the nail to grow from the cuticle if the nail was removed.[61,62]

CLINICAL POINT: When educating patients newly diagnosed with diabetes about checking their feet daily, remember to include complications with the toenails. Emphasize getting treatment early rather than waiting. ■

Check Your Progress: Section 40.9

1. What age-related physiologic changes increase the risk for fungal nail infections in older adults?
2. What are the risk factors for development of fungal nail infections?
3. Where is the best location for evaluation and treatment of nail injury?

CHAPTER SUMMARY

40.1 Chapter Overview and Case Studies

Differentiate acute from chronic skin conditions, and describe concepts related to acute disorders of the skin.

- Acute skin conditions are usually short-term and respond to treatment. Most of them respond to over-the-counter medications. Although anaphylaxis is possible with many of the conditions, the usual symptoms can be managed.
- If untreated, some of the skin conditions can become serious. There are acute skin conditions that can become chronic.

40.2 Bacterial Skin Infections

Differentiate the causes, classification, underlying pathogenesis, and clinical manifestations of bacterial skin infections and approaches to diagnosis and treatment of these conditions across the lifespan.

- Cellulitis is a painful inflammation from bacteria under the first layer of the skin. It is usually cause by *Staphylococcus aureus* or MRSA, which can be contracted from home. The extremities are the most common places to be affected, and cellulitis can occur from a simple cut as well as a more serious injury. Antibiotics and pain medication are usually the treatment.

- Impetigo is an acute highly contagious bacterial infection of the skin most commonly affecting children. *Streptococcus* or *S. aureus* are the most common organisms causing the infection. This condition causes a rash that occurs anywhere on the body but often on the face, around the mouth, and on the abdomen. Antibiotics are the treatment of choice.
- Folliculitis is an inflammation of the hair follicle caused by bacteria, fungi, a virus, or a parasite. *S. aureus, Candida albicans,* and *Pseudomonas aeruginosa* are the common causative organisms. Each area of folliculitis will look like a white pimple and may cause burning and pain.
- A furuncle is an extension of folliculitis and often called a boil. Carbuncles are clusters of infected hairs. *S. aureus* is the most common causative bacteria. A red, firm painful area is the identifying mark. Incision of the point, antibiotics, and pain medications are the treatment choices.

40.3 Fungal Skin Infections

Differentiate the causes, classification, underlying pathogenesis, and clinical manifestations of fungal skin infections and approaches to diagnosis and treatment of these conditions across the lifespan.

- Candidiasis is a condition caused thrush and is caused by *C. albicans*. It is a yeast infection that affects primarily the mouth, throat, folds of skin, lungs, bowel, and vaginal area. There will be a white appearance to the tongue and mouth or a white discharge. Thrush is often caused by antibiotics. Candida is normally not life threatening but can cause sepsis. Medications usually treat the infection but may require 7–10 days.
- Tinea infections are highly contagious and are named according to the area of the body that is affected. A common name for tinea infection is ringworm, though no worm is involved. A common symptom is itching. Tinea infections can be caused by many organisms and usually require treatment with medications.

40.4 Dermititis

Differentiate the causes, classification, underlying pathogenesis, and clinical manifestations of dermatitis and approaches to diagnosis and treatment of these conditions across the lifespan.

- Contact dermatitis is an allergic reaction when an individual directly comes into contact with an allergen or irritant. Many chemicals can cause contact dermatitis; latex is the most common cause in the hospital setting. Itching, redness, swelling and later a rash will typically appear. Contact dermatitis is a type IV hypersensitivity reaction. Avoiding the known allergen is the best plan. If symptoms occur, antihistamines and corticosteroids are used.
- Seborrheic dermatitis (SD) is a chronic skin inflammation that comes and goes. It is called cradle cap, dandruff, psoriasis, and eczema. Exfoliative dermatitis (ED) is a widespread skin inflammation that is caused by preexisting skin disorders, drugs, cancer, or unknown causes. SD causes lesions covered with scales, while ED occurs in patches.
- Urticaria, also known as hives, is welts on the skin that often itch. Causes may be drug related, contact, ingested or inhaled allergens, aquagenic, emotional or physical stimuli, serum sickness, insect bites, transfusion reactions, and certain medical conditions. Urticaria usually disappears by itself, but antihistamines and corticosteroids may be needed for symptom control.
- Lichen planus is an inflammatory disorder of the skin, mouth, nails, scalp, and mucous membranes. The cause is unknown. The condition is not harmful and can have many causes or triggers. The skin will have many flat-topped, reddish to purple firm bumps with symmetrical sides and sharp borders.

40.5 Life-threatening Inflammatory Disorders

Differentiate the causes, classification, underlying pathogenesis, and clinical manifestations of life-threatening inflammatory disorders and approaches to diagnosis and treatment of these conditions across the lifespan.

- Necrotizing fasciitis is a life-threatening skin disorder. It is also known as the "flesh-eating disorder" because it can cause necrosis of the skin. It should be treated rapidly, and management of symptoms includes pain relief. This condition causes intense swelling, redness to the skin, irritation, and immense pain. Surgical excision of the area is usually recommended to prevent gangrene.
- Stevens-Johnson syndrome is a rare skin disorder that causes the epidermis to separate from the dermis. It can be life threatening and has a high mortality rate. Often caused by medications, it is highly unpredictable and often idiopathic.
- Toxic epidermal necrolysis is an inflammation of the skin caused by a poison resulting in necrosis and dissolving of the tissue. It is idiosyncratic, not easily predicted, and a potentially life-threatening, even fatal, dermatologic disorder that is commonly caused by medications or other metabolites.

40.6 Stings and Bites

Differentiate the causes, classification, underlying pathogenesis, and clinical manifestations of insect stings and bites and approaches to diagnosis and treatment of these conditions across the lifespan.

- Wasp and bee stings are common in the United States. Most people feel the sting and may experience redness, swelling, and pain. OTC medications are usually helpful in the treatment. Bees sting one time; a wasp can sting multiple times. The stinger of the bee should be removed carefully. Both insects inject a venom that can cause anaphylaxis if the individual is allergic to the venom. Otherwise, the symptoms are usually treated at home.

- Tick bites are common and can occur anywhere on the body. The bite of a tick is usually minimal with treatable symptoms. However, certain ticks can carry diseases that can become chronic, such as Lyme disease. Swelling, itching, and burning are common symptoms. The tick should be removed without twisting so that the head will come out with the body.

40.7 Disorders Caused by Infestations

Differentiate the causes, classification, underlying pathogenesis, and clinical manifestations of disorders caused by infestations and approaches to diagnosis and treatment of these conditions across the lifespan.

- Pediculosis is a skin disorder caused by lice. Lice infestations usually involve the hairy parts of the body. Lice occupy the hair of the head, body, and pubic areas. Direct contact with someone with lice is usually the mechanism by which the pest is spread. OTC medications are used to kill the mites and live lice and requires retreatment in 7–10 days.
- Scabies is an intense pruritic rash caused by a parasitic mite that burrows in the skin. Lines in the crevices of the skin are usually seen. Small red bumps will appear on the skin, but not every bump is a mite. Scabies are highly contagious and require treatment of the individual, sex partners, and family members and the home environment. The most common symptom is a red rash that is most intense at night, disturbing sleep.
- Bedbugs are ectoparasites that live on human blood. They usually live in rugs, bedding, bed frames, and box springs. They are not a result of poor hygiene or unsanitary conditions. They are usually present where there is a rapid turnover of people using the same furniture. Typical symptoms include a red area that is darker in the middle that may sting or burn. An exterminator may be needed to rid the home of an infestation.

40.8 Disorders Associated with Adolescent/Adult Skin

Differentiate the causes, classification, underlying pathogenesis, and clinical manifestations of disorders associated with adolescent/adult skin and approaches to diagnosis and treatment of these conditions across the lifespan.

- Acne vulgaris is a common rash on the face, nest, chest, or back of adolescents. Although adults can acquire acne, the hormonal changes in adolescents account for the pimples, whiteheads, blackheads, and papules. Treatment by a dermatologist may involve an acne product or an antibiotic.
- Rosacea involves a rash on the face, which turns red with raised bumps and visible blood vessels. In later stages, the skin can thicken, and the nose may broaden, and eyes may become involved. A dermatologist is usually recommended, and rosacea medications or laser/light therapy may be applied.

40.9 Disorders of the Nail

Differentiate the causes, classification, underlying pathogenesis, and clinical manifestations of disorders of the nail and approaches to diagnosis and treatment of these conditions across the lifespan.

- Nails that are brittle are usually a sign of aging. The nail is soft and flexible and may split easily. Moisture and certain disorders of the thyroid are usual causes. Biotin taken for at least 6 months is the recommended treatment.
- Fungal nail infections usually involve one nail of the toes or fingers but may involve more than one. The infection causes the nail to become yellow, green, or black. Yeast, candida, or molds are usually the causative organism. People with conditions such as diabetes and poor circulation are more prone to fungal nail infections. Medications can be oral, topical creams, or a type of polish that is painted on the nail. The condition is hard to cure and may return.
- Trauma to the nail includes splitting, bruising, crushing, removal of the nail, injury from an accident, or smashing it with an object. Treatment may be complete removal of the nail or removal of part of the nail. If the nail can be sutured or treated and saved, the doctor will opt to save the nail. Infections can occur when the nail has been punctured or split. Throbbing pain if blood pools under the nail is the most common symptom.

REVIEW QUESTIONS

1. Which of the following is true about acne vulgaris?
   a. In adulthood, it is more common in men.
   b. Whiteheads are open comedones.
   c. Blackheads are open comedones.
   d. Open comedones lead to inflammatory acne.
2. A 41-year-old woman complains of nails that crack easily. She receives a diagnosis of brittle nails (onychoschizia). The nurse anticipates that an evaluation will be performed for which of the following comorbidities?

a. Thyroid disorder, iron deficiency anemia, and arthritis
b. Iron deficiency anemia, arthritis, and rosacea
c. Arthritis, folate deficiency, and Stevens-Johnson syndrome

3. A new mother brings her newborn baby to the clinic. She is concerned because the baby's scalp is covered with white scales that appear greasy, and the hospital told her that the baby had cradle cap. Nursing education includes telling the mother that:
   a. cradle cap is a serious infection that will require hospitalization for treatment.
   b. this is a rare condition that will require specialist care.
   c. the baby has cradle cap because of unhygienic care in the hospital.
   d. cradle cap is a minor skin condition easily managed with shampoo and topical medication.

4. Your adolescent client has been on sulfonamide antibiotic treatment for a urinary tract infection for the past 4 days. Today, she has returned to the clinic because a burning, painful rash has developed on her face and upper chest. The nurse practitioner diagnosis Stevens-Johnson syndrome and has the nurse make arrangements to admit the child to the hospital. The teen's mother is upset, asking why hospitalization is necessary. How does the nurse respond?
   a. "This is not a simple rash from antibiotic allergy. It can progress to serious skin loss and involvement of the eye, so hospitalization is necessary for appropriate care."
   b. "The rash means that the sulfonamide antibiotic is not working, and her urinary tract infection requires hospital care."
   c. "Hospitalization is necessary because she cannot be cared for properly at home."
   d. "The rash means that she was misdiagnosed and given the wrong medication."

5. A middle-aged woman was brought to the emergency department by ambulance after having been stung by a wasp. Her family called the ambulance because she fainted and had difficulty breathing after the wasp sting. They are wondering why she is having such a severe reaction to a simple wasp sting. The client's history includes having reacted to ant bites with foot swelling and redness several years ago. Which of the following is true?
   a. The client is experiencing anaphylaxis to the wasp sting because she has a known allergy to venom.
   b. The client's previous reaction to the ant bite has nothing to do with her current reaction to the wasp sting.
   c. This type of reaction is minor, and the ambulance wasn't needed.
   d. The client's symptoms are all due to fear of wasps and are purely psychologic.

6. An older nursing home client has just been admitted to the hospital with a diagnosis of cellulitis of the right leg. The client's family asks the nurse why this infection developed and why hospitalization is necessary. Which of the following explanations is appropriate?
   a. "This is the fault of the nursing home for having too little staff and delivering substandard care."
   b. "In older adults, diminished immune function, poor circulation, and skin changes increase the risk for cellulitis."
   c. "Cellulitis is a minor condition and should have been managed in the nursing home."
   d. "The condition probably developed because the client refused her medications."

7. A teenage boy was helping his father fix the deck of their house and accidentally hit his own large toe with a hammer. He is in the emergency department and complains of severe pain. A subungual hematoma has developed. The nurse should anticipate preparing the client for which procedure?
   a. Surgical removal of the nail
   b. Suture repair of the nail
   c. Applying a dressing and then discharge to home
   d. Boring a hole in the nail to release trapped blood

8. A nurse is working at a health insurance help line when a 30-year-old woman calls complaining of hives on her face after dusting her home during spring cleaning. The nurse asks whether this has happened in the past, and the woman remembers it happening the year before. The nurse asks the client whether she is experiencing shortness of breath or lip swelling. The client denies any symptoms other than the hives. The nurse then provides appropriate advice as follows:
   a. "This is serious, and immediate emergency care is needed."
   b. "Hives are a common reaction to inhaled allergens in dust, and the condition may be managed with over-the-counter antihistamines and topical cortisone."
   c. "Hives can turn into infection, and antibiotics will be needed now to prevent this complication."
   d. "Simply keep scratching the hives if they are itchy, and they will resolve faster."

ANSWERS

Answers to Review Questions can be found in Appendix A. Answers to Case Study and Check Your Progress questions are available on the faculty resources site. Please consult with your instructor.

RECOMMENDED WEBSITES

American Academy of Dermatology
https://www.aad.org/public

DermNet New Zealand
https://www.dermnetnz.org

Mayo Clinic: Diseases and Conditions
https://www.mayoclinic.org/diseases-conditions

Merck Manuals: Skin Disorders
https://www.merckmanuals.com/home/skin-disorders

REFERENCES

1. Raph, A., & Kroshinsky, D. (2016). Cellulitis: A review. *JAMA, 316*(3), 325–337.
2. Mayo Clinic Staff. (2015). *Cellulitis*. Available at http://www.mayoclinic.org/diseases-conditions/cellulitis/basics/definition/con-20023471
3. Dhar, A. D. (n.d.). Cellulitis. *Merck manual: Consumer version*. Available at http://www.merckmanuals.com/home/skin-disorders/bacterial-skin-infections/cellulitis
4. LeMone, P., Burke, K., Bauldoff, G., & Gubrud, P. (2015). *Medical-surgical nursing: Clinical reasoning in patient care*. Hoboken, NJ: Pearson.
5. Adams, M., & Urban, C. (2016). *Pharmacology: Connections to nursing practice* (3rd ed.). Upper Saddle River, NJ: Pearson.
6. Lewis, L. S. (2016). Impetigo. *EMedicineHealth*. Available at http://emedicine.medscape.com/article/965254-overview#a2
7. American Academy of Pediatrics. (2015). *Impetigo*. Available at https://www.healthychildren.org/English/health-issues/conditions/skin/Pages/Impetigo.aspx
8. Satter, E. K. (2017). Folliculitis. *EMedicineHealth*. Available at http://emedicine.medscape.com/article/1070456-overview#a6
9. Medline Plus. (2016). *Folliculitis*. Available at https://medlineplus.gov/ency/article/000823.htm
10. Jalalat, S., Hunter, L., Yamazaki, M., Head, E., & Kelly, B. (2014). An outbreak of candida albicans folliculitis masquerading as Malassezia folliculitis in a prison population. *Journal of Correctional Health Care, 20*(2), 154–162.
11. Mayo Clinic Staff. (2014). *Folliculitis*. Available at http://www.mayoclinic.org/diseases-conditions/folliculitis/basics/definition/con-20025909
12. Miquel-Gomez, L., Vano-Galvan, S., Perez-Garcia, B., Carrillo-Gijon, R., & Jaen-Olasoio, P. (2015). Treatment of folliculitis decalvans with photodynamic therapy: Results in 10 patients. *Journal of the American Academy of Dermatology, 72*(6), 1085–1087.
13. Dhar, A. D. (2017). Furuncles and carbuncles. *Merck manual: Professional version*. Available at http://www.merckmanuals.com/professional/dermatologic-disorders/bacterial-skin-infections/furuncles-and-carbuncles
14. Mayo Clinic Staff. (2017). Boils and carbuncles. Available at http://www.mayoclinic.org/diseases-conditions/boils-and-carbuncles/home/ovc-20214754
15. Centers for Disease Control and Prevention. (2017). *Candidiasis*. Available at https://www.cdc.gov/fungal/diseases/candidiasis
16. Hildalgo, J. A. (2016). Candidiasis. *Medscape*. Available at http://emedicine.medscape.com/article/213853-overview#a5
17. Revankar, S. G., & Sobel, J. D. (2014). Candidiasis (invasive). In *Merck manual: Professional version*. Available at http://www.merckmanuals.com/professional/infectious-diseases/fungi/candidiasis-invasive
18. University of Maryland Medical Center. (2015). *Candidiasis*. Available at http://umm.edu/health/medical/altmed/condition/candidiasis
19. MedlinePlus. (2017). Tinea infections. Available at https://medlineplus.gov/tineainfections.html
20. American Academy of Pediatrics. (2015). *Tinea infections (ringworm, athlete's foot, jock itch)*. Available at https://www.healthychildren.org/English/health-issues/conditions/skin/Pages/Tinea-Infections-Ringworm-Athletes-Foot-Jock-Itch.aspx
21. American Osteopathic College of Dermatology. (2016). *Fungus infections*. Available at http://www.aocd.org/?page=FungusInfections
22. University of Maryland Medical Center. (2016). *Dermatitis*. Available at https://www.umm.edu/health/medical/altmed/condition/dermatitis
23. Hogan, D., & James, W. (2016). Allergic contact dermatitis. *Medscape*. Available at https://www.emedicine.medscape.com/article/1049216
24. Occupational Safety & Health Administration. (2017). Latex allergy. Available at https://www.osha.gov/SLTC/etools/hospital/hazards/latex/latex.html
25. Handler, M.Z.. (2017). Seborrheic dermatitis. *Medscape*. Available at http://emedicine.medscape.com/article/1108312-overview
26. Vearrier, D. (2017). Exfoliative dermatitis. *Medscape*. Available at http://emedicine.medscape.com/article/762236-overview
27. American Academy of Dermatology. (2017). *Hives*. Available at https://www.aad.org/public/diseases/itchy-skin/hives
28. Page, E. (2016). Urticaria (hives; wheals). In *Merck manual: Professional version*. Available at https://www.merckmanuals.com/professional/dermatologic-disorders/approach-to-the-dermatologic-patient/urticaria
29. American College of Allergy, Asthma, and Immunology. (2014). *Hives (urticaria)*. Available at http://acaai.org/allergies/types/skin-allergies/hives-urticaria
30. Mayo Clinic Staff. (2017). *Lichen planus*. Available at http://www.mayoclinic.org/diseases-conditions/lichen-planus/home/ovc-20188519
31. March of Dimes. (2014). Isotretinoin and other retinoids during pregnancy. Available at http://www.marchofdimes.org/pregnancy/isotretinoin-and-other-retinoids-during-pregnancy.aspx
32. Centers for Disease Control and Prevention. (2017). *Necrotizing fasciitis: A rare disease, especially for the healthy*. Available at http://www.cdc.gov/features/necrotizingfasciitis
33. Dhar. D. (2017). Necrotizing subcutaneous infection (necrotizing cellulitis or fasciitis). *Merck manual: Professional version*. Available at http://www.merckmanuals.com/

professional/dermatologic-disorders/bacterial-skin-infections/necrotizing-subcutaneous-infection
34. Oakley, A. (2017). Stevens Johnson syndrome/toxic epidermal necrolysis. *DermNet New Zealand*. Available at www.dermnetnz.org/topics/stevens-johnson-syndrome-toxic-epidermal-necrolysis
35. Mayo Clinic Staff. (2017). *Stevens-Johnson syndrome*. Available at http://www.mayoclinic.org/diseases-conditions/stevens-johnson-syndrome/basics/definition/con-20029623
36. Harris, V., Jackson, C., & Cooper, A. (2016). Review of toxic epidermal necrolysis. *International Journal of Molecular Sciences, 17*(12), 2135.
37. Cohen, V. (2016). Toxic epidermal necrolysis. *Medscape*. Available at emedicine.medscape.com/article/229698-overview
38. eMedicineHealth. (2017). *Bee and wasp stings*. Available at www.emedicinehealth.com/bee_and_wasp_stings/article_em.htm#bee_and_wasp_stings_overview
39. Roth, E. (2017). Wasp stings: Reaction, symptoms, and treatment. *Healthline*. www.healthline.com/health/wasp-sting#Overview1
40. Centers for Disease Control and Prevention. (2017). *Ticks*. Available at https://www.cdc.gov/ticks/index.html
41. MedlinePlus. (2017). *Tick bites*. Available at https://medlineplus.gov/tickbites.html
42. Dowshen, S. (2014). First aid: Tick bites. *KidsHealth*. Available at kidshealth.org/en/parents/tick-bites-sheet.html
43. Centers for Disease Control and Prevention. (2017). *Lyme disease*. Available at https://www.cdc.gov/lyme/index.html
44. Centers for Disease Control and Prevention. (2017). *Rocky mountain spotted fever (RMSF)*. Available at https://www.cdc.gov/rmsf/index.html
45. Bergen, T. (2017). Pubic lice infestation. *Healthline*. Available at www.healthline.com/health/std/pubic-lice
46. Centers for Disease Control and Prevention. (2017). *Parasites: Lice*. Available at https://www.cdc.gov/parasites/lice/head/epi.html
47. Sullivan, D. (2017). Body lice infestation. *Healthline*. Available at www.healthline.com/health/body-lice#Overview1
48. DeVore, C. D., & Schutze, G. E. (2015). Head lice. *Pediatrics*, 135(5). Available at http://pediatrics.aappublications.org/content/135/5/e1355
49. Mayo Center Staff. (2015). *Scabies*. Available at www.mayoclinic.org/diseases-conditions/scabies/basics/definition/con-20023488
50. MedlinePlus. (2017). *Scabies*. Available at https://medlineplus.gov/scabies.html
51. Stöppler, M. C. (2016). What is "Norwegian scabies"? *MedicineNet.com*. Available at http://www.medicinenet.com/what_is_norwegian_scabies/views.htm
52. American Academy of Dermatology. (2017). *Scabies: Overview*. Available at https://www.aad.org/public/diseases/contagious-skin-diseases/scabies
53. MedlinePlus. (2017). Lindane. Available at https://medlineplus.gov/druginfo/meds/a682651.html
54. Mayo Clinic Staff. (2017). *Bedbugs*. Available at www.mayoclinic.org/diseases-conditions/bedbugs/basics/definition/con-20026119
55. Rao, J., & James, W. (2016). Acne vulgaris. *Medscape*. Available at emedicine.medscape.com/article/1069804-overview
56. Mayo Clinic Staff. (2017). *Rosacea*. Available at http://www.mayoclinic.org/diseases-conditions/rosacea/home/ovc-20235169
57. International Rosacea Foundation. (2017). *Adult acne rosacea*. Available at www.international rosaceafoundation.org/acne_factor.php
58. Stöppler, M. C. (2017). Brittle nails. *MedicineNet*. Available at www.medicinenet.com/brittle_nails/symptoms.htm
59. MedlinePlus. (2015). *Nail abnormalities*. Available at https://medlineplus.gov/ency/article/003247.htm
60. Khan, A., & Dock, E. (2015). Fungal nail infection. *Healthline*. Available at www.healthline.com/health/fungal-nail-infection#Overview1
61. MedlinePlus. (2017). *Nail injuries*. Available at https://medlineplus.gov/ency/patientinstructions/000800.htm
62. Rehmus, W. (2017). Fingernail and toenail injury. *Merck manual: Consumer version*. Available at https://www.merckmanuals.com/home/skin-disorders/nail-disorders/fingernail-and-toenail-injury

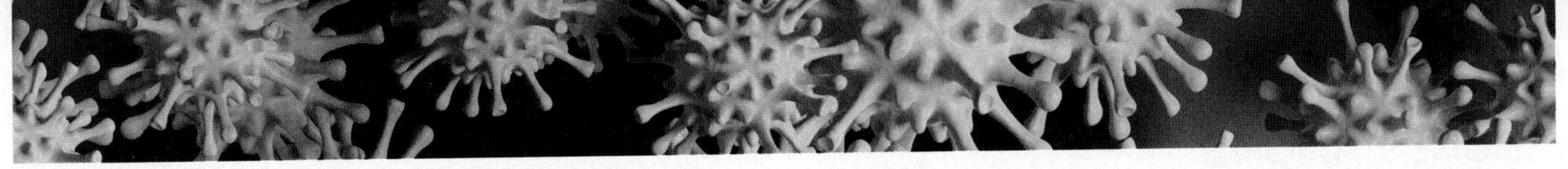

Chapter 41

Chronic Skin Disorders

Patricia Caudle

Chapter Outline and Learning Outcomes

41.1 Chapter Overview and Case Studies

Differentiate acute from chronic skin conditions and describe concepts related to chronic disorders of the skin.

41.2 Viral Skin Infections

Differentiate the causes, classification, underlying pathogenesis, and clinical manifestations of viral skin infections and approaches to diagnosis and treatment for those conditions across the lifespan.

41.3 Skin Disorders with a Genetic Basis

Differentiate the causes, classification, underlying pathogenesis, and clinical manifestations of skin disorders with a genetic basis and approaches to diagnosis and treatment for those conditions across the lifespan.

41.4 Benign Neoplasms of the Skin

Differentiate the causes, classification, underlying pathogenesis, and clinical manifestations of benign neoplasms of the skin and approaches to diagnosis and treatment for those conditions across the lifespan.

41.5 Skin Cancer

Differentiate the causes, classification, underlying pathogenesis, and clinical manifestations of skin cancer and approaches to diagnosis and treatment for those conditions across the lifespan.

41.6 Changes in Pigmentation of the Skin

Differentiate the causes, classification, underlying pathogenesis, and clinical manifestations of changes in pigmentation of the skin and approaches to diagnosis and treatment for those conditions across the lifespan.

41.7 Disorders of the Hair and Scalp

Differentiate the causes, classification, underlying pathogenesis, and clinical manifestations of disorders of the hair and scalp and approaches to diagnosis and treatment for those conditions across the lifespan.

KEY TERMS

Acrochordons, 1025
Actinic keratosis (AK), 1024
Alopecia areata (AA), 1033
Anagen, 1033
Anogenital herpes, 1013
Atopic dermatitis (AD), 1018
Atypia, 1017
Autoinoculation, 1014
Basal cell carcinoma (BCC), 1027
Café au lait macules or spots (CALMs), 1031
Catagen, 1033
Dermatome, 1013
Dermatosis, 1024
Dysuria, 1014
Eczema, 1018
Eczematous, 1018
Epidermal inclusion cysts (EICs), 1027
Excoriations, 1018
Exogen, 1033
Exudative, 1019
Flare-up, 1018
Hemangiomas, 1025
Herpes labialis, 1013
Herpes simplex virus (HSV), 1013
Herpes zoster (HZ), 1015
Hidradenitis suppurativa (HS), 1021
Hyperkeratosis, 1022
Hyperplasia, 1022
Incubation period, 1014
Lichenification, 1018
Lipoma, 1026
Melanoma, 1029
Moles, 1025
Nevi, 1025
Paresthesias, 1014
Photodermatitis, 1024
Phototherapy, 1021
Plaques, 1020
Prodrome, 1014
Pruritus, 1018
Psoriasis, 1019
Skin tags, 1025
Solar lentigo, 1031
Squamous cell carcinoma (SCC), 1028
Telangiectases, 1027
Telogen, 1033
Teratogenic, 1021
Urticaria, 1024
Vesicles, 1014
Vitiligo, 1030
Warts, 1016
Xerosis, 1018

ABBREVIATIONS

AA—alopecia areata
AD—atopic dermatitis
AK—actinic keratosis
AT—alopecia totalis
AU—alopecia universalis
BCC—basal cell carcinoma
CALMs—café au lait macules or spots
DFA—direct fluorescent antibody testing
EICs—epidermal inclusion cysts
HS—hidradenitis suppurativa
HPV—human papillomavirus
HSV—herpes simplex virus
HZ—herpes zoster or shingles
IL—interleukin
MRSA—methicillin-resistant *Staphylococcus aureus*
PCR—polymerase chain reaction
PHN—postherpetic neuralgia
PMLE—polymorphous light eruptions
PUVA—psoralen plus ultraviolet A light
SCC—squamous cell carcinoma
TNF—tumor necrosis factor
TYR—gene that encodes tyrosinase; associated with vitiligo
UV—ultraviolet light
VZV—varicella-zoster virus

41.1 Chapter Overview and Case Studies

Unlike acute skin conditions that respond readily to treatment and are short lived, chronic skin conditions are long-term, relapsing disorders that may or may not resolve. In this chapter, chronic skin disorders are the focus. Selected chronic skin disorders included in this chapter may be caused by viral infection, abnormal immune responses, or genetic changes. In addition, benign neoplasms, skin cancers, changes in pigmentation, and disorders of the hair and scalp are included.

Concepts Related to Chronic Skin Disorders

Chronic skin disorders may result from viral infections that challenge the immune system or from alterations in immunity and genetic susceptibility to autoimmune disease. The immune system alterations occur in both the cell-mediated and the humoral immune systems, ultimately causing chronic dermatologic disorders such as atopic dermatitis, hidradenosis suppurativa, psoriasis, vitiligo, or alopecia areata. These conditions are not often life threatening but the inflammation that results from changes in the immune system cause itching, pain, and disfigurement that result in loss of sleep, lower self-esteem, and depression (**Figure 41.1**).

Case Studies

The following cases are addressed throughout the chapter to assist in application of chapter content to clinical situations that involve individuals with chronic skin disorders.

Jessica Kimberlain: Introduction

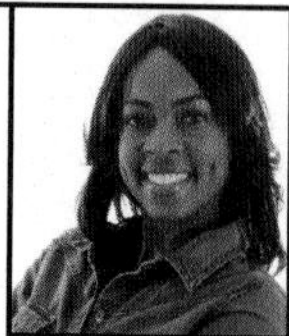

Jessica Kimberlain, age 25, is in Miami for her 2-week honeymoon. She has come to the clinic because she has developed a painful rash on her vulva and she is unable to urinate because of the pain. Ms. Kimberlain has always been healthy, not even a "cold sore" in her history. She tells the advanced practice registered nurse (APRN) that she has had three sexual partners in her lifetime, including her new husband, Richard. She and Richard have been going together for about a year and had decided together not to have sex until they were married.

Richard, age 27, tells the APRN that he had one episode of genital herpes at age 17, after his first sexual encounter. He has never had a recurrence or any other sexually transmitted infection. He denies any visible lesions on his genitals or any systemic symptoms.

1. Given that Jessica has had three sexual partners in her lifetime, would you consider her presenting symptoms to be part of an acute or chronic condition? Why?
2. Does Richard's single episode of genital herpes at age 17 make him the most likely source of Jessica's current symptoms? Why or why not?

Karen McKendrick: Introduction

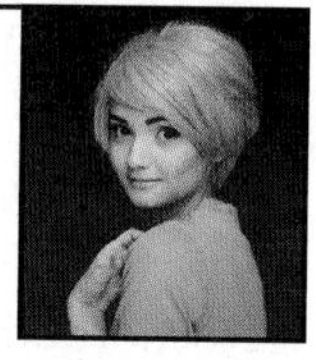

Karen McKendrick, age 25, is a fashion model who has moderate to severe plaque psoriasis. She was diagnosed when she was 17. Her mother, Jane, age 45, also has psoriasis and recently developed psoriatic arthritis. Jane has aided her daughter in developing self-help skills that have helped to keep the psoriasis under control so that she could pursue her modeling career. However, about 6 months ago, Ms. McKendrick experienced a sudden worsening of the psoriasis that was worse than any she had ever had.

1. What characteristics of Ms. McKendrick's plaque psoriasis classify it as a chronic condition?
2. Under which category of etiology would Ms. McKendrick's plaque psoriasis be listed? Why?

Check Your Progress: Section 41.1

1. What are the most common causes for chronic skin disorders?
2. Give three examples of chronic dermatologic disorders.
3. Regardless of the skin disorder, what are the most common symptoms experienced by patients?

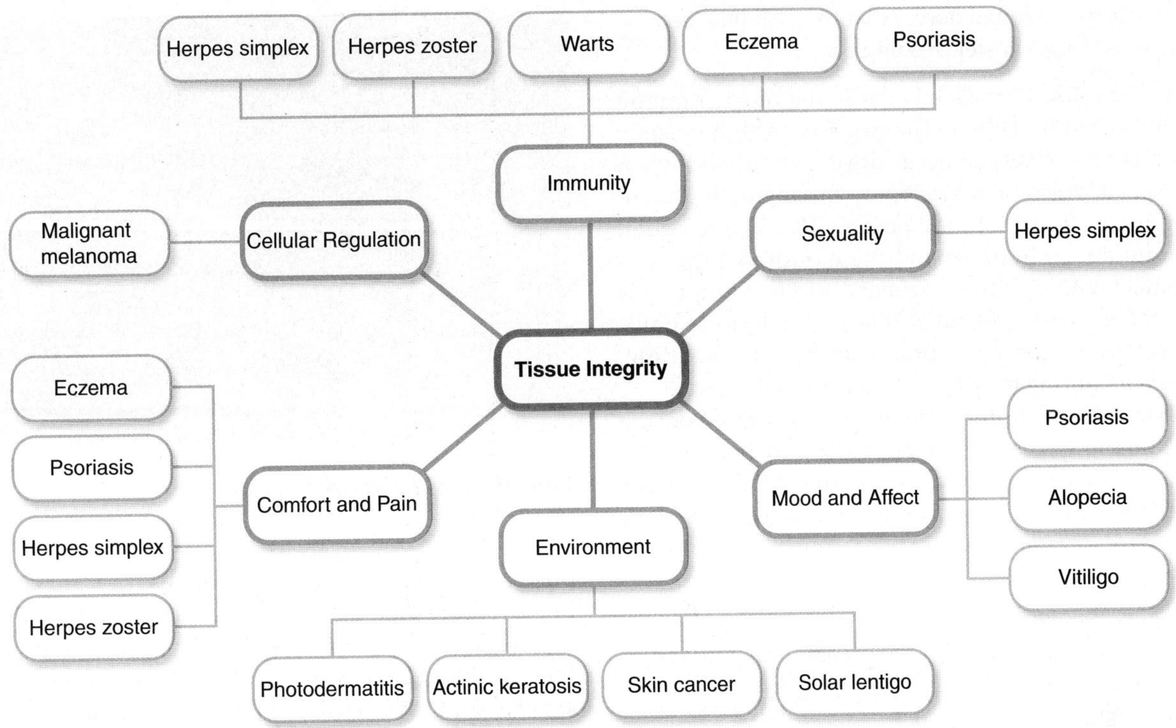

Figure 41.1 ■ Concepts related to chronic skin disorders.

41.2 Viral Skin Infections

There are many viruses that cause skin manifestations, but only a few that will cause chronic skin conditions. The focus of this section is on the most common chronic viral skin infections, including those caused by herpes simplex virus, varicella-zoster virus, and human papillomavirus. These chronic skin conditions may affect persons in any age group. Some of the lesions are disfiguring and benign whereas others may lead to oropharyngeal and anogenital cancers.

Herpes Simplex Virus Types 1 and 2

Herpes simplex virus (HSV) is a common infection of the skin and mucous membranes. The most common lesion caused by herpes simplex virus type 1 (HSV-1) is **herpes labialis** (herpes infection of the lips; cold sores), although it can cause infections in several different areas of the body. Herpes simplex virus type 2 (HSV-2) causes most **anogenital herpes** (herpes infection of the genitals, perineum, or anus) infection that is sexually transmitted. While HSV-1 is more likely to cause "cold sores," there are a growing number of HSV-2 infections in these areas. HSV-2 is less likely to cause recurrent outbreaks in or around the mouth.[1] Other nonoral and nongenital HSV-1 infections include herpetic keratitis (infection of the eye), herpetic whitlow (lesions on the digits or hands), herpes gladiatorum (infection on the torso of wrestlers), and herpetic sycosis (infection of the follicles of the beard).

HSV-1 infection is usually contracted during childhood and recurrences persist into old age. Based on United States population data, about 57.7 per 100,000 persons have serum antibodies of HSV-1.[1] HSV-2 is more likely to be contracted in adolescence or young adulthood via sexual contact. It is estimated that 1 in 6 adolescents and adults of both genders are infected with HSV-2.[2] HSV-2 is considered the fifth most common occurring sexually transmitted infection in the United States.[2]

Etiology and Pathogenesis

HSV-1 and HSV-2 are viruses. Viruses are intracellular parasites that contain cellular materials needed for survival in the host. Viruses require host cell nucleus materials in order to replicate. (Review Chapter 13 for the characteristics of viruses.) HSV-1 and HSV-2 are herpesviruses, part of a family of large DNA viruses that are covered by a glycoprotein coat that helps them attach to a host cell.[3] It is the glycoprotein G surrounding HSV that activates the formation of antibodies via the humoral immune system.[4] The preferred host cells for HSV are neurons and epidermal and dermal cells that either do not divide or are slow to replicate. The virus enters the skin or mucous membrane via a microscopic tear and travels to a sensory root ganglion where it becomes a dormant and permanent resident.[1] When triggered by forces that affect the cell-mediated immune system, the virus will be activated and will travel from the neuron to the skin that the neuron innervates. There the virus will enter the dermal and epidermal cells and replicate, causing a recurrent outbreak of the rash. It is because HSV-1 and HSV-2 cause a vesicular rash that erupts in a **dermatome** (area of skin innervated by a single sensory spinal nerve) that the rash may be misdiagnosed as herpes zoster or shingles.

Herpes Labialis. Herpes labialis is the most common infection caused by HSV-1. The primary or first-episode infection is most likely to occur during childhood when the virus is acquired via kissing or sharing eating utensils or linens with an infected person. This first infection erupts into a rash in or around the mouth in 2–20 days after contact with the virus.[1] Primary infection eruption is usually the most severe and will last from 10 to 14 days. The infection is most contagious during viral shedding, which occurs during the first 60–96 hours of infection.[1]

Recurrent eruption of the lesions occurs when the host's immune system is suppressed or may be triggered by stress, fever, sun exposure, or trauma.[1] Oral infections emerge from the trigeminal sensory ganglia and recur from one to six times a year.[1] Recurrent outbreaks are shorter and less severe.

The primary concern with recurrent herpes labialis among older adults is the spread of the virus from the lip lesion to the eyes or genitals, called **autoinoculation** (self-infection). ■

Genital Herpes. Genital herpes is more likely to be caused by HSV-2, although the incidence of cases caused by HSV-1 is increasing among adolescents and young adult females.[4] HSV-2 is spread via oral, vaginal, or anal sexual contact with an individual who is shedding the virus.[2] The virus enters via a small laceration in the skin or mucous membrane, causing the primary outbreak. The **incubation period** (time between contracting the virus and appearance of symptoms) is 2–12 days, with an average of 4 days. Anogenital herpes will move to the sacral ganglion and reside there in a dormant state.[1]

Many individuals have asymptomatic HSV-2. That is, the serum antibody is present, but the individual has never had symptoms. It is important to recognize that periodic viral shedding may occur even when there are no skin lesions.[2]

Like herpes labialis, a recurrence of genital herpes may be brought on by stress, trauma, fever, ultraviolet light exposure, or immunosuppression. Recurrent outbreaks of the lesions are shorter and less severe than the primary outbreaks. Interestingly, recurrences of genital herpes are more likely if caused by HSV-2.

Women with primary genital infection with HSV-1 or HSV-2 at the time of birth have a 57% risk for transmitting the virus to the neonate.[4] Although rare, neonatal herpes has a high mortality rate. Infants who survive neurologic or disseminated herpes are severely affected. ■

Clinical Manifestations

Both HSV-1 and HSV-2 primary infection will usually begin with a **prodrome** (an early set of symptoms that may indicate the start of disease before specific symptoms appear) of fever or flu-like symptoms. This is followed by the eruption of painful **vesicles** (small, fluid-filled sacs or blisters) on a red, swollen area of skin or mucous membrane (**Figure 41.2** ■). The regional lymph nodes will swell. The lesions open, leaving painful ulcers. The ulcers will then crust and begin to heal.[1,2] Many individuals will have asymptomatic herpes or a mild fever that they think is flu and no lesions. Primary genital herpes may cause **dysuria** (painful urination) and the pain will cause urinary retention, especially in women.[4]

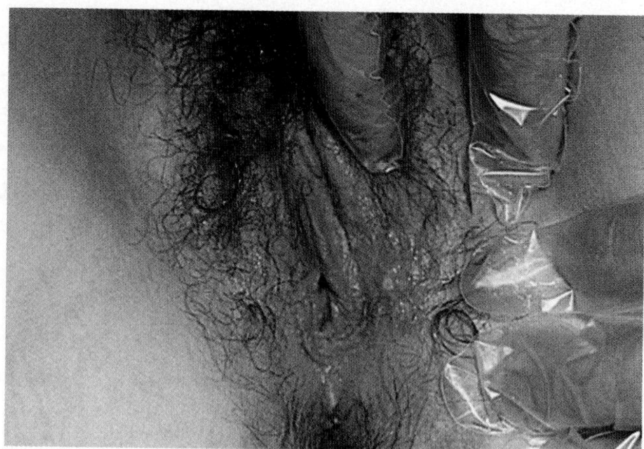

Figure 41.2 ■ Genital herpes simplex.

Recurrent herpes outbreaks will have a prodrome of pain, itching or **paresthesias** (tingling, prickling, or burning, or "pins and needles" felt after a limb "goes to sleep"). The vesicles on the red base appear in the same area as the primary outbreak according to the ganglion where it has been residing. The vesicles will become ulcers and crust more rapidly than in the primary infection and will heal in about a week.[1]

Jessica Kimberlain: Application

Ms. Kimberlain's vital signs are: pulse 60, respirations 14, temperature 101.3°F (38.5°C), blood pressure 110/70.

Chest and heart examinations are normal. Abdominal examination is negative except for a full bladder and right inguinal lymphadenopathy. Her right vulva is swollen, red, and there are several vesicles and small ulcers on the vulva and at the introitus near the urinary meatus.

A pregnancy test is negative and the herpes simplex virus/polymerase chain reaction (HSV PCR) is positive for genital herpes. The CBC is normal except for increased lymphocytes. Electrolytes show mild dehydration.

The diagnosis is first-episode genital herpes, urinary retention, and dehydration. Ms. Kimberlain is admitted for catheterization, IV fluids, and 24-hour observation. Her medications include valacyclovir (an antiviral medication) 1 g orally twice a day for 10 days, 1000 mL lactated Ringer's every 8 hours (to replace fluids and electrolytes lost to dehydration; to flush the bladder), and Toradol 30 mg IM every 4 to 6 hours prn for pain. The nurses are also instructed to keep track of fluid intake and output, offer cool compresses for the vulva, and provide lukewarm sitz baths (a shallow bath for cleansing the perineum).

On admission, the nurse notices that Ms. Kimberlain looks sad and withdrawn. Her husband is with her and is very attentive and loving. She is not responding to him until the nurse is preparing to place the catheter. Ms. Kimberlain turns to her husband and tells him to go back to the hotel and leave her alone.

3. Besides the positive HSV PCR test result, what clinical findings for Jessica are consistent with the presence of genital herpes?
4. What is the primary reason for the use of valacyclovir in treating Jessica's genital herpes?

Linking Pathophysiology to Diagnosis and Treatment

Diagnosis of many herpes simplex lesions can be done clinically, based on patient history and observation of the lesions. If there is a question about the diagnosis, or if a partner of an asymptomatic person develops the infection, then there are laboratory tests that help diagnose the condition. Viral culture taken from opened vesicles is a very accurate test during the time that the lesions are vesicular or ulcerative. Viral culture is limited, however, by the short amount of time the virus sheds and the low number of viral particles that can be obtained as the lesions heal or during recurrent outbreaks.[2] It takes at least 48 hours for results from culture.

Antigen testing (microscopic examination of fluid from lesions for antigens, such as glycoprotein G, found on the viral cells) is more rapid than culture, taking only 2–12 hours for results. There are more false positives (positive test results that are inaccurate) with this test than other options.[2,5] Direct fluorescent antibody (DFA) testing (cells obtained from the lesion are stained with antibodies and a dye that sticks to the viral cell antigen and causes it to glow when viewed with a special microscope) is used both to diagnose HSV and to distinguish between HSV-1 and HSV-2.[2] This test takes 2–3 hours to perform. Polymerase chain reaction (PCR) assays (technique for reproducing DNA or RNA from minute quantities of DNA or RNA) for HSV DNA are very sensitive and specific. PCR tests are used for testing lesions and is the preferred test for finding HSV in spinal fluid.[2] These tests can also be used to detect asymptomatic viral shedding.[5]

Serologic tests are blood tests used to detect antibodies to HSV that develop in response to the viral antigen. These antibodies take several weeks to develop, but will persist over a lifetime. Specific serologic tests can be used to detect antibodies specific to HSV-1 and HSV-2. These tests are most useful when there are recurrent lesions with negative culture results, a sexual partner with primary herpes, or as part of an evaluation of persons with other sexually transmitted disorders.[2]

Antiviral mediations are used to control symptoms, but do not cure the disease. Antivirals such as acyclovir, valacyclovir, and famciclovir are used to shorten duration and decrease the severity of primary and recurrent outbreaks. They work best when started within the first 72 hours of the symptoms. Antivirals are also used to suppress recurrent episodes.[2]

Pain or itching of the lesions can be alleviated with oral analgesics such as acetaminophen or ibuprofen. Topical application of cool compresses will soothe the burning pain of the rash. Sitz baths are recommended for women with genital herpes who are having difficulty urinating. The bath will dilute urine and decrease the burning when the urine touches the lesions.

Jessica Kimberlain: Outcome

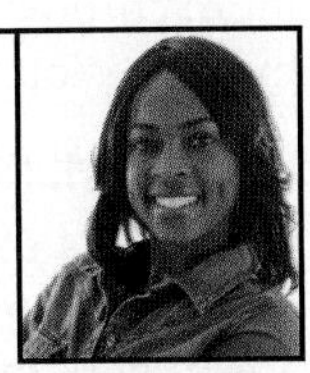

Ms. Kimberlain is able to urinate and is feeling much better 24 hours later so she is discharged with instructions to continue the valacyclovir and return to the clinic in 3 days, sooner if she begins to feel worse instead of better. She is scheduled for education and counseling concerning genital herpes as a chronic, recurring disorder. Reassurance that stress reduction and a healthy lifestyle can help control recurrences are explained. Planned pregnancy with good outcomes is possible for the Kimberlains with good obstetric care. Ms. Kimberlain and her husband have made peace with each other and have been talking but continue to have issues to resolve. Their minister or a marriage counselor is recommended.

5. Does the use of antiviral medications such as valacyclovir cure Mrs. Kimberlain of her genital herpes? Why or why not?
6. What measures can Mrs. Kimberlain take to decrease the recurrence of genital herpes?

Herpes Zoster

Herpes zoster (HZ) or *shingles* is a chronic viral skin condition caused by the varicella-zoster virus (VZV), the same virus that causes chickenpox. HZ affects about 1 million people per year in the United States.[6] The incidence is higher in adults 60 years or older where 10 cases per 1,000 population has been reported.[6] It is estimated that 1 in 3 people in the United States will develop HZ in their lifetime.[6] HZ cases are increasing in the United States and around the world. One theory for the reason for this increase is that more people are living longer and there is a larger pool of individuals over age 40 who have had chickenpox. One population study revealed that 99% of adults 40 years and older who were studied had serum antibodies specific for VZV.[7]

Etiology and Pathogenesis

VZV is a member of the herpesvirus family. It is a large DNA virus enveloped by a glycoprotein coat.[3] The first infection with this virus will cause chickenpox, a disease marked by fever and the eruption of a skin rash. Each lesion will have viral particles that will move to the sensory dorsal-root ganglia or a cranial nerve and become dormant for life.[8] Cell-mediated immunity prevents the virus from reactivation in the form of HZ.[7] As a person ages, cell-mediated immunity decreases, thereby increasing the risk for reactivation of VZV in the form of HZ.[6–8] HZ occurs when latent VZV is reactivated in a cranial nerve or dorsal-root ganglia and spreads via the sensory nerve to the dermatome and is released into the skin where it replicates and produces the painful rash.[7] The most frequently affected dermatomes are the thoracic, trigeminal, lumbar, and cervical dermatomes.[8]

Children who contract VZV in utero or during the first months after birth are at risk for HZ during childhood or adolescence.[8] ■

The primary risk factor for HZ is age. Other risk factors include female gender, white race, immunocompromise, psychologic or physiologic stress, trauma, immunosuppressant drugs, family history, and comorbidities (two or more chronic diseases present at the same time) such as hypertension, diabetes, and hyperlipidemia.[7,8]

Clinical Manifestations

Shingles is usually preceded by a prodrome of malaise, fever, chills, myalgia, headache, or nausea. In addition, the area where the rash will erupt will tingle, itch, burn, feel numb, or be painful or very sensitive to touch.[7,8] This prodromal pain may be severe, and depending on its location it may cause misdiagnosis. For instance, pain in a thoracic dermatome may lead to tests for myocardial infarction.

The rash of HZ begins as macules and papules on erythematous base and progresses to vesicles spread over the dermatome. All the vesicles do not erupt at once. The rash is usually on one side of the body or head in one or, less often, more than one dermatome (**Figure 41.3** ■). The vesicles will open then crust. The shedding or the VZV peaks at the time the vesicles rupture. Usually these very painful skin lesions resolve in 10–15 days, although some individuals will have the shingles for as long as a month.[6,8]

CLINICAL POINT: If the ophthalmic division of the trigeminal nerve is affected, then the eye will become inflamed and vision may be compromised. Vesicles on the tip of the nose indicate HZ ophthalmicus, an emergency condition requiring ophthalmologist care.[7,8] ■

Another cranial nerve that may be affected is the facial nerve (CN7). This will cause Ramsay-Hunt syndrome or HZ oticus. Symptoms include severe ear pain, one-sided facial muscle paralysis, and rash on the external ear or tympanic membrane.[7] This condition needs to be treated promptly to decrease the risk of hearing loss or permanent facial weakness.

The most common complication of HZ is postherpatic neuralgia (PHN). This is severe pain and sensitivity at the site of the rash that persists for more than a month after the rash erupts.[6–8] Other complications of HZ include transient ischemic attack (TIA), stroke, encephalitis, aseptic meningitis, chronic eye disorders, bacterial superinfection of the lesions, cranial or peripheral nerve palsies (paralysis accompanied by involuntary tremors), pneumonitis, hepatitis, and retinal necrosis. Persons who are immunocompromised are more likely to have the more severe complications.[6–8]

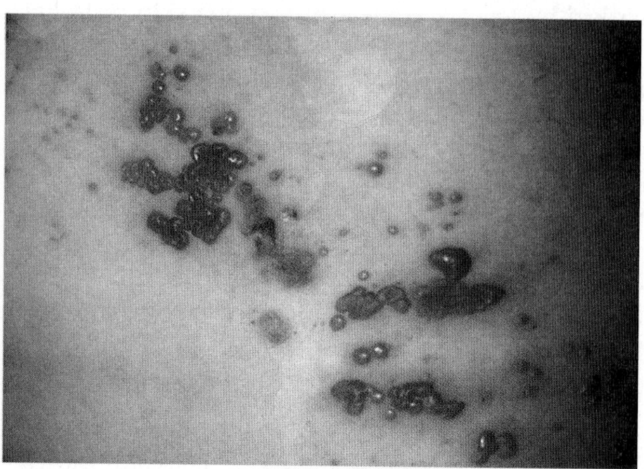

Figure 41.3 ■ Shingles (herpes zoster).

Linking Pathophysiology to Diagnosis and Treatment

Most cases of HZ can be diagnosed based on the patient's history and physical examination, especially after the rash appears. Atypical rashes or rashes that recur more than three times may require laboratory testing to differentiate the viral cause. Direct immunofluorescent assay for VZV antigen or PCR assay for VZV DNA in cells from the lesions are sensitive and specific tests for VZV. Of the two, PCR is considered the most reliable.[7]

Treatment for HZ begins with antiviral therapy, especially with valacyclovir and famciclovir, the most bioavailable of the antivirals. Antiviral therapy will shorten the duration, decrease the formation of new lesions, and decrease the severity of HZ if started within 72 hours of the first lesions.[7,8] Antivirals started later may benefit patients over age 50, patients with continued new lesion formation, and any patient with skin, motor, neurologic, or ocular complications.[7] There is no evidence that antiviral mediations will prevent postherpetic neuraligia (PHN).

Some clinicians will treat HZ by adding glucocorticoids such as prednisone in an effort to decrease pain and hasten healing in patients over 50 years old who have no contraindications such as diabetes, peptic ulcer, or osteoporosis. There is no evidence that the addition of this drug will hasten healing or prevent PHN.[7,8]

The pain may be treated with over-the-counter analgesics such as acetaminophen or ibuprofen. If the pain is severe, prescription analgesics will be needed. The rash can be soothed with cool compresses soaked in water mixed in equal parts with white vinegar.[9]

Warts

Warts are common skin lesions caused by a variety of human papillomavirus (HPV) types. Warts may occur anywhere on the skin or mucous membranes, including the mouth, upper respiratory system of a newborn, genitals, perineum, and anorectal areas. Most lesions caused by HPV are benign; however, there are HPV types that are linked to dysplasia (abnormal cell growth or development; earliest form of precancerous lesion) and cancer.

Common cutaneous warts occur most often in children and teens, but they are not a reportable disease in the United States.[10] Genital HPV, however, is considered the most frequently occurring sexually transmitted infection in the United States.[11] It is estimated that about 79 million Americans are infected with at least one type of genital HPV type.[12] Approximately 33,200 individuals develop HPV-associated cancers in the United States.[13] It is thought that HPV in combination with tobacco or alcohol causes about 90% of cervical and anal cancers, 70% of vaginal and vulvar cancers, 60% of penile cancers, and 70% of oropharyngeal cancers.[13] Genital HPV is covered in detail in Chapter 49, Sexually Transmitted Infections.

Etiology and Pathogenesis

Human papillomavirus is in the *Papillomaviridae* family of double-stranded DNA viruses.[14] Over 100 HPV types that have been identified; however, knowing the type does not change the treatment for warts or their sequelae.[15] HPV is very specific to humans and does not infect other species. The virus enters the skin via small openings and infects the epidermal basal layer. Viral replication occurs in the cell nucleus, where HPV will cause a change that will result in nuclear **atypia** (structural abnormality in a cell). This change in an epidermal cell will trigger replication and hyperproliferation of keratinocytes that will form the wart.[10]

HPV is spread via skin-to-skin or mucosa-to-mucosa contact. In addition, the virus may live on inanimate objects for long periods of time and can infect susceptible persons.[15] The incubation period for HPV infection may range from 3 weeks to 8 months.[10] For instance, people who walk barefoot frequently are at increased risk for plantar warts. Autoinoculation is frequently seen. Cell-mediated immunity helps protect against HPV. Individuals with cell-mediated immune deficiency are very susceptible to this virus, and the lesions they develop are difficult to treat.[10]

Clinical Manifestations

HPV is selective, that is, specific serotypes affect specific areas. The HPV that infects the hands and cause common warts are not the same as the HPV that infects the moist mouth and upper respiratory system. Consequently, the lesions produced are different. Nongenital skin warts may be flat, papular, or pedunculated (**Figure 41.4** ■). Flat warts are smooth papules on the face or backs of hands or along scratch marks. Papular warts are solid raised lesions with distinct borders and without a stalk. The peduculated type is attached to tissue via a stalk and is usually topped with a cauliflower-like cluster of keratinocytes. Nongenital mucosal warts may appear in the mouth as flat lesions or as respiratory papillomas (benign epithelial growth).[10,14]

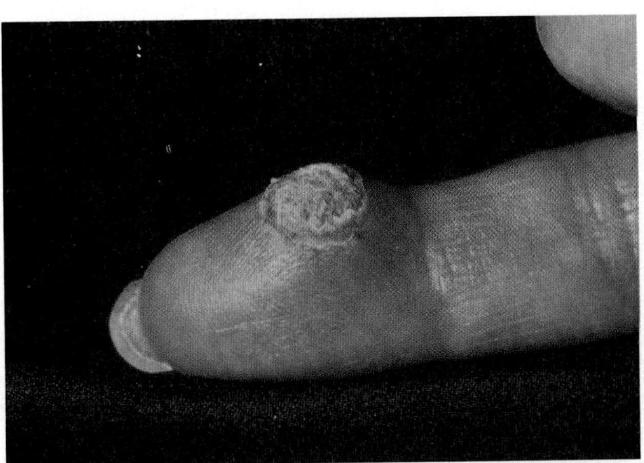

Figure 41.4 ■ Common wart.

Plantar warts look like a callus on the sole of the foot under pressure points such as the heel or metatarsal heads and can be very painful. Other types of warts include:[14,15]

- Filiform or digitate warts, which occur in clusters on the face and neck
- Intermediate warts, which are a combination of common and flat warts
- Mosaic warts, which are closely grouped sets of plantar warts
- Periungual or subungual warts, which are painful, thick warts around or under the nails.

HPV may be transmitted to the fetus from an infected maternal perineum during birth. This infection of the newborn may cause recurrent respiratory papillomas or anogenital warts.[14] ■

Linking Pathophysiology to Diagnosis and Treatment

Diagnosis of external cutaneous warts can be done via physical examination. HPV cannot be cultured.

Treatment of cutaneous warts will not eradicate the virus or prevent viral transmission.[15] Studies have shown that about half of cutaneous warts will resolve without treatment within 1 year. HPV does not respond to antiviral medication such as acyclovir. First-line treatment for simple warts is salicylic acid, a topical keratolytic agent that chemically destroys the wart.[15,16] Other agents used to remove warts include antiproliferative topical agents such as podophyllin and chemodestructive agents such as trichloroacetic acid.[10] Second-line treatment includes cryotherapy to freeze and destroy infected tissue.[16] Electrosurgery and simple surgical excision are used if the warts are particularly large or do not respond to topical treatment.

Check Your Progress: Section 41.2

1. What is the underlying physiologic change that occurs that allows the varicella-zoster virus (VSV) to manifest itself as herpes zoster (HZ) or shingles at a later time in a person's life?
2. What are the common clinical manifestations associated with HZ?
3. Since HPV disorders do not respond to antiviral medications, what are the first- and second-line treatments used to address this condition?

41.3 Skin Disorders with a Genetic Basis

It has long been known that the most important risk factor for certain chronic skin diseases is family history. More recently there has been an information explosion about how genetic factors influence the development of disease. This section discusses three chronic skin disorders that have a genetic pathogenesis: atopic dermatitis, psoriasis, and hidradenitis suppurativa.

Atopic Dermatitis

Eczema is a general term that describes inflammatory skin disorders. The most severe form of eczema is **atopic dermatitis (AD)**, a chronic, recurring, itchy, inflammatory disorder that is associated with increased serum immunoglobulin E (IgE). In addition, individuals who have AD often have other atopic disorders such as asthma or allergic rhinitis, or there is a family history of these disorders.[17]

AD most often affects children, although the disorder may persist into adulthood. Rarely, it will begin during the adult years. It is estimated that AD affects about 25% of children between ages 3 months and 5 years.[17,18] The disorder usually disappears by early adulthood. The incidence of AD is increasing worldwide. AD affects all races and is equally distributed between genders.[18]

Etiology and Pathogenesis

The complex pathogenesis of AD involves genetic, immunologic, and environmental factors that combine to cause a disorder of the epidermal barrier and changes in the immune system.[17] About 70% of individuals affected by AD have a family history of atopic diseases. Studies have shown that the children who have one parent with an atopic disorder are two to three times more likely to develop AD. If both parents have an atopic disorder, the odds increase to three to five times.[17]

The most frequently identified gene mutation seen in AD patients is in the *FLG* gene that is responsible for filaggrin (proteins that bind keratin to the epidermis). Filaggrin is necessary for the formation of the epidermal barrier and for the natural moisturizing factor.[17] Loss of filaggrin will lead to loss of the barrier function in skin, allowing transdermal water loss, the penetration of antigens, and increased inflammation.[18]

This gene mutation, however, is not the full answer to what causes AD. Some studies show that many patients who have AD do not have the *FLG* mutation. Conversely, there are many individuals with normal skin who do have the *FLG* mutation. Even with this conflicting data, *FLG* gene mutation is considered the highest genetic risk factor for AD.[17,18] Genomewide association studies (GWAS) performed on European and Japanese families have revealed linkage with AD on 1 chromosomes, with the 3p24 locus being the most replicated. None of these, however, are specific for AD.[19]

Immune dysfunction in the humoral, cell-mediated, and innate systems is evident in AD. In the humoral system, there are increased amounts of IgE and increased IgE sensitization in patients with AD.[17,18] Immune dysfunction in the cell-mediated system is in the form of an imbalance of T-cell subsets with a predominance of Th2 cells. Th2 cells produce inflammatory cytokines such as interleukin (IL)-4, IL-5, and IL-13, which play a significant role in the inflammation of AD. Recently, increased amounts of Th17 have been found in patients with AD. It is not yet clear whether this is significant.[18] Filaggrin mutations may influence the development of inflammation by causing the release of thymic stromal lymphopoietin (TSLP; a protein belonging to the cytokine family), IL-25, and IL-33. The innate system is also changed. There are increased numbers of eosinophils and mast cells, a reduction in antimicrobial peptides, less movement of neutrophils to the skin, and toll-like receptor defects in patients with AD.[18,19]

There are several environmental factors that aggravate AD. Climate extremes of heat, cold, or low humidity will cause exacerbations or **flare-ups** of the disorder. Low humidity is especially irritating because of the low moisture levels in the skin of patients with AD.[18]

Dysfunction of the epidermal barrier and the immune systems make AD patients more susceptible to bacterial, viral, and fungal infection. The skin of individuals with AD is often colonized with *Staphylococcus aureus*, both in skin lesions and in normal-appearing skin.[19] It is thought that *S. aureus* may be a cause or co-factor of AD because the toxins that the bacteria secretes have superantigenic properties.[18,19] Individuals with AD are also more susceptible to infection by MRSA (methicillin-resistant *S. aureus*) and other pathogens. Those with AD are also more susceptible to localized and disseminated HSV infections. Eczema herpeticum that occurs in patients with AD will present as vesicles in the eczematous areas that spread rapidly to normal skin.[18] Individuals with the worst cases of widespread HSV will need to be hospitalized for care. HSV in individuals with AD will recur, just as it does in patients with normal skin. In addition, fungal infections occur more frequently and are more severe in individuals with AD.

Clinical Manifestations

Pruritus (itching) is the prevailing symptom in AD. The incessant itching is what makes AD such a burden for children and adults with this ailment. In fact, AD has been called the "itch that rashes" because the itching will precede the **eczematous** (eruption of an itchy, red, weeping, crusting patch on skin) rash (**Figure 41.5** ■).[20] AD is exacerbation and remission of dry, itchy, red skin that begins in infancy. The constant pruritus will cause the person to scratch and rub the area, and **excoriations** (surface injury to skin that removes cell layer) and eventually **lichenification** (thick, leathery skin) will result. **Xerosis** (abnormal dryness) and crusting of lesions are also common features of AD.

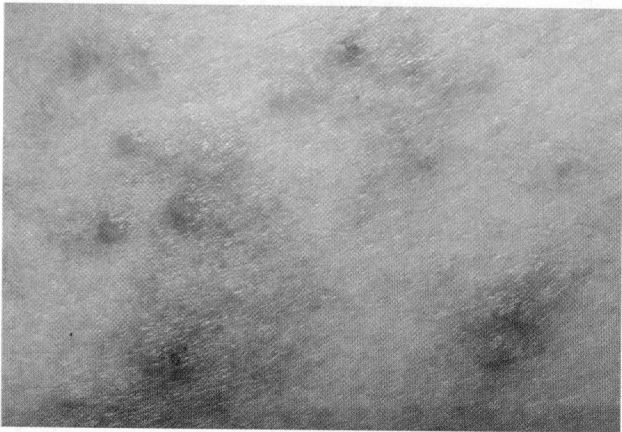

Figure 41.5 ■ Atopic dermatitis.

Periods of acute worsening of symptoms interspersed with periods of few symptoms is characteristic of AD. These periods of worsening of itching and eczematous skin rash are called flare-ups.[21] These periods of acute symptoms are not life threatening unless associated with complications such as bacterial or herpes infection. Nevertheless, flare-ups are very uncomfortable.

The cause of flare-ups is often unexplained. However, flare-ups have been associated with seasonal or climate changes, sweat, staphylococcal infection, food allergies, contact allergies, and stress.[18,21]

During infancy, AD begins with xerosis during the first months of life followed by eczematous skin lesions on the face, scalp, and antecubital and popliteal fossae. These lesions usually spare the diaper area and nose.[18] Constant pruritus causes irritability, poor feeding, and sleep disturbance.

During childhood, skin dryness covers the body. The skin for AD sufferers is flaky and rough. Repeated rubbing and scratching produces patches of lichenification, especially in skinfolds, over the knees and elbows, and on the forehead. Fresh lesions are **exudative** (oozing of fluid) and should not be confused with bacterial infection. The child's face is usually pale and there is redness and scaling around the eyes. Exacerbation, or flare-ups, and remission patterns will persist into the teen years and, in some individuals, into adulthood.[18] ■

Adults affected with AD continue to have dryness and scaling, but in fewer areas of the body. Some adults will have a brown macular discoloration around the neck.[18]

The quality of life of individuals with AD is severely affected. Sleep disturbances, poor memory, poor school and work performance, and depression have all been associated with AD.[17]

Linking Pathophysiology to Diagnosis and Treatment

There are currently no reliable biomarkers for AD. There are no laboratory tests that can diagnose the condition.[17] Diagnosis is based on clinical findings including history, the appearance and distribution of the rash, and associated signs and symptoms. The diagnostic criteria for AD established by the American Academy of Dermatology[17] are:

- Features that must be present: pruritus, eczema (typical distribution and configuration), chronic with recurring flare-ups
- Supporting signs: early age at onset, personal or family history of atopy or immunoglobulin E reactivity, xerosis
- All other possible skin conditions have been excluded.

AD is usually treated with topical agents. Severe flare-ups are also treated with topical agents, but may also need systemic anti-inflammatory medication or phototherapy to control the symptoms.[17] Topical agents for AD include moisturizers, corticosteroids, and topical calcineurin inhibitors (TCIs). TCIs are a second class of anti-inflammatory topical medication. Anti-inflammatory topical agents may be used alone or in combination. Treatment regimens depend on the particular drug and whether it is being used for acute flare-up or for prevention of flare-ups.[22]

Xerosis is a constant problem for patients with AD, and moisturizers are mandatory. In fact, moisturizers applied often and liberally will reduce inflammation and frequency of flare-ups.[22] Other strategies to decrease dryness include lukewarm water baths to remove scale, crusts, and allergens, followed while wet with the application of moisturizers; and cool-mist humidifiers used year round.

Wet-wrap therapy is used for significant flare-ups. Topical corticosteroid medication is applied and the medicated areas are wrapped with saline-soaked tubular bandages or gauze that is then covered with a dry outside layer.[22] This approach helps the absorption of the corticosteroids, decreases water loss via the skin, and provides a barrier against scratching.

Psoriasis

Psoriasis is a chronic, complex, multifactorial, inflammatory skin disease that is immune-mediated. The most common type of psoriasis is plaque psoriasis. It affects 85–90% of persons who have psoriasis.[23] About 80% of persons with psoriasis have mild to moderate disease; 20% have moderate to severe disease.[24] Even mild psoriasis can have a significant psychologic impact. Psoriasis has many different variations in skin lesion presentation and severity,[25–28] which are outlined in **Table 41.1** ■.

Psoriasis affects 7.4 million Americans[23] and about 2% of the world population.[24] More women than men are affected. The disorder can begin at any age; however, there are two peaks of age of onset: The first is between ages 15 and 30 years and the second is 50–60 years.[24] Whites are affected more often than people of color, and psoriasis is less likely to occur in a warm, humid climate.[26]

Table 41.1 Types and Presentation of Psoriasis

Type of Psoriasis	Presentation
Plaque psoriasis	Most common type, manifesting as raised, inflamed lesions covered with silvery scale
Scalp psoriasis	Affects about 50% of patients; manifests as raised plaques with silvery scale on the scalp
Inverse psoriasis	Less scaly and occurs in skinfolds; contributors are heat, trauma, and infection
Erythrodermic psoriasis	Least common form of psoriasis, covering up to 90% of body surface with redness and scaling; may occur abruptly or slowly and may be started by abrupt removal of corticosteroid medication
Pustular psoriasis	Manifests as sterile pustules on hands and soles; the severe acute form may cause life-threatening complications
Guttate psoriasis	Common in younger patients; manifests as pink papules with fine scaling that appear after group A beta-hemolytic streptococcal upper respiratory infection
Psoriatic onychodystrophy	Nail disorder common to psoriasis; manifests as pitting, hyperkeratosis under nails, lysis of nails
Psoriatic arthritis	Seronegative inflammatory arthritis that may develop about 12 years after onset of skin psoriasis; men and women are equally affected

Etiology and Pathophysiology

Psoriasis lesions are characterized by hyperproliferation of keratinocytes and a decrease in epidermal cell turnover rate and inflammation.[26] The keratinocytes will proliferate and the dermis and epidermis will thicken. New dermal vessels will form and neutrophils and lymphocytes will migrate to the area, causing inflammation. This multifactorial disorder has combined genetic and environmental causation. Heritability (proportion of differences in a trait among people of a population that are due to genetic differences) for psoriasis is high, at about 60–90%.[24] There have been about 40 genetic loci (specific location of a gene) for psoriasis identified. There are nine chromosomal segments linked to psoriasis susceptibility, with PSORS1 showing the highest risk for heritability.[24] The PSORS1 region contains the HLA-Cw6 allele that is found in many populations and is thought to be the most likely to cause psoriasis.[24,26] Human leukocyte antigen (HLA)-Cw6 is involved in antigen-presenting cells and in T-cell activation so that a genetic mutation in this gene would lead to the cell-mediated immune dysregulation seen in psoriasis.

Immunologic and genetic studies have also identified the interleukin (IL)-23/T-helper (Th)17 pathway as important in the pathogenesis of psoriasis. IL-23 promotes the growth and survival of Th17 cells that release cytokines and tumor necrosis factor.[24] Abnormal IL-23 signaling and Th17 release of cytokines are major factors in the chronic inflammation of psoriasis. Tumor necrosis factor alpha (TNFα) is increased in the dermis and in circulation. TNFα inhibitors used to control psoriasis are often successful because they will lower the TNFα.[26]

Innate immunity genetic variants also have roles in the pathogenesis of psoriasis. One aspect of the variants identified is the change in the expression of antiviral genes that cause an overproduction of cytokines. This alteration in antimicrobial function is considered a major contributor to the development of psoriasis.[24]

Gene deletions have been found that explain some of the skin barrier dysfunction in psoriasis. These gene mutations have been linked to poor skin repair after injury that allows antigen penetration. Poor skin repair sets up the chronic inflammation of the skin barrier seen in psoriasis.[24] Tissue and wound healing is covered in detail in Chapter 39.

Onset of psoriasis in a genetically susceptible person may occur without any apparent trigger or after a stressful event, direct skin trauma, streptococcal pharyngitis, viral infection, immunization, or the use of drugs such as antimalarials, beta-blockers, aspirin, or nonsteroidal anti-inflammatory drugs (NSAIDs).[26,27] In addition, smoking, obesity, and alcohol use have been shown to increase the risk of psoriasis exacerbations and to make the disease more severe.[27]

Clinical Manifestations

Most persons affected have plaque psoriasis. The skin lesions in these cases are usually round or oval, well-demarcated **plaques** (solid, raised, flat-topped lesions greater than 1 centimeter in diameter with a definite border that separates lesion from normal skin) of differing size covered with silvery scale (**Figure 41.6** ■). These lesions occur on the elbows, knees, scalp, buttocks, and trunk.[27] The face is usually not affected.[28] Patients with psoriasis develop the Koebner phenomenon, in which injury to normal skin will lead to plaque formation.[27,28] Sunburn and viral rashes may also cause a psoriatic lesion to appear. Increased vascularization of the lesions leads to Auspitz sign, in which pinpoint bleeding will occur when the scale is lifted.[28] Psoriatic lesions may itch, burn, or cause skin pain, especially when the scalp is involved.[28]

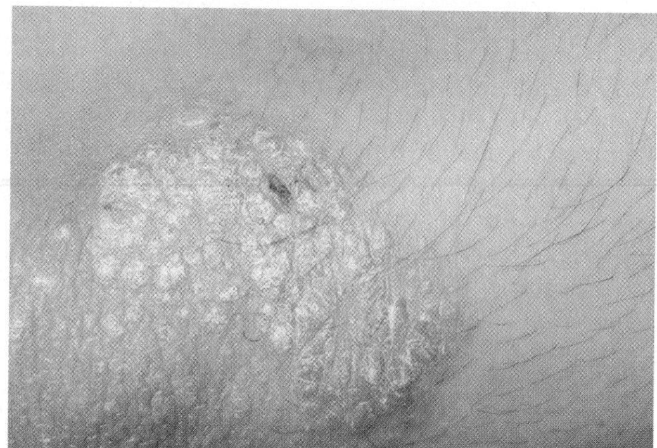

Figure 41.6 ■ Psoriasis.

Studies show that up to 42% of persons affected by plaque psoriasis will develop psoriatic arthritis within 5 to 12 years after onset of the skin lesions.[27,29] This form of arthritis usually affects the hands and feet, but may also involve medium and larger joints. Signs and symptoms include stiffness, pain, and progressive joint damage, and, if not treated, loss of function.[26,28]

Nail psoriasis occurs in about 50% of persons with plaque psoriasis and about 90% of psoriatic arthritis patients (**Figure 41.7** ■).[28] Nail psoriasis will manifest as abnormal nail plate growth that results in large deep pitting, proliferation of keratinocytes under the nail, and onycholysis (lifting of the end of the nail plate).[27,28]

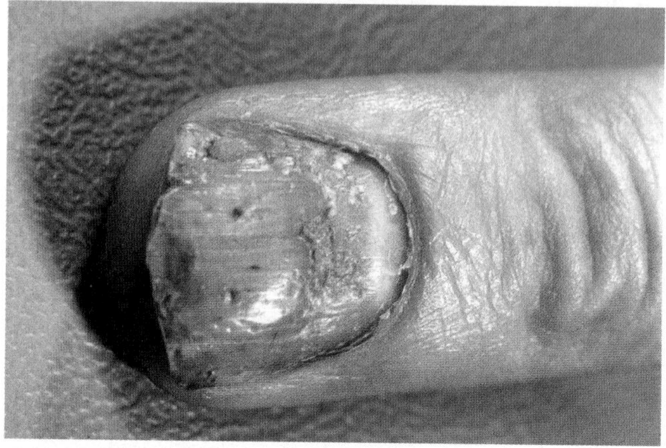

Figure 41.7 ■ Psoriasis of the nails.

Psoriasis exacerbations or flare-ups may occur spontaneously or be triggered by stress; trauma to the skin; infection; sunburn; and use of drugs such as antimalarials, beta-blockers, aspirin, or NSAIDs. Flare-ups are disfiguring and uncomfortable for the patient. During these episodes, the disease may spread and worsen. Careful treatment can increase the time of relatively normal skin between flare-ups.[27]

Karen McKendrick: Application

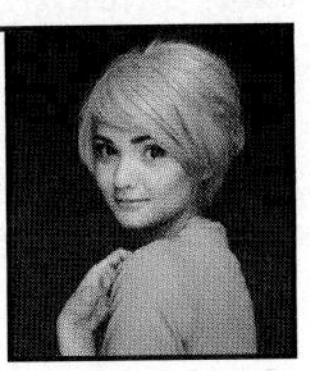

Ms. McKendrick's dermatologist suggests that she consider using ustekinumab (Stelara), a monoclonal antibody that targets the p40 subunit of IL-12 and IL-23. Ms. McKendrick consents after learning all about the drug and its side effects.

Ms. McKendrick's test for HLA-Cw6 is positive. Other baseline laboratory tests reveal:

CBC with differential: no anemia or sign of infection

Liver function tests: within normal limits (WNL)

Ms. McKendrick's history is negative for any serious infections or other chronic disease. She had tested negative for tuberculosis earlier and her immunizations are up to date. She is ready to start the medication.

3. Since Ms. McKendrick's plaque psoriasis is chronic, how will the ustekinumab (Stelara) help her deal with this condition?
4. Besides the medication prescribed above, what other preventive measures should Ms. McKendrick be advised to follow in order to prevent flare-ups?

Linking Pathophysiology to Diagnosis and Treatment

The diagnosis of psoriasis is based on the appearance of the lesions. Biopsy is rarely needed to make a diagnosis.[27] No biomarkers specific for psoriasis have been identified. Some skin lesions of psoriasis and psoriatic arthritis may mimic other disorders. This will necessitate laboratory testing to rule out other conditions before the diagnosis can be made.[26–28]

Treatment of psoriasis includes a variety of options for the different forms and severity of the disease. Mild psoriasis that involves less than 5% of the body surface and not the face, genitals, hands, or feet is treated topically with corticosteroids, vitamin D analogs, retinoids, or calcineurin inhibitors.[25]

- Corticosteroid therapy is the use of a rapid acting anti-inflammatory agents to control flare-ups. It is recommended that corticosteroid therapy be gradually tapered and discontinued after symptoms improve.[27,28] Symptoms will improve in a few weeks or months after corticosteroid use.
- Vitamin D analogs (decrease keratinocyte hyperproliferation and inflammation[3]) are well tolerated and have a slower onset of action than corticosteroids. They can be introduced into treatment before corticosteroids are tapered and may be continued afterward to give a longer time of remission than corticosteroids.[27]
- Topical retinoids (vitamin A derivative that reduces skin cell proliferation and reduces inflammation[3]) are **teratogenic** (cause fetal death or anomalies) and often cause itching and burning when applied. Topical retinoids are used in combination with corticosteroids or used every other day. These agents will also prolong the remission period.[27,28]
- Calcineurin inhibitors (immunomodulating agents that block chemical that activates inflammation[3]) improve symptoms without the atrophy and other side effects seen with corticosteroids. These agents are preferred for facial lesions and lesions in skinfolds.[27]

Moderate to severe psoriasis treatment requires systemic therapy in combination with **phototherapy** (exposing skin to ultraviolet light on a regular basis) or psoralen plus ultraviolet A (PUVA), in which a lotion is applied that will enhance the ultraviolet A rays. Systemic therapy requires baseline and periodic screening for serious side effects. Examples include methotrexate, cyclosporine, and biologic agents. Methotrexate has been used for over 50 years in the treatment of psoriasis with good results. It is given weekly. Cyclosporine gives rapid relief during flare-ups and from severe psoriasis, but side effects are severe. It is often given to suppress a crisis as slower-acting medications are introduced and take effect.[27]

Biologic agents include tumor necrosis factor inhibitors and the newer interleukin inhibitors. Genetic information is used to identify patients who are most likely to respond to biologic agents. For example, patients who are HLA-Cw6 positive are more likely to have a rapid decrease in skin lesions in response to ustekinumab (Stelara).[24]

Complications related to psoriasis and treatments for the disease include secondary infection, increased risk for lymphoma and squamous cell carcinoma, metabolic syndrome, ischemic heart disease, peripheral artery disease, stroke, kidney disease, arthritis, social isolation, depression, and suicide.[26,27,29] Therapies for moderate to severe psoriasis that affect the function of the immune system increase the risk for severe infection and other potentially dangerous side effects.

Karen McKendrick: Outcome

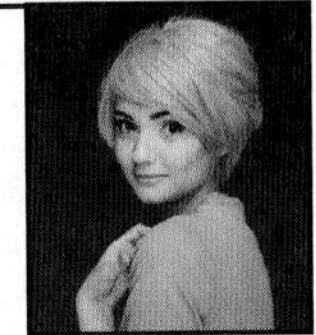

Ustekinumab is administered subcutaneously when the tests are completed, then repeated 4 weeks later. Ms. McKendrick now goes to her dermatologist every 12 weeks for an injection. She is monitored for infection and liver changes every 6 months. The psoriasis is well controlled and she continues to be a top model.

5. With her moderate to severe plaque psoriasis, what other treatment options does Ms. McKendrick have available in the event that ustekinumab stops working?
6. Even with good medication control, what complications related to psoriasis and the treatments could Ms. McKendrick be vulnerable to later in life?

Hidradenitis Suppurativa

Hidradenitis suppurativa (HS), also called *acne inversa*, is a painful, recurring, chronic inflammatory skin disease that involves the hair follicles in apocrine sweat gland areas such as the axilla and groin. Prevalence for this painful disease ranges from 0.53 to 4.1% of the general population.[30,31] In a survey of medical records in Olmsted County, Minnesota, an incidence of 6 per 100,000 of the general population was revealed. The age- and gender-adjusted data for this population showed that the highest incidence, 18.4 per 100,000, occurred among women age 20–29.[32] This finding supports other studies that have shown that women are more often affected than men by a 3:1 ratio.[31,33] HS develops during adolescence or the early 20s, becomes more severe after about 6–7 years, then decreases in severity until complete remission between the ages of 35 and 49.[30,32,33] Rarely, the disorder will continue into old age. All races are equally affected.[33]

Etiology and Pathogenesis

HS produces painful nodules, abscesses, and sinus tract formations in skinfold areas The basic lesion begins with occlusion of the hair follicle via infundibular **hyperkeratosis** (abnormal increase in keratin causing thickening in the funnel-like cavity that houses the hair follicle) and **hyperplasia** (abnormal increase in epithelial cells) of the follicular epithelium.[31,33] The occlusion is followed by collecting cellular wastes that cause a cyst to form in the apocrine sweat gland adjacent to the hair follicle. The nodule does not drain as a boil would, but opens under the skin and spreads laterally. This may be followed by abscess formation, and eventually by sinus tract (a tunneling wound in soft tissue) formation and keloid-like scarring.

The pathogenesis of HS appears to be multifactorial and includes genetic, immunologic, hormonal, and environmental factors. In about 40% of persons, there is a family history of HS, especially among female patients.[31,33] There is also evidence that HS is passed to offspring via an autosomal dominant route with variable penetrance (extent to which a gene is expressed in a person who is carrying the gene).[31] Several gene loci are associated with HS, but no specific gene has been proven causative. Mutations of gamma-secretase genes have been identified in families of individuals affected with HS.[31] Presence of these genes partially explains the changes seen in the hair follicle and the apocrine gland response.

An abnormal immune response is evident in HS. There is chronic inflammation without pathogenic bacteria, occasional incidence of biomarker-negative arthritis, and an association with Crohn disease in patients with HS. Studies have shown that an abnormal innate immune system is most evident since several inflammatory and anti-inflammatory cytokines have been found in HS lesions, including TNFα. Conversely, Th1, Th17, and Th22 cells are unchanged in blood samples from patients with HS.[31,34]

Hormonal factors, particularly androgen, have been proposed as causative factors in HS. This proposal is based on observations that HS does not occur until after puberty, affected women have exacerbations or flare-ups premenstrually, women may be in remission during pregnancy and breastfeeding, and symptoms go into total remission with menopause.[31,33] Despite these observations, plasma levels of androgen are the same for women with or without HS.[31] However, HS may be the result of increased sensitivity to androgen in the hair follicles and apocrine glands.[34]

Smoking cigarettes may trigger or exacerbate HS and increase the severity of the disease.[30–34] Studies of individuals with HS have demonstrated that 60–90% were active smokers and 5–15% were ex-smokers.[31] Nicotine from smoking can be found in axillary sweat for about 8 days after smoking. Nicotine promotes inflammatory responses, including mast cell degranulation and an increase in neutrophils to the axilla.

Obesity is also a factor in HS pathogenesis, although there are some patients with HS who are not obese. Obesity is associated with increased levels of TNFα and interleukins in blood and in the lesions of obese individuals with HS. These pro-inflammatory substances are produced in part by adipocytes (fat cells). In addition, overweight and obese persons have deeper skinfolds that produce more sweat and increase skin-on-skin friction. It is thought that the mechanical force of the friction produces small tears in the hair follicles of susceptible persons that initiate the HS lesions.[31]

Bacterial cultures of HS lesions are usually either sterile or filled with bacteria that are considered normal flora, such as *Staphylococcal epidermidis*.[31,34] This would indicate that bacterial infection, when it occurs, is secondary to the HS lesion, not causative. Superinfection will worsen HS.

There are several disorders that have been reported as comorbidities with HS. Severe, scarring acne; dissecting cellulitis of the scalp (rare disorder in which pus-filled lumps develop on the scalp and cause permanent hair loss); pilonidal cysts (painful boil that occurs over the end of the tailbone); and sinuses have been seen in many patients who also have HS.[31,34] Crohn disease has been seen as a comorbidity, although some sources argue that cutaneous manifestations of Crohn disease in the perianal area could be misdiagnosed as HS.[34,35] Peripheral joint arthritis triggered during flare-ups has been associated with HS, particularly in African American men.[31,34] Squamous cell carcinoma has occurred in HS lesions in the perineal and buttocks area. This comorbidity occurs most often in men, with a 4:1 ratio of men to women.[35] Thick, rope-like scars in the axilla frequently occur in HS and can limit arm movement. Lastly, HS patients are often socially isolated, depressed, and at risk for suicide.[31–34]

Clinical Manifestations

Men and women affected by HS will have painful nodules that develop in the skinfolds and evolve into abscesses, draining sinus tract formation, scarring, and fibrosis (**Figure 41.8** ■). These lesions do not cause fever, swollen lymph glands, or septicemia.[34] The lesions in men are more likely to occur on the axilla, buttocks, and perianal area. The lesions in women are more frequently seen in the axilla, inguinofemoral and pubic areas, vulva, and under the breasts.[31,32,34]

Unlike boils, HS nodules are deep, subcutaneous nodules that do not open to the skin surface. Instead, the

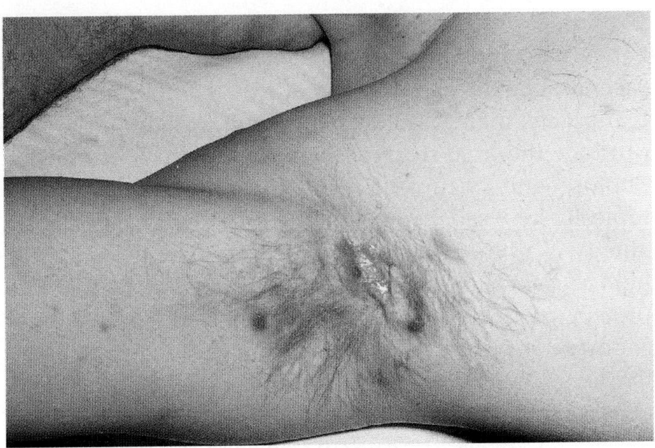

Figure 41.8 ■ Hidradenitis suppurativa lesions in the axilla.

nodule will open under the skin and the fluid from the cyst will spread subcutaneously in a lateral pattern and set up an inflammatory reaction that continues to be very active and growing.[34] Secondary lesions that form over the linear nodules are open double or tombstone comedones (open, multiheaded blackheads).[31,35] HS lesions occur intermittently with acute exacerbations that are variable in occurrence. The lesions may appear in one or more areas of the body. The worst lesions are painful, long, deep, draining sinus tracts with odorous discharge. These severe lesions are more likely to occur in men on the buttocks and perianal area. Diagnostic criteria for HS have been recommended by the Second International HS Research Symposium. These include[34,35]:

1. Typical lesions are either deep painful nodules (blind boils) in early primary lesions or abscesses, draining sinuses, bridged scars, and tombstone open comedones in secondary lesions
2. Typical topography includes axillae, groin, genitals, perineal and perianal region, buttocks, and infra- and intermammary folds
3. Chronicity and recurrences.

Linking Pathophysiology to Diagnosis and Treatment

Diagnosis of HS is made based on clinical presentation using Hurley staging[33–35]:

- *Stage I:* Solitary or multiple, isolated abscess formation without scarring or sinus tracts
- *Stage II:* Recurrent abscesses, single or multiple widely separated lesions, with sinus tract formation
- *Stage III:* Diffuse or broad involvement, with multiple interconnected sinus tracts and abscesses.

Patients with Hurley stages II and III HS may require culture and sensitivity testing to identify secondary infections. Occasionally it is necessary to biopsy lesions to rule out other possible causes.[30]

Treatment of HS begins with general care guidelines including instructions to stop using tobacco products; avoid dairy products; choose a low glycemic diet; maintain ideal weight; avoid scrubbing lesions; reduce trauma and friction to lesion areas; avoid overheating and sweating; wear loose, cool clothing; and use an antiseptic wash only if lesions are draining.[35,36] These general measures should be followed regardless of the Hurley stage of HS.

Medical care when the lesions are in Hurley stage I with few flare-ups annually may include use of clindamycin lotion in lesion areas twice a day to decrease inflammation. Other antibiotics that decrease inflammation are the tetracyclines and rifampin. Zinc supplements are encouraged to further control inflammation. In some cases, a corticosteroid may be injected into the lesions to reduce inflammation locally.[34]

Patients with Hurley stage II HS are treated with oral clindamycin and rifampin for 3 months. In addition to reducing inflammation, combined use of these antibiotics reduces superimposed infection. After 3 months, a maintenance dose of tetracycline is given. Oral zinc is recommended. Acute lesions may be injected with a medium-strength corticosteroid. Unroofing (removing the top from the lesions) is done and the wounds are left to heal. Care is taken not to squeeze or traumatize the wound further.[34]

Patients with Hurley stage III HS are treated with clindamycin plus rifampin, oral corticosteroids, or an immune suppressant such as cyclosporine. TNFα inhibitors like infliximab and etanercept that have been used for Crohn disease control also improve HS.[34] Medical care in these cases is intended to prepare the patient for extensive surgery to remove the deep lesions. Extensive surgery in stage III is the only permanent cure.[34]

Check Your Progress: Section 41.3

1. According to studies done on hidradenitis suppurativa (HS), what factors have been identified as having an influence on the development and proliferation of this condition?
2. What is unique about nodules that form during an episode of HS?
3. Regardless of the Hurley stage, what general care guidelines should patients be instructed to follow in order to decrease the clinical effects of HS?

41.4 Benign Neoplasms of the Skin

Benign neoplasms (abnormal cells that either multiply more than normal or do not die when they should) are noncancerous types of tissue proliferation. A few examples include moles, lipomas, and actinic keratosis. These benign lesions rarely cause problems unless they are in areas where they are rubbed or they enlarge to compress other organs. Some may be mistaken for cancer or may be premalignant. This section focuses on various types of benign neoplasms of the skin.

Photodermatitis and Actinic Keratosis

Photodermatitis or photosensitivity occurs when the immune system reacts to ultraviolet (UV) light after exposure to sunlight or tanning devices. It may affect anyone, but individuals with fair skin are the most sensitive.[37] There are several different forms and variations of photodermatitis, including solar **urticaria** (pale, raised plaques or welts on the skin; hives), drug-induced photosensitivity, phototoxicity, photoallergy, and polymorphous light eruption.[38] UV exposure will cause a photosensitivity reaction in individuals with preexisting autoimmune systemic lupus erythematosus or porphyria, an enzyme deficiency that allows heme (an iron-containing pigment) to accumulate.[37,38]

Actinic keratosis (AK) is a thick, rough, or scaly skin lesion that develops after chronic sun exposure, extensive exposure to x-rays, or to some industrial chemicals.[39,40] AK is a **dermatosis** (a skin disease that does not involve inflammation). It is most likely to affect people 50 years of age or older; however, individuals in their 20s who have had chronic exposure to UV rays may be affected. Persons with weakened immune systems, such as those undergoing cancer chemotherapy, those who have an organ transplant, or persons with HIV/AIDS, are also at risk. About 58 million people in the United States have AK.[40] Slightly more men than women are affected.

Etiology and Pathogenesis

Photodermatitis is an immune response to UV rays. UV exposure amounts and skin reactions differ depending on the person's skin type and other factors that make the skin more sensitive. Factors that make the skin more sensitive include an inherited tendency, preexisting diseases, about 100 different drugs, and exposure to certain plants or chemicals.[37,38] A few examples of substances that have caused photodermatitis include:

- Antibiotics, such as tetracyclines
- Antifungals, such as griseofulvin
- Coal tar and other topical skin products used in psoriasis
- Retinoids used for acne
- Nonsteroidal anti-inflammatory drugs
- Chemotherapy agents
- Antimalarials
- Antipsychotics
- Diuretics
- Antidepressants
- Fragrances
- Aftershave lotion
- Sunscreens with PABA
- Industrial cleaners that contain salicylanilide
- Lavender lotions, soaps
- Furocoumarin-containing plants such as limes, celery, and parsley.

The photodermatitis cutaneous reaction to sunlight may also be idiopathic (of unknown cause).

Sun exposure may inactivate or destroy epidermal Langerhans cells that supply some skin immunity. In the case of solar urticaria, skin cells may function as photoallergens that cause mast cell degranulation that will produce the hive reaction in sun-exposed areas only.[38] Photosensitivity-causing drugs that are ingested or used topically may cause photoallergy or phototoxicity. Photoallergy is a type IV cell-mediated response in which UV light causes changes in the drug that allow it to bind to cell protein, producing a complex allergenic. In this case, prior exposure to the drug-induced allergen is needed. Photoallergy may extend to non-UV-exposed skin. Phototoxicity occurs when UV light generates free radicals and inflammatory mediators that cause tissue damage, pain, and redness in sun-exposed skin.[38]

Polymorphous light eruptions (PMLEs) are reactions to light that are not associated with drugs or systemic disease. These eruptions will appear on sun-exposed areas in 30 minutes to several days after exposure. PMLEs are more common in women in colder climates. The lesions will disappear after a few days, or in some cases after a couple of weeks.[38]

Cumulative sun or tanning-device damage to the skin is the primary cause of AK. Even brief exposures to UV rays add to the total exposure over a lifetime. Consequently, AK is more likely to be seen in older skin. In fact, some dermatologists believe that everyone over 80 years of age will have AK.[40] AK is the result of keratinocyte changes that occur in response to chronic exposure to UV rays. About 10% of AKs will progress to squamous cell carcinoma. Conversely, about 40–60% of squamous cell carcinomas began as untreated AK.[40]

Clinical Manifestations

Signs and symptoms of photodermatitis include urticaria that develops in sun-exposed skin that is sometimes associated with wheezing, dizziness, or fainting, as well as erythema, pruritus, papules, vesicles, eczema, skin pain, chills, headache, fever, and nausea.[37,38] Chronic effects may include skin thickening and scarring.

AK are thick, rough, crusting or scaly areas on the bald head, face, ears, lips, backs of the hands and forearms, shoulders, neck, and other areas exposed to UV rays (**Figure 41.9** ■). Some are very small and roughened, like sandpaper. Some AK will grow to a centimeter in diameter. Some will be red, whereas others are light or dark tan, pink, or the same color as the skin. Sometimes, AK will itch.[40]

Linking Pathophysiology to Diagnosis and Treatment

Diagnosis of photodermatitis and AK is made according to clinical presentation. In some cases, phototesting may be needed to determine if the lesions can be reproduced by light exposure.[38]

Treatment of photodermatitis depends on the presenting history and manifestations. Solar urticaria may be treated with antihistamines, antimalarial drugs, topical corticosteroids, sunscreens, or psoralen plus ultraviolet A (PUVA) light. Psoralen is a plant-derived topical

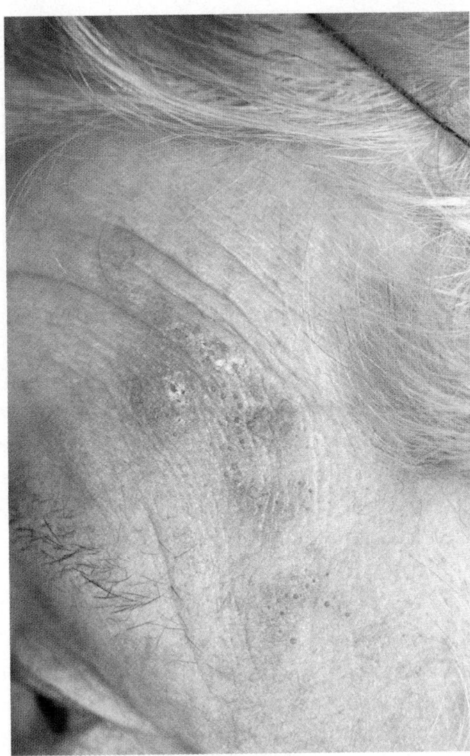

Figure 41.9 ■ Actinic keratosis.

compound applied to the skin and followed by exposure to UVA radiation.[38]

Photosensitivity secondary to drug use is treated with topical corticosteroids and avoidance, when possible, of the drug that caused the reaction.[38] PMLE may be self-limited or severe. For less severe reactions, topical corticosteroids are used with success. For the more severe cases, desensitization by phototherapy with PUVA may be used. Debilitating PMLE may require oral corticosteroids or immunosuppressive drugs.[38]

The treatments for AK are all aimed at destroying the lesions. Office procedures to remove the lesions include cryotherapy, chemical peel, curettage, and laser resurfacing.[39] There are several medications that patients with AK can apply themselves, including 5-fluorouracil (5-FU) cream, diclofenac sodium gel, imiquimod cream, and ingenol mebutate gel.[39] **Table 41.2** ■ describes how these medications work and the potential side effects.[38–41]

Table 41.2 Patient-Applied Medications to Treat Actinic Keratosis

Medication	Action	Side Effects
5-fluorouracil (5-FU) cream	Topical chemotherapy; causes inflammatory reaction	Redness, swelling, crusting
Diclofenac sodium gel	Nonsteroidal anti-inflammatory drug	Inflammation, irritation, pain, tingling, or blistering
Imiquimod cream	Immune modulator; stimulates production of interferon	Redness, ulceration
Ingenol mebutate gel	Immune modulator; works in 2–3 days	Redness, flaking, scaling, swelling, pain

Hemangiomas, Moles, and Skin Tags

Hemangiomas are congenital lesions that occur in 10–12% of all infants (**Figure 41.10** ■).[42] By age 7, about 70% of hemangiomas will have disappeared without treatment.[42]

Moles, also called **nevi**, may be congenital or may occur later in life. Moles are usually benign, but may change into cancer. Once formed, moles tend to stay for life, changing as the body grows.[42]

Skin tags, also called **acrochordons**, are soft papules on a stalk found in areas of the body where skin rubs on skin, such as the neck, axillae, and groin. Acrochordons are more prevalent in obese persons, pregnant women, and older men and women.[43,44] In fact, studies have shown that about 59% of persons have skin tags by the time they are 70 years old.[44]

Etiology and Pathogenesis

Hemangiomas are made up of extra blood vessels concentrated in an area within or just under the skin.[45] These lesions tend to grow during the first year of life then slowly disappear as the child grows. Hemangiomas may develop in the liver, around the eye, or in the nose or throat. Hemangiomas in these areas can be problematic if they block vision or compromise breathing.[42] Lesions that grow in the liver rarely require intervention.

Moles are made up of altered melanocytes that proliferate and grow in clusters.[43] Most people have moles. Many factors contribute to mole growth including age, race, genetics, and environment. Sun exposure can cause changes in moles that may lead to cancer.

It was once thought that skin tags are caused by a loss of elastin in skin. However, that theory has been disproven.[44] Friction between skin layers seems the most probable cause. Studies have shown that skin tags are often associated with insulin resistance, dyslipidemia, hypertension, and an elevated C-reactive protein.[44]

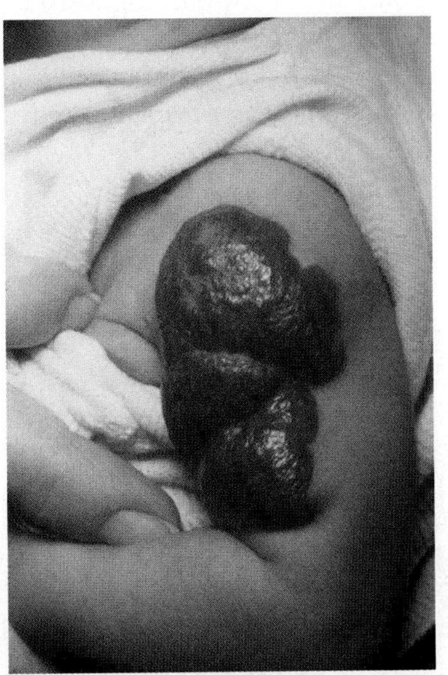

Figure 41.10 ■ Infantile hemangioma of the arm.

Clinical Manifestations

Hemangiomas are bright red, slightly raised lesions that are often referred to as strawberry birthmarks.[45] If the lesion is under the skin, it will appear bluish. More than 50% of hemangiomas occur on the head and neck, although they can appear anywhere on the body.[42] Rarely, these lesions will open and bleed slightly, requiring wound care. Hemangiomas that occur close to the eye may be large enough to block vision. Lesions that occur in the nose or throat may grow enough to affect breathing.

Moles or nevi are brown, yellow, red, black, tan, or flesh-colored macules, papules, or small plaques.[43] Mole size varies from small dots to an inch in diameter. Moles may be round, oval, flat, raised, smooth, rough, or have hair growing from them.[42] Moles may appear anywhere on the body. These lesions usually begin during childhood and grow during adolescence with body growth and remain on the skin for life. Typical moles are symmetric and have regular borders. Atypical moles (dysplastic nevi) are more likely to be multicolored, asymmetric, and have an irregular shape. These moles may have been exposed to ultraviolet sunlight and become dysplastic or there may be a hereditary tendency. Atypical moles may further evolve into melanomas, a severe skin cancer.[42,43] Warning signs of melanoma are described in Section 41-5.

Moles may normally darken during pregnancy. ■

Skin tags are pedunculated papules that may be flesh colored or darkly pigmented. Skin tags usually develop on the neck, axillae, or other areas where skin rubs on skin (**Figure 41.11** ■). Although unattractive, skin tags are not painful unless they are rubbed and irritated enough to bleed.[42,44]

Linking Pathophysiology to Diagnosis and Treatment

Hemangiomas, moles, and skin tags are easily identified on inspection and do not require diagnostic testing. Atypical moles are usually biopsied.

Hemangiomas usually disappear without intervention. In fact, scarring after surgical removal would be worse than the small lesion.[45] Hemangiomas that encroach on vision or breathing may be removed with laser treatments. Corticosteroids may be given to shrink the hemangioma before laser treatment.[42]

Most noncancerous moles do not need any treatment unless they are in an uncomfortable position or are cosmetically unattractive. These typical moles can be removed under local anesthetic using a scalpel.[42] Atypical moles should be inspected closely via dermoscopy by a dermatologist to be sure of the borders before removing the entire lesion for histologic study.[42,43]

Skin tags are not troublesome unless they are rubbed and irritated or the patient considers them unattractive. Under these conditions, the skin tags can easily be removed via cryotherapy, cutting them with scissors or a scalpel, or burning them via electrodesiccation (electric needle used to coagulate or burn a lesion).

Lipomas

Lipomas are common, benign lumps that grow under normal skin in subcutaneous tissues.[46] Lipomas may be single or multiple. About 80% are single.[47] Single lipomas are more common in women while multiple lipomas are more likely to occur in men.[46,47] Most lipomas are discovered between the ages of 40 and 60; however, they may arise during the second decade of life. An estimated 1 per 1000 persons per year develop lipoma.[47]

Etiology and Pathogenesis

Lipomas arise from the mesoderm (middle layer of the embryo) and are made of mature adipose cells within a fibrous sheath.[46,47] Solitary lipomas have been linked to changes in chromosome 12. Multiple lipomas do not show the same chromosomal changes; however, a familial tendency exists.[43]

Clinical Manifestations

Lipomas are smooth, usually soft, doughy, rubbery, painless masses in subcutaneous tissue (**Figure 41.12** ■).[42,46,47] Single lipomas are usually found on the trunk, upper arms, or neck. The size of single lipomas vary from less

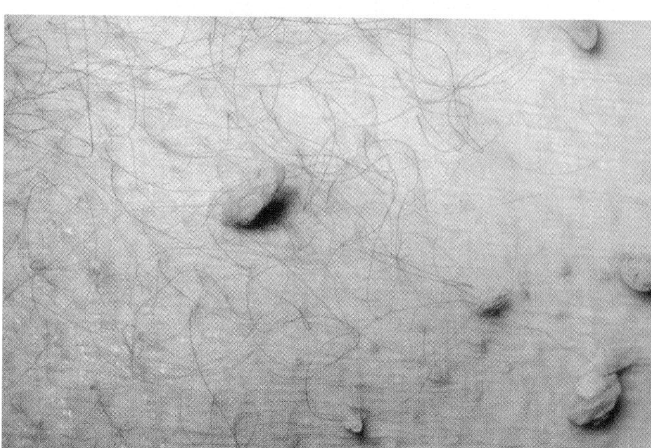

Figure 41.11 ■ Skin tags.

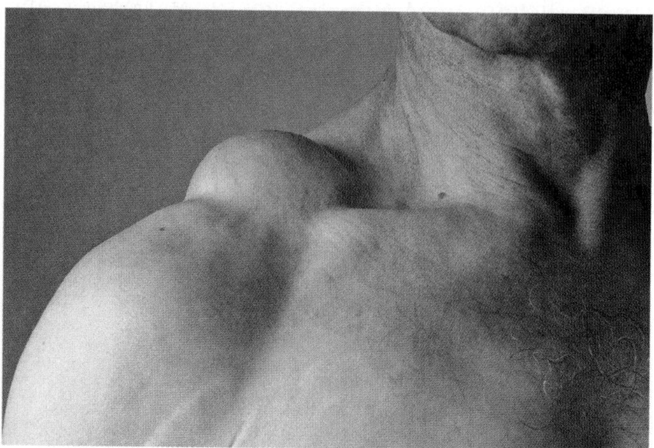

Figure 41.12 ■ Lipoma.

than 5 centimeters to as large as 20 centimeters in diameter.[47] About 80% of single lipomas are less than 5 centimeters in diameter.[47]

Linking Pathophysiology to Diagnosis and Treatment

Lipomas are easily diagnosed based on clinical presentation alone. No treatment is needed unless the lipoma is bothersome, tender, or pressing on other structures, or begins to change dramatically. In these cases, the lipoma can be reduced by liposuction or surgically removed.[43]

Epidermal Inclusion Cysts

Epidermal inclusion cysts (EICs) are common skin nodules that appear in adults between the ages of 30 and 49.[48] EICs are twice as common in men and occur in all races.

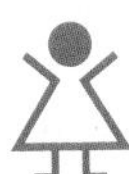

These lesions also occur as milia (very small, superficial EICs) in newborns. ■

Etiology and Pathogenesis

EICs are benign lesions that result from squamous epithelium of the epidermis being trapped or implanted in the dermis. This trapped epiderm forms a cavity that is filled with kerotinocytes and debris.[43,48] The origin of the epidermis is from around hair follicles. Some studies have shown that human papillomavirus and exposure to UV rays may be involved in the genesis of EICs, however, this has not been proven. Occasionally, skin cancers will arise from EICs. The cause of this change has not been fully explained.[48]

Clinical Manifestations

EICs are flesh-colored, firm nodules with a central punctum (sharp tip or point).[43] EICs are usually found on the face, scalp, neck, and trunk in adults.[48] The distribution of milia in the newborn is over the cheeks, forehead, nose, and nasolabial folds.[49]

Linking Pathophysiology to Diagnosis and Treatment

EICs are diagnosed based on clinical presentation. EICs do not need treatment unless they rupture under the skin. The material released from the cyst will cause inflammation or may become secondarily infected. These complications may require incision and drainage or antibiotics. Cysts may be surgically removed. Care must be taken to be sure that all of the cyst is removed or it will regrow from a leftover fragment.[43,48]

> **Check Your Progress: Section 41.4**
>
> 1. What characteristic makes actinic keratosis different from the majority of chronic skin disorders?
> 2. What is considered the primary cause of actinic keratosis (AK) and what age population does it mainly affect?
> 3. Although hemangiomas are often clinically benign, in what two regions of the body are they most worrisome and why?

41.5 Skin Cancer

Skin cancer is the most common cancer in the United States. In fact, more individuals are diagnosed with skin cancer each year than breast, prostate, lung, and colon cancers combined.[50] About 1 in 5 Americans will be diagnosed with skin cancer during their lifetime. In the past 30 years, the incidence of skin cancer has risen dramatically, probably due to the use of tanning devices and more leisure time spent in sunlight.[51] There are several forms of skin cancer. In this section, the focus is on the two most common forms of skin cancer, basal cell carcinoma and squamous cell carcinoma, and the one most dangerous, melanoma.

Basal Cell Carcinoma

Basal cell carcinoma (BCC) is the most frequently seen skin cancer, affecting about 2.8 million Americans annually.[52] About 80% of skin cancers diagnosed are BCC.[51,52] BCC is a slow-growing cancer and rarely metastasizes. However, if left untreated, BCC can cause significant disfigurement and in rare cases it can spread to bone.[51] BCC often recurs after treatment and 50% of persons with one BCC will have another within 5 years.[51] Risk factors for BCC include ultraviolet light exposure; radiation therapy as a child; having light-colored skin; personal history of skin cancer; older age; male gender; exposure to arsenic, coal tar, some pesticides, or oils; long-term or severe inflammatory skin disease; burn injury; treatment with PUVA; and reduced immunity.[51,53]

Etiology and Pathogenesis

BCC arises from the bottom layer (base) of cells of the epidermis, hair follicles, and eccrine sweat glands, usually in sun-exposed areas. Most BCC is caused by early (childhood), repeated, or prolonged exposure to ultraviolet light (UV) A and B rays from the sun or tanning devices. UV rays damage the DNA within the cell nucleus, thereby causing damage to genes that control skin cell growth.[51] One mutated gene that has been found in BCC most often is the "patched" (*PTCH*) gene. *PTCH* is a tumor-suppressor gene that is part of the "hedgehog" signaling pathways in cells.

Clinical Manifestations

BCC develops most often on sun-exposed areas including the face, ears, neck, scalp, shoulders, back, and hands (**Figure 41.13** ■).[52–54] BCC may also appear on skin exposed to arsenic and radiation, within areas of chronic inflammation, burn scars, or tattoos. Very rarely, BCC will appear in areas that are not sun exposed. BCC may be flat, firm, pale areas or small, raised pink or red, translucent, shiny, pearly bumps that bleed easily. The lesions may have **telangiectases** (spider veins; dilated capillaries at the surface of the skin) on or near them, a lower center area, and the color may be blue, brown, or black. Some BCC lesions may look like open sores or sores that will not heal. Large BCC lesions may have oozing or crusting at the center.[51–54] There have been six different histologic types of BCC identified.[53,54] **Table 41.3** ■ lists and describes these types.

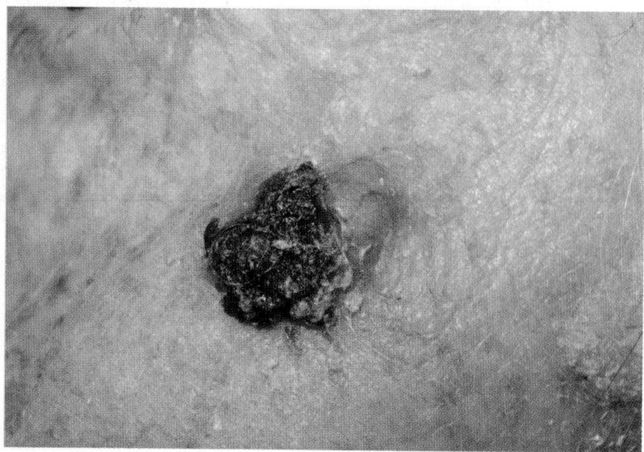

Figure 41.13 ■ Basal cell carcinoma.

Table 41.3 Histologic Types of Basal Cell Carcinoma

Histologic Type	Description
Mixed pattern	• Contains two or more of the following types • Occurs most often
Nodular	• Round, pearly, flesh-colored with telangiectases • Second most common, after mixed • May ulcerate
Superficial	• Reddened patch with whitish scale • Seen on upper trunk, shoulders • Grows slowly • Least invasive
Micronodular	• Yellow-white when stretched • Firm to touch • Aggressive
Morpheaform	• Flat, firm, white, waxy, toughened • Resembles a scar • Uncommon
Infiltrative	• Tumor infiltrates dermis • Margins less apparent • High recurrence rate

Linking Pathophysiology to Diagnosis and Treatment

Diagnosis of BCC begins with the inspection of the lesion and a high suspicion based on the lesion's appearance. Dermatologists may use a dermascope for magnification and a closer look at the lesion. Definitive diagnosis is made via biopsy. Biopsy may be done by shave technique, punch biopsy, incision, or excision.[51,53]

Treatment usually entails surgical removal of the lesion. There are several procedures that may be used to remove BCC. Most can be done in an office setting under local anesthesia. Procedures to remove BCC include curettage and electrodesiccation, cryosurgery, Mohs micrographic surgery for large or deep lesions, and excision. Excision of the entire lesion will result in a cure rate of 95%, while Mohs micrographic surgery has a cure rate of 99%.[51,52]

Topicals—such as 5-fluorouracil, diclofenac, and Picato—may be used, but they are reserved for early lesions and the recurrence rate is high when these medications are used for BCC. The immune modulator imiquimod has been used in early BCC but it is not as effective as surgery or other topical medication. In those rare cases of metastatic BCC, a targeted drug called vismodegib is used. This drug targets the "hedgehog" pathway proteins.[51]

Squamous Cell Carcinoma

Squamous cell carcinoma (SCC) is the second most common skin cancer, affecting approximately 1 million Americans per year.[50] The incidence of SCC has increased 200% in the past 30 years. SCC is more likely than BCC to metastasize. In 2012, 4000 to nearly 9000 persons died from SCC.[50]

Usually, SCC is a disease of persons 50 years or older, but the increased incidence in the past three decades affects 20- and 30-year-olds, particularly women. These changes in demographics probably reflect the increased use of tanning devices.[55] Women are more likely than men to use indoor tanning.

CLINICAL POINT: Use of tanning beds increases the risk for developing SCC and other skin cancers by 2.5 times.[55] Education of the public about the dangers of these devices is important, especially for teenagers. African Americans may also develop SCC, particularly if they have a preexisting inflammatory skin disorder such as psoriasis or burn scars. More Latinos are being diagnosed with SCC also.[55] ■

Etiology and Pathogenesis

SCC arises from damaged, unrepaired DNA in the nucleus of squamous cells of the epidermis. The cause of SCC is cumulative UV light exposure; that is, the more UV exposure, the higher the risk for SCC. Sunburn during childhood and the teen years is particularly high risk. UV radiation triggers cancerous transformation of keratinocytes. As these affected keratinocytes grow, they extend into the dermis. Once growing into the dermis, the lesion is considered SCC.[53] Metastasis occurs in about 5% of cases of SCC. Usually, lesions larger than 2 centimeters in diameter or SCC in immunocompromised persons is the reason for metastasis.[53]

TP53, a tumor-suppressor gene, has been identified as the gene most often mutated in SCC.[51] Mutation of *TP53* causes the damaged cells to live and grow longer and become malignant.

Risk factors for developing SCC include cumulative UV exposure; fair skin; light hair and eye color; outdoor occupation; personal history of BCC or SCC; male gender; older age; first-degree relative with SCC; chronic skin infection or inflammation; arsenic, coal tar, or oil exposure; immune deficiency; chemotherapy; PUVA treatment; antirejection drugs used in organ transplants; preexisting AKs; exposure to iodizing radiation; and smoking.[51,53,55] Individuals who have organ transplants and take antirejection drugs are 250 times more likely to develop SCC up to 20 years after the transplant.[55] AK are often precursors to SCC. Some dermatologists consider AK the earliest form of SCC.[55] It is estimated that 40–60% of SCCs begin as untreated AK.[40,55]

Clinical Manifestations

Squamous cell carcinoma appears as firm, smooth, or hyperkeratotic papules or plaques with an ulcer in the center on sun-exposed skin (**Figure 41.14** ■).[53] Often, SCC is a

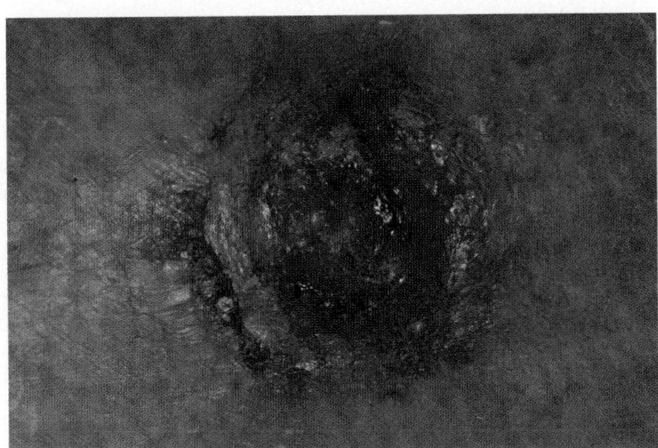

Figure 41.14 ■ Squamous cell carcinoma.

nonhealing sore that bleeds easily. SCC may also present as a large wart, a cutaneous horn, or as a slow-growing, scaly, red plaque. Sun-exposed areas where SCC usually appear include the rim of the ear, lower lip, face, balding scalp, neck, hands, arms, and legs.[55] SCCs may also occur in areas of the body that are not sun exposed, such as the genitals, mucous membranes, scars, or inflamed skin.[51]

Linking Pathophysiology to Diagnosis and Treatment

Diagnosis of SCC begins with clinical assessment of the lesions and is confirmed by biopsy. Use of dermoscopy assists dermatologists to differentiate SCC from other lesions. Biopsy is usually done in an office setting under local anesthesia. Procedures used for biopsy include shave, punch, incision, or excision of the entire lesion.

Treatment of SCC after confirmed diagnosis is usually surgery to remove the lesion. There are several options for surgical removal available, including curettage and electrodesiccation, Mohs micrographic surgery, and excision with a wide margin.[53] Topical chemotherapy may be employed for surface SCC, but would not be appropriate for deeper, larger lesions.[51] In cases in which metastasis has occurred, radiation or chemotherapy will be needed.

Melanoma

Melanoma is the most dangerous of the skin cancers. The incidence of this potentially deadly skin cancer is increasing. In 2014, an estimated 76,000 were expected to be diagnosed with melanoma. It was predicted that 9700 persons would die of melanoma during that same year.[56] This means that one person dies of melanoma every hour in the United States.[50] More men than women are affected by melanoma and men are more likely to die from the disease. However, in persons who develop melanoma before age 49, women outnumber men. Even though older age is a risk factor, melanoma occurs among individuals under 30 years of age. In fact, melanoma is one of the most common cancers in this age group.[50] Melanoma is 20 times more likely to occur in whites than in African Americans. Conversely, when melanomas do occur in African Americans, it is usually more advanced when diagnosed and the survival rate is much lower than in whites.[50]

Etiology and Pathogenesis

Melanomas originate in melanocytes in the lowest layer of the epidermis. Because of the pigment-producing properties of melanocytes, melanomas often look like moles and in some cases, melanoma will develop from moles.[56,57] The exact reason some moles change and others do not become malignant is not fully understood. Like other skin cancers, most melanomas develop because of unrepaired DNA damage to melanocytes that cause these cells to multiply rapidly and form cancerous tumors.[56,57] Some melanomas, however, occur in areas that are not exposed to sunlight. There are gene mutations that may be inherited. Usually familial melanomas will have changes in *CDKN2A* or *CDK4*, two tumor-suppressor genes.[56] Another gene mutation that has been discovered in melanomas involves the *BRAF* oncogene. This mutation is not inherited. Risk factors for the development of melanoma include UV light exposure, especially frequent sunburn as a child; moles, especially when there are more than 100 moles; familial moles or familial melanoma; fair skin; freckling; light hair; personal history of melanoma; immune suppression; age; and male gender.[56,57]

Clinical Manifestations

Most melanomas are brown or black; however, some melanomas do not make melanin and will be tan, pink, red, purple, blue, or white (**Figure 41.15** ■).[56,57] Melanomas may occur anywhere on the skin or mucous membranes. Melanomas are more likely to grow on the trunk in men and on the legs in women.[57] Melanomas may appear as unusual sores, lumps, spread of pigmented areas, new moles after age 30, color changes in the skin, or changes in an existing mole. Warning signs of changes to existing moles can be remembered using the mnemonic **ABCDE**:

Asymmetry: Asymmetric appearance; the two halves are different in shape
Borders: Irregular borders; uneven, notched, or scalloped
Color: Color changes within a mole; unusual color, multicolored
Diameter: More than $\frac{1}{4}$ inch wide, the size of a pencil eraser
Evolving: New mole in an individual over age 30, a changing mole, or an "ugly duckling" mole that is different from all the others

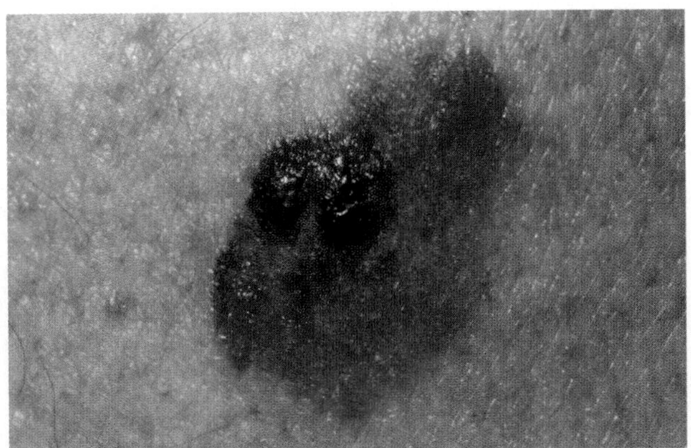

Figure 41.15 ■ Malignant melanoma.

Linking Pathophysiology to Diagnosis and Treatment

Most melanomas are discovered after the patient brings a skin change or lesion to the attention of a doctor. Most general practice doctors will refer the patient to a dermatologist if a melanoma is strongly suspected. The dermatologist will conduct a dermoscopic examination and proceed to biopsy or to complete excision with wide margins to effect both a biopsy and a cure.[56,57] If the melanoma has spread to lymph nodes, then those nodes will be removed for biopsy.

Treatment depends on the stage and size of the melanoma. Treatment methods may include surgery, immunotherapy, targeted therapy, chemotherapy, and radiation. Early melanomas will need to be excised. If the melanoma has spread, immunotherapy to boost the T-cell immune response may be used. Ipilimumab is a man-made antibody that targets and blocks *CTLA4*, thereby boosting the T-cell response to the tumor. This drug does not cure metastatic melanoma, but it does prolong life.[56]

Targeted therapy for melanoma has been developed for cells with the mutated *BRAF* gene. About half of all melanomas have these mutated genes. Vemurafenib is one *BRAF* inhibitor that will shrink the tumor and prolong the time before it grows again. Unfortunately, it will not cure advanced melanoma.[56] For melanomas that develop on the palms, soles, under the nails, or on mucosal surfaces, a drug that has been used in other forms of cancer is being studied. Imatinib targets the mutated *C-KIT* gene found in some melanomas.

Check Your Progress: Section 41.5

1. How does chronic UV exposure trigger the development of basal cell carcinoma?
2. What is the standard treatment intervention for lesions that have been diagnosed as squamous cell carcinoma?
3. In evaluating a mole that is suspicious for being melanoma, what mnemonic is useful in helping to make a clinical determination?

41.6 Changes in Pigmentation of the Skin

Pigmentary changes in the skin are permanent changes that are often associated with or serve as markers for other autoimmune disease or inherited autosomal disorders. Pigmentary changes do not itch or hurt and they are not life threatening. However, they can be cosmetically distressing. Pigmentary changes have the potential for affecting self-esteem, confidence, and emotional health. In fact, some cultures will marginalize people with pigmentary changes causing them to feel isolated and to have difficulty in finding a mate.[58] This section focuses on two forms of pigmentary changes: vitiligo and café au lait spots.

Vitiligo

Vitiligo is an acquired pigmentary disorder in which patches of skin, hair, or mucous membranes lose color. Vitiligo affects about 2% of the world's population and about 1% of the population of the United States.[58,59] The disorder affects men and women equally; however, women are more likely to seek medical care because of the cosmetic effect. The average age at onset is 20 years, with a range of 10–30 years.[59]

Etiology and Pathogenesis

Vitiligo is a multifactoral disorder involving genetic and environmental elements. The exact cause is unknown. There are several theories concerning causation listed in **Table 41.4** ■.[59,60]

The principal defect is the loss of functional melanocytes in areas of the skin, hair, or mucous membranes.[59] In about 30% of vitiligo cases, there is a first-degree relative with vitiligo or other autoimmune diseases.[60] Jin et al. identified genes associated with vitiligo, including *TYR* and several other genes associated with autoimmune disease.[61] The *TYR* gene region on chromosome 11 encodes tyrosinase, an enzyme needed for melanin biosynthesis. *TYR* is also a major autoantigen in vitiligo. In this study, there were 10 susceptibility loci identified that had associations with vitiligo and autoimmune diseases such as type 1 diabetes mellitus.[61]

Table 41.4 Theories for Causation of Vitiligo

Theory	Description
Autoimmune	• Alteration in humoral immunity • Circulating antibodies lead to destruction of melanocytes
Cytotoxic	• Destruction of melanocytes by abnormal CD8 T cells • Melanocyte-specific T cells found in blood samples of persons with vitiligo • Lymphocytes found in depigmented skin may be involved in melanocyte destruction
Intrinsic defect of melanocytes	• Preexisting defect in melanocytes that leads to early death
Oxidant/antioxidant system disturbance	• Increased free radicals that are toxic to melanocytes • Affected skin has oxidized substance that causes accumulation of hydrogen peroxide that destroys melanocytes
Neural theory	• Some cases of vitiligo occur after nerve injury • One form of vitiligo occurs in a dermatomal pattern • Toxic substances from nerves may interfere with melanin production

Other studies have revealed that autoimmune comorbidities to vitiligo occur in 25–55% of patients.[58,60] Comorbidities include thyroid disorders, psoriasis, pernicious anemia, alopecia areata, inflammatory bowel disease, and systemic lupus erythematosus. Consequently, vitiligo is considered a marker for some autoimmune disorders and clinicians will screen for thyroid disorders, diabetes, or other disorders when a patient presents with vitiligo.[58,60]

Clinical Manifestations

Vitiligo lesions are milky-white or chalk-white hypopigmented macules or patches on the skin that are well demarcated and surrounded by normal skin (**Figure 41.16** ■). Most of these lesions are round, oval, or linear and less than ¼ inch to more than 5 inches in diameter. Vitiligo lesions grow from the center out, spreading at an unpredictable rate. The distribution of vitiligo includes the hands, arms, feet, trunk, and face. On the face, the hypopigmentation often circles the eyes or the mouth.[59] Vitiligo may be localized, generalized, or universal:

- Localized:
  - Focal—one area affected
  - Segmental—one or more hypopigmented areas in a dermatome; seen more often in children
  - Mucosal—only the mucous membranes are affected
- Generalized:
  - Acrofacial—seen on fingertips and around the eyes and mouth
  - Vulgaris—scattered patches on much of the body
  - Mixed—combination of generalized or localized types
- Universal: Complete to nearly complete depigmentation of the skin.

Some forms of vitiligo may occur where there has been injury to the skin or begin as an inflammation.[59,60]

Linking Pathophysiology to Diagnosis and Treatment

Diagnosis of vitiligo is based on inspection of the skin and, occasionally, a biopsy to verify the diagnosis. There are many treatments for vitiligo, but not one that will restore skin color in all patients. Patients are encouraged to use high–sun protection factor (SPF) sunscreen to both protect the depigmented skin and reduce tanning of the unaffected skin. Sunburn can stimulate spread of the depigmentation process.[60]

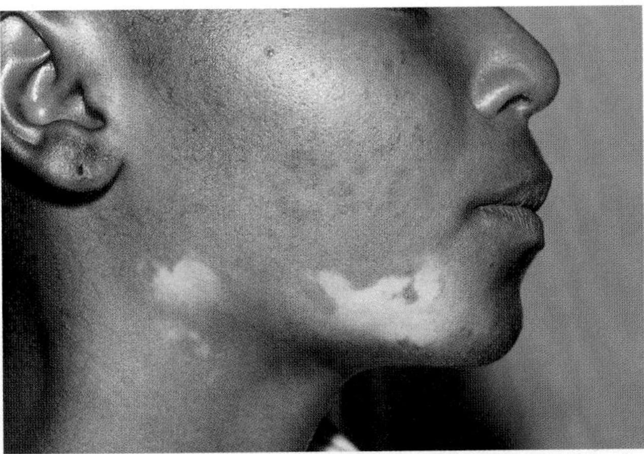

Figure 41.16 ■ Trichrome vitiligo.

Many patients with vitiligo prefer cosmetic cover-ups to give their skin an even color. There are several products available for vitiligo sufferers, such as Dermablend and C-ESTA Make-up for Vitiligo.[60] Only dermatologists offer the many treatment options available. Treatment must be individualized and many of the treatments for vitiligo have associated risks. Treatment options for vitiligo include systemic phototherapy, laser therapy, steroid therapy, topical tacrolimus ointment, and depigmentation therapy.

Café au Lait Spots

Café au lait spots or macules (CALMs) are hyperpigmented spots on the skin that are the color of "coffee with milk." When these brown spots occur singly, they are considered to be birthmarks. CALMs are seen in all races, but occur more often in blacks.[62] Both genders are equally affected. Multiple CALMs may indicate genetic disorders. The genetic disorder most often associated with CALMs is neurofibromatosis type 1 (NF1), an autosomal dominant disorder with high penetrance and variable expressivity, or it may occur because of a new germ cell mutation.[63,63] NF1, or von Recklinghausen disease, occurs in 1 of 2500–3000 individuals.[64] Of those with NF1, 95% will have CALMs.[62]

Etiology and Pathogenesis

CALMs occur because of an increase in melanin in spots on the skin. CALMs are usually benign. In persons with NF1, giant melanosomes (organelles where synthesis, storage, and transport of melanin occur) and stem cell factor cytokines are found within the CALM.[62] CALMs may also be seen in other inherited disorders such as NF2, Fanconi anemia, tuberous sclerosis, and Gaucher disease.

Clinical Manifestations

CALMs are flat, light brown or dark brown lesions that are have irregular or smooth borders and vary in size from a few millimeters to 10 centimeters or more (**Figure 41.17** ■). These hyperpigmented lesions are present at birth and darken with age. CALMs may appear on the trunk, buttocks, face, or limbs. The more CALMs present on the skin, the higher the likelihood of NF1. Axillary and inguinal CALMs are often diagnostic for NF1.

Linking Pathophysiology to Diagnosis and Treatment

CALMs may be diagnosed by inspection and do not require medical care. If the CALMs are associated with NF1 or another genetic disorder, other manifestations of the disorders will require medical care.

Solar Lentigo

A **solar lentigo** (plural is *lentigines*) is a benign, sun-induced lesion commonly known as age spots or liver spots.[65,66] Solar lentigines are seen in about 90% of American Caucasians over age 60 and in about 20% of Caucasians 35 years or younger.[65] These lesions are most

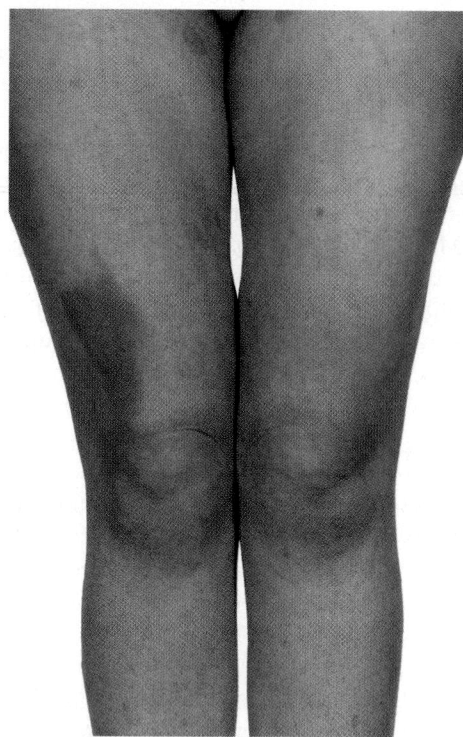

Figure 41.17 ■ Café au lait spots.

common among fair-skinned persons and are considered a sign of aging. Solar lentigines serve as a marker for ultraviolet skin damage and increased risk for skin cancer.[66]

Etiology and Pathogenesis

Ultraviolet light exposure induces hyperplasia of the epidermis where increased pigmentation occurs secondary to melanocytes replacing keratinocytes in the basal layer.[65,66] This change gives the solar lentigines their characteristic tan-brown to black color.

Clinical Manifestations

Solar lentigines are tan-brown or black macules that are well demarcated and surrounded by normal skin (**Figure 41.18** ■). Their size varies from 5 to 20 millimeters in diameter and they are irregular in shape. Multiple smaller lesions may grow together to form patches.[67] Solar lentigines are found on sun-exposed skin of the hands, forearms, face, neck, and shoulders.

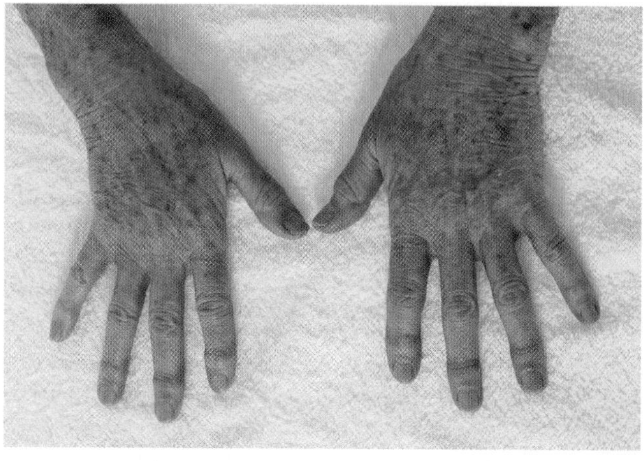

Figure 41.18 ■ Solar lentigo.

Linking Pathophysiology to Diagnosis and Treatment

Solar lentigines are diagnosed based on their appearance. Clinicians may use dermoscopy or biopsy to rule out lentigo maligna, a precancerous lesion, or melanoma.[67]

Solar lentigines are benign and do not require treatment, but many people do not like the cosmetic effect. Consequently, there are several modes of treatment available to fade or remove solar lentigines. Treatments available for solar lentigines include hydroquinone and tretinoin creams used as bleaching agents; antioxidants such as alpha hydroxyl acid, vitamin C, and azelaic acid; chemical peel with phenol; cryotherapy; and laser treatments.

Solar lentigines may be decreased or prevented by avoiding ultraviolet exposure from the sun or tanning devices. The use of sunscreen and protective clothing are recommended for those who must be in sunlight and want to avoid sunburn.

Check Your Progress: Section 41.6

1. What are the defining clinical manifestations of vitiligo lesions and how are they distributed throughout the body?
2. How are café au lait spots characterized?
3. Because of their cosmetic impact, solar lentigines, or age spots, are best treated using which interventions?

41.7 Disorders of the Hair and Scalp

Hair loss can be very worrisome for individuals experiencing it or parents of children who are losing hair. Hair loss may be associated with infection, systemic disease, stress, autoimmune disorders, or mental health problems. This section focuses on general hair loss, alopecia, and autoimmune hair loss, alopecia areata.

Alopecia

Alopecia is baldness or loss of hair from the scalp or body. Hair loss may indicate systemic disease and it can have a profound effect on the patient's self-esteem and emotional health.[68] The most common form of alopecia is androgenic alopecia, a genetic type of baldness related to the hormone androgen. Androgenic baldness affects men and women. Approximately 60–80% of Caucasian men will develop androgenic or male-pattern baldness.[69] About 20% of these men will develop this type of baldness during the late teens or early 20s, while 50% will develop baldness by age 50.[69] White men are more likely than black or Asian men to develop male-pattern baldness. It has been estimated that 40% of women older than age 70 will develop androgenic alopecia in female-pattern baldness.[69] Female-pattern hair loss may also occur among women with metabolic syndrome or polycystic ovary syndrome.[70]

Etiology and Pathogenesis

Hair follicles continually go through growth phases, including **anagen** (long growing phase), **catagen** (brief transitional phase), **telogen** (short resting phase), and **exogen** (hair falls out or sheds at end of resting phase).[68–70] In fact, hair follicles are the only organs that are continually changing and growing throughout life. Usually, 85–90% of hairs are in anagen growth, which varies in length from 1 to 8 years; 10–15% are in telogen rest that lasts for months; and less than 1% are in catagen transition that lasts for a few weeks.[68] Normal scalp hair will shed 50–100 hairs every day.

There are several causes of alopecia, and they are classified as scarring or nonscarring. Some of the scarring causes are acne keloidalis nuchae, chronic cutaneous lupus, and dissecting cellulitis of the scalp. Some of the nonscarring causes are anagen effluvium (caused by agents such as chemotherapy disrupting the anagen phase of hair growth), primary hair shaft disorders, trichotillomania (obsessive–compulsive hair pulling), androgenic alopecia, and alopecia areata.

Androgenic alopecia, the most common cause of baldness, is related to androgen, especially dihydrotestosterone. One gene that has been associated with androgenic alopecia is the androgen receptor gene, which provides instruction for making androgen receptors. For reasons not yet understood, the androgen receptors in the scalp hair follicles of men and women with androgen alopecia cause an excess of androgen in the hair follicles. This leads to a shorter hair growth cycle and shorter, thinner hair. Eventually, the hair follicles affected will stop replacing lost hair.[71]

Pregnancy usually produces a prolonged anagen phase, followed in postpartum by a prolonged telogen phase; telogen effluvium may persist for up to 1 year.[70] ■

Clinical Manifestations

The signs and symptoms of alopecia depend on the cause. Androgenic alopecia begins with hair loss around the temples and progresses to hair loss over the top of the scalp (**Figure 41.19** ■).

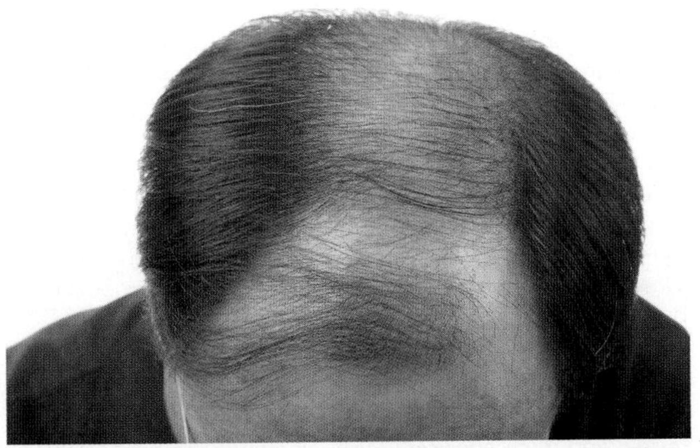

Figure 41.19 ■ Male-pattern androgenic alopecia.

Linking Pathophysiology to Diagnosis and Treatment

Diagnosis of alopecia is based on history and physical findings. Occasionally, a biopsy is needed to fully diagnose the cause.

Treatment of alopecia depends on the cause of the problem. For androgenic alopecia, minoxidil is a topical medication that helps with hair regrowth by prolonging the growth phase and producing mature hair in about 30–40% of patients who use it.[68] However, when the patient stops using minoxidil, alopecia returns. Finasteride is an oral medication that has been used for male-pattern baldness. It blocks the conversion of testosterone to dihydrotestosterone. It takes 6–8 months to work fully and there are some serious side effects. Like minoxidil, when finasteride is discontinued, the hair loss returns. Finasteride is not used in women and is considered teratogenic.[68] Hormonal modulators such as birth control pills or spironolactone help relieve female-pattern alopecia.

Alopecia Areata

Alopecia areata (AA) is a fairly common autoimmune disorder that causes chronic, relapsing, inflammatory-induced, nonscarring hair loss and nail changes.[72–74] AA affects about 4.5 million Americans of all ages and all colors of hair.[73] The prevalence of AA in the world's general population is 0.1–0.2%.[73,74] Men and women are equally affected. The earlier the age at onset of AA, the more severe the disease is.

Children who are affected by AA comprise about 20% of AA cases and up to 66% of cases occur in persons under age 30.[73,74] ■

Etiology and Pathogenesis

Hair follicles are continuously in transformation to produce and shed hairs. Anagen-phase hair follicles that contain proliferating keratinocytes and melanocytes are the major site of inflammatory attack in AA due to loss of immune privilege that usually shields the hair follicle.[73] This suggests that autoantigens are present only in the anagen phase. Inflammatory cells—including CD8+ T-cells, NK cells, eosinophils, and mast cells—attack anagen hair follicles, causing them to move into the catagen phase early. This weakens the hair shaft and hair breaks at or near the surface of the skin. As the hair enters telogen phase, the fragile hair falls out.[74] In AA, the process does not cause scarring so the hair follicle will be able to regenerate and continue the hair growth cycle spontaneously. However, relapsing inflammation may occur at any time.[73]

AA has a strong genetic connection, although cases do occur in persons with no family history of the disorder. A family history of AA is more often associated with more aggressive, severe cases with resistance to treatment.[73] In addition, family history of AA is often accompanied by history of other autoimmune disease, especially thyroid disorders, vitiligo, and atopy.[74] (See the Impact of Current Research on Clinical Practice feature.) Studies of families with AA have shown susceptibility loci on chromosomes 6, 10, 16, and 18.[73,74] Chromosome 6 has an HLA locus that may partially explain the onset of autoimmunity.

The chromosome 16 region in AA overlaps with a region near the susceptibility locus for Crohn disease. Chromosome 18 contains a psoriasis susceptibility region.[73] In patients with severe AA, cytotoxic T-lymphocyte–associated antigen 4 (*CTLA4*) has been identified and is also seen in patients with psoriasis.

Clinical Manifestations

AA is loss of hair in patches that are well demarcated on the scalp or beard (**Figure 41.20** ■). It begins suddenly and can progress to alopecia totalis (AT) or complete baldness of the scalp. In fewer cases, the hair loss may extend to the entire body, which is called *alopecia universalis (AU)*. The patches of hair loss may be single or multiple and are asymmetric over the head and face. There are no obvious changes in the underlying skin. Almost 90% of cases of AA seen by dermatologists involve only the scalp and about 5% of cases will involve the entire scalp or body.[74]

Occasionally, the underlying skin will be pink or peach colored. Inside the patch or at the borders "exclamation point" hairs will be seen.[74] These are short hairs that taper to a smaller base because of the arrest of growth in the anagen phase. There is no itching, burning, or pain with AA. The hair may begin to grow back spontaneously or it may start to grow with treatment. On recovery the hair is likely to be hypopigmented but will return to the original color in time.

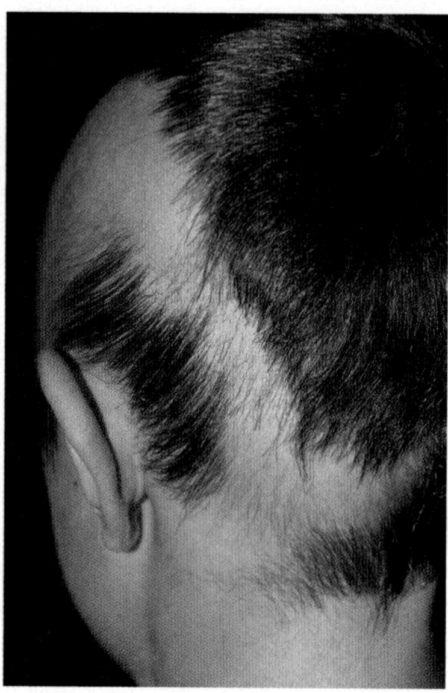

Figure 41.20 ■ Alopecia areata.

Around 50% of patients with AA will recover in a year without treatment.[74] Unfortunately, AA relapses are common. The more widespread the hair loss and the longer it persists, the more likely the baldness will be permanent. If the patient has a relative with AA, another autoimmune disorder, atopy, nail involvement, or is very young at onset of the disorder, the more likely the baldness will persist. In fact, less than 10% of patients with AT or AU will grow hair again.[74]

Nail changes related to AA have been reported in 7–66% of the patients studied.[74] The most commonly related nail dystrophy is pitting. Nail changes before, during, or after hair loss due to AA have occurred.

Linking Pathophysiology to Diagnosis and Treatment

AA can be diagnosed on inspection, and other testing is rarely needed. Routine screening for other autoimmune diseases is not indicated, even though thyroid disorders have been associated with AA in as many as 28% of AA patients.[74]

There are several treatments for AA, but there is no one treatment that will cure or prevent recurrence.[75] Treatments include topical corticosteroids plus minoxidil, intralesional corticosteroid injections, and topical immunotherapy. There is a high rate of spontaneous recovery.

Check Your Progress: Section 41.7

1. Which type of alopecia is the most common cause of baldness and how does it trigger this process?
2. What is the mechanism by which hair loss occurs in alopecia areata?
3. What are the most common treatments used to treat alopecia areata?

Impact of Current Research on Clinical Practice

Common Pathophysiologic Pathways

Description: Mohan and Silverberg conducted a meta-analysis to compare the prevalence of atopic dermatitis (AD) among participants who have early- or late-onset vitiligo and/or with alopecia areata (AA). They searched MEDLINE, EMBASE, Cochrane Library, and Google Scholar, and did a manual search of 12 additional journals in any language for research that explored the presence of AD among persons with vitiligo and AA reported between 1946 and April 5, 2014. Their search resulted in 16 studies of vitiligo patients and 17 studies of AA patients in 11 different countries that could be used for the meta-analysis. Data from the studies demonstrated that patients with early-onset vitiligo or alopecia totalis or alopecia universalis have an increased probability for AD. The studies reviewed did not specify whether the AD or vitiligo or AA came first.

Clinical Practice: Understanding that persons with early-onset vitiligo and alopecia totalis and alopecia universalis may also have AD suggests there may be common pathophysiologic pathways for developing these disorders. The common pathways suggested for study by the authors included Th17 and thymic stromal lymphopoietin. There may also be shared genetic pathways such as the filaggrin gene mutation. Knowing more about the commonalities of pathogenesis of AD, vitiligo, alopecia totalis, and alopecia universalis will be integral to the development of better treatments and, possibly, a cure for these disorders.

Research Study:

Mohan, G.C., & Silverberg, J.I. (2014). Association of vitiligo and alopecia areata with atopic dermatitis: A systematic review and meta-analysis. *JAMA Dermatology*; doi:10.1001/jamadermatol.2014.3324

CHAPTER SUMMARY

41.1 Chapter Overview and Case Studies

Differentiate acute from chronic skin conditions and describe concepts related to chronic disorders of the skin.

- Chronic skin disorders, unlike acute skin problems, are often incurable. Chronic skin disorders result from viral infection or alterations in immunity and genetic susceptibility to autoimmune disease.

41.2 Viral Skin Infections

Differentiate the causes, classification, underlying pathogenesis, and clinical manifestations of viral skin infections and approaches to diagnosis and treatment for those conditions across the lifespan.

- Herpes simplex type 1 is a viral infection that causes a painful vesicular rash. The most common site of this infection is the lips and mouth, but it can occur anywhere on the skin. This infection is treated but not cured with antiviral medications.
- Herpes simplex type 2 is a viral infection that causes a painful vesicular rash most often on the genitals. This infection is treated but not cured with antiviral medications.
- Herpes zoster or shingles is caused by the varicella-zoster virus that also causes chickenpox. The virus is able to live in the sensory dorsal nerve root ganglia or cranial nerves and erupt later in life as a painful, vesicular rash along a dermatome. Shingles may result in postherpetic neuralgia. The infection is treated with antivirals. Shingles may be prevented by vaccination.
- Warts are caused by the human papillomavirus. Warts may occur on the skin or mucous membranes. There are about 100 different human papillomaviruses, some of which have been linked to cancers of the throat, cervix, and anorectal areas.

41.3 Skin Disorders with a Genetic Basis

Differentiate the causes, classification, underlying pathogenesis, and clinical manifestations of skin disorders with a genetic basis and approaches to diagnosis and treatment for those conditions across the lifespan.

- Atopic dermatitis (AD) is an IgE-mediated atopic disorder that causes a chronic, relapsing, inflammatory, very pruritic skin disorder. AD may flareup for no apparent reason. Treatment of AD includes anti-inflammatory medications, immunomodulators, and moisturizers.
- Psoriasis is a chronic, relapsing, inflammatory, immune-mediated skin disorder with a high rate of heritability. Psoriasis will flare up periodically in response to stress or infection or other environmental triggers. Psoriasis is treated with anti-inflammatory drugs, antimetabolites, immunomodulators, and TNF inhibitors.
- Hidradenitis suppurativa (HS) is a recurrent, chronic inflammatory skin disease that involves the hair follicle in apocrine sweat glands in the axilla, pubic, and perineal areas. The lesions are nodules, abscesses, and sinus tracts under the skin. Keloid-like scarring is also seen. HS is treated by anti-inflammatory antibiotics, anti-androgens, immunosuppressants, and surgery.

41.4 Benign Neoplasms of the Skin

Differentiate the causes, classification, underlying pathogenesis, and clinical manifestations of benign neoplasms of the skin and approaches to diagnosis and treatment for those conditions across the lifespan.

- Photodermatitis occurs when an individual's immune system reacts to UV light with solar urticaria or other forms of allergic reactions. Actinic keratosis (AK) is a scaly, rough skin lesion that is caused by chronic sun exposure. AK is most likely to occur in older skin; however, increased UV exposure is causing AK to occur in some as young as 20 years old. AK is sometimes a precursor to squamous cell carcinoma.
- Hemangiomas are bright red growths made of capillaries that grow in or under the skin. Hemangiomas are usually benign, occur in newborns, and disappear without treatment by age 7.
- Moles or nevi are common benign hyperpigmented growths made up of proliferating melanocytes. Atypical moles may become cancerous.
- Skin tags or acrochordons are soft, flesh-colored, or pigmented papules with stalks that attach them to skin. These benign lesions are usually found where skin rubs on skin or on clothing and increase in number in obesity or pregnancy.
- Lipomas are common benign lumps made of adipose tissue that grow under the skin. Treatment is not indicated unless the lumps are large and bothersome. In these cases, the lipoma may be removed by liposuction or surgery.
- Epidermal inclusion cysts are skin nodules in which squamous epithelium of the epidermis is trapped or implanted into the dermis and are filled with keratinocytes and other debris. No treatment is indicated unless the cysts are secondarily infected.

41.5 Skin Cancer

Differentiate the causes, classification, underlying pathogenesis, and clinical manifestations of skin cancer and approaches to diagnosis and treatment for those conditions across the lifespan.

- Basal cell carcinoma (BCC) is the most frequently occurring skin cancer that develops in sun-exposed skin. BCC is unlikely to metastasize, but is disfiguring and is often removed surgically.
- Squamous cell carcinoma (SCC) is the second most common skin cancer and is more likely than BCC to metastasize. Treatment is surgery to remove the lesion.
- Melanoma is the most dangerous of the skin cancers. It originates in sun-damaged melanocytes in the basal epidermis and may develop from moles. Treatment depends on the stage and size of the melanoma.

41.6 Changes in Pigmentation of the Skin

Differentiate the causes, classification, underlying pathogenesis, and clinical manifestations of changes in pigmentation of the skin and approaches to diagnosis and treatment for those conditions across the lifespan.

- Vitiligo is an acquired disorder in which patches of skin lose color as melanocytes stop functioning. The exact cause is unknown but probably involves heredity, autoimmune mechanisms, and nerve injury. There is no single therapy for vitiligo that will cure the disorder.
- Café au lait spots or macules (CALMs) are hyperpigmented areas of the skin the color of coffee with milk. CALMs are often seen as single lesions and are considered benign birthmarks. If there are large numbers of CALMs, then neurofibromatosis type 1, an autosomal dominant disorder, should be suspected. There is no treatment needed for CALMs alone; however, any underlying genetic disorder will require medical treatment.
- Solar lentigines, also called age spots or liver spots, are very common. They are pigmented macules that occur in sun-exposed areas, usually in older people. Topical creams or chemical peels may be used to lighten solar lentigo.

41.7 Disorders of the Hair and Scalp

Differentiate the causes, classification, underlying pathogenesis, and clinical manifestations of disorders of the hair and scalp and approaches to diagnosis and treatment for those conditions across the lifespan.

- Alopecia is hair loss. There are many causes of hair loss. The most frequent cause is androgenic in both men and women. Treatment depends on the cause of the baldness.
- Alopecia areata is an autoimmune disease that causes nonscarring hair loss.

REVIEW QUESTIONS

1. A 6-month-old infant is brought into the emergency department by her parents. The mother reports that her daughter has been progressively developing patches of extreme dryness, particularly on her face, scalp, and antecubital regions. In addition, she has been really irritable, not feeding well, and has difficulty sleeping. After examining the infant, what treatment strategies would you advise the parents to follow at home?
   a. Bland diet, calamine lotion, liquid ibuprofen
   b. Cold-water baths, baby aspirin, clear liquids
   c. Hydrocortisone cream, soy formula, electric fan
   d. Lukewarm-water baths, moisturizers, cool-mist humidifiers
2. What key finding is usually observed in melanomas that is not found with basal and squamous cell carcinomas?
   a. The occurrence of a high fever
   b. The presence of lumps in areas not exposed to sunlight
   c. The chronic pruritus throughout the trunk region
   d. The dispersion of crusted lesions over the face and scalp
3. Which of the following medications should be administered to a patient who will be undergoing laser treatment for the removal of a hemangioma?
   a. Corticosteroids
   b. Antibiotics
   c. Antihistamines
   d. Topical retinoids
4. You are the nurse caring for a 16-year-old patient who was recently diagnosed with guttate psoriasis. The patient is curious and asks you what could have caused this condition to develop. How would you respond?
   a. "This condition is often associated with exposure to hazardous chemicals."
   b. "This condition has been linked to the consumption of uncooked meat."
   c. "This condition is usually seen after having a severe upper respiratory infection."
   d. "This condition develops in response to a really humid environment."

5. What is the definitive treatment for epidermal inclusion cysts that have not ruptured?
   a. Surgical excision
   b. Antibiotics
   c. Low-dose diuretics
   d. No treatment is required
6. A 68-year-old patient presents with a couple of non-healing sores on his neck that bleed very easily. What diagnostic test would be useful in identifying the origin of these sores?
   a. Skin biopsy
   b. CT scan
   c. Ultrasound
   d. Gamma scan
7. Postherpatic neuralgia, a common complication following shingles, is manifested as:
   a. a significant change in visual acuity with associated eye pain.
   b. a transient loss of sensation to all extremities.
   c. a precipitous drop in blood pressure with accompanied dizziness.
   d. a continuation of pain and sensitivity around the site of the initial shingles rash.
8. In caring for an adult patient with atopic dermatitis, how would you evaluate the effectiveness of the medications administered for a flare-up of this disorder?
   a. Increase in red blood cell count
   b. Decrease in serum immunoglobulin E (IgE) levels
   c. Decrease in neutrophil count
   d. Increase in T-cell lymphocyte count

ANSWERS

Answers to Review Questions can be found in Appendix A. Answers to Case Study and Check Your Progress questions are available on the faculty resources site. Please consult with your instructor.

RECOMMENDED WEBSITES

American Academy of Dermatology
https://www.aad.org/for-the-public

Centers for Disease Control and Prevention: Shingles (Herpes Zoster)
www.cdc.gov/shingles/

Hidradenitis Suppurativa Foundation, Inc.
www.hs-foundation.org

National Institute of Arthritis and Musculoskeletal and Skin Diseases
www.niams.nih.gov/Health_Info/

National Psoriasis Foundation
https://www.psoriasis.org

REFERENCES

1. Usatine, R. P., & Tinitigan, R. (2010). Nongenital herpes simplex virus. *American Family Physician*, 82(9):1075–1082.
2. Centers for Disease Control and Prevention (CDC). (2014). Self-study STD modules for clinicians: Genital herpes simplex virus (HSV) infection. Retrieved from www2a.cdc.gov/stdtraining/self-study/herpes/default.htm
3. Adams, M. P., Holland, L. N., & Urban, C. (2017). *Pharmacology for nursing: A pathophysiologic approach* (5th ed.). Hoboken, NJ: Pearson Education.
4. Stephenson-Famy A., & Gardella, C. (2014). Herpes simplex virus infection during pregnancy. *Obstetrics and Gynecology Clinics of North America*, 41:601–614.
5. Salvaggio, M. R., & Bronze, M. S. (2016). Herpes simplex workup. *Medscape*. Retrieved from http://emedicine.medscape.com/article/218580-workup.
6. Centers for Disease Control and Prevention (CDC). (2016). Shingles (herpes zoster): For Health Care Professionals: Clinical Overview. Retrieved from www.cdc.gov/shingles/hcp/clinical-overview.html.
7. Wilson, D. D. (2014). Herpes zoster: A rash demanding careful evaluation. *The Nurse Practitioner*, 39(5):31–36.
8. Cohen, J. I. (2013). Herpes zoster. *New England Journal of Medicine*, 369:255–263.
9. Mayo Clinic. (2016). Shingles. *Diseases and conditions.* Retrieved from http://www.mayoclinic.org/diseases-conditions/shingles/basics/definition/con-20019574
10. Gearhart, P. A. (2016). Human papillomavirus. *Medscape Reference*. Retrieved from http://emedicine.medscape.com/article/219110-overview#a0156.
11. Centers of Disease Control and Prevention (CDC). (2014). Reported STDs in the United States. Retrieved from www.cdc.gov/std/stats14/std-trends-508.pdf.
12. Centers of Disease Control and Prevention (CDC). (2016). Genital HPV infection: Fact sheet. Retrieved from www.cdc.gov/std/hpv/stdfact-hpv.htm.
13. Centers of Disease Control and Prevention (CDC). (2016). HPV-associated cancer statistics. Retrieved from www.cdc.gov/cancer/hpv/statistics/.
14. Blair, G. (2013). Warts. In T. M. Buttaro, J. Trybulski, P. P. Bailey, & J. Sandberg-Cook (Eds.),. *Primary care: A collaborative practice* (pp. 300–302). St. Louis, MO: Elsevier.

15. Mulhem, E., &, Pinelis, S. (2011). Treatment of nongenital cutaneous warts. *American Family Physician*, 84(3):288–293.
16. Dall'oglio, F., D'Amico, V., Nasca, M., & Micali, G. (2012). Treatment of cutaneous warts: An evidence-based review. *American Journal of Clinical Dermatology*, 13(2):73–96.
17. Eichenfield, L. E., Tom, W. I., Chamlin, S. I., et al. (2014). Guidelines of care for the management of atopic dermatitis: Section 1. Diagnosis and assessment of atopic dermatitis. *Journal of the American Academy of Dermatology*, 70:338–351.
18. Kim, B. S. (2016). Atopic dermatitis. *Medscape*. Retrieved from http://emedicine.medscape.com/article/1049085-overview #aw2aab6b2b2.
19. Boguniewicz, M., & Leung, D. Y. M. (2011). Atopic dermatitis: A disease of altered skin barrier and immune dysregulation. *Immunological Reviews*, 242:233–246.
20. Knee, N. W. (2013). Eczematous dermatitis (atopic dermatitis). In T. M. Buttaro, J. Trybulski, P. P. Bailey, & J. Sandberg-Cook (Eds.), *Primary care: A collaborative practice* (pp. 263–265). St. Louis, MO: Elsevier.
21. Eichenfield, L. E., Tom, W. I., Chamlin, S. I., et al. (2014). Guidelines of care for the management of atopic dermatitis: Section 4. Prevention of disease flares and use of adjunctive therapies and approaches. *Journal of the American Academy of Dermatology*, 71:1218–1233.
22. Eichenfield, L. E., Tom, W. I., Chamlin, S. I., et al. (2014). Guidelines of care for the management of atopic dermatitis: Section 2. Management and treatment of atopic dermatitis with topical therapies. *Journal of the American Academy of Dermatology*, 71:116–132.
23. Rachakonda, T. D., Schupp, C. W., & Armstrong, A. W. (2014). Psoriasis prevalence among adults in the United States. *Journal of the American Academy of Dermatology*, 70(3):512–516.
24. Mahil, S. K., Capon, F., & Barker, J. N. (2015). Genetics of psoriasis. *Dermatology Clinics*, 33:1–11.
25. Menter, A., Korman, N. J., Elmets, C. A., et al. (2011). Guidelines of care for the management of psoriasis and psoriatic arthritis: Section 6. Case-based presentations and evidence-based conclusions. *Journal of the American Academy of Dermatology*, 65:137–174.
26. Meffert, J. (2016). Psoriasis. *Medscape*. Retrieved from http://emedicine.medscape.com/article/1943419-overview.
27. Weigle, N., & McBane, S. Psoriasis. (2013). *American Family Physician*, 87(9):626–633.
28. Lo Sicco, K., Camisa, C., & Grandinetti, L. (2013). Psoriais. Cleveland Clinic Center for Continuing Education. Retrieved from www.clevelandclinicmeded.com/medicalpubs/diseasemanagement/dermatology/psoriasis-papulosquamous-skin-disease/.
29. Mease, P. J., & Armstrong, A. W. (2014). Managing patients with psoriatic disease: The diagnosis and pharmacologic treatment of psoriatic arthritis in patients with psoriasis. *Drugs*, 74:423–441.
30. Earwood, J. S., & Thompson, T. D. (2016). Hidradenitis suppurativa. *Essential Evidence Plus*. Retrieved from www.essentialevidenceplus.com.frontier.idm.oclc.org/content/eee/740.
31. Deckers, I. E., van der Zee, H. H., & Prens, E. P. (2014). Epidemiology of hidradenitis suppurativa: Prevalence, pathogenesis, and factors associated with the development of HS. *Current Dermatology Reports*, 3:54–60.
32. Vazquez, B. G., Alikhan, M. D., Weaver, A. L., et al. (2013). Incidence of hidradenitis suppurativa and associated factors: A population-based study of Olmsted County, Minnesota. *Journal of Investigatory Dermatology*, 133(1):97–103.
33. McAllister M. (2013). Hidradenitis suppurativa (acne inversa). In T. M. Buttaro, J. Trybulski, P. P. Bailey, & J. Sandberg-Cook (Eds.), *Primary care: A collaborative practice* (pp. 272–274). St. Louis, MO: Elsevier; 2013.
34. Danby, F. W., & Margesson, L. J. (2010). Hidradenitis suppurativa. *Dermatology Clinics*, 28:779–793.
35. Fimmel, S., & Zouboulis, C. C. (2010). Comorbidities of hidradenitis suppurativa (acne inversa). *Dermato-endocrinology*, 2(1):9–16.
36. Ngan, V., & Oakley, A. (2015). Hidradenitis suppurativa. *DermNet NZ*. Retrieved from http://dermnetnz.org/acne/hidradenitis-suppurativa.html.
37. University of Maryland Medical Center. (2015). Photodermatitis. Retrieved from http://umm.edu/health/medical/altmed/condition/photodermatitis.
38. MacNeal, R. J. (2016). Overview of effects of sunlight. Retrieved from www.merckmanuals.com/professional/dermatologic_disorders/reactions_to_sunlight/overview_of_effects_of_sunlight.html.
39. American Academy of Dermatology. (2016). Actinic keratosis. Retrieved from https://www.aad.org/dermatology-a-to-z/diseases-and-treatments/a—d/actinic-keratosis.
40. Skin Cancer Foundation. (2016). Actinic keratosis (AK). Retrieved from www.skincancer.org/skin-cancer-information/actinic-keratosis.
41. RxList. (2016). Voltaren gel. Retrieved from http://www.rxlist.com/voltaren-gel-drug.htm.
42. Aaron, D. M. (2016). Overview of skin growths. Retrieved from http://www.merckmanuals.com/home/skin_disorders/noncancerous_skin_growths/overview_of_skin_growths.html.
43. Woodhouse, J. G. (2010). Common benign growths. Retrieved from http://www.clevelandclinicmeded.com/medicalpubs/diseasemanagement/dermatology/common-benign-growths/.
44. Schwartz, R. A. (2016). Acrochordon. Retrieved from http://emedicine.medscape.com/article/1060373-overview#a0199.
45. Storey, L. (2012). *Pathophysiology: A practical approach*. Sudbury, MA: Jones & Bartlett Learning.
46. Moraru, R. A. (2016). Cutaneous lipomas. Retrieved from http://emedicine.medscape.com/article/1057855-overview.
47. Wolter, B. (2016). Lipoma. *Essential Evidence Plus*. Retrieved from www.essentialevidenceplus.com.frontier.idm.oclc.org/content/eee/746.
48. Fromm, L. J. (2016). Epidermal inclusion cyst. Retrieved from http://emedicine.medscape.com/article/1061582-overview.
49. Blackburn, S. J. (2013). *Maternal, fetal, and neonatal physiology: A clinical perspective*. Maryland Heights, MO: Elsevier/Saunders.
50. Skin Cancer Foundation. (2017). Skin cancer facts & statistics. Retrieved from www.skincancer.org/skin-cancer-information/skin-cancer-facts.
51. American Cancer Society. (2016). Skin cancer basal and squamous cell. Retrieved from www.cancer.org/cancer/skincancer-basalandsquamouscell/detailedguide/index.
52. Skin Cancer Foundation. (2016). Basal cell carcinoma (BCC). Retrieved from www.skincancer.org/skin-cancer-information/basal-cell-carcinoma.
53. Firnhaber, J. M. (2012). Diagnosis and treatment of basal cell and squamous cell carcinoma. *American Family Physician*, 86(2):161–168.
54. Bader, R. S. (2016). Basal cell carcinoma clinical presentation. Retrieved from http://emedicine.medscape.com/article/276624-clinical#aw2aab6b3b2.
55. Skin Cancer Foundation. (2016). Squamous cell carcinoma (SCC). Retrieved from www.skincancer.org/skin-cancer-information/squamous-cell-carcinoma.
56. American Cancer Society. (2016). Melanoma skin cancer. Retrieved from www.cancer.org/cancer/skincancermelanoma/detailedguide/index.
57. Skin Cancer Foundation.(2016). Melanoma. Retrieved from www.skincancer.org/skin-cancer-information/melanoma.
58. Sheth, V. M., Guo, Y., & Qureshi, A. A. (2013). Comorbidities associated with vitiligo: A ten-year retrospective study. *Dermatology*, 227:311–315.
59. Groysman, V. (2016). Vitiligo. Retrieved from http://emedicine.medscape.com/article/1068962-overview.

60. McAllister, M. (2013). Pigmentation changes (vitiligo). In T. M. Buttaro, J. Trybulski, P. P. Bailey, & J. Sandberg-Cook (Eds.), *Primary care: A collaborative practice* (pp. 281–284). St. Louis, MO: Elsevier.
61. Jin, Y. (2010). Variant of TYR and autoimmunity susceptibility loci in generalized vitiligo. *New England Journal of Medicine*, 362:1686–1697.
62. James, W. D. (2016). Café au lait spots. Retrieved from http://emedicine.medscape.com/article/911900-overview.
63. Beery, T. A., & Workman, M. L. (2012). *Genetics and genomics in nursing and health care*. Philadelphia: F.A. Davis.
64. McBride, M. C. (2016). Neurofibromatosis. Retrieved from www.merckmanuals.com/professional/pediatrics/neurocutaneous_syndromes/neurofibromatosis.html?qt=cafe%20au%20lait&alt=sh.
65. Schwartz, R. A. (201). Lentigo. Retrieved from http://emedicine.medscape.com/article/1068503-overview.
66. Ngan, V. Lentigo. Retrieved from www.dermnetnz.org/lesions/lentigines.html.
67. Knott, L. (2016). Lentigo. Retrieved from www.patient.co.uk/doctor/lentigo.
68. Levinbook, W. S. (2016). Alopecia. Retrieved from www.merckmanuals.com/professional/dermatologic_disorders/hair_disorders/alopecia.html.
69. McLellan, F. (2015). Alopecia and baldness. Retrieved from www.essentialevidenceplus.com.frontier.idm.oclc.org/content/eee/721.
70. Knott, L. (2016). Alopecia. Retrieved from www.patient.co.uk/doctor/Alopecia.htm.
71. Genetics Home Reference. (2016). Androgenic alopecia. Retrieved from http://ghr.nlm.nih.gov/condition/androgenetic-alopecia.
72. Mohan, G. C., & Silverberg, J. I. (2015). Association of vitiligo and alopecia areata with atopic dermatitis: A systematic review and meta-analysis. *JAMA Dermatology*, 151(5):522–528.
73. Gilhar, A., Etzioni, A., & Paus, R. (2012). Alopecia areata. *New England Journal of Medicine* 366:1515–1525.
74. Alkhalifah, A., Alsantali, A., Wang, E., et al. (2010). Alopecia areata update: Part I. Clinical picture, histopathology, and pathogenesis. *Journal of the American Academy of Dermatology*, 62:177–188.
75. Alkhalifah, A., Alsantali, A., Wang, E., et al. (2010). Alopecia areata update: Part II. Treatment. *Journal of the American Academy of Dermatology*, 62:191–202.

Unit XIII

Disorders of Digestion, Metabolism, and Elimination

Disorders of digestion, metabolism, and elimination are many and varied, and their causes range from structural alterations to diet, immobility, side effects of medication, infection, inflammation, and pregnancy.[1] The digestive system is responsible for preparing ingested foods and fluids for either absorption or elimination. The system is made up of the gastrointestinal (GI) tract as well as accessory organs of digestion. When functioning optimally, the gastrointestinal system allows for the ingestion and movement of food and fluid boluses throughout the GI tract. The upper GI system secretes mucus, water, and enzymes at various points to aide in mechanical and chemical digestion; whereas the lower gastrointestinal system absorbs the nutrients and fluids and eliminates the wastes. Disorders arising from the GI tract may cause alterations and impairment to one or more of these functions.

The clinical manifestations of gastrointestinal system disorders are often nonspecific and may be due to a number of impairments. Patients with disorders that alter the GI system present with any combination of the four cardinal signs and symptoms: pain (the concept of pain and comfort), altered ingestion (the concept of digestion and nutrition), altered motility (the concept of elimination), and bleeding (the concept of perfusion).

The accessory organs of the gastrointestinal tract are the liver, gallbladder, and pancreas. The liver produces bile that is stored in the gallbladder. The liver is also responsible for numerous other functions within the body, including synthesis of plasma proteins, metabolism and elimination of drugs and toxins, as well as the storage of vitamins, glucose, and blood. The exocrine pancreas aids in the digestion of carbohydrates, fats, and proteins with the production of enzymes, as well as bicarbonate that is needed to neutralize chyme in the duodenum. These three accessory organs each contribute a distinct aspect of the digestive process, yet all work together to get their secretions to the duodenum to assist with digestion.

The liver is a metabolically complex and vascular organ that has a direct impact on all other organs and tissues within the body. The liver is involved in the regulation of coagulation and nutrition, and it plays a major role in the metabolism and excretion of medications. Considering the importance of this organ, any deterioration in function can have significant consequences for health.

The kidneys are responsible for homeostasis via urine production and elimination, as well as numerous endocrine functions. Blood pressure (BP), electrolyte and acid–base balance, red blood cell (RBC) production, and even bone health all rely on kidney function to maintain well-being. The maintenance of homeostasis depends on the kidneys to filter, save, or excrete waste products and hormones. Compensation is often noted when one of the other body systems fail, causing the kidney to alter its work to maintain a constant internal environment.

A number of different disorders or systemic alterations can cause alterations to digestive, metabolic, or eliminatory functions. Three common culprits are obstruction, volume depletion, and inadequate perfusion.

In some clients with disorders in digestive, metabolic, or elimination processes, clinical manifestations may be nonspecific or, in the case of a chronic disorder with a slow onset, may take months to appear. Adults who can report symptoms and respond with clarity to questions and physical examination assist clinicians to narrow the focus of the examination and selection of diagnostic tools. Infants and toddlers, however, lack the ability to do this. Crying, irritability, and poor feeding are common distress signals for this age group and unfortunately are associated with many disorders, including infection and anxiety. Careful assessment of very young children is important.[2]

References

1. Cleveland Clinic. (2013). Gastrointestinal disorders. Retrieved from http://my.clevelandclinic.org/health/articles/gastrointestinal-disorders
2. Ball, J.W., Bindler, R.C., Cowen, K., & Shaw, M. (2017). *Principles of Pediatric Nursing: Caring for Children* (7th ed.). Hoboken, NJ: Pearson Education.

Liver Failure
• Clinical manifestations
– Portal hypertension
– Esophageal varices
– Ascites
– Hepatic encephalopathy
• Common causes of liver failure
– Viral hepatitis
– Alcoholic liver disease
– Autoimmune hepatitis
– Acute liver failure

Disorders of the Upper and Lower GI System
• Disorders of the esophagus
• Disorders of the stomach
• Disorders of the small intestine, large intestine, and rectum

Cardinal Signs and Symptoms of GI Disorders
• Pain
– Heartburn
– Chest (esophageal) pain/pressure
– Dyspepsia
– Odynophagia
– Globus sensate
• Altered ingestion
– Regurgitation
– Reflux
– Vomiting
– Dysphagia
• Altered motility
– Diarrhea
– Constipation
• Bleeding
– Hematemesis
– Melena
– Hematochezia
– Occult blood

Acute Kidney Injury and End-Stage Kidney Disease
• Acute kidney injury (AKI)
– Acute onset
– Acute, reversible increase in serum creatinine
– Normal hemoglobin, renal size
• Chronic kidney disease (CKD)
– Slow onset
– Chronic, irreversible increase in serum creatinine
– Low hemoglobin
– Reduced renal size
– Renal osteodystrophy
– Peripheral neuropathy

Disorders of the Exocrine, Pancreatic, and Hepatobiliary Systems
• Disorders of the liver
– Cancer of the liver
– Cirrhosis and metabolic disorders
• Disorders of the gallbladder
– Cholelithiasis
– Cholangitis
– Cholecystitis
– Cancer of the gallbladder
• Disorders of the pancreas
– Acute pancreatitis
– Chronic pancreatitis
– Pancreatic cysts
– Cancer of the pancreas

Disorders of the Kidney and Urinary Tract Structure and Function
• Glomerular disorders
• Diabetic neuropathy
• Hypertensive neuropathy
• Urinary tract infection
• Renal calculi
• Urinary incontinence
• Benign tumors and malignancies of the kidney and bladder

Chapter 42

Disorders of Upper and Lower Gastrointestinal Systems

Susan M. Krawczyk

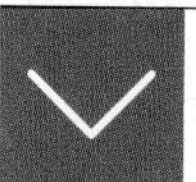

Chapter Outline and Learning Outcomes

42.1 Chapter Overview and Case Studies

Outline the four cardinal symptoms of disorders of the upper and lower gastrointestinal systems and concepts related to GI alterations.

42.2 Disorders of the Esophagus

Differentiate the causes, classification, underlying pathogenesis, and clinical manifestations of disorders of the esophagus and approaches to diagnosis and treatment of these conditions across the lifespan.

42.3 Disorders of the Stomach

Differentiate the causes, classification, underlying pathogenesis, and clinical manifestations of disorders of the stomach and approaches to diagnosis and treatment of these conditions across the lifespan.

42.4 Disorders of the Small Intestines, Large Intestines, and Rectum

Differentiate the causes, classification, underlying pathogenesis, and clinical manifestations of disorders of the small and large intestines and the rectum and approaches to diagnosis and treatment of these conditions across the lifespan.

KEY TERMS

Acid pocket, 1051
Adenocarcinoma of the esophagus, 1053
Appendicitis, 1060
Barrett esophagus (BE), 1052
Bowel obstruction, 1060
Coffee ground appearance, 1045
Colon cancer, 1063
Constipation, 1044
Crohn disease (CD), 1058
Diarrhea, 1044
Diverticula, 1062
Diverticulitis, 1062
Diverticulosis, 1062
Dyspepsia, 1044
Dysphagia, 1044
Dysphonia, 1052
Esophageal cancer, 1053
Esophageal chest pain, 1044
Esophageal diverticula, 1048
Esophageal perforation, 1049
Esophageal ring, 1045
Esophageal web, 1046
Esophagitis, 1046
Gastric outlet obstruction, 1056
Gastritis, 1055
Gastroesophageal reflux disease (GERD), 1051
Globus sensation, 1044
Heartburn, 1044
Helicobacter pylori (*H. pylori*), 1053
Hematemesis, 1045
Hematochezia, 1045
Hemorrhoid, 1062
Hiatal hernia, 1049
Infantile hypertrophic pyloric stenosis (IHPS), 1056
Inflammatory bowel disease (IBD), 1058
Irritable bowel syndrome (IBS), 1062
Melena, 1045
Occult blood/bleeding, 1045
Odynophagia, 1044
Peptic ulcer disease (PUD), 1054
Rectal cancer, 1063
Reflux, 1044
Reflux esophagitis, 1051
Regurgitation, 1044
Squamous cell carcinoma (SCC), 1053
Stomach cancer, 1057
Transient LES relaxation (TLESR), 1051
Ulcer, 1051
Ulcerative colitis (UC), 1059
Vomiting, 1044

ABBREVIATIONS

BE—Barrett esophagus
CD—Crohn disease
CRC—colorectal cancer
EoE—eosinophilic esophagitis
GEJ—gastroesophageal junction
GERD—gastroesophageal reflux disease
GI— gastrointestinal
GIT—gastrointestinal tract
HSV—herpes simplex virus
IBD—inflammatory bowel disease
IBS—irritable bowel syndrome
IHPS—infantile hypertrophic pyloric stenosis
LES—lower esophageal sphincter
NSAIDs—nonsteroidal anti-inflammatory drugs
PPI—proton pump inhibitor
PUD—peptic ulcer disease
SBO—small bowel obstruction
SCC—squamous cell carcinoma
TLESR—transient LES relaxation
UC—ulcerative colitis

42.1 Chapter Overview and Case Studies

The digestive system is responsible for preparing ingested foods and fluids for either absorption or elimination. The system is made up of the gastrointestinal (GI) tract (the mouth, esophagus, stomach, duodenum, small intestine, large intestine, rectum, and anus) and accessory organs of digestion (the tongue, salivary glands, liver, pancreas, and gallbladder). When functioning optimally, the GI system allows for the ingestion and movement of food and fluid boluses throughout the GI tract (GIT). The upper GI system secretes mucus, water, and enzymes at various points to aid in mechanical and chemical digestion; the lower GI system absorbs the nutrients and fluids and eliminates the wastes. Disorders arising from the GIT may cause alterations and impairment to one or more of these functions. This chapter focuses on common pathophysiologic conditions associated with the organs of the GIT and their effects on normal function.

Concepts Related to Disorders of the Gastrointestinal System

The clinical manifestations of GI system disorders are often nonspecific and may be related to a number of impairments. Patients with disorders that alter the GI system present with any combination of the four cardinal signs and symptoms: pain (the concept of pain and comfort), altered ingestion (the concept of digestion and nutrition), altered motility (the concept of elimination), and bleeding (the concept of perfusion) (**Figure 42.1** ■).

Pain

Heartburn is discomfort or a burning sensation behind the sternum that originates from the epigastrium. Heartburn is

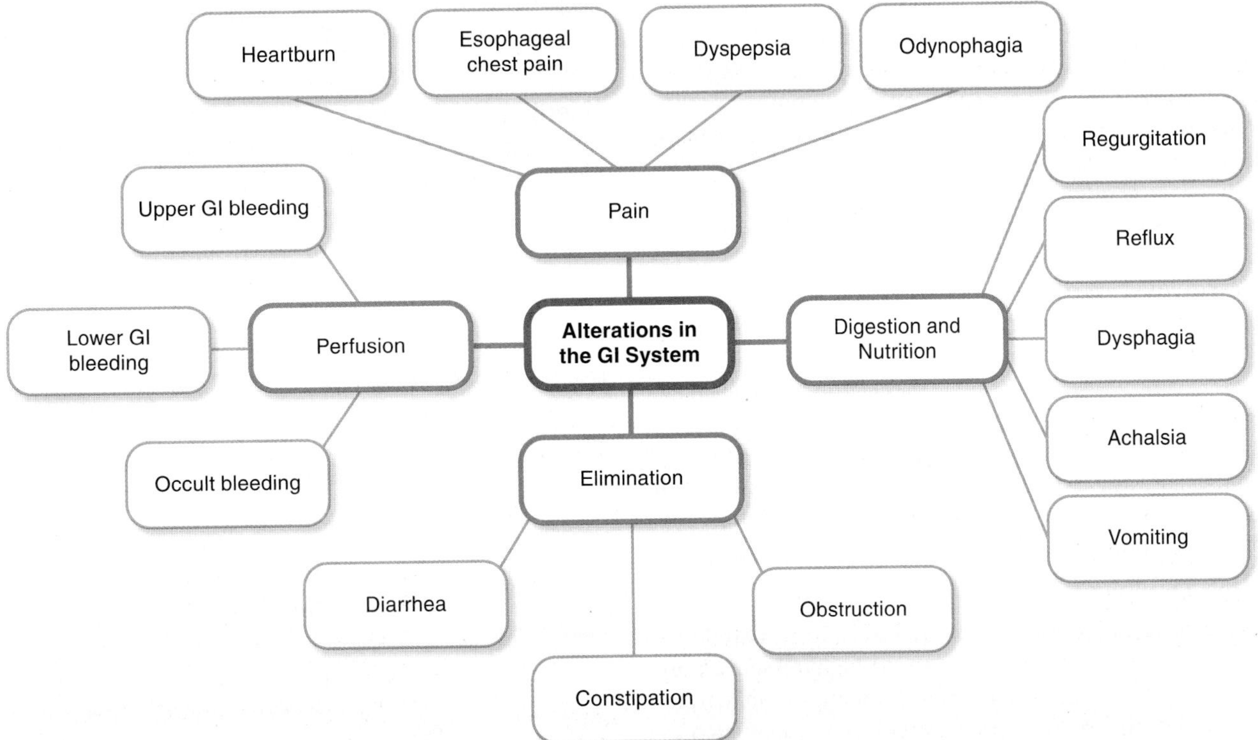

Figure 42.1 ■ Concepts related to alterations of the gastrointestinal system.

an intermittent symptom and is commonly experienced after eating, during exercise, and while in the lying in the supine position.[1] It is the most common esophageal symptom.[1]

Esophageal chest pain, like heartburn, is experienced as a pressure-like sensation felt in the midchest. What differentiates esophageal chest pain from heartburn is its likeness to cardiac chest pain, in that it may radiate to the back, arms, and jaw. Its similarity to chest pain of a cardiac nature is most likely due to the two organ systems sharing the same nerve plexus. Gastroesophageal reflux is the most common cause of esophageal chest pain and heartburn.[1]

In addition to painful sensations, patients may experience **dyspepsia**, uncomfortable feelings associated with pathophysiology of the upper GIT such as mild, gnawing discomfort of the chest or upper abdomen, fullness, bloating, early satiety, and nausea. **Odynophagia** is pain caused by swallowing. **Globus sensation**, also known as globus pharyngis, is a fullness or a lump in the throat.

Altered Ingestion

Regurgitation is the effortless return of food and fluids into the pharynx without nausea or retching. Maneuvers that increase intra-abdominal pressure can induce regurgitation; these include overdistending the stomach (as with overeating), bending, and belching. Patients complain of a burning sensation in the throat and a sour taste in the mouth. They may report undigested food returning to the mouth. Clinically, patients may present with halitosis (bad breath).

Reflux, an involuntary process, is the backwards movement of GI contents at any point in the GIT. **Vomiting** is the forceful evacuation of gastric contents. It is frequently preceded by the sensation of nausea.

Dysphagia, difficulty swallowing food and liquids, is often described as the feeling of food "sticking" in the throat or chest. Dysphagia may be described as episodic versus continuous, progressing versus stable, and dysphagia for solids versus dysphagia for solids and liquids.

Dysphagia for solids is often a symptom of an obstructive lesion, such as a tumor, a ring or web, or a stricture. It may occur at any level of the esophagus: upper, mid, or lower. Dysphagia for solids and liquids is often a symptom of a motor disorder. Dysphagia for solids and liquids can be further divided into upper esophageal dysphagia and lower esophageal dysphagia. Upper esophageal (or oropharyngeal) dysphagia is due to striated muscle dysmotility and is seen in conditions such as myasthenia gravis and stroke.[2] Lower esophageal dysphagia is due to smooth muscle dysmotility and is associated with conditions such as systemic sclerosis, limited scleroderma (CREST syndrome), and achalasia (a rare disorder that prevents relaxation of the esophageal sphincter).[2]

Altered Motility

Because bowel elimination patterns vary from person to person, alterations in motility should be assessed on an individual basis. Generally, normal eliminations range from infrequent (one elimination per week) to frequent (two to three eliminations per day).

Table 42.1 Major Causes of Diarrhea

Cause	Explanation
Large-Volume Diarrhea	
Osmotic causes	Nonabsorbable substances in the lumen of the bowel draw water into the bowel (e.g., ingestion of synthetic sugars, such as sorbitol or full-strength tube feeding formulas).
Secretory causes	Excessive mucosal secretion interferes with chloride and sodium transport, decreasing water absorption (e.g., bacterial and viral infections).
Small-Volume Diarrhea	
Inflammatory bowel	Inflammation causes smooth muscle contraction, cramping, urgency, and frequency of elimination (e.g., ulcerative colitis, Crohn disease).
Motility causes	Excessive motility decreases mucosal surface contact time, decreasing opportunity for absorption (e.g., short bowel syndrome, laxative abuse).

Diarrhea is an increase in stool content, volume, and weight as well as an increase in the frequency of evacuations of stool per day. Diarrhea may be classified two ways: as large-volume diarrhea, which is, generally, an increase in the volume of stool, or small-volume diarrhea, which is associated not with increased volume of stool but rather with increased intestinal motility. **Table 42.1** ■ lists the major causes of diarrhea by classification and provides examples of each type.

Constipation is difficult or infrequent evacuation, including reports of passage of hard stools, straining, or a sense of incomplete evacuation. Constipation is more common in women, young children, and older adults.[3] It is not considered significant until it causes health risks or impairs the patient's quality of life. Constipation may be classified as primary or secondary. **Table 42.2** ■ describes the classifications of constipation.

Bleeding

Upper GI bleeding is bleeding from the esophagus, stomach, or duodenum. It may present as blood in the patient's vomitus, known as **hematemesis**. Hematemesis may contain frank, bright red (undigested) blood or dark, grainy

Table 42.2 Classifications of Constipation

Classification	Description
Primary constipation	Normal transit: normal rate of stool passage but difficulty with evacuation; commonly due to low-fiber diets, sedentary lifestyle Slow transit: involves impaired colonic motor activity with infrequent evacuations Pelvic floor dysfunction: difficulty evacuating stool owing to pelvic floor muscle failure
Secondary constipation	Neurogenic causes: stroke, spinal cord injury, multiple sclerosis Pharmacologic causes: opioids, calcium carbonate or aluminum hydroxide antacids Endocrine or metabolic causes: hypothyroidism, diabetes mellitus Mechanical causes: weakness, frailty, pain

(digested) blood, described as having a **coffee ground appearance**. Upper GI bleeding may also present as blood in the patient's stool, known as melena. **Melena** is black, tarry stools caused by digestion of blood in the GIT.

Lower GI bleeding is bleeding from the small intestine, large intestine, colon, or rectum. Blood in the stool from lower GI bleeding presents as black, tarry stools (melena) or frank, bright red blood in the stool (**hematochezia**).

Both upper and lower GI bleeding may present as occult bleeding. **Occult blood** is due to slow, chronic bleeding and is not detectable by routine inspection of the stool or gastric secretions. Occult blood is detected only through a guaiac test, which uses samples of stool collected at home or during a rectal examination by a healthcare provider.

Case Studies

The following cases will be addressed throughout the chapter to assist in application of chapter content to clinical situations that involve individuals with disorders of the upper and lower GI systems.

Greg Ross: Introduction

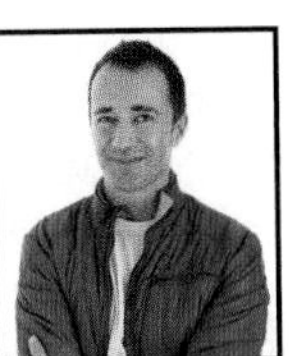

Greg Ross is 44 years old and has a history of inflammatory bowel disease, specifically ulcerative colitis. He works as a sales representative and travels frequently as part of his job. Recently, while on vacation, he began to experience significant abdominal pain. At first, he associated the pain with the stresses of traveling and his inability to maintain an appropriate diet. He has now been experiencing abdominal pain and diarrhea for the past 5 days.

1. Which of the four cardinal signs and symptoms of GI system disorders is Mr. Ross experiencing?
2. Is Mr. Ross more likely to be experiencing small-volume or large-volume diarrhea?

Pam Allen: Introduction

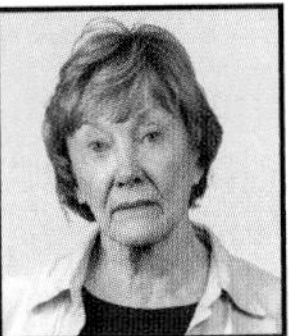

Pam Allen is 65 years old and considers her health to have been "good" for most of her life. She has a prior medical history of endometrial cancer at age 50, and she underwent a total hysterectomy with bilateral removal of the ovaries. She has ongoing issues with constipation with a sense of fullness in the rectum. She has begun to experience increased fatigue over the past month.

1. Which of the four cardinal signs and symptoms of GI system disorders is Ms. Allen experiencing?
2. Given Ms. Allen's history, why are her symptoms of concern?

Check Your Progress: Section 42.1

1. What differentiates esophageal chest pain from heartburn?
2. What is the difference between regurgitation and vomiting?
3. Differentiate the appearance of bleeding from the upper and lower GI tracts.

42.2 Disorders of the Esophagus

After entering the mouth, food and liquids are masticated and mixed with salivary enzymes and, under voluntary control, are positioned at the back of the throat for entry into the esophagus. With the last effort of voluntary control, foods and liquids are pushed into the esophagus for involuntary transit to the stomach. While in transit, ingested materials may encounter various defects in the esophagus, commonly causing three of the four cardinal symptoms of GI disorders: pain, alteration in ingestion, and bleeding (see **Table 42.3** ■).

Rings and Webs

An **esophageal ring** is a circumferential, nondistendable narrowing of the lumen of the esophagus. Most commonly, rings appear membranous and occur within the mucosa at the level of the gastroesophageal junction (GEJ). These narrowings are called B rings. A Schatzki ring is the name given to a symptomatic (causing dysphagia) B ring. Less commonly, rings may occur higher up in the lower esophagus and appear muscular in nature. These are called A rings.[4]

An **esophageal web** is a thin, membranous tissue that occupies the lumen of the esophagus, decreasing the diameter of the lumen. Esophageal webs may be congenital or acquired. Acquired webs are more common than congenital webs and occur in women twice as often as in men.

Etiology and Pathogenesis

The etiology of esophageal rings is unknown. A Schatzki ring appears to be associated with a decreased incidence of Barrett esophagus, although it does not seem to protect

Table 42.3 Esophageal Diseases by Defect

Etiology	Examples
Structural	
Acquired	Rings and webs Diverticula Tumors Hiatal hernia
Congenital	Webs Esophageal atresia
Traumatic	Esophageal perforation Mallory-Weiss tear Foreign bodies Food impaction
Functional	
Motility	Dysphagia Achalasia Diffuse esophageal spasms
Mucosal integrity	Gastroesophageal reflux disease (GERD) Barrett esophagus Esophagitis (eosinophilic, infectious, radiation, corrosive)
Manifestations of systemic diseases	Scleroderma esophagus Dermatologic diseases

against reflux.[4] Schatzki rings are also associated with eosinophilic esophagitis, particularly in children.[4]

Congenital webs result from improper union of embryonic esophageal structures in utero. The etiologies of acquired esophageal webs are complex. Esophageal webs and iron deficiency anemia in middle-aged women are a part of a condition known as Plummer-Vinson syndrome. Esophageal webs have been associated with some dermatologic disorders.

Clinical Manifestations

The clinical manifestations of esophageal rings and webs are related to the narrowing of the esophageal lumen. Schatzki B rings (**Figure 42.2** ■) occur in approximately 10–15% of the general population and are typically asymptomatic. When the esophageal lumen decreases to fewer than 13 millimeters in diameter, patients report symptoms of dysphagia for solids.[4] This dysphagia is often chronic and episodic. A Schatzki ring is the most common cause of acute food impaction; typically, pieces of meat become impacted in the ring. Additionally, patients may have associated symptoms of gastroesophageal reflux disease such as heartburn or regurgitation.

Most patients with esophageal webs are asymptomatic; however, the typical presenting symptom is dysphagia for solids. Dysphagia can begin in infancy or early childhood years in patients with congenital esophageal webs. As the esophageal lumen diameter narrows, patients may present with acute food impaction. Additionally, patients may experience nasopharyngeal reflux, aspiration, and spontaneous perforation.[4]

Linking Pathophysiology to Diagnosis and Treatment

In patients with long-standing dysphagia, despite dietary restrictions, diagnosis may be made with radiologic studies, such as a barium swallow study. Upper endoscopy is indicated to determine the optimal treatment strategy. For esophageal rings and webs, first-line treatment is endoscopic dilation therapy. In some cases, resistant rings may require dilation combined with endoscopic incisional therapy, in which the stricture is incised to open the esophageal lumen.[5]

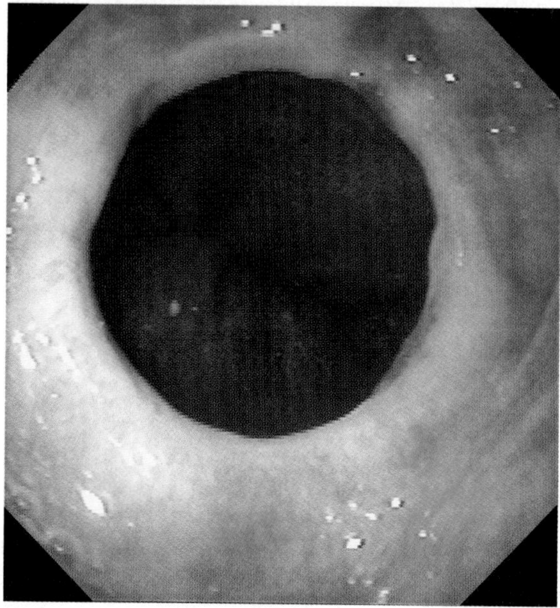

Figure 42.2 ■ Esophageal B (Schatzki) ring.

Esophagitis

Esophagitis is the general term to describe irritation to and inflammation of the tissues of the esophagus that may lead to damage to the esophagus. Esophagitis has many types and causes. Types of esophagitis include eosinophilic, infectious, radiation, corrosion, and pill esophagitis.

Eosinophilic esophagitis (EoE) is an allergic esophagitis, characterized by histologic evidence of eosinophil induced inflammation and clinical symptoms of esophageal dysfunction. It is being progressively more recognized in adults and children in the United States and around the world. EoE affects males more than females, with a ratio of approximately 3:1, and presents in childhood or during the third or fourth decade. Although EoE affects all racial and ethnic groups, it occurs most frequently in Caucasians.[6]

Infectious esophagitis, once noted to be a complication of AIDS, is now seen in more patient populations, owing to the increased use of immunosuppressant drug therapy for chronic inflammatory diseases and organ transplants. Infectious esophagitis may be focal or may affect the whole length of the esophagus. Esophagitis may also occur as the result of iatrogenic injury (radiation esophagitis) or mechanical injury (corrosive and pill esophagitis).

Etiology and Pathogenesis

The cause of EoE is unknown, although it is likely to be multifactorial with a genetic predisposition.[6] With EoE, eosinophils are recruited to the esophagus (esophageal eosinophilia) during inflammatory or infectious processes and after exposure to food and environmental allergens. Risk factors for EoE include gastroesophageal reflux disease (GERD), food allergy, and genetic predisposition. GERD is frequently associated with EoE, as is the presence of atopic conditions such as allergic rhinitis, eczema, and asthma.[7]

A large number of parasites, viruses, fungi, and bacteria can cause infections in the esophagus. Infectious esophagitis is most commonly caused by herpes simplex virus (HSV), cytomegalovirus, and *Candida*.

Radiation esophagitis may occur when the esophagus is intentionally or unintentionally irradiated in the treatment of thoracic cancers. The condition is exacerbated by the use of chemotherapeutic agents that sensitize the cancer to radiation (radiosensitizers); these include doxorubicin, bleomycin, cyclophosphamide, and cisplatin.[1]

Corrosive esophagitis occurs as the result of accidental or intentional ingestion of strong alkaline (e.g., lye) or acid (e.g., hydrogen chloride) substances. In children, ingestion of caustic substances is primarily accidental; in the United States, 5000 cases of accidental corrosive injuries in children are reported annually.[8] In adulthood, ingestion of caustic substances may be accidental but is most often done in an attempt at suicide.

Pill esophagitis occurs when a swallowed pill lodges transversely in the lumen of the esophagus, causing inflammation. A number of medication are notorious for lodging in the esophagus, the most common being doxycycline, tetracycline, quinidine, phenytoin, potassium chloride, ferrous sulfate, nonsteroidal anti-inflammatory drugs (NSAIDs), and bisphosphonates.[1]

Clinical Manifestations

While some patients with EoE may be asymptomatic, the most commonly reported symptoms are dysphagia (93%), food impaction (62%), and heartburn (24%).[7] Additionally, patients may experience GERD-like symptoms, upper abdominal pain, and globus sensation.

Patients with infectious esophagitis usually present with dysphagia, chest pain, and odynophagia. Fever and malaise may be present in immunocompromised patients with HSV-induced esophagitis. Some patients, particularly those with *Candida*-induced esophagitis, may be asymptomatic.

Both radiation esophagitis and corrosive esophagitis can cause the esophageal mucosa to become edematous, ulcerate, and become friable. In addition to dysphagia and odynophagia, patients may experience chest pain and esophageal bleeding, which can present as hematemesis or melena. In severe cases, patients can present with esophageal perforation.

In patients with pill esophagitis, pain is often sudden chest pain accompanied by odynophagia.

Linking Pathophysiology to Diagnosis and Treatment

A thorough history in patients who present with dysphagia and pain—whether it is heartburn, chest pain, and/or odynophagia—will lead the practitioner to the appropriate differential diagnosis, the proper diagnostic examinations, and best treatment for the patient.

Patients who present with dysphagia and food impactions should be suspected of having EoE. EoE is diagnosed via clinical symptoms, endoscopy, and pinch biopsy of the proximal and distal esophagus. Histologically, a finding of 15 or more eosinophils per high-power field confirms the presence of eosinophils in the esophageal epithelium. Additionally, upper GI contrast studies, peripheral eosinophil count, and skin-prick testing or immunoglobulin E blood test for allergens may provide supportive information for the diagnosis of EoE.

Motivated patients may consider dietary modifications for the treatment of EoE. Histologic remission rates have been noted with an elemental diet (90.8%), the six-food elimination diet (72.1%), and allergy testing-directed food elimination diets (45.5%).[9]

Steroids, both systemic and swallowed topical, are useful in reducing the eosinophil count and decreasing inflammation but are not recommended for long-term use. Medications to reduce gastric acid may be helpful in reducing the symptoms of associated conditions. For the treatment of esophageal narrowing and food impaction, esophageal dilation may be necessary.

The presentation of EoE in children may include chest or abdominal pain, nausea, vomiting, and food aversion.[1] Specific antigen removal or elemental diets have been proven effective therapies in children.[6,8] As in adults, systemic and swallowed topical steroids may be helpful in treating acute symptoms but are not recommended for long-term use. Esophageal dilation may be necessary to restore the esophageal lumen diameter in some patients.[6,8] ■

Patients with a history of immunosuppression and complaints of dysphagia, chest pain, and odynophagia should be suspected of having infectious esophagitis. Patients are typically diagnosed on the basis of history and physical examination and confirmation with endoscopy. Treatment is aimed at the specific pathogen: antifungal medication for *Candida*, oral antiviral medication for HSV, and intravenous antiviral medication for cytomegalovirus.

Clinical symptoms related to radiation esophagitis may last for weeks to months after radiation therapy. Patients who present with dysphagia and odynophagia with a history of radiation therapy to the chest or neck within the past year should be suspected of having radiation esophagitis. Confirmation of diagnosis may be made with endoscopy, but extreme care must be taken to prevent further damage to the esophageal mucosa. Treatment is supportive. If strictures develop, esophageal dilation may be necessary.

Corrosive esophagitis is suspected when symptoms accompany a history of ingestion of a known or unknown substance. Knowing what type of substance was ingested is helpful, as alkaline substances are more caustic than acidic ones are. Chest imaging is necessary to rule out pulmonary infiltrates and evidence of perforation, such as pneumomediastinum and subcutaneous emphysema. Endoscopy may be used to confirm diagnosis and grade the severity of the injury. Severely corrosive esophagitis is a medical emergency and requires intravenous therapy, total parenteral nutrition, and antibiotics. Glucocorticoids have not been shown to improve clinical outcomes and are not recommended.[1] After the esophagus has healed, barium studies may be necessary to determine the degree of esophageal narrowing that has resulted from the injury. Repeated esophageal dilations are often necessary.

When a thorough history reveals that the patient is taking medications that are known to lodge in the throat, sudden onset of chest pain with odynophagia may lead the practitioner to suspect pill esophagitis. After other differential diagnoses have been ruled out, treatment for pill esophagitis is supportive, and endoscopy is not necessary. Patients typically recover within a few weeks of discontinuing the offending pill.

Esophageal Diverticula

Esophageal diverticula are outpouchings of the esophagus that may be located in the upper, middle, or lower esophagus. Esophageal diverticula in the upper esophagus are termed hypopharyngeal diverticula. The most common type is Zenker diverticulum, which occurs at the junction between the pharynx and the esophagus in an area known as the Killian triangle (**Figure 42.3** ■). Midesophageal diverticula occur at the level of the bifurcation of the trachea.

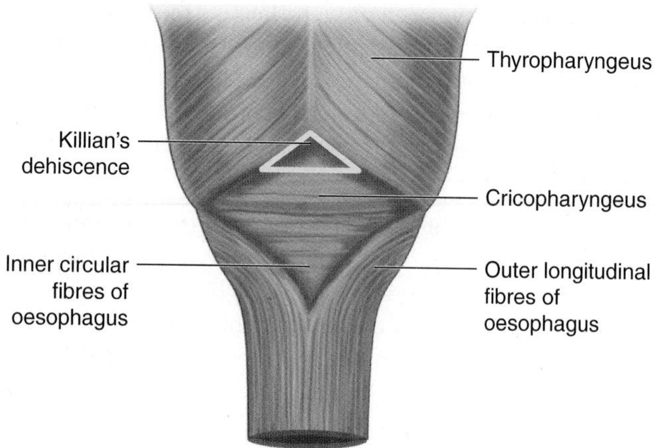

Figure 42.3 ■ Killian triangle.

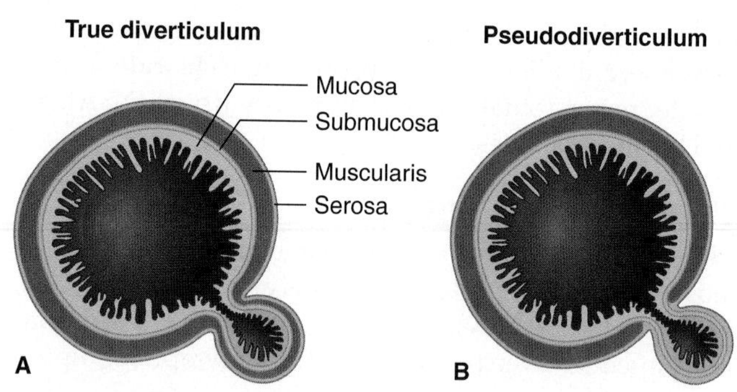

Figure 42.4 ■ True and false (pseudodiverticula) diverticula of the esophagus.

In the lower esophagus, epiphrenic diverticula occur at the distal esophagus and are often associated with hiatal hernia.

Etiology and Pathogenesis

Esophageal diverticulum is an acquired, non–gender-specific condition that usually affects middle-aged and older adults. Most commonly, diverticula occur as a result of increased pressure in the lumen of the esophagus caused by impairment in esophageal motility. The increased pressure pushes esophageal mucosa through weaknesses in the esophageal wall, causing outpouching. Hypopharyngeal diverticulum and epiphrenic diverticulum occur in this way. Additionally, these types are grouped as pulsion diverticula because of the nature of herniation and pseudodiverticula as only the mucosal and submucosal layers of the esophagus become herniated.

In the case of midesophageal diverticula, weaknesses in the esophageal musculature are due to traction on the esophagus caused by inflammatory diseases of the mediastinum, such as tuberculosis, and are termed traction diverticula. Midesophageal diverticula are considered true diverticula, as all layers of esophageal become herniated through the weakened esophageal wall. The differences between true and false or pseudodiverticula are shown in **Figure 42.4** ■.

Clinical Manifestations

Most esophageal diverticula are asymptomatic. However, when large enough to hold undigested food and fluids, hypopharyngeal diverticula present with symptoms that affect the upper esophagus and airway. Patients complain of dysphagia and heartburn and may experience a gurgling sound during swallowing. When the diverticulum is sufficiently large, a neck mass may develop. Regurgitation of undigested food is characteristic of hypopharyngeal diverticula, and patients present with halitosis. Regurgitation may lead to laryngitis and pulmonary aspiration.

Midesophageal diverticula occur infrequently and are mostly asymptomatic. Epiphrenic diverticula are symptomatic in relation to associated conditions, such as hiatal hernia, with patients experiencing symptoms of hiatal hernia.

Linking Pathophysiology to Diagnosis and Treatment

Regurgitation of undigested food and fluids is characteristic of hypopharyngeal diverticula. Furthermore, borborygmus (bowel sounds) auscultated at the neck, with or without the presence of a palpable lump, nearly certainly indicates Zenker diverticulum.

Diagnosis is made via radiologic studies, including chest and abdominal x-rays and barium swallow studies. Continuous dynamic fluoroscopy is preferred to assess for smaller diverticula that are not readily seen on static images.[10] Esophagoscopy may be used to evaluate for esophagitis. Esophageal manometry is used to diagnosis conditions of impaired motility.

Small esophageal, midesophageal, and epigastric diverticula do not usually require intervention. When the diverticula are large and symptomatic, surgical intervention may be necessary. Surgical interventions for diverticulectomy include an open approach, in which an incision in made externally on the neck, and an intraoral approach with either a rigid or a flexible endoscope.[10] Additionally, if there is impaired esophageal motility because of strictures, a myotomy, an incision in the esophageal musculature to release strictures, may be necessary.

Esophageal Perforation

An **esophageal perforation** is a tear or rupture that creates a hole through the layers of the esophagus. Most cases of esophageal perforation have iatrogenic causes, such as endoscopy or insertion of nasogastric tubes. While uncommon, perforations usually occur at places where the esophagus naturally narrows, such as at the cricopharyngeus muscle (upper esophagus), at the aortic knob (middle esophagus), and at the gastroesophageal junction (distal esophagus).[11] However, an esophageal perforation may occur at any point in the esophagus where the luminal wall has become weakened.[11]

A Mallory-Weiss tear is a spontaneous tear in the mucosa of the proximal stomach and distal esophagus caused by severe retching.[2] It is seen in patients who vomit frequently and forcefully, such as patients with alcoholism and bulimia.

Boerhaave syndrome is a spontaneous rupture of the distal esophagus that is most often due to endoscopy (75%)

but may also be caused by the forceful retching that occurs in bulimia.[2]

Etiology and Pathogenesis

Most commonly, esophageal perforations occur at sites of luminal narrowing and frequently have iatrogenic causes, such as endoscopy and nasogastric tube insertion. Boerhaave syndrome accounts for 15% of cases of perforation. Esophageal perforations may also be due to foreign body or caustic substance ingestions, blunt or penetrating trauma, intraoperative injuries, esophageal malignancy, and infection.[11] Conditions that may contribute to impaired esophageal wall strength and are associated with esophageal perforation include malignancy, gastroesophageal reflux disease, achalasia, stricture (e.g., caustic, benign, anastomotic), scleroderma, and hiatal hernia.

Clinical Manifestations

Patients presenting with esophageal perforation most frequently complain of pain. When the injury is located in the upper esophagus, patients present with dysphagia or neck pain with flexion. If the perforation is in the mid-esophageal region, patients report pain in the chest, back, or epigastrium. If the perforation is in the lower esophagus, patients report abdominal pain or epigastric pain with radiation to the shoulders when the diaphragm is irritated.

Pneumomediastinum (free air in the thoracic cavity) may ensue as air disperses subcutaneously. Crepitus of the chest or neck may be palpable because of subcutaneous emphysema, and a crunching sound (Hamman sign) may be heard on auscultation. Additionally, patients may have signs and symptoms of systemic infection or septic shock, including fever, tachycardia, and hypotension.

Patients with Mallory-Weiss tear classically present with hematemesis. Boerhaave syndrome classically presents as chest pain and dyspnea following forceful vomiting.

Linking Pathophysiology to Diagnosis and Treatment

A thorough history helps to confirm the presence of an esophageal tear or rupture. A tear or rupture should be highly suspected in patients who present with the aforementioned signs and symptoms combined with a recent history of upper endoscopy and the presence of a condition associated with esophageal perforation.

Diagnosis is confirmed with chest radiography and swallow studies. Because most perforations have iatrogenic causes, care should be taken in doing repeat endoscopy for diagnostic purposes. Computed tomography may be necessary to establish the extent of extraesophageal involvement.

Patients with esophageal perforations can quickly develop septic shock; therefore, treatment needs to be initiated promptly. Broad-spectrum antibiotics should be administered early. A chest tube may need to be placed to drain pleural effusions. Until enteral nutrition can be resumed, plans for parenteral nutrition should be made.

Approximately 25% of patients may be managed nonsurgically if they meet specific criteria such as having a recent, well-circumscribed perforation that does not leak into the abdominal cavity. Nonsurgical management includes NPO status (no food or fluids by mouth), decompressive therapies, and an endoscopically placed esophageal stent.[11]

Abdominal esophageal perforations should be managed surgically. Surgical interventions include drainage of the contaminated space, debridement and repair of the perforation, esophageal diversion and delayed repair, and esophagectomy.

Hiatal Hernia

A **hiatal hernia** is a herniation of the stomach through the esophageal hiatus of the diaphragm. Hiatal hernias are classified in two divisions: sliding and paraesophageal. Their structure and severity are further categorized by type, ranging from type I to type IV, as shown in **Table 42.4** ■).

Etiology and Pathogenesis

The cause of hiatal hernia may be multifactorial and may be due to a widening of the diaphragmatic hiatus, shortening of the esophagus and pulling up on the stomach, and/or increased intra-abdominal pressure pushing the stomach upward.[12] Additionally, a genetic link has been proposed.[12]

Clinical Manifestations

Many patients with hiatal hernias are asymptomatic. However, when symptomatic, patients most frequently report symptoms of gastroesophageal reflux, such as heartburn, nocturnal epigastric distress, and a sour or acidic taste at the back of the throat. Patient experience the symptoms of acid reflux because of the distortion of the gastroesophageal junction and, more important, the distortion of the lower esophageal sphincter (LES).

The LES is the body's most effective defense against acid reflux. It is the distalmost portion of the esophagus and makes up the esophageal portion of the GE junction. It is reinforced by the crural portions of the diaphragm, and it is able to change its pressure in relation to the patient's intragastric pressure. That is, as the patient's intragastric pressure increases, the LES tone increases, preventing acid and partially digested food from reentering the esophagus. As the diaphragm widens around the GEJ, as the GEJ is pulled cephalad from its original position, or as the stomach herniates alongside the GEJ, the LES becomes less effective and permits the reflux of gastric contents. With type IV paraesophageal hernias, patients may experience dyspnea, reduced exercise tolerance, and possible syncope. Bowel sounds may be audible at the left lung base.

Linking Pathophysiology to Diagnosis and Treatment

Because patients with hiatal hernias may be asymptomatic or only mildly symptomatic, many hiatal hernias are found incidentally on chest radiography films. Chest films can reveal soft tissue changes associated with hiatal hernia. Additionally, hiatal hernia is diagnosed with contrast swallow studies and endoscopy.

Treatment for hiatal hernia begins with pharmacologic treatment of symptomatic gastric reflux. Surgery is indicated when the hernia, either sliding and paraesophageal, is symptomatic or when a paraesophageal hernia may be at risk for strangulation or gastric volvulus.

Table 42.4 Classifications and Anatomic Features of Hiatal Hernias

Type	Description
Sliding Hiatal Hernia	
Type I 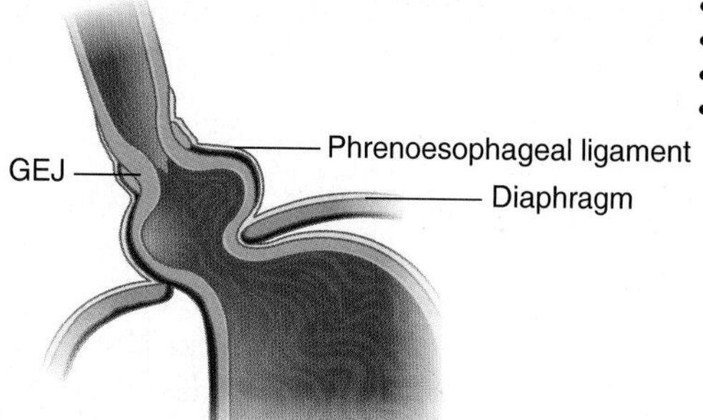 	• The GEJ migrates above the diaphragm. • The stomach remains in longitudinal alignment with the fundus below the GEJ. • The sliding mechanism is dynamic and changes as the patient's position changes. • More than 95% of all hiatal hernias are type I.
Paraesophageal Hiatal Hernia	
Type II 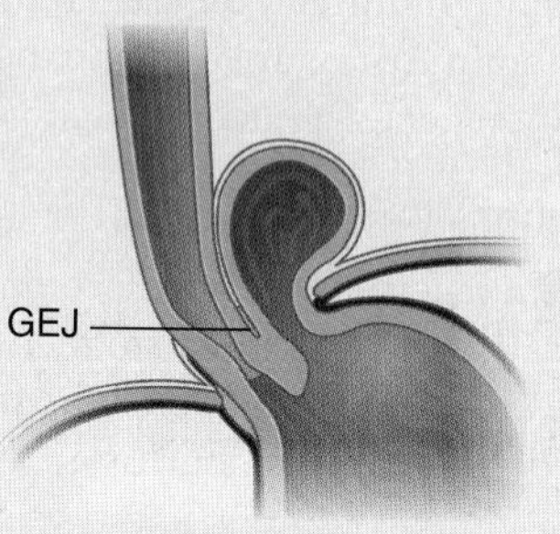 	• The GEJ remains in the normal anatomic position. • A portion of the fundus herniates through the diaphragmatic hiatus.
Type III 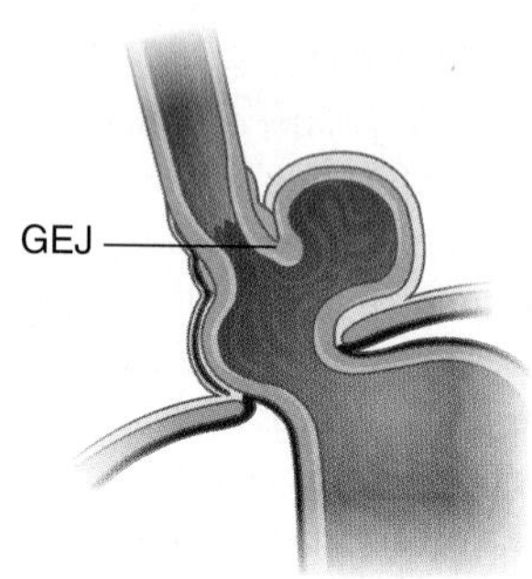 	• Occurs as the result of mixed hiatal hernia types I and II. • The GEJ and the fundus of the stomach herniate through the diaphragmatic hiatus. • The fundus pushes above the GEJ. • 90% of all paraesophageal hiatal hernias are type III.
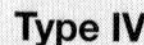**Type IV** 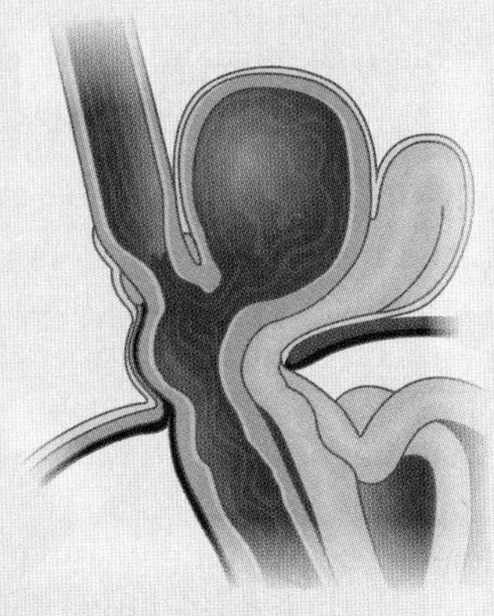	• The herniation contains other abdominal structures, such as the omentum, colon, or small bowel.

SOURCE: Kohn, G. P., Price, R. R., Demeester, S. R., et al. (2013). *Guidelines for the management of hiatal hernia*. Available at http://www.sages.org/publications/guidelines/guidelines-for-the-management-of-hiatal-hernia

Gastroesophageal Reflux Disease

Reflux of gastric contents into the esophagus is a common physiologic occurrence; however, with increased frequency and damaging effects, chronic reflux becomes referred to as gastroesophageal reflux disease. **Gastroesophageal reflux disease (GERD)** is more than esophagitis caused by the reflux of gastric contents (**reflux esophagitis**); it is a multifactorial condition resulting in a constellation of esophageal and extraesophageal symptoms. The prevalence of GERD in North America is estimated to be between 8.8% and 27.8%.[13,14] Risk factors for GERD include the following:

- Decreased LES tone
- Surgical vagotomy, decreased endogenous gastrin levels
- Pregnancy
- Impaired esophageal motility
- Obesity.

GERD has been associated with asthma, atrial fibrillation, and lower systolic blood pressure measurements.

Etiology and Pathogenesis

Normally, reflux of gastric contents into the esophagus is prevented at the GEJ by the LES and crural portion of the diaphragm. The LES receives signals when the esophagus is actively transporting solids and liquids to the stomach and relaxes to allow the substances to pass. Conversely, when there are solids and liquids in the stomach to be digested, the LES receives signals (both chemical and physical) and becomes tighter (i.e., it increases its tone) to prevent gastric contents from reentering the esophagus. During periods when intragastric pressure may override the LES (e.g., straining, overdistention of the stomach), the crural diaphragm cinches inward, reinforcing the LES. The LES and crural diaphragm are considered the internal and external sphincters of the GEJ and act synergistically to prevent reflux.[14] GERD occurs when these protective mechanisms chronically fail and allow acid, pepsin, and bile to reflux and linger in the esophagus, causing erosions and ulcerations. An **ulcer** is an area of the mucosal layers of the gastrointestinal tract that becomes damaged with erosion and fails to heal. Factors that may cause chronic failure of the LES and crural diaphragm include transient LES relaxation, hiatal hernia, acid pocket, obesity, and ineffective esophageal clearance.

Gastric reflux occurs primarily during periods of transient LES relaxation. **Transient LES relaxation (TLESR)**, a means for the stomach to vent excessive gas, is a motor pattern triggered by vagal afferents in the stomach (usually in response to gastric distention) that causes rapid relaxation of the LES, esophageal shortening, and inhibition of the crural diaphragm.[14] TLESRs are common after a meal. TLESRs occur in healthy individuals as well as patients with GERD; however, acid reflux during TLESRs is twice as likely in people with GERD.[15] The distortion of the LES and malalignment of the crural diaphragm caused by some hiatal hernias increase the likelihood of gastroesophageal reflux. In addition to TLESRs, a number of factors affect the LES tone. **Table 42.5** lists these factors.

Although food has been thought to buffer gastric acid, recent research has shown that a pocket of gastric acid floats on top of ingested meals.[14] These **acid pockets** occur in healthy individuals as well as people with GERD. In those with GERD, acid pockets are larger and closer to the GEJ. If the acid pocket is located above the diaphragm, as in the case of hiatal hernia, acid becomes the major component of refluxed content, predisposing the esophagus to erosive changes.

Obesity contributes to GERD by chronically increasing intra-abdominal pressure and the pressure gradient across the LES. When gastric contents reach the esophagus, rapid return to the stomach is essential for reducing damage to the esophageal lining. This is achieved by secondary esophageal peristalsis and gravity and is aided by pH buffering from saliva. Reflux clearance may be impaired by the supine position, reduced saliva production, decreased secondary peristalsis, and disorders of esophageal motility. Prolonged exposure to the esophageal lining allows gastric content to cause erosion and ulceration.

Clinical Manifestations

Typically, patients with GERD present with heartburn, epigastric pain, and regurgitation, often after meals. Most patients with GERD have mild to moderate symptoms; however, increased exposure to gastric contents may lead to more serious complications, such as erosive esophagitis, Barrett esophagus, peptic strictures, and even esophageal cancer.[14]

Patients may also present with a number of extraesophageal symptoms, including acid injury to tooth enamel, sore or burning throat, hoarseness, **dysphonia** (difficulty in speaking as a result of a condition of the mouth, throat, or vocal cords), excessive throat clearing, chronic cough, globus, and dysphagia.[15]

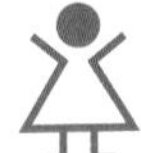

In infants, symptoms are unreliable but may include recurrent vomiting or regurgitation; cough, stridor, or wheezing due to aspiration; failure to thrive; and, in rare cases, apneic spells. As a result of acid-related symptoms, infants may experience sleep disturbances, irritability,

Table 42.5 Factors That Affect LES Tone

Factors	Increase Tone	Decrease Tone
Endocrine/paracrine	Gastrin, motilin, substance P, histamine	Cholecystokinin, somatostatin, vasoactive intestinal peptide (VIP)
Neural agents	Alpha-adrenergic agonists, beta-adrenergic antagonists, cholinergic agonists	Beta-adrenergic agonists, alpha-adrenergic antagonists, anticholinergic agents, serotonin
Food and liquids	Protein meal	Fat, chocolate, peppermint, alcohol, coffee, tea
Medications	Antacids, metoclopramide, domperidone, cisapride, baclofen	Meperidine, morphine, dopamine, calcium channel–blocking agents, barbiturates, theophylline, nitrates, sildenafil, albuterol

and difficulty feeding or refusal to eat.[16] Older children may present with symptoms of abdominal pain or describe heartburn-like symptoms, regurgitation, and cough. ■

Linking Pathophysiology to Diagnosis and Treatment

Because the symptoms of GERD are quite characteristic, diagnosis can usually be made with a thorough history and physical examination, along with a successful trial of empiric therapy. However, care must be taken to differentiate the symptoms from those of the various other conditions that cause esophagitis or esophagitis-like symptoms, such as infectious, pill, or eosinophilic esophagitis. It is especially important to consider coronary artery disease in differential diagnosis. Studies that are used to confirm diagnosis include esophageal pH monitoring, endoscopy, and manometry studies.

Treatment for GERD includes nonpharmacologic and pharmacologic measures. Nonpharmacologically, patients may be taught lifestyle modifications, which include diet changes and adoption of behaviors that may minimize reflux. Diet changes include avoiding foods and drinks that are known to lower LES tone and avoiding acidic foods. Behavior changes include weight loss in obese patients, smaller meals, and avoidance of the supine position immediately after meals.

The predominant pharmacologic approach to treating GERD is control of acid production and secretion. Proton pump inhibitors (PPIs) are the most potent antisecretory agents in use, followed by histamine 2 (H2) receptor antagonists.

A surgical approach may be an appropriate alternative to chronic pharmacologic treatment in some patient populations. A Nissen fundoplication is a surgical procedure in which the proximal stomach is wrapped around the distal esophagus, creating a physical antireflux mechanism.

Older patients are more prone to GERD because of age-related changes in their esophageal physiology, including decreased sensation to reflux (preventing early detection) and poor primary and secondary peristalsis (allowing acid to remain in the esophagus) and because of the likelihood of various comorbidities that may require medications that reduce LES tone.[17] The comorbidities as well as atypical GERD symptoms (anorexia, weight loss, anemia, vomiting, and dysphagia) found in older patients make diagnosis and treatment of GERD more challenging.[17] Treatment of older patients is similar to younger patients, and includes PPI and H2 blocker therapy and possibly antireflux surgery. Older patients are at increased risk of complications from medical and surgical interventions. ■

Barrett Esophagus

Barrett esophagus (BE), also known as Barrett metaplasia, is a metaplastic change in the lining of the esophageal mucosa in which normal esophageal, squamous epithelium begins to resemble gastric, columnar epithelium. Barrett esophagus is a complication of GERD. Based on a retrospective cohort study of nearly 500,000 patients, researchers found the incidence of BE to be 10.1% in patients with uncomplicated GERD.[18] In addition to GERD, the risk factors of BE include age over 50 years, male gender, obesity, being Caucasian, and family history.[19]

Etiology and Pathogenesis

The cause of BE is long-standing GERD. Injury to the esophageal mucosa from chronically refluxed acid, pepsin, and bile cause acute and chronic inflammatory changes. In response, esophageal stem cells at the GEJ respond by developing gastric-like columnar cells. The metaplasia will regress if the reflux is halted. If it is not halted, metaplasia may lead to dysplasia, which can lead to carcinoma.

Clinical Manifestations

Because gastric-like cells grow up and into the esophagus, refluxed materials, which may once have caused the common symptoms of GERD, are now tolerated in the esophagus, and many patients are asymptomatic. However, patients who present with symptoms often report heartburn and regurgitation.

Linking Pathophysiology to Diagnosis and Treatment

Even though many patients with BE are asymptomatic, routine screening is generally not recommended. Screening may be considered for patients with multiple risk factors. Diagnosis of BE is made with macroscopic visualization with upper GI endoscopy and histologic confirmation of metaplasia changes.

First and foremost, the treatment for BE consists of the aggressive treatment of GERD, including pharmacologic measures (PPIs) and possibly surgical measures. Endoscopic surveillance and biopsies are generally recommended because of the risk of progression to carcinoma. If dysplasia is present, therapy includes endoscopic eradication therapy and intensive surveillance. Endoscopic eradication therapy includes radiofrequency ablation and photodynamic therapy. Additionally, endoscopic mucosal resection may be effective for the treatment of early esophageal adenocarcinomas or dysplasia. Surgery to remove the diseased esophagus (esophagectomy) is indicated with early adenocarcinoma that has extended into the esophageal submucosa.

Esophageal Cancer

Esophageal cancer is a malignant growth or tumor resulting from the division of abnormal cells in the esophagus. There are two main types of esophageal cancer: squamous cell carcinoma (SCC) and adenocarcinoma. Together, they make up 95% of esophageal cancers. Other, rarer cancers of the esophagus include small cell carcinoma and nonepithelial cell cancers such as lymphomas, sarcomas, and metastatic tumors. Esophageal cancer is rare in young adults. The incidence of esophageal cancer increases with age, peaking in the sixth to eighth decades of life. In recent years, the rate of adenocarcinoma has risen, and the rate of SCC has decreased.[20]

Adenocarcinoma of the esophagus is defined as a carcinoma displaying glandular differentiation that arises in the esophagus.[2] It is the most common esophageal cancer in the United States. Risk factors of adenocarcinoma include BE and obesity. It usually occurs in Caucasian men aged 50–60 years.

Squamous cell carcinoma (SCC) is a malignant neoplasm of the esophagus with squamous differentiation, usually with signs of keratin.[2] It is the most common esophageal cancer in developing countries. Any factor that may cause chronic irritation and inflammation of the esophagus is a risk factor for SCC; these factors include smoking and alcohol use, achalasia, dysphagia, Plummer-Vinson syndrome, and caustic ingestions. The sex distribution is more equal with SCC, and it usually occurs in the sixth and seventh decades of life.

Etiology and Pathogenesis

No definitive cause of esophageal carcinoma has been identified. The cause is most likely multifactorial, incorporating environmental factors such as repeated exposure to irritants (e.g., smoking, alcohol, chronic GERD) in combination with genetic factors. Population-based case–control and cohort studies indicate that the main risk factors are GERD, cigarette smoking, and obesity.[20]

The rising incidence of adenocarcinoma has been hypothesized to be related to the increasing prevalence of GERD and obesity with GERD combined with the decline of *Helicobacter pylori* infection.[20] ***Helicobacter pylori (H. pylori)*** is a gram-negative bacterium that causes gastritis and ulcers. *H. pylori* infection may be somewhat protective in that the intragastric bacterial infection leads to gastritis and gastric atrophy, which reduces gastric acid production. Decreased acid production leads to decreased esophageal exposure to gastric acid, reducing the risk of BE and thus adenocarcinoma.

Several individual observational studies have shown a significant association between treatment with PPIs, aspirin and NSAIDs, and statins and a decreased risk of dysplasia and adenocarcinoma in patients with BE.[20]

Clinical Manifestations

The clinical presentations of esophageal adenocarcinoma and SCC are similar. Patients present with progressive dysphagia for solids, weight loss, and heartburn that is unresponsive to medical treatment. Less common symptoms include hoarseness, dry cough, and pneumonia related to laryngeal nerve involvement and odynophagia.

Linking Pathophysiology to Diagnosis and Treatment

Patients over the age of 55 years who present with dyspepsia should be considered for endoscopy for evaluation. Patients with persistent new-onset symptoms or those with alarm features at any age should undergo endoscopy.[21] Alarm features include anemia, dysphagia, weight loss, and persistent vomiting.

Diagnosis is made with upper endoscopic evaluation and biopsy. The endoscopic appearance of the two types of cancer are similar; however, they may be differentiated by their location in the esophagus. Adenocarcinoma lesions are usually found in the distal esophagus. SCC is more frequently found in the proximal to middle esophagus.[20] Endoscopic ultrasonography and positron-emission tomography are utilized for advanced screening of the cancer.

For small, asymptomatic tumors (< 2 centimeters in diameter) that are noncircumferential, treatment may include endoscopic mucosal resection. This approach is usually combined with endoscopic ablation of the remaining BE lesion. For locally advanced tumors, treatment consists of chemotherapy, radiation, and surgical resection (esophagectomy).[20] For tumors that are too advanced to be surgically treated, obstructive symptoms can be treated with palliative endoscopic esophageal stenting.

Check Your Progress: Section 42.2

1. While in transit, ingested materials may encounter esophageal defects, leading to which of the cardinal signs and symptoms of GI disorders?
2. How do the causes of structural esophageal disorders and functional esophageal disorders differ?
3. Describe the anatomic characteristics of a type II hiatal hernia.

42.3 Disorders of the Stomach

Bolused foods and liquids enter the stomach from the esophagus for the purpose of advancing digestion. Normally, potent gastric acid is kept in balance by various defenses, including feedback mechanisms and protective barriers in the gastric lining. However, when imbalances occur, patients may present with any of the four cardinal GI symptoms: pain, altered ingestion, altered digestion, and GIT bleeding. Specific to the stomach, patients are at risk for disorders of secretion and disorders of motility (see **Table 42.6** ■).

Peptic Ulcer Disease

Peptic ulcer disease (PUD), also known as acid peptic disease or ulcer disease, is a condition of chronic erosion, destruction, and ulceration in the lining of the stomach and

Table 42.6 Disorders of the Stomach

Type of Disorder	Examples
Disorders of secretion	Peptic ulcer disease Ulcers Gastrinoma Gastritis Stomach cancer
Disorders of motility	Gastroparesis Gastric outlet obstruction Pyloric stenosis

duodenum. Typically, patients with peptic ulcer disease present with mild gnawing or burning chest or abdominal pain resulting from ulcers in the lining of the stomach or the duodenum. See **Table 42.7** for a comparison of the features of gastric and duodenal ulcers.

Etiology and Pathogenesis

Erosion and ulceration in the GIT may be due to transient imbalances between the potent agents necessary for digestion—hydrochloric acid and pepsinogen/pepsin—and the protective mucosal barriers in the lining of the GIT. When the GIT is exposed to a causative agent, transient imbalances become persistent imbalances because of increased gastric acid secretion or a weakened mucosal barrier, and the person develops peptic ulcer disease.[22]

Mucosal erosion is distinguished from mucosal ulceration by the depth of the damage. Mucosal inflammation and erosion affect the mucosal and submucosal layers of the GIT; mucosal ulcerations penetrate the mucosal layers and begin to erode the muscular layers of the GIT. When eroded through and through, the GIT wall is said to be perforated (**Figure 42.5**).

The agents that contribute most notably to PUD are *H. pylori* infection and NSAIDs. Other, less common causes are Zollinger-Ellison syndrome, anastomosis ulcer after subtotal gastric resection, tumors (gastric, lymphoma, lung), Crohn disease of the stomach or duodenum, acute and chronic gastritis, viral infections (cytomegalovirus or HSV infection) in immunocompromised patients, and severe systemic disease (extensive burns causing Curling ulcer or head injury causing Cushing ulcer).[22] Several patient-related risk factors that are noted to contribute to ulcer formation are smoking, excessive alcohol use, drug use, emotional stress, and psychosocial factors; however, none of these are noted to cause ulcer formation on their own.[22]

Clinical Manifestations

Most commonly, patients with PUD present with epigastric pain and dyspepsia, although some patients may be asymptomatic. Although the incidences of complications related to PUD have been on the decline since the identification and treatment of *H. pylori* and the reduction of NSAID use in susceptible patient populations, the most common complications have not changed. GI bleeding remains the most common complication of PUD; the next most common is perforation, then GI obstruction.[23] Patients who are experiencing any of these three complications are considered to be suffering from complicated PUD.

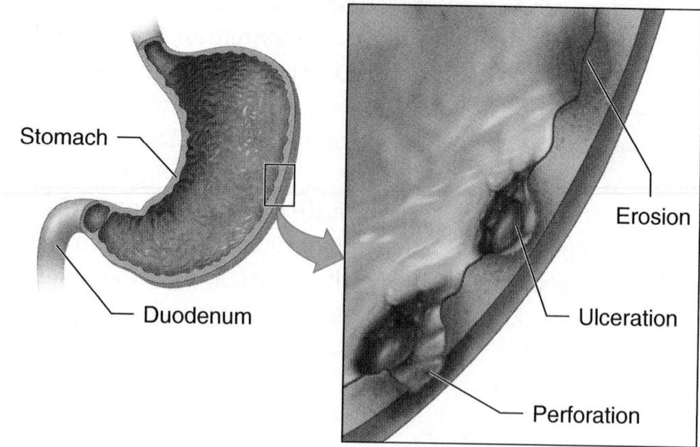

Figure 42.5 Degrees of mucosal injury seen in peptic ulcer disease.

Linking Pathophysiology to Diagnosis and Treatment

On the basis of clinical presentations, including dyspepsia, relation of pain to meal/pain at night that is relieved by food of antacids, and/or GI bleeding, clinicians may suspect PUD. Because of its ability to directly visualize the GI mucosa, obtain tissue samples, and perform therapeutic interventions, upper GI endoscopy is performed more commonly than upper GI x-rays and is used for diagnosis and prognosis of PUD.[24] Identifying the causative factor is important, and since *H. pylori* ulcers cannot be differentiated from NSAID-induced ulcers, additional testing for *H. pylori* is essential for all patients who present with the symptoms of PUD.

In uncomplicated PUD, upper GI endoscopy is used to confirm the diagnosis and rule out malignancy.[24] In complicated PUD, upper GI endoscopy is used for the diagnosis, prognosis, and treatment of bleeding ulcers and gastric outlet obstruction. Endoscopy should not be used in cases of perforated ulcers.[24]

If the ulcer is *H. pylori* positive, the treatment of choice is *H. pylori* eradication with a combination of acid-inhibiting therapy for 10–14 days. Treatments may be either triple therapy (PPIs, clarithromycin, and amoxicillin or

Table 42.7 Distinguishing Features of Gastric and Duodenal Ulcers

Type	Incidence	Pathology	Pathophysiology	Presentation
Gastric ulcers (GUs)	Occur later in life with peak incidence in the sixth decade	GUs more likely to represent a malignancy; benign GUs most often found in or near the antrum of stomach	*H. pylori* and NSAID induced; associated with normal to decreased gastric acid secretion	Burning or gnawing discomfort; may be precipitated by food; nausea and weight loss frequently accompany GU
Duodenal ulcers (DUs)	Estimated to occur in 6–15% of Western population; treatment of *H. pylori* and reduction of NSAIDS have reduced rates of DU greatly	Most often occur in the first portion of the duodenum; usually ≤ 1 cm in diameter but may reach 3–6 cm (giant ulcer); malignant DUs are rare	*H. pylori* and NSAID induced; associated with increased basal and nocturnal gastric acid secretion and decreased bicarbonate secretion in duodenal bulb	Burning or gnawing discomfort; occurs with an empty stomach and during the night and is usually relieved by food or antacids; patients frequently report being awakened at night by pain

metronidazole) or quadruple therapy (PPIs, bismuth salts, tetracycline, and metronidazole), depending on the prevalence of antibiotic resistance in an area.[22]

If the ulcer is NSAID induced, more than 90% of gastric or duodenal will heal with approximately 2 months of a standard-dose H2 receptor antagonists and cessation of the NSAID.[22] If the NSAID is continued, PPIs have shown to be more effective than H2-receptor antagonists in healing gastric ulcers.

Gastritis

Gastritis is a condition of gastric mucosal irritation or injury that results in histologically confirmed inflammation. A gastric mucosal disorder that does not produce inflammation is called *gastropathy*. Gastritis can be classified in numerous ways: by time course, by histologic features, and by anatomic distribution (see **Table 42.8**).

Etiology and Pathogenesis

Acute gastritis most often has infectious causes, *H. pylori* being the most common infectious agent.[25] Less commonly, acute gastritis may be caused by other bacterial infections or viral, parasitic, or fungal infections. Ulcerohemorrhagic gastritis is seen in critically ill patients and is due to physiologic stress and ischemic changes caused by shock, hypotension, or the release of vasoactive substances.[25] Drug-induced gastritis may be caused by a number of medications, most notably NSAIDs, steroids, some chemotherapeutic agents, alcohol, and iron supplements.

The pathogenesis of acute gastritis is an acute imbalance between mucosal injury and repair mechanisms leading to mucosal hyperemia and erosive changes with histologic presence of inflammation.[25]

Chronic gastritis is often caused by infectious agents, primarily bacteria, specifically *H. pylori*, but it may also be caused by viral, parasitic, and fungal infections. Chemical and caustic agents such as NSAIDs and excessive alcohol ingestion may case chronic gastritis, as can radiation exposure. Chronic gastritis may also be the consequence of autoimmune diseases such as Crohn disease, Wegener granulomatosis, and sarcoidosis.

Chronic gastritis begins with mucosal injury and impaired restorative mechanisms, and the condition may then progress. In the early phase, superficial gastritis, inflammation is limited to the surface of the mucosa. In the subsequent stage, atrophic gastritis, the inflammatory changes extend deeper into the mucosa, damaging gastric secretory glands. Damaged secretory glands lead to decreased acid production and decreased intrinsic factor production. Intrinsic factor is necessary for intestinal absorption of vitamin B_{12}; without it, patients develop vitamin B_{12} deficiency (pernicious anemia).[26] In the final stage, gastric atrophy, gastric glandular structures are lost and/or converted to intestinal phenotypes (metaplasia). This is a precursor to gastric cancer.

Clinical Manifestations

Most often, patient with gastritis do not report symptoms or may complain of mild dyspepsia. The symptoms of gastritis may be masked by an underlying or more pressing medical condition. Symptoms may include abdominal pain or upset, burning sensation in chest or upper abdomen, feeling of fullness, bloating, belching, and reflux. More severe symptoms include, nausea, vomiting, GI bleeding, fever, and weight loss.

Linking Pathophysiology to Diagnosis and Treatment

Diagnosis is made with upper GI endoscopic exam and biopsies from multiple sites in the stomach for both acute and chronic gastritis. Specific causes of the gastritis may be determined by the microscopic features of the biopsies.

For both acute and chronic gastritis, treatment begins with elimination of the causative agent or exacerbating factors. If the cause is related to *H. pylori*, eradication of the infection is indicated. For treatment of the dyspeptic symptoms, medications to reduce gastric acid production, such as a PPI or a histamine blocker, are indicated in acute gastritis. In chronic gastritis, medications that act to enhance mucosal protection, such as sucralfate and misoprostol, are effective in reducing dyspeptic symptoms. Acupuncture has also been used effectively for the treatment of symptoms of chronic gastritis. In both acute and chronic gastritis, surgery is indicated for treatment of GI bleeding.

Gastric Outlet Obstruction

Epigastric pain and postprandial vomiting may be due to a mechanical obstruction in the pyloric region. In adults, this is often termed gastroduodenal outlet obstruction or **gastric outlet obstruction**. Infants are known to suffer from a type of gastric outlet obstruction known as pyloric stenosis.

Etiology and Pathogenesis

Gastric outlet obstruction may be due to gastric pathology, duodenal pathology, and/or extraluminal pathology. Peptic

Table 42.8 Categories of Gastritis, Definition, and Causes

Category	Definition	Causes
Acute or erosive gastritis	Gastritis that presents with sudden onset and results from acute mucosal injury and inadequate mucosal repair	Causative mechanisms include infection, ulcerohemorrhagic causes, and effects of drugs and caustic injury
Chronic gastritis	Gastritis associated with infiltration of chronic inflammatory cells into the gastric mucosa, causing inflammation, atrophy, and/or metaplasia	Nonatrophic: infectious related/*H. pylori* related; location: antral-predominant Atrophic: autoimmune; location: body-predominant Special types: chemical or reactive, eosinophilic, lymphatic

ulcer disease was once the predominant cause of gastric outlet obstruction; however, with the identification and treatment of *H. pylori*, that is no longer true.[27] In recent decades, more cases are attributable to malignancies of the pancreas, stomach, duodenum, and biliary tract and metastatic cancer.[28] Less common causes include chronic GI conditions, such as Crohn disease and pancreatitis, caustic injuries, and postsurgical or postinterventional complications.

In the case of malignancy, tumors are the cause of the obstruction. With the chronic GI conditions and caustic injuries, obstruction is caused by inflammation, edema, and tissue deformation followed by chronic scarring and tissue remodeling due to the process of healing. Surgical- and interventional-induced obstructions are due to slippage or malpositioned tubes and stents or to bariatric or stomach-reducing surgeries.

Clinical Manifestations

Patients with gastric outlet obstruction may present with abdominal pain, distention or bloating, vomiting, dehydration, and weight loss.[27] Patients may also experience early satiety and feelings of nausea.

Linking Pathophysiology to Diagnosis and Treatment

If gastric outlet obstruction is suspected, a succussion splash should be performed. With a stethoscope placed over the stomach (upper abdomen), the patient logrolls back and forth. A splashing sound indicates retained gastric contents. If it occurs more than 3 hours after a meal, it suggests gastric outlet obstruction. Diagnosis is confirmed with radiologic evaluation, including abdominal x-rays, contrast studies, and upper GI endoscopy.

For benign cases of gastric outlet obstruction, treatment initially consists of medical management: nasogastric tube suction, medications to suppress gastric acid production, IV fluid and electrolyte replacement, and nutritional supplementation. After a period of time, a liquid diet may be tried. Patients who fail the initial medical management may require endoscopic balloon dilation or surgery.

For cases due to malignancy, the treatment depends on the underlying cause. Therapeutic procedures may include stenting, chemotherapy, endoscopic balloon dilation, or surgery. Palliative procedures, such as surgical bypass or placement of an endoscopic enteral stent, may be the best options for advanced cancers.

Infantile Hypertrophic Pyloric Stenosis

Infantile hypertrophic pyloric stenosis (IHPS) is a condition that frequently affects young infants. It is characterized by hypertrophy of the pylorus muscle leading to eventual gastric outlet obstruction.[29]

Etiology and Pathogenesis

The exact etiology of IHPS is unknown. However, it is most likely due to a number of factors, including genetic and environmental factors, such a maternal smoking, bottle feeding, and the administration of macrolide antibiotics within the first 2 weeks of life.[29]

Normally, the stomach contents easily pass to the duodenum via the pylorus. In IHPS, the pylorus becomes progressively obstructed as a result of hypertrophy of the pyloric muscles.

Clinical Manifestations

The classic presentation of IHPS includes gradual onset of worsening nonbilious projectile vomiting beginning at 4–6 weeks of age, dehydration or weight loss, and possibly visible peristalsis in the upper abdomen.[30] The typical clinical feature is that the baby is hungry after vomiting and eager to feed. Laboratory findings include hypochloremia, hypokalemia, and metabolic alkalosis. On physical examination, some infants may have a palpable olive-sized mass in the right upper quadrant.

Linking Pathophysiology to Diagnosis and Treatment

IHPS is suspected when a baby presents with projectile, nonbilious vomiting, visible peristalsis, and hyperchloremic metabolic alkalosis. Diagnosis may be reinforced with the palpation of the small olive-sized mass in the right upper quadrant, if appreciated. Ultrasound is preferred to confirm diagnosis and to evaluate pyloric muscle thickness and pyloric canal length.[30]

The definitive treatment for IHPS is surgery. If the infant is well hydrated with normal electrolytes, the surgery may take place on diagnosis. If the infant is dehydrated or has electrolyte abnormalities, surgery is delayed to optimize the patient's fluid and electrolyte status. ■

Stomach Cancer

Stomach cancer refers to tumors or neoplasms in the stomach that arise from the gastric mucosa (adenocarcinoma), the connective tissue of the gastric wall (GI stromal tumors or GISTs), neuroendocrine tissues (carcinoid tumors), or lymphoid tissues (lymphomas).[31] About 85% of stomach cancers are adenocarcinomas, and 15% are other types. See **Table 42.9** ■ for the Lauren Classification of Adenocarcinoma of the Stomach.

Etiology and Pathogenesis

Stomach cancer is the fourth most common cancer among men and the fifth most common cancer among women worldwide.[31] Globally, it accounts for 8% of total number of cancer cases and 10% of deaths annually.

Risk factors for the development of gastric cancer include *H. pylori* infection, cigarette smoking, high levels of alcohol ingestion, excessive dietary salt, inadequate fruit and vegetable consumption, and pernicious anemia.

Ingestion of high concentrations of nitrates appears to be associated with a higher risk of stomach cancer. The nitrates found in preserved foods (dried, smoked, and salted foods) are believed to be converted to carcinogenic nitrites by bacteria. Such bacteria may be introduced through the ingestion of partially decayed foods, which are consumed in abundance worldwide by people at lower socioeconomic levels. The chronic inflammation caused by *H. pylori* also contributes to this effect by causing atrophic gastritis, which

Table 42.9 Lauren Classification of Adenocarcinoma of the Stomach

Subtype	Pathology	Prognosis
Intestinal (most common type)	• Cohesive neoplastic cells • Form glandlike structures or masses • Well differentiated • Associated with the presence of *H. pylori* infection	Associated with better prognosis than diffuse adenocarcinoma
Diffuse	• Absent neoplastic cell cohesion • Individual cells infiltrate and thicken the stomach wall, throughout the whole stomach • No mass forms • Often preceded by a prolonged precancerous process, such as *H. pylori* infection	Results in loss of distensibility of the gastric wall (*linitis plastica*, or "leather bottle" appearance) Associated with poorer prognosis than intestinal adenocarcinoma
Intermediate (least common type)	• Uncommon histology • Includes mixed carcinoma, SCC, parietal cell carcinoma, undifferentiated carcinoma, mixed adenoneuroendocrine carcinoma	Depends on type

SOURCE: Berlth, F., Bollschweiler, E., Drebber, U., Hoelscher, A. H., & Moenig, S. (2014). Pathohistological classification systems in gastric cancer: Diagnostic relevance and prognostic value. *World Journal of Gastroenterology, 20*(19), 5679–5684. doi:10.3748/wjg.v20.i19.5679

results in loss of gastric acidity, leading to intestinal metaplasia, dysplasia, and then cancer.[32]

Clinical Manifestations

Weight loss and abdominal pain are the most common symptoms of stomach cancer at initial diagnosis. Abdominal pain tends to be vague and mild early in the disease and worsens as the disease progresses such that, at the time of presentation, most patients with stomach cancer already have advanced disease. Patients may present with dysphagia from tumors of the gastroesophageal junction or proximal stomach or gastric outlet obstruction from tumors of the distal stomach. Other manifestations include nausea, early satiety, and occult GI bleeding. A mass may be palpable in the upper right quadrant of the abdomen. Together, these clinical manifestations make up a set of features known as alarm features of stomach cancer; when they are noted, the healthcare provider should consider gastric cancer.[31]

Linking Pathophysiology to Diagnosis and Treatment

Stomach cancer is suspected if a patient over the age of 55 years presents with new-onset dyspepsia and alarm symptoms. Diagnosis is confirmed with upper GI endoscopy and biopsy. In cases of stomach cancer, upper endoscopy may help to diagnosis, stage, treat, and perform palliative procedures. Depending on the stage of the cancer, treatment may range from endoscopic resection and follow-up to radiation and chemotherapy and surgical resection.

Check Your Progress: Section 42.3

1. Describe the differences in clinical presentation between a gastric ulcer and a duodenal ulcer.
2. What are the risk factors for the development of stomach cancer?
3. What clinical manifestations suggest that a baby has infantile hypertrophic pyloric stenosis?

42.4 Disorders of the Small Inestines, Large Intestines, and Rectum

Materials enter the small bowel via the duodenum in the form of chyme. The body must now move the slurry through the bowel for the absorption of nutrients, vitamins, electrolytes, and water. Motility is an essential feature, and failure results in malabsorption, malnutrition, and dehydration. Patients with pathology in the small and large intestines and in the rectum most often suffer from the following cardinal GI symptoms: altered motility, pain, and bleeding. The disorders of the small and large intestines and the rectum can be grouped by etiology. **Table 42.10** shows the etiologies of the most prevalent disorders.

Inflammatory Bowel Disease

Inflammatory bowel disease (IBD) is a chronic inflammatory disorder involving the GIT. The two major disorders in this category are ulcerative colitis and Crohn disease.

Ulcerative colitis (UC) is a chronic inflammatory condition limited to the mucosal layers of the colon. It is characterized by relapsing and remitting episodes of inflammation.

Table 42.10 Etiology of Disorders of Small and Large Intestines and the Rectum

Etiology	Selected Disorders
Intestinal inflammation	Inflammatory bowel disease Appendicitis
Disorders of motility	Bowel obstruction Irritable bowel syndrome
Disorders of intestinal structure	Diverticular disease Hemorrhoidal disease
Neoplasm	Colon Rectum

It usually involves the rectum and may extend proximally and in a continuous fashion to involve other portions of the colon.

Crohn disease (CD) is a chronic inflammatory condition that may involve any portion of the GIT. It is characterized by transmural inflammation of the bowel and most commonly affects the ileum and proximal colon. Lesions are not always continuous, as seen in UC, and are therefore referred to as skip lesions.

Etiology and Pathogenesis

The pathogenesis of IBD is incompletely understood. Environmental factors, microbial imbalance in the gut, genetic susceptibility, and an inappropriate immune response all appear to play roles in the pathogenesis of these diseases, leading to inflammation and destruction of the bowel.[33]

In UC, inflammation is limited to the mucosal and submucosal layers of colon. A continuous lesion of inflammation may extent into the proximal colon and, in some cases, may affect the whole colon (pancolitis). Changes in the bowel include epithelial damage, inflammation, crypt abscesses, and loss of goblet cells.

In CD, inflammation extends through the layers of the bowel and may result in fissures and fistulas within the affected bowel. CD affects any segment of the bowel and may skip from segment to segment. Changes in the bowel include bowel wall thickening, ulcerations, and submucosal thickening, leading to cobblestone patterns of the mucosa. **Figure 42.6** ■ illustrates the effects of each disease on the bowel.

Clinical Manifestations

IBD is an intermittent disease. When active, IBD may cause a wide array of symptoms ranging from mild to severe that depend on the segment of the bowel that is affected. When IBD is in remission, symptoms may decrease and even disappear. General symptoms associated with both UC and CD include fever, loss of appetite, weight loss, fatigue and night sweats.

Symptoms of UC include bloody and/or mucoid diarrhea, dehydration, and anemia. Patients frequently experience crampy abdominal pain as well as pain with defecation and tenesmus (a sense of urgency and a feeling of incomplete bowel evacuation) due to involvement of the rectum. Involvement of the rectum may also lead to constipation.[34] UC is associated with an increased risk of intestinal cancer.

Patients with UC may develop a rare condition known as toxic megacolon. This condition is a life-threatening emergency characterized by dilation of the colon and excessive episodes of bloody diarrhea that may lead to the need for blood transfusions. If this condition cannot be managed with aggressive medical treatment, emergent bowel surgery may be indicated.[34]

Symptoms of CD include nausea, vomiting, and diarrhea with or without blood. Patients with CD also experience abdominal pain and pain with defecation due to anorectal fissures. Complications of CD include bowel strictures and obstructions. Patients may develop perforations in the bowel and intra-abdominal abscesses. If the disease cannot be managed with medical treatment, surgery may be indicated.[34]

IBD is associated with extraintestinal (other than bowel) manifestations in up to 25% of patients and primarily affects the skin, joints, eyes, and liver.[34,35] See **Table 42.11** ■ for a list of extraintestinal manifestations.

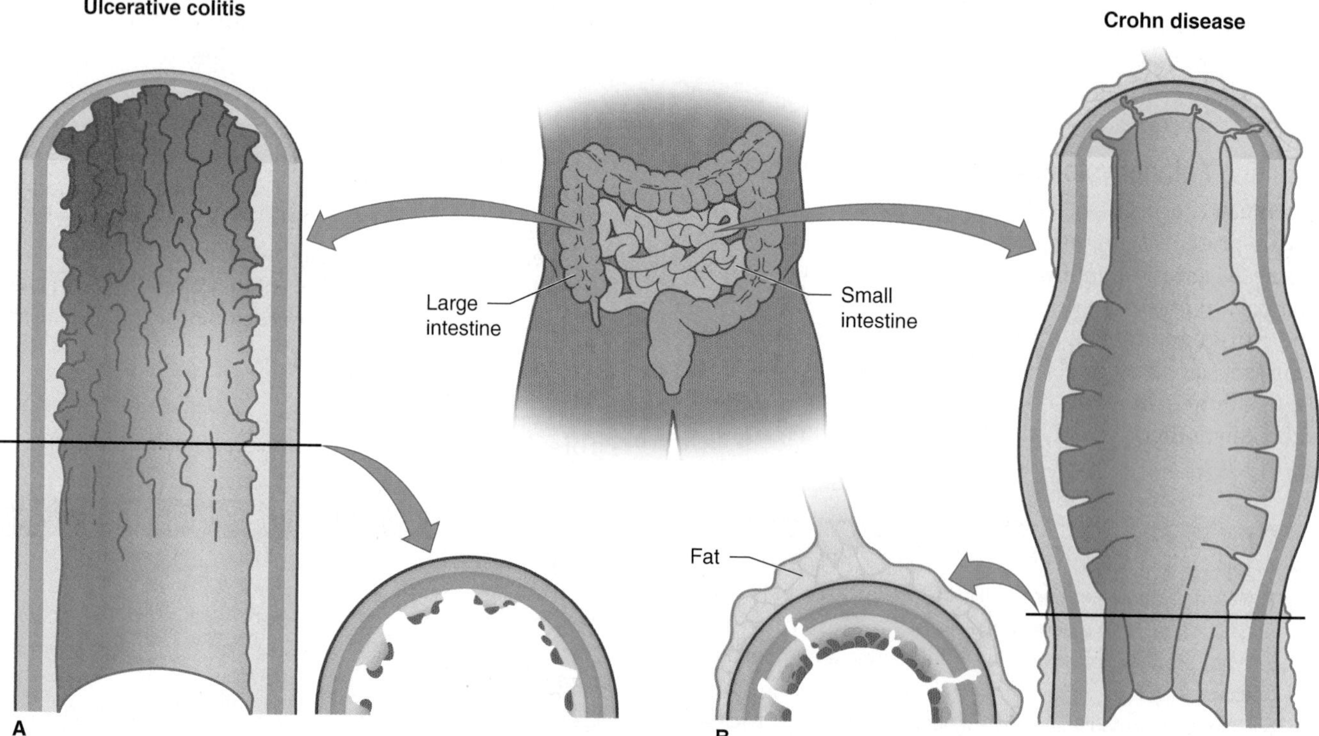

Figure 42.6 ■ Comparison of **A.** ulcerative colitis and **B.** Crohn disease.

Table 42.11 Extraintestinal Manifestations of IBD

Location	Manifestations
Skin	Pyoderma gangrenosum Erythema nodosum
Joints and bone	Arthritis Ankylosing spondylitis Osteoporosis
Eyes	Iritis Uveitis Episcleritis
Organs	Primary sclerosing cholangitis Nonalcoholic fatty liver disease (NAFLD) Nephrolithiasis in CD Gallstones in CD
Vascular	Venous thromboembolism Avascular necrosis Ischemic arterial events
Other	Depression Anxiety

SOURCES: Bernstein, C. N., Fried, M., Krabshuis, J. H., et al. (2010). World Gastroenterology Organization practice guidelines for the diagnosis and management of IBD in 2010. *Inflammatory Bowel Diseases, 16*(1), 112–124. doi:10.1002/ibd.21048. Feuerstein, J. D., & Cheifetz, A. S. (2014). Ulcerative colitis: Epidemiology, diagnosis, and management. *Mayo Clinic Proceedings, 89*(11), 1553–1562. doi:10.1016/j.mayocp.2014.07.002

Greg Ross: Application

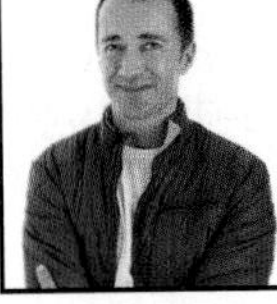

On examination, Mr. Ross's vital signs are temperature 101°F, blood pressure 146/96 mmHg, heart rate 100, respirations 20. He has been experiencing diarrhea (more than six stools per day) accompanied by abdominal pain for the past 5 days. He reports drinking "some" fluids but has eaten little food, as he lacks appetite and has nausea.

3. What findings suggest that Mr. Ross is dehydrated?
4. For what potentially life-threatening condition should Mr. Ross be monitored?

Linking Pathophysiology to Diagnosis and Treatment

The diagnosis of UC and CD is based first on clinical symptoms. Patients with bloody or mucoid diarrhea and cramping abdominal pain should undergo stool sampling to rule out infectious causes of diarrhea (infectious enterocolitis) and to determine whether markers of intestinal inflammation are in the stool. Serum assays such as C-reactive protein and erythrocyte sedimentation rate may provide evidence and degree of inflammation. A complete blood count identifies the presence of anemia. Diagnosis is confirmed with lower endoscopy studies to visualize and biopsy the bowel tissues. Radiologic studies such as barium studies may be indicated for evaluating segments of the bowel that might not be reached with lower endoscopy.

The management goals of IBD are optimizing the patient's quality of life by treating acute processes, inducing and maintaining remission, and decreasing the use of corticosteroids. Wholesome nutrition and healthy lifestyle habits are utilized along with medical management.

Medical therapy for IBD includes anti-inflammatory agents (5-aminosalicylic acid and corticosteroids), immunosuppressants (cyclosporine, methotrexate, and theopurines), anti–tumor necrosis factor agents, antibiotics, and probiotics.

Surgery is indicated in UC for UC that does not respond to medical management or for the presence of dysplasia in the bowel; 25–30% of UC patients may require surgery, and surgery is considered curative.[34] Surgery is indicated in CD for disease that does not respond to medical management; 70–75% of CD patients may require surgery at some point to relieve symptoms. However, surgery is rarely curative in cases of CD, owing to the "skip" nature of the disease.[34]

Greg Ross: Outcome

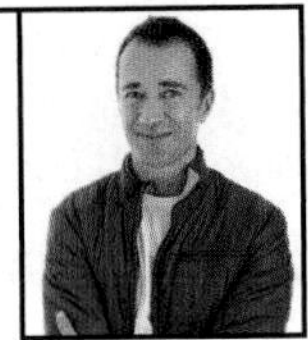

Mr. Ross, presented with a complaint of abdominal pain and diarrhea over past 5 days. He reports that fatigue has developed over the past 3 days, and his oral intake has been minimal, consisting mostly of fluids. He has a prior medical history of mild ulcerative colitis treated by dietary restrictions and takes no medications except during periods of disease exacerbation.

Laboratory findings include the following:

RBC (red blood cells): 3.5 million cells/μL

Hemoglobin: 9.2 g/dL

Erythrocyte sedimentation rate: 40 mm/hour

C-reactive protein: 130 mg/L

Mr. Ross is displaying exacerbation of UC. The elevated erythrocyte sedimentation rate and C-reactive protein are consistent with increased disease activity. The decrease in red blood cells and hemoglobin reflect GI bleeding and are common findings during periods of disease exacerbation. Mr. Ross's heart rate is elevated as a result of the anemia tied to blood loss. Disease exacerbation is typically treated with corticosteroid therapy and sulfasalazine. Mr. Ross is not expected to require ongoing pharmacologic therapy after treatment of the exacerbation.

5. Which laboratory tests should be monitored during Mr. Ross's treatment to determine whether inflammation is decreasing?
6. Identify realistic treatment goals for Mr. Ross.

Appendicitis

Appendicitis is an infectious process that causes inflammation of the vermiform appendix. It may be caused by an obstruction of the appendix by a fecalith (a hard mass of feces), a mass, or a foreign body. Appendicitis without complications (e.g., gangrene, perforation, or abscess) is classified as simple; appendicitis is classified as complicated when it involves any one of the noted complications. If an infected appendix ruptures, peritonitis and death may result.

Etiology and Pathogenesis

The etiology of appendicitis is still not completely understood. It has long been believed that the process occurs as a result of an appendiceal obstruction with a fecalith that causes distention, bacterial overgrowth, increased intraluminal pressure, and progressive tissue compromise.[35] However, mounting evidence shows that increased intraluminal pressure and fecaliths are not present in all cases of appendicitis, and not all cases of appendicitis result in perforation.[36] Obstruction remains a leading premise in the pathogenesis of appendicitis.

Obstruction is thought to lead to bacterial overgrowth and luminal distention. Increased intraluminal pressure and/or excessive inflammation can inhibit blood flow, causing vascular compromise to the affected tissue. In some cases, the appendix becomes gangrenous and may rupture.

Clinical Manifestations

Patients with appendicitis may present with crampy and steady central abdominal pain that migrates to the right lower quadrant of the abdomen. The pain is usually vague at first, increasing in intensity as the condition progresses. The classic signs of appendicitis include the cramping abdominal pain, tenderness with palpation of the right lower quadrant of the abdomen, nausea or vomiting, increased white blood cell count, and a low-grade fever.

Linking Pathophysiology to Diagnosis and Treatment

When a patient presents with the classic symptoms of appendicitis, imaging studies such as abdominal ultrasound and CT scan can assist in making a definitive diagnosis. Treatment is aimed at medical stabilization with intravenous fluids, electrolyte replacements, and antibiotics. While some practitioners may advocate for purely medical management for some cases of simple appendicitis,[36] surgery—most often laparoscopic surgery—remains the gold standard for treatment of simple and complicated appendicitis.

Appendicitis is the most common nonobstetric surgical emergency during pregnancy. It occurs in approximately 1 in 800–1500 pregnancies. However, preoperative diagnosis is inaccurate up to 50% of the time, owing to the physiologic changes associated with pregnancy, such as displacement of the appendix by the gravid uterus, leukocytosis, and pregnancy-related nausea and vomiting.[37] While maternal risk is nearly zero, the risk of fetal loss is increased in cases of perforated appendix and when an appendectomy is performed on a nondiseased appendix (negative appendectomy). Imaging is critical for assisting in an accurate diagnosis. In 2011, the American College of Radiology Appropriateness Criteria indicated ultrasound as the initial imaging study of choice in this patient population.

In 2015, Theilen, Mellnick, Longman, Tuuli, Odibo, Macones, and Cahill published the findings of their 5-year retrospective cohort study (n = 171) of pregnant women who underwent MRI for suspected appendicitis.[37] They found that MRI yielded a high rate of appendix visualization and diagnostic accuracy for appendicitis in pregnancy. As in other imaging studies, they noted that the rate of appendix visualization with MRI decreased in later trimesters. They concluded that use of MRI in pregnant women was valuable in ruling in or ruling out the diagnosis of appendicitis as well as ruling in differential diagnosis and guiding subsequent treatment. ■

Bowel Obstruction

Bowel obstruction, or intestinal obstruction, is a blockage of the intestinal tract. Eighty percent of bowel obstructions occur in the small bowel[38] and are called small bowel obstructions (SBOs). Partial obstructions are called low-grade obstructions; complete obstructions are called high-grade obstructions. Bowel obstruction is also commonly described as either simple or strangulated; in strangulated obstructions, vascular insufficiency and intestinal ischemia are evident. Functional obstruction, also known as ileus and pseudo-obstruction, is the absence of bowel motility rather than a physical blockage. All obstructions may become strangulated if vascular insufficiency and intestinal ischemia develop.

Etiology and Pathogenesis

Seventy-five percent of SBOs are due to adhesions.[39] Adhesions are fibrous bands (scar tissue) that form between tissues and organs and commonly occur after abdominal surgery. Other common causes are tumors, hernias, and intrinsic defects. The mnemonic HANG IV[40] may be used to recall the causes of SBO:

Hernia
Adhesions
Neoplasm/tumor
Gallstone ileus
Intussusception
Volvulus.

Hernias result when the bowel protrudes through a weakness or defect in the abdominal wall and becomes pinched, compromising gastric motility and blood flow. Adhesions are the result of intraperitoneal scar tissue. Intussusception results when a portion of the intestine slides, or telescopes into itself, causing impaired motility and circulation. Volvulus results when the bowel twists around a focal point on the mesentery. **Figure 42.7** ■ provides examples of herniation, adhesions, intussusception, and volvulus.

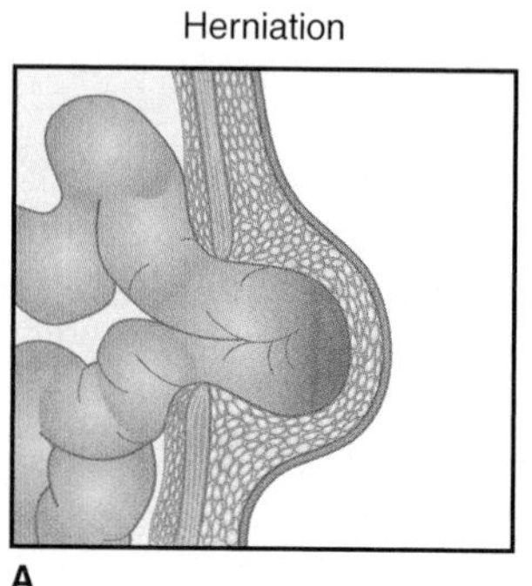

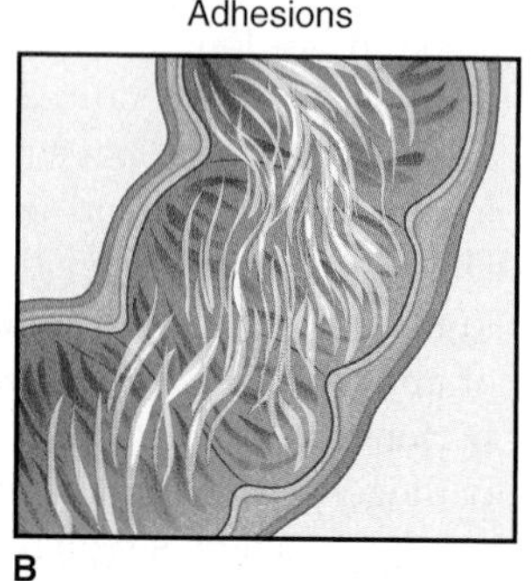

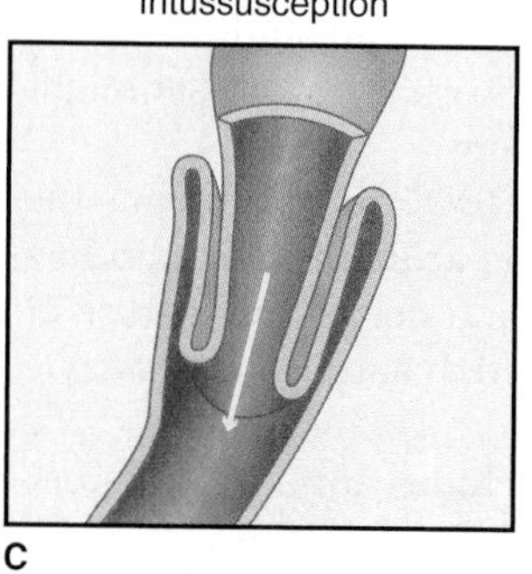

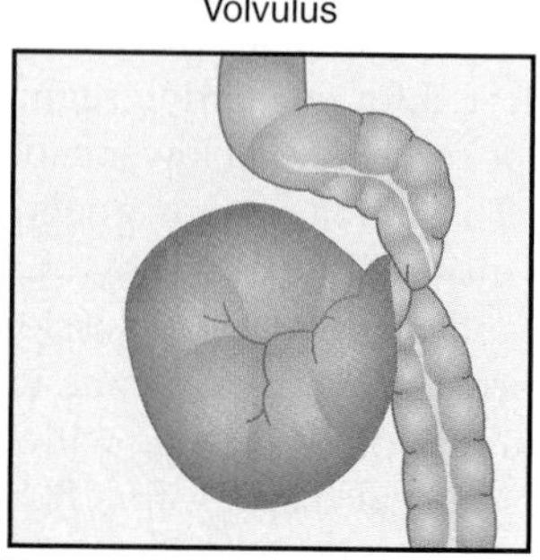

Figure 42.7 ■ Types of bowel obstruction. **A.** Herniation. **B.** Adhesions. **C.** Intussusception. **D.** Volvulus.

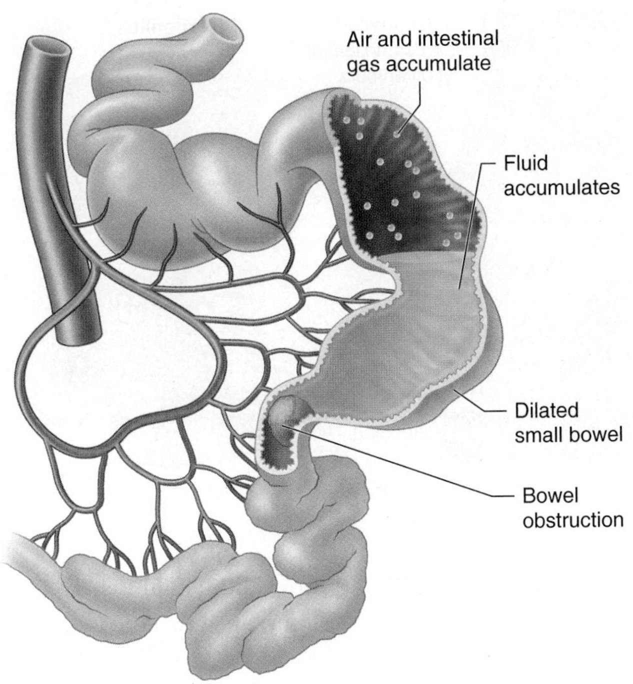

Figure 42.8 ■ Pathogenesis of bowel obstruction.

As the bowel obstructs, the bowel becomes dilated proximal to the blockage, as shown in **Figure 42.8** ■. Swallowed air and normal intestinal gas are unable to pass and accumulate, adding to bowel distention. Sensing stalled motility, the body pulls fluid into the lumen of the bowel to help push contents along, causing further distention and bowel edema and impairing the absorptive function of the bowel. With proximal bowel obstruction, distention is relieved with vomiting. Vomiting leads to further fluid losses and electrolyte abnormalities, causing hypovolemia and metabolic alkalosis.

Clinical Manifestations

The classic signs and symptoms of SBO are abdominal pain, nausea, vomiting, and abdominal distention.[39] Additionally, patients report the inability to satisfactorily pass gas or stool.

On physical examination, patients with SBO demonstrate hyperactive, high-pitched bowel sounds ("rushes and tinkles"); an absence of bowel sounds is noted with an ileus.

SBO is associated with serious complications, including strangulation in 30% of cases and bowel necrosis in 15% of cases. These complications may lead to bowel perforation, sepsis, and death and are worsened by advanced age, comorbid illness, and delayed diagnosis.[39]

Linking Pathophysiology to Diagnosis and Treatment

In patients with the classic signs of SBO, CT of the abdomen and pelvis should be performed to make a diagnosis. MRI and ultrasound may serve as alternatives to CT scan but have limitations. When patients fail to improve after a trial period of nonoperative management, a water-soluble contrast study should be considered to aid in diagnosis as well as treatment.[41]

Patients without clinical or radiologic signs and symptoms of bowel ischemia can safely undergo medical management with gastric decompression, intravenous fluids, and serial physical and serum evaluations. Medical management is successful in 65–80% of cases.[41] If the symptoms do not resolve in 3–5 days, the patient should undergo surgery.

Patients with signs of strangulation and bowel ischemia (fever, leukocytosis, tachycardia, continuous pain, metabolic acidosis, peritonitis) should undergo emergent surgery because of the increased risk of morbidity and mortality. Imaging studies will assist in diagnosis and detection of most patients who need early operative intervention.[41]

Irritable Bowel Syndrome

Irritable bowel syndrome (IBS) is defined as abdominal discomfort associated with altered bowel habits.[42,43] IBS can be subdivided into IBS with a prevalence for constipation (IBS-C), IBS with a prevalence for diarrhea (IBS-D), IBS with mixed constipation and diarrhea (IBS-M), and an unclassified category (IBS-U).

Etiology and Pathogenesis

IBS is a disorder of motility that has been attributed to abnormal gut motor and sensory activity, central neural dysfunction, psychologic disturbances, mucosal inflammation, stress, and luminal factors. However, no pathognomonic abnormalities have been identified.[43]

IBS is not associated with abnormal radiologic findings or endoscopic abnormalities; nor is it associated with a reliable biomarker. Diagnosis currently rests entirely on clinical findings.

Clinical Manifestations

The clinical manifestations of IBS are vague and include abdominal pain, cramps, or discomfort; change in bowel habits; and bloating. Patients may indicate that their symptoms are triggered after eating. Symptoms may also include nausea, lethargy, backache, and bladder symptoms.

Linking Pathophysiology to Diagnosis and Treatment

The diagnosis of IBS relies exclusively on the recognition of positive clinical features and elimination of other organic diseases. According to the Rome III classification, the diagnosis of IBS is made when the patient experiences recurrent abdominal pain or discomfort at least 3 days per month in the last 3 months associated with two or more of the following:

1. Improvement with defecation
2. Onset associated with a change in frequency of stool
3. Onset associated with a change in form (appearance) of stool.[42]

Treatment for IBS depends on the type and severity of the disorder. Treatment often involves education, reassurance, and dietary/lifestyle changes. For patients with IBS-D, treatment includes pharmacologic agents such as antispasmodics, antidiarrheals, bile acid binders, and gut serotonin modulators. For patients with IBS-C, treatment includes increased fiber intake and the use of osmotic agents. For patients with IBS involving predominantly gas and bloating,

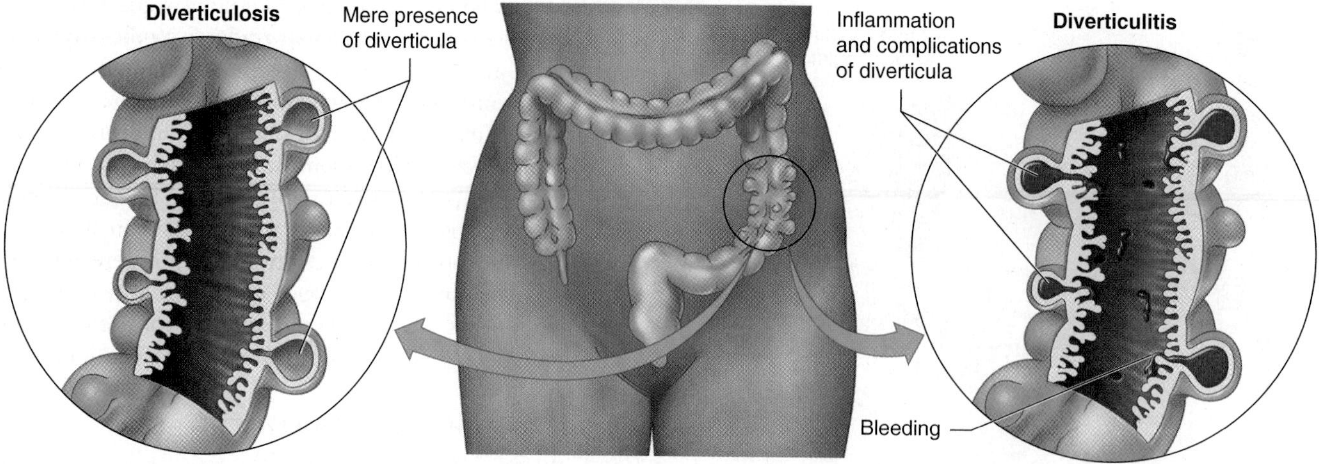

Figure 42.9 ■ Diverticulitis and diverticulosis of the bowel.

treatment includes dietary modifications. A small proportion of patients with IBS have severe and refractory symptoms and should be referred to specialists. Antidepressants and other psychologic treatments have been recommended for this group of patients.

Diverticular Disease

Diverticula are small outpouchings, or herniations, of the colonic mucosa through the muscle layers of the colon wall (**Figure 42.9** ■). **Diverticulosis** refers to diverticula without evidence of inflammation. **Diverticulitis** refers to inflamed diverticula.

Etiology and Pathogenesis

Diverticula can occur anywhere in the GIT but are found predominantly in the descending colon. Diverticulosis in the colon results from increased intraluminal pressure and weakness of the bowel wall. Associated factors include alterations in colonic wall resistance, alterations in colonic motility, and low-fiber diets. NSAIDs increase the risk of developing diverticulosis, as do advanced age, obesity, and lack of exercise.[44]

Diverticula typically occur at any point where a feeder artery penetrates through the muscle layer, resulting in a break of colonic wall integrity. High-amplitude contractions, caused by the need to evacuate high-fat and low-fiber stool, at an area of weakness result in herniation of the mucosa. Consequently, the feeder artery may become compressed or eroded, leading to perforation or bleeding. Chronic low-grade inflammation results. This is termed uncomplicated diverticulosis. Diverticulitis develops as a result of obstruction, stasis, altered local bacteria, and ischemia of the diverticula. Complicated diverticulitis is inflammation associated with formation of an abscess, fistula, obstruction, bleeding, or a perforation.[44]

Clinical Manifestations

Patients may present with sudden and constant abdominal pain in the left lower quadrant. Additionally, patients may report abdominal distention, nausea, diarrhea, constipation, and decreased appetite. Vital signs may reveal fever, tachycardia, and hypotension.[44]

Linking Pathophysiology to Diagnosis and Treatment

For patients with mild symptoms, imaging is not necessary. For complicated diverticulitis, CT scan, ultrasound, and MRI are useful to confirm the diagnosis and determine the severity of the disease.

Blood should be collected for a complete blood count to assess leukocytosis and a basic metabolic panel to assess electrolytes and renal function. Urine should be collected for urinalysis to rule out urinary tract infection and for a human chorionic gonadotropin urine test to rule out pregnancy in premenopausal women. Stool should be tested for occult GI bleeding.

Most patients (94%) can be treated on an outpatient basis.[44] Outpatient management includes a clear liquid diet, oral broad-spectrum antibiotics, and follow-up. For patients with signs of peritonitis or with a high suspicion of complicated diverticulitis, treatment is on an inpatient basis and includes no food or drink by mouth, intravenous fluids, and intravenous antibiotics. Approximately 25% of patients who are admitted with acute diverticulitis will require a surgical or procedural intervention.[44]

Hemorrhoidal Disease

The anus contains three vascular mucosal cushions (hemorrhoidal cushions), which assist with anal continence. **Hemorrhoids** are abnormal engorgements of these cushions. They may be classified as internal (originating above the dentate line) or external (originating below the dentate line), as shown in **Figure 42.10** ■. The dentate line represents the site where two different embryonic origins, the endoderm and the ectoderm, meet. Being from different embryonic origins, internal and external hemorrhoids have distinctly different vascular supply, epithelialization, and innervation. External hemorrhoids are usually uncomfortable or painful, whereas internal hemorrhoids are not.[45]

Etiology and Pathogenesis

Engorgement and straining lead to prolapse of this tissue into the anal canal. Over time, the anatomic support system of the hemorrhoidal complex weakens, exposing this tissue

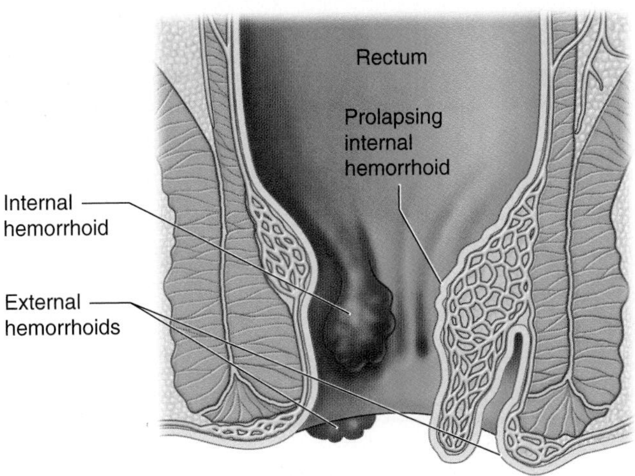

Figure 42.10 ■ Internal and external hemorrhoids.

to the outside of the anal canal, where it is susceptible to injury. Risk factors include conditions that increase intra-abdominal pressure and/or impede venous return, such as pregnancy or portal hypertension.

As the supporting tissues of anal cushions weaken, abnormal downward displacement of the cushions (prolapse) causes venous dilation, resulting in swelling and repeating tissue damage. Additionally, pathologic changes in the cushions contribute to swelling and prolapse, including abnormal venous dilation, vascular thrombosis, degenerative changes in collagen and elastin fibers and tissues, and distortion and rupture of anal musculature.

Clinical Manifestations

Patients present with hematochezia (approximately 60%), itching (approximately 55%), perianal discomfort (approximately 20%), and soiling (approximately 10%).[45] The bleeding usually occurs with defecation and is noticed on the toilet paper or in the toilet water. Large hemorrhoids may produce a feeling of rectal fullness or of incomplete evacuation.

Linking Pathophysiology to Diagnosis and Treatment

Diagnosis is typically made from the patient's report of symptoms. Examination of the anus, digitally and visually, and of the pelvic region is necessary for accurate diagnosis. Anoscopy is the procedure of choice for evaluation of internal hemorrhoids and to rule out anal prolapse.

The severity of the hemorrhoid is determined by a standard grading scale: Stage I involves enlargement with bleeding, stage II involves protrusion with spontaneous reduction, stage III involves protrusion requiring manual reduction, and stage IV involves irreducible protrusion.[46]

Based on the severity of the disease, treatment ranges from diet modification, topical glucocorticoids, vasoconstrictors, analgesics, and sclerotherapy (stages I and II) to procedural interventions, such as hemorrhoidal banding and surgical hemorrhoidectomy (stages III and IV).[45,46]

Cancer of the Colon and Rectum

Colon cancer is a malignant growth or tumor resulting from the division of abnormal cells in the ascending, transverse, or descending colon. **Rectal cancer** is a malignant growth or tumor occurring up to 15 cm from the anal opening.[47] The most recent estimates from the American Cancer Society estimates that over 135,000 cases of colorectal cancer will be diagnosed in the year 2017.[48] When these two diseases are combined together as colorectal cancer (CRC), the American Cancer Society estimates that over 50,000 men and women will die from the cancers. CRC remains the third most common cause of cancer death in the United States among both men and women. The incidence of CRC has been decreasing since the 1980s, owing to changes in modifiable risk factors (in particular, smoking and NSAIDs) and increases in screening among adults starting at the age of 50 years. However, the rates for adults younger than 50 years of age has been slowly increasing. Overall, mortality rates have been decreasing.[48]

Adenomas (or polyps) of the colon are benign tumors formed from glandular structures in the intestinal mucosal epithelium. Adenomas may be flat or sessile (raised), or they may have a stalk (pedunculated) (**Figure 42.11** ■). They are the precursors to most of CRCs and are estimated to be present in 20–53% of the U.S. population older than 50 years of age. In adults under 60 years of age, slightly more than half of adenomas are located in the distal colon. In adults over the age of 60, they are more likely found in the proximal colon.[47]

Etiology and Pathogenesis

CRC develops as the result of genetic abnormalities combined with environmental factors. Sequencing studies have found that, most commonly, conventional adenomas and sessile serrated polyps develop into cancer through either the chromosomal instability pathway or the microsatellite instability pathway. In both pathways, a number of genes become the major drivers of the CRC cancer; they include mutated tumor suppressor genes and mutated oncogenes. **Table 42.12** ■ briefly explains the pathways to CRC.[47] Risk factors that increase the risk of malignant features of adenomas include large size of the polyp, older age, a history of smoking, a family history of cancer, and nonuse of NSAIDs.[49]

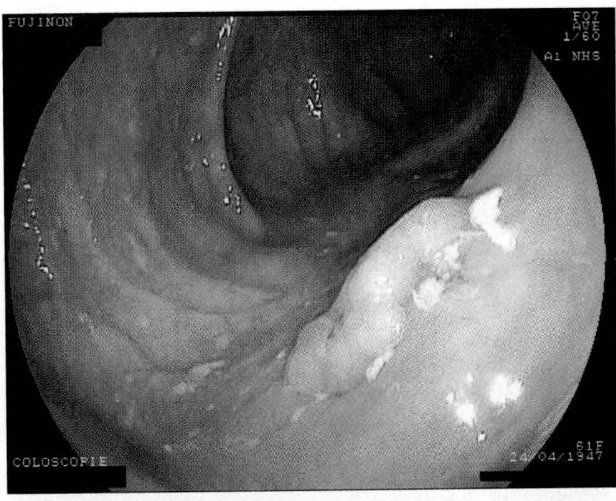

Figure 42.11 ■ Sessile adenoma seen in the colon of a woman in her 60s.

Table 42.12 Pathways to CRC

Pathway	Type of CRC	Gene Mutations	Location
Chromosomal instability	Familial adenomatous polyposis Sporadic CRC	APC mutation K-ras overexpression COX-2 and EGFR promote tumor growth	Left colon, distal colon
Microsatellite instability	Autosomal dominant hereditary nonpolyposis (HNPCC) Sporadic CRC	Mutation of DNA mismatch repair genes COX-2 promotes tumor growth	Right colon, proximal to splenic flexure
CpG island methylation pathway	Sporadic CRC	Early mutation of MMR genes Then becomes the microsatellite instability pathway	

NOTE: APC, a tumor suppressor gene; K-ras, a proto-oncogene (promotes cell growth); MMR, mutation mismatch repair; COX-2, cyclooxygenase-2; CpG, cytosine–phosphodiester bond–guanine DNA region.

Modifiable factors that increase risk of CRC include obesity, a sedentary lifestyle, smoking, moderate to heavy alcohol ingestion, and a diet that that is heavy on red and processed meats and light on fruits and vegetables.[48] Modifiable factors that decrease the risk of CRC include a diet that is rich in whole-grain fiber and the use of NSAIDs, such as aspirin.

Hereditary and medical factors that increase risk include a family history of CRC and/or polyps, some genetic factors, inflammatory bowel disease (ulcerative colitis or Crohn disease), and type 2 diabetes mellitus. The risk of CRC increases with age.[48]

Clinical Manifestations

Early CRC typically does not have symptoms. However, when symptomatic, patients present with a complaint of hematochezia and change in bowel habits. Other complaints may include fatigue, weight loss, generalized or localized abdominal pain, and symptoms of anemia.[48]

Advanced disease will have unique manifestations based on the location of the cancer. Right-sided cancers (ascending colon) are usually silent and may evolve to pain with a palpable mass in the right lower quadrant. Tumors stay to one side of the colon wall, and obstruction is not likely. Blood in stool is dark red in color.[47] Left-sided tumors (descending colon) grow circumferentially around the colon and may lead to intestinal obstruction. Stools may become long and pencil-like, and blood, when present, is bright red.[47]

On physical examination, patients may have a distended abdomen. On palpation, lymph nodes may be enlarged, and there may be a palpable mass in the abdomen. If the cancer is rectal, a mass may be palpable with digital examination.

Pam Allen: Application

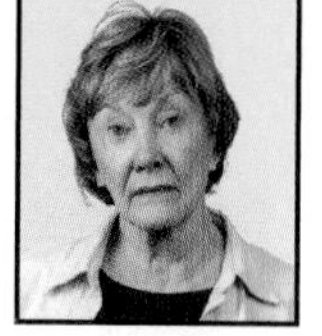

Ms. Allen is experiencing increased fatigue with constipation. After defecating, she noted reddish-brown spots within her stools. On physical examination, a palpable mass is noted, and a stool sample tests positive for occult blood. Given her prior history of cancer, Ms. Allen is concerned about the possibility of another tumor.

3. In view of Ms. Allen's findings on physical examination, what is the likely location in the colon for tumor growth?
4. If Ms. Allen has colon cancer and it is detected early, what are her 5-year survival statistics?

Linking Pathophysiology to Diagnosis and Treatment

Because there are very few signs in early CRC, early detection is essential. Screening should begin at age 50 for men and women.[48] Screening should begin sooner for individuals with predisposing genetic factors. Lower GI endoscopy can detect adenomas, biopsy tissue, and remove the adenomas in the same procedure. Screening may also include fecal tests for occult blood and DNA testing for mutant genes from the pathways.[49]

Staging of CRC may be made by endoscopy or with surgery for advanced stages. The National Cancer Institute classification is simplified below and shown in **Figure 42.12**[47]:

Stage 0: In situ, mucosal lining only
Stage I: Extension to middle layer of colon wall; no spread to lymph tissue

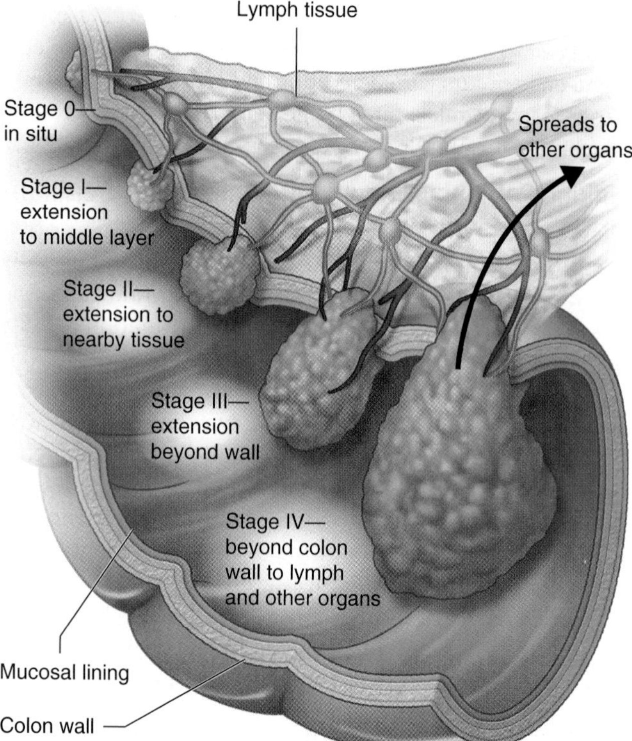

Figure 42.12 Staging of colorectal cancer.

Stage II: Extension beyond colon wall to nearby tissues; no spread to lymph tissue
Stage III: Extension beyond colon wall to nearby tissues/organs or peritoneum; includes spread to lymph
Stage IV: Beyond colon wall; includes lymph; has spread to other organs.

Staging usually includes the TNM (tumor, lymph nodes, and metastases) classification for more precise medical management

Although adenomas may be removed during endoscopy, surgery is the most common treatment for CRC that has not spread. When the cancer has extended beyond the wall of the bowel, chemotherapy or both chemotherapy and radiation are administered before or after surgery. For cancer that has spread to other parts of the body and organs, treatment usually includes chemotherapy and organ- or tissue-specific therapy.[48]

The survival rates for CRC are 65% at 5 years and 58% at 10 years. If the cancer is caught early, survival at 5 years can increase to 90%.[48]

The majority of colorectal cancers are asymptomatic until late. The cancer often involves the colon and rectum and results in GI bleeding and fatigue associated with chronic blood loss. Diagnosis is made through evaluation of polyps found during a colonoscopy. A biopsy of the polyp can identify whether the polyp is cancerous and capable of dissemination. Small polyps may also be removed during the colonoscopy. Further identification of a mass on diagnostic imaging can identify a tumor that requires removal and biopsy. Found early, these cancers are readily treatable. Once the tumor has begun to disseminate out of the colon, the course of treatment is often more complex with a poorer prognosis. Surgery revision of the rectum and colon may be necessary, and depending on the stage of the tumor, radiation and chemotherapy may be necessary.

Pam Allen: Outcome

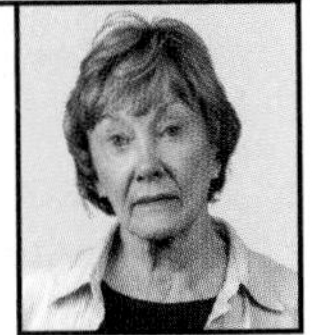

Ms. Allen's CT scan confirms the presence of colorectal cancer. Surgical revision of the tumor will involve a colectomy with establishment of a colostomy. Lymph nodes in the region of the cancer will be harvested for biopsy to determine the extent of the tumor. Depending on the biopsy results, chemotherapy with radiation may be indicated.

5. If Ms. Allen's tumor is found to be confined to the mucosal lining of the colon with no spread to the lymph nodes, at what stage will her cancer be classified?
6. What is the typical treatment for Stage 0–I colon cancer?

Check Your Progress: Section 42.4

1. What are the risk factors for diverticular disease?
2. Describe the Rome III classification for making a diagnosis of irritable bowel syndrome.
3. What are the classic clinical manifestations of small bowel obstruction?

CHAPTER SUMMARY

42.1 Chapter Overview and Case Studies

Outline the four cardinal symptoms of disorders of the upper and lower gastrointestinal systems and concepts related to GI alterations.

- The four cardinal signs and symptoms of disorders of the GI system are pain, altered ingestion, altered motility, and bleeding.
- Altered ingestion includes regurgitation, reflux, vomiting, and dysphagia.
- Large-volume diarrhea is due to forces pulling more volume into the intestinal lumen; small-volume diarrhea is due to faster intestinal motility.
- Primary constipation is due to stool composition and impaired muscles of evacuation; secondary constipation is due to a secondary cause impairing the muscles of evacuation, such as a neurogenic, pharmacologic, or metabolic cause.
- Upper GI bleeding presents as hematemesis, bright red blood in vomitus or "coffee ground" emesis and melena, black tarry stools. The dark brown and black colors found in coffee ground emesis and melena are due to digested blood.
- Lower GI bleeding presents as melena or hematochezia; hematochezia is bright red blood in stool.
- GI bleeding may be occult, which means that it is not detectable by visual inspection. Guaiac testing is needed to detect occult blood.

42.2 Disorders of the Esophagus

Differentiate the causes, classification, underlying pathogenesis, and clinical manifestations of disorders of the esophagus and approaches to diagnosis and treatment of these conditions across the lifespan.

- Esophageal webs are remnants of embryonic tissue and are associated with other conditions such as some dermatologic disorders and Plummer-Vinson syndrome, a condition of iron deficiency anemia in middle-aged women.
- Esophagitis is irritation and inflammation of the esophagus; it is caused by allergies, infection, radiation, caustic ingestion, and mechanical means (e.g., a pill lodged in the esophagus).

- Eosinophilic esophagitis results after exposure to a food or environmental allergen and is associated with other atopic (allergy-related) conditions such as eczema and asthma. Eosinophilic esophagitis in children presents as chest or abdominal pain, nausea, vomiting, and food aversion.
- Pill esophagitis develops when a swallowed pill does not clear the esophagus and becomes lodged in the esophagus, perhaps at an esophageal ring or web. Pill esophagitis is more common in older adults and with larger pills, such as antibiotics, quinidine, phenytoin, potassium, ferrous sulfate, NSAIDs, and bisphosphonates.
- Esophageal diverticula located in the upper esophagus are called hypopharyngeal diverticula and Zenker's diverticula; they are associated with the retention of undigested food, regurgitation, and aspiration. Diverticula in the esophagus present singularly, whereas diverticula in the colon present as a number of small diverticulum.
- A hiatal hernia occurs when a portion of the stomach migrates up through the esophageal hiatus of the diaphragm and enters the thoracic cavity. There are four types of hiatal hernia; 95% of individuals will develop a type I (sliding hiatal) hernia.
- The lower esophageal sphincter (LES) is the most reliable feature of the esophagus in preventing gastric reflux. Its ability to open to allow food and liquids to enter the stomach and tighten up when food and fluids have entered, when digestion is taking place, and whenever the pressure in the stomach (intragastric pressure) increases makes the LES the ultimate gatekeeper between the two organs.
- When intragastric pressure rises above the LES tone, erosive materials (acid, pepsin, bile) reflux into the esophagus. GERD is a condition in which this occurs chronically, resulting in inflammation, erosion, and ulceration of the esophagus. In adults, this typically causes heartburn; in infants, chronic regurgitation may produce pulmonary symptoms such as cough, stridor, or wheezing.
- A major complication of GERD is Barrett esophagus (BE). In BE, the epithelial cells of the distal esophagus change to resemble the columnar cells of the stomach. If left untreated, this metaplasia (abnormal change in tissue) can lead to adenocarcinoma of the esophagus.
- Ninety-five percent of esophageal cancers are squamous cell carcinoma and adenocarcinoma. The most common signs and symptoms of esophageal cancer are heartburn, dysphagia for solids, and weight loss.

42.3 Disorders of the Stomach

Differentiate the causes, classification, underlying pathogenesis, and clinical manifestations of disorders of the stomach and approaches to diagnosis and treatment of these conditions across the lifespan.

- Peptic ulcer disease (PUD) is caused by imbalances between the potent agents of digestion and the protective mucosal barriers of the lining of the GIT. PUD most commonly results in duodenal ulcers but may also result in gastric ulcers. Gastric ulcers are more often associated with malignancy.
- Duodenal and gastric ulcers have various stages: (1) Erosion occurs as inflammation affects the mucosal and submucosal layers only, (2) ulceration occurs as the damage penetrates the muscular layers of the GIT, and (3) perforation results as the damage erodes through all of the GIT layers.
- Irritation or injury to the gastric mucosa that does not produce inflammation is called gastropathy. When inflammation is involved, it is called gastritis; it may be classified as acute or chronic.
- In chronic gastritis, a condition commonly seen in older adults, inflammation destroys the glandular function of the gastric mucosa. The stomach is unable to produce appropriate levels of gastric acid, nor can it produce intrinsic factor, an essential substance for the intestinal absorption of vitamin B_{12}. Without vitamin B_{12}, the body suffers from pernicious anemia. The metaplasia of chronic gastritis is a precursor to gastric cancer.
- Gastric outlet obstruction may be due to gastric pathology, duodenal pathology, or extraluminal pathology (factors affecting GIT motility at the pylorus outside of the GIT, such as intestinal adhesions or volvulus).
- A common cause of gastric outlet obstruction in infants is infantile hypertrophic pyloric stenosis (IHPS), a condition of severe pyloric thickening and aggressive narrowing of the pylorus (the exit from the stomach to the duodenum) that requires urgent surgical intervention to prevent malnutrition and dehydration in young infants.
- Worldwide, stomach cancer is the fourth leading cause of cancer among men and the fifth leading cause of cancer in women. Risk factors include *H. pylori* infection, cigarette smoking, high levels of alcohol ingestion, and chronic gastritis.

42.4 Disorders of the Small Intestines, Large Intestines, and Rectum

Differentiate the causes, classification, underlying pathogenesis, and clinical manifestations of disorders of the small and large intestines and the rectum and approaches to diagnosis and treatment of these conditions across the lifespan.

- Inflammatory bowel disease (IBD) is a chronic inflammatory condition involving the lower GIT that usually develops in young adulthood (20–30 years of age). IBD is an intermittent disease that alternates between remissions and active disease states. IBD is associated with extraintestinal manifestations that may or may not coincide with the active and remissive states of the disease.
- Ulcerative colitis (UC) is an IBD that often affects the rectum and colon. UC develops as a continuous lesion;

when indicated, surgical resection is curative. Crohn disease (CD), an IBD, may develop all along the GIT, from the mouth to the anus, but usually affects the portion of the bowel where the small intestine and large intestine meet. CD may develop in various areas, and lesions are not continuous. Surgery for CD is not curative for the disease but is restorative for bowel function.

- UC is associated with more emergent infectious complications than CD and is more often associated with cancer, particularly colorectal cancer.
- Appendicitis is the infectious inflammation of the vermiform appendix. Appendicitis is the most common nonobstetric surgical emergency in pregnant women. There is a high risk of fetal loss with nonobstetric perinatal surgeries, and there is a higher risk of fetal loss with the surgical emergency that accompanies a ruptured appendix. While ultrasound is the gold standard for evaluating this patient population, a recent study found MRI more reliable for ruling in appendicitis in early parturients.
- Intestinal obstruction or bowel obstruction is the blockage of the intestinal tract by causes within the bowel (intraluminal), by causes outside of the bowel (extraluminal), and by forces that inactive the bowel. The mnemonic HANG IV can remind the clinician of the causes of bowel obstruction: herniation, adhesions, neoplasm, gallstone ileus, intussusception, and volvulus.
- Diverticula in the lower GIT most often occur in the colon. Diverticulosis is the presence of diverticula in the colon. Diverticulitis is the inflammation of diverticula.
- Colon cancer and rectal cancer, together called colorectal cancer (CRC), is the third leading cause of cancer related death in men and women in the United States. As a result of attention to modifiable risk factors and early detection, incidences have been decreasing.
- Progression to CRC is complex; the cancer develops in a sequential manner from the formation of adenomas (polyps) in the colon and the rectum. Genetic and environmental factors play a large role in the development of CRC from polyp.

REVIEW QUESTIONS

1. The nurse is caring for a patient with chronic gastritis. Which vitamin should the nurse anticipate administering to the patient?
   a. Vitamin A
   b. Vitamin B_{12}
   c. Vitamin C
   d. Vitamin D

2. Which of the following diets should the nurse recommend to a patient with diverticulosis?
   a. High-protein diet
   b. Low-cholesterol diet
   c. High-fiber diet
   d. Low-carbohydrate diet

3. The nurse on the GI unit is caring for a patient with pain on defecation from an anorectal fissure. Which of the following conditions does the patient most likely have?
   a. Crohn disease
   b. Ulcerative colitis
   c. Gastroesophageal reflux disease
   d. Colon cancer

4. The nurse is teaching a class in the community about colon cancer prevention and detection. Which of the following should the nurse teach about modifiable risk factors?
   a. Eat a diet that is rich in fiber.
   b. Avoid nonsteroidal anti-inflammatory drugs.
   c. Remove skins from fresh fruits.
   d. Limit fat intake.

5. A patient with hemorrhoids has frank bright red blood in his stool. The nurse documents this finding as:
   a. occult blood.
   b. melena.
   c. hematemesis.
   d. hematochezia.

6. A patient with small bowel obstruction exhibits fever, tachycardia, and continuous pain. Laboratory findings reveal leukocytosis and metabolic acidosis. Which of the following is the priority action for the nurse?
   a. Medicate the patient for pain.
   b. Contact the physician immediately.
   c. Repeat the laboratory tests in 6 hours.
   d. Administer acetaminophen for fever.

7. A patient is admitted with appendicitis. Which of the following manifestations is the nurse most likely to assess?
   a. Steady central abdominal pain that migrates to the right lower quadrant of the abdomen
   b. Steady central abdominal pain that migrates to the right upper quadrant of the abdomen
   c. Intermittent central abdominal pain that migrates to the right lower quadrant of the abdomen
   d. Intermittent central abdominal pain that migrates to the right lower quadrant of the abdomen

8. Which of the following findings are most likely to be assessed in a patient with stomach cancer?
   a. Ascites, nausea, and abdominal pain
   b. Nausea, early satiety, and occult blood in stool
   c. Hematochezia, early satiety, and weight gain
   d. Weight loss, constipation, and hematemesis

ANSWERS

Answers to Review Questions can be found in Appendix A. Answers to Case Study and Check Your Progress questions are available on the faculty resources site. Please consult with your instructor.

RECOMMENDED WEBSITES

American College of Gastroenterology
http://patients.gi.org

GIKids
http://www.gikids.org

Society of Gastroenterology Nurses and Associates
https://www.sgna.org

REFERENCES

1. Kahrilas, P. J., & Hirano, I. (2015). Diseases of the esophagus. In D. Kasper, A. Fauci, S. Hauser, D. Longo, J. Jameson, & J. Loscalzo (Eds.), *Harrison's principles of internal medicine* (19th ed.). New York, NY: McGraw-Hill.
2. Goljan, E. F. (2014). Gastrointestinal disorders. In E. F. Goljan (Ed.), *Rapid review pathology* (4th ed., pp. 419–466). Philadelphia, PA: Elsevier Saunders.
3. Sommers, T., Corban, C., Sengupta, N., Jones, M., Cheng, V., Bollom, A., Nurko, S., Kelley, J., & Lembo, A. (2015). Emergency department burden of constipation in the United States from 2006 to 2011. *American Journal of Gastroenterology, 110*, 572–579. doi:10.1038/ajg.2015.64
4. Liu, J. J, & Kahrilas, P. J. (2006). Pharyngeal and esophageal diverticula, rings, and webs. *GI Motility Online*. Available at http://www.nature.com/gimo/contents/pt1/full/gimo41.html#relatedcontent
5. de Wijkerslooth, L. R. H., Vleggaar, F. P., & Siersema, P. D. (2011). Endoscopic management of difficult or recurrent esophageal strictures. *American Journal of Gastroenterology, 106*, 2080–2091. doi:10.1038/ajg.2011.348
6. Liacouras, C. A., Furuta, G. T., Hirano, I., et al. (2011). Eosinophilic esophagitis: Updated consensus recommendations for children and adults. *Journal of Allergy and Clinical Immunology, 128*(1), 3–20. doi:10.1038/ajg.2013.71
7. Dellon, E. S., Gonsalves, S., Hirano, I., Furuta, G. T., Liacouras, C. A., & Katzka, D. A. (2013). ACG clinical guideline: Evidence based approach to the diagnosis and management of esophageal eosinophilia and eosinophilic esophagitis (EoE). *American Journal of Gastroenterology, 108*, 679–692. doi:10.1038/ajg.2013.71
8. Papadopoulou, A., Koletzko, S., Heuschkel, R., et al. (2014). Management guidelines of eosinophilic esophagitis in childhood. *Journal of Pediatric Gastroenterology and Nutrition, 58*(1), 107–118. doi:10.1097/MPG.0b013e3182a80be1
9. Arias, A., Gonzalez-Cervera, J., Tenias, J., et al. (2014). Efficacy of dietary interventions for inducing histologic remission in patients with eosinophilic esophagitis: A systematic review and meta-analysis. *Gastroenterology, 146*, 1639–1648. doi:10.1053/j.gastro.2014.02.006
10. Law, R., Katzka, D. A., & Baron, T. H. (2014). Zenker's diverticulum. *Clinical Gastroenterology and Hepatology, 12*, 1773–1782.
11. Nirula, R. (2014). Esophageal perforation. *Surgical Clinics of North America, 94*, 35–41. doi:10.1016/j.suc.2013.10.003
12. Gordon, C., Kang, J. Y., Neild, P. J., et al. (2004). Review article: The role of the hiatus hernia in gastroesophageal reflux disease. *Alimentary Pharmacology & Therapeutics, 20*, 719–732. doi:10.1111/j.1365-2036.2004.02149.x
13. El-Serag, H. B., Sweet, S., Winchester, C. C., & Dent, J. (2014). Update on the epidemiology of gastro-oesophageal reflux disease: A systematic review. *Gut, 63*, 871–880. http://dx.doi.org/10.1136/gutjnl-2012-304269
14. Boeckxstaens, G. E., & Rohof, W. O. (2014). Pathophysiology of gastroesophageal reflux disease. *Gastroenterology Clinics of North America, 43*, 15–25. doi:10.1016/j.gtc.2013.11.001
15. Madanick, R. D. (2014). Extraesophageal presentations of GERD: Where is the science? *Gastroenterology Clinics of North America, 43*, 105–120. doi:10.1016/j.gtc.2013.11.007
16. Rosen, R. (2014). Gastroesophageal reflux in infants: More than just a phenomenon. *JAMA Pediatrics, 168*(1), 83–89.
17. Achem, S. R., & DeVault, K. R. (2014). Gastroesophageal reflux disease and the elderly. *Gastroenterology Clinics of North America, 43*, 147–160. doi:10.1016/j.gtc.2013.11.004
18. Kramer, J. R., Shakhatreh, M. H., Naik, A. D., et al. (2014). Use and yield of endoscopy in patients with uncomplicated gastroesophageal reflux disorder. *JAMA Internal Medicine, 174*(3), 462–465.
19. Fitzgerald, R. C., di Pietro, M., Ragunath, K., et al. (2014). British Society of Gastroenterology guidelines on the diagnosis and management of Barrett's oesophagus. *Gut, 63*(1), 7–42. doi:10.1136/gutjnl-2013-305372
20. Rustgi, A. K., & Hashem, B. E. Esophageal carcinoma. (2014). *New England Journal of Medicine, 371*, 2499–2509. doi:10.1056/NEJMra1314530
21. Allum, W. H., Blazeby, J. M., Griffin, S. M., Cunningham, D., Jankowski, J. A., & Wong, R. (2011). Guidelines for the management of oesophageal and gastric cancer. *Gut, 60*(11), 1449–1472. doi:10.1136/gut.2010.228254
22. Malfertheiner, P., Chan, F., & McColl, K. (2009). Peptic ulcer disease. *Lancet, 374*, 1449–1461. doi:10.1016/S01406736(09)60938-7
23. Wang, Y. R., Richter, J. E., & Dempsey, D. T. (2010). Trends and outcomes of hospitalizations for peptic ulcer disease in the United States, 1993 to 2006. *Annals of Surgery, 251*, 51–58. doi:10.1097/SLA.0b013e3181b975b8
24. The Standards of Practice Committee of the American Society for Gastrointestinal Endoscopy. (2010). The role of endoscopy in the management of patients with peptic ulcer disease. *Gastrointestinal Endoscopy, 71*(4), 2010. doi:10.1016/j.gie.2009.11.026
25. Gregory, Y., Lauwers, G. Y., Fujita, H., Nagata, K., & Shimizu, M. (2010). Pathology of non-Helicobacter pylori gastritis: Extending the histopathologic horizons. *Journal of Gastroenterology, 45*, 131–145. doi:10.1007/s00535-009-0146-3
26. Hernandez, C. M. R., & Oo, T. H. (2015). Advances in mechanisms, diagnosis, and treatment of pernicious anemia. *Discovery Medicine, 19*(104), 159–168.
27. Yusuf, T. E., & Brugge, W. R. (2006). Endoscopic therapy of benign pyloric stenosis and gastric outlet obstruction. *Current Opinion in Gastroenterology, 22*, 570–573. doi:10.1097/01.mog.0000239874.13867.41

28. Tendler, D. A. (2002). Malignant gastric outlet obstruction: Bridging another divide. *American Journal of Gastroenterology, 97*, 4–6. doi:10.1111/j.1572-0241.2002.05391.x
29. Eberly, M. D., Eide, M. B., Thompson, J. L., & Nylund, C. M. (2015). Azithromycin in early infancy and pyloric stenosis. *Pediatrics, 135*, 483–488. doi:10.1542/peds.2014-2026
30. Kundal, V. K., Gajdhar, M., Shukla, A. K., & Kundal, R. (2013). Infantile hypertrophic pyloric stenosis in twins. *BMJ Case Reports*. doi:10.1136/bcr-2013-008779
31. Thrumurthy, S. G., Chaudry, M. A., Hochhauser, D., Ferrier, K., & Mughal, M. (2013). The diagnosis and management of gastric cancer. *BMJ, 347*, f6367. doi:10.1136/bmj.f6367
32. Chung, H. W., & Lim, J. B. (2014). Role of the tumor microenvironment in the pathogenesis of gastric carcinoma. *World Journal of Gastroenterology, 20*(7), 1667–1680. doi:10.3748/wjg.v20.i7.1667
33. Lobat, T., Vermeire, S., Van Assche, G., & Rutgeerts, P. (2014). Review article: Anti-adhesion therapies for inflammatory bowel disease. *Alimentary Pharmacology & Therapeutics, 39*, 579–594. doi:10.1111/apt.12639
34. Bernstein, C. N., Fried, M., Krabshuis, J. H., et al. (2010). World Gastroenterology Organization practice guidelines for the diagnosis and management of IBD in 2010. *Inflammatory Bowel Diseases, 16*(1), 112–124. doi:10.1002/ibd.21048
35. Feuerstein, J. D., & Cheifetz, A. S. (2014). Ulcerative colitis: Epidemiology, diagnosis, and management. *Mayo Clinic Proceedings, 89*(11), 1553–1562. doi:10.1016/j.mayocp.2014.07.002
36. Flum, D. R. (2015). Acute appendicitis: Appendectomy or the "antibiotics first" strategy. *New England Journal of Medicine, 372*, 1937–1943. doi:10.1056/NEJMcp1215006
37. Theilen, L. H., Mellnick, V. M., Longman, R. E., et al. (2015). Utility of magnetic resonance imaging for suspected appendicitis in pregnant women. *American Journal of Obstetrics & Gynecology, 212*, 345.e1–345.e6. doi:10.1016/j.ajog.2014.10.002
38. Jacobs, D. O. (2015). Acute intestinal obstruction. In D. Kasper, A. Fauci, S. Hauser, D. Longo, J. Jameson, & J. Loscalzo J. (Eds.), *Harrison's principles of internal medicine* (19th ed. New York, NY: McGraw-Hill.
39. Taylor, M. R., & Lalani, N. (2013). Adult small bowel obstruction. *Academic Emergency Medicine, 20*, 528–554. doi:10.1111/acem.12150
40. O'Handley, J. (2002). Diary from a week in practice. *American Family Physician, 65*(7), 1313–1314.
41. Maung, A. A., Johnson, D. C., Piper, G. L., et al. (2012). Evaluation and management of small-bowel obstruction: An Eastern Association for the Surgery of Trauma practice management guideline. *Journal of Trauma and Acute Care Surgery, 73*(5), S362–S369. doi:10.1097/TA.0b013e31827019de
42. Ford, A. C., Moayyedi, P., Lacy, B. E., et al. (2014). American College of Gastroenterology monograph on the management of irritable bowel syndrome and chronic idiopathic constipation. *American Journal of Gastroenterology, 109*, S2–S26. doi:10.1038/ajg.2014.187
43. Owyang, C. (2015). Irritable bowel syndrome. In D. Kasper, A. Fauci, S. Hauser, D. Longo, J. Jameson, & J. Loscalzo. (Eds.), *Harrison's principles of internal medicine* (19th ed., New York, NY: McGraw-Hill.
44. Wilkins, T., Embry, K., & George, R. (2013). Diagnosis and management of acute diverticulitis. *American Family Physician, 87*(9), 612–620.
45. Jacobs, D. (2014). Hemorrhoids. *New England Journal of Medicine, 371*, 944–951. doi:10.1056/NEJMcp1204188
46. Ahmed, R., & Gearhart, S. L. (2015). Diverticular disease and common anorectal disorders. In D. Kasper A. Fauci, S. Hauser, D. Longo, J. Jameson, & J. Loscalzo (Eds.), *Harrison's principles of internal medicine* (19th ed.). New York, NY: McGraw-Hill.
47. Doig, A. K., & Huether, S. E. (2014). Alterations of digestive function. In K. L. McCance & S. E. Huether (Eds.), *Pathophysiology: The biological basis for disease in adults and children* (7th ed., pp. 1423–1485). St. Louis, MO: Elsevier Mosby.
48. American Cancer Society. (2017). *Colorectal cancer facts & figures*. Retrieved from https://www.cancer.org/research/cancer-facts-statistics/colorectal-cancer-facts-figures.html
49. Williamson, B., & Strum, W. B. (2016). Colorectal adenomas. *New England Journal of Medicine, 374*, 1065–1075. doi:10.1056/NEJMra1513581

Chapter 43

Disorders of the Exocrine Pancreatic and Hepatobiliary Systems

Martha Olson

Chapter Outline and Learning Outcomes

43.1 Chapter Overview and Case Studies

Describe the normal function, epidemiology of alterations, and concepts related to the exocrine pancreatic and hepatobiliary systems.

43.2 Disorders of the Liver

Differentiate the causes, classification, underlying pathogenesis, and clinical manifestations of disorders of the liver and approaches to diagnosis and treatment of these conditions across the lifespan.

43.3 Disorders of the Gallbladder

Differentiate the causes, classification, underlying pathogenesis, and clinical manifestations of disorders of the gallbladder and approaches to diagnosis and treatment of these conditions across the lifespan.

43.4 Disorders of the Pancreas

Differentiate the causes, classification, underlying pathogenesis, and clinical manifestations of disorders of the pancreas and approaches to diagnosis and treatment of these conditions across the lifespan.

KEY TERMS

Acute pancreatitis, 1088
Ascites, 1073
Asterixis, 1082
Biliary colic, 1085
Caput medusa, 1082
Cholangitis, 1085
Cholecystitis, 1087
Choledocholithiasis, 1085
Cholelithiasis, 1083
Chronic pancreatitis, 1090
Cirrhosis, 1078
Cullen sign, 1089
Esophageal varices, 1082
Grey-Turner sign, 1089
Hepatomegaly, 1072
Icteric sclera, 1077
Jaundice, 1073
Pancreatic cysts, 1090
Paresthesia, 1089
Spider angioma, 1082
Steatorrhea, 1085
Steatosis, 1078

ABBREVIATIONS

AFP—alpha-fetoprotein
ALP—alkaline phosphatase
ALT—alanine aminotransferase
AST—aspartate aminotransferase
GGT—gamma-glutamyl transferase
LUQ—left upper quadrant
PERRLA—pupils equal, round, react to light accommodation
RFA—Radiofrequency ablation
RUQ—right upper quadrant
SIRS—systematic inflammatory response syndrome

43.1 Chapter Overview and Case Studies

The accessory organs of the gastrointestinal tract are the liver, gallbladder, and pancreas (**Figure 43.1** ■). The liver produces bile, which is stored in the gallbladder. The liver is also responsible for numerous other functions in the body, including synthesis of plasma proteins, metabolism and elimination of drugs and toxins, and storage of vitamins, glucose, and blood. The exocrine pancreas aids in the digestion of carbohydrates, fats, and proteins with the production of enzymes as well as bicarbonate, which is needed to neutralize chyme in the duodenum. Each of these three accessory organs contributes a distinct aspect of the digestive process; all work together to get their secretions to the duodenum to assist in digestion.

Concepts Related to the Exocrine Pancreatic and Hepatobiliary Systems

The liver is a metabolically complex and vascular organ that has a direct impact on all other organs and tissues in the body. As a result, the liver has the ability to interrelate many concepts, such as immunity, infection, metabolism, hemostasis, elimination, comfort, nutrition, energy balance, environment, and inflammation and oxidative stress. The pancreas and gallbladder play an important role in the digestive process and in nutrition, comfort, and metabolism. These concepts will be discussed as they relate to the pathogenesis of the exocrine pancreatic and hepatobiliary systems. See **Figure 43.2** ■ for selected concepts related to disorders of the hepatobiliary system, and see Figure 44.1 in Chapter 44 for concepts related to liver failure.

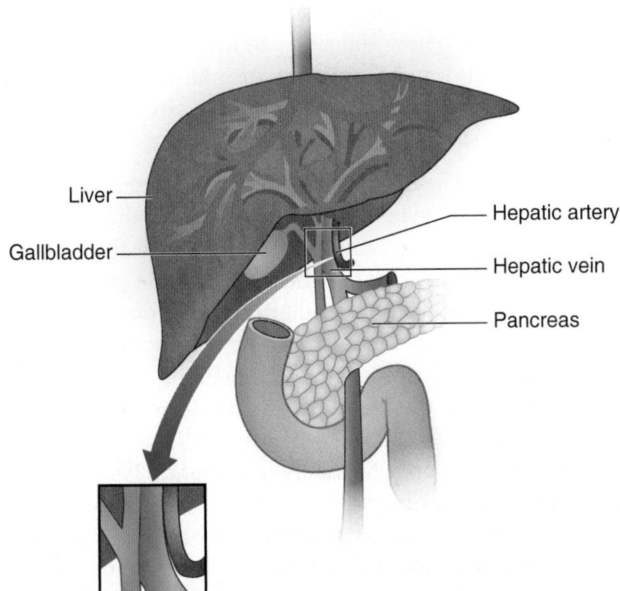

Figure 43.1 ■ Accessory organs of digestion.

Case Studies

The following cases will be addressed throughout the chapter to assist in applying chapter content to clinical situations that involve individuals with disorders of the exocrine pancreatic and hepatobiliary systems.

Jack Birkland: Introduction

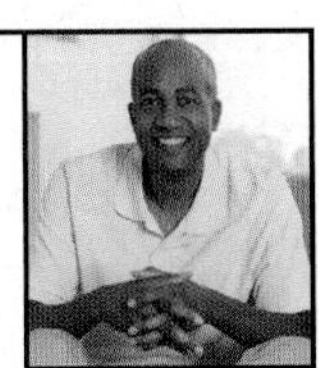

Jack Birkland is a 60-year-old male. He comes to the walk-in-clinic accompanied by his wife, Judy. His chief complaint is pain to his right upper quadrant of the abdomen that has been getting progressively worse for 2 weeks. He has experienced some weight loss and has not been eating much at meals, often feeling bloated and nauseated. The primary healthcare provider completes the assessment, noting mild jaundice, abdominal tenderness, and distention. Mr. Birkland weighs 126 kilograms, down from 132 kilograms at his last visit. A liver scan is ordered. The healthcare provider also orders the following laboratory tests: liver function tests, complete blood count, international normalization ratio, alkaline phosphatase, and alpha fetoprotein. A urine specimen is collected for analysis.

1. Mr. Birkland complains of right upper quadrant abdominal pain. What organs and structures are found in that area of the body that may contribute to his symptoms?
2. Based on Mr. Birkland's symptoms and clinical findings at his first clinic visit, alpha-fetoprotein testing is ordered. An elevation in this test would suggest what liver pathology?
3. For patients with unexplained weight loss, evaluation should include diagnostic testing to rule out what condition?
4. Mr. Birkland's initial presentation included abdominal distention. What is a possible cause of this abdominal distention?

Helen Martin: Introduction

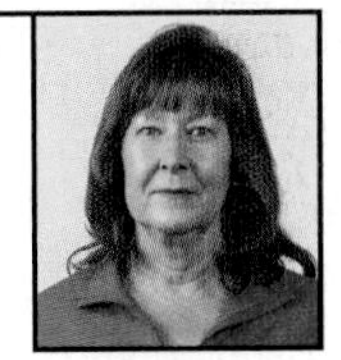

Helen Martin is a middle-aged female who is experiencing perimenopause. She is obese and diets frequently to lose weight. Recently, she has been experiencing indigestion after eating. She and her husband Gil live in a blended household that includes several family members, a situation that contributes to her stress and anxiety.

Mrs. Martin experiences right upper quadrant pain. She is seen by her primary healthcare provider for complaints of digestive disturbances and abdominal pain after meals, especially fatty meals. Fat intolerance is reported with abdominal pain and then "greasy-looking stools." Mrs. Martin reports that her stool this morning appeared light colored. A urine specimen of dark amber urine is collected.

Assessment findings are a 48-year-old female who is alert and oriented. Vital signs are pulse 102, respirations 22, temperature 99.6°F (37.5°C), blood pressure 126/66. Saturation level is 96% on room air. Skin is warm and dry but noted to be jaundiced. Apical pulse is strong and regular. Abdomen is distended and tender. An abdominal ultrasound is ordered.

1. On physical examination, Mrs. Martin appears to be jaundiced. This yellowing of the skin and sclera of the eyes is caused by what substance and suggests initial thoughts of pathology in which organ(s)?
2. What elements of the history suggest possible gallbladder disease in this patient?
3. Why would Mrs. Martin have greasy stools?
4. Mrs. Martin reports light-colored stools. What the pathophysiologic process would cause this symptom?

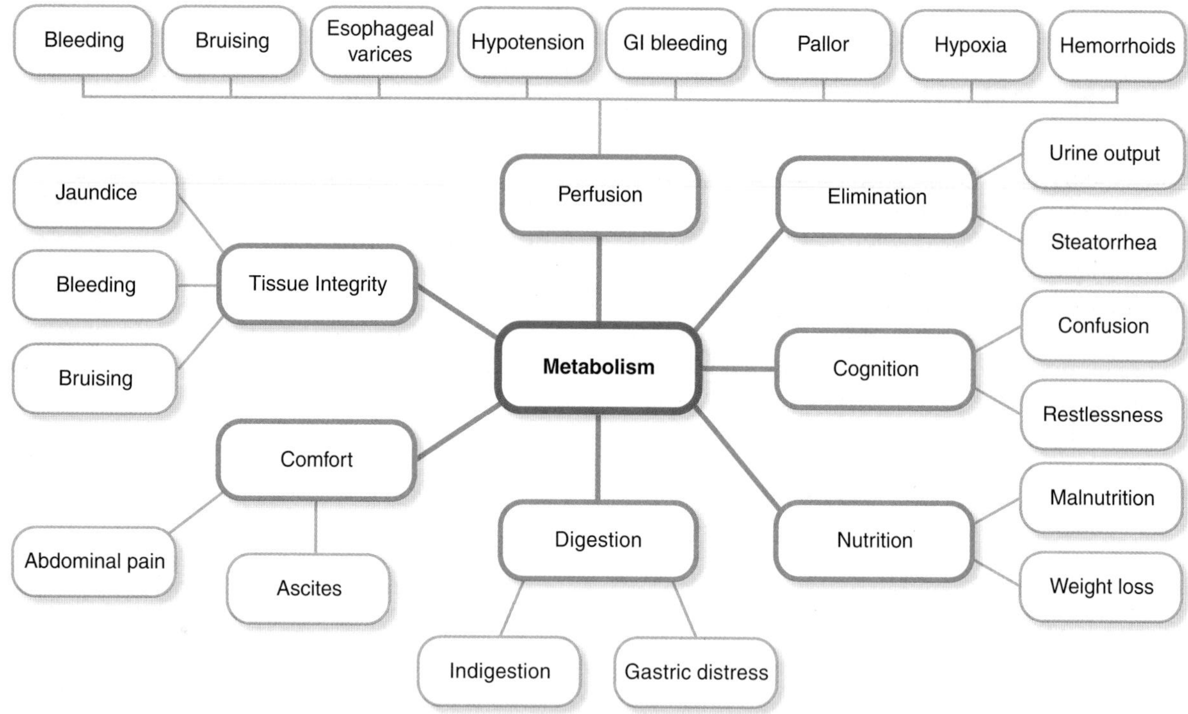

Figure 43.2 ■ Concepts related to hepatorenal syndrome.

Jimmy Gerde: Introduction

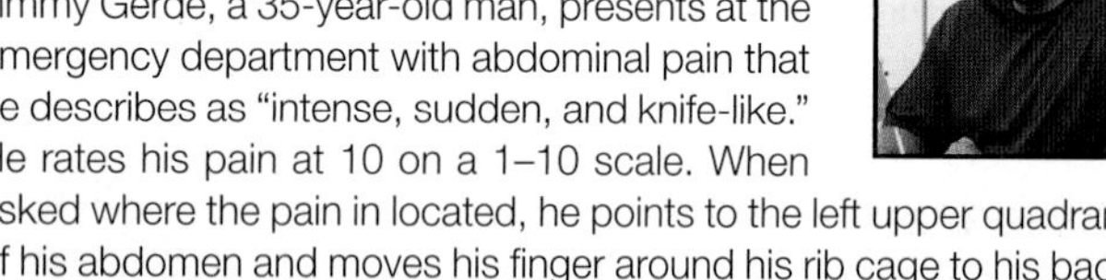

Jimmy Gerde, a 35-year-old man, presents at the emergency department with abdominal pain that he describes as "intense, sudden, and knife-like." He rates his pain at 10 on a 1–10 scale. When asked where the pain in located, he points to the left upper quadrant of his abdomen and moves his finger around his rib cage to his back and shoulder. He is diaphoretic and anxious appearing as a result of the pain. His prior medical history is significant for alcohol abuse.

1. Sudden, intense left upper abdominal pain that radiates to the back and sometimes the shoulder suggests inflammation of what organ?
2. In observing Mr. Gerde, you notice he appears anxious and is sweating. His pain assessment is 10 on a 1–10 scale. What alterations in vital signs might be expected?
3. Mr. Gerde has severe pain as part of his clinical presentation. What pathologic processes are causing his pain?

Check Your Progress: Section 43.1

1. What are the accessory organs of digestion?
2. What substance is produced by the liver and stored in the gallbladder?
3. The pancreas produces what substance that neutralizes chyme?

43.2 Disorders of the Liver

The liver is a solid organ located in the upper abdomen (see Figure 43.1). The largest organ of the abdomen, the liver has the unique ability to regenerate. It has four lobes: the right and left lobe, divided by the falciform ligament, and the caudate lobe and quadrate lobe, which are smaller lobes of the larger right lobe. This large vascular organ sits under the diaphragm, protected by the rib cage. Located in the right upper quadrant (RUQ) of the abdomen, the lower edge of the liver is normally located at the costal margin.[1] **Hepatomegaly** (an abnormally enlarged liver) is often a sign of liver disease, with palpation below the costal margin and percussion below the costal margin or above the fifth or sixth intercostal space.[1]

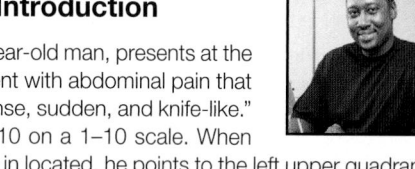

The infant's liver is a relatively large organ in the abdomen, occupying a larger portion of the abdomen than it does in adults. As a result, the liver extends farther below the rib cage than it does in adults. Because the abdominal muscles of infants are weak, the abdomen normally tends to protrude. The weak abdominal muscles make palpation of the liver easier.[2] ■

The liver lobule is the structural unit for the liver, containing the hepatocytes or specialized cells of the liver. The hepatocytes produce enzymes that catalyze the various chemical reactions, making the liver capable of a variety of specific functions. The capillaries of the liver lobule are called sinusoids and are located between the hepatocytes. The role of the sinusoids is to receive blood from both the hepatic artery and the portal vein and to remove foreign materials from the blood.

The blood supply to the liver is unique because 75% of the blood comes from a vein and the remaining 25% is supplied from the hepatic artery, which brings oxygen-rich blood from the abdominal aorta to the liver via the visceral branch to the celiac trunk (see Figure 43.1).[3] The hepatic portal vein is responsible for bringing nutrient-rich blood from the digestive system to the liver. The superior mesenteric vein brings blood to the liver from the small intestine and the ascending and transverse sections of the large intestine as well as the stomach. Blood flow from the splenic vein flows from the spleen and pancreas. The inferior mesenteric vein collects blood from the descending region of the large intestine and the rectum to contribute to the hepatic portal system. The inferior mesenteric vein and the splenic vein connect with the larger superior mesenteric vein to form the hepatic portal vein.[4] This series of blood vessels brings a significant amount of blood to the liver.

In the liver, the central veins join to become the hepatic veins, moving blood out of the liver to the inferior vena cava and back to the heart. The liver requires a higher volume of blood supply to accomplish numerous functions in the body, including storage, excretion, metabolism, digestion, glucose regulation, detoxification, and hematology. Vascular functions include storage of blood for use as needed by the body during hemorrhage or hypovolemia. Fat-soluble vitamins (A, D, E, and K), vitamin B12, the minerals iron and copper, and glucose and fat are stored in the liver and used to maintain homeostasis. Glycogen storage in the liver helps the body regulate the blood sugar with the conversion of glycogen to glucose.

The liver is also responsible for filtration of the blood. The rich blood supply via the portal vein brings drugs, bacteria, pathogens, toxins, and other foreign substances from the gastrointestinal system to the liver, where filtration takes place.[5] The phagocytic cells, called Kupffer cells, line the sinusoids to remove the bacteria and foreign material from the blood.

Metabolism of carbohydrate, protein, and fat occurs in the liver, along with the production of proteins involved in coagulation. The liver is responsible for the synthesis of clotting factors I (prothrombin), II (fibrinogen), VII, IX, and X from amino acids. Indeed, all plasma proteins except the gamma globulins are made in the liver. Albumin and globulin are other major proteins that the liver is responsible for producing. Albumin maintains the osmotic pressure; globulins are used for cellular enzymatic reactions.[5,6]

Bile, a yellow-green thick fluid, is made up of water, bile acids, bile salt, mucus, cholesterol, phospholipids, electrolytes, and the pigments bilirubin and biliverdin. Bile production is completed in small bile ducts called bile canaliculi. Daily bile production is 600–1000 mL. Bilirubin is a brownish-yellow substance that is produced when the liver breaks down red blood cells. Biliverdin is the pigment that gives bile its greenish color.

Bile leaves the liver in the common hepatic duct and goes to the cystic duct of the gallbladder. Bile is stored and concentrated in the gallbladder. It is released via the common bile duct to the duodenum. Food entering the small intestine stimulates the hormone secretin in the duodenum to produce bile. Bile breaks fat into small globules, thus making more surface area available for chemical digestion to finish the digestive process.

Bilirubin is secreted and conjugated in the liver. Excretion of bilirubin and cholesterol is completed with bile transport to the feces, where the substances are eliminated from the body. Detoxification of substances in the liver can cause damage to the hepatocytes. The liver breaks down and detoxifies many substances, including medications, steroid hormones, and alcohol. The damage is often first noted by way of abnormal laboratory values. Liver function tests are often ordered as a panel to help get an overall laboratory analysis of the liver function. This panel includes albumin, bilirubin, aspartate aminotransferase (AST), alanine aminotransferase (ALT), gamma-glutamyl transferase (GGT), and prothrombin (**Table 43.1** ■).

Albumin, which is produced in the liver, is essential for maintenance of the oncotic pressure, thus helping to maintain the vascular system. With liver damage, albumin production stops, resulting in the body fluid leaking out of the vessels into the interstitial spaces and peritoneal cavity, causing edema and **ascites** (an abnormal collection of fluid in the peritoneal cavity) (**Figure 43.3** ■).

Ammonia is a by-product of protein metabolism that is converted to urea in the liver. The kidneys are responsible for the elimination of urea from the body. With liver dysfunction, the liver is not able to convert ammonia to urea; as a result, toxic levels of ammonia accumulate in the blood, causing systemic damage.[7]

The bilirubin level is also an indicator of liver and pancreatic dysfunction. **Jaundice** (a yellowish discoloration of the whites of the eyes, skin, or mucous membranes caused by the bile salts in the tissues) is one clinical symptom of an elevated bilirubin level (**Figure 43.4** ■). Bilirubin is the waste product of red blood cell destruction. This form of bilirubin is lipid soluble and must be transformed to a water-soluble product to be excreted. Albumin carries unconjugated bilirubin to the liver, where it detaches from the albumin and is then conjugated to a water-soluble product. Removal of this conjugated bilirubin is accomplished with bile salts that enter the intestine from the common bile duct. From the intestines, the bilirubin is broken down to urobilinogen, which is mostly eliminated in the feces (40–280 mg/day). A small part of the urobilinogen is directed back to the blood,

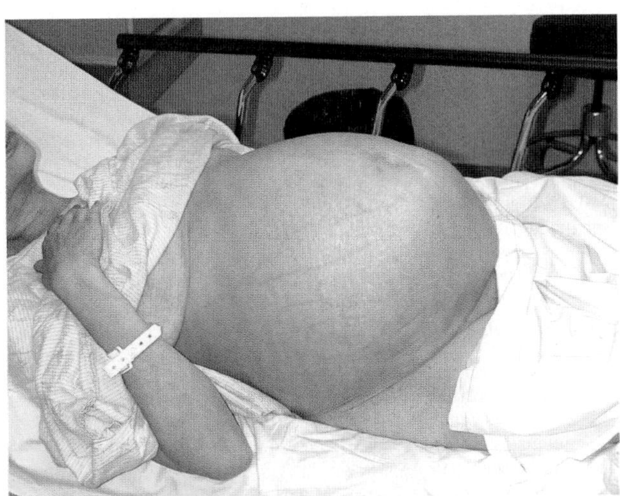

Figure 43.3 ■ In ascites, serous fluid collects in the abdominal cavity, causing uniform distention.

Table 43.1 Common Diagnostic and Laboratory Tests of Hepatic and Exocrine Function

Test with Description and Reference Values	Expected Abnormality	Used to Diagnose
Alanine aminotransferase Alanine aminotransferase (ALT)/serum glutamic pyruvic transaminase (SGPT) is an enzyme found primarily in the liver cells. It is effective in diagnosing hepatocellular destruction. It is also found in small amounts in the heart, kidney, and skeletal muscle. ***Reference Values*** Adult: 10–35 unit/L; 4–36 unit/L at 37°C (SI units). *Male:* Levels may be slightly higher. Child: *Infant:* Could be twice as high as adult. *Child:* Similar to adult. Older adult: Slightly higher than adult.	Increased or decreased	Increased values indicate damage to the liver. Hepatitis and infection are the most common reasons. Certain medications can also increase values. Decreased values can occur from long-term infectious hepatitis or malnutrition.
Albumin Albumin, a component of proteins, makes up more than half of plasma proteins. Albumin is synthesized by the liver. It increases osmotic pressure (oncotic pressure), which is necessary for maintaining the vascular fluid. A decrease in serum albumin will cause fluid to shift from within the vessels to the tissues, resulting in edema. ***Reference Values*** Adult: 3.5–5.0 g/dL; 52–68% of total protein. Child: *Newborn:* 2.9–5.4 g/dL. *Infant:* 4.4–5.4 g/dL. *Child:* 4.0–5.8 g/dL.	Increased or decreased	Increased values indicate dehydration. Decreased values can reflect liver damage or issues with nutritional absorption and malnutrition.
Alkaline phosphatase Alkaline phosphatase (ALP) is an enzyme produced mainly in the liver and bone; it is also derived from the intestine, kidney, and placenta. The ALP test is useful for determining liver and bone diseases. The ALP level may be only slightly elevated in cases of mild liver cell damage, but it could be markedly elevated in acute liver disease. Once the acute phase is over, the serum level will decrease promptly, whereas the serum bilirubin will remain increased. ***Reference Values*** Adult: 42–136 unit/L; ALP[1]: 20–130 unit/L; ALP[2]: 20–120 unit/L. Child: *Infant and Child (aged 0–12 years):* 40–115 unit/L. *Older Child (13–18 years):* 50–230 unit/L. Older adults: Slightly higher than adult.	Increased or decreased	Increased values indicate biliary obstruction or tissue damage. Certain medications can also increase values. Decreased values indicate malnutrition and forms of anemia. Oral contraceptives can also decrease values.
Ammonia Ammonia, a by-product of protein metabolism, is formed from bacterial action in the intestine and from metabolizing tissues. Most of the ammonia is absorbed into the portal circulation and is converted in the liver to urea. With severe liver decompensation or when blood flow to the liver is altered, the plasma ammonia level remains elevated. ***Reference Values*** Adult: 15–45 mcg/dL, 11–35 μmol/L (SI units). Child: *Newborn:* 64–107 mcg/dL. *Child:* 29–70 mcg/dL; 29–70 μmol/L(SI units).	Increased	Increased values indicate liver damage. Also associated with kidney failure and select genetic syndromes.
Aspartate aminotransferase Aspartate aminotransferase/serum glutamic oxaloacetic transaminase (AST/SGOT) is an enzyme found mainly in the heart muscle and liver, with moderate amounts in skeletal muscle, the kidneys, and the pancreas. Its concentration is low in the blood except when there is cellular injury, and then large amounts are released into circulation. ***Reference Values*** Adult: *Average range:* 8–35 unit/L 5–40 unit/mL (Frankel), 4–36 international unit/L, 15–50 unit/mL at 30°C (Karmen), 8–33 unit/L at 37°C (SI units). Female values may be slightly lower than those of males. Exercise tends to increase values. (Values can vary among institutions.) Child: *Newborn:* Four times the normal level. *Child:* Similar to adults. Older adults*:* Slightly higher than adults.	Increased	Increased values indicate tissue inflammation. Such inflammation can be associated with cardiac or skeletal issues. More helpful when viewed in contrast to other laboratory values to aid in distinguishing possible source of inflammation.

Test with Description and Reference Values	Expected Abnormality	Used to Diagnose
Lactic dehydrogenase Lactic dehydrogenase (LDH) is an intracellular enzyme that is present in nearly all metabolizing cells, the highest concentrations being in the heart, skeletal muscle, liver, kidney, brain, and red blood cells. LDH has two distinct subunits: M (muscle) and H (heart). These subunits are combined in different formations to make five isoenzymes. ***Reference Values*** Adult: *Total LDH:* 100–190 IU/L, 70–250 unit/L. Values can differ according to the method used. Isoenzymes: LDH_1, 14–26%; LDH_2, 27–37%; LDH_3, 13–26%; LDH_4, 8–16%; LDH_5, 6–16%. Differences of 2–4% are considered normal. Child: *Newborn:* 300–1500 IU/L. *Child:* 50–150 IU/L; 110–295 IU/L.	Increased	Increased values of isoenzymes 4 and 5 indicate liver damage.
Gamma-glutamyl transpeptidase The enzyme gamma-glutamyl transferase (GGT) is found primarily in the liver and kidney, with smaller amounts in the spleen, prostate gland, and heart muscle. GGTP is sensitive for detecting a wide variety of hepatic (liver) parenchymal diseases. The serum level will rise early and will remain elevated as long as cellular damage persists. ***Reference Values*** 0–45 unit/L (overall average) Adult: *Male:* 4–23 IU/L, 9–69 unit/L at 37°C (SI units). *Female:* 3–13 IU/L, 4–33 unit/L at 37°C (SI units). Values differ among institutions and methods used. Child: *Newborn:* 5 times higher than adult. *Premature:* 10 times higher than adult. *Child:* Similar to adult. Older adult: Slightly higher than adult.	Increased	Increased values aid in determining the presence of biliary duct disorders or obstruction. Often evaluated in chronic alcohol abuse.
Red Blood Cell Measures		
Bilirubin Bilirubin is formed from the breakdown of hemoglobin by the reticuloendothelial system and is carried in the plasma to the liver, where it is conjugated (directly) to form bilirubin diglucuronide and is excreted in the bile. There are two forms of bilirubin in the body: the conjugated, or direct-reacting (soluble), and the unconjugated, or indirect-reacting (protein bound). If the total bilirubin level is within normal range, direct and indirect bilirubin levels do not need to be analyzed. If one value of bilirubin is reported, it represents the total bilirubin. ***Reference Values*** Adult: *Total:* 0.1–1.2 mg/dL, 1.7–20.5 μmol/L (SI units). *Direct (conjugated):* 0.1–0.3 mg/dL, 1.7–5.1 μmol/L (SI units). Child: *Newborn: Total:* 1–12 mg/dL, 17.1–205 μmol/L (SI units). *Child:* 0.2–0.8 mg/dL. Panic Level: 15 mg/dL.	Low	Anemia
Prothrombin Prothrombin (factor II of the coagulation factors) is synthesized by the liver and is an inactive precursor in the clotting process. Prothrombin is converted to thrombin by the action of thromboplastin, which is needed to form a blood clot. The prothrombin time (PT) measures the clotting ability of factors I (fibrinogen), II (prothrombin), V, VII, and X. Alterations of factors V and VII will prolong the PT for about 2 seconds, or 10% of normal. In liver disease, the PT is usually prolonged because the liver cells cannot synthesize prothrombin. ***Reference Values*** Adult: 10–13 seconds (depending on the method and reagents used) or 70–100%. *For Anticoagulant Therapy:* 1.5–2.0 times the control in seconds or 20–30%. International normalization ratio: 2.0–3.0. Child: Same as adult.	Increased	Indicates that the liver is unable to make clotting factors. Usually found in cases of liver damage or cirrhosis.

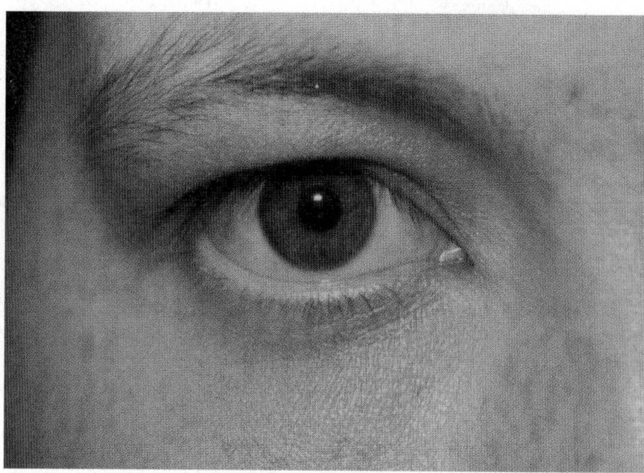

Figure 43.4 ■ Jaundice in a light-skinned patient.

where it is either eliminated in the urine (0.4–1 mg/day) or moved back to the liver. The dark color of the feces is from the bilirubin; when bilirubin is absent, the stools are often clay colored.[7]

The digestive enzymes amylase and lipase help with diagnosis of disorders to the accessory organs of digestion. Amylase is a digestive enzyme that breaks down starch to disaccharides. Lipase, from the pancreas, assists with fat digestion to produce fatty acids and glycerol from triglycerides.

Hemolysis of the red blood cells in a newborn is common after birth. Normally, the red blood cells of the newborn have a shorter lifespan (60–90 days compared to 120 days in the adult). An increased total bilirubin in the newborn can be attributed to either hemolysis that is occurring faster than normal or the liver of the newborn being slower to conjugate the bilirubin. The liver of the newborn takes longer to remove the bilirubin from the blood because it takes a few days to produce glucuronyl transferase, an enzyme needed to convert unconjugated bilirubin to conjugated bilirubin. This can result in newborn physiologic jaundice. Another factor contributing to newborn physiologic jaundice is that intestinal flora in newborns is slower to convert bilirubin to urobilinogen, thus putting bilirubin back into the circulation. Because of these physical changes, about 60% of full-term newborns experience physiologic jaundice starting 24 hours after birth. The rate of jaundice is even higher in preterm infants.[7] ■

Liver disorders often manifest with common symptomatology. Abdominal pain and indigestion are early, vague symptoms that are easily ignored or dismissed by the patient. Abdominal pain is often dull and diffuse across the abdomen. When more serious symptoms appear, such as jaundice or ascites, the liver disorder is often at an advanced stage, often making the prognosis and outcome less favorable. This section focuses on alterations in the liver from cancer and cirrhosis.

Cancer of the Liver

Liver cancer, also called hepatoma or hepatocellular carcinoma, has a poor survival rate. As well as being the fifth most commonly diagnosed cancer, liver cancer is the second most common cause of death worldwide in men.[8] The incidence of liver cancer is increasing, and the liver is one of the top ten sites for new cancer cases and deaths. Liver cancer is responsible for 35,660 new cases each year. This type of cancer is more prevalent in males with an average age of 63 years.[9] Asians and Pacific Islanders have rates three times higher than that of whites.[8] Hepatocellular carcinoma is the most commonly found liver cancer; 80% of the liver cancer cases are of this type. Rates of intrahepatic cholangiocarcinoma, the second most common type of liver cancer, are also increasing.[10]

Individuals with cirrhosis, hemochromatosis, and carriers of hepatitis B or hepatitis C virus have a higher risk of hepatocellular carcinoma. Other risk factors related to lifestyle are excess alcohol consumption, coffee consumption, exposure to aflatoxins, obesity, and oral contraceptive use.[7,10–13]

Inflammation and hepatocyte regeneration, seen in chronic liver disease, precede pathophysiologic changes, important factors in the development of liver cancer. Hepatitis is one such chronic liver disorder, known to cause liver cancer in up to 85% of patients with hepatocellular carcinoma.[13] The hepatitis B virus causes liver cancer by damaging the cells and their DNA. Worldwide, hepatitis B accounts for 23% of liver cancer. In the United States, hepatitis C is responsible for the increased rates and incidence of liver cancer and mortality in recent years.[14]

Besides hepatitis, causes of liver cancer are linked to the damaging effects of drinking alcohol, exposure to aflatoxins produced by molds, or consuming aflatoxin-contaminated foods.[15]

The majority of liver cancer cases are in developing countries. Asia and Africa have the highest incidence; Europe, Latin America, and the Caribbean have the lowest rates.[15] Rates of obesity, hepatitis C, and alcoholism are increasing in Western countries, thus contributing to the higher rates of liver cancer in this part of the world.[10]

Older adults are vulnerable to liver disease, especially as they age. Important considerations for cellular senescence of the older adult are how cumulative life events have contributed to inflammation and other potential sources of tissue damage, leading to an increased risk of metastatic liver cancer. ■

Etiology and Pathogenesis

Primary tumors of the liver are not as common as metastatic tumors. The liver is vascular; therefore, it is affected by the spread of diseases and disorders, including cancer, from other organs and tissues. A liver biopsy is often needed to help distinguish and confirm primary from metastatic liver cancer.[16]

Inflammation, a result of the initiation of the immune response from the damage caused by the toxins in the liver, begins the process of cellular transformation. Cirrhosis remains one of the major risk factors for hepatocellular carcinoma because the constant tissue necrosis and damage to the hepatocytes leave the cells damaged and at risk for mutations.[10] Aflatoxins are chemicals that are produced from *Aspergillus flavus* and *Aspergillus parasiticus*, mold fungi found on corn (maize), most often during hot, dry conditions when the corn is in the final stages of filling before production.[17] Gradual accumulation of mutations in the host and the genetic changes to the DNA contribute to the malignant cell transformation.[10]

Clinical Manifestations

Early symptoms of hepatocellular cancer are often vague. Weakness, weight loss, and bloating are signs that people often ignore until later, when more serious symptoms appear that prompt medical attention. Abdominal discomfort is often described as aching or a feeling of fullness. This type of pain stems from tissue stretching with the beginning of abdominal ascites and liver enlargement. If present, jaundice is mild.[18]

Jaundice is best assessed in natural daylight. The sclera of the eye is often the first place the yellow discoloration is noted in patients with fair skin; this is called **icteric sclera** (see Figure 43.4). Dark-skinned patients will show the change initially in the inner canthus of the eye or the mucous membranes of the hard palate. Assessment of jaundice also includes the palms of the hands and the plantar surfaces of the feet. The discoloration of the skin and sclera of the eye result from the increased unconjugated bilirubin. When the bilirubin level is 2–4 milligrams in older children and adults, the symptoms of jaundice are noted.[7]

Liver dysfunction, as noted in liver cancer, is responsible for many other conditions, such as disturbances in clotting factors and hormones. Hypoprothrombinemia might be noted as a result of the lack of bile salts that contribute to emulsification of fat-soluble vitamins, such as vitamin K, and their absorption in the intestine. Without sufficient vitamin K in the bloodstream, the liver cannot make enough prothrombin, which is needed for blood clotting.[7] As a result, bleeding and easy bruising might be noted on assessment of patients with liver dysfunction, including liver cancer.

Jack Birkland: Application

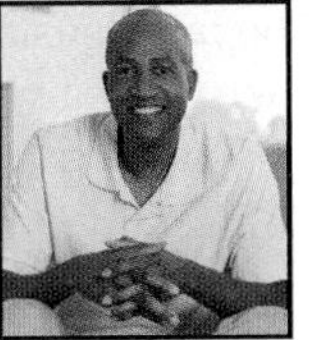

Mr. Birkland tells the primary healthcare provider that he works for a grain elevator company that purchases and stores corn and soybeans. He has worked at this job for over 35 years, and it often involves loading moldy grain that has been stored before shipment. The laboratory test results show the presence of abnormally high levels of alpha-fetoprotein. The midstream urine specimen was dark brown.

The liver scan is the initial diagnostic test, and results indicate an abnormally large liver mass with uneven contour in the abdomen. The radiologist report diagnoses a primary hepatocellular carcinoma after a liver biopsy is completed.

Mr. Birkland is admitted to the medical–surgical unit for consultation with a specialist and further testing. The admitting nurse completes the admission with physical assessment and past medical history. Abnormal findings on assessment include jaundice. Pupils are equal and round, and they react to light accommodation (PERRLA) with icteric sclera. Mr. Birkland also complained of "itchy skin."

5. What occupational hazard may be responsible for Mr. Birkland's developing liver cancer?
6. The liver scan shows a single large mass with irregular borders, and a biopsy is performed to make the definitive diagnosis. At the same time, the elevated alpha-fetoprotein result is obtained. What diagnosis does this suggest?
7. Why is it important to obtain an occupational history from patients even if they are healthy?

Linking Pathophysiology to Diagnosis and Treatment

The blood flow to the liver helps to support the many functions that occur in this organ. The blood supply comes from both the portal circulation and a direct extension off the aorta. Because of this, the liver is exposed to many pathogens, drugs, toxins, and malignant cells that cause changes to the microenvironment as well as damage in the form of hypoxia, inflammation, or oxidative stress, which set the stage for carcinogenesis and tumor initiation.[5,10] Carcinogenesis is the transformation of normal cells to abnormal cells that have an unlimited ability to proliferate, thus forming malignant tumors that develop resistance to many therapies. Liver cancer is believed to be caused by both infiltration of immune cells and oxidative stress. The release of cytokines and chemokines from Kupffer cells contributes to the inflammatory process in the liver as well as the deregulation of liver cell proliferation.[10] Insulin plays a role in liver cancer for the obese patient by several methods. Insulin resistance causes increased levels of pro-inflammatory cytokine (tumor necrosis factor and interleukin 6) that contribute to hepatic steatosis and inflammation. Also, high levels of insulin upregulate insulin-like growth factor 1, a protein that stimulates mechanisms of cellular proliferation and inhibits other mechanisms of programmed cellular death. An association between elevated body mass index (BMI) and primary liver cancer has been established. When the patient has a BMI of 25–30, the risk of liver cancer increases 17% in comparison to an individual of normal weight; in a patient with a BMI greater than 30, the increased risk of primary liver cancer is 90% when compared to an individual of normal weight.[19]

Tumor development is thought to result from the environmental factors that cause the initiation of signaling pathways. One gene, glutathione *S*-transferase (*GST*), is responsible for detoxification and plays an important role in cellular protection. Malfunction in this isoenzyme renders the body less able to detoxify toxins and carcinogens that may contribute to carcinogenesis.[13]

Liver cancer is suspected when the following laboratory values are elevated: alkaline phosphatase (ALP), GGT, acid phosphatase, AST, ALT, and lactic dehydrogenase (LDH). Alpha-fetoprotein (AFP) can help to diagnose primary hepatoma of the liver as well as testicular cancer.[7] This test lacks specificity; only half of patients with hepatocellular carcinoma have elevated AFP levels. An accurate diagnosis of liver cancer requires other abnormal test results.

AFP is normally found in the blood of a newborn but decreases to trace amounts after birth and is just slightly detected at age 2 years. ■

When liver metastasis is suspected, a liver and spleen scan can be completed in 10–15 minutes following the IV injection of the radionuclide. The confirmation of the diagnosis is made with a liver biopsy performed with either computed tomography (CT) or ultrasound guidance if the patient does not have ascites or bleeding problems.[7] The risk of developing hepatocellular carcinoma can be decreased through sustained abstinence from alcohol, avoidance of exposure to carcinogens such as aflatoxin in the environment, and prophylaxis for hepatitis.[11]

Treatment depends on the stage and size of the tumor. Surgery offers a chance for a cure. For tumors that are 10 centimeters in diameter or larger, hepatic resection is the preferred method of treatment. There is a high incidence of morbidity and recurrence following this surgical procedure.[20] Transplantation is the other surgical option.

Local therapy can result in a cure if lesions are smaller and complete ablation is achieved. Local therapies include radiofrequency ablation (RFA) and cryotherapy. Regional therapy includes the transcatheter arterial chemoembolization, percutaneous ablation, or external beam radiation therapy. Chemoembolization is a procedure that uses chemotherapy and embolization to inject anticancer drugs directly into the blood vessel that directly feeds the tumor.[20,21] RFA is now an important tool that is used to treat both nonresectable and resectable tumors of the liver.[22]

Early recurrence by daughter lesions often occurs in the same area of the liver after an ablation procedure (72%), the later new growths occurring in areas other than where the ablation was originally complete. Following ablation, contrast-enhanced ultrasound, CT, and magnetic resonance imaging (MRI) are done to detect recurring tumors.[22]

Sorafenib or doxorubicin is used as systemic therapy that uses molecular targeting. A protein kinase inhibitor, sorafenib was approved by the U.S. Food and Drug Administration in 2005 for primary kidney cancer and in 2007 for advanced primary liver cancer. In 2013, it was approved to treat thyroid cancer that is resistant to treatment with radioactive iodine.[23]

Response to the treatment involves noting the clinical markers and progression of the tumor as well as the recurrence of the tumor and progression of the underlying disease. The lesion size may actually increase after treatment. Assessment findings also help to make determinations about the response to treatment, including ascites, coagulopathy, pleural effusion, and lymphadenopathy.[24] Liver cancer continues to have a poor prognosis, owing to the vagueness of early symptoms, which delays diagnosis, and to the complex nature of the liver.

Jack Birkland: Outcome

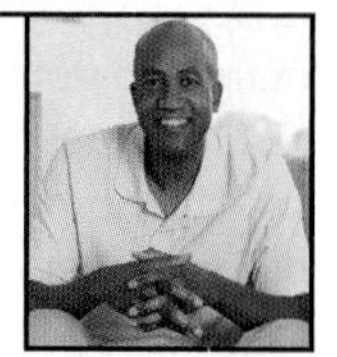

Mr. Birkland has a laparoscopic liver biopsy that confirms hepatocellular carcinoma. The surgical oncologist documents in the diagnostic report that Mr. Birkland's tumor is greater than 5 centimeters in diameter and that his cancer is likely directly related to occupational exposure to aflatoxins. Treatment options are discussed with the Birklands, and they agree with the decision to use image-guided ablation. Chemotherapy using sorefenib will be implemented after the ablation. Mr. Birkland's ablation is successful with minimal postprocedure complications. His jaundice, pruritus, and ascites improve over the next several months, and his laboratory values for bilirubin, AST, and ALT improve following treatment. Contrast-enhanced ultrasound is scheduled to assess for reoccurring tumors. Abdominal CT and MRI will also be done at regular intervals to watch for any spread of the tumors to other segments of the liver. Mr. Birkland has retired from his job and is now enjoying time with his family.

8. On physical examination, Mr. Birkland is noted to be jaundiced. Although his sclerae are icteric, his eye exam is otherwise normal. He complains of itchy skin and has dark urine. What substance is responsible for all of these abnormal findings and symptoms?
9. After ablation treatment, why is a contrast-enhanced ultrasound ordered? Should additional imaging studies be ordered for Mr. Birkland in the future?
10. What is the significance of the improvement in Mr. Birkland's liver panel blood tests?

Metabolic Disorders

Cirrhosis is a late stage of scarring of the liver and affects millions of people worldwide. The most common cause of cirrhosis is alcohol consumption; it can also be caused by hepatitis or chronic obstruction of the bile ducts. The liver is the organ responsible for alcohol metabolism. Alcoholic liver disease may cause either an acute or a chronic condition. Alcoholic hepatitis is acute damage; cirrhosis, steatosis, steatohepatitis, or fibrosis contributes to chronic liver damage.[11] Other causes of cirrhosis include chronic viral hepatitis, bile duct disease, genetic diseases such as Wilson disease, hemochromatosis, glycogen storage disease, alpha-1 antitrypsin deficiency, and autoimmune hepatitis.[25]

Rates of cirrhosis are higher in males and in countries with higher absolute alcohol consumption per capita, such as France and Spain, where more than 30 per 100,000 deaths per year are related to cirrhosis.[13] Mortality rates as high as 50% are noted for patients with severe acute alcoholic hepatitis. Survival is only 1–2 years for patients with advanced cirrhosis.[11]

Etiology and Pathogenesis

Liver disease can result from hepatocellular damage, inflammation, and obstruction, which may cause damage to the hepatocytes and surrounding tissues (**Figure 43.5** ■). Damage to the liver is a serious concern because of the many specialized functions performed by the hepatocytes. Alcohol is especially damaging to the hepatocytes and contributes to progressive deterioration of the liver cells, starting with a condition known as fatty liver. Alcohol is catalyzed by enzymes in the body. The first enzyme, alcohol dehydrogenase, converts small amounts of alcohol to a toxic substance called acetaldehyde. Aldehyde dehydrogenase, the second enzyme, converts acetaldehyde to acetate. Once alcohol has been broken down, the liver uses these enzymes to make fatty acids that accumulate in the liver as fat. The early stage of fatty liver disease is called **steatosis**. A fatty liver will heal if the person stops drinking at this stage; it will progress to fibrosis or cirrhosis if the drinking continues, damaging the hepatocytes.[7]

Consumption of larger amounts of alcohol can cause the liver to use a different method of metabolism called the microsomal ethanol-oxidizing system. In this system, different enzymes are typically used for metabolizing drugs and foreign substances. No matter the method of alcohol metabolism, the end result is triglycerides or fat deposits in the liver.

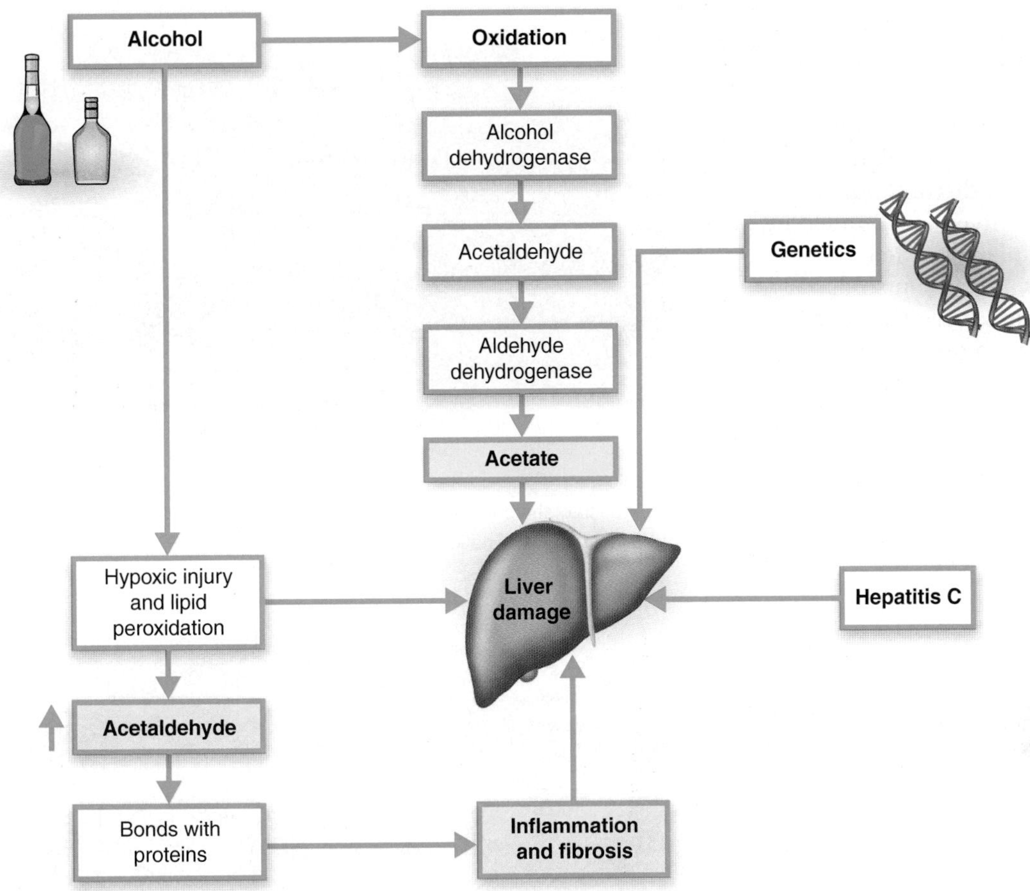

Figure 43.5 ■ The pathogenesis of alcohol-associated liver damage.

Cirrhosis is more serious than fatty liver because the hepatocytes are replaced as scar tissue, causing metabolic functions in the liver to be impaired. Inflammation from the toxic effects of alcohol cause excess collagen formation that eventually becomes scar tissue, compromising the liver's ability to metabolize, detoxify, regenerate, and store.[7]

The fibrous connective tissue of cirrhosis becomes damaged with the constriction of blood and bile flow in the liver lobules. This constriction forces blood out of the liver in vessels that have a lower pressure, thus contributing to portal hypertension. Blood is shunted to the spleen, causing splenomegaly. White blood cells (WBCs), red blood cells, and platelets are damaged in this engorged spleen, contributing to systemic effects from leukopenia, anemia, and thrombocytopenia, respectively.[25]

Dyspnea is often noted on patient assessment and is caused by ascites related to portal hypertension. The increased abdominal fluid puts pressure on the diaphragm, making it difficult for the person to breathe, even at rest. The abdomen appears swollen and protrudes as a result of the accumulation of fluid (**Figure 43.6** ■). Congestive heart failure, nephrosis, peritonitis, and neoplastic cancer are other causes of ascites.[1,11]

Many factors contribute to the severity of alcohol-induced liver disease and play a part in the outcome for the patient. Factors include the pattern of drinking, the amount of alcohol consumed, and how many years the person has been drinking alcohol. Someone who consumes alcohol on a regular basis has a higher risk of liver cirrhosis than does someone who drinks alcohol intermittently. Liver damage is a complex process that is affected by such factors as the person's immunity, humoral disorders, genetic and biochemical makeup, and overall nutrition, diet, and health status. The patient with metabolic syndrome and obesity has an increased risk of damage because the liver is aggravated by the higher caloric intake, which naturally leads to the fat deposits.[11]

The liver damage can be managed or even repaired if alcohol consumption is eliminated through abstinence. If drinking continues, inflammation of the liver cells causes fibrosis and further damage of the liver tissue and to the cell membranes and organelles, including the mitochondria. Finally, the liver shrinks and takes on a nodular appearance. The damage at this stage is not reversible.[5,11] Liver failure is often manifested in multisystem effects, making treatment decisions more complex (See Chapter 44 for more detail).

Clinical Manifestations

The vascular and regenerative abilities of the liver, as well as its deep location in the abdominal cavity, tend to delay diagnosis of liver damage. The patient with steatosis is usually asymptomatic with slightly elevated liver function tests (AST and ALT). Palpation to the abdomen reveals an enlarged liver (often found by chance during a routine examination). RUQ discomfort is reported as a nonspecific or dull feeling.[5,13]

With continued drinking and damage to the liver, the patient will begin to experience weakness, nausea, anorexia,

Normal liver

The liver contains multiple lobules made up of plates of hepatocytes, the functional cells of the liver, surrounded by small capillaries called sinusoids. These sinusoids receive a mixture of venous and arterial blood from branches of the portal vein and hepatic artery. Blood from the sinusoids drains into the central vein of the lobule. Hepatocytes produce bile, which drains outward to bile ducts.

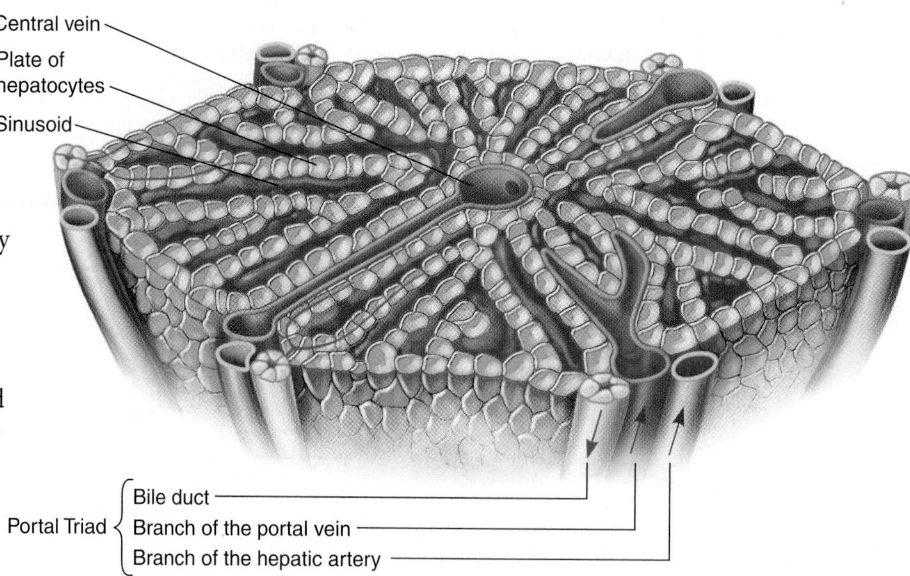

Fatty liver

Ingested alcohol is primarily metabolized in the liver. Acetaldehyde, formed when alcohol is metabolized, damages hepatocytes and impairs the oxidation of fatty acids. As a result, fat accumulates within hepatocytes and liver lobules. Other alcohol metabolism by-products, including oxygen free radicals, promote inflammation and may stimulate autoantibody production.

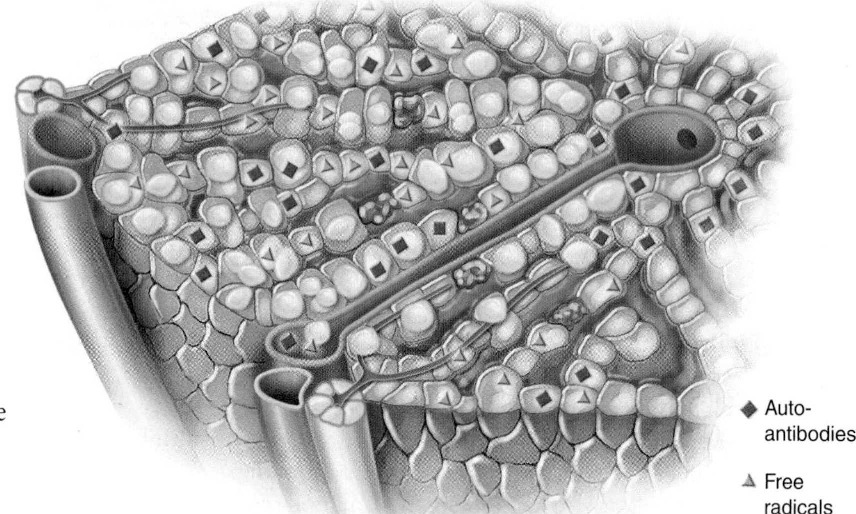

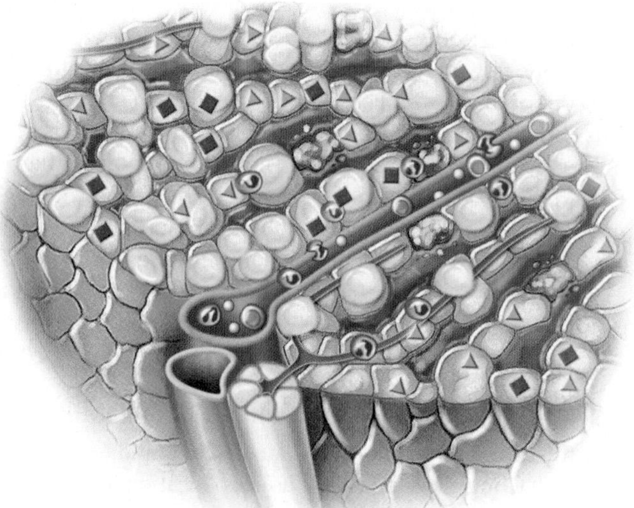

Alcoholic hepatitis

With continued alcohol intake, liver cells degenerate and spotty cellular necrosis occurs. Inflammatory cells such as polymorphonuclear leukocytes and lymphocytes infiltrate the lobule.

Figure 43.6 ■ The pathophysiology of cirrhosis and portal hypertension.

(Continued)

Alcoholic cirrhosis

Cellular necrosis and inflammation transform some liver cells into fibroblasts that produce and deposit collagen. Weblike bands of connective tissue develop around the portal triads and central vein, eventually connecting with one another. Small islands of liver cells continue to regenerate, forming nodules. Hepatocyte destruction outpaces regeneration. As a result of cell loss, fibrosis, and scarring, the liver shrinks and becomes hard and nodular.

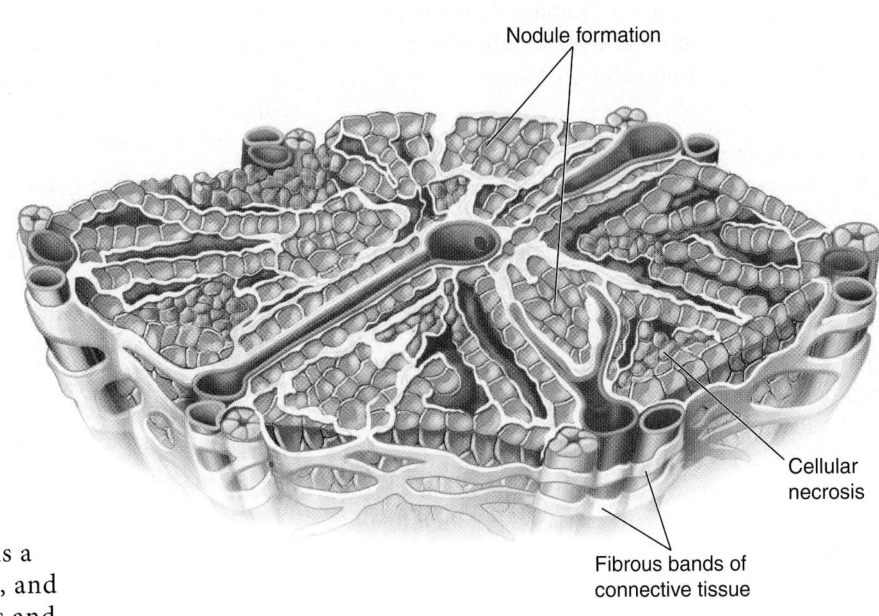

Portal hypertension

Bands of fibrotic scar tissue obstruct the sinusoids and blood flow from the portal vein to the hepatic vein. Pressure in the portal venous system, which drains the gastrointestinal tract, pancreas, and spleen, increases. This increased pressure opens collateral vessels in the esophagus, anterior abdominal wall, and rectum, allowing blood to bypass the obstructed portal vessels. Prolonged portal hypertension leads to the development of (1) varices (fragile, distended veins) in the lower esophagus, stomach, and rectum; (2) splenomegaly (an enlarged spleen); (3) ascites (accumulation of fluid in the abdomen); and (4) portal systemic encephalopathy (disrupted CNS function with altered consciousness).

Fibrous bands of connective tissue

Esophageal varices
Splenomegaly
Nodular cirrhosis
Ascites
Hemorrhoids

Figure 43.6 ■ *Continued*

weight loss, jaundice, and icterus. Damage to the hepatocytes is suspected with abnormal liver function tests. The prolonged prothrombin time can be deduced from easy bruising and bleeding.

CLINICAL POINT: Noting the skin color is often one of the first assessments to be done. Many liver disorders cause jaundice. Hemochromatosis, a genetic disorder, is unique because it causes the skin to have a bronze color from excessive absorption of iron that accumulates in the liver (**Figure 43.7** ■). ■

Portal hypertension causes the shifting of fluids within body compartments, such as ascites and generalized edema. Hypoalbuminemia contributes to ascites of the abdomen because of the loss of colloid osmotic pressure of plasma. Normally, proteins such as albumin keep the fluid in the intravascular spaces instead of allowing this plasma-rich fluid to leak into the extravascular spaces. Hyperaldosteronism also encourages excess body fluid resulting from the retention of sodium and water. This extra fluid contributes to both pitting edema and ascites.[5,11]

CLINICAL POINT: Morbidly obese patients without other disease conditions may have ascites as a result of the pressure on the abdominal blood vessels causing portal hypertension.[1] ■

Patients with hepatic encephalopathy or portal systemic encephalopathy will show neurologic changes that result from the buildup of toxins and fluid, affecting cognition. Restlessness is a vague, early symptom of systemic toxicity for the nurse to note. The patient may also initially manifest with agitation or impaired judgment, progressing to confusion, disorientation, and decreased cognition with increased cerebral edema. The pressure inside the cranium continues to increase, causing cerebral hypoxia that will manifest in changes to cognitive status.[5]

Ammonia is a waste product of protein metabolism made by bacteria in the intestines. Ammonia is converted to urea in the liver and eliminated by the kidneys. Without the conversion to urea in the liver, ammonia remains in the blood as a toxin. Medications can also accumulate to toxic levels without the liver to metabolize them.[5,11]

Gynecomastia in men with liver disease is due to the inability of the liver to degrade estrogens and the effects of phytoestrogens in alcohol that inhibit testosterone production, causing an imbalance of the hormones testosterone and estrogen. Physiologic gynecomastia normally affects half of adolescent males starting at age 13 and 65% of males age 50–80 years as a result of changes in testosterone and estrogen levels.[26]

Physiologic gynecomastia is a normal assessment finding in newborns due to maternal hormonal influence. Male newborns often have breast tissue that is palpable as a result of the estrogen from the mother that crosses the placenta, causing the male breast tissue to swell. This condition, found in 90% of newborn boys, will resolve within a month. Changes in estrogen-to-testosterone levels also cause breast tissue enlargement in males during puberty and as part of the aging process after age 50.[26] ■

Further liver failure will manifest with portal hypertension that contributes to asterixis, spider angioma, and caput medusa. **Asterixis** is a muscle tremor that causes the downward flap of the hand when the arm is extended and dorsiflexed at the wrist. This can also be noted in the feet or tongue of the patient with portal hypertension.[5]

Spider angioma, also called spider telangiectasis or nevus, is a discoloration of the skin (**Figure 43.8** ■). The dilated arteriole is seen as a small red dot with tiny, fragile veins surrounding it, giving it a spiderweb appearance. These are most commonly found on the face, neck, and upper trunk. The cause of this is the liver's not metabolizing estrogens.[3]

Caput medusa is another abnormal assessment finding in the patient with portal hypertension. The abdomen has bluish veins just under the skin that radiate out across the umbilicus as a result of ascites and increased abdominal pressure.

Esophageal varices, another abnormal finding, is swollen esophageal veins that are the result of increased pressure in the vessels due to portal hypertension from liver scarring.[27] Esophageal varices can cause the patient to have symptoms ranging from hematemesis to frank bleeding. Hemorrhage to these fragile vessels can happen suddenly and without warning. The lack of vitamin K metabolism and storage in the liver contributes to the clotting problems, making bleeding esophageal varices a very serious condition.

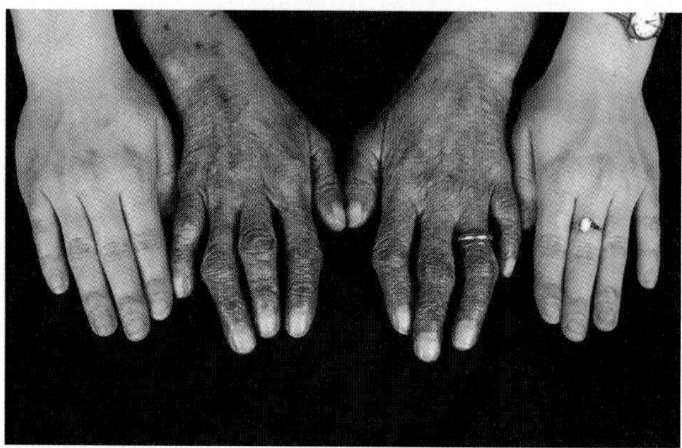

Figure 43.7 ■ The distinct bronze skin color of a patient with hemochromatosis.

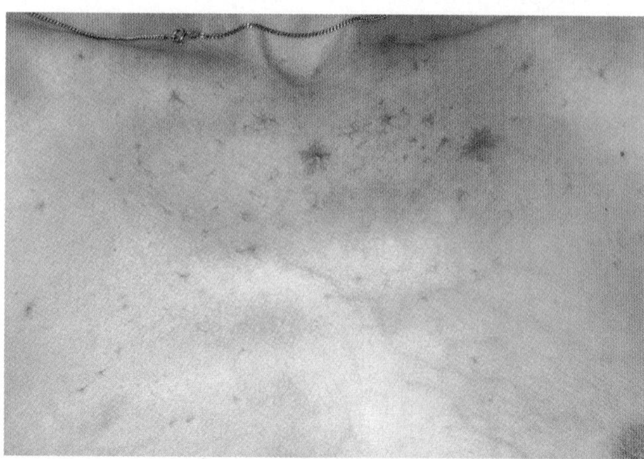

Figure 43.8 ■ Spider angioma, also called spider telangiectasis or nevus, is a small red dot with tiny, fragile veins surrounding it, giving it a spiderweb appearance. It is caused by the liver's failure to metabolize estrogens.

Linking Pathophysiology to Diagnosis and Treatment

Diagnosis of liver disease will consist of the patient's report of symptoms, abnormal laboratory values, and noninvasive sonography and transient elastography. Liver biopsy, still considered the gold standard for diagnosis, can help to determine whether the patient has simple steatosis or a more serious condition, such as cirrhosis.[20] Other noninvasive methods, such as blood markers and instrumental methods, have been used to make the diagnosis.[8]

The most important treatment for liver disease is abstinence from alcohol. Abstinence improves the prognosis in any stage of the disease, as long as the abstinence is sustained. Liver transplant is an option only for patients who have maintained sobriety. Liver transplantation removes the diseased liver and replaces it with a donor liver, requiring immunosuppressant drugs that will be taken for the rest of the person's life to prevent organ rejection.

Treatment also includes improving overall health and nutrition. Malnutrition is considered to indicate a rather poor prognosis for patients with liver disease. Changes in diet include the addition of lean protein as well as polyunsaturated fatty acids and phytochemicals. Resveratrol is one such phytochemical that is being researched because it has the ability to neutralize free radicals and inflammatory cytokines, thus reducing oxidative stress.[11]

Prevention of more serious complications that result from pathologic changes, including hemorrhage from esophageal varices, infection to the peritoneal cavity, fluid and electrolyte shifts with ascites, and confusion manifested by hepatic encephalopathy, also need to be addressed.[11] Treatment to prevent bleeding of esophageal varices may include medications to reduce blood pressure in the portal vein or a surgical procedure of band ligation. Bleeding varices are a medical emergency. Treatment includes band ligation, medications to slow blood flow, or placement of a shunt to divert blood away from the portal vein.[27] Stool softeners are given to prevent damage to the swollen rectal veins. A hemorrhoidectomy can also be performed on the swollen rectal vessel. Abdominocentesis is completed by removal of the ascitic fluid with a needle. A shunt can also be implanted to help remove the fluid but retain the albumin in the body.

Similar symptoms and physical changes in the liver from liver cancer were discussed previously. Liver disease is a complex illness because it necessitates the management of the multisystem effects (**Figure 43.9** ■).

Check Your Progress: Section 43.2

1. Which cells of the liver remove bacteria and foreign material from the blood?
2. In liver damage, liver inflammation, or liver obstruction pathologies, what diagnostic tests on the liver panel will show an elevation?
3. What pathologic process increases the risk of liver cancer in patients infected with hepatitis B virus or hepatitis C virus?

43.3 Disorders of the Gallbladder

The gallbladder, a small accessory organ of the digestive system the size of a kiwi fruit, is responsible for the storage of about 70 mL of bile. Made in the liver, bile is stored and concentrated in the gallbladder.[6] The gallbladder is located on the right side of the inferior border of the liver. **Cholelithiasis**, or stone formation, is the most common disorder of the gallbladder.[3] The presence of stones in the gallbladder often contributes to the other disorders seen in the gallbladder, such as choledocholithiasis, cholangitis, cholecystitis, and cancer of the gallbladder (**Figure 43.10** ■).

Cholelithiasis

Cholelithiasis affects 10–15% of the population in the United States.[5] Changes in diet, including type of food and fluid consumed and amount of fat and cholesterol, as well as obesity have a direct impact on stone formation in the gallbladder and biliary tract.

Etiology and Pathogenesis

The presence of fatty chyme in the duodenum causes smooth muscular contraction to release bile. The hormone cholecystokinin from the duodenal mucosa is the stimulus for the gallbladder and pancreas to contract, releasing their digestive juices bile and pancreatic juices, as well as the relaxation of the hepatopancreatic sphincter of Oddi.

Disorders of the gallbladder most often result from gallstone formation and blockage of bile, causing inflammation and tissue damage. Although much less common, gallbladder cancer can be caused from the damage caused by gallstones in the gallbladder and biliary tract.

Most stones form in the gallbladder and then migrate to the bile ducts, causing an obstruction and inflammation. Stones in the gallbladder obstructing flow are formed from cholesterol or pigment, 80% of the stones being formed from cholesterol.[5,29] Excess cholesterol is noted in obesity, in patients whose diets are high in fat and cholesterol, and in patients who take medications that lower serum cholesterol. Precipitating factors in the formation of gallstones include changes in metabolism, biliary stasis, obstruction, hypertriglyceridemia, and infection. Risk factors specific for women include multiparous, use of estrogen replacement therapy, oral contraceptives, and the **FIVE F'S**:

1. Female
2. Fair
3. Fat
4. Fertile
5. Forty

Other risk factors include a sedentary lifestyle, diabetes mellitus, regional enteritis, and having family members who have had cholelithiasis.[29]

Children with hemolytic diseases such as sickle cell disease may develop gallstones. These stones are more likely to be acalculus. ■

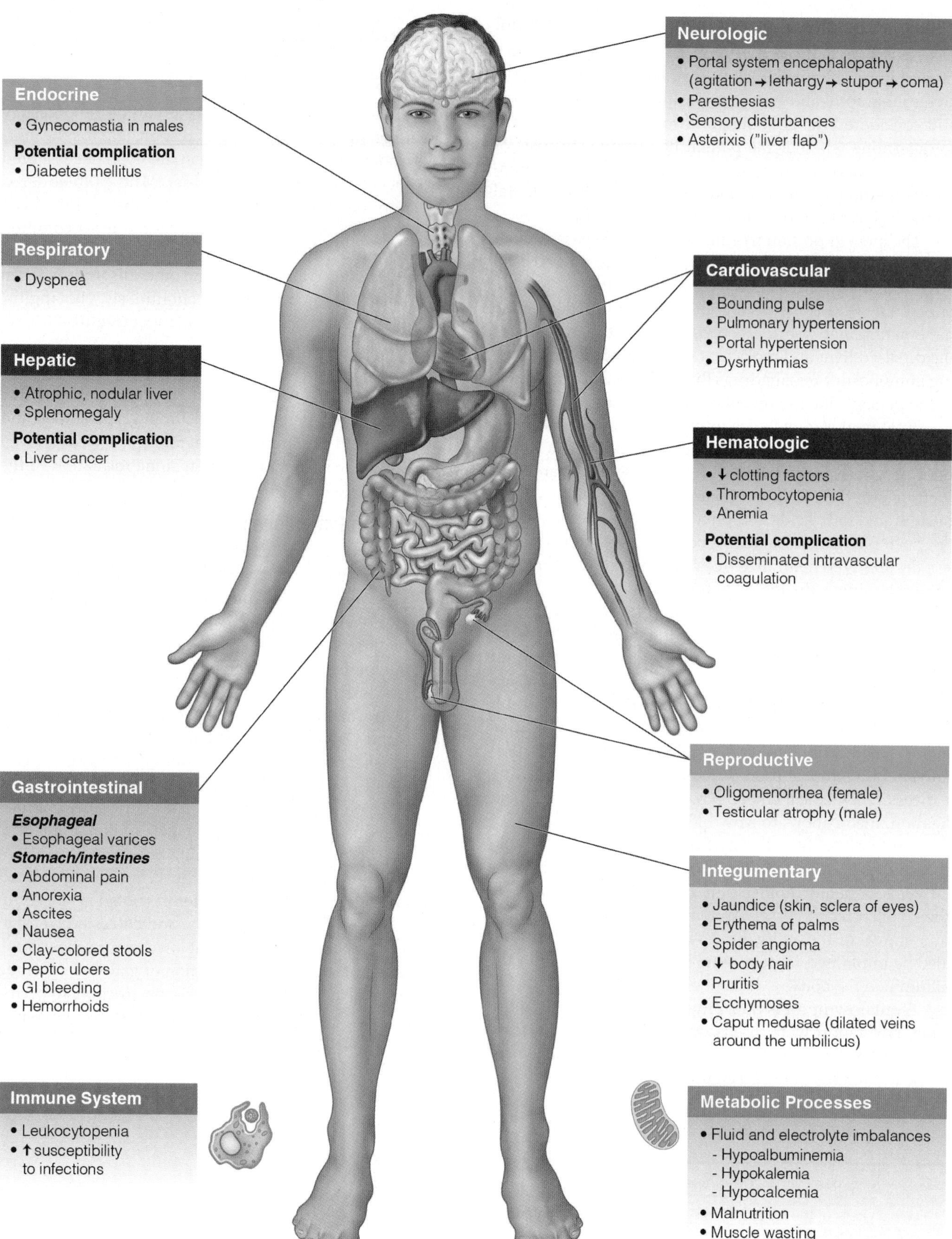

Neurologic
• Portal system encephalopathy (agitation → lethargy → stupor → coma)
• Paresthesias
• Sensory disturbances
• Asterixis ("liver flap")
Endocrine
• Gynecomastia in males
Potential complication
• Diabetes mellitus
Respiratory
• Dyspnea
Cardiovascular
• Bounding pulse
• Pulmonary hypertension
• Portal hypertension
• Dysrhythmias
Hepatic
• Atrophic, nodular liver
• Splenomegaly
Potential complication
• Liver cancer
Hematologic
• ↓ clotting factors
• Thrombocytopenia
• Anemia
Potential complication
• Disseminated intravascular coagulation
Reproductive
• Oligomenorrhea (female)
• Testicular atrophy (male)
Gastrointestinal
Esophageal
• Esophageal varices
Stomach/intestines
• Abdominal pain
• Anorexia
• Ascites
• Nausea
• Clay-colored stools
• Peptic ulcers
• GI bleeding
• Hemorrhoids
Integumentary
• Jaundice (skin, sclera of eyes)
• Erythema of palms
• Spider angioma
• ↓ body hair
• Pruritis
• Ecchymoses
• Caput medusae (dilated veins around the umbilicus)
Immune System
• Leukocytopenia
• ↑ susceptibility to infections
Metabolic Processes
• Fluid and electrolyte imbalances
- Hypoalbuminemia
- Hypokalemia
- Hypocalcemia
• Malnutrition
• Muscle wasting

Figure 43.9 ■ Multisystem effects of liver disease.

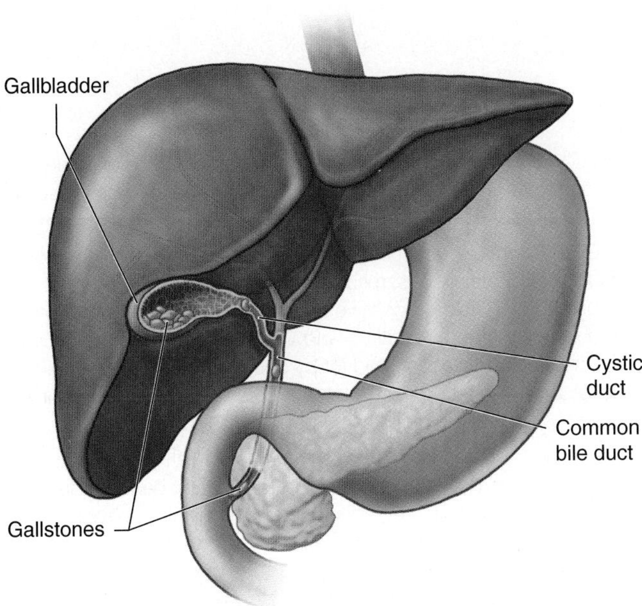

Figure 43.10 ■ Common location of gallstones.

Clinical Manifestations

Early signs of gallstones are often vague, with nonspecific complaints of indigestion or mild gastric distress after consumption of fat in the diet. The stone can become lodged in the duct, causing a severe and sudden onset of midepigastric pain that radiates to the RUQ and right subscapular region and to the back or shoulder. **Biliary colic** (painful spasms to the RUQ that accompany obstruction in the cystic duct by a stone) is due to the distention and pressure to the gallbladder when the bile is not allowed to flow in the duct.[29] The patient often experiences nausea, vomiting, sweating, and tachycardia, which are typically noted with severe pain. If the bile is able to reflux into the liver, jaundice, pain, and damage to the hepatocytes can occur. If the obstruction is located in the common bile duct, the pancreas can also be involved. Pancreatic enzymes reflux to the pancreas, causing pancreatitis.[5,29]

The patient with gallstones obstructing bile could have further complications, including bleeding and easy bruising related to the lack of bile causing impaired digestion of fats. The patient is unable to absorb fat-soluble vitamins, including vitamin K. When increased bilirubin is eliminated by the kidneys, the urine is a dark tea color. **Steatorrhea** (greasy, foulsmelling feces containing undigested fats) is often reported and results from the lack of bile to digest the fat in the duodenum. Bile salts that accumulate in the blood are finally eliminated via the integumentary system, causing pruritus.

Gallstones are not uncommon in pregnancy. Rates of gallstone formation increase throughout the peripartum period from 5.2% in the second trimester to 10.2% at 6 weeks postpartum.[29] ■

Helen Martin: Application

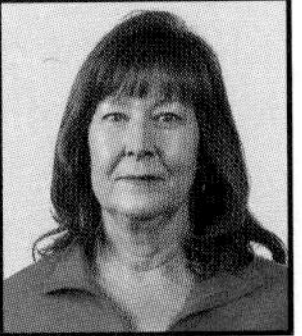

Mrs. Martin is overweight and has been trying different diets to lose weight. She has a stressful family life and is also experiencing perimenopause with hot flashes and weight gain. Her indigestion is not relieved by antacids. When she experiences RUQ abdominal pain without relief for a couple of hours, she schedules an appointment to see her family physician, Dr. Rowe.

Mrs. Martin has an ultrasonography procedure done the next day. The results confirm the presence of several gallstones in both the gallbladder and the biliary tract. Mrs. Martin discusses with Dr. Rowe the options for treatment, which include either surgery of modification of her diet. Mrs. Martin decides to try changing her diet instead of surgery. A referral to a dietitian at the Neighborhood Patient Education Center is arranged. The dietitian educates Mrs. Martin about eating low-fat and low-calorie foods to promote weight loss and manage her symptoms.

5. Treatment options provided to Mrs. Martin included dietary management. If this approach does not prove successful in eliminating her gallstones, what are some of the factors that are likely to contribute to the lack of success?
6. Why might patients think they are having a heart attack instead of a gallbladder attack?
7. In addition to ultrasound, what imaging studies are available to help make a definitive diagnosis of Mrs. Martin's condition?

Linking Pathophysiology to Diagnosis and Treatment

The gallbladder concentrates the bile by absorbing some of the water and ions. From the time when the bile enters the gallbladder until its release, the bile becomes 10 times more concentrated.[4] This concentrated bile tends to form stones.

Obstruction of the common bile duct causes bile to reflux back into the liver, causing damage to the hepatocytes. The pancreas can also be damaged by this obstruction in the common bile duct from enzymes that cause autodigestion. Lab values for amylase and lipase are elevated, demonstrating involvement of the pancreas.

Diagnosis is based on symptomatology. Diagnostic tests may include an abdominal x-ray, ultrasound, oral cholecystogram, or a gallbladder scan. The conjugated bilirubin may be elevated if there is bile obstruction. Inflammation and infection would be noted in the elevated WBC.

Treatment is conservative if the patient is asymptomatic and has a low risk of complications from the presence of stones. Medications such as ursodiol and chenodiol can be used to decrease cholesterol production in the liver and dissolve the stone. This form of treatment can take up to 2 years to dissolve the stone, and the stones can reoccur once the medication has been discontinued. Symptomatic patients require surgical intervention with either a laparoscopic cholecystectomy or an open cholecystostomy not only to remove the gallbladder, but also to explore the common bile duct with possible placement of a T-tube to maintain patency of the common bile duct as a result of inflammation.[5] When a cholecystectomy is performed, the hepatic duct is connected to the common bile duct, thus allowing the bile to flow into the duodenum directly from the liver.

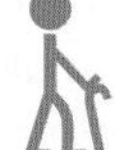

The incidence of cholelithiasis increases with age. At age 75, almost 50% of women and 20% of men will have gallstones.[30] ■

Choledocholithiasis and Cholangitis

Choledocholithiasis is a gallstone in the common bile duct. **Cholangitis** is inflammation of the common bile duct (see

Impact of Nutrition in Clinical Practice

The Role of Dietary Factors in Cholelithiasis

Joanne Kouba

It is estimated that 20–25 million adults in the United States are afflicted with cholelithiasis (CL).[1] The pathophysiology of CL formation includes lithogenic (stone-forming) bile resulting from hypersecretion of cholesterol into bile, reduced cholesterol crystallization time, gallbladder dysmotility, hypertriglyceridemia, hyperinsulinemia, and/or insulin resistance.[2] Approximately 80% of CL is categorized as cholesterol CL. Established modifiable risk factors for CL include diet, lack of physical activity, rapid weight loss, obesity, and dyslipidemia.[2]

Epidemiologic evidence links CL with eating patterns that are characterized by high intakes of refined carbohydrates and fat and low intake of fiber.[2] A high fiber intake may protect against CL formation by accelerating intestinal transit, which decreases the formation of secondary bile acids and attenuates cholesterol saturation in bile. An inverse relationship between caffeine and protein intakes with CLL have been reported. Caffeine stimulates gallbladder motility, which may explain its protective role. By contrast, individuals who have received total parenteral nutrition experience gallbladder stasis and increased risk of CLL.[2]

Excess energy intake also plays a role in CL risk in both youths and adults because it leads to obesity, which is associated with increased cholesterol production, biliary cholesterol secretion, and cholesterol supersaturation.[2,3,4] The risk of CLL in adults was approximately double for those who were obese and approximately 45–65% greater for those who were overweight compared to adults of a healthy weight.[3] A case-control study reported that children admitted for CL were 5.78 times more likely to be obese than were those admitted for appendicitis. The study also reported that for every 1 *z*-score increase in body mass index, the CL risk creased by 79%.[4] The incidence of CL after bariatric surgery, accompanied by rapid weight loss, ranges from 30% to 70%.[2] Various reports have suggested that this relationship is strongest in both genders, North American Indians, individuals with adolescent obesity, and those who consume more than 2500 calories daily.[5] Inconsistent findings may be attributable to methodologic issues in energy intake by self-report.

Dyslipidemias, particularly hypertriglyceridemia and low high-density lipoprotein levels, result in increased cholesterol saturation of bile and CL risk.[2] A positive relationship between both type 1 and type 2 diabetes mellitus and CL has been reported. While this may be partly accounted for by obesity, it has also been suggested that genetic dysregulation, which is known to occur in diabetes, increases the bile acid pool and CL risk.

Current research is also investigating the relationship between genetic factors and the gut microbiota in CL pathogenesis. Current evidence supports CL prevention through modifiable behaviors such as maintaining a healthy weight, regular physical activity, and establishing eating patterns consistent with the *Dietary Guidelines for Americans*, which are plant-based and include generous amounts of fiber and modest fat intake. A little caffeine might also be beneficial.

References

1. Stinton, L. M., & Shaffer, E. A. (2012). Epidemiology of gallbladder disease: Cholelithiasis and cancer. *Gut and Liver*, *6*(2), 172–187.
2. O'Connell, K., & Brasel, K. (2014). Bile metabolism and lithogenesis. *Surgical Clinics of North America*, *94*, 361–375.
3. Acosta, A., & Camilleri, M. (2014). Gastrointestinal morbidity in obesity. *Annals of the New York Academy of Sciences*, *1311*, 42–56.
4. Fradin, K., Racine, A. D., & Belamarich, P. F. (2014). Obesity and symptomatic cholelithiasis in childhood: Epidemiologic and case-control evidence for a strong relationship. *Journal of Pediatric Gastroenterology and Nutrition*, *58*, 102–106.
5. Cuevas, A., Miquel, J. F., Reyes, M. S., et al. (2004). Diet as a risk factor for cholesterol gallstone disease. *Journal of the American College of Nutrition*, *23*(3), 187–196.

Figure 43.10). A stone located in the common bile duct can also cause complications for the liver and pancreas.

Etiology and Pathogenesis

Stones found in the common bile duct most often originate in the gallbladder, but a stone can also form in the common bile duct. Cholangitis is a serious condition in which the gallstone becomes impacted in the bile duct with resulting inflammation. Untreated, this impacted stone can cause bacteremia and septicemia and is associated with a higher mortality rate when diagnosis and treatment are delayed.[31] Secondary pancreatitis is also a concern, as the obstruction causes chemical damage from reflux of bile and pancreatic digestive juices to the pancreas.

Clinical Manifestations

Patients with choledocholithiasis and cholangitis present with symptoms similar to those of cholelithiasis and acute cholecystitis, which is covered below. Clinical symptoms include RUQ pain, fever, jaundice, abdominal tenderness, and pruritus.[5] As a result of the elevated bilirubin, the patient will have dark-colored urine and clay-colored stools. The patient with advanced cholangitis will have clinical signs consistent with sepsis, such as hypotension and changes in mental status.[31]

Linking Pathophysiology to Diagnosis and Treatment

Several tests can be completed to diagnose inflammation and obstruction in the bile ducts. Serum tests include an increased alkaline phosphatase and GGT as well as supporting laboratory tests of elevated AST, ALT, bilirubin, amylase, and lipase.[7] Leukocytosis will be noted with cholangitis.

Several diagnostic tests can be completed by using contrast dye to visualize the obstruction. An intravenous cholangiogram visualizes the blood through the liver and is excreted with bile to the gallbladder. When the dye is injected directly into the biliary tree through the abdominal wall, this test is percutaneous transhepatic cholangiography. In an endoscopic retrograde cholangiopancreatography (ERCP), the dye is inserted from the sphincter of Oddi. The advantage of the ERCP is that the opening of the sphincter of Oddi can be enlarged, allowing the stone to pass out of the common bile duct. When the dye is ingested in the form of a tablet in order to observe the excretion of the bile, this is an oral cholecystography.[30]

Surgical treatment is a choledocholithotomy to remove the stone with an incision into the common bile duct. Supportive therapy includes analgesics, antihistamines, nutrition, antibiotics, and antiemetics.[5] Early intervention with antibiotics and fluids to treat sepsis is needed to improve patient outcomes associated with cholangitis.

Cholecystitis

Cholecystitis is an acute or chronic inflammation of the gallbladder, often resulting from gallstones or other conditions that damage the walls of the gallbladder.

Etiology and Pathogenesis

Cholecystitis is most often caused by a cystic duct stone; other, less common causes include trauma, infection of the gallbladder, and sepsis.[31] The inflammation is caused by both the stone and digestive juices. The gallstone irritates the walls of the gallbladder, causing inflammation and thickening.[31] The increased pressure in the gallbladder from the buildup of bile causes chemical damage to the gallbladder, resulting in tissue ischemia. The result is damage to the walls of the gallbladder and surrounding mucosa that can lead to perforation of the gallbladder and necrosis.[5]

Acute cholecystitis results from the blockage of the cystic duct, causing pain and biliary colic. Without treatment, the gallbladder becomes scarred with fibrosis, leading to chronic cholecystitis. Bile may contain bacteria with chronic cholecystitis, contributing to an infectious process. Other, more serious conditions that develop from impaired circulation and edema are gangrene, abscess or fistula formation, and perforation with peritonitis and sepsis.[5] Perforation is a serious complication that can also occur without treatment of cholecystitis.

Clinical Manifestations

History includes intolerance of dietary fat with epigastric heaviness or RUQ abdominal pain after eating. The patient may complain of flatulence, belching, and regurgitation. Colicky pain is caused by the obstruction of bile flow. These symptoms can last up to 18 hours and are often more vague with chronic cholecystitis.[5] Biliary obstruction causes clay-colored stools or steatorrhea, the urine color is amber, and the patient may experience bleeding, jaundice, and pruritus.[31] Fever and chills accompany cholecystitis as a result of inflammation of the gallbladder and possible sepsis.

Linking Pathophysiology to Diagnosis and Treatment

Diagnosis includes the use of reported symptoms, along with CT scans, ultrasound, and a cholescintigraphy. Highly reliable, the cholescintigraphy is a nuclear scan that uses an injected radionuclide, technetium-99m, to obtain images within several minutes. It is also known as a hepatobiliary iminodiacetic acid scan. Treatment includes laparoscopic cholecystectomy and antibiotics.[31]

Helen Martin: Outcome

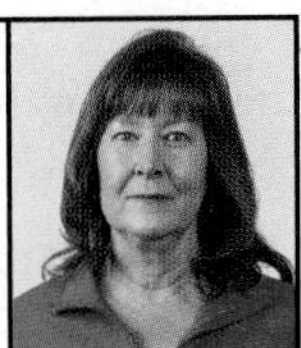

Mrs. Martin is noncompliant with her diet, especially given the stress of her home life. When Mrs. Martin experiences chest pain and dyspnea, she attributes this to her continued gastrointestinal symptoms. Finally, when the pain becomes intense and her heart is racing, Mrs. Martin decides that it is time for surgery to remove her gallbladder. A laparoscopic cholecystectomy is completed. Mrs. Martin initially experiences postoperative pain and nausea, but she recovers quickly and is discharged home the following day. She acknowledges the importance of discharge instructions about restricting her fat intake. She is also aware that removal of the gallbladder will not have adverse consequences on her lifespan.

8. Because Mrs. Martin has cholelithiasis and possible cholangitis, what laboratory test results might be elevated on diagnostic blood work?
9. If Mrs. Martin had not undergone cholecystectomy but instead remained untreated and her cholelithiasis had caused cholecystitis, what possible complications might have occurred?
10. If Mrs. Martin's gallstones had not been treated and remained in place, irritating the lining of her gallbladder, what is one possible adverse outcome that would cause early mortality?

Cancer of the Gallbladder

Cancer of the gallbladder is similar to liver and pancreatic cancer in that diagnosis is often delayed because the early symptoms are vague. Only 20% of cases of cancer of the gallbladder are diagnosed in the early stages before metastasis has occurred.[32]

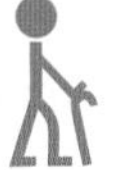

Older adults are most often affected by cancer of the gallbladder, with higher rates in the seventh decade of life.[16] ■

Cancer of the gallbladder and the connecting bile ducts accounts for over 10,000 new cases a year, women being affected more often than men. Survival, as in many other types of cancer, depends on the stage of cancer at diagnosis.[33] In stage I, this form of cancer is found only in the gallbladder with a survival rate of 50% at 5 years. When the lymph nodes are involved, the 5-year rate of survival drops to only 7%; it is less than 5% if the spread is to other parts of the body.[33]

Etiology and Pathogenesis

Cancer of the gallbladder and bile ducts originates in the surface lining or epithelium more than 80% of the time. When the origin is the biliary tract, known as cholangiocarcinoma, the prognosis is less favorable because this type of aggressive cancer penetrates the walls of the bile duct or gallbladder. A more superficial adenocarcinoma found in the lumen of the biliary tract, known as biliary papillomatosis, has a better prognosis.[34]

Damage to the inner mucosal lining of the gallbladder or bile ducts from gallstones, toxins, bacteria, or parasites can predispose a patient to cancer (see Impact of Current Research on Clinical Practice). Gallstones are the main risk factor, found in 80% of the patients with cancer of the gallbladder, especially large stones that cause discomfort.

Gallstones can cause damage in the form of calcification to the walls of the gallbladder. Finally, benign polyps are also considered a risk factor.[34]

Clinical Manifestations

Early symptoms are often subtle and hard to distinguish from other abdominal disorders. Cholelithiasis often accompanies gallbladder cancer and is believed to contribute to the development of cancer from the chronic irritation to the mucosal tissue of the gallbladder.[16] Late symptoms include intense RUQ abdominal pain, jaundice, and weight loss. The gallbladder will be palpable at this time.

Linking Pathophysiology to Diagnosis and Treatment

Early diagnosis improves the outcome. Serum CA19-9 will often be elevated in patients with bile duct cancer and other cancers, so a definitive diagnosis must be made by a more invasive method to directly obtain cells. The use of cytopathology with either fine-needle aspiration or biopsy is considered the gold standard for the diagnosis. Fine-needle aspiration acquires the cells for microscopic examination from an endoscope. Biopsy of the cells from a laparotomy using general anesthesia can also be used to obtain cells to make a definitive diagnosis. Treatment for gallstones with a cholecystectomy is often how cancer of the gallbladder is initially and often unexpectedly discovered.[16]

Cure is best obtained with surgical removal of the carcinoma by a laparoscopic cholecystectomy or by an open cholecystectomy when a larger, advanced tumor must be removed. When the cancer has spread, a Whipple resection will be done to remove diseased tissues of the bile duct, ampulla of Vater, head of the pancreas, gallbladder, or proximal duodenum.[34]

> **Check Your Progress: Section 43.3**
>
> 1. Which is the most common disorder of the gallbladder?
> 2. What parasite is known to increase the risk of gallbladder cancer, biliary tract cancer, and liver cancer?
> 3. Are there medications that can dissolve gallstones?

43.4 Disorders of the Pancreas

The pancreas, a yellow gland shaped like a triangle, is located in the upper abdomen, posterior to the stomach (see Figure 43.1). The pancreas is divided into three sections (the head, midsection, and tail) and is responsible for making digestive enzymes in the exocrine cells and hormones in the endocrine cells. Disorders of the pancreas include acute and chronic pancreatitis, pancreatic cysts, and cancer of the pancreas.

Acute Pancreatitis

Acute pancreatitis is inflammation or necrosis of the pancreas (**Figure 43.11** ■). It is most often a mild disease known as edematous pancreatitis. Acute pancreatitis can contribute to pancreatic ischemia. The more serious and often painful inflammation of the pancreatic tissue happens in 20% of cases of pancreatitis.[35] Early treatment is essential to prevent serious complications.

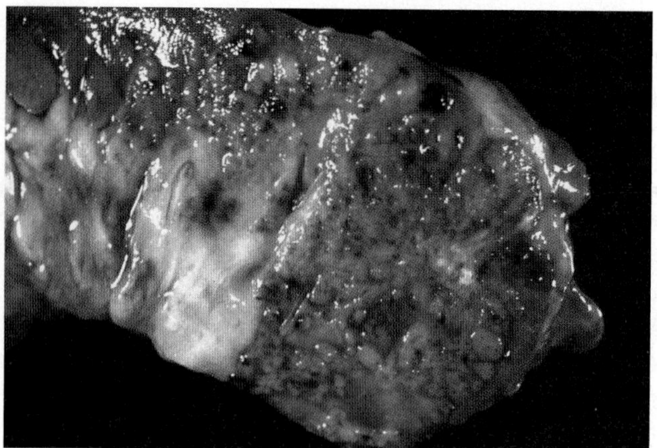

Figure 43.11 ■ Gross clinical specimen of a pancreas affected by acute pancreatitis. Pseudocyst, a pus-filled bleb see as the yellow area (lower left center), is a potential complication of pancreatitis.

Etiology and Pathogenesis

Alcohol abuse and gallstones are the most common causes of acute pancreatitis. Other causes are viral infections, trauma, abdominal surgery, hyperlipidemia, and some medications such as acetaminophen or thiazide diuretics.[1,16]

By stimulating pancreatic secretions, alcohol initiates pancreatitis when the ethanol is metabolized, injuring the tissues with the toxic metabolites that release activated enzymes. The result is partial sphincter obstruction and tissue irritation.[16,35] Pancreatitis that results from gallstone obstruction of the pancreatic ducts causes trapped digestive enzymes, usually trypsin, to autodigest the pancreatic tissue, activating an acute inflammatory response.[7,35] Trypsin activates other enzymes, including lipase, elastase, and chymotrypsin. Pain results from the stretching of the edematous tissues, enzymatic chemical irritation, and obstruction of the biliary tract.[35] The inflammatory process can progress beyond the pancreas to other organs, creating conditions for systematic inflammatory response syndrome (SIRS) and multiple organ failure.[16] Inflammatory mediators are released, causing an increase vascular permeability and vessel dilation. The result is leaking of fluid into the peritoneal cavity, which initiates a series of events in the entire body. Hypovolemia contributes to decreased perfusion to the organs, causing decreased renal blood flow with resulting lower urine output and renal failure if not corrected. Multiple organ failure and SIRS are very serious, contributing to most of the deaths from acute pancreatitis.[35]

Clinical Manifestations

Inflammation of the pancreas usually manifests with pain to the upper abdomen with a knifelike pressure. The pain is often deep epigastric pain or is referred to the umbilical, chest, or flank area. Abdominal distention and tenderness

Impact of Current Research on Clinical Practice

Cultural Impact or Food Safety Impact?

Description: Parasitic infections contribute to cancer of the liver and gallbladder as well as the bile ducts. Prevalent in Far Eastern countries such as Japan, *Clonorchis sinensis*, the Chinese liver fluke, infects humans when they eat raw or undercooked freshwater fish that contains the *Clonorchis* cyst parasite. The parasite becomes a fluke and travels from the duodenum up the common bile duct, where maturation takes place. The worms thrive in this internal environment by consuming bile, growing to 1 centimeter in length in only 1 month. The mature parasite hooks onto the epithelial lining with its sucker, causing irritation and damage to the tissue, eventually causing scar tissue formation. Obstruction of the bile ducts leads to the symptoms of abdominal pain, nausea, diarrhea, and eventually inflammation when not treated. The risk of biliary tract cancer increases significantly as a result of this uninvited guest. Diagnosis is most often the result of testing a stool sample that contains the eggs. The cysts would show up on a CT or MRI scan.

Clinical Practice: This type of parasitic infection can be prevented by avoiding consumption of raw fish and killing the parasites by cooking fish to an internal temperature of at least 145°F (63°C). The treatment of choice to eliminate the infection is praziquantel or albendazole.

Research Study:

Johns Hopkins Pathology. (2016). *Gallbladder and bile duct cancer*. Available at http://pathology.jhu.edu/gbbd/disease_info.cfm

often accompany acute pancreatitis. Changes in vital signs related to pain and fluid shifts include tachycardia and hypotension. Fever results from the inflammatory process. Jaundice, which is common in accessory organ dysfunction, is caused by the obstruction of the bile duct.

Paresthesia, a prickly pins-and-needles sensation, is noted most in alcoholics and is related to vitamin B1 deficiency affecting the feet, toes, and legs. Without treatment, the paresthesia progresses gradually to a burning sensation and eventual loss of function from atrophy. Thiamine supplements help to reverse these symptoms.

Hemorrhagic pancreatitis causes bruising and edema to the subcutaneous tissue surrounding the umbilicus, known as **Cullen sign**. **Grey-Turner sign** is another specific clinical sign in which the flank area appears bruised with bluish discoloration from bleeding behind the peritoneum.[2] Steatorrhea from decreased or absent lipase is noted in pancreatic disease.[35]

Warning signs of a more serious condition include low urine output, hypoxemia, restlessness, confusion, and worsening tachypnea and tachycardia. The loss of vascular fluid volume with the leaking into the abdominal, retroperitoneal, and peripancreatic space contributes to hypovolemic shock.[16]

Jimmy Gerde: Application

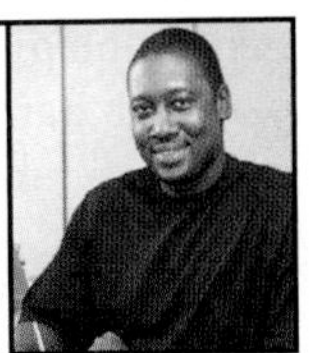

A systems assessment is completed, and Mr. Gerde is noted to be alert with restlessness. He reports constant nausea and two episodes of vomiting with frequent retching within the past 24 hours. His abdomen is distended and tender to palpation. The abdomen has a greenish discolored area around the umbilicus. Bowel sounds are hypoactive in all quadrants. Extremities are without edema, but he does report that he has had an abnormal pins-and-needles feeling in his feet for several months. Vital signs are pulse 122 and bounding, respirations 24 and irregular, temperature 100.2°F (37.8°C), blood pressure 108/72. Color is pale. Saturation level is 96% on room air. Mr. Gerde is 187.9 centimeters tall and weighs 67.1 kilograms. He is admitted to the hospital with a diagnosis of acute pancreatitis.

4. Because Mr. Gerde has a distended, tender abdomen with a greenish discoloration around his umbilicus, you suspect what underlying pathology?
5. On the basis of the presenting signs and symptoms, what other physical sign might be found in Mr. Gerde?
6. When Mr. Gerde is admitted to the hospital, he is placed on a telemetry unit. Why should he need telemetry for his cardiac status when his problem is gastrointestinal?
7. You notice that Mr. Gerde exhibits restlessness. This makes you aware that he is at risk for what complication?

Linking Pathophysiology to Diagnosis and Treatment

Acute pancreatitis is initially diagnosed on the basis of abnormal laboratory results. Amylase and lipase are the results that help to guide early diagnosis because they are often elevated to 3 times the normal limit.[35] Serum amylase lacks specificity; therefore, lipase is often collected with amylase to help make a diagnosis of pancreatitis. Serum amylase levels increase in just 3–6 hours after an attack of pancreatitis, peaking in 20–30 hours. The duration of the increase is 2–3 days. Lipase levels rise later than amylase levels in pancreatitis.[7]

Other enzymes that will be elevated include alkaline phosphatase, AST, ALT, and LDH. Elevated WBC and bilirubin are also noted in the patient with an acute condition. CT scans and dynamic contrast-enhanced CT help with diagnosis and identify necrosis or fluid accumulation in the pancreas.

CLINICAL POINT: The severity of acute pancreatitis does not necessarily correlate with the degree of elevation noted in the serum lipase and amylase levels.[16] Normal amylase levels can be found in patients with fatal pancreatitis.[7] ■

Treatment of acute pancreatitis depends on the severity of the inflammation and damage to the surrounding tissues as well as the patient's response. Immediate management includes pain relief, intravenous fluid replacement, and allowing the pancreas to rest by keeping the patient NPO to decrease the production of digestive enzymes. Nasogastric suctioning may be ordered to prevent stimulation of the digestive processes. Meperidine is often a preferred analgesic for management of severe pain because it causes fewer spasms to the pancreatic duct sphincters than morphine. If the patient has fluid loss into the peritoneal cavity, IV colloid solutions help to maintain the colloid osmotic pressure.[16]

Jimmy Gerde: Outcome

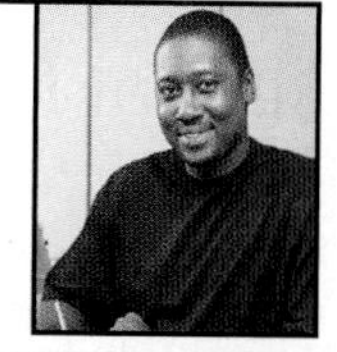

Mr. Gerde has significantly elevated amylase and lipase levels. He is admitted to the medical unit with orders for telemetry monitoring, intravenous fluid, and electrolyte replacement at 150 mL/hour. He is NPO with a nasogastric tube to low suction. Pain control is with meperidine via patient-controlled analgesia. Mr. Gerde's blood sugar is monitored every 6 hours with point-of-care testing. He is also monitored for alcohol withdrawal by using the Clinical Institute Withdrawal Assessment of Alcohol Scale. He continues to have intense abdominal pain. Famotidine, a histamine H_2-*receptor* blocker, is ordered to help reduce the gastric acid secretions. Thiamine injections are ordered for the paresthesia.

Mr. Gerde remains NPO with the nasogastric tube to low suction for 36 hours. Once the acute pain and ileus resolve, the nasogastric tube is removed, and his diet is progressed slowly, starting with clear liquids. The IV rate is slowed to 75 mL/hour and eventually converts to a saline lock once his intake is adequate. Mr. Gerde is referred for alcohol rehabilitation upon discharge on day 6.

8. Why is thiamine ordered as a treatment for Mr. Gerde's paresthesias?
9. Nursing care of Mr. Gerde includes monitoring for alcohol withdrawal using the Clinical Institute Withdrawal Assessment of Alcohol Scale. Why is it necessary to monitor him in this way?
10. After Mr. Gerde's initial medical event is resolved, he is referred to alcohol rehabilitation on hospital discharge. Why is this important?

Chronic Pancreatitis

Chronic pancreatitis is similar to acute pancreatitis except that the chronic pain is often less severe, but the tissue damage is irreversible. Alcoholism is the most common cause of this permanent, chronic condition.[16]

Etiology and Pathogenesis

Besides alcoholism, any condition that causes an obstruction or strictures of the pancreatic duct can cause chronic pancreatitis, including calculi (stones), pseudocysts, or tumors. Other causes of pancreatic dysfunction include smoking, cystic fibrosis, primary sclerosing cholangitis, exposure to toxic metabolites, and inflammatory bowel disease.[16,36] Genetics can contribute to chronic pancreatitis with familial hyperlipidemia.[37] The tissues of the pancreas experience irreversible damage, which causes pancreatic dysfunction, increasing the risk for future pancreatic cancer.

Clinical Manifestations

Common symptoms of chronic pancreatitis are weight loss and abdominal pain. Weight loss results from anorexia and malabsorption of fats and proteins, causing steatorrhea. Dull, constant abdominal pain to the left upper quadrant (LUQ) or epigastric area is a common clinical symptom. Patients with chronic pancreatitis often experience pain caused by ductal pressure that contributes to increased pressure and autodigestion. Alcohol is often a precipitating factor in the pain. Treatment of chronic pain associated with chronic pancreatitis often results in chemical addiction.

Linking Pathophysiology to Diagnosis and Treatment

Treatment of chronic pancreatitis includes elimination of alcohol and smoking. A low-fat diet is recommended because the patient lacks pancreatic enzymes. Enzyme deficiencies are corrected with oral replacements, such as pancreatin or pancrelipase, taken just before and during a meal. Insulin injections are often needed to control blood sugars in the absence of islet cell insulin production. Surgery can be done to relieve obstructions, prevent cyst rupture, or resect the pancreas. Pain control might include a surgical nerve block to the splanchnic or celiac ganglion nerve.[36]

Pancreatic Cysts

Commonly found in the general population, **pancreatic cysts** are small, fluid-filled sacs. Most cysts are asymptomatic. They are typically found incidentally when abdominal imaging is done for other causes.

Etiology and Pathogenesis

Most pancreatic cysts are asymptomatic. Prevalence of pancreatic cysts increases with age, almost a quarter of autopsy results demonstrating pancreatic cysts.[38,39]

Cysts vary in their epithelial lining and the ability to become malignant. Pseudocysts, or false cysts, and serous cystadenomas are more commonly found and are most often noncancerous.[40] Without an epithelial lining, this type of cyst is found on or around the pancreas, often encapsulated. Pseudocysts are filled with enzymatic fluid from the pancreas, and the pseudocyst wall is inflamed and fibrotic as a result of the damage to the tissue.[40]

Mucinous cysts, the more serious type of pancreatic cyst, are often malignant. These include intraductal papillary mucinous neoplasms, peripheral mucinous cystic neoplasms, and cystic islet-cell neoplasms.[41] They have the potential to become malignant, prompting treatment with surgical intervention.[41] There is a lack of consensus in the professional community about treatment and follow-up, owing to treatment costs, availability of cross-sectional imaging, and exposure to ionizing radiation and invasive procedures once the cysts have been identified. This is further complicated by the fact that more cysts are being identified as imaging techniques improve.[40] Risk factors include previous damage to the pancreas by acute or chronic pancreatitis or abdominal trauma.[40]

Clinical Manifestations

Most cysts are asymptomatic, found often when imaging tests such as CT or MRI are done for other reasons. When the patient does have symptoms, they are often related to where the cysts are exerting pressure on the surrounding tissues and the size of the cyst. As the cyst enlarges, the symptoms become more prominent. Half of the pseudocysts can be palpated in the epigastric area. Pain in the epigastric region often radiates to the back. Nausea, vomiting, jaundice, and abdominal fullness are symptoms that are seen in pancreatic disorders, including cysts.[40] Obstructive jaundice is caused by the pressure on the bile duct created by the cysts located in the head of the pancreas.

Linking Pathophysiology to Diagnosis and Treatment

Pancreatic cysts are often found on advanced abdominal imaging; up to 3% of abdominal computer tomography scans reveal cysts. Ultrasound-guided fine-needle aspiration allows the cystic fluid to be analyzed to identify the type of cyst present and tumor markers.[38] This information will help determine if the benign cyst will be monitored or a more aggressive treatment is needed for a malignant cyst. Next-generation sequencing is being used to assist with clinical diagnosis, especially with detecting malignancy.[39] Cystic neoplasms are the most common type of lesion. This type of cyst is benign and will be monitored for changes that would require treatment.[40] Intraductal papillary mucinous neoplasms and mucinous cystic neoplasms can become malignant cysts. Therefore, treatment is needed because they have the potential to invade surrounding tissues and become a pancreatic adenocarcinoma.[39]

Serious complications can develop, many related to the corrosive action of the pancreatic enzymes. Obstruction, fistula, and abscess formation can result from the tissue damage. Hemorrhage from the rupture of the cyst can also occur.

Surgery is often completed on solid-appearing cysts.[40] Skin damage is common after surgery in which a sump drainage tube removes the pancreatic secretions Most of the pancreatic cysts are small, benign, and asymptomatic and require monitoring only. When a pancreatic cyst is possibly malignant or a complication develops, surgical intervention is needed. Today, with the number of cysts that are identified, the challenge is to find a way to accurately monitor them safely and cost-effectively once they have been identified.[40]

Cancer of the Pancreas

Pancreatic cancer is considered relatively rare but is ranked fourth for cancer deaths because of its aggressive nature.[41] Survival rates remain low with mortality at almost 100%. Diabetes mellitus, obesity, and an aging population are all contributing to the increasing incidence of this deadly form of cancer.[3,36] Research is focusing on finding the cause and early detection. Diagnostic markers in the blood and new treatments are being developed to help improve early detection and survival.[42]

Etiology and Pathogenesis

The cause of pancreatic cancer remains unknown; however genetics and lifestyle are associated with this cancer. Lifestyle factors include diet, obesity, and cigarette smoking. Diets that include nitrates, preservatives, and high fat, which are characteristic of processed meats such as bacon, are associated with higher rates of pancreatic cancer.[3,36] Cigarette smoking, the most significant risk factor, doubles the risk of pancreatic cancer.[16,41] Patients who have diabetes mellitus and chronic pancreatitis have a higher incidence of pancreatic cancer. Genetic predisposition accounts for about 10% of cases of pancreatic cancer.[3,41] Most pancreatic tumors (95%) are found in the exocrine cells.[3,41] Ductal adenocarcinomas can occur in any part of the pancreas.

Tumors in the pancreatic head in the RUQ spread quickly, causing an obstruction of the common bile duct and portal vein. When the common bile duct is obstructed, the reflux of bile flow damages the liver, contributing to jaundice.[3,39]

The pancreatic body and tail reach into the LUQ . Pain is noted when the cancer is located in the body of the pancreas, owing to the involvement of the celiac ganglion. Tumors in the body and tail spread quickly and easily to the posterior abdominal wall. Pancreatic cancer spreads easily with early invasion to the lymphatic system. Infiltration to the major vessels, including the aorta, mesenteric artery, and vena cava, further contribute to the spread of this cancer and metastasis to other sites in the body, including the liver. Obstruction of the veins contributes to the development of ascites.[3,36] Another contributing factor is that the pancreas does not have a well-developed capsule, allowing the surrounding organs, such as the stomach and duodenum, to be affected by a pancreatic tumor.[6]

Clinical Manifestations

Symptoms of pancreatic cancer are slow to develop, contributing to the delay in diagnosis and treatment. Vague abdominal discomfort and weight loss are often observed first. However, it is the jaundice from the bile duct obstruction that often causes the person to initially seek medical care. Back pain is noted to be worse when the person is lying supine; it is often accompanied by nausea, vomiting, and dull epigastric discomfort that radiates to the back.

Dark urine, steatorrhea, jaundice, and pruritus result from the obstruction of the bile duct. Steatorrhea is a result of the malabsorption of fat in the duodenum. Bile salt buildup causes the toxins to be excreted from the skin, causing itching or pruritus. The production of pancreatic enzymes fails, causing malabsorption and weight loss.

Diabetes mellitus is a risk factor for pancreatic cancer but can also be caused by pancreatic cancer. Damage to the beta cells causes decreased insulin production. Older adults with new-onset diabetes should be evaluated for pancreatic cancer.

Late stages of pancreatic cancer involve ascites, hepatomegaly, splenomegaly, and esophageal varices from increased pressure causing portal vein hypertension.[3] The clinical presentation will depend on the size and extent of the cancer and whether there is metastasis to other organs and tissue.

Linking Pathophysiology to Diagnosis and Treatment

Early diagnosis is critical to improve the survival rates from pancreatic cancer, yet no routine screening test is available. Researchers have identified a possible biologic marker that is expected to help with early detection of pancreatic cancer. Exosomes are released by all cells, including cancerous cells. These circulating vesicles release the protein glypican-1 (encoded by the *GPC1* gene), which is specific to pancreatic cancer. The presence of this exosome should help to improve early detection of this devastating cancer.[42]

Diagnosis is usually made with the use of endoscopic ultrasound and contrast-enhanced CT scans. These diagnostic tools can detect smaller tumors that might be missed with percutaneous fine-needle aspiration.[16,36]

Several options are available for the treatment of pancreatic cancer. Surgically, a cholecystojejunostomy or gastrojejunostomy can be performed, but the surgeon may elect to complete a pancreatectomy in an effort to remove the numerous lesions and improve the outcome.[36] A radical antegrade modular pancreatosplenectomy is a new procedure in which dissection proceeds from right to left; in the traditional distal pancreatosplenectomy, the tumor is removed from left to right. Complete tumor resection is considered essential for a cure.[43]

Radiochemotherapy is another treatment choice. Gemcitabine has been the main drug used for more than 20 years. A new chemotherapy option approved is irinotecan liposome used in combination with fluorouracil and leucovorin when gemcitabine treatments are no longer effective.[41] Pancreatic cancer continues to challenge healthcare professionals because its insidious and vague nature, as well as metastasis, contributes to the poor prognosis.

Check Your Progress: Section 43.4

1. Fluid loss into the peritoneum may require administration of which intravenous solution?
2. Which two diagnostic blood tests are used to help make the diagnosis of pancreatitis?
3. What is one complication of pain management for chronic pancreatitis?

CHAPTER SUMMARY

43.1 Chapter Overview and Case Studies

Describe the normal function, epidemiology of alterations, and concepts related to the exocrine pancreatic and hepatobiliary systems.

- The accessory organs of the gastrointestinal tract work together to aid digestion. A complication in one organ often affects the other organs in the hepatobiliary system.
- Concepts related to disorders of the exocrine pancreatic and hepatobiliary systems include immunity, infection, metabolism, hemostasis, elimination, comfort, nutrition, energy balance, environment, and inflammation and oxidative stress.

43.2 Disorders of the Liver

Differentiate the causes, classification, underlying pathogenesis, and clinical manifestations of disorders of the liver and approaches to diagnosis and treatment of these conditions across the lifespan.

- The liver is a metabolically active and vascular organ that affects every other body system. Liver dysfunction causes symptoms and complications in multiple body systems.
- The liver is the largest organ of the abdomen, with cells that have a unique ability to regenerate.
- Liver cancer has a high mortality rate.
- Inflammation and initial damage precede the development of symptoms by a significant amount of time.
- Metabolic disorders of the liver include cirrhosis, caused by hepatitis or alcohol abuse.

43.3 Disorders of the Gallbladder

Differentiate the causes, classification, underlying pathogenesis, and clinical manifestations of disorders of the gallbladder and approaches to diagnosis and treatment of these conditions across the lifespan.

- The gallbladder, a small organ that is used to store bile, contributes to many serious hepatobiliary complications, most often from cholelithiasis.
- Cholelithiasis is stones in the gallbladder. This is a common disorder found most often in females over the age of 40 years who are fair complexioned and overweight.
- Choledocholithiasis is gallstones in the common bile duct leading to an obstruction of the duct, preventing the movement of bile. This leads to chemical damage of surrounding tissues.
- Cholangitis is acute or chronic inflammation of the bile duct, most often resulting from an infection.
- Cholecystitis is acute or chronic inflammation of wall of gallbladder. It results primarily from the formation of a stone and can lead to chemical damage of tissue as a result of accumulating bile.
- Cancer of the gallbladder is often discovered late in the disease course.

43.4 Disorders of the Pancreas

Differentiate the causes, classification, underlying pathogenesis, and clinical manifestations of disorders of the pancreas and approaches to diagnosis and treatment of these conditions across the lifespan.

- Pancreatic disorders result in tissue damage due to the caustic nature of pancreatic enzymes.
- Acute pancreatitis is inflammation or necrosis of the pancreas. It can lead to ischemic damage of the pancreas.
- Chronic pancreatitis is similar to acute pancreatitis except that the chronic pain is often less severe but the tissue damage is irreversible.
- Pancreatic cysts are small fluid-filled sacs in the pancreas. Most are benign and asymptomatic, but some types can become malignant.
- Pancreatic cancer has a high mortality associated with the vague symptoms that contribute to the late diagnosis.

REVIEW QUESTIONS

1. To maintain nutritional status, enzymes from the exocrine pancreas aid in the digestion of which macronutrient? (Select all that apply.)
   a. Fats
   b. Carbohydrates
   c. Proteins
   d. Lipids

2. A new mother brings her infant to the clinic for evaluation because she could feel a mass in the RUQ of the baby's abdomen while she was bathing the baby. She is worried that this is a cancer. The baby has normal eating, defecation, and urination patterns and appears active and responsive. Since birth, the infant has gained weight and height appropriately for age. When the mass is palpated, the infant does not exhibit any distress. What is the most likely reason for this abdominal finding?
   a. Enlarged gallbladder
   b. Severe constipation and large stool mass
   c. Normal finding of the liver extending below the right lower rib cage
   d. Hernia of the abdomen

3. Which of the following is true about neonatal physiologic jaundice?
   a. The neonate's liver is slower to conjugate bilirubin, resulting in impaired excretion and buildup of this substance, causing jaundice.
   b. Only a small percentage of full-term infants develop physiologic jaundice.
   c. Neonatal physiologic jaundice occurs at a higher rate in the premature infant than in the full-term infant.
   d. The red blood cells of newborns have a longer lifespan than those of adults.

4. Which of the following is NOT true about liver cancer?
   a. Liver cancer is more common in developed (industrialized) nations.
   b. Risk factors for liver cancer include obesity, alcoholism, and hepatitis virus infection.
   c. Hepatic cirrhosis is one of the most important risk factors for development of liver cancer.
   d. Primary hepatocellular cancer is more common than metastatic liver cancer.

5. An individual who has suffered alcoholism for many years comes into the emergency department with a complaint of vomiting blood. On physical exam, he is found to have caput medusa, asterixis, and multiple spider angiomas of the face and neck. Which of the following statements is NOT true?
   a. The hematemesis may be due to esophageal varices that developed as a result of portal hypertension.
   b. Abstention from alcohol can improve the individual's prognosis.
   c. Because of the stage of liver damage, there is a reduced risk of development of ascites.
   d. There is a risk of peritonitis.

6. A client has been told that her generalized easy bruising is due to her cholelithiasis, and client education is provided regarding treatment for this symptom. The nurse is aware that:
   a. gallbladder dysfunction causes abdominal pain and elevated blood pressure, causing the bruising.
   b. digestive function is impaired with reduced absorption of vitamin K needed for synthesis of clotting factors.
   c. digestive function is impaired with reduced absorption of protein from the diet, resulting in lack of hemoglobin.
   d. gallbladder dysfunction can cause pancreatitis, which is associated with easy bruising.

7. In the initial management of the individual with acute pancreatitis and absent or hypoactive bowel sounds, why is the individual kept NPO and a nasogastric tube inserted for suctioning?
   a. Keeping the client NPO will reduce the need for changing bed linens that are soiled from vomiting.
   b. NG suctioning will remove the blood from pancreatic hemorrhage.
   c. Medications can be delivered via NG tube to avoid the need for intravenous fluids.
   d. The pancreas needs to rest, and being NPO as well as using nasogastric tube suctioning will reduce digestive stimulation of pancreatic activity.

8. Which of the following is true about pancreatic cysts?
   a. Most pancreatic cysts are highly symptomatic.
   b. Obstructive jaundice occurs with cysts present in the tail of the pancreas.
   c. Noninvasive ultrasound, MRI, or CT scans can determine the type of cyst fluid in order to guide treatment.
   d. Obstruction, fistula, abscess formation, and hemorrhage are possible complications of pancreatic cysts.

ANSWERS

Answers to Review Questions can be found in Appendix A. Answers to Case Study and Check Your Progress questions are available on the faculty resources site. Please consult with your instructor.

RECOMMENDED WEBSITES

Pancreatic Cancer Risk Factors
http://www.cancercenter.com/pancreatic-cancer/risk-factors

Cancer Prevention and Control
https://www.cdc.gov/cancer

Cancer Fact Sheet
http://www.who.int/mediacentre/factsheets/fs297/en

REFERENCES

1. D'Amico, D., & Barbarito, C. (2012). *Health & physical assessment in nursing* (2nd ed.). Upper Saddle River, NJ: Pearson.
2. Dillon, P. (2016). *Nursing health assessment* (3rd ed.). Philadelphia, PA: F.A. Davis.
3. Capriotti, T., & Frizzell, J. (2015). *Pathophysiology: Introductory concepts and clinical perspectives*. Philadelphia, PA: F.A. Davis.
4. Marieb, E., & Hoehn, K. (2015). *Human anatomy & physiology* (10th ed.). San Francisco, CA: Pearson.
5. Pearson. (2018). *Nursing: A concept-based approach to learning* (Vol. 1, 3rd ed.). Hoboken, NJ: Pearson Education.
6. Sole, M., & Klein, D. (2013). *Introduction to critical care nursing* (6th ed.). St. Louis, MO: Elsevier.
7. Corbett, J. (2013). *Laboratory tests and diagnostic procedures with nursing diagnosis* (8th ed.). Upper Saddle River, NJ: Pearson.
8. Altekruse, S., Henley, J., Cucinelli, J., & McGlynn, K., (2014). Changing hepatocellular carcinoma incidence and liver cancer mortality rates in the United States. *American Journal of Gastroenterology, 109*, 542–553. doi:1038/ajg.2014.11
9. American Cancer Society. (2015). *How many people get liver cancer?* Available at http://cancer.org/cancer/livercancer/overviewguide/liver-cancer-overview-key-statistics
10. Aravalli, R., Cressman, E., & Steer, C. (2013). Cellular and molecular mechanisms of hepatocellular carcinoma: An update. *Archives of Toxicology, 87*, 227–247. doi:10.1007/s00204-012-0931-2
11. Bruha, R., Dvorak, K., & Petrtyl, J. (2012). Alcoholic liver disease. *World Journal of Hepatology, 4*(3), 81–90. Available at http://www.ncbi.nlm.nih.gov/pmc/articles/PMC3321494/
12. Duqum, M., & McCullough, A. (2015). Diagnosis and management of alcoholic liver disease. *Journal of Clinical and Translational Hepatology, 3*(2), 109–116. doi:10:14218/JCTH.2015.00008
13. Shen, Y., Chen, S., Peng, Y., Shi, Y., Huang, X., Yang, G. H., Ding, Z. B., Yi, Y., Zhou, J., Qiu, S. J., Fan, J., & Ren, N. (2014). Quantitative assessment of the effect of glutathione S-transferase genes GSTM1 and GSTT1 on hepatocellular carcinoma risk. *Tumor Biology, 35*, 4007–4015. doi:10.1007/s13277-013-1524-2
14. American Cancer Society (2015). *Hepatitis B virus*. Available at http://www.cancer.org/acs/groups/content/@research/documents/webcontent/acspc-045101.pdf
15. American Cancer Society. (2016). Liver cancer risk factors. Retrieved from https://www.cancer.org/cancer/liver-cancer/causes-risks-prevention/risk-factors.html
16. American Cancer Society. (2016). Tests for liver cancer. Retrieved from https://www.cancer.org/cancer/liver-cancer/detection-diagnosis-staging/how-diagnosed.html
17. Tanaka, S., Iimuro, Y., Hirano, T., Hai, S., Suzumura, K., & Fujimoto, J. (2015). Outcomes of hepatic resection for large hepatocellular carcinoma: Special reference to postoperative recurrence. *American Surgeon, 81*(1), 64–73.
18. American Cancer Society. (2016). Early detection, diagnosis, and staging. Retrieved from https://www.cancer.org/content/dam/CRC/PDF/Public/8700.00.pdf
19. Wang, Y., Wang, B., Shen, F., Fan, J., & Cao, H. (2012). Body Mass Index and Risk of Primary Liver Cancer: A Meta-Analysis of Prospective Studies. *The Oncologist, 17*(11), 1461–1468. http://doi.org/10.1634/theoncologist.2012-0066
20. Munkvold, G., Hurburgh, C., & Meyer, J. (2012). *Aflatoxins in corn*. Iowa State University. Available at https://store.extension.iastate.edu/Product/pm1800-pdf
21. Duan, F., Yu, W., Wang, Y., Liu, F., Wang, Z., Yan, J., Yuan, K., & Wang, M. (2015). Trans-arterial chemoembolization and external beam radiation therapy for treatment of hepatocellular carcinoma with a tumor thrombus in the inferior vena cava and right atrium. *Cancer Imaging 15*(1), 7. doi:10.1186/s40644-015-0043.3
22. Catalano, O., Izzo, F., Vallone, P., Sandomenico, F., Albino, V., Nunziata, A., Fusco, R., & Perillo, A. (2014). Integrating contrast-enhanced sonography in the follow-up algorithm of hepatocellular carcinoma treated with radiofrequency ablation: Single cancer center experience. *Acta Radiologica, 56*(2), 133–142. doi:10.1177/0284185114521108
23. National Cancer Institute. (2013). FDA approval for sorafenib tosylate. Retrieved from https://www.cancer.gov/about-cancer/treatment/drugs/fda-sorafenib-tosylate
24. Patel, T., & Harnois, D. (2014). Assessment of response to therapy in hepatocellular carcinoma. *Annals of Medicine, 46*, 130–137.
25. American Liver Foundation (2015). *Cirrhosis*. Available at http://www.liverfoundation.org/abouttheliver/info/cirrhosis
26. Dickson, G. (2012). Gynecomastia. *American Family Physician, 85*(7), 716–722. Available at http://www.aafp.org/afp/2012/0401/p716.html
27. Mayo Clinic. (2017). Esophageal varices. Retrieved from http://www.mayoclinic.org/diseases-conditions/esophageal-varices/diagnosis-treatment/treatment/txc-20206471
28. Steel, P. A. D. (2017). Acute cholecystitis and biliary colic. *Medscape*. Retrieved from http://emedicine.medscape.com/article/1950020-overview
29. Penn State Hershey. (2016). Gallstones and gallbladder disease. Retrieved from http://pennstatehershey.adam.com/content.aspx?productId=10&pid=10&gid=000010
30. Siddiqui, A. A. (2016). Choledocholithiasis and cholangitis. *Merck Manual*. Retrieved from http://www.merckmanuals.com/professional/hepatic-and-biliary-disorders/gallbladder-and-bile-duct-disorders/choledocholithiasis-and-cholangitis
31. Medline Plus. (2017). Acute cholecystitis. Retrieved from https://medlineplus.gov/ency/article/000264.htm
32. American Cancer Society. (2015). *Gallbladder cancer*. Available at http://www.cancer.org/cancer/gallbladdercancer/detailedguide/gallbladder-key-statistics
33. Cancer Net. (2015). *Gallbladder cancer: Statistics*. Available at http://www.cancer.net/cancer-types/gallbladder-cancer/statistics
34. John Hopkins Pathology. (2016). *Gallbladder and bile duct cancer*. Available at http://pathology.jhu.edu/gbbd/disease_info.cfm
35. Tang, J. C. F. (2017). Acute pancreatitis. *Medscape*. Retrieved from http://emedicine.medscape.com/article/181364-overview
36. Huffman, J. L. (2016). Chronic pancreatitis. Medscape. Retrieved from http://emedicine.medscape.com/article/181554-overview
37. Nakai, Y., Iwashita, T., Park, D., Samarasena, J., Lee, J., & Chang, K. (2015). Diagnosis of pancreatic cysts: EUS-guided, through-the-needle confocal laser-induced endomicroscopy

and cystoscopy trial: DETECT study. *Gastrointestinal Endoscopy, 81*(5), 1204–1214.

38. Nikiforova, M., Khalid, A., Fasanella, K., et al. (2013). Integration of KRAS testing in the diagnosis of pancreatic cystic lesions: A clinical experience of 618 pancreatic cysts. *Modern Pathology, 26*, 1478–1487.
39. Nougaret, S., Reinhold, C., Chong, J., Escal, L., Mercier, G., Fabre, J. M., Guiu, B., & Molinari, N. (2014). Incidental pancreatic cysts: Natural history and diagnostic accuracy of a limited serial pancreatic cyst MRI protocol. *European Radiology, 24*, 1020–1029. doi:10.1007/s00330-014-3112-2
40. Cleveland Clinic. (2014). Pancreatic cysts and pseudocysts. Retrieved from https://my.clevelandclinic.org/health/articles/pancreatic-cysts-and-pseudocysts
41. Cancer Treatment Centers of America. (n.d.). *Pancreatic cancer.* Available at http://www.cancercenter.com/pancreatic-cancer/risk-factor
42. National Cancer Institute. (n.d.). *Pancreatic cancer study finds possible diagnostic marker in blood.* Available at http://www.cancer.gov/news-events/cancer-currents-blog/2015/pancreatic-exosomes
43. Murakawa, M., Aoyama, T., Asari, M., et al. (2015). The short- and long-term outcomes of radical antegrade modular pancreatosplenectomy for adenocarcinoma of the body and tail of the pancreas. *BioMedicalCentral Surgery, 15*(120), 1–6. doi:10.1186/s12893-015-0107-0

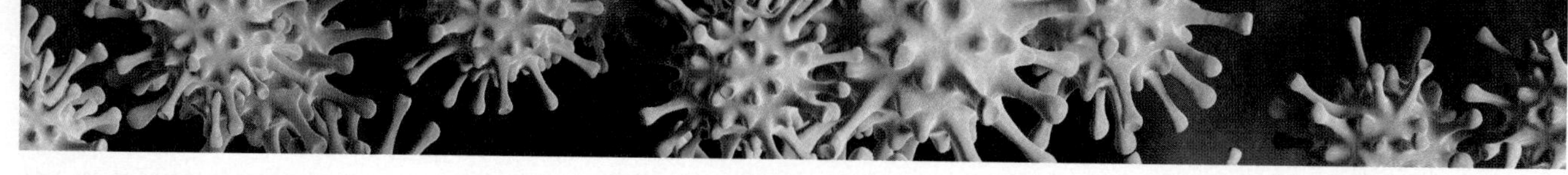

Chapter 44
Liver Failure

Carolyn Driscoll

Chapter Outline and Learning Outcomes

44.1 Chapter Overview and Case Studies

Define liver failure, including populations most at risk and key pathologic concepts related to failure.

44.2 The Normal Liver

Outline the normal function of the liver.

44.3 Clinical Manifestations and Complications of Liver Failure

Differentiate underlying pathogenesis of liver failure and common complications in the context of approaches to treatment and diagnosis across the lifespan.

44.4 Common Causes of Liver Failure

Differentiate the causes, classification, underlying pathogenesis, and clinical manifestations of disorders causing liver failure and approaches to diagnosis and treatment of these conditions across the lifespan.

KEY TERMS

Acute liver failure, 1110
Alcoholic liver disease, 1107
Ascites, 1100
Autoimmune hepatitis, 1109
Ballooning degeneration, 1107
Bilirubin, 1102
Cholestasis, 1102
Cirrhosis, 1097
Conjugated bilirubin, 1102
Esophageal varices, 1100
Hepatitis, 1103
Hepatocytes, 1098
Hepatomegaly, 1108
Hepatopulmonary syndrome (HPS), 1101
Hepatorenal syndrome (HRS), 1101
Icterus, 1102
Jaundice, 1102
Mallory bodies, 1107
Nonalcoholic fatty liver disease (NAFLD), 1109
Portal hypertension, 1099
Portopulmonary syndrome, 1102
Portosystemic shunt, 1100
Splanchnic circulation, 1098
Steatohepatitis, 1107
Steatosis, 1105
Unconjugated bilirubin, 1102

ABBREVIATIONS

cccDNA—covalently closed circular DNA
HAV—hepatitis A virus
HBV—hepatitis B virus
HCC—hepatocellular carcinoma
HCV—hepatitis C virus
HDV—hepatitis D virus
HEV—hepatitis E virus
HLA—human leukocyte antigen
HPS—hepatopulmonary syndrome
HRS—hepatorenal syndrome
NAFLD—nonalcoholic fatty liver disease
NASH—nonalcoholic steatohepatitis
TIPS—transjugular intrahepatic portosystemic shunt

44.1 Chapter Overview and Case Studies

The liver is the largest solid organ in the body and has a multitude of functions. It is involved in the regulation of coagulation and nutrition and plays a major role in the metabolism and excretion of medications. Considering the importance of this organ, any deterioration in its function can have significant consequences for health. The loss of liver function is referred to as failure. A number of clinical conditions are associated with the development of acute or chronic liver failure. Both acute and chronic failure result in a several clinical signs and symptoms. Understanding the signs and symptoms of liver failure and the underlying pathogenesis will enhance identification and management of this serious condition.

There are several potential causes of liver failure, ranging from substance ingestion to viral etiologies. Excessive consumption of alcohol is the major cause of chronic liver disease around the world.[1] Alcohol-related liver failure is considered the third most preventable cause of death in the United States alone. Exposure to a particular virus (hepatitis C), is another leading cause of liver disease across the globe. Liver damage and ultimately failure are therefore serious, life-threatening conditions.

Concepts Related to Liver Failure

The liver is a complex organ with many functions, including detoxification, storage, metabolism, and production of many substances. As a result, liver failure can manifest with a myriad of symptoms and associated conditions. However, understanding the underlying pathophysiology of liver failure will allow differentiation between acute liver failure and **cirrhosis** (scarring of the liver associated with poor liver function). Acute liver failure is more commonly associated with elevated liver tests resulting from inflammation or hepatocyte destruction. This is associated with laboratory changes, such as prolonged coagulation, and clinical symptoms such as altered mental status due to decreased toxin clearance. In contrast, liver failure associated with cirrhosis may have similar symptoms but is often commonly found also to have systemic changes associated with portal hypertension. Concepts related to liver failure are shown in **Figure 44.1** ■.

Case Studies

The following cases are addressed throughout the chapter to assist in application of chapter content to clinical situations that involve individuals with liver failure.

Henry Winston: Introduction

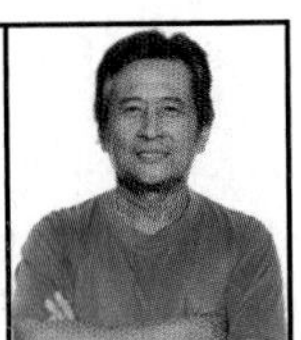

Henry Winston, age 59, is seen by his primary care provider after learning that he had elevated liver function tests during his annual work physical at his employee health clinic. He states that he has been doing fine. Mr. Winston last saw his primary care provider 5 years earlier, so a comprehensive history and physical examination are performed. Mr. Winston denies any current alcohol or drug use but admits to a history of intravenous drug use in his 20s. His physical exam is within normal parameters except for an enlarged liver that is palpable.

1. What risk factors does Mr. Winston have for liver disease?
2. What role does the liver play in Mr. Winston's health?

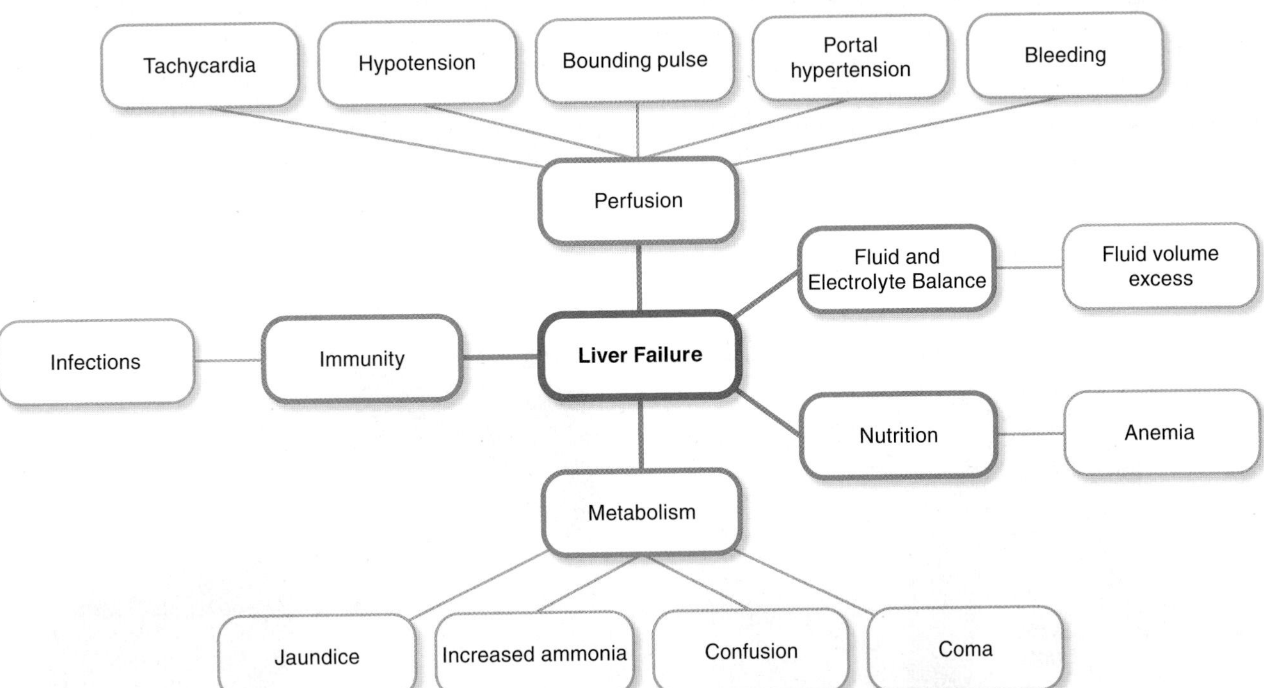

Figure 44.1 ■ Concepts related to liver failure include metabolism, perfusion, fluid and electrolyte balance, nutrition, and immunity, among others. Signs and symptoms of these alterations in these related concepts are shown in the outer ring on the map.

Sylvia St. John: Introduction

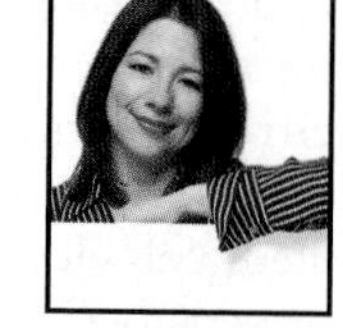

Sylvia St. John, age 48, visits her primary care provider for an annual evaluation. She had been feeling well until 4–5 months earlier, when she developed nausea with occasional vomiting on awakening in the morning. She complains of mild shortness of breath and feels that she has been more forgetful lately.

1. Which of Ms. St. John's manifestations may indicate liver disease?
2. What is the most common cause of chronic liver disease?

Check Your Progress: Section 44.1

1. What is the leading cause of liver disease worldwide?
2. What is acute liver failure?
3. What is cirrhosis?

44.2 The Normal Liver

The liver is the largest solid organ in the body. It is located in the right upper quadrant of the abdomen and weighs between 1200 and 1600 grams. It is a complex organ with many functions, including bile production; detoxification; storage of certain vitamins and minerals; production of proteins; and metabolism of carbohydrates, proteins, and fat. It acts as the intersection of the **splanchnic circulation** (circulation of the gastrointestinal organs, including the small intestines, colon, pancreas, stomach, liver, and spleen) and systemic circulation.

The liver has two lobes, the right and left, defined by the right and left portal veins, which supply them. The liver is attached to the diaphragm and abdominal wall by the falciform ligament, which separates the two lobes (**Figure 44.2** ■). The right lobe is further divided into the caudate and quadrate lobes. A covering of connective tissue, called the Glisson capsule, surrounds the entire liver and contains nerves, blood vessels, and lymphatics. Distention of the capsule from an enlarged liver may cause pain or result in the release of fluid into the abdominal cavity from the lymphatic system.[2]

The lobes of the liver are made up of numerous functional units called lobules. A lobule consists of cords of **hepatocytes** (hepatic cells) arranged in a radial pattern around a central vein from the hepatic venous system (**Figure 44.3** ■). The parenchyma closest to the central vein is known as the centrilobular parenchyma. The next section is the midzonal parenchyma, and furthest away from the central vein is the periportal area, which borders the portal tract. Portal tracts are in the periphery and composed of a terminal bile duct, hepatic artery, and portal vein. Many types of hepatic injury demonstrate a zonal distribution of damage. Between the hepatocytes are sinusoids, which are lined with Kupffer cells that destroy bacteria and other foreign material in the blood. As blood passes through the sinusoids, oxygen is extracted, foreign material is removed, and nutrients are absorbed by the hepatocytes for metabolism.[2]

Also located in the lobule are bile canaliculi and the spaces of Disse. The hepatocytes produce bile, which drains into the tiny bile ducts (canaliculi) located between the cords of hepatocytes. Bile from the canaliculi drains into the terminal bile ducts leading to the right and left hepatic ducts. The spaces of Disse are located between the sinusoids and the hepatocytes. As blood flows through the sinusoids, substances can pass freely from the blood into the spaces of Disse. Excess fluid in this space is drained by the lymph system.[2]

The liver has a dual blood supply, composed of the hepatic artery and the portal vein, which carry approximately 25% of the body's total cardiac output. The hepatic artery, which supplies approximately 30% of the blood to the liver, branches from the aorta and supplies oxygenated blood. The portal vein, which supplies approximately 70% of the blood to the liver, provides primarily deoxygenated, nutrient-rich blood from the splenic vein and the inferior and superior mesenteric veins. Blood from the hepatic artery and the portal vein mix and enter the sinusoids of the liver lobules. Blood leaves the liver through the hepatic vein to the inferior vena cava for recirculation.[2]

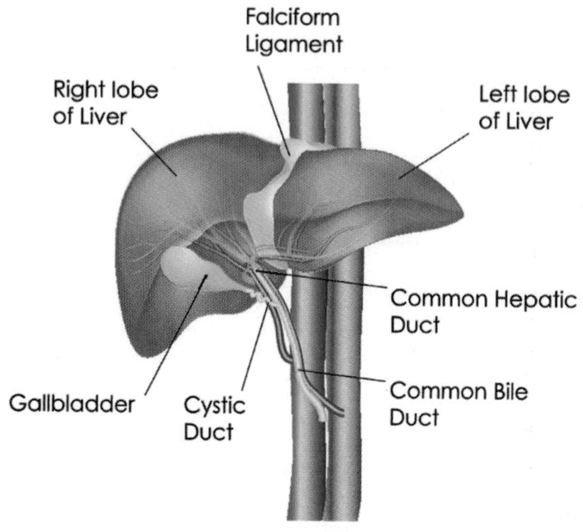

Figure 44.2 ■ Anatomy of the liver.

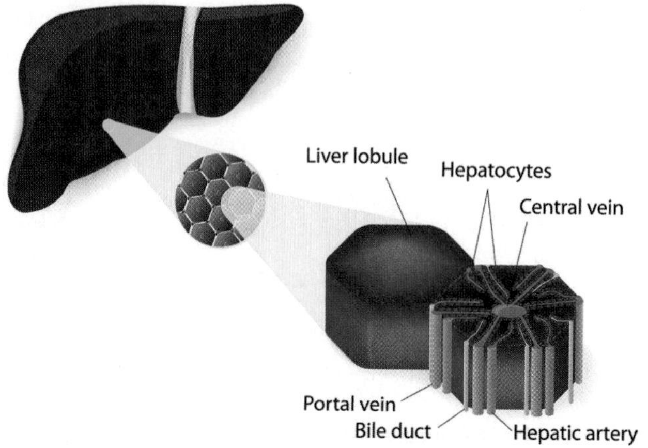

Figure 44.3 ■ Structure of the liver lobule.

Check Your Progress: Section 44.2

1. Describe the function of the Kupffer cells.
2. Which structure of the liver aids in draining excess fluid?
3. Trace the flow of blood through the liver.

44.3 Clinical Manifestations and Complications of Liver Failure

Liver failure is associated with many clinical manifestations that affect the liver as well as other organs. These clinical consequences may develop as a result of progressive chronic liver disease or from acute liver disease (**Figure 44.4** ■). More than 80–90% of hepatic function must be compromised before hepatic failure is evident. The most common complications of chronic liver failure include portal hypertension, which is associated with splenomegaly, esophageal varices, and ascites, and hepatic encephalopathy. Less common complications include hepatopulmonary syndrome, portopulmonary hypertension, hepatorenal syndrome, hyponatremia, and hepatic pleural effusion.[2] Acute liver failure is associated with hepatic encephalopathy and coagulopathy in a noncirrhotic liver.[3]

Portal Hypertension

Portal hypertension is the result of increased resistance to blood flow through the portal venous system (**Figure 44.5** ■). It is defined as increased portal venous pressure demonstrated by a portal pressure gradient greater than 5 mmHg. Normal portal pressure is approximately 3 mmHg. Hepatic venous pressure measurements greater than 10 mmHg are typically associated with the

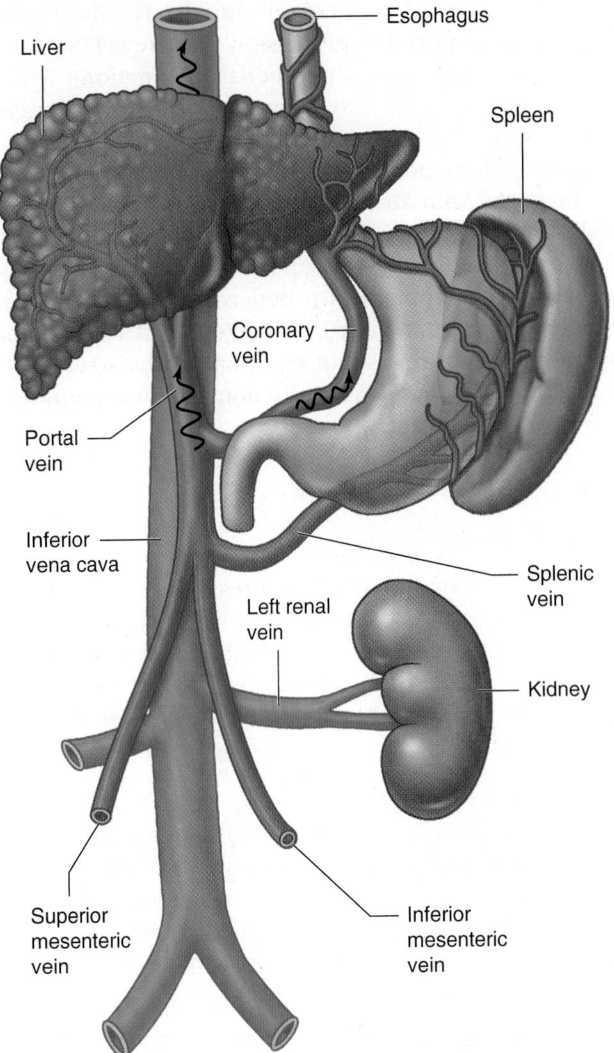

Figure 44.5 ■ Portal hypertension.

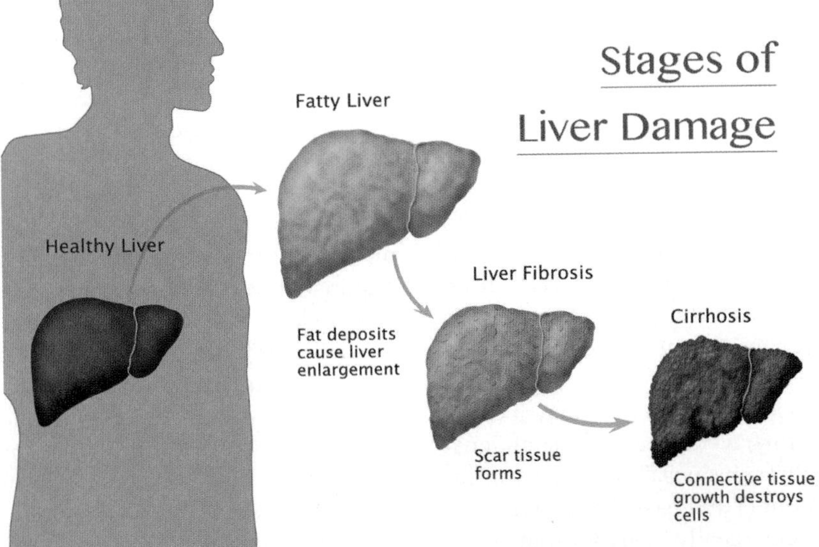

Figure 44.4 ■ Changes in the liver that occur with progressive damage from a variety of liver conditions. Each panel shows histologic changes with increasing fibrosis leading to cirrhosis.

clinical manifestation of complications.[4] The most common cause of portal hypertension is cirrhosis (scarring of the liver associated with poor liver function), which results in decreased intrahepatic blood flow. Noncirrhotic causes of portal hypertension include prehepatic causes, such as portal vein thrombosis and narrowing of the portal vein, or posthepatic causes, such as severe right-sided congestive heart failure and hepatic vein outflow obstruction.[5] Increasing portal pressure is associated with the development of a hyperdynamic circulation, esophageal varices and hemorrhage, rectal varices, and splenomegaly. Ascites and encephalopathy develop as a result of systemic circulatory abnormalities and/or a **portosystemic shunt**.[4]

Esophageal Varices

Etiology and Pathogenesis

Esophageal varices develop as a result of increased portal hypertension. As the portosystemic gradient increases, there is decreased flow through the liver, resulting in increased pressure in the blood vessels lining the esophagus. As the size of the blood vessels increases, so does the risk of bleeding.[4]

Clinical Manifestations

Classic symptoms of acute bleeding from esophageal varices may include melena, hematemesis, or bright red blood from the rectum. Slow bleeding may result in a progressive decline in the hemoglobin and hematocrit levels, leading to symptoms of dyspnea and fatigue with or without the presence of melena.[6]

Linking Pathophysiology to Diagnosis and Treatment

Bleeding from esophageal varices is a leading cause of hospital admission that develops from a combination of erosion by gastric acid or certain medications (in particular, nonsteroidal anti-inflammatory drugs) and increasing portal pressure.[7] The annual rate of bleeding for esophageal varices is estimated at 5–15%.[7] The risk increases with increasing portal pressure and increasing size of the varices. Acute bleeding from ruptured esophageal varices is a clinical emergency and requires immediate hospitalization as significant blood loss leading to shock may occur. It is associated with a 20% risk of death within 6 weeks of a bleed. The 1-year mortality rate after an acute esophageal bleed ranges from 20% to 60%, with greater mortality in the setting of higher portal pressure.[7] Less commonly, bleeding may develop from gastric varices, typically seen as hematemesis or melena, or from rectal varices, which may present as large amounts of bright red blood from the rectum.

Treatment of acute esophageal bleeding may include the use of vasoconstrictors, venodilators, esophageal band ligation, and blood transfusions. Transjugular intrahepatic portosystemic shunt (TIPS) has also been used to decrease portal pressure emergently. Long-term management includes recurrent esophageal band ligation until varices are eradicated, the use of nonselective beta blockers, and TIPS.[8]

Ascites

Etiology and Pathogenesis

Ascites, which is the abnormal collection of excess fluid in the abdominal cavity, is the most common complication of cirrhosis, occurring in about 10% of patients.[9] Development of ascites is an indicator of poor prognosis that is associated with increased mortality—56% within 3 years—and morbidity, such as the development of spontaneous bacterial peritonitis or hepatorenal syndrome.[9] The underlying pathogenesis of ascites formation is complex and thought to be the result of peripheral arterial vasodilation. Portal hypertension leads to arterial vasodilation of the splanchnic circulation, which results in decreased systemic vascular resistance. In addition, vasodilator factors such as nitric oxide, carbon monoxide, and endogenous cannabinoids have demonstrated increased activity and production. Spontaneous portosytemic shunts also develop as portal hypertension develops, leading to the redirection of blood and vasodilators from the splanchnic to the systemic circulation. Capillary permeability and lymph formation increase in the splanchnic organs, and ascites develops when the body can no longer absorb this fluid.[9]

Clinical Manifestations

Clinical manifestations of ascites include increased abdominal girth, weight gain, bulging flanks, and shifting dullness. With significant ascites, patients may also experience decreased appetite, abdominal discomfort, and dyspnea due to pressure from the abdominal fluid.[6]

Linking Pathophysiology to Diagnosis and Treatment

Addressing the underlying liver disease may help to improve ascites. For example, when patients with alcoholic cirrhosis stop drinking, their ascites may improve or go away completely. However, in most cases, treatment is targeted at reducing the amount of ascites. The most common treatment approach involves the use of diuretics and sodium restriction. The target sodium intake is less than 2000 mg a day. The most common oral diuretic regimen is single morning doses of both spironolactone and furosemide. The use of both diuretics helps to minimize the hyperkalemia associated with spironolactone. Use of furosemide alone is less efficacious than use of spironolactone alone.[10] Electrolytes (sodium and potassium) and creatinine levels should be monitored during diuretic treatment.

Refractory ascites, which is fluid that is resistant to maximal diuretic doses and a sodium restricted diet, may require frequent large-volume paracentesis (a procedure in which a large volume of ascites is drained from the abdominal cavity) (**Figure 44.6** ■). This procedure can be done in the outpatient setting. Monitoring of vital signs, ascites output, electrolytes, creatinine, and fluid cell count to evaluate for infection is part of the procedural care. Patients from whom more than 5 liters of ascites fluid is drained should receive intravenous 25% albumin at an amount equivalent to 8 g/L fluid removed.[9,10]

Shunts have been used to decrease portal pressure. A TIPS may be beneficial for some patients with refractory ascites. The TIPS is usually inserted by an interventional

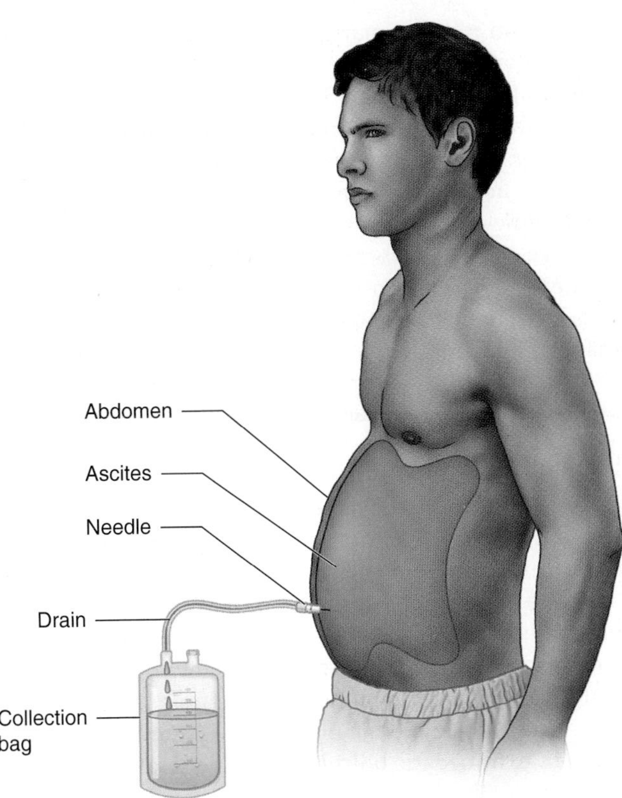

Figure 44.6 ■ Paracentesis.

radiologist and bridges the portal vein and hepatic vein, allowing approximately 70% of inflowing blood to bypass the liver. This reduces portal pressures, resulting in decreased ascites formation. The most common complication of a TIPS is the development of moderate to severe hepatic encephalopathy.

Sylvia St. John: Application

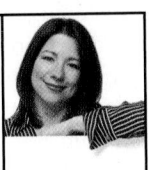

Ms. St. John admits to drinking two to three glasses of wine a day and says that her father is an alcoholic. Her physical examination reveals an obese woman with a respiratory rate of 22, O_2 saturation of 94%, and decreased breath sounds in the lower half of her right lung. Her abdomen is distended, with fluid present. Laboratory tests are ordered to further assess Ms. St. John's liver function.

3. What clinical manifestations may Ms. St. John expect if her condition is due to ascites?
4. How might abstention from alcoholic beverages affect Ms. St. John's condition?

Hepatorenal Syndrome

Etiology and Pathogenesis

Hepatorenal syndrome (HRS), which is defined as functional renal failure, develops as a result of portal hypertension and the associated systemic circulatory changes.[11] It develops almost exclusively in patients with ascites. Type 1 HRS develops as a result of the significant reduction of circulating volume associated with excessive splanchnic arterial vasodilation and decreased cardiac output. It is a rapidly progressing condition in which the serum creatinine level increases over 2.5 mg/dL within 2 weeks. Median survival is 1 month.[12] Type 2 HRS has a better prognosis. This functional renal failure occurs in patients with cirrhosis and ascites with a serum creatinine level over 1.5 mg/dL. The median survival is 6.7 months. The main mechanism of renal dysfunction develops from renal arterial resistance, which leads to renal hypoperfusion, and from arterial hypotension. The underlying pathophysiology of HRS develops as a result of the portal hypertension changes, including decreased peripheral vascular resistance, leading to vasodilation, central hypervolemia, increased cardiac output and compensatory mechanisms that affect the sympathetic nervous system and the renin–angiotensin–aldosterone system that stimulates increased resorption of sodium in the proximal tubule.[11]

Clinical Manifestations

In the clinical presentation of hepatorenal syndrome, serum creatinine is elevated without other evidence of underlying renal disease, shock, or nephrotoxic drugs. However, there is no specific test to diagnose hepatorenal syndrome. Ascites is typically present.[11,12]

Linking Pathophysiology to Diagnosis and Treatment

Liver transplantation is the preferred treatment for hepatorenal syndrome, after which there is a return of renal function in patients without other renal disorders.[7] Other treatments for hepatorenal syndrome are focused on delaying progression. Albumin infusions are used to expand the circulatory blood volume. Vasoconstrictors, such as terlipressin, are used to constrict blood flow in the splanchnic bed. This corrects the underlying vasodilation and decreased cardiac output. Renal replacement therapy may be used for life-threatening electrolyte imbalance, metabolic acidosis, or volume overload and as a bridge to liver transplantation.[9,11]

Hepatopulmonary Syndrome

Etiology and Pathogenesis

Hepatopulmonary syndrome (HPS) is a common complication of cirrhosis resulting in arterial hypoxemia. The pathophysiology of HPS in humans is incompletely understood. However, it is recognized that intrapulmonary vasodilation can lead to hypoxemia. Nitric oxide and pulmonary angiogenesis are both proposed mechanisms.[13]

Clinical Manifestations

Clinical findings are often nonspecific but may include dyspnea, which is a common complaint with many etiologies, or clubbing of the fingers, which may be seen when HPS has been present for a longer time. Pulse oximetry can be used to screen for HPS. SaO_2 levels less than 97% can detect patients with HPS and a PaO_2 less than 70 mmHg. An SaO_2 level less than 94% identifies more severe hypoxemia with a PaO_2 less than 60 mmHg with high reliability and specificity.[13]

Linking Pathophysiology to Diagnosis and Treatment

Liver transplantation is the only treatment that reliably improves oxygenation in patients with HPS. However, other treatments have been tried, including agents that affect the nitrous oxide pathway, somatostatin, almitrine (a pulmonary vasoconstrictor), propranolol (reduce portal hypertension), cyclooxygenase inhibitors, antibiotics (gut decontamination), pentoxifylline (tumor necrosis factor alpha [TNF-α] inhibitor), and garlic. Responses to these treatments vary. Supplemental oxygen may also be used, although improvement in dyspnea or quality of life has not been demonstrated.[13]

Portopulmonary Syndrome

Portopulmonary syndrome is a serious complication of portal hypertension from cirrhotic and noncirrhotic causes. It is defined as the presence of pulmonary artery hypertension that develops as a consequence of portal hypertension.

Etiology and Pathogenesis

The underlying pathophysiology leading to portopulmonary syndrome remains unclear without an apparent relationship between the severity of the pulmonary hypertension and the underlying liver disease.

Clinical Manifestations

Patients with portopulmonary syndrome may experience dyspnea at rest or with exertion. Chest pain or syncope may be seen with severe portopulmonary syndrome. Less frequently seen signs include a hyperdynamic precordium, an accentuated second heart sound, or a systolic murmur caused by tricuspid regurgitation. Jugular vein distention, peripheral edema, ascites, and an S3 may be found in patients with severe portopulmonary syndrome. Mild hypoxemia may be present, but clubbing of the nails and cyanosis are not common. Diagnostic criteria for portopulmonary syndrome include the following:

- Portal hypertension
- Mean pulmonary artery pressure greater than or equal to 25 mmHg
- Pulmonary vascular resistance greater than 240 dyne/s/cm^{-5}
- Pulmonary capillary wedge pressure 15 mmHg or less
- Transpulmonary gradient greater than 12 mmHg.

Severity is determined based on the mean pulmonary artery pressure: mild (more than 24, less than 35 mmHg), moderate (35 or more to less than 45 mmHg) or severe (more than 45 mmHg). Portopulmonary syndrome is characterized by pulmonary obstructions resulting in increased pressure, in contrast to HPS, which is associated with vasodilation. This difference is particularly pertinent in terms of liver transplantation, as moderate to severe portopulmonary syndrome may be an exclusion to liver transplantation, while HPS can be an indication for liver transplantation.[14,15]

Linking Pathophysiology to Diagnosis and Treatment

The treatment goal for portopulmonary syndrome is to improve pulmonary hemodynamics by reducing the obstruction to pulmonary arterial flow. Medications that result in vasodilation, antiplatelet aggregation, and antiproliferative effects may be used. Liver transplantation may also potentially cure portopulmonary syndrome. However, an inability to reduce the pulmonary artery pressure below transplant center guidelines may be a contraindication for liver transplantation.[14] Previous studies have shown 100% mortality if the mean PAP is over 50 mmHg, 50% of mortality if the mean PAP is between 35 and 50 mmHg, and 0% mortality if the mean PAP is less than 35 mmHg.[15]

Jaundice and Cholestasis

Etiology and Pathogenesis

Bilirubin is produced as the final product in the degradation of heme from natural destruction of red blood cells, premature destruction of newly formed red blood cells in the bone marrow, and turnover of hepatic heme or hemeproteins. Elevated levels of bilirubin can result in **jaundice** (yellowing of the skin) or **icterus** (yellowing of the sclerae of the eyes), as well as **cholestasis**, the systemic retention of excess bilirubin and other bile solutes (**Figure 44.7** ■). Once formed, extrahepatic bilirubin binds with albumin and is delivered to the liver, where it undergoes glucuronidation in the endoplasmic reticulum, resulting in the excretion of water-soluble, nontoxic bilirubin glucuronides into the bile. Gut bacteria then deconjugate the bilirubin into colorless urobilinogens that are excreted with any remaining intact bile pigments in the feces. Some of these products may be resorbed and excreted in the urine. This process results in the formation of both conjugated and unconjugated bilirubin.

There is an important difference between unconjugated and conjugated bilirubin. **Unconjugated bilirubin** is tightly bound to serum albumin and is essentially insoluble in water. Therefore, this type of bilirubin cannot be excreted in the urine. In contrast, **conjugated bilirubin** is loosely bound to albumin, nontoxic, and water soluble. Consequently, this form of bilirubin can be excreted in the urine. See **Table 44.1** ■ for causes of jaundice.[16–18]

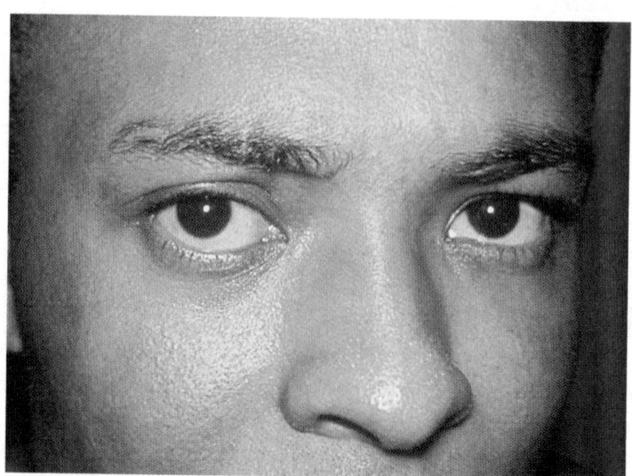

Figure 44.7 ■ Jaundice.

Table 44.1 Causes of Jaundice

Primarily Unconjugated Hyperbilirubinemia	Primarily Conjugated Hyperbilirubinemia
Gilbert syndrome	Dubin Johnson syndrome
Crigler Najjar type I	Impaired bile flow
Crigler Najjar type II	
Hemolytic anemias	
Resorption of blood from hemorrhage	
Thalassemia	
Pernicious anemia	
Neonatal jaundice	

Cholestasis can develop as a result of hepatocellular dysfunction or biliary obstruction from intrahepatic or extrahepatic causes. Severe hepatic dysfunction from acute liver failure or advanced chronic liver disease and cirrhosis can result in hyperbilirubinemia and cholestasis. Drug-induced liver disease[16] and sepsis[17] may also cause cholestasis. Hepatocellular damage and obstruction of bile canaliculi interfere with the normal process of bilirubin uptake, glucuronidation, and excretion, resulting in increases in conjugated and unconjugated bilirubin.

Extrahepatic obstructive cholestasis may develop as a result of obstruction of the common bile duct from a tumor, a gallstone, or compression from other etiologies such as pancreatitis. The liver continues to conjugate the bilirubin, which cannot pass through the liver to the duodenum for excretion in the feces. Instead, the water-soluble conjugated bilirubin enters the bloodstream and is excreted in the urine.[18]

Clinical Manifestations

Yellowing of the skin and icterus are the most common signs of jaundice. As bilirubin levels increase, urine may become darker in color (tea colored), and stools become lighter in color (clay colored). This occurs as the excretion of bilirubin is shifted. Pruritus is a common symptom associated with hyperbilirubinemia as a result of deposition of bile acids in peripheral tissues, including the skin. Levels of serum alkaline phosphatase and gamma glutamyl transpeptidase (GGT) may also be elevated. Xanthomas, which are lipid deposits in the skin typically seen around the eyes, may also be seen in some cholestatic disorders. Reduced bile flow results in decreased intestinal absorption, so deficiencies of fat-soluble vitamins such as A, D, and K may be seen. Fever, chills and right upper quadrant abdominal pain may be present in cholecystitis or infectious causes of hyperbilirubinemia.[18]

Linking Pathophysiology to Diagnosis and Treatment

Treatment of jaundice and cholestasis varies according to the underlying etiology. Some conditions, such as Gilbert syndrome, do not require intervention. Similarly, jaundice associated with resorption of a hematoma does not require intervention and symptoms improve with time. In a similar fashion, neonatal jaundice generally does not require treatment, but phototherapy may be used to help break down the bilirubin accumulated in the skin. Pruritus associated with jaundice can be symptomatically treated with several different types of medications, including bile salt resins, rifampin, opioid antagonists, and sertraline.[19] Obstructive jaundice may respond to insertion of a biliary stent or surgery (e.g., cholecystectomy).[20]

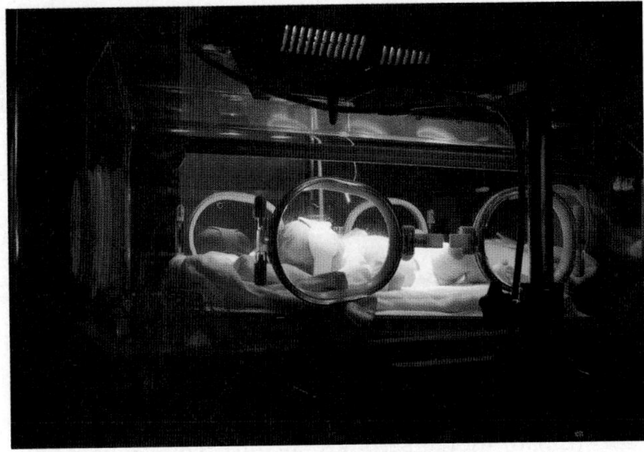

Figure 44.8 ■ Treatment for neonatal jaundice.

Neonatal jaundice is treated with special light therapy. If the neonate does not respond, further investigation is required (**Figure 44.8** ■). ■

> **Check Your Progress: Section 44.3**
>
> 1. What are the clinical manifestations of esophageal varices?
> 2. What are the consequences of elevated bilirubin levels?
> 3. Describe the difference between unconjugated and conjugated bilirubin.

44.4 Common Causes of Liver Failure

Viral Hepatitis

Viral **hepatitis** comprises a number of viruses that primarily affect the liver, although they may also have extrahepatic manifestations. The most common types of viral hepatitis are hepatitis A (HAV), hepatitis B (HBV), hepatitis C (HCV), hepatitis D (HDV) (or delta hepatitis), and hepatitis E (HEV). An additional blood-borne virus is hepatitis G, which typically is not a cause of significant disease. It is possible to have more than one strain of viral hepatitis at a time. In addition, patients with HBV, HCV, or HDV may be coinfected with human immunodeficiency virus (HIV) because the routes of transmission are the same. See **Table 44.2** ■ for virus characteristics.[21–23]

Etiology and Pathogenesis

Hepatitis A. HAV is a member of the picornavirus family. It is spread through contaminated water or food via fecal–oral transmission. It is a self-limited virus without chronicity. It is shed through stool for 2–3 weeks before and 1 week after

Table 44.2 Characteristics of Types of Viral Hepatitis

	HAV	HBV	HCV	HDV	HEV
Type of virus	RNA	DNA	RNA	RNA	RNA
Mode of transmission	Fecal–oral	Parenteral, sexual, perinatal	Parenteral	Parenteral, sexual, perinatal	Fecal–oral
Incubation	30 days	28–180 days	35–72 days	30–180 days	15–60 days
Onset	Acute	Insidious	Insidious	Insidious	Acute
Chronic infection	No	Yes	Yes	Yes	No

the onset of jaundice. It is more common in the setting of substandard hygiene and sanitation. Outbreaks commonly occur in institutional settings, such as schools, or where overcrowding is prevalent. Hepatitis A may also be spread by eating contaminated shellfish such as oysters, mussels, or clams that are raw or undercooked or via infected workers in the food industry.[21]

Hepatitis B. Hepatitis B is a member of the *Hepadnaviridae* family. It is transmitted through contact with infected blood and body fluids. Sexual transmission and perinatal transmission also occur.[24] Younger age at time of infection is associated with a higher likelihood of developing a chronic infection.[25] Three types of particles are present in patients with HBV infection. The largest particle, known as a Dane particle, is 42 nm in diameter and represents the intact virion. It has a lipid bilayer. The outer lipid bilayer is composed of host hepatocytes and is studded with hepatitis B surface antigen (HBsAg). This surrounds the inner layer, which contains hepatitis B core antigen (HBcAg). In the inner layer are the HBV genome and viral polymerase. The other two particles appear as small, round particles or as filaments and are composed of host lipids and HBsAg. They do not have any of the HBV genome and are not considered infectious. A serologic assay is used to detect the presence of HBsAg and diagnose HBV.[24]

Infection of a hepatocyte with HBV is initiated by the attachment of a mature Dane particle to the hepatocyte. The Dane particle becomes internalized in the cytoplasm, and the lipid bilayer and nucleocapsid are dissolved. The partially double-stranded DNA is conveyed to the nucleus and repaired, and covalently closed circular DNA (cccDNA) is formed. This serves as the template for transcription of the viral mRNAs, which are transported to the cytoplasm and translated into viral proteins, leading to ongoing replication.[24] Ongoing replication of HBV requires cccDNA. Immature viral nucleocapsids may be transported back to the nucleus to replenish the cccDNA, which remains very stable in the hepatocyte. It can persist even after antiviral therapy and clearance of HbsAg, contributing to the possibility of disease reactivation after stopping antiviral treatment, following withdrawal of immunosuppression, de novo infections from HBcAb-positive organ transplantation, or development of drug resistance.[24]

HBV infection has been classified into three phases: immune tolerant, immune active, and inactive (**Table 44.3** ■). The immune tolerant phase occurs as a result of vertical transmission from a mother who is HBsAg and HBeAg positive to her infant in the perinatal period. The immune active phase may also be referred to as chronic HBV. During this phase, the patient is HBsAg positive and may be either HBeAg positive or HbeAg negative. HBeAg-positive patients typically have elevated ALT levels and HBV DNA levels greater than 20,000 IU/mL. HBeAg-negative patients usually have lower ALT and HBV DNA levels. The inactive phase is characterized by loss of HBeAg and development of HBeAb with normal ALT levels and HBV DNA less than 2000 IU/mL. Clearance of HBV infection is demonstrated with loss of HBsAg and development of HBsAb. HBcAb remains positive in all phases.[22,23,25]

Hepatitis C. Hepatitis C is a major cause of liver disease affecting approximately 3% of the world population. HCV is a member of the *Flavivirdae* family. It is a small, enveloped, single-stranded, RNA virus. Seven major genotypes exist. However, genotype 1a or 1b is the most common in the United States followed by genotypes 2 and 3. HCV levels begin to rise within days of infection. Elevation in the transaminases occurs about 8–12 weeks after infection. The incubation period is 2–26 weeks, with a mean of 6–12

Table 44.3 Characteristics of Different Phases of HBV Infection

	Immune Tolerant	Immune Active	Inactive	Resolved
ALT	Normal	Elevated	Normal	Normal
HBsAg	Positive	Positive	Positive	Negative
HBcAb	Positive	Positive	Positive	Positive
HBeAg	Positive	Positive or Negative	Negative	Negative
HBeAb	Negative	Positive or Negative	Positive	Positive
HBV DNA	> 200,000 copies IU/mL	> 2000 copies IU/mL	< 2000 copies IU/mL	Undetectable
Liver histology	No or minimal activity	Mild to severe disease	Mild or minimal activity	Varies

weeks. Most infections become chronic (75–80%).[23,26] Acute infection with HCV is often asymptomatic. Development of HCV antibodies occurs 3–6 weeks after exposure. Unfortunately, the antibodies are not protective and do not indicate eradication of the virus.

The clinical course for chronic HCV can vary. Approximately 17% of patients progress to cirrhosis, while more than 80% may have mild disease to bridging fibrosis.[23,25] HCV in the setting of obesity, diabetes, or chronic heavy alcohol use is associated with more advanced disease. Histologic features common to HCV are epithelial damage of small bile ducts, formation of lymphoid aggregates, and **steatosis** (fatty deposits in the liver as a result of the accumulation of lipid droplets).[21] HCV has also been associated with many other clinical conditions, and findings including extrahepatic manifestations. These include autoimmune hepatitis, cryoglobulinemia, membranoproliferative glomerulonephritis, porphyria cutanea tarda, lichen planus, and lymphoproliferative disorders.[23,27]

Hepatitis D. Hepatitis D occurs only in people who have the HBV infection. HDV is a small RNA virus that uses HBsAg for transmission and packaging. Only a small percentage of people with HBV have also been exposed to HDV: approximately 15 million of the 340 million HBV cases worldwide. Simultaneous acquisition of HDV and HBV is associated with more severe acute hepatitis and death as well as an increased likelihood of progression to cirrhosis. People who clear the HBV virus also simultaneously clear the HDV virus. In HDV/HBV coinfection, HBV viral titers are often low as the HDV virus suppresses replication of HBV. Eight HDV genotypes have been identified. Genotype 1, the most common, is associated with more severe disease. Genotype 3 is also associated with more severe disease. Milder disease is associated with genotype 2.[22]

The knowledge of the pathogenesis of HDV is limited. Cellular immune responses are thought to contribute to control of HDV infection. It has also been shown that the endogenous interferon system is highly activated. Peripheral HDV-specific T-cell responses declined during interferon treatment and correlated with response. Altered immune responses against HBV in coinfected patients has also been identified. HDV suppresses both HBV and HCV infection.[28]

Hepatitis E. HEV is a single-stranded, nonenveloped RNA virus. The mechanism by which is enters hepatocytes is unknown. Four of the identified five genotypes can infect humans. Genotypes 1 and 2 are the most common cause of classic epidemic HEV. Transmission is fecal–oral, and waterborne outbreaks are common. The waterborne form of HEV typically affects adolescents and young adults and is associated with a high rate of jaundice and cholestasis. Infection from genotypes 3 and 4, which are more common in the United States, may be asymptomatic or have more transient symptoms. This type of infection can become chronic in immunocompromised patients. The incubation period is 3–8 weeks, after which symptoms and elevated ALT may develop.[22]

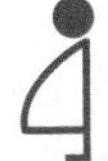

The mortality rate is high for pregnant women with HEV, possibly owing to the hormonal and immunologic changes associated with pregnancy. ■

Clinical Manifestations

The clinical symptoms of the different types of viral hepatitis have a similar pattern of presentation. The pattern seen in acute hepatitis includes three phases: prodromal, icterus, and recovery. The prodromal phase typically begins about 2 weeks after the initial exposure and continues until the development of jaundice. Symptoms in the prodromal phase are often vague and nonspecific and may be seen in many different types of viral illness. They may include fatigue, malaise, nausea, vomiting, low grade fever, cough, and anorexia. Weight loss may occur during this phase. A small percentage of people may experience additional symptoms, such as arthralgias, rash, purpura, or nephritis (with HBV or HCV). The desire to smoke or drink may diminish. During this phase, the patient is highly infectious.

The icteric phase typically begins within 2 weeks after the prodromal phase and can last for up to 6 weeks. Jaundice develops as a result of damage to the hepatocytes and stasis of bile in the intrahepatic bile ducts, leading to elevated bilirubin levels that are composed primarily of conjugated bilirubin. Jaundice is also associated with darker urine (tea or cola colored) and lighter stools (clay colored), as the bilirubin is no longer excreted through the bile ducts to the intestines. Instead, the kidneys begin to excrete bilirubin but are not as efficient. The liver is enlarged and may be tender. Serum bilirubin rises and may be between 5 and 10 mg/dL. The liver transaminases may be markedly elevated: in the hundreds or even the thousands. PT/INR may also be prolonged. During this phase, patients may feel better than they did during the prodromal phase, as gastrointestinal and respiratory symptoms abate. However, they look sicker because of the jaundice.

The final phase is the recovery or posticteric phase. This begins as the jaundice starts to resolve, typically 6–8 weeks after exposure. The liver may continue to be enlarged and tender. However, the transaminases begin to improve, and the liver profile typically returns to normal within 12 weeks after the onset of jaundice.

Infections that do not resolve within 6 months after exposure are considered chronic viral hepatitis. HAV and HEV do not become chronic infections. HBV, HCV, and HDV, however, may develop into chronic infections. Interestingly, some patients with chronic hepatitis may not have experienced these acute hepatitis phases and are surprised to find out they have a chronic infection.[21,22,25,26]

Linking Pathophysiology to Diagnosis and Treatment

Vaccines exist for HAV and HBV but not for the other types of viral hepatitis. Since the HAV vaccine became available in 1995, the number of acute HAV infections has dropped markedly. Since 2006, it has been given as part of the routine vaccination series for newborns. The HBV vaccine was licensed in 1983, and its use increased around 1987, initially for healthcare workers and men who have sex with men. It was also incorporated into the series of vaccines for newborns around 1993 and then for adolescents around 1997. As a result of the increased use of this vaccine, the number of acute HBV infections has decreased dramatically since the mid-1980s. Currently, it is recommended that patients with any type of liver disease be offered the HAV and HBV vaccines to prevent these infections in the setting of other liver disease. A combination vaccine exists for patients who need to be vaccinated against both HAV and HBV.[29] Serologic testing exists for each viral hepatitis infection (see **Table 44.4** ■).

Hepatitis A. Diagnosis of acute HAV is confirmed by the presence of a positive serum HAV IgM antibody. This response declines over a few months and is followed by the development of HAV IgG antibodies, which indicate immunity. Treatment is focused on symptom management with rest, nutrition, and fluid management. Healthy individuals between 1 and 40 years of age who have been exposed to HAV can receive a single dose of the HAV vaccine for prophylaxis. Immunoglobulin can be administered for those with chronic health conditions or those outside the range of 1–40 years.[21]

Hepatitis B. Diagnosis of HBV is made through serologic testing. Acute infection is characterized by the presence of HBsAg and HBcAg IgM. The presence of HBsAg for more than 6 months indicates a chronic infection. Loss of HBsAg and development of HBsAb indicates resolved infection (see Table 44.4). Treatment of HBV is determined by disease severity. Immune active patients are typically treated if their HBV viral load and ALT are elevated.[25,26]

Table 44.4 Serologic Testing for Viral Hepatitis

Infection	Tests
HAV	HAV IgM indicates current infection. HAV IgG indicates immunity.[21]
HBV	HBsAg indicates active infection. HBsAb indicates immunity (past infection or vaccination). HBcAb indicates past exposure or infection. HBeAg indicates high viral replication and infectivity. HBeAb indicates low viral replication and low risk of transmission. HBV DNA measures the amount of virus in the blood.[24] HBsAg is a surrogate marker as decreasing HBsAg titers signal viral clearance.[28]
HCV	HCV antibody indicates exposure and usually signifies infection. This must be confirmed by viral testing. HCV PCR measures the amount of virus in the blood and confirms the presence of infection. HCV genotype specifies the subtype of HCV and guides treatment options.[26]
HDV	HDV IgM indicates acute infection. HDV IgG indicates prior exposure. It persists in chronic infections and may decline or persist with viral clearance. HDV RNA indicates active infection.
HEV	HEV IgM indicates acute infection and can persist for months. HEV IgG indicates prior exposure and can persist for years. HEV PCR measures the amount of virus in the blood and confirms the presence of infection.[29]

Hepatitis C. The initial screening test for HCV is the HCV antibody. In approximately 85% of cases, this indicates an active infection as the antibody is not protective. Confirmatory testing is performed by sending an HCV PCR viral load. If positive, active infection is confirmed. An HCV genotype should then be sent. Six genotypes have been identified. In the United States, genotype 1 is the most common. Also seen are genotypes 2 and 3. The remaining three genotypes are seen less often in the United States. Treatment length and medication are determined on the basis of genotype. In the past, interferon-alfa–based regimens were the backbone of HCV treatment. Recently, however, oral-based therapies have been approved. These treatment regimens have fewer side effects, and most have greater than 90% efficacy. As a result, treatment recommendations are evolving.[26] Genotype 2 is considered the easiest to treat. Liver biopsy is the gold standard to determine disease extent and severity. Noninvasive methods of assessing fibrosis have started to become more acceptable as well.[26]

Hepatitis D. All patients with HBV should be tested for anti-HDV antibodies followed by HDV RNA confirmation if they are present. Acute HDV/HBV infection may cause severe hepatitis, and there is a risk of fulminant liver failure. Despite this, up to 90% of adults clear the infection. If HDV RNA is positive, liver biopsy should be considered to grade and stage disease activity, to determine whether there is a need to monitor for hepatocellular carcinoma, and for consideration of antiviral treatment. Pegylated interferon-alfa has been effective in sustained viral clearance of HDV in approximately 25% of patients. Patients coinfected with HBV and/or HCV should be monitored over time to determine which virus is dominant, and treatment should be directed toward the dominant virus.[28]

Hepatitis E. Good hand hygiene and supportive care make up the primary treatment for acute HEV. For the small percentage of chronic HEV infections, which often occur in immunocompromised individuals such as organ transplant recipients or patients with HIV, reduction in immunosuppression has resulted in clearance in some cases. Treatment with pegylated interferon with or without ribavirin has been used for chronic infections as well.[22]

Henry Winston: Outcome

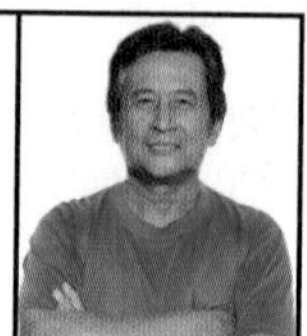

Mr. Winston underwent laboratory tests and an ultrasound of the liver. The results were as follows:

- Hepatic panel (normal values are in parentheses): AST 97 (0–34), ALT 121 (0–37), alkaline phosphatase 67 (25–130), total bilirubin 0.8 (0.3–1.3), conjugated bilirubin 0.2 (0–0.3), albumin 4.2 (3.5–4.5)
- INR: 0.8 (0.8–1.1)
- HAV antibody negative, HBsAg negative, HBsAb positive, HCV antibody positive, HCV PCR viral load 6.7×10^6 copies, HCV genotype 2a, HIV negative
- Ultrasound of the liver: Enlarged liver with smooth contour. No splenomegaly. No ascites.

These tests reveal that Mr. Winston has inflammation in his liver demonstrated by elevation of his AST and ALT. The pattern of ALT > AST suggests etiologies that include viral hepatitis. On the basis of Mr. Winston's history of IV drug use in his 20s, the primary care provider orders several viral hepatitis studies as well as an HIV test. These tests show that Mr. Winston is not immune to HAV and does not have hepatitis B (HBsAg negative) but may have been exposed in the past, as he is immune (HBsAb positive). He does have a positive HCV antibody and a positive HCV PCR viral load, which confirm that he has HCV. He does not have HIV, which can be transmitted similarly to HBV and HCV. His HCV genotype is 2a, and that will direct the type of treatment he should receive. Because of the enlarged liver on physical exam, an ultrasound of the liver was performed. It revealed an enlarged liver with a smooth contour, no splenomegaly or ascites. This suggests that Mr. Winston does not have cirrhosis of the liver. The enlargement is from chronic viral HCV. Mr. Winston is referred to a hepatologist for treatment options.

3. What are the viral characteristics (type of virus, mode of transmission, incubation, onset, and chronic infection) of Mr. Winston's HCV?
4. What is the significance of the results of the HCV PCR and HCV antibody serologic tests?

Alcoholic Liver Disease

Ingestion of alcohol has many harmful consequences and affects many body systems. **Alcoholic liver disease** is defined as damage to the liver and its function due to alcohol abuse. Toxicity from alcohol is the third most common cause of morbidity worldwide, and alcohol-related morbidity is the third most common cause of preventable death in the United States.[30]

Etiology and Pathogenesis

The association between liver disease and alcohol consumption is well described. Interestingly, only a small proportion of people who drink heavily develop significant liver disease. Although many variables exist, it has been found that men who drink more than 30 g of alcohol a day and women who drink more than 15 g of alcohol a day are at greater risk of developing signs of hepatotoxicity. Those who drank more than 120 g of alcohol a day were most likely to develop cirrhosis. Older age and gender are also associated with alcoholic liver disease. Most people who are hospitalized with alcoholic liver disease are between 46 and 64 years of age. Although women are more susceptible to damage from alcohol ingestion, men are much more likely to develop alcoholic liver disease.[31]

The histologic findings associated with alcoholic liver disease include steatosis, steatohepatitis, ballooning degeneration, Mallory body formation, regeneration, and fibrosis with progression to cirrhosis. Steatosis is the accumulation of lipid droplets in the cytoplasm of the liver cells. This occurs as a byproduct of alcohol metabolism. The normal metabolic pathway uses cytosolic alcohol dehydrogenase to convert alcohol to acetaldehyde and acetaldehyde dehydrogenase, which then converts to acetate. The acetate can be broken down into fatty acids, which eventually form triglycerides. The lipid droplets seen in steatosis contain not only triglycerides, but also free fatty acids, monoglycerides, and diglycerides. Normally, the liver does not store lipids, but after even moderate alcohol ingestion, lipid droplets begin building up in the liver. Initially, these droplets are small (microvesicular), but over time, they coalesce, forming larger droplets (macrovesicular).[32]

Chronic alcohol exposure also affects the cytochrome p450 system. CYP2E1 is induced, leading to increased catabolism in the endoplasmic reticulum, which increases reactive oxygen species, leading to lipid peroxidation and acetaldehyde protein adducts. Impaired methionine metabolism also occurs, resulting in decreased intrahepatic glutathione levels, which increases the oxidative injury in the liver from microsomal and peroxisomal metabolism of alcohol.[32]

Swelling of hepatocytes is termed **ballooning degeneration** and is the result of severe cell injury. Cell death can occur in the most severe instances. This finding, although common in alcoholic liver disease, is not specific to alcoholic liver disease. It may also be seen in other forms of hepatic toxicity, including alcoholic hepatitis, ischemic injury, and cholestasis. Cell necrosis is the end point of ballooning degeneration, at which point the cellular contents are released. This is a hallmark of steatohepatitis.

Mallory bodies are damaged filaments in the liver that accumulate in alcoholic liver disease as well as other forms of liver disease such as nonalcoholic steatohepatitis, primary biliary cirrhosis, and Wilson disease. They are the result of misfolding or amassing of keratins. They are often surrounded by neutrophils and may contribute to ongoing inflammation and damage to the hepatocytes.[32]

Inflammation is multifactorial in alcoholic liver disease and is often seen in the setting of steatosis; therefore, it is known as **steatohepatitis**. Neutrophils and lymphocytes can be seen wrapped around ballooned hepatocytes containing Mallory bodies. Inflammation in the portal areas can result from accumulation of lymphocytes, plasma cells, macrophages, neutrophils, eosinophils, and mast cells. Kupffer cells, which make up 80% of the systemic host mononuclear phagocytic system, are found on the luminal side of the sinusoidal epithelium to capture microorganisms and other matter as it arrives from the splanchnic circulation. Gut permeability increases with alcohol ingestion, increasing hepatic exposure to gut-derived bacterial degradation products such as endotoxin. This activates Kupffer cells, which then release proinflammatory cytokines such as TNF-α, interleukin 2 (IL-2), and IL-12. Multiple events occur in the setting of alcoholic liver disease, including endotoxin, proinflammatory cytokines, fat metabolism, and free radical generation.[32]

Alcohol-induced damage leads to hepatocellular death as a result of damage to and disruption of proteins (cytoplasmic, nuclear and organelle) and DNA. Oxygen free radicals and toxic cytokines (TNF-α) are released, resulting in tissue damage that is made worse by an increase in other inflammatory cells. Nitric oxide is released by endothelial cells and potentiates hepatocellular necrosis.[32]

Clinical Manifestations

Alcoholic liver disease represents a spectrum of damage ranging from mild to alcoholic cirrhosis. Included in this spectrum is acute alcoholic hepatitis, which is an acute form of liver injury from substantial alcohol consumption over time. Symptoms of alcoholic hepatitis can vary from mild to severe. Mild symptoms may be nonspecific and can include nausea, vomiting, fever, anorexia, weight loss, abdominal pain, and fever. Encephalopathy and hepatic failure represent the other end of the spectrum. Physical examination findings can include **hepatomegaly** (enlarged liver), jaundice, ascites, encephalopathy, and spider angiomata (a collection of swollen blood vessels with a central red spot and additional vessels spread out around it like a spiderweb).[33] Laboratory results typically show a 2:1 ratio between the aspartate aminotransferase (AST) and alanine aminotransferase (ALT), although in more severe cases, the AST may be as much as 6 times greater than the ALT. Leukocytosis may be present as well. GGT was thought to be a marker of alcoholic hepatitis; however, it has also been reported that it has low sensitivity and specificity.[34]

Physical examination findings for patients with alcoholic cirrhosis are the same as one might find in any patient with cirrhosis from any cause. These may include ascites, jaundice, hepatic encephalopathy, splenomegaly, hepatomegaly, spider angiomata, and palmar erythema. The AST/ALT ratio is also usually 2:1. Leukocytosis is not common in alcoholic cirrhosis, and as in alcoholic hepatitis, GGT has not been shown to be useful.[34]

Linking Pathophysiology to Diagnosis and Treatment

Several calculations exist for evaluating the severity of alcoholic hepatitis. A variety of clinical methods are used to identify the patients who are most likely to benefit from select courses of treatment. Depending on the scoring system, the patient may receive a 4- to 6-week course of corticosteroidal therapy. Medications other than corticosteroids may be used in the treatment of alcoholic hepatitis. Pentoxyfylline for 28 days has been shown to improve survival, with rates similar to those of corticosteroids, and is an alternative to corticosteroid treatment.

CLINICAL POINT: The most important component of treatment of alcoholic liver disease is abstinence from alcohol. ■

Improvement in liver function can be seen with abstinence from alcohol, including resolution of complications such as ascites. However, abstinence can be difficult. Participation in a rehabilitation program (inpatient or outpatient), counseling, or attendance at sobriety meetings such as Alcoholics Anonymous can aid in maintaining long-term sobriety. Medications such as disulfiram and acamprosate have been used to support abstinence after detoxification.[33]

Nutritional support is also necessary, as malnutrition is fairly common. The patient should be assessed for deficiencies of vitamins and minerals such as thiamine and folate as well as protein malnutrition. Small, frequent meals including higher amounts of protein and calories are helpful as the patient recovers.

Liver transplantation is an option for treatment of alcoholic cirrhosis. However, the patient must have maintained complete abstinence for a minimum of 6 months for most programs. Long-term outcomes for this option are good as long as the patient remains abstinent indefinitely. In contrast, liver transplantation for acute alcoholic hepatitis has not been considered a standard treatment option. However, emerging data suggest beneficial outcomes for patients with a single episode of acute alcoholic hepatitis who underwent liver transplantation.[35]

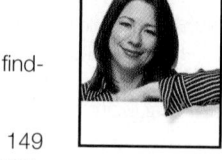

Sylvia St. John: Outcome

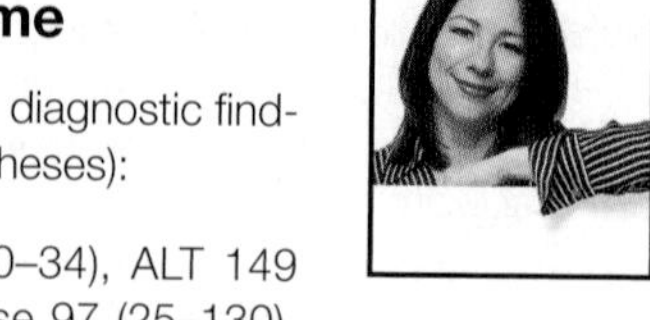

Sylvia St. John had the following diagnostic findings (normal values are in parentheses):

- Hepatic panel: AST 171 (0–34), ALT 149 (0–37), alkaline phosphatase 97 (25–130), total bilirubin 2.7 (0.3–1.3), conjugated bilirubin 2.1 (0–0.3), albumin 3.2 (3.5–4.5), GGT 145 (5–27)
- INR: 1.8 (0.8–1.1)
- Basic metabolic panel: Na 132 (135–145), K 4.2 (3.5–5.0), creatinine 1.19 (0.6–1.2)
- Ultrasound of the liver: Large volume abdominal ascites; liver with nodular contour, no focal masses; spleen enlarged
- Chest x-ray: moderate size pleural effusion on the right side.

These findings demonstrate elevated liver enzymes (AST and ALT), indicating ongoing inflammation. The pattern of AST > ALT is commonly seen in alcoholic liver disease. The elevated total bilirubin, decreased albumin, and elevated INR suggest damage to the liver. These tests represent the function of the liver as the liver clears bilirubin and produces albumin and clotting proteins. The elevated conjugated bilirubin is consistent with damage to the liver as the cause of the elevation. The elevated GGT suggests alcohol as the underlying etiology. The results of the basic metabolic profile show mild hyponatremia, which may be seen in cirrhosis. The ultrasound of the liver describes a nodular contour of the liver, which is consistent with cirrhosis. There is also a large amount of ascites, which is a consequence of portal hypertension and cirrhosis. Splenomegaly is also seen with portal hypertension from cirrhosis.

Treatment for Ms. St. John will focus on complete abstinence from alcohol. This may allow the liver to repair itself over time. However, the underlying cirrhosis will not resolve. Therefore, Ms. St. John will now need ongoing monitoring for complications of cirrhosis such as esophageal varices and hepatocellular carcinoma. The recent ultrasound of the liver reveals no masses in the liver. Ultrasound should be repeated every 6 months. An endoscopic gastroduodenoscopy should be ordered to screen for esophageal varices.

Treatment for Ms. St. John's pleural effusion may include a thoracentesis if her symptoms of dyspnea are severe, or diuretics such as furosemide and spironolactone may help. Ascites is commonly seen in patients with pleural effusion. Diuretics can help to improve symptoms. Large-volume paracentesis may be performed to drain the fluid if Ms. St. John has substantial distention and discomfort or if the diuretics are not effective in controlling the ascites fluid.

5. What is the most important component of Ms. St. John's treatment?
6. What pharmacologic and nonpharmacologic therapies can help Ms. St. John abstain from alcohol over the long term?

Nonalcoholic Fatty Liver Disease

The prevalence of obesity has increased significantly across the world. This increase in obesity is also associated with increased prevalence of other medical conditions such as diabetes, hypertension, and dyslipidemia. In addition to these conditions, obesity is also strongly linked to the development of **nonalcoholic fatty liver disease (NAFLD)** in adults and children. Interestingly, however, NAFLD may also be seen in nonobese individuals as well.[36]

Etiology and Pathogenesis

NAFLD is a spectrum of liver diseases ranging from simple steatosis to nonalcoholic steatohepatitis (NASH) and is the most common chronic liver disease worldwide (**Figure 44.9** ■). It is characterized by the deposit of lipids in the liver and is histologically similar to alcoholic liver disease without the presence of chronic alcohol use. On one end of the spectrum is simple steatosis, a mild liver disease that is defined as more than 5% hepatic lipid accumulation and rarely progresses to advanced liver disease. In contrast, NASH represents the other end of the spectrum of NAFLD and has a component of inflammation and damage to hepatocytes with the potential to progress to cirrhosis.[34] The pathogenesis of NAFLD is complex with genetic, environmental, psychosocial, and behavioral factors.[35,36] Adipose tissue remodeling occurs in the presence of obesity, leading to dysfunctional adipocytes, abnormal cytokine production, and chronic low-grade inflammation.

Insulin resistance is the key abnormality associated with obesity-related NAFLD. The fatty liver becomes insulin resistant and overproduces glucose, very low-density lipoprotein, C-reactive protein, and interleukin-6, leading to hyperglycemia, dyslipidemia, and hyperinsulinemia, which are components of metabolic syndrome.[34] Both metabolic syndrome and insulin resistance are important components associated with the development of NASH.[37] See Chapter 5 for more information on metabolic syndrome.

Clinical Manifestations

Few symptoms are present in the presence of NAFLD. Liver transaminases may be elevated, AST levels typically being higher than ALT levels. Symptoms of metabolic syndrome, such as obesity, diabetes, or dyslipidemia, may be present.[36]

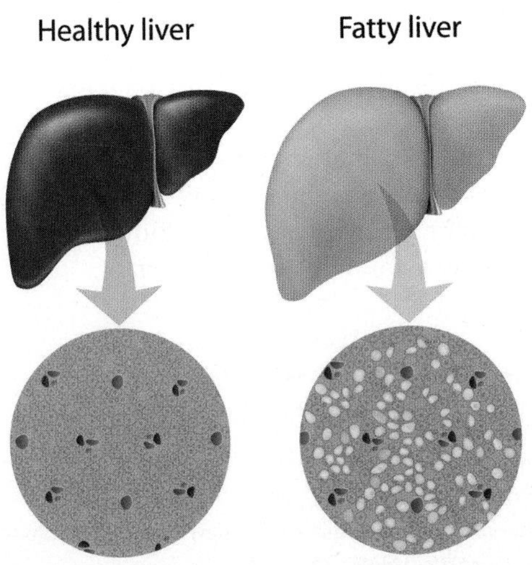

Figure 44.9 ■ Changes seen with fatty liver disease.

Linking Pathophysiology to Diagnosis and Treatment

Obesity and insulin resistance are the most important factors underlying NAFLD. Unfortunately, few medical treatments exist for NAFLD other than optimizing management of other coexisting conditions such as diabetes or dyslipidemia. The one exception is vitamin E, which improved both histology and liver enzymes in nondiabetic patients with biopsy-proven NASH.[34] However, other treatments such as oral hypoglycemics, statins, orlistat, and ursodeoxycholic acid have not been found to be effective and are not recommended as primary treatment. Weight loss remains the best way to improve NAFLD, yet behavior modification targeting weight loss and exercise has had limited benefit. In contrast, bariatric surgery has been shown to be effective in achieving weight loss and subsequent improvement of NAFLD.[36]

Obesity and diabetes are also associated with an increased risk of hepatocellular carcinoma, most likely in the setting of NASH-related cirrhosis. Recently, however, hepatocellular carcinoma (HCC) has been reported in NAFLD patients without cirrhosis or fibrosis.[37] Screening for HCC in NASH-cirrhotic patients should follow routine guidelines. However, no guidelines have yet been developed for screening of HCC in noncirrhotic NAFLD patients.

Autoimmune Hepatitis

Autoimmune hepatitis is a progressive inflammatory liver disease characterized by significantly elevated serum immunoglobulin levels. It is more common in women than in men. Although chronic autoimmune hepatitis is the typical presentation, acute autoimmune hepatitis may also develop. Medications and infections may initiate autoimmune hepatitis.[38] Circulating autoantibodies are positive, and interface hepatitis is seen on histology.

Etiology and Pathogenesis

Genetic and environmental triggers for autoimmune hepatitis have been identified. Specific human leukocyte antigen (HLA) haplotypes have been associated with autoimmune hepatitis. Haplotypes such as HLA DR3 or HLA DR4 may have a more aggressive disease course or increased extrahepatic manifestations, respectively. Gene deletions have also been linked with disease progression in younger women.[38] Additional genes associated with susceptibility to autoimmune hepatitis include *CTLA-4*, *TNS-α*, *TBX21*, *TGF*-β1, *Fas*, and *VDR*. Left untreated, autoimmune hepatitis is likely to progress to cirrhosis and liver failure requiring transplantation.[39]

Clinical Manifestations

The clinical presentation of autoimmune hepatitis is variable and insidious. Progressive fatigue, recurring jaundice, amenorrhea, weight loss, and in some cases arthralgias may be present. However, approximately 25% of patients experience no symptoms and are diagnosed after an incidental finding of elevated transaminases. Approximately 30% of patients have cirrhosis at time of diagnosis, indicating that the disease has been present for a long time.

There are two types of autoimmune hepatitis. In type 1, ANA and/or antismooth muscle antibody are positive. Patients with type 2 have a positive anti-liver kidney microsomal type 1 antibody and/or an anti-liver cytosol type 1 antibody. Type 2 autoimmune hepatitis is more common in children. The most common laboratory abnormality is elevation of the transaminases. A cholestatic pattern with elevated bilirubin and alkaline phosphatase is less likely and should raise suspicion for another etiology. Serum globulins are usually elevated

A liver biopsy is important in confirming the diagnosis of autoimmune hepatitis. Interface hepatitis, which is hepatitis at the portal–parenchymal interface, is typical of autoimmune hepatitis, although it can be seen in other conditions. Lymphocytes, plasma cells, and histiocytes surround dying hepatocytes in this area. The severity of the histologic appearance suggests prognosis. Inflammatory changes around the bile ducts may be seen in an overlap syndrome with primary sclerosing cholangitis.[40]

Linking Pathophysiology to Diagnosis and Treatment

Immunosuppression is the treatment for autoimmune hepatitis. First-line therapy is corticosteroids such as prednisone or prednisolone, with or without azathioprine. Approximately 80% of patients respond to this treatment. Normalization of transaminases occurs before histologic response, which is slower. Long-term treatment with azathioprine alone helps maintain remission. For patients who have not achieved remission on this treatment, other medications such as methotrexate, cyclosporine, mycophenolate mofetil, cyclophosphamide, and UDCA have been tried. Lack of response to immunosuppressive treatment is typically associated with disease progression leading to cirrhosis, liver failure, and liver transplantation.[39]

Acute Liver Failure

Acute liver failure is the loss of hepatocyte function affecting almost the entire liver without the presence of cirrhosis. The damage occurs over days or weeks and is characterized by the hallmark signs of altered mental status and coagulopathy. Approximately 2000 people a year in the United States experience acute liver failure.

Etiology and Pathogenesis

The leading cause of acute liver failure is drugs, accounting for about 60% of the cases. Acetaminophen, the most common cause of drug-induced acute liver failure, is responsible for approximately 80% of these cases. The remaining cases of drug-induced acute liver failure are the result of idiosyncratic drug reactions. Other causes of acute liver failure include viruses, toxins, and an autoimmune response. Before the 1990s, however, hepatitis B was the leading cause of acute liver failure.[3]

Massive hepatic necrosis affecting 80–90% of the liver occurs before signs and symptoms are visible. The mechanism of cell injury may be direct toxic damage or a combination of toxic damage and inflammation associated with immune-mediated destruction of hepatocytes. Mortality from acute liver failure is high (70–95%). Patients with a milder presentation may recover, but for the most severe cases, liver transplantation is the only intervention.[3]

Clinical Manifestations

Coagulopathy and altered mental status are the hallmark clinical signs of acute liver failure. Jaundice may also occur, but it is not universal. Acute liver failure from acetaminophen is characterized by marked elevation in transaminases (> 3500 IU/L) with a relatively low total bilirubin level (< 5). Acute kidney injury is also common in patients with acetaminophen-induced acute liver failure, affecting approximately 70% of patients with massive hepatic necrosis and encephalopathy. Acute liver failure from other causes, such as viruses or other drug-induced liver injury, is more likely to have an elevated total bilirubin level (> 5) and may have lower transaminases. In the most severe cases, hepatic coma or cerebral edema is present.[3]

Linking Pathophysiology to Diagnosis and Treatment

CLINICAL POINT: Acute liver failure is a serious injury that requires immediate attention. Supportive care in an intensive care unit is typically required for patients with encephalopathy and is often considered for patients with profound coagulopathy that may progress to encephalopathy. ■

The head of the bed is elevated to minimize the risk of aspiration in the setting of altered mental status. Frequent neurologic checks are necessary to monitor for additional changes in mental status. Dehydration is common, and volume resuscitation is initiated. Patients with acetaminophen-induced acute liver failure should receive N-acetylcysteine (NAC), an acetaminophen antidote. However, NAC has also been used for patients with drug-induced liver injury from other causes with improvement in spontaneous recovery and transplant-free survival.

Hepatic encephalopathy is often associated with elevated ammonia levels. In acute liver failure, although there is a loose correlation between the degree of encephalopathy and ammonia levels, this link is not as strong as in chronic liver failure. In the setting of acute kidney injury, elevated ammonia levels and cerebral edema are more common. In the absence of acute kidney injury, elevated ammonia levels are rarely seen. The use of lactulose for treatment of hepatic encephalopathy in acute liver failure has not been shown to be effective and may negatively impact surgical interventions related to possible colonic distention.[3] Trials are underway with a novel agent, L-ornithine phenylacetate, as an alternative ammonia-lowering agent.[3,41]

Check Your Progress: Section 44.4

1. What are typical laboratory test findings in alcoholic liver disease?
2. What is the correlation between insulin resistance and obesity-related NAFLD?
3. What are the hallmarks of acute liver failure?

CHAPTER SUMMARY

44.1 Chapter Overview and Case Studies

Define liver failure, including populations most at risk and key pathologic concepts related to failure.

- The liver is the largest solid organ in the body.
- A loss of liver function is referred to as failure.
- There are several potential causes of liver failure, ranging from alcohol to viruses.
- Liver failure can be either acute or chronic. Acute liver failure is tied to elevated liver function tests. Chronic liver failure will lead to elevated laboratory values but presents additional symptoms such as portal hypertension.

44.2 The Normal Liver

Outline the normal function of the liver.

- The liver is in the right upper quadrant of the abdomen.
- The functions of the liver include bile production, detoxification, storage of certain vitamins and minerals, production of proteins, and metabolism of carbohydrates, proteins, and fat.
- The liver is the intermediary between gastrointestinal and systemic circulation.
- The lobes of the liver are made up of numerous functional units called lobules.
- Many types of hepatic injury demonstrate a zonal distribution of damage.
- Between hepatocytes are sinusoids, which are lined with cells that destroy bacteria and other foreign material. As blood passes through the sinusoids, oxygen is extracted, foreign material is removed, and nutrients are absorbed by the hepatocytes
- Hepatocytes produce bile, which drains into the tiny bile ducts.
- The liver receives blood from the hepatic artery and the portal vein, which carry approximately 25% of the body's total cardiac output.

44.3 Clinical Manifestations and Complications of Liver Failure

Differentiate underlying pathogenesis of liver failure and common complications in the context of approaches to treatment and diagnosis across the lifespan.

- More than 80–90% of hepatic function must be compromised before failure is evident.
- Portal hypertension results from increased resistance through the venous system of the gastrointestinal tract.
- The most common cause of portal hypertension is cirrhosis. Portal hypertension can be caused by issues related to the portal system (prehepatic) or systemic issues such as heart failure (posthepatic).
- Portal hypertension can lead to ascites and varices.
- Esophageal varices are dilated vessels in the esophagus. These vessels dilate as a result of increased pressure and are prone to rupture. Acute bleeding from esophageal varices may manifest as melena, hematemesis, or bright red blood from the rectum.
- Slow seepage of blood can result in declining hemoglobin and hematocrit levels, leading to symptoms of anemia.
- Treatment of acute esophageal bleeding may include the use of vasoconstrictors, venodilators, esophageal band ligation, and blood transfusions.
- Ascites, an abnormal collection of excess fluid in the abdominal cavity, is the most common complication of cirrhosis. The pathogenesis is thought to be the result of peripheral arterial vasodilation. Ascites manifests with increased abdominal girth, weight gain, bulging flanks, and shifting dullness. Addressing the underlying liver disease may help to improve ascites.
- Refractory ascites often requires drainage through catheters inserted through the wall of the abdomen.
- The loss of circulating volume in individuals with ascites can result in hepatorenal syndrome, which results in increased serum creatinine. Liver transplantation is the preferred treatment for hepatorenal syndrome.
- Jaundice is a yellowing of the skin from elevated levels of bilirubin. Yellowing of the skin and sclerae of the eyes are the most common signs of jaundice. Treatment of jaundice and cholestasis varies, depending on the underlying etiology.

44.4 Common Causes of Liver Failure

Differentiate the causes, classification, underlying pathogenesis, and clinical manifestations of disorders causing liver failure and approaches to diagnosis and treatment of these conditions across the lifespan.

- Viral hepatitis is a term referring to a number of viruses that primarily affect the liver. The most common types of viral hepatitis are hepatitis A, B, C, D, and E. It is possible to have more than one strain of viral hepatitis at a time.
- Patients with HBV, HCV, or HDV may be coinfected with human immunodeficiency virus (HIV) because the routes of transmission are the same.
- Hepatitis A is spread through contaminated water or food via fecal–oral transmission. It is a self-limited virus. Hepatitis B is transmitted through contact with infected blood and body fluids. Hepatitis C is a major cause of liver disease, affecting approximately 3% of the world population.

- Acute infection with HCV is often asymptomatic. HCV in the setting of comorbid disease is associated with more advanced disease.
- Hepatitis D occurs only in people who have HBV infection.
- HDV is a small RNA virus that uses HBsAg for transmission and packaging. Acquiring HDV and HBV at the same time is associated with significantly worsened hepatitis.
- Hepatitis E is usually transmitted through the fecal–oral route, and waterborne outbreaks are common.
- The clinical symptoms of the different types of viral hepatitis have a similar pattern of presentation. Symptoms in the prodromal phase are often vague and nonspecific and may be seen with many different types of viral illness. They include fatigue, malaise, nausea, vomiting, low grade fever, cough, and anorexia.
- The icteric phase typically begins within 2 weeks of the prodromal phase and can last for up to 6 weeks. Jaundice develops as a result of damage to the hepatocytes and stasis of bile in the intrahepatic bile ducts, leading to elevated bilirubin levels.
- Infections that do not resolve within 6 months after exposure are considered chronic viral hepatitis. HAV and HEV do not become chronic infections. HBV, HCV, and HDV may develop into chronic infections.
- Vaccines exist for HAV and HBV but not for the other types of viral hepatitis.
- Alcoholic liver disease is defined as damage to the liver and its function due to alcohol abuse.
- Inflammation is multifactorial in alcoholic liver disease and is often seen in the setting of steatosis, so it is therefore known as steatohepatitis.
- Alcohol-induced damage leads to hepatocellular death as a result of damage to and disruption of proteins (cytoplasmic, nuclear, and organelle) and DNA. Oxygen free radicals and toxic cytokines (tumor necrosis factor alpha) are released, resulting in tissue damage, which is made worse by an increase in other inflammatory cells.
- Alcoholic liver disease represents a spectrum of damage ranging from mild to alcoholic cirrhosis. Physical examination findings can include hepatomegaly (enlarged liver), jaundice, ascites, encephalopathy, and spider angiomata.
- Several calculations exist for evaluating the severity of alcoholic hepatitis. Depending on the scoring system, the patient may receive corticosteroid therapy.
- The most important component of treatment of alcoholic liver disease is abstinence from alcohol.
- Liver transplantation is an option for treatment of alcoholic cirrhosis. However, patients must have maintained complete abstinence for a minimum of 6 months.
- Nonalcoholic fatty liver disease (NAFLD), which is common around the world, is characterized by the deposit of lipids in the liver and is histologically similar to alcoholic liver disease without the presence of chronic alcohol use. Few symptoms are present in most individuals with NAFLD.
- Acute liver failure occurs over days or weeks and is characterized by the hallmark signs of altered mental status and coagulopathy. The leading cause of acute liver failure is drug usage, with acetaminophen overuse being the most common cause.
- Massive hepatic necrosis affecting 80–90% of the liver occurs before signs and symptoms are visible.
- Acute liver failure is a serious injury that requires immediate attention.

REVIEW QUESTIONS

1. Which of the following findings would the nurse expect to assess in a client with portal hypertension?
   a. Esophageal varices
   b. Rectal varices
   c. Splenomegaly
   d. All of the above
2. Which of the following nursing actions is a priority in the client who just had 5 liters of ascites fluid removed through paracentesis?
   a. Monitor vital signs every 4 hours.
   b. Monitor intake and output every shift.
   c. Infuse intravenous 25% albumin equal to 8 g/L fluid removed.
   d. Increase sodium intake to 2500 mg/day.
3. Nutrition education in the client with alcoholic liver disease should include instructions to:
   a. increase vitamin and mineral intake.
   b. eat large meals.
   c. reduce protein intake.
   d. reduce caloric intake.
4. The nurse should question which of the following orders for the client with acute liver failure?
   a. Perform frequent neurologic checks.
   b. Increase intravenous fluids.
   c. Administer acetaminophen as needed for pain.
   d. Elevate the head of the bed.
5. The client in the prodromal phases of acute hepatitis will most likely have which of the following findings?
   a. Jaundice, low-grade fever, malaise
   b. Dark urine, light clay-colored stools, tender liver
   c. Jaundice, prolonged INR, tender liver
   d. Fatigue, low-grade fever, and malaise

6. Which recommendation for hepatitis vaccination should the nurse follow?
   a. Clients at risk for HVC should be vaccinated.
   b. Clients with liver disease should receive HAV and HBV vaccines.
   c. Clients over age 50 who have been exposed to HAV can receive a single dose of HAV for prophylaxis.
   d. Two-year-olds should receive HAV and HBV vaccines.
7. Which of the following statements made by a client with HDV indicates that the client does not understand the disorder?
   a. "HDV will not develop into a chronic infection."
   b. "HDV suppresses both HBV and HCV infections."
   c. "HDV IgM shows that I have an acute infection."
   d. "Acute HDV/HBV infection can cause severe hepatitis."
8. The nurse teaches a client who is at risk for hepatitis that which form of hepatitis may be transmitted by sexual contact?
   a. HAV
   b. HBV
   c. HCV
   d. HEV

ANSWERS

Answers to Review Questions can be found in Appendix A. Answers to Case Study and Check Your Progress questions are available on the faculty resources site. Please consult with your instructor.

RECOMMENDED WEBSITES

Alcoholics Anonymous
www.aa.org

American Gastroenterological Association
www.gastro.org

American Liver Foundation
http://www.liverfoundation.org

Chronic Liver Disease Foundation
http://www.chronicliverdisease.org

REFERENCES

1. Gao, B., & Bataller, R. (2011). Alcoholic liver disease: Pathogenesis and new therapeutic targets. *Gastroenterology, 141*, 1572–1585.
2. McCuskey, R. (2012). Anatomy of the liver. In T. D. Boyer, M. R. Manns, & A. J. Sanyal (Eds.), *Zakim and Boyer's hepatology* (6th ed., pp. 3–19). Philadelphia, PA: Saunders.
3. Lee, W. (2013). Drug-induced acute liver failure. *Clinical Liver Disease, 17*, 575–586.
4. Albilllos, A., & Garcia-Tsao, G. (2011). Classification of cirrhosis: The clinical use of HVPG measurements. *Disease Markers, 31*, 121–128.
5. Khanna, R., & Sarin, S. K. (2014). Non-cirrhotic portal hypertension: Diagnosis and management. *Journal of Hepatology, 60*:421–441.
6. Wilkins, T., Khan, N., Nabh, A., & Schade, R. R. (2012). Diagnosis and management of upper gastrointestinal bleeding. *American Family Physician, 85*, 469–476.
7. Kumar, S., Asrani, S. K., & Kamath, P. S. (2014). Epidemiology, diagnosis and early patient management of esophagogastric hemorrhage. *Gastroenterology Clinics of North America, 43*(4), 765–782. doi:10.1016/j.gtc.2014.08.007
8. American Association for the Study of Liver Diseases. (2007). *Prevention and management of gastroesophageal varices and variceal hemorrhage in cirrhosis*. Available at http://www.aasld.org/practiceguidelines/pages/guidelinelisting.aspx
9. Gordon, F. D. (2012). Ascites. *Clinical Liver Disease, 16*, 285–299.
10. Runyon, B. A. (2009). Management of adult patients with ascites due to cirrhosis: An update. *Hepatology, 49*, 2087–2107.
11. Lata, J. (2012). Hepatorenal syndrome. *World Journal of Gastroenterology, 18*, 4978–4984.
12. Mindikoglu, A., & Weir, M. R. (2013). Current concepts in the diagnosis and classification of renal dysfunction in cirrhosis. *American Journal of Nephrology*, 2013, *38*, 345–354.
13. Koch, D. G., & Fallon, M. B. (2014). Hepatopulmonary syndrome. *Clinical Liver Disease, 18*, 407–420.
14. Cartin-Ceba, R., & Krowka, M. J. (2014). Portopulmonary hypertension. *Clinical Liver Disease*, 2014, *18*, 421–438.
15. Fritz, J. S., Fallon, M. D., & Kawut, S. W. (2013). Pulmonary vascular complications of liver disease. *American Journal of Respiratory and Critical Care Medicine, 187*, 133–143.
16. Padda, M. S., Sanchez, M., Akhtar, A. J., & Boyer, J. L. (2011). Drug induced cholestasis. *Hepatology, 53*, 1377–1387.
17. Kosters, A., & Karpen, S. J. (2010). The role of inflammation in cholestasis-clinical and basic aspects. *Seminars in Liver Disease, 30*, 86–194.
18. Peter, L. M., Jansen, U. B., Ronald, P. J., & Oude, E. (2012). Mechanisms of bile secretion. In T. D. Boyer, M. R. Manns, & A. J. Sanyal (Eds.), *Zakim and Boyer's hepatology* (6th ed., pp. 47–63). Philadelphia, PA: Saunders.
19. Imam, M. H., Gossard, A. A., Sinakos, E., & Lindor, K. D. (2012). Pathogenesis and management of pruritus in cholestatic liver disease. *Journal of Gastroenterology and Hepatology, 7*, 1150–1158.
20. Fang, Y., Gurusamy, K. S., Wang, Q., et al. (2012). Pre-operative biliary drainage for obstructive jaundice. *Cochrane Database of Systematic Reviews, 9*, CD005444. doi:10.1002/14651858.CD005444.pub3
21. Matheny, S. C., & Kingery, J. E. (2012). Hepatitis A. *American Family Physician, 86*, 1027–1034.
22. Price, J. (2014). An update on hepatitis B, D, and E viruses. *Topics in Antiviral Medicine, 5*, 157–163.
23. Fiel, M. I. (2010). Pathology of chronic hepatitis B and chronic hepatitis C. *Clinical Liver Disease, 14*, 555–575.
24. Doo, E. D., & Ghany, M. G. (2010). Hepatitis B virology for clinicians. *Clinical Liver Disease, 14*, 397–408.

25. McMahon, B. J. (2010). Natural history of chronic hepatitis B. *Clinical Liver Disease, 14*, 381–396.
26. Chan, J. (2014). Hepatitis C. *Disease-a-Month, 60*, 201–212.
27. Zignego, A. L., Gragnani, L., Giannini, C., & Laffi, G. (2012). The hepatitis C virus infection as a systemic disease. *Internal and Emergency Medicine, 3* (Suppl.), S201–S208.
28. Wedemeyer, H. (2011). Hepatitis D revival. *Liver International, 31* (Suppl. 1), 140–144.
29. Voise, N., & Advisory Committee on Immunization Practices (ACIP) of the Centers for Disease Control and Prevention. (2011). A shot at hepatitis prevention. *Journal of the American Osteopathic Association, 10* (Suppl. 6), S13–S16.
30. National Institute on Alcohol Abuse and Alcoholism. (2014). *Alcohol facts and statistics*. Available at http://www.niaaa.nih.gov/alcohol-health/overview-alcohol-consumption/alcohol-facts-and-statistics
31. Schwartz, J. E., & Reinus, J. F. (2012). Prevalence and natural history of alcoholic liver disease. *Clinical Liver Disease, 16*, 659–666.
32. Crawford, J. M. (2012). Histologic findings in alcoholic liver disease. *Clinical Liver Disease, 16*, 699–716.
33. Sohail, U., & Satapathy, S. K. (2012). Diagnosis and management of alcoholic hepatitis. *Clinical Liver Disease, 16*, 717–736.
34. Tynjala, J., Kangestupa, P., Laatikanen, T., Aalto, M., & Niemela, O. (2012). Effect of age and gender on the relationship between alcohol consumption and serum GGT: Time to recalibrate goals for normal ranges. *Alcohol and Alcoholism, 47*, 558–562.
35. Singal, A. K., Chaha, K. S., Rasheed, K., & Anand, B. S. (2013). Liver transplantation in alcoholic liver disease current status and controversies. *World Journal of Gastroenterology, 19*, 5953–5963.
36. Yilmaz, Y., & Younossi, Z. M. (2014). Obesity-associated nonalcoholic fatty liver disease. *Clinical Liver Disease, 18*, 19–31.
37. Goodman, Z. D. (2014). The impact of obesity of liver histology. *Clinical Liver Disease, 18*, 33–40.
38. Imam, M. H., Talwalkar, J. A., & Lindor, K. D. (2013). Clinical management of autoimmune biliary diseases. *Journal of Autoimmunity, 46*, 88–96.
39. Liberal, R., Grant, C. R., Mieli-Vergani, G., & Vergani, D. (2013). Autoimmune hepatitis: A comprehensive review. *Journal of Autoimmunity, 41*, 126–139.
40. Liberal, R., Grant, C. R, Longhi, M. S., Mieli-Vergani, G., & Vergani, D. (2014). Diagnostic criteria of autoimmune hepatitis. *Autoimmunity Reviews, 13*, 435–440.
41. Jalan, R., & Lee, W. M. (2009). Treatment of hyperammonemia in liver failure: A tale of two enzymes. *Gastroenterology, 136*, 2048–2051.

Chapter 45

Disorders of Kidney and Urinary Tract Function

Tammy Poma and Martha Olson

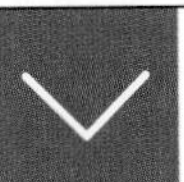

Chapter Outline and Learning Outcomes

KEY TERMS

Acute kidney injury (AKI), 1116
Chronic kidney disease (CKD), 1116
Cryptorchidism, 1117
Cystitis, 1125
Diabetic nephropathy, 1122
End-stage renal disease (ESRD), 1116
Epispadias, 1117
Focal segmental glomerulosclerosis (FSGS), 1121
Glomerular crescents, 1121
Glomerulonephritis (GN), 1118
Hemolytic uremic syndrome (HUS), 1121
Hydronephrosis, 1125
Hypertensive nephropathy, 1124
Hypospadias, 1117
Immunoglobin A nephropathy (IgAN), 1121
Membranous glomerulonephritis, 1121
Nephritic syndrome, 1119
Nephrolithiasis, 1127
Nephrotic syndrome, 1120
Nocturnal enuresis, 1128
Postinfectious glomerulonephritis (PIGN), 1121
Proteinuria, 1118
Pyelonephritis, 1126
Rapidly progressive glomerulonephritis (RPGN), 1121
Renal calculi, 1127

Key Terms continue on next page.

Renal cell carcinoma (RCC), 1129
Thrombotic thrombocytopenic purpura, 1122
Urinary incontinence, 1127
Urinary tract infection (UTI), 1125
Vesicoureteral reflux (VUR), 1127
Wilms tumor, 1129

ABBREVIATIONS

ACE—angiotensin-converting enzyme
AKI—acute kidney injury
ANCA—antineutrophil cytoplasmic antibodies
ARB—angiotensin receptor blocker
CKD—chronic kidney disease
ESRD—end-stage renal disease
FSGS—focal segmental glomerulosclerosis
GBM—glomerular basement membrane
GN—glomerulonephritis
HUS—hemolytic uremic syndrome
IgAN—immunoglobin A nephropathy
PIGN—postinfectious glomerulonephritis
RAAS—renin-angiotensin-aldosterone system
RCC—renal cell carcinoma
RPGN—rapidly progressive glomerulonephritis
UTI—urinary tract infection
VUR—vesicoureteral reflux

45.1 Chapter Overview and Case Studies

The urinary tract produces, stores, and eliminates urine and is composed of two kidneys, two ureters, the bladder, and the urethra. Kidneys are responsible for homeostasis via urine production and elimination, as well as numerous endocrine functions. Blood pressure (BP), electrolyte and acid–base balance, red blood cell (RBC) production, and even bone health all rely on kidney function to maintain well-being. **Acute kidney injury (AKI)** is a rapid decrease in kidney function, whereas **chronic kidney disease (CKD)** presents as a loss of kidney function over time resulting in a failure of the body to remove waste products. Without intervention and treatment, the result can be **end-stage renal disease (ESRD)**. Therefore, kidney disease usually manifests as a systemic illness.[1]

As with adults, children experience kidney disorders such as glomerular diseases and neoplasms, but some diseases are more common in children. Kidney diseases in children may be inherited or acquired, and **Table 45.1** ■ lists inherited kidney disorders.[2] Improved urologic care and management of congenital pediatric kidney diseases and uropathy has improved, allowing delayed time for initial renal transplantation, along with improved graft and patient survival.[3] ■

This chapter briefly reviews the normal anatomy and physiology of the kidney and then delves into the pathophysiology of the kidneys and urinary tract. The focus is on glomerular disorders; diabetic nephropathy, which is the most common type of nephrotic syndrome and leading cause of end-stage renal disease (ESRD)[4]; hypertensive nephropathy; urinary tract infections; renal calculi; and malignancy across the lifespan. Diabetic nephropathy, hypertensive nephropathy, and many of the glomerular diseases all fall under the umbrella of CKD, which, along with AKI and ESRD, are explained in more detail in Chapter 46.

Although children may experience diabetes and hypertension, these comorbidities are not usually associated with CKD in a child, as both result in progression of CKD over a period of years. The usual etiology of CKD in children is congenital, such as obstructive uropathy, vesicoureteral reflux (VUR), autosomal recessive polycystic kidney disease, or glomerular diseases with increasing age. Children who have CKD that progresses to ESRD usually start dialysis and then eventually receive a kidney transplant.[2] ■

Table 45.1 Characteristics of Selected Inherited Disorders that May Affect the Kidneys

Inherited Disorders	Characteristics
Autosomal dominant polycystic kidney disease	Usually presents in adulthood
Autosomal recessive polycystic kidney disease	A leading cause of CKD in children younger than age 12
Medullary cystic kidney/autosomal dominant interstitial kidney disease	Early-onset gout
Von Hippel-Lindau disease	Multiple tumors/renal cell carcinomas
Tuberous sclerosis	Skin tumors, seizures, cognitive impairment
Sickle cell nephropathy	Papillary necrosis/focal segmental glomerulosclerosis
Alport syndrome	Visual/auditory loss, basement membrane disease
Familial thin-membrane disease	Common cause of hematuria

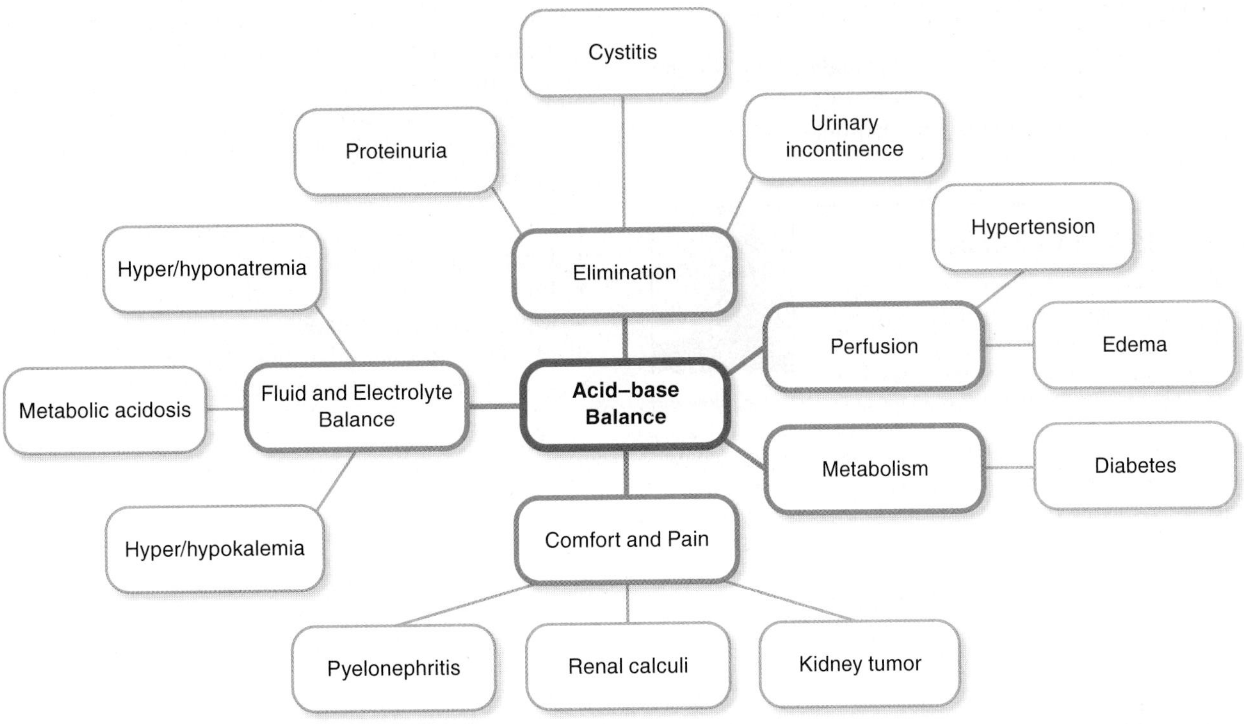

Figure 45.1 ■ Concepts related to disorders of the kidney and urinary tract function.

Concepts Related to Disorders of Kidney and Urinary Tract Function

Concepts related to the function of the kidney include fluid and electrolyte balance, acid–base balance, elimination, pain, perfusion, tissue integrity, and health promotion (see **Figure 45.1** ■). The maintenance of homeostasis depends on the kidneys to filter, save, or excrete waste products and hormones. Compensation is often noted when one of the other body systems fails, causing the kidneys to alter their work to maintain a constant internal environment.

Elimination of waste products depends on adequate perfusion to the kidney. Without blood flow to the vascular kidneys, urine output decreases. Pain can be noted in several kidney disorders, including urinary calculi and urinary tract infection. Asymptomatic kidney disorders such as hypertensive nephropathy can cause extensive damage that progresses to CKD. Urinary incontinence can contribute to problems with tissue integrity as the urea and other waste products break down tissue. Health promotion includes drinking water and other fluids to flush toxins and other wastes from the urinary system as well as regular elimination patterns. Controlling blood pressure is also important for kidney health.

The kidneys are responsible for acid–base balance; bicarbonate acts as a buffer maintaining blood pH in a narrow therapeutic range of 7.35–7.45. In acidotic states, the kidneys prevent bicarbonate losses by actively reabsorbing filtered bicarbonate in the proximal tubule. Hydrogen ions or acid is also excreted in the urine from the collecting ducts. Thus, more bicarbonate is generated, and more $NH3$ buffer is formed. In an alkalotic state, the kidney excretes more bicarbonate, and there is reduced secretion of hydrogen ions.[1,5]

Hypospadias, epispadias, and cryptorchidism are common abnormalities in the male newborn. **Hypospadias** is a congenital abnormality of the location of the male urethral meatus. The meatus develops on the ventral (underneath) side of the penis and can be anywhere from the glans to the perineum (**Figure 45.2** ■). **Epispadias** is a congenital abnormality in which the urethral opening is on the dorsal (upper) surface of the penis.[4] **Cryptorchidism** is failure of the testicles to descend into the scrotum.[6] Surgery is indicated for correction of these abnormalities and is usually done before or around 1 year of age. ■

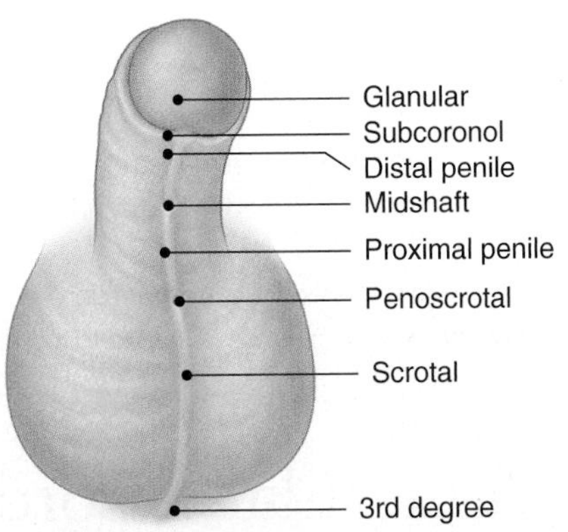

Figure 45.2 ■ Potential anatomic locations of hypospadias.

Case Studies

The following cases are addressed throughout the chapter to assist in application of chapter content to clinical situations that involve individuals with disorders of kidney and urinary tract function.

Donald Clark: Introduction

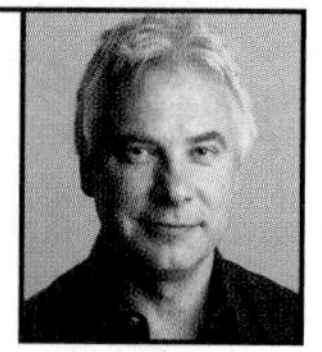

Donald Clark, age 60, presents to the emergency department (ED) with complaints of dark red urine and decreased urine output, fatigue, and edema. Mr. Clark reports that he started feeling more tired than usual about 7 days ago. He noticed the changes in his urine and his ankle edema about 3 days ago. He has a past medical history significant for hypertension for 20 years, which is well controlled with hydrochlorothiazide (Microzide), and osteoarthritis, for which he reports taking over-the-counter ibuprofen as needed. He denies any recent illness. Mr. Clark's blood pressure in the ED is 182/100. He is in no acute distress. His physical exam is unremarkable with the exception of 2+ dependent edema bilaterally in the lower extremities.

1. Of the symptoms Mr. Clark was experiencing at home that caused him to go to the ED, what ones are of concern to you and may be related to disorders of the kidney?
2. Mr. Clark has a 20-year history of hypertension and is taking a prescribed medication. He also has osteoarthritis and takes an over-the-counter NSAID to control his symptoms. In the ED, Mr. Clark's blood pressure was 182/100 mmHg. Explain how an elevated BP might affect urine flow, urine output, and kidney function.

Yvonne Johnson: Introduction

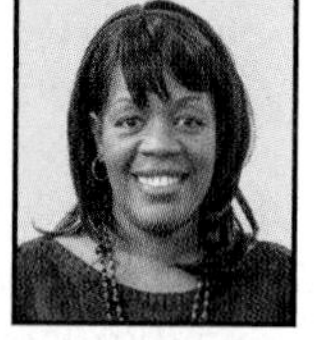

Yvonne Johnson, age 38, presents to your office with complaints of burning on urination; cloudy, pinkish, malodorous urine; and a suprapubic pain level of 3 on a 0–10 scale. She has a past medical history significant for systemic lupus erythematosus, antiphospholipid antibody syndrome, and hypertension. Her current medications are warfarin, hydroxychloroquine, prednisone, lisinopril, and chlorthalidone. Ms. Johnson's vital signs are pulse 96, respirations 12, temperature 99.1°F, blood pressure 138/78. She appears to be in no acute distress. The physical exam is unremarkable except for some suprapubic pain on palpation. Costovertebral tenderness is absent.

1. Ms. Johnson complains of suprapubic pain. What kidney dysfunctions might be present with this type of pain?
2. What is the role of kidney function in the body?

Check Your Progress: Section 45.1

1. Describe the parts and function of the urinary tract.
2. Compare and contrast acute kidney injury and chronic kidney disease.
3. What concepts are related to kidney function?
4. Explain how acid–base balance is related to kidney function.

45.2 Glomerular Disorders

Glomerulonephritis (GN) is inflammation of glomeruli and capillaries. It is characterized by proteinuria, hematuria, and edema. **Proteinuria** is defined as persistent urinary excretion of protein. Glomerular disorders are the primary cause for AKI and CKD. There are multiple glomerular disorders, which are classified on the basis of urinalysis, the patient's age, and histologic findings (see **Table 45.2** ■).

Primary GN is limited to the kidneys and includes the following disorders:

- Membranous glomerulonephritis
- Focal segmental glomerulosclerosis
- Immunoglobin A nephropathy
- Minimal change disease
- Membranoproliferative glomerulonephritis
- Crescentic glomerulonephritis.

Secondary GN is usually the result of another systemic illness, such as diabetes mellitus, and includes the following disorders:

- Lupus nephritis
- Diabetic nephropathy
- Postinfectious glomerulonephritis
- Antineutrophil cytoplasmic antibodies (ANCA)–associated vasculitis
- Antiglomerular basement membrane syndrome.

As with adults, there are many causes of pediatric glomerular diseases, both primary and secondary. The most common primary glomerular disorder seen in children is idiopathic nephrotic syndrome, attributed to minimal change nephrotic syndrome. Children will present with edema and usually respond to prednisone, but relapses are common. Postinfectious glomerulonephritis has been decreasing in industrialized nations, and the prognosis for children is excellent.[7] ■

Table 45.2 Specific Glomerular Disorders

Glomerular Disorders	Etiology/Features/Symptoms
Primary	
Membranous glomerulonephritis	Usually idiopathic
Focal segmental glomerulosclerosis	Idiopathic or genetic, more in African Americans
IgA nephropathy	Follows upper respiratory tract infection
Minimal change disease	Similar to focal segmental glomerulosclerosis; glomeruli may appear normal in some situations
Membranoproliferative glomerulonephritis	Immune complex and complement mediated
Crescentic glomerulonephritis	Glomerular injury that appears crescent-shaped
Secondary	
Lupus nephritis	Increased risk of thrombotic event
Diabetic nephropathy	Albuminuria present
Postinfectious glomerulonephritis	Beta-hemolytic streptococci infection
ANCA-associated vasculitis	Vasculitis of smaller blood vessels
Antiglomerular basement membrane	Idiopathic, vasculitis, autoantibodies attack glomerular basement membrane

Etiology and Pathogenesis

Immune complex deposits in the glomerulus are the source of many glomerulopathies (**Figure 45.3** ■). Etiology of glomerular disease could also be postinfectious, systemic disease, exposure to toxins, thrombosis, or even genetic.

Clinical Manifestations

A patient with glomerular disease typically presents with hematuria, proteinuria, edema, or hypertension. Some glomerular disorders are considered mild, possibly going undetected for months or even years; some can cause severe, acute illness.[1] **Nephritic syndrome** refers to the clinical presentation of hematuria, mild proteinuria, RBC casts, and even the presence of RBCs that are dysmorphic (**Figure 45.4** ■). When approximately fewer than half of the glomeruli biopsied are diseased, nephritic syndrome is called focal. When most or all biopsied glomeruli are diseased, nephritic syndrome is called diffuse, and the patient is more likely to present with kidney dysfunction.[8] Kidney biopsy is indicated when the cause cannot be determined with less invasive methods, symptomatology suggests a kidney disease that can be diagnosed with a biopsy, and the differential diagnosis includes diseases that are managed differently or have different potential outcomes.[4]

Acute glomerulonephritis causes changes because of the antigen–antibody deposits that get into the glomerular membrane. The usual causes of the formation of antigen–antibody complexes are external antigens from bacteria such as *Streptococcus*, internal causes such as systemic lupus erythematosus (SLE), or foreign protein.[6] Patients with acute nephritis typically present with hematuria, RBC casts, edema, hypertension, pyuria, and decreased renal function. Examples of acute nephritis are lupus nephritis, postinfectious glomerulonephritis, antiglomerular basement

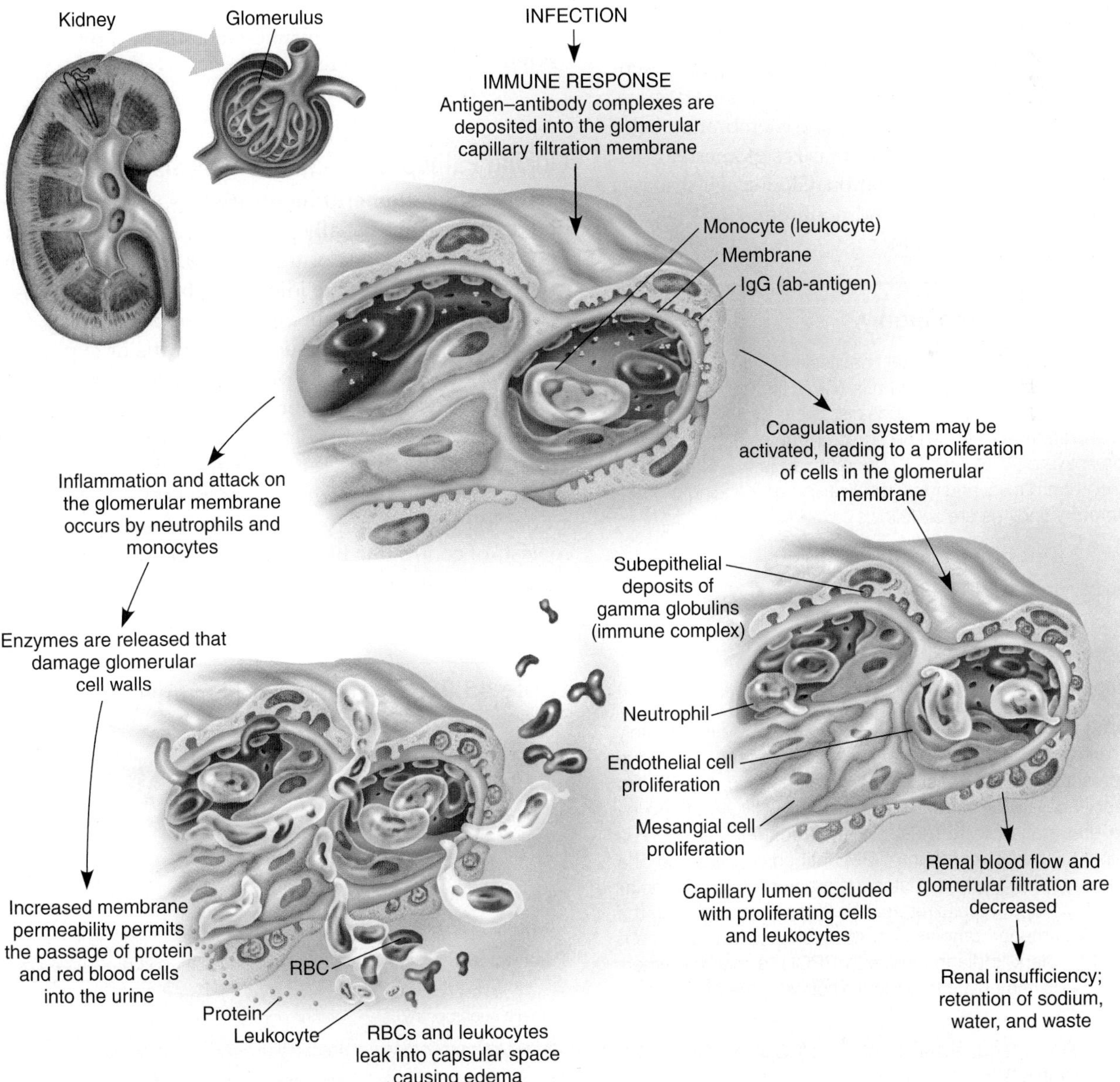

Figure 45.3 ■ Pathophysiology of acute postinfectious glomerulonephritis.

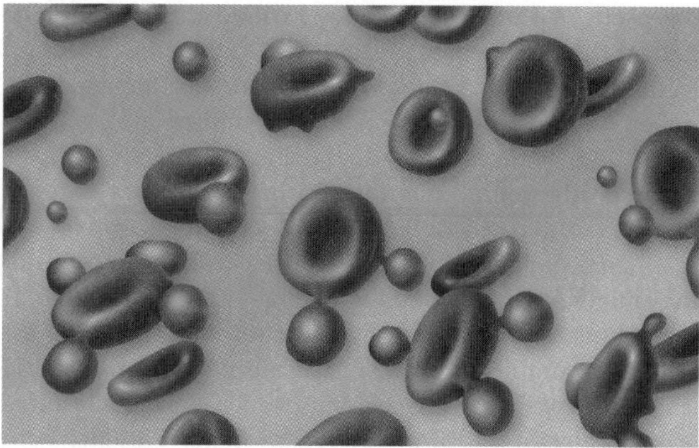

Figure 45.4 ■ Dysmorphic urinary RBCs.

membrane disease, and immunoglobin A nephropathy. When proteinuria is greater than 3 grams/day, the syndrome is termed nephrotic. In **nephrotic syndrome**, hyperlipidemia, hypoalbuminemia, edema, and urinary fatty casts are usually observed, but RBCs and RBC casts are typically absent (**Figure 45.5** ■). Examples of nephrotic syndromes are diabetic nephropathy, minimal change disease, focal segmental glomerulosclerosis, and membranous glomerulonephritis. **Table 45.3** ■ summarizes glomerular disorders and their clinical presentation. Glomerular diseases can present as both nephritic and nephrotic, but typically one predominates over the other.

Donald Clark: Application

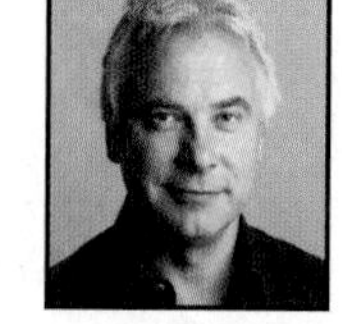

Mr. Clark is admitted to the hospital, manifesting rapidly progressive glomerulonephritis (RPGN) and hypertension. New orders include discontinuing the ibuprofen and starting an angiotensin-converting enzyme (ACE) inhibitor. The rationale is that NSAIDs are considered nephrotoxic, and Mr. Clark is also experiencing proteinuria. Laboratory findings are as follows:

Creatinine 3.2 mg/dL (baseline: 0.9 mg/dL)

Blood urea nitrogen (BUN) 42 mg/dL

Hemoglobin 9.2 g/dL

Urinalysis revealed 2+ protein.

Microscopy revealed dysmorphic RBCs and RBC casts.

Mr. Clark's lab results indicate AKI as evidenced by the acutely elevated creatinine and BUN. Hematuria is present, and urine has the presence of RBC casts, which are nephritic. Mr. Clark's coagulation labs are ordered, and he is made NPO (nothing by mouth) in preparation for a renal biopsy. Additional lab work is ordered, including ANCA and anti-GBM antibodies. Because of a high suspicion of RPGN, corticosteroids are administered empirically before the biopsy results return. The kidney biopsy shows the deposition of immune complexes in the glomeruli with crescent formation. Mr. Clark is diagnosed with RPGN, a medical emergency that needs immediate treatment to prevent the progression to ESRD.

3. What signs and symptoms of RPGN is Mr. Clark demonstrating?
4. Why was a kidney biopsy performed on Mr. Clark?

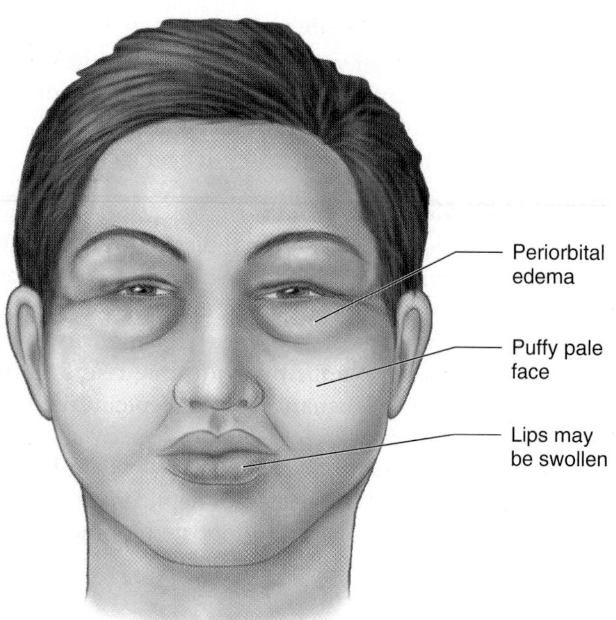

Figure 45.5 ■ Clinical manifestations of nephrotic syndrome include severe edema.

Linking Pathophysiology to Diagnosis and Treatment

Membranous glomerulonephritis, also called membranous nephropathy, usually presents as a primary glomerular disorder and is one of the leading causes of nephrotic syndrome. Most cases are idiopathic, but some are considered secondary, as the etiology may be malignancy, SLE, medications, or infection such as hepatitis or syphilis. In membranous glomerulonephritis, the podocytes of the glomerular basement membrane (GBM) become damaged by an antigen–antibody complex, and proteinuria ensues. The patient usually presents as nephrotic with hyperlipidemia, hypertension, edema, and possibly hypercoagulation. Management of membranous glomerulonephritis consists of controlling blood pressure and proteinuria with an angiotensin-converting enzyme (ACE) inhibitor or

Table 45.3 Glomerular Disorders and Their Clinical Presentation

Glomerular Disorders	Clinical Presentation	Typical Age at Onset
Membranous glomerulonephritis	Nephrotic	Adult
Focal segmental glomerulosclerosis	Nephrotic	Child/adult
IgA nephropathy	Nephritic/nephrotic	Adult
Postinfectious glomerulonephritis	Nephritic	Child
Diabetic nephropathy	Nephrotic	Adult
Minimal change disease	Nephrotic	Child
Crescentic glomerulonephritis	Nephritic	Adult

an angiotensin II receptor blocker (ARB) and controlling hyperlipidemia with statins. Most patients are managed conservatively for 6 months with ACE inhibitors and ARB therapy. Carefully selected high-risk patients might benefit from immunosuppressive therapy with alkylating agents and steroids.[9] If proteinuria is excessive (more than 4 grams/day), then immunosuppressive treatment is initiated. See **Table 45.4** ■ for a list of ACE inhibitors and ARBs.

CLINICAL POINT: ACE inhibitors and ARBs are classified as antihypertensives, but they also play a crucial role in treating proteinuria in glomerular disorders. ■

Focal segmental glomerulosclerosis (FSGS) is a group of syndromes that have podocyte injury in both focal and segmental scarring occurring in the glomerulus. The term focal segmental glomerulosclerosis indicates that the scarring involves some (focal) but not all glomeruli and that the scarring is seen in only a portion (segmental) of the glomerulus.

Primary or idiopathic FSGS is not well defined but continues to be a main type of primary glomerulonephritis, contributing to 4% of cases of ESRD in the United States.[10] Primary FSGS is usually idiopathic, whereas secondary FSGS may be caused by genetic factors, viruses, medications, or loss of nephrons. Histology reveals multiple variants of FSGS, but all have a consistent form of podocyte abnormality. Podocytes are unique cells that have permselectivity (selective permeation for certain molecules) for glomerular filtration. A circulating permeability factor or toxin has been identified in some cases of FSGS, resulting in podocyte injury. Once the podocytes have been injured, their slitlike filters allow the passage of proteins and nephrotic syndrome develops. The unaffected glomeruli tend to hypertrophy, and hyperfiltration ensues.

Treatment of primary FSGS consists of immunosuppressive therapy for more severe cases; BP control, usually with an ACE inhibitors or ARBs; and management of hyperlipidemia with statins as indicated. Secondary FSGS is not usually treated with immunosuppression but by treating the primary cause and slowing down proteinuria. FSGS can recur, and patients who advance to ESRD and receive a kidney transplant usually undergo plasmapheresis to promote remission.[11]

Immunoglobin A nephropathy (IgAN) is the leading cause of GN in the world, affecting Caucasian and Asian males more often. There is mesangial deposition of IgA in the glomerulus, and crescents are seen in some of the glomeruli. Fibrin plays a role in the pathogenesis of **glomerular crescents**, in which there is a space or hole in the GBM; macrophages and other cells proliferate, crowding the space; and a crescent-shaped scar forms. Patients typically present with hematuria following an upper respiratory tract infection. As with many types of GN, biopsy is the only method to conclusively diagnose IgAN. Mild IgAN is typically treated with ACE inhibitors for BP control and statins as indicated. For patients with a rising serum creatinine level, immunosuppression may be indicated.[12]

Postinfectious glomerulonephritis (PIGN) usually presents as acute antibody-mediated nephritis and follows an infection, typically a beta-hemolytic streptococcal infection. The frequency of PIGN has decreased in the United States, but it is still prevalent globally. Although nephritic symptoms can persist for prolonged periods, most patients recover. **Rapidly progressive glomerulonephritis (RPGN)** is a syndrome that presents as AKI and is a medical emergency. Biopsy is indicated, and the majority of the glomeruli present with crescents. The etiology is either idiopathic, the result of anti-GBM antibodies, immune complex mediated (IgAN, PIGN), or pauci-immune type.

Anti-GBM antibody disease can also affect the pulmonary system, and the patient may present with hemoptysis. Pauci-immune type disease manifests without anti-GBM antibodies or immune complexes, but antineutrophil cytoplasmic antibodies (ANCA) are present in the majority of cases. Positive ANCA pauci-immune patients will typically have symptoms of systemic vasculitis. Clinically, a distinctive feature is the small vessel vasculitis that spreads to many organ systems.[13] There are multiple forms of systemic vasculitic diseases that present as glomerulonephritis, as shown in **Table 45.5** ■.

Hemolytic uremic syndrome (HUS) is one of the main causes of AKI in children and is usually acquired. Thrombocytopenia, hemolytic anemia, and renal failure with proteinuria are seen, and symptoms are usually preceded by a bout of bloody diarrhea. A Shiga toxin–producing *Escherichia coli* infection is usually the cause. Treatment is typically supportive. Research discusses the use of eculizumab, the C5 monoclonal antibody, in the treatment of HUS.[14] ■

When this rare but acute disease is seen in adults, it may include neurologic manifestations and thrombotic microangiopathies and would then be referred to as **thrombotic thrombocytopenic purpura**.[15]

ANCA-associated pauci-immune GN is the most common biopsy result in elderly patients with progressive kidney dysfunction. Renal biopsy helps with diagnosis and prognosis and can prevent unnecessary treatments in older adults, as well as in all other age groups. Increased age should not be the only contraindication for the use of renal biopsy.[16] ■

Table 45.4 Common ACE Inhibitors and ARBs

Angiotensin-Converting Enzyme (ACE) Inhibitors	Angiotensin II Receptor Blockers
Benazepril	Candesartan
Captopril	Eprosartan
Enalapril	Irbesartan
Fosinopril	Telmisartan
Lisinopril	Valsartan
Ramipril	Losartan

Donald Clark: Outcome

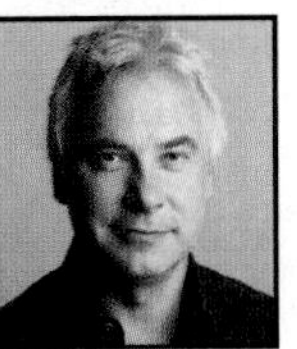

Mr. Clark's BP and laboratory values improve throughout his hospital stay. His current BP is 146/90. His urine output has increased, and the urine is now dark amber in color. Edema to the

Table 45.5 Systemic Vasculitis with Renal Involvement

Types of Systemic Vasculitis	Characteristics	Treatment
Polyarteritis nodosa	Fever, weight loss, joint pain, pericarditis, seizures	Prednisone, cyclophosphamide; plasmapheresis if hepatitis B
Henoch-Schönlein purpura	Presents as IgAN with skin involvement	Supportive
Granulomatosis with polyangiitis	Affects respiratory tract and kidneys; more common in Caucasians; ANCA-positive	Prednisone, cyclophosphamide

lower extremities is 1+, and Mr. Clark is feeling more energetic, sitting up in the chair for meals. He has developed a dry cough but otherwise is feeling better. Laboratory findings are as follows:

Creatinine 1.0 mg/dL (baseline: 0.9 mg/dL)

BUN 28 mg/dL

Hemoglobin 10.2 g/dL

Urinalysis revealed 1+ protein.

Microscopy revealed no dysmorphic RBCs or RBC casts.

Mr. Clark is switched to an ARB, candesartan, because of the cough that started after he began taking the ACE inhibitor; cough is a common side effect of this class of drugs. A conservative management plan will be followed because the protein level in Mr. Clark's urine has remained below 4 grams/day and he is showing improvement in his symptoms.

5. What is proteinuria?
6. Mr. Clark is being treated with an antihypertensive medication (an ARB). What therapeutic effect does an ARB have on kidney function?

Check Your Progress: Section 45.2

1. How are glomerular disorders classified?
2. What are the signs and symptoms of nephritic syndrome?
3. Why might a renal biopsy be an intervention for older adults?

45.3 Diabetic Nephropathy

Etiology and Pathogenesis

Diabetic nephropathy is a hyperglycemic-induced glomerulosclerosis that results in eventual hyperfiltration, proteinuria, and CKD. It is the leading cause of ESRD.[1,4] One third of the population either have diabetes or are prediabetic. Today, 26 million people in the United States are diabetic, and obesity is the major risk factor.[17] Risk factors for developing diabetic nephropathy are poor glycemic control, uncontrolled hypertension, obesity, smoking, race, and genetic factors.[18] Blacks, Hispanic, American Indian, and Asian individuals are more likely to develop diabetic nephropathy compared to other ethnic and racial groups. Much of what is known about the progression of diabetic nephropathy has come from studying type 1 diabetics, as their age at the onset of the disease is known. Persistent mild albuminuria is considered an early indication of diabetic nephropathy and typically occurs 10–15 years after the diagnosis of diabetes.[19]

Table 45.6 Classification of Albuminuria

Class	24-Hour Timed	Albumin/Creatinine Ratio (Spot Check)
Normal	$<$ 30 mg	$<$ 30 mg
Moderate albuminuria	30–300 mg	30–300 mg
Severe albuminuria	$>$ 300 mg	$>$ 300 mg

CLINICAL POINT: Individuals with diabetes are at increased risk for developing contrast-induced nephropathy. Therefore, exposure to contrast should be minimized, and nephrotoxic agents (metformin and NSAIDs) should be stopped before contrast administration.[1] ■

Proteinuria, which is defined as the persistent urinary excretion of protein, can result from glomerular injury when the glomerular capillaries are not able to filter out macromolecules, such as albumin in the glomerulus (see **Table 45.6** ■).[4] There are various types of proteinuria; when there is glomerular damage, it appears as albuminuria and can usually be detected with a dipstick assessment. Smaller proteins in the urine may indicate tubular proteinuria and usually do not appear with a dipstick assessment. Aggressive management has been shown to decrease or even reverse the advancement of diabetic nephropathy.

CLINICAL POINT: The hematologic cancer multiple myeloma is associated with CKD. The usual pathogenesis is excessive monoclonal immunoglobulin production, which leads to light-chain deposition, affecting the kidney tubule.[20] ■

Diabetic nephropathy begins with hyperglycemia leading to polyuria and increased renal blood flow, glomerular hypertrophy, glomerular hypertension, and hyperfiltration. Hyperglycemia is considered the driving force behind nephropathy development.[21] Prolonged hyperglycemia results in the glycosylation of amino acids, which leads to the development of advanced glycosylation end products, which can accumulate in tissues, causing microvascular complications. The resulting hypoxia and increased oxidative stress cause the glomeruli to lose their selective permeability, and proteinuria ensues.[21] The histologic findings with diabetic nephropathy include glomerular hypertrophy, GBM widening, expansion of the mesangium, and podocytopenia that eventually leads to nodular glomeruloscloerosis (**Figure 45.6** ■).[22]

Clinical Manifestations

Manifestations of diabetic nephropathy are albuminuria and hyperfiltration, and hypertension is usually present. Mild albuminuria is usually the earliest indicator of diabetic nephropathy; it can progress to severe albuminuria

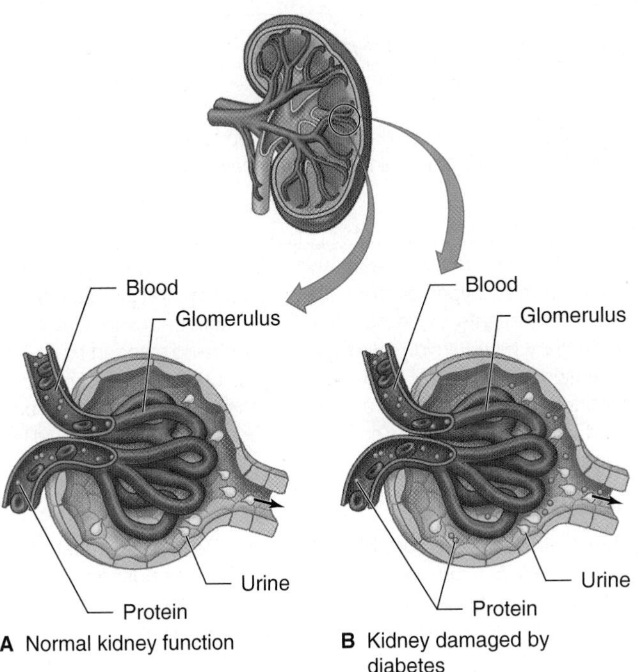

Figure 45.6 ■ Diabetic nephropathy.

(nephrotic) if left untreated, and it is also a risk factor for cardiovascular morbidity and mortality. Normally, systolic BP decreases at night, but there has been an association between diabetics who do not experience this decrease in nocturnal BP and the development of albuminuria.[20] Patients with diabetes who have been diagnosed with CKD, which is an irreversible loss in kidney function, can attribute the CKD to diabetes if there is albuminuria with retinopathy. Also, if a patient has been a type 1 diabetic for more than 10 years and has mild albuminuria, this indicates that the etiology for CKD is diabetic nephropathy.

Linking Pathophysiology to Diagnosis and Treatment

A biopsy is not usually indicated unless the patient exhibits additional symptoms that are not typically associated with diabetic nephropathy. For instance, the presentation of urinary RBC casts may indicate another glomerular disorder; or a rapid decline in kidney function or increase in hypertension after initiation of an ACE inhibitors or ARB may be a sign of renal artery stenosis. For ideal glycemic control, diabetics should target a hemoglobin A1C (A1C) of less than 7%, and ideally, their BP should be less than 140/90 mmHg.[23] Lifestyle modifications, glycemic control, BP control, and management of dyslipidemia all play roles in the management of diabetic nephropathy (**Table 45.7** ■).[1]

Older adults should not be overly aggressive with BP and glycemic control, since they are at increased risks for falls and other deleterious outcomes. For patients 60 years of age and older who do not have CKD or diabetes, current recommendations are for a target BP less than 150/90.[23] ■

There is compelling evidence that diabetics with hypertension be should be treated with ACE inhibitors or ARBs and that more than one agent will probably be required to achieve a BP lower than 140/90 mm Hg.[23] Diabetics who do not have hypertension but who do have albuminuria should also be treated with ACE inhibitors or ARBs. Screening of diabetics for nephropathy should occur annually and should include assessing for proteinuria and calculating estimated glomerular filtration rate) with serum creatinine, albumin to creatinine ratio, A1C lower than 7%, BP management of less than 140/90 as a target for all patients. Statin therapy is also indicated.[24] Patients who are started on ACE inhibitors or ARBs should have their potassium and creatinine levels assessed after initiation of treatment and during treatment, as either hyperkalemia or a decrease in renal function can occur after starting therapy. See the Impact of Current Research box for more information on treating hyperkalemia.

Table 45.7 Recommendations for Lipid Management in Patients with Diabetes

	LDL	HDL	Triglycerides
Goal	< 100 mg/dL	Women: > 50 mg/dL Men: > 40 mg/dL	< 150 mg/dL
Diabetics with additional cardiac risk factors	< 70 mg/dL		

CLINICAL POINT: The concurrent use of ACE inhibitors and ARBs is no longer recommended.[24] Cough is the most common side effect reported with ACE inhibitors.[1] ■

ACE inhibitors and ARBs are contraindicated in pregnancy, and alternative antihypertensives should be considered if a woman is planning pregnancy. ■

Check Your Progress: Section 45.3

1. What are the risk factors for developing diabetic nephropathy?
2. What ethnic and racial groups are more likely to develop diabetic nephropathy?
3. Treatment of diabetic nephropathy consists of what interventions?
4. What medications are contraindicated in treatment of pregnant individuals diagnosed with diabetic nephropathy?

45.4 Hypertensive Nephropathy

Hypertensive nephropathy is CKD resulting from longstanding hypertension. Hypertension is the second leading cause of ESRD, second to diabetes, and it affects not only the glomerulus, but also the tubules and vasculature of the kidneys, leading to nephrosclerosis. Risk factors for the development of hypertensive nephropathy are genetic, having diabetes, having another renal disorder, markedly elevated blood pressure, and race. African Americans are

Impact of Current Research on Clinical Practice

Novel Treatment for Hyperkalemia

Description: Hyperkalemia is a life-threatening condition that can result in cardiac arrhythmia and sudden cardiac death. Hyperkalemia is usually caused by the kidneys' inability to excrete potassium, impairment of mechanisms that transport potassium into cells as in diabetes, or a combination of the two factors. Medications may also contribute to the formation of hyperkalemia. ZS005 is a global, multicenter trial designed to investigate the long-term safety and efficacy of ZS-9 for patients with hyperkalemia (potassium levels > 5.0 mEq/L). ZS-9 is an insoluble, nonabsorbed zirconium silicate designed to preferentially trap potassium ions in order to lower and maintain control of serum potassium levels. ZS-9 is passed through the digestive tract and eliminated in the stool.

Patients with hyperkalemia were given ZS-9 10 g TID during the 24- to 72-hour acute phase of the study. Those who achieved normokalemia were then given 5 g once daily with the ability to titrate dose in 5-g increments or decrements, if needed, to maintain normokalemia. The primary end point was safety and tolerability; the secondary end point was the proportion of patients with an average serum potassium of 5.1 mEq/L or less between months 3 and 12.

In patients with hyperkalemia, ZS-9 rapidly normalized serum potassium levels and maintained serum potassium levels at 4.6 mEq/L with once daily treatment for up to 52 weeks, and more than 90% of patients maintained these levels with 5 or 10 grams of ZS-9.

Clinical Practice: Hyperkalemia is a life-threatening problem for patients with kidney disease and those with diabetes. Current treatments for hyperkalemia include IV calcium and insulin, which requires patients to be hospitalized. Cation–ion exchange has potentially harmful side effects and is contraindicated in multiple scenarios. Dialysis will treat hyperkalemia but is an invasive procedure. The availability of a treatment that is easily administered and tolerated for hyperkalemia should decrease patient morbidity while saving money.

Research Study:

Tumlin, J. A., Kosiborod, M., Pergola, P., Qunibi, W., Packham, D., Roger, S., Lerma, E., Fishbane, S., Rasmussen, H., & Spinowitz, B. (2015). Long-term (52-week) efficacy and safety of ZS-9 in the treatment of hyperkalemia: Interim results from a phase 3 open-label, multi-center, multi-dose maintenance study. Poster Presentation, ASN Kidney Week, Nov 7, 2015, Chattanooga, TN.

at significantly increased risk to develop CKD and ESRD from hypertension.[25]

CLINICAL POINT: Monotherapy using ACE inhibitors and ARBs in African Americans is not as efficacious as in other groups. An additional agent is usually required for this population.[25] ■

Etiology and Pathogenesis

The kidney has been implicated in the pathogenesis of hypertension, but hypertension in turn can cause CKD. There are numerous etiologies of essential hypertension; genetics, lifestyle choices and diet, activation of the renin-angiotensin-aldosterone system (RAAS), arterial stiffness, and the sympathetic nervous system have all been implicated. Hypertension as a result of kidney failure is secondary hypertension.[1] In normal individuals, the kidneys can maintain a normal BP even with an increase in sodium intake. But in some people, the increased intake of sodium can lead to hypertension. African Americans are affected disproportionately more than other populations.[25] This impaired natriuresis, or "salt sensitivity," appears to be genetic. Activation of the RAAS is a main cause of primary hypertension that may lead to the progression of CKD.[26] Hypertension increases the development of atherosclerosis in the afferent and efferent arterioles of the kidney, leading to plaque obstructions. Fragile capillaries are damaged by excessive blood pressure. These changes lead to a buildup of waste products from the damage; this causes a decrease in the glomerular filtration rate, leading to proteinuria and microalbuminuria.[4]

The sympathetic nervous system causes activation of the RAAS, starting with renin production by the kidney. Atherosclerosis is the primary cause of RAAS activation, which leads to a reduction in blood flow to the glomeruli, constant secretion of renin, and the kidney responds with by increasing the systemic blood pressure. This may become a vicious cycle, leading to the development of malignant hypertension.[4] Hypertension leads to medial hypertrophy and thickened glomerular walls. There is loss of nephrons, hyperfiltration, hypertrophy, and sclerosis.[4]

Clinical Manifestations

Classifications of hypertension are covered in detail in Chapter 23. Long-standing hypertension may lead to the development of left ventricular hypertrophy, and this finding would manifest on electrocardiography. Ophthalmoscopic examination in a patient with long-standing hypertension can reveal changes such as arteriovenous nicking or retinal hemorrhage. Patients with chronic hypertension that progresses to nephrosclerosis may manifest with mild proteinuria, and blood urea nitrogen (BUN) and creatinine will increase gradually over time.

Hydronephrosis, or dilation of the renal pelvis, may develop with ureteropelvic junction obstruction and can be detected even with antenatal ultrasound. Pyeloplasty is a surgical procedure that may be indicated for treatment of ureteropelvic junction obstruction.[27] The embryonic development of posterior urethral valves in males can lead to problems with bladder compliance and capacity and is the most important cause of end stage renal disease in young boys.[28] ■

Linking Pathophysiology to Diagnosis and Treatment

For patients with CKD or diabetes, the target BP is less than 140/90 mmHg. Lifestyle modifications are encouraged, such as regular exercise, smoking cessation, restriction of dietary sodium to less than 2.4 grams/day, moderate alcohol consumption if the patient drinks alcohol, and maintaining a body mass index (BMI) below 25. CKD is a compelling indication to use ACE inhibitors or ARBs for management of BP, especially when there is proteinuria.

CLINICAL POINT: Patients with renal artery stenosis can experience a decrease in the estimated glomerular filtration rate when treatment with ACE inhibitors or ARBs is initiated. ■

Women who have kidney disease before becoming pregnant are at increased risk for developing preeclampsia during their pregnancy. Preeclampsia is a systemic disease that manifests with hypertension, proteinuria, edema, and possibly liver dysfunction with coagulation derangements with advanced disease. ■

The incidence of renal artery stenosis increases with age, and all patients should be medically managed, but surgical options are angioplasty with or without stenting. ■

Check Your Progress: Section 45.4

1. What are the risk factors for developing hypertensive nephropathy?
2. How does hypertension increase the development of atherosclerosis in the kidneys?
3. What are treatment interventions for hypertensive nephropathy in individuals living with CKD or diabetes?

45.5 Urinary Tract Infections

Urinary tract infection (UTI) is infection of the lower urinary tract of the bladder, the upper urinary tract, or the kidney.

Cystitis

Cystitis is infection of the bladder (**Figure 45.7** ■). It is the most common bacterial infection. The majority of cases are classified as acute uncomplicated and usually occur in healthy, sexually active women with normal genitourinary tracts. Diabetes mellitus, familial predisposition, obstruction, neurogenic bladder, and the use of spermicides and diaphragms have been associated with increased risk of developing cystitis. Cystitis is classified as complicated when the urinary tract is abnormal; when the patient is pregnant, immunocompromised, or male; when the patient has had recent invasive procedures performed on the urethra; or when the etiology of the UTI is likely to result in failure of therapy.[1] Urethritis is infection and inflammation of the urethra and is usually associated with sexually transmitted disease in men.[29]

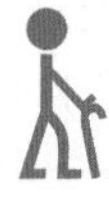

The risk of a UTI in older adult men can be related to issues with the prostate. Men 73 years of age and older have a higher incidence of UTI. ■

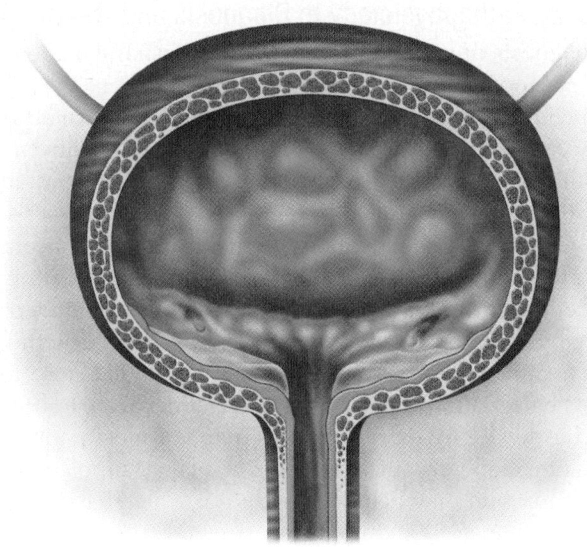

Figure 45.7 ■ Bladder wall affected by cystitis.

Etiology and Pathogenesis

Cystitis develops from the ascension of bacteria through the urethra to the bladder. The majority of infections are caused by *Escherichia coli* (*E. coli*), a fecal pathogen. Obstruction in the flow of urine and residual urine contribute to the development of UTIs.

Children with obstructive disease are more predisposed to developing a UTI. Some additional risk factors for a UTI are being an uncircumcised male younger than 3 months of age and being a female younger than 4 years of age. It is important to include UTI in the differential diagnosis of a febrile infant, as many children with fevers have pyelonephritis, and it can be difficult to differentiate between cystitis and pyelonephritis in a child. Urinary stasis is considered the most important factor that contributes to UTI.[30] ■

Pregnant women should be screened for asymptomatic cystitis, as urinary tract infection during pregnancy is associated with premature birth and low birth weight.[30] ■

Clinical Manifestations

Most patients with cystitis present with complaints of dysuria, urgency, and frequency. Asymptomatic cystitis is bacteria in the urine, but no signs or symptoms are reported by the patient. Asymptomatic cystitis, or asymptomatic bacteriuria, is usually not treated unless the patient is pregnant or otherwise considered to be at high risk.[30] Painful bladder syndrome, also known as interstitial cystitis, mimics the symptoms of UTI in the absence of infection or pathology.[31]

Advanced age, complications of the cardiovascular and neurologic systems, as well as diabetes and health conditions that impair mobility increase the risk for urinary tract infections.[32]

Older adults may manifest confusion as the presenting symptom of a UTI. Frequent UTIs in older adults may be managed with long-term treatment with trimethoprim 100 mg daily.[1] ■

Linking Pathophysiology to Diagnosis and Treatment

A diagnosis of uncomplicated cystitis is usually made on the basis of clinical symptoms, and the patient may be treated empirically without a urine culture, but urinalysis may rule out bacteriuria. A urine culture with sensitivities should be obtained for recurring infections, treatment failure, or pyelonephritis and in complicated cases of cystitis.

Current recommendations for the treatment of uncomplicated acute cystitis are to treat with nitrofurantoin, trimethoprim-sulfamethoxazole, or fosfomycin. Cranberry juice has been reported as an effective preventive method and treatment for cystitis because one of its ingredients prevents bacteria from adhering to the bladder wall, but few studies have proven it to be effective. For most patients, drinking cranberry juice or taking cranberry supplements can't hurt and may help.[33] Because it is a bladder irritant, cranberry juice should not be consumed by patients with interstitial cystitis.[1] Prophylactic use of antibiotics is recommended for recurrent cystitis and can be administered daily or after sexual intercourse.

Yvonne Johnson: Outcome

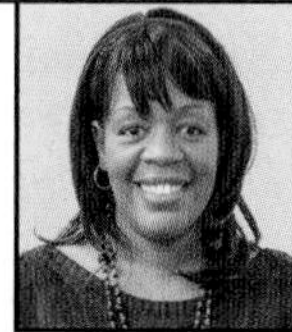

A urine culture with antimicrobial susceptibility and relevant labs are ordered. Final laboratory findings include the following:

Hg 13.2 g/dL

WBC 13,200

Creatinine 0.8 mg/dL

INR 4.2

Urine culture positive for *E. coli* susceptible to ciprofloxacin and 2+ blood detected.

Because Ms. Johnson is immunosuppressed, given her diagnosis of SLE, her UTI is considered complicated, and a fluoroquinolone antibiotic is indicated. Ms. Johnson described her urine as pinkish, and blood was detected, which could be explained by the supratherapeutic INR. Ms. Johnson's warfarin dose was adjusted appropriately, and she was encouraged to follow up with her primary care provider in 3 days for another INR evaluation. She was also advised to report to the emergency department if she notices gross hematuria.

3. Why is Ms. Johnson's UTI considered complicated cystitis?
4. Besides the antibiotic, decreased dose of warfarin, and follow-up in 3 days, what health promotion strategies might have been offered to Ms. Johnson?

Pyelonephritis

Pyelonephritis is infection of the renal pelvis and parenchyma of the kidney.[4] Like cystitis, pyelonephritis is classified as uncomplicated or complicated on the basis of the presence of anatomic or functional abnormalities, pregnancy, recurrence, or pathogen. The majority of infections are seen in females, and the usual pathogen is *E. coli.*

Vesicoureteral reflux (VUR) can occur in infants and children because of incompetency of the vesicoureteral valve mechanism. VUR, coupled with infected urine, is the most common cause of chronic pyelonephritis. The ureter lengthens with age, increasing the competence of the vesicoureteral valve mechanism, resulting in a decrease of reflux. Usually, the reflux of urine improves with age, and many children will outgrow the reflux. Surgery may be an option for VUR in children, and prophylactic antibiotics are frequently used to prevent upper UTI.[30] ■

Risk factors for pyelonephritis include the following:

- Female gender, including whether the woman is sexually active, the type of contraception used (diaphragm and/or spermicide), and whether she is pregnant
- Abnormal genitourinary tract as a result of cystic disease, obstruction, neurogenic bladder, or the presence of catheters or stents
- Immunocompromised host, such as the recipient of a kidney transplant
- Diabetes mellitus.

Obstruction can result from congenital or acquired causes. Ureteropelvic junction obstruction is the most common type of obstructive uropathy in children and has a wide range of manifestations from normal renal parenchyma to extensive tubulointerstitial injury. (Note that it can also occur in adults.) Laparoscopic pyeloplasty is a surgical option to treat this condition.[34] Some congenital obstructive reflux processes will improve as the child ages. ■

Etiology and Pathogenesis

Pyelonephritis usually develops as the pathogen ascends from the bladder through the ureter to the kidney, but it can also be the result of bacteremia (**Figure 45.8** ■). Obstructive processes (stones and papillary necrosis) or instrumentation (catheters and stents) contribute to pyelonephritis. Pyelonephritis can be acute or chronic; chronic pyelonephritis usually results from obstructive processes. A cause of chronic pyelonephritis, **vesicoureteral reflux (VUR)** is the abnormal backflow of urine from the bladder to the kidney,[30] which

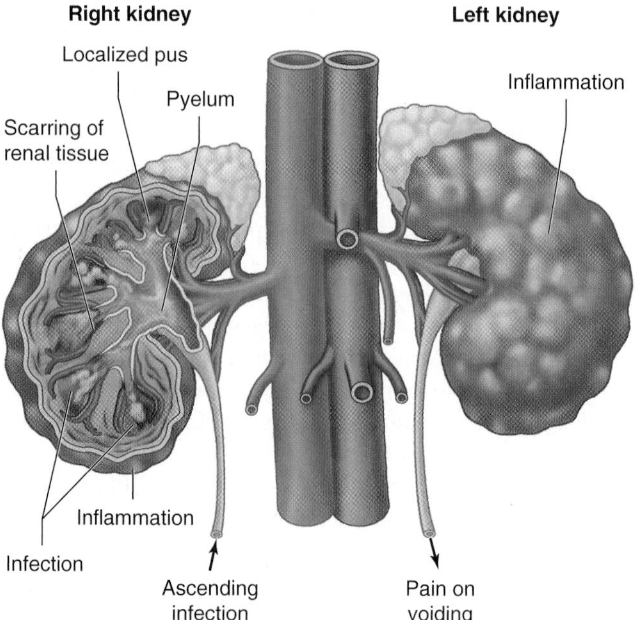

Figure 45.8 ■ Pyleonephritis.

can lead to renal scarring and ESRD. VUR is usually the result of a congenital abnormality or obstruction. Sepsis and septic shock are often caused by an infection in the urinary tract; up to 30% of sepsis cases are attributed to infection from the renal system.[35]

Older adults often present with atypical signs of infection, such as confusion, decreased appetite, and unsteady gait, making early detection of sepsis more difficult. Mortality rates for older adults with sepsis remain high; early identification and prompt treatment are essential for survival.[36] Cystitis left untreated or undertreated can progress to pyelonephritis and eventually bacteremia and sepsis.[32] ■

Clinical Manifestations

Patients with acute pyelonephritis usually complain of costovertebral angle pain, chills, and fever and may also have lower UTI symptoms.

Linking Pathophysiology to Diagnosis and Treatment

A urine culture with sensitivities is recommended and possibly computed tomography (CT) scanning to rule out any obstruction. The recommendations for treatment of pyelonephritis are more aggressive than those for cystitis and include treating with broad-spectrum antibiotics until the results of the urine culture are available and a more specific antibiotic can be started.

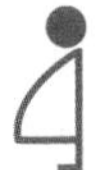

Pregnant patients with pyelonephritis should not be treated with fluoroquinolones, as there is positive evidence of fetal risk based on adverse reaction data. ■

Check Your Progress: Section 45.5

1. What are risk factors for developing cystitis?
2. What is the pathophysiology of cystitis?
3. What are the clinical manifestations of cystitis?
4. What are the types of cystitis?
5. What are the risk factors for pyelonephritis?

45.6 Renal Calculi

Renal calculi, also known as kidney stones or **nephrolithiasis**, result from the formation of urinary crystals into larger stones. Renal calculi are a common obstructive ailment usually affecting white males more than other populations. Renal calculi disease that recurs tends to reappear in younger, white males, which may be from a genetic component and therefore best practice is to identify the type of stone and initiate preventive treatment.[1] Risk factors associated with renal calculi include having a previous stone, dehydration, hypercalcuria, hyperoxaluria, and a high-sodium diet.[6]

Etiology and Pathogenesis

The majority of renal calculi are calcium based. Uric acid, struvite, and cysteine stones can also form but are seen much less frequently. Stone formation usually involves damage to the lining of the urinary tract, decreased amounts of substances that allow crystals to aggregate, and slow urine flow that allows urine to crystallize.[1] Stone formation begins with the inability of crystals to dissolve because of their high concentration, also called supersaturation. The excretion of large amounts of calcium by the kidney, urinary pH, and a lack of inhibitors all promote stone formation. The supersaturation results in the aggregation of crystals, leading to nuclei formation and eventual stone development (**Figure 45.9** ■).[1]

Clinical Manifestations

Most patients with renal calculi present with an acute onset of unilateral flank pain, nausea, and vomiting. The pain can be mild or severe and can come and go; it is referred to as renal colic. Hematuria is usually present.

Linking Pathophysiology to Diagnosis and Treatment

Diagnosis of renal calculi is usually made by clinical presentation; ultrasound and plain x-ray films may confirm the presence of stones, but CT scan may be required for confirmation. Acute management starts with pain control and hydration. If the patient can tolerate oral intake, the condition can usually be treated in an outpatient clinic. Thiazide diuretics and allopurinol have been shown to be effective in promoting stone expulsion.[1] If the patient has uncontrollable pain, infection, declining kidney function, bilateral obstruction, or only one kidney, hospital admission is usually required, with a urology consult.

All patients with renal calculi should strain their urine to try to capture the stone, as the majority of stones pass spontaneously, especially if they are smaller than 4 millimeters in diameter. Surgery may be required, depending on the type of stone and its location. Surgical options for renal calculi include flexible ureteroscopy and shock wave lithotripsy; in the case of large stones, percutaneous nephrolithotomy may be indicated.[37] Prevention of calcium oxalate stones includes increasing the factors that help to prevent stone formation, such as citrate and decreasing the levels of oxalate in the urine.

Check Your Progress: Section 45.6

1. What are risk factors for development of renal calculi?
2. Explain the pathogenesis and etiology of stone formation?
3. How is the presence of renal calculi generally diagnosed?

45.7 Urinary Incontinence

Urinary incontinence, the involuntary leakage of urine, is a symptom, not a diagnosis.[38] The condition is more common in women than in men. Up to 45% of women have some form of urinary incontinence.[38] Therefore, the International Urogynecological Association and the International Continence Society published a joint report standardizing incontinence terminology in women as outlined below[39]:

- *Stress:* Involuntary loss of urine with physical activity or sneezing/coughing

- *Urgency:* Involuntary loss of urine with feeling of urgency
- *Postural:* Involuntary loss of urine with position change
- *Nocturnal enuresis:* Involuntary loss of urine during sleep
- *Mixed:* Involuntary loss of urine with physical activity or sneezing/coughing and feelings of urgency
- *Continuous:* Complaint of continuous loss of urine
- *Insensible:* Complaint of incontinence but the woman is unaware that it happened or how it occurred because it was not felt
- *Coital:* Involuntary loss of urine with coitus.

Nocturnal enuresis is the involuntary loss of urine while sleeping (bedwetting). It is common in young children but becomes concerning if the child was previously continent. Most children become continent by the age of 5. Multiple factors can contribute to nocturnal enuresis, such as UTI, genetics, increased urinary output, sleep apnea, neurologic abnormalities, and constipation. Psychologic issues are not usually the cause but can exacerbate the problem.[30] ■

In addition to being a Caucasian female, risk factors for urinary incontinence include pregnancy; older age; obesity; hypertension, smoking; alcohol consumption; postmenopausal diabetes mellitus; and neurologic disease such as Parkinson disease, multiple sclerosis, and stroke.[1,38]

Etiology and Pathogenesis

An increase in intra-abdominal pressure, pelvic floor weakness, detrusor muscle dysfunction (urgency urinary incontinence), and urethral sphincter incompetence (stress urinary incontinence) have been implicated in urinary incontinence.[4] Bladder contractility may be impaired secondary to neuropathic causes.

Age-related barriers to toileting, such as changes in mobility, dexterity, sensory capacity, and cognition, contribute to incontinence in older patients. Men who have undergone prostate surgery or instrumentation are at risk for developing urinary incontinence.[1] ■

Stress incontinence is likely to develop during pregnancy. Having a higher BMI at term has been associated with sustained stress incontinence even after delivery.[30] ■

Clinical Manifestations

Stress urinary incontinence is the most common form of urinary continence, and patients usually complain of loss of urine with coughing or sneezing. Patients should have a thorough history and physical examination and a urinalysis. Additional assessment measures include a pelvic exam, and a voiding diary for 3 days to identify the time and frequency of incontinence and the impact of incontinence on the patient's quality of life.[38]

Urinary incontinence should not be considered a normal part of aging. Older adults should be screened for incontinence, as it is underreported and is treatable.[1] ■

Linking Pathophysiology to Diagnosis and Treatment

Weight loss, bladder training, pelvic floor muscle training, a pessary (an intravaginal support device), medications, and surgery have all been shown to be effective in the treatment of incontinence.[1] Antimuscarinics/anticholinergics, which are indicated for overactive bladder and urge incontinence, act on detrusor muscle receptors, decreasing bladder pressure. Pessaries that support the pelvic floor are used to treat stress incontinence; they should be fitted by an experienced practitioner.

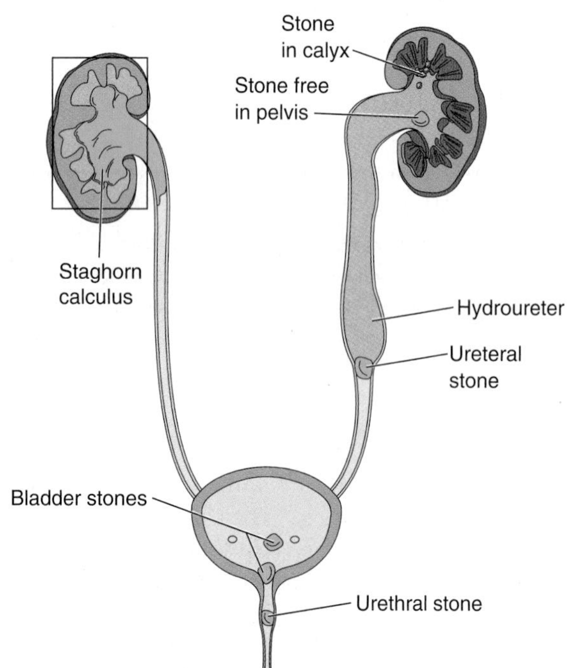

Figure 45.9 ■ Development and location of calculi within the urinary tract.

Check Your Progress: Section 45.7

1. What are the types and definitions of female urinary incontinence as determined by the International Urogynecological Association and the International Continence Society?
2. What are risk factors for developing urinary incontinence?
3. What type of assessment should be done for individuals with urine leakage?

45.8 Benign Tumors and Malignancies of the Kidney and Bladder

Kidney Tumors

Tumors involving the kidneys may be benign or malignant. Characteristics of benign tumors of the kidney and bladder are outlined in **Table 45.8** ■. If a mass is detected, it can be

Table 45.8 Benign Tumors of the Kidney and Bladder

Classification	Characteristic
Renal papillary adenoma	Hereditary proximal tubule
Oncocytoma	Well encapsulated, difficult to differentiate from malignancy
Angiomyolipoma	Associated with tuberous sclerosis

difficult to determine whether it is benign or malignant; a biopsy or active surveillance may be indicated.

Renal cell carcinoma (RCC) is the most common malignant neoplasm of the kidney. Its incidence is increasing, especially among African Americans. Risk factors for RCC are hypertension and obesity, and there is a higher incidence of RCC in men than in women.[1]

The most common kidney cancer in children is nephroblastoma, or **Wilms tumor**, which is associated with many genetic abnormalities. Most cases are diagnosed when the child is younger than 5 years old, and they usually manifest with an abdominal mass or abdominal swelling. The majority of cases are unilateral, and the survival rate is about 90%. Surgery, chemotherapy, and radiation are all treatments for Wilms tumor.[30,40] ■

Etiology and Pathogenesis

Approximately 85% of kidney neoplasms are RCC that rise from the renal cortex; the remainder originate from the renal pelvis and are considered urothelial or transitional cell cancers (**Figure 45.10** ■). Urothelial cancers arise from the epithelial lining of the urinary tract; therefore, renal pelvis cancers and bladder cancers are treated similarly. RCCs are classified on the basis of pathology and the most common is clear cell RCC. Less common types of RCC include papillary, chromophobic, and collecting duct tumors. Approximately 33% of patients with Von Hippel-Lindau disease, which is an inherited disease manifested by the presence of tumors, develop RCC. Genetic abnormalities have been identified in the pathogenesis of RCC but are not completely understood.

Clinical Manifestations

Symptoms of RCC may include hematuria, abdominal mass, weight loss, and dull, aching pain. However, these tumors are rather insidious, which delays diagnosis. Many patients are asymptomatic, and the diagnosis of a kidney tumor is an incidental finding.[1]

Linking Pathophysiology to Diagnosis and Treatment

Surgery is indicated for the treatment of RCC and is considered curative if the disease has not metastasized. Surgery may result in a radical nephrectomy, a highly vascular surgery that has the potential for increased blood loss during surgery.[1] Thermal ablation may be considered in nonsurgical candidates. Immunotherapy and molecularly targeted therapies (antiangiogenic and mTor inhibitors) are being used to treat advanced RCC.[41–43] Cancer staging involves the location of the primary tumor (T), tumor size and extent of tumors, lymph node involvement (N), and whether there is metastasis (M) of the primary tumor.[1,4]

Bladder Cancer

Bladder cancer is the most common urinary tract cancer and occurs three times more often in men than in women. As with RCC, smoking has been identified as the most important risk factor for the development of bladder cancer; industrial exposure to aromatic amines is another major risk factor. Indwelling catheter use is also considered to contribute to the development of cancer in the bladder.[4,44]

Etiology and Pathogenesis

Bladder cancer can be superficial and not invade the muscle, or it can invade the muscle. It can also go beyond the muscle, metastasizing to lymph nodes or other organs, usually the lungs, liver, or bone (**Figure 45.11** ■). Exposure to known carcinogens from smoking or environmental factors has been shown to alter the epithelial lining, resulting in transitional cell cancer. Genetic alterations in the epithelial cells have also been identified as contributing to bladder cancer formation.[4]

Clinical Manifestations

Symptoms of bladder cancer include hematuria (which may be microscopic) and complaints of urgency, frequency, and dysuria. In the absence of glomerular bleeding, hematuria is suggestive of urothelial cancer in adult patients.

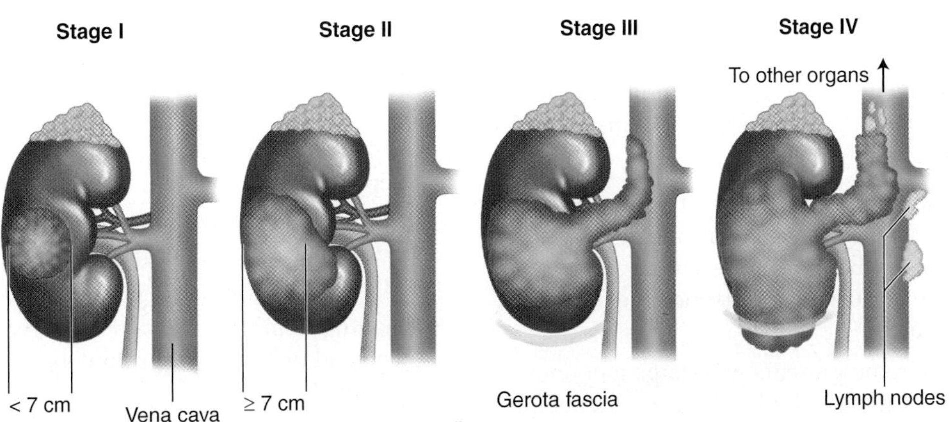

Figure 45.10 ■ Staging of renal cell carcinoma.

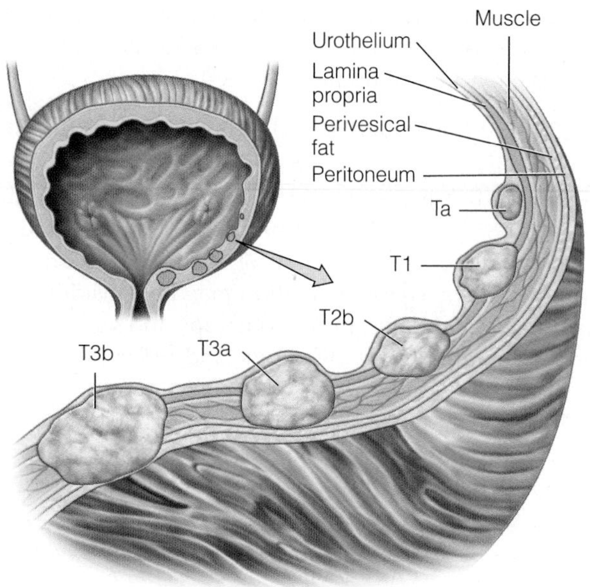

Figure 45.11 ■ Stages of bladder tumor development and invasiveness.

Linking Pathophysiology to Diagnosis and Treatment

Cystoscopy with urine cytology is indicated for evaluation of symptoms. If there is evidence of disease, patients should undergo further evaluation for metastatic disease and continue with transurethral resection of bladder tumor, which is used for staging and to manage tumors that have not invaded the muscle layer. Bladder cancer is staged by using the tumor, node, metastasis classification system.

Radical cystectomy with urinary diversion or partial cystectomy is indicated for bladder cancer that has invaded the muscle. Urinary diversion options are the creation of a urostomy or an internal reservoir, which may require self-catheterization.

Chemotherapy and radiation are options for the treatment of bladder cancer that has invaded the muscle, as are the more invasive transurethral resection of the tumor and radical cystectomy.[4] Use of molecular markers to evaluate immunohistochemistry is being studied as a possible means to provide a reliable risk assessment tool for recurrence and progression of bladder cancer.[44]

Check Your Progress: Section 45.8

1. What are risk factors for renal cell carcinoma (RCC)?
2. Describe the etiology and pathogenesis of RCC.
3. Explain the etiology of bladder cancer.
4. What are the symptoms of bladder cancer?

CHAPTER SUMMARY

45.1 Chapter Overview and Case Studies

Describe the role of the kidneys, and discuss concepts related to kidney and urinary tract function.

- The kidneys are responsible for acid–base balance and homeostasis.
- The kidneys possess endocrine functions.
- The kidneys regulate blood pressure.

45.2 Glomerular Disorders

Differentiate the causes, classification, underlying pathogenesis, and clinical manifestations of glomerular disorders and approaches to diagnosis and treatment of these conditions across the lifespan.

- In primary glomerular disorders, the glomeruli are affected, and there is no other systemic disease causing the disorder, as there is with secondary glomerular disease, which is caused by systemic illness, such as diabetes mellitus.
- Nephrotic syndrome presents with large amounts of proteinuria ($>$ 3 g/day), hyperlipidemia, hypoalbuminemia, and edema. Urinary fatty casts are usually observed, but RBCs and RBC casts are typically absent.
- Nephritic syndrome presents with hematuria, mild proteinuria, hypertension, urinary RBC casts, and dysmorphic RBCs.
- Kidney biopsy is the gold standard for diagnosing glomerular disorders.
- RPGN is a syndrome that presents as nephritic. Kidney dysfunction and crescentic glomeruli are typically seen.

45.3 Diabetic Nephropathy

Differentiate the causes, classification, underlying pathogenesis, and clinical manifestations of diabetic nephropathy and approaches to diagnosis and treatment of this condition across the lifespan.

- Mild albuminuria is an early indicator of diabetic nephropathy.
- In the majority of diabetics, the target hemoglobin A1C is less than 7%, and target BP readings are lower than 140/90 mmHg.
- Tight glycemic control and management of hypertension and proteinuria can slow the progression of CKD in diabetics.
- ACE inhibitors and ARBs are recommended for treatment of BP and proteinuria in diabetics.

- Most diabetics manifest with hypertension and usually require more than one antihypertensive to manage it effectively.

45.4 Hypertensive Nephropathy

Differentiate the causes, classification, underlying pathogenesis, and clinical manifestations of hypertensive nephropathy and approaches to diagnosis and treatment of this condition across the lifespan.

- Hypertensive nephropathy is preventable in most cases.
- The target BP is lower than 140/90 mmHg but is lower than 150/90 mmHg in adults over 60 years of age without compelling indications such as CKD or diabetes.
- The recommended treatment of hypertensive nephropathy begins with ACE inhibitors or ARBs.
- African Americans are at greater risk of developing hypertensive nephropathy and typically need an additional agent along with an ACE inhibitors or ARB.

45.5 Urinary Tract Infections

Differentiate the causes, classification, underlying pathogenesis, and clinical manifestations of urinary tract infections and approaches to diagnosis and treatment of these condition across the lifespan.

- Cystitis is the most common bacterial infection and usually affects sexually active women.
- Cystitis is classified as acute uncomplicated or complicated; the two types are treated differently empirically.
- The majority of UTIs are the result of infection with *E. coli*, which is a fecal pathogen.
- Asymptomatic cystitis is usually not treated in healthy women.
- Pyelonephritis usually results from the ascension of bacteria to the kidneys but can also result from bacteremia.
- Sexually active women are more likely to develop pyelonephritis.
- Pyelonephritis usually presents with fever, chills, flank pain, nausea, and vomiting.
- Antimicrobial therapy for acute pyelonephritis is longer in duration than cystitis treatment.

45.6 Renal Calculi

Differentiate the causes, classification, underlying pathogenesis, and clinical manifestations of renal calculi and approaches to diagnosis and treatment of this condition across the lifespan.

- Renal calculi, or kidney stones, are a common cause of urinary obstruction.
- Males are more likely to develop renal calculi, which tend to recur.
- The majority of renal calculi are calcium oxalate, and prevention includes lowering urinary oxalate and adding citrate to inhibit stone formation.
- Hydration is important in treating and preventing renal calculi.

45.7 Urinary Incontinence

Differentiate the causes, classification, underlying pathogenesis, and clinical manifestations of urinary incontinence and approaches to diagnosis and treatment of this condition across the lifespan.

- Stress and urge incontinence are the most common types of urinary incontinence; mixed incontinence is a combination of the two.
- Older adults should be screened for incontinence, as it is underreported.
- Incontinence should not be considered a normal part of aging, and it is treatable.

45.8 Benign Tumors and Malignancies of the Kidney and Bladder

Differentiate the causes, classification, underlying pathogenesis, and clinical manifestations of benign tumors and malignancies of the kidney and bladder and approaches to diagnosis and treatment of these conditions across the lifespan.

- Kidney tumors are often discovered inadvertently. All kidney tumors should be treated as malignant unless proven otherwise, as they are difficult to differentiate with imaging.
- Surgery is indicated for RCC and is considered curative if the disease has not metastasized.
- Symptoms of bladder cancer include hematuria (which may be microscopic) and complaints of urgency, frequency, and dysuria. In the absence of glomerular bleeding, hematuria is suggestive of urothelial cancer in adult patients. Smoking and being male are risk factors associated with bladder cancer, which tends to recur.

REVIEW QUESTIONS

1. In a client with glomerular disease, a kidney biopsy is:
   a. not indicated if you are able to determine nephrotic or nephritic syndrome.
   b. indicated when the cause cannot be determined through less invasive methods.
   c. indicated if the client has long-standing diabetes mellitus.
   d. indicated only if the patient has hematuria.

2. The recommended target BP, hemoglobin A1C, and lipid levels (LDL, HDL, triglycerides) in a female diabetic are:
   a. 128/70 mmHg, 7.1%, 100 mg/dL, 68 mg/dl, 160 mg/dL.
   b. 138/72 mmHg, 6.2%, 72 mg/dL, 48 mg/dL, 148 mg/dL.
   c. 146/82 mmHg, 8.8%, 52 mg/dL, 68 mg/dL, 150 mg/dL.
   d. 120/62 mmHg, 6.8%, 32 mg/dL, 60 mg/dL, 156 mg/dL.
3. Mr. Clark returns to the clinic and reports a persistent cough. The nurse suspects that which of the following is contributing to his cough?
   a. Allergic reaction to trimethoprim-sulfamethoxazole
   b. Von Hippel-Lindau disease
   c. Benazepril
   d. Nephroblastoma
4. An 87-year-old female with incontinence was recently admitted to the hospital with a new onset of confusion. The most likely explanation for her confusion is:
   a. dementia.
   b. membranous glomerulonephritis.
   c. UTI.
   d. postinfectious glomerulonephritis.
5. The prophylactic use of antibiotics in women with recurrent cystitis is:
   a. contraindicated.
   b. acceptable only if the patient is not sexually active.
   c. prescribed for daily or postcoital use.
   d. discouraged, as it may lead to dependence.
6. The bacteria most likely to cause cystitis are:
   a. *Helicobacter pylori.*
   b. *Streptococcus.*
   c. *Clostridium tetani.*
   d. *Escherichia coli.*
7. A 62-year-old Caucasian male with a past medical history of renal calculi is seen in the office with complaints of mild right-sided flank pain that started suddenly today and nausea without vomiting. The nurse knows that acute management in the clinic involves:
   a. scheduling a CT scan.
   b. scheduling an ultrasound and plain X-ray films.
   c. having the client drink fluids, take pain medication, and strain the urine.
   d. sending the client to the emergency department.
8. A female client reports leakage of urine whenever she coughs or sneezes and says that she occasionally has the sudden urge to urinate but does not make it to the toilet. The nurse recognizes the symptoms as what type of urinary incontinence?
   a. Stress
   b. Nocturnal enuresis
   c. Insensible
   d. Mixed

ANSWERS

Answers to Review Questions can be found in Appendix A. Answers to Case Study and Check Your Progress questions are available on the faculty resources site. Please consult with your instructor.

RECOMMENDED WEBSITES

National Comprehensive Cancer Network
https://www.nccn.org/default.aspx

National Kidney Foundation
https://www.kidney.org

National Institute of Diabetes and Digestive and Kidney Diseases: Kidney Disease
https://www.niddk.nih.gov/health-information/kidney-disease

REFERENCES

1. Pearson Education. (2015). *Nursing: A Concept-Based Approach to Learning* (2nd ed.). Hoboken, NJ: Pearson Education.
2. Harambat, J., van Stralen, K. J., Kim, J. J., Tizard, E. J. (2012). Epidemiology of chronic kidney disease in children. *Pediatric Nephrology, 27*(3), 363–373.
3. Bagga, H. S., Lin, S., Williams, A., Schold, J., Chertack, N., Goldfarb, D., & Wood, H. (2016). Trends in renal transplantation rates in patients with congenital urinary tract disorders. *Journal of Urology, 195*(4, Pt. 2), 1257–1262. doi:10.1016/j.juro.2015.10.004

4. Capriotti, T. & Frizzell, J. (2016). *Pathophysiology: Introductory concepts and clinical perspectives.* Philadelphia, PA: F.A. Davis
5. Hamm, L., Nakhoul, N., & Hering-Smith, K. (2015). Acid-base homeostasis. *Clinical Journal of the American Society of Nephrology, 10*(12), 2232–2242.
6. Sommers, M., & Fannin, E. (2015). *Diseases and disorders: A nursing therapeutics manual* (5th ed.). Philadelphia, PA: F.A. Davis.
7. Dagan, R., Cleper, R., Davidovits, M., Sinai-Trieman, L., & Krause, I. (2016). Post-infectious glomerulonephritis in pediatric patients over two decades: Severity-associated features. *Israel Medical Association Journal, 18*(6), 336–340.
8. Kwiatkowski, S., Kwiatkowska, E., Rzepka, R., et al. (2016). Development of a focal segmental glomerulosclerosis after pregnancy complicated by preeclampsia: Case report and review of literature. *Journal of Maternal-Fetal & Neonatal Medicine, 29*(10), 1566–1569. doi:10.3109/14767058.2015.1053865
9. Tran, T. H., Hughes, G. J., Greenfeld, C., & Pham, J. T. (2015). Overview of current and alternative therapies for idiopathic membranous nephropathy. *Pharmacotherapy, 35*(4), 396–411. doi:10.1002/phar.1575
10. Kim, J. S., Han, B. G., Choi, S. O., & Cha, S. (2016). Secondary focal segmental glomerulosclerosis: From podocyte injury to glomerulosclerosis. *Biomedical Research International, 2016*, 1–7. doi:10.1155/2016/1630365
11. Schachter, M. E., Monahan, M., Radhakrishnan, J., et al. (2010). Recurrent focal segmental glomerulosclerosis in the renal allograft: Single center experience in the era of modern immunosuppression. *Clinical Nephrology, 74*(3), 173–181.
12. Wyatt, R. J., & Julian, B. A. (2013). IgA nephropathy. *New England Journal of Medicine, 368*(25), 2402–2414.
13. Lionaki, S., & Boletis, J. N. (2016). The prevalence and management of pauci-immune glomerulonephritis and vasculitis in western countries. *Kidney Diseases (Basel, Switzerland), 1*(4), 224–234. doi:10.1159/000442062
14. Keir, L. S. (2015). Shiga toxin associated hemolytic uremic syndrome. *Hematology/Oncology Clinics of North America, 29*(3), 525–539. doi:10.1016/j.hoc.2015.01.007
15. Scully, M., & Goodship, T. (2014). How I treat thrombotic thrombocytopenic purpura and atypical haemolytic uraemic syndrome. *British Journal of Haematology, 164*(6), 759–766. doi:10.1111/bjh.12718
16. Sumnu, A., Gursu, M., & Ozturk, S. (2015). Primary glomerular diseases in the elderly. *World Journal of Nephrology, 4*(2), 263–270. doi:10.5527/wjn.v4.i2.263
17. Blair, M. (2016). Diabetes mellitus review. *Urologic Nursing, 36*(1), 27–36. doi:10.7257/1053-816X.2016.36.1.27.
18. Narres, M., Claessen, H., Droste, S., Kvitkina, T., Koch, M., Kuss, O., & Icks, A. (2016). The incidence of end-stage renal disease in the diabetic (compared to the non-diabetic) population: A systematic review. *Plos One, 11*(1), e0147329. doi:10.1371/journal.pone.0147329
19. Bakris, G. L., & Molitch, M. (2014). Microalbuminuria as a risk predictor in diabetes: The continuing saga. *Diabetes Care, 37*(3), 867–875.
20. Leung, N., Gertz, M., Kyle, R. A., Fervenza, F. C., Irazabal, M. V., Eirin, A., Kumar, S., Cha, S. S., Rajkumar, S. V., Lacy, M. Q., Zeldenrust, S. R., Buadi, F. K., Hayman, S. R., Nasr, S. H., Sethi, S., Ramirez-Alvarado, M., Witzig, T. E., Herrmann, S. M., & Dispenzieri, A. (2012). Urinary albumin excretion patterns of patients with cast nephropathy and other monoclonal gammopathy-related kidney diseases. *Clinical Journal of the American Society of Nephrology, 7*(12), 1964.
21. Sun, Y., Su, Y., Li, J., & Wang, L. (2013). Recent advances in understanding the biochemical and molecular mechanism of diabetic nephropathy. *Biochemical and Biophysical Research Communications, 433*(4), 359–361. doi:10.1016/j.bbrc.2013.02.120
22. Lizicarova, D., Krahulec, B., Hirnerova, E., Gaspar, L., & Celecova, Z. (2014). Risk factors in diabetic nephropathy progression at present. *Bratislavske Lekarske Listy, 115*(8), 517–521.
23. James, P. A., Oparil, S., Carter, B. L., et al. (2014). 2014 evidence-based guideline for the management of high blood pressure in adults: Report from the panel members appointed to the Eighth Joint National Committee (JNC 8). *JAMA, 311*(5), 507–520.
24. Kowalski, A., Krikorian, A., & Lerma, E. V. (2014). Diabetic nephropathy for the primary care provider: New understandings on early detection and treatment. *Ochsner Journal, 14*(3), 369–379.
25. Cohen, D. L., & Townsend, R. R. (2013). Is it variants in the apolipoprotein L1 gene, or blood pressure control, that predicts progression of nondiabetic hypertensive nephropathy in African Americans? *Journal of Clinical Hypertension, 15*(7), 445–446. doi:10.1111/jch.12126
26. Yamout, H., Lazich, I., & Bakris, G. L. (2014). Blood pressure, hypertension, RAAS blockade, and drug therapy in diabetic kidney disease. *Advances in Chronic Kidney Disease, 21*(3), 281–286. doi:10.1053/j.ackd.2014.03.005
27. Khoder, W., Alghamdi, A., Schulz, T., et al. (2016). An innovative technique of robotic-assisted/laparoscopic re-pyeloplasty in horseshoe kidney in patients with failed previous pyeloplasty for ureteropelvic junction obstruction. *Surgical Endoscopy, 30*(9), 4124–4129. doi:10.1007/s00464-015-4678-8
28. Matsell, D. G., Simon, Y., Morrison, S. J., & Yu, S. (2016). Antenatal determinants of long-term kidney outcome in boys with posterior urethral valves. *Fetal Diagnosis & Therapy, 39*(3), 214–221. doi:10.1159/000439302
29. Workowski K. A., & Bolan, G. A. (2015). Sexually transmitted diseases treatment guidelines, 2015. *Morbidity and Mortality Weekly Report (MMWR), 64*(RR3), 1–37. Retrieved from http://www.cdc.gov/mmwr/preview/mmwrhtml/rr6403a1.htm
30. Perry, S., Hockenberry, M., Lowdermilk, D., & Wilson, D. (2014). *Maternal child nursing care* (5th ed.). St. Louis, MO: Elsevier.
31. Anderson, R., & Zinkgraf, K. (2013). Use and effectiveness of complementary therapies among women with interstitial cystitis. *Urologic Nursing, 33*(6), 306–311.
32. Freeman-Jabson, J., Rogers, J., & Ward-Smith, P. (2016). Effect of an education presentation on the knowledge and awareness of urinary tract infection among non-licensed and licensed health care workers in long-term care facilities. *Urological Nursing, 36*(2), 67–71.
33. Cleveland Clinic. (2015). Health essentials: Can cranberry juice stop your UTI? Available at https://health.clevelandclinic.org/2015/10/can-cranberry-juice-stop-uti
34. Powell, C., Gatti, J. M., Juang, D., & Murphy, J. P. (2015). Laparoscopic pyeloplasty for ureteropelvic junction obstruction following open pyeloplasty in children. *Journal of Laparoendoscopic & Advanced Surgical Techniques, Part A, 25*(10), 858–863. doi:10.1089/lap.2015.0074
35. Wagenlehner, F. M., Lichtenstern, C., Rolfes, C., Mayer, K., Uhle, F., Weidner, W., et al. (2013). Diagnosis and management for urosepsis. *International Journal of Urology, 20*(10), 963–970.
36. Umberger, R., Callen, B., & Brown, M. L. (2015). Severe sepsis in older adults. *Critical Care Nursing Quarterly, 38*(3), 259–270. doi:10.1097/CNQ.0000000000000078
37. Palmero, J. L., Duran-Rivera, A. J., Miralles, J., Pastor, J. C., Benedicto, A. (2016). Comparative study for the efficacy and safety of percutaneous nephrolithotomy (PCNL) and retrograde intrarenal surgery (RIRS) for the treatment of 2–3,5 cm kidney stones. *Archivos Españoles de Urología, 69*(2), 67–72.
39. Ostle, Z. (2016). Assessment, diagnosis, and treatment of urinary continence in women. *British Journal of Nursing, 25*(2), p. 84–91.
39. Haylen, B. T., de Ridder, D., Freeman, R. M., et al. (2010). An International Urogynecological Association (IUGA)/International Continence Society (ICS) joint report on the terminology

for female pelvic floor dysfunction. *Neurourology and Urodynamics, 29*(1), 4–20.

40. Dome, J. S., Graf. N., Geller, J. I., Fernandez, C. V., Mullen, E. A., Spreafico, F., Van den Heuvel-Eibrink, M., & Pritchard-Jones, K. (2015). Advances in Wilms tumor treatment and biology: Progress through international collaboration. *Journal of Clinical Oncology*, 33(27), 2999–3007.
41. Motzer, R. J., Escudier, B., McDermott D. F., et al.. (2015). Nivolumab versus Everolimus in advanced renal-cell carcinoma. *New England Journal of Medicine, 373*(19), 1803–1813.
42. Molina, A. M., & Motzer, R. J. (2011). Clinical practice guidelines for the treatment of metastatic renal cell carcinoma: Today and tomorrow. *Oncologist, 16*(Suppl. 2), 45–50.
43. National Comprehensive Cancer Network. (2016). Kidney cancer: NCNN guidelines. Available at https://www.nccn.org/professionals/physician_gls/f_guidelines.asp#site
44. Sanguedolce, F., Bufo, P., Carrieri, G. & Cormio, L. (2014). Predictive markers in bladder cancer: Do we have molecular markers ready for clinical use? *Critical Reviews in Clinical Laboratory Sciences, 51*(5), 291–304.

Chapter 46

Acute Kidney Injury and Chronic Kidney Disease

Tammy Poma and Martha Olson

Chapter Outline and Learning Outcomes

46.1 Chapter Overview and Case Studies

Describe the role of the kidneys, and discuss concepts related to acute kidney injury and chronic kidney disease.

46.2 Acute Kidney Injury

Differentiate the causes, underlying pathogenesis, and clinical manifestations of acute kidney injury and approaches to diagnosis and treatment of the condition across the lifespan.

46.3 Chronic Kidney Disease

Differentiate the causes, classification, underlying pathogenesis, and clinical manifestations of chronic kidney disease and approaches to diagnosis and treatment of the condition across the lifespan.

KEY TERMS

Acute interstitial nephritis, 1142
Acute kidney injury (AKI), 1137
Acute tubular necrosis (ATN), 1137
Albumin:creatinine ratio, 1151
Albuminuria, 1146
Anuric, 1142
Azotemia, 1137
BUN:creatinine ratio, 1152
Chronic kidney disease (CKD), 1144
Chronic kidney disease–mineral and bone disorder (CKD-MBD), 1149
Contrast-induced nephropathy (CIN), 1141
End-stage renal disease (ESRD), 1142
Erythropoietin, 1149
Fractional excretion of sodium (FE_{Na}), 1143
Fractional excretion of urea (FE_{urea}), 1143
Glomerulosclerosis, 1146
Hemodialysis, 1154
Hydronephrosis, 1144
Hyperkalemia, 1150
Hypervolemia, 1150
Intrinsic AKI, 1138
Ischemic ATN, 1140
Metabolic acidosis, 1147
Nephrotoxic ATN, 1140
Nonoliguric, 1142
Oliguric, 1142
Peritoneal dialysis, 1154
Polycystic kidney disease (PKD), 1146
Postrenal AKI, 1139
Prerenal AKI, 1138
Renal transplantation, 1154
Uremia, 1150

ABBREVIATIONS

AKI—acute kidney injury
AKIN—Acute Kidney Injury Network
ATN—acute tubular necrosis
BUN—blood urea nitrogen
CIN—contrast-induced nephropathy
CKD—chronic kidney disease
CKD-MBD—chronic kidney disease–mineral and bone disorder
ESRD—end-stage renal disease
FE_{Na}—fractional excretion of sodium
FE_{urea}—fractional excretion of urea
GFR—glomerular filtration rate
HUS—hemolytic-uremic syndrome
KDIGO—Kidney Disease Improving Global Outcomes
KDOQI—Kidney Disease Outcomes Quality Initiative
PKD—polycystic kidney disease
PTH—parathyroid hormone
RAAS—renin–angiotensin–aldosterone system
RIFLE—Risk, Injury, Failure, Loss, End-Stage Renal Disease
RPGN—rapidly progressive glomerulonephritis

46.1 Chapter Overview and Case Studies

The kidneys regulate body fluids and electrolytes and excrete waste products, which is essential to maintain normal physiologic function. A decline in kidney function, either acute or chronic, can be life-limiting and life-threatening. Although clinical manifestations of acute kidney injury (AKI) may be quickly noted, manifestations of chronic kidney disease (CKD) may be silent for many years. Prompt identification of AKI can result in the preservation of normal kidney function. CKD can be controlled through monitoring and treatment of conditions that contribute to the progression of this disorder.

Kidney function affects many physiologic processes. Alteration of kidney function results from both acute and chronic disorders. Acute kidney injury (AKI) occurs on a continuum from risk of injury to overt kidney failure. Recent consensus on the definition of AKI with the Risk, Injury, Failure, Loss, End-Stage Renal Disease (RIFLE), the Acute Kidney Injury Network (AKIN) criteria, and the Kidney Disease Improving Global Outcomes (KDIGO) classification systems will result in better identification of AKI in patients and facilitate AKI research, providing established and accurate definitions needed for publishing results and studies that can be compared with one another.

The aims of this chapter are threefold. The first is to identify the causes, underlying pathophysiologic processes, and clinical manifestations of AKI, as well as differentiating the types of AKI so that prompt and appropriate treatment can be initiated. The second is to explain the major etiologies of CKD, discuss preventable causes, and describe measures to prevent disease progression. Finally, systemic manifestations and management of end-stage renal disease will be addressed.

Concepts Related to Acute Kidney Injury and Chronic Kidney Disease

Concepts related to acute kidney injury and chronic kidney disease include acid–base balance, fluid and electrolyte balance, perfusion, stress and coping, and pain. Each concept relates to the importance of the kidney's ability to regulate fluid volumes and maintain healthy electrolyte levels along with controlling the blood pressure (**Figure 46.1** ■).

The kidneys help to maintain internal homeostasis and volume by regulating the hormones and substances that the body eliminates or retains. This is accomplished through adequate perfusion to the nephrons. Acute kidney injury is often the result of infection or inflammation, such as urinary tract infections or nephrolithiasis, and can usually be reversed if treated early. Chronic kidney disease is often vague and asymptomatic early in the disease process and is the result of long-term damage to the kidney from diseases such as untreated hypertension or diabetes mellitus (DM) or medications and other drugs. Acute kidney injury can progress to chronic kidney disease.

Case Studies

The following cases are addressed throughout the chapter to assist in application of chapter content to clinical situations that involve individuals with disorders of the kidneys.

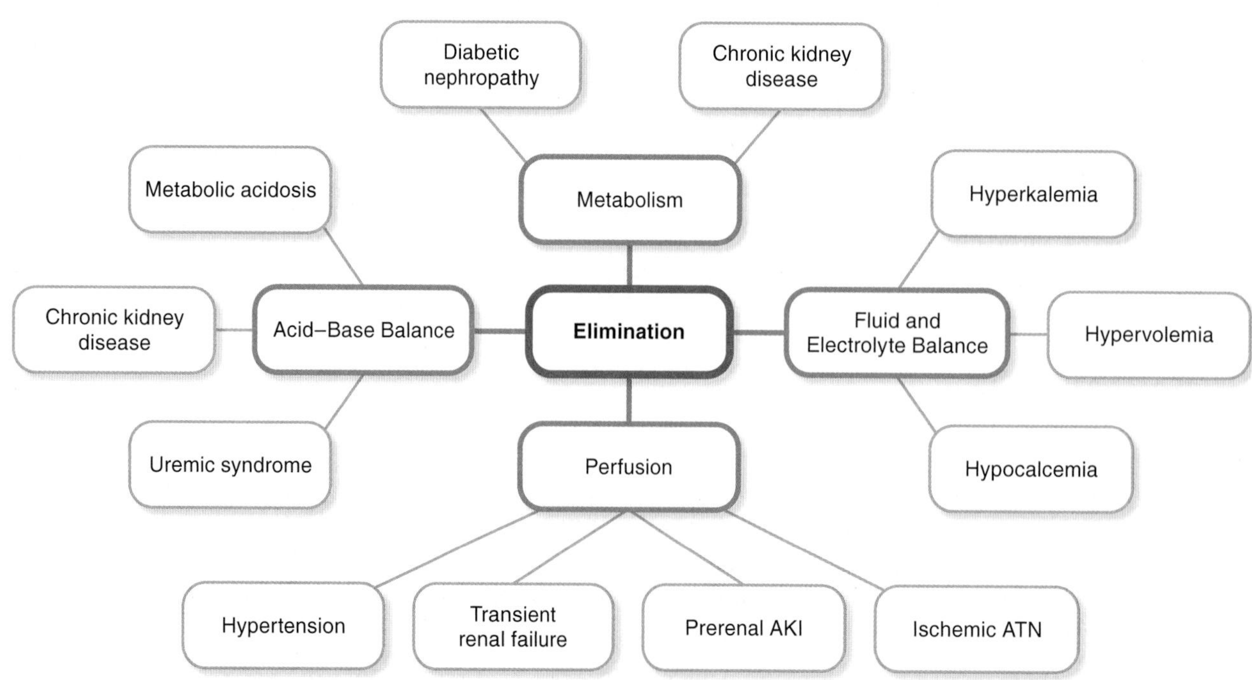

Figure 46.1 ■ Concepts related to acute kidney injury and chronic kidney disease.

Steven Marshall: Introduction

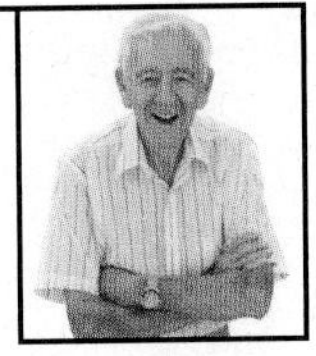

Steven Marshall, age 82, lives in an assisted living facility. He is taken to the emergency department with altered mental status and hypotension. Mr. Marshall's past medical history is significant for DM, hypertension, benign prostatic hypertrophy, and cerebral vascular accident with right hemiparesis. Despite his comorbid conditions, he is alert and oriented and does well in his assisted living environment.

1. What potential risk factors does Mr. Marshall have for kidney disease?
2. On the basis of Mr. Marshall's history, is it likely that he has acute or chronic kidney disease?

Yvonne Johnson: Reintroduction

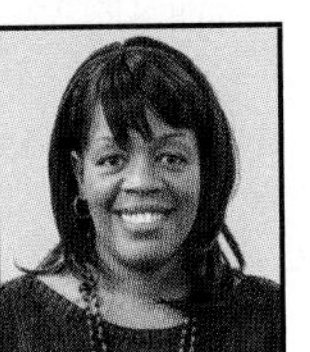

We introduced Yvonne Johnson in Chapter 45. She was 38 years old with a past medical history significant for systemic lupus erythematosus (SLE), antiphospholipid antibody syndrome, and hypertension. Ms. Johnson's SLE has been complicated with generalized joint pain, which she has been treating with over-the-counter ibuprofen. Ms. Johnson, now 43, has not seen a rheumatologist in a few years. Her primary care physician has been refilling Ms. Johnson's medications since her rheumatologist retired. Ms. Johnson has been managing well until she noticed some alopecia and an increase in her joint pain, which prompted her to go to the urgent care clinic.

1. What factors in Ms. Johnson's history increase her risk for kidney disease?
2. On the basis of Ms. Johnson's history, is it likely that she has acute or chronic kidney disease?

Check Your Progress: Section 46.1

1. What is the function of the kidneys?
2. Compare the causes of acute and chronic kidney disease.
3. Why is scientific consensus on the definition of acute kidney disease so important?

46.2 Acute Kidney Injury

Acute kidney injury (AKI) is an abrupt reduction in kidney function that is often reversible.[1] AKI is characterized by the accumulation of nitrogenous wastes such as creatinine and blood urea nitrogen (BUN), called **azotemia**.[1] The term *AKI* has replaced the use of the term *acute renal failure* and is generally accepted as representing most types of acute kidney disease,[1] but if the acute kidney injury is advanced and renal replacement therapy is required, the term *acute renal failure* may be utilized. **Acute tubular necrosis (ATN)**, a histologic finding, is the most common cause of acute injury.[1]

All types of AKI are potentially reversible, but AKI is associated with long-term problems and increases the risk for death.[2] Because of the continuum of kidney damage that can occur in AKI and the lack of consensus on a definition, in 2004 the Acute Dialysis Quality Initiative Group developed the Risk, Injury, Failure, Loss, End-Stage Renal Disease (RIFLE) criteria to standardize the diagnosis and treatment of AKI (**Figure 46.2** ■).[3] **RIFLE** stands for

Risk
Injury
Failure
Loss
ESRD

In 2007, The Acute Kidney Injury Network (AKIN) expanded on the RIFLE criteria by including patients who experienced a ≥ 0.3 mg/dL increase in the serum creatinine in a 48 hour period.[4] In 2012 the Kidney Disease Improving Global Outcomes (KDIGO) classification system expanded on the RIFLE criteria and provided guidelines for the definition, risk assessment, evaluation, prevention, and treatment of AKI.[5] The RIFLE, AKIN, and KDIGO staging systems utilize the current kidney function indices of serum creatinine levels and urinary output to identify the level of injury or failure. The accumulation of serum creatinine signifies an excess of nitrogenous waste products, and urinary output reflects the ability of the kidney to remove waste products and maintain fluid balance (see **Table 46.1** ■).

The glomerular filtration rate (GFR), which is an estimation of kidney function, is determined by using an equation and may involve serum creatinine and the patient's age, gender, and race.[6] The Cockcroft-Gault equation, which preceded the Modification of Diet in Renal Disease (MDRD) equation, may overestimate creatinine clearance. The MDRD is the equation that many laboratories still utilize when reporting GFR as part of the basic metabolic panel, but in 2009, the National Kidney Foundation recommended the Chronic Kidney Disease-Epidemiology Collaboration (CKD-EPI) equation to estimate the GFR. The CKD-EPI is preferred for better prediction of CKD risk and is more accurate when the GFR is normal or only mildly decreased.[7] **Table 46.2** ■ compares three GFR equations. Further discussion of GFR and biomarkers is found later in the chapter, in the discussion of diagnosis of AKI. A common definition is helpful in AKI case identification. Standardized definitions and staging criteria and their link to individual morbidity and mortality have improved the management of individuals with AKI.[8] RIFLE, AKIN, and KDIGO criteria will affect AKI research, as they have provided a standard definition that can be used in clinical trials to improve classifications of individuals with AKI. The criteria also highlight the continuum of AKI from increased risk to persistent failure and thus may affect treatment and clinical outcomes.

The incidence of AKI with even small increases in creatinine levels is greater in critically ill individuals and plays a major role in their clinical outcomes. Creatinine levels can rise more slowly, thus contributing to a delay in accurate diagnosis of AKI.[8] AKI that progresses to CKD alters the patient's overall health, lifestyle, and expected lifespan.[9]

RIFLE Criteria for Classification of Acute Kidney Injury

	Nonoliguria	Oliguria
Risk	Abrupt (1–7 days) decrease in GFR (> 24%) or Serum creatinine increased x 1.5 sustained	Decreased urine output relative to fluid input or Urine output < 0.5 mL//kg/hr for 6 hr
Injury	GFR decreased by 50% or Serum creatinine increased x 2	Urine output < 0.5 mL/kg/hr for 12 hr
Failure	GFR decrease by 75% or Serum creatinine increased x 3 or Serum creatinine > 4 mg/dL with acute rise > 0.5 mg/dL	Urine output < 0.3 mL/kg/hr for 24 hr or Anuria for 12 hr
Loss	Irreversible AKI or persistent AKI > 4 weeks	
ESRD	ESRD > 3 months	

Figure 46.2 ■ RIFLE classification of acute kidney injury.

Table 46.1 AKI Criteria Comparison Based on Serum Creatinine Level

	RIFLE	AKIN	KDIGO
AKI diagnosis	↑ in serum creatinine > 50% over < 7 days	↑ in serum creatinine of 0.3 mg/dL or a 50% ↑ over < 48 hours	↑ in serum creatinine of 0.3 mg/dL over 48 hours or a 50% ↑ over 7 days
Staging AKI			
RIFLE-Risk AKIN/KDIGO stage 1	↑ in serum creatinine > 50% over < 7 days	↑ in serum creatinine of 0.3 mg/dL or > 50%	↑ in serum creatinine of 0.3 mg/dL or > 50%
RIFLE-Injury AKIN/KDIGO stage 2	↑ in serum creatinine > 100%	↑ in serum creatinine > 100%	↑ in serum creatinine > 100%
RIFLE-Failure AKIN/KDIGO stage 3	↑ in serum creatinine > 200%	↑ in serum creatinine > 200%	↑ in serum creatinine > 200%
RIFLE-Loss	Requires renal replacement therapy > 4 weeks		
RIFLE-ESRD	Requires renal replacement therapy > 3 months		

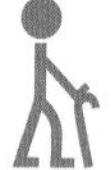

In older adults, AKI incidence increases as renal function declines with age. Older individuals who develop AKI are also at risk for CKD.[9] ■

The incidence of AKI in the pediatric population has increased, particularly among hospitalized children.[10] A common cause of AKI in young children is hemolytic-uremic syndrome (HUS) and glomerulonephritis Most cases of HUS in children result from diarrhea-producing *Escherichia coli* infections caused by contaminated food.[11] Dehydration and poor perfusion contribute to transient renal failure.[12] A modified version of the RIFLE criteria for pediatric patients, known as pRIFLE, takes into account GFR changes rather than changes in creatinine (**Figure 46.3** ■).[13] ■

AKI has three main etiologies; these are classified as prerenal, intrinsic (intrarenal), and postrenal (**Figure 46.4** ■). Prerenal disorders are the most common cause of acute kidney injury and are responsible for about 60% of AKI.[1]

- **Prerenal AKI** is usually reversible and characterized by increases in serum creatinine and BUN and a reduction in urine output, referred to as oliguria. A reduction in renal perfusion causes a reduction in the GFR.
- **Intrinsic AKI** may be related to diseases in one of several renal anatomic structures: the glomeruli, tubules,

Table 46.2 GFR Calculation Equations

Name	Formula	Comparisons
Cockcroft-Gault	Creatinine clearance = (140 − age) × (weight in kg)/(creatinine mg/dL) × 72 (multiply by 0.85 if female)	Not adjusted for body surface area. Less accurate when the GFR is normal.
MDRD	GFR = 186 × $(\text{creatinine})^{-1.154}$ × $(\text{age})^{-0.203}$ × (0.742 if female) × (1.212 if African American)	Used by many labs when reporting GFR; accounts for race and sex.
CKD-EPI	GFR = 141 × min (creatinine/κ, $1)^{\alpha}$ × max(S_{cr}/κ, $1)^{-1.209}$ × 0.993^{age} × 1.018 (if female) × 1.159 (if African American)	Works well at higher GFRs, better prediction of risk in comparison to other equations.

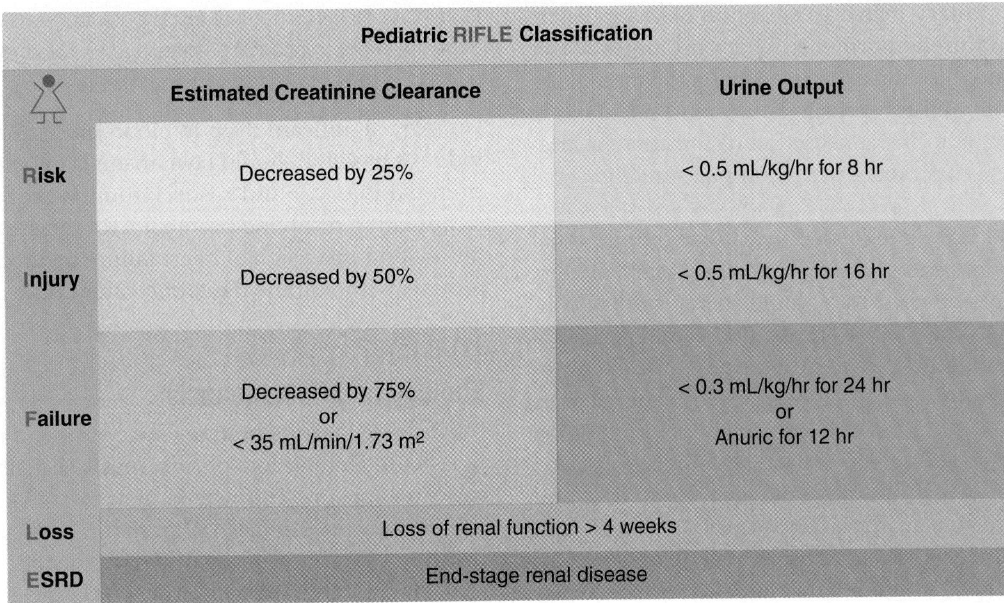

Pediatric RIFLE Classification		
	Estimated Creatinine Clearance	Urine Output
Risk	Decreased by 25%	< 0.5 mL/kg/hr for 8 hr
Injury	Decreased by 50%	< 0.5 mL/kg/hr for 16 hr
Failure	Decreased by 75% or < 35 mL/min/1.73 m^2	< 0.3 mL/kg/hr for 24 hr or Anuric for 12 hr
Loss	Loss of renal function > 4 weeks	
ESRD	End-stage renal disease	

Figure 46.3 ■ Pediatric RIFLE.

interstitium, and blood vessels. Vascular disease can involve the large renal vessels but is more likely to involve the microvasculature.

- **Postrenal AKI** is most commonly caused by obstruction within the kidney itself, bilateral ureteral obstruction, or urethral obstruction.

Prerenal AKI

Etiology and Pathogenesis

Prerenal AKI occurs for two primary reasons:

- Reduced blood flow to the kidney due to intravascular volume depletion from nausea, vomiting, diarrhea, or aggressive diuresis
- Reduced effective arterial blood volume from shock, related to heart failure, hypovolemia, or sepsis.[1] Reduced blood flow to the kidneys occurs for a variety of reasons. However, medications that reduce blood pressure also reduce perfusion to the kidneys, resulting in prerenal AKI. Prerenal AKI is reversible if volume is quickly replaced or hemodynamic pressure is returned to normal, thus avoiding kidney injury. If prerenal AKI is not treated promptly, intrinsic AKI can occur and can potentially lead to CKD.

The renal response to intravascular volume depletion involves the activation of two neurohormonal systems: the sympathetic nervous system and the renin–angiotensin–aldosterone system (RAAS). When intravascular volume depletion occurs, the juxtaglomerular cells sense a drop in blood pressure and secrete renin, which promotes the production of angiotensin I. Angiotensin-converting enzyme (ACE) converts angiotensin I to angiotensin II, a potent vasoconstrictor. Angiotensin II constricts the efferent arterioles and, to a lesser extent, the afferent arterioles, thus maintaining glomerular blood pressure and GFR. Angiotensin II also stimulates the adrenal cortex and the posterior pituitary. Stimulation of the adrenal cortex increases aldosterone secretion and enhances the resorption of sodium and water in the distal convoluted tubule. Stimulation of

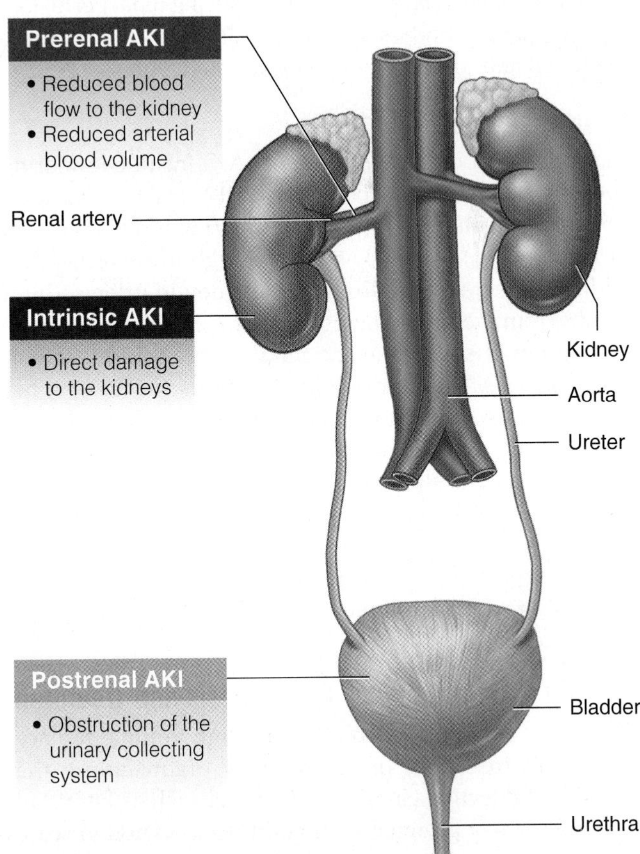

Figure 46.4 ■ AKI is classified into prerenal, intrinsic, and postrenal causes. Renal causes of AKI should be considered under the different anatomic components of the kidney (vascular supply, glomerular, tubular, and interstitial disease).

the posterior pituitary increases secretion of vasopressin, also called antidiuretic hormone, which promotes water resorption in the collecting duct. In addition, dilation of the afferent arteriole through prostaglandin and nitric oxide activation along with the constriction of the efferent arteriole work to maintain renal perfusion pressure and renal blood flow.[1]

Renal blood flow is regulated by cardiac output, renal perfusion pressure, and glomerular hemodynamic factors. Cardiac output is affected by volume status, cardiac contractility, and sodium and water retention. Renal perfusion pressure is regulated by mean arterial pressure. (Refer to Chapter 23 for information on calculating mean arterial pressure.) Glomerular filtration rate is affected by vasodilation or vasoconstriction of the afferent and efferent arterioles.[1] The kidneys can usually autoregulate renal blood flow and function when the mean arterial pressure is between 70 and 105 mmHg.[14] However, when the mean arterial pressure falls below 70 mmHg, autoregulation is impaired. Medications can also interfere with autoregulation of renal blood flow and GFR and can provoke prerenal AKI. Individuals who are treated with ACE inhibitors or diuretics for hypertension can experience prerenal AKI through a further reduction in blood pressure. ACE inhibitors also relax the efferent arteriole, which in turn decreases the GFR. Nonsteroidal anti-inflammatory drugs (NSAIDs) can reduce the vasodilatory properties of the afferent arteriole, reducing renal perfusion, and thwart the body's response to intravascular volume depletion and/or reduction in mean arterial pressure.[15]

Clinical Manifestations

Classic clinical features of prerenal AKI include low urine sodium concentration (< 20 mmol/L), fractional excretion of sodium (FE_{Na}) ($< 1\%$), and fractional excretion of urea (FE_{urea}) ($< 35\%$) as well as high urine osmolality and specific gravity (1.030).[16] A reduction in urine sodium results from the activation of aldosterone, which causes the absorption of sodium in the tubules. In addition, activation of the RAAS may result in oliguria as well as a higher concentration of urine as the body retains volume to correct the reduced renal blood flow. An individual's risk for AKI should be evaluated to prevent AKI. Past medical history should be evaluated as well as the procedure type; for instance, cardiovascular surgery increases the risk for AKI. Preoperative hypovolemia should be corrected, and postoperative fluid volume should be monitored to prevent hypovolemia.

Linking Pathophysiology to Diagnosis and Treatment

Treatment of volume depletion through volume replacement and treatment of the primary organ failure that decreased effective circulating volume, such as heart failure, can correct prerenal AKI. Fluid resuscitation in sepsis is geared toward maintenance of organ perfusion, including the kidneys. Vasoactive medications that improve cardiac output in heart failure can reverse prerenal AKI. Improvement in urine output and serum creatinine signal reversal of the prerenal condition.

CLINICAL POINT: Prerenal AKI is potentially reversible. Therefore, diligence in observation of patients and knowledge of their baseline blood pressure and kidney function are vital. ■

Any significant drop in blood pressure from the individual's baseline should be managed aggressively to avoid prerenal injury. Fluid resuscitation is the most common treatment in resolving prerenal AKI. Overdiuresis of heart failure and provision of heart failure medications for individuals with volume depletion can initiate prerenal AKI.

Intrinsic AKI

Etiology and Pathogenesis

Intrinsic AKI results from several causes and include vasculitis, acute glomerulonephritis, sepsis, ischemia, and nephrotoxin exposure. Intrinsic kidney injury is different from prerenal and postrenal AKI in that it does not necessarily result in prompt recovery of renal function. As was previously mentioned, intrinsic AKI affects the anatomic structures of the kidney; the glomeruli, tubules, interstitium, blood vessels, and the kidney structure itself are affected. Typically, both the BUN and creatinine levels rise in intrinsic AKI. Ischemic insult may result from a prolonged prerenal condition, leading to ATN. ATN seen in intrinsic AKI mostly results from ischemic causes, but toxins, whether medications or endogenous toxins, also contribute to ATN. Nephrotoxic agents, such as aminoglycoside antibiotics, can accumulate in the kidney cortex and damage the proximal tubules, manifesting as muddy brown urinary casts. Glomerulonephritis refers to inflammation of glomeruli and capillaries, and immune complex deposits are the cause of many glomerulonephropathies. Glomerulonephritis is discussed in detail in Chapter 45.

The clinical course of ATN can be variable, lasting anywhere from weeks to months. Initially, there is an oliguric phase, although some individuals remain nonoliguric throughout the course of illness. The oliguric phase is followed by a diuretic phase, which indicates recovery of renal function. Mortality associated with ATN is high, with rates reported as high as 50–70%. Many of these individuals manifest one or more comorbidities that place them at additional risk. Although the majority of individuals recover renal function, CKD can occur.[17] **Ischemic ATN** can result from prerenal hypoperfusion that is not readily treated. Prolonged hypoperfusion from sepsis, surgery, or unresolved heart failure results in a loss of autoregulation that further enhances renal vasoconstriction. Risk factors for the development of ischemic ATN include preexisting CKD, atherosclerosis, DM, hypertension, advanced malignancy, and poor nutritional status.[18] Acute tubular necrosis is also associated with several disturbances that contribute to tubular necrosis, including endothelial and epithelial cell injury, intratubular obstruction, and an inflammatory response (**Figure 46.5** ■). Scientists are still in the process of understanding inflammatory mediators and potential treatment options to stop renal tubular damage.

Nephrotoxic ATN occurs as a result of direct toxic damage to the renal tubules. Medications that can cause

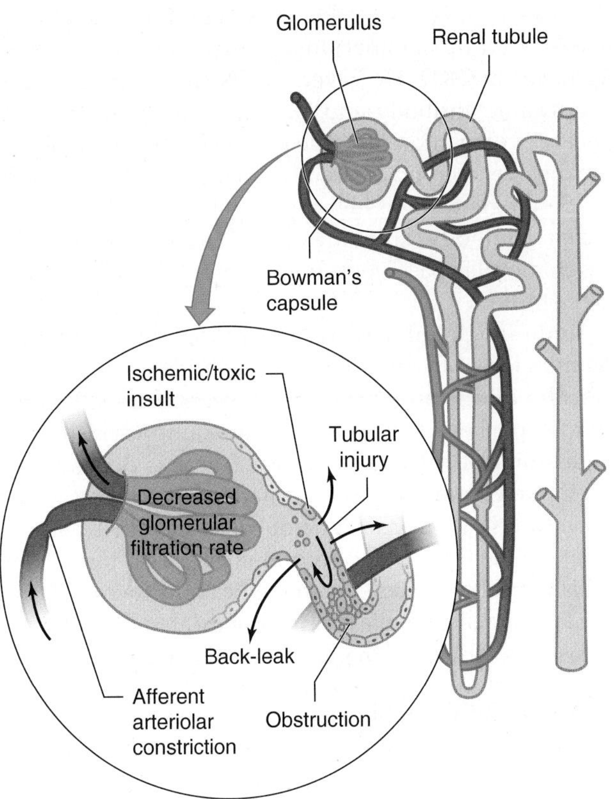

Figure 46.5 ■ Acute tubular necrosis.

toxic tubular damage include aminoglycoside antibiotics, amphotericin B, chemotherapeutic agents, and calcineurin inhibitors (cyclosporine). Damage can also occur related to massive hemolysis from blood transfusion reactions and myoglobin pigments from rhabdomyolysis, the result of breakdown of skeletal muscle fibers. Usually, removal of the causative agent, such as the aminoglycoside, results in return to normal renal function. **Contrast-induced nephropathy (CIN)** is a significant cause of nephrotoxic ATN. Typically, individuals who receive IV radiocontrast agents have a rise in serum creatinine within 24 hours after the iodinated contrast medium is given. The risk is highest in older adults and in individuals who are dehydrated, take nephrotoxic medications, and have a history of renal damage [9] Increased mortality, both during hospitalization and after discharge, is attributed to hospital-acquired contrast-induced nephropathy.[19]

Contrast-induced nephropathy can cause AKI in older adults, especially those with preexisting risk factors (CKD, diabetic nephropathy, decreased effective arterial blood volume, and the use of NSAIDs).[19] ■

Sepsis-induced ATN combines sepsis and AKI and is associated with a 70% mortality rate.[20] Sepsis is the most common cause of AKI in hospitalized individuals. Both ischemia from hypotension and toxic damage from endotoxins, a type of toxin contained in the cell wall secreted by mainly gram-negative bacteria, contribute to tubular damage. Endotoxins promote activation of inflammatory mediators, which produces a systemic response.[21]

Multiple pathophysiologic processes occur in both ischemic and nephrotoxic ATN that contribute to tubular injury and result in decreased GFR. In ischemic ATN, there are both microvascular (glomerular vascular and medullary vascular) and tubular components that result in ATN. An initial injury, often prolonged prerenal ischemia or a profound episode of hypotension, disrupts both glomerular and medullary microvascular blood flow and disrupts autoregulation of renal blood flow. This results in decreased renal perfusion, renal hypoxia, tubular epithelial cell ischemia, and decreased GFR. The reduction in glomerular and medullary blood flow occurs secondary to increased vasoconstriction and decreased vasodilation. Increased vasoconstriction results from an increase in endothelin, a potent vasoconstrictor produced by renal endothelial cells, as well as other vasoconstrictive agents such as angiotensin II and sympathetic nervous system activation. Decreased vasodilation results from a decrease in nitric oxide, which is released from renal endothelial cells, as well as other vasodilatory substances including prostaglandin E_2, acetylcholine, and bradykinin. Paradoxically, the molecular mediators discussed above, which are produced in response to renal ischemia and hypoxia, produce hemodynamic alterations that further increase ischemia and decrease the GFR.[1,22,23]

Continued vasoconstriction leads to structural damage to endothelial and vascular smooth muscle cells. Continuing hypoxia following the initial ischemic event results in an inflammatory response. Following AKI, the ability of the renal cells to repair is linked to alterations in hypoxia.[24] Leukocytes are activated by pro-inflammatory mediators, including cytokines, reactive oxygen species, and eicosanoids, which enhance adhesion of leukocytes to the endothelium. Reactive oxygen species can also cause endothelial and vascular smooth muscle cell injury. Additional pro-inflammatory cytokines, such as interleukin 1 (IL-1) and tumor necrosis factor alpha (TNF-α), also help to sequester leukocytes. The resulting accumulation of leukocytes can lead to vascular obstruction, a further decrease in renal blood flow, and more inflammation.

Diminished renal blood flow, renal hypoxia, and pro-inflammatory and vasoactive mediators promote renal tubular epithelial cell injury. Further release of pro-inflammatory and vasoactive mediators follows, thus amplifying the preexisting inflammatory milieu. Ischemia results in breakdown of the cytoskeleton, which provides a framework needed to maintain cell shape and allow rapid changes in cell structure. Dysfunction of the sodium–potassium pump results in cell edema and an increase in intracellular calcium, which activates numerous proteolytic enzymes, causing tubular cell necrosis. Apoptosis also plays a role in the loss of renal tubular cells. Dead tubular cells slough off into the lumen of the tubule. Damaged tubular epithelial cell remnants or casts in the tubular lumen obstruct the flow of filtrate, leading to decreased urine output.[25] Eventually, epithelial and endothelial cells undergo repair, and recovery of renal function occurs. This time frame is referred to as the maintenance and recovery phase. Full recovery may take weeks to months; however, CKD can still occur, depending on the extent of tubular damage. Some individuals never recover renal function and reach the terminal renal stage, or **end-stage renal disease (ESRD)**, requiring permanent renal replacement therapy. Considered an important risk factor for ESRD, survival of AKI has increased the need for dialysis from 2.4 per 100,000 population to 19.4. It has been estimated that approximately 25% of ESRD patients on dialysis had AKI before becoming dialysis-dependent.[26] AKI is more prevalent in patients with underlying CKD; conversely, patients with CKD are more vulnerable to AKI.[5] Also it has been reported that even mild AKI cases can develop into CKD, and recovery time is a predictor of who will develop CKD. The severity of the AKI increases the risk for incomplete recovery, resulting in CKD and progression to ESRD.[26,27] **Table 46.3** ■ outlines the differences between AKI and CKD.

Acute interstitial nephritis is AKI resulting from inflammation of the interstitial tissue of the kidney including the tubules, usually from a reaction to a medication. Medications commonly associated with acute interstitial nephritis include penicillin, NSAIDs, and proton pump inhibitors.[28,29] Acute interstitial nephritis usually presents with rash, fever, and eosinophilia. Urinary findings in acute interstitial nephritis include sterile pyuria, white blood cell casts, nonnephrotic-range proteinuria, hematuria, and eosinophiluria.[30] Some individuals may have severe proteinuria. Eosinophils are granulocytes that are seen in allergic reactions. However, not all individuals have symptoms, so diagnosis may not occur for several months. Renal biopsy is the gold standard for diagnosis.

Acute glomerulonephritis and rapidly progressive glomerulonephritis (RPGN) are two of the more common glomerular disorders that produce AKI. Both disorders involve inflammation of the glomerulus, usually as a result of an immune response. Antibody deposition in the kidney is the precipitating event and involves both humoral and cell-mediated immunity. The complement cascade is activated in the glomeruli, activating chemotactic and proinflammatory molecules that damage glomerular epithelial, endothelial, and mesangial cells. Inflammation within the glomerulus and damage from macrophages cause functional and structural damage to the kidney, including disruption of the glomerular basement membrane and the capillary wall.[9,31]

Table 46.3 Differentiation between AKI and CKD

Signs/Symptoms	AKI	CKD
History of onset	Short (days to weeks)	Long (months to years)
Hemoglobin concentration	Normal	Low
Renal size	Normal	Reduced
Renal osteodystrophy	Absent	Present
Peripheral neuropathy	Absent	Present
Serum creatinine concentration	Acute reversible increase	Chronic irreversible

Rapidly progressive glomerulonephritis is usually due to postinfectious glomerulonephritis and typically does not result in CKD. However, RPGN from antineutrophil cytoplasmic antibody and Goodpasture syndrome may quickly evolve into CKD. The pathologic feature of RPGN is extensive necrotic crescent formations in the glomerulus. Serologic tests to identify the etiology include antinuclear antibody, antineutrophil cytoplasmic antibody, antiglomerular basement membrane titers, and complement studies.

Immunoglobulin A (IgA) nephropathy is the most common form of acute glomerulonephritis worldwide and typically affects adults age 20–30 years.[32] Usually, gross microscopic hematuria is noted after an upper respiratory or gastrointestinal viral infection. There is deposition of IgA in the glomerulus, and formation of crescents is seen in some of the glomeruli. Macrophages and other cells proliferate in the hole, and a crescent-shaped scar forms. Mild IgA is typically managed with medications for blood pressure and hyperlipidemia control as indicated.[32] Glomerular diseases are discussed in greater detail in Chapter 45.

Clinical Manifestations

Clinical manifestations of the initial phase of intrinsic AKI are not immediately apparent except for the changes in urine output and serum creatinine. Individuals in the maintenance phase who become oliguric may manifest symptoms of fluid overload, including peripheral edema and pulmonary edema. As kidney function worsens, increases in creatinine and urea occur. In addition, excess sodium may be noted in the urine. Hypocalcemia, hyperphosphatemia, and hyperkalemia can occur. Metabolic acidosis can occur as a result of retention of hydrogen ions. Individuals can become uremic, with alterations in mental status, including seizures. Prerenal and postrenal causes of AKI are more likely reversible; therefore, clinical manifestations of AKI that lead to CKD usually result from intrinsic causes. The clinical course of intrinsic AKI consists of three phases and is primarily attributed to ATN. The initial phase is the time from the initial insult to kidney tissue and identification of a reduction in renal function. If identified early, renal damage may be reversed. The second phase is the maintenance phase. This phase can last from a few days to a few weeks to 2 months, and the serum creatinine level can continue to rise. Individuals in this phase may be **anuric** (no urine output), **oliguric** (urine output less than 400 milliliters in 24 hours), or **nonoliguric** (urine output greater than 400 milliliters in 24 hours). Nonoliguria is a more promising sign for renal recovery. The recovery phase highlights the return of serum creatinine toward the normal range and can last from 3 to 12 months. These individuals may experience polyuria, which can result in fluid and electrolyte abnormalities.[9,33]

CLINICAL POINT: Although there are many causes of intrinsic AKI, including prerenal and postrenal causes, the most common are ischemic and toxic causes. It is the intrinsic damage to the nephron and its structures, especially the tubules, that leads to permanent kidney damage. ■

Linking Pathophysiology to Diagnosis and Treatment

Laboratory tests, including urinalysis, can assist in differentiating prerenal AKI from intrinsic AKI. Once AKI occurs, clinicians can globally assess the degree of renal dysfunction by using the GFR. A reduced GFR suggests that underlying injury has developed or that a new acute or chronic injury has occurred. For multiple reasons, the serum creatinine level may not increase immediately in AKI; therefore, GFR may not be the best indicator for AKI. Studies are under way to establish early detection of AKI, evaluating novel urinary and serum biomarkers such as serum cystatin C, neutrophil-gelatinase–associated lipocalin, insulin-like growth factor–binding protein 7, and tissue inhibitor of metalloproteinases 2 are all potential biomarkers of kidney damage.[34] These biomarkers may be diagnostic for kidney damage before elevations in serum creatinine levels are seen.

The serum creatinine and BUN levels are also markers for kidney injury. Both markers estimate accumulation of toxins that occurs in AKI. However, both tests are nonspecific in relation to actual kidney injury. The serum creatinine and BUN levels can be significantly elevated even in mild AKI. Most experts agree that the serum creatinine and GFR estimations are valuable in the acute setting when individuals have stable kidney function. If baseline kidney function is unknown, the estimation equations may be less useful.[9]

Diagnostic testing is one way to differentiate the actual cause of AKI. Urinalysis is one of the most common and inexpensive tests used to provide important information in determining the etiology of AKI (**Table 46.4** ■).

Measurement of the urine sodium concentration is helpful in distinguishing prerenal disease from ATN. In prerenal acute renal failure, the RAAS is activated to retain sodium and water and maintain intravascular volume. This results in less sodium and water excretion and concentrated (increased osmolality) urine. When the renal tubules are damaged in ATN, the tubules cannot retain sodium and water; therefore, urine characteristically has more sodium and is more dilute. The urinary **fractional excretion of sodium (FE_{Na})** can be calculated to differentiate prerenal AKI from ATN and is expressed as a percentage. A value below 1% suggests prerenal disease, and a value above 2% is indicative of ATN. FE_{Na} is most accurate in severe AKI and may be less accurate in individuals who are receiving diuretics, as they change the concentration and amount of sodium excreted. A low FE_{Na} is not unique to prerenal disease and can occur with normal tubular function and a low GFR. Glomerulonephritis, CIN, and rhabdomyolysis can present with a low FE_{Na}. For individuals on diuretics, the **fractional excretion of urea (FE_{urea})** can be calculated, as urea excretion is not affected by diuretics and is retained in prerenal states. A FE_{urea} value below 35% is indicative of prerenal AKI, and a FE_{urea} value above 50% is indicative of ATN (**Table 46.5** ■).

Measures to prevent CIN include use of nonionic contrast agents and adequate hydration with intravenous saline as important interventions. Sodium bicarbonate and oral N-acetylcysteine have frequently been used prophylactically to prevent CIN, but there is no strong evidence for their use.[35] Avoidance of contrast in individuals with CKD is encouraged, as is the avoidance of other nephrotoxic medications such as NSAIDs and aminoglycoside antibiotics. It is the standard of care to withhold oral diabetic medications and NSAIDs for a minimum of 48 hours after CIN is administered or until baseline kidney function returns. Any potential hypoxic event, such as hypotension and acute respiratory hypoxia, should be identified and aggressively treated.[9]

CLINICAL POINT: Patients with CKD and older adults are at higher risk of developing AKI during hospitalization and when taking medications such as NSAIDs that can precipitate decreased perfusion to the kidneys. Once a decrease in GFR or urine output or a rise in creatinine is noted, looking for potential causes and obtaining urinary testing can assist in reversing AKI. ■

Postrenal AKI

Etiology and Pathogenesis

Postrenal AKI results from obstruction of the urinary collecting system resulting in cessation of urinary flow and azotemia. Obstruction may occur within the kidney or at the level of the ureters, urethra, or bladder. Ureteral or kidney tissue obstructions are usually due to tumors or renal stones. Obstruction must be bilateral in the kidney or ureters to cause AKI. Obstruction in only one kidney means that the other kidney functions normally; therefore, it is possible that the AKI will go undetected unless the individual has a solitary kidney. Most kidney stones are calcium-based, usually calcium oxalate. Struvite stones are also possible and typically form secondary to bacterial infection.[36] In adult women, retroperitoneal and pelvic malignancies are the most frequent causes of obstruction. In men, prostatic disease is the most typical etiology.

Common causes of obstruction in children include congenital ureteral strictures. ■

Table 46.4 Urinalysis in Acute Kidney Injury

Acute Renal Disease	Urinary Characteristics
Acute glomerulonephritis	Hematuria with red blood cell casts, dysmorphic red blood cells, proteinuria
Acute interstitial nephritis	Leukocyturia with leukocyte casts or urinary eosinophils
Acute tubular necrosis	Renal tubular epithelial cells and muddy brown casts
Prerenal disease, urinary tract obstruction	Few cells with little or no casts or proteinuria

Table 46.5 Differentiating Prerenal and Intrinsic (ATN) Causes of AKI

Diagnostic test	Prerenal	ATN
FE_{Na}	< 1%	> 2%
FE_{urea}	< 35%	> 50%

Clinical Manifestations

Postrenal AKI can present as partial or complete obstruction. Complete obstruction is manifested by anuria or sudden cessation of urine. Obstruction of urine flow can occur anywhere from the kidney to the urethral meatus. Obstruction of the ureters can lead to **hydronephrosis**, or swelling of the kidney. Partial obstruction may lead to frequency, hesitancy, nocturia, or incomplete emptying of the bladder. Symptoms such as hematuria, abdominal or flank pain, renal colic, or pelvic fullness can occur.

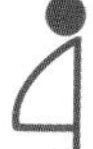

Postrenal etiologies can occur in pregnancy, as the fetus may obstruct urine flow. Relief of the obstruction usually results in return of normal kidney function. ■

Steven Marshall: Application

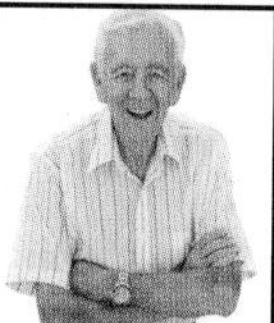

Mr. Marshall's vital signs are pulse 110, respirations 18, temperature 97.2°F, blood pressure 80/55. He is alert and oriented to person only. Mr. Marshall is admitted to the medical ICU, and his laboratory work returns the following results:

- Creatinine 3.2 mg/dL (baseline: 1.3 mg/dL)
- BUN 92 mg/dL
- Hemoglobin 12.2 g/dL
- Urine dipstick nitrite-positive, suggesting the presence of bacteria
- Microscopic urinalysis shows bacteria, tubular epithelial cells, and muddy brown casts
- $FE_{Na} > 2\%$
- FE_{urea} 60%
- Urine and blood cultures pending.

Despite fluid resuscitation, Mr. Marshall's creatinine level continues to rise, reaching 5.6 mg/dL, and he meets RIFLE/AKIN criteria for AKI. His urine output has been 300 mL/24 hours (oliguric). All of these signs are significant for ATN. Fluids are continued to try to flush damaged tubular epithelial cells to treat tubular obstruction and maintain blood pressure, being mindful of fluid overload. Mr. Marshall does not respond to diuretics and is becoming fluid overloaded. He is also noted to be acidotic, so a temporary dialysis catheter is inserted in his femoral vein, and dialysis is initiated to correct acidosis and fluid overload. Antibiotics are administered empirically until cultures return; all medications are renally adjusted.

3. With a blood pressure of 80/55, what is the ability of Mr. Marshall's kidneys to autoregulate renal blood flow?
4. How do Mr. Marshall's FE_{Na} and FE_{urea} values support a diagnosis of ATN?

Linking Pathophysiology to Diagnosis and Treatment

Ultrasound imaging is a standard, noninvasive method to diagnose many postrenal obstructions. Dilation of the collecting system is typically seen with obstructions. If obstruction is detected, correction of the causative agent is imperative to avoid infection or kidney injury, which could potentially lead to ESRD. Postrenal obstructions are typically treated on an outpatient basis, unlike prerenal and interstitial AKI.[37] Nephrolithiasis is discussed in greater detail in Chapter 45.

Steven Marshall: Outcome

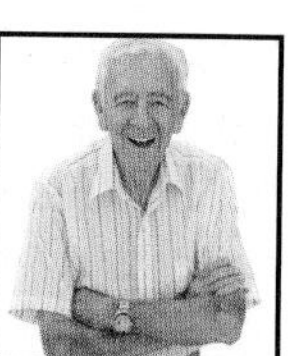

Mr. Marshall's urine culture and blood cultures grow *Escherichia coli*, which is susceptible to cefazolin. He receives cefazolin dosed for GFR of 9 mL/min/1.73 m^2. Mr. Marshall's serum creatinine level continues to rise, reaching 7.0 mg/dL, but with appropriate treatment for his infection, his blood pressure and mental status improve. Mr. Marshall is eventually discharged to a rehabilitation facility and continues to require dialysis therapy. After 4 weeks, his serum creatinine has decreased to 3.5 mg/dL, and his urine output has increased to 1,000 mL/8 hours. His nephrologist closely monitors Mr. Marshall's progress, and at 2 months, his creatinine level is 2.0 mg/dL, his urine output is back to baseline, and he no longer requires hemodialysis.

5. Because of Mr. Marshall's history of ATN, what precautions should be taken if he were to need a scan involving contrast media?
6. How might Mr. Marshall's history of benign prostatic hypertrophy affect his kidney function?

Check Your Progress: Section 46.2

1. What common indices are utilized by RIFLE, AKIN, and KDIGO to diagnose AKI?
2. Describe the mechanism for AKI to go unnoticed in the person with postrenal obstruction.
3. Describe the role of urine sodium concentration in distinguishing prerenal disease from ATN.

46.3 Chronic Kidney Disease

Chronic kidney disease (CKD) is defined as either kidney damage or GFR less than 60 mL/min/1.73 m^2 for 3 months or more. Kidney damage is defined as pathologic abnormalities or markers of damage in blood or urine tests and imaging studies.[38] According to the National Kidney Foundation practice guidelines, CKD is a worldwide public health problem.[6] The incidence and prevalence continue to increase in the United States and worldwide, especially among older adults. The number of people with ESRD has been projected to increase, and 25% of those starting on dialysis will die within the first year of treatment.[9] In 2013, the ESRD program was treating approximately 661,000 dialysis and kidney transplant patients, and the incident rate of ESRD has remained relatively stable over the past few years.[39] African Americans and native Americans have a higher incidence of CKD than Caucasians, and Hispanics also have a higher incidence than non-Hispanics.[39] Compared to European Americans, African Americans are 4–5 times more likely to develop ESRD independent of socioeconomic status. African Americans, compared to the general population, also progress more rapidly to ESRD with consideration for age-associated progression.[40] Outcomes of CKD include complications of decreased kidney function, which include anemia, uremia, derangements of bone and mineral metabolism, cardiovascular disease (CVD), and the potential to progress to ESRD. Hypertension contributes to and complicates CKD or can result from CKD. Cardiovascular disease is the leading cause of death for people with CKD. Increasing evidence suggests that some of the adverse outcomes can be delayed by early prevention and treatment of CKD.[9] Chronic kidney disease can progress to ESRD rapidly, over a few months, or slowly over many years with the deterioration related to the cause. Management of CVD risk factors reduces the risk of progression.[1]

To improve identification, prevention, and treatment of CKD, the Kidney Disease Outcomes Quality Initiative (KDOQI) published guidelines that outline goals for CKD. These goals include (1) defining CKD and classifying stages of the disorder regardless of cause, (2) evaluating laboratory measurements for the clinical assessment of CKD, (3) associating the level of kidney function with complications of CKD, and (4) stratifying the risk for loss of kidney function with development of CVD.[41] The KDOQI guidelines note that early detection of CKD can be accomplished through routine laboratory tests such as creatinine and GFR.[41] The presence and stage of CKD should be established, regardless of the etiology, on the basis of level of kidney damage and evaluation of kidney function by GFR as described in **Table 46.6** ■.

Table 46.6 Stages of Chronic Kidney Disease

Stage	Description	GFR (mL/min/1.73 m²)
1	Kidney damage with normal or ↑ GFR	≥ 90
2	Kidney damage with mild ↓ GFR	60–89
3	Moderate ↓ GFR	30–59
4	Severe ↓ GFR	15–29
5	Kidney failure (ESRD)	<15 or dialysis

SOURCE: National Kidney Foundation.

Yvonne Johnson: Application

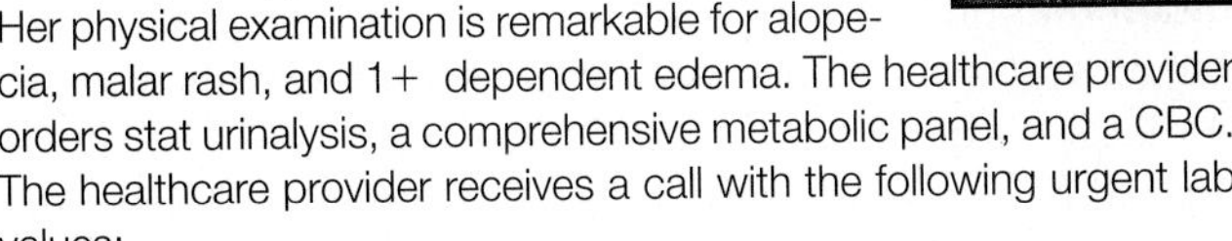

Ms. Johnson's vital signs are pulse 96, respirations 18, temperature 98.1°F, blood pressure 168/98. She appears to be in no acute distress. Her physical examination is remarkable for alopecia, malar rash, and 1+ dependent edema. The healthcare provider orders stat urinalysis, a comprehensive metabolic panel, and a CBC. The healthcare provider receives a call with the following urgent lab values:

- Creatinine 3.8 mg/dL
- GFR 16 mL/min/1.73 m^2
- BUN 36 mg/dL
- Hemoglobin 7.8 g/dL
- Potassium 5.1 mg/dL
- Nephrotic range proteinuria.

The healthcare provider contacts Ms. Johnson and instructs her to go to the emergency department because of her her abnormal labs. In the emergency department, Ms. Johnson is seen by a nephrologist, who assumes CKD as a result of SLE and the utilization of NSAIDs compounding the kidney disease. A kidney biopsy is performed after holding Coumadin and bridging with heparin. The nephrologist's suspicions are confirmed: Ms. Johnson has lupus nephritis. Immunosuppressive therapy of prednisone and mycophenolate mofetil are initiated to treat her SLE. She is discharged on immunosuppressive therapy and instructed to avoid nephrotoxic agents and to follow up with a nephrologist and a rheumatologist.

3. On the basis of a GFR of 16 mL/min/1.73 m^2, what is Ms. Johnson's stage of chronic kidney disease, according to the National Kidney Foundation?
4. What is the correlation between Ms. Johnson's hemoglobin of 7.8 g/dL and CKD?

Etiology and Pathogenesis

Most CKD arises from three main etiologies: diabetic nephropathy, hypertensive nephrosclerosis, and chronic glomerulonephritis.[39] All individuals should be assessed for risk of kidney disease during routine health encounters. DM, hypertension, relevant family history, and history of AKI are some of the clinical risk factors for CKD. Being older than 65 years of age, African American, Native American, Hispanic, Asian, and/or of a low socioeconomic level are some of the sociodemographic risk factors. Identification of risk factors can prevent the progression of CKD to ESRD. With the recent stabilization of the number of new ESRD cases, the continuing rise in ESRD prevalence is attributed mainly to the longer survival of patients with ESRD.[39]

Loss of nephrons occurs as people age, so a reduction in GFR is seen in older adults.[42] The prevalence of CKD increases by 1% each year over the age of 40. Obesity, hypertension, and DM, which are risk factors for other related disorders, also increase the risk of CKD.[43] The GFR should be monitored in people who are administered nephrotoxic medications such as NSAIDs and calcineurin inhibitors.[44] ■

Children may develop CKD early in life. Nephrotic destruction occurs despite the child's being asymptomatic. Signs and symptoms occur later, when renal damage has advanced. Congenital renal disorders are frequently caused by obstructive uropathy, vesicoureteral reflux that causes urinary tract infections, and birth defects. Growth is affected by chronic renal failure, especially in the preadolescent child.[12] ■

Chronic kidney disease is a multifactorial disorder with genetic and environmental factors that affect the development and progression of the disease. Early stages of CKD have similar rates among different racial, ethnic, and socioeconomic groups; however, the rate of end-stage renal disease is greater for minorities.[45] The most important risk factors for developing CKD are DM, hypertension, and the presence of a positive family history. Assessment of susceptibility genes for CKD is currently in progress. People who have risk factors for CKD need frequent screening and education about modifiable risk factors. Modifiable risk factors include hypertension, hyperglycemia, dyslipidemia, obesity, excessive protein and sodium intake, and exposure to nephrotoxic agents such as radiocontrast dyes. Individuals with a family history of CKD need to be more aware of modifiable factors because of the increased risk signaled by the history.[9] Nonmodifiable risk factors include age, premature birth, heredity, and ethnicity. Heredity and genetic predisposition are primary reasons for early intervention to prevent CKD. Early diagnosis of CKD can lead to interventions that may slow progression of the disease and permit identification and treatment of complications and comorbidities of CKD.

The relationship between CVD and CKD needs to be evaluated. Reduced kidney function is associated with increased levels of inflammatory factors, which are also thought to be associated with CVD. Abnormal lipid profile and endothelial dysfunction, which can lead to atherosclerosis, are increased with reduced kidney function.[1]

Yvonne Johnson: Application

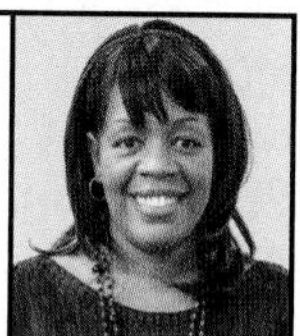

Ms. Johnson has several risk factors for CKD. Her African American ethnicity, which increases her risk for CKD, is a nonmodifiable risk factor. However, her hypertension and SLE are modifiable.

5. How are the rates of occurrence of early and late CKD affected by ethnicity?
6. How do Ms. Johnson's modifiable risk factors affect treatment of her CKD?

Diabetic Nephropathy. Diabetic nephropathy is the most frequent cause of CKD in patients who develop ESRD, accounting for more than 50% of new ESRD cases. CKD occurs in 30% of people with type 1 diabetes mellitus (T1D) and in 25–40% of people with type 2 diabetes mellitus (T2D) regardless of glucose control, highlighting the familial predisposition. Although DM is associated with hyperglycemia, hypertension, and altered lipids, most people with diabetes do not develop nephropathy; genetic factors may be responsible for these differences. Moderately increased **albuminuria** (albumin in the urine) is an early indicator of diabetic nephropathy. Clinically, diabetic nephropathy is characterized by a reduced GFR, hypertension, severely increased albuminuria, and a high risk of CVD. The changes in the kidney include basement membrane thickening, mesangial expansion, increased glomerular permeability, and decreased GFR.[9] Diabetic nephropathy is discussed in further detail in Chapter 45.

Hypertensive Nephrosclerosis. In T2D, the prevalence of hypertension is increasing with the higher incidence of diabetes and obesity. Hypertension increases the incidence of ESRD and has increased in recent years, disproportionately affecting African Americans.[46]

Over time, impaired renal autoregulation occurs. Increasing pressure in the glomerulus leads to damage of glomerular cells, ultimately resulting in **glomerulosclerosis** (scarring of the glomerulus). Chronic hypertension damages the small arteries and arterioles in the kidney. Inadequate blood supply to the nephron narrows the arterial and arteriolar lumens, which decreases blood flow to the glomeruli and causes sclerosis. The remaining nephrons that are not damaged compensate by hyperfiltration, which leads to increased glomerular filtration and thickening of the glomerular vessels.[1] Hypertension leads to initiation of the RAAS, resulting in retention of sodium and water. Research suggests that this increase in sodium and water retention also causes vascular remodeling and glomerular fibrosis. Significant hypertension is a key predictor of accelerated progression of renal dysfunction and failure. Hypertensive nephrosclerosis is discussed in further detail in Chapter 45.

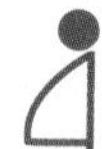

Severe pre-eclampsia leads to hypertension and larger glomeruli from hyperfiltration and increased pressure. It usually reverses after delivery. ■

Chronic Glomerulonephritis. Inflammation of the glomerulus is one of the top three leading cause of CKD. Initiating factors, genetic predisposition, and progression of the disease can lead to different outcomes. However, glomerulonephritis can progress, leading to chronic consequences of hypertension and proteinuria that promote continuing kidney damage.[47] Glomerulopathies involve direct injury to the glomerulus. Because of the insidious nature of this disorder, many patients with glomerulonephritis are not diagnosed until the disease is clinically advanced.[47] Almost all forms of glomerulonephritis can advance to CKD. Inflammation and activation of molecular mediators, similar to the process of diabetic nephropathy, lead to progressive glomerular and tubulointerstitial fibrosis and a reduction in GFR.

Chronic glomerulonephritis usually begins similarly to acute glomerulonephritis: with antibody deposition that results in glomerular inflammation. However, in chronic glomerulonephritis, the inflammatory process is chronic, and nephron units are destroyed over time. Activation and proliferation of mesangial cells promote inflammation through the release of chemokines and cytokines as well as the development of glomerulosclerosis.[1]

There are two general patterns in glomerular disease. One is a nephritic pattern, which is associated with inflammation and produces an active urine sediment with red cells, white cells, granular cell casts, and often red cell and other casts with a variable degree of proteinuria. The other pattern is a nephrotic pattern, which is associated not with inflammation but with proteinuria, often in the nephrotic range, and inactive urine sediment with few cells or casts. A diagnosis of chronic glomerulonephritis usually requires a renal biopsy to identify the precise etiology. Glomerular diseases are detailed further in Chapter 45.

Polycystic Kidney Disease. Polycystic kidney disease (PKD) is another cause of CKD and globally is the third most common cause of ESRD. Hypertension usually develops early in the disease process, but the pathogenesis is different in PKD.[48] Cysts usually develop from the collecting duct of the nephron and are highly focal in nature. The cysts increase in number and size as an individual ages (**Figure 46.6** ■). The cysts encroach on normal renal tissue, causing macrophage infiltration, neovascularization,

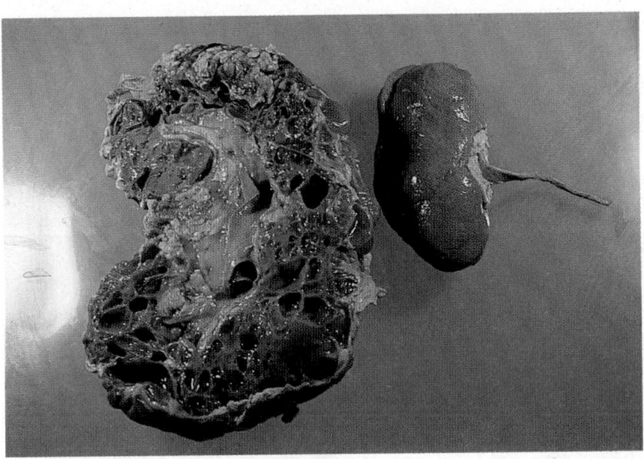

Figure 46.6 ■ A polycystic kidney. The functional tissue of the kidneys is gradually destroyed and replaced with fluid-filled cysts.

SOURCE: A. Glauberman / Photo Researchers, Inc.

progressive fibrosis, and a slow deterioration in renal function. Apoptotic loss of renal tubular epithelial cells and release of inflammatory mediators have been targeted as causes of the destruction of normal renal tissue. Approximately 90% of cases are caused by a mutation of the *PKD1* gene with an onset starting at 30 years of age.[49]

Clinical Manifestations

A review of the functions of the kidney can elucidate the chronic systemic effects that occur in CKD. Excretory functions of the kidney include removal of the waste products of metabolism such as urea and creatinine, removal of excess fluid, regulation of acid–base balance, and regulation of electrolyte levels. Secretory functions include regulation of blood pressure via the RAAS system, red blood cell mass through erythropoietin, and calcium metabolism through activation of vitamin D.[1] Patients with CKD may present with edema, fatigue, and anorexia or may exhibit no clinical manifestations except when detected from laboratory studies (**Figure 46.7** ■).

Cardiovascular Disease. Cardiovascular disease is the most common cause of death in individuals with CKD and ESRD.[50] The risk of CVD occurs early in the progression of CKD. Individuals on dialysis often die from cardiovascular causes, and cardiac disease is identified as the leading cause of death for the person with ESRD.[9] Not only do hypertension and dyslipidemia contribute to CVD in CKD, but a chronic inflammatory state manifested by increased levels of C-reactive protein may indicate increased risk of CVD. Cardiovascular causes of death can include acute myocardial infarction and heart failure.

Hypertension, especially when poorly controlled, can lead to CKD. It can also be a consequence of CKD, since hypertension increases as the GFR decreases. Hypertension contributes to a reduction in renal function by impairment of renal autoregulation and the transmission of elevated pressures to the glomerulus and endothelial, mesangial, and epithelial cell injury. On the other hand, CKD adversely affects blood pressure. Sympathetic hyperactivity results from stimulation of the RAAS system, which results in increased angiotensin II. Angiotensin II stimulates the release of aldosterone, promoting sodium and water retention. Angiotensin II also results in higher calcium levels. Increases in sodium and calcium lead to vasoconstriction and elevation of blood pressure. Albuminuria is also a significant predictor of CVD in CKD.

Whether hypertension is a cause or a result of CKD, it can lead to other cardiovascular and cerebrovascular disorders. Hypertension can lead to left ventricular hypertrophy. Prolonged hypertrophy can result in heart failure. The presence of left ventricular hypertrophy in individuals with CKD is high in all age groups, begins early in the disorder, and progresses as renal function declines. It is associated with a poor prognosis. Adverse effects noted include heart failure, ventricular arrhythmias, reduced left ventricular ejection fraction, sudden death, myocardial infarction, and stroke. The use of medications that block the RAAS and decrease blood pressure, such as ACE inhibitors and angiotensin receptor blockers (ARBs), as well as statins and antiplatelet therapy are used to reduce cardiovascular disease risk and slow the progression of CKD.[47]

Dyslipidemia occurs with CKD and accelerate its progression. Dyslipidemia occurs early in CKD and worsens as kidney function declines. Multiple types of lipid abnormalities can occur in CKD; they include elevated total cholesterol and triglycerides, increased low-density lipoprotein (LDL) cholesterol, and decreased high-density lipoprotein (HDL) cholesterol. Patients with nephrotic syndrome (proteinuria greater than 3.5 g/dL) tend to have higher total cholesterol and LDL levels. This may be due to the increased production and decreased catabolism of lipoproteins. Hypertriglyceridemia is thought to occur as a result of decreased catabolism of triglycerides. HDL cholesterol decreases and LDL cholesterol increases as kidney function worsens. Thus, proteinuria potentiates dyslipidemia, which can lead to further decline in kidney function and even more proteinuria. Dyslipidemia is also a risk factor for CVD. Higher levels of LDL cholesterol and triglycerides and lower levels of HDL cholesterol create an increased risk for development or worsening of CVD.[47]

Metabolic Acidosis. Chronic kidney disease is the most common cause of chronic **metabolic acidosis**. In CKD, the kidneys tend to retain hydrogen ions. This leads to a progressive metabolic acidosis, which is especially prominent in stages 4 and 5 CKD.[9] As the number of functioning nephrons declines, the acid–base balance is maintained by renal excretion of ammonia. Ammonium excretion falls as the GFR is reduced to 40–50 mL/min. Thus, retention of hydrogen ions occurs.

Normally, the proximal convoluted tubule resorbs approximately 80% of the filtered sodium bicarbonate. This resorption is reduced in CKD. Mortality is increased in CKD when the bicarbonate is less than 22 mmol/L. Metabolic acidosis can produce or exacerbate existing bone disorders and accelerate muscle degradation and loss.

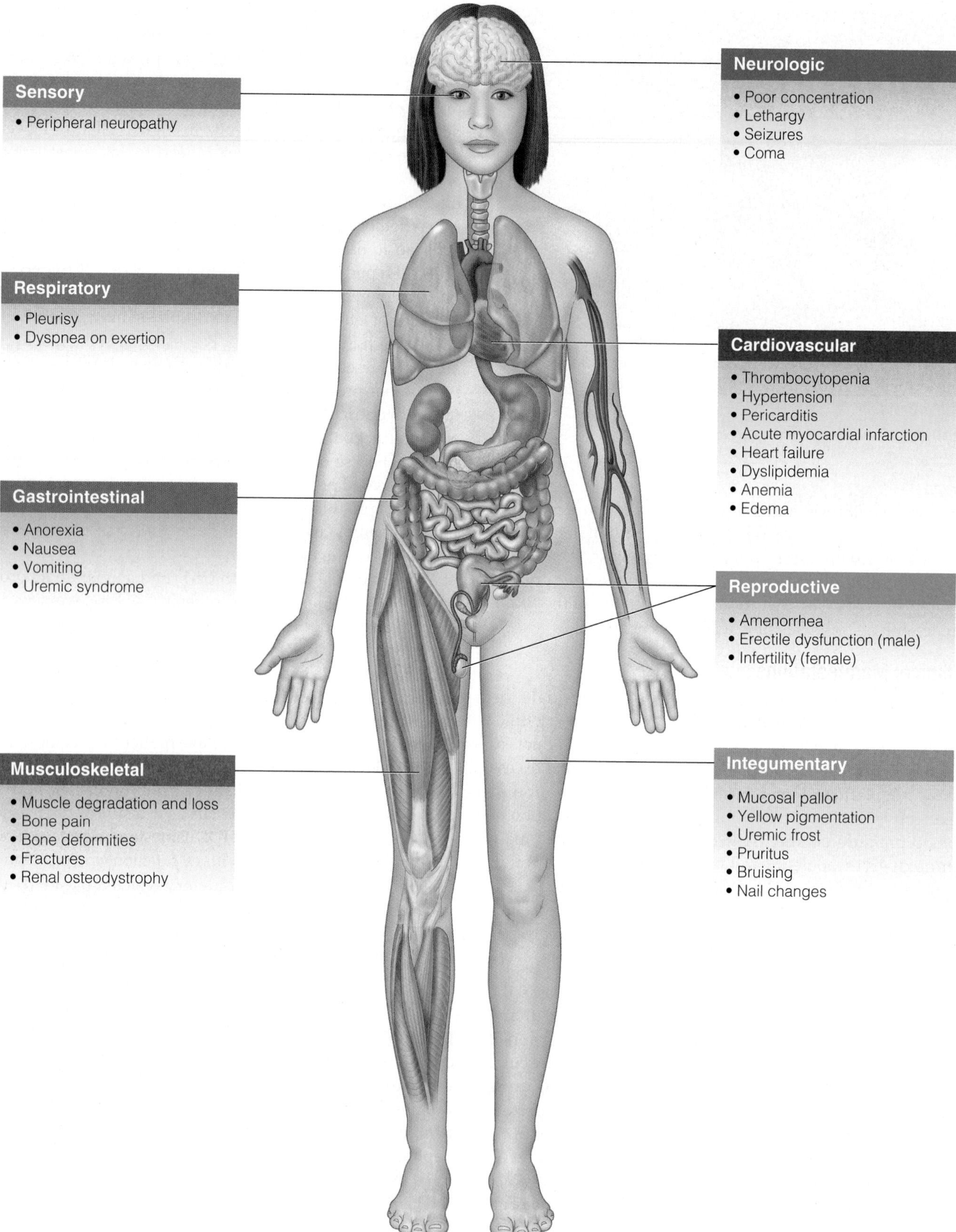
Sensory
• Peripheral neuropathy
Neurologic
• Poor concentration
• Lethargy
• Seizures
• Coma
Respiratory
• Pleurisy
• Dyspnea on exertion
Cardiovascular
• Thrombocytopenia
• Hypertension
• Pericarditis
• Acute myocardial infarction
• Heart failure
• Dyslipidemia
• Anemia
• Edema
Gastrointestinal
• Anorexia
• Nausea
• Vomiting
• Uremic syndrome
Reproductive
• Amenorrhea
• Erectile dysfunction (male)
• Infertility (female)
Musculoskeletal
• Muscle degradation and loss
• Bone pain
• Bone deformities
• Fractures
• Renal osteodystrophy
Integumentary
• Mucosal pallor
• Yellow pigmentation
• Uremic frost
• Pruritus
• Bruising
• Nail changes

Figure 46.7 ■ Multisystem effects of chronic kidney disease.

In children with CKD, chronic metabolic acidosis, renal osteodystrophy, dietary restrictions leading to inadequate nutrition, and anemia can retard growth.[12] ■

Chronic Kidney Disease–Mineral and Bone Disorder. **Chronic kidney disease–mineral and bone disorder (CKD-MBD)** is the term used to describe the bone disease process in CKD that results from mineral and hormonal changes.[51] These changes typically become apparent in stage 3 CKD. Individuals can experience bone pain, deformities, and fractures as long-term complications. The kidneys have a major role in calcium and phosphate regulation. Normally, as serum calcium levels fall, parathyroid hormone (PTH) is secreted by the parathyroid gland. This causes the kidneys to produce activated vitamin D (calcitriol), resulting in increased absorption of calcium by the small intestine and release of calcium from bone. Additionally, calcium is retained by the kidneys, and phosphorus is excreted. The result is a normal calcium level.

In CKD, however, the kidney function is diminished, and retained phosphorus may bind with calcium. Trying to control elevated phosphorus, fibroblast growth factor 23 inhibits calcitriol synthesis, which also contributes to a decrease in calcium.[52] The lack of calcitriol and the binding of phosphorus with calcium result in hypocalcemia. PTH is produced initially and removes calcium from bone to maintain normal levels. However, high phosphorus binding to calcium continues as the CKD progresses, PTH levels rise, and secondary hyperparathyroidism results. Eventually, PTH becomes less responsive to calcitriol and calcium. Bone also becomes less responsive, so higher levels of PTH are required for normal bone turnover to replace old bone with new bone. As a consequence, an abnormally high level of bone turnover occurs; hypocalcemia, hyperphosphatemia, and hyperparathyroidism continue; and MBD progresses.[52] Weakened bones and fractures can result. Phosphorus–calcium complexes that result from hyperphosphatemia result in soft tissue (cornea, conjunctiva, muscles, lungs, gastrointestinal tract, skin) and vascular calcifications. Vascular calcifications have been implicated in death from CVD and may preclude a patient from receiving a kidney transplant.[53] See Impact of Nutrition in Clinical Practice for a discussion of dietary phosphorus and CKD.

Anemia. Healthy kidneys produce **erythropoietin**, a hormone that stimulates production of red blood cells in the bone marrow. In CKD, the production of erythropoietin is reduced, and anemia of CKD occurs. The anemia usually becomes more profound as CKD worsens. Evaluation of anemia should occur when the hemoglobin level is less than 12 mg/dL in females and less than 13.5 mg/dL in males. Diagnosis of anemia due to CKD is made by excluding other causes of anemia, including gastrointestinal losses, iron, folate, and serum transferrin deficiencies.

Hemodynamic adaptations occur as the kidneys become unable to produce erythropoietin. Increased cardiac preload and reduction in afterload result in a high cardiac output. This mechanism of adapting to anemia results in cardiac remodeling as evidenced by left ventricular

Impact of Nutrition in Clinical Practice

Dietary Phosphorus and Chronic Kidney Disease

Joanne Kouba

When the GFR falls below 60 mL/min, which is approximately CKD stage 3, hyperphosphatemia and hyperparathyroidism are common.[1] These physiologic abnormalities are linked with increased mortality in patients with CKD.[1] Early in the progression of CKD, monitoring of serum phosphorus, calcium, and PTH is advised.[1] Individualized treatment recommendations for patients with CKD stages 3–5 on chronic dialysis often include phosphorus restriction as an adjunct to phosphate-binding medications, supplemental calcium, and vitamin D while maintaining adequate intake of other key nutrients such as calories and protein.[2,3] The risk for chronic CKD–MBD and soft tissue calcification increases with chronic hyperphosphatemia.

Prevention of CKD–MBD includes a combined approach of phosphorus and calcium regulation, often including vitamin D supplementation.[2,3] The Academy of Nutrition and Dietetics Evidence Analysis Library recommends restriction of phosphorus to 800–1000 mg/day if serum phosphorus levels are elevated, or 10–12 mg phosphorus per gram of dietary protein.[2] Like many other "diet orders," this is easier to dispense than to live with, especially over the long term. Phosphorus is widespread in the food supply and concentrated in high-protein sources (e.g., meat, poultry, milk, legumes, nuts).[3] Traditionally, advice for limiting phosphorus intake has been to control intake of dairy products and meat while still consuming adequate amounts of protein.[3] For example, a diet that contains 70 grams of protein will contain approximately 1000 milligrams of phosphorus.

Recently, attention to dietary phosphorus has widened to include processed foods with phosphate additives, such as sodium, calcium, and magnesium phosphate.[4] These additives not only are in foods that that are typically *not* considered high-phosphorus sources, but also are more readily absorbed than phosphorus that is naturally found in meat and whole-grain cereals. Phosphate additives are often found in processed meat (e.g., chicken nuggets), baking mixes (e.g., biscuit, pancake, and cake mixes), frozen baked goods, instant puddings, and cereal bars.[4,5] Food manufacturers use phosphate additives to enhance the consistency and appearance of foods, such as boxed or frozen macaroni and cheese. The contribution of daily dietary phosphorus from such additives is estimated to be 1000 mg/day, the same amount that many CKD patients are advised to consume for the entire day.[4] In the United States, the Nutrition Facts Label is not required to, but may, list the phosphorus content per serving of a food product.[3,5] Patients with CKD should be advised to check the Nutrition Facts Label for phosphorus content and read ingredient labels to avoid products with phosphate additives. The phosphorus content of some common foods is listed below.[6] Equally important in phosphorus regulation of patients with CKD is regular use of phosphate-binding medications to reduce gastrointestinal absorption of dietary phosphorus.[1,2]

(*Continued*)

Impact of Nutrition in Clinical Practice *Continued*

Food	Amount	Phosphorus (mg)
Pizza	1 slice	380
Chocolate pudding: instant mix made with milk	1 cup	340
Chicken: white meat	3 ounces	290
Milk: whole, low-fat, or nonfat	1 cup	240
Cheese: cheddar, mozzarella, provolone	1 ounce	150
Waffle, frozen	1 square	150
Pasta or noodles: plain	1/2 cup	60
Soda: cola or other dark type	12 fluid ounces	50
Bread: white	1 slice	30–40
Apple: raw	1 cup	13
Fats and oils such as butter, margarine	1 tablespoon	< 5
Soda: lemon-lime	12 fluid ounces	0

References

1. Kidney Disease: Improving Global Outcomes (KDIGO) CKD–MBD Work Group. (2009). KDIGO clinical practice guideline for the diagnosis, evaluation, prevention, and treatment of chronic kidney disease–mineral and bone disorder (CKD–MBD). *Kidney International*, 76(Suppl. 113), S1–S130.
2. American Dietetic Association. (2017). Chronic kidney disease: Evidence-based nutrition practice guidelines. *Evidence Analysis Library.* Available at http://www.andeal.org/topic.cfm?menu=5303
3. Beto, J. A., Ramirez, W. E., & Bansal, V. K. (2014). Medical nutrition therapy in adults with chronic kidney disease: Integrating evidence and consensus into practice for the generalist. *Journal of the Academy of Nutrition and Dietetics*, *114*, 1077–1087.
4. Takdea, E., Yamamoto, H., Yamanake-Okumura, H., & Taketani, Y. (2014). Increasing dietary phosphorus intake from food additives: Potential for negative impact on bone health. *Advances in Nutrition*, *5*, 92–97.
5. Academy of Nutrition and Dietetics. (2017). Renal. *Nutrition care manual.* Available at https://www.nutritioncaremanual.org/topic.cfm?ncm_category_id=1&lv1=5537&ncm_toc_id=5537&ncm_heading=&page
6. U.S. Department of Agriculture, Agricultural Research Service. (2007). *USDA national nutrient database for standard reference* (Release 27). Available at http://w222.ars.usda.gov/ba/bhnrd/ndl

hypertrophy and dilation of the left ventricle. Activation of the RAAS system and subsequent increased afterload also contribute to left ventricular hypertrophy and CVD. Anemia has also been implicated as an additional risk factor for stroke.[54]

Hyperkalemia. Hyperkalemia usually develops during ESRD as oliguria develops (**Figure 46.8** ■). Hyperkalemia may result from decreased aldosterone secretion and decreased excretion of potassium by the renal tubules. Other factors include a high-potassium diet, increased tissue breakdown, impaired cell uptake of potassium, and potassium-sparing diuretics.

Hypervolemia. Normal intravascular volume is usually maintained until the GFR falls below 10–15 mL/min. Once the GFR falls to this level, decreased renal excretion of sodium and water occurs, resulting in **hypervolemia**. This hypervolemia exacerbates left ventricular hypertrophy and CVD.[55] Individuals with CKD and hypervolemia generally respond to diuretics and sodium restriction.

Uremia. As waste products such as urea accumulate in CKD, individuals can develop uremia. **Uremia** is a syndrome that affects every organ system and is a result of a combination of factors in ESRD. Individuals usually become symptomatic when the GFR is less than 10 mL/min. Urea accumulation in the blood can cause symptoms of fatigue, nausea, vomiting, and headache.

Gastrointestinal disturbances are among the earliest and most common signs of the uremic syndrome. A metallic taste and loss of appetite lead to anorexia, nausea, vomiting, and weight loss, which can improve once dialysis has been initiated. Individuals are also more prone to gastrointestinal disorders, including gastritis, peptic ulcer formation, and arteriovenous malformations.

Central nervous system manifestations frequently occur in uremic syndrome. Lethargy, irritability, encephalopathy, asterixis, and seizures are late manifestations of uremia. Edema may lead to peripheral neuropathy. Reduced deep tendon reflexes, restless leg syndrome, and foot drop may also be present.

Skin changes in uremic syndrome include pruritus and yellow pigmentation. Pruritus (itchy skin) is a common complaint and may resolve with dialysis. An increased yellowish hue is a result of retained liposoluble pigments, such as lipochromes and carotenoids.

Metabolic acidosis becomes severe in uremic syndrome. An elevated anion gap metabolic acidosis is present. Hyperkalemia, hypervolemia, and hypocalcemia can lead to hemodynamic instability and arrhythmias. Cardiovascular disturbances include left ventricular hypertrophy, which may result in heart failure. Heart failure may lead to pulmonary edema or congestive heart failure as hypervolemia increases pulmonary venous pressures. Cardiac arrhythmias may also present, and pericarditis can occur as a result of inadequate dialysis.

Linking Pathophysiology to Diagnosis and Treatment

Diagnostic Tests. Because of the lack of awareness among patients and even healthcare providers of existing CKD and the insidious onset that many patients experience, routine screening for kidney disease is recommended.[44]

- ***Blood and urine tests.*** Estimates of GFR are the best overall indices of kidney function[9] as highlighted in **Table 46.7** ■. Providers can estimate the GFR from one of the prediction equations discussed earlier; the CKD-EPI, MDRD, or Cockcroft-Gault equation. The equations are useful estimates of the GFR in adults and are all easy to calculate by using online websites.

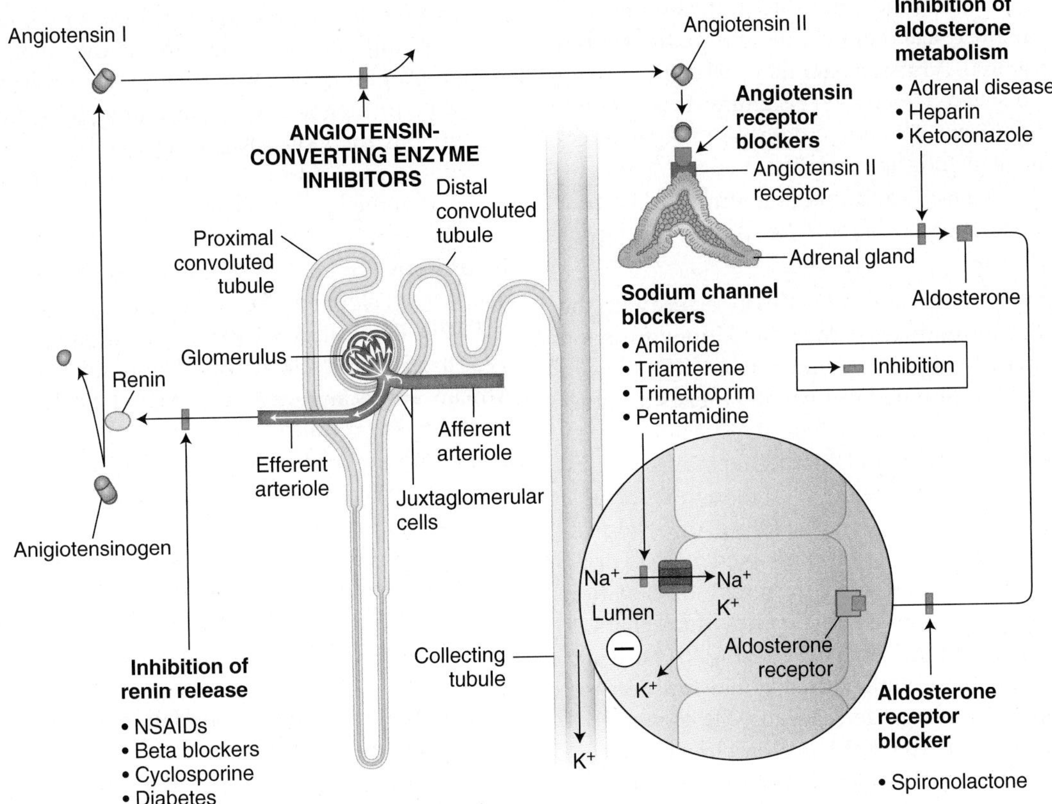

Figure 46.8 In the renin–angiotensin–aldosterone cascade, aldosterone stimulates sodium resorption in the collecting duct, which, in turn, generates a lumen-negative potential. The luminal electronegativity serves as a driving force for potassium excretion. Drugs that interfere with this process are depicted according to mechanism of action. Use of these agents in the setting of chronic renal insufficiency can predispose to the development of hyperkalemia.

The GFR decreases with age and decreased GFR in older adults is predictive of adverse outcomes. The GFR peaks at age 30, with a continued loss of function each year. By 70 years of age, the GFR is 70 mL/min. Levels less than 60 mL/min are associated with CKD and its complications.[1]

— Albuminuria is a principal marker of kidney damage. Protein levels are monitored in disorders that can lead to CKD such as DM, hypertension, and chronic glomerular disorders. The **albumin:creatinine ratio** is the gold standard for measurement of albuminuria. A ratio greater than 30 mg/g in a spot urine

Table 46.7 Diagnostic & Laboratory Tests for CKD

Test with Description, Rationale, and Normal Values	Expected Abnormality	Use to Diagnose
Serum creatinine becomes elevated with kidney damage; useful in calculating GFR. Normal is 0.6–1.2 mg/dL in males and 0.5–1.1 mg/dL in females	Serum creatinine usually increases gradually in CKD.	CKD
BUN is increased in kidney disease but is influenced by other factors; high-protein diet or liver disease may affect BUN. The BUN:creatinine ratio is normally around 10:1.	BUN will rise with AKI or CKD. The BUN:creatinine ratio will increase	Prerenal AKI when the BUN:creatinine ratio is > 20:1
Serum phosphorus becomes elevated as GFR declines; diseased kidneys are unable to excrete excess phosphorus. Normal phosphorus is 2.5–4.5 mg/dL	Serum phosphorus > 4.5 mg/dL	CKD-MBD; usually hyperphosphatemia is apparent CKD stage 3.
PTH becomes elevated in response to increasing phosphorus and decreasing calcium. Normal PTH is 10–55 pg/mL	As kidney function declines, the acceptable range for PTH increases	Secondary hyperparathyroidism, CKD-MBD
Serum potassium becomes elevated in CKD; may result in profound weakness and fatal dysrhythmias. Normal potassium is approximately 3.5–5.0 mEq/L (depending on the laboratory reference range)	Serum potassium > 5.0 (or greater than the laboratory reference range)	Advanced CKD, decreased aldosterone

sample indicates moderately increased albuminuria and that glucose and blood pressure control should be monitored. A ratio greater than 300 mg/g is diagnostic of severely increased albuminuria and represents significant glomerular damage. Other markers of damage include abnormalities in urine sediment, urine chemistries, and imaging studies. The first void in the morning should be used in testing for albuminuria.

— The serum creatinine level varies inversely with the GFR. For individuals with stable kidney function who have normal kidney function or CKD, a rise in the serum creatinine level usually means a reduction in the GFR. However, the compensatory hyperfiltration that occurs in DM and hypertension may blunt the rise in creatinine even though damage is occurring in the nephron. Therefore, other indicators of disease progression, such as changes in urine sediment, a rise in protein excretion, or elevation in blood pressure, must be pursued. Small changes in serum creatinine level (0.9–1.2 mg/dL) are significant for people with normal kidney function and can represent a large decrease in GFR. However, if an individual with CKD has a baseline creatinine level of 4.0 mg/dL, an increase to 6.0 mg/dL represents a smaller decrease in GFR, as the GFR is already reduced.

— Blood urea nitrogen (BUN) is another parameter that is evaluated in CKD. The BUN level also rises as the GFR falls. The BUN level can rise more rapidly in AKI than in CKD. The **BUN:creatinine ratio** is useful to diagnose hypovolemia. A normal BUN:creatinine ratio is about 10:1; but a ratio greater than 20:1 may signal hypovolemia. In addition, approximately 40–50% of the filtered urea is passively resorbed in the renal tubules; thus, in cases of hypovolemia, more urea is resorbed. The BUN will therefore rise disproportionately to the GFR. This is why the greater than 20:1 BUN:creatinine ratio can be helpful in diagnosing prerenal AKI.

— Routine urinalysis can reveal advanced kidney disease. A low specific gravity or abnormal numbers of white or red blood cells, bacteria, or protein indicate renal abnormalities. A low specific gravity can signal tubular damage and an inability to concentrate urine. Increased white blood cells may be due to chronic pyelonephritis or other infection. Red blood cells may signal glomerulonephritis. Casts are not typically noted in CKD.[56]

- ***Additional laboratory tests.*** A liver profile, thyroid function tests, and other electrolytes (calcium, magnesium, bicarbonate) indicate other abnormalities in kidney function. Further discussion of renal diagnostic testing is found in the discussion of the systemic effects of ESRD.
- ***Imaging.*** Radiologic studies evaluate the size and function of the kidneys and can assist in determining a cause for CKD. Radiologic films of the kidneys, ureters, and bladder; renal ultrasound; renal scan; renal arteriogram; abdominal computed tomography (CAT) scan; or magnetic resonance imaging (MRI) can identify obstructions, CKD, PKD, or birth defects.[56] A renal biopsy is performed to verify the cause of CKD or to determine if the cause is unknown.

Treatment. Treatment of CKD focuses on reduction of risk factors, slowing of disease progression, and treatment of ESRD. Clinical predictors of accelerated progression of CKD to ESRD include increased albuminuria, hypertension, African American race, lower serum HDL levels, and lower levels of serum transferrin. The degree of proteinuria and tubulointerstitial damage predicts progression to ESRD. Cases of focal segmental glomerulosclerosis from hypertension and nephrotic syndrome occur in African Americans at higher rates. ESRD in African Americans is being researched with the apolipoprotein L-1 (*APOL1*) allele located on chromosome 22 for younger African Americans with a family history of ESRD. Genetic studies continue to assess for links to ESRD.[40]

The National Kidney Foundation has developed guidelines to identify people who are at increased risk of CKD.[6] All individuals should be assessed at routine health encounters to determine their risk of CKD. Individuals at risk should have testing to evaluate markers of kidney damage and GFR. Specific interventions are based on the stage of CKD. Disorders that can lead to CKD such as hypertension and DM need to be evaluated and controlled (see **Table 46.8** ■). A review of systems by the healthcare provider can identify urinary symptoms to assess for infection or obstruction and skin rash or arthritis, which may suggest an autoimmune disorder. Chronic disorders that can result in reduced effective arterial blood volume, such as heart failure, cirrhosis, or GI fluid losses, should be identified. Any previous urologic evaluations should be discussed. A family history of kidney disorders, such as PKD, may underscore genetic factors that may result in CKD.[45]

Individuals who have been diagnosed with CKD need interventions at various stages of the disease. **Table 46.9** ■ lists the stages of CKD along with actions to be taken by the healthcare provider at each stage. Starting treatment at the right point in the CKD progression is essential to prevent adverse outcomes. Individuals who have been diagnosed with DM and started on the antihypertensive medications, such as ACE inhibitors and ARBs, manifest a reduction of CVD events and slower progression to ESRD. These medications lower blood pressure by reducing the effects of the RAAS and sympathetic nervous system activation on renal perfusion. They also reduce albuminuria; therefore, there is a slower reduction of the GFR. In T2D, prevalence of hypertension is 82.1%.[57] Treatment of hyperlipidemia with lipid-lowering medications such as a hydroxymethylglutaryl-coenzyme A inhibitor to reduce cholesterol levels can also reduce cardiovascular events.

Nephrology consultations should be obtained when the GFR is severely decreased to less than 30 mL/min, which is

Table 46.8 Treatment of Common Systemic Disorders in Chronic Kidney Disease and End-Stage Renal Failure

Condition	Treatment
CVD	Control hypertension and dyslipidemia Smoking cessation
Hypertension	Treat initially with ACE/ARB medications Add other antihypertensives as needed
Dyslipidemia	Treat patients with diet management and statin therapy
CKD-MBD	Decrease elevated phosphorus with diet and phosphorus binders Maintain normal calcium Treat abnormal PTH levels by adding vitamin D analog and/or calcimimetic
Anemia	Erythropoeitin, supplemental iron as needed
Hyperkalemia	Renal replacement therapy Reduced used of potassium-sparing diuretics Discontinue ACE inhibitors Potassium binders (cation exchange resin, patiromer)
Hypervolemia	Diuretic therapy with thiazide and loop diuretics Use caution with potassium-sparing diuretics Sodium restriction depending on urinary sodium loss Renal replacement therapy in stage 5 CKD
Protein calorie malnutrition	Maintain nutrition and appetite
Uremia	Renal replacement therapy

SOURCES: Kidney Disease: Improving Global outcomes (KDIGO) CKD Workgroup. (2013). KDIGO 2012 clinical practice guideline for the evaluation and management of CKD. *Kidney International*, 3(Suppl.), 1–150. Inker, L., Astor, B., Fox, C., et al. (2014). KDOQI US Commentary on the 2012 KDIGO Clinical Practice Guideline for the Evaluation and Management of CKD. *American Journal of Kidney Disease, 63*(5), 713–735.

stage 4 CKD. Some other indications for nephrology referral are uncontrolled hypertension or hyperkalemia.[44] In stage 4, the discussion for treatment options of advanced CKD are started; these options include conservative management, renal replacement therapy, and kidney transplantation.

CLINICAL POINT: CKD is a result of both genetic and environmental factors. People with a genetic predisposition to CKD should monitor their kidney function on a yearly basis. People who develop CKD should identify risk factors, especially hyperglycemia and hypertension, and should implement lifestyle changes to prevent progression of the disease. ■

Anemia in chronic kidney disease is treated with oral or intravenous iron if the patient is not iron replete. However, if the patient is iron replete and no other cause of anemia has been identified, such as gastrointestinal losses, the treatment for anemia includes replacement of endogenous erythropoietin with injectable erythropoietin-stimulating agents to avoid blood transfusions. Correction of anemia in the CKD population is intended not to attain a normal hemoglobin level but to keep the hemoglobin level greater than 10 mg/dL and less than 11.5 mg/dL.[58] Therapy should be individualized, weighing risks against benefits, as there have been increased risks of stroke or thrombosis in clinical trials. Erythropoietin-stimulating agents are contraindicated in certain cancers because of the possibility that they promote of cancer growth.

Derangements in CKD-MBD are common and usually become apparent at CKD stage 3. An elevated phosphorus level is treated with diet restrictions and oral phosphorus binders, which are taken with meals; they bind with phosphorus in food in the gastrointestinal tract and exit the body via stool, therefore not increasing phosphorus in the blood. Elevated PTH is treated with active vitamin D analogs, which suppress PTH levels. Serum calcium levels may also rise with active vitamin D use, and a calcimimetic is a novel medication to treat secondary hyperparathyroidism, usually used in stage 5 CKD. Calcimimetics bind with the calcium-sensing receptors and lower PTH levels.

The presence of uremia with its adverse effects is usually the catalyst to begin dialysis. Individuals with pericarditis, persistent hyperkalemia, intractable gastrointestinal symptoms, or encephalopathy should be started on dialysis even if their GFR does not meet ESRD levels. The type of dialysis selected is individualized and depends on sociodemographic factors. Conservative care is also an option for patients with advanced CKD who do not want renal replacement therapy or do not qualify for kidney transplantation. This includes management of symptoms, palliative care, and planning for advanced care.[44]

Table 46.9 CKD Interventions Grouped by CKD Stages

Stage	Description	GFR (mL/min/1.73 m^2)	Interventions
1	Kidney damage with normal or increased GFR	> 90	Diagnosis and treatment of etiology, CVD risk reduction
2	Kidney damage with mildly decreased GFR	60–89	Estimate and slow progression, control BP and DM, avoiding nephrotoxins
3	Kidney damage with moderately decreased GFR	30–59	Evaluating and treating complications (hyperphosphatemia, anemia)
4	Kidney damage with severely decreased GFR	15–29	Preparation for renal replacement therapy (hemodialysis access if planning hemodialysis, peritoneal dialysis catheter placement, or initiating a kidney transplantation workup)
5	Kidney failure	< 15	Renal replacement therapy (if uremia present) or conservative management (controlling hyperkalemia, hypervolemia, metabolic acidosis)

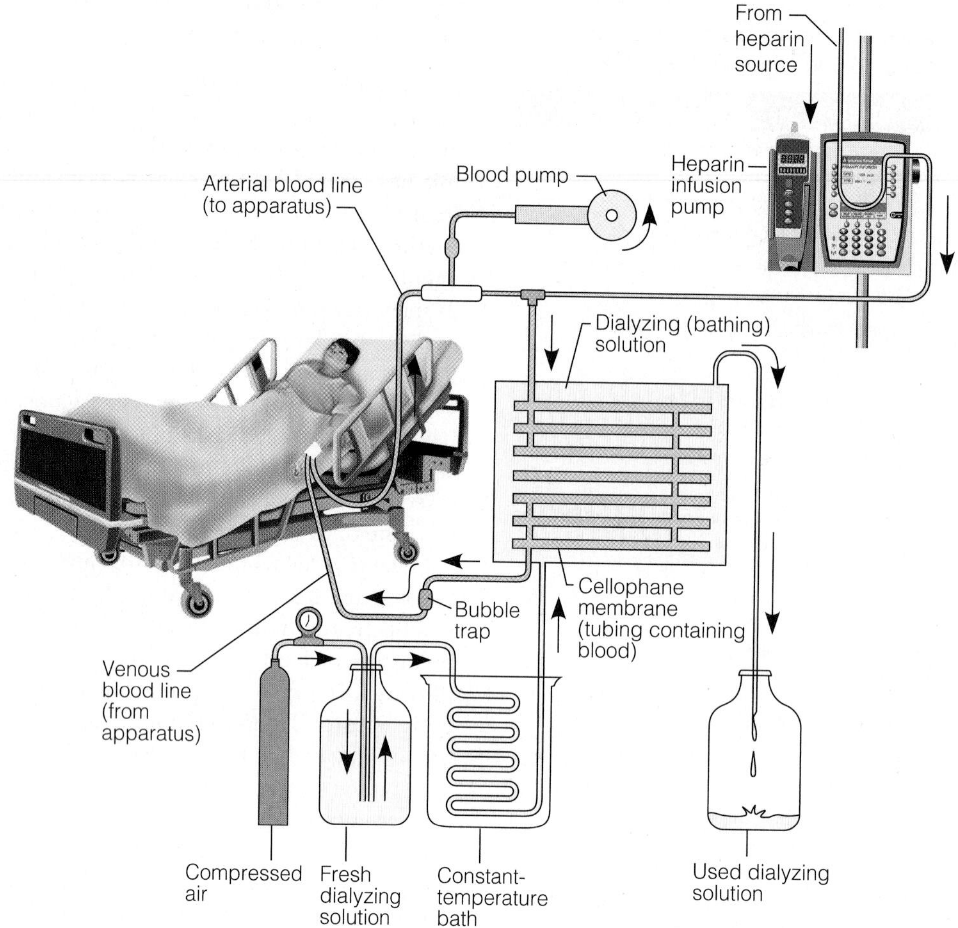

Figure 46.9 ■ Hemodialysis.

Most individuals who choose renal replacement therapy initiate hemodialysis. **Hemodialysis** involves removal of toxins (urea, potassium) and accumulated fluid from the blood. Access to the bloodstream through a surgically created arteriovenous shunt or central venous catheter is required (**Figure 46.9** ■). Blood leaves the patient and enters a dialyzer, where diffusion, ultrafiltration, and convection occur. Solutes and fluid move across a semipermeable membrane in the dialyzer, with blood on one side and dialysate on the other, but they never mix and they flow in opposite directions (countercurrent flow). Diffusion occurs when solutes move across the dialyzer membrane from a higher to a lower concentration. Ultrafiltration is the movement of fluid across the dialyzer membrane. Convection is the movement of solutes with fluid during ultrafiltration across the membrane and is independent of concentration gradients. Blood is returned to the patient, and the net loss of solutes and fluid corrects uremia and restores electrolyte balance and euvolemia.[9]

Peritoneal dialysis removes toxins by utilizing the peritoneum, a semipermeable abdominal membrane (**Figure 46.10** ■). A catheter is inserted into the peritoneal space, and dialysate fluid is infused and allowed to dwell for the time prescribed by the physician. The fluid, called peritoneal effluent, is then drained, and toxins and fluids are removed from the body with the fluid. New fluid is infused, and the process is repeated. Most exchanges occur at night using a machine called a cycler, and patients can sleep during the process.[9]

Renal transplantation is encouraged for patients who have the potential for a good quality of life after a transplantation. CKD patients need to complete a thorough evaluation for candidacy before undergoing transplantation. Active infection, recent malignancy, and strong noncompliance are some contraindications to transplantation. The transplanted kidney, which can come from a live or deceased donor, is transplanted into the lower abdomen, and the recipient's native kidneys are left intact (**Figure 46.11** ■). To maintain the graft, recipients are required to maintain immunosuppression, which results in increased risk for infection and malignancy.[41]

Yvonne Johnson: Outcome

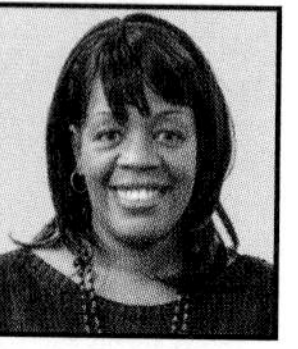

Despite treatment with multiple immunosuppressive therapies, Ms. Johnson experiences no clinical response to treatment and eventually needs to initiate dialysis. She chooses in-center

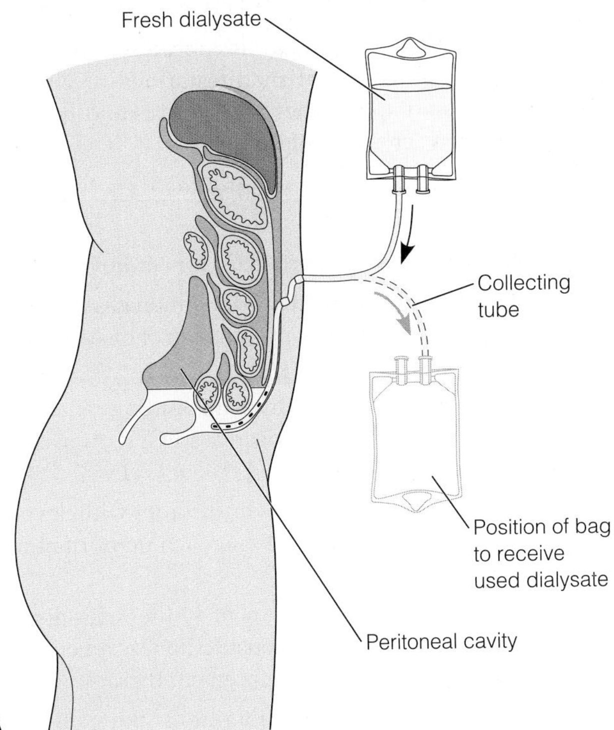

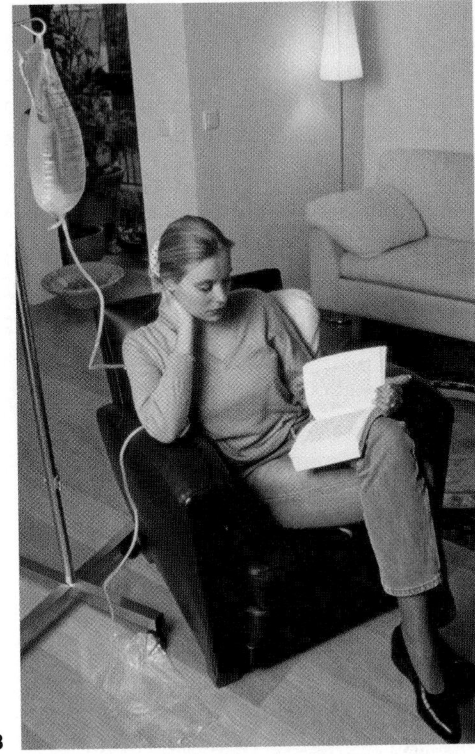

Figure 46.10 ■ Peritoneal dialysis.

hemodialysis. A referral is made for a hemodialysis access, and a forearm fistula is created in her nondominant arm. Ms. Johnson begins hemodialysis and is also in the process of completing her kidney transplant workup. She is fortunate, as some members from her church have offered to be tested as potential kidney donors.

7. What is the goal of hemodialysis for Ms. Johnson?
8. What factors make Ms. Johnson a good candidate for transplantation?

Check Your Progress: Section 46.3

1. What is a key early indicator of diabetic neuropathy?
2. Describe the appropriate interventions for a person with CKD and a GFR of 15–29 mL/min/1.73 m^2.
3. What is the difficulty in using BUN for diagnosing CKD?

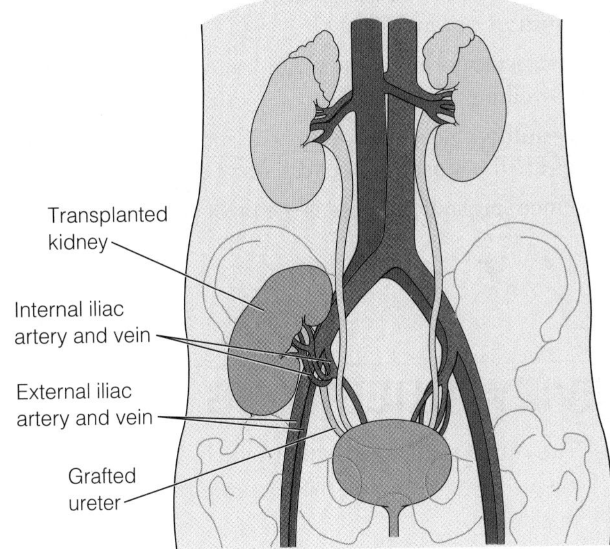

Figure 46.11 ■ Kidney transplantation.

CHAPTER SUMMARY

46.1 Chapter Overview and Case Studies

Describe the role of the kidneys, and discuss concepts related to acute kidney injury and chronic kidney disease.

- The kidneys regulate body fluids and electrolytes and excrete waste products.
- A decline in kidney function, either acute or chronic, can be life-limiting and life-threatening.
- Although clinical manifestations of acute kidney injury (AKI) may be quickly noted, manifestations of chronic kidney disease (CKD) may be silent for many years.
- Prompt identification of AKI can result in the preservation of normal kidney function.

46.2 Acute Kidney Injury

Differentiate the causes, underlying pathogenesis, and clinical manifestations acute kidney injury and approaches to diagnosis and treatment of the condition across the lifespan.

- Prerenal AKI is the most prevalent form of AKI and may be reversible.
- Reduction of urine output, increased creatinine, and low sodium excretion are clinical features of prerenal AKI
- Fluid resuscitation is the most common treatment of prerenal AKI.
- The two most common etiologies of intrinsic AKI are ischemic and nephrotoxic AKI.
- Prerenal AKI that progresses to ATN is the most common cause of intrinsic AKI.
- Sepsis has characteristics of both ischemic and nephrotoxic ATN, and there is a high mortality rate when both occur.
- Postrenal AKI results from obstruction of the urinary collecting system, which causes cessation of urinary flow and azotemia.
- Ureteral or kidney tissue obstructions are usually due to tumors or renal stones.
- Obstruction of the ureters can lead to hydronephrosis or swelling of the kidney.
- In adult women, retroperitoneal and pelvic malignancies are the most frequent causes of obstruction.
- In men, prostatic disease is the most typical etiology.

46.3 Chronic Kidney Disease

Differentiate the causes, classification, underlying pathogenesis, and clinical manifestations of chronic kidney disease and approaches to diagnosis and treatment of the condition across the lifespan.

- Incidence and prevalence of CKD are increasing worldwide.
- CKD is a strong predictor for cardiovascular disease.
- The National Kidney Foundation has developed stages of CKD to identify progression of disease and treatment goals.
- Diabetic nephropathy is the leading cause of ESRD and is characterized by decreased GFR, hypertension, proteinuria, and increased risk of CVD.
- PKD is a primary genetic disorder with development of fluid-filled cysts that encroach on normal renal tissue and function.
- Stages of progression of kidney disease should be assessed to initiate consultation by a nephrologist and initiation of renal replacement therapy.
- The albumin:creatinine ratio is the gold standard for measurement of urine protein.
- Derangements in bone and mineral metabolism are common in CKD and manifest as hyperphosphatemia, secondary hyperparathyroidism, and hypocalcemia.
- Anemia in CKD results from decreased production of erythropoietin.
- Hyperkalemia develops with increased oliguria and can prompt initiation of renal replacement therapy.
- Renal replacement therapy is initiated when uremic symptoms occur.

REVIEW QUESTIONS

1. The nurse understands that which of the following clients has the greatest risk for chronic kidney disease (CKD)?
   a. A Hispanic woman of low socioeconomic status
   b. A European American woman of low socioeconomic status
   c. A 75-year-old Caucasian woman
   d. A 75-year-old African American man

2. Which of the following clients does the dialysis nurse recognize as being at stage 4 CKD?
   a. The client with an elevated glomerular filtration rate (GFR)
   b. The client with a GFR greater than 90 mL/min/1.73 m^2
   c. The client with a GFR of 75 mL/min/1.73 m^2
   d. The client with a GFR of 20 mL/min/1.73 m^2

3. The nurse is preparing to admit a patient with immunoglobulin A nephropathy to the nursing unit. Which of the following will the nurse expect to find?
   a. A recent upper respiratory viral infection
   b. Pain on urination
   c. A 50-year-old client
   d. A recent bacterial skin infection

4. Which laboratory values would be expected in the client with nephrotic syndrome?
   a. Low total cholesterol and LDL levels
   b. Low triglycerides and high LDL levels
   c. High HDL and high LDL levels
   d. High total cholesterol and high LDL levels

5. Which of the following statements by a client undergoing peritoneal dialysis indicates that more teaching is needed?
   a. "I will perform peritoneal dialysis at night."
   b. "I will need to care for a fistula in my arm."
   c. "My peritoneum acts as a membrane to filter toxins."
   d. "The dialysate will dwell in my peritoneum for a few hours."
6. The nurse is caring for a client who has been vomiting for 24 hours. The client has poor skin turgor, a heart rate of 120 beats/min, and a blood pressure of 88/60 mmHg. The nurse assesses that this client is at risk for:
   a. chronic kidney disease.
   b. prerenal AKI.
   c. intrinsic AKI.
   d. postrenal AKI.
7. The nurse is preparing a client for hemodialysis. Which of the following occurs during hemodialysis?
   a. Urea and potassium are removed from the blood.
   b. A dialysate is infused into the client.
   c. Blood and dialysate are mixed in the dialyzer.
   d. Solutes move from a lower to a higher concentration.
8. Which of the following clients is a likely candidate for renal transplantation?
   a. A client with ongoing urinary infections
   b. A client with concurrent lymphoma
   c. A client who refuses to follow the medical regimen
   d. A client with a good social support system

ANSWERS

Answers to Review Questions can be found in Appendix A. Answers to Case Study and Check Your Progress questions are available on the faculty resources site. Please consult with your instructor.

RECOMMENDED WEBSITES

Acute Kidney Injury Network
http://www.akinet.org

American Nephrology Nurses Association
https://www.annanurse.org

Kidney Disease: Improving Global Outcomes
http://kdigo.org

Kidney Early Evaluation Program Publications
https://www.kidney.org/news/keep

Medscape Nephrology Center
http://www.medscape.com/nephrology

The National Kidney Foundation
https://www.kidney.org

The National Kidney Foundation Kidney Disease Outcomes Quality Initiative (NKF KDOQI)
https://www.kidney.org/professionals/guidelines

The Nephron Information Center
http://nephron.com

REFERENCES

1. Capriotti, T., & Frizzell, J. (2016). *Pathophysiology: Introductory concepts and clinical perspectives*. Philadelphia, PA: F.A. Davis
2. Singbartl, K., & Kellum J. A. (2012). AKI in the ICU: Definition, epidemiology, risk stratification, and outcomes. *Kidney International, 81*(9), 819–825. doi:10.1038/ki.2011.339
3. Ratanarat, R., Skulratanasak, P., Tangkawattanakul, N., & Hantaweepant, C. (2013). Clinical accuracy of RIFLE and Acute Kidney Injury Network (AKIN) criteria for predicting hospital mortality in critically ill patients with multi-organ dysfunction syndrome. *Journal of the Medical Association of Thailand (Chotmaihet Thangphaet), 96*(Suppl. 2), S224–S231.
4. Lopes, J., & Jorge, S. (2013). The RIFLE and AKIN classifications for acute kidney injury: A critical and comprehensive review. *Clinical Kidney Journal, 6*(1), 8–14.
5. Kidney Disease: Improving Global Outcomes (KDIGO) Acute Kidney Injury Work Group. (2012). KDIGO clinical practice guideline for acute kidney injury. *Kidney International*, 2(Suppl.), 1–138.
6. National Kidney Foundation. (n.d.). *Glomerular filtration rate*. Available at https://www.kidney.org/atoz/content/gfr
7. National Kidney Foundation. (2009). *CKD-EPI creatinine equation*. Available at https://www.kidney.org/content/ckd-eip-creatinine-equation-2009
8. Thomas, M. E., Blaine, C., Dawnay, A., et al. (2015). The definition of acute kidney injury and its use in practice. *Kidney International, 87*(1), 62–73. doi:10.1038/ki.2014.328
9. Ignatavicius, D., & Workman, M. (2013). *Medical-surgical nursing: Patient-centered collaborative care* (8th ed.). St. Louis, MO: Elsevier.
10. Sutherland, S., Byrnes, J., Kothari, M., et al. (2015). AKI in hospitalized children: Comparing the pRIFLE, AKIN, and KDIGO definitions. *Clinical Journal of the American Society of Nephrology, 10*(4), 554–561. doi:10.2215/cjn.01900214

11. Loirat, C., Fakhouri, F., Ariceta, G., et al. (2015). An international consensus approach to the management of atypical hemolytic uremic syndrome in children. *Pediatric Nephrology, 31*(1), 15–39. doi:10.1007/s00467-015-3076-8
12. Perry, S., Hockenberry, M., Lowdermilk, D., & Wilson, D. (2014). *Maternal child nursing care* (5th ed.). St. Louis, MO: Elsevier.
13. Soler, Y., Nieves-Plaza, M., Prieto, M., García-De Jesús, R., & Suárez-Rivera, M. (2013). pRIFLE (pediatric risk, injury, failure, loss, end stage renal disease) score identifies acute kidney injury and predicts mortality in critically ill children: A prospective study. *Pediatric Critical Care Medicine, 14*(4), e189–e195. doi:10.1097/PCC.0b013e3182745675
14. Burke, M., Pabbidi, M., Farley, J., & Roman, R. (2014). Molecular mechanisms of renal blood flow autoregulation. *Current Vascular Pharmacology, 12*(6), 845–858. doi:10.2174/15701611113116660149
15. Lameire, N., Van Biesen, W., & Vanholder, R. (2005). Acute renal failure. *Lancet, 365*(9457), 417–430. doi:10.1016/s0140-6736(05)17831-3
16. Pahwa, A., & Sperati, C. (2015). Urinary fractional excretion indices in the evaluation of acute kidney injury. *Journal of Hospital Medicine, 11*(1), 77–80. doi:10.1002/jhm.2501
17. Chu, R., Li, C., Wang, S., Zou, W., Liu, G., & Yang, L. (2014). Assessment of KDIGO definitions in patients with histopathologic evidence of acute renal disease. *Clinical Journal of the American Society of Nephrology, 9*(7), 1175–1182. doi:10.2215/cjn.06150613
18. Turner, J., & Coca, S. (2014). Acute tubular injury and acute tubular necrosis. *National Kidney Foundation primer on kidney diseases* (6th ed., pp. 304–311). Philadelphia, PA: Elsevier Saunders.
19. Traub, S. J., Kellum, J. A., Tang, A., Cataldo, L., Kancharla, A., & Shapiro, N. I. (2013). Risk factors for radiocontrast nephropathy after emergency department contrast-enhanced computerized tomography. *Academic Emergency Medicine: Official Journal of the Society for Academic Emergency Medicine, 20*(1), 40–45. doi:10.1111/acem.12059
20. Schrier, R., & Wang, W. (2004). Acute renal failure and sepsis. *New England Journal of Medicine*, 351(2), 159–169. doi:10.1056/nejmra032401.
21. Dirkes, S. (2013). Sepsis and inflammation: Impact on acute kidney injury. *Nephrology Nursing Journal, 40*(2), 125–132.
22. Rodriguez, F., Bonacasa, B., Fenoy, F. J., & Salom, M. G. (2013). Reactive oxygen and nitrogen species in the renal ischemia/reperfusion injury. *Current Pharmaceutical Design, 19*(15), 2776–2794.
23. Meola, M., Nalesso, F., Petrucci, I., Samoni, S., & Ronco, C. (2016). Pathophysiology and clinical work-up of acute kidney injury. *Contributions to Nephrology, 188*, 1–10. doi:10.1159/000445460
24. Maringer, K., & Sims-Lucas, S. (2016). The multifaceted role of the renal microvasculature during acute kidney injury. *Pediatric Nephrology (Berlin, Germany), 31*(8), 1231–1240. doi:10.1007/s00467-015-3231-2
25. Xu, Y., Ruan, S., Wu, X., Chen, H., Zheng, K., & Fu, B. (2013). Autophagy and apoptosis in tubular cells following unilateral ureteral obstruction are associated with mitochondrial oxidative stress. *International Journal of Molecular Medicine, 31*(3), 628–636. doi:10.3892/ijmm.2013.1232
26. Macedo, E., & Mehta, R. L. (2014). Targeting recovery from acute kidney injury: Incidence and prevalence of recovery. *Nephron. Clinical Practice, 127*(1–4), 4–9. doi:10.1159/000363704
27. Heung, M., Steffick, D., Zivin, K., et al. (2016). Acute kidney injury recovery pattern and subsequent risk of CKD: An analysis of Veterans Health Administration data. *American Journal of Kidney Diseases*, 67(5), 742–752. doi:10.1053/j.ajkd.2015.10.019
28. Blank, M., Parkin, L., Paul, C., & Herbison, P. (2014). A nationwide nested case-control study indicates an increased risk of acute interstitial nephritis with proton pump inhibitor use. *Kidney International, 86*(4), 837–844. doi:10.1038/ki.2014.74
29. Muriithi, A. K., Leung, N., Valeri, A. M., Cornell, L. D., Sethi, S., Fidler, M. E., & Nasr, S. H. (2015). Clinical characteristics, causes and outcomes of acute interstitial nephritis in the elderly. *Kidney International, 87*(2), 458–464. doi:10.1038/ki.2014.294
30. Perazella, M. A. (2014). Diagnosing drug-induced AIN in the hospitalized patient: A challenge for the clinician. *Clinical Nephrology, 81*(6), 381–388. doi:10.5414/CN108301
31. Thurman, J. M., & Le Quintrec, M. (2016). Targeting the complement cascade: Novel treatments coming down the pike. *Kidney International, 90*(4), 746–752. doi:10.1016/j.kint.2016.04.018
32. Brake, M., & Batuman, V. (2016). IgA nephropathy. *Medscape*. Available at http://emedicine.medscape.com/article/239927-overview\#a6
33. Kashani, K., & Kellum, J. A. (2015). Novel biomarkers indicating repair or progression after acute kidney injury. *Current Opinion in Nephrology & Hypertension, 24*(1), 21–27. doi:10.1097/MNH.0000000000000090
34. Kimmel, M., Shi, J., Latus, J., et al. (2016). Association of renal stress/damage and filtration biomarkers with subsequent AKI during hospitalization among patients presenting to the emergency department. *Clinical Journal of the American Society of Nephrology, 11*(6), 938–946. doi:10.2215/cjn.10551015
35. Weisbord, S., & Palevsky, P. (2016). Prevention of contrast-associated acute kidney injury: What should we do? *American Journal of Kidney Diseases, 68*(4), 518–521. doi:10.1053/j.ajkd.2016.05.005
36. El-Zoghby, Z., Lieske, J., Foley, R., et al. (2012). Urolithiasis and the risk of ESRD. *Clinical Journal of the American Society of Nephrology, 7*(9), 1409–1415. doi:10.2215/cjn.03210312
37. Faubel, S., Patel, N., Lockhart, M., & Cadnapaphornchai, M. (2013). Renal relevant radiology: Use of ultrasonography in patients with AKI. *Clinical Journal of the American Society of Nephrology, 9*(2), 382–394. doi:10.2215/cjn.04840513
38. Delanaye, P., Glassock, R. J., Pottel, H., & Rule, A. D. (2016). An age-calibrated definition of chronic kidney disease: Rationale and benefits. *Clinical Biochemist. Reviews/Australian Association of Clinical Biochemists, 37*(1), 17–26.
39. US Renal Data System. (2016). 2015 Annual data report: Epidemiology of kidney disease in the United States. *American Journal of Kidney Diseases, 67*(3, Suppl. 1), 1–S434. doi:10.1053/j.ajkd.2015.12.015
40. Anyaegbu, E. I., Shaw, A. S., Hruska, K. A., & Jain, S. (2015). Clinical phenotype of APOL1 nephropathy in young relatives of patients with end-stage renal disease. *Pediatric Nephrology (Berlin, Germany), 30*(6), 983–989. doi:10.1007/s00467-014-3031-0
41. Inker, L., Astor, B., Fox, C., et al. (2014). KDOQI US commentary on the 2012 KDIGO clinical practice guideline for the evaluation and management of CKD. *American Journal of Kidney Disease, 63*(5), 713–735. doi:10.1053/j.ajkd.2014.01.416
42. Alvis, B. D., & Hughes, C. G. (2015). Physiology considerations in geriatric patients. *Anesthesiology Clinics, 33*(3), 447–456. doi:10.1016/j.anclin.2015.05.003
43. McMahon, G., Hwang, S., & Fox, C. (2016). Residual lifetime risk of chronic kidney disease. *Nephrology Dialysis Transplantation*, gfw253. doi:10.1093/ndt/gfw253
44. Kidney Disease: Improving Global Outcomes (KDIGO) CKD Workgroup. (2013). KDIGO 2012 clinical practice guideline for the evaluation and management of CKD. *Kidney International*, 3(Suppl.), 1–150.
45. Nicholas, S. B., Kalantar-Zadeh, K., & Norris, K. C. (2013). Racial disparities in kidney disease outcomes. *Seminars in Nephrology, 33*(5), 409–415. doi:10.1016/j.semnephrol.2013.07.002
46. Randall, O., Kwagyan, J., Retta, T., et al. (2013). Effect of intensive blood pressure control on cardiovascular remodeling in hypertensive patients with nephrosclerosis. *International Journal of Nephrology, 2013*, 120–167. doi:10.1155/2013/120167
47. McLaughlin, M., & Courtney, A. E. (2013). Early recognition of CKD can delay progression. *Practitioner, 257*(1758), 13.
48. Torres, V., Abebe, K., Chapman A., et al. (2014). Angiotensin blockade in late autosomal dominant polycystic kidney disease. *New England Journal of Medicine, 371*(24), 2267–2276. doi:10.1056/nejmoa1402686

49. Sommers, M., & Fannin, E. (2015). *Diseases and disorders: A nursing therapeutics manual* (5th ed.). Philadelphia, PA: F.A. Davis.
50. Chang, T. I., Tabada, G. H., Jingrong, Y., Tan, T. C., Go, A. S., & Yang, J. (2016). Visit-to-visit variability of blood pressure and death, end-stage renal disease, and cardiovascular events in patients with chronic kidney disease. *Journal of Hypertension, 34*(2), 244–252. doi:10.1097/HJH.0000000000000779
51. Cozzolino, M., Ureña-Torres, P., Vervloet, M. G., et al. (2014). Is chronic kidney disease-mineral bone disorder (CKD-MBD) really a syndrome? *Nephrology, Dialysis, Transplantation: Official Publication of the European Dialysis and Transplant Association–European Renal Association, 29*(10), 1815–1820. doi:10.1093/ndt/gft514
52. Jovanovich, A., Bùzková, P., Chonchol, M., et al. (2013). Fibroblast growth factor 23, bone mineral density, and risk of hip fracture among older adults: The cardiovascular health study. *Journal of Clinical Endocrinology and Metabolism, 98*(8), 3323–3331. doi:10.1210/jc.2013–1152
53. Fang, Y., Ginsberg, C., Sugatani, T., Monier-Faugere, M., Malluche, H., & Hruska, K. (2014). Early chronic kidney disease mineral bone disorder stimulates vascular calcification. *Kidney International, 85*(1), 142–150. doi:10.1038/ki.2013.271
54. Kaiafa, G., Savopoulos, C., Kanellos, I., et al. (2017). Anemia and stroke: Where do we stand? *Acta Neurologica Scandinavica, 135*(6), 596–602. doi:10.1111/ane.12657
55. Sole, M., Klein, D., & Moseley, M. (2013). *Introduction to critical care nursing* (6th ed.). St. Louis, MO: Elsevier.
56. Van Leeuwen, A., & Bladh, M. (2015). *Comprehensive handbook of laboratory and diagnostic tests with nursing implications* (6th ed.). Philadelphia, PA: F.A. Davis.
57. Iglay, K., Hannachi, H., Joseph Howie, P., et al. (2016). Prevalence and co-prevalence of comorbidities among patients with type 2 diabetes mellitus. *Current Medical Research and Opinion, 32*(7), 1243–1252. doi:10.1185/03007995.2016.1168291
58. Kidney Disease: Improving Global Outcomes (KDIGO) Anemia Work Group. (2012). KDIGO clinical practice guideline for anemia in CKD. *Kidney International, 2*(Suppl.), 279–335.

Unit XIV

Disorders of Sexuality and Reproduction

Disorders of the male and female reproductive systems and sexually transmitted infections (STIs) share some commonalities in that they:

- Are often not discussed outside healthcare circles thus many people outside the healthcare field have a limited knowledge about them
- Cause an array of symptoms depending on etiology and location, but generally always result in some degree of anxiety and/or pain or physical discomfort
- Often result in unexpected healthcare costs for the individuals experiencing them.

In addition, terminology used in the care and treatment of these types of disorders can often be confusing for patients. For example, clinically adenomyosis is considered a benign condition, but a woman with adenomyosis who experiences painful intercourse and painful menstrual periods may not be as inclined to consider the condition "benign."

Disorders of the reproductive system (male or female) and STIs often have a psychosocial aspect. Sexuality is an important part of being a human being and is important to health and quality of life. The idea of some aspect of sexuality being affected by a life-altering illness or an STI can cause anxiety in the individual who is diagnosed as well as among partners and family members. In the care of patients who may have or who have been diagnosed with cancer, anxiety and distress can arise related to anything from anxiety over a diagnostic procedure to fear of treatment side effects and concern over the ability to continue to perform important roles, such as those of spouse, parent, or caregiver.[1] Infertility is very stressful for couples. Going through any of the reproductive technologies that treat infertility can be a complicated process.

Patients with reproductive disorders or STIs are often embarrassed to discuss their symptoms and reproductive and sexual health. Care of these patients requires compassion and a respectful, nonjudgmental attitude on the part of the provider using terms that the patient can understand.[2,3] Education and counseling for those at risk of these disorders as well as early identification and treatment are necessary to prevent long-term or life-threatening sequelae. Untreated STIs and untreated disorders of the reproductive system can have long-term consequences. For example, untreated chlamydia can cause pelvic inflammatory disease and chronic pelvic pain in women. Both men and women can experience sterility as a result of untreated chlamydia.[4] Any cancer that goes unchecked can result in continued cell growth and possible mortality.

In addition to providing respectful nursing care and promoting early identification and treatment, nurses working with patients at risk for or with an identified reproductive disorder or STI implement patient teaching and other interventions that:

- Promote patient safety and comfort
- Promote healthy behaviors
- Empower patients to reduce risk for recurrence or complications.[3]

References

1. National Comprehensive Cancer Network. (2017). NCCN Guidelines for Patients: Distress. Retrieved from https://www.nccn.org/patients/guidelines/distress/files/assets/common/downloads/files/distress.pdf
2. Centers for Disease Control. (2017). 2015 Sexually Transmitted Diseases Treatment Guidelines: Clinical Prevention Guidance. Retrieved from https://www.cdc.gov/std/tg2015/clinical.htm
3. Potter, M. L., & Moller, M. D. (2016). *Psychiatric–Mental Health Nursing: From Suffering to Hope.* Hoboken, NJ: Pearson Education.
4. U4 Cincinnati Children's Hospital. (2014). Sexually transmitted infections. Available at https://www.cincinnatichildrens.org/health/s/std

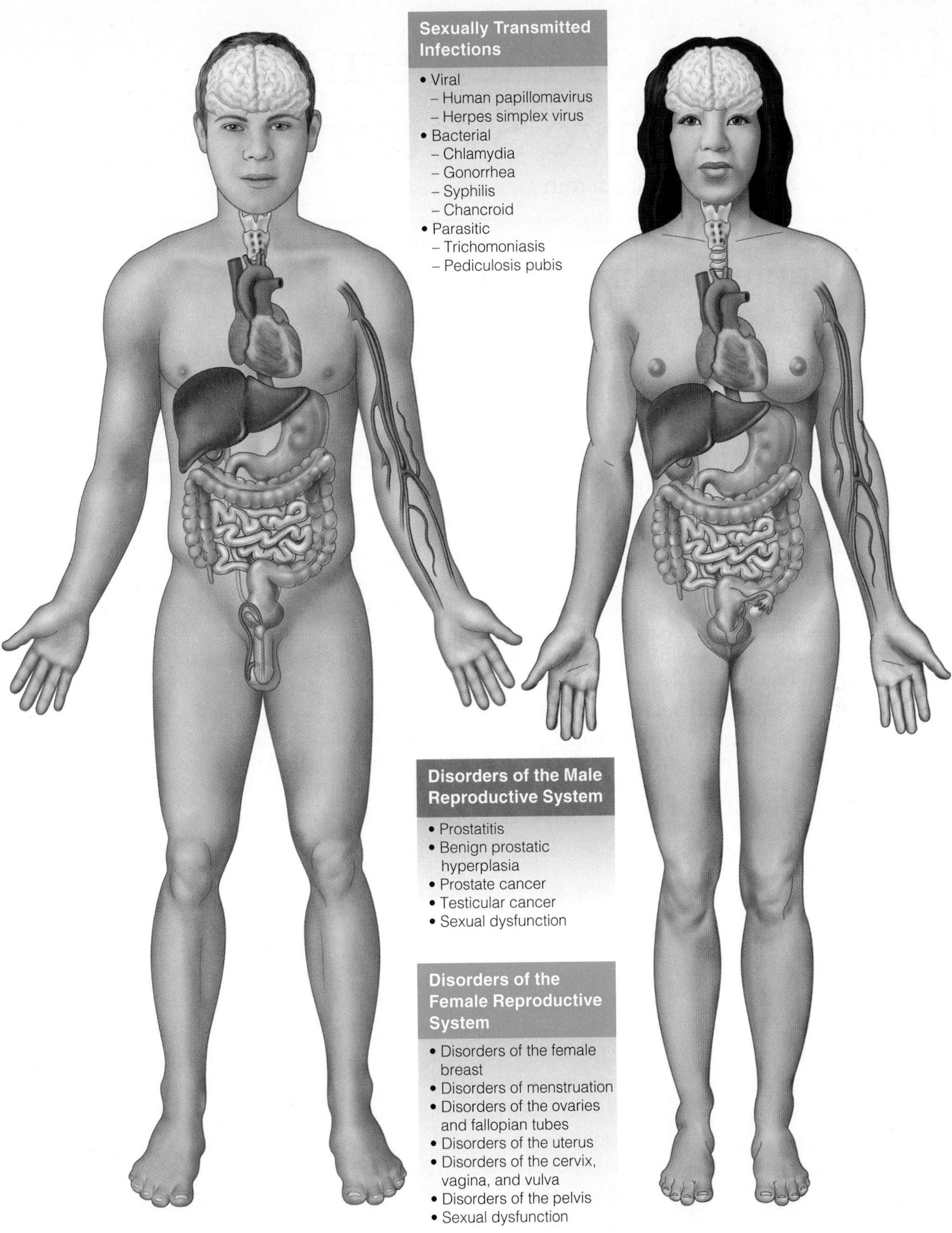
Sexually Transmitted Infections
• Viral
– Human papillomavirus
– Herpes simplex virus
• Bacterial
– Chlamydia
– Gonorrhea
– Syphilis
– Chancroid
• Parasitic
– Trichomoniasis
– Pediculosis pubis
Disorders of the Male Reproductive System
• Prostatitis
• Benign prostatic hyperplasia
• Prostate cancer
• Testicular cancer
• Sexual dysfunction
Disorders of the Female Reproductive System
• Disorders of the female breast
• Disorders of menstruation
• Disorders of the ovaries and fallopian tubes
• Disorders of the uterus
• Disorders of the cervix, vagina, and vulva
• Disorders of the pelvis
• Sexual dysfunction

Chapter 47

Disorders of the Female Reproductive System

Marcia Stout and Jennifer Eisenstein

Chapter Outline and Learning Outcomes

47.1 Chapter Overview and Case Studies

Describe the normal female reproductive system and concepts related to disorders of the female reproductive system.

47.2 Disorders of the Female Breasts

Differentiate the causes, classification, underlying pathogenesis, and clinical manifestations of disorders of the female breasts and approaches to diagnosis and treatment of these conditions across the lifespan.

47.3 Disorders of Menstruation

Differentiate the causes, classification, underlying pathogenesis, and clinical manifestations of disorders of menstruation and approaches to diagnosis and treatment of these conditions across the lifespan.

47.4 Disorders of the Ovaries and Fallopian Tubes

Differentiate the causes, classification, underlying pathogenesis, and clinical manifestations of disorders of the ovaries and fallopian tubes and approaches to diagnosis and treatment of these conditions across the lifespan.

47.5 Disorders of the Uterus

Differentiate the causes, classification, underlying pathogenesis, and clinical manifestations of disorders of the uterus and approaches to diagnosis and treatment of these conditions across the lifespan.

47.6 Disorders of the Cervix, Vagina, and Vulva

Differentiate the causes, classification, underlying pathogenesis, and clinical manifestations of disorders of the cervix, vagina, and vulva and approaches to diagnosis and treatment of these conditions across the lifespan.

47.7 Disorders of the Female Pelvis

Differentiate the causes, classification, underlying pathogenesis, and clinical manifestations of disorders of the female pelvis and approaches to diagnosis and treatment of these conditions across the lifespan.

47.8 Disorders of Fertility

Differentiate the causes, classification, underlying pathogenesis, and clinical manifestations of disorders of female fertility and approaches to diagnosis and treatment of these conditions across the lifespan.

47.9 Sexual Dysfunction

Differentiate the causes, classification, underlying pathogenesis, and clinical manifestations of disorders of sexual dysfunction and approaches to diagnosis and treatment of these conditions across the lifespan.

KEY TERMS

Adenomyosis, 1175
Amenorrhea, 1170
Bartholinitis, 1179
Benign breast disease (BBD), 1165
Benign ovarian cysts, 1174
Breast cancer, 1167
Cervical cancer, 1180
Cervicitis, 1178
Dysfunctional uterine bleeding (DUB), 1171
Dysmenorrhea, 1169
Dyspareunia, 1184
Ectopic pregnancy, 1174
Endometrial cancer, 1177
Endometrial polyps, 1175
Endometriosis, 1176
Galactorrhea, 1166
Infertility, 1182
Leiomyomas, 1176
Mastitis, 1166
Orgasmic dysfunction, 1183
Ovarian cancer, 1174
Pelvic inflammatory disease (PID), 1181

Pelvic organ prolapse, 1181
Polycystic ovary syndrome (PCOS), 1173
Premenstrual syndrome (PMS), 1172
Vaginal cancer, 1180
Vaginismus, 1183
Vaginitis, 1178
Vulvar cancer, 1181
Vulvovestibulitis, 1179

ABBREVIATIONS

BBD—benign breast disease
DUB—dysfunctional uterine bleeding
HCG—human chorionic gonadotropin
HPV—human papillomavirus
OCP—oral contraceptive pill
PCOS—polycystic ovary syndrome
PID—pelvic inflammatory disease
PMS—premenstrual syndrome

47.1 Chapter Overview and Case Studies

Disorders of the female reproductive system can involve multiple reproductive organs including the ovaries, fallopian tubes, uterus, cervix, vagina, or breasts. Disorders may present as an alteration in menstruation, pelvic pain, or infertility. Cancers that affect the reproductive tissues generally occur in the later reproductive years or after menopause. Female reproductive disorders can also stem from diseases that originate in other body organs such as the brain, pituitary, hypothalamus, thyroid, adrenals, liver, and kidney. The female reproductive system has five primary hormones that affect female reproductive health: estrogen, progesterone, gonadotropin-releasing hormone, follicle-stimulating hormone, and luteinizing hormone, all of which are affected by aging and disease. Alterations in these hormones can lead to loss of bone mass (osteoporosis), inflammation, and atrophy of estrogen-deprived tissues (atrophic vaginitis) as well as alterations in cardiovascular function. An increase in hormones may increase risk for the development of cancer. Diagnosis and treatment of reproductive system disorders are complicated by societal attitudes, behaviors surrounding reproductive health, healthcare providers' avoidance of discussing sexual problems, and patients' delaying treatment because of denial, fear, embarrassment, or guilt.[1]

Concepts Related to Sexuality

Sexuality can influence every aspect of life. Sexuality does not merely refer to whether an individual is a male or female or to a specific sexual behavior. Perceptions related to sexuality begin early in life and develop throughout childhood and puberty as the individual learns to relate to the world. Gender identity and sexuality can influence choices of careers, partners, friends, interests, and self-image. Socially rooted beliefs of cultural and faith, emotional and physical stressors, abuse, illness, and medical and surgical treatments can influence frequency and severity of issues related to an individual's sexual identity and response. It is estimated that 35–45% of women experience some type of sexual disorder in their lifetime, most frequently a low sex drive. A woman's sexual desire can be biologically based. An imbalance of excitatory and inhibitory processes mediated by neurotransmitters in the brain may also have an effect on sexual drive.[2] Some of the concepts related to disorders of the female reproductive system are mapped in **Figure 47.1** ■.

Case Studies

The following cases are addressed throughout the chapter to assist in application of chapter content to clinical situations that involve individuals with disorders of the female reproductive system.

Midge Palmer: Introduction

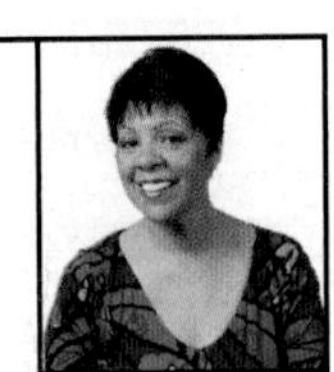

Midge Palmer, age 58, comes in for a screening mammogram. Mrs. Palmer says that her mother and maternal grandmother both had breast cancer. She confirms she has been postmenopausal for 2 years and has a past medical history of type 2 diabetes mellitus, hypertension, dyslipidemia, and obesity. Her obstetric history is G1P1 (gravida 1, para 1). She was 31 years old when her son was born, and she never breastfed. She is concerned because she has been able to feel a mass on her right breast and a lump in her right axilla that she never noticed before. Mrs. Palmer tells you that for many years, her breasts have felt tender and lumpy, particularly around the time of her periods. She explains that the two newly detected masses are different; they are not tender and have gotten significantly larger over the past several months. She appears very anxious and asks whether this is something serious. She has also heard that there is a link between diabetes and breast cancer and would like more information.

1. What information from Mrs. Palmer's family history may point to an increased risk of breast cancer?
2. What additional information about Mrs. Palmer's lifestyle is important to obtain so that you can assess her modifiable risk factors of breast cancer?

Yaira Gomez: Introduction

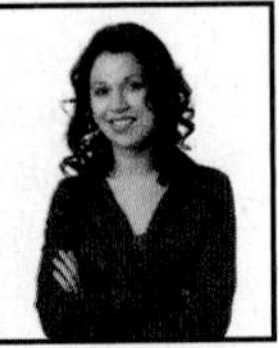

Yaira Gomez, age 35, is referred to the gynecologist by her primary care provider after she complains of lower back pain, irregular menstrual

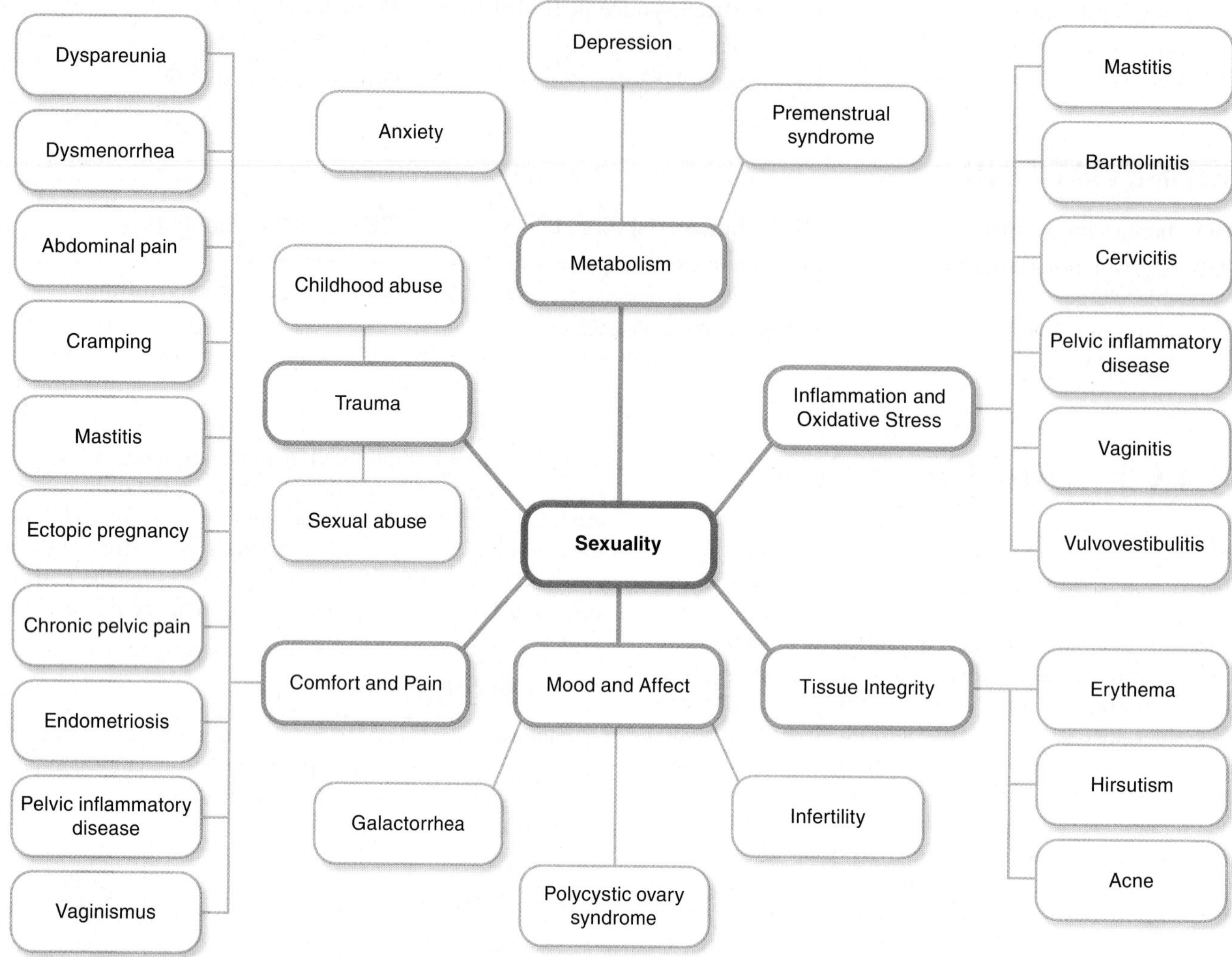

Figure 47.1 Concepts related to disorders of the female reproductive system.

cycles, and abdominal pain with cramping. She states that the pain begins 5–7 days before her cycle. She has menstrual cycles that last 5 days with heavy bleeding and clotting on days 1–3. Mrs. Gomez and her husband have been trying to conceive for 4 years with no success. Her husband's sperm count and motility test are within normal limits for fertility. Mrs. Gomez is anxious to start a family. She is frustrated by her infertility feels guilty and depressed because she thinks it's "her fault." She currently works as a flight attendant and finds that her issues are beginning to affect her job. This is the first time she has contacted a specialist about her issue.

1. What cultural factors might influence Mrs. Gomez's perceptions about her reproductive issues?
2. What information about the impact of her reproductive issues reflect how significant they are to her?

Check Your Progress: Section 47.1

1. Disorders of the female reproductive system commonly present with which symptoms?
2. What are the five primary hormones that affect female reproductive health?
3. What is the most common type of female sexual disorder?

47.2 Disorders of the Female Breasts

Disorders of the female breasts range from benign, noncancerous lesions to malignant or cancerous abnormalities that are detected by palpation or imaging. Most women will experience some type of breast changes at some point in their life (**Figure 47.2**). Generally, these are noncancerous and are not life threatening. Breast changes may be related to age, hormone levels, and certain medications. Local breast tissue changes may be a palpable mass, changes in breast skin appearance, or nipple discharge of fluid that is not breast milk. Many women fear that these changes could be related to breast cancer. In reality, only a small percentage of breast changes indicate cancer. Of course, malignant disorders, once confirmed, require prompt treatment and may involve loss of breast tissue or possibly even loss of life. Early recognition and intervention are important. It is estimated that one in eight women in the United States will have a diagnosis of breast cancer in their lifetime. Proper follow-up with a practitioner should be encouraged to help

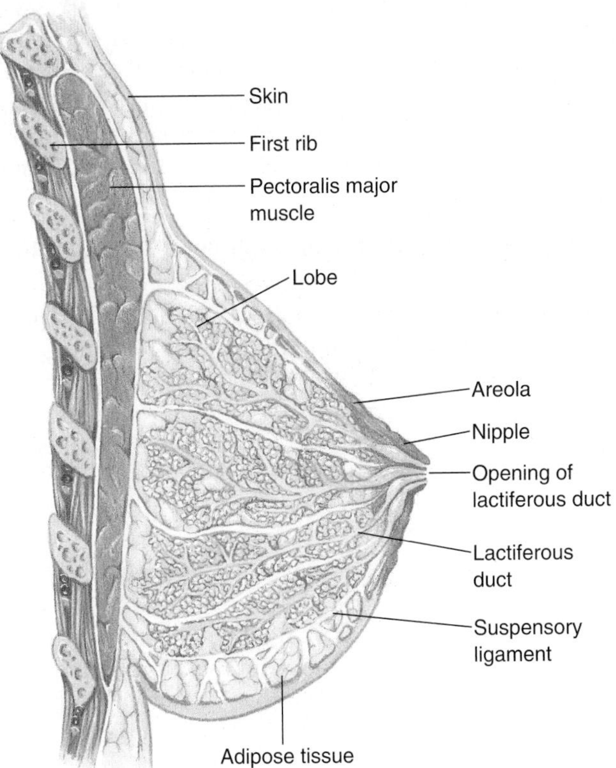

Figure 47.2 ■ Structure of the female breast.

the woman with diagnosis, treatment, and her emotional response to breast disorders.

Benign Breast Disease

Benign breast disease (BBD) is defined as all noncancerous ailments of breast tissue. BBD consists of an assorted group of lesions, including developmental abnormalities, inflammatory lesions, epithelial and stromal proliferations, and neoplasms. Contrary to popular belief, most abnormalities of the breast are benign, not cancerous. All noncancerous breast lesions are included in the BBD category. Common benign breast masses include fibrocystic disease, fibroadenoma, intraductal papilloma, and abscess.

Etiology and Pathogenesis

There are three main tissues in the breast that are related to most of BBD cases. These are the stroma, epithelium, and fat. The breast tissue also contains Cooper ligaments, which are composed of connective tissue and help to give shape to the breast. In BBD, there can be dimpling of these ligaments due to a growth beneath the breast surface.[3] Breast tissue can change throughout the month in conjunction with a woman's menstrual cycle and hormonal changes, causing the breast tissue to feel larger and more painful than it would during the rest of the month. These changes are not part of any disease process. BBD is based on cellular changes of the breast tissue and can be categorized as either proliferative or nonproliferative disease. If the issue is categorized as proliferative BBD, there is an increase in cell production, resulting in a benign breast tumor. Proliferative masses can carry an increased risk of subsequent breast cancer. Nonproliferative BBD involves no increase in cellular production and does not carry an increased risk of subsequent cancer.[3]

Clinical Manifestations

The most common clinical manifestations of BBD are pain in the breast, a palpable mass, and nipple discharge. Cyclic breast pain is often linked to the menstrual cycle, starting 2 weeks before the cycle and returning at the same time every month. Noncyclic pain of the breast occurs most often in postmenopausal women and can be traced to certain medications such as hormone therapy, antidepressants, digoxin, and thiazide diuretics. The diagnostic methods will be dictated by whether the pain is associated with a mass or occurs by itself.[4] Many patients with BBD have an accompanying palpable mass in the breast. Depending on the type of mass, there might be a change to the woman's monthly menstrual cycle. These types of masses are usually benign and may come and go as well as change in size throughout the month. A mass can be solid or fluid-filled. Nipple discharge in the absence of breastfeeding can be alarming. Many BBDs can cause some form of discharge. The discharge can range in color from milky white to yellow or green. Certain medications can cause nipple discharge; these include oral contraceptives, antidepressants, and any other medications that alter the dopamine levels in the brain.[5]

Linking Pathophysiology to Diagnosis and Treatment

The patient's chief complaint at the time of the visit will often dictate the methods that the practitioner uses to diagnose and treat the BBD. The practitioner will first examine the breast using visualization and examination by touch and feel of the breast tissue. Other methods that might be used include ultrasound, mammography, and biopsy. Ultrasound is used to visualize the mass and cellular changes of the tissue. Mammography provides a more detailed image of the breast, and the mammogram allows the practitioner to detect changes in the tissue that may occur in the fat, stroma, and epithelium of the breast (**Figure 47.3** ■). Biopsies are

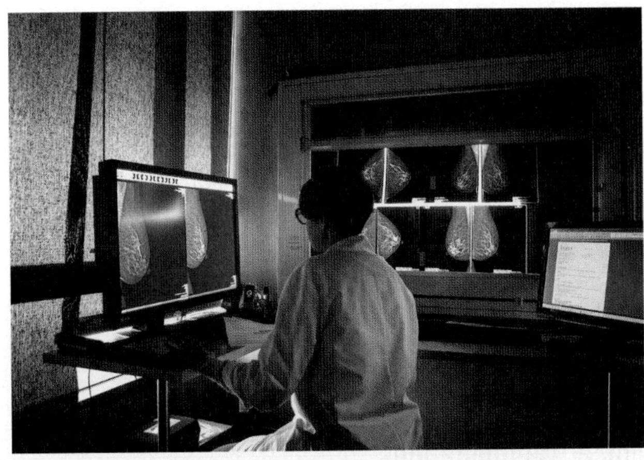

Figure 47.3 ■ A radiologist studies mammograms, looking for changes in the tissue.

used to differentiate the content of the mass.[6] Treatment of BBD depends on a number of factors. Practitioners evaluate not only the signs and symptoms, but also any likelihood that a cancer might develop. Often, treatment is not needed, but BBD causes a great deal of anxiety for women, so the importance of educating females on breast self-examination, proper follow-up for any physical changes, and what they can do to prevent cancer cannot be overstated.

It is estimated that 50% of women will develop some form of BBD in their lifetime; it generally starts in the second decade of life and tends to peak after menopause. In contrast to malignant breast cancers, the incidence of BBD is highest in the fourth and fifth decades of life but has a reduced rate after menopause.[6]

Galactorrhea

Galactorrhea is a discharge of milk or any milklike substance from the breast in the absence of pregnancy or beyond a 6-month postpartum period in a woman who did not breastfeed. The flow of the milk can be continuous or intermittent, in trace amounts or abundant, expressible or free flowing, and unilateral or bilateral.[7]

Etiology and Pathogenesis

Galactorrhea has eight different etiologies: medications, tumors on either the pituitary or hypothalamic and pituitary stalk, thyroid disorders, chronic renal failure, neurogenic causes, neonatal galactorrhea, injury, idiopathic cases. Medications that stimulate galactorrhea are often ones that cause changes in hormones such as dopamine and estrogen levels, which then can stimulate lactotrophs and induce lactation. Examples of these medications are oral contraceptives, psychiatric medications, and some pain medications such as codeine and morphine. The most common pathologic cause of galactorrhea is pituitary tumors. These tumors cause lactation by producing prolactin and/or by blocking the channel of dopamine from the hypothalamus to the pituitary gland. Hypothyroidism, although rare, can stimulate lactation in both adults and children. In most cases, galactorrhea is related to an increase in thyrotropin-releasing hormones, which can stimulate a release of prolactin, causing lactation. Up to 30% of patients with chronic renal failure will experience galactorrhea sometime during their illness.[8] Decreases in kidney clearance could account for higher prolactin levels, which would induce lactation. Neurogenic causes of galactorrhea could come as a result of breast stimulation during sexual activity. Injuries to the chest wall from surgeries or burns and spinal cord injuries can also cause a prolactin-stimulated release.

Neonatal galactorrhea is caused by elevated levels of estrogen in the intrapartum period resulting in breast engorgement and lactation in neonates of either gender. Also known as "witch's milk," this issue usually clears on its own in the neonatal period. ■

Clinical Manifestations

A history and physical examination should be performed on all patients. Common patient complaints are headache, visual issues, changes in appetite, weight gain or loss, amenorrhea, new use of medication (especially antipsychotics, antidepressants, and some antihypertensives), and a family history of thyroid disease or endocrine neoplasia.[7] Physical findings on exam might include poor growth, gigantism, bradycardia or tachycardia, deficits in visual fields, hirsutism, and acne.

Linking Pathophysiology to Diagnosis and Treatment

Three tests are used for diagnosing galactorrhea: prolactin levels, thyroxine (T4) and thyroid-stimulating hormone (TSH) levels, and computed tomography (CT) or magnetic resonance imaging (MRI). Elevated levels of prolactin, typically greater than 5 times the normal range, indicate a prolactin-secreting pituitary tumor. Drug treatment is used in most cases to shrink the tumor. Serum gonadotropin and estradiol levels are either low or in the normal range in women with hyperprolactinemia. Primary hypothyroidism is ruled out by an elevated serum level of TSH. If the level of TSH is not elevated, further testing is needed to rule in a different causative reason for galactorrhea. CT or MRI is the method of choice in identifying microadenomas, which are tumors less than 10 mm in diameter.[8] Treatment for galactorrhea will include a dopamine agonist such as bromocriptine, cabergoline, or quinagolide. Medication is dosed low and can be titrated in increments on a weekly basis to the desired dose. Prolactin levels are measured to assess efficacy of the medication. Considerations for determining a medication regimen are pregnancy, breastfeeding, and being an older adult with kidney disease.[9]

Older adults with chronic renal failure, hypothalamic-pituitary disorders, hypothyroidism, or those taking certain herbal medications may experience galactorrhea. ■

Mastitis

Mastitis is a localized erythematous and painful inflammation of the breast. It involves infection of the breast tissue and most often develops during breastfeeding. It can occur any time during breastfeeding, but most cases of mastitis occur around the sixth to twelfth week postpartum.

Etiology and Pathogenesis

Mastitis can be triggered by nipple irritation, breast tissue trauma, or chafing as a result of inappropriate infant latch during breastfeeding related to poor technique or abnormalities of the infant's mouth, including cleft palate. Other contributing factors may be nipple fissures through which bacteria can enter the breast tissue, yeast infections, and nipple piercings, which can provide a pathway for bacteria to infect the breast. Plugged milk ducts or galactoceles may result in inadequate milk drainage from the breast. Tight-fitting bras and carrying heavy bags may also restrict milk flow. The prolonged engorgement from plugged ducts or pressure can lead to mastitis. Fatigue, stress, poor nutrition, and a previous history of mastitis have also been noted as contributors.

Clinical Manifestations

Symptoms of mastitis most often appear within 4–6 weeks after childbirth. Clinical manifestations include local tenderness, swelling, warmth, and erythema in one breast with a consistent or intermittent burning sensation during breastfeeding. Flulike symptoms of fever 101°F (38.3°C) or greater, chills, malaise, body aches, headache, and loss of appetite may also be experienced.

Linking Pathophysiology to Diagnosis and Treatment

Breast infections are divided into lactational and nonlactational or into puerperal and nonpuerperal if the process is not associated with lactation or pregnancy. The pathophysiology involves a localized cellulitis that has developed in the skin. Mastitis is diagnosed clinically from the characteristic presentation of the sudden onset of breast tenderness, warmth, inflammation, and induration generally in one breast only. Treatment of mastitis includes improving breastfeeding technique with the help of a lactation specialist, specifically to improve position and latching. Use of cold compresses to reduce pain and swelling is generally recommended, along with over-the-counter acetaminophen and ibuprofen. Adequate rest, a healthy diet, and good hydration are all important for mastitis management. If the mastitis does not resolve, it can develop into an abscess, and then treatment is more aggressive. Lancing and draining the abscess surgically or by needle aspiration would be considered. Depending on the severity of the abscess, using appropriate antibiotics might be effective. The most common organisms responsible for mastitis are *Staphylococcus aureus*, *S. epidermidis*, and streptococci.[10] An early prescription of appropriate antibiotics reduces the incidence of abscess development. Mastitis typically responds to antibiotic treatment within 24 hours.[11]

Mastitis will not spread to an infant: nor does breastfeeding in the presence of mastitis pose a risk to the infant. Drainage of milk from the affected breast is encouraged through continuing breastfeeding or pumping to relieve engorgement and to maintain the mother's milk supply. ■

Peripheral nonlactating breast abscesses can be associated with diabetes, rheumatoid arthritis, steroid treatment, trauma, and granulomatous lobular mastitis. These may present as a cellulitis or abscess and are often associated with obesity, large breast, and poor hygiene.[12]

Breast Cancer

Breast cancer is a malignant tumor that originates in the cells of the breast. Breast cancer is the most commonly diagnosed cancer in women. Risk factors for breast cancer include age, gender, a family history of breast cancer in a first-degree relative under the age of 50, and having a *BRCA1* or *BRCA2* gene mutation.[13] Other risk factors include menarche before age 12, menopause after age 55, and previous breast issues such as BBD or breast cancer. Obesity raises the risk of breast cancer after menopause, particularly with fat accumulation in the abdominal area. Environmental risks for breast cancer include smoking, overuse of alcohol, and exposure to radiation.[14]

Etiology and Pathogenesis

Current research on the etiology of cancer emphasizes the series of changes at the molecular level of the cell. Breast cancer begins when the cells of the breast begin to grow at a rapid rate and do not die off as regular developing cells do. When normal breast cells experience damage to their DNA, it creates a risk for becoming cancerous. If cancer is not present in the damaged DNA, the cells will simply die off. But if the breast cells are cancerous, they will continue to regenerate, producing abnormal cancerous cells and using up all the resources meant for healthy cell growth. The breast cancer develops into a malignant tumor over time and can spread to other areas of the body. New subtypes of breast cancers are being discovered on an ongoing basis. The current classifications of breast cancers are broken down on the basis of the presence or absence of estrogen receptors, progesterone receptors, and human epidural growth factor receptor 2 (HER2).[13,15]

Carcinoma of the breast is the most common malignancy of women in the United States. It is associated with ovarian hormonal function, a high-fat diet, a family history of disease, and a possible link to hormone replacement therapy. Malignant breast disease encompasses many histologic types that include, but are not limited to, infiltrating ductal or lobular carcinoma, in situ ductal or lobular carcinoma, and inflammatory carcinoma. The main concern for most women presenting with any breast changes or a breast mass is the likelihood of a cancer being present. Fortunately, most breast masses are benign.

Clinical Manifestations

In the early stages of breast cancer, a patient may be asymptomatic with no signs of breast changes or pain. When symptoms are present, they may include changes in the size or shape of the breast, skin changes such as dimpling; inverted nipple; thickening of the skin; or a red, scaly, rash-like appearance. Symptoms that are concerning can include blood-tinged nipple discharge; red, scaly nipples; ulceration of the breast tissue; and a mass that can be felt in the breast tissue or axillary region that is hard, fixed, and nonmobile on palpation.[16]

Midge Palmer: Application

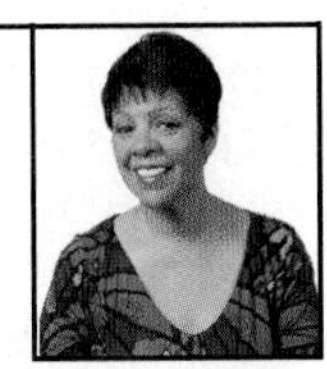

On examination of Mrs. Palmer's right breast, you are able to palpate a mass measuring approximately 4 × 3 cm in diameter; it is a firm, irregular mass at the 1:00 position on the breast. You note no skin changes, no dimpling, and no nipple discharge. The mass is fixed and nonmobile. The left breast exam shows no palpable masses. You also note a palpable lymph node in right axilla that is concerning. When the mammogram is read, there is a density in Mrs. Palmer's medial right breast that is suspicious for malignancy. There are also faint calcifications in the same position on the left breast. A chest x-ray is done to rule out lung metastasis; the x-ray is within normal limits. Laboratory tests ordered by Mrs. Palmer's oncology team include a CMP 12 (comprehensive metabolic panel). The results are normal except for the fasting glucose, which is elevated; the levels of estrogen receptors, which are mildly elevated; and the progesterone receptors, which are negative.

3. What additional laboratory testing is indicated in the workup of Mrs. Palmer's prognosis?
4. Why is a palpable lymph node in Mrs. Palmer's right axilla concerning?

Linking Pathophysiology to Diagnosis and Treatment

Diagnosis for breast cancer is based on clinical and diagnostic testing. Practitioners use the triple assessment for diagnosis of breast cancer. This method includes clinical examination, imaging of the breast using mammography and/or ultrasound, and needle biopsy for examination of cells and tissue. The clinical breast exam will assess changes in the breast as well as the location, size, and shape of the mass and any nodular involvement. Breast tissue spans the area from the clavicle to the sternum and from the sternum to the axilla.

Mammography and ultrasound will guide biopsies and aid in staging of the cancer.[17,18] Staging of the cancer is done by using the TNM system, which involves measuring the size of the primary tumor (T), determining how many nodes (N) are involved locally and regionally from the breast, and whether there is metastasis (M) in any other areas of the body.[19] This will help to guide the treatment plan. The cancer is staged as 0–IV (**Figure 47.4** ■). Other factors that are included in determining treatment are whether the woman has reached menopause, assessment of her hormone receptor status to guide the medication regimen, her baseline health status, and the risk for recurrence (including the patient's *BRCA1* or *BRCA2* status).

The hormone receptor assay is included in pathology reports that suggest the possibility of breast cancer. Hormone receptors are proteins found in and around breast cells. They pick up hormone signals that tell the cells to grow. A cancer is called estrogen receptor positive (ER+) if it has receptors for estrogen. Cancer cells, like normal breast cells, get signals from estrogen to promote growth. The cancer is progesterone receptor positive (PR+) if it has progesterone receptors; the cells respond to progesterone to promote growth. The hormone receptors guide the oncologist's treatment decisions for hormone therapy that can block or lower the specific hormone in the body, stopping or at least slowing the growth of the cancerous cells. If no receptors are present, hormone therapy would not be effective, and another treatment is chosen.[14,15]

Once the cancer has been staged, surgery (either lumpectomy or mastectomy), radiation, and/or chemotherapy is initiated. Metastatic breast cancer is treated with additional hormones and chemotherapy. Selective estrogen receptor modulators, tamoxifen, and raloxifene have been approved for and are used to reduce the breast cancer in high-risk patients.[14,16]

Breast masses in children and adolescents are uncommon. If they do occur, they are most often benign. Breast masses in the pediatric and adolescent population include intraductal papillomas, phyllodes tumors, primary breast cancer, and metastatic lesions. Unlike breast cancer in adults, pediatric and adolescent breast cancer is more often a secretory type and is unlikely to be metastatic. However, cases of inflammatory and medullary breast cancers have been noted to occur in young girls, and these cancers can be aggressive. Radiation treatment is used cautiously because of its effect on breast development and increased risk of cancer development later in life. Routine axillary node dissection in children has been found to be unnecessary. Sentinel node biopsy is preferred, with axillary dissection only if lymph nodes are positive.[20] ■

Midge Palmer: Outcome

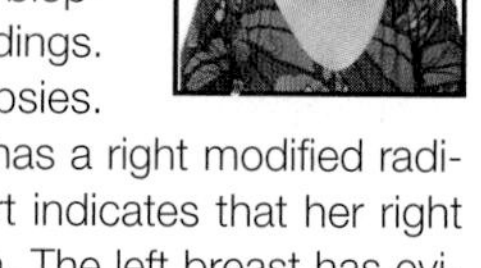

Plans for surgery have been discussed with Mrs. Palmer and her family. She consents to be biopsied and to have surgery based on the findings. Her surgeon performs bilateral breast biopsies. On the basis of the findings, Mrs. Palmer has a right modified radical mastectomy. The final pathology report indicates that her right breast had extensive intraductal carcinoma. The left breast has evidence of fibrocystic disease, which Mrs. Palmer had noted as part

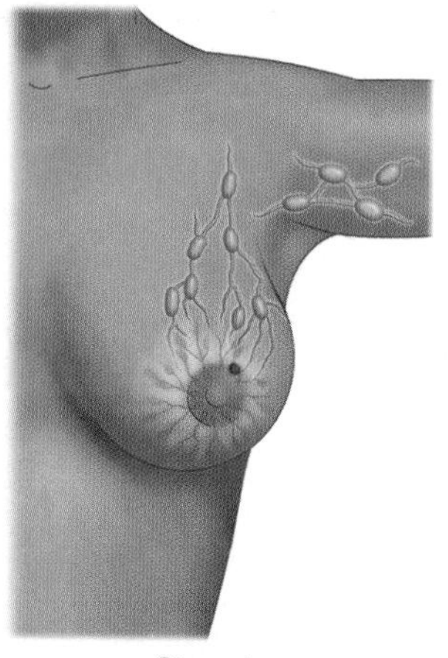

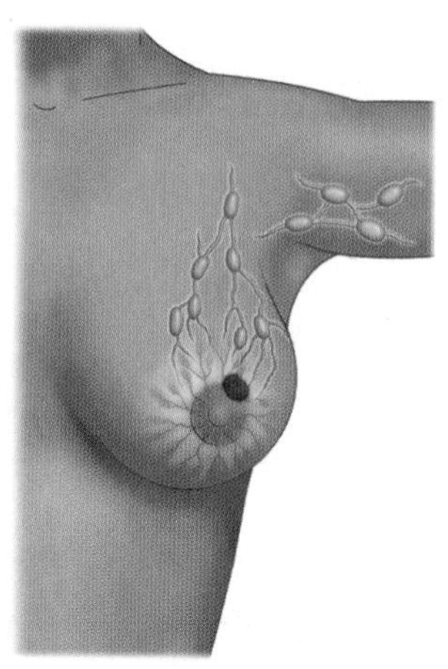

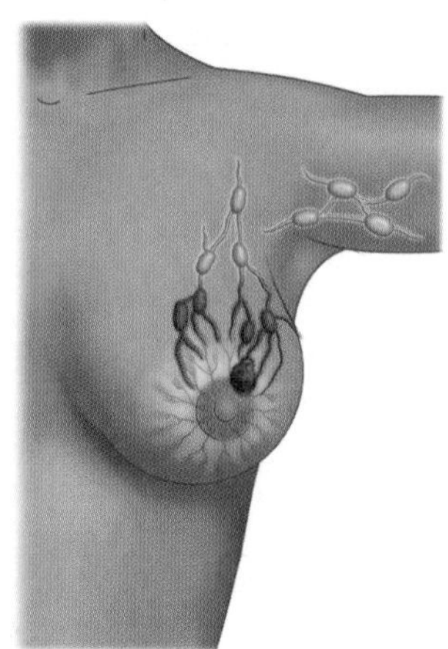

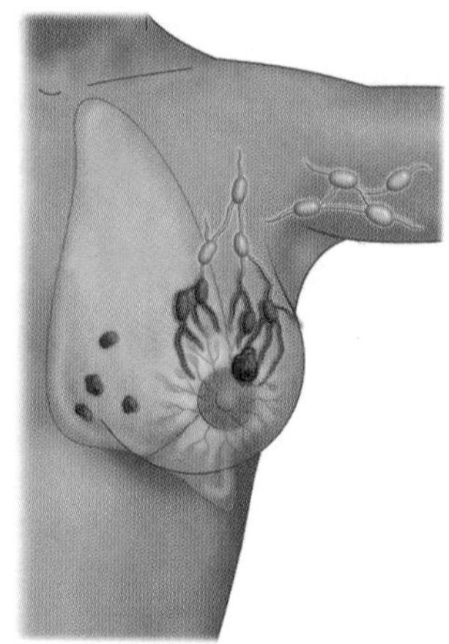

Figure 47.4 ■ Breast cancer staging.

of her medical history in her initial visit. Ten axillary lymph nodes are also removed; they are negative for metastases. The tumor that is removed is 2.1 cm in diameter. Three courses of chemotherapy using Cytoxan (cyclophosphamide) and Adriamycin (doxorubicin) are ordered after surgery. These take 3–6 months to complete with a period of days off during the treatment course to allow Mrs. Palmer to recover from the chemotherapy. Mrs. Palmer works with the oncology team to determine the form of hormone therapy that will be most effective in blocking the growth of new cancer cells. The hormone receptor status is an important part of her prognosis discussion. ER+ tumors tend to have better survival rate. With the help of her oncology nurse navigator, Mrs. Palmer tolerates her oncology therapy well, her cancer is in remission, and she has made a commitment to properly manage her diabetes and overall health with the support of the oncology team.

5. What are the modifiable risk factors that may reduce the risk of recurrence for Mrs. Palmer?
6. Why is hormone therapy used after surgery and chemotherapy treatment?

Check Your Progress: Section 47.2

1. Most cases of benign breast disease are related to which three tissues in the breast?
2. What are the eight different etiologies for galactorrhea?
3. Breast cancer classifications are based on what characteristics of the cells?

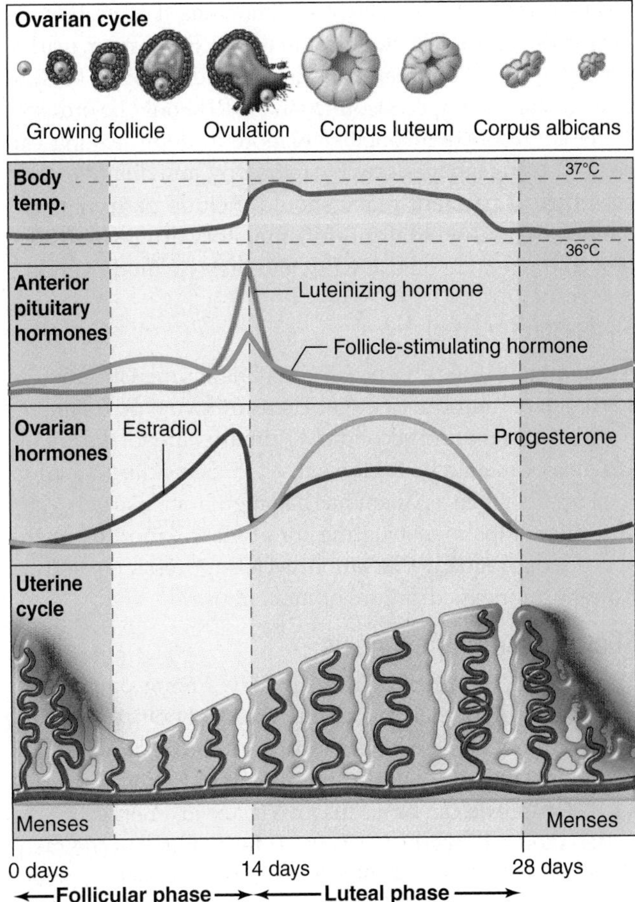

Figure 47.5 ■ The normal menstrual cycle.

47.3 Disorders of Menstruation

The menstrual cycle is the monthly cycle of changes in the ovaries and uterus that produces an ovum making pregnancy possible. Menstruation is the endpoint of that process if the egg is not fertilized. In menstruation, the blood and muscosal lining that has built up in the uterus is discharged through the vagina. The normal menstrual cycle is illustrated in **Figure 47.5** ■.

Dysmenorrhea

Dysmenorrhea is a condition that causes painful uterine cramping during menstruation. Dysmenorrhea is categorized as primary or secondary depending on clinical features, signs, and symptoms. Primary dysmenorrhea is a painful menstrual cycle in the absence of pelvic disease. Secondary dysmenorrhea is menstrual pain that is a result of underlying disease such as endometriosis or pelvic inflammatory disease (PID), both of which are discussed in detail later in this chapter.

Etiology and Pathogenesis

During menstruation, a female's body releases prostaglandins from the shedding of the endometrial cells in the lining of the uterus. This event leads to the uterine contraction of the myometrium, obstruction of blood flow, and vasoconstriction. Prostaglandins tend to be at their highest level in the first few days of the menstrual cycle causing pain and discomfort for patients who suffer from dysmenorrhea.[21] In a woman with primary dysmenorrhea, the menstrual cycle is regular and ovulation occurs monthly. The discomfort is caused by the elevated prostaglandin levels. In secondary dysmenorrhea, the pain is often related to an underlying uterine condition such as PID or a sexually transmitted infection (STI).[22] (STIs are covered in detail in Chapter 49.)

Clinical Manifestations

Patients with primary dysmenorrhea will present with symptoms that begin about 6 months after menarche. The duration can be anywhere from 48 to 72 hours. The pain is described as high-intensity cramping. The patient may also have lower back pain with radiation to the upper back and one or both thighs. Pelvic examination is often unremarkable. Secondary dysmenorrhea affects patients in their second and third decades of life. The patients may have had normal pain-free menstrual cycles until this point. Clinically, they present with heavy flow or irregular bleeding, painful intercourse, vaginal discharge, and poor response to pain medication or oral contraceptives.[23]

Linking Pathophysiology to Diagnosis and Treatment

A history and physical examination should be completed with a full inspection of the genitalia, including the vaginal vault, cervix, and rectum. No specific laboratory tests are used to diagnose primary dysmenorrhea. For secondary diagnosis, a complete blood count (CBC), STI testing, urinalysis, quantitative human chorionic gonadotropin (HCG) to rule out pregnancy, ultrasound, and MRI should be ordered. If the lab tests are inconclusive, more in-depth testing can be done using laparoscopy, hysteroscopy, and dilatation and curettage. Treatment plans should include pain management with nonsteroidal anti-inflammatory drugs (NSAIDs), oral contraceptive pills (OCPs), and lifestyle modification.

Amenorrhea

Amenorrhea is the absence of spontaneous menstruation in a woman of reproductive age. There are two types of amenorrhea: primary and secondary. Primary amenorrhea is the absence of menarche by the age of 15. Secondary amenorrhea occurs when a patient has had regular menstrual cycles and then stops menstruating for at least 3 months in the absence of pregnancy, lactation, cycle suppression resulting from hormone medication, or menopause.

Etiology and Pathogenesis

The etiology of amenorrhea can vary among patients. In adolescents, hypothalamic amenorrhea and polycystic ovary syndrome (PCOS) are often the cause of the disorder. (PCOS is covered in detail later in this chapter.) Eating disorders such as anorexia can be a causative factor in amenorrhea. To understand amenorrhea, it is important to look at the menstrual cycle and the physiology of the hormones involved. Gonadotropin-releasing hormone starts off the menstrual cycle stimulation with the release of luteinizing hormone (LH) and follicle-stimulating hormone (FSH). The FSH prepares the follicle for ovulation, and the LH surge causes ovulation. After this preparation of the follicle, the corpus luteum forms to allow for implantation of a fertilized ovum. If implantation does not occur after 14 days, the corpus luteum is shed and menstruation begins. When the cycle is disrupted at any point, a patient may experience amenorrhea.[24]

Clinical Manifestations

The patient with amenorrhea presents with complaints of absence of menstruation. A history and physical examination help to guide the practitioner toward diagnosis. If the patient is being seen for primary amenorrhea, the exam should focus on pubertal development and the possibility of an obstruction in the vagina. Tanner staging of the breasts and pubic hair should be documented (**Figure 47.6**). An examination of the genitalia should include visualization and patency of the hymen. Factors that contribute to amenorrhea are high levels of stress, excessive exercise, PCOS, medications such as OCPs, antipsychotic medications, malnutrition, and obesity.[25]

Linking Pathophysiology to Diagnosis and Treatment

To treat amenorrhea, the underlying cause has to be diagnosed. In primary amenorrhea, hormones are usually the underlying cause. Laboratory tests should be done to evaluate the patient's progesterone, LH, FSH, and prolactin levels. It is important for the practitioner to stage the patient's sexual characteristics. If a patient has gone through puberty, pregnancy should be ruled out as a causative factor. The causes of primary amenorrhea include but are not limited to chronic illness, pregnancy, ovarian failure, and eating disorders. Treatment for primary amenorrhea depends on the causative factors. Hormonal lab results guide the treatments if hormone insufficiency is evident. For chronic illness and ailments such as anorexia, bulimia, and obesity, psychologic evaluation and treatment are recommended. The goal of treatment of primary amenorrhea is to support the patient in having normal sexual development.

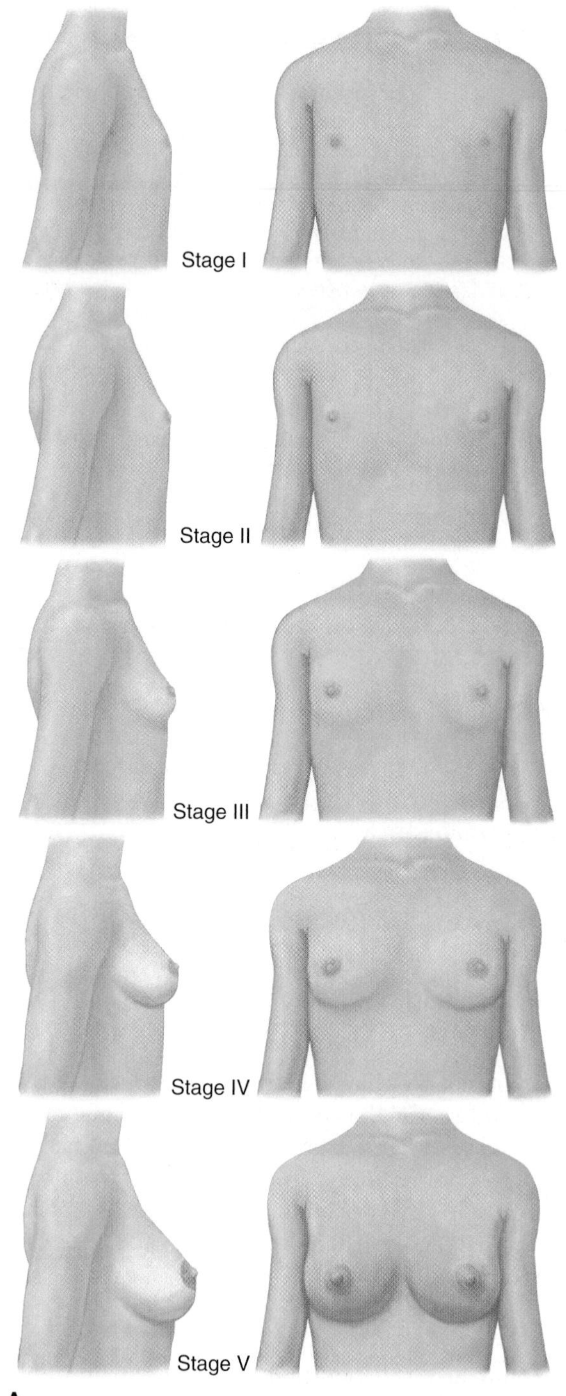

Figure 47.6 Tanner staging of **A.** breasts and **B.** pubic hair (on facing page.)

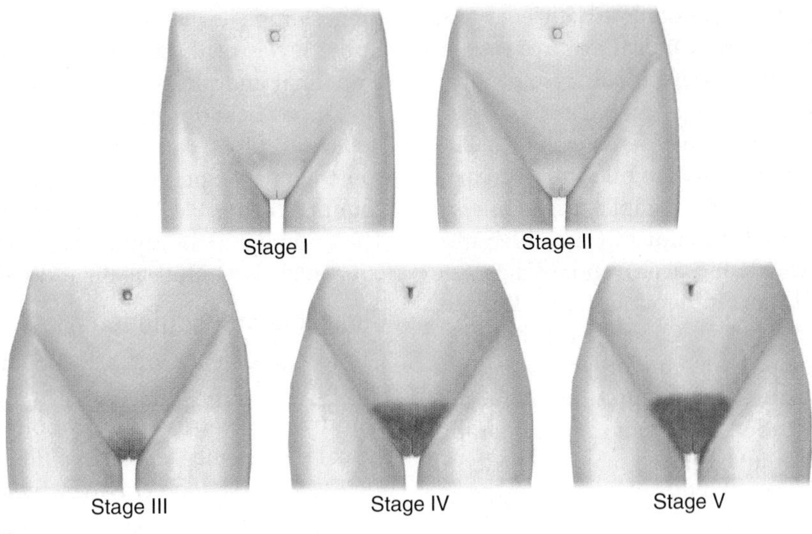

Diagnosis of secondary amenorrhea also requires laboratory evaluation to rule out thyroid disease, pregnancy, or hyperprolactinemia. Further testing with CT or MRI may be needed if lab tests are within normal limits and pituitary or reproductive tumors need to be ruled out. The goals of treatment of secondary amenorrhea are to help the patient preserve fertility and to prevent complications from disruptive hormones.[26]

Irregularities in the menstrual cycle are very common in the adolescent years. This is especially true in the first 2–3 years after menarche. ■

Dysfunctional Uterine Bleeding

Dysfunctional uterine bleeding (DUB) is any abnormal bleeding from the uterus not associated with a physical lesion such as a tumor, inflammation, or pregnancy.

Etiology and Pathogenesis

In the luteal phase of a normal menstrual cycle (see Figure 47.5), the progesterone levels increase and levels of estrogen, LH, and FSH decline. If there is not implantation of an ovum, the lining of the uterus that has been built up is shed, and normal menses begins. Aberrations or irregularity of the menstrual cycle causing DUB stems from hormonal insufficiency caused by an increase in endogenous or exogenous estrogen production. Those affected tend to be women who have just started their menstrual cycles and those who are either perimenopausal or in the menopause phases of their life.[27] If left without diagnosis and treatment, the lining of the uterus can thicken, causing hyperplastic cells and possible malignancy.

Clinical Manifestations

Patients with DUB present with complaints of bleeding that occurs at different times throughout the month. There are six main categories of DUB:

1. Menorrhagia: abnormally heavy bleeding
2. Intermenstrual bleeding: bleeding that occurs between normal cycles
3. Metrorrhagia: irregular and frequent bouts of bleeding that are noncycle related
4. Menometrorrhagia: excessive bleeding over a prolonged period of time at irregular intervals
5. Polymenorrhea: bleeding that occurs at intervals of 21 days or less
6. Dysmenorrhea: painful menstruation (covered in the previous section).[27]

Yaira Gomez: Application

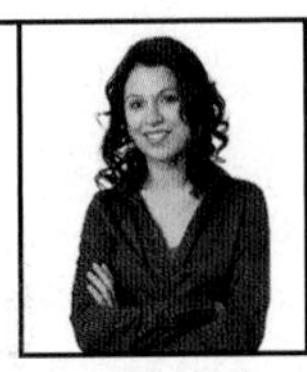

Mrs. Gomez states that she has suffered from numerous issues surrounding her menstrual cycle since she was in her early 20s. She has painful menstrual periods every month with heavy bleeding that often soaks through more than two pads in an hour on days 1–3. She is experiencing pelvic pain that radiates into her abdomen and lower legs. She also complains of urinary frequency and urgency that are worse during her cycle. She has a feeling of abdominal fullness with bloating and excessive gas. Dyspareunia (difficult or painful sexual intercourse) is especially uncomfortable with penetration. She tells you that she has been unable to get pregnant in spite of frequent unprotected sexual intercourse during charted ovulation. She is often incapacitated for at least 2–5 days out of the month from her symptoms. On examination, Mrs. Gomez's vital signs are pulse 65, respirations 18, temperature 98.6°F, blood pressure 100/78. She is currently on day 2 of her cycle. Her abdomen is soft and tender with tender painful palpable masses along the uterosacral ligaments, the posterior uterus, and the posterior cul-de-sac. An ultrasound and blood work are ordered.

3. A decrease in which two hormones causes the follicular stage in which menstruation occurs?
4. What categories of DUB is Mrs. Gomez describing?

Linking Pathophysiology to Diagnosis and Treatment

For a patient with DUB, a complete history and physical exam should be performed. The goal of the history is for the practitioner to gain a better understanding of the symptoms, the amount and severity of bleeding, its frequency, and the time between cycles. These should all be carefully documented. Patients often suffer from iron deficiency anemia related to heavy blood flow. Clinical features such as bruising, hirsutism, acne, and obesity should also be taken into consideration, since a hormone imbalance can also cause these issues. Blood tests to be ordered include a CBC to check for underlying anemia, HCG to rule out pregnancy, progesterone levels if the patient is complaining of anovulation, testosterone levels to rule out PCOS (which also causes excessive hair growth and acne), and TSH to rule out a thyroid disorder. If more in-depth testing is needed, an ultrasound, endometrial biopsy, CT, and MRI should be ordered. Treatment is guided by the underlying causes.

Pharmacologic measures are the first-line approach in treating DUB and include NSAIDs, hormone therapy, and iron therapy. Surgical intervention may be needed if all other measures fail to get the bleeding under control. Hysterectomy is reserved for the most severe cases that do not respond to other treatment.[27]

CLINICAL POINT: Because of the permanence of hysterectomy, counseling and education by the nursing and the medical team are needed to support patients in making informed decisions about this treatment. ■

Yaira Gomez: Application

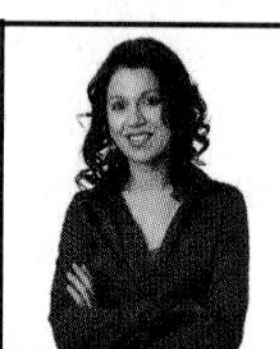

Mrs. Gomez returns to the clinic for her follow-up appointment. Laboratory findings include a CBC showing leukocytosis indicating iron deficiency anemia, Hb 9 g/dL, HCT 28%, and WBC 15,000. Ultrasound findings are inconclusive. Laparoscopy is ordered to aid in diagnosis. Biopsy samples are taken from endometrial tissues. Several lesions are found during laparoscopy in multiple sites involving the uterus, ovaries, bladder, and ureters. These findings are congruent with a diagnosis of stage IV endometriosis.

5. Mrs. Gomez's hemoglobin level is consistent with her history of which disorder?
6. Pharmacologic treatment for DUB would include what classes of medications?

Premenstrual Syndrome

Premenstrual syndrome (PMS) is a complex of symptoms affecting women of childbearing age that can cause a variety of physical and psychologic symptoms.

Etiology and Pathogenesis

The definitive cause of PMS is unknown. Current research has disproved many of the earlier theories and provides strong evidence to support serotonin deficiency as possibly influencing symptoms of PMS. Symptoms of PMS respond well to selective serotonin reuptake inhibitors (SSRIs), which increase the amount of circulating serotonin. Magnesium and calcium deficiencies are also thought to play a role in PMS symptomatology. Studies that have evaluated the effects of calcium and magnesium supplements indicate improved physical and emotional symptoms.[28] Women with PMS have been found to have the same estrogen and progesterone levels as those without PMS, but rapid shifts in the levels of these hormone promote the pronounced emotional and physical responses. Another theory is that alterations in endorphins (peptides in the body that act on opiate receptors, causing a natural pain-killing effect) that some women experience during menses may increase discomfort during PMS because of lower levels of peptides. The gamma-aminobutyric acid system and hypoprolacteinemia may also influence the PMS response.[29]

Clinical Manifestations

Clinical manifestation of PMS may include emotional symptoms of mood swings, irritability, anxiety, social withdrawal, poor concentration, insomnia, changes in sexual desire, and depression. Physical symptoms include increased thirst, food cravings, breast tenderness, bloating, weight gain, headache, fatigue, swelling of hands and feet, skin problems, gastrointestinal problems, and abdominal pain. Depression and anxiety disorders are common in PMS; approximately half of women seeking treatment for PMS will have at least one of these disorders.

Linking Pathophysiology to Diagnosis and Treatment

To diagnose PMS, a pattern of symptoms must be confirmed. Symptoms must be present for five days before the menstrual period begins and should persist for at least three consecutive menstrual cycles. Symptoms must clearly interfere with normal activities of life and end within 4 days after the menstrual cycle begins. Treatment includes simple changes in diet such as adding complex carbohydrates and calcium-rich foods; reducing fats, sugars, and salt; avoiding caffeine and alcohol; and eating smaller meals to keep blood levels stable for mood symptoms and food cravings. Medications that can be used to treat PMS symptoms include SSRIs to improve mood in some women, NSAIDs for generalized menstrual discomfort and cramping, diuretics for water retention, and hormonal contraceptives to lesson physical symptoms.

Check Your Progress: Section 47.3

1. What is the cause of discomfort in primary dysmenorrhea?
2. What are common causes of primary amenorrhea?
3. Which hormone is involved in the underlying etiology of irregular menstrual cycles causing dysfunctional uterine bleeding?

47.4 Disorders of the Ovaries and Fallopian Tubes

The area between the lateral pelvic wall and the cornu of the uterus is called the adnexal space. The structures within this space are called the adnexa and include the ovaries, fallopian tubes, the upper portion of the broad ligament, and remnants of the embryonic Mullerian duct

(**Figure 47.7** ■). Of these organs, the most commonly affected by disease are the ovaries and the fallopian tubes. Because the adnexal space is located near the urinary and gastrointestinal organs, disorders of these organs may cause symptoms in the pelvic area and need to be distinguished from gynecologic disorders. A complete pelvic exam is needed for full evaluation.

Polycystic Ovary Syndrome

Polycystic ovary syndrome (PCOS) is a disorder in which a woman's hormones are out of balance. Specifically, the metabolism of estrogen and androgen is abnormal. PCOS often causes many small cysts to grow on the ovaries.

Etiology and Pathogenesis

PCOS can result from abnormal function of the hypothalamic–pituitary–ovarian axis, which is outlined in **Figure 47.8** ■. Elevated hormones or androgens cause cessation of menses and irregular periods.

Clinical Manifestations

The major features of PCOS are menstrual dysfunction, anovulation, and signs of hyperandrogenism, including hirsutism (increased facial hair) and acne. Other effects of PCOS are infertility, irregular menses, obesity, metabolic syndrome, diabetes, and obstructive sleep apnea.

Linking Pathophysiology to Diagnosis and Treatment

On examination, findings in women with PCOS may include virilizing signs (excess facial hair, acne), acanathosis nigricans (dark, velvety discoloration in body folds and creases often linked to diabetes), enlarged ovaries, and hypertension. A diagnosis is made by excluding all other disorders that could result in menstrual irregularity and hyperandrogenism, including adrenal or ovarian tumors, thyroid dysfunction, congenital adrenal hyperplasia, hyperprolactinemia, acromegaly, and Cushing syndrome. Treatment includes the use of hormonal contraceptives to treat the hyperandrogenism, hirsutism, and acne. For treatment of infertility, clomiphene is the first-line treatment of choice.[30]

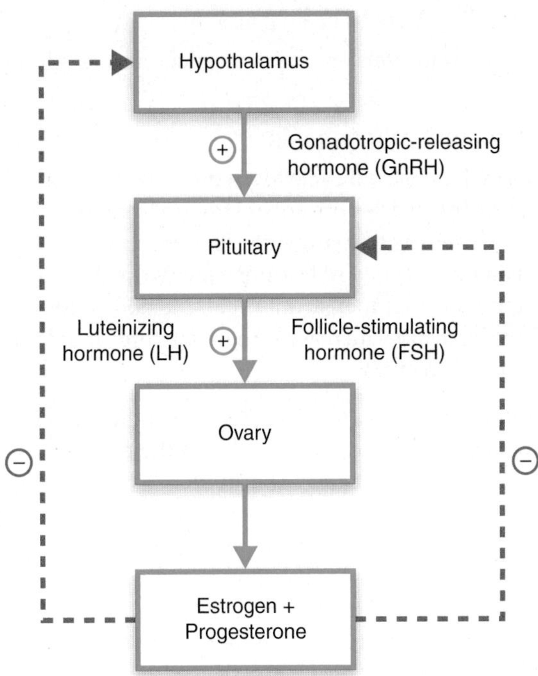

Figure 47.8 ■ The hypothalamic–pituitary–ovarian axis.

4 Women with PCOS are at a higher risk for cardiac, metabolic, oncologic, psychologic and obstetric complications throughout life.[31] In women with PCOS, gestational diabetes mellitus is the most common pregnancy complication. Risk for pregnancy-induced hypertension is also increased, as is risk for miscarriage. ■

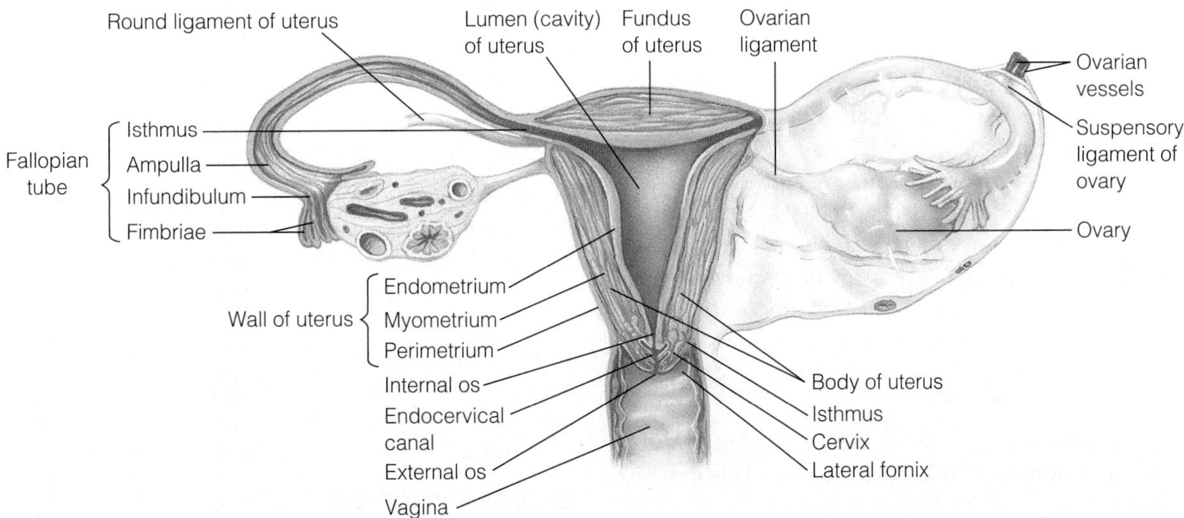

Figure 47.7 ■ The female reproductive organs, including the adnexal space.

Benign Ovarian Cysts

Benign ovarian cysts are any noncancerous cysts found on the ovaries

Etiology and Pathogenesis

In a normal menstrual cycle in a woman with optimal ovarian health, the ovaries produce estrogen from the dominant follicle. This leads to a surge of LH, which results in ovulation. If an interruption of hormone levels occurs at any time during the normal menstrual cycle, the ability for cysts to form on the ovaries increases. There are three main types of benign ovarian cysts:

- Follicular cysts form during the follicular phase of the cycle. These cysts form when the ovum fails to be released. Often, there is a surge of FSH and a lower level of LH before ovulation occurs, causing cyst formation.
- Corpus luteal cysts form in the absence of a pregnancy. If the corpus luteum does not dissolve as it is supposed to after 14 days, it can form a cyst.
- Theca lutein cysts are caused by excessive amounts of HCG. These cysts are often caused by multiple gestations or ovarian hyperstimulation.[32]

Clinical Manifestations

Patients with benign ovarian cysts can present with pelvic or abdominal pain, painful intercourse, a disruption in normal menstrual cycle, a sensation of pressure in the lower abdomen, polyuria, urgency with urination, abdominal distention, an increase in size of the lower abdomen in the absence of pregnancy, and a reduction in appetite and feeling of fullness without eating a lot of food.[33]

Linking Pathophysiology to Diagnosis and Treatment

Treatment for benign ovarian cysts is based on findings from the physical examination, ultrasound, and laboratory testing. Laboratory testing to rule out ovarian cancer is done by using the CA-125 tests. Patients with positive results should be immediately referred for further testing and follow-up.[34] Asymptomatic patients who have cysts that are smaller than 5 cm in diameter can be followed up with ultrasound after 4 months to determine whether there is any change in the size of the cysts. Cysts that are greater than 5 cm in diameter often do not resolve on their own, and the patient should be referred for further care, as the patient is at greater risk for complications such as cystic rupture or ovarian torsion. Treatment may involve pharmacologic therapy such as OCPs. Laparoscopy is considered for persistent cysts that fail to respond to hormone therapy. A bilateral oophorectomy in conjunction with a hysterectomy is considered for postmenopausal patients who have not responded to less invasive treatments.[32]

Ectopic Pregnancy

Ectopic pregnancy is any gestation that occurs in a location other than the endometrial lining of the uterus. This implantation can take place in the fallopian tubes, cervix, ovary, or abdominal or pelvic cavity. For an ectopic pregnancy to take place, there must be a fertilization of the ovum as well as an abnormal implantation.

Etiology and Pathogenesis

Several risk factors predispose a woman to developing an ectopic pregnancy: damage to the fallopian tubes, a history of ectopic pregnancies, smoking, a history of infertility treatment with hormonal medication, multiple sex partners, advanced maternal age, and a positive history for STIs. An ectopic implantation most commonly occurs in one of the fallopian tubes, and an ovum implanted there can continue to grow between 6 and 16 weeks' gestation. After this point, rupture of the fallopian tube is likely unless the ectopic pregnancy is caught earlier and can be removed. Ectopic ruptures place a patient at great risk for hemorrhage and, without proper treatment, can result in death.[32]

Clinical Manifestations

Ectopic pregnancies often present with a triad of clinical symptoms: abdominal pain, amenorrhea, and vaginal bleeding. Other complaints can be dizziness, weakness, fever, flu-like symptoms, vomiting, syncope, and in rare cases cardiac arrest. On examination, the patient may present with guarding, rigid abdomen, tenderness on palpation in the abdominal area, orthostatic blood pressure, and tachycardia.[35]

Linking Pathophysiology to Diagnosis and Treatment

Diagnosis of ectopic pregnancy is made by using the serum B-HCG testing for the presence of HCG in the blood. HCG levels in an ectopic pregnancy tend to be lower than those in a normal uterine implantation and are used to determine a normal versus abnormal pregnancy. Ultrasound is needed to determine placement of the ectopic pregnancy as well as the level of pelvic fluids and whether there is evidence of bleeding. There are two choices for treatment of an ectopic pregnancy. Methotrexate, a chemotherapy drug that can stop cells from dividing, can be administered for a smaller and nonruptured ectopic pregnancy. Surgical intervention is often use to remove the ectopic pregnancy. The placement and size of the gestation will determine whether the fallopian tube can be preserved. Practitioners consider the patient's age, the possibility of fertility preservation, and the patient's desire for future children before surgical intervention. Follow-up for ectopic pregnancy includes blood work to ensure a decline in HCG levels, Rh status to determine the need for immunoglobulin treatment, and a CBC to ensure the patient's stability.[36]

Ovarian Cancer

Ovarian cancer is a form of cancer that presents with malignant lesions of the ovaries. It includes primary lesions from normal structures within the ovary and secondary lesions from cancers arising in other parts of the body. Ovarian cancer is the most common cause of cancer death from gynecologic tumors in the United States. It is estimated that more than 200,000 women develop ovarian cancer every year globally and about 100,000 die from the disease. The lifetime risk of a woman developing epithelial ovarian cancer is 1 in 70.[37]

Etiology and Pathogenesis

The precise cause of ovarian cancer is unknown, but several reproductive and genetic contributing factors have been identified. New evidence on the pathophysiology of ovarian cancer indicates that the tumors that were once thought to originate on the ovary actually originate in the fimbria of the fallopian tube (see Figure 47.7). Metastases to the ovaries can occur frequently. Most of the cancers that metastasize to the ovaries originate in the endometrium, breast, colon, stomach, and cervix.

Clinical Manifestations

Early in the disease, ovarian cancer causes minimal, nonspecific, or no symptoms. Because of this, most cases are diagnosed in the advanced stage when the disease has spread beyond the ovaries. Clinical manifestations include abdominal bloating, pelvic or abdominal pain, trouble eating but feeling full, urinary frequency, fatigue, back pain, pain with intercourse, constipation, and weight loss. The prognosis in ovarian cancer is closely related to the stage of the disease at diagnosis, but the overall prognosis for patients with ovarian cancer is poor unless there is early detection.

Linking Pathophysiology to Diagnosis and Treatment

Standard treatment includes aggressive debulking surgery (to reduce the tumor) and chemotherapy. The use of neoadjuvant chemotherapy (chemotherapy before surgery) has recently increased as a treatment measure; it appears to offer improved morbidity and survival rates.[38]

The incidence of ovarian cancer increases with age and peaks in the eighth decade of life. Management of older patients tends to be less aggressive, and treatment is often inadequate. ■

Check Your Progress: Section 47.4

1. The etiology of PCOS is caused by dysfunction of what hormonal axis?
2. A benign ovarian cyst that develops during the follicular phase of the cycle is due to what physiologic alteration?
3. Which disorder involves gestation in a location other than the endometrial lining of the uterus?

47.5 Disorders of the Uterus

Disorders of the uterus can stem from multiple causes, including abnormalities that may have been present since birth. Past surgeries may affect fertility, and exposure to certain drugs before birth, such as diethylstilbestrol (DES), can cause uterine deformities.

Endometrial Polyps

Endometrial polyps are hyperplasic overgrowth of the endometrial glands and stroma. Endometrial polyps are typically localized to the uterus and can be seen as a single polyp or multiple growths ranging in size from a few millimeters to several centimeters in diameter.

Etiology and Pathogenesis

The exact etiology of endometrial polyps is not known. An imbalance of the hormones estrogen and progesterone are causative factors for polyp growth.[39] The polyps are composed of fibroblast-like spindle cells and large blood vessels with thick walls. The epithelium of the polyp may be active, pseudostratified, or flat.[40]

Clinical Manifestations

Endometrial polyps occur in women over the age of 20 until after completion of menopause. Clinical signs and symptoms can be abnormally heavy uterine bleeding, pain in the abdominal cavity, bleeding after completion of menopause, a history of amenorrhea, infertility or trouble maintaining a pregnancy after conception, and use of medications such as tamoxifen. Uterine prolapse can also occur with the presence of large endometrial polyps.[40]

Linking Pathophysiology to Diagnosis and Treatment

Diagnosis of endometrial polyps is made by using ultrasound or hysteroscopy with guided biopsy. Most endometrial polyps are not malignant. In many cases, management with no medical intervention can be done if malignancy is ruled out and the polyps do not cause any symptoms. When medical management is needed, pharmacologic treatment includes hormonal medications. Surgical treatment includes surgical excision of the polyps and possible resection. The only way to guarantee that a patient will be free of all polyps is to undergo a hysterectomy. This should be done only for patients who do not wish to preserve fertility and when all other methods have been exhausted.[41]

Endometrial polyps can sometimes cause problems with fertility and even cause miscarriage. The polyps are overgrowths that affect the lining of the uterus, and a normal uterine cavity and endometrial lining are needed to conceive and maintain pregnancy. ■

Endometrial polyps are common in older adults. Most are asymptomatic with a low risk of malignancy. Patients need to be aware that the risk factors for endometrial cancers are age, obesity, and long-term treatment with estrogens. ■

Adenomyosis

Adenomyosis is a condition in which the glandular endometrial tissue invades the uterine myometrium. Adenomyosis is a benign condition and can affect the entire uterus or just a part of it. In this condition, the endometrial tissue invades the myometrium lining, producing enlargement of the uterus.

Etiology and Pathogenesis

The endometrial tissue invasion causes an inflammatory response and allows for reproduction of the tissues at an accelerated rate.[42] The specific cause of adenomyosis is unknown. It is hypothesized that pregnancy-related issues such as cesarean birth, abortion, curettage, and any other invasive techniques involving the uterus can disrupt the endometrial–myometrial margin, allowing tissue from the endometrial glands and stroma to cross into the myometrium.[43]

Clinical Manifestations

Patients who are affected by adenomyosis are typically between the ages of 30 and 50 and tend to be obese, have had multiple children, have had early onset of menstruation, or have a history of uterine surgical interventions. Patients present with menorrhagia, pelvic pain, dyspareunia (painful or difficult sexual intercourse, which is discussed in detail later in this chapter), and dysmenorrhea. Diffuse pain is felt with uterine palpation, and the enlarged abdomen can be the size of a 12-week pregnancy. Recent studies have shown that patients with a history of depression with antidepressant use have an increased risk of adenomyosis, as do patients using Tamoxifen for breast cancer treatment.[42]

Linking Pathophysiology to Diagnosis and Treatment

Diagnosis of adenomyosis is made based on history and physical examination as well as laboratory testing, CT, ultrasound, and MRI. Diagnostic criteria for adenomyosis can be made when there is evidence of myometrial invasion at 2.5 mm or one half of a low-power microscopic field from the endometrial border.[44] Treatment includes hormonal supplementation with OCPs, either combined or progesterone-only, which thins the endometrial lining and reduces inflammation, or gonadotropin-releasing hormone agonists, which slow the progression of adenomyosis by decreasing the estrogen levels and decreasing the affected areas in the uterus. The Mirena intrauterine device has also been used for treatment of adenomyosis, as it thins the endometrial lining and provides 5 years of contraception. Follow-up is required for medication regimens because the symptoms will return once medications have been discontinued. Hysterectomy is reserved for patients for whom all other treatments have failed and no further pregnancies are desired.[43]

Adenomyosis can cause pregnancy concerns for women who are trying to become pregnant as endometrial tissue begins to grow into the muscle layers of the uterus. ■

Leiomyomas

Leiomyomas, also known as fibroids or myomas, are benign soft tissue tumors resulting from an overproduction of smooth muscle cells surrounded by compressed muscle fibers.

Etiology and Pathogenesis

Precise causes of leiomyomas are unknown, but there have been advances in the understanding of hormonal, genetic, and growth factors as well as the cell structure of these benign tumors. Both estrogen and progesterone promote the growth of myomas. Leiomyomas are not often noted before puberty and are most prevalent during a woman's reproductive years. Leiomyomas generally regress after menopause because of the drop in estrogen. Women are most likely to be diagnosed during their 40s; this relates to hormonal changes and increased fibroid growth during this time.

Clinical Manifestations

Clinical manifestations of leiomyomas may include abnormal uterine bleeding or menorrhagia, pelvic pressure or pain, dysmenorrhea, menstrual periods lasting more than a week, dyspareunia, frequent urination, constipation, and back and leg pain. Leiomyomas can range in size from small, undetectable lesions to bulky masses of benign soft tissue that can distort and enlarge the uterus.[45]

Linking Pathophysiology to Diagnosis and Treatment

During a pelvic bimanual examination, uterine leiomyomas (fibroids) may be detected incidentally. There may be palpable irregularities in the shape of the uterus. A transabdominal or transvaginal ultrasound can be ordered to confirm a diagnosis and provide measurements of the fibroids. Blood work is also ordered to rule out anemia, bleeding, or thyroid disorders. Many treatment options exist, depending on the presenting symptoms. If there are no symptoms, monitoring the fibroids is considered the best approach to care.[46]

Fibroids usually develop before pregnancy and are detected with the routine ultrasound or examination. Pregnancy complications in general are minimal, but risks of miscarriage and prematurity increase slightly. If fibroids are blocking the cervical opening, there will be an increased chance for a cesarean delivery. ■

Endometriosis

Endometriosis is the presence and growth of functioning endometrial tissue in places other than the uterus. It affects 6–10% of all women, 25–50% of infertile women, and 75–80% of women with chronic pelvic pain.[47]

The average age of diagnosis of endometriosis is 27 years, but the condition also occurs in adolescents.[47] ■

Etiology and Pathogenesis

The exact cause of endometriosis is unknown. It is hypothesized that in endometriosis the endometrial cells move from the uterus and become implanted in ectopic sites. Transport of the cells could be through the menstrual tissue, known as retrograde menstruation, in which cells move through the fallopian tubes and are transported by the endometrial cells into the intra-abdominal space, causing the lymphatic and circulatory system to transport the cells to distant sites such as the pleural cavity. The most common sites for ectopic endometrial tissue to grow are in the dependent portions of the female pelvis, including the fallopian tubes, vagina, cervix and the uterosacral ligaments. But all other organs have the potential for abnormal endometrial growth. An increased incidence of endometriosis in women who have a first-degree relative with endometriosis has been seen, which suggests that there is a hereditary component to the disorder.[47]

Clinical Manifestations

Pelvic pain is one of the first complaints that many patients have in endometriosis. Pain is likely to occur before or during the menstrual cycle and during sexual intercourse. Patients may also complain of an inability to get pregnant. Bleeding between periods may be seen in some patients. Dysmenorrhea is an excellent diagnostic clue for practitioners to rule in a diagnosis of endometriosis. Pelvic examination may be completely normal or can include an enlarged uterus, an ovarian mass felt on palpation, or a thickness in the rectovaginal septum.[47]

Yaira Gomez: Application

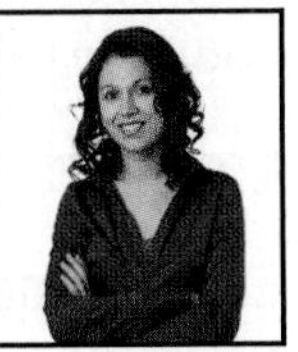

Because of her age and her desire for pregnancy, fertility preservation is imperative in Mrs. Gomez's case. A conservative approach to treatment must be started to give her the best chance of conception. Mrs. Gomez is prescribed iron for her anemia and NSAIDs for pain and discomfort. In consultation with her healthcare team, Mrs. Gomez chooses surgical resection with ablation of endometrial tissue as the best way to preserve the functionality of her uterus.

7. What is the purpose of ablation of endometrial tissue to treat endometriosis?
8. Mrs. Gomez asks you whether the endometriosis will cause complications in getting pregnant. What is your best response?

Linking Pathophysiology to Diagnosis and Treatment

Initial diagnosis can be made on the basis of clinical symptoms but must be confirmed with a biopsy of the endometrial tissues. Biopsy is obtained through a pelvic laparoscopic procedure. Imaging testing can be done by using ultrasound, barium enemas, CT, and MRI scanning. Endometriosis is classified in four stages (**Figure 47.9** ■). Stage I involves minimal invasion of the endometrial tissue. Stage II involves deeper implantation into the endometrial tissue. Stage III is moderate and involves many deep implants into the tissue with endometriomas on one or both of the ovaries as well as some adhesions. Stage IV, the most severe stage of endometriosis, involves many deep implants with large endometriomas on one or both ovaries as well as deep adhesions that can grow into the rectum on the backside of the uterus. Treatment for endometriosis involves pain medication, hormones to suppress ovarian function and reduce endometrial tissue growth, and possibly surgical interventions to reduce tissue overgrowth. Hysterectomy may be performed depending on the patient's age, the stage of the endometriosis, and the patient's desire for fertility. Conservative methods of treatment will keep endometriosis under control, but if medication is stopped, most endometrial overgrowth will reoccur within 6 months to a year.[48]

Endometriosis can affect adolescent girls. Those with a first-degree relative with the condition have an increased chance of developing this condition. ■

Endometriosis makes getting pregnant a challenge, as adhesions and scarred pelvic tissue can block the fallopian tubes. But it is important to let patients know that not all women with endometriosis are infertile. ■

CLINICAL POINT: Educating the patient and reassuring her that a life-threatening situation does not exist may help her to accept a conservative and progressive treatment for endometriosis. Nurses can give important psychologic support to patients who experience some of the side effects of endometriosis, such as disabling pain, sexual dysfunction secondary to dyspareunia, and possible infertility. Nurses should educate themselves on preoperative and postoperative measures for endometriosis so that they can provide accurate information to their patients. ■

Yaira Gomez: Outcome

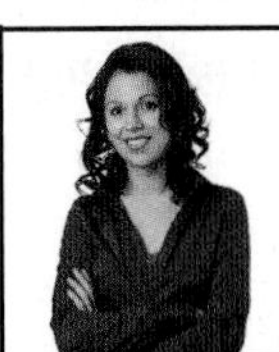

Mrs. Gomez undergoes surgery for endometriosis, and it is successful. She is then referred to a fertility specialist. After 1 year of in vitro fertilization treatments, she is able to conceive and carry a twin gestation to term. Her children are born via cesarean delivery at 36 weeks without complications. One year after the birth of her twins, Mrs. Gomez's endometriosis returns. Ovulation-suppressing medications are used for 6 months after the relapse without success. Mrs. Gomez then opts for a total abdominal hysterectomy with bilateral salpingo-oophorectomy. She is prescribed hormone replacement therapy and is symptom free after the surgery.

9. Mrs. Gomez asks you what would happen if she discontinued her hormone therapy. What is your best response?
10. Why is hormone replacement therapy necessary after total abdominal hysterectomy?

Endometrial Cancer

Endometrial cancer is cancer of the endometrial lining of the uterus. According to the National Institutes of Health (NIH) and the American Cancer Institute, endometrial cancer is the most common gynecologic malignancy in the United States. In 2016, there were 60,050 cases and 10,470 deaths from endometrial cancer.

Etiology and Pathogenesis

There are two types of endometrial cancer. Type I is estrogen dominated, and type II is non–hormone related.[49] Risk factors for endometrial cancer include obesity, diabetes, a

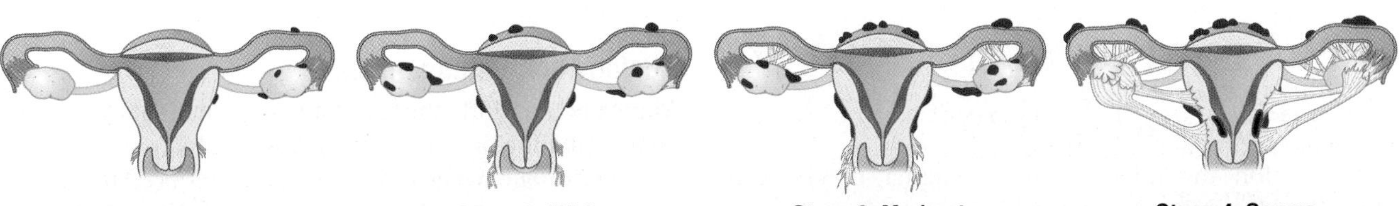

Figure 47.9 ■ Staging of endometriosis.

high-fat diet, increased exposure to hormones such as estrogen, early onset of menarche, a history of anovulation, infertility, and nulliparity (never having given birth or carried a pregnancy).[50]

Clinical Manifestations

According to the American Cancer Society, approximately 90% of women with endometrial cancer will have some form of vaginal bleeding. Irregular vaginal bleeding is one of the earliest signs of endometrial cancer. Bleeding can occur between periods, after sexual intercourse, or after menopause when a woman has experienced no bleeding for at least a 1 year. Abnormal vaginal discharge may also occur. Complaints of pelvic pain, a feeling of fullness in the pelvic area, and weight loss without dieting can be signs of a tumor in the endometrium.[51]

Linking Pathophysiology to Diagnosis and Treatment

Diagnosis of endometrial cancer is done by using transvaginal ultrasound or via histologic evaluation of the endometrial tissue which can be performed in a gynecology office. Endometrial cancer is classified into stages. In stage I, the cancer is growing only in the body of the uterus. In stage II, the cancer has spread from the uterus and is growing outside in the connective tissue of the cervix. In stage III, the cancer has spread outside the uterus into the tissues of the pelvic area.[52,53] Treatment involves surgery followed by chemotherapy with or without radiation. Lymph node metastasis is an important concern, particularly with advanced endometrial cancers; a lympadenectomy may be performed for patients who are at high risk for advanced disease.[54]

Gynecologic malignancies are most often diagnosed in postmenopausal women, but these malignancies can also occur in premenopausal women for whom issues of fertility are a concern. Women are waiting longer to have children, and many of the standard treatments for cancers result in permanent sterility. It is important to let patients know about fertility data and to discuss surgical-sparing procedures for younger patients who may still wish to conceive. ■

Check Your Progress: Section 47.5

1. What are the tissue characteristics of endometrial polyps?
2. What condition results when glandular endometrial tissue invades the uterine myometrium?
3. What are the two types of endometrial cancer?

47.6 Disorders of the Cervix, Vagina, and Vulva

Inflammation and infection of the vagina, cervix, and vulva tend to occur when natural immune defenses of lactobacillus and acid vaginal secretions maintained by sufficient estrogen levels are disrupted. OCPs, antibiotics, and corticosteroids can alter vaginal pH and trigger an overgrowth of organisms. Resistance may decrease with aging and poor nutrition. Most lower genital tract infections are related to sexual intercourse resulting in transmission of organisms, tissue trauma, and alteration of the vaginal acid–base balance.

Cervicitis

Etiology and Pathogenesis

Cervicitis is an inflammation of the cervix that can be caused by infection or other vaginal issues. The most common cause of infectious cervicitis is chlamydia or gonorrhea. It can also be related to trichomoniasis or genital herpes. Noninfectious cervicitis may result from trauma to the cervix, radiation treatments, systemic inflammation, and malignancy. Because of the anatomic placement of the cervix deep inside the vaginal canal, it is a natural host environment for inflammation. When infection does occur, edema of the subepithelial stroma will cause an increase in lymphocyte and plasma cells. The blood vessels dilate, and the surface columnar and glandular epithelium of the cervix becomes irritated, distended, and inflamed. An increase in cervical secretions results, with mixed blood and malodorous mucopurulent drainage. The vaginal discharge that originates at the cervical os is known as leukorrhea and is one of the diagnostic signs of infection.[55]

Clinical Manifestations

The most common clinical manifestations of cervicitis are vaginal discharge and vaginal bleeding between menses or after sexual intercourse. Other symptoms include pruritus, a burning sensation, inner and outer vaginal irritation, dysuria, and dyspareunia. Fever, cervical motion tenderness, and hemorrhages on the cervix may be present. Although cervicitis can be painful, most patients do not experience pain.[56]

Linking Pathophysiology to Diagnosis and Treatment

Because of the relationship between cervicitis and STIs, all patients with cervicitis and their partners should be tested for STIs. Because the cervix is connected to the uterus, all patients should also be tested for PID because the infection can migrate toward the uterus and ovaries. If an infection is present, antibiotic treatment will be started. If symptoms persist, testing for *Mycoplasma genitalium*, a persistent bacterial infection with a long incubation, is warranted because it has been found to cause cervicitis.[57] Practitioners should encourage treatment of patients and all of their sex partners.

Vaginitis

Etiology and Pathogenesis

Vaginitis is an inflammation of the vagina that causes discharge, itching, and pain. Vaginitis results from a change in the normal balance of bacteria and infection. It can also be a result of reduced estrogen levels after menopause. It is the most common gynecologic condition seen in adult women. Bacterial vaginosis constitutes 40–50% of vaginitis cases, vaginal candidiasis accounts for 20–25% of the cases, and 15–20% are caused by trichomoniasis.[58]

Clinical Manifestations

Bacterial vaginitis is asymptomatic in up to 50% of women. Any discharge is thin, malodorous, and grayish white or yellow in color. Pruritus may be present, but vaginal pain or irritation is uncommon.

Linking Pathophysiology to Diagnosis and Treatment

A complex balance of microorganisms maintains the vaginal flora. Vaginal organisms include lactobacilli, corynebacteria, and yeast. Factors that change the flora include age, sexual activity including abuse, hygiene, immune status, and underlying skin diseases. The normal vaginal pH is 3.9–4.2. At this pH, the growth of pathogenic organisms is inhibited. Disturbance of normal vaginal pH leads to overgrowth of pathogens. Factors that alter the vaginal flora include contraceptives, feminine hygiene products, vaginal medications, antibiotics, STIs, sexual intercourse, and stress. The overgrowth of normally present bacteria, viruses, and an infecting bacteria can cause symptoms of vaginitis.

The age of the female affects the anatomy and physiology of the vagina. Vaginitis is uncommon in prepubertal girls. Prepubertal children have a more alkaline vaginal pH than do pubertal and postpubertal adolescents and women. ■

In the United States, an average of 16% of pregnant women have bacterial vaginosis.[59] ■

Vulvovestibulitis

Vulvovestibulitis, also called *vulvar vestibulitis*, is pain or irritation in the vestibule, the area that surrounds the opening of the vagina (**Figure 47.10** ■). The pain can occur during any attempted vaginal entry, including sexual intercourse, tampon insertion, and gynecologic examinations.

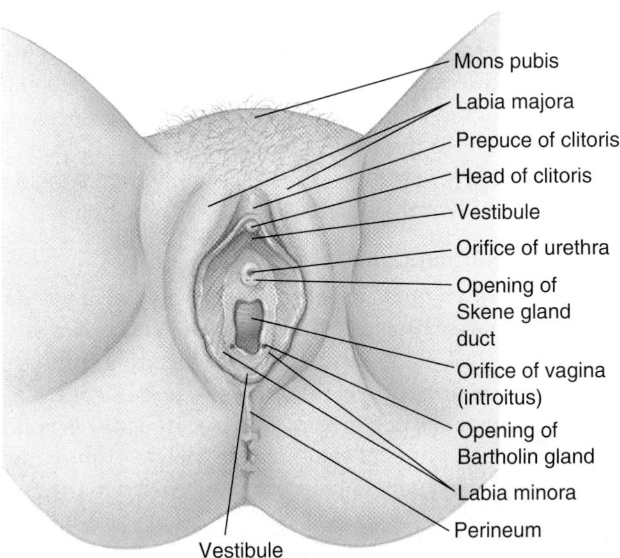

Figure 47.10 ■ The external organs of the female reproductive system.

Etiology and Pathogenesis

The women who are affected by vulvovestibulitis are generally young and sexually active. Most patients have had symptoms for several months, have tried multiple remedies, but have had no improvement. Vulvovestibulitis may be primary or secondary. Primary vulvovestibulitis is characterized by the presence of pain at initiation of sexual activity. It can also start from insertion of a tampon or vaginal speculum during a gynecologic exam. Secondary vulvovestibulitis develops after a period of comfortable sexual activity, and tolerance for tampon, and speculum insertion.

Clinical Manifestations

Symptoms of vulvovestibulitis include pain, soreness, and burning with any kind of touch or pressure on the vestibule. In addition to intercourse, tampons, and vaginal examinations, the pain can be caused by wearing tight clothes, riding a bicycle, or even sitting for too long. The pain is not constant, but any attempt to enter the vagina causes pain.

There may be small areas of erythema where the pain is located.

Linking Pathophysiology to Diagnosis and Treatment

Standard pelvic examination of women with vulvovestibulitis typically reveals no physical findings. During the pelvic exam, even gentle pressure with a cotton-tipped applicator at the vestibule or the base of the hymenal ring will elicit significant pain. Treatment includes the use of topical medications such as A&D ointment (usually used for diaper rash), lidocaine gel, witch hazel pads (Tucks pads), steroid ointments applied in a thin layer to areas of discomfort, and trichloroacetate acid, which chemically destroys the affected areas so that new tissue can replace unhealthy skin. Oral medications, biofeedback, and physical therapy are sometimes prescribed, and surgery or laser treatment has been recommended as a last resort.

Bartholinitis

Etiology and Pathogenesis

Bartholinitis is an inflammation of the Bartholin gland (see Figure 47.10). The Bartholin glands are located on either side of the posterior vaginal opening in the labia minora. The glands, which are typically nonpalpable, play a key role in vaginal lubrication and mucus secretion. When a buildup of mucus occurs, it can lead to inflammation and cyst formation.[60] Most cases of bartholinitis are in the form of a cyst or abscess and occur in women of childbearing age. When the ostium of the Bartholin duct becomes obstructed, the fluid builds up and leads to distention of the gland. The cause of cyst formation often nonspecific inflammation or physical trauma, and the cyst can range in size from 1 to 3 cm in diameter. Abscesses of the gland are caused by infection. In rare cases, inflammation of the glands can be the result of an adenocarcinoma.[61]

Clinical Manifestations

Patients with bartholinitis present with complaints of a unilateral mass in the labial minora area of the vagina. The mass can be tender and fluid-filled. Erythema and edema can be localized to the mass or may encompass the surrounding vaginal tissues.[61]

Linking Pathophysiology to Diagnosis and Treatment

Because most abscesses are caused by polymicrobial organisms, it is rare for bartholinitis to be related to STIs. Nonetheless, all patients should undergo testing for STIs as a precautionary measure. In the case of suspected carcinoma, patients should be referred for biopsy and possible excision of the mass. For uncomplicated cysts, patients can use a sitz bath to help reduce the size of the cyst and cause eventual rupture and resolution of the symptoms. Patients who present with abscesses will need excision and drainage of the gland to reduce the symptoms. Antibiotics and analgesics are prescribed to prevent infection and deliver pain relief.[62]

Cervical Cancer

Etiology and Pathogenesis

Cervical cancer is a form of cancer that invades the cells of the cervix. Cervical cancer is the third most common cancer diagnosed in women in the United States and worldwide. Except in rare cases, the human papillomavirus (HPV) causes cervical cancer. While it is possible to transmit HPV without sexual contact, a majority of HPV cases originate from some type of sexual interaction. The risk factors for contracting HPV are initiation of sexual contact at a young age, multiple sex partners, and a history of STIs. Positive cases of HPV placed a woman at risk for HIV and other sexually transmitted diseases. Cervical cancer occurs only in women who have had an HPV virus.[63]

Clinical Manifestations

Patients with cervical cancer may present with abnormal vaginal bleeding. This bleeding may occur after sexual intercourse or between menstrual periods. Regional discomfort can also occur either with sexual contact or at any other time. Some patients may complain of malodorous discharge from the vaginal area. Dysuria is also seen in some patients. If treatment is sought at a later time, the cervical cancer tumors can grow, extending past the epithelial surfaces of the cervix and invading the squamous and glandular tissues. The cancer cells will extend toward the endometrial cavity and extend through the vaginally epithelial tissues as well as into the pelvic wall. The cells can also invade the bladder and rectum, which can lead to constipation, hematuria, fistulas, and a blockage in the urethra.[64]

Linking Pathophysiology to Diagnosis and Treatment

Initial evaluation for cervical cancer is made by using Papanicolaou smear testing (Pap). Pap smear testing allows for analysis of the cervical cells and helps to guide the practitioner toward further testing for treatment and evaluation. The staging of the cancer will determine the treatment and can range from biopsy to radiation and chemotherapy. The prognosis for cervical cancer is based on staging and has a 5-year survival rate of 30–90% survival rate depending on the stages (I–IV).[64]

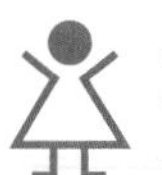

An HPV vaccination is now available for women 9–26 years of age. It has been recommended for prevention of cervical cancer as well as genital warts. All women should undergo Pap smear testing beginning at age 21 or within 3 years of initiating sexual activity. Pap smear testing at regular scheduled intervals has been proven to prevent HPV infections from resulting in cervical cancer. ■

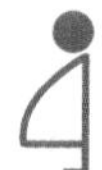

HPV infection during pregnancy can require the patient to undergo a cesarean birth for protection of the fetus during delivery. ■

According to the CDC, an increase in HPV is being seen in Americans age 65 years and older, particularly those in retirement communities who are having unprotected sex. For this reason, it is important to continue pelvic exams and Pap smear testing through at least age 65 and older if the person's symptoms and lifestyle warrant it. ■

Vaginal Cancer

Etiology and Pathogenesis

Vaginal cancer is a rare type of cancer in which malignant cancer cells form in the vagina. It occurs most often in women age 60 years and older and is more prevalent in women who had HPV. HPV infection is associated with the pathogenesis of squamous cell vaginal carcinoma. Risk factors for vaginal cancer include being age 60 or older, having been exposed to DES before birth, and having a history of abnormal cervical cells or cervical cancer. Vaginal cancer is not common. There are two main types of vaginal cancer: squamous cell carcinoma and adenocarcinoma of the vagina.

Squamous cell carcinoma forms in the squamous cells lining the vagina. It spreads slowly and generally stays locally in the vagina but can metastasize to the lungs and liver. This form is most commonly found in women age 60 and older. Adenocarcinoma of the vagina affects the glandular cells in the vaginal lining. These cells release the fluids and mucus in the vagina. Adenocarcinoma is found in women age 30 or younger and is more likely to spread to the lungs and lymph nodes.[65]

Clinical Manifestations

Symptoms of vaginal cancer are not always evident, particularly in its early stages. Cancer in later stages can cause symptoms such as abnormal vaginal bleeding, difficulty or pain when urinating, pain during sexual intercourse, a lump in the vagina, pelvic pain, pain in the back or legs, and leg swelling. A physical examination, pelvic examination, Pap smear, biopsy, and colposcopy can be used to diagnose vaginal cancer.

Linking Pathophysiology to Diagnosis and Treatment

Treatment options for vaginal cancer include surgery, internal and external radiation therapy, and chemotherapy. The prognosis depends on the stage of the cancer, whether it has spread, the size of the tumor, the grade of the tumor cells, whether there are symptoms, where the cancer is in the vagina, whether the patient is in general good health, the patient's age, and whether the cancer is newly diagnosed or has reoccurred.[65]

The squamous cell form of vaginal cancer affects women age 60 and older. Practicing safe sex to protect against HPV is important at all ages. Having regular Pap tests and quitting smoking can also be beneficial. ■

Vulvar Cancer

Etiology and Pathogenesis

Vulvar cancer is a form of cancer that occurs on the outer surface area of the female genitalia. It can occur at any age but is most commonly seen in women age 70 years or older. Vulvar cancer in women younger than 40 years accounts for approximately 15% of cases. As the population ages, the incidence of vulvar cancer may be increasing. In most cases, an extended delay in diagnosis occurs because the patient does not seek medical advice for many months or the lesion is not biopsied early enough for a definitive diagnosis.[66]

Clinical Manifestations

Vulvar cancer commonly forms as a lump or sore on the vulva, causing itching. The cancer can appear on any part of the vulva but most occurs on the labia. The more rare forms occur as Bartholin gland carcinomas. Metastasis to inguinal lymph nodes may occur early in the process.

Linking Pathophysiology to Diagnosis and Treatment

Vulvar cancer is diagnosed by biopsy and possibly imaging tests such as CT and MRI. Treatment includes surgery to remove the cancer and a small amount of surrounding tissue.[67]

CLINICAL POINT: Nurses have the opportunity to educate women about common genital conditions and how to reduce their risks. Helping women to recognize symptoms that might indicate a problem supports women in their decision to seek timely care. It can be difficult to discuss problems related to sexual intercourse or genital disease, but a nonjudgmental attitude can make woman feel more comfortable discussing their concerns, and can encourage them to seek more accurate information about their health. When a diagnosis of a condition of the genitals is made, it is important for the nurse to ensure that the patient fully understands the treatment measures, medication dosages, and optimal dosing times, such as the nighttime administration of vaginal creams to ensure a longer exposure time. Using models to teach and demonstrate proper technique can improve understanding. ■

Check Your Progress: Section 47.6

1. What is the most common cause of infectious cervicitis?
2. What is the main cause of bartholinitis?
3. HPV infection is a risk factor for what type of vaginal cancer?

47.7 Disorders of the Female Pelvis

In women, the pelvic floor involves the muscles, ligaments, connective tissue, and nerves that support the bladder, uterus, vagina, and rectum and assists these pelvic organs to function. According to the NIH, almost one quarter of women have pelvic floor disorders at some point in their lives. The study noted that women of all ages from 20 to 80 years can be affected by some form of pelvic floor disorder.[68]

Pelvic Inflammatory Disease

Pelvic inflammatory disease (PID) is an infection caused by bacteria that originates in the vagina or cervix and is carried to the uterus, fallopian tubes, and ovaries.

Etiology and Pathogenesis

The etiology of PID includes multiple sex partners, early sexual activity, young age for first intercourse, and use of an IUD for contraception. Some surgeries may put women at risk of PID, including total abdominal hysterectomy and bilateral tubal ligation. An infection caused by bacteria is carried into the uterus, fallopian tubes, and ovaries.

Clinical Manifestations

Patients with PID may be asymptomatic but more often have pain and tenderness in the lower abdomen, fever, chills, and an elevated white blood cell count and erythrocyte sedimentation rate. The pain is described as dull, crampy, bilateral, and constant. It begins a few days after the onset of the last menstrual period and can increase with motion, exercise, or intercourse. Pain can last from 7 days to 3 weeks. Vaginal discharge can occur, as can postcoital vaginal bleeding. Fever, nausea, and vomiting can occur late in the clinical course.

Linking Pathophysiology to Diagnosis and Treatment

Common bacteria involved in PID are those that cause chlamydia and gonorrhea. Treatment includes a combination of IV and oral antibiotics, bedrest, possible surgery to drain abscesses if they occur, removal of adhesions, and repair of damaged fallopian tubes. PID can lead to increased risk for ectopic pregnancy or infertility.[68]

CLINICAL POINT: Priorities in nursing care for patients with PID include focusing on managing symptoms and teaching the patient about the disease. Ensure that pain management is a priority. Instruct the patient about possible causes of PID, and teach her to avoid sexual activity that puts her at risk for PID. Communicate nonjudgmentally to build trust. Arrange for follow-up care or support group referrals. ■

Pelvic Organ Prolapse

Etiology and Pathogenesis

Pelvic organ prolapse is drop of pelvic organs when pelvic floor muscles weaken or become injured (**Figure 47.11** ■). Pelvic floor defects may be created as a result of childbirth

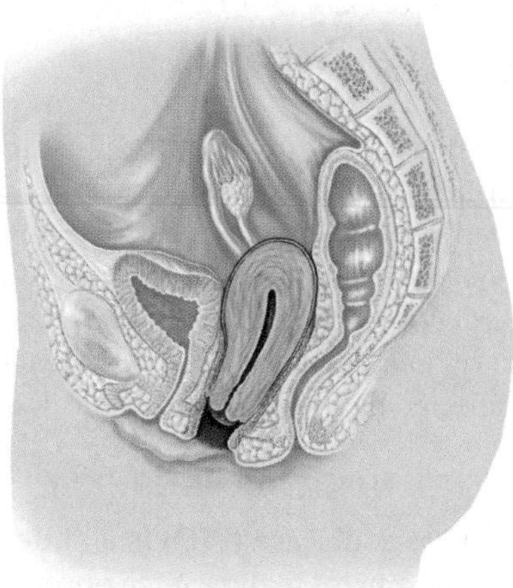

Figure 47.11 ■ Example of pelvic organ prolapse.

and are caused by stretching and tearing of the fascia and muscles. Pregnancy without vaginal birth has been noted to be a risk factor also. Because of the nerve impairment to the pelvic floor muscles, tone decreases, leading to sagging and stretching. Multiparous women (women who have had multiple births) are at particular risk for pelvic organ prolapse. Genital atrophy, decreased estrogen, and being postmenopausal may also contribute to prolapse. The exact mechanism is not completely understood. Prolapse may also result from pelvic tumors, sacral nerve disorders, diabetic neuropathy, and conditions that increase pelvic pressure, such as obesity, chronic pulmonary disease, smoking that produces a chronic cough, chronic constipation, and rare connective tissue disorders such as Marfan disease, which is linked to pelvic organ prolapse.

Clinical Manifestations

Symptoms of pelvic organ prolapse may include a sensation of vaginal fullness or pressure, sacral back pain with standing, vaginal spotting from ulceration of the protruding cervix or vagina, coital difficulty, discomfort in the lower abdomen, and voiding and defecating difficulties. Typically, the patient feels a bulge in the lower vagina or the cervix protruding through the vaginal introitus.[69] Voiding difficulties, urinary frequency, urgency, or incontinence are common symptoms associated with pelvic organ prolapse. Voiding dysfunction is common for patients with advanced degrees of pelvic organ prolapse. The urethra may become kinked, causing urinary retention because of the obstruction. This advanced prolapse can lead to lower urinary tract dysfunction or more serious kidney issues such as hydronephrosis and obstructive nephropathy. A thorough evaluation and understanding of all support defects are of critical importance because most women with pelvic organ prolapse have multiple defects.

Linking Pathophysiology to Diagnosis and Treatment

A postvoid residual for urine volume test can be done to determine whether there is obstruction as a result of urethral kinking or incomplete emptying related to poor bladder contractility. Treatment may include pessaries inserted vaginally to support the bladder, vagina, uterus, and rectum. Pelvic floor exercises (also known as Kegel exercises) can be helpful. Surgery to attach a surgical sling to support the pelvic organs may be required.[69]

Older women may be reluctant to get help for problems related to prolapse when they do not fully understand what is happening to them. Also, they may think that surgery is the only possible intervention. Patients should be referred to a urogynecology specialist to determine all treatment options, including pessaries and pelvic floor exercises. ■

Check Your Progress: Section 47.7

1. What is the term for a bacterial infection in the vagina or cervix that is carried to the uterus, fallopian tubes, and ovaries?
2. What laboratory findings are consistent with pelvic inflammatory disease?
3. In pelvic floor prolapse, why is a postvoid residual test is performed?

47.8 Disorders of Fertility

Infertility is the inability to conceive after having regular unprotected sexual intercourse. It can refer to the inability to contribute to conception or the inability to carry a pregnancy to full term. An infertility assessment is usually initiated after 1 year of regular unprotected intercourse in women under age 35 and after 6 months of unprotected intercourse in women age 35 and older. Evaluation may be initiated sooner in women with irregular menstrual cycles or in those who have risk factors for infertility such as endometriosis, a history of PID, or reproductive tract malformations. Infertility affects 10–20% of women of reproductive age.

Etiology and Pathogenesis

The etiology of female infertility is multifactorial and can arise from various parts of the reproductive system:

- Cervix: Cervical stenosis or abnormalities of the interaction between cervical mucus and sperm
- Uterus: Congenital or acquired defects of the uterus
- Ovaries: Failure to ovulate, which is the most common infertility problem
- Fallopian tubes: Abnormalities or damage to the fallopian tubes
- Peritoneum: Anatomic defects, infection, adhesions, or adnexal masses in the peritoneum.

Treatment plans are based on the etiology, the number of years of infertility, and a woman's age. Underlying factors affecting fertility may be managed by medical treatment, pharmacotherapy, or surgical interventions.

It should be noted that men can also have or contribute to infertility issues. When a couple is having difficulty conceiving, men are tested early in the process of infertility evaluation.

Clinical Manifestations

Changes in the menstrual cycle and ovulation may be symptoms of a disease related to infertility. Symptoms include abnormal periods, with heavier or lighter bleeding than usual; irregular periods in which the number of days in between periods varies; no periods or the woman has never had a period; or periods that have stopped. Female infertility may be related to hormonal problems that cause skin changes such as acne; changes in sex drive; dark hair growth on the lips, chest, or chin; loss or thinning of hair; weight gain; milky discharge from nipples that is not related to lactation; and painful intercourse.

Linking Pathophysiology to Diagnosis and Treatment

A diagnosis of infertility is made if there is a failure to conceive, regardless of the cause, after 1 year of unprotected intercourse. Basic assessments are usually performed by a gynecologist, and then a referral is made to a reproductive specialist. Testing for couples may include hormone testing, genetic testing, imaging, ovulation testing, ovary reserve testing, hysterosalpingography, and other specialized testing. Treatment consists of reproductive technologies to treat infertility and may include in vitro fertilization, gamete intrafallopian transfer, zygote intrafallopian transfer, intracytoplasmic sperm injection, intrauterine insemination, or oocyte or embryo cryopreservation.[70]

CLINICAL POINT: Infertility can be very stressful for couples. Using any of the reproductive technologies that treat infertility can be a complicated process. Infertility nurses come from a variety of training backgrounds but may have had previous experience in women's healthcare. The infertility nurse will work closely with a couple to help execute treatment plans, provide teaching on subcutaneous and IM injections, and support the couple going through the challenging journey from diagnosis to fertility treatment to pregnancy. ■

Check Your Progress: Section 47.8

1. What condition is characterized by the inability to conceive after having regular unprotected sexual intercourse?
2. What is the most common problem of the reproductive organs associated with infertility?
3. At what point are men assessed during the infertility evaluation?

47.9 Sexual Dysfunction

About 30–50% of women have sexual problems at some point during their lifetime. If the problems are severe enough to cause distress, they may be considered sexual dysfunction. Sexual dysfunction can be described and diagnosed in terms of the specific problems, such as lack of interest or desire, difficulty becoming aroused or reaching orgasm, pain during sexual activity, involuntary tightening of the muscles around the vagina, or persistent and unwanted genital arousal. Almost all women with sexual dysfunction have features of more than one specific problem. For example, women who have difficulty becoming aroused may enjoy sex less, have difficulty reaching orgasm, or even find sex painful. These women and most women who have pain during sexual activity often understandably lose their interest and desire for sex. Many factors cause or contribute to various types of sexual dysfunction.[71]

Vaginismus

Vaginismus is vaginal tightness that causes discomfort, burning, pain, penetration problems, or complete inability to have intercourse. Painful spasmodic contraction of the vagina in response to physical contact or pressure during sexual intercourse, gynecologic exams, and even tampon insertion is painful.

Etiology and Pathogenesis

The exact etiology of vaginismus is unknown. It is usually linked to female anxiety or fear of intercourse, but it is not clear which precipitated initially: the vaginismus or the anxiety. Some women have vaginismus in all situations and with anything that is inserted vaginally. Others have pain only in certain circumstances, with one partner and not another, or only with sexual intercourse but not with tampons or gynecologic examinations.[72]

Clinical Manifestations

Pain with sexual intercourse is usually the woman's first sign that she has vaginismus. Pain happens only with penetration and usually, but not consistently, resolves with withdrawal. Women describe the pain as a tearing sensation. Often, women may feel discomfort when inserting a tampon or during a pelvic exam.

Linking Pathophysiology to Diagnosis and Treatment

Many healthcare providers are not familiar with vaginismus. Diagnosis involves a thorough history, including questions on penetration problems, underlying medical problems, and avoidance of intercourse with a partner due to pain, after childbirth, and for no identifiable physical cause. Physical therapists have a growing number of specialists treating pelvic floor and sexual pain disorders. Many physical therapists set up home programs so that women can work at their own pace. Women with vaginismus can do exercises privately, learning to control and relax the muscles around the vagina. Psychotherapy is usually recommended for women whose vaginismus is related to fear or anxiety.[73]

Orgasmic Dysfunction

Orgasmic dysfunction is a condition that occurs when there has never been an experience of orgasm, difficulty reaching orgasm, or substantially decreased intensity of orgasm even when there is arousal and sexual stimulation. In women, this condition is known as female orgasmic dysfunction. Men can also experience orgasmic dysfunction, but it is much less common.

Etiology and Pathogenesis

Female orgasmic disorder, defined as persistent or recurrent delay or absence of orgasm after a normal excitement phase, occurs in 3.4–5.8% of U.S. women. It can be either primary, in which the patient has never achieved orgasm, or secondary, which results from another sexual dysfunction, typically a hypoactive sexual desire disorder. Primary disorders can be genetic but are often associated with a history of trauma or abuse.

It can be difficult to determine the underlying cause of orgasmic dysfunction. Women may have difficulty reaching orgasm for multiple physical, emotional, or psychologic reasons. Other contributing factors may include age, medical conditions such as diabetes, history of gynecologic surgeries, taking medications such as SSRIs for depression, cultural or religious beliefs, embarrassment or shyness, guilt about enjoying sexual activity, a history of sexual abuse, mental health issues such as depression or anxiety, stress, poor self-esteem, relationship issues, or lack of trust. A combination of these factors may lead to difficulty achieving orgasm.

Clinical Manifestations

The main symptom of orgasmic dysfunction is the inability to achieve a sexual climax regardless of the stimulus. The inability to reach orgasm can lead to distress, which may make achieving orgasm in the future even more difficult. Having unsatisfying orgasms and/or taking longer than normal to achieve an orgasm are also symptoms. Women with orgasmic dysfunction may have difficulty achieving orgasm during either sexual intercourse or masturbation.

Linking Pathophysiology to Diagnosis and Treatment

Generally, primary orgasmic dysfunction does not resolve without treatment. Psychotherapy and counseling for the woman and her partner may help with primary orgasmic disorder, particularly if it is associated with abuse. No effective therapy exists for unexplained primary orgasmic disorder in which the patient has never achieved orgasm, even with masturbation. Secondary orgasmic disorder often resolves with treatment of the primary dysfunction. Adjunctive education on masturbation techniques may also be helpful.[74]

Dyspareunia

The term **dyspareunia** is broadly defined as episodes of pain with intercourse. With that definition, as many as 60% of women in the United States have probably experienced dyspareunia.[75] A much smaller group of women have symptoms severe enough to require medical attention. Too often, women with persistent symptoms do not seek medical care.

Etiology and Pathogenesis

Dyspareunia is painful or difficult sexual intercourse with genital pain experienced just before, during, or after sexual intercourse. Etiology may include inadequate lubrication, atrophy, vaginismus, vulvodynia, or vulvovestibulitis. Other etiologies are endometriosis, pelvic congestion, adhesions or infections, and adnexal pathology. Other urethral disorders such as cystitis and interstitial cystitis may also cause painful intercourse. There is no single etiology for the origins of the pain. This contributes to diagnostic difficulty.

Clinical Manifestations

Clinical manifestations of patients with dyspareunia include pain with coitus, but in some women, pain can occur after coitus. There are no consistent characteristics of women with dyspareunia. The incidence of dyspareunia is not associated with age, parity, marital status, race, income, or educational level. Pain before coitus may be associated with irritation of the vaginal tissues.[76]

Linking Pathophysiology to Diagnosis and Treatment

Dyspareunia has historically been defined by psychologic theories, but the current treatment approach favors identification of causative factors to reach a definitive diagnosis.[77,78] Treatment for dyspareunia depends on the origins of the issue. The diagnosis should begin with an extensive history, including a sexual health history and an obstetric history. Questions are asked that can help guide the diagnosis of dyspareunia. The physical examination should include examination of all vaginal structures and tissues. The healthcare provider should note any areas of dryness, areas of skin breakdown, erythema in vaginal tissues, or discharge from the cervix. Lubrication can reduce issues of dryness and alleviates superficial cases of dyspareunia. Patients should be encouraged to try different sexual positions that may alleviate pain. Assessment for STIs is included in the exam, and antibiotics are initiated for positive cultures. For postmenopausal women, topical estrogens can be prescribed to help reduce symptoms of dryness and atrophy. If a mass is felt on palpation, ultrasound can be ordered. If the pain is not relieved with treatments, stronger pain control methods could be initiated, or a referral to a pain specialist may be necessary. If sexual abuse is suspected in the patient's history, a mental health provider should be recommended.[77,78]

CLINICAL POINT: Nurses need to be aware of the high prevalence of sexual problems in women in the United States. Approximately 40% of women have sexual concerns, and 12% report distressing sexual problems. The origin of the word *dyspareunia* means "bad or difficult mating." The etiology of these problems ranges from simple anatomic problems to complex psychosocial or biologically based issues. The intricate balance of anatomic, physiologic, and psychologic factors contribute to painful intercourse. ■

Check Your Progress: Section 47.9

1. What symptoms characterize vaginismus?
2. What are the broad reasons of orgasmic dysfunction?
3. How does the diagnostic process of dyspareunia begin?

CHAPTER SUMMARY

47.1 Chapter Overview and Case Studies

Describe the normal female reproductive system and concepts related to disorders of the female reproductive system.

- Disorders of the female reproductive system can involve multiple reproductive organs, including the ovaries, fallopian tubes, uterus, cervix, vagina, or breasts. Disorders may involve an alteration in menstruation, pelvic pain, or infertility.
- The female reproductive system has five primary hormones that affect female reproductive health: estrogen, progesterone, gonadotropin-releasing hormone, follicle-stimulating hormone and luteinizing hormone, all of which are affected by aging and disease.
- Diagnosis and treatment of reproductive system disorders are complicated by societal attitudes, behaviors surrounding reproductive health, and healthcare providers' avoidance of discussing sexual problems. Treatment may be delayed because of denial, fear, embarrassment, and guilt.
- Concepts related to disorders of the female reproductive system include, but are not limited to, comfort and pain, inflammation and oxidative stress, trauma, metabolism, mood and affect, and tissue integrity.

47.2 Disorders of the Female Breasts

Differentiate the causes, classification, underlying pathogenesis, and clinical manifestations of disorders of the female breasts and approaches to diagnosis and treatment of these conditions across the lifespan.

- Benign breast disease encompasses a range of disorders that may be discovered as a palpable lesion or on imaging. After the lesion is determined to be benign, treatment is focused on symptom relief and patient education. Some benign lesions such as atypical hyperplasia can be considered risk markers for potential development of breast cancer in the future and can be used as such to guide prevention measures.
- Galactorrhea is a milky nipple discharge unrelated to normal milk produced during breastfeeding. Galactorrhea is not a disease but could be a sign of an underlying problem. It usually occurs in women who have never had children and can occur after menopause. Excessive breast stimulation, medication side effects, birth control, cocaine, chronic kidney disease, spinal cord injury, or pituitary disorders that increase the level of prolactin, a milk-stimulating hormone, can be the cause. The condition may resolve, or the underlying condition may need to be treated.
- Mastitis is inflammation of the breast tissue that may be accompanied by infection and may respond to antibiotics. Breastfeeding should be continued to relieve engorgement and mastitis symptoms in a lactating female. Mastitis does not always occur during lactation. Forms of nonlactational mastitis include periductal mastitis and idiopathic granulomatous mastitis.
- Breast cancer is a malignant tumor that originates in the cells of the breast. To date, breast cancer is the most commonly diagnosed cancer among women. Epidemiologic studies have found that certain risk factors contribute to a greater percentage of developing breast cancer; these include age, gender, and a family history of breast cancer in first-degree relatives under the age of 50.

47.3 Disorders of Menstruation

Differentiate the causes, classification, underlying pathogenesis, and clinical manifestations of disorders of menstruation and approaches to diagnosis and treatment of these conditions across the lifespan.

- Dysmenorrhea or painful menstruation is one of women's most common gynecologic problems. Prostaglandins, which form in the lining of the uterus during menstruation, cause muscle contractions in the uterus, increasing pain and decreasing blood flow and oxygen to the uterus. They also contribute to the nausea, diarrhea, fatigue, headache, fatigue some women experience. Symptoms vary in type and severity, as does treatment.
- Amenorrhea is the absence of menses. This can be transient, intermittent, or a permanent condition as a result of a hypothalamus, pituitary, ovarian, uterus, or vaginal dysfunction. It is classified as either primary, which is the absence of menarche by age 15, or secondary, which is an absence of menses for more than 3 months in girls or women who previously had regular menstrual cycles.
- Dysfunctional uterine bleeding (DUB) is menstrual bleeding of abnormal quantities, duration, or schedule. It occurs in 10–35% of women as a common gynecologic problem. Chronic prolonged uterine bleeding can result in anemia, can interfere with daily activities, and can raise concerns about uterine cancer. Menorrhagia is a common reason for referral to a gynecologist, and iron deficiency anemia may develop in 21–67% of these cases. Most DUB can be managed in outpatient setting, but if it is severe enough, it may necessitate emergency medical care.
- Premenstrual syndrome (PMS) refers to a group of physical and behavioral symptoms that occur during the second half of the menstrual cycle. Symptoms

may include mood swings, anxiety, irritability, anger, decreased interest in usual activities, concentration difficulty, fatigue, back pain, changes in appetite, breast tenderness, swelling, headaches, weight gain, and feelings of being overwhelmed and out of control.

47.4 Disorders of the Ovaries and Fallopian Tubes

Differentiate the causes, classification, underlying pathogenesis, and clinical manifestations of disorders of the ovaries and fallopian tubes and approaches to diagnosis and treatment of these conditions across the lifespan.

- Polycystic ovary syndrome (PCOS) is a condition that occurs in 5–10% of women. Elevated hormones or androgens cause cessation of menses and irregular periods, along with symptoms of facial hair, acne, and male-pattern hair thinning.
- Benign ovarian cysts are fluid-filled sacs that develop in or on the ovary. Cysts can range from 0.5 inches to 4 inches in diameter but are not considered cancerous.
- Ectopic pregnancy is an extrauterine pregnancy. It generally occurs in the fallopian tube; other sites include the cervix, the proximal segment of the fallopian tube (cornual), on a cesarean scar (hysterotomy), intramural, ovarian, abdominal, and rarely both uterine and extrauterine (heterotopic). Diagnosis is made by measurement of the human chorionic gonadotropin (HCG) and findings on ultrasound. Options for treatment depend on the site and may include surgery or methotrexate therapy.
- Ovarian cancer is the second most common cancer of the female reproductive organs in the United States. The average age of women affected is 63 years. Epithelial ovarian cancer, the most common type, is treatable with surgery and chemotherapy.

47.5 Disorders of the Uterus

Differentiate the causes, classification, underlying pathogenesis, and clinical manifestations of disorders of the uterus and approaches to diagnosis and treatment of these conditions across the lifespan.

- Endometrial polyps are localized tumors in the mucosa of the uterine cavity. They are common findings in women both with and without symptoms. Most endometrial polyps are asymptomatic. Symptomatic premenopausal women with endometrial polyps suffer from abnormal bleeding, spotting, or menorrhagia. Risks include advanced age, hypertension, obesity, and use of tamoxifen.
- Adenomyosis is a benign condition that can affect the entire uterus or just a part of it. In this condition, the endometrial tissue invades the myometrium lining, producing enlargement of the uterus.
- Leiomyomas are also known as fibroids or myomas. They are benign soft tissue tumors resulting from an overproduction of smooth muscle cells surrounded by compressed muscle fibers. Abnormal uterine bleeding or menorrhagia, pelvic pressure or pain, and dysmenorrhea can occur. The size of the fibroids varies; the larger the fibroid, the more symptoms.
- Endometriosis is the presence and growth of functioning endometrial tissue in places other than the uterus. The exact cause of endometriosis is unknown. It is hypothesized that in endometriosis, the endometrial cells move from the uterus and become implanted in ectopic sites.
- Endometrial cancer is cancer of the endometrium lining of the uterus. According to the NIH and the American Cancer Institute, endometrial cancer is the most common gynecologic malignancy in the United States.

47.6 Disorders of the Cervix, Vagina, and Vulva

Differentiate the causes, classification, underlying pathogenesis, and clinical manifestations of disorders of the cervix, vagina, and vulva and approaches to diagnosis and treatment of these conditions across the lifespan.

- Cervicitis is an inflammation of the cervix that can be caused by infection or other vaginal issues. The most common cause of infectious cervicitis is sexually transmitted chlamydia or gonorrhea.
- Vaginitis is an inflammation of the vagina resulting in discharge, itching, and pain. Vaginitis results from a change in the normal balance of bacteria and infection. It can also be a result of reduced estrogen levels after menopause.
- Vulvovestibulitis is characterized by severe pain during attempted vaginal entry, including intercourse or tampon insertion. Women who are affected are usually young and sexually active.
- Bartholinitis is an inflammation of the Bartholin gland. The Bartholin glands are located on either side of the posterior vaginal opening in the labia minora. The glands, which are typically nonpalpable, play a key role in vaginal lubrication and mucus secretion.
- Cervical cancer is the third most common cancer diagnosed among women in the United States and worldwide. Except in rare cases, cervical cancers are caused by the human papillomavirus (HPV). While it is possible to transmit HPV without sexual contact, a majority of HPV cases come from some type of sexual interaction.
- Vaginal cancer is a rare type of cancer in which malignant cancer cells form in the vagina. It presents more often in women age 60 years and older and in adults who have a history of HPV.
- Vulvar cancer is a form of cancer that occurs on the outer surface area of the female genitalia. Vulvar cancer commonly forms as a lump or sore on the vulva, causing itching. It can occur at any age but is most commonly seen in older women age 70 years or older.

47.7 Disorders of the Female Pelvis

Differentiate the causes, classification, underlying pathogenesis, and clinical manifestations of disorders of the female pelvis and approaches to diagnosis and treatment of these conditions across the lifespan.

- Pelvic inflammatory disease (PID) is an infection caused by bacteria that originates from the vagina or cervix and is carried to the uterus, fallopian tubes, and ovaries. The main risk factors are multiple sex partners, early sexual activity, young age for first intercourse, and use of an intrauterine device for contraception.
- Pelvic organ prolapse is drop of pelvic organs when pelvic floor muscles weaken or become injured. Multiparous women are at particular risk for pelvic organ prolapse.

47.8 Disorders of Fertility

Differentiate the causes, classification, underlying pathogenesis, and clinical manifestations of disorders of female fertility and approaches to diagnosis and treatment of these conditions across the lifespan.

- Disorders of female fertility involve the inability to conceive after having regular unprotected sexual intercourse. Infertility can involve the inability to contribute to conception or to the inability to carry a pregnancy to full term. Infertility can stem from irregular menstrual cycles or as a result of known risk factors for infertility, such as endometriosis, a history of pelvic inflammatory disease, or reproductive tract malformations.

47.9 Sexual Dysfunction

Differentiate the causes, classification, underlying pathogenesis, and clinical manifestations of sexual dysfunction and approaches to diagnosis and treatment of these conditions across the lifespan.

- Vaginismus is a condition in which women experience vaginal tightness, pain, and penetration problems. Treatment includes pelvic floor exercises, insertion and dilation training, pain elimination techniques, and exercises to help the woman identify and resolve contributing emotional factors.
- Orgasmic dysfunction is characterized by a recurrent delay or absence of orgasm following sexual arousal and stimulation. Symptoms include significant distress and interpersonal difficulty. Treatment for female orgasmic disorder consists principally of education and psychosocial interventions.
- Dyspareunia is pain during or after intercourse; often accompanied by vaginismus, which is a tightening of vaginal muscles during penetration. Pain from dyspareunia may involve the vagina, clitoris, or labia.

REVIEW QUESTIONS

1. Which type of breast mass is a form of breast cancer?
   a. Fibrocystic disease
   b. Lobular carcinoma
   c. Fibroadenoma
   d. Intraductal papilloma

2. A new mother who is breastfeeding has a sudden onset of breast tenderness, warmth, inflammation, and induration of her right breast and is diagnosed with mastitis. When she asks whether she should continue to breastfeed her infant, which of the following is the most appropriate response from her nurse?
   a. "Continue breastfeeding only from the left breast."
   b. "Discontinue breastfeeding until after the infection has cleared."
   c. "Continue breastfeeding from both breasts."
   d. "Stop breastfeeding and pumping from the right breast."

3. A 50-year old female with galactorrhea is found to have decreased levels of T4. The nurse is confident that the client understands the reason for the galactorrhea when the client says which of the following?
   a. "The release of prolactin from the pituitary tumor is blocking the secretion of dopamine."
   b. "Decreased clearance of prolactin from my kidneys is causing lactation from my breasts."
   c. "The increase in thyrotropin-releasing hormones is stimulating release of prolactin."
   d. "An increase in estrogen and oxytocin, due to my age, is causing lactation."

4. A 40-year old female with a family history of breast cancer asks the nurse about her risk factors for the disease. Which of the following statements reflects appropriate understanding of her risk of having breast cancer?
   a. "I understand that my risk is higher because my mother was diagnosed before age 50."
   b. "I'm at high risk even though my great-grandmother died of breast cancer at age 80."
   c. "I have a very low risk because I have the *BRCA1* gene mutation."
   d. "Just because I've had benign breast disease in the past doesn't mean I'm at higher risk."

5. A 45-year old perimenopausal female complains of profuse bleeding with blood clots during her last three periods. She is diagnosed with dysfunctional uterine bleeding and is wondering whether she really needs

treatment. She asks about common complications of this disorder and what may result if she doesn't have treatment. Which of the following would be the most appropriate response from the nurse?

a. "It is common to have vaginal dryness in between periods, which could lead to discomfort during sex."
b. "The amount of blood loss is not usually enough to cause iron deficiency anemia, but you'll need to eat lots of green leafy vegetables."
c. "The low levels of estrogen production can lead to osteoporosis and bone fractures."
d. "The lining of the uterus can thicken, causing hyperplastic cells and possible malignancy."

6. A 32-year old female with a history of undergoing infertility treatment with hormonal medication presents with abdominal pain and vaginal bleeding that has soaked her underwear. Her blood pressure is 128/80, her heart rate is 92, and her respiratory rate is 20. She states that she is 10 weeks' pregnant and terrified of losing the baby. What is the initial priority assessment that should be performed to evaluate the need for emergent treatment?
   a. Orthostatic blood pressure to examine fluid status
   b. Pelvic ultrasound to evaluate for ectopic rupture
   c. Serum beta-HCG level to determine the viability of her pregnancy
   d. Rh status to evaluate for the need to administer immunoglobulin

7. A 36-year old female was recently diagnosed with cervical cancer. Which of the following statements by the clients reflects appropriate understanding of the cause of cervical cancer?
   a. "I shouldn't have used tampons during my periods."
   b. "I've never had a sexually transmitted disease."
   c. "The cancer was caused by having multiple sex partners."
   d. "Human papillomavirus caused the cervical cancer."

8. Which of the following statements is *correct* regarding the cause of sexual dysfunction?
   a. Sexual dysfunction is always associated with loss of interest in and desire for sex.
   b. Psychologic and physiologic factors can contribute to sexual dysfunction.
   c. Female sexual dysfunction is due to anxiety or fear of intercourse.
   d. Vaginismus, involuntary tightening of vaginal muscles, is a major cause of sexual dysfunction.

ANSWERS

Answers to Review Questions can be found in Appendix A. Answers to Case Study and Check Your Progress questions are available on the faculty resources site. Please consult with your instructor.

RECOMMENDED WEBSITES

American Association of Sexuality Educators, Counselors and Therapists
https://www.aasect.org

American Cancer Society
https://www.cancer.org

The American Congress of Obstetricians and Gynecologists
https://www.acog.org

Association of Women's Health, Obstetric and Neonatal Nurses
https://www.awhonn.org

Centers for Disease Control and Prevention: Women's Reproductive Health
https://www.cdc.gov/reproductivehealth/womensrh

Foundation for Women's Cancer
http://www.foundationforwomenscancer.org

National Breast Cancer Foundation
http://www.nationalbreastcancer.org

National Cancer Institute
https://www.cancer.gov

National Institutes of Health Office of Research on Women's Health
https://orwh.od.nih.gov

Nurse Practitioners in Women's Health
https://www.npwh.org

Office on Women's Health, U.S. Department of Health and Human Services
https://www.womenshealth.gov

REFERENCES

1. Taylor, A, & Gosney, M. A. (2011). Sexuality in older age: Essential considerations for healthcare professionals. *Age and Ageing, 40*(5), 538–543. doi:10.1093/ageing/afr049
2. Barth, C, Villringer, A., & Sacher, J. (2015). Sex hormones affect neurotransmitters and shape the adult female brain during hormonal transition periods. *Frontiers in Neuroscience, 37*(9), 1–20. doi:10.3389/fnins.2015.00037
3. Pearlman, M. D., & Griffin, J. L. (2010). Benign breast disease. *Obstetrics and Gynecology, 116*(3), 747–758. doi:10.1097/AOG.0b013e31881ee9fc7
4. Lee, E. (2009). Evidence based management of benign breast diseases. *American Journal for Nurse Practitioners, 13*(7–8), 22–31.
5. Santen, R. J. (2014). Benign breast disease in women. [Updated 2014 Feb 22]. In L. J. De Groot, G. Chrousos, K. Dungan, et al., (Eds.), *Endotext*. South Dartmouth, MA: MDText.com. Available at https://www.ncbi.nlm.nih.gov/books/NBK278994
6. Hartmann, L. C., Degnim, A. C., Santen, R. J., Dupont, W. D., & Ghosh, K. (2015). Atypical hyperplasia of the breast: Risk assessment and management options. *New England Journal of Medicine, 372*, 78–89. doi:10.1056/NEJMsr1407164
7. Huang, W. (2012). Evaluation and management of galactorrhea. *American Family Physician, 85*(11), 1073–1080.
8. Patrascu, O. M., Chopra, D., & Dwivedi, S. (2015). Galactorrhoea: Report of two cases. *Maedica: A Journal of Clinical Medicine, 10*(2), 136–139. Available at https://www.ncbi.nlm.nih.gov/pmc/articles/PMC5327809
9. Yang, L., Wu, D., & Fan Z. M. (2015). Retrospective analysis of pathologic nipple discharge. *Genetics and Molecular Research, 14*(1), 1443–1449. doi:10.4238/2015.february.13.23.
10. Jahanfar, S., Ng, C. J., & Teng, C. L. (2013). Antibiotics for mastitis in breastfeeding women. *Cochrane Database Systematic Review, 28*(2), CD005459. doi:10.1002/14651858
11. Dixon, M. (2011). Treatment of breast infection. *British Medical Journal, 342*, d396. doi:10.1136/bmj.d396
12. Shaw, R. W., Luesley, D., & Monga, A. K. (2011). *Gynaecology*. Edinburgh, UK: Churchill Livingstone/Elsevier.
13. Cashin-Garbutt, A., & Mandal, A. (2013). Breast cancer pathophysiology. *News-Medical.Net*. Available at http://www.news-medical.net/health/Breast-Cancer-Pathophysiology.aspx
14. Chalasani, P., & Harris, J. E. (2016). Breast cancer. *Medscape*. Available at http://emedicine.medscape.com/article/1947145-overview
15. Sazman, B., Fleegle, S., & Tully, A. (2012). Common breast problem. *American Family Physician, 86*(4), 343–349. Available at http://www.aafp.org/afp/2012/815/p343.html
16. Miller, J. W., Royalty, J., Henley, J., White, A., & Richardson, L. C. (2015). Breast and cervical cancers diagnosed and stage at diagnosis among women served through the National Breast and Cervical Cancer Early Detection Program. *Cancer Causes & Control Cancer Causes Control, 26*(5), 741–747. doi:10.1007/s10552-015-0543-2
17. Chelbowski, R. T., & Budoff, M. J. (2016). Changing adjuvant breast-cancer therapy with a signal for prevention. *New England Journal of Medicine, 375*, 274–275. doi:10.1045/NEJMe1606031
18. Klukin, L. M., & Morozov, S. Y. (2014). Analysis of modern methods for breast cancer diagnosis. *Biomedical Engineering, 48*(3), 164–167. doi:10.1007/s10527-014-9444-z
19. Lonzetta, N., Tortorelli, C. L., & Nassar, A. (2010). Clinicians guide to imaging and pathologic findings in benign breast disease. *Mayo Clinic Proceedings, 85*(3), 274–279. doi:10.4065/mcp.2009.0656
20. Kennedy, R. D., & Boughey, J. C. (2013). Management of pediatric and adolescent breast masses. *Seminars in Plastic Surgery*, 27(1), 19–22. doi:10.1055/s-oo33-1343991
21. Perry, M. (2012). Treatment options for dysmenorrhoea. *Practice Nursing, 23*(4), 195–198. doi:10.12968/pnur.2012.23.4.195
22. Iacovides, S., Avidon, I., & Baker, F. C. (2015). What we know about primary dysmenorrhea today: A critical review. *Human Reproduction Update, 21*(6), 762–778.
23. Sasaki, K. J., & Zuckerman, A. L. (2012). Menstruation disorders in adolescents: Background, pathophysiology, etiology. *Medscape*. Available at http://emedicine.medscape.com/article/953945-overview
24. Golden, N. H., & Carlson, J. L. (2008). The pathophysiology of amenorrhea in the adolescent. *Annals of the New York Academy of Sciences, 1135*(1), 163–178. doi:10.1196/annals.1429.014
25. Heinman, DL. (2010). Amenorrhea. *Primary Care Clinic Office Practice, 36*, 1–17. doi:10.1016/j.pop.2010.10.005
26. Polotsky, A. J. (2010). Amenorrhea caused by extremes of body mass: Pathophysiology and sequelae. *Contemporary OB/GYN, 55*(8), 18(6). Available at http://contemporaryobgyn.modernmedicine.com/%5Bnode-source-domain-raw%5D/news/modernmedicine/modern-medicine-now/amenorrhea-caused-extremes-body-mas?page=full
27. Felix, H. M., & Cervonka, D. (2012). Dysfunctional uterine bleeding from the primary care perspective. *Journal of the American Academy of Physician Assistants, 25*(4), 47–49. doi:10.1097/01720610-201204000-00009
28. Raines, K. (2010). Diagnosing premenstrual syndrome. *Journal for Nurse Practitioners, 6*(3), 224–225. doi:10.1016/j.nurpra.2009.12.013
29. Cunningham, J., Yonkers, K. A., O'Brien, S., & Eriksson, E. (2011). Update on research and treatment of premenstrual dysphoric disorder. *Harvard Review of Psychiatry, 12*(2), 120–137. doi10.1080/10673220902891836
30. Legro, R. S., Arslanian, S. A., Ehrmann, D. A., et al. (2013). Diagnosis and treatment of polycystic ovary syndrome: An Endocrine Society clinical practice guideline. *Journal of Clinical Endocrinology and Metabolism*, 98(12), 4565–4592. doi:10.1210/jc.2014–2350
31. Palomba, S., Santagni, S., Falbo, A., & Battista La Sala, G. (2015). Complications and challenges associated with polycystic ovary syndrome: Current perspectives. *International Journal of Women's Health, 7*, 745–763. doi:10.2147/IJWH.S70314
32. Grabosch, S. M., & Helm, W. (2016). Ovarian cysts. *Medscape*. Available at http://emedicine.medscape.com/article/255865
33. Oliver, A., & Overton, C. (2014). Detecting ovarian disorders in primary care. *Practitioner, 258*(1769), 15–19. Available at http://www.thepractitioner.co.uk
34. Royal College of Obstetricians & Gynecologists. (2011). *Management of suspected ovarian masses in premenopausal women*. Available at https://www.rcog.org.uk/globalassets/documents/guidelines/gtg_62.pdf
35. Sepilian, V. P., & Wood, E. (2016). Ectopic pregnancy. *Medscape*. Available at http://emedicine.medscape.com/article/2041923-overview
36. Dulay, A. T. (2016). Ectopic pregnancy. *Merck Manual*. Available at http://www.merckmanuals.com/professional/gynecology-and-obstetrics/abnormalities-of-pregnancy/ectopic-pregnancy
37. Tew, W. P., & Moore, K. M. (2016). The approach to ovarian cancer in older women. *UpToDate*. Available at https://www.uptodate.com/contents/the-approach-to-ovarian-cancer-in-older-women

38. Prat, J. (2012). New insights into ovarian cancer pathology. *Annals of Oncology, 23*(Suppl. 10), 111–117. doi:10.1093/annonc/mds300
39. American Association of Gynecologic Laparoscopists. (2012). AAGL practice report: Practice guidelines for the diagnosis and management of endometrial polyps. *Journal of Minimally Invasive Gynecology, 19*(1), 3–10. doi:10.1016/j.jmig.2011.09.003
40. Ünal, B., Doğan, S., Karaveli, F., et al. (2014). Giant endometrial polyp in a postmenopausal woman without hormone/drug use and vaginal bleeding. *Case Reports in Obstetrics and Gynecology, 2014*, 518398. doi:10.1155/2014/518398
41. Annan, J. J., Registrar, S., et al. (2012). The management of endometrial polyps in the 21st century. *The Obstetrician & Gynaecologist, 14*(1), 33–38. doi:10.1111/j.1744-4667.2011.00091.x
42. Taran, F., Stewart, E., & Brucker, S. (2013). Adenomyosis: Epidemiology, risk factors, clinical phenotype and surgical and interventional alternatives to hysterectomy. *Geburtshilfe und Frauenheilkunde, 73*(9), 924–931. doi:10.1055/s-0033-1350840
43. Cockerham, A. Z. (2012). Adenomyosis: A challenge in clinical gynecology. *Journal of Midwifery & Women's Health, 57*(3), 212–220. doi:10.1111/j.1542-2011.2011.00117.x
44. Levgur, M. (2007). Diagnosis of adenomyosis: A review. *Journal of Reproductive Medicine, 52*, 177–193.
45. Vilos, G. A., Allaire, C., Laberge, P. Y., & Leyland, N. (2013). The management of uterine leiomyomas. *Journal of Obstetrics and Gynaecology Canada, 37*(2), 157–178. doi:10.10116/S1701-2163(15)30338-8
46. American Association of Gynecologic Laparoscopists. (2012). Advancing minimally invasive gynecology worldwide. AAGL practice report: Practice guidelines for the diagnosis and management of submucous leiomyomas. *Journal of Minimally Invasive Gynecology, 19*, 152–171.
47. Eisenberg, E. (2016). Endometriosis. *Merck Manual*. Available at http://www.merckmanuals.com/professional/gynecology-and-obstetrics/endometriosis/endometriosis
48. Davila, W., Rivlin, M., & Alderman, E. (2016). Endometriosis: Practice essentials, Pathophysiology, etiology. *Medscape*. Available at http://emedicine.medscape.com/article/271899-overview
49. Al-Talib, A., Nezhat, F., & Tulandi, T. (2012). Etiology and fertility preservation treatment for young women with endometrial cancer. *Journal of Gynecologic Surgery, 28*(4), 280–287. doi:10.1089/gyn.2011.0019
50. Holland, A. C., Hodges, A., Catron, K. S., Bevis, K. S., Berman, N. R., & Meneses, K. Endometrial cancer: Using evidence to impact practice and policy. *Journal for Nurse Practitioners, 12*(6), 395–402. doi:10.1016/j.nurpra.2016.04.006.
51. National Cancer Institute. (2017). *Endometrial cancer treatment (PDQ®): Patient version*. Available at http://www.cancer.gov/types/uterine/patient/endometrial-treatment-pdq
52. Committee on Practice Bulletins—Gynecology and the Society of Gynecologic Oncology. (2015). ACOG guidelines at a glance: Endometrial cancer. *Contemporary OB/GYN*. Available at http://contemporaryobgyn.modernmedicine.com/contemporary-obgyn/news/acog-guidelines-glance-endometrial-cancer
53. Xin, L., & Ruijin, S. (2014). PCOS and obesity: Insulin resistance might be a common etiology for the development of type I endometrial carcinoma. *American Journal of Cancer Research, 4*(1), 73–79. Available from: Academic Search Complete, Ipswich, MA.
54. Pinkerton, J. V. (2016). Polycystic ovary syndrome (PCOS). *Merck Manual Professional Version*. Available at https://www.merckmanuals.com/professional/gynecology-and-obstetrics/menstrual-abnormalities/polycystic-ovary-syndrome-pcos
55. Centers for Disease Control and Prevention. (2015). *Diseases characterized by urethritis and cervicitis*. Available at http://www.cdc.gov/std/tg2015/urethritis-and-cervicitis.htm
56. Soper, D. E. Cervicitis. (2016). *Merck Manual Professional Version*. Available at http://www.merckmanuals.com/professional/gynecology-and-obstetrics/vaginitis,-cervicitis,-and-pelvic-inflammatory-disease-pid/cervicitis
57. Ollendorff, A. T. (2017). Cervicitis: Background, etiology, epidemiology. *Medscape*. Available at http://emedicine.medscape.com/article/253402-overview
58. Kumar, N., Behera, B., Sairi, S. S., Pal, K., Ray, S. S., & Roy, S. (2011), Bacterial vaginosis: Etiology and modalities of treatment. *Journal of Pharmacy and BioAllied Sciences, 3*(4), 496–503. doi:10.4103/0975-7406.90102
59. U.S. Preventive Services Task Force. (2016). Evidence summary: Bacterial vaginosis in pregnancy to prevent preterm delivery: Screening. Retrieved from https://www.uspreventiveservicestaskforce.org/Page/Document/evidence-summary12/bacterial-vaginosis-in-pregnancy-to-prevent-preterm-delivery-screening
60. Lee, M. Y., Dalpiaz, A., Schwamb, R., Miao, Y., Waltzer, W., & Khan, A. (2015). Clinical pathology of Bartholin's glands: A review of the literature. *Current Urology, 8*(1), 22–25. doi:10.1159/000365683.
61. Quinn, A. (2016). Bartholin gland diseases. Practice essentials, pathophysiology, epidemiology. *Medscape*. Available at http://emedicine.medscape.com/article/777112-overview
62. Barroso dos Reis, H. L., Petillo de Pinho, C. R., & de Carvalho Ferreira, D. (2014). Diagnosis and management of acute puerperal bartholinitis caused by Escherichia coli. *Revista da Sociedade Brasileira de Medicina Tropical, 47*(6), 814. doi:10.1590/0037-8682-0160-2014
63. Koeneman, M. M., Kruse, A. J., Kooreman, L. F. S., et al. (2016). TOPical imiquimod treatment of high-grade cervical intraepithelial neoplasia (TOPIC trial): Study protocol for a randomized controlled trial. *BMC Cancer, 16*(1). doi:10.1186/s12885-016-2187-3
64. Boardman, C., Huh, W., & Matthews, K. (2016). Cervical cancer. Practice essentials, background pathophysiology. *Medscape*. Available at http://emedicine.medscape.com/article/253513-overview
65. Bardawi, T., & Manetta, A. (2015). Vaginal cancer. *Medscape*. Available at http://emedicine.medscape.com/article/269188-overview
66. Alkatout, I., Schubert, M., Garbrecht, H., et al. (2015). Vulvar cancer: Epidemiology, clinical presentation, and management options. *International Journal of Women's Health, 7*, 305–313.
67. Creasman, W. T., Buchanan, R., Talavera, F., et al. (2016). Malignant vulvar lesions. *Medscape*. Available at http://emedicine.medscape.com/article/264898-overview
68. Shepard, S. M., Karjane, N., & Rivlin, M. E. (2016). Pelvic inflammatory disease treatment & management. *Medscape*. Available at http://emedicine.medscape.com/article/256448-treatment
69. Lazarou, G., Bogdan, A. G., & Strohbehn, K. (2016). Pelvic organ prolapse. *Medscape*. Available at http://emedicine.medscape.com/article/276259-overview
70. Rebar, R. W. (2016). Overview of infertility. *Merck Manual Professional Version*. Available at https://www.merckmanuals.com/professional/gynecology-and-obstetrics/sexual-dysfunction-in-women/orgasmic-disorder
71. Hayslett, R. L., & Nykamp, D. (2015). Sexual dysfunction in women. *US Pharmacist, 40*(9), 46–49. Available at http://www.medscape.com/viewarticle/852664
72. Basson, R. (2013). Vaginismus. *Merck Manual Professional Version*. Available at https://www.merckmanuals.com/professional/gynecology-and-obstetrics/sexual-dysfunction-in-women/vaginismus
73. Basson, R. (2013). Orgasmic disorder. *Merck Manual Professional Version*. Available at https://www.merckmanuals.com/professional/

gynecology-and-obstetrics/sexual-dysfunction-in-women/orgasmic-disorder

74. Preda, A., & Bienenfeld, D. (2015). Female orgasmic disorder. *Medscape*. Available at http://emedicine.medscape.com/article/2185837-overview
75. Edwards, A., & Bowen, M. (2010). Dyspareunia. *Practice Nurse, 39*(6), 26–30. doi:10.1016/j.mpmed.2010.03.001
76. Stoelting-Gettelfinger, W. (2010). A case study and comprehensive differential diagnosis and care plan for the three Ds of women's health: Primary dysmenorrhea, secondary dysmenorrhea, and dyspareunia. *Journal of the American Academy of Nurse Practitioners, 22*(10), 513–522. doi:10.1111/j.1745-7599.2010.00544.x
77. Garard, R., Vancaille, T., & Farrell, E. (2011). Pelvic pain: A diagnosis in itself. *Australian Nursing and Midwifery Journal, 21*(3), 36–39. doi:10.1055/b-0036-134932
78. Mayo Clinic. (2015). *Painful intercourse (dyspareunia): Definition.* Available at http://www.mayoclinic.org/diseases-conditions/painful-intercourse/basics/definition/con-20033293

Chapter 48

Disorders of the Male Reproductive System

Shari Lynn

Chapter Outline and Learning Outcomes

48.1 Chapter Overview and Case Studies

Describe the male reproductive system, disorders related to it, and the concepts integral to managing those disorders.

48.2 Disorder of the Prostate

Differentiate the causes, classification, underlying pathogenesis, and clinical manifestations of disorders of the prostate and approaches to diagnosis and treatment of these conditions.

48.3 Disorders of the Testicles

Differentiate the causes, classification, underlying pathogenesis, and clinical manifestations of disorders of the testicles and approaches to diagnosis and treatment of these conditions across the lifespan.

48.4 Disorders of the Penis

Differentiate the causes, classification, underlying pathogenesis, and clinical manifestations of disorders of the penis and approaches to diagnosis and treatment of these conditions across the lifespan.

KEY TERMS

Androgen, 1195
Benign prostatic hyperplasia (BPH), 1195
Cryptorchidism, 1200
Digital rectal examination (DRE), 1195
Dihydrotestosterone (DHT), 1195
Dysuria, 1195
Epididymis, 1198
Epididymitis, 1198
Epispadias, 1201
Erectile dysfunction, 1201
Gynecomastia, 1200
Hydrocele, 1198
Hypospadias, 1200
Nocturia, 1195
Orchiectomy, 1200
Orchitis, 1198
Paraphimosis, 1201
Peyronie disease, 1201
Phimosis, 1201
Priapism, 1201
Prostate cancer, 1196
Prostate specific antigen (PSA), 1194
Prostatitis, 1194
Spermatocele, 1198
Testicular cancer, 1199
Testicular torsion, 1198
Testosterone, 1195
Varicocele, 1198
Watchful waiting, 1196

ABBREVIATIONS

BPH—benign prostatic hyperplasia
DHT—dihydrotestosterone
DRE—digital rectal exam
PSA—prostate specific antigen

48.1 Chapter Overview and Case Studies

The male reproductive system involves many different anatomic parts, each of which can develop its own problems. Men's reproductive health and sexuality are closely related. Multiple disorders can result in erectile dysfunction, which is the inability to maintain an erection, and infertility. These are often difficult subjects for men to discuss, so they sometimes delay needed visits to a healthcare provider when issues arise.

Concepts Related to the Male Reproductive System

There are many physiologic disorders that relate to male reproductive health, and these disorders also have a psychologic aspect. A young man who receives a diagnosis of testicular cancer and is facing an orchiectomy may also be concerned about his ability to start a family. A man who receives a diagnosis of prostate cancer may be afraid that his life will soon end. Sexuality is an important part of being a human being and is important to health and quality of life, and it can be affected by disorders of the reproductive system. The thought of a life cut short by a diagnosis of cancer has a huge psychologic impact, as do issues that may affect sexual function. Healthcare providers should give the psychologic aspects of reproductive disorders the same priority as the physiologic aspects. Holistic treatment of patients with reproductive disorders includes discussing treatment options and exploring patients' emotions related to diagnosis and treatment.

Physical factors that may affect the male reproductive system include aging, chronic disease, poor perfusion, sexually transmitted infections (STIs), and inflammation. Individuals with mobility issues related to musculoskeletal or neurologic disabilities may have difficulty with sexual relations and sexual responses. The proximity and interrelatedness of the sexual organs and the organs of elimination may lead to difficulties such as urinary tract infections (UTIs), urinary retention, ejaculatory issues, or anal and rectal problems and constipation. In some cases, patients who suffer from urinary or bowel problems may experience alterations in sexual function because of anxiety, embarrassment, or physical limitations related to these problems.

Because sexuality affects so many aspects of human health, nurses must be well versed in the possible causes, signs, symptoms, and results of alterations in male reproductive organs. Good communication skills are essential, as sexuality is a difficult or taboo topic for many patients to discuss. Nurses can strengthen the therapeutic relationship by remaining sensitive to and nonjudgmental of patients' sexuality while at the same time providing education and support.

Concepts related to male reproductive disorders are shown in **Figure 48.1** ■.

Case Studies

The following cases are addressed throughout the chapter to assist in application of chapter content to clinical situations involving individuals with disorders of the male reproductive system.

Mark Embers: Introduction

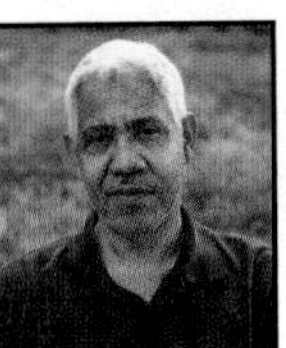

Mark Embers, age 63, presents to his healthcare provider with the complaint of waking up frequently during the night to urinate and then having trouble beginning to urinate. He states that he

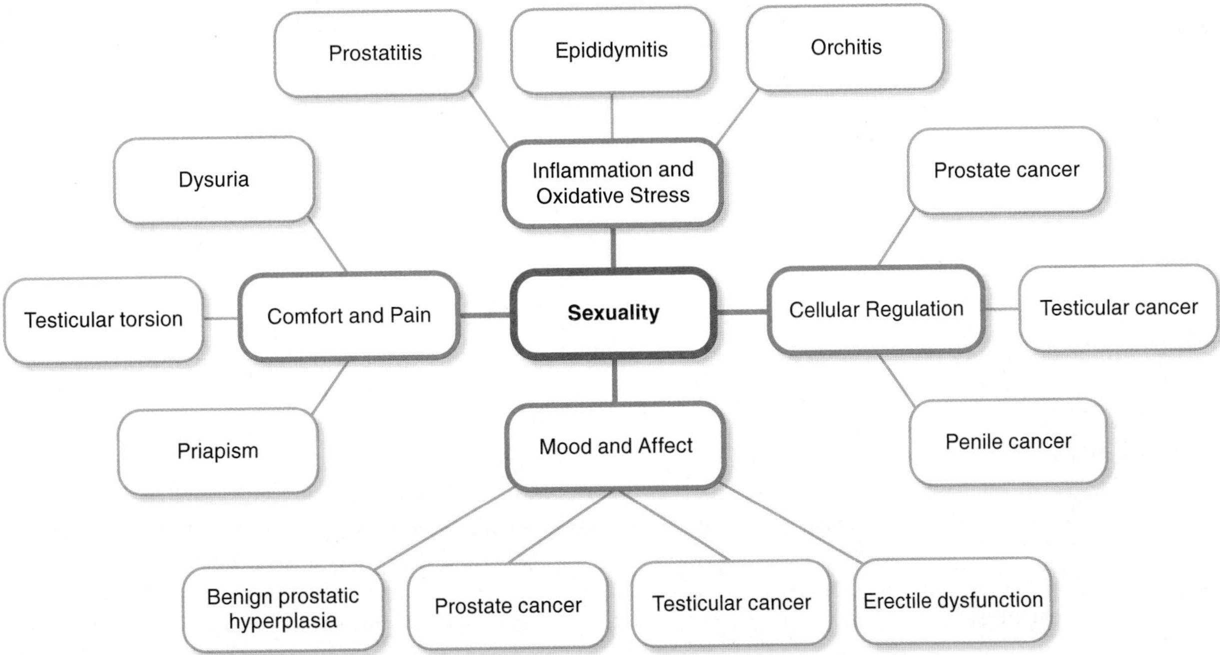

Figure 48.1 ■ Concepts related to disorders of the male reproductive system.

often feels as though he hasn't completely emptied his bladder and notices that some urine "dribbles out" on occasion.

1. What four symptoms does Mr. Embers verbalize?
2. How might these problems be affecting Mr. Embers's lifestyle?

Bart Howard: Introduction

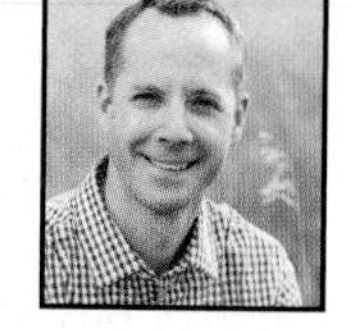

Bart Howard, age 41, visits his healthcare provider with the complaint of a dull ache in his right testicle. He reports that he is an avid equestrian and, while training his horse for jumps, came down quite hard in the saddle. He figured that the ache was due to this trauma, and he did not ride for a few days. This morning, he noticed that his testicle felt swollen, and he decided that it needed to be checked out.

1. What problem is Mr. Howard describing?
2. How can trauma be a possible cause of Mr. Howard's symptoms?

Check Your Progress: Section 48.1

1. Why do many men wait to present symptoms of reproductive system disorders to a healthcare provider?
2. What physical factors can affect the male reproductive system?
3. How can nurses create a therapeutic environment for discussing reproductive issues with men?

48.2 Disorders of the Prostate

The prostate gland is donut shaped and surrounds the urethra. It is about the size of a walnut and is located underneath the bladder and in front of the rectum (**Figure 48.2** ■). The prostate's main function is to produce some of the seminal fluid necessary for ejaculation. In this fluid is **prostate specific antigen (PSA)**, a protein that helps to liquefy semen and assists in motility of sperm. At the time of ejaculation, the seminal vesicles contract, together with the prostate, to expel seminal fluid through the urethra.

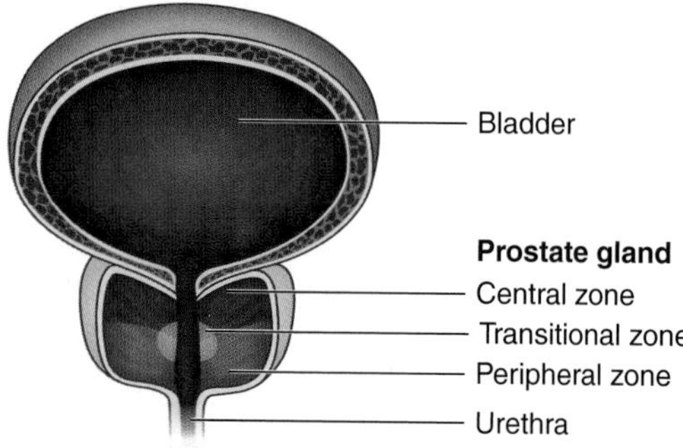

Figure 48.2 ■ The prostate gland and surrounding structures.

Prostatitis

Prostatitis is inflammation of the prostate gland. When the prostate becomes enlarged, it pinches the urethra, interfering with the flow of urine from the bladder through the urethra, which passes through the prostate.

Prostatitis results in approximately 2 million medical visits per year in the United States. It is diagnosed in approximately 25% of males who present with genitourinary symptoms, and approximately 8.2% of males will have prostatitis at some point. Chronic prostatitis/chronic pain syndrome accounts for 90–95% of all cases of prostatitis. Acute bacterial prostatitis and chronic bacterial prostatitis each account for 2–5% of cases.[1]

Etiology and Pathogenesis

The risk of prostatitis increases in men who have recently had infections of the urethra or bladder, those who have recently had a catheter inserted into the urethra, and those who do not empty their bladder completely or often enough. Prostatitis may stem from rigorous exercise such as bicycling, horseback riding, jogging, or heavy lifting, trauma; dehydration; urethral stricture; prostatic calculi; STIs; HIV infection; sexual abstinence; performing activities on a full bladder; or transrectal biopsy.[1]

There are four categories of prostatitis as designated by the National Institutes of Health[2]:

I. ***Acute bacterial prostatitis.*** This is the least common type, but it is the easiest to diagnose and is usually caused by gram-negative bacteria such as *Escherichia coli, Pseudomonas, Klebsiella,* or *Proteus.* It causes severe prostatitis symptoms, systemic infection, and acute bacterial UTI.

II. ***Chronic bacterial prostatitis.*** Chronic bacterial infection of the prostate occurs with or without symptoms of prostatitis, often with recurrent UTIs caused by the same bacterial strain, associated with episodes of urethritis, epididymitis, or acute prostatitis. Common infecting bacteria include *Escherichia coli, Enterobacter,* and *Klebsiella.*

III. ***Chronic prostatitis/chronic pelvic pain syndrome.*** This is the most common type of prostatitis, and it may be part of an autoimmune response. It is sometimes broken down into IIIA (inflammatory with presence of WBCs) and IIIB (noninflammatory, no WBCs present). Symptoms include chronic pelvic pain and possible voiding symptoms in the absence of a UTI. It may be caused by urinary tract abnormalities, neurologic or psychiatric disorders, trauma, or a local irritation that results in pelvic floor neuromuscular dysfunction.

IV. ***Asymptomatic inflammatory prostatitis.*** Prostate inflammation without genitourinary tract symptoms, usually found during examination for other conditions (e.g., infertility, prostate cancer) when samples of semen or a prostate biopsy produces inflammatory cell or leukocytes with no associated pain or discomfort.

Clinical Manifestations

Symptoms of acute bacterial prostatitis include fever, chills, arthralgia, low back pain, pelvic pain, abdominal pain, perineal fullness, **dysuria** (painful urination), urinary frequency and urgency usually at night, painful ejaculation, foul-smelling urine, urinary obstruction, blood-tinged urine, and/or semen-tinged urine. Symptoms of chronic bacterial prostatitis include intermittent obstructive urinary tract symptoms, recurrent UTIs, intermittent dysuria, and constipation usually without systemic symptoms. Symptoms of chronic prostatitis include painful ejaculation; dysuria; blood-tinged urine; blood-tinged semen; and pain in the perineal, suprapubic, coccygeal, rectal, urethral, testicular, and scrotal areas.[1]

Linking Pathophysiology to Diagnosis and Treatment

Diagnosis of prostatitis includes a **digital rectal examination (DRE)**, during which the clinician palpates the prostate through the rectum. An enlarged, boggy, tender prostate may be an expected finding. There may also be tenderness of the groin lymph nodes and scrotum, warmth, and swelling. Diagnostic tests may include urinalysis and triple void urine samples, urine culture for detection of white blood cells (WBCs) and bacteria, measurement of urine output, and semen analysis to detect elevated WBCs and decreased sperm motility as well as decreased sperm count. Additional tests may be ordered, including CT scan, intravenous urography, cystoscopy, voiding cystourethrography, ultrasonography, or needle biopsy to obtain an abscess culture for acute bacterial prostatitis. Healthcare providers should also use the National Institute of Health (NIH) Chronic Prostatitis Symptom Index.

Treatment of prostatitis includes antibiotics, anticholinergics, alpha blockers, stool softeners, analgesics, muscle relaxants, and antipyretics according to the type of prostatitis diagnosed. Patients should be advised to drink plenty of water, and pelvic floor exercises may help to reduce urinary symptoms. Integrative therapies in the form of supplements and herbal remedies may also be used. These may include cernilton (rye grass), quercetin (a chemical found in green tea, onions, and other plants), saw palmetto, zinc, selenium, and vitamin C. Mind–body therapies such as acupuncture also may be helpful.[3]

Benign Prostatic Hyperplasia

Benign prostatic hyperplasia (BPH), also known as *benign prostatic hypertrophy*, is a nonmalignant enlargement of the prostate (**Figure 48.3** ■).

BPH is considered a normal part of aging; it is noted in 50% of men by age 60 and in 90% of men by age 85.[4] Although an enlarged prostate can cause many problems, it is not a form of cancer. ■

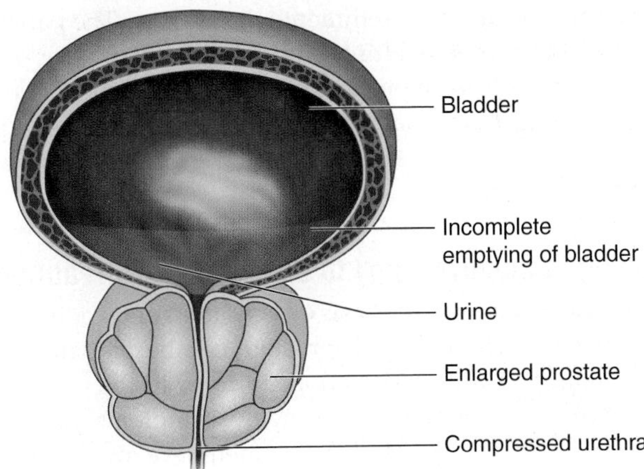

Figure 48.3 ■ In benign prostatic hyperplasia, the prostate enlarges, compressing the urethra. This can cause incomplete emptying of the bladder.

Etiology and Pathogenesis

An **androgen** is a type of hormone that stimulates the development and maintenance of male sex characteristics. The androgen **testosterone** signals the prostate to produce **dihydrotestosterone (DHT)**, which mediates prostatic growth. Although androgen levels decrease in aging men, the aging prostate appears to become more sensitive to available DHT. Estrogen, produced in small amounts in men, appears to sensitize the prostate gland to the effects of DHT. Increased estrogen levels associated with aging or a relative increase in estrogen related to testosterone levels contributes to prostatic hyperplasia.

The two main risk factors for developing BPH are age and the presence of testosterone. BPH rarely causes symptoms before age 40, but more than 50% of males have some symptoms of lower urinary tract symptoms by their sixth decade. The National Institute of Diabetes and Digestive and Kidney Diseases, a division of the NIH, predicts that up to 90% of men over the age of 80 will experience symptoms of BPH and almost all men will develop BPH if they live long enough.[5] Racial background may play a role in BPH. Black and Hispanic or Latino men develop symptoms earlier than Caucasian men, and Asian men develop symptoms later than Caucasian men.[4]

Clinical Manifestations

Clinical manifestations of BPH relate to obstruction and include difficulty starting the flow of urine even with straining, hematuria (from straining), a weak stream of urine, multiple interruptions during urination, feeling that the bladder is full, feeling that the bladder has not completely emptied, **nocturia** (urinating during the night), and dribbling once urination is complete. As the bladder becomes more sensitive to the retention of urine, incontinence may result. The inability to empty the bladder completely may result in the need for catheterization, which is placement of a catheter through the urethra into the bladder. The patient may experience bedwetting and the inability to respond quickly enough to the need to urinate. Urethral obstruction or enlarged prostate that is left untreated may result in infection, bladder stones, and increasing pressure that may damage the kidneys.

Linking Pathophysiology to Diagnosis and Treatment

Diagnosis is made on the basis of symptoms and confirmed with a DRE. The enlarged prostate can be palpated on examination. A urinalysis is done to rule out the presence of an infection that may be causing the symptoms. In addition, a PSA level is checked. Many men have low levels of PSA, and an elevated PSA may be indicative of prostate cancer. The American Urological Association has a Prostate Symptom Index that healthcare providers can use to help determine the diagnosis.

CLINICAL POINT: Infection may also increase PSA levels, so it is important to note that PSA levels cannot be used to distinguish between cancer and benign prostatic hyperplasia. ■

The least invasive treatment for BPH is **watchful waiting**, or *active surveillance*. This approach is used for patients who have minimal symptoms and minimal enlargement of the prostate. Patients who opt for watchful waiting receive yearly examinations with evaluation using DRE. During this period, the patient should avoid tranquilizers and over-the-counter medications that contain decongestants, as these medications can worsen obstructive symptoms. In addition, patients should avoid excess fluids in the evening to decrease the chances of nocturia.

Pharmacologic treatment may also be an option for BPH. Types of drugs currently being used are 5-alpha-reductase inhibitors and alpha blockers. It is not possible to predict which drug will work best for any particular patient; however, these drugs appear to improve selected symptoms in up to 80% of men who take them.[4] Alpha blockers act on the alpha receptors in the prostate, causing the smooth muscles of the prostate to relax. Relaxation of these muscles decreases constriction of the urethra. It may take 2 weeks to 4 months to notice symptom improvement. This class of drugs includes alfuzosin (UroXatral), doxazosin (Cardura), indoramin (Doralese), prazosin (Minipress), tamsulosin (Flomax), and terazosin (Hytrin). The patient needs to be aware of adverse effects such as headache, nasal congestion, dizziness, drowsiness, postural hypotension, reflex tachycardia, and retrograde or delayed ejaculation. Although some patients may prefer to try herbal remedies before pharmacologic therapies, there is insufficient evidence to support the use of alternative therapies to treat BPH, with the exception of *Pygeum africanum*.[6]

Some men experience better results with a combination of alpha blockers and 5-alpha reductase inhibitors. This combination has been shown to delay clinical progression by as much as 67%, although other men do not achieve better results from a combination of the two drugs. The pharmacologic approach is quite specific to the patient. If the patient with BPH has an overactive bladder, an anticholinergic to relax bladder smooth muscle such as oxybutynin, may be added.

If medication is not an effective treatment and the patient is not a candidate for surgery, then incontinence caused by obstruction of the urethra secondary to prostate enlargement can be managed through intermittent catheterization of the bladder or by using an indwelling catheter or suprapubic catheter, a catheter placed through the abdominal wall into the bladder. The indwelling catheter can stay in place permanently to be changed monthly or according to protocol.[5]

There are a number of surgical options if pharmacologic treatment is not effective and the patient is a good candidate for surgery. These include transurethral resection of the prostate, in which the entire inner prostate is removed, leaving the outer layer intact; transurethral incision of the prostate, in which two small incisions are made in the prostate to relieve compression of the urethra; and open prostatectomy, for patients with a very large prostate who are experiencing complications such as bladder stones, in which the prostate is removed through an abdominal incision. Laser surgery, microwave therapy, water thermotherapy, ablation, and stents are also used to treat BPH.[5]

Mark Embers: Outcome

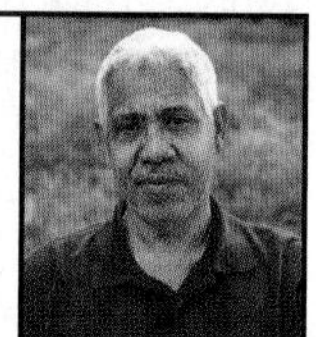

Mr. Embers is diagnosed with BPH. When asked how severe he feels his symptoms are, Mr. Embers states that they are annoying but he does not consider them severe. The healthcare provider tells Mr. Embers that he is most likely experiencing benign prostatic hyperplasia. Mr. Embers says that he has heard of this and agrees to have a PSA test. The healthcare provider explains that this is not a definitive test but it is appropriate as a screening tool and for establishing a baseline for monitoring purposes. After a digital rectal examination, the healthcare provider recommends that Mr. Embers take a watchful waiting approach, as his prostate has minimal enlargement at this time. Mr. Embers is instructed to return to the provider if his symptoms increase in frequency or severity.

3. What clinical reasoning was used to prescribe the PSA lab test and the watchful waiting?
4. For what other options is Mr. Embers a possible candidate to treat his symptoms?

Prostate Cancer

Prostate cancer is the second most common cancer in men (after skin cancer). The American Cancer Society estimates that in 2017, there were over 160,000 new cases of prostate cancer and more than 26,000 deaths from prostate cancer.[7] Prostate cancer is a slow-growing cancer. It remains difficult to diagnose, as there are no extraordinary warning signs.

Prostate cancer is often considered a cancer of older men. The median age of men diagnosed with prostate cancer is 69 years. Many patients, particularly those who have cancer that is localized, die of other diseases without ever knowing that they had prostate cancer.[8] ■

The American Cancer Society recommends that men have a DRE annually beginning at the age of 50. The recommendation changes to age 45 for African American men and those with a first-degree relative with prostate cancer and to age 40 for those with more than one first-degree relative with prostate cancer.[9] Benefits of early screening of PSA levels are unclear. There have been many instances of men with elevated PSA levels who do not have prostate cancer and men with normal readings who do have prostate cancer.

Etiology and Pathogenesis

The three areas of the prostate are the central, transition, and peripheral zones (see Figure 48.2). The peripheral zone, located at the back of the prostate, is most susceptible to prostate cancer. Tumors that develop in the prostate tend to develop on the periphery of the gland and do not obstruct the passage of urine; hence, they go unnoticed until there is associated pain. Prostate cancer will often metastasize to lymph nodes and the lungs and then progress to other organs. Prostate cancer is usually curable when it is localized, and it responds to treatment even when widespread. When prostate cancer has metastasized to the bone, patients may still experience an extended survival rate.

Clinical Manifestations

Men with local prostate cancer may have no symptoms or may experience frequent urination, weak urine flow, blood in the urine, the urge to urinate frequently especially at night, blood in the semen, erectile dysfunction, pain or burning on urination, and/or discomfort while sitting.[10]

If the cancer has spread outside of the prostate, symptoms may include pain in the bones of the back, hip, thighs, and shoulders; edema in the legs or feet; unexplained weight loss; fatigue; and change in bowel habits.[10]

Linking Pathophysiology to Diagnosis and Treatment

The patient who is found to have prostate cancer is diagnosed further by using various scoring systems and staging methods. One of the scoring systems is the Gleason Scoring System.[11] This system differentiates the diagnosis of prostate cancer into five different grades. In grade 1, the tissue is well differentiated, and the patient is most likely to have a good prognosis with the greatest chance of a cure. A grade 5 classification would be a poorly differentiated cancer with a poor prognosis. Tissue samples from two different sites are graded separately, and the two scores are added together. The highest score possible on the Gleason scale is a 10 if each of the two sites tested is graded as a 5.

There are various treatment options for prostate cancer. One option is surgery. In radical prostatectomy, the patient's prostate and seminal vesicles are removed. If it is deemed necessary, the surgeon may also remove pelvic lymph nodes.

Radiation is a nonsurgical option for patients who would like to avoid surgery and who the physician feels may benefit from this form of treatment. Radiation also may be used after surgery if there is evidence that the cancer has metastasized. The two options for radiation treatment include the use of an external beam of radiation that is aimed at the tumor and surgical implantation of small radioactive pellets into the prostate.

Another treatment for prostate cancer is cryotherapy. Liquid nitrogen is delivered into the prostate through the perineum using metal probes to freeze the prostate. This treatment is not used often, as it has a low success rate; usually needs to be repeated; and may result in impotence, incontinence, and rectal complications.

Ablative hormone therapy is often used for men whose cancer has metastasized into the lymph nodes or bones. The term *ablative* (which mean "suppression of") refers to suppression of testosterone. Testosterone is an androgen, and androgens can promote the growth of tumors. Suppression of these hormones may lead to slowing of tumor growth and to symptom relief. This type of treatment is referred to as neoadjuvant therapy when it is used to shrink the prostate before radiation treatment.

For advanced prostate cancer, the patient may receive chemotherapy. It is often used for men who have hormone-refractory prostate cancer, that is, they no longer respond to ablative hormone therapy. Chemotherapy is given in pill form or intravenously and is administered in cycles, with a treatment period followed by a rest period. These cycles may be daily, weekly, or every 3–4 months.

The patient with prostate cancer has many decisions to make. If he will need radiation and/or chemotherapy, the hospital stay and adverse effects of treatment will require more extensive education and care. Some studies have associated an increased risk of prostate cancer with a high consumption of calcium. The nurse can educate the patient about foods that contain high levels of calcium and possible alternatives. Eating certain plant foods that contain selenium and animals that eat plants containing selenium has been shown to offer some hope for prostate cancer prevention. There has also been evidence showing an increase in prostate cancer in men who took more than seven multivitamins a week.[12] Even though these studies are not conclusive, the information can be part of patient education.

Check Your Progress: Section 48.2

1. At what age should screening begin for prostate cancer?
2. Why is localized prostate cancer often diagnosed late?
3. What are the types of treatment for prostate cancer?

48.3 Disorders of the Testicles

The testicles (testes) are the male gonads; they are central to the male reproductive system and endocrine system. The anatomy of the testicles is shown in **Figure 48.4** ■. The testicles are contained in the scrotum, and their primary function is to produce sperm and testosterone.

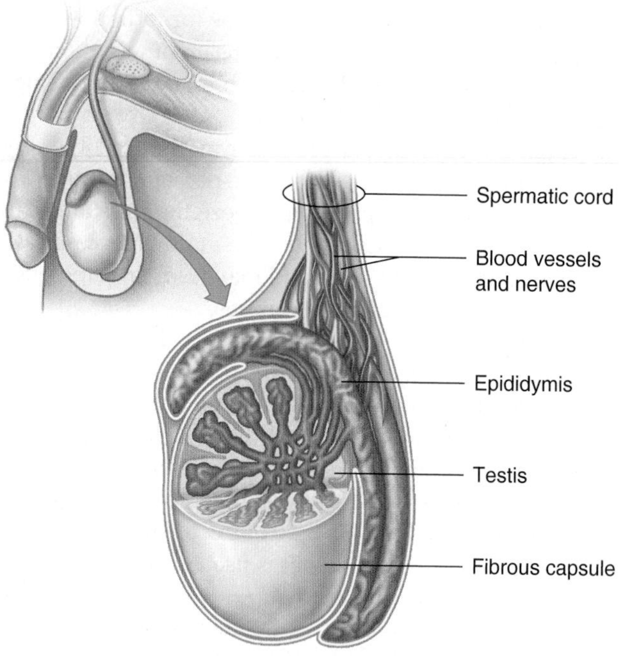

Figure 48.4 ■ The testicles are encased in the scrotum, hanging outside of the body.

Varicocele, Hydrocele, and Spermatocele

A **varicocele** is an enlargement of the veins in the scrotum, similar to varicose veins in the legs. Most varicoceles develop slowly over time and cause few, if any, symptoms. However, they can cause low sperm production and decreased sperm quality, both of which are factors in infertility. Varicoceles can be surgically repaired if necessary.[13]

A **hydrocele** is a fluid-filled sac that surrounds a testicle, causing swelling. In older boys and men, hydroceles can develop as a result of injury and inflammation of the scrotum. The swelling is usually painless and may appear on one or both testicles. Pain increases with the size of the swelling. Hydroceles are usually not dangerous, but they can be associated with underlying conditions such as an infection, a tumor, or an inguinal hernia.[14]

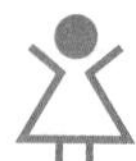
Hydroceles are common in newborns. They usually disappear in the first year of life without any treatment. ■

A **spermatocele** is a cyst that forms in the epididymis, the tube that collects and transports sperm. These cysts are not cancerous and are usually painless. They do not usually affect fertility and rarely grow large enough to cause discomfort or require surgery.[15]

Epididymitis and Orchitis

The **epididymis** is the tube that collects and transports sperm. It is a curved structure located along the posterior of the testis (see Figure 48.3). **Epididymitis**, inflammation of the epididymis, is the fifth most common urologic diagnosis in men age 18–50. It may be acute or chronic.[16] **Orchitis** is inflammation of one or both testicles and is usually caused by a viral or bacterial infection. Bacterial orchitis often develops from a case of epididymis and can also be caused by STIs. Most cases of bacterial orchitis occur in sexually active men or in men with BPH.[17]

Etiology and Pathogenesis

Epididymitis is often an infectious process, but cultures often fail to show an identifiable infectious agent. Severe epididymitis that extends to the testicle is called acute epididymo-orchitis.[16]

Bacterial orchitis often develops from a case of epididymis and can also be caused by STIs. Most cases of bacterial orchitis occur in sexually active men or in men with BPH. Viral orchitis is usually caused by the mumps virus. One third of adolescent and adult males who contract mumps after puberty will develop orchitis 4–7 days after the onset of the infection.[17]

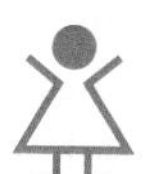
Most cases of orchitis in children are caused by mumps. ■

Clinical Manifestations

Symptoms of acute epididymitis include pain and swelling over several days. Chronic epididymitis is pain and swelling that lasts for more than 6 weeks; it may be accompanied by scrotal induration (hardening of the scrotum). Complications can include scrotal abscess, testicular infarction or atrophy, fertility problems, and recurrence.[16]

Signs and symptoms of orchitis usually develop suddenly and include swelling in one or both testicles, pain, tenderness, fever, nausea, and vomiting. The pain may range from mild to severe. Men who are experiencing such symptoms should see their healthcare provider immediately. Orchitis can cause infertility, especially if both testicles are affected.[17]

Linking Pathophysiology to Diagnosis and Treatment

Tests for diagnosing epididymitis and orchitis include STI screening, urinalysis, and an ultrasound or nuclear scan to rule out testicular torsion. Both epididymitis and bacterial orchitis are treated with antibiotics. Patients should be tested for comorbid STIs, and they and their sexual partners should be treated accordingly. Patients should rest, support the scrotum with an athletic strap, and use ice packs and pain medication as needed. Treatment of viral orchitis is supportive, including the measures used for epididymitis. It can take several weeks for the tenderness to subside.[16,17]

Testicular Torsion

Testicular torsion occurs when the spermatic cord structures twist within the testicle, causing loss of blood supply to the ipsilateral testis (**Figure 48.5** ■). Testicular torsion is a medical emergency. Failure to treat this condition promptly can cause loss of fertility and/or loss of the testicle.

Etiology and Pathogenesis

Testicular torsion may be intravaginal or extravaginal. Intravaginal torsion occurs when the tunica vaginalis in the testicle is attached too high, allowing the spermatic cord to

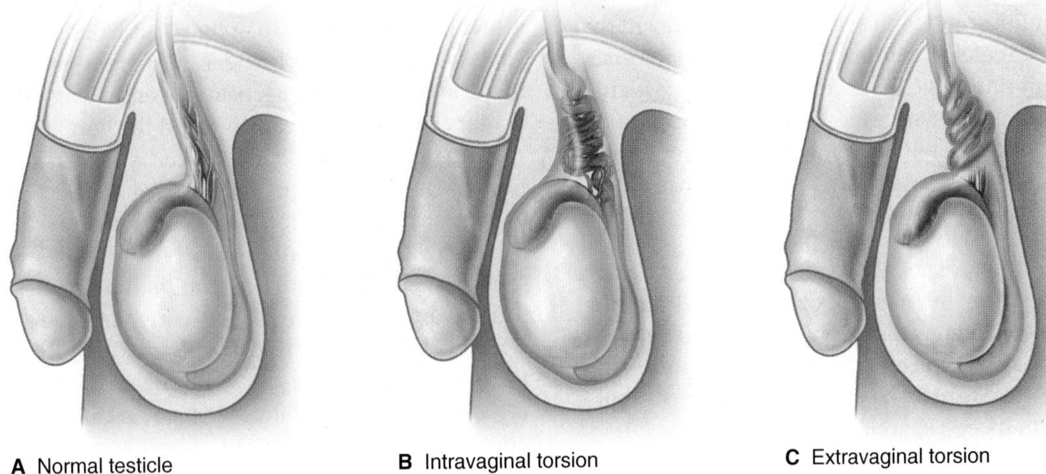

Figure 48.5 ■ The normal testicle **A** compared with intravaginal torsion **B** and extravaginal torsion **C**.

rotate. This is a congenital deformity. Torsion can occur during sports, be related to trauma, or occur spontaneously.[18]

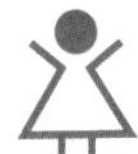

Intravaginal torsion occurs most commonly in adolescents, probably as a result of the weight of the testicles after puberty. ■

Extravaginal torsion occurs when the tunica vaginalis is not yet firmly secured, so the tunica vaginalis and spermatic cord twist as a unit.[18] The torsion of the testicle causes venous occlusion and engorgement along with arterial ischemia. The amount and duration of the torsion influence the ability to salvage the testicle.

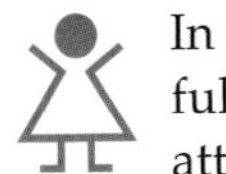

In newborns, the testicles may not have descended fully into the scrotum and therefore may become attached to the tunica vaginalis, predisposing them to torsion. Extravaginal torsion occurs most often in newborns and can even occur months before birth, although it is typically diagnosed in the first 7–10 days of life. ■

Clinical Manifestations

The clinical manifestation of testicular torsion is severe unilateral scrotal pain followed by swelling. About one third of patients experience nausea and vomiting. Patients usually have no trouble urinating. Most patients have a high position of the testicle.[18]

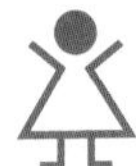

In newborns, testicular torsion presents as a firm, hard, scrotal mass that is fixed to the scrotal skin. ■

Linking Pathophysiology to Diagnosis and Treatment

If history and physical examination suggest testicular torsion, laboratory and imaging tests are not usually necessary. The Testicular Workup for Ischemia and Suspected Torsion (TWIST) scoring system can be used. This scoring system, which assigns points for testis swelling, hard testis, absent cremasteric reflex, nausea/vomiting, and high-riding testis, has been well validated. Patients with low TWIST scores do not have torsion, those with intermediate scores are sent for ultrasound evaluation, and those with high scores are sent directly to surgery.[18]

To salvage the testicle, surgical repair must happen within 6 hours of the onset of symptoms. If surgical treatment is delayed, the patient may have decreased fertility or require an orchiectomy (removed of the testicle). The surgical procedure to correct torsion anchors the testis to the scrotal wall.[18]

Testicular Cancer

Testicular cancer is a rare form of cancer usually found in males between the ages of 15 and 34. Approximately 8000 men in the United States are diagnosed with testicular cancer each year, and 400 of them will die from the disease.[19] Testicular cancer is usually curable; cure rates are 90% and higher. The U.S. Preventive Services Task Force (USPSTF) recommends against testicular cancer screening, citing the rarity of the disease, lack of evidence that showed substantial accuracy of self-examination or clinical examination, and highly favorable outcomes from treatment. The recommendation of the USPSTF is for clinicians to consider testicular cancer in their differential diagnosis for patients who present with testicular symptoms.[20]

Etiology and Pathogenesis

The exact cause of testicular cancer is unknown, but it is believed that the primordial cells do not follow the normal pattern of development, which would be progression into spermatogonia. These cells are thought to remain in their undifferentiated state, becoming carcinoma in situ, and may then develop into an invasive cancer. Most testicular tumors are of germ cell origin and fall into one of two classifications: either seminomas (containing 100% seminoma) or nonseminomas (composed of more than one type of cancer cell).

There are certain risk factors associated with testicular cancer, including having had mumps, low weight at birth, trauma to the testes, a family history of testicular cancer,

cryptorchidism (the absence of one or both testes from the scrotum, also referred to as undescended testes), age, congenital abnormalities, and white ethnicity. It is believed that men born with Klinefelter syndrome had abnormal testicular development and have an increased risk of testicular cancer; males with this syndrome have an abnormality of chromosome 48. Males with cryptorchidism may have a 10–40% increased chance of getting testicular cancer.[21]

Clinical Manifestations

Signs and symptoms of testicular cancer may include a dull ache in the groin; the presence of a painless lump that may be associated with swelling, enlargement, or hardening of the testes; and **gynecomastia** (breast swelling). Men with metastatic disease may experience shortness of breath, masses located in the neck, and back pain.

Linking Pathophysiology to Diagnosis and Treatment

Early diagnosis and treatment are keys to curing testicular cancer. Physical assessment should include thorough and careful palpation of the testes, the abdomen, and any lymph nodes. It is important that a firm mass not be mistaken for epididymitis. For clarification, a testicular ultrasound can be used to evaluate the mass (**Figure 48.6** ■).

Tumor markers are essential indicators of testicular cancer. These tumor markers include alpha-fetoprotein, human chorionic gonadotropin, and lactate dehydrogenase. The blood tests are important in diagnosing and monitoring testicular cancer. These serum markers may detect testicular cancer even before a small tumor is evident.

If ultrasound shows a testicular tumor, additional diagnostics such as chest x-ray and CT scan of the abdomen and pelvis will be performed to determine whether there is metastasis. For testicular tumors confirmed by ultrasound, a radical **orchiectomy**, removal of the testicle, will most likely be performed. A testicular needle biopsy would be contraindicated, as this increases the chance of metastasis.

Classification is important in identifying and treating testicular cancer. It is important to know whether the tumor is single cell or multiple cell. Knowing the cell type is important for treating the tumor and estimating the risk of metastasis. Staging is important to understand how far the cancer has spread. Stage I testicular cancer is limited to the testes. Stage II testicular cancer involves one or both testes and the retroperitoneal and para-aortic lymph nodes. If there is involvement of more than five lymph nodes or if the diameter of any of the lymph nodes is greater than 2 centimeters, there is an increased risk of recurrence. Stage III is any testicular cancer that spreads beyond the lymph nodes.

Treatment of testicular cancer is related to the type of tumor. The three stages of testicular cancer require different surgical interventions, including removal of the testicle or removal of the testicle and lymph nodes in combination with chemotherapy and radiation. Some surgery can be done by using laparoscopy, which has the advantage of a shorter recovery period. Males who have been cured of testicular cancer have a 2% cumulative risk of developing testicular cancer in the other testicle during the 15 years after the initial diagnosis.[19]

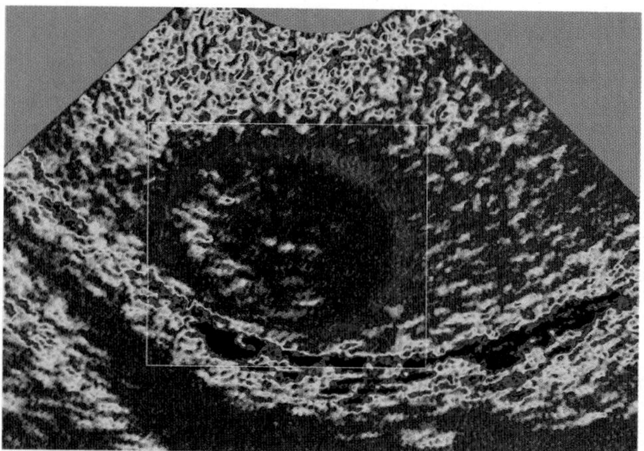

Figure 48.6 ■ Testicular cancer shown on ultrasound.

Bart Howard: Outcome

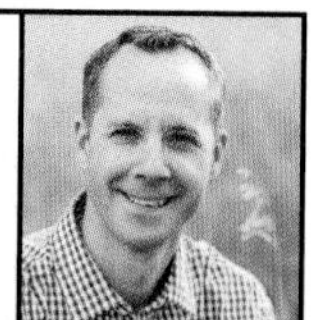

Mr. Howard is examined by his healthcare provider, who follows up with an ultrasound. Blood tests are done to check tumor markers. It is determined that Mr. Howard has stage I seminoma testicular cancer. His healthcare provider recommends that Mr. Howard donate sperm samples for possible future use in starting a family. An orchiectomy is also recommended, along with chemotherapy and radiation. When Mr. Howard asks what caused the cancer, he is told that the cause is unknown but that there is a 95% cure rate.

3. What risk factors for testicular cancer does Mr. Howard have?
4. What are the clinical manifestations of testicular cancer?

Check Your Progress: Section 48.3

1. What test can differentiate between a testicular tumor and epididymitis?
2. What are the tumor markers for testicular cancer?
3. Why is it important for the nurse to understand classification and staging of the tumor in testicular cancer?

48.4 Disorders of the Penis

The penis is the external male genital organ through which the urethra passes. The penis is used both for elimination of urine and as the sexual organ. The anatomy of the penis is shown in **Figure 48.7** ■. Disorders of the penis may be congenital (such as hypospadias and epispadias), inflammatory (such as balanitis), structural (such as phimosis), or cancerous. Penile cancer is rare in the United States, with about 2000 new cases diagnosed each year.[22]

Hypospadias and Epispadias

Hypospadias and epispadias are congenital abnormalities found in newborn males. **Hypospadias** is an abnormality of the location of the male urethral meatus. The meatus develops on the ventral (underneath) part of the penis and can be anywhere from the glans to the perineum (see Figure 45.2 in Chapter 45). This abnormality

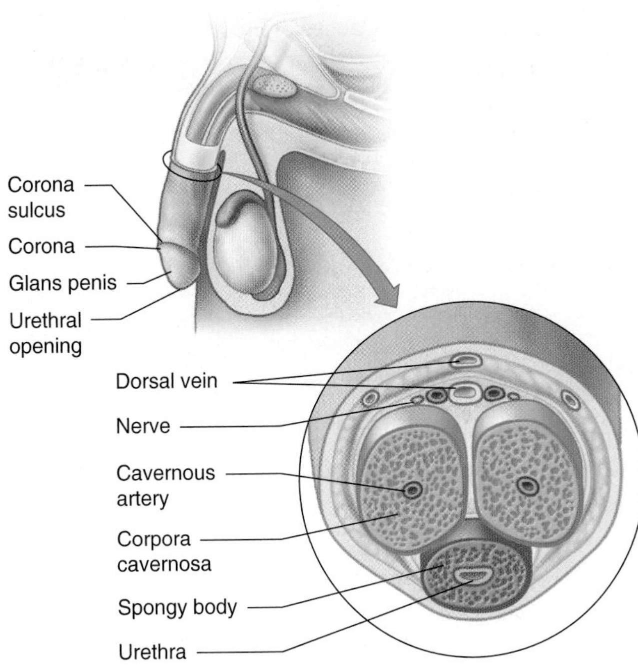

Figure 48.7 ■ The anatomy of the penis.

occurs in up to 4 of every 1000 newborn boys.[23] **Epispadias** is a rare defect in which the urethral opening is on the dorsal (upper) surface of the penis. It occurs in 1 in 117,000 boys.[24] Both conditions can be surgically repaired, usually when the child is between 6 months and 2 years of age. Boys with these conditions should not be circumcised at birth. ■

Phimosis and Paraphimosis

Phimosis and paraphimosis are disorders of the foreskin of the penis. **Phimosis** is a condition in which the foreskin cannot be retracted over the glans penis. It can occur naturally in newborns or later after the foreskin was previously retractable, usually as a result of scarring of the foreskin. Physiologic phimosis occurs when adhesions form between the epithelial layers of the inner prepuce and glans. The adhesions dissolve as the male grows and the foreskin is intermittently retracted with erections. Pathologic phimosis is caused by poor hygiene or recurrent episodes of infection of the glans penis (balanitis) leading to scarring.[25] Pathologic phimosis causes painful erections, hematuria, recurrent UTIs, and a weak urinary stream.

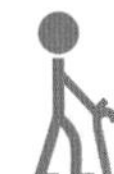

Older men are at risk of phimosis because of the loss of skin elasticity and infrequent erections. ■

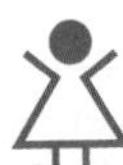

Phimosis in infants is usually noted by parents who have difficulty retracting the foreskin during bathing. ■

Paraphimosis occurs in uncircumcised or partially circumcised males when the retracted foreskin is trapped behind the coronal sulcus. Patients with either physiologic or pathologic phimosis are at risk for developing paraphimosis.[25] Paraphimosis manifests as a swollen, painful glans penis in a patient who is uncircumcised or partially circumcised. It is seen in adolescents or adults after participation in vigorous sexual activity.[25]

Older men with indwelling catheters are at risk for paraphimosis when caregivers do not replace the foreskin after catheterization or cleaning. ■

Paraphimosis is a medical emergency—failure to resolve the problem can lead to necrosis and gangrene of the glans penis. The goal is to reduce the foreskin to its naturally occurring position over the glans penis. This can be done in a variety of ways, including manual reduction, which may include using osmotic methods, puncture, or aspiration; vertical incision; or emergent circumcision.[25]

Priapism

Priapism is a prolonged erection that continues for hours. Ischemic priapism is a painful condition caused by blood not being able to leave the penis. It is an uncommon disorder in the general population but is more common in men with sickle cell disease. Nonischemic priapism, which is usually painless, happens when penile blood flow is not regulated properly.[26]

Causes of priapism include blood disorders such as sickle cell disease or leukemia, prescription medications such as antidepressants and blood thinners, erectile dysfunction treatments including injected and oral medications, alcohol and drug use, injury, spider bites, scorpion stings, metabolic disorders such as gout, spinal cord injury, and penile cancer.

Diagnostic tests are used to determine the type of priapism; these may include blood gas measurements, complete blood count, ultrasound, and toxicology screens.

Ischemic priapism is a medical emergency that requires immediate treatment. Blood is drained from the penis, and medications are injected to constrict the blood vessels that carry blood into the penis. Nonischemic priapism often resolves on its own. Ice packs and pressure on the perineum can help to end the erection.[26]

Peyronie Disease

Peyronie disease is a caused by fibrous plaque that affects the tunica albuginea, causing the penis to curve or bend. Peyronie disease affects as many as 23% of men age 40–70 but is rare in younger men. The etiology of the plaque formation is unknown but may involve prior injury to the penis or an autoimmune disorder. The presence of the hard, fibrous plaque causes the penis to bend, which in turn causes painful, bent erections. Symptoms may be mild or severe, and they may appear slowly or quickly. Peyronie disease sometimes resolves on its own or may be treated with oral or injected medications, medical therapies such as ultrasound to break up the plaque, or surgery as a last resort.[27]

Erectile Dysfunction

Erectile dysfunction (ED) is the most common male sexual disorder. In basic terms, ED is the inability to attain or maintain an erection sufficient to permit mutually satisfactory sexual intercourse with a partner. ED may involve a total inability to achieve erection, an inconsistent ability to achieve erection, or the ability to sustain only brief erections. In some cases, the penis may become semierect but lack sufficient rigidity for intercourse.

Erectile dysfunction occurs in men of all ages and can be chronic, intermittent, or episodic. Some men experience primary ED, meaning that they have had trouble achieving erection throughout their life. Others experience secondary ED, meaning that their problems began after a period of normal erectile function. Still other men experience situational ED, in which they have erectile difficulties only in specific circumstances.

The incidence of ED is difficult to estimate because affected men might not report the disorder and because there are differing views on how long a man must be affected before a diagnosis can be made.

Etiology and Pathogenesis

Physiologically, ED involves a disruption in the normal process by which an erection occurs. An erection is a neurovascular event that requires functional autonomic and somatic nerves, smooth and striated muscles in the penile shaft and pelvic floor, and adequate arterial blood flow. The erectile reflex to sexual stimulation occurs when the chambers in the erectile tissue of the penis become filled with blood via arterioles that dilate in response to nitric oxide. At the same time, pelvic muscle contractions help to increase penile rigidity, and the veins of the penis constrict, blocking blood outflow until orgasm or removal of the sexual stimulus occurs.[28]

A range of factors may disrupt any of the mechanisms in the erectile process, resulting in ED. These factors are broadly classified as either psychologic or physical; physical causes of ED can then be further described as vascular, neurologic, urologic, endocrine, respiratory, iatrogenic, or lifestyle related. The most common psychologic and physical causes of ED are shown in **Table 48.1** ■. All of the causes listed in the table can also be considered risk factors for the development of ED.

In addition to the factors listed in Table 48.1, the aging process itself increases the risk for erectile dysfunction. As a man ages, the collagen in his penis becomes less elastic, leading to decreased distensibility. This interferes with the veno-occlusive mechanism, which prevents blood from prematurely "leaking" out of the penis and into the general vasculature. Problems with this mechanism result in incomplete erections. The skin's ability to sense vibrotactile stimulation also declines with age, which may in part explain why some older men require a longer period of stimulation to achieve an erection. In addition, many older men are affected by hypogonadism, which results in decreased testosterone and may contribute to erectile problems. Finally, age increases a man's likelihood of suffering from chronic conditions such as diabetes, kidney disease, alcoholism, atherosclerosis, and vascular disease, all of which are linked to ED, either because of the changes they cause in the body or because of the therapeutic interventions they require. ■

Table 48.1 Common Causes of Erectile Dysfunction

Cause	Examples
Vascular	Atherosclerosis Heart disease Hyperlipidemia Hypertension Metabolic syndrome Stroke
Neurologic	Multiple sclerosis Nerve disease Parkinson disease Spinal cord injury
Urologic	Direct injury to the penis that affects the nerves or vascular supply Hypospadias and epispadias Kidney failure Peyronie disease
Endocrine	Abnormal prolactin levels Diabetes mellitus Hypogonadism Low testosterone levels Thyroid disease
Respiratory	Chronic obstructive pulmonary disease Obstructive sleep apnea
Iatrogenic	*Medications including:* Antidepressants Antihistamines Antihypertensives Appetite suppressants Cimetidine Tranquilizers *Procedures including:* Bladder surgery Colon surgery Pelvic radiation or surgery Radical prostatectomy Spinal cord surgery
Lifestyle related	Alcohol use Excessive caffeine use Illicit drug use Lack of physical activity Obesity/overweight Tobacco use
Psychologic	Anxiety Depression Fatigue Fear of sexual failure Guilt Low self-esteem Relationship problems Stress

SOURCES: American Psychiatric Association. (2013). *Diagnostic and statistical manual of mental disorders* (5th ed.). Arlington, VA: American Psychiatric Association; Gerber, D. (2014). Sexual problems. In B. A. Magowan, P. Owen, & A. Thomson (Eds.), *Clinical obstetrics and gynaecology* (3rd ed., pp. 191–202). Philadelphia, PA: Elsevier Health; Mayo Clinic. (2015). Erectile dysfunction: Causes. Available at http://www.mayoclinic.org/diseases-conditions/erectile-dysfunction/basics/causes/con-20034244

Clinical Manifestations

A medical diagnosis of ED requires that the problem be present for at least 3 months; a psychiatric diagnosis of ED requires that the problem persist for 6 months or longer.[29,30] Overall, about 52% of men report at least occasional erectile difficulties. Older men are affected at higher rates. Whereas about 40% of men experience occasional ED at age 40, roughly 70% of men are affected by age 70. Rates for chronic or complete ED are lower than those for occasional ED, but they too increase with age, going from about 5% at age 40 to about 15% at age 70.[26]

Linking Pathophysiology to Diagnosis and Treatment

Prevention of ED is aimed at mitigation of risk factors. Regular exercise, eating a balanced diet, maintaining a healthy body weight, and abstaining from alcohol and tobacco use are steps that can reduce any man's likelihood of ED. Other prevention strategies are specific to the physical or psychologic risk factors experienced by particular patients. For example, men with diabetes can reduce their chances of erectile difficulties by maintaining appropriate blood glucose levels, and men with depression or relationship problems can reduce their risk of ED by seeking counseling. However, many medications used in the treatment of various conditions that have been linked to ED, such as heart disease and depression, can themselves produce erectile problems as a side effect.

Pharmacologic treatment of ED includes medications such as sildenafil (Viagra) and tadalafil (Cialis) that enhance the effects of nitric oxide to increase blood flow to the penis. Other medications are self-injected into the base or side of the penis. Penis pumps and surgical implants may also be considered.[31]

Check Your Progress: Section 48.4

1. Why is paraphimosis a medical emergency?
2. What are the possible causes of priapism?
3. What oral medications are often prescribed for erectile dysfunction?

CHAPTER SUMMARY

48.1 Chapter Overview and Case Studies

Describe the male reproductive system, disorders related to it, and the concepts integral to managing those disorders.

- The male reproductive system involves many different anatomic parts, each of which can develop problems of its own. Men's reproductive health and sexuality are closely related.
- Although there are many physiologic disorders that relate to male reproductive health, these disorders also have a psychologic aspect. Selected concepts related to male reproductive disorders include sexuality, inflammation, infection, elimination, and mood and affect.

48.2 Disorder of the Prostate

Differentiate the causes, classification, underlying pathogenesis, and clinical manifestations of disorders of the prostate and approaches to diagnosis and treatment of these conditions.

- The prostate gland is donut shaped and surrounds the urethra. It is about the size of a walnut and is located underneath the bladder and in front of the rectum.
- Prostatitis is inflammation of the prostate gland. When the prostate becomes enlarged, it pinches the urethra, interfering with the passage of urine from the bladder through the urethra, which passes through the prostate to the bladder. There are four types of prostatitis: acute bacterial prostatitis, chronic bacterial prostatitis, chronic prostatitis/chronic pelvic pain syndrome, and asymptomatic inflammatory prostatitis.
- Benign prostatitis (BPH) is a nonmalignant enlargement of the prostate. The two main risk factors for developing BPH are age and the presence of testosterone. Clinical manifestations of BPH relate to obstruction and include difficulty starting the flow of urine. The least invasive treatment for BPH is watchful waiting.
- Prostate cancer is the second most common cancer in men and is usually a very slow-growing cancer. It remains a difficult cancer to diagnose, as there are no extraordinary warning signs.

48.3 Disorders of the Testicles

Differentiate the causes, classification, underlying pathogenesis, and clinical manifestations of disorders of the testicles and approaches to diagnosis and treatment of these conditions across the lifespan.

- A varicocele is an enlargement of the veins in the scrotum, similar to varicose veins in the legs. Most varicoceles develop slowly over time and cause few, if any, symptoms.
- A hydrocele is a fluid-filled sac, usually painless, that surrounds a testicle, causing swelling. In older boys and men, hydroceles can develop as a result of injury and inflammation of the scrotum.
- A spermatocele is a cyst that forms in the epididymis, the tube that collects and transports sperm. These cysts are not cancerous and are usually painless.
- Epididymitis (inflammation of the epididymis) is the fifth most common urologic diagnosis in men ages 18–50. It may be acute or chronic. Symptoms include pain and swelling.
- Orchitis is inflammation of one or both testicles and is usually caused by a viral or bacterial infection. Symptoms develop suddenly and involve swelling, pain, tenderness, fever, nausea, and vomiting.
- Testicular torsion occurs when the spermatic cord structures twist within the testicle, causing loss of blood supply to the ipsilateral testis. Testicular torsion is a medical emergency requiring surgery. Failure to treat this condition promptly can cause loss of fertility and/or loss of the testicle.
- Testicular cancer is a rare cancer usually found in males between the ages of 15 and 34. The exact cause of testicular cancer is unknown. Signs and symptoms of testicular cancer may include a dull ache in the groin, the presence of a painless lump that may be associated with swelling, enlargement or hardening of the testes, and gynecomastia.

48.4 Disorders of the Penis

Differentiate the causes, classification, underlying pathogenesis, and clinical manifestations of disorders of the penis and approaches to diagnosis and treatment of these conditions across the lifespan.

- Hypospadias is a congenital abnormality of the location of the male urethral meatus. The meatus develops on the ventral side of the penis and can be anywhere from the glans to the perineum.
- Epispadias is a rare congenital defect in which the urethral opening is on dorsal surface of the penis.
- Phimosis is a condition in which the foreskin cannot be retracted over the glans penis. It can occur naturally in newborns or later after it was previously retractable, usually as a result of scarring of the foreskin.
- Paraphimosis occurs in uncircumcised or partially circumcised males when the retracted foreskin is trapped behind the coronal sulcus.
- Priapism is a prolonged erection that continues for hours. Ischemic priapism is a painful condition caused by blood not being able to leave the penis. It is an uncommon disorder in the general population but is more common in men with sickle cell disease.
- Peyronie disease is a caused by fibrous plaque that affects the tunica albuginea of the penis, causing it to curve or bend.
- Erectile dysfunction (ED), the most common male sexual disorder, is the inability to attain or maintain an erection sufficient to permit mutually satisfactory sexual intercourse with a partner.

REVIEW QUESTIONS

1. What is cryptorchidism?
   a. Inflammation of the testicles
   b. Undescended testicles
   c. Removal of both testicles
   d. Herniation of the right testicle
2. A client presents to the emergency department with pain, saying that "the pain is everywhere between my lower abdomen and scrotum." The client also complains of difficulty urinating and blood-tinged urine. A urinalysis shows no evidence of a UTI. What should the nurse anticipate as the diagnosis?
   a. Acute bacterial prostatitis
   b. Chronic bacterial prostatitis
   c. Chronic prostatitis/chronic pelvic pain syndrome
   d. Asymptomatic inflammatory prostatitis
3. A client is diagnosed with BPH. Which statement, made by the nurse, is correct regarding the next step in the process?
   a. "The next step is for you to have blood drawn to check for tumor markers."
   b. "The next step is for you to donate sperm before the surgery, which will be an orchiectomy."
   c. "You should expect to develop cancer related to the BPH. I am so sorry."
   d. "If your symptoms become worse, you may need further follow-up with a urologist."
4. In what part of the prostate does prostate cancer most often develop?
   a. Central zone
   b. Transition zone
   c. Peripheral zone
   d. Medial zone
5. Where is the most frequent site of metastasis for prostate cancer?
   a. Lymph nodes
   b. Bloodstream
   c. Bone marrow
   d. Spinal fluid
6. What is removed when a radical prostatectomy is performed?
   a. The prostate and epididymis
   b. The prostate and seminal vesicles
   c. The prostate and testes
   d. The prostate and ureters
7. Enlargement of the prostate can cause constriction of what part of the reproductive system?
   a. Ureters
   b. Bladder
   c. Urethra
   d. Penis
8. Saw palmetto is an example of what type of treatment?
   a. An herbal treatment
   b. A surgical procedure
   c. A prescribed medication
   d. An over-the-counter treatment

ANSWERS

Answers to Review Questions can be found in Appendix A. Answers to Case Study and Check Your Progress questions are available on the faculty resources site. Please consult with your instructor.

RECOMMENDED WEBSITES

CancerCare: Prostate Cancer
https://www.cancercare.org/diagnosis/prostate_cancer

National Institute of Diabetes and Digestive and Kidney Diseases
https://www.niddk.nih.gov

NIH Chronic Prostatitis Symptom Index
http://www.prostatitis.org/symptomindex.html

Patient Information: Testicular Self-Examination
http://www.cancernetwork.com/testicular-cancer/patient-information-self-examination-testes

Prostatitis Foundation
http://www.prostatitis.org

The Testicular Cancer Resource Center
http://tcrc.acor.org

Urology Care Foundation
http://www.urologyhealth.org

REFERENCES

1. Turek, P. J. (2017). Prostatitis. *Medscape*. Available at http://emedicine.medscape.com/article/785418-overview
2. Krieger, J. N., Nyberg, L., Jr., & Nickel, J. C. (1999). NIH consensus definition and classification of prostatitis. *JAMA, 282,* 236–237.
3. University of Maryland Medical Center. (2016). *Prostatitis.* Available at http://www.umm.edu/health/medical/altmed/condition/prostatitis
4. Deters, L. A. Benign prostatic hypertrophy. *Medscape.* Available at http://emedicine.medscape.com/article/437359-overview#a1
5. National Institute of Diabetes and Digestive and Kidney Diseases. (2014). *Prostate enlargement: Benign prostatic hyperplasia.* NIH Publication No. 14–3012. Available at http://www.niddk.nih.gov/health-information/health-topics/urologic-disease/benign-prostatic-hyperplasia-bph
6. National Center for Complementary and Integrative Health. (2016). Benign prostatic hyperplasia and complementary and integrative approaches. *NCCIH Clinical Digest.* Available at https://nccih.nih.gov/health/providers/digest/BPH
7. American Cancer Society. (2017). *Key statistics for prostate cancer.* Available at https://www.cancer.org/cancer/prostate-cancer/about/key-statistics.html
8. Prostate Cancer Foundation. (2017). *Risk factors.* Available at https://www.pcf.org/risk-factors/
9. American Cancer Society. (2017). *American Cancer Society recommendations for prostate cancer early detection.* Available at https://www.cancer.org/cancer/prostate-cancer/early-detection/acs-recommendations.html
10. Cancer.net Editorial Board. (2017). *Prostate cancer: Symptoms and signs.* Available at http://www.cancer.net/cancer-types/prostate-cancer/symptoms-and-signs
11. American Cancer Society. (2017). *Understanding your pathology report: Prostate cancer.* Available at https://www.cancer.org/treatment/understanding-your-diagnosis/tests/understanding-your-pathology-report/prostate-pathology/prostate-cancer-pathology.html
12. National Cancer Institute. (2017). *Prostate cancer, nutrition, and dietary supplements.* Available at https://www.cancer.gov/about-cancer/treatment/cam/hp/prostate-supplements-pdq
13. Mayo Clinic Staff. (2017). *Varicocele: Diseases and conditions.* Available at http://www.mayoclinic.org/diseases-conditions/varicocele/basics/definition/con-20024164
14. Mayo Clinic Staff. (2014). *Hydrocele: Diseases and conditions.* Available at http://www.mayoclinic.org/diseases-conditions/hydrocele/basics/definition/con-20024139
15. Mayo Clinic Staff. (2014). *Spermatocele. Diseases and conditions.* Available at http://www.mayoclinic.org/diseases-conditions/spermatocele/basics/definition/con-20024190
16. Kim, D. Epididymitis. *Medscape.* Available at http://emedicine.medscape.com/article/436154-overview#a4
17. Mayo Clinic Staff. (2014). *Orchitis. Diseases and conditions.* Available at http://www.mayoclinic.org/diseases-conditions/orchitis/basics/definition/con-20032815
18. Kim, E. D. (2016). Testicular torsion. *Medscape.* Available at http://emedicine.medscape.com/article/2036003-overview
19. National Cancer Institute. (2017). *Testicular cancer.* Available at https://www.cancer.gov/types/testicular
20. U.S. Preventive Services Task Force. (2011). *Testicular cancer: Screening.* Available at https://www.uspreventiveservicestaskforce.org/Page/Document/UpdateSummaryFinal/testicular-cancer-screening
21. American Cancer Society. (2016). *What are the risk factors for testicular cancer?* Available at https://www.cancer.org/cancer/testicular-cancer/causes-risks-prevention/risk-factors.html
22. American Cancer Society. (2017). *What are the key statistics about penile cancer?* Available at https://www.cancer.org/cancer/penile-cancer/about/key-statistics.html
23. U.S. National Library of Medicine. (2015). Hypospadias. *MedlinePlus.* Available at https://medlineplus.gov/ency/article/001286.htm
24. U.S. National Library of Medicine. (2015). Epispadias. *MedlinePlus.* Available at https://medlineplus.gov/ency/article/001285.htm
25. Ghory, H. Z. (2016). Phimosis and paraphimosis. *Medscape.* Available at http://emedicine.medscape.com/article/777539-overview#a5
26. Mayo Clinic Staff. (2016). *Priapism.* Available at http://www.mayoclinic.org/diseases-conditions/priapism/home/ovc-20208946
27. National Institute of Diabetes and Digestive and Kidney Diseases. (2014). *Penile curvature (Peyronie's disease).* Available at https://www.niddk.nih.gov/health-information/urologic-diseases/penile-curvature-peyronies-disease
28. Levin, R. J. (2015). Anatomy and physiology in the male. In K. R. Wylie (Ed.), *ABC of sexual health* (3rd ed., pp. 7–11). Hoboken, NJ: Wiley.
29. Lakin, M., & Wood, H. (2012). Erectile dysfunction. Available at http://www.clevelandclinicmeded.com/medicalpubs/diseasemanagement/endocrinology/erectile-dysfunction
30. American Psychiatric Association. (2013). *Diagnostic and statistical manual of mental disorders* (5th ed.). Arlington, VA: American Psychiatric Association.
31. Mayo Clinic Staff. (2017). *Erectile dysfunction.* Available at http://www.mayoclinic.org/diseases-conditions/erectile-dysfunction/home/ovc-20314087

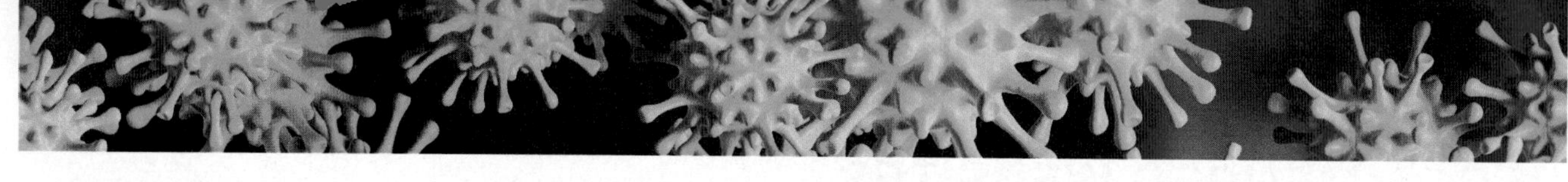

Chapter 49
Sexually Transmitted Infections

Daniel Mead, Christina Lattner, and Matthew Sorenson

Chapter Outline and Learning Outcomes

49.1 Chapter Overview and Case Studies

Discuss the epidemiology and prevalence of sexually transmitted infections and concepts related to sexually transmitted infections.

49.2 Viral STIs

Differentiate the causes, classification, underlying pathogenesis, and clinical manifestations of viral STIs and approaches to diagnosis and treatment of these conditions across the lifespan.

49.3 Bacterial STIs

Differentiate the causes, classification, underlying pathogenesis, and clinical manifestations of bacterial STIs and approaches to diagnosis and treatment of these conditions across the lifespan.

49.4 Parasitic STIs

Differentiate the causes, classification, underlying pathogenesis, and clinical manifestations of parasitic STIs and approaches to diagnosis and treatment of these conditions across the lifespan.

KEY TERMS

Chancre, 1213
Chlamydia, 1211
Genital warts, 1209
Gonorrhea, 1212
Herpes simplex virus (HSV), 1210
Human papillomavirus (HPV), 1208
Pediculosis pubis, 1215
Pelvic inflammatory disease, 1211
Pyogenic, 1212
Sexually transmitted disease (STD), 1207
Sexually transmitted infection (STI), 1207
Syphilis, 1213
Trichomoniasis, 1214

ABBREVIATIONS

HPV—human papillomavirus
HSV—herpes simplex virus
STD—sexually transmitted disease
STI—sexually transmitted infection

49.1 Chapter Overview and Case Studies

The term **sexually transmitted infection (STI)** is used to describe a number of infections resulting from sexual contact. These infections are caused by a variety of bacteria, fungi, viruses, and parasites, and most can be readily cured. Although *sexually transmitted infection* is the more recent term for these disease states, there is a difference between an STI and a **sexually transmitted disease (STD)**. The latter term is used more commonly to refer to infections that cannot be readily cured, such as herpes simplex virus. Regardless of the distinction, many sources use the terms STI and STD interchangeably.

The incidence of STI has continued to increase over the past several years. It is estimated that 357 million new cases of readily curable STIs occur each year worldwide.[1] In the United States alone, over 20 million new cases of STI occur yearly, 50% of them affecting individuals between the ages of 15 and 24.[2] There are some gender differences in that females experience more cases of gonorrhea while males have higher rates of chlamydia and syphilis.[3] Long-term complications can occur in both genders and include effects on reproductive function and fertility.[2]

Although most STIs are acquired through sexual contact with an infected individual, some STIs can be passed from mother to infant during childbirth. Exposure to infection can also occur through sharing of needles for injecting drugs and through blood transfusion. Risk factors include low socioeconomic status, low levels of education, use of substances such as alcohol and drugs, multiple sex partners, and the exchange of sex for money or services.[4] There are thus a number of activities by which infection may be transmitted. This highlights the need for prevention education on the part of the nursing profession. Several STIs can be readily treated with antibiotics, but many individuals are asymptomatic or do not display symptoms of disease until years after they are infected. Thus, early detection and treatment can be difficult. This chapter provides an overview of some of the major STIs caused by viruses, bacteria, and parasites.

Concepts Related to STIs

Cultural and media representations of sexual behavior and peer pressure can influence sexual expectations and the sexuality of an individual. In turn, sexuality affects relationships, self-image, mood and affect, and sexual behavior. The surrounding environment also influences the possibility of engaging in sexual behavior that may lead to STIs. The presence of an intact immune system may aid in providing a degree of defense or influence initial responses to an infectious agent. When an STI is contracted, it may produce physiologic symptomatology or it may remain asymptomatic for a significant period of time. Symptoms may affect elimination and tissue integrity. The presence of an STI may have lasting effects on reproductive health and, if not treated, may be transmitted from a mother to her infant. Concepts related to STIs are shown in **Figure 49.1** ■.

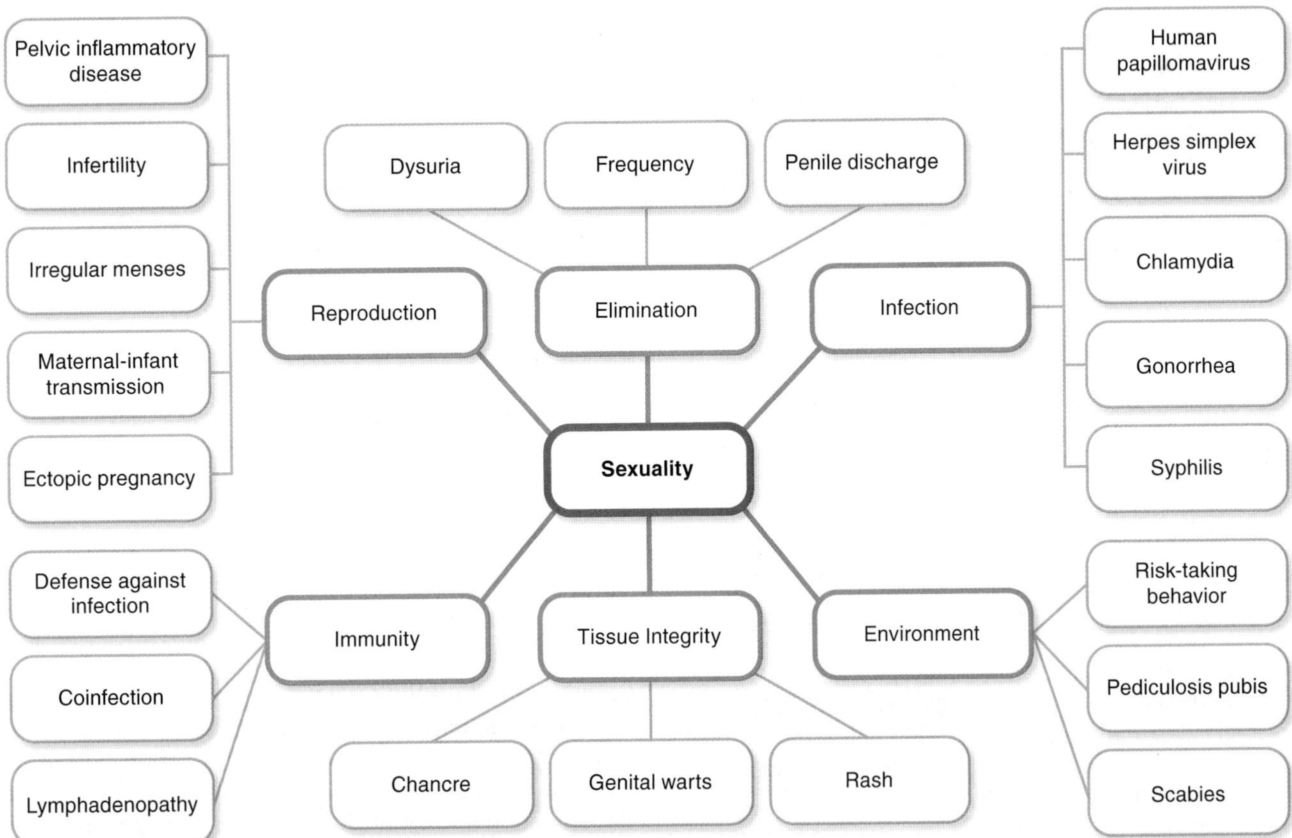

Figure 49.1 ■ Concepts related to sexually transmitted infections.

The presence of asymptomatic infections increases the possibility of maternal-infant transmission. In the absence of symptoms, the mother is less likely to be tested. This has led to a recommendation that all pregnant women be tested for STIs. ■

CLINICAL POINT: It is important to remember, for both your patients and yourself, that most STIs can be prevented. Know the methods of preventing STIs, use them yourself, and teach them to your patients (**Figure 49.2** ■). ■

Case Studies

The following cases are addressed throughout the chapter to assist in application of chapter content to clinical situations that involve individuals with sexually transmitted infections.

Nicole Thomas: Introduction

Nicole Thomas is a 29-year-old female who works as a real estate agent. She has come to the clinic for evaluation, as she is concerned about some bumps her boyfriend has on his penis. On history, she reports that her boyfriend was treated approximately 2 years ago for genital warts.

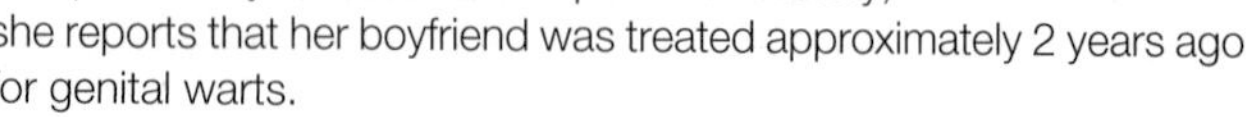

1. What information would be important to obtain about Ms. Thomas's sexual behavior that may affect her risk of acquiring a sexually transmitted infection?
2. What additional information about Ms. Thomas's sexual history would be important to obtain, and why?

Kristina Martin: Introduction

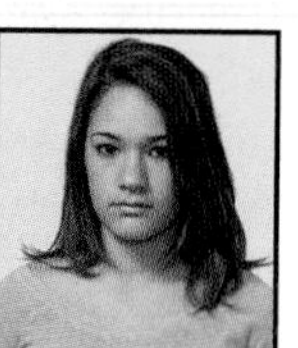

Kristina Martin is a 17-year-old high school junior. She has been dating a couple of boys but has one she favors, and she has been trying to gain his attention by dating others to make him jealous. She gets a text message from this boyfriend saying that they need to talk. He reveals that he has been diagnosed with chlamydia.

1. What risk factor does Ms. Martin have that increases her chance of getting an STI?
2. Of the number of new STIs diagnosed each year, what percentage is diagnosed in Ms. Martin's age group?

Check Your Progress: Section 49.1

1. What is the difference between a sexually transmitted infection and a sexually transmitted disease?
2. What types of sexually transmitted infections are more common in males?
3. What are some of the potential physiologic consequences of sexually transmitted infections?

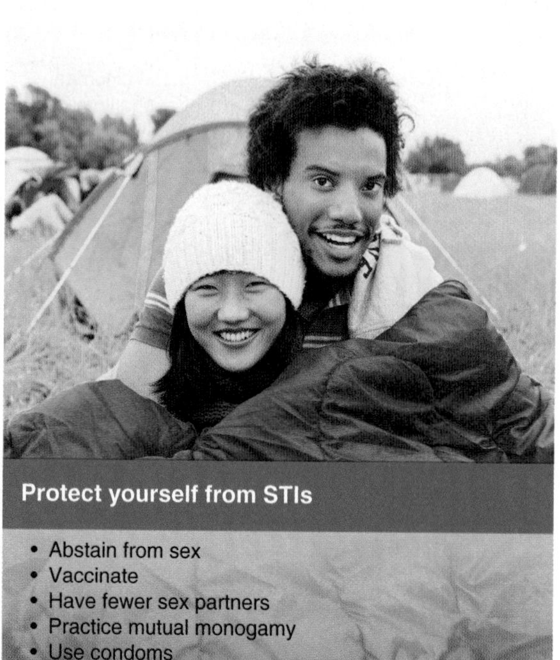
Protect yourself from STIs
• Abstain from sex
• Vaccinate
• Have fewer sex partners
• Practice mutual monogamy
• Use condoms

Figure 49.2 ■ Methods for protecting yourself from STIs include abstinence from sexual activity, vaccination for hepatitis B and HPV, limiting the number of sex partners you have, practicing mutual monogamy, and using condoms.

SOURCE: Centers for Disease Control and Prevention. (2016). *How you can prevent sexually transmitted diseases.* Available at https://www.cdc.gov/std/prevention

49.2 Viral STIs

Several viruses are known to be associated with sexually transmitted infections. Certain viral infections such as hepatitis B or C and HIV can have lifelong ramifications. Other viral infections can be treated with some success or prevented through vaccination. This section focuses on two common viral STIs: human papillomavirus and herpes simplex virus. Of the two, HPV can be prevented through vaccination.

Human Papillomavirus

Human papillomavirus (HPV) is the most prevalent of all sexually transmitted infections; reports indicate that nearly 80 million people are currently infected in the United States. The virus goes undetected in a majority of cases because most people are asymptomatic; however, HPV is the most common cause of many types of cancers, primarily cervical cancer. Besides education on general risk and prevention of STI, vaccination is available for protection against HPV.[5]

Etiology and Pathogenesis

Human papillomaviruses are small, double-stranded DNA viruses that infect cutaneous and mucosal epithelial tissues of the anogenital tract. Infection can also include areas of the hands and the feet. To date, over 100 different viral types have been identified, and about one third of these infect epithelial cells in the genital tract. A subset of HPV types are the causative agents of cervical cancer, since 99% of tumors are positive for HPV DNA. HPVs that infect the genital tract are sexually transmitted, and it is estimated that about two thirds of individuals who have sexual relations with an infected partner will themselves become infected.[6]

Infection of the genital tract by HPVs can initially result in lesions called *dysplasias* or *cervical intraepithelial neoplasia grade I*. These lesions exhibit only mildly altered patterns of differentiation, and many of them are cleared by the immune system in less than a year without causing further illness. The mechanisms by which the cellular immune response clears HPV infections are not completely understood. Lesions that are not cleared by the immune system often persist for several decades before being detected. Persistence of infection by high-risk HPV types is the greatest risk factor for development of genital malignancies such as squamous cell carcinoma. An individual can be infected with multiple types of HPV at the same time.[6]

High-risk types of HPVs are associated with the development of anogenital cancers, including cancers of the cervix. By contrast, infections by the low-risk HPVs induce only benign genital warts. High-risk types include HPV-16, HPV-18, HPV-31, HPV-33, and HPV-45. Low-risk types are HPV-6 and HPV-11. The human papillomavirus capsid lacks an envelope, which makes this viral organism extremely stable and resistant to various medical treatments. Serologic typing is unavailable because of the lack of consistency in methods of in vitro culture. Distinguishing types of HPV is based on genotyping, which is used to generally determine the molecular hybridization using molecular cloned HPV DNA.[6]

Clinical Manifestations

HPV is the most common STI in women. Up to 79% of sexually active women acquire some form of genital HPV infection during their lifetime. However, the infection is usually transient and asymptomatic. Genital warts (**Figure 49.3** ■), which are the most visible manifestation of the HPV infection, occur in only about 1% of the sexually active American population. Patients who present with clinical symptoms represent only a small part of a vast population of infected individuals.[7]

Infection with HPV may be latent, subclinical, or clinical, depending on the genotype in an infected person. The HPV infection may take the pathway of low viral load infection without clinical disease presentation, or high viral load infection with clinical disease presentation. HPV infections that manifest as genital warts are typically seen as low- or high-grade intraepithelial lesions. In women, up to 30% of cases of genital warts will spontaneously regress within 4 months if left untreated.

Up to 90% of women infected with high- or low-risk HPV may clear the infection within 2 years. It is not clear whether an immune-mediated regression of low- or high-grade intraepithelial lesions eliminates the infection or suppresses it permanently, but in either event, the virus ceases to manifest lesions. The average time to clearance of genital warts after a course of medical treatment is about 6 months. A small minority of infected individuals fail to clear the infection; these individuals are at risk of progression to malignancy, primarily in the anogenital or cervix area.[7]

HPV infection in women is most common in their early 20s. After 20 years of age, the prevalence of HPV has a steady decline. Recently, a second peak of prevalence has been occurring in postmenopausal women. The second peak of HPV may be attributed to an existing viral persistence or to a new acquisition of the viral infection. The typical interval between infection with HPV to a diagnosis of malignant cancer cells is 10–20 years, which is often about 40 years of age. Because the diagnosis of cervical cancer caused by HPV does not appear until many years after the initial infection, testing for HPV infection in sexually active women is most useful between 20 and 40 years of age. Cervical cancer is a primary concern in women with HPV infection; there are also other, rarer HPV-induced cancers of the vagina, vulva, anus, and penis.[7]

Low-risk HPV types (HPV-6 and HPV-11) cause 90–95% of anogenital lesions, commonly referred to as **genital warts**. Genital warts appear as recurrent papules or cauliflower-like, flat lesions also referred to as *condyloma planum*. Lesions can appear as slightly raised, papular or macular, with or without keratinization and may have brown, gray, or blue pigmentation. In laboratory testing, genital warts often turn white with application of a 3–5% acetic acid solution, however, this test is nonspecific.[7]

High-risk HPV types, particularly HPV-16 and HPV-18, account for 70% of cervical cancers. High-risk HPV types tend to persist longer than low-risk types. High-risk HPV often results in 95% of all diagnosed cervical dysplasias. HPV-16 causes 50% of squamous cell cervical cancers, and HPV-18 is responsible for 20% of adenocarcinoma. Adenocarcinoma is a less common cancer; however, it is aggressive and arises from the glandular epithelium of the endocervical canal.[7]

Individuals can become infected with multiple high-risk types of HPV. Multiple high-risk types of HPV act

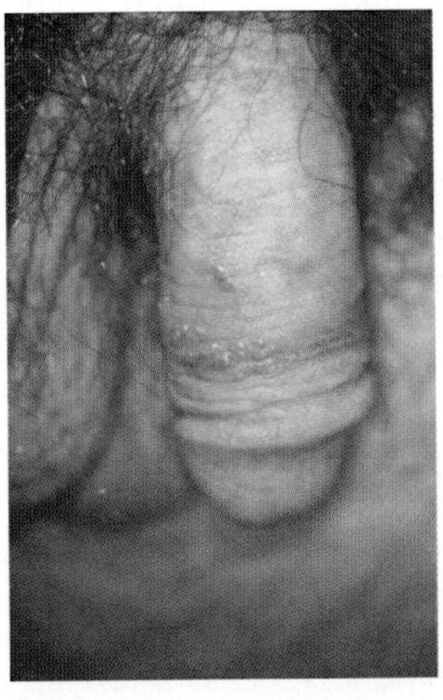

A

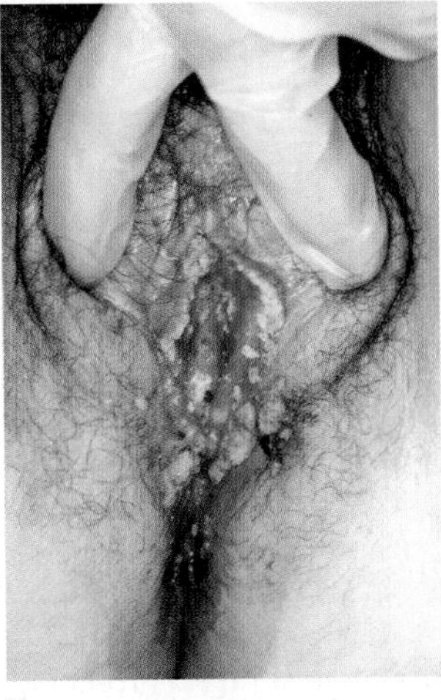

B

Figure 49.3 ■ Genital warts on **A.** the penis and **B.** the vulva.

synergistically in cervical carcinogenesis. Grade 1 cervical intraepithelial neoplasia (CIN 1) indicates an active HPV infection. CIN 2 is considered a high-grade lesion but may regress spontaneously in 40% of infected women.[7]

Age-related physiologic changes put older women at increased risk for STIs. Decreased estrogen production after menopause results in a thinner vaginal wall lining that is more prone to tearing and abrasion during intercourse. ■

Nicole Thomas: Application

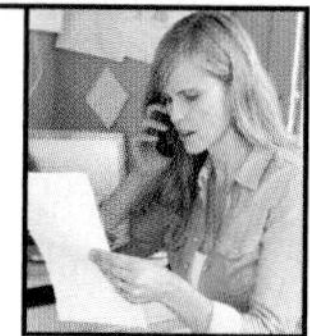

On physical examination, multiple small raised lesions are found in Ms. Thomas's perineal area. A biopsy is taken of one of the growths. The results indicate that the lesions are genital warts, and Ms. Thomas is diagnosed with HPV.

3. How should you respond when Ms. Thomas asks, "When will the genital warts go away?"
4. What educational needs may Ms. Thomas have regarding the diagnosis of HPV?

Linking Pathophysiology to Diagnosis and Treatment

HPV infections are detected through polymerase chain reaction testing or DNA testing. DNA tests detect only high-risk HPV types. Testing for low-risk HPV types has no clinical benefit because of the lack of correlation between low-risk HPV and cervical cancer. Current testing with the Digene HPV Test or Hybrid Capture 2 has a sensitivity of approximately 90% for high-risk HPV types.

HPV infection can be detected and managed in various ways. The Papanicolaou test (commonly known as the Pap smear) is the gold standard of primary screening for cervical dysplasia. Research shows that low-risk HPV is associated with 10–25% of abnormal cervical smears. The basis of cell morphology does not allow the cytologist or pathologist to differentiate smears obtained in a Pap smear to be associated with low-risk HPV from those associated with high-risk HPV. Abnormal cervical smears require additional testing for definitive results. Patients with any lesions that are suspected of being high grade or cancerous should be sent for biopsy.

Treatment of infection with human papillomavirus consists of ruling out other possible associated STIs and includes detailed exploration of the patient's sex partner(s). The treatment plan for each patient is determined by a series of factors, which include the following:

- The number, size, and anatomic distribution of the lesions
- Lesion extension, grade of keratinization, time of development, and resistance to other treatments
- The patient's immunologic state
- The effectiveness, availability, and ease of application of the most desirable therapeutic method along with the patient's preference and previous experience
- Toxicity and cost of treatment
- The patient's age.[7]

Although the possibility of spontaneous regression may exist in certain types of HPV, the general tendency is to treat the lesions in order to control disease spread, relieve the patient's anxiety, and improve the patient's general self-esteem.

Therapeutic methods often prescribed for patients to self-administer include 0.5% podophyllotoxin solution or gel applied topically to the lesions twice a day for 3 consecutive days, followed by 4 days without treatment. This regimen is repeated for up to 4 weeks.

Imiquimod 5% cream is a family of molecules (imidazoline heterocyclic amines) that work not by destroying the lesions but rather by inducing the local synthesis of cytokines, mainly interferon alpha, thus modifying the immunologic response of the organism infected by HPV and eliminating the lesions.[7]

Therapeutic methods administered by health professionals include cryotherapy with liquid nitrogen, 10–25% podofilox resin or surgical extirpation with cold scalpel, and electrocoagulation. CO_2 laser treatment is typically done for infection in areas such as the urethral meatus or the anal canal.

HPV-related cancers and STIs are considered vaccine-preventable illnesses. The Centers for Disease Control and Prevention's Advisory Committee on Immunization Practices currently recommends that all males and females be vaccinated with the three-dose HPV vaccine starting at age 10–12 years. The two vaccines currently available to prevent HPV infection are Gardasil and Cervarix. Gardasil's labeled use is to protect against cancer of the cervix, vagina, and vulva in girls and to protect against warts in the anal and genital region of males age 9–26 years. Cervarix is approved and labeled for protection of females only against cancer of the cervix age 10–25 years.

The most pressing need for HPV vaccination is in the developing world, where most women never receive Papanicolaou testing and cervical cancer is a major cause of death. Approximately 80% of cases of cervical cancer occur in the developing world. Globally, 529,000 women are diagnosed with cervical cancer every year, and 275,000 deaths are attributed to cervical cancer.[5] A vaccine that is effective against the four or five most common high-risk HPV types could prevent 80–90% of cervical cancers worldwide.

Nicole Thomas: Outcome

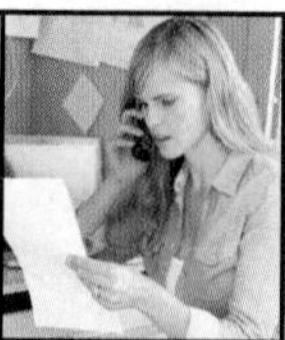

Ms. Thomas's warts are removed by cryosurgery, and a vaccine is administered to protect her against other types of HPV. She is educated about the prevention of exacerbations and the need to follow up in 6 months.

5. Ms. Thomas asks how her lesions were tested to rule out high-risk HPV types. How would you respond?
6. What information should be given to Ms. Thomas's boyfriend?

Herpes Simplex Virus

There are two forms of **herpes simplex virus (HSV)**: HSV-1 and HSV-2. Both forms can be associated with genital infection, but HSV-1 is more commonly associated with infections around the mouth, typically manifesting as cold sores. HSV-2 is more commonly associated with genital infection and can manifest as blisters around the genital area. Each type can exist without the appearance of related symptoms. Both forms are transmitted by direct contact with the bodily fluids of an infected individual. Most commonly, such transmission occurs through sexual contact and can occur even while the infected individual is asymptomatic.[8]

Etiology and Pathogenesis

After infection, HSV enters nerve cells and resides in the cellular ganglion. Its location in the ganglion aids in protecting the virus from being cleared by the immune system. HSV is generally latent in the nerve cell and can be reactivated by periods of physical or psychologic stress. Viral reactivation can result in the appearance of characteristic symptoms.[9]

The appearance of HSV infection is more common in young adult populations and often tied to early sexual experiences and a relatively high number of sex partners. It is estimated that one out of every six individuals between 14 and 49 years of age in the United States has been exposed to HSV.[8] The lack of symptoms in some individuals aids in transmission of the virus.

Clinical Manifestations

Orofacial manifestations of HSV appear as erythematous papules that develop into vesicles within a short period of time. The appearance of orofacial lesions is typically preceded by pain or a burning sensation at the site of lesion development.[10]

Genital manifestations of HSV include small vesicles located in the genital area that are often accompanied by pain (**Figure 49.4** ■). For males, lesions typically manifest on the glans or shaft of the penis. In females, lesions appear primarily on the external genitalia such as the labia. For both genders, lesions may persist for 4–15 days. Anal lesions may result from anal intercourse.

In cases of genital HSV infection, lesions may be preceded by headache, fever, and myalgia. Constitutional symptoms generally appear for less than 1 week. Genital lesions may be preceded by burning or paresthesia at the lesion site before the lesions develop. It is important to remember that most primary infections are asymptomatic.[10]

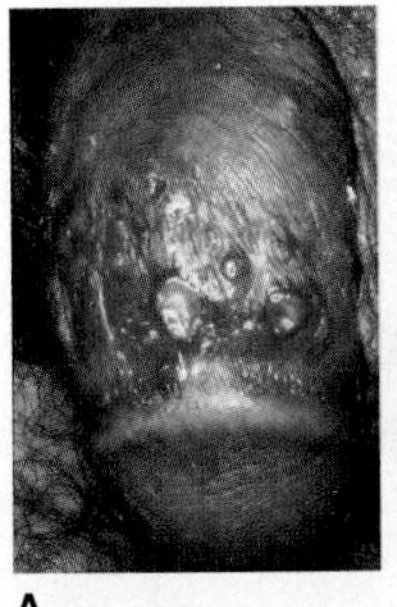

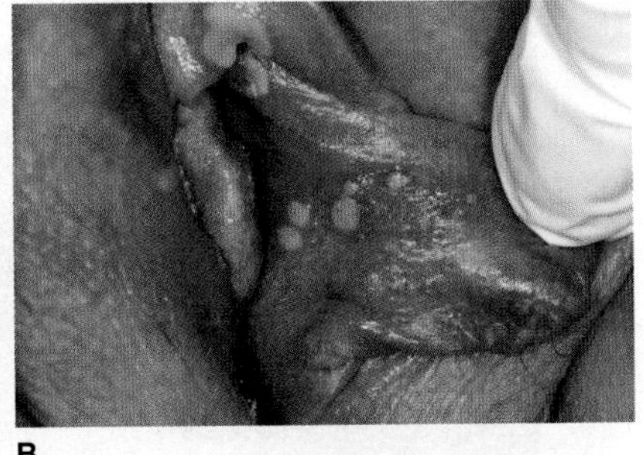

A **B**

Figure 49.4 ■ Genital herpes on **A.** the penis and **B.** the vulva.

Linking Pathophysiology to Diagnosis and Treatment

The most effective means of treating HSV is preventing transmission (see Figure 49.2). There is no curative agent, and the location of the virus in cells of the nervous system aids in ensuring the survival of the virus. Current therapeutic approaches are designed to shorten the periods of exacerbation and symptomatology and to lessen the severity of these episodes. Antiviral therapies are the mainstay of pharmacologic treatment; some evidence supports the use of such agents to prevent viral transmission.[11]

Check Your Progress: Section 49.2

1. What are the low-risk types of HPV that are usually responsible for genital warts?
2. If a patient decides to have sexual relations with a person infected with HPV, what is the risk of transferring the infection?
3. Which type of herpes simplex virus is more commonly associated with infections around the mouth?

49.3 Bacterial STIs

Pelvic inflammatory disease (an infection of a woman's reproductive organs, including the ovaries, fallopian tubes, uterus, and cervix), vaginosis (bacterial overgrowth in the vagina), and epididymitis (inflammation of the epididymis in men) are disease states associated with bacteria exposure. These conditions are but a sample of STIs tied to bacterial infection. However, when the topic of bacterial STIs arises, most people think of chlamydia, gonorrhea, and syphilis. Each of these STIs has a long history, and they are still relatively common today. The section provides a brief overview of these bacterial STIs.

Chlamydia

Chlamydia is caused by the bacterium *Chlamydia trachomatis*, which has multiple strains associated with eye disease and genital tract infections. The infection is usually spread through sexual contact.

There is a high rate of maternal transmission of chlamydia to the infant during birth. It may result in conjunctivitis or pneumonia in the infant. ■

Etiology and Pathogenesis

Chlamydia is the most common bacterium STI in the United States and is often found in combination with gonorrhea. Approximately 3 million new cases of chlamydia occur each year in the United States, primarily in the adolescent and young adult populations. The prevalence of chlamydia is believed to be significantly underestimated, as most infections are asymptomatic. This can lead to delay in seeking treatment and may result in complications such as infertility and ectopic pregnancy.[12] In men, chlamydia is often asymptomatic as well and can lead to the development of a form of arthritis.[12]

Chlamydia infects mainly the genital tract, with a particular affinity for columnar epithelial cells. Initial exposure results in an inflammatory response that can result in tissue damage and the production of antibodies. While the body produces antibody to chlamydia, it does not prevent reinfection. Chlamydia depends on the host for nutrients and survival. The bacterium is able to manufacture its own DNA and RNA but requires energy from the host cell.[13]

Asymptomatic infection still elicits an inflammatory response that can lead to scarring and damage to the reproductive system of both males and females. In males, the infection can extend to the prostate and testes. Chlamydia can affect the structure and function of sperm, resulting in malformation of sperm and reduced motility. In females, the infection can extend into the fallopian tubes and uterus, resulting in pelvic inflammatory disease leading to scarring and tissue damage.[13,14]

Clinical Manifestations

The most common site of chlamydia infection is the urinary tract. Most chlamydia infections are asymptomatic. Common symptoms that may indicate infection in males include dysuria and urethral drainage that is yellow in color. Scrotal pain and swelling may also be seen. In females, vaginal discharge and abnormal vaginal bleeding may result. Pain on urination and on intercourse is common.[14]

Kristina Martin: Application

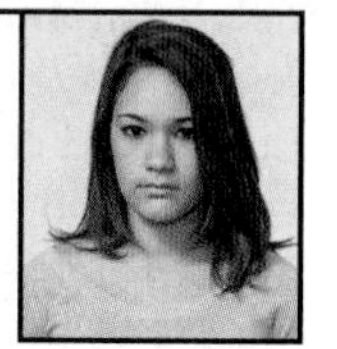

Ms. Martin goes to a community health center in her neighborhood. She says that she has not usually used protection while having sex and that she has had three sex partners. She denies the presence of any lower urinary tract symptoms and is surprised to hear that she might have an STI. She is given an oral course of azithromycin.

3. What area of the body is susceptible to infection with chlamydia?
4. What type of symptoms might Ms. Martin describe if she is infected with chlamydia?

Linking Pathophysiology to Diagnosis and Treatment

A common diagnostic measure for chlamydia is the evaluation of a urine sample. The organism is excreted in the urine and can be isolated for testing. Vaginal swabs are also an effective means of sample collection with high sensitivity. Considering the high rate of coinfection, empiric treatment may be provided before diagnostic results are available if the individual is symptomatic. The primary means of treatment is providing a single dose of azithromycin or doxycycline for 1 week. Both sex partners should be treated at the same time. Sexual activity should not be resumed until treatment has been completed.[12]

Kristina Martin: Outcome

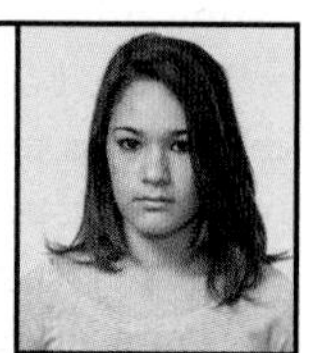

Ms. Martin is concerned about the possibility of developing an STI in the future. She is given appropriate education by the community health nurse, and she is supported regarding the need to notify her sex partners about the possibility of their having developed chlamydia. Ms. Martin acknowledges the need to use precautions from now on.

5. What complications might Ms. Martin have if the chlamydia is left untreated?
6. What other types of precautions should the nurse discuss with Ms. Martin?

Gonorrhea

Gonorrhea is caused by a pyogenic bacterium known as *Neisseria gonorrhoeae*, a gram-negative diplococcus. The term **pyogenic** refers to the production of pus. A pyogenic bacterium is then one associated with the development and expression of pus. In the case of gonorrhea, this refers to purulent discharge from the urethra or vagina. There are approximately 900,000 new cases of gonorrhea in the United States each year, and it is often a coinfection with chlamydia.[15]

Etiology and Pathogenesis

Neisseria gonorrhoeae has surface pili, which are small extensions along the surface membrane. The presence of these pili prevents the organism from being phagocytized by neutrophils. A protease that is present on the surface of the pili facilitates attachment of the organism to the wall of the urethra or vagina. *Neisseria gonorrhoeae* also has the ability to attach to spermatozoa, which allows for effective transmission.

Clinical Manifestations

As with other STIs, a significant percentage of the individuals with gonorrhea are asymptomatic until later stages of the disease. In males, symptoms include dysuria and purulent penile discharge (**Figure 49.5** ■). Females with gonorrhea exhibit dysuria, purulent vaginal discharge, and pain during intercourse. Without treatment, the infection may progress to pelvic inflammatory disease and a form of acute perihepatitis.[15]

Gonococcal infection can extend to the eye and the pharynx. Pharyngitis may be asymptomatic or can manifest with lymphadenopathy. Ocular manifestations generally present with unilateral purulent discharge.

Linking Pathophysiology to Diagnosis and Treatment

As with other bacterial STIs, a urine sample can be cultured for the presence of *Neisseria gonorrhoeae*. If pharyngeal involvement is suspected, the throat should be cultured as

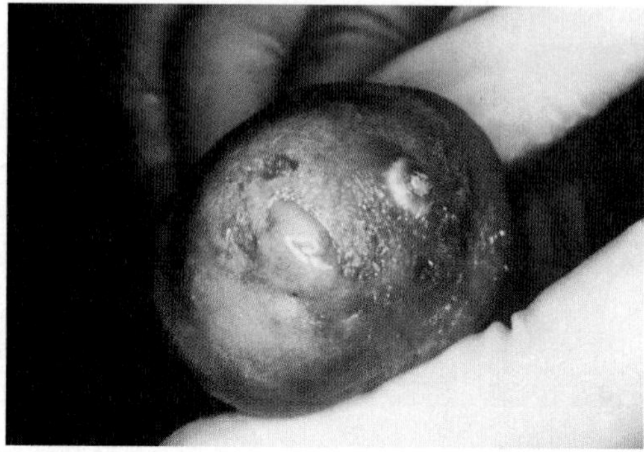

Figure 49.5 ■ Purulent penile discharge resulting from gonorrhea.

well. Because the organism resides within cells, any culture should include cells.

Treatment guidelines recommend the use of two antibiotics: an intramuscular injection of ceftriaxone and an oral dose of azithromycin. As with chlamydia, all sex partners of the infected individual should be treated at the same time. Sexual activity should not be resumed until treatment has been completed.[15]

Syphilis

Syphilis is an STI acquired through direct sexual contact with an infected individual or through blood transfusion.

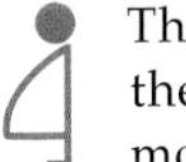

There is a congenital form of syphilis in which the infection can be passed to a fetus from the mother. ■

Etiology and Pathogenesis

Spirochetes are double-membraned anaerobic bacteria with helical cells. Three main families or genera of spirochetes are known to cause infections in human populations. One of these families, *Treponema*, is associated with syphilis, in particular *Treponema pallidum*. Transmission results from contact with open lesions known as **chancres**.[16]

After infection, the spirochetes rapidly disseminate systemically, traveling through the blood and lymphatic systems. The incubation period averages approximately 3 weeks and can range from 10 to 90 days. During this time, the spirochetes penetrate the central nervous system. The characteristic lesion or chancre reflects underlying inflammation and infiltration of tissue by leukocytes. The inflammatory response can also lead to damage to the inner lining of peripheral arteries that can result in vessel occlusion.

Without appropriate intervention, syphilis will progress through four stages: primary, secondary, latent, and tertiary; each stage is associated with characteristic symptomatology. Without treatment, syphilis causes cardiovascular and neurologic damage, resulting in death.

During 2014, there were approximately 63,000 new cases of acquired syphilis in the United States. Men who had sex with other men accounted for over 80% of all new cases.

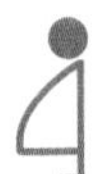

The incidence of congenital syphilis was far lower than that of acquired syphilis; 458 cases of congenital syphilis were reported in the United States in 2014.[16] ■

Clinical Manifestations

Clinical manifestations of syphilis change as the infection progresses through the four stages:

- ***Primary syphilis*** is associated with the development of a lesion, or chancre (**Figure 49.6** ■), often considered characteristic of the disease. Whether or not the patient receives treatment, the lesion will resolve within 3 months and may even go unnoticed.
- ***Secondary syphilis*** reflects the systemic distribution of the spirochetes and can have variable symptomatology. Manifestations that are common in this state include alopecia, fever, arthralgia, lymphadenopathy, and rash. The rash is most likely to be on the soles of the feet or palms of the hands. The secondary stage typically appears 1–3 months after infection, and manifestations will generally last for 4–6 weeks.[17]
- ***Latent syphilis*** reflects a period of asymptomatic infection. The manifestations of the primary and secondary stage have resolved. Certain individuals will continue to experience the development of the characteristic skin lesion or chancre, but most will be asymptomatic.
- ***Tertiary syphilis*** reflects the accumulation of damage to the arterial lining and nervous system. Cardiovascular manifestations are generally related to damage to the lining of the ascending aorta that may result in development of an aneurysm. Neurologically, meningitis may occur and reflects not only the presence of infection but also damage to the arterial lining. Confusion, vision disturbance, and hearing loss are not uncommon.[17]

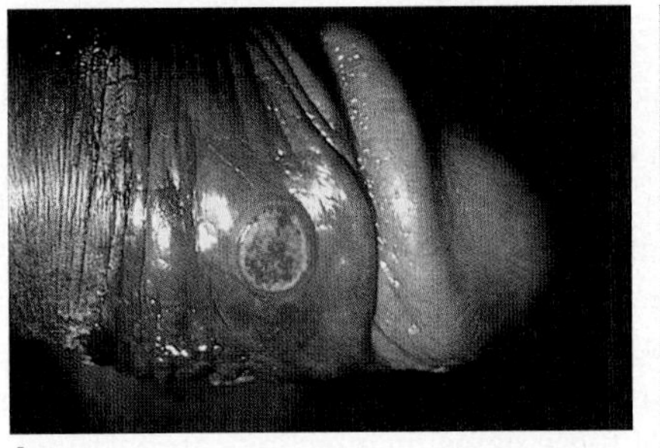

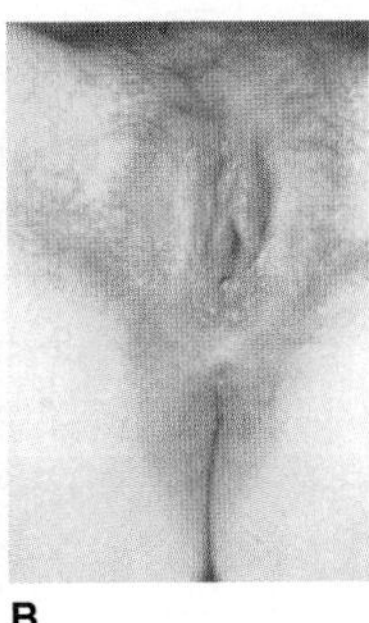

A B

Figure 49.6 ■ Chancre of primary syphilis on **A.** the penis and **B.** the vulva.

Linking Pathophysiology to Diagnosis and Treatment

Early diagnosis of syphilis is imperative, given the serious nature of the disease, especially the danger of progression to tertiary syphilis. Initial screening is based on the patient's history and the development of ulcerative lesions (chancre) on the penis or external labial surfaces. *Treponema pallidum* cannot be cultivated in the laboratory setting, and the small size of this organism makes microscopic detection unlikely. Serologic screening is considered the most appropriate means of testing. Point-of-care blood tests have been developed in recent years to aid with identification in the clinical or outpatient setting.[17]

Pharmacologic treatment remains the main approach, intramuscular penicillin being the antibiotic of choice. For patients who are allergic to penicillin, alternative medications include cephalosporin and erythromycin. As with most STIs, prevention is the optimal means of restricting the incidence of syphilis.

Check Your Progress: Section 49.3

1. Why should an individual who is being treated for chlamydia also be treated for gonorrhea?
2. What are the associated symptoms of primary syphilis?
3. Cardiovascular and neurologic manifestations of syphilis are present in which stage?

49.4 Parasitic STIs

Parasites are small organisms that can live on the outside surface of the skin or burrow underneath the skin surface. Pediculosis pubis is a common disease brought about through contact with a member of the lice family. It is particularly noted for living on pubic hair but can extend to hair on other parts of the body. Trichomoniasis is a disease brought up by a protozoan that infects vaginal surfaces or the urethra. Both of these parasitic infections are relatively common and are acquired through sexual contact.

Trichomoniasis

Etiology and Pathogenesis

Trichomoniasis is a parasitic STI known colloquially as "trich." It is transmitted by the protozoan *Trichomonas vaginalis* (**Figure 49.7** ■). Trichomoniasis can infect a human host by itself; however, there is an increasing prevalence of coinfection throughout the world.[18] Much like other STIs, trichomoniasis can increase a patient's risk of contracting and developing an HIV infection, leading to AIDS. Trichomoniasis is thought to be underdiagnosed in general for a host of reasons, including lack of specific symptoms, asymptomatic patient carriers, and poor sensitivity (50–70%) of the wet mount diagnostic technique.[19] The usual pathogenesis of a trichomoniasis infection is sexual contact and sometimes through fomites. The prevalence of trichomoniasis in the United States is estimated at 8 million cases yearly. However, this is likely not an accurate estimate because trichomoniasis infection is not a reportable infectious disease. The World Health Organization estimates the prevalence of trichomoniasis infection in the world to be greater than 200 million cases annually.[18,20]

Clinical Manifestations

Trichomonal infection is asymptomatic in roughly 50% of female patients and nearly 90% of male patients. This is one of the many reasons why trichomoniasis spreads quickly. Males and females may have varying nonspecific clinical manifestations.[21] Females exhibit symptoms ranging from asymptomatic carrier states to full-blown severe pelvic inflammatory disease. Acute infections involve all or some of the following symptoms[19,20]:

- Vulvar itching, burning, soreness, swelling, and redness
- White, grayish-green, or yellow discharge that sometimes has a frothy characteristic
- Musty or fishy smelling odor of the discharge
- pH of discharge greater than 5
- A "strawberry cervix" pelvic exam (named for the cervical petechiae and friability of the cervix)
- Dyspareunia
- Dysuria
- Sometimes postcoital bleeding and lower abdominal pain.

Chronic trichomoniasis can involve large amounts of discharge consistent with the above characteristics but slight to no vaginal mucosal inflammation. Chronic trichomoniasis is less likely to involve dyspareunia, a strawberry cervix, and postcoital bleeding.

A male infected with *Trichomonas vaginalis* can be an asymptomatic carrier, may have mild symptomatic disease, or may have acute trichomoniasis. These three categories span the symptoms from asymptomatic to severe urethritis complicated by prostatitis. If there are symptoms, they will include some or all of the following: purulent discharge, mucoid discharge, dysuria, urethritis, testicular pain, and lower abdominal pain. Most symptomatic infections in males are intermittent and self-limiting; however, a male partner should always be treated, owing to the high likelihood of being an asymptomatic carrier.

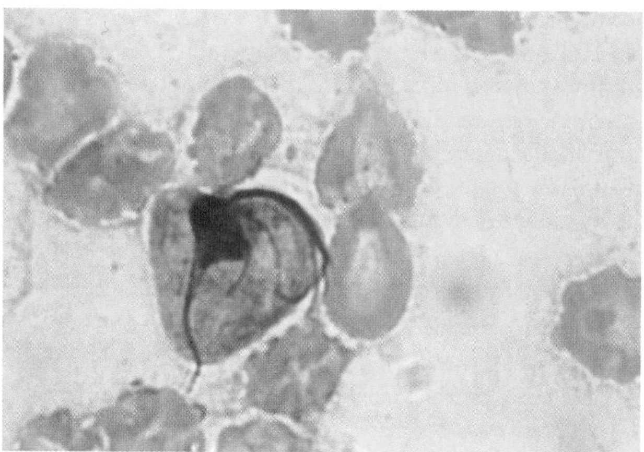

Figure 49.7 ■ Micrograph of a *Trichomonas vaginalis* parasite.

Linking Pathophysiology to Diagnosis and Treatment

The history and physical examination of a woman with trichomoniasis might involve a foul, watery discharge, which is likely to be green in color and possibly frothy, and a strawberry cervix. However, because many cases of trichomoniasis have mild or nonspecific symptoms or are asymptomatic, the physical examination and history will not necessarily provide conclusive evidence of infection. A laboratory test will be needed to confirm the diagnosis.

The diagnosis of trichomoniasis is generally made by placing a small amount of vaginal drainage (wet mount) on a microscope slide and then examining the slide under a microscope. The key feature is microscopic identification of gyrating motile protozoan parasites. These are generally identifiable by ameboid-type movement, four flagella protruding from one side of the round or pear-shaped body of the protozoan, and one single undulating membrane extending backward from the four flagella.[19,20]

Other tests include pH testing of the vaginal or seminal fluid, which will reveal a pH of 5.0–6.0; however, this is not conclusive of trichomoniasis, as bacterial vaginosis often has this characteristic as well. The "whiff test" entails placing several drops of KOH prep solution onto the specimen. A positive result will be a fishy odor from the sample. Again, this is not conclusive of trichomoniasis, as bacterial vaginosis also has this characteristic. A standard culture can be completed when a specimen was not found to have identifiable *Trichomonas vaginalis* protozoan on a wet mount but the healthcare provider remains suspicious of trichomoniasis. The standard culture is highly sensitive but costlier and takes longer to complete than the traditional saline wet mount.[19,20]

All sex partners should be treated if one partner is positive for *Trichomonas vaginalis*. Without concurrent treatment, the patient will likely be reinfected even after one event of sexual contact. The first-line treatment for trichomoniasis is oral metronidazole. The second-line treatment includes a higher dose and/or longer treatment duration of metronidazole or use of other 5-nitroimidazole medications such as tinidazole and clotrimazole. It is important to teach safe sexual practices and to instruct the patient to avoid sexual intercourse until the treatment regimen has been completed.

Pediculosis Pubis

Pediculosis pubis, also known as *Pthirus pubis,* louse (singular) or lice (plural), or the street term "crabs," is an ectoparasite (parasite that live on the outside of the body) that is spread through sexual contact, sharing of undergarments, or living in very close quarters with many other individuals, especially in unsanitary conditions.

Etiology and Pathogenesis

Individuals who practice safe sex with condoms are not safe from infestation with pubic lice, as condoms do not stop the spread of the parasite. However, the lice cannot be spread by a toilet seat, as is a common myth, as they cannot live for a long time without a warm human host body, and they have trouble moving along flat, smooth surfaces because of their anatomy.[22,23]

A female louse can lay up to three to six eggs daily, which can result in a massive infestation in a short time. The *Pthirus pubis* is whitish-gray and oval-shaped, with a short broad body and large front claws, which contribute to the street name of "crabs." The louse uses these large claws to grasp coarse hair mainly in the groin, perianal, and/or axillary areas of the body (**Figure 49.8** ■).

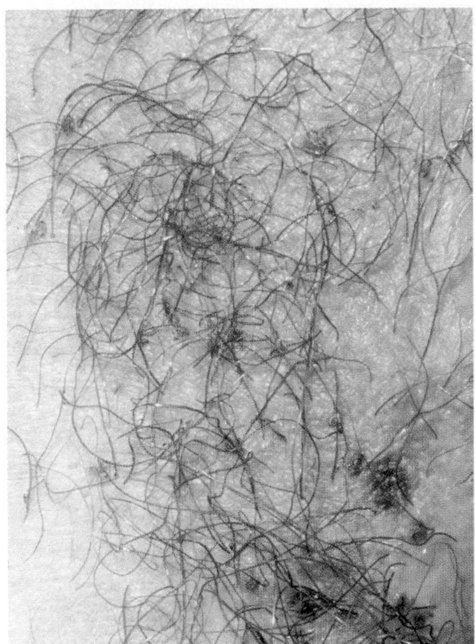

Figure 49.8 ■ Pubic lice on the mons pubis of a woman.

The nits (eggs) of the louse attach to hair shafts and/or the fibers of clothing and bed linens with a strong, durable, insoluble cement, which contributes to failures in treatment and reinfestation in individuals. Much like trichomoniasis, pediculosis pubis is not a reportable disease, so accurate numbers are difficult to obtain.[22,23]

Clinical Manifestations

Clinical manifestations of pediculosis pubis are similar in males and females, the predominant symptom being pruritus in the affected area or areas, which usually include the groin and the perianal and anal areas. The parasite can also spread to other regions of the body. Usually, the pruritus or spotting of the parasite or nits (eggs) is the principal reason for a patient to seek healthcare advice and treatment. Excoriations commonly accompany the pruritus. Another clinical finding in patients with a pubic louse infection is the presence of maculae ceruleae, which are pathognomonic for pubic lice. A maculae ceruleae is a bluish-gray macule that signifies a bite from the louse on the skin. Crusts and pinpoint blood staining of the underwear can also be noted, with or without the presence of maculae ceruleae. Other, less common signs and symptoms include inguinal lymphadenopathy and axillary lymphadenopathy.[22,23]

Linking Pathophysiology to Diagnosis and Treatment

The principal diagnostic finding of pediculosis pubis is microscopy of the louse, *Pthirus pubis*. It is important to note that the microscopy of nits is not diagnostic of an active infestation; however, if nits are found in or near a hairy region on the patient, active infestation is likely. Cellulose tape can be applied over an infested area to pick up lice and nits for microscopic examination. A Wood light examination can be done on infested areas to illuminate lice and nits, which will glow a yellow-green color.[21,23]

Typically, pediculosis pubis can be treated with over-the-counter permethrin (usually 1%) lotion and sometimes a mousse-type application with a combination of medications. Permethrin is highly effective against live lice; however, it will not penetrate unhatched nits. A second treatment with permethrin is recommended roughly 9 days after the first treatment to kill any newly hatched nits to prevent another life cycle. Delaying or omitting this second treatment can lead to the new lice laying more nits, which will contribute to reinfestation.[24]

In addition to pharmacologic intervention, infested areas should be washed and towel dried to kill nits and stray lice. Towels, clothing, and even bedding from the patient's environment used within 2–3 days before treatment should be machine-washed in water of at least 130°F and dried on the hot setting in a dryer to kill the remaining lice and nits. Any items that cannot be washed need to be disposed of or placed in a garbage bag for a period of no less than 2 weeks. This will kill the remaining lice and nits within the soiled cloth.[24]

Check Your Progress: Section 49.4

1. What symptoms are most commonly associated with trichomoniasis in males?
2. Which three types of tests are used to detect trichomoniasis infection?
3. Which type of methods are used to identify infection with *Pthirus pubis*?

CHAPTER SUMMARY

49.1 Chapter Overview and Case Studies

Discuss the epidemiology and prevalence of sexually transmitted infections and concepts related to sexually transmitted infections.

- The term *sexually transmitted infection (STI)* is used to describe a number of infections resulting from sexual contact that are caused by various bacteria, fungi, viruses, and parasites. Most of these infections can be readily cured.
- Concepts related to STIs include sexuality, reproduction, tissue integrity, infection, and environment.

49.2 Viral STIs

Differentiate the causes, classification, underlying pathogenesis, and clinical manifestations of viral STIs and approaches to diagnosis and treatment of these conditions across the lifespan.

- Human papillomaviruses (HPVs) are small, double-stranded DNA viruses that infect cutaneous and mucosal epithelial tissues of the anogenital tract, infecting nearly 80 million people in the United States.
- High-risk types of HPVs are associated with the development of anogenital cancers, including cancers of the cervix. Infections by the low-risk HPVs induce only benign genital warts.
- Therapeutic methods often prescribed for patients with HPV to self-administer include 0.5% podophyllotoxin solution or gel applied topically to the lesion twice a day for 3 consecutive days, followed by 4 days without treatment.
- There are two forms of herpes simplex virus. HSV-1 is more commonly associated with infections around the mouth, typically manifesting as cold sores; HSV-2 is more commonly associated with genital infection and can manifest as blisters around the genital area.
- After infection, HSV enters nerves cells and resides in the cellular ganglion, where the virus is protected from being cleared by the immune system.
- Orofacial manifestations appear as erythematous papules that develop into vesicles within a short period of time. Genital manifestations include small vesicles located in the genital area, often accompanied by pain.
- The most effective means of treating HSV is preventing transmission.

49.3 Bacterial STIs

Differentiate the causes, classification, underlying pathogenesis, and clinical manifestations of bacterial STIs and approaches to diagnosis and treatment of these conditions across the lifespan.

- Pelvic inflammatory disease (an infection of a woman's reproductive organs, including the ovaries, fallopian tubes, uterus, and cervix), vaginosis (bacterial overgrowth in the vagina), and epididymitis (inflammation of the epididymis in men) are disease states associated with bacteria exposure.
- Chlamydia is an STI caused by the bacteria *Chlamydia trachomatis*, which has multiple strains associated with eye disease and genital tract infections.
- Chlamydia is the most common bacterial STI in the United States. It is often found in combination with gonorrhea. Most chlamydia infections do not result in symptoms.
- A common diagnostic measure for chlamydia is the evaluation of a urine sample; the primary means of treatment is providing a single dose of azithromycin or doxycycline for 1 week.
- Gonorrhea is an STI caused by a pyogenic bacterium known as *Neisseria gonorrhoeae*.
- *Neisseria gonorrhoeae* has surface pili that prevent the organism from being phagocytized by neutrophils.
- Treatment guidelines for gonorrhea recommend the use of two antibiotics: an intramuscular injection of ceftriaxone and an oral dose of azithromycin.
- Syphilis is an STI acquired through direct sexual contact with an infected individual or through blood transfusion.
- The spirochete *Treponema*, in particular *Treponema pallidum*, causes infection as a result of contact with open lesions known as chancres.

- Without appropriate intervention, syphilis will progress through four stages: primary, secondary, latent, and tertiary.
- Pharmacologic treatment remains the main approach, intramuscular penicillin being the antibiotic of choice.

49.4 Parasitic STIs

Differentiate the causes, classification, underlying pathogenesis, and clinical manifestations of parasitic STIs and approaches to diagnosis and treatment of these conditions across the lifespan.

- Trichomoniasis is a parasitic STI, known colloquially as "trich," that is transmitted by the protozoan *Trichomonas vaginalis*. Trichomonal infection is often asymptomatic, so laboratory tests are needed to confirm diagnosis.
- The first-line treatment of trichomoniasis is oral metronidazole. The second-line treatment includes a higher dose and/or longer treatment duration of metronidazole or use of other 5-nitroimidazole medications such as tinidazole and clotrimazole.
- Pediculosis pubis, also known as *Pthirus pubis*, louse (singular) or lice (plural), or the street term "crabs," is an ectoparasite (parasite that live on the outside of the body) that is spread through sexual contact, sharing of undergarments, or living in very close quarters with many other individuals, especially in unsanitary conditions.
- Clinical manifestations of pediculosis pubis are similar in males and females, the predominant symptom being pruritus in the affected area or areas.
- Typically, pediculosis pubis can be treated with over-the-counter permethrin (usually 1%) lotion and sometimes a mousse-type application with a combination of medications.

REVIEW QUESTIONS

1. A 37-year-old woman who is pregnant for the first time comes to the clinic for her regular checkup. She is informed about the need for routine testing for sexually transmitted infections. She replies, "I've been married for 15 years. Do I really need to be tested?" What should your response be?
   a. "We will perform the testing only if you are having symptoms."
   b. "Many sexually transmitted infections do not cause symptoms."
   c. "Sexually transmitted infections cannot be transmitted to an infant."
   d. "Since the risk is small, you likely don't need to be tested."

2. Which of the following is the most accurate description of syphilis?
   a. A double-stranded DNA virus that infects epithelial cells of the anogenital tract
   b. A bacterial infection of columnar epithelial cells of the urinary tract causing dysuria
   c. A spirochete that penetrates the central nervous system and results in chancres
   d. An ectoparasite that is whitish-gray and oval-shaped with a short, broad body and large front claws

3. A 23-year-old woman presents to the clinic with complaints of pain with urination and intercourse and discharge coming from her vagina. What is the most likely cause of her symptoms?
   a. Chlamydia
   b. Gonorrhea
   c. Syphilis
   d. Pediculosis pubis

4. A 76-year-old man presents to the clinic and is diagnosed with secondary syphilis. What symptoms is he most likely to experience during this stage?
   a. Fever, severe abdominal pain, diarrhea, loss of appetite, nausea, and vomiting
   b. Symptoms of meningitis, blurred vision, and confusion
   c. Severe fatigue and headaches,
   d. Fever, alopecia, arthralgia, lymphadenopathy, and rash on the palms of the hands

5. A 35-year-old woman is diagnosed with high-risk human papillomavirus. The warts are removed by using cryosurgery, and she is given an HPV vaccine. How would you prepare her, in terms of education and follow-up, to monitor for the potential complications of this condition?
   a. She will require follow-up in 6 months to screen for the possible development of genital malignancies.
   b. She will not require any additional routine screening.
   c. She will need to monitor for eruption of small vesicles around the genital area that are painful.
   d. She will require follow-up in 1 year to assess for the presence of chancres and meningitis.

6. A 30-year-old man presents with small vesicles over the shaft of his penis. He states that the previous week, he experienced a fever, headache, and general muscle aches for a few days before the eruption of the vesicles. What is the most appropriate information for you to provide as part of the education about his treatment?
   a. "You will be given an intramuscular injection of an antibiotic to treat the lesions."

b. "The lesions will need to be treated with cryotherapy to make them go away."
c. "You will need to continue taking antiviral medication to control the infection."
d. "The lesions will be treated with oral antibiotics, which will also relieve the general symptoms."

7. A 17-year-old male is diagnosed with pediculosis pubis. What information is most appropriate for you to provide as part of his education?
a. "You will need to apply only one treatment, but make sure that you wash all clothes and linens."
b. "It is important to apply a second treatment 9 days after the first, and you must wash all clothes and linens."
c. "After the dose of antibiotics, you will need to be rechecked in another month for reinfection."
d. "There is a very low risk that you will transmit the parasite to others after the first treatment."

8. A 20-year-old male is diagnosed with chlamydia and prescribed treatment with doxycycline for 1 week. His sex partner is also notified and prescribed treatment. What is the appropriate response when the client asks you when he can resume having sex?
a. "You can resume having sex as soon as you start the treatment."
b. "You should not resume having sex until 1 month after treatment."
c. "The treatment will require a follow-up visit to verify that the infection is cured before you can resume having sex."
d. "You can resume having sex after you and your partner have completed the treatment."

ANSWERS

Answers to Review Questions can be found in Appendix A. Answers to Case Study and Check Your Progress questions are available on the faculty resources site. Please consult with your instructor.

RECOMMENDED WEBSITES

Centers for Disease Control and Prevention: Sexually Transmitted Diseases (STDs)
https://www.cdc.gov/std/default.htm

The STI Foundation
http://www.stif.org.uk

World Health Organization: Sexual and Reproductive Health
http://www.who.int/reproductivehealth/topics/rtis/en

REFERENCES

1. World Health Organization. (2016). *Sexually transmitted infections (STIs)*. Available at http://www.who.int/mediacentre/factsheets/fs110/en
2. Centers for Disease Control and Prevention. (2015). *Reported STDs in the United States: 2014 national data for chlamydia, gonorrhea, and syphilis*. Available at https://www.cdc.gov/std/stats14/std-trends-508.pdf
3. Centers for Disease Control and Prevention. (2016). *2015 sexually transmitted diseases surveillance*. Available at https://www.cdc.gov/std/stats15/default.htm
4. Centers for Disease Control and Prevention. (2017). *Sexually transmitted disease: Fact sheets*. Available at http://www.cdc.gov/std/healthcomm/fact_sheets.htm
5. Centers for Disease Control and Prevention. (2016). *United States cancer statistics: 1999–2013 incidence and mortality web-based report*. Available at https://nccd.cdc.gov/uscs
6. Longworth, M. S., & Laimins, L. A. (2004). Pathogenesis of human papillomaviruses in differentiating epithelia. *Microbiology and Molecular Biology Reviews, 68*(2), 362–372. http://doi.org/10.1128/MMBR.68.2.362-372.2004
7. Juckett, G., & Hartman, H. (2010). Human papillomavirus: Clinical manifestations and prevention. *American Family Physician, 82*(10), 1209–1214.
8. Centers for Disease Control and Prevention. (2017). *Genital herpes—CDC fact sheet*. Available at http://www.cdc.gov/std/herpes/stdfact-herpes.htm
9. Bradshaw, M. J. & Venkatesan, A. (2016). Herpes simplex virus-1 encephalitis in adults: Pathophysiology, diagnosis, and management. *Neurotherapeutics, 13*, 493. doi:10.1007/s13311-016-0433-7
10. Jerome, K. R., & Morrow, R. A. (2015). Herpes simplex viruses and herpes B virus. In J. H. Jorgensen, K. C. Carroll, G. Funke, et al. (Eds.), *Manual of clinical microbiology* (11th ed., pp. 1687–1703). Washington, DC: ASM Press. doi:10.1128/9781555817381.ch98
11. Patel, R., Alderson, S., Geretti, A., Nilsen, A., Foley, E., Lautenschlager, S., Green, J., van der Meijden, W., Gomberg, M., & Moi, H. (IUSTI/WHO Europe). (2011). European guideline for the management of genital herpes. *International Journal of STD and AIDS, 22*(1), 1–10. doi:10.1258/ijsa.2010.010278. PubMed PMID: 21364059
12. Office on Women's Health. (2015). *Chlamydia*. Available at http://www.womenshealth.gov/publications/our-publications/fact-sheet/chlamydia.html
13. Bender, N., Herrmann, B., Andersen, B., et al. (2011). Chlamydia infection, pelvic inflammatory disease, ectopic pregnancy and infertility: Cross-national study. *Sexually Transmitted Infections, 87*, 601–608.

14. Kalwij, S., Macintosh, M., & Paraitser, P. (2010). Screening and treatment of chlamydia trachomatis infections. *British Medical Journal, 340*: c1915. doi:10.1136/bmj.c1915
15. Centers for Disease Control and Prevention. (2016). *Gonorrhea—CDC fact sheet (detailed)*. Available at http://www.cdc.gov/std/gonorrhea/stdfact-gonorrhea-detailed.htm
16. Centers for Disease Control and Prevention. (2017). *Syphilis—CDC fact sheet (detailed)*. Available at http://www.cdc.gov/std/syphilis/stdfact-syphilis-detailed.htm
17. Hicks, C. B., & Clement, M. (2017). Syphilis: Treatment and monitoring. *UpToDate*. Available at http://www.uptodate.com/contents/syphilis-treatment-and-monitoring
18. World Health Organization. (2017). *Sexually transmitted infections (STIs)*. Available at http://www.who.int/go/sti/en
19. Smith, D. (2016). Trichomoniasis. *Medscape*. Available at http://emedicine.medscape.com/article/230617-overview
20. Centers for Disease Control and Prevention. *Trichomoniasis—CDC fact sheet*. Available at https://www.cdc.gov/std/trichomonas/stdfact-trichomoniasis.htm
21. Dains, J. E., Baumann, L. C., & Scheibel, P. (2016). *Advanced health assessment & clinical diagnosis in primary care* (5th ed.). St. Louis, MO: Elsevier.
22. Guenther, L. (2016). Pediculosis and pthiriasis (lice infestation). *Medscape*. Available at http://emedicine.medscape.com/article/225013-overview
23. Centers for Disease Control and Prevention. (2016). Pediculosis. *DPDx—Laboratory identification of parasitic diseases of public health concern*. Available at https://www.cdc.gov/dpdx/pediculosis/index.html
24. Centers for Disease Control and Prevention. (2015). *2015 sexually transmitted diseases treatment guidelines*. Available at https://www.cdc.gov/std/tg2015/ectoparasitic.htm

Unit XV
Trauma and Multisystem Conditions

Trauma can be generally defined as a serious or life-threatening physical or psychological injury. However, specific definitions of trauma can vary by agency or organization. The World Health Organization often uses the terms "injury" and "trauma" interchangeably.[1] The American Psychiatric Association classifies trauma as experiencing or witnessing a serious or life-threatening injury or incident of violence to self or another.[2] Emergency medical systems (EMS) classify trauma according to the mechanism and severity of injury. For example, field triage guidelines of U. S. EMS systems recommend that the highest level of trauma care be provided to patients whose Glasgow Coma Scale scores are ≤ 13; or who have a systolic blood pressure of < 90 mmHG; or who have a respiratory rate < 10 or > 29 breaths per minute or need ventilator support.[3]

It can be argued that severity of trauma is indicated by three factors: the extent to which the injury or incident threatens ability, functioning, or life; the extent to which the individual perceives the injury or incident as a threat to ability, functioning, or life; and the length and severity of the time and effort required to recover from the trauma and any resulting sequelae (such as the eventual loss of a limb if perfusion to the area cannot be restored). Context (such as whether the injury occurred as an accident or as an act of violence) also matters, as does the individual's personal resilience, degree of support, and access to resources.[4]

In addition to a disabling or life-threatening injury, exposure to a hazardous material can also initiate a traumatic event. Patients exposed to biologic, chemical and radiologic materials are not only at risk for significant illness or injury themselves but in many cases, they also pose a threat to those who seek to care for them. Daily, emergency departments (EDs) see patients exposed to these substances as a result of industrial and transportation incidents, with injuries ranging from minor to life-threatening.

Trauma care is provided to individuals experiencing acute, life-threatening or disabling injuries until their condition becomes sufficiently stable to transfer to a medical-surgical unit, a rehabilitation facility, or to discharge to home. Trauma care emphasizes addressing physiologic instability first, followed by managing psychosocial and spiritual needs as the patient's condition permits. The goal of trauma care is to maintain life and restore function to the greatest degree possible.

In contrast, palliative care is the total care provided to patients experiencing life-threatening, progressive illness. Palliative care emphasizes control of distressing symptoms with attention to physiological, psychosocial, and spiritual needs.[5] The goal of palliative care is the attainment of the highest possible quality of life for patients and their families. In the context of both of these types of care, nurses provide a variety of interventions, including therapeutic communication, ongoing monitoring, medication reconciliation and administration, pain and comfort management, and patient and family teaching to reduce fear and increase participation in the treatment plan.

Nurses in all settings will find themselves working with patients who have experienced trauma of one kind or another. The term *trauma-informed care* refers to care that recognizes the experiences, signs, and symptoms of trauma (regardless of how long ago the patient experienced the trauma); responds using policies and practices that are informed by an understanding of the physiologic, psychologic, neurologic, and other consequences of trauma; and seeks to avoid retraumatizing the patient.[6] The principles of trauma-informed care include safety, trustworthiness and transparency, collaboration, and empowerment, among others.[6]

References

1. World Health Organization. (2014). Injuries and violence: The facts. Available at http://apps.who.int/iris/bitstream/10665/149798/1/9789241508018_eng.pdf?ua=1&ua=1&ua=1
2. American Psychiatric Association. (2013). *Diagnostic and Statistical Manual of Mental Illness* (5th ed.). Washington, DC: Author.
3. Sasser, S. M., Hunt, R. C., Faul, M., Sugarman, D., Pearson, W. S., et al. (2011). Guidelines for Field Triage of Injured Patients: Recommendations of the National Expert Panel on Field Triage, 2011. Retrieved from https://www.cdc.gov/mmwr/preview/mmwrhtml/rr6101a1.htm
4. Potter. M. P., & Moller, M. D. (2016). *Psychiatric–Mental Health Nursing: From Suffering to Hope.* Hoboken, N. J: Pearson Education.
5. World Health Organization. (2017). WHO definition of palliative care. Retrieved from http://www.who.int/cancer/palliative/definition/en/
6. Substance Abuse and Mental Health Services Administration. (2015). Trauma-informed approach and trauma-specific interventions. Retrieved from https://www.samhsa.gov/nctic/trauma-interventions

Types of Traumatic Injury

- Blunt trauma
- Penetrating trauma
- Thermal injury
- Chemical burns
- Electrical injuries

Blunt Trauma

- Acceleration/deceleration injuries
- Abrasions
- Contusions
- Lacerations
- Fractures

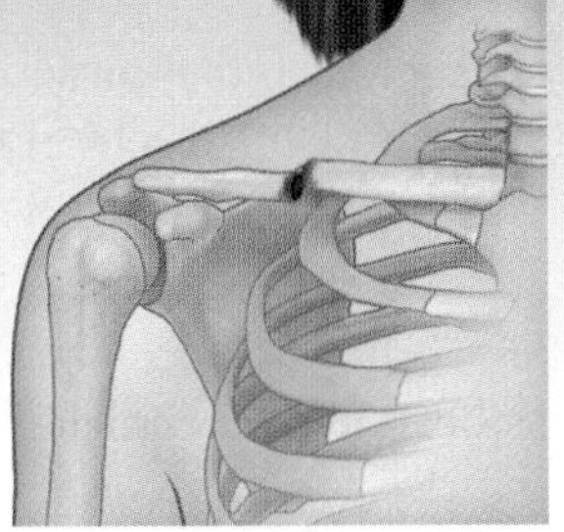

Penetrating Trauma

- Lacerations and punctures
- Bites
- Fractures
- Missile injuries (bullet wounds)

Biologic, Chemical and Radiologic Agents

- Act to reduce ongoing exposure
- Causative agent may not be confirmed for several days
- Response may be local or systemic

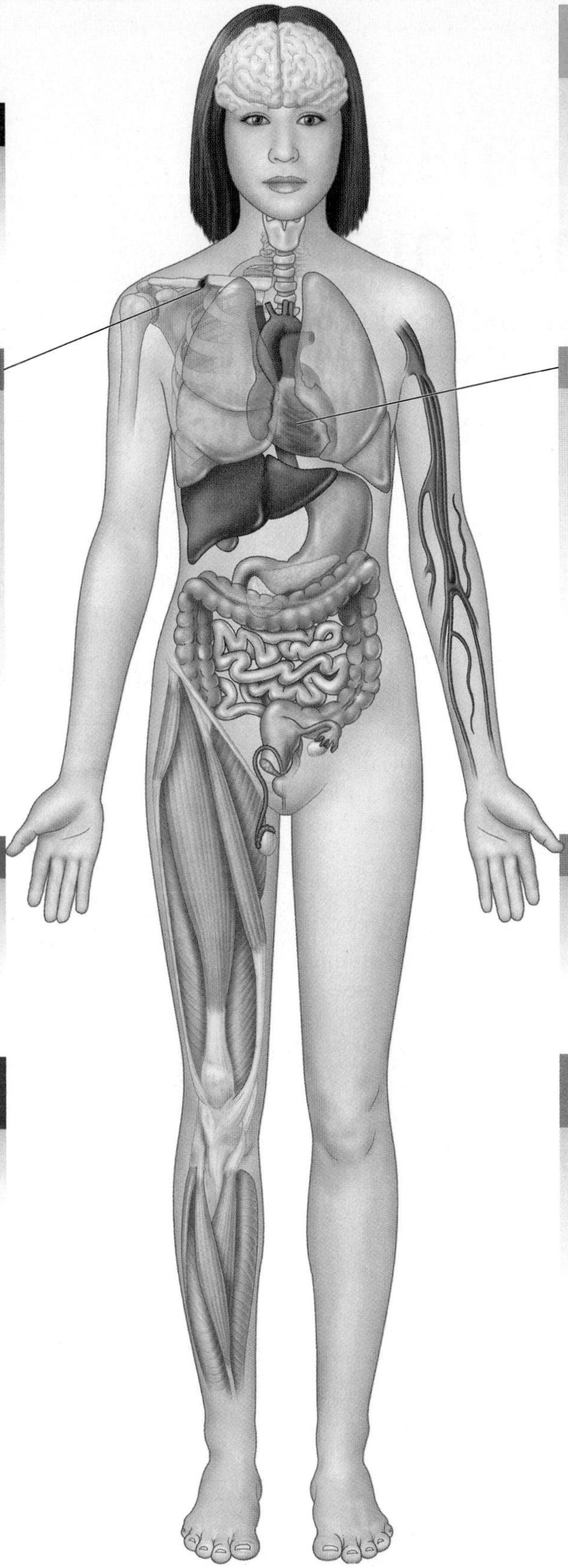

Primary and Secondary Traumatic Injury

Primary survey

- **A**irway and c-spine stabilization
- **B**reathing
- **C**irculation
- **D**isability (neurologic) status
- **E**xpose and **E**nvironment

Secondary survey

- Head-to-toe assessment

Lethal Triad of Trauma

Hypothermia

Lethal triad

Acidosis

Traumatic coagulopathy

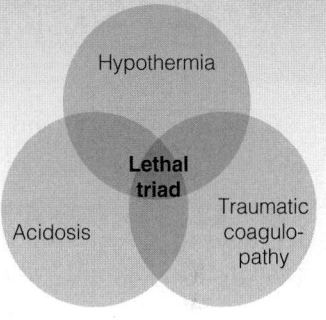

Palliative Care

Emphasizes

- Physical comfort
- Physiologic needs
- Psychosocial needs
- Spiritual needs

Pathophysiology at the End of Life

- Pain
- Dyspnea, cough
- Excessive secretions
- Nausea, vomiting
- Anorexia, cachexia
- Fatigue
- Constipation, urinary incontinence
- Delirium

Chapter 50

Mechanisms of Traumatic Injury

Kyle Bergan, Adam Boise, and Vicki Keough

Chapter Outline and Learning Outcomes

50.1 Chapter Overview and Case Studies

Describe the epidemiology of traumatic injury and concepts related to trauma.

50.2 Modern Trauma Care

Outline the team approach to trauma care and the ABCDE approach to trauma care.

50.3 Blunt Trauma

Differentiate the causes, classification, and clinical manifestations of injuries caused by blunt trauma and approaches to diagnosis and treatment of those injuries across the lifespan.

50.4 Penetrating Trauma

Differentiate the causes, classification, and clinical manifestations of injuries caused by penetrating trauma and approaches to diagnosis and treatment of those injuries across the lifespan.

50.5 Thermal Injury

Differentiate the causes, classification, and clinical manifestations of thermal injuries and approaches to diagnosis and treatment of those injuries across the lifespan.

50.6 Chemical Burns

Differentiate the causes, classification, and clinical manifestations of chemical burns and approaches to diagnosis and treatment of those injuries across the lifespan.

50.7 Electrical Injuries

Differentiate the causes, classification, and clinical manifestations of electrical injuries and approaches to diagnosis and treatment of those injuries across the lifespan.

50.8 Lethal Triad of Trauma

Differentiate the causes, classification, underlying pathogenesis, and clinical manifestations of the lethal triad of trauma and approaches to diagnosis and treatment of those conditions across the lifespan.

50.9 Trauma Deaths and Trauma Prevention

Describe the trimodal distribution of trauma deaths and the four-step process for trauma prevention.

KEY TERMS

Abrasion, 1227
Blunt trauma, 1226
Contusion, 1227
Electrical burn, 1236
Full thickness burn, 1232
Laceration, 1228
Lethal triad of trauma, 1223
Partial thickness burn injury, 1232
Rule of Nines, 1233

ABBREVIATIONS

ABCDE—airway, breathing, circulation, disability, environment/exposure
ATCN—Advanced Trauma Core Nursing
ATLS—Advanced Trauma Life Support

50.1 Chapter Overview and Case Studies

Trauma is the leading cause of death in the United States for individuals under 46 years of age.[1] The largest increase in trauma deaths has come in the baby boomer generation, or individuals born between 1946 and 1964. Trauma deaths of young adults occur at a time when they would become productive members of society.[2–4] This loss costs society approximately $260 billion annually.[3] Although trauma is often seen as a disease of the young, it knows no boundaries when it comes to age, culture, sex, or economic status.[3] This chapter presents an overview of mechanisms of traumatic injuries, the three peak times of death due to trauma, and the lethal triad. The **lethal triad of trauma** is the interrelated development of hypothermia, acidosis, and coagulopathy.

Concepts Related to Traumatic Injury

Traumatic injury can result in numerous physiologic disruptions, several of which constitute a triad of lethality (described in fuller detail later in this chapter). Traumatic injury can result in damage to blood vessels, resulting in a loss of blood volume with a corresponding reduction in tissue perfusion. Compensatory mechanisms lead to tachycardia as the body tries to maintain cardiac output. The loss of volume can also cause shifts in fluid and electrolyte balance. The destruction of skin surface through the experience of burns can further contribute to the loss of fluid. Sepsis and other complications can lead to shifting of fluid into interstitial spaces (third spacing), leading to a further reduction in blood volume. The resultant loss of volume leads to a decrease in the available number of erythrocytes, contributing to anemia. Destruction of skin surface and tissue results in issues of thermoregulation. Without an adequate protective skin layer, an adequate body temperature cannot be maintained. As the patient begins to experience hypothermia, the body responds with shivering, which increases oxygen consumption in skeletal muscle and metabolic demand. The increased metabolic demand in conjunction with decreased volume and perfusion problems leads to issues with acid–base regulation, ultimately resulting in metabolic acidosis. Associated with the acidotic state are high levels of lactic acid, which in combination with loss of thrombocytes can lead to coagulopathy (**Figure 50.1** ■).

Case Studies

The following cases will be addressed throughout the chapter to assist in application of chapter content to clinical situations that involve individuals with traumatic injuries.

Jaylen Henderson: Introduction

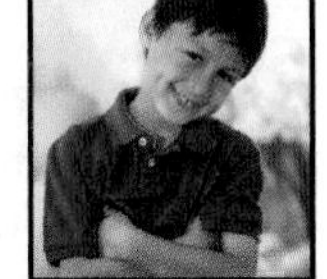

Jaylen Henderson is an 8-year-old boy who was riding his bicycle when he was struck by two stray bullets. Paramedics identify three wounds. There are two entrance wounds to the anterior thorax and an exit wound to the left flank. The patient is transported to the pediatric trauma center for further assessment.

1. On the basis of the paramedics' observations, which of Jaylen's organs might be affected by the mechanism of injury?
2. Why is it important to transport Jaylen to a pediatric trauma center rather than a closer community hospital?

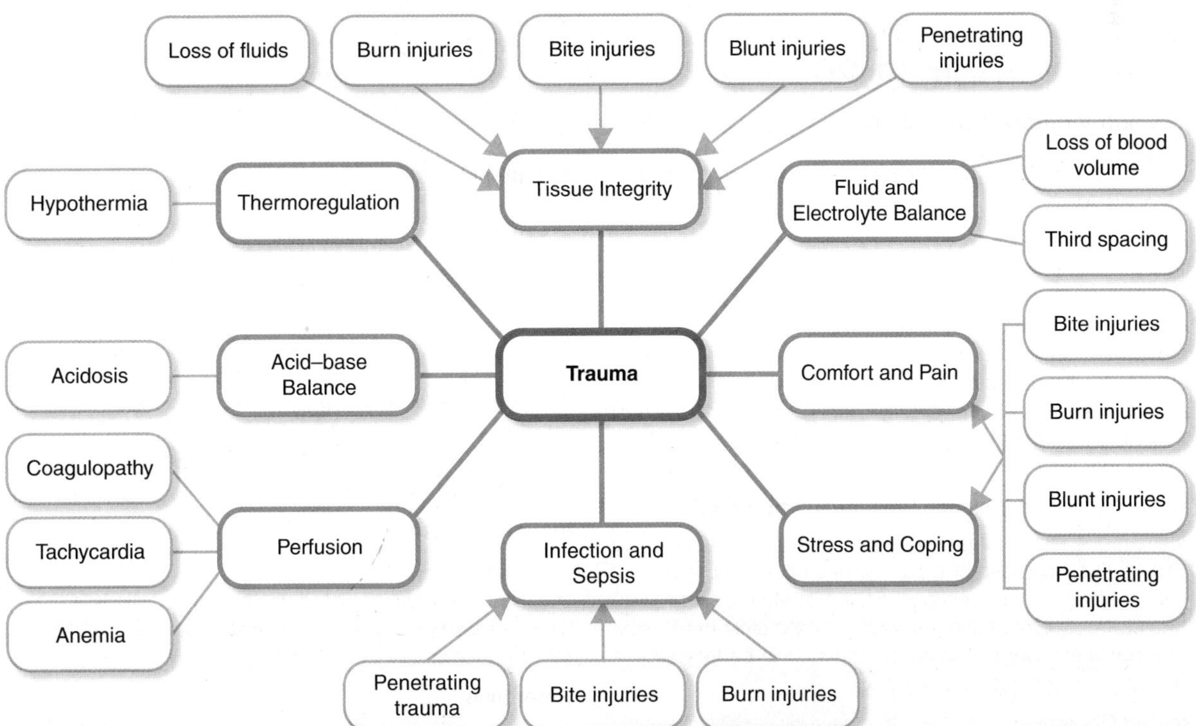

Figure 50.1 ■ Concepts related to traumatic injury.

Linda Dickson: Introduction

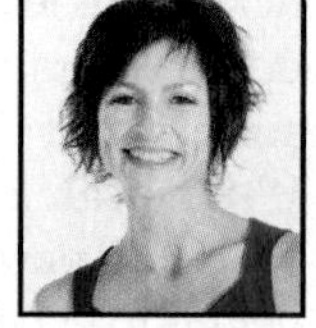

Linda Dickson, age 43, was asleep when her home caught fire. She was quickly overcome by smoke and lost consciousness. Firefighters were able to rescue her from the building after searching for approximately 20 minutes. Ms. Dickson is transported to the burn center for treatment.

1. Why is the time interval noted in the situation important to know?
2. What type of injuries might you expect to see in Ms. Dickson?

Check Your Progress: Section 50.1

1. What are the three parts of the lethal triad of hypothermia?
2. How can a large area of skin loss from a traumatic injury such as a major burn contribute to the lethal triad of hypothermia?
3. How can the body lose blood volume in trauma?

50.2 Modern Trauma Care

Violence and resulting injuries have been part of the human experience since the beginning of the human race. Wars have played an important role in injury management, forcing healthcare practitioners to discover new ways in which human life can be saved after devastating injuries. If anything good ever came from wartime injuries, it may be the current trauma care system in use today, which was based on the mobile army surgical hospital (MASH) philosophy first used in the Korean War. The basis of this approach to wound management was to first identify and treat all life-threatening injuries and to get the soldier to a definitive healthcare environment where skilled surgeons could perform immediate interventions. The current trauma system espouses this same philosophy and subsequently has built a science around advancing trauma care across the nation and around the world.[5]

Trauma may be classified in many ways. Trauma can be designated by location of injury, injury severity, intentional/nonintentional injury, and the manner in which injuries occurred. However, the most common classification for trauma is the mode in which the injury occurred. This mode includes blunt trauma, penetrating trauma, thermal trauma, electrical trauma, and chemical trauma.[6]

The Office of Disease Prevention and Health Promotion, which is part of the U.S. Department of Health and Human Services, has identified injury and violence prevention as one of its topics for *Healthy People 2020*.

Trauma Centers

The management of severely injured patients requires a well-organized, well-educated, and highly skilled trauma team and trauma care system to maximize the outcome for trauma patients. In 1991, the U.S. Congress passed the Trauma Care Systems Planning and Development Act, which required the development of a Model Trauma Care System Plan that each state was to use for a model of trauma care. All states were to identify a system of trauma care and

Healthy People 2020

Injury and Violence Prevention

Goal: Prevent unintentional injuries and violence, and reduce their consequences.

Overview: Injuries and violence are widespread in society. Unintentional injuries and those caused by acts of violence are among the top 15 killers of Americans of all ages. Many people accept them as "accidents," "acts of fate," or "part of life." However, most events that result in injury, disability, or death are predictable and preventable. The Injury and Violence Prevention objectives for 2020 represent a broad range of issues that, if adequately addressed, will improve the health of the nation.

Why Are Injury and Violence Prevention Important?

Injuries are the leading cause of death for Americans ages 1 to 44, and a leading cause of disability for all ages, regardless of sex, race/ethnicity, or socioeconomic status. More than 180,000 people die from injuries each year, and approximately 1 in 10 sustains a nonfatal injury that is serious enough to be treated in a hospital emergency department.

Selected Objectives: There are 43 objectives in *Healthy People 2020*, broken into three categories. Selected objectives include the following.

Intentional Injury

1. Reduce fatal and nonfatal injuries.
2. Reduce fatal and nonfatal traumatic brain injuries.
3. Reduce fatal and nonfatal spinal cord injuries.
4. Increase access to trauma care.

Unintentional Injury

13. Reduce motor vehicle crash-related deaths.
23. Prevent an increase in fall-related deaths.
24. Reduce unintentional suffocation deaths.
26. Reduce sports and recreation injuries.

Violence Prevention

29. Reduce homicides.
30. Reduce firearms-related deaths.
31. Reduce bullying among adolescents.
40. Reduce sexual violence.

Reference

1. U.S. Department of Health and Human Services. (2017). *Injury and violence prevention*. Available at https://www.healthypeople.gov/2020/topics-objectives/topic/injury-and-violence-prevention

categorize hospitals on the basis of their ability to deliver appropriate care to trauma patients. Hospitals were categorized as Level I to Level V trauma centers (**Table 50.1** ■).

The Level I category is the highest level of care with around-the-clock trauma surgery immediately available along with the ability to assess and treat all life-threatening injuries. Prehospital providers are trained in how to identify and evaluate trauma patients, determine which patients need to be brought to Level I trauma centers, and determine the most appropriate hospital according to the severity of injuries. The American College of Surgeons has developed a set of criteria that hospitals must meet to qualify as a Level I, Level II, Level III, Level IV, or Level V trauma center. The American College of Surgeons' Committee on Trauma designed a course entitled Advanced Trauma Life Support (ATLS), which is available to physicians, nurse practitioners, and physician assistants who treat trauma patients.[7] In parallel with Advanced Trauma Life Support is the course Advanced Trauma Core Nursing (ATCN). While the didactic portion of the two courses is identical, the practical sessions are specific to the role of each provider on the trauma team. These courses are designed to educate medical professionals in how to approach trauma care in an organized, systematic manner and cover optimal treatment guidelines for seriously injured patients.[7,8] Additional trauma programs available for nurses include the Trauma Nurse Core Curriculum and the Certified Advanced Trauma Nurse course offered by the Emergency Nurses Association and Trauma Nurse Specialist courses that are specific to various states throughout the country.

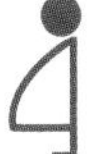

Traumatic injuries are the most common cause of death of pregnant women not directly related to gestation. Trauma is also the most common reason for fetal demise.[9] All women between the ages of 10 and 50 years should be screened for pregnancy on presentation to the trauma bay.[9] While the standard ABCDE (airway, breathing, circulation, disability, and environment/exposure) method of the primary survey must be followed, it is critical to understand that a woman's anatomy and physiology undergo multiple changes during pregnancy. The overarching principle is to aggressively resuscitate the woman to maximize the opportunity for fetal survival. If pregnancy has been detected, monitoring of the fetal heartbeat should be initiated and should continue for 4–6 hours after the injury.[10]

The physiologic changes in pregnancy may alter how traumatic injuries affect the mother and fetus. Pregnant women experience a 45% increase in plasma volume.[9] This volume expansion allows for women to lose up to 35% of their blood volume before showing any signs of hypovolemic shock. Note, however, that in a hypovolemic state, the body shunts blood to essential organs and away from nonessential organs, including the uterus. There can be extensive fetal compromise before the mother shows any signs of shock. Because pregnant women show signs of shock later than nonpregnant women, early fluid resuscitation is especially critical to preventing decompensation in pregnant women. If blood is to be administered and the rhesus (Rh) status of the mother is unknown, Rh-negative blood should be used to avoid producing antibodies that could harm the fetus.[9]

The vital signs of pregnant women also differ from those of women who are not pregnant. Because of the additional fluid volume and additional thyroxine, the woman's heart rate may increase by 10–15 beats per minute.[9] Pregnant women usually have normal to low blood pressures due to higher levels of circulating estrogen. This mild tachycardia and physiologic hypotension must be accounted for in managing pregnant trauma patients.

The enlarging uterus presents multiple issues in managing the trauma patient. The blood flow through the uterus is 100 times greater at term when compared to the prepregnancy state.[9] The enlarging uterus can also displace the woman's heart and compress the inferior vena cava and other large veins.[9] To counteract the compression of the vena cava and subsequent decrease in venous return, the patient should be wedged to the left to displace the uterus and prevent supine hypotension. Care should be taken that the tilting of the patient does not compromise appropriate spinal precautions.

Direct injury to the uterus or fetus must also be considered. The Kleihauer-Betke test is used to detect fetal blood in circulation.[9] This can be an indication of fetal hemorrhage. Deceleration injuries can also cause placental abruption. Placental abruption is the partial or complete separation of the placenta from the uterine wall. Up to 50% of pregnant women with significant trauma and 5% with minor trauma will experience a placental abruption.[10]

In managing the pregnant trauma patient, it is important to realize that two patients are being cared for. The best way to ensure survival of the fetus is to aggressively resuscitate the mother and prevent hypotension. Emergent

Table 50.1 Trauma Center Levels of Care

Category	Key Features
Level I	• Trauma care is available at all hours with specialty surgical services available. • Has a system in place for substance abuse screening and intervention. • Provides system leadership and oversight. • Provides education to the surrounding community on trauma and injury prevention.
Level II	• Trauma care is available at all hours with specialty surgical services available. • Provides education on trauma and injury prevention to institutional staff. • May need to refer patients to a Level I facility after initial stabilization.
Level III	• Is able to provide basic trauma emergency services with around-the-clock laboratory services. • Has a relationship in place with a higher level of care facilities to aid in patient transfer and treatment.
Level IV	• Is able to provide basic trauma emergency services with around-the-clock laboratory services. • May not be able to provide 24-hour coverage in terms of surgical services.
Level V	• Is able to provide basic trauma level services. • May not have 24-hour coverage in terms of surgical services. • Generally is not involved in continuing or community-level educational activities.

cesarean delivery should be considered when there is maternal or fetal distress. To be viable, the fetus must be at least of 26 weeks' gestation and have a detectable heartbeat.[11] Even with prompt emergency cesarean birth, one study still found a 25% mortality rate for infants delivered by using this method.[11] ■

Children who have sustained traumatic injuries present many unique challenges to the trauma team. While the primary management of the pediatric trauma patient follows the same approach as of the adult patient, multiple anatomic and physiologic differences must be considered. Vital signs vary by age and may differ greatly from the values that are expected in an adult patient. Also, because of the proportionally larger head, children will experience a different injury pattern in comparison to adults with the same mechanism of injury. The cause of injury must also be considered. Abuse must be considered as a possible mechanism when the injury pattern does not match the described mechanism. Early transfer to a pediatric trauma center should be considered, especially when operative intervention is not immediately indicated but may become needed if injuries progress. ■

It is estimated that by 2050, 20% of United States population will 65 years of age or older.[12] Modern medical advances have not only extended life, but also enabled older adults to be more active. Although traditional thinking deemed trauma to be a "young person's" disease, older adults are more and more affected by injuries. Older adults usually have more comorbid conditions that must be treated concurrently with the traumatic injuries, but preexisting comorbidities are not considered independent risk factors for mortality of the geriatric trauma patient.[12] The most frequent mechanisms of injury for older adults include falls and motor vehicle crashes.[12] Elder abuse should also be considered as a potential cause of injury.

An additional consideration in managing older trauma patients is the polypharmacy that is frequently part of the healthcare regimen of older adults. For example, beta-blocker medications for hypertension slow the heart rate and do not allow the patient to compensate for shock by becoming tachycardic. This coupled with being hypertensive at baseline may cause the patient to have "normal" vital signs even in the setting of severe shock. Anticoagulants are frequently prescribed to older adults for atrial fibrillation and after cerebral vascular attacks. Treatment with anticoagulants complicates injuries by increasing bleeding time and leading to more blood loss than would occur in a non-anticoagulated patient.[13] Reversal of anticoagulants depends on the specific agent being used. Warfarin is reversed by administering vitamin K, fresh frozen plasma, and four-factor prothrombin complex (Kcentra or PCC).[13] Direct factor Xa inhibitors such as rivaroxaban and apixaban as well as direct thrombin inhibitors such as dabigatran do not have any specific antidote. For rivaroxaban, four-factor prothrombin complex has shown some activity in reversing the drug, but there is not enough data to formally recommend routine PCC use for reversal.[13] ■

Trauma Teams

Using a team approach to trauma care is the international standard method of caring for an injured patient. The trauma team usually consists of some combination of the following: a trauma surgeon, trauma nurse practitioners or physician assistants, emergency medical services personnel, emergency nurses, emergency physicians, anesthesiologists, radiology technicians, critical care personnel, and rehabilitation teams.[14] The trauma team operates according to well-developed and well-organized standards. These guidelines offer direction and assist in establishing priorities for treating even the most complicated trauma patients.

In trauma care, as in emergency care in general, life-threatening injuries are assumed to be present until proven otherwise.[7,14] The ABCDE (airway, breathing, circulation, disability, and environment/exposure) approach to trauma care forces the trauma team to discover all life-threatening injuries in an organized fashion and prevents the team from being distracted from other, often gruesome injuries that may not be life-threatening. **ABCDE** stands for the following:

Airway/C-spine control
Breathing
Circulation
Disability (neurologic deficit)
Exposure/Environment

For example, orthopedic injuries are often very painful and appear very serious; however, the trauma team should not attend to any less serious, though obvious injuries until all life-threatening injuries have been ruled out.[7,8] In keeping with the ABCDE approach to trauma care, the pathophysiology of traumatic injuries will be discussed by using this same approach.[7,14]

Check Your Progress: Section 50.2

1. How do trauma centers improve outcomes for severely injured patients?
2. Why would a fetus be more susceptible to shock in a traumatically injured pregnant woman even though she has 45% more plasma than a nonpregnant woman?
3. Explain why older adults are more susceptible to trauma injuries when compared to the younger adult population.
4. What special characteristics of children make them more vulnerable to the effects of trauma?

50.3 Blunt Trauma

Blunt trauma is caused by an impact that does not result in an object's entering the body. Motor vehicle crashes, falls, assaults, and athletics-related accidents are some of the most common mechanisms of blunt trauma. These mechanisms often result in a compression or crushing type injury. As with all trauma, patients who have experienced a blunt mechanism should be evaluated by using the ABCDE method to rapidly identify any potentially life-threatening

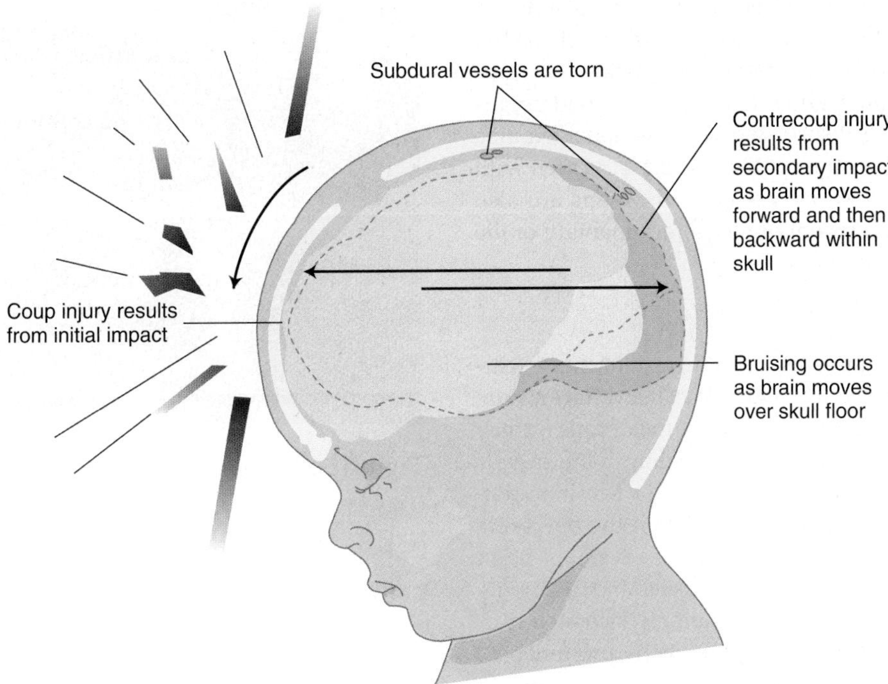
Subdural vessels are torn
Contrecoup injury results from secondary impact as brain moves forward and then backward within skull
Coup injury results from initial impact
Bruising occurs as brain moves over skull floor

Figure 50.2 ■ Brain injury in children and adults can result from a direct blow to the head (coup injury) or the acceleration–deceleration movement of the brain (contrecoup injury). The inertial forces that result when the head and skull stop moving allow the brain tissue to continue moving within the skull. This results in tearing of nerves, fibers, and blood vessels.

injuries. The most common internal injuries associated with blunt trauma are injuries to the liver, spleen, and small intestine.

Acceleration–Deceleration Injury

Blunt trauma commonly occurs as a result of an acceleration–deceleration injury from a fall or motor vehicle crash.[15] In collision type injuries, there are three basic mechanisms that result in damage to tissues. The first type of impact occurs when the vehicle is struck by another vehicle or strikes a fixed object, such as a tree) and results in direct injuries. The second type of impact occurs when one or more parts of the motor vehicle (e.g., the dashboard, mirror, or steering wheel) strike the patient. The third type of impact occurs when internal parts of the body (e.g., the brain, lungs, heart, and/or kidney) strike the internal structures of the body (e.g., the brain strikes the inside of the skull or internal organs strike the chest or abdominal wall) or other outside objects (i.e. the dashboard or the road) and result in internal injuries (**Figure 50.2** ■).[16] These injuries typically result in abrasions, contusions, or lacerations from a crushing type injury.

Abrasions

Abrasions occur when the superficial layers of the skin are damaged as a result of friction or pressure from being rubbed or scraped along a fixed object. Abrasions are often referred to as rug burn, road burn, or road rash.[6] When the body tissues meet a solid object such as the road, gravel, or the ground under force, as when a person is thrown from a motorcycle or a car, the epidermis and dermis are torn in a shearing fashion, leaving the dermal and subcutaneous structures exposed (**Figure 50.3** ■). When only the dermis and subcutaneous tissues are involved, the tissues will normally heal very well as long as no infection occurs. However, if the abrasion extends to the muscle or bone, serious permanent injuries can occur that may require extensive surgeries or skin grafting.[6]

Contusions

Contusions occur when blunt force is applied to the tissues causing underlying blood vessels to tear, resulting in ecchymosis or purple discoloration of the skin due to blood seeping into the subcutaneous tissues. Very often, this

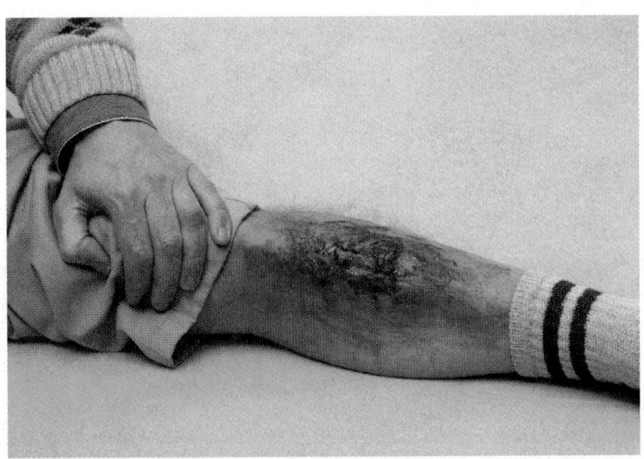

Figure 50.3 ■ Abrasion.

contusion lies below a superficial abrasion. As blood vessels are disrupted when a contusion occurs, the damaged area appears dark red or purple with well-defined margins within the first 48 hours. After 48 hours, the blood begins to break down and be absorbed, giving the damaged area a yellow or brown appearance (**Figure 50.4** ■).[6] Often with a contusion, the underlying tissues and organs are also injured, causing a permanent or temporary inability of the involved organ to function properly.

Lacerations

When a blunt force injures tissue to the extent that a tearing of the tissue occurs, the injury is called a **laceration**. The laceration or tear may involve only the dermis or may pass through all layers of skin to the underlying organs (**Figure 50.5** ■). Blunt force may also cause a tear in underlying blood vessels and organs even when the overlying skin structures are intact. For example, as a result of blunt trauma, bridging veins that lie under tissues and organs are often torn. Tissues that are most commonly lacerated during a blunt force are those located over bony prominences such as such as the skull, knees, elbows, and eyebrows.[17] The margins of the injury often involve areas of nonviable crushed skin, which would not be suitable for suturing and often involve a complicated wound repair and debridement.

Check Your Progress: Section 50.3

1. A 20-year-old college football player collides head first into another player, causing the first player to briefly lose consciousness. Describe the three different impacts that occurred during the collision and how the player's helmet may have helped to reduce the force of impact.
2. A 40-year-old woman is pushed through an older plate glass window during an argument. What type(s) of soft tissue injuries might you expect to see?
3. An EMS unit reports that they are transporting a 75-year-old male who has fallen down several steps of a wooden stairway. What type of soft tissue injury would you suspect?

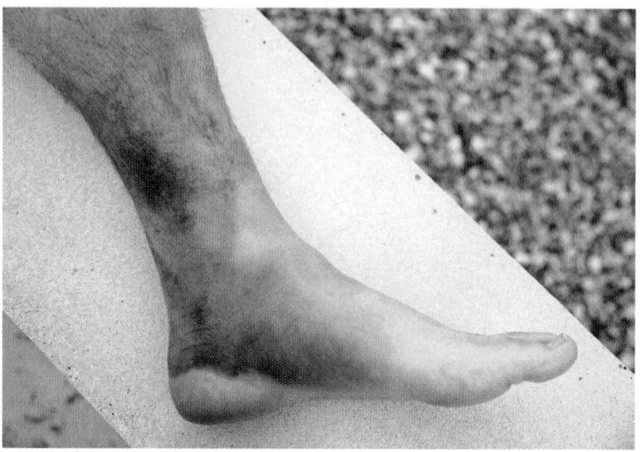

Figure 50.4 ■ Contusion.

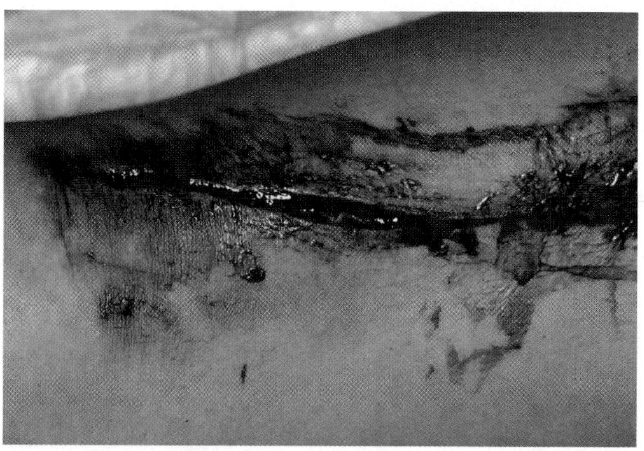

Figure 50.5 ■ Laceration.

50.4 Penetrating Trauma

Unlike blunt trauma, in which there is no entry of the body by an object, penetrating trauma results from an impact that violates the skin. Mechanisms of penetrating trauma include stabbings, gunshot wounds, and impalements. A foreign body may or may not be left in the victim. Prompt management of penetrating trauma victims is needed to minimize blood loss and prevent infection.

Lacerations and Puncture Wounds

Injury inflicted to any area of the body with a sharp instrument is called a stab wound, incisional wound, or puncture. Incisional wounds are longer than they are deep and have distinct edges. Stab wounds are injuries that are deeper than they are long. Puncture wounds are caused by a sharp point without any distinct wound edges (**Figure 50.6** ■). The cutting pattern varies depending on the instrument causing the injury; however, the healthcare professional must consider the size and shape of the instrument when assessing tissue and organ injury from penetrating trauma. In contrast to blunt trauma, penetrating trauma generally does not involve crush type injuries that cause damage to underlying vessels. Instead, penetrating injuries cause severing of underlying tissue, vessels, nerves, and direct injury to underlying organs.

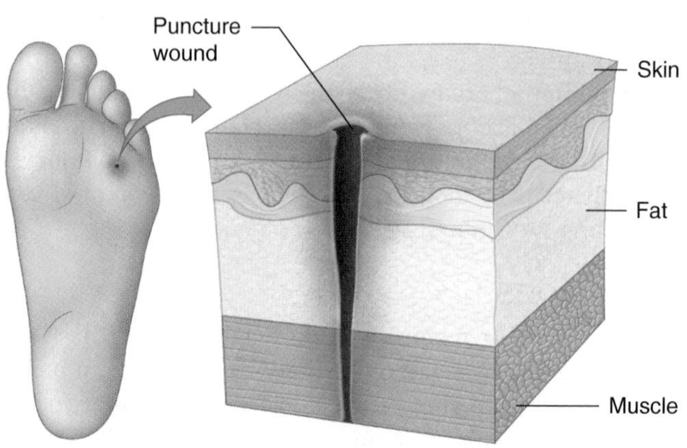

Figure 50.6 ■ Puncture wound.

Bite Injury

Dog, Cat, and Human Bites

Bites occur when tissue is damaged as a result of contact with human or animal mouth and teeth (**Figure 50.7** ■). Bite injuries from dogs are one of the most common types of bite injury in the United States, with children ages 5–9 experiencing the highest rates of dog bite injuries.[18] Saliva and debris from the mouth should also be considered in examining a bite injury; this will give the healthcare practitioner an idea about what foreign body contamination, such as soil or vegetation, might have been introduced into the tissues. Bite marks are typically categorized by degree of severity:

- ***Mild.*** First degree: extends through the epidermis and part of the dermis
- ***Moderate.*** Second degree: extends through the epidermis and dermis
- ***Severe.*** Third degree: extends through the epidermis, dermis, and subcutaneous tissues, resulting in blood loss.

During bite injuries, tissue often undergoes several types of trauma, including contusions, lacerations, and cuts. To prevent further infection, appropriate antimicrobial therapy must be administered and is based on the species that caused the bite. Immunoglobulin therapy against rabies should be considered if the bite is from a high-risk species and the animal is not available for testing.[19]

A primary survey must be completed to determine whether the bite has caused any life-threatening injuries. Once immediate life-threatening injuries have been ruled out, the healthcare provider must be concerned about infection to the injured tissues. Meticulous irrigation and debridement of any foreign material and saliva must be undertaken. If foreign material is suspected, an x-ray must be ordered to determine whether there is material involved in the wound. If the wound appears clean and there is little risk of contamination, it can be sutured. However, if there is concern about infection or wound contamination, the wound should be left open to close by secondary intention. The general rule of thumb is that bite wounds that cause deep penetrating injuries, wounds that are more than 6 hours old, and wounds of the hand and foot should not be sutured immediately after injury but should be closed by secondary intention. Although dog bites carry about a 6–7% risk of infection, cat bites carry a greater risk of infection. This higher rate of infection from cats is primarily due to their sharper teeth and ability to bite deeper into the tissues and deposit bacteria deep within the wound.[20]

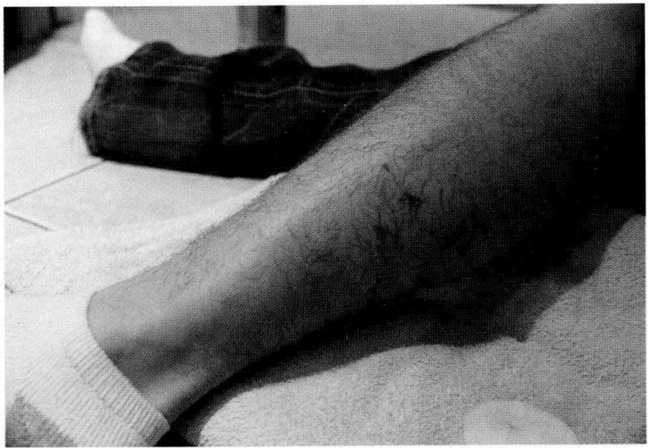

Figure 50.7 ■ Dog bite injury.

Human bites rank as the third leading type of bite resulting in visits to emergency departments. Infections occur in approximately 10–15% of human bite wounds.[21] Clenched-fist injury results when the knuckle of one person's fist comes into contact with another person's front tooth, causing a small, open wound of up to 8 mm in length on the first person's hand. Occlusive bites are those with sufficient force to break the skin. Careful wound cleaning and debridement are necessary to reduce the risk for infection. Prophylactic antibiotics are necessary.[21]

The highest risk for infection from a human or animal bite is in the hand. The small size of the wound and the tight spaces through which bacteria can travel make these wounds difficult to irrigate, increasing the risk for infection.[20,21]

Snake Bites

The bite of a snake can produce physical damage from the fangs puncturing skin and blood vessels. The bite itself is often not the major concern, as fangs are often not long enough to penetrate to major vessels. Rather, the major issue is the presence of snake venom. Snake venom can vary in potency and effect depending on the combination of peptide components. These peptides often bind to physiologic receptors and can cause neuromuscular blockade or cardiovascular consequences.

The local tissue damage can result in ecchymosis or bruising along with edema of tissue. Tissue edema can be exacerbated through changes in the permeability of capillary walls, leading to leakage of fluid and blood into tissue. Depending on the nature of the venom, more severe reactions such as hemolysis and coagulative disruption can occur.

Several rating scales exist for determining the degree of envenomation (injection of venom). The ratings can vary widely depending on the potency of the venom. For instance, snake bites can be categorized as causing mild, moderate, or severe reactions.

- ***Mild reactions*** include scratches or small lacerations from the physical fangs. These reactions are not accompanied by any systemic responses beyond the possibility of minor localized edema caused by the puncture or laceration of the skin.
- ***Moderate reactions*** include extension of edema beyond the site of the bite. These reactions are not considered to be life threatening.
- ***Severe reactions*** emerge from anaphylactic responses to snake venom or from physiologic receptor blockade. Select venoms can result in coagulopathy, leading to thrombocytopenia and excessive bleeding. Bleeding

Table 50.2 Reactions to Insect and Spider Bites

	Manifestations	Mechanisms of Action	Commonly Associated Insects or Spiders
Minor	Localized edema, erythema, and pruritus	Localized	Mosquitoes
Severe	Laryngeal edema with wheezing and dyspnea.	Allergic reaction to components in the venom	Bees, fire ants, wasps
Toxic	Inflammation or necrosis at the site of the bite or sting; development of a disease as a result of bacteria or virus	In particular, spider venom can contain toxins that cause neuromuscular blockade or cellular apoptosis, resulting in necrosis.	Brown recluse or black widow spider, some members of the scorpion family

into tissue and significant edema lead to a reduction in circulatory volume. The lack of adequate circulating volume then contributes to hypotension and possibly shock. Hypotension in combination with hemolysis can then contribute to the development of acute renal failure. Treatment of severe snake bite involves management of hypovolemia and shock. Receptor blockade requires the administration of specific antivenom.

Insect and Spider Bites and Stings

Regardless of location, insect and spider bites are commonplace. The majority of exposures result in short-term inflammation and skin irritation. These reactions are typically treated with topical corticosteroids to alleviate localized skin inflammation. Some bites or stings can result in more serious manifestations due to the presence of toxins or diseases (such as malaria transmitted by mosquitoes) that can be transmitted through the bite or sting. At times, scratching an inflamed area can result in a secondary infection.

Emergency measures may be necessary to treat anaphylaxis brought about by allergic responses to components in the bite or sting (as with bee stings) or to treat a transmitted disease (**Table 50.2** ■).

Missile Injuries (Bullet Wounds)

For the year 2015, firearms were the leading cause of death for individuals ages 15 and up, with homicide by firearm being the leading cause of death among those ages 15 to 34, and suicide by firearm the leading cause of deaths for those age 35 and older.[15] Entrance of the missile or bullet is usually marked by a circumferential area of abrasion to the skin where the bullet penetrated. In contrast, the exit wound does not have an area of initial blunt contact with the missile and will have no area of abrasions (**Figure 50.8** ■). The entrance wound must be observed for evidence of gunpowder residue and should be documented and photographed before the area is cleansed because the information may be needed as evidence during legal proceedings. The identification of the entrance and exit of the bullet path is important for the practitioner to predict injured organs in the path of the bullet. Bullets will follow the path of least resistance and will bounce off hard, bony structures toward soft, pliable substances, damaging tissues, vessels, nerves, and organs along the way. In considering the path of the bullet, it is important to know the force with which the bullet entered, how close the victim was to the bullet, and the type of bullet.

The physical characteristics of the bullet are important to consider in treating bullet injuries. The bullet mass refers to the diameter and length of the bullet and will help to predict how much damage the bullet did after entering the tissues. A very long lead bullet will penetrate deeper into body tissues than a hollow-point bullet. Another important characteristic of the bullet is whether it is made of solid lead or has a partial metal jacket covering the lead component or a full metal jacket. Bullets with a full metal jacket have an outer covering on the bullet tip and penetrate deep within the body without deforming. The jacket rarely separates from the bullet tip; however, if it does separate, it can cause as much damage as a leaded bullet. Civilians often use hollow-point bullets, which flatten out when they come into contact with a solid structure and form a mushroom-like shape. This means that there is more of a mass to cause destruction to surrounding tissues and therefore the damage to the tissues is greater. The velocity with which the bullet entered the tissues is also a very important determinant of the degree of damage to the body.[22,23]

Another important consideration in evaluating a bullet injury is the type of tissue the bullet contacts during its journey through the body. When a bullet hits hard, bony matter, it has a tendency to deflect toward softer tissue; when a bullet enters tissues, blood vessels, or soft organs (e.g., lungs, myocardium), it easily destroys the soft tissues. Bullets also are made to twist during travel and therefore will tumble as they pass through the body, marking a line of destruction along the bullet's path known as cavitation. Cavitation along the path of the bullet may cause more damage to surrounding tissues as the width of the bullet itself, especially if the resulting cavity fails to recoil and the affected tissue becomes permanently

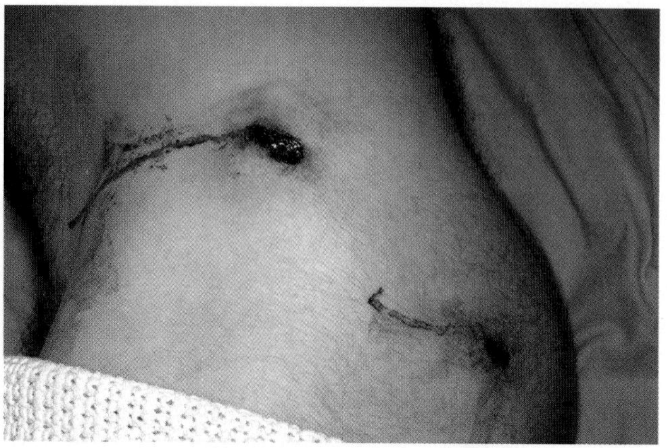

Figure 50.8 ■ Gunshot wound showing entry (middle of photo) and exit (lower right) of the bullet.

damaged (**Figure 50.9** ■).[23] Most vulnerable to this path of destruction are tissues in organs such as the brain, myocardium, liver, and spleen.

Another consideration in evaluating bullet wounds is the degree of fragmentation of the bullet. For example, shotgun shells used by most hunters consist of plastic tubes filled with gunshot, which is made up of many small metal balls. When the target is hit, the tiny metal balls travel through the tissues, damaging tissues that are in their path. Other fragments that can be associated with bullet wounds is fragments of bone or body tissues and bacteria from organs (e.g., the colon) that are projected through the body by the bullets along with fragments of metal that separate from the bullet during impact or fragments of foreign objects that the bullet has passed through on the way to the body.

CLINICAL POINT: The locations of a bullet's entrance and exit wounds will not be reliable indicators of the path of destruction. The healthcare provider must be alert to other possible injuries caused by a deflection of the bullet off bony or ligamentous structures through soft tissues. ■

Jaylen Henderson: Outcome

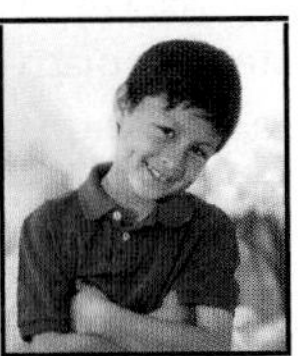

At the Level I pediatric trauma center, Jaylen is lethargic and disoriented. Vital signs are temperature 98.8° F, pulse 150 (strength 1/4), respirations 36, blood pressure 64/40. He is diaphoretic with signs of cyanosis around the mouth and increased nail bed refill time. An endotracheal tube is placed, an intravenous access route is established. Jaylen begins to exhale a fine mist of blood and is placed on a ventilator. A thoracotomy is performed to remove blood from the lung, and a tube is left in place to provide a means of draining the area. He is moved into the surgical suite for repair of injures to the lung and thoracic area.

3. In addition to what was noted in the scenario, what findings might the trauma team record that would assist in investigation of the crime?
4. In addition to the lung injury, what major injury should be suspected, especially given Jaylen's vital signs?

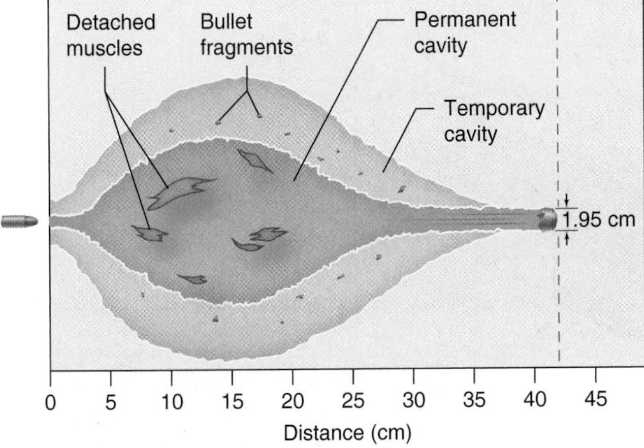

Figure 50.9 ■ Cavitation of bullet injury.

Check Your Progress: Section 50.4

1. Contrary to popular belief, most snake bites are not life threatening. However, if someone is bitten by a snake, what findings would suggest that the patient has become seriously ill?
2. A 7-year-old boy was bitten in the face and neck by a dog. What would be your most immediate concerns about his injuries?
3. How do the shape and composition of a bullet relate to the amount of tissue damage that occurs when a person is shot?

50.5 Thermal Injuries

Types and Incidence of Burns

Burns occur when soft tissue is exposed to high-energy heat-producing elements (fire or heated objects), chemicals, and electrical energy.[16] Approximately 480,000 Americans are treated for burn injuries each year in the United States.[24] Burns are categorized according to the severity of the burn, which is determined by the depth of the injury (determined by the layer of skin involved), the size of the injury relative to body surface area, and whether there are complicating injuries. Depending on the severity of the burn, permanent scars may result. These scars can be disfiguring and may lead to body image consciousness in burn survivors.

The skin has several functions that are important for maintaining homeostasis in the body. The first function is to provide protection to the underlying structures of the body, preventing injury and providing protection against pathogens. The second function of skin is to control body temperature and excretion of water from the body. Finally, the skin provides sensation, alerting the body to invasion of foreign objects, disruption to the integrity of the skin, or injury. When the skin is compromised, all the functions of the skin become impaired, and the body is at risk for infection, disorders of temperature and water regulation, and loss of sensation to the affected body part.

When tissue is burned, cells in the tissues become compromised, and their ability to regulate water absorption and excretion is lost. When cellular destruction occurs, the sodium pump begins to fail, there is an influx of intracellular water, and sodium and potassium are lost. As water and electrolytes leak from the body, there is a massive loss of circulating blood volume, and cardiovascular compromise quickly ensues unless life-saving interventions are initiated. Acid–base disturbances progress, and lactic acidosis will occur if the patient is left untreated. Added to this loss of circulatory volume, severe burns result in a decrease in cardiac contractility and thus in cardiac output.[16]

Along with a disruption in the fluid and electrolyte balance after a severe burn injury, fluid loss also leads to an increased hematocrit and increased blood viscosity due to hemoconcentration. Anemia will occur if erythrocytes are destroyed by the burn injury or if there is a resultant blood loss due to associated trauma.

The gastrointestinal system is often adversely affected as part of the systemic complications of a burn injury. Because large quantities of narcotic medications are often required along with the fluid shifts, patients often develop an ileus. This will result in the inability to feed patients, who may then require total parental nutrition to meet caloric needs to facilitate wound healing. Ulcers are often associated with burns and are the result of the body's stress response. As fluid shifts, the plasma volume decreases, causing ischemia and necrosis of the duodenum. This results in a Curling ulcer. This in part is why burn patients are often given prophylactic proton pump inhibitors.

As physical destruction of tissues and cells progresses following a severe burn injury, a systemic reaction occurs that is known as the systemic inflammatory response. Typical systemic reactions include hypothermia, hypovolemia, and infection. This response involves the release of cellular mediators that have the ability to disrupt every system of the body and can lead to death if it progresses.[16] See Chapter 11 for a complete discussion of the systemic inflammatory response.

Depth and Extent of Burns

The depth of a burn injury is determined by the layers of tissue involved in the burn and is classified as superficial, superficial partial thickness, deep partial thickness, or full thickness (**Figure 50.10** ■). Superficial injury (formerly known as a first-degree burn) involves damage to the epidermal layer of skin. The most common example of a superficial burn injury is a sunburn. The burned skin is reddened and painful but usually heals with no intervention within 7 days.

Partial thickness burn injuries (formerly known as second-degree burns) are further classified as superficial partial thickness burns or deep partial thickness burns. In superficial partial thickness burns, the epidermis and the papillary dermis are burned.[25,26] Blistering usually occurs, and the dermis is red and moist with good capillary refill. These burns are very painful. The burn usually heals in 14–21 days with little scarring. Deep partial thickness burns involve damage to the epidermis, papillary dermis, and reticular layer of the dermis. The reticular layer involves injury to the hair follicles and the sweat and sebaceous glands. The root of the hair follicles and the sweat and sebaceous glands are usually spared and, once healed, return to normal functioning. Skin is usually blistered, and the exposed dermis is whitish to yellow, does not blanch, and does not have good capillary refill. There is usually no pain sensation to the area of deep partial thickness burns. Healing typically occurs within 3 weeks to 2 months, and permanent scars will result.

A **full thickness burn** (formerly known as a third-degree burn) involves injury to epidermal, all the dermal layers and structures, and subcutaneous tissues. Full-thickness burns may even extend into muscle, bone, or organs. The skin is charred, pale, and painless and has a leathery appearance. There is no capillary refill and no blanching. These burns will not heal without surgical intervention, and scarring is always involved.[16,25]

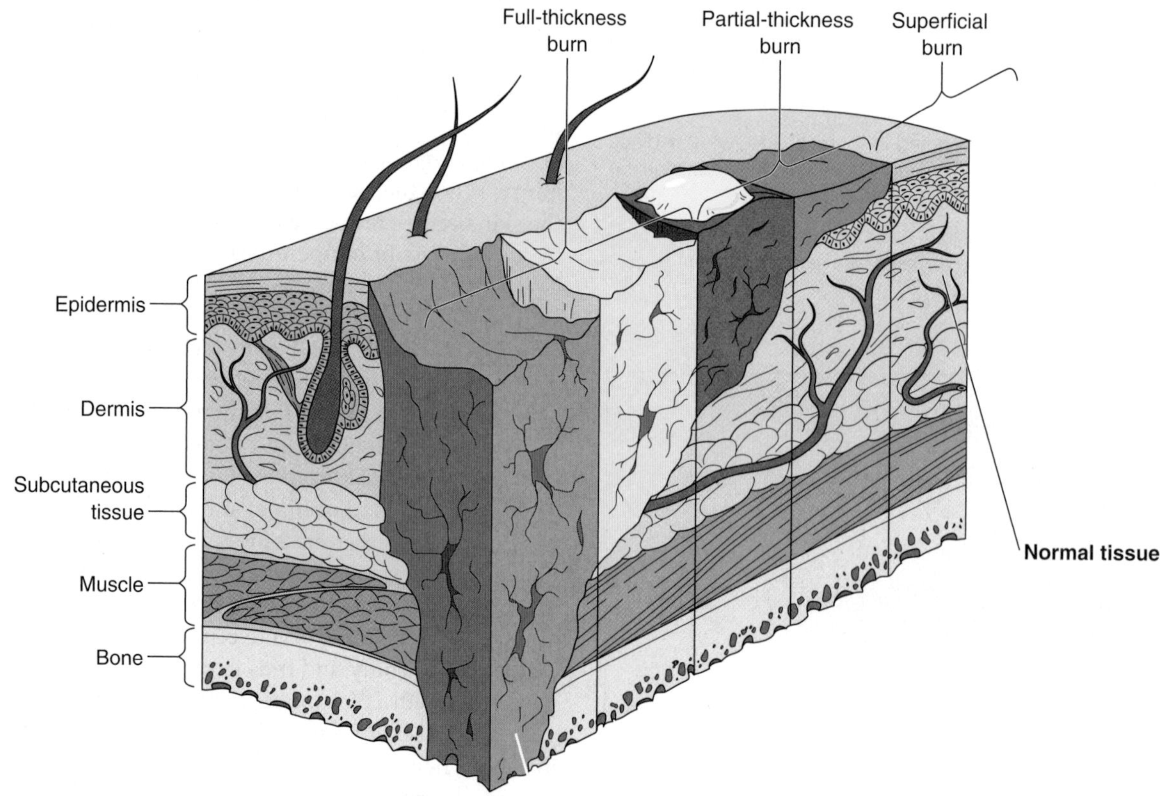

Figure 50.10 ■ Depth and extent of burn wounds.

An additional consideration in evaluating burn injury is the area of the body that is burned. Skin thickness varies in different areas of the body. The skin is very thick on the palms of the hands, the soles of the feet, and the upper part of the back. Therefore, in comparison to thinner skin, these areas can be exposed to higher heat for a longer period of time before injury will occur.[22,23] Degradation of the skin can leave the burn victim at severe risk of infection. This risk is even greater in the pediatric and geriatric populations. The burn also leads to loss of the normal protective flora that assists in preventing opportunistic infections from infecting the patient.

When the skin is exposed to heat, three zones of injuries occur (**Figure 50.11** ■).[24,25] The most severe damage occurs when there is total decimation of the tissue resulting in necrosis and charring of the tissue, causing a full-thickness burn. This area is the center of the zone and is considered nonviable; it is referred to as the zone of coagulation or zone of necrosis. The area surrounding the zone of coagulation is the zone of stasis or zone of ischemia. This area involves cells that are severely damaged but may be viable. Fibrin deposits, vasoconstriction, and thrombosis occur throughout this area, making the surrounding tissues vulnerable to necrotic death. This usually occurs in areas of mild to deep dermal burns where there is compromised blood flow. The outermost zone is called the zone of hyperemia, where there is minimal cell damage but vasodilation occurs as a result of the release of mediators to the adjacent area. Typically, this tissue will recover fully.

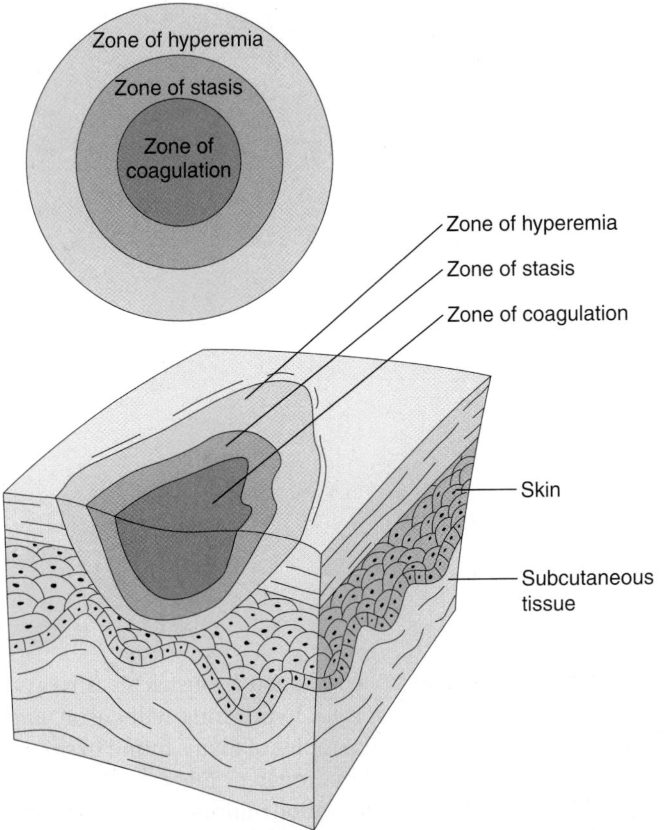

Figure 50.11 ■ Zones of burn injury.

CLINICAL POINT: Determining an accurate percentage of body surface area burned is essential in estimating fluid loss and fluid replacement needs for the patient with acute burn injury. ■

The **Rule of Nines** gives a rough estimate of body surface area (BSA) burned by assigning 9% to each body area. The Rule of Nines for an adult patient is as follows:

9% is assigned to the head (front and back together)
9% for EACH arm (front and back)
18% for EACH leg (front and back)
18% for front torso
18% for back torso (includes buttocks)
1% for genitalia.[22]

The Rule of Nines for a pediatric patient is as follows:

18% is assigned to the head (front and back)
9% for each arm (front and back)
36% for the torso (front and back)
14% for each leg (front and back)
1% for the genitals.

If the burns are patchy in distribution, the Rule of Palm may be used. In the Rule of Palm, the patient's palm without the fingers represents approximately 1% of the patient's body surface area. The Rule of Nines and the Rule of Palm are used most often by emergency medical services to convey the extent of injury to the receiving hospital.

In the hospital or burn center, more sophisticated calculations are used, such as the Lund-Browder method (**Figure 50.12** ■).

Linda Dickson: Application

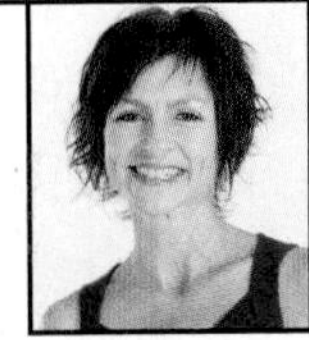

On arrival at the emergency department, Ms. Dickson remains unconscious. Partial thickness burns are found on her head and upper body. In particular, partial thickness burns cover much of her thoracic and abdominal region. Her Lund-Browder score is as follows: head 7%, neck 2%, and chest and back 26% for a total of 35% total BSA burned. Ms. Dickson's vital signs are pulse 110, respirations 28, blood pressure 100/50. Oxygen saturation as determined by pulse oximetry is 88%. As part of initial stabilization, two intravenous access routes are established for administration of fluid.

3. On the basis of Ms. Dickson's vital signs, in what physiologic condition does she present?
4. What is the priority of care at this time?

There are several formulas for estimating initial fluid replacement requirements for the severely burned patient. The most commonly used is the Parkland formula:

$$4\text{ mL} \times \text{weight in kilograms} \times \%\text{ BSA burned} = \text{amount of fluid over 24 hours}$$

The formula is used to determine the amount of lactated Ringer's solution that should be infused over the first 24 hours, the first half being infused over the first 8 hours and the second half being infused over the next 16 hours.[16]

Complicating injuries, which are common among burn patients, can be more life threatening than the burn itself. Inhalation injuries that result from burn injury to the lungs

Area	Age (years)					%	%	%	%
	0–1	1–4	5–9	10–15	Adult	1°	2°	3°	Total
Head	19	17	13	10	7				
Neck	2	2	2	2	2				
Ant. trunk	13	13	13	13	13				
Post. trunk	13	13	13	13	13				
R. buttock	2½	2½	2½	2½	2½				
L. buttock	2½	2½	2½	2½	2½				
Genitalia	1	1	1	1	1				
R.U. arm	4	4	4	4	4				
L.U. arm	4	4	4	4	4				
R.L. arm	3	3	3	3	3				
L.L. arm	3	3	3	3	3				
R. hand	2½	2½	2½	2½	2½				
L. hand	2½	2½	2½	2½	2½				
R. thigh	5½	6½	8½	8½	9½				
L. thigh	5½	6½	8½	8½	9½				
R. leg	5	5	5½	6	7				
L. leg	5	5	5½	6	7				
R. foot	3½	3½	3½	3½	3½				
L. foot	3½	3½	3½	3½	3½				
					Total				

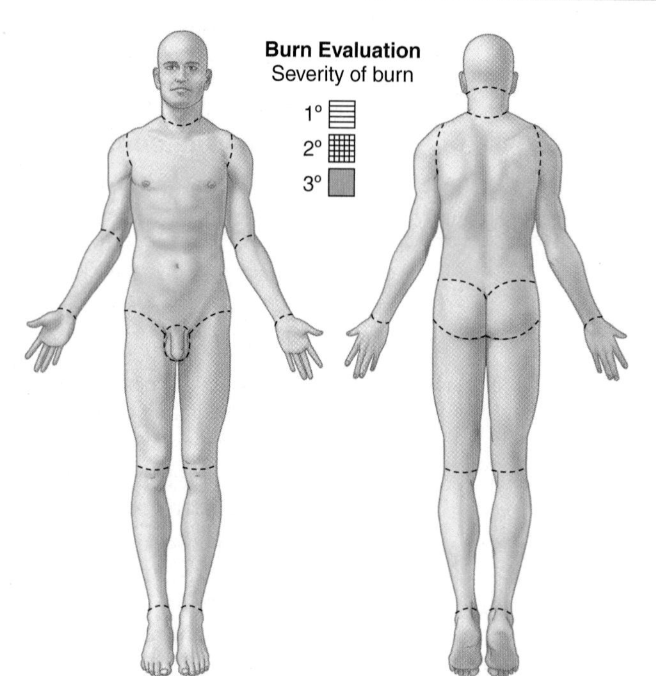

Figure 50.12 ■ Lund-Browder formula.

are the main cause of mortality in the burn patient. Smoke inhalation injuries are the leading cause of death due to fire in the United States.[27] Inhalation injuries are generally associated with fires that occur in closed spaces such as bedrooms and storage rooms. Smoke contains particles that are extremely toxic to the lung tissues. As these particles reach the bronchioles, an inflammatory response is triggered, causing bronchospasms, edema, and constricted airways. If this process is not reversed, hypoxemia will ensue, and death can occur quickly. Examples of toxins found in smoke are carbon monoxide and hydrogen cyanide.[27]

Many patients with inhalation injuries go on to develop acute respiratory distress syndrome (which is covered in Chapter 17) from the toxins and the inflammatory response triggered by the pulmonary parenchyma. Emergency treatment possibilities for inhalation injuries include intubation with 100% humidified oxygen; frequent monitoring of arterial blood gases; cardiac monitoring; fluid resuscitation; and the prevention, early identification, and treatment of pneumonia. Additional interventions may be necessary depending on the nature of the toxins inhaled.[27]

Because of the massive cellular destruction and fluid and electrolyte abnormalities caused by burn injuries, the body enters a severely hypermetabolic state. Energy expenditure by a burn patient often exceeds 200% of that of a normal person, resulting in depletion of carbohydrate, fat, and protein stores. As a result of this severe increase in energy expenditure, the patient is at risk for immunosuppression; wound healing will be impaired; and muscle, bone, and tissue growth will be delayed. Without appropriate treatment, this hypermetabolic state can result in increased risk for infection, multi-organ dysfunction, and even death. Therefore, close attention must be paid to replacing the severely burned patient's energy stores. Sophisticated measurements of energy expenditure and requirements are available in most intensive care units. Early interventions that include continuous enteral feeding can help enhance patients' metabolic states and reduce risk for further deterioration.[28,29] This enhanced rate of metabolism will also decrease the duration of effectiveness of medications. For example, burn patients require large quantities of pain medications, and the metabolic processes that break the drug down are greatly accelerated.

Treatment of burn injuries in the emergency department focuses on fluid resuscitation, prevention of infection, wound care, and pain control. Burn injuries can be extremely painful, and pain control must be given high priority in the treatment of burn patients. Frequent, standardized pain assessment and documentation are necessary. Most burn patients benefit from a combination of pharmalogic and nonpharmalogic pain therapies.[29,30]

Linda Dickson: Outcome

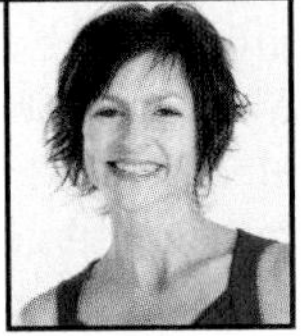

Ms. Dickson is hospitalized for 20 days with treatment focusing primarily on the effects of smoke inhalation and postexposure pneumonia. Because of the composition of the smoke to which she was exposed, she is at long-term risk for development of respiratory disease or worsening of her pre-existent asthma. A periodic assessment of pulmonary function will be necessary, and a bronchoscopy may have to be done to evaluate the extent of tissue damage.

It is possible for partial thickness burns to heal without scarring, depending on the depth of the burn, but complete healing of the skin will take up to 70–80 days. Before Ms. Dickson is discharged, an education plan needs to be established that covers dressing changes and the need to ensure proper aseptic technique before dressings are changed. Depending on the depth of Ms. Dickson's burn, there may be need for debridement or skin grafting, in which case, pain management before treatment may be a significant component of her care.

5. What is the potential impact of burn scarring on Ms. Dickson's emotional well-being?
6. What potential adverse effects does Ms. Dickson face in regards to pain management?

Check Your Progress: Section 50.5

1. Which skin functions can be compromised in a large partial or full thickness burn?
2. You are evaluating a serious scald burn on a 2-year-old child. You note that much of her head and chest and both her arms were affected. What is your estimate of total body surface area affected by the injury?
3. A 45-year-old male was trapped briefly in his bedroom during a house fire. You see no signs of burns, but he is covered in soot, coughing up black sputum, and wheezing. What do you suspect is happening to the patient?

50.6 Chemical Burns

Etiology and Pathogenesis

Chemical burns occur when corrosive (caustic) substances such as strong acids or bases come into contact with skin or mucous membranes or are inhaled or ingested. Corrosive bases are present in household products such as oven cleaners that contain potassium or sodium hydroxide and in bleach. Various household products contain corrosive acids, including drain, tile, toilet, and metal cleaners. Although chemical burns may occur in the home as a result of accidental exposure to these products, life-threatening chemical burns are more likely caused by accidents in workplaces where large amounts of corrosive chemicals are used or as a result of assault with a chemical.

Clinical Manifestations

Local manifestations at the site of a chemical burn on the skin or mucous membranes include pain, erythema, burning sensation, numbness, blisters, and necrotic tissue. Chemical burns of the eye can cause visual impairment and blindness. If vapor from a corrosive chemical is inhaled, it causes coughing and dyspnea and can burn the lining of the respiratory tract. If the vapor reaches the alveoli, it can injure the alveolar–capillary membrane, resulting in pulmonary edema and impaired gas exchange. If a corrosive chemical is swallowed, it can burn the mouth, esophagus, stomach, and intestines. Scar tissue formation can result from chemical burns and may impair function; for example, scar tissue in the esophagus from swallowing a corrosive chemical can impair swallowing. There are specific hazards that may vary depending on the specific chemical to which the patient is exposed. When a patient with a chemical burn presents for treatment, a materials safety data sheet (MSDS) should be obtained for information that includes first aid measures, effects on the body, and any special precautions that must be taken to protect staff members from exposure. A chemical burn can cause systemic manifestations through direct toxicity and by causing fluid shifts. These symptoms may include hypotension, headache, dizziness, and dysrhythmias. If they are left untreated, severe chemical burns may be lethal.

Linking Pathophysiology to Treatment

The primary prevention of chemical burns can be accomplished through education on the safe handling of chemical products. The risk of harm can be greatly reduced by keeping potentially dangerous chemicals out of the reach of children and following the manufacturer's recommendations. The risk of accidental inhalation of caustic chemicals can be reduced by using them in a well-ventilated area or outdoors. Chemicals should never be mixed, as chemical reactions may release harmful substances. Finally, using the recommended protective equipment will minimize the contact exposure risk.

Corrosive chemicals will continue to cause damage as long as they are in contact with tissue. Therefore, it is important to remove any clothing that has been contaminated with the chemical and to irrigate the burned area of the body with large amounts of water, saline, or lactated Ringer's solution. If the patient was exposed to a powdered chemical, excess material should be brushed off the patient before irrigation. A guiding principle in patient decontamination should be preventing the contamination of staff members or of areas of the patient that were not exposed to the chemical. A patient who is grossly contaminated may require a deluge shower for decontamination. Special attention should be paid to containing the runoff water. This water should be considered contaminated, to be disposed of as hazardous waste.

Once the patient has been decontaminated and is no longer an exposure risk to staff members, the ABCDE approach to trauma resuscitation should be followed. Depending on the extent of the patient's burns and the patient's hemodynamic status, fluid resuscitation similar to that used in treating a flame- or heat-related burn might be required. Sterile dressing should be applied to the affected areas. Opioid analgesics will likely be required for pain control. If there are extensive burns, debridement of necrotic tissue may be required.

Check Your Progress: Section 50.6

1. A farm worker comes to the emergency department waiting room covered in insecticide dust. He is coughing and drooling, and he has abdominal cramping. What would be your first priority?
2. You are an occupational health nurse at a high-tech manufacturing facility. You are notified over a two-way radio that a chemical liquid splashed onto a worker and soaked her. What instructions would you provide to the on-scene personnel as you respond to the incident?

50.7 Electrical Injuries

Electrical Burns

Electrical burns account for approximately 1000 deaths a year with a mortality rate of 3–15%.[31] The three populations that are most at risk for electrical burns are toddlers, adolescents, and electrical workers.[32] Electrical burns from either electricity or lightning bolts can be very deceiving. They may produce very little evidence of external damage; however, there is internal damage along the path of the electrical charge as it passes through the body, burning and destroying tissues and organs along its path. Seven factors contribute to the degree of damage to the body:

1. Type of current
2. Amount of current
3. Voltage
4. Pathway of current
5. Duration of current
6. Area of contact
7. Resistance of the body.[16,33]

Electrical current is the movement of electrical energy, called current. The flow of current is measured in amperes. This flow can be changed by the degree of resistance applied to the current, hence resulting in various amperes. The type of current may be either direct current (DC) or alternating current (AC). Direct current means that the electrical flow is in one direction; alternating current means that the electrical flow periodically reverses the direction of the current. Most household electricity in the United States is alternating current.

Toddlers are particularly at risk of injury from electricity. As they explore their world and place objects in their mouth, toddlers can chew on an electrical cable or place metal objects in electrical sockets. These injuries can result in exposure to temperatures in excess of 3000°C.[32] Injuries from chewing on an electrical wire often result in the need for reconstructive surgery and can cause lifelong dental problems. ■

Injuries resulting from voltages of less than 1000 volts are considered low-voltage injuries; high-voltage injuries are those resulting from voltages greater than 1000 volts. Most household electrical outlets provide 110 volts of AC electricity. Power lines typically contain 720 volts. Because household voltage is so low, burns from household electrical injuries are usually minor; however, 110 volts is enough to cause ventricular fibrillation and cardiac arrest. Pulses from Taser guns contain approximately 50,000 volts but have very low amperage and low energy. They are designed to stimulate contraction of voluntary muscles and paralyze the victim temporarily while the muscle recuperates.

Materials that enhance the flow of electrical current are called conductors; materials that slow or stop the conduction of electrical current are called insulators. Most of the tissues of the body are conductors, easily allowing the flow of electrical current through body tissues. Although bone will still conduct current, it has a higher resistance than other tissues in the body. Water is a conductor of electricity, and since the body is composed mainly of water, electricity tends to flow readily through the body. For example, dry skin has some resistance to electricity, but wet skin will easily conduct electricity.

Because electricity follows the path of least resistance, the practitioner must consider the path of the electrical injury as it bounces off hard surfaces such as bone toward soft tissues such as arteries, muscles, and organs. Damage does not necessarily follow a straight path; however, the damage will follow a path parallel to that of the electricity conducted through the body. High-voltage injuries typically result in systemic manifestations. Tissue and even limb necrosis is possible. Extravasion of fluids occurs as injured tissues become more permeable, reducing intravascular volume and requiring IV Ringer's solution.[33]

Rescue workers must be cautious when resuscitating patients with high-voltage electrical injuries. Power lines, the ground, the patient, and objects on the ground may be excellent conductors of electrical current that can then flow to the rescue personnel. Only adequately insulated materials should be used to rescue victims of high-voltage electrocution. The best initial treatment is to make sure the power is turned off. Until the power is confirmed to be off, all electrical wires and devices should be considered live and should not be approached by rescuers.

When a patient comes to the emergency department with an electrical injury, the healthcare provider must be alert for signs of cardiac and neurologic injury. Patients who have any symptoms of cardiac or neurologic injury such as shortness of breath, chest pain, palpitations, loss of consciousness, or any transthoracic injury must be placed on a cardiac monitor, and a thorough neurologic workup must be completed. Spinal precautions must be utilized until spinal injuries have been ruled out. If large muscle groups or severe extremity injuries are noted, the patient must be screened for rhabdomyolysis, the breakdown of muscle cells that produces toxic myoglobin, which in large amounts will destroy the kidneys. A very careful physical examination should be done to determine all serious life-threatening injuries and secondary complications that may have resulted from the electrical injury. Several complications of electrical injuries must be considered during the initial evaluation, such as cardiac conduction defects, central nervous system injury, spinal cord injury, peripheral nerve injury, wounds, bone injury, blast injury, inhalation injury, eye injury, auditory system injury, oral burns, GI injuries, vascular and muscle injury, and disseminated intravascular coagulation.[33]

Lightning Burns

Although it is exceedingly rare to be struck by lightning, the event is potentially lethal. There are four mechanisms of lightning strike. The first is a direct strike in which the patient is hit directly from a cloud. This injury pattern accounts for 3–5% of lightning strike incidents and is frequently lethal.[34] In a contact injury, the person is touching an object that is struck, and the object carries the current to the person; the contact mechanism accounts for approximately 5% of lightning strike injuries. A splash strike occurs when one object is struck and the current then is transferred to another object that the patient is touching; 35% of lightning strike injuries are caused by splash strikes.[35] The final mechanism of lightning strike is a ground strike, in which the lightning is conducted through a surface leading to the injury; approximately 55% of lightning strikes are ground strikes.

Death from lightning strike is usually due to simultaneous cardiac and pulmonary arrest.[35] The high voltage and amperage associated with lightning causes asystole as well as paralysis of the respiratory center in the brain. Rapid recognition of the cardiopulmonary arrest is critical to patient survival. The respiratory center is slower to recover from such an injury, and the patient may regain a pulse before beginning to breathe spontaneously.[35] With the need for rapid intervention to initiate cardiopulmonary resuscitation, bystanders play an important role in rapid recognition of the patient's status and in initial resuscitation efforts.

All patients who sustain a lightning injury that includes a direct strike, loss of consciousness, neurologic deficits, chest pain, dyspnea, multiple trauma, concurrent pregnancy, or burns over more than 10% of the BSA are considered to be at high risk for morbidity and mortality.[35] Screening echocardiography and 12-lead electrocardiography should be performed.[35] Arrhythmias may range from transient atrial fibrillation to ST segment changes to complete collapse of the cardiac electrical system.[35] Because of the high morbidity and mortality associated with lightning strikes, all injuries with this mechanism meet criteria for transfer to a certified burn center.

Check Your Progress: Section 50.7

1. You stop at the scene of a motor vehicle crash where a power pole has been heavily damaged. A power line is draped across the roof of the car. The driver is sitting in the car and appears to be alert and uninjured. Bystanders are urging him to get out of the vehicle before it "blows up." What should you do?
2. A 55-year-old man is electrocuted while working on a 220-volt clothes dryer. He has contact burns to his left hand and left foot. He presents to your urgent care clinic after his partner insists that he should be evaluated. The patient says that he feels fine and does not want to be seen. What should you tell him?
3. A sudden summer storm occurs during a golf tournament. Before some of the players and spectators can seek shelter, lightning strikes a tree near them. Several victims are lying on the ground unconscious; others are complaining of a burning sensation, tingling, and ringing ears. Who should you help first? Why?

50.8 Lethal Triad of Trauma

Many trauma deaths can be attributed to the lethal triad of trauma. The lethal triad represents three interdependent factors that lead to increased bleeding, worsening shock, and ultimately death. The three components of the lethal triad are hypothermia, coagulopathy, and acidosis. If these factors are reversed, the patient's chances of survival can be improved (**Figure 50.13** ■).

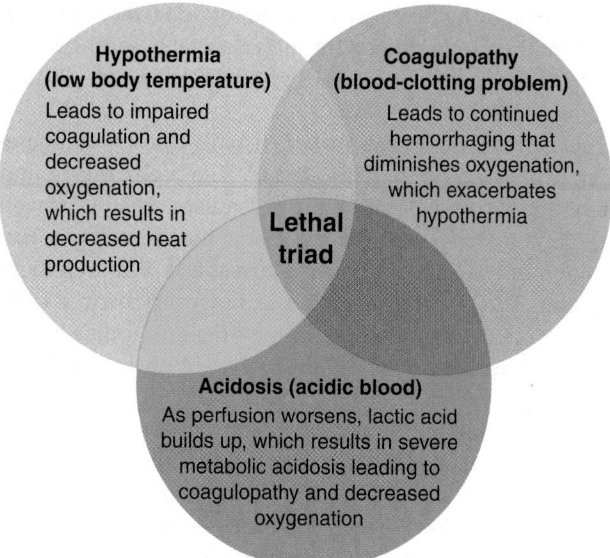

Figure 50.13 ■ Lethal triad of trauma.

Relative hypothermia leads to impaired perfusion, which is compounded by the trauma patient's hypovolemic state. This decrease in perfusion leads to decreased oxygenation and decreased heat production. This leads to worsening hypoxia. Also, the body's clotting factors are less active at lower body temperatures, leading to further blood loss.

Hypothermia can result from both nonmedical and medical causes. Patients may become hypothermic after an injury in even relatively warm climates. Also, immersion in water less than 80°F may lower the patient's core temperature. Wintertime trauma can serve as a significant source of hypothermia that should be reversed as early as possible during the evacuation process. Care must be taken throughout the resuscitation and operative processes to ensure that the patient is not allowed to become chilled. This includes warm resuscitation rooms or operating rooms, applying warmed blankets to the patient, and infusing warmed intravenous fluids and blood products.

Acidosis also leads to coagulopathy. With the decreased perfusion, waste products including lactic acid build up in the tissues, and serum pH decreases. Damaged cells release toxins that can lead to further acidosis. Clotting factors cannot work as efficiently when the serum pH is not within the normal physiologic range of 7.35–7.45; if the function of clotting factors is impaired, a feedback loop is created that leads to worsening bleeding as the metabolic acidosis progresses.

As packed red blood cells and saline are administered, platelets and coagulation factors are diluted. Current guidelines call for a replacement of red blood cells, platelets, and fresh frozen plasma in a 1:1:1 ratio in an attempt to replace all blood components that are lost as a result of bleeding. These products should be warmed before administration, as they are usually kept refrigerated; hypothermia may be worsened if they are not warmed. It should also be noted that normal saline and other crystalloid solutions do not offer any oxygen-carrying capacity. ATLS guidelines suggest administration of blood for hypotension after a 2000-mL bolus of crystalloid.

Check Your Progress: Section 50.8

1. A male gunshot victim is brought to the trauma center by EMS. You note several penetrating wounds to his chest and abdomen. His skin is pale, cool, and diaphoretic. He is exposed to his underwear, and he is shivering and appears to be short of breath. What should be the initial actions of the trauma team?
2. A woman who is 26 weeks pregnant is struck by a car as she attempts to cross a street. She is suspected to have both a pelvic fracture and a left femur fracture. Her vital signs include a heart rate of 140 beats per minute and a blood pressure of 84/60. She is breathing at 30 breaths per minute. How can her presentation lead to the triad of trauma?
3. At what point should a trauma team switch from using crystalloid fluids to blood-based products in a hypovolemic trauma patient?

50.9 Trauma Deaths and Trauma Prevention

Trimodal Distribution of Trauma Deaths

The basis for the current trauma systems is the knowledge that there are three peak times during which trauma patients are most likely to die. This is known as the trimodal distribution of trauma death (**Figure 50.14** ■).[8,26] The first peak of trauma deaths is those that occur instantly, at the scene of the injury. An example of this would be death from a massive head injury or penetrating wound to the heart or aorta, which would cause immediate exsanguination. The only way to save these patients is through aggressive prevention strategies such as helmet laws and highway and automobile safety.

The second peak of trauma deaths occurs in the early minutes and early hours of injury. Most of these deaths occur from major injuries to the head, chest, and abdomen.

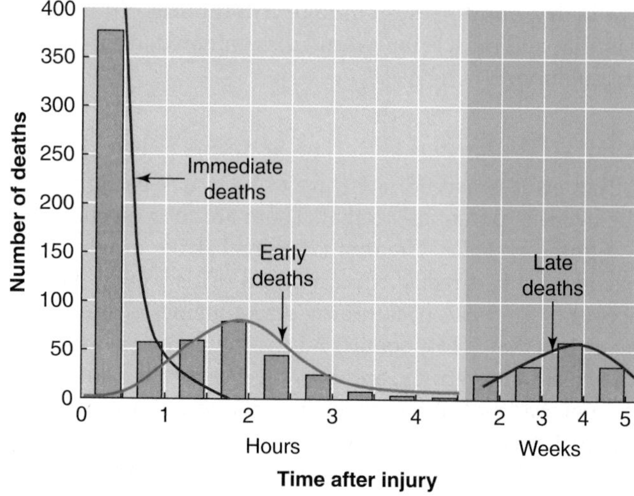

Figure 50.14 ■ Trimodal distribution of trauma deaths.

Deaths during this peak of trauma can be decreased by enforcing a trauma system that accurately identifies these vulnerable patients and quickly transports them to an appropriate trauma center that is staffed with qualified surgeons, nurses, and operating room personnel. Improvements in the identification, rapid treatment, and evaluation of life-threatening injuries affect the number of deaths during this phase of trauma.

The third peak of trauma deaths occurs when trauma patients die in the hospital, usually in the intensive care unit. These deaths occur when the organ damage that occurred during the initial injury and the resuscitation phase begins to fulminate or when sepsis develops. Multiple organ failure begins to occur, often resulting in shock and death, usually days or weeks after the initial injury. Aggressive resuscitative care, prompt recognition of early signs of shock and organ ischemia, and early treatment of these injuries are paramount in the ongoing treatment of acutely injured patients.[16]

Trauma Prevention

Trauma care has developed into a well-researched, well-developed science across the United States. Quick response to trauma from highly educated personnel in the field as well as in emergency departments has escalated the survival rates of all trauma patients. To increase survival for trauma patients, many public and private agencies have come together to provide governmental response teams, governmental financial support to trauma researchers and trauma response teams, healthcare worker education and training, and education and training of transport agencies across the nation. In spite of all the major advances in the understanding and treatment of the severely injured trauma patient, injury prevention remains the only true cure for this devastating disease. In 1972, William Haddon developed the well-known Haddon Matrix, which helped to emphasize the impact of traffic on traumatic injuries and provided a framework of 10 strategies that helped to guide government agencies to begin measures to promote highway safety.[16] As a result, there are far fewer trauma fatalities today than there were in the 1950s. Many agencies, including the Centers for Disease Control and Prevention, now use a four-step public health approach to violence prevention:

1. Define the problem.
2. Identify causes and risk factors.
3. Develop and test interventions.
4. Implement effective interventions and evaluate their impact.[36]

Nurses are integral members of the trauma team and can have a dramatic impact on the manner in which trauma care is addressed and trauma prevention strategies are employed. A thorough understanding of the physiology underlying traumatic injuries provides the foundation on which trauma interventions are built and from which new intervention strategies emerge. Nurses who are dedicated to the prevention, recognition, and emergent treatment of traumatic injuries will be instrumental in molding the future of trauma care.

Check Your Progress: Section 50.9

1. What strategies would help to reduce morbidity during the third phase of the trimodal distribution of trauma deaths?
2. There has been a recent spate of children drowning in swimming pools in your community. You have been asked to serve on a committee that is tasked with formulating recommendations to reduce the incidence. Using Kellerman and Houry's four-step process toward trauma prevention, how would you approach this problem?

CHAPTER SUMMARY

50.1 Chapter Overview and Case Studies

Describe the epidemiology of traumatic injury and concepts related to trauma.

- Trauma is the leading cause of death in the United States for people under 46 years of age.
- Traumatic injuries costs society approximately $260 billion annually.
- Traumatic injury respects no boundaries in terms of age, culture, sex, or economic status.
- There are several trauma classification systems based on location or manner of injury. The most common injury classification is the mode of injury: blunt trauma, penetrating trauma, thermal trauma, electrical trauma, and chemical trauma.
- There are five levels of trauma care; Level I systems represent the highest level of care and system leadership.
- Traumatic injuries are the most common cause of death in pregnant women not directly related to gestation. Trauma is also the most common reason for fetal demise.
- Pregnancy-associated expansion of blood volume allows for the loss of 35% of blood before the woman exhibits signs of hypovolemic shock. With a later onset of symptom presentation as a result of blood loss in the pregnant patient, early fluid resuscitation is critical.

50.2 Modern Trauma Care

Outline the team approach to trauma care and the ABCDE approach to trauma care.

- Pregnancy results in an elevation of the heart rate and a slight decrease in blood pressure. These changes need to be kept in mind during patient assessment.
- Consideration of abuse as a mechanism is needed when the injury pattern does not match the described mechanism of injury in children and older adults.
- Polypharmacy may complicate management of the geriatric patient.
- Anticoagulant use in older adults mandates careful assessment of any bleeding.
- The ABCDE method refers to airway, breathing, circulation, disability and exposure.

50.3 Blunt Trauma

Differentiate the causes, classification, and clinical manifestations of injuries caused by blunt trauma and approaches to diagnosis and treatment of those injuries across the lifespan.

- Blunt trauma is caused by an impact that that does not result in an object's entering the body.
- Motor vehicle crashes, falls, assaults, and athletics-related accidents are some of the most common mechanisms of blunt trauma.
- Most blunt trauma results from compressing or crushing types of injury.
- The most common type of blunt trauma occurs as a result of an acceleration–deceleration injury.
- Mechanisms of acceleration–deceleration often results in more than one injury as a result of initial impact and from a recoiling or ricochet of internal contents.
- Abrasions are damage to the superficial layers of the skin as a result of friction or pressure.
- Contusions occur when blunt force is applied to the tissues causing underlying blood vessels to tear, resulting in ecchymosis or purple discoloration of the skin due to blood seeping into the subcutaneous tissues.
- Lacerations are a tearing of tissue that may involve only the dermis or may pass through all layers of skin to the underlying organs.

50.4 Penetrating Trauma

Differentiate the causes, classification, and clinical manifestations of injuries caused by penetrating trauma and approaches to diagnosis and treatment of those injuries across the lifespan.

- Penetrating trauma results from an impact that violates the skin. Mechanisms of penetrating trauma include stabbings, gunshot wounds, and impalements.
- Incisional wounds are longer than they are deep and have distinct edges.
- Stab wounds are deeper than they are long.
- Puncture wounds are caused by a sharp point without any distinct wound edges.
- Penetrating injuries cause severing of underlying tissue, vessels, nerves, and direct injury to underlying organs.
- Bites occur when tissue is damaged as a result of contact with human or animal mouth and teeth.
- Bite marks are typically categorized by depth of penetration into tissue.

50.5 Thermal Injuries

Differentiate the causes, classification, and clinical manifestations of thermal injuries and approaches to diagnosis and treatment of those injuries across the lifespan.

- Burns are categorized according to the severity of the burn, which is determined by the depth of the injury (determined by the layer of skin involved), the size of the injury according to body surface area, and any complicating injuries.
- When the skin is compromised, all the functions of the skin become impaired, and the body is at risk for infection, problems with temperature regulation and water regulation, and loss of sensation to the affected body part.
- As water and electrolytes leak from the body, there is loss of circulating blood volume, and cardiovascular compromise can quickly ensue unless life-saving interventions are initiated.
- Severe burns can stimulate release of myocardial depressant factor, which causes a decrease in cardiac contractility and thus in cardiac output.
- The loss of fluid related to severe burn leads to a dilutional increase in hematocrit and blood viscosity.
- Systemic inflammatory response can follow a severe burn injury. This involves the release of cellular mediators that lead to multiple system disruption.
- Superficial injury (formerly known as a first-degree burn) involves damage to the epidermal layer of skin.
- Partial thickness injuries (formerly known as second-degree burns) are further divided into superficial partial thickness burns and deep partial thickness burns.
- In superficial partial thickness burns, the epidermis and the papillary dermis are burned. Blistering usually occurs, and the dermis is red and moist with good capillary refill.
- Deep partial thickness burns involve damage to the epidermis, papillary dermis, and reticular layer of the dermis.
- Full thickness burns (formerly known as third-degree burns) involve damage to the epidermis, all the dermal layers and structures, and subcutaneous tissues.

50.6 Chemical Burns

Differentiate the causes, classification, and clinical manifestations of chemical burns and approaches to diagnosis and treatment of those injuries across the lifespan.

- Local manifestations at the site of a chemical burn on the skin or mucus membranes include pain, erythema, burning sensation, numbness, blisters, and necrotic tissue.

- If vapor from a corrosive chemical is inhaled, it causes coughing and dyspnea and can burn the lining of the respiratory tract. If the vapor reaches the alveoli, it can injure the alveolar–capillary membrane, resulting in pulmonary edema and impaired gas exchange.
- A chemical burn can cause systemic manifestations through direct toxicity and by causing fluid shifts. These symptoms may include hypotension, headache, dizziness, and dysrhythmias.

50.7 Electrical Injuries

Differentiate the causes, classification, and clinical manifestations of electrical injuries and approaches to diagnosis and treatment of those injuries across the lifespan.

- The three populations that are most at risk for electrical burns are toddlers, adolescents, and electrical workers.
- Electrical burns are often very deceiving, producing little external damage while resulting in significant internal damage along the path of the electrical charge.
- Ventricular fibrillation and cardiac arrest can result from exposure to as little as 110 volts. Hence, while low-voltage sources such as household currents might not result in burn, they can still elicit a cardiac effect.
- The nurse must be alert to the possibility of neurologic or cardiac damage resulting from an electrical burn.
- If large muscle groups or severe extremity injuries are noted, the patient must be screened for rhabdomyolysis, the breakdown of muscle cells that produces toxic myoglobin, which in large amounts will destroy the kidneys.
- Patients who experience lighting strikes that result in loss of consciousness, neurologic deficits, chest pain, dyspnea, and multiple trauma, pregnancy, or burns over more than 10% of the BSA are considered to be at high risk for morbidity and mortality.

50.8 Lethal Triad of Trauma

Differentiate the causes, classification, underlying pathogenesis, and clinical manifestations of the lethal triad of trauma and approaches to diagnosis and treatment of those conditions across the lifespan.

- The lethal triad is a constellation of three interdependent components—hypothermia, coagulopathy, and acidosis—that lead to increased bleeding, worsening shock, and ultimately death.
- Hypothermia leads to impaired perfusion, which is compounded by the trauma patient's hypovolemic state. The decrease in perfusion leads to decreased oxygenation and decreased heat production. This leads to worsening hypoxia. Also, the body's clotting factors are less active at lower body temperatures, leading to further blood loss.
- As packed red blood cells and saline are administered, platelets and coagulation factors are diluted. Current guidelines call for a replacement of red blood cells, platelets, and fresh frozen plasma in a 1:1:1 ratio in an attempt to replace all blood components that are lost as a result of bleeding.

50.9 Trauma Deaths and Trauma Prevention

Describe the trimodal distribution of trauma deaths and the four-step process for trauma prevention.

- The trimodal distribution of trauma death states there are three peak times during which trauma patients are most likely to die.
- The first peak reflects deaths that occur instantly or at the scene of the injury.
- The second peak of trauma death occurs in the early minutes and hours after injury. Most of second peak deaths occur from major injuries to the head, chest, and abdomen.
- The third peak reflects deaths in the hospital setting, usually in the intensive care unit. Third peak deaths occur when the organ damage that occurred during the initial injury and the resuscitation phase begins to fulminate or sepsis develops. Multiple organ failure begins to occur, often resulting in shock and death, usually days or weeks after the initial injury.

REVIEW QUESTIONS

1. A fall from a second story window would be classified as which type of injury?
   a. Penetrating
   b. Crushing
   c. Hematoma
   d. Blunt
2. Which of the following clients would be most likely to overcome injuries from a serious car crash?
   a. A 12-year-old female
   b. A 37-year-old male
   c. A 69-year-old female
   d. A 78-year-old male

3. A 27-year-old female at the beginning of her third trimester of pregnancy trips and falls onto the sidewalk. She has swelling and pain to her left wrist but is able to wriggle her fingers without difficulty. Her blood pressure is 104/70, and her heart is beating at 100 times per minute. Which of the following statements best explains her vital signs?
   a. She is bleeding internally into her uterus, which is causing her blood pressure to fall and her heart rate to rise.
   b. These vital signs are consistent with a woman in the third trimester of pregnancy.
   c. The pain in her wrist is causing her heart rate to rise significantly, which in turn is causing her blood pressure to fall.
   d. There is less blood volume in the mother as the blood is shifted toward the fetus during pregnancy, causing blood pressure to decrease and heart rate to increase.
4. A 74-year-old female is brought to the emergency department by EMS after she fell off a toilet, striking the side of her head. Which of the following medical history findings would be of most immediate concern?
   a. She takes a calcium channel blocker and Coumadin daily.
   b. She has a history of high blood pressure and atrial fibrillation.
   c. She is allergic to several medications, including penicillin.
   d. She was in a serious car crash 20 years ago.
5. A young child is scalded on his arm after pulling a pot of boiling water off a stove. The skin is open and reddened, and blisters have formed in several places. The child is crying and in pain. How would you classify this burn?
   a. Superficial injury
   b. Superficial partial thickness injury
   c. Deep partial thickness injury
   d. Full thickness injury
6. Several workers from a nearby industrial plant come into your clinic waiting area after a toxic chemical release. They are coughing and complaining of burning sensations to their eyes, noses, and throats. Your immediate action is to:
   a. take vital signs and document them for record keeping.
   b. keep the workers in the waiting area and call for assistance.
   c. initiate intravenous access for each client and administer fluids.
   d. look up the MSDS information about the chemical involved.
7. Hypothermia in a trauma patient contributes to impaired perfusion, which can lead to an increase in:
   a. the rate of blood clotting.
   b. serum pH.
   c. acidosis.
   d. heat production.
8. A 20-year-old male was shot with a small caliber handgun. There is a single penetrating wound in the right upper quadrant of his abdomen. There is minimal external bleeding. He is awake, anxious, and complaining of abdominal pain and shortness of breath. His heart rate is 130, and his respiratory rate is 28. His skin feels cold, and he appears pale and diaphoretic. His lung sounds are clear and equal bilaterally. Which of the following injuries is most likely?
   a. A collapsed right lung
   b. A liver injury
   c. Bleeding from the stomach
   d. A spinal cord injury

ANSWERS

Answers to Review Questions can be found in Appendix A. Answers to Case Study and Check Your Progress questions are available on the faculty resources site. Please consult with your instructor.

RECOMMENDED WEBSITES

American Trauma Society
http://www.amtrauma.org

Brain Injury Alliance: About Brain Injuries
https://biau.org/about-brain-injuries

The Brain Injury Guide & Resources: Mechanisms of Injury
http://braininjuryeducation.org/TBI-Basics/Mechanisms-of-Injury

World Health Organization: Guidelines for Essential Trauma Care
http://apps.who.int/iris/bitstream/10665/42565/1/9241546409_eng.pdf

REFERENCES

1. Rhee, P., Joseph, B., Pandit, V., Aziz, H., Vercruysse, G., Kulvatunyou, N., & Friese, R. (2014). Increasing trauma deaths in the United States. *Annals of Surgery, 260*(1), 13–21.
2. Centers for Disease Control and Prevention (CDC). (2017). Deaths and mortality. *National Center for Health Statistics.* Retrieved from https://www.cdc.gov/nchs/fastats/deaths.htm.
3. Carrico, C. J., Holcomb, J. B., Chaudry, I. H., PULSE Trauma Work Group. (2002). Scientific priorities and strategic planning for resuscitation research and life saving therapy following traumatic injury: Report of the PULSE team work group. *Shock 17,* 165–168.
4. Nichols, H. (2017). The top 10 leading causes of death in the Unity States. *Medical News Today.* Retrieved from http://www.medicalnewstoday.com/articles/282929.php.
5. Ravage, B. (2006). As real as it gets: The evolution of trauma care and emergency medicine. *The Safety Net.* Retrieved from http://essentialhospitals.org/wp-content/uploads/2014/01/Evolution.pdf.
6. National Association of Emergency Medical Technicians. (2016). *PTHLS: Prehospital trauma life support* (8th ed.). Burlington, MA: Jones & Bartlett.
7. American College of Surgeons Committee on Trauma. (2017). *Advanced trauma life support* (10th ed.). Chicago, IL: American College of Surgeons..
8. Tintinalli, J.E. (2016). *Emergency medicine: A comprehensive study guide* (8th ed.). New York, NY: McGraw-Hill.
9. Battaloglu, E., Battaloglu, E., Chu, J., & Porter, K. (2014). Obstetrics in trauma. *Trauma, 17*(1), 1–7.
10. Mendez-Figueroa, H., Dahlke, J. D., Vrees, R. A., et al. (2013). Trauma in pregnancy: An updated systematic review. *American Journal of Obstetrics & Gynecology, 209*(1), 1–10.
11. Morris, J., Rosenbower, T., Jurkovich, G., et al. (1996). Infant survival after cesarean section for trauma. *Annals of Surgery, 223*(5), 481–491.
12. Hashmi, A., Ibrahim-Zada, I., Rhee, P., Aziz, H., Fain, M., Friese, R., & Joseph, B. (2014). Predictors of mortality in geriatric trauma patients: A systematic review and meta-analysis. *Journal of Trauma and Acute Care Surgery, 76*(3), 894–901.
13. Gordon, J. L., Fabian, T. C., Lee, M. D., & Dugdale, M. (2013). Anticoagulant and antiplatelet medications encountered in emergency surgery patients: A review of reversal strategies. *Trauma and Acute Care Surgery, 75*(3), 475–486.
14. Dries, D. J. (2017). Initial evaluation of the trauma patient. Retrieved from: http://emedicine.medscape.com/article/434707-overview#a2
15. Centers for Disease Control. (2016). Injury and Prevention Control: Web-Based Injury Statistics and Reporting System. Retrieved from: https://www.cdc.gov/injury/wisqars/facts.html
16. Bledsoe, B. E., & Cherry, R. A. (2017). *Paramedic Care: Principles and Practice.* (5th ed.). New York, NY: Pearson.
17. Rozzi, H. V. (2014). Laceration or incised wound: Know the difference. Retrieved from http://www.acepnow.com/article/laceration-incised-wound-know-difference/
18. Centers for Disease Control. (2015). Preventing dog bites. Retrieved from https://www.cdc.gov/features/dog-bite-prevention/
19. World Health Organization. (2013). Animal bites. Retrieved from http://www.who.int/mediacentre/factsheets/fs373/en/
20. Ellis, R., & Ellis, C. (2014). Dog and Cat Bites. *American Family Physician, 90*(4): 239–243.
21. Barrett, J. (2016). Human Bites. Retrieved from http://emedicine.medscape.com/article/218901-overview#a2
22. American Association of Neurological Surgeons. (2017). Gunshot Wound Head Trauma. Retrieved from http://www.aans.org/en/Patients/Neurosurgical-Conditions-and-Treatments/Gunshot-Wound-Head-Trauma
23. Murphy, P., Colwell, C., Bryan, T., & Pineda, G. (2010). Shootings: What EMS providers need to know. Retrieved from http://www.emsworld.com/article/10319706/gunshot-wounds
24. American Burn Association. (2016). Burn Incidence and Treatment in the United States: 2016. Retrieved from http://www.ameriburn.org/resources_factsheet.php
25. Huether, S. E., McCance, K. L., Brashers, V. L., & Rote, N. S. (2017). Understanding pathophysi-ology, 6th ed. St. Louis, MO: Elsevier.
26. Kearns, R. D., Holmes, J. H., & Cairns, B. A. (2013). Burns injury: what's in a name? Labels used for burn injury classification: a review of the data from 2000–2012. Annals of Burns and Fire Disasters, 26(3), 115–120.
27. Lafferty, K. A. (2016). Smoke inhalation injury. Retrieved from http://emedicine.medscape.com/article/771194-overview
28. Williams, F. N., Bransky, L. K., Jeschke, M. G., & Herndon, D. N. (2011). What, How, and How Much Should Burn Patients Be Fed? *Surgical Clinics of North America, 91*(3), 609–629.
29. Rowan, M. Cancio, L. C., Elster, E. A., Burmeister, D. M., Rose, L. F., Natesan, F., Chan, R. K., Christy, R. J., & Chung, K. K. (2015). Burn wound healing treatment: review and advancements. *Critical Care, 19*(243). Retrieved from: https://ccforum.biomedcentral.com/articles/10.1186/s13054-015-0961-2
30. Girtler, R., & Gustorff, B. (2011). Pain management of burn injuries. *Anesthesist, 60*(3), 243–50.
31. Edlich, R. F., Farinholt, H. M., Winters, K. L., Britt, L. D., & Long, W. B. (2005). Modern concepts of treatment and prevention of electrical burns. *Journal of Long-Term Effects of Medical Implants, 15,* 511–532.
32. Pontini, A., Reho, F., Giatsidis, G., Bacci, C., Azzena, B., & Tiengo, C. (2015). Multidisciplinary care in severe pediatric electrical oral burn. *Burns, 41*(3), E41–-E46.
33. Edlich, R. F. (2016). Electrical Burn Injuries. Retrieved from http://emedicine.medscape.com/article/1277496-overview#a2
34. Cooper, M. A. (2016). Lightning injuries. Retrieved from: http://emedicine.medscape.com/article/770642-overview
35. Russell, K., Cochran, A., Mehta, S., Morris, S., & McDevitt, M. (2014). Lightning burns. *Journal of Burn Care & Research, 35*(6), 436–-438
36. Centers for Disease Control and Prevention. (2015). The public health approach to violence prevention. Retrieved from https://www.cdc.gov/violenceprevention/overview/publichealthapproach.html

Chapter 51

The Pathophysiology of Primary and Secondary Traumatic Injury

Adam Boise, Kyle Bergan, and Vicki Keough

Module Outline and Learning Outcomes

51.1 Chapter Overview and Case Study

Describe the primary survey and application to traumatic injuries in the context of the A (Airway), B (Breathing), C (Circulation), D (Disability), E (Exposure) approach to trauma.

51.2 The Primary Survey and Injury

Describe the primary survey and differentiate the underlying pathogenesis of traumatic injuries.

51.3 The Secondary Survey and Injury

Describe the secondary survey and application to pathogenesis of traumatic injuries.

KEY TERMS

Airway obstruction, 1249
Anterior cord syndrome, 1252
Brown-Séquard syndrome, 1252
Central cord syndrome, 1252
Cerebral contusion, 1259
Cerebral perfusion pressure (CPP), 1257
Cricothyroidotomy, 1250
Diffuse axonal injury (DAI), 1260
Epidural hematoma, 1259
Flail chest, 1254
Genitourinary trauma, 1263
Glasgow Coma Scale (GCS), 1245
Hemothorax, 1253
Intracranial pressure (ICP), 1257
Jefferson fracture, 1252
Life-threatening injury, 1245
Mean arterial pressure (MAP), 1257
Monro-Kellie hypothesis, 1257
Myocardial contusion, 1261
Open pneumothorax, 1254
Peritoneal bleed, 1256
Pneumothorax, 1253
Primary survey, 1245
Secondary survey, 1245
Spinal shock, 1251
Subdural hematoma (SDH), 1260
Tension pneumothorax, 1254
Traumatic brain injury (TBI), 1257

ABBREVIATIONS

CPP—cerebral perfusion pressure
DAI—diffuse axonal injury
DPL—diagnostic peritoneal lavage
FAST—Focused Assessment with Sonography for Trauma
GCS—Glasgow Coma Scale
HI—head injury
ICP—intracranial pressure
MAP—mean arterial pressure
SDH—subdural hematoma
TBI—traumatic brain injury

51.1 Chapter Overview and Case Study

Trauma is one of the most devastating diseases, causing loss of life and disability to patients during the most productive years of their lives. Traumatic injuries cross all boundaries of age, gender, race, culture, and socioeconomic status. Healthcare providers who care for trauma patients need to have a great deal of knowledge about the physiology and pathophysiology of trauma to understand the science behind the primary and secondary surveys and the need for timely life-saving interventions among this unique group of patients.

Trauma care requires an exquisite understanding of anatomy and physiology and of the alterations in normal physiology that occur in response to injury. Trauma resuscitation is based on standards and guidelines that offer patients the best chance to survive even the most devastating injuries. All resuscitation efforts begin with a **primary survey**, or primary assessment, during which all life-threatening injuries are discovered and managed before moving on to less serious (but sometimes more distracting) injuries. A **life-threatening injury** is one that is likely to result in death, permanent disfigurement, or permanent loss of function or impairment of function to a body part or mental ability.

In the moments immediately after a traumatic event such as a motor vehicle crash or a fall from a height, some life-threatening injuries may be quickly and easily observed. Others, such as some blunt traumas, might not be easily assessed. It is critical that healthcare providers who work with trauma patients consider the cumulative effects of trauma, regardless of the type or mechanism of injury. The U.S. Guidelines for Field Triage of Injured Patients provides an algorithm that is useful in assisting providers to quickly determine the likelihood that a patient has a life-threatening injury (**Figure 51.1** ■). For example, step 1 calls for field providers to immediately transport a patient to a trauma center if the patient has a compromised level of consciousness as exhibited by a Glasgow Coma Scale score below 14, low systolic blood pressure, and compromised airway or respiratory function, regardless of all other criteria.[1]

The guidelines also provide another important reminder: Context matters. While this chapter provides an overview of specific life-threatening injuries that must be identified and managed as part of the primary survey, nurses and other healthcare providers must remember that these injuries occur in the context of the individual patient's medical history and anatomic variations, the mechanism of the injury, and other injuries sustained—the total context of the patient's trauma experience. For instance, suppose paramedics are on the scene of a motor vehicle crash involving two passengers. Passenger A does not meet the criteria for immediate transport to a trauma center as outlined in step 1 in Figure 51.1, but Passenger B died on impact. Because the impact of the crash was sufficient to kill Passenger B, the paramedics and subsequent providers caring for Passenger A should assume and assess for life-threatening injuries until Passenger A has been thoroughly evaluated and all assessments and diagnostics have been completed.

Once all life-threatening injuries have been identified and treated during the primary survey, providers continue with a **secondary survey**, which assists in identifying less severe injuries and in continuing to develop a thorough understanding of the patient's needs and treatment plan.

The primary assessment or survey is also known as the **ABCs** of initial trauma care, and begins with the following:

Airway and cervical spine stabilization
Breathing
Circulation.

The airway is assessed for any compromise to the patient's ability to take in oxygen. While the airway is assessed, the cervical spine is examined for injury. When the healthcare provider is confident that the airway and cervical spine have been stabilized, severe bleeding is stopped, and then breathing is assessed and managed, followed quickly by assessment and management of circulation.

Once the ABCs of the primary assessment have been evaluated and treated, the healthcare provider proceeds to assess the full **ABCDEs:**

Disability (neurologic status)
Expose (undress) and Environment (temperature control).

Assessment of neurologic status generally begins with the **Glasgow Coma Scale (GCS)**, a tool for evaluating level of consciousness (**Table 51.1** ■). A GCS score below 9 indicates severe head trauma and is considered a neurologic emergency. Finally, the primary assessment is completed by exposing the patient, looking for all life-threatening injuries that may have been missed, and addressing the physiologic importance of warming or cooling the patient as needed.

The primary assessment ends with the healthcare provider taking a complete set of vital signs and preparing to conduct a secondary assessment. Note, however, that the steps of primary assessment take place within a very short period of time and that some components may be done simultaneously. For example, the initial assessment of the patient's airway and spinal stability may allow the provider to determine the patient's neurologic status; a patient who is alert and oriented and able to speak clearly and without obstruction presents differently on assessment than the patient who is unconscious.

The secondary assessment begins once the patient is stabilized, while the healthcare provider continuously assesses for any change in the primary survey. The secondary assessment includes an evaluation of all anatomic and physiologic systems in order to find all injuries and to plan for interventions to address them. Traumatic injuries to children and older adults as well as pregnant women are of special concern, and these patients will have specific physiologic responses to injuries. Throughout this chapter, alterations in patterns of injuries and the response to traumatic injuries for these populations are highlighted.

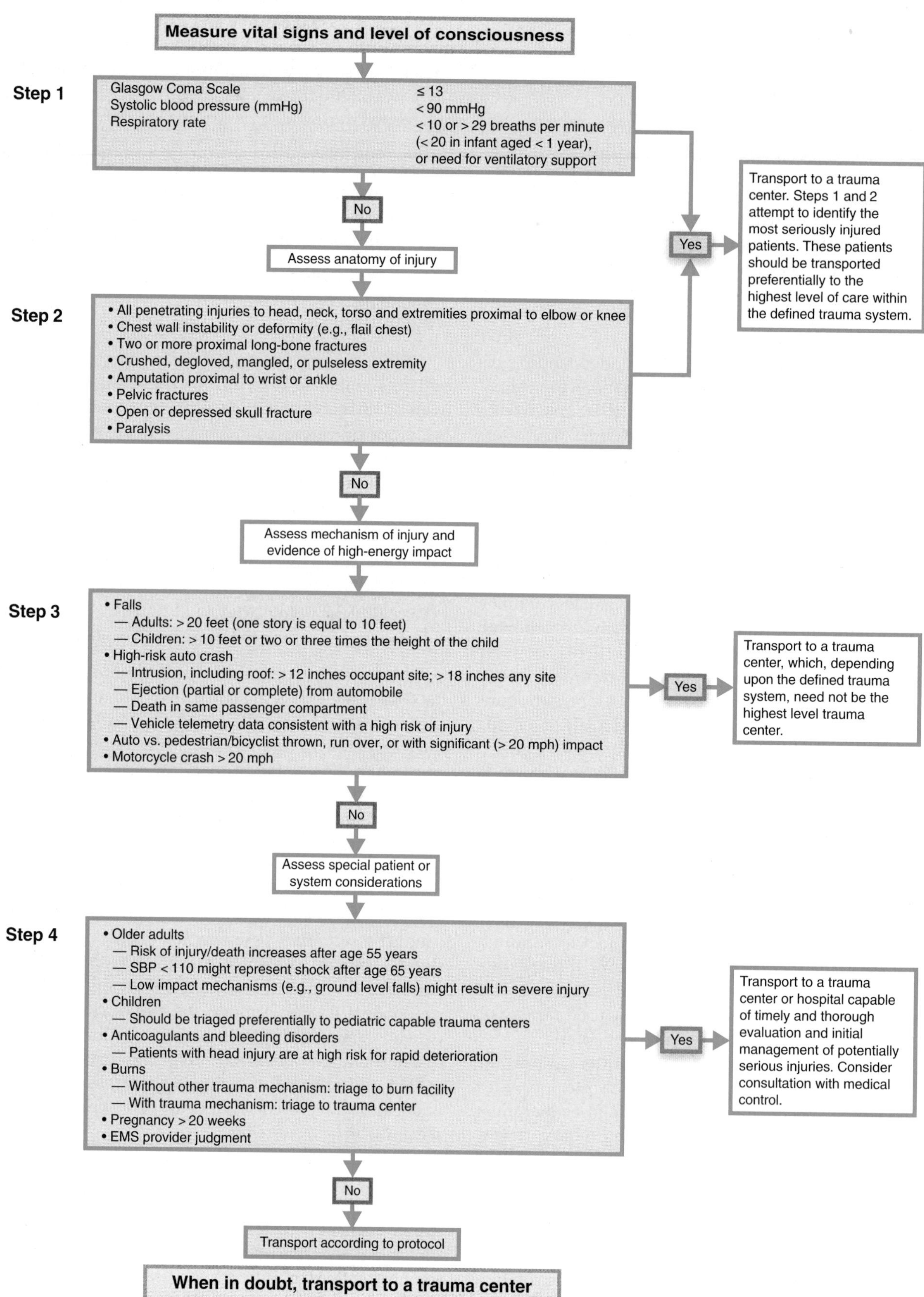

Figure 51.1 Guidelines for field triage of injured patients, United States, 2011.

SOURCE: Centers for Disease Control and Prevention. (2012). Guidelines for field triage of injured patients: Recommendations of the national expert panel on field triage 2011. *Morbidity and Mortality Weekly Report*, *61*(RR01), 1–20. Available at https://www.cdc.gov/mmwr/preview/mmwrhtml/rr6101a1.htm

Table 51.1 Glasgow Coma Scale

Assessment	Response	Score
Eyes open (Record *C* if eyes are closed by swelling.)	Spontaneously To speech To pain No response	4 3 2 1
Best motor response (Record best upper arm response.)	Obeys commands Localizes pain Flexion-withdrawal Abnormal flexion Abnormal extension No response	6 5 4 3 2 1
Best verbal response (Record *T* if an endotracheal or tracheostomy tube is in place.)	Oriented Confused Inappropriate words Incomprehensible sounds No response	5 4 3 2 1
Total score can range from 3 to 15: (A higher score indicates a higher level of functioning.)		

Because the blood volume of pregnant women is increased by approximately 30% throughout the pregnancy, the physiologic response to blood loss will be delayed in pregnant women. ■

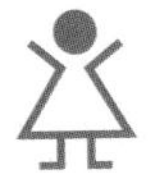

It is estimated that one in four children require medical care for an unintentional injury every year.[2] ■

Older adults have a narrowed tolerance for alterations in blood volume and will demonstrate very different signs of hypovolemic shock from those of younger adults. ■

Concepts Related to Trauma

The experience of multiple trauma can lead to the disruption of several body systems as a result of a single incident. Depending on the nature of injury, different body systems may be involved. An example of how traumatic injury can influence different systems is provided in the concept map in **Figure 51.2** ■. A motor vehicle crash can result in a traumatic injury from the head striking some part of the vehicle. In turn, a concussion may lead to inflammation within the cranial vault. Depending on the severity of concussion, blood seeping into the brain can lead to increased pressure within the cranial vault that compresses brain tissue, causing further injury. The experience of a concussion can result in motor weakness, leading to issues with mobility and sensory challenges such as peripheral neuropathy or dysthesia. The cognitive effects of concussion are well established and can include difficulty with memory retrieval and performance of executive functions. Damage to the medulla can lead to suppression of respiratory drive that could interact with a spontaneous pneumothorax resulting from trauma to the chest experienced during the accident. The appearance of the pneumothorax manifests in dyspnea with adverse effects on oxygenation that can result in a respiratory acidosis, a disruption of acid–base balance. Trauma-associated bleeding can result in hypovolemia from blood loss, leading to a hypoxic state that is worsened by the oxygenation issues tied to a pneumothorax. The presentation of numerous injuries requires careful evaluation of the trauma patient, rapid intervention, and close monitoring post injury.

Case Study

The following case is addressed throughout the chapter to assist in application of chapter content to clinical situations that involve an individual experiencing traumatic injury.

Judi Stone: Introduction

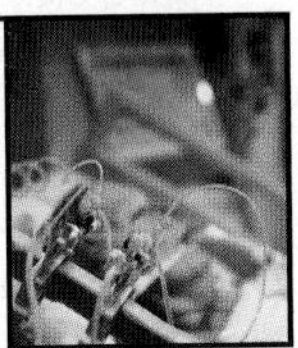

Judi Stone is a 50-year-old female who jumped out of her second-floor window trying to escape a house fire and fell to the concrete sidewalk. Paramedics find her with an altered level of consciousness, and she alternates between being combative and unresponsive. When she is unresponsive, her respirations range between 4 and 8 breaths per minute. The paramedics note a puncture wound to her left upper chest wall with subcutaneous emphysema, or air trapped under the skin. She has no air movement from the puncture wound. Because of the patient's respiratory compromise, the paramedics decide to take control of her airway and intubate her at the scene. They use a technique called rapid sequence intubation, which consists of a sedative, a paralytic agent, and rapid placement of an oral endotracheal tube. The paramedics place a 6.5-centimeter endotracheal tube and connect the bag-valve-mask to 100% oxygen so that they can ventilate her on the way to the emergency department (ED). They immobilize Ms. Stone's cervical spine (c-spine) using a hard cervical collar and then roll her onto a backboard to move her to the ambulance cot. Spinal motion restriction is implemented.

Following intubation, Ms. Stone has a normal rise and fall of her chest wall upon bagging, and she has equal and full breath sounds bilaterally. The paramedics transport her to the ED. They report the following to the ED staff:

Airway/c-spine: Ms. Stone's cervical spine was immobilized with a hard collar and backboard. Before being sedated and intubated, she was able to move all extremities.

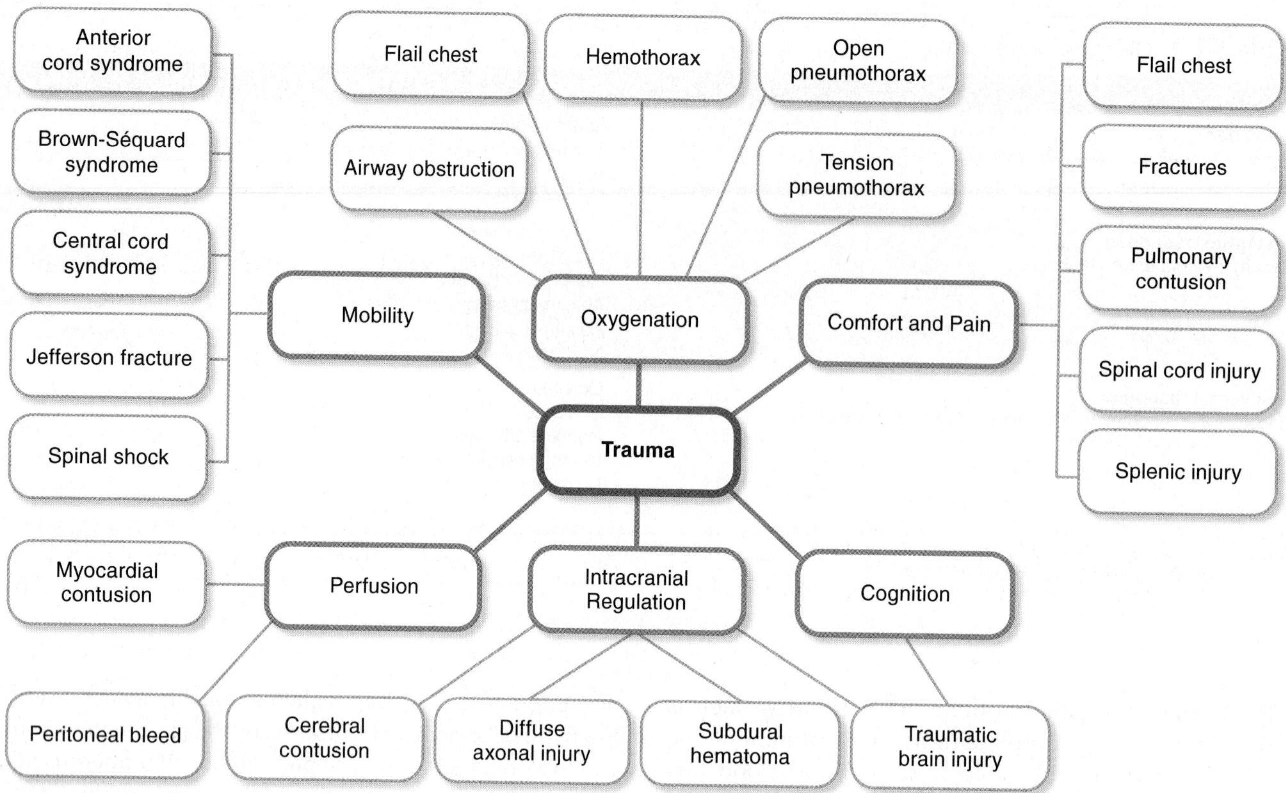

Figure 51.2 ■ Concepts related to traumatic injury.

Breathing: Her respirations were assisted with bag-valve-mask ventilation, her breath sounds were clear bilaterally, and she had good bilateral chest movement. Subcutaneous emphysema to her left chest wall was noted. An occlusive dressing was placed over the puncture wound.

Circulation: Ms. Stone's pulses were of good quality and regular; skin pink, warm, and dry; no active external bleeding; no jugular venous distention or tracheal deviation

Deficits (neurologic): She did not open her eyes, follow commands, or respond to verbal or painful stimuli; pupils were equal and reactive to light.

Expose/warm: No other areas of active bleeding or gross deformities were found to her front or back; temperature 97°F axillary.

1. Why was it important for the paramedics to intubate Ms. Stone?
2. What was the rationale for placing Ms. Stone into spinal restrictions?

Check Your Progress: Section 51.1

1. What does the ABCDE approach to trauma describe?
2. Why should the ABCDE approach be followed in order?
3. Must each step of the ABCDE process be completed before the next is performed? Why or why not?

51.2 The Primary Survey and Injury

The primary survey consists of an initial assessment of the trauma patient during which all life-threatening injuries are identified and treated on the basis of their severity. The ABCD approach makes the primary survey relatively easy to remember, which is important during a highly stressful, critical period of care.[3–5] This system of rapid assessment and resuscitation begins on arrival of the emergency medical response team at the patient's side or when the patient enters the emergency department (ED). The primary assessment continues until all life-threatening injuries have been identified and treated. Some examples of specific lethal injuries that are immediately addressed by following the ABCD approach are as follows:

- Airway: airway obstruction
- Breathing: tension pneumothorax, flail chest, open chest wound
- Circulation: massive external hemorrhage
- Disability: head injury, spinal cord injury.

Older adult patients who live with chronic illness may have little reserve capacity with which to combat a traumatic injury. It is often difficult for healthcare providers to determine the health status of the older adult trauma patient in the few moments they have to complete the primary and secondary trauma assessments. At the same time, the frail older trauma patient will not survive if quick and immediate interventions are not provided. This is a constant challenge for trauma practitioners, since research has shown that when older adults come to the hospital in severe shock, fatality rates can reach as high as 100%.[6–9] ■

A: Airway Stabilization and Compromise

Inspecting the airway has the highest priority in the care of the trauma patient because, although the airway might not appear to be the worst injury for a trauma patient, death will follow very quickly without an adequate airway. During assessment of the airway, the trauma team is searching for any signs of airway compromise. The healthcare provider needs to monitor for signs of impaired oxygenation such as bluish color to the skin, capillary refill greater than 3 seconds, and oxygen saturation below 95%. For a severely injured trauma patient with hypothermia (temperature less than 30°C), the pulse oximetry reading will not be reliable because little hemoglobin is available to transport the oxygen. In these patients, the healthcare provider must look for other signs of oxygenation.[10] If any signs of airway compromise are noted, the first step is to open and maintain the airway and provide adequate oxygenation.[11] The airway must be managed before moving on to breathing and the rest of the assessment.

Etiology and Pathogenesis

One of the life-threatening dangers in opening an airway is that the maneuver could cause an unstable cervical spine fracture to further injure the spinal cord. When a fracture to the bone is such that the layers of the bone are separated and the bone is in danger of becoming disrupted or separating, an unstable fracture exists. An in-line fracture, or stable fracture, is one that occurs within the bone structure and the bone remains strong and intact. Cervical vertebrae 3, 4, and 5 house the nerves in the spinal column that are responsible for normal respiration. If this area of the spinal cord is compromised, the patient will not be able to breathe. Therefore, cervical spine stability must be maintained constantly while the airway is inspected. For that reason, "A" represents airway *and* cervical spine immobilization as the highest priority in trauma care.[2,3,12,13]

The cranium is much larger in relation to the neck in infants than in adults. Therefore, there is a natural passive flexion of the cervical spinal column in infants. To prevent further flexion to the cervical spine, the healthcare provider must be cautious not to hyperextend the neck when opening the pediatric airway.[14] The pediatric trauma patient should be kept parallel to the backboard and should be placed in the "sniffing position" during airway control.[2] ■

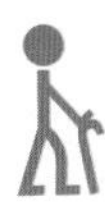

When attempting to intubate an older adult, the healthcare provider must determine whether the patient suffers from cervical stenosis or cervical osteoarthritis. If cervical disease is present, hyperextension of the neck to foster tracheal intubation could cause a serious cervical spine fracture and must not be attempted. Osteoarthritis and osteoporosis make the bones of the spine brittle, putting older adults at risk for vertebral fractures and resultant spinal cord injuries.[15] ■

Linking Pathophysiology to Diagnosis and Treatment

Airway obstruction, a blockage of the airway that prevents air from getting into the lungs, presents an imminent threat to life. The most common obstruction in the airway of a trauma patient is the tongue. If the hypoglossal or glossopharyngeal nerves are injured, the movement of the tongue is compromised, and the tongue often falls back into the oral pharynx and obstructs the larynx. Other causes of airway obstruction in trauma patients include (in order of frequency) blood, loose teeth, vomitus, and foreign objects. Multiple facial fractures, especially Le Fort type fractures (facial fractures that cause a separation of the facial bones), could cause either a complete or partial airway obstruction. To clear the airway, a jaw-thrust maneuver is recommended because this has been proven to cause the least manipulation to the cervical spine. The jaw-thrust maneuver is accomplished by placing the fingers of one hand under the mandible and gently lifting the mandible in an upward position while using the thumb on the other hand to gently push the lower lip downward to open the mouth (**Figure 51.3** ■).[10,11] If a patent airway cannot be established with the jaw-thrust maneuver, lift the chin and tilt the head just enough to establish air flow. This is known as the head-tilt/chin-lift maneuver and must be done very carefully, as it could worsen any spinal injury.

Any compromise to the airway must be immediately cleared, and if the patient cannot protect his or her own airway, then airway control must be obtained. If the patient answers in a clear, normal voice, the healthcare provider can assume that the airway is patent. However, any sign of vocal difficulties suggests a compromise to the vocal cords and may be a sign of airway compromise.[10,11]

If the patient is unable to sustain adequate ventilation, the easiest way to obtain control of the airway is by inserting a nasal or oral airway to assist with the manual airway maneuver. A nasal airway is best used for patients who are conscious; an oral airway is recommended for unconscious patients because it is very uncomfortable and often stimulates a gag response in conscious patients. If airway and breathing are both compromised, then immediate intubation and ventilatory support are required.[2,11,13]

According to the American College of Surgeons Committee on Trauma, the decision to intubate the trauma patient is based on the presence of one of the following clinical signs and symptoms[2]:

- Apnea
- Inability to maintain patent airway
- Need to protect the lower airway from aspiration of blood or vomitus
- Impending or potential compromise of the airway

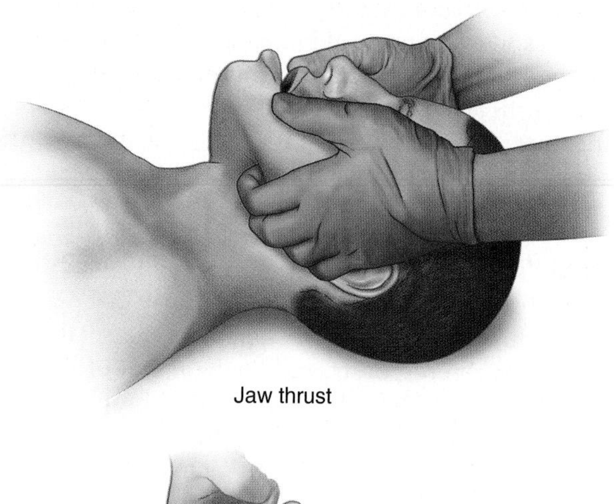

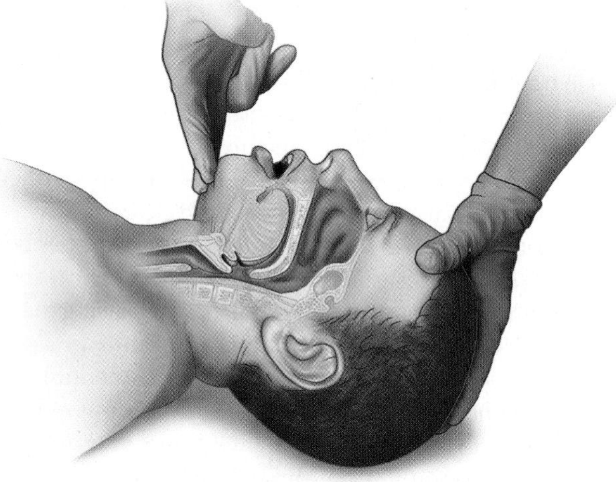

Figure 51.3 ■ The jaw-thrust maneuver and the Head-tilt/chin-lift maneuver are used to open the airway.

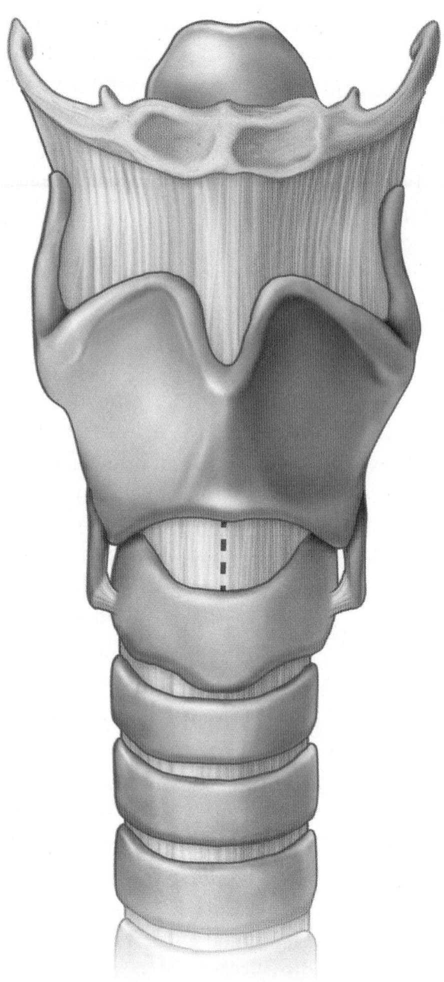

Figure 51.4 ■ A cricothyrotomy is an incision made through the skin and cricoid membrane to establish an airway.

- Presence of a closed head injury (GCS < 8) (See Table 51.1.)
- Inability to maintain adequate oxygenation by face mask oxygen supplementation.

The most successful technique for intubating a patient is by using a rapid sequence endotracheal intubation. Rapid sequence intubation consists of administering high-flow oxygen via a nonrebreather mask or bag-valve-mask. After the patient is pre-oxygenated, a sedative is administered intravenously followed by a paralytic agent (i.e., succinylcholine), at which time the patient can be intubated. If this technique is not successful, then manual ventilations must be immediately resumed. If the patient cannot be ventilated while paralyzed, a surgical airway must be rapidly obtained.[16]

A **cricothyroidotomy** is the most common procedure for obtaining a surgical airway. A cricothyroidotomy is performed by making an incision through the cricothyroid membrane and placing an endotracheal tube or cuffed tracheostomy tube through the cricothyroid membrane into the trachea (**Figure 51.4** ■).[2]

If an oral airway is not obtainable in the infant or child, a surgical airway, while not routinely recommended, can be used as a last resort. The cricothyroid membrane is slit just like that of an adult. However, very often, the cricothyroid membrane can be accessed with a 14 gauge or 16 gauge IV catheter in a pediatric trauma patient until a definitive airway can be obtained.[17,18] The patient may then be attached to a jet insufflator to provide ventilator support while further attempts to establish a definitive airway are made. ■

Once the patient is intubated, a carbon dioxide detector, also known as a colorimetric CO_2 monitoring device, should be attached to confirm that the endotracheal tube has been placed properly into the lung and not erroneously into the esophagus.[19]

CLINICAL POINT: If an airway is difficult to obtain, ventilating the patient with a bag-valve-mask will provide continuous oxygenation to the lungs and tissues unless there is a complete airway obstruction, which is rare. A supraglottic airway, such as a laryngeal mask airway, may also provide support until a more definitive airway can be established in patients without complete obstruction.[17] ■

Spinal Cord Injury

Spinal cord injuries are among the most devastating injuries in trauma patients. There are approximately 12,000 new spinal cord injuries in the United States each year.[16] Spinal cord injuries also carry a high mortality rate, often reaching 50%. The vast majority of these deaths are attributed to high-level spinal cord injuries.[20]

Etiology and Pathogenesis

Spinal cord injuries occur primarily as a result of five mechanisms:

- Flexion injuries
- Extension injuries
- Lateral extension injuries
- Axial loading injuries
- Penetrating injuries.[20–22]

A review of the anatomy and physiology of the spinal column is important to understand this very complicated injury.

Immediately after a spinal cord injury, a series of physical, chemical, and biochemical changes occur that result in an array of clinical manifestations. Once the spinal cord has been injured, there is an uncoupling of oxidative phosphorylation and a shift to anaerobic glycolysis.[21,23] As adenosine triphosphate (ATP) is depleted, the calcium-dependent ATPase, which is necessary to control intracellular levels of calcium, becomes inactivated. This results in a sharp increase in intracellular calcium, which causes calcium-dependent phospholipase A2 to be activated and arachidonic acid to be released. Once the arachidonic acid cascade has been stimulated, lipid peroxides, unsaturated fatty acids, and other free radicals accumulate in the cells and become toxic to cell membranes. The protein and phospholipid bilayers of the cells in the spinal cord are destroyed; free water, sodium, lactate, norepinephrine, dopamine, and histamine accumulate in the cell; and potassium becomes depleted. As cells in the spinal cord begin to die, further damage to the spinal cord results, causing secondary injury to the spinal cord and extending the degree of damage in an ascending pattern.[21–24]

Once the cord has been injured, the physiologic responses initiate an ascending pattern of injury up the spinal column, resulting in further injury. For this reason, patients with spinal cord injury must be closely monitored for further ascending deterioration of the spinal cord.[20,22]

CLINICAL POINT: Because edema will progress in an upward fashion throughout the spinal column, a patient who came in with a C7 injury could rapidly progress to a high cervical spine injury as the secondary cord injury ascends the spinal canal. Because C3, C4, and C5 are involved in respiration, monitoring the peak airway flow of the patient will be a good indicator as to the progression of respiratory weakness, indicating the progression of the spinal injury. ■

Clinical Manifestations

Clinical manifestations of spinal cord injury depend on the location of the injury and the degree of injury. With a complete spinal cord injury, the spinal vertebrae completely crush or lacerate the spinal cord, and all motor and sensory function below the level of the spinal cord injury is lost. As the descending autonomic pathways become injured, spinal shock ensues. **Spinal shock** is the temporary loss of all or most spinal reflex activity below the level of the injury. Other injuries of the spinal cord result in "incomplete" cord injuries and are related to the specific region of the cord injured. Whether the cord lesions are complete or partial (incomplete) cannot be determined until spinal shock has resolved.[21–24]

The spinal column consists of an anterior, a middle, and a posterior column (**Figure 51.5** ■). The middle and

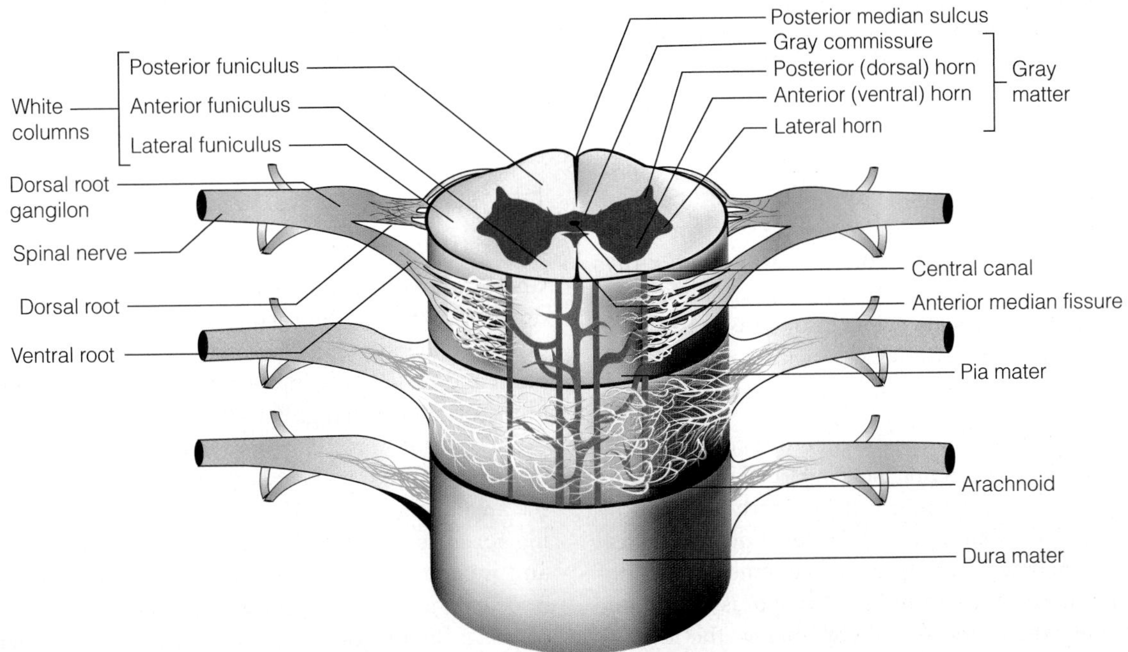

Figure 51.5 ■ The structure of the spinal cord.

posterior columns are most instrumental in maintaining spinal cord stability. It is usually injuries to the posterior column that result in devastating neuromuscular deficits because of the close proximity of the nerve bundles in the posterior spinal column.[21–24]

Anterior Cord Syndrome. **Anterior cord syndrome** results from damage to the corticospinal and spinothalamic pathways, although there is preservation of the posterior column. Patients will present with a loss of motor function, pain, and temperature sensation distal to the lesion with a preservation of vibration, crude touch, and position. Anterior cord syndrome typically occurs as a result of a flexion injury or direct injury to the anterior spinal column.[21–25]

Central Cord Syndrome. **Central cord syndrome** usually occurs when there is damage to the central portion of the cord and less injury to the peripheral cord. Typically, this occurs as a result of a hyperextension injury in older patients who have preexisting cervical spondylosis. Patients typically have decreased strength, pain, and temperature sensation to the upper extremities with a lesser degree of involvement in the lower extremities.[21–25]

Brown-Séquard Syndrome. **Brown-Séquard syndrome** typically occurs from a direct penetrating injury to the cord that causes a hemisection of the spinal cord. This lesion causes ipsilateral loss of motor function, proprioception, and vibratory sensation, as well as contralateral loss of pain and temperature.[21–25]

Jefferson Fracture. A **Jefferson fracture** indicates a fracture of C1 which involves both the anterior and posterior arches results from axial loading onto the spinal column. This is usually a stable fracture. Dislocations involving C1 on C2 are also rare. A more common cervical spine fracture is that seen with high-speed head-on motor vehicle crashes with rapid cervical hyperextension. This typically consists of fractures of C2 and C3 with soft tissue swelling, and the spinal cord is usually intact.[20] Any injury to the spinal column must be carefully examined radiologically before a spinal cord fracture can be ruled out. It is also very important that the cervical spine is palpated for any pain and obvious abnormalities or irregular bone formations found around bony prominences that will indicate the presence of a bony fracture. Criteria that indicate that cervical spine x-rays may not be warranted include absence of posterior midline cervical spine tenderness, no evidence of intoxication, alert mental status, no focal neurologic deficits, and no painful distracting injuries.[26]

Spinal Shock. One of the most dangerous complications of spinal cord injuries is spinal shock. Spinal shock occurs when there is an interruption of sympathetic outflow pathways after a spinal injury at the level of the cervical or thoracic vertebrae. There is loss of visceral and peripheral autonomic control and uninhibited parasympathetic impulses. Reflexes in the spinal cord below the level of transection are depressed, while reflexes in the cranial part remain intact. A loss of alpha-adrenergic tone and dilation of the arterial and venous vessels cause hypotension. Lack of sympathetic innervation to the myocardium results in a paradoxical bradycardia with loss of cutaneous vasoconstriction and of bladder control.

Linking Pathophysiology to Diagnosis and Treatment

Recommended therapies include fluid bolus, vasopressor administration, and atropine if bradycardia continues.[21–23] Continued monitoring is necessary, as the trauma patient with suspected spinal shock may be suffering from hypovolemia from traumatic bleeding, which can lead to hypovolemic shock.

The secondary injury that occurs as a result of spinal cord injury can be as devastating to the viability of the spinal cord as the initial injury. Ischemia, inflammation, and cellular necrosis result from the secondary injury cascade that occurs after the initial insult to the spinal cord.

In comparison to adults, infants and children have a much larger head in proportion to the body, and their spine has increased ligamentous laxity and differently shaped facets, making it more susceptible to cervical injuries. Because of the laxity to the ligaments in the cervical spine, it is possible for an infant to have a spinal cord injury without radiologic abnormality because the pediatric vertebral column is vulnerable to deformation without fracture. Children below the age of 8 years are most at risk for this injury.[2,20,22,23] ■

Judi Stone: Application

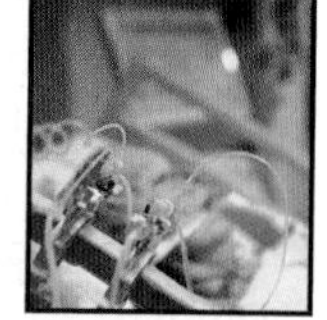

On admission to the ED, Ms. Stone is placed on a ventilator and given 100% oxygen while her primary survey is completed. Her vital signs on admission to the ED are as follows: pulse 118, respirations rate 8, blood pressure 148/88. Her GCS score is 3T (she was pharmacologically paralyzed and sedated en route to the ED). Laboratory studies and CT scans of her head, cervical spine, chest, abdomen, and pelvis are ordered.

3. What is the status of Ms. Stone's ABCDs?
4. What is the focus of the trauma team's efforts at this point?

B: Breathing—Chest Trauma and Respiratory Status

Chest trauma accounts for approximately 25% of all trauma deaths[27–29] and is the second leading cause of traumatic deaths, following head injuries. Chest injuries can result from blunt and penetrating injuries; however, blunt chest injuries are associated with higher morbidity and mortality rates.

The correct procedure for identifying all life-threatening injuries is to first inspect and then auscultate and palpate the area being examined. Breathing is assessed by examining for a rise and fall of the chest, pink color to the skin and mucous membranes, good capillary refill (less than 3 seconds in adults), and normal oxygen saturation (SaO_2 of 95%). Breath sounds are evaluated for symmetry, fullness, and respiratory effort. Any abnormal signs must be addressed quickly, and high-flow oxygen should be delivered to all trauma patients. If there is any sign of abnormal breathing or diminished oxygenation, the trauma patient must be examined for the presence of life-threatening chest injuries that would compromise breathing. The first step is to determine whether the injury is a result of penetrating or blunt chest trauma.[2,10,28]

Etiology and Pathogenesis

Three populations of trauma patients may demonstrate breathing patterns and oxygen values different from those of other populations: pediatric, pregnant, and older adult patients.

Infants have varied breathing patterns, and it is common to find irregular rate and depth of breathing among infants. Unlike adults, infants are diaphragmatic breathers; therefore, any compromise to the infant's abdomen may result in difficulty breathing. Because children's bones are more pliable, pediatric patients are more likely to suffer from blunt lung injuries without bony abnormalities usually found in the adult population.[15,27,29] ■

In pregnant women, breathing patterns differ as the pregnancy progresses. As the uterus expands, the diaphragm becomes elevated, and the woman's normal tidal volume increases by as much as 40% with a decrease in residual volume by approximately 25%. The functional residual capacity of the pregnant woman also decreases, and the woman compromises by increasing the respiratory rate. Because the respiratory rate is increased, the woman tends to hyperventilate, resulting in a higher pH (respiratory alkalosis). The kidneys will compensate for the respiratory alkalosis to maintain a normal serum pH.[30–32] ■

Older adults experiencing trauma are more susceptible to the development of hypoxia resulting from diminished reserve capacity in the lungs. Older adults have less pliable lung tissue, and this diminished elasticity results in a reduction in pulmonary compliance and diminishes their ability to compensate for invading organisms. They also experience changes in the total surface area of the lung as alveoli and small airways reduce in mass with age.[5,33] It is not unusual to find a PaO_2 of 80 mmHg as a normal value among older adult trauma patients.[34] ■

When penetrating trauma invades the pleura, a pneumothorax or hemothorax is likely to occur from the laceration of parenchymal tissue and the disruption of the negative pressure in the thoracic cavity allowing an escape of air into the thorax (**Figure 51.6** ■). A **hemothorax** is a type of pleural effusion in which blood accumulates in the pleural cavity (see Figure 51.6A). A **pneumothorax** is a collapsed lung that occurs when air leaks into the space between the lung and chest wall. Both conditions cause the lungs, heart, and great vessels to be compressed if not released. The vast majority of these patients can be managed with a chest tube decompression of the thoracic cavity, and fewer than 20% of these patients will require surgery.[2,27,29,35]

CLINICAL POINT: When caring for a patient with penetrating chest trauma, it is important for the healthcare provider *not* to remove the penetrating object. Once the patient has been evaluated, the surgeon must decide whether the object is penetrating major organs such as the heart, lungs, and diaphragm. If any of these organs have been penetrated, the object must be removed in the operating room in a controlled environment where surgeons can carefully remove the object and stop any bleeding and repair tissue damage. ■

In caring for a pregnant woman with a penetrating chest trauma, consideration must be given to the displacement of the diaphragm. Because the diaphragm of the pregnant woman is elevated, if the pregnant trauma patient should need a thorocostomy tube or open thorocostomy, the healthcare provider must remember that the diaphragm may be elevated as much as 4 centimeters from its nongravid position.[30–32] ■

Blunt chest trauma, by contrast, usually entails a series of injuries resulting from a powerful force to the thorax.

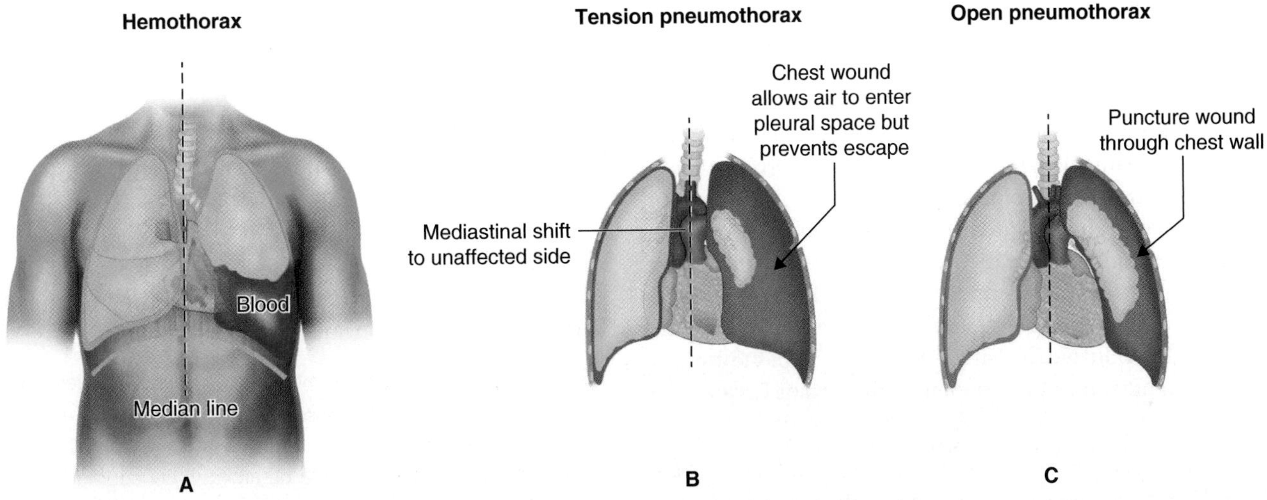

Figure 51.6 ■ Types of hemothorax and pneumothorax: **A.** Hemothorax. **B.** Tension pneumothorax. **C.** Open pneumothorax.

Blunt chest trauma can result in rupture injuries to the lungs, myocardium, and vessels; direct trauma injuries to the lungs, myocardium, ribs, blood vessels, muscles, and tissues; or soft tissue injuries. The severity of the injury will predict the course of hospitalization and clinical outcomes for these patients.[29]

Clinical Manifestations and Treatment

Tension Pneumothorax. A **tension pneumothorax** occurs when the pleural space becomes disrupted and the negative pressure in the pleural cavity is broken, allowing atmospheric air to enter the pleural space, where it becomes trapped and compresses the adjacent lung tissue (see Figure 51.6B). If the air is allowed to continue entering the pleural space, the pleura will soon fill with air pressure, displacing the great vessels and compressing the myocardium, resulting in hypoxemia and diminished cardiac output. Without prompt intervention, cardiac arrest will occur. Clinical signs of a tension pneumothorax include dyspnea, hypoperfusion, distended neck veins, diminished or absent breath sounds on the affected side, a hyperresonant percussion note on the affected side due to the entrapment of air, and tracheal deviation to the opposite side. Hyperexpansion of the chest wall may also be noted on the affected side. Intervention involves rapidly inserting a small cannula (typically a 3-inch-long 14 gauge IV catheter) through the chest wall into the pleural space at the second intercostal space at the midclavicular line to convert the tension pneumothorax to an open pneumothorax, immediately relieving the compression of the heart and great vessels. As soon as the initial survey has been completed, a chest tube must be inserted on the side of the tension pneumothorax before the first x-ray is taken.[2,27,28,36]

Open Pneumothorax. When there is a penetrating trauma to the outer chest wall that causes a temporary invasion of the pleural space, an **open pneumothorax** occurs (Figure 51.6C). If the opening to the chest wall is more than two thirds the size of the trachea, air will preferentially flow through the defect in the chest wall and compromise oxygenation.[10,36] This opening into the pleural space causes respiratory distress because the patient is unable to ventilate the affected side of the lung. As air moves from the outside into the pleural space, a "sucking" sound occurs, which is why an open pneumothorax is often called a "sucking chest wound." Definitive treatment will require a chest tube thoracotomy; however, a traditional emergency treatment is application of an occlusive dressing that is taped to the chest on three sides, allowing air to escape from one side of the dressing. This will stop the air leak and prevent air from entering the thoracic cage and expanding to a tension pneumothorax. If a three-sided occlusive dressing is used to control the air leak, careful monitoring of the patient is important because the covered wound could trap air inside the pleura and result in a tension pneumothorax.[2,28,29,36]

Flail Chest. Another common chest injury is a **flail chest** (**Figure 51.7** ■), which occurs when a segment of the rib cage breaks as a result of trauma and becomes detached from the rest of the thorax. The free-floating segments of rib cause a ventilation–perfusion mismatch and can result in severe pain and respiratory distress. A paradoxical chest wall movement or uneven movement of the chest wall with respiration is noted upon physical examination, and jugular venous distention may be evident on the affected side. Breaths sounds are diminished on the affected side. Respiratory failure that is associated with flail chest is treated with intubation, mechanical ventilation, and pain control.[27–29]

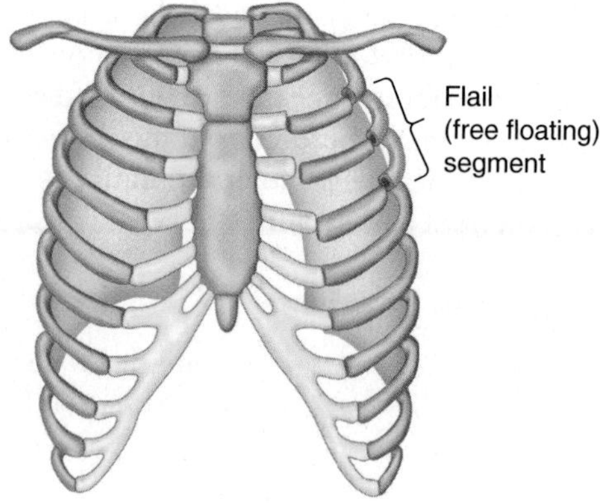

A Fracture pattern of flail chest

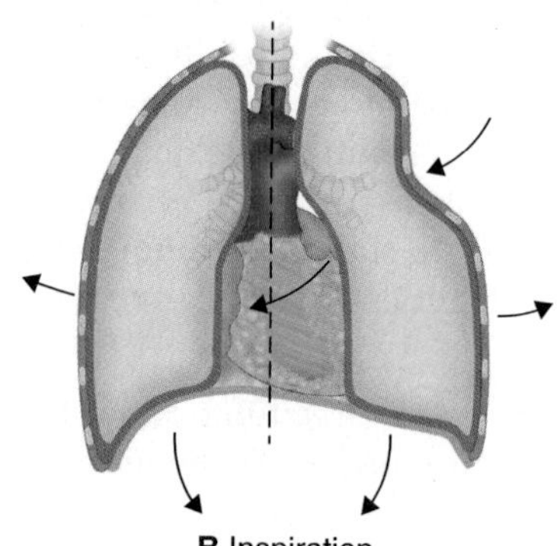

B Inspiration

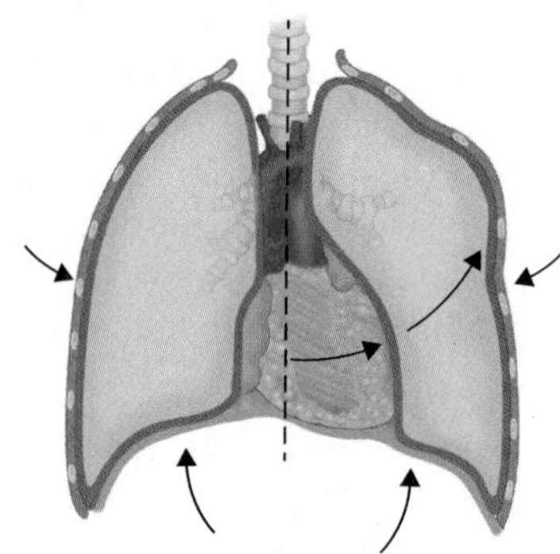

C Expiration

Figure 51.7 ■ Flail chest with paradoxical chest wall movement.

CLINICAL POINT: A patient with a flail chest should receive aggressive pain control because this very painful condition can lead to hypoventilation as the patient attempts to self-splint the injury. The goal of treatment is to facilitate breathing by encouraging frequent pulmonary exercises, such as incentive spirometry. Because breathing causes severe pain for these patients, pain control takes high priority.[27] ■

Other chest injuries that may be noted during the primary survey include rib fractures, lung injury, and soft tissue injuries. Some life-threatening injuries, though originating in the chest, result in circulatory compromise and are discussed in the next section.

Lung injury may be severe enough to require intubation and mechanical ventilation. The healthcare provider should be quick to intubate the severely injured trauma patient. Indications for ventilatory support include a respiratory rate greater than 30–35 breaths per minute, a vital capacity of less than 10–15 mL/kg, and/or a negative inspiratory force of less than 25–30 cm H_2O.[11,27,28]

C: Circulation—Bleeding and Shock

Etiology and Pathogenesis

When there is sufficient injury to the vessels and organs to cause bleeding that compromises perfusion and oxygenation to tissues, the patient is at risk for developing hypovolemic shock. If a trauma patient arrives in the ED with signs of circulatory shock (e.g., unstable vital signs, altered level of consciousness, and pale, cool, or diaphoretic skin), the healthcare provider must consider the strong possibility that the patient has undiscovered, uncontrolled bleeding. If the patient continues to bleed and hypovolemic shock progresses without immediate intervention, the results can be devastating. When patients progress from class I shock (approximately 15% blood loss) to class IV shock (about 40% blood loss), it is considered unsurvivable. Although patients in class IV shock might not die immediately, the damage to the cells, organs, and tissues result in secondary trauma. This secondary injury often results in death from multiple organ failure days to weeks after the original trauma. (See Chapter 28 for a complete discussion of the cellular and systemic changes that occur as a result of hypovolemic shock.) For this reason, the trauma team's first priority is to identify the source of uncontrolled bleeding and stop the bleeding while at the same time supporting the patient's compensatory mechanisms in combating and preventing irreversible shock.[2,36–38] Because bleeding in the pericardial, pleural, or pericardial space might not be easily identifiable, use of a FAST exam (Focused Assessment with Sonography for Trauma) in the field or at the bedside may help the healthcare provider to determine the presence of internal bleeding.

As the circulation is being assessed, all signs of external bleeding must be stopped. In addition, radial, carotid, and femoral pulses are assessed, and the blood pressure is noted. Heart tones are assessed to determine whether the heart is compromised in any way, such as by cardiac tamponade. Intravenous lines are initiated; usually, a large-bore IV catheter is used so that large volumes of fluid and blood can be infused over a short period of time, and blood is sent to the lab for analysis. Hypovolemia is treated with infusions of warm crystalloids; a 2-liter bolus is the usual volume initiated. A determination must be made about transfusion of matched or unmatched blood.[2]

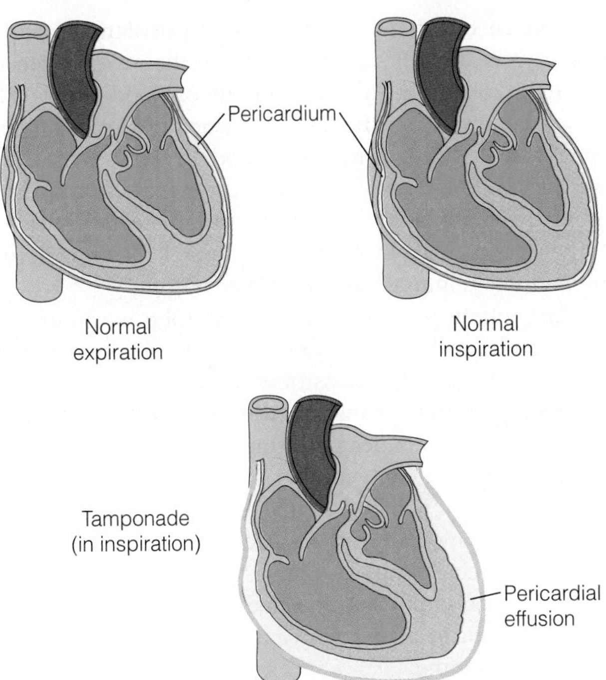

Figure 51.8 ■ In pericardial tamponade, fluid in the pericardial sac prevents the heart from fully expanding or contracting, reducing cardiac output.

Clinical Manifestations and Treatment

Pericardial Tamponade (Cardiac Tamponade). Any type of trauma that causes blood to accumulate in the pericardial sac will cause a pericardial tamponade (**Figure 51.8** ■). As the pericardial sac fills with blood, the heart is unable to fully expand or contract; this dramatically reduces the cardiac output until compensatory mechanisms are no longer able to sustain life, at which time a cardiac arrest will ensue. Signs and symptoms of a pericardial tamponade, known as Beck's triad, include hypotension, distended neck veins, and muffled heart tones. These symptoms are similar to a tension pneumothorax except that breath sounds are usually clear with a cardiac tamponade. If there is any doubt that a pericardial tamponade exists, a bedside ultrasound will reveal fluid in the pericardial sac if present. If nothing is done to relieve the pressure in the pericardial sac, death will follow the cardiac arrest.[27,35,38]

The initial treatment of a pericardial tamponade is an emergency pericardiocentesis, during which a needle inserted into the pericardial sac drains the blood and fluid, relieving pressure. Once the pericardial sac has been drained, signs and symptoms should resolve at once. Immediately after the bedside emergency pericardiocentesis, preparations must be made to bring the patient to the operating room for a definitive pericardial window procedure.[2,27,38]

Massive Hemothorax. If the lung or the vessels supplying oxygen and nutrients to the lung are injured, large amounts of blood can accumulate in the thorax. The thorax can hold approximately 50% of the circulating blood volume. A massive hemothorax for an adult is defined as a 1500-mL blood loss and is a life-threatening condition as a result of three separate mechanisms. First, acute hypovolemia occurs, causing a reduction in preload due to the massive bleed. This hypovolemia reduces the amount of blood returned to the left ventricle, causing a rapid reduction in cardiac output. Second, as the accumulated blood compresses the lung, and the lung collapses, causing acute hypoxia and shortness of breath. Finally, as blood and air accumulate in the thorax, the heart and great vessels are compressed, resulting in further reduction in preload and cardiac output.[27,35,36,38]

Immediate placement of a chest tube is required if the hemothorax becomes life-threatening. The patient will require a surgical thoracostomy as soon as he or she is stable enough to be transported to the operating room.[27] Emergent thoracotomies performed in the ED have a very low survival rate.[39] A hemothorax is considered nonemergent when there is blood drainage of less than 100 mL/h for 6 hours or more, or if there is less than 600 mL of initial drainage. If rebleeding or ongoing bleeding occurs, a surgical thoracotomy may be indicated, although conservative management can often resolve the injury with a bedside tube thorocostomy.[2,27,35]

Aortic Dissection. Traumatic rupture of the thoracic aorta is highly associated with immediate death. The most common mechanism of injury causing a tear to the thoracic aorta results from the shearing force of an acceleration–deceleration injury. During an acceleration–deceleration injury the aortic isthmus is torn from its attachment at the aortic arch and the descending aorta. When this tear occurs, the layers of the aorta are torn away. The aorta has three layers; the innermost layer is the intima, the media lies next to the intima, and the adventitia is the least elastic outer layer. If all three layers are torn, blood leaks from the great vessel, causing rapid and severe blood loss. Death ensues within minutes. A less severe injury to the thoracic aorta occurs when not all layers of the vessel are torn. Patients who typically survive a thoracic aortic injury generally have preserved the integrity of the adventitia layer of the artery or have formed a perivascular hematoma around the injury site and make it to the ED in very fragile condition. If these injuries are not discovered quickly, the patient will die in the ED. Clinical signs and symptoms of a thoracic aorta disruption include chest pain, midscapular back pain, and shortness of breath. Stridor, hoarseness, and dysphagia may be present as a result of compression of the laryngeal nerve and esophagus. Generalized hypertension may occur as a result of the stimulation of aortic stretch receptors that result in compensatory hypertension. A harsh systolic murmur may be heard over the precordium, and precordial ecchymosis may be present. A chest x-ray will typically demonstrate a widened mediastinum, a shift of the trachea to the right, a downward shift of the left mainstem bronchus, and an obliteration of the aortic arch. If a confirming CT scan is positive, an immediate life-saving surgical procedure is necessary.[2,27,38]

Peritoneal Bleeding. Ruptured vessels and organs in the abdominal region (a **peritoneal bleed**) can result in massive blood loss and death. For this reason, any patient that presents in hypovolemic shock must have a thorough assessment of the abdomen. A bedside ultrasound is currently the gold standard to evaluate for intra-abdominal bleeding. Any signs of active bleeding into the peritoneal space, such as positive peritoneal tenderness to palpation, an observable intra-abdominal mass, or an observable pulsatile mass along with unstable vital signs, requires the surgeon to immediately take the patient to the operating room to tamponade or control the bleeding and restore adequate perfusion. Bleeding into the retroperitoneum, such as the kidneys, will not be demonstrated by positive peritoneal signs and can be deceiving to the healthcare provider.

Damage control surgery is a resuscitative measure that is used when a patient is determined to have severe life-threatening, intra-abdominal hemorrhage requiring immediate surgical intervention. Damage control surgery enables the surgeon to open the abdomen to quickly tamponade bleeding by packing the wound and then send the patient back to the ICU for continued resuscitation. The surgery is completed when the patient is more stable and able to tolerate a longer operative procedure.[3,38] IV resuscitation with crystalloids or blood while the patient is waiting for surgery facilitates perfusion.[2,36,40] Trauma patients who suffer penetrating chest injuries with concomitant hypovolemic shock are likely to have intrathoracic injuries such as injuries to the lung, heart, or great vessels or injuries to intercostals or intermammary arteries. Blunt chest injuries associated with hypovolemic shock include pelvic or extremity fractures, intra-abdominal injuries, and intrathoracic bleeding.

CLINICAL POINT: If any signs of external bleeding are found, proximal pressure is applied prior to placement of a tourniquet to stop the bleeding. ■

An increased heart rate is the most important early indication of hypovolemia in infants and children. This increase in heart rate can maintain adequate circulatory volume until the blood and fluid loss exceeds 45%. For this reason, blood pressure is a poor sign of hypovolemia in the pediatric population. ■

The myocardium stiffens with age, causing a decrease in cardiac output with each contraction. An 80-year-old patient will normally have about 50% of the cardiac output of a healthy 20-year-old patient. Therefore, when there is a circulatory compromise, the older adult is unable to compensate quickly for low blood volume. Given the significant presence of hypertension among older adults, an older patient with a normal heart rate and normal blood pressure may indeed be in hypovolemic shock. A decrease from the baseline blood pressure of the older adult patient may serve as a sensitive indicator of hypotension leading to shock that may be easily missed.[7] ■

Pregnant women may experience up to 45% increase in blood volume throughout their pregnancy. In addition, the normal heart rate during pregnancy increases by approximately 10–20 beats, and the systolic and diastolic pressure decreases by about 10–15 mmHg. The cardiac output also increases by 1.0–1.5 L/min during pregnancy. This hyperdynamic and hypervolemic state may be misleading for the healthcare provider. A pregnant woman may lose up to 35% of her blood volume before signs of shock are apparent.[30,31] ■

Judi Stone: Application

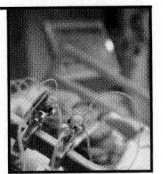

The trauma team continues to evaluate the Ms. Stone, focusing on her chest. The chest rises and falls equally. Lung sounds are significantly decreased over the injured side when compared to the opposite side. Palpating the chest wall reveals no obvious crepitus. Percussing the chest results in normal resonance. The subcutaneous air pockets first reported by the paramedics have not changed. Neck veins are nondistended. Ms. Stone's pulse is full, equal, and regular. Her heart sounds are normal. Skin color is pink, skin is dry, and capillary refill is less than 3 seconds. There are no obvious signs of internal bleeding. On the basis of these findings, no circulatory compromise is immediately found. Two large-bore IVs are started in Ms. Stone's right and left antecubital area, and blood is sent for analysis, including a type and cross-match.

5. According to these findings, which chest injuries can be effectively ruled out?
6. Which intervention might the trauma team be considering performing?

D—Disability: Neurologic Assessment

A rapid neurologic assessment is performed as part of the primary survey. The GCS (see Table 51.1) is used throughout the United States as a means to quickly evaluate patients with suspected head injuries and determine what level of trauma care they will require. It is important to note that this is only one aspect of the neurologic exam and is meant to be used as a quick indicator of gross brain injury. **Traumatic brain injury (TBI)** is the disruption of normal brain function caused by a bump, blow, jolt, or penetrating injury to the head.

The GCS is based on an assessment of three factors: eye opening, motor response, and verbal response. The GCS score has a range of 3 (severe deficit in each category) to 15 (normal neurologic exam). Patients who come to the ED with a GCS score less than 15 and an appropriate mechanism of injury are assumed to have a head injury until proven otherwise. For nonintubated, nonsedated patients, GCS scores indicate the following:

- **Severe TBI:** GCS score below 9
- **Moderate TBI:** GCS score from 9 to 13
- **Mild TBI:** GCS score from 14 to 15.[41]

Neurologic deficit can result from any number of etiologies. This section focuses on head trauma and issues related to perfusion to the brain.

Etiology and Pathogenesis

Head trauma is very commonly seen and treated in emergency departments and is responsible for about 33% of all injuries.[42] About 10% of trauma patients with head injury (HI) die before reaching the hospital. Of those who reach the hospital, approximately 80% will have a mild HI, 10% will have a moderate HI, and the remaining 10% have a severe HI. HI may cause TBI, which usually occurs from a blow to the head causing either blunt or penetrating trauma to the brain. The peak incidence of TBI is among males between ages 15 and 24, although intoxicated individuals, older adults, and children are also at high risk for TBI as a result of social and physiologic factors.[2,43]

As in adults, HI accounts for the majority of trauma deaths among the pediatric population. Because infants' and children's heads are larger in proportion to the rest of their body than is the case for adults, the head is the most likely part of the child's anatomy to be injured. For infants, the most common cause of HI is from a fall; for children, the most common cause of HI is child abuse. Child abuse should always be a consideration in caring for a pediatric patient with a HI that does not fit the parent's or caregiver's description of the incident.[2,42,44,45] ■

Acute brain injury is categorized into two phases: primary and secondary. Primary brain injury occurs when the brain is initially injured on impact, usually by blunt or penetrating trauma. The resulting damage to the brain tissues and structures is known as the primary injury. Secondary brain injury occurs as the injured brain cells begin to swell and reduce the available blood supply to the cells, robbing vital brain cells of life-saving oxygen, causing secondary cellular brain death.[46,47]

Although the brain accounts for only about 2% of total body weight, it consumes approximately 20% of the body's total oxygen and 15% of total cardiac output.[42,46] Because the brain has high oxygen consumption, when brain perfusion is compromised, brain cells die rapidly. For this reason, blood perfusion to the brain, commonly known as **cerebral perfusion pressure (CPP)**, must be maintained if secondary brain injury is to be prevented. Many factors determine CPP; two of these are the **intracranial pressure (ICP)** (pressure within the brain) and the **mean arterial pressure (MAP)** (pressure within the cardiovascular system). To understand these pressure variations in the brain, an understanding of the Monro-Kellie hypothesis is paramount.

The **Monro-Kellie hypothesis** states that the total volume of the intracranial contents remains constant. Because the cranial vault is composed of hard fused bones, the cranial vault is a closed system. Inside this vault lie three major components: brain mass, intracerebral spinal fluid, and blood volume. For homeostasis to be maintained within the brain, all three components must be adequately perfused with oxygen-rich blood, and stable pressures must exist within the cranial vault. If any of the contents of the cranial vault swell or diminish, pressures in the other two components will change to compensate. The three major pressure systems in the brain are the ICP, the CPP, and the

MAP. To understand the concept of secondary brain injury, an understanding of the three pressure systems is necessary.

Intracranial pressure represents the pressure measured inside the cranial vault. If the ICP rises, the brain mass and blood flow will diminish. On the other hand, if the brain mass swells, the ICP will also rise, and cerebral blood flow and cerebral perfusion to the cells will diminish. Adequate perfusion to the brain cells must be maintained to avoid brain cell death. Therefore, the CPP must be preserved if secondary brain injury is to be prevented.[2,42,48]

Normal ICP in adults is less than 15 mmHg. When ICP rises above 15 mmHg, undue pressure is placed on the blood vessels that perfuse the brain, causing blood flow to be diminished. Therefore, when ICP rises, CPP falls. When CPP falls, blood flow to the brain cells is diminished, and cell death ensues.[2,42,48]

CPP is described as the difference between blood flowing into the brain and blood flowing out of the brain, which is responsible for the cerebral blood flow. CPP can be calculated by taking the mean arterial pressure minus the intracranial pressure (MAP – ICP). The recommendation is that the CPP should be at a level of 60–70 mmHg to maintain cerebral cellular oxygenation.[2,42,48]

CLINICAL POINT: To calculate MAP, use this formula:

$$\text{MAP} = \text{diastolic BP} + \frac{\text{systolic BP} - \text{diastolic BP}}{3}.$$ ■

If cerebral perfusion is compromised immediately after a primary head injury, brain cells begin to decompensate very quickly. Immediately after an acute brain injury, ATP production is decreased, resulting in a depletion of cellular energy. Once the cellular energy stores are exhausted, normal cellular metabolism is compromised, and the cells go into a crisis state. As a result, there is an influx of sodium and water that leads to cellular edema, cellular acidosis, and an influx of calcium. Cell death ensues. When the brain cells are reperfused, cellular damage is accelerated, resulting in a reperfusion injury. Oxygen free radicals produce oxidative stress, causing further damage to the already compromised brain cells. When cells begin to die, the body naturally releases cytokines to the area of damage. As the release of cytokines accelerates, there is also a migration of neutrophils, monocytes, and macrophages to the injury site, causing further edema, decreasing CPP, and accelerating secondary brain injury. For this reason, the primary treatment to prevent secondary brain injury among trauma patients remains prevention of increased ICP, preservation of CPP, and prevention of ischemia and hypoxia.[2,6,42,43,45–49]

Aggressive fluid resuscitation may be necessary to prevent hypotension. MAP should be maintained above 90 mmHg (systolic BP of approximately 120–140 mmHg) to achieve adequate brain perfusion along with adequate oxygenation and blood volume.[2,42,43,48]

CLINICAL POINT: In cases of increased ICP, it may be necessary to induce a hypervolemic and hypertensive state to normalize the CPP in an effort to prevent secondary brain injury. ■

Clinical Manifestations

The spectrum of TBI ranges from mild to severe. Mild TBI includes any trauma patient who reports a loss of consciousness, amnesia or loss of memory to the event, any change in mental status at the time of the event, and/or persistent or transient focal neurologic deficit, such as weakness to one side of the body. A GCS score of 13–15 would fall into the classification of mild TBI.[2,42,48]

Moderate TBI encompasses patients with a GCS score of 9–12 and accounts for about 10% of all TBI. Although mortality rates for these patients are very low, long-term disabilities among this group can be as high as 50%.[42,43]

Patients diagnosed with severe TBI have a GCS score less than 9. Mortality rates among this group are as high as 40%, and fewer than 10% of these patients will make even a moderate recovery.[42,43]

Linking Pathophysiology to Diagnosis and Treatment

The three cornerstones in treating patients with TBI include identification of other life-threatening injuries, prevention of further secondary brain injury, and identifying treatable mass lesions.[42,43,48] Observing for signs and symptoms of increasing ICP and decreasing CPP is important in the initial resuscitation phase, and the healthcare provider must be aware of these symptoms because invasive monitoring is rare in the initial resuscitation phase. The Brain Trauma Foundation in conjunction with the American Association of Neurological Surgeons has established guidelines for the management of TBI.[50] The guidelines indicate that monitoring of intracranial pressure is needed for patients with a severe TBI (as evidenced by a postresuscitation GCS score of 3–8) and an abnormal CT scan and patients with severe TBI whose CT scans are normal but who have at least two of the following: unilateral or bilateral motor posturing, systolic BP less than 90 mmHg, or age older than 40 years. Treatment recommendations direct healthcare providers to ensure that the patient maintains a systolic BP greater than 90 mmHg and an oxygen saturation greater than 90%.

Skull Fractures. All patients with suspected skull fractures must have a CT of the head to determine whether there are underlying injuries. There are three basic types of skull fractures: linear, comminuted, and basilar skull fractures (**Figure 51.9** ■).

Linear and comminuted fractures are isolated fractures involving a break in the skull that either follows a straight line or involves multiple fractures in the same area. These fractures may be involved with lacerations or may be closed. Each fracture must be evaluated independently. If the fractures are stable, they may be treated with pain medication and serial CT scans to ensure that there are no resultant hematomas. If the fracture is unstable, surgery may be indicated.[42]

Basilar skull fractures often involve a fracture into the temporal bone, which houses the external auditory canal and the tympanic membrane.[42] This type of fracture is commonly associated with a torn dura, leading to CSF leakage from the ear. Signs and symptoms associated with a basilar skull fracture include CSF otorrhea or rhinorrhea, mastoid ecchymosis (Battle sign), periorbital ecchymosis (raccoon

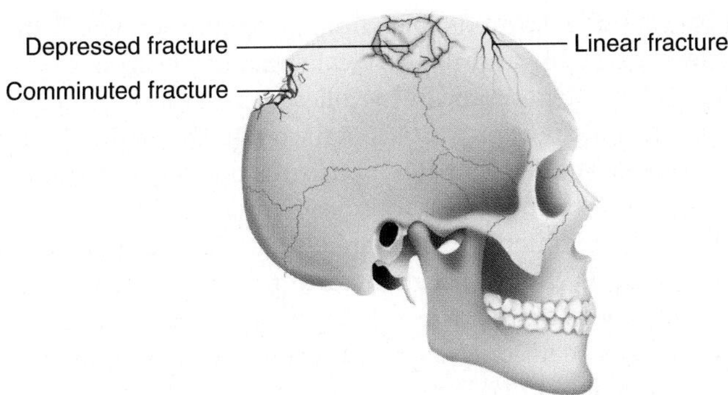

Figure 51.9 ■ Types of skull fractures include depressed, comminuted, and linear.

eyes), hemotympanum (blood in the tympanic cavity of the middle ear), vertigo and decreased hearing or deafness, and damage the cranial nerve VII resulting in seventh nerve palsy (also called Bell palsy), which causes paralysis of the muscles on one side of the face.[42,51]

Brain Herniation. There are four major types of brain herniation: uncal transtentorial, central transtentorial, cerebellotonsillar, and upward posterior fossa. These herniations occur when the swelling in the brain causes such severe pressure that brain tissues press on the fossa in the brain, causing the brain to extend outside its normal boundary and herniate, usually in a downward fashion. Because the skull is fixed at the superior aspect of the brain and prevents the brain from moving upward, the brain has only one place to expand: inferiorly toward the foramen magnum. Of these four types of brain herniations, the most common is the uncal transtentorial herniation, which leads to a compression of the third cranial nerve (oculomotor), causing an ipsilateral fixed and dilated pupil. As the herniation progresses, the pyramidal tract is compressed, leading to contralateral motor paralysis.[42,43,51]

Central transtentorial herniation causes bilateral pinpoint pupils, bilateral Babinski sign, and increased muscle tone. As the herniation continues, fixed midpoint pupils are followed by hyperventilation and decorticate posturing (**Figure 51.10** ■).

Cerebellotonsilar herniation occurs when the cerebellar tonsils herniate through the foramen magnum, causing pinpoint pupils, flaccid paralysis, and sudden death. The fourth type of brain herniation, upward posterior fossa herniation, occurs from a posterior fossa lesion and results in a conjugate downward gaze with absence of vertical eye movements, pinpoint pupils, and rapid death.[51,52]

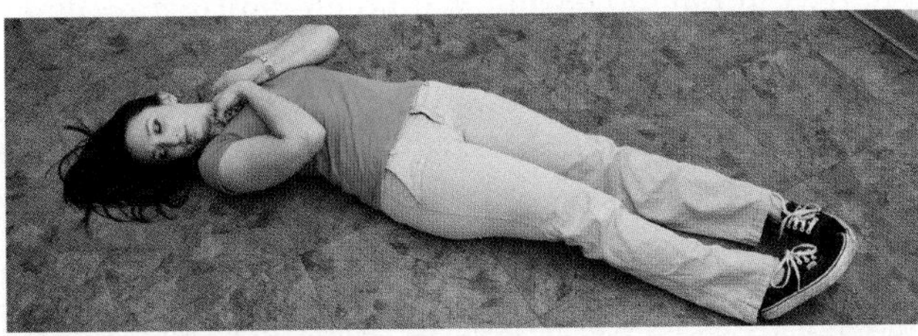

Figure 51.10 ■ Decorticate posturing is characterized by rigid flexion.

CLINICAL POINT: As the level of brain herniation progresses downward, the patient will begin with decorticate posturing, progressing to decerebrate posturing and finally to flaccidity. ■

Cerebral Contusions and Intracerebral Hemorrhage. One of the most common brain injuries seen in EDs across the United States is a **cerebral contusion**. A cerebral contusion occurs when the brain matter directly below the injured skull is bruised. Depending on its severity, a cerebral contusion can result in a full range of brain injuries from a mild concussion to severe injury to the axons of the brain cells causing severe brain injury.

One type of cerebral contusion is the coup-contrecoup injury, which results from both a direct injury to the brain (coup) and the resulting injury to the opposite side of the brain (contrecoup) as the brain bounces off the skull on the side opposite to the primary injury (**Figure 51.11** ■).[42,43,52,53]

Intracerebral hemorrhages can occur at the site of the coup-contrecoup injury as brain tissues and small blood vessels are damaged (**Figure 51.12** ■). Because this intracerebral hemorrhage may take hours or days to reveal itself, patients are often discharged home before the final extent of the brain injury is known.

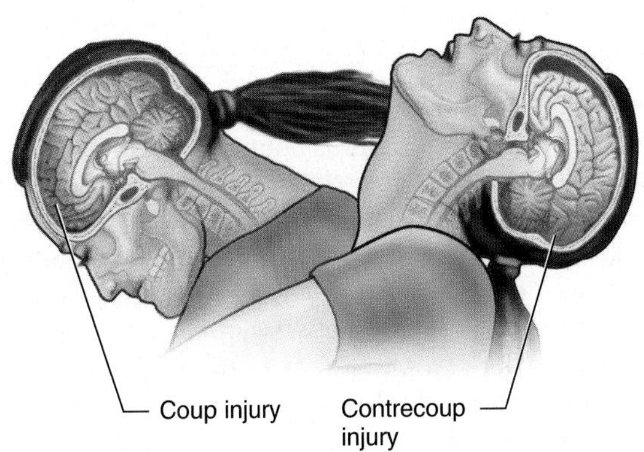

Figure 51.11 ■ Coup and contrecoup injuries.

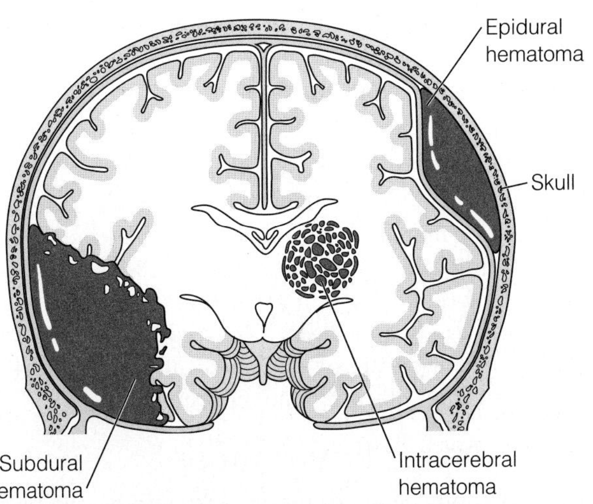

Figure 51.12 ■ Types of hematomas include epidural, subdural, and intracerebral.

Subarachnoid Hemorrhage. When the subarachnoid vessels are injured and bleed, blood leaks into the subarachnoid space, causing a traumatic subarachnoid hemorrhage. As the subarachnoid space fills with blood, blood is found in the CSF. Patients will often complain of photophobia (eyes irritated by light) and mild meningeal signs such as headache. When a traumatic subarachnoid hemorrhage occurs, the patient has a dramatically increased likelihood of death and disability. For this reason, a CT is always required when any sign of subarachnoid hemorrhage is discovered, and an immediate neurosurgical consultation and admission to an ICU are vital.[42,48,51]

Epidural Hematoma. When a head injury causes blood to leak between the skull and the dura mater, an **epidural hematoma** will occur (see Figure 51.12). Most epidural hematomas occur from a blunt trauma to the temporal or temporoparietal area and are often associated with a skull fracture and middle meningeal arterial disruption. On CT scan, an epidural hematoma appears biconvex (football shaped). The hallmark sign of an epidural hematoma is a blunt head injury resulting in a brief loss of consciousness followed by a lucid period and then unconsciousness. Because an epidural hematoma is caused by an arterial bleed, brain herniation can occur within hours and must be diagnosed and treated early if secondary brain injury is to be prevented.[2,43,48,52]

Subdural Hematoma. When the brain injury is severe enough to cause the brain to bounce around the skull, a tearing or shearing of the bridging veins often occurs, resulting in formation of a blood clot between the dura and the arachnoid mater. This clot is better known as a **subdural hematoma (SDH)** (see Figure 51.12). Patients with brain atrophy (usually older adults and patients who abuse alcohol) have more room for clots to form in the dura and are more susceptible to SDH. Because this is a venous bleed, the bleeding is slower, and it may take days or weeks for the full extent of the injury to be revealed. For that reason, SDH is classified as acute (signs and symptoms occur within 14 days of the injury) or chronic (signs and symptoms occur at least 2 weeks after injury). The CT scans of patient with SDH show a crescent-shaped lesion. Treatment depends on the degree of secondary brain injury and the signs and symptoms displayed by the patient.[42,43,48]

Older adults who experience trauma are at a higher risk for developing a subdural hematoma. There are three reasons for this: With aging, the brain atrophies, leaving more room for slow venous bleeding to occur and less tamponading of slow bleeds. Older adults also have friable bridging veins and small vessels, which tend to shear more easily and bleed. Older adults are also more likely to be taking anticoagulant medications, putting them at greater risk for bleeding into the brain.[9,54] ■

E: Exposure/Environment

During this final stage of the primary survey, the patient is exposed so that all areas of the body can be observed for other hidden injuries such as bruises, lacerations, impaled objects, bullet wounds, bleeding, or open fractures. If the ABCs are stable and the cervical spine has been immobilized, the patient should be logrolled onto his back for examination of the posterior aspect of the body. The environment must be controlled so that hypothermia does not complicate the patient's recovery. Continuous temperature monitoring should be initiated. Warm blankets should be applied and warm fluids should be initiated to prevent hypothermia, which would further exacerbate shock. Once the primary survey has been completed and all life-threatening injuries have been identified, a more thorough secondary survey is conducted.[2]

Judi Stone: Application

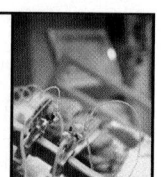

Ms. Stone has a GCS score of 3 on admission because she was chemically sedated, paralyzed, and intubated. Ms. Stone also has ecchymosis to her right parietal area and chin, along with bleeding from her left tympanic membrane. When the trauma team exposes the rest of her body, the only other injury they discover is pale, mottled feet bilaterally. Warm blankets, warming lights, and warm IV fluids are applied.

7. What head injury should be suspected on the basis of these findings?
8. What will be the team's focus in managing this injury?

Check Your Progress: Section 51.2

1. In assessing the airway of a trauma patient, what other structure must be considered at the same time?
2. How do mean arterial pressure, cerebral perfusion pressure, and intracranial pressure relate to the Monro-Kellie hypothesis?
3. A 10-year-old child is kicked by a horse during riding lessons. There are no outward signs of injury. However, the child is tachycardic and hypotensive with cool, pale skin. Which body cavity should be carefully assessed for internal bleeding?

51.3 The Secondary Survey and Injury

Once all life-threatening injuries have been identified and treated, a thorough head-to-toe assessment is done to determine whether any additional injuries need to be managed. The healthcare provider must be careful to go back and conduct the primary survey every few minutes throughout the secondary survey to ensure that no life-threatening complications arise.[2] Selected trauma injuries will be discussed below using a head-to-toe approach.

Head Injury

Etiology and Pathogenesis

Diffuse Axonal Injury. When the axonal fibers in the white matter and brainstem become sheared, a **diffuse axonal injury (DAI)** occurs. DAI injuries can be one of the most devastating brain injuries because although the patient has a totally normal CT scan, the cells in the brain have sheared and cellular death has occurred. Typically, this injury results from a rapid acceleration–deceleration injury such as a motor vehicle crash or shaken baby syndrome. When DAI occurs, there is an immediate increase in ICP, and the patient becomes unconscious. The CT is often normal, but in some cases, deep hemorrhagic injuries may be noticed. Very often, patients with DAI remain in a persistent vegetative state until death. Treatment options for DAI are very limited, but prevention of secondary brain injury remains a mainstay of therapy.[42,43,48]

Mild Traumatic Brain Injury (Concussion). A diagnosis of mild traumatic brain injury, commonly known as concussion, is made when any alteration in cerebral function is caused by a traumatic injury to the head and results in one of the following: a brief loss of consciousness, light-headedness, vertigo, headache, nausea, vomiting, photophobia, cognitive and memory dysfunction, tinnitus, blurred vision, difficulty concentrating, amnesia, fatigue, personality change, or a balance disturbance. Approximately 50% of patients with a concussion will experience some symptoms at least 3 months after the injury, and approximately 20% will experience symptoms for 6 months or more.[55] This persistence of symptoms is referred to as *postconcussive syndrome*, and it may occur after a TBI of any severity. Patients with severe symptoms or symptoms lasting more than a few days should be referred to a neurologist for long-term care.[52,55]

Neck Trauma

Etiology and Pathogenesis

Because the neck contains so many vascular, digestive, glandular, and spinal structures that are relatively close to the skin, trauma to the neck can result in many life-threatening injuries. Typically, the neck is divided into three zones (**Figure 51.13** ■).

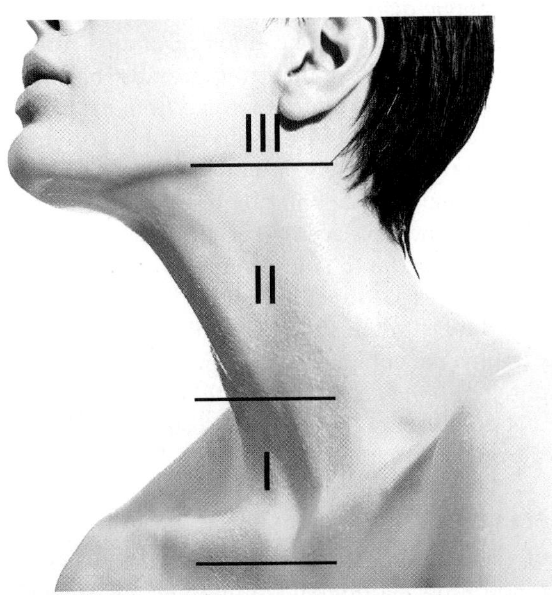

Figure 51.13 ■ Zones of neck injuries.

- *Zone I* extends from the vertebral and proximal carotid arteries and includes the major thoracic vessels, superior mediastinum, lungs, esophagus, trachea, thoracic duct, and spinal cord.
- *Zone II* extends from the inferior margin of the cricoid cartilage to the angle of the mandible. Injuries in zone II may involve the carotid vertebral arteries, jugular veins, esophagus, trachea, larynx, and spinal cord.
- *Zone III* is located between the angle of the mandible and the base of the skull and includes the distal carotid and vertebral arteries, pharynx, and spinal cord.

Penetrating injuries to the neck most often result from a stab wound, gunshot wound, or sharp instrument. Blunt neck trauma is rare because the head, shoulders, and chest offer protection to the neck. Some blunt neck injuries are attributed to hyperextension, hyperflexion, rotation, and direct blows to the neck. Shearing forces that cause neck injuries result from seat belts and objects that strike the neck, such as stationary cords (e.g., electrical cord, clothesline). These injuries are often associated with lacerations to the esophagus and laryngotracheal injuries. Although blunt neck injuries are rare, they can be fatal.[1,55–57]

Thoracic Trauma

Once all life-threatening chest injuries have been identified and managed, the secondary survey consists of inspecting, auscultating, and palpating the chest to discover any further injuries. A discussion of specific injuries resulting from chest trauma follows.

Hemothorax

As described earlier, a hemothorax is considered nonemergent when there is blood drainage of less than 100 mL/h for 6 hours or more or less than 600 mL initial drainage. If ongoing bleeding occurs, a surgical thorocotomy may be indicated.

Cardiac Contusion

Myocardial contusion may occur in patients who suffer blunt chest trauma. The severity of myocardial injury varies widely from a minor area of bruising on the myocardium to severe, massive damage resulting in necrosis and myocardial stunning. If the myocardium is stunned, it will not contract efficiently enough to maintain a cardiac output that can sustain life, and this relatively small group of patients will not survive a severe myocardial contusion.[11] Complications that can occur as a result of damage to the myocardium include thromboembolism from mural thrombus, myocardial rupture, cardiac tamponade, ventricular aneurysm, and pericarditis.[2,13,27]

Signs and symptoms of myocardial contusion include nonpleuritic chest pain, ecchymosis, and redness to the chest wall (73%). Tachycardia is the most common sign of cardiac contusion and is present in approximately 70% of patients diagnosed with a cardiac contusion. Electrocardiography is recommended but is not specific for cardiac contusion. Cardiac enzymes are also not specific for cardiac contusions; however, there is some evidence that an increased level of cardiac troponin indicates myocardial injury. A bedside echocardiogram will detect myocardial wall motion abnormalities.

A young, healthy trauma patient suffering a mild myocardial contusion will usually survive with no cardiac sequelae. The routine treatment for such a patient consists of cardiac monitoring for at least 12–24 hours. This has proven to be the time when dysrhythmias are most likely to occur, and virtually no life-threatening injuries have been reported more than 12 hours after injury. The patient who is asymptomatic and has no complications can often be discharged from the ED. However, if any signs of myocardial compromise exist, the patient must be admitted to a monitored bed. Finally, in the most severe cases, when the myocardium is stunned or bruised to the point of pump failure or cardiac cellular necrosis, treatment includes myocardial rescue, hyperperfusion to drive the cardiac output, and inotropic pharmacologic support. These patients have a grave prognosis.[2,27,28]

Pulmonary Contusion

Bruising of the lung occurs in 30–72% of all patients suffering from blunt chest trauma.[13] This injury usually occurs when the chest strikes a steering wheel, car door, or air bag in a motor vehicle crash. Falls, blast injuries, and high-velocity missile wounds can also cause a pulmonary contusion. When the blunt trauma is severe enough to damage the alveolar–capillary walls, intra-alveolar and interstitial hemorrhage occur. As a result of the blood and fluid accumulating in the alveoli and bronchi, mucus begins to accumulate, and increased capillary permeability occurs, resulting in decreased lung compliance, increased pulmonary vascular resistance, and increased alveolar–arterial oxygen difference. Signs and symptoms of a pulmonary contusion range from shortness of breath, cough, and mild tachypnea to hypoxia, hypoxemia, and respiratory arrest. Physical examination reveals decreased breath sounds to the area of injury. Chest x-ray will demonstrate patchy, irregular infiltrates over the area of injury. Often, radiographic findings do not reveal any injuries until 12–24 hours after the incident.

Treatment of a pulmonary contusion is directly related to the severity of the injury. In mild cases of pulmonary contusion in a young, healthy, stable patient, the patient can simply be observed for any signs of compromise. More aggressive treatment of pulmonary contusion consists of pulmonary support, aggressive pulmonary toileting, and pain management. Respiratory support can include supplemental oxygen by face mask, a continuous positive airway pressure or bilevel positive airway pressure device, or mechanical ventilation. However, careful fluid resuscitation is important, as overhydration can cause further injury.[2,27,28]

CLINICAL POINT: Pulmonary contusions can progress to acute respiratory distress syndrome (ARDS). During the acute stages of ARDS, aggressive pulmonary therapies are employed to sustain oxygenation to the vital organs. Some of these aggressive therapies include high-pressure ventilation, hypercapneic ventilation, prone positioning, use of high-frequency oscillating ventilation, and extracorporeal membrane oxygenation. ■

Clavicular Fracture/Dislocation

Clavicular fracture is generally secondary to blunt trauma, often as a result of a fall or acceleration–deceleration injury. The most common area of clavicular injury is in the middle third of the clavicle. The injury is associated with a pneumothorax or hemothorax in 3% of cases and then is nearly always associated with multiple ipsilateral rib fractures. Clavicular fractures that are not associated with ligamentous or vessel injury often can be treated with a sling or figure eight brace.[58]

Judi Stone: Application

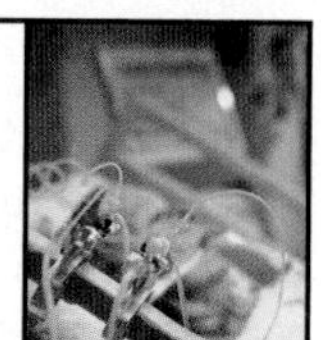

During the secondary survey, no further head or neck trauma is identified. Ms. Stone's pupils are reactive to light at 2–3 centimeters. She is unable to follow commands for extraocular movements. She has no jugular venous distention or signs of facial or neck injuries. Her cervical spine is palpated, and no deformities are found. Her clavicle is palpated and found to be uneven and deformed. Her ribs are palpated, and no deformities are noted. Her breasts are inspected and palpated, and no abnormalities are noted.

9. What do the pupillary findings suggest in relation to a brain injury?
10. On the basis of these findings, can Ms. Stone's spinal restrictions be removed?

Abdominal Injury

The word *abdomen* is derived from a Latin word meaning "to hide," and that is exactly what occurs with abdominal trauma: The injury is hidden in the abdomen. For this reason, patients who suffer injuries to the abdomen present a difficult diagnostic challenge to healthcare providers. It is imperative to consider underlying structures in determining the specific injuries resulting from abdominal trauma.

The most frequently injured abdominal organ is the spleen (46%), followed by the liver (33%).[59,60] Concomitant injuries closely associated with intra-abdominal injuries include pelvic disruption, abdominal wall injury, femoral fracture, hip dislocation, head injury, or any intrathoracic injury.[3,59,60] Intra-abdominal trauma must be considered with any penetrating injuries located from the pelvis up to the fourth intercostal space anteriorly, the sixth intercostal space laterally, and the scapular tip posteriorly. Penetrating abdominal injuries typically result from stab wounds, gunshot wounds, or lacerations. However, blunt abdominal trauma is by far the most common cause of abdominal injuries. Causes of abdominal trauma include motor vehicle crashes, blows to the abdomen, falls, and sports injuries. Any trauma patient with a blunt injury occurring below the diaphragm to the pelvic rim should be considered to have intra-abdominal trauma until diagnostic tests either confirm or rule out such trauma [3,59,60]

Liver Injury

The liver is the most common organ injured as a result of penetrating abdominal trauma and the second most common organ injured with blunt trauma. Patients with enlarged liver (hepatomegaly) or chronic obstructive pulmonary disease may be at greater risk for traumatic liver injuries because the enlarged liver will protrude from the costovertebral borders. The severity of the liver injury depends on the mechanism or injury and the hemodynamic instability that follows. In blunt trauma injuries, massive blood losses may occur, resulting in hypovolemic shock and instability. Liver injuries are graded according to degree of injury (on a scale of 1 to 6). Types of liver injuries range from a small hematoma or laceration to intraparenchymal hematoma, subcapsular hematoma, contusion, vascular damage, biliary duct transaction, or complete hepatic avulsion.[56] When major hepatic vessels are involved, massive blood loss will result. Treatment varies according to the severity of the injury.[2,59–61]

Splenic Injury

The most common cause of injuries to the spleen is a motor vehicle crash. However, the spleen may also be injured as a result of contact sports and direct blows to the abdomen.[59,61]

In the case of severe splenic injury, the patient will typically present with hemodynamic instability, including tachycardia, hypotension, dizziness, syncope, nausea, abdominal pain, and left upper quadrant tenderness. Kehr sign (referred pain to the right shoulder) may also be present.[59] Splenic injury is diagnosed on the basis of the CT scan and is graded on a scale of 1 to 5 depending on the severity of the injury. Injuries can range from parenchymal laceration to contusion or fracture. Pedicular vessels may also be torn and disrupted, causing massive bleeding. Conservative management of splenic injuries is recommended because of the risk of overwhelming postsplenectomy infection, a rare disorder with a high mortality rate that can occur when the spleen is removed.

Hollow Viscus Injuries

Hollow viscus injuries to the stomach, duodenum, small bowel, and colon usually occur as a result of a penetrating injury. They also can result from a shearing or tearing force due to a rapid acceleration–deceleration injury or from a severe increase in intraluminal pressure due to an external force such as a seat belt in a high-speed motor vehicle crash. The most common organ involved in a hollow viscus injury is the colon. When injuries to the stomach and duodenum occur, pneumoperitoneum (an abnormal presence of air in the peritoneal cavity) often occurs as well as blood in the peritoneum and blood in the NG tube. The healthcare provider should consider multiple hollow viscus lacerations as a result of penetrating trauma. Blunt trauma can result in mucosal tears, contusions, lacerations, or transections to hollow organs.[1,60,62]

Signs and symptoms of hollow viscus injury include early signs of peritoneal irritation such as mild, diffuse tenderness. Diagnosis may be made on the basis of a CT scan, diagnostic peritoneal lavage (DPL), or water-soluble gastrointestinal contrast studies. Early CT scans might not be useful in detecting hollow organ injury; a FAST scan or DPL will be more helpful in diagnosing a hollow organ injury. If the patient is unstable, operative exploration should be expedited in lieu of definitive diagnosis.[2,59,63]

Diaphragmatic Rupture

Diaphragmatic ruptures are one of the most challenging injuries to diagnose in trauma care and are often not discovered in the initial resuscitation phase. The mechanism of injury usually involves a crush injury to the chest wall or a penetrating trauma that produces small perforations. If the rupture is large enough, abdominal contents may herniate into the chest cavity or even strangulate through the diaphragmatic opening. If a liver or spleen laceration is present, the defect allows blood to accumulate in the thoracic cavity, compromising respiratory function and leading to a massive hemothorax. If the diaphragm is ruptured, the chest x-ray will demonstrate blurring of the diaphragm, a small pleural effusion, or an orogastric tube in the hemithorax. The injury may also be diagnosed by a CT scan. Treatment always requires surgical repair of the diaphragm.[2,59,62]

Genitourinary Trauma

Genitourinary trauma is typically referred to as trauma to any of the following structures: kidneys, ureters, bladder, or urethra. A direct blow to the back or flank, lower abdominal quadrant, or pelvis or any penetrating injury to the back, flank, lower abdomen, or pelvic area should alert the healthcare provider to the possibility of a genitourinary (GU) injury. Because most of the GU organs are located in the retroperitoneal space, it is often difficult to diagnose these hidden injuries. Evidence of hematuria or frank blood at the meatus are positive signs of GU trauma. However, most GU injuries are not that easily identified.[59,61,63]

Because the kidneys are highly vascular and are responsible for filtering all the blood that flows through the body, the trauma patient is at great risk for hemorrhagic shock when one or both kidneys are injured. For this reason, caregivers must pay close attention to signs of renal injury. Specific injuries to the kidneys can result in contusions, lacerations, fragmentation, and pedicle injuries; however, 85% of all renal injuries occur in the parenchyma. Renal vascular injuries are the most immediate life-threatening injury that occurs in GU trauma. Because the renal vascular structures are not fixed, they tear and shear easily with trauma, causing massive bleeding into the abdomen.[64]

The diagnostic study of choice to detect acute renal trauma is the FAST exam, as it can be performed at the bedside and will give a gross indication of active bleeding. The FAST exam will also detect injuries to the ureters, urethra, and bladder. Other tests include the IV contrast-enhanced CT scan, BUN and creatinine studies, and urinalysis. Urinalysis allows for assessment of the degree of hematuria, which is directly related to the degree of renal injury. The presence of hematuria greater than 100 red blood cells per high power field accompanied by hypotension is a significant finding and may indicate the presence of an urgent life-threatening GU injury. Uncomplicated microscopic hematuria will usually resolve with little or no intervention.[64]

Judi Stone: Application

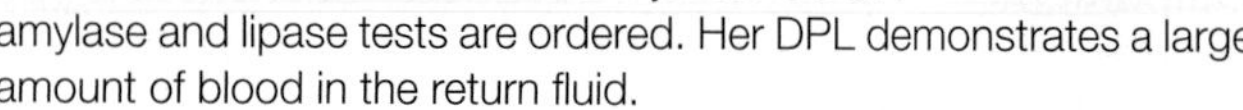

Ms. Stone's abdomen is soft and flat to palpation. Bowel sounds are audible. Because she is unresponsive to pain, a DPL is performed to further evaluate for intra-abdominal injuries. Serum amylase and lipase tests are ordered. Her DPL demonstrates a large amount of blood in the return fluid.

11. What do these findings suggest?
12. What steps would the team take next to further evaluate and manage this situation?

Pelvic Injuries

Because the pelvis is one of the strongest structures in the human body, injury to the pelvis requires a significant force, usually from a high kinetic energy transfer such as a motor vehicle crash, a fall from a distance, or a crushing blow to the pelvis.[63] Motor vehicle crashes account for approximately 60% of pelvic injuries, and falls are the second leading cause of pelvic fractures in adults. Consequently, pelvic fractures are associated with a high degree of morbidity and mortality due to injuries in the pelvis and concomitant injuries associated with pelvic fractures. Patients who suffer pelvic fractures have a significantly increased mortality rate when they present with the following concomitant findings: abdominal injuries requiring laparotomy (52% mortality), head injury requiring neurosurgery (50% mortality), and hypotension at the time of admission (42% mortality). Patients with an anteroposterior pelvic fracture have an 800% increased rate of aortic rupture. Patients who present to the ED with hypotension must be immediately evaluated for sources of active bleeding.

The pelvis consists of the sacrum and three innominate bones (the ileum, ischium, and pubis), which constitute the pelvic ring (**Figure 51.14** ■). The innominate bones connect anteriorly at the symphysis pubis. The sacrum is joined to each innominate bone by the sacroiliac joints. There are many ligamentous complexes that support the pelvis (see Figure 51.14). This strong structure provides protection to the lower abdominal and pelvic organs and is an important load-bearing structure in the skeletal system. The pelvis also contains a rich source of blood, housing the iliac and hypogastric arteries and the gluteal, obturator, and internal pudendal arteries.[2,65,66] With this rich supply of arterial and venous vessels surrounding and within the pelvic ring, it is understandable that a shearing injury or major disruption of the pelvic ring, causing a laceration to the many vessels in the pelvis, would provide a major source of blood loss. Ninety percent of hemorrhage from a pelvic fracture results from venous bleeding from bony structures.[65,66] Other injuries associated with pelvic fractures include gastrointestinal, GU, and spinal cord injuries.

Extremity Injuries

Four major extremity injuries that result from trauma include arterial bleeding, fractures, dislocations, and soft tissue injuries. The goal of treatment is to first stop any bleeding, preserve optimal function of the extremities, and maintain the integrity of the extremity. Many extremity injuries can be cared for during the secondary survey. However,

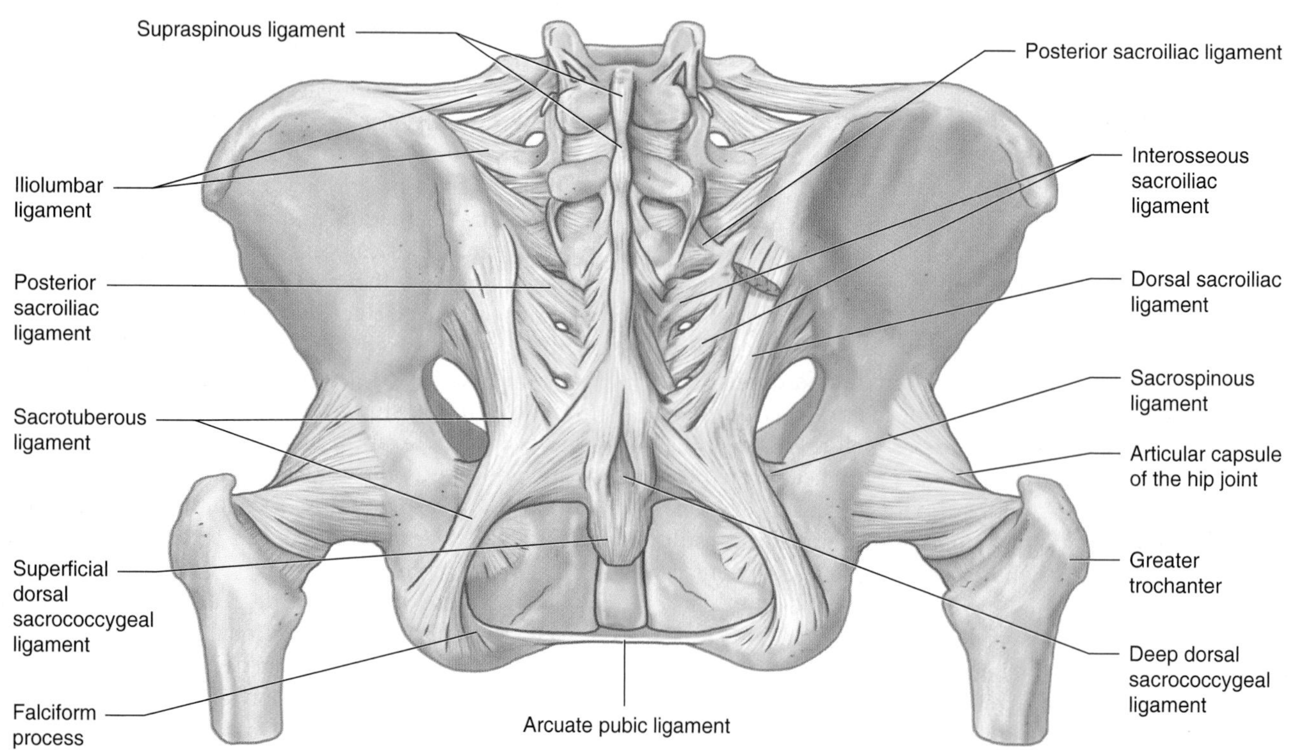

Figure 51.14 ■ The bones and ligaments of the pelvis.

when the extent of the extremity injury threatens life (such as major arterial injuries or life-threatening blood loss), care of the extremity injury becomes part of the primary resuscitation effort.[2,67]

Arterial Bleeding in the Extremities

Displaced fractures along with penetrating injuries can result in major arterial and venous bleeding in the extremities. Significant hemorrhage can result as the patient bleeds either externally through an open wound or internally into the soft tissues. All extremities should be observed for any signs of internal or external bleeding. The presence and quality of pulses should be assessed in all extremities. Any sign of vascular injury, such as a cold, pale, or pulseless extremity or an expanding hematoma, indicates a vascular emergency, and immediate consultation with a vascular surgeon is required.[2,67]

Extremity Fractures

A fracture is defined as any break in the cortex of the bone. Fractures are usually caused by a traumatic injury; however, there are several disease states that can result in extremity fractures. Fractures resulting from trauma are usually associated with soft tissue injuries. The specific type of fracture is named according to its appearance on x-ray.[67] Refer to Chapter 35, and especially Figure 35.3, for more information on fractures.

CLINICAL POINT: The reason this determination is so important is that open fractures put the patient at risk for osteomyelitis, an infection of the bone, which can cause months and years of pain, disability, medical and surgical therapies, and possibly, as a last resort, amputation. ■

Fractures in children are a particular problem in trauma care because children's bones have more elasticity and may have end plates that have not finished growing and are not fused (epiphyses). Severe disruptions in the epiphyses can disrupt bone growth development and may result in lack of growth or in deformities. ■

The primary diagnostic test of an extremity injury is to visually examine the injured extremity, palpate for tenderness or deformity, perform a thorough physical examination, and obtain radiologic tests. Orthopedic consults should be requested early and before any extensive diagnostic tests have been ordered.[2]

The mainstay of treatment for an extremity injury in trauma care revolves around one major concept: Save the patient's life first, and then save the limb—hence the saying "Life over limb."[2,41,67] If the severity of injury to the limb is causing life-threatening hypovolemia, then the limb must be sacrificed. However, barring any life-threatening injury, preservation of the limb and of functional abilities is the next priority. Once pain management has been initiated and the pain is under control, the limb must be stabilized and immobilized, and swelling must be controlled. Definitive therapies depend on diagnostic findings and can range from splinting and outpatient follow-up to emergent vascular and bony surgical repairs.[2,41,67,68]

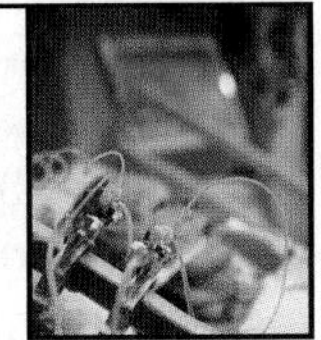

Judi Stone: Outcome

A head CT reveals that Ms. Stone has a left subdural hematoma along with a contusion to her left temporal and parietal lobe. She also has a left temporoparietal skull fracture with air leaking into the brain (pneumocephalus), which has caused a midline shift of the brain to the right. Ms. Stone also has a basilar skull fracture, a zygoma fracture, mastoid and temporal bone fractures, and a displaced left clavicular fracture.

Her DPL is positive for blood, so she is taken to the operating room for definitive care. The neurosurgical team joins the trauma team there. While the neurosurgical team evacuates the subdural hematoma and plates the skull fractures, the trauma team explores the abdomen for any intra-abdominal injuries. Ms. Stone is found to have a grade IV splenic laceration that requires a splenectomy.

Along with a clavicular fracture, her chest x-ray shows a questionable mediastinal widening. Aortography is performed; it is negative for an aortic tear. Ms. Stone also has a 15% pneumothorax to the left upper thorax for which a chest tube is placed.

After surgery, Ms. Stone is taken to the trauma ICU. She has serial CT scans of her head to look for any changes and continuous IPC and CPP monitoring. Her pneumothorax resolves after 4 days, and her chest tube is removed without complication. She is successfully weaned from the ventilator 6 days after sustaining her injuries. After spending 21 days in the hospital and an additional 30 days in a rehabilitation center, Ms. Stone goes on to make a full recovery.

13. How did the actions of the paramedics and the trauma team influence the patient's outcome?

Check Your Progress: Section 51.3

1. What injuries can result in major blood loss, causing a shock condition to occur?
2. Why is genitourinary trauma difficult to detect?
3. A 75-year-old male is involved in a head-on motor vehicle crash. He was driving an older car with no air bag installed. There is bruising to his chest wall that looks as though it came from contacting the steering wheel. He is complaining of shortness of breath and heavy chest pressure. What thoracic injuries should be considered in evaluating this patient?

CHAPTER SUMMARY

51.1 Chapter Overview and Case Study

Describe the primary survey and application to traumatic injuries in the context of the A (Airway), B (Breathing), C (Circulation), D (Disability), E (Exposure) approach to trauma.

- The purpose of the primary survey is to identify and treat all life-threatening injuries immediately as the patient arrives in the emergency department.
- The first three systems to be assessed during the primary survey are the systems that will threaten life emergently: Airway (including cervical spine), Breathing, and Circulation (ABC).
- Once the ABCs of the primary assessment have been evaluated and treated, the healthcare provider proceeds to assess Disability (neurologic status) and Expose (undress) and Environment (temperature control).
- Assessment of the airway includes checking that the airway is open and looking for signs of adequate oxygenation such as skin color, capillary refill, and oxygen saturation.

51.2 The Primary Survey and Injury

Describe the primary survey and differentiate the underlying pathogenesis of traumatic injuries.

- If the airway is compromised, the healthcare provider must take measures to immediately correct the problem, such as preparing for immediate intubation, delivering oxygen via a bag-valve-mask, or providing positive pressure ventilation.
- The cervical spine is assessed during the airway assessment because of the anatomic proximity of the cervical spine to the airway and because of the neurologic association of cervical vertebrae 3, 4, and 5 necessary to maintain adequate respiration.
- Spinal cord injuries vary by degree of damage to the spinal cord and can range from a complete spinal cord dissection to partial transection. Clinical neurologic signs of spinal cord injury can be traced to the anatomic spinal cord injury.
- Traumatic injuries that compromise breathing can result from a head injury, a spinal cord injury, chest injuries, or injuries to the circulatory system.
- Traumatic injuries that cause an opening into the thorax will compromise the closed negative pressure system in the thorax that facilitates expansion of the lungs and will allow air to rush into the thorax. This invasion of air into the thorax is called a pneumothorax and will cause the lungs to collapse.
- Bleeding into the lungs, known as a hemothorax, can also result in a collapse of the lungs and will compromise breathing.
- The Glasgow Coma Scale (GCS) is used as a means to quickly evaluate patients with suspected head injuries and to determine what level of trauma care they will require.
- The brain injury is classified as severe if the GCS score is less than 9 on arrival at the emergency department, moderate if the GCS score is 9–12, and mild if the GCS score is 13–15.
- The Monro-Kellie hypothesis centers on the concept that the brain resides inside a fixed skull and that the total volume of the intracranial contents (brain mass, intracerebral spinal fluid, and cerebral blood volume) remains constant. For homeostasis to be maintained, the three components must be adequately perfused with oxygen-rich blood, and stable pressures must exist within the cranial vault. If any of the contents of the cranial vault swell or diminish, pressures in the other two components will change to compensate.
- The three critical pressure systems in the brain structure that affect brain oxygenation are intracerebral pressure (CICP), mean arterial pressure (MAP), and cerebral perfusion pressure (CPP).
- Basilar skull fractures are commonly associated with a torn dura and are often associated with CSF otorrhea or rhinorrhea, mastoid ecchymosis (Battle sign), periorbital ecchymosis (raccoon eyes), hemotympanum, and vertigo.
- Brain herniations occur when the swelling in the brain causes such severe pressure that brain tissues press on the fossa in the brain, causing the brain to extend outside its normal boundary and herniate, usually downward.
- There are three major sites of brain herniation: uncal transtentorial, central transtentorial, cerebellotonsillar, and upward posterior fossa.
- A cerebral contusion is a bruising of the brain and can result in a full range of brain injuries from a mild concussion to a severe brain injury.
- A coup-contrecoup injury is an injury that results from both a direct injury to the brain (coup) and the resultant injury to the opposite side of the brain (contrecoup) as the brain bounces off the skull on the opposite side of the primary injury
- Brain hemorrhage is classified according to the dural membrane in which the bleeding occurs: subdural hematoma, epidural hematoma, or subarachnoid bleed.
- When pressure builds in the thorax, whether it comes from air or blood flowing into the thorax or both, it can cause a collapse of the lungs and the heart. This is a life-threatening condition called a tension pneumothorax.
- When the anterior ribs are fractured in a way that causes a free-floating rib segment in the thorax, there is

a disruption in the physiologic rise and fall of the chest, resulting in a ventilation–perfusion mismatch and lack of adequate oxygenation.

- Excessive injury to the circulatory system that results in either internal or external bleeding can cause hypovolemic shock, a potentially life-threatening situation.
- Injury to the heart that causes bleeding into pericardium is called a pericardial tamponade and will cause the accumulating blood to collapse the heart, leading to cardiac arrest.
- Injury to the heart that causes bleeding into the thorax can also cause the lungs and heart to collapse, resulting in cardiac arrest.

51.3 The Secondary Survey and Injury

Describe the secondary survey and application to pathogenesis of traumatic injuries.

- When the axonal fibers in the white matter and brainstem become sheared, a diffuse axonal injury (DAI) occurs.
- A concussion occurs when there is an injury to the brain resulting in mild traumatic brain injury and one or more symptoms such as light-headedness, vertigo, nausea, vomiting, photophobia, blurred vision, and difficulty concentrating. Bruising to the heart is called a cardiac contusion and is a common finding among trauma patients and can range in severity.
- Bruising of the lung is called a pulmonary contusion and results from blunt trauma to the chest. When the blunt trauma is severe enough to damage the alveolar–capillary walls, intra-alveolar and interstitial hemorrhage occurs.
- Abdominal trauma presents difficult diagnostic challenges because of the potential for hidden injuries in the peritoneum and retroperitoneum. Blunt trauma is the most common cause of abdominal trauma.
- Patients with a history of hepatomegaly or chronic obstructive pulmonary disease are at increased risk for liver injury because the liver protrudes from the protection of the costovertebral border.
- Bleeding from the liver and spleen can be so severe that the patient suffers hypovolemic shock.
- Hollow viscus injuries are common in blunt abdominal trauma. The most common site of hollow viscus injuries is the colon.
- Ruptures to the diaphragm are very difficult to diagnose and often are discovered when abdominal contents are noted on the chest x-ray or CT scan. Diaphragmatic ruptures always require immediate surgical repair.
- Genitourinary trauma usually results in bleeding into the retroperitoneum and is difficult to diagnose. Hematuria or frank blood in the urine or bleeding at the urinary meatus are all signs of genitourinary trauma.
- Patients with pelvic fractures have an increased rate of morbidity and mortality if the pelvic fracture injury is associated with an abdominal or head injury that requires surgery or with hypotension on admission.
- Significant hemorrhage can result from an extremity injury, as the patient may either bleed externally through an open wound or internally into the soft tissues.

REVIEW QUESTIONS

1. While working with an industrial press, an adult female accidentally crushes her arm in the machine. The extremity is misshapen, with several lacerations seen. Bleeding is continuous. Which of the following steps should be performed first?
   a. Check for a radial pulse.
   b. Control the bleeding.
   c. Apply a splint.
   d. Straighten the arm.

2. An adult male is struck by a car while walking across the street. The force of the impact causes him to strike the windshield with his face. He responds to a physical pain stimulus by drawing his arms toward his chest. There are numerous abrasions and lacerations to his face, and his jaw appears to be fractured. Loose and missing teeth are noted, and blood is coming from his mouth and nose. You can hear gurgling as he breathes, and his pulse rate is slow. Of the following steps in managing this client which is the most critical?
   a. Evaluate the mean arterial pressure to determine whether it is high enough to overcome increased intracranial pressure.
   b. Cover the lacerations with sterile gauze to prevent infection.
   c. Suction the airway to eliminate gurgling and possible aspiration.
   d. Apply a rigid cervical collar to reduce the possibility of a spinal cord injury.

3. A 15-year-old baseball pitcher was struck in the left temporal region of his head by a line drive from the

batter. Witnesses report that the client was immediately unconscious and they observed a brief period of seizure activity. On evaluation, the client's pupils are constricted. He is hyperventilating and hypertensive. Babinski reflexes can be seen in both feet. Which of the following herniation patterns should be suspected?
a. Cerebellotonsillar
b. Central transtentorial
c. Uncal transtentorial
d. Upward posterior fossa

4. A young man was shot in the left lateral chest during a fight. He is anxious and confused, and his skin is pale and diaphoretic. He has asymmetric chest rise, with the left side of the chest larger than the right. His neck veins are distended. He is hypotensive and bradycardic. Which of the following procedures is most important to do?
a. Decompress the left side of the chest.
b. Provide artificial ventilation.
c. Cover the wound with an occlusive dressing.
d. Establish large bore intravenous access.

5. An older female falls down a flight of stairs. She is awake but confused, complaining of chest and abdominal pain. Her skin is pale, cool, and clammy. She is breathing rapidly, and you can detect a weak, rapid pulse. Her blood pressure is 92/60 mmHg. Lung sounds are clear, and her neck veins are nondistended. Which of the following injuries is most likely, given the client's presenting signs and symptoms?
a. Abdominal bleeding
b. Pericardial tamponade
c. Tension pneumothorax
d. Spinal cord injury

6. A 35-year-old female comes to the emergency department complaining of a headache, nausea, and vomiting for the past 6 hours. Her husband reports that she was in a minor motor vehicle crash 2 days ago, in which she struck the left side of her head against the side window. She felt fine immediately after the crash, but over the last 12 hours, she has been feeling increasingly weak and unsteady on her feet. The workup is focused on determining whether she is bleeding into her brain. What type of hematoma should be suspected?
a. Epidural
b. Subdural
c. Coup-contrecoup
d. Intracerebral

7. An adolescent female is stabbed during a fight. The knife is impaled in the chest, just above the right breast. She is awake, in severe pain, and having difficulty breathing. Which of the following actions should be performed?
a. Remove the knife and control the bleeding.
b. Remove the knife and cover the wound with an occlusive dressing.
c. Keep the knife in place and evaluate lung sounds.
d. Keep the knife in place and place a seal around it.

8. An adult male is constructing a bomb in his garage when some of the material unexpectedly explodes. He is thrown several feet and lands on the garage floor. He is alert, in pain, and complaining of severe pain to his chest. There is no evidence of burns to his face. He is tachypneic and tachycardic and has pale, cool skin. His blood pressure is normal. Lung sounds are diminished bilaterally, and his chest wall is tender to palpation without crepitus or subcutaneous emphysema. Which of the following procedures is *not* indicated at this time?
a. Administer a large amount of intravenous fluids.
b. Prepare to artificially ventilate the client.
c. Monitor oxygenation levels in the blood.
d. Order an x-ray of the chest wall.

ANSWERS

Answers to Review Questions can be found in Appendix A. Answers to Case Study and Check Your Progress questions are available on the faculty resources site. Please consult with your instructor.

RECOMMENDED WEBSITES

Eastern Association for the Surgery of Trauma
http://www.east.org

European Society for Trauma & Emergency Surgery
http://www.estesonline.org

Society of Trauma Nurses
http://www.traumanurses.org

Trauma.Org
http://www.trauma.org

REFERENCES

1. Centers for Disease Control and Prevention. (2012). Guidelines for field triage of injured patients: Recommendations of the national expert panel on field triage 2011. *Morbidity and Mortality Weekly Report, 61*(RR01), 1–20.
2. American Academy of Pediatrics Committee on Pediatric Emergency Medicine; Council on Injury, Violence, and Poison Protection; Section on Critical Care; Section on Orthopaedics; Section on Surgery, et al. (2016). Management of pediatric trauma. *Pediatrics*. Available at http://pediatrics.aappublications.org/content/early/2016/07/21/peds.2016-1569
3. American College of Surgeons Committee on Trauma. (2017). *Advanced trauma life support* (10th ed.). Chicago, IL: American College of Surgeons.
4. Maerz, L. L., Davis, K. A., & Rosenbaum S. H. (2009). Trauma. *International Anesthesiology Clinics, 47*, 25–36.
5. Salomone, J. P., & Salomone, J. A. (2013). Prehospital care. In K. L. Mattox, E. E. Moore, & D. V. Feliciano (Eds.), *Trauma* (7th ed.). New York, NY: McGraw-Hill.
6. Berry, S. D., Ngo, L., Samelson, E. J., & Kiel, D. P. (2010). Competing risk of death: An important consideration in studies of older adults. *Journal of the American Geriatric Society, 58*, 783–787.
7. Bartley, M. K., & Shiflett, L. A. (2010). Handle older trauma patients with care. *Nursing, 40*, 24–29.
8. Nirula, R., & Gentilello, L. M. (2004). Futility of resuscitation criteria for the "young" old and the "old" old trauma patient: A national trauma data bank analysis. *Journal of Trauma, Injury, Infection, and Critical Care, 57*, 37–41.
9. Weber, J. M., Jablonski, R. A., & Penrod J. (2010). Missed opportunities: Under-detection of trauma in elderly adults involved in motor vehicle crashes. *Journal of Emergency Nursing, 36*, 6–9.
10. Codner, P. A., & Brasel, K. J. (2013). Initial assessment and management. In K. L. Mattox, E. E. Moore, & D. V. Feliciano (Eds.), *Trauma* (7th ed.). New York, NY: McGraw-Hill.
11. Toschlog, E. A., Sagraves, S. G., & Rotondo, M. F. (2013). Airway management. In K. L. Mattox, E. E. Moore, & D. V. Feliciano (Eds.), *Trauma* (7th ed.). New York, NY: McGraw-Hill.
12. Cameron, P., & Knapp, R. J. (2016). Trauma in adults. In J. E. Tintinalli, J. S. Stapczynski, O. J. Ma, D. M. Cline, & G. D. Meckler (Eds.), *Emergency medicine: A comprehensive study guide* (8th ed.). New York, NY: McGraw-Hill.
13. Emhoff, T. A. (2011). Initial assessment and management of the trauma victim. In R. V. Aghababian (Ed.), *Essentials of emergency medicine* (2nd ed.). Sudbury, MA: Jones & Bartlett.
14. Roskind, C. G., Dayan, P. S., Klein, B. L. (2016). Acute care of the victim of multiple trauma. In R. M. Kliegman, J. W. Stanton, N. F. St. Geme, N. F. Schor, & R. E. Behrman (Eds.), *Nelson textbook of pediatrics* (20th ed.). Philadelphia, PA: Elsevier Saunders.
15. Yelon, J. A. (2013). The geriatric patient. In K. L. Mattox, E. E. Moore, & D. V. Feliciano (Eds.), *Trauma* (7th ed.). New York, NY: McGraw-Hill.
16. National Spinal Cord Injury Center. (2014). Spinal cord injury facts and figures at a glance. *Journal of Spinal Cord Medicine, 37*, 117–118.
17. Coté, C., & Hartnick, C. (2009). Pediatric transtracheal and cricothyrotomy airway devices for emergency use: Which are appropriate for infants and children? *Pediatric Anesthesia, 19*, 66–76.
18. Nazarcy, P. P., &, Hirsh, M. (2011).Pediatric injuries. In R. V. Aghababian (Ed.), *Essentials of emergency medicine* (2nd ed.). Sudbury, MA: Jones & Bartlett.
19. Kortbeek, J. B., Al Turki, S. A., Ali, J., et al. (2008). Advanced trauma life support, 8th edition, the evidence for change. *Journal of Trauma, 64*, 1638–1650.
20. Kim, N. H. (2011). Spine injuries. In R. V. Aghababian (Ed.), *Essentials of emergency medicine* (2nd ed.). Sudbury, MA: Jones & Bartlett.
21. Sheerin, F. (2005). Spinal cord injury: Acute care management. *Emergency Nurse, 12*, 26–34.
22. Bawa, M., & Fayssoux, R. (2013). Vertebrae and spinal cord. In K. L. Mattox, E. E. Moore, & D. V. Feliciano (Eds.), *Trauma* (7th ed.). New York, NY: McGraw-Hill.
23. Go, S. (2016). Spine trauma. In J. E. Tintinalli, J. S. Stapczynski, O. J. Ma, D. M. Cline, & G. D. Meckler (Eds.), *Emergency medicine: A comprehensive study guide* (8th ed.). New York, NY: McGraw-Hill.
24. Kwon, B. K., Tetzlaff, W., Grauer, J. N., Beiner, J., & Vaccaro, A. R. (2004). Pathophysiology and pharmacologic treatment of acute spinal cord injury. *Spine Journal, 4*, 451–464.
25. Mistovich, J. J., Limmer, D., & Krost, W. S. (2004). Incomplete spinal cord injuries. *Emergency Medical Services, 33*, 56–58.
26. Hoffman, J. R., Mower, W. R., Wolfson, A. B., et al. (2000). Validity of a set of clinical criteria to rule out injury to the cervical spine in patients with blunt trauma. *New England Journal of Medicine, 343*, 94–99.
27. Bernardin, B., & Troquet, J. M. (2012). Initial management and resuscitation of severe chest trauma. *Emergency Medicine Clinics of North America, 30*, 377–400.
28. Jones, D., Nelson, J., & Ma, O. J. (2016). Pulmonary trauma. In J. E. Tintinalli, J. S. Stapczynski, O. J. Ma, D. M. Cline, & G. D. Meckler (Eds.), *Emergency medicine: A comprehensive study guide* (8th ed.). New York, NY: McGraw-Hill.
29. DuBose, J. A., O'Connor, J. V., & Scalea, T. M. (2013). Lung, trachea, and esophagus. In K. L. Mattox, E. E. Moore, & D. V. Feliciano (Eds.), *Trauma* (7th ed.). New York, NY: McGraw-Hill.
30. DeLorio, N. M. (2016). Trauma in pregnancy. In J. E. Tintinalli, J. S. Stapczynski, O. J. Ma, D. M. Cline, & G. D. Meckler (Eds.), *Emergency medicine: A comprehensive study guide* (8th ed.). New York, NY: McGraw-Hill.
31. Criddle, L. M. (2009). Trauma in pregnancy. *American Journal of Nursing, 109*, 41–47.
32. Chames, M. C., & Pearlman, M. D. (2008). Trauma during pregnancy: Outcomes and clinical management. *Clinical Obstetrics & Gynecology, 51*, 398–408.
33. Fleischmann, R .J., & Ma, O. J. (2016). Trauma in the elderly. In J. E. Tintinalli, J. S. Stapczynski, O. J. Ma, D. M. Cline, & G. D. Meckler (Eds.), *Emergency medicine: A comprehensive study guide* (8th ed.). New York, NY: McGraw-Hill.
34. Keough, V., & Letizia, M. (1998). Blunt cardiac injury in the elderly trauma patient. *International Journal of Trauma Nursing, 4*, 38–43.
35. Limmer, D., Mistovich, J. J., & Krost, W. S. (2004). Penetrating chest trauma. *Emergency Medical Services, 33*, 44–47.
36. Bonatti, H., & Calland, J. F. Trauma. (2008). *Emergency Medicine Clinics of North America, 26*, 625–648.
37. Emhoff, T. A. (2011). Shock in the trauma victim. In R. V. Aghababian (Ed.), *Essentials of emergency medicine* (2nd ed.). Sudbury, MA: Jones & Bartlett.
38. Wall, M. J., Tsai, P., & Mattox, K. L. (2013). Heart and thoracic vascular injuries. In K. L. Mattox, E. E. Moore, & D. V. Feliciano (Eds.), *Trauma* (7th ed.). New York, NY: McGraw-Hill.
39. Hunt, P. A., Greaves, I., & Owens, W. A. (2006). Emergency thoracotomy in thoracic trauma: A review. *Injury, 37*, 1–19.
40. Hirshberg, A. (2013). Trauma laparotomy. In K. L. Mattox, E. E. Moore, & D. V. Feliciano (Eds.), *Trauma* (7th ed.). New York, NY: McGraw-Hill.
41. Codner, P. A., & Brasel, K. J. (2013). Initial assessment and management. In K. L. Mattox, E. E. Moore, & D. V. Feliciano (Eds.), *Trauma* (7th ed.). New York, NY: McGraw-Hill.
42. Wright, D. W., & Merck, L. H. (2016). Head trauma. In J. E. Tintinalli, J. S. Stapczynski, O. J. Ma, D. M. Cline, & G. D. Meckler (Eds.), *Emergency medicine: A comprehensive study guide* (8th ed.). New York, NY: McGraw-Hill.
43. Post, A. F., Boro, T., & Ecklund, J. M. (2013). Injury to the brain. In K. L. Mattox, E. E. Moore, & D. V. Feliciano (Eds.), *Trauma* (7th ed.). New York, NY: McGraw-Hill.

44. Alexiou, G. A., Sfakianos, G., & Prodromou, N. (2011). Pediatric head trauma. *Journal of Emergencies, Trauma and Shock, 4*(3), 403–408.
45. Tuggle, D. W., & Kreykes, N. S. (2013). The pediatric patient. In K. L. Mattox, E. E. Moore, & D. V. Feliciano (Eds.), *Trauma* (7th ed.). New York, NY: McGraw-Hill.
46. Okonkwo, D. O., & Stone, J. R. (2003). Basic science of closed head injuries and spinal cord injuries. *Clinics in Sports Medicine, 22*, 467–481.
47. Jeremitsky, E., Omert, L., Dunham, C. M., Protetch, J., & Rodriguez, A. (2003). Harbingers of poor outcome the day after severe brain injury: Hypothermia, hypoxia, and hypoperfusion. [see comment]. *Journal of Trauma, Injury, Infection, & Critical Care, 54*, 312–319.
48. Post, A. F., Boro, T., & Ecklund, J. M. (2013). Injury to the brain. In K. L. Mattox, E. E. Moore, & D. V. Feliciano (Eds.), *Trauma* (7th ed.). New York, NY: McGraw-Hill.
49. Greve, M. W., & Zink, B. J. (2009). Pathophysiology of traumatic brain injury. *Mount Sinai Journal of Medicine, 76*, 97–104.
50. Brain Trauma Foundation. (2007). Management and prognosis of severe traumatic brain injury. *Journal of Neurotrauma, 24*, S1–S106.
51. Hall, W. (2011). Head injuries. In R. V. Aghababian (Ed.), *Essentials of emergency medicine* (2nd ed.). Sudbury, MA: Jones & Bartlett.
52. Nolan, S. (2005). Traumatic brain injury: A review. *Critical Care Nursing Quarterly, 28*, 188–194.
53. Hunt, J. P., Marr, A. B., & Stuke, L. E. (2013). Kinematics. In K. L. Mattox, E. E. Moore, & D. V. Feliciano (Eds.), *Trauma* (7th ed.). New York, NY: McGraw-Hill.
54. Scheetz, L. J. (2011). Life-threatening injuries in older adults. *AACN Advanced Critical Care, 22*, 128–139.
55. Arciniegas, D. B., Anderson, C. A., Topkoff, J., & McAllister, T. W. (2005). Mild traumatic brain injury: A neuropsychiatric approach to diagnosis, evaluation, and treatment. *Neuropsychiatric Disease and Treatment, 1*(4), 311–327.
56. Bean, A. (2016). Trauma to the neck. In J. E. Tintinalli, J. S. Stapczynski, O. J. Ma, D. M. Cline, & G. D. Meckler (Eds.), *Emergency medicine: A comprehensive study guide* (8th ed.). New York, NY: McGraw-Hill.
57. Tisherman, S. A., Bokhari, F., Collier, B., et al. (2008). Clinical practice guideline: Penetrating zone II neck trauma. *Journal of Trauma, 64*, 1392–1405.
58. Khan, L. K., Bradnock, T. J., Scott, C., & Robinson, C. M. (2009). Fractures of the clavicle. *Journal of Bone and Joint Surgery. American Volume, 91*(2), 447–460.
59. Simon, B. J. (2011). Abdominal injuries. In R. V. Aghababian (Ed.), *Essentials of emergency medicine* (2nd ed.). Sudbury, MA: Jones & Bartlett.
60. French, L. K., Gordy, S., & Ma, O. J. (2016). Abdominal trauma. In J. E. Tintinalli, J. S. Stapczynski, O. J. Ma, D. M. Cline, & G. D. Meckler (Eds.), *Emergency medicine: A comprehensive study guide* (8th ed.). New York, NY: McGraw-Hill.
61. Wisner, D. H. (2013). Injury to the spleen. In K. L. Mattox, E. E. Moore, & D. V. Feliciano (Eds.), *Trauma* (7th ed.). New York, NY: McGraw-Hill.
62. Kleinman, M. E., Chameides, L., Schexnayder, S. M., et al. (2010). Part 14: Pediatric advanced life support: 2010 American Heart Association Guidelines for Cardiopulmonary Resuscitation and Emergency Cardiovascular Care. *Circulation, 122*, S876.
63. McStay, C., Ringwelski, A., Levy, P., & Legome, E. (2009). Hollow viscus injury. *Journal of Emergency Medicine, 37*, 293–299.
64. Simon, B. J. (2011). Genitourinary injuries. In R. V. Aghababian (Ed.), *Essentials of emergency medicine* (2nd ed.). Sudbury, MA: Jones & Bartlett.
65. Frakes, M. A., & Evans, T. (2004). Major pelvic fractures. *Critical Care Nurse, 24*, 18–30.
66. Torres, U. (2011). Hip and pelvic fracture. In R. V. Aghababian (Ed.), *Essentials of emergency medicine* (2nd ed.). Sudbury, MA: Jones & Bartlett.
67. Emhoff, T. A. (2011). Upper and lower extremity injuries. In R. V. Aghababian (Ed.), *Essentials of emergency medicine* (2nd ed.). Sudbury, MA: Jones & Bartlett.
68. Menkes, J. S. (2016). Initial evaluation and management of orthopedic injuries. In J. E. Tintinalli, J. S. Stapczynski, O. J. Ma, D. M. Cline, & G. D. Meckler (Eds.), *Emergency medicine: A comprehensive study guide* (8th ed.). New York, NY: McGraw-Hill.

Chapter 52

Biologic, Chemical, and Radiologic Agents of Disease

Will Chapleau and Peter Pons

Chapter Outline and Learning Outcomes

52.1 Chapter Overview and Case Studies

Describe dissemination of, current threats from, and concepts related to disorders caused by biologic, chemical, and radiologic agents.

52.2 Biologic Agents

Differentiate the causes, classification, underlying pathogenesis, and clinical manifestations of disorders caused by biologic agents and approaches to diagnosis and treatment of these conditions across the lifespan.

52.3 Chemical Agents

Differentiate the causes, classification, underlying pathogenesis, and clinical manifestations of disorders caused by chemical agents and approaches to diagnosis and treatment of these conditions across the lifespan.

52.4 Radiologic and Nuclear Devices

Differentiate the causes, classification, underlying pathogenesis, and clinical manifestations of disorders caused by radiologic and nuclear devices and approaches to diagnosis and treatment of these conditions across the lifespan.

KEY TERMS

Acute radiation syndrome (ARS), 1286
Anhydrous ammonia, 1283
Anthrax, 1272
Asphyxiants, 1284
Botulinum toxin, 1272
Bubonic plague, 1277
Chlorine, 1272
Cyanide, 1272
Dirty bomb, 1272
Lewisite, 1272
Mustard gas, 1272
Nerve agents, 1272
Phosgene, 1272
Plague, 1272
Pneumonic plague, 1277
Pulmonary agents, 1272
Radiologic dispersal device, 1272
Ricin, 1272
Riot control agents, 1272
Sarin, 1272
Septicemic plague, 1277
Smallpox, 1272
Soman, 1281
Tabun, 1281
Vesicants, 1272
VX, 1272

ABBREVIATIONS

ARS—acute radiation syndrome
Bq—Becquerel
Ci—Curie
Gy—Gray
rad—radiation absorbed dose
rem—roentgen equivalent man
Sv—Seivert

52.1 Chapter Overview and Case Studies

Over the past decade, the chances of nurses having to deal with biologic, chemical, or radiologic hazards has greatly increased. The news is replete with stories about individuals manufacturing chemical or biologic agents designed to inflict harm to large numbers of people. The possibility of various factions employing biologic or radiologic weapons as acts of terrorism also seems a very real possibility. However, it is more common to see patients exposed to these substances as a result of industrial and transportation incidents. Patients who have been exposed to biologic, chemical, or radiologic materials are not only are at risk for significant illness or injury themselves but, in many cases, also pose a threat to the people who care for them. This chapter is designed to give healthcare providers information about these threats as a way of not only providing care to patients, but also protecting themselves against risk.

Some general precautions applicable to the agents discussed in this chapter include ensuring that patients who have been exposed to any of these agents be immediately undressed to remove any residual agent that might remain on clothing in order to minimize the likelihood of ongoing exposure. Removing clothing from a contaminated patient removes approximately 80–90% of residual contaminant. The next step is to decontaminate the patients by having them shower using copious amounts of water. If available, soap can be used as well, but there should be no delay in showering while trying to find soap. Once decontaminated, the patients should be observed for the development of any symptoms or signs of ongoing exposure that would indicate incomplete decontamination or should be counseled as to how to proceed, depending on the suspected agent involved.

Nurses are trained to take the appropriate steps to protect themselves and others from exposure to infectious diseases. Personal protection from exposure to released intentionally biologic agents is no different from the precautions taken for any other infectious diseases that a healthcare provider may encounter. The principles of treatment for these patients will be the same, regardless of the cause of the exposure. What needs to be emphasized is that the nurse should always consider the potential for an intentional exposure even when it might not be readily apparent.

The identification of, protection from, and treatment for exposure to chemical agents depend in large part on being able to recognize the clinical presentation that various chemical agents produce. In most cases, specific laboratory studies to formally identify the chemical are not available, or a prolonged amount of time would be required for results to be returned.

Radiologic exposures present one of the more difficult challenges because radiologic agents are difficult to identify without specific detection equipment. Teamwork and communication between public safety responders at the scene of the initial incident or exposure and the staff at the receiving hospital are key to optimal management of these victims.

Common Biologic, Chemical, and Radiologic Agents

Biologic agents include bacteria, viruses, and biologic toxins.[1,2] The common bacterial agents that have been weaponized include **anthrax** (*Bacillus anthracis*), **plague** (*Yersinia pestis*), tularemia (*Francisella tularensis*), glanders (*Burkholderia mallei*), brucellosis (four different types of *Brucella* species), and Q fever (*Coxiella burnetii*). Anthrax and plague are perhaps the most common potential bacterial agents and will be discussed in more detail later in this chapter. Common viral agents that can be used as potential weapons include **smallpox** (variola virus), Venezuelan equine encephalitis (V.E.E. virus), and the viral hemorrhagic fevers (e.g., Ebola, Marburg, Crimean-Congo hemorrhagic fever, dengue). The common toxins that are potential weapons include **botulinum toxin** and **ricin**.

Chemical agents are classified into several groups on the basis of either their chemical nature or the effect that they produce clinically.[1] These categories are the **cyanides**, **nerve agents** (**sarin**, **VX**), lung toxicants (choking or **pulmonary agents** such as **phosgene**, **chlorine**, and ammonia), **vesicants** (blistering agents such as **mustard gas** and **Lewisite**), incapacitating agents (BZ and opiates), lacrimating agents (**riot control agents** such as tear gas and pepper spray), and vomiting agents.

Radiologic exposures, although rare, can result from accidental or intentional events. Exposure can come from the detonation of a nuclear weapon (which would be unlikely), a **dirty bomb** or **radiologic dispersal device**, an accident or sabotage at a nuclear facility, or the mishandling of nuclear materials or waste.

Concepts Related to Disorders Caused by Biologic, Chemical, and Radiologic Agents

There are a number of important considerations regarding biologic agents and the diseases that they produce. The first is the identification and management of patients who have been exposed to any of these disease-causing agents. The definitive diagnosis of the specific cause typically takes time, in some cases several days. Therefore, the healthcare provider must be able to recognize the presenting symptom and signs as representative of the syndrome caused by a particular agent or class of agents and then must intervene accordingly, even before the formal diagnosis has been confirmed. Second, some of these biologic agents are transmissible from person to person, and some are not. Unfortunately, all of the diseases caused by these agents initially present in similar fashion with a flulike syndrome. Until the definitive cause has been identified, the healthcare provider will usually not know whether the biologic agent is transmissible. Therefore, every patient must be handled with full infectious disease precautions until the causative agent is known.

Exposure to chemical or biologic agents and to sources of radiation can have similar effects on health. The inhalation of nerve agents and chemicals and exposure to radiation can damage lung tissues, resulting in an inability to effectively oxygenate the blood, leading to overall hypoxia. Chemical exposure and high doses of radiation can lead to skin ulceration, contributing to a loss of tissue integrity and possible issues with thermoregulation. Biologic agents can lead to significant fluid shifts, contributing to issues with edema along with fluid and electrolyte balance considerations. Chemical and biologic agents can cause esophageal trauma, as can radiation, resulting in nutritional deficits. Chemical agents and radiation can result in neutropenia and other cellular deficits, leading to a reduction in immunologic function. Each of these agents can result in tracheal damage and edema, leading to respiratory difficulties and compromised oxygenation. Hormonal regulation through the thyroid can be adversely affected by radiation exposure contributing to a disruption of reproductive capability (**Figure 52.1** ■).

Case Studies

The following cases are addressed throughout the chapter to assist in application of chapter content to clinical situations that involve individuals with exposure to a chemical, biologic, or radiologic agent.

James Jerome: Introduction

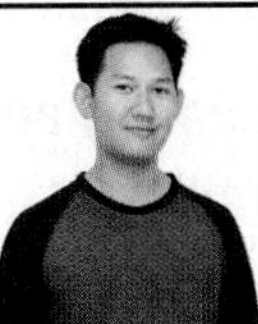

James Jerome, age 37, presents to the hospital complaining of fever, chills, and multiple aches and pains. He reports that he first became ill approximately 3 days ago and treated himself symptomatically, thinking that he had the flu. He said he felt better after about 36–48 hours but now is feeling much worse. He says that he now feels short of breath, is coughing, and feels nauseated in addition to all of the previously mentioned symptoms.

1. What would be your initial impression of Mr. Jerome's presenting symptoms?
2. What personal protective precautions might you consider when managing this patient?
3. What other questions might you consider asking during your evaluation?

Kasey Robinson: Introduction

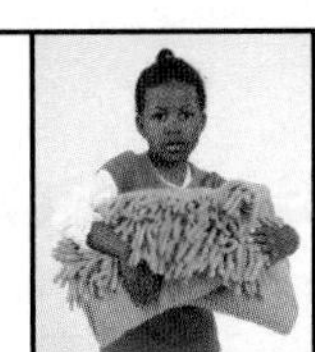

Kasey Robinson is an 8-year-old girl who was participating in a large celebration with her parents after their favorite sports team won the national championship. As the celebratory group became larger and larger, a number of the participants, who appeared to be intoxicated, starting to turn over parked vehicles and set a number of garbage receptacles on fire. To stop the now out-of-control group, the police fired canisters of tear gas at the crowd. Kasey immediately noticed a burning sensation in her eyes with copious tearing, burning in her nose with the onset of runny secretions from both nostrils, and similar burning in her throat with coughing. When paramedics arrive at the scene, Kasey continues to have these complaints and is transported to the local emergency department.

1. What is your initial suspicion of the cause for Kasey's chief complaints?
2. Given the mechanism of injury, what safety concerns do you have?
3. What would you do first in managing Kasey's conditions?

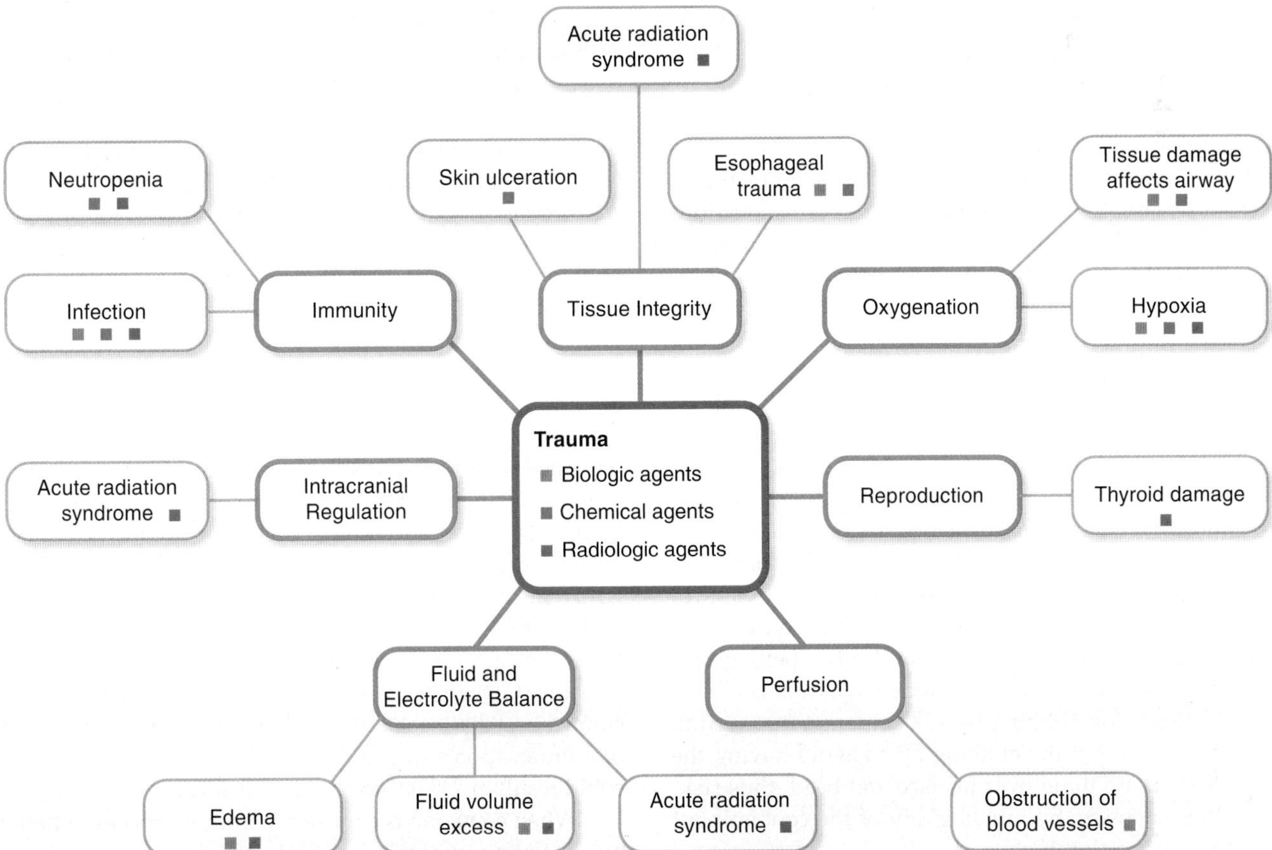

Figure 52.1 ■ Concepts related to exposure to biologic, chemical, and radiologic agents.

Check Your Progress: Section 52.1

1. What is your greatest concern about managing patients who have been affected by biologic, chemical, or radiologic agents?
2. Why do healthcare providers often miss the initial signs and symptoms of a biologic agent exposure?
3. What would be the best way to protect yourself from unnecessary exposure to biologic, chemical, or radiologic agents?

52.2 Biologic Agents

Infectious disease agents may pose a threat to the well-being of healthcare workers and other people who come into contact with the infected patient. The weaponizing of biologic agents and intentional exposure of individuals to these agents adds complexity to the healthcare system's capability to identify the specific cause of an infectious disease and to limit further exposures in a timely manner. Because all of the biologic agents are odorless, colorless, and tasteless, it is both more difficult and more crucial to identify the agent in such a situation as soon as possible. While protecting ourselves and others from contamination due to biologic agents is not more complicated than using the standard PPE precautions that are commonplace in all hospitals, the primary problem is that the specific agent is typically not identified for several days after the exposure. As a result, all patients who present with symptoms and signs of biologic agent exposure must be treated as if they are infectious and pose a risk of disease transmission. The importance of using proper PPE with all patients before ruling out transmissible disease cannot be overstated.

Intentional exposure to a biologic agent can occur in a number of ways, including both overt and covert methods. An overt release involves direct contact with the infectious substance, as in the anthrax-contaminated letters in the 2001 biologic attacks. Another method of release could involve aerosolizing the biologic agent using some sort of spraying device. This latter method of dispersal has the advantage (from the perpetrator's point of view) of wider dissemination and the potential for a greater number of casualties. In both cases, contamination and exposure occur either by direct contact with the substance or by inhalation of the infectious agent. Until the victim and anything else that came into contact with the substance has been decontaminated, other people who are in close contact with the victim or the scene are at risk of exposure as well. Therefore, appropriate PPE must be used by all who come into contact with the patient, the patient's clothing and other belongings, or anything else at the scene that may have been contaminated. In removing clothing from a contaminated victim, it is important to cut the clothing off to avoid having the victim pull off anything over his face and head, thus risking further exposure by inhaling any of the contaminant remaining on the clothing.

The second type of exposure is a remote or covert terrorist exposure. In this case, the infectious material could be released into the ventilation system of a building, allowing unsuspecting victims to inhale the agent. Another possibility involves a terrorist who intentionally inoculates himself or herself with a biologic agent to expose other people with whom the terrorist comes into contact.

One other method of exposure is secondary infection from an infected individual who was unknowingly exposed to the biologic agent days earlier and is now ill with the disease. This poses a risk to any family members, coworkers, and hospital staff who come into contact with the victim. This, of course, presumes that the selected agent results in a disease that is transmissible from person to person, which is not the case for every biologic agent. A review of specific biologic agents follows this section.

Anthrax

Bacillus anthracis is the spore-forming bacterium responsible for anthrax.[1–8] Anthrax spores can be found in the soil of every continent and are most prevalent in countries with inadequate infrastructure and healthcare systems.

Etiology and Pathogenesis

Anthrax exposure typically occurs in one of three ways: ingestion leading to gastrointestinal anthrax, skin inoculation causing cutaneous anthrax, and inhalation leading to inhalation anthrax.[1–3] Before the 20th century, the disease was most commonly spread by infected livestock that humans then consumed or by individuals who worked with animals and were exposed to their skin, wool, meat, or body fluids and developed the cutaneous form of the disease (hence the name *woolsorter's disease*). Gastrointestinal exposure is rare in modern times; most cases now come through contact with broken skin (95%) or inhalation (5%). Gastrointestinal anthrax accounts for fewer than 1% of the cases today. Just 20 years ago, inhalation anthrax resulted in death in over 90% of cases. Today, with prompt recognition and aggressive treatment, the mortality rate can fall to less than 50%.[3] With proper treatment, cutaneous infections are fatal in fewer than 1% of cases, but the mortality rate can rise to 20% without treatment. Gastrointestinal anthrax has a mortality of approximately 50%.

Anthrax was first weaponized by Japan in the 1930s; it has since been prepared as a potential biologic weapon by a number of other countries.[1] Accidental release of aerosolized anthrax spores at a Russian military facility in 1979 caused 79 individuals to become infected with pulmonary anthrax; 68 of them died. In 2001, elected officials in Washington, D.C., and several news outlets received letters in the mail that contained anthrax spores, resulting in 22 cases of infection and 5 deaths.[1] Of these, 11 were pulmonary infections, and 11 were cutaneous. It has been estimated that a release of 220 pounds of anthrax spores over a city the size of Washington, D.C., could result in 130,000 to 3 million deaths.

When someone is exposed to anthrax spores, whether by inhalation, ingestion, or skin inoculation, a number of pathophysiologic events begin. Anthrax spores, which are the inactive form of the *Bacillus anthracis* bacteria, can survive a very long time (decades) in a wide variety of conditions. When the spores enter the exposed individual, they are attacked by macrophages in an attempt to defend against the infection and are often carried to regional lymph nodes. The spores then germinate within the macrophage and produce the active or vegetative bacteria, leading to the destruction of the macrophage and the release of the bacteria, which then multiply. The active bacteria produce three proteins that together act as toxins that cause the symptoms and signs of clinical anthrax. These three compounds are called the *edema factor*, *lethal factor*, and *protective antigen*. Protective antigen binds to the surface of cells and creates the opening in the cell membrane that allows the other two factors to enter. It then combines with the other two factors to allow them to function. Edema factor causes swelling of the affected cell, and lethal factor leads to necrosis and death of the cell (see **Figure 52.2** ■). Anthrax is not transmissible from person to person, with the exception of the cutaneous form, which can be spread to another person if the anthrax lesion has any discharge from it.

Clinical Manifestations

The symptoms and signs of anthrax relate to the route of exposure and result from the actions of the factors described above.

Cutaneous Anthrax. Spores that enter through a break in the skin result in a localized infection and response. The initial finding is a raised papule or blister. The initial lesion may be pruritic, but it is typically painless. As the papule enlarges, it becomes more swollen (edema factor) and will ulcerate and progress into a dry, black necrotic eschar (lethal factor)[1–3] (**Figure 52.3** ■). Even if this form of anthrax goes untreated, the mortality rate is less than 1%.[3]

Gastrointestinal Anthrax. When anthrax spores are ingested, macrophages attempt to prevent the infection by attacking the spores and carrying them to the regional lymph nodes, in this case along the gastrointestinal tract into the neck and abdomen. The same sequence of events occurs as in inhalation anthrax, leading to fever and chills, malaise, headache, sore throat, pain and difficulty in swallowing, nausea, vomiting (which may be hemorrhagic), bloody diarrhea, and acute abdominal pain.[1,2] Mortality rates are much higher for gastrointestinal anthrax than for cutaneous anthrax, reaching as high as 60% if untreated.[3]

Inhalation or Pulmonary Anthrax. Spores inhaled into the lungs will end up in the alveoli, where they are attacked by the macrophages. They will be carried to the regional lymph nodes, in this case in the mediastinum of the exposed victim. When the bacteria produce the toxins, the result is swelling of the mediastinal lymph nodes, causing an acute hemorrhagic mediastinitis (**Figure 52.4** ■). Within several days to a week of exposure (though some individuals have had latent periods for as long as 60 days), patients present initially with a nonspecific flulike syndrome that includes fever, chills, dyspnea, cough, chest pain, headache, and vomiting. After

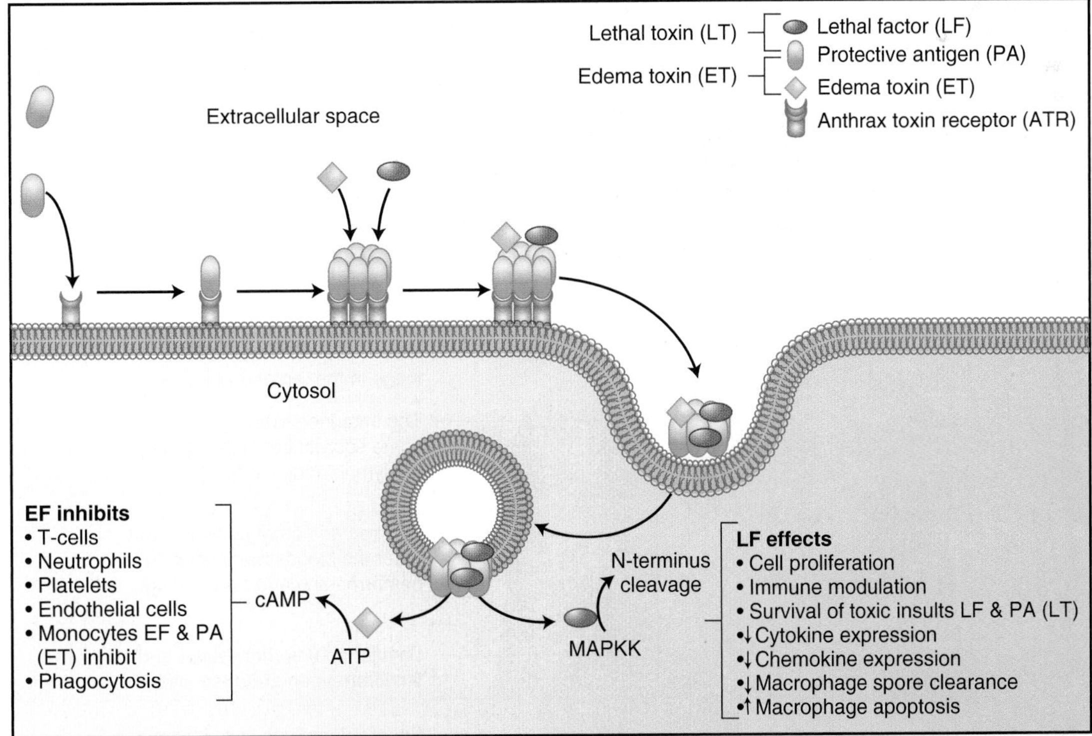

Figure 52.2 ■ Formation and activity of anthrax toxins. ATP = adenosine triphosphate, ATR = anthrax toxin receptor, cAMP = cyclic adenosine monophosphate, ET = edema toxin, LF = lethal factor, LT = lethal toxin, MAPKK = mitogen-activated protein kinase, PA = protective antigen.

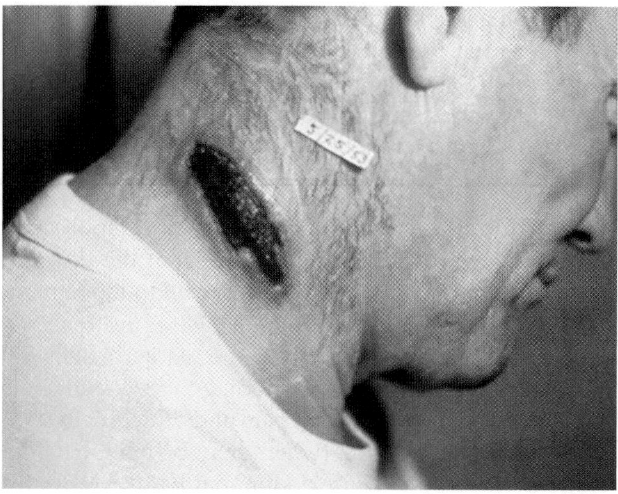

Figure 52.3 ■ Cutaneous anthrax of the neck. Note the central area of necrosis with surrounding edema.

a couple of days, the patient will improve and feel better only to rapidly deteriorate into fever, dyspnea, diaphoresis, shock, and death.[1,2] It is important to remember that patients with inhalation anthrax are not contagious and do not pose a risk to caregivers. However, this can be considered only after the formal diagnosis has been made, as several other biologic agents that are highly transmissible can present in similar fashion. Traditionally, the mortality rate for inhalation anthrax was considered the highest (at 90%), but advances in medical care have reduced that percentage to 45.[3]

James Jerome: Application

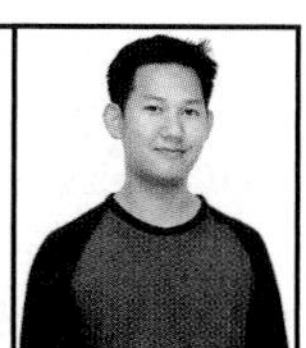

On arrival at the emergency department, Mr. Jerome appears to be in moderate respiratory distress. His vital signs are pulse 108, respirations 32, temperature 38.9°C (102°F), blood pressure 116/74, and oxygen saturation 89%. On further history, Mr. Jerome reports that he works for the federal government and that a number of his coworkers in the same office have also become ill with similar symptoms. As his evaluation and workup continue, a chest x-ray reveals that his mediastinum appears widened and he has some pleural effusion. The emergency physician suspects that this could be anthrax and calls the public health department to initiate an investigation. Blood cultures and sputum cultures are obtained and sent to the lab. With the application of oxygen, Mr. Jerome's oxygen saturation improves to 93%. Antibiotics are begun in the emergency department, and Mr. Jerome is admitted to the intensive care unit.

4. What is the likely route of attack for the presumed anthrax spores?
5. What is the possibility that Mr. Jerome's condition is the result of an organized attack?
6. Should you take any significant protective precautions as you manage Mr. Jerome?

Linking Pathophysiology to Diagnosis and Treatment

Anthrax can be prevented by administration of the anthrax vaccine. However, vaccination is currently recommended only for military personnel and lab and industrial workers who are at risk for exposure. The vaccine requires a series of injections that include the initial dose; follow-up injections

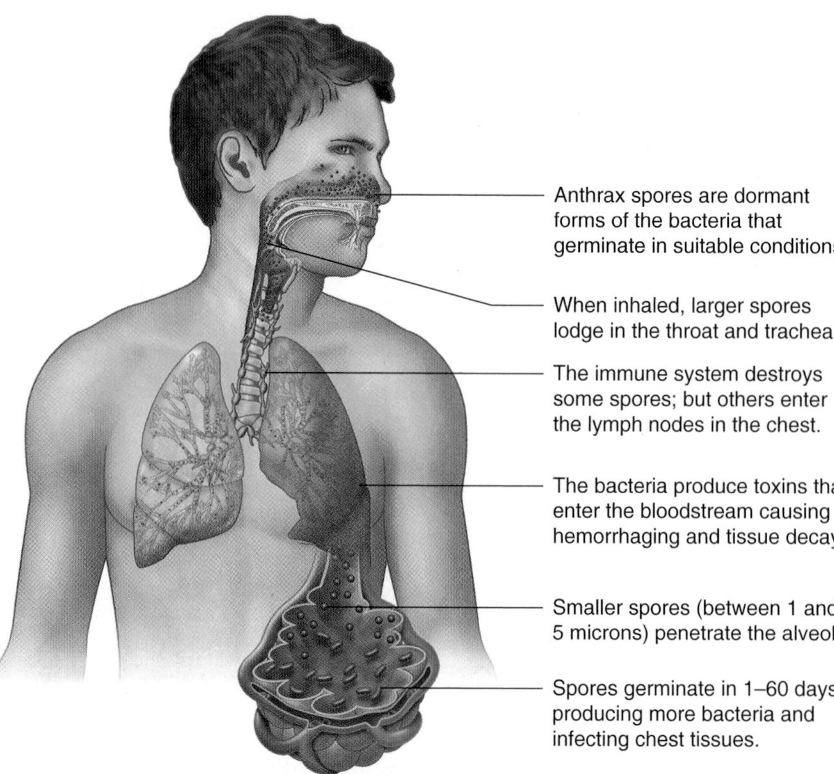
Anthrax spores are dormant forms of the bacteria that germinate in suitable conditions.
When inhaled, larger spores lodge in the throat and trachea.
The immune system destroys some spores; but others enter the lymph nodes in the chest.
The bacteria produce toxins that enter the bloodstream causing hemorrhaging and tissue decay.
Smaller spores (between 1 and 5 microns) penetrate the alveoli.
Spores germinate in 1–60 days, producing more bacteria and infecting chest tissues.

Figure 52.4 ■ The pathogenesis of inhalation anthrax.

at 1 month, 6 months, and 1 year; and annual boosters after that. The vaccine is recommended for prophylaxis only and not for treatment of patients with active disease.

If an exposure is known to have occurred, treatment for both adults and children includes prophylaxis with the vaccine with the initial injection and repeat doses at 2 and 4 weeks in addition to 60 days of antibiotic administration.[6] Current antibiotic recommendations are oral doxycycline or quinolone (ciprofloxacin or levofloxacin).

Once overt inhalational disease has developed, treatment involves multiple antibiotic administration and aggressive intensive and respiratory care.[4] In addition, two antitoxins are now available that help to prevent the protective antigen from facilitating the entry of edema factor and lethal factor into cells and could be used for both prophylaxis and treatment after exposure.[4] Treatment of cutaneous anthrax involves single antibiotic administration.

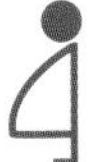

Pregnant women who contract cutaneous anthrax have high rates of maternal and fetal death.[3] ■

James Jerome: Outcome

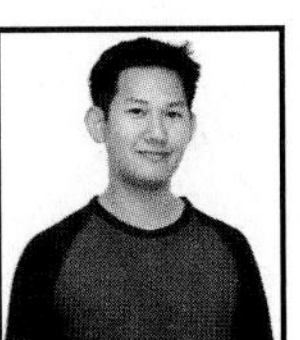

Over the course of the next 24 hours, Mr. Jerome's condition deteriorates. His oxygen saturation decreases to 84%, and he has to undergo endotracheal intubation and is placed on mechanical ventilation. The public health department investigation reveals that some threats had been made against Mr. Jerome's office and that all of the sick coworkers had similar symptoms. The public health department agrees with the concern about anthrax exposure and infection. The laboratory evaluation eventually confirms the presence of anthrax bacilli in the cultures and that the bacteria are susceptible to the antibiotics that were selected. In addition, the Centers for Disease Control and Prevention makes the antitoxin available, and a dose is administered to Mr. Jerome. Over the next several days, Mr. Jerome shows gradual improvement. Unfortunately, several of his coworkers are not as fortunate, and two die of the disease. The criminal investigation into the source of the bacteria and the identity of the perpetrator continues.

7. What preventive strategies could have been used to reduce the level of impact of this exposure?
8. What other activities should the public health department perform during this time period?
9. Which oral antibiotics could be used during the initial response to an inhalational anthrax exposure?

Plague

Plague can present in several ways, depending on the route of infection. Plague is the famous "Black Death" that resulted in the death of 20–30 million people in 1346. Plague is caused by the *Yersinia pestis* bacteria.[1,3,9] Naturally occurring plague is carried by fleas and rodents and is found across the United States west of the Mississippi River and around the world. In fact, there is an average of 6–10 cases of plague annually in the United States. Plague has been weaponized for military use, and it is estimated that a release of 110 pounds as an aerosol over a city of 5 million could result in 150,000 cases of plague, resulting in 36,000 deaths.

Etiology and Pathogenesis

Naturally occurring plague results when an individual is bitten by a flea that became infected with plague after it bit an infected animal, typically a prairie dog or other rodent.[1,9] When the flea bites a human, it regurgitates some of its stomach contents, which contain the plague bacteria, into the bite. The bacteria then travel through the lymphatic system to the regional lymph nodes, where they are attacked by white blood cells and phagocytes attempting to defend against the infection. The white blood cells are usually successful in destroying the plague bacteria; however, those that are ingested by phagocytes multiply, destroy the phagocyte, and are released. This process results in enlargement and eventually necrosis of the lymph nodes. This is known as **bubonic plague** (a bubo is a swollen lymph node). Symptoms of infection typically occur within 2–8 days of the flea bite.

Two other forms of plague may occur after exposure: pneumonic plague and septicemic plague.[9] Intentional or terrorist exposure could involve an aerosolized release of plague bacteria which ensures that the pathogen would be inhaled, thus causing **pneumonic plague**. Pneumonic plague can also result from inhaling the respiratory droplets from an infected animal or person. Pulmonary infection with plague results in edema in the alveoli of the lungs and marked pulmonary congestion. Symptoms begin within 1–6 days of exposure, and if treatment is delayed, death results 2–6 days after respiratory symptoms develop.[3]

Septicemic plague can be either primary or secondary. In the primary form of the disease, the bacteria enter the circulatory system directly from the lymphatic system, leading to a sepsis syndrome with multiple organ failure and shock. The secondary form of septicemic plague can result from either the bubonic or pneumonic form of the disease when bacteria enter the circulation (**Figure 52.5** ■).

Clinical Manifestations

Regardless of the mode of exposure, the initial presentation of the patient with plague is the same. As with anthrax (and most other biologic agents), the patient develops a flulike syndrome with high fever, chills, headache, and malaise.[1,3,9]

When plague is caused by the bite of an infected flea, the incubation period is 2–8 days, during which time the patient will present with flulike complaints. There may also be vomiting and abdominal pain. Then, within a day or two, acutely swollen lymph nodes (buboes) in the neck, groin, and axillae will be noted (see **Figure 52.6** ■). The location of the buboes depends on the site of the flea bite; lower extremity bites lead to inguinal buboes, upper extremity bites cause axillary buboes, and bites of the head and neck result in cervical buboes. Approximately 10% of patients with bubonic plague will develop secondary pneumonic plague, with chest pain, dyspnea, cough, and hemoptysis. Bubonic plague has a fatality rate greater than 50% if the disease is not recognized and immediately treated. Cases of untreated bubonic exposure can progress to systemic illness and death with a fatality rate of almost 100%. With prompt treatment, however, the death rate associated with bubonic plague decreases to less than 5%.

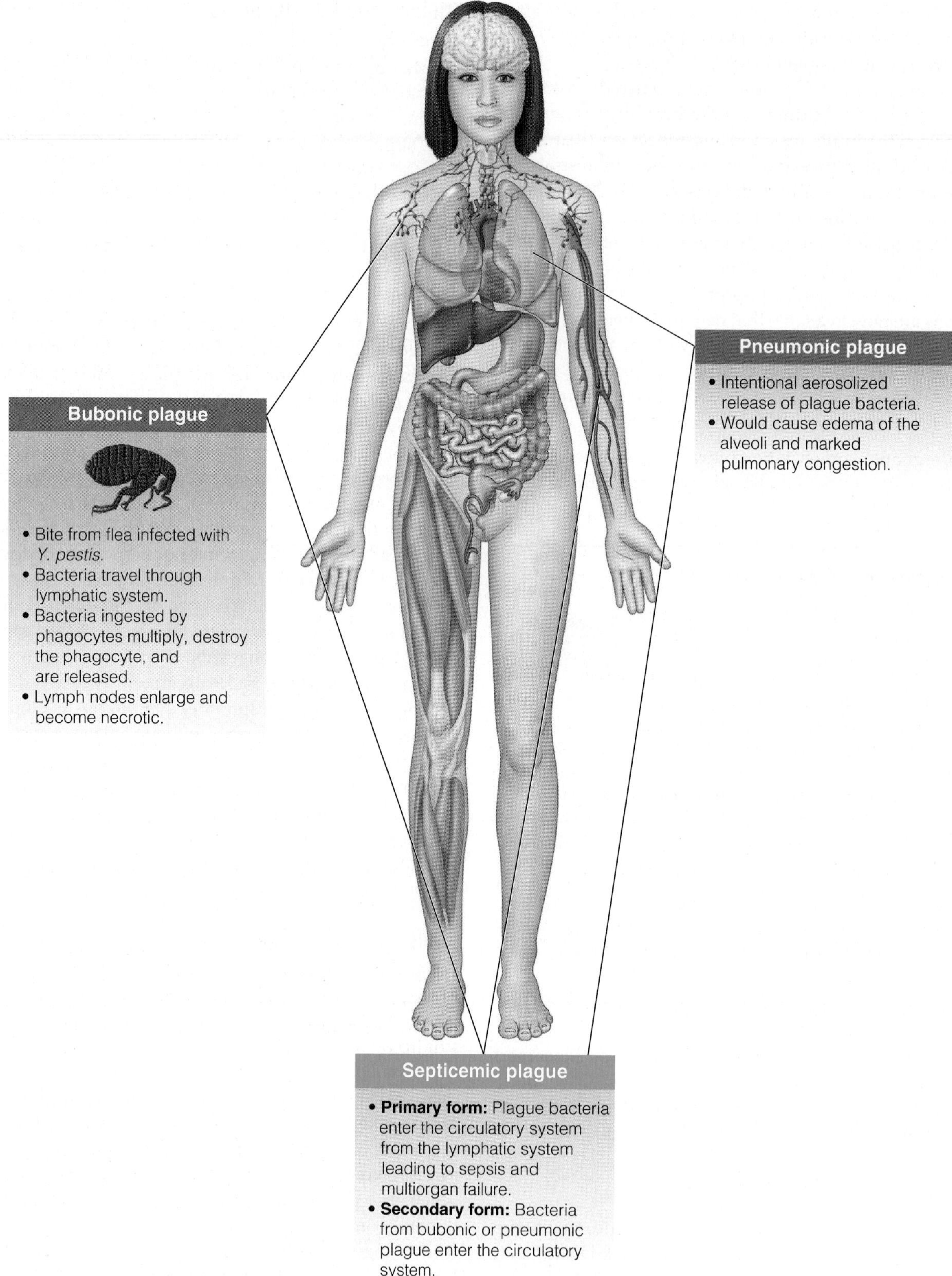

Pneumonic plague
• Intentional aerosolized release of plague bacteria.
• Would cause edema of the alveoli and marked pulmonary congestion.
Bubonic plague
• Bite from flea infected with Y. pestis.
• Bacteria travel through lymphatic system.
• Bacteria ingested by phagocytes multiply, destroy the phagocyte, and are released.
• Lymph nodes enlarge and become necrotic.
Septicemic plague
• Primary form: Plague bacteria enter the circulatory system from the lymphatic system leading to sepsis and multiorgan failure.
• Secondary form: Bacteria from bubonic or pneumonic plague enter the circulatory system.

Figure 52.5 ■ Syndromes produced by plague infection.

Intentional or terrorist exposures to plague would be delivered as an aerosol inhaled by the exposed victim, causing pneumonic plague.[1,3,9] The incubation period is shorter; symptoms develop within 1–2 days. Patients will present with fever, cough, chest pain, and dyspnea with bloody or watery sputum.[3,9] They may also have nausea, vomiting, diarrhea, and abdominal pain. Buboes are typically not seen. Without prompt treatment (within 24–48 hours of symptom onset), the mortality rate approaches 100%. Of particular importance is the fact that, unlike anthrax,

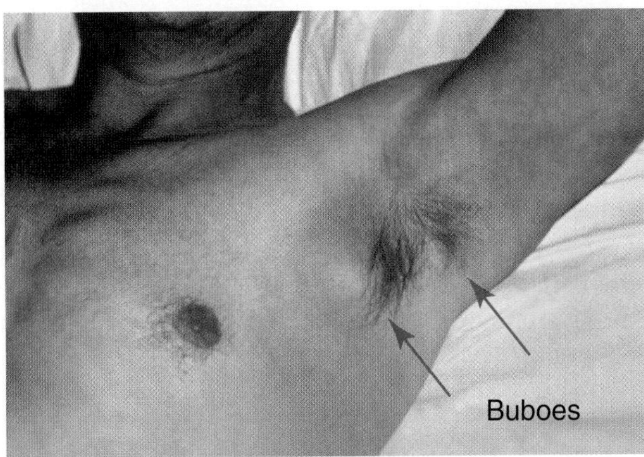

Figure 52.6 ■ A man with bubonic plague and two buboes in the axilla.

pneumonic plague is transmissible from person to person. Therefore, appropriate infection control precautions must be taken in evaluating and treating these patients.

In the pneumonic and septicemic forms of the disease, the spread of plague through the body can lead to obstruction of the small blood vessels of parts of the body and necrosis of areas of skin and distal locations such as the fingers, toes, ears, and nose. Medically, this is referred to as acral necrosis. In medieval Europe, this disease was called the Black Death in reference to these areas of dead tissue (see **Figure 52.7** ■).

Linking Pathophysiology to Diagnosis and Treatment

Antimicrobial treatment and supportive therapy are the cornerstones of treatment for infected patients. Prompt initiation of antibiotic treatment is essential if death is to be avoided. Recommended antibiotics for both adult and pediatric patients include streptomycin, gentamycin, ciprofloxacin, levofloxacin, doxycycline, and chloramphenicol.[3,9] Prophylactic treatment with doxycycline or ciprofloxacin is recommended for anyone who has had unprotected contact with infected individuals or exposure to an intentional release of the bacteria.

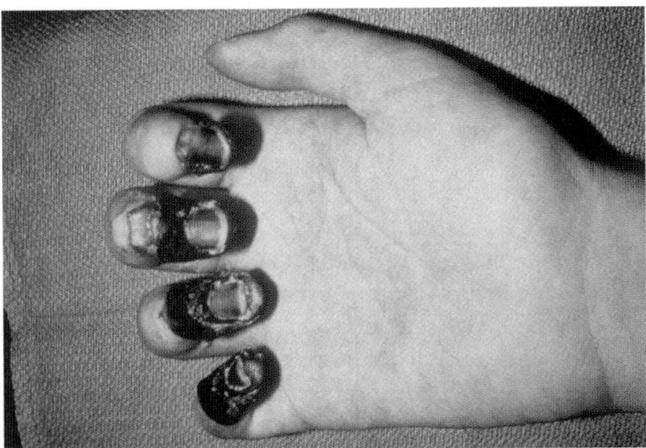

Figure 52.7 ■ Acral gangrene resulting from systemic plague infection.

A number of vaccines have been developed in an effort to prevent plague infection. Unfortunately, to date, none of them have been proven to be particularly efficacious. Given the short incubation period and long time required for immunity to develop after vaccination, there appears to be limited utility for a vaccine in an acute plague incident.[9]

Smallpox

Smallpox has been known to exist for over 3000 years. Thanks to an intensive global vaccination effort, naturally occurring smallpox disease was declared eradicated in 1977.[1,3] However, at least two samples of the smallpox virus still exist in laboratories. One is located at the Centers for Disease Control and Prevention (CDC) in the United States, and the other is in Russia. The former Soviet Union was suspected of weaponizing smallpox in 1980, and there is concern that this virus may have changed hands when the Soviet Union came apart.

Before being eradicated, smallpox had a mortality rate of approximately 30–50%.[1,3] The disease is highly contagious and can be transmitted by becoming airborne from coughing or sneezing patients or as a surface contaminant spread by clothing and linens.[1–3]

Etiology and Pathogenesis

Smallpox is caused by the variola virus. There are two varieties that have been named on the basis of the severity of the infection they produce: variola major (30% mortality) and variola minor (1% mortality).[1,3] Viruses related to smallpox include monkeypox, cowpox, and vaccinia, which can all infect humans.

The virus typically infects by entering through the oropharynx and infecting the mucous membranes, although it can also enter through the skin or the conjunctiva of the eye. The virus has a 7- to 17-day incubation period before symptoms arise. During this time, the virus first spreads to the regional lymph nodes, where it propagates itself. After about 4 days, it spreads further to other lymph nodes, the spleen, and bone marrow. Approximately 1 week after infection, the virus spreads systemically, and the initial symptoms of fever, chills, headache, and vomiting (flulike syndrome) develop. The virus then localizes in the small blood vessels of the skin, where it causes full-thickness damage by creating vesicles and pustules that heal over the course of the next several weeks by scarring the skin.

Clinical Manifestations

Twelve to 14 days after exposure and infection, the patient will present with fever, malaise, headache, and a backache. Once the fever develops, the patient is considered infectious. Within a day or two, this is followed by the development of a maculopapular rash that begins in the oral mucosa, quickly progressing to a generalized skin rash with round, tense vesicles and pustules. One of the means of distinguishing smallpox from chickenpox is that lesions associated with chickenpox start and are more densely populated

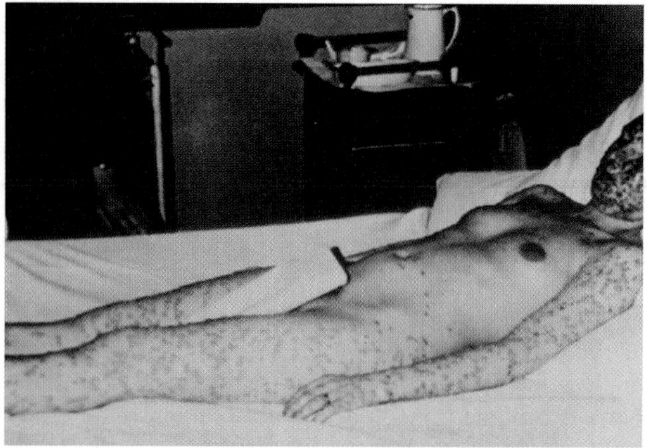

Figure 52.8 ■ A woman with characteristic smallpox lesions.

on the trunk with lesions in various stages of development. In smallpox, the lesions are usually more densely situated on the head and shoulders with uniform development (**Figure 52.8** ■). In addition, smallpox lesions often involve the palms of the hands and the soles of the feet, whereas chickenpox does not.

Linking Pathophysiology to Diagnosis and Treatment

Smallpox is highly contagious, being spread primarily by droplets in coughs and sneezes. Contact infection can also occur, and there is some evidence for airborne spread. Therefore, full infection control precautions—including airborne, droplet, and contact—must be used in dealing with these patients.[1,3] Patients with smallpox should be kept in isolation from other patients. It would be wise to limit the treatment team to individuals who have previously been vaccinated.

Treatment for smallpox is primarily supportive. Because the patient can have large fluid shifts into the developing vesicles, maintaining proper hydration is important. The skin lesions can be quite painful, so provision of analgesia as necessary is required. Skin care is also important, as the lesions can become secondarily infected with bacteria. The administration of antiviral medications to treat smallpox holds some promise for the future. However, since smallpox no longer occurs as a natural disease, there is no experience with these medications to determine how effective they will prove to be if used.

Prevention of smallpox is the mainstay of care if a smallpox outbreak should occur. The smallpox vaccine, which actually uses the vaccinia virus, if given within 4 days of exposure to smallpox, is generally effective in preventing or reducing the severity of the disease, given the rather long incubation period of smallpox.[1,3]

Toxins

Toxins are naturally occurring chemicals produced by biologic agents such as bacteria or plants that cause illness or injury when taken internally.[10,11] The naturally occurring toxins are in many cases much more dangerous than any of the human-made chemicals. The good news about toxins (if there is any good news) is that, with very rare exceptions, they are not transmissible from person to person and are not absorbed through intact skin.

The bacterium *Clostridium botulinum* produces the most toxic substance known. The botulinum toxin is 15,000 times more toxic than the nerve agent VX and 100,000 times more toxic than the nerve agent sarin. There are three natural occurring forms of botulism: wound, food-borne, and intestinal.[3] Wound botulism results when the bacteria enter a dirty wound or are injected during illicit drug use and then produce the toxin; food-borne botulism comes from improperly prepared or home-canned foods in which the bacteria grow and produce toxin; and intestinal botulism, which is rare and more common in infants, occurs when the bacteria are ingested, colonize the intestine, and then produce the toxin. The weaponized delivery of botulism would result from either inhalation of aerosolized botulinum toxin or ingestion of food that has intentionally been contaminated with the toxin.[3] Finally, an extremely rare and unusual method of exposure to botulinum toxin would be inadvertent overdose with Botox, a commercial form of botulinum toxin that is used medically for a variety of indications.

Infant botulism, first described in 1976, is the most common presentation of botulism in the United States, with about 100 cases annually. Sources of infant botulism may include raw honey, soil and dust from construction sites, and items found in various infant foods such as powdered milk, cereal, and corn syrup.[4] ■

Ricin is a protein that is produced in the seeds of the castor oil plant and as a by-product of processing castor beans into castor oil. Natural exposure to ricin has occurred from eating castor beans, but it rarely leads to fatalities because of the small amount present in the beans. Weaponized ricin is known to have been used for at least one assassination and has been investigated for larger delivery systems, but it is not practical for large exposures. Ricin is effective by inhalation, ingestion, or injection.

Etiology and Pathogenesis

Botulinum toxin has eight slightly different subtypes, which have been labeled A through H.[3] Regardless of the route of exposure, botulism results when the toxin gets absorbed into the bloodstream and is carried to the nerves of the body. In all of its forms, botulinum toxin is a nerve agent that binds irreversibly with the neuromuscular junction, preventing the normal release of the neurotransmitter acetylcholine, bringing about a descending flaccid paralysis.

To understand how the toxin works, a review of normal neurologic function is appropriate. When a neural impulse is transmitted down a nerve cell, it reaches the end of the neuron, where acetylcholine is released to cross the synaptic gap and stimulate the target receptor. Once the desired effect has occurred, acetylcholinesterase is released to break down the acetylcholine and stop any further stimulation of the target receptor. Botulinum toxin binds irreversibly with the end-plate of the neuron and prevents the release of acetylcholine. The target neurons for botulinum toxin are the ones that mostly innervate the muscles of the body. As a result, the victim develops paralysis. In contrast, ricin acts as a direct cellular poison that inhibits the synthesis of proteins with the cells. This leads to cellular death and necrosis of the involved tissues and organs.

Clinical Manifestations

The clinical symptoms and signs of botulism poisoning can come on within a few hours or a few days, depending on the dose of toxin received.[1,3] The patient first presents with multiple cranial nerve deficits, including diplopia (double vision), difficulty seeing, difficulty swallowing, and difficulty speaking.[3] The patient will complain of being fatigued from the gradually increasing muscle weakness. As the disease progresses, the patient can lose the gag reflex and suffer paralysis of the muscles that support ventilation, resulting in respiratory failure. The classic botulism triad is as follows:

- Descending flaccid paralysis
- Lack of fever
- A clear sensorium.

Symptoms and signs of ricin poisoning depend on the route of exposure and the organs involved. Inhalation of ricin causes sudden congestion of the upper air passages, including the nose and throat. The patient develops a necrotizing tracheitis and pneumonitis with severe pulmonary edema leading to death. Ingestion of ricin results in acute onset of nausea, vomiting, diarrhea, and abdominal pain with subsequent ulceration and necrosis of gastrointestinal structures. Injection of ricin causes pain at the site of injection, followed by liver and renal failure.

Linking Pathophysiology to Diagnosis and Treatment

Care of both adult and pediatric patients with botulism is administration of the botulinum antitoxin, which is available from the CDC, and supportive care, particularly as it relates to the patient's respiratory status. The antitoxin is a heptavalent product that will inactivate the toxin from the A–G subtypes.[3] No antidote is known for subtype H. The progression of respiratory muscle weakness can be gradual and requires careful monitoring; many patients will require endotracheal intubation and mechanical ventilation to support their breathing. Because the toxin binds irreversibly with the neurons, the administration of antitoxin does not reverse neurologic effects that have already developed, but it prevents further progression of the symptoms. Existing neurologic deficits will resolve only when the neurons generate new nerve endings. This regenerative process can take weeks to several months.

Management of patients with ricin poisoning is purely supportive care. Victims of ricin inhalation require ventilatory support. Patients who ingested ricin are treated with activated charcoal and intravenous fluid and electrolyte replacement. Victims who were injected with ricin require symptomatic support.

Check Your Progress: Section 52.2

1. What is a differential sign or symptom between exposure to a biologic agent and exposure to a toxin?
2. You are evaluating a 5-year-old girl who presents with a fever, nausea and vomiting during the past 36 hours, and a painful rash on her chest and arms. Her mother reports that the girl had not been immunized for childhood diseases. What could be causing her presentation?
3. An 8-month-old infant is short of breath and is drooling but has no fever. While he is awake, his arms and legs appear to be limp. During history taking, the mother indicates that she had been feeding him a mixture of raw honey and herbs to help build his immune system. What might you suspect?

52.3 Chemical Agents

Patients can be exposed to chemical agents in intentional terrorist events, but exposure occurs more commonly in the manufacture, transport, and legitimate use of dangerous chemicals.[1,12–14]

Nerve Agents

Originally developed as insecticides, nerve agents had a surge in development as weapons during the early and mid-1900s once it became clear that they were as effective on humans as on insects. Nerve agents now can be found in military stockpiles all over the world.[12–14] Examples of nerve agent use in modern times include a release in the Tokyo subway system in 1995[1] and use in the Syrian civil war in 2013 and again in 2017. The nerve agents fall into two categories: G agents and V agents.[1,14] The G agents were developed in Germany; the V agents were first developed in Great Britain. An important difference between these two groups of nerve agents is how long they persist once released. The G agents are considered nonpersistent, meaning that they disperse readily. The V agents are oily in consistency and therefore persist much longer.

The G agents include GA (**tabun**), GB (sarin), GD (**soman**), and GF (cyclosarin). Of this group of chemicals, sarin is the most volatile. The V agents include VE, VG, VM, and VX. These agents can kill at very low dosages and are usually delivered as a vapor. Even a drop of VX the size of a head of a pin on the skin surface could result in death.

Etiology and Pathogenesis

The nerve agents are all liquids with varying degrees of volatility. When they volatilize, they turn into a vapor. Thus, the nerve agents pose a risk from both dermal contact and inhalation.

Nerve agents work by blocking the action of the enzyme acetylcholinesterase.[1,13,14] This enzyme is necessary to inhibit the action of acetylcholine, a neurotransmitter that stimulates cholinergic receptors, many of which are found in smooth and skeletal muscles and glands. If acetylcholine is not inactivated, the result is overstimulation of the receptor organs.

There are two types of acetylcholine receptors: muscarinic and nicotinic. The effect of overstimulation of the muscarinic receptors, which are mostly secretory organs and smooth muscles in the body, can be remembered by the mnemonic DUMBELS:

Diarrhea
Urination
Miosis
Bradycardia
Emesis
Lacrimation
Salivation.

Stimulation of the nicotinic receptors, which represent autonomic nervous system and voluntary muscle effects, will cause another set of symptoms captured by the mnemonic MTWHF:

Mydriasis
Tachycardia
Weakness
Hypertension/hyperglycemia
Fasciculations.

Clinical Manifestations

Clinical manifestations depend on the route of exposure and dose.[1,13,14] Inhalation of nerve agent typically causes symptoms within seconds to minutes, whereas with dermal exposure, the onset of symptoms can take as long as 18 hours. In small amounts, vapor exposure results in irritation to the eyes, nose, and airways. Marked secretions including salivation and bronchorrhea along with urination and diarrhea are seen with larger doses. Bronchospasm can occur and may be quite severe, mimicking a critical asthma attack. Loss of consciousness, seizures, apnea, and muscular flaccidity will result from inhalation of large doses. Liquid exposure on the skin typically results in localized sweating and muscle fasciculations at the site of exposure. With larger exposures, gastrointestinal symptoms develop; with severe exposure, seizures, loss of consciousness, and respiratory arrest occur.

Linking Pathophysiology to Diagnosis and Treatment

Contamination of an individual with nerve agent poses a serious risk of secondary contamination of rescuers and healthcare providers. Clothing that may have been contaminated with any nerve agent should be removed and appropriately secured. Victims need to be decontaminated with copious washing with water before they can be cared for. Dilute bleach solution, which is commonly recommended as a decontamination solution, is not really necessary, and attempts to prepare it only delay the decontamination effort. Once decontamination has been accomplished, a primary assessment is performed, antidotes are administered, and supportive therapy is provided. The effect of nerve agents on the airways and breathing may make it difficult to assist ventilations, and the patient is likely to need frequent suctioning for the copious secretions and may require endotracheal intubation and positive pressure mechanical ventilation.

The effects of nerve agents can largely be reversed with the administration of antidote.[1,13,14] There are three drugs that are useful:

- Atropine is an anticholinergic medication that will reverse most of the muscarinic effects. It is used to help dry up the secretions, particularly those in the pulmonary system, and to help relieve the bronchospasm that occurs. It is given in 2-mg doses that are repeated until the oral and bronchial secretions dry up and ventilation is eased. Dosages are adjusted accordingly for pediatric patients.
- Pralidoxime chloride (2-PAM chloride) uncouples the bond between the nerve agent and acetylcholinesterase, reactivating the enzyme, thus reducing the effect of the nerve agent on the nicotinic receptors. Of note, the bond between the nerve agent and acetylcholinesterase will be become permanent over time. This is referred to as *aging*. Once aging has occurred, pralidoxime will no longer be effective. The amount of time necessary for aging depends on the particular nerve agent used. For sarin, the bond becomes permanent in approximately 5–6 hours; for both tabun and VX, aging occurs after about 40 hours; for soman, the bond is fixed in 2 minutes.
- Diazepam (Valium) is used to control seizures and limit brain injury. Intravenous delivery is preferred, since intramuscular injection is subject to erratic absorption of the medication.

All three of these medications are available as autoinjectors, thus speeding the time to administration of the antidote and minimizing the need to draw up the medication or calculate a dosage.

Vesicants

Vesicants, also referred to as blister agents, have been stockpiled by military forces around the world since World War I. Sulfur mustard (mustard gas) is an example of this type of agent that has been in use since World War I. It was used by Iraq against the Kurds in 1980, during the Iran–Iraq war of the mid-1980s, and by the terrorist organization Islamic State against the residents of Aleppo, Syria, in 2015. An oily, clear to yellow-brown liquid, sulfur mustard can be aerosolized in a bomb blast or sprayed. It has low volatility and can persist on surfaces for a week or more. Lewisite, another vesicant, has effects similar to those of sulfur mustard but a much quicker onset of symptoms.[1,13]

Etiology and Pathogenesis

Sulfur mustard is absorbed through the skin and mucous membranes, causing cell damage within 3–5 minutes of contact.[1,13,15–17] Unfortunately, the onset of symptoms of exposure is delayed and may take as little as 1 hour or as many as 12 hours but usually occurs within 4–6 hours. Therefore, victims may not be aware of their exposure and the need for decontamination for quite some time.[1] By the time symptoms develop, the damage from the sulfur mustard has already occurred. Moist areas of the body are where sulfur mustard will often concentrate and facilitate absorption, so the mucous membranes, groin, and axillary regions of the body are areas of particular concern. Sulfur mustard acts by damaging cellular DNA. This DNA damage is of particular concern in tissues of the body that have rapidly dividing cells, such as the bone marrow.

Lewisite is a vesicant developed by the United States during World War I that was never actually used. Unlike sulfur mustard, Lewisite causes symptoms immediately on exposure. It also does not have the bone marrow effects of sulfur mustard.[13]

Clinical Manifestations

The injury caused by either sulfur mustard or Lewisite is similar in nature to a burn of the exposed tissues. Manifestations can be found in the eyes, skin, and upper airways and range from mild erythema to edema and full thickness necrosis, depending on the amount of exposure.[15–17] In high doses, exposure to sulfur mustard can cause nausea, vomiting, and bone marrow suppression. Lewisite, unlike sulfur mustard, does not cause the bone marrow depression.

Linking Pathophysiology to Diagnosis and Treatment

There are no antidotes for sulfur mustard, so care is primarily supportive.[1,13] Of particular importance is the role of decontamination (**Figure 52.9** ■). While decontamination will not change the course of the illness experienced by the exposed individual, since the cellular DNA damage occurs within a few minutes of exposure, it will prevent contamination of responders and healthcare providers who come into contact with the victim. The skin damage mimics that of a thermal burn; therefore, care of the patient to minimize the risk of secondary infection is important.[17]

Lewisite, unlike sulfur mustard, does have an antidote: British Anti-Lewisite (BAL or dimercaprol). BAL binds to the arsenic molecule in the Lewisite to help diminish its toxic effects. As with sulfur mustard, decontamination should occur as soon as possible. Care is primarily supportive with the subsequent administration of BAL.

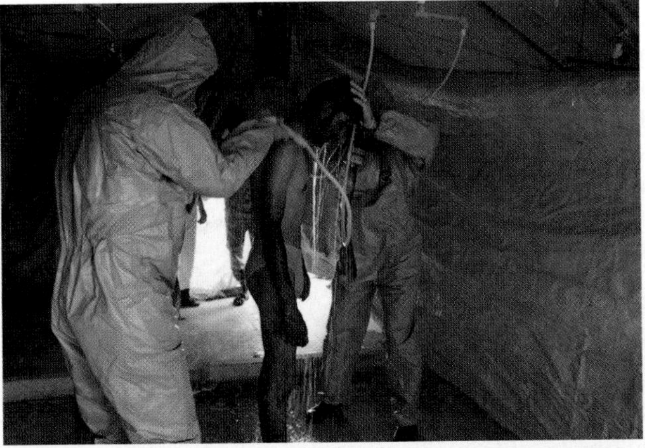

Figure 52.9 ■ A resident of Aleppo, Syria, is decontaminated after a mustard gas attack by terrorists on September 1, 2015.

Pulmonary Agents

The pulmonary agents are a group of chemicals that all produce direct irritation of and corrosive effects on the moist tissue surfaces with which they come into contact.[1,12,13,18] The primary chemicals in this class are chlorine, **anhydrous ammonia**, and phosgene. While many of these chemicals can be and have been used as weapons, they are far more commonly encountered in industry and manufacturing processes.[12] In fact, large quantities of these chemicals are transported daily on our highways and railways. In addition, riot control agents such as tear gas (CS) and pepper spray fall into this category, but they have little corrosive effect. Riot control agents are solid chemicals that are aerosolized to produce the sensation of burning in the eyes, nose, mouth, and airways and a feeling of chest tightness. They typically do not result in any permanent damage.

Etiology and Pathogenesis

The pulmonary irritant chemicals constitute a diverse group of compounds:

- Chlorine is a gas that is cooled and compressed into a liquid for transport. When it is released, it quickly converts into a gas. When chlorine gas comes into contact with the moist mucous membranes and skin of the body, it will react to form hypochlorous and hydrochloric acid. The acid causes coagulation necrosis of the tissues with which it comes into contact. While the damage from exposure can be quite severe, the fact the injury is a coagulation necrosis helps to limit the degree of tissue penetration of the acid.
- Anhydrous ammonia is an extremely concentrated form of ammonia. As with chlorine, it is compressed into liquid form into the transport containers and readily converts into a gas when released. It has no water in it (anhydrous) but when water is added or when it comes into contact with the moist mucous membranes and skin of the body, it reacts quickly, forming ammonium hydroxide, which is a strong alkali or base and highly caustic. When ammonium hydroxide comes into contact with human tissue, it causes liquefaction necrosis of the tissues. This process allows the ammonium hydroxide to penetrate deeply into tissues.
- Phosgene is a chemical that is widely used in the manufacture of plastics and pesticides.[18] Like chlorine and ammonia, phosgene is cooled and compressed into liquid form for transport. It also readily converts into a gas once it is released. Phosgene reacts with the moisture in mucous membranes to form hydrochloric acid.

The site of action of these chemicals depends in large part on the degree to which they are soluble in water.[1,12,13] Ammonia is highly water soluble, chlorine is moderately water soluble, and phosgene is slightly water soluble. Therefore, ammonia will react quickly with the moisture in the nose and upper air passageways. Chlorine, being less soluble, will be able to penetrate deeper into the respiratory tract and will affect both upper and lower pulmonary structures. Phosgene, the least water soluble, will penetrate deeply into the lungs and alveoli and cause damage at that level. Phosgene will cause damage to the alveolar–capillary membrane, and large amounts of fluid will leak into the alveoli from the circulatory system, producing noncardiogenic pulmonary edema. The amount of fluid lost via the lungs can be substantial, leading to volume depletion and signs of hypovolemia.

Clinical Manifestations

The symptoms and signs of exposure to the pulmonary irritants depend in large part on the water solubility of the chemical. Those that are highly water soluble, such as ammonia, will cause symptoms very quickly, mostly in the upper air passages. The victim will note a burning sensation of the mucous membranes and conjunctivae, there will be copious mucus production and rhinorrhea, and upper airway swelling may occur along with stridor and hoarseness. Chemicals such as chlorine that are less water soluble will affect both the upper airways, with findings similar to those of ammonia, and also the lower airways, producing bronchial irritation and wheezing. Dermal contact with both of these chemicals can lead to tissue necrosis. Phosgene, which is the least water soluble, will penetrate deeply into the lungs. Because it is poorly soluble, the onset of symptoms is often delayed as much as 24 hours. Phosgene will cause bronchospasm and give an asthma-like presentation with wheezing, and the alveolar injury will result in diffuse rales. The noncardiogenic pulmonary edema can result in the production of large amounts of pink, frothy sputum.

The riot control agents all result in a similar clinical presentation. They will cause a sense of burning in all exposed mucous membranes and the conjunctivae. The burning sensation in the eyes will lead to blepharospasm (tight closing of the eyelids). In addition, they cause profound tearing (lacrimation) and secretions in the nose (rhinorrhea) and salivation. Fortunately, life-threatening complications and permanent injury are extremely rare and usually result from exacerbation of underlying disease processes, particularly pulmonary problems such as asthma.

Kasey Robinson: Application

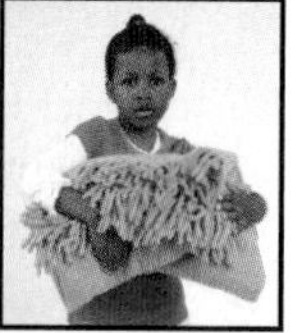

On arrival at the emergency department, Kasey is noted to have both eyes tightly closed with profuse tearing coming from both eyes. When she is asked to open her eyes, the conjunctivae in both eyes are markedly injected and red. She has some mild erythema of the skin of her face along with a runny nose. Examination of her lungs reveals that both of them are clear without any wheezes, rhonchi, or rales. The remainder of her physical exam is unremarkable. Within several minutes of entering the room with Kasey, you note the onset of mild burning in both of your eyes along with some rhinorrhea.

4. Given your developing signs and symptoms, what should you do next?
5. What is the likelihood that Kasey's condition will worsen?
6. What is course of treatment for Kasey?

Linking Pathophysiology to Diagnosis and Treatment

Because the effects of the pulmonary agents relate to ongoing exposure and inhalation of the toxic gases, the most important initial action is to remove the patient from the location and source of the exposure. Clothes that have been contaminated with any of the chemicals should be removed and appropriately discarded. Skin that came into contact with these chemicals should be copiously washed and irrigated. Exposure to ammonia, given its mechanism of action of liquefaction necrosis, requires prolonged washing and irrigation. Eyes must be irrigated for a minimum of 15 minutes and then be checked with pH paper to ensure restoration of a normal pH.

There is no specific treatment for the respiratory symptoms beyond symptomatic support.[1,12,13] If the patient demonstrates signs of hypoxia and respiratory failure, supplemental oxygen and ventilatory support, including endotracheal intubation and mechanical ventilation, will be required. Bronchospasm is treated in standard fashion with inhaled beta agonists.

The primary treatment for exposure to the riot control chemicals is time. The effects of these agents typically wear off between 15 and 60 minutes after exposure. If the symptoms are severe, irrigation of the eyes and skin may help to reduce some of the symptoms.

Kasey Robinson: Outcome

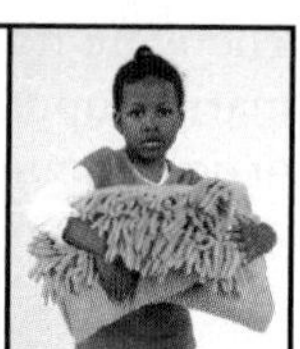

Realizing that your symptoms of exposure to the riot control agent are likely due to some residual contamination on Kasey's clothing and skin, you immediately cut off Kasey's clothing and double-bag it. You first anesthetize both Kasey's eyes and then gently irrigate them to help reduce the irritation. You then take Kasey to the shower room to wash off her skin. You observe her for the next 2 hours and note that her symptoms resolve. After a total of 2 hours, she is discharged home with her parents.

7. If Kasey had been exposed to a more significant pulmonary irritant such as phosgene, what signs and symptoms would you expect to see?
8. What other class of agent could cause excessive tearing in the eyes, among other more serious symptoms?
9. If one of these nerve agents was involved, what medications could be used to treat the symptoms?

Asphyxiants

Asphyxiants are chemicals that interfere with oxygen transport or metabolism in the body. Simple asphyxiants replace oxygen in the air that is inhaled, thus effectively making the exposed victim hypoxic. Systemic asphyxiants interfere with the transport of oxygen by hemoglobin or with its use in cellular metabolism, specifically in the cytochrome system of mitochondria, interfering with cellular energy production.

Etiology and Pathogenesis

Cyanide is an example of a systemic asphyxiant. Cyanide poisoning can result from exposure to chemicals such as hydrogen cyanide or cyanogen chloride.[1,13] Cyanide toxicity can result from either inhalation or ingestion, either as a result of intentional exposure or accidentally from such incidents as fires involving combustion of common items such as carpets, plastics, insulation, home furnishings, and a variety of other products.[19]

The mitochondria of every cell are the energy-producing structures. They will use glucose and oxygen and metabolize them via the Krebs cycle to make ATP, which stores energy for use in all other cellular processes. When the cyanide is introduced, the cyanide binds with cytochrome a3 in the mitochondria and prevents the use of oxygen. This interrupts aerobic metabolism and leads to anaerobic metabolism. Oxygen is no longer being extracted from the hemoglobin in the red blood cells for energy production. As a result, lactic acid accumulates, leading to a metabolic acidosis.

Clinical Manifestations

The clinical findings of cyanide poisoning relate to the fact that the patient has become functionally hypoxic at the cellular level, even though the blood is fully saturated with oxygen. Therefore, the initial response will be to increase respirations to try to get more oxygen to the cells. At the same time, the cardiovascular system will respond by increasing the heart rate and blood pressure. With lower doses of cyanide, the victim may complain of headache, anxiety, weakness, lightheadedness, vertigo, and ataxia. At larger doses, the patient will progress rapidly (in some cases in as little as 20–30 seconds) to convulsions, muscle rigidity with opisthotonus and trismus, decerebrate posturing, respiratory depression and arrest (1–2 minutes), and cardiac dysrhythmias, including bradycardia, hypotension, and finally cardiac arrest.

Linking Pathophysiology to Diagnosis and Treatment

The key to the diagnosis of cyanide exposure is to recognize that the patient is manifesting signs of profound oxygen deficit even though blood taken for laboratory studies appears bright red in color. This is because the exposed victim, in reality, has more than adequate amounts of oxygen in the blood but simply cannot use it at the cellular level.

Treatment is aimed at removing the cyanide. Fortunately, cyanide's binding with cytochrome a3 is not irreversible. There is an antidote that will remove cyanide from the cytochrome system and allow reactivation of energy production.[1,19,20] The antidote is hydroxocobalamin (Cyanokit), which is a precursor of vitamin B_{12}, given in a dose of 5 grams intravenously over 15 minutes. When hydroxocobalamin is administered, it combines with the cyanide to form cyanocobalamin, which is vitamin B_{12}, thus rendering the cyanide nontoxic.

Check Your Progress: Section 52.3

1. Certain nerve agents will affect nicotinic receptor sites. What signs and symptoms would you expect to see in a person who has been exposed to such a nerve agent?
2. How do pulmonary agents such as chlorine and anhydrous ammonia cause their effects?
3. Why do victims of cyanide poisoning appear to suffocate, even though there is plenty of oxygen in their bloodstream?

52.4 Radiologic and Nuclear Devices

Basics of Radiation

Radiation exposure results when matter gives off energy in the form of either high-speed particles or rays. This energy can be alpha or beta radiation, gamma rays, or neutrons. Regardless of the form the energy takes, it is capable of interacting with molecules in living cells to break down chemical bonds and displace electrons from atoms, resulting in chemical changes that can lead to short- and long-term damage to the body.

Effects of Ionizing Radiation on Humans

Alpha Radiation. Alpha particles are energized particles that are released from a radioactive source. They have a very limited ability to penetrate objects with which they come into contact and can be stopped by a single sheet of paper or a few inches of air. However, they do pose a risk to humans if they are inhaled or ingested into the body.

Beta Radiation. Beta particles are similar to electrons. They are lighter and smaller than alpha particles; as a result, they can penetrate more deeply into tissue. Beta particles will travel several feet in air and can be stopped by a thin sheet of metal or plastic or a block of wood.

Gamma Rays. Gamma rays are highly energized waves that travel at the speed of light, cover great distances, and have great penetration capability. To stop gamma rays, several feet of concrete or several inches of lead are needed.

Neutrons. Neutrons are extremely high-energy particles with marked penetration capability. Because they are so high energy, they can make target objects radioactive. Several feet of concrete, water, or lead are required to protect against neutron particles.

Radiation Doses

There are four ways in which radiation is measured that are related but vary in their reported units and effects:

- The radioactivity of a particular substance represents the amount of radiation being given off by the material and includes all of the various forms of radiation, including alpha, beta, gamma, x-rays, and neutrons. The amount of radioactivity is reported in curies (Ci) or becquerels (Bq).
- Exposure to radiation refers to the amount of radiation that is traveling through air and is measured in roentgens (R) or coulombs per kilogram (C/kg).
- The amount of radiation absorbed by a person exposed to a radioactive source is measured as the radiation absorbed dose (rad) or gray (Gy).
- The combination of the absorbed dose of radiation and its effect medically is the roentgen equivalent man (rem) or sievert (Sv).

From a practical perspective when dealing with these various measurements, 1 roentgen is the same as 1 rad, which, is the same as 1 rem. In addition, 100 rad = 1 gray, and 100 rem = 1 sievert.

Types of Radiation Exposure

An individual can be exposed to radioactive materials through irradiation, contamination, or incorporation.

Irradiation. Irradiation occurs when either part or all of the body is exposed to a radiation source and x-rays or gamma rays penetrate the exposed area. This is similar to getting an x-ray in a medical facility. In this instance, the radiation passed through the body but the exposed part does not become radioactive and does not pose any threat to subsequent healthcare providers who come into contact with the victim.

Contamination. Contamination refers to the deposition of radioactive material either on or in the victim. For example, if some radioactive material was included in a bomb that detonated, individuals near the site of explosion may get covered with dust and debris from the explosion. That dust and debris may be contaminated with some of the radioactive material, which is now on the victim's skin. In addition, if the individual breathes in or ingests some of the radioactive material or perhaps a piece of the radioactive material became a piece of shrapnel that was embedded in a victim, internal contamination can result.

Incorporation. Incorporation refers to the process of the cells of certain organs taking up the radioactive materials, incorporating them into the organ itself, and concentrating the radioactive material in the organ. This can lead to prolonged exposure of the organ and nearby anatomic structures to the radioactive material, leading to problems such as cancer in the future.

Dispersion of Radiation

Exposure to radiation can occur in a number of different ways, some intentional, some unintentional.

Simple Radiologic Device. Exposure via a simple radiologic device occurs when someone is exposed to a radioactive element or source. This method of exposure generally requires close proximity to the radiation source to receive larger doses of radiation.

Radiologic Dispersal Devices (Dirty Bomb). Explosions involving radiation and radioactive materials can take several forms. The easiest and one of significant national security concern is the radiologic dispersal device, also referred to as a dirty bomb. In this situation, a conventional explosive such as dynamite is combined with some radioactive material and then detonated. This will not result in a nuclear explosion but will disperse the radioactive material over a large area. From a health risk perspective, the likelihood of significant radiation exposure is quite small; the major effect will be psychologic, such as producing widespread panic. To expose large numbers of people to large doses of radiation, the detonation of either an improvised nuclear device or a formal nuclear bomb would be necessary. In either case, while radiation exposure would be a significant concern, the initial, overwhelming medical disaster would involve the thousands of victims who sustained thermal burns and trauma.

Nuclear Reactor Accident or Incident. Rare but not unheard of incidents involving nuclear reactor accidents and meltdowns can result in the release of large amounts of radiation and radioactive material.

Acute Radiation Syndrome

Acute radiation syndrome (ARS) is the spectrum of disorders that occur after exposure to radiation. ARS is also often referred to as radiation sickness. The onset of symptoms and the specific organ systems that are affected depend on the dose of radiation received as well as the time frame in which it was received. The tissues and cells most susceptible to the effects of radiation are those that are rapidly dividing and immature. However, damage to any and all tissues and organs of the body can result.

Etiology and Pathogenesis

Exposure to radiation, whether the energized particles or the energy waves, results in damage to cellular proteins, particularly DNA. In addition, free radicals are produced within the cells that lead to further damage. This damage may become manifest rapidly as cells die, or it may take weeks, months, or even years to become evident.

Clinical Manifestations

The clinical findings associated with radiation exposure follow a relatively predicable course and time frame. There are four phases of radiation sickness and four syndromes of disease:

1. *Prodrome:* The onset of this phase is related to the total dose of radiation and can begin minutes to hours after exposure. This phase is characterized by fever, nausea, vomiting, and anorexia. At doses below about 500 rads, it lasts approximately 2–4 days. At higher doses of radiation, this phase may be persistent with increasing severity.
2. *Latent:* This phase follows the prodromal phase and lasts for a few days to 2–3 weeks depending on the total dose of radiation. During this time, the patient typically looks and feels better. However, critical cell populations (leukocytes, platelets, and gastrointestinal cells) are decreasing as a result of radiation injury to the bone marrow and gastrointestinal tract.
3. *Illness:* In this phase of illness, the four primary disease syndromes manifest themselves:
   - *Hematologic:* This results from damage to the bone marrow. The marrow becomes suppressed, leading to decreased circulating white blood cells and platelets. This impairs the ability of the body to resist infection and also leads to hemorrhage.
   - *Gastrointestinal:* Radiation exposure leads to destruction of the gastrointestinal tract, resulting in nausea, vomiting, diarrhea, gastrointestinal hemorrhage, fluid and electrolyte disorders, and

opportunistic infection with gastrointestinal flora that can lead to sepsis and death.

- *Central nervous system:* Large doses of radiation will affect the brain and neural tissues, leading to cerebral edema, increased intracranial pressure, seizures, herniation, and death.
- *Cutaneous:* The effects of radiation on the skin include a burnlike appearance with erythema, skin blistering, hair loss, and possible full thickness necrosis.

4. *Recovery or death:* The ultimate outcome of the exposed victim depends on the total dose of radiation received, the organs damaged as a result, and the availability of critical care medical services and interventions. Even if the patient recovers from the acute illness phase, the patient must be monitored over many years for possible development of chronic problems such as radiation-related cancers.[21,22]

The dose effect of radiation exposure is summarized in **Table 52.1** ■.

Linking Pathophysiology to Diagnosis and Treatment

Because radiation affects tissues that are dividing rapidly, the onset of the prodrome is a clue to the severity of the exposure and the dose received. The faster that a patient develops nausea and vomiting, the more likely it is that a large dose of radiation was received. The onset of the prodrome also has implications as to likely survival; individuals whose symptoms begin more than 2 hours after exposure have a reasonable chance of surviving.

The effect of radiation of the bone marrow can also be followed to help determine the patient's prognosis. The bone marrow suppression will lead to a decrease in circulating lymphocytes. Depending on the extent to which the lymphocyte count falls over the first 48 hours after exposure, a reasonable estimate of survival can be made. Patients whose absolute lymphocyte count remains above 1200 are likely to survive, whereas those whose count falls below 300 are likely to die.

Treatment of radiation-exposed patients is focused on the effects of the radiation. Fluid and electrolyte balance must be maintained. Precautions against infection are key. A new class of medications called colony-stimulating factors has been developed in an attempt to stimulate the bone marrow to recover function and help promote the production of white blood cells. In addition, a number of steps can be taken to help minimize the risk of incorporation of radioactive materials in target organs and increase the likelihood of excreting the material. If the specific radioactive agent is identified, some medications are available to limit the uptake or facilitate the removal of the radioactive material.

Table 52.1 Dose Effect of Radiation Exposure

Radiation Dose (rad)	Onset of Nausea, Vomiting	Acute Radiation Syndrome Organ Systems Affected
1000	< 30 minutes	Hematologic, gastrointestinal, central nervous system
400	30 minutes to 2 hours	Hematologic
200	2–6 hours	Hematologic
50	> 6 hours	

Check Your Progress: Section 52.4

1. List the different types of radiation, from least to most powerful.
2. How is a radiologic dispersal device designed to work?
3. What is the relationship between the amount of radiation that a person receives and the time of onset of the initial signs and symptoms?

CHAPTER SUMMARY

52.1 Chapter Overview and Case Studies

Describe dissemination of, current threats from, and concepts related to disorders caused by biologic, chemical, and radiologic agents.

- Exposure to biologic, chemical, or radiologic agents places not only the exposed victim at risk of illness or injury but also, in many cases, the healthcare provider.
- Individuals who have been exposed acutely to biologic, chemical, or radiologic agents should be immediately undressed and decontaminated using copious amounts of water (with or without soap).
- Removal of an exposed victim's clothing removes approximately 80–90% of any residual contamination.
- Diagnosis of exposure to chemical, biologic, and radiologic agents depends in large part on recognition of the presenting clinical syndrome.

52.2 Biologic Agents

Differentiate the causes, classification, underlying pathogenesis, and clinical manifestations of disorders caused by biologic agents and approaches to diagnosis and treatment of these conditions across the lifespan.

- Personal protective equipment and body substance isolation for biologic agents is the same as that used daily in hospitals for routine management of infectious diseases.
- Although some biologic agents are not transmissible from person to person, the initial presentation for all of them is essentially the same; therefore, appropriate precautions must be taken with each and every patient.

Identification of the specific causative biologic agent usually takes several days. Therefore, initial management of the patient must be based on the presenting findings.

52.3 Chemical Agents

Differentiate the causes, classification, underlying pathogenesis, and clinical manifestations of disorders caused by chemical agents and approaches to diagnosis and treatment of these conditions across the lifespan.

- Exposure to liquid chemicals poses a risk of secondary contamination of healthcare workers. Therefore, decontamination is an important priority.
- Diagnosis of chemical exposure depends on recognition of the presenting symptoms and the organ systems involved.
- The antidotes atropine and pralidoxime for nerve agents and hydroxocobalamin for cyanide are available and should be administered on the basis of the presenting symptoms and signs.
- Care for patients who have been exposed to a pulmonary toxicant is primarily supportive.

52.4 Radiologic and Nuclear Devices

Differentiate the causes, classification, underlying pathogenesis, and clinical manifestations of disorders caused by radiologic and nuclear devices and approaches to diagnosis and treatment of these conditions across the lifespan.

- Exposure to radiation can result from irradiation, contamination (external or internal), or incorporation.
- The rapidity of onset of nausea and vomiting provides a strong clue as to the dose of radiation that has been absorbed.
- The most susceptible organs and tissues of the body are those with rapidly dividing cells and immature cells, such as the bone marrow.

REVIEW QUESTIONS

1. A 35-year-old female complains of a fever, nausea and vomiting for 24 hours, and increasing shortness of breath. She mentions that an envelope containing a powdery substance was found at her workplace a few days ago. How should you modify your personal protection approach?
   a. Seal off the area, and request emergency first responders to manage the incident.
   b. Use standard personal precautions, and continue to evaluate the client.
   c. Step out of the room, and don a gown, mask, and face shield.
   d. Have the client disrobe and take a shower to wash off any residue.

2. A terrorist group decides to introduce weaponized anthrax into the air circulation system of a large building that houses a bank and other corporate offices. What method of intentional exposure would this be?
   a. Direct contact
   b. Secondary
   c. Covert
   d. Overt

3. A 65-year-old male presents with fever and reports increasing bouts of shortness of breath for the past 2 days. He has experienced nausea, vomiting, and diarrhea in the past 12 hours and has been coughing up blood-tinged sputum. Physical exam findings include auscultation of fluid in both lungs and nontender lymph nodes in the neck. Your greatest suspicion is that the client has:
   a. pneumonic plague.
   b. bubonic plague.
   c. inhalational anthrax.
   d. smallpox.

4. A 5-year-old boy is brought to the clinic by his parents. They state that over the past 48 hours, their son has had difficulty seeing and speaking clearly and has experienced worsening shortness of breath. The child is afebrile, and he was not ill before the start of this event. Which of the following conditions is most likely cause of the client's presenting signs and symptoms?
   a. Ricin exposure
   b. Botulism
   c. Smallpox
   d. Meningitis

5. A farm worker is brought to the emergency department by EMS. They report that the victim had been spraying crops for several hours when the fumes overcame him and he collapsed. His signs include abdominal cramping, diarrhea, vomiting, excessive tearing, and salivary secretions. Which nervous system receptor is most likely involved in this exposure?
   a. Nicotinic
   b. Sympathetic
   c. Muscarinic
   d. Dopaminergic

6. Several workers at a manufacturing plant were overcome by fumes that were released during an accidental spill of a liquid chemical. They are complaining of a severe burning sensation in their eyes and throat. A

few of them are having difficulty breathing, hoarseness, and wheezing. Which of the following treatments would most likely be used in the more severely injured clients but not the others?

a. Copious flushing of the eyes with water
b. Supplemental oxygen
c. Inhaled beta agonists
d. Washing the skin to remove direct contamination

7. A worker from a nearby manufacturing plant is profoundly short of breath. Coworkers report that the victim had been rinsing electronic boards in a chemical bath when it spilled, splashing him with the fluid. He is confused and breathing rapidly. His lung sounds are clear, and his blood appears to be fully saturated with oxygen. Which of the following chemicals could he have been exposed to?
   a. Chlorine
   b. Cyanide
   c. Anhydrous ammonia
   d. Phosgene

8. A laboratory technician is being evaluated for radiation sickness after discovery that radioactive material in her work area was not properly covered for an unknown period. She says that about a week ago, she had what she thought were coldlike symptoms: She felt run down, had a fever, and had a day's worth of nausea and some vomiting. However, she felt better within a couple of days and went back to work. Which of the following phases of radiation sickness might the client be in at the moment?
   a. Illness
   b. Prodrome
   c. Latent
   d. Recovery

ANSWERS

Answers to Review Questions can be found in Appendix A. Answers to Case Study and Check Your Progress questions are available on the faculty resources site. Please consult with your instructor.

RECOMMENDED WEBSITES

CDC: Emergency Preparedness and Response
https://emergency.cdc.gov/bioterrorism

Chemical Warfare Mass Casualty Management
http://emedicine.medscape.com/article/831375-overview

Clinical Framework and Medical Countermeasure Use During an Anthrax Mass-Casualty Incident
https://www.cdc.gov/mmwr/pdf/rr/rr6404.pdf

MedicineNet: Bioterrorism
http://www.medicinenet.com/bioterrorism/article.htm

Radiation Emergency Medical Management
https://www.remm.nlm.gov

REFERENCES

1. Joseph, B., Brown, C. V., Diven, C., Bui, E., Aziz, H., & Rhee, P. (2013). Current concepts in the management of biologic and chemical warfare casualties. *Journal of Trauma and Acute Care Surgery, 75*(4), 582–589.
2. Christian, M. D. (2013). Biowarfare and bioterrorism. *Critical Care Clinics, 29*(3), 717–756.
3. Adalja, A. A., Toner, E., & Inglesby, T. V. (2015). Clinical management of potential bioterrorism-related conditions. *New England Journal of Medicine, 372*, 954–962.
4. Waseem, M. (2015). Pediatric botulism. *Medscape*. Available at http://emedicine.medscape.com/article/961833-overview
5. Centers for Disease Control and Prevention Expert Panel Meetings on Prevention and Treatment of Anthrax in Adults. February 2014. Available at https://wwwnc.cdc.gov/eid/article/20/2/13-0687_article
6. Bradley, J. S., Peacock, T., Krug, S. E., William A. Bower, W. A., Cohn, A. C., Meaney-Delman, D., Pavia, A. T., AAP Committee on Infectious Diseases, & Disaster Preparedness Advisory Council. (2014). Pediatric anthrax clinical management. *Pediatrics, 133*, e1411–e1436.
7. Kamal, S. M., Rashid, A. K., Bakar, M. A., & Ahad, M. A. (2011). Anthrax: An update. *Asian Pacific Journal of Tropical Biomedicine, 1*(6), 496–501.
8. Doganay, M., & Demiraslan, H. (2015). Human anthrax as a re-emerging disease. *Recent Patents on Anti-Infective Drug Discovery, 10*(1), 10–29.
9. Center for Infectious Disease Research and Policy. (2013). *Plague*. Available at http://www.cidrap.umn.edu/infectious-disease-topics/plague
10. Pita, R., & Romero, A. (2014). Toxins as weapons: A historical review. *Forensic Science Review, 26*(2), 85–96.
11. Anderson, P. D. (2012). Bioterrorism: Toxins as weapons. *Journal of Pharmacy Practice, 25*(2), 121–129.
12. Tomassoni, A. J., French, R. N., & Walter, F. G. (2015). Toxic industrial chemicals and chemical weapons: Exposure, identification,

and management by syndrome. *Emergency Medical Clinics of North America, 33*(1), 13–36.
13. Anderson, P. D. (2012). Emergency management of chemical weapons injuries. *Journal of Pharmacy Practice, 25*(1), 61–68.
14. Bailey, A. M., Baker, S. N., Baum, R. A., Chandler, H. E., & Weant, K. A. (2014). Being prepared: Emergency treatment following a nerve agent release. *Advanced Emergency Nursing Journal, 36*(1), 22–33
15. Razavi, S. M., Ghanei, M., Salamati, P., & Safiabadi, M. (2013). Long-term effects of mustard gas on respiratory system of Iranian veterans after Iraq-Iran war: A review. *Chinese Journal of Traumatology, 16*(3), 163–168.
16. Batal, M., Boudry, I., Mouret, S., Cléry-Barraud, C., Wartelle, J., Bérard, I., & Douki T. (2014). DNA damage in internal organs after cutaneous exposure to sulphur mustard. *Toxicology and Applied Pharmacology, 278*(1), 39–44.
17. Jenner, J., & Graham, S. J. (2013). Treatment of sulphur mustard skin injury. *Chemico-Biological Interactions, 206*(3), 491–495.
18. Hardison, L. S., Jr., Wright, E., & Pizon, A. F. (2014). Phosgene exposure: A case of accidental industrial exposure. *Journal of Medical Toxicology, 10*(1), 51–56.
19. Anseeuw, K., Delvau, N., Burillo-Putze, G., De Iaco, F., Geldner, G., Holmström, P., Lambert, Y., & Sabbe, M. (2013). Cyanide poisoning by fire smoke inhalation: A European expert consensus. *European Journal of Emergency Medicine, 20*(1), 2–9.
20. Bebarta, V. S. (2013). Antidotes for cyanide poisoning. *European Journal of Emergency Medicine, 20*(1), 65–66.
21. Kamiya, K., Ozasa, K., Akiba, S., Niwa, O., Kodama, K., Takamura, N., Zaharieva, E. K., Kimura, Y., & Wakeford, R. (2015). Long-term effects of radiation exposure on health. *Lancet, 386*(9992), 469–478. doi:10.1016/S0140-6736(15)61167-9
22. Schubauer-Berigan, M. K., Daniels, R. D., Bertke, S. J., Tseng, C. Y., & Richardson, D. B. (2015). Cancer mortality through 2005 among a pooled cohort of U.S. nuclear workers exposed to external ionizing radiation. *Radiation Research, 183*(6), 620–631.

Chapter 53
Pathophysiology at the End of Life

Diane Klein and MariJo Letiza

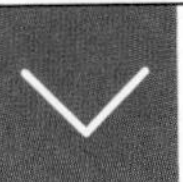

Chapter Outline and Learning Outcomes

53.1 Chapter Overview and Case Studies

Differentiate palliative care from curative care and describe the settings in which palliative care is delivered, and explain how the concept of oxygenation is related to symptoms experienced near the end of life that require palliative care.

53.2 Pain

Recognize the importance of pain assessment and management for individuals with terminal illness.

53.3 Dyspnea

Analyze the pathophysiologic mechanisms that are responsible for a patient's dyspnea on the basis of the disease processes that are present and the patient's description of the difficulty in breathing, and relate the pathophysiology to treatment.

53.4 Cough

Explain the factors that trigger the cough reflex in terminal illness, the potential complications of coughing, characteristics of coughing that should be assessed, and pharmacologic and nonpharmacologic treatment strategies.

53.5 Excessive Secretions

Attribute the production and signs of excessive airway secretions in terminal illness and treatment strategies to the underlying pathophysiology.

53.6 Nausea and Vomiting

Discriminate the characteristics of nausea and vomiting and the factors that trigger the emetic response, and relate the prevention and treatment of nausea and vomiting to the underlying cause.

53.7 Anorexia and Cachexia

Explain the pathophysiologic mechanisms involved in anorexia and cachexia and the clinical manifestations, treatment, and interrelationship of anorexia and cachexia occurring near the end of life.

53.8 Fatigue

Explain the pathophysiologic mechanisms involved in fatigue and the multifactorial causes of fatigue in terminal illness and its management.

53.9 Constipation

Describe the multifactorial causes of constipation associated with terminal illness, and explain prevention of and treatment strategies for underlying causes.

53.10 Urinary Incontinence

Differentiate the causes, underlying pathogenesis, clinical manifestations, diagnosis and treatment approaches of transient urinary incontinence from those in chronic urinary incontinence (stress, urge, overflow, and functional types).

53.11 Delirium

Explain factors that contribute to delirium at the end of life, its various manifestations, diagnosis, and treatment strategies.

53.12 Last Expected Changes at the End of Life

Attribute the underlying pathophysiologic mechanisms to the clinical manifestations that occur in the active phase of dying and the indicators of somatic death.

53.13 Pediatric Considerations

Compare pediatric palliative care to adult palliative care with regard to causes of terminal illness, symptoms experienced near the end of life, and approaches to assessment of symptoms.

KEY TERMS

Active phase of dying, 1309
Algor mortis, 1309
Anorexia, 1303
Asthenia, 1303
Brain death, 1310
Cachexia, 1303
Cheyne-Stokes breathing, 1309
Confusion Assessment Method (CAM), 1309
Constipation, 1306
Cough, 1298
Death rattle, 1299
Delirium, 1308
Dyspnea, 1295
Emetic response, 1300
Fatigue, 1305
Hospice, 1292
Karnofsky Performance Status Scale, 1293
Livor mortis, 1310
Nausea, 1300
Palliative care, 1292
Palliative sedation, 1310
Rigor mortis, 1310
Somatic death, 1309
Urinary incontinence, 1307
Vomiting, 1300

ABBREVIATIONS

ACE—angiotensin-converting enzyme
ATP—adenosine triphosphate
CAM—confusion assessment method
COPD—chronic obstructive pulmonary disease
CTZ—chemoreceptor trigger zone
GABA—gamma-aminobutyric acid

53.1 Chapter Overview and Case Studies

Palliative care is care provided to patients experiencing life-threatening, progressive illness that focuses on providing effective relief of symptoms rather than on curing the illness. Chronic life-threatening conditions that commonly affect adults include heart disease, cancer, cerebrovascular disease, chronic obstructive pulmonary disease (COPD), Alzheimer disease, diabetes mellitus, and liver disease. Life-threatening conditions that affect children and the associated palliative care considerations are addressed in section 53.13. Palliative care emphasizes control of distressing symptoms with attention to the patient's physiologic, psychosocial, and spiritual needs.[1] The goal of palliative care is to attain the best possible quality of life for patients and their families. Palliative care begins when the illness is diagnosed and continues through the bereavement period. Palliative care is planned and delivered through the collaborative efforts of an interdisciplinary team that includes doctors, nurses, pharmacists, dietitians, chaplains, psychologists, and social workers.

Hospice is a formal program that delivers palliative care, rather than curative treatment, to patients who are near the end of life. Hospice care exists under the umbrella of palliative care services. Both palliative care and hospice are provided to patients across clinical settings including the patient's home, nursing homes, outpatient clinics, adult and pediatric intensive care units, and other hospital units. Palliative care is increasingly being integrated with curative care[2] (**Figure 53.1** ■), and healthcare professionals are being educated to improve their ability to deliver palliative care in clinical settings such as ambulatory care,[3] intensive care units,[4,5] and emergency departments as well as in hospice settings.

There is evidence supporting the benefits of palliative care. For example, a study of 151 patients recently diagnosed with lung cancer who were randomly assigned to receive palliative care integrated with standard cancer care found that after 12 weeks, the patients who received the integrated care had a statistically significant improvement in quality of life and a decrease in depression.[6] Furthermore, they lived 3 months longer than patients who received standard cancer care alone. These findings demonstrate the importance of incorporating palliative care to enhance the quality of life of patients with advanced, noncurable illness.

This chapter addresses the most common symptoms that patients receiving palliative care experience. These symptoms include pain, dyspnea, cough, excessive secretions, nausea and vomiting, anorexia, cachexia, fatigue, constipation, urinary incontinence, and delirium. Each symptom has the potential to cause distress for both patients and their family members. The chapter presents the pathophysiology of each of these symptoms, associated typical clinical manifestations, and an overview of treatment options linked to the underlying pathophysiology. Interventions are considered in the plan of care when their benefit outweighs the burden of the intervention on the patient.

Dying patients and their families have questions, concerns, and fears about the dying process. Because most people have not seen someone die, patients and family members are taught about the process of normal dying and what is likely to occur in the absence of aggressive interventions. They are reassured when they learn that most symptoms experienced at the end of life can be anticipated and well managed.

At the end of life, patients often experience multiple symptoms resulting from multiple causes. In addition to determining the presence of symptoms, nursing

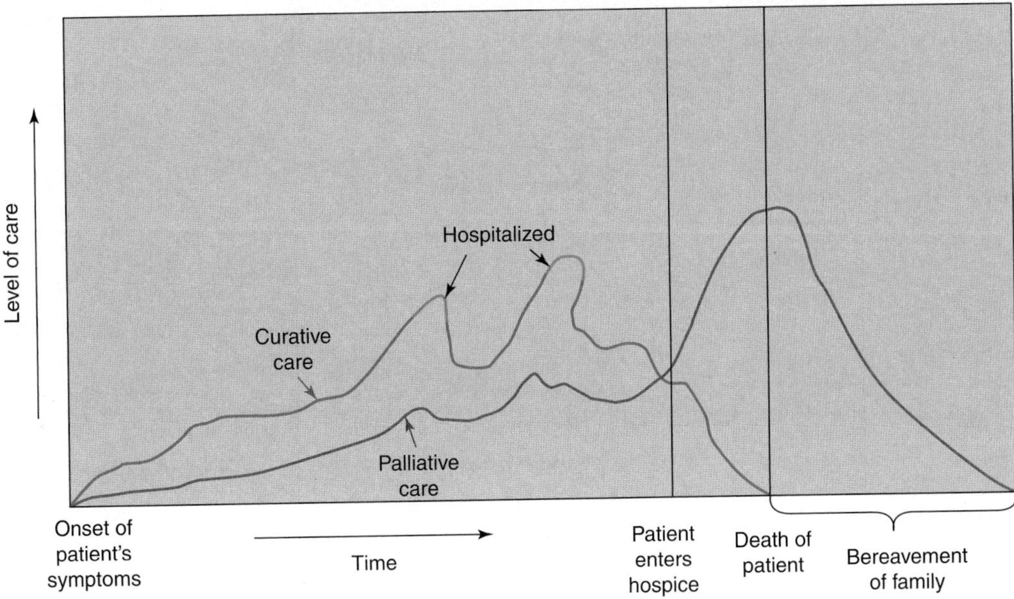

Figure 53.1 ■ Integrated model of palliative care. Palliative care for individuals with a chronic life-threatening illness should begin with the onset of symptoms and take place concurrently with curative care. The levels of curative and palliative care vary over time depending on the patient's needs. When curative care is no longer effective or its burden on the patient outweighs its benefit, the focus shifts to mainly palliative care. The palliative care team continues to support the patient's family through the bereavement period after the death of their loved one.

assessments are aimed at identifying underlying causes of symptoms and whether the symptoms are creating discomfort or distress for the patient. Patients cannot experience an acceptable quality of life or a good death if physiologic symptoms are not well controlled. The patient's overall condition and expected prognosis also determine the appropriateness of interventions. For example, the healthcare team will review medication profile carefully to decide which drugs remain suitable as the patient enters the dying process. Medications that patients were taking earlier in the progression of their diseases can actually contribute to problems during the dying phase; therefore, unnecessary medications are stopped. Laboratory, radiologic, and other diagnostic tests are not typically performed in the care of the terminally ill patient unless the results of such testing will change the management plan and benefit the patient.

The **Karnofsky Performance Status Scale**, created in 1949 and still in use today, allows patients to be classified according to their functional impairment (**Table 53.1** ■).[7] This scale can be used to compare the effectiveness of different therapies and to assess the patient's prognosis. The lower the Karnofsky score, the worse the patient's functional status and survival.

Table 53.1 Karnofsky Performance Status Scale

Performance Level	Score	Description of the Score
Able to carry on normal activity and to work; no special care needed	100	Normal, no complaints; no evidence of disease
	90	Able to carry on normal activity; minor signs or symptoms of disease
	80	Normal activity with effort; some signs or symptoms of disease
Unable to work; able to live at home and care for most personal needs; varying amount of assistance needed	70	Cares for self; unable to carry on normal activity or to do active work
	60	Requires occasional assistance but is able to care for most personal needs
	50	Requires considerable assistance and frequent medical care
Unable to care for self; requires equivalent of institutional or hospital care; disease may be progressing rapidly	40	Disabled; requires special care and assistance
	30	Severely disabled; hospital admission is indicated although death not imminent
	20	Very sick; hospital admission necessary; active supportive treatment necessary
	10	Moribund; fatal processes progressing rapidly
	0	Dead

SOURCE: Karnofsky, D. A., & Burchenal, J. H. (1949). The clinical evaluation of chemotherapeutic agents in cancer. In C. M. McLeod (Ed.), *Evaluation of chemotherapeutic agents* (p. 196). New York, NY: Columbia University Press.

Concepts Related to the Pathophysiology of End of Life

Impaired cellular oxygenation resulting in a deficit of adenosine triphosphate (ATP) production is the fundamental mechanism responsible for death from all causes. Although impaired oxygenation is not the only factor responsible for symptoms experienced near the end of life, it is a mechanism that is common to many symptoms linked to the interrelated concepts depicted in **Figure 53.2** ■, such as mobility, cognition, perception, inflammation, and

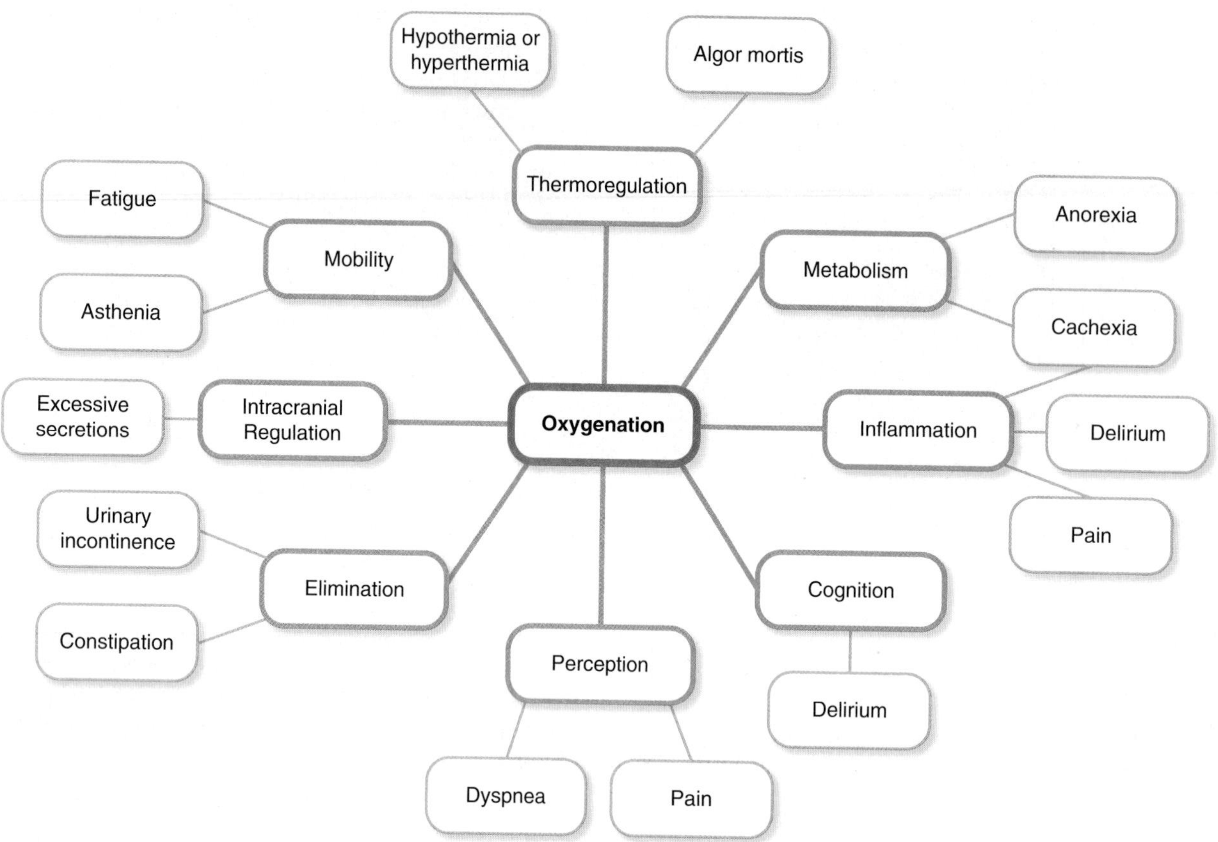

Figure 53.2 At the end of life, impaired oxygenation adversely affects the related concepts of neural regulation, mobility, thermoregulation, metabolism, inflammation, cognition, perception, and elimination, resulting in the symptoms commonly experienced near the end of life (shown in the outer boxes).

metabolism. These concepts will be addressed in the description of the pathogenesis of symptoms throughout the chapter.

Case Studies

The pathophysiology involved and the clinical significance of the symptoms experienced by the individuals in the following cases will be addressed throughout the chapter to assist in applying chapter content to clinical situations involving individuals with terminal illness.

Irene Rollins: Introduction

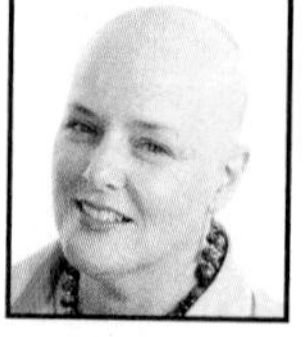

Irene Rollins is a 67-year-old woman with metastatic ovarian cancer that was diagnosed 16 months ago. She has been admitted to the emergency department with symptoms of bowel obstruction. Ms. Rollins reports pain, dyspnea, anorexia, nausea, and moderate vomiting two to three times daily over the past 2 days. She states that she has no appetite and is taking only occasional sips of liquids. She indicates that abdominal bloating had increased over the past week and that she has not had a bowel movement or passed flatus (gas) for the past 4 days. Although she feels quite fatigued, she denies chills, fever, or night sweats, so her fatigue is not likely due to an infection.

On her admission to the emergency department, Ms. Rollins's blood pressure is 94/62 when supine, and it decreases to 80/55 when standing. Her heart rate is 110, her pulse is thready, and her respiratory rate is 24 and shallow. Though alert and oriented, Ms. Rollins is in obvious distress with restlessness and frequent repositioning to try to get comfortable. Her intact buccal mucosa is notably dry with visible longitudinal furrows in the tongue.

The fluid wave test for ascites (accumulation of fluid in the abdominal cavity) is positive. Ms. Rollins has tenderness and guarding to light palpation across the abdomen. It is not possible to palpate her liver, spleen, and kidneys because of abdominal pain and distention. Rectal examination reveals no impacted stool, and testing was negative for occult blood. Ms. Rollins has 4+ pitting ankle edema bilaterally and slightly limited ankle range of motion. Radiographic films of her abdomen demonstrate loops of intestine distended with gas, which is indicative of obstruction.

1. Which of the clinical findings clearly indicate that Ms. Rollins has evidence of dehydration?
2. What is the most likely cause of Ms. Rollins's bowel obstruction?

William Thompson: Introduction

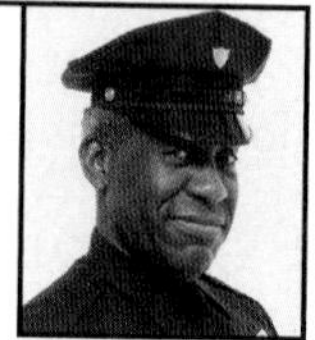

William Thompson, a 54-year-old police sergeant, was diagnosed 8 months ago with advanced stage bronchogenic lung cancer. Although he received chemotherapy and radiation after this diagnosis, he was later found to have metastasis to the brain, clavicle, and adrenal glands. At the time of his admission to a hospice program, he has progressively worsening dyspnea and has lost 40 pounds over the prior 3 months. He also expresses having a very poor appetite and debilitating fatigue. The hospice team uses the Karnofsky Performance

Status Scale (see Table 53.1) to classify his functional impairment and estimate expected survival. Mr. Thompson scores 40 out of a possible 100 on the day of admission to hospice care.

During Mr. Thompson's admission to hospice, his family expresses concern that he has "given up hope" and is "not fighting hard enough" against the disease. His children believe that more physical activity and a better appetite will improve his overall condition. The family is also distressed by Mr. Thompson's lack of interest in watching his favorite television shows, reading the newspaper, and participating in family conversations.

1. Do Mr. Thompson's weight loss and nutritional ambivalence technically meet the definitions of anorexia and cachexia?
2. What techniques can the family use to improve Mr. Thompson's quality of life?

Is there one cause or are there multiple causes of the symptoms experienced by the patients in these two cases? Is suffering caused by a variety of symptoms an inevitable consequence of terminal illness, or can understanding of the underlying pathophysiologic mechanisms guide appropriate therapy resulting in patient comfort and a peaceful death? Can you answer questions that patients and family members have about the causes and treatment of symptoms experienced near the end of life?

Check Your Progress: Section 53.1

1. Differentiate palliative care from hospice care.
2. Explain how the Karnofsky Performance Status Scale is used in the management of patients with terminal illness.

53.2 Pain

Because the pathophysiology of pain is extensively covered in Chapter 32, this chapter will discuss pain briefly and then focus in more depth on other symptoms that can be equally or more debilitating for patients receiving palliative care.

Causes of pain associated with terminal illness are multifactorial. Nociceptive pain results from stimulation of nociceptors (pain receptors) in body tissues or organs by pressure, extremes of temperature, or release of chemicals from tissues injured by hypoxia, trauma, or inflammation. Neuropathic pain results from injury to or malfunction of sensory nerves or the pathways that process pain. For example, pain in an individual with terminal cancer can be caused by pressure from the enlarging cancerous tumor on nociceptors or pressure on a hollow organ such as the intestines resulting in obstruction and distention. Cancer-induced pain is also caused by the inflammation that occurs in response to injury as cancer cells invade previously healthy organs and tissues. Another common cause of pain is impaired oxygenation resulting, for example, from a chronic lung disease or pulmonary edema and subsequent tissue injury and inflammation.

Comprehensive pain assessment is essential, with particular attention given to the patient's self-report of pain, including location, intensity, quality, pattern, and effects on function. The healthcare team notes factors that exacerbate or alleviate the pain and incorporates these findings into the plan of care.

Nonopioid analgesics such as ibuprofen, opioid analgesics such as morphine, and adjuvant analgesics, which are medications that are used primarily to treat other conditions but help to relieve certain types of pain, are used along with nonpharmacologic interventions that promote comfort. For patients experiencing chronic pain, long-acting medications are provided around the clock; short-acting medications are also made available for breakthrough pain. As the dying process progresses, the patient may be unable to swallow medications, and alternative routes of administration must be used.

Irene Rollins: Application

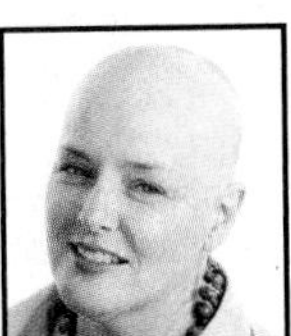

Ms. Rollins states that she has had cramping, nonradiating, central abdominal pain that she rates as 9 out of 10 in severity for the past 3 days. The pain occurs on and off with nothing specific that exacerbates or alleviates it. Because Ms. Rollins has metastatic ovarian cancer and radiographic films of the abdomen demonstrate loops of intestine that are distended with gas, her pain is likely due to her markedly distended abdomen and distended and obstructed intestines caused by growth of the cancer in the abdominal area. Evidence of abdominal distention and intestinal obstruction also include the following assessment findings. Her flanks are bulging bilaterally when she is supine, and her umbilicus is slightly everted. Her abdominal skin is glistening and taut with striae and prominent dilated veins. Bowel sounds are hypoactive. Ms. Rollins's pain is treated with two opioid analgesics. A transdermal fentanyl (Sublimaze, Duragesic) patch is placed on the skin to provide continuous pain relief, and morphine sulfate is ordered to be injected subcutaneously every 2 hours for breakthrough pain that is not relieved by medication released from the transdermal patch.

3. What nutrition choices should be considered for Ms. Rollins at this point in her condition?
4. How does the injectable morphine sulfate differ from the transdermal fentanyl patch in terms of action and impact?

Check Your Progress: Section 53.2

1. List the four major causes of pain associated with terminal illnesses.
2. What is the most comprehensive means of assessing pain?
3. Identify the three classes of pain medications used for terminally ill patients and provide an example of each.

53.3 Dyspnea

Dyspnea is defined by the American Thoracic Society as "a subjective experience of breathing discomfort that consists of qualitatively distinct sensations that vary in intensity."[8] In patients with advanced disease, the sensation of dyspnea is disproportionate to the patient's level of activity. Up to 70% of dying patients experience dyspnea.[9,10] It is a frightening problem for both patients and family members that should never be ignored.

Etiology and Pathogenesis

Several mechanisms underlie the dyspnea that palliative care patients experience.[8,11,12] Chemical and mechanical receptors in the lungs and chest wall send afferent signals to the brain about the patient's need to breathe, and efferent signals to the muscles of respiration are involved in the ability to breathe. An imbalance between the need to breathe and the ability to breathe results in dyspnea. The receptors and neural pathways involved in dyspnea are depicted in **Figure 53.3** ■.

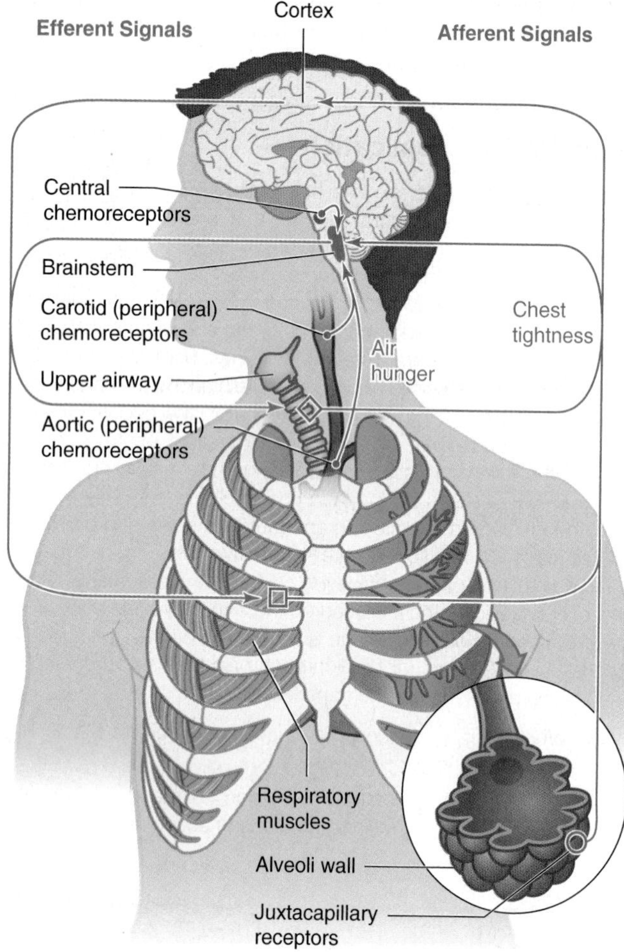

Figure 53.3 ■ Mechanisms involved in dyspnea. Central and peripheral chemoreceptors detect indicators of inadequate ventilation, such as decreased oxygen and increased carbon dioxide and hydrogen ion levels in the blood. They relay such findings to the cerebral cortex, leading to the sensation of dyspnea. Three types of mechanical receptors also provide information about the adequacy of ventilation to the cerebral cortex by way of the vagus nerve: (1) Stretch receptors in the airways, lungs, chest wall, and pulmonary vessels are stimulated by inflammatory processes, tumors, pulmonary emboli, and pulmonary hypertension. (2) Irritant receptors in the epithelial tissue of the airways are stimulated when chemicals, tobacco smoke, gas, and dust are inhaled. (3) The juxtacapillary receptors located in the c-fibers of the vagus nerve in the alveoli are stimulated by edema, effusion, and emboli. Additionally, the vagus nerve communicates ventilatory impedance (resistance to air flow), increased ventilatory demand, and abnormal respiratory muscle functioning to the cerebral cortex, leading to the sensation of dyspnea.

Several underlying disease processes directly affect the mechanisms of breathing, contributing to dyspnea. Pulmonary conditions include obstruction of a bronchus or upper airway by a primary or metastatic tumor; pleural effusion (excessive fluid in the pleural space) from a lung tumor, lymphoma, or infection; COPD; aspiration or infectious pneumonia; radiation- and chemotherapy-induced lung toxicity; pulmonary embolus; and pneumothorax (accumulation of air in the pleural space compressing the lung). Other pulmonary problems such as asthma, bronchitis, emphysema, tuberculosis, and cystic fibrosis also may contribute to dyspnea in terminally ill patients. Examples of cardiovascular conditions that cause dyspnea include pericardial effusion from a tumor invading or irritating the pericardium and superior vena cava syndrome resulting from an underlying lung tumor compressing or obstructing the superior vena cava. Comorbidities such as heart failure, dysrhythmia, pulmonary hypertension, and severe anemia also contribute to dyspnea. Examples of neuromuscular conditions that impair ventilation and cause dyspnea include amyotrophic lateral sclerosis, muscular dystrophy, and myasthenia gravis. Obesity, ascites, and hepatomegaly can cause pressure on the lungs, and dehydration may lead to thick, tenacious secretions. Fear and anxiety about the underlying disease process can further compound the labored breathing.

Clinical Manifestations

Patients can experience acute or chronic dyspnea. In both types, a patient's self-report of difficult breathing provides the most reliable data. When referring to their dyspnea, patients use a variety of terms, known as descriptors, such as "shortness of breath," "breathlessness," and others that may reflect the underlying cause. These descriptors might express the rate or depth of breathing, the effort it takes to breathe, the phase of the respiratory cycle that is affected (inspiration or expiration), and associated sensations, such as suffocation or chest tightness. Descriptors that are distinct for each underlying cause of dyspnea have not been found; however, some descriptors are used more frequently by patients with certain conditions.[12] For example, patients with chronic obstructive pulmonary disease often use a descriptor that reflects impaired exhalation, such as "my breath does not go out all the way," which describes the result of air trapping in the alveoli resulting in lung overinflation. Patients with asthma are more likely to use descriptors such as "my chest feels tight" or "my chest feels restricted," which is the result of bronchoconstriction.

Additional factors that must be assessed include the intensity of the dyspnea, the quality and effects on the patient's ability to function, and exacerbating and alleviating factors. Several validated instruments are available that patients can use to rate these factors.[13,14]

The presence of distended neck veins, skin pallor or cyanosis, tachycardia, tachypnea, or abnormal lung sounds should be noted during the physical assessment, since they can help in determining the underlying cause of dyspnea, particularly in patients who cannot communicate verbally about their difficulty breathing.

Linking Pathophysiology to Diagnosis and Treatment

The diagnosis of dyspnea is based on observation of the patient's breathing and the self-report of difficulty breathing. Dyspnea is evident to the observer who notes gasping breaths, use of accessory muscles to breathe, stridor (high-pitched sound caused by obstruction in the trachea or larynx), restlessness, agitation, and facial grimacing.

CLINICAL POINT: Objective findings such as respiratory rate, hemoglobin saturation with oxygen, pulmonary function testing, and arterial blood gas results often do not predict the patient's experience of dyspnea or correlate with the patient's self-report of dyspnea.[15] ■

Opioid medications, such as morphine, are highly effective in treating dyspnea.[16–18] Opioid medications cause venous dilation, reducing blood return to the heart and therefore cardiac preload (volume load), oxygen consumption, demand for ventilation, and central perception of breathlessness.[17] Opioid medications are therefore the cornerstone of treatment for end-stage dyspnea. Additional medications are effective for certain causes of dyspnea. Inhaled bronchodilators are often effective in relieving bronchospasm in patients with asthma or COPD. Corticosteroids improve airflow by reducing airway inflammation and may be helpful for patients with inflammatory disorders, such as asthma, that are contributing to dyspnea. For patients with dyspnea related to anxiety, benzodiazepines are appropriate because of their sedative effect. Diuretics, which increase urine output, may be provided to patients who are experiencing fluid overload and pulmonary edema contributing to dyspnea. If anemia is an underlying cause of dyspnea, blood transfusion or erythropoietin injections, which increase red blood cell production in the bone marrow, can be used. Pulmonary infections contributing to dyspnea may be treated with appropriate antibiotic, antifungal, or antiviral medications.

Several nonpharmacologic approaches can be employed to alleviate dyspnea. Patients are taught to use diaphragmatic and pursed-lip breathing to prevent small airway collapse and to improve elimination of carbon dioxide.[17,19] Assuming the supine position with the head elevated promotes lung expansion. Alternating periods of rest and activity help to conserve energy and decrease ventilatory demand, as do relaxation techniques. When thick secretions are contributing to dyspnea, increasing the humidity level of the environment and increasing oral intake of liquids as tolerated may help. Supplemental oxygen can be administered; however, not all patients with dyspnea are hypoxic, and for those who are hypoxic, the oxygen therapy may not reverse the hypoxia or relieve the dyspnea if disease prevents the additional oxygen from reaching the alveoli or diffusing into the blood. Particularly in advanced disease states, oxygen may not be more effective than a fan, open window, or cool air placed near the patient's face.[20] Stimulation of receptors along the trigeminal nerve in the face has a central inhibitory effect on the sensation of dyspnea. Air movement across the face produced by a fan, for example, can help to relieve dyspnea.[8,21] Keeping the room temperature cool and eliminating environmental irritants are other helpful interventions to include in the plan of care.

Other treatment options are considered when their benefit outweighs their burden on the patient. For example, a course of radiation to reduce tumor size may be appropriate for patients with dyspnea resulting from airway obstruction by a tumor. Aspiration of pericardial effusion fluid to enhance cardiac performance or aspiration of pleural effusion to enhance lung expansion may be beneficial; likewise, paracentesis may help the patient in whom ascites fluid limits lung expansion. For dyspnea caused by stenosis (narrowing) of the trachea or main bronchi that is unrelieved by other interventions, an airway stent can be inserted.[22,23] Stents are inserted by a bronchoscopy tube into the occluded airway (see **Figure 53.4** ■). Although stent placement can provide immediate relief of dyspnea due to airway occlusion and can improve the individual's quality of life, the procedure does not necessarily prolong survival. Also, airway stenting has potential complications, including respiratory infection, tissue injury and hemorrhaging, impaired clearance of mucus, and stent migration to a site where it is no longer effective.[22,23]

Irene Rollins: Application

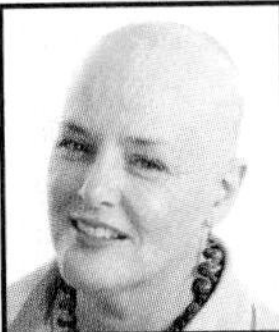

When Ms. Rollins was admitted to the emergency department, one of her complaints was difficulty breathing. Her dyspnea is likely a result of impaired movement of the diaphragm, the major muscle of respiration, due to abdominal distention secondary to her ascites and large tumor burden in the abdominal cavity. When Ms. Rollins was started on opioid medications to control her pain, the opioids also provided some, but not total, relief of her dyspnea. A fan was brought into her room and positioned to produce airflow across her face to stimulate the trigeminal nerve. This intervention provided some additional relief but not total relief of her dyspnea, which she finds very distressing.

5. Would the use of diuretics be beneficial for Ms. Rollins's dyspnea? Why or why not?
6. Which body position would help Ms. Rollins with her difficulty in breathing?

William Thompson: Application

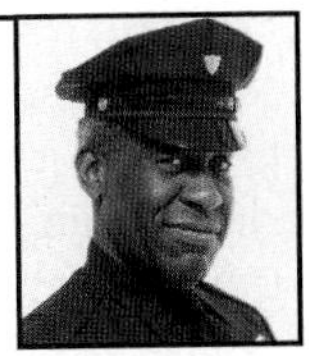

Mr. Thompson had severe dyspnea when he was admitted to the hospice program. Factors contributing to his dyspnea include lung cancer cells growing into the bronchi and obstructing airflow and his cachexia- and anorexia-induced loss of skeletal muscle mass causing respiratory muscle weakness. The dyspnea is contributing to Mr. Thompson's worsening functional impairment. A trial of oxygen therapy does not provide any relief from the dyspnea. However, administration of an opioid medication around the clock provides enough relief that Mr. Thompson now states that the dyspnea is tolerable.

3. How does opioid medication help Mr. Thompson better tolerate his dyspnea?
4. What is the main reason why the oxygen therapy did not provide any dyspnea relief for Mr. Thompson?

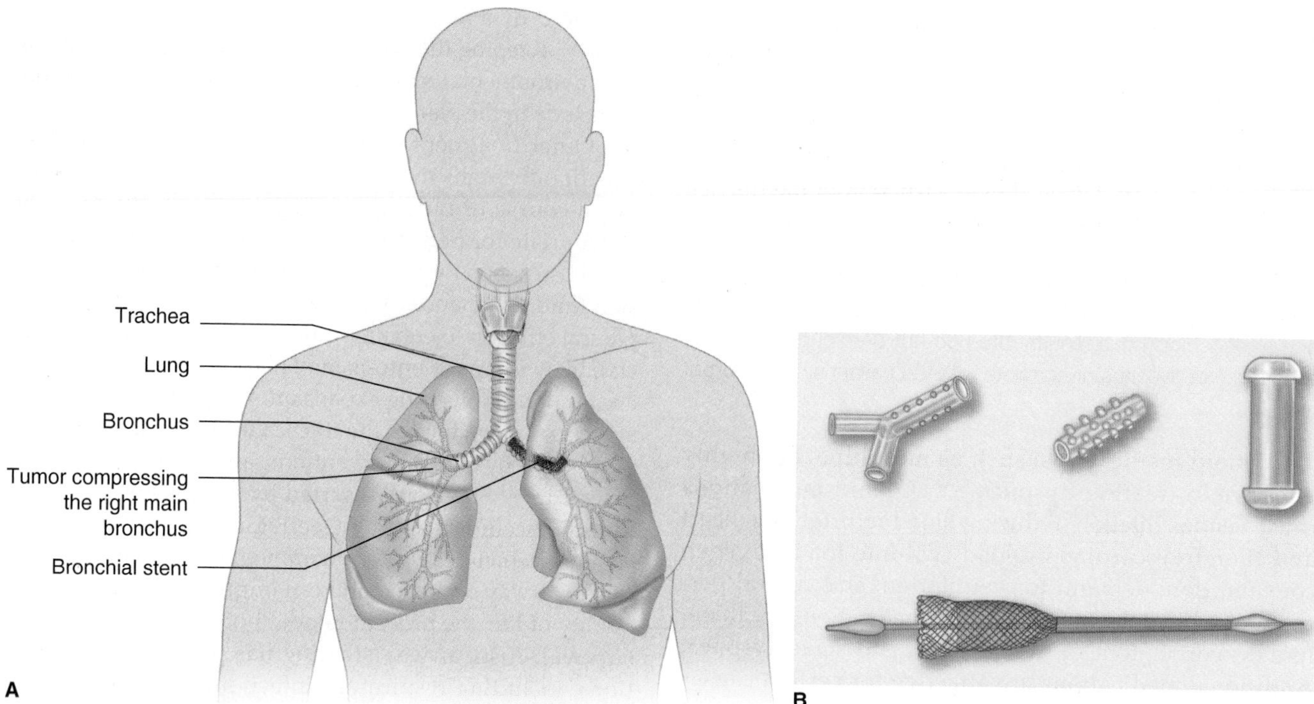

Figure 53.4 ■ **A**. Bronchial stents, also called tracheobronchial prostheses, are tubes inserted into an airway to widen a section that has been narrowed, for example, by compression from a tumor. The increased airway patency improves airflow and decreases dyspnea. The trachea and the right or left main bronchus are common stent placement sites. **B**. Bronchial stents are made of silicone or a metal mesh and are available in a variety of lengths and diameters in either a straight or a Y shape.

Check Your Progress: Section 53.3

1. Explain the pathogenesis of dyspnea.
2. Describe the clinical manifestations of dyspnea, and list some terms that patients commonly use to describe their difficulty in breathing.
3. Explain the pharmacologic and nonpharmacologic approaches to the management of dyspnea.

53.4 Cough

Cough is the forceful release of air through the trachea and mouth. In the last year of life, 40–70% of palliative care patients experience coughing.[24] Although it can be a defense mechanism that clears the airways of excessive secretions or inhaled foreign substances, it can also be maladaptive and lead to pain, fatigue, impaired sleep, interruption of speech, fractured ribs, anorexia, vomiting, and urinary incontinence.[25] Cough also it serves as a disturbing reminder of disease to patients and their families.

Etiology and Pathogenesis

The cough reflex involves activation of cough receptors located in the respiratory tract and other organs that send afferent nerve signals to the cough center in the medulla, which then sends efferent nerve signals to muscles of respiration, resulting in a forceful expulsion of air.[26] The cough reflex is depicted in **Figure 53.5** ■.

Underlying respiratory conditions that cause coughing include cancer, pulmonary embolus, infection, aspiration, asthma, COPD, pneumonia, bronchitis, and postnasal drip. Cardiac conditions such as heart failure, which can cause edema in the airways, and gastrointestinal conditions such as gastroesophageal reflux disease, in which gastric acid can become aspirated into the airways, also may lead to coughing. Many medications can cause cough; prime culprits include angiotensin-converting enzyme (ACE) inhibitors, which decrease the breakdown of bradykinin and can therefore cause edema in the airways. Often, a patient's coughing will have more than one cause.

Clinical Manifestations

Coughing is diagnosed on the basis of the clinical manifestations described in the previous section. Diagnostic tests may be indicated if the underlying cause of the coughing is unknown. For example, a chest x-ray could be performed and a sputum sample obtained. If a respiratory infection is the suspected cause of the cough.

Cough can be classified as acute (lasting up to 3 weeks), chronic (lasting longer than 3 weeks), or nocturnal (occurring at night). The cough can be described as hacking, hoarse, barking, or bubbling. Particular focus is placed on reports of dry versus productive cough; with productive coughs, the color, thickness, and amount of sputum are documented. Patients are asked about their level of distress with the cough and factors that exacerbate their coughing, such as activity and weather.

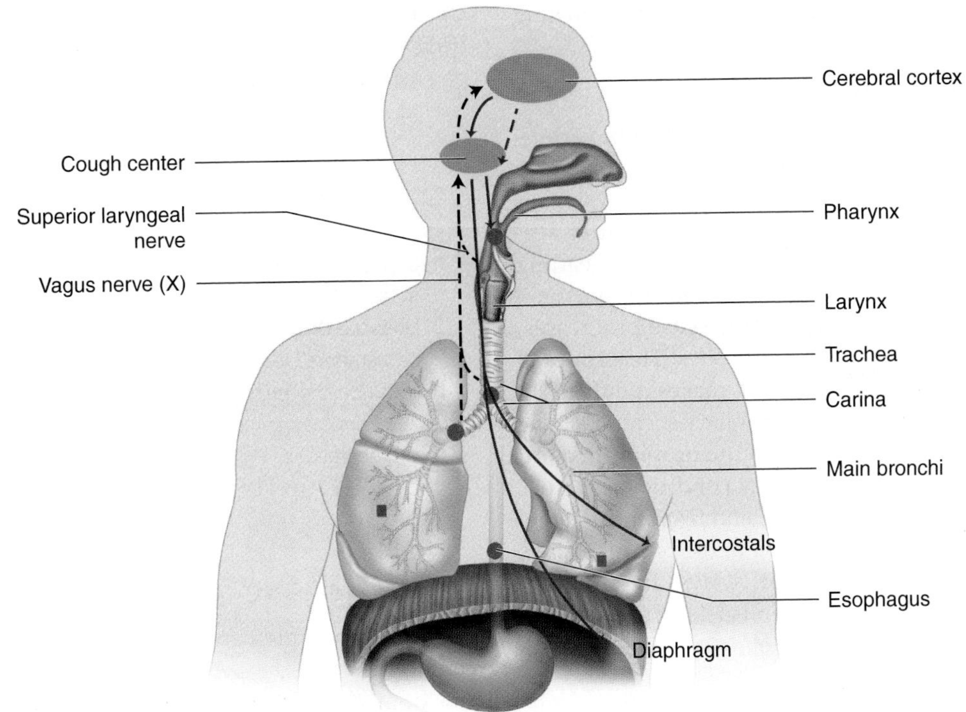

Figure 53.5 ■ The cough reflex is activated by stimulation of two types of receptors on sensory nerve endings. Mechanical receptors located primarily in the upper respiratory tract are stimulated when tissues are irritated, stretched, inflamed, or displaced. Chemical receptors located primarily in the lower respiratory tract are stimulated on exposure to irritants such as smoke, noxious gases, blood, purulent secretions, and mucus. Afferent vagal stimulation originating in the auditory meatus, esophagus, diaphragm, and stomach also contributes to coughing. Afferent nerve signals from the cough receptors are transmitted to the cough center in the medulla. Efferent motor fibers of the vagus (cranial nerve X), trigeminal (V), glossopharyngeal (IX), and phrenic nerves from the cough center innervate the larynx, abdominal muscles, and intercostal muscles. The cough reflex involves a deep inspiration followed by contraction of expiratory muscles with air forced out against a closed glottis that quickly opens, resulting in a forceful exhalation (cough).

Linking Pathophysiology to Diagnosis and Treatment

The treatment choice for coughing depends on the underlying etiology. Antibiotics, mucolytics, and expectorants are used if the cough is thought to be related to a bacterial lung infection. If bronchospasm is a causative factor, inhaled bronchodilators are used to relax the smooth muscles of the airway. Corticosteroids are used for patients with airway restriction, obstruction, or inflammation. If fluid overload is a contributing factor, diuretics are prescribed to increase fluid excretion by the kidneys. Antitussive medications (cough suppressants), including opioids, anticholinergics, and local anesthetics, are particularly effective at bedtime to help the patient achieve rest. When possible, medications that are thought to be inducing cough are discontinued, or the dose is decreased.

Nonpharmacologic interventions for cough include increasing the humidity in the environment and keeping the patient well hydrated if possible to decrease the viscosity of respiratory secretions. Chest physiotherapy can be helpful in mobilizing accumulated secretions. Patients who experience hemoptysis (coughing up blood) may be sedated to relieve distress; family members are taught to use dark towels to help lessen the disturbing visual effects of bloody secretions. Other interventions include aspiration of pleural effusion fluid and radiation therapy to decrease the size of enlarging tumors that are causing airway obstruction leading to cough.

Check Your Progress: Section 53.4

1. Contrast the benefits and the harmful effects of coughing.
2. How do the characteristics of a cough help to determine its cause and treatment?
3. Describe the pharmacologic and nonpharmacologic approaches to treatment of coughing.

53.5 Excessive Secretions

At the end of life, oscillating movements of secretions in the upper airway may lead patients to experience a gurgling sound in the throat, which is called the **death rattle** because its onset generally precedes death by about 48 hours.[27] Such terminal congestion occurs in 23–92% of dying patients.[28] The rattle can be distressing to family members because of the perception that the patient is suffocating or drowning in his own secretions.

Etiology and Pathogenesis

Excessive secretions in dying patients result from various factors. As the brain becomes deoxygenated in the dying patient, regulation of the autonomic nervous system is lost, resulting in the release of the neurotransmitter acetylcholine, which activates muscarinic receptors, leading to an increase in salivary, bronchial, and gastrointestinal secretions. As a patient's underlying disease progresses, her level of consciousness often diminishes. This, coupled with increasing generalized weakness, makes it difficult to swallow saliva and expectorate pulmonary secretions. The result is retained secretions in both the oropharynx and the bronchial tree. Cardiopulmonary conditions, such as pleural effusion, pulmonary edema, and respiratory infection, also lead to fluid accumulation in the bronchial tree. Dehydration is another contributor because the resultant increase in the thickness and tenaciousness of mucus compromises the patient's ability to mobilize and clear secretions out of the airways.

Clinical Manifestations

Patients with excessive retained secretions have usually progressed in the dying process to the point at which they cannot verbally communicate about this and other symptoms. Objective signs of excessive secretions include audible gurgling, rattling, or crackling sounds in the upper airway with each breath.

Linking Pathophysiology to Diagnosis and Treatment

Diagnosis of the death rattle does not require auscultation with a stethoscope. The gurgling sound can be heard a few inches from the patient's chest in most cases to several feet away in more severe cases.

Because of the involvement of muscarinic receptors in the production of secretions, antimuscarinic medications are the drugs of choice for patients with the death rattle.[29,30] These medications do not eliminate existing accumulated secretions, so they must be initiated at the first sign of the death rattle. Other medications also may be considered in the plan of care, depending on the presumed etiology of the secretions. For example, antibiotics can be given for secretions related to pulmonary bacterial infections, and diuretics can be given to increase urine output, thereby reducing lung and bronchial fluid accumulation.

The patient's head should remain elevated, and the patient can be turned from side to side to help mobilize secretions and interrupt the rattle temporarily. Oropharyngeal suctioning is usually not recommended because this procedure causes discomfort, is ineffective if secretions are beyond the reach of the catheter, and does not correct the underlying problem. It is essential that nurses reassure relatives that once the patient's level of consciousness has diminished enough that the patient no longer has an active cough or gag reflex, the patient is unlikely to be aware of, or distressed by, the excessive secretions.

CLINICAL POINT: It is important to recognize that patients with decreasing levels of consciousness are likely to have an impaired gag reflex and can experience aspiration into the lungs if they are fed foods or fluids. Therefore oral intake should be stopped. ■

Check Your Progress: Section 53.5

1. Explain the pathogenesis of excessive secretions that occur at the end of life.
2. Does the death rattle cause distress for patients and/or family members? Why or why not?
3. Describe the pharmacologic and nonpharmacologic treatment approaches to the prevention and treatment of excessive secretions.

53.6 Nausea and Vomiting

Nausea is an unpleasant sensation that can precede vomiting and is often described by patients as feeling "sick to my stomach" or "queasy." **Vomiting**, which is also called emesis, is a neuromuscular reflex that results in forceful expulsion of gastric contents through the oral or nasal cavity. Nausea and vomiting often occur together; however, some patients experience nausea without ever vomiting, while others vomit without experiencing preceding nausea. Nausea occurs more frequently than vomiting, and up to 70% of hospice and palliative care patients experience one or both of these distressing symptoms.[31] Nausea and vomiting can significantly compromise quality of life and are among the most difficult symptoms to manage in this patient population. Vomiting can lead to dehydration, electrolyte deficits, metabolic alkalosis from loss of gastric acid, and fatigue due to decreased caloric intake.

Etiology and Pathogenesis

Although nausea and vomiting are considered gastrointestinal symptoms, they involve both the brain and abdominal organs. The **emetic response** (vomiting reflex) occurs as a result of the transmission of neural impulses by one of four pathways to the vomiting center located in the medulla (**Figure 53.6** ■). Stimuli originating in the cerebral cortex and the vestibular system directly activate the vomiting center and stimuli from the gastrointestinal tract and blood activate the vomiting center indirectly by first activating the chemoreceptor trigger zone (CTZ), which then activates the vomiting center. Efferent motor and parasympathetic neural impulses from the vomiting center coordinate the emetic response by innervation of the abdominal muscles, stomach, and diaphragm.

CLINICAL POINT: A variety of neurotransmitters and their respective receptors are involved in the emetic response (see Figure 53.6). Antiemetic medications block one or more of these receptors. Decisions about the most effective antiemetic medication for a particular patient are based on the neural pathway and receptors involved in that patient's nausea and vomiting. ■

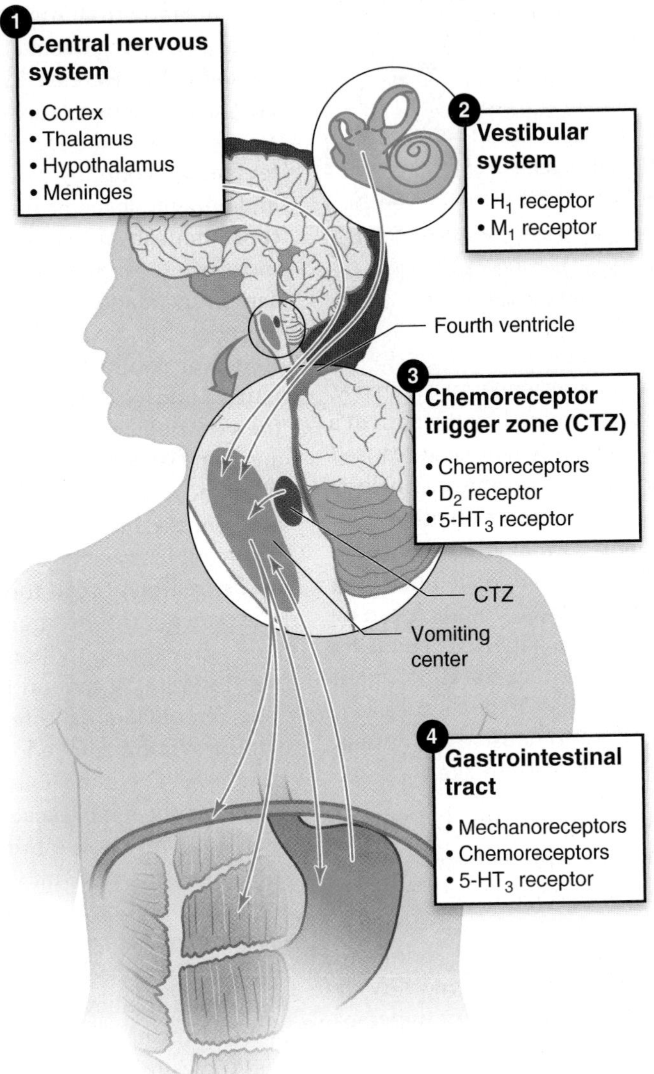

Figure 53.6 ■ Four pathways transmit afferent impulses to the vomiting center and trigger the emetic response.

1. **Central nervous system:** Information from the cerebral cortex directly activates the vomiting center in the medulla. Sensory information, such as unpleasant odors or sights and pain, as well as anxiety, fear, stress, and anticipation of an unpleasant event are common triggers of nausea and vomiting by way of the cerebral cortex. Increased intracranial pressure from a brain tumor affects this pathway.
2. **Vestibular system:** Stimulation of receptors in the vestibular system of the inner ear can lead to nausea and vomiting by directly stimulating the vomiting center. Examples include rapid position changes and medications such as aspirin, opioids, and drugs with ototoxic effects (harmful to the eighth cranial nerve or the organs involved in hearing or balance). Movement-associated problems, such as vestibular disease, and inner ear diseases, such as ear infections, are underlying etiologies that stimulate the vestibular system. The neurotransmitters acetylcholine and histamine are involved in this pathway and stimulate muscarinic type 1 and histamine type 1 receptors, respectively.
3. **Chemoreceptor trigger zone (CTZ) and the vomiting center:** Input from the vestibular apparatus and sensory input from the cerebral cortex directly activate the vomiting center in the brainstem. Other triggers, such as vagal afferent nerves from the stomach and some blood-borne emetic chemicals, activate the CTZ first, which then relays the signal to the vomiting center. The CTZ is on the floor of the fourth ventricle in the brain. Because it is outside the blood–brain barrier, it can be activated by substances that do not enter the brain to any significant extent. It is in contact with cerebrospinal fluid, which is in equilibrium with contents in the blood. Medications that can activate the CTZ include nonsteroidal anti-inflammatory, opioid, steroid, antibiotic, antineoplastic (anticancer), and anticholinergic medications. Metabolic changes that activate the CTZ include uremia, hypercalcemia, hyponatremia, hypoxia, and ketoacidosis. Toxins that accumulate as a result of liver disease, tumors, and metastatic cancers also produce nausea and vomiting associated with the CTZ. Neurotransmitters and their respective receptors involved in this pathway include serotonin (5-HT_3), dopamine, opioids, and neurokinin.
4. **Gastrointestinal tract:** Nausea and vomiting can result from peripheral pathway stimuli. The vagus and other visceral nerves convey afferent signals from the gastrointestinal tract to the vomiting center when there is a gastrointestinal infection or when abdominal organs are overstretched. Causes of such stretching include overdistention from hepatomegaly, ascites, constipation, and delayed gastric emptying, as well as obstruction from a tumor, adhesions, inflammation. These mechanical forces stimulate the release of neurotransmitters involved in vomiting, including serotonin. Efferent neural output from the vomiting center to the stomach, diaphragm, and abdominal muscles causes the forceful stomach contraction that is responsible for vomiting.

Irene Rollins: Application

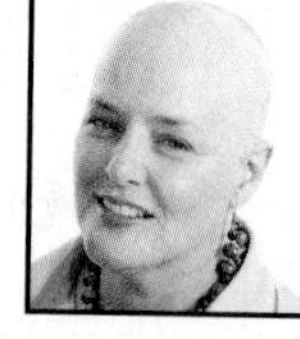

As a result of obstruction from cancer growth, neural signals from Ms. Rollins's overdistended abdominal organs to the vomiting center in her brain is the mechanism that is likely to be responsible for the nausea and vomiting she has been experiencing.

7. What are the untoward consequences of persistent vomiting?
8. Besides medications, what measures could Ms. Rollins use to minimize episodes of nausea and vomiting?

Clinical Manifestations

Because nausea is a subjective experience, its intensity, duration, and distress are best determined by the patient's self-report. Common accompaniments to nausea are caused by activation of the autonomic nervous system and include diaphoresis (profuse sweating), increased salivation, dizziness, and loss of interest in surroundings. Patients may report that particular odors, body position changes, and food intake stimulate nausea. In contrast, vomiting can be observed and measured. Because the pattern of vomiting can vary in frequency and quality, its onset, duration, quantity, and character are carefully assessed. Patients are asked about the relationship of vomiting to nausea, abdominal pain, medication administration, and food intake.

Linking Pathophysiology to Diagnosis and Treatment

The diagnosis of nausea and vomiting is based on the patient's self-report and clinical manifestations. Physical examination done to diagnose the underlying cause of nausea and vomiting includes examination of the abdomen, which may reveal changes in gastrointestinal motility or obstruction indicated by distention, inaudible or hyperactive bowel sounds on auscultation, and tenderness on palpation. If a cerebral component of nausea and vomiting is suspected, neurologic and fundoscopic eye examinations may indicate increased intracranial pressure. Treatment approaches for nausea and vomiting are directed at the underlying etiology of these symptoms. Because there may be more than one etiology, a multiple-treatment approach is often used. When possible, reversible causes of nausea and vomiting are aggressively treated. For example, if the suspected cause is constipation, a bowel program that includes laxatives is implemented. For patients with gastrointestinal stasis not associated with full bowel obstruction, prokinetic agents are given to stimulate intestinal motility. For patients with complete bowel obstruction, the somatostatin analogue octreotide (Sandostatin) decreases gastrointestinal secretions and stimulates absorption of water and electrolytes, helping to dry up secretions in the gastrointestinal tract. Antimicrobial medications for gastrointestinal infections can eradicate the infection and the nausea and vomiting that causes it. Medications that decrease gastric acid secretion, such as histamine receptor antagonists and proton pump inhibitors, along with cytoprotective agents are used to treat nausea and vomiting that result from gastric irritation. Nonsteroidal anti-inflammatory medications, such as aspirin and ibuprofen, are avoided because they can cause gastric irritation. If the suspected cause of nausea and vomiting is inflammation from tumor activity, corticosteroids are helpful in decreasing edema in and around the tumor. Corticosteroids also decrease intracranial pressure, which when elevated is another cause of nausea and vomiting.

Because of the significant influence of neurotransmitters on the vomiting center, the basis for many antinausea and antiemetic medications is blocking of the receptors for those neurotransmitters. The medications that are used most often for this purpose are dopamine antagonists, serotonin antagonists, histamine antagonists, and anticholinergics.[32] For example, medications that block histamine type 1 or cholinergic receptors are effective for treating nausea and vomiting that arise from conditions affecting the vestibular system. Dopamine and serotonin receptor antagonists block receptors in the CTZ and the gastrointestinal tract and are used, for example, to treat antineoplastic drug-induced nausea and vomiting.

Nonpharmacologic approaches are essential to include in the treatment plan for nausea and vomiting. Palliative care patients are encouraged to attempt to ingest fluids and foods that appeal to them and that they believe they may best tolerate. A general recommendation is to eat bland food at room temperature. Small, frequent meals are served, while environmental odors are controlled and relaxation is promoted. Dietitians may have other helpful suggestions, including the use of palatable nutritional supplements.

More aggressive interventions, such as insertion of a nasogastric tube, may be necessary for patients with intractable nausea and vomiting.[33] For patients with a gastric obstruction, a venting gastrostomy tube allows for drainage and prevents vomiting. Palliative surgery may be performed to alleviate bowel obstruction. Radiation may be used for nausea and vomiting related to underlying gastrointestinal and brain tumors to reduce tumor size.

Irene Rollins: Application

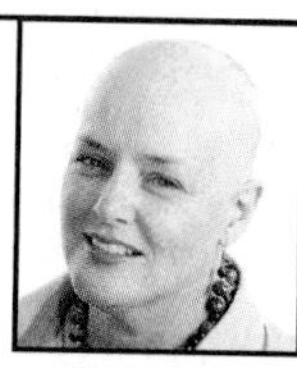

Ms. Rollins demonstrates clinical manifestations of a patient with advanced ovarian cancer, including nausea and vomiting. From the initial workup, she was diagnosed with a bowel obstruction secondary to cancer. The oncologist meets with Ms. Rollins and her family to discuss the progression of her disease and to develop an appropriate and acceptable plan of care. The initial management plan involves no oral intake to provide bowel rest and a nasogastric (NG) tube to provide continuous suction and intravenous fluid replacement. While an NG tube can achieve decompression and drainage, the insertion of a venting gastrostomy tube can be a more effective palliative treatment strategy. A venting gastrostomy consists of a tube placed through the skin into the stomach to allow air and liquid to escape into a drain. The tube can be used both for decompression and as a means of providing nutrition when the obstruction resolves. This procedure is attempted for Ms. Rollins on the day after her admission to the hospital, but it is unsuccessful because the tumor burden in her abdominal cavity prevents the team from being able to visualize the stomach wall.

A hospice team member evaluates Ms. Rollins, who is admitted to the program after being discharged to home following a 4-day hospitalization. At discharge, Ms. Rollins's IV fluids are discontinued, but the NG tube remains in place because her obstructive symptoms have not subsided. At intervals throughout the day, a member of Ms. Rollins's family disconnects the suction on the NG tube, and during that time, she is able to take and tolerate small amounts of clear liquids. Attaining comfort is a primary goal of care. Careful skin, oral, and nasal hygiene is maintained.

9. What should the hospice team instruct the family to do if Ms. Rollins experiences nausea while the NG tube is still in place?
10. What are the key assessment findings that indicate that Ms. Rollins's bowel obstruction has gotten progressively worse?

Check Your Progress: Section 53.6

1. Differentiate the characteristics of nausea from those of vomiting.
2. Explain the emetic response (vomiting reflex).
3. What is the basis for antinausea and antiemetic medications? List the four major categories of these medications.

53.7 Anorexia and Cachexia

Anorexia is loss of the desire to eat leading to decreased intake of foods and fluids. **Cachexia** is skeletal muscle wasting and involuntary weight loss resulting from both metabolic abnormalities and a lack of nutrition.[34,35] A patient may experience anorexia without cachexia; however, anorexia is often one of the underlying causes of cachexia. These two symptoms are commonly associated with advanced disease; they occur in 70–80% of patients at the end of life.[36] Because of related weight loss, both anorexia and cachexia serve as visible reminders of a patient's disease and therefore are often particularly disturbing problems for family members of terminally ill patients. Relatives may interpret a patient's refusal to eat as "losing hope" or "giving in to the disease." They also may mistakenly believe that the only way for the patient to improve is by eating.

William Thompson: Application

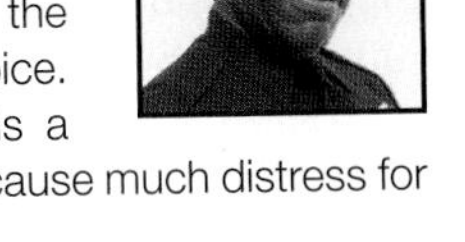

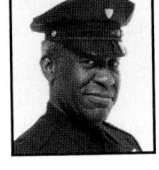

Mr. Thompson has had an unintentional weight loss of 40 pounds that occurred over the 3 months before he was admitted to hospice. This weight loss and his anorexia, which is a contributing factor, and the resultant fatigue cause much distress for both Mr. Thompson and his family.

5. How did Mr. Thompson's anorexia eventually lead to the fatigue he subsequently developed?
6. What strategy could the nurse use to help the family cope with this visible change in Mr. Thompson's physical appearance?

Etiology and Pathogenesis

Many factors contribute to anorexia at the end of life. Disease-related problems include oral or systemic infections, poorly fitting dentures, pain or difficulty swallowing associated with eating, physical obstruction to dietary intake, and impaired absorption of dietary nutrients. Progression of the underlying disease itself may contribute to anorexia. For example, in end-stage chronic obstructive pulmonary disease, the increased work of breathing may leave few energy reserves for the effort required to eat and digest food. Treatment-related contributors to anorexia include adverse effects of radiation and chemotherapy such as stomatitis and gastritis. Nutritional deficiencies ultimately produce ketosis, leading to a lack of interest in food.[37] Certain medications may cause problems by inducing changes in taste, nausea, appetite suppression, delayed gastric emptying, and constipation. Depression, anxiety, and delirium are among the many comorbidities that can contribute to anorexia and cachexia.

Cachexia is a complex process resulting from changes in carbohydrate, lipid, and protein metabolism (**Figure 53.7** ■). These metabolic changes lead to weight loss, adipose tissue loss, and skeletal muscle wasting. **Asthenia**, a loss or lack of physical strength, is a consequence of skeletal muscle wasting. In patients with cancer and other inflammatory conditions, the immune system produces chemical mediators that lead to these changes. Specific mediators, called proinflammatory cytokines, include tumor necrosis factor, interleukin-1, interleukin-6, and interferon. These mediators also may contribute to anorexia by acting on the hypothalamus to decrease hunger sensation. Unlike starvation, in which there is depletion of adipose tissue to spare skeletal muscle protein, in cachexia both adipose tissue and skeletal muscle are depleted. In cachexia, there is a shift from normal daily synthesis of skeletal muscle proteins to muscle protein degradation to provide substrates for enhanced hepatic synthesis of acute-phase proteins involved in the inflammatory response.[35,38]

Clinical Manifestations

Objective manifestations of cachexia include unintentional weight loss of at least 5% from the pre-illness weight within a 6-month period.[39] Decreased fat stores and loss of muscle mass and asthenia are other hallmark features. A thorough physical examination may reveal loose skin turgor, dry mouth and thirst, confusion and drowsiness, difficulty clearing pulmonary secretions, abdominal discomfort, and decreased urine output. Subjectively, along with stating a decreased or lack of appetite, patients may complain of fatigue, diminished overall body strength, and pain with eating.

Linking Pathophysiology to Diagnosis and Treatment

The diagnosis of anorexia is based on the patient's report of diminished appetite and observations of decreased food intake. The diagnosis of cachexia is based on the clinical manifestations described in the previous section. In addition, the patient's serum albumin level is expected to be low as a result of protein malnutrition.

Every effort is made to make appealing foods and fluids available to palliative care patients (see the Impact of Nutrition in Clinical Practice feature). The healthcare team is sensitive to the concerns of family members who may feel that they are failing or abandoning the patient by not feeding him. It is helpful to inform them that decreased intake of foods and fluids can lead to ketosis and subsequent release of endorphins that contribute to an enhanced sense of well-being and diminished discomfort.[27] Family members can be assisted in redirecting their expression of care and concern away from food to other measures that provide comfort to the patient.

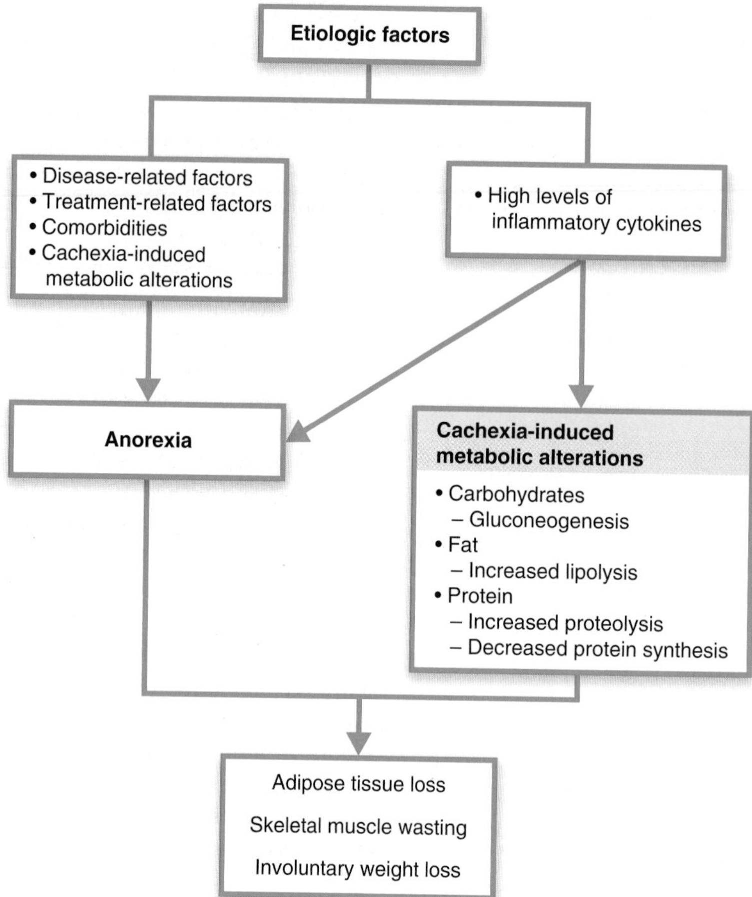

Figure 53.7 ■ Anorexia contributes to cachexia; however, it is not the only factor involved. Chronic high levels of inflammatory cytokines shift metabolism toward increased degradation of protein and fat and increased production of glucose to provide substrates for synthesis of acute phase proteins, which are involved in the inflammatory response. Anorexia and cachexia both contribute to involuntary weight loss, loss of adipose tissue, and skeletal muscle wasting.

In certain situations, interventions can be attempted to alleviate anorexia. For example, anxiety, nausea, dehydration, constipation, and oral infections can be managed, which may help to increase the patient's desire for food. A trial of medications can also be attempted to increase appetite. Corticosteroids such as dexamethasone and prednisone may help to increase appetite and physical strength for a short time. Medications with effects similar to those of progesterone may improve appetite, with effects evident after 1–2 weeks of treatment. Prokinetic agents, such as metoclopramide (Reglan), increase the rate of gastric emptying; this in turn can reduce the feeling of abdominal fullness that some patients with decreased appetite experience.

Impact of Nutrition in Clinical Practice

Nutrition at the End of Life

Joanne Kouba

At the end of life, the goal is for the patient to eat for pleasure and satisfaction. Dietary restrictions are eliminated, and patients are encouraged to eat and drink whatever foods and fluids appeal to them. Patients and family members must receive information about anorexia and cachexia as an expected consequence of end-stage disease. They should be informed that better care or increased effort to feed the patient will not reverse cachexia because the process of muscle protein degradation is not due just to decreased caloric intake and therefore does not respond to interventions such as supplemental nutrition or high-calorie foods. Enteral feedings via gastrostomy or nasogastric tubes are limited to patients who state that they are hungry but do not have the mechanical ability to eat.

Artificial hydration and nutrition at the end of life is a subject of considerable controversy. The benefits must be weighed against the burdens of such treatment, including the associated risks of fluid overload, peripheral and pulmonary edema, electrolyte imbalances, infection, and aspiration into the lungs. A decrease in food and fluid intake is part of the normal process of dying; as death approaches, parenteral and enteral feeding does not improve symptoms or prolong life.

Check Your Progress: Section 53.7

1. Differentiate the characteristics of anorexia, cachexia, and asthenia.
2. What clinical manifestations are commonly seen in patients with anorexia and cachexia?
3. Why doesn't increased nutritional intake alone reverse cachexia?

53.8 Fatigue

Fatigue is a pervasive feeling of tiredness and lack of energy that is not relieved by rest. Fatigue is present in 60–90% of patients with life-limiting illnesses.[11,40] While fatigue is associated with other symptoms such as anorexia and cachexia, correcting those symptoms generally does not reverse the fatigue that palliative care patients experience. Asthenia, a loss or lack of physical strength, is another symptom that is connected closely to fatigue. Fatigue and asthenia can significantly impair the quality of life of patients and their family caregivers.

Etiology and Pathogenesis

Fatigue is frequently a multidimensional symptom involving physiologic, cognitive, and psychosocial factors. Specific underlying pathophysiologic mechanisms for fatigue have yet to be fully uncovered. In patients with cancer, researchers are closely investigating the relationship between proinflammatory cytokines and fatigue.[41,42] At the end of life, fatigue can result from immobility resulting in loss of muscle mass and muscle deconditioning as well as sleep disruption, inadequate rest, nutritional deficiencies, and unrelieved symptoms such as pain or cough. Many medications that are used to treat hospice and palliative care patients have a sedative effect that can contribute to fatigue; these include anticholinergics, antihistamines, benzodiazepines, and anticonvulsants. Metabolic abnormalities that may lead to fatigue include electrolyte and acid–base imbalances, uremia, malnutrition, dehydration, infection, and fever. Preexisting or co-existing diseases also play a role; these include anemia, depression, hypothyroidism, infection, sleep disorders, heart failure, and chronic obstructive pulmonary disease. Radiation therapy and antineoplastic medications are treatment-related factors that are linked to causing fatigue.

Clinical Manifestations

Patients may express feeling tired while participating in activities of daily living and activities such as walking and socializing. Other symptoms related to fatigue include decreased muscle strength, difficulty concentrating, confusion, limited mobility, and reduced independence. Factors that alleviate and exacerbate fatigue are important to note.

Linking Pathophysiology to Diagnosis and Treatment

A patient's self-report of tiredness not relieved by rest is a crucial piece of data in diagnosing fatigue. The Karnofsky Performance Status Scale (see Table 53.1) can be used to assess the severity of fatigue and its response to interventions.[11]

For all patients experiencing fatigue, energy conservation is necessary, with rest and activity balanced according to the patient's response Family members may interpret fatigue as a sign that the patient is giving up or not trying hard enough to stay well. In the terminal phase of care, patients and family members are taught that fatigue is an expected and generally uncontrollable consequence of progressive disease; relatives are encouraged to avoid pressuring the patient to be more involved or more energetic than she can be.

Patients with fatigue related to uncontrolled symptoms such as pain and dyspnea are likely to have more energy when interventions successfully alleviate such problems. Techniques that help a patient achieve sleep are also important. They include reducing caffeine intake as bedtime approaches, positioning for comfort, and providing a calm and quiet environment.

Pharmacologic interventions may also be beneficial. A short course of corticosteroids may improve the patient's appetite and increase energy and well-being. Psychostimulants may effectively reduce sedation and increase energy during the daytime (see the feature on Impact of Current Research on Clinical Practice). Patients with significant anemia may benefit from erythropoietin administration, which stimulates red blood cell production in the bone marrow, or from packed red blood cell transfusions. If fatigue is associated with depression, a trial of antidepressants is indicated.

William Thompson: Outcome

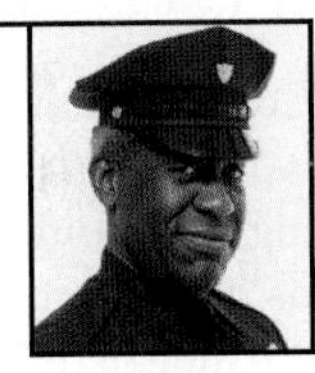

Mr. Thompson experiences debilitating fatigue near the end of his life. In addition to completing the Karnofsky Performance Status Scale, the hospice team needs to further assess Mr. Thompson's report of fatigue and anorexia to develop an appropriate plan of care. In doing so, they rule out correctable causes of these symptoms. Team members meet with Mr. Thompson and his family to discuss the likelihood that the symptoms he is experiencing relate directly to his underlying advanced stage of cancer. They note that attempting aggressive interventions to correct these symptoms will not change the course of the disease. At that meeting, Mr. Thompson and his family begin to acknowledge the possibility of his imminent death.

Mr. Thompson's family receives information about comfort measures that they can provide, which include giving Mr. Thompson foods and fluids that he enjoys or requests while not pressuring him to maintain a certain level of nutrition. They learn about methods to promote Mr. Thompson's energy conservation and begin to feel more comfortable about letting him rest as needed. As they become more accepting of the terminal nature of his condition, family members refocus their efforts on providing Mr. Thompson with conditions for a peaceful and dignified death.

7. What are some correctable metabolic causes that could lead to the development of fatigue and anorexia?
8. What evidence confirms that the family has accepted the inevitable outcome of Mr. Thompson's disease?

Impact of Current Research on Clinical Practice

Treatment of Fatigue with a Central Nervous System Stimulant

Description: Fatigue and depression are common near the end of life and have a negative effect on the person's quality of life. In a double-blind investigation in which neither clinicians nor patients knew whether the patient received the investigational medication or placebo, 30 hospice patients in either inpatient or outpatient settings were randomly assigned to receive treatment with either methylphenidate (Metadate, Ritalin), a mild central nervous system stimulant that increases the levels of norepinephrine and dopamine in the brain, or a placebo. The placebo was a tablet that looked identical to methyphenidate but contained starch instead of the medication. The research study nurse conducted the physical assessments and administered the symptom assessment scales. While all patients reported fatigue, no differences in severity scores were observed between the treatment and placebo groups at the beginning of the study.

Clinical Practice: A statistically significant decrease in the severity of fatigue was observed by day 14 in the group treated with methylphenidate. No improvement in fatigue was experienced by patients in the placebo group. Patients treated with methylphenidate who had clinically significant depression at the beginning of the study experienced improvement in depression based on three depression self-report scales; less improvement was noted in the placebo group. These results support the use of the central nervous system stimulant methylphenidate to improve the quality of life of patients experiencing fatigue or depression associated with terminal illness.

Research Study:

Kerr, C., Drake, J., Milch, R., et al. (2012). Effects of methylphenidate on fatigue and depression: A randomized, double-blind, placebo-controlled trial. *Journal of Pain and Symptom Management*, *43*(1), 68–77.

Check Your Progress: Section 53.8

1. Describe the etiologic factors involved in causing fatigue near the end of life.
2. What are the clinical manifestations that often accompany fatigue?
3. Describe the pharmacologic and nonpharmacologic approaches to management of fatigue.

53.9 Constipation

Constipation is the infrequent passage of small amounts of hard, dry stool. This common yet underrecognized distressing symptom occurs in an estimated 51–84% of hospice and palliative care patients; the incidence and severity increase as the time of death approaches.[43,44,45] Constipation can contribute to other symptoms, including pain and vomiting.

Etiology and Pathogenesis

Peristaltic muscle contractions in the gastrointestinal tract mix intestinal contents, aiding in digestion and the movement of unabsorbed content onward to the rectum for excretion. In constipation, this transit time is prolonged. At the end of life, constipation often results from several factors, including the primary disease that is causing the terminal illness, concurrent diseases, treatment-related variables, medications, dietary factors, and physical inactivity. Disease-related conditions that contribute to constipation in terminally ill patients include primary and metastatic tumor growth, spinal cord compression, ascites, and hypercalcemia. Concurrent diseases, including chronic neurologic and neuromuscular conditions, diabetes, hypothyroidism, and diverticular disease, can slow bowel motility. Treatment-related variables include bowel adhesions from surgery and radiation-induced fibrosis. Medications that frequently lead to constipation include antidepressants, anticholinergics, anticonvulsants, calcium-channel blockers, muscle relaxants, and opioids. Palliative care patients are frequently prescribed opioid medications to control pain and/or dyspnea. However, these drugs bind to intestinal opioid receptors and slow peristalsis, as well as causing an increase in anal sphincter tone, leading to constipation.[45] In contrast to other therapeutic and adverse effects of opioids, tolerance to the constipating effects of these medications does not develop.

CLINICAL POINT: Because of the constipating effects of opioid medications, all patients on long-term opioid therapy should be placed on a preventive protocol for constipation, including a laxative. ■

Terminally ill patients are also predisposed to constipation because their typical diet is inadequate in both fluid, leading to increased fluid absorption from intestinal contents and harder stool, and fiber, decreasing the bulk of stool and peristalsis. These patients also become physically inactive and develop general debility with muscle weakness. Generalized pain, diminished consciousness, loss of normal bowel routine, and inadequate privacy during toileting due to need for assistance are other factors that may contribute to constipation.

Clinical Manifestations

In evaluating a patient for constipation, it is important to first ask about the patient's normal bowel pattern, including the typical frequency, amount, characteristics, and time of bowel movements. Patients with constipation often report abdominal cramping, pain, and bloating; nausea; straining on attempting a bowel movement; and rectal pressure. On physical examination, common findings include abdominal distention, hypoactive bowel sounds, and hemorrhoids. The rectal examination may reveal fecal impaction.

Linking Pathophysiology to Diagnosis and Treatment

The diagnosis of constipation is based on the frequency of bowel movements and the consistency of fecal matter. The optimal management approach for constipation is to anticipate and prevent this symptom. Regardless of the expected change in oral intake with disease progression, patients should have a bowel movement at least every 72 hours. Patients who have experienced constipation before the terminal phase of their illness may have followed an effective bowel program so it is important to ask about that and help them continue it when possible.

Patients who are taking opioid medications must also be provided with daily laxatives, and the dose of the laxative must be titrated upward when the dose of the opioid is increased. In palliative care, stimulant laxatives are generally the drugs of choice; they increase gastrointestinal motility and reduce fluid absorption from the colon. A common recommendation is to combine a stimulant laxative with a stool softener to increase water penetration in the bowel and produce a moister stool. Bulk and osmotic laxatives can be used if the patient is able consume and tolerate a sufficient oral intake. Prokinetic medications increase peristaltic activity; however, they cannot be used in patients with complete bowel obstruction because they can cause cramping and intestinal rupture. Lubricant laxatives, such as glycerin suppositories, reduce friction and facilitate stool passage; they are alternatives for patients who no longer can safely swallow an oral laxative. Nonpharmacologic approaches for constipation are also included in the plan of care. Increased fluid intake and the addition of high-fiber foods are encouraged for patients who can tolerate them. When possible, toileting is scheduled at regular times, and the patient is assured that assistance is available and privacy will be maintained when the patient has the urge to have a bowel movement. Manual disimpaction and enemas are treatments for patients who develop impaction; patients are premedicated with an analgesic before these uncomfortable procedures.

Check Your Progress: Section 53.9

1. Explain the disease-related and treatment-related factors that contribute to the etiology of constipation in terminally ill patients.
2. Describe the clinical manifestations that often accompany constipation.
3. What are the pharmacologic and nonpharmacologic approaches to the management of constipation?

53.10 Urinary Incontinence

Urinary incontinence is loss of bladder control that results in involuntary leakage of urine. Prevalence rates among patients with terminal illness range from 29–72%.[46] This problem often develops in the late phase of illness when family caregivers are becoming overwhelmed.[47] New onset of urinary incontinence is a visible indication to patients of loss of control and can be a source of great embarrassment for them.

Etiology and Pathophysiology

Urinary incontinence can occur transiently or as a chronic condition. Transient urinary incontinence can result from acute delirium, impaired or restricted mobility, particular medications, infection, or stool impaction. Chronic urinary incontinence can be further classified as follows.

- *Stress urinary incontinence:* During normal urination, the detrusor muscle contracts while the urethral sphincter relaxes following input from the pelvic nerves to the cerebral cortex. Weakened pelvic floor muscles, neurologic lesions of the lower spine, neuromuscular diseases, or surgical procedures such as radical hysterectomy and prostatectomy can compromise the nerves or muscles necessary for closure of the urethral sphincter. The result is urinary leakage when bladder and intra-abdominal pressure exceeds the strength of the urethra to remain closed.
- *Urge urinary incontinence:* This type develops when overactivity of the detrusor muscle leads to involuntary bladder contractions. Common contributors to urge urinary incontinence include urinary tract infection, bladder tumor, and effects of cancer treatment.
- *Overflow urinary incontinence:* Incomplete emptying of the bladder during voiding can lead to urinary retention and bladder overdistention, resulting in leakage of urine. Common contributing factors include weakened bladder muscle, spinal injury and pelvic nerve damage, and conditions that block the urethra, such as stones, tumors, and an enlarged prostate.
- *Functional urinary incontinence:* Fatigue and deficits in mobility, dexterity, or cognition can contribute to incontinence because the patient cannot reach or use the bedside commode or toilet.

Clinical Manifestations

The patient with stress urinary incontinence typically experiences involuntary urine leakage during strenuous activities such as coughing, laughing, sneezing, or physical exertion. The patient with urge incontinence experiences an uncontrollable involuntary urine leakage immediately following a very strong urge to urinate. Dysuria (painful urination), hematuria (blood in the urine), and nocturia (excessive urination during the night) are important findings to note. The patient should also be asked about his sense of the fullness of the urinary stream and about any sense of incomplete bladder emptying after voiding.

Linking Pathophysiology to Diagnosis and Treatment

The diagnosis of the type of urinary incontinence is based on the clinical manifestations described previously. Measuring a postvoid residual urine volume is useful in determining the need for catheterization because of incomplete bladder emptying or urinary retention. A postvoid residual urine of 25% or less of the voided volume is generally considered indicative of acceptable bladder emptying. In designing interventions for palliative care patients who are experiencing urinary incontinence, attention focuses on helping them achieve death with dignity. Treatment involves identifying the cause of the incontinence and eliminating precipitating factors when possible. Consideration should be given to the many medications that can contribute to urinary incontinence, including antidepressants, sedative-hypnotics, antihistamines, and opioids.

An anticholinergic medication may be helpful for patients who are experiencing urge incontinence. Anticholinergics suppress bladder contractions and allow for a more complete bladder emptying upon voiding. If urinary tract infection is a suspected cause of a new onset of urinary incontinence, consideration can be given to a course of antibiotics. While exercises to strengthen pelvic floor muscles have been demonstrated as effective for stress incontinence in other patient populations, hospice and palliative care patients may be unable to perform these exercises. Urinary incontinence in terminally ill patients can be treated with behavioral methods; one approach is to establish a voiding schedule for patients who can tolerate movement using a bedpan, bedside commode, or toilet. Adjustment of oral intake is indicated if the type and timing of beverages are contributing to a new onset of urinary incontinence. For example, patients may find that limiting intake of beverages with a diuretic effect, such as those containing caffeine, throughout the day and minimizing fluid intake before bedtime improve symptoms.

Persistent incontinence may require placement of an indwelling, intermittent, or external bladder catheter. Urinary catheters are often helpful for terminally ill patients who are immobile or experience pain when being repositioned. For all patients who are experiencing urinary incontinence, a care priority is keeping the skin clean and dry to prevent breakdown. Diapers and incontinence pads are frequently used at the end of life.

Check Your Progress: Section 53.10

1. Differentiate the causes, pathogenesis, and clinical manifestations of transient urinary incontinence from those of chronic urinary incontinence (stress, urge, overflow, and functional urinary incontinence).
2. What diagnostic approaches are used to determine the type of urinary incontinence that is present in a patient?
3. Describe the pharmacologic and nonpharmacologic approaches for managing urinary incontinence.

53.11 Delirium

Delirium is an acute and usually fluctuating change in cognition or awareness that can be reversible and is unrelated to preexisting dementia, which develops gradually and gets progressively worse. Delirium is a common symptom affecting hospice and palliative care patients; the incidence is as high as 80%.[48–50] Delirium is one of the most difficult symptoms to treat at the end of life. It impairs the ability of patients to interact with others, make decisions, and describe their symptoms and response to treatment.

Etiology and Pathogenesis

Delirium often results from more than one factor. It involves neurotransmitters and neuropathologic processes, although specifics of the alterations are not well understood. Three neurotransmitters play a role in cognitive function: dopamine, acetylcholine, and gamma-aminobutyric acid (GABA). Dopamine has an excitatory effect on neurons that is countered by the two other neurotransmitters. An imbalance in the levels of these three neurotransmitters leads to changes in neurotransmission and subsequent delirium.[51] This imbalance can result from disease processes, metabolic changes, and certain medications.

Clinical factors that contribute to delirium include uncontrolled pain, fever, dehydration, hypoxia, urinary retention, fecal impaction, organ failure, and infection. Vitamin deficiencies and metabolic changes leading to hypoglycemia, hypercalcemia, hyponatremia, and uremia are other factors to consider. Direct central nervous system causes of delirium are brain tumors, seizure activity, and cerebrovascular disease. Medications can be a prime culprit in causing delirium in this patient population. For example, impaired renal clearance of the opioid medications commonly used in palliative care combined with dehydration can cause active metabolites of morphine to accumulate and lead to symptoms of delirium. Other medications that contribute to delirium include steroids, benzodiazepines, anticholinergics, and antineoplastics.

Clinical Manifestations

Delirium is a change in mental status that develops suddenly with the clinical manifestations and severity typically fluctuating over time. Manifestations include a reduced ability to focus and appropriately shift or sustain attention, disturbance in memory, disorientation, fluctuating level of consciousness, and perceptual disturbances such as hallucinations. There are three forms of delirium: agitated delirium, hypoactive delirium, and a mixed form. In agitated delirium, anxiety with motor and sensory excitement may be seen, including rapid and incoherent speech. These changes may be more pronounced in the evening. As the patient approaches death, a type of agitated delirium called terminal delirium is also common. Symptoms include aggressive behavior and verbal communication; auditory, visual, and tactile hallucinations; difficulty concentrating or falling asleep; and agitation, restlessness, disorientation, and moaning. In contrast, hypoactive delirium often manifests as increased drowsiness and disturbances in the sleep–wake cycle. In the mixed form of delirium, manifestations of hyperactive and hypoactive delirium can be present at various times.

The following manifestations are also considered in the patient who is experiencing delirium, because they can point to an underlying cause: fever, signs of dehydration, bowel impaction, and an oxygen saturation level that demonstrates hypoxemia. Diagnostic tests that can be done to determine underlying factors of delirium include a metabolic panel and complete blood count to rule out anemia, infection, and electrolyte imbalance; urinalysis to rule out a urinary tract infection; and a chest x-ray to rule out pneumonia.

Linking Pathophysiology to Diagnosis and Treatment

Delirium is diagnosed by comparing the patient's mental status before and after the onset of new symptoms. This information is often obtained from individuals who are familiar with the patient before such change, such as family members. Early detection of delirium is essential; failure to diagnose this condition can lead to further morbidity. The **Confusion Assessment Method (CAM)** is a delirium rating scale that is recommended for use in detecting delirium and differentiating it from dementia.[52] The diagnosis of delirium using CAM is based on the presence of an acute onset of change in mental status with fluctuations in severity throughout the day plus impaired ability to focus attention. In addition to those two manifestations, either disorganized thinking or an altered level of consciousness must be present.

Delirium in the final stages of life is generally irreversible; it is important that this be communicated to the patient's family members so that they do not have unrealistic expectations for reversal of the problem. However, efforts are directed at identifying and eliminating any correctable causes of delirium. For example, unnecessary medications are discontinued; others may be reduced in dose or frequency of administration. If delirium is thought to be related to opioid use, a different opioid medication can be substituted; this strategy is called opioid rotation. Infection can be treated with the appropriate antimicrobial medication, and electrolyte imbalances can be corrected. Environmental approaches are critical components in the plan of care for patients experiencing delirium. A priority is providing a safe physical environment. The patient's room should be calm, quiet, and well lit. Familiar people, music, sounds, objects, and photos may help to reorient the patient. Reestablishment of a normal sleep–wake cycle can also be helpful.

Haloperidol (Haldol) is an antidopaminergic medication that is often effective for delirious patients who are experiencing agitation and hallucinations.[53] Benzodiazepines, such as lorazepam (Ativan) are considered second-line treatment for agitated delirium; they act at the gamma-aminobutyric acid receptor sites to enhance the inhibitory effects on nerve cell firing at those sites. Benzodiazepines decrease anxiety, relax smooth muscle, and provide sedation. However, benzodiazepines should not be used alone for treatment of agitated delirium because they can cause disinhibition and increased agitation.[54] In contrast, for patients who are experiencing hypoactive delirium, a psychostimulant such as methylphenidate (Metadate, Ritalin) may help to increase the level of alertness.

Check Your Progress: Section 53.11

1. Distinguish delirium from dementia, and explain the screening scale that can be used to differentiate these conditions.
2. Differentiate the clinical manifestations of agitated delirium, hypoactive delirium, and mixed delirium.
3. Describe the pharmacologic and nonpharmacologic approaches to management of agitated and hypoactive delirium.

53.12 Last Expected Changes at the End of Life

Although death can occur suddenly and unexpectedly, most people die following an illness that leads to a gradual deterioration of body systems. The final days of that process is the **active phase of dying**. During that time, physiologic changes lead to expected symptoms until death occurs. Interventions continue to focus on patient comfort, and the multidimensional plan of care continues to address the patient's and family's psychosocial and spiritual issues.

Pathogenesis

In the active phase of dying, the major organs lose function. Dehydration from an inability to swallow and severe muscle weakness affect the cardiac system. Decreased blood volume and diminished cardiac contractility lead to decreased delivery of oxygenated blood to cells. Hypotension further diminishes perfusion, leading to a decline in mental status, a cooling of the extremities, and decreased urine output. The pulse becomes irregular and weak. Decreased venous return to the heart results in increased capillary hydrostatic pressure and low protein intake decreases capillary colloid osmotic pressure. Both of these alterations increase fluid leakage out of capillaries, leading to pleural effusion, abdominal ascites, and peripheral edema. Blood begins to pool in dependent areas, causing mottling, a purplish discoloration, of the soles of the feet and the hands, which is a sign of imminent death. Impaired cardiac function also leads to pulmonary congestion and changes in ventilation and perfusion that impair gas exchange. The subsequent hypercapnia and hypoxia result in slowed mentation, confusion, disorientation, restlessness, hypersomnolence, and coma. Carbon dioxide retention leads to respiratory acidosis, and decreased tissue oxygenation leads to metabolic acidosis.

Clinical Manifestations

Clinical manifestations of the active phase of dying include use of accessory muscles to breathe and **Cheyne-Stokes breathing**, which is characterized by a waxing and waning of the depth of breathing with regularly recurring intervals of apnea. Cheyne-Stokes breathing is a sign of imminent death. Brain hypoxia occurs because of decreased cerebral blood flow due to poor cardiac function, metabolic imbalances, toxin accumulation, and renal and hepatic failure. Changes in the thermoregulatory system can result in either hyperthermia or hypothermia.

Death of the whole person, in contrast to death of individual cells, is called **somatic death**. Signs of somatic death include fixed and dilated pupils; cessation of heartbeat, respiration, movement, and reflexes; and relaxation of muscles and sphincters. Shortly after death, the patient's jaw becomes relaxed and open. The pronouncement of death is made when there is an absence of heart sounds, spontaneous respirations, and pupillary light reflex. **Algor mortis** is the drop in body temperature that begins immediately after death and is due to cessation of heat-producing metabolic reactions and regulation of body temperature. Body temperature continues to decline until it reaches that of the environment within about 24 hours after death. **Rigor mortis** is the stiffening of body muscles that begins within 2–3 hours after death. It occurs because calcium leaks into the cell cytoplasm from disintegrating organelles where calcium had been stored. Since cells are no longer producing ATP, the calcium cannot be pumped out of the cytoplasm, and the excess calcium causes cross-bridging between the actin and myosin muscle filaments, resulting in contraction. The lack of ATP prevents muscle relaxation, which is an active process. Rigor mortis reaches a peak at about 12 hours after death, and then over the next few days, as body tissues decompose, muscle fibers are degraded and muscles relax.[55] When the heart is no longer pumping blood throughout the body, blood settles in the dependent parts of the body, resulting in a purple-red discoloration of those areas called **livor mortis**.

Linking Pathophysiology to Diagnosis and Treatment

After a terminal illness, the manifestations described previously are sufficient for the pronouncement of death. However, in some other situations, determination of brain death is necessary. **Brain death** is the irreversible cessation of cerebral and brainstem function.[56] Determination of brain death may be required in situations, such as traumatic brain injury, stroke, or rupture of a cerebral aneurysm, in which technology such as mechanical ventilation has been used as artificial life support when the brain is no longer regulating bodily functions. Even though the brain is not functioning and therefore the lungs are no longer receiving signals to breathe, the heart may continue contracting because of its inherent pacemaker activity as long as it receives an adequate supply of oxygen and nutrients. When a decision is made to no longer use artificial life support technology, brain death is determined by neurologic examination and sometimes additional tests. There are evidence-based clinical guidelines for determination of brain death in adults[56] and in infants and children.[57] Determination of brain death is most often based on findings from neurologic examination, including coma, absence of reflexes such as pupil constriction in response to light, the gag and corneal reflexes, the cough reflex in response to tracheal stimulation, and the withdrawal reflex in response to a pain stimulus. Additional diagnostic tests to determine brain death include measurement of cerebral electrical activity with an electroencephalogram, tests of cerebral blood flow, and the apnea test.[56] The apnea test is done to determine whether an individual can breathe on her own when removed from a ventilator. Carbon dioxide accumulates when the patient is removed from the ventilator; if the chemoreceptor reflex is intact, it should stimulate breathing when the partial pressure of carbon dioxide in the arterial blood ($PaCO_2$) is greater than 60 mmHg, or more than 20 mmHg above the person's baseline $PaCO_2$.[56,57] Factors that depress central nervous system function and impair the accurate interpretation of assessments used to determine brain death need to be ruled out or reversed. These include hypothermia, medications that cause neuromuscular blockade, and drug overdoses and other poisonings.

In the active phase of dying, patients require an intensive level of care. Because they are bedbound with little or no active movement, they need frequent repositioning and attention to keeping the skin clean and dry to prevent breakdown and discomfort. Dehydration requires careful mouth care. Because the patient is unable to safely swallow, an alternative to the oral route of administration is selected for medications that are necessary for symptom control and comfort. In rare cases in which a terminally ill patient's symptoms are refractory to available standard interventions, palliative sedation is a treatment option.[58,59] According to the American Academy of Hospice and Palliative Medicine, **palliative sedation** is "the intentional lowering of awareness towards, and including, unconsciousness for patients with severe and refractory symptoms."[60] Medications that are used to achieve palliative sedation have a rapid onset of action and short duration and include benzodiazepines, barbiturates, opioids, and anesthesia-induction agents. The medications are administered by continuous or intermittent intravenous or subcutaneous infusion and are titrated to the desired effect, and then the lowest effective dose is used.[58,59] The option of palliative sedation should be discussed with the patient and family before it is needed in order to obtain consent for its use and to relieve concerns that severe, unrelieved suffering might occur before death.

At the time of the patient's death, a member of the healthcare team asks relatives whether they want to participate in postmortem care. Care of the body is in accordance with the family's cultural and religious practices and traditions. Assisting with funeral arrangements and initiating bereavement services are other crucial roles of the healthcare team after the death of the patient.

In the case of death from an acute event, such as trauma or a myocardial infarction, or upon termination of artificial life support when the individual is a potential organ donor, care is required to maintain viability of organs for transplantation. The lack of regulation of the function of multiple organs in patients with brain death who are on artificial life support results in hemodynamic instability with fluctuations in blood pressure and heart rate, fluid and electrolyte imbalances, and inability to control body temperature. Diabetes insipidus is common in these patients, owing to brain hypoxia causing a deficiency of antidiuretic hormone, and leads to a large urine output with resultant dehydration, hypernatremia, and a decreased circulating blood volume.[61] If the patient is a potential organ donor, these conditions need to be managed to maintain organ viability until the organs designated for donation are removed.

Irene Rollins: Outcome

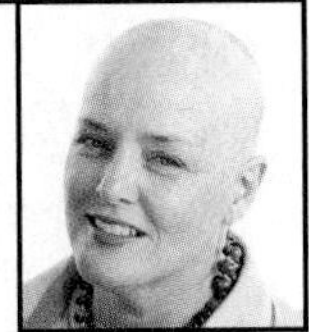

As Ms. Rollins entered the active phase of dying, the hospice nurse removed her NG tube, since Ms. Rollins no longer wants to ingest even clear liquids. Several weeks ago, when Ms. Rollins and her family decided that she would spend her last weeks of life at home, the hospice team discussed the option of administering palliative sedation if her symptoms, such as pain, nausea, or dyspnea, became unbearable. They all agreed to that option. Since Ms. Rollins has begun to experience intractable suffering and is increasingly agitated, she is started on palliative sedation to decrease her awareness of symptoms. The next day, Ms. Rollins dies comfortably and peacefully in her home, surrounded by her family.

11. What was the purpose of palliative sedation for Ms. Rollins?

12. How can the family be involved in the active phase of dying?

Check Your Progress: Section 53.12

1. What major changes occur during the active phase of dying?
2. Describe the indicators that are used to determine somatic death.
3. What indicators and diagnostic tests are used to determine brain death?

Table 53.2 Ten Leading Causes of Death in Infants and Children*

Leading Causes of Neonatal and Infant Deaths	Leading Causes of Deaths Ages 1–19 Years
1. Congenital malformations and chromosomal abnormalities	1. Unintentional injuries (trauma)
2. Disorders related to prematurity and low birth weight	2. Assault/homicide
3. Sudden infant death syndrome	3. Intentional self-harm (suicide)
4. Newborn affected by maternal complications of pregnancy	4. Cancer
5. Unintentional injuries (trauma)	5. Congenital malformations and chromosomal abnormalities
6. Newborn affected by complications of placenta, umbilical cord, and membranes	6. Heart diseases
7. Bacterial sepsis	7. Influenza and pneumonia
8. Infant respiratory distress syndrome	8. Chronic lower respiratory diseases
9. Disease of the circulatory system	9. Cerebrovascular diseases
10. Neonatal hemorrhage	10. Sepsis

*Conditions are listed with the most common cause first and others in order of decreasing frequency. Source: Data from Hamilton, B., Hoyert, D., Martin, J., et al. (2013). Annual summary of vital statistics: 2010–11. Pediatrics, 131(3), 548–558; Friebert, S. (2009). NHPCO facts and figures: Pediatric palliative and hospice care in America. Alexandria, VA: National Hospice and Palliative Care Organization; National Consensus Project for Quality Palliative Care. (2103). Clinical practice guidelines for quality palliative care (3rd ed.). Available at http://www.nationalconsensusproject.org/Guidelines_Download2.aspx.

53.13 Pediatric Considerations

Terminal illness resulting in death is less common during childhood than during adulthood. There are some differences in the conditions that affect pediatric populations, the way symptoms are assessed, and the length of time that palliative care services are needed.[62] According to the 2013 Annual Summary of Vital Statistics, 23,907 neonates and infants and 20,192 children and adolescents aged 1–19 years died in the United States in 2011, the most recent year for which data had been analyzed when this chapter was written.[63] Leading causes of death for neonates (birth to 1 month of age) and infants (1 month to 1 year of age) and for children ages 1–19 years that would require palliative care are listed in **Table 53.2**. Although there are different clinical practice guidelines for adult and pediatric palliative care, their basic goals are similar and include total care of the child's physiologic, psychologic, and spiritual needs provided by a multidisciplinary team that also provides support to the child's family.[64]

Common symptoms experienced by children with terminal illness are similar to those experienced by adults and include the same kinds of physiologic and psychologic symptoms. Fatigue is especially distressing to children, who are normally full of energy and engaging in activities with siblings and friends at home and school. Fatigue prevents the child from interacting with other children in physical activities and contributes to feelings of isolation.

Because neonates, infants, and children under the age of 3 years do not have the verbal skills to accurately self-report symptoms, parental reports, assessment of physiologic and behavioral changes, and special assessment tools are used. For example, the CRIES scale can be used for assessment of pain in full-term neonates.[65] This scale uses behavioral indicators such as crying, sleeplessness, facial expressions, and physiologic indicators, such as heart rate and blood pressure, in the assessment of pain. For older children, there are scales such as the Oucher Scale, with faces depicting mild to severe levels of distress caused by pain that the child can point to in assisting nurses in assessment of the child's pain severity. Instruments for assessment of several other symptoms in children are also available. For example, the Children's Fatigue Scale assesses the impact of fatigue on factors such as the child's ability to engage in play or run, length of sleep, and feeling tired during the day. The Memorial Symptom Assessment Scale scores the physical and psychologic aspects of several symptoms.[62]

While adults with terminal illness are often admitted to specialized palliative care services such as hospice within days to months before death, children with terminal illness often have an extended need for palliative care services lasting for years. Parents may continue to hope for a miracle cure for their terminally ill child and be reluctant to stop aggressive and invasive therapy. Parents may view palliative care, with its focus on relieving distressing symptoms, as being opposed to care that is focused on cure and prolongation of life. They may need reassurance that palliative care and curative care are not mutually exclusive and that a goal of palliative care is to improve the child's quality of life. ■

Check Your Progress: Section 53.13

1. Explain whether the goals of palliative for children are similar to or different from those for adults.
2. What are the leading causes of terminal illness in neonates and infants compared to children age 1–19 years?
3. Explain differences in the way in which symptoms may need to be assessed in children compared to adults.

CHAPTER SUMMARY

53.1 Chapter Overview and Case Studies

Differentiate palliative care from curative care and describe the settings in which palliative care is delivered and the functions of hospice, and explain how the concept of oxygenation is related to symptoms experienced near the end of life that require palliative care.

- Palliative care is healthcare devoted to controlling a patient's symptoms regardless of the patient's prognosis as well as promoting psychosocial and spiritual well-being.
- Hospice is a formal program consisting of a multidisciplinary team of healthcare providers who deliver palliative care for individuals near the end of life.
- Palliative care takes place in a variety of settings, including the patient's home, outpatient clinics, nursing homes, intensive care units, and emergency departments.
- Conditions that are common causes of terminal illness in adults include cardiovascular disease, cancer, COPD, Alzheimer disease, and diabetes mellitus.
- In cases of terminal illness, diagnostic tests usually are limited to those whose results will help in making in making decisions about the best interventions to benefit the patient's symptoms.
- Impaired cellular oxygenation resulting in a deficit of adenosine triphosphate (ATP) production is the fundamental mechanism responsible for death from all causes.

53.2 Pain

Recognize the importance of pain assessment and management for individuals with terminal illness.

- Pain is a common symptom near the end of life that is very distressing to patients and contributes to anorexia, sleep impairment, delirium, and decreased mobility.
- Assessment of the patient's self-report of pain is essential and should include the location, intensity, and quality of the pain and factors that exacerbate and alleviate the pain.
- Long-acting medications are administered to relieve chronic pain around the clock. Short-acting medications can be administered for breakthrough pain.

53.3 Dyspnea

Analyze the pathophysiologic mechanisms that are responsible for a patient's dyspnea on the basis of the disease processes that are present and the patient's description of the difficulty in breathing, and relate the pathophysiology to treatment.

- Dyspnea is a sensation of difficulty in breathing.
- The individual's self-report is the most useful piece of assessment data for patients who are experiencing dyspnea.
- Patients' descriptions of their difficulty breathing, such as "my breath does not go out all the way" or "my chest feels tight," can help to differentiate the underlying cause.
- Activation of chemoreceptors in the arteries or brain by alterations in the oxygen, carbon dioxide, or hydrogen ion content of the blood as well as activation of mechanical receptors in the lungs by stretch, irritants, or pressure are involved in causing dyspnea.
- The mainstay treatment of dyspnea in patients who are receiving palliative or hospice care is opioid medications, which decrease the perception of dyspnea.
- Additional medications, such as bronchodilators, anti-inflammatory drugs, and diuretics, are used to target the underlying cause of dyspnea.

53.4 Cough

Explain the factors that trigger the cough reflex in terminal illness, the potential complications of coughing, characteristics of coughing that should be assessed, and pharmacologic and nonpharmacologic treatment strategies.

- Excessive coughing can impair sleep and speech as well as causing pain, fatigue, fractured ribs, and urinary incontinence.

- The cough reflex is activated by stimulation of mechanical receptors in the upper airways by displacement or inflammation or by stimulation of chemical receptors in the lower airways by noxious gases, smoke, blood, or excessive secretions.
- To help determine the cause of coughing, the following should be assessed: the duration of the cough; its time of occurrence; whether it is a productive or nonproductive cough; and whether it sounds hacking, barking, hoarse, or bubbling.
- Medications that are used to treat excessive coughing depend on the underlying cause and include antimicrobials, mucolytics, expectorants, bronchodilators, and anti-inflammatory drugs.
- Increasing environmental humidity and ensuring good hydration help to decrease the viscosity of respiratory secretions, and chest physiotherapy is used to loosen secretions so that they can more easily removed from the airways.

53.5 Excessive Secretions

Attribute the production and signs of excessive airway secretions in terminal illness and treatment strategies to the underlying pathophysiology.

- Movement of secretions retained in the upper airways near the end of life produce a gurgling sound called the death rattle.
- These secretions accumulate because of neural dysregulation resulting in release of acetylcholine, which stimulates muscarinic receptors, resulting in excessive salivary and bronchial secretions.
- Patient weakness and difficulty swallowing and coughing up secretions contribute to their accumulation.
- This symptom can be particularly distressing for patients' family members.
- Antimuscarinic medications are used to block muscarinic receptors, thereby decreasing production of excessive secretions.
- Elevating the patient's head and frequent turning help to mobilize secretions.

53.6 Nausea and Vomiting

Discriminate between the characteristics of nausea and vomiting and the factors that trigger the emetic response, and relate the prevention and treatment of nausea and vomiting to the underlying cause.

- Nausea is the unpleasant sensation that often precedes vomiting, which is a forceful expulsion of gastric contents through the mouth or nose.
- The emetic response is a reflex involving transmission of neural impulses arising from sensory input, the vestibular system, or the gastrointestinal tract. Many medications can also cause nausea and vomiting as an adverse effect.
- Several neurotransmitters, including histamine, serotonin, dopamine, and acetylcholine, are involved in the various pathways of activation of the emetic response. The choice of medication to treat nausea and vomiting is based on the pathways and neurotransmitter involved.

53.7 Anorexa and Cachexia

Explain the pathophysiologic mechanisms involved in anorexia and cachexia and the clinical manifestations, treatment, and interrelationship of anorexia and cachexia occurring near the end of life.

- Anorexia is a loss of the desire to eat that can be caused by infection, difficulty swallowing, ketosis, nausea, inflammatory cytokines, and certain medications and that results in involuntary weight loss.
- Cachexia is skeletal muscle wasting caused by metabolic derangements and deceased nutritional intake or absorption.
- Asthenia is the loss or lack of physical strength caused by skeletal muscle wasting occurring as a result of anorexia or cachexia.
- Appealing foods are made available to patients with anorexia and cachexia; however, increased caloric intake does not reverse cachexia.
- Anorexia, cachexia, and asthenia are common at the end of life and do not respond well to medical interventions.

53.8 Fatigue

Explain the pathophysiologic mechanisms involved in fatigue and the multifactorial causes of fatigue in terminal illness and its management.

- Fatigue is a pervasive feeling of tiredness and lack of energy that is not relieved by rest.
- Causes of fatigue near the end of life are multifactorial and include sleep impairment, muscle deconditioning from lack of physical activity, decreased muscle mass from anorexia and cachexia, anemia, heart failure, depression, electrolyte and acid–base imbalances, and impaired tissue oxygenation.
- A balance of activity and rest is important to prevent worsening of fatigue. Symptoms such as pain and dyspnea that contribute to fatigue should be treated.

53.9 Constipation

Describe the multifactorial causes of constipation associated with terminal illness, and explain prevention and treatment strategies for underlying causes.

- Constipation is the infrequent and difficult elimination of hard stool, making defecation uncomfortable.
- Factors that contribute to constipation in terminal illness include impaired neuromuscular function, dehydration, lack of fiber intake, tumor compression of the intestinal tract, and physical inactivity.

- Medications, such as opioids, anticholinergics, muscle relaxants, and anticonvulsants, can impair gastrointestinal motility, resulting in constipation.
- Laxatives are administered daily to prevent medication-induced constipation.
- Increased intake of fluids and foods that are high in fiber can relieve or help to prevent constipation.

53.10 Urinary Incontinence

Differentiate the causes, underlying pathophysiology, clinical manifestations, and treatment approaches of transient urinary incontinence from those in chronic urinary incontinence (stress, urge, overflow, and functional types).

- Urinary incontinence (loss of bladder control) is an embarrassing problem for patients.
- Factors contributing to transient urinary incontinence include delirium, impaired mobility, urinary tract infections, and certain medications, such as diuretics.
- Stress incontinence is a type of chronic urinary incontinence characterized by leakage of urine when intra-abdominal or bladder pressure exceeds the ability of the urethral sphincter to remain closed, as occurs with coughing, laughing, and physical exertion. Pelvic floor strengthening exercises are helpful for stress incontinence; however, terminally ill patients may not have the strength to perform these exercises.
- Urge incontinence is a type of chronic urinary condition characterized by involuntary bladder contractions and can be caused by bladder infection or tumors.
- Overflow incontinence is a chronic condition characterized by incomplete bladder emptying resulting in urinary retention and bladder overdistention, leading to leakage of urine. It is often caused by bladder muscle weakness or impaired innervation of the bladder.
- Functional urinary incontinence occurs when the individual cannot get to the bathroom or a bedside commode fast enough because of weakness, confusion, or immobility.
- Care of the patient with urinary incontinence revolves around maintaining the patient's dignity and keeping the skin warm, clean, and dry to prevent breakdown, with specific therapy directed by the type of urinary incontinence.

53.11 Delirium

Explain factors that contribute to delirium at the end of life, its various manifestations, diagnosis, and treatment strategies.

- Delirium is a potentially reversible fluctuating impairment in cognition caused by alterations in neurotransmission in the brain.
- Delirium can be caused by fever, uncontrolled pain, acid–base or electrolyte imbalances, hypoglycemia, brain tumors, and cerebrovascular disease.
- There are three forms of delirium: agitated delirium, hypoactive delirium, and mixed delirium.
- Antidopaminergic medications and benzodiazepines are used to treat agitated delirium. Psychostimulant medications are used to treat hypoactive delirium.
- Provision of a safe physical environment with familiar objects is a priority for patients with delirium.

53.12 Last Expected Changes at the End of Life

Attribute the underlying pathophysiologic mechanisms to the clinical manifestations that occur in the active phase of dying and the indicators of somatic death.

- The active phase of dying occurs in the final days of that process during which multiple organ systems fail.
- The exact time of expected somatic death, which is death of the individual rather than death of only some cells in the body, cannot be predicted in a patient with a terminal illness. However, decreasing urine output, mottled extremities, abnormal breathing patterns, and decreased level of consciousness indicate imminent death.
- Somatic death is pronounced when there is absence of cardiorespiratory functions, including lack of heart sounds and spontaneous respirations.
- Shortly after death, the resultant impaired perfusion of tissues and organs leads to cessation of function of all organs; lack of movement and reflexes such as the pupillary light reflex; algor mortis, which is a decline in body temperature; rigor mortis, which is stiffening of body muscles; and livor mortis, which is the red to purple discoloration of dependent body parts.
- Brain death is the irreversible cessation of cerebral and brainstem functioning and is determined by neurologic examination and sometimes additional tests such as those of cerebral blood flow or cerebral electrical activity or the apnea test to check for spontaneous breathing after removal from a ventilator.
- Determination of brain death is required when technology, such as mechanical ventilation, has been used to sustain organ functions when the brain is no longer functioning to regulate body systems.

53.13 Pediatric Considerations

Compare pediatric palliative care to adult palliative care with regard to causes of terminal illness, symptoms experienced near the end of life, and approaches to assessment of symptoms.

- The leading causes of life-threatening conditions in neonates and infants are congenital malformations, chromosomal abnormalities, and complications associated with premature birth.
- Trauma and cancer are the leading causes of life-threatening conditions in children ages 1–19 years.

- Symptoms experienced by children near the end of life are the same as those experienced by adults, including pain, dyspnea, cough, fatigue, anorexia, cachexia, nausea, vomiting, and impaired elimination.
- Parental reports of symptoms and age-appropriate assessment tools must be used for young children to determine characteristics of their symptoms and the response to interventions.

REVIEW QUESTIONS

1. Pleural effusion and pulmonary edema make it more difficult for clients to breathe comfortably because these conditions:
   a. stimulate the brain to release increased amounts of serotonin.
   b. alter the inspiratory to expiratory ratio from 1:2 to 1:1.
   c. contribute directly to the amount of excessive secretions already present.
   d. inhibit the phrenic nerve from innervating the diaphragm.
2. Mr. Sims is a 78-year-old client who had a prostatectomy procedure 6 months ago to relieve the effects of an enlarged prostate. Since then, he reports that he frequently "pees" in his underwear even when his bladder is not full. What type of urinary incontinence does this represent?
   a. Stress
   b. Overflow
   c. Functional
   d. Urge
3. A client with a reported pain level of 9 out of 10 and associated symptoms such as anxiety and intractable discomfort would benefit most from which medications?
   a. Antibiotics
   b. Opioids
   c. Corticosteroids
   d. Antipyretics
4. The leading causes of death in children ages 1–19 years are:
   a. chromosomal abnormalities and congenital malformations.
   b. metabolic disorders and seizures.
   c. food contamination and lead poisoning.
   d. trauma and cancer.
5. What role does calcium play in the development of rigor mortis?
   a. It triggers cross-bridging of actin and myosin filaments, resulting in a sustained contraction.
   b. It promotes the movement of fluid from the intravascular space into muscle tissue, leading to stiffness.
   c. It blocks the reuptake of acetylcholine, thereby preventing muscle relaxation.
   d. It signals the brain to reflexively contract all muscles as a defense mechanism.
6. Which of the following outcomes would indicate effective palliative sedation?
   a. The client does not respond to verbal or physical stimuli.
   b. The client is fully alert and is still experiencing distress symptoms.
   c. The client is partially awake and is constantly moaning.
   d. The client can respond to verbal cues and is not in major distress.
7. A 63-year-old client with end-stage lung cancer has had a persistent and productive cough for the past 3 weeks and has not slept well. She denies any fever, chills, or night sweats. Which intervention would likely provide the most relief?
   a. Antihistamines
   b. Antibiotics
   c. Antitussives
   d. Antipyretics
8. Which of these factors is known to contribute to the development of constipation in a client with a terminal illness?
   a. Laxatives
   b. Physical inactivity
   c. Fruits and vegetables
   d. Increased fluid intake

ANSWERS

Answers to Review Questions can be found in Appendix A. Answers to Case Study and Check Your Progress questions are available on the faculty resources site. Please consult with your instructor.

RECOMMENDED WEBSITES

American Academy of Hospice and Palliative Medicine
www.aahpm.org

American College of Critical Care Medicine: Recommendations for end-of-life care in the intensive care unit
http://www.learnicu.org/SiteCollectionDocuments/EOL.pdf

End of Life Nursing Education Consortium
www.aacn.nche.edu/elnec

Hospice and Palliative Nurses Association
www.hpna.org

National Consensus Project for Quality Palliative Care. Clinical practice guidelines for quality palliative care, 2nd edition (2009).
http://www.nationalconsensusproject.org/Guideline.pdf

National Hospice and Palliative Care Organization
www.nhpco.org

Promoting Excellence at the End of Life
www.promotingexcellence.org

Society of Critical Care Medicine
www.sccm.org

REFERENCES

1. World Health Organization. (2013). *WHO definition of palliative care.* Retrieved from http://www.who.int/cancer/palliative/definition/en/.
2. Lanken, P., Terry, P., DeLisser, H., et al. (2008). An official American Thoracic Society Clinical Policy Statement: Palliative care for patients with respiratory diseases and critical illnesses. *American Journal of Respiratory and Critical Care Medicine, 177,* 912–927.
3. Griffith, J., Lyman, J., & Blackhall, L. (2010). Providing palliative care in the ambulatory care setting. *Oncology Nursing Forum, 14*(2), 171–175.
4. Truog, R., Campbell, M., Curtis, J., et al. (2008). Recommendations for end-of-life care in the intensive care unit: A consensus statement by the American College of Critical Care Medicine. *Critical Care Medicine, 36*(3), 953–963.
5. Mosenthal, A., Weissman, D., Curtis, J., et al. (2012). Integrating palliative care in the surgical and trauma intensive care unit: A report from the Improving Palliative Care in the Intensive Care unit (IPAL-ICU) Project Advisory Board and the Center to Advance Palliative Care. *Critical Care Medicine, 40*(4), 199–1206.
6. Temel, J., Greer, J., Muzikansky, A., et al. (2010). Early palliative care for patients with metastatic non -small-cell lung cancer. *New England Journal of Medicine,* 363(8):733–742.
7. Girgis, A., & Waller, A. (2015). Palliative care needs assessment tools. In N. Cherney, M. Fallon, S. Kaasa, R. K. Portenoy, & D. C. Currow (Eds.): *Oxford Textbook of Pallative Medicine* (5th ed.). New York, NY: Oxford University Press.
8. Parshall, M., Schwartzstein, R., Adams, L., et al. An official American Thoracic Society Statement: Update on the mechanisms, assessment, and management of dyspnea. *American Journal of Respiratory and Critical Care Medicine, 185*(4), 435–452.
9. Currow, D., Davidson, P., Newton, P., et al. (2010). Do the trajectories of dyspnea differ in prevalence and intensity by diagnosis at the end of life? A consecutive cohort study. *Journal of Pain and Symptom Management, 39*(4), 680–690.
10. Emanuel, E. J. (2015). Palliative and end-of-life care. In D. Kaspar, A. Fauci, S. Hauser, & D. Longo (Eds.), *Harrison's online principles of internal medicine* (19th ed.). New York, NY: McGraw-Hill.
11. Burki, N., & Lee, L.-Y. (2010). Mechanisms of dyspnea. *Chest, 138*(5), 1196–1201.
12. Schwartzstein, R. M. (2015). Dyspnea. In D. Kaspar, A. Fauci, S. Hauser, & D. Longo (Eds.), *Harrison's online principles of internal medicine* (19th ed.). New York, NY: McGraw-Hill.
13. Galbraith, S., Fagan, P., Phys, D., et al. (2010). Does the use of a handheld fan improve chronic dyspnea? A randomized, controlled, crossover trial. *Journal of Pain and Symptom Management, 39*(5), 831–838.
14. Dorman, S., Byrne, A., & Edwards, A. (2007). Which measurement scale should we use to measure breathlessness in palliative care? A systematic review. *Palliative Medicine, 21,* 177–191.
15. Meek, P., Banzett, R., & Parshall, M., et al. (2012). Reliability and validity of the multidimensional dyspnea profile. *Chest, 141*(6), 1546–1553.
16. Luce, J. M., & Luce, J. A. (2001). Management of dyspnea in patients with far-advanced lung disease: Once I lose it, it's kind of hard to catch it. *Journal of the American Medical Association, 285,* 1331–1337.
17. Jennings, A., Davies, A., Higgins, J., et al. (2002). A systematic review of the use of opioids in the management of dyspnea. *Thorax, 57*(11), 39–944.
18. Mahler, D., Selecky, P., Harrod, C., et al. (2010). American College of Chest Physicians consensus statement on management of dyspnea in patients with advanced lung or heart disease. *Chest, 137*(3), 674–691.
19. Currow, D., McDonald, C., Oaten, S., et al. (2011). Once-daily opioids for chronic dyspnea: A dose increment and pharmacovigilance study. *Journal of Pain and Symptom Management, 42*(3), 388–399.
20. Marciniuk, D., Goodridge, D., Hernandez, P., et al. (2011). Managing dyspnea in patients with advanced chronic obstructive pulmonary disease: A Canadian Thoracic Society clinical practice guideline. *Canadian Respiratory Journal, 18*(2), 69–78.
21. Booth, S., & Wade, R. (2003). Oxygen or air for palliation of breathlessness in advanced cancer. *Journal of the Royal Society of Medicine, 96*(5), 215–218.
22. Bandyopadhyay, D., & Induru, R. (2011). Role of palliative tracheobronchial stenting in hospice patients: Boon or bane? *American Journal of Hospice & Palliative Medicine, 28*(6), 445–448.
23. Liu, Y.-H., Wu, Y., Hsieh, M.-J., et al. (2011). Straight bronchial stent placement across the right upper lobe bronchus: A simple alternative for the management of airway obstruction around the carina and right main bronchus. *Journal of Thoracic and Cardiovascular Surgery, 141*(1), 303–305.
24. Edmonds, P., Karlson, S., Khan, S., & Addington-Hall, J. (2001). A comparison of the palliative care needs of patients dying from chronic respiratory disease and lung cancer. *Palliative Medicine, 12,* 245–254.
25. Chan, K-S., Tse, D., & Sham, M. M. K. Dyspnoea and other respiratory symptoms in palliative care. In N. Cherney, M. Fallon, S. Kaasa, R. K. Portenoy, & D. C. Currow (Eds.): *Oxford Textbook of Palliative Medicine* (5th ed.). New York, NY: Oxford University Press.

26. Chung, K., & Pavord, I. (2008). Prevalence, pathogenesis, and causes of chronic cough. *Lancet, 371,* 1364–1374.
27. Ferris, F. D., von Gunten, C. F., & Emmanuel, L. L. (2003). Competency in end-of-life care: Last hours of life. *Journal of Palliative Medicine, 6,* 605–613.
28. Wee, B., & Hillier, R. (2012). Interventions for noisy breathing in patients near to death. *Cochran Library, 3,* 1–17.
29. Prommer, E. (2012). Anticholinergics in palliative medicine: An update. *American Journal of Hospice & Palliative Medicine, 30*(5), 490–498.
30. Wildiers, H., Dhaenekint, C., Demeulenacre, P., et al. (2009). Atropine, hyosine butybromide, or scopolamine are equally effective for the treatment of death rattle in terminal care. *Journal of Pain and Symptom Management, 38,* 124–133.
31. Hardy, J. R., Glare, P., Yates, P., & Mannix, K. (2015). Palliation of nausea and vomiting. In N. Cherney, M. Fallon, S. Kaasa, R. K. Portenoy, & D. C. Currow (Eds.): *Oxford Textbook of Palliative Medicine* (5th ed.). New York, NY: Oxford University Press.
32. Basch, E., Prestrud, A., Hesketh, P., et al. (2011). Antiemetics: American Society of Clinical Oncology practice guideline update. *Journal of Clinical Oncology, 29,* 4189–4198.
33. Glare, P., Miller, J., Nikolva, T., & Tickoo, R. (2011). Treating nausea and vomiting in palliative care: A review. *Clinical Interventions in Aging, 6,* 243–259.
34. Tsoli M., & Robertson G. (2013). Cancer cachexia: Malignant inflammation, tumorkines, and metabolic mayhem. *Trends in Endocrinology and Metabolism, 24*(4), 174–183.
35. Baracos, V. E., Watanabe, S. M., & Fearon, K. C. H. (2015). Aetiology, classification, assessment, and treatment of the anorexia-cachexia syndrome. In N. Cherney, M. Fallon, S. Kaasa, R. K. Portenoy, & D. C. Currow (Eds.): *Oxford Textbook of Palliative Medicine* (5th ed.). New York, NY: Oxford University Press.
36. Wallengren, O., Lundholm, K., & Bosaeus, I. (2013). Diagnostic criteria of cancer cachexia: Relation to quality of life, exercise capacity and survival in unselected palliative care patients. *Supportive Care in Cancer, 21,* 1569–1577.
37. Frederich, M. (2002). Artificial hydration and nutrition in the terminally ill. *AAHPM Bulletin, 2002,* 8–13.
38. Suzuki, H., Asakawa, A., Amitani, H., et al. (2013). Cancer cachexia: Pathophysiology and management. *Journal of Gastroenterology, 24,* 574–594.
39. Inui, A. (2002). Cancer anorexia-cachexia syndrome: Current issues in research and management. *CA: A Cancer Journal for Clinicians, 52,* 72–91.
40. Ross, D., & Alexander, C. (2001). Management of common symptoms in terminally ill patients: Part 1. *American Family Physician, 64*(5), 807–814.
41. Yennurajalingam, S., & Bruera, E. (2015). Fatigue and asthenia. In N. Cherney, M. Fallon, S. Kaasa, R. K. Portenoy, & D. C. Currow (Eds.): *Oxford Textbook of Palliative Medicine* (5th ed.). New York, NY: Oxford University Press.
42. Norheim, K., Jonsson, G., & Omdal, R. (2011). Biological mechanisms of chronic fatigue. *Rheumatology, 50,* 1009–1018.
43. McMillan, S., & Small, B. (2002). Symptom distress and quality of life in patients with cancer newly admitted to hospice home care. *Oncology Nursing Forum, 29*(10), 1421–1428.
44. Clark, K., Smith, J., & Currow, D. (2012). The prevalence of bowel problems reported in a palliative care population. *Journal of Pain and Symptom Management, 43*(6), 993–1000.
45. Selvaggi, K., & Abraham, J. (2012). Symptom management in palliative medicine. *ACP Medicine, 2012,* 1–20. doi:10.2310/7900.1095.
46. Flaherty, J. (2004). Urinary incontinence and the terminally ill older person. *Clinics in Geriatric Medicine, 20,* 467–475.
47. Baker, B., & Ward-Smith, P. (2011). Urinary incontinence nursing considerations at the end of life. *Urologic Nursing, 31*(3), 169–172.
48. Hosie, A., Davidson, P., Agar, M., et al. (2012). Delirium prevalence, incidence, and implications for screening in specialist palliative care inpatient settings: A systematic review. *Palliative Medicine, 27*(6), 486–498.
49. Esper, P., & Heidrich, D. (2005). Symptom cluster in advanced illness. *Seminars in Oncology Nursing, 21*(1), 20–28.
50. Smith, J., & Adcock, L. (2011). The recognition of delirium in hospice inpatient units. *Palliative Medicine, 26*(3), 283–285.
51. Zaal, I., & Slooter, A. (2012). Delirium in critically ill patients: Epidemiology, pathophysiology, diagnosis and management. *Drugs, 72*(11), 457–1471.
52. Wong, C., Holroyd-Leduc, J., Simel, D., & Straus, S. (2010). Does this patient have delirium? Value of bedside instruments. *JAMA, 304*(7), 779–786.
53. Prommer, E. (2012). Role of haloperidol in palliative medicine: An update. *American Journal of Hospice & Palliative Medicine, 29*(4), 295–301.
54. Agar, M., Alici, Y., & Breitbart, W. S. (2015). Delirium. In N. Cherney, M. Fallon, S. Kaasa, R. K. Portenoy, & D. C. Currow (Eds.): *Oxford Textbook of Palliative Medicine* (5th ed.). New York, NY: Oxford University Press.
55. Saladin, K. (2012). Muscular tissue. In K. Saladin, *Anatomy & physiology: The unity of form and function* (6th ed., pp. 404–440). New York, NY: McGraw-Hill.
56. Wijdicks, E., Varelas, P., Gronseth, G., & Greer, D. (2010). Evidence-based guideline update: Determining brain death in adults. *Neurology, 74,* 1911–1918.
57. Nakagawa, T., Ashwal, S., Mathur, M., et al. (2012). Guidelines for the determination of brain death in infants and children: An update of the 1987 Task Force Recommendations—Executive Summary. *Annals of Neurology, 71* 573–585.
58. Krakauer, E. (2015). Sedation at the end of life. In N. Cherney, M. Fallon, S. Kaasa, R. K. Portenoy, & D. C. Currow (Eds.): *Oxford Textbook of Palliative Medicine* (5th ed.). New York, NY: Oxford University Press.
59. Mercadante, S., Intravaia, G., Villari, P., et al. (2009). Controlled sedation for refractory symptoms in dying patients. *Journal of Pain Symptom Management, 37,* 771–779.
60. American Academy of Hospice and Palliative Medicine. (2014). *Statement on palliative sedation.* Retrieved from at http://aahpm.org/positions/palliative-sedation.
61. Rincon, F. (2014). Neurologic criteria for death in adults. In J. Parrillo & R. Dellinger (Eds.), *Critical care medicine: Principles of diagnosis and management in the adult* (4th ed., pp. 1098–1105). Philadelphia, PA: Elsevier.
62. Collins, J. J., Campbell, K., Edmonds, W., Frost, J., Mherekumombe, M. F., & Samy, N. (2015). Care of children with advanced illness. In N. Cherney, M. Fallon, S. Kaasa, R. K. Portenoy, & D. C. Currow (Eds.): *Oxford Textbook of Palliative Medicine* (5th ed.). New York, NY: Oxford University Press.
63. Hamilton, B., Hoyert, D., Martin, J., et al. (2013). Annual summary of vital statistics: 2010–2011. *Pediatrics, 131*(3), 548–558.
64. World Health Organization. (2013). *WHO definition of palliative care for children.* Available at http://www.who.int/cancer/palliative/definition/en/.
65. Krechel, S. W., & Bildner, J. (1995). CRIES: A new neonatal postoperative pain measurement score: Initial testing of validity and reliability. *Paediatric Anaesthesia, 5,* 53–61.

Appendix A

Answers to Review Questions

Note: Rationales for the answers can be found in the eText and in the Instructor Resources; consult your instructor to access the rationales.

Chapter 1

1. a
2. d
3. c
4. b
5. c
6. a
7. c
8. c

Chapter 2

1. a
2. c
3. b
4. a
5. b
6. a
7. b
8. a

Chapter 3

1. b
2. b
3. d
4. a
5. a
6. c
7. a
8. c

Chapter 4

1. b
2. d
3. a
4. a
5. b
6. c
7. c
8. d

Chapter 5

1. a
2. d
3. c
4. c
5. d
6. b
7. c
8. c

Chapter 6

1. d
2. b
3. a
4. c
5. a
6. c
7. c
8. a

Chapter 7

1. c
2. a
3. d
4. d
5. d
6. a
7. d
8. c

Chapter 8

1. d
2. b
3. c
4. c
5. c
6. b
7. c
8. d

Chapter 9

1. c
2. a
3. c
4. d
5. b
6. c
7. d
8. d

Chapter 10

1. b
2. a
3. a
4. d
5. b
6. c
7. c
8. a

Chapter 11

1. c
2. d
3. d
4. c
5. a
6. b
7. c
8. b

Chapter 12

1. d
2. b
3. c
4. b
5. a
6. d
7. c
8. c

Chapter 13

1. b
2. d
3. b
4. a
5. b
6. c
7. b
8. b

Chapter 14

1. a
2. b
3. d
4. c
5. b
6. a
7. b
8. b

Chapter 15

1. c
2. d
3. c
4. c
5. d
6. a
7. b
8. b

Chapter 16

1. a
2. d
3. c
4. d
5. a
6. a
7. c
8. b

Chapter 17

1. a
2. b,c,e
3. b
4. a
5. a
6. b,c,e
7. b,c,e
8. a

Chapter 18

1. c
2. a,c
3. a
4. c,e
5. b,d
6. a,b,e
7. a,b,c
8. c

Chapter 19

1. b
2. c
3. d
4. b
5. a
6. c
7. d
8. c

Chapter 20

1. a
2. c
3. d
4. b,d,e
5. b
6. a
7. b
8. d

Chapter 21

1. b
2. d
3. c
4. b
5. a
6. b
7. d
8. c

Chapter 22

1. a
2. d
3. d
4. c
5. d
6. a,b,c
7. a
8. b

Chapter 23

1. c
2. a
3. b
4. d
5. d
6. d
7. d
8. b

Chapter 24

1. c
2. a,b
3. a
4. c
5. b,c
6. c
7. d
8. b

Chapter 25

1. a
2. b,c,e
3. b
4. c
5. a
6. b
7. d
8. a

Chapter 26

1. d
2. b
3. c
4. a,b,c,d
5. b
6. a,b,d
7. a,c
8. c

Chapter 27

1. c
2. b
3. d
4. a
5. d
6. c
7. b
8. a

Chapter 28

1. b
2. c
3. a
4. a
5. d
6. b
7. a
8. c

Chapter 29

1. c
2. b
3. a
4. d
5. c
6. a
7. c
8. a

Chapter 30

1. a
2. d
3. b
4. b
5. a
6. d
7. b
8. a

Chapter 31

1. a,c,d
2. a,d
3. c
4. a
5. a,c
6. a,b,d
7. a,b,e
8. b,c,e

Chapter 32

1. d
2. b
3. d
4. d
5. a
6. c
7. a
8. a

Chapter 33

1. b
2. c
3. d
4. b
5. a
6. d
7. a
8. c

Chapter 34

1. c
2. c
3. d
4. a,c,d
5. a
6. d
7. d
8. d

Chapter 35

1. d
2. b
3. d
4. a
5. c
6. c
7. b
8. a

Chapter 36

1. b
2. d
3. d
4. c
5. a
6. c
7. a
8. a

Chapter 37

1. b
2. a
3. d
4. b
5. b
6. c
7. a,b,c,e
8. b

Chapter 38

1. b
2. d
3. c
4. a
5. c
6. c
7. b
8. a

Chapter 39

1. a
2. c
3. b
4. d
5. a
6. d
7. b
8. a

Chapter 40

1. c
2. a
3. d
4. a
5. a
6. b
7. d
8. b

Chapter 41

1. d
2. b
3. a
4. c
5. d
6. a
7. d
8. b

Chapter 42

1. b
2. c
3. a
4. a
5. d
6. b
7. a
8. b

Chapter 43

1. a,b,c,d
2. c
3. a
4. d
5. c
6. b
7. d
8. d

Chapter 44

1. d
2. c
3. a
4. c
5. d
6. b
7. a
8. b

Chapter 45

1. b
2. b
3. c
4. c
5. c
6. d
7. c
8. d

Chapter 46

1. d
2. d
3. a
4. d
5. b
6. b
7. a
8. d

Chapter 47

1. b
2. c
3. c
4. a
5. d
6. b
7. d
8. b

Chapter 48

1. b
2. c
3. d
4. c
5. a
6. b
7. c
8. a

Chapter 49

1. b
2. c
3. b
4. d
5. a
6. c
7. b
8. d

Chapter 50

1. d
2. b
3. b
4. a
5. b
6. b
7. c
8. b

Chapter 51

1. b
2. c
3. b
4. a
5. a
6. b
7. c
8. a

Chapter 52

1. b
2. c
3. a
4. b
5. c
6. c
7. b
8. c

Chapter 53

1. c
2. a
3. b
4. d
5. a
6. d
7. c
8. b

Glossary

Abrasion Damage to the superficial layer of skin that is usually caused by a grinding of tissue.

Absence seizures Seizure activity characterized by a loss of consciousness without change in muscle activity.

Absolute refractory period The period after the firing of a nerve fiber during which the nerve fiber cannot be stimulated, regardless of the strength of the stimulus that is applied.

Accidental hypothermia An unintended fall in core temperature to hypothermic levels that typically occurs in association with exposure to cold or traumatic conditions.

Acid A substance that dissociates into an H^+ and a conjugate base.

Acidosis A condition of below-normal blood pH due to an excess of acid relative to base.

Acid pocket A pocket, or reservoir, of gastric acid that floats on top of a recently ingested meal in the stomach.

Acne vulgaris The formation of comedones papules, pustules, nodules, or cysts when hair follicles and sebaceous glands become inflamed because of obstruction; most often seen in adolescents.

Acoustic trauma The damage to hearing that results from exposure to an intense impulse noise.

Acquired (adaptive) immunity Acquired immunity is a form of immunity that is continually refined throughout the life of the individual and is highly specific to a pathogen. Acquired immunity allows an individual, once exposed to a pathogen, to have long-lasting protection against that particular pathogen.

Acquired immunodeficiency syndrome (AIDS) The most advanced stage of HIV infection; characterized by severe immunodeficiency (i.e., CD4 + T-lymphocyte count < 200 cells/mm^3), opportunistic infections, and/or malignancies.

Acrochordons Skin tags that are soft, flesh-colored, or pigmented papules with stalks that attach them to skin.

Acropachy Soft-tissue swelling and clubbing in hands and fingers found in patients with Graves disease.

Actinic keratosis (AK) Thick, rough, or scaly skin lesions that develop after chronic sun exposure, extensive exposure to x-rays, or exposure to some industrial chemicals

Active immunity Resistance to infectious disease that develops as a result of activation of the host's own immune system; may occur by either natural or artificial means.

Active phase of dying The phase of dying that occurs during the final days of an illness and leads to a gradual deterioration of body systems and organ failure, resulting in death.

Active transport A transport system that requires energy in the form of ATP to allow electrons to flow uphill.

Acute bronchitis A very common, self-limited lower respiratory tract inflammation; often referred to as a "chest cold."

Acute coronary syndrome (ACS) A clinical presentation that includes non–ST-segment elevation acute coronary syndrome (non–ST-segment elevation myocardial infarction and unstable angina) and ST-segment elevation myocardial infarction.

Acute interstitial nephritis Acute kidney injury resulting from inflammation of the interstitial tissue of the kidney, including the tubules, usually caused by a reaction to a medication.

Acute kidney injury (AKI) A rapid decline of kidney function that occurs over hours to days.

Acute liver failure The loss of hepatocyte function affecting almost the entire liver without the presence of cirrhosis.

Acute lymphocytic leukemia (ALL) A form of acute leukemia characterized by the overproduction of lymphoblasts.

Acute myelogenous leukemia (AML) A form of leukemia characterized by the rapid growth of white blood cells; also known as *acute myeloid leukemia.*

Acute otitis media (AOM) An infection of the middle ear with acute onset.

Acute pain Pain resulting from traumatic damage or inflammation of tissue with resolution of the pain on repair or recovery of the tissue.

Acute pancreatitis Inflammation or necrosis of the pancreas.

Acute phase response The physiologic changes that occur shortly after an injury or beginning of an infectious process that results from cytokine-induced systemic reactions.

Acute radiation syndrome (ARS) A clinical disease caused by radiation exposure, includes four phases: prodrome, latent, illness, and recovery or death.

Acute respiratory distress syndrome (ARDS) A severe form of acute respiratory failure characterized by noncardiac pulmonary edema and progressive refractory hypoxemia (the decrease of arterial oxygen despite the administration of oxygen at high flow rates).

Acute tubular necrosis (ATN) A histologic finding involving damage to or death of the tubular cells lining the renal tubules; presents with muddy brown casts.

Adam forward bend test A test used to screen for scoliosis.

Adaptation The physiologic and psychologic processes used in response to stress.

Adaptive (acquired) immune system A system of antigen-specific defense mechanisms that, on activation, require several days to become host-protective.

Addison disease This disorder occurs when the adrenal gland is unable to produce sufficient amounts of adrenocortical hormones despite sufficient amounts of ACTH; it is also referred to as *primary adrenal insufficiency*.

Adenocarcinoma of the esophagus A carcinoma displaying glandular differentiation that arises in the esophagus.

Adenoma A benign tumor of glandular origin.

Adenomyosis Invasion of the uterine myometrium by glandular endometrial tissue.

Adhesive capsulitis Acute inflammation of the ligaments in the shoulder joint; also known as *frozen shoulder*.

Adipocytes Cells that produce and store fat.

Adult congenital heart disorder (ACHD) Structural disorders of the heart in adults.

Advanced COPD In the GOLD classification system, the end stage (stage 4) of COPD, in which the FEV_1/FVC is less than 70%, the FEV_1 is less than 30% of predicted, or the FEV_1 is less than 50% of predicted with chronic respiratory failure.

Afterload The amount of pressure the heart needs to pump blood out of the ventricle.

Agonist A substance that combines with a receptor and initiates a physiologic response.

AIDS-related lymphoma A heterogeneous collection of B-cell malignancies that occur in extranodal sites, including the central nervous system, gastrointestinal tract, and liver.

Air trapping Mechanism by which airway obstruction prohibits expiration of pulmonary gases; may produce lung hyperinflation.

Airway obstruction A blockage of the airway that prevents air from getting into the lungs.

Alarmone A chemical messenger that halts bacterial metabolic processes and can lead to death of the bacteria or cessation of spore formation.

Albumin:creatinine ratio The gold standard for measurement of albuminuria; useful for screening for kidney disease.

Albuminuria Albumin in the urine; an indicator of kidney disease.

Alcohol Generally refers to grain alcohol, or ethanol, rather than other types of alcohol (such as wood or isopropyl alcohol) that are too toxic to be drinkable.

Alcoholic liver disease Damage to the liver and its function due to alcohol abuse.

Alcohol intoxication Blood alcohol content sufficient to produce physical abnormalities consistent with behavioral changes.

Alcohol overdose Blood alcohol content sufficient to produce impairments that increase the risk of harm, including death.

Alcohol use disorder A pattern of alcohol intake that is characterized by difficulty in controlling alcohol intake, preoccupation with alcohol, continued use of alcohol despite the fact that it is causing problems, needing more alcohol to get the same effect, or having withdrawal symptoms when rapidly decreasing or stopping alcohol consumption.

Alcohol withdrawal syndrome Severe, life-threatening symptoms that tend to occur 24–72 hours after cessation of drinking or reduction of alcohol use.

Aldosterone A mineralocorticoid secreted from the adrenal gland in response to hemodynamic changes; directly opposes atrial natriuretic peptide.

Algor mortis The drop in body temperature that begins immediately after death and is due to cessation of heat-producing metabolic reactions and regulation of body temperature.

Alkalosis A condition of above-normal blood pH due to a deficit of base relative to acid.

Allele Alternative forms of an individual gene.

Allergen Another term for antigen. Any substance that may cause signs and symptoms of allergies.

Allergic reactions Another term for a hypersensitivity reaction.

Allodynia Pain from a nonnoxious stimulus that normally does not produce pain.

Allostasis A method of viewing internal regulation similar to homeostasis. Differs from homeostasis in that body systems are seen as being in a state of dynamic fluctuation without the need for a set point.

Allostatic load The consequence of exposure to recurrent or long-term hormonal or catecholamine release as a result of stress.

Alopecia areata (AA) Fairly common autoimmune disorder that causes chronic, relapsing, inflammation-induced, nonscarring hair loss and nail changes

Alveolar-arterial O_2 gradient (A-a gradient) A measure of the difference between the alveolar concentration of oxygen and the arterial concentration of oxygen.

Amblyopia A condition in which one or both eyes cannot see clearly despite corrective lenses and a normal, healthy ocular appearance.

Amenorrhea Absence of menstruation.

Aminoglycoside antibiotics Medications used to treat infections caused by gram-negative bacteria and administered either intramuscularly or intravenously.

Amyotrophic lateral sclerosis (ALS) A progressive neurodegenerative disease that causes weakness, disability, and eventual death in 3–5 years; also known as *Lou Gehrig's disease.*

Anabolism The process through which complex molecules are synthesized from less complex precursors.

Anagen The long growing phase of hair follicles.

Anaphylactic shock Shock resulting from a systemic vascular response to a hypersensitivity reaction referred to as anaphylaxis. Triggered by an allergic reaction to an antigen such as insect venom, foods, medications, blood transfusion, and vaccines following a previous exposure resulting in IgE production.

Anaphylaxis A systemic life-threatening type I hypersensitivity reaction.

Androgen A type of hormone that stimulates the development and maintenance of male sex characteristics.

Anemia Condition in which the amount of oxygen carried by red blood cells is reduced because of either a decrease in cell size or a decreased number of cells.

Anemia of chronic disease (ACD) Form of anemia found in patients with chronic disease; also known as *anemia of chronic inflammation.*

Aneuploidy An abnormal chromosome number; can involve a gain or a loss of chromosome(s).

Aneurysm A bulging out of a weak arterial wall; plaque and hypertension are the primary causes.

Angina Chest pain, discomfort, pressure, and/or squeezing symptoms of coronary artery disease when the myocardium is not experiencing enough blood perfusion.

Angiogenesis The formation of new blood vessels; also referred to as neovascularization.

Angioplasty A procedure used to open an occluded artery with a balloon catheter; usually includes stent placement to keep the vessel open.

Anhydrous ammonia Concentrated ammonia that has not been diluted with water.

Anion An ion that carries a negative charge.

Anion gap $Na^+ - (Cl^- + HCO_3^-)$; used to detect the presence of an increase level of anions produced from nonvolatile acids.

Anogenital herpes Herpes infection of the genitals, perineum, or anus, caused by HSV-2

Anorexia Loss of the desire to eat leading to decreased intake of foods and fluids.

Anorexigenic Appetite suppressant.

Anterior cord syndrome A condition that results from damage to the corticospinal and spinothalamic pathways, although there is preservation of the posterior column.

Anthrax A disease caused by the bacterium *Bacillus anthracis*; it has three clinical forms: cutaneous, gastrointestinal, and inhalational.

Antigen A toxin or other foreign substance that induces an immune response in the body, especially the production of antibodies.

Antigenic drift In relation to influenza, characterized by minor changes in the structure of viral hemagglutin in A and neuraminidase, which may result in an influenza epidemic.

Antigenicity The ability to stimulate the formation of antibodies.

Antigenic shift In relation to influenza, characterized by a major genetic change that enables the influenza virus to jump from one species to another.

Antioxidants Natural and synthetic molecules that either inhibit the reactions responsible for production of reactive oxygen species (ROS) or neutralize ROS.

Antiport A transport molecule that moves two different electrolytes in opposite directions across a cell membrane.

Antiretroviral therapy (ART) Medications used in the treatment of HIV to suppress viral replication.

Antisense oligonucleotide A sequence of complementary nucleotides that can bind directly to a target gene sequence to block production of the gene product.

Anuric No passage of urine.

Anxiety An emotion that helps individuals adapt to a perceived challenge or threat but that can also create sustained apprehension such that the individual develops avoidant patterns as a means of coping with distress.

Aplastic anemia Disorder that occurs when the body stops producing enough new blood cells.

Apnea–hypopnea index (AHI) The average number of apneas and hypopneas per hour of sleep.

Apoptosis Genetically programmed cell death; programmed cell death that prevents a cell with abnormal DNA from replicating.

Appendicitis An infectious process that causes inflammation of the vermiform appendix.

Arterial blood gases A measure of the pH, $PaCO_2$, PaO_2, and bicarbonate in the arterial blood.

Arterial dissection Separation or dissection of the walls of a blood vessel resulting from a tear in the tunica intima in which the blood vessel splits and blood goes between the inner and outer layers.

Arteriosclerosis A disorder of the arteries characterized by thickening, loss of elasticity, and calcification of arterial walls.

Arteriovenous malformation (AVM) An abnormal connection between arteries and veins that bypasses the capillary system.

Ascites Abnormal collection of fluid in the peritoneal cavity.

Asphyxiants Chemicals that interfere with oxygen transport or metabolism in the body.

Aspiration The entry of secretions or foreign material into the trachea and lungs.

Assistive listening device Devices such as amplified telephones and televisions as well smoke detectors and other warning devices that assist people with hearing deficits.

Asterixis A muscle tremor when the extremity is extended and dorsiflexed; also called *liver flap* or *flapping tremor*. Noted in the hands, feet, and tongue.

Asthenia The loss or lack of physical strength as a consequence of skeletal muscle wasting.

Asthma Chronic inflammatory disorder of the airways characterized by recurrent episodes of reversible airway obstruction and hyperreactive airways.

Astigmatism A refractive error in which the eye has an elliptical shape rather than a spherical shape; as a result, light focuses on two different points in the eye.

Atelectasis Partial lung collapse or inadequate inflation of a portion of the lung; also may refer specifically to alveolar collapse.

Atheroma A fatty deposit, or plaque, on the endothelium of an artery due to arteriosclerosis.

Atherosclerosis The buildup of plaque, which is made up of cholesterol (fatty) deposits, in the coronary arteries, leading to narrowing and reducing blood flow to the myocardium.

Atopic A predisposition to develop hypersensitivity to common environmental allergens mediated by an IgE–mast cell reaction.

Atopic dermatitis (AD) Most severe form of eczema; AD is a chronic, recurring, itchy, inflammatory disorder that is associated with increased serum immunoglobulin E.

Atopy Genetic predisposition toward developing allergies.

Atrial fibrillation Dysrhythmia causing the atria (upper chambers of the heart) to beat at a rapid, irregular rate, which can lead to pooling and clotting of blood and increased risk for acute events such as myocardial infarction or stroke.

Atrial natriuretic peptide (ANP) A natriuretic peptide produced by atrial cells in response to atrial stretching and/or fluid overload.

Atrial septal defect (ASD) A congenital heart defect in which a hole in the wall (septum) between the atria allows oxygenated blood from the left atrium to flow (shunt) to the right atrium, whereupon it moves through the tricuspid valve to the right ventricle and on to the pulmonary system.

Atrioventricular valves The valves between the atria and the ventricles; the mitral valve is on the left, and the tricuspid valve is on the right.

Atrophy A decrease in cell size.

Attention-deficit/hyperactivity disorder (ADHD) A neurodevelopmental disorder that is usually first diagnosed in childhood and often lasts into adulthood, typically manifested as having trouble paying attention, difficulty controlling impulsive behaviors, or being overly active.

Atypia Structural abnormality in a cell.

Aura A perceptual disturbance that may precede the onset of seizure activity.

Autism spectrum disorder (ASD) A mental condition, present from early childhood, characterized by difficulty in communicating and forming relationships with other people and in using language and abstract concepts.

Autoantibody An antibody that is active against tissues, cells, or cell components of the individual who produces it.

Autoimmune hepatitis A progressive inflammatory liver disease characterized by significantly elevated serum immunoglobulin levels.

Autoinoculation Self-infection, such as touching a lesion then touching the eyes or genitals.

Automaticity The ability of specialized myocardial cells, or pacemaker cells, to generate an electrical impulse (depolarization) to regulate the heart rate in accordance to the body's needs.

Autophagy A normal physiologic process in the body that deals with the destruction of cells within the body.

Autoregulation The constant regulation of local blood flow through a tissue such as the myocardium despite changes in perfusion pressure.

Azotemia Elevated levels of nitrogenous waste in the blood.

Bacteria Small unicellular organisms that are important causes of infectious disease in humans; informally categorized on the basis of their staining with the Gram stain, shape, and distinctive physiologic characteristics.

Ballooning degeneration Swelling of hepatocytes from severe cell injury.

Barr body The inactivated X chromosome in each cell.

Barrett esophagus A metaplastic change in the lining of the esophageal mucosa in which normal esophageal squamous epithelium begins to resemble gastric columnar epithelium.

Bartholinitis Inflammation of the Bartholin gland.

Basal cell carcinoma (BCC) Most frequently occurring skin cancer, which develops in sun-exposed skin; it is unlikely to metastasize, but is disfiguring and is often removed surgically

Base An H^+ acceptor.

Base excess (BE) A measure of all bases in the blood, including bicarbonate, phosphate, and proteins such as albumin and hemoglobin; the test detects either a base excess or a base deficit.

Benign A growth of tissue that does not spread to other parts of the body or invade and destroy surrounding tissue.

Benign breast disease (BBD) Noncancerous ailments of the breast tissue.

Benign ovarian cysts Noncancerous cysts found on the ovaries.

Benign prostatic hyperplasia (BPH) Nonmalignant enlargement of the prostate.

Benzodiazepines A class of psychoactive drugs that enhance the effect of the neurotransmitter gamma-aminobutyric acid (GABA), resulting in sedative, hypnotic, anxiolytic, anticonvulsant, and muscle relaxant effects.

Bicarbonate (HCO_3^-) A weak base that can combine with free H^+ to form carbonic acid, which is a weak acid.

Biliary colic Painful spasms to the right upper quadrant of the abdomen that accompany obstruction in the cystic duct by a stone, causing the gallbladder to contract and cause pain.

Bilirubin A yellowish pigment found in bile.

Binge drinking A pattern of drinking that brings the blood alcohol concentration (BAC) levels to 0.08 g/dL.

Biofilm A community of bacteria that colonize together within a sticky web of extracellular material; develops on surfaces within the host and serves to protect the microorganisms from host elimination and antibiotic treatment.

Biopsy A sample of tissue removed to review for suspicious and or abnormal changes.

Bipolar disorders A group of mood disorders that are characterized by manic, hypomanic, and depressive episodes.

Bipolar I disorder A mood disorder that consists of one or more manic or mixed episodes and in which the course of illness is usually accompanied by major depressive episodes.

Bipolar II disorder A mood disorder that consists of one or more major depressive episodes accompanied by at least one hypomanic episode.

Bleb A small, thin-walled, air-filled sac on the surface of the lung.

Bleeding precautions A set of health education instructions given to patients who are at risk for a bleeding disorder.

Blood alcohol concentration (BAC) The percentage of ethanol in the blood in units of mass of alcohol per volume of blood.

Blood–brain barrier Specialized endothelium present in brain capillaries that permits selective entry of substances into the brain.

Blunt trauma Injury caused by an object that does not enter the body.

Body mass index Ratio of weight to height that is calculated by dividing weight (kilograms) by the square of one's height (meters) and used as an indicator of body mass status (underweight, normal, obese).

Botulinum toxin A neural toxin formed by the bacterium *Clostridium botulinum*.

Bowel obstruction Partial or complete blockage of the intestinal tract.

Bradycardia An abnormally slow heart rate that is lower than a normal resting rate, generally less than 60 beats per minute in an adult; also called *bradydysrhythmia*.

Brain death The irreversible cessation of cerebral and brainstem function.

Brain natriuretic peptide (BNP) A natriuretic peptide originating from the ventricle in response to ventricular stretching and/or fluid overload; particularly helpful in diagnosing or monitoring heart failure exacerbation and/or renal failure.

Breakthrough pain Transient exacerbation or flare-up of pain in an individual with continuous stable pain.

Breast cancer A form of cancer that affects the cells of the breast tissue.

Brittle nails Nails that easily become cracked, chipped, split, or peeled.

Bronchiectasis Obstructive lung disorder characterized by irreversibly dilated bronchi that readily collapse and cause airway obstruction and frequent infections.

Bronchiolitis A condition characterized by inflammation of the bronchioles.

Bronchoconstriction Narrowing of airways caused by contraction of smooth muscle in bronchial and bronchiolar walls.

Bronchodilation Widening of airways caused by relaxation of smooth muscle in bronchial and bronchiolar walls.

Brown-Séquard syndrome A condition caused by direct penetrating injury to the spinal cord that involves a hemisection of the cord.

Bruxism Grinding one's teeth during sleep.

Bubonic plague A type of plague infection resulting from the bite of an infected flea that causes infection with the bacterium *Yersinia pestis* and produces swelling of the regional lymph nodes.

Buffer system A chemical system consisting of a weak acid and a weak base that reacts almost immediately to minimize a change in H^+ concentration in body fluids.

Built environment The human-made (rather than natural) conditions of housing and other buildings, transportation of goods and people, physical safety hazards, and accessibility to recreational venues.

Bulla A large blister.

BUN:creatinine ratio A useful ratio to diagnose hypovolemia.

Bursitis Inflammation of a fluid-filled sac that cushions muscles, tendons, and bony prominences.

Cachexia Skeletal muscle wasting and involuntary weight loss resulting from both metabolic abnormalities and a lack of nutrition.

Café au lait spots or macules (CALMs) Hyperpigmented spots on the skin that are the color of "coffee with milk."

Calcium A mineral; a positively charged electrolyte.

Cancer General term encompassing more than 200 diseases that occur at different ages with distinct rates of growth, differentiation, detection evasiveness, capacities to spread to adjacent tissue and/or metastasize to distant sites, treatment responses, and prognoses.

Candidiasis A fungal infection caused by *Candida albicans*.

Cannabis A complex combination of over 400 chemicals of which about 70 are unique to the cannabis plant and are called cannabinoids; one of the most pharmacologically active of these is delta-9-tetrahydrocannabinoid (THC).

Cannabis use disorder The development of tolerance and cravings for cannabis and the development of withdrawal symptoms, inability to sleep, restlessness such as nervousness, anger, or depression within a week of ceasing heavy use.

Caput medusa Distended, engorged veins that radiate across the abdomen.

Carbonic acid (H_2CO_3) A volatile acid produced in the body that dissociates into CO_2 and H_2O. It is the acid component of the bicarbonate (HCO_3^-) buffer system.

Carbon monoxide (CO) A tasteless, odorless, colorless gas that causes more than half of all deaths from poisoning.

Carbuncle A group of infected hair follicles.

Carcinogenesis The three-step process of initiation, promotion, and metastasis by which normal cells transform into cancer cells.

Cardiac index The value obtained when the cardiac output is divided by the body surface area.

Cardiac output (CO) The amount of blood pumped from the left or right ventricle determined by stroke volume (SV) and heart rate (HR) represented by the equation $CO = SV \times HR$ and measured in liters per minute.

Cardiac remodeling The changes in size, shape, structure, and physiology of the heart that develop after injury.

Cardiac tamponade A life-threatening condition of increased pericardial pressure as a result of blood or fluid buildup between the myocardium and the pericardium.

Cardinal signs of inflammation Redness (rubor), heat (calor), swelling (tumor), pain (dolor), and loss of function.

Cardiogenic shock Shock resulting from decreased cardiac output that cannot meet tissue metabolic needs. Causes include heart failure, heart attack, and cardiac tamponade.

Cardiovascular disease (CVD) A pathologic process that causes disease of the heart or coronary and systemic circulation; includes diagnoses such as stroke, transient ischemic attack, claudication, and limb ischemia in addition to heart-related angina pectoris, myocardial ischemia, and ischemia.

Carpal tunnel syndrome Irritation of the nerves that pass through the tunnel through which the flexor tendons and median nerves pass between the wrist and the hand.

Catabolism The process through which complex molecules are broken down into smaller units.

Catagen The brief transitional phase of hair growth.

Cataplexy A condition characterized by sudden loss of muscle tone, usually resulting in a fall, caused by strong emotions such as anger, fear, or surprise.

Cataract A cloudy or opaque discoloration of the otherwise clear lens.

Catecholamines Biologic amines derived from tyrosine with a catechol group attached that function as neurotransmitters or hormones.

Cation A positively charged electrolyte; monovalent (+) or divalent (2+).

Cauda equina A portion of the spinal cord that resembles a horse's tail.

CD4 receptor Site for the major histocompatibility complex class II molecule on antigen-presenting cells.

Cell cycle The period of time from one cell division to the next.

Cell cycle checkpoints Control mechanisms that function to ensure that the process of DNA replication occurs in the correct sequence, that errors are corrected, and that one event is completed before the next is started.

Cellular adaptation Changes that occur in cell structure or function in response to stressors that support cell survival.

Cellulitis A diffuse painful inflammation of the skin and subcutaneous layers.

Central cord syndrome A condition that occurs when there is damage to the central portion of the spinal cord and less injury to the peripheral cord.

Central dogma The process of conversion of DNA to RNA to Protein.

Central pain Regional pain caused by a primary lesion or dysfunction of the central nervous system that persists after resolution of the initial inflammation or trauma.

Central pain syndrome A disorder that is a result of damage to or dysfunction of the CNS, including the brain, brainstem, and spinal cord.

Central sleep apnea (CSA) A pause in breathing during sleep resulting from decreased respiratory center output.

Central tolerance The elimination of self-reactive T cells and B cells in the central lymphoid organs.

Cerebral autoregulation A process that aims to maintain adequate cerebral blood flow.

Cerebral blood flow The blood supply to the brain in a given time, typically 750 milliliters per minute, or 15% of the cardiac output in an adult.

Cerebral contusion Bruising of the brain matter directly below a skull injury.

Cerebral perfusion pressure (CPP) Blood perfusion of the brain.

Cerebrospinal fluid (CSF) A clear, colorless body fluid found in the brain and spinal cord that is produced by the choroid plexus and acts as a cushion for the brain cortex, provides immunologic protection inside the skull, and serves a vital function in cerebral autoregulation.

Cervical cancer A form of cancer that invades the cells of the cervix.

Cervicitis Inflammation of the cervix.

Chancre A painless open lesion, especially one that develops on the penis, primarily as a result of a sexually transmitted infection.

Channelopathies Mutations in proteins that are part of an ion channel and are responsible for a variety of genetic and acquired disorders.

Chemokine receptors G-protein–coupled receptors whose activation mediates leukocyte extravasation and migration.

Chemokines Chemokines are a class of cytokines that attract leukocytes to areas of inflammation as well as performing various other functions. Examples of chemokines include CXC chemokines and CC chemokines.

Chemotaxis The process of attracting macrophages and neutrophils.

Chemotherapy Drugs that arrest cellular proliferation by interfering with DNA synthesis and replication of both normal and malignant cells.

Cheyne-Stokes breathing Breathing characterized by a waxing and waning of the depth of breathing with regularly recurring intervals of apnea; often a sign of imminent death.

Chill phase The phase of fever in which there is mild to severe shivering, vasoconstriction, and an uncomfortable sense of cold, which are thermoregulatory responses that generate and conserve heat to adjust the body temperature to the new higher set point.

Chlamydia A sexually transmitted infection caused by the bacteria *Chlamydia trachomatis.*

Chloride An anion that occurs naturally in the human body.

Chlorine A chemical agent commonly used in industry that can also be used as a chemical weapon.

Cholangitis Acute or chronic inflammation of the bile duct.

Cholecystitis Acute or chronic inflammation of the wall of the gallbladder.

Choledocholithiasis Gallstones in the common bile duct.

Cholelithiasis Stones in the gallbladder.

Cholestasis Impairment of the flow of bile from the liver to the duodenum.

Chromosome The long DNA double helix combined with proteins called histones and compacted. Each chromosome contains a large amount of DNA and many genes.

Chromosome nondisjunction Failure of chromosomes to separate properly during cell division.

Chromosome translocation The occurrence when a piece of one chromosome breaks off and fuses to another chromosome.

Chronic bronchitis Form of chronic obstructive pulmonary disease; characterized by persistent, inflammation-induced narrowing of the airways, copious mucus production, and chronic productive cough.

Chronic kidney disease (CKD) A loss of kidney function over time. Kidney damage or glomerular filtration rate less than $60\ \text{mL/min}/1.73\ \text{m}^2$ for 3 months or more.

Chronic kidney disease–mineral and bone disorder (CKD-MBD) The bone disease process in CKD that occurs as a result of mineral and hormonal changes.

Chronic lymphocytic leukemia (CLL) A form of leukemia characterized by the overproduction of B cells.

Chronic myelogenous leukemia (CML) A form of leukemia characterized by overproliferation of mature granulocytes.

Chronic obstructive pulmonary disease (COPD) An umbrella term for progressive lung disorders such as chronic bronchitis and emphysema.

Chronic otitis media (COM) Consistent infection of the inner ear, typically greater than 6 weeks, with persistent effusion in the middle ear space.

Chronic pain Pain that persists longer than 6 months after an acute disease or injury. It is associated with a chronic pathologic process in the peripheral and/or central nervous system.

Chronic pancreatitis A disorder that is similar to acute pancreatitis except that the chronic pain is often less severe, but the tissue damage is irreversible.

Chronic venous disease (CVD) Chronic vascular conditions that affect veins.

Chronic venous insufficiency (CVI) A disorder of inadequate venous return over a prolonged period due to vein blockage or valve leakage in the leg veins.

Chvostek sign Ipsilateral twitching or spasms of the muscles of the face in response to percussive tapping of the facial nerve. A positive finding is indicative of hypocalcemia and/or hyperphosphatemia.

Chylothorax A collection of dietary fat in the pleural cavity due to thoracic duct disruption.

Circadian rhythm A pattern based on a 24-hour cycle, especially the repetition of certain physiologic phenomena.

Cirrhosis Serious largely irreversible and frequently deadly disease in which liver cells are replaced by fibrous tissue, resulting in inadequate liver function; usually caused by chronic heavy alcohol use.

Claudication Leg pain that is induced by exercise, typically caused by decreased arterial blood flow.

Clinical manifestations The signs and symptoms typically associated with a disease state, including alterations in diagnostic tests such as imaging studies and biochemical analyses of bodily fluids.

Clonal disease Disease in which all malignant cells derive from a single errant cell.

Clonic phase A phase of seizure activity characterized by intermittent muscular contraction and relaxation.

Closed-angle glaucoma The type of glaucoma that occurs when the angle between the iris and cornea is blocked; this condition is treated as an emergency; also called *narrow-angle glaucoma.*

Cluster headache (CH) A sudden unilateral severe pain that occurs in clusters and is associated with ipsilateral autonomic symptoms.

Cluster of differentiation A cell surface marker used to identify leukocytes in the laboratory; frequently used to designate cell type in hematologic malignancies such as leukemia or lymphomas.

Coagulopathy A bleeding disorder associated with an impairment of clotting mechanisms.

Coarctation of aorta (COA) A congenital heart defect in which there is narrowing of the aorta, usually around the area of the arch and most commonly in the thoracic area.

Cochlear implant A device implanted in the cochlea to stimulate it to cause hearing.

Cochleotoxic Medications that damage the sensory cells of the cochlea, resulting in sensorineural hearing loss.

Codon Every three nucleotides grouped together in mRNA, corresponding to a specific amino acid.

Coffee ground appearance The dark, grainy appearance of digested blood; may be found in vomitus, gastric secretions, or stool.

Cognition The way in which people acquire, store, learn, use and communicate information.

Cognitive-behavioral therapy (CBT) A treatment for anxiety disorders in which the individual learns to identify and challenge fearful automatic and catastrophic thoughts.

Collagen A fibrous protein that imparts great strength to tendons, ligaments, and fascia.

Colloid osmotic pressure The concentration of proteins, particularly albumin, that gives rise to water-pulling forces of a particular compartment; also known as *oncotic pressure.*

Colon cancer A malignant growth or tumor resulting from the division of abnormal cells in the colon.

Colonization High concentration of organisms at a site where they can be detected but the person has no signs or symptoms.

Commensal microorganism Harmless nonpathogenic flora that typically populate the human host.

Compensation The state in which various chemical buffers and renal or respiratory function return the pH closer to or actually back within the normal range; however, the underlying disease process responsible for the acid–base imbalance is still present.

Complement proteins Proteins found in the blood that assist in fighting infection.

Complex regional pain syndrome (CRPS) Chronic regional pain that follows an injury to a major nerve or limb. CRPS Type I was previously called *reflex sympathetic dystrophy (RSD).* CRPS type II was previously called *causalgia.*

Conditioned response An automatic response to an otherwise benign stimulus; also known as *classical conditioning.*

Conditioned stimulus The beginning of the fear conditioning pathway in which stimuli trigger apprehensions.

Conductive hearing loss Hearing loss that occurs due to problems that affect the outer and middle ear system structures that prevent sound from traveling normally to the inner ear.

Confusion Assessment Method (CAM) A delirium rating scale that is recommended for use in detecting delirium and differentiating it from dementia.

Congenital adrenal hyperplasia (CAH) A form of adrenal insufficiency in which the enzyme that produces cortisol and aldosterone is deficient.

Congenital heart defect (CHD) A gross structural abnormality of the heart or intrathoracic great vessels that is actually or potentially of functional significance.

Conjugated bilirubin A water-soluble form of bilirubin that can be excreted in the urine.

Conjunctivitis Inflammation of the conjunctiva.

Consolidation The process by which an individual's brain labels an event as threatening and to be feared.

Constipation The infrequent passage of small amounts of hard, dry stool.

Contact dermatitis An eruption of skin related to contact with an irritating substance or allergen.

Continuous positive airway pressure (CPAP) A flow of air at a preset pressure, which acts as a splint to hold the airway open.

Contractility The strength of muscular contraction in the heart muscle.

Contraction alkalosis A state of below-normal pH due to loss of extracellular fluid volume without comparable loss of bicarbonate, which increases the concentration of bicarbonate.

Contracture An abnormal, usually permanent condition of a joint, characterized by flexion and fixation.

Contrast-induced nephropathy (CIN) Acute kidney injury as a result of the administration of intravenous contrast.

Contusion An area of tissue injury in which capillaries leak blood, leading to the formation of a bruise.

Coping The dynamic process through which individuals apply psychologic and behavioral measures to handle internal and external stress demands.

Corneal abrasion A scratch or cut that causes a defect on the surface of the cornea.

Coronary angiogram An invasive diagnostic or interventional procedure performed in a special laboratory that is used to confirm the diagnosis of coronary artery disease after noninvasive tests have been inconclusive or in the presence of life-threatening coronary symptoms; also known as *coronary angiography* or *arteriography.*

Coronary artery disease (CAD) A condition of reduced blood flow through coronary arteries to the myocardium, leading to reduced supplies of oxygen and nutrients; often caused by atherosclerosis.

Coronary collateral circulation The adaptation of collateral vessels that anastomose (branch) to reroute blood flow to the myocardium when a coronary artery is blocked.

Coronary heart disease (CHD) A term that is used interchangeably with *coronary artery disease* to describe the buildup of plaque in the coronary arteries that leads to reduced blood flow to the myocardium.

Coronary microvascular disease Damage to the walls and inner linings of small coronary arteries that can lead to narrowing, spasms, and decreased blood flow; also known as *cardiac syndrome X* or *nonobstructive coronary heart disease* because the coronary arteries do not appear to have atherosclerotic plaque.

Coronary perfusion pressure Pressure of blood through coronary circulation as a result of the pressure gradient between the aortic pressure and the right atrial pressure.

Correction In an acid–base imbalance, the state that occurs when the condition responsible for the imbalance is controlled or no longer present and the pH is within the normal range.

Cortisol A glucocorticoid hormone with significant effects on metabolism, glucose regulation, and immune function.

Cough The forceful release of air through the trachea and mouth.

Counterregulatory hormones A group of hormones whose functions are antagonistic to insulin. These hormones include glucagon, epinephrine, cortisol, and growth hormone.

C-reactive protein (CRP) A protein found in plasma that increases in response to inflammation. Measuring changes in CRP over time can be helpful in monitoring disease progression or response to treatment.

Crepitus Crackling or grating of a joint.

Cricothyroidotomy A procedure in which a surgical incision is made through the cricothyroid membrane so that an endotracheal tube can be placed to obtain an airway.

Critical congenital heart disease (CCHD) A group of serious congenital heart defects that usually require surgical correction within the first year of life.

Crohn disease (CD) A chronic inflammatory condition that is characterized by transmural inflammation of the bowel and most commonly affects the ileum and proximal colon; it is considered to be an *inflammatory bowel disease.*

Croup An acute viral infection of the upper respiratory tract commonly caused by parainfluenza viruses that spread through children younger than 5 years of age in daycare centers, families, and hospitals; also called *laryngotracheobronchitis.*

Cryptorchidism The absence of one or both testes from the scrotum, also referred to as *undescended testes.*

Cullen sign Bruising and edema of the subcutaneous tissue surrounding the umbilicus caused by hemorrhagic pancreatitis.

Cushing disease A disorder characterized by increased secretion of adrenocorticotropic hormone (ACTH) from the anterior pituitary.

Cushing syndrome A clinical condition that results from chronic exposure to excess glucocorticoids; can be the result of exogenous pharmacologic doses of corticosteroids or endogenous sources of cortisol.

Cyanide A chemical agent, a common by-product of combustion, that is a cellular asphyxiant preventing the utilization of oxygen at the cellular level.

Cyclothymic disorder A mood disorder in which the patient has chronic, fluctuating mood disturbance involving numerous periods of hypomanic symptoms and numerous periods of depressive symptoms.

Cystic fibrosis (CF) Recessive genetic disorder that inhibits sodium reabsorption in skin sweat ducts but enhances sodium transport across epithelial cells in the respiratory system, pancreas, bile ducts, and sperm ducts.

Cystitis Infection of the bladder.

Cytogenetics The study of chromosome number and structure.

Cytokine Proteins involved in cell-to-cell communication, coordinating antibody and T-cell immune interactions, and amplifying immune reactivity.

Cytomegalovirus (CMV) A double-stranded DNA virus that is carried by the majority of the general population but replication of which is normally inhibited by the immune system; found in blood, saliva, semen, cervical secretions, and urine.

Death rattle A gurgling sound caused by oscillating movements of secretions in the upper airway, the onset of which generally precedes death by about 48 hours.

Decreased pulmonary blood flow defects A category of congenital heart defects in which obstruction to pulmonary blood flow decreases the flow of blood to in pulmonary circulation, which increases pressure on the right side of the heart.

Deep vein thrombosis (DVT) A blood clot in a vein deep in the body.

Defervescence phase The phase of fever that occurs when the pyrogen level subsides, the temperature set point stabilizes to lower levels, febrile temperatures feel uncomfortably hot, and sweating becomes profuse.

Delayed cerebral ischemia (DCI) A clinical syndrome of focal neurologic deficits, cognitive deficits, or both that occurs in approximately 30% of patient during the initial 3–14 days following hemorrhage.

Delayed union Fracture healing that takes longer than expected.

Delirium An acute and usually fluctuating change in cognition or awareness that can be reversible.

Dementia A chronic or persistent disorder of the mental processes caused by brain disease or injury and marked by memory disorders, personality changes, and impaired reasoning.

Demyelination Damage to the myelin sheath that surrounds nerve axons and leads to slowing or cessation of nerve impulses.

Dendritic cells Antigen-presenting cells, such as Langerhans cells, involved in the early phase of adaptive host defense that engulf or phagocytose microbial antigen.

Deoxyribonucleic acid (DNA) A sequence of molecules that form a genetic code used to create each specific gene sequence, considered the building block of genetic material.

Depressant A group of drugs that generally depress the central nervous system and at high doses induce sleep; includes alcohol, barbiturates, and other sedative hypnotic drugs.

Depression A pervasive mental illness that is a debilitating condition that includes feelings of sadness, hopelessness, guilt, and restlessness; difficulty concentrating, sleeping; decreased energy; and thoughts of death or suicide. It creates a serious negative impact on functioning and interpersonal relationships.

Dermal papillae Elevation in the dermis, as seen in fingerprints on the surface of the skin.

Dermatome Area of skin innervated by a single sensory spinal nerve.

Dermatosis Skin disease that does not involve inflammation

Dermis The layer of the skin just below the epidermis, consisting of papillary and reticular layers.

Dermopathy A noninflamed, indurated plaque with a deep pink or purple color and an orange skin appearance seen in patients with Graves disease.

Development The ability to adapt to the environment; refers to behavioral aspects of growth such as talking, walking, and running.

Developmental potential The "ability to think, learn, remember, relate, and articulate ideas appropriate to age and level of maturity," as defined by Aboud and Yousafzai.

Dextroscoliosis A right thoracic curve.

Diabetic ketoacidosis (DKA) A state of absolute or relative insulin deficiency that is typically characterized by hyperglycemia, metabolic acidosis, and ketonemia; most commonly caused by underlying infection, disruption of insulin treatment, and new onset of T1D.

Diabetic nephropathy Hyperglycemic-induced glomerulosclerosis that results in eventual hyperfiltration, proteinuria, and CKD.

Diabetic peripheral neuropathy (DPN) Peripheral nerve damage associated with diabetes as a result of hyperglycemia and impaired blood supply.

Diabetic retinopathy Damage to the retina in individuals with diabetes in which the blood vessels in the retina change; may be nonproliferative or proliferative.

Diarrhea An increase in stool content, volume, and weight.

Diastolic heart failure A condition with normal contractility of the heart but abnormal relaxation of the heart; referred to as heart failure with preserved ejection factor.

Differentiated cancers Cancers that are composed of more mature cells and tend to be less aggressive than undifferentiated cancers.

Differentiation The maturation of a normal cell to one with distinct morphology and specialized functions.

Diffuse axonal injury (DAI) A brain injury that occurs when the axonal fibers in the white matter and brainstem become sheared.

Diffusion The net movement of a substance, such as solutes, from a region of greater concentration to a region of lower concentration.

Digital rectal examination (DRE) Digital palpation of the prostate through the rectum to determine its size and condition.

Dihydrotestosterone (DHT) An androgen that mediates prostatic growth.

Diploid cells Cells that contain two of each chromosome type for a total of 46 chromosomes.

Dirty bomb A conventional explosive to which a radioactive substance has been added in order to disperse it over a wide area and create panic and psychologic distress and fear; also referred to as a radiologic dispersal device.

Discectomy Surgery to remove a disc.

Disease An impairment of some functional ability that results in the appearance of symptoms.

Dislocation An injury in which the ends of the bones are moved out of the normal position, causing a loss of joint attachment.

Disorder A synonym for disease, more commonly used in relation to psychologic health; can refer to lasting physiologic consequences resulting from a disease.

Disseminated intravascular coagulation (DIC) A life-threatening condition that occurs when a pattern of systemic clotting is activated.

Distal symmetric polyneuropathy One of the most common forms of HIV-associated peripheral neuropathy; a sensory axonal neuropathy that typically involves the toes and soles of the feet, although the fingers and hands may become involved over time.

Distributive shock Shock resulting from inadequate tissue perfusion (blood delivery to tissues) following a pattern of extensive vasodilation. It is often associated with a lack of normal responsiveness of blood vessels to vasoactive agents. It causes include systemic inflammatory responses, conditions tied to sepsis, and anaphylaxis.

Diverticula Small outpouchings, or herniations, of gastrointestinal mucosa through the muscular layers of the gastrointestinal tract; most commonly found in the esophagus and the colon.

Diverticulitis Inflamed diverticula.

Diverticulosis Diverticula without evidence of inflammation.

DNA replication The process whereby double-stranded DNA copies itself, resulting in two double-stranded DNA molecules.

Dopamine A neurotransmitter that is found in the basal ganglia and other regions of the brain; a precursor to epinephrine involved in cognition and motivation.

Dose–response relationship Increased risk of toxicity as the dose of a substance increases.

Double helix The double-stranded helical structure of DNA.

Down syndrome A genetic disorder caused by trisomy of chromosome 21, resulting in miscarriage or in a live-born child with a combination of birth defects, characteristic facial features, and variable degrees of cognitive impairment.

Dressler syndrome Pericarditis that occurs about 1 week to a few months after a myocardial infarction; also known as *post-MI syndrome*.

Dry macular degeneration The more common and less severe type of macular degeneration, in which the symptoms are a blurry or "wavy" central vision with normal peripheral vision.

Dysfunctional uterine bleeding (DUB) Any abnormal bleeding from the uterus not associated with a physical lesion such as a tumor, inflammation, or pregnancy.

Dysmenorrhea Painful menstruation.

Dysoxia An imbalance between oxygen supply and oxygen demand.

Dyspareunia Painful or difficult sexual intercourse.

Dyspepsia Generalized, uncomfortable feelings including mild, gnawing discomfort in the abdomen or chest, bloating, early satiety, and nausea.

Dysphagia Difficulty in swallowing food and liquids.

Dysphonia Difficulty in speaking as a result of a condition of the mouth, throat, or vocal cords.

Dysplasia Deranged cell growth of specific tissue that results in cells that vary in size, shape, and organization.

Dyspnea The subjective experience of difficulty breathing; often used interchangeably with the term *shortness of breath*.

Dysrhythmia An abnormal heart rhythm that can be irregularly slow or fast; also known as an *arrhythmia*.

Dysthymia A depressed mood (feeling sad or down) that occurs on more days than not and occurs for most of the day; also called *persistent depressive disorder*.

Dysuria Painful urination.

Ecchymoses Bruises that may occur after relatively minor trauma.

Eccrine sweat A clear, odorless, and dilute solution that is secreted from millions of eccrine sweat glands that cover most of the body. The evaporation of sweat promotes cooling of skin surfaces and makes it effective as a heat defense thermoeffector.

Ectopic pregnancy Gestation that occurs anywhere other than the uterus.

Eczema Eruption of an itchy, red, weeping, crusting patch on the skin

Edema: The accumulation of interstitial fluid volume.

Effusion Fluid in a joint.

Eicosanoids Signaling molecules derived from omega-3 and omega-6 fatty acids that are involved in several different pathways. Types of eicosanoids include prostaglandins, prostacyclins, thromboxanes, and leukotrienes. Depending on the type of eicosanoid, they may promote inflammation or inhibit it. Drugs such as NSAIDs and aspirin act by affecting eicosanoid production.

Ejection fraction The volume of blood the heart pumps out during a beat divided by the volume of blood in the ventricle when filled.

Elastin A protein that forms the principal substance of elastic connective tissue fibers.

Electrical burn Tissue damage resulting from the flow of electricity through the body.

Electrocardiogram A recording of cardiac activity.

Electroencephalogram A recording of the electrical activity of the brain.

Electrolyte A substance that dissociates into ions in water.

Electromyelogram A recording of muscle tension and relaxation.

Electro-oculogram A recording of the electric currents produced by eye movements.

Embolism A condition in which an embolus (a substance or foreign matter) travels via the bloodstream and subsequently lodges in a blood vessel, creating a partial or complete obstruction of blood flow through the affected vessel.

Embolus A mass in the bloodstream that may be a blood clot, foreign material such as air or gas bubble, fat droplet, or clump of bacteria; the plural form is *emboli*.

Emerging infectious disease A disease that is newly identified in a population or one that has significantly increased in incidence or geographic range.

Emetic response The vomiting reflex that occurs as a result of the transmission of neural impulses by one of four pathways to the vomiting center located in the medulla.

Emphysema Form of chronic obstructive pulmonary disease; characterized by the irreversible loss of walls between alveoli with no evidence of fibrosis.

Empyema A collection of pus in the pleural cavity.

Endolymph A fluid that is very high in potassium and fills the scala media in the cochlea.

Endometrial cancer Cancer of the lining of the uterus.

Endometrial polyps Hyperplasic overgrowth of the endometrial glands and stroma.

Endometriosis The presence and growth of functioning endometrial tissue in places other than the uterus.

Endotoxemia The presence of a high level of endotoxin in the bloodstream.

Endotoxin Lipopolysaccharide molecule located within the cell wall of gram-negative bacteria; integral to the inflammatory process as well as to the pathogenesis of sepsis and septic shock caused by gram-negative bacteremia.

End-stage renal disease (ESRD) Renal failure along with chronic renal insufficiency that results in the failure of the body to remove waste products.

Engineering controls A set of methods to control exposures by modifying the source of contaminants or reducing the quantity of contaminants released into the environment.

Enthesitis Areas around a joint where the ligaments and tendons attach to the bone in the knee, foot, or hip.

Enuresis Urination or incontinence of urine, especially nocturnal bed-wetting.

Environmental hazard A substance, state, or event that potentially threatens the health or safety of people or the environment.

Environmental health According to the National Environmental Health Association, "the science and practice of preventing human injury and illness and promoting well-being by identifying and evaluating environmental sources and hazardous agents and limiting exposures to hazardous physical, chemical, and biological agents in air, water, soil, food, and other environmental media or settings that may adversely affect human health."

Ephaptic crosstalk Depolarization of a demyelinated neuron from electrical potentials that jump from adjacent nerve fibers.

Epidemic A widespread outbreak of an infectious disease in which many people are infected simultaneously.

Epidemiology A field of study that investigates the occurrence and patterns of health and disease.

Epidermal inclusion cysts (EICs) Benign lesions that result from squamous epithelium of the epidermis being trapped or implanted in the dermis

Epidermis The visible, upper layer of skin composed of multiple layers of stratified squamous epithelial cells called *keratinocytes*.

Epididymis The anatomic tube that collects and transports sperm.

Epididymitis Inflammation of the epididymis.

Epidural hematoma A condition that occurs when a head injury causes blood to leak between the skull and the dura mater.

Epigenetics The study of genetic and genomic modifications that have occurred to a particular cell.

Epigenome The collection of the chemical compounds (not part of genomic DNA) that instruct the genome where and when genes are expressed within a cell.

Epigenomics The area of study that focuses on the complete set of modifications to cellular DNA. The study of the chemical compounds that instruct the genome where and when genes are expressed within a cell.

Epiglottitis A rapidly progressive inflammation of the epiglottis and adjacent structures that may cause airway obstruction; most often caused by bacterial infection, including *Haemophilus influenzae* type b (Hib).

Epilepsy A collection of neurologic conditions characterized by seizure activity.

Epispadias A congenital abnormality of the location of the male urethral meatus in which the urethral opening is on the dorsal (upper) surface of the penis.

Erectile dysfunction The inability to attain or maintain an erection sufficient to permit mutually satisfactory sexual intercourse with a partner.

Erythrocytes Red blood cells.

Erythropoietin Hormone produced by the kidneys that regulates the production of red blood cells.

Esophageal cancer A malignant growth or tumor resulting from the division of abnormal cells in the esophagus.

Esophageal chest pain A pressure-like sensation felt in the midchest that may radiate to the back, arms, and jaw.

Esophageal diverticula Acquired outpouchings of the esophagus located in the upper, middle, or lower esophagus.

Esophageal perforation A tear or rupture that creates a hole through the layers of the esophagus.

Esophageal ring A circumferential narrowing of the lumen of the esophagus.

Esophageal varices Enlarged blood vessels in the esophagus as a result of portal hypertension.

Esophageal web A thin, membranous tissue that occupies the lumen of the esophagus, decreasing luminal diameter.

Esophagitis Irritation and inflammation of the tissues of the esophagus; may be due to allergic reactions, infections, radiation, ingestion of corrosive substances, or improper passage of a pill.

Essential (primary) hypertension Elevated blood pressure that does not have an identifiable cause.

Etiology The cause of a disease or injury.

Eukaryote Any cell that contains a distinct nucleus and membrane-enclosed organelles.

Eukaryotic cell Cell with a true nucleus.

Euthyroid Normal thyroid function.

Evidence-based practice (EBP) The conscientious, explicit, and judicious use of current best evidence in patient care decision making; includes integrating clinical expertise with consideration paid to the patient's values and preferences.

Evisceration The protrusion of an internal organ through a wound or surgical incision, especially in the abdominal wall.

Exacerbation An increase in the severity or intensity of a disease.

Excitotoxicity A pathologic process in which neurons are damaged and killed by overactivation of receptors for the excitatory neurotransmitter glutamate, which allows calcium influx into cells that activates enzymes that cause cell damage.

Excoriations Surface injury to skin that removes cell layers.

Exercise A subcategory of physical activity that is planned, structured, and repetitive, with a goal of improvement or maintenance of one or more components of physical fitness.

Exfoliative dermatitis (ED) An inflammation of skin characterized by erythema involving loss of exfoliated skin.

Exogen Shedding at end of resting phase of hair growth

Exons The coding portion of the gene.

Exophthalmos A forward displacement or "bulging" of the eyeball.

Exotoxin Polypeptide proteins that are produced primarily by gram-positive bacteria; also may be produced by some forms of gram-negative bacteria.

Extinction The process by which a new association forms between a conditioned stimulus and a conditioned response.

Extracellular fluid (ECF) The fluid found outside of the cells; accounts for approximately one third of total body fluid.

Extracellular matrix A substance containing collagen, elastin, proteoglycans, glycosaminoglycans, and fluid, in which connective tissue cells are embedded.

Exudate Fluid produced as the result of an inflammatory process; contains water, cells, large amounts of protein, and other materials.

Exudative Condition involving the oozing of fluid

Fatigue A pervasive feeling of tiredness and lack of energy that is not relieved by rest.

Fear-centered anxiety disorders Anxiety disorders such as panic disorder and social anxiety disorder that may occur following a situation that the mind associates with overwhelming negative consequences.

Febrile seizure Seizure activity brought about through increased bodily temperature.

Femtoliter (fL) Unit of measurement equal to 1 mm^3.

Fetal alcohol syndrome Prenatal alcohol exposure can cause a number of physical, behavioral, cognitive, and neural impairments, collectively known as *fetal alcohol spectrum disorders (FASD).*

Fever A systemic host response that produces an elevated body temperature by raising the thermoregulatory set point control levels in the hypothalamus. Molecular mechanisms that elevate temperature also boost immune responses but are also responsible for the accompanying distress and malaise of fever.

Fibrinous inflammation Inflammation associated with increased vascular permeability that allows fluid with large proteins (e.g., fibrinogen) to leak out of the blood vessels into the surrounding tissue.

Fibroblasts An undifferentiated cell in the connective tissue that gives rise to precursor cells such as the chondroblast, collagenoblast, and osteoblast, which form the fibrous, binding, and supporting tissue of the body.

Fibromyalgia (FM) A disorder characterized by chronic widespread pain in multiple tender points lasting longer than 3 months and accompanied by nonrestorative sleep patterns, fatigue, and cognitive impairment.

Fibronectin A glycoprotein that spans the external cellular membrane and binds with membrane components associated with cellular adhesion.

First-order neuron A neuron that conducts a noxious stimulus from a peripheral receptor to the second-order neuron in the dorsal horn.

First-pass effect The biotransformation of ingested substances the first time they are transported to the liver via the hepatic portal vein.

Flail chest A chest injury that occurs when a segment of the rib cage breaks as a result of trauma and becomes detached from the rest of the thorax.

Fluorescence in situ hybridization (FISH) A test using fluorescent probes to detect chromosome number and target specific DNA sequences on chromosomes.

Focal segmental glomerulosclerosis (FSGS) A group of syndromes that have podocyte injury in which the scarring involves some (focal) but not all glomeruli and the scarring is seen in only a portion of the glomerulus (segmental).

Folate B vitamin necessary for the production of erythrocytes.

Folic acid Synthetic form of folate found in supplements.

Folliculitis An inflammation of the hair follicle.

Fomite Inanimate object or substance by which an infectious organism can be transmitted from one individual to another.

Fractional excretion of sodium (FE_{Na}) The percentage of sodium filtered by the kidney that is excreted in the urine; useful to determine classification of acute kidney injury.

Fractional excretion of urea (FE_{urea}) The percentage of urea filtered by the kidney that is excreted in urine; useful when the patient is on diuretics.

Fracture A break in the continuity of a bone.

Frostbite Localized injury that occurs to the skin and underlying structures when the person is exposed to freezing temperatures. It results from extracellular fluids forming ice crystals that disrupt the osmotic gradient across cell membranes, causing water to move from the cells into the extracellular fluid, raising the concentration of electrolytes in the cells, which initiates cell death, or intracellular fluids freeze and their subsequent expansion mechanically destroys cells.

Full thickness burn Destruction of all dermal layers and structures along with destruction of subcutaneous tissues.

Full thickness wound A wound in which the epidermis and the entire thickness of the dermis are lost or destroyed.

Fungi Any member of a large group of spore-producing eukaryotic organisms that includes microorganisms (e.g., yeasts, molds, and mushrooms).

Furuncle A deep folliculitis consisting of a pus-filled mass that is painful and firm; also known as an *abscess* or *boil*.

Galactorrhea Spontaneous inappropriate flow of milk from the nipple.

Gamma-aminobutyric acid (GABA) A primary inhibitory amino acid neurotransmitter that is widely distributed in the central nervous system.

Gangrene A mass of necrotic tissue.

Gastric outlet obstruction A mechanical obstruction in the pyloric region of the stomach.

Gastritis Inflammation of the gastric mucosa.

Gastroesophageal reflux disease (GERD) A constellation of esophageal and extraesophageal symptoms associated with chronically refluxed gastric contents.

Gene A segment of DNA that codes for the production of a certain protein.

Gene amplification An increase in the number of gene copies.

Gene product A protein that is the end product of gene expression, which includes DNA transcription and RNA translation into protein.

General adaptation syndrome A physiologic response pattern to stress consisting of three stages (alarm, exhaustion, resistance).

Generalized anxiety disorder (GAD) A state of excessive worrying that interferes with daily function.

Generalized seizure Seizure activity involving both hemispheres of the brain.

Genetic imprinting The differential expression of genes based on whether they are inherited from the mother or the father.

Genetics The study of individual genes and their impact on inheritance and single-gene and chromosomal disorders.

Genital warts A soft, raised growth on the outer surface of the skin in the genital area; also referred to as *condyloma planum*.

Genitourinary trauma Trauma to the kidneys, ureters, bladder, or urethra.

Genome-wide association studies (GWAS) A genomic test that is used both in research, such as in the Human Genome Project, and in clinical practice to identify relationships between common genome variation and particular traits of interest.

Genomics The study of the function of sets or groups of genes. Generally, focuses on examining the genome of an individual cell.

Genotype The actual genetic code in a person.

Germ line mutations A disease causing changes in the inherited DNA transmitted via the egg or sperm cells that join to form an embryo. This is passed on to offspring.

Gestational diabetes mellitus (GDM) A condition in which the onset of DM is first diagnosed during pregnancy.

Ghon's complex A lesion consisting of a granuloma with an associated lymph node that signals an immune response to *M. tuberculosis* bacilli.

Glasgow Coma Scale (GCS) A neurologic scoring system that is used to quickly evaluate level of consciousness.

Glaucoma A group of diseases characterized by an increase in intraocular pressure leading to a slow, painless, and progressive loss of vision.

Globus sensation The feeling of fullness or a lump in the throat.

Glomerular crescents Fibrin deposition that occurs as a result of severe glomerular injury and appears histologically as crescents.

Glomerulonephritis (GN) Inflammation of glomeruli and capillaries that is characterized by proteinuria, hematuria, and edema.

Glomerulosclerosis Scarring of the glomerulus, seen in diabetes mellitus.

Gluconeogenesis The formation of glucose or glycogen from noncarbohydrate sources.

Glucosuria The excretion of glucose into the urine.

Glutamate The predominant excitatory neurotransmitter in the CNS; binds to the a-amino-3-hydroxy-5-methyl-4-isoxazolepropionic acid and NMDA receptors.

Glycosaminoglycans (GAGs) Polysaccharides that are highly polar and attract water to the ECM.

Glycogen The storage form of glucose that is primarily located in skeletal muscle and the liver.

Glycogenolysis The process through which liver and muscle glycogen are converted to glucose.

Glycolysis The breakdown of carbohydrate.

Goiters An abnormal enlargement of the thyroid gland.

Gonadal cells Egg and sperm cells.

Gonorrhea A sexually transmitted infection caused by the bacteria *Neisseria gonorrhea.*

Gout A disease process that causes accumulation of uric acid crystals.

Gram-negative bacteria Bacteria with a cell wall composition that does not retain the crystal violet stain after acid washing.

Gram-positive bacteria Bacteria with a cell wall composition that retains the crystal violet stain after acid washing, resulting in a purple coloration.

Granulation tissue Soft pink fleshy tissue that forms during the healing process of a wound.

Granuloma A mass of fused macrophages that sequester persistent infectious agents and prevent their activation and dissemination.

Graves disease A type of autoimmune disorder that causes hyperthyroidism.

Graves ophthalmopathy An eye disease that is present in Graves disease and is characterized by lid lag and retraction, periorbital edema, exophthalmos, diplopia, corneal involvement, and visual loss.

Grey-Turner sign Bruising of the flank area with bluish discoloration from bleeding behind the peritoneum, often noted in pancreatitis.

Growth factor A protein that stimulates growth, division, and differentiation of specific types of cells.

Gynecomastia Swelling of the male breasts.

Hallucinogen persisting perception disorder (HPPD) Disorder in which hallucinations occur unpredictably, interfere with daily activities, and cause anxiety and depression.

Haploid cells Cells that contain one of each chromosome type, for a total of 23 chromosomes.

Hashimoto thyroiditis An autoimmune disease that results in hypothyroidism; also known as *chronic lymphocytic thyroiditis.*

Health A state of normative physiologic or psychologic function.

Healthcare-associated infections Infections that are acquired within a hospital or other healthcare setting.

Healthcare-associated pneumonia (HCAP) A classification of pneumonia in which the infection develops (a) following hospitalization in an acute care hospital for two 2 or more days within 90 days of developing the infection; (b) subsequent to residency in a long-term care facility or nursing home; (c) within 30 days of receiving intravenous antibiotic medications, chemotherapy, or wound care; or (d) after attending a hospital or hemodialysis clinic.

Hearing aid Small device that fits in or on the ear to amplify sound.

Heartburn Discomfort or a burning sensation behind the sternum, originating from the epigastrium.

Heart failure (HF) A condition caused by an inability of the heart to pump enough blood to meet the body's metabolic needs.

Heat exhaustion A milder form of heat-related illness than heat stroke but considered to be on the same continuum; causes malaise, headache, and nausea.

Heat stress The point at which the net heat load to which a person is exposed begins to overcome the body's means of controlling it.

Heat stroke An uncompensated conflict between homeostatic thermoregulatory drives to lose heat by increasing skin blood flow and cardiovascular drives to maintain blood pressure; a medical emergency.

Helicobacter pylori (H. pylori) A gram-negative bacterium that causes gastritis and ulcers.

Helminths Parasitic worms (e.g., nematodes, flukes, and tapeworms).

Hemangiomas Congenital lesions that are made up of extra blood vessels concentrated in an area within or just under the skin

Hematemesis Bright red blood in vomitus.

Hematochezia Bright red blood in stool.

Hematocrit The proportion of red blood cells in a volume of blood.

Hematoma A collection of blood within tissue that forms after damage to the integrity of blood vessels.

Hematopoiesis The process behind the formation of blood cells.

Hemodialysis Removal of fluid and solutes from blood across a semipermeable membrane in a dialyzer.

Hemoglobin Protein containing iron that allows for the transportation of oxygen.

Hemoglobin A1C A blood test that provides information about a person's average blood glucose level over the past 3 months.

Hemolytic uremic syndrome (HUS) A disorder usually acquired from Shiga toxin–producing *Escherichia coli* infection resulting in acute kidney injury and microangiopathic lesions.

Hemophilia A hereditary genetic bleeding disorder resulting from the loss of select clotting factors.

Hemoptysis Expectoration of blood from the airways caused by an erosion through a pulmonary or bronchial blood vessel wall.

Hemorrhage Bleeding from a ruptured blood vessel.

Hemorrhagic stroke A stroke resulting from hemorrhage within the brain leading to increased pressure within the skull.

Hemorrhoid Abnormal engorgement of the hemorrhoidal cushions of the anus.

Hemostasis The termination of bleeding; consists of vasoconstriction, platelet aggregation, and thrombin and fibrin synthesis.

Hemothorax A type of pleural effusion in which blood accumulates in the pleural cavity.

Hepatitis Inflammation of the liver with characteristic changes in the number of inflammatory cells; may be caused by viruses, autoimmune reactions, or substances such as alcohol.

Hepatocytes Cells in the liver that are involved in synthesis, detoxification, and storage functions.

Hepatomegaly An abnormally enlarged liver.

Hepatorenal syndrome (HRS) Progressive renal failure in a patient with cirrhosis in the setting of normal kidney histology.

Herd immunity Immunity that is occurs when a significant portion of a population is immunized, thus reducing the number of susceptible hosts enough to slow or halt the spread of an infectious agent.

Herniated/ruptured disc A condition in which the disc between two vertebrae ruptures, allowing the disc fluid to leak and impinge on the nerves.

Herpes labialis Herpes infection of the lips, also knowns as a "cold sore," caused by HSV-1

Herpes simplex virus (HSV) A sexually transmitted virus that causes painful sores around the mouth and genitals.

Herpes zoster (HZ) Chronic viral skin condition caused by varicella-zoster virus (VZV), the same virus that causes chickenpox; also called *shingles*

Heterozygous A genetic term used to describe a pair of genes that are present at corresponding loci of homologous chromosomes.

Hiatal hernia Herniation of the stomach through the hiatus of the diaphragm.

Hidradenitis suppurativa Painful, recurring, chronic inflammatory skin disease that involves the hair follicles in apocrine sweat glands in areas such as the axilla and groin; also called *acne inversa*.

High-density lipoproteins (HDLs) Complexes in the blood that clear cholesterol from the arteries and transport it to the liver for excretion.

Highly active antiretroviral therapy (HAART) The use of a combination of antiretroviral medications to suppress replication of HIV while simultaneously helping to prevent the occurrence of viral resistance to the medications.

Histamine An important mediator of both acute and chronic inflammation as well as hypersensitivity responses. It influences several functions of cells involved in regulating the immune response. Histamine is produced by mast cells and is stored in connective tissue near sites where injury is most likely to occur, such as the nose, blood vessels, and stomach lining.

HIV-associated lipodystrophy syndrome (HALS) A collection of morphologic and metabolic abnormalities associated with HIV, including insulin resistance, glucose intolerance, dyslipidemia, and fat redistribution.

Hodgkin lymphoma (HL) A form of lymphoma that is characterized by the presence of an abnormal form of lymphocytes known as *Reed-Sternberg cells*.

Homeostasis A conceptual model of a state of balance maintained by a coordinated regulation of body systems. Often includes the idea of a set point at which a response is required to return the body to a state of balance.

Homeostatic mechanism The physiologic processes that detect changes from a set baseline.

Homozygous Identical alleles for a given gene.

Honeymoon period A temporary period of endogenous insulin secretory recovery that follows overt development of T1D.

Hordeolum A tender, red, often pus-filled bump that develops along the edge of the eyelid; also called a *stye*.

Hospice A formal program that delivers palliative care, rather than curative treatment, to patients who are near the end of life.

Hospital-acquired pneumonia (HAP) A classification of pneumonia in which the infection (a) was not incubating at the time of hospital admission; and (b) develops 48 hours or more following after hospital admission.

Host An organism that harbors another organism.

Human immunodeficiency virus (HIV) A retrovirus that infects key cells in the immune system and induces defects in cellular and humoral immunity; the causative agent of AIDS.

Human papillomavirus (HPV) A sexually transmitted virus that causes genital warts.

Huntington disease (HD) An inherited progressive, incurable, neurodegenerative disease of the brain that causes uncontrolled, involuntary movements, dementia, and behavioral changes.

Hyaline An alteration within the cells or in the extracellular space.

Hyaluronan A polysaccharide found in the ECM that serves as a binding, lubrication, and protection agent.

Hydrocele A fluid-filled sac that surrounds a testicle, causing swelling.

Hydrocephalus An abnormal accumulation of cerebrospinal fluid within the ventricles of the brain resulting in increased pressure within the skull.

Hydronephrosis Dilation of the renal pelvis, usually a result from an obstruction in the urinary tract.

Hydrostatic pressure The pressure of fluids or to their properties when in equilibrium.

Hyperalgesia An exaggerated and prolonged perception of pain.

Hypercalcemia An abnormally high plasma concentration of calcium ions.

Hypercapnia Increase in arterial carbon dioxide levels.

Hyperchloremia An abnormally high plasma concentration of chloride ions.

Hyperchloremic metabolic acidosis Acidosis in which increased chloride levels cause metabolic acidosis when the chloride accumulates because it results in increased renal excretion of the base HCO_3^-.

Hyperglycemia High serum glucose level.

Hyperinflation Overexpansion of the lungs due to air trapping; often associated with obstructive respiratory disorders such as emphysema, asthma, and cystic fibrosis.

Hyperinsulinemia Increased insulin secretion relative to the plasma glucose.

Hyperkalemia An abnormally high plasma concentration of potassium ions.

Hyperkeratosis Abnormal increase in keratin causing thickening.

Hyperlipidemia An elevated level of lipids in the blood.

Hypermagnesemia An abnormally high plasma concentration of magnesium ions.

Hypernatremia An abnormally high plasma concentration of sodium ions.

Hyperopia A refractive error in which an eye has a short axial length, causing light to focus "behind" the retina; also called *farsightedness*.

Hyperphosphatemia An abnormally high plasma concentration of phosphate ions.

Hyperplasia An increase in the number of cells in an organ or tissue.

Hyperreactivity An exaggerated response to a stimulus.

Hypersensitivity reaction Disorders caused by inappropriate immune response.

Hypertension (HTN) A condition in which systolic blood pressure is higher than normal, which is less than 120/80 mmHg.

Hypertensive emergency (HTN-E) A condition that occurs when diastolic pressure exceeds 120 mmHg and there is evidence of target-organ damage.

Hypertensive nephropathy Chronic kidney disease resulting from long-standing hypertension.

Hypertensive urgency A condition in which the patient presents with severe hypertension but no evidence of organ damage.

Hyperthermia An unregulated temperature elevation involving dysfunctional thermoregulatory mechanisms; most frequently caused by exertional heat illness, exertional rhabdomyolysis (muscle cell destruction), malignant hyperthermia, or direct damage to thermoregulatory control centers in the brain.

Hyperthyroidism A group of disorders characterized by a greater than normal amount of thyroid hormones; also known as *thyrotoxicosis*.

Hypertonic Having a greater osmotic pressure than a reference solution that is ordinarily assumed to reflect blood plasma or interstitial fluid; fluid in which cells shrink.

Hypertrophic scar Scarring caused by excessive formation of new tissue in the healing of a wound.

Hypertrophy An increase in cell size that is coupled with an increase in the amount of functioning tissue mass.

Hyperventilation Increased alveolar ventilation in excess of carbon dioxide production as a result of an increased rate and/or depth of breathing.

Hypervolemia Fluid overload that occurs once the GFR falls below 10–15 mL/min, causing decreased renal excretion of sodium and water.

Hypnagogic hallucination A vivid image that occurs while one is falling asleep.

Hypnogram A summary of time spent in each stage of sleep; also called a *sleep histogram*.

Hypnopompic hallucination A vivid dreamlike hallucination that occurs on awakening.

Hypocalcemia An abnormally low plasma concentration of calcium ions.

Hypochloremia An abnormally low plasma concentration of chloride ions.

Hypochloremic metabolic alkalosis Chloride deficit contributing to alkalosis.

Hypochromia Condition in which red blood cells are pale in color because of a deficit of hemoglobin.

Hypocretin A neuropeptide hormone that is produced in the lateral and posterior hypothalamus and plays a key role in wakefulness and regulation of appetite. Also called *orexin*.

Hypodermis A layer of connective tissue between the dermis and underlying tissues and organs.

Hypoglycemia Low serum glucose level.

Hypokalemia An abnormally low plasma concentration of potassium ions.

Hypomagnesemia An abnormally low plasma concentration of magnesium ions.

Hypomania A less extreme form of mania that is not severe enough to markedly impair functioning or require hospitalization.

Hyponatremia An abnormally low plasma concentration of sodium ions in the blood.

Hypophosphatemia An abnormally low plasma concentration of phosphate ions.

Hypoplastic left heart syndrome (HHLS) A congenital heart condition in which the left side of the heart does not fully develop during gestation, including many or all of the left side structures such as the left ventricle, mitral valve, aortic valve, and ascending portion of the aorta.

Hypopnea A transient drop in the SO_2.

Hypospadias A congenital abnormality of the location of the male urethral meatus in which the urethral opening is on the ventral (underneath) surface of the penis.

Hypothermia A condition of mild to profound heat loss in which the body is unable to maintain the lower limits of the core temperature set point range that are required for metabolic, enzymatic, and other physiologic functions. A core body temperature below 36°C.

Hypothyroidism A group of disorders characterized by a less than normal amount of thyroid hormones.

Hypotonic Having a lesser degree of tension. A lesser osmotic pressure than a reference solution, which is ordinarily assumed to be blood plasma or interstitial fluid; more specifically refers to a fluid state in which cells would swell.

Hypoventilation Inadequate alveolar ventilation and ventilation-perfusion mismatches.

Hypovolemic shock Shock resulting from a loss of fluid volume associated with significant blood and/or extracellular fluid loss. Causes include trauma, ruptured ectopic pregnancy, excessive or protracted vomiting and diarrhea, and inadequate fluid intake.

Hypoxemia Decrease in arterial oxygen level.

Hypoxia Inadequate oxygenation of tissues.

Iatrogenic The etiology of conditions that are caused unintentionally by a treatment or diagnostic procedure or an error caused by a healthcare provider.

Iatrogenic hypothermia The inadvertent heat loss associated with anesthesia, convective air flow, or evaporation of solutions from the skin during treatments; also called *nosocomial hypothermia*.

Icteric sclera Yellow coloration of the sclera of the eye.

Icterus Yellowing of the sclerae of the eyes.

Ideal cardiovascular health The American Heart Association's term for the absence of cardiovascular disease with the presence of ideal levels, rather than poor or intermediate levels, of seven graded key health indicators called "Life's Simple 7."

Idiopathic Any disease or condition for which the etiology cannot be determined.

Idiopathic interstitial pneumonia A classification of interstitial lung disease that includes all related disorders for which no cause has been identified, such as idiopathic pulmonary fibrosis.

Idiopathic pulmonary fibrosis A respiratory disease of unknown cause in which pulmonary tissue becomes stiff and noncompliant, leading to decreased oxygenation and decreased perfusion of lungs.

Illness The presence of a disease or other disruption of normative function.

Immune response The coordinated and collective response of the immune system's cells and molecules in the body. This is how the body recognizes and defends against bacteria and viruses along with both foreign and harmful substances.

Immunity Protection from infectious disease.

Immunodeficiency A weakened immune response as a result of a defect in one or more components of the immune system.

Immunoglobin A nephropathy (IgAN) Mesangial deposition of IgA in the glomerulus, and crescents are seen in some of the glomeruli.

Immunologically ignorant A form of self-tolerance in which reactive lymphocytes and their target antigen are both detectable in an individual, yet no autoimmune attack occurs.

Impaired fasting glucose (IFG) A condition in which the fasting blood glucose level or hemoglobin A1C is higher than normal but not diagnostic of DM.

Impaired glucose tolerance (IGT) A condition in which the blood glucose level 2 hours after an oral glucose load is higher than normal but is not diagnostic of DM.

Impetigo A highly contagious superficial skin infection that is initially seen as red pimples and fluid-filled blisters, and later changes to yellow crusted lesion.

Impingement syndrome An injury in which tendons of the shoulder muscles are trapped under the acromion.

Inadvertent hypothermia Unintended heat loss that occurs in homes or institutional settings and often involving vulnerable infants, ill individuals, or those with impaired thermoregulation.

Incidence The number of new cases of a disease or condition that occur during a specified period of time in a population that is at risk for developing the disease or condition.

Increased pulmonary blood flow defects The most common category of CCHD and includes four different types of defects, all of which increase the blood flow to the pulmonary system.

Incubation period The elapsed time between exposure to an infectious agent and the appearance of signs or symptoms of illness or disease.

Industrial hygiene The science related to anticipating, recognizing, controlling, and evaluating hazards that arise in or from the workplace that may affect the health and well-being of workers and members of the community.

Infantile hypertrophic pyloric stenosis (IHPS) A condition that frequently affects young infants and is characterized by hypertrophy of the pylorus muscles leading to eventual gastric outlet obstruction.

Infant respiratory distress syndrome (IRDS) Disorder that occurs in premature newborns whose lungs have not fully developed and therefore have a deficiency of surfactant due to either the immature lung's inability to produce enough surfactant or a genetic mutation of the SP-B surfactant protein; also called *neonatal respiratory distress syndrome.*

Infarction Complete obstruction of a blood vessel.

Infectious disease A disorder caused by invasion of a host organism by a pathogen.

Infertility The inability to achieve clinical pregnancy after 12 or more months of regular unprotected sexual intercourse.

Inflammasome Complex proteins that promote the production of pro-inflammatory cytokines such as IL-1 β, IL-18, and IL-33.

Inflammation The immune response of tissues to bodily injury (e.g., trauma, heat, radiation, chemicals) or foreign substances such as infectious agents or allergic antigens. Inflammation may be acute or chronic.

Inflammatory bowel disease (IBD) A chronic inflammatory disorder of the gastrointestinal tract.

Influenza A highly contagious viral infection that sweeps through a geographic region as an epidemic that lasts 6 to 8 weeks during the winter months.

Initiation The first step in the carcinogenesis model in which irreversible changes occur in the genotype of the cell, resulting in malignancy.

Injury Damage caused to the body by an external force.

Innate (natural) immune system A system of antigen-nonspecific defense mechanisms that respond quickly after exposure to an infectious agent; this is the immunity one is born with and is the initial response by the body to prevent infection.

Innate immunity Innate immunity occurs naturally and is the body's first line of defense against an injury or foreign substance.

Insomnia The inability to fall sleep or to remain asleep throughout the night.

Insulin resistance The inability of insulin to achieve its expected biological response as the cells fail to respond to the normal actions of insulin.

Integrase An enzyme that facilitates integration of viral DNA into the nuclear DNA of a host cell.

Integrins Receptors in the ECM that facilitate cell-to-cell communication.

Intercostal retraction Retraction of muscles between the ribs when breathing.

Intervertebral disc degeneration A health problem caused by drying out or degeneration of the pads between the vertebrae.

Intracellular fluid (ICF) The fluid found in the cells of the body; accounts for about two thirds of total body fluid.

Intracranial pressure (ICP) The pressure exerted by the contents of the cranium: brain tissue, blood, and cerebrospinal fluid.

Intractable seizure Seizure activity that is resistant to pharmacologic treatment.

Intrinsic AKI Acute kidney injury affecting one or several renal anatomic structures: glomeruli, tubules, interstitium, and blood vessels.

Introns Noncoding sequences in genes.

Ionizing radiation Radiation that has enough energy to eject electrons that are tightly bound to atoms, producing positively and negatively charged ions.

Iron Nutrient necessary for the formation of hemoglobin.

Iron deficiency anemia Anemia that occurs when blood lacks adequate healthy red blood cells owing to a lack of iron.

Irritable bowel syndrome (IBS) A disorder of motility causing abdominal discomfort and altered bowel habits.

Ischemia A restriction of blood supply in the tissues that causes a shortage of oxygen and glucose needed for cellular metabolism.

Ischemic ATN Prerenal hypoperfusion resulting in endothelial and epithelial cell injury, intratubular obstruction, and an inflammatory response.

Ischemic stroke A stroke that develops as a result of ischemia damage.

Isotonic Property of solutions in which the concentration of sodium in fluid is equally to the concentration of sodium in the cell; results in a situation in which cells neither swell nor shrink.

Jaundice A yellowish discoloration of the whites of the eyes, skin, or mucous membranes caused by the bile salts in the tissues.

Jefferson fracture A fracture of all four rings of C1 that results from axial loading onto the spinal column.

Jet lag A temporary mismatch between the person's circadian rhythm and local time caused by rapid travel across several time zones.

Juvenile dermatomyositis (JDM) An inflammatory disease that causes muscle weakness and a skin rash on the eyelids and knuckles.

Juvenile idiopathic arthritis (JIA) A chronic inflammatory juvenile autoimmune disorder.

Kaposi sarcoma (KS) The most common AIDS-associated malignancy; caused by human herpesvirus 8, this disorder most commonly produces skin tumors but may also produces tumors in the oral cavity, gut, lymph nodes, brain, and visceral organs.

Karnofsky Performance Status Scale A tool that allows patients to be classified according to their functional impairment and can be used to compare effectiveness of different therapies and to assess the prognosis in individual patients.

Karyotyping A test used to examine the visual appearance of chromosome structure and number.

Keloid An overgrowth of collagenous scar tissue at the site of a skin injury, particularly a wound or surgical incision.

Keratinization A process by which epithelial cells lose their moisture and are replaced by horny tissue.

Keratinocyte An epidermal cell that synthesizes keratin.

Ketogenesis The production of ketones, which are important sources of energy for peripheral tissues such as muscle.

Ketonemia The presence of ketone bodies in the blood.

Ketonuria The presence of ketone bodies in the urine.

Kinins Proteins in the blood that promote inflammation. They increase blood flow, promote repair of damaged tissue, stimulate pain receptors, and enhance the ability of fluids to pass through small vessels.

Kussmaul respirations Deep labored breathing often associated with diabetic ketoacidosis.

Kyphoscoliosis A combination of outward and lateral spine curves.

Kyphosis A convex spinal column.

Laceration A cut or tear in skin tissue, usually extending deeper than the superficial layer of the skin.

Laminectomy Removal of the lamina.

Laminin A glycoprotein in the basement membrane that provides adhesion of cells above and below it.

Laminotomy Partial removal of the lamina.

Latent viral state A condition in which a virus is not eliminated from the body but remains present in an inactive form that, under certain conditions, can be reactivated and cause illness.

Lead A heavy metal that occurs naturally as part of the earth's crust and can be toxic to most organs.

Left-sided heart failure A condition in which the left side of the heart is unable to pump enough blood to meet the needs of the body.

Leg ulcers Sores on the skin caused by chronic venous insufficiency that persist for more than 6 weeks.

Leiomyomas Benign tumors, also known as uterine fibroids, that develop from an overgrowth of smooth muscle and connective tissue in the uterus.

Lentiviruses A family of viruses that infect cells of the immune system and cause immunodeficiency; includes HIV.

Lethal triad of trauma The developing of hypothermia, acidosis, and coagulopathy resulting from traumatic injury.

Leukemia A hematologic malignancy originating in the bone marrow or blood.

Leukocyte A white blood cell.

Leukocytosis An increase in circulating white blood count above normal range.

Leukotrienes A type of eicosanoid mediators produced by leukocytes and usually accompanied by the production of histamine and prostaglandin. One of their major roles is triggering contraction of the smooth muscle lining of the bronchioles, which is associated with asthma.

Levoconvex Curvature of the spine to the left.

Lewisite A vesicant or blister chemical weapon that causes a chemical burn. Symptoms of exposure typically occur immediately on contact.

Lichenification Thick, leathery skin; result of constant scratching

Lichen planus (LP) An inflammatory skin lesion that is pruritic and has an unknown cause.

Life-threatening injury An injury that is likely to result in death, permanent disfigurement, or permanent loss of function or impairment of function to a body part or mental ability.

Lipemia Excess lipids in the blood.

Lipofuscin A granular yellow-brown pigment composed of lipidcontaining residues of lysosomal digestion.

Lipolysis The process through which triglycerides are hydrolyzed to fatty acids and glycerol.

Lipoma Common, benign lumps that grow under normal skin in subcutaneous tissues

Livor mortis The purple-red discoloration that occurs after death when the heart is no longer pumping blood throughout the body and so blood settles in dependent parts of the body.

Long terminal repeats (LTRs) Control centers for gene expression; structures that contain binding sites for viral proteins that regulate replication.

Lordosis A concave spinal column.

Loss of heterozygosity A common event in the development of inherited cancer that occurs with loss of the somatic wild-type allele.

Low-density lipoproteins (LDLs) Lipoproteins that are the primary carriers of cholesterol.

Lower back pain A common health problem that causes stiffness, mobility changes, and possible long-term health problems.

Lymphoma A hematologic malignancy originating in the lymphatic tissues.

Macrocytic Form of anemia characterized by large erythrocytes, defined as greater than 100 fL.

Macrovascular disease Disease of large vasculature; diabetic macrovascular disease includes coronary artery disease, peripheral arterial disease, and stroke.

Macular degeneration A condition in with the macula (the central part of the retina) degenerates resulting in distortion or loss of central vision; also called *age-related macular degeneration*.

Major depressive disorder (MDD) A clinical syndrome involving alterations in mood and characterized by the presence of one or more depressive episodes in an individual's lifetime.

Major depressive episode A clinical syndrome involving a depressed mood (anhedonia) that lasts for 2 weeks in addition to other symptoms.

Major histocompatibility complex (MHC) proteins Cell surface peptide-presenting proteins that allow natural killer cells to distinguish normal cells from target cells.

Malignant Aberrant, uncontrolled invasive cell growth with the potential to become life threatening.

Malignant hyperthermia A rare genetic condition associated with uncontrolled heat production caused by a mutation in a type of ryanodine receptor that causes intracellular Ca^{2+} release channels in skeletal muscle to react when a susceptible individual receives inhalation anesthetics or depolarizing muscle relaxants.

Mallory bodies Damaged filaments found in the liver, most commonly associated with alcoholic liver disease.

Malunion A bone fracture in which the bone fragments join in a position that is not anatomically correct.

Mania A mood state characterized by an abnormal and persistently elevated, expansive, or irritable mood and increased energy (or activity) present for most of the time, nearly every day, or a week or more.

Marfan syndrome A genetic disorder in which a mutation in a connective tissue gene causes pathogenic skeletal, ocular, and cardiac features.

Marijuana The dried leaves, flowers, stems, and seeds of the hemp plant. The plant contains the mind-altering chemical delta-9-tetrahydrocannabinol (THC) and related compounds. Extracts with high amounts of THC can also be made from the cannabis plant.

Mastitis Inflammation and infection of breast tissue, typically due to bacterial infection from a break in the skin or nipple or a blocked mild duct.

Maturity-onset diabetes of the young (MODY) DM that first occurs in children or adolescents and is characterized by mild hyperglycemia.

Mean arterial pressure (MAP) Pressure within the cardiovascular system.

Mean corpuscular hemoglobin (MCH) Measurement of the average concentration of hemoglobin in red blood cells.

Mean corpuscular volume (MCV) Measurement of the average red blood cell size; a standard measurement that aids in the classification of anemia.

Megakaryocytopoiesis The production of thrombocytes by the megakaryocyte; also referred to as *thrombopoiesis*.

Meiosis A cell division process that produces four haploid daughter cells (egg and sperm) needed for reproduction.

Melanin A nonhemoglobin brown-black pigment synthesized in melanocytes.

Melanocyte A cell that produces the dark pigment melanin.

Melanoma Most dangerous of the skin cancers, which originates in sun-damaged melanocytes in the basal epidermis and may develop from moles.

Melatonin peptide hormone produced in pineal gland in response to darkness which sets circadian rhythm.

Melena Black, tarry stool.

Membranous glomerulonephritis A glomerular disorder in which the podocytes of the glomerular basement membrane (GBM) become damaged from an antigen–antibody complex and proteinuria ensues; usually idiopathic but can be secondary; also called *membranous nephropathy*.

Ménière disease An inner ear disorder that manifests in both auditory and vestibular symptoms.

Mesolimbic pathway A group of dopamine-containing neurons that have their cell bodies in the midbrain and their terminal in the forebrain on various structures associated with the limbic system; believed to be important for many types of behavioral reinforcement.

Messenger RNA (mRNA) The template for protein synthesis.

Metabolic acidosis A state of H^+ excess, bicarbonate deficit, and decreased blood pH, and a decreased ratio of bicarbonate to carbonic acid below 20:1 caused by accumulation of nonvolatile (fixed) acids or excessive loss of the base bicarbonate.

Metabolic alkalosis A state of H^+ deficit, bicarbonate excess, increased blood pH, and an increased ratio of bicarbonate to carbonic acid above 20:1 caused by excessive loss of nonvolatile (fixed) acids or excessive accumulation of the base HCO_3^-.

Metabolic equivalent of task (MET) The ratio of metabolic rate (rate of energy consumption) during a specific physical activity to a reference rate of metabolic rate at rest.

Metabolic syndrome A cluster of risk factors occurring together that increase the risk for cardiovascular disease.

Metaplasia A reversible change in which one adult cell type, such as the epithelial or mesenchymal, is replaced by another.

Metastasize To spread from a primary site to another part of the body.

Microcytic Form of anemia characterized by small erythrocytes, defined as less than 80 fL.

microRNAs Very small pieces of noncoding RNA that control gene expression in many cellular processes.

Microvascular disease Disease of smaller vasculature; diabetic microvascular disease includes diabetic nephropathy, neuropathy, and retinopathy.

Middle ear effusion Serous or mucoid fluid found in the middle ear in acute otitis media.

Migraine headache A pulsatile, unilateral headache that is frequently accompanied by nausea, vomiting, photophobia, and phonophobia; can be preceded by a visual or sensory aura.

Missense mutation A point mutation resulting in a change in amino acid sequence, which often results in production of an abnormal protein.

Mitochondrial DNA (mtDNA) DNA located in the mitochondria, organelles in eukaryotic cells that convert chemical energy from food into adenosine triphosphate (ATP).

Mitochondrial dysfunction Damage to the mitochondria of the cell that causes damage that leads to abnormal functioning.

Mitosis The process of cell division used to create identical copies of a cell.

Mixed acid–base imbalance Two or more types of acid–base imbalance present in an individual at the same time.

Mixed blood flow defects Congenital heart defects in which oxygenated and deoxygenated blood become mixed because of the structural defect, resulting in either increased or decreased pulmonary blood flow or obstructed systemic flow.

Mixed hearing loss Hearing loss that has both conductive and sensorineural components.

Mode of transmission The way in which microorganisms are transferred from their source to a host.

Modifiable risk factor A risk factor that the individual can change, such as diet or smoking.

Modulation The process by which peripheral and central neurotransmitters and other substances enhance or dampen the transduction and transmission of a noxious stimulus.

Moles Altered melanocytes that proliferate and grow in clusters; they are usually benign, but may change into cancer; also called *nevi*.

Monogenic Involving a single gene.

Monro-Kellie hypothesis The hypothesis that the total volume of intracranial contents (the brain mass, intracerebral spinal fluid, and blood volume) remains constant.

Morbidity A departure from physiologic or psychologic well-being, encompassing disease, injury, and disability.

Mortality The number of deaths in a given population.

Mosaicism The presence of more than one genetic cell line in a person.

Multiple myeloma A cancerous condition involving active B cells referred to as plasma cells that accumulate in multiple locations.

Multiple organ dysfunction syndrome (MODS) A condition characterized by progressive organ dysfunction of two or more organ systems.

Multiple sclerosis (MS) A chronic, inflammatory, demyelinating and axonal degenerative disorder of the CNS in which disease progression ranges from benign and relatively stable to devastating with rapid deterioration and early death.

Mustard gas A vesicant or blister chemical weapon that causes a burn. Symptoms of exposure typically are delayed for several hours.

Mutation A permanent alteration in the DNA sequence of a gene that adversely affects gene function.

Mutator genes DNA repair genes.

Mutualism A relationship between a host and one or more organisms in which both the microorganisms and the host derive benefits from one another.

Mycobacteria A category of bacteria called acid-fast bacteria because they cannot be decolorized easily with acid solutions.

Myocardial contusion Bruising of the myocardium.

Myocardial infarction (MI) The formation of an area of necrosis (tissue death) related to obstructed blood flow to the myocardium commonly caused by a thrombus; also known as a *heart attack*.

Myocardial ischemia Restriction of blood supply to heart muscles tissues causing a shortage of oxygen and nutrients needed for cellular function and survival.

Myofascial pain syndrome A regional pain syndrome characterized by discrete trigger points of localized areas of deep muscle tenderness or hyperirritability and a pattern of referred pain that may be localized or remote from the trigger point.

Myopia A refractive error that is caused by an eye that has a long axial length; also called *nearsightedness*.

N1 Stage 1 of nonrapid eye movement sleep, characterized by low-amplitude mixed-frequency EEG activity and slow rolling movements of the eyeballs.

N2 Stage 2 of nonrapid eye movement sleep, characterized on EEG by sleep spindles and K complexes; also called *light sleep*.

N3 Stage 3 of nonrapid eye movement sleep, called *deep sleep* or *slow wave sleep* because of the delta wave forms on EEG of this stage.

Naloxone An opioid antagonist designed to rapidly reverse opioid overdose.

Narcolepsy A syndrome characterized by sudden sleep attacks, cataplexy, sleep paralysis, and visual or auditory hallucinations at the onset of sleep.

Natural immunity Resistance to infectious disease that results from exposure to a pathogen and subsequent formation of immune memory cells that are capable of responding readily to this specific infectious agent on reexposure to the same agent.

Nausea An unpleasant sensation that can precede vomiting and is often described by patients as feeling "sick to my stomach" or "queasy."

Necrosis Cell death caused by injury in an organ or tissue that is still part of a living organism.

Necrotizing fasciitis (NF) A rare but serious infection of the subcutaneous tissue and fascia that is rapidly progressive and destructive.

Neonatal diabetes mellitus (NDM) DM that first occurs in newborns and young infants.

Neoplasia The process of abnormal growth of cells.

Neoplasm An abnormal growth of cells; also called a *tumor*.

Nephritic syndrome Glomerular disease characterized by hematuria, mild proteinuria, RBC casts, and even the presence of dysmorphic RBCs.

Nephrolithiasis The formation of urinary crystals into larger stones; also known as *renal calculi* or *kidney stones*.

Nephropathy Damage to the kidneys; diabetic nephropathy is kidney damage caused by diabetes.

Nephrotic syndrome Glomerular disease characterized by severe proteinuria, hyperlipidemia, hypoalbuminemia, edema, and urinary fatty casts but usually no RBCs or RBC casts.

Nephrotoxic ATN Direct toxic damage to the renal tubules, usually from medications such as nonsteroidal anti-inflammatory drugs and antibiotics.

Nerve agents A group of chemicals, originally designed as insecticides, that block the action of acetylcholinesterase, leading to the cholinergic syndrome.

Neuralgia Pain that follows the distribution of a nerve.

Neuritis Inflammation of a nerve.

Neurocognitive disorders (NCDs) Disorders whose primary features are cognitive impairments.

Neurodegeneration Progressive damage and death of neurons that can cause neurologic dysfunction such as cognitive, motor, and sensory disturbances.

Neurodevelopmental disorders Impairments of brain function that occur as the brain develops and usually manifest before a child enters kindergarten.

Neurofibromatosis An autosomal dominant genetic condition that causes progressive neurocutaneous lesions.

Neurogenic shock Shock resulting from a loss of vascular tone; associated with a disruption of sympathetic function often as a result of injury or damage to the central nervous system.

Neuroleptic malignant syndrome A relatively rare and potentially lethal response to neuroleptic drugs. No laboratory tests can specifically diagnose the disorder. However, when cardinal signs of severe muscular rigidity, elevated body temperature above 38°C, autonomic instability, and cognitive changes occur with the start of neuroleptic therapy, the disorder is suspected. Fever, muscle rigidity, and neurologic changes may progress to rhabdomyolysis and death.

Neuropathic pain Pain caused by dysfunction of the peripheral or central nervous system.

Neuropathy Damage to nerves; diabetic neuropathy is nerve damage caused by *diabetes mellitus*.

Neurotoxins Natural or artificial substances that destroy all or part of a neuron.

Neurotransmitter Chemicals that are released from neurons at the presynaptic nerve and cross the synapse, where they join with receptors to initiate an electrical event, such as depolarization (i.e., excitatory postsynaptic potentials) or hyperpolarization (i.e., inhibitory postsynaptic potentials).

Nevi Altered melanocytes that proliferate and grow in clusters; they are usually benign, but may change into cancer; also called *moles*

Night terrors A form of dissociated sleep, usually in children, in which there are episodes of abrupt awakening from sleep with signs of panic and anxiety; also known as *sleep terrors*.

Nociceptive pain Pain caused by activation of nociceptive afferent fibers secondary to tissue trauma or inflammation.

Nociceptive-specific (NS) neuron A second-order neuron with a small receptive field that responds only to nociceptive stimuli.

Nociceptors Sensory receptors at the free endings of peripheral nerves, specifically Aß and C fibers, that are sensitive to noxious stimuli.

Nocturia Frequent urination at night in response to polyuria.

Nocturnal enuresis The involuntary loss of urine while sleeping.

Noise-induced hearing loss (NIHL) Hearing loss that results either from prolonged exposure to a high-intensity noise, such as a jackhammer or leafblower, or from a single exposure to a brief but intense impulse sound, such as a gunshot close to the ear or a fireworks explosion.

Nonalcoholic fatty liver disease (NAFLD) A spectrum of liver diseases ranging from simple steatosis to nonalcoholic steatohepatitis; the most common chronic liver disease worldwide. One of a group of liver abnormalities associated with obesity.

Nonalcoholic steatohepatitis A cause of fatty liver, characterized by accumulation of fat in the liver and not associated with alcohol use.

Nonatherosclerotic peripheral arterial disease (NAPAD) A disorder in which blood flow is decreased for reasons other than plaque buildup.

Non-Hodgkin lymphomas (NHLs) A collection of varied cancers leading to lymphoma characterized by overproduction of B cells, T cells, or natural killer cells.

Nonionizing radiation Radiation that has enough energy to cause atoms to vibrate but not enough to eject electrons.

Nonmodifiable risk factor A risk factor that an individual cannot change, such as age, race, and genetic variables.

Nonnociceptive pain Pain that results from nerve cell dysfunction in the peripheral nervous system and/or the central nervous system.

Nonoliguric Maintenance of urine output, urine output greater than 400 milliliters in 24 hours.

Nonproliferative diabetic retinopathy Damage to the retina that occurs when blood glucose levels are elevated for a prolonged period in an individual with diabetes.

Non–rapid eye movement sleep (NREM sleep) Periods of sleep in which the eyeballs move either very slowly or not at all; the majority of sleep time and with distinctive characteristics on the EEG.

Nonsense mutation A point mutation that causes a premature stop codon, resulting in a truncated protein product.

Non–ST-segment elevation acute coronary syndrome (NSTE-ACS) A term that encompasses non–ST-segment elevation myocardial infarction and unstable angina as a condition characterized by the clinical signs and symptoms of myocardial ischemia in the absence of ST-segment elevation on electrocardiogram.

Non–ST-segment elevation myocardial infarction (NSTEMI) A condition characterized by the clinical signs and symptoms of myocardial ischemia in the absence of ST-segment elevation on electrocardiogram but the presence of elevated biomarkers of necrosis.

Nonsyndromic genetic hearing loss Hearing loss that results from a specific genetic alteration that causes hearing loss only, with no other physical changes in the individual.

Nonunion A bone fracture that shows no sign of healing for at least 3 months.

Nonvolatile acid Acids that are not gases and therefore cannot be eliminated by the lungs and are eliminated mainly by the kidneys; also called *fixed acids*.

Norepinephrine (NE) A catecholamine with multiple roles, including those as a hormone and neurotransmitter; it is secreted in the central nervous system, at the nerve endings of the sympathetic nervous system, and by the adrenal gland. It is the hormone and neurotransmitter that is most responsible for vigilant concentration and is considered important for regulating waking and appetite.

Normochromic Term used to describe red blood cells that are normal in color.

Normocytic Term used to describe red blood cells that are normal in size.

Normothermia The usual range of core body temperature, which is between 36°C and 38.5°C for adults.

Nucleotide The building block of DNA consisting of a phosphate, a deoxyribose, and one of four nitrogenous bases (adenine, guanine, cytosine, or thymine).

Nystagmus A rapid, involuntary eye movement.

Obesity Abnormal or excessive fat accumulation.

Obligate intracellular parasite A microorganism that can replicate only inside a host cell.

Obstructed systemic blood flow defects A type of congenital heart disorder in which pulmonary blood flow is obstructed, resulting in little or no blood reaching the lungs to get oxygenated.

Obstructive shock Shock resulting from obstruction of major blood vessels or obstruction of the cardiac pumping action. Causes include cardiac tamponade and pulmonary embolism.

Obstructive sleep apnea (OSA) A type of sleep apnea involving physical obstruction in the upper airways that decreases or prevents air flow to the lungs.

Occult blood/bleeding Blood or bleeding that is not detected by visualization.

Odynophagia Pain caused by swallowing.

Oliguria Urine output less than 400 milliliters in 24 hours.

Oncogene A gene that may become cancer causing as a result of a permanent gene alteration (mutation).

Oogenesis The process of making egg cells.

Open-angle glaucoma The most commonly diagnosed form of glaucoma, in which the trabecular meshwork channels are open but the aqueous humor does not drain fast enough.

Open pneumothorax A condition that occurs when penetrating trauma to the outer chest wall causes a temporary invasion of the pleural space.

Ophthalmopathy Eye changes seen in patients with Graves disease, including lid lag and retraction, periorbital edema, exophthalmos, diplopia, corneal involvement, and visual loss.

Opioid use disorder A chronic, relapsing illness of a pattern of opioid use that is associated with negative health consequences.

Opportunistic infection (OI) An infection that occurs with increased frequency or greater severity as a result of the host's weakened or compromised immune response.

Opportunistic pathogens A microorganisms that use the opportunity to infect a host that has weakened defense mechanisms, such as an individual with AIDS, a transplant recipient, an individual with an autoimmune disease, or one who is on immunosuppressive therapy.

Opsonization The process by which a pathogen is marked by complement proteins for ingestion and destruction by phagocytic cells.

Orchiectomy Surgical removal of a testicle.

Orchitis Inflammation of one or both testicles.

Orexigenic Appetite-stimulating.

Orgasmic dysfunction The inability of an individual to reach orgasm during sexual stimulation.

Osmolality Osmotic concentration; number of osmoles of a solute per kilogram of solvent (water); molecules per weight of water; measures the number of milliosmoles per kilogram (mOsm/kg) of water.

Osmosis The net movement of water through a selectively permeable membrane (impermeable to one or more of the solutes) separating two aqueous solutions with different concentrations.

Osseointegrated hearing implants Assistive devices that are surgically implanted and use bone conduction of sound to stimulate the inner ear, thus bypassing the conductive component of the hearing loss caused by otosclerosis.

Osteoarthritis (OA) The most common form of arthritis, affecting 50% of the world's population age 65 years and older; it develops as wear and tear on the joints break down the cartilage in the joint, causing bone to rub on bone.

Osteocalcin level A blood test that measures osteoclastic activity.

Osteolysis Bone breakdown.

Osteomalacia Softening of the bones.

Osteomyelitis Bone infection.

Osteonecrosis A disease caused by reduced blood flow to joints, causing the bones within the joint to die and break down.

Osteopenia Decreased bone density.

Osteoporosis Low bone density caused by low intake of nutrients for bone growth or increased bone resorption.

Otitis media (OM) An inflammation of the middle ear space often associated with Eustachian tube dysfunction.

Otosclerosis Abnormal bone growth in the middle ear space.

Ototoxic Medications that can damage the sensory cells of the inner ear.

Ovarian cancer A form of cancer that originates in the ovaries.

Oxidative stress An imbalance between the production of reactive oxygen species and the ability of the body to counteract, or detoxify, their harmful effects through neutralization by antioxidants.

Paget disease A disease that causes bones to overgrow and become weak.

Pain An unpleasant sensory and emotional experience associated with actual or potential tissue damage or described in terms of such damage.

Pain threshold The lowest level of pain that a patient can recognize.

Pain tolerance The greatest level of pain that a patient can tolerate.

Palliative care Care provided to patients experiencing life-threatening, progressive illness that focuses on providing effective relief of symptoms with attention to physiologic, psychosocial, and spiritual needs.

Palliative sedation Defined by the American Academy of Hospice and Palliative Medicine as "the intentional lowering of awareness towards, and including, unconsciousness for patients with severe and refractory symptoms."

Pancreatic cysts Small, fluid-filled sacs in the pancreas.

Pancytopenia A reduction in the three cell populations that are produced in the bone marrow: erythrocytes, leukocytes, and thrombocytes.

Pandemic A widespread outbreak of an infectious disease that affects a region, a continent, or the world; represents expansion of an epidemic.

Panic breathing A fast, shallow, ineffective breathing pattern that results when the person has the sensation of air hunger.

Panic disorder A condition characterized by sudden episodes of intense fear that often results in increased sympathetic function.

Pannus Overgrowth of synovial membrane.

Paraneoplastic syndromes A rare and benign group of symptoms associated with an altered immune system that accompanies, but is not due to, a malignancy.

Paraphimosis A condition found in uncircumcised or partially circumcised males in which the retracted foreskin is trapped behind the coronal sulcus.

Parasomnia Abnormal behaviors during sleep, such as movement, sensations, or autonomic activity.

Paresthesia A sensation or feeling of tingling, tickling, pricking, or burning without a physical cause. The tingling, prickling, burning, or "pins and needles" sensation felt after a limb "goes to sleep"

Parkinson disease (PD) An idiopathic, chronic, progressive and degenerative disorder of the central nervous system with classic motor symptoms of tremors, bradykinesia, rigidity, and postural instability.

Parkinsonism A symptom complex including tremors, bradykinesia, rigidity, and postural instability that is found in patients with Parkinson disease and other disorders of motor function.

Paroxysmal nocturnal dyspnea Sudden shortness of breath while sleeping.

Partial seizure Seizure activity that occurs when abnormal electrical activity is contained within a limited area of the brain; also known as *focal seizure*.

Partial thickness burn injury Classified as either superficial or deep, depending on the depth of damage to the epidermis or dermis.

Partial thickness wound A wound in which the epidermis and all or a portion the dermis remain intact.

Passive immunity The provision of temporary protection from an infectious agent by the administration of exogenous antibody to a recipient.

Patent ductus arteriosus (PDA) A congenital heart defect in which the connection present in utero allows blood to bypass the lungs after right ventricular ejection; because of high pulmonary pressures the connection remains open and continues to shunt blood to the aorta.

Pathogen Microorganism that harms the host or produces disease.

Pathogen-associated molecular pattern Structures within antigens that are recognized by the innate immune system.

Pathogenesis The sequence of events in response to one or more etiologic agents involving structural and/or functional alterations in cells, tissues, or organs that result in disease.

Pathology A medical discipline focused on structural alterations in tissues and organs.

Pathophysiology The study of functional alterations that occur at the molecular, cellular, tissue, and organ system levels that are involved in disease states.

Pattern-recognition receptors Receptors present on host defense cells, such as phagocytic and dendritic cells, that recognize pathogen-associated molecular patterns and mediate an instant response against the invading microorganism.

Pectus carinatum A congenital disorder that causes a convex appearance to the anterior chest wall; also called *pigeon chest*.

Pectus excavatum A congenital disorder that causes a concave appearance of the anterior chest wall; also known as a *sunken chest* or *funnel chest*.

Pediculosis An infestation of the skin or hair by lice.

Pediculosis pubis An ectoparasite that is spread through sexual contact, sharing of undergarments, or living in very close quarters with many other individuals, especially in unsanitary conditions; also known as *Pthirus pubis*, louse (singular) or lice (plural), or the street term "crabs."

Pedigree A graph of several generations of a family that allows the pattern of genetic diseases to be visualized.

Pelvic inflammatory disease An infection of a woman's reproductive organs, including the ovaries, fallopian tubes, uterus, and cervix, often caused by chlamydia.

Pelvic organ prolapse The abnormal descent or herniation of the pelvic organs from the normal attachment sites or positions in the pelvis.

Penetrance The proportion of individuals who inherit a mutation that will have clinical symptoms.

Peptic ulcer disease (PUD) A condition of chronic erosion, destruction, and ulceration of the lining of the stomach and duodenum.

Perception The cognitive appreciation of a noxious stimulus; involves the somatosensory cortex and limbic structures and includes the subjective, sensory, and emotional aspects of pain.

Pericarditis Swelling and inflammation of the pericardium, the thin double-layered sac surrounding the heart, often causing chest pain as irritated layers rub against one another.

Perilymph Fluid that is very high in sodium and very similar to cerebrospinal fluid that fills the canals within the cochlea.

Peripheral artery disease (PAD) A category of circulation disorders that occur when pathologic changes (arteriosclerosis and atherosclerosis) impair blood supply to peripheral arteries.

Peripheral neuropathy Constant or intermittent burning, aching, or lancinating limb pain due to lesions or dysfunction of peripheral nerves.

Peripheral tolerance The mechanisms that take place outside the primary lymphoid tissues to prevent lymphocytes from initiating potentially dangerous immune responses against the body's own tissues or against other harmless materials such as food or commensal organisms.

Peripheral vascular disease (PVD) A category of circulation disorders that occur when pathologic changes impair blood supply to peripheral arteries or veins.

Peritoneal bleed Bleeding from ruptured vessels and organs into the abdominal region.

Peritoneal dialysis Removal of fluid and solutes from blood across the peritoneum.

Permanent threshold shift (PTS) A condition where hearing fails to recover completely between exposures to noise and then does not recover at all.

Persistent depressive disorder A condition characterized by a depressed mood (feeling sad or down) that occurs on more days than not and occurs for most of the day; also called *dysthymia*.

Persistent postsurgical pain (PPSP) Pain that persists more for than 2 months after a surgical procedure that cannot be attributed to other causes.

Pertussis A highly contagious respiratory infections usually caused by *Bordetella pertussis* which has been controlled in children with through pertussis vaccination; also known as *whooping cough*.

Peyronie disease A disorder of the penis that is caused by fibrous plaque that affects the tunica albuginea and causes the penis to curve.

pH The negative logarithm or power (the *p* in "pH") to which the number 10 must be raised in order to equal the concentration of H^+ (the *H* in "pH") in mEq/L/liter.

Phantom limb pain (PLP) Pain that is perceived to be coming from a surgically removed limb or body part.

Pharmacogenomics The study of how genetic variants affect an individual's responses to medications.

Phenotype The clinical expression of the genotype.

Pheochromocytoma A catecholamine-secreting tumor that may precipitate life-threatening hypertension.

Phimosis A condition in which the foreskin of the penis cannot be retracted over the glans penis.

Phosgene A chemical commonly used in industry that can be used as a chemical weapon; its primary effect is on the pulmonary system.

Phosphorus A naturally occurring element in the human body that plays a role in bone formation.

Photodermatitis Immune response to UV rays causing skin reactions that differ depending on the person's skin type and other factors that make the skin more sensitive

Phototherapy Exposing skin to ultraviolet light on a regular basis for medical purposes

Physical dependence The presence of a consistent set of symptoms when a drug is stopped. These withdrawal symptoms imply that homeostatic mechanisms of the body had made adjustments to counteract the drug's effect.

Physical environment The places where people live, work, and play.

pKa The dissociation constant of a weak acid.

Plague A bacterial infection caused by *Yersinia pestis* that resulted in the deaths of 20–30 million people in medieval times.

Plaque A buildup of cholesterol, calcium, and other substances that harden on arterial walls, causing them to narrow. Lesions found in patients with multiple sclerosis that develop at different times and in different locations throughout the CNS and typically occur in the periventricular white matter, optic nerve, brainstem, and cerebellum. Solid, raised, flat topped lesion greater than 1 centimeter in diameter

Plateau phase The phase of fever in which body temperature reaches the new set point and thermoregulatory warming responses are no longer stimulated

Platinum-based antineoplastic medications One of the most widely used chemotherapy drugs today.

Pleural effusion A collection of excess fluid in the pleural space.

Pneumonia An inflammation of the lung parenchyma that is typically characterized by lung consolidation with alveoli filled with exudate.

Pneumonic plague One type of plague infection characterized by the inhalation of the bacterium *Yersinia pestis*, leading to pneumonia.

Pneumothorax The presence of air between the visceral and parietal pleurae that compresses lung tissue and compromises lung function.

Poikilothermia A condition of disrupted body temperature regulation in which the individual has lost the ability to maintain internal body temperature within the thermoeffector threshold zone. Skin temperature that is the same as room temperature.

Point mutation A change in one nucleotide of a gene sequence.

Polycystic kidney disease (PKD) An inherited kidney disease in which fluid-filled cysts enlarge and damage the kidneys.

Polycystic ovary syndrome (PCOS) A treatable condition in which a woman has an imbalance of estrogen and progesterone characterized by irregular or no menstrual periods, acne, and excess hair growth.

Polycythemia vera Disorder of the bone marrow in which too may red blood cells are produced; white blood cells and platelets may increase as well.

Polydipsia Excessive thirst.

Polygenic Involving multiple genes.

Polymorphisms The presence of two or more alternative forms of a gene that are present at stable frequencies with a population.

Polyphagia Excessive hunger.

Polysomnography The polygraphic recording during sleep of multiple physiologic variables that are both directly and indirectly related to the state and stages of sleep.

Polyuria Excessive urination.

Portal hypertension Increased pressure in the portal vein and its branches as a result of blockage in blood flow through the liver.

Portal of entry The means by which a pathogen enters the host.

Portal of exit The means by which a pathogen exits a reservoir.

Portopulmonary syndrome Pulmonary hypertension in a person with portal hypertension.

Portosystemic shunt A vascular abnormality that diverts blood from the abdominal viscera to the heart, bypassing the liver.

Postherpetic neuralgia (PHN) A painful peripheral neuralgia caused by the varicella zoster virus.

Postictal period A period of postseizure activity characterized by a loss or alteration of consciousness.

Postinfectious glomerulonephritis (PIGN) An acute antibody-mediated glomerular disease that usually follows a beta-hemolytic streptococcal infection.

Postrenal AKI Acute kidney injury caused by obstruction within the kidney itself, bilateral ureteral obstruction, or urethral obstruction.

Postural instability A feeling of imbalance that occurs as a result of the loss of postural reflexes.

Potassium A positively charge element in the human body. This ion is the predominant cation in the intracellular fluid.

Precautionary principle The assertion that interventions must be taken when an environmental threat to human health is feasible even if scientific evidence is not conclusive.

Prediabetes A term that is used to identify people who are at increased risk for developing DM.

Preimplantation genetic diagnosis The screening of embryos that are produced through in vitro fertilization for the presence of genetic or chromosome abnormalities.

Preload The amount of blood present in the ventricle at the end of diastole.

Premenstrual dysphoric disorder A clinical syndrome that is a severe form of PMS (premenstrual syndrome) in which typical prementrual symptoms appear but are so severe that they affect the woman's mental health, resulting in depression or anxiety.

Premenstrual syndrome (PMS) Any complex of physical and mood disturbances experienced by some women in the days immediately before menstruation.

Prerenal AKI A reduction in renal perfusion that causes a reduction in glomerular filtration rate; usually caused by hypovolemia.

Presbycusis Hearing loss due to aging.

Presbyopia A refractive error in which the ciliary muscle that controls the shape of the lens is no longer able to function properly, resulting in a decline in the accommodative (focusing) ability of the eye.

Pressure equalization (PE) tubes Hollow plastic or metal cylinders that are inserted during surgery to allow normal aeration of the middle ear space until the Eustachian tube is functional.

Pretibial myxedema Thickening of the skin over the pretibial area.

Prevalence The number of people in a specific population who have a certain disease or condition at a point in time or during a period of time.

Priapism A prolonged erection that continues for hours.

Primary hyperaldosteronism An endocrine disorder characterized by excessive secretion of the hormone aldosterone from the adrenal glands; also referred to as *Conn syndrome.*

Primary hypothyroidism Common endocrine disorder that results from inadequate production of thyroid hormones.

Primary immune response Occurs when an antigen comes into contact with a immune system for the first time. During this time, the immune system has to learn to recognize antigen and how to make antibodies, and it eventually produces memory lymphocytes.

Primary immunodeficiencies (PIs) A heterogeneous group of genetic disorders affecting all components of immune system function, including phagocytic and complement activity as well as B-lymphocyte, T-lymphocyte, and natural killer cell function.

Primary intention Healing that occurs in wounds that involve minimal loss of tissue and in which the edges of the wound can be approximated.

Primary survey A trauma assessment during which all life-threatening injuries are discovered and managed before moving on to less serious (but sometimes more distracting) injuries.

Primary tumor A tumor that grows at the site where the cancer originated.

Prion A nonliving particle that is transmitted to mammals and causes neurodegenerative disease.

Prodrome Early set of symptoms that may indicate the start of disease before specific symptoms appear

Progeny Descendant cells.

Progression The third and final step in the carcinogenesis model, with invasion and metastasis of malignant cells.

Prokaryote Any cell that does not have a nucleus, distinct membrane-bound cell organelles, or mitochondria.

Proliferation Unregulated cell growth.

Proliferative diabetic retinopathy (PDR) Later stage of diabetic retinopathy where tiny new vessels grow from the retina into the vitreous humor, clouding vision. In severe PDR, the presence of new vessels can also signal proliferation of fibrovascular tissue, creating traction on the retina that leads to retinal detachments and blindness.

Promotion The second step of the carcinogenesis model, with the introduction of cancer-causing agents (carcinogens). Promoters bind to receptors on the cell surface to affect signaling pathways within the cell that promote the proliferation and immortalization of the altered cell, resulting in large numbers of daughter cells with the malignant mutation.

Prostate cancer A usually slow-growing cancer of the prostate gland.

Prostate specific antigen (PSA) A protein that helps to liquefy semen and assists in motility of sperm.

Prostatitis Inflammation of the prostate gland.

Protective factors Factors that decrease the risk of disease or injury.

Proteinuria Persistent protein in the urine, usually a symptom of kidney disease.

Proteolytic stress An imbalance between the synthesis and clearance of unwanted proteins within the cell that causes excess formation of unwanted proteins or impaired protein degradation, leading to accumulation and aggregation of proteins. These protein aggregates can interfere with normal ubiquitin–proteasomal system function, which can impair critical cellular processes.

Proto-oncogene A gene that regulates cell proliferation and may be a transcription factor, growth factor, or other growth-promoting agent. A normal gene involved in cell division that has the potential for mutation and conversion to an oncogene.

Protozoa Unicellular, eukaryotic microorganisms that include the familiar amoeba and paramecium; typically acquired through contaminated food or water or the bite of an infected arthropod such as a mosquito.

Provirus Viral DNA that is integrated into the genetic material of a host cell; may be transmitted from one cell generation to the next without causing cellular death.

Pruritus Itching.

Psoriasis Skin lesions characterized by hyperproliferation of keratinocytes and a decrease in epidermal cell turnover rate and inflammation.

Psychoactive drugs A drug that acts primarily on the central nervous system, where it alters brain function, resulting in changes in perception, mood, consciousness, and behavior.

Psychogenic pain Physical pain caused by emotional or mental stress and is not associated with any somatic or visceral inflammation or trauma.

Psychologic dependence The formation of positive memories and reinforcement for continued substance use that develops through consistent and frequent exposure to a stimulus.

Psychoneuroimmunology The study of how emotional and psychologic states influence body systems, particularly the immune and neurologic systems.

Psychosis Abnormal thought processes that interfere significantly with perceptions of reality and are usually manifested in odd or disturbed speech or behaviors.

Pterygium A benign growth that develops on the conjunctiva.

Public health The science of protecting and improving the health of families and communities through promotion of healthy lifestyles, research for disease and injury prevention, and detection and control of infectious diseases

Pulmonary acini Functional units of the lung in which gas exchange occurs; specifically, the respiratory bronchioles and their associated alveolar ducts and alveolar sacs.

Pulmonary agents A group of chemical agents that cause irritation and damage to the pulmonary system. Chemicals include ammonia, chlorine, and phosgene.

Pulmonary arterial hypertension (PAH) A primary disorder of increased blood pressure in the pulmonary arteries; characterized by an increased pulmonary arterial resistance in the absence of left ventricular failure or chronic thromboembolism.

Pulmonary edema Accumulation of fluid in the tissue and air spaces of the lungs leading to impaired gas exchange and possible respiratory failure.

Pulmonary embolism (PE) A blockage in a pulmonary artery caused, in most cases, by a blood clot that has traveled to the lungs.

Pulmonary granulomas Small, localized collections of macrophages that form in response to an inhaled antigen that cannot be degraded or an autoimmune disorder.

Pulmonary hypertension (PH) Increased blood pressure in the pulmonary arteries; may occur as a primary disorder or secondary to a primary disease process.

Pulmonary stenosis A congenital heart defect in which narrowing of the pulmonary valve results in decreased pulmonary blood flow.

Pulmonary vascular resistance The resistance to flow of blood generated by blood vessels in the pulmonary circulation.

Punnett square A graph used to determine the probability of the genotype that children will inherit based on the genotype for a particular trait of the parents.

Purpura Bleeding on the skin in the form of tiny pinprick hemorrhages.

Purulent (suppurative) inflammation Inflammation characterized by the formation of pus, which contains many neutrophils, cellular debris, and edema fluid.

Pyelonephritis Infection of the renal pelvis and parenchyma of the kidney.

Pyogenic Producing pus.

Pyogenic cocci Spherical bacteria that can cause suppurative (pus-producing) infections.

Pyrogen Any agent that causes fever.

qSOFA Quick version of the Sequential Organ Failure Assessment (SOFA) tool used to assess sepsis.

Radicular pain Pain caused by inflammation or compression of a spinal nerve root; radiates along the sensory distribution of the nerve.

Radiculopathy Loss of sensory and/or motor function as a result of impaired conduction block in a spinal nerve or its roots. Symptoms include numbness and weakness in the distribution of the affected nerve.

Radiologic dispersal device A conventional explosive to which a radioactive substance has been added to disperse the substance over a wide area and create panic and psychologic distress and fear; also referred to as a *dirty bomb*.

Rapid cycling A symptom of the bipolar disorders in which the person experiences four or more depressive and/or manic episodes within 12 months. Each episode must be of appropriate duration (at least 1 week for manic or hypomanic episodes, 2 weeks for depressive episodes), and there must be either a period of remission in between the episodes or a switch to the opposite mood .

Rapid eye movement sleep (REM sleep) The phase of sleep characterized by rapid characteristic eye movements, low-amplitude mixed-frequency EEG, and relaxation of all skeletal muscles, associated with dreaming.

Rapidly progressive glomerulonephritis (RPGN) A glomerulonephritis syndrome that presents as acute kidney injury and considered a medical emergency; etiology is either idiopathic, the result of anti-GBM antibodies, immune complex mediated, or pauci-immune type.

Raynaud disease A disorder in which the small arteries in the fingers and toes spasm and cause blood flow to be restricted.

Reactive oxygen species Oxygen-containing molecules that include free radicals such as superoxide and hydroxyl radicals and nonradicals such as hydrogen peroxide.

Reconsolidation The process in the brain by which an older memory is activated and once again consolidated or reinforced.

Rectal cancer A malignant growth or tumor resulting from the division of abnormal cells in the rectum.

Reepithelialization A process whereby epithelial cells migrate to the area and replicate by mitosis.

Referred pain Pain that is perceived as occurring in a region of the body distant from the actual source.

Reflux The involuntary backwards movement of gastrointestinal contents.

Reflux esophagitis Inflammation of the esophagus caused by the reflux of gastric contents.

Regurgitation The effortless return of food or fluids into the pharynx without nausea or retching.

Remission A reduction or abatement of disease over a particular period of time.

Renal calculi The formation of urinary crystals into larger stones; also known as nephrolithiasis or kidney stones.

Renal cell carcinoma (RCC) Malignant neoplasm of the kidney.

Renal transplantation Transplant of a healthy kidney from a live or deceased donor into someone with advanced chronic kidney disease.

Renin–angiotensin–aldosterone system (RAAS) A complex regulatory system for hemodynamic changes in the body.

Replicative senescence The limitation in the number of times cells can divide.

Reservoir An environment in which microbial pathogens may live, grow, and multiply; a source of infection to humans.

Respiratory acidosis A state of elevated CO_2 (hypercapnia) and carbonic acid and decreased blood pH.

Respiratory alkalosis A state of decreased CO_2 (hypocapnia) and carbonic acid and increased blood pH.

Respiratory failure An inadequate gas exchange that is demonstrated by hypoxemia with or without hypercapnia.

Restless legs syndrome (RLS) A condition characterized by an irritating sensation of uneasiness, tiredness, itching, or pain deep within the muscles of the leg during sleep and accompanied by twitching.

Retinopathy Any disorder of, or damage to, the retina.

Retrovirus Any category of viruses for which replication involves insertion of a DNA copy of the viral genome into the host cell; for example, HIV.

Reverse transcriptase A viral polymerase that generates two copies of DNA using the viral RNA as a template.

Reward pathway The brain structures including the ventral tegmental area (VTA), the nucleus accumbens, and the prefrontal cortex that are activated by a rewarding stimulus (such as drugs).

Rhabdomyolysis Muscle cell destruction resulting from severe injury in which skeletal muscle cells release toxic intracellular substances into circulating blood. The resulting rise in calcium levels in the cytoplasm causes skeletal muscle contraction, which accelerates heat production, induces mitochondrial dysfunction, and increases reactive oxygen species, leading to skeletal muscle cell death. While exertional rhabdomyolysis is possible with overexertion in warm conditions, rhabdomyolysis can also occur when a susceptible individual is exposed to specific anesthetics or neuroleptic drugs.

Rheumatoid arthritis (RA) A chronic systemic autoimmune disorder that produces a response against the body's own cells and tissues, resulting in damage to the tissues.

Rhinoconjunctivitis Characterized by one or several of the following symptoms: nasal congestion, runny nose, postnasal drip, sneezing, red eyes, and itching of the nose or the eyes. It may be, but is not always, allergic in origin.

Rhinorrhea A condition characterized by profuse, watery nasal discharge; commonly known as a runny nose.

Ribonucleic acid (RNA) A single-stranded molecule that is implicated in coding, decoding, regulation, and expression of genes.

Ribosomal RNA (rRNA) Functions to produce ribosomes, which are the machinery for protein formation to occur.

Ricin A chemical by-product of castor oil production from castor beans; a cellular poison.

Right-sided heart failure A condition in which the right side of the heart is unable to pump enough blood to meet the needs of the body.

Rigor mortis The stiffening of body muscles that begins within 2 to 3 hours after death.

Riot control agents A group of chemical agents that cause irritation of the mucous membranes and conjunctiva.

Risk assessment An assessment of the potential adverse health effects on humans as a consequence of exposures to hazardous substances or situations.

Risk factor Anything that puts a person at a greater risk for developing a particular disease.

Rosacea A chronic rash that involves the central part of the face and is characterized by its red color.

Rotoscoliosis Curvature of the vertebral column turned on its axis.

Route of exposure The route by which a contaminant contacts or enters the human body, which can be through inhalation, ingestion, dermal absorption, or transplacentally.

Rule of Nines Calculation that gives a rough estimate of body surface area (BSA) burned by assigning 9% to each body area.

Sarcoidosis A systemic disease of unknown origin that is characterized by formation of chronic noncaseating (solid) granulomas.

Sarin A nonpersistent nerve agent.

Satiety The feeling of being full after eating.

Scabies A parasitic infestation caused by a mite.

Scarring Replacement of epithelial cells by fibroblasts after significant tissue damage.

Schizophrenia A long-term mental disorder involving a breakdown in the relationships between thought, emotion, and behavior, leading to faulty perception, inappropriate actions and feelings, withdrawal from reality and personal relationships into fantasy and delusion, and a sense of mental fragmentation.

Sciatica Irritation or compression of all or part of the sciatic nerve.

Scoliometer A device used to measure the degree of scoliosis.

Scoliosis Lateral (sideways) curve of the spine.

Seborrheic dermatitis (SD) An acute inflammation of skin from an unknown cause that usually begins on the scalp and has rounded, irregular lesions and yellow scales.

Secondary adrenal insufficiency Disorder caused by dysfunction of the anterior pituitary leading to loss of ACTH production resulting in deficiency of adrenocortical hormones.

Secondary hyperaldosteronism Disorder that occurs when aldosterone is stimulated by excess secretion of renin by the juxtaglomerular apparatus of the kidney; it is a response to hypovolemia as seen in renovascular hypertension and with diuretic therapy.

Secondary hypertension High blood pressure due to an identifiable cause.

Secondary immune response Occurs each subsequent time a person is exposed to the same antigen. At this point, immunologic memory has been established, and the immune system can start making antibodies immediately.

Secondary immunodeficiency An acquired immunodeficiency.

Secondary intention Healing that occurs when a full thickness wound is allowed to heal without a closure attempt.

Secondary survey A trauma assessment that is done after the primary survey to identify less severe injuries and continue to develop a thorough understanding of the patient's needs and treatment plan.

Secondhand smoke (SHS) Smoke inhaled from tobacco that is being smoked by someone else.

Second-order neuron A neuron that transmits a noxious stimulus from the dorsal horn of the spinal cord to the thalamus.

Seizures A pattern of unregulated electrical discharge across part of the brain resulting in alteration of consciousness or uncontrolled motor activity.

Selective serotonin reuptake inhibitor (SSRI) A 5-HT-enhancing drug that is widely prescribed for the treatment of anxiety.

Self-tolerance The physiologic state that exists in an organism when its immune system has proceeded far enough into the process of self-recognition to lose the capacity to attack and destroy its own bodily constituents.

Sensorineural hearing loss Hearing loss in which sound is transmitted normally to the cochlea but the characteristics of the incoming sound—including the frequency and intensity—can no longer be accurately processed and/or transmitted to the auditory cortex.

Sentinel health event An event that heralds an environmental health problem not just for an individual, but also potentially for others in the home, work, and community environments.

Septicemic plague In the primary form of this type of plague, the bacteria enter the circulatory system directly from the lymphatic system, leading to a sepsis syndrome with multiple organ failure and shock; the secondary form can result from either the bubonic or pneumonic form of the disease when bacteria enter the circulation.

Septic shock Shock resulting from a pattern of systemic vasodilation in response to systemic inflammation; often occurs after infectious exposure and septicemia.

Sequential Organ Failure Assessment (SOFA) Tool for the clinical assessment of sepsis.

Seroconversion The point in time at which a particular antibody becomes detectable in the plasma.

Serotonin (5-HT) A neurotransmitter found in the raphae nuclei (cluster of nuclei found in the brainstem) derived from tryptophan that is involved in sleep, depression, memory, and other neurologic processes.

Serous inflammation Inflammation that is characterized by fluid accumulation that contains proteins but not many cells and is a result of tissue injury.

Sexually transmitted disease (STD) A term used to describe sexually transmitted infections that are not readily curable.

Sexually transmitted infection (STI) A term used to describe sexually transmitted infections that are viewed as curable.

Shift to the left An increased level of immature neutrophils in the circulation.

Shift work disorder Sleepiness during a work shift accompanied by daytime insomnia, experienced by people who have difficulty adapting to working at night.

Shivering The primary thermoeffector response to generate heat, which involves involuntary motor activity generating heat by friction produced as a result of aerobic muscle contractions.

Shortness of breath The subjective experience of breathlessness; often used interchangeably with the term *dyspnea*.

Sickle cell disease (SCD) Cluster of autosomal recessive disorders that results in misshapen forms of hemoglobin that resemble a sickle in shape.

Sign An objective indication of disease that is observable by on physical assessment.

Silent mutation A point mutation that does not change the amino acid sequence.

Simple acid–base imbalance The presence of one type of acid–base imbalance.

Single-nucleotide polymorphism (SNP) A nucleotide change that is present in more than 1% of the population.

Skin tags Soft papules on a stalk found in areas of the body where skin rubs on skin such as the neck, axillae, and groin; also called *acrochordons*

Sleep A a reversible state of detachment from the environment in which the individual neither senses nor responds to the surroundings.

Sleep-disordered breathing Disruption of respiratory airflow as a result of either airway constriction or airway collapse (obstructive sleep apnea, OSA) or secondary to impaired neurologic control of respiration (central sleep apnea, CSA).

Sleep latency The period of time before falling asleep after going to bed.

Sleep paralysis A temporary inability to move the voluntary muscles that occurs during transition between sleep and wake.

Sleep phase delay A shift in circadian rhythm experienced in adolescence in which the individual goes to sleep later and, consequently, wakes up later when permitted.

Smallpox A highly contagious disease caused by the variola virus that is characterized by high fever and the development of skin vesicles and pustules.

Smokeless tobacco A type of tobacco that is not burned to provide its effect, such as various forms of chewing tobacco and snuff.

Social anxiety disorder (SAD) A condition characterized by periods of significant fear resulting from a feeling of being judged that leads to significant impairment of daily function.

Social environment Both social and psychosocial factors in the environment such as gender, education, employment status, social networks, and interpersonal interactions.

Sodium A metallic element; primary cation in the extracellular fluid.

Solar sentigo Benign, sun-induced lesion commonly known as age spots or liver spots.

Soman A nonpersistent nerve agent.

Somatic cells All cells other than germ cells.

Somatic death Death of the whole person, in contrast to death of individual cells.

Somatic mutations A change in DNA sequence of body cells (except sperm and eggs) that can affect the progeny of that non–germ line cell. These mutations are not inherited by the next generation of children.

Somatic pain Pain arising from the skin, muscles, and joints; usually discrete and intense.

Somnambulism Sleepwalking.

SOREMPs Sleep onset REM periods, in which a person with narcolepsy goes directly from wakefulness to REM sleep.

Spermatocele A cyst that forms in the epididymis.

Spermatogenesis The process of making sperm.

Spherocytosis Hemolytic anemia is which the erythrocytes are sphere shaped.

Spider angioma Swollen superficial blood vessels that give the appearance of a spiderweb; also known as telangiectasis.

Spinal fusion Surgery to join two or more vertebrae together using bone grafts, screws, and rods.

Spinal shock The temporary loss or all of most spinal reflex activity below the level of the injury.

Spinal stenosis Narrowing of the spinal column.

Spirillia Spiral-shaped bacteria that possess flagella.

Spirochete A thin, flexible spiral-shaped bacterium that has endoflagella, which are made up of axial filaments.

Splanchnic circulation Circulation in the gastrointestinal organs, including the small intestines, colon, pancreas, stomach, liver, and spleen.

Splicing The process of removal of noncoding parts of messenger RNA (introns) and joining together of the coding parts (exons) to produce the instructions to make a protein.

Spondyloarthropathies A group of diseases that affect the joints, including ankylosing spondylitis, reactive arthritis, psoriatic arthritis, and enteropathic arthritis (joint problems that occur with inflammatory bowel disease).

Spore A highly resilient dehydrated structure that represents a dormant or nonvegetative state of bacteria; formed when bacteria are nutrient-deprived and/or in harsh environmental conditions, such as extremes of temperature or osmolarity.

Sprain Stretching or tearing of ligaments around a joint.

Squamous cell carcinoma (SCC) A malignant neoplasm of the esophagus with squamous differentiation, usually with signs of keratin. Second most common skin cancer and is more likely than BCC to metastasize; treatment is surgery to remove the lesion

Stable angina Chest pain, discomfort, pressure, and/or squeezing symptoms that often occurs with increased myocardial oxygen demand and reduced blood flow during exertion or emotional stress; often relieved by rest and/or administration of nitroglycerin.

Stage I shock The first stage of shock; also called *early, reversible,* or *compensated shock*. In this stage, a number of compensatory systems are activated to maintain or restore perfusion when low blood flow is initially detected. The patient in this stage of shock has a strong chance of recovery with proper treatment.

Stage II shock The second stage of shock; also called *progressive* or *intermediate shock*. In this stage, the compensatory mechanisms begin to fail. The resulting decrease in perfusion leads to cellular hypoxia with accompanying hypoxic tissue injuries. Stage II shock is reversible with promptly instituted appropriate treatment.

Stage III shock The third stage of shock; also called *irreversible* or *refractory shock*. In this stage, poor perfusion has persisted for long enough that it begins to take a permanent toll on the body's organs and tissues. The endpoint of stage III shock is patient death due to multiple organ dysfunction.

Stapedectomy A surgery that involves removal of a diseased stapes bone and attachment of a prosthetic stapes in its place.

Status epilepticus Unremitting seizure activity or recurrent seizure activity across a span of 30 minutes during which the individual is unable to recover.

Steatohepatitis Liver inflammation in the setting of steatosis.

Steatorrhea Greasy, foul-smelling feces containing undigested fats.

Steatosis Early stage of fatty liver disease. Fatty deposits in the liver that result from the accumulation of lipid droplets.

Stevens-Johnson syndrome (SJS) A rare but serious disorder of the skin and mucous membranes in which cell death causes the epidermis to separate from the dermis.

Stomach cancer A malignant growth or tumor resulting from the division of abnormal cells in the stomach.

Strabismus A condition in which one or both eyes turns in, out, up, or down.

Strain Injury to a muscle or muscle-tendon unit caused by overstretching.

Stratum basale Also called the *basal layer*, the deepest of the five layers of the epidermis, composed of a single layer of germ cells.

Stratum corneum The horny, outermost layer of the skin, composed of dead flat cells converted to keratin that continually flakes away.

Stratum granulosum One of the layers of the epidermis, situated just below the stratum corneum except in the thick skin of the palms of the hands and soles of the feet, where it lies just under the stratum lucidum.

Stratum lucidum One of the layers of the epidermis, situated just beneath the stratum corneum and present only in the thick skin of the palms of the hands and soles of the feet.

Stratum spinosum One of the layers of the epidermis, composed of several layers of spiky-shaped cells.

Stress The physiologic or psychologic response to an event that is perceived as a threat or challenge.

Stressor An event or trigger that results in stress.

Stroke Loss of brain function due to a disturbance in the blood supply to the brain caused by ischemia or hemorrhage.

Stroke volume (SV) The amount of blood pumped from the ventricle during one contraction measured in volume per heartbeat.

Structural heart disorder defect (SHD) A group of structural abnormalities that occur during gestation, resulting in abnormal blood flow through the heart in the postnatal period.

ST-segment elevation myocardial infarction (STEMI) A more precise definition of the common term *heart attack*, which occurs when obstruction of blood flow to the myocardium results in necrosis and clinical signs and symptoms of myocardial infarction, ST-segment elevation on electrocardiogram, and elevated biomarkers.

Stump pain Pain at the site of an extremity amputation.

Stye A tender, red, often pus-filled bump that develops along the edge of the eyelid; also called a *hordeolum*.

Subdural hematoma (SDH) A condition that occurs when a brain injury is severe enough to cause the brain to bounce around the skull, tearing or shearing the bridging veins, resulting in a formation of a blood clot between the dura and arachnoid mater.

Subluxation An injury in which the joint bones remain in partial contact.

Sudomotor Any stimulus that activates or regulates the sweat glands.

Superantigen A specialized toxin that is present on the cellular surface of certain bacteria; activates T lymphocytes, leading to massive production of cytokines that damage host tissues.

Suppuration The process of pus formation.

Suprachiasmatic nucleus (SCN) The body's "master clock," located in the anterior hypothalamus; it regulates the circadian rhythm.

Surveillance An important public health function in which health data on populations are systematically collected, analyzed, and interpreted on an ongoing basis and used to design and implement interventions to prevent and control health problems.

Susceptibility A key vulnerability factor that denotes characteristics including age, gender, race/ethnicity, stage of development, and genetic predisposition that increase the risk of individuals for environmental disease or injury.

Symport A transport molecule that moves two different electrolytes in the same direction across a cell membrane.

Symptom A subjective sensation indicative of disease that is perceived by the affected individual but not observable on physical examination.

Syndrome A collection of symptoms associated with particular disease.

Syndromic hearing loss A genetic hearing loss in which the individual has a pattern of other clinical abnormalities as well.

Syphilis A sexually transmitted infection caused by the bacteria *Treponema pallidum*.

Systemic inflammatory response syndrome (SIRS) An inflammatory state, related to sepsis, that affects the entire body in which there is abnormal regulation of cytokines. Criteria for diagnosis of SIRS in adults include demonstrating at least two of the following: (1) body temperature less than 36°C or more than 38.5°C, (2) heart rate greater than 90 beats per minute, (3) tachypnea greater than 20 breaths per minute or arterial partial pressure of carbon dioxide less than 32 mmHg, (4) white blood cell count less than 4000 cells/mm^3 or greater than 12,000 cells/mm^3 or the presence of more than 10% immature neutrophils.[1]

Systemic lupus erythematosus (SLE) An inflammatory connective tissue disease that is often held to be an autoimmune disease. It occurs chiefly in women and is characterized especially by fever, skin rash, and arthritis, often by acute hemolytic anemia, by small hemorrhages in the skin and mucous membranes, by inflammation of the pericardium, and in serious cases by involvement of the kidneys and central nervous system.

Systemic vascular resistance (SVR) Resistance to forward flow of blood generated by the blood vessels in the systemic circulation.

Systolic heart failure A condition in which the contraction of the heart muscle is impaired; referred to as *heart failure with reduced ejection factor*.

Tabun A nonpersistent nerve agent.

Tachycardia An abnormal rapid heart rate that exceeds a normal resting rate, generally more than 100 beats per minute; also called *tachydysrhythmia*.

Targeted therapy Treatments that inhibit or block the targeted receptor or pathway, thus preventing cell growth and promoting death of the immortalized malignant cell.

Telangiectases Spider veins; small dilated capillaries at the skin surface

Telogen Short resting phase of hair growth

Temporary threshold shift (TTS) A temporary loss of hearing followed by a recovery of hearing if no repeated exposure occurs.

Tension pneumothorax A condition that occurs when the pleural space becomes disrupted and the negative pressure in the pleural cavity is broken, allowing atmospheric air to enter the pleural space, which becomes trapped and compresses the adjacent lung tissue.

Tension type headache A pericranial myofascial pain.

Teratogenic Anything that causes fetal death or anomalies.

Tertiary intention Healing that occurs when would closure is delayed.

Testicular cancer Cancer of the testicle, a rare form of cancer that is usually found in males between the ages of 15 and 34.

Testicular torsion A condition that occurs when the spermatic cord structures twist within the testicle, causing loss of blood supply to the ipsilateral testis.

Testosterone A hormone produced mainly in the testes that stimulates the development of secondary sexual characteristics in males.

Tetany A constellation of symptoms caused by hypocalcemia that is characterized by painful carpal spasms and laryngeal stridor.

Tetrahydrocannabinol (THC) The most potent active chemical found in cannabis.

Tetralogy of Fallot (TOF) A compilation of four congenital heart defects: a ventricular septal defect, pulmonary stenosis, right ventricular hypertrophy, and an overriding aorta.

Thalassemia Genetically transmitted blood disorder associated with an inability to properly form hemoglobin.

Therapeutic hypothermia The deliberate lowering of body temperature to decrease the oxygen requirements of vital tissue, particularly those of the brain and heart.

Thermoeffector responses Involuntary responses to heat and cold stimuli that combine both physiologic and physical processes to either conserve heat within or promote the transfer of heat away from the body's most vulnerable regions.

Thermoeffector threshold zone The zone in the brain that defines the acceptable core temperature range of 36–38.5°C. A set point mechanism, like your home thermostat, is thought to keep core temperature levels within this range.

Thermoneutral zone A dynamic state in which body temperature is stable and does not require any regulatory changes in heat production or heat loss.

Thermoreceptors Peripheral and central warm or cold sensors that monitor the core temperature.

Thermoregulation The regulation of body temperature.

Third-order neuron A neuron that transmits noxious impulses from the thalamus to the primary somatosensory areas for perception of pain.

Third spacing The accumulation of fluid in areas that normally have no fluid or a minimal amount of fluid. Examples of third spacing include ascites and edema that is associated with burns.

Thoracentesis Removal of accumulated fluid from the pleural space using either a needle or a small catheter.

Thoracic outlet syndrome (TOS) A disorder that occurs when the thoracic outlet narrows, the blood flow and nerves become restricted, and function is compromised in the arms and fingers.

Thrombocytes Cellular fragments known as platelets that are involved in coagulation.

Thrombocythemia An excess of platelets that can cause spontaneous blood clot formation.

Thrombocytopenia A reduction in the number of platelets in the blood.

Thromboembolism The blocking of a blood vessel by a particle formed from a thrombus or part of a thrombus.

Thrombopoiesis The production of thrombocytes; also referred to as *megakaryocytopoiesis*.

Thrombosis The process of formation of a blood clot (thrombus) that obstructs blood flow to organs depending on where it forms; when formed in coronary artery, the blockage can cause a myocardial infarction, or heart attack.

Thrombotic thrombocytopenic purpura A rare but acute disease that manifests with renal and neurologic involvement, purpura, hematuria, and epistaxis and may present secondary to thrombocytopenia.

Thyroiditis An inflammation of the thyroid gland.

Thyroid nodule Abnormal growth of thyroid cells that forms a lump within the thyroid gland.

Thyroid scintigraphy A nuclear medicine procedure that visually identifies the functional status (e.g., hyperfunctioning or hypofunctioning) thyroid tissue on the basis of the selective uptake of various radionuclides.

Thyroid storm A life-threatening condition characterized by an exacerbation of all of the signs and symptoms of hyperthyroidism; also called *thyrotoxicosis*.

Thyrotoxicosis A life-threatening condition characterized by an exacerbation of all of the signs and symptoms of hyperthyroidism; also called *thyroid storm*.

Tinea Superficial fungal infection of the skin.

Tinea corporis Fungal infection of the body.

Tinea cruris Fungal infection of the groin that may extend to the inner thighs and buttocks.

Tinea pedis Fungal infection of the soles of the feet and the space between the toes and/or toenail.

Tinnitus The subjective experience of hearing a noise such as ringing, buzzing, or hissing in the head or ears in the absence of any external noise.

Tobacco use disorder A disorder characterized by the harmful consequences of persistent tobacco use, a pattern of compulsive tobacco use, and (sometimes) physiologic dependence on tobacco (i.e., tolerance and/or withdrawal).

Tolerance Reduced effectiveness of a drug after repeated administration.

Tonic–clonic seizure The most common type of seizure, characterized by alternating repetitive tonic–clonic activity.

Tonic phase A phase of seizure activity characterized by muscle rigidity.

Total anomalous pulmonary venous return (TAPVR) A congenital heart defect in which the pulmonary veins drain into the right side of the heart instead of the left side, as normally occurs.

Total CO_2 (TCO_2) A measure of carbon dioxide in the form of HCO_3^- ions, H_2CO_3, and CO_2 attached to proteins such as hemoglobin as well as the CO_2 dissolved in plasma.

Toxicant Any toxic substance.

Toxic epidermal necrolysis (TEN) An inflammation of the skin caused by a poison and resulting in necrosis and dissolving of the tissue.

Transcription The process of "reading" a gene to creating a chain of mRNA from a template strand of DNA.

Transcription factor modulators Medications that affect the levels of gene transcription in the body.

Transcription factors Regulatory proteins that bind to the promoter region at the beginning of a gene, thereby activating the gene.

Transduction The conversion of a noxious thermal, mechanical, or chemical stimulus into a nerve impulse.

Transfer RNA (tRNA) A type of RNA that carries appropriate amino acids to the template mRNA strand so that protein formation can occur.

Transient ischemic attack (TIA) A temporary interruption of blood flow and oxygen to the brain in which symptoms resolve within 24 hours.

Transient LES relaxation (TLESR) A motor pattern triggered by vagal afferents in the stomach causing rapid relaxation of the LES, esophageal shortening, and inhibition of the crural diaphragm; a means for the stomach to vent excess gas.

Translation The conversion of messenger RNA into a series of amino acids, which are then used to synthesize a protein product.

Transmission The passage of a pathogen from an infected host to a previously noninfected host via direct or indirect contact; the transfer of a noxious peripheral stimulus to the CNS.

Transmitted drug resistance (TDR) The transmission of drug-resistant forms of HIV.

Transport media The means through which environmental hazards are transported to people, including via air, soil, water, and food.

Transposition of the great arteries A congenital heart defect in which the pulmonary artery arises from the left ventricle (in the normal heart, it arises it from the right ventricle) and the aorta arises from the right ventricle (it normally arises from the left ventricle).

Transudate A collection of watery, low-protein fluid in the tissues or extravascular space due to increased membrane permeability; usually not caused by an inflammatory process.

Traumatic brain injury (TBI) The disruption of normal brain function caused by a bump, blow, jolt, or penetrating injury to the head.

Trichomoniasis A parasitic sexually transmitted infection that is transmitted by the protozoan *Trichomonas vaginalis*; known colloquially as "trich."

Trigeminal neuralgia (TN) Sporadic, sudden burning or shock-like neuropathic pain of the face and head associated with injury or damage to the trigeminal nerve.

Trigger A stimulus that precipitates or incites a physiologic response.

Triploidy An extra set of chromosomes resulting from the fertilization of one egg by two sperm or the fertilization of an egg that then divides into two, resulting in an embryo with 69 chromosomes; generally incompatible with life.

Tropism The degree to which a potential host is susceptible to infection by a specific pathogen. The preference of a virus to bind to specific targets or host cells.

Trousseau sign Contraction of the arm and hand elicited by occluding the arterial blood flow of the arm for 5 minutes, usually with a blood pressure cuff. A positive Trousseau sign is indicative of hypocalcemia and/or hyperphosphatemia.

Tuberculosis (TB) A pulmonary infection caused by *Mycobacterium tuberculosis*, an acid-fast bacillus that is transmitted through aerosolized droplets; hallmarks of this disorder include formation of granulomas in the alveolar macrophages.

Tumor An abnormal growth of cells; also called a *neoplasm*.

Tumor markers Substances normally found in the blood, urine, or other body fluids that can be produced in greater amounts as a tumor grows. Laboratory tests may be used to evaluate the status of tumor growth.

Tumor necrosis factor A cytokine secreted by macrophages that causes cell death; also known as *cachectin*.

Tumor suppressor gene A gene that codes for a product that controls cell growth. A normal gene that slows cell division to repair DNA errors and directs programmed cell death. When these genes are mutated, normal cells are transformed to immortalized malignant cells.

Type I respiratory failure A condition that results from a low level of oxygen in the blood (hypoxemia) without an increased level of carbon dioxide in the blood (hypercapnia); also known as *hypoxemic respiratory failure*.

Type II respiratory failure A condition that results from inadequate alveolar ventilation, causing an increased level of carbon dioxide in the blood (hypercapnia) with or without a low level of oxygen in the blood (hypoxemia); also known as *hypercapnic respiratory failure* or *ventilatory respiratory failure*.

Ulcer Damage and erosion of the mucosal layers in the gastrointestinal tract that fail to heal.

Ulceration A local defect caused by necrosis of cells and sloughing of necrotic tissue resulting from very severe inflammation.

Ulcerative colitis (UC) A chronic inflammatory condition limited to the mucosal layers of the colon characterized by relapsing and remitting episodes of inflammation; it is considered to be an *inflammatory bowel disease.*

Unconjugated bilirubin An insoluble form of bilirubin that cannot be excreted in the urine.

Undifferentiated cancer Cancers that are composed of immature cells; tend to be more aggressive than differentiated cancers.

Union A bone fracture that heals without difficulty.

Unstable angina A condition of chest discomfort related to lack of blood flow through coronary arteries to the myocardium that is less predictable than stable angina and may occur at rest.

Upper respiratory tract infection (URI) An acute infection of one or more structures of the upper respiratory tract, including the nose, paranasal sinuses, pharynx, larynx, trachea, and bronchi.

Uremia Elevated urea and other nitrogenous waste products in the blood; can lead to nausea, vomiting, and malaise.

Urinary incontinence Loss of bladder control that results in involuntary leakage of urine.

Urinary tract infection (UTI) Infection of the lower urinary tract of the bladder, the upper urinary tract, or the kidney.

Urticaria Pale, itchy plaques or welts on the skin; hives.

Vaccination (immunization) The administration of an infectious agent or its components to an individual with the purpose of inducing an immune response and forming memory cells to this infectious agent, hence protecting the individual on future exposure.

Vaginal cancer A rare cancer that occurs in the cells lining the vagina.

Vaginismus Painful spasmodic contraction of the vagina in response to physical contact or pressure during sexual intercourse, gynecologic exams, manual penetration, or insertion of tampons.

Vaginitis Inflammation of the vagina caused by infection, poor hygiene, or medical conditions and resulting in discharge, itching, and pain.

Valvular disorder Abnormal functioning of one or more of the four heart valves such as regurgitation, prolapse, or stenosis; also known as *heart valve disease* or *valvular heart disease.*

Vaping Inhalation and exhalation of the vapor produced by an electronic cigarette or similar device.

Variable expressivity Differing degree of clinical phenotypes in individuals with mutations in the same gene.

Varicocele An enlargement of the veins in the scrotum.

Varicose veins Veins that have become enlarged and twisted as a result of the rupture of valves.

Vascular pain Pain that results from severe vasospasm, usually in response to cold and/or increased activity of the SNS.

Vasodilation Enlargement of vessel wall lumen, often occurring as part of the inflammatory cascade, permitting increased blood flow to the injured area.

Vasospasm A spasm, or sudden constriction, of a blood vessel that decreases the diameter of the vessel and subsequently decreases blood flow.

Vector Living intermediaries that convey an infectious agent from its reservoir to a susceptible host.

Vehicle A nonliving intermediary that conveys an infectious agent from its reservoir to a susceptible host.

Venous blood gases A measure of the pH, $PaCO_2$, PaO_2, and bicarbonate in the venous blood.

Ventilator-associated pneumonia (VAP) A classification of pneumonia in which the individual develops pneumonia more than 48 to 72 hours after tracheal intubation.

Ventricular aneurysm A defect in the left or right ventricle wall in which there is bulging outward, usually as a result of weakened tissue from myocardial ischemia or infarction.

Ventricular septal defect (VSD) A congenital heart defect in which there is a hole in the wall (septum) between the ventricles; accounts for one quarter of all CCHDs.

Ventricular septal rupture A type of ventricular septal defect in which there is an abnormal opening between the left and right ventricles, which causes mixing of oxygenated blood (from the left ventricle) with deoxygenated blood (from the right ventricle).

Vertigo A false sensation of rotation of oneself or one's environment that is often accompanied by intense nausea and vomiting.

Vesicants A group of chemical agents that cause a clinical picture similar to a burn with redness and blistering of skin and damage to other exposed tissues.

Vesicles Small, fluid-filled sacs or blisters

Vesicoureteral reflux (VUR) The abnormal backflow of urine from the bladder to the kidney; can lead to renal scarring and ESRD.

Vestibulotoxic Medications that can damage the sensory cells of the peripheral balance system.

Viral set point In reference to HIV, the stabilized amount of virus remaining in the body after the initial immune response.

Virulence The degree to which a microorganism is capable of causing infectious disease.

Virulence factors Substances that enhance the pathogenicity of microorganisms.

Virus An infectious organism that typically consists of a nucleic acid molecule in a protein coat and is capable of replication only when inside the living cells of a host environment.

Visceral adiposity Central fat distribution.

Visceral pain Diffuse and poorly localized pain, frequently referred to as a somatic site.

Vitiligo Multifactoral disorder involving genetic and environmental elements resulting in the loss of functional melanocytes in areas of the skin, hair, or mucous membranes

Volatile acid An acid that can dissociate, forming a gas that is eliminated by the lungs.

Volkmann contracture Deformity of the wrist, hand, and fingers caused by ischemia to the forearm.

Vomiting A neuromuscular reflex that results in forceful expulsion of gastric contents through the oral or nasal cavity; also called emesis.

von Willebrand disease (vWD) A common hereditary bleeding disorder caused by defects in the genetic expression of the glycoprotein von Willebrand factor.

Vulnerability The diminished capacity of an individual or a population to withstand adverse health risks from environmental exposures based on several factors including: differential exposure, the interrelated factors of preparedness and ability to recover, and susceptibility.

Vulnerable plaque Plaque that has a thin fibrous cap that is susceptible to rupture and thrombosis.

Vulvar cancer A form of cancer that occurs on the outer surface area of the female genitalia.

Vulvovestibulitis A syndrome characterized by inflammation and pain in the vaginal opening and surrounding tissues.

VX A persistent nerve agent; the most lethal of the nerve agents.

Warts Common skin lesions caused by a variety of human papillomavirus types

Watchful waiting The least invasive treatment for benign prostatic hyperplasia, involving yearly examinations with evaluation using digital rectal examination; also known as *active surveillance.*

Wernicke-Korsakoff syndrome Injury to the brainstem and areas near the third and fourth ventricles of the brain resulting in double vision, ataxia, hyperactivity, confusion, delirium, and anxiety. Occurs after heavy alcohol use over a long time.

Wet macular degeneration The more severe form of macular degeneration, in which new blood vessels from the underlying retinal layer, called Bruch's membrane, grow around the macula and cause bleeding, scarring, and photoreceptor atrophy.

Wheeze An abnormal breath sound associated with obstruction of airflow though bronchial tubes.

Wide dynamic range (WDR) neuron A second-order neuron located in the dorsal horn of the spinal cord and responsive to all peripheral thermal, chemical and mechanical stimuli.

Wilms tumor The most common kidney cancer in children; associated with many genetic abnormalities; also called *nephroblastoma*.

Window period The period between infection with HIV and the appearance of neutralizing antibodies.

Wind-up Increased excitability of second-order wide dynamic range neurons in the dorsal horn in response to repeated noxious inputs from first-order neurons.

Worry-centered anxiety disorders Anxiety disorders such as GAD that occur when the mediating neural structures that should be able to process a presenting threat are functioning suboptimally.

Wound An injury that disrupts the normal structure and function of a tissue or organ.

Xenobiotics Exogenous (not produced in the body) chemical agents.

Xerosis Abnormal dryness

Zeitgeber An environmental cue, such as light or activity, that resets the circadian clock in the brain.

Zoonosis Any disease that can be passed from animals to humans.

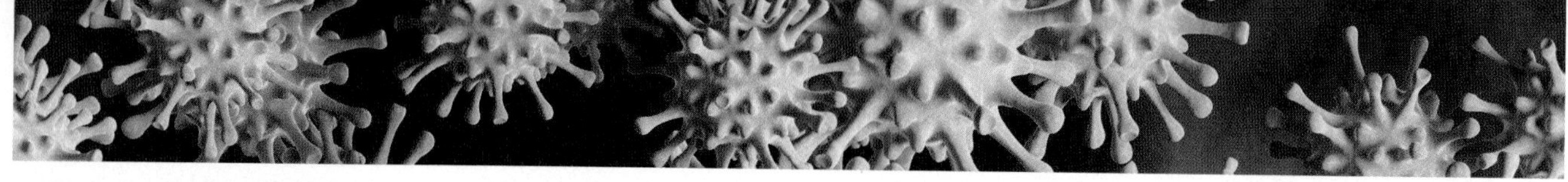

Credits

Cover images: Fox Studio/Shutterstock; Elizaveta Lavrik/Shutterstock; National Institutes of Health.

Frontmatter images: Xi, Eleonora_os/Shutterstock; Xi, Wavebreak Premium/Shutterstock; Xi, PT Images/Shutterstock; xi Michael Jung/Shutterstock; Xii, Lisa F. Young/Shutterstock; Xii, Fox Studio/Shutterstock; Xviii, Colorado Springs Gazette/Tribune News Service/Getty Images.

Chapter opening banner: Fox Studio/Shutterstock.

Chapter 1: 8, 13, 17, Case Study 1, Fotoluminate LLC/Shutterstock; 9, Fig. 1.4B Michael jung/Shutterstock; 9, Fig 1.4C Vitalinka/123RF.com; 17, Evidence Based Medicine: What it is and What it isn't" by David L Sackett, William M C Rosenberg, J A Muir Gray, R Brian Haynes and W Scott Richardson in British Medical Journal, Volume 312, pp. 71–72. Published by BMJ Publishing Group Ltd, © 1996.

Chapter 2: 24, 34, 38, 39, Case Study 1,Wavebreak Premium/Shutterstock; 25, 38, Case Study 2, Auremar/123RF.com; 25, 40, Case Study 3, Amble Design/Shutterstock; 26, Fig. 2.4, BALL, JANE W.; BINDLER, RUTH C.; COWEN, KAY J., CHILD HEALTH NURSING, 3rd Ed., © 2014. Reprinted and Electronically reproduced by permission of Pearson Education, Inc., New York, NY; 35, Fig 2.15, DenKuvaiev/iStock/Getty Images; 35, Fig 2.16A, Hercules Robinson/Alamy Stock Photo; Fig 2.16B, Girand/BSIP SA/Alamy Stock Photo; 40, Fig 2.21, Mediscan/Alamy Stock Photo; 27, From "Genes, Genetics, and Epigenetics: A Correspondence" by C. Wu and J. R. Morris in Science, Vol. 293, Issue 5532, pp. 1103–1105. Published by American Association for the Advancement of Science, © 2001.

Chapter 3: Case Study 2, Centers for Disease Control and Prevention (CDC); Case Study 3, Rafal Trubisz/Pearson Education, Inc.; 48, National Environmental Health Association,(2013).New Perspectives on Environmental Health: The approval of new definitions. Journal of Environmental Health, 76(3), 72-73; 49, From Social Determinants of Health, Healthy People 2020. Published by U.S. Department of Health and Human Services. 65, From ""Endocrine Disruptor Induction of Epigenetic Transgenerational Inheritance of Disease"", by Michael K. Skinner in Molecular and Cellular Endocrinology, Vol. 398, Issues. 1–2, pp. 4–12. Published by Elsevier Ireland Ltd, © 2014; 63-64, Levy BS, Wegman DH, Baron SL, Sokas RK. Occupational and Environmental Health: Recognizing and Preventing Disease and Injury (6th ed). 2011. New York: Oxford University Press.

Chapter 4: 78, 81, 84, 89, Case Study 1, James Peragine/Shutterstock; 79, 81, 90, Case Study 2, PeopleImages/DigitalVision/Getty Images.

Chapter 5: 102, 108, 113, Case Study 1,Michael Jung/Shutterstock; 103, 108, 113, Case Study 2, Christopher Oates/Shutterstock; 111, Fig 5.7, Sebastian Kaulitzki/Shutterstock; 112, Fig 5.8, Txking/iStock/Getty Images; 112, Fig 5.9, Benedicte Desrus/Alamy Stock Photo; 113, Fig 5.10, ChooseMyPlate.gov. Published by United States Department of Agriculture; 114, Fig 5.11, Colorado Springs Gazette/Tribune News Service/Getty Images; 114, From "Physical Activity, Exercise, and Physical Fitness: Definitions and Distinctions for Health-Related Research" by Carl J. Caspersen, Kenneth E. Powell, Gregory M. Christenson in Public Health Reports, Vol. 100, No.2, pp. 126–31. Published by Sage Publications, © 1984.

Chapter 6: 122, 126, 137, Case Study 1,Fritzphoto/Shutterstock; 122, 129, 130, Case Study2, Bikeriderlondon/Shutterstock; 132, Fig 6.5, AmpH/E+/Getty Images.

Chapter 7: 147, 150, 154, 155, Case Study 1, Mike Flippo/123RF.com; 147, 157, 159, Case Study 2, Arina P Habich/Shutterstock; 147, 161, 162, Case Study 3,Tyler Olson/Shutterstock; 146, Fig 7.1, From Buysse DJ. (2014). Sleep health: Can we define it? Does it matter? Sleep, 37(1):9-17; 153, Fig 7.11, LifeJourneys/iStock/Getty Images; 158, Fig 7.16,Brian Chase/Shutterstock.

Chapter 8: 171, 187, Case Study 1, Kurhan/Shutterstock; 172, 179, 180, 187, Case Study 2, Monkey Business Images/Shutterstock; 181, Fig 8.8, Maridav/iStock/Getty Images.

Chapter 9: 199, 217, 218, Case Study 1, Amble Design/Shutterstock; 199, 210, 220, 221, Case Study 2, Leungchopan/Shutterstock; 199, 214, 222, 225, 226, Case Study 3, Gareth Boden/Pearson Education, Inc.

Chapter 10: 239, 247, Case Study 1, Barbs images/Shutterstock; 239, 252, 253, Case Study 2, Jeff Cleveland/Shutterstock; 254, Fig 10.12, LSOphoto/iStock/Getty Images.

Chapter 11: 273, 281, 282, 285, Case Study 1, Kurhan/Shutterstock; 273, 284, Case Study 2, Andy Dean Photography/Shutterstock.

Chapter 12: 296, 307, 312, 313, 318, Case Study 1,Warren Goldswain/123RF.com; 296, 303, 312, 314, 318, Case Study 2,Racorn/Shutterstock; 310, Fig 12.15, Ulrich Baumgarten/Getty Images; 314, Table 12.3, Republished with permission of American College of Surgeons, from AJCC Cancer Staging Manual, 8e edited by Mahul B. Amin, Stephen B. Edge, Frederick L. Greene, David R. Byrd, Robert K. Brookland, Mary Kay Washington, Jeffrey E. Gershenwald, Carolyn C. Compton, Kenneth R. Hess, Daniel C. Sullivan, J. Milburn Jessup, James D. Brierley and Lauri E. Gaspar © 2016; permission conveyed through Copyright Clearance Center, Inc.

Chapter 13: 328, 333, 336, Case Study 1, Alan Bailey/Shutterstock; 329, 342, 344, 345, Case Study 2, Andrej Andic/Shutterstock; 338, Fig 13.4A, KTSDESIGN/SCIENCE PHOTO LIBRARY/Getty Images; 338, Fig 13.4B, IiLexx/iStock/Getty Images; 344, Fig 13.7, Nicholas Mayeux/Stocktrek Images Inc./Alamy Stock Photo; 350, Fig 13.9, PeopleImages/iStock/Getty Images; 354, Fig 13.12,Ricardo Funari/BrazilPhotos/Alamy Stock Photo.

Chapter 14: 366, 370, 374, Case Study 1, Creatista/Shutterstock; 369, Fig 14.5, Mediscan/Alamy Stock Photo.

Chapter 15: 383, 391, 392, Case Study 1, Roi Brooks/Shutterstock; 383, 384, 391, Case Study 2, Jon Barlow/Pearson Education, Inc.; 392, Fig 15.7, Mediscan/Alamy Stock Photo.

Chapter 16: 403, 405, Case Study 1, Ariwasabi/Shutterstock; 403, 407, 408, Case Study 2, Jose Manuel Gelpi Diaz/123RF.com; 403, 411, Case Study 3, Aigars Reinholds/123RF.com; 401, Fig 16.1, Alila Medical Media/Shutterstock; 406, Roberto Biasini/123RF.com; Fig 16.3, 408, Fig 16.4, Stacy Howard/Centers for Disease Control and Prevention (CDC); 413, Fig 16.5, Mediscan/Alamy Stock Photo; 416, Fig 16.6 Cavallini James/BSIP SA/Alamy Stock Photo.

Chapter 17: 427, 429, Case Study 1, PT Images/Shutterstock; 427, 430, 431, Case Study 2, Michaeljung/Shutterstock.

Chapter 18: 441, 446, 449, 450, Case Study 1, RSnapshot-Photos/Shutterstock; 450, Fig 18.6, Jacopin/BSIP SA/Alamy Stock Photo; 460, Fig 18.14, Cavallini James/BSIP SA/Alamy Stock Photo.

Chapter 19: 466, 470, 471, Case Study 1, Michael Jung/Shutterstock; 466, 478, 481, Case Study 2, Lord and Leverett/Pearson Education, Inc.; 477, Fig 19.4, BINDLER, RUTH C.; COWEN, KAY J., PRINCIPLES OF PEDIATRIC NURSING: CARING FOR CHILDREN, 5th Ed., © 2012. Reprinted and Electronically reproduced by permission of Pearson Education, Inc., New York, NY; 478, Fig 19-5, George Dodson/Pearson Education, Inc.

Chapter 20: 496, 498, 501, Case Study 1, Pathdoc/Shutterstock; 496, 499, 509, Case Study 2, Kiselev Andrey Valerevich/Shutterstock.

Chapter 21: 514, Fig 21.1, Image Source/Alamy Stock Photo; 515, 518, 526, Case Study 1, Gareth Boden/Pearson Education, Inc. 515, 519, 528, Case Study 2, Lord and Leverett/Pearson Education, Inc.; 518, Fig 21.4, Westminster Hospital/Science Source; 520, Fig 21-5, Martin M. Rotker/Science Source; 534, Fig 21.7, Sciepro/Science Photo Library/Getty Images.

Chapter 22: 536-537, Fig 22.1, MARTINI, FREDERIC H.; OBER, WILLIAM C.; NATH, JUDI L.; BARTHOLOMEW, EDWIN F.; PETTI, KEVIN, VISUAL ANATOMY & PHYSIOLOGY (SUBSCRIPTION), 2nd Ed., © 2015. Reprinted and Electronically reproduced by permission of Pearson Education, Inc., New York, NY; 538, 543, Case Study 1, Domenicogelermo/123RF.com; 538, 547, Case Study 2, Piotr Marcinski/Shutterstock; 540-541, Fig 22.3, MARTINI, FREDERIC H.; OBER, WILLIAM C.; NATH, JUDI L.; BARTHOLOMEW, EDWIN F.; PETTI, KEVIN, VISUAL ANATOMY & PHYSIOLOGY, BOOKS A LA CARTE EDITION, 2nd Ed., © 2015. Reprinted and Electronically reproduced by permission of Pearson Education, Inc., New York, NY.

Chapter 23: 554, 557, 558, Case Study 1, Alexander Raths/Shutterstock; 554, 561, 562, Case Study 2, ZouZou/Shutterstock; 554, 565, 567, Case Study 3, Peter Bernik/Shutterstock; 559, Fig 23.5, Richard Newton/Alamy Stock Photo; 560, Fig 23.7, Mediscan/Alamy Stock Photo; 561, Fig 23.8, Mark Boulton/Alamy Stock Photo.

Chapter 24: 574, 580, 591, 593, Case Study, Andrey Arkusha/Shutterstock; 576, Fig 24.2, From "Heart Disease and Stroke Statistics—2015 Update A Report From the American Heart Association", by Dariush Mozaffarian, Emelia J. Benjamin, Donna K. Arnett, Michael J. Blaha, Mary Cushman, Sarah de Ferranti; et al.in Circulation, Vol. 131, Issue 4, pp. e29–e322. Published by American Heart Association, © 2015; 589, Fig 24.14, Biophoto Associates/Science Source; 590, Fig 24.15A, SCIEPRO/Science Photo Library/Getty Images; 590, Fig 24.15B, Zephyr/Science Photo Library/Getty Images; 602, Fig 24.17, Cavallini James/BSIP SA/Alamy Stock Photo.

Chapter 25: 613, From "Congenital Heart Disease in 56, 109 Births Incidence and Natural History", by S. C. Mithell, M.D,S. B. Korones and H.W. Berendes in Circulation, Volume 43, Issue 3, pp.323–332. Published by American Heart Association, © 1971; 614, 617, 618, 622, Case Study 1, Eleonora_os/Shutterstock; 614, 631, 632, Case Study 2, Studio 8/Pearson Education, Inc.

Chapter 26: 638, 648, 649, 651, Case Study 1, Lisa F. Young/Shutterstock; 639, 648, 650, 651, Case Study 2, Michael Puche/Shutterstock; 641, Table 26.1, Data from Yancy, CW, Jessup, M, Bozkurt, B, et al. 2013 ACCF/AHA Guideline for the management of heart failure. Journal of the American College of Cardiology. 2013; 62(16): e147-239. doi: 10.1016/j.jacc.2013.05.019; 642, Table 26.2, From "Treatment of Myocardial Infarction in a Coronary Care Unit: A Two Year Experience with 250 Patients" by Thomas Killip and John T Kimball in The American Journal of Cardiology, Vol. 20, pp. 457–64. Published by Elsevier Inc., © 1967; 645, Table 26.3, Data from Lough, ME. Hemodynamic Monitoring: Evolving Technologies & Clinical Practice. 1st ed: Elsevier; 2016; Miller, LR, Hemodynamic monitoring. In: Burns,S, ed. AACN Essentials of Critical Care Nursing. 3rd ed. McGraw-Hill; Edwards Lifesciences. Normal Hemodynamic Parameters and Laboratory Values. Accessed from http://ht.edwards.com/scin/edwards/sitecollectionimages/edwards/products/presep/ar04313hemodynpocketcard.pdf; 649, Fig 26.7, JFsPic/iStock/Getty Images.

Chapter 27: 662, 664, 665, 668, 670, 674, Case Study 2, Yaromir/Shutterstock; 668, Fig 27.9, Scott Camazine/Alamy Stock Photo; 675, Fig 27.14, Callista Images/Cultura RM/Alamy Stock Photo.

Chapter 28: 682, 689, 690, Case Study 2, Monkey Business Images/Shutterstock; 687, Table 28.1, Data from American College of Surgeons. (2017). Advanced trauma life support (10th ed.). Chicago, IL: American College of Surgeons.

Chapter 29: 703, 721, 722, Case Study 1, Awesomeshotz/123RF.com; 704, 710, 712, Case Study 2, Arek Malang/Shutterstock; 713, Table 29.2, Data from American Psychiatric Association. (2013). Diagnostic and statistical manual of mental disorders (5th ed.). Washington, DC: American Psychiatric Association Publishing.

Chapter 30: 733, 741, Case Study 3, Rob Judges/Pearson Education, Inc.; 734, From "Very Early Childhood Development" by Frances E Aboud and Aisha K Yousafzai in Reproductive, Maternal, Newborn, and Child Health: Disease Control Priorities, 3e by Robert Black, Ramanan Laxminarayan, Marleen Temmerman and Neff Walker. Published by The World Bank, © 2016; 734, From "The Effect of Breastfeeding on Neuro-Development in Infancy" by Cathal McCrory and Aisling Murray in Maternal and Child Health Journal, Vol. 17, 2013. Published by Springer Science+Business Media, © 2012; 736, Fig 30.2, POTTER, MERTIE L.; MOLLER, MARY D., PSYCHIATRIC-MENTAL HEALTH NURSING: FROM SUFFERING TO HOPE, 1st Ed., © 2016. Reprinted and Electronically reproduced by permission of Pearson Education, Inc., New York, NY; 738, Fig 30.3, Ellepigrafica/Alamy Stock Phot; 739, Fig 30.3, Scott Camazine/Alamy Stock Photo; 742,

Fig 30.5, Tetra Images/Alamy Stock Photo; 743, Fig 30.6, Rick's Photography/Shutterstock; 737, From Dementias, Including Alzheimer's Disease. Published by U.S. Department of Health and Human Services.

Chapter 31: 752, 758, Case Study 1, Julie Campbell/Shutterstock; 752, 763, Case Study 2, Privilege/Shutterstock; 753, 769, 770, Case Study 3, J Creation/Shutterstock; 757, Fig 31.5, Mediscan/Alamy Stock Photo; 767, Fig 31.9, Mark Waugh/Alamy Stock Photo; 769, Fig 31.10, Lucia Lanpur/Alamy Stock Photo.

Chapter 32: 779, From IASP Taxonomy. Published by International Association for the Study of Pain, © 2015; 780, 790, 792, Case Study 1, AJR_photo/Shutterstock; 780, 790, 796, Case Study 3, Gareth Boden/Pearson Education, Inc.; 790, Fig 21.11A, From Wong's Essentials of Pediatric Nursing, Volume 1, 6e by Donna L Wong, Marilyn Hockenberry-Eaton and Patricia Schwartz. Copyright © 2001 by The Wong-Baker FACES™ Foundation. Used by permission of The Wong-Baker FACES™ Foundation; 798, Fig 32.15, Dr. Baumgärtner Martin/ImageBROKER/Alamy Stock Photo.

Chapter 33: 817, 823, 828, Case Study 1,Darren Brode/Shutterstock; 817, 831, Case Study 2, Suzanne Tucker/Shutterstock; 817, 832, 833, Case Study 3, Duncan Noakes/123RF.com; 828, Fig 33.6, Annie Griffiths Belt/National Geographic/Getty Images.

Chapter 34: 844, 847, Case Study 1, PT Images/Shutterstock; 844, 850, 853, Case Study 2, Kiselev Andrey Valerevich/Shutterstock; 845, Fig 34.3, Biophoto Associates/Science Source/Getty Images; 847, Table 34.1, Data from Hoehn, M.M. & Yahr, M.D. (1967). Parkinsonism: Onset, Progression, and Mortality. Neurology, 17:427; 850, Fig 34.7, From Types of MS. Published by National Multiple Sclerosis Society, © 2000; 852, Fig 34.9, Living LLC/Science Source/Getty Images; 852, Table 34.2, Data from Diagnostic criteria for multiple sclerosis: 2010 revisions to the McDonald criteria. Annals of Neurology, 69(2): 292 – 302; 854, Table 34.3, From "A Proposed Staging System for Amyotrophic Lateral Sclerosis" by Jose C. Roche, Ricardo Rojas-Garcia, Kirsten M. Scott, William Scotton and Catherine E. Ellis in Brain, Vol. 135, pp. 847–852. Published by Oxford University Press; 855, Fig 34.10, Biophoto Associates/Science Source/Getty Images; 855, Table 34.4, Data from Vonsattel, J.P., Myers, R.H., Stevens T.J., Ferrante, R.J., Bird, E.D., & Richardson, E.P., Jr. (1985). Neuropathological Classification of Huntington's Disease. Journal of Neuropathology and Experimental Neurology, 44(6): 559 – 577.

Chapter 35: 864, 874, Case Study 2, Elena Elisseeva/Shutterstock.

Chapter 36: 884, 886, 888, Case Study 1, Christine Langer-Pueschel/Shutterstock; 890, Fig 36.4, George Dodson/Pearson Education, Inc.; 892, Fig 36.6, Muzayan Fakhoury/Alamy Stock Photo; 894, Fig 36.7, BURGER/Phanie/Alamy Stock Photo.

Chapter 37: 906, 907, 921, Case Study 1, Cherry-Merry/Shutterstock; 906, 907, 928, Case Study 2, Pearson Education, Inc.; 907, 908, 918, Case Study 3, Ffoto29/Shutterstock; 907, 908, 918, Case Study 4, Michael Jung/Shutterstock; 909, Fig 37.2, Zuzanae/Shutterstock; 918, American Diabetes Association. Classification and Diagnosis of Diabetes. Diabetes Care 2015; 38 Suppl:S8-S16; 923, Fig 37.16, Bilous, R. W., Donnelly, R., & Williams, G. (2010). (4th ed.). Hoboken, NJ: Wiley-Blackwell; 925, Brownlee, M. (2001). Biochemistry and molecular cell biology of diabetic complications. Nature, 374, 813–820.; 927, Fig 37.21, Kokel/BSIP SA/Alamy Stock Photo.

Chapter 38: 934, 937, 939, 940, Case Study 1, Marie C Fields/Shutterstock; 937, Fig 38.5, Chris Pancewicz/Alamy Stock Photo; 938, Fig 38.6, Medicshots/Alamy Stock Photo.

Chapter 39: 955, 962, 968, 972, 976, Case Study 1, Nolte Lourens/Shuttertsock; 956, 975, Case Study 2, Sirtravelalot/Shutterstock; 960, Fig 39.7, Jacopin/BSIP SA/Alamy Stock Photo; 967, Fig 39.12, Davor Lovincic/iStock/Getty Images; 970, Fig 39.15A, Scott Camazine/Science Source; Fig 39.15B, Biophoto Associates/Science source; Fig 39.15C, SPL/Science Source; Fig 39.15D, SPL/Science Source; 973, Fig 39.16, Mediscan/Alamy Stock Photo; 974, Fig 39.17, Biophoto Associates/Science Source/Getty Image; 974, Fig 29.18, Biophoto Associates/Getty images; 977, Table 29.1, Stages 1, 2, 3, Mediscan/Alamy Stock Photo;Stage 4, Dr P. Marazzi/Science Source; Unstageable, BSIP/ContributoUniversal Images Group/Getty Images; Deep tissue injury, Dr M.A. Ansary/Science Source.

Chapter 40: 983, 991, 992, Case Study 1,Minerva Studio/Shutterstock; 984, 995, Case Study 2, Gelpi JM/Shutterstock; 985, Fig 40.2,Scott Camazine/Alamy Stock Photo; 986, Fig 40.3, Scott Camazine/Alamy Stock Photo; 987, Fig 40.4, Cavallini Jame/Bsip Sa/Alamy Stock Photo; 988, Fig 40.5, Robert Lind/Alamy Stock Photo; 989, Fig 40.6, Mediscan/Alamy Stock Photo; 990, Fig 40.7, Ted Foxx/Alamy Stock Photo; 991, Fig 40.8, Custom Medical Stock Photo/Alamy Stock Photo; 992, Fig 40.9, Blickwinkel/Fotototo/Alamy Stock Photo; 993, Fig 40.10, Mediscan/Alamy Stock Photo; 994, Fig 40.11, Mendil/Bsip Sa/Alamy Stock Photo; 996, Fig. 40.12, PJF Military Collection/Alamy Stock Photo; 998, Table 40.1, Data from Centers for Disease Control and Prevention. (2016). Tickborne diseases of the United States. Available at https://www.cdc.gov/ticks/diseases; 999, Fig 40.13, Kevin Shields/Alamy Stock Photo; 1000, Fig 40.14, Naomi Aylott/Alamy Stock Photo; 1001, Fig 40.15,Ian West/Alamy Stock Photo; 1002, Fig 40.16, Kuttig - RF - Kids/Alamy Stock Photo; 1003, Fig 40.17, Milan Lipowski/Alamy Stock Photo.

Chapter 41: 1012, 1014, 1015, Case Study 1, Pruitt/123RF.com; 1012, 1021, Case Study 2, Sheftsoff Women Girls/Shutterstock; 1014, Fig 41.2, Biophoto Associates/Science Source; 1016, Fig 41.3, Centers for Disease Control and Prevention (CDC); 1017, Fig 41.1, Dr. P. Marazzi/Science Source; 1018, Fig 41.5, Pan Xunbin/Shutterstock; 1019, Eichenfield LE, Tom, WI, Chamlin SI, et al. (2014). Guidelines of Care for the Management of Atopic Dermatitis: Section 1. Diagnosis and Assessment of Atopic Dermatitis. J Am Acad Dermatol. 70:338-351; 1020, Fig 41.6, Olavs/Shutterstock; 1020, Fig 41.7, Mediscan/Alamy Stock Photo; 1023, Fig 41.8, Mediscan/Alamy Stock Photo; 1025, Fig 41.9, Mediscan/Alamy Stock Photo; 1025, Fig 41.10, Centers for Disease Control and Prevention (CDC); 1026, Fig 41.11, Mediscan/Alamy Stock Photo; 1026, Fig 41.12, Christopher Marsh/Alamy Stock Photo; 1028, Fig 41.13, Dr. P. Marazzi/Science Source; 1029, Fig 41.14, Dr. P. Marazzi/Science Source; 1030, Fig 41.15, Dr. P. Marazzi/Science Source; 1031, Fig 41.16, MD. John F. Wilson/Science Source; 1032, Fig 41.17, Mediscan/Alamy Stock Photo; 1032, Fig 41.18, Chassenet/BSIP SA/Alamy Stock Photo; 1033, Fig 41.19, Gang Liu/Shutterstock; 1034, Fig 41.20, Dr. Harout Tanielian/Science Source.

Chapter 42: 1045, 1059, Case Study 1, Alexandre Nunes/Shutterstock; 1046, Fig 42.2, M.D. David M. Martin/Science Source; 1050, Table 42.2, Data from Kohn GP, Price RR, Demeester SR, et al. Guidelines for the management of hiatal hernia. SAGES Online. http://www.sages.org/publications/guidelines/guidelines-for-the-management-of-hiatal-hernia/.

Reviewed and approved on April 2013. Accessed October 10, 2015; 1057, Table 42.9, Data from Berlth F, Bollschweiler E, Drebber U, Hoelscher AH, Moenig S. Pathohistological classification systems in gastric cancer: Diagnostic relevance and prognostic value. World J Gastroenterol. 2014; 20(19): 5679-5684. doi: 10.3748/wjg.v20.i19.5679.; 1063, Fig 42.11, Belmonte/BSIP SA/Alamy Stock Photo.

Chapter 43: 1071, 1077, 1078, Case Study 1, Sockbroker/ 123RF.com; 1072, 1089, 1090, Case Study 3, Lisa F. Young/ Shutterstock; 1073, Fig 43.3, Charles Stewart MD FACEP, FAAEM; 1076, Fig 43.4, Garry Watson/Science Source; 1082, Fig 43.7, Clinical Photography, Central Manchester University Hospitals NHS Foundation Trust, UK/Science Source; 1082, Fig 43.8, Mediscan/Alamy Stock Photo; 1088, Fig 43.11, CNRI/Science Source.

Chapter 44: 1092, 1106, Case Study 1, Naluwan/ Shutterstock; 1098, 1101, 1108, Case Study 2, Andy Dean Photography/Shutterstock; 1098, Fig 44.2, Snapgalleria/ Shutterstock; 1098, Fig 44.3, Designua/Shutterstock; 1099, Fig 44.4, Monica Schroeder/Science History Images/Alamy Stock Photo; 1102, Fig 44.7, Dr. Thomas F. Sellers/Emory University/Centers for Disease Control and Prevention (CDC); 1103, Fig 44.8, Cindy Minear/Shutterstock; 1109, Fig 44.9, Alila Medical Media/Shutterstock.

Chapter 45: 1118, 1120, 1121, Case Study 1, Doglikehorse/ Shutterstock; 1127, Data from Haylen BT, de Ridder D, Freeman RM, et al. (2010). An International Urogynecological Association (IUGA)/International Continence Society (ICS) joint report on the terminology for female pelvic floor dysfunction. Neurourology and Urodynamics. 2010; 29(1):4-20.

Chapter 46: 1137, 1144, Case Study 1, Aastock/Shutterstock; 1145, Table 46.6, Data from National Kidney Foundation. (n.d.). Glomerular filtration rate. Available at https://www.kidney .org/atoz/content/gfr; 1147, Fig 46.6, Arthur Glauberman/ Science Source; 1155, Fig 46.10B, Philippe Garo/Science Source.

Chapter 47: 1163, 1167, 1168, Case Study 1, Peter Weber/ Shutterstock; 1163, 1171, 1172, 1177, Case Study 2, Claudia Veja/Shutterstock; 1165, Fig 47.3, AMELIE-BENOIST/BSIP SA/Alamy Stock Photo; 1182, Fig 47.11, TriFocal Communications/Stocktrek Images/Alamy Stock Photo.

Chapter 48: 1193, 1196, Case Study 1, Rob Marmion/ Shutterstock; 1194, 1200, Case Study 2, Arina Habich/ 123RF.com; 1200, Fig 48.6, Cavallini James/BSIP SA/Alamy Stock Photo.

Chapter 49: 1208, 1210, Case Study 1, Stockbroker/ 123RF.com; 1208, Fig 49.2, A J James/DigitalVision/Getty Images; 1209, Fig 49.3A,B, Centers for Disease Control and Prevention (CDC); 1211, Fig 49.4A, Centers for Disease Control and Prevention (CDC); Fig 49.4B, Dr P. Marazzi/ Science Source; 1212, Fig 49.5, Centers for Disease Control and Prevention (CDC); 1213, Fig 49.6A, Biophoto Associates/Science Source; Fig 49.6B, Centers for Disease Control and Prevention (CDC); 1214, Fig 49.7, BSIP SA/Alamy Stock Photo; 1214, Data from Smith, D. (2016). Trichomoniasis. Medscape. Retrieved from http://emedicine.medscape.com/ article/230617-overview; Centers for Disease Control and Prevention. Trichomoniasis – CDC fact sheet. Retrieved from https://www.cdc.gov/std/trichomonas/stdfact-trichomoniasis.htm; 1215, Fig 49.8, Mediscan/Alamy Stock Photo.

Chapter 50: 1223, 1231, Case Study 1, Digital Media Pro/ Shutterstock; 1224, 1233, 1235, Case Study 2,Michael Jung/ Shutterstock; 1225, Table 50.1, From Injury and Violence Prevention. Published by U.S. Department of Health and Human Services; 1227, Fig 50.3, Kuttig - People/Alamy Stock Photo; 1228, Fig 50.4, Paul cox/Alamy Stock Photo; 1228, Fig 50.5, Hercules Robinson/Alamy Stock Photo; 1229, Fig 50.7, Kathie Nichols/Alamy Stock Photo; 1230, Fig 50.8, Mediscan/Alamy Stock Photo.

Chapter 51: 1246, Fig 51.1, From "Guidelines for Field Triage of Injured Patients: Recommendations of the National Expert Panel on Field Triage 2011" in MMWR, Vol. 61, Issue: RR01, pp. 1–20. Published by Centers for Disease Control and Prevention; 1247, 1252, 1257, 1260, 1262, 1264, 1265, Case Study, Amelie Benoist/BSIP SA/Alamy Stock Photo; 1249, Data from American Academy of Pediatrics. (2016). Committee on Pediatric Emergency Medicine; Council on Injury, Violence, and Poison Protection; Section on Critical Care; Section on Orthopaedics; Section on Surgery, et al. Management of pediatric trauma. Pediatrics. Retrieved from http:// pediatrics.aappublications.org/content/early/2016/07/21/ peds.2016-1569; 1261, Fig 51.15, Steve Kraitt/Cultura RM/ Alamy Stock Photo.

Chapter 52: 1273, 1276, 1277, Case Study 1, Ijansempoi/ Shutterstock; 1273, 1284, Tudor Photography/Pearson Education, Inc.; 1276, Fig 52.3, Centers for Disease Control and Prevention (CDC); 1279, Fig 52.6, Margaret Parsons/Dr. Karl F. Meyer/Centers for Disease Control and Prevention (CDC); 1279, Fig 52.7, William Archibald/Centers for Disease Control and Prevention (CDC); 1280, Fig 52.8, Jr. Dr. Charles Farmer/ Centers for Disease Control and Prevention (CDC); 1283, Fig 52.9, Mamun Ebu Omer/Anadolu Agency/Getty Images.

Chapter 53: 1293, Table 53.1, From Evaluation of Chemotherapeutic Agents: Symposium Held at the New York Academy of Medicine by David A. Karnofsky; 1294, 1295, 1297, 1302, 1311, Case Study 1, Lisa F. Young/Shutterstock; 1294, 1297, 1303, 1305, Case Study 2, XiXinXing/Shutterstock; 1295, From "An Official American Thoracic Society Statement: Update on the Mechanisms, Assessment, and Management of Dyspnea"", by Mark B. Parshall, Richard M. Schwartzstein, Lewis Adams, Robert B. Banzett, Harold L. Manning, Jean Bourbeau, Peter M. Calverley, Audrey G. Gift, Andrew Harver, Suzanne C. Lareau, Donald A. Mahler, Paula M. Meek, and Denis E. O'Donnell in American Journal of Respiratory and Critical Care Medicine, Vol 185, Issue 4, pp 435–452. Published by American Thoracic Society, © 2012; 1310, From Statement on Palliative Sedation. Published by American Academy of Hospice and Palliative Medicine, © 2014; 1311, Table 53.2, Data from Hamilton B, Hoyert D, Martin J,et al. Annual summary of vital statistics: 2010-11. Pediatrics 2013; 131(3):548-558 and Friebert S. NHPCO Facts and Figures: Pediatric Palliative and Hospice Care in America. Alexandria, VA: National Hospice and Palliative Care Organization, April 2009. http://www.nationalconsensusproject.org/ Guidelines. Accessed September 21, 2014.

Index

*Page numbers with *b* indicate boxes; *f*, figures, and *t*, tables.

A

F

G

H

I

J

K

O

P

S

T

U

V

Special Features

Genetics and Genomics for Clinical Practice

Healthy People 2020

Impact of Current Research on Clinical Practice